1973 The first two programs to be accredited by the AVMA are those at Michigan State University and Nebraska College of Technical Agriculture.

The Association of Animal Technician Educators (AATE) is formed at the third Symposium on Animal Technician Training.

The AVMA House of Delegates passes a resolution proposing "registration" but not "licensing" of animal technicians. The Committee on Accreditation for Training of Animal Technicians changes its name to the Committee on Animal Technician Activities and Training.

1975 The Washington State Association of Veterinary Technicians (WSAVT) is established.

The AATE constitution is adopted and the first officers are elected.

1976 CATAT is recognized by the U.S. Office of Education as the accrediting body for animal technician training programs.

The first professional journal for veterinary technicians, *Methods: The Journal for Animal Health Technicians,* is published.

The Veterinary Technicians and Assistants Association of Pennsylvania (VTAAP) is created.

1977 The first written state examination for animal health technicians in the state of New York is administered.

1978 The Virginia Association of Licensed Veterinary Technicians is established.

1978 The AVMA adds a continuing education section for veterinary technicians to its program at the annual convention in Dallas, Texas.

The Alberta Association of Animal Health Technologists is formed.

1980 *The Compendium on Continuing Education for the Animal Health Technician* (later called *Veterinary Technician*) is first published.

At the annual AVMA convention, members of an ad hoc committee composed of representatives from the United States and Canada discuss the idea of forming a United States–Canadian veterinary technicians' association.

Association des Techniciens en Sante Animale du Québec (ATSAQ) begins with 25 members.

1981 The North American Veterinary Technician Association (NAVTA) is organized.

The Association of Zoo Veterinary Technicians is formed.

The Veterinary Hospital Managers Association is formed.

1982 CALAS creates a plan for the voluntary registration of laboratory animal technicians.

NAVTA adopts *The Compendium on Continuing Education for the Animal Health Technician* (later called *Veterinary Technician*) as its first official journal.

1984 *The Compendium on Continuing Education for the Animal Health Technician* is changed to *Veterinary Technician.*

NAVTA adopts a national code of ethics for veterinary technicians.

1985 The AVMA Executive Board establishes the Animal Technician Testing Committee, which generates the Animal Technician National Examination (ATNE) in conjunction with Professional Education Services (PES).

The Association of Animal Technician Educators (AATE) changes its name to the Association of Veterinary Technician Educators (AVTE).

1986 The first ATNE is given in Maine.

1988 In Canada, the Eastern Veterinary Technician Association (EVTA) is established with 30 members.

CALAS implements a testing and registration plan for laboratory animal technicians.

The AVMA votes against a resolution that would change terminology from "animal technician" to "veterinary technician."

1989 The Canadian Association of Animal Health Technologists and Technicians (CAAHTT) is formed.

The AVMA House of Delegates approves the use of the term "veterinary technician," which replaces "animal technician." Consequently:

- The Committee on Animal Technician Activities and Training (CATAT) is changed to the Committee on Veterinary Technician Education and Activities (CVTEA).
- The Animal Technician Testing Committee (ATTC) is changed to the Veterinary Technician Testing Committee (VTTC).
- The Animal Technician National Examination is renamed the Veterinary Technician National Examination (VTNE).

1990 NAVTA adopts its official mission statement and begins a strategic planning process. NAVTA produces "The World of the Veterinary Technician" video.

The Ontario Association of Animal Health Technicians (OAAHT) establishes a registry.

McCurnin's

CLINICAL TEXTBOOK *for* VETERINARY TECHNICIANS

McCurnin's

CLINICAL TEXTBOOK *for* VETERINARY TECHNICIANS

Seventh Edition

Joanna M. Bassert, VMD
Professor and Director
Program of Veterinary Technology
Manor College
Jenkintown, Pennsylvania

Dennis M. McCurnin, DVM, MS, Dipl ACVS
Professor of Surgery and Management
Director of Continuing Education
Veterinary Clinical Sciences
School of Veterinary Medicine
Louisiana State University
Baton Rouge, Louisiana

With 1770 illustrations

SAUNDERS

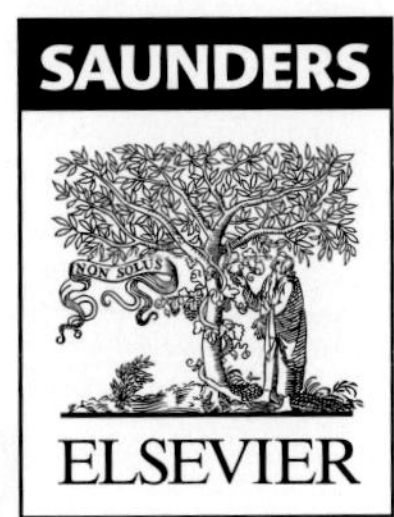

ELSEVIER

SAUNDERS
ELSEVIER

11830 Westline Industrial Drive
St. Louis, Missouri 63146

CLINICAL TEXTBOOK FOR VETERINARY TECHNICIANS 978-1-4160-5700-0

Notice

Knowledge and best practice in this field are constantly changing. As new research and experience broaden our knowledge, changes in practice, treatment, and drug therapy may become necessary or appropriate. Readers are advised to check the most current information provided (i) on procedures featured or (ii) by the manufacturer of each product to be administered, to verify the recommended dose or formula, the method and duration of administration, and contraindications. It is the responsibility of the practitioner, relying on their own experience and knowledge of the patient, to make diagnoses, to determine dosages and the best treatment for each individual patient, and to take all appropriate safety precautions. To the fullest extent of the law, neither the Publisher nor the Editors assumes any liability for any injury and/or damage to persons or property arising out of or related to any use of the material contained in this book.

The Publisher

Library of Congress Cataloging-in-Publication Data
Bassert, Joanna M.
McCurnin's clinical textbook for veterinary technicians/Joanna M. Bassert, Dennis M. McCurnin.–7th ed.
p. ; cm.
Rev. ed. of: Clinical textbook for veterinary technicians/Dennis M. McCurnin, Joanna M. Bassert. 6th ed. 2006.
Includes bibliographical references and index.
ISBN 978-1-4160-5700-0 (hardcover : alk. paper) 1. Veterinary medicine. I. McCurnin, Dennis M. II. McCurnin, Dennis M. Clinical textbook for veterinary technicians. III. Title. IV. Title: Clinical textbook for veterinary technicians.
[DNLM: 1. Veterinary Medicine. 2. Animal Diseases–nursing. 3. Animal Technicians. SF 745 B318m 2010]
SF745.C625 2010
636.089–dc22
2008024803

Vice President and Publisher: Linda Duncan
Publisher: Penny Rudolph
Managing Editor: Teri Merchant
Developmental Editor: Shelly Stringer
Publishing Services Manager: Catherine Jackson
Project Manager: Rachel E. McMullen
Design Direction: Paula Catalano
Cover Designer: Paula Catalano

Printed in China

Last digit is the print number: 9 8 7 6 5 4 3 2

Dennis Michael McCurnin, DVM, MS, DACVS

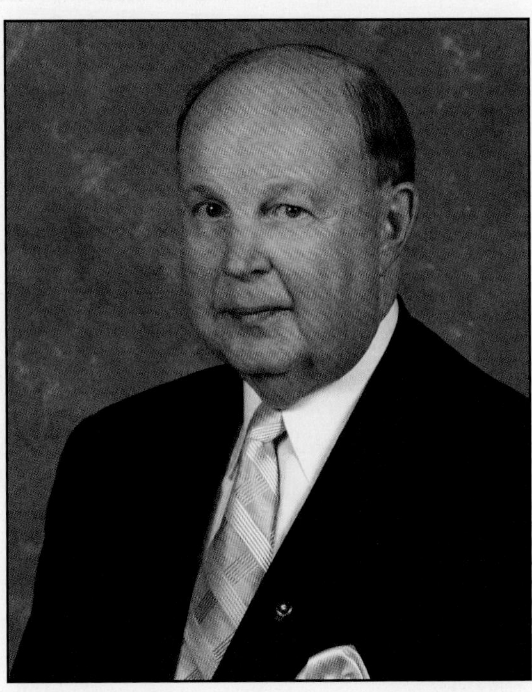

Dr. Dennis McCurnin started the first edition of the *Clinical Textbook for Veterinary Technicians* more than 28 years ago. Now, on the eve of his retirement as editor, it is fitting to dedicate this page and this edition to him. It has been my good fortune to work with Dr. McCurnin on the last three editions, and during this time he has taught and guided me through every aspect of the editing process. I am therefore indebted to him and feel honored to write this dedication.

Dr. McCurnin is famously hardworking. Few can surpass him in energy or in his ability to carry out multiple tasks at once. During the early part of his career, Dr. McCurnin became a boarded veterinary surgeon. He has held faculty positions in three different veterinary medical colleges: Iowa State, Colorado State, and Louisiana State Universities. In addition, he has taught in the Agricultural College at Arizona State University. A prolific writer, he has produced eight textbooks; 12 shorter works; and 155 articles, including 16 in refereed journals; and made several instructional recordings and videos. His professional speaking has led him to 43 different states and 30 countries around the world, where he has given hundreds of presentations (480 seminars between 1970 and 2007).

Dr. McCurnin possesses the gifts of foresight and vision, which have benefited the many organizations he has helped guide. He is able to motivate the masses as well as individuals in ways known only to great leaders—combining straightforward and positive communication with a genius for interpersonal sensibilities. Dr. McCurnin has dedicated long hours to veterinary medicine as a member and officer of committees in many national, state, and regional organizations. Most notable among these is his leadership in the American Veterinary Medical Association, American Animal Hospital Association, National Commission on Veterinary Economic Issues, and American College of Veterinary Surgeons. Dr. McCurnin is not afraid to speak his mind even when his opinions are unpopular. He publicly advocated for the education and licensure of veterinary technicians, for example, at a time when most veterinarians were not ready to embrace the idea. In these ways and many others, both the professions of veterinary medicine and veterinary technology have thrived under his influence.

When Dr. McCurnin prepared the first edition of the *Clinical Textbook for Veterinary Technicians* in 1985, veterinary technicians were struggling to gain recognition within the profession and among state legislatures. The National Association of Veterinary Technicians in America (NAVTA) was only just taking form. Even the term *veterinary technician* struggled to emerge from what is now the archaic *animal health technician.* In this context, the first edition of the *Clinical Textbook for Veterinary Technicians* was one of few texts produced to educate veterinary technicians. It contained 24 chapters and about 500 pages. Since then, the text has more than doubled in size with 39 chapters and 1400 pages. Dr. McCurnin was committed to using authors who were specialists in their field, experts who normally wrote veterinary medical texts for veterinary medical students rather than for undergraduates. As veterinary technology programs made use of the early editions, veterinary technicians transitioned from being "trained" to being "educated."

The importance of understanding physiology and pathogenesis, and the technician's ability to think critically became clear as veterinary medicine increased its demands on the veterinary health care team, leading to greater distinction between the veterinary technician and other staff members.

In countless ways both large and small, veterinary medicine has benefitted from Dr. McCurnin's extraordinary efforts. Through teaching, writing, and speaking, Dr. McCurnin has helped move the profession forward, and this in turn has led to the most important outcome of all—improved medical care for animals. Dennis, on behalf of all of us, human and otherwise, who have been touched by your hard work, passion, and wisdom, I extend my deepest appreciation.

Thank you.
Joanna M. Bassert, VMD

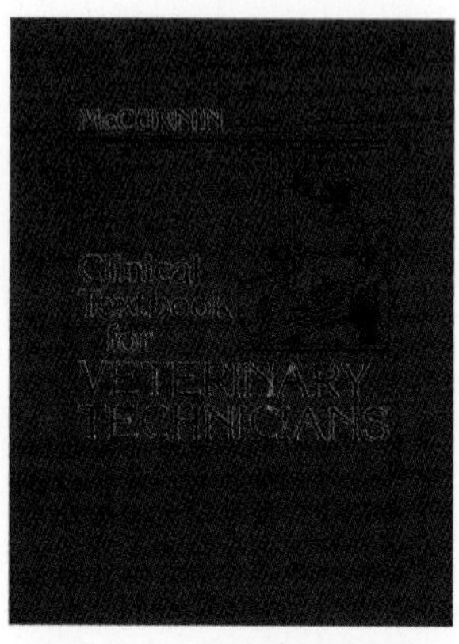

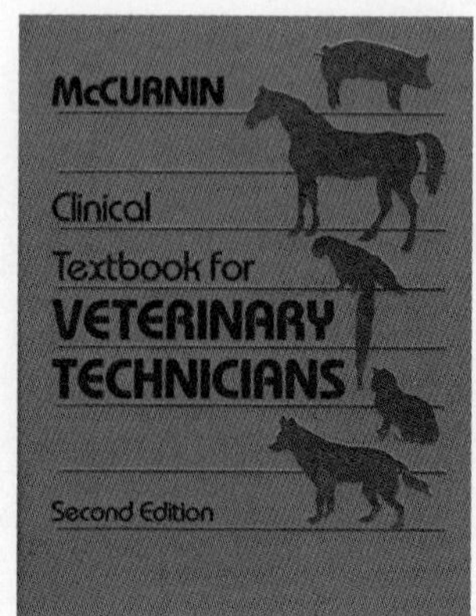

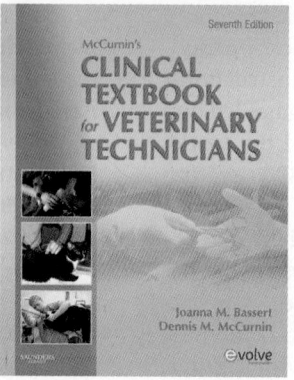

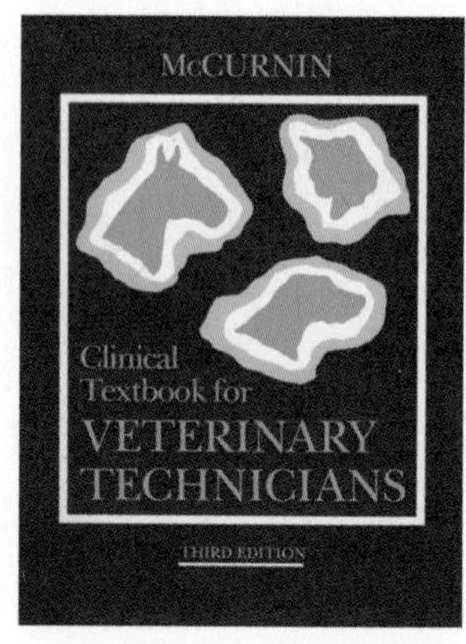

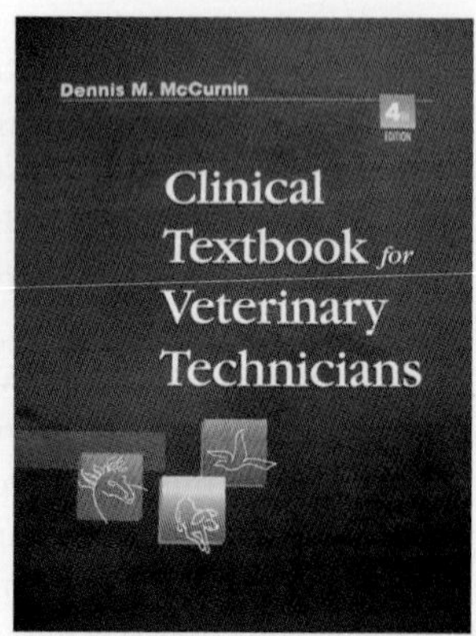

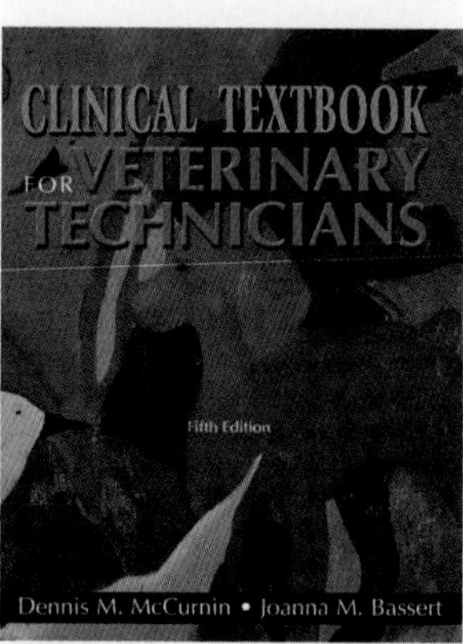

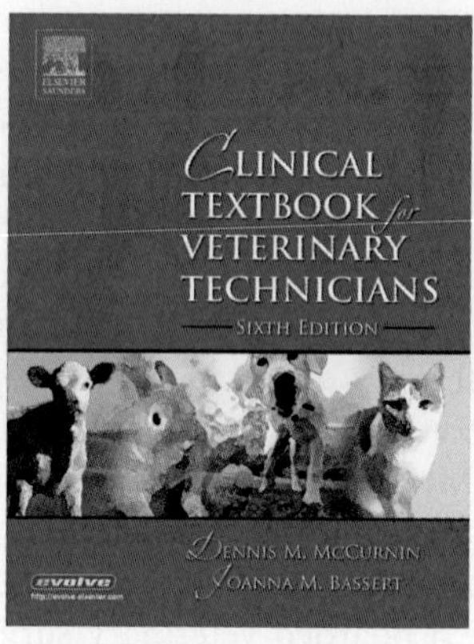

To all my family, but especially my wife, Jeri; son, Brad; and grandson, Evan, for their support of my professional activities by sometimes giving up their own plans and activities so that I might complete my professional journey.
Thank you and I love you all.

DMM

For Ed,
with love and gratitude.

JMB

Vet Tech Threads

With this edition of *Clinical Textbook for Veterinary Technicians,* we are inaugurating a set of features and design elements that will be shared with other vet tech titles on the Mosby and Saunders lists. The purpose of the "Vet Tech Threads" is to make it easier for students and instructors to incorporate multiple books into the fast-paced and demanding vet tech curriculum.

The shared features in *Clinical Textbook for Veterinary Technicians,* seventh edition, include the following:

- Cover and internal **design similarities:** the colorful, student-friendly design encourages reading and learning of this core content.
- Lists of **Objectives** begin each chapter.
- **Clinical Application** boxes demonstrate clinical relevance of chapter topics.
- **Key Terms** are in bold the first time they appear in the chapter.
- An extensive **Glossary** of the key terms is at the end of the text.

Contributors

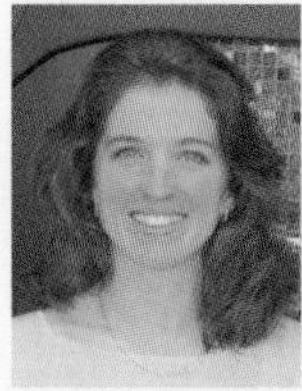

Caroline Adamson Adrian, MS, PT, CCRP
Director, Physical Therapy Services
Alameda East Veterinary Hospital
Denver, Colorado

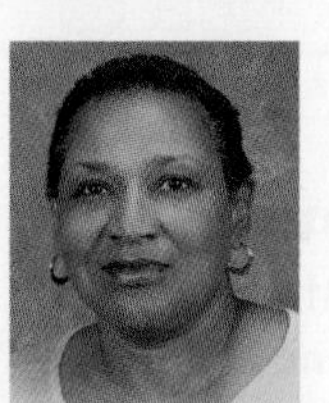

Marvene Augustus, PharmD
Pharmacy Manager Emeritus
Veterinary Teaching Hospital and Clinics
School of Veterinary Medicine
Louisiana State University

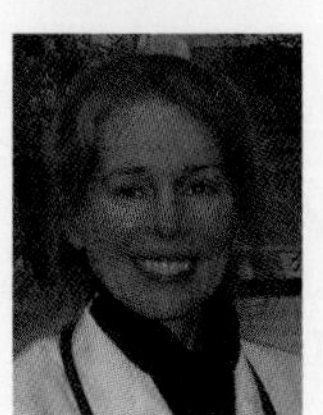

Joanna M. Bassert, VMD
Program Director and Professor
Program of Veterinary Technology
Manor College
Jenkintown, Pennsylvania

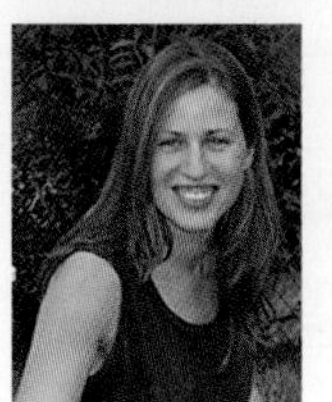

Amy I. Bentz, VMD, Dipl ACVIM
NRSA Postdoctoral Fellow
University of Pennsylvania
Philadelphia, Pennsylvania

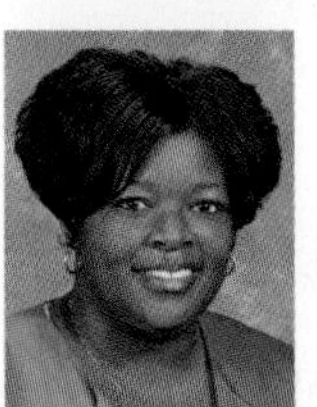

Sonya Bremer Boss, RPh
Assistant Pharmacy Manager
Veterinary Teaching Hospital and Clinics
School of Veterinary Medicine
Louisiana State University
Baton Rouge, Louisiana

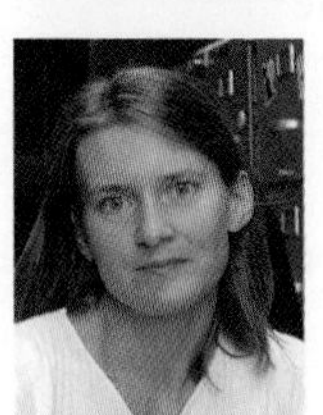

Loretta J. Bubenik, DVM, MS, Dipl ACVS
Assistant Professor, Companion Animal Surgery
Veterinary Clinical Sciences
School of Veterinary Medicine
Louisiana State University
Baton Rouge, Louisiana

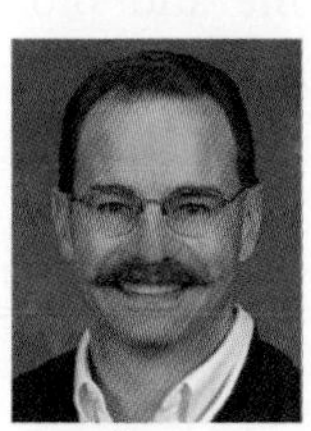

Daniel J. Burba, DVM, Dipl ACVS
Professor of Equine Surgery
Veterinary Clinical Sciences
School of Veterinary Medicine
Louisiana State University
Baton Rouge, Louisiana

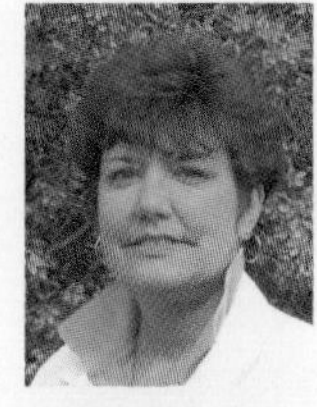

Vickie Byard, CVT, VTS (Dentistry)
Dentistry Department Coordinator
Rau Animal Hospital
Glenside, Pennsylvania

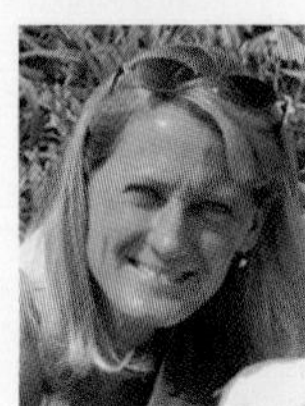

Mary Tefend Campbell, CVT, VTS (ECC)
Shorter, Alabama

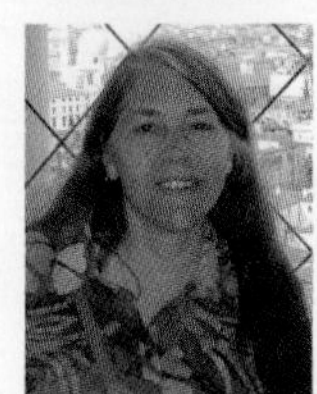

Margret L. Casal, Dr med vet, PhD, Dipl ECAR
Assistant Professor of Medical Genetics
Department of Clinical Studies
University of Pennsylvania
Philadelphia, Pennsylvania

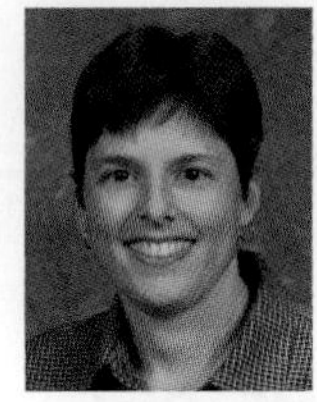

Jacqueline R. Davidson, DVM, MS, Dipl ACVS
Professor, Companion Animal Surgery
Veterinary Clinical Sciences
School of Veterinary Medicine
Louisiana State University
Baton Rouge, Louisiana

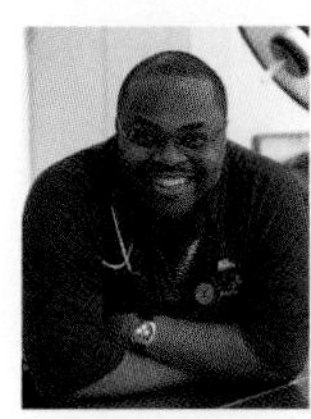

Harold Davis, BA, RVT, VTS (ECC) (Anesth)
Manager, Emergency and Critical Care Service
Veterinary Medical Teaching Hospital
School of Veterinary Medicine
University of California
Davis, California

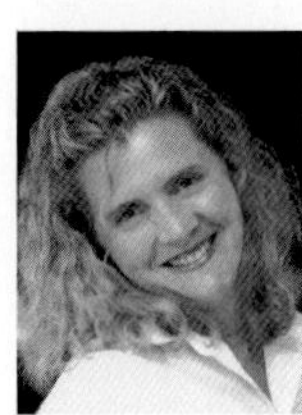

Lee Ann Eddleman, CVT, VTS (ECC)
Head Nurse, Recovery and Intensive Care Unit
Veterinary Teaching Hospital and Clinic
School of Veterinary Medicine
Louisiana State University
Baton Rouge, Louisiana

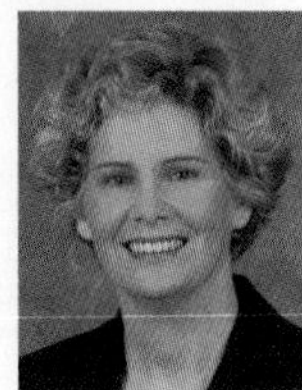

Susan M. Eddlestone, DVM
Associate Professor
Veterinary Clinical Sciences
School of Veterinary Medicine
Louisiana State University
Baton Rouge, Louisiana

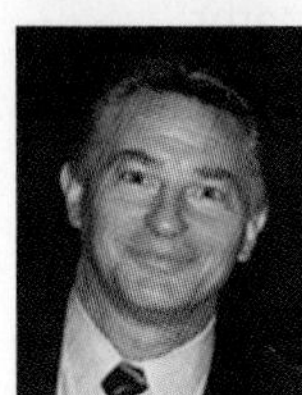

Bruce Edward Eilts, DVM, MS, Dipl ACT
Professor of Theriogenology
Veterinary Clinical Sciences
Louisiana State University
Baton Rouge, Louisiana

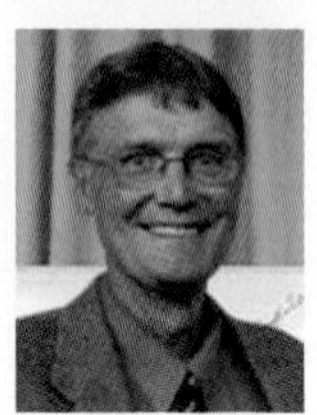

Dennis D. French, DVM
Professor and Section Chief
Farm Animal Health Management
Veterinary Clinical Sciences
School of Veterinary Medicine
Louisiana State University;
Professor, Veterinary Science
Louisiana State University AgCenter
Baton Rouge, Louisiana

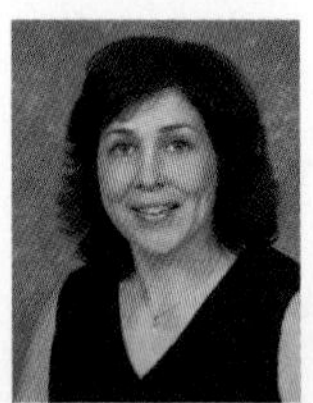

Lorrie Gaschen, PhD, Dr habil, DVM, Dr med vet, Dipl ECVDI
Associate Professor
Veterinary Clinical Sciences, Radiology
School of Veterinary Medicine
Louisiana State University
Baton Rouge, Louisiana

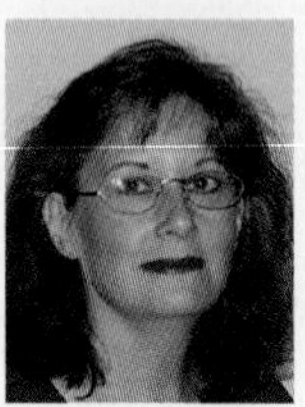

Marjorie S. Gill, DVM, MS, Dipl ABVP
Professor, Farm Animal Health Management
Veterinary Clinical Sciences
School of Veterinary Medicine
Louisiana State University
Baton Rouge, Louisiana

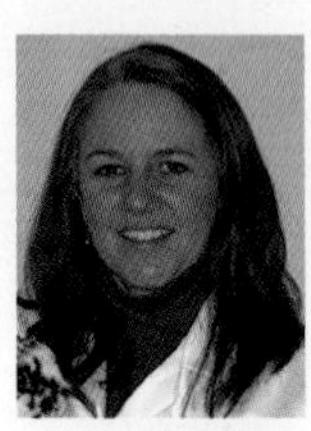

Tamara Grubb, DVM, MS, Dipl ACVA
Director, Veterinary Anesthesia and Analgesia Specialists
Uniontown, Washington

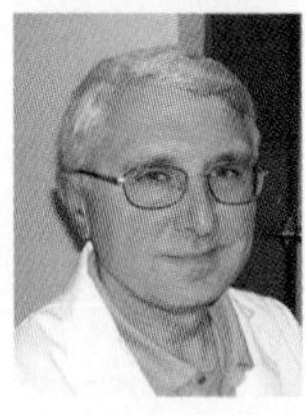

Perry L. Habecker, VMD, Dipl ACVP
Chief, Large Animal Pathology Service
Department of Pathobiology
School of Veterinary Medicine
University of Pennsylvania
Philadelphia, Pennsylvania

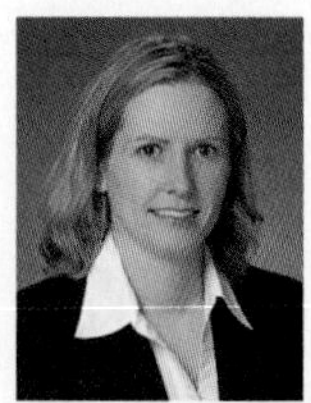

Carolyn J. Hammer, DVM, PhD
Director, Equine Studies
Department of Animal Sciences
North Dakota State University
Fargo, North Dakota

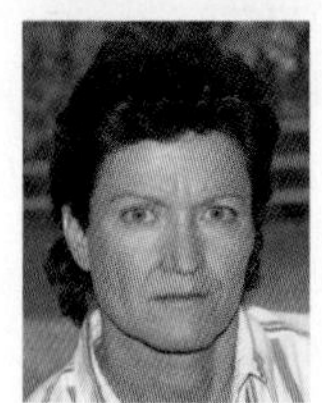

Elizabeth A. Hanie, DVM, MS
Honors College
University of North Carolina at Charlotte
Charlotte, North Carolina

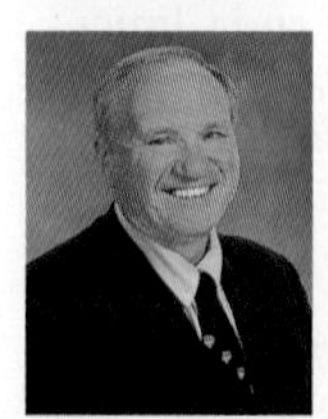

Charles M. Hendrix, DVM, PhD
Professor, Department of Pathobiology
College of Veterinary Medicine
Auburn University
Auburn, Alabama

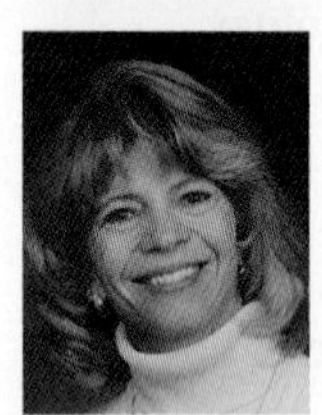

Suzanne Hetts, PhD, CAAB
Co-Owner and President
Animal Behavior Associates, Inc.
Littleton, Colorado

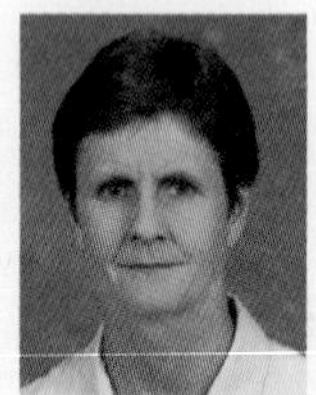

Giselle Hosgood, BVSc, PhD, FACVSc, Dipl ACVS
Professor of Veterinary Surgery
Veterinary Clinical Sciences
School of Veterinary Medicine
Louisiana State University
Baton Rouge, Louisiana

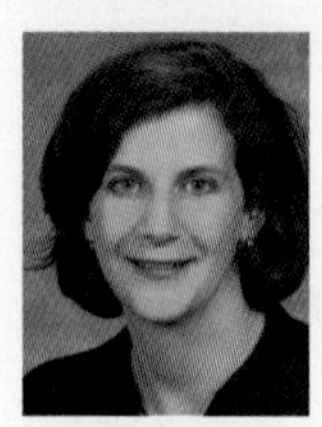

Stephanie W. Johnson, MSW, LCSW
Instructor, Veterinary Clinical Sciences
School of Veterinary Medicine
Louisiana State University
Baton Rouge, Louisiana

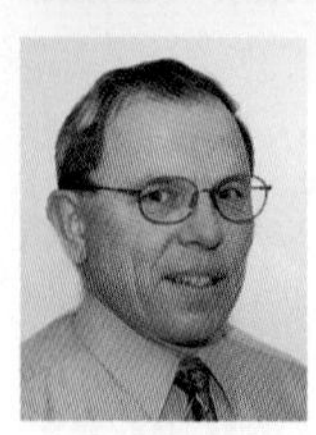

Robert L. Jones, DVM, PhD, Dipl ACVM
Professor, Microbiology
Department of Microbiology, Immunology, and Pathology
College of Veterinary Medicine and Biomedical Sciences
Colorado State University
Fort Collins, Colorado

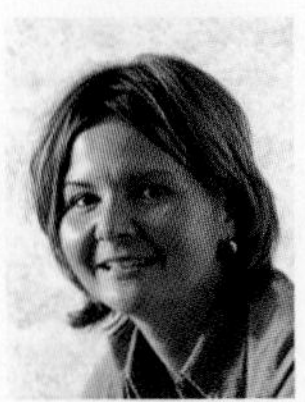

Christine Jurek, DVM
Associate Veterinarian
TOPS Veterinary Rehabilitation
Grayslake, Illinois

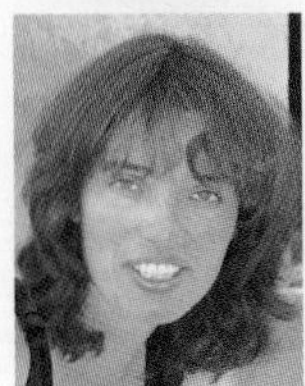

Susanne K. Lauer, Dr med vet, Dipl ACVS, ECVS
Assistant Professor
Veterinary Clinical Sciences
School of Veterinary Medicine
Louisiana State University
Baton Rouge, Louisiana

Teresa A. Lazo, Esquire, JD
Assistant Counsel
Pennsylvania Office of General Counsel
Department of State
State Board of Veterinary Medicine
Harrisburg, Pennsylvania

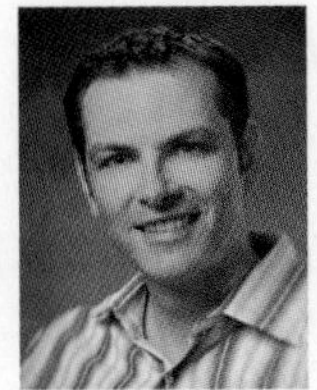

Phillip Lerche, BVSc, PhD, Dipl ACVA
Assistant Professor
Department of Veterinary Clinical Sciences
The Ohio State University
Columbus, Ohio

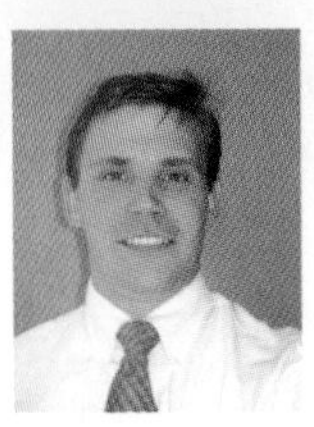

John R. Lewis, VMD, FAVD, Dipl. AVDC
Assistant Professor
Dentistry and Oral Surgery
Department of Clinical Studies
School of Veterinary Medicine
University of Pennsylvania
Philadelphia, Pennsylvania

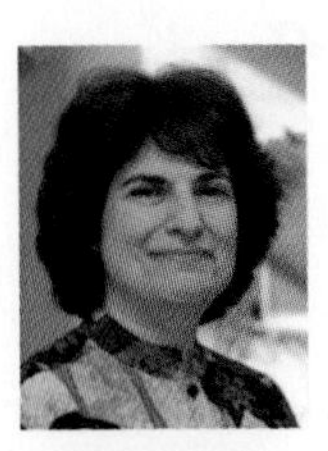

Meryl P. Littman, VMD, Dipl ACVIM
Associate Professor of Medicine
Department of Clinical Studies
School of Veterinary Medicine
University of Pennsylvania
Philadelphia, Pennsylvania

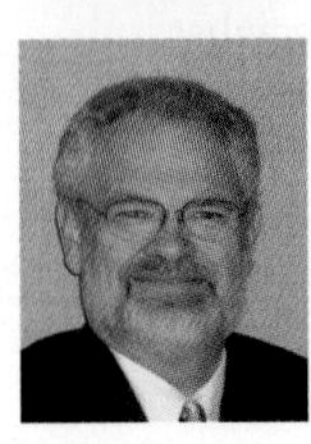

Roger L. Lukens, MS, DVM
Professor Emeritus
Veterinary Technology Program
School of Veterinary Medicine
Purdue University
West Lafayette, Indiana

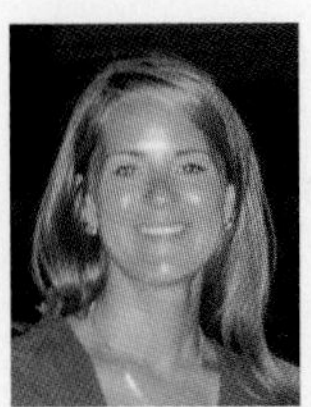

Rebecca B. Marquardt, CVT
Ward Supervisor, Department of Nursing
School of Veterinary Medicine
University of Pennsylvania
Philadelphia, Pennsylvania

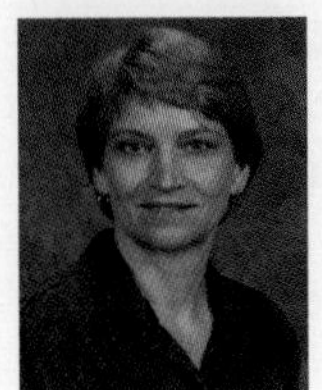

Glenna E. Mauldin, DVM, MS, Dipl ACVIM (Oncology) and ACVN
Cancer Centre for Animals
Western Veterinary Specialist Centre
Calgary, Alberta

G. Neal Mauldin, DVM, Dipl ACVIM (Internal Medicine and Oncology) and ACVR (Radiation Oncology)
Cancer Centre for Animals
Western Veterinary Specialist Centre
Calgary, Alberta

Charles T. McCauley, DVM, Dipl ABVP (Food Animal Practice), ACVS
Assistant Professor of Equine Surgery
Veterinary Clinical Sciences
Louisiana State University
Baton Rouge, Louisiana

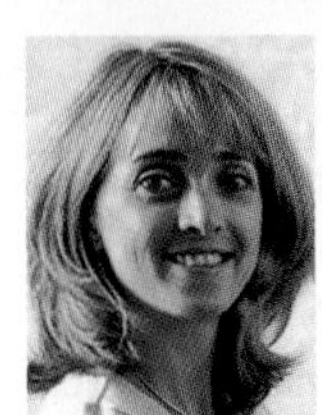

Laurie McCauley, DVM
Medical Director
TOPS Veterinary Rehabilitation
Grayslake, Illinois

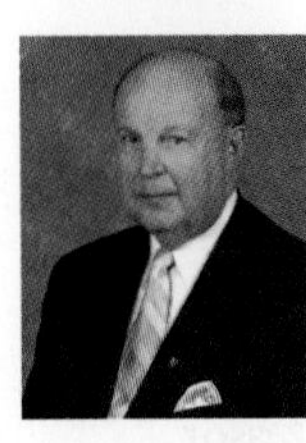

Dennis M. McCurnin, DVM, MS, Dipl ACVS
Professor of Surgery and Management
Director of Continuing Education
Veterinary Clinical Sciences
School of Veterinary Medicine
Louisiana State University
Baton Rouge, Louisiana

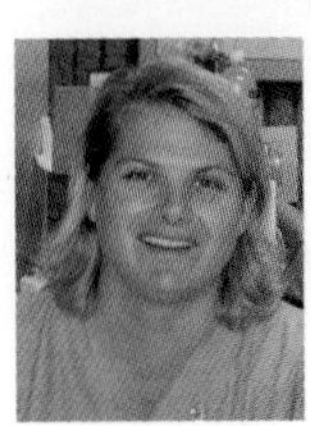

Kristin Miguel, BS, RVT, VTS (LA Internal Medicine)
Supervisor, Large Animal Intensive Care and Isolation
William R. Pritchard Veterinary Medical Teaching Hospital
School of Veterinary Medicine
University of California
Davis, California

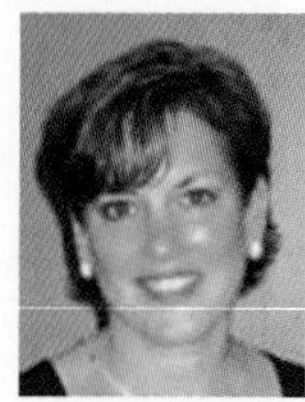

Bonnie R. Miller, RDH, BS
Dentistry and Oral Surgery
School of Veterinary Medicine
University of Pennsylvania
Philadelphia, Pennsylvania

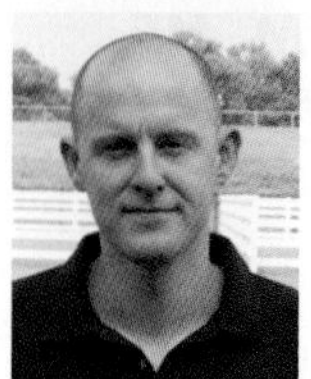

Colin F. Mitchell, BVM&S, MS, Dipl ACVS
Assistant Professor, Equine Surgery
Veterinary Clinical Sciences
School of Veterinary Medicine
Louisiana State University
Baton Rouge, Louisiana

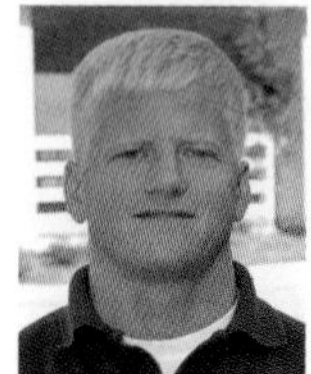

Rustin M. Moore, DVM, PhD, Dipl ACVS
Department Chair, Bud and Marilyn Jenne Professor
Department of Veterinary Clinical Science
College of Veterinary Medicine
The Ohio State University
Columbus, Ohio

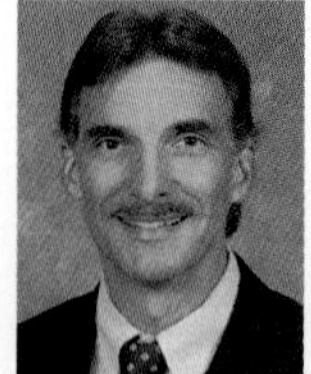

Dale L. Paccamonti, DVM, MS, Dipl ACT
Professor, Theriogenology
Department of Veterinary Clinical Sciences
School of Veterinary Medicine
Louisiana State University
Baton Rouge, Louisiana

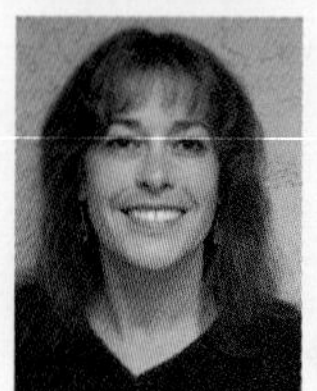

Marika Pappagianis, BS, RVT, VTS (LA Internal Medicine)
Large Animal Clinic Nursing Manager
William R. Pritchard Veterinary Medical Teaching Hospital
School of Veterinary Medicine
University of California
Davis, California

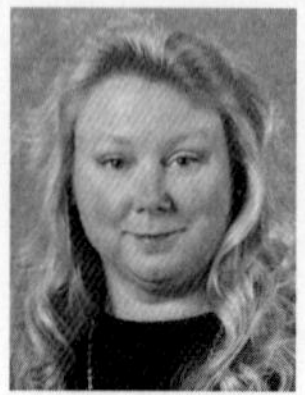

Beth Paugh Partington, DVM, MS, Dipl ACVR
Adjunct Clinical Associate Professor
Veterinary Clinical Sciences
School of Veterinary Medicine
Louisiana State University
Baton Rouge, Louisiana

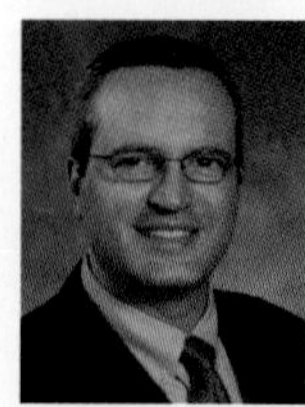

Carlos R.F. Pinto, MedVet, PhD, Dipl ACT
Assistant Professor
Population Health and Pathobiology
College of Veterinary Medicine
North Carolina State University
Raleigh, North Carolina

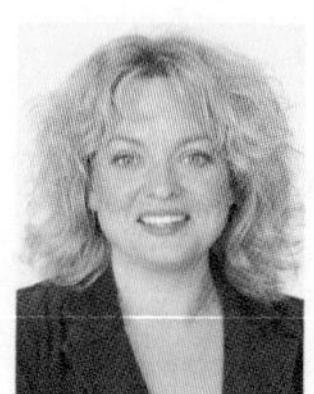

Jill A. Richardson, DVM
Consultant, Technical Services and Marketing
Lloyd Labs, Inc.
Shenandoah, Iowa

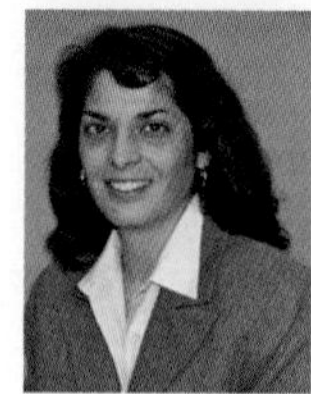

Darlene L. Riel, RVT, VTS (Small Animal Internal Medicine)
Manager, Ira M. Gary Gourley Clinical Teaching Center
Academic Programs
School of Veterinary Medicine
University of California
Davis, California

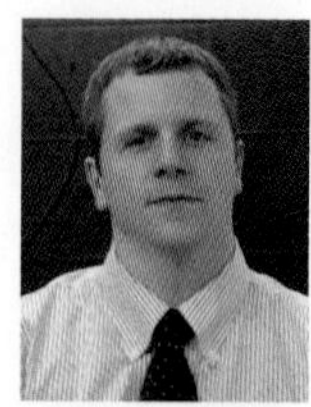

Mark P. Rondeau, DVM, Dipl ACVIM (Small Animal)
Department of Clinical Studies
School of Veterinary Medicine
University of Pennsylvania
Philadelphia, Pennsylvania

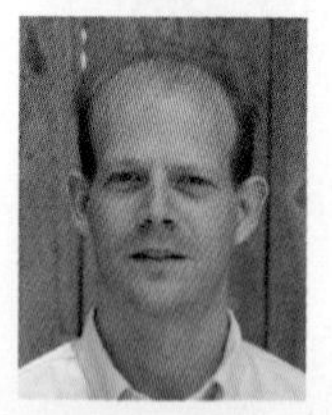

Kirk Ryan, DVM, Dipl ACVIM (Small Animal)
Assistant Professor
Department of Veterinary Clinical Sciences
School of Veterinary Medicine
Louisiana State University
Baton Rouge, Louisiana

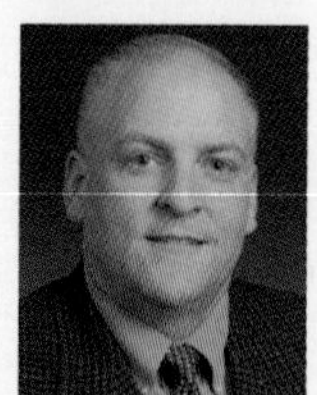

William D. Schoenherr, PhD
Principal Nutritionist
Pet Nutrition Center
Hill's Pet Nutrition, Inc.
Topeka, Kansas

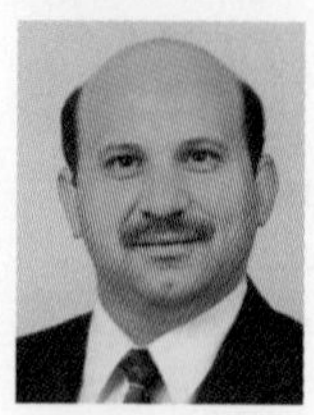

Philip J. Seibert, Jr., CVT
Consultant, SafetyVet
Calhoun, Tennessee

Nancy Shaffran, CVT, VTS (ECC)
Senior Veterinary Nursing Specialist
Veterinary Specialty Team
Pfizer Animal Health
New York, New York

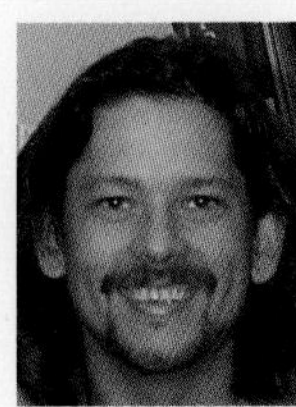

Jeffrey R. Sirninger, DVM, PhD, Dipl ACVP
Assistant Professor of Veterinary Clinical Pathology
Department of Pathobiology
School of Veterinary Medicine
Louisiana State University
Baton Rouge, Louisiana

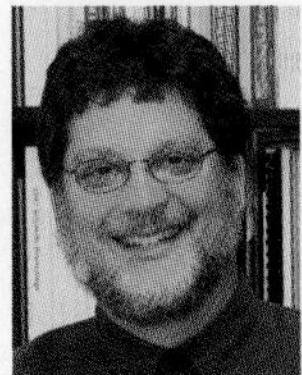

Joseph Taboada, DVM, Dipl ACVIM
Associate Dean, Student and Academic Affairs
Professor, Small Animal Internal Medicine
Veterinary Clinical Sciences
School of Veterinary Medicine
Louisiana State University
Baton Rouge, Louisiana

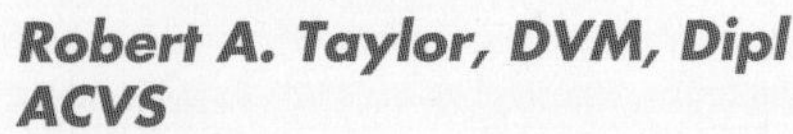

Robert A. Taylor, DVM, Dipl ACVS
Alameda East Veterinary Hospital
Denver, Colorado

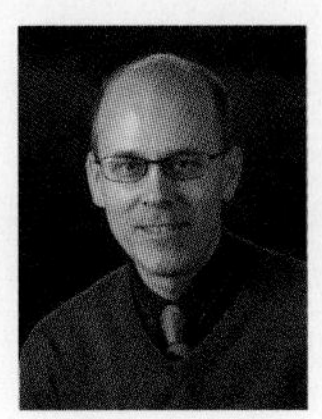

John A. Thomas, DVM
Assistant Professor, Veterinary Technology
Cuyahoga Community College
Cleveland, Ohio

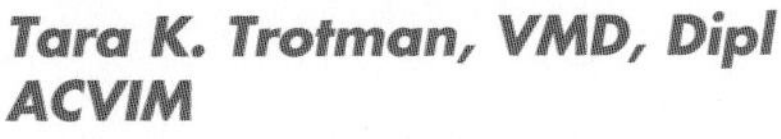

Tara K. Trotman, VMD, Dipl ACVIM
Staff Veterinarian, Internal Medicine
Department of Clinical Studies
Matthew J. Ryan Veterinary Hospital
University of Pennsylvania
Philadelphia, Pennsylvania

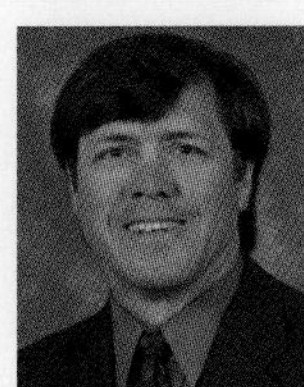

Thomas N. Tully, Jr., DVM, MS, Dipl ABVP (Avian), ECAMS
Professor Zoological Medicine
Veterinary Clinical Sciences
School of Veterinary Medicine
Louisiana State University
Baton Rouge, Louisiana

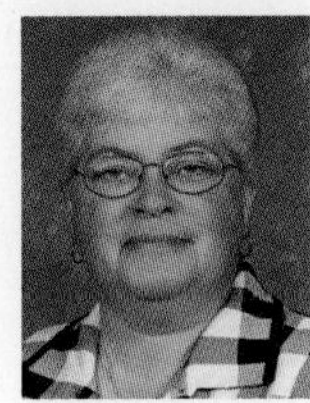

Jan L. VanSteenhouse, DVM, PhD, Dipl ACVP
Director of Clinical Pathology
Department of Clinical Pathology
MPI Research
Mattawn, Michigan

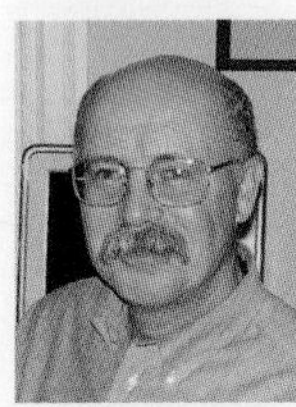

Thomas J. Van Winkle, VMD, Dipl ACVP
Professor, Department of Pathobiology
School of Veterinary Medicine
University of Pennsylvania
Philadelphia, Pennsylvania

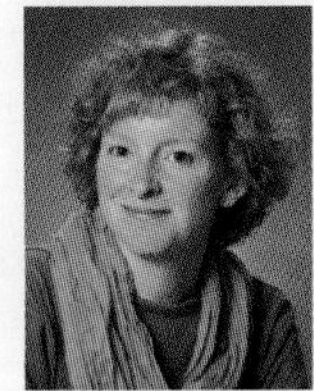

Sarah A. Wagner, DVM, PhD, Dipl ACVCP
Assistant Professor of Veterinary Technology
Department of Animal Sciences
North Dakota State University
Fargo, North Dakota

Preface

The spectrum of knowledge and skills required of a veterinary technician today requires increasing knowledge of current practice, self-evaluation, and clinical competence. Today's veterinary technician must have critical thinking abilities when problem-solving or making legal and ethical decisions.

A career as a veterinary technician is challenging and rewarding. The veterinary technician has emerged as a critical component of the veterinary health care team. Like the registered nurse in the field of human health care, the veterinary technician supports the clinical activities of the supervising doctor. However, unlike registered nurses, veterinary technicians are expected to perform the duties of radiology and laboratory technicians as well as those of medical, surgical, and anesthesia nurse. In addition, veterinary technicians must be prepared to work with multiple species rather than just one. Thus the veterinary technician has a surprisingly broad range of clinical responsibilities.

It is with pleasure that we present the seventh edition of the *Clinical Textbook for Veterinary Technicians.* Over the years, the text has come to figure prominently in the education of veterinary technicians, not only in the United States and Canada, but in many countries around the world. Keeping the material current and consistent with the changing trends in veterinary practice has been a key goal for us, and we therefore have been committed to generating a new edition every 4 years.

KEY FEATURES

Like prior editions, this new text is filled with updates, additions, and the presentation of emerging fields. There are 24 new contributors, each one an expert in his or her chosen field. The talent of these authors brings particular value to the textbook, particularly in light of the development of nursing specialties.

As always, the technician's role in every procedure is emphasized to enable students to focus on their responsibilities in every aspect of practice.

This edition is lavishly illustrated with hundreds of photographs and line drawings in full color, and includes more tables and boxes than ever before. Of the text's 39 chapters, five are new chapters and nine have been completely rewritten. Each chapter begins with a list of **key terms** and a series of **learning objectives. Technician notes** continue to be a helpful study tool for students. A comprehensive **glossary** has been assembled from the key terms and appears at the end of the text.

NEW FEATURES

The seventh edition features **increased coverage of large animals**—including history and physical exam, preventive health, diagnostic sampling, pain management, anesthesia, surgical assistance, dentistry, emergency nursing, and wound management—integrated into existing chapters, providing students with more in-depth information on large animal procedures, assessment, and treatment.

Many chapters also contain **new case presentations**—scenarios of actual patient situations and outcomes that link chapter information to relevant, real-life situations and help students reinforce book knowledge with practical experience.

Students and instructors will value the new student-friendly features throughout each chapter. An outline, key terms, and learning objectives begin each chapter. These, along with an introduction that synthesizes the material and explains its significance and the Technician Tips throughout the chapters, help students navigate through the chapters and focus their learning.

ORGANIZATION

At first glance, you will see that the text has been completely reorganized and divided into eight sections that are delineated by different colored pages.

- Part One is an introduction to the profession, and focuses on practice management, computer applications, medical records, and health and safety. A new chapter, "Laws, Regulations, and Ethics," has been added to this section to give students a foundation for making legal and ethical decisions.
- Part Two transitions into basic nursing topics such as restraint, handling, physical examination, and preventive health medicine.
- Part Three covers clinical sciences including diagnostic imaging. The parasitology chapter includes all new color photographs of both internal and external parasites.
- Part Four, Medical Nursing, includes diagnostic sampling and therapeutic techniques—a chapter that has been expanded to include large animal procedures and sequential illustrations of techniques, which emphasize the role of the vet tech in collecting specimens. This part also includes small animal medical nursing, and alternative medicine, and a new chapter, "Large Animal Medical Nursing." Another new chapter, "Physical Therapy and Rehabilitation," enables students to integrate the basics of physical rehabilitation into patient care.

- Part Five presents pharmacology, pain management, and anesthesia. The pain management chapter emphasizes the key role of the vet tech as a patient advocate in pain management. The anesthesia chapter, in addition to integrating large animal anesthesia, describes the role of the vet tech in patient preparation, monitoring, administration, care of equipment, and anesthetic emergencies.
- Part Six, Surgical Nursing, includes topics in surgery, surgical assisting, and dentistry. Oral surgery and equine dentistry have been added to the new dentistry chapter. "Large Animal Surgical Nursing" is a new chapter.
- Part Seven, Emergency and Critical Care, contains an expanded emergency and critical care chapter that now includes large animal emergency care. Wound healing, wound management and bandaging, and toxicology are also covered.
- Part Eight, End of Life, brings together oncology, a new chapter on **Geriatric and Hospice Care,** bereavement, and necropsy.

This new organizational scheme is illustrated in the simplified Table of Contents, which allows the reader to quickly locate desired topics. Cross referencing has been expanded and included in every chapter to direct the reader to related topics in other chapters.

THE LEARNING PACKAGE

The seventh edition of *Clinical Textbook for Veterinary Technicians* is designed as a comprehensive learning package.

The student package includes:
- The textbook
- Student Workbook
- Evolve website

The faculty package includes:
- The textbook
- TEACH Instructor Resources
- Student Workbook
- Evolve website

The entire package has been designed with the student and educator in mind. The ease of reading each comprehensive chapter and the additional materials provides students with the maximum opportunity to learn. The driving force in the development of this package was the creation of a proficient veterinary technician.

Student Workbook

The student workbook is designed to be a supplement to the learning process. The content of the workbook matches the book chapter by chapter to help students master and apply key concepts and procedures in a clinical situation. Included are multiple choice questions, matching exercises, photo quizzes, labeling exercises, crossword puzzles, and other activities to help in the studying process.

TEACH Instructor Resources

Available in print format and electronically on Evolve, TEACH Instructor Resources are designed to save the instructor time and take the guesswork out of classroom planning and preparation. It includes the Chapter focus, teaching tips, lesson plans, answers to the Workbook exercises, and an updated Test Bank.

Evolve Website

Elsevier has created a website dedicated solely to support this learning package: http://evolve.elsevier/com/Bassert/McCurnin/. The website includes both a Student site and an Instructor site.

Student site resources include:
- Sneak preview of workbook activities
- Medical Record Forms: 25 medical records that correlate directly with the medical records chapter in the book. These are full size forms that can be printed and used. They are listed alphabetically.
- Student activities
  - Crossword Puzzles: created for each chapter using the key words from the text
  - Picture-it Exercises: drag-and-drop activities that help identify labels on critical illustrations
  - Hangman: word-building activity
  - Quiz Shows: may be played as a group activity or individually

Faculty site resources include:
- TEACH Instructor Resources
  - Lesson Plans
  - PowerPoint Lecture Presentations
  - Test Bank in Examview 6 including 2000 questions
  - Answer Key: contains answers to the questions included in the workbook
- Image collection: contains all of the images from within the book, plus some additional images
- Access to all the student resources

SUPPORT

If you have questions or need assistance with ordering or adopting the *Clinical Textbook for Veterinary Technicians* learning package, contact Faculty Support at 1-800-222-9570 or via e-mail at sales.inquiry@elsevier.com.

We wish you professional fulfillment and pride in your career as a veterinary technician. So without further ado, it gives us great pride to present the seventh edition of *Clinical Textbook for Veterinary Technicians.*

Joanna M. Bassert
Dennis M. McCurnin

Acknowledgments

As with all large texts, this one would not be possible without the team effort of many people. In addition to our talented contributors, we are grateful to the many veterinary technicians in the greater Philadelphia area who graciously allowed Dr. Bassert to photograph them while they completed their clinical work. Among these, in particular, we are grateful to Karen Gries, CVT, for her support and assistance on the long but incredibly fun days of photojournalism at the small and large animal hospitals of the University of Pennsylvania. We are grateful to Harry Cowgill at Louisiana State University and Don O'Connor at Elsevier for performing their usual magic in the production of beautiful photographs and illustrations, respectively. Finally, and most important, we would like to acknowledge the leadership and skill of Teri Merchant at Elsevier, who encouraged and cajoled and managed this book through every stage of development and saw it to completion. Her contributions are without measure. Without Teri, this text would exist, but the journey would not have been such a grand adventure.

Joanna M. Bassert
Dennis M. McCurnin

Contents

How to Use This Learning Package

Clinical Textbook for Veterinary Technicians is the ultimate learning package for preparing students to become veterinary technicians. It provides a solid foundation for the basic and advanced clinical skills students must master to achieve competence, and its student-friendly style clarifies even the most complex concepts and procedures to help prepare for the VTNE and certification.

TEXTBOOK FEATURES

A simple chapter outline introduces you to the chapter material as a whole, allowing you to see at a glance how the subject material is organized. It also helps you focus on one topic at a time by showing you the relationship to other topics in the chapter.

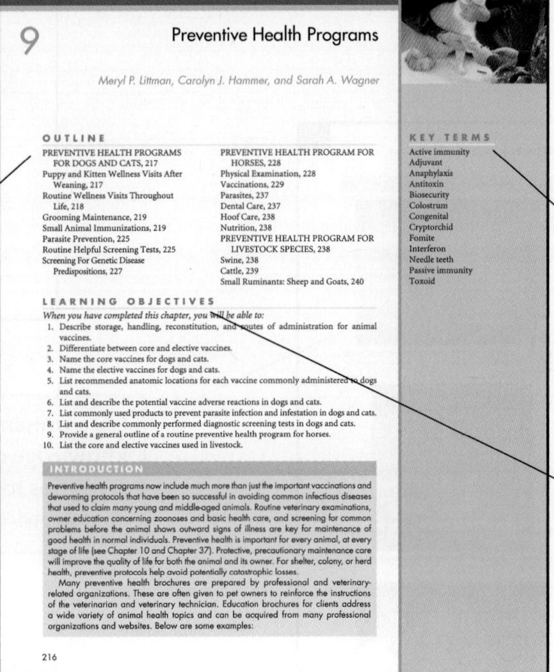

9

Preventive Health Programs

Meryl P. Littman, Carolyn J. Hammer, and Sarah A. Wagner

OUTLINE

PREVENTIVE HEALTH PROGRAMS FOR DOGS AND CATS, 217
Puppy and Kitten Wellness Visits After Weaning, 217
Routine Wellness Visits Throughout Life, 218
Grooming Maintenance, 219
Small Animal Immunizations, 219
Parasite Prevention, 225
Routine Helpful Screening Tests, 225
Screening For Genetic Disease Predispositions, 227
PREVENTIVE HEALTH PROGRAM FOR HORSES, 228
Physical Examination, 228
Vaccinations, 229
Parasites, 237
Dental Care, 237
Hoof Care, 238
Nutrition, 238
PREVENTIVE HEALTH PROGRAM FOR LIVESTOCK SPECIES, 238
Swine, 238
Cattle, 239
Small Ruminants: Sheep and Goats, 240

KEY TERMS

Active immunity
Adjuvant
Anaphylaxis
Antitoxin
Biosecurity
Colostrum
Congenital
Cryptorchid
Fomite
Interferon
Needle teeth
Passive immunity
Toxoid

LEARNING OBJECTIVES

When you have completed this chapter, you will be able to:

1. Describe storage, handling, reconstitution, and routes of administration for animal vaccines.
2. Differentiate between core and elective vaccines.
3. Name the core vaccines for dogs and cats.
4. Name the elective vaccines for dogs and cats.
5. List recommended anatomic locations for each vaccine commonly administered to dogs and cats.
6. List and describe the potential vaccine adverse reactions in dogs and cats.
7. List commonly used products to prevent parasite infection and infestation in dogs and cats.
8. List and describe commonly performed diagnostic screening tests in dogs and cats.
9. Provide a general outline of a routine preventive health program for horses.
10. List the core and elective vaccines used in livestock.

INTRODUCTION

Preventive health programs now include much more than just the important vaccinations and deworming protocols that have been so successful in avoiding common infectious diseases that used to claim many young and middle-aged animals. Routine veterinary examinations, owner education concerning zoonoses and basic health care, and screening for common problems before the animal shows outward signs of illness are key for maintenance of good health in normal individuals. Preventive health is important for every animal, at every stage of life (see Chapter 10 and Chapter 37). Protective, precautionary maintenance care will improve the quality of life for both the animal and its owner. For shelter, colony, or herd health, preventive protocols help avoid potentially catastrophic losses.

Many preventive health brochures are prepared by professional and veterinary-related organizations. These are often given to pet owners to reinforce the instructions of the veterinarian and veterinary technician. Education brochures for clients address a wide variety of animal health topics and can be acquired from many professional organizations and websites. Below are some examples:

216

Key Terms listed on the chapter opening page reinforce new terminology.

Learning Objectives help you focus on key concepts and procedures for mastery on completion of the chapter.

Introduction gives an overview of the chapter that distills the key points and focuses your study.

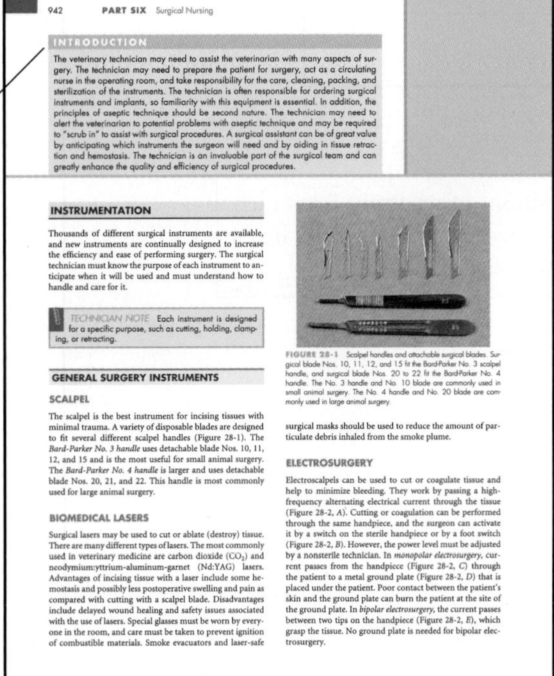

942 PART SIX Surgical Nursing

INTRODUCTION

The veterinary technician may need to assist the veterinarian with many aspects of surgery. The technician may need to prepare the patient for surgery, act as a circulating nurse in the operating room, and take responsibility for the care, cleaning, packing, and sterilization of the instruments. The technician is often responsible for ordering surgical instruments and implants, so familiarity with this equipment is essential. In addition, the principles of aseptic technique should be second nature. The technician may need to alert the veterinarian to potential problems with aseptic technique and may be required to "scrub in" to assist with surgical procedures. A surgical assistant can be of great value by anticipating which instruments the surgeon will need and by aiding in tissue retraction and hemostasis. The technician is an invaluable part of the surgical team and can greatly enhance the quality and efficiency of surgical procedures.

INSTRUMENTATION

Thousands of different surgical instruments are available, and new instruments are continually designed to increase the efficiency and ease of performing surgery. The surgical technician must know the purpose of each instrument to anticipate when it will be used and must understand how to handle and care for it.

TECHNICIAN NOTE Each instrument is designed for a specific purpose, such as cutting, holding, clamping, or retracting.

GENERAL SURGERY INSTRUMENTS

SCALPEL

The scalpel is the best instrument for incising tissues with minimal trauma. A variety of disposable blades are designed to fit several different scalpel handles (Figure 28-1). The *Bard-Parker No. 3 handle* uses detachable blade Nos. 10, 11, 12, and 15 and is the most useful for small animal surgery. The *Bard-Parker No. 4 handle* is larger and uses detachable blade Nos. 20, 21, and 22. This handle is most commonly used for large animal surgery.

BIOMEDICAL LASERS

Surgical lasers may be used to cut or ablate (destroy) tissue. There are many different types of lasers. The most commonly used in veterinary medicine are carbon dioxide (CO_2) and neodymium:yttrium-aluminum-garnet (Nd:YAG) lasers. Advantages of incising tissue with a laser include some hemostasis and possibly less postoperative swelling and pain as compared with cutting with a scalpel blade. Disadvantages include delayed wound healing and safety issues associated with the use of lasers. Special glasses must be worn by everyone in the room, and care must be taken to prevent ignition of combustible materials. Smoke evacuators and laser-safe surgical masks should be used to reduce the amount of particulate debris inhaled from the smoke plume.

FIGURE 28-1 Scalpel handles and attachable surgical blades. Surgical blade Nos. 10, 11, 12, and 15 fit the Bard-Parker No. 3 scalpel handle, and surgical blade Nos. 20 to 22 fit the Bard-Parker No. 4 handle. The No. 3 handle and No. 10 blade are commonly used in small animal surgery. The No. 4 handle and No. 20 blade are commonly used in large animal surgery.

ELECTROSURGERY

Electroscalpels can be used to cut or coagulate tissue and help to minimize bleeding. They work by passing a high-frequency alternating electrical current through the tissue (Figure 28-2, *A*). Cutting or coagulation can be performed through the same handpiece, and the surgeon can activate it by a switch on the sterile handpiece or by a foot switch (Figure 28-2, *B*). However, the power level must be adjusted by a nonsterile technician. In *monopolar electrosurgery*, current passes from the handpiece (Figure 28-2, *C*) through the patient to a metal ground plate (Figure 28-2, *D*) that is placed under the patient. Poor contact between the patient's skin and the ground plate can burn the patient at the site of the ground plate. In *bipolar electrosurgery*, the current passes between two tips on the handpiece (Figure 28-2, *E*), which grasp the tissue. No ground plate is needed for bipolar electrosurgery.

Technician Notes are interspersed throughout each chapter to help you retain key information related to the technician's role.

FIGURE 26-6 Administering transmucosal buprenorphine to cat. Transmucosal delivery of buprenorphine is extremely efficacious in the cat and provides up to 8 hours of pain relief in the hospital or at home.

TECHNICIAN NOTE Butorphanol should not be used as the sole analgesic unless mild pain of short duration (less than 1 hour) is expected.

Opioid Reversal

Naloxone hydrochloride (pure opioid antagonist). One of the reasons that makes opioid use safe is the ability to rapidly reverse sedation and adverse side effects. Antagonists work by blocking opioid action at the receptors. Onset of reversal occurs within 1 to 2 minutes of IV administration and can last for 1 to 4 hours. Treatment may be repeated when reversing narcotics with a longer duration. Typical dosage is 2 μg/kg IV. **Butorphanol tartrate (torbugesic) (mu antagonist).** See preceding comments.

Synthetic Opioid

Tramadol. Tramadol is a synthetic drug with opioid-like analgesic effects, but fewer side effects. Tramadol has opioid-like activity at the mu receptor and appears to be quite effective in controlling moderate pain, especially when used in conjunction with an NSAID. It is available in oral form making it suitable for long-term at-home management of postoperative, cancer, orthopedic, and other chronic pain. A wide variety of dosages have been tried and reported in both the dog and the cat. Current dosing recommendation is for 4 mg/kg PO b.i.d. to t.i.d. in the dog and cat. It is also unscheduled, an additional benefit. Tramadol may be effective in management of long-term cancer patients, problem osteoarthritis cases, or postoperative prolonged pain.

α_2-Agonists

Xylazine, medetomidine (Domitor), and dexmedetomidine (dexdomitor) are α_2-agonists widely used in veterinary medicine. Dexdomitor is the most potent and selective α_2-agonist and is playing an ever-increasing role in pain management and sedation. α_2-Agonists, which are nonnarcotic and nonscheduled agents, can be useful as adjuncts in a balanced analgesic protocol. The main effect is to produce significant sedation accompanied by visceral and somatic analgesia. There are a variety of new ways to use this drug class as a premedication, rough recovery rescue and ongoing management of in-hospital pain and anxiety. α_2-Agonist combinations are also extremely effective in cats for a variety of surgical and nonsurgical procedures.

α_2-Agonists inhibit release of the excitatory neurotransmitter norepinephrine to produce analgesia and sedation. α_2-Agonists are short-duration analgesics and can be rapidly reversed with α_2-antagonists. This characteristic makes these drugs suitable for procedures requiring short-term restraint and analgesia. α_2-Agonists may bind to the same receptors as opioids and act synergistically with them. The dosages of other analgesic and anesthetic agents can be significantly reduced if given concurrently with α_2-agonists. α_2-Agonists can have profound effects on the cardiovascular and nervous systems, but these adverse events can be minimized by using low dosages. Bradycardia and vomiting are the most common side effects with α_2-agonists.

TECHNICIAN NOTE α_2-Agonists cause vasoconstriction and, like kinking a water hose, the narrowed vessels result in increased blood pressure or hypertension. Because heart rate normally goes up when blood pressure is low and down when pressure is high, slowed heart rate is expected. Bradycardia is considered a normal finding when using α_2-agonists.

Advantages of α_2-Agonists Over Other Sedatives

Other commonly used sedatives (e.g., acepromazine and diazepam) do not provide pain relief. The analgesia achieved with α_2-agonists is of moderate intensity and moderate duration. Even more importantly, α_2-agonists work synergistically with opioids (such as butorphanol or morphine) and improve both the intensity and the duration of pain relief. Other advantages are that the degree of sedation can be "tailored" or "titrated" by using different dosages and/or different drug combinations to provide mild to profound sedation and that α_2-agonists are reversible. Antisedan (atipamezole) is most commonly used to reverse Dexdomitor. Antisedan is the safest of all of the reversal agents because it works almost exclusively by simply displacing Dexdomitor from the α_2-receptors so that the nerve function can return to normal. After the administration of Antisedan, patients usually awaken in about 5 to 10 minutes and are able to stand or walk in less than 10 minutes. α_2-Agonists, are used in a variety of ways to provide patient comfort including as premedicant before surgery combined with an opioid, as a stand-alone sedative or analgesic for short procedures, such as x-rays, and as a rescue drug for patients experiencing rough recovery from anesthesia. The most common use of α_2-agonists in cats is in a combination called "kitty magic," which consists of an α_2-agonist,

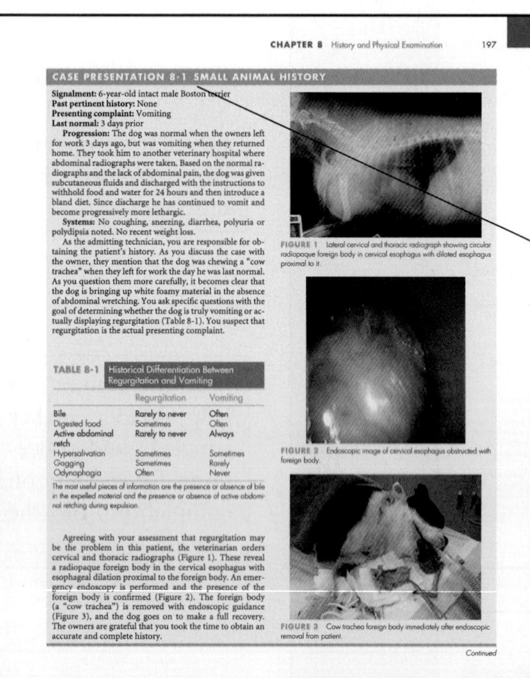

CHAPTER 8 History and Physical Examination 197

CASE PRESENTATION 8-1 SMALL ANIMAL HISTORY

Signalment: 6-year-old intact male Boston terrier
Past pertinent history: None
Presenting complaint: Vomiting
Last normal: 3 days prior

Progression: The dog was normal when the owners left for work 3 days ago, but was vomiting when they returned home. They took him to another veterinary hospital where abdominal radiographs were taken. Based on the normal radiographs and the lack of abdominal pain, the dog was given subcutaneous fluids and discharged with the instructions to withhold food and water for 24 hours and then introduce a bland diet. Since discharge he has continued to vomit and become progressively more lethargic.

Systems: No coughing, sneezing, diarrhea, polyuria or polydipsia noted. No recent weight loss.

As the admitting technician, you are responsible for obtaining the patient's history. As you discuss the case with the owner, they mention that the dog was chewing a "cow trachea" when they left for work the day he was last normal. As you question them more carefully, it becomes clear that the dog is bringing up white foamy material in the absence of abdominal wretching. You ask specific questions with the goal of determining whether the dog is truly vomiting or actually displaying regurgitation (Table 8-1). You suspect that regurgitation is the actual presenting complaint.

TABLE 8-1 Historical Differentiation Between Regurgitation and Vomiting

	Regurgitation	Vomiting
Bile	Rarely to never	Often
Digested food	Sometimes	Often
Active abdominal retch	Rarely to never	Always
Hypersalivation	Sometimes	Sometimes
Gagging	Sometimes	Rarely
Odynophagia	Often	Never

The most useful pieces of information are the presence or absence of bile in the expelled material and the presence or absence of active abdominal retching during expulsion.

Agreeing with your assessment that regurgitation may be the problem in this patient, the veterinarian orders cervical and thoracic radiographs (Figure 1). These reveal a radiopaque foreign body in the cervical esophagus with esophageal dilation proximal to the foreign body. An emergency endoscopy is performed and the presence of the foreign body is confirmed (Figure 2). The foreign body (a "cow trachea") is removed with endoscopic guidance (Figure 3), and the dog goes on to make a full recovery. The owners are grateful that you took the time to obtain an accurate and complete history.

FIGURE 1 Lateral cervical and thoracic radiograph showing circular radiopaque foreign body in cervical esophagus with dilated esophagus proximal to it.

FIGURE 2 Endoscopic image of cervical esophagus obstructed with foreign body.

FIGURE 3 Cow trachea foreign body immediately after endoscopic removal from patient.

Continued

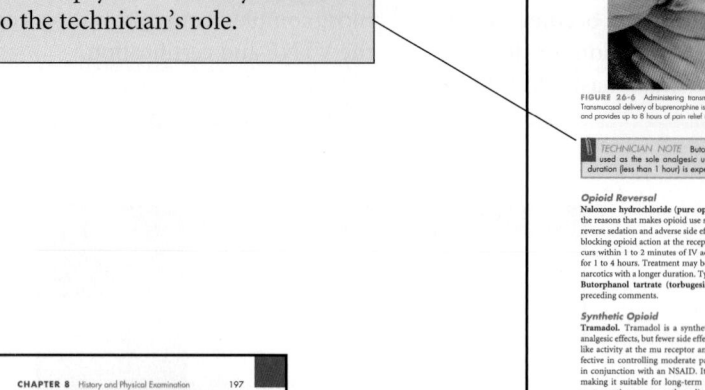

Case presentations challenge you to apply your knowledge of chapter content to realistic clinical scenarios to solve problems and make appropriated decisions.

Glossary

Abaxial Facing away from the axis of an organ
Abdominal pinging Technique of identifying abdominal gas accumulations by simultaneous percussion and auscultation of the abdominal wall
Abdominocentesis The insertion of a needle (attached to a syringe) into the abdominal cavity using sterile technique to obtain free abdominal fluid for evaluation
Abomasopexy Surgical fixation of the abomasum to the body wall
Abomasum The "true stomach" of the ruminant; secretes acids, mixes and contracts ingesta, and moves liquid chyme into the small intestine.
Abrasion Tooth wear associated with chewing on objects, such as rocks, ice cubes, toys, and bones in an area where skin has been scraped
Abscess Localized collection of pus in part of the body, formed by tissue disintegration usually resulting from bacterial infection and surrounded by an inflamed area
Absorption The uptake of substances into or across tissue
Acanthocephalan A "thorny-headed" worm. *Macracanthorhynchus hirudinaceus* is a "thorny-headed" worm parasite found in the small intestine of pigs.
Acanthocytes RBCs with multiple, irregularly spaced, club-shaped projections from the cell surface
Acariasis Infestation by either mites or ticks
Acarines Parasites that are either mites or ticks. *Demodex canis*, the follicular mite, and *Rhipicephalus sanguineus*, the brown dog tick, are classified as acarines.
Accessory motion Refers to the spin, roll, and gliding motions of one joint surface on another
Accounts receivable Money that is due to the practice from the sale of goods or services
Acid-Base Metabolic status associated with pH of blood or tissue
Acidemic Serum pH above the reference interval
Acid-Fast stain A useful differential staining procedure that specifically stains all members of the genus *Mycobacterium*. The high lipid and wax content of the mycobacterial cell walls is thought to be the reason that the cells will resist decolorization with acid alcohol and stain red, the color of the initial stain carbol fuchsin.
Acidosis Elevated levels of metabolic acids within the blood or tissue
Acids Compounds whose water-based solutions have a sour taste, turn blue litmus paper red, and can combine with metals to form salts and yield hydrogen ions or protons when dissolved in water
Acoustic impedance Attenuation of the energy of the ultrasound beam as it passes through different tissues. It is specific for each tissue type (fluid, air, bone, fat, etc.).
Acoustic shadow Ultrasound beam interaction with a highly reflective surface, such as bone, foreign material, or gas, causing a high degree of attenuation of the beam and blocking of the pathway of the beam to deeper tissue
Active assisted range of motion (AAROM) Patient is assisted manually or mechanically to achieve a normal range of motion when the prime muscle mover is weak or injured
Active listening skills A combination of acutely paying attention to what another is saying plus demonstrating that focused attention through body language and verbal feedback while maintaining a nonjudgmental attitude
Active range of motion (AROM) Ability of a patient to voluntarily move a limb through a range of motion
Acupuncture The use of needles (or injection of fluid, laser, ultrasound, surgically implanted material, and electrical stimulation) to stimulate specific predetermined "acupuncture" points in the body to produce chemical or physiologic changes in the body. It is combined with herbs and massage to make up traditional Chinese medicine (TCM).
Acute radiation toxicity Side effects caused by radiotherapy that occur between day 1 (the start of radiotherapy) and day 90. They are characterized by toxicity to rapidly proliferating normal tissues, such as skin, mucous membranes, intestinal tract, and bone marrow, and often resolve within days to weeks.
Adaptation Adjustment of a dental instrument that accounts for curvature of the tooth
Adjunctive agent Medications other than those commonly used that may help primary treatment
Adjuvant therapy Cancer treatment that is given in addition to the primary or initial treatment. The most common examples are radiotherapy that is given to treat residual cancer remaining after an incomplete surgical resection or postoperative chemotherapy that is administered to prevent or treat systemic metastasis. The overall purpose of adjuvant therapy is to decrease the likelihood of cancer recurrence.
Adrenocortical Pertaining to the cortex or outermost layer of the adrenal gland
Adsorbent Solid substance that attracts and holds a substance to its surface
Adulticide A therapeutic compound that will kill the adult stages of a parasite
AE title The name assigned to each modality so it can communicate electronically with the PACS in digital imaging
Aerobe An organism that can live and grow in the presence of oxygen. An organism that can use oxygen as a final electron acceptor in a respiratory chain. Obligate aerobes cannot grow anaerobically.
Aerophagia Swallowing an excessive volume of air
Agammaglobulinemic Description of a pathologic condition in which the body forms few or no γ-globulins or antibodies
Agglutination Clumping of blood. Agglutinated RBCs tend to appear as clumps secondary to strong specific antibody cross-linking of RBCs; will not dissociate upon addition of saline

1361

Glossary with definitions of key terms from each chapter reinforces new terminology and helps you comprehend the reading material.

STUDENT WORKBOOK

The Workbook, sold separately, includes review exercises for all chapters, including definitions of key terms, matching, fill-in-the-blank, short answer, true-false, review questions, photo quizzes, word searches, superclues, and crossword puzzles.

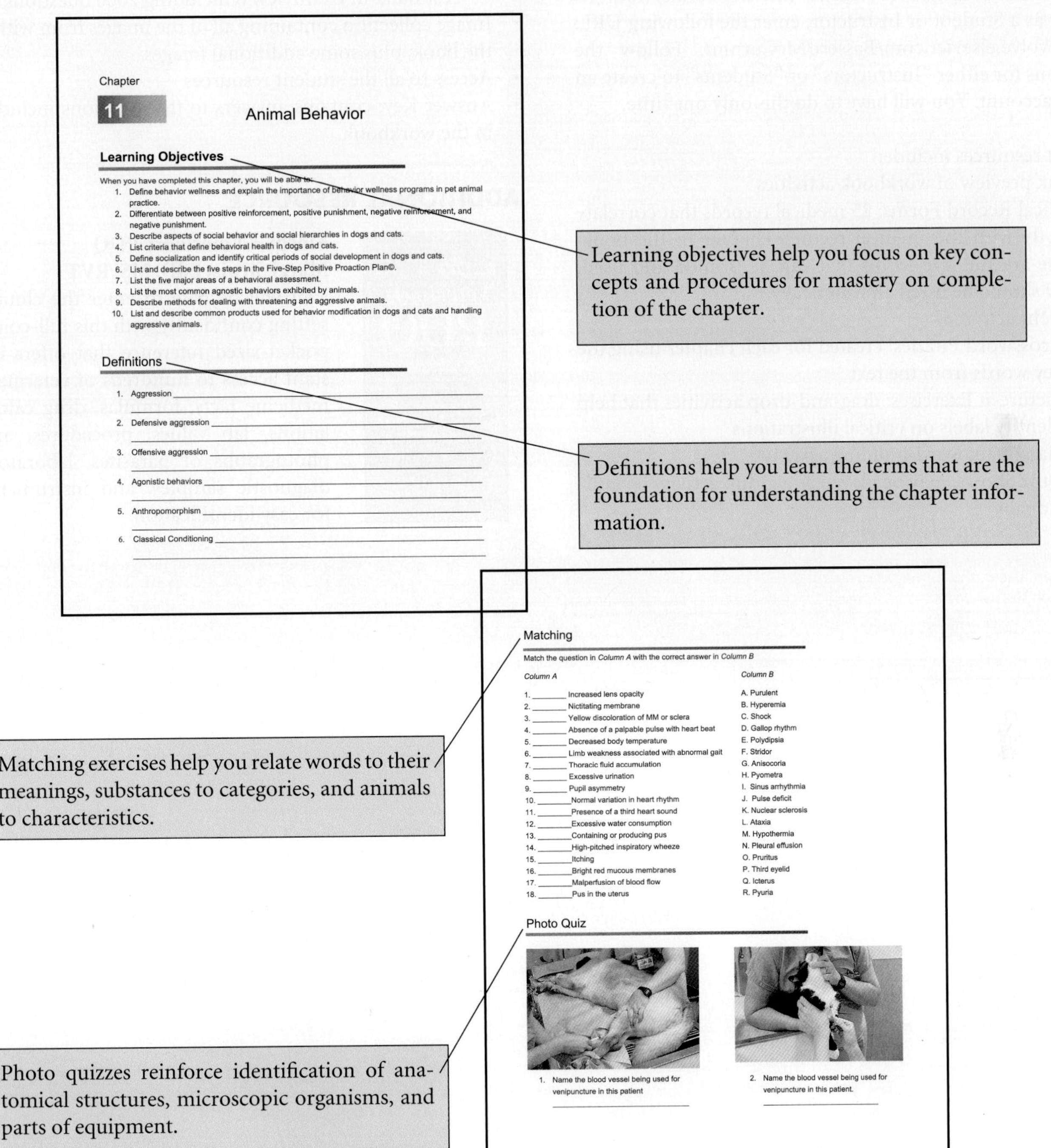

Chapter 11 Animal Behavior

Learning Objectives

When you have completed this chapter, you will be able to:

1. Define behavior wellness and explain the importance of behavior wellness programs in pet animal practice.
2. Differentiate between positive reinforcement, positive punishment, negative reinforcement, and negative punishment.
3. Describe aspects of social behavior and social hierarchies in dogs and cats.
4. List criteria that define behavioral health in dogs and cats.
5. Define socialization and identify critical periods of social development in dogs and cats.
6. List and describe the five steps in the Five-Step Positive Proaction Plan©.
7. List the five major areas of a behavioral assessment.
8. List the most common agnostic behaviors exhibited by animals.
9. Describe methods for dealing with threatening and aggressive animals.
10. List and describe common products used for behavior modification in dogs and cats and handling aggressive animals.

Definitions

1. Aggression
2. Defensive aggression
3. Offensive aggression
4. Agonistic behaviors
5. Anthropomorphism
6. Classical Conditioning

Matching

Match the question in *Column A* with the correct answer in *Column B*

Column A	*Column B*
1. ______ Increased lens opacity	A. Purulent
2. ______ Nictitating membrane	B. Hyperemia
3. ______ Yellow discoloration of MM or sclera	C. Shock
4. ______ Absence of a palpable pulse with heart beat	D. Gallop rhythm
5. ______ Decreased body temperature	E. Polydipsia
6. ______ Limb weakness associated with abnormal gait	F. Stridor
7. ______ Thoracic fluid accumulation	G. Anisocoria
8. ______ Excessive urination	H. Pyometra
9. ______ Pupil asymmetry	I. Sinus arrhythmia
10. ______ Normal variation in heart rhythm	J. Pulse deficit
11. ______ Presence of a third heart sound	K. Nuclear sclerosis
12. ______ Excessive water consumption	L. Ataxia
13. ______ Containing or producing pus	M. Hypothermia
14. ______ High-pitched inspiratory wheeze	N. Pleural effusion
15. ______ Itching	O. Pruritus
16. ______ Bright red mucous membranes	P. Third eyelid
17. ______ Malperfusion of blood flow	Q. Icterus
18. ______ Pus in the uterus	R. Pyuria

Photo Quiz

1. Name the blood vessel being used for venipuncture in this patient

2. Name the blood vessel being used for venipuncture in this patient.

Learning objectives help you focus on key concepts and procedures for mastery on completion of the chapter.

Definitions help you learn the terms that are the foundation for understanding the chapter information.

Matching exercises help you relate words to their meanings, substances to categories, and animals to characteristics.

Photo quizzes reinforce identification of anatomical structures, microscopic organisms, and parts of equipment.

EVOLVE WEBSITE

The Evolve website includes free learning resources available to instructors and students using *McCurnin's Clinical Textbook for Veterinary Technicians.* At the front of this textbook is a page introducing the Evolve site. All you need to get started is a computer with an internet connection. To register as a Student or Instructor, enter the following URL: http://evolve.elsevier.com/Bassert/McCurnin/. Follow the directions for either "Instructors" or "Students" to create an Evolve account. You will have to do this only one time.

Student resources include:

- Sneak preview of workbook activities
- Medical Record Forms: 25 medical records that correlate directly with the medical records chapter in the book. These are full size forms that can be printed and used. They should be listed alphabetically.
- Student activities
  - Crossword Puzzles: created for each chapter using the key words from the text
  - Picture-it Exercises: drag-and-drop activities that help identify labels on critical illustrations
  - Hangman: word-building activity
  - Quiz Shows: may be played as a group activity or individually

Instructor resources include:

- TEACH Instructor Resources
  - Lesson Plans
  - PowerPoint Lecture Presentations
  - Test Bank in Examview 6 including 2000 questions
- Image collection containing all of the images from within the book, plus some additional images
- Access to all the student resources
- Answer Key: contains answers to the questions included in the workbook

ADDITIONAL RESOURCE

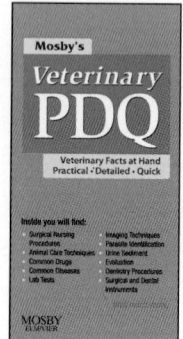

Mosby's Veterinary PDQ
Margi Sirois, EdD, MS, RVT
You will be able to enter the clinical setting confidently with this full-color, pocket-sized reference that offers instant access to hundreds of veterinary medicine facts, formulas, drug calculations, lab values, procedures, and photographs of parasites, laboratory diagnostic samples, and instruments for easy identification.

An Introduction to Veterinary Technology

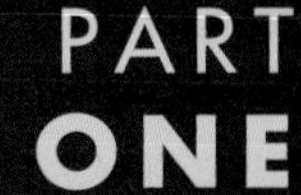

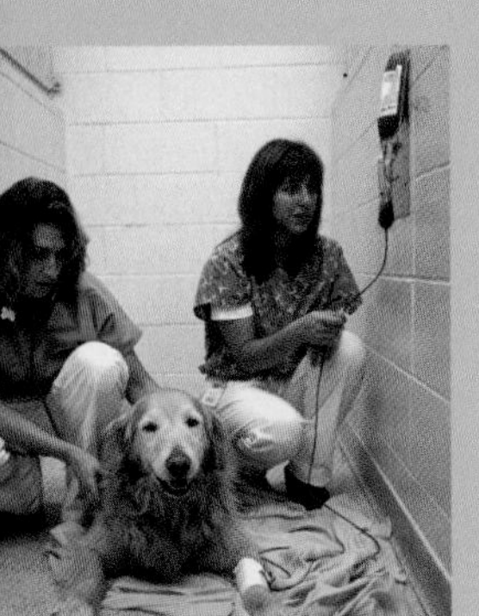

Veterinary Technology: An Overview

1

Joanna M. Bassert

KEY TERMS

CAAHTT
IVNTA
NAVTA
Veterinarian
Veterinary assistant
Veterinary technician
Veterinary technician specialist
Veterinary technologist
Veterinary technology
VTNE
Walter E. Collins, DVM

OUTLINE

LEARNING OBJECTIVES

When you have completed this chapter, you will be able to:

1. Name the organizations represented by the acronyms AVMA, CVMA, CVTEA, NAVTA, and AAVSB and describe their roles in the education and credentialing of veterinary technicians.
2. List the members of the veterinary health care team.
3. List the roles and responsibilities of the veterinary technician in a variety of clinical settings.
4. List the recognized veterinary technician specialty academies and describe the general process for obtaining a veterinary technician specialist (VTS) credential.
5. Describe the purpose of the VTNE and the AALAS examinations.
6. List and describe the aspects of professionalism for veterinary technology.
7. Describe the components of a properly written professional letter.
8. List the components commonly found in a résumé.
9. List the aspects of preparing for an interview.
10. Describe workplace stressors and methods for reducing stress.

I solemnly dedicate myself to aiding animals and society by providing excellent care and services for animals, by alleviating animal suffering, and by promoting public health.

I accept my obligations to practice my profession conscientiously and with sensitivity, adhering to the profession's Code of Ethics, and furthering my knowledge and competence through a commitment to lifelong learning.

Veterinary Technician Oath

INTRODUCTION

The veterinary technician has emerged as a critical component of the veterinary health care team. Like the registered nurse in the human health care field, the veterinary technician supports the clinical activities of the supervising veterinarian. However, unlike registered nurses, veterinary technicians are expected to perform the duties of a radiology and laboratory technician and those of a medical, surgical, and anesthesia nurse (Figure 1-1). In addition, veterinary technicians must be prepared to work with multiple species rather than just one. Thus the veterinary technician has a surprisingly broad range of clinical responsibilities. Over the past 55 years, veterinary medicine has become highly sophisticated. Many veterinarians find that they can no longer meet their practice goals, in terms of both providing a high level of medical care and attaining acceptable profit margins, without the skilled assistance of veterinary technicians. In addition, the development of veterinary-centered television programs has given the public a look into the inner workings of the animal hospital. For the first time, the public is able to see the important role that veterinary technicians play in the real-life drama of saving animal's lives. Thus there is heightened awareness of veterinary technology and an increased expectation, for both the practitioner and the pet owner, that animal patients will receive excellent veterinary nursing care. This introduction presents an overview of the profession of veterinary technology. It discusses the profession's history, educational requirements, range of duties, salaries, specialties, professional organizations, and expectations for professional conduct. In Chapter 2, the laws and ethics that define the profession of veterinary technology will be discussed.

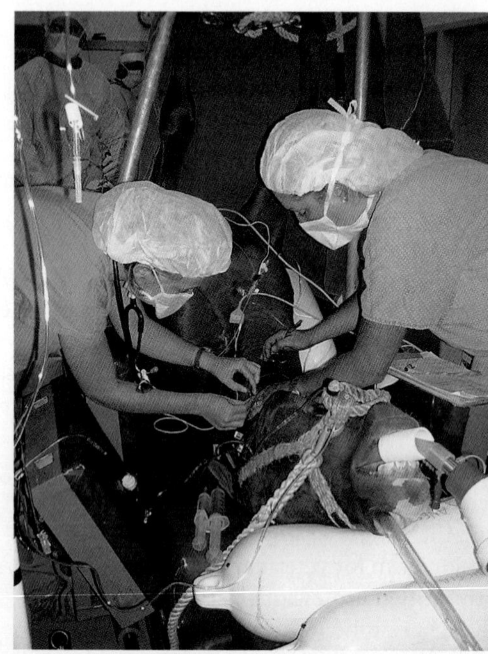

FIGURE 1-1 The veterinary technician has emerged as a critical component of the veterinary health care team. These veterinary technicians work at the New Bolton Center, University of Pennsylvania School of Veterinary Medicine. (Courtesy Dr. Joanna Bassert.)

HISTORY OF VETERINARY TECHNOLOGY

Historically, many veterinarians practiced independently and performed many of the laboratory and nursing duties themselves. Often spouses and other laypersons served as veterinary assistants, receptionists, and office managers. Today many practices employ multiple veterinarians and require a staff of veterinary technicians, assistants, receptionists, and kennel workers to carry out the many duties required in running a successful practice. This team approach is a fundamental part of veterinary practice management today, and the veterinary technician often serves as an important link between the veterinarian and support personnel.

The profession of veterinary technology began to take form in the early 1960s with the establishment of the first formal university-level program for the education of animal health technicians. The period that followed 1960 is rich with the accomplishments of dedicated veterinarians and veterinary technicians whose professional developments are listed on the inside cover of this book. Of particular importance are the accomplishments of Dr. Walter E. Collins (Box 1-1), who is now considered the father of veterinary technology. Veterinary technicians were first called "animal health technicians." The adjective "veterinary" referred exclusively to veterinarians until 1989 when the term "veterinary technician" was approved for use by the American Veterinary Medical Association's (AVMA) House of Delegates. As of this printing, there are more than 178 accredited programs of veterinary technology in Canada and the United States, though this number is steadily increasing. Current listings of these programs can be found at www.avma.org for programs accredited by the AVMA and at www.caahtt-acttsa.ca for programs accredited by the Canadian Veterinary Medical Association (CVMA) and by the Ontario Association of Veterinary Technicians (OAVT). Thousands of individuals have graduated from these programs, and the number of veterinary technology programs continues to grow as the demand for educated, skilled personnel increases.

THE VETERINARY TECHNICIAN TODAY

Veterinary technicians work in a wide range of facilities, perform many different kinds of tasks, and may encounter all manner of animal species. For example, veterinary technicians may work in private veterinary practices, such as companion animal, equine, food animal, or mixed practices. (A mixed practice is one that treats both farm and companion animals.) Veterinary technicians may also work in zoos, aquariums, wildlife rehabilitation centers, and research facilities. In addition, they may work for pharmaceutical companies as sales representatives of veterinary products, or they may become entrepreneurs by establishing their own kennel facility or pet-sitting businesses. Qualified veterinary technicians may also become instructors in veterinary technology programs or other academic programs. The range of job opportunities for the veterinary technician today is broader than ever before (Table 1-1 shows the income estimates from the 2006 U.S. Department of Labor, Bureau of Labor Statistics).

Within this diverse array of opportunities, veterinary technicians may also narrow their field of work and concentrate on specific areas. For example, a technician working in a practice that treats exotic species, such as birds and reptiles, will develop skills and knowledge particular to that aspect of veterinary medicine. In addition, some veterinary practices are called "specialty" or "referral" practices because they employ veterinarians who have completed special training in a particular aspect of veterinary medicine, such as dermatology, surgery, internal medicine, radiology, or ophthalmology. The veterinary hospitals associated with schools of veterinary medicine are examples of large specialty practices.

BOX 1-1 Walter Emmett Collins, DVM, The Father of Veterinary Technology

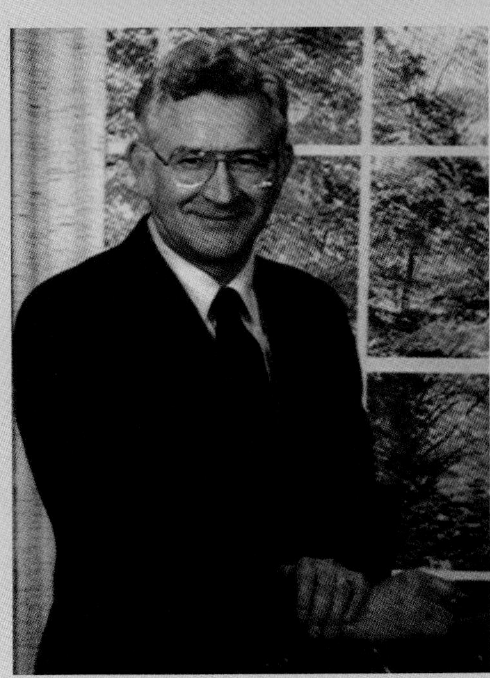

On November 19, 1930, Dr. Walter Collins was born on a small farm in Milford, N.Y. Like many children reared in a bucolic setting, Dr. Collins grew to love the expansive fields of crops and the many farm animals that were part of his young life. In 1948 after graduating from high school, his interest in agriculture led him to the State University of New York (SUNY) at Delhi, where he studied general agriculture for 2 years. Afterward, he served as a dairy herd improvement supervisor for 2 years before entering the U.S. Air Force. Dr. Collins believed that he was fortunate to be assigned to the Veterinary Department at Webb Air Force Base in Big Spring, Tex., where he worked under the direction of three "understanding and stimulating" veterinarian commanding officers who encouraged him to pursue a career in veterinary medicine. When his tour ended in the spring of 1956, Dr. Collins moved to Ithaca, N.Y., where he studied preveterinary science and subsequently attended New York State College of Veterinary Medicine at Cornell University. He graduated and received a doctor of veterinary medicine (DVM) degree in June 1961 and later returned to Delhi, where he joined a large animal practice. After 1 year, he opted to establish his own private veterinary practice in Delhi.

In the fall of 1964, while still practicing part time in Delhi, Dr. Collins became a teacher for the first time by joining the faculty of the Animal Science Technology Program. He was hired by Dr. Winfield Stone, the director of the program, who soon became an important mentor and friend. Several years later, in 1967, after Dr. Stone accepted another position on campus, Dr. Collins became the new program director at Delhi. During his tenure as director, Dr. Collins was awarded, as administrator, a grant from the U.S. Department of Health, Education, and Welfare to develop a model curriculum guide for training animal health technicians. From 1969 to 1975, Dr. Collins authored or coauthored several significant publications and the model curriculum.

In the early 1970s, Delhi's faculty was anxious to prove that the program was meeting real needs of New York practitioners. Dr. Collins decided to survey veterinarians and presented his findings at the 62nd New York State Conference for Veterinarians. Dr. Collins wrote, "For myself, I had felt the veterinary practitioner employer could use his/her new technician employee to relieve them of many non-professional duties as was already being accomplished similarly in human medicine. Both, my staff and I were gratified at the time by this small sampling survey which certainly hinted that we were on the right track!"

After leaving Delhi, Dr. Collins served as program director for 1 year at Mountain View College in Dallas. He subsequently became an associate professor and coordinator of the Veterinary Technology Program at Michigan State University, where he stayed from 1977 until his retirement in 1990. In Michigan, he served on the Michigan Veterinary Medical Association (MVMA) Veterinary Technician Committee, which assisted in the development of legislation that defined veterinary technology for Michigan.

When asked about the important events occurring in his professional life, Dr. Collins readily recalled his involvement in the formation of the Association of Animal Technician Educators (now the Association of Veterinary Technician Educators [AVTE]). In addition, he remembered well his service during the formative years on AVMA's Committee on Animal Technician Activities and Training (now called the Committee on Veterinary Technician Education and Activities) and on the National Veterinary Technician Testing Committee, which was charged with developing the Veterinary Technician National Examination. Finally, Dr. Collins was proud to host the 1981 AVTE Symposium at Michigan State University, which gave rise to the first professional organization for veterinary technicians, the North American Veterinary Technician Association (now known as the National Association of Veterinary Technicians in America).

For these efforts and a lifetime of commitment to the development of the profession, Dr. Collins is considered to be the "father of veterinary technology in the United States."

TABLE 1-1 U.S. Bureau of Labor Statistics 2006

National Estimate and Mean Wage Estimate

Employment No.	Average Hourly Wage	Average Annual Income
69,700	$13.34	$27,750

Percentile Wage Estimates

Percentile	10%	25%	50% (median)	75%	90%
Hourly wage	$8.79	$10.44	$12.88	$15.77	$18.68
Annual wage	$18,280	$21,720	$26,780	$32,800	$38,850

Top Paying States

State	Employment	Hourly Mean Wage	Annual Mean Wage
Connecticut	1010	$16.18	$33,650
Illinois	2660	$15.66	$32,570
Michigan	1710	$15.54	$32,310
Massachusetts	1780	$15.39	$32,020
California	8180	$15.08	$31,380

Top Paying Metropolitan Areas

Metropolitan Area	Employment	Hourly Mean Wage	Annual Mean Wage
Lake County-Kenosha County, Illinois-Wisconsin Metropolitan Division	390	$21.88	$45,510
Lansing and East Lansing, Mich	200	$19.11	$39,750
Jefferson City, Mo	8	$18.26	$37,970
Danbury, Conn	40	$18.18	$37,460
Poughkeepsie-Newburgh Middletown, NY	140	$18.01	$37,460

They are also the hospitals where most veterinary specialists complete their specialty training. Veterinarians who are general practitioners and not specialists may refer particularly challenging or difficult cases to specialty practices. Veterinary technicians who work in specialty practices see unusual cases and become skilled in addressing the particular needs of these critically ill patients. It is not uncommon for specialty practices to share their facility with an emergency and trauma practice. Some veterinary technicians prefer the challenge and excitement of emergency practice, rather than general practice, and have dedicated their careers to this aspect of veterinary technology.

Recently veterinary technicians have also been given the opportunity to become specialists recognized by the National Association of Veterinary Technicians in America (NAVTA). Refer to the discussion of veterinary technician specialists in this chapter for additional information.

JOB PROSPECTS, SALARIES, AND ATTRITION

Presently there are widespread shortages of veterinary technicians nationwide, and graduates of veterinary technology programs are finding ample job opportunities. Although job opportunities are bright, salaries vary depending on the field of interest and the level of experience (see Table 1-1). For example, in 2006 the U.S Bureau of Labor Statistics reported that the average salary for veterinary technicians nationwide was $27,750 per year. However, the level of experience, location of work, and field of interest have an impact on income potential. For example, technicians working in metropolitan areas earn more, on average, than those working in rural areas. Similarly, technicians working in industry and sales earn more than technicians working in companion animal practices. An experienced graduate veterinary technician, particularly one with management and technical responsibilities, working in a metropolitan setting may earn from $35,000 to $60,000 per year. Income for an experienced VTS, the highest paid cohort working in clinical practice, may range from $45,000 (suburbs) to $80,000 (New York City) for those working in large specialty practices. Recent graduates may earn far less than experienced graduates who have had time to develop expertise and skill in particular areas of practice. Overall, however, from 2003 to 2006, the U.S. Bureau of Labor Statistics reported a 10.6% increase in the average salary of the veterinary technician (from $24,200 to $26,780). One can extrapolate a 3.5% annual increase since 2006 to estimate the average salary of veterinary technicians today.

In addition to salary compensation, many employers offer a range of benefits, including health care coverage, retirement plans, and payment of continuing education (CE) and professional membership fees. Large companies or practices are generally better equipped to provide more complete benefits packages than small private businesses. Some pharmaceutical companies offer educational packages that finance continued education in a related field. In this way, bachelor's and master's degrees have been financed by some corporate employers.

The profession of veterinary technology has a high rate of attrition, estimated to range from 45% to 55% after only 4 years of employment. Graduate technicians report leaving the profession because of a lack of appreciation and underutilization by their employer, low pay, and lack of advancement opportunities. Attrition from the profession is a critical part of the current shortage problem. Many states have shortages of veterinarians and veterinary assistants as well as technicians.

The National Commission on Veterinary Economic Issues (NCVEI) has established a website to help guide practice owners, practice managers, and staff toward more efficient management protocols (refer to www.ncvei.org). Because employee attrition is costly, both fiscally and in terms of the morale and efficiency of the veterinary health care team, improved staff management is particularly critical to the health of the practice. With improved understanding of the abilities of credentialed veterinary technicians, it is hoped that practices will more fully use their skill. Statistics gathered by NCVEI indicate that the most financially sound practices are those that make full use of their staff. Veterinarians in these well-run practices complete only those tasks, which by law, they alone are permitted to do. All other animal care tasks are completed by veterinary technicians and veterinary assistants.

EDUCATION

Programs of Veterinary Technology

Like nursing schools in the human health care field, programs of veterinary technology may include 2, 3, or 4 years of undergraduate study and may result in either an associate degree (2 or 3 years) or a baccalaureate degree (4 years). Programs in the United States are accredited by the Committee on Veterinary Technician Education and Activities (CVTEA), which is under the auspices of the AVMA. Programs in Canada are accredited by the Animal Health Technology/Veterinary Technician Program Accreditation Committee (AHT/VT PAC), which is under the auspices of the CVMA (though programs in Ontario are accredited by the OAVT). For accreditation by the CVTEA, a program must meet 11 essential criteria for curricula, faculty, facility, and admissions requirements. Each program must submit reports to the accrediting body for review semiannually, annually, or biannually depending on the age and stability of the program. In addition, the accrediting body carries out on-site visits of each program. Based on the on-site evaluation, recommendations by the accrediting body are classified into three categories: critical, major, and minor recommendations. Programs must document in reports to the accrediting body progress made in addressing the deficits cited by the on-site review committee.

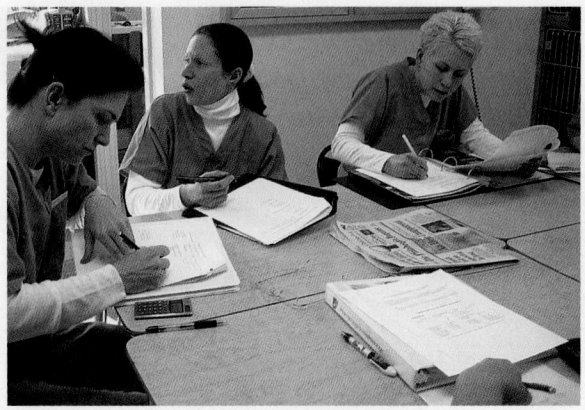

FIGURE 1-2 Students in AVMA-accredited programs of veterinary technology must complete hands-on training. In this clinical laboratory at Manor College, students calculate preoperative drug and anesthetic dosages before anesthetizing a cat. (Courtesy Dr. Joanna Bassert.)

Two- and Four-Year Programs

The curriculum of veterinary technology programs includes general college-level courses, such as biology and chemistry, and courses specific to clinical practice, such as veterinary parasitology, medicine, and clinical chemistry. There are almost 350 "essential" and "recommended" tasks listed in the *Accreditation Policies and Procedures Handbook* of the CVTEA, which constitutes the foundation of the hands-on curriculum for laboratories and practical training (Figure 1-2). Many 4-year programs include the same veterinary technology curriculum as 2-year programs with greater numbers of liberal arts courses. A few 4-year programs include advanced veterinary technology courses in the junior and senior years in addition to the standard curriculum required by the CVTEA. As the profession continues to grow, greater numbers of 4-year programs are expected to form, and some of these programs will offer increasing numbers of advanced veterinary technology courses. Refer to Box 1-2 for a list of courses typically offered in veterinary technology programs.

Standard Criteria

Through the development of standard criteria for each required task, programs ensure consistency of standards among various faculty members, classroom sections, and distance education versus traditional courses. In addition, programs are required to document that every student successfully completes each of the required tasks before graduation.

Distance Education

Although most veterinary technology programs are offered to students in the traditional on-campus fashion, some programs are available via distance education using the Internet and teleconferencing. Distance education programs offered via the Internet provide educational opportunities to students around the world. The courses are rigorous and

BOX 1-2 Types of Courses Required in Veterinary Technology Programs

Basic Math and Science Courses

Technical math
Biology
Chemistry
Microbiology
Comparative mammalian anatomy and physiology
Medical terminology
Computer science

Veterinary Technology Courses

Introduction to veterinary technology
Veterinary practice management
Animal management and nutrition
Farm animal clinical procedures
Companion animal clinical procedures
Laboratory animal science
Animal medicine
Veterinary radiology
Animal parasitology
Veterinary hematology
Veterinary clinical chemistry and urinalysis
Veterinary surgical assisting
Veterinary pharmacology and anesthesiology

require a high degree of self-discipline from students who often must work independently, though communication with teachers and classmates is encouraged via threaded discussions and e-mail list servers. The flexibility of distance education programs makes them particularly well suited for mature students who are already working in veterinary practices and who may not live near a college or university with a traditional program.

Many distance education programs require that students work in veterinary practices while completing the online course work. This enables the student to be supervised by an employer or other mentor while completing required hands-on skills. In addition, it offers ready access to many of the materials and animals needed to complete the required clinical tasks. As documentation, distant students are often asked to film themselves successfully completing tasks in keeping with the program's standard criteria and AVMA requirements. They may also be asked to turn in the results of projects, such as blood films, radiographs, and lab results, in addition to completing the usual written assignments and examinations that traditional students complete.

As of this printing, the following distance programs have been accredited by the AVMA:

Blue Ridge Community College, Virginia—www.br.cc.va.us

Cedar Valley College, Texas—ollie.dcccd.edu/vettech

Jefferson State Community College, Alabama—www.jeffstateonline.com/veta/

Northern Virginia Community College, Virginia—www.nvcc.edu

Penn Foster College, Arizona—www.pennfostercollege.edu

Purdue University, Indiana—www.vet.purdue.edu/vettech/

St. Petersburg College, Florida—www.spcollege.edu/hec/vt/

San Juan College, New Mexico—www.sjc.cc.nm.us/pages/1.asp

Continuing Education

Most states require veterinary technicians to attend CE lectures and workshops to maintain licensure, certification, or registration. These lectures are available at various national, regional, and local professional conferences and workshops throughout the United States, Canada, and through AVMA- and CVMA-accredited programs of veterinary technology. CE is also available online through the websites of many professional associations and veterinary information centers. Refer to the list of professional associations and veterinary information links at the end of this chapter. As veterinary medicine rapidly progresses and changes, it is particularly important for veterinary technicians to commit themselves to a career of lifelong learning.

THE VETERINARY TECHNICIAN NATIONAL EXAMINATION

After completing the requirements to graduate from a program of veterinary technology, most students prepare to take the Veterinary Technician National Examination (VTNE), which is required in most states and provinces. The VTNE is developed under a contractual agreement between the American Association of Veterinary State Boards (AAVSB) and the Professional Examination Service (PES). The AAVSB is represented by the Veterinary Technician Testing Committee (VTTC), which is composed of veterinarians and veterinary technicians who are engaged in clinical practice, national practice associations, AVMA-affiliated specialty boards, and academia. Members of the committee are appointed by the executive boards of AVMA, NAVTA, AVTE, and the Canadian Association of Animal Health Technologists and Technicians (CAAHTT). The PES provides the committee with two draft examinations for their review and validation. These drafts are developed from a computerized bank of questions, originally written by veterinarians and veterinary technicians from all aspects of the veterinary medical profession. The questions are reviewed independently for accuracy, relevance to the field of veterinary technology, and level of difficulty. In addition, the questions are further screened for grammar, style, and conformity to psychometric principles. Each state licensing board is responsible for the administration of the examination and establishes the location, date, and time when it is offered. Although PES provides test scoring services, the state boards are responsible for reporting the scores to the veterinary technician candidates.

The examination is offered in many states and Canadian provinces on the third Friday in June and the third Friday in

January of every year. It is composed of 200 multiple-choice questions that cover the following seven primary areas or domains within the profession of veterinary technology:

1. Pharmacy and pharmacology
2. Surgical preparation and assisting
3. Laboratory procedures
4. Animal nursing
5. Radiology, ultrasound, and other electronic imaging
6. Anesthesia
7. Office and hospital procedures

On a scale from 200 to 800, each state determines the passing score, which can be found in the "data resource" section of the website of the AAVSB at www.aavsb.org. A total score and a locally derived scale score may also accompany the test results report that is sent to each candidate. Candidates who need to have their VTNE scores sent to multiple state boards must register with the Interstate Reporting Service. There is a fee for registration with the Interstate Reporting Service and a second fee for each transfer. Notice that the term registered does not mean that the credentialing process is the same in all of the states that register veterinary technicians. Similarly the process is not the same in all states that certify technicians. Each state dictates its own approach toward credentialing and determines the terminology to be used. This can be particularly confusing to veterinary technicians who are relocating to another state.

> *TECHNICIAN NOTE* Candidates have 4 hours to complete the VTNE. Because candidates receive no additional penalties for incorrect responses, test takers are encouraged to answer all the questions, even if it means guessing.

SCOPE OF PRACTICE

As the sophistication of veterinary medicine has increased, the responsibilities of the veterinary technician in clinical practice have broadened. Veterinarians are rapidly moving away from doing the nursing and laboratory tasks themselves and are delegating these tasks to veterinary technicians. However, there is much variability among veterinary practices in the way in which veterinary technicians are employed. In a well-managed practice, veterinary technicians perform all the duties associated with the care and treatment of animal patients except those tasks that by law can only be performed by the veterinarian. In addition, they are empowered to delegate appropriate tasks to veterinary assistants. Although the state laws that define veterinary medicine differ (see Chapter 2), it is widely accepted and proposed by both the AVMA and the AAVSB that *only* veterinarians may do the following:

1. Prescribe
2. Diagnose
3. Prognose
4. Perform surgery

Veterinary technology typically includes the remaining animal care–related duties, but they may also be involved in nonclinical tasks, such as personnel management, management of facilities and equipment, client education, and inventory control. Veterinary practices are organized into distinct working areas. A veterinary technician, depending on his or her job description and the size of the practice, may work in all, a few, or only one of the areas discussed in the following sections.

> *TECHNICIAN NOTE* In a well-managed practice, veterinary technicians perform all the duties associated with the care and treatment of animal patients except those tasks that by law can only be performed by the veterinarian.

RESPONSIBILITIES OF THE VETERINARY TECHNICIAN

Reception Area

Although many practices hire receptionists, and not veterinary technicians, to work in the reception area, it is important for the clinical staff to be cross-trained in this aspect of the practice so that important information can be accessed easily when the receptionist is not available, such as during a weekend emergency. The veterinary technician should be familiar with the computer network system and practice management software used by the practice. This will facilitate obtaining existing records, creating new patient records, and accessing medical histories and billing information during emergencies that may occur after hours.

Examination Rooms and Outpatients

The veterinary technician ensures that office visits are handled in an efficient and professional manner. This involves directing clients to the appropriate examination room or treatment area, obtaining a brief history, weighing the patient, and acquiring the necessary vaccines, instruments, and materials needed for the visit. The veterinary technician may also draw blood at this time and obtain skin scrapings and fecal, urine, and cytology samples for laboratory testing. In addition, the veterinary technician provides important information to clients regarding preventive care, diet, behavior modification, medication, discharge instructions, and spay and neutering procedures for their animals.

Because pet owners often feel more at ease talking to the veterinary technician than to the veterinarian, the technician can be a valuable support person for bereaved or worried pet owners. In addition, the veterinary technician answers clients' questions both in person and over the telephone and occasionally must address difficult or angry pet owners.

Laboratory and Pharmacy

The veterinary technician has the skills to perform all of the routine laboratory tests used in the practice (Figure 1-3). The number of the laboratory tests actually performed on site varies from practice to practice. In veterinary hospitals that make full use of these skills, veterinary technicians

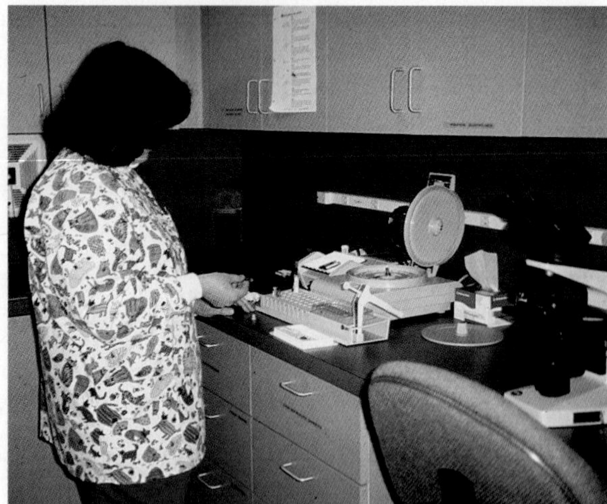

FIGURE 1-3 A veterinary technician completes laboratory tests using automated analyzers. (Courtesy Dr. Joanna Bassert.)

perform complete blood counts, differential counts, and morphologic examinations of blood. They perform urinalysis, including examination of urine sediment, and fecal analysis for evidence of parasites. Veterinary technicians are skilled in the use of enzyme-linked immunosorbent assay (ELISA) test kits, dextrometers, refractometers, and dry chemistry analyzers. In addition, veterinary technicians are familiar with interpreting common cytologic preparations, such as ear swabs and vaginal smears.

Once a diagnosis is made, the veterinarian prescribes, either in writing or orally, a treatment for the animal patient. The veterinary technician interprets the prescription language, then fills and dispenses the medication to the pet owner with instructions for its use. In addition, veterinary technicians are often responsible for ensuring that the pharmacy is well stocked, that expired drugs are discarded, and that controlled substances are handled appropriately.

Radiology

The x-ray (also known as a radiograph) is an important diagnostic tool in veterinary medicine. Veterinary technicians are skilled in radiographic techniques, including positioning of the patient, making the proper settings, and taking exposures at the appropriate times. In addition, veterinary technicians are skilled in both manual and automatic development techniques and in troubleshooting technical errors. If an x-ray service is not employed by the practice, veterinary technicians may be responsible for maintaining the development and fixative solutions and for keeping the x-ray screens and other equipment clean and in good working order. In addition, technicians ensure that the hospital staff members protect themselves from harmful radiation by wearing appropriate protective clothing, such as lead aprons, gloves, and thyroid shields, and that dosimeters are used routinely to monitor x-ray exposure. Often technicians are responsible for managing the ordering and mailing of the dosimeters. Finally, veterinary technicians may conduct special imaging and contrast studies, such as ultrasound and endoscopic studies and those in which gas, barium sulfate, or other contrast agents are used.

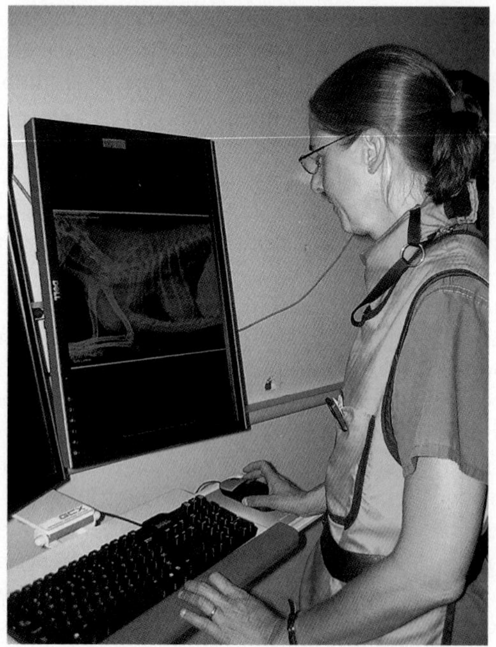

FIGURE 1-4 Veterinary technicians are skilled in the use of radiographic equipment. Today digital radiographs, as shown, have proved to be quick to generate and easy to store. (Courtesy Dr. Joanna Bassert.)

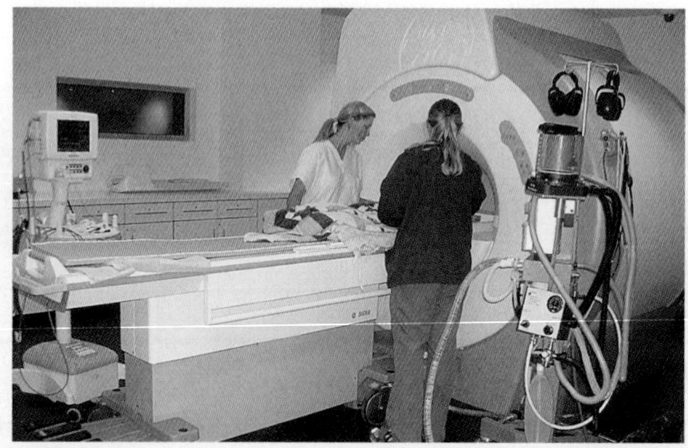

FIGURE 1-5 Advanced imaging techniques, such as the use of MRI, as shown, are becoming an important diagnostic tool in veterinary medicine today. (Courtesy Dr. Joanna Bassert.)

Many veterinary technology programs are also teaching students to use digital radiographic equipment and to employ the corresponding software that allows for the adjustment of the image to maximize accurate interpretation by the veterinarian (Figure 1-4). Digital imaging has many advantages over standard radiographic techniques. It is faster to produce, easier to adjust, and convenient to store. In addition, the images can be sent electronically via e-mail to specialists for a second opinion or to referring veterinary hospitals. Similarly, advanced imaging techniques, such as the use of computed tomography (CT) and magnetic resonance imaging (MRI), are being used with increasing frequency in veterinary medicine (Figure 1-5), particularly in specialty

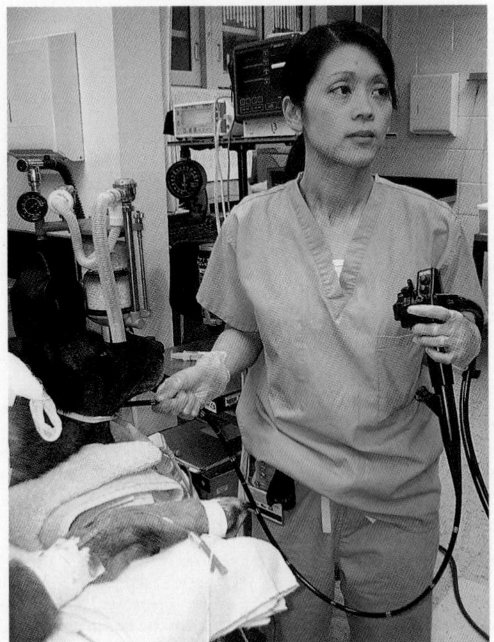

FIGURE 1-6 This veterinary technician works at the Mathew Ryan Veterinary Hospital of the University of Pennsylvania, where she has become proficient in using fiber-optic endoscopes. (Courtesy Dr. Joanna Bassert.)

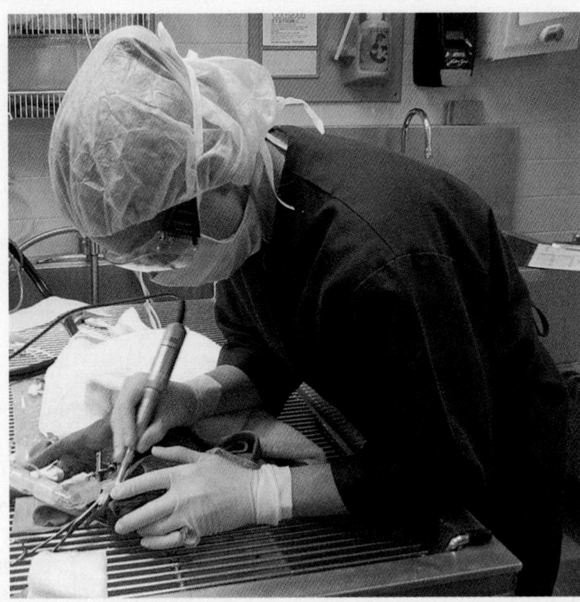

FIGURE 1-7 Performing oral examinations, dental charting, and prophylactic teeth cleanings are important aspects of veterinary technology. (Courtesy Dr. Joanna Bassert.)

practices and veterinary teaching hospitals. In addition, veterinary technicians are playing a greater role in collecting images using ultrasound and endoscopy (Figure 1-6). As in the human medical field, technicians can acquire digital images, using these special imaging techniques, that are subsequently interpreted by a radiologist.

Treatment Room

Most veterinary hospitals have a treatment room where patients are brought for various procedures and where animals are prepped for surgery. In more contemporary hospital designs, the treatment area is a large central room that may include a bank of cages for the postoperative and critical care patients. This arrangement facilitates the monitoring of in-house patients and enables the technical staff to be more efficient in completing important treatment duties. Dental operatories and procedure sinks may also be part of the main treatment room where dentistry and minor surgical procedures are completed.

Veterinary technicians are responsible for carrying out treatment orders given by the supervising veterinarian. This involves giving medications by all routes (e.g., orally, intramuscularly, intravenously). It may also involve setting up and monitoring intravenous fluids. Small amounts of blood may be collected every few hours, and the animal may be routinely checked for alertness, temperature, pulse, respiration, urination, and defecation. For critical cases, treatment may include changing bandages; lavaging open wounds; placing and monitoring nasal oxygen; and maintaining chest, tracheal, urethral, or abdominal tubes. Veterinary technicians are responsible for recording all treatments, data, and physical findings in the patient's record. The patient record is an important legal document and a means of ensuring that errors in treatment are not made.

The veterinary technician prepares the patient before it enters the operating room. This involves ensuring that the animal has not had anything to eat or drink and that the animal urinates before surgery. The technician is responsible for weighing the animal and then calculating and administering preoperative anesthetic agents. In many veterinary practices, the veterinary technician is responsible for induction and maintenance of anesthesia. Although there are many ways to anesthetize an animal, this usually involves placing an intravenous catheter, setting up fluids, placing an endotracheal tube, and administering intravenous and/or gas anesthetic agents. Monitoring equipment, such as a pulse oximeter, esophageal stethoscope, Dinamap monitor, Doppler ultrasonography machine, or oscilloscope, may be used by the technician to assist in monitoring the anesthetized patient. Before moving the patient to the operating room, the technician clips hair from the region of the animal that will undergo surgery and performs an initial cleansing of the area.

Often a technician is responsible for performing routine dental prophylactic procedures, which must be done while the animal is anesthetized (Figure 1-7). In this situation, the technician must perform two important jobs at once: namely, monitor the patient under an anesthetic, and clean and polish the animal's teeth. The veterinary technician must be prepared for an anesthetic emergency and should be familiar with the emergency drugs and procedures needed to resuscitate animals in crisis.

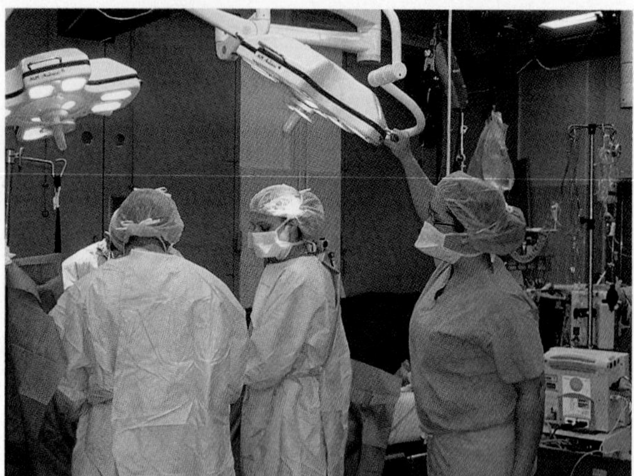

FIGURE 1-8 A veterinary technician adjusts operating lights for the surgeon and surgical assistants. (Courtesy Dr. Joanna Bassert.)

> *TECHNICIAN NOTE* Often a technician is responsible for performing routine dental prophylactic procedures, which must be done while the animal is anesthetized. In this situation, the technician must perform two important jobs at once: namely, monitor the patient under an anesthetic, and clean and polish the animal's teeth.

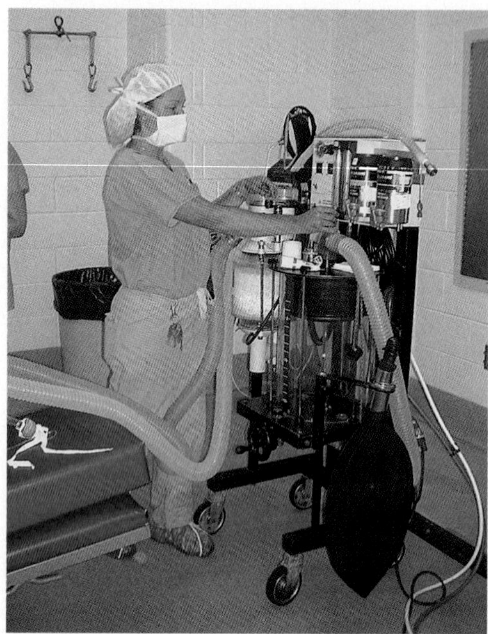

FIGURE 1-9 Administering anesthetics and monitoring anesthetized patients is one of the most challenging aspects of veterinary technology and is associated with a high level of responsibility for the life of the patient. (Courtesy Dr. Joanna Bassert.)

Operating Room

The operating room (OR) technician, or circulating nurse, positions the animal patient on the operating table and completes the final surgical scrub. Instruments, equipment, and materials needed by the surgeon are made available. In addition, the technician retrieves any additional materials requested during the procedure, adjusts surgery lights, tilts the surgery table, and in general, does whatever is necessary to support the comfort of the surgeon (Figure 1-8). In some practices, the technician acts simultaneously as both anesthetist and circulating nurse. Occasionally, technicians are asked to assist during a particularly challenging operation and must be skilled in proper sterile techniques, including gloving and gowning. After the procedure, the technician washes and dries the surgical instruments and reorganizes them into surgical packs for sterilization. The technician may also perform the duties of the postoperative care nurse for the recovering patient.

Being an anesthetist is one of the most important duties of the veterinary technician. In some practices, veterinary technicians are responsible for completing the dosage calculations for preoperative, postoperative, and intraoperative drugs. The technician is also responsible for induction and intubation of the patient and for intraoperative monitoring of blood pressure and heart and respiratory rates. A negative change in vital signs might require the veterinary technician to give compensational and resuscitative drugs. Though modern anesthetic agents are considered safe to use, there continues to be risk whenever an anesthetic is administered. Unexpected reactions to the anesthetic agents, surgical complications, and human error can be fatal to a patient. Anesthesia technicians must be meticulous about checking and rechecking the functionality of the anesthesia machine. Valves, tubing, vaporizer, oxygen levels, and rebreathing bags must be in impeccable condition and working order. The technician therefore is responsible for checking and rechecking the equipment before commencing to anesthetize a patient. Refer to Chapter 27 for more information about anesthesia and the role of the veterinary technician in its administration (Figure 1-9).

Wards

Veterinary technicians play an important role on the wards, not only in ensuring that treatments are given correctly and in a timely manner but also in providing animals with compassion and a gentle touch. Nurturing animals when they are sick is an important part of their recovery. Even healthy animals that are being boarded benefit from special care and reassurance from the technical staff.

The veterinary technician is often the first to observe a patient in distress or pain (Figure 1-10). Difficulties with intravenous lines, infusion pumps, or monitoring equipment are also first noticed by the veterinary technician. Thus the veterinary technician serves as the eyes and ears of the veterinarian. Immediate correction of problems are carried out by the technician when appropriate, recorded in the medical record, and communicated to the veterinarian. Sometimes the veterinarian is needed to assess a changing status of a patient, issue new treatment orders, or make other adjustments in the patient's care. The veterinary technician is responsible for monitoring and assessing the level of pain in patients and ensuring that appropriate pain management is provided.

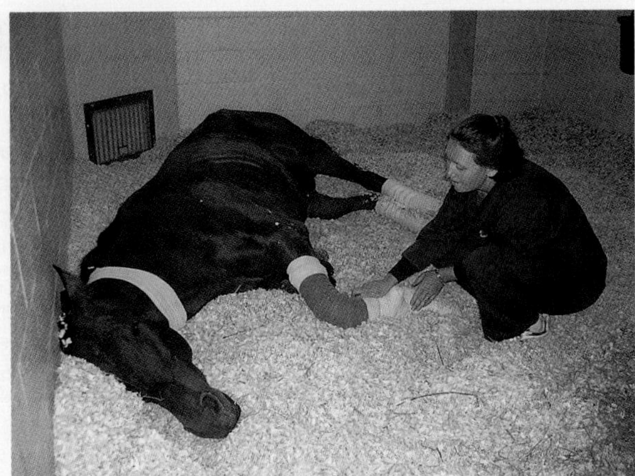

FIGURE 1-10 Veterinary technicians monitor hospitalized patients and are often the first to notice an animal in pain or distress. Technicians are responsible for alerting the attending veterinarian and ensuring that patients receive effective pain management and treatment. (Courtesy Dr. Joanna Bassert.)

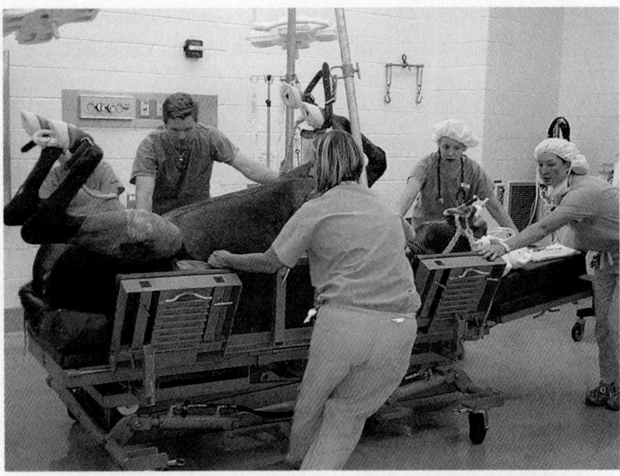

FIGURE 1-11 The veterinary health care team must work collaboratively to provide the best possible veterinary medical care. Here a veterinary team rushes an anesthetized horse to recovery. (Courtesy Dr. Joanna Bassert.)

BOX 1-3 American Veterinary Medical Association Nomenclature

Nomenclature

Veterinary technology is the science and art of providing professional support to veterinarians. AVMA accredits programs in veterinary technology that graduate veterinary technicians and/or veterinary technologists.

A **veterinary technician** is a graduate of an AVMA- or CVMA-accredited program in veterinary technology. In most cases, the graduate is granted an associate degree or certificate.

A **veterinary technologist** is a graduate of an AVMA- or CVMA-accredited program in veterinary technology that grants a baccalaureate degree.

Veterinary assistant: The adjectives animal, veterinary, ward, or hospital combined with the nouns attendant, caretaker, or assistant are titles sometimes used for individuals whose training, knowledge, and skills are less than that required for identification as a veterinary technician or veterinary technologist.

From: The Committee on Veterinary Technician Education and Activities: Accreditation policies and procedures, 2007.

Hospital Management

Veterinary technicians, particularly those with an interest in business, may pursue additional training in hospital management and become employed as a hospital manager. They may oversee the veterinary staff and assist with scheduling, hiring, personnel, client management, bookkeeping, and inventory control. Increasingly, veterinary technicians, particularly in large practices, are drawn into some management duties, such as management of technical staff and ordering supplies. In some states, where it is legal for nonveterinarians to own veterinary practices, veterinary technicians have become practice owners and managers.

TERMINOLOGY AND THE VETERINARY HEALTH CARE TEAM

A productive and efficiently managed veterinary practice depends on the dedication of a team of veterinary professionals and support personnel (Box 1-3). As described in the following sections, each member of the team plays a collaborative role in helping to provide quality health care for the animal patient (Figure 1-11).

Veterinarian

A veterinarian typically completes 4 years of study at an AVMA- or CVMA-accredited school of veterinary medicine after completing 4 years of undergraduate study. Graduates of veterinary medical schools are distinguished by the initials DVM after their names, unless they have graduated from the University of Pennsylvania, in which case they will have the initials VMD after their name. To practice, veterinarians must be licensed by the state in which they work. Typically, this requires successful completion of national and state examinations and the payment of a licensing fee. In addition, graduates of foreign veterinary medical colleges that are not accredited by the AVMA are eligible to apply for licensure in most states following certification by the Educational Commission of Foreign Veterinary Graduates (ECFVG). There are about 28 American and 5 Canadian colleges of veterinary medicine, though this number is increasing. For a current listing of accredited colleges of veterinary medicine in the United States and Canada, go to www.avma.org and www.cvma.org, respectively.

In some states, exceptions for licensure are made to veterinarians who are employed in university veterinary teaching hospitals.

TECHNICIAN NOTE Veterinary technicians must take responsibility for their own safety. The first step involves having personal health care coverage and always staying up to date with rabies and tetanus immunizations.

Veterinary Technician Specialist

In February 1994, NAVTA formed the Committee on Veterinary Technician Specialties (CVTS) to address a growing interest among veterinary technicians who wanted to attain higher levels of skill and knowledge in a particular aspect of veterinary technology. For this reason, CVTS established

BOX 1-4 What Does it Take to Become a Specialist?

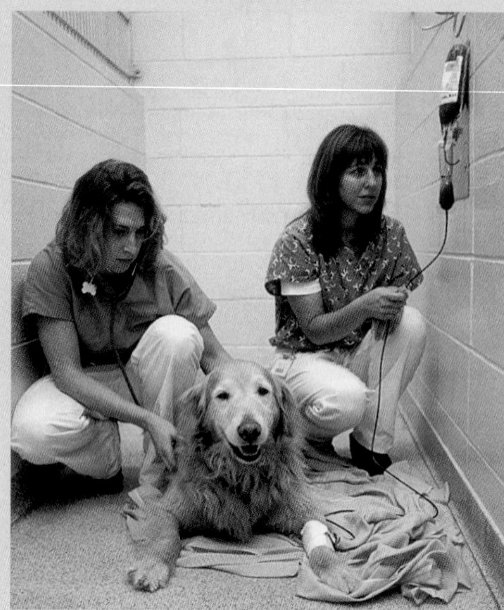

Each academy develops its own requirements for acquiring a certificate in a particular specialty. The specific requirements can be found on each of the academy websites (refer to the end of this chapter for the links to these sites). The Academy of Emergency and Critical Care Technicians (AVECCT) is the first to be recognized by NAVTA and is the first to reach full academy status.

AVECCT requires:

1. Completion of 5760 hours (3 years full-time) work experience in the field of veterinary emergency and critical care nursing. The work experience must be completed within a 5-year period before the application.
2. Completion of a minimum of 25 hours of continuing education in the field. The education must be completed within a 5-year period before the application and must be completed at a nationally recognized conference or program. Proof of attendance is required.
3. Completion of the advanced veterinary emergency critical care nursing skills form, which documents that the candidate has mastered required emergency critical care nursing tasks at an advanced level.
4. Completion of a case record log that spans a 1-year time frame from Jan. 1 to Dec. 31 immediately preceding the submission of the application. A minimum of 50 cases is required (more are recommended because some cases will not be accepted).
5. The log entry for each case should include: the date, patient identification, signalment, weight, diagnosis, length of care, final outcome, and summary of nursing care techniques and procedures performed by the applicant on the patient.
6. Four cases selected from the record log must be submitted as case reports, each one of no more than five pages in length. The case reports must demonstrate expert management of four veterinary patients that required emergency critical care.
7. Letters of recommendation from an AVECCT member or a veterinarian who is a diplomate of the American College of Veterinary Emergency and Critical Care or a member of the Veterinary Emergency Critical Care Society. (Until there are sufficient numbers of the aforementioned, letters of recommendation will be accepted from the following: non-VECCS emergency practice veterinarians and board certified specialists in anesthesia, internal medicine, or surgery.)

Modified from the AVECCT website. Additional information can be found at www.avecct.org.
For information about becoming a veterinary technician specialist in dentistry, anesthesia, internal medicine and behavior, go to www.navta.net/career_dev/specialties.php.

a process and a list of criteria for the formation of academies in specialized fields of veterinary technology.

The first step in the process of forming a specialty is for a group of veterinary technicians who share an interest in a particular field of veterinary technology to establish a professional society or association. After the society has grown in size, it may then petition CVTS for recognition as an academy. The organizing committee of the proposed academy together with CVTS establishes the advanced requirements and examination process for becoming a VTS in the field of interest. As of this printing, NAVTA has recognized five areas of specialty in veterinary technology. These fall under the auspices of the following academies:

The Academy of Veterinary Emergency and Critical Care Technicians (AVECCT)* (Box 1-4)
The Academy of Veterinary Technician Anesthetists (AVTA) (Figure 1-12)
The Academy of Veterinary Dental Technicians (AVDT)
The Academy of Internal Medicine for Veterinary Technicians (AIMVT)
The Academy of Veterinary Behavior Technicians (AVBT)

Thus the VTS is a veterinary technician who has reached a higher level of skill and understanding in a particular field of veterinary technology. The VTS must meet the following criteria:

- He or she must be a graduate of an AVMA-accredited program of veterinary technology and/or be legally credentialed to practice veterinary technology in his or her respective state, province, or country.
- Successfully complete the education, training, and experience requirements established by the respective academy of specialists.
- He or she must be reviewed and approved for specialist status by the academy.

In addition, it is strongly recommended that applicants be a member of national, state, and local veterinary technician associations and a member of the specialty society.

*NAVTA has granted full academy status to AVECCT and provisional academy status to AVTA, AVDT, AIMVT, and AVBT.

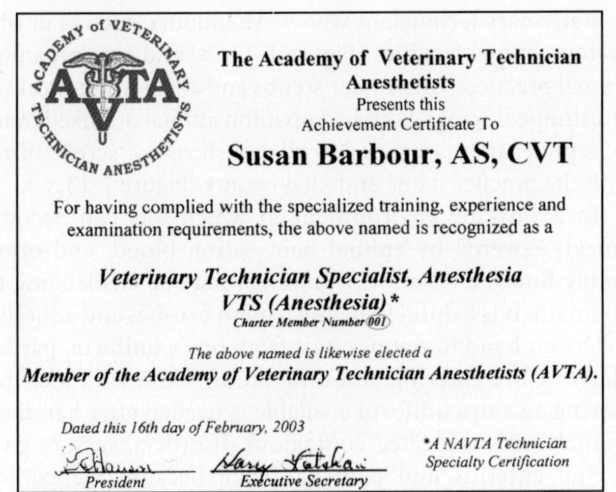
ACADEMY of VETERINARY TECHNICIAN ANESTHETISTS
AVTA
The Academy of Veterinary Technician Anesthetists
Presents this
Achievement Certificate To
Susan Barbour, AS, CVT
For having complied with the specialized training, experience and examination requirements, the above named is recognized as a
Veterinary Technician Specialist, Anesthesia
VTS (Anesthesia) *
Charter Member Number 001
The above named is likewise elected a
Member of the Academy of Veterinary Technician Anesthetists (AVTA).
Dated this 16th day of February, 2003
*A NAVTA Technician Specialty Certification
President
Executive Secretary

FIGURE 1-12 The first certificate awarded by the Academy of Veterinary Technician Anesthetists was given to Susan Barbour, AS, CVT, in February 2003.

Veterinary technicians who have achieved specialty status are signified by the initials VTS (and their field of specialty in parentheses) after their names. For example, the technician Mary Jones, CVT, VTS (dentistry), is a specialist in veterinary dentistry.

The VTS often works in specialty and referral veterinary hospitals and in teaching hospitals associated with universities. In these environments, the VTS can concentrate on his or her field of interest and share knowledge with veterinary medical and veterinary technology students.

Veterinary Technologist

In the United States, the veterinary technologist holds a bachelor of science (BS) degree in veterinary technology from a 4-year, AVMA-accredited program. The veterinary technologist works in positions that may require a greater level of education than the veterinary technician, such as project leader, practice supervisor, or teacher in a veterinary technology program. Some veterinary technologists, particularly those employed in teaching hospitals of veterinary medical schools, may become highly skilled in a particular aspect of veterinary technology. Some institutions and practices use the term veterinary technologist to refer to a veterinary technician who holds a BS degree in any field.

In Canada, the term veterinary technologist is synonymous with veterinary technician.

Veterinary Technician

A veterinary technician is a person who has earned an associate of science (AS) degree in veterinary technology from a 2-year or 3-year, AVMA-accredited program of veterinary technology. In many states, veterinary technicians are required to complete national and state examinations before they can be licensed, registered, or certified. Frequently, veterinary technicians are required to pay a fee to the state or state veterinary association to receive a license, certification, or registration.

Veterinary Assistant

The term veterinary assistant is used to describe those individuals involved in the care of animals who are not veterinary technicians, laboratory animal technicians, or veterinarians. Typically, veterinary assistants are responsible for assisting the veterinary technician and the veterinarian by restraining animals, setting up equipment and supplies, cleaning and maintaining practice and laboratory facilities, and feeding and exercising patients. Most veterinary assistants are trained on the job by a supervising veterinary technician or veterinarian, but some assistants complete 4 to 6 months of training in a formal course of study.

The profession of veterinary technology started to take form in the early 1960s. Before this time, veterinary technicians, as defined today, did not exist, and veterinary practices depended exclusively on the skill of on-the-job–trained veterinary assistants. Today veterinary assistants continue to constitute a large and important portion of the work force in veterinary practices nationwide. Veterinary technicians and veterinary assistants work together in many veterinary practices, and although the AVMA and NAVTA make clear distinctions between the two groups, some states have confused these distinctions.

As the number of traditional and distance AVMA-accredited programs grows, education in the field of veterinary technology becomes increasingly more accessible to veterinary support staff members who wish to become veterinary technicians.

Veterinary Nurse

The term veterinary nurse rather than veterinary technician is used in European countries.

LABORATORY ANIMAL TECHNICIANS

The American Association for Laboratory Animal Science (AALAS) and the Canadian Association of Laboratory Animal Science (CALAS) have established a certification program that certifies the following three levels of animal technicians:

- Assistant laboratory animal technician (ALAT)
- Laboratory animal technician (LAT)
- Laboratory animal technologist (LATG)

AALAS- and CALAS-certified animal technicians care for the laboratory animals used in research facilities and teaching institutions. These facilities are registered by the U.S. Department of Agriculture (USDA) and may be located in pharmaceutical companies, universities, and colleges. A technician does not need to be a graduate of an AVMA- or CVMA-accredited program of veterinary technology to be eligible for AALAS or CALAS certification; however, many are graduates. Graduates of AVMA- and CVMA-accredited programs must complete 6 months of additional training in a registered facility before they are eligible for the level one ALAT examination.

Like the VTNE, AALAS certification examinations are developed and administered by the PES, but they fall under the auspices of AALAS rather than the AAVSB. All three levels of examinations are multiple choice, but each level becomes more rigorous and asks more questions. For example, the ALAT examination is composed of 100 questions; the LAT examination, 125 questions; and the LATG examination, 150 questions. Candidates must complete a specified amount of on-the-job experience to qualify for the next level of AALAS or CALAS certification.

PROFESSIONALISM

As with all professions, veterinary technology is best represented by the excellent skill, ethical conduct, and passion of its members. Veterinary technicians are bound by a code of ethics and ideals established by NAVTA (see Chapter 2) and by our societal expectations of what constitutes professionalism. Though the ethics and ideals of veterinary technology may be clearly defined in writing, the nuances of professional conduct may be less clear, much like the subtleties of social interpersonal conduct. Programs of veterinary technology are therefore challenged to instill in their diverse student body a common understanding of professional manners. To this end, programs may have mandatory dress codes and rules about comportment on campus and particularly in the classroom. A portion of a lab grade, for example, may assess the professional conduct of the student. Did the student come to class on time, in uniform, and with a positive attitude? Did the student work well with classmates and teachers? These assessments help guide and prepare the student for work in a clinical environment in which they will be judged by pet owners and the employer.

The following guidelines outline the principle aspects of professionalism in veterinary technology.

PROFESSIONAL APPEARANCE

The initial impression a veterinary technician makes is usually based simply upon how he or she looks. Neat, clean, well-fitted, and ironed uniforms are essential. Long hair should be pulled back, fingernails kept short, and there should be little to no jewelry, makeup, or perfume worn. Tattoos should be covered, if possible, and facial body piercings (such as those in the tongue, nose, and eyebrow) should be devoid of studs or rings.

Uniform

Veterinary technicians wear a variety of "uniforms" depending upon the field in which they work. In an equine practice, for example, many technicians wear collared shirts; khaki pants; and solid, protective footwear, which have proved to be durable, warm, and practical in the rugged and often unheated setting of hospital barns (Figure 1-13, *A*). Sturdy, leather boots, in particular, are important to protect the feet from fracturing under the weight of a shod hoof. Clearly, sneakers, sandals, and other open-toed shoes would be inappropriate in a barn. Technicians who work in bovine practices are likely to wear insulated coveralls and weatherproof boots to stay warm while working in muddy cattle pens.

Veterinary technicians who work indoors, such as in laboratory animal facilities (Figure 1-13, *B*) and in companion animal practices, often wear scrubs and clean white sneakers or orthopedic clogs. Some companion animal or mixed practices prefer the staff to wear collared shirts (or scrub shirts) with the practice name and khaki pants (Figure 1-13, *C*).

In a working environment in which one can become quickly covered by animal hair, saliva, blood, and other bodily fluids, a clean, neat uniform may be challenging to maintain. It is helpful to have garment brushes and adhesive rollers on hand to remove hair from one's uniform, particularly before entering an examination room with a client. Having an extra uniform available is needed after handling animals with suspected contagious disorders, such as parvoviral enteritis and panleukopenia because the pathogens can be transmitted to other animals by contaminated clothing.

Uniforms must be clean and ironed; they must also fit well. In other words, bending over should not reveal either cleavage or a backside. To instill this message in its students, one veterinary technology program uses the slogan "say no to crack, front and back." Thus maintaining a professional appearance for many technicians includes wearing white crew-neck T-shirts under a V-neck scrub shirt, for example, or scrub pants with elastic waistbands rather than drawstrings. The pants should be hemmed to an appropriate length so that there is no risk of tripping (Figure 1-13, *D*).

Veterinary technicians are encouraged to wear professional pins on their shirts and the name tag or practice logo required by the practice. Many programs of veterinary technology award college or university pins to graduating students. These pins bear the veterinary caduceus and the name of the college or university. In addition, NAVTA awards pins to its longtime members as does several state veterinary technician associations. Though college rings are not acceptable, because they are prohibited in the operating room, pins are encouraged symbols of the profession.

Finally the uniform of all veterinary technicians, regardless of field of interest, must include a watch with a second hand. Vital signs and appropriate patient assessment, which is an important part of veterinary nursing, cannot be completed without a suitable watch. Other items, such as a functional pen and a stethoscope, are also critical tools for the veterinary technician to have readily available at all times. It should be noted that Zebra pens are particularly helpful in the practice because they are able to work continuously when writing on vertical surfaces.

Hands and Nails

It is well known in the health industry that contagions can be spread from one patient to another on the hands, especially under the nails, of health care workers. For this reason, it is important to make a habit of washing hands several times a day, particularly between contacts with different animals. In addition, fingernails should be kept as short as possible and free of nail lacquer, which can chip off into sterile surgical fields. Not only can long nails harbor infectious agents, but

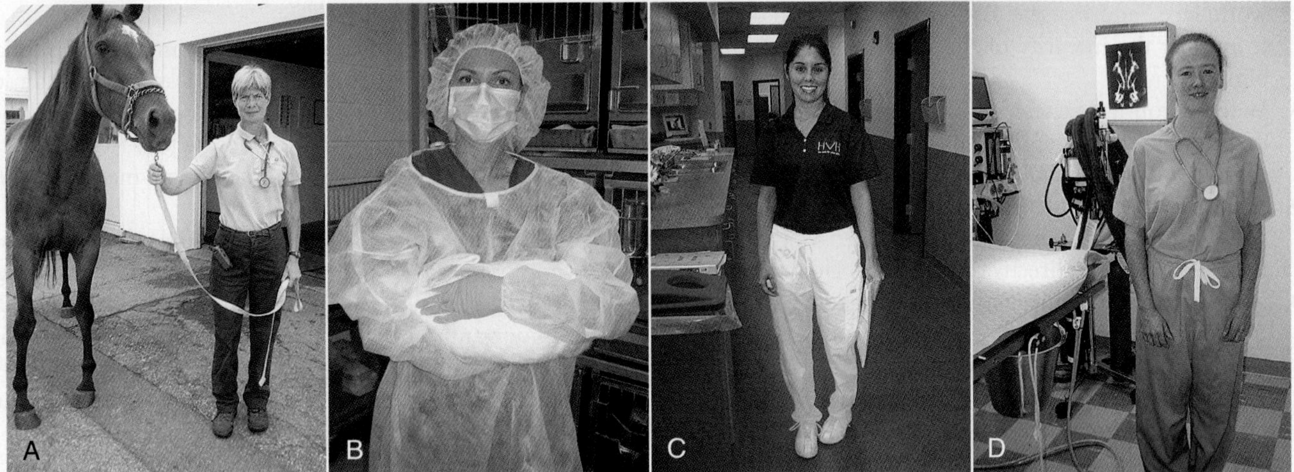

FIGURE 1-13 A, Many veterinary technicians who work in equine practice wear collared shirts, pants, and solid protective boots, which have proved to be practical in the rugged setting of hospital barns. B, A technician who works in a laboratory animal facility must wear gloves and protective gowns to ensure that contagions are not transmitted to the animals in the vivarium. C, Some veterinary technicians working in companion animal practice wear collared shirts that carry the practice name and logo. D, An operating nurse wears clean scrubs and is equipped with a watch and stethoscope to evaluate the status of anesthetized and recovering patients. (Courtesy Dr. Joanna Bassert.)

BOX 1-5 NAVTA's Professional Ideals

NAVTA

National Association of Veterinary Technicians in America

1. Veterinary technicians shall strive to participate in defining, upholding, and improving standards of professional practice, legislation, and education.
2. Veterinary technicians shall strive to contribute to the profession's body of knowledge.
3. Veterinary technicians shall strive to understand and support the attachment between a person and his or her companion animal.

they also interfere with daily nursing tasks, such as scruffing cats, putting on surgical gloves, and placing IV catheters.

Jewelry, Face, and Hair

Veterinary technicians must be proficient in and prepared to restrain animals. Risk of injury to the technician and other staff members is increased if jewelry and long hair can be caught up in the fury of claws and flailing limbs. Necklaces, dangling earrings, and loose bracelets are particularly dangerous for technicians to wear. In addition, small items, such as studs, earrings, earring backs, and individual hairs, can accidentally fall into sterile surgical fields or, worse, into open surgical incisions. Veterinary technicians must wear their hair pulled back and remove all jewelry, including studs, before working. Finally, because of the close working conditions of most operating rooms and ward facilities, veterinary technicians should avoid chewing gum and wearing strong cologne, which may be offensive to co-workers and to pet owners.

PROFESSIONAL CONDUCT

The way in which a veterinary technician behaves represents the most important aspect of his or her professionalism. Technicians, like many health care professionals, are held to a high standard of conduct. For this reason, NAVTA developed the list of professional ideals listed in Box 1-5. Below are specific guidelines for professional conduct both in and outside the workplace.

In the Workplace

1. Be honest and forthright in communications with co-workers and clients. Take responsibility for making a mistake and, if possible, take immediate action to correct the error.
2. Maintain a positive attitude and an even, controlled disposition. Be respectful of co-workers and pet owners at all times. Avoid expressing anger, sarcasm, and cynicism because this has a demotivating effect on the veterinary health care team and often worsens the situation.
3. Be tactful and careful in both verbal and written communication. Avoid saying all that is thought and felt. Be considerate of the time, place, and quality of a query when asking questions.
4. Be a collaborative, team player. Provide the ideas and positive energy needed to help improve the efficiency of the health care team and the quality of the medical services it provides.
5. Be attentive to the concerns and needs of both co-workers and pet owners. Avoid mentally tuning out. Take initiative to pitch in and help where needed.
6. Respect the veterinarian-client relationship. Keep in mind that there are communications most appropriately delivered to clients by the veterinarian.
7. Be aware of the clinical and professional competence of others. When concerned about incompetence in the

workplace, address the issue promptly and tactfully to protect the integrity of the practice. Do not turn a blind eye.
8. When a conflict arises, address it promptly, privately, and calmly with those directly involved. Avoid drawing those not directly involved into the conflict.
9. Maintain the confidentiality of professional and personal information about clients and co-workers that was learned either directly or indirectly. Do not gossip.
10. Be committed to being competent and skilled. Be receptive to new ideas and suggestions for improvement. Be enthusiastic about teaching others.
11. Be aware of and abide by the laws that define the scope of practice in your state.

Outside of the Workplace

1. Join and participate in national, state, and local professional organizations.
2. Participate in high school career days and give presentations about the profession when the opportunity arises.
3. Attend national, state, and local veterinary conferences. Stay current on issues affecting the profession.
4. Support legislation in your state that better defines and strengthens veterinary technology.
5. Maintain state licensure, certification, or registration.

PROFESSIONAL COMMUNICATION

Verbal Communication

Clear and frequent communication with co-workers and clients is an important part of an efficient health care team. Veterinary technicians should be sure to use correct grammar, articulated speech, and avoid using words that might offend. For some who are accustomed to speaking in an informal manner, cleaning up one's language can be a challenge. To expedite the cleanup process, some veterinary technology programs penalize the professionalism portion of a student's grade for using inappropriate words and expletives in class. Cursing is universally considered to be unprofessional communication.

Written Communication

Medical Records

The medical record is a legal document owned by the veterinary practice or supervising institution. It can be subpoenaed by a court of law and subject to detailed scrutiny. Errors in the document can render the medical record invalid, and this could have adverse legal ramifications for the practice. In addition, medical records of animals used for teaching in veterinary technology programs and in schools of veterinary medicine are examined by the USDA inspector who could cite deficiencies during an inspection if the written record contains errors. Using correct spelling and grammar is important in these legal documents. Refer to Chapter 5 for additional information about errors in medical records.

E-mail

E-mail is a common form of written communication today, and though they are often considered less formal than letters, use of correct spelling and grammar are important when e-mailing clients and colleagues. It is helpful to get into the habit of doing the following when sending e-mails to professional contacts.

1. Begin with a salutation that includes the person's name to whom you are writing (i.e., "Dear Mary" or "Good Evening Dr. Brown"). E-mail accounts can be shared, and it is important to be clear about for whom the e-mail is intended. Salutations may not be necessary during frequent exchanges, but should be included when first making contact.
2. Write a concise e-mail that is grammatically correct. Use a spell-checker.
3. Keep in mind that e-mail can be forwarded and that the tone can be misinterpreted. *Never* write an angry e-mail or one that is critical of a colleague or co-worker. Be careful with the use of humor lest it be misinterpreted.
4. Always end with a closing and your name. Many professionals program their computers to automatically end each e-mail with a prewritten closing. Typically, this includes the person's full name, title, address, and telephone number.
5. Maintain an e-mail address that does not leave a bad impression. Silly, cute, and animal-related e-mail addresses, such as bunnyluvr@comcast.net or pintaday@msn.com, are not helpful toward the development of a professional image. A simple e-mail that includes your first initial and last name works well. Similarly, make sure that recorded answering machine greetings are appropriate for professional colleagues, particularly if you are actively searching for a new position and expect potential employers to call.

> TECHNICIAN NOTE Keep in mind that e-mail can be forwarded and that the tone can be misinterpreted. Never write an angry e-mail or one that is critical of a colleague or co-worker.

Letters and Résumés

Entire books have been written about the many ways in which professional letters and résumés can be written. For the purpose of brevity, I will describe only one way. It is not necessarily "the best" way, but it is a commonly used approach.

Getting started. The quality of stationery used to send a letter and résumé is the first nonverbal communication made between the writer and the recipient. If the paper is lined student paper or printer paper, for example, the nonverbal message to the recipient is "I do not take pride in preparing this letter" or worse "I do not know how to send a proper business letter because I am not particularly well educated." Either message is bad. To make the best impression, use a good quality stationery *with matching envelopes.* The best papers have watermarks and contain a high percentage of cotton. These can be purchased in the business, résumé, or

Jean Cynthia Rondinello
642 Wambler Road
Newark, NJ 14335
H: (253) 487-2298
C: (267) 345-8763
jrondinello@aol.com

January 30, 2010

Dr. Ronald Smith
Smith Animal Hospital
3 Kingston Highway
Newark, NJ 14335

Dear Dr. Smith:

I am a graduate of the Program of Veterinary Technology at Burbecker College and am seeking full-time employment as a veterinary technician this summer. I live in Newark and am familiar with your practice, because my mother is one of your clients. You may recall our cat "Perry" who has been your patient since he was a kitten.

I am looking forward to working in a clinical setting where I can make full use of the skills and concepts that I have learned in school. I was struck by the progressive nature of your practice when I last visited and am convinced it would offer opportunities for professional growth. I am enclosing my resume for your review. Please feel free to call me on my cell phone if you have any questions.

I look forward to hearing from you.

Respectfully yours,

Jean C. Rondinello

JR
Enclosure

FIGURE 1-14 A business letter that accompanies a résumé is called a cover letter. Its purpose is to introduce the applicant.

stationery sections of any office supply store, such as Staples and Office Max. Light gray, ivory, or white paper is preferable to brightly colored paper.

Next, generate a name and address graphic for the top of the letter and résumé. You may use the same graphic for both the letter and the résumé. If you are using a résumé wizard, you can select from a variety of graphic designs. Some include lines that separate the name and address, which is at the top of the page, from the text of the letter or résumé below.

A professional letter. A letter that accompanies a résumé is called a cover letter (Figure 1-14). It is used only when the résumé is being mailed, either via the postal service or via the Internet. Its purpose is to introduce the applicant and highlight important points that may not be obvious in the résumé. Cover letters are not given to employers at interviews because the applicants are present in person to introduce themselves and to present their qualifications.

Professional letters should always be typed. It is best to start with a size 12 print with single spacing. If the text of the letter is too long or too short to center on one page, the size of the print and spacing can be adjusted to achieve the best visual effect. There are many acceptable format styles for business letters; however, in this case a standard block format will be used. This means that all of the text except the name and address heading will be aligned to the left. Do not tab to indicate a new paragraph; instead leave one space between each paragraph.

Contents of the letter

1. Date:
   Under the graphic heading allow two or more spaces and then enter the date. Do not abbreviate anything in a formal letter including months of the year. Write out the full word "February" rather than "Feb." In general, do not use contractions in formal letters. Write out "cannot" rather than saying "can't."
2. Name and address of the recipient:
   Under the date leave one or two spaces, then enter the name of the recipient. If the letter is being sent to a veterinarian, be sure to write either "Dr. Douglas Browne" or "Douglas Browne, DVM." Do not write "Dr. Douglas Browne, DVM" because this is redundant.

3. The salutation:
   Begin the letter by writing "Dear Dr. Browne." Note that in business letters a colon is used, not a comma. Do not write "Dear Mr. Browne" if he is a veterinarian. Do not write "Dr. Browne:" without the word "Dear."
4. The text:
   Leave one space between the salutation and the text. When writing the text use simple, grammatically correct language and keep the letter concise and specific to the job at hand. Emphasize the positive, but do not sound arrogant, insincere, or inflationary. For example, do not say "I am an extremely fast learner." Instead simply say "I am a fast learner." If you find yourself using a lot of adjectives, such as "very," "extremely," and "super," you probably sound as though you are exaggerating or trying to impress the recipient. Let your references do the bragging for you.

Some other pitfalls to avoid when writing the text are:

- Do not begin the letter by saying "My name is…" This sounds silly because it is obvious from the signature who is sending the letter.
- Do not say, "throughout my entire life, I have always had animals." This sounds as though you are making a big deal about being a pet owner. If you mention owning animals, make a statement that augments your preparedness for the job to which you are applying. For example, "I have owned a wide variety of animal species including some exotics," or "I have enjoyed the three dogs that I have owned. They have taught me about loyalty and compassion."
- Remember that the words veterinary technician, veterinary assistant, and veterinarian are not capitalized. In general, the only words that you should capitalize are proper nouns (names and titles).
- Also keep in mind that the word veterinary is an adjective and veterinarian is a noun. For example, be sure to say veterinary hospital, not veterinarian hospital.
- Do not give your life history and future long-term career plans. Keep the letter specific only to the job at hand. Do not say, for example, that you want to go into a master's degree program and then to veterinary school since this is not related to the position and indicates that you may not stay in practice for long.
- Avoid repeating everything that is in your résumé and try not to be long winded. Do not say in three sentences what you can say in one. Remember that the reader is busy and is thinking "get to the point … get to the point … GET TO THE POINT! … and the point is?"

5. Closing:
   End the text of the letter with a formal closing. These include the following: Yours truly, Very truly yours, Yours very truly, Respectfully, and Respectfully yours. Notice that only the first letter of the first word in the closing is capitalized. Do not use informal closings, such as Love, Cheers, Sincerely, Sincerely yours, Cordially, or Cordially yours.
6. Signature and credentials:
   After the closing, allow three lines for your signature. Your full name should be typed on the fourth line after the closing. You may use your middle initial here, but do not write out your middle name. After your name, list your highest degree, followed by your veterinary technician credentials. Keep in mind that you should not list every degree that you have earned. The credentials that you list after your name should *not* reflect your entire educational history, rather they indicate the highest level acquired in each professional and academic field. If you have earned multiple bachelor of science degrees, for example, you would list "BS" only once. Similarly, if you are certified, registered or licensed as a veterinary technician in multiple states, list the credential pertinent to where you are currently living. Do not list every state in which you are credentialed. You will do this in your résumé. If you live in a state such as Pennsylvania that requires veterinary technicians to be graduates of AVMA-accredited programs, then it is assumed that you have an associate in science degree and therefore you would not list the degree.
   Below are some examples:

1. Correct: Cindy Stark, CVT (PA) or Cindy Stark, CVT; Incorrect: Cindy Stark, AS, CVT (PA)
2. Correct: Bruce Wills, BS, CVT; Incorrect: Bruce Wills, AS, BS, CVT
3. Correct: Mary Welden, RVT, VTS (ECC), MS; Incorrect: Mary Welden, AS, AS , BS, MS, CVT, RVT, VTS (ECC)
4. Correct: Sandra Reynolds, DVM, PhD; Incorrect: Sandra Reynolds, BS, DVM, PhD, PhD
5. Correct: Hannah Geisburg, LVT, JD; Incorrect: Hannah Geisburg, BS, LVT, JD

At the bottom left corner of the page write the initials of the person who typed the letter in capitals followed on the next line by the word "Enclosure." If there is no enclosure, do not add this word.

> *TECHNICIAN NOTE* The credentials that you list after your name should NOT reflect your entire educational history, rather they indicate the highest levels acquired in academia and in each professional field.

Writing a résumé. If you are sending a résumé to a large corporation that receives hundreds of thousands of job applications, you want to be sure that your résumé is no longer than a single page. Résumés sent to large businesses are often read by computers searching for key words.

If you are applying to a veterinary practice for a position, do not worry that your résumé will be lost in a sea of applicants because veterinary practices in general are suffering from staff shortages and receive relatively few résumés. Therefore if you believe that you need to go beyond one page, that would be fine, but do not staple the pages together. This is considered improper. Figure 1-15 gives an example of one type of résumé.

A résumé should consist minimally of the following sections:

1. Objective
2. Education (including academic awards and honor society memberships)
3. Experience
4. Credentials (licensure, registration, certification)
5. Volunteer experience
6. Professional memberships

The following sections may also be included where appropriate:

1. Summary or profile: This section would be placed after the objective to give the reader a quick summary of the applicant. It should not be more than one sentence.
2. Skills: This section highlights specific technical skills in which the applicant is proficient. It should be included only if the applicant has little employment experience.
3. Publications: This section lists journal articles, book chapters, and textbooks authored or edited by the applicant.
4. Activities and interests: This section lists musical, artistic, sports, and animal-related activities.
5. Professional awards and honors: This section lists entries in *Who's Who* publications and awards from professional organizations.
6. Professional presentations: This section lists any lectures and presentations made to clubs, schools, and at professional conferences.
7. Grants: This section lists any meritorious awards or grants received by the applicant.
8. Languages: This section lists languages spoken fluently other than English. Do not list languages that you studied in school. List only those that you can speak as a second language.

Jean Cynthia Rondinello
642 Wambler Road
Newark, NJ 14335
H: (253) 487-2298
C: (267) 345-8763
jrondinello@aol.com

Objective: To obtain a position as a veterinary technician in a progressive companion animal practice.

Education: **Burbecker College,** Stanton, NY
Program of Veterinary Technology
Degree: A.S. May, 2010

Mount Holly High School, Mount Holly, NJ
Diploma: June 2007

Employment: Veterinary Assistant — June to August, 2009
Maplewood Veterinary Hospital, Newark, NJ
Duties:
- Assisted veterinary technicians with the administration of medications to hospitalized patients
- Restrained cats and dogs for physical examination
- Prepared and sterilized surgical packs
- Maintained sanitation of examination, OR, and treatment rooms
- Performed fecal analysis and completed heartworm ELISA tests

Kennel Assistant — June 2007 to June 2009
Folkways Animal Clinic, Mount Holly, NJ
Duties:
- Prepared regular and prescription diets for boarding dogs and cats
- Cleaned and maintained dog and cat kennels and hospital ward cages
- Walked dogs and transported cats to and from play room
- Attended and participated in monthly staff meetings

Credentials: Certified Veterinary Technician (Pennsylvania)

Professional Memberships: NAVTA, NYVTA

A

FIGURE 1-15 Sample résumé **(A)** and reference list **(B)**. There are many different types of résumés. Regardless of the format used, make sure that the résumé contains accurate, current information; is grammatically correct; and is free of spelling, punctuation, and capitalization errors.

Continued

Jean Cynthia Rondinello
642 Wambler Road
Newark, NJ 14335
H: (253) 487-2298
C: (267) 345-8763
jrondinello@aol.com

List of References

Miriam Williams, DVM
Maplewood Veterinary Hospital
534 Red Rover Drive
Newark, NJ 28765
Work: (564) 234-1876
E-mail: mwilliams@msn.com

Jose Binidos, LVT
Folkways Animal Clinic
30 Baltimore Road
Mount Holly, NJ 65419
Work: (324) 897-2654
E-mail: JNBINIDOS@Verizon.net

Ms. Cynthia Moore
Windy Way Street
Mirror Lakes, NJ 32876
Work: (876) 893-1873
E-mail: cmoore@pfizer.com

B

FIGURE 1-15—cont'd

Résumé components in detail

Objective. The objective is the first statement in a résumé that tells the reader concisely what type of position the applicant is immediately seeking. An example of an objective would be: "To obtain a position as a veterinary technician in a progressive companion animal practice." Do not give your life plans, such as "to graduate from college, work in companion animal practice for awhile, move to Australia, and then establish a zoo for endangered marsupials."

Education. Be sure to list the dates attended, field of study, full name of school, town, and state where the school is located. Leave a space between each school entry. It is often effective to bold the name of the school.

Example:
Brubecker College, Windsor, Minnesota
Program of Veterinary Technology
AS: May, 2007
Abington High School, Abington, Minnesota
Diploma: June, 2004

Refer to Box 1-6 for a list of commonly acquired degrees. Notice that the degree awarded to most veterinary technicians who graduate from a 2-year program is an associate in science degree.

Experience. In this section of your résumé, list the most recent experience first. If you have a great deal of experience, you may not want to include all of it, but be sure to list experience that is relevant to the job for which you are applying.

BOX 1-6 Commonly Awarded Degrees

Associate Degrees
AS—Associate in science
AA—Associate in arts
AAS—Associate in applied science
ADN—Associate degree in nursing

Baccalaureate Degrees
BS—Bachelor of science
BA—Bachelor of arts
AB—Artium baccalaureus
BSN—Bachelor of science in nursing

Master's Degrees
MS—Master of science
MA—Master of arts
MFA—Master of fine arts
MBA—Master of business administration

Doctoral Degrees
DVM—Doctor of veterinary medicine
VMD—Veterinariae medicinae doctoris
PhD—Doctor of philosophy
JD—Jurum doctor (doctor of jurisprudence)

For example, if you worked with horses 20 years ago, you should consider listing it because it has relevance to a position in a veterinary practice. List the job title first followed by the date. On a second line, you can add the name of the employer, town, and state. Under this, you can bullet duties and responsibilities. Use the present verb tense if you are currently employed in the position; otherwise, use the past tense. Be sure to use the same layout, format, and sentence structure as you describe your various employment experiences.

Example:
Veterinary Assistant ***June 2001-2003***
Cat Clinic of Titerton, Titerton, Colorado

- Assisted with the administration of medication to hospitalized patients
- Restrained animals for examination
- Cleaned surgical instruments
- Exercised kenneled dogs

Notice that each bulleted point begins with a verb in past tense.

Veterinary Technician Specialist (Anesthesia) ***June 2008 to present***
Burns Veterinary Associates, Maplewood, California

- Perform preoperative and postoperative nursing care of surgical patients
- Oversee implementation of pain management protocols
- Induce anesthesia
- Maintain and monitor anesthetized patients

Here, notice that the technician is currently employed at this practice, so the bulleted points are in present tense.

Credentials. List all of the states in which you are licensed, registered, and certified. If you are a specialist, give the dates when you received your specialty certificates followed by the field of specialty. If you have received certificates in special programs, such as in acupuncture, practice management, and nutrition, be sure to list these certificates followed by who awarded them and where and when they were awarded.

Continuing education (CE). If you are credentialed in a state that mandates continuing education, it is assumed that you are completing CE credits by attending professional conferences and lectures. You do not need to list all of the CE classes that you have attended. This is dull. However, if you have attended advanced CE classes in your area of specialty, this would be important to list.

Volunteer experience. For those with little paid experience, this is a good way to list pet-sitting experience, community outreach, shelter work, and so on. It can be a valuable section to add for new graduates.

Professional memberships. This is a good place to list the professional associations of which you are a member.

References. Often résumés state "references available upon request" at the end of the résumé. When you are asked to give references, it is best to do so in writing on a separate page. Be sure to list at least three references. Select persons who have worked with you, taught you, and mentored you. Do not select friends and family members because these references are viewed as biased and unreliable. Once you have selected a list of persons to serve as references on your behalf, you must call them and acquire permission to use their name. This is also a good opportunity to let your references know about the positions to which you are applying. It is also a good time to collect the current address, telephone number, and e-mail address of the referring person and to confirm the correct spelling of their name.

THE JOB INTERVIEW

The interview is an excellent opportunity for an applicant to gain greater insight into the strengths and weaknesses of a potential job. It also gives the potential employer a chance to get to know the applicant and to gain an impression of the applicant's suitability for the position. In this way, interviews are valuable for both the employer and the applicant. An excellent interview can tip the scales in favor of the applicant. This is particularly true if the applicant possesses good interpersonal skills in spite of limited experience. Keep in mind that well-run veterinary practices seek employees that work collaboratively, so the value of an applicant who is a team player with no experience may be greater to a practice than a highly experienced applicant who has difficulty working with others. Although the interview is an opportunity to impress the employer and to present oneself as a self-assured professional, a poor impression can be made as immediately as a good one (Box 1-7). Therefore it is important for the applicant to be fully prepared for the interview.

Preparing for an Interview

1. **Prepare what you are going to wear well in advance** to allow time to have clothes dry-cleaned, if necessary. Make sure that your shoes are clean, polished, and in good condition. Iron your clothes. Plan on wearing dressy casual clothes to most interviews in companion animal practice (skirt or dress pants and blouse for women and sports jacket and tie for men). If you are asked to have a working interview, you should wear matching scrubs and white sneakers. For interviews in equine practices, khaki pants, collared shirts, and leather shoes work well. Interviews in pharmaceutical or pet food corporations would require formal business attire (business suit with conservative dress shoes).
2. **Prepare your résumé.** Make sure your résumé is current and printed on good quality stationery. Take three copies of your résumé to the interview.
3. **Practice shaking hands and greeting someone.** Your posture, handshake, and facial expressions are the first nonverbal communications made when greeting someone for the first time. Make sure that you communicate confidence, integrity, and strength. To do this, simply do what our mothers have been telling us for centuries: "Stand up straight with shoulders back, look the person in the eye, *smile*, and shake their hand *firmly*." Always shake hands using your *right* hand.
4. **Prepare your answers to commonly asked interview questions** (Box 1-8). Review and consider questions that you might be asked in an interview. Writing out your answers is an excellent way to organize your thoughts

BOX 1-7 The Dos and Don'ts of Interviewing

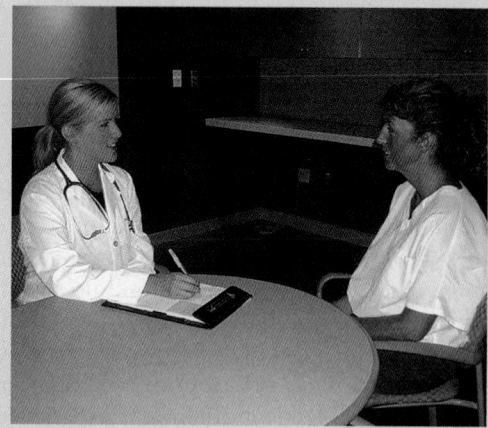

Do

1. Make sure you are dressed appropriately for the interview. Arrange your hair neatly and pulled back. Be sure to have short, clean fingernails with no nail polish. Remove all jewelry from body piercings and wear clothes that cover tattoos. Examine yourself carefully in the mirror with a critical eye, including your shoes.
2. Expect to be given a tour of the facility as part of the interview. Wear shoes that are comfortable and quiet when walking.
3. Arrive 10 minutes early. If you arrive on time, a person who advances his watch by 5 minutes will perceive you as being late.
4. Give nonverbal cues of possessing self-confidence by standing up straight, making good eye contact, smiling, and giving a firm handshake.
5. Employ your best manners. Wait to be seated until directed to do so, cover your mouth if you cough or sneeze, say please and thank you, etc.
6. Bring three copies of your résumé and have them stored in a folder or brief case.
7. Bring a pencil or pen and a writing tablet so that you are prepared to write down important bits of information.
8. Bring a list of three references with the associated contact information.
9. Be prepared to ask at least three excellent questions.
10. Sit up straight, smile, speak clearly and with articulation. Avoid "mall speak." If asked how you are, answer "well," not "good."
11. Show respect for the interviewer and do not presume to be chummy, even if you are friends.
12. *Always* tell the truth, even if you are asked directly about a previous difficult situation.
13. Have a positive outlook.
14. At the end of the interview, shake hands and thank the interviewer. Ask when you can expect to hear from him or her.
15. After the interview, write a letter of thanks and mail it to the interviewer. Use the business letter format on good stationery. Do not send the letter via e-mail. Written thank you letters help your candidacy stand out from the others.

Don'ts

1. Don't wear excessive amounts of makeup, perfume, and jewelry.
2. Don't leave in a tongue stud because you think no one will see it.
3. Don't chew gum. Don't smoke, and don't smell of smoke.
4. Don't wear a hat.
5. Don't wear clothing that conveys professional immaturity, such as platform shoes, fishnet stockings, short skirts, low-cut blouses, tank tops, tight sweaters, flip-flops, jeans, T-shirts, excessively high-heeled shoes, or any shoes that make a lot of noise when you walk or that make you look fragile and helpless.
6. Don't be late.
7. Don't give a weak handshake.
8. Don't look at the interviewer furtively or have eyes fixed on your hands or on the floor.
9. Don't have extraneous actions that communicate nervousness, such as jiggling your knee or foot, touching your face, repeatedly readjusting your position, giggling, and playing with your hair or with something in your hands.
10. Don't say "umm" or "uhhh" before answering a question. Avoid "mall speak." Don't use the words: like, totally, awesome, wow, and cool.
11. Don't be too serious. It is important to smile, appear relaxed, and have some humor.
12. *Never* criticize anyone in an interview. Do not deprecate your high school, your college, your teachers, previous bosses, co-workers, or even your parents.
13. *Never* gossip (positively or negatively).
14. *Never* lie. Do not assume the interviewer does not know what you know about a previously embarrassing event. Keep in mind that good judgment comes from experience, and experience comes from bad judgment.
15. Don't attempt to negotiate compensation or benefits until after you have been offered the position.

and articulate your answers clearly. Always be honest and never brag or self-deprecate.

5. **Prepare no less than three brilliant questions.** At the end of the interview, you will invariably be asked if you have any questions. *Never* say no. This is an excellent opportunity to show your interest and enthusiasm for the position and to illuminate your knowledge of veterinary technology. Review the practice's website, and consider the areas that are of particular interest to you. Formulate informed, intelligent, and well-worded questions.
6. **Confirm directions and time of arrival.** Some applicants feel more confident by driving to the site of the interview a day or 2 in advance. This enables the applicant to determine the travel time and to identify any pitfalls that may arise, such as highway construction or detours. It also confirms the accuracy of the directions.
7. **Add the telephone number of the practice to your cell phone.** In the event of emergency, it will be necessary to notify the veterinary practice as soon as possible. Use of a cell phone facilitates this process.

BOX 1-8 Commonly Asked Interview Questions

Employers will often ask a series of standard questions in interviews to help guide the discussion and ensure that important topics are not overlooked. You can improve your performance in an interview if you anticipate and consider the questions ahead of time. Here are some examples of commonly asked questions:

1. What do you perceive as your greatest strengths and weaknesses?
2. Why are you applying for this position?
3. What did you like and dislike about your previous positions?
4. What was your most valuable professional experience and why?
5. What was your worst professional experience and why?
6. On a scale from 1 to 10, how would you characterize yourself in the following areas?
   a. Neatness
   b. Organizational skills
   c. Ability to work with difficult people
   d. Tendency to gossip
   e. Efficiency
   f. Ability to generate creative, new ideas
   g. Ability to adapt to change
   h. Ability to work collaboratively
   i. Awareness and sensitivity toward others
   j. Level of clinical competence
   k. Your performance as a student in college
7. What are your long- and short-term goals?
8. Do you have any particular clinical interests?
9. Do you have experience working with the public? What was that like for you?
10. How do you feel about teaching technician students, interns, and co-workers?
11. Do you have any questions?

TECHNICIAN NOTE Although the interview is an opportunity to impress the employer and to present oneself as a self-assured professional, a poor impression can be made as immediately as a good one. Therefore it is important for the applicant to be fully prepared for the interview.

STRESS IN THE WORKPLACE

Veterinary technology, like other health care professions, includes a fair degree of stress. Veterinary technicians who work in clinical practices are on their feet for the vast majority of the day. Many technicians believe that they have little time for lunch or other breaks and are challenged to keep up with the pace of a busy practice. Animals can be uncooperative, and their owners, who may be stressed themselves (particularly if their pet is ill), can be difficult at times. In addition, the closely knit staff that comprises many veterinary health care teams can be particularly vulnerable to stress if conflict arises within the team. Finally, pet loss from euthanasia and illness, particularly unexpected deaths, can bring sadness and lower morale, which in turn exacerbates an already stressful working environment. With time, experienced technicians learn to pace themselves and recognize and address potentially stressful situations as they arise. Nevertheless, stress is an all too common aspect of working in veterinary technology. It is important for clinical supervisors to recognize stress among staff members and to understand the toll that it can bring upon the mental and physical well-being of those that carry it, particularly for long periods of time.

THE PHYSIOLOGY OF STRESS

The body responds to stress via a three-phase physiologic event called the *general adaptation syndrome* (GAS). The first phase is an *alarm reaction* in which a cascade of hormones is released from the hypothalamus and pituitary gland and subsequently from the adrenal glands. Epinephrine, released from the adrenal gland, increases respiration and heart rates and increases muscle tension. Elevated blood pressure, dry mouth, and chest contractions can follow. The adrenal gland also releases increased levels of glucocorticoid hormones, which lowers the body's immune response. Concurrent stimulation of the autonomic nervous system affects the digestive system and exacerbates muscle tension (Figure 1-16). Gastric reflux, ulcers, and nausea together with muscle aches and pains can ensue.

The second part of the GAS stress response is called the *adaptive phase*. During this time, the body tries to adjust to elevated levels of stress hormones and to changes in the autonomic nervous system. If the stress persists for a prolonged period of time and is then hammered with additional unexpected stressors, the body can lose its ability to adapt and may enter the *phase of exhaustion*. This final stage, as its name implies, can culminate in psychological and physical exhaustion. Cumulative changes occur in the brain as stress is prolonged, which increasingly sensitizes the person to additional stressors. Anxiety, depression, and anger are common psychological responses, and as the stress continues, a person becomes less able to cope.

PERSONALITY AND STRESS

Not all people will experience all three phases of GAS. Whether or not a person can adapt to stress depends upon the situation, the level and duration of the stress, and upon the personality of the individual. Some personality types are susceptible to stress, whereas others are stress resistant. People who have a tendency to be competitive, perfectionists, and often angry are also people who are more vulnerable to stress. They are called type A personalities. Type A persons appear to suffer from "hurry sickness." They tend

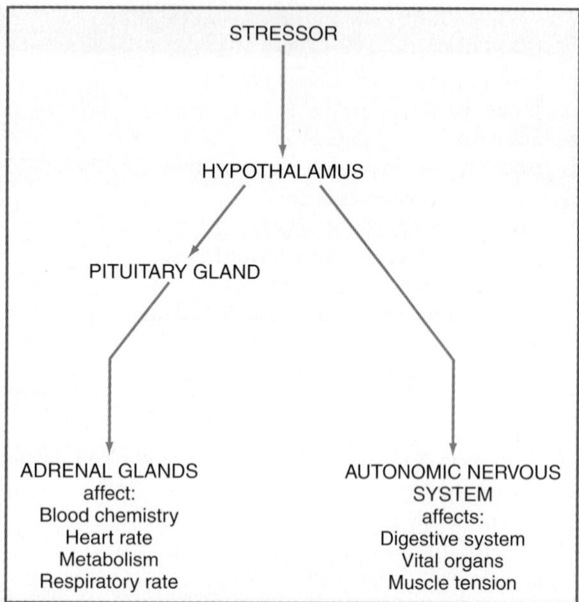

FIGURE 1-16 Stress induces a cascade of hormones, which affect the adrenal glands and autonomic nervous system. This sequence of physiologic events is part of the general adaptation syndrome (GAS), which can lead to illness and exhaustion if stress is prolonged. (From McCurnin DM, Bassert JM: *Clinical textbook for veterinary technicians*, ed 6, St. Louis, 2002, Saunders.)

to walk and talk quickly, are impatient, and feel insecure. They set deadlines and schedules for themselves and feel guilty when they relax. In contrast, type B personalities are stress resilient. They tend to have realistic expectations of what they can accomplish and are not worried about failure. They approach experiences with the belief that they are in control of their own life and destiny and take responsibility for what happens to them. They attempt to understand the people and activities in their lives and do not withdraw from situations. Finally, stress-resilient people find change exciting and conducive to personal growth. They have strong spiritual convictions, though they are not necessarily affiliated with any religious institution. Are you more of a type A or type B personality? Test yourself using the quiz in Figure 1-17.

STRESSORS

The extent to which a person is self-confident and possesses self-esteem is also important in the level of stress experienced by the person. For example, an individual who is confident in her abilities, intelligence, and organizational skills may be relatively calm while planning a wedding, working full-time, and volunteering to run the community fundraiser. On the other hand, a less confident individual might feel tremendously stressed when performing the simplest tasks.

Previous experiences, personal backgrounds, and the circumstances of one's living situation can make an individual more or less resilient to the stress of clinical practice. Life events play a key role in the performance of workers and in the level of stress that they experience. A person who feels supported by family and friends, for example, is more stress resilient in the workplace than someone who does not have support. Stress can come from both positive events, such as getting married, and from negative events, such as experiencing the death of a loved one. Both are stressful. An employee who has overextended himself or herself in his or her activities outside of the workplace may feel tired and short tempered, even though the activities are designed to be fun. Thus moderation is an important part of a balanced and happy life. As evident in Box 1-9, there is often a fine line between good stress and bad stress.

Thomas Holmes and Richard Rahe created a scale to measure the impact of 43 life events (Table 1-2). Individuals at risk for stress-related illness are those who experience more than 300 life change units in a year. For individuals who accrue less than 150 life change units, only a slight risk of illness is expected. The scale is helpful in estimating levels of stress, but the actual amount of stress experienced by an individual is based on personality, background, and other circumstances as mentioned.

REDUCING STRESS IN THE WORKPLACE

Veterinary technicians who are leaders within the veterinary health care team can help to create a positive working environment for the team by minimizing stress and by building a culture of collaboration. Insisting on no gossip, for example, and removing staff members who incite conflict can alleviate a huge source of stress for the team. Technicians can help to create an environment in which staff members feel free to admit mistakes and where individuals are not singled out and shamed. Finally, veterinary technician leaders can decrease stress within the veterinary health care team through regular, open, and clear communication with team members.

Below are five steps for reducing stress in clinical practice:

1. Plan for the unexpected.
   a. Keep time slots free for emergencies and delays.
   b. Arrange for emergency backup personnel in the event that a team member unexpectedly cannot work and when more emergencies than expected arrive for treatment.
   c. Cross-train staff.
   d. Have backup generators that keep the practice (and the computer system) functional during power failures.
   e. Prepare written standard operating procedures and review them with the staff.
2. Create reasonable work schedules.
   a. Avoid scheduling excessively long hours.
   b. Insist that each member of the health care team takes at least one break per 8-hour period.
   c. Schedule and take vacation time.

Statement	Disagree	Cannot say	Agree
I never seem to have enough time to accomplish my goals.			
I totally understand people who become so impatient in traffic that they start honking.			
I have to make it into the top 10% or else people won't respect me.			
I find it difficult and useless to confide in someone.			
A driver's license should be more difficult to get in order to avoid having all those idiots on the road.			
It really bothers me if I cannot finish what I planned for the day.			
I often choose not to spend time with my friends or family if I have something important to do.			
I am hardly ever satisfied with my achievements.			
I get a lot of pleasure out of acquiring things.			
It is not easy for me to express my feelings.			
People who don't know what they want get on my nerves.			
When I finish my task, I feel good about myself.			
I function best under stress or pressure.			
Talking about emotions is a sign of weakness and can be used by others to get you later.			
If everybody did their job properly, my life would be much easier.			
I think hobbies such as fishing or bowling are just a waste of time.			
Total points	**Type B = (maximum score = 16)**		**Type A = (maximum score = 16)**

FIGURE 1-17 Chart used to determine a personality type. Respond to each of the following statements and then total your points at the bottom of the chart.

3. Create a culture of collaboration, trust, and mutual support (rather than of gossip, blame, and finger pointing).
   a. Model professional behavior and respect for co-workers.
   b. *Never* reprimand a staff member in front of others.
   c. Keep emotions under control at all times.
4. Recognize and counsel staff members who are particularly stressed.
5. Provide clear communication with staff members.
   a. Have regular staff meetings.
   b. Support open communication, but at the same time, limit complaining.

BOX 1-9 Examples of Good and Bad Stressors

Good Stress	Bad Stress
Starting a new job	Your spouse is laid off
Completing a fun assignment	Taking a comprehensive verbal examination
The birth of a child	Getting divorced
Attending to an emergency when you feel prepared and competent	Trying to treat a patient when the needed drugs are not available
Starting a romantic relationship	Being raped
Designing your own project	Maintaining someone else's poorly executed project
Buying a new house	Having severe financial problems

SUBSTANCE ABUSE AND STRESS

The combination of a stressful workplace and the availability of various drugs in veterinary practice puts veterinary personnel at risk for engaging in illegal drug use. Since the nervous system, brain, and emotions are dependent on the normal action of neurotransmitters, some individuals suffering from stress may turn to drugs and alcohol, almost as a form of self-medication. Alcohol and drugs can enhance, distort, or even eliminate information normally exchanged by the nerve cells. There seems to be evidence that indicates that there may be a genetic vulnerability to substance abuse. Substance abuse and dependence seem to run in families. Some cultural groups have established patterns of use, and some age groups seem to be vulnerable. In studies comparing occupations, physicians and health care professionals have been found to be more vulnerable than other occupations. When the individual has knowledge about the drug(s) and access to the drugs, the individual is at risk. In general, a veterinarian or veterinary staff member with a substance abuse problem will exhibit a change in behavior. Their behavior in the practice may change so that they neglect duties, appear disorganized, or exhibit poor judgment in the practice of veterinary medicine. Other signs may include prescriptions written for themselves, friends, or family, or there may be missing drugs from the practice during the hours in which they were on duty. They may reveal the presence of financial or legal problems. There may be unexplained absences, conflicts with others, and career instability.

Some kind of intervention and action is needed anytime substance abuse interferes with practice as described. Client, patient, and co-worker safety is of primary importance. The entire practice may be at risk for malpractice as a result of the substance abuser. In every state, there is a board of veterinary medicine that awards, reviews, and can suspend licenses for veterinarians of that state. Most governing boards for health care professionals have stipulations upon continued licensing in which impairment of the professional prevents renewal. Generally speaking, the impaired professional should be confronted, preferably by a peer or superior, and asked to seek treatment. Many situations end happily with successful remedial action and/or treatment.

All 50 states have resources and guidance for the impaired veterinary professional, either through the governing board or their state professional association. Most states have a list of qualified counselors and treatment centers that have successfully worked with other impaired professionals. The counselor will do an evaluation to determine what type of treatment is recommended.

PROFESSIONAL ORGANIZATIONS

As the profession of veterinary technology matures, there are increasing numbers of professional organizations forming at the national, state, or provincial and local levels. These organizations support the education, professional interests, and activities of the veterinary technician. NAVTA and CAAHTT, for example, represent the professional foundation of veterinary technology in the United States and Canada, respectively. But there are also numerous national organizations forming based on the special interests of their members. Examples include: the Association of Zoo Veterinary Technicians, the Society of Veterinary Behavior Technicians, and the American Association of Equine Veterinary Technicians. Continued growth of veterinary technology depends heavily on the efforts of individuals within these and other professionally related organizations. Graduate veterinary technicians can assist in advancing their profession by joining and being active members. A full listing of veterinary technician and affiliated organizations is located at the end of this chapter.

NATIONAL ASSOCIATION OF VETERINARY TECHNICIANS IN AMERICA

NAVTA has been a particular leader in shaping and supporting the profession of veterinary technology in the United States. It has written the code of ethics, the veterinary technician oath, and the veterinary technician portion of the model practice act and has brought about important changes in the profession's terminology. In addition, NAVTA is an important source of support and information for veterinary technicians. It publishes *The NAVTA Journal* and has

TABLE 1-2 Social Readjustment Rating Scale

Life Event	Number of Life Changes
Death of a spouse	100
Divorce	73
Marital separation	65
Jail term	63
Death of close family member	63
Personal injury or illness	53
Marriage	50
Fired at work	47
Marital reconciliation	45
Retirement	45
Change in family member's health	44
Pregnancy	40
Sex difficulties	39
Gain of new family member	39
Business readjustment	39
Change in financial state	38
Death of close friend	37
Change to different line of work	36
Change in number of arguments with spouse	35
Mortgage of $100,000	31
Foreclosure of mortgage or loan	30
Change in work responsibilities	29
Son or daughter leaving home	29
Trouble with in-laws	29
Outstanding personal achievement	28
Spouse begins or stops work	26
Begin or end school	26
Change in living conditions	25
Revision of personal habits	24
Trouble with boss	23
Change in work hours or conditions	20
Change in residence	20
Change in schools	20
Change in recreation	19
Change in church activities	19
Change in social activities	18
Mortgage or loan less than $100,000	17
Change in sleeping habits	16
Change in number of family get-togethers	15
Change in eating habits	15
Vacation	13
Christmas	12
Minor violations of the law	11

Modified from Holmes TH, Rahe R: *J Psychosom Res* 11:213, 1967; with permission.

established a website at www.navta.net (Figure 1-18, *A* and *B*). The website contains a plethora of information, ranging from important credentialing information for technicians relocating to another state to promotional materials for National Veterinary Technician Week. Therefore it is not surprising that NAVTA's mission statement is: "to represent and promote the profession of veterinary technology. NAVTA provides direction, education, support, and coordination for its members and works with other allied professional organizations for the competent care and humane treatment of animals." In addition, the goals of NAVTA are to help its members do the following:

1. Influence the future of veterinary technology.
2. Be part of the decision-making process that affects veterinary technology.
3. Foster high standards of veterinary care.
4. Promote the veterinary health care team.

To be an active member of NAVTA, you must live in the United States; be a graduate of an AVMA-accredited program of veterinary technology; or be licensed, certified, or registered as a veterinary technician. In addition, associate members include veterinarians, veterinary technicians who live outside the United States, and veterinary assistants. Associate members may serve on committees, but may not vote or hold an elected office.

The Canadian Association of Animal Health Technologists and Technicians/Association Canadienne des Techniciens et Technologists en Santé Animale.

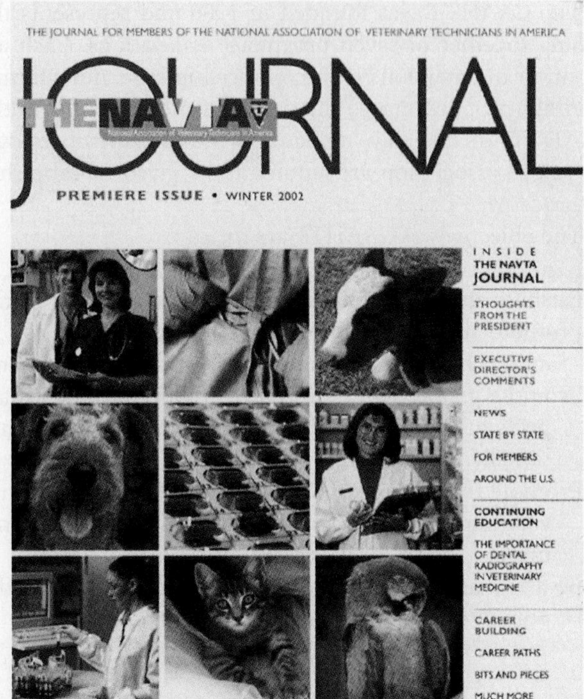

FIGURE 1-18 A, The cover of the premier issue of *The NAVTA Journal* (Winter 2002).

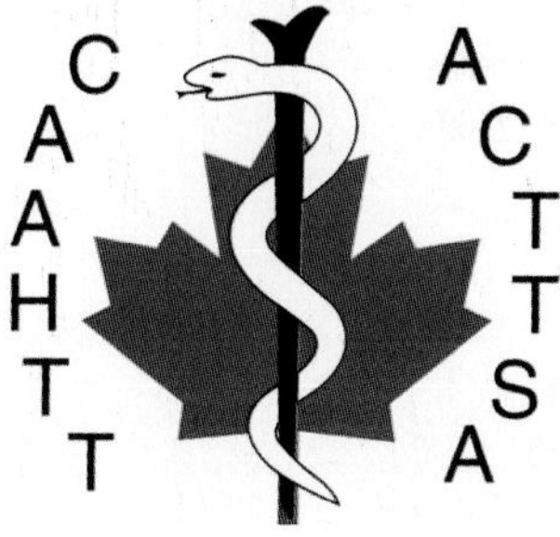

The CAAHTT was founded in 1989 and represents the joining together of seven provincial associations. Each association maintains its own membership base and submits funding (proportional to the size of its membership) to the CAAHTT. In this way, individuals who are members of a provincial association are automatically given membership in the CAAHTT.

The objectives of CAAHTT are to:

- Establish and maintain a national standard of membership.
- Promote and assist in providing continuing education to animal health technologists and veterinary technicians.
- Promote greater communication among the various aspects of the profession, both nationally and internationally.
- Promote the profession of animal health technology and veterinary technology within the animal health community and to the general public.
- Be a resource to members of the profession and to the public regarding national and international issues.

> *TECHNICIAN NOTE* NAVTA and CAAHTT have designated the third week in October as National Veterinary Technician Week! Mark your calendars! For more information, check www.navta.net or www.caahtt-acttsa.ca.

Directory of Professional Associations

International Veterinary Nurses and Technicians Associations

International Veterinary Nurses and Technicians Association (IVNTA)
Website: www.vetweb.co-uk/sites/ivnta

Australia
Veterinary Nurses Council of Australia
PO Box 2233
North Ringwood, Victoria 3134, Australia

Canada
Canadian Association of Animal Health Technologists and Technicians (CAAHTT)
Phyllis Mierau, Executive Director
PO Box 91
Grandora, SK, Canada SOK 1VO
Phone: 306-329-4956; fax: 306-329-4700
E-mail: s.vettech@sasktel.net, phyllis.caahtt@sasktel.net
Website: www.caahtt-acttsa.ca

Denmark
Ms. Jannie Larssen
Veterinaersygeplejerske Association
Christoffers Alle 86, st. mf., 2800
Lyngby, Denmark

Finland
Ms. Jaana Lindfors
Felina Kissaklinikka (Cat Clinic)
Tyomiehenkatu 4C, 00180
Helsinki, Finland

Germany
Ms. Barbara Johnson
Mittlestrasse 28a, 52072
Aachen, Germany

Ghana
Mr. K. Tetteh Alorbu
PO Box 1341
Tema, Ghana

Japan
Ms. Chiharu Ishida, AHT, JVNTA
33 Kalesukuri-cho
Wakatama-shi, Wakayama-ken, 640 Japan

Netherlands
VEDIAS, Schaepmanstratt 121, 6702 AS
Wageningen, Netherlands
Phone: 0 317 419 101
Fax: 0 317 419 101

New Zealand
Ms. Kathryn Ching
22 Box Hill
Khandallah, Wellington, New Zealand

Norway
Ms. Anita Granum
Norwegian Veterinary Nursing
FD TA, NVH, PB 8156 Dep, 0033
Oslo, Norway

South Africa
Matron Linda Muller
PO Box 12924
Onderstepoort, 0110, South Africa

Sweden
Ms. Helen Wallin, VT, RAID
Stromsholm Referral Animal Hospital
73040 Kolback, Sweden

United Kingdom
British Veterinary Nurses Association
Ross White, Dipl. AVN (Surg), VN, President
Level 15, Terminus House, Terminus Street
Harlow, Essex, CM20 1XA
Phone: 01279 450567
Fax: 01279 420866
E-mail: bvna@bvna.co.uk
Website: www.bvna.org.uk

United States of America
National Association of Veterinary Technicians in America (NAVTA)
Andrea Ball, Executive Director
50 S. Pickett Street, Ste. 110
Alexandria, VA 22304
703-740-8737

Fax: 703-823-7237
E-mail: navta@navta.net
Website: www.navta.net

Academies of Recognized Veterinary Technician Specialties in the United States

Academy of Veterinary Emergency and Critical Care Technicians (AVECCT)
Organizing Committee, c/o VECCS
15729 San Pedro, San Antonio, TX 78232
Phone: 210-826-1488
Website: www.avecct.org

Academy of Veterinary Dental Technicians (AVDT)
Vickie Byard, CVT, VTS (Dentistry)
551 Creek Rd
Warminster, PA 18974
Website: www.avdt.us
Contact: Sara L. Sharp, CVT, AVDT Secretary
E-mail: DBLTRBSLS@aol.com

Academy of Veterinary Technician Anesthetists (AVTA)
Sharon Johnston, LVT, VTS (anesthesia)
205 Alender Way
Simpsonville, SC 29681
Phone: 864-884-6065
Website: www.avta-vts.org

Academy of Internal Medicine for Veterinary Technicians (AIMVT)
Website: www.aimvt.com

Veterinary Technician Education and Testing

Academy of Veterinary Behavior Technicians (AVBT)
Website: www.svbt.org

Association of Veterinary Technician Educators (AVTE)
Terry Teeple, DVM
Pierce College
9401 Farwest Drive SW
Tacoma, WA 98498
Phone: 253-964-6668; fax: 253-964-6599
Website: www.avte.net

Committee on Veterinary Technician Education and Activities (CVTEA)
American Veterinary Medical Association (AVMA)
Suite 100, 1931 North Meacham Road
Schaumburg, IL 60173
Phone: 847-925-8070; fax: 847-925-1329
Website: www.avma.org

Northeast Veterinary Technician Educators Association (NEVTEA)
Amy Shields, CVT, UTS (ECC)
Director of Nursing and Critical Care Veterinary Referral Center
340 Lancaster Avenue
Fraser, PA 19355
Phone: 610-674-2950

Professional Examination Service (PES)
475 Riverside Drive
New York, NY 10115-0089
212-367-4200
Website: proexam.org
(For information regarding the VTNE or the AALAS Animal Technician Certification Program)

Important Related Professional Organizations

American Animal Hospital Association (AAHA)
PO Box 150899
Denver, CO 80215-0899
Phone: 303-986-2800; fax: 303-986-1700

American Association of Veterinary State Boards (AAVSB)
3100 Main Street, Suite 208
Kansas City, MO 64111
Phone: 816-931-1504; fax: 816-931-1604
Website: www.aavsb.org

American Veterinary Medical Association (AVMA)
Suite 100, 1931 North Meacham Road
Schaumburg, IL 60173
Phone: 847-925-8070; fax: 847-925-1329
Website: www.avma.org

British Small Animal Veterinary Association
Dr. Ed Hall, BSAVA Congress
Woodrow House
1 Telford Way
Waterwells Business Park
Quedgeley, Gloucester, GL24AB
Website: www.bsava.com

Canadian Veterinary Medical Association/Association canadienne des médecins veterinaries
CVMA/ACMV and the Animal Health Technology/Veterinary Technician Program Accreditation Committee AHT/VTPAC
339 Rue Booth St.
Ottawa ON K1R 7K1
www.canadianveterinarians.net or www.animalhealthcare.ca

LINKS TO RELATED PROFESSIONAL ORGANIZATIONS

AAAHT—The Alberta Association of Animal Health Technologists www.aaaht.com
AAEP—American Association of Equine Practitioners www.aaep.org
AAEVT—American Association of Equine Veterinary Technicians www.AAEVT.org
AAFP—American Association of Feline Practitioners www.aafponline.org
AAHA—American Animal Hospital Association www.aahanet.org or www.healthypet.com
AALAS—The American Association for Laboratory Animal Science www.aalas.org
AAVSB—American Association of Veterinary State Boards www.aavsb.org
ACLAM—The American College of Laboratory Animal Medicine www.aclam.org
AHTA—Animal Health Technologists Association of British Columbia www.ahta.bc.ca
AIMVT—Academy of Internal Medicine for Veterinary Technicians www.AIMVT.com

AMCNY—Animal Medical Center of New York www.amcny.org
ASLAP—The American Society of Laboratory Animal Practitioners www.aslap.org
ASVCP—American Society for Veterinary Clinical Pathology www.asvcp.org
ASVDT—American Society of Veterinary Dental Technicians www.asvdt.org
ATASQ—Association des Techniciens en Santé Animale du Québec www.atsaq.org
AVDS—American Veterinary Dental Society www.avds-online.org
AVDT—Academy of Veterinary Dental Technicians www.avdt.us
AVECCT—Academy of Veterinary Emergency and Critical Care Technicians www.avecct.org
AVTA—Academy of Veterinary Technician Anesthetists www.avta-vts.org
AVTE—Association of Veterinary Technician Educators www.avte.net
AZVT—Association of Zoo Veterinary Technicians www.azvt.org
CALAM—Canadian Association for Laboratory Animal Medicine www.uwo.ca/animal/website/CALAM
CALAS—Canadian Association for Laboratory Animal Science www.calas-acsal.org
CVDT—Canadian Veterinary Dental Technician Program www.sl.on.ca
EVTA—Eastern Veterinary Technician Association Ltd. of the Atlantic Provinces www.evta.ca
MAHTA—Manitoba Animal Health Technologists Association Inc. www.mahta.ca
NCVEI—National Commission on Veterinary Economic Issues www.ncvei.org
OAVT—Ontario Association of Veterinary Technicians www.oavt.org
SAVT—Saskatchewan Association of Veterinary Technologists www.savt.ca
SVBT—Society of Veterinary Behavior Technicians www.svbt.org
AVH—The Academy of Veterinary Homeopathy www.theavh.org
VECCS—Veterinary Emergency and Critical Care Society www.veccs.org
VHMA—Veterinary Hospital Managers Association Inc www.vhma.org
VOTS—Veterinary Opthalmic Technician Society www.votsweb.com
VIN—Veterinary Information Network www.vin.org
VSPN—Veterinary Support Personnel Network www.vspn.org
Check www.theagapecenter.com/organizations for further listings that may be of interest.
Check NetVet—find anything to do with animals at netvet.wustl.edu/e-zoo.htm.

COMMON ACRONYMS

Veterinary Health Care Team
ACT—Animal Care Technician
AHT—Animal Health Technician
CVPM—Certified Veterinary Practice Manager
CVT—Certified Veterinary Technician
DVM—Doctor of Veterinary Medicine
LVT—Licensed Veterinary Technician
OJT—On-the-job–Trained (veterinary assistant)
RAHT—Registered Animal Health Technician
RVT—Registered Veterinary Technician
VA—Veterinary Assistant
VHM—Veterinary Hospital Manager
VMD—Veterinary Medical Doctor (Univ. of Penn)
Laboratory Animal Technology
AALAS—American Association of Laboratory Animal Science
ALAT—Assistant Laboratory Animal Technician
LAT—Laboratory Animal Technician
LATG—Laboratory Animal Technologist
CALAS—Canadian Association of Laboratory Animal Science
RLAT—Registered Laboratory Animal Technician
RLAT (Res)—Registered Laboratory Animal Technician in Research
RMLAT—Registered Master Laboratory Animal Technician
RMLAT (Res)—Registered Master Laboratory Animal Technician in Research
Organizations, Associations, and Committees
AALAS—American Association of Laboratory Animal Science
AAVDT—American Association of Veterinary Dental Technicians
AAVLD—American Association of Veterinary Laboratory Diagnosticians
AAVMC—American Association of Veterinary Medical Colleges
AAVSB—American Association of Veterinary State Boards
AAZVT—American Association of Veterinary Zoo Technicians
ACVECC—American College of Veterinary Emergency and Critical Care
ACVIM—American College of Veterinary Internal Medicine
ACVS—American College of Veterinary Surgeons
AVDT—Academy of Veterinary Dental Technicians
AVECCT—Academy of Veterinary Emergency and Critical Care Technicians
AVMA—American Veterinary Medical Association
AVTA—Academy of Veterinary Technician Anesthetists
AVTE—Association of Veterinary Technician Educators
BVNA—British Veterinary Nurses Association
BSAVA—British Small Animal Veterinary Association
CAHLN—Canadian Animal Health Laboratorians Network

CCAC—Canadian Council on Animal Care
CDC—Centers for Disease Control
CFIA—Canadian Food Inspection Agency
CVMA—Canadian Veterinary Medical Association
CVMA AHTVT PAC—Canadian Veterinary Medical Association Animal Health Technology/Veterinary Technician Program Accreditation Committee
CVTEA—Committee on Veterinary Technician Education and Activities (AVMA committee)
CVTS—Committee for Veterinary Technician Specialties
FDA—Food and Drug Administration
FECAVA—Federation of European Companion Animal Veterinary Association
IVECCS—International Veterinary Emergency and Critical Care Symposium
IVNTA—International Veterinary Nurses and Technicians Association
NAFTA—North American Free Trade Agreement
NAHLN—National Animal Health Laboratory Network
NAVLE—North American Veterinary Licensing Exam
NAVTA—National Association for Veterinary Technicians in America
NBVME—National Board of Veterinary Medical Examiners
NEVTEA—Northeast Veterinary Technician Educators Association
NCVEI—National Commission on Veterinary Economic Issues
NOC system—National Occupational Classification system
OSHA—Occupational Safety and Health Administration
PES—Professional Examination Service
USDA—United States Department of Agriculture
VECCS—Veterinary Emergency and Critical Care Society
VHMA—Veterinary Hospital Managers Association, Inc.
VIN—Veterinary Information Network
VSPN—Veterinary Support Personnel Network
VTAS—Veterinary Technician Anesthetist Society
VTNE—Veterinary Technician National Examination
VTS—Veterinary Technician Specialist
VTTC—Veterinary Technician Testing Committee
WSAVA—World Small Animal Veterinary Associations

RECOMMENDED READING

The NAVTA Journal
Quarterly publication by NAVTA
PO Box 224, Battleground, IN 47920
Phone or fax: 765-742-2216
E-mail: navta@navta.net

TECHNEWS-The Official Journal for Canadian Veterinary Technicians
Publication by the Ontario Association of Veterinary Technicians in association with CAAHTT
c/o OAVT Ontario Agricentre, Suite 104, 100 Stone Road West
Guelph ON NIG 5L3
Phone: 519-836-4910
Fax: 519-836-3638
www.oavt.org

The Veterinary Technician
Professional journal by Veterinary Learning Systems
780 Township Line Road, Yardley, PA 19067
Phone: 800-426-9119, Ext. 2447

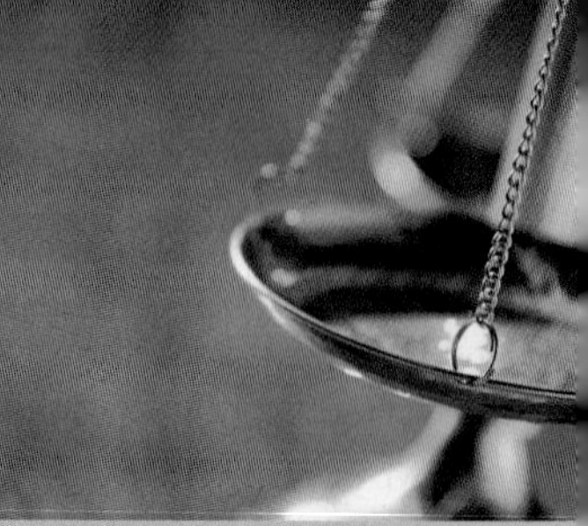

2 Laws, Regulations, and Ethics

Teresa A. Lazo

OUTLINE

KEY TERMS

Conviction
Crimes of depravity
Crimes of moral turpitude
Felony
Interference with justice
Malpractice
Perjury
Prosecution
Statute
The Board
Tort

LEARNING OBJECTIVES

When you have completed this chapter, you will be able to:

1. Name the laws and regulations that govern the practice of veterinary medicine.
2. Differentiate between laws and regulations.
3. Describe the components of veterinary practice acts.
4. Describe the term specialty academy and explain the role of the academy in the credentialing of veterinary professionals.
5. List the specialty academies recognized by NAVTA.
6. Describe the nomenclature used for credentialed veterinary technicians in various locales.
7. Describe requirements for the credentialing of veterinary technicians.
8. Describe the roles of the state boards of veterinary medicine in the credentialing of veterinary professionals.
9. Define ethics and name the organizations that develop ethical guidelines for veterinary professionals.
10. List the tasks that veterinary technicians are not permitted to perform.

INTRODUCTION

This chapter discusses the laws and regulations that govern the practice of veterinary technology. Laws are also called statutes or acts. The United States Constitution reserves for the federal government legal and regulatory authority over only those matters considered of nationwide impact and importance. The practices of professions and occupations, such as dentistry, engineering, and veterinary technology, are considered matters to be governed by the states. Therefore the majority of laws and regulations that govern the practice of veterinary technology are state based. However, veterinary medical practice is also regulated at the federal level. For example, the Occupational Safety and Health Act (enforced by the Occupational Safety and Health Administration [OSHA]) requires that guidelines be met in the workplace to protect the health and safety of workers; both federal and state laws and regulations direct how drugs and medical devices may be handled and disposed of, and both federal and state laws affect the practice of veterinary medicine on production animals. A veterinary technician does not need to be an expert in all of the federal and state laws that affect the profession; however, a veterinary technician should have a strong grasp of the state law that provides for the licensing, professional conduct, and discipline of technicians and veterinarians. In addition, a veterinary technician should be familiar with some of the areas governed by federal law so that if a question arises, the technician will know where to look for further information.

This chapter will also discuss professional conduct and ethics. In the practice of the healing arts, practitioners are frequently faced with situations where the right course of conduct is not immediately apparent. To some extent, this is magnified in veterinary medicine because veterinarians and technicians are responsible not only for the care of a patient, but also have responsibilities to the animal's owner and, in some cases, to the general public. For this reason, when considering the question of "right conduct," one must first ask "right for whom?" This chapter will give the technician an example of a decision-making process that will guide the technician in working through difficult professional conduct and ethical issues.

LAWS AND REGULATIONS GOVERNING THE PRACTICE OF VETERINARY MEDICINE AND VETERINARY TECHNOLOGY

LAWS VERSUS REGULATIONS

State laws are "enacted"—written and passed by the legislature and signed into law by the governor (Refer to Box 2-1 National Association of Veterinary Technicians in America's [NAVTA] Model Practice Act and to Appendix A American Veterinary Medical Association's [AVMA] Model Practice Act). Regulations are "promulgated"—written by executive branch or independent agencies and reviewed by a variety of entities. The review process by which an agency, such as a state board of veterinary medicine, promulgates a regulation varies from state to state; however, regulations generally do not have to be approved by either the legislature or the governor. Laws are often general mandates or prohibitions, whereas regulations more specifically describe required or prohibited conduct.

The public may have input into both laws and regulations. The public may influence laws by providing information and opinions to their legislators. The public may affect regulations by providing information and opinions to the state agency that is promulgating the regulation. You may influence regulations that affect your practice by providing information and your opinion to your state board of veterinary medicine.

Regulations are said to have the "force and effect" of law because they must be followed or the violator will be subject to sanction (Box 2-2). Violation of a law may subject the violator to monetary penalties, imprisonment, or both. Violation of a regulation may also subject the violator to monetary penalties, but will not subject the violator to imprisonment. Regulations promulgated by an agency with the authority to regulate a profession may subject a violator to sanctions against the violator's license. These sanctions include the imposition of a reprimand, a monetary penalty, restrictions placed on a license, suspension of a license, or revocation of a license. Most licensing agencies also have the authority to impose sanctions designed to remediate the conduct of the violator. Remedial sanctions may include requiring that an individual practice with monitoring or complete additional continuing education. Sanctions imposed by the licensing agency will be discussed more fully later in this chapter.

TECHNICIAN NOTE Veterinary technicians should have copies of their state's veterinary medicine practice act and regulations of their state licensing board and keep the copies updated as the act and regulations are amended.

PRIMARY LAW GOVERNING THE PRACTICE OF THE PROFESSION

The primary law that governs the practice of the profession is called the "practice act." Every state has a practice act that governs the practice of veterinary medicine, and most states also govern the practice of veterinary technology under the state's veterinary medicine practice act. The practice act creates the administrative agency that governs the practice of veterinary medicine and technology in each state. The formal name of this administrative agency may vary from state to state; names such as "Board of Veterinary Medical Examiners," "State Board of Veterinary Medicine," or "Licensing Board of Veterinary Medicine" are common. This administrative agency is commonly referred to as "the board."

The practice act usually defines the practice of veterinary medicine and veterinary technology, although in some states the board has been left to define the practice of veterinary technology. Some states do not license veterinary technicians or regulate the practice of veterinary technology. The definition of the practice is important not only because it informs veterinarians and technicians of the practices in which they may engage, but because by defining the practice, persons who are not veterinarians or veterinary technicians are prohibited from practicing veterinary medicine or veterinary technology. The unlicensed practice of veterinary medicine or veterinary technology will subject the unlicensed individual to sanction by the board and, in most states, is also a crime that may subject an unlicensed individual to criminal penalties, including imprisonment. The practice act also may set general or specific parameters for entry into practice and grounds for disciplining veterinarians and technicians. The practice act creates the board and authorizes it to oversee and regulate the professions. Refer to Box 2-3 and Appendix A.

BOX 2-1 Model Practice Act for Veterinary Technicians

Section I. Title

This act shall be known and may be cited as the "Model Practice Act."

Section II. Legislative Intent and Purpose

The practice of veterinary technology is a privilege granted by legislative authority to maintain public health, safety and welfare and to protect the public from being misled by unauthorized individuals.

Section III. Definitions

When used in the text that follows, except where otherwise indicated by context the words and phrases below shall have the following meanings:

Animal—Any mammalian animal other than man, and any avian, amphibian, fish or reptile, wild or domestic.

Board—The State Board of Veterinary Medical Examiners or Board of Governors.

Veterinary Technology—The science and art of providing all aspects of professional medical care and treatment for animals with the exception of diagnosis, prognosis, surgery and prescription.

Emergency—When an animal has been placed in a life-threatening condition and immediate treatment is necessary to sustain life; or where death is imminent and action is necessary to relieve pain or suffering.

Licensed Veterinarian—An individual who is validly and currently licensed by the Board to practice veterinary medicine in ____.

Veterinary Technician (Licensed, Registered or Certified)—An individual who has graduated from a veterinary technology program that is accredited according to the standards adopted by the American Veterinary Medical Association's Committee on Veterinary Technician Education and Activities and who has passed the examination requirements as prescribed by the Board in _____ shall be known as a licensed, registered or certified veterinary technician.

Section IV. Tasks

Certain tasks may be performed ONLY by a licensed veterinarian OR licensed, registered or certified veterinary technician under the direction, supervision and control of a veterinarian licensed to practice in the state of _____.

See the Rules and Regulations Document for a list of tasks.

Section V. Examination for Licensure, Registration or Certification

Veterinary technicians applying for licensure, registration or certification shall be required to pass the Veterinary Technician National Examination, with scores as set by the Board before licensure, registration or certification.

See the Rules and Regulations Document for a list of tasks.

Section VI. Continuing Education

All licensed, registered or certified veterinary technicians shall be required to continue their professional education as a condition of maintenance of his/her status in the state of _____.

See the Rules and Regulations Document for a list of tasks.

Section VII. Denial, Suspension, or Revocation of Veterinary Technician Licenses, Registrations or Certifications

The Board may suspend, revoke or deny the issuance or renewal of license, registration or certification of any veterinary technician if after a hearing by his/her peers, he/she has been found guilty of any of the following:

Fraud or misrepresentation in applying for license, registration, or certification.

Criminal offense relating to veterinary medicine.

Any violation of the Uniform Controlled Substances Act or the Legend Drug Act.

Convicted of cruelty to animals.

Violation of any of the rules or regulations stated in the Rules and Regulations Document.

From the American Veterinary Medical Association (AVMA) membership directory.

TECHNICIAN NOTE Only individuals who have been granted entry into a NAVTA-recognized academy may use the term "specialist" or the initials "VTS."

TERMINOLOGY

Boards

Do not confuse the state board that governs the practice of the profession with academic specialty groups for veterinarians and technicians, which are also referred to as "boards" or "specialty boards." A specialty board may also be called an "academy" or "college." A specialty board in human and veterinary medicine is an organization that confers specialty status on a physician or veterinarian who has completed an educational program and examination in a particular medical or veterinary medical specialty. In veterinary medicine, the specialty boards are associated with the AVMA. A veterinarian may, for example, become board certified in surgery by the specialty organization known as the American College of Veterinary Surgeons (ACVS). A board certified veterinarian is permitted to use the initials "ACVS" behind her name and to advertise as a "specialist" in surgery. To maintain the specialty certification, the veterinarian must complete continuing education in her specialty as mandated by the specialty board. Board certified veterinarians often practice in groups in referral hospitals, where they primarily see patients referred by other practicing veterinarians for a second opinion or for performance of more complex diagnostic, surgical, and therapeutic procedures.

Veterinary Technician Specialist

Veterinary technicians also have specialty boards. Technicians' specialty boards are associated with NAVTA. NAVTA has adopted the term "academy" to refer to a group that has received recognition as a specialty (Box 2-4). NAVTA has given full academy status to the Academy of Veterinary Emergency and Critical Care Technicians

BOX 2-2 NAVTA Model Rules and Regulations for Veterinary Technicians

I. Licensed, Registered or Certified Veterinary Technician Activities

Tasks

Levels of supervision defined

Immediate supervision—A licensed veterinarian is within direct eyesight and hearing range

Direct supervision—A licensed veterinarian is on the premises, and is readily available

Indirect supervision—A licensed veterinarian is not on the premises, but is able to perform the duties of a licensed veterinarian by maintaining direct communication

The following tasks may be performed ONLY by a licensed, registered or certified veterinary technician (or licensed veterinarian) under the direction, supervision and control of a veterinarian licensed to practice in ____ provided said veterinarian makes a daily physical examination of the patient treated:

Immediate supervision

Induction of anesthesia

Dental extraction not requiring sectioning of the tooth or the resectioning of bone

Surgical assistant to a licensed veterinarian within the rules and regulations issued by the Board of Veterinary Medical Examiners and the laws of the state of ______

Direct supervision

Euthanasia

Blood or blood component collection, preparation and administration

Application of splints and slings

Dental procedures including, but not limited to the removal of calculus, soft deposits, plaque and stains; the smoothing, filing and polishing of teeth; or the flotation or dressing of equine teeth

Indirect supervision

Administration and application of treatments, drugs, medications and immunological agents by parenteral and injectable routes (subcutaneous, intramuscular, intraperitoneal and intravenous) except when in conflict with government regulations

Initiation of parenteral fluid administration

Intravenous catheterizations

Radiography including settings, positioning, processing and safety procedures

Collection of blood; collection of urine by expression, cystocentesis or catheterization; collection and preparation of tissue, cellular or microbiological samples by skin scrapings, impressions or other non-surgical methods except when in conflict with government regulations

Routine laboratory test procedures

Supervision of the handling of biohazardous waste materials

Other

Services which a licensed, registered or certified veterinary technician is competent to perform under the appropriate degree of supervision

Under conditions of emergency, a licensed, registered or certified veterinary technician may render the following life-saving aid and treatment:

Application of tourniquets and/or pressure bandages to control hemorrhage

Administration of pharmacological agents and parenteral fluids shall only be performed after direct communication with a veterinarian authorized to practice in _____ and such veterinarian is either present or en route to the location of the distressed animals

Resuscitative procedures

Application of temporary splints or bandages to prevent further injury to bones or soft tissue

Application of appropriate wound dressings and external supportive treatment in severe wound and burn cases

External supportive treatment in heat prostration cases

HOWEVER, nothing shall be construed to permit a licensed, registered or certified veterinary technician to do the following:

Make any diagnosis or prognosis

Prescribe any treatments, drugs, medications or appliances

Perform surgery

II. Examinations

Examinations of applicants for licensure, registration or certification as a veterinary technician in ______ shall be held at least annually at a time, place and date set by the Board no later than ninety (90) days before the scheduled examination.

An applicant shall be required to pass the Veterinary Technician National Examination (VTNE) with scores as set by the Board before licensure, registration or certification.

III. Continuing Education Requirements for Licensed, Registered or Certified Veterinary Technicians

All licensed, registered or certified veterinary technicians shall be required to continue their professional education as a condition of maintaining his/her license of veterinary technology in the state of _____ with hours of continuing education required annually.

Continued

BOX 2-2 NAVTA Model Rules and Regulations for Veterinary Technicians—cont'd

IV. Removal of Veterinary Technician Licenses, Registrations or Certifications

All licenses, registrations or certifications issued to veterinary technicians in the state of _____ shall expire on _____ of every year unless renewed.

All license, registration or certification holders shall submit renewal fees and a current mailing address by the dates determined by the Board on a renewal form that shall be provided by the Board and mailed to all license, registration or certification holders.

All license, registration or certification holders will be required to submit evidence of the necessary amount of continuing education in the fields of veterinary medicine to the Board as required by the Board for license, registration or certification renewal.

Failure to submit the appropriate license, registration or certification renewal fee by the dates determined by the Board shall result in forfeiture of all privileges and rights extended by the license, registration or certification and the license, registration or certification holder must immediately cease and desist in engaging further in the performance of veterinary technician activities under the veterinary practice act until payment of delinquency fee in addition to the license, registration or certification renewal fee had been received by the Board.

From the American Veterinary Medical Association (AVMA) membership directory.

BOX 2-3 American Association of Veterinary State Boards (AAVSB)

Veterinary Technology State Practice Act Model Language Concerning Veterinary Technicians

Veterinary Technician means:

A person who is duly licensed to practice veterinary technology under the provisions of this Act.

The Practice of Veterinary Technology means:

Any person practices veterinary technology with respect to animals when such person performs any one or more of the following:

(a) Provides professional medical care, monitors and treats animals, under supervision of a licensed Veterinarian;
(b) Represents oneself directly or indirectly, as engaging in the practice of veterinary technology; or
(c) Uses any words, letters or titles under such circumstance as to induce the belief that the person using them is qualified to engage in the practice of veterinary technology, as defined. Such use shall be prima facie evidence of the intention to represent oneself as engaged in the practice of veterinary technology.

Nothing in this section shall be construed to permit a Veterinary Technician to do the following:

(a) Surgery.
(b) Diagnosis and prognosis of animal diseases.
(c) Prescribing of drugs, medicine and appliances.

Regulations Defining Tasks of Veterinary Technicians:

The board shall adopt regulations establishing animal healthcare tasks and an appropriate degree of supervision required for those tasks that may be performed only by a Veterinary Technician or a Veterinarian.

BOX 2-4 NAVTA-Recognized Academies

For more information about veterinary technician specialties, visit the following academy websites.

* Academy of Veterinary Emergency and Critical Care Technicians (AVECCT) www.avecct.org
* Academy of Veterinary Technician Anesthetists (AVTA) www.avta-vts.org
* Academy of Veterinary Dental Technicians (AVDT) www.avdt.us
* Academy of Internal Medicine Veterinary Technicians (AIMVT) www.aimvt.com
* Academy of veterinary Behavior Technicians (AVBT) www.avbt.org

(AVECCT) and has given provisional academy status to the Academy of Veterinary Technician Anesthetists (AVTA), the Academy of Veterinary Dental Technicians (AVDT), and the Academy of Internal Medicine for Veterinary Technicians (AIMVT). Technicians who have earned academy status may use the name "Veterinary Technician Specialist" or the initials "VTS" followed by their specialty, such as "anesthesia," or "ECC" (emergency and critical care). NAVTA also recognizes specialty societies.

NAVTA defines a society as a group of individuals, veterinary technicians, hospital staff, and veterinarians who are interested in a specific discipline of veterinary medicine. NAVTA currently recognizes one society: the American Association of Equine Veterinary Technicians (AAEVT). A technician who is a member of a society should not use the term "specialist" in describing their practice, and in some states, the use of the term "specialist" is forbidden by the practice act or the state board's regulations.

A VTS is a veterinary technician who has attained a higher level of knowledge and skill in a particular field. Each academy sets forth the criteria for certification, which may include formal course work, on-the-job training, and completion of a certain number of tasks. In addition, the work of the individual seeking specialty certification must be reviewed and approved before academy status is granted. Although many VTSs practice in specialty or referral hospitals or in teaching hospitals where they can concentrate on their field of interest, a VTS can be a valuable part of the veterinary medical team in any veterinary hospital by bringing a higher level of technician expertise to the practice.

Veterinary Technologist and Veterinary Technician

A "veterinary technologist" holds a bachelor's degree in veterinary technology from a 4-year, AVMA-accredited program at a college or university. A veterinary technician holds an associate degree in veterinary technology from a 2- or 3-year, AVMA-accredited program. Whereas these terms are used in some veterinary practices and in academia, no state law recognizes a distinction between the graduate of a 2-, 3-, or 4-year AVMA-accredited program. In all states that license technicians, all graduates of AVMA-accredited veterinary technology programs are eligible to sit for the national licensure examination, the Veterinary Technician National Examination (VTNE), and upon passing the examination, are eligible for licensure as a veterinary technician. For an example of an application for licensure, see the Evolve site at http://evolve.elsevier.com/McCurnin/vettech/.

Veterinary Assistant

"Veterinary assistant," "animal assistant," and "caretaker" are some of the titles given to individuals who work in veterinary hospitals but are not licensed to practice veterinary technology in their state. Some states have, through regulations promulgated by the state board, set forth a scope of practice for veterinary assistants. Veterinary assistants are usually not permitted to perform all of the functions of a veterinary technician and often must have a higher level of supervision by a veterinarian when performing functions in the hospital.

ENTRY INTO PRACTICE

LICENSES, CERTIFICATES, AND REGISTRATIONS

The state organization charged with the responsibility of regulating the practice of the profession and the conduct of licensed professionals is called the state board. Because the practice of veterinary technology is regulated by each state, there is some variety in the terminology used to designate an individual that the state board has authorized to practice. This area can seem confusing because one state may issue a license, whereas another may issue a certificate. The grant of a license by a state board implies that the board has reviewed and approved the qualifications of the individual to practice (Figure 2-1). The grant of a certificate implies that some other entity has reviewed and approved the qualifications of the individual to practice and has certified that the person is competent to practice. However, some states issue a license but call a technician certified (e.g., in Pennsylvania, technicians' qualifications are reviewed by the board, and the board issues a license bestowing the title "Certified Veterinary Technician"). Some states "register," rather than license, technicians. The term registered implies that neither the state board nor an independent entity has reviewed and approved the qualifications of the technician to practice; however, to lawfully practice veterinary technology, the individual must register and provide information to the state board. Some state boards that refer to registration actually do review and approve the qualifications of technicians. A technician should check with their state's board before

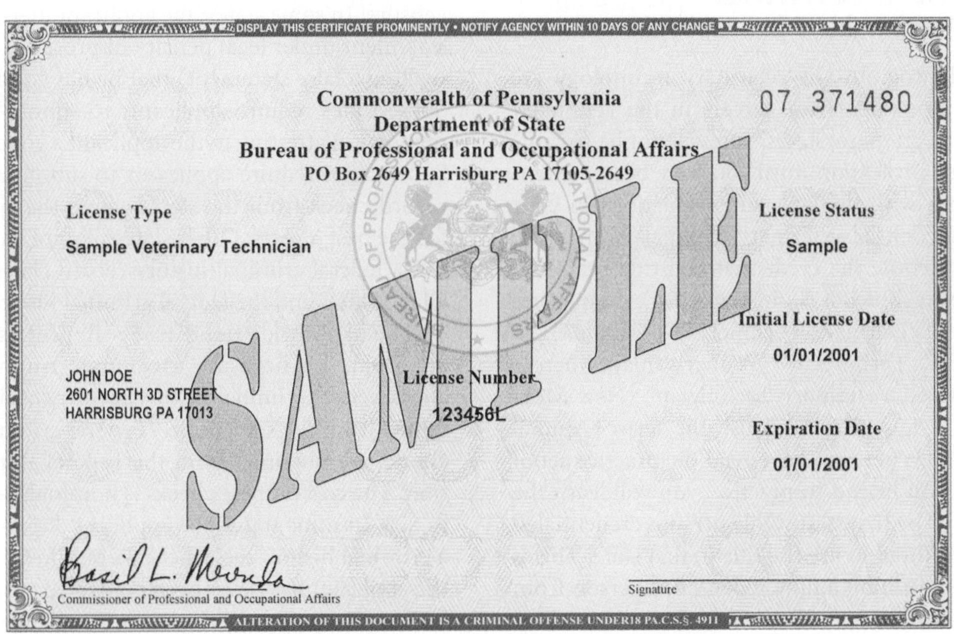

DISPLAY THIS CERTIFICATE PROMINENTLY • NOTIFY AGENCY WITHIN 10 DAYS OF ANY CHANGE

07 371480

Commonwealth of Pennsylvania
Department of State
Bureau of Professional and Occupational Affairs
PO Box 2649 Harrisburg PA 17105-2649

License Type
Sample Veterinary Technician

License Status
Sample

Initial License Date
01/01/2001

JOHN DOE
2601 NORTH 3D STREET
HARRISBURG PA 17013

License Number
123456L

Expiration Date
01/01/2001

SAMPLE

Commissioner of Professional and Occupational Affairs

Signature

ALTERATION OF THIS DOCUMENT IS A CRIMINAL OFFENSE UNDER 18 PA.C.S.S. 4911

FIGURE 2-1 Sample of a license to practice veterinary technology from the state of Pennsylvania.

BOX 2-5 Credentialling by State

States Boards That License Veterinary Technicians:
Alabama, Alaska, California, Delaware, Georgia, Illinois, Indiana, Iowa, Kansas, Kentucky, Michigan, Missouri, Nebraska, Nevada, New Jersey, New York, North Carolina, North Dakota, Ohio, Oklahoma, Pennsylvania, South Carolina, South Dakota, Tennessee, Texas, Virginia, West Virginia, Washington, Wisconsin, Wyoming
State Boards That Offer Certification, but Do Not Require It:
Arizona, Arkansas, Colorado, Idaho, Louisiana, Maine, Maryland, Minnesota, New Mexico, Oregon
States Boards That Do Not License or Certify Veterinary Technicians: (Registration may be available through private organizations.)
Connecticut, Florida, Hawaii, Massachusetts, Mississippi, Montana, New Hampshire, Rhode Island, Utah, Vermont

beginning practice to ensure that the technician has obtained the proper authorization to practice.

The terminology used in the state in which you plan to practice is not as important as the distinction made between a person who has been authorized by the state to practice and one who has not been authorized by the state to practice. In most states, only a person who has been issued some credential by a state may perform the functions that the state defines as the practice of veterinary technology. In this chapter, the term "license" will be used to denote the authorization to practice conferred by a state board, and the term "licensed veterinary technician" will be used to denote an individual whose qualifications to practice have been reviewed and approved by a state board (Box 2-5).

OBTAINING THE CREDENTIALS THAT AUTHORIZE YOU TO PRACTICE

AVMA-accredited programs of veterinary technology are designed to prepare students for careers in the veterinary health care industry. In many states, you will not be permitted to practice your profession until you have been credentialed in accordance with the laws and regulations in your state. States that credential veterinary technicians may use different terms to denote the credential and title bestowed upon the veterinary technician. Some states, for example, use the term "Licensed Veterinary Technician" (Alabama), or "Certified Veterinary Technician" (Pennsylvania), whereas others use "Registered Veterinary Technician" (New Mexico). In addition, a few states still use the term "Animal Health Technician." When you have read the practice act of the state in which you intend to practice, you will learn the title that is conferred by that state. Only persons credentialed by the state are permitted to use the title in that state. This is because most states prohibit a noncredentialed person from "holding himself out" as a credentialed veterinary technician, even if that person has completed the same amount of education and has successfully completed the VTNE. In other words, to be a credentialed veterinary technician, you must submit the appropriate paperwork required by the state and pay the necessary fees. Licensed veterinary technicians must complete an application for licensure, which is subsequently reviewed and approved by the state board. If this is not done, a veterinary technician cannot call herself a *LICENSED* veterinary technician, even if she is a graduate of an AVMA-accredited program and has passed the VTNE. Refer to http://evolve.elsevier.com/Bassert/McCurnin/ for an example of an application for licensure.

TECHNICIAN NOTE For more information about the VTNE, see the website for the American Association of Veterinary State Boards (AAVSB) at www.aavsb/org/TIVA. The Technician Information Verifying Agency (TIVA) is the AAVSB's service for verifying the credentials of veterinary technicians. The VTNE Candidate Information Booklet is available on the website, as is further information about fees for the examination and a list of examination locations.

Each state's practice act and/or regulations of the board set forth the qualifications for entry into the practice of veterinary technology. In most states, these qualifications include successful completion of an AVMA-accredited program of veterinary technology and the VTNE. In addition, many states require that applicants demonstrate good moral character.

GOOD MORAL CHARACTER AND CRIMINAL CONVICTIONS

States vary widely in how the board determines whether an applicant possesses the good moral character required for licensure. In some states, the applicant merely verifies (signs a statement under legal penalty of prosecution for perjury, or making a false statement) that he has good moral character. Some states require applicants to submit letters of recommendation attesting to the applicant's good moral character. Some states require applicants to submit a criminal history record check from the states where the applicant has lived for the past 5 years. Other states require an applicant to submit a federal criminal history record check, which includes all the states and the federal criminal justice system.

The nationwide trend across all professions is to require applicants for licensure to submit criminal history record checks. State criminal history record checks are usually obtained from the state police. Federal criminal history record checks are obtained from the Federal Bureau of Investigation. The cost of these checks is nominal, usually around $10 to $25. In some states, the applicant does not have to submit a criminal history record check, but does have to verify that the applicant has never been convicted of a crime.

Remember that citations for "underage drinking," "disorderly conduct," and driving while under the influence of alcohol or driving while intoxicated (DUI or DWI) are crimes that must be reported on your application for licensure. Generally, traffic offenses, such as "speeding" or "failure to yield," do not need to be reported. Read the application carefully and err on the side of reporting any criminal convictions you believe you may have. If the board does not have the authority to refuse to issue a license based on the crime you have committed, the board will disregard the information.

How does a board view an applicant with a criminal record? To some extent, the answer to this question varies from state to state. Some states have absolute bars to licensure, meaning that if a person has been convicted of certain crimes, they may not be issued a license. It is rare to find a state that has an absolute lifetime bar to licensure regardless of the crime that the applicant has committed; to do so would be contrary to the theory that a person who has committed a crime can be rehabilitated. It is not unusual, however, to see 5- and 10-year bars to licensure. For example, in some states, a person who has been convicted of a felony-level criminal offense involving drugs may be barred from licensure for 10 years. In other states, a person who has been convicted of any violent crime may be barred from licensure for 5 years.

> TECHNICIAN NOTE Report any criminal convictions to the board when you apply for a license, even if you do not think it is a reason for the board to refuse to issue you a license. The board will be able to determine whether the conviction prohibits you from licensure.

State boards may use an applicant's criminal convictions to support the board's finding that the applicant does not have good moral character and may then refuse to bestow licensure. The most common criminal convictions that lead boards to refuse to license an applicant are convictions involving ***crimes of moral turpitude.*** A crime of moral turpitude is a crime that involves dishonesty or deception, a crime that evidences immorality or depravity, or a crime that involves interference with justice. All theft offenses, such as shoplifting, theft by unlawful taking, theft by deception, and embezzlement and false swearing, are considered crimes of moral turpitude because they involve dishonesty. Crimes such as forgery and writing bad checks are considered crimes of moral turpitude because they involve dishonesty. ***Crimes of depravity*** include murder, rape, and distribution of drugs, but also include misdemeanor offenses, such as stalking, harassment, and assault. Crimes that involve ***interference with justice*** include eluding a police officer or interference with the conduct of a criminal investigation.

If you have a criminal conviction in your background, you should read the practice act and regulations of the board in the state in which you plan to practice to determine whether the conviction will bar you from being licensed in that state. Remember that not all criminal convictions bar licensure; in many cases, the board may exercise its discretion to determine whether a particular individual should be granted a license. When faced with a decision on whether or not to license a person who has a criminal conviction in their background, the board will seek to determine whether the person is rehabilitated (unlikely to commit further criminal offenses). Positive indications of rehabilitation include no additional criminal convictions, steady work history, admission of responsibility for the crime, and positive outlook toward the future. Check with your veterinary technician program advisor and with the legal counsel to the board in the state in which you wish to practice to determine the impact a criminal conviction may have on your ability to obtain licensure.

If you have a criminal history, you must report it to the board at the time you apply for licensure. Do not make the mistake of thinking that the board will not find out about your conviction. Should the board discover the conviction after you have been issued a license, your license will be subject to discipline not only on the basis of the conviction, but on the further grounds of committing fraud or deceit in the application for licensure. The latter is considered a serious offense that most likely will lead to the denial of your application for licensure. It is much better to deal with your past head-on than to try to hide it.

Other information commonly required on an application for licensure includes whether the applicant has held any other professional license in any state, whether the applicant has ever had a license disciplined by a state, and whether the applicant is now or has ever been addicted to alcohol or drugs. In most states, the simple fact that a person has held a professional license that has been subject to discipline is a legal ground to deny the application for licensure. However, all state boards view applications on a case-by-case basis, so prior disciplinary history will not necessarily be a bar to licensure. A veterinary technician in one state who had his or her license revoked for stealing drugs from the practice will not likely be granted a veterinary technician license in another state. A nurse who abused patients may not be granted a license to practice veterinary technology. A notary public who failed to complete continuing education required for his or her licensure renewal is likely to be granted a license to practice veterinary technology. In any case, a state board will be looking at the information provided by the applicant with the goal of determining whether granting the applicant a license will put the citizens of the state at risk.

IMPAIRED PROFESSIONALS

For persons who currently have or have previously had addiction or impairment issues, many states offer treatment and monitoring programs that allow professionals to continue practicing while receiving treatment and while being monitored. In many cases, these treatment and monitoring programs are confidential. Some states limit the admission of persons into a confidential treatment and monitoring program to those individuals who have not been convicted of a crime related to their impairment. DUI may not be considered a crime that would preclude an individual from participating in a confidential program; however, distribution of narcotics is a crime that is likely to preclude an individual from a confidential program. Most states also have "public" treatment and monitoring programs. To say that a treatment and monitoring program is public means that the individual's license will be placed on probationary status until the person has completed the requirements of the program. Any member of the public may find out that a professional licensee is on probation. In some states, a member of the public may even read the board's written decisions in disciplinary cases directly from the board's website.

> TECHNICIAN NOTE It is your responsibility to renew your license whether or not you receive notice from the licensing board that your license is about to expire.

MAINTAINING YOUR LICENSE IN GOOD STANDING

Every state that issues a license to practice veterinary technology requires that the license be renewed. The length of time that a license is valid varies from state to state; some states require annual renewal, others require biennial or triennial renewal. In most states, you will be able to renew your license online. Online renewal is faster and more cost-effective.

To renew your license, you will be required to fill out a renewal application and pay a renewal fee. Refer to http://evolve.elsevier.com/Bassert/McCurnin/ for an example of an application for license renewal. Although renewal applications vary from state to state, the common theme of renewal applications is to determine whether the licensee remains fit to hold the license. Therefore common questions on renewal applications will require you to inform the board if you are licensed in any other state, if you have had any disciplinary action taken by your own state board or any other state board, if you have any criminal charges pending, or if you have been convicted of any crime. The state is asking these questions to determine if you are suitable for continued licensure.

Some states (e.g., New Mexico) require veterinary technicians to annually register with the state board and inform the board of their employment. In addition, a technician may be required to inform the board whenever the technician changes employment to another veterinarian.

Most states require professional licensees, including veterinary technicians, to complete continuing education to renew their licenses. The number of hours of continuing education required for licensure renewal varies from state to state. Be sure to check with the board in the state in which you intend to practice for detailed information about the state's continuing education requirements.

State requirements as to the type of activities that can be used to fulfill the continuing education requirement also vary. A common scheme used by many states is to have a list of continuing education providers who offer continuing education programs that are acceptable in the state. For example, many states consider all continuing education programs offered by the state's schools of veterinary technology, all programs offered by the AVMA or state veterinary medical association, all programs offered by NAVTA or state technician association, and all programs approved by the Registry of Continuing Education (RACE) of the AAVSB to be acceptable. This approval list will encompass most of the large national veterinary medical conferences, such as the Western States Veterinary Conference and the Atlantic Coast Veterinary Conference. Some states limit the number of continuing education hours that may be earned from "distance learning" sources, which usually include Internet-based courses, teleconferences, and journal articles with test questions that are mailed to the journal's publisher.

> TECHNICIAN NOTE Be sure to check your state board's regulations to ensure that the continuing education courses you plan to take will be counted toward the continuing education requirement for licensure renewal.

Many states also permit technicians to obtain board approval for other educational activities so that these activities may count toward meeting the continuing education requirement for licensure renewal. Board approval for a nontraditional educational activity must be obtained in advance of the end of the renewal period. This can be an excellent way to earn continuing education credits. For example, many larger veterinary hospitals offer in-house lunch-and-learn programs for their veterinarians and veterinary technicians. Conducting research on a topic of particular interest and writing an article for a peer-reviewed journal may also be used to meet the continuing education requirement in many states. Attendance at conferences sponsored by specialty organizations, such as homeopathic veterinary medicine or animal behavior, may also be approved by a state board. A state board will approve an educational program for credit when it appears that the program will enhance the technician's knowledge and skills and advance the practice of veterinary technology. If you have an interest in a specialized field of study, be sure to work with your state board if you would like to have your educational activities in the field credited for meeting the state's continuing education requirement.

> TECHNICIAN NOTE Careful planning of your continuing education will allow you to demonstrate expertise in a subject area of particular interest and may further your employment prospects.

DISCIPLINARY ACTION

The grounds for which a state licensing board may discipline a veterinary technician's license will vary from state to state; however, all states permit a board to discipline a licensee for certain core reasons. The two most important grounds for discipline for purposes of this chapter are practicing beyond the scope of the license granted by the state and negligence (or malpractice) in carrying out the duties of the license. Licensing boards are composed of members of the profession; veterinary licensing boards generally consist of five to seven veterinarians, one or two veterinary technicians, and one or two members of the public. Because licensing boards are composed of members who practice the profession that they are regulating, the laws that authorize these boards give them broad discretion to determine whether a licensee has committed a violation of the practice act and to determine the appropriate disciplinary sanction that should be imposed on the licensee. Although sanctions may vary slightly from state to state, the most common disciplinary sanctions that may be imposed by a board include revocation, suspension, probation, reprimand, and civil penalty.

PROCEDURE IN DISCIPLINARY MATTERS

The fifth amendment of the United States Constitution provides that a person may not be deprived of life, liberty, or property without due process of law. The United States Supreme Court has determined that individuals have a constitutionally protected property interest in a professional license. Thus when a licensing board asserts that an individual is subject to the discipline of the individual's license (through revocation or suspension), the licensing board is threatening to deprive the licensee of property and may only do so if the board provides the licensee with appropriate due process protections. State constitutions also protect an individual's professional license as property. Because there is a property interest in a professional license, a board may not discipline the licensee without providing the licensee with due process of law. What process is due may vary slightly depending on how the courts have interpreted the different aspects of due process protection in various contexts and in different jurisdictions. But the core concepts of due process are the same everywhere: due process requires notice and an opportunity to be heard.

> *TECHNICIAN NOTE* The legal procedure used to conduct a disciplinary hearing is designed to provide the board with all the facts needed to reach a fair decision.

NOTICE

Notice means that the authority considering "taking" a person's property, in this case by disciplining the person's professional license, must notify the licensee of the reasons that the authority is considering disciplinary action. This notice is provided in writing and sets forth specific factual allegations. For example, a state may allege that a technician is subject to discipline under the practice act because the technician has been convicted of a crime, and a particular section of the practice act gives the board the authority to take disciplinary action against licensees who have been convicted of certain crimes. The notice is usually sent by certified mail, return receipt requested, but may also be sent by first class mail. In some cases, a board will have the notice delivered to the accused licensee by personal service (i.e., hand delivery). If the board cannot locate the licensee because the licensee has moved and has not notified the board of the licensee's forwarding address, notice may be accomplished by publishing an announcement in a publication of legal record within the state. (This publication is generally the same publication in which a board publishes notice of new regulations governing the practice of the profession.)

In addition to setting forth the factual allegations that give rise to the action against the licensee, the notice will also inform the licensee that he or she has a right to a hearing to defend himself or herself against the allegations and tell his or her side of the story. The hearing may be held before an administrative law judge or hearing officer or may be held before one or more members of the licensing board.

The licensee is not required to be represented by an attorney at a disciplinary hearing before a licensing authority. There is no "right" to an attorney in disciplinary matters, as there is in criminal matters; therefore the state will not appoint (and pay for) an attorney to represent you if you cannot afford legal representation, a concept you are likely familiar with from television shows depicting the criminal legal process. However, an attorney is likely to tell you that you should have an attorney to represent you because the disciplinary action before the board is a legal proceeding and attorneys have expertise in the law. The administrative law judge or hearing officer will often assist an unrepresented licensee in the technical aspects of presenting their evidence. Although it is not necessary to retain legal counsel, it is advisable.

OPPORTUNITY TO BE HEARD

The opportunity to be heard requires that a licensing authority hold a hearing so that the licensee can present evidence and provide responses to the allegations. Hearings are matters of public record, which means that the public may come to a hearing or may obtain a transcript of the hearing. In lieu of a hearing on the alleged violations of the practice act, the state's attorney may offer the licensee a settlement (or consent) agreement. Settlement agreements are documents wherein the licensee admits that he violated the practice act and agrees to a sanction set forth in the agreement. In some cases, more lenient sanctions are offered if the licensee will agree to settle the matter through agreement because this resolution of a case saves the state time and money by not requiring the formal presentation of evidence at a hearing. The state board must approve the agreement before it is considered final.

> *TECHNICIAN NOTE* The board needs to know the technician's decision-making process to determine whether the imposition of a disciplinary sanction is necessary and to determine the proper sanction to impose.

AT A HEARING

A hearing generally begins with an announcement of the time and location that the hearing is being held and an introduction of the officials present. There will generally be a presiding officer, whether an administrative law judge or hearing officer. A prosecuting attorney who works for the state will represent the state (the state's attorney). The licensee may have legal counsel or may proceed without legal counsel. The state's attorney will proceed first because it bears the responsibility for demonstrating that the licensee has committed a violation of the law or regulations. She may call witnesses, including the licensee, and may present documents. The licensee, in turn, may question the state's witnesses. Following the presentation of the state's case, the licensee will have an opportunity to call witnesses and produce documents. The state's attorney may question the licensee's witnesses. The hearing officer or any board member may also question any witness. The hearing usually concludes with closing arguments. Each side makes a statement about what they believe the evidence introduced at the hearing has shown and whether or not they believe the licensee has violated the licensing law or regulations. The state's attorney and the licensee may also make recommendations regarding the disciplinary sanction, if any, that they believe should be imposed. Following the hearing, the parties are generally given an opportunity to file a written argument regarding what they believe the evidence has shown. The board will issue a written opinion at a later date, generally anywhere from 2 months to a year after the hearing. The written opinion issued by the board will set forth what the board believes happened and whether the licensee is subject to discipline. If the board finds that the licensee is subject to discipline, the written opinion will include an order setting forth the disciplinary sanction imposed by the board.

DISCIPLINARY SANCTIONS THAT MAY BE IMPOSED BY A BOARD

Revocation

Revocation of a license is considered the most severe sanction that a board may impose. In some states, revocation is the permanent preclusion of an individual from the practice of a profession. In other states, an individual may apply for relicensure after 5 or 10 years. To be relicensed, the individual must demonstrate all the qualifications for licensure, including good moral character. To demonstrate good moral character, an applicant for relicensure must demonstrate both that the applicant has rehabilitated himself and that the grant of relicensure will not create an unacceptable risk of harm to the public. In addition, because following revocation the individual's application is considered anew, the individual must meet all other qualifications for licensure, including retaking the licensure examination.

Suspension

Suspension is also considered a severe sanction that may be imposed by a board because a suspension prohibits the sanctioned individual from practicing the profession. A suspension may be imposed for an indefinite period of time, with the suspension lifted when the licensee has completed specific tasks assigned by the board. For example, in a disciplinary case where the board found that the technician exceeded the scope of practice of the profession, the board might require the technician to complete continuing education in the role of a veterinary technician and a continuing education course in the state's law governing veterinary technicians. A license suspension may also be for a definite period of time (e.g., 6 months). When the sanctioned technician is permitted to return to practice, the board may further limit the technician by means of terms of probation.

Probation

A licensing board may place a licensee on probation. A licensee who is on probationary status with the board is permitted to practice the profession; however, boards generally place limits on the practice of an individual who is on probation. Limits may include ongoing continuing education, practicing under a higher level of supervision, or restriction from performing specific tasks. For example, a technician who made an error in administering an anesthetic may be required to observe the administration of an anesthetic during 10 surgical procedures and then be directly monitored by another technician for 10 surgical procedures before being able to resume normal practice.

Reprimand

A reprimand is a public censure of a licensee without attendant suspension or probation. This sanction is generally reserved for matters that are more serious than a violation warranting only a civil penalty or for repeated violations that warrant more than a civil penalty.

Civil Penalty

A civil penalty is a fine paid to the licensing board. Civil penalties are often levied in addition to a suspension of a license. Virtually every state has statutory limits on the amount of the civil penalty that may be imposed for a violation of the state's licensing laws. Although this varies from state to state, common caps are at $1000 (Pennsylvania), $5000 dollars (Illinois), and $10,000 (Connecticut) per violation. Some boards permit licensees who have been sanctioned with a civil penalty to make installment payments on the penalty.

GROUNDS FOR DISCIPLINARY ACTION BY A BOARD

The grounds for which a board may discipline a licensee (or refuse to grant an application to an applicant for licensure) are set forth in the state practice act. Additional grounds for discipline may also be set forth in the state board's regulations. Some violations of the practice act are spoken of as ***technical violations.*** The so-called technical violations include practicing on a lapsed license, failing to complete mandatory continuing education, a criminal conviction that is not related to the practice of the profession, or discipline by another state's licensing board. These violations are considered technical violations because there is no direct link between the licensee's misconduct and harm to an animal. It is important to note that in virtually every state, a licensee may be prosecuted and disciplined for misconduct, even if the licensee's misconduct did not cause any harm to an animal.

The so-called substantive violations of the practice act and regulations are violations that bear directly on the licensee's conduct in practicing the profession. Common grounds for discipline include unprofessional conduct, malpractice, incompetence, deviation from the standards of acceptable and prevailing practice, practicing beyond the scope of practice authorized in the state, violating any rules of the board or any rules set forth in the practice act, engaging in acts of moral turpitude, fraud or deceit in the practice of the profession or entry into the practice of the profession, misrepresentation, animal abuse, animal neglect or animal cruelty, engaging in any act that is illegal related to the profession, aiding another person to violate the practice act, impairment by reason of addiction to drugs or alcohol or by mental disease that prevents safe practice, and a criminal conviction.

> *TECHNICIAN NOTE* The board may only discipline a licensee for conduct charged in the formal prosecution document.

A licensee may be prosecuted and disciplined for violating any rule of the board or any rule set forth in the practice act that is not otherwise specifically mentioned in the enumerated grounds for discipline. Examples of misconduct that might be prosecuted and disciplined under a section such as this include: failing to properly display a professional license and holding oneself out as a specialist without having the proper credentials to use the title.

A licensee may be prosecuted and disciplined for committing fraud or deceit in the practice of the profession or entry into the practice of the profession. This includes falsifying information submitted on an application for licensure, omitting requested information on an application, and cheating on the licensure examination. It also includes conduct such as falsifying a health certificate or other document and signing a form for the veterinarian that the veterinarian is required to sign. Finally, violations under this section may include fraudulent or deceitful conduct related to the client, such as charging for services not performed, and may include fraudulent or deceitful conduct related to the technician's employer, such as stealing from the practice.

In some states, a licensee may be prosecuted and disciplined for engaging in acts of moral turpitude and engaging in immoral conduct. Because "moral turpitude" is a well-defined term in criminal law, a licensing board will usually look to the criminal law in its state to determine what conduct by a licensee involves moral turpitude. (Refer to the earlier discussion regarding disclosing your criminal history on the application for licensure for additional information on crimes involving moral turpitude.) In addition to being authorized to discipline a licensee who has been convicted of a crime of moral turpitude, a licensing board may have the authority to discipline a licensee for engaging in acts of moral turpitude, even if the licensee was not convicted of a crime related to the conduct. Some state practice acts include a definition of immoral conduct, some reference criminal statutes for the definition of immoral conduct, and some do not specify what kind of conduct is considered immoral conduct.

> *TECHNICIAN NOTE* If a client asks you for medical advice, you must refer the client to the veterinarian. Technicians may not diagnose or give a prognosis.

A licensee may be prosecuted and disciplined for misrepresentation. Misrepresentation is saying something that is not accurate. Telling a client that you are a specialist when you do not hold the state-recognized credentials that entitle you to call yourself a specialist is one example of misrepresentation. Telling a client that a certain treatment will cure a patient is also misrepresentation because virtually nothing in medicine is an absolute certainty and a technician may not give a prognosis. However, it is not a violation to say:

> "From the sample that we were able to obtain from your pet, it appears that your pet is suffering from a particular kind of infection. The medication that the veterinarian prescribed for your pet usually takes care of this type of infection. It is important that you follow the veterinarian's instructions on how to give the medication and that you bring your pet back for the veterinarian to examine at the time the veterinarian requested, so that the veterinarian can check your pet and determine whether the treatment has worked in your pet's case. If you have any problems or notice any changes, especially these particular warning signs, be sure to call us and we'll get your pet in for a re-check right away."

A licensee may be prosecuted and disciplined for animal abuse, animal neglect, or animal cruelty. States vary on whether the abuse, neglect, or cruelty applies to any animal or only animals that are under the care of the technician. In some states, the board considers abuse, neglect, or cruelty to be a deviation from the standards of acceptable and prevailing practice, rather than a separate offense.

A licensee may be prosecuted and disciplined for engaging in an illegal act that is related to the profession. For example, a licensee who provides a performance-enhancing drug to a competition animal could be prosecuted for engaging in an illegal act related to the profession. The "related to the profession" prong may be met by the technician's knowledge that a drug enhances performance, by the technician's access to the drug, or by the relationship of the profession or offense to animal care.

A licensee may be prosecuted and disciplined for aiding another person to violate the practice act. If you were to give unauthorized assistance to another person in taking the licensing examination, you would be guilty of aiding another person to violate the practice act. The most common example of this misconduct occurs when an unlicensed person is working in a veterinary practice and the licensed persons in the practice know, or even instruct, the unlicensed person to perform acts that only licensed persons are allowed to perform. This situation occurs fairly often when veterinarians who are licensed to practice in another country come to the United States and become employed as noncredentialed veterinary assistants. It may take a year or longer for them to become licensed veterinarians in the United States. However, because they may have been practicing veterinary medicine outside the United States for a number of years, they may appear to be competent to perform a wide variety of tasks within a hospital. It is important to remember that unlicensed, noncredentialed individuals are limited to performing only those tasks that the statute and board regulations authorize, regardless of the knowledge or skill level of the individual. Any licensed person who assists an unlicensed person in performing tasks that the statute includes as the practice of the profession may be aiding unlicensed practice.

Licensees may be prosecuted and disciplined for an impairment from the addiction to drugs or alcohol or by mental disease. This in turn prevents them from practicing competently and safely. Most states require licensees to report to the board any other licensee that they believe is impaired and unable to practice safely. As noted earlier in this chapter, state licensing boards may permit a licensee to continue to practice while the licensee is being treated for the impairment. The licensee must practice under supervision and must actively participate in treatment. In addition, the licensee must submit random observed urine samples that are tested for drugs of abuse, including alcohol.

> *TECHNICIAN NOTE* The most common reason that a technician is disciplined by a licensing board is that the technician has exceeded the scope of practice authorized by law.

Practicing Beyond the Scope of Practice Authorized by Licensure

A licensee may be prosecuted and disciplined for practicing beyond the scope of practice authorized in the state. This violation is considered among the most serious misconduct that may be committed by a licensee because it demonstrates either a fundamental misunderstanding of the role of the licensee or a deliberate disregard for the role of the licensee.

Most states prohibit veterinary technicians from performing surgery, diagnosing an animal's ailment, attesting to an animal's health status, offering a prognosis for the animal, and prescribing treatments or drugs. In addition, states often limit the practice of veterinary technicians in specific areas, such as the administration of an anesthetic, by requiring that the technician practice only when supervised by a veterinarian. The level of supervision required for a technician to be authorized to perform any particular task is generally set forth in the regulations of the state board.

There are a wide variety of state regulations on the authorized scope of practice of veterinary technicians, especially in particular areas. One such area that has recently undergone intense scrutiny by licensing boards nationwide is the appropriate scope of practice for technicians performing dental procedures. States range from permitting technicians to perform only cleaning and polishing without subgingival scaling to permitting technicians to perform certain types of extractions. Massachusetts permits a veterinary technician to clean and polish teeth under direct veterinary supervision. Georgia permits a veterinary technician under the direct supervision of a veterinarian to remove calculus, soft deposits, polish stains, smooth and file teeth, and perform dental extractions that do not require sectioning of the tooth or resectioning bone.

At a hearing before a licensing board where the allegation against the licensee is that the licensee practiced beyond the authorized scope of practice, the board will attempt to discern whether the licensee committed the violation because the licensee did not understand the proper role of a technician or because the licensee disregarded the proper role. If the latter is found, the board will further attempt to discern the licensee's rationale for the misconduct. The board's findings on these key issues will determine the degree of culpability (guilt) of the licensee, which, in turn, will influence the disciplinary sanction imposed by the board.

If the technician is found to have deliberately practiced beyond the scope of practice authorized by the state, it is likely that the sanction imposed will be severe. The theory behind imposing a severe sanction, such as revocation or suspension of a license, is that the public can only be protected by prohibiting the individual from practicing. If, on the other hand, the board determines that the technician did not understand his role in the delivery of veterinary health care, the board is more likely to impose a sanction that seeks to educate the technician about the proper role of a technician and impose a probationary period during which the technician must practice under more intense monitoring and supervision to ensure that the technician does not err again.

> *TECHNICIAN NOTE* A technician must know what tasks the technician is permitted to perform under the state's licensing law and regulations.

Unprofessional Conduct, Malpractice, Incompetence

A licensee may be prosecuted and disciplined for unprofessional conduct. Unprofessional conduct usually refers to conduct that disparages the profession in the eyes of the public.

A licensee may also be prosecuted and disciplined for malpractice (also called negligence). Malpractice refers to the deviation from or failure to conform to the acceptable standards of practice. Licensing law borrows the concept of a "tort" from civil law; in civil law, a tort is a wrong or injury for which a court will provide a remedy. The usual remedy in a tort action is the award of monetary damages. For a person to recover damages for the infliction of a negligent tort, the person must prove the existence of a legal duty owed to the person by another, the other's breach of the duty, a causal relationship between the breach and the person's injury, and damages suffered by the person. In the laws governing professionals (unlike in civil lawsuits), the state's prosecuting attorney need only establish a duty to the patient and a breach of the duty by the licensed practitioner. The patient does not have to suffer any injury for the professional to be disciplined for malpractice. An additional difference is that a state board does not award monetary damages to the animal's owner; the state board's authority is limited to imposing disciplinary sanctions on the professional.

Finally a licensee may be prosecuted and disciplined for incompetence. Incompetence is conduct that increases the risk that negligence will occur, even if negligence has not yet actually occurred. For example, sloppy laboratory practices, incomplete record keeping, or improper sanitation may demonstrate incompetence because they increase the risk that something could go wrong. For example, sloppy laboratory practices increase the risk of tainted samples and misdiagnoses; incomplete record keeping increases the risk for an animal to be given the wrong medication; and improper sanitation increases the risk that animals (or humans) may be inflicted with a virus or infection.

A veterinary technician should be able to identify the substances in a veterinary office that are hazardous and should know how to properly handle these substances. Refer to Chapter 6 for more information about hazards in the workplace. A veterinary technician should know how to properly handle and dispose of infectious waste, sharps, and other medical waste. Safety for the animals, clients, and employees of a veterinary hospital must always be made a priority of every staff member.

Responsibility for Actions

As a credentialed professional, a veterinary technician is responsible for his or her conduct. Because a technician is employed by and acts under the supervision and direction of a veterinarian, the veterinarian is also responsible for the conduct of the technician. For this reason, as a general rule, whenever a veterinary technician is disciplined by a licensing board for exceeding the technician's authorized scope of practice, incompetence, or negligence or malpractice, the veterinarian responsible for supervising the technician may also be disciplined by the board.

ETHICS

Ethics is defined as:

"(a) the discipline concerning what is good and bad or right and wrong or with moral duty and obligation; (b) a group of moral principles or set of values; (c) the principles of conduct governing an individual or a profession; (d) standards of behavior." (From *Webster's Third New International Dictionary,* unabridged, 1971, G & C Merriam.)

How does one determine what is good and what is bad and what is right and what is wrong? Is the technician's primary concern the animal, the client, or the employer?

When asking these questions in the context of ethics for the veterinary technician, it is important to start with the law and regulations that govern the practice of veterinary technology. As discussed earlier, these rules may vary from state to state, so every veterinary technician must understand the rules that govern the practice in the state in which the technician plans to practice. When reading the veterinary medical practice act and rules of the board, remember that the overriding purpose of the board is to protect the public—you are likely to find the rules easier to understand if you remember the purpose of the rules. Also remember that you are required to follow the law.

Veterinary technicians should also consider the rules or guidelines set forth by the profession of veterinary technology (professional ethics). These guidelines are often set forth as goals, rather than mandates. However, because neither the legislature nor the board can anticipate every situation that will arise in practice, the ethical guidelines of a professional organization, such as NAVTA, will often be of assistance to the technician when faced with situations where there is no clear answer in the rules of the board. Refer to Box 2-6 for NAVTA's veterinary technician code of ethics.

Finally the technician must consider his or her own personal ethics. In cases when the technician's personal ethics conflict with the mandates of the law or regulations of the board or with the guidelines set forth by NAVTA, the best course of action may be for the technician to withdraw from the case (Box 2-7).

If a particular course of conduct is required or prohibited by the practice act and regulations of the state board, a technician cannot act contrary to the act and regulations without facing disciplinary sanction by the technician's state board. Sometimes, however, the practice act and regulations will not address the question facing the technician or may be unclear. The technician may write to the state board and ask for clarification of the rules and guidance. The board should also be able to inform the technician if other laws or regulations (e.g., regulations of the state department of agriculture related to rabies disclosure) affect the particular question facing the technician. The technician may also consult model acts and regulations of organizations for additional guidance. Model acts and regulations are not mandatory. In addition, the technician may consult codes of professional ethics set forth by professional organizations, such as the AVMA and the NAVTA for guidance. Finally the technician will need to determine if acting or not acting in a certain manner will conflict with the technician's personal ethics.

Ethical questions are often complicated in veterinary medicine because veterinarians and technicians serve not only the patient, but also the client. Conflicts may arise when the recommendations of the veterinary medical team are not adopted by the client. The veterinary medical team must work within the limits set by the client, who is often balancing the desire to provide the best care for the animal with the constraints of financial, work, and familial commitments, which may or may not be known by the veterinary medical team. It is important in such situations to remember that, in every state, the client is the owner of the animal and as such has the ultimate decision-making authority over the care provided to the animal.

BOX 2-6 NAVTA's Veterinary Technician Code of Ethics

Introduction

Every veterinary technician has the obligation to uphold the trust invested in the profession by adhering to the profession's Code of Ethics.

A code of ethics is an essential characteristic of a profession and serves three main functions:

1. A code communicates to the public and to the members of the profession the ideals of the profession.
2. A code is a general guide for professional ethical conduct.
3. A code of ethics provides standards of acceptable conduct that allow the profession to implement disciplinary procedures against those who fall below the standards.

No code can provide the answer to every ethical question faced by members of profession. They shall continue to bear responsibility for reasoned and conscientious interpretation and application of the basic ethical principles embodied in the Code to individual cases.

Ethical standards are never less than those required by law; frequently they are more stringent.

Preamble

The code of ethics is based on the supposition that the honor and dignity of the profession of veterinary technology lies in a just and reasonable code of ethics. Veterinary technicians promote and maintain good health in animals; care for diseased and injured animals; and assist in the control of diseases transmissible from animals to human. The purpose of this code of ethics is to provide guidance to the veterinary technician for carrying out professional responsibilities so as to meet the ethical obligations of the profession.

Code of Ethics

1. Veterinary technicians shall aid society and animals by providing excellent care and services for animals.
2. Veterinary technicians shall prevent and relieve the suffering of animals with competence and compassion.
3. Veterinary technicians shall remain competent through commitment to life-long learning.
4. Veterinary technicians promote public health by assisting with the control of zoonotic diseases and educating the public about these diseases.
5. Veterinary technicians shall colloborate with other members of the veterinary medical profession in efforts to ensure quality health care services for all animals.
6. Veterinary technicians shall protect confidential information provided by clients, unless required by law or to protect public health.
7. Veterinary technicians shall assume accountability for individual professional actions and judgments.
8. Veterinary technicians shall safeguard the public and the profession against individuals deficient in professional competence or ethics.
9. Veterinary technicians shall assist with efforts to ensure conditions of employment consistent with the excellent care for animals.
10. Veterinary technicians shall uphold the laws/regulations that apply to the technician's responsibilities as a member of the animal health care team.
11. Veterinary technicians shall represent their credentials or identify themselves with specialty organizations only if the designation has been awarded or earned.

Ideals

In addition to adhering to the standards listed in the Code of Ethics, veterinary technicians must also strive to attain a number of ideals. Some of these are:

- Veterinary technicians shall strive to participate in defining, upholding, and improving standards of professional practice, legislation, and education.
- Veterinary technicians shall strive to contribute to the profession's body of knowledge.
- Veterinary technicians shall strive to understand, support, and promote the human-animal bond.

BOX 2-7 Queries to Help Determine What Is a Good Course of Conduct

1. Do the practice act and the regulations of the state board require that the technician act in a certain manner or prohibit the technician from acting in a certain manner?
2. Do the ethics of the profession of veterinary medicine or veterinary technology require that the technician act in a certain manner or prohibit the technician from acting in a certain manner?
3. Do the individual technician's personal ethics require that the technician act in a certain manner or prohibit the technician from acting in a certain manner?

The most meaningful discussion of professional ethics is provided by considering examples of situations that technicians frequently encounter in practice and by applying ethical queries to help resolve the dilemmas. Later, you will find two scenarios for classroom discussion. Use the reference material available in this chapter and its appendices to assist you during your discussion of these scenarios.

CASE SCENARIOS

Scenario One. Six weeks ago you learned that you had passed the VTNE, and yesterday you received your state credentials. Today, you received a call from a busy four-veterinarian practice where you interviewed last week. They congratulate you and tell you that they have decided to hire you as a technician beginning tomorrow. On your first day at work, you are assigned to shadow Annette. Annette is introduced to you as the "head technician," and you are told that she has been working at the practice for 9 years and that she will show you how things are done in the "real world." Annette's name tag identifies her as "technician" and "behavior specialist."

Annette takes you to the back and introduces you to Beatrice, a young basset hound that was dropped off that morning to be spayed. Annette takes the dog's vital signs and listens to her heart. Annette tells you that everything is normal and that there is no need to do preoperative blood work, which will make the owner happy when she gets her bill. Annette directs you to administer preanesthetic medications to Beatrice and then carry her into the surgical room. Annette then administers IV medication to Beatrice, scrubs, clips and drapes her, and tells you to call Dr. White on his cell phone and let him know that Beatrice is ready for surgery. Dr. White is just pulling up to the hospital when he takes your call and tells you he will be right in. When Dr. White arrives, he asks Annette how everything is; Annette says everything is okay. Dr. White begins the surgery, but Beatrice loses her heartbeat and is unable to be revived. A necropsy reveals that Beatrice had a serious heart condition that should have been audible on auscultation. Do you have any legal or ethical responsibilities in this situation?

Scenario Two. You have an employment interview scheduled with a veterinarian who has been in practice for 30 years. The veterinarian had told you that he has no other employees and is looking for someone to be his "right hand." Upon entering the practice, you notice a strong odor of urine, and your feet even stick to the floor as you walk through the facility. The veterinarian does not have equipment that you have been trained on (e.g., there is no oxygen in the facility and no gas anesthesia machine).

APPENDIX A AVMA-Model Veterinary Practice Act

Section 1—Title

This act shall be known as the [name of state] Veterinary Practice Act. Except where otherwise indicated by context, in this act the present tense includes the past and future tenses and the future tense includes the present, each gender includes both genders, and the singular includes the plural, and the plural the singular.

Section 2—Definitions

When used in this act these words and phrases shall be defined as follows:

1. "Abandoned" means to forsake entirely, to neglect or refuse to provide or perform legal obligations for the care and support of an animal, or to refuse to pay for treatment or other services without an assertion of good cause. Such abandonment shall constitute the relinquishment of all rights and claims by the client to such an animal.
2. "Accredited college of veterinary medicine" means any veterinary college, school, or division of a university or college that offers the degree of Doctor of Veterinary Medicine or its equivalent and that is accredited by the Council on Education of the American Veterinary Medical Association (AVMA).
3. "Accredited program in veterinary technology" means any postsecondary educational program that is accredited by the Committee on Veterinary Technician Education and Activities of the AVMA.
4. "Animal" means any animal other than a human.
5. "Board" means the [State Board of Veterinary Medicine].
6. "Client" means the patient's owner, owner's agent, or other person responsible for the patient.
7. "Complementary, alternative, and integrative therapies" means a heterogeneous group of preventive, diagnostic, and therapeutic philosophies and practices, which at the time they are performed may differ from current scientific knowledge, or whose theoretical basis and techniques may diverge from veterinary medicine routinely taught in accredited veterinary medical colleges, or both. These therapies include, but are not limited to, veterinary acupuncture, acutherapy, and acupressure; veterinary homeopathy; veterinary manual or manipulative therapy (i.e., therapies based on techniques practiced in osteopathy, chiropractic medicine, or physical medicine and therapy); veterinary nutraceutical therapy; and veterinary phytotherapy.
8. "Consultation" means when a licensed veterinarian receives advice in person, telephonically, electronically, or by any other method of communication, from a veterinarian licensed in this or any other state or other person whose expertise, in the opinion of the licensed veterinarian, would benefit a patient. Under any circumstance, the responsibility for the welfare of the patient remains with the licensed veterinarian receiving consultation.
9. "Credentialed veterinary technician or technologist" means a veterinary technician or veterinary technologist who is validly and currently registered, certified, or licensed by the Board.
10. "Direct supervision" means a licensed veterinarian is readily available on the premises where the patient is being treated.
11. "ECFVG® certificate" means the certificate issued by the Educational Commission for Foreign Veterinary Graduates® of the AVMA indicating that the holder has demonstrated knowledge and skill equivalent to that possessed by a graduate of an accredited college of veterinary medicine.
12. "Extralabel use" means actual use or intended use of a drug in an animal in a manner that is not in accordance with the approved labeling. This includes, but is not limited to, use in species not listed in the labeling, use for indications (disease or other conditions) not listed in the labeling, use at dosage levels, frequencies, or routes of administration other than those stated in the labeling, and deviation from the labeled withdrawal time based on these different uses.
13. "Impaired veterinarian" means a veterinarian who is unable to practice veterinary medicine with reasonable skill

Continued

APPENDIX A AVMA-Model Veterinary Practice Act—cont'd

and safety because of a physical or mental disability as evidenced by a written determination from a competent authority or written consent based on clinical evidence, including deterioration of mental capacity, loss of motor skills, or abuse of drugs or alcohol of sufficient degree to diminish the person's ability to deliver competent patient care.

14. "Indirect supervision" means a veterinarian has given either written or oral instructions for treatment of the patient and is readily available by telephone or other form of communication.
15. "Informed consent" means the veterinarian has informed the client, in a manner that would be understood by a reasonable person, of the diagnostic and treatment options, risk assessment, and prognosis, and has provided the client with an estimate of the charges for veterinary services to be rendered and the client has consented to the recommended treatment.
16. "Licensed veterinarian" means a person who is validly and currently licensed to practice veterinary medicine in this state.
17. "Patient" means an animal that is examined or treated by a veterinarian.
18. "Person" means any individual, firm, partnership (general, limited, or limited liability), association, joint venture, cooperative, corporation, limited liability company, or any other group or combination acting in concert; and whether or not acting as a principal, partner, member, trustee, fiduciary, receiver, or as any other kind of legal or personal representative, or as the successor in interest, assignee, agent, factor, servant, employee, director, officer, or any other representative of such person.
19. "Practice of veterinary medicine" means:
    a. To diagnose, treat, correct, change, alleviate, or prevent animal disease, illness, pain, deformity, defect, injury, or other physical, dental, or mental conditions by any method or mode; including:
        i. the prescription, dispensing, administration, or application of any drug, medicine, biologic, apparatus, anesthetic, or other therapeutic or diagnostic substance or medical or surgical technique, or
        ii. the use of complementary, alternative, and integrative therapies, or
        iii. the use of any manual or mechanical procedure for reproductive management, or
        iv. the rendering of advice or recommendation by any means including telephonic and other electronic communications with regard to any of the above.
    b. ***To represent, directly or indirectly, publicly or privately, an ability and willingness to do an act described in subsection 19(a).***
    c. To use any title, words, abbreviation, or letters in a manner or under circumstances that induce the belief that the person using them is qualified to do any act described in subsection 19(a).
20. "Practice of veterinary technology" means:
    a. To perform patient care or other services that require a technical understanding of veterinary medicine on the basis of written or oral instruction of a veterinarian, excluding diagnosing, prognosing, surgery, or prescribing drugs, medicine, or appliances.
    b. To represent, directly or indirectly, publicly or privately, an ability and willingness to do an act described in subsection 20(a).
    c. To use any title, words, abbreviation, or letters in a manner or under circumstances that induce the belief that the person using them is qualified to do any act described in subsection 20(a).
21. "Veterinarian" means a person who has received a professional veterinary medical degree from a college of veterinary medicine.
22. "Veterinarian-client-patient relationship" means that all of the following are required:
    a. The veterinarian has assumed the responsibility for making clinical judgments regarding the health of the animal and the need for medical treatment, and the client has agreed to follow the veterinarian's instructions.
    b. The veterinarian has sufficient knowledge of the animal to initiate at least a general or preliminary diagnosis of the medical condition of the animal. This means that the veterinarian has recently seen and is personally acquainted with the keeping and care of the animal either by virtue of an examination of the animal, or by medically appropriate and timely visits to the premises where the animal is kept.
    c. The veterinarian is readily available or has arranged for emergency coverage for follow-up evaluation in the event of adverse reactions or the failure of the treatment regimen.
23. "Veterinary medicine" means all branches and specialties included within the practice of veterinary medicine.
24. "Veterinary premises" means any premises or facility where the practice of veterinary medicine occurs, including but not limited to a mobile clinic, outpatient clinic, satellite clinic, or veterinary hospital or practice, but shall not include the premises of a veterinary client, research facility, a federal military base, or an accredited college of veterinary medicine.
25. "Veterinary prescription drug" means a drug that may not be dispensed without the prescription of a veterinarian and that bears the label statement: "CAUTION: Federal law restricts this drug to use by or on the order of a licensed veterinarian."
26. "Veterinary specialist" means that a veterinarian has completed all of the requirements to become a Diplomate within an AVMA-recognized veterinary specialty organization.
27. "Veterinary technician" means a graduate of a two- or three-year accredited program in veterinary technology.
28. "Veterinary technologist" means a graduate of a four-year accredited program in veterinary technology.

APPENDIX A AVMA-Model Veterinary Practice Act—cont'd

Section 3—Board of Veterinary Medicine

1. A Board of Veterinary Medicine shall be appointed by the governor and shall consist of five licensed veterinarians, one credentialed veterinary technician or technologist, and one member of the public who is not a veterinarian or veterinary technician or technologist. All persons appointed to the Board shall have been residents of this state for at least the two years immediately preceding appointment. Each member shall be appointed for a term of five years or until a successor is appointed, except that the terms of the first appointees may be for shorter periods to permit a staggering of terms. Members of the Board appointed under the chapter that this act replaces may continue as members of the Board until the expiration of the term for which they were appointed. Vacancies due to death, resignation, or removal shall be filled for the remainder of the unexpired term in the same manner as regular appointments. No person shall serve more than two consecutive full terms.
   a. A licensed veterinarian shall be qualified to serve as a member of the Board if he has been licensed to practice veterinary medicine in this state for the five years immediately preceding the time of his appointment. A credentialed veterinary technician or technologist shall be qualified to serve as a member of the Board if he has been credentialed in this state for the five years immediately preceding his appointment.
   b. Each member of the Board shall be paid for each day or substantial portion thereof if he is engaged in the work of the Board, in addition to such reimbursement for travel and other expenses as is normally allowed to state employees.
   c. Any member of the Board may be removed in accordance with the Administrative Procedures Act of this state or other applicable laws.
2. The Board shall meet at least once each year at the time and place fixed by rule of the Board. Other necessary meetings may be called by the Board by giving notice as may be required by rule. Except as may otherwise be provided, a majority of the Board constitutes a quorum. Meetings shall be open and public except that the Board may meet in closed session to prepare, approve, administer, or grade examinations, or to deliberate the qualification of an applicant for license or the disposition of a proceeding to discipline a licensed veterinarian.
3. The Board shall annually elect officers from its membership as may be prescribed by rule. Officers of the Board serve for terms of 1 year and until a successor is elected, without limitation on the number of terms an officer may serve. The duties of officers shall be prescribed by rule.
4. The Board shall have the power to:
   a. Adopt, amend, or repeal all rules necessary for its government and all regulations necessary to carry into effect the provisions of this act, including the establishment and publication of standards of practice and professional conduct for the practice of veterinary medicine.
   b. Adopt, promulgate, and enforce rules and regulations relating to specific duties and responsibilities; certification, registration, or licensure; and other matters pertaining to veterinary technicians, veterinary technologists, or nonlicensed persons consistent with the provisions of this act.
   c. Initiate disciplinary procedures, hold hearings, reprimand, suspend, revoke, or refuse to issue or renew credentials, and perform any other acts that may be necessary to regulate veterinary technicians and technologists in a manner consistent with the provisions of this act applicable to veterinarians.
   d. Examine by established protocol the qualifications and fitness of applicants for a license to practice veterinary medicine in the state.
   e. Issue, renew, or deny the licenses and temporary permits to practice veterinary medicine in this state.
   f. Limit, suspend, or revoke the licenses of disciplined veterinarians or otherwise discipline licensed veterinarians consistent with the provisions of the act and the rules and regulations adopted thereunder.
   g. Establish and publish annually a schedule of fees for licensing, certification, and registration.
   h. Conduct investigations of suspected violations of this act to determine whether there are sufficient grounds to initiate disciplinary proceedings. All investigations shall be conducted in accordance with the Administrative Procedures Act of this state or other applicable laws.
   i. Inspect veterinary premises and equipment, including practice vehicles, at any time in accordance with protocols established by rule.
   j. Hold hearings on all matters properly brought before the Board and in connection thereto to administer oaths, receive evidence, make necessary determinations, and enter orders consistent with the findings. The Board may require by subpoena the attendance and testimony of witnesses and the production of papers, records, or other documentary evidence and commission depositions. The Board may designate one or more of its members to serve as its hearing officer or may employ a hearing officer defined by state law. All hearings shall be conducted in accordance with the Administrative Procedures Act of this state or other applicable laws.
   k. Employ full or part-time personnel necessary to effectuate the provisions of this act and purchase or rent necessary office space, equipment, and supplies.
   l. Appoint from its own membership one or more members to act as representatives of the Board at any meeting within or outside the state where such representative is deemed desirable.
   m. Bring proceedings in the courts against any person for the enforcement of this act or any regulations made pursuant thereto.
5. The powers enumerated above are granted for the purpose of enabling the Board to effectively supervise the practice

Continued

APPENDIX A AVMA-Model Veterinary Practice Act—cont'd

of veterinary medicine and veterinary technology and are to be construed liberally to accomplish this objective.

Section 4—License Requirement

No person may practice veterinary medicine in the state who is not a licensed veterinarian or the holder of a valid temporary permit issued by the Board unless otherwise exempt pursuant to Section 6 of this act.

Section 5—Veterinarian-Client-Patient Relationship Requirement

1. No person may practice veterinary medicine in the state except within the context of a veterinarian-client-patient relationship.
2. A veterinarian-client-patient relationship cannot be established solely by telephonic or other electronic means.

Section 6—Exemptions

This act shall not be construed to prohibit:

1. Any employee of the federal, state, or local government performing his official duties.
2. Any person who is a student in an accredited college of veterinary medicine or an accredited program in veterinary technology performing duties or actions assigned by instructors or working under the direct supervision of a licensed veterinarian.
3. Any person advising with respect to or performing acts that the Board has designated by rule as accepted livestock management practices.
4. Any person providing consultation to a licensed veterinarian in this state on the care and management of a patient.
5. Any member in good standing of another licensed or regulated profession within any state, or any member of an organization or group approved by the Board within the rules and regulations, providing assistance requested by a veterinarian licensed in the state, acting with informed consent from the client, and acting under the direct or indirect supervision and control of the licensed veterinarian. Providing assistance involves hands-on active participation in the treatment and care of the patient. The licensed veterinarian shall maintain responsibility for the veterinarian-client-patient relationship.
6. Any veterinarian employed by an accredited college of veterinary medicine providing assistance requested by a veterinarian licensed in the state, acting with informed consent from the client, and acting under the direct or indirect supervision and control of the licensed veterinarian. Providing assistance involves hands-on active participation in the treatment and care of the patient. The licensed veterinarian shall maintain responsibility for the veterinarian-client-patient relationship.
7. Any pharmacist, merchant, or manufacturer selling at his regular place of business medicines, feed, appliances, or other products used in the prevention or treatment of animal diseases as permitted by law.
8. Any person lawfully engaged in the art or profession of horseshoeing.
9. Any person rendering advice without expectation of compensation.
10. Any owner of an animal and any of the owner's regular employees caring for and treating the animal belonging to such owner, except where the ownership of the animal was transferred for purposes of circumventing this act. Notwithstanding the provisions of this subsection 10, a veterinarian-client-patient relationship must exist when prescription drugs or nonprescription drugs intended for extralabel use are administered, dispensed, or prescribed.
11. Any person who provides appropriate training for animals that does include diagnosing or the prescribing or dispensing of any therapeutic agent.
12. Any instructor at an accredited college of veterinary medicine or accredited program in veterinary technology performing his regular functions or any person lecturing or giving instructions or demonstrations at an accredited college of veterinary medicine or accredited program in veterinary technology or in connection with a veterinary or veterinary technology continuing education course or seminar.
13. Any person selling or applying pesticides, insecticides, or herbicides as permitted by law.
14. Any person engaging in bona fide scientific research that reasonably requires experimentation involving animals.
15. Any credentialed veterinary technician, veterinary technologist, or other employee of a licensed veterinarian performing duties other than diagnosis, prognosis, prescription, or surgery under the direction and supervision of such veterinarian who shall be responsible for the performance of the employee.
16. Any graduate of a non-accredited college of veterinary medicine who is in the process of obtaining an ECFVG® certificate and is performing duties or actions assigned by instructors in an accredited college of veterinary medicine.
17. Any person who, without expectation of compensation, provides emergency veterinary care in an emergency or disaster situation.
18. Any animal shelter employee acting under the supervision of a licensed veterinarian or authorized by the Board to perform euthanasia in the course and scope of employment.

Section 7—Veterinary Technicians and Technologists

1. No person may practice veterinary technology in the state who is not a veterinary technician or technologist credentialed by the Board.
2. A veterinary technician or technologist who performs veterinary technology contrary to this act shall be subject to disciplinary actions in a manner consistent with the provisions of this act applicable to veterinarians.
3. Credentialed veterinary technicians and technologists shall be required to complete continuing education as prescribed by rule to renew their credentials.

Section 8—Status of Persons Previously Licensed

Any person who holds a valid license to practice veterinary medicine in this state on the date this act becomes effective shall be recognized as a licensed veterinarian and shall be entitled to retain this status so long as he complies with the provisions of this act, including periodic renewal of the license.

APPENDIX A AVMA-Model Veterinary Practice Act—cont'd

Section 9—Application for License: Qualifications

1. Any person desiring a license to practice veterinary medicine in this state shall make written application to the Board. The application shall show that the applicant is a graduate of an accredited college of veterinary medicine or the holder of an ECFVG® certificate. The application shall also show that the applicant is a person of good moral character and such other information and proof as the Board may require by rule. The application shall be accompanied by a fee in the amount established and published by the Board.
2. If the Board determines that the applicant possesses the proper qualifications, it shall admit the applicant to the next examination, or if the applicant is eligible for license by endorsement under Section 11 of this act, the Board may forthwith grant him a license. If an applicant is found not qualified to take the examination or for a license by endorsement the Board shall notify the applicant in writing within 30 days of such finding and the grounds therefore. An applicant found unqualified may request a hearing on the questions of his qualifications under the procedure set forth in Section 16.

Section 10—Examinations

1. The Board shall provide for at least one examination for licensing, certification, or registration during each calendar year and may provide for such additional examinations as are necessary. The Board shall give public notice of the time and place for each examination at least 120 days in advance of the date set for the examination or in compliance with state law. A person desiring to take an examination shall make application at least 60 days before the date of the examination.
2. The preparations, administration, and grading of examinations shall be governed by rules prescribed by the Board. Examinations for veterinary licensure shall be designed to test the examinee's knowledge of and proficiency in the subjects and techniques pertaining to the practice of veterinary medicine commonly taught in an accredited college of veterinary medicine. The passing score for the examination shall be established by the testing entity. The Board may adopt and use the results of the examinations prepared by the National Board of Veterinary Medical Examiners.
3. After examination, each examinee shall be notified of the result of the examination, and the Board shall issue a certificate of registration to the new licensees. Any person who fails an examination may be admitted to any subsequent examination on payment of the application fee.

Section 11—License By Endorsement

1. The Board, in its sole discretion, may issue a license by endorsement to a qualified applicant who furnishes satisfactory proof that he is a graduate of an accredited college of veterinary medicine or holds an ECFVG® certificate. The applicant must also show that he is a person of good moral character, and:
   a. is currently licensed to practice veterinary medicine in at least one state, territory, or district of the United States and has practiced veterinary medicine in one or more of those states without disciplinary action by any state or federal agency for at least the three years immediately before filing the application, or
   b. has within the three years immediately before filing the application passed the licensing examination prepared by the National Board of Veterinary Medical Examiners.
2. The Board may, in its sole discretion, issue a limited license by endorsement to a qualified applicant who furnishes satisfactory proof that he currently holds a license to practice in at least one state, is an active diplomate in an AVMA-recognized veterinary specialty organization, and will limit his practice to his certified specialty.
3. At its sole discretion, the Board may examine any person qualifying for licensing under this Section.

Section 12—Temporary Permit

The Board, in its sole discretion, may issue a temporary permit to practice veterinary medicine in this state:

1. To a qualified applicant for license pending examination, provided that such temporary permit shall expire the day after the notice of results of the first examination given after the permit is issued and provided that the grantee is under indirect supervision of a licensed veterinarian. No temporary permit may be issued to any applicant who has previously failed the examination in this state or in any other state, territory, or district of the United States or a foreign country.
2. To a nonresident veterinarian who is a graduate of an accredited college of veterinary medicine or an ECFVG® certificate holder validly licensed in another state, territory, or district of the United States or a foreign country who pays the fee established and published by the Board, provided that such temporary permit shall be issued for a period of no more than 60 consecutive days and that no more than one permit shall be issued to a person during a calendar year. A temporary permit may be summarily revoked or limited by the Board without a hearing.

Section 13—License Renewal

1. All licenses shall expire periodically but may be renewed by registration with the Board and payment of the registration renewal fee established and published by the Board. At least 30 days in advance, the Board shall mail a notice to each licensed veterinarian that his license will expire and provide him with a form for re-registration. The Board shall issue a new certificate of registration to all persons registering under this act.
2. The Board shall establish the continuing education requirements that must be met for license renewal. The Board shall also define the types of continuing education that will meet its requirements.
3. Any person who shall practice veterinary medicine after the expiration of his license and willfully or by neglect fail to renew such license shall be practicing in violation of this act. Any person may renew an expired license within five years of the date of its expiration by making written application for renewal, paying the current renewal fee plus all delinquent renewal fees, and complying with current continuing education requirements.

Continued

APPENDIX A AVMA-Model Veterinary Practice Act—cont'd

4. The Board may by rule waive the payment of the registration renewal fee of a licensed veterinarian during the period when he is on active duty with any branch of the armed services of the United States.

Section 14—Discipline of Licensees

Upon written complaint sworn to by any person the Board, in its sole discretion, may, after a hearing, revoke, suspend, or limit for a certain time the license of, or otherwise discipline, any licensed veterinarian for any of the following reasons:

1. The employment of fraud, misrepresentation, or deception in obtaining a license.
2. The inability to practice veterinary medicine with reasonable skill and safety because of a physical or mental disability, including deterioration of mental capacity, loss of motor skills, or abuse of drugs or alcohol of sufficient degree to diminish the person's ability to deliver competent patient care.
3. The use of advertising or solicitation that is false or misleading.
4. Conviction of the following in any federal court or in the courts of this state or any other jurisdiction, regardless of whether the sentence is deferred.
   a. Any felony
   b. Any crime involving cruelty, abuse, or neglect of animals, including bestiality
   c. Any crime of moral turpitude
   d. Any crime involving unlawful sexual contact; child abuse; the use or threatened use of a weapon; the infliction of injury; indecent exposure; perjury, false reporting, criminal impersonation, forgery and any other crime involving a lack of truthfulness, veracity, or honesty; intimidation of a victim or witness; larceny; or alcohol or drugs.
5. For the purposes of subsection 4, a plea of guilty or a plea of nolo contendere accepted by the court shall be considered as a conviction.
6. Incompetence, gross negligence, or other malpractice in the practice of veterinary medicine.
7. Aiding the unlawful practice of veterinary medicine.
8. Fraud or dishonesty in the application or reporting of any test for disease in animals.
9. Failure to report, as required by law, or making false or misleading report of, any contagious or infectious disease.
10. Failure to keep accurate and comprehensive patient records as set by rules promulgated by the Board.
11. Dishonesty or gross negligence in the performance of food safety inspections or the issuance of any health or inspection certificates.
12. Failure to keep veterinary premises and equipment, including practice vehicles, in a clean and sanitary condition as set by rules promulgated by the Board.
13. Failure to permit the Board or its agents to enter and inspect veterinary premises and equipment, including practice vehicles, as set by rules promulgated by the Board.
14. Revocation, suspension, or limitation of a license to practice veterinary medicine by another state, territory, or district of the United States on grounds other than nonpayment of registration fee.
15. Loss or suspension of accreditation by any federal or state agency on grounds other than nonpayment of registration fees or voluntary relinquishment of accreditation.
16. Unprofessional conduct as defined in regulations adopted by the Board.
17. The dispensing, distribution, prescription, or administration of any veterinary prescription drug, or the extralabel use of any drug in the absence of a veterinarian-client-patient relationship.
18. Violations of state or federal drug laws.
19. Violations of any order of the Board.
20. Violations of this act or of the rules promulgated under this act.

Section 15—Impaired Veterinarian

1. The Board shall establish by rule a program of care, counseling, or treatment for impaired veterinarians.
2. The program of care, counseling, or treatment shall include a written schedule of organized treatment, care, counseling, activities, or education satisfactory to the Board, designed for the purposes of restoring an impaired person to a condition whereby the impaired person can practice veterinary medicine with reasonable skill and safety of a sufficient degree to deliver competent patient care.
3. All persons authorized to practice by the Board shall report in good faith any veterinarian they reasonably believe to be impaired as defined in Section 2, subsection 13.

Section 16—Hearing Procedure

All hearings shall be in accordance with the Administrative Procedures Act of this state or other applicable state law.

Section 17—Appeal

All appeals shall be in accordance with the Administrative Procedures Act of this state or other applicable state law.

Section 18—Reinstatement

Any person whose license is suspended, revoked, or limited may be reinstated at any time, with or without an examination, by approval of the Board after written application is made to the Board showing cause justifying relicensing or reinstatement.

Section 19—Veterinarian-Client Confidentiality

1. No licensed veterinarian shall disclose any information concerning the licensed veterinarian's care of a patient except on written authorization or by waiver by the licensed veterinarian's client or on appropriate court order, by subpoena, or as otherwise provided in this Section.
2. Copies of or information from veterinary records shall be provided without the owner's consent to public, animal health, animal welfare, wildlife, or agriculture authorities, employed by federal, state, or local governmental agencies who have a legal or regulatory interest in the contents of said records for the protection of animal and public health.
3. Any licensed veterinarian releasing information under written authorization or other waiver by the client or under court order, by subpoena, or as otherwise provided by this Section shall not be liable to the client or any other person.

APPENDIX A AVMA-Model Veterinary Practice Act—cont'd

4. The privilege provided by this Section shall be waived to the extent that the licensed veterinarian's client or the owner of the patient places the licensed veterinarian's care and treatment of the patient or the nature and extent of injuries to the animal at issue in any civil criminal proceeding.

Section 20—Immunity from Liability

Any member of the Board, any witness testifying in a proceeding or hearing authorized under this act, any person who lodges a complaint pursuant to this act, and any person reporting an impaired veterinarian shall be immune from liability in any civil or criminal action brought against him for any action occurring while he was acting in his capacity as a Board member, witness, complainant, or reporting party, if such person was acting in good faith within the scope of his respective capacity.

Section 21—Cruelty to Animals—Immunity for Reporting

Any veterinarian licensed in this state who reports, in good faith and in the normal course of business, a suspected incident of animal cruelty, as described by law, to the proper authorities shall be immune from liability in any civil or criminal action brought against such veterinarian for reporting such incident.

Section 22—Abandoned Animal

1. Any animal placed in the custody of a licensed veterinarian for treatment, boarding or other care, which is unclaimed by the client for more than ten days after written notice by certified mail, return receipt requested, or US priority mail, confirmation of receipt, is sent to the client at the client's last known address shall be deemed to be abandoned. Such abandoned animal may be turned over to the nearest humane society or animal shelter, or otherwise disposed of or destroyed by the licensed veterinarian in a humane manner.
2. If notice is sent pursuant to subsection 1 of this Section, the licensed veterinarian responsible for such abandoned animal is relieved of any further liability for disposal. If a licensed veterinarian follows the procedures of this Section, the veterinarian shall not be subject to disciplinary action under Section 14 of this Act, unless such licensed veterinarian fails to provide the proper notification to the client.
3. The disposal of an abandoned animal shall not relieve the client of any financial obligation incurred for treatment, boarding, or other care provided by the licensed veterinarian.

Section 23—Enforcement

1. Any person who practices veterinary medicine without a valid license or temporary permit issued by the Board shall be guilty of a criminal offense and upon conviction for each violation shall be fined [an appropriate amount of money according to the Board or the laws of the state] or imprisoned [an appropriate amount of time according to the Board or the laws of the state], provided that each act of such unlawful practice shall constitute a distinct and separate offense.
2. Any person not licensed under this act is considered to have violated this act and may be subject to all the penalties provided for such violations if he:
   a. Performs any of the functions described as the practice of veterinary medicine as defined in this act, or
   b. Represents, directly or indirectly, publicly or privately, an ability and willingness to perform any of the functions described as the practice of veterinary medicine as defined in this act, or
   c. Uses any title, words, abbreviation, or letters in a manner or under circumstances that induces the belief that the person using them is qualified to perform any of the functions described as the practice of veterinary medicine as defined in this act.
3. The Board may bring an action to enjoin any person from practicing veterinary medicine without a currently valid license or temporary permit issued by the Board. If the court finds that the person is violating or is threatening to violate this act, it shall enter an injunction restraining him from such unlawful acts.
4. Not withstanding other provisions of this act, the Board may take immediate action if there is an imminent threat to the health, safety, or welfare of the public. The Board shall find that this action is necessary for the protection of the public and necessary to effectively enforce this act. If the Board takes immediate action pursuant to this subsection 4, efforts shall be made as soon as possible to proceed in accordance with a hearing pursuant to Section 16 of this act.
5. In addition to any other penalty or remedy provided by law, the Board shall have the authority to implement a system of Cite and Fine procedures for licensed and nonlicensed persons who violate the state veterinary practice act. The Board may also impose a civil penalty, upon conviction, for each separate violation. This civil penalty shall be in an amount not to exceed [dollar amount] for each violation and shall be assessed by the Board in accordance with the provisions set forth in Section 16 of this act.
6. The success or failure of an action based on any one of the remedies set forth in this Section shall in no way prejudice the prosecution of an action based on any other of the remedies.

Section 24—Severability

If any part of this act is held invalid by a court of competent jurisdiction, all valid parts that are severable from the invalid part remain in effect.

Section 25—Effective Date

This act shall become effective on –1st, 20–. This act does not affect rights and duties that matured, penalties that were incurred, and proceedings that were begun before its effective date.

Approved by the AVMA Executive Board, November 2003. Courtesy of Dr. Beth Sabin.

3 Veterinary Practice Management

Dennis M. McCurnin and Roger L. Lukens

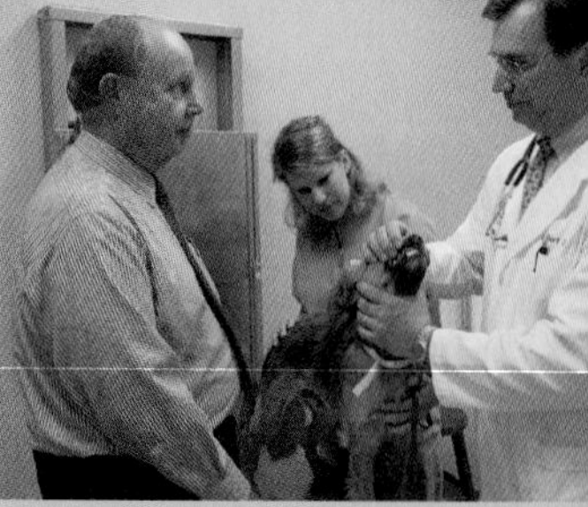

OUTLINE

KEY TERMS

Accounts receivable
Appointment system
Cash flow
Consultation
FIFO
Gross income
Haul-in facility
Inpatient
Marketing
NCVEI
Net income
Nonshopped fees
Outpatient
Petty cash
Shopped fees
Traffic flow
Travel sheet
Veterinary team
Walk-in system

LEARNING OBJECTIVES

When you have completed this chapter, you will be able to:

1. List the terms used to describe various types of veterinary facilities.
2. Describe the components and management issues related to the inpatient, outpatient, surgical, and support areas of the small animal hospital.
3. List and explain the requirements for maintenance in a veterinary facility.
4. List the roles and responsibilities of each member of the veterinary health care team in a variety of practice settings.
5. List and describe the steps in the hiring process and appropriate questions to ask potential employees during an interview.
6. Describe the components of an effective inventory control program.
7. Name the components to consider in setting fees for practice services.
8. Describe procedures related to collections, billing, and cash flow.
9. Describe the components of effective communication with clients and methods of handling difficult clients.
10. List the components related to marketing of the veterinary practice services and products.

INTRODUCTION

Each veterinary practice is a professional business that offers medical care to animals with their owners' consent. Only willing owners consent to pay a fee for professional services provided by the veterinary team. The total cost of operating a medical business providing these services is paid by the gross income of the practice. Marketing efforts must effectively attract (and retain) sufficient clients to each practice or it will go bankrupt. No professional veterinary business will survive if it is not profitable.

The highest quality of care possible for the animals must be offered to their owners in a cost-effective (not cost-cutting) manner; this is extremely important to both patients and their owners. A high-quality practice requires keeping up with the latest medical knowledge and technologies. It also requires the most effective and caring communication possible with owners by the entire veterinary team. Quality communication is absolutely necessary to inform, educate, and obtain owner compliance for the veterinarian's recommendations to benefit the animal.

The profitability of the practice and the care of the client's animal are at risk if the veterinary team fails to deliver quality medical care for the animal coupled with caring effective communication with the owner. The services of the veterinary team are not successful unless the patient is helped and the client understands the service, the client is pleased with the caring attitude of the team, the client tells others of his or her enthusiasm for that practice, and the client wants to return for future veterinary care of pets. Veterinary technicians are important to the success of the veterinary team in accomplishing these goals. Effective management of the veterinary practice as a business is also necessary because of increased competition, growing malpractice threats, new technology, new Internet information, Internet pharmacies, shifting client expectations, and continuing inflation of medical equipment, supply, and personnel costs. All these risks and challenges must be well managed to enhance both productivity and the quality of patient care. It has been said, "What is good business may be bad medicine, and what is good medicine may be bad business." Veterinary practice represents the art of balancing both business and medicine to meet the needs of patients, clients, and the veterinary team.

VETERINARY PRACTICE MANAGEMENT AREAS

Veterinary students are naturally interested in managing the nursing care of patients. They must realize the necessity of effective communication with clients to benefit the patient and begin to understand the business side of medicine. This develops only after gaining significant experience in a veterinary practice. Managing the equipment, facility, and staff and marketing is not of much interest until the student has experienced problems or limitations in these areas that have a negative impact on patient care (or the technician's salary).

Each of these management areas (Box 3-1) must be coordinated with the other areas to meet the veterinary team's goals for the operation (mission statement and strategic plan). A successfully managed practice enjoys success and accomplishment with people, both internally and externally. Failure to properly manage patients, people, and the business ultimately leads to a reduction in the quality of service rendered, staff dissatisfaction, staff turnover, a disorganized practice, dissatisfied clients, and decreasing business.

VETERINARY FACILITIES

The type of practice facility will vary greatly according to the needs of the clients and the species of animals served by the practice staff. Facility design must accommodate the needs of the patients, the number of clients served, the interests of the veterinarians, the level of care to be provided, and the financing available for investing in the facility. Many facilities are simply expanded and remodeled as the practice grows and demands change. Occasionally the existing facility is totally replaced with one redesigned to meet the practice's goals.

BOX 3-1 Management Areas

- Facility design
- Patient care
- Client communications
- Human resources
- Finance
- Marketing
- Building
- Equipment
- Medical records
- Inventory control
- Computerization

The practice may limit veterinary service to a single species (feline, equine, swine, cattle), to small animals (dogs, cats, exotic pets), to large animals (any livestock, horses), to exotic animals, or to a mixed practice (all species). Each type of practice has unique requirements for a facility that is designed to accommodate their patients and clients. Large animal and mixed practices may provide all veterinary services on the owner's premises, have haul-in facilities for these species, or provide both options as a convenience to the client.

The majority of practicing veterinarians are general practitioners who offer primary care level of services. They increasingly refer problem cases to specialists at referral practices (secondary care providers) or veterinary schools (tertiary care providers). These specialists are board certified in surgery, internal medicine, dermatology, ophthalmology, or other areas. Once treatment by the specialists is finished, the patient and client are transferred back to the primary care provider. Primary care providers are also able to use the skills of consultant specialists to read x-rays, ultrasound images, and electrocardiograms (ECGs) or consult with specialists by telephone or via the Internet without referring the case.

Many diseases are not fully understood because diagnostic methods are unavailable, clinical treatments are inadequate, and prevention is not yet possible. Therefore this network of referring practitioners not only is providing the best quality of care possible, but it also is the foundation of supporting clinical research at the tertiary care centers at the veterinary schools. Both clinical and basic science research is absolutely necessary to discover the pathogenesis of unsolved diseases, new and effective diagnostics, effective treatments, and ultimately, the preventative steps necessary to prevent patient death and client despair.

FACILITY NOMENCLATURE

Numerous terms are applied to veterinary facilities. The American Veterinary Medical Association (AVMA) has developed guidelines (Box 3-2) for consistency in naming

BOX 3-2 Veterinary Facility Nomenclature

Office
Room where limited or consultative type of practice is conducted

Mobile Facility
A vehicle for making house or farm calls or a vehicle equipped with special medical and/or surgical facilities; both must have a permanent base of operations (published address and telephone number)

Clinic
Outpatient practice facility not offering overnight patient confinement

Hospital
Inpatient practice facility offering overnight hospitalization of patients; sometimes called primary care facility

Emergency Facility
Emergency practice facility that focuses primarily on treating and monitoring emergencies with veterinarian and staff who are always available (during specified hours of operation) and is equipped to provide timely and appropriate level of emergency care

On-Call Emergency Service
Veterinarians and staff who are not on premises all the time but are available via on-call basis to handle emergency calls

Referral Center
Staff of board certified specialist veterinarians who receive referrals from the primary care practitioners of the above facilities; sometimes called secondary care facility

Animal Medical Center
A large facility (veterinary teaching hospitals, large corporate practices) offering consultative, clinical, and hospital services to referred clients and their local veterinarian; also performs significant research on animal health problems and conducts advanced professional education programs; sometimes called tertiary care facility

veterinary facilities to prevent confusion by the general public. In addition, many state practice acts and regulations not only have been updated to specify standards of practice and professional competency for both veterinarians and technicians, but also have adopted facility and equipment requirements and hired inspectors to ensure that these standards are being met. The American Animal Hospital Association (AAHA) also has extensive standards of excellence that cover most of the management areas listed in Box 3-1. These must be met to have the hospital accredited by AAHA.

MANAGEMENT OF HOSPITAL AREAS

The small animal hospital (see Box 3-2) is the most complete facility for primary care practice for small animals. It provides the best model for discussing location, function, and management of each of the facility areas in this chapter. Good management of hospital areas is the foundation of understanding the principles of improving the efficiency of any practice. Conversely, lack of attention to facility area management ultimately leads to inefficiencies, disorder of the practice, staff frustration, loss of income, and a decrease of the quality of client service and patient care.

Small animal hospital facilities are designed to provide overnight hospitalization, complete surgical facilities, and sufficient examination rooms to provide outpatient services. They also must have ancillary support areas to provide reception, laboratory, pharmacy, imaging, diagnostic procedures, treatment, and inpatient ward space. The appropriate size and location of each area in the hospital are related to the number of veterinarians and support staff in the practice and the number of clients and patients served.

Patient management and possibly client management are obviously the most interesting and necessary management topics for entry-level veterinary technicians. It often takes more experience and a desire for advancement before veterinary technicians become interested in the other areas of practice management (see Box 3-1). Students need to develop a working knowledge of the principles of management of hospital areas to be effective technicians and to prepare for future advancement in the veterinary technology profession. This understanding is also critical for assessing practice differences when searching for the best employment opportunity (see self-marketing section at the end of this chapter).

Outside Areas

Location is the primary factor (other than referrals from satisfied clients) in attracting new clients. Location will often dictate slow or rapid practice growth. Location provides visibility for potential clients and allows existing clients to easily find the practice. Prime locations within shopping centers and on main streets are expensive during the initial investment period, but will repay the investment by increasing practice growth and increasing real estate value. The location of the facility should also be considered by veterinary technicians when selecting a practice for employment.

Further, the practice sign must be evaluated for visibility and professional appearance. The optimal sign would be a well-placed, neat professional sign that allows the client clear visibility and direction (Figure 3-1). The sign becomes even more important during an emergency. Some form of lighting will allow clients to identify the building entrance after dark. A lit sign is also an excellent marketing tool at night.

Attention must be given to the parking lot area. Litter must be picked up, and plants and grass must be tended. The parking lot entrance and exit should be clearly marked by signs. Parking spaces should be reserved for clients only, with employee parking behind the building or in a remote area away from the building entrance (Figure 3-2).

The entrance to the veterinary facility should be in full view and well marked to allow easy access by clients. If more than one entrance is available (i.e., small animal and large animal or canine and feline), each entrance should be well marked. To prevent client congestion, the entrance and exit should be separate. Practice employees should not use the public entrance of the building. Further, those with routine

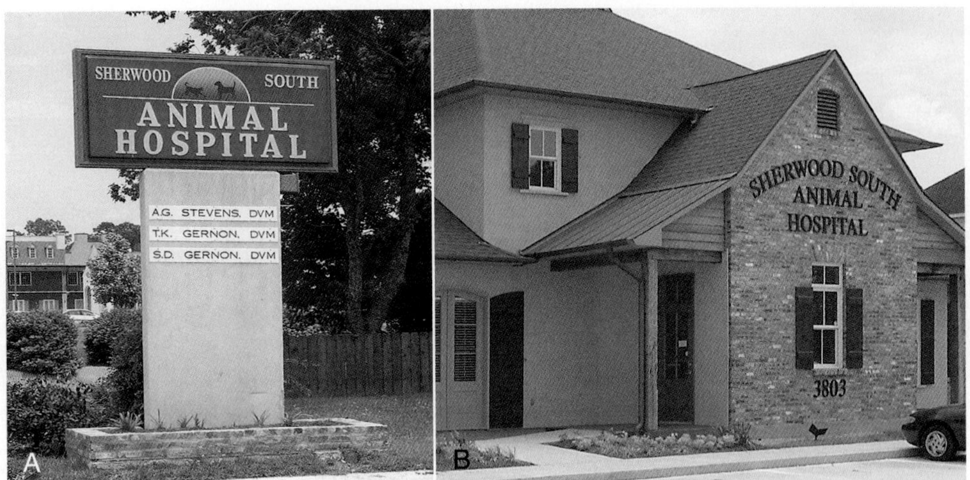

FIGURE 3-1 A, Hospital signs should be professional and clearly visible from the street. B, Signs directly on the building may also be used.

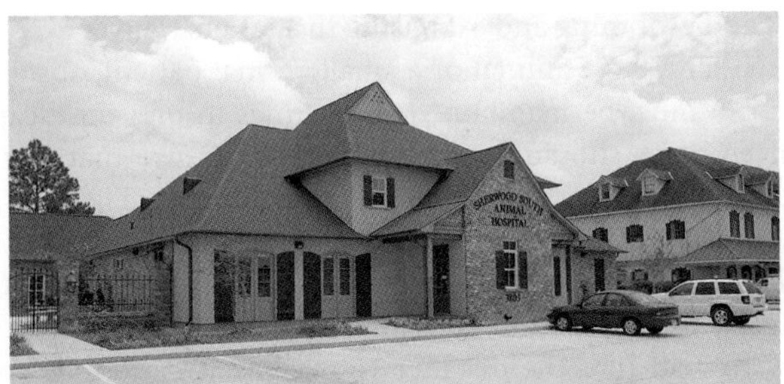

FIGURE 3-2 Client parking lot should be clearly designated and clean.

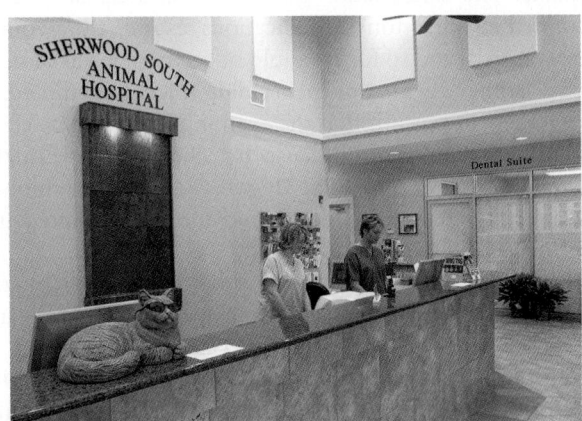

FIGURE 3-3 Reception area should give a warm, comfortable feeling to clients and staff.

deliveries and service activities should enter and exit the building away from client contact when possible.

Professional activities within a veterinary hospital can be grouped into four areas: outpatient, inpatient, surgical, and support. Depending on the practice size and type, the veterinarian, technician, or both may work in all four areas or focus on one or more areas. Effective management of each of these areas is needed to improve service, patient care, and profitability.

> *TECHNICIAN NOTE* Animal security within the hospital must always be a high priority. Animals that escape are the legal responsibility of the hospital.

Outpatient Area

The first area to be discussed is the outpatient area. This area is composed of the reception area, examination rooms, laboratory, pharmacy, and public restrooms. Most commonly, clients will only have access to this area of the hospital. Special attention must be paid to maintain the outpatient area in a clean, organized, quiet, and odor-free condition. Because the client's first contact is with the outpatient area, lasting impressions are made that may raise or lower the overall client confidence in the quality of care. A disorganized, dirty, smelly, noisy area will be remembered just that way. Veterinarians, technicians, and other staff must be well groomed, clean, and professionally attired. A professional appearance is mandatory for a professional image. All personnel in the outpatient area should also refrain from smoking, eating, and drinking when clients are present.

The reception area should always be considered by all hospital employees as a reception or client greeting area and not as a waiting room. The reception area should be comfortable and project a feeling of warmth, not a sterile feeling. Plants will help to create this warm feeling, but they must be well cared for. Dead or dying plants in the reception area will not send a positive message to the client. Warm colors will also help to brighten the area. Reading material, if present, should be complete and not torn or half missing. A bright reception area with attractive wall hangings and plants will help relax clients (Figure 3-3).

The clients should spend only a short period of time in the reception room before they are escorted to one of the examination rooms. This requires effective appointment scheduling and dedication to timely service. As a general rule, two examination rooms should be available in the outpatient area for each veterinarian. Therefore in the typical

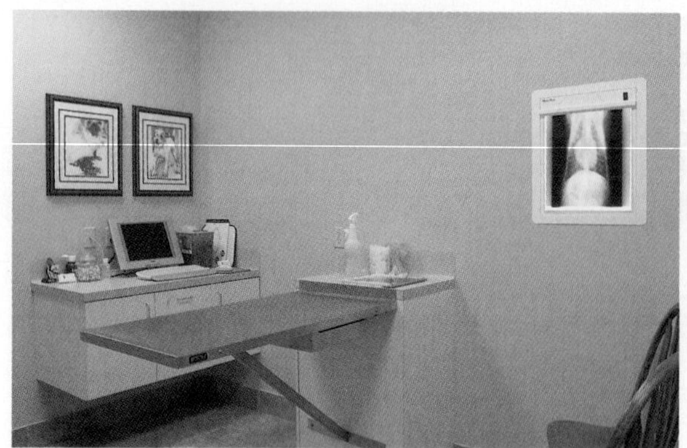

FIGURE 3-4 Examination rooms should be warmly decorated, clean, and in excellent condition.

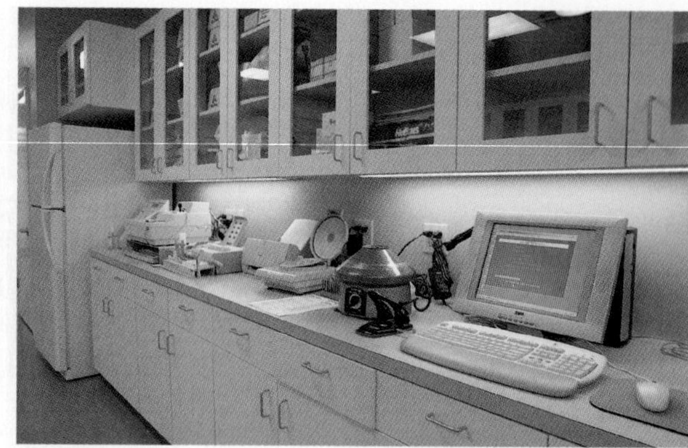

FIGURE 3-5 The laboratory is located just beyond the examination rooms.

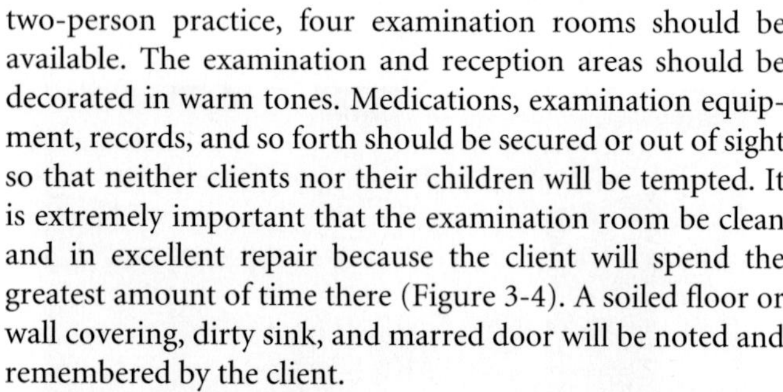

two-person practice, four examination rooms should be available. The examination and reception areas should be decorated in warm tones. Medications, examination equipment, records, and so forth should be secured or out of sight so that neither clients nor their children will be tempted. It is extremely important that the examination room be clean and in excellent repair because the client will spend the greatest amount of time there (Figure 3-4). A soiled floor or wall covering, dirty sink, and marred door will be noted and remembered by the client.

The laboratory and pharmacy should be well organized and clean. Clients will only occasionally visit these areas and should always be accompanied by a hospital employee. In some practices, the laboratory and pharmacy will be combined for more efficient use of floor space. They are usually located behind the examination rooms and accessible to the inpatient treatment areas (Figure 3-5). The pharmacy may also have Occupational Safety and Health Administration (OSHA)-required material safety data sheet (MSDS) files and an eyewash station (Figure 3-6). The public restrooms should be cleaned and inspected regularly and should be conveniently located for client use.

Inpatient Area

The second work area is the inpatient area, consisting of a treatment area, patient wards and/or large animal stalls, isolation area, exercise area, an area in which necropsy is performed, a kitchen, and a bathing and grooming area. The client has much less contact with this area than with the outpatient area, but constant attention must be given to maintain a clean, odor-free environment to prevent nosocomial infections of patients (Box 3-3).

Kennels, runs, and stalls must be cleaned several times during the day. Hospitalized patients must have closer attention than animals who are just boarding. Sick animals often cannot control urination and defecation; therefore more frequent attention to these areas will be required. Some pets are not used to eliminating indoors and will be reluctant to urinate and defecate unless they are in an exercise run. To maintain a quiet environment in public areas of the hospital, patient wards must be well insulated to reduce noise.

If large animals are hospitalized, adequate holding stalls will be necessary, with regular attention given to cleaning the stall and grooming and exercising the patient. When exercising either a large animal or a small animal patient, absolute security must be maintained at all times to prevent escape. Fenced areas should always be used to ensure that in the event of escape the animal will still be contained (Figure 3-7). The veterinarian, hospital, or both assume all liability for an animal entrusted to them. Few experiences will match the helpless feeling of watching an escaped dog, cat, horse, or cow run off into the distance (especially if close to a busy street or highway).

Because of the security problem, the ward or stall area of the hospital should be adjacent to the exercise area with an escape-proof fence or walls connecting the two. Exercise areas for small animals ideally should be located within a well-insulated area of the hospital in which the temperature and humidity can be maintained at a constant level. Most city zoning laws will allow a small animal hospital to be located in proximity to residential areas because modern construction techniques use totally enclosed, attractive, and well-insulated designs.

> *TECHNICIAN NOTE* Animal security within the hospital must always be a high priority. Animals that escape are the legal responsibility of the hospital.

Large animal or mixed hospitals (caring for both large and small animals) will usually be required to locate in a less-developed area of a city to allow exercise areas and odors to be properly addressed. Fewer veterinary hospitals now board animals on a regular basis. When boarding is offered, it should be explained to the client as "veterinary-supervised boarding." The recent trend has been away from construction of large boarding facilities as part of an animal hospital. Because of both the cost of construction and the cost of hospitalization, most veterinary practices work on an outpatient basis whenever possible. Construction and labor costs have made long-term hospitalization a financial burden to both client and veterinarian.

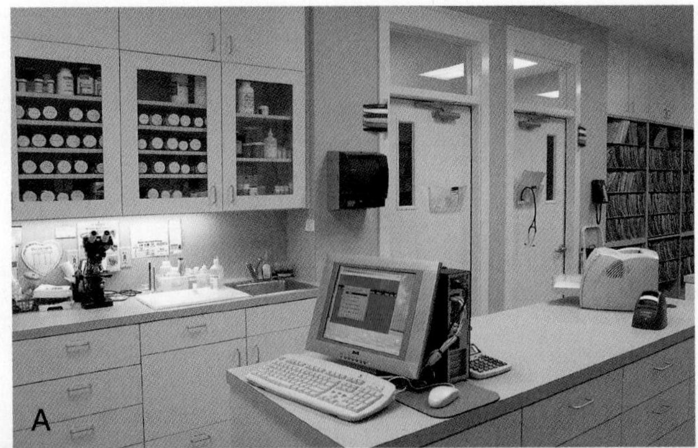

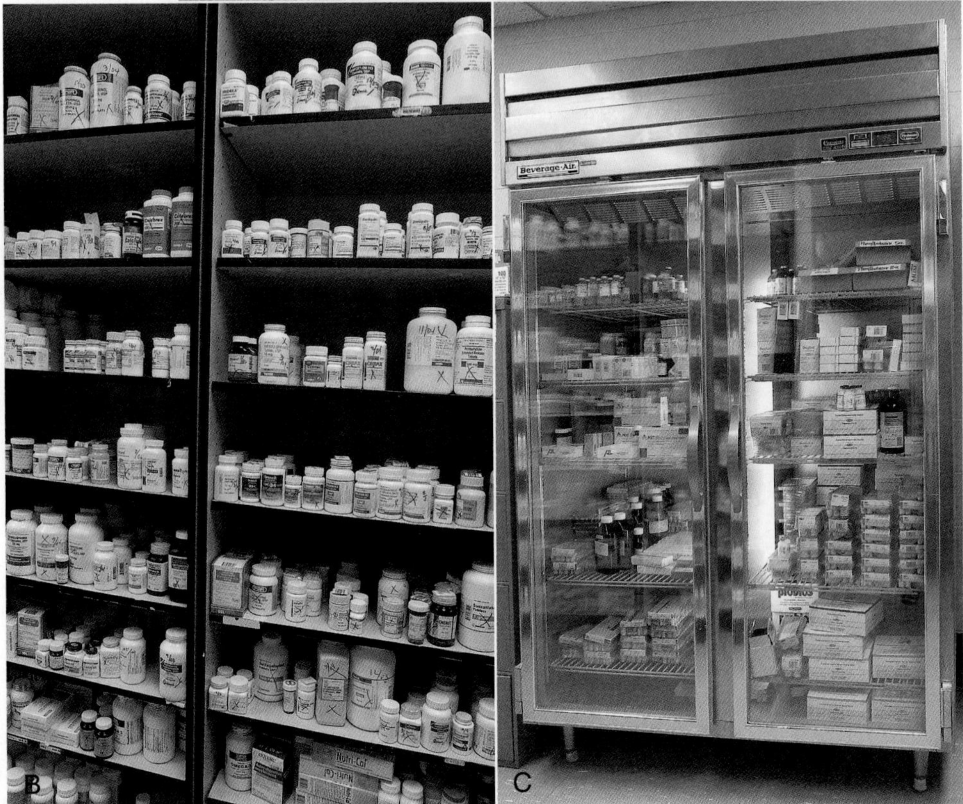

FIGURE 3-6 **A,** Pharmacy is located near examination rooms and inpatient treatment area. **B,** Drug shelf storage in pharmacy. **C,** Glass door refrigerator for storage of vaccines and biologics.

In certain instances, animals with infectious diseases must be hospitalized. Adequate isolation facilities must be available before a patient with an infectious disease is admitted. The isolation area should have only one entrance and exit with proper disinfectant and clothing protection available. The air-handling system for the isolation area must be separate from the remainder of the building to prevent aerosol transmission of contagious disease organisms. In the event adequate isolation facilities are not available on the premises, the case should be referred to a veterinarian who has the proper facility. All treatments and handling of the infectious patient should be done by one or two persons only. The patient should be treated within the isolation facility and should not be taken to the main treatment room. The staff must be trained to follow stringent isolation protocols to prevent nosocomial infections (see Box 3-3).

The treatment area should be the central hub of the hospital (Figure 3-8). Patients from both the wards (inpatients) and examination rooms (outpatients) will be moved to this area for diagnostic procedures, medication administration, and recheck procedures (cast, bandage, or splint changes or removal). Certified veterinary technicians are increasingly performing the prescribed medical treatment and other nursing procedures, and the veterinarian is performing surgery or seeing outpatients. One of the technical staff should have the primary responsibility for organization and cleanliness of the treatment room.

On occasion, clients may accompany the patient to the treatment area to assist with a bandage change or other minor procedure. The area therefore must be presentable at all times. In addition to the routine treatment functions carried out in the treatment room, many hospitals also use this

BOX 3-3 Nosocomial Infections

Definition: Nosocomial infections are new infections acquired by patients in the veterinary facility.

Examples of Nosocomial Infection Sources

Staff: Unwashed hands; contaminated equipment, including dirty needles, clothing, and boots; inadequate cleaning and disinfecting protocols; breaks in aseptic technique

Other patients: Direct contact, airborne droplets, hair, excrement, blood

Environment: Cages, drains, floors, walls, feed or water pans, dust, bedding

Staff Prevention

Always wash hands between patients.

Always wear clean clothing and boots.

Always follow established cleaning, disinfecting, sterilizing, and aseptic protocols.

Train the staff in preventive protocols.

NOTE: Recent studies indicate that human hospital workers wash their hands less than one half of the time before touching human patients; this is one factor in the recent increase of nosocomial infections in human patients.

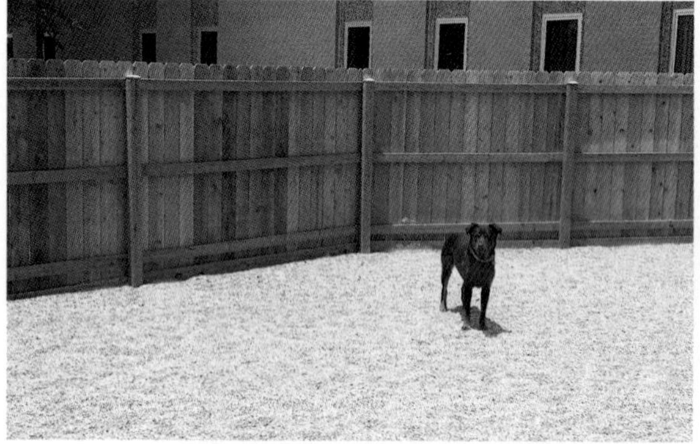

FIGURE 3-7 For security, fenced enclosures should always be used for outside exercise.

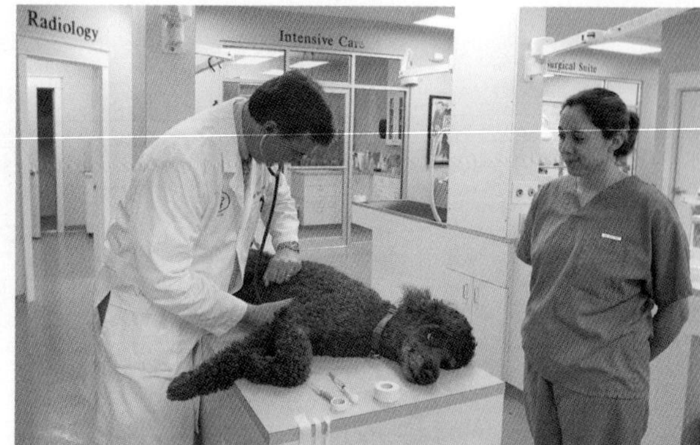

FIGURE 3-8 Centralized treatment area accommodates both outpatient and inpatient treatment.

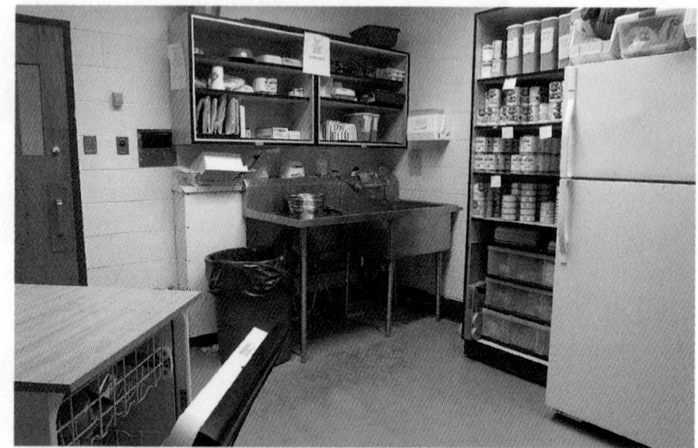

FIGURE 3-9 Hospital kitchen should contain diet materials, dishwasher, counter space, and refrigerator.

room for preparation of the surgical patient. In the smaller practice, the treatment room may also contain x-ray facilities, laboratory equipment, or both. Because of the high traffic volume in the treatment area, hair and other debris will build up rapidly and should be removed with a vacuum cleaner on a regular basis to prevent nosocomial infections.

The kitchen in a small animal hospital should be an area in which animal food is stored and prepared. Usually, both canned and dry foods are available, and it should be stored in dry, rodent-proof containers. An automatic dishwasher is of great value if any quantity of dirty pans must be cleaned on a daily basis. It will also sanitize the pans with very hot water and remove soap and significant residues that cause digestive problems in sensitive patients. Hot and cold running water, a sink, countertop space, and a refrigerator should be available in the kitchen (Figure 3-9). Human food and drinks must not be stored in this refrigerator (OSHA regulations).

In the large animal hospital, the feed room will usually contain several grain mixtures and ration supplements. All materials must be stored in dry, rodent-proof containers. Grass hay, alfalfa, and bedding straw should be stored in a dry area protected from the weather to prevent mold and mildew. Moldy hay or alfalfa should never be fed to an animal because of possible toxicity and allergies.

The bathing-grooming area in the small animal hospital will usually consist of a raised bathroom tub (elevated about 60 to 90 cm [Figure 3-10]), a combing table, and a dryer cage. It is critically important that all patients dismissed from the hospital be clean and dry. Grooming services within the hospital may not be offered, but attention to daily grooming of all patients by all employees is necessary. Attention to grooming is also important for the equine patient and is usually done in the stall on a daily basis.

The final area to be discussed within the inpatient work area of the hospital is the necropsy area. The veterinary technician is able to perform a prosection (initial dissection) for the veterinarian to quickly inspect all organs for lesions and decide what specimens should be collected (see Chapter 39). The technician will collect, properly prepare, and ship the designated specimens to a diagnostic laboratory with the history (see Chapter 20). The necropsy area should be located in an isolated place in the building and is well lighted and well ventilated. Hot and cold running water and a drain should also be present. Necropsy tables or racks are used for small animals, whereas the necropsy floor is usually used for

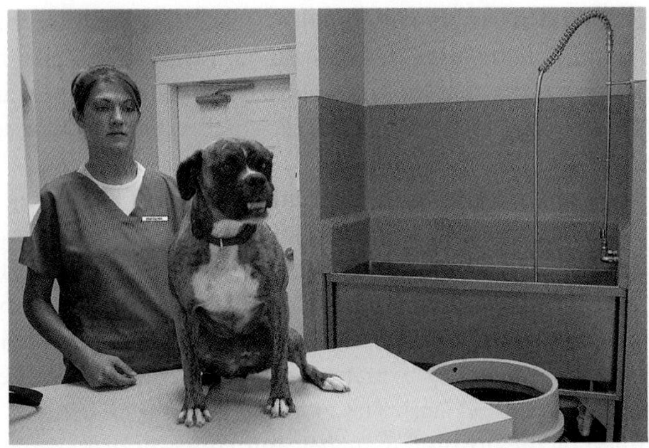

FIGURE 3-10 Custom pet-bathing tub in background designed to aid in controlling animal during bath.

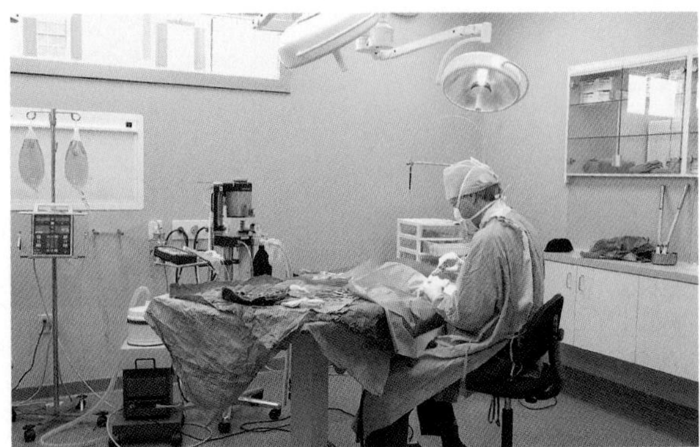

FIGURE 3-11 Surgical room with one door for both entrance and exit, ceiling-mounted lights, and minimal countertops.

dissecting large animals. Gloves, boots, and aprons should be available in addition to specific necropsy instruments and specimen bottles. The availability of a 35-mm camera, digital camera, or video camera is helpful to record specific lesions.

Acceptable carcass disposal, preferably cremation, must be offered to owners. The body may also be released to the owner for burial.

In conclusion, the hospital inpatient area is the most labor-intensive section because of patient contact. Most hospitals expend the greatest amount of effort in maintaining this area. Most employees spend their greatest amount of time in this area performing direct animal care, diagnostic procedures, and nursing treatments. The outcome of most cases will also be determined here.

Surgical Area

The third work area in the hospital is the surgical area, which consists of the preparation room, operating rooms (ORs), radiology section, and recovery room. All four areas in the surgical section must be in close proximity to one another. Frequently the surgeon may need to obtain a postoperative radiograph of a fracture reduction to determine bone alignment or implant placement. When neurosurgery is to be performed, the surgeon may request a myelogram just before surgery; this requires that the patient be moved from the preparation room to the radiology area, back to the preparation room, and then into surgery.

As stated earlier, the preparation room may also be the treatment room. All presurgical preparation of the patient, surgeon, and technician should take place outside the OR. Instrument preparation and sterilization usually will be completed in the preparation room. Clipping and scrubbing the patient and hand scrubbing of the surgeon and technician should be done before entering the OR. A vacuum cleaner should be available in the preparation room to remove all loose hair from the patient, table, and floor.

The OR itself should be a "dead-end" room with only one entrance-exit (Figure 3-11). Dust-carrying bacteria are easily stirred into the air when people walk through the room and will settle into the open surgical incision. No one should enter the OR without proper clothing, shoes, cap, and mask. The OR should be used only for surgical procedures and must not double as a treatment or examination room. Storage cabinets should be kept to a minimum and should contain only items that are used in surgery. Items used elsewhere in the hospital should not be stored in the OR. Countertops should be kept to a minimum because flat surfaces collect dust and must be wiped down daily. Some flat surface is desirable to allow the opening of packs and layout of instruments.

> *TECHNICIAN NOTE* The OR must be used only for surgery and cannot be used as an examination or treatment room.

Wall-mounted radiographic viewers (or digital monitors) should be present to allow several views of a body part to be observed at once. Surgery lights, oxygen outlets, and patient monitors should be ceiling- or wall-mounted when possible. The floors, walls, and ceiling should be washable, smooth, and seam free to allow complete and easy cleaning. Cleaning under the surgery table base, the top of surgical lights, the floor, and flat surfaces (window ledges, countertop, etc.) should be performed daily. The air-handling system for the OR should be separate and should create a slight positive pressure to prevent dust and other debris from entering the room from other rooms when the door is opened.

All cleaning materials and utensils used in the OR should be restricted to use in this room. Mops and sponges that are used elsewhere in the building and then used in the OR will bring additional contamination into the room. The cleanliness of the OR should be everyone's concern to prevent a nosocomial infection of the surgical patient.

The radiology area should be located near the OR, the preparation room, and the treatment area (for diagnostic work-ups). The radiology section should not be visited by clients during film exposure because of potential radiation exposure. Protective aprons, gloves, and film exposure badges should always be worn by all personnel in radiology. The technician will usually be responsible for equipment maintenance, exposure, developing, and filing radiographs

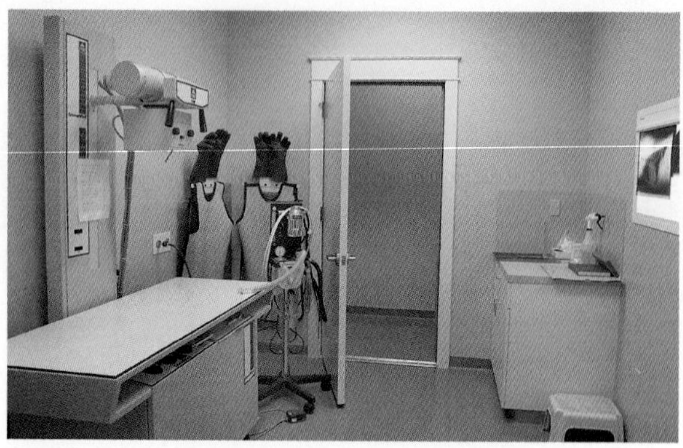

FIGURE 3-12 Radiology room with x-ray machine and protection equipment hanging on the wall. The automatic film processor is not visible through the open door.

(Figure 3-12). In most surgical orthopedic cases, the radiology area will be visited after surgery (or intraoperative digital films taken during surgery) to evaluate bone alignment or a metal implant placement or both before placing the patient in the recovery room.

The surgical patient in the recovery area should be monitored at all times by a technician until the endotracheal tube has been removed. The recovery area may be in a room adjacent to the treatment room or behind a glass partition in the treatment room, or the recovery process may occur on a blanket on the treatment room floor. Whenever surgical recovery occurs, the patient should be closely monitored by the technical staff. Under no circumstances should any patient recovering from anesthesia be left unattended in the ward, in a stall, or elsewhere with an endotracheal tube in place.

In review, the surgical work area is a technical and equipment-oriented area. Clients will not be permitted in this area except in unusual circumstances. The skill level of technical support in this area must be high, requiring familiarization with anesthesia (induction and administration), emergency procedures, radiology, surgical assisting, medical-surgical nursing, use of fiber-optic equipment, sterile technique, sterilization, monitoring equipment hookup, electrosurgical equipment, and necropsy techniques.

Support Area

The fourth work area of the hospital is the hospital support area. This area contains, somewhat by default, some of the "leftovers," but it also contains the planning and management areas of the hospital. The support area contains the professional offices, business management office, library, employee lounge, and storage-inventory areas. In smaller practices, the professional office, business management office, and library will be in one room.

> *TECHNICIAN NOTE* The support area of the hospital contains the professional offices, business management office, library, employee lounge, and storage areas.

In some multiperson practices, each veterinarian may have an office or large desk area in addition to the hospital manager's office. Larger practices may also have a library and conference room combination in which weekly staff meetings and conferences can be held.

The role of the hospital manager will vary according to practice size and management philosophy, but his or her office will usually be in proximity to the admissions-discharge functions of the hospital. Credit policy, accounts receivable, inventory control, purchasing, receiving orders, accounts payable, computer information management, management reports, personnel activities, and so forth will usually be handled by the hospital manager. In many practices, some of these functions are divided among the staff, and the veterinarian or veterinarians will assume the overall management role. For most veterinary technicians, some management skills will be required for advancement. Hospital management is now developing into a specialty area of veterinary medicine for nonveterinarians.

The professional office of the veterinarian functions as a client consultation area, a medical management area for discussing new products with drug company salespeople, and a professional management area for writing medical records, contacting clients, and discussing difficult or interesting cases with other veterinarians or staff. Many office hours are spent by the practicing veterinarian studying and reading textbooks, journals, Internet articles, and reference materials and evaluating computer management information. Veterinary technicians must also keep up with the latest advances in animal nursing, imaging, laboratory procedures, and management issues. Most states also require a minimum number of hours of approved continuing education for both certified veterinary technicians and licensed veterinarians.

The last portion of the support area is storage. From the management viewpoint, hospital storage space is the most expensive floor space in the building because this space produces the least income. Therefore the storage areas must be given close attention so that this valuable space will function as efficiently as possible. Supplies and equipment that are no longer used or usable should be removed to make room for the essential items. Inventory control (avoiding overstocking or understocking) and space organization will ensure maximal use. Items that can be hung on the wall or ceiling should be removed from the floor. Metal or wooden shelving will organize space for bulk drugs, food, and cleaning supplies. Flammable or toxic materials should be safely marked and stored away from food or drugs (see Chapter 6).

In summary, the four major hospital work areas (outpatient, inpatient, surgery, support) are somewhat separate in function, but are related in patient care and support. The smaller the practice, the less distinct the areas will be. Further, the smaller the practice, the fewer the number of technical staff and assistants, resulting in less opportunity for the veterinary technician to focus on one work area. This is not to imply that the smaller practice is less desirable. Sometimes the small practice can provide more personal satisfaction because of closer contact with the entire operation and a diversification of job roles. Each technician and each veterinarian need to choose the type of practice with staffing use patterns that provide the greatest personal and professional satisfaction.

TRAFFIC FLOW

The four work areas that have been discussed are important from both client-patient and hospital organization viewpoints. The client wants personalized and professional service that is efficient, thorough, and cost-effective. If each employee fully understands and enjoys his or her work area, the client and patient will usually experience satisfaction if all communicate effectively. However, the veterinary team must be efficient at handling the necessary number of patients to provide the needed cash flow required to stay in business. An efficient traffic flow (i.e., the movement of the client and patient from admission to dismissal) becomes important to accommodate the required number of clients each day.

LARGE ANIMAL FACILITIES

Whereas about 75% of veterinarians practice in small animal facilities, about 4% of the practices in the United States are equine and 10% are primarily food animal (swine, dairy, and/or beef) practices. A decreasing number (less than 10%) are mixed practices in which veterinarians see both large animal and small animal patients. If the livestock population is high in an area, a group practice may have several large animal veterinarians, each focusing on a specific species for providing diagnostic, treatment, and surgical services and preventive medicine consultation.

LARGE ANIMAL MOBILE UNITS

Veterinary diagnostic and preventive medicine services for a herd of animals require the veterinarian to visit the owner's facility on the farm or in the stable. The large animal practice often makes use of a mobile facility (Figure 3-13) for conducting these farm visits. These visits require stringent sanitary precautions to prevent transmitting disease among animal facilities. Washing hands, changing to clean coveralls, chemical disinfecting of boots, and cleaning of equipment between farm calls are paramount to prevent disease transmission among farms and to gain and keep the confidence of the livestock owner.

Mobile facilities used to serve large animal patients and clients may vary from a car with a few portable "grips" in the trunk, to a van with a set of drawers and containers, to a specially designed mobile truck unit. The truck units are usually fully equipped with refrigeration for biologics plus hot water and a supply of disinfectants, drugs, vaccines, medical supplies, restraints, diagnostic and treatment equipment, and sometimes even mobile x-ray units. Everything needed for a series of planned visits plus unexpected emergencies must be on board. The water supply and disinfectants are used to clean and disinfect hands, boots, and equipment after every farm call. A portable cattle chute may be also pulled behind the mobile unit to the farm to process herds of cattle (Figure 3-14).

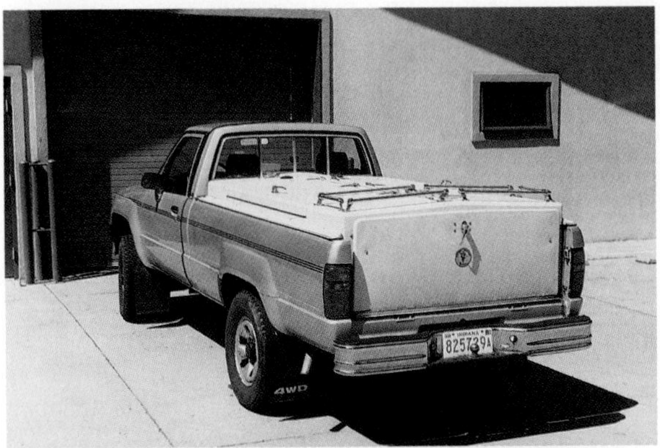

FIGURE 3-13 A veterinary mobile unit is equipped with hot water, a refrigerator, and many compartments for equipment and supplies.

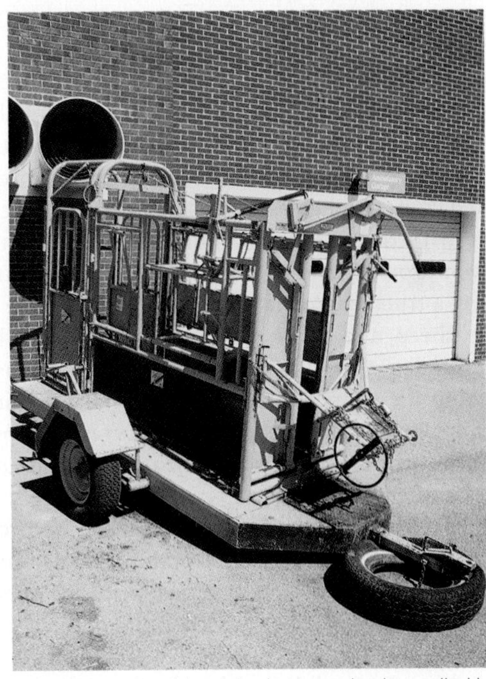

FIGURE 3-14 A portable cattle chute on wheels is pulled behind the ambulatory truck to the farm. It has a head table on front for head work and a palpation cage on back for reproductive examinations.

A veterinary technician may be responsible for stocking, organizing, and maintaining the large animal mobile unit. The mobile unit inventory will vary depending on the nature of the practice, the preferences of the veterinarian, and the species served. Preparing inventory lists and organizational charts for this daily activity ensures that the veterinarian will have what is needed on every call. Obviously, there is a wide range of specific supplies necessary for the routine practice of large animal veterinary medicine. This inventory must be replenished frequently, organized for easy and quick access, and cleaned and disinfected on a daily basis and after every farm call. Many technicians desire to assist veterinarians on farm calls and become efficient at maintaining and organizing the mobile unit.

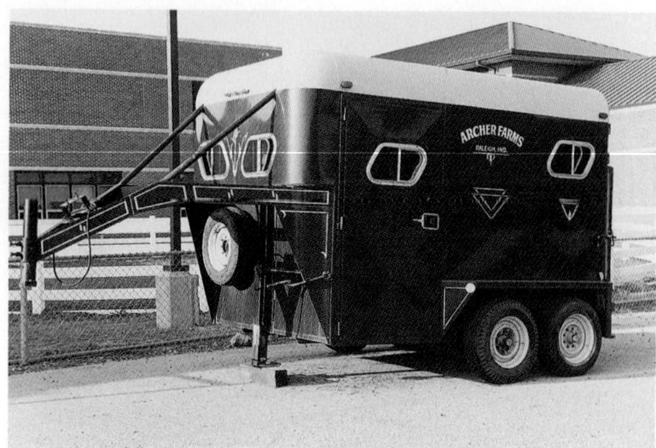

FIGURE 3-15 A stock trailer is used by animal owners to transport farm animals to the large animal hospital for treatment.

LARGE ANIMAL HAUL-IN FACILITIES

Some veterinarians with mixed and large animal practices provide haul-in facilities for individual patients to be trucked or brought by trailer into the practice (Figure 3-15). Unloading chutes and gates for cattle trucks and stock trailers are provided at the large animal outpatient entrance. A few even provide holding corrals and squeeze chutes for processing a truckload of cattle or sheep. Unloading chutes for cattle, sheep, and swine must adjust to different heights to accommodate the trucks, pickups, and trailers used for transporting the animals. It is paramount that fencing and panel arrangements be constructed to prevent escape from the premises if the animal escapes from the head-catch or alleyway or when unloading.

When haul-in facilities for large animals are provided, each of the areas previously discussed for a small animal facility will be present for serving large animal patients. They may be in separate or combined rooms. In larger facilities, they will often be separate from the small animal areas. Frequently, some areas will be used for both small animal and large animal service (e.g., the reception area, laboratory, conference rooms, pharmacy, public restrooms). Large mixed hospitals often have a separate pharmacy for large animal supplies, separate public restrooms, and possibly a separate reception area. The nature of the large animal facilities of each practice is quite variable depending on the needs of the livestock population and owners served by the practice.

The large animal inpatient treatment area may be the same as the outpatient examination area for large animal patients. An alleyway with a head-catch or squeeze chute is used for bovine patients, a stock is used for equine patients, and pigs or sheep may be treated in their stall. When haul-in facilities are available for large animals, patient wards with a few stalls (Figure 3-16) are usually provided. These will often be indoors to protect the patients from bad weather, although outdoor pens may be used in good weather. Isolation areas in a different barn are sometimes necessary to prevent the spread of infectious disease.

Examination rooms are always separate because large animal examinations require stocks for horses (Figure 3-17), a squeeze chute and head-catch for cattle, and large special examination tables for restraining cattle on their side for hoof work or minor surgery. Cattle chutes (see Figure 3-14) are manual or hydraulic squeeze chutes located at the end of an alleyway. A head-catch on the front of an alleyway will

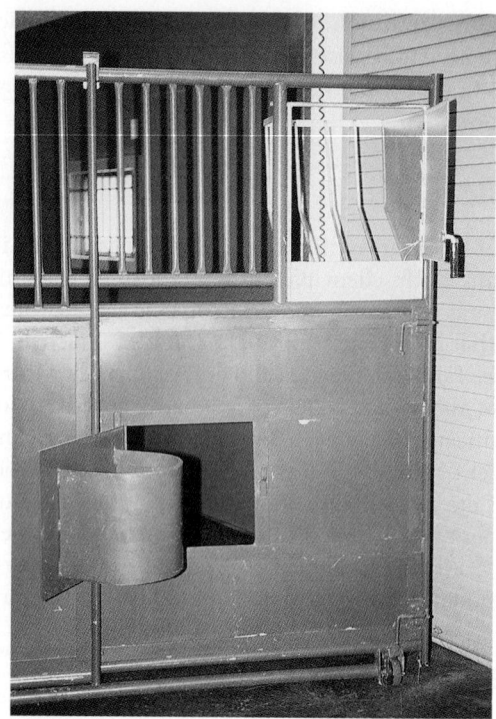

FIGURE 3-16 Large animal stall door has minidoors to feed and water large animal patients without having to enter the stall.

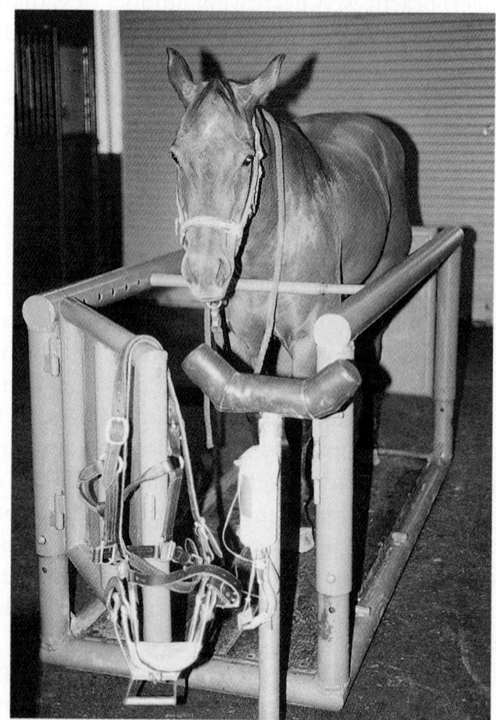

FIGURE 3-17 Horse in stocks with bar in front of chest to keep horse back against rear door. Mouth speculum is used to perform equine dental procedures.

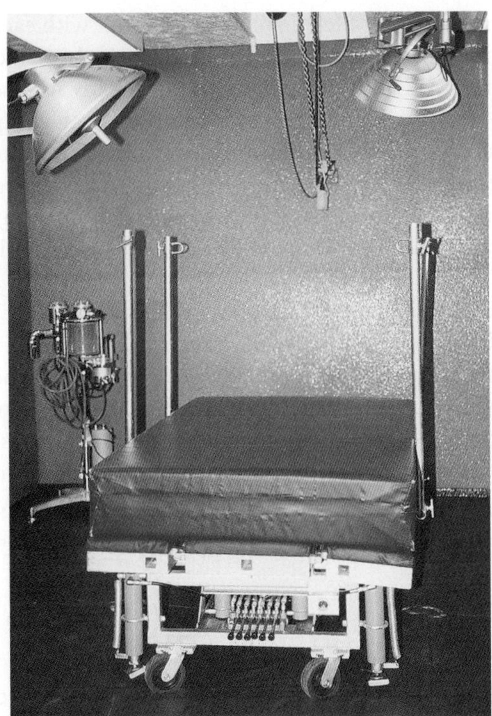

FIGURE 3-18 Large animal surgery table with anesthesia machine and padded walls of recovery room for recovering anesthetized horses.

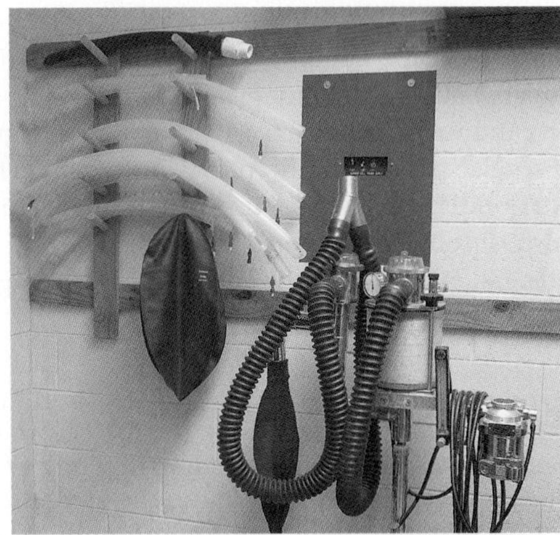

FIGURE 3-19 Large animal endotracheal tubes, rebreathing bags, and related anesthesia equipment stored on a rack for quick access.

suffice for some cattle examinations and procedures. The alleyways leading to the chutes are sometimes arranged in a circular manner to facilitate easier cattle movement to the examination area. Because of the size of these species, the staff should be well trained in restraint and safety procedures; this ensures protection for the large animal patients, owners, and staff. A variety of restraint procedures are used (see Chapter 7).

Most food animal practices also use the treatment area as a minor, nonsterile surgical room. Because of the large patient size and the extensive amount of hair and excrement large animals bring to these areas, high-pressure hoses and disinfectant systems are necessary along with removable floor drain traps. Most mixed practices use the same support areas for small and large animal clients and patients with the exception of storage of cleaning equipment, lawn mowers, large animal hoof equipment, general supplies, and bulk pharmacy items.

The surgical room in the equine practice facility is organized to provide the same stringent asepsis as provided in a small animal surgery. However, because the patient is much larger, mechanical or hydraulic equipment designed to lift the horse is provided. Larger equine practices have an induction room (may also be the treatment and minor surgery area), an OR with a large animal radiology machine, and a padded recovery room. The surgical area is equipped with a surgical table on which the horse is placed after the induction of general anesthetic (Figure 3-18). Anesthesia is maintained with an equine gas anesthesia machine (Figure 3-19).

An area where a necropsy can be appropriately performed must also be available (see Chapter 5). Necropsies are more frequently performed when a large animal dies than for a small animal. Because of the economic value of large herds or flocks, necropsies of dead animals are often done to determine if the rest of the herd or flock is threatened. Confirmation of the diagnosis will often require the submission of specimens to a state or university diagnostic laboratory for testing and review by a board certified pathologist. Sometimes necropsy of several animals may be done (more common in sheep, pigs, and poultry) to determine which of several concurrent diseases is the probable cause of death.

Necropsies are valuable as a preventive measure to stop the spread of a disease and prevent it in the future. They are also a great learning tool for the veterinary staff to become better prepared to recognize similar cases in the future.

Traffic flow patterns in large animal and mixed practices vary greatly. Facilities that primarily serve small animal patients with a moderately used large animal facility attached have some mixing of traffic from both groups. In some facilities, a practice that has many large animal patients may be organized with more separation to reduce crossover of traffic patterns of the small and large animal clients. Obviously, if it is an exclusive large animal facility (e.g., an equine practice), these areas are similar to a small animal practice in name, but the arrangement and size will depend on the type of horses routinely presented for treatment.

BUILDING MAINTENANCE

The building, land, and equipment in a veterinary hospital require a large capital investment. Maintenance of this investment requires significant management attention to maximize its effective use for client service and to provide a reasonable financial return on the investment. It is easy to ignore routine maintenance because the team gets busy with clients and patients and becomes used to the working environment. Therefore routine maintenance must be assigned to someone so that a regular schedule of preventive maintenance will be followed.

Clients often initially evaluate the level of patient care by the appearance of the building and grounds. This requires professional landscaping and proper parking lot surfacing. The continual maintenance of building and grounds through regular painting and repair is important. The care of the exterior of the building along with the meticulous care of the lawn, shrubs, trees, and flowers often conveys an initial impression of a well-organized and caring feeling to the client.

GENERAL MAINTENANCE

General maintenance within the building is an ongoing challenge. The floors, flat surfaces, walls, cages, runs, and stalls must be kept sparkling clean and odor free. The counters, magazine racks, and pictures need to be organized and dusted frequently. The reception room, examination rooms, and public bathrooms must be inspected and cleaned regularly throughout each day. Some of this general maintenance needs to be scheduled on a regular basis. However, to reach the "cleanliness is next to godliness" goal, everyone in the practice must assume some of the cleaning responsibility. An old adage for new graduates is that "veterinary medicine is 90% cleanup and 10% medical practice." No one should look for someone else to clean up a fresh urine or fecal deposit. It is usually quicker and easier to clean it up yourself.

One of the reasons cleanup in a veterinary practice is so challenging is the larger quantity of hair shed by animals than humans. Hair is such a major problem that a vacuum system needs to be available and used before general mopping; otherwise, there is a buildup of hair that is simply moved around the facility. Some practices have been built with a central vacuum system to improve the efficiency of hair reduction from the floors. The removal of hair from the environment is extremely important for the proper care of electronic equipment and computers.

Clients notice hospital cleanliness. The lack of it can result in complaints or nosocomial infections. When one client actually complains, there are probably many other clients quietly forming a negative impression of the practice. If the veterinary hospital is to be considered a modern and progressive medical facility, all personnel must rigidly monitor odors and sanitation. Whenever a pet soils an area or cage, it must be cleaned quickly and thoroughly. Appropriate disinfectants need to be used to prevent odor buildup. Deodorizers may be of benefit to help clean the area, but should not be used to cover up a sanitation problem. The ventilation system should be capable of exhausting all air within the building within 15 to 20 minutes to facilitate odor control. In addition to exhaust fans in the wards, fans can also be useful in the examination rooms and laboratory areas.

MANAGING EQUIPMENT MAINTENANCE

Cleaning equipment must be an ongoing activity. Each major piece of equipment should be assigned to a specified member of the hospital team to keep it well maintained. It is recommended that the person most familiar with each piece of equipment be assigned to maintain it. If this is done, all equipment will last longer and always be ready for use when needed for quality patient care. Nonmedical equipment, such as typewriters, calculators, computers, air conditioning and heating units, lawn mowers, and related general maintenance equipment, should also have maintenance responsibility assigned to those who are most responsible for its use.

Major equipment items should have a specific documented maintenance schedule to ensure proper servicing (e.g., anesthetic machines, endoscopes, ultrasound machines, x-ray developer solutions, automatic processors, autoclaves, microscopes, clinical pathology laboratory analyzers, computer terminals, central vacuum systems, furnaces, hot water heaters, air conditioners). Computer software is available to organize these efforts for equipment, facility areas, and vehicles.

MANAGING ELECTRICAL EQUIPMENT

Supervisors should take the time to teach staff members about electrical safety and how to check equipment to ensure that it is in proper working order with no frayed electrical cords (see Chapter 6). This can prevent tragic electrocution accidents to both the patient and staff.

Veterinary technicians, animal handlers, and veterinarians should be aware of some easy-to-follow rules to minimize macroshock hazards (Box 3-4). Too often people become careless when working around electricity on a continuous basis from either habit or haste.

A file of warranties, service, and repair representatives for each item of major equipment should be maintained. The file should also include the instruction manuals that must be read to chart the needed schedule of required maintenance. This scheduled maintenance chart should be initialed when each maintenance is performed. Failure to do required maintenance often violates warranties and results in a shorter life of this costly equipment. Many items need to be cleaned or serviced after each use. These include electric clippers, surgical instruments, endoscopes, otoscopes, ophthalmoscopes, instrument trays, and oxygen tanks (gas levels).

To be efficient, all team members must learn to complete the last step of the action cycle (Figure 3-20) immediately after every event in the hospital. Otherwise, records are not up to date and the area or equipment is not ready when needed for the next patient. Unfinished paperwork, lack of needed cleanup, and forgotten follow-up on cases stack up and require part of the evening to finish or are forgotten. Encourage the staff to be list makers and checkers to complete all the action cycles during a busy day. Tasks will be forgotten when staff members are interrupted before finishing all the follow-up tasks. Much of the disarray of a busy practice often comes from the frequent lack of completion of the action cycle by one or more members of the staff team.

BOX 3-4 Electrical Equipment Safety Rules

The Patient

Avoid touching the animal and any conductive metal surface of an electrical instrument at the same time.

Be sure all electrical equipment in the vicinity of or attached to the animal is effectively grounded with three-wire power cords, and do not allow any equipment with two-prong plugs in the animal's vicinity.

When two or more electrical instruments are used near a patient, connect them to the same wall outlet. Remove all unnecessary electrical equipment from the patient's environment.

Always plug electrical equipment into the wall outlet with the equipment power switch off.

Power Cords

Avoid using extension cords with any patient instrumentation and never use a two-prong to three-prong cheater adapter on two-wire outlets.

Keep electrical cords out of well-traveled pathways and do not step on or roll equipment over electrical cables.

Plug and unplug the power cord of the equipment by holding onto the plug firmly and straight.

Before power cords and their connectors are used, carefully check for intermittent or loose connections, frayed wires, cracked connectors, and overall quality.

Appliances

Check all electrical appliances (especially motorized devices) periodically for current leakage and ground wire continuity.

If performance of an instrument is unsatisfactory or a tingling sensation is felt from it, remove it from use and have it checked.

Keep fluids, chemicals, spillable products, and heat away from electrical equipment and cables.

General

Know the location of circuit breakers for each wall outlet serving clinical areas.

Remember that body moisture or perspiration lowers electrical resistance and permits greater current to flow.

Use common sense when working with electrical equipment.

Remember that the patient is in the electrical environment and could become part of an unsuspected circuit.

Modified from Swift C, Carithers R: Electrical safety for the veterinarian: macroshock hazards, *J Am Vet Med Assoc* 172:903, 1978.

VETERINARY HEALTH CARE TEAM

Whereas the majority of veterinary practices were one-person practices in the twentieth century, a major shift has been occurring recently toward larger groups of veterinarians and support staff working in the same facility. This shift to increase the size of veterinary teams is being driven by an explosion of veterinary information, a demand for more and better pet health care by pet owners, and the need for a more economic and efficient delivery of veterinary services.

The team approach to veterinary practice allows different members of the team to focus on the areas of responsibility for which they have been trained and should leverage an increase of the veterinarians' effectiveness and productivity. It has also increased the demand for certified veterinary technicians. Although each member of the veterinary health care team has a different role, members must be hired and organized to work together efficiently as an effective team rather than as competing or isolated individuals.

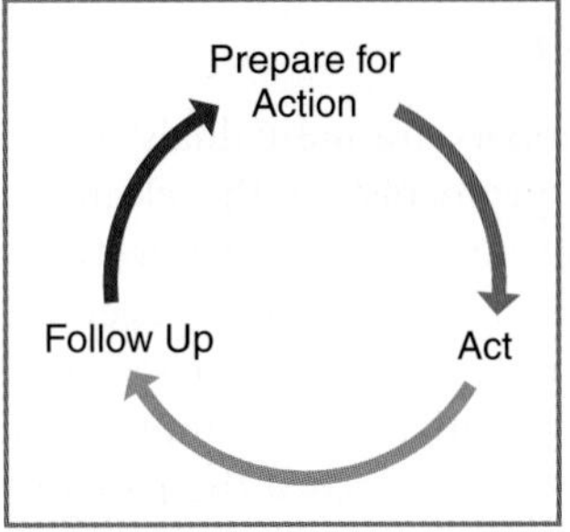

FIGURE 3-20 Action cycle.

The veterinary health care team is composed of the veterinarian(s), practice manager, veterinary technician(s), veterinary technologist(s), veterinary technician specialist(s), veterinary assistant(s), ward staff, and receptionist(s). Refer to the introduction for a description of team members except for practice manager, ward staff, and receptionist, which will be discussed here.

VETERINARY PRACTICE MANAGER

Veterinarians also managed their practices through most of the last century when one-person practices were prevalent. An increasing number of veterinarians (especially in group practices) are delegating the business management responsibilities to a practice manager. Medium-sized practices may divide these duties between several members of their veterinary team. In large practices, a full-time, bachelor of science (BS)–trained individual may serve as the veterinary practice manager (VPM).

Because veterinary practices are small businesses, the practice manager's role is to facilitate an efficiently operated and profitable medical business. The duties of the manager usually include hiring, supervising, and terminating personnel; managing inventory; handling client financial issues; facilitating accounting procedures needed for case control; analyzing progress toward goals; and developing and initiating new protocols for areas of hospital operation.

The owners in concert with the hospital manager and other team members must develop the mission statement and strategic plan for growth or change. The practice manager is delegated the responsibility for making day-to-day management decisions to meet these goals for the business. The practice manager must also unite the team of veterinarians and support staff to work well together to meet the practice goals. Another management challenge necessary for business is the development of a marketing plan for the practice (discussed at the end of this chapter).

WARD STAFF

Ward staff members are individuals trained on the job to follow specific protocols for the cleaning and sanitation required to prevent nosocomial infections. They perform the basic husbandry required for keeping patients clean, groomed, fed, watered, and exercised with the safety and comfort of each patient taken into consideration. Ward staff must observe and record the patient's appetites, attitudes, bowel movements, and urinary output and alert the staff about observed abnormal behavior. They also move patients from the wards to the treatment area, to the reception area for discharge, or to surgery. They may also be assigned basic janitorial duties in the rest of the hospital. Ward staff can also double as veterinary assistants through cross-training.

RECEPTIONISTS

Receptionists facilitate client service, communicate a sense of friendliness and helpfulness, and organize appointments so that clients do not have to wait an unreasonable amount of time. The receptionist is a key position in any hospital operation. The "life blood" of the practice (clients) must filter through the receptionist via the telephone and one-on-one contact in the reception area. The old adages that "you don't have a second chance to make a first impression" and "the receptionist will make or break the practice" are key issues for selecting receptionists.

Receptionists have the critical role of handling the fee payments, billings, and daily cash records. These duties must be performed effectively to keep the business running smoothly, clients happy, and the rest of the veterinary team aware of what is happening with clients and their pets. Receptionists are often the last person communicating with the client at checkout and can assess the general client satisfaction level when clients leave the premises. The business needs satisfied clients who will return as continuing clients and refer their friends and associates. The receptionist's effectiveness is key to practice growth and happy clients. The receptionist may also be referred to as a client relations specialist.

PERSONNEL MANAGEMENT

Personnel management is important because the greatest percentage of overhead is in personnel. All personnel must work as a team to ensure productivity. Working with someone is always better than working for someone. All practice employees (including veterinarians) must be as productive as possible to provide a profitable and pleasant work environment. Veterinarians and technicians are usually not professionally trained to be managers. Both must work together to have a successfully managed practice, which will result in greater career satisfaction, not just a job.

Regardless of the size of the practice and how it is managed, each position within the practice should have a backup person who is cross-trained in that area to take over when sickness, vacation, and emergencies arise. Without a cross-training plan, the practice may become crippled when one person is gone. This is especially true in smaller practices. In most practices, the staff duties can be divided into the following job areas: (1) reception; (2) examination room or outpatient duties; (3) inpatient duties; and (4) building, kennel, and barn maintenance. The reception area is staffed and operated by one or more receptionists.

They must be friendly and caring people. The entire mood of the practice and, to a great extent, the attitude of the client will be determined by the communication skills and judgment of the receptionist. For example, the receptionist should screen patients and schedule undiagnosed medical problems or cases requiring radiography earlier in the day so that the client will have a diagnosis before the day's end. Emergencies obviously need immediate attention. The receptionist greets clients, starts the medical record by obtaining some history, answers questions by telephone, makes appointments, handles the records for patient dismissal, answers general medical questions, quotes certain fees, maintains a schedule of all veterinarians, handles money and bank deposits, and manages accounts receivable and other duties as assigned. In short, an effective receptionist in most practices is a superperson.

A veterinary technician is usually assigned to examination room duties. In some practices, the receptionist and examination room duties will be performed by one person. The role of this individual may include backup or fill-in for the receptionist in addition to assisting in the examination rooms; obtaining medical histories; filling prescriptions; restraining patients; administering medications; demonstrating treatment techniques to clients; obtaining blood samples; performing laboratory work; escorting patients to the wards; dismissing patients; maintaining the examination, laboratory, and pharmacy areas in a clean and orderly manner; and other duties necessary for a smooth patient flow in the public areas of the hospital. Efficiency is enhanced with multiple examination rooms and an assistant or orderly assigned to assist both the technician and veterinarian. Every patient must be examined by a veterinarian to make the diagnosis to ensure that existing problems are not overlooked (e.g., hernias, retained testicles, heart murmurs, external parasites). Patients should not be admitted unless a veterinarian has had contact with the patient and client to establish a legal client-patient-veterinarian relationship.

The duties in the inpatient area are more isolated, and there is usually less client contact. Most of these duties are performed by a team of technicians and assistants. These duties include administering anesthetic or monitoring anesthesia, preparing patients for surgery, monitoring surgical and postsurgical patients; surgical assisting; collecting laboratory samples; performing dental cleanings; administering and monitoring treatments; exposing and developing radiographs; performing laboratory tests; maintaining medical records; maintaining surgical and anesthesia logs; providing direct medical and surgical nursing care; and maintaining the surgery, treatment, and radiology areas.

Maintaining the building, barn, and wards in a clean and orderly manner and other duties necessary for hospitalized patients to be well cared for are usually delegated to assistants and caretakers and supervised by a veterinary technician. Animal caretakers and ward staff clean, bed, and feed patients, allowing the veterinary technician to perform additional technical support functions. The role of the technician is determined by the staffing and delegation patterns and the size and type of practice.

A veterinary technician must be able to work in all areas of the hospital. The most common technical support use in veterinary practices involves the generalist type of veterinary technician. For a technician to function effectively as a generalist, a broad base of information and techniques must be mastered and maintained with cross-training in all technical areas. Being a high-quality generalist is not an easy task.

Large private and institutional teaching hospital practices have the caseload to allow the technical staff to become skilled in one area. Examples of these areas would be surgery, intensive care, anesthesiology, cardiology, internal medicine, ophthalmology, dermatology, radiology, clinical pathology, and office management. Specialty societies and certifications for veterinary technicians are now available in critical care, dentistry, anesthesia, behavior, and management (Box 3-5).

BOX 3-5 Societies With or Developing Specialty Certification Programs

Academy of Veterinary Emergency and Critical Care Technicians (AVECCT) www.avecct.org: AVECCT members can be certified as veterinary technician specialists in emergency and critical care and will use VTS (Emergency/Critical Care) after their name and state certification [i.e., Jane Doe, RVT, VTS (Emergency/Critical Care)].

Academy of Veterinary Dental Technicians (AVDT) www.avdt.us

Academy of Veterinary Technician Anesthetists (AVTA) www.avta-vts.org

Society of Veterinary Behavior Technicians (SVBT) www.svbt.org

Veterinary Hospital Managers Association, Inc. (VHMA) www.vhma.org: To be certified, a VHMA member must be actively employed as a veterinary practice manager (not necessarily a technician or DVM), achieve 18 college credit hours in business management, pass VHMA written and oral examinations, and participate in 6 days of management continuing education every 2 years. The designation of certified veterinary practice manager (CVPM) is conveyed to successful applicants (i.e., Jane Doe, CVPM; if a registered technician, Jane Doe, RVT, CVPM).

DELEGATION PRINCIPLES

Personnel costs may be reduced by hiring the correct personnel for the job and delegating properly. Too many practices are still trying to hire a new veterinarian to perform veterinary technician duties. Many also hire veterinary technicians to perform non–income-producing duties of assistants and caretakers. Consequently the practice spends more money than necessary on personnel and frustrates a new veterinarian or technician in the process in addition to limiting income produced.

Both veterinarians and veterinary technicians should be paid according to gross income produced; therefore aides and assistants hired at near minimum-wage levels should be relied on as much as possible to perform most non–income-producing tasks, such as restraint, general cleaning, and animal husbandry. Veterinarians should focus on making diagnoses, prescribing treatments, and performing surgery and delegate billable treatments, such as anesthesia, dental prophylaxes, imaging, and laboratory procedures, to certified veterinary technicians. The delegation of routine examination and/or communication procedures to the veterinary technician in the examination room allows the veterinarian to greatly increase efficiency.

JOB DESCRIPTIONS

Regardless of position in the hospital setting, all personnel should have a detailed job description. A job description will allow both the employee and management to maintain a clear understanding of current and new areas of responsibility. Job descriptions are also useful when hiring new employees or replacing employees.

Through the use of job descriptions (expectations) and periodic performance evaluations, employees can be rewarded according to their performance, poor workers can be guided and encouraged to improve, and chronically poor workers can be discharged. One of the most common mistakes in personnel management is to put off regular employee evaluations. Personnel problems resulting from poor work performance do not just go away; they only become worse. A job evaluation system that is applied equally and fairly to all employees needs to be maintained. Employees cannot improve their performance unless they are given an opportunity to identify shortcomings. If improvement is not observed within a reasonable period of time, both the practice and employee will probably be better off with employee dismissal.

HIRING PROCEDURES

When hiring a new employee, it is important that all employees have input into the decision if teamwork is to be expected. This is an important decision. The cost of selection, training, and adaptation can equal 1 year's salary. A bad choice means disruption, turnover, and a loss of thousands of dollars to the practice.

A simple method of candidate evaluation that will satisfy most employees is to have two or three employees interview each candidate first and make recommendations to the veterinarian. The screening committee should establish some specific questions for each interviewer to ask each candidate using the job description prepared for that specific job. The recommendations made to the veterinarian should include job suitability, personality, professionalism, knowledge, experience, dress, and other interview assessments. The veterinarian should have the final word on hiring and firing unless a practice manager has been hired for personnel management.

The major steps in the hiring process are as follows:

1. Analyze personnel requirements.
2. Develop a specific job description.
3. Develop a set of interview questions.
4. Announce and advertise the position.
5. Review the applications and résumés.
6. Rank the candidates for interview.
7. Check references.
8. Interview the top-ranked two to four candidates.
9. Make a final selection.
10. Offer the job to the best candidate and set salary.
11. Establish a starting date.
12. Provide full orientation on the first workday.

The analysis of personnel requirements will be done by the veterinarian or office manager based on the needs of the practice or business. Once the general need for the position or positions has been established (or replacement approved), a detailed job description must be prepared or the previous job description updated. The job description is usually developed on one page and consists of four or five job functions outlined in one or two sentences each. Each job function is then assigned a percentage of time. Once the job description is developed or updated, it can be used to write the advertisement to search for a specific individual. To prepare for the interview, a set of interview questions needs to be developed.

Some interview questions are unlawful or discriminatory and must not be asked (e.g., questions on race, religion, national origin, gender, handicaps, marital status). Questions should always be open ended (Box 3-6) and allow the candidates to express themselves. The following requests and questions could be considered when preparing interview questions:

1. Please review your previous position.
2. Describe your best boss.
3. Describe your worst boss.
4. What did you like best about your last position?
5. What did you like least about your last position?
6. What specific skills and abilities do you have that apply to this particular position?
7. What are your short-range and long-term employment goals?
8. What accomplishments have made you most proud?
9. What type of working relationships do you want to cultivate?
10. How do you feel about constructive criticism and formal performance evaluation?
11. How do you feel about being on call several times per month?
12. Do you have any questions you would like to ask?

BOX 3-6 Communication Techniques for Interviewing Client

- Open-ended (or probing) questions
  Who?
  How?
  What?
  When?
  Where?
- Leading (yes/no) questions
  Did (this happen, you like it, etc.)?
  Was it (good, bad, etc.)?
- Answers will be yes or no even if client is not sure.
- Answers will be detailed descriptions.

One-Word Acknowledgement

Use one word (e.g., oh, OK, yes) with eye contact and voice inflection that imply you understand and want him or her to continue talking. This can be done with eye contact, nonverbal signs of active listening, and verbal silence with some clients.

Accent Questions

Restate one or two words used by the client in a questioning tone, which serves to request the client to elaborate on the description of events or signs.

Paraphrasing

Restate client statements (in your own words) to check with the client whether you understand what the client is trying to say before going on in the interview. Use paraphrasing periodically in each segment of the interview to give the client an opportunity to clarify or confirm your understanding.

Summarizing

Restate main points at the end (or at end of major segments) to emphasize key points and inform the client about what is going to happen next.

During the interview, the evaluator should ask each candidate the same questions so the responses can be objectively compared. The interview period is the time to evaluate motivation, personal appearance, and personal hygiene. The job description, salary, and benefits should be reviewed. Each interviewer or interview team should limit their part of the interview to 30 minutes.

After the interview, personal references should be checked and past supervisors contacted. When all the above material has been collected and weighed, the individual who is the best person (and match) for the position should be offered the job.

When the final selection has been made, the most common initial contact will be by telephone. During the telephone call, the job description should be reviewed, salary and benefits discussed, and starting date established. When the above steps are followed, the best candidate should be more easily identified and successfully hired. Other candidates should be notified that the position has been filled with the applicant who best matched the position.

A potential problem in personnel management is inadequate internal communication. To avoid internal disputes, weekly (or monthly) staff meetings should be held to update all employees on various aspects of hospital operation. Often, notes on a blackboard just do not do the job. These meetings can also be used to develop teamwork via group problem-solving techniques and role playing in communication skills.

> TECHNICIAN NOTE Practice staff meetings should be held at least once per month to ensure open communication.

ROLE OF VETERINARY TECHNICIANS AND VETERINARIANS IN MANAGEMENT

Technicians have an ever-increasing role in practice management. In most practice situations, technicians will be involved in the management of the patient, client, equipment, and inventory. They may also be involved in staff, facility, and business management. To develop management skills, one must be willing to assume increasing levels of responsibility. As the practice changes in staffing, number of cases, facility, type of clients, new technologies, and so forth, the veterinary technician must adapt his or her management skills to these changes.

The role of the veterinary technician in management will vary depending on the type of practice and the previous experiences of the technician and the veterinarian. The technician who can (1) conceptualize the vision and goals set by the veterinarian for the practice, (2) efficiently organize each area in which he or she is given responsibility, (3) become a productive team player and a good communicator, and (4) develop the ability to solve problems constructively to enhance both patient care and the veterinary team will usually be given a greater role in practice management.

To be effective, the veterinarian-owner must act as the overall hospital chief executive officer (CEO) and delegate appropriate areas of responsibility to the veterinary technician and to other members of the team. The effective delegation of responsibility to the technician must include billable (income-producing) technical procedures of medical and surgical nursing. Ideally, veterinarians diagnose, prescribe, and perform surgery; technicians perform venipunctures, laboratory tests, and prescribed treatments; expose and develop radiographs; and anesthetize, prepare, and manage recovery of surgical patients. The veterinary technician should also delegate most non–income-producing tasks to lower-paid aides, assistants, or animal caretakers. Clinic aides restrain, move, feed, and exercise the animals and assist both technicians and veterinarians when needed. Receptionists handle scheduling, receiving, discharging, billing, and related front office duties. There should be a direct relationship between the salary level paid and the income produced (productivity) for each veterinary technician and veterinarian in a practice if effective delegation is occurring.

> TECHNICIAN NOTE The veterinary technician should delegate most non–income-producing tasks to assistants or aides.

Practice management efforts are necessary in all types of practice. To be effective, the veterinarian and veterinary technician must be human resources managers. This requires both excellent communication skills and a policy and procedures manual for the practice team. It involves hiring, training, and scheduling performance appraisals and the discharge of staff. The veterinarian and technician must work together with the rest of the staff as both a management team and a medical team. Unfortunately, most colleges provide little training in hospital or people management for either technicians or veterinarians because it takes students so much time and effort to gain the medical expertise, technical skills, and confidence necessary to succeed medically. However, there are many new resources available to meet this need for management training after graduation, including continuing education short courses, books, journals, organizations, Internet courses (i.e., veterinary information network–www.vin.com), and consultants.

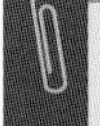

> TECHNICIAN NOTE Never argue with a dissatisfied client.

PATIENT MANAGEMENT

Patient management and client management go hand in hand. Both should be handled together, but for the sake of this discussion they are treated separately.

Patient management can best be described by outlining the typical case as it moves through the hospital. The first contact is with the receptionist. The receptionist should move the patient and client as quickly as possible into an examination room. A patient presented as an emergency should receive priority. An emergency case is always any case that the owner believes is an emergency. Most of these cases are not emergencies, but each should be managed as if it were to ensure client satisfaction with quality of service.

In many practices, the patient will be escorted into the examination room by a veterinary technician. The technician will continue to develop the medical record by obtaining the temperature, pulse, respiration, and weight of the patient. Additional informational questions are asked to establish a preliminary history, and a brief physical examination may also be helpful to the veterinarian (see Box 3-6).

Once the veterinarian enters the examination room, the patient and owner should be introduced to the veterinarian by the technician. Name tags should be worn by all personnel to help clients remember who they have met and who is the veterinarian. A veterinary assistant or technician should assist the veterinarian in the physical examination by restraining the patient as necessary. If blood, urine, or skin specimens are needed, the technician should usually take the patient to the treatment room and conduct these procedures away from the client with the help of an assistant while the veterinarian is seeing another client and patient. Once a diagnosis has been made by the veterinarian, the patient will either be treated and released or hospitalized.

If the patient is to be treated and released, the technician will often administer the treatment and will prepare prescriptions as needed. The technician will explain (or demonstrate) how to administer home medications or treatments and will then escort the client to the receptionist for dismissal and fee payment.

When the patient is to be hospitalized, the assistant or technician will escort the patient to the ward and ensure that the necessary items are present to make the patient comfortable. The veterinarian will establish each treatment regimen and evaluate its success. During hospitalization, the technician will maintain and manage most routine treatments, therapy, laboratory tests, and medical records and delegate exercise, feeding, restraint, and grooming to assistants or animal caretakers. Often the daily telephone contact with the client will be through the technician. A blackboard or bulletin board in the treatment room can be used to remind personnel of the diagnostic, treatment, and surgery schedules for hospitalized patients. All patients should be evaluated several times each day, and these evaluations should be documented with appropriate entries into the medical record. Walking through daily ward rounds can be helpful to all personnel to keep everyone updated on each case.

The dismissal of a hospitalized patient is similar to that of the outpatient except that dispensed medications and patient cleanup must be completed before the owner's arrival. When dismissing a hospitalized patient, the following points should be considered:

- An itemized fee statement should be ready at the time the owner is called to pick up the animal.
- All medications should be dispensed in child-proof containers with proper labels.
- The veterinarian should be available for consultation with the client.
- The technician should be available to demonstrate treatment and home-care techniques with handout instructions for home reference.
- Fee collection should take place.
- The next appointment or recheck should be scheduled.
- The patient should be presented dry, clean, and odor free.

Some conditions dictate that the patient be presented before fee collection and the scheduling of the next appointment. When this occurs, someone should be available to hold or control the animal until the client has completed the dismissal process. The technician can be extremely valuable during the dismissal process by explaining to the client what to do if specific events occur (through reinforcement of directions given by the veterinarian). Clients will often ask technicians questions that they forgot or were afraid to ask the veterinarian.

Most clients will judge the medical care an animal has received by the condition and appearance of the animal at dismissal. The patient should always be as clean or cleaner than when admitted. If an animal soils itself just before dismissal, always clean or bathe the animal before sending it home, even if the client has to wait a few minutes longer. The client should be informed that the animal has accidentally soiled itself and that you are cleaning it up: "We certainly do not want him to leave dirty." When dismissing surgical patients, in addition to the animal itself being clean, the surgical incision, bandages, splint, or cast must be clean and dry. The surgery technique will often be judged by the neatness of hair removal at the surgical site and the appearance of the incision.

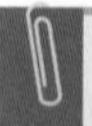

TECHNICIAN NOTE Never send a patient home that has soiled itself or has an unpleasant odor.

INVENTORY MANAGEMENT

The purpose of inventory management and control is to always have every drug, vaccine, or supply item available when needed for use (or sale) yet not waste money acquiring and storing extra supplies that are not needed in the near future. This is a delicate balance because the amount and selected use of drugs and supplies can change rapidly. Close attention to inventory levels of surgical supplies, pet food, pharmaceuticals, vaccines, x-ray film, and other items will ensure that an adequate stock is maintained without oversupply if an effective inventory control system is being used to reorder and replenish items before they are gone.

If too much stock is on hand, extra money and storage space are committed and the stock will be paid for long before the last of it is used. If too little is kept on hand, needed items will sometimes not be available to provide the preferred treatment for the patient or an opportunity for profiting from the sale of a product will be missed. If the right amount is on hand, the veterinarians and staff always have what is needed, large amounts do not have to be ordered and stored, and much of it is used before the payment to the supplier is due, creating the needed cash flow to pay the supplier.

Inventory is the second largest expense area of operating a veterinary practice. Drugs should be used and be replaced about every 45 to 60 days (a turnover rate of six to eight times per year). The formula that is used for computing turnover rate is listed in Box 3-7. Turnover can be computed for every item in the inventory, averaged for the total inventory, or focused on the 20% of the items that account for the majority (80%) of uses (Pareto's law). Some inventory items will naturally turn over every 2 to 3 weeks (12 to 18 times per year), such as pet food, and often much or all of the item will be sold, generating income before the supplier requires payment.

Practice managers, sometimes veterinary technicians or a veterinarian, and occasionally reception staff or an assistant will be assigned responsibility for inventory control.

BOX 3-7 Inventory Management Formulas

Turnover rate* of an item = yearly inventory expense for item ÷ average cost of item on hand at any one time

Average cost of inventory on hand at one time = (inventory at midyear + inventory at year's end) ÷ 2

Modified from Lukens RI, Landon RM: *Effective inventory control,* West Chester, Pa, 1993, SmithKline Beecham.

*Pareto's law, or the 80/20 rule, states that 20% of the items account for 80% of the annual inventory expenses; this suggests that the above formulas should be used to evaluate and adjust the turnover rate of the biggest expense items to attain the "ideal turnover rate."

Sometimes the responsibilities are divided among several staff members. One person should be the primary person placing orders, making sure that what is received is what was ordered and/or billed, and authorizing payment for the shipments. It is also important to set up an inventory master list of all items in stock in the hospital; keep a pharmacy library of all company product inserts, catalogs, and ordering procedures; and keep a file of MSDSs for all products as required by OSHA.

Considerable money is involved in inventory purchases. Much can be lost through inadequate inventory control procedures. This loss may occur because the business was billed for materials that were never shipped or never received at the practice, or the business was double billed for one shipment, billed for damaged goods, or billed for more or different items than were received. Back orders that are not canceled when the product is reordered elsewhere double the inventory. Losses also occur because of ordering too many months' supply of perishable vaccines, biologics, antibiotics, and reagents that deteriorate beyond the printed expiration date on the container and are no longer effective or legally safe to use. Oversupply also crowds the shelf and storage space and leads to more misplacement and overordering or loss from not rotating new items to the back and oldest products forward to be used first. The best stock rotation system is "first in, first out" (FIFO).

The sales representative's responsibility is to sell their product and "deals" that may provide more product than can be used in 1 or 2 months. It makes little sense to buy and store a year's supply of an item, no matter how much the price has been reduced. On the other hand, during a seasonal increase of use of a product, it will make sense to buy a large supply instead of the normal 1-month supply, particularly if the price has been cut significantly.

There are many computerized and manual inventory systems available for upgrading a current practice's procedures for inventory control. Because computerized systems require the input of everything that is sold and used to be accurate, they are only moderately successful in providing all the inventory control information needed (see Chapter 4). Manual procedures, such as identifying minimum stock reorder points on the shelf, posting want lists or reorder bins for all staff to use, and taking frequent inventory count of all supplies, can go a long way to help the computerized inventory control process be a success.

An effective inventory control system should be easy to use, ensure that all medications and supplies are available when needed, and reduce expenses by achieving a turnover rate of 8 to 12 times per year. It should provide a signal when each item needs to be reordered, track seasonal variations, track past usage rates, and provide purchase cost information to keep the pricing and supply of products current. It should ensure that ordered items are actually received and back-ordered items are tracked so that overordering does not occur. It should also be easy to account for when and where items are used so that cost can be allocated to various profit centers within the practice. It should ensure proper monitoring and handling of Drug Enforcement Agency (DEA) controlled substances, provide a procedure for checking invoices to make sure they are accurate for amounts ordered and prices quoted, and periodically assess the value of the inventory. It should also reduce the cost of ordering the supplies by taking advantage of minimum orders for prepaid shipments and discounts for early payments when available. The inventory control system should also allow the practice to obtain the best prices available, identify expired or outdated items for prompt removal and return to suppliers for credit if provided, and enable the manager to detect staff pilferage if it occurs.

All of these desirable results of managing inventory will not occur if someone is not put in charge of inventory control and given adequate time and support by all members of the veterinary team to accomplish the assignment.

CLIENT MANAGEMENT

The most important person in any practice is each client. The practice of veterinary medicine is truly a people business. Everyone in the practice must enjoy working with and problem solving for the clients served by the practice. Veterinarians and technicians who do not like working with clients and their animal problems should not be employed in practice because they are ineffective with client communication. Many other professional careers are now available for individuals who desire less public contact.

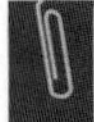

TECHNICIAN NOTE The most important person in any practice is each client.

VALUE OF THE CLIENT

The availability of veterinary services in the United States appears to be at an all-time high. New schools of veterinary medicine and expanded enrollment at existing schools have resulted in this increased availability of graduate veterinarians. The net result of the increasing supply of veterinary practitioners is increased competition for clients among established and new practices.

The practices that will financially survive must offer expanded services that are competitive. Practices can become more cost-effective by using both technicians and assistants effectively to leverage the veterinarians' productivity while expanding service.

How valuable is each client? The practice will collapse unless old clients are retained and new clients are continually entering the practice. Clients are the lifeblood of the practice. Everyone in the practice works for the client. Some practices would like to think that they control their clients, but client loyalty is seldom mandated. Loyalty is won with hard work and dedicated caring service to each client. The only unique product that a veterinary practice has to offer is service. If everyone in the practice understands that his or her primary role is to provide the finest quality medical care possible to the patient with the end result being a pleased and informed client, the practice will grow. If the staff attitude becomes one of negative feelings toward clients (e.g., not another one of these!), the practice clientele will dwindle. A practice's facilities, equipment, and techniques may be the finest available, but they will remain unused until enough clients willingly authorize or request that practice's services.

CLIENT SELECTION OF A VETERINARIAN

How does a client select a veterinarian? Most clients with small animals will select a veterinarian because the practice location is convenient. Following closely after practice location, recommendations from friends are ranked next. Once a practice is selected, the individual veterinarian will be evaluated in the following areas: friendly and caring personality, gentleness in handling the animal, communication skills, and professional knowledge. In the selection process, it becomes readily apparent that practice location, facility appearance, and recommendations from satisfied clients are extremely important to practice growth.

Once the client enters the hospital, the ability of the veterinarian and staff to project a concerned, caring personality; the expertise used in carefully handling the animal; and the clarity of the communication are the most important determining factors. It is interesting to note that professional knowledge falls to the bottom of the list. The general public has a limited informational basis by which to judge the professional knowledge of a physician, dentist, attorney, or veterinarian.

TECHNICIAN NOTE Practice location and personal referrals are the two most common methods by which new clients find a veterinarian.

When does the veterinary technician have an impact on the client selection process? Clients always view the hospital staff as an extension of the veterinarian. A friendly personality, gentle patient-handling techniques, and caring communication skills become critically important in this whole process.

Clients with large animals usually select a veterinarian based on recommendations from others. Once the veterinarian arrives at the farm or ranch, the retention and satisfaction issues are the same as the ones used by small animal owners with the addition of economic return. In food animal practice, the veterinarian must become an economic asset to the overall farm profitability or the client cannot afford to seek veterinary services. Companion animal practice (i.e., small animal, horse) has some economic limits, but the sentimental and emotional attachment (human-animal bond) of the client to the animal is relied on to extend that economic limit, which the food animal client may not do.

EVALUATION OF THE CLIENT

The technician's attitude toward himself or herself will be reflected in how clients are handled. People who are happy and positive about themselves and what they are doing will find that this attitude dominates client relations. One of the most contagious attitudes is enthusiasm. Enthusiastic people turn other people on! Enthusiasm is caught, not taught. The client must be handled effectively so that staff members do not cause a positive client to become negative. Conversely, veterinary personnel should deal with a negative client in a friendly and positive manner, identifying his or her concerns and needs, and trying to help find a solution.

Generally, after working with a client for a short period of time, a staff member will get enough feedback to make some judgments about the client's expectations. These expectations are in the form of client-pet relationships, client-hospital relationships, and one-on-one personal relationships. One should not judge clients by their outward appearance only. Clients who appear to have nothing materially may value their animal highly and spend their resources to support veterinary care. In contrast, clients who drive up in a luxury car and have expensive clothes may not have the animal's best interests in mind and may be financially overextended. You cannot always judge a book by its cover, and you cannot judge people by their appearance.

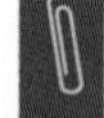

TECHNICIAN NOTE Do not judge the client's ability to pay by his or her appearance.

In most instances, the technician and veterinarian will have to discuss the perceived pet's value with the client and give the client the opportunity to express himself or herself. One of the most important roles in communication with clients is to establish the value of the animal within the client-pet relationship. Some clients will be difficult to really figure out, and veterinary personnel may never believe that they understand the client's intent or interest level.

CLIENT TRAFFIC FLOW PATTERNS

When the client first enters the reception area, the admission process begins. The receptionist initiates the proper business and medical records for each case. The client is escorted into one of the examination rooms. A preliminary history and examination (including temperature, pulse, and respiration [TPR]) may be taken by the technician before the veterinarian arrives. After examination and consultation with the veterinarian, either the client will leave the animal (hospitalization for further diagnostic tests, treatment, surgery, or observation) or the patient will be treated and, if necessary, medication will be dispensed before the patient returns to the receptionist for dismissal. In the event the patient is dismissed (outpatient), the client settles the account and is scheduled to return for a reexamination or to call with a follow-up report. During the routine outpatient visit, the client usually only contacts the outpatient work area. The client's traffic pattern for an outpatient visit is reception to admission to examination (to pharmacy to laboratory) to dismissal.

If the patient is hospitalized, the client may have some contact with the inpatient area in addition to the outpatient area. A typical client traffic pattern in the hospitalized case would be reception to admission to examination to treatment area or surgical area to hospitalization to admission (discussion of dismissal and payment-credit policy). The client would leave the hospital and return to the reception area on the day of dismissal.

On dismissal of hospitalized cases, the client enters the reception area and usually receives the patient's information from the receptionist or technician. The client proceeds to the examination room for a brief consultation with the veterinarian followed by home-care instructions and demonstrations from the technician (Figure 3-21). To reduce confusion at dismissal, it is advisable for the client to return to the dismissal area and settle the account before the patient is presented. Once the patient has been returned to the client, communication may be difficult during the reunion process.

In addition to the routine and outpatient client traffic pattern, a third type of contact exists when the client visits a hospitalized patient. In this event, the client usually makes an appointment with the receptionist to visit the animal at a specific time that is convenient to both the client and the hospital operation. When the client arrives, he or she will proceed directly to the examination or treatment room. Visiting patients in the ward is usually discouraged because other patients in the ward are disturbed. During the visit with the animal, a technician (or veterinarian) should be present to answer questions concerning care and progress made by the patient. The client should always visit with the veterinarian at some point in the examination room or the treatment room or in the veterinarian's private office.

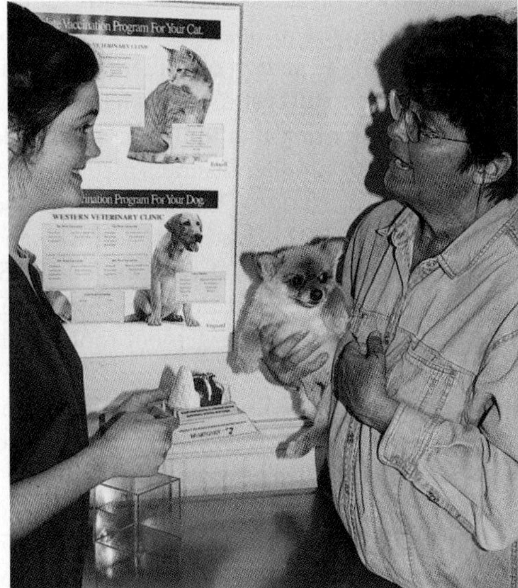

FIGURE 3-21 Veterinary technician uses a heartworm model to enhance client understanding of the impact of heartworm disease.

Client visits are often beneficial for both the hospitalized patient and the client. The mental attitudes of client and patient can be strengthened, and communication can be improved between the veterinarian and client. Client visits should be encouraged rather than discouraged.

OFFICE PROCEDURES

General office procedure knowledge is required of all staff in a veterinary practice. The staff (veterinarians, technicians, assistants, office managers) needs to have a working knowledge of how appointments are made, personnel staffed, fees developed and collected, inventory ordered and controlled, and pet insurance used. Most practices have a limited number of staff positions; everyone must have the ability to perform basic office procedures. The ability to perform other jobs is obtained through cross-training.

The additional information needed to perform the work of others is acquired by being cross-trained through working in different jobs while being trained in one's new job. This allows most jobs to be temporally performed by different people when a person is out sick or on vacation. In small businesses, this ability to fill in with other staff is essential to maintain a smooth-running business.

APPOINTMENTS

Companion animal practices can operate either through the use of an appointment or a walk-in system. Each system has advantages and disadvantages, but the appointment system is preferred by most veterinarians. Appointments allow the practice to control the flow of clients and patients into specific time periods that will improve the efficiency of the work schedule. When more clients are scheduled, more staff can be made available during the busier periods; on the other hand, when no appointments are scheduled, staff numbers can be reduced.

The appointment system usually functions around the scheduling of consultation times (office visits) in 15-, 20-, or 30-minute blocks. When 15-minute blocks are used, then four appointments per hour can be scheduled. Companion animal practices usually schedule 3 or 4 hours of appointment times in the morning and afternoon. A typical appointment period might be from 8 AM to 12 PM and 3 PM to 6 PM. Between noon and 3 PM, case work-ups, treatments, and surgery are performed.

Because of clients' work schedules, practices are now scheduling consultations in the evening to help meet the needs of the working family. Several evenings may be scheduled from 6 PM to 8 PM. Saturdays are also becoming more important to many clients because Monday through Friday are filled with work and family activities. In many practices, Saturday is becoming the busiest day of the week.

The walk-in practice is the other method of scheduling. When using this work schedule, clients simply come in whenever they want and wait to be seen. The advantages to the client are not having to make an appointment and the ability to drop in at the practice when it is convenient. The disadvantages are the length of wait time and the congestion when several clients come in at the same time. For the practice, the major disadvantage is not having the ability to plan and somewhat control and spread the workload to prevent several people coming at the same time.

To change from a walk-in practice to an appointment schedule requires planning and communication with the client. The first step is to set up 1 hour for appointments in the morning and 1 hour for appointments in the afternoon. As clients come into the practice for service or call the practice, explain that for the convenience of the client the practice has changed to an appointment schedule. Each client should be encouraged to use the appointment system the next time. As more and more clients are educated about the use and convenience of the appointment system, the 1-hour periods are expanded. Eventually, only 30 minutes of unscheduled time is left in the morning and afternoon for walk-ins and semiemergencies.

Emergency cases are accepted at any time and are given priority over all appointments. However, if a client with an appointment and a walk-in client come into the practice at the same time, the client with the appointment is always given preference. Walk-in clients are always serviced, but they should not be given priority over a client with an appointment unless it is a true emergency. Walk-in clients should never be turned away just because they do not have an appointment.

PRACTICE SCHEDULING

More and more people are now employed outside the home, so clients often have difficulty in visiting the practice between 8 AM and 5 PM Monday through Friday. To help solve this problem, many practices now are expanding their consultation hours in the evening and on Saturdays. Some practices also offer early drop-off or late pickup service. This requires the veterinarian to communicate directly with the owner before the pickup or drop-off time. Cell phone use has greatly improved communication directly with the client.

The technician will also need to be able to discuss the case with the owner when he or she arrives at the practice during these extended hours since the veterinarian may not always be available.

In addition to extending the hours, the staff must be scheduled to provide coverage during all practice hours. If the practice is open 6 days per week and operates 10 hours per day, support staff must be limited to a work schedule of 40 hours per week so that overtime can be kept at a minimum. Veterinarians who are nonowners are usually scheduled between 38 and 45 hours per week.

The larger the number of employees in the practice, the more scheduling flexibility is available. Early morning, late evening, and Saturday periods are usually rotated so that everyone shares in these hours. If part-time employees are used, they could be scheduled into these extended hours and relieve the full-time staff. The use of part-time employees greatly increases the flexibility to cover the expanded hours necessary to meet clients' needs. Part-time employees are more available now for both professional and support staff and can be readily used for coverage of extended hours.

PROFESSIONAL FEES

The only money available for funding a veterinary practice is collected from the clients as professional fees for professional medical services and products purchased. Loans from a bank will have to be obtained to cover deficits when there are more expenses than income. The veterinary business is vulnerable to failure if sufficient income is not received from enough clients to pay the operating costs of the business.

There are no government subsidies, few if any donations, and small amounts of money from pet insurance companies paid to veterinary practices. All employees must understand that their salary level is directly related to the health of the business and their productivity in generating income from billable tasks and product sales. Health care teams must be effectively organized with this principle in mind or the business will deteriorate.

Each veterinary practice should set fees based on what it costs to deliver services. However, the methods used for determining fees vary from practice to practice just like the cost of land and staffing of the facilities will vary. Methods used to set fees vary from accounting methods for establishing fees based on the cost of offering the service to a competitive guess of trying to match or undercut the price that other practices charge to just estimating what each client can afford. Only the accounting method is an acceptable business procedure. In 2002 another business method of evaluating fees was developed (National Commission of Veterinary Economic Issues [NCVEI]). This online service can be accessed by any AVMA member at www.ncvei.org. Specific fees can be observed based on national, regional, and state data. There are currently 38 management tools available at NCVEI.

Many veterinarians try to discount fees to a level that they think the client can afford. However, it is impossible to accurately judge what a client can afford and is willing to spend. Only the client can freely decide what the animal means to him or her and what he or she is willing to pay. Discounting fees will eventually lead to reducing the quality of medical service, and that is unfair to the patient. It may also expose the team to charges of negligence and legal liabilities if the quality of care is below the accepted standard of care offered in similar practices in the area.

The practice manager or accountant must be able to identify the indirect costs and direct costs of operating the business via the financial reports to set or adjust the fees. Several steps are required to arrive at the appropriate fee for each procedure based on the cost of providing that service or product. First, direct costs are identified for each procedure related to the expendables used (drugs, bandages, film, etc.). Amortization of equipment costs over the equipment's expected useful life is also computed. For example, depreciating an x-ray machine over 7 years of useful life requires determining the number of x-rays taken per year from the radiology records. This will allow one to calculate the amount that must be included in the radiology fee for each x-ray taken. The machine will be paid for in the 7 years if the projected number of x-rays is taken (i.e., if the projected number of radiograph exposures is accurate).

The indirect costs (overhead) of operating a business must be computed. These include the purchase or rental of the land, construction or rental of the building, monthly cost of the utilities, facility upkeep, taxes, and interest on the debt. A new furnace, remodeling costs, and additions to the facility are either included as an annual cost or spread over several years. This cost of operation is added to each fee assessed as a percentage of overhead expense. It is spread over the number of expected client transactions in each fee to recover the indirect costs of overhead.

The biggest cost of running a professional business is the payroll for the staff. Veterinarians' salaries, whether they are owners or employees, and the salaries of the rest of the veterinary team must all be prorated to each fee. The accountant does this for each procedure based on time input for each of the team members. Therefore an estimate of the normal time the receptionist, veterinarian, veterinary technician, and veterinary assistant spend to support each service must be computed. Time is valued per minute using each salary level and adding the payroll overhead costs (often 30% or more of salary). This is multiplied by the average time each person spends on the procedure and added to that fee. Once computed, all fees should be reviewed semiannually and adjusted as cost increases occur because of inflation. Obviously, fees must be refigured if anything major changes with the staff's time, the length of the procedure, or the purchase of new equipment.

The goal is to charge fair and equitable fees to cover the practice's cost of providing each service to clients. The fees should support using modern equipment, paying appropriate salaries to keep an effective team employed, and providing a fair return on the investment to the owners for taking business risks.

Fees fall into two groups: shopped fees or nonshopped fees. The shopped fees (examination fee, vaccination fee, and elective surgery fees: neuter, spay, declaw, etc.) should be competitive with other area practices. The level of shopped fees should be controlled by the going rate of other practices in the immediate practice area. Clients will judge the level of all practice fees by how competitive the shopped fees seem to them when they call and shop your practice.

The other group of fees are the nonshopped fees (clients do not call and shop these services), which include all other services in the practice. Examples of nonshopped fees are treatment for diarrhea or vomiting, fracture repair, chest x-ray, complete blood count, general anesthesia, cystotomy, angiogram, and cataract surgery. Most fees in a practice are nonshopped. The practice can assess a fair fee for any of these services without concern about what other local practices are charging. The only fees that must be competitive are the shopped fees.

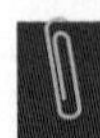
TECHNICIAN NOTE The only fees that must be competitive are the shopped fees.

The nonshopped fees should be increased by the inflation rate on at least an annual basis. If the annual inflation rate reaches 6%, the nonshopped fees should be adjusted on a quarterly or monthly basis. The rate of medical inflation can be estimated by multiplying the consumer price index (CPI) by a factor of 2 to 3. Smaller, regular increases are not noticed by the client as much as one large annual increase. The major fees that attract client attention are the shopped fees, and these are only adjusted when local area practices adjust theirs. Computerization allows fee adjustments to be made easily and quickly even when done on a monthly basis.

Practice computerization (see Chapter 4) has allowed practices to have a much more detailed listing of fees for services and products. Fee codes can easily run into the thousands, but are carefully adjusted and accounted for by the computer. This allows the client to receive a detailed invoice at the conclusion of the practice visit. Computer software can also provide the client with a detailed fee estimate before service. This allows the client to make an informed decision about the level of service desired before the service is actually provided. This level of communication with the client is necessary to control collections and monthly billing.

Practice managers, owners, and the accountants that set up the accounting system of the practice will use monthly and yearly statistical summaries of incomes and expenses for evaluating changing trends for different procedures in all areas of the hospital, including profit centers. The trends of change from month to month and year to year are easy to track and recognize. The productivity of each veterinarian and veterinary technician can also be tracked, with computerization software and salaries adjusted up or down based on productivity. In general, the software should provide the business reports containing necessary information to make management decisions on what fees should be raised or lowered. This system enhances and rewards motivation and helps manage change. In summary, the accounting procedure for setting professional fees provides the basis for managing an effective business that will change as costs and demand for services change. The fees should be evaluated and adjusted at least twice yearly as appropriate to keep the fees in line with the costs and practice goals.

COLLECTIONS AND BILLINGS

Most practices have a standard payment policy of payment in full at the time service is provided. Cash payment is always the best method of payment. However, some services can be expensive, and payment in full may not be possible at the time the service is rendered. Alternative payment plans are usually required if the service is to be provided.

Alternative payment plans include the use of bank credit cards (Master Card, Visa, Discover, American Express, etc.), medical credit cards (Care Credit), local bank credit, pet insurance, and practice credit accounts. After all of the above payment plans are discussed, the practice credit account should always be used as the last option. When internal credit is provided, specific controls must be in place. The usual controls for practice credit include approval of a credit application, a 50% deposit (initial payment) at the time the fee estimate (treatment plan) is given, the balance to be paid in three or four monthly payments, 1.5% per month interest charge on the unpaid balance, and payment of a monthly billing fee (usually \$3 to \$8). The monthly billing fee covers the cost of billing each client (computer time, personnel time, stationery, envelopes, postage).

The collection of a 50% initial payment based on the treatment plan at the time of admission is the standard way of determining how the client will pay the account. All hospitalized cases should have a written treatment plan prepared before service. Routine outpatient services usually do not receive a written treatment plan. True emergency cases are an exception to the written treatment rule because of the critical nature of the case. When a written treatment plan is prepared on a hospitalized case, the client will be informed by the business manager, technician, or veterinarian that it is hospital policy to collect a 50% initial payment before performing the requested services, and the balance of the account will be payable at dismissal. This allows the client and the practice the opportunity to discuss case finances before the service.

If the client determines the estimated services are too costly, the veterinarian will have an opportunity to recommend another possible treatment or method that is less costly or discuss credit options. By making routine use of a written treatment plan and 50% initial payment, the level of practice credit can be carefully controlled. The level of accounts receivable (practice credit) in a practice should not exceed 25% of the average of 1 month's gross income. As an example, the level of accounts receivable should not exceed \$25,000 in a practice grossing \$100,000 per month (\$1,200,000 annual gross income). If the level of accounts receivable goes beyond 25%, a more strict credit policy needs to be put in place or enforced.

Effective communications related to collecting the fee from the client begin with confident receptionists, technicians, and veterinarians who understand how the fee is computed and are confident that it is deserved and fair and truly represents the quality of service provided. An educated staff is more confident, positive, and informed in discussing fees with clients, whether at the time of the initial written treatment plan or at the time of payment or billing.

Billings charged by clients for future payments are called accounts receivable. The more accounts receivable grow, the less cash is available to pay ongoing expenses that include the payroll of the practice. The goal must be to collect (not charge) a fee according to a defined practice policy in a business manner that does not offend or alienate clients.

Most companion animal veterinarians attempt to collect all fees and not allow clients to charge. Increased credit card availability has allowed most clients to delay actual payments by transferring the charges to a credit card. This provides almost immediate payment to the business by the credit card company and prevents the practice from losing a significant amount of money from clients who will not or cannot pay their bills in the future. Credit card payment allows money to be immediately available to pay inventory purchases, apply to payroll, or pay other bills.

If credit is provided, the practice manager should be involved before the services are provided to approve the client's credit application, establish initial payment amounts, and develop a repayment schedule. The charging of fees and sending monthly billings by mail are more common with large animal practices. Established clients with excellent credit who have a large number of animals may negotiate a monthly payment instead of a payment for each service rendered.

CASH CONTROL

Cash control is best accomplished using some form of fee slips in triplicate that are numbered serially. One copy is kept in the examination room, one stays with the daybook ledger of income received, and one is given to the client. With this method, if someone's payment is unintentionally (or intentionally) omitted from being recorded in the daybook ledger, the numbered fee slip can be traced back to determine who that client was and what happened. This system allows errors to be corrected, prevents embezzlement, and provides a way to track clients who may have forgotten to check out and pay for a service. Computerized systems should also have these and other cash control features.

Petty cash is often needed by staff to purchase stamps and incidental supplies from local businesses. A procedure must be set up to track petty cash to prevent embezzlement and meet U.S. Internal Revenue Service (IRS) business deductibility rules. Generally a cash box accessible to approved staff for petty cash is set up with a set amount of cash (e.g., \$100). The petty cash box must always contain \$100 made up of the total value of signed and dated purchase receipts, cash, and temporary IOUs made out by the person as he or she removes petty cash to get supplies. When the person returns, his or her receipt plus change must equal the IOU, which is removed and replaced by the change and signed receipt. When petty cash gets low, the receipts are taken out of the box, totaled, and entered into business records as petty cash expenses. A check for expenses is made out for that amount and cashed, and that amount of cash is returned to the petty cash box. This prevents suspicion of embezzlement if every person follows this procedure, preferably overseen by the practice manager. It also makes sure all expenses are accounted for when monthly and annual reporting is due.

The staff and veterinarians should record all supplies and products taken from the practice for personal use even when these are provided free as a staff benefit. This prevents embezzlement and pilferage, accounts for the level of benefit actually provided, and keeps everyone honest and above suspicion by management, co-workers, and the IRS. It encourages honesty, prevents destructive suspicions, and promotes trust if followed by all employees, including practice owners. Consulting accountants, owners, and the practice manager have resources to set up standard business procedures for the receptionist and staff to follow to develop a smooth-operating veterinary business.

BUSINESS MANAGEMENT

Professionals as a whole would often like to abstain from the business side of practice and concentrate exclusively on professional (medical) activities. In reality, without the business side of any profession, there would be few opportunities to practice that profession. The business management aspects of practice can become as challenging as patient management. The lack of available time and interest and minimal experience are limiting factors. Clinical signs of poor business management are lax credit policies, increasing accounts receivable (total dollars clients owe), reduced operating capital, lowered gross income, lowered net income, increasing personnel costs, increasing overhead, reduced client numbers, and reduced average transaction fee per patient. Tests used to identify problems of poor business management include complete review of monthly business information to establish trends, comparison of this month's data with the same month 1 year ago, comparison with NCVEI national and state data, review of the fee schedule, review of the credit policy, review and comparison of inventory levels, and turnover rates.

The prognosis is generally good once the diagnosis of poor business management has been supported by a review of the diagnostic tests. The treatment will usually need to continue for the life of the practice. Some recommended treatments for the poor business management syndrome follow:

- Establish a firm, written credit policy.
- Make use of a written fee estimate sheet to itemize all patient charges.
- Before admission, have the owner sign and retain one copy of the treatment plan (estimate sheet).
- The credit policy should be clearly stated on the written treatment plan (see an example of a fee estimate form in Chapter 5).
- Make use of appointment systems to schedule clients for the most efficient use of time.

The practice fee schedule should be reviewed and updated at least every 3 to 6 months, and a current printed fee schedule should be available near each telephone. Accounts receivable need to be monitored monthly, with legally appropriate follow-up telephone calls and letters to stimulate payment in a timely manner.

Accounts payable should be handled in a way to obtain discounts for prompt payment. Accounts that do not provide discounts should be paid near the due date to conserve working capital. No account should be allowed to become past due. A poor credit image for the practice is difficult to remove.

One tool for analyzing and correcting poor business management is the office computer. The office computer can provide online storage and have information readily available at the push of a button. The computer can provide income analysis, accounts receivable information, inventory control, client information analysis, patient diagnosis analysis, online medical records, and so forth. Computerization is becoming increasingly cost-effective, and well-designed programs are now available through several vendors. Additional information about computers in veterinary medicine is found in Chapter 4.

If these treatments are properly applied, the prognosis for "poor business management syndrome" should be complete recovery. The result of improved management is a sound and stable veterinary practice that pays dividends to clients, patients, employees, and owners.

PET INSURANCE

Health insurance has had a significant role in funding the costs of human medicine for several decades as a third-party payer insulating patients from most of the medical and surgical costs. Dental insurance has also had a positive impact on dental practice. Pet insurance (veterinary pet insurance [VPI]) was introduced into veterinary medicine about 1982. Most pet insurance policies will cover specified services, have limits, co-payment levels, and deductibles, similar to human medicine policies. Some policies provide wellness benefits that include routine vaccinations, physical examinations, and dental services.

Recently, more companies have been encouraged to offer pet insurance because more pet owners value their pet as a member of the family and want some protection against catastrophic costs from unexpected accidents and disease. If these policies increase in number, they may help the business of veterinary practice. More patients will have major unexpected costs covered, wellness programs will be supported for saving money by preventing some costly treatments, and fewer owners will choose unnecessary euthanasia of their animals. Thus everyone benefits including the animal when the client has pet insurance. Approximately, 2% of the U.S. population is covered by pet insurance as compared with 50% of the population in Sweden.

CLIENT COMMUNICATION

Excellent interpersonal communication skills can serve to develop and expand veterinary service markets. Improved communication between client and veterinarian results in more personalized professional care. Reduction in the spendable income of clients may reduce demand for elective procedures, but this can be offset by providing a more comprehensive preventive medicine program through improved communication skills. Clients are unable to make service selections until they fully understand all their options.

Common courtesy and genuine concern affect all professions and businesses. It has been said, "I don't care how much you know until I know how much you care!" The world as a whole is becoming more depersonalized. When a veterinary practice loses sight of the individual client, the personal service feeling is lost to both the client and patient. Courtesy begins with acknowledging clients as soon as they enter the reception room, carefully explaining why an appointment is helpful, calling clients by name, asking about the clients' families—in short, treating clients as important guests in your practice.

Courtesy also extends to telephone manners. All calls should be answered by the third ring; the caller should be greeted by "Good morning, this is ABC Animal Hospital; this is Kathy speaking. How may I help you?" The caller immediately knows he or she has reached the correct hospital, and Kathy is there to help. Telephone courtesy is just as important as personal courtesy because most clients have their first contact with the hospital by telephone.

> *TECHNICIAN NOTE* All telephone calls should be answered by the third ring, although callers prefer the telephone to be answered on the first ring.

If the veterinary staff of a hospital treats each caller and each client with common courtesy, the impression the client will receive is genuine concern. A lack of concern for people and their pets' problems is a common complaint voiced by some clients of veterinary practices. If veterinary personnel treat each client as they would like to be treated when selecting or securing service, the result will be more happy clients who experience courtesy and concern.

Closely accompanying the issue of courtesy and concern is effective communication. The majority of complaints against veterinarians are the result of ineffective or misunderstood communication between veterinarian or the staff and client. To communicate completely, staff members must have concern for both the animal and client. In addition, they must learn to listen to the client and then communicate a caring attitude and information that is understandable and effective. Most people hear other people talking, but few people have developed the ability to listen effectively to what is communicated. The successful veterinary team must develop this ability.

To ensure effective communication consider these four rules:

1. Use terminology the client will understand; scientific terms can be confusing to the client.
2. Do not rush through the information just because you are hurried or because it appears to be "common knowledge" to you, or the client will feel "brushed off."
3. Do not assume a superior manner or tone to the extent the client feels "put down."
4. Use effective communication techniques for obtaining a history (see Box 3-6).

In short, show concern and respect. Attempt to treat each client with respect, honesty, and as a special person, even if you do not agree with him or her. If the communication is open, honest, and caring, it will be effective, and most problems can be prevented. One of the most common reasons for veterinarians to refer clients to other veterinarians is because of the failure to communicate effectively with the client.

> *TECHNICIAN NOTE* About 40% of all communication is verbal; 60% is body language and environmental factors.

Listening is an extremely important communication skill. The skill of listening must be practiced on a regular basis to become effective. Many people would rather talk than listen. Often, the client will assist in the diagnosis by providing important clues in the history if only someone will listen. Active listening involves listening to clients and then verbally rephrasing their messages back to them for verification. This technique (active listening) ensures that the client was heard correctly and the technician or veterinarian received the entire message.

Listening requires understanding both the "music" and the "words." The correct words must be sent and received. In addition, the nonverbal music (facial expressions, hand gestures, body stance, etc.) must also be observed and understood to allow complete communication.

CLIENT EXPECTATIONS

Most clients expect the following five things during a consultation with a veterinarian: examination of the animal, diagnosis (cause if possible), prognosis (predicted outcome), treatment plan, and fee estimate. Communication of the prognosis, treatment plan, and fee estimate is difficult for most veterinarians. Clients believe that they are unprepared to make judgments without this information and often complain if complications occur. Malpractice (professional negligence) concerns can be virtually eliminated if these areas are effectively handled with the client. The veterinary technician should be part of the communication team in these areas. Clear, effective communication is a team effort and absolutely necessary for the client's compliance and quality patient care.

COMMON COMPLAINTS FROM CLIENTS

When dealing with a cross section of the public, as most practices do, the goal of complete satisfaction for all clients can never be obtained. However, when clients do have complaints, careful attention must be given to them. Each client has the right to expect a certain level of service and the

BOX 3-8 Client's Bill of Rights

Every client is always right.
Every client deserves a 100% clean hospital.
Every client has the right to complain.
Every client has the right to a greeting and thank you.
Every client has the right to a treatment plan (estimate).
Every client has the right to quality service and referral when necessary.

"Bill of Client's Rights" is found in Box 3-8. To reduce the number of complaints from clients, several potential problem areas will be addressed. The more common areas of the client's complaints are fees, courtesy and concern, communication, appointment schedule, sanitation, and the quality of patient care.

Every client deserves a complete explanation and breakdown of all anticipated costs of each service to be performed. Whenever communication is incomplete, complaints will result. One of the most sensitive issues practitioners deal with is financial estimates. Quoted fees must be written down and honored unless revised with the full consent of the owner. The most common complaint of clients will concern fees. The use of a treatment plan (fee estimate sheet) and upfront, open communication will eliminate most fee complaints.

Another common area of clients' complaints centers on the quality of care offered to the patient and client. Often, animal owners are hesitant to accept one veterinarian's opinion. As in human medicine, seeking multiple opinions on a case has become routine. Specialists have become more common in veterinary practice, and veterinary clients are requesting second and third opinions. Multiple opinions have been good for both the patient and client, but they require veterinarians to be thorough and up to date with their information and techniques.

THE DIFFICULT CLIENT

Some clients remain difficult to deal with regardless of the best efforts of everyone in the practice. Some of these difficult people actually enjoy being difficult. The attitude of the difficult client toward the technical and reception staffs may be different from the attitude toward the veterinarian. A difficult, demanding person can suddenly become quite reasonable when the veterinarian enters the room. When this happens, the technician should not believe that he or she has failed but rather should work a little harder to understand and win the client's trust.

In dealing with someone who is politely complaining, listen to their perceptions and feelings and attempt to convey that you understand the problem (you will appear to be agreeing; this will help to reduce the level of the confrontation). A good example would be the common complaint that fees are too high, which can be answered by, "Yes, fees are high. Everything seems high these days."

In situations in which the client appears to be unreasonable about the complaint, establish the specific problem (i.e., fees, unsatisfactory treatment result, poor communication) and indicate to the client that you would like for him or her to speak to the veterinarian. Once the unreasonable client has been identified, escort the client out of the reception room and into an examination room away from other clients; then the veterinarian can handle the problem as quickly as possible.

The most difficult people to reason with are people who have been drinking or are on drugs. Be careful how you handle these people. Do not argue or confront them because they could become violent and uncontrollable. In situations in which drugs or alcohol have been consumed to excess, law enforcement officials should be contacted to handle the situation.

Never argue with a dissatisfied client. The client is "always right, even when wrong." In other words, clients have a real concern that must be acknowledged and understood. If a client leaves angry, 10 other people are told how terrible you, your veterinarian, and your hospital are. When the client leaves the practice enthusiastically, he or she will only tell three other people. We cannot have clients leaving angry. Sometimes we must all "eat a little crow" to keep the client's good will. In the long run, this will benefit all concerned. Sometimes eating crow will taste pretty good.

PROFESSIONAL MARKETING

Some professionals feel uncomfortable with the idea of marketing because the scope of marketing activity has been poorly understood. Often, the connotation of marketing is advertising. However, advertising is only a small portion of the total marketing picture for a professional business.

Professional marketing has numerous definitions, but the one that will be used here is "the communication of professional services and goods offered to existing and potential clients." The veterinary technician must understand marketing principles to be an effective communicator of professional services and goods offered by the practice.

Definition

Professional marketing consists of all activities that increase the client's awareness of professional services and goods. Marketing occurs through effective relations with clients; professional appearance of the hospital, clinic, or ambulatory vehicle; listening to owners' opinions; a convenient practice location; a polite support staff; offering full-service care; sending clients service reminders; being neat and clean; using business cards; sending clients educational newsletters or e-mail notes; providing nutritional counseling and dietary management; providing emergency service; offering pet and livestock supplies; giving career talks at high schools; leading 4-H, Future Farmers of America (FFA), or scouting groups; attending dog, cat, and horse shows; having producer or client education nights; being involved in a community service club; setting up a website on the Internet; advertising in the yellow pages of the telephone book; providing handout material to clients; having an attractive and well-located building sign; sending thank-you and sympathy cards to appropriate clients; appearing as a guest on radio and television shows; writing a newspaper animal column; using attractive letterhead stationery; becoming active in professional associations; and group advertising in the newspaper about the annual rabies vaccination clinic.

Animals are totally dependent on their owner's awareness of health care needs. Professional marketing should be designed to help more animals by informing and serving more clients. If successful, it will result in an increased practice income through increasing the number of clients, the revisit rate, or the amount of each client transaction. It requires balancing improved animal health and public health with the needs and goals of the practice. One of the most critical questions a veterinarian should ask is "What business am I in?" To be able to conduct a successful professional business, one must be clear about the specific business objectives. Some practitioners believe as long as high-quality medical and surgical skill is delivered, the client will continue to use their service based on the quality of service alone. Fortunately, clients today are usually well-informed consumers and are looking for both quality and value. The average client lacks the professional background to accurately judge the quality of medical or surgical services performed. However, clients do have the ability to judge the quality of caring communication that they received personally, which influences their perception of the value of the professional service received. Clients' perceived value of services is their reality of the practice's quality.

Veterinary medicine is in the people-service business. The profession cares for animals, but provides professional service to their owners. Patients cannot come to the practice without the owners. If each staff member understands that she or he is in the people-service business, a completely different orientation will take place. When clients call on the telephone, for example, they are not interrupting the veterinarian's or technician's time in the examination room or surgery room; they are the reason for the existence of the examination room and surgery room. Veterinary practices do provide high-quality professional service to animals, but only after the agreement and financial support of the owner. Only satisfied clients return and refer others.

> *TECHNICIAN NOTE* Clients' telephone calls are not an interruption because clients are the reason for the existence of the practice.

The professional success of most veterinarians and technicians is the result of interpersonal skills, rather than strictly clinical skills. The ability to relate well to people and their problems will allow the practice the opportunity to provide high-quality veterinary medicine (Figure 3-22).

Once the practice is viewed as a people-service business, marketing of those services becomes possible. The product to be marketed is high-quality, people-oriented, professional veterinary medical service.

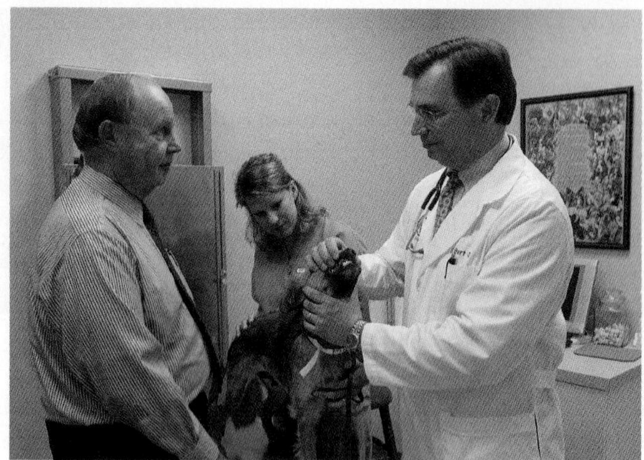

FIGURE 3-22 Client, technician, and veterinarian communicate as a team about patient care.

Marketing techniques must benefit the profession as a whole to achieve maximal success. The overall program must promote the benefits of veterinary services rather than the specific service.

If one were to compare the benefits of a program of immunization with one that sold a vaccination, the long-term effects are evident. A program that details the benefits of immunization can build a preventive medicine program through a physical examination, dental care, nutritional management, and so forth on an annual basis. The approach of selling a vaccination is just that—promoting a vaccine.

The program of promoting the benefits of a high-quality, people-oriented, professional veterinary medical service must be the end goal.

Marketing techniques will not overcome the effects of poor relations with clients within a practice. Unless effective communication with the client and orientation of the client are practiced on a client-by-client basis, marketing will be unsuccessful.

Practice Marketing

The first step in a marketing plan is to determine the client's needs. One must listen closely to the services that are requested by each client and determine what service trends are going on within the practice in response to the economic growth of the community. As an example, both spouses usually work. This results in some people being unable to seek veterinary care during the traditional 8 AM to 5 PM period. The typical client also has less free time to devote to shopping around at several stores for items when all items could be purchased at one convenient location. By listening to clients and observing service needs, the practitioner may opt to extend the practice hours two evenings per week and open later in the mornings on those days. The practice may also expand services to include veterinary-supervised boarding and offer selected nonprofessional supplies, such as grooming aids.

The practice owner must determine the direction of the marketing plan by listening to the client's needs and gathering additional facts concerning community trends. The marketing process will then be guided by current facts and psychodemographic information.

Specific Marketing Techniques

Professional marketing can be divided into internal and external marketing. Internal marketing techniques are the day-to-day activities that occur within each practice, whereas external marketing involves techniques used outside the practice. The purpose of both internal and external techniques is to enlarge the number and size of the client's transaction.

Internal Marketing

Internal marketing is aimed primarily at the existing client base. Internal marketing techniques attempt to educate and inform current clients about the various veterinary services and service programs available. They also should generate enthusiasm for the practice. The following methods are meant to serve as an idea base and not as a complete listing of techniques for internal marketing.

Client Relationships

The most important technique to use in any marketing program is personalized, sincere care of the client. Most clients require as much attention and care as the patient. Clients today want both high technology and high touch. Personalized service that emphasizes each individual client will allow the opportunity for excellent communication to be established. Both the veterinarian and technician must be skilled communicators and technically skilled professionals. The staff must support these efforts.

Practice Appearance

The visual appearance of the clinic, hospital, or ambulatory vehicle is the first outward signal to the client concerning the potential quality of service. One must consider the appearance of the building (repair, paint, cleanliness) and the grounds (Figure 3-23). Plants and grass must be neat and trimmed and the parking lot clean and well signed for parking. The interior of the building must also be clean, well cared for, and odor free. Silent but powerful marketing messages are sent to clients through the appearance of the facility.

A practice facility does not have to be new or have the latest equipment to project a positive professional image. The older facility that has been given proper care and maintenance will exhibit a strong marketing message of "we care" to people passing by each day.

Support Staff Utilization

Most internal marketing carried on within a practice will be through the veterinary team members. Support staff activities will augment the efforts of the veterinarian in relations with clients and personal appearance. Primarily, veterinary technicians and receptionists will be responsible for recommending services or goods and following up on hospital programs that require appointments or individual contact with the client. These team members are regarded as an extension of the veterinarian and must have a professional approach to the management of the client.

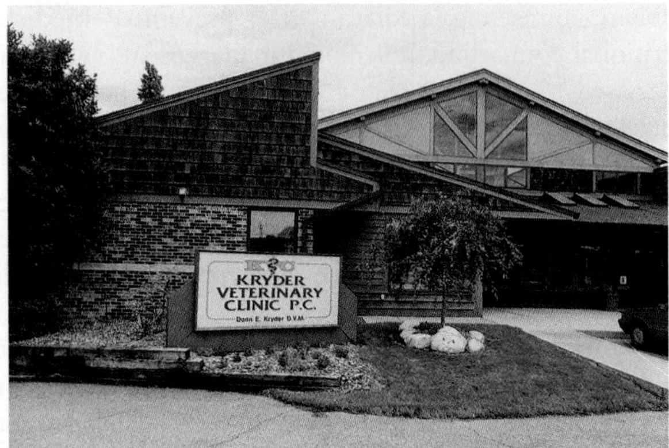

FIGURE 3-23 Exterior appearance of the hospital should provide a positive image.

The technical staff will usually deliver the majority of education to the client with the assistance of receptionists. Handout materials, visual aids, and video (Internet) presentations will help the staff in their educational efforts. The staff will need detailed information concerning the various preventive health programs from the veterinarian. To be able to promote the product, everyone needs to be clear about the product. The veterinarian and the support staff must work together as a service team, all delivering the same high-quality service.

Professional sales point displays can add another level of service for clients. These displays need continuous monitoring by the support staff to provide "on-the-spot" professional information. Areas in which the support staff should have in-depth knowledge include nutrition, parasite control (internal and external), grooming aids, dental care, immunization programs, obedience training, and rearing orphan animals. In addition, the support staff must be on the constant lookout for new clients and additional services. Staff members who are active in dog or horse clubs have continual access to new potential clients. New clients may not be aware of services offered, so all staff members must be willing to provide program information at any time. When certain key support staff members are given a small percentage of income from all new services and new clients they provide the practice as an incentive, a new wave of enthusiasm may develop in everyone.

Full-Service Care

Listening to the needs of the client will verify that clients want full-service care when possible. People are exposed to 1-hour photo processing, 1-hour eyeglasses, 7-Eleven, fast-food restaurants, K-Mart, Wal-Mart, drive-through banking, and so forth. Convenient, fast, economic, one-stop shopping is the rule for single-parent families and families in which both husband and wife work. People are now asking for this same type of convenient service in their veterinary care. In a small animal practice, full-service care would include prepurchase counseling concerning pets, human-animal bond and behavioral problem counseling, pediatric care, preventive medicine, nutritional counseling, nutritional management, veterinary-supervised boarding, geriatric care, dentistry, bereavement counseling, cremation service, and full routine veterinary care. The service would extend from birth to death.

In a full-service practice, various programs can be packaged for marketing. The goal of marketing is to sell a program, not an individual service. The emphasis of a quality practice is to provide preventive health care, not just disease treatment. A small animal practice must develop a complete health-maintenance (wellness) program for new puppies and kittens in addition to puppy-training classes. This program carries into adulthood and on into the geriatric period. The wellness program could include annual physicals, periodic routine blood screens, nutritional counseling, dental care, and immunizations. Nutritional counseling would include pediatric, adult, and geriatric care as the patient matures. As clients continue their regular contact with the practice to purchase food, the practice has a regular opportunity to review the medical record and to market other health preventive care services.

Client Reminders

One of the more successful early attempts at practice marketing was through the use of a vaccination reminder system for small animals. During the early discussions on the use of a recall system, many practitioners believed that it was unprofessional to send a reminder card to clients because it was advertising. No one was considering the service provided to the client and animal. Most veterinarians thought only of how it would appear to other veterinarians.

Charles, Charles and Associates discovered that sending vaccination reminders was even more important to clients than having boarding facilities or an attractive building. Clients want to be reminded when specific services are to be done. However, clients prefer to receive reminders by regular mail or e-mail rather than by telephone.

TECHNICIAN NOTE Clients now expect the practice to send annual service reminders.

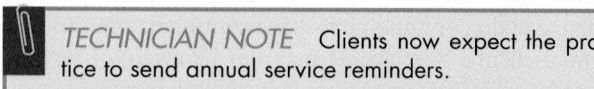

A reminder system is a major marketing feature of most practice management computer software packages. A system that has the capacity to generate only one reminder is not nearly as valuable as a system that will produce a second and third reminder if the client does not respond. Using a system that will generate an additional second or third notice to be sent will greatly increase the service return rate.

Most practices now accept the use of a reminder system as a valuable marketing tool for routine immunizations. The reminder system must be expanded to include other routine services for clients. The additional use in small animal practice could be in the areas of dental hygiene (routine cleaning), annual physical examination, geriatric care, hip-dysplasia evaluations, follow-up laboratory testing, heartworm evaluation, and so forth. The suggestion of an annual physical examination may appear on the surface to be a poor recommendation in light of physicians now recommending fewer annual physicals. However, considering that the dog and cat age seven to nine times as rapidly as humans and that the diligent veterinarian and technician are able to find a potential problem on almost every physical examination, many clients will take advantage of the service when offered. When performing the examination, the veterinarian and technician must explain and demonstrate the findings to the client (i.e., potential problems with ears, eyes, teeth, anal sac, hair coat, obesity) (Figure 3-24).

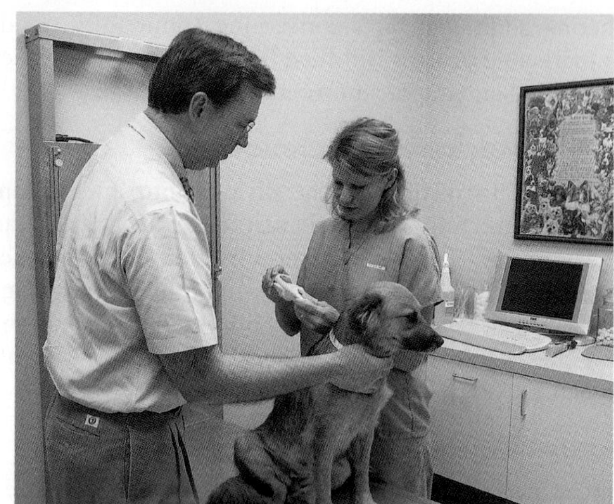

FIGURE 3-24 Technician explaining a diagnosis to client using visual aid.

Small animal geriatric care is another relatively untapped market area. When patients reach a specific age (i.e., 7 to 8 years of age), a reminder letter could be sent to the client providing information on specific conditions to be monitored. The letter could approach the client in the following way: "Blackly has now reached a senior age status and now requires that certain diseases and organ functions are monitored on a regular basis to help increase his life expectancy." This letter could be developed and recalled by the computer at a specific age and use the correct name and sex to personalize it. Another area in which a reminder system could be used is to recall young animals that have been previously vaccinated, but not yet neutered. The recall of unneutered animals is an opportunity to market ovariohysterectomy and castration services. This reminder may attract some clients who would otherwise go to a low-cost spay and neuter clinic. A personalized letter could detail the specific features of the service, which is not possible from the spay and neuter clinics.

The use of a recall system allows the market to be segmented (targeted). An example of market segmentation would be to send all feline owners a reminder about leukemia vaccination.

Personal Appearance

The personal appearance and hygiene of each staff member reflect the quality of the practice. Many clients relate personal appearance to the sanitation and level of quality of the

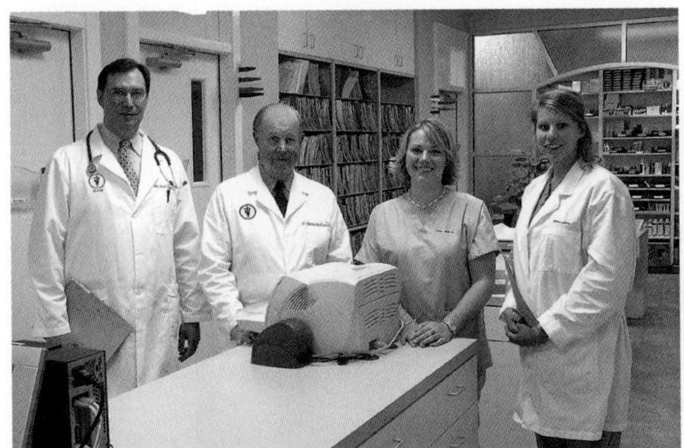

FIGURE 3-25 A professional appearance is a marketing tool that projects quality.

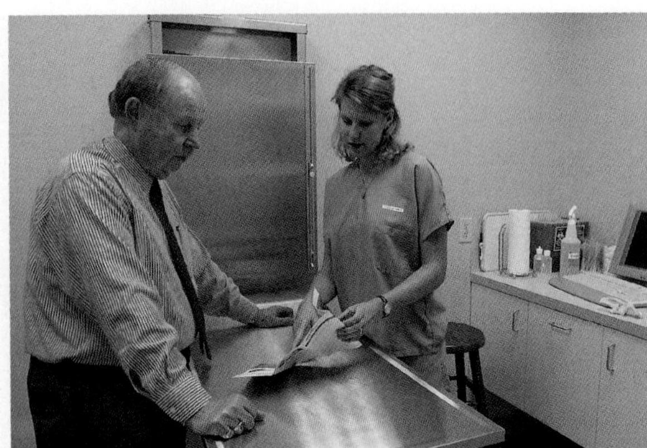

FIGURE 3-26 Technician explaining and providing a handout to client.

practice. If someone does not care enough to change a dirty smock, coveralls, or boots, why should he or she care enough to provide the highest-quality service? Not only should handwashing occur between all patients, but also it should be practiced in front of the client. This enhances the client's awareness of disease-prevention efforts. Personal appearance marketing works just like building appearance—an outward signal of internal quality (Figure 3-25). A professional image is perceived by the client when all hospital members have a professional appearance. Staff uniforms, shirt and tie, dress, and smocks for veterinarians are recommended.

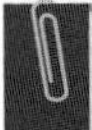

TECHNICIAN NOTE Personal appearance is a direct reflection of practice quality.

Handout Materials

Marketing with handout materials has been used for a number of years. The quantity and quality of commercially available handouts are excellent. Most commercial companies realize the value of client-oriented professional literature. These pieces should be carefully reviewed by the practice so that only acceptable material is made available to clients. Once the material has been reviewed and useful pieces selected, the staff must be made familiar with how and when they should be used. A professional rubber stamp (or printed stick-on labels) can be purchased with the practice name, location, and telephone number on it and used to personalize all commercial handout materials. A professional print shop may also be used to imprint the practice information on all brochures. The handout material must be handed directly to the client by the veterinarian or technician to be most effective (Figure 3-26). The handout materials displayed in the reception room for clients to pick up are often not well used. Clients will pick up material from a display rack and take it home, but few will ever read it.

In addition to commercial handouts, materials may be purchased from veterinary organizations. AVMA, the American Association of Equine Practitioners, and AAHA, among others, provide useful handout materials for clients.

Practices may also produce their own informational material. Quality handouts on whelping, ovariohysterectomy, cystic calculi, colic, mastitis, and so forth can be easily prepared on the computer. Discharge instruction handouts are effective because clients often forget verbal explanations and instructions. Practice information brochures can also be produced to more fully explain practice hours, services, equipment, facilities, and the staff's function (Figure 3-27). Other forms of handout materials used on a regular basis are business cards and letterhead stationery. They are effective forms of marketing. Remember that business cards have both a front and back to each card that can be used for your message. Business cards should be made available to clients from both veterinarians and key support staff, especially certified veterinary technicians and receptionists.

Sympathy and Thank-You Communications

A personal marketing approach is to appropriately use sympathy and thank-you types of communication. One may choose to use commercially prepared cards or develop a letter format on the computer that can be personalized. Regardless of the format used, the use of personal messages to specific clients for specific purposes has an everlasting positive effect. In the case of clients newly referred by current clients, a note or card to both the referring client (thanking them for the referral) and the new client (welcoming them to the practice) is appropriate. As the use of the Internet becomes more common, e-mail notes could also be used.

The sympathy card or personal note is helpful when a pet dies to demonstrate open concern for the feelings of the client during his or her emotional loss. The expression helps the client deal with the loss and allows the client to understand the "I care" attitude of the practice for both the client and pet.

Newsletter or E-mail

The use of newsletters will increase client activity through improved understanding and education about veterinary services. Educational goals for newsletters should be to inform animal owners of the signs of illness, to make seasonal animal health care recommendations (i.e., heat stroke in summer), to review health care programs, and to introduce key staff members. Many clients do not understand how to

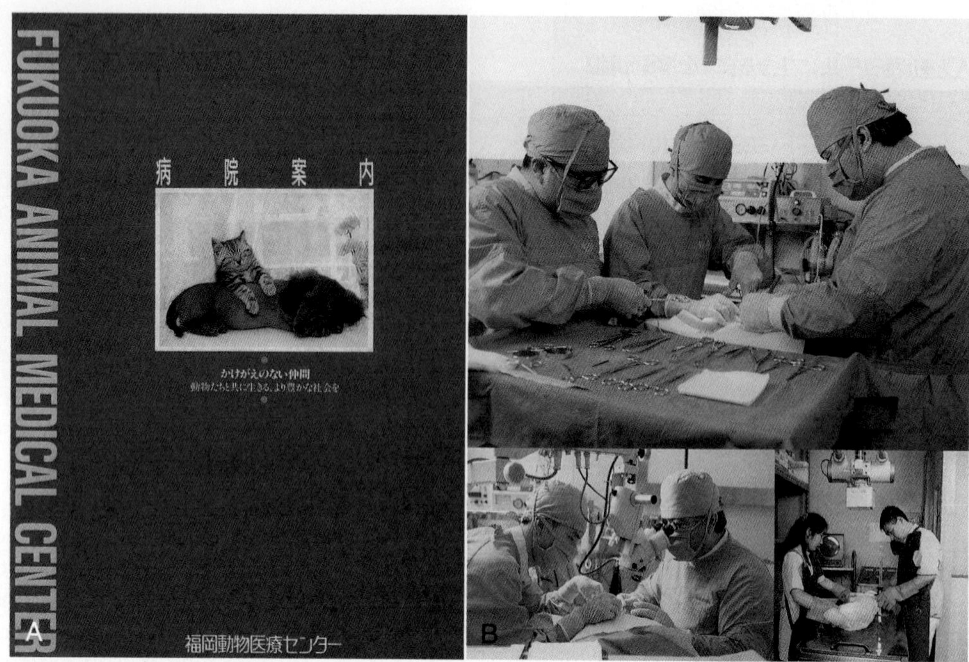

FIGURE 3-27 Practice information pamphlet. **A**, Cover. **B**, Inner page. (Courtesy Fukuoka Animal Medical Center, Fukuoka, Japan.)

tell when an animal is ill or in serious condition. This lack of knowledge is especially true for cat and horse owners.

Newsletters will allow the client to be exposed to specific pieces of information that will help owners to know when to call a veterinarian for help. Total health care plans can also be explained to allow the owner to be aware of full-service health care that extends beyond vaccinations. The newsletter should help market the benefits of healthy animals. The newsletter can also refer the reader to the practice's website for further information on a specific subject found in the electronic library of the website.

Newsletters can be sent to specific segments of clients in the practice computer base; however, they can also be provided through a hand-generated list or passed out to all clients as they enter the practice. Most veterinarians do not have the experience or time to compose a complete newsletter three or four times per year. The practice manager, veterinary technicians, and receptionists may develop articles for a practice newsletter, or consideration can be given to purchasing a professionally edited newsletter service. Newsletters are also available from Veterinary Information Network (www.vin.com).

Each newsletter should be personalized by the practice to allow the reader easy access to the practice's location and telephone number. Another advantage newsletters have in overall marketing is the ability to reach the nonuser. If the client receiving the newsletter passes it on to a nonclient friend, the nonclient has an opportunity to be exposed to various veterinary services offered by the practice.

A spinoff use of the newsletter could be through the use of news notes or Internet letters. News notes are postcard-size updates mailed to the client three or four times per year. As more clients become connected to the Internet, short e-mail letters can be used in place of newsletters sent by regular mail. The Internet notes allow rapid and economical communication.

Special Services

Practices can either expand existing services or add new services to increase their market share. In a small animal practice, market expansion might be in the areas of birds and exotic service, bereavement counseling, prepurchased evaluation of pets to determine suitability for family, behavior counseling, nutritional counseling (i.e., puppy, adult, senior), dental care (i.e., endodontics, periodontics, orthodontics), geriatric care, cremation service (Figure 3-28), emergency care, and intensive-acute care unit. Because most small animal practices cater to dogs, many cat owners do not feel welcome or comfortable in an environment with dog pictures on the walls and barking dogs in the reception area. Practices that want to increase feline clients might be well rewarded by considering the needs of cats and cat owners when remodeling. Having a separate reception area for cats and keeping cats in a separate ward (cat condos) should be a starting point. A previous lack of recognition of these needs may be the primary reason for serving fewer cat owners than dog owners with professional veterinary care.

Sales Point Displays

When displays are being considered as an internal marketing technique, several important points must be contemplated if they are to be successful. First, the practice must define the clients' needs. The specific products must be carefully selected and priced. An appropriate location or locations must be established in the clinic or hospital that may be monitored at all times by the technical staff (Figure 3-29). The products must be attractively arranged and kept neat and clean. Prices must be clearly marked on all products.

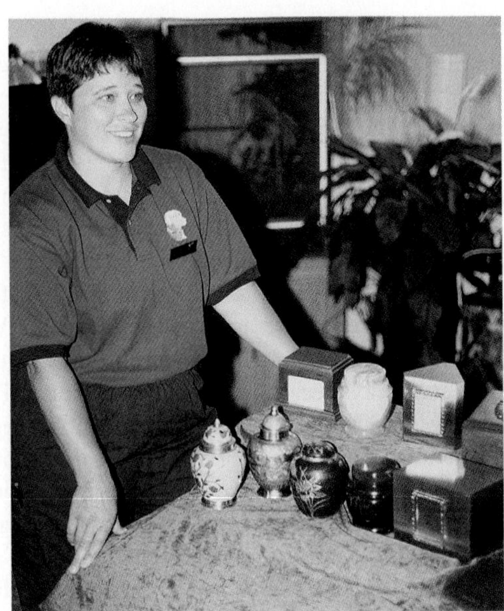

FIGURE 3-28 Veterinary technician shows a variety of urns for ashes of cremated patient. These services and compassion for the family's grief are greatly appreciated by clients.

The most important difference between a hospital or clinic display and a retail store display is the professional advice that is provided with each item sold. Professional counseling is not available at the feed store, pet shop, grocery store, department store, Internet shops, or mail-order outlet. The technical staff will play a key role in providing product information for the client.

Professional displays may include limited product lines confined to the examination rooms, a specific area of the reception room, or a special room adjacent to the reception room.

Animal Care Talks

Veterinary technicians and veterinarians can both become involved in providing veterinary medical care talks to grade school and high school students and to adult clients. The most effective and unique visual aid is a live animal. These presentations can provide information on routine animal health care, first-aid activities, signs to look for when an animal is ill, and general information on the educational requirements of veterinarians and technicians. These presentations will also help to change the established norms about animal care.

When a presentation has become polished, service clubs in the community make excellent audiences. Talks to service clubs are helpful to enhance the awareness of quality medical care provided by the individual practice and the profession. A PowerPoint computer presentation that features both the veterinarian and technician in their team roles is effective.

The veterinary technician could present information on the care of the new puppy or kitten, exotic pets and birds, first aid, feeding the pet, behavior control, whelping and queening, hip dysplasia, parasite control, pet obedience training, and pet selection. Education programs for clients should be given on a regular basis and offered at convenient times. Attendees should be provided with handout material to take home for future reference.

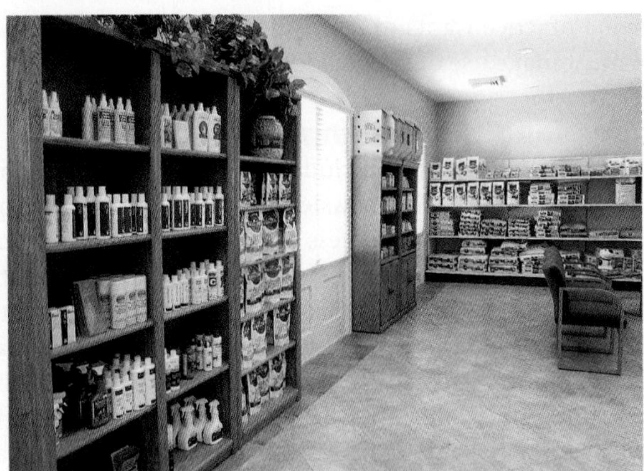

FIGURE 3-29 Professional display in reception area.

> *TECHNICIAN NOTE* Technicians can present education programs for clients to expand professional services for preventive medicine.

When the education program is held at the practice, a complete tour of the facilities should be planned. Clients are interested in seeing hospital equipment and understanding more about hospital care. An annual hospital open house is an excellent image builder for clients. Having a "behind-the-scenes" tour is something that most clients have not had an opportunity to experience. Many will be "amazed" to see x-ray, anesthesia, surgery, and laboratory equipment "just like in a human hospital." Children are especially impressed with show-and-tell demonstrations using live animals.

By providing educational opportunities for clients, the client becomes more bonded to the practice. When veterinary problems arise, the client is more apt to contact the practice that has provided an inside look and veterinary medical information.

External Marketing

Most external marketing activities are aimed at expanding current client activity and identifying new nonclient activity. External marketing can be carried out by an individual practice, group practice, organized veterinary medicine, and commercial companies. Institutional advertising is now regularly done on television for specific drug products that commercial companies are promoting and then stating that these products are available from your veterinarian or physician (when it is a human product being advertised).

Some types of external marketing are currently being used in many practices. The use of an Internet website, newsletters (direct mail to nonclients), telephone yellow page advertising, building signs, nights for educating clients, community service activities, and AVMA's National Pet Week materials expands the image of the practice to clients and nonclients.

When a practice wants to penetrate into the nonclient base, one must make use of selected forms of advertising.

Professional Advertising

Professional advertising includes hospital signs, telephone book listings, practice newsletters, vaccination reminders, and professional business cards. However, the focus on advertising in this discussion will center more on the more hard-core forms of advertising: yellow pages of the telephone book, newspapers, magazines, radio, direct mail, and telephone. Attitudes concerning advertising differ between the professional and the consumer. A great majority of professionals (physicians, dentists, attorneys, veterinarians) are against advertising for a variety of reasons: it seems to be unprofessional and unethical, and it lowers status, credibility, and the sense of dignity. Just as professionals feel strongly negative toward advertising, consumers feel strongly positive. Consumers generally believe advertising by a professional would not compromise that professional's credibility, status, image, or dignity as long as it is honest and not misleading. Most consumers believe that advertising by professionals would help them make a more intelligent choice.

Telephone Yellow Pages

When a yellow page advertisement is deemed to be appropriate for external marketing purposes, several guidelines should be followed. First, the advertisement should not be larger than one fourth of a page; advertisements larger than one fourth of a page are perceived as being more unprofessional by the consumer. Second, the advertisement should be set in one color (preferably black). The use of multiple colors (e.g., red, green) is perceived by the consumer as being less professional. Finally the advertisement should provide as much information as possible about the practice and its services. Yellow page advertising appears to be most affective in rapidly growing areas or when a new practice first opens. The established practice does not benefit as much from yellow page advertising.

Internet Web Page

Web pages are the newest form of marketing for veterinary practices and organizations. Many practices are using their own website to provide public access to information about the practice, its staff, pet care, and services provided, and often include pictures for a virtual tour of the medical facility and procedures. A Web page may also provide the practice clientele with the ability to make an appointment online and provide quality information about pet selection, training, feeding, and selected medical conditions. The practice Web page can be updated frequently and may replace the need for practice newsletters and some practice brochures. Other quality sources for veterinary-related information on the Internet can be reviewed and approved and set up as a link to the practice Web page (see www.avma.org for initial links to the Virtual Library, PetVet, Care for Pets, and the Electronic Zoo on the Internet).

Newspapers

Newspaper advertising, like telephone yellow page advertising, is useful for an initial impact when opening or expanding a practice. Many professionals will have a newspaper listing when opening a new practice, when relocating an existing practice, or when adding new associates to an existing practice. The continual use of newspaper advertising for veterinarians has been largely prohibited by cost.

Probably the best form of newspaper advertising for veterinarians is the "animal care information" format. Weekly animal care information columns are a public service, and newspapers are always seeking educational material. Pet columns have become popular reading as the public begins to acknowledge and understand the human-animal bond. To address the need for weekly newspaper columns, several private column services have sprung up that will provide the practitioner with 52 professionally written articles on animal care each year. This service can be purchased by individual veterinarians or through associations.

Radio and Television

Veterinary associations can obtain air time essentially free by participating in talk shows. The subject of animals, animal care, and animal behavior is a fascinating subject to most listening and viewing audiences. A number of the larger radio and television markets have regularly scheduled talk shows (some hosted by veterinarians) that have a question-and-answer format devoted to animal care. The talk show format is an excellent opportunity for associations that have articulate and knowledgeable veterinarians and technicians to sell veterinary medicine for the profession as a whole.

Recently, popular television programs, such as *Animal Planet* and *Emergency Vets,* have had a large impact on marketing the veterinary profession. Likewise, the earlier James Herriot books and televised Public Broadcasting System (PBS) series attracted many animal lovers to the profession. All these media events help public awareness of the high level of medical care provided by the veterinary profession.

Community Activities

Veterinary practices that engage in community activities have a much wider client base.

Veterinarians and technicians should become involved in community service through Girl Scouts, Boy Scouts, 4-H Veterinary Science Leader, school boards, humane societies, country clubs, Rotary clubs, Lions clubs, and church activities. Potential contacts with clients are made in the course of being involved and contributing to these organizations. In addition, one becomes more knowledgeable about the species, breed, and show-circuit problems when participating in animal breed clubs.

One should not join a community activity only to make contacts with clients. Practice is too time consuming for both the veterinarian and technician to become involved in too many activities or activities that are not personally rewarding. However, a reasonable involvement in some of these activities is an important marketing tool in addition to being necessary for supporting the community.

GRADUATE TECHNICIAN SELF-MARKETING

Veterinary technicians must learn to choose employment in practices in which veterinarians will delegate sufficient billable technical tasks to allow the technician to also generate income. This must be sufficient for adequate leveraging of the veterinarian's productivity to provide the technician an adequate salary sufficient to stay in the veterinary technology profession. The IAMS publication, *How to Market Yourself: A Veterinary Technician Placement Program,* is an excellent resource to plan this critical choice. Also see Recommended Reading at the end of this chapter.

> TECHNICIAN NOTE Leveraging the veterinarian's productivity through delegation of billable tasks to the technician should provide adequate salary support for the technician.

The second phase of technician marketing occurs after the initial adjustment period of employment. Once a technician is a productive and trusted part of the veterinary team, strategies must be undertaken to improve and enhance the technician's productive role on the veterinary team. "I can do that" spoken at appropriate times is one of many ways to encourage greater delegation. Keeping a log of technical duties performed by the veterinarian and preparing an analysis of potential time (and money) that could be saved through delegation can also be effective. The same process can be applied to tasks performed by the technician that could be economically done by an entry-level assistant. Additional information concerning the financial rewards of the use of the veterinary technician is available at www.ncvei.org.

Obviously, there must be some role delineation between technicians and assistants and between veterinarians and technicians while maintaining the most productive teamwork possible. In general, tasks should be delegated to the lowest paid person who can perform them correctly, especially when other income-producing tasks are available. We need everyone on the team to get the job done.

SUMMARY

Practices that will flourish in the twenty-first century will be those that integrate well-trained technicians with responsible communication with clients, deliver high-quality medicine and surgery, maintain excellent client-patient and personnel-business management, fully use current technology, practice in attractive facilities aided by a good location, and practice preventive maintenance on the facility, equipment, and grounds. These flourishing practices will be exciting and rewarding for clients, patients, the staff, and owners.

RECOMMENDED READING

Ackerman L: *Business basics for veterinarians,* Lincoln, Neb, 2002, ASJA Press.

American Veterinary Medical Association: *Your professional image,* Schaumburg, Ill, 2000, American Veterinary Medical Association.

Fassig SM: *Associate's survival guide.* Lakewood, Colo, 2005, AAHA Press.

Gerson RF: *Beyond customer service: keeping clients for life.* Schaumburg, Ill, 1993, American Veterinary Medical Association.

Haberer JB, Webb MW: *Teamwork: 50 ways to make it work in your practice.* Schaumburg, Ill, 1996, American Veterinary Medical Association.

Heinke ML, McCarthy JB: *Practice made perfect, a guide to veterinary practice management.* Lakewood, Colo, 2001, AAHA Press.

Wise JK: *US pet ownership and demographics sourcebook.* Schaumburg, Ill, 2002, American Veterinary Medical Association.

Manuals and Directories

AAHA hospital standards and accreditation manual. Denver, 2008, American Animal Hospital Association.

2008 AVMA membership directory and resource manual. Schaumburg, Ill, 2008, American Veterinary Medical Association.

How to market yourself: a veterinary technician placement program. Dayton, Ohio, 2000, IAMS.

Journals

DVM Newsmagazine, Cleveland, Advantstar Communications, monthly.

Trends, Denver, American Animal Hospital Association, monthly.

Veterinary Economics, Lenexa, Kan, Veterinary Medicine Publishing Group, monthly.

Veterinary Practice News, BowTie, Mission Viejo, Calif, monthly.

Management Short Courses

Veterinary Management Development School, Denver. Contact AAHA for details.

Veterinary Management Institute at Purdue University. Contact AAHA for details.

Internet Sites

www.avma.org (information on veterinary medicine and links to pet care sites)

www.avma.org/navta/ (veterinary technology profession information)

www.ncvei.org (financial information for the veterinary profession)

4 Computer Applications in Veterinary Practice

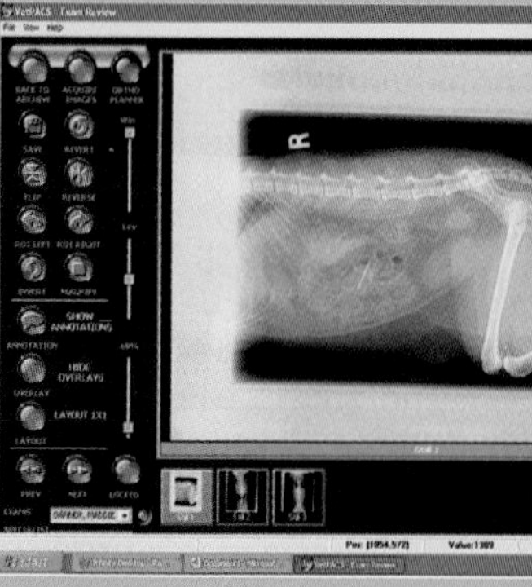

Vickie Byard

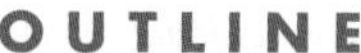

OUTLINE

KEY TERMS

American Animal Hospital Association (AAHA)
Application software
Digital Imaging and Communications in Medicine (DICOM)
Hardware
Network
Operating software
Software

LEARNING OBJECTIVES

When you have completed this chapter, you will be able to:

1. Differentiate between operating software and application software.
2. Describe methods to research, select, and purchase hardware and software.
3. List routine maintenance needs for computer hardware.
4. Define the terms server, network, and database.
5. Describe the types of data included in the veterinary practice database.
6. List the advantages of computerized scheduling and name common features of scheduling software programs.
7. List the advantages of electronic medical records and describe common components of an electronic medical record.
8. Describe common features of inventory software systems.
9. Describe common features of billing software systems.
10. List and describe computer applications and websites related to veterinary research and education.

INTRODUCTION

Much of what we do in our daily lives involves some sort of computer technology. Many individuals rise in the morning to drink their first cup of coffee while reading their e-mail. When you stop at the bank machine on the way to work, a computer hands you money and automatically deducts that amount from your bank account. If you self-checkout at a grocery store, the computer reads the bar codes on those selected items and then charges you appropriately. If you charge the amount to a credit card, the computer reads your personal information from the magnetic strip on your card then sends the information electronically to gain approval for the transaction. Once approved, the system requests your signature, and you are on your way. All of this could have taken place before you even entered the front door of the veterinary practice where you work. We have entered a time in which computers play an integral part in all of our lives. This technology is efficient, cost-effective, and dramatically reduces human error.

Since the onset of the 1990s, veterinarians began to introduce computers into their practices. Initially, they were used for invoicing and bookkeeping tasks. With the introduction of software specifically designed for veterinary practices, innovative veterinarians and practice managers began to realize the potential these systems offered.

Well into the year 2008, the integration of computers into the veterinary setting is necessary, if not vital. Now most practices depend on computers for appointment scheduling, medical records management, inventory management, payroll, marketing, data collection, and accounting. As technology advances, so does the role of the computer. This chapter will introduce the reader to the usual computer applications and stimulate some thought on innovative and practical uses to make the practice of veterinary medicine more exciting and ultimately more productive.

COMPUTER HARDWARE AND SOFTWARE

This discussion about the specifics of computer hardware and software assumes a certain amount of basic computer knowledge. *Computer hardware* relates to the parts of the system that you can touch: the monitor, the hard drive, the mouse, the printers, the modem, the disks, the scanner, and more (Figure 4-1). *Software* relates to the computer instructions contained within the hardware or added to the hardware. An important distinction should be made between *operating software* and *applications software.* The operating software tells the different parts of the hardware how to communicate with each other. For instance, the operating system translates strikes on the keyboard to letters seen on the screen. It monitors and organizes files and directories, and it controls peripheral devices, such as printers, scanners, and disk drives. Some commonly recognized operating systems are DOS, OS/2, Windows, Macintosh, UNIX, and LINUX. Application software is programs that help a user perform certain tasks. Some common examples of application software include word processing software, bookkeeping software, and practice management information systems.

Veterinary software products are becoming faster and more flexibile. The software programs offer users the ability to import results from certain laboratory equipment and allow multiple employees to manipulate data from different workstations simultaneously. Veterinary practice management software also provides a revision history feature. This means that all changes to the medical record are tracked. This is vital when considering a "paperless environment" in the event of litigation.

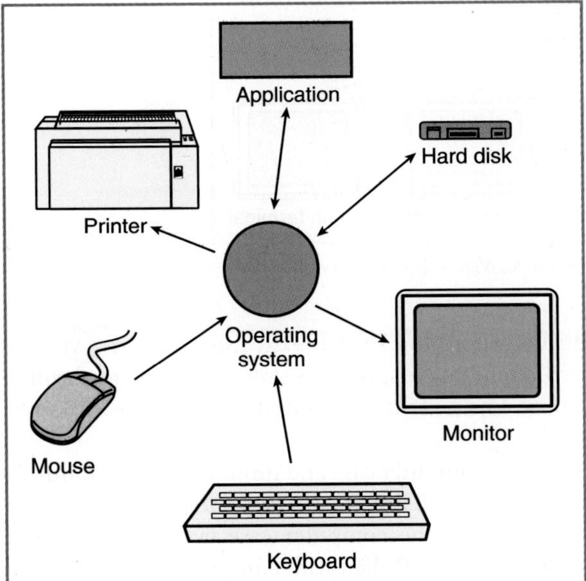

FIGURE 4-1 This diagram depicts the function of the operating system and the flow of the information (direction) by and among peripheral devices.

COMPUTER CONFIGURATIONS

A solo veterinarian may require a computer terminal in the reception station, one in the pharmacy, one in the examination room, and one in the business and/or her office. These terminals would all be connected through a *server,* that manages the network of computer stations. The veterinary software is stored on the server in addition to the associated patient-client database. There are various configurations of networks found in veterinary hospitals depending on the complexity and functions of the system and on the needs of the practice (Figure 4-2).

Today's veterinary environment supports many large practices staffed with general clinicians and specialists of various disciplines, multiple support staff, and a space occupying large square footage. In this type of setting, the above described network would not suffice. It is not unusual to see a terminal in each exam room, two to three terminals in the operating-treatment room, two to three terminals in the administrative offices, and two to three terminals in the reception area. Printers of differing types are scattered throughout these practices: a pharmacy label printer, a laser printer in reception, a printer for the bookkeeper, a printer for the administrator, and a printer in the laboratory. All of this hardware would be linked together through the network operating system, and the server manages the veterinary management software.

Recently, Tablet PCs have entered the veterinary arena. These are a type of notebook computer that has an LCD screen on which the user can write using a stylus. The handwriting is digitalized then converted to standard text. Tablets are wireless, affording the user the ability to take this technology wherever needed. Much of the information entered is accomplished through touching selected menus on the screen with the stylus. Many of the newer bundled packages come with supplemental software, such as anatomic diagrams, feeding recommendations, or drug formularies. With a touch to the screen, the staff can send home a patient health report card and customized client education materials while speaking with the client.

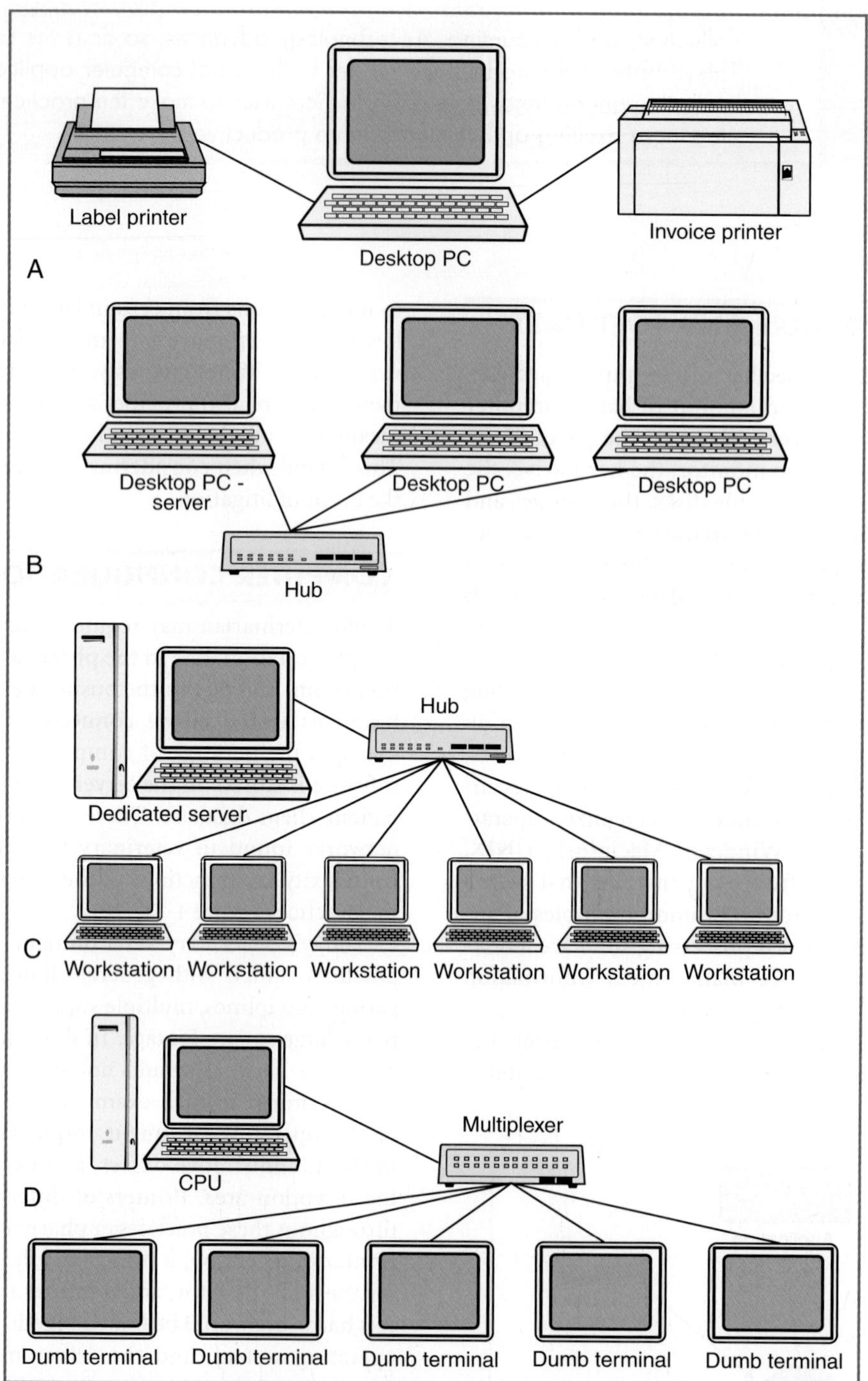

FIGURE 4-2 **A,** Single station system. **B,** Multistation system with nondedicated server. **C,** Multistation system with dedicated server. **D,** A configuration with one central processing unit (CPU) and "dumb" terminals attached. *PC,* Personal computer.

Do not avoid computerizing a practice or increasing the system's capabilities for fear that medicine will become less personalized. These systems should enable better time management so that quality time can be spent with each client and better care can be afforded to each patient.

MAINTENANCE TIPS

Make sure the computer case has plenty of room. The microprocessor, the motherboard, and other parts of the hardware accumulate heat. Computer cases have a cooling fan and slots where the air can exit. Especially in a veterinary environment, make sure these slots are not clogged with hair and dust. Ensure that the computer is in an area with plenty of cool air.

Dust the computer case and monitor once a month. Dust left unchecked will find its way into the computer.

Clean inside the computer case every 2 to 3 months. This can be accomplished with compressed air (Figure 4-3). It may be wiser to contract a computer repair company to regularly perform this function. Even the smallest amount of static electricity can ruin vital parts of the hardware.

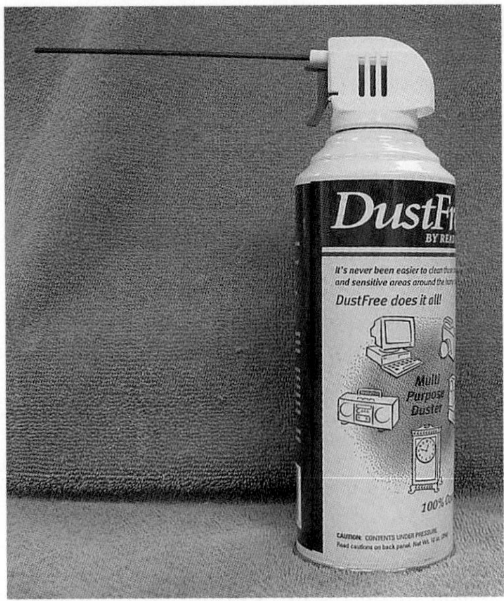

FIGURE 4-3 This is an example of compressed air for routine computer maintenance.

Regardless of the size of the system chosen, it is recommended that an electrical surge protector be provided for the system together with a battery backup. If not properly protected, vital information can be lost in the event of an electrical surge or a complete power outage.

Although initially expensive, it is wise to consider redundant (or mirrored) hard drives. When information is saved, it is saved to two or three hard drives. In the event that one crashes, at least one additional drive would contain all of the current practice information.

> *TECHNICIAN NOTE* Although initially expensive, it is important to back up information on multiple hard drives. In the event that one crashes, at least one additional drive would contain all of the current practice information.

HOW TO RESEARCH, SELECT, AND PURCHASE HARDWARE AND SOFTWARE

When deciding to purchase a computer system for the veterinary practice, one must consider a number of factors.

- What is the flow of client traffic within the practice?
- What are the uses for the system?
- Who is responsible for entering data?
- What do you envision for the future of the practice?

After these questions have been answered, it is time to begin researching the various veterinary software companies. Most of the software programs available have similar features. The differences may be the ease of use, ability of the program to integrate with other equipment within the practice, and flexibility for the future.

The American Animal Hospital Association (AAHA) publishes a trends survey every 2 years of what software programs are being used and how they are rated. In addition, many of the software vendors demonstrate their products at the national meetings. This is a great venue because you can compare and contrast different features of a number of competing products within one room. Contact the companies and discuss your needs. The vendors will assist you in deciding on what computer configuration is recommended to run their program and what the approximate costs will be. Some vendors also have demo CDs available so that you can investigate the program thoroughly.

Once you have narrowed down the search, there are some additional factors to consider:

- How long has the company been in business?
- How many systems have they sold?
- Can they provide references from practices employing this software?
- Are both hardware and software included in the support contract?
- What kind of staff training is provided and for how long?
- What is the anticipated cost of updates?
- If hardware is purchased from a separate vendor from the software, what support, warranties, and equipment loans do they offer?

As technology advances, it is reasonable for practices to replace hardware and/or software every 5 to 10 years. Although purchasing the components to computerize a practice is initially expensive, the following sections will demonstrate that savings to the practice will justify the costs.

TYPICAL USES OF COMPUTERS IN VETERINARY PRACTICE

The current trend in veterinary medicine is for veterinarians to practice as a group. Large practice groups offer veterinarians flexible schedules and no initial outlay of capital to establish a practice. As the client base of the practice grows, the number of veterinarians and support staff increases. This increase of human resources creates the need to manage information and communication between staff members, departments, and shifts. This trend would not be possible if veterinarians were not employing computers to help manage all of that increased information (Box 4-1).

DATA COLLECTION

Data is simply pieces of information. When a client enters a veterinary practice for the first time, the receptionist asks them to fill out a new client-patient form with their personal information on it. This information will include their name, address, home telephone number, work telephone number, possibly even their e-mail address. All of this information, or data, is keyed into the computer. The form will ask for information regarding the patient: pet name, species, breed, age, color, etc. The receptionist will also enter this information, thus creating a virtual record for that client and patient (Figure 4-4).

BOX 4-1 Computer Applications in Veterinary Practice

- Demographic data collection
- Name, address, phone number of the client
- Name, age, gender, species, breed, color of the patient
- Scheduling
- Client appointment by veterinarian
- Boarding reservations
- Vacation scheduling
- Conference scheduling
- Billing
- Accounts receivable
- Accounts payable
- Mass mailings
- Monthly statements
- Newsletters and client information
- Reminders
  - Vaccinations, fecal or dental examinations, heartworm tests
  - Rechecks and follow-ups
- Inventory management
- Drugs, controlled substances
- Supplies
- Financial
- Cash drawer reconciliation
- Deposit slips automatically generated
- Payment records: cash, check, credit card receipts
- Payroll calculations
- Profit and loss reports
- Productivity reports: areas making or losing money
- Fee code entry to keep track of clients' and patients' bill status
- Income analysis
- Practice profile and analysis
- Medical records
- Patient's history
- Daily progress reports and treatment records
- Laboratory data storage and retrieval
- Surgical procedures
- Diagnostic codes: storage and retrieval
- Physical examination results
- Fee code entry to keep track of prescriptions and treatments completed
- Certificates and forms
  - Vaccinations, rabies tag number tracking
  - Spay/neuter
  - Euthanasia
  - Release forms: surgery
- Communication
- Patient's medical and financial records available to all staff at any time
- Security: who can and cannot access certain data
- Diagnostic aids
- Diagnostic programs
- Drug formulary
- Remote modem communication
- Home to hospital
- Ranch or farm to hospital
- Satellite clinic to hospital
- Meeting or conference to hospital
- Cellular phone to hospital

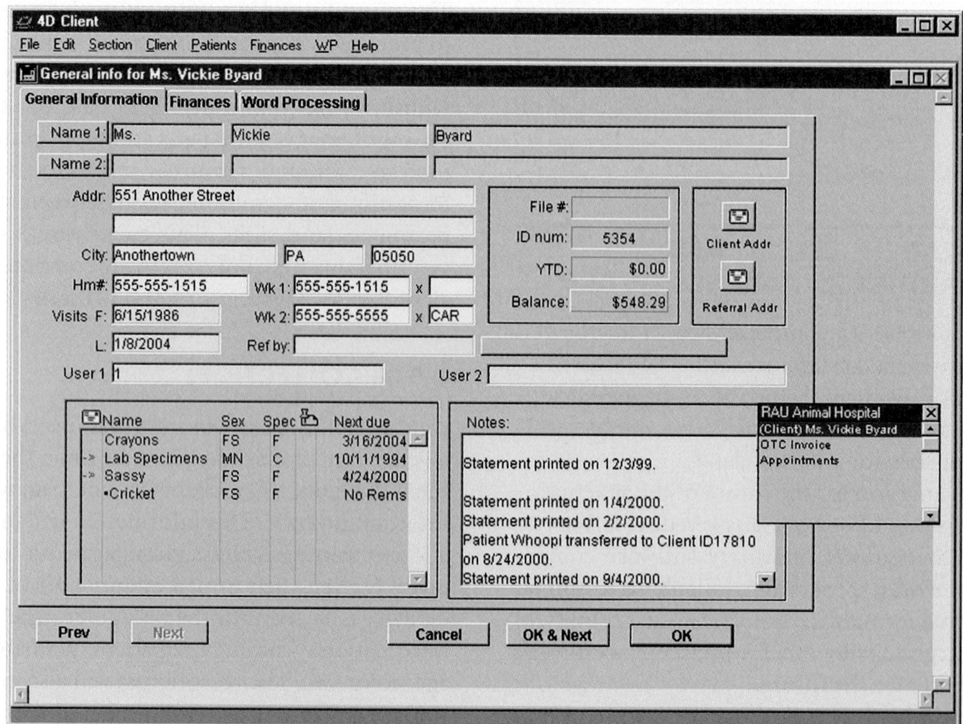

FIGURE 4-4 An example of a client data screen.

As the client moves from the waiting room to the exam room, the technician continues to gather information. The weight of the patient is obtained and entered into the patient record. Any past inoculations and the dates last administered are entered into the record. Any past medical problems will be keyed into the computer. This data is stored in a *database*.

Through a *query* screen, the user can request a patient's record by a variety of parameters: client last name, patient name, telephone number, or address. If the last name of the client is a common one, such as Smith, the computer would produce a long list. In that case, it would be easier to change the query parameter to *Patient Name* and enter the name, "Sassy." The result will be a shorter list of all of the patients in the database by that name.

Data collection is important in a multitude of ways. The computer is capable of producing a list of all patients that are due to be inoculated in the month of June in the year 2008. This list can be used to produce the vaccination reminders that are to be mailed out, thus prompting next year's appointments.

The computer can produce a list of all patients that received recommendations for dentistry. It can even identify the practice's top 1000 income-generating clients so that you can send them the practice's newsletter. All of these functions can be accomplished in a matter of minutes with the use of a computer compared with the amount of time it takes to generate any of these lists by hand.

SCHEDULING

When evaluating veterinary software, an important feature is the appointment scheduler. When the appointment book is not computerized, only one staff member can manipulate the schedule at a time. Computers make it possible for multiple staff members to be able to add or delete appointments concurrently. The veterinarian can schedule an appointment while speaking to the client, and the technician can schedule a recheck appointment while discharging the patient from surgery. Ideally the appointment schedule should be available at a variety of workstations. This feature alone decreases the chaos at the front desk created when all client contact requires a receptionist.

Some veterinary software synchronizes the appointment scheduler with the client-patient medical records. When you are in the patient record, a drop-down menu will offer a link to the appointment scheduler. When a time and date are selected, the patient name, client last name, and telephone number is automatically put in that slot. Another element of a computerized appointment scheduler is the "find next appointment" feature. If a client has forgotten when his or her appointment is scheduled, the receptionist may enter the patient record, drop down a menu, gain access to the appointment scheduler, and select "find next appointment." The computer will then search and display the appointment. This would be a tedious task without the help of a computer.

Some appointment schedulers are capable of appointment time customization. Identified tasks can be assigned specific lengths of time. Instead of scheduling a standard 15- or 20-minute appointment for suture removal, it could be customized to a 5- or 10-minute appointment. Some schedulers track and identify clients that have missed previous appointments. This enables the reception staff to confirm those appointments with a telephone call.

Seventy percent of all scheduled appointments are generated from reminders. Some powerful veterinary software will display vaccine alerts prompting multiple pet visits, rather than just scheduling the appointment driven by the mailed reminder.

> *TECHNICIAN NOTE* Computers simplify the scheduling of appointments and ensure the transfer of client information. For example, when an appointment is scheduled, client information is automatically transferred from the electronic medical record to the newly scheduled time slot.

BILLING

Older systems depend on the use of a "travel sheet." This is a sheet that has a list of *line items* on it. The term line item refers to any product or service within the practice that has a price attached to it. As services are rendered, the staff member highlights the line item on that patient's travel sheet. At the end of the day, a staff member enters those line items into the patient's invoice.

Systems that employ the use of a "travel sheet" inevitably lead to lost income. Traditionally, these are two-sided sheets, and it is possible in a rushed moment to forget to input charges highlighted on the back. It is easy to forget to highlight a product dispensed. It is not unusual for there to be a $20,000 to $50,000 loss of income per full-time veterinarian per year with charges that are not captured.

With newer veterinary software, as staff members perform medical tasks, they enter those services directly into the computer. An invoice is created as a patient enters the practice. When the veterinarian examines a pet, they enter a code for "office visit." A window then opens for them to enter their SOAP notes. When they close that window, they select a code for the next service (e.g., "in-house serum chemistry and CBC"). The veterinary software handles updating the invoice. As the services increase, so does the invoice.

Veterinary software does not come with predetermined prices of products and services. As the software is introduced, the administrators of the practice input set prices for each service or product. When computers were not employed, veterinarians were aware of the costs to the client. They tended not to charge for services out of a sense of guilt and/or discomfort. Invoice totals were lower, thus cutting the profit to the practice. With the use of advanced systems, the staff is less aware of the prices accruing as they render medical treatment. This feature alone is largely responsible for practices being able to afford more professional staff, thus increasing the standard of care and decreasing staff burnout.

MEDICAL RECORDS

Chapter 5 specifically discusses medical records. The discussion here is meant to highlight the benefits of electronic medical records.

In the past, when medical records were made of paper, only the person handling the record could gain access to the information. With computerized medical records, staff in different rooms of the practice can see the information simultaneously.

Paper medical records could be found in a variety of places: in the file, in a stack of records awaiting communications, in a pile of records on the bookkeeper's desk, in a pile waiting to be refiled, or even in a box in the attic as a result of inactivity. Because paper medical records "walk," they are often difficult to find. Computers allow us to retrieve vital information immediately.

Computerization has also improved the quality of the information. The information is legible and more organized. With the use of templates, the different parts of the exam are listed, defaulting to "nothing abnormal seen." When notable findings are made, the veterinarian can either type in the information or select a finding from a menu.

It is also true that many veterinarians are not typists. Voice recognition software is not out of the realm of possibility within the near future. The medical findings are spoken into a microphone, which then translates the sound of a voice into words on a word processor. These notes can then be cut and pasted into the medical record.

Advanced veterinary software permits documents, such as referral reports, electrocardiogram strips, radiographs (Figure 4-5), photos (Figure 4-6), and more to be scanned or imported directly into the patient's medical record. This reduces staff time searching for reports, pulling radiographs, and subsequent refiling.

Some programs are capable of maintaining a digital photo of the client on the record. Upon retrieval of the patient file, there may be a photo of the patient. A digital camera can be used to take images of lesions or teeth (Figure 4-7), or it can be attached to a microscope for images of cytology or hematology slides (Figure 4-8). These images can be imported right into the patient's electronic medical record for future use or e-mailed to a referral specialist.

CLIENT COMMUNICATIONS AND MASS MAILINGS

As discussed in the Data Collection section, information that is entered into the record can be retrieved later for marketing purposes. Vaccination reminders are printed and mailed

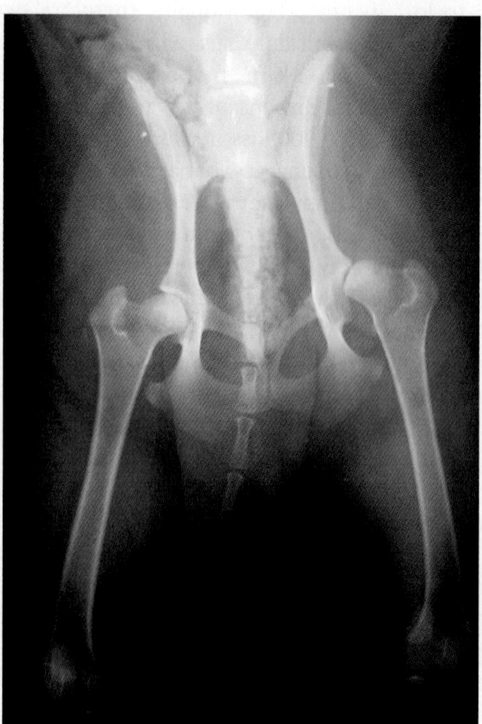

FIGURE 4-5 An example of a digital pelvic radiograph of a dog with evidence of two BBs.

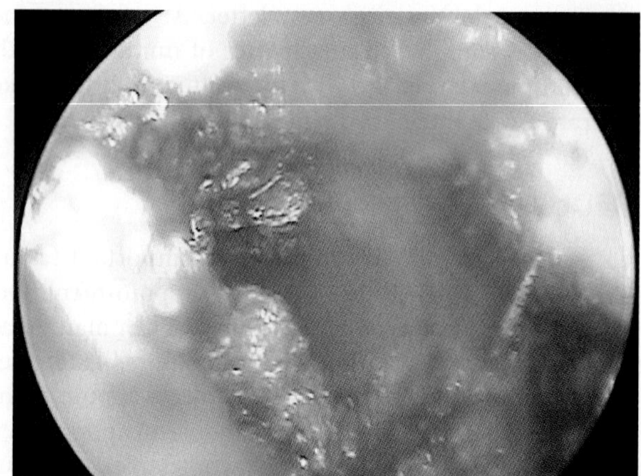

FIGURE 4-6 A digital image of an ear canal before an ear flush. This image was obtained with a video otoscope.

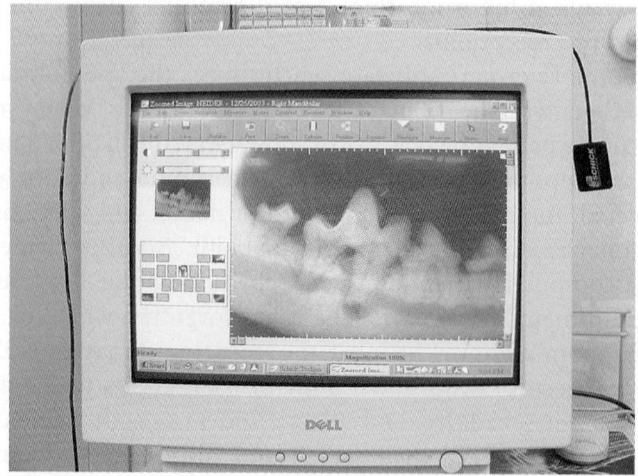

FIGURE 4-7 This photograph shows an intraoral radiograph taken with a digital sensor (to the right of the monitor) and a dental x-ray unit.

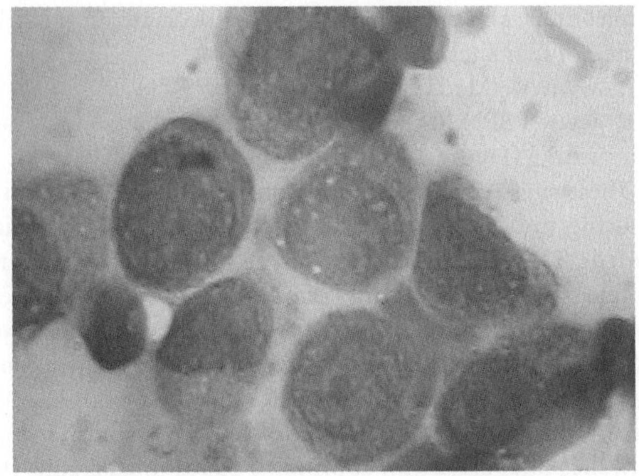

FIGURE 4-8 An image of a cytology slide taken with a digital camera attached to a microscope.

out monthly. Recommendations made in patients' records can be tracked. The practice can then prepare and send mass mailings extolling the benefits of senior-wellness packages, dental cleanings, and other services. Once the list is created, address labels can be printed, and new business is only days away.

INVENTORY MANAGEMENT

With most veterinary software, inventory management is a module of the program. Because the nature of practice, this module of veterinary software is not without its problems. If all of the inventory for the practice was ordered, received, stocked, prescribed, and sold, the inventory management would be easily handled by the computer. Unfortunately, catheters, tape, syringes, needles, cleaning supplies, and sterilization supplies constitute items that are used within the practice on a regular basis, but are separately billed therefore making them difficult to track. Not every intravenous catheter attempt is successful, yet the client is only charged for one. Dispensable items, such as medication, food, shampoo, etc., can be tracked. Levels can be set within the system, and weekly order reports can be generated by the computer as levels get low. Presently, computerized inventory management is almost always coupled with a manual system for all usable items.

ACCOUNTING AND PRACTICE MANAGEMENT

As medical services are added to the medical record, charges are added to the invoice. When the receptionist cashiers out the client, the payment is recorded on the invoicing-payment screen. If there is a balance on the account, the veterinary software keeps track of the accounts receivable.

The practice administrator sets a time within the system when accounts are considered overdue (30 days, 60 days, and 90 days). Monthly bills can then be sent out to all past due accounts. The software is also capable of adding a late fee depending on the length of delinquency.

Today's software also makes it possible to block a client from charging fees in the event that they are habitually negligent in paying their bills. Without alerts and blocks, accounts receivable could get prohibitively high.

Another aspect of the veterinary software is the ability to track income production for each veterinarian. Some practices pay their veterinarians a base salary plus compensation based on production. As entries are made within the medical record, the veterinarian that ordered the service is credited with the production of that fee. Even if the veterinarians are not compensated for production, this gives management valuable information. For instance, if Drs. A and B are able to produce a consistent percentage of the gross annual income by generating dentistry but Dr. C's production is much lower, management can have an educated discussion about making appropriate recommendations for care.

Practices will need to supplement with separate accounting software to complement the data gathered within the veterinary software. Products such as Peachtree Accounting or QuickBooks are commonly used. Bookkeepers input information gained from the billing and invoicing features of the veterinary software to manage the financial aspects of the business. This financial software manages accounts payable, prints checks, and tracks expenses. It tracks financial information and prepares tax information for the accountant. There are even programs currently available that allow practices to handle all of this online.

Accounting software, whether it is part of the veterinary software or a supplemental software package, is essential for evaluation and management of the practices' *profit centers.* Profit centers are specific components of a practice that generate income. For instance, boarding is a profit center within the practice. There are costs incurred by the practice to provide boarding services, and there is income generated. Evaluation of the profit-to-loss ratio aides practice managers in decisions regarding that profit center (i.e., staffing, equipment, supplies, etc.). To attempt to get this information without the use of a computer would be difficult and time consuming.

> *TECHNICIAN NOTE* As medical services are added to the medical record, charges are automatically added to the invoice. This facilitates billing and reduces the potential for lost revenue.

IMPLICATIONS FOR THE FUTURE

PAPERLESS VERSUS LESS PAPER

The term *paperless* applies to a business that manages all of its information on one computer system. Currently, most veterinary practices are considered to be "less-paper" practices rather than "paperless." The typical computerized veterinary practice still generates literally tons of information on paper and media that are not being stored in the computer. X-rays, consent forms, travel sheets, time cards, faxes, admission forms, referral letters, anesthesia-surgery logs, controlled substances logs, etc., are all still produced on a daily basis. A *paperless* office is not a pipe dream any longer. Scanners and CD-Rom technology are readily available and affordable. Information stored electronically is safer than printed media. Ten CDs can store approximately hundreds of thousands of documents. All of that information can easily be carried out of the practice and stored off of the premises. The loss of information in the event of a fire can be catastrophic in a conventional veterinary setting.

Some practice managers hesitate to convert to a paperless system for legal reasons. To date, it appears that no paperless case has gone to court. Yet the concerns are that medical records must be protected from alteration afterward. Proof of electronic medical record security can be provided by backing up the records on a monthly basis and storing them with a data storage facility. Comparison can then be made by the court that both copies match, ensuring the information contained within has not been corrupted.

OTHER APPLICATIONS FOR COMPUTER USE IN THE VETERINARY PRACTICE

The previous sections involved discussions about the software available to manage many of the business aspects of veterinary medicine. Technicians will find that computers will play an ever increasing role in their daily professional lives.

Continuing education is a good example. There are websites on the Internet dedicated to providing technicians a venue to ask questions, research information, read recent publications, and have direct access to specialists in the field. Some popular sites for technicians are:

- www.VetMedTeam.com (Figure 4-9)
- www.VSPN.org (veterinary support personnel network) (Figure 4-10)

These sites require no more than a brief registration form ensuring the site that you are a technician or a technician student. They are free and encourage your participation and professional growth. Both sites have message boards on every discipline: anesthesia, animal behavior, avian and exotics, clinical pathology, dentistry, emergency and critical care, practice management, and other topics. They both have libraries with search engines to narrow the information search. Both sites offer classes for continuing educational credits (fee associated), and both have chat rooms used for classes.

There are other veterinary-related websites:

- www.avma.org (American Veterinary Medical Association [AVMA])
- www.vin.com (Veterinary Information Network)

The AVMA site is open to anyone who wants to visit the site, including pet owners. There is a special section of the website called NOAH. Access to this area is gained with a membership number (dues required) and a password. Vin.com is a site "for veterinarians by veterinarians." There are membership costs for veterinarians, and technicians are not permitted on this site. VSPN.org is the technician subsidiary of this site.

These sites are all beneficial because they offer veterinary professionals a means of discussing cases and sharing information. Each *message board* is monitored or edited by veterinarians or technicians that are either board certified specialists or hold a certain degree of expertise in a given discipline.

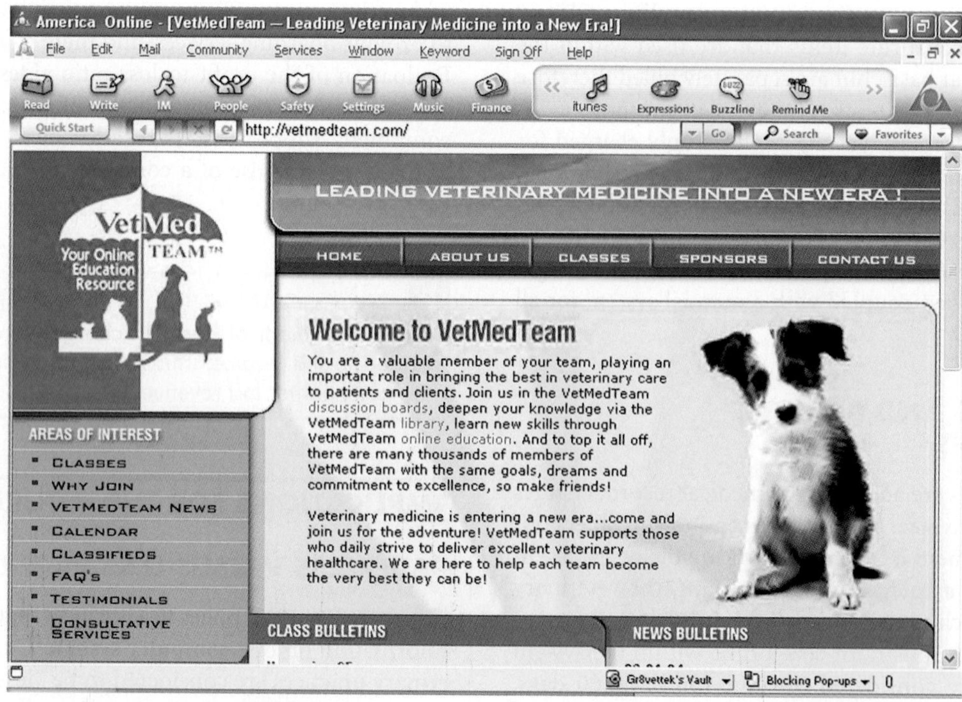
America Online - [VetMedTeam — Leading Veterinary Medicine into a New Era!]
File Edit Mail Community Services Window Keyword Sign Off Help
Read Write IM People Safety Settings Music Finance
itunes Expressions Buzzline Remind Me
Quick Start
http://vetmedteam.com/
Go
Search
Favorites
LEADING VETERINARY MEDICINE INTO A NEW ERA !
VetMed TEAM™
Your Online Education Resource
HOME
ABOUT US
CLASSES
SPONSORS
CONTACT US
Welcome to VetMedTeam
You are a valuable member of your team, playing an important role in bringing the best in veterinary care to patients and clients. Join us in the VetMedTeam discussion boards, deepen your knowledge via the VetMedTeam library, learn new skills through VetMedTeam online education. And to top it all off, there are many thousands of members of VetMedTeam with the same goals, dreams and commitment to excellence, so make friends!
Veterinary medicine is entering a new era...come and join us for the adventure! VetMedTeam supports those who daily strive to deliver excellent veterinary healthcare. We are here to help each team become the very best they can be!
AREAS OF INTEREST
CLASSES
WHY JOIN
VETMEDTEAM NEWS
CALENDAR
CLASSIFIEDS
FAQ'S
TESTIMONIALS
CONSULTATIVE SERVICES
CLASS BULLETINS
NEWS BULLETINS
Gr8vettek's Vault
Blocking Pop-ups
0

FIGURE 4-9 The VetMedTeam.com homepage.

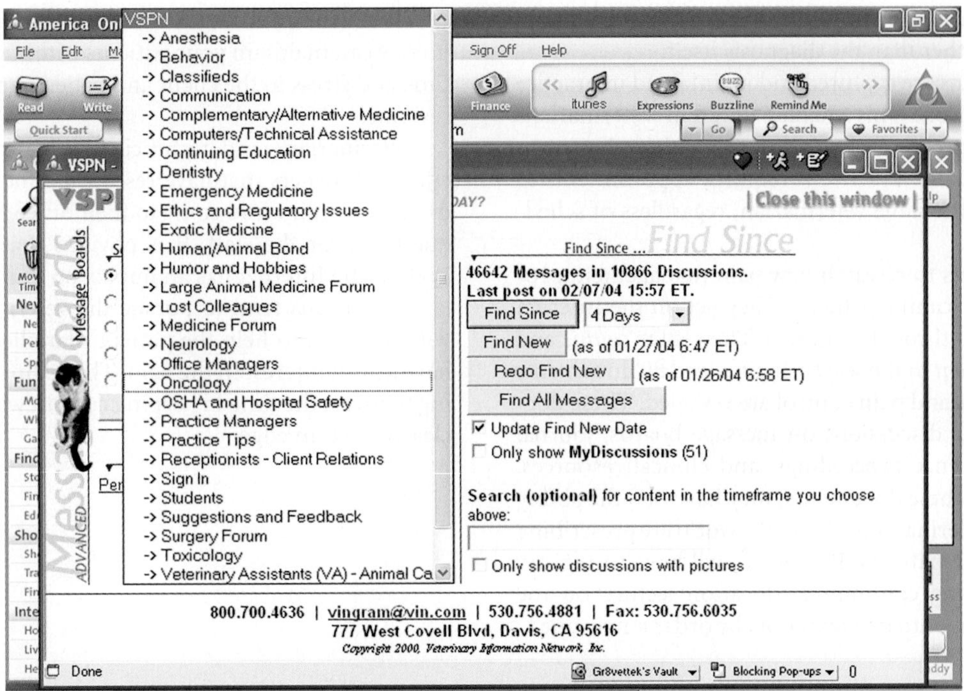

FIGURE 4-10 This shows the VSPN.org list of message boards in which technicians can participate.

It is not unusual to see digital photographs of lesions, unusual ECG strips, even digital radiographs posted within a discussion. This technology brings the case before many people from all over the world to gain varying ideas and options regarding treatment plans. The caveat to any information obtained on the Internet is this: there are no governing bodies regulating what is written or said on the World Wide Web. These websites have disclaimers reminding the reader that, regardless of the recommendations, the veterinarians are ultimately responsible for the care of their patients. Consider and confirm the information read on the Internet before employing it.

THE FUTURE IS NOT FAR AWAY

All of the discussed technology costs the practice money. But money invested upfront provides a greater return on investment in the long run. Some of the equipment available today for veterinarians is:

- Digital cameras
  - For capturing images of lesions, teeth, etc.
  - Able to be adapted to microscopes for slide imaging
  - Can capture image of radiographs
- Flatbed scanners
  - Expensive but capable of scanning conventional radiographs
- Digital radiology
  - Both regular and intraoral
- An affordable means of capturing and organizing dental radiographs
- DICOM (**D**igital **I**maging and **C**ommunications in **M**edicine) technology: a standard for handling, storing, and transmitting medical imaging. DICOM images can only be transmitted to entities that can receive DICOM images. The image will contain the patient's data, such as patient ID, so that the information about the patient and the image can never be separated.
- Computerized digital otoscope or endoscope
- Video capture systems for ultrasonography

Let us consider some of the ways that computer-related technology can help us provide more efficient and cost-effective medical care for our patients. In the following cases, practice A has various computer-related technologies, practice B does not.

1. A cat is admitted to practice A because of a misaligned bite. Practice A does not have a board certified veterinary dentist on staff. Instead, they take digital photos and digital radiographs and e-mail these images to a specialist. Within hours, practice A has heard from a board certified veterinary dentist as to whether or not referral holds any benefit to the patient. Practice B would have to copy and send the medical records along with the patient to the specialist for evaluation. These appointments can take weeks to months to obtain.
2. Practice A has provided training for technicians to obtain sonographic video images. These images can either be sent via the Internet to a medical consulting service, such as DarkHorse Telemedicine or a radiologist can come into the practice to review the tapes and provide diagnoses. Practice B will have to refer the patient to another practice that can provide these services.
3. Practice A can obtain images from cytology slides (see Figure 4-6) and maintains the images in a file. The samples are sent to an outside pathologist for review. When the report returns, the diagnosis is added to the file for

educational purposes within the practice. Practice B does not benefit further than the diagnosis itself.

4. Images of lesions are captured and maintained in practice A for comparison. This enables different veterinarians within the practice to evaluate progress without having to be present initially. Practice B requires appointments to be made with the same veterinarian, regardless of scheduling conflicts.
5. Practice A wants to research new pain management protocols for their canine patients. They get on the Internet and gain access through Vin.com. They enter *canine* and *pain management* in the search engine, and 80 documents relating to dogs and pain control are revealed. These documents include discussions on message boards, journal articles, conference proceedings, and clinical resources. After perusing these documents, they have had the ability to read what veterinarians all over the world are prescribing for their canine patients. Practice B will have to register for an upcoming continuing education lecture on the subject, read an outdated textbook, or order a new one.

These examples demonstrate how computer-related technology can maintain your patients within your practice, save time and stress to the client and patient, and overall increase revenue.

Veterinarians and technicians are surprised daily with educated owners that have researched their pet's symptoms or disease online and come to their office visit with educated questions for the staff. It is obvious that the World Wide Web or the Internet has an impact on our daily lives.

Technicians tend to pursue the veterinary field to work with animals, to help the patient's families, or because they have a keen interest in the field. The technicians that are willing to invest the time in keeping current with technology will clearly have an edge.

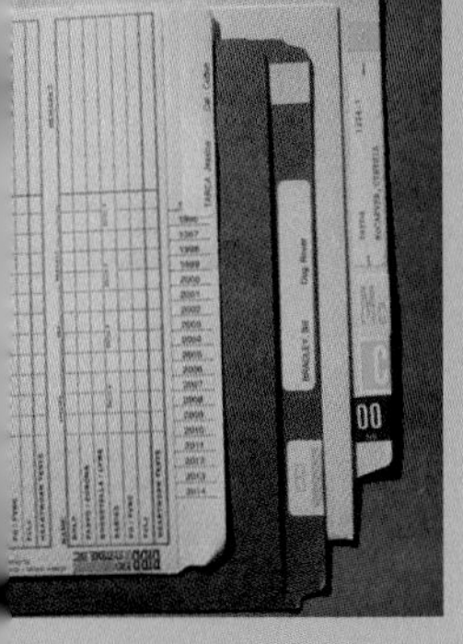

Medical Records

5

Joanna M. Bassert

KEY TERMS

Master problem list
Previous history
Problem-oriented medical record (POMR)
Progress notes
Recent history
Signalment
SOAP
Source-oriented medical record (SOMR)
Veterinary medical database
Working problem list

OUTLINE

LEARNING OBJECTIVES

When you have completed this chapter, you will be able to:

1. List and describe the primary and secondary purposes of the medical record.
2. Differentiate between letter-size, card file, and carbonized sheet medical records.
3. Differentiate between source-oriented and problem-oriented medical records.
4. List and describe the components of a problem-oriented veterinary medical record.
5. List the information recorded on a patient's medical history.
6. Define the SOAP process and explain the types of information included in each portion of the SOAP record.
7. List and describe the types of forms and logs commonly used in veterinary practice.
8. Describe the requirements of the Comprehensive Drug Abuse and Control Act.
9. List and describe the types of filing systems commonly used in veterinary practices.
10. Describe the ethical and legal issues related to the ownership of medical records, release of medical information, and maintenance of medical records.

INTRODUCTION

The keeping of medical records in veterinary practices has become increasingly more-sophisticated during the past several decades. Now with the use of computers, faxes, and e-mail, medical record keeping has taken on a new look and a greater level of complexity. Not surprisingly, even the term medical record keeping seems outdated because the phrase "veterinary medical health information management" more accurately describes the plethora of written and electronic records that are now routinely maintained by veterinary practices. Free from the confines of federal and state regulations that define medical record keeping in human hospitals, veterinary practices are able to apply a creative spectrum of approaches to record keeping. In this way, the individual needs of veterinary practices, in terms of business and medical information, may be effectively met by practice owners and managers.

Veterinary medical records include a wide range of forms and logs that document the treatment and care of animal patients. The results of physical examinations, laboratory tests, and diagnostic procedures, such as radiographic imaging, ultrasound, electrocardiograms, and endoscopy, are examples of information that is included in the record. In addition, medical records document treatment protocols, such as the administration of medication and intravenous fluids, surgery, wound care, and radiation or physical therapy. Medical records also describe the progress of patients, list daily observations, and chart vital signs and other monitoring data. Finally, medical records document euthanasia and postmortem examinations and include important authorization and consent forms.

The number and types of forms and logs that comprise medical records vary from practice to practice. Large teaching hospitals (e.g., those associated with schools of veterinary medicine) tend to have extensive medical records in which a separate form is used for each department, procedure, or study. Private companion animal practices, on the other hand, often employ shorter medical records that combine information into a concise chart or folder, which is easy to store and interpret. Finally, ambulatory food animal and equine practices often employ the most abbreviated form of medical record by using carbonized billing sheets as both medical record and invoice.

This chapter discusses the many approaches to medical record keeping that one sees in veterinary medicine. It offers a comprehensive "dissection" of the patient record, presents a variety of filing systems, and clarifies the ethical and legal issues that accompany the record keeping process.

FUNCTIONS OF THE MEDICAL RECORD

The Institute of Medicine has organized the functions of the medical record into two broad categories: primary purposes and secondary purposes. Primary purposes support the patient's medical care, such as the documentation of diagnostic procedures, diagnoses, prognoses, and treatment. Secondary purposes are not clinically based, but include evaluations of medical information for business, legal, and research purposes.

PRIMARY PURPOSES

Supports Excellent Medical Care

The medical record is a critical tool that enables and supports the effective treatment and care of animals, and it does this in many ways. First, it assists the veterinary health care team in correctly identifying the patient and the owner. There are, after all, many black Labrador retrievers that look alike and many owners named Smith, Jones, or Brown. In this way, the medical record helps to prevent confusion of the identities of the patients and their owners. Second, it helps in the generation of an effective diagnostic and treatment plan. It documents the veterinarian's physical examination findings, lists the diagnostic procedures and tests to be performed, and records the veterinarian's ideas regarding differential diagnoses. The medical record also enables practitioners to document the patient's responses to treatment, so plans may be adjusted as needed. As time passes and members of the health care team change, the medical record supports continuity of care. It helps practitioners, who are not familiar with the patient, to understand the medical history and conditions of the animal. In this way, it provides an avenue for communication between each of the members of the veterinary health care team so that treatment can be accurately and effectively administered.

Documents Communication

The medical record also documents communication with the client, which is particularly important when there are many members of the veterinary health care team assisting the same client. Take-home instructions, for example, will be included in the medical record, so any confusion about home care by the client (owner) can be quickly clarified. In addition, the medical record assists in the generation of reminder cards that help pet owners to stay current in their pet's preventive medical plan. In these ways, good communication is critical for providing a logical, continued plan of patient care for both the health care providers and for the pet owner.

Interactions with clients and their pets are also aided by the use of medical records. Financial limitations, for example, and the behavioral idiosyncrasies of the pet may be recorded. In addition, the veterinarian-client relationship can be further enhanced when the names of other family members and important family activities are noted in the record as reminders for future topics of informal discussion.

SECONDARY PURPOSES

Supports Business and Legal Activities

The medical record lists all of the services rendered to the pet owner, whether it is boarding a dog or spaying a cat. This documentation verifies billing and serves as legal evidence of services received by the owner. It can be used to assess the workloads of staff members, formulate income analysis, make budgetary plans, perform actuarial calculations, maintain inventory, and generate a marketing strategy. In addition, it plays an important role during hospital accreditations and helps assess compliance with standards of care.

The medical record is used as a legal document in a court of law and is valuable during litigation. It serves as evidence of procedures performed and treatments administered, and it provides specific dates and times of events. In this way, the medical record is critical in defending against malpractice suits. Special care must be taken to ensure that the record is complete and accurate. Keep in mind that in a court of law, the prevailing view is "not recorded, not done." In addition, insurance companies may require the medical record to assess whether a claim is to be paid.

Supports Research

The medical record is a key element in the preparation of case studies and presentations for conferences. Information from medical records is collected to develop registries

BOX 5-1 Summary Chart: Functions of the Medical Record

I. Primary Purposes
Supports Excellent Medical Care
A. Identifies correct patient and owner
B. Supports generation of diagnostic and treatment plans
C. Supports continuity of care
D. Supports communication
 1. Among health care team members
 2. With the owner
 3. Personalizes veterinarian-client relationship

II. Secondary Purposes
Supports Business and Legal Activities
A. Verifies billing
B. Supports actuarial calculations
 1. Income analysis
 2. Budgetary plans
 3. Staff workloads
C. Supports inventory maintenance
D. Supports formulation of marketing strategy
E. Supports hospital accreditation
F. Acts as a legal document
Supports Research
A. Case studies and presentations
B. Registries and databases
C. Education of veterinarians and veterinary technicians

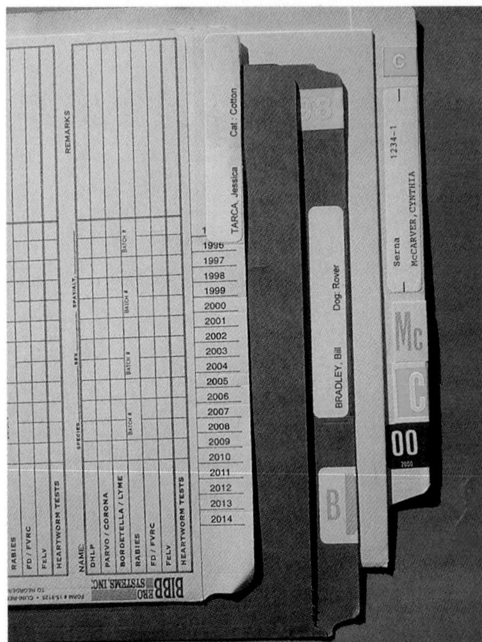

FIGURE 5-1 Shown are a variety of letter-size folders. The color and style of the folders can vary in addition to whether charting is stamped on the cover. Color-coded decals are placed on the edge of the folders to facilitate filing.

and databases, which assist in the conduction of retrospective studies and in predicting clinical outcomes. It is used to teach veterinary medical and veterinary technician students. To maintain confidentiality, all patient markers are removed from the record before they are used for any purpose other than patient care (Box 5-1).

TECHNICIAN NOTE A comprehensive medical record supports excellent medical care, research, and good business practices. It also helps to protect practices during malpractice litigation.

TYPES OF PATIENT RECORDS

With use of computers and veterinary practice management software, veterinary hospitals are managing information better and more efficiently than ever before. However, the vast majority of practices continue to employ hard copy, paper-based medical records in addition to using computers. This chapter concentrates on the written record, whereas Chapter 4 concentrates on the digital record and the use of computers in information management.

Medical records come in a variety of shapes and sizes. They typically appear as letter-size folders that contain a variety of forms and charts held in place by fixed clips. However, they can also come in the form of large index-type cards on which the veterinarian makes handwritten notes. In addition, ambulatory food or equine practices often carry simple carbonized forms that serve as both a record of the services rendered and the charges assigned. Let us examine each type of medical record in greater detail.

LETTER-SIZE FOLDERS

The vast majority of veterinary practices today make use of 8- × 10-inch folders in which medical information is stored and organized (Figure 5-1). Each patient has its own folder. Tabs are located at the edge of one end of the folder to facilitate the placement of color-coded decals. Some folders have grids printed on the outside of the cover on which critical information, such as the animal's immunization history, can be written. In this way, the staff can quickly visualize key pieces of information. More commonly, however, veterinary practices use folders with a plain Manila cover.

Letter-size folders are typically stored vertically on shelves, which are kept behind or near the receptionist's desk for easy retrieval. Some particularly large practices may have record rooms in which a mobile shelving system may be employed. In these systems, large shelves are mounted on tracks so that they can be moved easily from one location to another when pushed. Mobile shelving systems save space because shelves may be positioned up against one another when access to their records is not needed (Figure 5-2).

CARD FILES

To conserve space and cost, some veterinary practices use a card file system instead of maintaining letter-size folders. One type of card used is 5 × 8 inches, which is stored in a

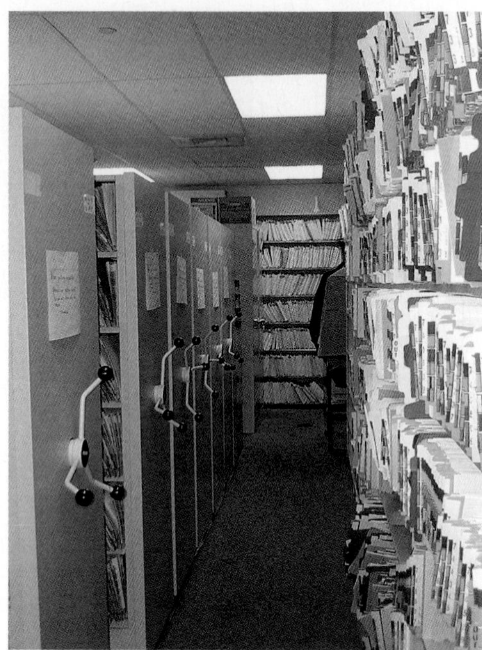

FIGURE 5-2 Mobile shelving creates more storage space for medical records. These shelves move on tracks that are fixed to the floor. Each shelf is moved by turning the wheel crank located on the side of the shelf.

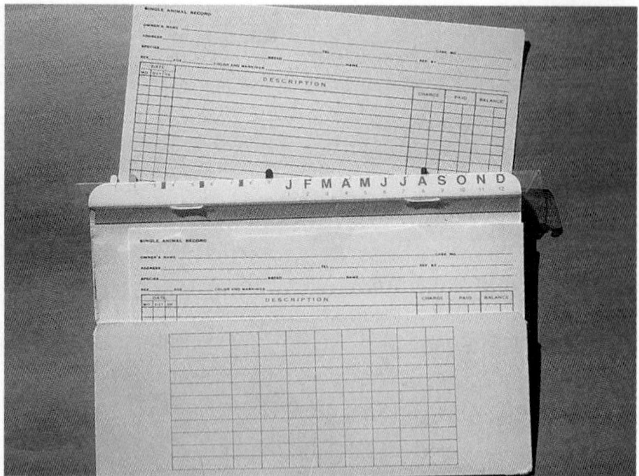

FIGURE 5-3 The card-style record with pocket folder, though once popular, is not as commonly used as the letter-sized folders.

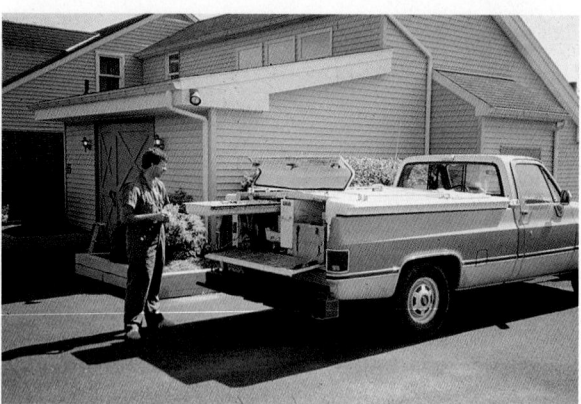

FIGURE 5-4 An ambulatory veterinarian has little room in his truck for cumbersome medical records.

file pocket (Figure 5-3). Laboratory data and other reports can also be stored in the pocket with the animal record. As more and more writing space is needed, additional cards can be stapled to the original card. If a family has more than one animal, there is a separate card for each patient, but the cards are often clipped together and filed as one unit.

Another card system involves the use of a 10- × 16-inch card, which can accommodate more information per card than the 5 × 8 system. The 10- × 16-inch card can be folded in half to facilitate handling.

Card files are typically stored in file drawers rather than on shelves and are generally organized in alphabetic order according to the first letter of the last name of the client.

A plastic strip along the top of the folder contains a letter for each month and numbers that help receptionists to keep track of when reminder cards should be mailed. In addition, the strip contains hooks that enable the file to be suspended on a rack in the file drawer.

As a result of their small size and limited writing space, information contained on cards is brief. The patient's information is usually entered in reverse chronologic order. The date and information regarding each appointment is entered on a separate line. Each card file must contain the owner's and patient's information along with sufficient data to allow the proper and adequate care of the animal. However, in our modern, litigious society, keeping thorough and complete records is increasingly more important because detailed medical information is often requested in a court of law. In addition, practices seeking accreditation by the American Animal Hospital Association (AAHA) are required to use letter-size folders. For these reasons, cards, though once popular, are not as commonly used today because letter-size folders can accommodate a more comprehensive animal health record.

CARBONIZED SHEETS (AMBULATORY LARGE ANIMAL PRACTICES)

Ambulatory food animal and equine practitioners work long hours and put many miles on their trucks as they travel from farm to farm (Figure 5-4). The use of lengthy medical records is impractical in a situation where there is little storage space (in the truck) and where paper might blow out the window. Many ambulatory practitioners make handwritten notes on carbonized invoice sheets that are loaded into a sturdy metal dispenser (Figure 5-5). Once procedures are performed, diagnostic and treatment notes and billing information may all be included on the invoice pages. A copy is given to the owner. Information from the sheets is typed into the computerized record keeping system at the practice's home office. A veterinarian who spends long days on the road might joke that this system is in keeping with the "Veterinary Medicine Paperwork Reduction Act," but it is also cost-effective and practical. Throughout the year, but particularly in the spring, during lambing and foaling season when practitioners receive remarkably little sleep, the carbonized sheets provide adequate documentation and communication in a time-efficient manner. This helps the veterinarian meet the heavy demands of ambulatory practice.

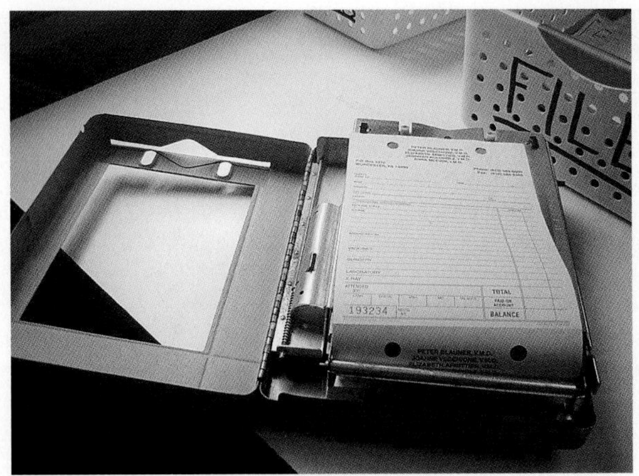

FIGURE 5-5 The carbonized billing sheet also serves as an accounting of the treatments performed during a farm call.

Many veterinarians have begun to use laptop computers in the trucks to assist with record keeping. In this situation, the practitioner enters diagnostic, treatment, and billing information into a portable laptop computer that can be plugged into the cigarette lighter or run on batteries. The data can later be transferred to the practice's networked computer system when the veterinarian returns to the office to restock the truck. Some ambulatory practitioners use an index of bar codes, each one representing a different diagnosis, procedure, or medication. The veterinarian scans the appropriate bar codes to create an invoice and to document the diagnosis and treatments rendered. Instructions to the owner might also be generated. A small portable printer carried in the truck would enable the document to be printed on-site and subsequently given to the owner. Wireless capabilities are also being explored by some progressive ambulatory practices.

It is impractical for food animal veterinarians, who are responsible for the health of entire herds of livestock, to maintain an individual record for every animal treated. In this situation, records are kept on the herd as a whole. Immunizations and reproductive histories are maintained for the group, although individual records may be generated for animals that have undergone special surgical or treatment procedures.

Large animal teaching hospitals and full-service equine practices commonly have hospitalized surgery, medicine, and neonatal patients and often employ the standard 8- × 10-inch file record system. In this situation, each patient has its own medical record. In-house treatments and procedures are recorded in the record by hospital staff members. An invoice is generated separately and is typically given to the owner for payment before the animal is allowed to be discharged and loaded onto the trailer.

FORMAT OF THE PATIENT RECORD

As mentioned, veterinary medical records are not subject to the federal and state regulations that one sees in the human medical field. Therefore there is a wide range of approaches to record keeping, which vary from practice to practice. Most methods, however, fall into one of three categories:

1. Source-oriented medical record (SOMR)
2. Problem-oriented medical record (POMR)
3. Combination of source- and problem-oriented medical records

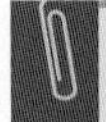

TECHNICIAN NOTE Most companion animal practices use a combination of SOMR and POMR.

SOURCE-ORIENTED MEDICAL RECORD

The source-oriented method is typically used in records that have limited space, such as in the card- or pocket-type records. Information comes from various sources and is entered chronologically by office visit or period of hospitalization. In this way, the most recent information is located last. Typically the date is entered in the far left-hand column of a line on the card, and the entry is made to the right of that. Physical exam findings, the database, diagnoses, and treatments are all listed. The veterinarian often makes entries in a "free form" that integrates information from various sources as it becomes available or comes to mind. The source-oriented method is easy to learn and takes little time to complete; however, it can lack detailed documentation, which may prove vital during litigation. Remember, "if it is not written down, it didn't happen."

PROBLEM-ORIENTED VETERINARY MEDICAL RECORD

The problem-oriented veterinary medical record (POVMR) is used in conjunction with the folder type of medical record and is used in teaching hospitals, AAHA-accredited hospitals, and many private companion animal practices, including specialty and emergency centers. The format helps to provide a whole view of the patient and supports a logical and organized approach to clinical medicine. It fosters excellent communication, team-oriented medical care, and rapid retrieval of information. Veterinary teaching hospitals find the POVMR particularly helpful when veterinary medical and veterinary technology students first learn to approach medical cases. The format provides a structured way to walk students through complicated cases, one problem at a time. In addition, a requirement for AAHA-accreditation is use of the problem-oriented format.

Though the components of the POVMR can vary somewhat, it most commonly includes the following:

1. Client and patient information
2. History
3. Physical examination
4. Master problem list and working problem list
5. Progress notes, assessment, and plan
6. Pertinent forms: surgery, anesthesia, radiography, special imaging, and laboratory reports
7. Case summary
8. Fee information

BOX 5-2 Standard Information for Veterinary Medical Records

Client Information
Name of owner
Address
Home phone number
Alternate phone number
If applicable, referring person
Additional information if co-owned

Patient Information
Name of animal
Signalment: species, breed, age, sex, and spayed or neutered
Color and markings
If applicable, tattoo, microchip number, and identification (ID) number

Pertinent History
Presenting complaint
Last normal
Frequency of episodes
Client observations and/or concerns
Current medications
Allergies
Current diet

Previous History
Previous problems
Previous treatments and responses (including transfusions)
Previous surgeries
Previous medications
Previous diagnostic tests
Immunization history
Environmental history
Travel history
Patient's weight history
Previous diet

Physical Examination Form
Master problem list and working problem list
Progress notes:
Date
Physical examination findings
Problems
Tentative diagnoses
Definitive diagnoses
Prognoses
Therapeutic plans
Changes in therapy
Medications administered and dispensed
Name of medication
Expiration date
Time
Date
Dosage and directions
Fluid rate
Route of administration
Frequency
Duration of treatment
Identification of individuals
Cautionary notes
Slaughter withdraw and/or milk withholding dates (food animal)
Procedures performed in chronologic order
Client communications

Pertinent Forms
Laboratory reports
Reports and assessments of diagnostic procedures (endoscopy, radiography, ultrasound, and special imaging)
Description of surgical and dental procedures, including duration of procedure and name of surgeon
Anesthesia record
Consultation reports with specialists or other referring veterinarians (dermatology, oncology, cardiology, ophthalmology, surgery, internal medicine, dentistry, and neurology)
Signed consent forms
Client waivers or deferrals of recommendations
Client phone log
Discharge instructions
Necropsy report

Financial Records

From Peden AH: *Comparative records for health information management,* Delmar, AVMA Guidelines for Basic Information for Records, and the American Animal Hospital Association Standards of Accreditation.

These components can be further subdivided into more specific units of information (Box 5-2).

COMPONENTS OF THE POVMR

CLIENT AND PATIENT INFORMATION

Typically the receptionist first takes the name, address, and telephone number of the client when the first appointment is made. This information is confirmed later when the owner arrives for the appointment. It is particularly important to record the correct spelling of the owner's first and last name. Even seemingly simple names such as Megan Brown may be spelled Meaghan Brown or Meghan Browne. Do not assume to know the correct spelling of the client's name; always confirm it. This will prevent subsequent filing and client-identity errors.

Cell phone numbers and e-mail addresses of the owner may also be important to obtain when the owner is in the office. In addition, the receptionist might want to have a general idea of the client's schedule for the day and where he or she can be reached at what time. This is particularly critical if the pet is undergoing surgery or a procedure that requires anesthesia. Unexpected events or findings can occur during clinical procedures, and the veterinarian may need to consult the owner immediately. Sometimes the owner must

DATE ____________ CASE NUMBER ____________

COMPANION ANIMAL CLIENT/PATIENT INFORMATION FORM

Please provide the following information for our records: **PLEASE PRINT!**

OWNER INFORMATION

OWNER'S NAME			SOCIAL SECURITY NUMBER
STREET ADDRESS			
CITY/STATE		ZIP CODE	PARISH OR COUNTY
TELEPHONE NUMBER(S) (Area Code, if long distance) →	HOME		BUSINESS
DRIVER'S LICENSE NUMBER	PLACE OF EMPLOYMENT		HOW LONG?

ANIMAL INFORMATION

ANIMAL SPECIES (Dog, Cat, Other)			BREED
ANIMAL'S NAME		SEX	HAS ANIMAL BEEN SEXUALLY ALTERED? ☐ Yes ☐ No
COLOR	BIRTHDATE (Month/year, or approximate)	The undersigned owner or agent certifies that the herein described animal has a maximum value of approximately $	

REFERRAL INFORMATION

WERE YOU REFERRED BY A VETERINARIAN? ☐ Yes ☐ No	IF YOU WERE REFERRED BY A VETERINARIAN, PLEASE COMPLETE THE FOLLOWING:
VETERINARIAN'S NAME	PHONE
STREET ADDRESS	
CITY/STATE	ZIP CODE

You will be advised of estimated cost and anticipated procedures. Please feel free to discuss the proposed treatment and its cost with the veterinarian. A minimum deposit of 50% of the initial estimated charges will be required for hospitalization of an animal patient.

STATEMENT OF OWNERSHIP AND CONSENT: I am the owner of the above described animal, or have authorization from the owner to consent to its treatment.

I hereby authorize the performance of professionally accepted diagnostic, therapeutic, anesthetic, and surgical procedures necessary for its treatment.

I accept financial responsibility for these services.

I have read the above consent and understand why the above procedures may be necessary. I also have been told of the possible complications and alternatives to the listed procedures.

PAYMENT CHOICE: ☐ Cash ☐ Check ☐ Bank Card

SIGNATURE (Owner/Agent)	DATE

FIGURE 5-6 Client and patient information form.

make important decisions over the telephone, such as the extent of treatment to be performed, while the animal is on the surgery table and/or under an anesthetic. In this situation, good communication and care for the patient is maximized if the client can be contacted.

In addition to the client information, the receptionist also records the age, breed, sex, and species of the patient. This information is collectively known as the signalment. In some veterinary practices, it is imprinted, together with the client information, on the top of each medical record form using a plastic hospital card. When using a wide range of forms, as is done in many veterinary teaching hospitals, it is important to always remember to stamp each and every form. Refer to Figure 5-6 for an example of a client-patient information form.

The signalment of the patient is the first critical bit of information that helps the veterinarian in problem solving. Cancerous tumors, for example, are less likely to occur in puppies than in older dogs. Similarly, congenital abnormalities, such as a cleft palate, are often first noticed in young animals, so it is rare to first diagnose them in older animals. Similarly, there are certain conditions that are typically seen in large breeds of dogs and rarely seen in small breeds. Disorders may typically be seen in cats, but not in dogs. In this way, the signalment immediately assists the veterinarian to hone in on certain disorders and rule out others.

HISTORY FORM

A comprehensive history includes both previous and recent history information. It is typically taken during each new-patient visit and during visits from those patients that have not been seen in several years. Some practices have two

VETERINARY HOSPITAL OF THE UNIVERSITY OF PENNSYLVANIA
3900 DELANCEY STREET
PHILADELPHIA, PA 19104

RABIES SUSPECT ? ___ YES ___ NO | CHANGES FROM LAST VISIT ___ NONE ___ AS NOTED

MANAGEMENT	BEHAVIOR
ORIGIN – GEOGRAPHIC LOCATION FROM WHOM – WHEN	USUAL DISPOSITION UNUSUAL BEHAVIOR PATTERN
STATES AND COUNTRIES KEPT IN	ENVIRONMENT
WHERE KEPT ALLOWED TO RUN FREE?	OTHER ANIMALS WITH HEALTH PROBLEMS
USUAL DIET	RELATED DISEASE (IN OWNER'S FAMILY)
PREVENTION	ALLERGIES / REACTIONS
	DIET
RABIES VACCINATION DATE GIVEN DATE DUE	MEDICATION / TREATMENT
COMBINATION VACC. DATE GIVEN	BLOOD COMPONENT THERAPY
________ VACC. DATE GIVEN	X-MATCHED
HEARTWORM Seasonal Y N	REPRODUCTIVE
BRAND ________ Year 'round Y N	NEUTERED
FLEA/TICK Seasonal Y N	LAST ESTRUS
BRAND ________ Year 'round Y N	
	BRED

PREVIOUS CONDITIONS, PROBLEMS, OR OPERATIONS (LIST, WITH DATE, IF KNOWN)

PRESENTING PROBLEM OR COMPLAINT (INCLUDE TREATMENT BY OTHER VETERINARIANS)

HISTORY

B-1
FORM CONTROL NO.

A

FIGURE 5-7 A, Example of a comprehensive history form.

history forms: one in which the previous history information is recorded and the other for recent history information. Figure 5-7, *A* shows an example of a history form in which both the previous and recent history information is recorded together.

Previous history information includes the following:

1. Origin: animal's birthplace and date
2. Preventive medicine program: immunizations, parasite control, dental care program, ear care program
3. Behavior: usual disposition and temperament, unusual behavioral events
4. Environment: kept indoors or outdoors, presence of other pets in the home, level of exposure to non–family-owned pets, travel history
5. Known allergies and reactions: atopy, food, contact with substances, medications, blood transfusions
6. Reproduction: neutered, estrus cycles, when bred, number of litters
7. Previous conditions, trauma, or surgical operations

Recent history information includes:

1. Presenting complaint and circumstances
2. Last normal
3. Frequency of episodes
4. Current medications
5. Treatment efforts
6. Comments and concerns of the owner
7. Current diet
8. Information from previous or referring veterinarian

PHYSICAL EXAMINATION FORM

The physical examination is one of the most important diagnostic procedures and, if performed carefully and systematically, can provide the clinician with the critical information that ultimately leads to a diagnosis. The physical examination

PHYSICAL EXAMINATION

Temp.	Pulse/min.	Resp./min.

Attitude at time of Exam (Circle one)
(Vicious, excited, alert, depressed, comatose, other________)
Nutritional state (Circle one)
(Obese, overweight, normal, underweight, cachectic)

State of Hydration: good, fair, poor. (Circle one) Weight (from scale) kg.

SYSTEMATIC EXAMINATION (Use space below as needed)

Oro-Pharyngeal

Eyes

Ears

Respiratory

Cardiovascular

Gastrointestinal and Anus

Rectal

Uro-Genital

Integument

Lymph Nodes

Musculo-Skeletal

Nervous

Physical Exam Performed By:

(Student's signature)

PROBLEMS:
1.
2.
3.
4.

B

FIGURE 5-7—cont'd B, This physical examination form is printed on the back of the comprehensive history form shown in Figure 5-5.

form is structured in such a way as to help the veterinarian and the veterinary technician to examine each anatomic system without overlooking anything. Notes are made directly on the form. "WLN," for example, may be written, which means "within normal limits," or "B & A" may be written, which means "bright and alert." There is a wide variety of abbreviations that clinicians use when completing medical record forms. Refer to Figures 5-7, *B* and 5-8 for examples of a physical examination form.

DATABASE

In the POVMR, the signalment, history, physical examination, and diagnostic tests are collectively known as the database. The database forms the foundation of information on which veterinarians are able to make their diagnoses and therapeutic plans. Each veterinary hospital, however, may have its own variation on the standard database. Animals admitted for either a routine visit or a hospital stay may have, for example, a complete blood count, urinalysis, and fecal analysis. In this way, the database can vary depending on the needs of the patient. The tests done on the first visit will be considered the original database, and any subsequent visits should provide data for current problems.

In many emergency and critical care units, the database is considered to include five or six important pieces of information that are key in treating the critical patient. These include the: packed-cell volume, total solids, potassium, blood urea nitrogen, dextrose, and urinalysis. These data can be

JONATHAN HART DVM 2441 TREASURE HILL BLVD HOUSTON, TEXAS 78550 210 389 4726	BERNARD DAVIS 66444 1087 TARA BLVD BATON ROUGE, LA 70825 CAN LAB F/S BO BLK 11/30/96

IMMUNIZATION PREVENTATIVE RECORD

DATE	5/10/03	6/14/04							
RABIES	X	X							
DA2PL	X	X							
PARVO	X	X							
FVRCP									
FELV VACC.									
FELV/FIV									
FECAL	neg.	neg.							
HEARTWORM	neg.	neg.							

PROBLEM LIST	DATE ENTERED	DATE RESOLVED
1. Elective Ovariohysterectomy	8/10/95	8/10/95
2. Malassezia-otitis externa	8/10/95	8/17/95
3. Dental prophylaxis	11/3/98	11/3/98
4. Gastroenteritis — small bowel diarrhea	3/15/99	3/18/99
5. Uncomplicated UTI	2/3/05	2/16/05
6. Recurrent UTI — E. Coli	3/14/05	3/28/05
7. Recurrent UTI	6/10/05	6/20/05
8. Right Renomegaly; Cystic kidney mass	6/20/05	
9. Right unilateral nephrectomy	6/23/05	6/23/05
10. Renal carcinoma	6/24/05	
11. Lethary, anorexia	7/2/05	7/5/05
12.		
13.		

BREED= SEX=

FIGURE 5-8 Immunization history record and master problem list.

acquired quickly with a small amount of blood, a countertop centrifuge and analyzer, and dipsticks.

MASTER PROBLEM LIST

A defining part of the POVMR is the problem list. The master problem list includes the major medical disorders experienced by a patient during its lifetime. These medical problems are listed in chronologic order, and a date is noted when and if they are resolved. In this way, the master problem list serves as a snapshot overview of the patient's medical history. At a glance, the clinician can determine what happened, when, and how long it lasted. See Figure 5-8 for an example of a master problem list. A summary of the preventive medical history may accompany the master problem list, which includes the dates when immunizations were administered and the results of fecal analysis and feline leukemia and heartworm tests.

> TECHNICIAN NOTE The working problem list helps the veterinarian to evaluate symptoms, think critically, and arrive at a final diagnosis.

WORKING PROBLEM LIST

The working problem list (Figure 5-9 and Table 5-1) is often used in veterinary teaching hospitals and assists the clinician and student in working through problems that are relevant to the current hospital stay. For example, if the patient is hospitalized and is subsequently diagnosed with autoimmune hemolytic anemia, the working problem list may list symptomatic problems initially until the final diagnosis is made.

Compare the working problem list with the master problem list. Notice that the master problem list is essentially a list of final diagnoses rather than a list of symptoms.

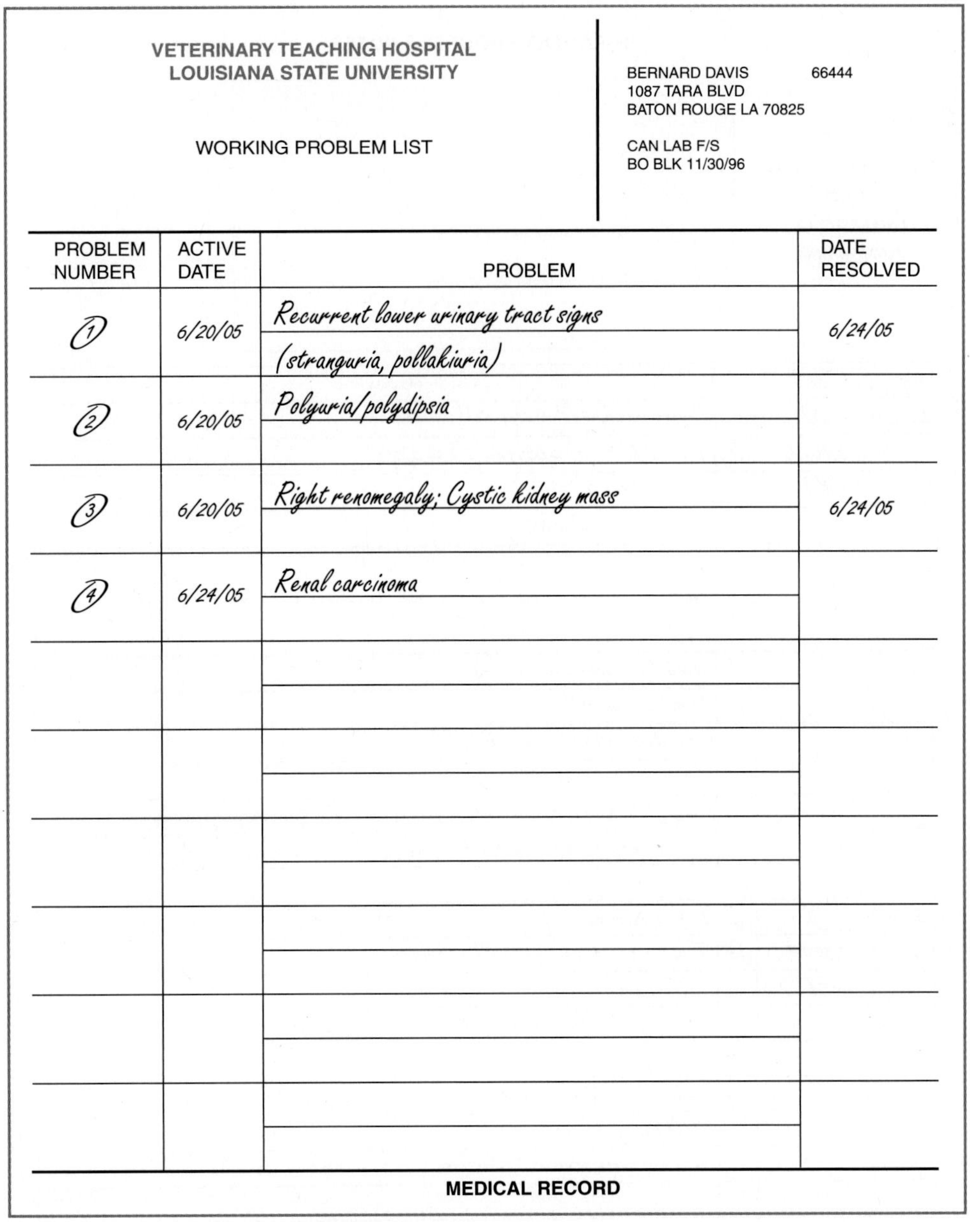

VETERINARY TEACHING HOSPITAL
LOUISIANA STATE UNIVERSITY

WORKING PROBLEM LIST

BERNARD DAVIS 66444
1087 TARA BLVD
BATON ROUGE LA 70825

CAN LAB F/S
BO BLK 11/30/96

PROBLEM NUMBER	ACTIVE DATE	PROBLEM	DATE RESOLVED
1	6/20/05	Recurrent lower urinary tract signs (stranguria, pollakiuria)	6/24/05
2	6/20/05	Polyuria/polydipsia	
3	6/20/05	Right renomegaly; Cystic kidney mass	6/24/05
4	6/24/05	Renal carcinoma	

MEDICAL RECORD

FIGURE 5-9 Working problem list.

TABLE 5-1 Working Problem List

Problem Number	Active Date	Problem
1	6/20/05	Depression/lethargy
2	6/20/05	Pale yellow mucous membrane
3	6/20/05	Mild tachycardia
4	6/21/05	Anemia
5	6/21/05	Icterus
6	6/22/05	Autoimmune hemolytic anemia

The working problem list helps the clinician to list clinical signs as they become apparent without offering a specific diagnosis. When a final diagnosis is reached, such as autoimmune hemolytic anemia in this case, the diagnosis can be added to the master problem list.

PROGRESS NOTES

The ongoing management of veterinary patients is documented in the progress notes (Figure 5-10). Each time a patient visits the veterinary hospital, notes are made to summarize the visit. The date of the appointment, physical examination findings, and the reason for the visit are noted. If the animal is sick, problems are listed and a tentative diagnoses or list of differential diagnoses is generated. If diagnostic procedures are performed, the findings are entered and a definitive diagnosis may be noted together with therapeutic plans, the medication given, and the patient's prognosis. Communications with the client and any changes in therapy are also noted.

When the patient is hospitalized, progress notes are used to record the daily events. In many practices and in teaching hospitals, the patient is examined carefully at the beginning

IN-PATIENT PROGRESS NOTES

VETERINARY HOSPITAL OF THE UNIVERSITY OF PENNSYLVANIA

DATE	PROBLEM NUMBER	S.O. A.P.	PROGRESS NOTES
03/06/05	①	S	Bright and alert (B + A), sternal recumbancy
	8:30 AM	O	T = 101.5°F P = 85 bpm RR = 30bpm
	JMB		CRT < 2 sec
			PCV = 42 TS = 6.8
			Incision looks clean and all sutures present. No evidence of seroma or discharge.
		A.	Normal post-operative recovery
		P.	Send home this PM
			disp. #20 250 mg Clavamox P.O. BID
	3:30 PM		"Misty" discharged to owner w/Clavamox as per JMB. Gave surgery discharge
	TNP		instruction sheet & reviewed it w/owner.
03/16/05	①	Ⓢ	B + A, standing
	1:30 PM	Ⓞ	T = 101.2 P = 90 bpm RR = panting
	WCT		CRT < 2 sec
			incision: excellent skin apposition & closure. 2 sutures missing.
		Ⓐ	Normal healing incision
		Ⓟ	Removed remaining sutures (9)
			No follow-up necessary
			— remind owner of annual visit in June

B - 9
FORM CONTROL NO.

FIGURE 5-10 Progress notes.

of each day. Therapeutic treatment and plans are evaluated and adjusted according to the progress of the patient. This process is called a morning SOAP. SOAP is an acronym for subjective, objective, assessment, and plan. In teaching hospitals, the SOAPs are typically performed by the veterinary medical students and residents. In private practices, veterinary technicians often complete the first half (S and O) of the SOAP, whereas the latter half (A and P) may be completed by the veterinarian. The subjective portion of the SOAP refers to the way the patient appears from the point of view of the casual observer. The patient, for example, may be "standing, panting, and wagging its tail," or the patient may be "awake, but in left lateral recumbency." Vocalizations, body posture, attitude, and positions are all noted as "subjective."

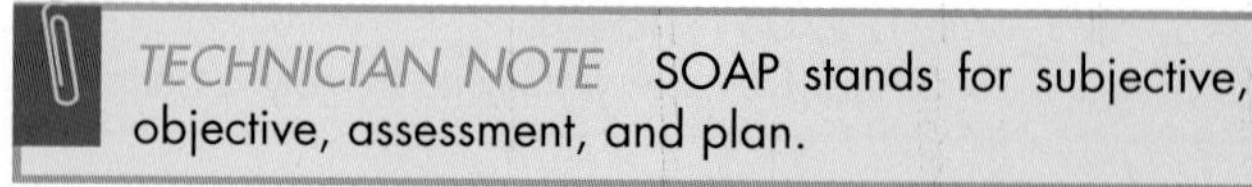

TECHNICIAN NOTE SOAP stands for subjective, objective, assessment, and plan.

The objective portion of the SOAP includes physiologic data, such as temperature, pulse, and respiration. The examiner would also note any vomitus, urination, and defecation and would describe the color and consistency of these, if applicable. If the patient were on intravenous fluid therapy, a small sample of blood would be drawn and the packed-cell volume, total solids, and results from the azodipsticks and dextrodipsticks would be recorded. Other easily accessible data, such as sodium and potassium values, might also be noted here. If the patient had surgery, notes regarding the surgical site, number of sutures present, and the level of swelling or drainage would also be made. If a urinary catheter and collection bag had been placed, urine output would be recorded.

Under the section assessment, the examiner would record the status of the patient. If the patient had undergone surgery, for example, the note might read "nonremarkable recovery postoperative" or "localized inflammatory response to suture material." An assessment for a medical case might read "polyuria and polydipsia noted with hyperglycemia. Diabetes mellitus likely."

Plan refers to the course of action that will be taken that day. Perhaps the patient will be discharged and given take-home medication, or perhaps the patient will undergo more diagnostic testing and observation. The medication to be given, procedures, and treatment plans to be performed are all described in this portion of the SOAP.

In teaching hospitals, an assessment and plan are sometimes written for each of the problems in the working problem list separately. Because this approach can lead to a lot of paperwork, an alternate method is to write an assessment and plan for the patient as a whole. Often the conditions and special circumstances of the case determine which approach is taken.

Any incoming information from a referring veterinarian or an animal's owner would also be placed in the progress notes section in chronologic order. Communication with the owner either in person, by telephone, or by e-mail is recorded in the progress notes in chronologic order.

> *TECHNICIAN NOTE* Be sure to initial the entries you make in the medical record. In a court of law, handwriting alone may be shown to be inadequate in identifying the author.

WARD TREATMENT SHEETS AND CAGE CARDS

Carrying out the treatments of hospitalized patients can be complicated, particularly in busy practices with heavy caseloads and in practices that treat emergency and critical care patients. To assist the veterinary health care team in carrying out the prescribed treatments efficiently, a treatment grid may be used. The grid may be part of a letter-size, ward treatment form that is kept in the patient's file (see the Evolve site at http://evolve.elsevier.com/McCurnin/vettech/), or it may be stamped on a card that is placed on the cage of the patient. The grid lists the treatments to be given and specifies the times throughout the day when each of the treatments should be completed. Specific doses, methods of administration, and cautionary notes should be noted. Examples of specialized ward treatment sheets for equine patients with colic (A) and diarrhea (B) and foals housed in the intensive care unit (C) can be found on the Evolve site at http://evolve.elsevier.com/McCurnin/vettech/. In most practices, the medications and supplies needed to complete the treatments are kept near the patient for convenience. Some practices store a patient's medications and treatment supplies in bins on a table or shelf along with the patient's medical record (Figure 5-11, *A*). Other practices prefer to use baskets that can be suspended from the patient's cage together with the ward treatment sheet (Figure 5-11, *B*). Hospitals for equine and food animal patients often maintain medications and supplies in treatment carts that can be wheeled easily in the barn aisles from stall to stall. Regardless of the approach used, it is important to label the medications and supplies clearly with the patient's name, signalment, and owner information.

Cage and stall cards are used to identify the patient and the reason for the hospitalization. The owner's and patient's information is stamped on the card. In some practices that do not use separate ward treatment sheets, the treatment grid is also stamped on the cage and stall card and lists the procedures to be performed. In some specialty practices, the color of the card may be used to indicate the hospital division that is treating the patient. A red card, for example, might indicate surgery, whereas a blue card might indicate internal medicine or cardiology.

PERTINENT FORMS

Depending upon the size and caseload of the veterinary practice, there may be separate forms for different hospital departments, specialists, or diagnostic procedures. Anesthesia, surgery, recovery, and pain management forms, for example, may all be pertinent to a patient that has undergone a surgical procedure (see the Evolve site at http://evolve.elsevier.com/McCurnin/vettech/). Similarly the results of diagnostic procedures, such as radiography and endoscopy, and laboratory tests may all be found in the medical record of an animal that had an esophageal foreign body (see the Evolve site at http://evolve.elsevier.com/McCurnin/vettech/).

LABORATORY DIAGNOSTIC SUMMARY AND FLOW SHEET

The laboratory diagnostic flow sheet is a compilation of laboratory data collected from an individual animal. It can be used for outpatients or inpatients. It shows at a glance the different laboratory values for the tests that have been performed on the patient. Specific values can be compared on the different dates for blood counts, chemistry panels, blood gases, urinalyses, and coagulation rates (see the Evolve site at http://evolve.elsevier.com/McCurnin/vettech/). This sheet is of particular value when evaluating internal medicine cases, such as animals with diabetes, anemia, chronic renal failure, hepatic failure, Addison's disease, and Cushing's disease. Two spaces at the bottom of the left column

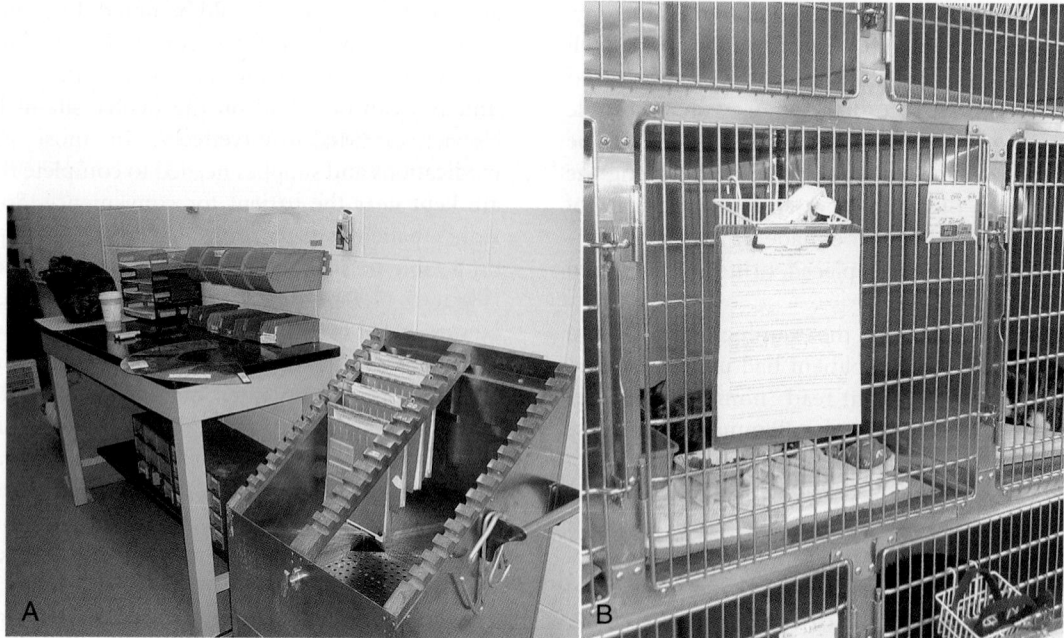

FIGURE 5-11 A, Some practices use individual bins to store the medications and supplies of each patient. These are kept near the medical record and are labeled with the patient's name. Notice that records kept on the wards are stored in protective metal holders. The record is removed from the holder before it is filed. B, Some practices store patient medications in wire baskets that can be attached directly to the door of the patient's cage. Medical records can also be attached to the cage. Both the record and the medications must be labeled clearly.

are reserved for additional laboratory data that is not already listed in the grid.

CONSULTANTS

Teaching and referral hospitals are often divided into departments. Specialties such as behavior, dermatology, medicine, neurology, nutrition, oncology, ophthalmology, orthopedics, and surgery are examples of the departments that can make up a large teaching and referral center. As cases are worked up, specialists may be consulted to address specific problems that the patient is experiencing. A consultation form would be employed, and the consulting veterinarian's findings, diagnosis, and recommendations would be recorded. Refer to the Evolve site at http://evolve.elsevier.com/McCurnin/vettech/. A copy of the consultation form is kept in the patient's record.

CASE SUMMARY AND DISCHARGE INSTRUCTIONS

When the patient is ready to be discharged, a summary of the case is written and discharge instructions are prescribed by the clinician. In some practices, the summary and home instructions are included on the same form. A copy of the form is given to the owner, and the veterinarian or veterinary technician reviews it with the owner before the animal leaves the hospital. In this way, the owner has a written account of the pet's diagnosis and treatment, which can be referred to frequently. The discharge instructions are written out clearly and reviewed directly with the owner (see the Evolve site at http://evolve.elsevier.com/McCurnin/vettech/). Often the clinician's name and contact information are included on the form so that the owner can call if questions or problems arise. If the animal was hospitalized at a specialty and referral center, the veterinarian often writes a formal letter to the referring veterinarian summarizing the case. In some veterinary practices, a copy of the case summary and discharge instructions form is mailed to the referring veterinarian in lieu of a formal letter.

Several days after a patient is discharged, the veterinarian often completes a follow-up call to the owner. This enables the clinician to assess the patient's progress at home and gives the owner an opportunity to ask questions. Pet owners are often grateful and appreciative of the special care that a follow-up call represents.

CONSENT AND AUTHORIZATION FORMS

Consent and authorization forms document in writing an understanding between the veterinary practice and the pet owner. The forms outline the specific conditions, risks of the procedure, and responsibilities of the two parties. In keeping with the doctrine of informed consent, completed authorization forms provide veterinary practices with legal evidence that the owner was informed of important information and that the owner agreed to pursue a particular course of action based on the circumstances and information given to him or her.

In many practices, consent forms are generated in those areas where there is the greatest potential for bad feelings as a result of poor communication. Obtaining authorizations to perform surgery, necropsy, and euthanasia are a few examples of situations where written owner permission and verbal communication are critical. During emergencies, for example, owners can be particularly emotional and may have difficulty making clear decisions. Owners who decide to euthanize their seriously injured pet may regret their decision later. They may blame the veterinary staff for feeling "pressured into it" or believe that they were not given all of the necessary information needed to make a sound choice. Authorization forms, such as the one posted on the Evolve site at http://evolve.elsevier.com/McCurnin/vettech/, verify the identity of the owner and free the practice of liability in performing euthanasia. Signed consent forms are part of the medical record and should be stored and filed with the medical records.

A common source of consternation in veterinary practices is miscommunication regarding the cost of services. Many veterinary hospitals have developed fee-estimation and consent-for-treatment forms (see the Evolve site at http://evolve.elsevier.com/McCurnin/vettech/). These forms give owners a written estimate of the cost of the procedures, verify ownership, and establish an agreement in the event that the animal is abandoned by the owner. This empowers the practice to take action in the event that the owner cannot meet his responsibility to pay for services and/or retrieve their pet.

Obtaining consent from the owner is recommended whenever there is an indication that a client might end up causing a problem. Often legal difficulties can be prevented by identifying potentially difficult clients in advance. Having the owner's written consent to restrain his or her own pet during an examination, for example, may protect the practice later if the client is bitten. Sometimes an owner that normally insists on holding their own pet during an office visit may decide not to after reading and signing a consent form that lists the risks of restraining an animal.

LOGS

In addition to the documents contained within the patient record, medical information is maintained continuously in logs that are located throughout the veterinary hospital. In many practices, there are logs for radiology and special imaging, surgery, anesthesia, controlled substances, ultrasound, clinical laboratory, and euthanasia. In addition, some practices have unexpected death, drug reaction, and medical waste logs. Any division of the veterinary hospital or specific activity could conceivably have a log that records the daily activity in that particular aspect of the hospital. Some large practices may have 8 to 12 different types of logs, whereas smaller practices may have two to four logs.

The logs serve two purposes:

1. They provide additional documentation for legal support.
2. They provide data for quick analysis and retrospective studies.

A practice that is interested in examining the average length of surgery, for example, can quickly calculate that figure based on data in the surgery log. In radiology, techniques could be evaluated by examining the recorded settings in the x-ray log. Typically, logs are kept in binders or bound composition books so that pages cannot be lost or discarded accidentally.

Some of the commonly used logs are listed below.

RADIOLOGY LOG

The radiology log records the technique used for every x-ray taken. It includes the following:

- Patient's name and identification (ID) number
- Client's name
- Date
- Study type
- Measurement of body thickness
- Technique used: milliamperes (mA), time, kilovolts peak (kVp)
- Radiographic findings or diagnosis

The radiology log is typically completed by the veterinary technician (Figure 5-12) and is particularly helpful when improved exposure technique is desired and repeat films are requested.

> *TECHNICIAN NOTE* The radiology log is especially helpful to technicians who wish to review and improve previous exposure techniques.

SURGERY LOG

Although there is much variation from practice to practice regarding the content and structure of the surgery log, most contain the following information:

- Date
- Animal and owner's name
- Case number
- Patient's weight
- Name of surgeon
- Surgical procedure
- Duration of surgery
- Complications

The surgery and anesthesia logs are particularly helpful when completing retrospective studies regarding the cost of performing each surgical procedure and regarding surgical complications (see the Evolve site at http://evolve.elsevier.com/McCurnin/vettech/). Some practices have separate surgery and anesthesia logs, whereas other practices combine the information to prevent redundancy.

ANESTHESIA LOG

The anesthesia log documents the anesthetic protocol used in surgical and nonsurgical procedures. Dental procedures, thorough ear examinations, and bone marrow aspirates are all examples of procedures that would require anesthesia

Radiology Log

Date	Case No.	Owner	Patient	Species	Study	Grid	Thickness (cm)	KVP	MA	Time Sec.	MAs	Tech. Initials
5/10/05	3246	Marshall	"Ed"	K-9	Abd.	Yes	21	90	300	1/30	10	cd
5/10/05	2671	Edward	"Wayne"	K-9	FR ext	No	6	60	100	1/20	5	df
5/10/05	6342	Kahn	"Nathanial"	Iguana	LF ext	No	1	50	100	1/20	5	cd
5/11/05	4563	Marshall	"Will"	Feline	Thorax	Yes	8	60	75	1/10	7.5	cd
5/12/05	4532	Pattison	"Hatchie"	Feline	Abd.	Yes	10	60	100	1/10	10	df
5/12/05	6543	Bassert	"Serena"	K-9	LH ext	No	6	60	100	1/20	5.0	cd
5/12/05	8964	Rose	"Suzie"	Feline	Thorax	Yes	8	60	75	1/10	7.5	df
5/12/05	8964	Rose	"Suzie"	Feline	Abd.	Yes	5	50	100	1/10	10	my
5/14/05	6751	Stern	"Gadget"	Snake	Skull	No	1	50	100	1/20	5.0	lb
5/14/05	7602	Berson	"Pete"	K-9	Adb.	Yes	14	76	300	1/40	7.5	cd
5/14/05	4398	Yates	"Mila"	K-9	Abd.	Yes	23	94	300	1/30	10	my
5/14/05	8743	Busch	"Abby"	K-9	Abd.	Yes	18	84	300	1/30	10	cd
5/14/05	4032	Brass	"Rose"	Feline	Thorax	Yes	8	60	75	1/10	7.5	lb
5/14/05	6302	Ash	"Sue"	K-9	Abd.	Yes	22	92	300	1/30	10	cd

FIGURE 5-12 Example of a radiology log.

but that might not be entered into the surgery log. Information contained in the anesthesia log might include the following:

- Patient's and owner's name
- Patient's weight
- Relative risk category or result of physical examination
- Anesthetic protocol, including type and dosage of each anesthetic agent
- Anesthesia start and end time
- Number of intubation attempts
- Surgical procedure and name of surgeon
- Anesthetist's name
- Complications

The anesthesia log complements the information entered on the anesthesia form (see the Evolve site at http://evolve.elsevier.com/McCurnin/vettech/). Some of the information is repeated and is found in both the log and the form. However, the advantage of the log is that it is easily accessible (the notebook often sits out) and represents a summary of all of the anesthesia cases. The anesthesia form, on the other hand, although it contains more detailed information, is not as accessible and contains information about one anesthesia case.

NECROPSY LOG

The necropsy log is a compilation of data regarding the death of animals. It includes the date and cause of death and type of necropsy performed (see the Evolve site at http://evolve.elsevier.com/McCurnin/vettech/). It also contains the owner's name, case number, species, name of the veterinarian performing the evaluation, histopathology and gross findings, and special tissue submitted. The log is typically kept in the necropsy area.

CONTROLLED SUBSTANCES LOG

The Comprehensive Drug Abuse and Control Act (the act) is federal law that was passed by Congress in 1970 and regulates the possession of drugs that have the potential to be abused. These drugs are called controlled substances. In the act, the drugs are categorized according to their potential for addiction. The categories range from Schedule I drugs, which are the most addictive, to Schedule V drugs, which are the least addictive. Schedule I drugs include LSD, heroin, crack cocaine, and peyote and have no accepted medical use. All of the other scheduled drugs (Schedules II, III, IV, and V) must be securely stored in a locked cabinet and inventoried separately from noncontrolled drugs. An inventory of all controlled substances must be made every 2 years, though most practices do this annually. The inventory should include the following:

1. Name, address, and DEA registration number
2. Date and time the inventory is performed
3. Contents of the inventory
4. Signature of the person taking the inventory

A separate inventory record must be kept for each Schedule II drug. The records for Schedule III, IV, and V drugs may be combined into one log, but must be kept separate from the other practice records. In addition, all drug-log information must be kept in a bound composition book or book in which the pages cannot be torn out without notice. Although specific requirements vary from state to state, a typical controlled substances log includes the following:

1. Date
2. Owner's and patient's name
3. Starting volume
4. Ending volume
5. Amount used
6. The initials of the person who used the drug

All inventory records must be kept for 2 years.

ORGANIZATION AND FILING

Many veterinary hospitals use a folder system that is developed specifically for veterinary medicine. There are a number of companies that make a variety of systems, so they are easy to acquire (you can order them from a catalog), and there is a wide selection of styles, sizes, and colors (see Figure 5-1). Most folders include internal flexible clips that hold forms in their correct order (Figure 5-13). In addition, the folders are designed to accommodate color-coded tabs or stickers (known as signaling devices) that are applied to the outer edge of the folder making filing more efficient and filing errors easier to identify.

ALPHABETIC

Colored stickers are sold separately, which allows the practice to choose the organizational scheme of the color-coding system. For example, it can be alphabetic, numeric, or a combination of both. In the alphabetic system, a different color is given to each letter of the alphabet. It is easy to learn and does not require cross-referencing with a master list of clients. The primary challenge of using the alphabetic system, however, is that the employee doing the filing must be careful to correctly apply the alphabetic order and spell the clients' names without exception. Unfortunately, errors in spelling and filing do occur from time to time, so misfiled records tend to be more common with the alphabetic system than with other systems.

NUMERIC

In the numeric system, each client is assigned a number. The number assigned to the file may be a hospital-generated number or the client's telephone or social security number. Each digit in the number has a different color, and the files are shelved from lowest to highest (Figure 5-14). In this way, it is easy to correctly sequence the files, and any misfiled records are easily identified because the file color sequence does not match those of the surrounding files. Can you see the misfiled record in Figure 5-15? To retrieve a particular file, the receptionist must first check a cross-reference that lists the client's name and the corresponding file number.

One of the advantages of the numeric filing system is that fewer filing errors occur because numbers are easier to read and interpret than letters, and spelling is not a factor. In addition, numeric filing systems are practical for large-volume practices because no file duplication occurs, whereas in the

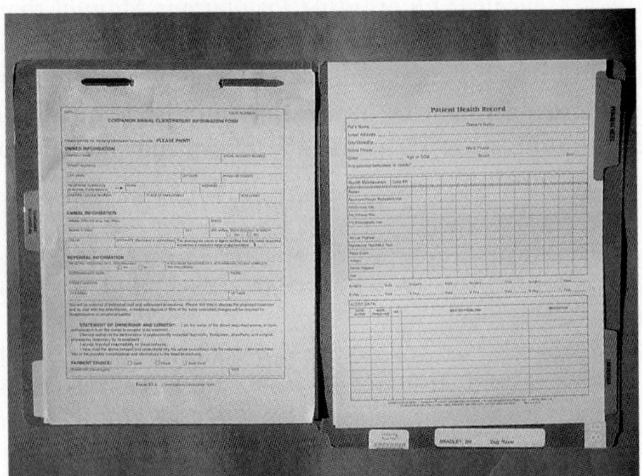

FIGURE 5-13 Letter-size folders contain flexible metal clips that hold forms in their correct order. Dividers allow for rapid retrieval of lab reports, operative notes, and progress notes.

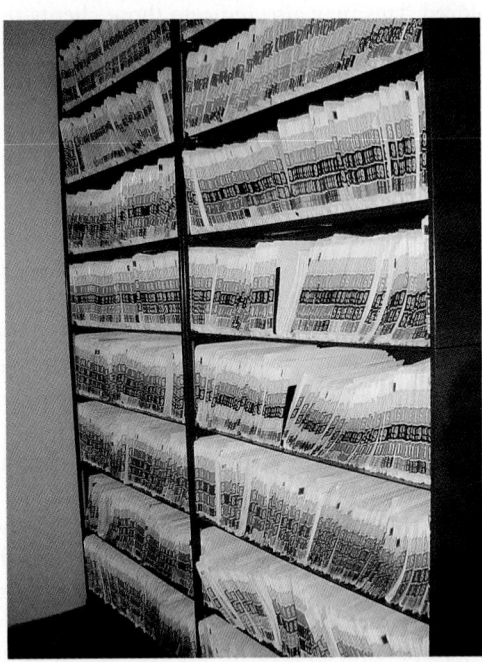

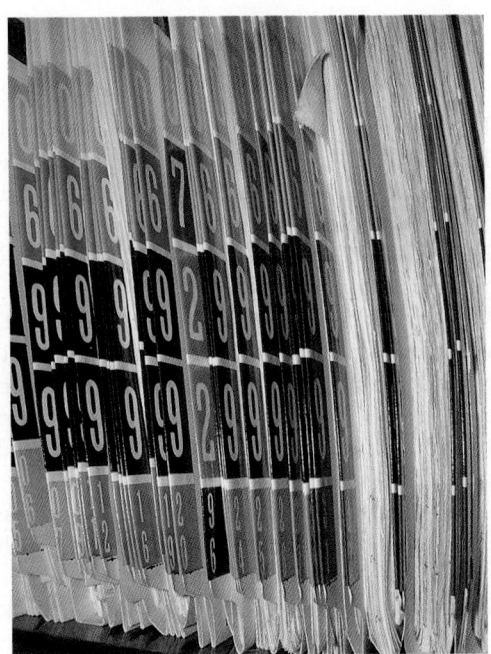

FIGURE 5-14 Numeric color-coding systems allow for rapid retrieval and filing.

FIGURE 5-15 Can you spot the filing error in these color-coded files?

alphabetic system, there may be many clients named Jones or Brown. The disadvantage of the numeric system, however, is that a cross-reference list must be generated and maintained. If telephone numbers are used, the files will have to be assigned a new number and refiled whenever a client moves or changes telephone numbers.

Additional colored tabs can be applied to files to alert the receptionist of specific client-patient issues. For example, the records of animals that need immunizations and worming can be flagged to indicate that reminders should be mailed out. Colored flags may also indicate those clients that have an outstanding bill or that have not returned to the practice in a long time. In this way, colored signaling devices can be added to identify groups of files that need attention.

FILE PURGING

Periodically the collection of medical records should be reviewed and purged of files that are not in current use. Each veterinary hospital has its own review and purging schedule; however, the following rules can be a helpful starting point:

1. The collection of medical records should be reviewed at least once per year.
2. Active records covering a 3-year period are maintained in the primary medical records collection.
3. Records that have been inactive for 4 years or more are moved to storage. Storage should be easily accessible.
4. Records 8 years old or older may be removed from storage and shredded.

Use of color-coded tabs with the year can be of particular value when completing the annual review of medical records. They enable the receptionist to quickly identify the 4-year-old and 8-year-old records by their specific colors.

LOST RECORDS

The risk of losing records in both a small and a large hospital is problematic. They can be lost through misfiling, incorrect spelling of names, or misplacement. At times even after an exhaustive search, the record continues to be missing. Sometimes the loss is not discovered until the animal comes back to the practice for a return visit.

It is best, in this case, to explain to the client that the record has been misplaced. A new record should be started and information requested from the client and veterinarian. In addition, copies of laboratory data, pathology reports, and radiologic information should be obtained and added to reestablish the file.

Although the problem of lost records is embarrassing to the practice and inconvenient to the client, it will happen with even the most elaborate record keeping system; however, every effort possible should be made to quickly and accurately file each record after each visit. Clients feel more at ease and welcomed if the record is complete and easily accessible.

ETHICAL AND LEGAL ISSUES

OWNERSHIP OF MEDICAL RECORDS

The laws concerning ownership of medical records vary from state to state. However, in general, the records made during the course of a patient's treatment are owned by the veterinary hospital or hospital owner. Although the client purchased the veterinary services that generated the medical information, the client is not, by law, the owner of the medical record. However, the owner may request a copy of the record at any time. It is customary for clients to request copies of their pet's medical record when they are moving and changing veterinary practices. This facilitates continued care of the patient and prevents repetition of immunizations or diagnostic tests. It is recommended that copies of medical records be mailed to the successive veterinarian and not hand delivered by the owner who may be apt to misinterpret the status of his or her animal's health. A cover letter should be included with the copy of the record so that the original veterinary hospital and veterinarian can be easily contacted, if necessary. A flat fee for copying the record may be charged, or the practice may levy a fee on a per-page basis.

RELEASE OF MEDICAL INFORMATION

A signed authorization form (see the Evolve site at http://evolve.elsevier.com/McCurnin/vettech/) or a written letter of request for record copies should be obtained from the animal's owner before any information is released to him or her, another veterinarian, or an insurance company. The practice owner should be the only person to authorize the release of information contained in the record. However, there is an exception to this rule. Local, state, and federal agencies require the reporting of certain diseases that may be dangerous to the public or to the widespread health of animals. These are called reportable diseases and include rabies, brucellosis, and equine encephalitis. Additional regulations regarding reportable diseases can be found in the *Animal Movement Quarantine Regulations Manual* that is published by the U.S. Department of Agriculture (USDA). In addition, physicians, animal control agencies, and the regional department of health may inquire about the rabies immunization status of an animal that has bitten a human.

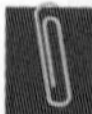

TECHNICIAN NOTE AVMA Ethics and Medical Records

A. Veterinary medical records are an integral part of veterinary care. The records must comply with the standards established by state and federal law.
B. Medical records are the property of the practice and the practice owner. The original records must be retained by the practice for the period required by statute.

Continued

C. Ethically the information within veterinary medical records is considered privileged and confidential. It must not be released except by court order or consent of the owner of the patient.
D. Veterinarians are obligated to provide copies or summaries of medical records when requested by the client. Veterinarians should secure a written release to document that request.
E. Without the express permission of the practice owner, it is unethical for a veterinarian (or veterinary technician) to remove, copy, or use medical records or any part of any record.

From: The principles of veterinary medical ethics. In AVMA membership directory and resource manual, 2007.

TECHNICIAN NOTE Errors should not be scratched out, erased, or blotted out. Instead, a single line should be drawn through the mistake and initialed. The correct information should then be written in the margin and initialed and dated next to the correction. Any erasure or blotting out may suggest tampering of the record and could render the document inadmissible in a court of law.

Example:

"Fluffy" exhibits moderate pain in the cranioventral abdomen. ~~Small~~ JMB 7/7/07 Firm oval mass palpable approx. 2 cm × 2.5 cm.

MEDICAL AND LEGAL REQUIREMENTS

It is important to keep in mind that the medical record is a legal document and could be used in a court of law. It is generated not only to ensure consistent and accurate veterinary care, but also to protect the veterinarian against potential malpractice litigation. Any written data contained in the medical record must be complete, accurate, and legible. An inaccurate, illegible, or incomplete record may be construed as evidence of professional incompetence and substandard care. Keep in mind that in a court of law, "if it was not written down, it didn't happen," and "if the writing is illegible, it was not written down." Below are some guidelines for generating clear, complete, and accurate records.

1. Entries should either be typed or written in black ink.
2. In a court of law, handwriting alone is not an adequate way to identify the author of a notation. Entries should be dated and initialed to identify the person making the entry. Additional validity to an entry can be made by entering the time and the date.
3. Errors should not be scratched out, erased, or blotted out. Instead, a single line should be drawn through the mistake and initialed. The correct information should then be written in the margin and initialed and dated next to the correction. Any erasure or blotting out may suggest tampering of the record and could render the document inadmissible in a court of law.
4. Only approved, standard abbreviations should be used.

The medical record is considered legal evidence of services and procedures performed by the veterinary health care team. In the event of litigation, such as during a malpractice or insurance suit, the record could be subpoenaed and admitted as evidence.

Legal guidelines for medical records vary from state to state and may dictate the type of information that should be included, how long the record should be kept, and restrictions on the release of medical information. It is recommended that all members of the veterinary health care team be familiar with the laws of the state in which they work.

VETERINARY MEDICAL DATABASE

The Veterinary Medical Database (VMDB) is a national data bank located at Purdue University. It contains computerized veterinary medical data supplied by 24 veterinary schools in the United States and Canada. Each institution submits data for the VMDB on a quarterly basis to a central processing center. The data consist of abstracted data from each clinical case seen at each teaching hospital. The national database allows studies of national trends in various animal diseases. It provides patient chart number, institution code, date of visit, length of stay, clinician code, gender, species, breed, discharge status, age, weight, diagnosis, and procedures for each animal. The VMDB is available for use in retrospective studies and in the evaluation of national and regional disease patterns.

COMPUTERS

Computers have become an integral part of veterinary practice management today. Software packages designed specifically for veterinary practices help organize a wide range of management issues, such as billing, reminders, scheduling, and inventory in addition to medical records. Chapter 4 addresses these and other topics regarding the use of computers in veterinary practice.

RELATED ASSOCIATIONS

American Animal Hospital Association, 12575 West Bayaud Ave., Lakewood, CO 80228

American Health Information Management Association, North Michigan Avenue, Suite 2150, Chicago, IL 60601-5800, www.ahima.org

American Veterinary Health Information Management Association, c/o Flo Nelson, University of Missouri, Veterinary Medical Teaching Hospital, 379 E. Campus Drive, Columbia, MO 65211

American Veterinary Medical Association, 1931 N. Meacham Road, Suite 100, Schaumburg, IL 60173-4360

RECOMMENDED READING

AAHA: *Standards of accreditation CD-ROM,* Lakewood, Colo, 2003, American Animal Hospital Association.

Allen DG: The problem-oriented approach. In *Small animal medicine,* Philadelphia, 1991, Lippincott.

Heinke ML, McCarthy JB: *Practice made perfect: a guide to veterinary practice management,* Lakewood, Colo, 2001, American Animal Hospital Association.

Johns ML: *Information management for health professions,* ed 2, 2002, Delmar.

Johns ML: *Health information management technology: an applied approach,* American Health Information Management Association.

Peden AH: Veterinary settings. In *Comparative records for health information management,* Delmar.

For access to all of the medical record forms discussed in this chapter, see the Evolve site at http://evolve.elsevier.com/McCurnin/vettech/.

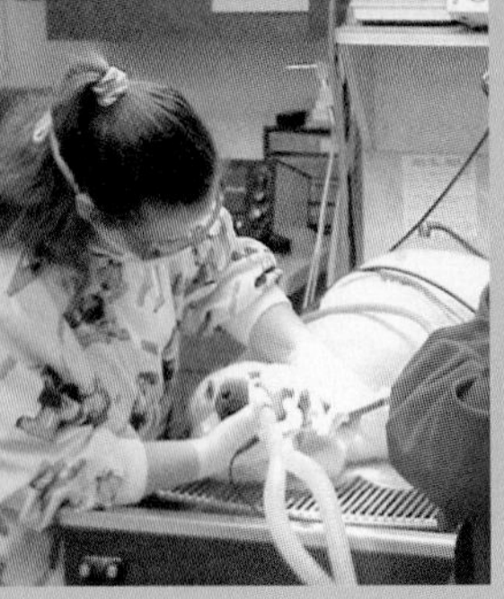

Occupational Health and Safety in Veterinary Hospitals

6

Philip J. Seibert, Jr.

KEY TERMS

Carpal tunnel syndrome
Centers for Disease Control & Prevention (CDC)
Coccidia
Cutaneous larval migrans
Ergonomic injury
Giardia
Hazardous chemical
Hazardous materials plan
Hazmat
Hospital Safety Manual
Lyme disease
Material safety data sheet (MSDS)
Occupational Safety and Health Act
Occupational Safety and Health Administration (OSHA)
Panleukopenia
Parvoviral enteritis
Personal protective equipment (PPE)
Rabies
Right to know law
Ringworm
Sarcoptic mange
Toxoplasmosis
Visceral larval migrans
Waste anesthetic gas
Zoonotic disease

OUTLINE

LEARNING OBJECTIVES

When you have completed this chapter, you will be able to:

1. Describe the role of OSHA in veterinary practice safety.
2. List the general requirements of the federal laws related to workplace safety.
3. Explain proper methods for lifting objects and animals.
4. List common workplace hazards in a veterinary facility.
5. Describe the requirements and the OSHA "right to know" law.
6. Explain the acronym MSDS and describe the components of an MSDS.
7. List the hazards associated with the use of ethylene oxide, formalin, glutaraldehyde, anesthetic gases, and compressed gases.
8. Define the term zoonotic disease and list common zoonotic diseases encountered in the veterinary practice.
9. List methods to minimize the hazards associated with animal handling.
10. Describe the proper handling of hazardous and medical wastes.

INTRODUCTION

Most people who work in the veterinary health care professions do so because of a love for animals and a desire to help them. Working as a veterinary technician and a part of the veterinary health care team can be deeply rewarding. However, with every reward comes responsibility. One of the responsibilities of a veterinary technician is to help ensure the safety of co-workers, patients, and clients and to ensure one's own safety. If you are hurt on the job, the injury incurred extends beyond the physical pain and disability you suffer. The hospital is also affected, both financially and operationally, because the veterinary health care team loses an important member—you. Other employees of the practice have to work harder to cover the personnel shortage. In addition, the quality of health care delivered to the animals may also be adversely affected by having less than a full team of caregivers.

As a staff member in a veterinary hospital, you are exposed to hazards in the day-to-day routine of clinical practice. These hazards include exposure to infectious diseases, harmful chemicals, radiation, and the risks of being scratched, bitten, shoved, stepped on, and kicked. That is the bad news. The good news is that these hazards, when properly identified, can be managed and the risk of injury minimized or even eliminated.

By reading this chapter and educating yourself about hazards in the veterinary health care field, you are taking the first step in minimizing your risk of injury and of contracting a contagious disease. Some of the topics discussed will be familiar to you, whereas others will be new. The important point is to remember that all of the topics presented in this chapter are true health risks for the veterinary technician in clinical practice.

The second step in minimizing health risks in the workplace is to integrate the safety procedures you learn in this chapter into the everyday habits of your job. You are the most important person in ensuring your safety on the job. As human beings, we operate from a set of habits for most of life's activities. Your safety should not be something you have to stop to think about—it should be automatic. The only way it becomes automatic is by developing and practicing good work habits.

SAFETY

OBJECTIVES OF A SAFETY PROGRAM

The purpose of any safety program is to reduce or eliminate the possibility of injuries or illnesses to employees. The Occupational Safety and Health Administration (OSHA) enforces federal laws that help to ensure a safe workplace for American workers. These laws require employers to have a safety program, which includes educating employees about the inherent risks in their jobs, providing them with appropriate safety equipment, and training them in safety procedures and the proper use of safety equipment. If you are receiving this training from your employer, she or he is fulfilling important OSHA requirements. If you are learning this material as a self-study program, you can take pride in the knowledge that you are becoming a "self-taught expert" in the field of occupational safety. Your knowledge and initiative will be a welcomed component to your veterinary health care team.

YOUR SAFETY RIGHTS

One can never eliminate every hazard completely, but each of us can minimize our exposure to them in most cases.

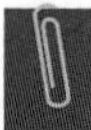

TECHNICIAN NOTE You have the right to expect your workplace to be reasonably free from hazards.

The ability to participate in a safety program at work is an important part of your rights. It is often assumed that the owner and/or manager of a business knows all that there is to know about the business. But too often it is the employee who first becomes aware of potential safety problems. As an employee, you have the right to bring those concerns to the attention of the employer without fear of reprisal. In most instances, the complaint is first presented to the immediate supervisor, but be aware that not all complaints will bring about changes to the operation of the practice. Some complaints stem from a lack of familiarity with standard safety procedures on the part of the employee, and in these cases, instruction by the employer is all that is needed to resolve the issue. However, if a complaint is not taken seriously by the employer or if there is a dangerous situation that is not adequately addressed, the employee has the right to bring the issue to the attention of the regional OSHA office.

When records, such as medical evaluations or radiation exposure reports, are collected by the veterinary hospital, the records must be made available to the employee for review. This does not mean that you are entitled to see private or sensitive information about other staff members, but it does mean that you are entitled to see data that is relevant to your safety. You are also entitled to know about the nature and type of accidents that have occurred in your hospital. If your practice employs more than 10 employees, you have the right to view the summary of work-related injuries and illnesses (OSHA form 300A), which should be posted on the employee bulletin board at certain times of the year.

YOUR SAFETY RESPONSIBILITIES

It is your responsibility to learn and follow the safety rules and practices that have been established for your position in the veterinary hospital. Even though OSHA will not cite or fine the employee directly for violations of these responsibilities, he or she is required under the Occupational Safety and Health Act (the act) to "comply with all occupational safety and health standards and all rules, regulations, and orders issued under the Act." This not only includes specific OSHA standards, but it also applies to workplace-specific rules established by the leadership in your hospital.

TECHNICIAN NOTE It is your responsibility to learn and follow the safety rules and practices that have been established for your position in the veterinary hospital.

Although you cannot be disciplined by your employer for exercising your rights under the act, you can be disciplined by your employer for willful violations of any safety rule or standard. In some cases, this discipline can be as simple as a verbal reprimand, but in severe or chronic situations, it can include termination. In most states, if you are terminated for the willful violation of safety rules, you will likely be denied unemployment benefits.

In addition to the responsibility to follow the rules, the act requires you to:

- Read the OSHA poster (Figure 6-1).
- Comply with all applicable standards.
- Wear or use prescribed personal protective equipment (PPE) while working.
- Report hazardous conditions to your supervisor.
- Report any job-related injury or illness to the proper person and seek treatment promptly.

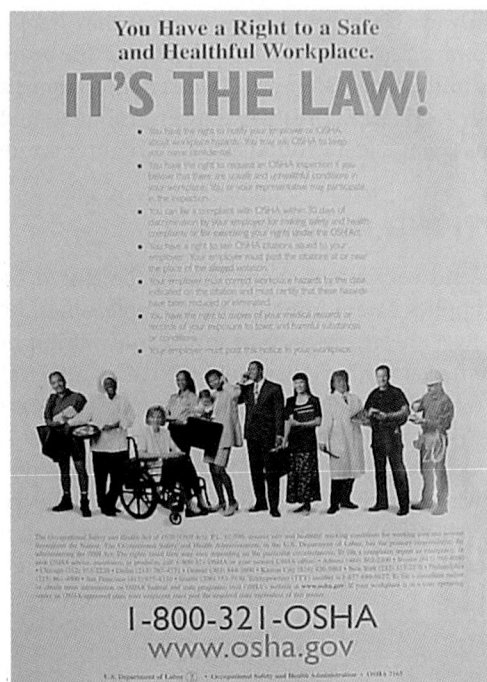

FIGURE 6-1 Locate and read all of the safety notices where you work.

THE LEADERSHIP'S RIGHTS

Although the act and OSHA require the leadership of a business to maintain safety standards, this is not meant to restrict their right to set rules of conduct or operation for its staff. The practice owner, for example, has the right to set and enforce rules for his or her own practice as long as those rules are consistent with federal safety laws.

Practice owners must have ample time to correct any safety-related problems. In other words, the employee should not rush off to file a grievance with the regional OSHA office without first giving the employer ample time to correct the deficiency.

In the event that a practice is inspected, the practice owner has the right to be present because the practice is considered his or her personal property. An employee is not authorized to admit an OSHA inspector to the practice in the absence of the employer (unless, of course, the employer specifically gives the employee the authority to act on his or her behalf). However, OSHA inspectors may enter a practice without the presence of the owner and without permission by the employee if the inspectors have a court order to do so.

THE LEADERSHIP'S RESPONSIBILITIES

The leadership of a veterinary practice is responsible for providing a safe work environment for the employees. This does not mean providing a facility with no hazards—that would be impossible. It means that the leadership must make a reasonable effort to identify the hazards present, correct the ones that can be eliminated, and control the ones that cannot be eliminated.

The practice must comply with the laws and regulations pertaining to safety and health by establishing safety procedures for the hospital, including emergency procedures for addressing employee's accidents. The leadership must enforce these rules as diligently as it would be expected to enforce any other rule in the practice.

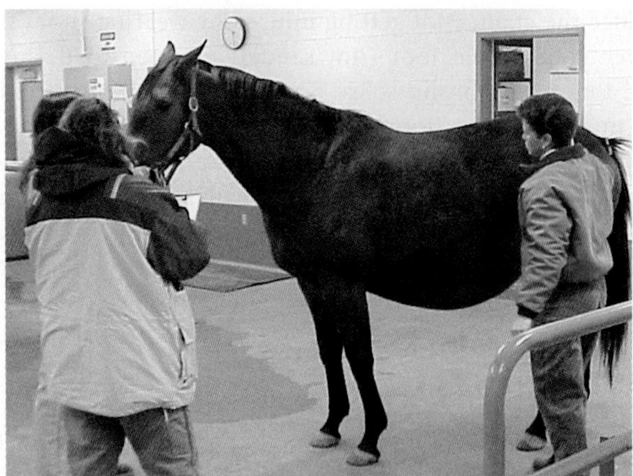

FIGURE 6-2 Safety training can be conducted in a formal session and enhanced by one-on-one discussions.

The employer is also responsible for providing practice-specific safety training to the employees (Figure 6-2). Even if a veterinary technician has years of prior experience, the practice is required to make sure that the technician is capable of doing her or his job safely. This training can be provided in a formal setting, such as in staff meetings or a continuing education course, or it can be given in the practice. A great deal of learning takes place in many practices every day. On-the-job training can be an effective way to obtain knowledge about safety, but be sure you know your limits and abilities. Ultimately, you are the best person to determine if you are competent to do a job safely. If you think you need extra safety training in an area, do not hesitate to ask for it. Tell your supervisor immediately so that arrangements can be made for the proper instruction.

GENERAL WORKPLACE HAZARDS

Every practice should have a collection of written safety-related policies known as the *Hospital Safety Manual.* You should know where the *Hospital Safety Manual* is located in your practice and take time to become familiar with it. Memorize the "do's and don'ts" for your particular veterinary hospital and always follow the safety rules. No one can protect you from an injury or illness better than you.

> *TECHNICIAN NOTE* Every practice should have a collection of written safety-related policies known as the *Hospital Safety Manual.*

DRESSING APPROPRIATELY FOR THE JOB

One of the first rules of safety is to dress appropriately for the job at hand. In the veterinary profession, this includes protective footwear and minimal, if any, jewelry. You can reduce the chances of getting injured by wearing shoes that cover your whole foot (not sandals or open-toed shoes) and that have nonslip soles. Be especially cautious walking on uneven or wet floors. Never run inside the hospital or on uneven footing. Excessive jewelry can present a hazard in many clinical situations, but particularly when an animal struggles during restraint and can inadvertently link an earring or necklace with a claw. This is definitely one of those circumstances when less is more.

SAVE YOUR BACK!

According to insurance statistics, back injuries account for one in every five workplace injuries among American workers. To minimize your chances of suffering one of these painful injuries, remember the rules for lifting: keep your back straight and lift with your legs (Figure 6-3). Never bend over at the waist to lift an object. That rule applies when lifting patients and inanimate objects, such as boxes or supplies. If your practice does not have a motorized lift table, get help when lifting patients more than 40 lb. Remember to follow sound ergonomic principles when positioning or restraining patients, especially when working with horses or food animals.

CASE PRESENTATION 6-1

A 22-year-old man has been a veterinary technician for 2 years. He has worked at a companion animal practice in the past, but has recently started working in an equine-only hospital. During his first week on the job, he suffered a debilitating back injury while trying to capture and restrain a fractious patient.

Since he has a background in companion animals, the technician viewed restraint as primarily a physical overpowering of the patient. Had he received proper training when he first started the job, he would have known that tranquilization and sedation are the primary methods of restraint for horses that become fractious when physical restraint (such as placement in a stock) is not practical.

The technician was confined to bed for 3 days by the physician and restricted in his physical activities for 2 weeks to overcome the muscle strain.

Because veterinary technicians perform such a variety of jobs in any given hour, it is rare for us to acquire the types of ergonomic injuries common in other industries (such as **carpal tunnel syndrome**). However, it is important to note that the best defense against almost all ergonomic injuries is to change your posture and routine frequently.

CLEAN UP AFTER YOURSELF

Some injuries are caused by cluttered or dirty work areas. In addition, clutter is known to contribute to the severity of accidents that otherwise would be minor. Cleanliness and organization are good business standards, especially in a health care facility. Always clean up spills as soon as they happen. You should always clean and return equipment to the proper storage place immediately after use. At least daily, remove all trash from your work area. Organize drawers, cabinets, and counters so that items can be found easily and clutter is reduced.

EVERYTHING IN ITS PLACE

Supplies and equipment should always be stored properly. Heavy supplies or equipment, for example, should be kept on the lower shelves to prevent unnecessary strain in trying to lift them overhead and to reduce the risk of material falling on your head. Never use stairways or exit hallways as storage areas. Do not overload shelves or cabinets (Figure 6-4). Store liquids in containers with tight-fitting lids and always replace the lids when finished using the product. Whenever possible, store chemicals on shelves at or below eye level; this will minimize the possibility of accidentally spilling the chemical

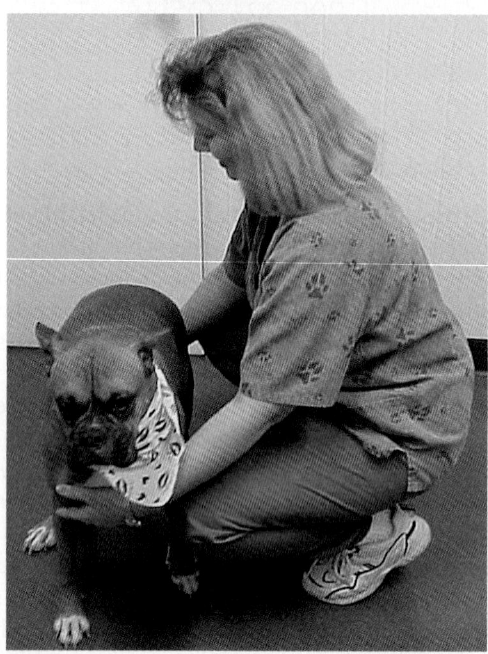

FIGURE 6-3 Remember to keep your back straight and lift with your legs.

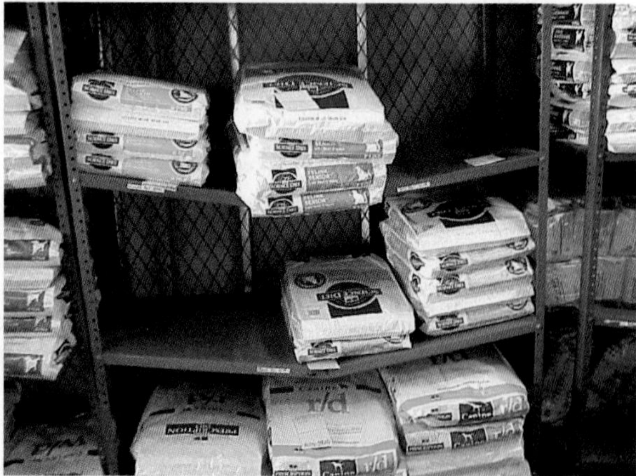

FIGURE 6-4 Improper storage of materials can lead to serious injury.

on you when getting or replacing a container. Never climb into or on cabinets, shelves, chairs, buckets, or similar items. Use an appropriate ladder or step to reach high locations.

BEWARE OF BREAK TIMES

The ingestion of pathogenic organisms or harmful chemicals while eating on the job is a possibility in veterinary hospitals. This is why it is important to eat and drink only in areas designated for staff breaks that are free of toxic and biologically harmful substances. This also applies to the preparation of food and beverages. Make sure coffeepots and utensils are well away from the sources that could contaminate food, such as laboratories and treatment and bathing areas. Check the cabinets or shelves above food preparation areas to ensure that no hazards could spill onto the area. Always store food, drinks, condiments, and snacks in a separate refrigerator from the one used to store biologic or chemical hazards, such as vaccines, drugs, and laboratory samples.

> *TECHNICIAN NOTE* Always store food, drinks, condiments, and snacks in a separate refrigerator from the one used to store biologic or chemical hazards, such as vaccines, drugs, and laboratory samples.

MACHINERY AND EQUIPMENT

Never operate machinery or equipment without all the proper guards in place. Equipment such as fans and cage dryers have moving parts that can severely hurt or even sever a finger. Long hair should be tied back or pinned up to prevent it from getting caught in fans or other moving parts. Avoid wearing excessively loose clothing or jewelry when working around machinery with moving parts.

When using equipment such as autoclaves, microwave ovens, cautery irons, or other heating devices, be sure to understand the proper rules for safe operation. Burns, especially from steam, are painful and serious and almost always can be prevented. Autoclaves also present a danger from the pressure that is used for proper sterilization. Before opening an autoclave, be sure to first release the pressure by activating the vent device, and at the same time keep your hands and face away from the steam. Let the steam dissipate completely before opening the door fully and be careful when removing the packs because they may still be hot. Always assume cautery devices and branding irons are hot, and use the insulated handle whenever you touch them. Never place heated irons on any surface where they could overheat and start a fire or where someone might accidentally touch them.

ELECTRICAL

Many procedures performed on a daily basis require the use of electricity. Although new equipment and buildings have many safety features built into the design, you must be conscious of preventing a situation that could cause a fire or physical harm to yourself, another person, or a patient.

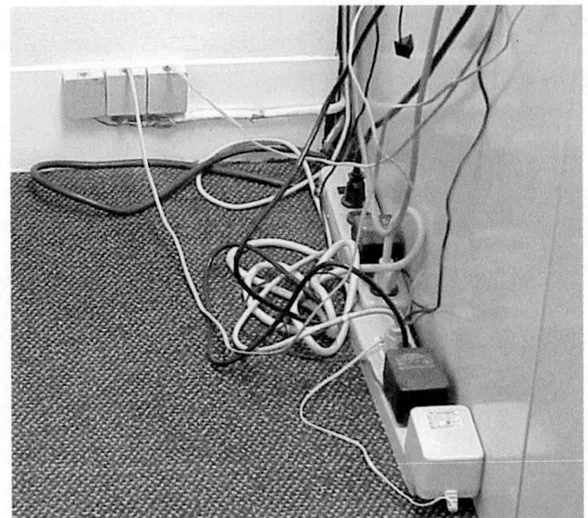

FIGURE 6-5 Overloaded surge suppressors or extension cords can start a fire.

Do not remove light switch or electrical outlet covers. Always keep circuit-breaker boxes closed and never block access by stacking supplies or equipment in front of them. Only persons trained to perform maintenance duties should repair electrical appliances, outlets, switches, fixtures, or breakers.

If you must use a portable dryer or other electrical equipment in a wet area, make sure it is properly grounded and only plugged into a ground-fault circuit interruption (GFCI) type of outlet. Extension cords should only be used for temporary applications and should always be of the three-conductor, grounded type. Never run extension cords through windows or doors that may close and damage the wires or across aisles or floors where a tripping hazard may be created.

Surge suppressors should only be used to protect sensitive electronic equipment and should never be overloaded (Figure 6-5). In addition, surge suppressors should never be used with portable heaters, autoclaves, or coffeepots because they may overheat and cause a fire.

Equipment with grounded plugs must never be used with adapters or nongrounded extension cords. Never alter or remove the ground terminals on plugs. Appliances or equipment with defective ground terminals or plugs should not be used until repaired.

When changing light bulbs (especially fluorescent bulbs), be careful to remove and replace the bulb without breaking it. Inoperable bulbs should be disposed of directly into the outside dumpster or inside of a container to keep the bulb from breaking.

FIRE AND EVACUATION

The potential for the dramatic loss of life (both human and animal) and the destruction of property make a hospital fire one of the most feared accidents imaginable. Fortunately,

BOX 6-1 Using a Fire Extinguisher

- If you must use a portable fire extinguisher, remember the word PASS:
  - Pull the pin: Some extinguishers require releasing a lock latch, pressing a puncture lever, or other motion. (Check your extinguishers to be sure.)
  - Aim low: Point the extinguisher (or its horn or hose) at the base of the fire.
  - Squeeze the handle: This releases the extinguishing agent.
  - Sweep from side to side at the base of the fire until it appears to be out.
  - Watch the fire area. If a fire breaks out again, repeat the use of the extinguisher.
  - Most portable extinguishers work according to these directions, but read and follow the directions on your specific extinguisher.

this danger can be significantly reduced by a few simple precautions.

Never use power adapters or surge suppressors as a substitute for permanent wiring. Overloaded or faulty electrical cords can overheat or short out and start a fire, even when the equipment is turned off.

Always store flammable liquids properly; many, such as gasoline, paint thinner, and ether, should never be stored inside the hospital except in an approved flammable storage cabinet. Some components of specialty dental and large animal acrylic repair kits are also flammable. Very small amounts of these components are usually not a problem, but always ensure that they are stored and used in an area with good ventilation and that the containers have tight-fitting lids that are replaced immediately after use.

Flammable materials, such as newspapers, boxes, and cleaning chemicals, must always be stored at least 3 feet away from an ignition source, such as a water heater, furnace, or stove. Always use extra care when using portable heaters. Never leave them unattended and always make sure they are placed no closer than 3 feet from any wall, furniture, or other flammable material.

Become familiar with the location of the emergency exits in your facility. Make sure the emergency exits are always unlocked and free from obstructions when you are in the building. If you must work in a building when security warrants that the doors be locked, make sure you have at least two clear exits from the building.

TECHNICIAN NOTE Become familiar with the location of the emergency exits in your facility. Make sure the emergency exits are always unlocked and free from obstructions when you are in the building.

Learn the emergency warning system in your hospital. If the facility is equipped with an electronic alarm system, be sure you know how to activate it manually. In the absence of an electronic alarm system, a verbal alarm is effective. You can use the telephone intercom feature to alert everyone that there is a fire in the building, or in small buildings, simply yell in a loud clear voice to get the message out.

Know your duties in the event of a fire. Remember, your first responsibility is to notify others about the fire and then to get out of the building safely if an evacuation is ordered. Leave the rescue duties to the professionals that are trained and equipped to handle this dangerous task. If you do evacuate the building, immediately report to the designated assembly area for accountability. This is important since others will assume you are trapped in the building if you are not present at the assembly area.

Know where the fire extinguishers are located and how to use them (Box 6-1). Most veterinary hospitals are equipped with dry-chemical type of fire extinguishers. But before you decide to use a fire extinguisher, make sure the alarm has been sounded, everyone has left the building (or is in the process of leaving), and the fire department has been called.

The National Fire Protection Association recommends that you never attempt to fight a fire if any of these conditions are true:

- The fire is spreading beyond the immediate area where it started or involves any part of the building or structure.
- The fire could block your escape route.
- You are unsure of the proper operation of the extinguisher.
- You are in doubt that the extinguisher you are holding is designed for the type of fire at hand or is large enough to suppress the fire.

DO NOT BECOME A VICTIM OF VIOLENCE

Just as in any occupation, you are at risk of injury from accidents not directly related to your job. Vehicle accidents, personal assault, robbery, and even natural disasters have resulted in veterinary technicians being injured while on duty. Although no one can prevent every possible scenario, preparation can certainly help and sometimes will minimize the injury. When outside of the hospital building, be aware of your environment and do your best to avoid placing yourself in a situation that could go bad.

Always keep the "nonclient" doors locked from the outside to prevent anyone from gaining unauthorized or undetected entry into the building (Figure 6-6).

If you work in a critical care or 24-hour practice, you should use the "barriers" that are usually available. Things such as buzzers to control access through the front door and one-way locks on the remaining doors (to let you out in case of an emergency, but keep the door locked from the outside) are essential in these environments, so do not prop doors open, disassemble the locking system, or turn the system off. In any business that keeps money or stores valuable items, there is a potential for robbery. If you ever find yourself in a situation where someone demands money, drugs, or other material items while threatening your personal safety—do

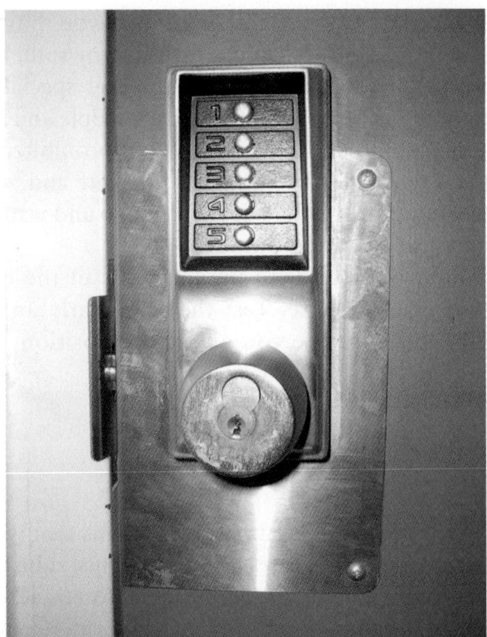

FIGURE 6-6 Personal safety includes the diligent use of locks and barriers to deter unauthorized persons from entering the facility.

not withhold the things they demand. As soon as safely possible, let everyone else know of the situation. You should attempt to contact the police if it can be safely done without the person's knowledge; otherwise, do it immediately after the person has left.

Cooperate with their demands and give them what they want, but do not go with the person. Resist physical assault or battery to the best of your abilities and preferably outside the building so that passersby can see what is happening and render assistance or call the police.

HAZARDOUS CHEMICALS: RIGHT TO KNOW

You may not think about it, but many products that you use every day can be hazardous. Every chemical, even common ones, such as cleaning supplies, have the potential to cause you harm. Some chemicals contribute to health problems, whereas others may be flammable and pose a fire threat. The most common chemicals in use in the veterinary practice are as follows:

- Cleaning and disinfecting agents
- Insecticides and pesticides
- Drugs and medications (including anesthetic gases)
- Sterilization agents
- Radiology processing fluids

Planning and training are the keys to safely handling any chemical. Every business, including your practice, must follow the requirements of OSHA's "right to know" law. This law requires you to be informed of all chemicals you may be exposed to while doing your job. The right to know law also requires you to wear all safety equipment that is prescribed by the manufacturer and the practice when using any product containing a hazardous chemical. The safety equipment must be provided to you at no cost, but it is not optional—you must wear what is prescribed.

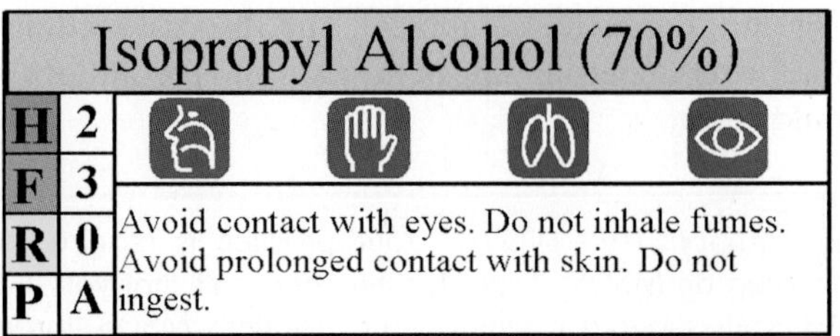

Isopropyl Alcohol (70%)

H	2	
F	3	
R	0	Avoid contact with eyes. Do not inhale fumes. Avoid prolonged contact with skin. Do not ingest.
P	A	

FIGURE 6-7 Example of a secondary container hazard warning label.

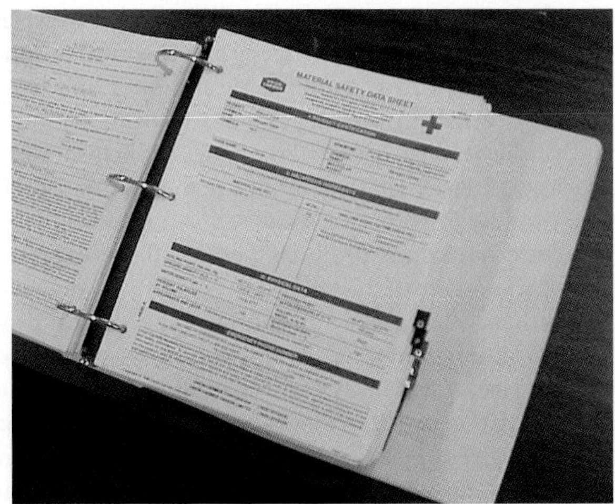

FIGURE 6-8 MSDSs contain safety information that may not be indicated on the product label.

A key component of the right to know law is the hazardous materials plan. The hazardous materials plan includes instructions for organizing and filing the practice "right to know" label, but that information is generally written for the average consumer who will have limited exposure using the product. When a product is used in a business, such as your veterinary practice, you may be exposed to that product more than the average consumer, so your risk may be different. Chemicals, such as alcohol, may be shipped in a large container by the manufacturer and subsequently transferred to smaller containers or spray bottles by hospital personnel to facilitate their use in the practice. It is important to remember to apply a secondary container hazard warning label (Figure 6-7) on the second container to ensure that the chemical is used safely. In addition, the manufacturer of a product that contains a hazardous chemical will prepare a material safety data sheet (MSDS) for that product. The MSDS will give you additional precautions, instructions, and advice for handling that product in the workplace (Figure 6-8). Your practice is required to keep an MSDS library for the chemicals that you use. Ask your supervisor where your hospital's MSDS library is located. Take the time to review the MSDSs for the products you use frequently. Although MSDSs may look complicated at first glance, the information that is important to you is easy to find: review the health, protective equipment, and disposal sections to gain a better understanding of the risks and precautions you should know.

> *TECHNICIAN NOTE* Your practice is required to keep an MSDS library for the chemicals that you use. Ask your supervisor where your hospital's MSDS library is located.

Working bottles of hazardous products should always have tight-fitting, screw-on lids. Always remember to replace the cap back on the bottle after using any chemical product. You should endeavor to store chemical bottles in a closed cabinet; this will help prevent animals from injury in the event that they escape. Ideally the cabinet or shelf should be at or below eye level. This will minimize the chances of spilling the product in your face if the cap is not secure. Never store or use hazardous products near food, beverages, or food preparation areas.

Be cautious when mixing or diluting any chemical product. Try to keep the material from splashing on your hands, clothes, or face. If it is likely that the product will splash on you, wear a pair of protective latex or nitrile gloves and some protective goggles or glasses. When making solutions from a concentrate, you should always start with the correct quantity of water then add the concentrate. Never add the water to the concentrate because the chemical may splash or react differently.

When two chemicals are mixed together, the result is seldom a simple mixture. It is often a new, sometimes different and possibly dangerous chemical. Never mix any chemicals unless directed to do so on the label or an MSDS.

Minor spills of most chemicals can be cleaned up with paper towels or absorbent (e.g., kitty litter) and disposed of in the trash; however, dangerous chemicals, such as mercury, require special procedures. Before you use a new chemical, review the MSDS and learn the procedures you must follow for cleaning up a spill. When cleaning up any spill, remember to wear protective gloves and any other special equipment required on the MSDS. Keep other people and animals away from the spill until it is safe. Unless prohibited by the instructions on the MSDS, wash the spill site and any contaminated equipment with a detergent soap and water—not a disinfecting soap (Box 6-2).

Familiarize yourself with the locations of the eyewash stations in your practice. Test them regularly and know how to use them before you are in the position to need them.

SPECIAL CHEMICALS

Ethylene Oxide

Many hospitals use gas sterilization for items that would be damaged by other procedures. Electrical drills, rubber products, and sharps are commonly exposed to ethylene oxide (EtO) as a sterilization agent in human and veterinary medicine. This method has distinct advantages, but since EtO is thought to be a human carcinogen, special precautions must be maintained.

- Read the MSDS carefully and follow all instructions.
- Store the ampules in a closed cabinet away from sources of heat.
- Only use approved devices for the procedure.
- Read, understand, and follow all the written procedures and safety precautions relevant to your practice.
- Know the emergency procedures to be performed in case of an accidental release of EtO.

Formalin

Historically, formalin has been used in the veterinary profession for tissue preservation, diagnostic tests (knott), and even sterilization. Since formaldehyde is also a suspected human carcinogen, OSHA takes its use seriously. The standards

BOX 6-2 Chemical Spill Cleanup

- Step 1. Keep unnecessary people and pets out of the area to prevent spreading the spilled material.
- Step 2. If the area is small or the fumes are extremely strong, increase ventilation by opening a window or turning on an exhaust fan. Do not use an electric exhaust fan or electric equipment and avoid turning switches on or off when cleaning up spilled flammable materials.
- Step 3. Put on a pair of protective latex or nitrile gloves. If it is likely that your clothing will become contaminated during the cleanup, put on a protective apron and protective eyewear.
- Step 4. As soon as possible, cover the spill with absorbent materials, such as paper towels or cat litter. Allow the absorbent material to fully collect the liquid.
- Step 5. Using a broom, gently sweep the saturated absorbent into a dustpan and deposit it in a plastic trash bag.
- Step 6. When all the material has been picked up, seal the trash bag and dispose of it as regular waste unless your institution, city, or county requires you to do otherwise.
- Step 7. Wash the contaminated area thoroughly with plain water or a detergent (not a disinfectant) soap if permissible by the instructions in the MSDS. Allow the area to air-dry.
- Step 8. Remove any protective equipment used during the cleanup. Dispose of single-use items as regular trash unless your institution, city, or county requires you to do otherwise.
- Step 9. Wash your hands thoroughly and change any clothing that has become contaminated during the cleanup process.
- Step 10. Replace used materials in the spill kit.

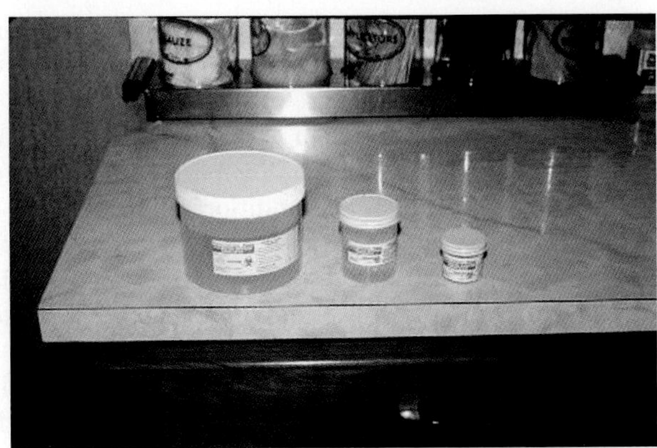
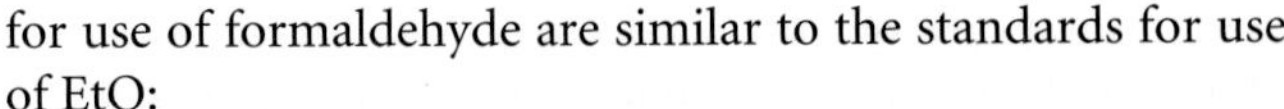

FIGURE 6-9 When possible, use only biopsy jars prefilled with formalin to prevent excessive exposure.

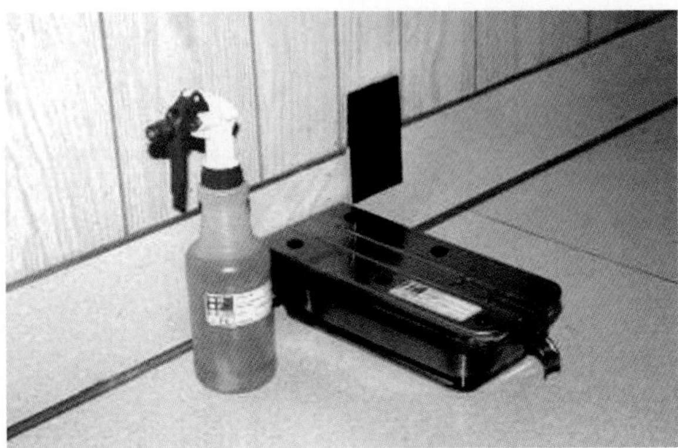

FIGURE 6-10 Disinfectants are designed to kill living organisms, so they must be handled safely.

for use of formaldehyde are similar to the standards for use of EtO:

- Read the MSDS carefully and follow all instructions.
- Store supplies safely; include museum jars.
- Use only with good ventilation in the room and avoid breathing vapors.
- Wear gloves and goggles to prevent skin and eye contact.

Whenever possible, you should obtain formalin in small, premeasured containers (also called biopsy jars) so that the serious risk is minimized (Figure 6-9). Often the diagnostic laboratory will supply prefilled biopsy jars at no charge, so be sure to ask.

Glutaraldehyde

Glutaraldehyde is a potent chemical used in the veterinary practice to sterilize hard instruments without the use of an autoclave. Because it is so effective at killing germs, it can also be harmful to other living organisms including you (Figure 6-10). Be sure to follow all the manufacturer's safe handling rules when using this "cold-sterilization" solution, including washing your hands after handling instruments exposed to the solution and keeping the trays covered to minimize evaporation.

MEDICAL AND ANIMAL-RELATED HAZARDS

We cannot forget that the overriding purpose of a veterinary practice is the care and treatment of animals. But sometimes handling our patients can be a hazard in itself. Anyone who has worked with animals under stress or in pain will relate personal accounts of injuries from patients. Insurance statistics show that animal-related accidents are the most common type of injury among workers in veterinary-related jobs, including veterinary technicians.

> *TECHNICIAN NOTE* Insurance statistics show that animal-related accidents are the most common type of injury among workers in veterinary-related jobs, including veterinary technicians.

Unfortunately, this hazard cannot be eliminated, so we have to do the next best thing—minimize it. The best way to protect yourself from this hazard is to obtain training and practice in animal restraint. The first safety rule when working around animals is to stay alert. Animals sometimes react to situations unexpectedly. Sudden noises, movements, or even light can be the stimulus that would cause an animal to react, so if you are the person responsible for restraining the animal, keep your attention focused on the animal's reactions and not on the procedure. You must learn the proper restraint positions for each of the species of animals with which you work. Refer to Chapter 7 for additional information about the restraint and handling of animals.

Remember that capture-restraint equipment is available if the animal is fractious or not cooperating; sometimes just a piece of rope to hobble a leg or a piece of gauze for a hasty muzzle will make all the difference. And do not forget that chemical restraint, rather than physical restraint, is often better for both you and the animal, but be sure to ask the veterinarian for approval before administering any medication to a patient.

Large animals, such as horses and cattle, are particularly dangerous and may severely injure or even kill a person when trying to escape restraint. Never put your hand, leg, or any other part of your body between the animal and the side of the enclosure or chute; use a hook or pole to pass ropes or belts through the chute. If you have to enter a stall, paddock, or trailer with a large animal, stay on the side of the animal nearest the door so that you can escape if the situation becomes hazardous. If you must capture a fractious animal from a cage or pen, make sure there is another person present that can assist you if you get into trouble.

If your job entails handling exotic or nondomestic animals, remember that they all have their own unique methods of defense. You should know and understand their possible reactions before you attempt to restrain or treat them.

NOISE

Dogs in cages will inevitably bark, and barking dogs can adversely affect your hearing, especially if you work in an indoor kennel. Noise levels in dog wards can reach as high as

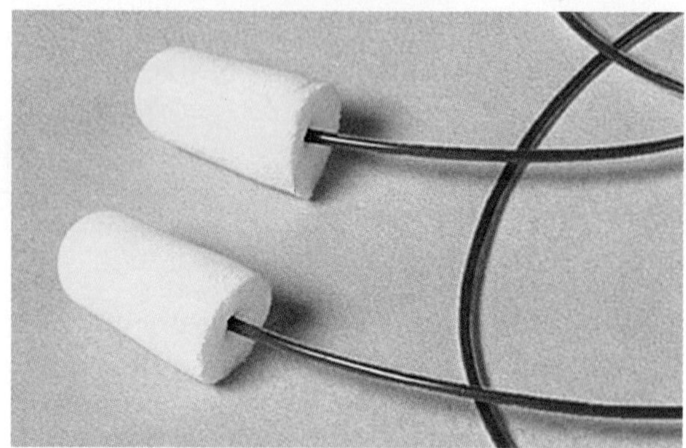

FIGURE 6-11 Hearing protectors should always be used in noisy kennels.

110 dB. Although relatively short-duration exposure to these noise levels, such as going into the kennel just to retrieve a patient, poses no serious damage to your hearing, chronic or long-term exposure can contribute to hearing loss. When working in noisy areas for extended periods of time (e.g., cleaning of cages), you must wear personal hearing protectors (Figure 6-11). It does not matter what style or type of hearing protectors you use (earplugs or muffs), as long as they are rated to filter the noise by at least 20 dB (the package will indicate the rating).

> *TECHNICIAN NOTE* Dogs in cages will inevitably bark, and barking dogs can adversely affect your hearing, especially if you work in an indoor kennel. Noise levels in dog wards can reach as high as 110 dB.

BATHING, DIPPING, AND SPRAYING AREAS

There is probably no area of an animal hospital with a greater risk for injury than in the bathing or insecticide application areas. Although newer parasite control products significantly reduce exposure to pesticides and insecticides, shampoos and medical dips are still a big concern.

The products used for bathing and dipping animals can be harmful to your health and the environment. Even the "all natural" shampoos can cause eye irritation, and you can develop sensitivities to even the mildest products if you are exposed often enough. Because it is impossible to prevent splashing and shaking, it is important to always wear protective glasses or goggles when bathing or dipping animals. In most cases, it is also important to wear gloves and a protective apron to prevent the product from getting on your skin or clothing; this minimizes the amount absorbed through the skin.

Bottles of dips, shampoos, and insecticides should be stored in a cabinet at or below eye level. The bottle should be properly labeled with the contents and any hazard warning that is appropriate (refer to the discussion on chemicals in this chapter for more details). Always replace the cap or lid on the container when you are finished using it to prevent accidental spillage. Plastic containers recycled from other areas can be used for diluted shampoos and dips; however, only use the ones that have a screw-on cap or lid.

Always use a ventilation fan to keep the fumes from shampoos and dips at a safe level. When exhaust fans are too large, they waste heating or air conditioning, so you may be hesitant to use them in some situations. If that is the case, ask your hospital administrator to have a smaller fan installed directly over the tub or area so that fumes can be exhausted without sacrificing the comfort in the room.

Make sure you know where the eyewash station for this area is located. Learn how to properly use the eyewash device before it is needed. If you ever splash a chemical in your eyes, do not rub your eyes with your hands. Immediately call out for help; there is usually someone nearby. With a coworker's assistance, go to the eyewash station and flush both eyes (even if only one eye is affected). Avoid using the spray attachments for tubs and sinks since the water pressure is unregulated and the streams of water from these devices can be fine enough to lacerate your cornea.

ZOONOTIC DISEASES

Infectious diseases that can be passed from animals to humans are known as zoonotic diseases. Some zoonotic diseases are not easily transmitted from animals to humans, whereas others are easily spread. You can be exposed to the organisms that cause disease by several means: inhalation, contact with broken skin, ingestion, contact with eyes and mucous membranes, and via accidental inoculation by a needle. There is a wide variety of zoonotic agents to which a veterinary technician may be exposed, certainly more than can be discussed in this chapter. However, some important ones are listed below.

Viral Infections

Rabies is a serious (almost always fatal) viral disease that can affect any warm-blooded animal (including humans). The virus is spread by contact with an infected animal's saliva. Usually the virus is transmitted through a bite, but it has also been transmitted by open wounds or mucous membranes coming in contact with virus-rich saliva.

Although the disease is ever present in wild animal populations (primarily bats, raccoons, and skunks in the United States), in recent years many states have confirmed record high numbers of rabies in domestic species, such as cats, dogs, horses, and cattle. Several university veterinary hospitals have also recorded cases of rabies in horses, cattle, and companion animals. Some of those animals were even adopted from pet shops. Although rare, it is possible that you will encounter a rabid pet at the veterinary hospital where you work.

It is important that you are aware of the prevalence of rabies and the incidence among wild species in your area because it varies in each region of the country. If you work in a high-risk environment, such as with unvaccinated, stray, and homeless animals in a shelter or with wild animals at a rehabilitation center, you should be immunized with preexposure prophylaxis. Ask your hospital administrator about the availability of these vaccines. They are often available through the occupational health divisions of regional human hospitals. When you must handle an unvaccinated, wild, or stray animal, wear protective (rubber or latex) gloves and wear protective gowns and goggles in cases where the procedure may be "messy."

Bacterial Infections

There is a wide variety of both pathogenic and nonpathogenic bacteria that you may be exposed to during your professional life. Some examples of pathogenic bacteria include *Salmonella* spp., *Pasteurella* spp., *E. coli*, and *Pseudomonas* spp. Bacteria can be transferred by direct contact with the animals and their exudates. This is particularly likely if you have any cuts or open sores. Some bacteria may be aerosolized and inhaled or absorbed through mucous membranes. The best protection against exposure to bacteria is simply good personal hygiene. Always follow the personal hygiene rules discussed later in this chapter.

Lyme Disease

Recently, **Lyme disease** has become a more serious concern for animals and people. When an infected deer tick bites a host (an animal or person) to feed, the bacteria *Borrelia burgdorferi* is transferred to the host. Lyme disease in humans is characterized by aches in the joints, fever, and a host of other flulike symptoms. The best defense against this disease is to check yourself daily for ticks and remove them promptly. If you work in a food- or mixed-animal practice, it is also a good idea to use an insect repellent when you go out into fields or woods to work.

Fungal Infections

Contrary to its name, **ringworm** is not a parasite or worm. It is an infection of the skin caused by a fungus know as *Microsporum* sp. Ringworm is passed between animals and humans. Cats and horses are particularly susceptible to ringworm infestations. The most effective protection from ringworm infection is to wear gloves when handling or treating animals diagnosed with the condition and to practice good personal hygiene. Be especially careful about preventing contamination of your clothing when treating patients with *Microsporum* sp. because it is believed that the fungal spores can be carried to other locations (such as your home) on clothing and infect other animals or other people.

Internal Parasites

When the eggs of common internal parasites, such as roundworms, infect humans, they usually do not mature into adult parasites, but they do cause other problems. Roundworm larvae can migrate to virtually any organ in the body and develop into a cystlike growth known as **visceral larval migrans.** These "cysts" are usually not clinically noticeable unless they develop in a vital organ such as the eye where they can do permanent damage to the retina and may cause blindness. Puppies almost always have some level of roundworm infestation because the passage of worms from the bitch to the fetus occurs through the placenta and via lactation. When the infected puppy defecates in soil, the roundworm eggs are able to survive for long periods of time until they are picked up and ingested by another mammal.

Another common internal parasite, hookworms, can also cause problems in humans by a condition known as **cutaneous larval migrans.** This condition is particularly prevalent in southern areas of the United States where there are warm, humid winters. Children who play barefoot where pets defecate frequently may be affected in addition to people who lie on the ground where dogs have defecated. Unlike the visceral cysts from roundworms, the cutaneous larval migrans are relatively easy to spot and appear as small, red lines in the regions where the parasite has burrowed into the skin from the soil. Often these marks are itchy and lengthen as the parasite moves from one part of the body to another, subcutaneously.

External Parasites

The irritating and itchy mite that causes **sarcoptic mange** can spread easily to humans from animals. Typically, this occurs in regions where there is tight clothing, such as along bra lines and waistbands. When treating animal patients for mange, always wear gloves and a protective gown and wash your hands thoroughly with disinfecting soap immediately after the procedure.

Protozoal Infections

Infestation with a protozoan known as *Toxoplasma gondii* is called **toxoplasmosis.** Although it is usually not harmful to most adults, it can have devastating effects on the development of a human fetus by causing hydrocephalus and mental retardation. Nonsporulated *Toxoplasma* eggs are shed in the feces of infected cats. The eggs subsequently sporulate approximately 2 to 4 days later. These 3-day-old, sporulated oocysts—if ingested by some pregnant women—are particularly dangerous to the fetus. Pregnant women can avoid potential exposure to *Toxoplasma* by taking the following steps:

1. Avoid cleaning cat litter pans when possible, particularly those that contain feces older than 2 days. If it is unavoidable, be sure to wear gloves when handling the litter box and wash your hands when you are finished.
2. Wash raw vegetables thoroughly (dirt on vegetables may contain oocytes).
3. Do not eat raw or uncooked meat, particularly lamb and pork, which can carry the encysted protozoan in the muscle tissue. Cook all meat thoroughly.
4. When gardening, wear gloves that can be removed easily. Under no circumstances should dirt accidentally enter your mouth (e.g., when removing a hair from your mouth).
5. Women in the veterinary profession are encouraged to have *Toxoplasma* titers evaluated before becoming pregnant, if at all possible. Your physician can give you more specific advice about *Toxoplasma* titers during your pregnancy.

Other zoonotic protozoal agents, such as ***Giardia*** and **coccidia,** cause diarrhea and gastrointestinal cramping in humans. These are typically spread to people from their contact with infected animals (particularly puppies and kittens), but they can also be acquired by drinking contaminated water.

Because you will probably come in contact with some of these diseases in your job, particular attention to personal hygiene and sanitary work practices is essential. Good personal hygiene includes making sure your clothes do not become soiled by chemicals or biologic material and, of course, regular hand washing. In general, you should wash your hands:

1. After handling medications or lab samples
2. After treating patients or cleaning cages
3. Before and after you use the restroom
4. Before lunch or meal breaks and before you leave work at the end of your shift

NONZOONOTIC DISEASES

Some infectious agents, such as **parvoviral enteritis** in dogs and **panleukopenia** in cats, are not a serious concern to human health, but they are so highly contagious that you can carry the live virus home to your pets on your clothes and shoes. For this reason, some technicians when working with parvoviral cases at work leave their shoes outside their front door and change their clothes immediately upon entering their home, and some even change clothes before they leave the hospital. In addition, technicians who work with cats that have certain viral upper respiratory conditions and chlamydia can themselves contract pinkeye or conjunctivitis. Therefore when treating cases with contagious diseases, be sure to wear a protective apron, surgical mask, examination gloves, and, when appropriate, eye protection. Thoroughly wash your hands with a disinfecting agent, such as chlorhexidine or povidone-iodine scrub, at the completion of the treatment and change your clothes before handling your own animals.

A DIRTY MOUTH? PRECAUTIONS FOR DENTISTRY OPERATIONS

Dental procedures that include use of a high-speed and ultrasonic scaler aerosolize oral microbes, making personal protection a necessity. One of the most common pathogens in the mouths of animals is *Pasteurella multocida,* an organism that has been linked to cardiac and pulmonary problems in humans and animals alike. Therefore when performing dental procedures, be sure to wear goggles, gloves, and a surgical mask (Figure 6-12).

RADIOLOGY

The ability to "see inside the body" is a great tool in medicine. In most cases, the method of choice is diagnostic radiography (x-rays). Short-duration, infrequent exposure to radiation, such as having radiographs taken of yourself, is considered an acceptable level of exposure (the benefits outweigh the risks). However, long-term exposure to low doses of radiation has been linked to many medical disorders. High-dose exposure can cause skin changes, cell damage, and gastrointestinal and bone marrow disorders that can be fatal. Fortunately, much is known about the properties of x-rays, and we are clear about the ways in which we need to protect ourselves. By following some simple safety precautions, you can safely use radiography in your practice.

Although modern radiographic machines have many safeguards integrated in their design, there is still the possibility of injury if these tools are used incorrectly. When you are taking x-rays, always wear a lead apron and lead gloves. Lead thyroid collars and lead glasses are also recommended, particularly during extensive studies, such as with fluoroscopy. Though restraint of animals during radiographic studies can be challenging, never place any part of your body, even a gloved hand, in the primary beam (Figure 6-13).

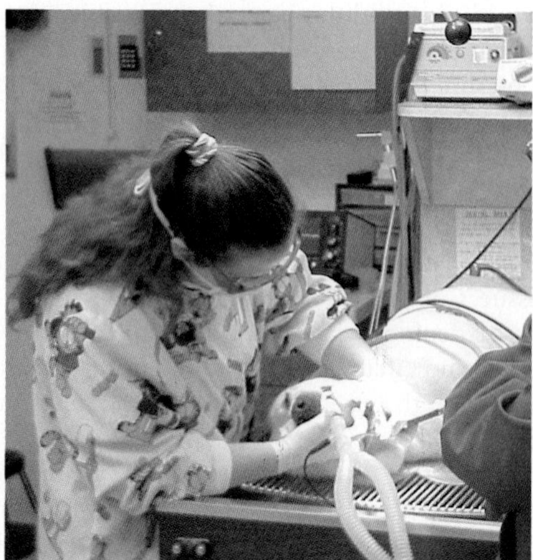

FIGURE 6-12 Always wear eye protection, a mask, and gloves when performing dental prophylactic procedures.

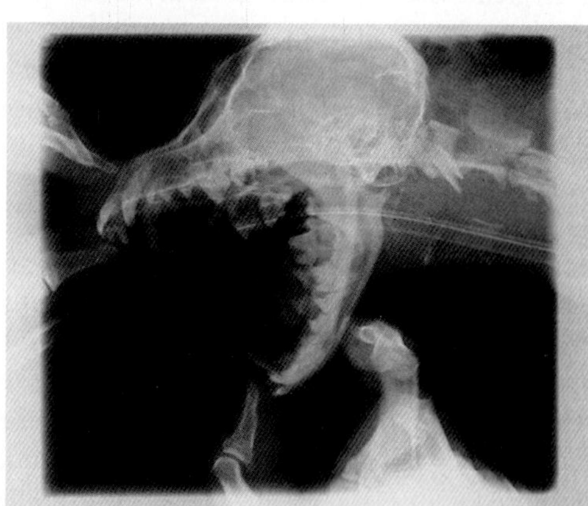

FIGURE 6-13 Never place your hand or any other part of your body in the primary beam when taking radiographs.

Before you use an x-ray machine, make sure you know the purpose of every knob and button. Always use the collimator to restrict the primary beam to a size smaller than the size of the cassette—in other words, "cone down" to the area to be radiographed so that scatter radiation is minimized. A properly collimated radiograph will have a small clear border around the entire film once developed.

Always follow the written operational and safety procedures from the hospital or machine manufacturer. If you have not already done so, make an exposure chart specific to your machine so that you can replicate the best techniques for various studies. By following a proven technique chart and positioning the patient correctly the first time, you will have fewer "retakes" and will therefore reduce unnecessary exposure.

CASE PRESENTATION 6-2

A 40-year-old veterinary technician has noticed dark colored spots on her hands that are not typical aging spots. A visit to her dermatologist revealed a diagnosis of skin cancer. It was later determined that the cancer was a type that is typical with exposure to radiation.

An investigation into the case revealed that the technician has worked at various veterinary hospitals and even in a research facility throughout her career. In most of those positions, her duties included the exposure and processing of radiographs. Because the technician was "small in size," she found the protective gloves used for the procedure bulky and cumbersome. Therefore she most often chose to restrain the patients without the gloves. At one job in a mixed-animal hospital, she even held the cassette for lameness evaluations with her bare hand. Her desire to help patients without regard to her own safety was compounded by the perpetual "hurry up and get it done" attitude that sometimes prevails in practice.

In this case, the damage was not evident, and there was no physical pain when the exposure happened, so the technician falsely assumed that the practice of taking radiographs without gloves was safe. Her failure to follow the instructions given when she was a technician student and the safety training that was continual throughout her career is the primary cause of her incurable condition.

Portable machines, such as those used in large animal and mobile practices, can be particularly dangerous because of their multipurpose abilities. These machines can be aimed in any direction, and because of their limited power, they must use longer exposure times to produce diagnostic images. When using a portable machine, always make sure no one is in the path of the primary beam (even at a distance). Always use a cassette-holding pole and never hold a cassette with your hands while the exposure is made—even with gloves. Remember to wear a lead apron and gloves when near the machine during exposure.

If you are involved in the exposure portion of radiography, you must have and use an individual dosimetry badge. This badge is worn on your collar outside your protective apron during radiographic procedures, not as protection, but as a measurement of any incidental radiation you may receive during the procedure. It is important to return the badge to the designated storage location (outside the x-ray area) when not in use. Unless you are taking radiographs, do not wear your badge outside because exposure to sunlight will result in false readings. As a result of the relatively low numbers of radiographs taken in most practices, safer machines, and the use of good protective equipment, most technicians receive little, if any, occupational exposure to radiation.

Radiographic processing chemicals (the developer and fixer) can be corrosive to materials and organic tissues so use protective gloves and goggles when mixing and pouring the chemicals. When using manual processing tanks, stir the chemicals with care and avoid splashing. After handling radiographic developing chemicals, always wash your hands. In addition, it is important to avoid breathing the fumes of the processing chemicals, so make sure there is adequate ventilation in the dark room; generally an exhaust fan is necessary.

Radiographic developing solutions can react dangerously with other chemicals. For this reason, never pour chemicals down the drain with developing solutions. Some liquid drain openers, when mixed with developer and fixer solutions, can produce toxic gases. Others can produce an exothermic reaction (generates high temperature) that can damage pipes.

ANESTHESIA

Anesthesia is as common to veterinary medicine as antiseptic wound care. The National Institute of Occupational Safety and Health (NIOSH) estimates that more than 250,000 U.S. workers are at risk from exposure to waste gases that are not metabolized by the patient. Long-term exposure to **waste anesthetic gases** (WAGs) has been linked to congenital abnormalities in children, spontaneous abortions, and even liver and kidney damage.

Although the recent development and use of improved WAGs have lowered risk to patients and health care workers, there is no chemical that is entirely without risk. We must therefore continue to take precautions to protect ourselves, even when using isoflurane and sevoflurane. OSHA has established a safe exposure limit for all halogenated anesthetic agents that is not to exceed 2 parts per million (ppm).

TECHNICIAN NOTE OSHA has established a safe exposure limit for all halogenated anesthetic agents that is not to exceed 2 parts per million (ppm).

Using a proper scavenging system is the single most effective means of reducing exposure to WAGs. There are three general types of scavenging systems: active scavenging, passive exhaust, and absorption. Each has a place, but rarely does one method fit all circumstances. Regardless of the system chosen, make sure it is fully operational and in use before turning on the anesthesia machine. If you use absorption canisters, be sure to check them (by weighing with a gram scale) regularly and replace them as needed. Once the canister becomes saturated with gas, it is ineffective.

According to some research, as much as 90% of the anesthetic gas levels found in the room during a procedure can be attributed to leaks in the anesthesia machine, so be sure to perform a leak check before use (Box 6-3 and Figures 6-14 to 6-17). Also make sure that the correct size hoses and rebreathing bags are used. Intubation tubes should be placed and the cuff inflated before connecting the animal to the anesthesia machine. Start the flow of anesthetic gases only after the patient is connected to the machine. When

BOX 6-3 Leak Check Your Anesthesia Machine Before Each Use

1. Assemble all hoses, canisters, valves, or tubes according to the manufacturer's instructions.
2. Turn on the oxygen supply to the machine.
3. Close the pressure relief (pop-off) valve (see Figure 6-14).
4. Use your thumb or palm to form a tight seal on the Y piece (the part of the hose that attaches to the patient's endotracheal tube) (see Figure 6-15).
5. Turn on the oxygen until the bag is slightly overinflated (or when the pressure on the manometer reaches the 20 mark), then close the valve (see Figure 6-16).
6. Observe the pressure in the system on the manometer and watch closely for any decrease. (If your machine is not equipped with a manometer, observe the size of the bag closely.) If the pressure remains constant, the machine is leak free. If the pressure drops, there is a leak (or leaks) in the system. The faster the pressure drops, the larger the leak(s) (see Figure 6-17).
7. If there is a leak, check the bag, hoses, and other rubber (plastic) parts for evidence of cracks or deterioration. Replace any parts that are damaged. Check all connections, especially the seals at the top and bottom of the soda lime canister and on the one-way valves (clear plastic domes). Tighten any loose connections you find.
8. After checking all connections and hoses, if there is still a leak, have the machine serviced by a qualified technician before use.
9. When the machine is leak free, reset the pressure relief (pop-off) valve to the proper position to use the machine normally.

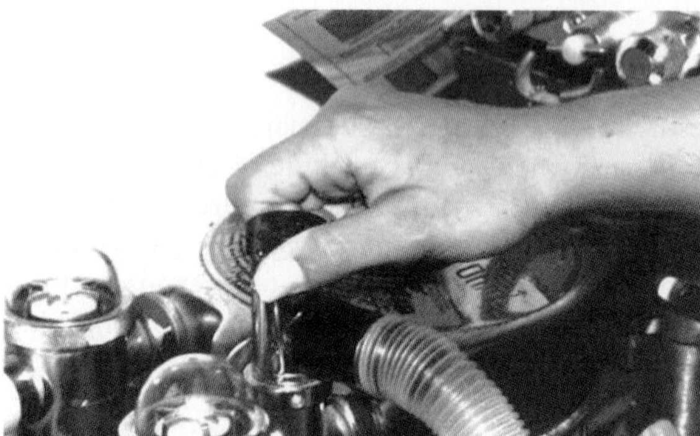

FIGURE 6-14 Step 3: Close the pop-off valve.

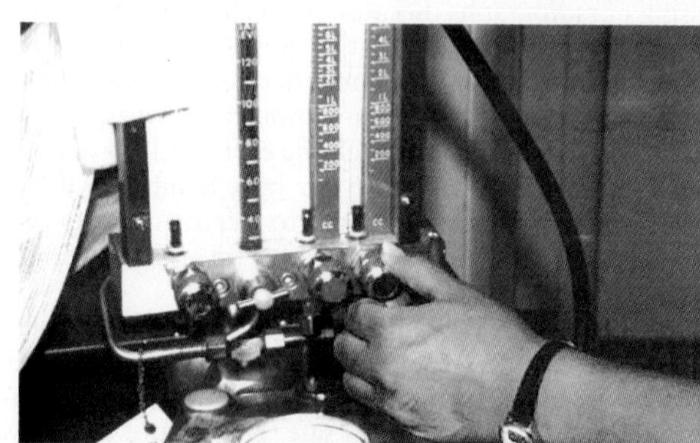

FIGURE 6-16 Step 5: Turn on the oxygen until bag is slightly overinflated.

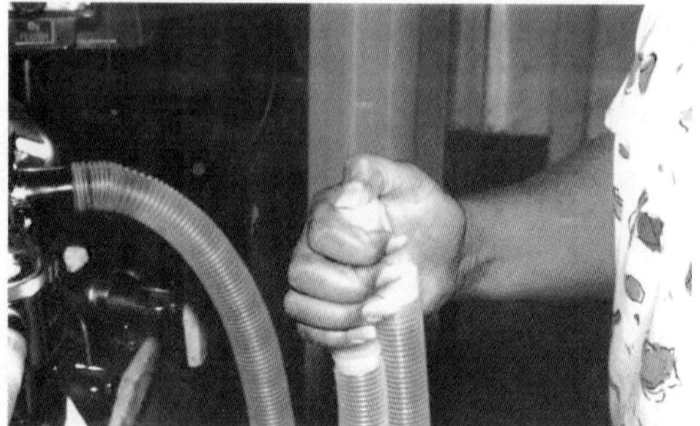

FIGURE 6-15 Step 4: Use your thumb or palm to form a tight seal on the Y piece.

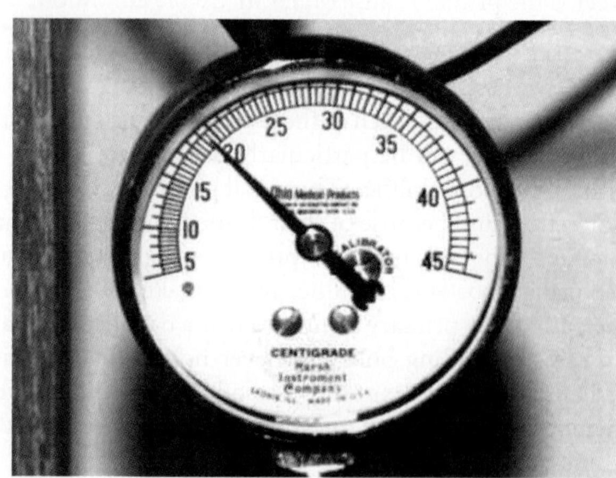

FIGURE 6-17 Step 6: Observe the pressure in the system on the manometer and watch closely for any decrease.

the surgical procedure is finished, turn off the vaporizer and increase the flow of oxygen to the patient. Be sure to use the "flush" feature to purge the circuit before disconnecting the patient.

Before filling the vaporizer, move the anesthesia machine to a well-ventilated area. Use a pouring funnel and be careful to avoid overfilling the vaporizer or spilling the liquid anesthetic. If you accidentally break a bottle of anesthetic, immediately evacuate all nonessential people from the area. Any windows in the area should be opened, and all exhaust fans should be turned on. Quickly control the liquid with a generous amount of kitty litter, and place a plastic bag over the spill to reduce evaporation. Pick up the absorbed liquid and kitty litter with a dust pan, and place it inside a plastic garbage bag. Seal the bag tightly and dispose of it in an outside trash can. Leave the exhaust fans on and the windows open until you are sure the gas level has been reduced to a safe level.

The anesthetic protocols that involve masking the patient or using a tank for induction are more likely to generate a larger amount of WAGs. When using these protocols, be sure to use an appropriate flow rate and proper reservoir bag for the size of the patient—do not turn up the oxygen flowmeter to maximum when masking a patient. Induction chambers should always be connected to the scavenging system or absorption canisters to reduce the levels of escaping gases. Make sure the ventilation in the room is good and use local exhaust fans when available.

Anesthetized animals do not metabolize all of the anesthetic gas that they have inhaled. They exhale some of it into the room after they have been extubated and while they are recovering. When monitoring patients during their recovery, you should avoid putting your face close to the animal's face. In addition, keep the number of recovering patients to an acceptable number based on the size of the area and ventilation system (Figure 6-18). As much as possible, delay extubation and allow the patient to recover while still connected to the anesthetic machine (oxygen only) and scavenging system.

> *TECHNICIAN NOTE* Anesthetized animals do not metabolize all of the anesthetic gas that they have inhaled. They exhale some of it into the room after they have been extubated and while they are recovering.

When changing the soda lime (carbon dioxide absorbent) in anesthetic machines, wear rubber or latex gloves. When the soda lime is wet, as is often the case from humidity in the system, it can be caustic to tissues and some metals. Dispose of the used soda lime granules in a plastic trash bag as regular trash.

Pregnant women should discuss the risks of exposure to anesthetic gases with their physician. In addition, they should inform their supervisor of their condition as soon as possible so that safety procedures can be reviewed and adjusted, if necessary.

COMPRESSED GASES

Every year, hundreds of workers are injured while working with compressed gas cylinders, usually because of improper storage or handling of these cylinders. Regardless of the size of the cylinder or whether the cylinder is empty, full, or in use, store them in a dry, cool place, away from potential heat sources, such as furnaces, water heaters, and direct sunlight. Always secure the tanks, even the small ones, in an upright position by means of a chain or strap (Figure 6-19). Cylinders that are stored inside a closet should also be secured since they can fall against the door and cause injury when you open the door. If the cylinder is equipped with a protective cap, they must be firmly screwed in place when the cylinder is not in use. If you have to move a large cylinder, do

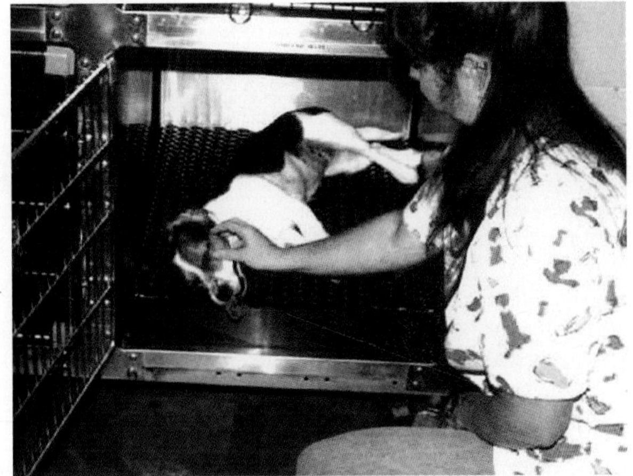

FIGURE 6-18 Monitor recovering anesthesia patients "at arms length" to minimize exposure to gases emitted during respiration.

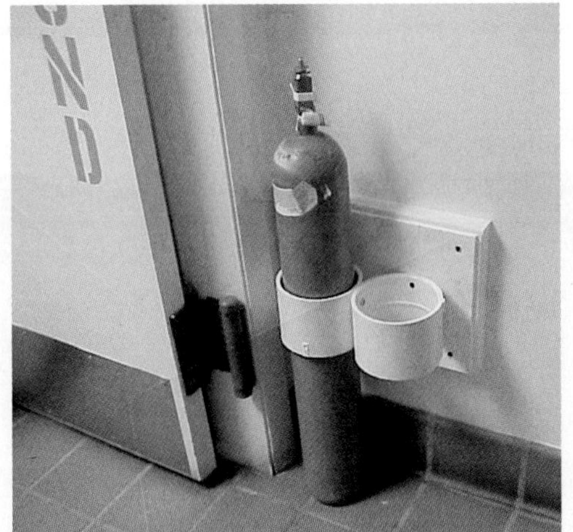

FIGURE 6-19 Small compressed-gas cylinders must be secured to prevent them from falling over.

not roll or drag it; always use a hand truck or handcart, and remember to strap the tank in.

SHARPS AND MEDICAL WASTE

The most serious hazard from needles or sharp objects in a veterinary medical environment is from the physical trauma (and possible bacterial infection) that is caused by a puncture or laceration. To prevent these types of accidents, always keep sharps, needles, scalpel blades, and other sharp instruments capped or sheathed until ready for use. Do not attempt to recap the needle after use unless the physical danger from sticks or lacerations cannot be prevented by any other means. When it is necessary to recap a needle, you should use the "one-handed" method (Box 6-4 and Figures 6-20 to 6-22). Although some practice is needed before the one-handed method becomes second nature, it is the safest and most practical approach for most veterinary situations.

Do not remove the needle from the syringe for disposal because this unnecessary handling often results in injuries. Whenever possible, the entire needle and syringe should be disposed of in the designated sharps containers immediately after use. Do not try to overfill a sharps container—when it is full, it is full! When the sharps container is full, seal it and replace it with a new one. Never open a sharps container that has already been sealed or stick your fingers into one for any reason.

Destroying the needle before disposal is not recommended because it may aerosolize the contents of the needle and increase your exposure. Likewise, you should not collect sharps in a smaller container and transfer them to a larger container for disposal. Of course, never throw needles or sharps directly into regular trash containers, regardless of whether or not they are capped.

Table 6-1 explains which materials are usually considered hazardous and which are not. Although this chart is essentially accurate, some states have special rules for discarding medical waste, so be sure to follow the rules prescribed by your state.

HAZARDOUS DRUGS AND PHARMACY OPERATIONS

Medicines are designed to cure diseases and make patients better, but it is important to remember that all medicines are chemicals and chemicals can be dangerous. In the veterinary pharmacy, you can be exposed to all kinds of drugs just by handling them. Liquids can splash in your eyes when you pour them or they can release vapors that you can inhale. Handling, crushing, or breaking tablets can leave powder residue on your hands that will be ingested next time you put your hands near your mouth or mucous membranes.

BOX 6-4 One-Handed Needle Recapping

- Step 1. Place the cap on a flat surface, such as the countertop or even the floor.
- Step 2. Using only one hand, hold the syringe in the tips of your fingers with the needle pointing away from your body (see Figure 6-20).
- Step 3. Place your fingertips on the flat surface so that the needle and syringe are parallel to and in line with the cap (see Figure 6-21).
- Step 4. You may then use your other hand to "seat" the cap firmly (see Figure 6-22).

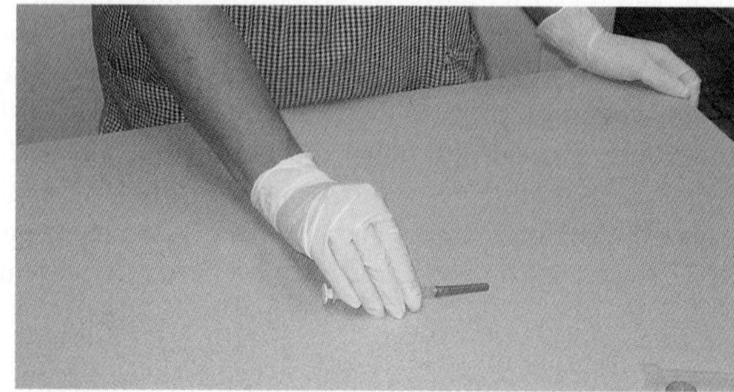

FIGURE 6-21 Step 4: Move your hand forward until the needle is inside the cap.

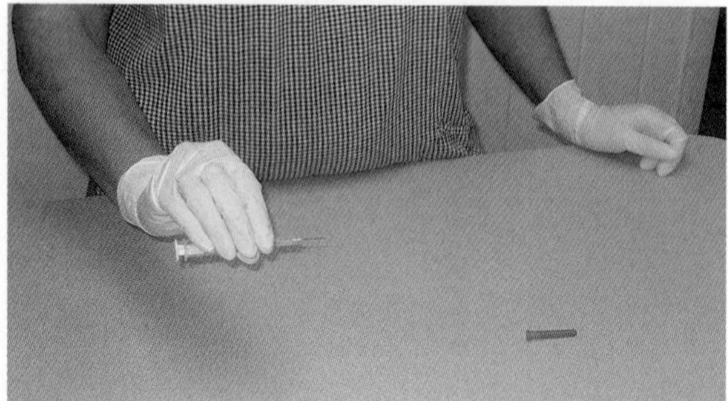

FIGURE 6-20 Using only one hand, hold the syringe in the tips of your fingers with the needle pointing away from your body.

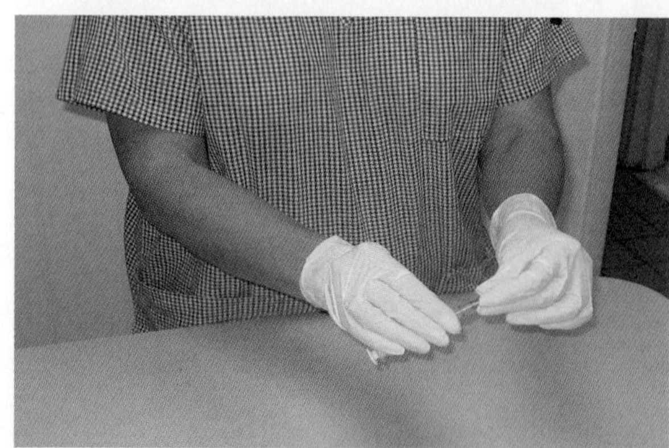

FIGURE 6-22 Final step: Use your other hand to "seat" the cap firmly.

TABLE 6-1 Typical Medical Waste Definitions

Material	Medical Waste	Normal Trash
Sharps (any device with characteristics that make it possible to puncture, lacerate, or penetrate the skin) Medical devices such as blood tubes, vials, catheters, IV tubes, etc.	Any used needles and scalpel blades Glass or hard plastic that is contaminated with a *human disease*–causing agent Considered biomedical waste only when they contain *human* pathogens or they have been used for chemotherapy	Glass or hard plastic that is not contaminated with *human disease*–causing agents can be disposed of as normal waste. Devices that simply contain or are contaminated with animal blood (except from primates) are normally not considered biomedical waste.
Animal blood or tissues	Only dead animals or animal parts that are infected with diseases that are communicable to *humans;* this includes but is not limited to rabies, brucellosis, systemic fungal diseases, tuberculosis, atypical mycobacteriosis, etc.	Tissues from routine surgical procedures (castration, ovariohysterectomy, etc) should be considered regular waste.
Laboratory cultures	Microbiologic cultures (bacterial, fungal, or viral) of *human* pathogens are considered biomedical waste	In some cases, culture media from negative tests may be considered regular trash, but it is probably wise to just classify all lab cultures as biomedical waste for simplicity.
Bandages/sponges	Used absorbent materials such as bandages, gauze, or sponges that are saturated with blood or body fluids that contain *human* pathogens that may splash or drip	Sponges or bandages used on animals not infected with a disease transmissible to humans.
Primate materials		Normally, waste generated from work on primates is considered regular waste *unless it fits in another category* (such as from research studies using human pathogens).
Animal waste	Waste from animals infected with a disease contagious to *humans* that can be transmitted by means of the waste. Waste from chemotherapy patients for up to 48 hours after the last treatment	Normally, waste from animals not infected with human disease–causing agents should be disposed of as regular trash.

Some drugs, such as the cytotoxic drugs (CDs) used to treat patients with cancer, are so potent even minute exposures can cause harm. When preparing CDs, always wear powder-free chemotherapy gloves and a disposable gown that is not used for any other purpose. Chemotherapy drugs should always be mixed inside of a biologic safety cabinet (Figure 6-23). Be sure to follow all of the instructions on the MSDS, package insert, and your practice's chemotherapy safety plan.

During the administration of CDs, expect the unexpected. Keep unnecessary people out of the area and wear protective equipment such as gloves, disposable aprons, surgical masks, and eyeglasses. You should avoid wearing contact lenses when preparing or administering CDs.

When handling patients that have received chemotherapeutic treatments, remember that some drugs are excreted in bodily fluids, so proper precautions are necessary when cleaning up their urine, feces, and other bodily excretions. Always wear powder-free chemotherapy gloves and avoid contaminating your clothes when cleaning cages or picking up waste from chemotherapy patients. Make sure you

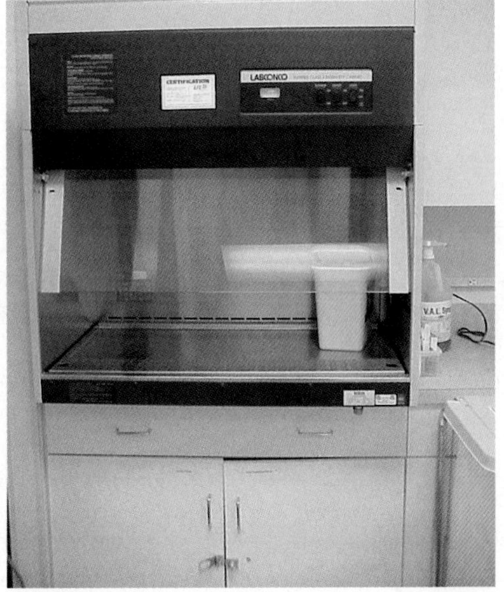

FIGURE 6-23 A biologic safety cabinet (BSC) is required when preparing cytotoxic drugs.

dispose of all soiled materials from these patients as medical waste and launder nondisposable items separately from general laundry.

The biggest rule to remember when handling any medication is to practice good personal hygiene, especially a thorough hand washing.

CASE PRESENTATION 6-3

A 25-year-old veterinary technician is working in private mixed-animal hospital. She and her husband have been trying to conceive a child for several years without success. Her obstetrician has suggested that her exposure to hazards at work may be contributing to her inability to conceive. After a thorough analysis of the chemicals, pathogens, and physical hazards she is exposed to at work, it was determined that her failure to use proper precautions when handling patient medications, in particular, chemotherapy drugs, contributed to unviable egg production.

After retraining and by practicing better personal hygiene when handling patients and medications, she became pregnant within a year.

SUMMARY

We all face dangers in life every day, but that does not mean we have to intentionally place ourselves in danger to get our job done. The successful person makes sure the reward for the action far outweighs the risk.

In this chapter, we discussed your rights and responsibilities in a safety program, the hazards associated with your job from both a general and medical perspective, and the actions you should take to protect yourself. Employing good safety practices should not be the cause for additional work. If a job is safely completed and the correct protocol is followed, then it is done properly. Occupational risks should not keep you from doing your job; they should motivate you to do your job better, to pay attention to what you are doing, and to comply with the standard operating procedures established in your practice. Employing good safety practices will enable you to remain healthy and will therefore allow you to continue to practice your career for a long time.

Have fun and be safe.

INTERNET RESOURCES/SUGGESTED READING

SafetyVet: www.safetyvet.com
OSHA: www.osha.gov
Canadian OSHA: www.canoshweb.org
National Institute of Occupational Safety and Health (NIOSH): www.cdc.gov/niosh
Centers for Disease Control and Prevention: www.cdc.gov
Canadian Centre for Occupational Health & Safety: www.ccohs.ca
The Veterinary Information Network (VIN): www.vin.com
The Veterinary Support Personnel Network (VSPN): www.vspn.org
Infection Control Today: www.infectioncontroltoday.com
The Virtual Anesthesia Machine: http://vam.anest.ufl.edu/
Lab Safety Supply: www.labsafety.com
Environmental Protection Agency: www.epa.gov
Department of Labor: www.dol.gov

Patient Management and Nutrition

PART TWO

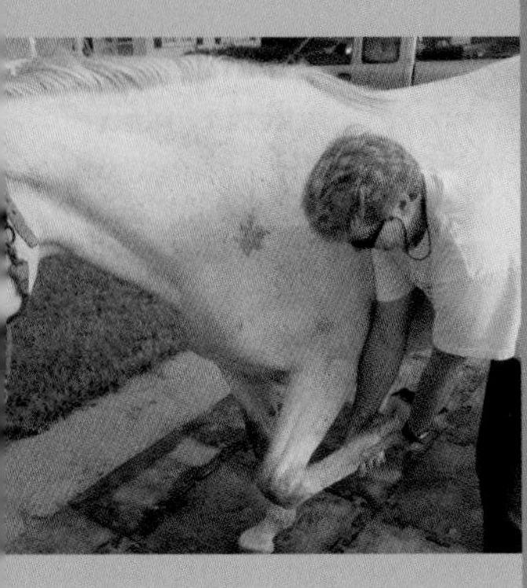

Restraint and Handling of Animals

7

Dennis D. French and Thomas N. Tully, Jr.

KEY TERMS

Agonistic behavior
Fear biting
Fight-or-flight response
Hobbles
Intermale aggression
Maternal aggression
Passerine
Psittacine
Raptorial species
Stocks
Tail tie
Territorial aggression
Tortoise
Turtles
Twitch

OUTLINE

LEARNING OBJECTIVES

When you have completed this chapter, you will be able to:

1. Discuss the indications for restraint of animals and behaviors exhibited by aggressive animals.
2. Explain the physiologic principles that affect animal perceptions and methods of restraint in small and large animals.
3. Describe the methods for approaching, haltering, tying, and leading equine patients.
4. Define twitch and describe various types of twitches and their uses in equine restraint.
5. Explain the methods used for lifting a horse's foot, applying a tail tie, and applying hobbles.
6. Describe the indications and procedures for the use of stocks in equine patients.
7. Describe the indications and procedures for moving cattle and sheep into pens and chutes.
8. Describe the procedures for tail jacking and casting of cattle.
9. Explain the methods of capturing individual sheep, goats, and pigs.
10. Describe the proper procedures for carrying and lifting large dogs, small dogs, and cats.
11. List and describe the types of muzzles and mouth gags that are used on dogs and cats and explain the proper procedures for their use.
12. Describe restraint and handling techniques used with birds, reptiles, and amphibians.
13. Describe restraint and handling techniques used with ferrets, rabbits, and rodents.
14. Discuss the indications for use of chemical restraint in animal patients.

INTRODUCTION

Most people entering the field of veterinary medicine have had experience with some animals, but few have had the experience necessary to deal with all the species that may be encountered. To assume all animals respond in the same manner is not correct and can be quite dangerous. Restraint techniques differ markedly among species, and the response of different animals to restraint is highly variable. The wise individual is able to ascertain what the body language of a particular animal means and respond appropriately to the actions of that animal.

This chapter is intended to be a guide to the behavior, handling, and restraint of animals commonly encountered in veterinary practice. It is not intended to be an exhaustive text, but rather to provide a range of techniques to build confidence and competence.

INDICATIONS FOR RESTRAINT

Competent restraint of animals is critical to a veterinary practice for the following reasons:

1. **To control an animal so that it can receive medical care.** Most animals resist physical examination and the administration of diagnostic and therapeutic procedures. Proper restraint of a sick animal may allow humans to save its life.
2. **To prevent the animal from harming itself while it is receiving medical care.** Animals must be restrained when panicked and trying to flee from, what they perceive as, a dangerous situation. Jumping off an examination table, attempting to crash through a fence or chewing the bars of a confinement are examples of fleeing behavior that can have disastrous results. Maintaining a safe environment, including well constructed stalls, cages and fencing is a critical part of protecting the animal from injury.
3. **To protect personnel.** The safety of veterinary personnel, clients and handlers is of the utmost importance. The injury and even death of individuals can devastate families, and veterinary practices. It can lead to the loss of wages, expensive litigation, anxiety, decreased morale, and loss of livelihood. Practice owners are responsible for any injuries incurred by veterinary personnel and clients during the performance of veterinary procedures. This liability begins when the client enters the practice or when the truck stops in the driveway. For this reason, many practitioners believe that a veterinary technician's ability to perform excellent animal restraint is the most important skill for a technician to master.

> *TECHNICIAN NOTE* Excellent skill in restraint is critical to ensure that the animal receives medical care without injury to the patient or the care givers.

ANIMAL PERCEPTION AND BEHAVIOR

Current studies in behavioral science and ethology provide us with information on animal-to-animal communication that aids in the understanding of how best to restrain various species. This data improves the ability of humans to assess animal responses and better understand how our interactions affect an animal's behavior. Animals employ their senses, such as sight, smell and hearing, in ways that are different from humans. Therefore, animal gestures, touches, smells and actions that provide important information to other animals is often missed or misinterpreted by humans. A veterinary technician's ability to correctly interpret these non-verbal, species-specific forms of communication is critical for implementation of effective and compassionate restraint.

SMELL

The sense of smell is well developed in all domestic mammals. The rabbit and cat have improved olfaction because of olfactory epithelium that is nearly 14 times more developed than in humans.

Horses will snort when faced with a smell with which they are unfamiliar. Bulls may react by pawing and blowing when they are faced with a different smell. We now are more aware of the chemical changes that occur in the human body which may cause changes in scent that communicate illness, stress and anxiety. Consider, for example, that we now train dogs to detect cancer in humans because the illness alters metabolic chemistry.

The language of smell undoubtedly has a more extensive vocabulary in animals than in humans. This is important to acknowledge when handling various species in a single hospital setting such as an exam room or treatment area. For example examinations of prey species such as rats, rabbits and mice should not be done in an area where a cat was recently examined. The finely tuned scent organs of the prey animals will detect the scent of a predator which may increase blood cortisol levels and alter heart and respiratory rates. Other odors to consider that may affect an animal's behavior are anal sac excretions, vaginal discharge from intact female dogs or urine from a mare in estrus.

HEARING

Domestic animals are able to move the external ear, or pinnae, with muscles, which enables them to focus on the source of the sound. This is advantageous because an approach by a handler is often observed. Slight sounds will elicit movement of the ears and allow the animal to become aware of the presence of someone new. Low, smooth, confidant tones will allow the animal to become comfortable with your presence. The response of the ear is important to assess the animal's attitude. The ears-back position in a horse or llama signals that the animal is upset or aggressive. A dog pricks its ears forward when alert or actively aggressive, whereas a submissive dog wrinkles and flattens its ears. Cats with their ears pinned back should be considered dangerous. Alterations in the shape and size of an animal's ears may decrease the ability of the handler to use ear position as a sole indicator of the animal's state of arousal.

VISION

The eyes of domestic animals focus by means of muscles controlling the shape of the lens through a process called accommodation. In small animals and pigs, accommodation is accomplished by increasing the dioptic power of the lens by changing the shape of the lens. Most animals accommodate the eye on near objects much less readily than do humans. It is known that the nearest point at which dogs can focus is about 30 cm, and this is most likely true for the pig. The dog's ability to discriminate form and pattern is thought to be poor when compared with human abilities. This is particularly important when dealing with those dogs that are noted to be "fear biters."

Cats have excellent night vision, which is consistent with their nocturnal habits. They are also acutely aware of a small movement, which facilitates the precision of their rush after stalking their prey. Unfortunately, this also enhances the ability of a fearful or painful feline patient to strike out against those humans who move too suddenly or come too close.

The pig has eyes that are directed more forward than the horse, but less than that of most dogs. The size of their binocular visual field could be as large as 30 degrees on either side of the midline. Ruminants have much less ability to accommodate with the lens of their eyes and will therefore have a much longer near-focus distance. Herbivorous animals have wide fields of vision enabling them to detect the encroachment of predators from various angles. This is particularly evident in the horse and rabbit, both of which enjoy nearly circumferential vision without moving the head. The horse has a particularly sluggish accommodation. What some handlers may perceive as fractious and spooky may in fact be nothing more than the horse attempting to visually accommodate. This is particularly noticeable when an already nervous human makes fast movements near a horse. The horse moves about in a rapid manner trying to ascertain what the human wants. Horses have acute vision at middle and far distances, which is not surprising for a prey species. Many of the behavioral displays of horses are visual in nature, and subtle movements by handlers at seemingly great distances will generate responses from horses. It is assumed that the binocular segment of the visual field for a ruminant is about 30 degrees on either side of the midline.

> TECHNICIAN NOTE With the exception of pigs, domestic animals have a special layer behind the lens called the *tapetum,* which permits them better vision in low light.

TOUCH

The sense of touch is becoming more important in the handling of animals. Numerous behaviorists and trainers are proponents of contact on different body parts to enhance communication between animals and among animals and humans. Contact behaviors that appear to result from or resolve conflict are the ones most described in handling. Dominant animals use biting, scratching, kicking, or striking to teach youngsters proper behavior. Horses kick or slam a shoulder into other horses to demonstrate dominance and make a point of their supremacy. Mares training youngsters in a herd will actually keep a particularly hardheaded yearling out of the herd by biting and kicking at it. This communication is species specific and it is best to avoid attempts to replicate these behaviors. It is important to remember that these behaviors occur in specific contexts and may relate to control of resources. Some people will use blows to correct unacceptable equine behavior. When using these techniques, the target must be carefully selected, and the individual must possess the physical strength to make the procedure effective. As a general rule, humans will end up hurting themselves much more than the horse they were trying to correct. It has also been shown that physical correction for behaviors can create fear, stress and anxiety for the animal in addition to damaging the human-animal bond.

The actual method of how to touch animals is a manner of skill. Tentative, light touches or repeated patting makes many species nervous and apprehensive. Steady, firm strokes are reassuring to most species. Watching animals in a natural setting provides the insight into how to most effectively touch them when they are nervous. You will never observe one animal slapping another to calm it down in a natural setting. Clever individuals learn to read the animals that they are asked to restrain and develop the touch necessary to keep them calm.

AGONISTIC BEHAVIORS

Agonistic behaviors are those associated with conflict. Many animals have to be maneuvered into a position in which restraint is possible, or they must be restrained from the outset as a safety measure. Such maneuvering is perceived by the animal as conflict (threat). To understand the principles of maneuvering each species, it is wise to become familiar with the prevalent forms of agonistic behavior in the different species. Agonistic behaviors cover the range of responses to conflict from passive avoidance to the extreme of aggression and fighting. In nature, overt aggressive attacks that lead to fights with other animals of the same or different species are not common outside of sexual or predatory behavior. Dominance and submissive behaviors represent the more common methods of resolving disagreement over resources such as food, territory, and reproduction. Chapter 11 gives additional information on animal behavior.

Fight or Flight

When a stranger approaches an animal, the same basic principles apply whether it is a domestic or wild animal. Each species in a given environment has its own degree of response, but the factors or cues giving rise to the response are common to all animals in varying degrees. Each animal has a fight-or-flight distance. When that space is invaded, the animal goes into a state of alert. The sympathetic nervous system releases epinephrine from the adrenal gland. This hormone causes increased heart rate and a subsequent increase in blood flow to the skeletal muscles, lungs, and brain. Further encroachment into the animal's space will lead to action that may take the form of avoidance (the cow or horse crash through a fence, the dog runs off down the road) or aggression (the dog bites, the cow runs over the stranger). This action is aptly termed the *fight-or-flight response.* The response will vary from animal to animal of the same species and may vary from time to time for the same animal. When this happens, it is difficult to come up with a good restraint plan.

AGGRESSIVE BEHAVIOR

Aggressive behavior is the form of agonistic or conflict behavior that leads to and includes fighting. Aggression is not the result of a single cause. The different forms of aggression are classified according to the stimuli or circumstances giving rise to the ferocity.

Irritable or Pain-Induced Aggression

Inevitably, pain-induced aggression is a common problem in the veterinary hospital and in field situations. Herd animals that have become incapacitated and are incapable of keeping up with the herd must resort to aggression to stay alive. Injections and certain manipulations, such as the treatment of wounds, cause pain and discomfort to animals. Even the initial injection of a local anesthetic can be most uncomfortable, no matter how skilled the anesthetist. The state of mind of the patient has a lot to do with an aggressive outcome. If the animal is initially apprehensive and nervous, the probability for aggression is high. This is the reason that calming and familiarization of the patient are practiced whenever possible. Sedation may also be indicated for certain patients.

Maternal Aggression

All female domestic animals that are suckling their young are sensitized to interference with their offspring by strangers. The calmest, old broodmare in the herd may be extremely protective of her new foal. The bitch can be aggressive with strangers and even family members if she perceives a threat to her pups. A sow within earshot of her piglets when they are being restrained can become one of the most dangerous animals encountered. All parties working within a farrowing house must exercise caution because the vocalization of any young piglet as it is manipulated can make all the sows in the house become sensitized.

> *TECHNICIAN NOTE* All female domestic animals that are suckling their young are sensitized to interference with their offspring by strangers.

Predatory Aggression

Aggressive activity displayed by chasing and killing prey is observed in predatory domestic animals, such as the dog and cat, and is called *predatory aggression*. This form of aggression does not usually pose a threat to the animal handler, although large dogs may pull the handler down if they feel the urge to chase a cat while on a leash.

Territorial Aggression

All domestic mammals have a degree of territorial domain. They will protect the area over which they range from intruders, and they may exhibit territorial aggression. Separate groups of horses may share feeding sites and watering holes, but they remain apart from one another and retain control of their own separate home range. The domestic dog may regard the yard, porch, or house as its territory. Strangers are treated with suspicion, and this suspicion may lead to barking or attack. Unfortunately, territorialism in dogs can be difficult to distinguish from behavior that has been conditioned, is related to fear, lack of socialization or lack of mental stimulation. Dogs that harass the mail carrier or meter reader are behaving within the norm of canine behavior. The female rabbit is strongly territorial in the captive situation. If a buck is taken to her cage, she will attack him aggressively, often causing serious injury. Thus the doe is always taken to the buck's cage for mating. This female territoriality may be associated with aggression that continues even when the nesting box is empty and can be directed at humans. Although the concept of an "attack rabbit" may seem humorous, it becomes less so when reaching into the cage of an old doe and being growled at, struck, and bitten.

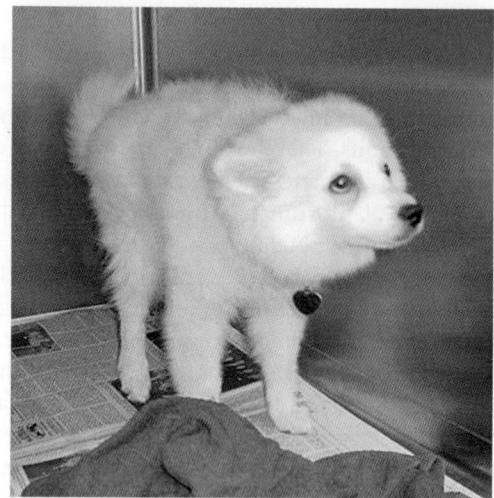

FIGURE 7-1 This dog demonstrates the posture of a classic "fear biter." Note the defensive stare with the ears laid back and the tail between the legs.

Fear-Induced Aggression

When an animal is terrified of an environment and the people in it and is not given an option to avoid the circumstances, it will resort to aggression. Fear is a common cause of aggression in dogs placed under such circumstances. Fear biting is the most commonly encountered type of attack in veterinary hospitals. The dog is usually giving classic signs of being intimidated: avoiding direct eye contact with the head down, lips pulled back horizontally, ears flattened, and the tail between the legs, which have been ignored or misinterpreted by human handlers (Figure 7-1). When the personal space of such a dog is encroached, a sudden attack may ensue. This is fear biting. The attack is usually confined to the proffered hand or forearm, and the purpose is simply to repel the invader.

Intermale Aggression

Aggression occurring between males can be a problem, particularly when stud animals are kept. Boars can be extremely vicious when confronting each other, and great care should be taken when handling them. Stallions can become extremely agitated when mixed with another stallion. Bulls spend a great deal of time head butting and pushing one another around to establish the dominance order when they are turned out together.

Dominance Aggression

In the past it was presumed that certain dogs would establish their authority over a human family, other animals, and strangers because of their heritage as pack animals. Alternatively a dog may accede to dominance from one family member, but attempt to assert itself aggressively with other family members. Current scientific data refutes such arguments. Past assumptions were made by observation of wolves which were then applied to domestic dogs. Animal behaviorists, both in veterinary medicine and university settings no longer use the term dominance aggression due to the incorrect assumptions of the past.

Information collected by modern day animal behaviorists and ethologists shows that dogs while genetically related to wolves, differ in behavior. The effects of years of domestication and breed selection for specific characteristics have yielded results that favor the dog's ability to live among humans. Additionally, original theories on dominance as a whole did not take into account how human interactions alter the behavior of domestic species. For example, old theories on dominance would say that when a dog jumped up on a human the dog was asserting its dominance. However, if the owner pets the dog when it jumps on them then the behavior is not dominant at all but has been conditioned of "trained" by the human. From the dog's perspective it jumps on the human in order to receive contact and be petted.

In today's world of veterinary behavior the term dominance aggression would most likely be related to a conflict between two animals regarding resources. Aggression would be the resulting behavior if neither animal was willing to give up the resource. An example of this would be two stallions competing for a band of mares.

TYPICAL BEHAVIOR OF DOMESTIC ANIMALS IN AGGRESSION AND AVOIDANCE

Cattle

The primary concern when dealing with cattle is bulls, regardless of size. Dairy breed bulls, such as the Jersey and Holstein, should be considered the most dangerous animal of all the species that veterinary personnel are asked to restrain or handle. They are powerful and unpredictable. Aggressive behavior is characterized by pawing the ground with the forefeet while holding the head with the frontal area nearly vertical with the ground and snorting. These bulls after charging and knocking the person down will make continued attempts to toss the victim, which will lead to goring if the bull still has horns. Bulls may also attempt to kneel on the victim or continually smash the victim with their foreheads. Little can be done to dissuade or thwart a bull once this activity begins. Front-end loaders and pickup trucks have been used to try to push these animals away from their targets without success. Bulls, particularly the dairy breed types, should always be treated with the utmost respect and with the appropriate means of restraint and containment. The likelihood of a snorting bull, posturing in an aggressive stance, hurting a handler is actually less than one that has been hand raised. The hand-raised bull may appear to be quite gentle and yet when approached may react aggressively. Special handling considerations are made for those who work with semen donors at bull studs. These bulls are selected for the high-quality genetic potentials, and their semen is worth considerable amounts of money. Insensitive handling before and during collection may give rise to reproductive behavior problems leading to decreased collection volumes and significant economic loss.

Aggressiveness in the heifer and cow seems to be directly related to breed and socialization. Dairy cows are generally docile, probably because they are handled a great deal. Beef cows that have been handled frequently in a quiet, professional manner are manageable. However, beef cattle that are raised on range with little human interaction or those that are handled with lots of whipping and shouting tend to be apprehensive and may become quite aggressive. This aggressiveness is compounded when they are nursing calves.

The fight-or-flight distance for a herd of cattle will vary depending on the previous degree and type of contact with humans. The handling of dairy cattle and beef cattle differs greatly. The flight distance for dairy cows is extremely short, with the animal veering off only when directly confronted by the handler. Most dairy cattle are used to a number of different people around them during milking time, and the introduction of someone new into the herd does not create stress or fear. This makes handling dairy cows easier for veterinary personnel. Beef cattle have a much larger flight space, which is accentuated when they sense a new presence in a field or pen. It is common for ranchers to be able to walk or drive among their cattle at close range. When a new pickup or person enters the pasture, the cattle's heads come up and they will gradually move further away. If the cattle are approached too quickly, they will break into a disorganized run, which makes them nearly impossible to maneuver. It is important to realize the impact that outsiders have on a herd of beef cattle before trying to handle and examine individuals. This is a common problem in "Penturbia," where owners get two pregnant cows to decorate their acreage (usually of 3 to 5 acre lots) and then need veterinary attention. Routinely, they do not have adequate handling facilities on site. It is extremely important for veterinary personnel to understand this before initiating procedures to capture the animals in a run-in shed or a makeshift corral.

A part of the secret of maneuvering cattle is using a body extension. Canes, stock whips, or wiffle paddles used by a person on foot are viewed by the cattle as an extension of the body. If the cattle can be kept calm, the visual barrier created by these devices allows the handler to maneuver the cattle from pen to pen. If cattle are accustomed to observation from horseback, maneuvering a herd can be quite easy for one or two riders. Mixing riders and walkers in a pasture

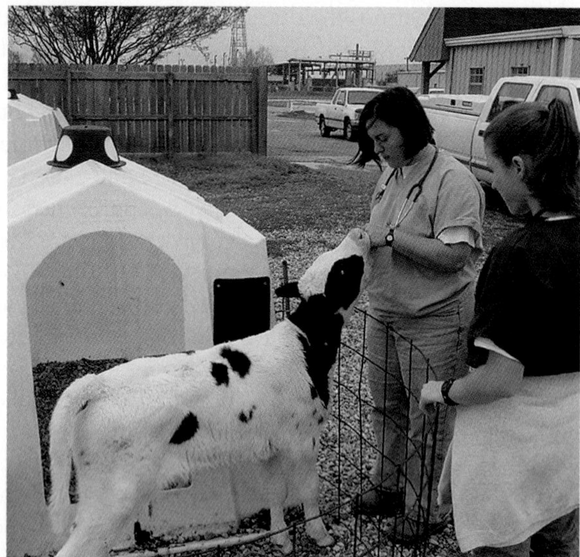

FIGURE 7-2 This Holstein calf demonstrates the curiosity that most bovids have at an early age. It has come up to the new handler without any reservations.

is not a good idea and should only be done as a last resort when trying to maneuver a herd of cattle. It should be made clear that maneuvering the herd (or all the animals that are housed together) is much easier than attempting to separate an individual.

> *TECHNICIAN NOTE* When dealing with food animals that are pets, move the entire herd into a small enclosure before attempting to separate an individual, even though only one of the individuals is affected.

Calves

Calves are inquisitive and will become attentive to the presence of someone new. The calf stretching its head or neck toward the new handler is the usual posture (Figure 7-2). Darting movements will cause the calf to panic, veer, and run away. The approach toward a calf should be slow and deliberate with the hands slightly away from the sides of the body. No loud noises are necessary, and movement of the hands and arms should be kept to a minimum. Using a fence line or wall, the handler should move to cut off escape routes and negotiate the calf into a corner and grab it with one arm under the jaw, and the other hand should reach and grab the tail.

Cats

Aggressive behavior in cats should never be underestimated. They can be formidable patients in situations of conflict because they will use the claws of all four feet, they have razor-sharp teeth, and when stressed they seem to have a spinal cord that is made much like a Slinky, which allows them to go in many different directions at once. It should be remembered that the cat stalks its prey and runs only short distances to pounce. It is a stealthy aggressor. The true speed of the cat never becomes apparent until it is actively avoiding conflict. It is the wise staff that closes all doors and windows before attempting to handle cats in any environment to prevent escape.

> *TECHNICIAN NOTE* When handling cats in any environment, close all doors and windows to prevent escape.

Dogs

Overtly aggressive behavior, although not a common problem in dogs, is a significant social problem and one that will present difficulties for veterinary personnel. Dominance and submission are important in communication between two dogs in a conflict situation. Fixing the other animal in a direct stare is a direct threat of aggression. The ears are raised and angled forward. The front end of the body is held high, and the hackles on the back of the neck are raised. The head is held up, and the lips curl to reveal the incisor and canine teeth. The tail will be raised. The clinical stare of veterinary personnel as they examine a dog can be taken as a threat of aggression by a dog.

Lowering the front end of the body and avoiding direct eye contact demonstrate the submissive behavior. Usually the tail will be held between the legs, and the dog may squat and urinate or defecate. The ears will flatten on the back of the head, and the lips may become pulled back at the corners of the mouth into a "grin." The spine may adopt an S shape, and the animal may lie down on its side or back, raising the legs and exposing the undefended belly. When dogs display this behavior it is similar to saying "take my keys and wallet, please don't hurt me." These behaviors are designed to appease an aggressor which would decrease or diffuse conflict between dogs. In the veterinary clinic this behavior is commonly demonstrated by fearful or anxious dogs.

When confronted by a person, the dog may demonstrate potential aggression by adopting the aggressive posture, or it may adopt a submissive stance. A dog in the active aggressive posture may attack if the threat is not removed from its fight-or-flight distance. A dog in this posture will bite if you attempt to encroach on its space. Dogs demonstrating submissive postures may also bite when handlers reach into their space or lean over them accidentally increasing the dog's fear. Some dogs may show active aggression only when the owner is present. The protectiveness may be possessiveness as the dog defends its own favored object, owner conditioned behavior, or specifically trained behavior (protection/security dogs). Removing the owner may resolve the conflict. The opposite may occur when handling dogs that have developed a bond with their usual handlers. These dogs may be quite fearful without their human partner in the examination room. Retrievers, herding dogs, and guard dogs that tend to associate closely with only one individual may be quite difficult to handle without their owner present.

Certain dogs do not attempt to resolve conflict by aggression, preferring to avoid it if at all possible. Those that skillfully avoid conflict are described as having a passive defense reflex. Dogs that tend to face conflict are said to have an active defense reflex.

Horses

Blatant aggressiveness in the horse is not common. However, certain horses can be nasty with their aggression. This is most commonly seen in horses that are stalled most of the time. Racehorses and breeding stallions seem to be the worst offenders. Aggressive behavior may be observed on broodmare farms with mares protecting new foals and stallions protecting their band of mares. Lunging forward and biting, kicking with the hind legs, and striking with the front legs characterize the aggressive acts of the horse. Although the field of vision of the horse is nearly 360 degrees, the binocular field of vision is only 60 degrees to 70 degrees in front of the animal. Binocular vision is required for judging distance; therefore vision outside this range requires movement of the head and sometimes the entire body to allow the horse to further investigate what it perceives as the threat.

The approach to a horse should not be made from the blind spot directly behind the horse. The horse, as it detects new objects or people in its environment, will raise its head and observe. If no threat is perceived, the horse resumes its previous activity. If the threat is perceived as real, the head turns toward the object, the neck is raised, and the ears will turn toward the object. The nostrils will become dilated to further evaluate the threat. The tail will also become elevated, and the muscles of the torso and lower limbs will become more rigid, ready for fight or flight. Occasionally the horse will snort, further alerting other horses to the presence of a threat. Mares with foals will usually nicker, and the foal will move to the other side of the mare. Further encroachment results in rapid movement away from the intruder. If the horse is in a stall, it will circle rapidly away, always keeping its hind end toward the intruder.

> *TECHNICIAN NOTE* The approach to a horse should not be made from the blind spot directly behind the horse.

Pigs

Aggressive behavior in the domestic pig has serious economic and physical consequences. Adult boars that are mixed together will circle and threaten each other with grunts and jaw snapping. Fighting commences in the side-to-side position with sideways pushing and slashing at one another with the tusks. Solid panels of plywood should be used to separate the combatants. Commercial pigs are reared in groups, which provide plenty of opportunity for fighting. When new pigs are introduced into a group, fighting will occur, especially if living space and trough space are limited. Introducing a sow into an established group may induce savage attacks and even deaths. Allowing more space and diversions for the group reduces aggression in pigs.

Large numbers of unfamiliar pigs adapt better than smaller numbers. There is less fighting, probably because dominance is more difficult to establish in the larger social groups. Avoidance behavior in young pigs in confined areas involves running into corners and huddling, shoving, and climbing over one another. This does not present a problem if small groups are huddled, but larger groups that pile up may produce traumatic lesions and in severe cases death from suffocation.

Remember that the lactating sow can be extremely dangerous because of maternal aggression. When handling suckling pigs, always remove the sow to a secure area out of earshot, if possible.

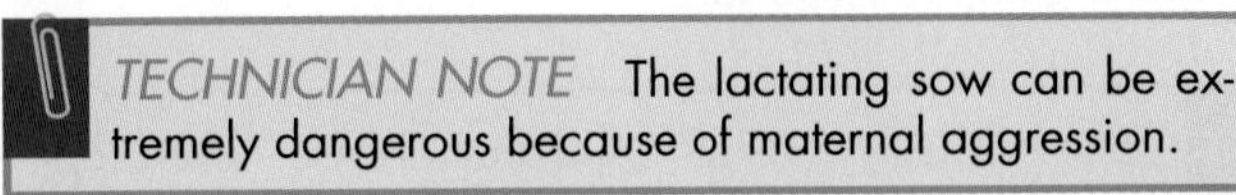
TECHNICIAN NOTE The lactating sow can be extremely dangerous because of maternal aggression.

Sheep

Avoidance behavior in sheep is the basis of maneuvering the flock. When sheep are approached, they will flock together and move as a single unit. This herding behavior is well understood by dogs. By carefully controlling their posture, speed of movement, and distance from the flock, the dog uses the sheep's avoidance behavior to maneuver the flock into an enclosure. This is one of the most fascinating and complex interspecies relationships in domestic animal management. Handling areas should be well lighted and free of objects that may project shadows into the sheep's visual path and should have solid sides.

Aggression between rams may lead to injuries between the combatants. Handling these rams may also be difficult because of the willingness of the ram to challenge the handler. Rams are most dangerous when they attempt to head butt and as such should be treated with respect.

MANAGEMENT ETHOLOGY

Ethology is the study of animal behavior (see also Chapter 11) Capture, handling, and restraint might be called management ethology, which is the study of animal behavior as a means of determining how best to maneuver and control animals. The approach and handling techniques that are described for each species are in harmony with the typical behavior of the animals that we are asked to restrain, and the physical techniques described are compatible with their anatomy. Humans have great powers of observation, and it is important for students of the animal industries to enhance their powers of observation about animal behavior. Knowledge of body systems and anatomic structure is clearly important, but there is no substitute for alertness, observation, and perception of how the animal is reacting to its environment and to the presence of veterinary personnel. Mental preparation must begin well in advance of any potentially dangerous restraint situation. Confidence and knowledge will be gained over time that ensures the handler of a correct assessment of any situation.

CAPTURE AND RESTRAINT OF HORSES

A cardinal rule when approaching any animal, *especially* a horse, is not to startle it. The handler should always make his or her presence known by talking or calling to the horse. Many horses have learned that capture leads to work or some sort of unpleasantness, and these type of horses will practice avoidance. Horses also do not like to be closely confined or "squeezed." Close quarters will make many horses anxious, and some will attempt to escape, which may result in injury to the horse and people involved. By calling to the horse, the handler begins to have an appreciation of how a particular animal is going to respond.

> TECHNICIAN NOTE A cardinal rule when approaching any animal, especially a horse, is not to startle it.

The normal flight distance of most horses is between 3 and 10 m. Events that occur outside this radius are of little concern to the horse. Once within this area, sudden movements or sharp noises may easily startle it. Always be sure that the horse is observing you as you approach. A horse that is looking at you is less likely to be startled than one looking off at some other object. Be aware that if the horse decides to become nervous the first evasive maneuver that it will perform is to wheel away, leaving you facing the hindquarters of the animal.

It should be obvious that approaching a horse from the rear should be avoided, if possible. Given the horse's zone of vision and its blind spot, the horse is not likely to see a person directly behind them. A horse's kicking zone extends 1.8 to 2.5 m behind it. The furthest extension of the heels is the most dangerous and is the area of potentially fatal kicks to the head or chest. Horses usually kick to the rear, rather than to the side, but many of them can "cow kick," or kick to the side well. It is wise to grant at least 3 m behind and to the side of a horse when dealing with the rear quarters of the horse. The other alternative is to stay in direct contact with the horse as you maneuver about the hind end (Figure 7-3). Staying close to the hindquarters will not allow the full force of a kick and will keep the force of the blow low on the recipient's anatomy. This does not mean that the blow will not be painful or damaging. However, a fractured tibia may be some consolation over a fractured skull. Grasping the tail may discourage some horses from kicking.

The prospective handler should also never stand directly in front of the horse. A horse that becomes agitated may strike out with a front foot and leg at any instant. Agitated horses also may decide to become carnivores at any time and attempt to bite the handler.

The initial approach to the horse is best accomplished from the front and left side (Figure 7-4). The left side in equine terminology is known as the *near side.* This is the side that the horse is accustomed to being handled from because of tradition and the fact that most people lead their horses with their right hand. The first point of contact for the handler on the horse should be the withers. The handler should have a slightly outstretched arm that is no higher than the handler's shoulder. The handler should make some low, confidence-building conversation as he or she moves toward the horse. This goes back to the natural behavior of the horse, from mares licking their foals to the social interaction between horses in which they will rub each other on the withers. If the horse moves away, the handler should stop and stay still until the horse has quieted again. Many times if the handler will turn slightly away from the horse and not look directly at it, the horse will turn back to the handler (Figure 7-5). This movement mimics the communication found in herds of horses when an outsider is finally "welcomed" into the herd. It is always wise to move in slow increments without raising your hands or voice.

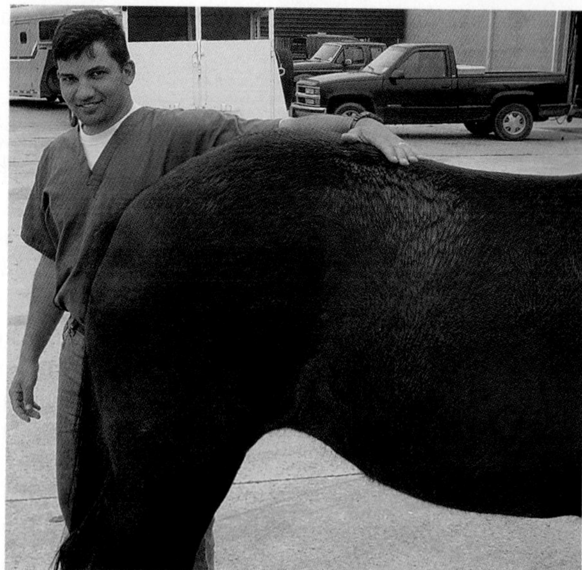

FIGURE 7-3 Note how the handler maintains contact with the horse as he begins to move from one side of the animal to the other. This is especially important since he is in the horse's blind spot.

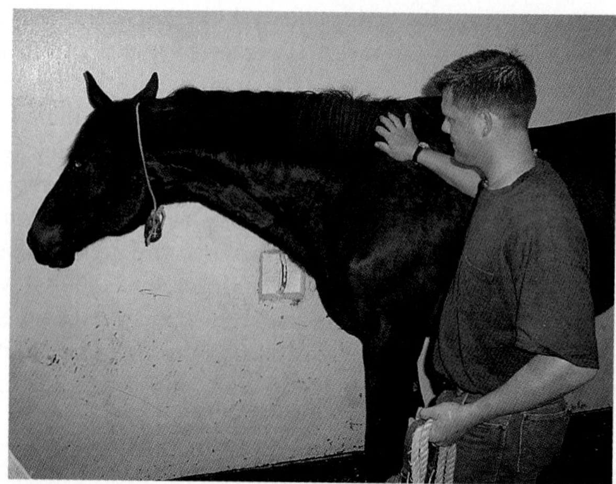

FIGURE 7-4 Initial approach to the horse should be from the left, or near, side. Note the right hand leads to touch the horse at the withers. The left hand holds the halter and lead rope low and to the handler's side.

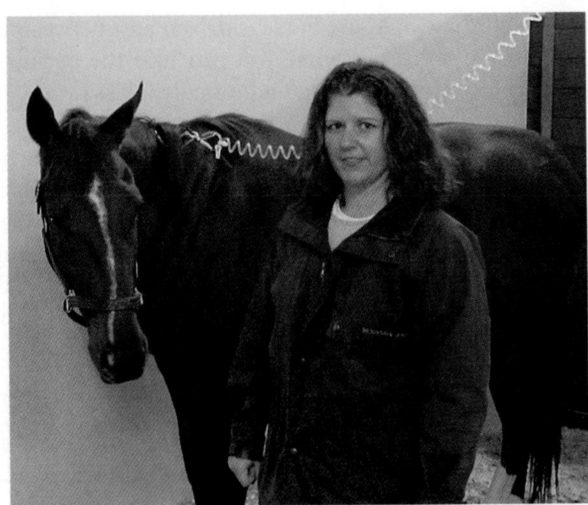

FIGURE 7-5 Note how the horse's ears and head are directed toward the would-be handler, almost as if the horse wants to know what is going to happen next.

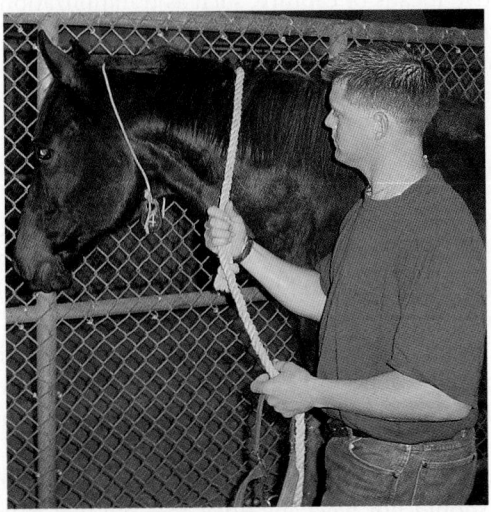

FIGURE 7-6 The use of a small rope looped over the horse's neck will aid in controlling the horse's head and allow the handler to place the halter over the nose.

Presenting the hands in an open and empty manner may help the horse to gain confidence. Sometimes it is beneficial to squat down. This works reasonably well with young foals and some horses. The shorter stature probably makes the figure less threatening and increases the horse's curiosity. Do not rush toward the horse at any time. Horses will assume you are giving chase and continue to move away, and some can become quite panicked. Once the would-be handler is behind the horse, the horse perceives even more of a threat since it cannot see the presumed intruder.

The approach to halter the horse should also be unhurried and without sudden movements. Keeping the lead rope or halter hidden by your side may assist in the capture of the skittish horse. A small-diameter catch rope may aid in the capture of the horse's neck (Figure 7-6). The rope may be carried up along the neck after gaining the horse's confidence at the withers by a moment of petting. If the horse moves away, attempt to stay with it by moving along side and holding onto the mane. Most horses will have sense enough to know that you mean business if you stay with them at this time.

When the horse is standing quietly, loop a rope around the neck by passing the rope over the horse's neck with the right hand and reaching under the neck to grab the free end with the left hand. When placing the rope over the neck, start as low on the back as possible. Remember that slow and steady movements are the key to success. Once the rope is around the neck, the horse may be held in the loop, and the rope can be maneuvered to the throatlatch area. The halter can be placed by sliding the noseband over the nose and passing the crown strap to the right hand and then bringing the strap over the horse's head for fastening.

The horse that does not respond to any of the above techniques becomes the biggest problem encountered in a field service practice. The arrival of veterinary personnel may trigger memories of previous contact that the horse does not want to have repeated. The usual reaction is for the horse to move off as far away from the handlers as possible. Of course, the simple solution is to have the horse caught before arrival of the veterinary team. However, this is not always possible. The usual solution to this problem is bribery with a handful or bucket of grain, which will entice the horse to approach or at least be approached. It is best to hold the bribe in the left hand and turn at right angles to the horse so that the neck is within easy reach for petting. As the horse gains confidence with some firm strokes along the shoulder, the right hand can then ease around the neck and allow capture. Many of these horses will attempt to wheel away when the arm is first placed over the neck, and this is where the small rope may be of assistance as a restraint aid. It is desirable to not allow horses to escape the first time because if they do it once they are likely to persist and become even harder to capture the second time. A horse that persists in whirling away becomes a candidate for trapping or, in extreme cases, roping.

Many horses that are impossible to catch in an open field will give up in an enclosed space. However, there are some that become exceptionally nervous in a small area and will kick or try to jump out when approached. The use of another haltered, calm horse within the stall to trap the nervous one will work in a majority of these cases. Similar to catching an unbroken foal, one handler will use the calm horse to trap the other in a corner. Then with slow and steady movements beginning at the withers, the second handler eases up the neck with a rope and makes the loop, which will allow temporary restraint of the nervous horse. A second technique that may be used is to have a solid panel that may be used to "squeeze" the horse into a corner. The panel needs to be sturdy enough to withstand the horse pushing against it and be movable enough to allow the handlers to back away in case the horse "blows up." This should be used as a last resort in attempting to capture the nervous horse. Remember that exciting a horse like this is self-defeating. Excited horses lose whatever sense they have and in fear will go over, under, or through whatever is attempting to contain them.

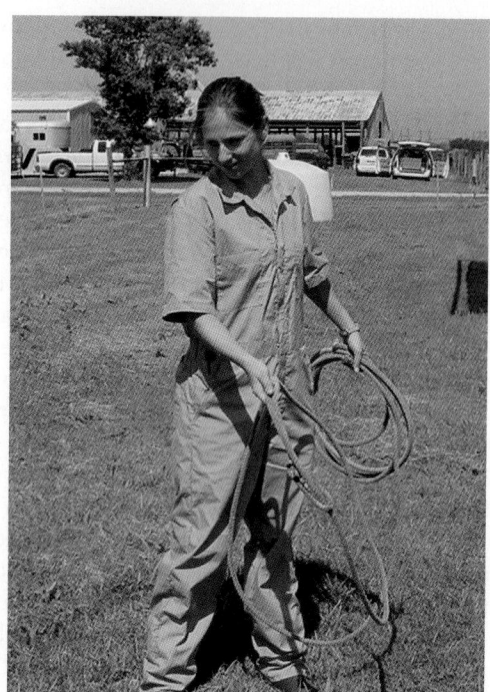

FIGURE 7-7 The method of holding the rope for a backhand throw.

> *TECHNICIAN NOTE* Attempting to lasso a horse with a rope is the last thing any sane individual wants to do.

It is nearly impossible to rope a horse in a field, and holding on to the horse after it has been successfully roped is also difficult. Dallying the rope off to the bumper of a truck is not an easy maneuver to accomplish, and the roper must be able to stay out of the way of the rope as the horse swings back and forth on the other end. If you must rope a horse, it should only be attempted in a small, sturdy enclosure, such as a wooden round pen. Do not use a round pen made of pipes. This is an invitation to disaster. It is better to leave the horse uncaught than to have to destroy it because it became hung up in pipes and fractured a leg. There are a multitude of trainers that are experienced in this arena, and the owner should be informed of their availability for hire. It is important to keep the horse as quiet as possible and to hide the rope as well as possible. If you are forced into a situation where veterinary care is absolutely necessary in an immediate fashion and the horse must be caught, the following techniques should be remembered. Whirling the rope overhead is not good form because the sound and sight of the rope will frighten most horses. A low, backhand technique is preferable to the cowboy throw. The loop is made so that it brushes the ground when the loop and rope are held at waist level (Figure 7-7). A generous amount of excess rope is played out from the coils, which should be held loosely in the off hand. The loop is held with the dominant hand and carried across the body in preparation for the backhand throw. The position of the roper should be about 3 m from a fence such that when the horse is driven past between the roper and the fence the horse will run into the backhand loop. This technique, although admittedly a last resort, can be extremely successful if all parties involved stay calm.

It should be emphasized that gloves should be worn when attempting to rope any animal. After the loop is over the horse's head, the coils will come off quickly. If the horse is charging through at such a rate that the rope cannot be held, release it before being jerked off balance and dragged in the dirt. The loose end of the rope can always be picked up from the ground after the horse has stopped running.

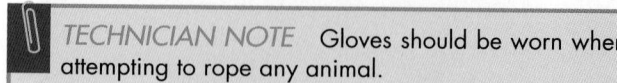

TECHNICIAN NOTE Gloves should be worn when attempting to rope any animal.

Horses that demonstrate signs of dangerous behavior or viciousness should not be given the opportunity to harm veterinary personnel by their physical proximity. There are alternative means of capture, such as tranquilization or anesthesia, that do not require closeness to the horse. Pole syringes, dart guns, and capture guns, although not common in equine practice, can save handlers from serious injury.

CAPTURE AND RESTRAINT OF FOALS

Newborn foals act from instinct in avoiding strange creatures and will hide behind the dam for safety. The capture of foals may be difficult and usually requires two people. Undoubtedly, these foals will not be halter broken, and if they are sick or injured, they do not need the increased stress that accompanies training to halter. The easiest way to capture a suckling foal is to first catch the mare and back her into a corner of a stout wall or solid fence, allowing her foal to come into the corner between the wall and the mare. The barrier should not have any holes that the foal may try to climb through. Flimsy barriers or barbed wire fences should never be used in an attempt to capture foals. The handler of the mare should realize that when the foal starts to struggle against the restraint, it may vocalize in fear and the mare might try to attack those who threaten her foal. The mare handler must be prepared to move the mare to a location away from the foal and handlers immediately following capture of the foal.

The mare should be positioned about the length of the foal away from the corner of the barrier, forming an open box in the corner of the barrier. One person then slowly goes behind the foal, and invariably the foal will cower to the hindquarters of the mare (Figure 7-8). The foal should be approached midway between the head and tail with the knowledge that once it senses hands or arms on it, it will try to escape by bolting, rearing, or kicking. Most commonly the foal will bolt forward into the mare's hindquarters, and the person should grab under the foal's neck and at the tail at this time. The tail should be held from underneath with the palm facing up. Grasping the tail is the most secure way to hold the hindquarters, even though the foal may be

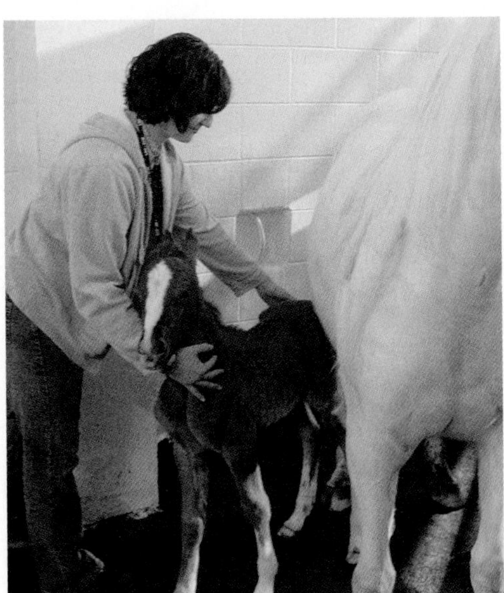

FIGURE 7-8 The mare is backed into a corner, and the foal is driven in beside her to safely capture the foal.

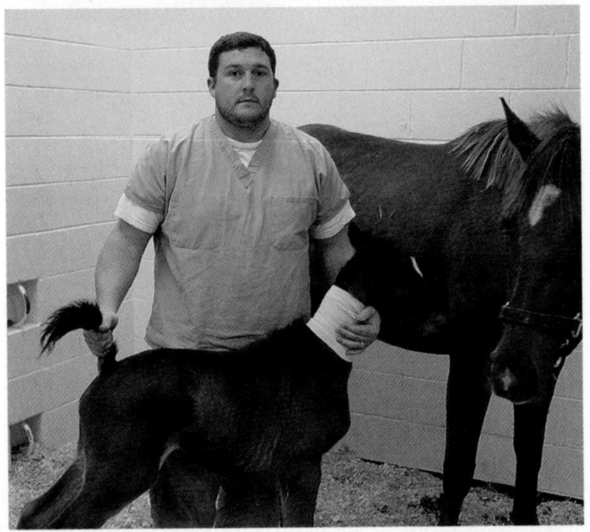

FIGURE 7-9 The handler must move in swiftly from the side of the foal and capture the tail first and sweep the arm under the neck of the foal. The mare handler must move her to a safe location at the same time.

uncomfortable. It is possible for one person to restrain the foal after this by grabbing the tail and holding it straight up over the back and keeping the other arm under the foal's neck (Figure 7-9). With bigger foals, two people are necessary for restraint, although the technique is similar. The first person advances toward the hindquarters of the foal as previously described and makes the initial contact with the hindquarters of the foal. The mare is then moved forward slightly, and the second person passes behind the mare and grabs under the foal's neck (Figure 7-10). Handlers may have to push the foal against a fence until the foal stops struggling. There is a tendency to lift small foals off the ground when accomplishing this task, which is poor form. When the foal loses its footing, it may become more frightened and struggle more vigorously and batter the shins of the handler.

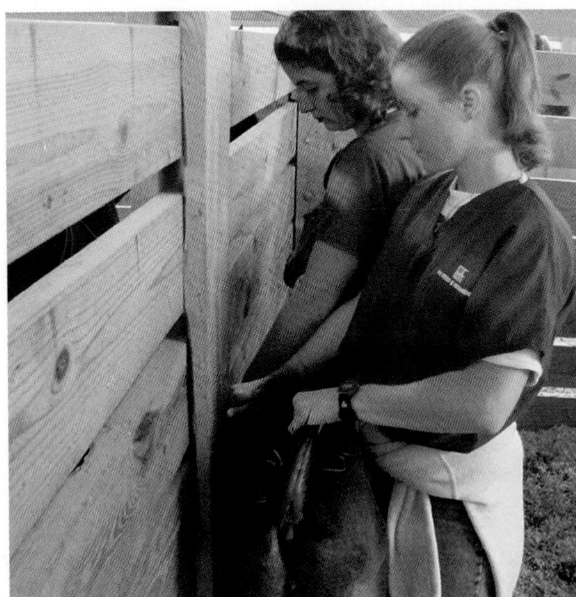

FIGURE 7-10 Two people may be necessary to capture larger foals. The first enters from the rear, and the second comes around behind the mare and grabs the foal under the neck. The foal is then moved toward a solid wall for support.

Attempts to capture foals only by the neck result in a rapid reverse by the foal and subsequent escape. Once a foal escapes, just as with adults, it becomes much harder to capture. Veterinary personnel should not contribute to the negative experiences of a foal. Extra care and gentle techniques should be employed to get the foal to develop trust in people as much as possible.

Following successful capture of the foal, it is usually in the best interest of all to position the mare and foal so that they face each other. They should be as close as possible without the mare becoming a nuisance for the procedure that is performed. It is generally not recommended to separate the mare and foal because they both will fret until rejoined.

HALTER AND LEADS

The halter is the basic restraint tool for horses, and the lead shank should always be attached to the halter. Horses should never be led by the halter alone; a lead should always be attached (Figure 7-11). The halter and rope shank may be inadequate for some tasks. Halters that have rings at the side of the nosepiece may be made more effective if a chain lead is passed from one side to the other. The lead is snapped on the side of the halter that is away from the handler after passing through the loop near the handler, usually on the near side. This arrangement allows finer control of the direction of the horse's nose and when snapped against the bridge of the nose, it reinforces the authority of the restraint because of the discomfort it causes. The chain lead should come in contact with the horse lightly, if at all, when leading the horse. Only when the horse misbehaves should the chain be used. Constant pressure is worrisome to the animal and does not leave the handler any reserve to use, if necessary.

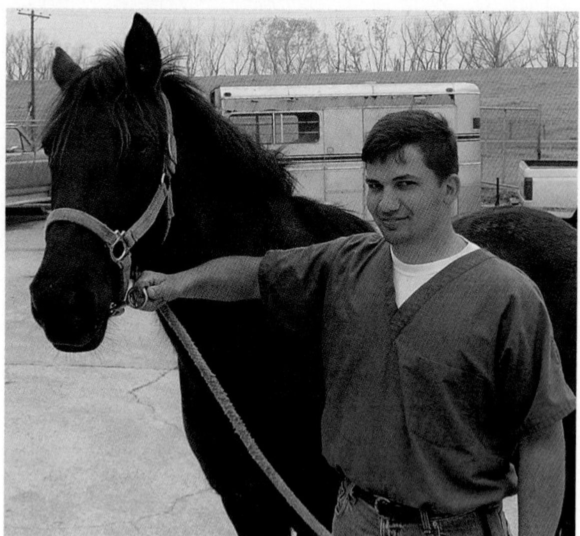

FIGURE 7-11 Halter and lead rope correctly placed on a horse. Note the position of the handler and the position of the arm. This allows the handler ample opportunity to sense impending movements.

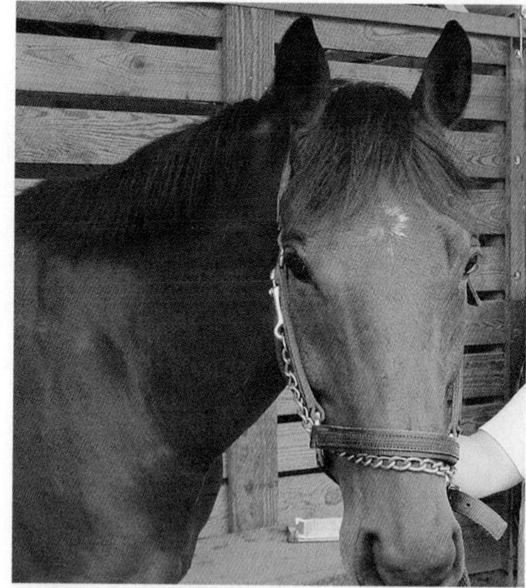

FIGURE 7-13 Lead shank across nose and then to the cheekpiece of the halter. This allows the handler much more control of a feisty horse.

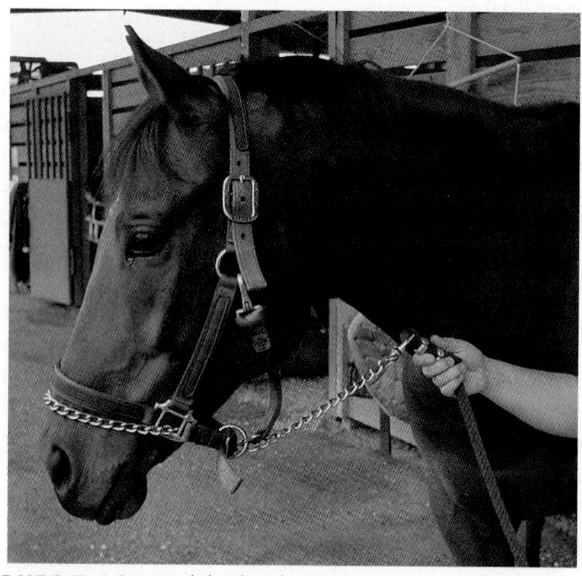

FIGURE 7-12 Lead shank with a chain positioned across the bridge of a stallion's nose to allow for more control.

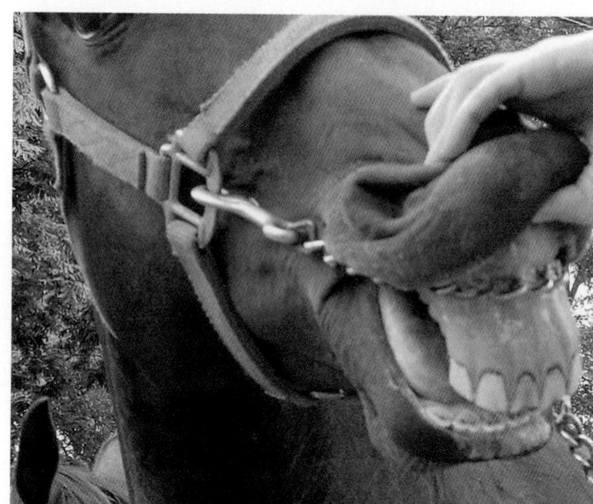

FIGURE 7-14 Lip chain added to the combination for restraint. This technique maximizes the control for the handler and replaces the use of a twitch in many instances.

There are three possible positions for the chain lead on the halter. The least authoritative is under the jaw, which causes a squeeze around the nose. Horses with tender chins or those that are not accustomed to a chain lead may throw their head or lunge backward when the lead is pulled. Horses that sense a squeezing of the nose as a signal to back up must be carefully restrained to respond correctly to this type of lead. It is often necessary to release pressure to allow the horse to stop its reverse. The chain over the nose is effective in controlling many horses (Figure 7-12). The top of a horse's nose is sensitive, and a pull on the lead with the chain across the nose will make the horse drop the nose and stop forward progress. Most stallions should be led with this technique. A variation of this technique is to carry the chain across the nose and then to the cheek piece connection of the halter (Figure 7-13). This gives the handler more control of the horse's head and nose. The most severe method of chain lead restraint is passing the chain over the upper lip and onto the gums of the upper jaw (Figure 7-14). This method works well with horses that have a bad attitude and need to be reminded about the "chain" of command. When using this technique, it is imperative that the chain is used only when the horse is misbehaving. When used correctly, this method of restraint replaces the use of a twitch and provides the handler with much more stopping power over the horse.

TYING THE HORSE

A horse should never be tied with a chain over or under the nose. This too is an invitation for disaster. Seldom will it be desirable for a handler to tie a horse to perform a procedure.

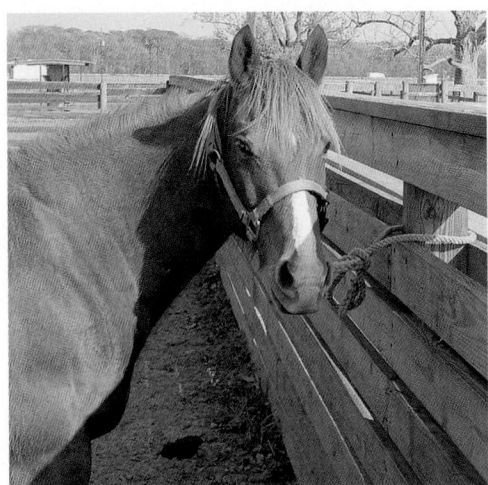

FIGURE 7-15 Properly tied horse at a rail. Note the level of the tie and the short amount of rope between the post and the halter.

When a horse must be tied, the equipment must be strong and sound. The halter, rope, and whatever the rope is tied to must be in premier shape. Snaps on a rope are always suspect because all but the heaviest will break when a horse jerks back on them. If something breaks (the rope, halter, or post), the horse will be free and has now learned to pull back as a means of escape whenever tied. Another serious problem that can result from the horse pulling back occurs when it goes over backward and sustains head or neck trauma on landing. A horse should be tied to objects that are at the level of its shoulder or higher to prevent it from pawing and getting a foot over the rope. This also prevents the horse from trying to graze and becoming entangled in the tie rope. Horses should also be tied short; only 60 cm of rope should be present from the halter to the post to prevent the horse from having too much play in the rope and getting in trouble (Figure 7-15). Once a horse is tied, care should be taken to prevent hazardous objects from arriving into the area that might spook the horse, and the horse should never be left unattended. The shorter the horse is tied, the less likely it is to get into trouble.

One technique that may be used to restrain (or train) a fitful horse is to place a cotton rope around the mid section of the horse just behind the rib cage and then pull it through between the front legs and through the bottom of the halter. This rope is tied slightly shorter than the halter rope. The basis of this technique is that the horse will hit the cotton rope first and feel the pull against its abdomen, causing it to move forward and release pressure on the rope (Figure 7-16).

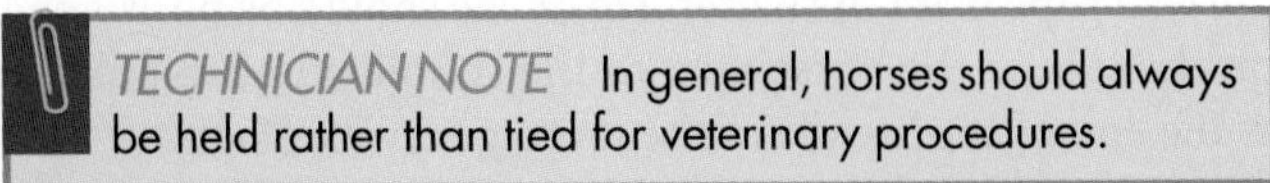
TECHNICIAN NOTE In general, horses should always be held rather than tied for veterinary procedures.

For veterinary purposes, it is generally preferable to hold a horse rather than tie it. It is imperative that the holder stand on the same side of the horse as the veterinarian so that the head may be directed toward the practitioner rather

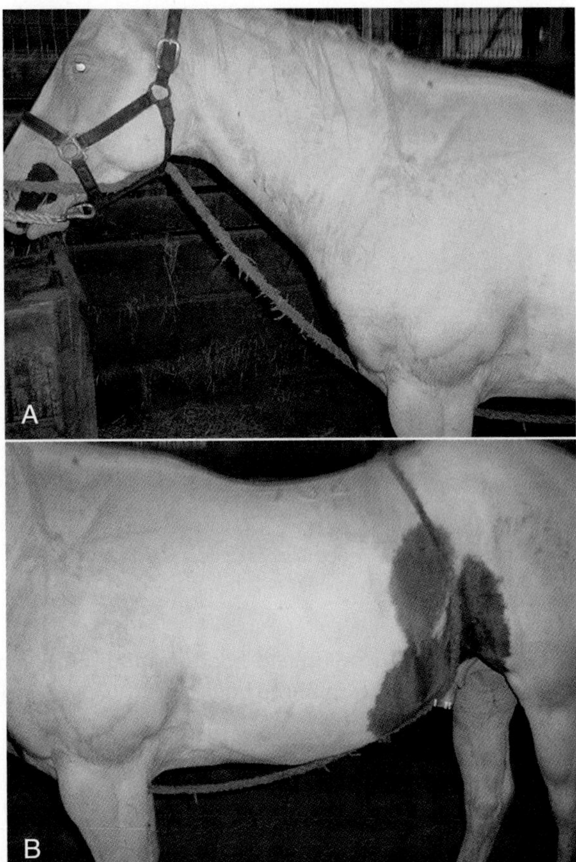

FIGURE 7-16 The technique necessary to place a belly rope on a horse that will not stand tied. **A,** A soft cotton rope is placed around the horse's abdomen and run between the front legs. **B,** The rope is run down the halter and tied slightly shorter than the halter rope.

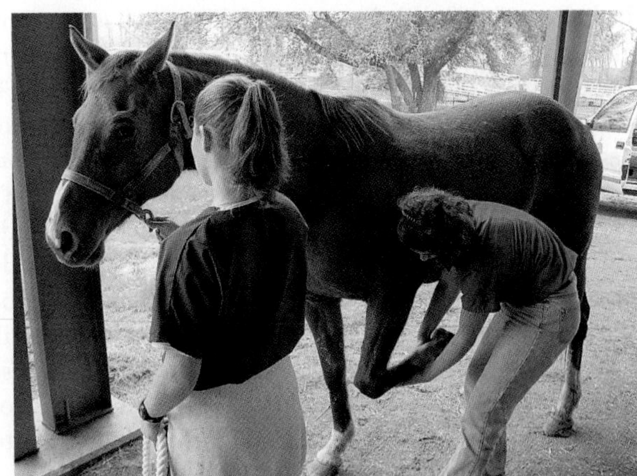

FIGURE 7-17 When handling horses for any procedure, it is necessary for the holder and the individual working on the horse to be on the same side of the animal.

than the body or hindquarters (Figure 7-17). If the handler is on the opposite side and the handler bails out, the head of the horse follows the handler, leaving the back end of the horse swinging directly into the veterinarian. When the head is controlled and the horse acts up, the worst that will happen is that the body of the horse will swing away from both handler and veterinarian. No matter what the circumstances,

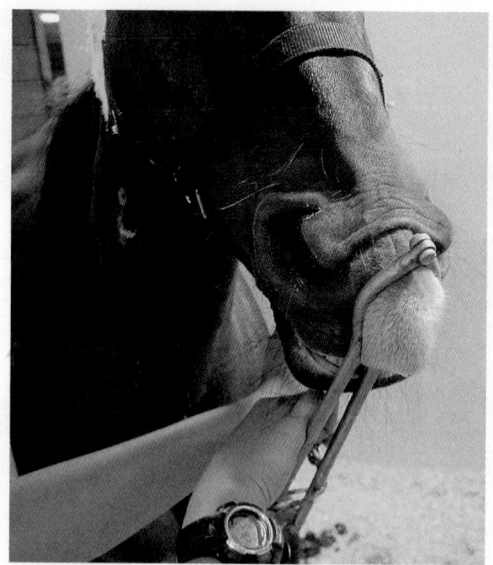

FIGURE 7-18 The humane twitch in place on a horse's lip.

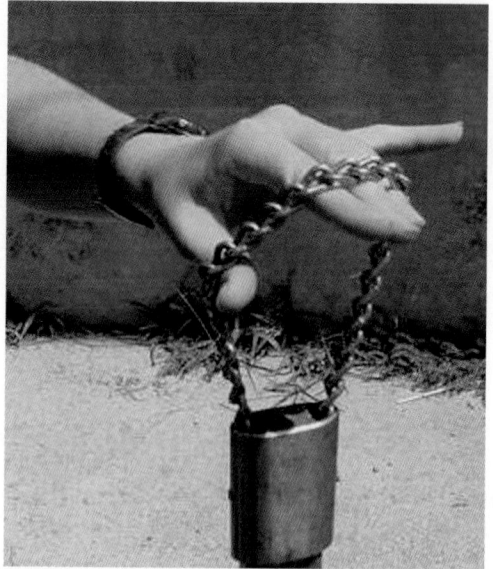

FIGURE 7-19 The proper placement of the fingers through the loop of chain before placing the twitch on a horse's nose.

this technique should be upheld because in an emergency situation, self-preservation of the holder will overcome protection of the practitioner.

THE TWITCH

The twitch is a nerve-stimulating device that may immobilize horses and can be helpful in equine restraint. Most twitches are applied to the upper lip of the horse. The most innocuous is the humane twitch, which is a hinged pair of long handles that squeeze down over the sides of the lip and may be secured at the bottom by a thong and snapped back to the halter. The major advantage of this twitch is that once applied it need not be held in place (Figure 7-18). Therefore one person may restrain a horse that is acting up. The disadvantage is that the pressure is fairly mild, and most horses ignore it. More traditional twitches rely on a loop and a leverage device. The loop is either of chain or rope and is placed on the lip and tightened by twisting the leverage device. The leverage may be from a piece of wood or pipe and is about 50 cm long. The loop needs to be seated on the lip behind the heavy gristle pad at the tip and ahead of the nostrils. This area may be hard to find on thick-nosed horses. Horses that have been twitched become quite wise and will throw their heads into the air and tighten their lips when attempts are made to apply the twitch.

The application of the twitch should be done with the calmness and assuredness of the initial capture of the horse. It is best to have an assistant holding the horse by a lead rope when the twitch is applied. The loop should be placed over the thumb and three fingers, leaving the little finger out so that the twitch does not slide down the hand or arm (Figure 7-19). Grasp the end of the horse's lip, raise the hand with the twitch on it, and slide it onto the horse's nose. The end of the handle should be held in the opposite hand, in case the horse throws its head. Twist the end of the handle until the twitch is snug and begins to elongate and distort the shape of the horse's upper lip. The twitch should be tightened until the horse responds by standing still. The average person cannot twist enough to damage the horse's nose. Once the twitch has been applied, the person holding it should also be holding the lead rope from the halter. He or she should be positioned on the side of the horse next to the shoulder and should be at the end of the handle of the leverage device (Figure 7-20). A number of handlerless twitches are now available for use in minor noxious procedures. These are placed on the horse's nose in the same fashion as previously described and secured to the halter as shown in Figure 7-21. In the absence of a twitch, it is possible for a person with a firm grip to hold the upper lip in their hand to accomplish a minor procedure. It

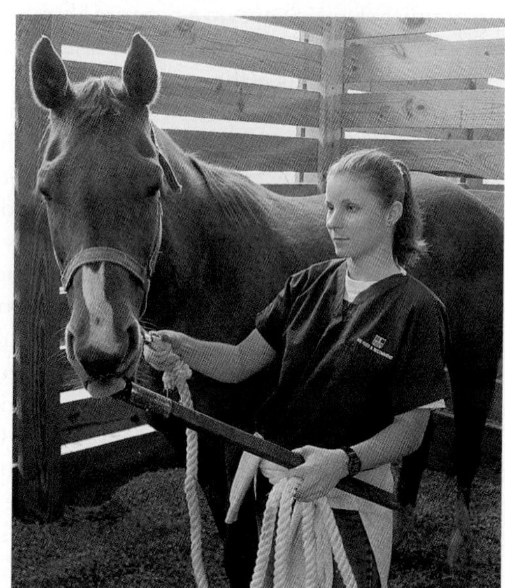

FIGURE 7-20 This handler demonstrates the proper positioning while holding the twitch and restraining the horse. Note that the horse is backed into a corner and there is still plenty of overhead space.

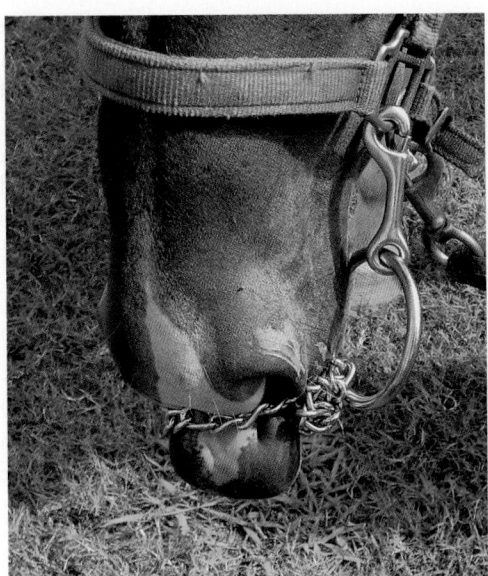

FIGURE 7-21 This is an example of a new "handlerless" twitch that may be attached to a horse's nose and secured to the horse's halter, allowing minor noxious procedures to be completed by one person.

should be remembered that horses are able to strike out with their front legs, and twitches may evoke this response. Never stand directly in front of the horse when applying or holding a twitch. As mentioned previously, the lip chain may be an alternative that will produce similar results without having to dodge the flying wooden handle of a twitch or the helicopter feet of a horse that has been stimulated to strike.

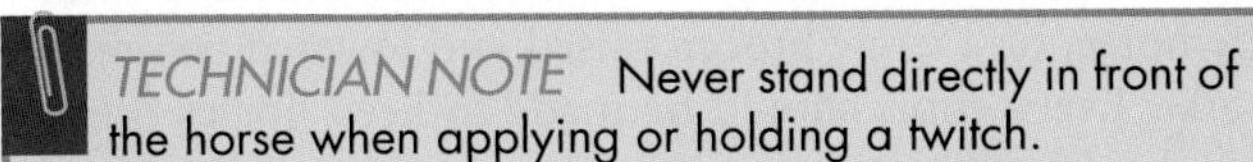

TECHNICIAN NOTE Never stand directly in front of the horse when applying or holding a twitch.

A skin twitch may be a more acceptable form of restraint for many owners. This technique may also help for those horses that seem to be "light" on their front feet, attempting to strike when a regular twitch is applied to their nose. Grabbing the skin of the neck just in front of the shoulder and rolling it around the clenched fist will make many horses stand still (Figure 7-22).

The old cowboy notion of twisting the horse's ear and biting down on it as a means of restraint is poor practice. The supporting structures of the ear may be damaged, and it is extremely common for the horse to become head shy following ear twisting. Owners are not keen on having this procedure done on their horses, and the handler risks a trip to the dentist after every attempt. Clearly, there are better forms of restraint available.

LIFTING THE FORELEG

Some horses will stand still if a foreleg is picked up and held. The theory is that with one leg in the air, the horse is less likely to leave the ground with the other three. To lift a horse's foreleg, face the rear and stand next to the horse slightly in front of the leg that is to be lifted (Figure 7-23). Bend from the waist and push your hips slightly into the horse as the hand closest to the horse squeezes the suspensory ligament. The suspensory ligament is immediately palmar to the third metacarpal bone. Squeezing the suspensory ligament will cause the horse to flex its fetlock joint, and cradling the anterior aspect of the fetlock as it flexes will allow the handler to pick up the foot.

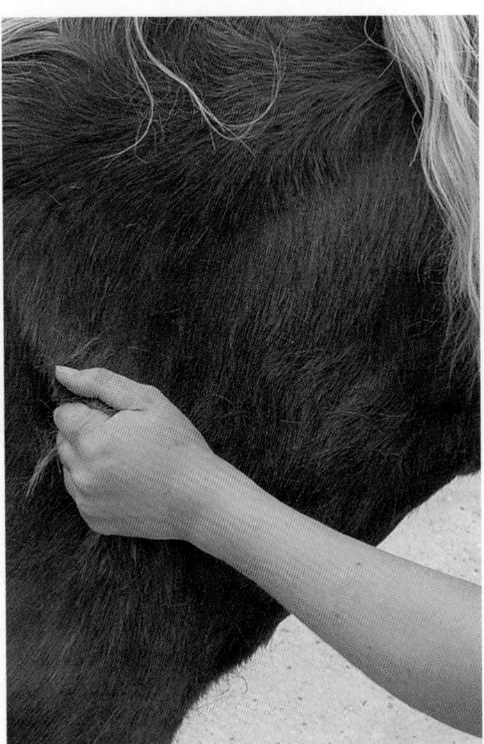

FIGURE 7-22 A skin twitch can be a powerful deterrent to an obnoxious horse. The skin just in front of the scapula is drawn into the clenched fist to accomplish this task.

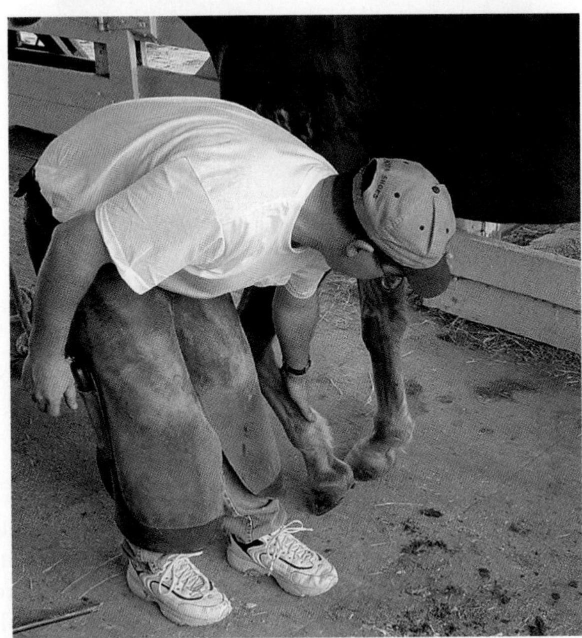

FIGURE 7-23 The proper foot positioning and bending at the waist to pick up a front foot of a horse. The inside hand is placed on the suspensory ligament of the horse's leg.

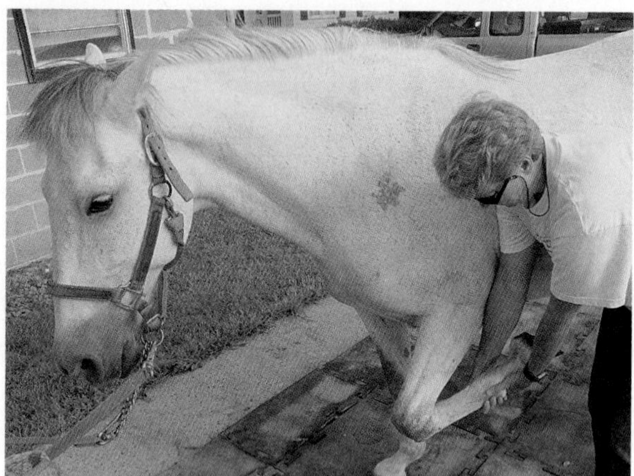

FIGURE 7-24 The handler is positioned properly to restrain the forelimb while a procedure is performed elsewhere.

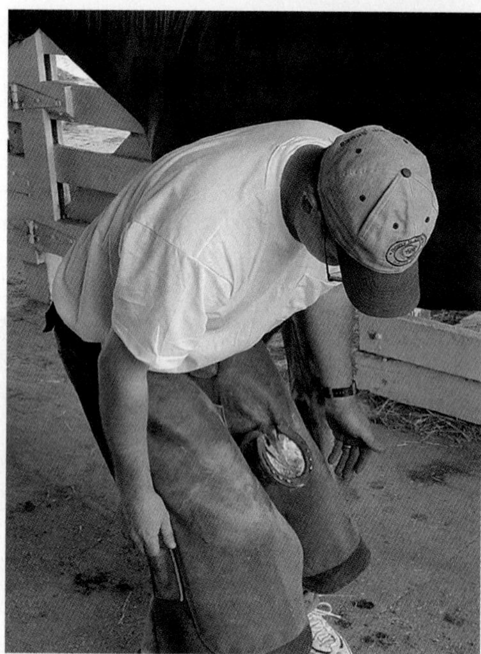

FIGURE 7-25 The hands-free stance while working on front feet. Note that the back is only slightly bent and the knees are directed together to hold the forelimb.

When holding the foot as a means of restraint, the handler should rotate and face forward with both hands supporting the foreleg (Figure 7-24). To handle the horse's hoof for procedures, the handler should face the rear of the horse. The foreleg should be placed between the handler's legs from the rear and held between the thighs just above the knees, freeing both hands to work on the foot (Figure 7-25).

LIFTING THE HIND LEG

Lifting the hind leg will only be done as part of an examination procedure, not as a means of restraint. To lift the hind leg, the handler stands near the flank area of the horse and bends from the waist with a hand palpating down the horse's rear limb. A slight lean into the horse will aid in elevating the limb off the ground, and the leg should be pulled upward toward the handler. Then the handler should walk under the limb, staying close to the horse's body until the leg is outstretched behind the horse with the foot resting on the inside thigh of the handler. The horse's hock should be at the level of the handler's waist and the tibial region snugly against the side of the back (Figure 7-26). The leg should stay braced in this position without the use of hands. If the horse should resist, the handler's arm should clamp down over the horse's hock joint and attempt to quiet the horse.

There are descriptions in the literature of how to tie the horse's legs up to examine them, but they have many disadvantages to both horse and handler. A horse with a leg tied up may fall and seriously injure itself. There are too many chemical mediators available in equine practice today to recommend rope restraints for lifting limbs.

STOCKS

The use of stocks for fitful horses is clearly the safest way to manage these horses. The best stocks are made of heavy pipes or poles, anchored well to the ground surface, with the horizontal pieces set at the level of the horse's shoulder (Figure 7-27). Stocks are used for many procedures, such as administration of fluids, dental work, nasogastric intubation, rectal palpations, and injections of jittery horses. Many horses will require some form of encouragement to get into the stocks. This can be done safely with voice commands, a slight raise of the arms by a second handler standing behind the horse, or a straw broom raised and lowered behind the horse. Every effort should be made to keep horses calm as they load into the stocks. Some horses have an innate fear of enclosure. These horses may do anything to get out of a set of stocks. Kicking, jumping, lunging, and striking are all ways in which the horse may try to escape. Therefore it is best to have a quick-release mechanism on the stocks, especially for the rear gate. The rear gate must be closed before tying the horse's head after loading a horse into the stocks. Once a horse is in the stocks, the same principles apply with regard to positioning of the handler. Do not assume that the horse cannot come over the front of the stocks because many have done so in the middle of a tantrum. Horses should never be left unattended in the stock.

> *TECHNICIAN NOTE* The use of stocks for fitful horses is clearly the safest way to manage these horses. Always close the rear gate before tying the horse's head.

The lack of a set of stocks presents a problem with restraint for more noxious veterinary procedures, such as dental work, nasogastric intubation, and rectal palpations. For dental work and nasogastric intubation without stocks, the horse should be backed into the corner of a secure and sturdy area and quieted. Make sure that the ceiling is not so low that if the horse rears it will hit its head. The handler

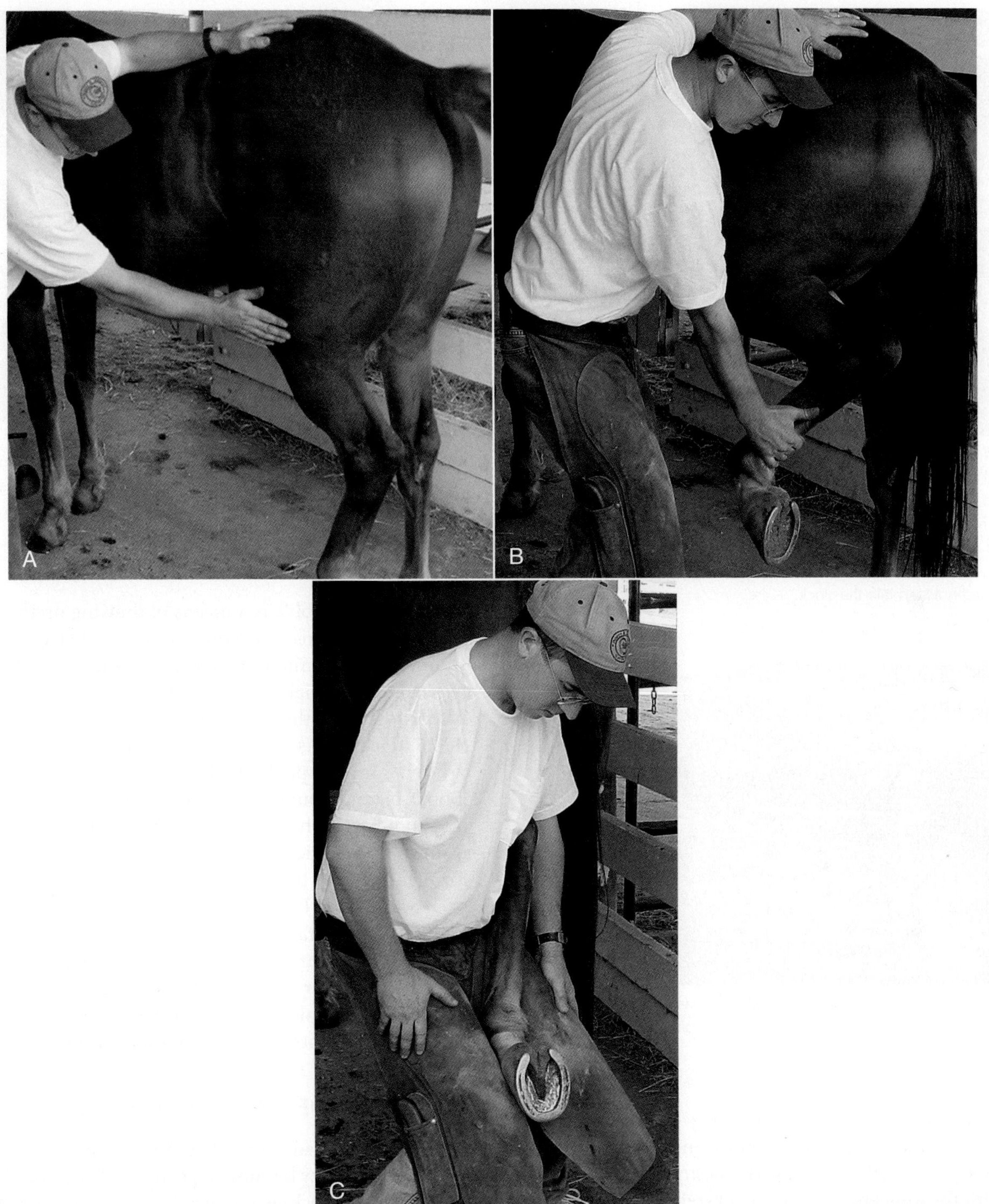

FIGURE 7-26 Lifting of the hind limb. **A,** The handler stands near the flank and palpates down the limb to give the horse knowledge of his presence. **B,** The leg is brought forward toward the handler before attempting to go out behind the horse. **C,** The handler walks in underneath the horse's leg, supporting the tibia on his hip and placing the hoof over the inside thigh to support the lower leg.

and the veterinarian should be located on the same side of the horse when performing the procedure (Figure 7-28). For palpation without stocks, the horse should be placed along a sturdy solid wall with the handler and veterinarian standing on the same side of the horse. The handler must "read" the horse, and everyone must have a clear idea of where the escape route is located when performing this procedure (Figure 7-29).

TAIL TIE

The horse's tail may be tied during rectal palpations, vaginal examinations, and minor obstetric procedures. This is accomplished by using a small rope or a roll of gauze tied into the hair of the tail. The tail should never be tied to anything but the horse. Tying the free end around the neck of the horse is best. Should a horse get loose with the tail

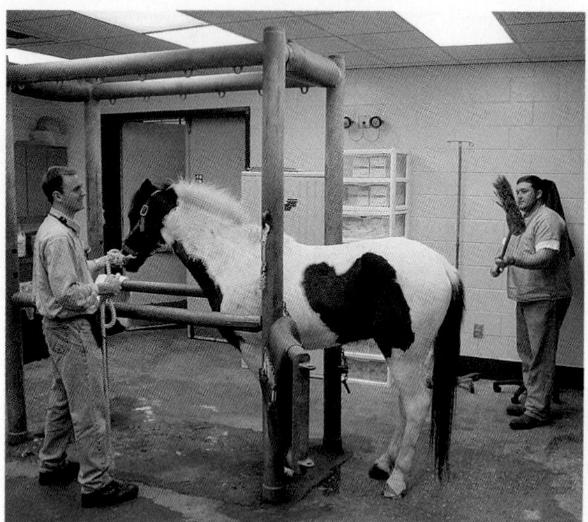

FIGURE 7-27 This horse is about to enter a set of pipe stocks. Note the height of the side pipes, about the level of the horse's shoulder and stifle joints. This stock is well anchored in cement to prevent unsteadiness once the horse is in the stock. The rear end of the horse must always be respected, and the back gate must be closed before securing the head of a horse in the stock. The judicious use of the broom helps get many horses to make the final step into the stock.

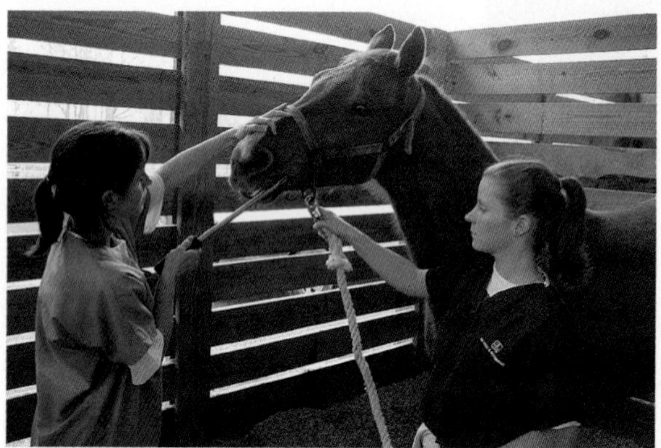

FIGURE 7-28 This horse is undergoing a dental procedure, and both the handler and the veterinarian are located on the same side of the horse for safety.

tied to a stationary object, serious injury could result. The tail tie is a simple quick-release knot using a rope or gauze placed across the tail just below the fleshy portion (Figure 7-30) with the long end tied in a quick-release knot around the neck.

HOBBLES

Horses are seldom hobbled or cast (thrown to the ground with the aid of ropes) since the advent of chemical restraint that is both powerful and short acting. Breeding hobbles are still commonly used on farms that have natural breeding operations. These hobbles prevent a mare from kicking effectively. They are fitted around the hocks with web or leather straps that are tied to a neck strap or rope after passing between the forelegs (Figure 7-31).

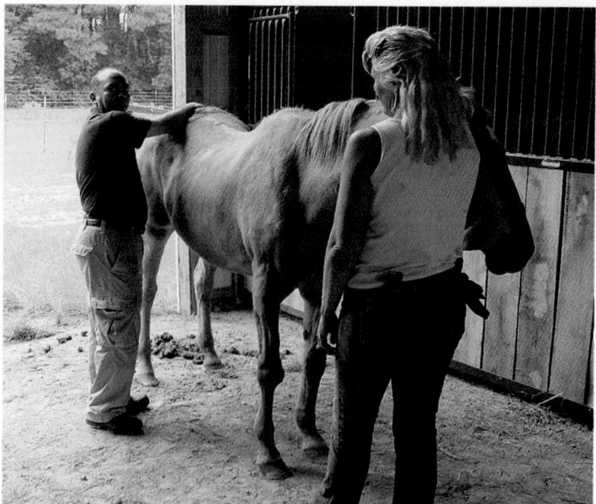

FIGURE 7-29 Positioning is extremely important when palpating horses without the use of stocks. Note the position of both the handler and the veterinarian on the same side of the horse with a wall on the opposite side of the horse to reduce the amount of space available for the horse to move away.

The scotch hobble is a means of drawing up the hind leg (Figure 7-32). This technique can be used as a form of restraint for the examination of the opposite forelimb. It works by keeping the weight on the hind leg of the side that is examined. Most often the scotch hobble will be used for holding the hind leg that is "up" out of the way during a castration. A heavy cotton rope should be used to prevent rope burn. A loop is placed around the horse's neck and tied with a bowline knot before the initiation of anesthesia. Once the horse is down in a surgical plane of anesthesia, the rope is passed through the loop behind the pastern area and then brought back to the loop. Pulling the end of the rope using the neck loop as a pulley draws the leg forward. Care must be taken to prevent a rope burn in the pastern area. Some people actually have a leather sheath with two loops on it that is used behind the pastern to allow the rope to slide around the leg without the potential of producing a rope burn.

RESTRAINT OF THE DOWN HORSE

Control of the head is the key to restraining a horse lying in lateral recumbency because to get up the head must be lifted. Kneeling on the neck near the head will keep most horses down. This should always be done from the back of the horse; any activities performed on a horse that is down must be done from the back. An approach from the belly side puts the handler in danger of thrashing legs and feet. To keep the horse from damaging the facial nerve and the down eye, the handler should cushion the lateral area of the face and orbital area. This may be done with a towel, inner tube, or foam mat placed under the head. If such a protection is not available and the horse is thrashing its head, pulling up on the nosepiece of the halter will elevate the nose and prevent the horse from moving the head and producing traumatic wounds to the eye and face.

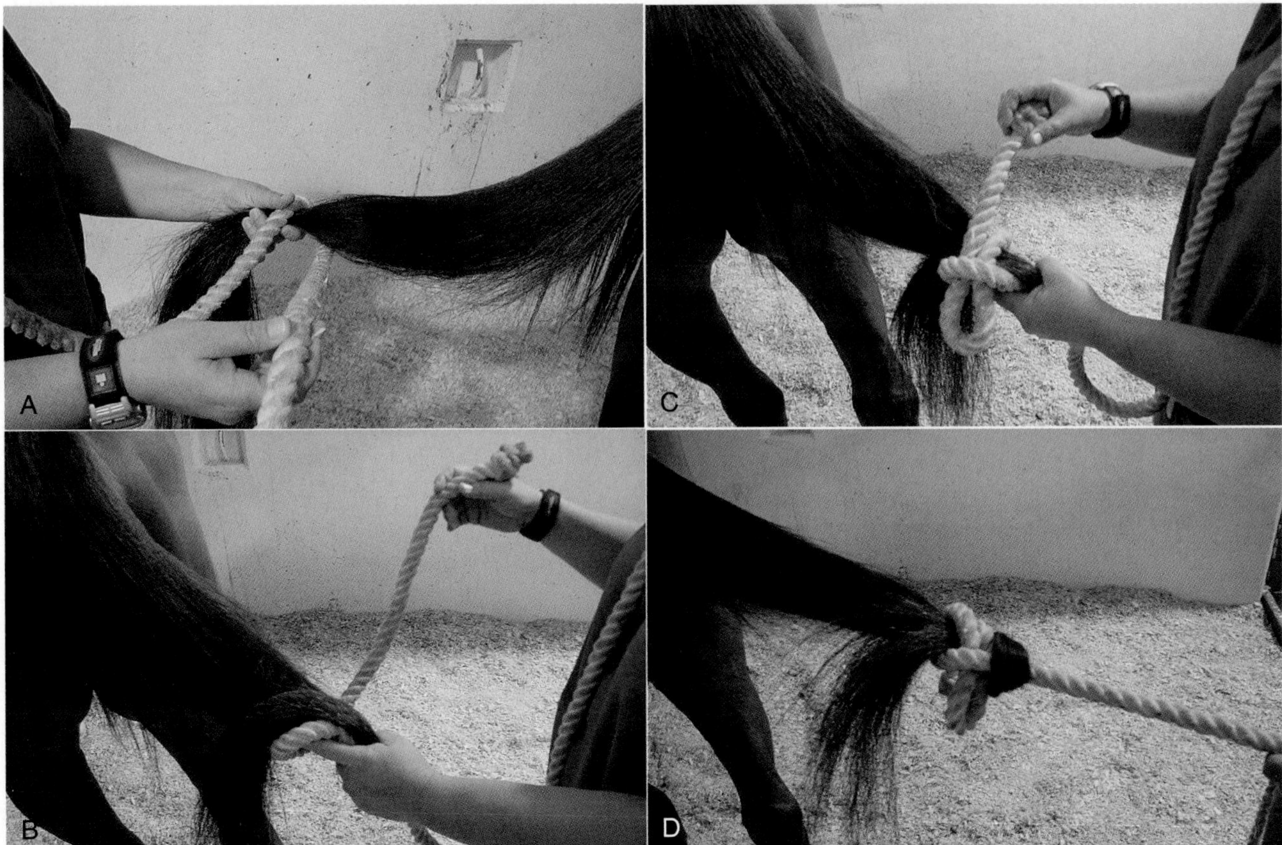

FIGURE 7-30 The steps in making a secure tail tie. **A,** The rope is placed around the tail. **B,** The tail is folded back on itself and on the rope. **C,** The short end of the rope passes over the folded tail, and a loop is pushed through the tail-encircling portion of the rope. **D,** Tension on the long end of the rope makes the knot snug. Pulling the short end of the rope will release the knot.

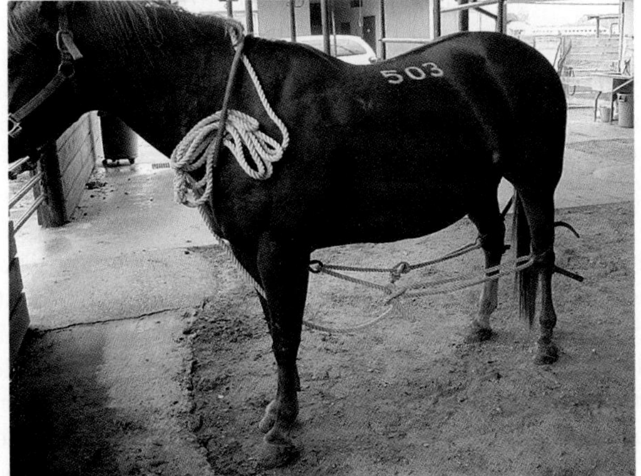

FIGURE 7-31 This is an example of breeding hobbles placed upon a mare before natural service to prevent her from kicking backward and potentially injuring the stallion.

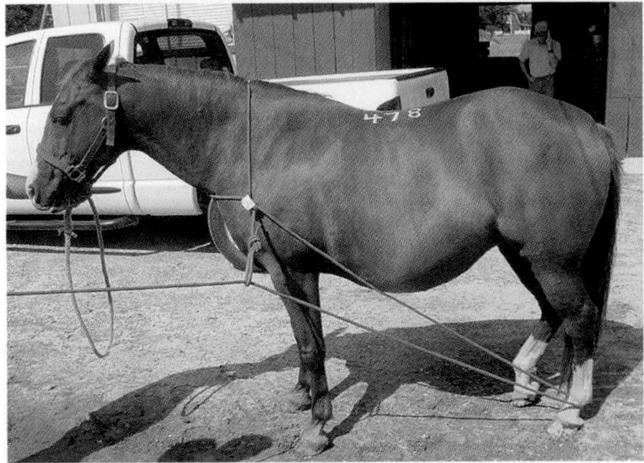

FIGURE 7-32 The scotch hobble on a standing horse.

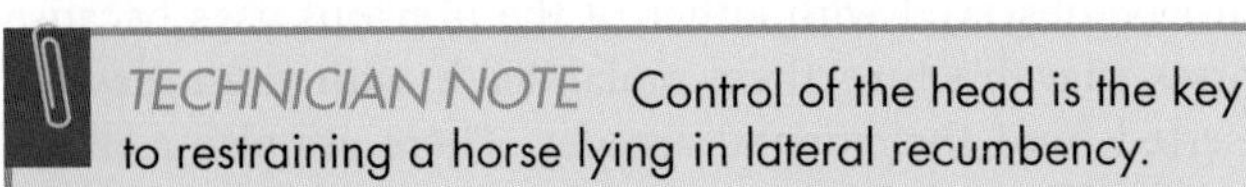

TECHNICIAN NOTE Control of the head is the key to restraining a horse lying in lateral recumbency.

OTHER HEAD AND MOUTH RESTRAINTS

Horses will sometimes tear at bandages. Devices are available that may be used to prevent this by restricting the horse's ability to move the head laterally. One such device is the cradle. It is made of wooden slats and leather straps with a buckle that goes over the horse's neck to secure the cradle and brace the neck in a straight line (Figure 7-33). This device prevents the lateral movement of the neck while allowing the horse to eat and drink. Another method of preventing the horse from chewing at bandages is to tether the horse to an overhead cable in the stall. Running the cable diagonally across the stall is the usual method. With this technique, the

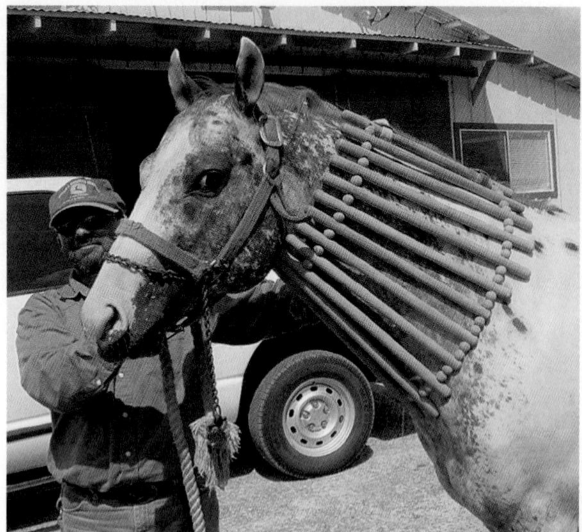

FIGURE 7-33 The horse wearing a neck cradle.

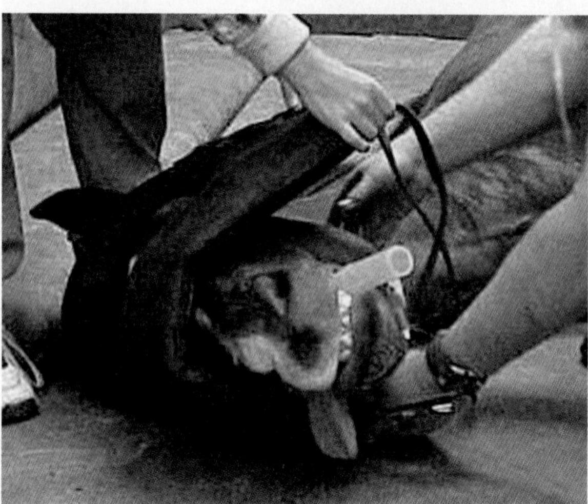

FIGURE 7-34 The handler is placing a protective foam and rubber helmet over the head of this anesthetized horse to protect the head during recovery from anesthesia.

horse is able to move about the stall freely, but cannot reach far enough laterally to gain access to the bandage.

Horses with severe pain, with neurologic disease, or undergoing anesthesia will frequently throw their heads, crashing into solid objects and mutilating themselves. To prevent this, there are foam rubber head protectors made to fit snugly over the head of the horse, much like a helmet (Figure 7-34). The use of these and padded stalls help to prevent self-inflicted trauma.

Wire or plastic muzzles are used frequently on horses that are to be held off feed and to prevent them from eating bedding while still allowing them access to water (Figure 7-35).

The examination of a horse's mouth and dental arcades may be accomplished by standing to the side of the horse's head and placing the hand of the arm more caudal to the mouth over the bridge of the horse's nose. The hand nearest the horse's nose is inserted into the interdental space

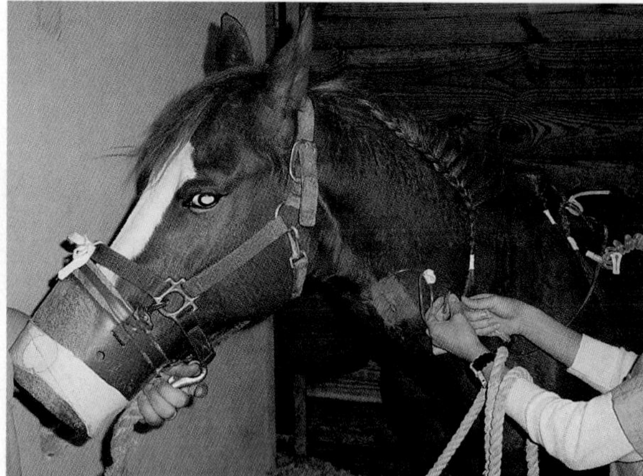

FIGURE 7-35 This horse is wearing a plastic muzzle to keep it from eating during the perioperative period. The muzzle does have holes to allow the horse access to water.

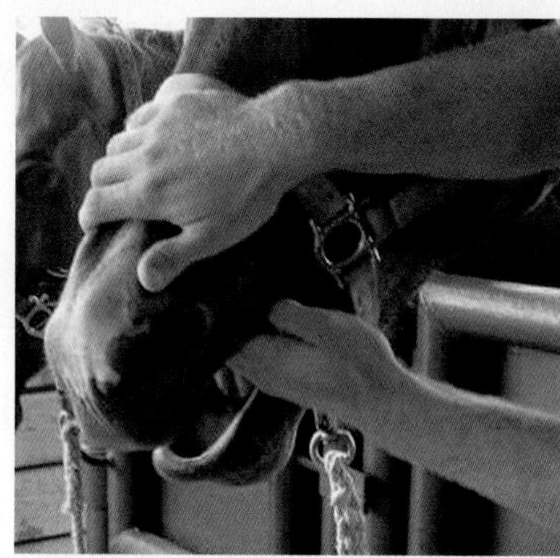

FIGURE 7-36 The handler is about to perform an oral and dental examination on this horse. It is critical that the examiner keep the hand in a vertical position while checking the teeth because the horse will bite down on a hand placed in a horizontal plane.

(Figure 7-36). The hand must be kept in a vertical position. The fingers are placed on the lingual surface of the dental arcade, and the thumb palpates the buccal surface. Following a dental examination, the tongue may be pulled out the side of the mouth through the interdental space. Mouth gags are available to allow for a more complete visual examination of horses' mouths. A simple wedge (Figure 7-37), which is pushed up between the upper and lower cheek teeth with the handle hanging out, is commonly used. A variation on this is a round gag, used in a similar fashion to the wedge. Caution must be observed with either of the previous gags because horses may fracture their molar teeth with these devices inserted onto their dental arcades. There are also a number of different large-hinged speculums that either fit over the upper and lower incisors or within the dental space and then are suspended from a halter (Figure 7-38). The mouth can then be cranked open, allowing examinations and procedures to be performed on the mouth. Although these devices are effective in getting the mouth open, it should be

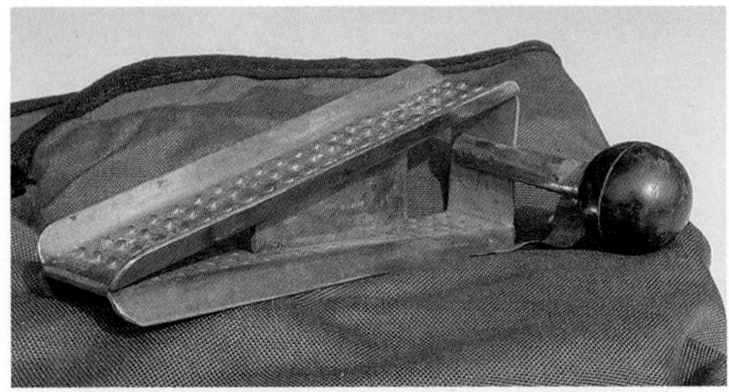

FIGURE 7-37 The wedge gag. The wedge is slid between upper and lower cheek teeth, and the handle comes out of the corner of the mouth.

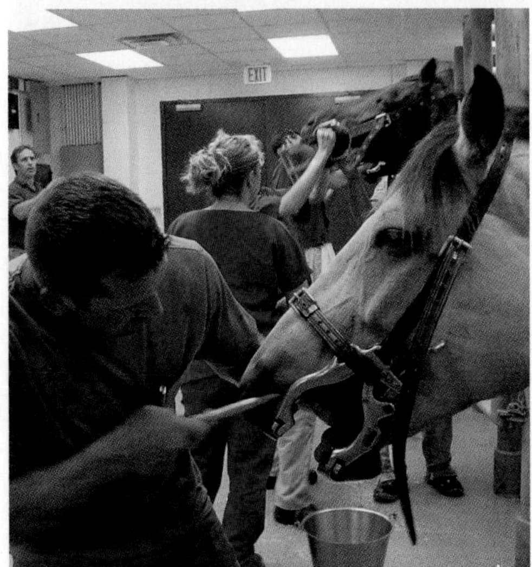

FIGURE 7-38 The position of the hinged speculum inside the horse's mouth to allow for visualization and work on the teeth of a horse.

remembered that they are heavy and cumbersome for both the handler and the horse. The use of any of these speculums is usually coincidental with the sedation of the horse.

MANUAL AND CHEMICAL RESTRAINT

The manual casting of horses to the ground has been replaced by chemical restraint and anesthesia. Casting always had inherent danger for both horse and handler. Musculoskeletal damage was always possible when the forefeet of the horse were pulled from under it. Once the horse was cast, the thrashing about caused a variety of injuries.

Chemical restraint is now widely accepted and practiced. Many different agents and combinations of agents are used. These are discussed in Chapter 27. Whenever a horse has been sedated, tranquilized, or anesthetized, it is important for veterinary personnel to stay with that horse until it is steady on its feet. When horses are tranquilized, handlers must remember to maintain a safe distance from the horse. When they are under deep sedation, tranquilization, or proceeding through stage 2 of anesthesia, horses may crash into an unwitting handler and cause significant injury to the person. Once the horse is down, make sure of the stage of anesthesia before placing restraint ropes or beginning surgical preparations. A slap to the flank of a horse awaiting castration may save damage from the kick of a partially anesthetized colt.

CAPTURE AND RESTRAINT OF CATTLE

Cattle are less difficult to capture than horses. They are also less discriminating than horses about what or whom they step on or run over. Generally, they are not directly approachable for haltering and leading. However, they are easier to drive into pens, alleyways, and chutes. Herds of cattle will vary in the amount of avoidance present. Some herds will allow a person to approach closely before moving away. It is preferable to have the herd begin to move when the handlers come within about 12 m of the herd. Cattle are herd oriented, so they will crowd and bunch together as they are driven, even climbing over other cows if they are driven too hard or fast. This should be avoided because bruising and other injuries are likely to occur.

It must be stressed that herding cattle into weak barriers must be avoided. Most beef cattle will walk through a barbed or smooth wire fence completely unconcerned and unscathed. Sometimes they even leave the wire in place, although much looser than it was. Calves become adept at slipping through the lower strands of pasture fences.

Cattle are usually less spooky than horses about strange surroundings, but they may balk and then bolt suddenly. Generally the balking occurs just as the cattle reach the open gate of a holding corral after being driven off of a pasture. The clever cattle rancher avoids the placement of strange things at the entrance to a corral, such as dogs, new people, or strange trucks. Veterinary personnel should remain out of sight unless the owner requests assistance in driving cows. Nothing aggravates a rancher more than having all the cows ready to go into the pen and having them spook at the last instant because something or somebody steps into their sight.

Once cattle are in the corral, they are funneled from larger areas into smaller pens and eventually into an alleyway leading to a chute. Usually, there is a system of gates that will allow the handler to block the cattle into these progressively smaller areas. These gates may be used to "cut" calves from cows to facilitate handling. It is best to work larger stock separately from the nursing calves. The handler must be careful in closing gates on a large group of cattle. If they get turned back toward the opening and hit the gate before getting it latched, there is a significant chance of injury to the handler.

The alleys leading to the chute should be built just wide enough for one animal to prevent attempts to turn around (Figure 7-39). People on foot may follow cattle in an alleyway to drive them toward the chute, but they should always be cautious and ready to climb out of the way. Never enter an alleyway that cannot be easily evacuated. The alleyway is usually arranged so that posts or boards may be slipped behind the cattle to prevent them from moving backward. "Tailing" may be used to push a cow ahead in the alley. Tailing is simply grasping the tail in the middle and twisting it

FIGURE 7-39 The alleyway that works best for moving cattle is only wide enough for one cow to pass through. Note that the alley is braced well with support posts and there are chains across the top of the alley to prevent it from spreading.

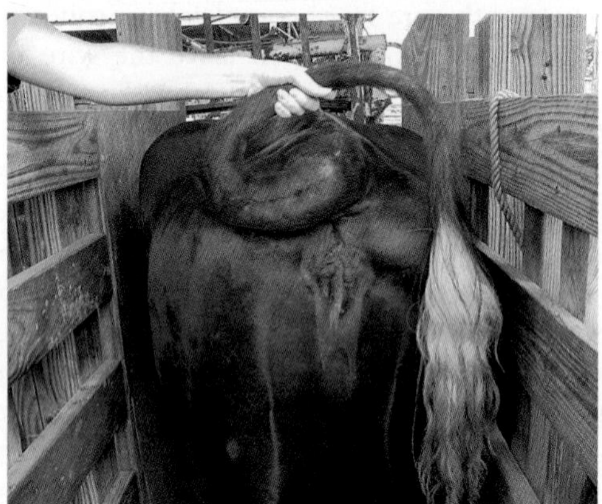

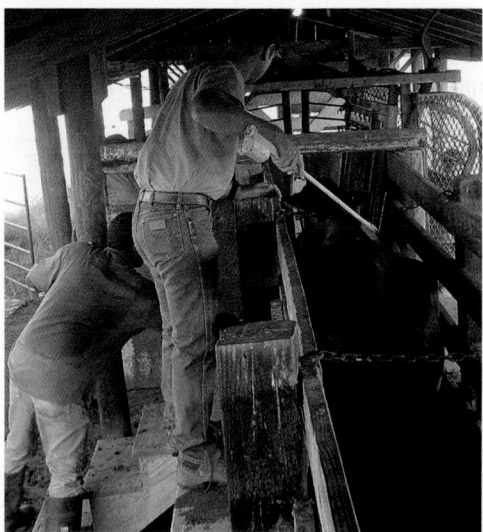

FIGURE 7-40 This is the tail twist method of pushing cattle into a space that they are reluctant to go. Care must be taken to not torque the tail so much as to cause a fracture of the coccygeal vertebrae.

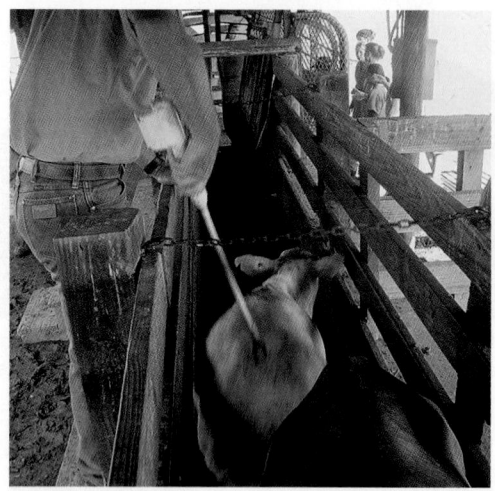

FIGURE 7-41 A "hot shot" with the proper positioning of the handler shown. These devices work well, but must be used judiciously to facilitate easy movement of cattle. The walkway that allows for human traffic above the cattle and outside the alleyway is evident just in front of the handler.

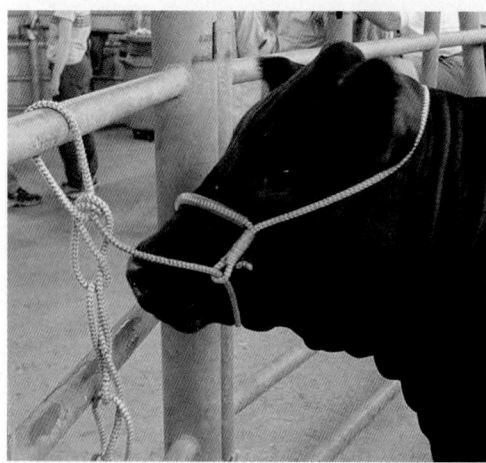

FIGURE 7-42 A rope halter placed correctly and tied to the pipe at an appropriate level to restrain this Angus heifer.

forward onto the cow's back (Figure 7-40). This provides discomfort to the cow, and the usual and expected response is for the animal to move forward. Never underestimate the ability of a cow to get frightened or balk and begin moving backward. This may cause serious injury to the unwise handler. Cattle prods, wiffle paddles, and electric "hot shots" are available and may be used from outside the alley. Many alleyways will have an elevated walkway that allows handlers to move the length of the alley to assist in moving cattle forward to the chute (Figure 7-41). If an alleyway and chute are not available, the next best solution is to run an individual cow into a gated corner. The handler must move quickly to get behind the animal and tail it to keep it from backing up. It may be necessary to rope a cow if no other method of restraint is possible, but this is not a technique that is advantageous or desirable in modern veterinary practice.

Once the animal has stopped moving, it is then possible to halter it and restrain it by the head. A single, calm cow restrained in a stall may be haltered without resorting to a chute. A bovine halter is all one piece and made from rope, as opposed to the equine halter. The halter is placed by loosening the nose loop first and then flipping the crown loop over the animal's ears. Once the crown loop is in place, the nose loop may be positioned and the slack in the free end of the rope taken up as the rope comes under the jaw (Figure 7-42). Always keep the cow's head at arm's length and bend forward from the waist because an animal that becomes nervous will throw its head and may catch the handler in a compromised position. Animals with horns may be restrained by placing a loop of rope around the base of both horns and then dallying off to a solid post.

Calves are captured in much the same manner as foals. If the calf is small enough, it may be "flanked" and placed in lateral recumbency (Figure 7-43). The dam of the calf deserves respect and must be observed for aggression.

Bulls must always be respected for the aggression that they possess. Extreme caution should be used if driving bulls on foot. The use of feed to entice bulls into a capture area

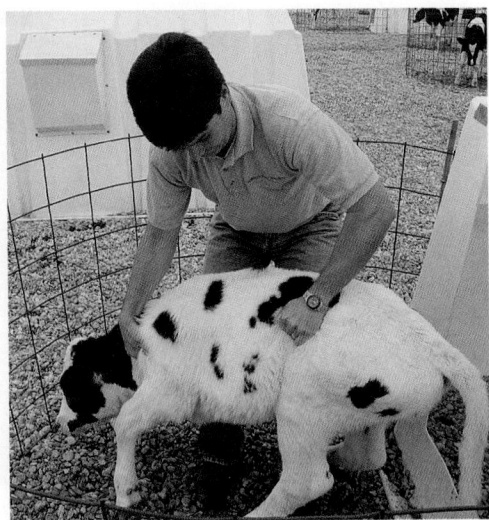

FIGURE 7-43 The proper positioning to "flank" a calf to the ground into lateral recumbency.

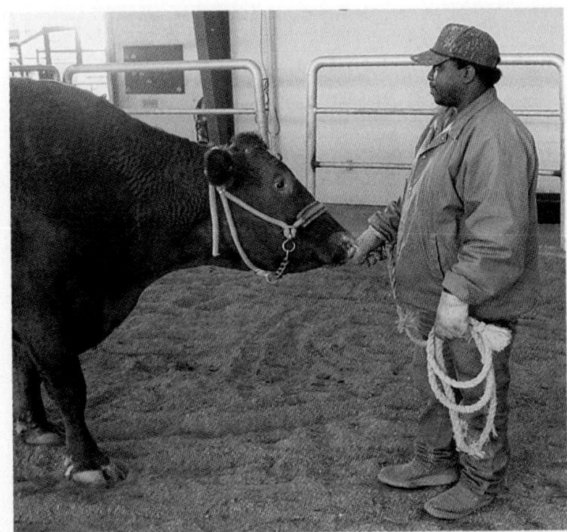

FIGURE 7-44 The handler has a long rope with a heavy snap in the nose ring of this bull and has also elected to hold the ring in his hand. The pipe arena that the bull is in provides additional safety for the handler.

is often necessary. Once the animal is in the enclosed area, gates may be used to squeeze the animal into a position that will allow restraint. Capturing the nose ring using a wire with a hook on the end and then snapping a long lead provide the necessary restraint for most bulls (Figure 7-44).

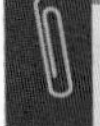

TECHNICIAN NOTE Extreme caution should be used if driving bulls on foot.

HEAD-CATCH

The head-catch or squeeze chute is the final capture and restraining device for cattle (Figure 7-45). Cattle usually do not willingly put their heads through the head-catch. It takes precise timing to close the head-catch following the presentation of the head and ears and before the shoulders. Once a bovid gets its shoulders through the head-catch, it will escape. Spring-loaded head-catches are available, but

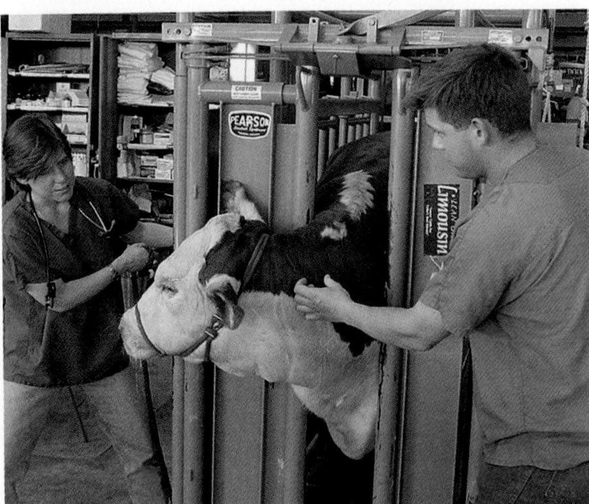

FIGURE 7-45 A chute with a Hereford cow captured inside of it. There are many varieties of chutes, and each has its own handling characteristics. They can be dangerous if the handler is unfamiliar with the use of the different type of pulls and levers.

their use is not as easy as the manufacturers would suggest. Most chutes also can squeeze the animal from side to side after the head is captured. This prevents the animal from moving about during an examination. Head-catches on manual or hydraulic chutes can be dangerous. Rapidly swinging handles or closing panels provide opportunity for the unfamiliar person to get hit. Take time to become familiar with the operation of any chute and head-catch before use.

RESTRAINT OF THE HEAD

Many different techniques may be used as an adjunct to the head-catch to restrain the animal for more invasive procedures than observation. Halters may be applied to pull the head to the side for exposure to the jugular veins. A strong person can grasp over the muzzle and place his or her hands into the mouth to allow for an oral examination. The nasal septum may be pinched between the thumb and forefingers, or nose tongs may be placed in the nose to stabilize the head. The horn or ear should be used to provide leverage for the handler. Care must also be taken to perform these techniques at arm's length to prevent a hit in the head as the animal throws its head up.

Grabbing the animal's tongue and moving it to one side of the mouth allows oral examinations in cattle. The handler makes life easier by grasping the tongue with a towel. Large, metal, hinged speculums may also be used in bovine oral examinations. These are placed and maintained as in the horse. Remember that cattle are not used to being restrained in the first place, and the use of additional hardware on the head may make them dangerous to the handlers should they become panicked or aggravated.

Mouth gags or speculums are used in cattle for the passage of orogastric tubes. The most common type is the Frick speculum (Figure 7-46). This is a stainless steel tube that is

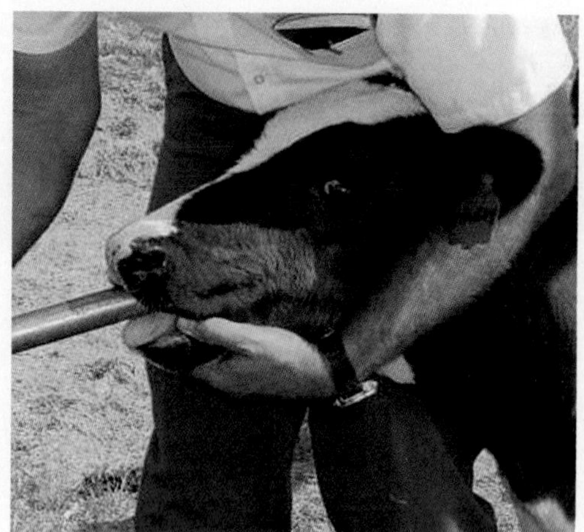

FIGURE 7-46 The handler is placing a Frick speculum into the oral cavity of this calf. The rear of the calf should be restrained in some manner before attempting this procedure, and great care should be taken to avoid advancing the speculum too far into the pharyngeal region.

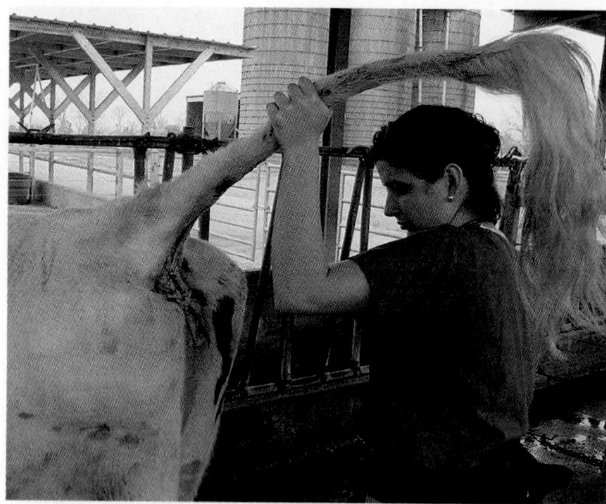

FIGURE 7-47 The tail "jack" technique. Handlers are reminded to keep the tail on the midline when pushing it forward and to keep their balance when pushing into the cow.

placed in the oral cavity, passed over the lingual bulla, and held in place while the tube is pushed through it into the esophagus. Care must be taken to ensure that the tube does not damage the pharyngeal mucosa. Another method that can be used is a block of wood that extends across the animal's mouth and has a hole in the center to allow for passage of the tube. The gag is placed in the interdental space and held by a strap placed behind the head.

TAIL RESTRAINT

The tail of a cow can be tied just like that of a horse, with the same precautions necessary about tying the tail to anything other than the cow. The tail of a cow may also be used for driving it as mentioned previously. "Jacking" the tail of a cow will also provide a means of restraint for short procedures. This technique involves pushing straight up and forward on the tail carrying it vertically in a plane directly over the cow's midline. The handler should remain balanced and have the tail about one third of the way down from the tail head (Figure 7-47). This technique works only when the tail is maintained vertically over the midline of the cow.

KICKING RESTRAINTS

Cattle usually kick to the side and forward with a hooking action rather than straight to the rear. Several commercial devices are available to prevent kicking and to restrain the hind legs. Milking hobbles are flat metal hooks with a chain in between that are placed over the tendons of the hind leg just above the hock. The open end of the hooks is to the inside of the leg, and the chain passes around the front of the limbs. Once the hooks are in place, the chain can be drawn up until the hocks are close together.

Pressure on the flank seems to discourage cows from kicking. A device shaped like giant ice tongs may be squeezed over the flank (Figure 7-48), or a rope may be tied snugly

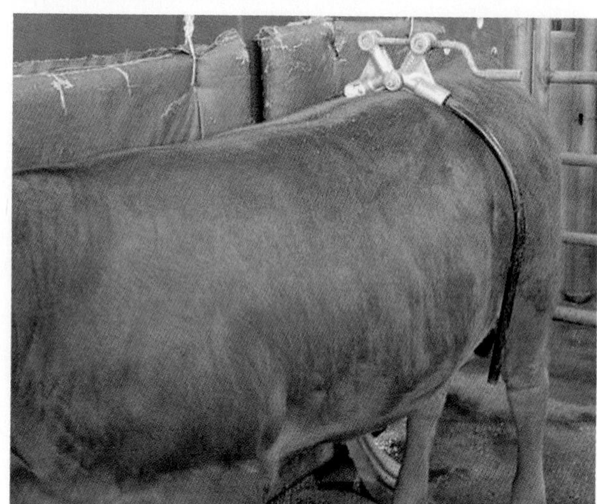

FIGURE 7-48 This commercially available restraint is known as the Can't Kick Device. The handle on the top turns to move the prongs of the device into the flanks of the cow for restraint and away from the flanks to remove.

around the abdomen just anterior to the udder or prepuce (Figure 7-49).

LIFTING FEET

Cattle are reluctant to lift up their feet, and to accomplish this in a standing animal without assistance requires great effort. The foreleg can be raised with a noose tied around the pastern and the free end of the rope passed over the back of the cow or around an overhead rail or pipe, which will then act as a pulley. The hind leg is more of a problem because there is no portion of the cow's anatomy that will act as a pulley. The limb may be tied to an overhead beam or rail following placement of a clove hitch around the animal's hock joint (Figure 7-50). Realize that most of the time this will be done in a chute or narrow area, and maneuvering space will be limited. However, the use of this procedure will allow for

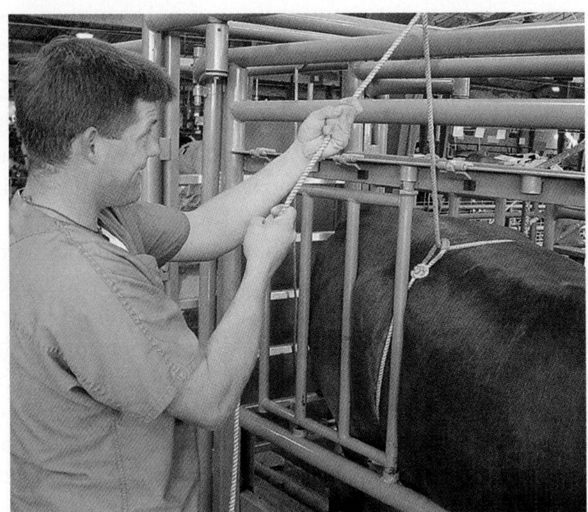

FIGURE 7-49 This technique involves the same concept as the Can't Kick Device, but provides more control of the animal by encompassing the entire abdomen. The rope can be cinched down as tightly as needed.

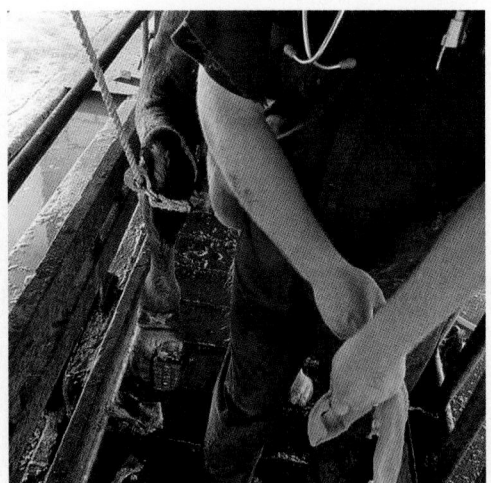

FIGURE 7-51 The person examining the foot and lower leg is not given much room in most chutes. The restraint of the limb by the clove hitch and rope elevation provides a good margin of safety for the examiner.

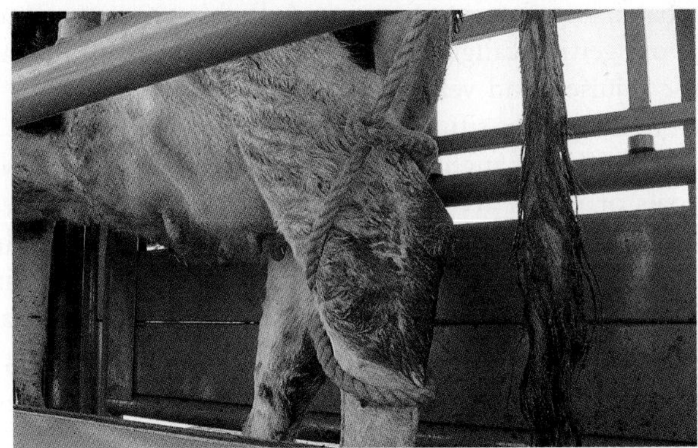

FIGURE 7-50 The hock of this cow is held by a clove hitch that has been placed in a sturdy rope. The rope restraint of the hock allows for the entire hind leg to be elevated by pulling the rope over a beam behind the cow.

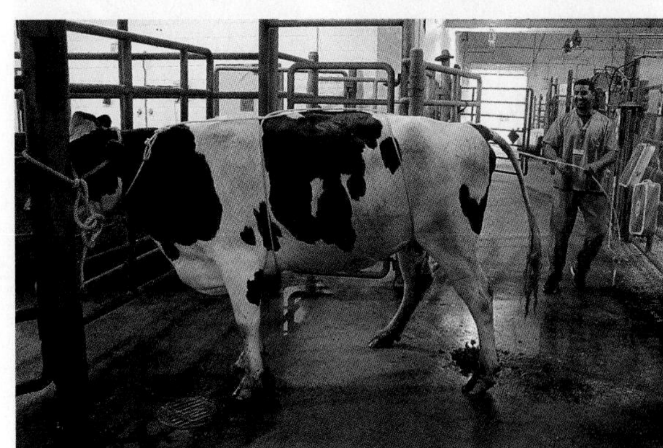

FIGURE 7-52 This is an example of the running W or double half-hitch technique of casting a cow. Care must be taken to ensure that the neck rope does not choke off the trachea; the thoracic portion is just behind the forelegs, and the abdominal portion of the rope is in front of the udder.

the visual and digital examination of the foot and interdigital space of all but the most recalcitrant cattle (Figure 7-51).

CASTING

The act of casting a bovid is quite simple. The animal must always be anchored to a sturdy post before placing one of the various rope harnesses on it. A sturdy halter is the first requirement for casting. The simplest harness technique consists of a noose around the neck, a half hitch around the girth, and a half hitch around the flank (Figure 7-52). Care should be taken to avoid incorporating the udder of a cow or the testicles of a bull into the flank rope. The free end of the rope comes off the animal's back with all knots positioned dorsally. Once the harness is secure, a strong pull toward the rear of the animal will make it lie down. One average-sized person can easily cast an adult cow in this manner.

The cow may be rolled onto her back if there are appropriate wedges available to keep her in dorsal recumbency. Square bales of hay may be used to wedge against the animal to keep it in position. The legs should be stretched to the front and rear with stout cotton rope. Cattle in sternal or dorsal recumbency are less likely to bloat than those in lateral recumbency when they are cast. A bovid that must be placed in lateral recumbency should be restrained on its right side (Figure 7-53). This allows the veterinary personnel to observe the rumen for any signs of bloat that may occur. If the bloat becomes large, the procedure should be terminated. Kneeling on the animal's neck may provide additional restraint for cattle in lateral recumbency. Standing cattle that are undergoing any procedure may go down at any time, for unspecified reasons. Restraint of the head should always be with a halter because a rope around the neck may tighten and strangle the cow and the use of nose tongs may lead to ripping out the nasal septum.

> *TECHNICIAN NOTE* A bovid that must be placed in lateral recumbency should be restrained on its right side.

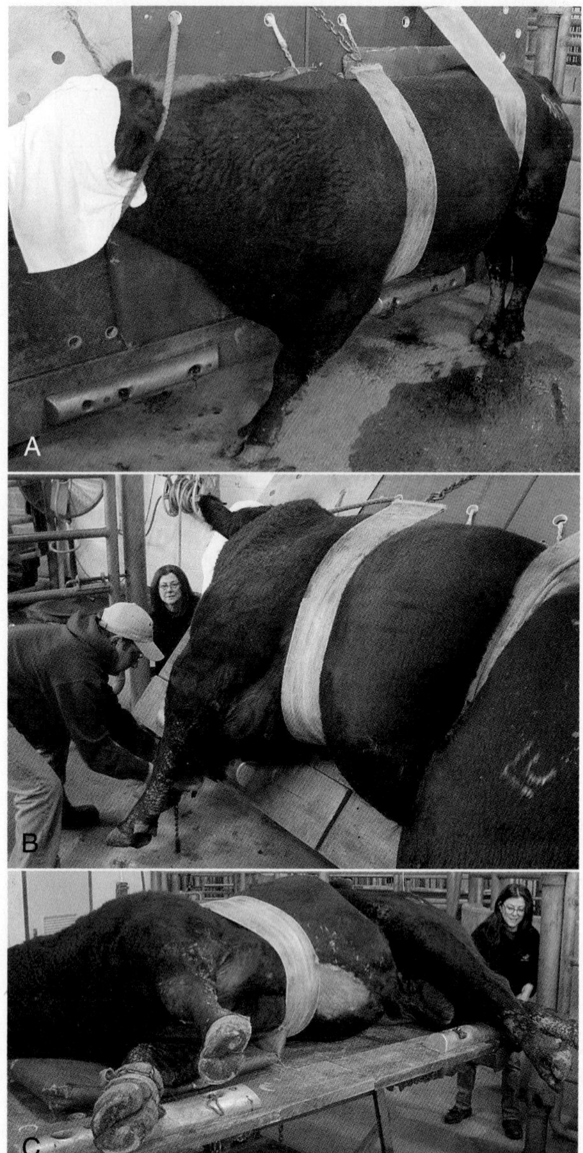

FIGURE 7-53 The techniques involved in tabling a ruminant. This bovine has been placed on a tilt table with the right side down so that constant observation of the left paralumbar fossa can be maintained. **A,** A towel is placed over the animal's eyes to minimize anxiety, and two bands are placed around the animal to initially restrain it to the table. **B,** The table is tilted slightly to raise the feet off of the ground, and the inside front leg is secured to the table with a wide band. **C,** The animal is then tilted into a horizontal position, and the rest of the legs will be restrained in a manner similar to the right foreleg.

Some dairy breed bulls and some beef bulls will have a nose ring. They are easily led with the ring, but care must be taken because the ring may break or pull through the nasal cartilage. Likewise, a bull should not be tied fast by the nose ring. A combination of a halter and nose ring may provide the most efficient means of leading a bull.

Chemical restraint is used for cattle; however, it must be remembered that ruminants are exquisitely sensitive to α_2-agonists, such as xylazine.

DRIVING SHEEP AND GOATS

Sheep and goats are more herd conscious than cattle and can be driven in bunches. Avoidance behavior in sheep is the basis of maneuvering the flock. When sheep are approached, they will flock together and move as a single unit. Taking advantage of their desire to escape is a fundamental part of successful handling. Dogs are an excellent adjunct in working sheep and some goat herds, although goats will occasionally challenge the dogs. Handling areas should be well lighted, have solid sides, and should be free of objects that may project shadows into the sheep's visual path. Sheep can be worked in alleyways, and although they tend to climb on and over each other more than cattle, they do less damage because of their smaller size. Sheep are much more athletic than cattle, yet they do not seem to want to climb out of enclosures or go over fences like cattle do. However, if driven hard, sheep may run through flimsy, temporary fencing, hang themselves, or break legs.

In addition, kids and lambs within a flock may be quite acrobatic, jumping into fences and climbing over structures to avoid getting caught. These activities may result in traumatic injuries, and veterinary personnel should be alert to prevent dangerous situations.

Sheep can be caught in small enclosures in the same way as foals or calves are caught, with a hand under the neck and one under the rump. It is important to remember that a sheep or mohair goat must not be restrained by grabbing the wool. The fleece may be damaged, or in meat animals, a subcutaneous bruise may develop at the site, damaging at least the aesthetics of the product.

CATCHING INDIVIDUAL SHEEP

Sheep are often set up on their rumps for several different procedures. There are several different ways to end up with the sheep on its rump with its back leaning against the holder for support. The handler may have to retain a grip on the forelegs for better support and control of the sheep (Figure 7-54). The easiest method is for the person to begin on the sheep's left side. Reach under the base of the neck with the left hand and over the back to the right hind leg with the right hand. The sheep is gently lifted off of the ground toward the right and upturned, as the right hind leg is lifted to get the animal's weight off of it. The right hand moves to the right foreleg as the left hand moves to the left foreleg, and the sheep is held on its rump facing away from the handler. One person can shear a sheep or perform other procedures unassisted with the sheep on its rump by steadying its upper torso between the arms and the lower torso between the legs as the person works.

The method of holding the legs of lambs for docking and castration is the same, whether they are held by the handler, laid on a bench, or placed over a fence. The holder grasps the parallel hind leg and foreleg, bringing the hind leg forward while holding between the hock and fetlock. The foreleg is held just below the elbow. One person can perform

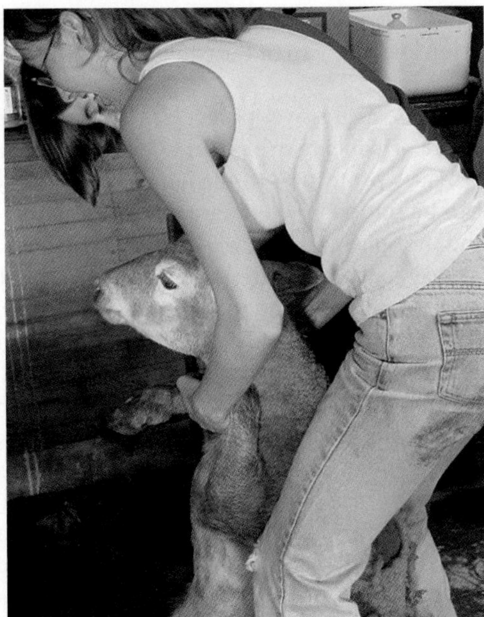

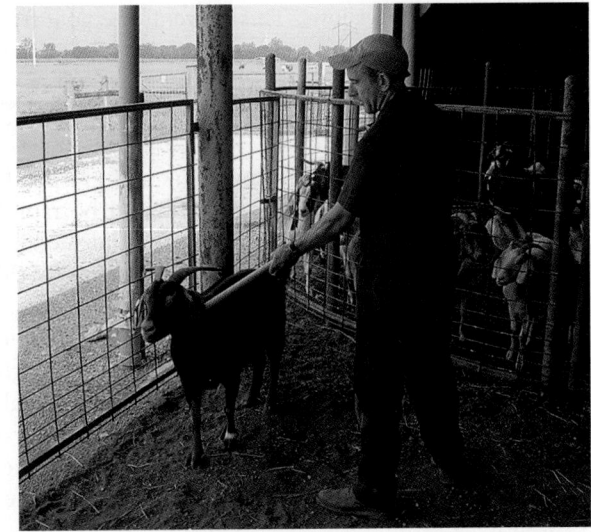

FIGURE 7-54 Holding the sheep set up on its rump. Note that the handler is supporting the sheep's head with one hand and the foreleg with the other. If the animal becomes more rambunctious, both forelegs can be grabbed and the sheep can be centered between the handler's legs for additional control.

drenching of oral fluids or medicines to a sheep. The sheep is backed into a corner as the handler straddles the sheep above its shoulders, squeezing slightly with the knees. The handler lifts the head by the lower jaw while holding loosely around the muzzle. The dose syringe is inserted into the interdental space on the opposite side of the mouth with the other hand. Do not lift the jaw above a line parallel to the ground surface and take care to administer the fluid slowly enough so that the sheep can swallow it. The nozzle of the syringe should be inserted well back into the mouth so that the fluid does not dribble out. Caution must be used to keep the animal's head under control so as not to traumatize the pharyngeal mucosa, as noted in the bovine section.

CATCHING INDIVIDUAL GOATS

When planning procedures that require physical restraint of goats, consideration of the layout and surrounding working facility, physical condition and temperament of the animals, and human and animal safety must be addressed. One person can easily restrain and carry out certain procedures on goats that have been handled frequently in a quiet, nonaggressive manner. However, when goats have had only occasional human contact, restraint and procedures should be performed with an assistant or many assistants (Figure 7-55). Patience and an easygoing manner of treatment often bring satisfactory results when handling goats.

A useful technique for capturing goats is the use of a shepherd's crook or cane. The goat can be hemmed in toward the fence, and the crook can be placed in the throatlatch area to catch the head (Figure 7-56). Care must be taken to prevent trauma to the trachea when using this technique.

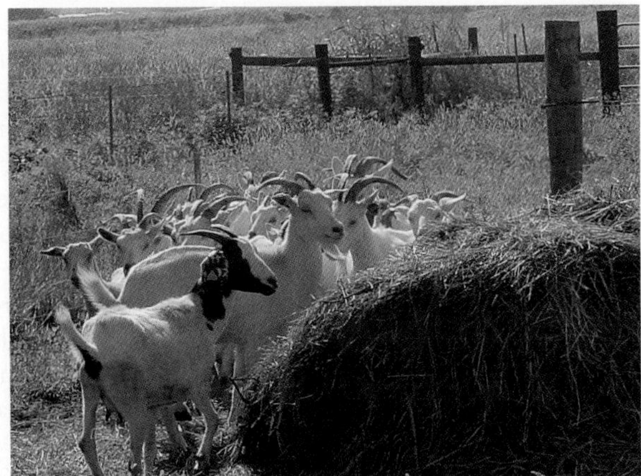

FIGURE 7-55 This photo represents a typical situation that veterinarians will be faced with when attempting to work a herd of goats. Note that the fences are thin, and there are obstacles in the pen. Care must be taken when approaching this herd to keep them all in the same location.

FIGURE 7-56 This photo demonstrates the use of a shepherd's crook or cane to capture a goat. Note the position of the handler in relation to the fence line.

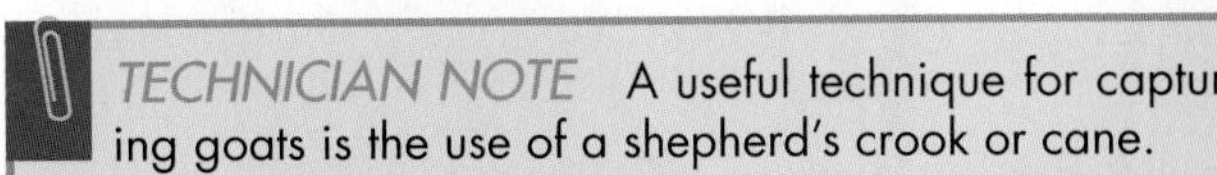

TECHNICIAN NOTE A useful technique for capturing goats is the use of a shepherd's crook or cane.

Equipment such as stanchions, tilt tables, and squeeze chutes can be used to assist in restraint. Realistically, these are rarely available in pet-goat households. Most procedures are accomplished by steadying the goat against a wall or fence by firmly holding a leg against the flank or thorax of the goat. A handler can also gently flip, place, and hold a goat in lateral recumbency by holding the legs and placing a knee on the neck of the goat. Another useful strategy is for a handler to straddle the goat and back it into a corner and firmly press their knees into the shoulders of the goat (Figure 7-57).

To restrain the head, one hand can be placed on each cheek with the fingers wrapped under the mandible. Be advised to avoid excessive pressure upon the trachea. The beard can also be grasped along with wrapping the other hand around the goat's neck. The horns may also be used to control the head, but this depends on the temperament of the goat and the strength and skill of the handler. Oral examinations are most efficiently accomplished using a speculum to ensure a clear view and protect the instruments and handler from being bitten by the goat.

When drenching, dispensing boluses, or passing an orogastric tube in a goat, the head should be held in a straight, natural position with the mandible parallel to the ground. The dose syringe should be inserted well back into the cheek pouch via the commissure of the lips. Give the goat time to swallow and dispense the fluid slowly because aspiration pneumonia can occur if fluids are exuberantly given or the head is tilted upward. A bolus can be administered by the use of a balling gun inserted over the base of the tongue, but not into the pharynx. Once the tablet or bolus is administered, the head position should be maintained with the mouth held closed until the goat swallows. This prevents the goat from spitting the bolus out.

CAPTURE AND RESTRAINT OF SWINE

Small piglets can be crowded into corners and grasped by a hind leg (Figure 7-58). The leg hold should be rapidly changed to holding the pig in both hands around the torso for the comfort of the pig (Figure 7-59). Obviously, this technique is not applicable to adult swine.

Veterinary personnel may be faced with the castration of large boars based on the owner's perception of when the signs are right. One technique that can be used on market-weight boars is to herd them to a corner and have two handlers grab the nearest hind leg. Following capture, the hind end is then elevated so that the pig is standing on his head in the corner.

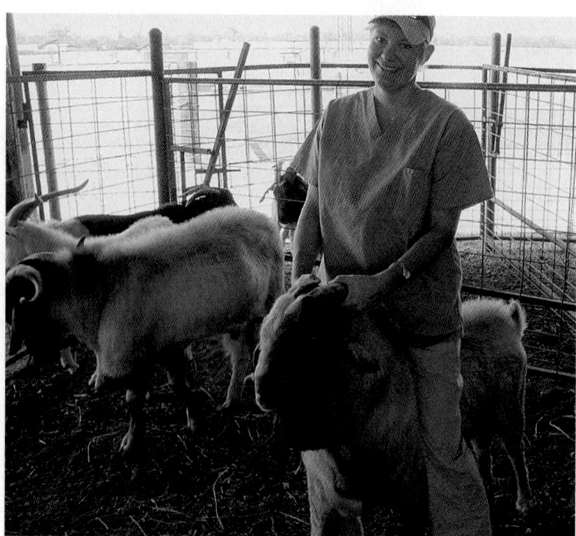

FIGURE 7-57 Restraint of an individual goat may be accomplished by straddling the goat and backing it into a corner while maintaining a grip on the horns and pressing the handler's knees into the thorax just behind the front legs.

This technique is not for the feint of heart; it requires the coordination and strength of the two handlers to accomplish the task.

Swine can be aggressive, particularly boars and nursing sows. A fence or panel may be used to "haze" them, and the barrier provides protection to the handler. When the panel is meant to be stationary, take care to push it all the way to the ground and plant it. Pigs will attempt to "root" underneath it. Always be aware of the escape route when entering a pen. Swine are intelligent and individualistic and may be difficult to direct in a large area. They tend to dart through small openings for escape. A cane is a valuable addition to a handler when attempting to drive and direct swine. Tapping them on the side of the neck and face with the cane while following on foot gives the handler some degree of "steering" capabilities.

Once pigs are inside a small enclosure, a snare may be used to catch them. A hog snare is an adjustable metal cable loop at the end of a rigid handle. The usual procedure in the capture of the pig is to push it into a corner and step in, tight to the flank area, and slip the snare loop over the upper

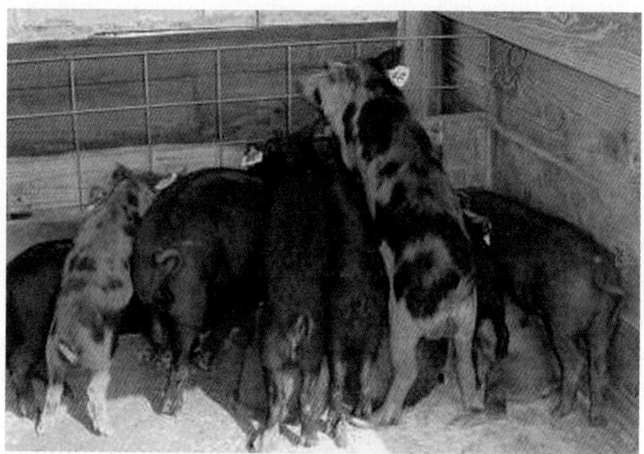

FIGURE 7-58 Piglets pile up in the corner when driven. It is easy to capture one by grabbing onto the hind legs that are presented.

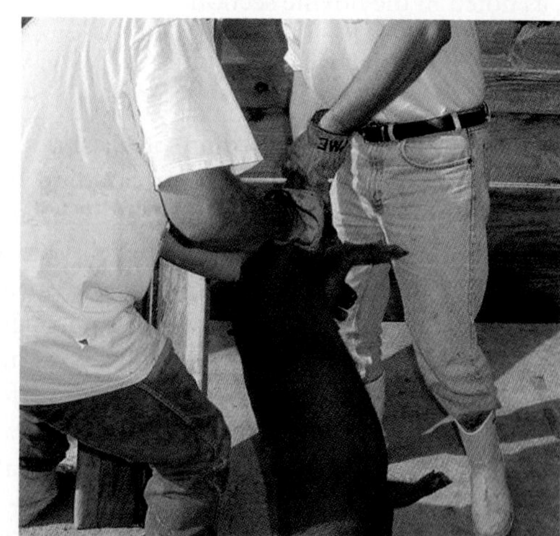

FIGURE 7-59 Two handlers have grabbed a piglet and are maneuvering it for a procedure. Many times this is all the restraint necessary for a procedure, especially on small pigs. This is not a recommended procedure for miniature or potbellied pigs because luxations of the hind limbs may occur.

jaw from behind. The loop is tightened after it is behind the incisors. The snare has a rigid handle that allows the handler to direct the snout after it is captured. Generally, swine will brace themselves by pulling backward when caught and are immobilized by its use (Figure 7-60). However, the discomfort of the snare usually results in nonstop squealing until it is removed. Handlers are encouraged to wear ear protection when performing any restraint on pigs.

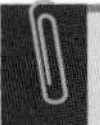
TECHNICIAN NOTE Handlers should wear ear protection when performing any restraint on pigs.

Pigs can be restrained on their backs in a trough, but find it unsettling and complain vocally (Figure 7-61). A sling of canvas with holes for the legs has been used with great success in laboratories and veterinary hospitals to cradle the pigs comfortably for certain procedures. The farrowing crate is the restraint device for sows, which keeps them from lying on their piglets.

Pigs can be restrained for castration or vaccination by holding them off the ground by the hind legs with their backs against the handler's legs. Large pigs will struggle less if their forefeet rest on the ground. Piglets receive oral administration by holding them up by the forelegs and leaning their backs against the handler's legs while they stand on their hind legs.

The pig is an intelligent animal that can be trained to tolerate minor discomforts; unfortunately, the time involved to train swine is often not profitable in agricultural animals. Miniature pigs, kept as pets, are most often seen these days in urban practices. Many of these are spoiled, willful creatures that dominate the household, and their owners are not impressed with rough handling. The support sling is the best method for restraint because it causes the animal no discomfort yet immobilizes well. Many pet pigs are fond of having people scratch their backs and may stand or lie quietly for an examination if this is done for them. Holding the pig cradled in the arms of a handler may seem a good idea until the pig struggles. Then the hind foot nearest the body will gouge the holder. Pigs also have powerful jaws and some will bite, especially if in pain. The examination of the mouth can be accomplished by the use of a U-shaped gag, which is placed into the mouth from the front to behind the canines; the gag is then rotated to spread the jaws. Never put fingers into the side of a pig's mouth since the cheek teeth are sharp.

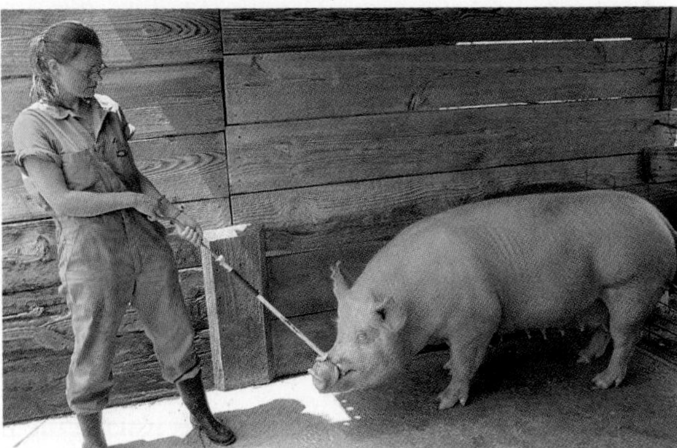

FIGURE 7-60 A handler with a hog snare has captured this pig by the upper jaw, just in front of the cheek teeth. It is obvious that the pig resents this and will resist by pulling back against the snare.

TECHNICIAN NOTE Many pet pigs are fond of having people scratch their backs and may stand or lie quietly for an examination if their backs are scratched.

Although a miniature pig may live in and control a house, it is still a pig. Pigs vocalize when they are uncomfortable or in pain. Do not be surprised when the cute little pig emits an ear-piercing shriek as it is picked up. This will continue until it is set free. Chemical agents for restraint are highly recommended for use on these animals.

CAPTURE AND RESTRAINT OF DOGS

CATCHING DOGS

The only time veterinary personnel should have to catch a dog that is not in a cage or run is if the animal has escaped. In a hospital, dogs are often motivated by fear, so personnel should learn to deal with the two types of behavior this produces. Avoidance with submissiveness when cornered is one, and the other is avoidance until cornered and then aggression, otherwise known as *fear biting*. Unfortunately, it may be difficult to discriminate between the two until the moment when hands are approaching the dog. It is the rare dog that will not snap at a handler that grabs it as it runs past, yet it is difficult to resist the temptation of doing so as a dog streaks past on its way to freedom.

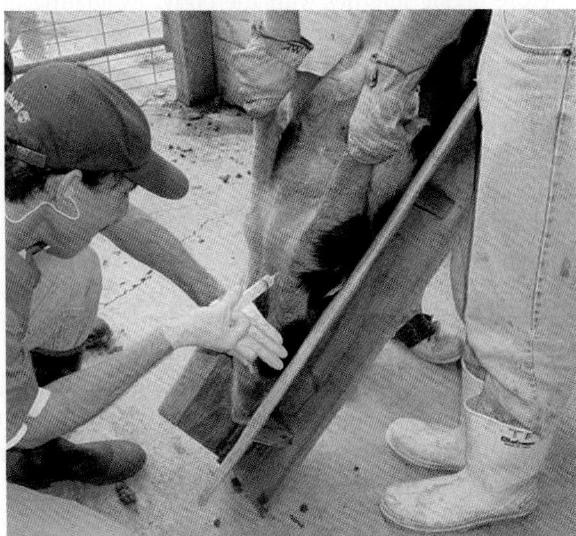

FIGURE 7-61 This pig is being restrained by both hind legs, and its back is supported by the V trough. Procedures such as ear notching and bleeding can be done with the pig in this position. The reader should note that the pig will squeal the entire time it is restrained in this fashion, and handlers should wear ear protection as is observed in the individual bleeding the pig.

Dogs that feel they are being chased will run, and a person is not going to outrun any but the smallest or most debilitated. It is best to try to keep the dog in sight until there is an opportunity to corner it. Sometimes it helps to have a canine companion to entice the dog to approach. In this situation, it will never hurt to have a pocketful of bait to gain the dog's favor. Most dogs respond favorably to voice reassurance, and a calm, friendly voice usually gets better results. With many dogs, squatting in front of them to appear less large and overbearing will help. Moving slowly and deliberately, offer the back of the hand at or below the level of the nose for the dog to sniff. The response to this action is the first indication of the tendency for the dog to try to bite. Never try to grab the dog's collar or pick it up until some reassurance is given to the animal. Do not confuse a wagging tail with friendliness in a dog with an unknown personality. Watch the ears, eyes, and face. It is not unusual for an aggressive dog to hold the tail erect with a tense, narrow, oscillating motion before biting, or for a fearful dog to suddenly snap as a hand is withdrawn or a collar grabbed.

The back of the hand is offered to the dog for two reasons. The first is that it is probably less threatening than the open palm, which may appear to the dog as an attempt to slap. Second, the fingers are out of the way, and the dog will be less likely to get the entire hand if it does bite. Caution should be exercised by all handlers in these situations because dogs bite with lightning speed, and the position of the hand may have little to do with the ability to withdraw from danger.

Some dogs are naturally gregarious and trusting and require little in the way of preliminary introduction. The trusting dog will sniff the hand, begin wagging the tail, and approach for more petting. It is a good idea for the handler to run the hands over the entire dog in a friendly fashion before taking liberties with the body. Evaluating dogs requires knowledge of the relationship of the dog with the owner. Some dogs have trained their owners rather than the opposite, and the handler must forge his or her own relationship with the dog.

Sometimes dogs act reasonably in an initial examination with the client present and then threaten to bite when approached after the client has gone. When faced with a dog that will bite if given the chance, the sensible approach is to keep your hands and body out of the way. Always remember to keep all outside gates and doors closed when working with difficult animals. The cage door should be held closed as much as possible when trying to catch these animals. They are trouble enough without trying to capture them after they have escaped. Small dogs may be managed by handling with heavy leather gloves. The dog will bite at the fingers of the glove of one hand while the handler picks up the animal under the chest with the other. A small fractious dog can also be picked up using a thick towel. Large dogs that want to bite are more concerning. The first step is to catch them by the neck. A lead rope with a slipknot can be tossed over a dog's head, but sometimes a rope or cable snare similar to a hog snare is required (Figure 7-62). Most dogs will relax or decrease aggressive behavior when caught by the neck. The truly vicious or confirmed fear biters will continue to attempt to bite and even attack. These animals will require a muzzle or rope with a pole to keep the teeth away from veterinary personnel. Often, chemical restraint is necessary for the safety of the patient and personnel.

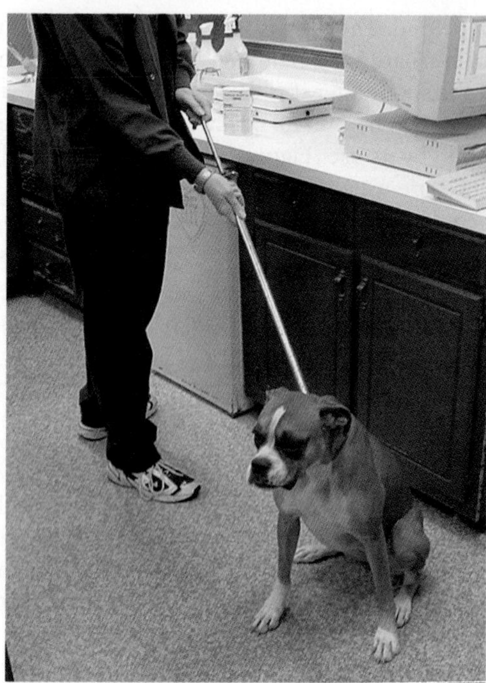

FIGURE 7-62 This dog has been captured with a cable snare. The steel handle allows the handler to keep the dog at a safe distance when maneuvering the animal.

> *TECHNICIAN NOTE* Often dogs act reasonably in an initial examination with the client present and then threaten to bite when approached after the client has gone.

A truly vicious large dog is a major challenge. These dogs must always be handled with at least one snare, possibly two if the dog is strong. Once captured, the dog is stretched between the snares for leading. Many of these dogs are used as guard animals, and only one person can handle them. The owner may be able to place the muzzle on the dog before bringing it into the practice. These dogs must always be treated with respect for their ability to harm the handler.

A dog at large that will not allow approach may require the use of a capture gun or pole syringe. Animal control officers are experienced with the use of these devices and may be able to provide assistance.

LIFTING DOGS

Lifting a dog onto the examination table is usually the first step in any examination or procedure. Grasping on either side of the thorax behind the elbows allows the handler to lift small dogs. Putting the arms around the front of the chest and behind the rump will allow a handler to easily lift a medium-sized dog. This technique places the handler in close proximity to the animal's teeth, so care must be taken to prevent being bitten by the frightened dog. Large dogs are harder to lift. Their weight may be prohibitive, their bulk makes them awkward, and they are not accustomed to being lifted. One person can lift a large dog by using a forklift technique, placing the arms behind the elbow and in front of the hind legs. If the animal struggles, there is danger that it will fall forward or backward. Two people can lift a dog together if one lifts the forequarters and the other person lifts the hindquarters. Both individuals should be on the same side, away from the table, to accomplish this technique. Some dogs object to being lifted from under the flank area, especially males. If this is the case, they definitely need two people to lift them, and the person in back should make sure the placement of the hand or arm is well forward on the abdomen. Many practices now have lift tables that allow dogs to be walked onto the table at floor level and elevated to a comfortable height for an examination (Figure 7-63). Keeping two hands on the dog while lift tables rise and lower is very important. Dogs may become nervous or frightened with the sounds associated with lift tables and decide to quickly leave. Handlers are cautioned that lifting dogs may result in a back injury. Lifting with the legs and keeping the back straight will help prevent muscle strains. Large dogs that are nervous about being lifted or react adversely to being on top of a table should be dealt with on the floor.

Never let a dog jump down from a table. Tables and floors have slick surfaces that invite slips and possibly fractures. Using commercially available bath mats, towels, or other nonskid surfaces can increase a dogs level of comfort with being on a table. Lift the dog off the table in the same manner as it was placed.

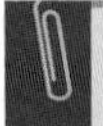

TECHNICIAN NOTE Never let a dog jump down from a table.

Injured or sick animals pose different problems in lifting. More support is required for patients with fractures or painful abdomens. A stretcher may be required for lifting a badly injured dog. Rational judgment should be used in all instances when lifting is required.

TABLE RESTRAINT

The degree of restraint required for a dog on the table depends on the procedure. The forequarters and hindquarters must be controlled at all times to prevent the dog from jumping or falling off the table. The form of restraint most commonly used is to have the arms either behind the rump or under the flank and in front of the chest pulling the dog inward in much the same manner as lifting. The head may be pulled toward the handler's chest and anterior shoulder (Figure 7-64). This is adequate restraint on most dogs for an examination and intramuscular or subcutaneous injections.

A rectal examination requires only slight adjustments for restraint. The holder's arm should not be behind the dog; it can be placed over the dog's back to stabilize lateral movement by drawing the body toward the handler. Often it is preferred to place the arm under the ventral abdomen to prevent the dog from sitting down. The size of the animal plays a role in which method is more effective.

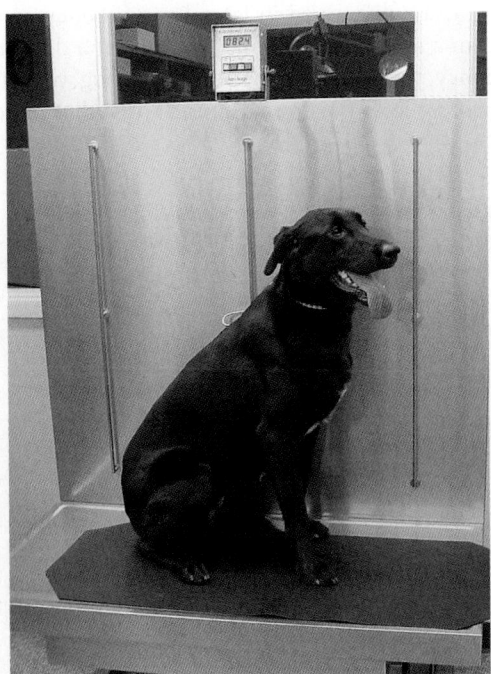

FIGURE 7-63 A stainless steel lift table that also has a self-contained scale. This allows large dogs or those that do not like to be picked up to step onto the table at floor level and be raised to a comfortable height for examination.

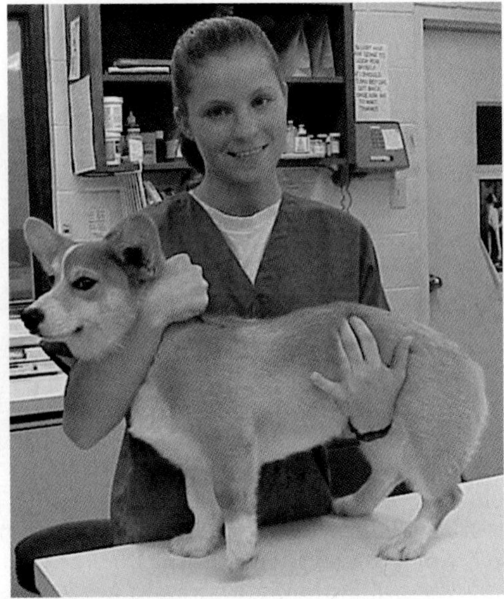

FIGURE 7-64 The handler is providing support for the dog and restraint for an examination at the same time. Note the placement of the arms in a forklift position under the neck and in front of the flank. The handler is positioned to draw the animal closer if serious anxiety develops.

Whenever procedures are done on puppies, it is wise to put the bitch into a crate or better, remove her to a kennel outside the room. Care must be taken when removing newborn pups from the bitch for the same reasons discussed previously.

RESTRAINT FOR VENIPUNCTURE

The dog must not be allowed to move during venipuncture because movement results in the perivascular placement of the needle. The primary reason for struggling and movement during venipuncture is anxiety. Calm, affectionate handling with petting and soothing words will help alleviate anxiety. The most painful portion of the venipuncture is the piercing of the skin and vessel, which is when the restraint must be most secure. Positioning is the most critical part of a venipuncture to allow for accurate location of the vessel. Diagnostic sampling is discussed in Chapter 20.

The holder must restrain the dog's body, present the forelimb, and occlude the vein to allow it to fill and be recognized under the skin for cephalic venipuncture. This can be performed with the dog in a sitting or standing position. Though many dogs feel comfortable on a table, large and giant breeds may be more comfortable on the floor. A muzzle to prevent biting should be used when necessary. The handler stands (or kneels) beside the dog facing the venipuncturist and places one arm under the dog's neck, using the hand of that arm to hold the dog's head against the anterior shoulder. At the same time, the handler wraps the other arm over the back of the dog and uses the hand of that arm to encircle the dog's forearm just below the elbow. The thumb is used to cover the cephalic vein on the medial side. The hand is then rotated to the lateral side pulling the skin and vessel as far to the outside as possible. Concurrently, the dog's elbow pushed forward to extend and stabilize the leg (Figure 7-65).

The handler must release the thumb when the person is ready to perform the injection. Failure to release the vessel will prevent the substance injected from reaching the general circulation and may result in the rupture of the vessel.

Kneeling or squatting behind a large dog that is sitting on the floor allows cephalic venipuncture to be performed in the same manner. Most dogs submit to cephalic venipuncture quite readily. Dogs that are gentle may allow cephalic venipuncture while sitting up.

Jugular venipuncture is sometimes needed. The handler stands (or kneels) alongside or behind the dog. One arm is placed around the neck of the dog and the hand is used to raise the chin so that the neck is extended and the dog's face is directed toward the ceiling. The fingers must not be placed too far caudally on the jaw, which may occlude the jugular vein and make it difficult to locate. The handler uses the other arm to encircle the dog's back and chest and hold the animal snuggly against the torso of the handler (Figure 7-66). The main advantage of this position is to provide a nearly straight plane from the angle of the jaw to the forefeet for easy access to the jugular vein. The correct position of the head should be no more than slightly above 90 degrees from the neck.

TECHNICIAN NOTE The saphenous vein, located on the lateral aspect of the hind leg, is an alternate venipuncture site for which the dog must be restrained in lateral recumbency.

The saphenous vein, located on the lateral aspect of the hind leg, is an alternate venipuncture site; for this procedure, the dog can be restrained in lateral recumbency or may be done from a standing position. To position a dog in lateral recumbency, the holder stands behind the dog with one forearm pressed across the animal's neck while that hand holds

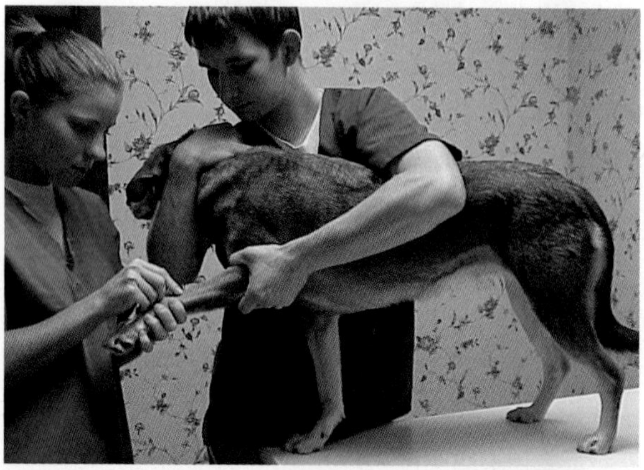

FIGURE 7-65 The correct positioning for obtaining blood samples from the cephalic vein. The handler has the dog well restrained, even though the dog remains standing, and has rolled the vein slightly outward to tighten the skin and provide easy access for the sample. If the dog becomes anxious, the handler will force the dog into sternal recumbency while maintaining the hold.

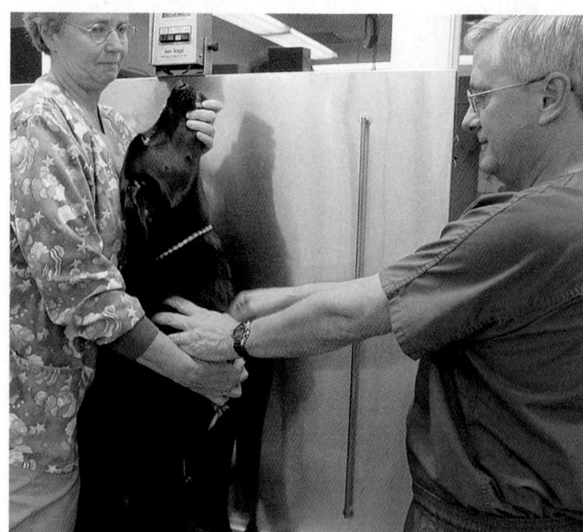

FIGURE 7-66 Method of holding the dog for jugular venipuncture. Note the straight line from the ramus of the mandible to the feet.

the forelegs with a finger between the legs. The other forearm presses across the dog's flank, and the hind legs are held in a similar manner. When venipuncture is performed, only the down leg is held; the person making the puncture stabilizes the other.

MUZZLES AND MOUTH GAGS

A dog's mouth can be restrained manually by bringing the hands forward from the rear on both sides of the face. The thumbs are placed on the forehead, and the fingers are looped under the mandibles. The palms of the hands should be below the ears. Concern for the owner's perception of this type of restraint and varying human hand sizes makes this method impractical and often unsafe.

Commercial muzzles are made of a variety of materials and come in various sizes. Several sizes should be available. Gauze or rope muzzles can be made, if necessary. Nylon rope slip leads are sometimes handy as muzzling devices for snapping dogs. Following capture of the dog, a loop of rope made with a single overhand knot is positioned from above the dog's nose until it is in place over the muzzle. This loop should be tightened quickly after it is positioned with the knot on top of the nose. Most dogs will try to push the rope loop off with their forepaw. The first knot must be held snugly while a second knot is made with the ends under the nose. The second knot may be a single overhand, or a square knot may be thrown. The two free ends are passed behind the dog's head and tied again. This knot is extremely important because it holds the muzzle in place, so it must be secure, yet it must be tied in such a manner to allow for quick release should the animal have difficulty breathing.

A gauze roll bandage (7.5 to 15 cm) may be used as a muzzle in the same fashion as the rope (Figure 7-67). Gauze is preferable to rope because it is less slick. However, it also makes a less rigid loop to apply to a recalcitrant dog. The piece of gauze should be cut at least 90 cm long for most dogs. It is important to have a sufficient length to begin with because there may be only one opportunity to muzzle the dog without a significant battle.

Brachiocephalic breeds are difficult to muzzle and can be determined biters. To muzzle them, the gauze bandage is first tied around the nose with the first knot tied underneath the jaw. The ends are then passed behind the head and tied with a square knot. Finally, one end is passed over the forehead and under the loop on top of the nose and then tied back to the other side. This keeps the loop from slipping off the top of the short nose. Commercial muzzles are now available for brachicephalic breeds.

The mouth of a dog can be examined in a variety of ways. The easiest, if the dog is a willing participant, is to open the mouth with the hands for a visual examination. Placing one hand on the upper jaw and the other on the lower and forcing the lips over the teeth will allow the handler to separate the jaws of the mouth (Figure 7-68). A variety of mouth gags can also be used on dogs. A simple wooden dowel may be pressed toward the back of the mouth to rest between the carnassial teeth. The dowel can be tied in place behind the ears, or it can be held by hand. Stomach tubes may be inserted with the dowel in place. The commercial spring mouth gag has a hole on either end for the canine teeth, and it is inserted on one side of the mouth for a variety of procedures. The disadvantage to this type of gag is that it hangs outside of the mouth, is heavy, and can fracture teeth to which it is attached. Concern for over-extension of the temporal mandibular joint should also be taken into account, especially when dealing with spring loaded mouth gags. A syringe case of appropriate size placed over the opposing canine teeth makes a lighter and safer gag, especially for use in dental work.

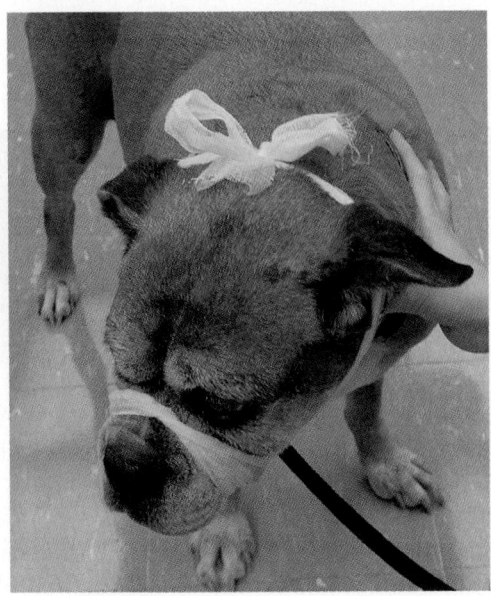

FIGURE 7-67 The gauze muzzle.

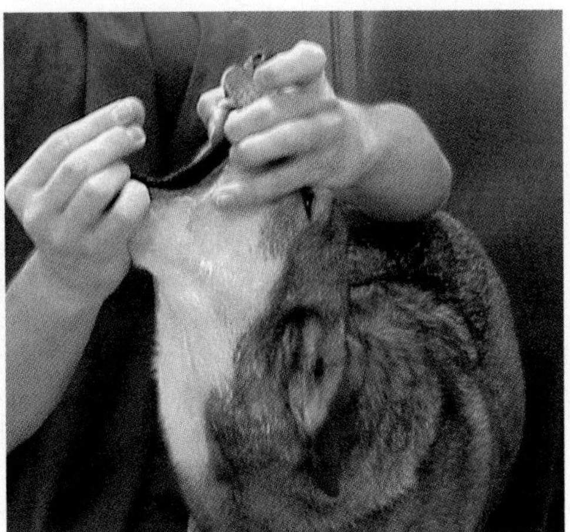

FIGURE 7-68 Technique for easy examination of the mouth. The lips of the upper jaw are pressed against the teeth by one hand while the lower lips are pressed into the teeth of the lower jaw. Forcing the lips apart opens the jaw.

MOBILITY-LIMITING DEVICES

Self-mutilation and tearing of bandages can be prevented with several devices. The most common is the Elizabethan collar. The concept is to place some type of stiff material extending from the collar area to the dog's nose so that it cannot chew or lick its body. Commercial plastic collars are available, or collars may be fabricated from buckets, large bottles, or heavy plastic sheets. It is most important to ensure that no sharp edges are present and that the collar is secured to the neck by gauze or the dog's collar. (It is not good for a veterinary practice if the dog traumatizes itself with the collar in a manner greater than the original lesion.) Attention must be given to the ability of the dog to eat and drink following the placement of these devices.

Fastening a pole along the body to a snug collar high on the neck makes another type of device that will limit movement of the head. This would mimic the cradle described for restraint of horses earlier in the chapter. Tape is usually used to keep the device from shifting. Commercial "neck braces" or cervical collars are also available that work in a similar manner by decreasing the ability to flex or turn the neck.

CHEMICAL RESTRAINT

Many drugs are available for chemical restraint and sedation for dogs. The main reason for tranquilization is to remove anxiety, which is one of the major reasons that dogs bite. However, the handler is cautioned that tranquilizing effects vary between dogs and that dogs are still capable of biting even when heavily tranquilized. Chapter 28 gives more information on the chemical agents of anesthesia.

CAPTURE AND RESTRAINT OF CATS

Cats are more apprehensive than dogs with strange people and surroundings. A cat that escapes will search out a hiding place, whereas a dog that escapes will look for room to run away. This may be due to the lower endurance that a cat has for running and the security that cats feel in an enclosed space. A cat that is trapped may respond with flattened ears, hissing, scratching, and biting at hands and extended fingers (Figure 7-69). Heavy leather gloves may be used to subdue these cats in the same manner as described for small dogs. Grasp the scruff of the neck to lift the cat (Figure 7-70). This may be followed by a rapid "stretch" restraint by also grasping the hind legs. One of the easiest ways to catch a cat is to force it into a box pushed into the cage. There are boxes available that will allow for anesthesia induction after the cat is captured without having to handle the cat at all. All escapes from the box are blocked once the cage is placed in the kennel until the cat is safely inside and the top is closed.

Squeeze cages are very helpful when working with cat that is extremely uncooperative. These can be constructed by cutting a board or thick Plexiglas the same size as the cage door and applying handles. The handles should be accessible through the front of the cage when the board is pressed against the back wall of the cage. A cat can then be safely brought to the front of the cage by pulling the handles forward placing the cat between the front of the cage and the squeeze board. Next, chemicals may be used to subdue the cat, either by oral spray or injection. The hindquarters will be accessible for intramuscular injections. This provides the greatest amount of safety for the handlers. Groups performing trap-neuter-release (TNR) will often have capture cages that contain squeeze devices built in to limit the possibility of a cat escaping during transport from capture cage to hospital kennel.

CARRYING CATS

Cats generally feel most secure in close quarters and seldom resist being put into a bag or rolled in a towel. They are best carried from place to place in a cat carrier or small cardboard box with a lid. They can also be carried with one arm if they are not particularly nervous. To carry a cat, its hindquarters are placed under the elbow area and pressed securely to the holder's body with the forearm (Figure 7-71). The cat lies in a sternal position along the forearm while the hand that has one finger between the legs holds the forelegs. The cat may

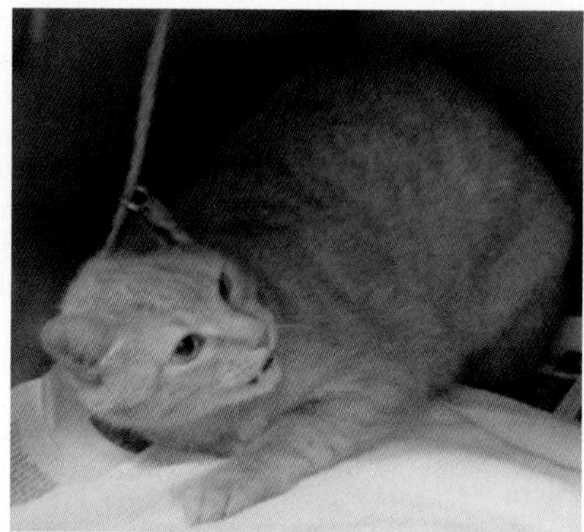

FIGURE 7-69 Trapped cats will display flattened ears and may hiss and growl before unleashing their claws.

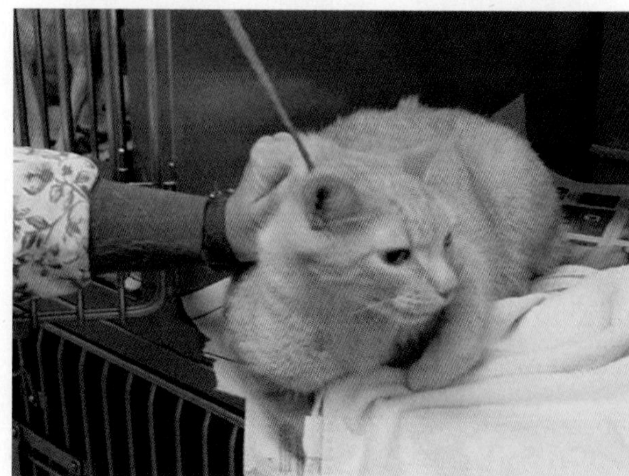

FIGURE 7-70 Capture of the head followed by grasping the scruff of the neck will restrain most cats.

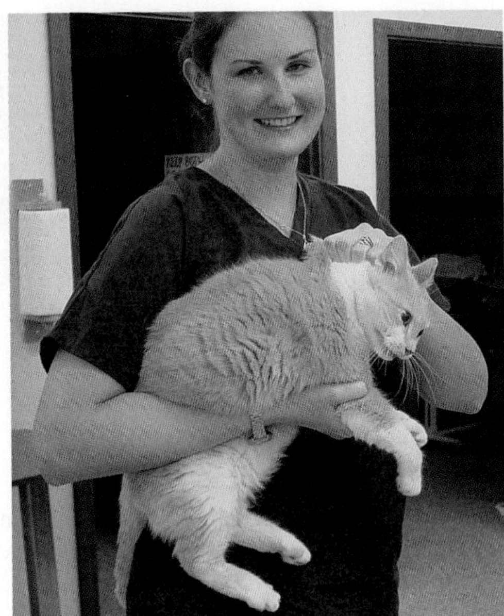

FIGURE 7-71 The proper carrying position for a cat. Note the support given to the abdomen, the grasp of the neck, and the restraint of both front feet.

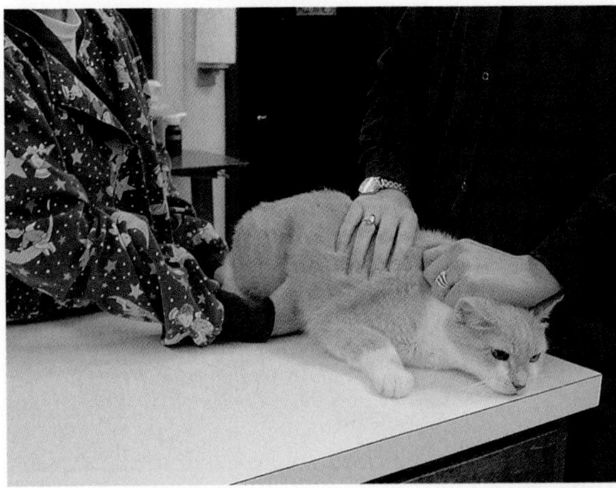

FIGURE 7-72 Restraint for examination of a cat. Note both the handler and examiner have on long-sleeved lab coats.

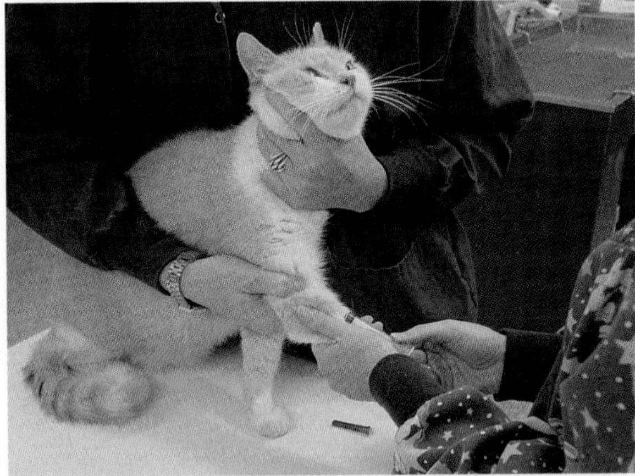

FIGURE 7-73 Proper restraint for cephalic venipuncture in the cat. The head, forearm, and back of the cat are all supported and well restrained by the handler.

still use the hind claws to gouge the abdomen of the holder, who must be ready to grab the scruff of the neck and hold the cat at arm's length if it panics. Quickly grasping the hind legs and pulling away from the scruff of the neck will effectively immobilize almost any cat. This is not a position of comfort for the cat, and the cat will object, but it is clearly safer for the holder.

> *TECHNICIAN NOTE* Cats usually feel most secure in close quarters, and they seldom resist being put into a bag or rolled in a towel.

RESTRAINT FOR EXAMINATION

Table restraint of cats is similar to that of dogs, except that cats tend to use their claws as their first line of defense (if they have them) rather than their teeth. Cats should be allowed supervised movement when it is not necessary for them to be still. Some cats are so terrified that they are best held or cuddled with the head buried under the holder's arm. Cats are not necessarily malicious when they climb onto a person's chest or clamp nails into a forearm, but their actions will hurt if the holder is not prepared. It is a good idea to wear protective gowns or laboratory coats with long sleeves when dealing with cats (Figure 7-72). Cat scratches are potentially dangerous to veterinary personnel, and care should be taken to avoid movements and behavior that will agitate the cat.

RESTRAINT FOR VENIPUNCTURE

Cephalic venipuncture restraint can be applied to cats much like it is applied to dogs (Figure 7-73). However, cats will tend to engage their claws and teeth in an effort to get away from the holder. When a cat becomes agitated, it seems to lose its spine and develops legs that swirl about like a Weedeater. Once cats develop this attitude, they are impossible to hold like dogs, and other restraint techniques must be employed. Jugular venipuncture may be more appropriate for some cats because the hold restrains the head and forefeet more securely than the cephalic technique (Figure 7-74). Wrapping the hind feet with a towel disarms all but the most persistent cat. The head is held with the hand over the top of the head, and the jaw or zygomatic arch is grasped with the thumb on one side and two or three fingers on the other side. The other hand restrains both forelimbs as in the dog.

There are other ways to hold a cat for jugular venipuncture. They involve the cat being placed on its back with the holder occluding the jugular vein and the person using the syringe pushing the chin down toward the table to make the head move backward to get a straight shot at the jugular. The holder can hold two legs in each hand with a finger between the legs while pushing the cat down on the table and using the little finger to press on the thoracic inlet to occlude the jugular vein. A cat can also be rolled in a towel or bag to engage the feet and legs. The holder need only steady the cat on its back and occlude the vessel.

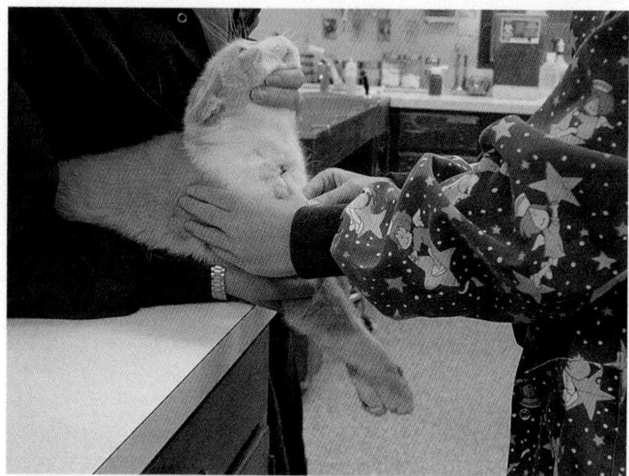

FIGURE 7-74 Restraint for jugular venipuncture in the cat. Note how the hind legs are tucked under the elbow of the handler and the forefeet are extended and held in one hand.

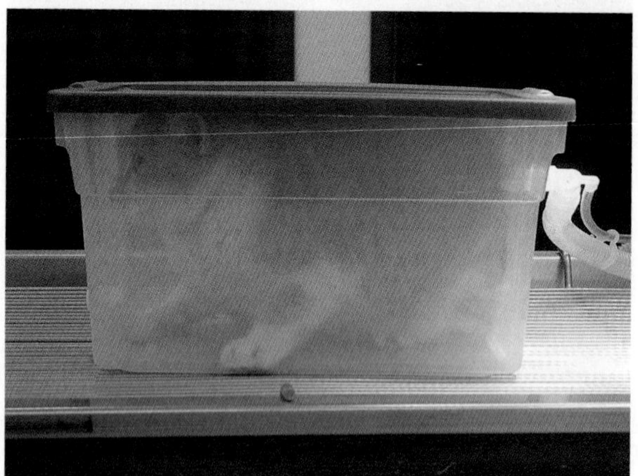

FIGURE 7-75 This cat is being restrained in a capture box that has inlet ports for inhalation anesthesia.

Cat bags are made with zippers so that a single limb may be withdrawn and used for cephalic venipuncture, and in a similar fashion, there are now restraint boxes made for cats that have different openings to allow for withdrawal of a limb (Figure 7-75).

Stretching a cat in lateral recumbency will provide access to the saphenous vein (Figure 7-76). Most cats do not seem to realize that they can use their forefeet to scratch the hand on the scruff of their neck when they are appropriately stretched. The medial saphenous vein can then be used for venipuncture by holding the hind leg that is up in a flexed position. The little finger can be used to hold off the vein on the down leg for the venipuncture. The person who is performing the venipuncture must restrain the down leg with one hand while handling the syringe with the other.

BATHING

Bathing a cat may be a trying experience for both the cat and the person. Most cats will try to climb up the person's arms to escape standing water or spray. Cats should be bathed on top of a screen suspended over a tub (a metal window screen

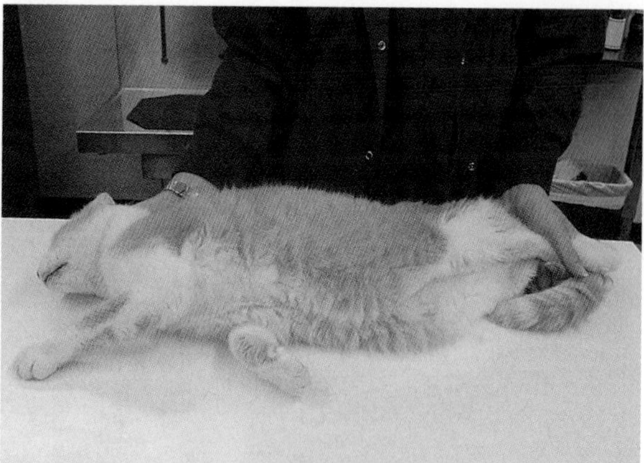

FIGURE 7-76 Stretching a cat on its side.

will suffice) and washed with a light spray of warm water. Almost all cats will clamp their claws into the screen and stand still for the entire bath when using this technique.

CHEMICAL RESTRAINT

The use of chemicals and anesthesia to restrain cats is common. The eyes should be treated with ophthalmic ointments to prevent corneal drying from the lack of blinking when these agents are used. See Chapter 27 for more information on anesthesia.

RESTRAINT OF EXOTIC ANIMALS

Minimal handling of all exotic animals is recommended and must be done efficiently, quietly, and confidently. The best method of learning restraint is by watching an experienced handler. Many clients judge the competency of veterinary professionals by how well they catch and handle the patient. Smooth handling and restraint of their animals reassure clients that the technician is well trained. It is often difficult to quantify the stress factor. The importance of fast, competent handling cannot be overemphasized. The sights, sounds, smells, and temperature of the strange environment will stress the exotic animal in a veterinary hospital. As a general rule, the more tame the animal, the better it will tolerate handling. However, do not underestimate the added stress of disease and trauma. Always discuss the risk of stressing an ill or traumatized nondomestic pet with the owner before handling begins. All treatment and testing material (culturettes, syringes) must be in place before the animal is restrained to minimize the stress. The patient work-up may have to be done incrementally because of the patient's poor physical condition or response to handling.

RESTRAINT OF BIRDS

Psittacine Species

When holding and examining a psittacine patient, the medical team should avoid the strong beak, jaws, wings, and feet. The feet usually have sharp, pointed claws, but the beak can cause the most harm to the handler. The equipment needed to capture and handle these patients will include towels or drapes, perches, and nets. Gloves should never be used with psittacine birds in the clinical setting. Gloves are not supple enough for handlers to feel the patient within their grasp and will not protect a finger or hand from the extreme pressure associated with a bite from these patients. Do not use gloves during stressful events with a pet bird because that bird will soon correlate the shape of the human hand with the negative experience of capture and restraint. The handler should first remove water bowls and perches from the cage or carrier. Room lights may be dimmed to take advantage of the bird's inability to rapidly accommodate to changes in lighting. The psittacine bird's primary weapon is the beak; therefore the head should be promptly secured. Placing a towel or drape over the bird's head and holding it with your hand is the best way to quickly secure the head. To prevent the bird from becoming afraid of the towel, you should come toward the bird with the towel covering the grasping hand in a manner in which the bird can see (Figure 7-77, *A* and *B*). By approaching the bird in a nonthreatening manner, you can often capture it with minimal stress. A wooden perch may be used to give the bird something to bite on other than fingers. The bird cannot bite the person attempting to catch it if it is chewing or biting the cage or carrier. If the bird is biting on the cage or carrier, this is an opportune time in which to quickly grab the head of a recalcitrant patient. Once the head is secured, the body is wrapped in the towel, the feet are held, and the bird is placed against the holder's body to control the wings. The towel or drape may be slowly removed from the patient's head for an examination, keeping the towel around the wings to secure them from flapping. Commercially available avian restraint boards allow for secure restraint with minimal risk to the patient or veterinary personnel (Figure 7-78, *A-C*). Care must be maintained to prevent restriction of the chest to allow the bird to properly breathe.

Passerine Species

Canaries and finches are the most common passerine species examined in veterinary offices. These birds are easily stressed under normal conditions and are even more sensitive when they are ill. Catching the patient for an examination must be done in a quick and efficient manner. For an attempt to catch a passerine patient, all lights should be turned off after the cage door is slowly lifted and the hand has been inserted into the cage door opening. Grab the patient with one hand and turn on the lights. To hold the bird for an examination, let the bird's head rest between the middle and index fingers while lying on its back. The fingers should not completely encircle the body but should stay on the sides of the bird. As with other avian species, do not put pressure on the breast, or the patient may suffocate (Figure 7-79). Care should be taken to hold the head straight so the thumb does not slip to the anterior part of the neck and occlude the trachea.

Raptorial Species

Birds of prey use their anatomic weapons in a different way than psittacine species. With raptors, it is of utmost importance for the handler to secure the talons. Although many raptors will bite, their jaws are not tremendously strong, and they do little damage with their beaks. The mouth is soft except the area close to the point of the beak, which the birds use for tearing flesh. The wings should also be considered a weapon and should be properly secured in a manner similar to that described for other avian species. The equipment necessary for restraining raptors includes towels or drapes, gloves of appropriate size and thickness, and hoods.

To approach a bird of prey using gloves, the handler should bend down low and quietly approach the patient. Dimming the lights may be a disadvantage for examining a species that hunts at night. The handler should present as little threat as possible to the raptor. As the handler places one hand in front of the raptor's face, the second hand should be brought in low toward the bird's feet. The upper hand should be held between the handler's face and the bird and may be used to distract the bird. The lower hand should quickly grasp the feet in an attempt to place the index finger between the bird's feet (Figure 7-80). The bird is smoothly and quickly pulled up out of the cage or off of the floor so

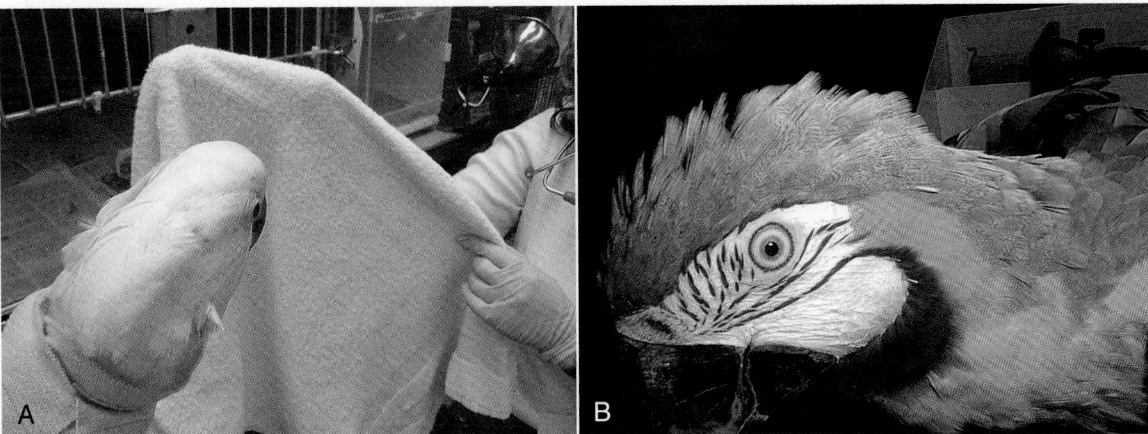

FIGURE 7-77 **A,** Preparing to restrain a cockatoo using a towel. **B,** Headfeathers up and marked constriction of pupils are indications that the patient is unwilling to be restrained.

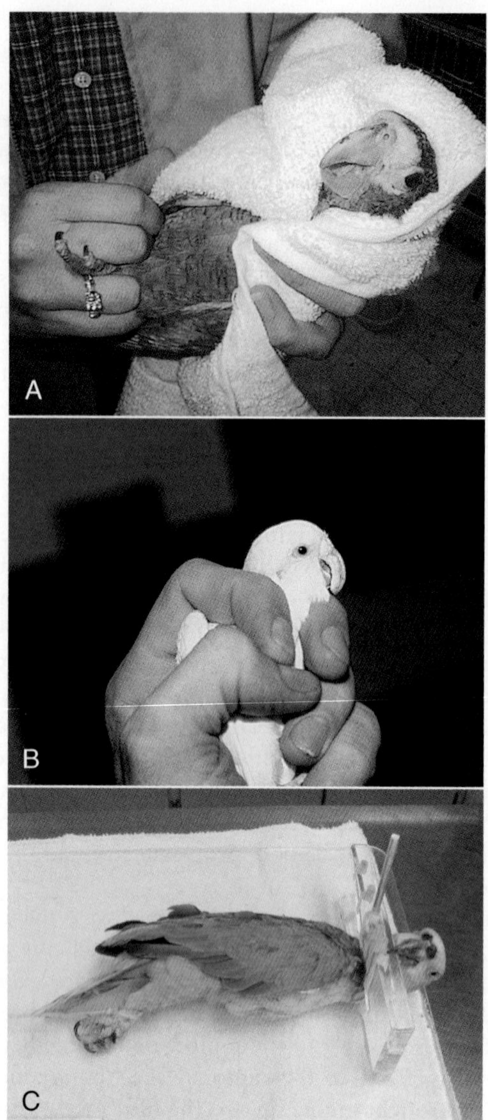

FIGURE 7-78 A, Restraint of a parrot with the use of a towel and an Elizabethan hand grip. B, One-handed restraint techniques can be used for a budgerigar. No pressure is being placed on the pectoral area to allow for breathing. C, Restraint with a commercial avian restraint board.

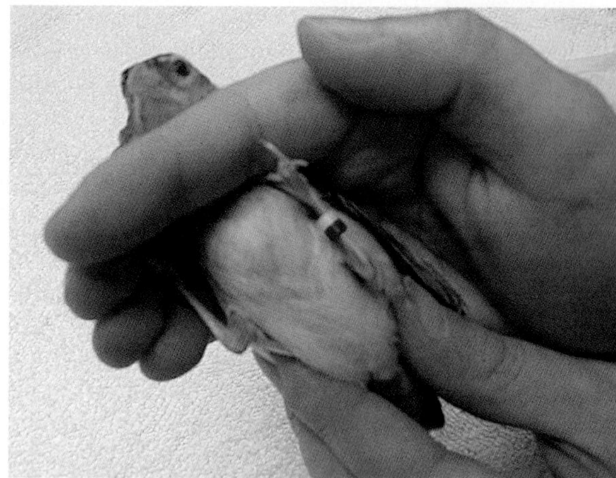

FIGURE 7-79 The proper technique for restraining a passerine for a physical examination.

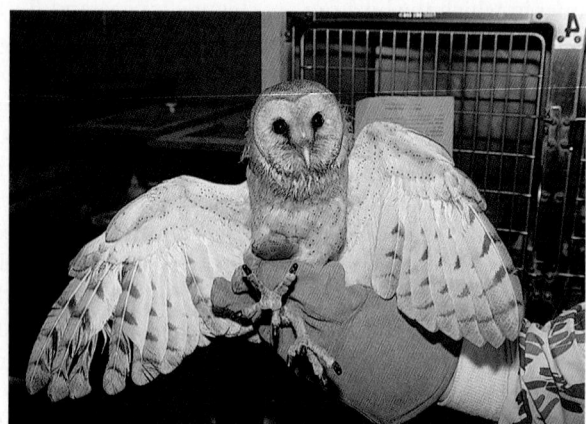

FIGURE 7-80 The restraint of a barn owl with the use of gloves. Note the restraint of the talons.

it does not beat its wings on any surfaces. It is important to hold the bird away from objects, such as the examining table or cage. The bird can be brought into a cradle position, with the wings secured between the handler's arm and body and the hood placed over the bird's head.

If hoods are not available, a towel may be draped over the bird's head, which will reduce visual and auditory stimuli and help to significantly calm the bird. An alternative approach to secure a bird of prey may be done with a towel or drape. The handler approaches the bird in the same manner, quietly and low, with the towel or drape spread in front with both hands. The handler moves in slowly until he or she is close enough to use the towel as a large glove completely covering the bird. The handler's hands should contact the bird at the level of the bird's shoulders. It is important to avoid simply throwing the towel because the bird will be able to dodge it or move from under it. The bird is pressed through the towel with enough pressure to make the bird push up, using its legs on the ground. The handler's hands are worked downward, alongside the wings, toward the legs, and the legs are grasped at the tarsometatarsus (below the hock). Once the bird is covered by the towel and its feet are secured, the handler lifts the bird up with the bird's back toward the handler's abdomen. A hood may replace the towel over the head. It is important never to release the feet of a bird of prey until someone else has secured them. A 10- to 15-cm long piece of 2.5-cm (1-inch) wide white cloth tape should be used to secure the talons to prevent accidents (Figure 7-81). If the bird's talons enter the flesh of a handler, the person restraining the bird must not try to pull away, but relax. The talons will grip a moving object tight, but relax when the object (e.g., arm, prey) is stationary. The taloned handler will have to have another person pry the talons away from their skin. Birds of prey under the control of a falconer are considered a different situation when examined because the

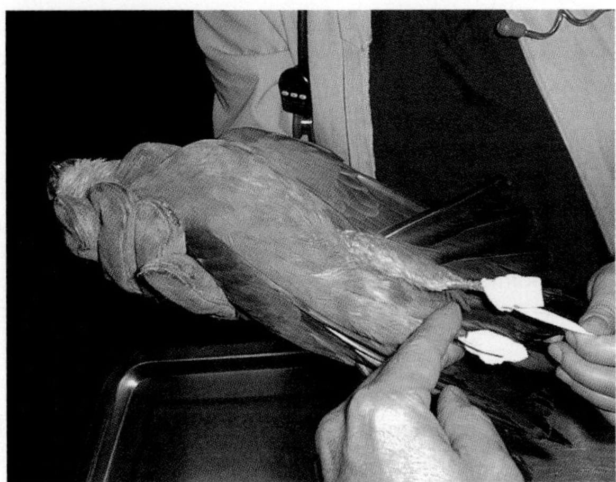

FIGURE 7-81 Taping the talons of raptors using 1-inch white adhesive tape will help protect the technician. Leaving a tab on the end of the taped talon, by folding over the tape, will aid in tape removal at the end of the procedure.

falconer is often adept at restraining the bird for a physical examination.

> *TECHNICIAN NOTE* A 10- to 15-cm long piece of 2.5-cm (1-inch) wide white cloth tape should be used to secure the talons to prevent accidents.

RESTRAINT OF REPTILES

Turtles and Tortoises

The veterinary technician should become as familiar as possible with the anatomic and physiologic adaptations of reptiles to handle them. Several sources of information are found in the recommended reading list at the end of this chapter. Restraint of turtles or tortoises should be done with caution. Some species of turtles have long necks and sharp powerful beaks (rhamphotheca) that can inflict a serious bite on the unwary handler. Some turtles may be able to extend their heads and necks nearly to the level of the hind limbs, two thirds of their body length. Many are quick and should be approached from the rear with the tail and legs securely held. Simply covering the head, neck, and forelimbs with a cloth towel is usually adequate to prevent injury to the turtle and handler. To prevent an animal from walking during an examination, the handler may place it on a broad-based object that will keep the chelonian limbs from touching the examination table surface (Figure 7-82). The legs may be kept in place by wrapping the shell, with the legs inside, with an elastic bandage. Straight ovoid delivery forceps or digital pressure may be used to remove a turtle's head from the shell for an examination (Figure 7-83). Care must be taken; and steady, gentle traction must be used without allowing the forceps to touch the eyes. The main force of the forceps' jaws should be applied away from the shell and not onto the head. Digital pressure is recommended to extend a turtle's or tortoise's head away from the shell over the use of delivery forceps.

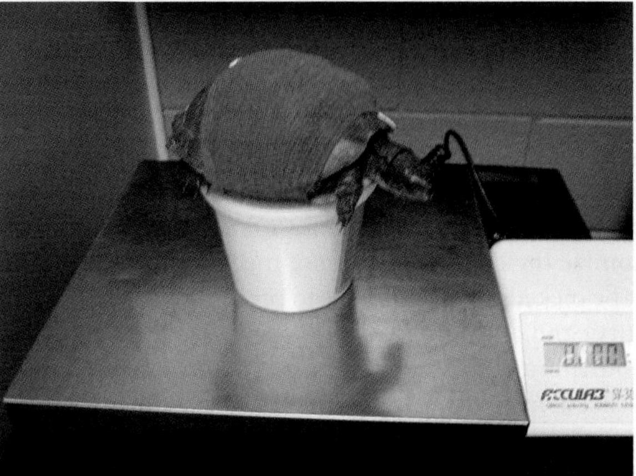

FIGURE 7-82 Placing a turtle or tortoise on a broad-based object will allow for easy handling and short-term restraint.

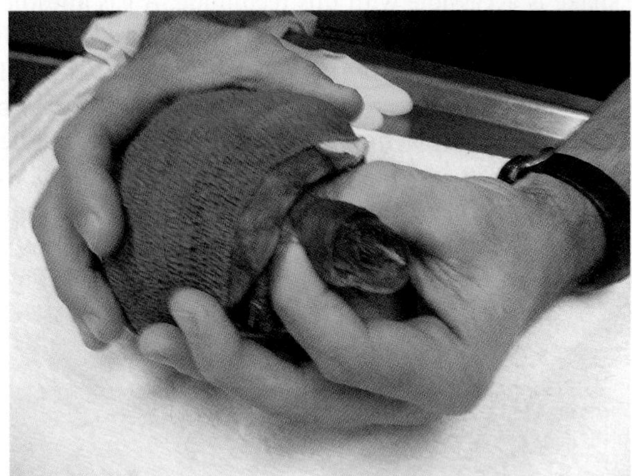

FIGURE 7-83 Gentle traction applied to the turtle's head with the thumb and forefinger is often effective in exposing the patient's head.

> *TECHNICIAN NOTE* Digital pressure is recommended to extend a turtle's or tortoise's head away from the shell over the use of delivery forceps.

Snakes

Snakes are usually more difficult to capture and restrain for the inexperienced technician. The equipment necessary may include Plexiglas shields, Plexiglas tubes, tongs, canvas bags or drapes, snake hooks, a gas anesthetic machine, and plastic bags.

The general approach to restraint of any snake is to immobilize the head and grasp it firmly with the hands at the base of the skull. Several methods may be used to immobilize the animal's head initially; a drape, piece of paper, or Plexiglas shield may be used to block the snake's vision while the hands grasp the animal behind the head (Figure 7-84, *A*). The Plexiglas shield can be held in one hand, pressing the head of the snake to the floor, while the other hand grasps the snake at the base of the skull as the shield is slowly moved rostrally off the body. A snake hook may be used to pin the head to the floor.

When a snake hook is used, a suitable soft and resilient padded surface is useful to prevent trauma to the snake. A hand then replaces the hook. It is possible to injure a reptile by applying too much pressure with the hook; only experienced technicians should use a snake hook on a client's animals. Most snakes can be easily maintained through hand control at the base of the skull. A few snake species can autotomize their tails as a defense mechanism. Snakes should not be picked up by their tails to prevent skin loss (degloving injury) and autotomization. Plexiglas tubes may be used in conjunction with a hook or pole. The hook is used to guide the snake into the Plexiglas tube, and the tube should be of a sufficiently small diameter to prevent the snake from turning around and coming back out. The aim is to get the snake to crawl up the tube; when it reaches the halfway point, the technician grasps the junction of the snake and the tube, trapping the snake's head within the tube. The caudal half of the snake is accessible with this technique. A gas anesthetic unit may be attached to the open end of the tube for further restraint. Plastic tubes are not generally recommended for many elapine snake species (e.g., coral snakes, cobras) because of their ability to turn around and injure the handler.

Placing snakes in a plastic bag or box and filling it with anesthetic gases may also induce anesthesia. After the induction of anesthesia, snakes are intubated and monitored on a gas anesthetic machine with intermittent ventilation (Figure 7-84, *B*). Snakes can be easily transported in canvas bags.

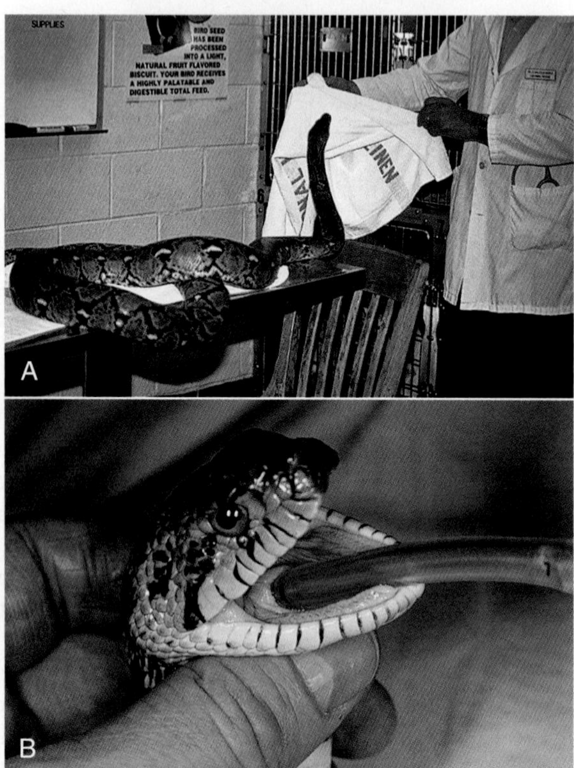

FIGURE 7-84 **A,** A towel may be used to block a snake's vision before grasping it from behind the head. **B,** Proper technique of holding a snake's head as an endotracheal tube is placed. These handlers are demonstrating restraint and passage of a stomach tube on a common boa constrictor.

When a snake is handled, its body should always be supported, and large species should always be handled by more than one person.

> *TECHNICIAN NOTE* It is possible to injure a reptile by applying too much pressure with the hook; only experienced technicians should use a snake hook on a client's animals.

Lizards and Crocodilians

Lizards and crocodilians may be restrained by using a combination of experience, snare poles, towels, drapes, nooses, or Plexiglas shields. All lizards will bite, and some have strong jaws and sharp teeth. Most lizards will also use their claws and tails as weapons. The approach for small-to-medium lizards is to attempt to block their vision with a towel or sheet of paper, make a quick grab around the shoulder girdle at the base of the skull with one hand, and restrain the pelvic girdle with the other hand. The tail may be tucked in against the body, under the arm (Figure 7-85).

A noose made of fine fish line at the end of a pole may be used for small lizards. The noose is lowered over the animal's neck, the pole is quickly lifted with the noose tightened, and the animal is lifted by the neck. The animal should be restrained and removed from the noose as quickly as possible. For a large lizard or crocodilian, it is important to block the animal's vision and quickly and safely immobilize the head and body simultaneously. This is best accomplished by grasping the animal at the base of the skull or neck with one or both hands, then sitting on it. Two or more people are needed to accomplish this task, and the animal's mouth should be taped shut as soon as it is restrained. A noose or rabies pole may be used to help control the mouth before attempts to restrain the head, legs, and tail are made. Crocodilians, most large lizards, and some chelonians can be immobilized for short periods (up to 30 seconds) by the application of gentle, inward pressure on their closed eyes for a few moments. The

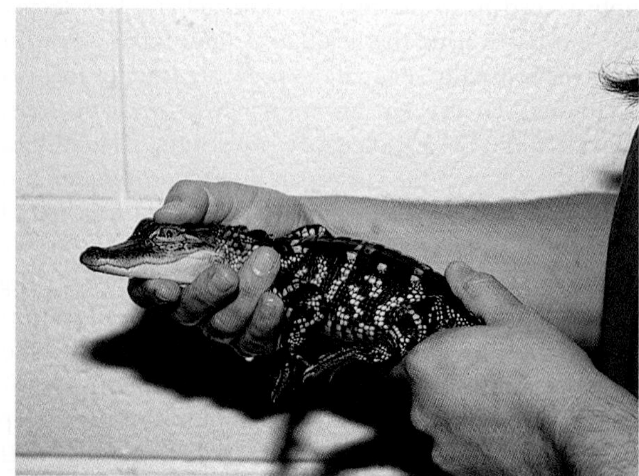

FIGURE 7-85 The proper restraint technique for a large lizard (tegu). One hand is placed firmly about the pelvis, and the other is about the shoulders and neck. The tail may be tucked beneath the elbow.

handler is cautioned that many lizards, particularly gecko species, have tails that autotomize when they are stressed or traumatized (Figure 7-86). Extreme caution should be used when lizard tails are handled.

> *TECHNICIAN NOTE* The handler is cautioned that many lizards, particularly gecko species, have tails that autotomize when they are stressed or traumatized (see Figure 7-86).

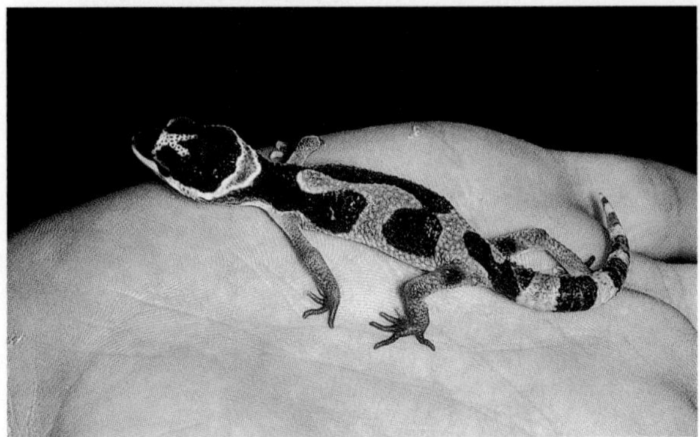

FIGURE 7-86 Great care must be used when restraining and treating patients that easily autotomize their tails, such as this gecko.

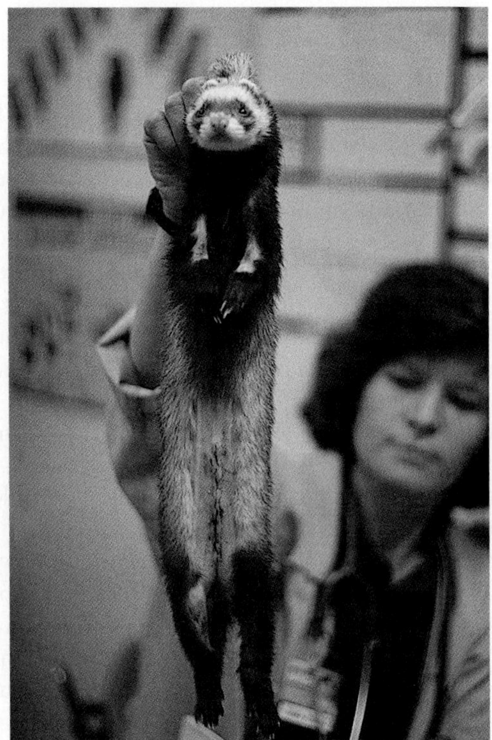

FIGURE 7-87 The proper technique to restrain a ferret. The scruff of the neck is held by one hand, and the other supports the body. Often this technique will elicit a "yawn," at which time the oral cavity may be examined.

RESTRAINT OF FERRETS

Ferrets that are not cooperative are a restraint challenge. Ferrets belong to the family group that includes weasels, and as such, they are quick, agile animals possessing sharp teeth. The ferret's primary weapons are its teeth, and when threatened, it will not hesitate to bite. Ferrets that are hand raised, which includes most pets, can make docile companion animals in the right circumstances. Proper precautions should be taken when restraining ferrets.

Primary restraint for a ferret is to secure the head and forelegs by gripping the animal by the skin in the dorsal cervical area (the scruff of the neck) (Figure 7-87). The other hand is used to support the bottom of the animal. For the highly aggressive ferret, a towel or drape may be placed over the animal to block its vision. The animal's head, neck, and shoulders can be grasped through the drape or towel. The handler may want to use gloves. Remember, it is not good for any pet animal to associate negative experiences with gloved hands. Once the animal is restrained with this method, the handler may alter the grip on the head to perform a thorough physical examination and other necessary diagnostic procedures. Ferrets may be "stretched" in a manner similar to that used for cats, or they may be grasped with both hands around the forequarters with one hand on the scruff of the neck and the other holding down the forelegs.

Ferrets are subject to hypnosis, although it is less likely to be effective when an animal is apprehensive in strange hands. For an attempt at hypnosis, a ferret is hung by the scruff with one hand and stroked around the entire length of its torso with the other hand. The susceptible ferret will begin to yawn, and its eyelids will droop or close after repeated stroking. The effect is not long lasting, and many ferrets will be easily startled out of the trance.

> *TECHNICIAN NOTE* Remember, it is not good for any pet animal to associate negative experiences with gloved hands.

RESTRAINT OF RABBITS

Proper rabbit restraint is important in reducing stress and injury to the patient (Figure 7-88, *A*). Rabbits have some peculiarities for restraint. Their muscle-to-skeleton ratio is high, and their bones are small and light for animals of their size. Rabbits also have extremely powerful hind legs. Restraint of rabbits without controlling their hind legs may precipitate a kicking episode that could result in a "broken back." This terminology is not precise because the bones of the back may not be fractured, but there is a definite loss of neural function in the hindquarters that results from trauma to the spinal cord. The hind legs become paralyzed, and bladder and anal tone are lost. The prognosis for recovery is poor in cases of total paralysis. Paralysis may be immediate

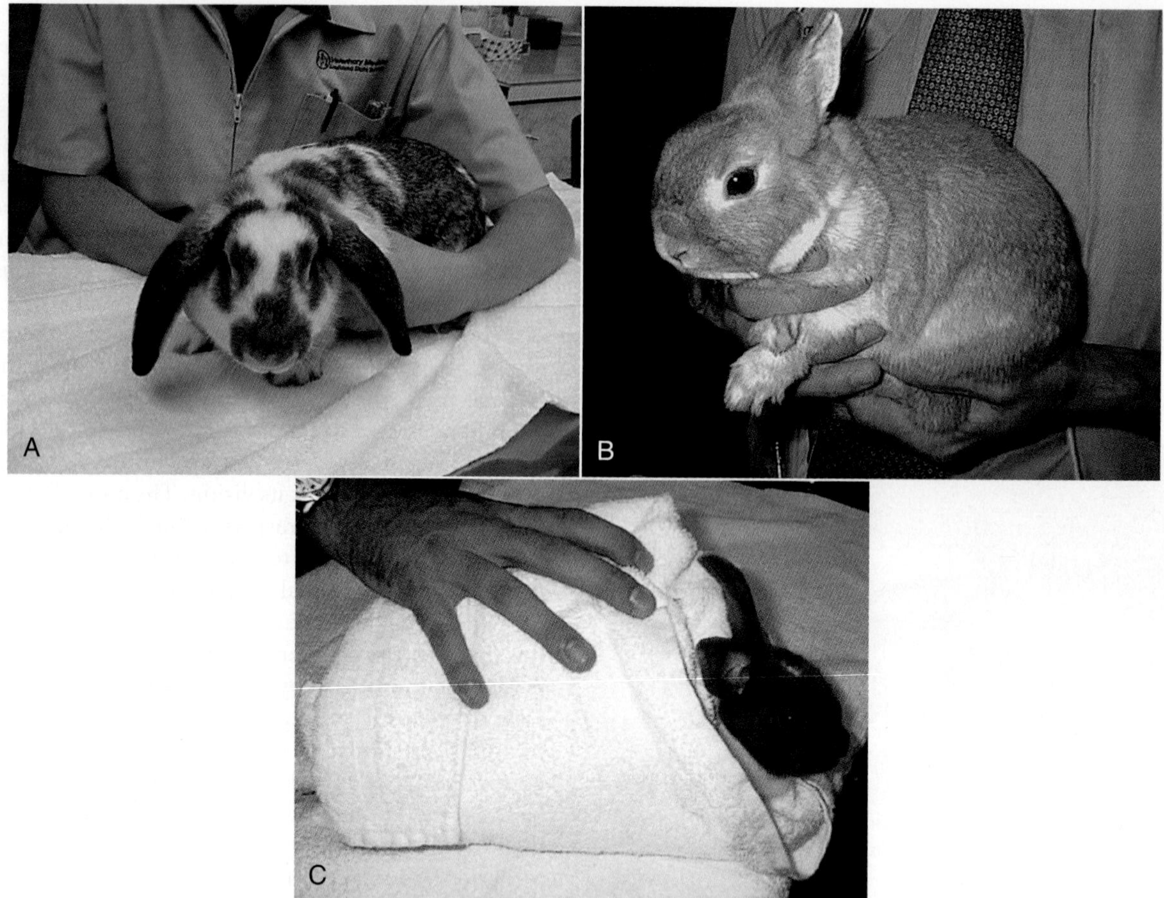

FIGURE 7-88 **A,** Proper holding technique for a rabbit undergoing a physical examination. **B,** The proper method of restraint for carrying a rabbit short distances. **C,** Wrapping a rabbit in a towel or "bunny burrito" is an effective way to restrain a fractious patient.

or delayed, depending on the amount of hemorrhage and edema that surrounds the spinal cord.

> *TECHNICIAN NOTE* Restraint of rabbits without controlling their hind legs may precipitate a kicking episode that could result in a "broken back."

To prevent this situation, never pick up, carry, or restrain a rabbit by its ears. To carry a rabbit short distances, grasp the nape of the neck skin with one hand while supporting the rear legs with the other (see Figure 7-88, *B*). The best way to re-place a rabbit in a cage is by holding its skin fore and aft, placing it well inside the cage facing outward, and pressing its body down to the floor for a few moments before releasing it. Use of this technique forces the rabbit to turn in its cage before leaping to the safety of the rear of the cage. The ears should never be used to lift a rabbit of any age. Small plastic pet carriers should be used when rabbits are carried for long distances. A towel can be placed around the rabbit to help with restraint when the animal is carried or examined (see Figure 7-88, *C*).

Rabbits do not like slick surfaces, and losing their footing agitates them. It is best to set them down on something on which they will have good traction, such as a rubber mat, during an examination or treatment. Pressing the rabbit to the table and pulling the hind feet to the rear allow for trimming of nails. The nails of the forefeet may be trimmed by lifting one foot at a time off the table while the rabbit is held to the surface. When on the examination table, rabbits must be secured at all times to prevent the patient from jumping off and being injured from the fall to the floor.

Rabbits have sensitive whiskers and will flinch whenever these hairs are touched or the mouth is approached. For an examination of the mouth, the head must be firmly held. To steady the head for an examination, the holder should place the rabbit facing away from his or her body with the forearms pressing down the entire length of the rabbit. The thumbs of the handler are placed behind the ears of the rabbit, and the fingers are used to lift the head from below the mandible. The incisor teeth may be trimmed, aural examinations may be conducted, and ear venipuncture may be performed with the rabbit in this position.

Rabbits will bite; therefore a conscious effort should be made to keep fingers away from the rabbit's mouth. Normally the fight goes out of even the most aggressive rabbit once its forequarters are pressed to the floor and the body is restrained from free movement.

> *TECHNICIAN NOTE* Rabbits will bite; therefore a conscious effort should be made to keep fingers away from the rabbit's mouth.

RESTRAINT OF RODENTS AND SMALL MAMMALS

Rodents and small mammals can be problematic to examine and treat because restraint without injuring such animals is difficult. These animals are generally small and may bite when placed in a stressful situation. Commercial restraint devices are available for small rodents, but it is difficult to perform a good external examination because of their design. To catch these small animals, a technician can use bare hands or leather gloves. However, the teeth of rodents will penetrate leather gloves, so protection is minimal and may be more psychologic than physical for the handler.

Cornering or encircling the animal with both hands will allow the handler to capture a large rodent. Both hands should be used to pick the animal up with the fingers underneath and the thumbs on top of the body. One hand should be behind the other to support the entire abdomen. Grasping the scruff of the neck and supporting the back legs provide restraint for larger rodents (e.g., guinea pigs, chinchillas, prairie dogs) (Figure 7-89). A large rodent that is standing on the examination table can also be restrained by wrapping a towel around its torso. Guinea pigs are different than most small mammals when restrained in that they can be quite vocal. Pregnant guinea pigs have pendulant bellies, and they may be lifted by grasping around the thorax with one hand and around the rump with the other to hold them up. The teeth of the guinea pig may be clipped by holding the head with one or two hands with the forefinger under the jaw and the thumb behind the head. The guinea pig tolerates being placed upside down in a trough with the legs tied down in the same fashion as swine.

> *TECHNICIAN NOTE* However, the teeth of rodents will penetrate leather gloves, so protection is minimal and may be more psychologic than physical for the handler.

Smaller rodents and mammals are initially restrained by grabbing the tail (e.g., mouse, rat) or the scruff of the neck (hamsters, sugar gliders, gerbils) (Figures 7-90 and 7-91).

Hedgehogs are covered with sharp spines, and most will require anesthesia when examinations need to be performed or diagnostic samples need to be obtained (Figure 7-92). Once restrained, these small patients are held by the scruff or around the neck with one hand while the other hand supports the body. Hamsters have a large amount of redundant tissue associated with the cheek pouches, and this must be gathered up in the hand to hold them. Most small rodents may be restricted from movement on a surface by placing a hand over them to form a cage with the head protruding between the first and second fingers. If a small rodent suddenly attempts to bite, it may be caught and restrained by driving it into a small tube. Rodent restraint tunnels are available in several sizes; usually they are made of Plexiglas and have several ports available for injection.

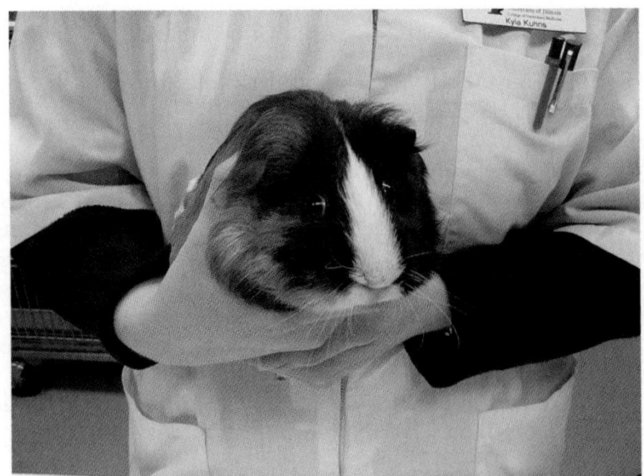

FIGURE 7-89 The proper restraint technique for a guinea pig.

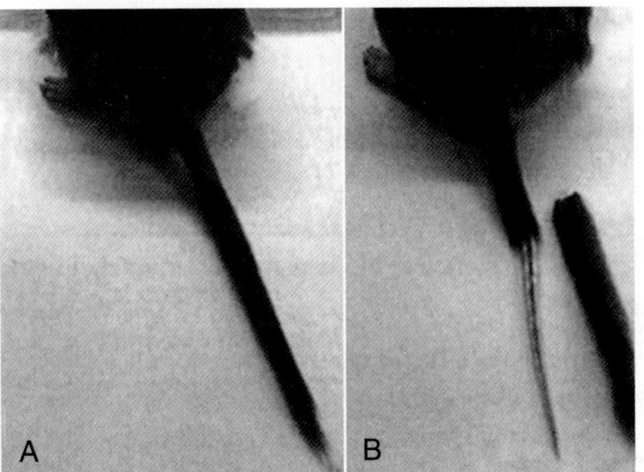

FIGURE 7-90 **A,** A normal gerbil tail, which should never be used to capture a gerbil. **B,** The skin has sloughed off the tail of this gerbil, which will require a surgical amputation to correct.

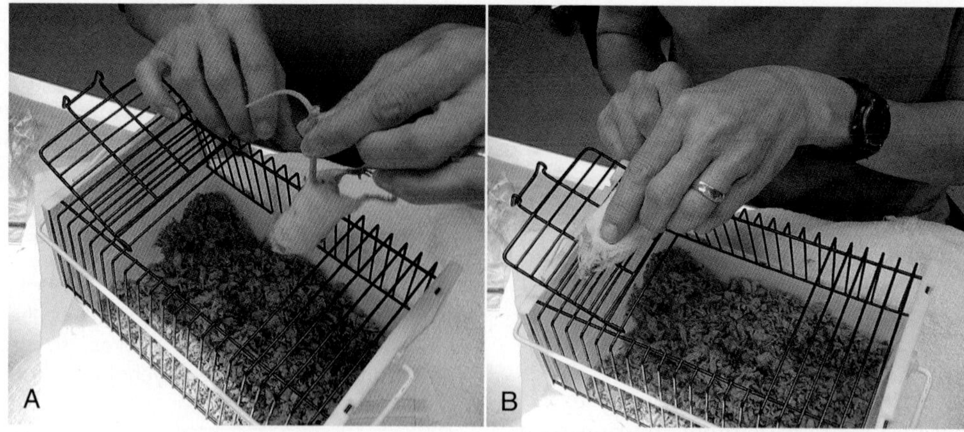

FIGURE 7-91 Grasping a mouse by the tail as it holds onto its cage (A) will allow one to grasp the back of the neck for adequate restraint (B).

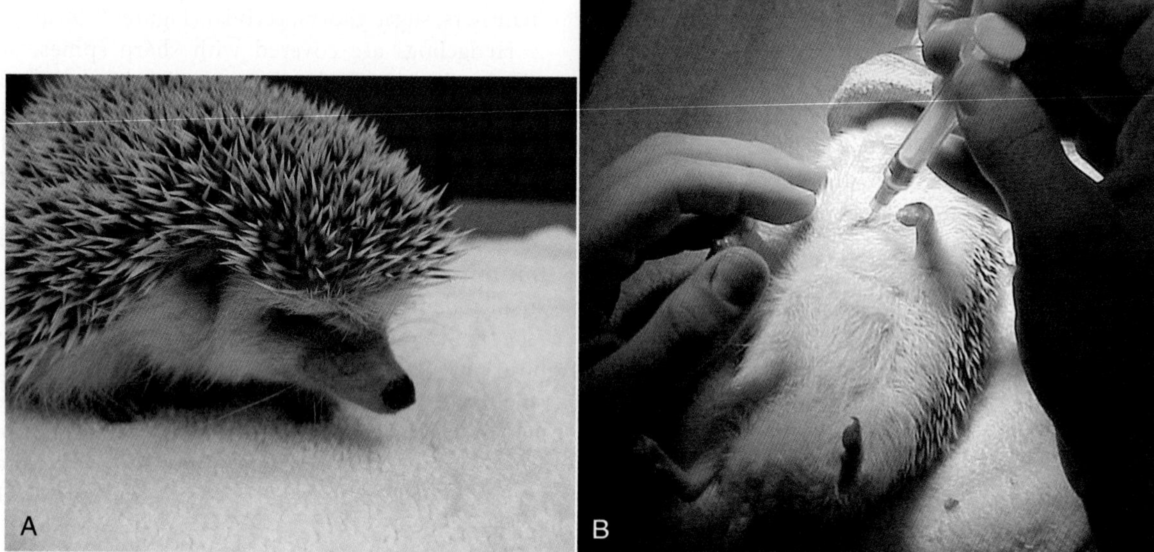

FIGURE 7-92 A, Hedgehogs are covered in sharp spines. B, They often need to be anesthetized for examination or handled with thin leather gloves.

RECOMMENDED READING

American Association for Laboratory Animal Science: *LATG Training Manual,* 2006, AALAS.

Beaver B: *Canine behavior: Insights and answers,* ed 2, Philadelphia, 2008, Saunders.

Beaver B: *Feline behavior: A guide for veterinarians,* ed 2, Philadelphia, 2003, Saunders.

Donaldson J: *The culture clash: A revolutionary new way to understanding the relationship between humans and domestic dogs,* Berkley, 1996, James and Kenneth Publishers.

Fowler ME: *Restraint and handling of wild and domestic animals,* ed 3, Ames, IA, 2008, Wiley-Blackwell.

Fraser AF: *Farm animal behavior and welfare,* ed 3, Oxfordshire, UK, 1996, CABI.

Keeling LJ, Gonyou, HW: Social behavior of farm animals, ed 1, Oxfordshire, UK, 2001, CABI

Kiley-Worthington M: *The behavior of horses in relation to management and training,* London, 1987, JA Allen.

Landsberg G, Hunthausen W, Ackerman L: Handbook of behavior problems in the dog and cat, ed 2, Philadelphia, 2004, Elsevier Ltd.

McGreevy P: Equine *Behavior: A guide for veterinarians and equine scientists,* Philadelphia, 2004, Saunders Ltd.

Pyror, K: *Don't shoot the dog,* New York, 1999, Bantam.

Roberts M: *The man who listens to horses,* New York, 1997, Random House.

Sheldon CC, Sonsthagen T, Topel JA: *Animal restraint for veterinary professionals,* St Louis, 2006, Mosby.

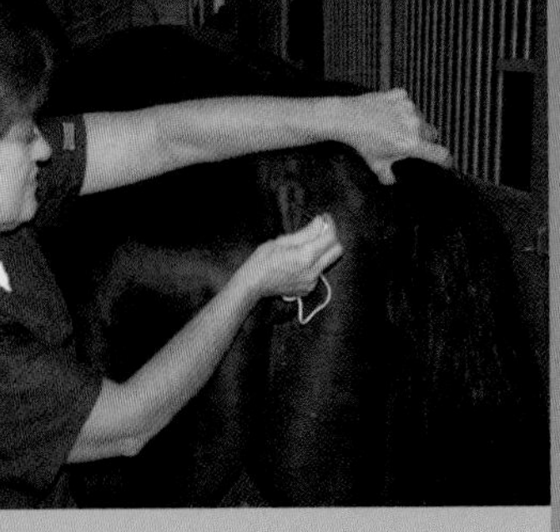

History and Physical Examination

8

Mark P. Rondeau, Rebecca B. Marquardt, and Elizabeth A. Hanie

KEY TERMS

Ataxia
Borborygmus
Colitis
Glucosuria
Hyperthermia
Hypothermia
Hypovolemia
Icterus
Ileus
Pleural effusion
Polydipsic
Pruritic
Shock
Signalment
Stertor
Stridor

OUTLINE

LEARNING OBJECTIVES

When you have completed this chapter, you will be able to:

1. Explain the role of the veterinary technician in obtaining the patient's medical history.
2. List questions commonly used to obtain a patient's medical history for small and large animals.
3. List the sections of information found in a medical history for small animal patients.
4. Describe the type of information contained in each section of the patient's medical history for small animals.
5. List the sections of information found in a medical history for large animal patients.
6. Describe the type of information contained in each section of the patient's medical history for large animals.
7. Describe the general procedures used to obtain a physical examination in dogs and cats.
8. Describe the general procedures used to obtain a physical examination in horses and cattle.
9. Discuss the methods for performing a comprehensive evaluation of each of the body systems.
10. List and describe unique procedures used in the examination of horses and cattle.

INTRODUCTION

History and physical examination are the first steps in the evaluation of any patient or group of patients. Information obtained from these processes provides the basis for all subsequent diagnostic and therapeutic plans. It is essential that veterinary technicians are able to obtain complete and accurate historical information in both individual patient and herd assessments. Similarly, good physical examination skills will allow rapid identification of significant problems and allow for appropriate therapeutic measures to ensue. This can be lifesaving in emergency situations. The following chapter will stress the importance of a systematic approach to both obtaining historical information and performing a physical examination. The use of such an approach will help ensure that all pertinent information and physical abnormalities will be identified in every case. There are significant differences in performing both a patient's history and physical examination between small animals and large animals. However, the basic premise that this information is an imperative part of the initial database in veterinary medicine holds true for all species.

HISTORY AND PHYSICAL EXAMINATION OF SMALL ANIMALS

HISTORY

Obtaining a complete history is the first step toward creating a diagnostic and therapeutic plan for most veterinary patients. Pertinent historical information is an important part of a complete and accurate assessment of the patient. The veterinary technician should be sure to ask questions that clarify the nature of current and previous clinical problems and that confirm the accuracy of the information. This may require asking the same question more than once and repeating responses back to the owner asking, "Do I have this correct?" Despite its importance, obtaining a thorough history is often overlooked by both veterinarians and veterinary technicians.

Obtaining a thorough history in a clear and organized manner is the foundation of a comprehensive patient's evaluation, but it can be challenging to do. For example, there are owners from whom it is difficult to extract information because they either say too little or talk incessantly about unrelated issues. In addition, the person presenting the patient to the practice may not be the patient's owner and may not know the answers to the questions you are asking. Finally, certain problems or disease states may require specifically tailored questions. The goal of this discussion is to present an organized approach for obtaining a complete and accurate history for each and every patient. This method serves as a foundation upon which questions, based on the owner's knowledge and the patient's specific complaints and preexisting diseases, can be added.

> *TECHNICIAN NOTE* Using a consistent, organized system for obtaining historical information about each and every patient is important to ensure that nothing is overlooked.

THE ROLE OF THE VETERINARY TECHNICIAN

The veterinary technician who is capable of obtaining a complete and accurate history can play a critical role in a busy veterinary practice. Obtaining information from clients is often time consuming, and veterinary technicians who can do this well free veterinarians to complete other work. The information that is obtained, however, is only useful if it is complete and accurate. Acquiring inaccurate information could be worse than obtaining no historical information at all. Faulty information might result in unnecessary diagnostic tests, treatments, and lost client trust. To optimize the likelihood that the information obtained is complete and accurate, technicians must gain the trust of the client.

Developing Rapport With the Client

When obtaining a medical history, the first step is to introduce yourself to the client and explain what you are doing so the client feels comfortable and is willing to share information with you. Always be certain to know the client's name and the pet's name and sex to prevent embarrassing mistakes when referring to the client or patient. In situations where the pet has been taken away from the client before obtaining the history (e.g., taken to the treatment area for cardiovascular stabilization following trauma), it is essential that you reassure the owner about the pet's status before asking questions. If the client is worried that his pet is in danger, he will not be able to focus on you and give you the information you need. Once you have established a rapport with the client, obtaining complete and accurate information will be easier. The next challenge is to ask questions in an effective manner.

Asking the Questions

The most important aspect of taking a history is to understand and respect the pet owner. Some owners have medical training and can be spoken to using medical jargon; however, the majority of owners do not understand medical terminology, and the veterinary technician must be careful to use simple language without belittling the client. For example, if the technician is doing a follow-up examination of a diabetic cat, whose owner is checking the urine daily for glucose, it would be inappropriate to ask, "Have you noted **glucosuria** since your previous visit?" It would be equally inappropriate to ask, "Is the little square pad on your dipstick changing color when you dip it in Fluffy's pee pee?" Finding words that are appropriate for the client is important so that he feels neither confused nor insulted. Technicians are safest asking "Has the urine strip been positive for sugar since your previous visit?" It is important to strike an appropriate balance and tailor your questions to the individual client to avoid losing trust.

It is also important to ask open-ended questions, rather than leading questions. An open-ended question is one that requires the client to fill in the information themselves, whereas a leading question is one that potentially guides her to an answer. For example, if you are trying to determine whether a pet is **polydipsic** it is best to ask the open-ended question, "Have you noticed any changes in his water intake during this illness?" rather than "Has he been drinking more water than usual?" When leading questions are asked, clients sense which response the interviewer prefers and are likely to give it; pet owners are anxious to help resolve their animal's problems. Needless to say, asking leading questions can generate inaccurate historical information.

When questioning clients, try to avoid being judgmental of their care and management of their pet because this may make them feel uncomfortable about giving truthful answers. The questions you ask should not show your biases or personal beliefs. For example, when questioning an owner about his dog that has acute vomiting and diarrhea, it would be unhelpful to ask, "You don't feed her table scraps, do you?" Faced with that question, an owner is likely to say, "No, of course not," even if she really does feed her pet table scraps. It would be better to ask, "What is her normal diet?" or "Did she eat anything outside of her normal diet recently?" or "What human food does she typically eat?" Making the client feel comfortable with their decisions will improve the chances that you receive accurate information.

> *TECHNICIAN NOTE* Explaining your position and role to clients and tailoring your questions to their level of understanding will allow you to gain the client's trust and obtain more detailed information.

Documenting the Information

Historical information is useless unless it is written carefully, neatly, and accurately in a structured medical record form. All veterinary hospitals should have a standardized history form as part of the medical record, which allows efficient recording of the information presented (see Figure 5-7, *A* in Chapter 5). This form should also provide prompts to remind you to obtain certain pieces of information. The information should be recorded in the medical record as it is obtained to prevent any subsequent misunderstanding. In addition, it should be written legibly or typed using appropriate medical terminology, and it should be clearly organized. Keep in mind that the medical record is a legal document, and, as such, should be written with the utmost care and precision. The medical history will provide a reference for the veterinary health care team as it implements and revises its diagnostic and treatment plans for the patient.

THE INFORMATION

The following sections provide a general listing of important information that should be obtained in most medical histories. Some additions or deletions may be appropriate in specific cases. This is meant to serve as a guideline to ensure that complete and accurate historical information is obtained in an efficient manner.

> *TECHNICIAN NOTE* The major focus of any medical history is the presenting complaint; however, it is equally important to obtain general background information.

Signalment

Every patient record should contain the pet's **signalment,** which includes age, breed (or dominant breed if mixed), sex, and reproductive status (spayed or neutered). It is important to confirm the signalment during the first meeting with the client because this information often provides important clues about the case. Certain diseases appear more commonly in animals of certain signalments. For example, congenital diseases are more likely to be diagnosed in very young patients than in very old patients.

Background Information

General Management

The background information should begin with a discussion of how long the pet has been owned and where and when it was obtained. Any previous medical problems should be recorded. If it was obtained from a breeder, it may be useful to note whether the client still has contact with the breeder and if she knows of any diseases present in related dogs. When discussing the pet's origins, ask if there has been any recent travel away from the pet's normal living areas. This information is most important when there is a suspicion of a disease that is endemic to a region where the pet has visited within the past 6 months.

This is also a good time to find out where the pet is kept during the day and what its normal routine is. If it is kept indoors, is it in a crate or restricted to a certain part of the home? If it is kept outdoors, is it in a fenced yard or allowed to run free? You should always get a thorough diet history at this time. This should include the type of food eaten, the amount, and the frequency. It is also important to note if there have been any recent changes in the diet or if the animal was fed anything unusual (or if it got into something it should not have) just before the onset of illness.

Preventive Medicine

Complete information regarding vaccination history should be obtained if the pet is not a previous patient. Note which vaccines were given, when they were given, and the expiration date of the vaccine. This is the time to also ask about other preventative medications, such as heartworm and flea and tick prevention. Information regarding the consistency with which these medications are given is important as is whether they are given year round or only during warmer months. When discussing flea and tick medication, it is also a good idea to ask whether the owner has seen fleas or ticks on the pet.

Behavioral Information

Ascertain what the pet's normal behavior is on a day-to-day basis and, more importantly, note any changes in the behavior relative to the illness. This is helpful in several ways. First, it lets you know if the pet is aggressive toward people or other animals, which may affect how you handle the animal when it comes time for a physical examination or hospitalization. Second, it allows you to determine if any behavior changes may explain the underlying illness, such as increased aggression, disorientation, unusual elimination habits, and so on.

Household Information

The health status of the other members of the patient's household can be important in determining the cause of the pet's illness, especially in cases of infectious disease. Determine to what extent the pet is exposed to other animals: what species, how many, and for what duration. You should also determine whether any of those animals are ill, regardless of whether the symptoms are similar to those of the presenting patient. Remember to ask questions about illnesses among the humans in the family. This is especially important in some cases of infectious dermatologic disease, such as sarcoptic mange, and may also provide information regarding the patient's exposure to toxins, such as medication belonging to family members.

Allergy History

Before instituting any medical therapy, it is important to note any known allergies or other adverse reactions to medications or food that the pet may have experienced. Even if these reactions have not been confirmed to be related to the exposure in question, they are important to note. Avoidance of medications to which there is even a suspicion of an allergy is sensible. At this time, also inquire about prior blood product transfusions and reactions. You should ask whether the pet has ever received a blood product transfusion. If they have, attempt to determine what product, when it was administered, if there was any adverse reaction, and if the pet's blood type is known. This information will help guide any subsequent blood product therapy.

Reproductive History

Although the current reproductive status of the patient will be noted in the signalment as discussed earlier, it is important to ask for historical information regarding the patient's prior reproductive history. If an animal is neutered, it is important to note at what age the procedure was performed. This information may pertain to disease prevalence. For example, mammary tumors are much more common in female dogs after they have gone through a single heat than if they are spayed before their first heat. If an animal is not neutered, you should ask if it is currently being bred and if it has previously been bred. The timing of the most recent heat cycle should be noted for all intact female dogs because **pyometra** occurs most commonly 2 weeks to 2 months following a heat cycle.

Past Pertinent Medical History

Identify any prior medical problems that the pet has experienced. Recurrent bouts of similar problems may represent a serious chronic disease. Some previous historical problems may be of no significance to the current presentation. Those problems can be ignored. However, if a problem sounds like it may be relevant to the current complaint, you will have the opportunity to question the owner more thoroughly about it.

Presenting Complaint

The presenting or chief complaint is the most important information to be addressed in the medical history. Every patient will have a presenting complaint, and owners are often anxious to discuss this. During emergencies, it is important to quickly obtain information regarding the presenting complaint before obtaining any background information because time is of the essence in treating life-threatening problems. The presenting complaint can be obtained simply by asking, "What brings you to the practice today?" A patient may have more than one presenting complaint. In this case it is best to record and discuss each complaint separately. Do not assume that all of the symptoms can be tied to one medical disorder.

> TECHNICIAN NOTE In emergency situations where rapid patient stabilization is necessary, information regarding the presenting complaint should always be obtained first to assist in generating an immediate treatment plan for the patient.

Last Normal

A good way to get a sense of the duration of a problem is to ask the client, "When would you say your pet was last normal?" This often helps the client recall a pleasant time when the pet was acting normally, which is easier than trying to remember how long the pet has been sick. The duration of each presenting complaint varies. Constructing a chronologic timeline is helpful to finding a diagnosis.

Progression

Once you have established a problem list, determine the order in which each problem appeared and how long each one lasted. Also ascertain how each problem has progressed. In other words, are the problems better, worse, or the same? This information may be helpful when constructing a diagnostic and therapeutic plan. A problem that is rapidly worsening may warrant a more aggressive course of therapy than a problem that is stable or improving.

Systems Review

The client should be asked a series of questions that reviews each of the pet's basic body systems. Some of these questions may have already been answered when discussing the presenting complaint, in which case they should not be repeated. However, some of the questions may provide information that would otherwise be overlooked by the owner because they are so focused on the presenting complaint. All clients should be asked about the presence of coughing, sneezing, vomiting, diarrhea, polyuria, and polydipsia. Current appetite and energy level should be addressed. Any perceived weight loss or weight gain should be noted.

Medications

Every client must be asked what medications, if any, they are currently giving their pet. This information should be as complete as possible. The goal should be to find out the following: type, dose and frequency for each medication, the duration for which it has been given, the reason it is being given, and whether it has provided benefit to the pet. In situations where all of this information is not known by the owner, you should obtain as much of the information as possible. In addition to conventional medication, you must always ask about any vitamins or dietary supplements that are given to the pet. Ask specifically about the use of topical eye and ear preparations and of medicated shampoos; some owners do not think of these as medications. Finally, be sure to review any preventative medications that are being given, such as heartworm and flea and tick products.

PHYSICAL EXAMINATION

A thorough physical examination is often the first and most important diagnostic test performed on a patient. Because we must rely on an owner's interpretation of their pet's illness and because the symptoms pets show are often vague, the physical examination may be more important than the medical history in determining the source of illness. The key to a good physical examination is to carefully complete all parts of the examination every time you perform it. You should perform all aspects of the physical examination in the same order in every patient. Developing this sort of routine will prevent you from forgetting to evaluate one area because you are overly focused on another. The routine you develop may need to vary slightly from patient to patient. You will find that certain areas of the examination will be covered more carefully in some patients than in others. For example, a complete neurologic examination may be unnecessary on a patient that is seen for coughing and is ambulating normally with no historical complaints about the nervous system. Similarly, in a patient that has hind limb paralysis, you may limit your respiratory examination to a brief auscultation and spend more time performing a complete neurologic examination, including reflex testing. The key is to perform some evaluation of every system during every examination. The guidelines in the following paragraphs provide one example of the method by which a physical examination could be performed, but you can develop your own routine as you become more experienced. As long as you follow the same routine every time you perform a physical examination, you can be sure that your examination will be thorough.

> TECHNICIAN NOTE As with the patient's history, following a consistent routine for every physical examination will prevent you from overlooking an important finding.

DOCUMENTING THE INFORMATION

As discussed for the medical history, the physical examination must be documented appropriately. All veterinary hospitals should have a standardized physical examination form as part of the medical record (see Figure 5-7, *B* in Chapter 5). This form should have areas for recording body weight, temperature, pulse rate, and respiratory rate. It should also provide prompts to remind you to examine each of the body systems discussed later and specified areas to record that information. As with any part of a medical record, the recorded information should be typed or legibly written, medical terminology should be used, and the content should always remain professional. Information should be documented in as much detail as possible so that the findings can be compared with those of future physical examinations.

> TECHNICIAN NOTE Historical and physical examination findings should be recorded thoroughly, professionally, and legibly in every patient's medical record.

SURROUNDINGS

Every physical examination should begin with a subjective assessment of the patient in its surroundings. Several pieces of useful information can be obtained just with a quick visual inspection of the animal from a distance as it behaves in the waiting room, examination room, or kennel. You can determine a general sense for the animal's **mentation.** Is the patient bright, alert, and responsive? Is the patient quiet but alert and responsive? These states may suggest a less emergent condition. Is the patient dull, depressed, or even unresponsive? These states could indicate more serious disease or neurologic dysfunction. In addition to the mentation, you can visually inspect the animal as it rests for increases in respiratory rate or effort. While the animal walks, quickly look for evidence of lameness, **ataxia,** or visual deficits. You may be able to identify any asymmetry or swelling of the patient. This is a good time to evaluate the body condition of the patient and assign a **body condition score**. The list of things that you can identify with a careful visual inspection is extensive. All of this information is important to determine before moving forward with the remainder of your physical examination.

> TECHNICIAN NOTE Taking a brief minute to observe the patient in its surroundings before performing a physical examination can provide important information.

TEMPERATURE, PULSE, AND RESPIRATION

The measurement of body temperature, pulse rate, and respiratory rate will be a part of every physical examination. Even if the veterinary technician will not be performing a complete physical examination, he or she will often be asked to obtain this information before the veterinarian's examination. For the veterinarian and veterinary technician, these values provide a quick reference to a substantial amount of information regarding the status of the patient. As mentioned previously, these values should be recorded in a dedicated area on the standard physical examination form.

The body temperature is optimally measured rectally using a rectal probe thermometer. Most rectal thermometers in current use report the temperature through a digital display window (Figure 8-1). These thermometers work quickly and are safe and accurate. Still available but less commonly used are the liquid-capillary thermometers, which rely on a column of liquid (usually alcohol or mercury) to rise inside the thermometer and be compared with a scale on the thermometer for temperature determination. Always use a protective cover with the thermometer to minimize disease transmission. Lubricating the probe will make insertion much easier. When using the liquid-capillary type of thermometer, remember to shake the thermometer with the insertion tip down so that the liquid level falls from where it was left following its most recent use. Forgetting this step could result in an inaccurate measurement. Whereas a rectal temperature measurement is optimal, an **axillary** or **aural** temperature measurement may be used in cases where the rectum or nearby anatomy is swollen or painful, such as severe **colitis** or a **perineal hernia.** These methods are less accurate than a rectal measurement and should only be used when necessary.

Variations from normal body temperature can be useful in determining the nature or severity of a patient's illness. An elevated body temperature (**fever** or **hyperthermia**) usually signifies the presence of infection, inflammation, or neoplasia. However, mild elevations may be noted secondary to the stress or anxiety associated with a visit to the practice. Significant true hyperthermia may occur when heat-dissipating mechanisms cannot overcome excessive ambient temperatures (heat stroke) or secondary to certain drugs. Severe elevations (>107° F) can lead to organ dysfunction and warrant initiation of gradual cooling mechanisms. Decreased body temperature (**hypothermia**) is seen less commonly and usually results from impaired thermoregulation in any sick animal, especially cats. Inability to maintain body temperature is more common in patients that are young, old, or thin. Conditions that commonly result in impaired thermoregulation include chronic renal failure, hypothyroidism, and CNS disease. Severe hypothermia (<90° F) can be life threatening and requires immediate attention. Normal body temperature ranges for dogs and cats are noted in Table 8-1.

Peripheral arterial pulses should be palpated to determine pulse rate and pulse quality in every patient. Pulses are generally palpated by way of the femoral artery, which is located high on the medial thigh of the animal. Digital pressure should be applied over the femoral artery using the tips of the fingers. Some degree of pressure will be required to feel the pulse, but excessive pressure could compress the vessel making the pulse difficult to feel. The degree of pressure needed will vary from patient to patient. The pulse rate (per minute) is calculated by counting the number of pulses palpated for 15 seconds and multiplying by 4. Normal pulse rates for the dog and cat are listed in Table 8-1. It is essential to auscult the heart while palpating pulses. The heart rate and pulse rate should be identical, and there should be a pulse of approximately equal quality produced by each heartbeat. The absence of a palpable pulse (or significant change in pulse quality) with an audible heartbeat is called a **pulse deficit.** Pulse deficits usually indicate an abnormal heart rhythm and warrant further evaluation, such as electrocardiography.

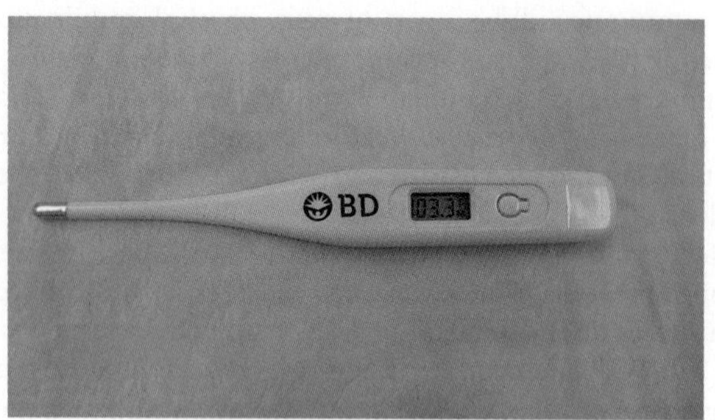

FIGURE 8-1 Digital rectal thermometer.

It is also important to determine the pulse quality when palpating peripheral arterial pulses. The pressure you feel when palpating a pulse is called the **pulse pressure.** Pulse pressure represents the difference between the systolic and diastolic arterial pressure. The intensity of the palpated pulse will vary depending on the body condition of the animal, appearing stronger in thin animals and weaker in obese or heavily muscled animals. Pulse quality is a subjective measurement and is likely to vary from technician to technician, given the level of experience and comfort in palpating peripheral pulses. An attempt should be made to describe the intensity of the pulse using terms such as weak, moderate, or strong. In general, a weak peripheral pulse is indicative of poor perfusion and may be caused by decreased cardiac output (as in congestive heart failure or **hypovolemia**) or increased peripheral resistance (as in **shock**). Pulses may also be described as slow to rise if the peak of intensity comes late in the pulse wave. This can be seen with obstruction to cardiac output, as is seen with **aortic stenosis.** A pulse that feels stronger than normal may also indicate a problem. These pulses may be described as bounding, tall, or hyperkinetic. Bounding pulses may be palpated in hyperdynamic states (early septic shock, anemia) or when there is a rapid drop-off in diastolic pressure (**patent ductus arteriosus).** Whenever pulse quality is abnormal, an evaluation of blood pressure using direct or indirect means is warranted.

The respiratory rate and effort should be noted in all patients. An initial notation of respiratory rate and effort should be performed before any stressful manipulation of the patient because stress will commonly cause an increase in those parameters. Respiratory rates are generally done visually first and then by auscultation to actually hear lung sounds. To calculate the respiratory rate (per minute), count the number of breaths for 15 seconds and multiply by 4.

TABLE 8-1 Normal TPR Values For Adult Small Animals

	Rectal Temperature °F	Heart Rate	Respiratory Rate
Dog	100.0-102.2	60-160/min (smaller breeds may have higher rates; puppies can have rates up to 200)	16-32/min
Cat	100.0-102.2	140-220/min	20-42/min

Normal respiration rates for the dog and cat are listed in Table 8-1. The determination of respiratory effort is more subjective. Animals respiring with normal effort should appear comfortable and lack any abdominal effort. If abnormal effort is detected, you should attempt to determine the phase of respiration during which effort is increased. Increased inspiratory effort may indicate an upper airway problem, especially if there is an associated noise, as with laryngeal paralysis. Increased expiratory effort may indicate a small airway obstructive disease, such as asthma. However, many patients will have an increased effort throughout respiration, which is less useful in determining the source of the problem and will be discussed in more detail later in the chapter.

SYSTEMS REVIEW

Following a visual inspection of the animal in its surroundings and the notation of temperature, pulse, and respiration, a more thorough examination of individual body systems is in order. As discussed earlier, the body systems examinations should be done in the same order in every patient to prevent overlooking any aspect of the physical exam. A consistent routine will ensure thorough physical examinations. However, the degree of detail with which you examine each system will vary from patient to patient based on their presenting complaint.

> *TECHNICIAN NOTE* Every major body system should be examined briefly in every patient. Special attention may be paid to specific systems depending on the individual patient.

Oropharyngeal System

Diseases of the oral cavity may cause loss of appetite, difficulty chewing, or **halitosis.** Dental disease (such as periodontal disease) is common in small animal patients. As such, a good oropharyngeal examination is an important part of the physical examination. An oral examination can be easily performed in most patients by lifting the lips with the mouth closed and by opening the mouth. However, caution should be taken during an oral examination, especially in uncooperative patients. Teeth should be examined visually for any evidence of discoloration, fracture, or excessive tartar formation. Abnormal teeth should be gently palpated to assess for pain and to determine if the tooth is loose (suggesting periodontal disease). Any missing teeth should be noted and recorded in the medical record. The gums should be examined for redness, which could indicate gingivitis, the precursor to periodontal disease. Any gingival swelling should be noted. Focal swellings could represent neoplastic masses or tooth root abscesses. More diffuse swelling can be seen with gingival hyperplasia. Gingival ulcers may be seen with renal disease, feline viral upper respiratory disease (herpesvirus, calicivirus), or ingestion of caustic substances. An examination with the mouth open will allow an inspection of the lingual surface of teeth and gums. This also allows an examination of the tongue for swelling, discoloration, or ulceration. You should always look under the tongue by pushing upward from under the jaw between the two rami of the mandible. An inspection under the tongue may reveal abnormalities, such as masses (sublingual squamous cell carcinoma [Figure 8-2]), swelling (a ranula or salivary mucocele), or foreign material (string around the base of a cat's tongue with a linear foreign body). An open-mouth examination also allows the inspection of the roof of the oral cavity (soft and hard palate) and the back of the oral cavity (pharynx, larynx). These areas should similarly be visually inspected for any swelling or mass, discoloration, or foreign material. Some pharyngeal masses may be large enough that they can be palpated externally by feeling the area just caudal to the mandible and cranial to the tracheal cartilage. More detail regarding an oropharyngeal examination and dental disease can be found in Chapter 32.

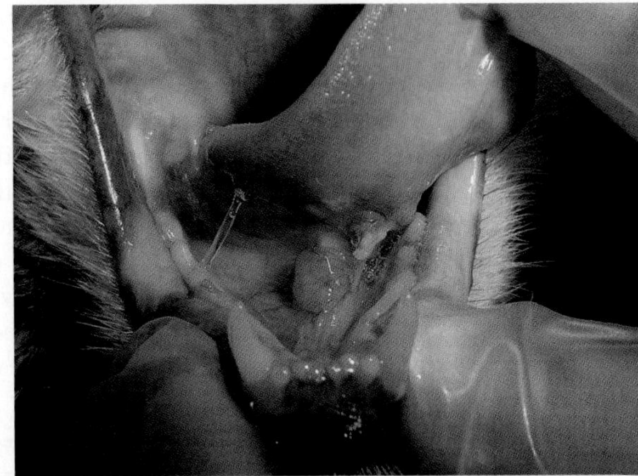

FIGURE 8-2 Sublingual squamous cell carcinoma visualized during an examination under the tongue of a cat.

> *TECHNICIAN NOTE* A thorough oropharyngeal exam should include an open- and closed-mouthed examination.

Eyes

A good initial ocular examination can be performed without any specialized equipment and should include an examination of the eyelids and external and internal structures of the eyes. It should also include an assessment of the patient's visual status. An examination of the eyelids should strive to identify any redness or swelling. The eyelid margins should be evaluated for evidence of masses or abnormal hairs (especially if they appear to be growing in toward the eye and causing irritation of the eye). Finally the position of the lower eyelid should be examined to see if the lower lid is rolling in toward the eye (entropion) or out away from the eye (ectropion) because both of these conditions can lead to ocular problems. Any ocular discharge should be noted and described in regard to symmetry (unilateral, bilateral) and character (serous, mucoid, purulent, hemorrhagic).

Excessive tearing or squinting of the eye may indicate irritation and should be noted. A general visual inspection of the globes should be performed to determine whether they are symmetrical and whether they are enlarged and/or protruding (as can be seen with glaucoma or lesions behind the eye) or sunken. The globes can be gently pressed with the thumbs over the eyelids. They may feel extremely firm when the intraocular pressure is high (such as with glaucoma) or soft when the intraocular pressure is low (such as with uveitis). If the eyes cannot be pushed backward (retropulsed) slightly, there may be a lesion (such as a mass) behind one or both eyes.

> *TECHNICIAN NOTE* Although a complete ocular examination requires specialized ophthalmologic equipment, a significant amount of information can be obtained with no equipment.

The external parts of the eye that can be evaluated include the conjunctiva, sclera, nictitating membrane, and cornea. The conjunctiva is the pink membrane that can be seen by pulling back the upper or lower eyelids and covers the outer part of the eye up to where the cornea begins. Redness of the conjunctiva (conjunctival hyperemia) is seen with many diseases of the external part of the eye, such as conjunctivitis. The sclera is the normally white part of the eye. It is an easy place to examine for the yellow discoloration seen with **icterus** (Figure 8-3). Redness seen in the sclera may be caused by conjunctival hyperemia (usually diffuse with small moveable blood vessels), episcleral injection (large straight blood vessels, often indicative of internal ocular disease), or subconjunctival hemorrhage (usually large, round to irregular blotches). Any eye redness should be recorded and reported to the veterinarian for further evaluation. The nictitating membrane (third eyelid) is usually not visible or only partially visible, and it rests beneath the lower eyelid on the medial aspect of the orbit. If the nictitating membranes are visible, that is abnormal and should be noted. If not, they can be briefly examined by pressing inward on the eye, causing the nictitating membrane to rise. They should be evaluated for swelling, redness, masses, or foreign material. The cornea is the transparent covering of the front of the eye, and it should be clear. It should be examined for cloudiness or other precipitates (such as pigment). Corneal ulcers are fairly common, and although fluorescein staining is usually required to recognize a corneal ulcer, deeper ulcers may be identifiable with only a visual inspection. A diseased cornea may have blood vessels growing into it (especially toward an area of ulceration to help with healing), and these should be noted.

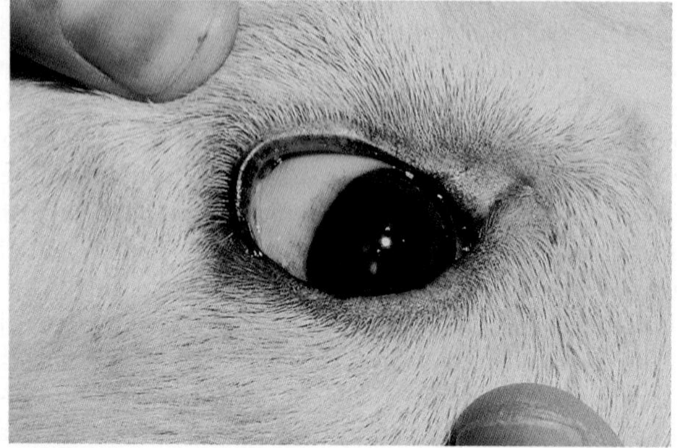

FIGURE 8-3 Yellow discoloration of the sclera seen with icterus.

The internal structures of the eye that can be evaluated without specialized equipment include the iris, lens, and anterior chamber. The iris is the colored part of the eye. It should be evaluated for swelling, discoloration, irregularity, or masses. The pupil is the opening of the iris. The pupils should always be evaluated for the degree of constriction or dilation and for symmetry of size. If the pupils are of differing sizes, this is referred to as anisocoria. The pupillary light response should be examined in all patients. When a light of sufficient strength is shone into one pupil, both that pupil and the opposite pupil should constrict. Anisocoria and abnormal pupillary light responses can indicate various ocular and neurologic diseases. The lens is the part of the eye responsible for focusing images onto the retina, and it is located inside the pupillary opening. In a normal patient, the lens is not visible without specialized equipment. However, increased lens opacity may be seen with nuclear sclerosis (a normal aging change seen commonly in dogs) or cataract formation. The anterior chamber is the part of the eye behind the cornea, but in front of the iris. This area should normally be clear, and there should be no difficulty in seeing the structures behind it. Cloudiness, pus, or blood may be present in the anterior chamber in association with severe ocular inflammation. Rarely, masses may be seen in the anterior chamber.

A simple evaluation of the patient's visual ability can be made as they are walking in or around the examination room. Most blind patients will have difficulty getting around in the unfamiliar setting of the veterinary hospital, even if they have accommodated for their blindness well at home. Another way to assess a patient's ability to see is to test their menace reflex by covering one eye (so you are testing only one eye at a time) and making a menacing gesture toward the other eye with your hand (being sure not to touch the patient or create excessive air movement that they could feel). A visual patient will close the eye in response to this gesture (assuming they are old enough to recognize that your gesture is menacing and that they have an intact facial nerve and are capable of blinking). You may also assess vision by dropping cotton balls in front of the patient from above their head and noting whether they visually follow the cotton balls as they pass by.

Ears

The examination of the ears should begin with the visualization and palpation of the pinnae. During visualization, the pinnae should be evaluated for symmetry (though in some patients asymmetry may be normal) and inspected inside and outside for swelling, redness, **alopecia,** crusting, or evidence of **excoriation.** Inside the pinnae is a common place to recognize **petechiation,** indicative of a primary hemostatic defect (such as thrombocytopenia) (Figure 8-4). Palpation of the pinnae will allow for recognition of focal swelling (such as with aural hematoma) or diffuse thickening (as might be seen with chronic otitis). Lifting and/or pulling back the pinnae will allow for a visual inspection of the external ear canal. The canine and feline ear canals consist of a vertical canal that opens to the external environment and runs inward parallel to the skull and a horizontal canal that is a short section between the vertical canal and eardrum, which runs more perpendicular to the skull. Only the vertical canal may be visualized without specialized equipment. This area should be evaluated for discharge, thickening and/or swelling, or masses. Aural discharge should be described in terms of amount (mild, moderate, severe) and appearance (waxy, black, hemorrhagic, purulent). The evaluation of the horizontal canal and eardrum requires the use of an otoscope.

TECHNICIAN NOTE An otoscopic examination is required to perform a thorough ear examination by visualizing both the vertical and horizontal canals.

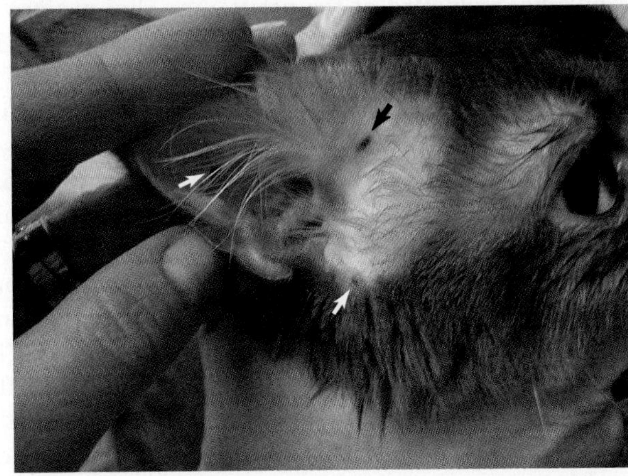

FIGURE 8-4 Petechiae *(arrows)* inside and in front of the pinna in a cat.

Most otoscopes found in veterinary practice will be wall mounted or portable. They typically consist of a handle, which allows the examiner to hold the instrument, and a head, through which the examiner visualizes the structures. For otoscopy, a cone is attached to the head. The cone is a gradually tapering tube, which fits nicely into the ear canal, through which the otoscope light shines to allow visualization. The majority of otoscopes can also be used as ophthalmoscopes by changing the head. Wall-mounted otoscopes usually have a base that plugs into an electrical outlet and hangs on the wall. The handle is attached to the base via a cord that supplies the power to light the otoscope. The handle is permanently attached to the base. The only assembly that is needed for use is to change the cone to match the size of the patient undergoing an examination. The cone should be large enough to allow a clear visualization of the structures inside the ear canal, but small enough so as not to cause the patient discomfort. The wall-mounted otoscopes have the advantage of always being ready for use and requiring little assembly, but they lack the flexibility of the portable units in terms of where the patient is positioned. For the wall-mounted units, the patient must be fairly close to the wall-mounted base, but for the portable units, the patient can be anywhere. The portable unit consists of a handle that contains a rechargeable battery to power the light source, a connecting piece that attaches the handle to the head, and the head (Figure 8-5). As with the wall-mounted unit, a cone must be attached to the head for an examination. The disadvantages of the portable otoscope are that the battery requires recharging and may not always be ready when needed and that the otoscope needs to be assembled before use.

To examine the horizontal canal and eardrum using an otoscope, the pinnae is first gently pulled upward (opposite the direction of the patient's legs) to lessen the angle between the vertical and horizontal canals. At this point, the otoscope cone is gently passed into the vertical canal while the examiner is looking through the head. The cone is gently advanced into the horizontal canal until the eardrum is

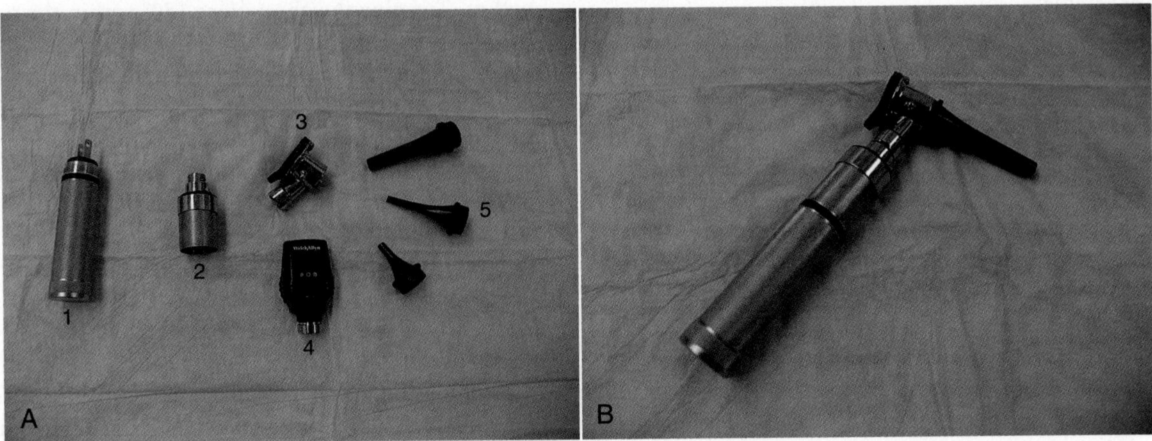

FIGURE 8-5 **A,** Components of a portable otoscope/ophthalmoscope. *1,* Handle. *2,* Connecting piece. *3,* Otoscope head. *4,* Ophthalmoscope head. *5,* Otoscope cones of varying size. **B,** Assembled portable otoscope.

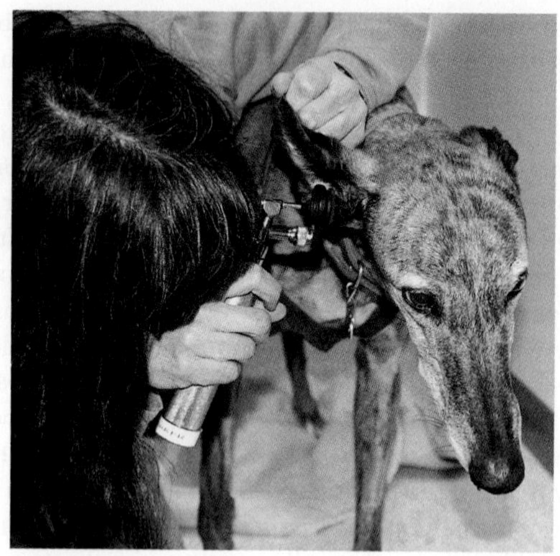

FIGURE 8-6 Technique for otoscopic examination.

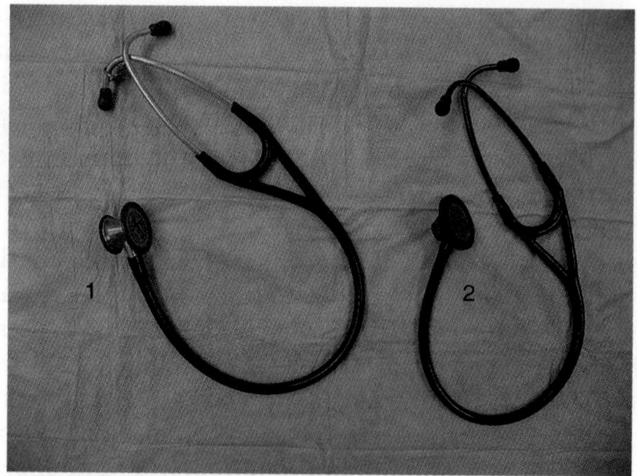

FIGURE 8-7 Stethoscopes. *1*, Chest piece with separate bell and diaphragm *2*, Chest piece with integrated bell and diaphragm.

visualized or until the patient shows evidence of discomfort (Figure 8-6). During passage of the otoscope through the vertical and horizontal canals, those areas should be examined for evidence of redness, swelling, masses, discharge, excess hair, or foreign material. The eardrum should appear as a grey to white, slightly transparent, round membrane separating the inner ear from the external ear canal. Abnormalities of the eardrum that should be noted include tears or perforation of the eardrum, increased thickness (or decreased transparency), or evidence of discharge behind the eardrum. It should be noted that an otoscopic examination is technically challenging and resisted by many patients. The visualization of the eardrum may be difficult for the novice technician, and only through frequent practice will the technique of otoscopy become comfortable.

Respiratory

The initial examination of a patient's respiratory status involves a visual determination of respiratory rate and effort as discussed previously. Patients in significant respiratory distress should be provided with supplemental oxygen and minimally stressed. The remainder of the physical examination should be brief or potentially postponed until the patient is more stable.

> TECHNICIAN NOTE Patients in significant respiratory distress should be placed in oxygen and stabilized before a complete respiratory examination is performed.

In a stable patient, an examination of the respiratory system should begin with the evaluation of the upper respiratory tract. The **nares** should be visually inspected to ensure symmetry and patency. Patency can be evaluated by holding a glass slide in front of the nares and looking for condensation to form from each nostril as the animal exhales. The nares should also be evaluated for normal opening size, especially in brachycephalic breeds of dogs, in which stenotic nares are common. Nasal discharge should be described in terms of symmetry (unilateral, bilateral), severity (mild, moderate, severe), and character (serous, mucoid, purulent, hemorrhagic). Opening the mouth and briefly visualizing the hard and soft palate at the roof of the mouth will allow a crude inspection of the nasopharynx for masses, which may appear as a bulging downward of the palate. Any clinical signs of upper airway disease noted during an examination should be recorded, such as sneezing, **stertor,** or **stridor.**

Auscultation using a stethoscope comprises the remainder of the respiratory examination. Most stethoscopes used in veterinary medicine are acoustic stethoscopes, which consist of a chest piece that contacts the patient and transmits sounds via hollow tubes to the examiner's ears (Figure 8-7). Electronic stethoscopes are less common. A stethoscope should be used such that the earpieces are pointing toward the examiner's nose when they are placed into the ears. The chest piece on most stethoscopes consists of two sides: a flat side called the diaphragm and a cup-shaped side called the bell. The diaphragm, which transmits high frequency sounds, is used most commonly and is appropriate for lung auscultation. The bell, which transmits low frequency sounds, is used less frequently and may enhance the ability to hear certain cardiac sounds, such as those associated with a gallop rhythm. Twisting the chest piece 180° within the tubing will change whether the bell or diaphragm is active. Some stethoscopes do not have a separate bell and diaphragm, but can function as both if the pressure with which the chest piece is applied to the patient is varied.

When performing respiratory auscultation, the patient should be in a quiet room. Many things can hamper your ability to effectively auscultate a patient, including ambient noise, the patient's movement (causing hair rubbing to be heard through the ear pieces), panting, or purring. The mouth should be held gently closed in a panting dog to improve auscultation. Attempts should be made to quiet a cat's purring, such as temporarily covering the nares, running water near the cat, or holding alcohol-soaked cotton to the nares. Once the conditions are optimal, respiratory auscultation should begin with the chest piece over

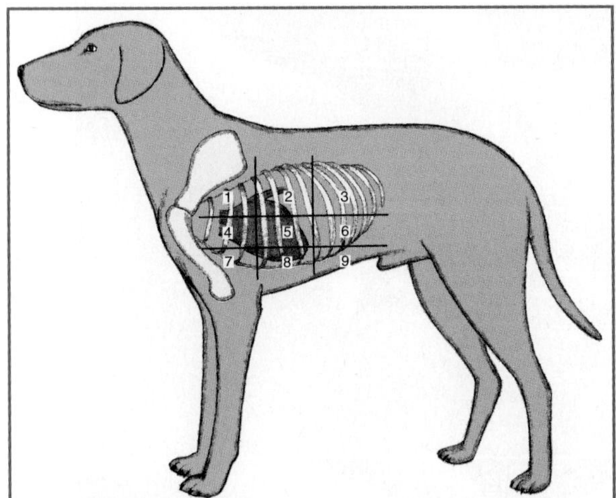

FIGURE 8-8 Division of the lungs into nine quadrants for auscultation and description of location of abnormal lung sounds. (From McCurnin DM, Poffenbarger EM: *Small animal physical diagnosis and clinical procedures*, St Louis, 1991, WB Saunders.)

the trachea. Normal tracheal airflow is turbulent, and the respiratory sounds should be loud and harsh. Abnormal sounds heard over the trachea suggest a problem in the upper airway (trachea or more cranial). For example, a high-pitched inspiratory sound may indicate partial upper airway obstruction, as can be seen with laryngeal paralysis. Although these abnormal upper airway sounds will likely be transmitted to the lungs and audible during lung auscultation, they do not indicate lung disease. The lungs should be auscultated on both sides of the patient, generally dividing the lung fields into nine quadrants on each side (Figure 8-8). Each quadrant should be auscultated through at least two to three respiratory cycles of inspiration and expiration. In a normal patient, air movement will be audible during both inspiration and expiration, but should be of minimal intensity. The intensity of normal lung sounds will vary with the body condition of the patient; the sounds are more intense in thin patients and less intense in obese or well-muscled patients. The most commonly identified abnormal lung sounds are crackles and wheezes. Inspiratory crackles usually indicate the presence of fluid within alveoli, as can be seen with **pulmonary edema.** Wheezes may occur during inspiration and/or expiration when air is moving through a narrowed airway, as can be seen with feline asthma. Failure to hear any air movement is also a sign of a problem. A lack of lung sounds occurring in the ventral lung fields in the standing animal usually indicates **pleural effusion** because the fluid tends to settle in the ventral areas. Conversely a lack of sounds in the dorsal lung fields often indicates a **pneumothorax** because the air will rise to the dorsal areas. Space-occupying masses and lung consolidation can also result in the absence of lung sounds. When abnormal lung sounds are auscultated (or lung sounds are absent), the technician should note whether they are occurring during inspiration or expiration and in which lung fields they were identified.

Cardiovascular System

The examination of the cardiovascular system begins with a look in the mouth. Rather than looking for specific oral pathologic conditions, we are looking at the gingival mucous membranes to gain an assessment of perfusion status. The gingival mucous membranes should be pink and moist, though some animals will have normally pigmented gingivae. Pallor of the mucous membranes usually indicates anemia or poor perfusion. Hyperemia of the mucous membranes can occur in stressed animals or can be seen in hyperdynamic states, such as the early phase of septic shock. If the mucous membranes are not moist but are dry or tacky, this is usually an early sign of dehydration. However, in a patient that is panting excessively, the mucous membranes will be dried by the air movement associated with panting, and mucous membranes will not be a good indicator of hydration status. The gingival mucous membranes are also used for measuring the capillary refill time, which serves as another indicator of perfusion. With the lip raised, the gingival surface is gently pressed with a finger to occlude blood flow until the color fades from the mucous membrane beneath the finger. The finger is removed, and the time it takes for the mucous membrane color to return to normal is measured (Figure 8-9). In a normal animal, this capillary refill time will be less than 2 seconds. Refill times longer than 2 seconds are indicative of poor perfusion, as can be seen with hypotensive states. Extremely rapid refill (<1 second) may be seen in stressed patients or in hyperdynamic states, such as the early phase of septic shock. The peripheral arterial pulse quality will also provide information regarding perfusion as discussed previously.

> *TECHNICIAN NOTE* A complete cardiac examination includes assessment of perfusion status, heart rate, heart rhythm, and heart sounds.

Cardiac auscultation will allow evaluation for abnormal heart rate, rhythm, and sounds. In dogs, the heart should be auscultated on each side of the chest around the level of the costochondral junction (just behind the level of the elbow when the patient is standing). By moving the chest piece around slightly, you will be able to auscultate in the vicinity of each heart valve. The pulmonic, aortic, and mitral valves can be auscultated best on the left side, whereas the tricuspid valve is auscultated best on the right side (Figure 8-10). Normal heart rates have been discussed previously. In cats, it is best to auscultate directly over the sternum initially and move the chest piece gradually up to the left side and back over to the right side. The valve positions are similar to the dog, but in cats, abnormal heart sounds are more commonly auscultated in the sternal area. The heart rhythm should be regular, meaning that each heartbeat is separated from the following one by an identical time interval. Dogs may normally have a slight variation in heart rhythm, such that the heart rate increases slightly during inspiration and decreases slightly during expiration. This is called respiratory sinus arrhythmia, and it is a sign that a dog has normal cardiac function.

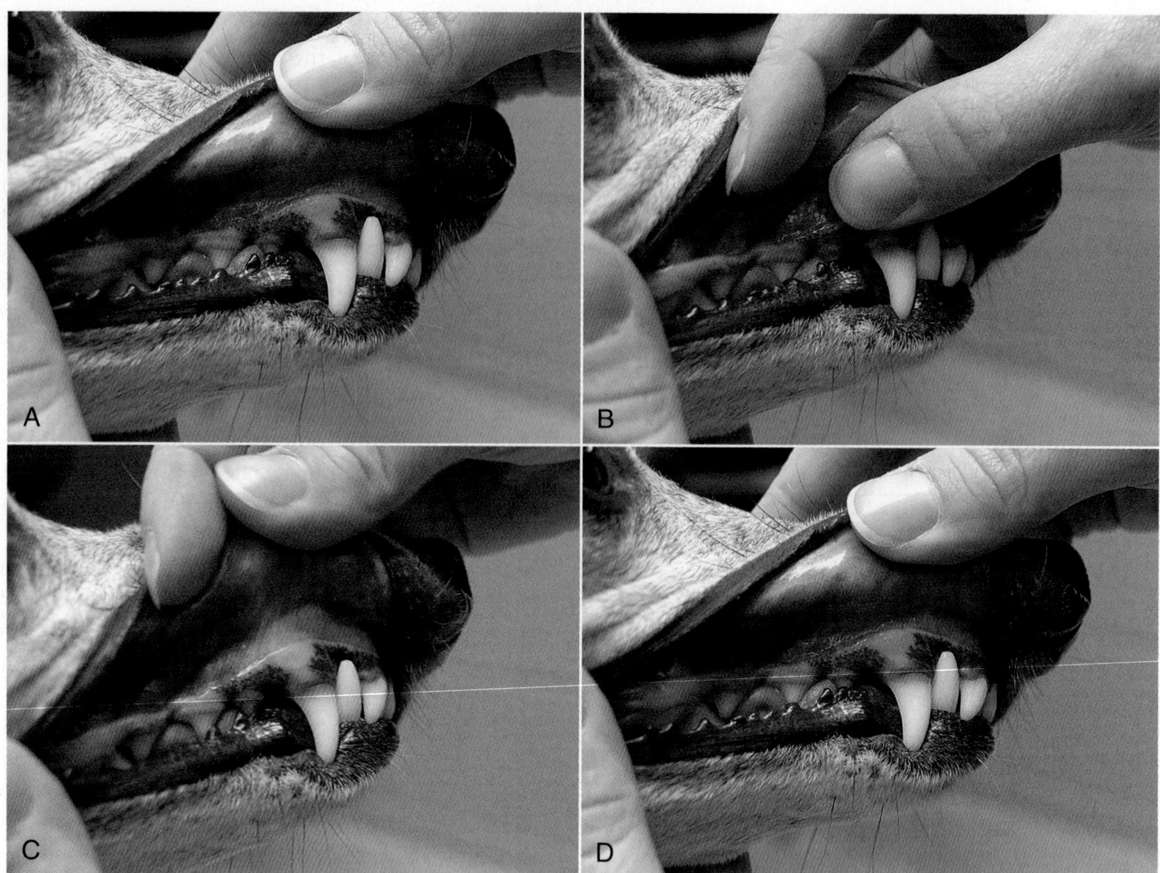

FIGURE 8-9 Assessing capillary refill time. **A,** Visualize the gingival mucous membranes by lifting the lip. **B,** Apply gentle pressure with the thumb onto the mucous membranes. **C,** Resultant area of pallor when the thumb is removed. **D,** Note time to return of normal mucous membrane color.

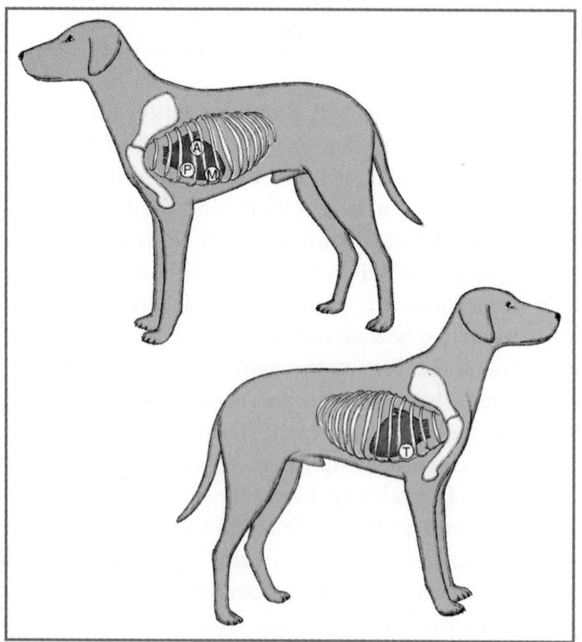

FIGURE 8-10 Location of heart valves as an aid in the determination of the origin of a heart murmur. *A,* Aortic; *M,* mitral; *P,* pulmonic; *T,* tricuspid. (From McCurnin DM, Poffenbarger EM: *Small animal physical diagnosis and clinical procedures,* St Louis, 1991, WB Saunders.)

To best evaluate the cardiac rhythm, the pulses must be palpated during auscultation. As discussed previously, there should be a pulse of approximately equal intensity generated with each heartbeat. In a patient with an abnormal heart rhythm or with pulse deficits, electrocardiography should be performed to determine the exact nature of the abnormality.

The heart sounds typically audible during auscultation in a normal patient are S_1 (the first heart sound), which is created by closure of the mitral and tricuspid valves at the start of systole, and S_2 (the second heart sound), which is created by closure of the aortic and pulmonic valves at the end of systole. These two short heart sounds result in the typical "lub-dub" sound of the normal heartbeat. The presence of a third heart sound is termed a gallop rhythm because the resulting heart rhythm sounds like the galloping of a horse. A gallop rhythm is not actually an abnormal rhythm in the sense of electrical activity, but is caused by an extra heart sound termed either S_3 or S_4. S_3 is usually associated with ventricular dilation, such as with dilated cardiomyopathy, whereas S_4 is usually associated with decreased ventricular compliance and hypertrophy, such as with hypertrophic cardiomyopathy. S_3 and S_4 cannot be differentiated via auscultation. Rarely the second heart sound (S_2) may be split and sound like a third heart sound. This phenomenon is uncommon.

TABLE 8-2 Grading of Heart Murmurs in Small Animals

Grade	Description
I	Very low intensity murmur that can only be heard in a quiet area
II	Murmur of soft intensity that can be heard immediately
III	Murmur of moderate intensity
IV	Loud murmur
V	Loud murmur with a palpable thrill on the body wall
VI	Loud murmur that can be heard with the stethoscope held some distance from the thoracic wall

A heart murmur is an abnormal sound caused by turbulent blood flow which typically sounds like a "swishing" noise. Identification of heart murmurs can indicate cardiac disease, though they can occur with noncardiac disease (such as with anemia) or can be normal in some young animals. Heart murmurs should be described by their intensity, when they occur in the cardiac cycle, and where they are heard loudest. The intensity of a heart murmur is typically graded on a scale from I to VI, as shown in Table 8-2. Systolic murmurs occur between S_1 and S_2 (i.e., during systole) or may mask those two sounds. Diastolic murmurs occur after S_2 and before the next S_1 (i.e., during diastole). A continuous murmur occurs throughout the cardiac cycle. The area on the chest where a murmur is loudest is termed the point of maximal intensity. For dogs, this point is usually identified in relation to the location of heart valves, as shown in Figure 8-10. For cats, this point may more easily be described in relation to the sternum (such as midsternum or left parasternum) since many feline murmurs are best auscultated in this area.

The final part of a thorough cardiovascular exam is evaluation of jugular veins. In a short-haired patient, the jugular veins can be visualized on either side of the trachea with the patient's muzzle lifted dorsally in a standing or sitting position. In animals with thicker or longer coats, the hair may need to be clipped or wet down to allow an evaluation. Normal patients should have jugular pulsations that do not extend more than one third up the neck. The jugular veins drain blood into the right atrium, and their pulsations and distension give a direct indication of right atrial pressure. Distended jugular veins extending farther up the neck can be seen in any disease causing elevated central venous pressure, especially those causing increased right atrial pressure, such as a pericardial effusion or pulmonic stenosis.

Gastrointestinal System

This section of the physical examination would more appropriately be called "abdominal palpation" because it actually involves the assessment of more than just the gastrointestinal (GI) tract. During abdominal palpation, other abdominal organs will be examined, including liver, spleen, kidneys, and urinary bladder. The technique of abdominal palpation can be difficult for the novice technician, but with practice, one can become quite proficient. As with the physical examination as a whole, following a consistent routine every time abdominal palpation is performed will ensure that nothing is missed. A thorough understanding of the anatomic location of the abdominal organs within the abdominal cavity is essential for effective palpation. Figure 8-11 shows the location of the abdominal organs within the abdomen. For the purposes of description, the abdomen can be divided into six sections (cranial-dorsal, cranial-ventral, middorsal, midventral, caudal-dorsal, caudal-ventral). For

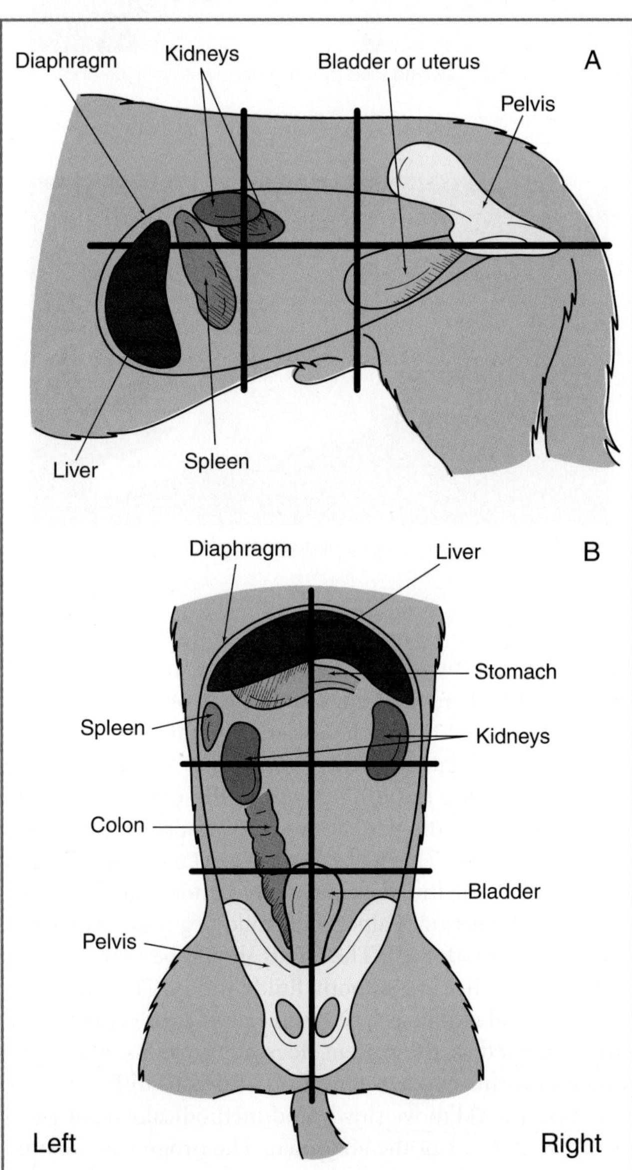

FIGURE 8-11 Location of internal organs within the abdominal quadrants. **A**, Lateral projection. **B**, Dorsoventral projection.

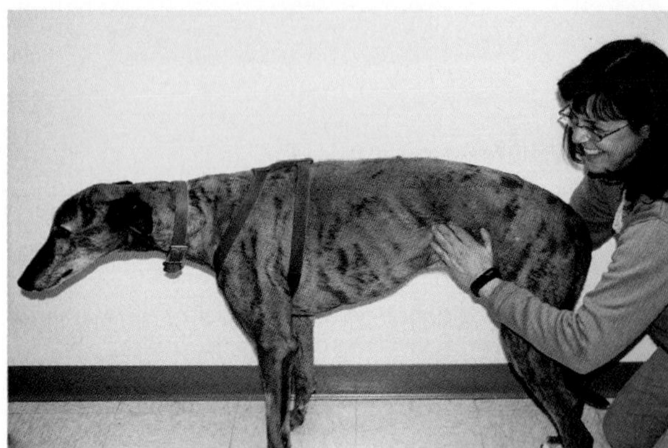

FIGURE 8-12 Two-handed abdominal palpation in the dog.

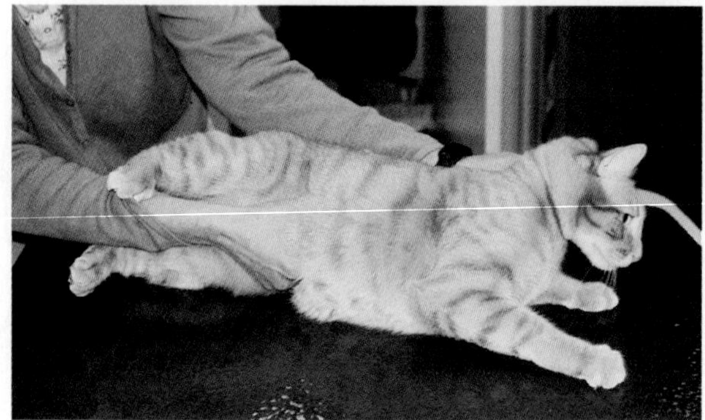

FIGURE 8-13 One-handed abdominal palpation in the cat.

most dogs, the two-handed technique is the best method (Figure 8-12). For small dogs and cats, a one-handed technique (Figure 8-13) may be easier, using the general principles discussed later for the two-handed technique. With the patient in the standing position, the examiner should stand just behind the patient or stand straddling the caudal end of the patient. This will allow the placement of one hand on either side of the abdomen. The hands should be in a flat, relaxed position. Palpation should begin in one section (such as cranial-dorsal). The hands should be moved gently toward each other in a smooth, fluid motion. The hands and fingers should remain relaxed, and excessive pressure should not be exerted so the patient does not tense its abdominal muscles (as this makes delineation of organs difficult). The palpation should move slowly and methodically through all the other sections of the abdomen. The progression should be the same each time you palpate a patient. Within each section, you should be noting any pain, swelling, firmness, or fluid. These findings should be recorded as to their severity and location (which section, left or right side). Be as specific as possible in your descriptions.

> *TECHNICIAN NOTE* Abdominal palpation should be performed using a consistent routine in every patient to avoid failure to evaluate any area.

Specific organs should be palpated in their respective regions. The liver should not be palpable in the normal animal, but if it is enlarged or contains a mass, it may be palpated in the cranial-ventral abdomen just caudal to the rib margin. The spleen is usually palpable in the cranial-ventral or midventral abdomen more on the left side. It should be gently palpated for enlargement or masses. The kidneys reside in the cranial-dorsal or middorsal abdomen and cannot be palpated in most dogs because they are encased in quite a bit of fat and are not moveable. However, they may be palpated in thin dogs or when there is **renomegaly.** Pain in those sections of the abdomen may represent renal pain. In cats, the kidneys are much more moveable and much more easily palpable. They are usually just caudal to the ribs in the dorsal abdomen and can be freely moved in most cats. They should be palpated for irregularities in size or shape and for evidence of pain. The urinary bladder can be easily palpated in the caudal-ventral abdomen, assuming it is not empty and that the patient is cooperative. Identification of the urinary bladder makes cystocentesis possible. The urinary bladder should also be palpated for distension or thickness. On rare occasions, bladder stones may be palpable on a physical examination. In male dogs, the prostate gland may be palpable in the caudal-dorsal abdomen, especially if it is significantly enlarged. However, the prostate is usually best examined via a rectal examination.

The GI tract can be examined during abdominal palpation to some extent. The stomach is usually not palpable if it is empty, but if there is gastric distension or a mass, it may be palpable in the cranial-dorsal abdomen (or farther caudal with severe distension). The small intestines are generally palpable as loops passing through your fingers in much of the midabdomen. It is not possible to delineate the different sections of small intestine by palpation. Small intestinal masses should be easily palpable, but other intestinal changes, such as wall thickening, are usually subtle and difficult to appreciate. The large intestine can usually be palpated in the middorsal and caudal-dorsal abdomen as it courses toward the rectum, assuming that it contains formed feces. If it is empty, it may not be as easily palpable. Good palpation may allow for identification of large intestinal masses or of constipation or obstipation. Remember that a complete GI examination includes an examination of the oral cavity, pharynx, rectum, and anus. The examination of these areas is discussed in other sections.

Rectal Examination

A rectal examination should be performed in almost every canine patient. In cats and small dogs, a rectal examination may be prohibitively painful and should only be performed in patients with a presenting complaint that may be referable to that area. A thorough rectal examination can be quick and provide a significant amount of useful information. The examination is typically performed using a well-lubricated, gloved index finger (though the pinkie finger can be used in smaller patients). Before examining the rectum, the perineal area and anus should be examined for redness,

CASE PRESENTATION 8-1 SMALL ANIMAL HISTORY

Signalment: 6-year-old intact male Boston terrier
Past pertinent history: None
Presenting complaint: Vomiting
Last normal: 3 days prior

Progression: The dog was normal when the owners left for work 3 days ago, but was vomiting when they returned home. They took him to another veterinary hospital where abdominal radiographs were taken. Based on the normal radiographs and the lack of abdominal pain, the dog was given subcutaneous fluids and discharged with the instructions to withhold food and water for 24 hours and then introduce a bland diet. Since discharge he has continued to vomit and become progressively more lethargic.

Systems: No coughing, sneezing, diarrhea, polyuria or polydipsia noted. No recent weight loss.

As the admitting technician, you are responsible for obtaining the patient's history. As you discuss the case with the owner, they mention that the dog was chewing a "cow trachea" when they left for work the day he was last normal. As you question them more carefully, it becomes clear that the dog is bringing up white foamy material in the absence of abdominal wretching. You ask specific questions with the goal of determining whether the dog is truly vomiting or actually displaying regurgitation (Table 8-1). You suspect that regurgitation is the actual presenting complaint.

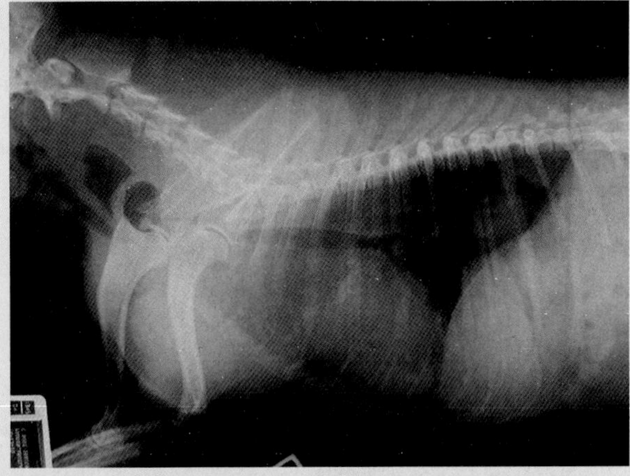

FIGURE 1 Lateral cervical and thoracic radiograph showing circular radiopaque foreign body in cervical esophagus with dilated esophagus proximal to it.

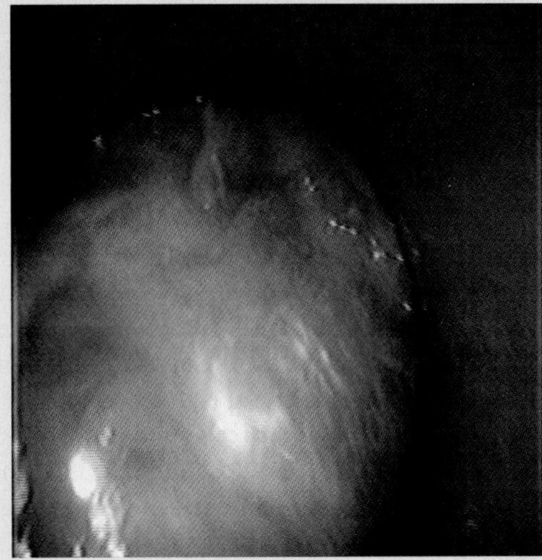

FIGURE 2 Endoscopic image of cervical esophagus obstructed with foreign body.

TABLE 8-1 Historical Differentiation Between Regurgitation and Vomiting

	Regurgitation	Vomiting
Bile	**Rarely to never**	**Often**
Digested food	Sometimes	Often
Active abdominal retch	**Rarely to never**	**Always**
Hypersalivation	Sometimes	Sometimes
Gagging	Sometimes	Rarely
Odynophagia	Often	Never

The most useful pieces of information are the presence or absence of bile in the expelled material and the presence or absence of active abdominal retching during expulsion.

Agreeing with your assessment that regurgitation may be the problem in this patient, the veterinarian orders cervical and thoracic radiographs (Figure 1). These reveal a radiopaque foreign body in the cervical esophagus with esophageal dilation proximal to the foreign body. An emergency endoscopy is performed and the presence of the foreign body is confirmed (Figure 2). The foreign body (a "cow trachea") is removed with endoscopic guidance (Figure 3), and the dog goes on to make a full recovery. The owners are grateful that you took the time to obtain an accurate and complete history.

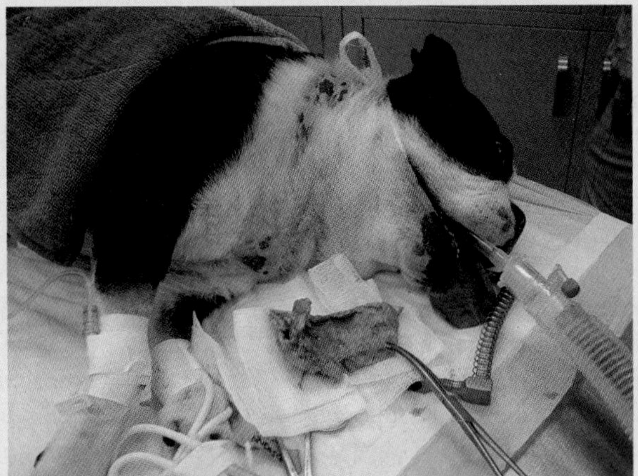

FIGURE 3 Cow trachea foreign body immediately after endoscopic removal from patient.

Continued

CASE PRESENTATION 8-1 SMALL ANIMAL HISTORY—cont'd

Summary: This is an example of how important good history-taking skills are. At the dog's initial visit, the individual obtaining the history was not able to discern that the dog was regurgitating. The erroneous historical diagnosis of vomiting resulted in the ordering of abdominal radiographs. This resulted in a missed diagnosis followed by inappropriate treatment. By taking the time to obtain a complete and accurate history, you will optimize the chances that the diagnostic and therapeutic plans will be appropriate.

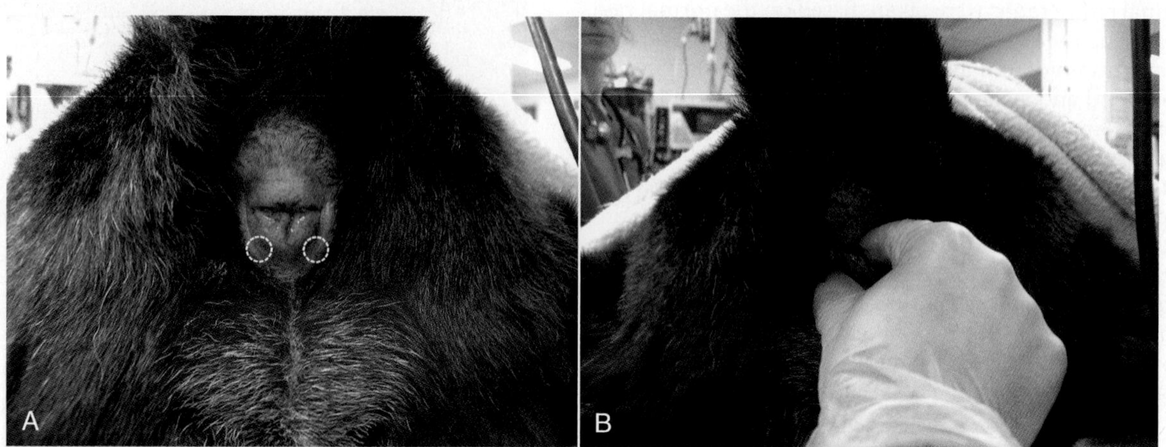

FIGURE 8-14 **A**, Approximate location of the anal sacs in a dog *(dotted circles)*. **B**, Technique for expression of the left anal sac in a dog.

swelling, masses, discharge, or other abnormalities. The finger is passed gently through the anal sphincter with the knuckles aimed dorsally. The finger is placed in as far as is comfortable for the patient, and structures are examined moving caudally. In the male dog, the prostate gland may be palpated ventral to the rectum cranial to the pelvic brim. It should be palpable in most intact dogs and in any dog with prostatomegaly. The normal gland is bilobed with a median raphe and should be smooth, symmetrical, and nonpainful. Enlargement or pain on palpation may be indicative of prostatic infection or neoplasia. Moving caudally, the urethra can be palpated ventral to the rectum as it courses caudally from the urinary bladder. Feel carefully for any irregularities (such as stones or masses). Dorsal to the rectum, the medial iliac lymph nodes are present to either side of the midline and may be palpated if they are enlarged. The inner mucosa of the rectum should be palpated during the examination by running the finger 360 degrees around the wall at various levels. The rectal wall should be evaluated for irregularity, thickness, or masses. The character of the stool within the rectum (if present) should be noted. If possible, a sample of stool should be removed with the gloved finger and examined. Finally the anal sacs can be palpated. The anal sacs lie just behind the anal mucosa with one on either side, located at approximately 5 and 7 o'clock (Figure 8-14, *A*). The anal sacs can be palpated by moving the finger within the rectum laterally and caudally while gently pressing with the thumb on the outside of the anus. Normal anal sacs should be small (<1 cm) and firm but slightly fluctuant. Distended anal sacs likely contain normal anal sac fluid, but could contain a mass. The sacs must both be fully expressed to confirm whether or not there is a mass present. This should be done in any patient with a palpably distended anal sac. Each sac opens at the rectal-anal junction adjacent to the location of the sac. The anal sacs are expressed by gently applying pressure with the thumb and finger during palpation (Figure 8-14, *B*). The anal sac fluid can vary in appearance from whitish to dark brown and can vary in consistency from watery to fairly thick. Evidence of blood or pus may indicate anal sac infection. Thick material can result in an anal sac impaction, which can be uncomfortable to the patient and lead to scooting of the rear end. Anal sac expression can be difficult in patients with an impaction and may require sedation.

TECHNICIAN NOTE The rectal examination provides an impressive amount of useful information and should be performed on every patient except those that will experience significant discomfort from the examination.

Urogenital

Much of the urinary system is evaluated during abdominal palpation and a rectal examination as discussed previously. The kidneys, urinary bladder, and proximal urethra have already been examined. The only part of the urinary system left to be evaluated is the distal urethra, which opens at the tip of the penis in the male and into the vestibule in the female. In male dogs, the penis should be gently extruded by pulling back the skin of the prepuce. Any discharge within the prepuce should be noted. The penis should be evaluated to ensure that the urethral opening is normal and appears patent. Any masses or wounds on the penis should be noted. Penile examination is not typically performed in the male cat except when the patient is sedated, such as would occur during urethral obstruction. Examination of the vagina and vestibule is not routinely performed in dogs and cats. In cases with a presenting complaint referable to the lower urinary tract, a vaginal examination may be indicated. A digital vaginal examination may be performed in the awake dog, but often sedation will be necessary. Sedation will always be required in the cat. In either case, the examiner should wear sterile gloves and use copious lubrication to prevent trauma and discomfort to the patient.

In the United States, the vast majority of dogs and cats are neutered. As such, an examination of reproductive organs is not commonly performed. In the intact male dog or cat, the testicles should be examined. The scrotum should be gently palpated to ensure that both testicles are present. Testicles should descend into the scrotum by 8 weeks of age in most patients and by 6 months in all patients. The testicles should be gently palpated to assess for any asymmetry in size, masses, heat, or pain. The penis should be extruded and examined as described earlier. In the intact female dog or cat, the reproductive organs are not as easily examined. A vaginal examination may be performed as described previously, but is not part of a routine examination. The uterus cannot be palpated during abdominal palpation unless it is enlarged, such as with pregnancy or **pyometra.** The ovaries cannot be palpated. It is good practice to palpate the mammary chains in all female dogs and cats, but it is especially important in sexually intact patients because they have a much higher risk of mammary cancer. Most dogs and cats will have five mammary glands on each side of the ventral abdomen. They should be gently palpated for heat, swelling, masses, or discharge. In lactating animals, milk should be expressed and examined.

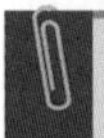

TECHNICIAN NOTE A urogenital examination is most important in patients who are sexually intact.

Integument

A complete evaluation of the integumentary system will include an examination of the hair, skin (including footpads and nails), and subcutaneous tissues. The character of the normal hair coat can vary greatly between breeds and between individual patients, but in general, it should be thick and shiny. Abnormal hair coats may be dull or greasy. They may contain scale (flakes of shed epidermis). The coat should be visually evaluated for areas of thinning or alopecia (Figure 8-15). If alopecia is noted, it should be described in terms of location (focal versus diffuse versus patchy, unilateral versus bilateral, symmetric versus asymmetric) and degree (partial versus complete). The coat should be inspected closely in alopecic areas. The examiner should look for evidence of broken hairs, which may indicate that the alopecia is caused by scratching or **barbering.** The skin should also be examined in the alopecic area for evidence of excoriation or underlying disease. The hair should be gently parted in several areas to look for evidence of ectoparasites, such as fleas.

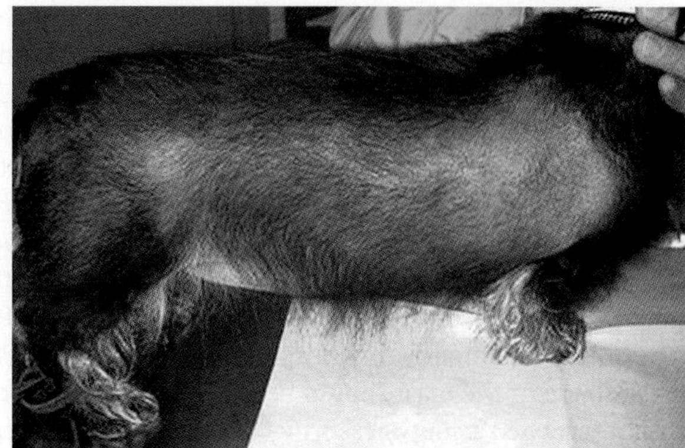

FIGURE 8-15 Bilaterally symmetric truncal alopecia in a dog with hyperadrenocorticism.

In highly suspicious cases, such as extremely **pruritic** animals, a flea comb can be used to improve the chances of identifying live fleas or their excrement.

TECHNICIAN NOTE Dermatologic diseases are common in small animal patients. A familiarity with the skin examination and terminology of skin lesions will be useful.

The extent to which the skin is directly examined will depend on the presenting complaint of the patient. A patient with no complaints referable to the skin (such as pruritus, flaking, or odor) need only have a cursory skin exam. Patients with complaints referable to the skin warrant a more thorough evaluation. In any patient lacking alopecia, the hair must be parted to allow an evaluation of the skin. The ventral caudal abdomen has a light covering of hair in many patients and is a good place to visualize the skin. Common abnormalities that can be identified on the skin include papules and pustules, which are seen commonly with a bacterial skin infection. A papule is a small pink or red elevated skin lesion smaller than 0.5 cm in diameter. A pustule is similar in size to a papule, but is a raised area containing pus, which usually has a pink or red base with a white tip. Scale and crusts are caused by any inflammatory process affecting the outer layers of skin. Both appear as flakes and contain shed epidermal cells, but crusts also contain inflammatory cells. They can be difficult to differentiate based on a visual inspection alone. Excoriations are areas of self-trauma caused by scratching in a pruritic animal. The skin is a good area to see petechiae and ecchymoses, which usually indicate a primary hemostatic defect. Erythema (redness) of the skin may be noted focally or diffusely. Nail beds and footpads should be examined, especially in patients with diseased skin, to evaluate for redness, discharge, or ulceration.

Masses are commonly found on the skin and within the subcutaneous tissues in veterinary patients. Most masses will be caused by benign neoplastic processes, though palpable masses may represent malignancy, vaccine reactions, abscesses, or swelling caused by trauma. It is important that any masses be noted in the medical record with great detail so that any changes in their size or appearance can be noted. Masses should be described based on their location, including whether they are on the surface of the skin (cutaneous) or under the skin (subcutaneous). Their exact location can be recorded in the medical record by using a body map. Such a map will allow for the precise marking of the location of the mass and is much more effective than written descriptions for comparisons with future examinations. The size and shape of the mass should be noted. The size is most precisely recorded using measuring calipers, though it can be estimated if calipers are not available. The mass should also be described as soft, fluctuant, or firm. Its adherence to underlying structures should be noted by recording whether it is moveable or fixed. Careful monitoring of cutaneous and subcutaneous masses is important in determining a diagnostic and therapeutic plan.

Lymph Nodes

In the normal patient, the peripheral lymph nodes that can be palpated are the mandibular, prescapular, and popliteal lymph nodes. Axillary and inguinal lymph nodes are typically only palpable when they are significantly enlarged. Similarly, enlarged medial iliac lymph nodes may be palpable via a rectal examination as discussed earlier. The mandibular lymph nodes are located on either side of the neck just caudal-dorsal to the ramus of the mandible and cranial-ventral to the mandibular salivary glands. They can be differentiated from the salivary gland because they tend to be more moveable, slightly firmer, and smaller (in the normal patient). The prescapular lymph nodes are located in the subcutaneous tissue just medial to the scapular-humeral joint on either side of the patient. These nodes are often encased in fat and may feel slightly softer than other normal nodes. The popliteal lymph nodes are located on the caudal aspect of each hind limb at the level of the stifle joint. The axillary lymph nodes, if palpable, will be located in the subcutaneous space on the lateral aspect of the ventral thorax under the arm. The inguinal lymph nodes are located in the most caudal part of the ventral abdomen, just medial to the thighs, on either side of the midline.

Lymph nodes should be palpated by gently isolating them between the thumb and index finger. Ideally the left and right lymph nodes are palpated simultaneously at each location to determine whether they are identical in size and shape. Normal lymph nodes are round to oval in shape, slightly moveable, and firm, but slightly compressible. Abnormal lymph nodes may be enlarged, firm, warm, or painful. The most common abnormality palpated is an enlarged lymph node. It should be noted that lymph nodes in young animals (less than 6 months of age) are normally mildly enlarged as compared with the size that they will be during adulthood. Lymph node enlargement may indicate that the node is infected, reacting to local inflammation, or neoplastic. Enlargement should be noted as focal (single node or single region) or generalized (all palpable nodes enlarged). The specific nodes that are enlarged should be noted and their size measured with calipers or estimated.

> *TECHNICIAN NOTE* The peripheral lymph nodes that should be palpable in every patient are the mandibular, prescapular, and popliteal lymph nodes.

Musculoskeletal System

The examination of the musculoskeletal system will vary greatly depending on the patient's presenting complaint. In a patient without symptoms referable to the musculoskeletal system (such as lameness, swelling, difficulty rising, or pain), the examination will be fairly cursory. Every patient should be observed as they walk around the examination room or waiting area for signs of lameness that the owner may not have perceived. In patients lacking lameness, the musculoskeletal examination should include a visual inspection of the standing animal for asymmetry of the limbs. This is followed by gentle palpation of each limb and the vertebral column over the neck and back. Initial palpation of limbs should be performed such that opposite sides are examined simultaneously (i.e., left and right forelimb, left and right hind limb). This will allow for a comparison with the opposite leg when evaluating swelling or pain.

In a patient that is seen with a complaint referable to the musculoskeletal system, such as lameness, or one in which the cursory musculoskeletal examination revealed an abnormality, a more thorough examination is indicated. This should start with observation of the animal walking or jogging on a lead for identification of lameness. Animals will put less weight on a painful limb when walking, shifting the weight to the good limb. This results in the patient putting their head down when stepping on the good limb and pulling the head up when stepping on the painful limb. Once the affected limb has been identified, the patient should be placed in lateral recumbency and each limb thoroughly examined one at a time. The soft tissues and long bones of the limb should be palpated with gradually increasing levels of pressure to identify swelling or pain. Then, starting at the toes, every joint should be put through a range of flexion and extension trying to isolate the examined joint and not move any other joints. It is important to examine all the limbs so that perceived discomfort in one limb can be compared with the opposite limb. If you identify pain in one limb and the patient does not show a similar response in the other limbs, you have likely identified a problem. The bones of the vertebral column should be palpated one at a time by pressing down on their dorsal surface on the animal's back. The neck should be put through a full range of motion and any pain noted.

> *TECHNICIAN NOTE* In a patient with lameness, all limbs should be thoroughly examined to allow comparisons to be made and isolate the affected area.

Nervous System

Similar to the musculoskeletal examination, the time allotted to the neurologic examination will vary greatly depending on the patient. The examination of every patient will include a subjective visual evaluation of mentation, visual acuity, and gait as it enters the examination room, as described in the section on observing patients in their surroundings. Most patients will have menace and pupillary light reflex testing performed as part of the eye examination. If these parameters are considered normal and the patient does not have any complaints that could be referable to the nervous system, the neurologic examination need not be any more extensive.

A patient with an abnormality noted on the cursory examination or one with a complaint that could be referable to the nervous system should have a more complete neurologic examination. Presenting complaints that could be referable to the nervous system include, but are not limited to, behavior changes, depression, lethargy, blindness, head tilt, circling, lameness, weakness, or paralysis. A complete neurologic examination includes an evaluation of mentation, gait and posture, muscle tone, cranial nerves, postural reactions, and reflexes. Mentation is assessed subjectively during visual observation of the patient and may be described as bright and alert, quiet, dull or obtunded (not interested in surroundings), stuporous (responsive only to noxious stimuli), or comatose (unresponsive to stimuli). The gait and posture are also observed. The patient should be walked or jogged on a lead and made to turn when assessing a gait. Although animals with neurologic disease can have a normal gait and posture, ataxia is a common gait abnormality in these patients. Ataxia is a term used to describe uncoordinated muscle movements when walking. When evaluating a patient's gait, ataxia is identified when you are unable to predict where the foot will fall on the patient's next step. Ataxia can vary in type and severity, and it is often confused with lameness by owners. Muscle tone is subjectively assessed by a visual inspection and palpation. The evaluation of muscle tone should include determination of anal sphincter tone. During a rectal examination, the anal sphincter muscles should tighten around your finger. Muscle atrophy or decreased tone may occur in denervated muscle.

A cranial nerve examination is an essential part of every complete neurologic examination. Cranial nerve reflex tests are summarized in Table 8-3. The olfactory nerve (cranial nerve I) is not routinely tested because a patient's response to

TABLE 8-3 Examination of the Cranial Nerves

		Test Response	
Nerve	Test	Normal	Abnormal
I. Olfactory	Volatile substance	Sniff, recoil, nose lick	No response
II. Optic	Menace	Blink	No blink
	Pupillary light reflex	Direct, consensual responses present	No direct or consensual responses
III. Oculomotor	Pupillary light reflex	Direct, consensual responses present	No direct response, consensual intact
	Observe eye follow an object	Normal eye movement	Impaired ocular movement in ventral, dorsal, and medial directions
IV. Trochlear	Observe	Normal eye position	Dorsomedial strabismus
	Palpate temporalis	Normal muscle tone	Muscle atrophy
	Corneal reflex	Eye blink	No blink
	Palpebral reflex	Eye blink	No blink
V. Trigeminal	Observe ability to chew	Normal jaw movement	Inability to chew
	Palpate masseter muscle	Normal muscle tone	Muscle atrophy
	Pupillary light reflex	Direct, consensual responses present	No direct or consensual response present
VI. Abducens	Observe	Normal eye position	Medial strabismus
VII. Facial	Observe	Facial symmetry	Lip droop
	Corneal reflex	Eye blink	No blink
	Palpebral reflex	Eye blink	No blink
	Menace	Eye blink	No blink
VIII. Acoustic	Hand clap	Startle response	No response
	Move head horizontally, vertically	Normal nystagmus	No response, resting or positional nystagmus
IX. Glossopharyngeal	Gag reflex	Swallow	No response
X. Vagus	Gag reflex	Swallow	No response
	Oculocardiac reflex	Bradycardia	No response
	Laryngeal reflex	Cough	No response
XI. Accessory	Palpate neck muscles	Normal muscle tone	Muscle atrophy
XII. Hypoglossal	Tongue stretch	Retraction of tongue	No response

From McCurnin DM, Poffenbarger EM: *Small animal and physical diagnosis and clinical procedures*, Philadelphia, 1991, WB Saunders.

scent is difficult to evaluate. The spinal accessory nerve (cranial nerve XI) is not evaluated. Lesions in this nerve cause atrophy of the trapezius muscle, which can be difficult to identify. As discussed in the section on the eye examination, the pupils should be evaluated for size and symmetry, and the menace and pupillary light reflex tests should be performed. These will evaluate the optic (cranial nerve II) and oculomotor nerves (cranial nerve III). The position of the eyes at rest and the doll's eye reflex (physiologic nystagmus) will evaluate the oculomotor, trochlear (cranial nerve IV), and abducens nerves (cranial nerve VI). The doll's eye reflex is performed by turning the patient's muzzle and head from left to right. As the head moves in one direction, the eyes should initially move to the opposite direction and then snap back to the center. The palpebral reflex is tested by tapping the medial and lateral canthus of the eye to induce a blink. The corneal reflex is tested by holding the eyelids open and gently touching the cornea with a wet cotton swab. Gently pinching the lips with a hemostat or placing the hemostat inside either nostril should cause the patient to move away and will evaluate the sensory portion of the trigeminal nerve (cranial nerve V). Facial symmetry should be assessed because a droop to one side compared with the other can indicate a lesion of the facial nerve (cranial nerve VII). The eyes should be examined for nystagmus, which can indicate a lesion in the vestibulocochlear nerve (cranial nerve VIII). The gag reflex is performed by pressing with a finger on the back of the patient's tongue; this should elicit contraction of the pharyngeal muscles. This evaluates the glossopharyngeal nerve (cranial nerve IX) and branches of the vagus nerve (cranial nerve X). A visual examination of the tongue for determination of deviation to one side or another can identify lesions of the hypoglossal nerve (cranial nerve XII).

TECHNICIAN NOTE A complete neurologic examination should include the evaluation of mentation, gait and posture, muscle tone, cranial nerves, postural reactions, and reflexes.

A neurologic examination of the limbs involves assessment of postural reactions, reflexes, and sensation. Conscious proprioception is tested in the standing patient by picking up one paw and placing its dorsal surface onto the floor. The normal patient will quickly lift and turn the foot so that the palmar or plantar surface is touching the floor. This test should be performed on each leg. Note that patients with significant muscle weakness may not have the strength to lift the limb to turn it, so you should help to support the patient's weight. Limb strength can be assessed by forcing the patient to hop on one limb at a time and comparing their strength to do so between limbs. In small patients, this can be easily done by supporting the weight of the other three limbs while the patient is moved from side to side on one limb. In larger dogs, it may be necessary to hold up only one forelimb and move the patient from side to side on the opposite forelimb while keeping the hind limbs fairly still. A similar technique can be used to evaluate the hind limbs. Reflex testing should be performed with the patient in lateral

TABLE 8-4 Grading of Reflex Responses

Grade	Description
0	No response
1	Hyporeflexia (less than normal response)
2	Normal response
3	Hyperreflexia (greater than normal response)
4	Clonus (repetitive response)

recumbency and relaxed. The forelimb reflexes to be tested include the withdrawal reflex, the biceps reflex, and the triceps reflex. Forelimb reflexes can be difficult to obtain, and the withdrawal reflex is the most reliable. It is performed by pinching the patient's toe, which should result in strong flexion of the limb. Hind limb reflexes are more reliable and include the withdrawal reflex, patellar reflex, and cranial tibial reflex. Reflex responses should be scored from 0 to 4, as described in Table 8-4. Although not a limb reflex, the cutaneous trunci reflex can provide information regarding the integrity of spinal segments. It is performed by gently pinching the skin on either side of the lateral thorax, which should cause a twitching of superficial muscles. Pinching the anal mucosa should result in a reflex contraction of the anal sphincter muscles (the perineal reflex). Sensation should be tested in paralyzed limbs by aggressively pinching the bones of the toes with a hemostat. The animal with intact sensation will vocalize or try to bite. Note that pulling the leg back in flexion does not indicate normal sensation, but rather indicates an intact withdrawal reflex. The absence of sensation suggests a more severe lesion. The results of the complete neurologic examination should allow for an anatomic localization of the source of neurologic symptoms.

HISTORY AND PHYSICAL EXAMINATION OF LARGE ANIMALS

When a large animal patient is presented for an evaluation, a database that will become part of the medical record is generated. The history and physical examination are the most important part of the database and serve as the starting point for identifying the patient's problems. After this initial information is collected, the database may be expanded to include laboratory tests, diagnostic imaging, and special examinations of body systems, depending on the purpose of the examination and the condition of the patient.

HISTORY

The husbandry practices, animal environments, and economic factors affecting large animals differ significantly from those of small animals; however, the basic approach to effective history taking is the same for both large and small animal patients. Experienced clients can provide an excellent history with little coaching, but most clients do not know how to give a concise, useful summary of their animal's condition. The technician will need to ask specific questions to obtain relevant information and keep the information on an organized timeline. Once the history is obtained, the accuracy of the information must be evaluated since owners may unknowingly give inaccurate information, believing it to be true. Occasionally, owners provide false information to spare embarrassment, not wanting to appear ignorant or admit that they may have made a mistake in management of their animals.

Even though the history will focus on the chief clinical problem of an animal or group of animals, it is essential for the technician to keep the bigger picture of herd health and husbandry in mind when taking a history of large animal patients.

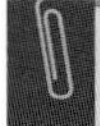

TECHNICIAN NOTE The history of an individual animal is not complete without herd health information.

OWNER/AGENT INFORMATION

It is common for large animals to be attended by a person (or persons) other than the owner, such as a trainer, groomer, farmhand, stable owner, or lessee (animal lease agreements are not uncommon). It is important to determine the identity of the person presenting the animal and establish his or her relationship to the animal. If the owner is not present, it is necessary to obtain appropriate contact information so that the veterinarian can communicate with the owner. It is also important to determine who has the decision-making responsibility for the animal since owners may entrust the trainer or agent to make decisions about their animal's treatment and care.

The insurance status of the animal should be determined. Although small animal insurance is becoming more commonplace, the economic value of certain large animals created a need many years ago for an insurance industry to protect owners' investments. In particular, equine insurance is widespread in the United States, and valuable ruminant breeding stock is also often insured. *Mortality insurance* covers the value of the animal in case of death. *Surgical insurance* covers specific costs of surgery and hospitalization with some limitations—similar to human health insurance policies. *Loss of use insurance* states specifically the intended use of the animal (breeding, racing, etc.), and if the animal cannot perform its intended use because of illness or injury, the owner may be reimbursed for lost potential income. The insurance company's and/or insurance agent's contact numbers should be noted in the medical record since they may be involved in the decision-making process for the affected animal. The type of insurance policy and estimated economic value of the animal should also be recorded since these factors often play an important role in the diagnostic and treatment options provided for the animal.

SIGNALMENT OF THE ANIMAL

The signalment of the animal typically includes age, sex, breed, color, and reproductive status. This information helps to formulate the patient's rule-out list of potential diagnoses since certain disease conditions have known predilections for subsets of the population according to signalment. For example, gray coat color in horses is associated with a higher incidence of melanomas than other coat colors; obstructive urolithiasis in ruminants is almost always associated with males; and β-mannosidase deficiency has only been reported in the Nubian breed of goats.

Another important part of the large animal signalment is the intended use of the animal; most large animals are kept for specific purposes, such as breeding, athletic performance, and commercial production of meat, milk, hair, or other products. The animal's occupation may predispose it to certain diseases or injuries, such as the increased occurrence of osteochondral "chip" fractures in race horses versus pleasure horses and the higher incidence of mastitis in dairy cattle than beef cattle.

The terminology used by clients with large animals to describe their animals is species specific, and the technician should be familiar with the commonly used terms for the sex, age, and reproductive status of large animal species (Tables 8-5 and 8-6).

INDIVIDUAL HISTORY AND CHIEF COMPLAINT

The history is usually obtained before beginning the physical examination since it may contain helpful information for the examiner. However, in emergency situations, it may be

TABLE 8-5 Age/Sex Terminology for the Horse

Foal	Young horse, from birth to weaning (weaning usually at 4-7 mo old)
Weanling	Young horse, from weaning to first birthday
Yearling	1 yr-1½ yr
Long Yearling	1½ yr to second birthday
Colt	Intact male between 2-3 yr old
Filly	Female between 2-3 yr old
Stallion	Intact male after third birthday
Mare	Female after third birthday
Gelding	Castrated male, of any age

TABLE 8-6 Age/Sex Terminology for Ruminants

Age	Cattle	Sheep	Goat
Parturition (freshening)	Calving	Lambing	Kidding
Neonate	Calf	Lamb	Kid
Male (<1yr)	Bull calf	Ram lamb	Buck kid
Female (<1yr)	Heifer calf	Ewe lamb	Doe kid
Immature female (has not given birth)	Heifer	Yearling ewe	Yearling doe
Mature female	Cow	Ewe	Doe (Nanny)
Mature male	Bull	Ram	Buck (Billy)
Castrated male	Steer	Wether	Wether

necessary to evaluate and stabilize the animal before proceeding with details about the animal's past. For example, an animal's vaccination and deworming history have little immediate value for an animal in need of treatment for severe shock.

> *TECHNICIAN NOTE* In an emergency situation, it may be necessary to perform the physical examination before taking a detailed history.

The individual history includes two major components: the history of the current problem and a general history of the animal. The history of the current problem is usually taken first and includes the client's chief complaint. The chief complaint is the primary reason for requesting an examination, though it is not always the animal's primary problem. It is important to listen to the client and avoid any perception of discounting or disregarding their concerns. Once the chief complaint has been determined, the technician can then begin a more directed line of questioning to accurately characterize the problem in terms of duration, progression, severity, frequency, and response to therapy (if attempted). Further questioning will focus on the specific body systems affected by the current problem; in an animal with respiratory disease, the presence and character of a cough, nasal discharge, or respiratory noise are important to determine. Information on appetite, dental care, abdominal pain, and fecal volume and consistency is important in assessing an animal with GI disease.

The general history includes information on the animal before the development of the current problem. Typically, this includes information on diet, exercise, preventative health maintenance, reproductive status, and previous medical problems and surgical procedures. Large animal clients are more likely than small animal owners to purchase and administer vaccines and deworming medications. Food animal producers commonly perform minor surgical procedures on their animals, such as dehorning, tail docking, and castration.

MEDICATION AND TREATMENT HISTORY

Most large animal facilities keep first-aid kits and pharmaceuticals on the premises, and animals are often treated before calling the veterinarian. This situation is fairly common in large animal practice, especially with production animals where economics often dictate whether or not the owner calls the vet immediately or attempts to solve the problem themselves. Owners may be reluctant to admit this information and may need to be asked specifically whether they have treated the animal and what they have attempted for treatment.

HERD HEALTH HISTORY

Large animals are seldom kept as isolated individuals and commonly share resources with other large animals. Similarly, animals often receive preventative health maintenance, such as vaccination, deworming, and external parasite control as a group. Therefore after obtaining the individual history, it may be important to gain information on the size and nature of the group or herd and the resources that they share. Resources include not only food and water, but also shelter facilities and common land areas, such as pastures and pens.

> *TECHNICIAN NOTE* Large animals often share resources, such as food, water, shelter, and turnout areas, with other animals.

Animals may be grouped randomly, but, more commonly, large animals are grouped by age, sex, reproductive status, or other common attributes. If other animals are affected, the signalment of those animals can hold vital clues to the nature of the problem. Shared food, water, and grazing sources allow ready transmission of infectious agents and the widespread distribution of parasites and toxins. Even horses that are housed in individual stalls are usually placed in common turnout areas for daily exercise, where they may contact other animals and/or their fecal material. Herd conditions may also create competition for food and water that prevents some individuals from getting adequate nutrition.

The source of feed, hay, bedding, and water may not always be the farm on which the animals are kept. Under pasture conditions, stream, creek, or pond water may provide water for the animals' use. The purity of such water sources may be affected by "upstream" agricultural activities and runoff. Commonly, feed, hay, and bedding are purchased and shipped to the farm from outside vendors, and their quality and content may not be guaranteed. For example, poisonous plants may be inadvertently harvested when hay is cut and baled, producing toxicity when animals consume it. In certain areas of the country, black walnut trees may be included in the production of wood shavings, but there are no labeling requirements for packaging; black walnut shavings may cause severe laminitis in horses when it is used for bedding.

A summary of basic large animals' history information is presented in Box 8-1.

BOX 8-1 Large Animal History

The following information should be obtained and recorded in the medical record:

Person Providing Information
Owner, agent, trainer, or farm employee

Insurance Information
Company Name, Contact Information
Policy Number
Type of Insurance

Patient Signalment
Age, sex, breed, color, and identifying markings

Diet
Feed Schedule
Forage/Hay
- Type
- Source

Grain
- Type
- Source

Supplements
Dietary Changes
- Intake: increased or decreased
- Change in appetite for certain foodstuffs
- Change in source of foodstuffs

Water
Sources
Availability

Housing Type

Reproductive Status

Vaccination History

Deworming History

Production History: Any Increase or Decrease in Production

Previous Illnesses/Surgical Procedures

Presenting (Chief) Complaint
Time of onset
Speed of onset: peracute, acute, or chronic
Duration
Progression of severity: improving, worsening, or static
Previous Treatments/Medications

Herd Information
Number of animals in herd
Number affected
Number of deaths

PHYSICAL EXAMINATION OF LARGE ANIMALS

Combined with a thorough history, the physical examination forms the basis for identifying a patient's true problems. Most clinicians use a problem-oriented approach to diagnosis and treatment; this provides a logical method to work through the simplest to most complicated medical and surgical cases. Regardless of the size or species of animal, developing a consistent and systematic approach to a physical examination will increase the proficiency of the examiner and decrease the likelihood of overlooking important findings.

PHYSICAL EXAMINATION OF THE EQUINE

When an animal is presented for veterinary evaluation of medical or surgical problems, a physical examination is performed for diagnostic purposes. The diagnostic physical exam may range from a basic "TPR" examination to a thorough multisystem or system-specific evaluation, depending on the patient's problems. In addition to the diagnostic type of physical examination, there are other types of "routine" physical examinations that horse owners may request for their horses. The *insurance examination* is required by the insurance company before a horse can receive insurance coverage. It may range from a basic physical exam to a thorough, in-depth examination of all body systems; the type of insurance and value of the animal will dictate the depth of exam required by the insurance company. The *prepurchase examination* is conducted before completing the sale of an animal and is a common procedure in equine practice. A seller and a buyer are identified, and the veterinarian performing the exam is presumed to be working in the buyer's best interest (the veterinarian is paid by the buyer). Like the insurance examination, the scope of the prepurchase examination is dictated by the intended use of the horse and its estimated value; it may be a simple physical examination or an in-depth exam, including biopsies, blood samples, endoscopy, EKG and/or echocardiogram, and diagnostic imaging. Prepurchase examinations are often a source of lawsuits against the veterinarian; therefore veterinarians go to great lengths to document the findings of prepurchase examinations and not to overstate their findings as predictions of future performance. The technician should understand the potentially sensitive nature of insurance and prepurchase examinations and help ensure the accuracy and privacy of the results.

TECHNICIAN NOTE Prepurchase examinations are a potential source of lawsuits, and examination results must be kept strictly confidential.

Getting Started

The basic physical examination always begins with observation of the animal from a distance. Good diagnosticians will take advantage of this opportunity to observe the animal before applying restraint and will consider the total picture of the horse and its environment. The attitude, alertness, and general body condition of the horse are noted. The movements of the horse provide an opportunity to observe lameness. If food and water are available, appetite, mastication, and swallowing reflexes can be observed. Interactions with other animals can also provide useful information.

After observing the horse and gauging its temperament, presence or absence of pain, and possible body systems that will need to be evaluated, the most appropriate method of physical restraint can be selected. All physical examinations begin with appropriate physical restraint. Physical restraint is necessary for the safety of personnel and the horse and facilitates the physical examination procedures. Depending on the body system (or systems) to be evaluated, the method of physical restraint may need to be changed during the examination. Chemical restraint may also need to be applied to supplement physical restraint of painful or uncooperative patients (refer to Chapter 7 for more information about restraint and handling of animals).

After proper restraint has been applied, the hands-on physical examination can begin. A basic physical examination typically includes temperature, pulse, and respiration ("TPR"); heart and lung auscultation; abdominal auscultation; hydration status; examination of mucous membranes; and height and weight measurement.

Body Temperature

A temperature is almost always taken rectally, using a standard mercury or digital thermometer. Rarely, a vaginal temperature may be used.

Although any thermometer may be used on large animals, thermometers designed strictly for large animals are commercially available. Large animal thermometers are typically 5 inches long and have a thicker glass casing than regular thermometers. In addition, they often include a "ring top", which allows the user to attach a short (<12 inches) string. Strings are helpful for managing two commonly encountered situations: aspiration of the thermometer into the rectum and pushing the thermometer out of the rectum. Some horses may pull the anus inward while the thermometer is in place; occasionally, this results in aspiration of the entire thermometer into the rectum. This is potentially serious if the thermometer breaks inside the rectum or if the horse strains to defecate; perforation of the rectum may occur and can be life threatening. The presence of the thermometer in the anus may also stimulate defecation; if this occurs, the thermometer will be passed out of the rectum, fall to the ground, and break. Broken thermometer glass can puncture hooves or skin or may be eaten as the horse browses for food. Because of these complications, it is common either to maintain a firm grip on the thermometer for the entire procedure or tie a string to the ring top and secure the string to the horse's tail hairs or hair coat (not the skin) with a clothespin or small alligator clamp. If the horse aspirates the thermometer, the string can be used to gently retrieve it or to follow the string manually into the rectum to retrieve it. If the horse pushes the thermometer out of the rectum, the secured string should prevent it from falling on the ground. Strings longer than 12 inches should be avoided; long strings allow the thermometer to dangle against the legs, which causes some horses to kick.

Inserting the rectal thermometer requires some tact. The thermometer should be lubricated with petroleum jelly, mineral oil, or water, but avoid dipping the thermometer in the horse's water bucket; this practice gives the impression of disregard for sanitary procedure. Even if the thermometer has been properly disinfected, it is viewed by owners as a piece of equipment that has been in other horses' rectums and has no place in their horse's water bucket.

To insert the thermometer, stand next to the horse's hindquarters, facing caudally (Figure 8-16). Never stand directly behind the horse. If the horse resists by kicking or appears agitated by manipulations of the tail and hindquarters, the technician can stand behind a stall door or a stack of hay bales for protection. Grasp the tail near the base and elevate it or push it to the opposite side of the horse; it is not necessary to force the tail into an extreme position, which will only be met with resistance by the horse. Move the tail only enough to get clear entrance to the anus (Figure 8-17). Some horses respond best to gentle rubbing of the perianal area before touching the anus with the thermometer, rather than thrusting the thermometer in the anus with no warning. The anal opening is identified either visually or by feel and the thermometer gently inserted with a twisting motion.

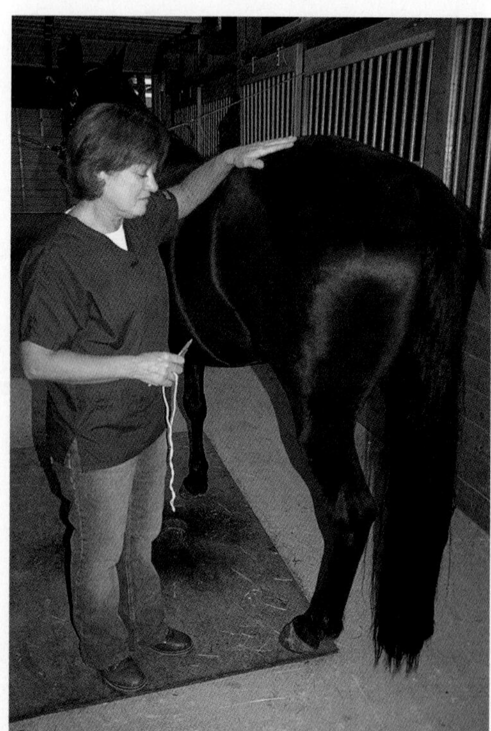

FIGURE 8-16 When taking rectal temperature, stand facing caudally, and maintain contact with the horse.

If the thermometer does not easily advance, never force it; the rectal wall may be perforated with little effort. If the horse strains in resistance, try distracting it by offering feed or having someone tap on the horse's forehead while the thermometer is being inserted. The thermometer usually enters horizontally, but some horses require tipping the thermometer slightly upward (dorsally) to enter the rectum.

> TECHNICIAN NOTE Rectal thermometers should be inserted and advanced into the rectum without using force.

The thermometer should be advanced several inches into the rectum, then either handheld or clipped to the tail hairs or coat hairs. It should be left in place for at least 60 seconds (mercury type) or until the audible or visual signal is heard or seen (digital type).

Normal rectal temperature varies by the age, breed, and environment of the animal. Body temperature is typically lowest in the morning. Normal rectal temperature of the adult horse at rest is 99.0° F to 101.5° F. From 101.5° F to 102.0° F is a "gray zone" and may be normal for some individuals, especially in hot weather. A temperature above 102.0° F is always suspicious, except following physical exercise, which can readily temporarily elevate temperature to this level and above. Normal values for TPR are given in Table 8-7.

Other factors may influence temperature. Large breeds and draft horses tend to have rectal temperatures at the lower end of the temperature range. Neonatal foals may lack the ability to generate body heat and often have low body temperatures immediately after birth. As heat-generating mechanisms develop, older foals may average approximately 1° higher than adults for the first few days to weeks after birth. Rectal procedures, such as a manual or endoscopic rectal examination, may allow air to enter the rectum, falsely lowering the rectal temperature; the temperature should be taken before any rectal procedure is performed.

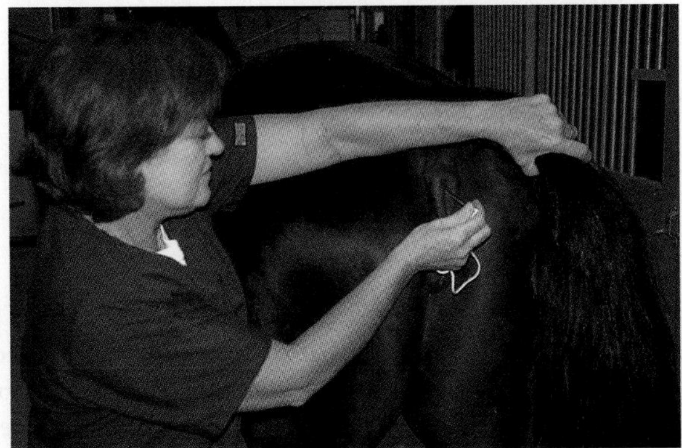

FIGURE 8-17 Grasp the tail at the base and move it gently to the side; the thermometer can then be inserted through the anus into the rectum.

If the rectum contains feces, the thermometer tip may sometimes be inadvertently inserted into a fecal ball. This is the most common cause of unexpectedly low readings. If this occurs, the procedure should be repeated.

Pulse Rate/Heart Rate

Strictly speaking, heart rate and pulse rate are not the same; heart rate refers to the number of heartbeats/min (beats/min [bpm]); pulse rate refers to the number of palpable arterial pulse waves/min. In normal animals, the heart rate and pulse rate are equal.

The pulse rate is taken by palpation of arteries. As blood passes from arteries through capillary beds, there is a dampening effect on arterial blood pressure fluctuations (waves); therefore veins do not have palpable pulses.

Auscultation of the heart is properly used for taking heart rate, not pulse rate. This is because some heart abnormalities may produce audible heart sounds that are not necessarily accompanied by an arterial pulse. For accuracy, when the heart is auscultated, the arterial pulse should be simultaneously palpated to be sure that every audible heartbeat is accompanied by a palpable pulse wave (Figure 8-18). If each audible heartbeat is not accompanied by a pulse wave, a condition called *pulse deficit,* the clinician should be notified.

Arterial pulses may be palpated at several locations. The most convenient location is over the facial artery where it courses across the ventral aspect of the mandible, rostral to the origin of the masseter muscle (Figure 8-19). Two or three fingers are lightly rolled back and forth across the ventromedial aspect of the mandible just rostral to the masseter muscle to identify the facial artery and facial vein; these vessels lie side by side and form a tubular, compressible type of structure. Once identified, the vascular bundle is firmly pressed against the mandible to feel the arterial pulse (Figure 8-20). If the bundle is pressed too tightly, the artery may be occluded and the pulse not easily felt. Large animal heart rates are much lower than their small animal counterparts, often requiring more patience to identify a palpable pulse.

TABLE 8-7 Normal TPR Values for Adult Large Animals

	Rectal Temperature °F	Heart Rate	Respiratory Rate
Horse	99.0-101.5	28-40/min	6-12/min
Cattle	101.5 (range 100.4-103.1)	40-80/min	10-30/min
Sheep	102.5 (range 102.0-104.0)	70-90/min	12-25/min
Goat	102.0 (range 101.5-104.0)	70-90/min	15-30/min

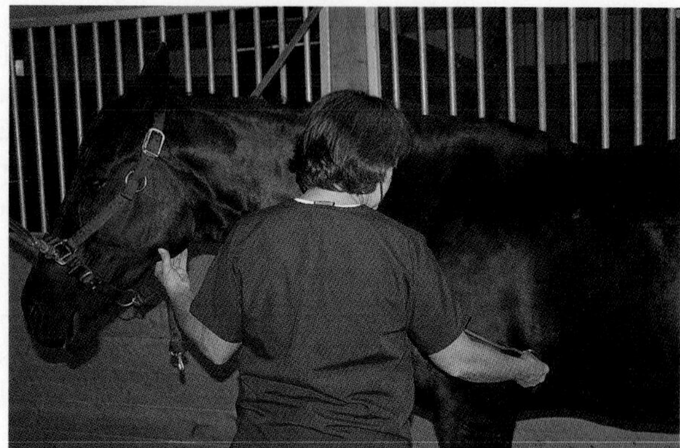

FIGURE 8-18 Simultaneous palpation of arterial pulse on the facial artery and auscultation of the heart for possible pulse deficit.

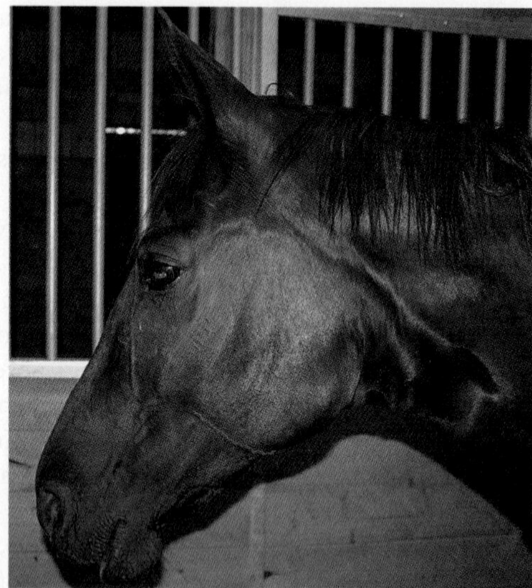

FIGURE 8-19 The facial artery courses along the rostral aspect of the masseter muscle and crosses the ventromedial aspect of the mandible.

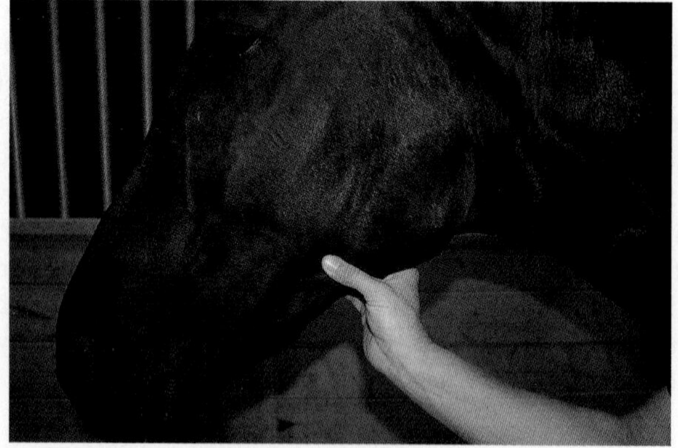

FIGURE 8-20 Press the vascular bundle firmly against the medial aspect of the mandible.

> *TECHNICIAN NOTE* The facial artery where it crosses the ventromedial aspect of the mandible is the most convenient location for obtaining the pulse rate.

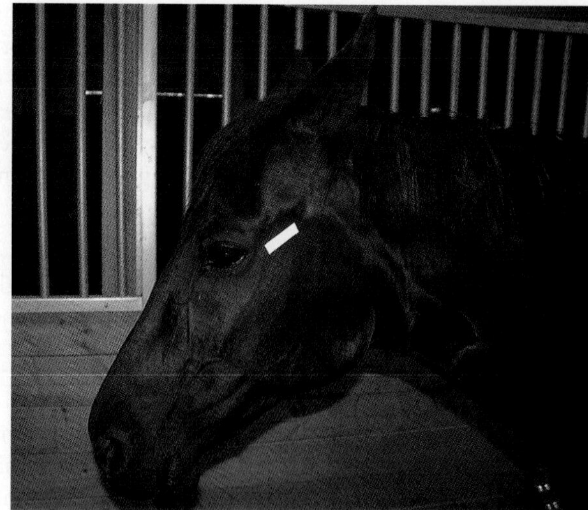

FIGURE 8-21 Location of the transverse facial artery.

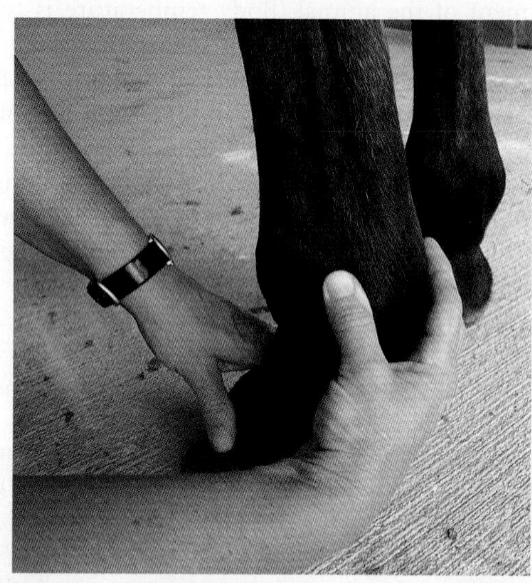

FIGURE 8-22 Palpation of the digital arteries over the proximal sesamoid bones.

Other arteries are available for obtaining pulse rates. The transverse facial artery is located in a horizontal depression about 1 inch caudal to the lateral canthus of the eye, just below the zygomatic arch (Figure 8-21). The coccygeal artery supplies the tail and is located along the ventral midline of the tail. The dorsal metatarsal artery is located between metatarsals 3 and 4 (cannon bone and lateral splint bone) on the hind limbs. The lateral and medial digital arteries can be palpated where they course over the abaxial aspect of the proximal sesamoid bones of each leg or just proximal to the collateral cartilages of each hoof (Figure 8-22). The carotid artery has a pulse wave, but it is difficult to accurately palpate in large animals because of its deep position and is seldom useful for palpation.

The main features of the pulse are rate and rhythm. The rate is recorded as number of beats/min (bpm). The pulse rate is normally 28 to 44 bpm in adult horses at rest. Foals have a rate of 60 to 80 bpm immediately after birth; this climbs to 75 to 100 bpm for the first week or 2 of life, then gradually declines toward the adult rate over the next several weeks to months. Athletically fit horses may normally have rates less than 28 bpm; 24 bpm is not uncommon in fit race horses.

The pulse rhythm is recorded as regular or irregular. Irregular rhythm likely indicates an arrhythmia of the heart. The most common cause of pulse irregularity in horses is second degree AV (atrioventricular) block, a heart arrhythmia caused by failure of the electrical current generated by the atria to reach the ventricles. There is an intermittent blockage of current at the AV node, resulting in "dropped" pulse beats. The dropped beats usually occur in *a regular pattern;* typically the dropped beat occurs every third or fourth heartbeat. Second degree AV block is readily identified by palpating the pulse. The regular rhythm is interrupted by a single "lost" (dropped) beat, with the "lost" beats occurring at regular intervals (beat-beat-beat-no beat-beat-beat-beat-no beat, etc.). Even though second degree AV block is usually considered to be a normal finding in horses, its presence should be noted in the medical record. Horses with this arrhythmia may have low resting heart rates, less than 28 bpm. Second degree AV block is more common in athletically fit horses and should disappear in any horse when the horse is exercised. It is believed to be caused by increased tone from the vagus nerve, part of the parasympathetic nervous system.

The pulse quality is often described as strong, bounding, weak, thready, or other nonspecific terms. The pulse quality is subjective; its usefulness depends on the experience of the person assessing the pulse and should not be overinterpreted.

Respiratory Rate

The number of respirations per minute can be counted several ways: (1) a stethoscope can be used to listen to air movements in and out of the trachea or chest; (2) a hand can be used to feel the movement of air in and out of a nostril; and (3) most commonly, visually counting chest excursions (rise and fall of the thoracic wall) per minute.

Respirations should be characterized by their effort and depth. Respirations may be described as shallow, deep, labored, gasping, and other nonspecific terms. Horses normally use a combination of thoracic and abdominal muscles to breathe; this is called costoabdominal breathing. Some painful conditions of the chest may lead to an increased use of the abdominal muscles to breathe, referred to as an *increased abdominal effort* in the respiratory pattern.

Normal horses cannot breathe through the mouth. If mouth breathing is observed, it should be noted and brought to the attention of the clinician.

Respiratory noises are not uncommon in horses and are often significant findings. Noises may be characterized as wheezing, whistling, honking, snoring, fluttering, etc. Noises may be heard only at rest or only during exercise. It is important to note the horse's activity at the time the noise is heard. Equally important is to note whether the noise occurs during inspiration, expiration, or both.

The normal respiratory rate of an adult horse at rest is 6 to 12 breaths per minute. The rate is higher during hot weather or following physical activity. Foals have a high respiratory rate at birth as a result of the residual fluid in the lower airways. Newborn foals may have a respiratory rate from 80 to 90; this will slow to 60 to 80 in the first 5 to 10 minutes after birth and gradually decrease to 20 to 40 for the first week or 2 of life.

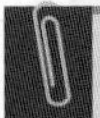
TECHNICIAN NOTE Respiratory noises should be characterized as inspiratory, expiratory, or both.

Heart Auscultation

Auscultation may be done on the left or right side of the chest, though most of the heart valves and sounds are heard best from the left side. However, the right side should not be overlooked; some murmurs are audible only on the right side and will be missed if the horse is auscultated only from the left.

Horses are athletes; the heart of the average horse may be as large as a basketball. The landmarks for basic auscultation of the heart are the same on either side of the chest. The landmarks for the dorsoventral position of the heart are the level of the shoulder joint for the heart base and the point of the elbow (olecranon) for the heart apex (Figure 8-23). The craniocaudal position is defined by the caudal border of the triceps muscle, which roughly divides the heart into cranial and caudal halves. Using these landmarks, the position of the heart can be estimated.

Usually, heart sounds are easier to hear when auscultation is performed cranial to the caudal border of the triceps muscle. However, the triceps muscle is too thick to allow any heart sounds to be heard through it; the head of the stethoscope must be placed directly against the chest wall. To expose the chest wall at this location, the triceps muscle can be gently elevated away from the chest wall before the stethoscope is positioned (Figure 8-24). Another approach is

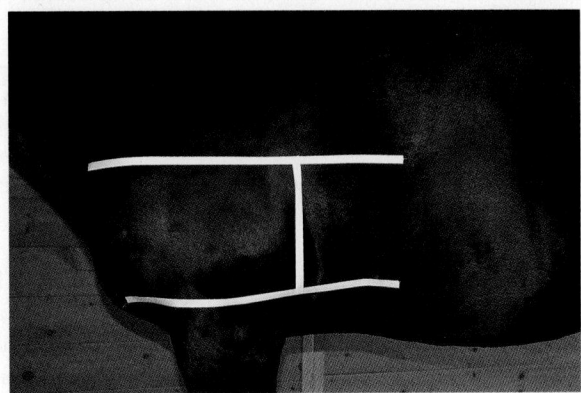

FIGURE 8-23 Landmarks for the heart: the horizontal marks indicate the level of the shoulder and elbow joints; the vertical mark indicates the caudal border of the triceps muscle.

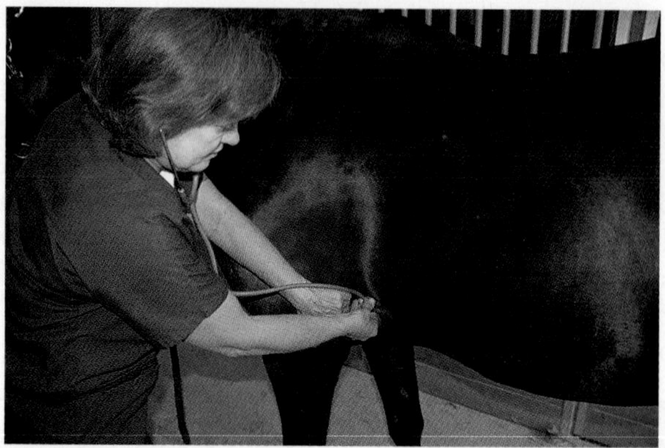

FIGURE 8-24 The triceps muscle is gently lifted away from the chest wall to provide access for the stethoscope.

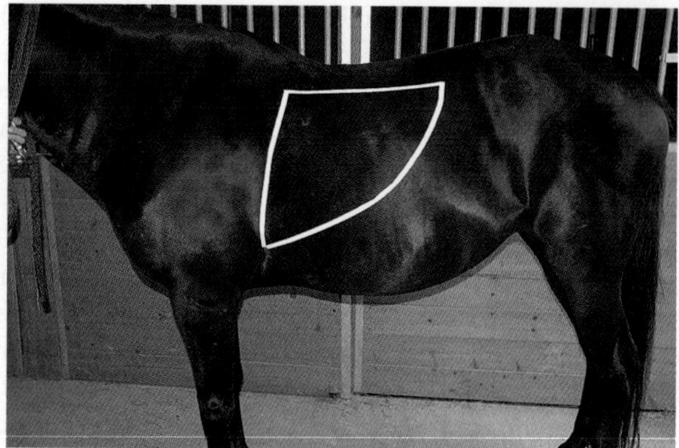

FIGURE 8-25 Borders of the left lung field for lung auscultation.

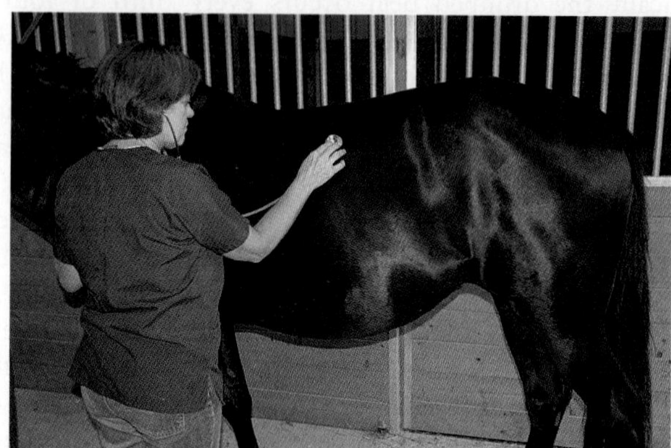

FIGURE 8-26 Auscultation of the left caudodorsal lung field.

to advance the forelimb to a more forward position, as if the horse were taking a step forward, which moves the triceps cranially. However, many horses are reluctant to hold this position for any length of time.

The heart rate is counted as beats per minute. The cardiac sounds S_1 (lub) and S_2 (dub) are components of one heartbeat. A common error, especially for those accustomed to small animal auscultation, is to count S_1 and S_2 as separate beats, essentially doubling the actual heart rate. The heart rate in large animals is slow, and the heart sounds are usually loud and distinct, leading to the possible confusion.

Auscultation is also used to detect abnormal heart sounds. Murmurs are not uncommon in horses, though most murmurs in the horse are actually normal heart sounds and are simply the result of large volumes of blood moving at high speeds through the heart valves. Because of the large heart size, these sounds are amplified and are referred to as *ejection murmurs*. Ejection murmurs are commonly heard in horses and should disappear when the horse is exercised. True cardiac disease is unusual in horses, but will usually be accompanied by murmurs or other abnormal sounds.

Heart murmurs are assessed for loudness, character, and the timing of the murmur in the cardiac cycle (systolic, diastolic, or continuous). The horse may be exercised to see if the abnormal sound disappears, stays the same, or gets louder with exercise. Using these initial criteria, the veterinarian decides whether further evaluation of the cardiovascular system is warranted.

> TECHNICIAN NOTE Ejection murmurs are commonly auscultated in the horse and are usually normal findings.

Lung Auscultation

Despite the large size of equine lungs, breath sounds may be difficult to hear. A quiet environment is important for an accurate evaluation. Lung auscultation should *always* be performed on *both* sides of the chest. Respiratory diseases do not necessarily affect both lungs and pleural cavities equally and can result in markedly different auscultation findings over the right and left lung fields of a single individual. Because of the large size of the lungs and possible uneven distribution of disease, auscultation findings may even vary over different areas of the same lung.

The borders of the lung fields are the same for the right and left sides of the chest and are outlined in Figure 8-25. The lung field basically consists of a cranioventral area and a caudodorsal area; a part of the cranioventral field is obscured by the shoulder musculature and cannot be heard. The stethoscope is placed in several locations within the lung field, listening to several breaths at each location (Figure 8-26). Normally, air movement in and out of the airways should be heard with each chest excursion; sounds may be amplified in foals, thin animals, and in any animal after exercise. Occasionally, it is desirable to induce deep breathing to accentuate lung sounds; this is easily accomplished by occluding the nostrils temporarily until the horse begins to object to the lack of air; at the first sign of discomfort, the examiner releases the nostrils and immediately moves to auscultate the chest. Abnormal respiratory sounds include wheezes, crackles, and gurgling, moist sounds; the absence of breath sounds may also be significant. The veterinarian should be alerted when abnormal sounds are detected.

Abdominal Auscultation

A stethoscope is used to listen to abdominal sounds, which are created by movements of the intestines. This is commonly referred to as *gastrointestinal motility* or *GI motility*. In reality, this term is a misnomer because some sounds are generated by the passive movement of gas and liquids in the intestines without actually being propelled by the intestinal musculature. It is not completely accurate to assume that all intestinal sounds are due to functional intestines. This becomes important in the patient with GI disease; diseased portions of intestine may have little or no purposeful motility, yet passive fluid and gas sounds may be heard. Experience is required to distinguish active motility from passive sounds.

Abdominal auscultation should be performed on both sides of the horse. Although auscultation can be performed at any location on the abdominal wall, the common sites for auscultation are in the areas known as the right and left "flanks." The flank is the slightly depressed area between the pelvis and the caudal margin of the rib cage. The point of the hip (tuber coxae) identifies the dorsal extent of the flank area (Figure 8-27). Horses may be sensitive in the flank and abdominal regions, so these areas should be approached slowly and gently. A good approach is to place the hand with the stethoscope on the horse's back and slowly slide it to the flank or lower abdominal area.

A standard four-point auscultation is sufficient for most patients. A stethoscope is used to auscultate the upper flank and the lower flank on both sides of the abdomen. The four points of auscultation are referred to as upper left, upper right, lower left, and lower right abdominal quadrants (Figure 8-28). Intestinal motility sounds, also called *borborygmi*, have been described as sounding like thunder rumbling or an approaching freight train. These sounds are usually associated with coordinated, normal patterns of large intestinal motility. The number of borborygmi per minute is counted in each abdominal quadrant; the stethoscope should be left in place for *at least 1 minute* at *each* of the four auscultation points to get an accurate count. "Normal" motility is considered to be one to three borborygmi per minute in each abdominal quadrant. More than this is considered to be hypermotility, and less than this rate is considered to be hypomotility. The complete absence of borborygmus is equated with "intestinal standstill," properly termed *ileus*. Ileus often indicates serious intestinal disease and is associated with increased morbidity and mortality in horses with colic. Auscultation in colic patients may be confusing because gas and fluid "tinkling" sounds may still be heard in horses with complete ileus. These are passive sounds and should not be confused with the motility of normally functioning intestines.

The findings of four-point abdominal auscultation are recorded in the medical record using the grid system in Box 8-2.

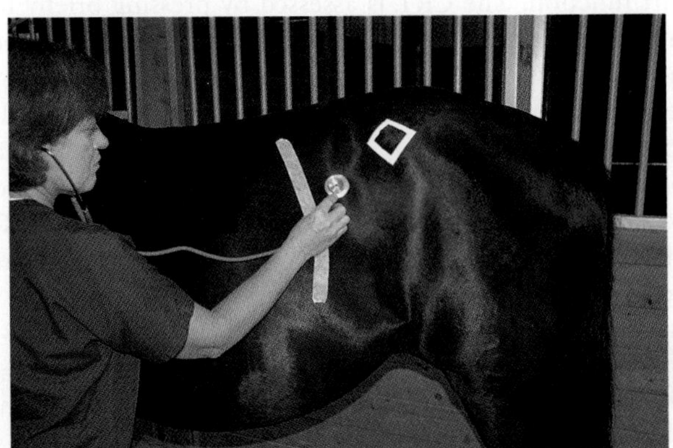

FIGURE 8-27 Landmarks for abdominal auscultation in the flank area are the point of the hip (tuber coxae) and the last rib.

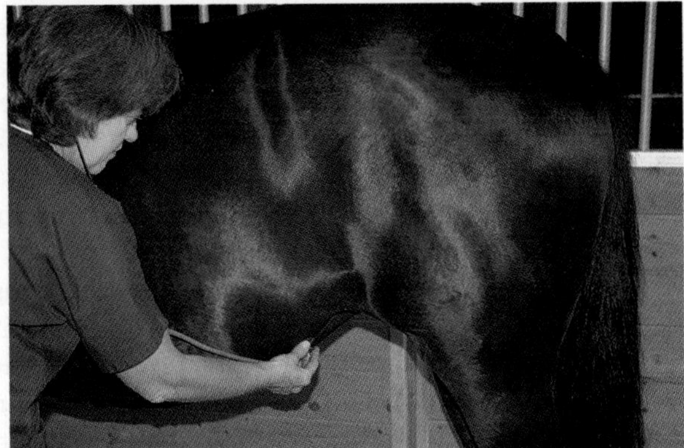

FIGURE 8-28 Auscultation of the lower left abdominal quadrant.

> *TECHNICIAN NOTE* The presence of intestinal sounds does not always indicate the presence of intestinal motility.

BOX 8-2 Four-Point Abdominal Auscultation

Findings from the four-point auscultation are recorded in the medical record using a grid that identifies each abdominal quadrant.

Upper Left Quadrant	Upper Right Quadrant
Lower Left Quadrant	Lower Right Quadrant

Results of auscultation at each location are recorded as follows:

0 = no motility heard
+1 = hypomotility (<1 borborygmus/min)
+2 = normal motility (1-3 borborygmi/min)
+3 = hypermotility (>3 borborygmi/min)

For example, a horse with hypomotility in the lower right quadrant and a normal number of borborygmi in all other quadrants would be recorded as follows:

+2	+2
+2	+1

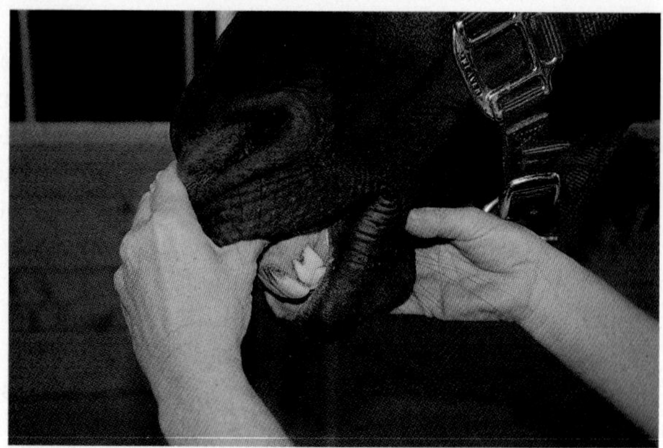

FIGURE 8-29 Examination of the gums. The upper lip is gently elevated to the extent necessary to see the gum tissue.

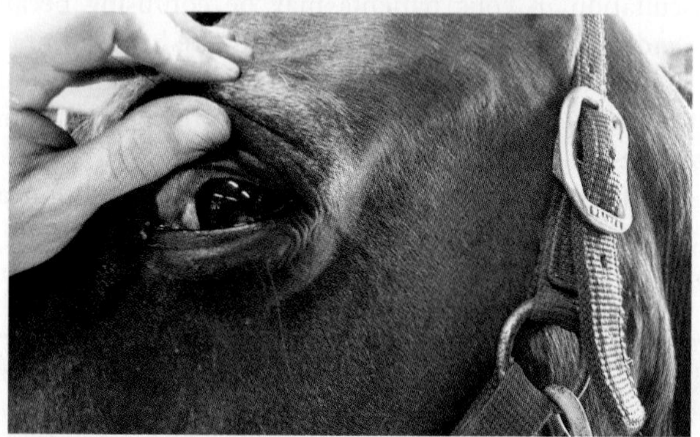

FIGURE 8-30 Examination of the conjunctiva. The upper lid is gently elevated upward, without pinching or pressing.

Mucous Membranes

Mucous membranes are tissues that have the ability to produce and secrete mucus. The mucous membrane color is helpful for disease diagnosis. There are several mucous membranes that are readily visible to the examiner: the gums (gingiva), conjunctiva of the eye, lining of the nostrils, and inner surfaces of the vulva in females (Figures 8-29 and 8-30). The inner surface of the ear pinna is not a mucous membrane, though it may be useful for detecting icterus and clotting disorders.

The mucous membrane color is usually light to dark pink. The color may change with abnormalities of blood perfusion and the oxygen content of the blood and other diseases. Cyanosis is a bluish tint that usually indicates extremely low oxygen content in the tissue. Brick red coloration indicates bacterial septicemia and/or septic shock. Endotoxic shock in the horse has the unique characteristic of producing a purple gum color that appears along the margin of the teeth and gums; this is commonly referred to as a *toxic line*. Yellowish coloring of the gums indicates icterus, usually resulting from liver dysfunction or abnormal hemolysis of red blood cells. Pale mucous membranes may indicate anemia or poor perfusion, though many normal horses have naturally pale pink gum color. Clotting disorders may produce visible hemorrhage in mucous membranes. Small pinpoint hemorrhages less than 1 mm in diameter are called *petechial hemorrhages* or *petechiae; ecchymotic hemorrhage* produces slightly larger hemorrhages 1 mm to 1 cm in diameter.

Mucous membranes are often assessed for moisture and are commonly described as moist, dry, tacky, or other subjective terms. This information is less useful than the membrane color.

Hydration Status

The hydration status of an animal is important information. It may be measured with laboratory tests or estimated from the physical exam. Two common methods of assessing the hydration of an animal on a physical examination are the skin turgor test and the capillary refill time.

The skin turgor is assessed by the *skin pinch* or *skin snap* test. The loose skin over the lateral aspect of the neck is briefly and firmly pinched with the fingers and allowed to retract back to its original position. In normally hydrated animals, the skin should return ("snap") promptly back to its original position in approximately 1 second or less. Dehydration (>5% dehydration) prolongs the response to greater than 1 second. Severely dehydrated animals may take 8 seconds or longer for the skin to retract. The skin turgor is less reliable in obese animals; fat in the cervical area may falsely improve the skin snap. Conversely, thin horses and horses older than 15 years may have delayed skin snap response, regardless of hydration status.

The capillary refill time (CRT) is a reflection of cardiac output, which is directly affected by hydration status. Prolonged CRT is usually associated with low cardiac output, which is most commonly caused by inadequate hydration of the animal. Low cardiac output can also result from decreased heart function. The CRT is assessed by pressing briefly but firmly on the gums with a fingertip to produce a "blanched" white spot. The time for the original gum color to return to the blanched spot is counted in seconds. The original color should return in less than 2.5 seconds. A CRT greater than 2.5 seconds is considered abnormally delayed. Dehydration and shock are the most common causes of a prolonged CRT in the horse. Severe dehydration and severe shock may produce a greatly prolonged CRT, from 5 to 8 seconds.

> *TECHNICIAN NOTE* The CRT is more accurate than the skin turgor in assessing an animal's hydration status.

Height/Weight Measurement

Height and weight measurements are needed for a variety of purposes. A height measurement may be required as part of an insurance or prepurchase examination, for breed registration, or for entry into certain horse show classes. The weight measurement is usually obtained for calculating the proper dose of drugs and therapeutic substances and for formulating the diet of the animal.

Height may be estimated or measured precisely. Rough estimates may be made with a height-weight tape. This instrument is essentially a tape measure, marked on one side for height measurement in hands (1 hand = 4 inches) and for weight measurement on the other side. Ideally the horse should stand on a firm, level surface with its weight distributed evenly on all four legs. The horse's head should not be elevated or lowered, but should be in a horizontal position with the neck parallel to the ground. One end of the measuring tape is held on the ground just behind the horse's forelimb. The tape is then stretched vertically to the withers and the height read at the level of the highest point of the withers. The tape gives an approximation of the animal's height.

For precise determination of height, commercially-made rigid measuring rulers are available. These rulers are made of metal and include bubble-style levels to ensure that the ruler is not tilted when the measurement is taken. The animal should stand squarely on a firm, level surface with the head and neck held parallel to the ground. The measurement is taken at the last mane hair or highest point of the withers, depending on the breed registry or rules of competition.

Weight may be roughly estimated with the height-weight tape or taken more precisely with a livestock scale. The height-weight tape has one side that is calibrated for weight measurement; the weight tick marks are based on measurements around the girth of the horse. The tape is applied to encircle the horse at its girth, which is the area caudal to the withers and just behind the forelimb (Figure 8-31). The weight tape is formulated from logarithms of "normal" animals and may be inaccurate for excessively thin or obese animals. The build of an animal may also affect the results. Height-weight tapes designed for cattle are not accurate for horses.

Precise weights for large animals may be obtained with livestock scales. Digital livestock scales have a walk-over design and are popular at many hospitals and practices. Traditional livestock scales are somewhat cumbersome to use and have largely been replaced by digital walk-over scales.

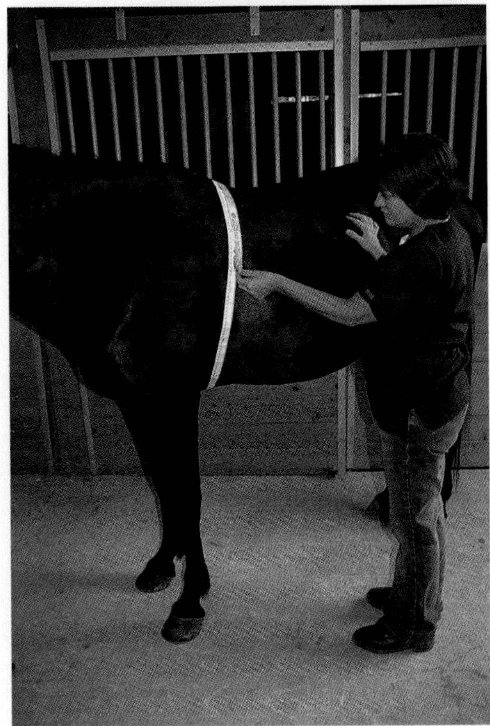

FIGURE 8-31 The weight tape is positioned around the thorax at the girth, just caudal to the withers.

PHYSICAL EXAMINATION OF RUMINANTS

The physical examination begins with an initial visual observation of the animal from a distance. The animal's posture, behavior, body condition, and alertness are easily observed. More specific signs, such as breathing pattern, respiratory noise, lameness, skin wounds, and muscle atrophy, may also be noted. When working with any species, some understanding of basic instincts and typical behaviors is essential to interpreting what is seen through observation. Although ruminants share many physiologic traits, they do not share a common "mentality," and the behavioral differences among the various ruminant species must be appreciated. This is especially important when observing an individual's interactions with the herd.

> *TECHNICIAN NOTE* Valuable information can be obtained by observing an animal from a distance before the physical examination.

The direct "hands-on" physical examination typically includes the "TPR," heart and lung auscultation, abdominal auscultation and assessment of rumen function, hydration status, and examination of mucous membranes. Animals must be adequately restrained for this portion of the physical examination, and the methods of restraint used for cattle, sheep, and goats are quite different. Cattle are typically restrained in a chute, whereas sheep and goats are usually restrained manually (see Chapter 7 for more information on restraint of large animals).

A temperature is taken rectally, similar to the procedure in horses. When taking the rectal temperature of the goat, a dark brown, waxy material may be seen near the anus; this is a normal secretion produced by sebaceous glands under the tail head. The pulse can be palpated readily at the facial artery; the coccygeal, median (forelimb), and great metatarsal (hind limb) arteries are also available (Figure 8-32). The femoral artery is useful in sheep and goats. The respiratory rate is best taken by counting chest excursions from a distance before herding or handling; the excitement and fear of herding and restraint can cause dramatic increases in respiratory rate,

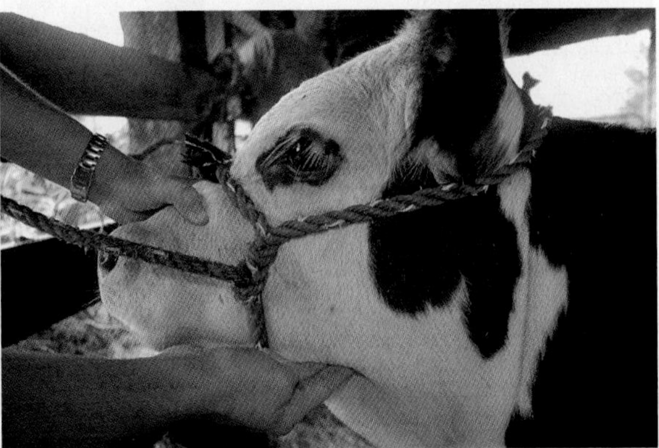

FIGURE 8-32 Palpation of the arterial pulse at the facial artery where it crosses the ventromedial aspect of the mandible.

especially in hot environmental temperatures, that will not reflect the true respiratory rate of the animal at rest. Ruminants, unlike horses, are capable of open-mouth breathing; when observed, it is usually considered to be a sign of distress or heat stress (usually when environmental temperature exceeds 85° F). Abdominal breathing is normal in ruminants. Normal values for TPR are given in Table 8-7.

Heart auscultation is performed using the same anatomic landmarks as in the horse. The shoulder joint and the olecranon indicate the dorsal-ventral position of the heart. The caudal border of the triceps muscle indicates the cranial-caudal position, generally corresponding to the fourth to fifth intercostal space. Auscultated cardiac sounds are normally only S_1 and S_2 in cattle (unlike the horse where any combination of S_3 and S_4 may accompany S_1 and S_2). The borders for lung auscultation in the ruminant are between the fifth rib cranially and the eleventh rib caudally. If it is necessary to induce deep breathing for lung auscultation, the nostrils and mouth (since ruminants can mouth breathe) can be held closed for about a minute to stimulate deeper breathing and a higher respiratory rate.

The mucous membranes should be pink and moist, with a CRT of 1 to 2 seconds (Figure 8-33). If it is necessary to fully open the mouth for an examination, placing the fingers into the interdental space and pressing on the hard palate encourages opening of the mouth; the tongue can be quickly grasped and brought to the side at the commissure of the lips, where it encourages the animal to keep the mouth open. Alternatively a mouth speculum may be used. The tongue of cattle has a single deep transverse groove across its dorsal surface; this groove is often mistaken for a laceration. The molars of ruminants may be sharp and jagged, and caution must be used whenever the hands are placed into the mouth. When examining the head and mouth area, be aware of the possibility of being struck with the head if it is not properly restrained. Adult cattle especially can cause serious injury from striking with the head.

When standing near a ruminant or when auscultating the thorax or trachea, occasional low-pitched fluttering sounds may be heard; this is eructation (burping), which is normal in ruminants. Eructation rates are approximately 18/hr in cattle, and 10/hr in sheep and goats.

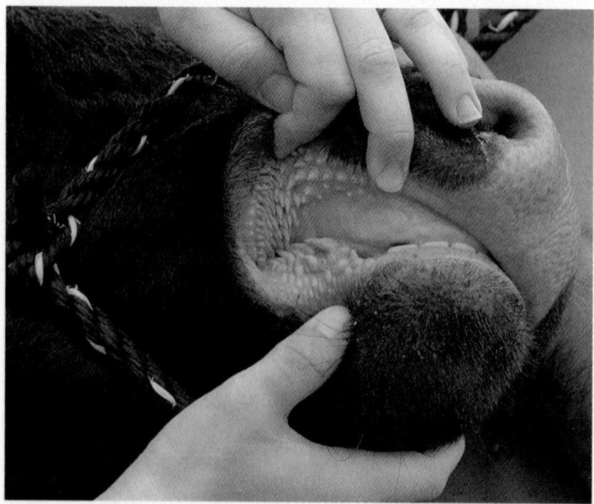

FIGURE 8-33 Normal mucous membranes in ruminants are pink and moist.

The evaluation of the ruminant abdomen includes an assessment of rumen contractions. The rumen occupies most of the left side of the abdominal cavity. The number of rumen contractions per minute may be counted by auscultation directly over the caudolateral rib cage or paralumbar fossa on the left side. Rumen contractions sound like a deep-pitched rumbling or "thunderstorm" noise, which gets gradually louder as the contraction wave approaches the stethoscope. Rumen contractions can also be counted by ballottement (palpation) by pressing both fists firmly into the left paralumbar fossa (use one fist in the sheep and goat). The fists are allowed to remain against the body wall for 1 minute. Each rumen contraction will be felt as a wave passing under the hands, pushing the hands slightly outward. The normal animal will have 1 to 2 contractions/min. Hypomotility and the absence of motility (ileus) are abnormal findings; hypermotility of the rumen is uncommon. Auscultation of the right side of the abdomen usually reveals few sounds; this is normal in ruminants.

The shape of the abdomen is observed by standing behind the animal, facing the head, and comparing the right and left abdominal outlines or "silhouettes." The overall shape of the right and left abdominal outlines should be similar, with the overall outline of the cow resembling a pear (wider at the lower flanks than at the paralumbar fossae) (Figure 8-34). The paralumbar fossae should be normally flat or slightly

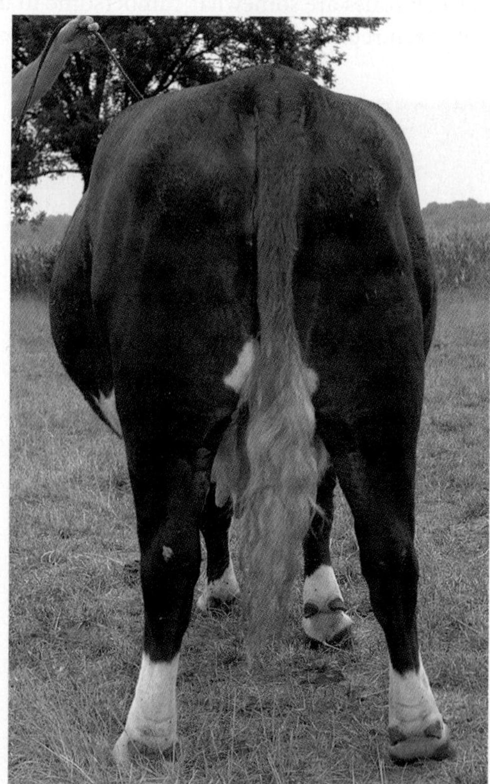

FIGURE 8-34 Normal "pear" abdominal shape of the cow as viewed from behind. As a result of the anatomic location of the rumen, the left side may appear slightly fuller than the right.

sunken. The accumulation of gas within certain portions of the GI tract (tympany or "*bloat*") can produce asymmetry and enlargement of the abdominal wall. The most common location for bloat, the rumen, appears as an enlargement of the left paralumbar fossa; this has been referred to as a "papple"-shaped abdomen, where the left side resembles an apple and the right side a pear. Severe abdominal gas accumulation can cause protrusion of the paralumbar fossa on both sides of the animal, changing the normal pear shape to one that resembles an apple.

> *TECHNICIAN NOTE* The abdominal "silhouette," viewed from behind the animal, provides useful diagnostic information for possible GI diseases.

Gas accumulations can also be detected by simultaneous percussion and auscultation, a technique commonly known as *abdominal pinging*. The stethoscope is held in place with one hand, while the other hand is used to snap a finger against the abdominal wall at several locations around the stethoscope head (Figure 8-35). Gas accumulations make a resonant tympanic "ping" sound, like a high-pitched drum. Pings are significant findings and generally indicate abnormal position or contents of one or more GI tract organs. Note that solid organs and non-GI organs cannot accumulate gas (with the exception of the uterus, which is extremely rare) and do not create pings. Pinging should be performed on both sides of the abdomen and may detect abnormalities before they are visible as external enlargement of the abdomen.

The character of feces and urine, if available for observation, should be evaluated. Fecal character varies among the ruminants. Cattle defecate 12 to 18 times/day; the feces have a semisolid "cow-plop" or "cow-pie" consistency, without distinct form. Goats produce well-formed feces in the shape of small, solid pellets. Sheep feces are also pelleted. The color of the feces depends on the diet, ranging from green to dark brown. Undigested roughage fibers in the fecal material are an abnormal finding and may indicate dysfunction of the rumen and/or reticulum.

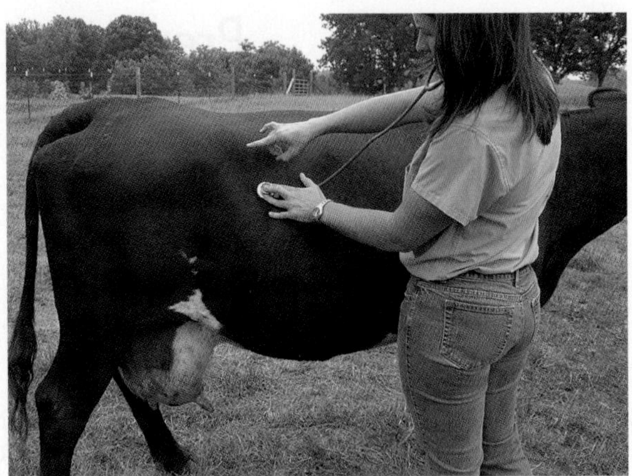

FIGURE 8-35 Proper technique for abdominal "pinging." The stethoscope is held in place while snapping a finger sharply against the abdominal wall in the vicinity of the stethoscope head.

SUGGESTED READING

Fubini SL, Ducharme NG: *Farm animal surgery*. Philadelphia, 2004, WB Saunders.

Hanie EA: *Large animal clinical procedures for veterinary technicians*. St Louis, 2006, Mosby.

McCurnin DM, Poffenbarger EM: *Small animal physical diagnosis and clinical procedures*. Philadelphia, 1991, WB Saunders.

Pugh DG: *Sheep and goat medicine*. Philadelphia, 2002, WB Saunders.

Smith MC, Sherman DM: *Goat medicine*. Baltimore, 1994, Williams & Wilkins.

Speirs VC: *Clinical examination of horses*. Philadelphia, 1997, WB Saunders.

9 Preventive Health Programs

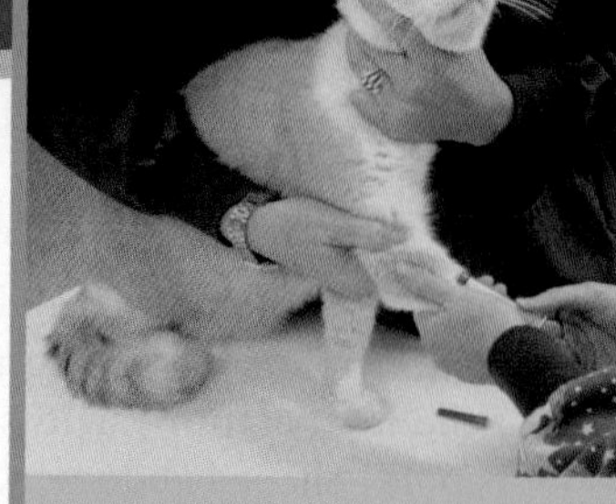

Meryl P. Littman, Carolyn J. Hammer, and Sarah A. Wagner

OUTLINE

KEY TERMS

Active immunity
Adjuvant
Anaphylaxis
Antitoxin
Biosecurity
Colostrum
Congenital
Cryptorchid
Fomite
Interferon
Needle teeth
Passive immunity
Toxoid

LEARNING OBJECTIVES

When you have completed this chapter, you will be able to:

1. Describe storage, handling, reconstitution, and routes of administration for animal vaccines.
2. Differentiate between core and elective vaccines.
3. Name the core vaccines for dogs and cats.
4. Name the elective vaccines for dogs and cats.
5. List recommended anatomic locations for each vaccine commonly administered to dogs and cats.
6. List and describe the potential vaccine adverse reactions in dogs and cats.
7. List commonly used products to prevent parasite infection and infestation in dogs and cats.
8. List and describe commonly performed diagnostic screening tests in dogs and cats.
9. Provide a general outline of a routine preventive health program for horses.
10. List the core and elective vaccines used in livestock.

INTRODUCTION

Preventive health programs now include much more than just the important vaccinations and deworming protocols that have been so successful in avoiding common infectious diseases that used to claim many young and middle-aged animals. Routine veterinary examinations, owner education concerning zoonoses and basic health care, and screening for common problems before the animal shows outward signs of illness are key for maintenance of good health in normal individuals. Preventive health is important for every animal, at every stage of life (see Chapter 10 and Chapter 37). Protective, precautionary maintenance care will improve the quality of life for both the animal and its owner. For shelter, colony, or herd health, preventive protocols help avoid potentially catastrophic losses.

Many preventive health brochures are prepared by professional and veterinary-related organizations. These are often given to pet owners to reinforce the instructions of the veterinarian and veterinary technician. Education brochures for clients address a wide variety of animal health topics and can be acquired from many professional organizations and websites. Below are some examples:

1. American Veterinary Medical Association: www.avma.org/communications/brochures/default.asp
2. Veterinary colleges: www.vet.cornell.edu/fhc/brochures/index.htm
3. The American Kennel Club: www.akc.org/public_education/health_overview.cfm
4. Industry: www.npwm.com/home.htm
5. Shelter medicine: www.sheltermedicine.com/portal/portal.shtml#top3

PREVENTIVE HEALTH PROGRAMS FOR DOGS AND CATS

PUPPY AND KITTEN WELLNESS VISITS AFTER WEANING

Multiple veterinary visits are important for puppies and kittens during the postweaning period (Tables 9-1 and 9-2). During these visits, the young animal is examined for abnormalities, including congenital problems. It is also dewormed and immunized, its growth and development charted, and the owner educated about pet-care issues including: parasite control, common behavioral and training techniques (refer to Chapter 11), nutrition and feeding schedules (refer to Chapter 12), neutering, exercise, and shelter requirements. Young pets must be protected from extremes of weather and the dangers of roaming. They must have fresh water available to them, and they should never be left in a car on a hot day, even for a few minutes, because they are particularly susceptible to heat stroke. Owners are grateful to be warned about common household exposures they may not realize could be dangerous for their pet. Examples of household dangers include: potentially toxic food items, such as grapes, raisins, chocolate, onions, and garlic; drugs, such as aspirin and acetaminophen; and poisons, such as antifreeze, rat poison, toxic plants, and lawn-care products. Refer to Chapter 35 for additional information about toxicology. When discussing nutrition, the veterinary health care team can inform owners about public health concerns regarding raw meat and diets or treats that can carry bacteria, such as *Salmonella*. The early visits are also an opportunity to talk about the pros and cons of neutering versus breeding (refer to Chapter 14 for more information about reproduction). Spaying female dogs prevents unwanted pregnancy, pyometra, ovarian cancer, helps prevent diabetes mellitus, and if done before the second heat, prevents mammary cancer. For breeds predisposed to gastric dilatation and volvulus, a preventive gastropexy may be done at the time of spaying. Spaying female cats not only prevents unwanted pregnancy, but also stops the almost incessant signs of heat because cats are induced ovulators. Neutering male dogs may prevent roaming, aggression toward other male dogs, prostatic hypertrophy, prostatic infections, and testicular cancer. Neutering male cats may prevent roaming, cat fight abscesses, and marking (spraying) of odiferous urine. Female dogs and cats are usually spayed at 6 months of age unless puppy vaginitis or vulvar conformation warrant going through one heat cycle.

TABLE 9-1 Canine Vaccination Protocol at the Matthew J. Ryan Veterinary Hospital

	Neonates*	Puppy Series			First Adult Booster	Adult Boosters	
Vaccines	*2-5 wk*	*6-8 wk*	*10-12 wk*	*13-16 wk§*	*15-16 mo*	*Every yr*	*Every 3 yr*
Core							
Rabies virus[K]				X†	X		X
Killed parvovirus[K]	X						
Distemper[ML,W]		X	X	X	X		X
Canine adenovirus type-2[ML,K]		X	X	X	X		X
Canine parainfluenza[ML]		X	X	X	X		X
Canine parvovirus[ML,K]		X	X	X	X		X
Non-core							
Leptospira[K] (optional)			X	X‡	X	X	
Bordetella[K,ML] (optional)			X	X‡	X	X	

Adapted from Bellwether 61:16, 2005 with gratitude to Dr. Margret Casal and with permission from the University of Pennsylvania School of Veterinary Medicine.

*A dog less than 6 wk of age that is lacking colostrum or is at high risk for infectious disease should be given a killed-parvovirus vaccine.

†Check the local laws in your area of practice for the age when rabies vaccine should be first given to puppies.

‡Because of the potential for allergic reactions, we recommend giving leptospirosis vaccine and a killed, injectable *Bordetella* vaccine 3-4 wk before the last vaccine in the puppy series. Boosters are subsequently given together with the last of the puppy series.

ML,K,W Available as modified-live (ML), killed (K), and/or W (virus vectored) vaccine.

§Try to give the last puppy booster at around 16 weeks of age.

TABLE 9-2 Feline Vaccination Protocol at the Matthew J. Ryan Veterinary Hospital

	Neonates*	Kitten Series		First Adult Booster	Adult Boosters	
Vaccines	*2-4 wk*	*6-8 wk*	*10-13 wk§*	*15 mo*	*Every yr*	*Every 3 yr*
Core						
Rabies virus[K,W]			X†	X	X‡	X‡
Feline viral rhinotracheitis[ML,K]	X	X	X	X		X
Panleukopenia[ML,K]	X	X	X	X		X
Feline calicivirus[ML,K]	X	X	X	X		X
Non-core						
Feline leukemia[K]		X	X	X	X	
Feline immunodeficiency virus[K]		X‖	X	X	X	

Adapted from Bellwether 61:17, 2005 with gratitude to Dr. Margret Casal and with permission from the University of Pennsylvania School of Veterinary Medicine.

*Give a few drops of the MLV (IN vaccine) in each eye and in each nostril as soon as the eyes open. Useful in catteries or during outbreaks in shelters. From 6-8 wk on, either the IN or the injectable FVRCP (feline viral rhinotracheitis, calicivirus, panleukopenia) can be used. Do not inject the IN vaccine.

†Check the local laws in your area of practice for the age when rabies vaccine should first be given to kittens.

ML,K,W Available as modified-live (ML), killed (K), and/or W (virus vectored) vaccine.

‡Repeat yearly if a recombinant vaccine is used.

§Try to give the last kitten booster at 13 weeks of age with the rabies booster.

‖A series of 3 vaccines are recommended between 6 and 12 weeks of age, at least 2 weeks apart.

Male dogs and cats are usually neutered at 6 to 8 months of age to prevent urinary marking, but large-breed dogs may be neutered later (up to 10 to 14 months of age) at their time of puberty. Cryptorchid dogs should be neutered early because an undescended testicle is at risk to develop cancer or torsion. Shelters advocate neutering puppies and kittens even before adoption, as early as 2 months of age, to help stop overpopulation; no adverse effects have been related to spaying and neutering at this young age.

Healthy visits are a good time to chat about common warning signs of problems that may occur in the course of a pet's life, such as a scooting dog rubbing its hind end on the floor may need its anal sacs emptied or may need to be treated for tapeworms. A thirsty dog may not be able to concentrate its urine, or a cat straining in the litter box may not be constipated, but may have a serious urethral obstruction that requires emergency care. The veterinary staff can also educate the owner about genetic predispositions for their pet's breed and how the staff can help screen or monitor for these.

In the past, after a pet's adolescent growth period, owners were likely to receive annual postcard reminders to schedule an appointment because annual booster vaccinations were due. Now we know that many of the vaccines we use for dogs and cats produce a longer duration of immunity than just 1 year, and the emphasis of preventive care has shifted from giving vaccines to the importance of routine visits for healthy animals before they become ill. History taking, a physical examination (Chapter 8), and education of the owner can be given the attention they truly deserve. Updates concerning nutrition, behavior, training, and screening for common diseases can be addressed on an individual basis based on the lifestyle and breeding of the animal.

ROUTINE WELLNESS VISITS THROUGHOUT LIFE

Wellness visits are an important part of preventive maintenance care, once or twice a year, throughout the pet's life (see www.npwm.com/home.htm). The pet's history needs to be updated concerning new potential health risks, such as those caused by lifestyle changes, travel, the addition of new pets to the home, the administration of new medications, or the development of disease among human family members. Vaccine protocols, nutrition, and parasite control may need adjustment, depending on the individual's needs. Screening tests and discussions about public health issues may be indicated because asymptomatic pets can be a source of illness for family members, particularly those who are immunocompromised or pregnant.

Subtle deteriorating health changes may be missed by owners. A complete physical examination may detect abnormalities or a change from the animal's previous "normal." By tackling problems early, before illness becomes obvious or more serious, intervention has its greatest advantage.

> *TECHNICIAN NOTE* After weaning, multiple visits every 3 to 4 weeks (until the puppy is 16 weeks or the kitten is 12 to 13 weeks old) are important for proper immunization, preventive care, and education of the owner. For adult animals, wellness visits every 6 to 12 months are recommended to update maintenance recommendations for the animal's needs and to prevent or treat problems before they become serious.

GROOMING MAINTENANCE

Pets are more comfortable when they are groomed and kept clean, and owners can better enjoy time with their pets. Bathing, ear cleaning, removing discharges and matted hair, nail trimming, and anal sac expression are common grooming procedures (see Chapter 8 for anal sacs; Chapter 21 for grooming). Preventive dental care is also important (see Chapter 32).

SMALL ANIMAL IMMUNIZATIONS

Immunity against disease can be acquired *passively* by maternal antibodies passing from mother to progeny via the placenta (in some species, but not dogs or cats) during gestation or via colostrum shortly after birth. Immunity can also be acquired *actively* as animals develop antibodies to antigens present in their environment. Antigens are usually proteins that are a part of the pathogenic organism. Vaccines include antigens from a pathogen that causes a particular disease. When the vaccine is introduced to the immune system, the animal forms antibodies to the antigen. If the immunization is successful, a protective level of humoral (B-cell) circulating antibodies and/or a cell-mediated (T-cell) lymphocyte response will be elicited. Subsequently, if the animal is exposed naturally to the pathogen, immunologic memory will cause a rapid and heightened immune response that protects the animal from illness.

MATERNAL ANTIBODY INTERFERENCE

Antibodies present in colostrum can be absorbed through the neonate's intestine for only about 1 day. Therefore it is important that neonates nurse within the first 24 hours of birth. The passive immunity gained from consuming colostrum wanes over time. For example, the half-life of maternal antibodies against distemper or the infectious hepatitis virus is roughly 8.5 days. In general, the neonate is protected against diseases by maternal antibodies for up to 14 to 16 weeks, depending upon the amount of colostrum the neonate ingests and the type and concentration of antibodies present in the colostrum. Interestingly, strong protective antibody titers in neonates render immunization ineffective. The passively acquired antibodies from the dam or queen block the neonate's ability to mount an active immune response from the vaccine. Without doing antibody titers on each young animal, we do not know how long the maternal antibodies are present for each disease in each individual. In addition, we do not know when the titer will still be high enough to interfere with the vaccine antigens, and most importantly, we do not know when the titer will be too low to protect the animal from disease due to natural exposure. We *do* know that there is a period when the antibody level is high enough to interfere with immunization yet, at the same time, is too low to be protective against environmental pathogens. This is a vulnerable and precarious time for the health of the young animal. For this reason, it is important to keep puppies and kittens away from other animals and their excrement until they have received a full series of immunizations. Thus the administration of a series of vaccinations every few weeks after weaning is recommended. In this way, immunization occurs during the earliest possible opportunity to confer active immunity (see Tables 9-1 and 9-2). Vaccinating more often than every few weeks is not recommended because of interferon interference (see later discussion). An adult animal, such as a stray, with no known history of being immunized does not need to complete a repetitive series of vaccines as does a puppy or kitten because adults lack maternal antibody interference. Adults without prior immunizations should receive two sets of vaccines given 3 weeks apart or may receive one set followed by natural exposure to the antigens, which acts as and has the same effect as the second set of immunizations. One year later, the animal may begin to receive adult boosters.

TYPES OF VACCINES

Vaccines work because they contain a pathogen that is either killed or altered. In this way, the vaccine is able to stimulate an immune response in an animal without actually causing the disease. Microbes are cultured, harvested, and inactivated by either killing them with heat or chemicals or modifying (attenuating) them by growing them in a nonhost species, such as birds (usually their eggs), or in the environment where the temperature is below body temperature. Vaccines do not need to include the entire pathogenic organism. Subunits of the organisms make effective antigens for use in vaccines. Modern vaccines may be produced using recombinant technology and include one or more synthesized antigens in each preparation. Viral- or DNA-vectored vaccines induce production of an antigen within the vaccinated animal's own cells because the DNA is incorporated within the host's genome and is transcribed.

Modified-live–virus (MLV) vaccines stimulate interferon production better than killed-virus vaccines do. Interferon helps protect the animal quickly, even before antibody production occurs. However, interferon from a previous vaccine may negate the animal's ability to mount a response to another vaccine if given within 2 weeks. That is why the 3- to 4-week interval between boosters for puppies and kittens is recommended. Theoretically the microbes in an MLV vaccine could be virulent if the attenuation process is incomplete or unsuccessful. In addition, the vaccine can be dangerous to immunosuppressed and pregnant animals. An MLV should only be given to healthy individuals that are not immunosuppressed or pregnant (fetuses may be affected). For example, a puppy recovering from a parvovirus is immunosuppressed because of its illness and should not receive an MLV distemper vaccine, lest it become ill from the distemper virus in the vaccine. Animals vaccinated with an MLV vaccine may shed virus particles for a few days. This can be beneficial because other animals in the house may be indirectly vaccinated, or it can be problematic because immunosuppressed and pregnant animals can be exposed. Immunosuppressed or pregnant animals can be safely vaccinated with killed-virus vaccines (if available), but the animals may not be able to mount protective titers. It is best to check the dam's or queen's vaccination status and boost if necessary before she is bred so that her colostrum will contain protective antibodies for the neonates. Bacterins (killed bacterial vaccines) in general do not stimulate immunity as well as MLVs, both in duration and efficacy. Bacterins tend to cause more postvaccinal side effects than MLVs because they possess a higher antigen load and contain adjuvants that, on one hand, enhance the immune response, but on the other hand, may be associated with more inflammation, including autoimmune, allergic, or even neoplastic complications.

STORAGE, RECONSTITUTION, AND ROUTE OF ADMINISTRATION

Vaccines need to be stored according to the manufacturer's directions (e.g., refrigerated). Lyophilized (freeze-dried) powders need to be reconstituted and gently mixed with the proper type and amount of diluent provided by the manufacturer. If an animal is to receive a DA_2PP *(distemper, hepatitis [adenovirus-2], parvovirus,* and *parainfluenza)* vaccine without adding a leptospirosis vaccine as the diluent, another sterile diluent should be used that is manufactured specifically for this purpose with the appropriate pH and preservatives.

The quantity of vaccine used for a small Chihuahua puppy is the same as for an adult Great Dane; vaccines should not be divided into smaller quantities because of the animal's age or size. Vaccines in multiuse vials must be gently mixed before drawn into a syringe, and care must be taken to ensure the continued sterility of the vial.

Most vaccines today are administered subcutaneously (SQ) rather than intramuscularly (IM), although some local laws require the rabies vaccine to be given IM in specific areas of the body. Refer to Chapter 20 for a description of injection techniques. When giving any SQ injection, make sure the vaccine is indeed placed SQ and not dripping down the side of the animal. It is not recommended to vaccinate in the tail or between the shoulder blades; there is poor drainage in the interscapular area, and if a postvaccinal lump develops, it is difficult to surgically remove it. Vaccines are generally given as SQ injections on the distal thigh or shoulder area so that if in the rare event a vaccine-induced mass should form at the injection site, amputation would be possible.

Transdermal vaccines are given without needles, using air-powered special devices, such as Merial's VET JET. Some vaccines are administered intranasally (IN) to stimulate the development of local mucosal immunoglobulins at the site where pathogens commonly gain entrance to the body. IN vaccines may overcome maternal antibody interference and may induce immunity faster, but for shorter duration. In addition, IN vaccines may have single or combined components. For example, an IN canine kennel cough complex includes a combination of modified-live adenovirus-2, parainfluenza, and *Bordetella.* An IN feline combination vaccine includes FVRCP (feline viral rhinotracheitis, calicivirus, and panleukopenia). IN-attenuated products may cause mild upper respiratory signs, such as sneezing for a few days, which assists the shedding of antigens to other animals. These vaccines should not be used in households with immunosuppressed or pregnant animals. These products are also available as SQ vaccines. An IN vaccine should never be injected SQ; animals where such a mix-up occurred have suffered severe illness, including hepatic necrosis.

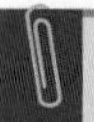

TECHNICIAN NOTE An IN vaccine should never be injected SQ.

CORE VERSUS ELECTIVE VACCINATIONS

Manufacturers have produced vaccines against more that 20 different types of infectious diseases in dogs and cats. In an effort to decrease possible side effects from overvaccinating, an individual's lifestyle and risk of exposure should be considered along with the benefits of vaccinating to design the best vaccination protocol for each animal. Elective vaccines may be indicated in some situations, but are not necessary for all dogs and cats. In contrast, core vaccines are necessary because they protect against highly contagious and dangerous viruses that are ubiquitous in the environment. Even indoor pets can become exposed to these dangerous viruses, and there is no specific therapy for viral infections. In addition, core vaccines are both safe and effective in preventing these illnesses. The core vaccines are listed below:

- Rabies vaccine (dogs and cats)
- DA_2PP combination vaccine (dogs)—Distemper, hepatitis (using adenovirus-2 vaccine), canine parvovirus, and parainfluenza
- FVRCP combination vaccine (cats)—Feline viral rhinotracheitis (herpesvirus), calicivirus, and panleukopenia (feline parvovirus)

DURATION OF IMMUNITY

Some vaccines produce long-acting immunity for 3 or more years, whereas others last only 6 to 12 months and even during this time may have questionable efficacy (Table 9-3). The DA_2PP and FVRCP vaccines work well and have a longer duration of immunity than previously thought. Although manufacturers' inserts may recommend annual boosters, the American Veterinary Medical Association (AVMA), American Animal Hospital Association (AAHA), and American Association of Feline Practitioners (AAFP) have established guidelines for the frequency of immunizations (refer to appendix). They recommend that canine DA_2PP and feline FVRCP combination boosters be given every 3 years rather than annually to adult pets that have received the puppy or kitten series and first adult booster.

SITES OF SUBCUTANEOUS VACCINE ADMINISTRATION

Because there is a small risk of the pet developing a localized vaccine reaction, the site of administration should always be recorded. A consensus of veterinary groups has

TABLE 9-3 Duration of Immunity and Efficacy for Canine Vaccines Commercially Available in the United States

Vaccine	Minimum Duration of Immunity	Estimate of Relative Efficacy (%)
Core		
Canine distemper	≥7 yr*	>90
Canine parvovirus-2	≥7 yr*	>90
Canine adenovirus-2	≥7 yr*	>90
Rabies virus	≥3 yr*	>85
Noncore		
Canine coronavirus	"Lifetime"‡,¶	—
Canine parainfluenza	≥3 yr*	>80
B. bronchiseptica	≤1 yr*,†	<70
L. canicola	≤1 yr†	≤50
L. grippotyphosa	≤1 yr§	—
L. icterohaemorrhagiae	≤1 yr†	≤75
L. pomona	≤1 yr§	—
B. burgdorferi (Lyme disease)	≥1 yr*	≤75
Giardia	≤1 yr§	—

*Experimental challenge studies and/or serologic studies have been performed. Field experience during outbreaks also confirm experimental challenge studies.

†Based on field experience and observations from outbreak studies and clinical records. Reliable experimental or controlled studies often not available.

‡Not available; cannot be determined. CCV has not been shown to cause significant disease.

§Vaccines recently licensed; information not available except from company data.

¶See text.

Reprinted with permission from www.ivis.org.

Schultz RD: Considerations in designing effective and safe vaccination programs for dogs. In Carmichael L, editor: *Recent advances in canine infectious diseases.* Ithaca, NY, 2000, International Veterinary Information Service (www.ivis.org). Document No. A0110.0500 available at http://www.ivis.org/advances/Infect_Dis_Carmichael/schultz/chapter_frm.asp?LA=1. Accessed October 4, 2008.

recommended that rabies vaccines be given SQ over the right rear leg area, the combination vaccines (DA_2PP, DA_2LPP, or FVRCP) should be given SQ over the right shoulder area, and elective vaccines should be given over the left rear leg. Should a lump, alopecia, or some other local problem appear, the specific vaccine involved is known.

> *TECHNICIAN NOTE* The sites for SQ vaccines for dogs and cats are the following:
> RH (right hind leg): Rabies (core for dogs and cats)
> Mnemonic and alliteration to remember: "Right rear-rabies—RRR"
> RF (right front leg): Combo DA_2PP or DA_2LPP (core for dogs)
> RF (right front leg): Combo FVRCP (core for cats)
> LH (left hind leg): Leptospirosis and/or *Bordetella* (elective for dogs)
> Mnemonic and alliteration: Left hind—Lepto
> LH (left hind leg): FeLV/feline immunodeficiency virus (FIV) (elective for cats)
> Mnemonic and alliteration: Left hind—Leukemia

IMMUNIZATIONS FOR DOGS

Rabies (Core Vaccine for Dogs and Cats)

Rabies is a most serious zoonotic rhabdoviral disease of all mammals that is usually transmitted by the saliva of an infected animal via a bite wound. The virus enters distal nerves near the wound and travels proximally toward the spinal cord and brain. This migration can take months during which time the animal is asymptomatic. Once in the brain and salivary glands, the infected animal generally dies of encephalitis within 10 days despite treatment. The clinical signs of rabies include 1 to 3 days of prodromal abnormal behavior followed by 3 to 4 days of hyperactivity, which may include aggressiveness, vicious behavior and biting ("furious" rabies), or motor neuron paralysis, which not only hampers normal movement in the legs, but also affects facial muscles and the ability to swallow (paralytic or "dumb" rabies). Dogs are more likely to become wildly aggressive and "foam at the mouth," whereas cats are more likely to have hind leg paralysis.

Rabies vaccine is a core vaccine for all dogs and cats. Proof of up-to-date rabies immunization is necessary for dog licensure in many locations. Rabies vaccines are killed-virus vaccines and may be approved as 1-year or 3-year vaccines. Local laws govern whether puppies require their first rabies vaccine at 13 weeks or 16 weeks and may require boosters more frequently than the manufacturer's recommendations. Local statutes may also insist on IM administration, which would override the manufacturer's recommendation for SQ administration. In areas where rabies is endemic in wildlife populations, such as among raccoons, skunks, and bats, additional protection may be warranted for the pet and the human family with which it lives. Giving a 3-year vaccine every 2 or 2.5 years may provide this added security. Stray animals with an unknown history of vaccination should receive a booster 1 year after the initial vaccine is administered. In some areas, stray animals are quarantined for a period of time since they could have been exposed to rabies and would be asymptomatic (and noninfectious) during an incubation period. Education is important for owners of new stray animals that have an unknown vaccination history and the possibility of previous bite wounds. There is no test available to diagnose rabies premortem.

Canine Distemper (Core Vaccine for Dogs)

Canine distemper (CD) killed countless numbers of puppies before vaccinations became available in the last century. It is caused by a paramyxovirus, which can be spread via direct contact between dogs or their excretions and by contact with wildlife reservoirs, such as coyote, wolf, raccoon, skunk, weasel, and otter. Because the disease is not easily treatable, this vaccine is considered a core vaccine. Clinical signs may include oculonasal discharge, coughing, dehydration, vomiting, diarrhea, seizures, and inflammation of the chorion and retina in the eye. Later-onset manifestations may include thickening of the footpads and planum nasale, enamel hypoplasia of the teeth, neurologic tics, or epilepsy. The CD paramyxovirus shares some antigens with the human measles virus; therefore a measles vaccine made for dogs can be used in young puppies because it can override colostral distemper antibodies and be protective. CD vaccines are currently modified-live or viral-DNA–vectored vaccines; the killed-virus CD vaccine proved ineffective and is no longer used. Remember that an MLV vaccine should not be given to immunosuppressed animals, such as puppies recovering from a parvovirus, lest they become sickened by the virus in the vaccine.

Infectious Canine Hepatitis (Core Vaccine for Dogs)

Adenovirus-1 causes infectious canine hepatitis, but it also causes a host of other problems, such as glomerulonephritis, vomiting, diarrhea, bleeding, and blue eye in dogs and wild canids. Unfortunately, the vaccine for adenovirus-1 could cause an immune-mediated side effect called "blue eye," which makes it unfavorable for use, and it is no longer recommended. The vaccine for adenovirus-2 (a virus in the kennel cough complex), on the other hand, does not cause blue eye and will confer protection against both adenovirus-1 and adenovirus-2. It is recommended as a core vaccine and is usually given SQ in combination with other vaccines, such as DA_2PP, or it is given IN together with kennel cough complex vaccines.

Canine Parvovirus (Core Vaccine for Dogs)

Parvovirus type-2 is now the most common viral cause of mortality in young dogs. The parvovirus particles are highly resilient in the environment and are not easily killed by common cleaning agents. They are ubiquitous and can be inadvertently brought into the home on the shoes and clothing of pet owners. In this way, even strictly indoor dogs can be exposed and succumb to this deadly disease. Kennels and contaminated areas, bedding, and clothing must be cleaned with either a 1:30 solution of bleach and water or with special parvocidal disinfectants. The illness causes vomiting, diarrhea (sometimes bloody, often foul smelling), fever, severe dehydration, and protein loss from the gastrointestinal tract. Infected animals have leukopenia with low neutrophil counts and are susceptible to secondary bacterial infections. Complete immunization confers a long duration of immunity (7 years or more). The virus in the MLV vaccine may be shed for a time and can cause a false-positive reaction on the fecal Parvocite test.

Parainfluenza (Core Vaccine for Dogs)

The canine parainfluenza virus, like the adenovirus-2, is one of the many viruses that make up the kennel cough complex. As with other viral diseases, it is not treatable with antibiotics, but fortunately does not cause a high degree of mortality, as does canine parvovirus. The vaccine is safe and effective (for 3 years or more) and is often given as a part of the core vaccine combo DA_2PP. It may also be given IN as part of the kennel cough complex vaccine.

Leptospirosis (Elective Vaccine for Dogs)

In many areas where leptospirosis is endemic, this vaccine is considered core. However, in hot, arid regions where leptospirosis is unlikely to occur, it should not be used because the vaccine has been associated with adverse reactions, such as anaphylaxis. These reactions are particularly prevalent among small-dog breeds and puppies under 12 weeks of age. Leptospirosis is caused by the bacteria *Leptospira* spp., which may induce acute or chronic disease in the kidney, liver, and eye. Any one of a number of types (serovars) of *Leptospira* spp. can cause disease in dogs. *L. canicola, L. icterohaemorrhagiae, L. pomona,* and *L. grippotyphosa* have been particularly implicated and the new four-serovar bacterins hope to protect against these bacterial types. Bivalent bacterins that protect against *L. canicola* and *L. icterohaemorrhagiae* do not protect against the other serovars and are no longer recommended. There are other pathogenic serovars against which there are no vaccines available; even the new four-serovars subunit vaccine is ineffective. Because the leptospirosis vaccines may not protect all dogs to the same extent, may not protect against the carrier state, and do not produce long-lasting immunity, they must be given annually. The vaccine comes as a liquid and can be given alone each year (over the left hind leg) or given as part of the combination vaccine DA_2LPP (over the right front leg). In the combination vaccine DA_2LPP, it is used as the diluent and is mixed with the lyophilized DA_2PP powder.

Leptospira spp bacteria are shed in the urine of affected animals, such as dogs, rats, cattle, and many types of wildlife. Infected animals can become carriers and shed the bacteria intermittently for years. Leptospirosis is a zoonotic disease and can cause illness in humans. It is important to protect yourself from exposure. Be sure to use universal precautions, such as wearing gloves when working with undiagnosed dogs with renal failure or icterus and those known to have leptospirosis.

Bordetella bronchiseptica (Elective Vaccine for Dogs)

This bacterium in the kennel cough complex is often given during the month before exposure (e.g., before the dog is boarded). Both killed bacterins are available, which are given SQ, and live-attenuated preparations, which are given IN. Immunization may not be completely effective in all vaccinates, and protection is not long lasting. Annual and biannual boosters therefore may be needed, depending upon the dog's risk for and frequency of potential exposures.

Other Elective Vaccines for Dogs

There are many elective annual boosters for dogs that are rarely necessary, controversial, or not recommended. The inactivated, *canine Giardia vaccine,* for example, does not protect against infection, but may help decrease shedding of oocysts. This vaccine may be useful in colony situations and may help decrease the risk of exposure to immunosuppressed owners or other animals. *Canine Lyme (Borrelia burgdorferi) vaccines* are either recombinant subunit OspA or killed bacterins and are controversial even in Lyme-endemic regions. One study showed that Lyme bacterin caused more adverse reactions than any other vaccine when used alone, including leptospirosis vaccine. The efficacy and duration of immunity are not strong, so annual boosters would be necessary. Because 95% of dogs exposed to *B. burgdorferi* remain asymptomatic, the use of Lyme vaccine appears unwarranted. Dogs with signs of Lyme-induced arthritis typically respond quickly to doxycycline. Rarely, dogs that may be genetically predisposed, such as Labradors, Golden retrievers, and Shetland sheepdogs, may acquire a serious form of protein-losing nephropathy called "Lyme nephropathy," which is an immune-mediated glomerulonephritis triggered by Lyme antigens. There are concerns that Lyme vaccines may sensitize an individual to this immune-mediated disease and may cause excessive amounts of antigen-antibody immune complexes to be deposited in glomeruli. Tick control is paramount in Lyme-endemic areas to prevent not only Lyme disease, but other tick-borne diseases, such as anaplasmosis, ehrlichiosis, Rocky Mountain spotted fever, babesiosis, and bartonellosis. *Canine coronavirus vaccine,* which is a killed-virus or MLV vaccine, is not recommended because the virus does not appear to cause disease in dogs by the age they would be seen for vaccination. Recommendations for other vaccines, such as *Crotalus atrox toxoid* (rattlesnake vaccine) and *Porphyromonas* sp. (periodontal disease vaccine) are still pending.

IMMUNIZATIONS FOR CATS

Feline Panleukopenia (Core Vaccine for Cats)

Panleukopenia is caused by a parvovirus that is similar, but not identical, to the one that infects dogs. Panleukopenia used to be called "feline distemper" because it was a common infectious feline disease when CD was a common infectious disease among dogs. Like canine parvoviral enteritis, panleukopenia causes severe dehydration, vomiting, diarrhea, fever, and leukopenia. It can also cause cerebellar hypoplasia in neonates if they are exposed during late gestation or early life. Killed-virus vaccines are safer to use than MLV vaccines in pregnant queens and immunosuppressed cats. Because viral particles can be shed from cats vaccinated with MLV vaccines, it is recommended that only killed-virus vaccines be used for animals that live with pregnant or immunosuppressed cats. Immunization with the kitten series followed by the first adult booster produces excellent protection and long-lasting immunity, probably as long as 7 years or more. This core vaccine is represented by the "P" (for "panleukopenia" or "parvo") in the FVRCP combination.

Feline Viral Rhinotracheitis (Herpesvirus) and Calicivirus (Core Vaccine for Cats)

These two viruses cause upper respiratory disease, including oculonasal discharges, ulceration of the mouth and nose (calicivirus), and sometimes serious ocular disease (herpes) or polyarthritis (calicivirus). The FVRCP combination vaccine can be given either SQ or IN and is produced as both an MLV or killed-virus product. The efficacy of the vaccine is not 100% because it may not protect against the carrier state and not all calicivirus vaccines protect against the rare serious systemic form of calicivirus. However, immunity lasts about 3 years in fully immunized adult cats. It is therefore recommended to be given every 3 years, not annually, after the kitten series and annual booster are completed. A risk factor worth noting is that vaccines for calicivirus may cause immune-mediated polyarthritis.

Feline Leukemia Virus (FeLV)) and Feline Immunodeficiency Virus (FIV) (Elective Vaccines for Cats)

These viruses are shed in the saliva and excretions of seropositive cats. The risk of exposure is greatest among young cats that go outdoors or that live in catteries. The FeLV virus is a retrovirus that can cause lymphoma, bone marrow dyscrasias, and immunosuppression in cats usually within 2 to 4 years of their becoming seropositive. The FIV is also a retrovirus and is responsible for causing "feline AIDS," characterized by immunosuppression and the predisposition for secondary infections. All cats should be tested for

FeLV and FIV before immunization. Ideally, cats would be quarantined for 8 weeks and would be tested at the beginning and at the end of this period before having contact with virus-free cats. The FeLV vaccine may be used to protect outdoor cats from sporadic exposure to the virus, but will not protect cats that have constant exposure such as those that live in the same home or cattery with one or more FeLV-positive cats. Vaccination with an FeLV vaccine does not interfere with testing for FeLV antigens. However, vaccination with FIV vaccine *does* interfere with FIV testing because the test screens for anti-FIV antibodies and cannot distinguish antibodies produced during immunization from those made in response to natural infection. Thus cats immunized against FIV will have a positive test result. It is recommended that FIV-immunized cats have an identity chip placed at the time of vaccination to facilitate identification and return of the cat to its home should it become lost. In this way, the cat would be spared euthanasia in a shelter or veterinary hospital that mistook it for an FIV-infected animal. The FIV and FeLV vaccines do not confer long-lasting immunity, so annual boosters are recommended for cats that go outdoors. Some veterinarians suggest that all cats receive the kitten and first adult FeLV boosters because exposure during early life is most problematic. In addition, adult cats may develop natural immunity to FeLV making it less important to vaccinate adult animals than cats less than 1 year old.

Other Elective Vaccines for Cats

The following vaccines are rarely necessary, controversial, or not recommended. They do not confer long-term immunity and must be given annually, if given at all. *Chlamydophila felis* (previously called *Chlamydia*) is a bacterial infection that causes upper respiratory disease and conjunctivitis. The disease is treatable with antibiotics and is not a common problem in cats in the United States. Thus vaccination with either the killed bacterin or attenuated vaccine is unnecessary unless cultures prove it is problematic in a particular cattery or colony. *Feline Bordetella* is also not a common pathogen among cats and may exist in normal flora of the feline respiratory tract. For this reason, the use of the attenuated vaccine is controversial. *Feline Giardia* killed-virus vaccine may help to decrease oocyst shedding and may be of use in catteries or in situations in which a *Giardia*-carrying cat lives with an immunosuppressed human. *Feline infectious peritonitis (FIP) vaccine* is a doubly mutated, modified-live coronavirus vaccine for cats that may induce a systemic sensitization to the virus and the local immunity it is designed to give. For this reason, it is a controversial vaccine. Circulating antibodies against FIP from first generation SQ vaccines were shown to cause increased immune-mediated vasculitis, faster illness, and death in vaccinates compared with nonvaccinates when both were challenged with a virulent FIP virus. *Feline ringworm (fungal) vaccine* is not currently available. This vaccine helped decrease skin lesions from ringworm in cats, but a cat could become an asymptomatic carrier and be a source of infection for owners or other animals.

POSTVACCINAL ADVERSE EVENTS

Postvaccinal adverse events should be reported both to the manufacturer and to the U.S. Pharmacopeia Veterinary Practitioner's Reporting Program (1-800-487-7776).

Anaphylaxis

Most postvaccinal side effects are not life threatening, such as local pain, transient swelling at the vaccination site, or mild systemic signs of lethargy or fever for a day or 2. However, sometimes an allergic reaction to microbial antigens, adjuvant, inactivators, or preservatives in a vaccine can cause severe reactions, such as anaphylaxis. Anaphylaxis is an immediate hypersensitivity response that may include respiratory arrest, cardiovascular collapse, and death within 30 minutes of immunization. Less severe, but still alarming symptoms are: hives, facial edema, and periocular swelling. Emergency treatment for anaphylaxis may include the administration of:

1. An antihistamine, such as Benadryl (diphenhydramine) at a dose of 2 to 4 mg/kg t.i.d. to q.i.d. PO, IM, or IV.
2. A short-term corticosteroid, such as dexamethasone at a dose of 0.25 mg/kg IV, or for milder reactions, discharge the animal with a short course of prednisone tablets at 0.5 to 1 mg/kg b.i.d. PO.
3. Severe cases may also require epinephrine at a dose of 0.5 to 1.5 ml IV of a 1:10,000 solution, to be repeated in 30 minutes.
4. Intravenous fluids and life support.

Sometimes it is difficult to determine the cause of the allergic reaction. For example, if a dog had a reaction after receiving a combined DA_2LPP and rabies vaccine, it is not clear which of the vaccines caused the problem. Because bacterins are most likely to cause anaphylaxis, and since they are elective vaccines, it is not necessary to subject an animal to the possibility of a second reaction by giving the product again. A prudent approach may be to give only the rabies vaccine as it is required by law and to pretreat the patient with a dose of antihistamine 30 minutes before the immunization is given. Close monitoring for 24 hours postinjection would also be needed. If there is no reaction, the DA_2PP vaccine without the leptospirosis bacterin might be administered at a later time using this pretreatment and monitoring protocol.

> TECHNICIAN NOTE Because anaphylaxis may occur within minutes of vaccine administration, the safest place to immunize is in a veterinary facility where emergency treatment and expertise is readily available.

Other Immune-Mediated Reactions

Delayed hypersensitivity reactions may occur days or weeks after vaccination, such as immune-mediated hemolytic anemia, immune-mediated thrombocytopenia, polyarthritis, hypertrophic osteodystrophy, or thyroiditis, possibly triggered by vaccine antigens in genetically predisposed individuals. Breeds with predispositions for vaccine reactions include small-dog breeds, white dogs, or dogs with a diluted coat color, Old English sheepdogs, Weimaraners, and Akitas. It is difficult to prove, but a causal relationship between an immune-mediated illness and the receipt of vaccine within 30 to 45 days has empirically been observed and has caused concern. Even harder to prove is immune-mediated damage to organs months to years after vaccination. For instance, when the FVRCP vaccination is administered SQ, but not IN, it has been shown to induce antibodies against feline kidney cells and against the vaccine viruses. This is not entirely surprising because the vaccine viruses are first grown in feline kidney cell cultures before they are inactivated or attenuated. Laboratory studies of renal function were not found to be impaired 56 weeks postvaccination, but more long-term studies are needed, particularly those that include vaccine boosters.

For animals that have had reactions to vaccines and for immunosuppressed animals that should not receive MLV vaccines, serologic titers for the core vaccine diseases, such as distemper, parvovirus, rabies, and FVRCP, can be quantified to offer some reassurance that an animal has protective humoral antibodies and does not need a booster. A negative titer does not necessarily mean that an animal is unprotected, since long-lasting immunity may exist as a result of cell-mediated immunity or local immunity, which are not easily measured.

Postvaccinal Sarcomas in Cats

A serious postvaccinal adverse effect is the development of fibrosarcoma at the injection site. Fortunately, this is fairly rare and occurs in 1 to 10 cats per 10,000 doses. It is usually associated with the administration of adjuvanted vaccines, such as rabies and FeLV vaccines. First described by veterinary pathologists Dr. Mattie Hendrick and Dr. Michael Goldschmidt at the University of Pennsylvania in 1991, this invasive cancer is the main reason why veterinarians have reevaluated and adjusted vaccine protocols for pets. Further scrutiny regarding the duration of immunity has led to triannual rather than annual protocols, checking titers, vaccinating at particular sites on the body, increased use of IN vaccines (despite postvaccinal sneezing or shedding), and the development of new nonadjuvanted vaccines.

The "1-2-3 rule" reminds us to carefully monitor lumps that occur at an injection site. Many masses are benign granulomas and resolve by 2 to 3 months postvaccination, but some may be serious invasive fibrosarcomas and need to be handled aggressively. All lumps should be recorded (location, size, shape) and assumed to be malignant until proven otherwise. A cytologic examination of an aspirate may not be definitive, so a biopsy or complete removal are recommended if the mass is still growing after 1 month, is greater than 2 cm in diameter, or if the mass persists for more than 3 months.

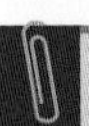
TECHNICIAN NOTE The "1-2-3" recommendations for a biopsy or removal of a postvaccinal mass are:
1. The mass is still growing after 1 month.
2. The mass is greater than 2 cm in diameter.
3. The mass persists for greater than 3 months.

PARASITE PREVENTION

The treatment of endoparasites and ectoparasites is further discussed in Chapter 17 and Chapter 25. Typically, all puppies are dewormed with a product such as pyrantel pamoate (Nemex) two to three times, 3 weeks apart, to treat roundworms and hookworms that may have been acquired from the mother. After treatment to prevent new infestations, owners are educated about how parasite eggs are shed in the feces of infected dogs and cats. They learn that the ova can be infective for many months, even after weather has removed the bulk of the feces in lawn areas and parks. To prevent reinfection, a monthly preventative may be used, which prevents both heartworm and a variety of intestinal parasite infections (Table 9-4). Flea bites may cause dermatitis, provoke allergies, cause blood loss, and may transmit infectious agents, such as *Bartonella, Mycoplasma,* and tapeworms. A variety of available flea-prevention products include insecticides that kill fleas, repellants that repel fleas, and growth inhibitors that render the flea unable to produce viable eggs after it has taken a blood meal (see Chapter 25). Tick exposure may transmit diseases, such as Lyme disease, anaplasmosis, babesiosis, ehrlichiosis, Rocky Mountain spotted fever, bartonellosis, and mycoplasmosis. Products available (see Table 9-4) include those that repel or prevent ticks from attaching and products that kill ticks within hours after they have attached. Since some types of organisms may be transmitted soon after tick attachment, products that prevent ticks from attaching may be preferred. Regional risks and the pet's lifestyle need to be considered. All topical products are somewhat waterproof in the rain or an occasional swim, but frequent shampooing decreases efficacy and may even require reapplication (e.g., imidacloprid products). Since products often distribute in the lipid layer of the skin, the application should not be done within a day of bathing. Products containing permethrins should not be used on or near cats. If a pet eats an amitraz collar, a special antidote called yohimbine needs to be administered.

ROUTINE HELPFUL SCREENING TESTS

SCREENING FOR REGIONAL INFECTIOUS DISEASES

In regions where certain infectious diseases are found, in-house screening tests may be a valuable aid to help monitor the prevalence of each disease, particularly occult disease that is not showing outward, clinical signs. See Table 9-5 for a list of recommendations for addressing positive and negative test results using the SNAP 4Dx (IDEXX) test.

Many cats carry *Bartonella henselae,* which is the causative agent of cat scratch fever in humans. Because of the potential health risk to owners, some veterinarians recommend that cats be tested for the presence of antibodies to *Bartonella* spp. A popular screening test for this purpose is the FeBart *Bartonella* Western blot (National Veterinary Laboratories, N.J.).

TABLE 9-4 Some Commonly Used Products for Prevention of Canine Parasites

	Heartworms	Ascarid Roundworms	Ancylostoma Hookworms	Trichuris Whipworms	Fleas	Ticks†	Otodectes (Ear Mites) & Sarcoptes (Scabies)	Mosquitoes
Heartgard Plus (oral ivermectin + pyrantel pamoate)	X	X	X					
Interceptor (oral milbemycin)	X	X	X	X				
Sentinel (Interceptor/Program) (oral milbemycin + lufenuron)	X	X	X	X	Eggs only			
Advantage Multi for dogs (topical imidacloprid + moxidectin)	X	X	X	X	X			
Frontline Top Spot Plus (topical fipronil + methoprene)					X	X		
Preventic collar* (amitraz collar)						X		
Advantage (topical imidacloprid)					X			
K9 Advantix* (topical imidacloprid + permethrin)					X	X		X‡
Vectra 3D* for dogs (topical permethrin + dinotefuran + pyriproxyfen)					X	X		X‡
Promeris for dogs* (topical metaflumizone + amitraz)					X	X		
Revolution for dogs (topical selamectin)	X				X		X	

*Repels as well as kills.
†Including ticks which can transmit Lyme disease, Ehrlichiosis, Anaplasmosis, Babesiosis, Rocky Mountain Spotted Fever, etc.
‡Repels most mosquitoes but should not be considered a heartworm preventive.

TABLE 9-5 Recommendations for Snap-4DX (IDEXX) Test Results

Case Signalment: 6 yr old Male Castrated Labrador Retriever
History: appears healthy to owner
Physical examination: no remarkable abnormalities

Possible Snap-4DX (IDEXX) Test Results and Recommendations				
	Heartworm Antigen +	*Borrelia burgdorferi* + (Lyme C6 Peptide Antibody Test)	*Ehrlichia canis* + Antibody test	*Anaplasma phagocytophilum* + Antibody test
Check for proteinuria	Yes*	Yes*	Yes*	Yes*
Check CBC	Yes	If proteinuric	Yes	Yes
Check Chemscreen	Yes	If proteiinuric	If proteinuric	If proteinuric
If no abnormalities on blood and urine tests and dog remains asymptomatic	Consider treatment with melarsomine or ivermectin; monitor for proteinuria	Monitor for proteinuria (treatment not always necessary)	Monitor for proteinuria and CBC changes (treatment not always necessary)	Monitor for proteinuria and CBC changes (treatment not always necessary)
Use Preventative	Yes	Yes	Yes	Yes
Treat with Doxycycline if dog is showing signs of disease or is proteinuric	Maybe (for Wolbachia) After chest radiographs, EKG, echocardiogram, consider melarsomine or ivermectin treatment. Check for antigen again 6 months posttreatment.	Yes Check Quantitative Lyme C6 Antibody level, pretreatment and 6-month posttreatment	Yes Check Quantitative *E. canis* titer, pretreatment and 6 month posttreatment	Yes Check Quantitative *A. phagocytophilum* titer, pretreatment and 6-month posttreatment

*Further recommendations concerning proteinuria:
1. Check for proteinuria (complete urinalysis plus E.R.D. [HESKA], microalbuminuria [MA] test, or urine protein/creatinine ratio). If negative, recheck periodically (2-4 times/year).
2. If proteinuric, monitor blood pressure measurements, check for target organ damage (retinal examination, etc), consider antihypertensive medication.
3. If very mildly proteinuric, recheck monthly for trend; quantify urine protein/creatinine ratio.
4. If moderately proteinuric, quantify, monitor, and investigate (consider diagnostic work-up including CBC, biochemical profile, urine culture, chest radiographs, abdominal ultrasound, tick serology, renal biopsy, etc). You are checking CBC and biochemical profile for changes associated with protein-losing nephropathy, anemia, leucopenia or thrombocytopenia due to immune-mediated or infectious disease, hypoalbuminemia, hypercholesterolemia, azotemia, etc. Consider checking for co-infections that may not be Doxycycline-responsive (e.g., *Babesia* spp., *Bartonella* spp., etc.).
5. If moderately proteinuric, intervene with treatment including an ACE (angiotensin-converting enzyme) inhibitor, omega-3 fatty acid supplement; if hypertensive, treat with amlodipine; if hypoalbuminemic, treat with an antithrombotic low dose of aspirin; consider immunosuppressive therapy for protein-losing nephropathy cases.
6. Educate owner about using better tick control products, landscaping techniques for tick avoidance, and public health issues. Monitor blood pressure measurements, blood and urine test results, posttreatment tick serology for new baseline values.

OTHER ANNUAL SCREENING TESTS

It is recommended that all pets be tested annually for proteinuria as a part of their wellness exam. Proteinuria can be quickly assessed by acquiring a free-catch urine sample and testing it for microalbuminuria using the in-house E.R.D. (HESKA) test or reference laboratory MA (microalbuminuria) test (Antech). This would be done in conjunction with a complete urinalysis. A thorough annual checkup would include a CBC, biochemical profile, and fecal examination. In addition, after 7 years of age, cats are typically screened for hyperthyroidism by requesting a serum T_4 test as a part of the annual routine blood work.

SCREENING FOR GENETIC DISEASE PREDISPOSITIONS

Every breed is somewhat inbred and predisposed to certain genetic problems. For a list of dog breeds and the diseases to which they are predisposed, refer to the Inherited Diseases in Dogs website at the University of Cambridge, School of Veterinary Medicine (www.vet.cam.ac.uk/idid/). In addition, the National Breed Club websites (available via the American Kennel Club at www.akc.org/clubs/search/index.cfm?action=national&display=on) have specific information about pet health and suggested screening tests for each breed. An ophthalmologic examination to check for congenital cataracts, PennHIP radiographs to check for hip dysplasia, and von Willebrand's testing for an abnormal tendency to bleed are examples of recommended screening tests for particular breeds. There are specific DNA tests available for a variety of genetic diseases. Testing laboratories are listed at www.akcchf.org/research/genetic_tests.pdf. For diseases in which a phenotypic change occurs (either grossly or by a laboratory abnormality), there may be a recommended age to check for it. Some breeds may have genetic predispositions with no age limit for when illness may occur. The Soft Coated Wheaten Terrier Club of America, for example, has an informative website (www.scwtca.org) that describes annual screening tests recommended for all Wheatens (Box 9-1).

Educating owners about their breed's predispositions helps them to avoid risky behavior and helps them be more observant for early warning signs of abnormalities. For instance, a dachshund is predisposed to intervertebral disk disease so catching objects in midair is not the best game to play with them. Screening tests that are available for genetic diseases should be done before breeding an animal, but it is also important for the individual so that intervention can be started as early in life as possible. For instance, Persian cats may have polycystic kidney disease (PKD), which can be detected after 10 months of age by ultrasonography, but otherwise would not be discovered for years because the average age of renal failure detection is at 7 years of age. Maine coon and rag doll cats may carry the gene for hypertrophic cardiomyopathy (with autosomal dominant inheritance). Therefore an annual echocardiogram is recommended in these breeds to detect it early before heart failure causes the cat distress.

PREVENTIVE HEALTH PROGRAM FOR HORSES

A preventive health program for horses should be designed to meet the specific needs of the individual animal or herd. Such programs generally vary from one stable to another and from one veterinary practice to another, depending on expected exposures, management styles, and personal preferences of attending veterinarians and horse owners.

An example of one preventive health program for horses is outlined in Box 9-2.

PHYSICAL EXAMINATION

All new additions to a stable or an established herd should have a negative Coggins test result for equine infectious anemia before arrival. Ideally upon arrival, the horse(s) should

BOX 9-1 Annual Screening Tests for Soft Coated Wheaten Terriers

Soft coated Wheaten terriers (SCWT) are predisposed to the following:

- Food allergies
- Inflammatory bowel disease (IBD)
- Protein-losing enteropathy (PLE)
- Protein-losing nephropathy (PLN)
- Renal dysplasia
- Addison's disease

Currently there are no predictive tests to detect which dogs will become affected in the future or which may be carriers. The SCWT Club of America (website: www.scwtca.org) recommends that all dogs (and especially breeding dogs) be screened annually with the following tests:

- CBC: to check for eosinophilia and other abnormalities
- Biochemical profile: to check for hypoalbuminemia, hypoglobulinemia, azotemia, hypocholesterolemia, or hypercholesterolemia
- Urinalysis: to check urine specific gravity, protein dipstick, sediment
- Urine E.R.D. (HESKA), MA (microalbuminuria), or urine protein/creatinine ratio
- Fecal α-1 proteinase inhibitor test (Texas A&M) to check for protein loss from the intestine (a sign of increased permeability, which may be seen with food allergies, IBD, PLE, but also may be seen with worms, enteritis, Addison's disease, etc.).
- In sick dogs, clinical signs of these genetic predispositions can mimic each other or be due to other canine diseases. A diagnostic work-up may require additional tests, such as abdominal ultrasound, a wedge renal biopsy to check for renal dysplasia, an ACTH stimulation test to rule out Addison's disease, endoscopy with biopsy of the intestine, etc.

BOX 9-2 General Outline of a Preventive Health Program for Horses

Spring

- Perform annual physical exam.
- Vaccinate all horses; vaccinate broodmares approximately 30 days before foaling.
- Obtain fecal egg count, deworm those with egg counts greater than 150 eggs/g.
- Perform annual dentistry exam, remove wolf teeth in 2-year-olds.
- Trim feet every 6-8 wk.

Summer

- Give booster vaccinations for herpesvirus and influenza in high-risk animals.
- Vaccinate foals beginning at 3-4 mo of age (can delay until 6 mo of age for foals born to vaccinated dams).
- Trim feet every 6-8 wk.
- Obtain fecal egg count, deworm those with egg counts greater than 150 eggs/g.

Fall

- Give booster vaccinations for herpesvirus and influenza in high-risk animals.
- Give booster vaccinations for equine encephalitis viruses (WEE, EEE, VEE) and WNV in endemic areas.
- Trim feet every 6-8 wk.
- Obtain fecal egg count, deworm those with egg counts greater than 150 eggs/g.
- Perform dentistry exam on horses under 5 yr of age and on horses with known dental problems.

Winter

- Trim feet every 6-8 wk.
- Deworm all horses with ivermectin-praziquantel or moxidectin-praziquantel to treat tapeworms and bots acquired over the summer and fall.

immediately be placed in quarantine for 1 month before entering the general population. During this time, the first physical examination of the preventive health program can be performed (refer to Chapters 8 and 22). If quarantine facilities are not available, at the very least, a thorough physical examination should be performed before the horse is allowed contact with any animals from the resident population. Any signs of illness or a parasite infection should be addressed before the new horse is turned in with resident horses.

VACCINATIONS

Vaccination schedules are based on the age of the horse, anticipated exposure to infectious organisms, and duration of immunity provided by the vaccine. Tables 9-6 and 9-7 list the vaccination guidelines provided by the American Association of Equine Practitioners. A variety of commercially available vaccines are approved for use in healthy horses, and the choice of product often depends on geographical location and personal experience and familiarity.

Young horses that are immunologically naive or any horse that has an unknown immunization history should receive an initial immunization followed by a second booster immunization. The length between initial and booster vaccinations can vary based on the type of vaccine and manufacturer, but is generally 4 weeks.

TECHNICIAN NOTE Young horses or those with an unknown vaccination history should receive an initial immunization followed by a booster in 4 weeks.

In rare instances, anaphylactoid reactions can occur with the use of any vaccine. These life-threatening crises must be handled quickly. Accordingly, it is essential that epinephrine be available for the treatment of anaphylactoid reactions. Other complications, such as fever, lameness, and swelling or abscess formation at the injection site, may also occur with the routine use of the vaccines. The horse owner should always be informed of these possibilities before any vaccine is administered.

Common diseases and vaccines used as an aid in disease prevention are discussed in the following sections.

TETANUS VACCINES

Tetanus, or lockjaw, is a disease characterized by muscular rigidity that may culminate in death from respiratory arrest or convulsions. Tetanus is caused by toxins produced by the anaerobic bacterium *Clostridium tetani.* Active immunity to tetanus is produced by the administration of a tetanus toxoid, which is a purified, inactivated toxin of *C. tetani. C. tetani* is routinely found in the environment, and yearly vaccinations are recommended for all horses. Tetanus toxoid booster vaccinations are also routinely given by many veterinarians when treating horses with penetrating injuries or at surgery.

Tetanus antitoxin is produced by hyperimmunization of donor horses with tetanus toxoid. Tetanus antitoxin provides protection by binding to the *C. tetani* toxin and can be used locally at the site of infection or given parenterally. The administration of tetanus antitoxin to unvaccinated horses induces immediate protection, which lasts approximately 2 weeks, but its use should be restricted to high risk cases because it can cause acute hepatitis.

Tetanus antitoxin and tetanus toxoid should never be mixed in the same syringe and should be injected at distant sites if administered at the same time.

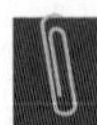

TECHNICIAN NOTE Tetanus antitoxin and tetanus toxoid should never be mixed in the same syringe.

WESTERN, EASTERN, AND VENEZUELAN ENCEPHALITIS VACCINES

Equine encephalomyelitis is a viral neurologic disease of horses caused by eastern, western, and Venezuelan viruses. These viruses are maintained in nature by bird and animal reservoirs and are transmitted to horses by biting insects. Venezuelan equine encephalomyelitis occurs primarily in South and Central America and has not been diagnosed in the United States for many years. The trivalent vaccine is commonly used for horses in states bordering Mexico to create a buffer zone, which may prevent the spread of Venezuelan equine encephalomyelitis into the United States.

The equine encephalomyelitis vaccines currently used for active immunization are inactivated-virus vaccines. They should be administered annually before the biting-insect season. Vaccine protection lasts approximately 6 to 8 months, and in areas where winter freezes are uncommon or in endemic areas, semiannual vaccinations are advisable.

EQUINE HERPESVIRUS VACCINES

Equine herpesvirus (EHV), also known as rhinopneumonitis, frequently causes respiratory disease, but can also cause abortion, neurologic disease, and neonatal illness. Although multiple herpesviruses have been identified, current vaccines offer protection against EHV-1 and EHV-4. These viruses cause respiratory disease; however, EHV-1 is also associated with infections of the central nervous system and the reproductive tract. EHV-4 is most frequently associated with upper respiratory tract disease in young horses and is rarely a cause of abortion.

Both inactivated and MLV vaccines are available for protection against the respiratory form of EHV; no currently available vaccines are licensed for protection against neurologic disease. Because the duration of immunity is short lived, high-risk animals should be vaccinated every 6 months. Pregnant mares should be vaccinated during the fifth, seventh, and ninth months of gestation with an approved vaccine to aid in the control of abortion.

Text continued on p. 236

TABLE 9-6 VACCINATIONS FOR FOALS[a,b]

CORE VACCINATIONS Protect Against Diseases that are Endemic to a Region, Those with Potential Public Health Significance, Required by Law, Virulent/highly Infectious, and/or Those Posing a Risk of Severe Disease. Core Vaccines have Clearly Demonstrated Efficacy and Safety, and thus Exhibit a High Enough Level of Patient Benefit and Low Enough Level of Risk to Justify Their Use in all Equids.

Disease	Foals and Weanlings (<12 months of age) *of mares vaccinated in the prepartum period for the disease*	Foals and Weanlings (<12 months of age) *of unvaccinated mare*	Comments
Tetanus	3 dose series: **1st** dose at 4-6 months of age **2nd** dose 4-6 weeks after the 1st dose **3rd** dose at 10-12 months of age	3 dose series: **1st** dose at 1-4 months of age **2nd** dose 4 weeks after the 1st dose **3rd** dose 4 weeks after 2nd dose	
Eastern/Western Equine Encephalomyelitis (EEE/WEE)	3 dose series: **1st** dose at 4-6 months of age[c] **2nd** dose 4-6 weeks after 1st dose **3rd** dose at 10-12 months of age, before the onset of the next vector season.	3 dose series: **1st** dose at 3-4 months of age[d] **2nd** dose 4 weeks after 1st dose **3rd** dose at 10-12 months of age, before the onset of the next vector season.	*Note:* Primary vaccination series scheduling may be amended with vaccinations administered earlier to younger foals that are at increased disease risk due to the presence of vectors. A foal born during the vector season may warrant beginning vaccination at an earlier age than a foal born before the vector season.
Rabies	3 dose series: **1st** dose at 6 months of age **2nd** dose 4-6 weeks after 1st dose **3rd** dose at 10-12 months of age	3 dose series: **1st** dose at 3-4 months of age **2nd** dose 4 weeks after 1st dose **3rd** dose at 10-12 months of age	
West Nile Virus (WNV)	*Inactivated vaccine*[e] 3 dose series: **1st** dose at 4-6 months of age **2nd** dose 4-6 weeks after 1st dose **3rd** dose at 10-12 months of age, before the onset of the next vector season	*Inactivated vaccine*[f] 3 dose series: **1st** dose at 3-4 months of age **2nd** dose 4 weeks after 1st dose **3rd** dose at 10-12 months of age, before the onset of the next vector season	*Note:* Primary vaccination series scheduling may be amended with vaccinations administered to younger foals that are at increased risk of exposure due to the presence of vectors. A foal born during the vector season may warrant initiation of the primary vaccination series at an earlier age than a foal born before the vector season.
	Recombinant canary pox vaccine 3 dose series: **1st** dose at 5-6 months of age **2nd** dose 4 weeks after 1st dose **3rd** dose at 10-12 months of age, before the onset of the next vector season	*Recombinant canary pox vaccine* 3 dose series: **1st** dose at 5-6 months of age **2nd** dose 4 weeks after 1st dose **3rd** dose at 10-12 months of age, before the onset of the next vector season	There is no data for the use of the recombinant or chimera product in foals < 5 months of age. If either product is administered to foals at < 5 months of age, the recommended primary schedule should still be completed.
	Flavivirus chimera vaccine 2 dose series: **1st** dose at 5-6 months of age **2nd** dose at 10-12 months of age, before the onset of the next vector season	*Flavivirus chimera vaccine* 2 dose series: **1st** dose at 5-6 months of age **2nd** dose at 10-12 months of age before the onset of the next vector season.	

TABLE 9-6 VACCINATIONS FOR FOALS[a,b]—cont'd

RISK-BASED VACCINATIONS Are Those Having Applications Which May Vary between Individuals, Populations, and Geographic Regions. Risk Assessment Should be Performed by, or in Consultation with, a Licensed Veterinarian to Identify Which Vaccines Are Appropriate for a given Horse or Population of Horses. The Listing of a Vaccine Here is **NOT** *a Recommendation for its Inclusion into a Vaccination Program. Vaccine Scheduling is Provided for Use After it has been Determined Which, if any, Risk-based Vaccines Are Indicated. Note: Vaccines Are Listed in this Table in Alphabetical Order, not in Order of Priority for Use.*

Disease	Foals and Weanlings (<12 months of age) *of mares vaccinated in the prepartum period for the disease*	Foals and Weanlings (<12 months of age) *of unvaccinated mare*	Comments
Anthrax	Not applicable. As it is not recommended to vaccinate mares during pregnancy there will be no foals of mares vaccinated prepartum.	No age specific guidelines are available for this vaccine. Manufacturer's recommendation is for primary series of 2 doses administered subcutaneously at a 2-3 week interval.	Antimicrobial drugs must **not** be given concurrently with this vaccine. Caution should be used during storage, handling, and administration of this live bacterial product. Consult a physician immediately should accidental human exposure (via mucus membranes, conjunctiva, or broken skin) occur.
Botulism	3 dose series: **1st dose** 2-3 months of age **2nd dose** 4 weeks after 1st dose **3rd dose** 4 weeks after 2nd dose	3 dose series: **1st dose** 1-3 months of age **2nd dose** 4 weeks after 1st dose **3rd dose** 4 weeks after 2nd dose	Maternal antibody does not interfere with vaccination; foals at high risk may be vaccinated as early as 2 weeks of age.
Equine Herpes Virus (EHV)	*Inactivated or modified live vaccine* 3 dose series: **1st dose** 4-6 months of age **2nd dose** 4-6 weeks after 1st dose **3rd dose** at 10-12 months of age Revaccinate at 6 month intervals	*Inactivated or modified live vaccine* 3 dose series: **1st dose** at 4-6 months of age **2nd dose** 4-6 weeks after 1st dose **3rd dose** at 10-12 months of age Revaccinate at 6 month intervals	
Equine Viral Arteritis (EVA)	**Colt (male) foals** Single dose at 6-12 months of age (see comments)	**Colt (male) foals** Single dose at 6-12 months of age (see comments)	**Before initial vaccination, colt (male) foals should undergo serologic testing** and be confirmed negative for antibodies to EAV. Testing should be performed shortly before, or preferably at, the time of vaccination. As foals can carry colostral derived antibodies to EAV for up to 6 months, testing and vaccination should NOT be performed before 6 months of age.

Continued

TABLE 9-6 VACCINATIONS FOR FOALS[a,b]—cont'd

Disease	Foals and Weanlings (<12 months of age) *of mares vaccinated in the prepartum period for the disease*	Foals and Weanlings (<12 months of age) *of unvaccinated mare*	Comments
Equine Influenza	*Inactivated vaccine* 3 dose series: **1st dose** at 6 months of age **2nd dose** 3-4 weeks after 1st dose **3rd dose** at 10-12 months of age	*Inactivated vaccine* 3 dose series: **1st dose** at 6 months of age **2nd dose** 3-4 weeks after 1st dose **3rd dose** at 10-12 months of age	An increased risk of disease may warrant vaccination of younger foals. Because some maternal anti-influenza antibody is likely to be present, a complete series of primary vaccinations should still be given after 6 months of age.
	Modified live vaccine 2 dose series Administered intranasally: **1st dose** at 6-7 months of age **2nd dose** at 11-12 months of age Revaccinate at 6 month intervals	*Modified live vaccine* 2 dose series Administered intranasally: **1st dose** at 6-7 months of age **2nd dose** at 11-12 months of age Revaccinate at 6 month intervals	
Potomac Horse Fever (PHF)	2 dose series: **1st dose** at 5 months of age **2nd dose** 3-4 weeks after 1st dose	2 dose series: **1st dose** at 5 months of age **2nd dose** 3-4 weeks after 1st dose	If risk warrants, vaccine may be administered to younger foals. Subsequent doses are to be administered at 4 week intervals until 6 months of age.
Rotavirus	Not recommended in foals	Not recommended in foals	
Strangles (*Streptococcus equi*)	*Killed vaccine* 3 dose series: **1st dose** at 4-6 months of age **2nd dose** 4-6 weeks after 1st dose **3rd dose** 4-6 weeks after 2nd dose	*Killed vaccine* 3 dose series: **1st dose** at 4-6 months of age **2nd dose** 4-6 weeks after 1st dose **3rd dose** 4-6 weeks after 2nd dose	Vaccination is NOT recommended as a strategy in outbreak mitigation. If risk warrants, the modified live vaccine (MLV) may be safely administered to foals as young as 6 weeks of age. However, vaccine efficacy in this age group has not been adequately studied. If MLV is administered to younger foals, a 3rd dose of vaccine should then be administered 2-4 weeks before weaning.
	Modified live vaccine 3 dose series Administered intranasally: **1st** dose at 6-9 months of age **2nd** dose 3-4 weeks after 1st dose **3rd** dose at 11-12 months of age	*Modified live vaccine* 3 dose series Administered intranasally: **1st** dose at 6-9 months of age **2nd** dose 3-4 weeks after 1st dose **3rd** dose at 11-12 months of age	

[a] **ALL** vaccination programs should be developed in consultation with a licensed veterinarian.
[b] The two categories (core and risk-based vaccinations) reflect differences in the foal's susceptibility to disease and ability to mount an appropriate immune response to vaccination based on the presence (or absence) of maternal antibodies derived from colostrum. The phenomenon of maternal antibody interference is discussed in the text portion of these guidelines.
[c] *Foals in the Southeastern USA:* The primary vaccination series should be initiated with an additional dose at 3 months of age due to early seasonal vector presence.
[d] *Foals in the Southeastern USA:* The primary vaccination series should be initiated at 3 months of age due to early seasonal vector presence.
[e] *Foals in the Southeastern USA:* Due to early seasonal vector presence, the primary vaccination series should be initiated earlier with the addition of a dose at 3 months of age.
[f] *Foals in the Southeastern USA:* Due to early seasonal vector presence, the primary vaccination series should be initiated at 3 months of age.

TABLE 9-7 VACCINATIONS FOR ADULT HORSES*

CORE VACCINATIONS Protect Against Diseases That Are Endemic to a Region, Are Virulent/Highly Contagious, Pose a Risk of Severe Disease, Those Having Potential Public Health Significance, and/or Are Required by Law. Core Vaccines Have Clearly Demonstrable Efficacy and Safety, with a High Enough Level of Patient Benefit and Low Enough Level of Risk to Justify Their Use in All Equids.

Disease	Broodmares	Other Adult Horses (>1 year of age) *previously vaccinated for the disease*	Other Adult Horses (>1 year of age) *unvaccinated or lacking vaccination history*	Comments
Tetanus	*Previously vaccinated*: Annual, 4-6 weeks prepartum *Previously unvaccinated or having unknown vaccination history*: 2 dose series **2nd** dose 4-6 weeks after 1st dose Revaccinate 4-6 weeks prepartum	Annual	2 dose series **2nd** dose 4-6 weeks after 1st dose Annual revaccination	Booster at time of penetrating injury or before surgery if last dose was administered over 6 months previously
Eastern / Western Equine Encephalomyelitis (EEE/WEE)	*Previously vaccinated*: Annual, 4-6 weeks prepartum *Previously unvaccinated or having unknown vaccination history*: 2 dose series **2nd** dose 4 weeks after 1st dose Revaccinate 4-6 weeks prepartum	Annual—spring, before onset of vector season	2 dose series **2nd** dose 4-6 weeks after 1st dose Revaccinate before the onset of the next vector season.	Consider 6 month revaccination interval for: 1. Horses residing in endemic areas 2. Immunocompromised horses
West Nile Virus (WNV)	*Previously vaccinated*: Annual, 4-6 weeks prepartum	Annual—spring, before onset of vector season	*Inactivated vaccine*: 2 dose series **2nd** dose 4-6 weeks after 1st dose Revaccinate before the onset of the next vector season.	When using the inactivated or the recombinant product consider 6 month revaccination interval for: 1. Horses residing in endemic areas 2. Juvenile (<5 yrs of age) 3. Geriatric horses (>15 yrs of age) 4. Immunocompromised horses
	Unvaccinated or lacking vaccination history: • It is preferable to vaccinate naïve mares when open. • In areas of high risk, initiate primary series as described for unvaccinated, adult horses.		*Recombinant canary pox vaccine*: 2 dose series **2nd** dose 4-6 weeks after 1st dose Revaccinate before the onset of the next vector season.	
			Flavivirus chimera vaccine: Single dose Revaccinate before the onset of the next vector season.	

Continued

TABLE 9-7 VACCINATIONS FOR ADULT HORSES*—cont'd

RISK-BASED VACCINES are Selected for Use Based on Risk Assessment Performed by, or in Consultation With, a Licensed Veterinarian. Use of These Vaccines May Vary between Individuals, Populations, and/or Geographic Regions. ‡

Disease	Broodmares	Other Adult Horses (>1 year of age) *previously vaccinated for the disease*	Other Adult Horses (>1 year of age) *unvaccinated or lacking vaccination history*	Comments
Rabies	Annual, 4-6 weeks prepartum or Before breeding (see comments)	Annual	Single dose: Annual revaccination	NOTE on before breeding: Due to the relatively long duration of immunity this vaccine may be given post foaling but before breeding and thus reduce the number of vaccines given to a mare prepartum.
Anthrax	Not recommended during gestation	Annual	2 dose series: **2nd** dose 3-4 weeks after 1st dose Annual revaccination	Do not administer concurrently with antibiotics. Use caution during storage, handling and administration. Consult a physician immediately if human exposure to vaccine occurs by accidental injection, ingestion, or otherwise through the conjunctiva or broken skin.
Botulism	*Previously vaccinated:* Annual, 4-6 weeks prepartum *Previously unvaccinated or having unknown vaccination history:* 3 dose series **1st** dose at 8 months gestation **2nd** dose 4 weeks after 1st dose **3rd** dose 4 weeks after 2nd dose	Annual	3 dose series: **2nd** dose 4 weeks after 1st dose **3rd** dose 4 weeks after 2nd dose Annual revaccination	
Equine Herpes Virus (EHV)	3 dose series with product labeled for protection against EHV abortion. Give at 5, 7, 9 months of gestation.	Annual (see comments)	3 dose series: **2nd** dose 4-6 weeks after 1st dose **3rd** dose 4-6 weeks after 2nd dose	Consider 6 month revaccination interval for: • Horses less than 5 years of age • Horses on breeding farms or in contact with pregnant mares • Performance or show horses at high risk
Equine Viral Arteritis (EVA)	Not recommended unless high risk	Annual **Stallions, teasers:** Vaccinate 2-4 weeks before breeding season **Mares:** Vaccinate when open	Single dose (See comments)	**Before initial vaccination, intact males and any horses potentially intended for export should undergo serologic testing** and be confirmed negative for antibodies to EAV. Testing should be performed shortly before, or preferably at, the time of vaccination.

Influenza	*Previously vaccinated:* *Inactivated vaccine:* Semiannual with one dose administered 4-6 weeks prepartum *Canary pox vector vaccine:* Semiannual with one dose administered 4-6 weeks prepartum *Previously unvaccinated or having unknown vaccination history:* *Inactivated vaccine:* 3 dose series **2nd** dose 4-6 weeks after 1st dose **3rd** dose 4-6 weeks prepartum *Canary pox vector vaccine:* 2 dose series **2nd dose** 4-6 weeks after 1st dose but no later than 4 weeks prepartum	Horses with ongoing risk of exposure: Semiannual Horses at low risk of exposure: Annual	*Modified live vaccine:* Single dose administered intranasally Revaccinate semiannually to annually *Inactivated vaccine:* 3 dose series **2nd** dose 4-6 weeks after 1st dose **3rd** dose 3-6 months after 2nd dose Revaccinate Semiannually to annually *Canary pox vector vaccine:* 2 dose series **2nd** dose 4-6 weeks after 1st dose Revaccinate Semiannually	
Potomac Horse Fever (PHF)	***Previously vaccinated:*** Semiannual, with one dose given 4-6 weeks prepartum ***Previously unvaccinated or having unknown vaccination history:*** 2 dose series **1st** dose 7-9 weeks prepartum **2nd** dose 4-6 weeks prepartum	Semiannual to annual	2 dose series **2nd** dose 3-4 weeks after 1st dose Semiannual or annual booster	A revaccination interval of 3-4 months may be considered in endemic areas when disease risk is high.
Rotavirus	3 dose series **1st** dose at 8 months gestation **2nd and 3rd** doses at 4 week intervals thereafter	Not applicable	Not applicable	
Strangles (*Streptococcus equi*)	***Previously vaccinated:*** *Killed vaccine containing M-protein):* Semiannual with one dose given 4-6 weeks prepartum ***Previously unvaccinated or having unknown vaccination history:*** *Killed vaccine containing M-protein):* 3 dose series **2nd** dose 2-4 weeks after 1st dose **3rd** dose 4-6 weeks prepartum	Semiannual to annual	*Killed vaccine containing M-protein:* 2-3 dose series **2nd** dose 2-4 weeks after 1st dose **3rd** dose (where recommended by manufacturer) 2-4 weeks after 2nd dose Revaccinate semiannually *Modified live vaccine:* 2 dose series administered intranasally **2nd** dose 3 weeks after 1st dose Revaccinate semiannually to annually	Vaccination is **not** recommended as a strategy in outbreak mitigation.

*ALL vaccination programs should be developed in consultation with a licensed veterinarian.
‡Note: Vaccines are listed in this table in alphabetical order, **not** in order of priority for use.

EQUINE INFLUENZA VACCINES

Equine influenza is a highly contagious viral disease with worldwide distribution. Influenza is contracted through inhalation and infects the upper and lower airways. Influenza is frequently seen in mobile populations of horses, and disease outbreaks usually occur in horses 1 to 3 years of age after mixing with infected horses at racetracks, training barns, or show grounds.

Both inactivated and MLV vaccines are available. MLV vaccines for influenza are administered IN and provide a greater duration of immunity. Booster vaccines are recommended every 6 months in high-risk animals.

STRANGLES VACCINES

Strangles is a respiratory disease caused by infection with the bacterium *Streptococcus equi*. Strangles is easily transmitted through direct contact with mucopurulent discharge from infected horses or from contaminated fomites, such as feeding utensils, buckets, or other equipment. Strangles is characterized by a sudden onset of fever and nasal discharge followed by acute swelling and abscess formation in submaxillary, submandibular, and retropharyngeal lymph nodes.

Several inactivated injectable vaccines and one low-virulence live strain IN vaccine are available to aid in the control and prevention of strangles. IM strangles vaccinations may cause postinjection reactions or abscesses at the site of administration. Because of these adverse effects, vaccination against strangles is recommended only for horses with a high likelihood of exposure. Vaccination is not 100% effective for preventing disease, but does often reduce the severity and incidence of disease. Purpura hemorrhagica (immune-mediated vasculitis) is a possible adverse effect of all strangles vaccines.

> *TECHNICIAN NOTE* Administration of IN vaccines often result in MLV contamination of hands and clothing. Therefore IN vaccines should be given last if a series of injections are being given, and hands should be washed thoroughly after administration.

EQUINE VIRAL ARTERITIS VACCINE

Equine viral arteritis (EVA) is a contagious viral disease. Although an infection is rarely serious in healthy adult horses, it is concerning to horse breeders because it can lead to abortion, neonatal death, and render stallions as permanent carriers of the virus.

Only one commercially available MLV vaccine is available against EVA. Vaccination is recommended for colts intended to be breeding stallions and for broodmares with no evidence of previous exposure to the virus before being bred to carrier stallions. Vaccination is tightly controlled in some states, and seropositive horses may have problems with import or export to certain countries.

POTOMAC HORSE FEVER VACCINES

Potomac horse fever (PHF) is caused by *Neorickettsia risticii* (formerly known as *Ehrlichia risticii*). It is most prevalent in the eastern United States, particularly near large waterways, but has been identified throughout the United States and in other countries.

Approved vaccines are available for use in the control and prevention of PHF, and their use should be considered in areas where the disease is known to occur. The antibody response to vaccination is reportedly poor; however, vaccinated animals may exhibit reduced severity of clinical signs.

BOTULISM VACCINE

Botulism is caused by toxins produced by the bacterium *Clostridium botulinum* and results in gradual progressive muscular weakness. Multiple types of *C. botulinum* exist, although type B is most common in horses and is associated with the consumption of decaying forage.

The currently available equine botulism vaccine is a *C. botulinum* type B toxoid and is recommended for use in endemic areas. This vaccine requires an initial three-dose series followed by annual vaccination. Foals from unvaccinated mares may benefit from vaccination beginning as early as 2 weeks of age.

ANTHRAX VACCINE

Anthrax is caused by the bacterium *Bacillus anthracis*. Infection results from ingestion of soil, forage, or water contaminated with spores.

The currently available vaccine is an avirulent live-spore vaccine. Because swelling and abscesses have been associated with vaccination, its use is generally limited to high-risk areas.

RABIES VACCINES

Rabies is a viral disease affecting the nervous system and resulting in death. Approved killed-virus vaccines are available for use in horses and should be used annually. Rabies vaccines induce a strong immunologic response; therefore only a single dose is required annually in adult horses.

WEST NILE VIRUS VACCINES

West Nile virus (WNV) was a foreign animal disease before 1999 when the disease was detected in humans and horses on the East Coast of the United States; however, WNV is currently prevalent throughout the United States. The disease is caused by a flavivirus that infects numerous species of birds and mosquitoes; humans and horses are dead-end hosts.

Several vaccines are available for protection against WNV. They should be administered annually before the biting-insect season. Vaccine protection lasts approximately

6 months, and in areas where winter freezes are uncommon, semiannual vaccinations are advisable.

PARASITES

A good preventive health program should also account for the control of internal and external parasites. Heavy parasite burdens decrease athletic and reproductive performance and can cause weight loss and colic. A good deworming program should target ascarids, small and large strongyles, bots, and tapeworms (see Chapter 17).

It is important that all horses maintained at a facility be on an effective deworming program. If all horses pastured together are not properly dewormed, the parasite control program for all horses will be ineffective. There is no standard program concerning the frequency of administration or anthelmintic of choice; therefore it is important to discuss available options with owners.

Although the standard has been to recommend deworming of all horses every 8 to 12 weeks, studies have demonstrated that a small number of horses on each farm are usually responsible for carrying the majority of all worms. Why some horses carry high worm burdens and some do not is still unknown. Although treating all horses similarly is easiest, it is not ideal. If possible, fecal flotations should be evaluated on 10% of the herd immediately before and 7 days after dewormer administration. Egg counts greater than 150 eggs/g before deworming indicate that the interval between treatments is too long. The presence of ova after treatment indicates resistance to the anthelmintic used.

> *TECHNICIAN NOTE* Developing deworming protocols based on fecal egg counts are generally more cost effective than "blanket deworming" all horses at set time periods.

A variety of anthelmintics are available, with benzimidazoles (fenbendazole, oxfendazole, and oxibendazole), pyrantel salts, ivermectin, and moxidectin as the most common. No anthelmintic is effective against all internal parasites, and a few differences should be pointed out:

1. Moxidectin and ivermectin are the only approved boticides.
2. Praziquantel is the only FDA-approved product for tapeworms and is available in combination with moxidectin and ivermectin.
3. Moxidectin and fenbendazole (fenbendazole given for 5 days at double dose) are approved for removing encysted small strongyles.

Daily deworming products are available that are added to a horse's grain and fed each day. The products currently available are ineffective at controlling all the species of internal parasites. Many horse owners incorrectly assume that because their horses are on daily dewormer internal parasites are not a problem.

Feed additives are also available that are lethal to developing housefly and stable fly larvae in treated horse feces (but not effective against existing adult flies). These types of feed additives should be used with caution because they are organophosphate larvicides with possible adverse effects if used concomitantly with other pharmaceutical products.

DENTAL CARE

The routine examination and care of the teeth is an important part of any horse's preventive health program. It is estimated that as many as 80% of horses have dental problems. Signs of a dental problem can range from obvious to subtle and include: weight loss, bad breath, excessive drooling, swelling of the face or jaw, dropping feed while eating, head tossing, excessive chewing of the bit, and problems while being ridden (bucking, tail ringing, fighting against the bit). The proper and thorough examination of the oral cavity usually requires sedation, a light source (such as headlamp or flashlight), and a mouth speculum.

In the horse, the teeth are continually erupting, and the lower jaw is narrower than the upper jaw. As the horse grinds its food from side to side, the teeth are worn down unevenly. The inside (near the tongue) of the upper teeth is worn as is the outside (near the cheek) of the lower teeth. Thus sharp points develop on the outside of the upper teeth and the inside of the lower teeth. These sharp enamel points can become severe and result in lacerations of the tongue and cheek. Most enamel points can be removed by floating (rasping). The cheek teeth of the upper jaw are often positioned slightly forward of the teeth in the lower jaw, and because of the offset positioning, hooks and ramps can form. Hooks are sharp points found on the first upper cheek teeth. Ramps are sharp points found on the last lower cheek teeth.

Wolf teeth are the small, pointed, rudimentary first premolars located just in front of the first cheek teeth. Wolf teeth do not appear in all horses, are more common in the upper jaw than in the lower jaw, and will vary in size. In some horses, the position of these teeth causes interference with the position and function of the bit. For this reason, wolf teeth are often removed before a horse enters training (around 12 to 18 months of age). Wolf teeth are generally removed while the horse is standing and sedated.

Normally the deciduous premolars are replaced by the permanent premolars between the ages of 2 to 4 years without a problem. Occasionally a deciduous premolar fails to fall out, a condition known as a retained cap. This can result in discomfort leading to decreased feed consumption and lowered performance. Caps are easily removed in standing, sedated horses.

Feed that becomes trapped around a tooth can lead to bacterial growth, resulting in an infection. Other causes of an infection are a fractured jaw and inflammation of the periodontal ligament (ligament that holds a tooth to the bone). An infected tooth usually leads to the more obvious clinical signs of dental disease, such as a swollen face or jaw, a draining abscess, trouble eating, and foul breath. Because the upper teeth are closely associated with the nasal sinuses, nasal discharge and sinusitis can also be a sign of an infection. Depending on the site of the infection and the length of the tooth root, the infected tooth may be pulled from the oral cavity or removed by accessing the roots via the maxillary sinus or mandible and driving the tooth forward into the oral cavity.

Routine dental maintenance can prevent or minimize many of the dental problems observed in horses. Yearly examinations are recommended for mature horses. Young horses (2 to 5 years) are losing deciduous teeth and gaining their permanent teeth. During this time, 24 teeth are lost and replaced, providing ample opportunity for dental problems to occur. Young horses should have a thorough dental examination before starting training and then twice yearly until all permanent teeth are in. Finally, horses with a history of dental problems should also have their teeth examined biannually or even more frequently if required.

> *TECHNICIAN NOTE* Young horses (under 5 years of age) and those with a history of dental problems should have their teeth examined biannually.

HOOF CARE

The role of the veterinarian and veterinary technician in hoof care is largely advisory for most routine hoof care is provided by farriers. However, education of the client on the importance of proper and frequent hoof care for the prevention of lameness is important.

Horse hooves grow an average of one quarter inch per month depending on ground surface, exercise frequency, nutrition, and individual growth rates. Based on the average growth rate, hooves should be trimmed every 6 to 8 weeks to maintain proper shape, balance, and movement. Keeping the hooves trimmed short and maintaining the correct hoof-pastern axis helps prevent excess stress on tendons and ligaments of the limb. In foals, some minor conformation problems, such as splayfoot or pigeon toe, can be corrected or minimized with frequent hoof trimming.

Cleaning out the bottom of the foot is also important. Hoof cleaning not only removes rocks and debris from the foot, but also helps in the prevention of thrush. Thrush is caused by anaerobic bacteria that grow in moist and dark conditions, such as in the sulci of the frog and under dirt that has accumulated and packed into the sole. Thrush appears as a moist, malodorous accumulation in the sulci of the frog and sometimes over the sole. Frequent cleaning removes dirt and exposes these bacteria to drying, aerobic conditions. Copper- or iodine-based solutions can be applied to the sulci and frog to treat thrush.

NUTRITION

Proper nutrition is the foundation for any preventive health program. Many health issues, such as laminitis, colic, and ulcers, can be directly related to nutritional problems. Owners should be encouraged to feed a balanced diet and to work closely with their veterinarian or equine nutritionist to develop proper diets for their horse(s). Equine nutrition is discussed in more detail in Chapter 13.

PREVENTIVE HEALTH PROGRAM FOR LIVESTOCK SPECIES

Preventive medicine is especially important in livestock to maintain the productivity of the herd. Management, nutrition, and vaccination each play a role in minimizing the incidence of disease in livestock species. This section is not intended to provide a comprehensive review of all of the vaccines available in livestock; the goal is to describe typical preventive management procedures and commonly used vaccination programs.

SWINE

BIRTH TO WEANING

Preventive medicine in swine herds begins with piglets, which must be kept in a warm, draft-free environment. When pigs are piled up on top of each other, they are too cold, and piling up increases the risk of rectal prolapse. Within the first week of life, piglets have their needle (canine) teeth trimmed and tails docked to decrease chewing on each other. Baby pigs are commonly given a shot of iron at the time of teeth and tail trimming, and male piglets that will not be used for breeding are castrated.

GROWING PIGS

Pigs are vaccinated against erysipelas at weaning, when they are removed from the sow and placed into groups of growing pigs. Erysipelas, which is caused by *Erysipelothrix rhusiopathiae,* is characterized by fever, skin lesions, and sudden death in infected pigs. Animals that survive the acute infection may develop chronic arthritis or endocarditis and consequently grow poorly. Pens into which weaned pigs are moved must be cleaned and disinfected, and they must be well ventilated without being cold or drafty. Newly grouped weaned pigs should not be mixed in pens or buildings with older pigs. Overcrowding must also be avoided. Because weaning is a stressful time for pigs, some farms will add antibiotics to the feed for a few weeks after weaning. Pigs may also be dewormed at weaning, if necessary, and some farms will vaccinate pigs at weaning against pathogens that may cause pneumonia, such as *Mycoplasma* bacteria.

Biosecurity (a protocol to prevent the introduction of disease organisms onto the farm) is practiced more commonly and more strictly in swine production than any other type of animal agriculture. On some farms, all visitors, including veterinarians and their staff, are asked to shower and change into clothing provided by the farm before coming into contact with any animals. The risk of spreading disease may also be minimized by working with the youngest pigs first then proceeding through progressively older groups of pigs.

BREEDING ANIMALS

Pigs are commonly vaccinated for leptospirosis, parvovirus, and again for erysipelas before entering the breeding herd. Leptospirosis, an infection with *L. pomona, L. bratislava,* or other members of the genus *Leptospira,* may cause infertility, abortion, stillbirth, or the birth of weak piglets. Animals purchased for breeding should be tested for brucellosis and pseudorabies if the animals are not from a pseudorabies-free area (most of the United States is now pseudorabies free). Brucellosis may cause abortion or infertility and it is zoonotic. Pseudorabies causes death in young pigs and respiratory disease with the possibility of chronic infection in older animals. Animals entering a herd free of porcine reproductive and respiratory syndrome (PRRS) should also be tested for the PRRS virus, which causes reproductive failure, respiratory disease, and chronic infections. Depending on their origin, animals may need to be treated for internal and external parasites. New additions to the herd should always be quarantined away from the herd for 30 days or more before introduction to the herd. Quarantine prevents new animals from spreading diseases they may have been carrying asymptomatically when they were purchased or diseases, such as pneumonia, that they may have developed during transport to the farm.

Sows in the breeding herd should have booster vaccinations against erysipelas and leptospirosis when their litters are weaned; boars may be given the same vaccines every 6 months. Sows and gilts (young sows) may also be vaccinated against *Escherichia coli* bacteria to diminish the occurrence of diarrhea in their offspring and against parvovirus, which may cause infertility and abortion.

> *TECHNICIAN NOTE* Because swine in modern production systems may never be outdoors, many pigs do not require deworming at any time.

CATTLE

Although beef and dairy production systems have many differences, they will be discussed together here because many of the principles of disease control and diseases of concern are the same in both systems.

BIRTH TO WEANING

Preventive medicine in cattle actually starts before birth because many pregnant cows are vaccinated against *E. coli,* rotavirus, and coronavirus to protect their calves from developing diarrhea. Colostrum from vaccinated cows provides extra protection to calves against diseases for which the cow has been vaccinated. Calves should be born into a dry, draft-free environment. It is essential that calves receive an adequate amount of good quality colostrum soon after birth. In beef herds, this is ensured by the frequent monitoring of cows during calving season, whereas dairy herds typically hand-feed colostrum to newborn calves. Dairy farms will keep frozen colostrum or colostrum replacer on hand to feed orphan calves or calves from dams that fail to produce adequate colostrum or leak colostrum before calving.

> *TECHNICIAN NOTE* The most important step in keeping calves healthy is ensuring that they receive an adequate amount of good quality colostrum shortly after birth.

Vaccination in beef calves should ideally begin before weaning because weaning is a stressful time for calves that increases their risk for developing disease. Weaning in dairy calves is done at a younger age than in beef calves (less than 2 months of age versus about 6 months), so vaccination is commonly delayed until after weaning. For any young cattle, vaccination at less than 3 months of age is likely to be incompletely effective as a result of interference from maternal antibodies obtained in colostrum. Calfhood vaccination programs usually include a clostridial vaccine, a viral respiratory and reproductive pathogen vaccine, and brucellosis vaccination (often called "Bangs" vaccination). Clostridial diseases, such as tetanus, blackleg, and malignant edema, are caused by bacteria from the genus *Clostridium,* occur primarily in young animals, and are often rapidly fatal. Viral respiratory and reproductive diseases are commonly included in one "five-way" or "six-way" product, usually with a brand name connoting strength rather than what the vaccine is designed to protect against. The viral reproductive and respiratory pathogens commonly included in combination vaccines are bovine diarrhea virus (BVD), which may cause diarrhea, mucosal ulcers, abortion, and immunosuppression, plus infectious bovine rhinotracheitis (IBR), parainfluenza 3 (PI3), and bovine respiratory syncytial virus (BRSV), which are primarily respiratory pathogens. These combination vaccines also frequently include the bacterial pathogens *Histophilus somnus,* which may cause sudden death or fever and depression, and/or *Leptospira* species, which cause infertility and abortion. Bangs vaccination protects against brucellosis, an infection with *Brucella abortus,* which is associated with abortion and infertility. Brucellosis vaccination is reported to the United States Department of Agriculture, and vaccinates are marked with an orange ear tag and tattoo in the right ear. Only heifers under 1 year of age may be legally vaccinated against brucellosis, and in some states, the maximum age for vaccination is less than 1 year. Vaccination against brucellosis is especially important for animals that may be sold as breeding stock. Special care is taken in the handling and administration of RB51, the brucellosis vaccine, because the vaccine contains live organisms and the disease is zoonotic. Unlike the clostridial and viral vaccines, the brucellosis vaccine is given only one time.

Animals that naturally have horns are commonly dehorned to protect other animals from injury. In dairy calves, this is usually done in the first few weeks of life, whereas in beef animals, dehorning may be done at the time of weaning.

> TECHNICIAN NOTE Cattle vaccines should be administered as labeled (IM or SQ) only in the neck region to maintain meat quality. In addition, most vaccines for food animals have withdrawal or withholding periods where the animal and its products (such as milk) may not be sold.

GROWING CATTLE

Disease in growing cattle is best prevented by appropriate nutrition and clean, well-ventilated housing (or good pasture) in addition to vaccination. Growing cattle that are at risk will need to be treated for external and internal parasites, as necessary. Adequate fly control will help prevent infectious bovine keratoconjunctivitis (pinkeye), an infection of the eye caused by *Branhamella ovis* and/or *Moraxella bovis* bacteria, which are carried between animals on flies. Heifers commonly receive another dose of viral respiratory and reproductive vaccine before being bred for the first time. Beef cattle are also typically given a repeat vaccination against viral respiratory pathogens upon entering the feedlot; in addition, such animals are commonly vaccinated against the bacterial respiratory pathogens *Histophilus somnus, Mannheimia hemolytica,* and *Pasteurella multocida.*

BREEDING ANIMALS

To protect the health of the herd, care must be taken when obtaining breeding bulls. Beef herds are more likely to purchase bulls because they generally employ natural breeding throughout the herd, whereas dairy herds tend to use artificial insemination extensively. In addition to a breeding soundness examination for fertility, purchased bulls should at least have a negative test result for BVD, which may cause infertility, abortion, diarrhea, death, or a chronic poor condition. It is also advisable to test bulls for the venereal disease trichomoniasis, which is passed to cows during breeding and causes fertility problems. It is preferable to purchase the bull from a herd that is free of Johne's disease, which causes chronic diarrhea and weight loss, and bovine leukosis virus, which causes cancer. Bulls should be vaccinated before the breeding season against the viral respiratory and reproductive pathogens; campylobacteriosis, which is passed to cows when breeding and causes infertility; and leptospirosis. Cows should also be revaccinated against these diseases before the breeding season.

> TECHNICIAN NOTE Nearly all adult cattle receive vaccinations against viral respiratory and reproductive pathogens (IBR, BVD, PI3, and BRSV), frequently combined with antigens for one or more bacterial pathogens, such as Pasteurella, Haemophilus, or Leptospira, at least once per year.

In dairy cows, mastitis (an infection of the mammary gland) is an important disease and a key focus of preventive efforts. Dairy cows are commonly vaccinated against mastitis caused by *E. coli*, which can be severe and life threatening. The vaccine does not prevent *E. coli* mastitis, but it does reduce the frequency and severity of the disease on the farm. Most mastitis cannot be prevented by vaccination; prevention relies on management steps. These include keeping cow housing and milking areas clean, cleaning the teats well before milking, dipping the teats into disinfectant before and after milking (called predipping and postdipping), and proper nutrition.

Only the most commonly used vaccines are mentioned previously, but many more are available. Not all available vaccines are considered effective. Vaccine protocols should be tailored to each herd specifically based on the needs and risks in the herd. It must also be kept in mind that even an excellent vaccination protocol cannot overcome poor management and nutrition.

Hoof trimming is especially important in dairy animals. They may not wear their hooves down as quickly as they grow, and animals that have suffered an episode of lameness may not wear their hooves evenly. Dairy cows should have their feet trimmed at least once a year and more often if problems develop. Because they walk more, beef animals do not usually need routine trimming, but it may be necessary for animals with abnormal hoof growth patterns, such as "corkscrew claws," in which the wall of the hoof spirals under the sole. This is thought to be a hereditary problem, so cows who display corkscrew claws should probably be removed from a breeding program.

As with bulls, purchased cows should be tested and quarantined before joining a herd. It is preferable to buy cows from a herd that is free of Johne's disease and bovine leukosis virus, and all animals should have a negative test result for BVD virus. In addition, the milk of purchased dairy cows should have a negative test result for the presence of contagious or incurable mastitis infections.

SMALL RUMINANTS: SHEEP AND GOATS

NEWBORN AND GROWING ANIMALS

As with cattle, preventive health programs for sheep and goats begin before birth, when pregnant ewes and does are vaccinated against *C. perfringens* type C and D and *C. tetani,* which cause the usually fatal diseases lamb dysentery, overeating disease, and tetanus. Protection for lambs and kids is provided through the colostrum of their vaccinated dams. Ewes and does should be vaccinated at least 4 weeks before their due date; if they have not previously been vaccinated against clostridial diseases, they should be vaccinated twice during pregnancy. If the ewes and does do not get vaccinated during pregnancy, kids or lambs should be vaccinated just after birth and again at 2 to 3 weeks of age, and tetanus antitoxin should be administered at the time of castration, dehorning, and tail-docking during the first week of life. The offspring of vaccinated dams should be vaccinated twice between 6 and 10 weeks of age. In selenium-deficient areas, ewes should be supplemented with selenium orally or by an injection to prevent weakness caused by selenium deficiency (white muscle disease) in the lambs.

> *TECHNICIAN NOTE* Diseases caused by bacteria of the genus *Clostridium* are especially dangerous in sheep and goats. Pregnant ewes and does should be vaccinated against clostridial diseases to protect their offspring.

Small ruminants may also be vaccinated against contagious ecthyma, also called orf or sore mouth. It is a viral disease that causes painful lesions of the skin on the mouth of young animals and the mouth and teats of ewes and does, resulting in decreased nursing by young animals. Sore mouth vaccination is performed by scratching the skin in an area without wool (inner ear or under the tail in older animals, inner thigh in young animals) and introducing a live virus into the scratch. This must be done well before lambing or kidding so that newborn animals will not be affected. In addition, great care must be taken by the person administering the vaccine because it contains a live virus and the disease is zoonotic. The vaccine should not be used in herds that have not had problems with the disease.

Coccidia are present in all sheep and goats, and they may cause diarrhea, weight loss, and illness in young animals under stress. Coccidia are controlled by management steps such as preventing overcrowding, good sanitation, and feeding off the ground. In addition, a coccidiostatic drug, such as lasalocid or decoquinate, may be added to the feed to help prevent outbreaks of coccidiosis.

THE BREEDING HERD

For small ruminants that are kept as pets, rabies vaccination is probably worthwhile, though it is not used in commercial flocks. As in other species, many other vaccines are available for use in sheep and goats; decisions about whether to use them in particular animals or herds should be made in consultation with a veterinarian and in light of specific needs and risks.

> *TECHNICIAN NOTE* Rabies vaccination is not practiced for all animals in commercial sheep and goat flocks, but it is a good idea for pet sheep and goats.

Parasitism is a serious problem in sheep and goats, particularly infestations with *Haemonchus contortus,* also called the barber pole worm. *H. contortus* attaches to the wall of the abomasum and consumes the animal's blood. If left untreated, infestation may lead to severe anemia and death. There is no strategy that completely eliminates internal parasites in sheep and goats, but there are a number of ways to reduce the burden. One aspect is good nutrition; well-nourished animals are less susceptible to parasitic illness. Animals should be fed off the ground in a trough into which young animals cannot climb to reduce the contamination of feed with feces. Goats that are able to browse plants above the ground, instead of just grazing as sheep do, will have reduced parasite burdens. Parasitism in sheep may be reduced by rotating them through pastures that have been kept empty or used by cattle or horses (not goats) or crops for the previous 3 to 6 months. Culling of animals with chronic severe parasitism is recommended because such animals have low parasite resistance, a trait that may be passed on to the offspring. Oral dewormers of the benzimidazole (e.g., thiabendazole) and avermectin (e.g., ivermectin) families are used in small ruminants, but these drugs must be used strategically because overuse promotes resistance. Some experts have recommended deworming only animals that show signs of disease. Sheep may also develop external parasites, such as ticks and lice, which should be treated as necessary with sprays, dips, or ivermectin-type drugs.

> *TECHNICIAN NOTE* Sheep may be examined for anemia caused by parasitism with *H. contortus* by examining the conjunctiva of the eyes. If it is white, not pink, the animal is likely to be anemic and heavily parasitized.

SUMMARY

There are many aspects of preventive medicine in livestock species. Vaccination is important, but it is not a substitute for proper management. Disease is also prevented through proper nutrition, good hygiene, appropriate housing, and parasite control. New animals must be tested for disease and quarantined before mixing them in with the herd to prevent the introduction of disease into the herd.

RECOMMENDED READING

Dogs and Cats

Kitchell BE: Feline vaccine-associated sarcomas, WSAVA Congress, 2005. Available at www.vin.com/proceedings/Proceedings.plx?CID=WSAVA2005&PID=10915&O=Generic. Accessed October 4, 2008.

Klingborg DJ, et al: AVMA council on biologic and therapeutic agents' report on cat and dog vaccines, *J Am Vet Med Assoc* 221:1401-1407, 2002.

Littman MP: The Lyme test is positive—now what? *Proc 25th Ann Vet Med Forum, ACVIM* pp 501-503, 2007.

Littman MP, et al: ACVIM small animal consensus statement on Lyme disease in dogs: diagnosis, treatment, and prevention, *J Vet Intern Med* 20:422-434, 2006.

Paul MA, et al: Report of the American Animal Hospital (AAHA) canine vaccine task force: 2006 AAHA canine vaccine guidelines, *J Am Anim Hosp Assoc* 42:80-89, 2006.

Richards JR, et al: The 2006 American Association of Feline Practitioners feline vaccine advisory panel report, *J Am Vet Med Assoc* 229:1405-1441, 2006.

Schultz RD: Considerations in designing effective and safe vaccination programs for dogs. In Carmichael L, editor: Recent advances in canine infectious diseases, Ithaca, NY, 2000, International Veterinary Information Service (www.ivis.org). Document No. A0110.0500 available at www.ivis.org/advances/Infect_Dis_Carmichael/schultz/chapter_frm.asp?LA=1. Accessed October 4, 2008.

Shelter medicine website from the University of California (Davis) Koret Shelter Medicine Program. Available at www.sheltermedicine.com/portal/is_vaccination.shtml#top3 and www.sheltermedicine.com/portal/portal.shtml#top3. Accessed October 4, 2008.

Horses

Ensminger ME, Hammer CJ: Ensminger's equine science, ed 8, Upper Saddle River, NJ, 2004, Pearson Prentice Hall.

Love S: Treatment and prevention of intestinal parasite-associated disease, *Vet Clin North Am Equine Pract* 3:791-806, 2003.

Smith BP: *Large animal internal medicine*, ed 4, St Louis, 2009, Mosby.

Livestock

Bagley CV: Vaccination program for beef calves. Available at http://extension.usu.edu/files/publications/factsheet/AH_Beef__40.pdf. Accessed October 4, 2008.

Bagley CV: Vaccination programs for dairy young stock. Available at http://extension.usu.edu/files/publications/factsheet/AH_Dairy_06.pdf. Accessed October 4, 2008.

Maryland small ruminant page: Available at www.sheepandgoat.com. Accessed October 4, 2008.

Tubbs RC: Herd health programs for swine seedstock production. Available at http://extension.missouri.edu/explore/agguides/ansci/g02508.htm. Accessed October 4, 2008.

Tubbs RC, Floss JL: Herd management for disease prevention. Available at http://extension.missouri.edu/explore/agguides/ansci/g02507.htm. Accessed October 4, 2008.

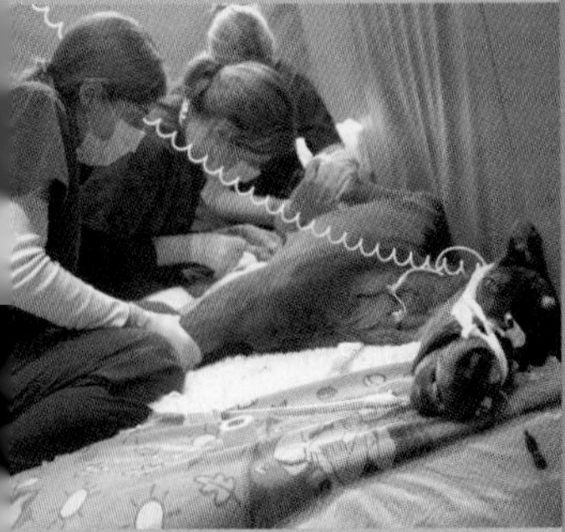

Neonatal Care of the Puppy, Kitten, and Foal

10

Margret L. Casal and Amy I. Bentz

KEY TERMS

Broodmare
Colt
Congenital
Dehydration
Filly
Foal
Gelding
Genetic
Hypoglycemia
Hypothermia
Mare
Neonatal period
Pediatric period
Stallion
Thermogenesis
Weanling
Yearling

OUTLINE

LEARNING OBJECTIVES

When you have completed this chapter, you will be able to:

1. Describe special requirements for examination of neonates.
2. List normal physiologic and behavioral parameters of neonatal puppies.
3. Describe diagnostic sampling techniques used for neonatal puppies.
4. Define hypothermia and describe problems related to hypothermia in neonatal puppies and kittens.
5. Explain how neonatal isoerythrolysis occurs and is managed in kittens.
6. List the symptoms, causes, and treatments of fading puppy or kitten syndrome.
7. Describe considerations for the care of orphan puppies and kittens.
8. Describe the care of the high-risk perinatal mare and list supplies needed to attend a high-risk foaling.
9. Describe the events that occur in each of the stages of labor in the mare.
10. Describe the normal development and routine nursing care, medical care, and diagnostic procedures in the neonatal foal.

INTRODUCTION

Human medicine is rich with volumes of books containing tables, graphs, and guidelines, such as the "Denver scores," that detail the normal and abnormal development of babies and that are readily available to clinicians for the assessment of their human pediatric patients. In contrast, veterinary medicine is challenged by diversity among species and breeds of animals and by the far broader ranges of what constitutes "normal" and "abnormal." Relatively speaking, veterinary personnel must rely on far fewer reference resources, making empirical experience and the observations of breeders critically important. Because the development of body systems continues well after birth, young animals are particularly vulnerable to age-related problems. A thorough history and physical examination are important to detect developmental complications and illnesses. This chapter addresses normal neonatal development and the most common reasons for illness in the puppy, kitten, and foal.

NEONATOLOGY OF PUPPIES AND KITTENS

HISTORY

Because of the unusual or nonspecific clinical signs associated with ill puppies and kittens, it is of great importance to obtain a comprehensive history not only of the patient, but also of the littermates, parents, and other relatives. The history should include: the number of ill animals, the method by which they were raised, their normal environment, behavior of each puppy or kitten within the litter, body weight curves, duration and type of clinical signs, and medications given. The queen's or bitch's history should include vaccination dates, estrous cycle (intervals and duration), breeding practice, medications or supplements given during pregnancy, and problems during pregnancy or birth. Has the disorder that the patient is experiencing been seen in previous litters or in any of the relatives? In certain cases, clients are advised to bring the whole litter or at least one healthy littermate including the mother so that the patient can be compared with its littermate(s). If the patient or its littermates have not been vaccinated, it may be better to have them come in the back door to prevent exposure to all the infectious diseases that may linger in the waiting room.

> *TECHNICIAN NOTE* Because of the unusual or nonspecific clinical signs associated with ill puppies and kittens, it is of great importance to obtain a comprehensive history not only of the patient, but also of the littermates, parents, and other relatives.

PHYSICAL EXAMINATION

The physical examination of the neonate and the juvenile patient can be challenging. Owners and littermates that were brought in for comparison can be quite distracting. Usually, one cannot expect cooperation from the youngest of our patients, especially those that are already aware of their surroundings. They are so distracted by the new environment that something as simple as a menace reflex is difficult to elicit. Whereas everyone knows how to perform a physical examination on an adult, the following two paragraphs focus on examination techniques for the neonate. Some specific examples are given, but keep in mind that the list is not complete. However, some of the developmental landmarks described later may be helpful in determining abnormalities.

For the physical examination of a neonate, a pediatric stethoscope with a 2-cm bell is helpful. In addition, a digital thermometer allows a rapid measurement of the body temperature, without causing great discomfort. Because the neonate can have a body temperature lower than 94° F, a digital thermometer that measures as low as 85° F is practical. Neonates cannot regulate their body temperature during the first 2 weeks of life. They should be examined on a warm, clean surface rather than the cold metal table. Checking the oral mucous membranes assesses hydration in the neonate because the skin turgor is not developed as it is in adults (Figure 10-1). Moist mucous membranes are present in an adequate state of hydration. The neonate is born with hair that covers most of the body except the ventral abdominal skin. A lack of hair or a sparse hair coat may indicate either a genetic abnormality of the skin or premature birth (Figure 10-2). The neonate normally has nonhaired, dark-pink, ventral abdominal skin. Bluish or dark red discolorations are indicative of a neonate in distress (cyanosis or sepsis, respectively). Other than urine and feces, a discharge from any orifice is abnormal in the neonate. The neonate's head, body, limbs, and tail are examined for symmetry and normal conformation. The head is specifically examined for open fontanelles, cleft palates, bulging eyes from behind closed eyelids (an infection behind closed eyelids), and formation of the nose and external ears. The presence of flattening or malformations of the chest are noted (e.g., swimmer syndrome, pectus excavatum) as are bulges in the neck area (e.g., gas in the esophagus, ectopic heart, goiter). Neonatal puppies are mildly pudgy, and neonatal kittens are generally

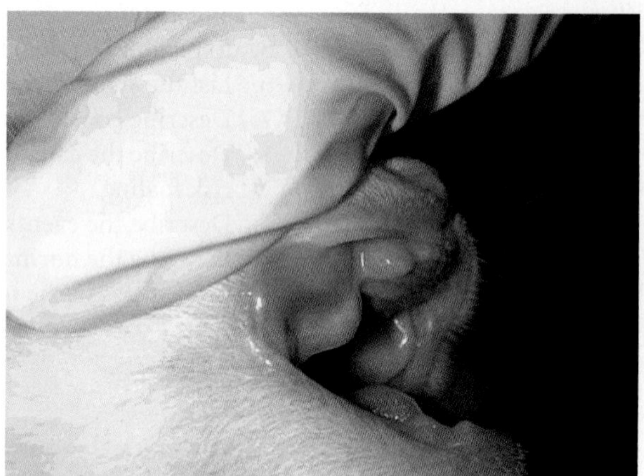

FIGURE 10-1 Mucous membranes in the mouth of a newborn kitten. Note the pale pink appearance, which is the normal color at this age.

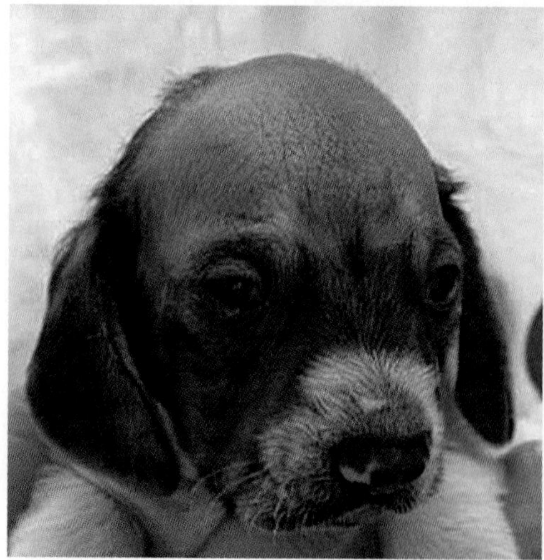

FIGURE 10-2 Two-week-old abnormal puppy displaying hairlessness and cloudy, slightly crusty eyes.

on the lean side. Neither of them should ever be bloated, which would be a sign of distress. The abdomen and urachus are especially examined for defects of the abdominal wall and ventral urine scalding, such as cannibalism as a result of an overzealous mother, ventral closure defects, and a persistent urachus. The genitals and the anus are checked for patency by stimulating urination and defecation using a moistened cotton ball. The presence of hair coat abnormalities over the dorsum may indicate the presence of a spina bifida. The tail is examined for muscle tone, length, curliness, and kinks. Abnormalities in tone may be indicators for associated defects or problems, such as abnormal innervation of the distal pelvis.

NORMAL DEVELOPMENT

During the first week of life, newborn kittens and puppies sleep throughout most of the day (80%) and nurse vigorously for a short period of time every 2 to 4 hours. Because the brain is not completely developed at birth, neuromuscular reflexes are missing and the only motor skills present are crawling, suckling, and distress vocalization. The neonates only respond to stimuli such as odor, touch, and pain. The queen or bitch initiates urination and defecation by licking the urogenital area. At 3 days of age, kittens and puppies should be able to lift their head and by 1 week crawl in a coordinated manner. Puppies and kittens are unable to maintain their body temperature during the first few days of life, and the shiver reflex does not develop until after the first week of life. Their body temperature at birth (94.5° F to 97.3° F) is lower than in adults and rises to 94.7° F to 100.1° F during the first week of life. Heart and respiratory rates may be irregular at birth (pulse [P] = 160 to 200 beats/min [bpm], respiration [R] = 10 to 20 breaths/min), and there is no abdominal component to their breathing. During the first week, the neonates begin to adjust to the new, extrauterine environment, and their physiology adjusts (P = 200 to 220 bpm, R = 16 to 35 breaths/min). The umbilical cord dries out during the first day of life and should have fallen off by day 2 to 3. The flexor tone present at birth switches over to extensor tone after the fourth day of life (Box 10-1). Although sex determination in normal newborn puppies is unambiguous, it can be challenging in kittens. The sex of kittens can be determined at birth by evaluating the anogenital distance, which is shorter in females (7.6 ± 1 mm) than in males (12.9 ± 1.5 mm). Male kittens are born with descended testicles, which are able to move freely in and out of the scrotum until 5 to 7 months of age. In dogs, the testicles do not descend until 6 weeks of age.

During the second week of life, kittens and puppies begin to crawl, and their body temperature slowly rises toward normal adult levels. Kittens and puppies will have doubled their birth weight by 7 to 10 and 10 to 12 days, respectively. They begin to open their eyes at 7 to 12 days of age, and the external ear canals open at 14 to 16 days of age. The iris is not well pigmented, has a blue-gray color, and the cornea is slightly cloudy as a result of an increased water content. Kittens may have divergent strabismus. By the end of 3 weeks of age, puppies and kittens are able to stand and have good postural reflexes. Refer to Box 10-2 for details about the development of specific organ systems.

BOX 10-1 Neurologic Examination of the Very Young Pediatric Patient

- Suckling reflex: Should be present at birth, puppy or kitten will try to suck or chew on a finger.
- Pressing reflex: Should be present at birth, puppy or kitten will press its head against a bowed hand.
- Flexor tone: Present until 3-4 days of age; when a puppy or kitten is held by the head, it will "roll up" and adduct its hind legs.
- Extensor tone: After 4 days of age, a puppy or kitten held by its head will stretch its back and hind legs.
- Lumbar reflex: Forcefully rubbing a healthy puppy or kitten in the lumbar region will result in vocalization and great activity.
- Extensor reflex: The patient is placed in dorsal recumbency, and a toe of a hind limb is pinched. If the puppy or kitten is less than 3 wk of age, it will adduct the other hind limb. Normal!
- Magnus reflex: The patient is placed in dorsal recumbency, and its head is bent toward one side. Under 3 wk of age, it will stretch its legs on this side and bend the ones on the other side.
- Tonic neck reflexes: The patient is held by the thorax, and its neck is bent toward one side; it should stretch the limbs on this side. The head is bent dorsally, the front limbs should be stretched, and the hind limbs adducted. Present until 3 wk of age.
- Hopping reflex: Is already present at 2-4 days of age.
- Anogenital reflex: If the patient's anogenital region is stimulated with a moist cloth or cotton, it should urinate or defecate. Present until 3-4 wk of age.
- Palpebral and corneal reflexes: Should be present as soon as the eyes are open.
- Menace reflex: Can be present as early as 2 wk of age, but usually not until 10-14 wk of age.

TECHNICIAN NOTE Although sex determination in normal newborn puppies is unambiguous, it can be challenging in kittens. The sex of kittens can be determined at birth by evaluating the anogenital distance, which is shorter in females (7.6 ± 1 mm) than in males (12.9 ± 1.5 mm).

DIAGNOSTICS

Blood can be easily obtained from the jugular vein in neonates. However, no more than 10% of the circulating volume should be drawn over the course of a week. In other words, if a neonate weighs 250 g, no more than 2.5 ml of blood should be drawn in 1 week. If a neonate remains in the hospital for several days, it may be worthwhile posting a chart next to the patient where every nurse can record the amount of blood drawn to prevent causing the patient to

BOX 10-2 Select Organ Development

- **Heart:** At birth, the right and left ventricles have approximately the same mass, changing to an ultimate adult ratio of 1:2 to 1:3 throughout puberty and change in the cardiac axis and shape. During this time, the canine heart changes from ellipsoid at birth to more globoid in adulthood. At 1 mo of age, puppies and kittens still have lower blood pressures, stroke volumes, and resistance in the peripheral vasculature than adults, but they have higher heart rates, cardiac outputs, and central venous pressure. Responses to cardiovascular drugs during the first weeks of life are less intense than in the adult. The development of the heart has been well studied in the dog, and it has been shown that normal adult values of the aforementioned parameters are reached by 7 mo of age. It is important to keep these differences in mind when evaluating chest radiographs, ECGs, and echocardiograms.
- **Immune system:** Virtually no antibodies are transferred in utero to canine and feline fetuses, and they are born immunologically immature. Puppies and kittens are dependent on the colostral transfer of antibodies (passive immunity) for postnatal protection against infectious diseases. In puppies and kittens, colostrum needs to be ingested within the first 24 and 16 hr of life, respectively, whereby mainly IgG and IgA are absorbed. Thereafter the gut seems to be closed for further absorption. Depending on the type of maternally derived antibodies, these may last from 6-16 wk after birth. Relative to the size of the puppy, the greatest size of the thymus is noted at birth, but its absolute size will be greatest at puberty, after which it begins to atrophy. Although the thymus and immune system are thought to be mature by 3-4 mo of age, puppies and kittens have the ability to produce functional IgM shortly before birth. Lymph node structure is normal at birth, but there are few lymphocytes, which increase in number during the first months of life. The lymph nodes should be palpable at birth, but the facial nodes are easier to palpate because of their increased reactivity.
- **Liver:** Drugs that require hepatic metabolism should only be carefully administered to neonatal patients because the liver does not reach full metabolic capacity until well after the neonatal period. Neonatal albumin and plasma protein levels are also significantly lower than in adults. Dosages of drugs that are bound to albumin or plasma proteins must be adjusted accordingly. The liver is also the site of the production of most coagulation factors. Because of its immaturity, many coagulopathies may be exacerbated during the neonatal age. Because growing requires rapid bone turnover, serum concentrations of ALP are often elevated, but they should never be increased more than twofold to threefold in healthy, growing animals. Serum alkaline phosphatase and GGT are not reliable indicators of liver disease during the first 2 wk of life because both are present in colostrum and are absorbed through the gut, increasing ALP and GGT levels greatly in the neonate. The lack of an increase in ALP and GGT in a less than 2-week-old puppy can be used as an indicator for not having received colostrum.
- **Kidney:** The neonate is particularly susceptible to dehydration because water makes up 82% of body weight, and water turnover is about twice that of an adult. Because of the neonate's limited ability to conserve fluid and the immaturity of the kidney, fluid requirements are high at 13-22 ml/100 g body weight per day. Nephrons are not completely formed until the third week of life, and glomerular filtration rates increase from 21% at birth to 53% by 8 wk of age. Whereas tubular secretion is generally thought to be mature by 8 wk of age, there are some reports that it takes 6 mo for the tubular function to be complete. Either way, this explains the low urine specific gravity until 8 wk old (1.006-1.017), increased concentrations of amino acids and proteins, and glucosuria, a common finding in neonates up to 2 wk of age. Given the immaturity of renal function, medications that affect kidney development should be avoided, and dosages of those that are excreted through the kidney must be adjusted to the patient's age.
- **Thyroid:** Serum thyroid hormones differ between puppies and kittens and their adult counterparts and also differ significantly with time during the first 12 wk of life. Therefore it is critical to know the exact age of puppies or kittens and not to use the standard reference range for adult normal dogs or cats, respectively. The lack of thyroid hormones in the neonate leads to much more serious disease than in the adult because of the involvement of the thyroid in development. Clinical signs in the affected puppies and kittens may be as mild as apathy and failure to thrive or as severe as joint and bone abnormalities, complete dullness, extremely stunted growth, and, in cats, constipation. Serum thyroid hormones should be determined at the slightest suspicion of hypothyroidism because the earlier treatment is initiated, the better the outcome. Therapy is performed as in adults, but thyroid levels should be checked frequently in young patients, and the results compared with normal values for the corresponding age group.
- **Gastrointestinal system:** The neonate is born with a sterile GI system, which will develop its own flora to aide in digestion during the first few days of life. The GI peristalsis is weaker (slower), there is lower intestinal blood flow, and the gastric fluid has a higher pH. It is clear that medication, changes in the environment, or disease will cause upset to this yet fragile system, which is most commonly apparent in the form of diarrhea. One of the most common causes for diarrhea in the orphaned neonate is overfeeding and inappropriate dilutions of milk replacer.

become anemic. This is especially helpful in neonates that cannot maintain proper blood glucose levels and need to be subjected to multiple blood draws (one drop of blood equals about 0.1 ml). Because of the small amount of sample drawn at a time, the appropriate-size collection tube should be used to ensure that the ethylenediaminetetraacetic acid (EDTA) does not dilute the sample resulting in false laboratory data.

To obtain urine samples, the neonate can simply be stimulated to urinate by gently rubbing the genital area with a moistened cotton ball. Alternatively the bladder can be carefully expressed. It is rarely necessary to obtain sterile urine samples by cystocentesis, which should be avoided because of the fragility of neonates' skin and organs.

Imagining techniques include radiography and ultrasonography. An ultrasound examination is best performed using a 7.5-MHz transducer, and neonates generally tolerate this imaging technique better than radiography. Radiography of neonates requires high-detail intensifying screens and single emulsion films. For optimal contrast, no whole body radiographs should be taken, and the kilovoltage should be reduced to half that of an adult because there is little body fat and poor mineralization at this age. If possible, a normal littermate should be radiographed for comparison.

COMMON CONCERNS AND DISORDERS IN THE PUPPY AND KITTEN (BOX 10-3)

Hypothermia

When puppies and kittens are born, they have almost no subcutaneous fat and thus little insulation. Initially, body heat is produced by brown fat metabolism, which is under the control of the sympathetic nervous system (nonshivering thermogenesis). Because of their relatively large surface area when compared with older animals, heat loss is much greater in neonates. As long as neonates are close to their dams and the mammary glands, there is not much heat loss, so they can maintain thermal balance. However, as the neonate begins to take up food, its metabolic rate increases, which in turn elevates its body temperature. Shivering and vasoconstrictive mechanisms may begin around 6 to 8 days, but by about 6 weeks, puppies and kittens are good homeotherms and have a body temperature that is similar to that of adults.

Hypothermia in the neonate is a serious problem. Gut motility slows with a decreasing body temperature, ultimately causing an ileus. When hypothermic neonates are tube fed, the milk replacer is either regurgitated and aspirated resulting in pneumonia, or the ingesta may ferment leading to bloat. This causes increased pressure to the thorax, which in turn causes labored breathing. Most neonates in pain or respiratory distress swallow air, which exacerbates a bloated condition. In this way, a downward spiral forms that ultimately results in circulatory collapse and death. Hypothermia also inhibits cellular immune functions, which may lead to an increased susceptibility to infections. A neonate is considered hypothermic if its body temperature drops below 94° F at birth, below 96° F at 1 to 3 days of age, or below 99° F at 1 week of age. Clinical signs in a chilled neonate with a body temperature above 88° F include restlessness, continuous crying, red mucous membranes, and skin that is cool to the touch. However, muscle tone is still good; the respiratory rate is greater than 40 breaths/min and the heart rate greater than 200 bpm. When the body temperatures fall into the range of 78° F to 85° F, the neonate appears lethargic and uncoordinated, but responsive. Moisture is seen around the corners of the lips, the heart rate drops below 50 bpm, and the respiratory rate is between 20 to 25 breaths/min. No abdominal sounds are heard, and metabolism is impaired, resulting in hypoglycemia (see later discussion). Below 70° F, the neonate appears to be dead. If extreme measures of arousal result in a response, treatment may be attempted. Hypoxia also contributes significantly to hypothermia. Therefore the neonate should be provided with proper ventilation or oxygen administration whenever possible.

BOX 10-3 Neonatal Illness That Needs Immediate Attention

- Hypothermia
- Dehydration
- Hypoglycemia
- Neonatal isoerythrolysis
- Malnutrition

The treatment consists of slowly (= 2° F/hr) reheating the patient by providing the appropriate ambient temperature and humidity. Heating pads, heat lamps, warm water gloves, rice bags, and incubators can be used, but it is essential that the temperature be controlled and monitored carefully, especially when using heating lamps or heating pads because the neonate cannot escape if the temperature is too warm. Warm air and oxygen in a human neonatal incubator or veterinary oxygen cage is optimal for rewarming the hypothermic neonate. Warm IV fluids can also be given, but at no more than 2° F above body temperature. Do not give anything orally until the patient has audible gut sounds and is moderately rewarmed. Rapid rewarming will result in heat prostration with increased respiratory rate and effort. Eventually the patient will become cyanotic and have diarrhea and seizures. Raising the neonatal body temperature more than 4° F is usually fatal because of delayed organ failure. Thermal burns may also occur if the surrounding temperature is not properly monitored.

> *TECHNICIAN NOTE* Hypothermia in the neonate is a serious problem. Gut motility slows with a decreasing body temperature, ultimately causing ileus. When hypothermic neonates are tube fed, the milk replacer is either regurgitated and aspirated resulting in pneumonia, or the ingesta ferments leading to bloat.

Dehydration

Any disease process or imbalance of fluids or electrolytes will quickly lead to dehydration in the neonate because of increased body water, increased water turnover, and immaturity of the renal system. As indicated before, checking the oral mucous membranes assesses hydration in the neonate because the skin turgor is not yet developed as it is in adults. Moist mucous membranes are present in an adequate state of hydration, but tacky to dry mucous membranes indicate 5% to 7% dehydration. At 10% dehydration, the mucous membranes are dry, and there is a noticeable decrease in skin elasticity.

Fluid requirements are high in neonates, but total volumes that can be given are low. All fluids should be warmed to 98° F to 99° F before administration unless the neonate is substantially colder. In that case, the fluids should be warmed to 2° F more than the current body temperature. Boluses can be given at 3.3 ml per 100 g of the kitten's weight over 5 to 10 minutes. The maintenance dose is 6 ml/kg/hr. To this, 50% of the deficit is added over 6 hours (deficit = body weight [BW] × % dehydrated). Fluids can be given intravenously (IV), intraosseously (IO), intraperitoneally (IP), or subcutaneously (SQ). It is often easiest to place a short 23- or 25-G catheter in the jugular vein for fluid administration. Another option is IO fluid delivery: the bone is still soft enough that an 18- or 19-G needle can be placed in the proximal tibia or proximal femur, and fluids are given at the same rate as IV fluids. It is important that each bone not be punctured more than once because the fluid will leak out of the other hole. Administering fluids at a constant rate is best accomplished by using either a syringe pump or a pediatric drip (60 drops/min). If IV or IO access is not available, fluids are given IP or SQ. However, absorption rates are slow with both routes, and they are not ideal for long-term fluid therapy. When giving fluids IP or SQ, the volume should be divided in 2 to 3 boluses per day. In many cases, the neonate is acidotic, but because of limited liver functions, the neonate has difficulty in metabolizing lactate into bicarbonate. In most cases, lactated Ringer's with 20 mmol/L of maintenance potassium is sufficient.

Hypoglycemia

The risk of hypoglycemia is great because the neonate is born with little glycogen stores and has poor gluconeogenesis in the liver. As long as the neonate is healthy, it can maintain normal blood glucose concentrations for up to 24 hours without nursing. However, the failure to suckle will result in hypoglycemia after 24 to 36 hours as a result of the depletion of hepatic stores. A variety of clinical signs may occur in the hypoglycemic (serum glucose <30 mg/dl) neonatal patient, including tremors, crying, irritability, increased appetite, dullness, lethargy, coma, stupor, and seizures.

The treatment consists of giving dextrose slowly IV or IO at 0.5 to 1 g/kg as part of a 5% to 10% dextrose solution in normal saline. Care should be taken giving 5% dextrose mixed with lactated Ringer's solution because the mixture will become hypertonic and volume replacement will have to be monitored carefully. Higher concentrations of IV dextrose should be avoided because of its irritant nature (phlebitis). Dextrose can be given at higher concentrations directly to the mucous membranes of the mouth if the neonate is not dehydrated or hypothermic (1 to 2 ml of a 5% to 15% dextrose solution). Dextrose solutions should never be given SQ because they may cause tissue damage. After the treatment, blood glucose levels should be monitored because of the risk of hyperglycemia as a result of poor regulatory mechanisms in the neonate.

Neonatal Isoerythrolysis in Kittens

Cats with blood type A have low titers of naturally occurring antibodies against blood type B red blood cells. Therefore blood type B kittens born to blood type A queens do not show any clinical signs of incompatibility reactions after the ingestion of colostrum-containing alloantibodies. However, all blood type B cats have high titers of naturally occurring antibodies against type A red blood cells. This may lead to incompatibility reactions when blood type A kittens receive colostral antibodies from a blood type B queen. Clinical signs are variable and range from jaundice and death within the first 2 days of life to no signs at all (which is rare). Sometimes the tail tip becomes necrotic and falls off at 10 to 14 days of life. Studies at the University of Pennsylvania indicate that kittens at risk for neonatal isoerythrolysis must be removed from their queens only during the first day of life.

The kittens can be tested at birth using handy blood-typing cards (DMS Laboratories, Flemington, N.J.), and if blood type B kittens are born to blood type A queens, they can be fostered to a blood type B queen or hand-raised during the first 24 hours of life. If kittens have neonatal isoerythrolysis during the first day of life, they should be removed from the queen for 24 hours and given supportive care.

Malnutrition

Many milk replacers can easily cover the daily caloric requirements of both puppies and kittens. However, it seems that the fluid requirements are not easily met. Regular feeding is important to maintain good hydration in the neonate. If only three feedings per day can be provided, then use a commercial milk replacer with a formulation that comes closest to the bitch's or queen's milk (Table 10-1) and provide the extra fluids SQ. Overfeeding or a high lactose content in the milk replacer often cause diarrhea. Nothing is better than mother's milk; it also contains bile-salt–activated lipase, which is necessary for proper digestion. After each meal, the neonate should be encouraged to urinate and defecate by stimulating the anogenital region with a moistened cotton ball. Neonates should be weighed daily on a suitable scale until 3 weeks of age to ensure proper weight gain.

Occasionally a neonate will not nurse from a bottle or will not gain the expected weight because of illness or malformations. Tube feeding is necessary in these cases. However, a puppy or kitten should never be tube fed if its body temperature is lower than normal for its age. If the body temperature is too low, the gut shuts down and the ingested material will start to form gas, which in turn will bloat the neonate and lead to serious distress. Tube feeding is performed by first measuring the distance from the tip of the neonate's nose to the end of the chest (Figure 10-3). Using a felt-tip pen or a piece of tape, a mark is made at 75% of this distance on the feeding tube measuring from the distal end of the feeding tube. Insert this length of a clean and dry feeding tube gently into the mouth of the neonate while holding the patient upright. No force is needed because most of the neonates will swallow the feeding tube easily. The syringe with the milk replacer is connected to the tube, and the plunger is pulled back gently. Negative pressure indicates that the feeding

TABLE 10-1 Requirements Overview and Milk Comparison

Age	Puppies kcal/100 g/Day	Kittens kcal/100 g/Day	Fluids for Both in ml/100 g
Week 1	13-15	<38 at birth; 28 thereafter	18 ml average
Week 2	15-20	28	Range 13-22
Week 3	20	27	Same
Week 4	≥20	25	Same

	Bitch's Milk	Queen's Milk	Cow's Milk‡	Goat's Milk‡
Fluid content	77	79	88	87
Fat%	9.5	8.5	3.5	4.1
Protein%	7.5	7.5	3.3	3.6
Lactose%	3.4	4.0	5.0	4.7
Calcium*	0.24	0.18	0.12	0.13
Phosphorus*	0.18	0.16	0.10	0.16
ME† kcal/100 ml milk	146	121	70	69

*g/100 ml
†Metabolizable energy
‡When mixing cow's or goat's milk as a milk replacer for neonates be aware that to cover the fat or protein requirements, the lactose concentrations will be far too high and cause diarrhea. Commercial milk replacers are a better choice.

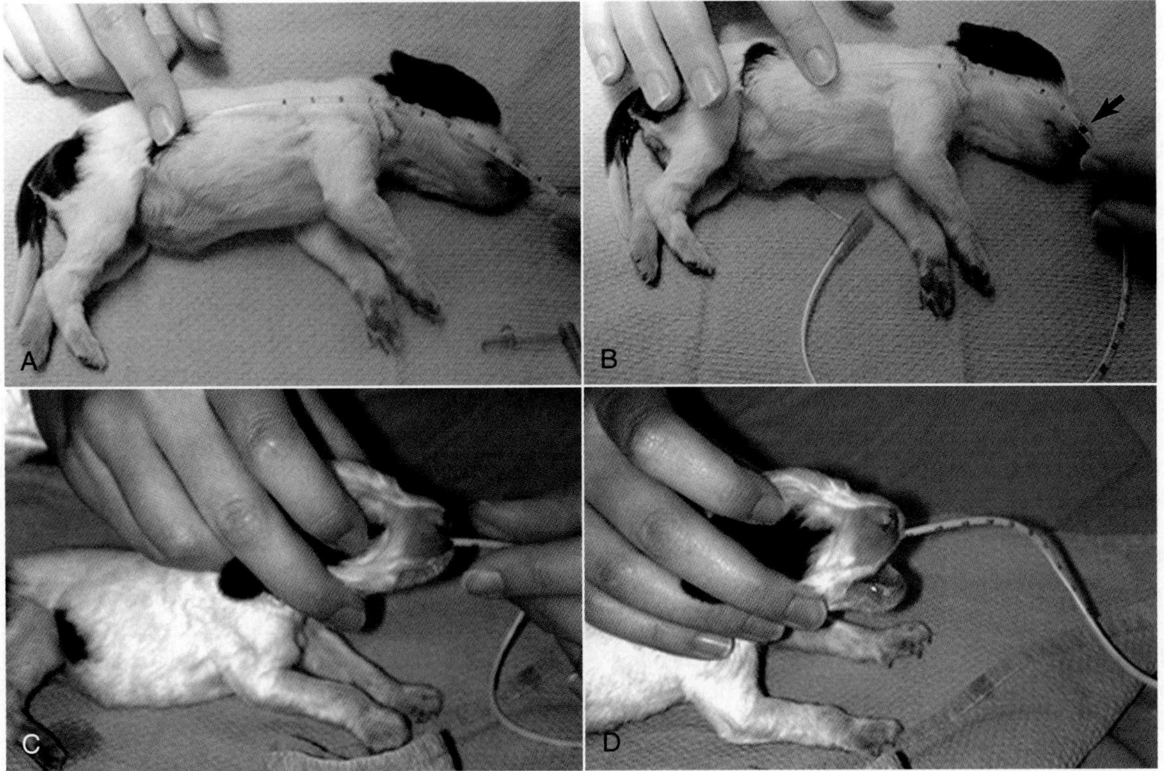

FIGURE 10-3 Tube feeding. **A,** Measure from the tip of the nose to the last rib. **B,** Make a mark at 75% length *(arrow)*. **C,** Insert tube gently to the mark. **D,** Check for negative pressure and give milk slowly.

tube is indeed in the lower esophagus and not in the lungs. When feeding milk replacer alone to puppies or kittens, use a 5-French feeding tube. As a rule of thumb, about 5 ml of milk replacer can be given per feeding to a 160-g puppy or kitten.

The Fading Puppy or Kitten Syndrome

The fading puppy or kitten syndrome is characterized by anorexia, lethargy, emaciation, death, and birth defects in cats and dogs. Kittens or puppies may be stillborn or born small, weak, and unable to nurse, resulting in dehydration,

BOX 10-4 Overview Neonatal Nutrition

- Puppies and kittens should be able to take up their daily requirements in 4-5 meals per day during the first few weeks of life.
- Puppies should gain 1 g for every 2-5 g milk intake.
- Kittens are born at 80-120 g and should gain between 70 and 100 g weekly.
- During the first week of life, kittens will only ingest 10%-15% of their body weight in milk. Thereafter this volume increases to 20%-25% of their body weight in milk (wk 1-4).
- Puppies get their energy from fat during the first weeks of life, whereas kittens get theirs from protein. Therefore milk replacer contents should be carefully reviewed before use.
- Many milk replacers can easily cover the daily caloric requirements of both puppies and kittens. However, it seems that the fluid requirements are not easily met. If only three feedings per day can be provided, then use one of the milk replacers, as outlined earlier, and provide the extra fluids SQ.

TABLE 10-2 Recipes for Homemade Milk Replacers

	Puppies		Kittens
Ingredient	Recipe 1	Recipe 2	Recipe 1
Skim milk	43.8 g	64 g	70 g
Low fat curd	40 g	15 g	15 g
Egg yolks	10 g	15 g	3 g
Vegetable oil	6 g	3 g	3 g
Lactose			0.8 g
Lean ground beef			8 g
Vitamin-mineral mix	0.2 g	2.5 g	0.2 g
Calcium carbonate		0.5 g	

hypothermia, hypoglycemia, and death within the first few days of life. Other neonates appear healthy during the first weeks of life; become weak, depressed. and anorectic; and die of starvation at the time of weaning.

Causes of neonatal deaths include poor management, malnutrition, inappropriate environmental conditions, congenital and genetic defects, and infections. Management and environmental problems can be easily detected by obtaining a detailed history or inspecting the facility. Problems may include poor hygiene, inappropriate temperature and humidity, overcrowding, frequent introduction of new animals, inappropriate use of medication, or exposure to chemical toxins. Nutritional deficiencies can be caused by inadequate diets for the mothers or the neonates. The treatment involves supportive care for the sickly neonate and removal of the inciting causes. If causes are not immediately apparent, necropsies of the neonates that have died are recommended.

Orphan Care

Fostering neonatal kittens and puppies is time consuming, considering that the neonate is completely helpless and requires almost 24-hour care. It is rewarding, however, once the happy, healthy puppy or kitten is ready for its new home. Materials needed are warm and clean bedding, milk bottles with a variety of different rubber nipples, feeding tubes, syringes, a gram scale, cotton balls, hand sanitizers, fur clippers, and the possibility to isolate the orphan from the other animals. Kittens or puppies need to be hand-raised because of maternal death or abandonment, a lack of milk in the mother, maternal aggression, large litter size, malformations, or trauma. When more than one neonate is taken care of, it is essential that each patient be uniquely identified so that progress can be assessed. Each orphan must be weighed daily, and records should be kept. An ambient temperature and humidity of 84° F to 90° F and 55% to 60%, respectively, should be provided during the first week of life, if possible. During the second week, the ambient temperature can be lowered to 79° F to 84° F and to 73.4° F to 79° F during the third week. Shivering reflexes will set in during the second week of life and will contribute to an increase in body temperature. The neonate must be kept warm and well hydrated at all times, following the principles outlined earlier. Proper nutrition or supplementation (Box 10-4) and clean and dry housing should be provided. After feeding, the orphan must be stimulated to urinate and defecate.

Common pitfalls are overfeeding and underfeeding. Overfeeding milk replacers often results in diarrhea and underfeeding in dehydration and a lack of weight gain. Homemade formulas are often deficient in growth factors, amino acids, and other nutrients essential for growth. Many of the commercial milk replacers are made using cow's milk as a base and are therefore not always complete. The energy density of the formula might be too high, and the fluid requirements will not be fulfilled and vice versa; the energy density is too low, and the stomach capacity is too small for the required amount. Therefore commercial milk replacers should be carefully evaluated, and homemade milk replacers should only be made using proven recipes (Table 10-2). Other problems that may arise are housing sick animals in the same room with orphans; overcrowding; improper hygiene (not washing hands between patients); too many fosters per person; damp blankets; and a cold, drafty environment. Lastly, because of the differences in physiology, medications will not be taken up and metabolized at the same rate as in adults. Care should be taken when choosing medications and administering them. Box 10-5 outlines the main physiologic differences between neonates and adults.

NEONATOLOGY OF FOALS

Breeding a mare and delivering a foal is an exciting time for many horse owners. Some clients will breed a mare they have owned for years and want to raise the foal for riding. Other owners will breed the mare to obtain a foal intended for racing. The desired outcome is the same in both instances: deliver a healthy foal and recognize when problems arise in the neonatal period. This section will focus on two critical

BOX 10-5 Considerations When Using Medication in the Pediatric Patient

- Total body water higher (up to 82% of body weight)
- Less fat
- Less muscle mass
- Muscle not well vascularized
- Plasma protein lower
- Gastric pH higher
- GI peristalsis weaker (slower)
- Lower intestinal blood flow
- Better intestinal absorption of proteins
- Not fully developed intestinal flora
- Blood-brain barrier not fully developed
- Liver: some enzymes need up to 4 mo to develop
- Kidney: glomerular filtration developed by 3-4 wk
- Kidney: tubular secretion developed by one-half yr
- Energy (cal) obtained through digestion of fat
- Sixty-five percent of fat is digested in stomach
- No lipase in milk—lower weight gain
- Milk curdles in stomach = normal!

High energy requirements—never fast a puppy or kitten.

areas: the perinatal period, as the late-term pregnant mare is preparing to deliver a foal, and the neonatal period, when the foal is prone to certain diseases. A foal's normal development will be discussed followed by a foal's potential diseases and referral for intensive care at a veterinary hospital. Sick foals referred to a veterinary hospital require a team approach, and the important role of the veterinary technician will be highlighted.

THE PERINATAL PERIOD AND THE HIGH-RISK MARE

Many mares have routine pregnancies and deliver healthy foals. However, sometimes the mare will develop a problem in late-term pregnancy and require treatment. These mares are referred to as "high-risk mares" and often exhibit early warning signs, indicating a problem with the pregnancy.

The average gestation's length in a mare is 340 days, but a normal gestation's length can range from 320 days to 400 days. When mares have multiple pregnancies, they often deliver around the same time each pregnancy, so this is an important part of the history to obtain. When a mare is bred, she will be evaluated at regular intervals by a veterinarian early in the pregnancy. The veterinarian will perform a rectal exam and transrectal ultrasound around 15 days, 30 days, and then 90 days. These examinations will ensure that the mare is retaining the embryo, check for the presence of twins, and evaluate amniotic and allantoic fluid levels surrounding the embryo. As long as the mare is maintaining the pregnancy and findings are within normal limits, she will be monitored closely for any changes, but will often not be evaluated again until the end of her pregnancy. In late-term pregnancy (7 to 10 months), the mare will be reevaluated by a veterinarian and closely watched for any abnormal signs. During this time, the mare should be comfortable, bright, alert, and eating readily. Exercise is important to maintain the mare's physical condition because delivery (parturition) is explosive in horses and the foal should be delivered within 30 minutes of stage 2 labor (water breaking). She should have no vaginal or udder discharge. If a vaginal discharge is present, it may indicate a problem, such as placentitis or urine pooling, and the mare needs to be evaluated. Toward the end of gestation, the mare's udder will slowly enlarge, and before delivery, beads of milk will appear on the end of her teats (waxing of teats). Unless delivery is imminent, the mare should not have milk dripping or streaming from her udder. There are three reasons for this clinical sign: twins, placentitis, or the owner calculated the wrong delivery date, and delivery actually is imminent.

A veterinarian needs to evaluate the mare to determine the cause for dripping milk. The most common reason is that the mare has an ascending placentitis, and subsequent inflammatory changes cause premature lactation. Older mares are especially prone to this problem as a result of poor vulvar conformation as they age. Performing a transrectal ultrasound will allow the veterinarian to evaluate the placental thickness near the cervical star (the area of placenta next to the cervix most often affected by ascending placentitis) and fetal fluid amount and appearance. The veterinarian can also evaluate gross fetal movement and measure the eye orbit to estimate fetal age. A transabdominal ultrasound will also aid in evaluating the foal and placenta and can provide valuable information.

A vaginal examination in a late-term pregnant mare is not recommended unless delivery is imminent because this can actually induce ascending placentitis. If the placenta appears thickened, detached, and/or the fetal fluid is more hyperechoic (more white noted on ultrasound from presence of cellular debris), the mare has placentitis and requires treatment. A typical treatment includes the use of broad-spectrum antimicrobials, such as trimethoprim sulfa, and nonsteroidal antiinflammatory medications, such as flunixin meglumine and progesterone (Regu-Mate is most commonly used in mares). This treatment is designed to kill any bacteria present, decrease the inflammation associated with placentitis, and help maintain the pregnancy until term. Many mares respond to this treatment quickly, and abnormal clinical signs, such as premature udder development and dripping milk, will resolve. If left untreated, most of these mares will deliver premature foals, with a poor chance for survival. If diagnosed and treated early enough, there may be no long-term effects on the foal, but this depends on how long the foal was affected and the extent of damage to the placenta. These mares are classified as "high risk" and need to be monitored closely for foaling. An attended foaling is important to ensure that the foal has the best chance for survival and to treat the foal quickly if any problems are noted. Other reasons for mares to be classified as "high risk" include the presence of twins and a prior history of foaling problems.

High-risk mares may be referred to a foaling facility or veterinary hospital to have an attended foaling and prompt delivery of medical care. Methods to monitor high-risk mares include a video camera placed in the stall to observe the mare's behavior without human interaction and telemetry to monitor the mare's and foal's heart rates. It is important for the mare to feel as comfortable as possible. Mares can begin stage 1 labor (exhibit behavioral changes indicating impending labor), but if they feel threatened, they can stop the labor and resume later. A video camera offers the optimal way to unobtrusively observe the mare's behavior. Telemetry to measure the foal's and mare's heart rates is a noninvasive way to assess fetal and maternal health. In late-term pregnancy, the foal will have a heart rate between 40 to 150 bpm. There will be periods when the foal's heart rate is low (e.g., 40 bpm) because the foal is sleeping and other times when the foal's heart rate is 120 bpm or higher during periods of exercise. The important point to note is that the foal should have a range of heart rates over time, not a sustained low or high heart rate, which can indicate that the foal is stressed in utero. Over the course of gestation, the resting fetal heart rate will gradually decrease and often stay around 40 to 80 bpm during periods of rest. A late-term pregnant mare should have a heart rate around 40 to 50 bpm with higher rates during periods of exercise (e.g., pasture turnout).

It is often difficult to predict exactly when a mare will foal. As parturition (foaling) approaches, the mare's udder will slowly enlarge and fill with milk, her vulva will lengthen, and pelvic ligaments will relax. Many mares will develop "wax" (drops of dried milk) on the tip of their teats. Often mares foal at night, when the stable is more quiet, but some mares will readily deliver a foal in the afternoon surrounded by noise. Knowing when a multiparous mare has foaled in the past is helpful, and they will often foal around the same date again. Also knowing her prior behavior changes will provide clues to when she might foal. A maiden mare (primiparous: mare has not foaled in the past) can be more challenging, but checking her vulvar relaxation, udder development, and the presence of wax on her teats will aid in predicting delivery. There are commercial kits available that measure the rise in calcium in the mare's first milk (colostrum) and accurately predict foaling in some normal mares. The rapid rise in colostral calcium represents one of the most consistent and significant changes before parturition. Calcium levels in colostrum samples can be rapidly measured in nearly every diagnostic laboratory or even just by the use of simple hard-water test kits. Colostral calcium levels above 10 to 12 mmol/dl are considered significant enough to predict parturition within the ensuing 24 hours. However, parturition in high-risk mares is often not reliably predicted by these kits. Despite the different methods available, the best choice for determining when a mare will foal is to have a well-trained staff monitor the mare's behavior 24 hours a day (especially by video camera in the stall) and note any changes. A docile mare may become cranky; an aggressive mare may become docile. Some mares drip milk from their udders just before foaling. Many mares show obvious stage 1 behavior changes: agitation, pacing, nickering, lifting the tail head (as a result of oxytocin release), turning and biting at her sides, and kicking her abdomen. If sweating around her shoulders is observed, the mare will foal within 30 minutes. As a veterinary technician at an assisted delivery, this time is crucial. It is best to notify the veterinarian, stay near the mare, ensure that all necessary equipment is present, and wrap the mare's tail with brown gauze to keep it clean and out of the way. Box 10-6 lists the equipment needed when attending a high-risk foaling.

BOX 10-6 Necessary Equipment for a High-Risk Attended Foaling

- Towels
- Stainless steel bucket
- Warm water
- Chains
- J-Lube (lubricant to aid in foal's delivery)
- One percent iodine solution to dip foal's umbilicus
- ECG machine to check foal's heart rate and rhythm
- Capnograph to measure foal's CO_2 level
- Endotracheal tubes (7, 8, and 9 mm) and 10-ml air syringe
- Ambu bag
- Oxygen supply
- IV catheter, prepared sterile scrub, sterile gloves, and suture
- IV fluids (5% dextrose in water [D_5W], Normosol R or Plasma-Lyte)
- Blood gas syringe (heparinized 3-ml syringe)
- Blood tubes, syringes, and needles
- Glucometer

Stage 2 in mares is explosive and starts when the mare's placenta ruptures and allantoic fluid escapes (water breaking). This is the actual labor, and the foal should be delivered within 30 minutes, but many foals are delivered within 10 to 15 minutes. If the foal is not delivered within 30 minutes, the foal will experience hypoxemia (low oxygen blood levels) and may have neurologic deficits or die. Therefore it is an emergency, and if the foal is unable to be delivered vaginally, a cesarean section is needed. If the foal's nose is protruding from the vulva, an endotracheal tube can be placed in the foal's trachea and breaths delivered via an Ambu bag. This will maintain the foal's oxygen needs and permit more time to prepare for a cesarean section. Stage 3 is when the mare passes her placenta. This can be painful, and many mares lay down to expel the placenta. The placenta should be collected, weighed, and evaluated to ensure that it is completely intact. If a piece is missing (often the tip of the placenta), the mare needs to be treated for a retained placenta. When the foal is delivered, the mare should show immediate interest in the foal by nickering and cleaning him. Before she stands, it is best to strip the umbilical cord of blood and gently break it near the foal's body, leaving a 2- to 3-inch remnant.

The mare will be thirsty and needs fresh, clean water. Additional bedding should be added to the stall because it will be slippery from fetal fluids. Many mares show mild discomfort (looking at her sides, kicking her abdomen), and a dose of a nonsteroidal antiinflammatory drug (NSAID), such as

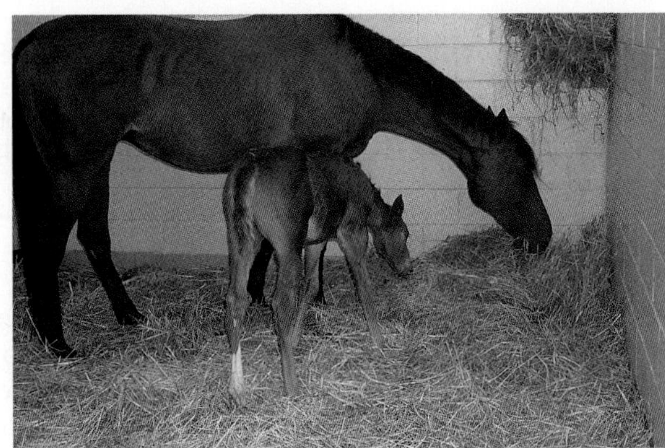

FIGURE 10-4 Mare and foal bonding in the stall.

flunixin meglumine, will often provide analgesia. Mares are often protective of newborn foals, so intervention should be minimized, and they should be left alone as much as possible to permit bonding (Figure 10-4). However, in the postpartum period, if the mare is not interested in the foal or appears to be in pain (e.g., rolling in the stall), intervention is necessary. Occasionally, mares will develop complications postpartum that require immediate treatment or else the foal may be rejected by the mare. Examples of complications include: mild colic, large colon volvulus, uterine artery hemorrhage, a retained placenta, and peritonitis. Depending on the problem, the foal may be able to stay with the mare or may need to be removed and either raised as an orphan (called a bucket baby) or "grafted" onto a nurse mare.

> *TECHNICIAN NOTE* High-risk mares should have an attended foaling at a veterinary hospital to ensure optimal survival of the mare and foal. Foaling equipment should be assembled and close to the mare's stall for easy access. Once stage 2 has started, a mare will normally deliver a foal within 30 minutes.

THE NEONATAL PERIOD: THE NORMAL FOAL

When a foal is born, many changes occur within the first 24 hours of life. In the wild, a foal must be able to stand, nurse, and run from predators within a short period of time or survival will be in jeopardy. Domesticated equine patients are similar, and a neonatal foal will develop rapidly. If not, the foal is often ill and requires treatment. Initial milestones for a foal after parturition include a suckle reflex shortly after birth (curling tongue and seeking to nurse), standing within 1 to 2 hours, and nursing successfully within 6 hours (often by 2 to 3 hours old). The first urination normally occurs around 12 hours. Foals pass meconium (black, sticky fecal material) within a few hours after birth, but some foals have difficulty and become uncomfortable, so they may require a warm-water, soapy enema. A typical enema for a 50-kg foal is 500 ml of warm water mixed with a small amount of Ivory soap. Within 24 hours of birth, the foal should be strong, alert, and capable of running. A nursing neonatal foal will urinate frequently. Urine will be dilute (specific gravity 1.001 to 1.006) because mare's milk is mostly water. Fecal material will be soft and yellow, and foals will defecate one to two times per day.

Observing the foal's behavior for a few minutes without human interaction is important to assess the foal's attitude and energy level. On a physical exam, a neonatal foal should be bright, alert, and responsive. A normal temperature, pulse, and respiration (TPR) at birth will be T = 99° F to 100° F (rectal temperature), P = 60 to 80 bpm, R = 10 to 20 breaths/min. The foal's heart rate will gradually increase to 120 bpm, and respiratory rate will gradually increase to 40 to 60 breaths/min. Mucous membranes will be pink and moist with a capillary refill time (CRT) less than 2 seconds. Eyes should be open and bright with no redness or discharge. Foals are born without a menace response, and it often takes a few weeks for a menace response to develop. The heartbeat should be strong and regular with a synchronous pulse. A quiet systolic murmur may be present (often a flow murmur), but will disappear over time. The respiratory rate and effort should be frequent and steady. Thoracic auscultation may initially sound moist, but will resolve over time. The foal's abdomen should not be swollen and the umbilical remnant clean and dry. The foal's legs will initially be weak, but after 24 hours, the foal should be able to stand readily and run quickly. There should be no joint swelling on palpation. A foal will quickly bond to his mother and follow at her flank. Neonatal foals will sleep about 10 to 20 minutes, then stand and nurse for 5 minutes, play, and sleep again. Normal nursing behavior includes the foal facing the mare's tail, bumping the udder to encourage milk let-down, then nursing for about 5 minutes. The foal should readily use both teats. Palpating the mare's udder after observing the foal nurse is important to ensure that the foal is nursing successfully from both sides of the udder. A healthy foal will nurse from both teats, and the mare's udder will contain minimal milk. A sick foal may appear to nurse, but when the udder is palpated, it is found to be engorged and painful to the touch. Healthy foals will gain an average of 2 to 4 lb a day (1 to 2 kg) and grow rapidly.

The neurologic system of a newborn foal is quite different from that of an adult horse. When the foal is standing for the first time, a basewide stance and exaggerated steps when ambulating are considered normal. An increased response to visual, auditory, and tactile stimuli and jerky movements are also normal. When the normal standing foal is restrained, it will initially struggle and fall limp, as if sleeping, into the arms of the handler. Loosening the restraint will cause the foal to support its weight again. This specific behavior must be kept in mind by people who are restraining standing foals for procedures, such as during the placement of an IV catheter.

Routine Neonatal Therapy

Routine care for all foals includes applying 1% iodine to the foal's umbilical remnant at birth and then three to four times daily for 2 days, monitoring the foal's attitude, appetite, urination, and fecal production. Foals from mares not vaccinated with tetanus toxoid in the last 4 to 6 weeks of gestation should receive 1500 international units (IU) of tetanus antitoxin intramuscularly. On some farms, an enema is routinely administered after birth.

It is important to measure the foal's antibody levels (IgG) approximately 12 hours after delivery. Foals are born without antibodies and need to drink colostrum within 12 to 24 hours after birth to gain antibodies. Colostrum contains antibodies from the mare, other proteins, growth factors, and opsonins to protect from bacterial infection. High-quality colostrum has a specific gravity of 1.080 or higher, and a sample taken shortly after parturition can be measured using a Colostrometer. Within the first 12 to 24 hours of life, the foal's gastrointestinal (GI) tract is able to absorb antibodies from colostrum. After 24 hours, the foal can no longer absorb the mare's antibodies. The IgG level should be greater than 800 mg/dl after 12 hours of age. The failure of passive transfer (FPT) of antibodies occurs when the foal's IgG level is less than 800 mg/dl after 24 hours old. Reasons include poor quality colostrum from the mare, a lack of colostrum as a result of milk dripping before parturition, the foal is too weak or has limb deformities, such as carpal contracture, which prevents the foal from standing to nurse. The FPT is associated with an increased susceptibility to an infection or sepsis, and these foals must be monitored carefully (e.g., daily weight and TPR recorded) to identify problems quickly.

Several tests are available to measure IgG levels, each with advantages and disadvantages. The radial immunodiffusion test is accurate but expensive with limited availability for routine screening. The commercial IgG screening kit with an enzyme-linked immunosorbent assay (ELISA), such as SNAP ELISA, (produced by Idexx Inc., Portland, Me.) is the most commonly used test because it is quick, accurate, easily performed, and readily available. Of the many rapid test methods including zinc sulfate turbidity, latex agglutination, glutaraldehyde coagulation test, and SNAP ELISA, only the SNAP ELISA has sensitivity (and specificity) in the 800-mg/dl range.

The FPT before 24 hours is treated by giving the foal high-quality colostrum from another mare via nasogastric intubation. After 24 hours, it is treated with IV administration of plasma from an appropriate donor. Commercial plasma is available (e.g., HiGamm by Lake Immunogenics, N.Y.), and although expensive, it is the safest and most reliable product. This plasma is harvested from hyperimmunized donors and has been shown to have IgG levels that far exceed normal plasma and is tested for antiequine antibodies. If fresh plasma is given from an on-site donor, a crossmatch should be performed to lessen the risk of a significant transfusion reaction. Plasma is administered via a sterile IV catheter. It is paramount to use a blood-administration IV line with a filter to strain out any large particles from the plasma. As a general rule, 1 L of commercial plasma raises the IgG level of a 45-kg foal by 200 mg/dl.

> *TECHNICIAN NOTE* A neonatal foal needs to be monitored closely for appropriate development milestones. An IgG level should be measured by 12 hours of age to ensure that the passive transfer of maternal antibodies has occurred.

Laboratory Evaluation

The laboratory parameters (hematology and serum chemistry values) of neonatal foals are distinctly different from those of adult horses. Coagulation values are initially different from adult horses. There are published references from the University of Florida, College of Veterinary Medicine, but because of variations in technique and equipment between different laboratories, reference ranges for values need to be established individually at each facility examining samples from veterinary patients. As foals age, many of their blood values will reach typical adult levels, so by 1 month, many parameters are similar to adult horse levels.

When evaluating a complete blood cell count (CBC), the packed cell volume of the normal foal during the first 24 hours of life (e.g., >40%) is greater than that of an adult horse. Subsequently a fall into the low normal range of an adult can be observed over the ensuing 2 weeks to 1 year. Band neutrophils are not normal in the healthy foal. Values of more than 100 to 150 band cells/dl are considered abnormal and usually indicate an acute infection, such as sepsis. Measuring plasma fibrinogen concentration can be helpful to evaluate the presence of active inflammation. Fibrinogen is an acute phase protein, produced by the liver in response to active inflammation. Fibrinogen levels vary between labs, but in general, will not exceed 420 mg/dl in foals up to 1 week of age. At birth, before the foal has nursed from the mare and has not absorbed immunoglobulins (IgG) from the mare's colostrum, the plasma protein concentration of an equine neonate is considerably lower than that of an adult horse (e.g., between 4 to 4.5 mg/dl). After a successful passive transfer of immunoglobulins from the mare's colostrum, the foal's total protein will increase to approximately 5.6 mg/dl, which is below the normal range for an adult horse.

The activities of various serum enzymes are distinctly different in foals than in adult horses. Alkaline phosphatase, gamma glutamyl transferase, sorbitol dehydrogenase, alanine transaminase, and glucose levels should be consistently higher in foals than in adults. An increase in alkaline phosphatase has been attributed to increased metabolic activities in bone, intestine, and liver. Increased gamma glutamyl transferase and sorbitol dehydrogenase activities are attributed to a greater activity in the liver in foals and may be associated with the greater mass of the liver in relation to total body mass. Changes in alanine transaminase levels are of questionable clinical significance because this enzyme has not been shown to be specific for a particular organ system in the horse. The serum glucose concentration in normal foals ranges from 60 to 120 mg/dl. A decrease in serum glucose concentration below the normal reference range is a concern and is indicative of an insufficient caloric uptake of the foal or metabolic derangements in the critically ill foal. In normal foals, the serum levels of creatinine and blood urea nitrogen are often above reference values for adults for the first 36 to 72 hours of life, but will gradually decrease to adult values.

THE NEONATAL PERIOD: THE SICK FOAL

Foals are born with minimal energy reserves, such as stored fat, and can quickly deteriorate with an infection. They also need to drink good-quality colostrum from the mare within 24 hours of delivery. If there is an FPT of maternal antibodies, foals are prone to infection. There are three main sites of entry for bacteria and viruses: GI tract, respiratory tract, and umbilicus. The foal is born with sterile GI and respiratory tracts. During the first week of life, foals will eat their mother's manure to colonize their GI tracts with proper bacteria. Since horses live in a dirty environment, foals are exposed to many pathogens. If foals are compromised for any reason, they are more likely to develop bacteremia (bacterial infection in the bloodstream) and sepsis.

Some foals develop infections as a result of their contaminated environment. Other foals are predisposed to developing infection from abnormal conditions in utero. Risk factors for compromised foals include prematurity, twin foals, a history of placentitis, the mare is sick and not producing much milk, or the foal is exhibiting abnormal behavior after delivery, such as weakness and inability to nurse, resulting in the FPT. Premature foals are born before they reach 320 days of gestational age. Signs of prematurity include low birth weight, weakness, silky hair coat, floppy ears, domed forehead, flexor tendon laxity, and angular limb deformities (e.g., incomplete ossification of cuboidal bones in the carpus and tarsus on radiographs). This incomplete ossification can result in crushing injuries of cuboidal bones from simple weight bearing, so these foals require extensive care for weeks and restrictive standing until the bones are completely ossified. The term dysmaturity usually refers to a large foal (e.g., >65 kg) with a longer than expected gestation (e.g., 400 days). The foal's hair coat will be coarse and long, and the incisor teeth will be erupted through the mucous membranes. The foal may be weak, unable to nurse correctly, and have angular limb deformities. Both of these types of foals are often products of their mare's abnormal placenta and have an increased susceptibility to disease and injury, requiring veterinary care.

Some foals have minor problems, such as orthopedic problems or an inguinal hernia, and require mild to moderate diagnostics and intervention. However, the classic early clinical signs of disease in critically ill foals are lethargy, depression, decreased suckle reflex, decreased nursing, and increased periods of recumbency and sleeping. Unfortunately, foals can quickly become critically ill and rapidly deteriorate, so they need to be monitored closely, especially in the first week of life. If a foal is developing any of these signs on the farm, the veterinarian needs to evaluate the foal and determine if a referral is needed for additional care. It is difficult to manage sick neonatal foals on the farm. They often require 24-hour care and extensive monitoring for optimal recovery. Sometimes, even despite the best care, critically ill foals do not survive. Since intensive care is expensive, the owner needs to decide about treatment options with the veterinarian's guidance and long-term goals for the foal.

Admitting the Critically Ill Foal

A neonatal team including a veterinarian, a veterinary technician, and assistants are vital to the initial evaluation and treatment of the critically ill foal. Many foals may require supportive care and recover quickly, but some will not survive without intensive management. A skilled veterinary technician plays an important role in treating these cases and recognizing when complications develop. There are numerous foal neonatal intensive care units (NICUs) providing quality care to these foals, and spending time in an NICU to gain experience is invaluable.

When a foal is admitted, triage by the veterinarian and veterinary technician is important to determine the initial diagnostic evaluation and treatment. A foal able to walk into the NICU will receive less intensive care than a hypothermic, recumbent foal. Initial triage includes obtaining a foal's history, weight, and a quick assessment of attitude, condition, TPR, and cardiovascular system (heart rate, rhythm, pulse, and limb temperature, which indicate perfusion). Ambulatory foals should be gently restrained during the examination to minimize stress and are usually stabled with their dams to permit normal nursing.

A comatose, recumbent foal should be evaluated rapidly and a treatment initiated, so many NICUs have standard protocols. Box 10-7 lists common diseases of neonatal foals. The foal is placed on a padded surface and eyes protected from trauma. At least three persons are needed to restrain the foal: one person holding the head, the second holding the front legs, and the third holding the hind legs. The foal's attitude is assessed, and a lack of response to stimuli indicates poor brain perfusion. Mucous membranes are often dark purple with prominent vessels (injected mucous membranes). Icterus (yellow color of mucous membranes and sclerae) is commonly noted in foals with sepsis. Petechiae may be noted (small areas of hemorrhage) on oral mucous membranes or on the foal's pinna (outer ear). The eyes may be sunken and entropion present (lower eyelids rolled inward) as a result of hypovolemia. The pupil size should be noted and eyes stained with fluorescein to check for corneal ulceration. Miotic (constricted) pupils often indicate sepsis. The foal may have tachycardia (e.g., >150 bpm) or bradycardia (e.g., <70 bpm), and the pulse may be bounding or difficult to palpate. The respiration may be fast (>60 breaths per minute) or slow (<20 breaths/min). Ribs should be carefully palpated, especially over the heart, to detect the presence of rib fractures. Auscultation of the GI tract may reveal audible borborygmi or the absence of GI sounds. The abdomen should be evaluated for distention and the umbilical remnant examined for discharge. Joints should be carefully

BOX 10-7 Common Diseases of Neonatal Foals

- Neonatal encephalopathy: "Dummy foal" or neonatal maladjustment syndrome resulting in abnormal behavior, poor nursing ability, weakness, and associated with other problems, such as sepsis, neonatal gastroenteropathy, and neonatal nephropathy.
- Neonatal gastroenteropathy: Abnormal GI tract motility and absorption leading to intolerance of enteral nutrition, such as reflux noted after feeding.
- Neonatal nephropathy: Renal insufficiency that may resolve or may be too severe for recovery.
- Neonatal isoerythrolysis: Acute, severe anemia caused by destruction of foal's red blood cells.
- Sepsis or septic shock: Acute, severe bacterial infection causing multiorgan dysfunction, including poor perfusion of the limbs, cardiovascular collapse, and metabolic derangements, such as profound hypoglycemia.
- Meconium retention: Meconium is retained in the colon, and the foal will display abdominal discomfort, such as tail flagging and rolling.
- Colitis: Foal develops acute diarrhea, often caused by infectious organism, such as rotavirus, *Salmonella* spp. or *Clostridium* spp. and requires immediate treatment in an isolated stall.
- Patent urachus: Foal's urachus is not closed and leaks urine.
- Ruptured bladder: Foal's urinary bladder or associated structures (e.g., ureters) develop(s) a tear, and urine leaks into the abdomen.
- Septic arthritis or septic physitis: Foal develops an infected joint or infected growth plate.
- Failure of passive transfer: Foal does not receive maternal antibodies from mare's colostrum within 24 hr of age.
- Musculoskeletal abnormalities (e.g., flexural deformities, angular limb deformities): Foal has tendon contracture, valgus, or varus problems causing deviated limbs.
- Prematurity: Foal is born before 320 days gestational age and exhibits typical signs, such as low birth weight, soft hair coat, floppy ears, domed head, and incomplete ossification of cuboidal bones.
- Dysmaturity: Very large foal is born at longer-than-expected gestational age (e.g., 400 days), long hair coat, erupted incisors, and often has limb deformities.
- Entropion: Lower eyelid rolls inward to cornea and causes corneal abrasion or ulceration.

palpated for swelling. Urine should be caught for a dipstick and specific gravity. Fecal matter should be examined, especially if diarrhea is present, for it often requires isolation of the patient. The limb temperature is important to assess. Often these foals will be hypothermic (T <99° F) and have poor perfusion to their limbs. Consequently the foal's legs will be cold, and pulses in the limbs will be difficult to feel. The median artery (on the medial upper forelimb near the elbow) and the great metatarsal artery (on the lateral distal hind limb) are two arteries frequently used to assess pulses and perform blood gas samples. The foal's blood pressure should be assessed.

Initial blood samples include drawing an arterial blood gas from the great metatarsal artery to assess oxygen and carbon dioxide levels. A venous sample can be taken at the time of catheter placement for a CBC, chemistry profile, glucose level, and blood culture. Typical blood work abnormalities of these critically ill foals include IgG less than 800 mg/dl, low white cell count (e.g., <5000 cells/µl), an increased fibrinogen concentration, profound hypoglycemia (<40 mg/dl), increased lactate, a low oxygen concentration, and increased carbon dioxide levels.

The initial treatment often entails administration of intranasal oxygen (oxygen insufflation), sterile placement of an IV catheter in the jugular vein, fluid therapy using crystalloid fluids (e.g., Normosol R), fluids containing dextrose (e.g., D_5W), and broad-spectrum antimicrobials. Placement of a jugular catheter requires aseptic technique. The area over the vein is clipped, and sterile scrub and sterile gloves are used to clean the area for 5 minutes. Masks for the foal handlers are also helpful to prevent contamination of the area. The placement of an IV catheter offers an ideal time to draw the first sample for a blood culture using a sterile syringe and sterile gloves. Whereas many critically ill foals may have sepsis, blood cultures are only positive about 30% of the time. In the past, sepsis was usually due to a gram-negative organism, but in recent years, gram-positive sepsis is on the rise. Antimicrobial therapy should be based on the isolation of infecting organisms and antimicrobial sensitivity testing. Special considerations need to be made regarding the physiologic features of the neonate, such as reduced hepatic activity and renal immaturity. However, antimicrobial therapy must be instituted as soon as sepsis is suspected, without waiting for culture results, which take a few days to finalize. In general, using ceftiofur sodium or a combination of penicillin and an aminoglycoside (e.g., amikacin) provides appropriate coverage. Shock therapy fluids can be administered at 20 ml/kg/hr for short periods, so many critically ill foals (e.g., 50-kg foal) will receive 3 L of fluid within the first 2 hours of admission.

Often after a few liters of IV crystalloid fluids and dextrose administration, the foal's perfusion will improve. The foal will appear more alert, sit up, and seek to nurse. To prevent corneal ulceration, ophthalmic ointment is placed in both eyes and entropion corrected if present. A hypothermic foal should be gradually warmed using blankets or forced-air warming units (Bair Hugger by Augustine Medical, Eden Prairie, Minn.). It is imperative to warm the foal slowly, or an increased metabolic demand will cause cardiovascular collapse. Blood pressure is monitored closely, and decreased blood pressure will be one of the first signs the foal is not responding to treatment. A foal's recumbency is changed every few hours to prevent decubital ulcers and permit expansion of the down lung. Glucose measurements using a Glucometer are frequently performed to ensure that the foal's glucose concentrations are within normal limits. If the foal remains hypoglycemic or hyperglycemic, the foal may have malmetabolism as a result of sepsis and requires close monitoring. Performing frequent urine dipsticks and assessing specific gravity will ensure that the foal is not losing glucose in the urine (glucosuria) and the kidneys are responding appropriately to fluid therapy.

Once the foal's cardiovascular system has stabilized, additional diagnostics can be performed. Thoracic radiographs and/or an ultrasound examination may be needed to assess for pneumonia or the presence of rib fractures. Abdominal ultrasound is often used to better assess the GI tract for meconium retention, evaluate the bladder to ensure that it is intact, and examine the internal remnant of the umbilicus. The external umbilical remnant is outside of the abdomen. It contains remnants of the urachus (which connects to the urinary bladder); two umbilical arteries, which travel caudally and insert in the bladder wall; and one umbilical vein, which courses cranially to the liver. Sick foals often develop a patent urachus and omphalitis (inflammation of the umbilicus). Externally the umbilical remnant will be moist and enlarged, and the foal will strain or dribble small streams when urinating. The examination of the urogenital system also includes palpation of the umbilical, inguinal, and scrotal areas for hernias and distention. If the foal has mild colic, he will often flag his tail when defecating. The foal may also roll onto his back and fold his front legs over his chest to indicate abdominal pain. When the foal's temperature is taken, fecal matter should be detected on the thermometer. If this does not occur and the foal exhibits signs of abdominal discomfort, the possibility of a nonpatent GI system caused by an anatomic abnormality (atresia ani, atresia coli) should be considered.

When additional venous blood samples are required, the cephalic and saphenous veins are ideal for collection, using the smallest needle and syringe possible, using a tuberculin syringe or 22-gauge, 1-inch needle and 3-ml syringe (Figure 10-5). Adequate restraint is paramount to successfully perform venipuncture in recumbent foals and usually requires three persons. Figure 10-5 depicts correct restraint of the recumbent neonatal foal to obtain a blood culture from the saphenous vein. Restraining the foal using bony areas, such as joints, offers the best approach to prevent harming soft tissue areas, such as the foal's abdomen. A foal's veins tend to roll, so clipping the area over the vein is helpful. After applying alcohol to the area, gently insert the needle at a 45 degree angle to obtain a blood sample. If additional arterial blood gas samples are required, the procedure is similar. Three persons are needed to restrain the foal. One person holds the foal's head and ensures that the eyes are protected from abrasion, the second holds the front legs, and the third person holds the hind legs. An area is clipped over the great metatarsal artery and alcohol applied. Arterial samples are painful, so infusing 0.1 to 0.2 ml of lidocaine in the area using a tuberculin syringe and needle is vital to collect the sample. It is important to use a specialized blood gas syringe to collect an arterial sample. Draw back on the plunger to 0.5 ml before taking the sample to ensure that the arterial blood can flow into the syringe. Palpate the arterial pulse and insert the needle gently at a 45 degree angle. Blood should immediately flow into the syringe and appear bright red. If the blood flows slowly and appears dark, it may be a venous sample. However, if the foal is comatose with extremely cold limbs and poor pulses, the sample may indeed be an arterial sample.

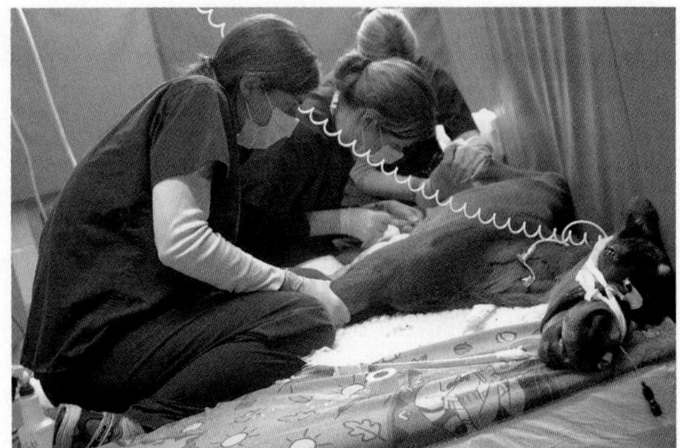

FIGURE 10-5 Correct restraint of the recumbent neonatal foal to obtain a blood culture from the saphenous vein. (Photo by Sabina Louise Pierce, University of Pennsylvania.)

Over the course of hospitalization, a foal may require additional treatment, including maintenance fluids, nutritional support, blood pressure support, treatment for orthopedic conditions, and a ventilator. Maintenance fluid rates can range from 90 to 150 ml/hr for the average 50-kg foal. Each case varies depending on the foal's illness and clinical course. Some foals with mild to moderate illness are only hospitalized for a few days and discharged on medication. Critically ill neonatal foals are often hospitalized for a few weeks, and the treatment is often expensive. Figure 10-6 depicts a typical IV fluid setup for a critically ill foal. The best outcome for a neonatal foal is early detection of disease on the farm and rapid intervention before the foal becomes critically ill.

> *TECHNICIAN NOTE* A critically ill neonatal foal should be evaluated and treated quickly by a veterinary team at a referral hospital for optimal outcome.

Monitoring and Nursing Care

Once the foal has been admitted to the veterinary hospital and initially examined, diligent monitoring is critical. Box 10-8 lists important considerations when monitoring the critically ill foal. The objective of frequent monitoring is to detect subtle changes signifying improvement or deterioration in the foal's condition. Complications during hospitalization include resistant nosocomial (hospital-acquired) infections, additional sites of infection (septic arthritis, osteomyelitis,

BOX 10-8 Monitoring the Critically Ill Foal

- Mentation: Bright and alert or depressed or comatose
- Oral mucous membranes: CRT <2 sec, pink and moist or dark red, injected and icteric, presence of petechiae
- Ocular: Presence of entropion, corneal ulceration, hyphema, miotic pupil, injected sclerae, icteric sclerae
- Jugular veins: Site of catheter placement has any signs of swelling or jugular vein thickening
- Cardiovascular: Pulses strong or weak, heart rate and rhythm consistent or changing to a faster or slower rate, stable blood pressure or consistently low blood pressure values
- Respiratory: Regular rate and effort or changing to a faster or slower rate and deeper or more shallow effort, periods of apnea (>20 sec of breath holding)
- GI tract: Presence or absence of borborygmi, frequency of bowel movements, signs of diarrhea or skin scalding, presence of abdominal distention, signs of colic
- Urinary: External umbilical remnant small and dry or moist and large, presence of abdominal distention, amount of urine produced daily
- Integument: Decubital ulcers, urine and/or fecal scalding, linear dermal necrosis over hocks, generalized edema
- Musculoskeletal: Joint swelling (effusion), acute lameness, joint contracture, incomplete ossification of cuboidal bones, and tendon and ligament laxity
- Thermoregulation: Able to maintain body temperature or consistently abnormal (hypothermic or febrile)
- Metabolic derangements: Foal's glucose levels within normal limits or consistently abnormal

thrombophlebitis, pneumonia), corneal ulcers, and decubital ulcers. The severity of the patient's illness will dictate the required frequency of monitoring. Parameters are recorded on a flow sheet for easy comparison at different time points. As a foal deteriorates, one of the earliest changes noted is decreasing blood pressure. Monitoring blood pressure frequently aids in detecting deterioration in the foal's condition and permits treatment changes before the case spirals downward. Performing regular TPRs will also aid in assessing the foal. A recumbent foal's temperature is often between 99° F and 101.5° F. A hypothermic foal is often unable to maintain a normal body temperature and often has a temperature less than 99° F, despite warming methods. A recumbent foal with a temperature greater than 102° F is febrile and may not be responding to the antimicrobial choice.

The hallmarks of nursing care for the foal are strict attention to asepsis and close observation of minor details. An experienced veterinary technician is invaluable and will often note changes in the foal before the veterinarian. If more than one foal is being treated by the technician, techniques, such as hand washing between patients, should be used to prevent cross contamination. Skin injections should be made only after the area has been cleaned with alcohol and dried. Intramuscular injections are limited to the semimembranosus region and should not be given in the neck, pectorals, or gluteal region. Figure 10-6 depicts a typical setup for continuous IV fluid administration in a critically ill foal. Fluid lines should be changed daily to prevent contamination. Major line changes should be performed every 3 days. If a fluid line is accidentally disconnected, it should be considered contaminated and must be replaced. All IV ports should be capped with injection caps and cleaned with alcohol swabs before a needle is inserted. Multidose vials of injectable drugs and injection caps or ports must be disinfected with an alcohol swab before needle insertion. Needles and syringes are not reused. If IV fluids are not attached continuously, catheters should be flushed with 3 ml of heparinized

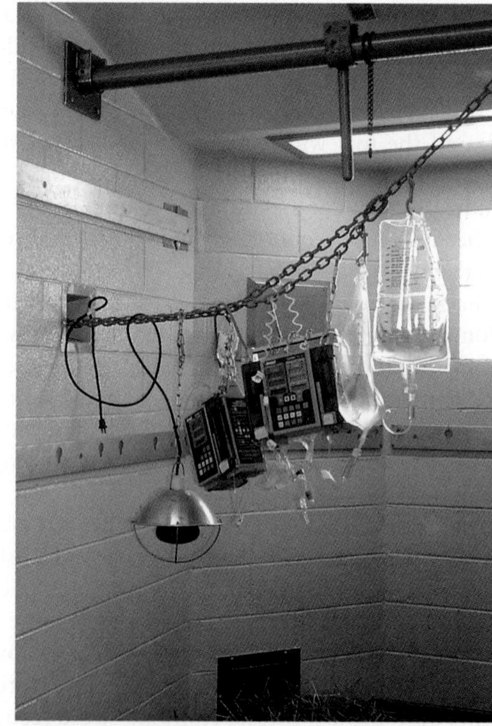

FIGURE 10-6 Typical IV fluid setup for a critically ill foal.

saline solution every 6 hours. It is important to avoid administering too much heparinized saline too frequently, or the foal may become heparinized. If IV fluids are attached continuously, 3 ml of sterile saline without heparin may be used to flush the catheter between medications. The interval for catheter changes depends on the type of catheter material used and the status of the vein. Teflon catheters should be removed and replaced within 72 hours. Silastic or polyurethane catheters are less thrombogenic and may remain in place for several weeks, but the catheter site should be monitored closely for swelling or thickening of the jugular vein. These catheters are expensive, but quickly become cost effective when compared with Teflon because of the extended time they can remain in place and the decreased likelihood of developing thrombophlebitis.

The foal should be kept clean, dry, and warm. Milk should be warmed to a tepid (not hot) temperature before it is fed to the foal. Performing physical therapy (passive range of motion) can be a helpful modality for recumbent foals, especially when one joint (often the fetlock joint) has a mild contracture. Foals should be kept in a sternal position to permit the adequate expansion of the lungs. This position can be attained by the use of pillows at the shoulder or wedge-shaped pads. Figure 10-7 demonstrates the correct positioning of a foal in sternal recumbency using a pillow at the foal's shoulder. The recumbent foal will require frequent turning from side to side every 2 hours to encourage complete ventilation of the lungs and to prevent decubital ulcers. Foals should be encouraged to stand and ambulate, when possible. This effort may range from the handler suspending the foal for a few minutes to the foal standing on his own once assisted.

Restraint should be safe for the foal, mare, and handlers. Ambulatory foals are usually restrained with one hand under the neck and the other surrounding the rump. It is not recommended to restrain a foal by his tail because the handler may inadvertently break the foal's tail. Bracing the foal against a wall provides more security and better control during a struggle. To lead a foal behind the mare, one person should walk the mare with a chain over her nose. The second person places a long cotton lead around the foal's chest and places the remaining rope around the rump. Holding the rope at the foal's withers, the person walks on the left side of the foal.

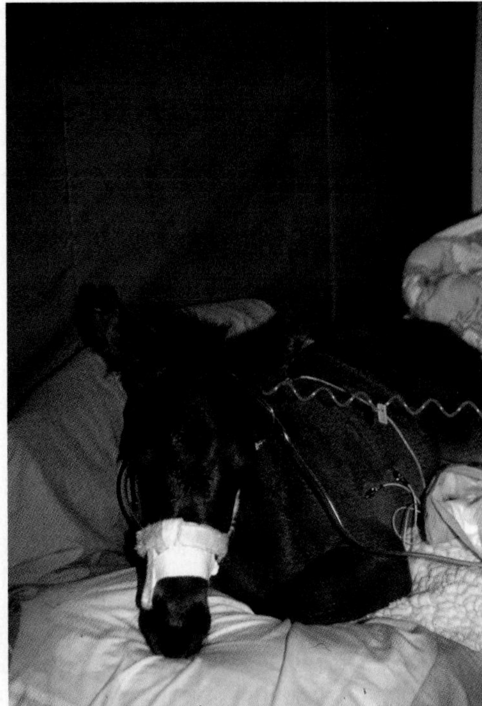

FIGURE 10-7 Correct sternal recumbency of a foal with a pillow placed at the foal's shoulder.

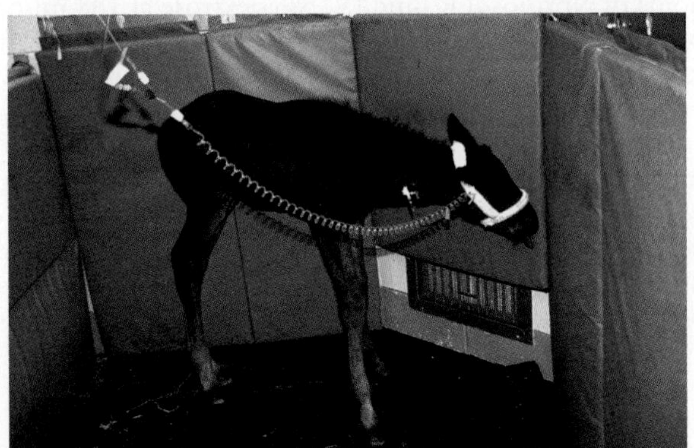

FIGURE 10-8 A foal with neonatal encephalopathy incorrectly seeking to nurse on a wall.

> *TECHNICIAN NOTE* A critically ill neonatal foal should be monitored closely for any changes in condition and treated appropriately. Blood pressure monitoring is vital to assess the foal's stability. A foal with decreasing blood pressure requires immediate attention.

NUTRITION OF THE NEONATAL FOAL

The healthy foal will nurse readily from the mare and receive adequate nutrition. Ideally a hospitalized foal is able to nurse from the mare to receive adequate nutrition. Some foals are unable to nurse because of different problems (e.g., neonatal encephalopathy, abnormal esophageal motility leading to aspiration pneumonia, and cleft palate). Figure 10-8 demonstrates a foal with neonatal encephalopathy incorrectly seeking to nurse on a wall. An indwelling nasogastric tube can be placed and taped to the foal's halter to permit feeding every 2 hours. It is an acquired skill to place these slender tubes because they can be difficult to palpate in the esophagus. These tubes can remain in place for weeks (or until the foal rubs it out and requires a new one). It is imperative to check a hospitalized foal's tongue daily. When foals are unable or reluctant to swallow and treated with antimicrobials, they are prone to develop oral candidiases. This yeast infection will coat the tongue with a white plaque and requires daily treatment (debulking the plaque with a dry 4 × 4 gauze, applying potassium permanganate topically and/or oral fluconazole).

To ensure that adequate nutrition is offered, the foal should be weighed daily. Foals with mild disease will usually gain 1 to 2 lb/day (0.5 to 1 kg). Alternate options for feeding foals are bottle feeding, bucket feeding, or bonding the foal to a nurse mare. Bottle feeding foals is labor intensive and must be done properly, or the foal may develop aspiration pneumonia. This method is often used when a foal is not able to nurse from his mare temporarily. Orphan foals are raised by giving milk in a bucket. Although this method is fine initially for many foals, often behavioral problems will develop, so these foals need to be handled properly to prevent problems.

CASE PRESENTATION 10-1 PREMATURE FOAL

A 20-year-old thoroughbred mare delivered a foal at day 318 of gestation, earlier than the owner expected. She exhibited stage 1 signs of labor, which included restlessness and pacing for a few hours. She advanced to stage 2 and delivered a foal within 10 minutes. The mare's placenta was delivered completely, but it seemed thick and heavier than normal (13 lb). The filly was small (85 lb, 39 kg) with a domed head, silky hair coat, and floppy ears (Figure 1). The foal had difficulty standing and was not able to nurse, so the owner shipped the mare and foal to an equine referral veterinary hospital. On the physical examination, the mare appeared healthy with no problems noted and did not require treatment. On the physical examination, the 15-hour-old foal was depressed and recumbent. She was tachycardic (HR = 140 bpm) and tachypneic (60 breaths/min) with mildly cool limbs and bounding pulses. As a result of her history and presentation, the foal was diagnosed as premature, and an ascending placentitis in the mare was considered a likely cause.

An IV catheter was placed in the foal's right jugular vein and blood samples taken for a CBC, chemistry profile, IgG, and blood culture. An arterial blood gas was also taken from the left great metatarsal artery. Blood work abnormalities included a low IgG (400 mg/dl), hypoglycemia (20 mg/dl), and hypoxemia (PaO_2 = 65 mm Hg). The initial treatment included intranasal oxygen insufflation at 3 L/min, a 2-L bolus of Normosol R fluid IV, 5% dextrose at 188 ml/hr to provide dextrose, antimicrobial medication (400 mg ceftiofur sodium IV q 6 hours), and 1 L of HiGamm plasma IV to provide antibodies because the foal was unable to nurse.

The foal became bright and alert a few hours after treatment and attempted to stand. Because she was premature, radiographs were taken to assess the ossification of her cuboidal bones (carpi and hocks). Her cuboidal bones were not completely ossified, so she was only permitted to stand briefly when changing position. During the first 48 hours of hospitalization, the foal responded quickly to treatment. Repeat blood work demonstrated resolution of the initial abnormalities, and no bacteria grew on the blood culture. The foal tolerated a few feedings of her mare's colostrum via nasogastric intubation with no reflux. The foal developed a normal suckle and was fed a few ounces of her mare's milk every 2 hours by bottle. She tolerated the feedings well with no sign of discomfort, so the amount was gradually increased.

Over the next week, the filly gradually became stronger, and IV fluids and oxygen therapy were discontinued. Her antimicrobial medication was changed to oral trimethoprim sulfa. The filly was allowed to stand for 10 to 20 minutes at a time, and repeat radiographs showed increased ossification of her cuboidal bones. By 4 weeks after her delivery, the foal was healthy, required no medication, and had normal ossification of her cuboidal bones (Figure 2). Her grateful owners took her home, and the filly and mare were placed in a small paddock every day, slowly increasing the turnout time over 2 weeks. The filly and mare had no subsequent problems.

The owners were instructed to send the mare to a hospital for an attended foaling in the future because the mare's age predisposes her to placentitis.

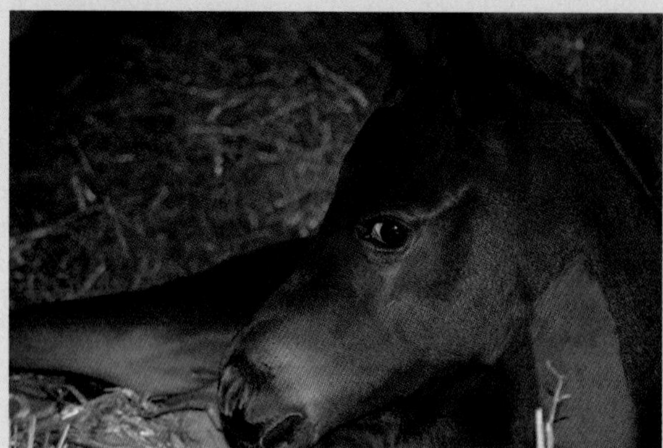

FIGURE 1 Premature foal with domed head and silky hair coat.

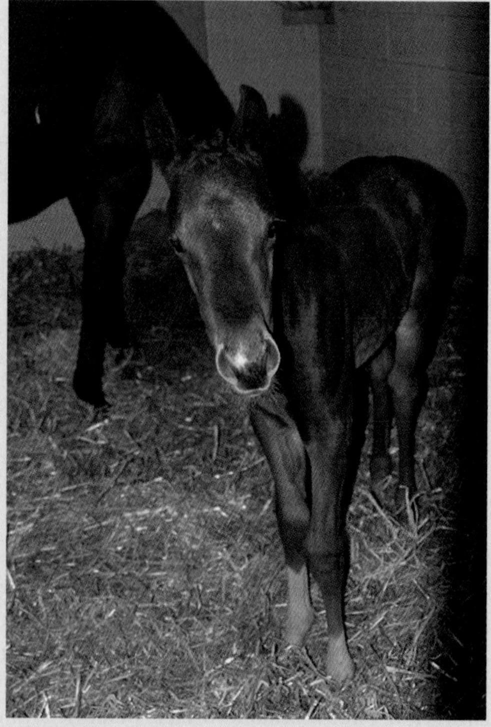

FIGURE 2 Healthy foal after treatment for prematurity.

The accepted energy requirement of the compromised equine neonate is 130 to 150 kcal/kg/day. To meet this requirement, a foal will consume approximately 20% of its body weight per day. Often critically ill foals lack a normal suckle reflex and have an abnormal GI tract. These foals will not tolerate large amounts orally, so feeding should start at 60 ml every 2 hours via a nasogastric tube. If the foal tolerates these feedings, the volume of milk may be gradually increased to 5% to 10% of its body weight, divided into 12 feedings every 2 hours. If the foal does not have reflux when passing a nasogastric tube, an indwelling nasogastric tube can be placed to feed the foal. The tube placement must be checked before each feeding to ensure proper positioning. If the tube has moved, aspiration pneumonia may result. The recumbent foal is placed in sternal recumbency, fed, and kept sternally for 20 minutes after feeding to prevent aspiration of milk.

Many critically ill foals will not initially tolerate enteral nutrition, so feeding should be discontinued if regurgitation, abdominal distention, colic, or severe diarrhea occurs. Additional calories are administered IV (parenteral nutrition) to offer a sufficient energy intake for the critically ill foal. There are two sources for parenteral nutrition, either commercial products or recipes using glucose, amino acids, lipids, trace minerals, and vitamins prepared for each foal. Since parenteral nutrition contains lipids and glucose, it is an optimal medium for bacterial growth. The IV bag and line must remain sterile at all times and IV line changes done every 3 days to eliminate problems with contamination.

Fresh mare's milk is the ideal source of oral nutrition for foals and is easily digestible. When available, mare's milk should be used to feed healthy and critically ill neonatal foals. If the foal's mare is in the hospital, she can be milked every 2 hours (with or without giving oxytocin before milking) to obtain milk for the foal. The mare's udder and the caretaker's hands should always be cleaned before milking to prevent mastitis. Proper restraint of the mare is important during milking. Lubricating the hand or udder with sterile lubricating jelly helps decrease chafing. Gentle massage or application of warm compresses before milking helps soften the udder and assist in milk expression. Milk can be collected by hand or by the use of an inverted 60-ml dosing syringe. Several alternatives to mare's milk are available, but all have their drawbacks. Milk replacers are readily available, but have high salt content, can be difficult for the foal to digest, and can cause diarrhea. Preparations formulated for enteral nutrition of other species are generally not suitable for the foal. Goat's milk is palatable, but causes some metabolic abnormalities and should not be used alone for extended periods. All utensils used for feeding foals should be thoroughly cleaned and disinfected before and after use because the GI tract is a potential portal for an infection. Once reconstituted, milk replacers should be kept refrigerated. The preparations should be discarded after 2 hours at room temperature.

SUMMARY

Working with neonatal foals can be rewarding. It is especially enjoyable to watch a pregnant mare deliver a healthy foal, see them bond, and eventually observe them running in the pasture together. When a foal becomes ill and requires intensive care, it can be challenging for the owner and the neonatal veterinary team to care for the foal. Figure 10-9 depicts the ultimate desired outcome for an NICU foal. Although some of these foals do not survive, many foals recover and lead normal lives as athletes, in great part because of the tremendous effort of many dedicated veterinary technicians. It is a privilege to work with many of these caring people who continue to move the veterinary profession forward.

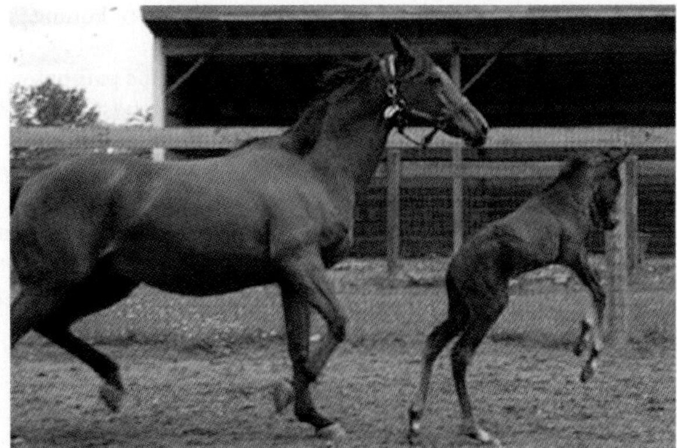

FIGURE 10-9 The ultimate desired outcome for an NICU foal.

RECOMMENDED READING

Section on Puppies and Kittens

Casal ML: Feline Paediatrics. In Raw ME, Parkinson TJ, editors: The Veterinary Annual, 35:210-235, 1995.

Davidson AP: Approaches to reducing neonatal mortality in dogs. In Concannon PW, England G, Verstegen III J et al, editors: Recent advances in small animal reproduction, Ithaca NY, 2003, International Veterinary Information Service.

Gunn-Moore D: Small animal neonatology: they look normal when they are born and then they die, Prague, Czech Republic, 2006, WSAVA Proceedings.

Hoskins JD: Veterinary pediatrics: dogs and cats from birth to six months. Philadelphia, 2001, WB Saunders.

Hotston Moore P, Sturgess CP: Care of neonates and young animals. In Simpson GM, England GC, Harvey MJ, editors: BSAVA manual of small animals, Cheltenham, United Kingdom, 1998, British Small Animal Veterinary Assoc.

Section on Neonatology in the Foal

Axon J, Palmer JE, Wilkins PA: Short and long term athletic outcome of neonatal intensive care unit survivors. In Proceedings of the annual American Association of Equine Practitioners convention, vol 45, Lexington, Ky, 1999.

Barton MH, Morris DD, Crowe N et al: Hemostatic indices in healthy foals from birth to one month of age, *J Vet Diagn Invest* 7:380-385, 1995.

Barton MH, Morris DD, Norton N et al: Hemostatic and fibrinolytic indices in neonatal foals with presumed septicemia. *J Vet Intern Med* 12:26-35, 1998.

Bentz AI, Wilkins PA, MacGillivray KC, et al: Thrombocytopenia in two thoroughbred foals with sepsis and neonatal encephalopathy, *J Vet Intern Med* 16:494-497, 2002.

Clabough DL: Disease of the equine neonate, *J Equine Vet Sci* 8(1): 5-10, 1988.

Drummond WH: Bridging the gap between the human and equine neonate. In Rossdale PD, editor: *The application of intensive care therapies and parenteral nutrition in large animal medicine,* Deerfield, Ill, 1986, Travenol Labs.

Koterba AM: IV fluid therapy and nutritional support in the sick neonate. *Equine Vet Educ* 3(1):33-39, 1991.

Koterba AM, Drummond WH, Kosch PC editors: *Equine clinical neonatology,* Philadelphia, 1990, Lea and Febiger.

Madigan JE, editor: *Manual of equine neonatal medicine,* ed 3, Woodlawn, Calif, 1997, Live Oak Publishing.

Marsh PS, Palmer JE: Bacterial isolates from blood and their susceptibility patterns in critically ill foals: 543 cases (1991-1998). *J Am Vet Med Assoc* 218:1608-1610, 2001.

McClure JT, Miller J, Deluca JL: Comparison of two ELISA screening tests and a non-commercial glutaraldehyde coagulation screening test for the detection of failure of passive transfer in neonatal foals.

In Proceedings of the annual American Association of Equine Practitioners convention, vol 49, Lexington, Ky, 2003.

McKenzie III HC, Furr MO: Equine neonatal sepsis: the pathophysiology of severe inflammation and infection, *Compend Contin Educ Pract Vet* 23:661-670, 2001.

Paradis MR: Update on neonatal sepsis, *Vet Clin North Am Equine Pract* 10(1):109-135, 1994.

Peek SF, Semrad S, McGuirk SM et al: Prognostic value of clinicopathologic variables obtained at admission and effect of antiendotoxin plasma on survival in septic and critically ill foals, *J Vet Intern Med* 20:569-574, 2006.

Pierce SW: Foal care from birth to 30 days: a practitioner's perspective. In Proceedings of the annual American Association of Equine Practitioners convention, vol 49, Lexington, Ky, 2003.

Vaala WE, House JK, Madigan JE: Initial management and physical examination of the neonate. In Smith BP, editor: *Large animal internal medicine: diseases of horses, cattle, sheep, and goats,* ed 3, St Louis, 2002, Mosby.

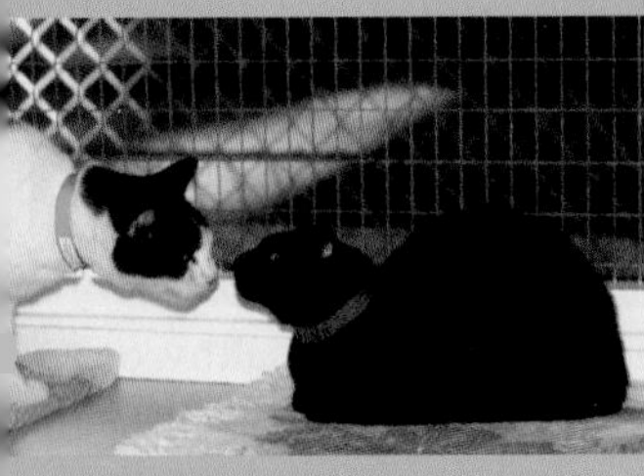

Animal Behavior

11

Suzanne Hetts

KEY TERMS

Active listening skills
Aggression
Agonistic behaviors
Anthropomorphism
Behavior wellness
Behavior wellness care
Behavior wellness programs
Behavioral needs
Classical conditioning
Displacement behavior
Dominance aggression
Dominant role
Operant conditioning
Negative punishment
Negative reinforcement
Nonthreatening greeting behaviors
Positive punishment
Positive reinforcement
Social hierarchies
Socialization
Species-typical behavior
Submissive behaviors
Subordinate role
Threatening behavior
Timeout from reinforcement

OUTLINE

LEARNING OBJECTIVES

When you have completed this chapter, you will be able to:

1. Define behavior wellness and explain the importance of behavior wellness programs in pet animal practice.
2. Differentiate between positive reinforcement, positive punishment, negative reinforcement, and negative punishment.
3. Describe aspects of social behavior and social hierarchies in dogs and cats.
4. List criteria that define behavioral health in dogs and cats.
5. Define socialization and identify critical periods of social development in dogs and cats.
6. List and describe the five steps in the Five-Step Positive Proaction Plan.
7. List the five major areas of a behavioral assessment.
8. List the most common agnostic behaviors exhibited by animals.
9. Describe methods for dealing with threatening and aggressive animals.
10. List and describe common products used for behavior modification in dogs and cats and handling aggressive animals.

INTRODUCTION

Most veterinary technicians do not need to be convinced how important understanding behavior and preventing and resolving behavior problems are to veterinary medicine. Multiple studies have shown that behavior problems are one of the most common reasons that dogs and cats are surrendered to shelters. Most dogs in shelters have not had basic training, and dogs that have been to basic training classes are less likely to be surrendered (Patronek et al, 1996a, 1996b; Salman et al, 1998). In addition, when owners have received advice about behavior problems that was not helpful or not tried, their pets are at greater risk for surrender. Understanding the communication signals and social behaviors of the species for which technicians provide care will allow you to handle and restrain them more safely and humanely.

WHY BEHAVIOR WELLNESS?

Many owners who relinquish their pets have tolerated problems for months or years, often unable to find effective help (DiGiacomo et al, 1998). Owners often ignore or tolerate problems, such as inappropriate elimination, phobias, or family pets not getting along, until the problem worsens or there is a lifestyle change that makes resolution of the problem a priority. For example, a couple might tolerate a pet's occasional or frequent house soiling until they learn that they are expecting a baby. Concern about the baby crawling on the soiled carpet in the future threatens the pet's continued presence in the home. Problems are usually much more difficult to resolve under these conditions—a long-standing problem and owners unrealistically demanding a quick solution—than if intervention had been obtained earlier.

In many cases, a window of opportunity for the prevention and detection of problems and for providing timely intervention exists, but owners and veterinary care providers are not taking full advantage of it. In the general practice of veterinary medicine, a pet's behavior is most often attended to during puppyhood and kittenhood, if the animal's behavior presents a problem at the veterinary hospital, and when the owner mentions a problem. Making behavior wellness care an integral part of the delivery of pet health care services is more beneficial than a narrow focus on problem resolution, which is often sought at a crisis moment, as in the earlier example.

WHAT IS BEHAVIOR WELLNESS?

Behavior wellness is the condition or state of normal and acceptable pets' conduct that enhances the human-animal bond and the pet's quality of life (Hetts, Heinke, Estep, 2004).

Behavior wellness care is the planned attention to a pet's conduct and the active integration of behavior wellness programs into the delivery of pet-related services, including routine veterinary medical supervision. Ten components to behavior wellness care have been suggested (Hetts, Heinke, Estep, 2004) and are listed in Box 11-1.

BOX 11-1 Components of Behavior Wellness Care

1. Promoting criteria for behaviorally healthy animals
2. Promoting helpful attitudes and realistic expectations
3. Promoting understanding of the behavioral needs of animals
4. Providing pet-selection information
5. Promoting socialization of young animals
6. Promoting a positive plan for proaction to create good behavior
7. Conducting regular assessments of behavioral health
8. Making the veterinary hospital a behaviorally friendly place
9. Offering proactive programs and presentations, such as preparing pets for a baby, for moving, or the addition of another pet
10. Providing timely referrals when needed

Behavior wellness programs are protocols, procedures, services, and systems that educate pet owners and professionals about what constitutes the behaviorally healthy or well pet; promote behavioral wellness through positive proaction, behavior assessments, early intervention, and timely referrals; and decrease unrealistic human expectations and interpretations of a pet's behavior.

TECHNICIANS CAN PLAY A STRATEGIC ROLE IN BEHAVIOR WELLNESS CARE

When given sufficient education in behavior and behavior wellness care, including direction and support from the veterinarian, veterinary technicians can be the most strategically positioned individuals on the veterinary health care team to deliver many behavior wellness services.

> *TECHNICIAN NOTE* The technician is often the first person owners ask about why their pets behave the way they do.

The technician is often the first person owners ask about why their pets behave the way they do, how to prevent problems, and what to do once their pets' behavior has become a problem. Technicians are usually best positioned to have the first contact with clients during scheduled appointments. With the support of the veterinarian, technicians can use these opportunities to deliver the appropriate elements of behavior wellness care. Elements of behavior wellness care are listed in Box 11-1.

Practice management consultants are emphasizing the importance of veterinarians delegating health care tasks to their support staff when such tasks do not require the veterinarian (Wood, 1997). The increased use of technicians in history taking, nutrition, prophylactic dental services, and general clients' education has set precedents that provide the veterinary technician with an opportunity to play a leading role in the delivery of behavior wellness care. Doing so is beneficial to the technician, the practice, and to pets and their owners (Box 11-2).

The advantages of providing behavior wellness care can extend beyond even these beneficiaries to communities and society at large. A decrease in dog bites could be seen if more veterinary hospitals:

1. Offered puppy socialization classes or routinely encouraged and referred puppy owners to them while puppies are still in the sensitive socialization period between 4 to 12 weeks of age.
2. More often used nonconfrontational handling and restraint techniques so as not to contribute to defensive aggressive behavior.
3. Discouraged the use of dangerous and harmful procedures, such as scruff shakes and "alpha rolls."
4. Provided behaviorally sound advice about how to help dogs fit into the social fabric of the family to counter the likening of families to wolf packs, as is common in popular media.

> TECHNICIAN NOTE **Behavior wellness programs have the potential to decrease the frequency of bites from dogs and cats.**

BEHAVIOR EDUCATION FOR TECHNICIANS

Technicians who deliver behavior wellness care must give up-to-date, scientifically accurate information. Scientific knowledge must replace nonscientific interpretations of behavior and information based solely on personal experience and beliefs.

Historically, most of the emphasis on continuing veterinary education in animal behavior has been on problem resolution. Lectures on resolving separation anxiety, aggression problems in both dogs and cats, and fears and phobias are common in veterinary technicians' continuing education programs. Time spent on these topics has often come at the expense of basic education in behavior.

As in other aspects of veterinary technicians' education, foundational skills must be acquired first. Whether within the veterinary technician's curriculum or through continuing education, technicians must become familiar with basic concepts in applied ethology and animal learning. The former should include knowledge of species-specific communication signals and body postures, and the latter must include principles of operant and classical conditioning.

Continuing education opportunities focused on implementation of behavior wellness services, including implementing puppy classes in the veterinary practice, are now available[*,†,‡,§] (Hetts and Estep, 1999). Technicians can also consider continuing education opportunities other than or in addition to those traditionally provided within the field. National humane organizations, animal-control associations, and dog-training associations conduct training conferences that would be beneficial to technicians delivering behavior wellness services. For example, the Association of Pet Dog Trainers 2007 Annual Conference included presentations on puppy classes and training, dog bites, shelter dogs, critical thinking and understanding the difference between true, junk, and pseudoscience, and one by a veterinarian on balancing disease prevention and a puppy's socialization.

Resolving behavior problems requires the most advanced and complex skill set, which in turn requires the most education and experience to acquire. Technicians should first build a solid education in the sciences of ethology and animal learning and have experience with other aspects of behavior wellness care before participating in problem-resolution activities.

BOX 11-2 Benefits of Providing Behavior Wellness Care

- The technician's job can be more rewarding and interesting.
- The technician and the practice will better understand and meet both the clients' and the patients' needs. It is clear from the studies of animal shelters that the need for behavioral services is not being met.
- A behavior wellness program can help to make a visit to the practice less stressful and more enjoyable for patients. This in turn can result in better health care for the pet. Many owners put off visiting the veterinarian if they know from past experience that this will be stressful and unpleasant for the animal.
- Pets become safer and easier to handle, and fewer staff members are bitten.
- A behavior wellness program increases the number of clients' visits per year.
- A program adds a significant dollar amount to the bottom line each year.
- A program attracts and retains a top-of-the-line staff: the most motivated and best educated.
- A program decreases frustration in dealing with problem owners and problem pets because the technician can now provide them with services that can prevent pets from becoming difficult patients.

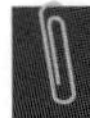

> TECHNICIAN NOTE **Resolving behavior problems requires the most advanced and complex skill sets.**

A CHANGE IN PERSPECTIVE

Providing behavior wellness care requires that the technician not only react to questions when they are asked, but also take a proactive approach and make behavior a part of every nonemergency appointment. This means initiating discussions about the pet's behavior, whether the owner does or not.

Veterinary technicians who do not take the lead in asking questions about behavior are missing the point of behavior wellness. As will be seen throughout this chapter, pet owners do not know what they do not know and are therefore unlikely to initiate discussions about behavior until a problem exists. This guarantees that opportunities for the promotion of good behavior and early detection of problems that are at the core of behavior wellness will be missed.

Providing behavior wellness is another example of providing preventive care. Just as vaccinations prevent contagious diseases and specific medications prevent parasite infestations, behavior wellness programs can prevent behavior problems and promote healthy behaviors.

[*] Hetts S, Estep DQ: Implementing puppy classes in the veterinary practice: a two-day workshop, Littleton, Colo, 2002, Animal Behavior Associates, Inc.
[†] Hetts S, Heinke ML: Implementing behavioral wellness services workshop, Lakewood, Colo, American Animal Hospital Association, 2000.
[‡] *Applied animal behavior for veterinary technicians,* Denver, Colo, 2004, Bel-Rae Institute of Animal Technology.
[§] Dogs! course, West Lafayette, Ind, 2004, Animal Behavior Clinic, School of Veterinary Medicine, Purdue University.

BEFORE IMPLEMENTING BEHAVIOR WELLNESS CARE

Before offering any kind of behavioral information, technicians should clarify their role with the practice owner or their designated supervisor. Veterinarians usually determine what medical information or advice they wish technicians to impart to clients, and the same procedure should be followed when it comes to behavior.

When technicians' roles are not clearly defined, they may feel pressured and resentful of the time spent answering behavioral questions because this prevents them from completing other assigned tasks. On the other hand, if technicians spend significant time on behavior issues that is not charged to the client, this sets a dangerous precedent for the practice. It is one of the reasons that veterinarians believe, often erroneously, that providing behavior services is not financially feasible.

Behavior services should be professionally delivered so that their value is fully recognized and they benefit not only clients and their pets, but also the practice. The Society of Veterinary Behavior Technicians promotes and encourages the training of technicians in behavior and their appropriate involvement in the delivery of behavior services, making this organization an invaluable resource (Price, 2001). Information about the society can be found at the website listed in Box 11-3.

> *TECHNICIAN NOTE* The first component of a behavior wellness program is defining characteristics of behaviorally healthy pets.

REQUISITE KNOWLEDGE

Any technician who wants to advise clients about promoting healthy behaviors or changing unwanted behavior patterns *must* have at least a rudimentary understanding of some aspects of learning theory and *must* be familiar with the ethology of the species they work with, including species-typical behavior patterns. In-depth coverage of these topics is beyond the scope of this chapter. However, to help technicians better understand and more effectively use the Five-Step Positive Proaction Plan discussed later in this chapter and to compensate for the dangerous misinformation regarding "dominance" and social hierarchies in both dogs and cats, an overview of these topics will be provided. Technicians are referred to the Further Readings Section at the end of this chapter for more information.

BOX 11-3 Useful Organizational Websites

- www.veterinarybehaviorists.org—website of the American College of Veterinary Behaviorists
- www.animalbehavior.org—website of the Animal Behavior Society (ABS, the organization that certifies Applied Animal Behaviorists)
- www.certfiedanimalbehaviorist.com—website of Certified Applied Animal Behaviorists (with links to the ABS website)
- www.ccpdt.org—website of the Certification Council for Professional Dog Trainers (CCPDT)
- www.apdt.com—website of the Association of Pet Dog Trainers (will also take you to the CCPDT site)
- www.svbt.org—website of the Society of Veterinary Behavior Technicians
- www.deltasociety.org—website of the Delta Society from which the document Professional Standards for Dog Trainers: Effective, Humane Principles can be obtained

An Overview of Operant Conditioning

Operant conditioning is only one type of learning that is important in behavior modification. Operant conditioning is based on the fact that the consequences of a behavior will influence its frequency. Behavior that is rewarded will increase in frequency, whereas behavior that causes unpleasantness to the animal will decrease. Technicians must not forget that rewards and punishments can be both external and internal to the animal and not always under the control of a trainer or handler.

> *TECHNICIAN NOTE* Operant conditioning is based on the fact that the consequences of a behavior will influence its frequency.

Operant conditioning allows for four behavioral consequences, which are diagrammed in Table 11-1. To better understand these consequences, technicians must remember to think of "positive" and "negative" in the mathematic sense of adding and subtracting. Remember that by definition reinforcement increases behavior and punishment decreases it, regardless of whether each is positive or negative.

Thus positive reinforcement increases behavior because something *pleasant* is *added* following a behavior. Positive punishment decreases behavior because something *unpleasant* is *added* following a behavior.

Negative punishment decreases behavior because something *pleasant* is *taken away (subtracted)* following a behavior. Negative reinforcement increases behavior because something *unpleasant* is *taken away or avoided (subtracted)* following a behavior. Box 11-4 gives examples of each of these consequences.

TABLE 11-1 Behavioral Consequences in Operant Conditioning

Type of Event or Stimulus	Add or Give	Take Away, Subtract, or Avoid
Something pleasant	Positive reinforcement	Negative punishment
Something unpleasant	Positive punishment	Negative reinforcement

An Overview of Social Behavior and Social Hierarchies in Dogs

For many years, in the popular literature and to some degree the professional literature, the dog's relationship to its human family has been likened to the social structure within a wolf pack. There are many problems with this model including misconceptions about a wolf's social behavior and that it does not take into account significant differences in behavior between wolves and dogs. A few of these differences are listed in Box 11-5.

Technicians will often encounter dog owners who say they have a "dominant dog," and this fact is the source of the dog's problems. This comment is incorrect in many respects, one of which is that it mistakenly implies that "dominance" is a personality trait, rather than the role a dog assumes in a relationship. A dog may assume a dominant role in a relationship with one individual and a subordinate role in another. Roles may change over time, based on who the social partners are and the context in which the interaction or conflict occurs.

For example, a dog may give up his resting place on his favorite chair when dog A or person A asks him to, but not when person B does. If dog B is clearly in a subordinate role with the dog on the chair, dog B will not even ask.

The function of social hierarchies is to prevent conflicts over resources from occurring in a social group. Many behaviors that have been attributed to "dominance problems" have nothing to do with resource allocation and roles and relationships. Examples of these are given in Box 11-6. Dog owners are often instructed to withhold certain privileges (such as sleeping on the bed) and to establish strict rules (never step over your dog, make your dog move out of your way) to establish their "dominance" over their dogs. The fallacies with these recommendations are that most dogs do not view these interactions as competitions, and they confuse "dominance" with obedience.

A dog owner may have little control over her dog (the dog does not respond to "commands," jumps on people, dashes through the door in front of her, pulls on the leash, barks at the door, even growls at visitors), but still be in a dominant role with her dog (she can easily take food and other items away from the dog, move the dog from the bed or furniture, pet and groom the dog, etc.).

Many dogs are mislabeled as "dominant" when they actually are quite fearful. This was the case with 9-month-old Zeke, a neutered male vizsla that was growling at his male owner when he tried to move him off the bed. Rather than using positive reinforcement techniques to teach the dog to get off the bed, the owner had been grabbing for the dog's collar and yanking him off the bed. The dog's body postures while growling were clearly fearful—ears back, head lowered, and eyes dilated—as he sought to defend himself from being manhandled. The confrontation was not about getting off the bed, but one of self-defense.

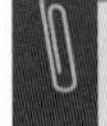

TECHNICIAN NOTE Many dogs are mislabeled as "dominant" when they are actually quite fearful.

Similar problems can develop when owners use "scruff shakes," and "alpha rolls" (throwing and pinning their dogs to the floor) to "discipline" their dogs. Technicians should avoid recommending these procedures and counsel dog owners about these dangers. These techniques do *not* mimic a dog's or wolf's behavior. Although a dog may voluntarily

BOX 11-4 Examples of Behavioral Consequences in Operant Conditioning

Positive reinforcement—Cat is given a piece of tuna immediately after scratching on his post (while still at the post).

Positive punishment—Cat is squirted with water while scratching the stereo speakers.

Negative reinforcement—Dog learns to stop at an electronic fence boundary to avoid being "shocked."

Negative punishment—Owner covers bird cage with a towel and leaves the room when bird screams for attention.

BOX 11-5 Examples of Differences Between Wolves and Dogs

A wolf pack is a closed social group—it does not accept "outsiders." Dogs maintain open social groups—both with people and other dogs.

A wolf pack is a group of related individuals. Social groupings in dogs are rarely related.

Parental care from both dam and sire and other relatives is common in wolves. In dogs, it is rare for any animal but the dam to provide parental care.

Female wolves come into season once/yr; most dogs (one exception is the basenji) come into season twice/yr.

The social hierarchy in a wolf pack is based on a breeding pair that occupy dominant social roles. There is no similar foundation for social hierarchies between dogs or between dogs and people. Relationships in a wolf pack are intraspecific (within the species). Obviously, social relationships between people and dogs are interspecific (between species).

BOX 11-6 Behaviors and Behavior Problems Erroneously Linked to Social Hierarchies ("Dominance Problems")

- Slow response to commands, refusal to obey commands, general disobedience
- Destructive behavior
- Aggression to strangers and children
- Pulling on leash
- Door dashing
- Excessive barking
- Marking and inappropriate elimination
- Coprophagy
- Excessive licking of people
- Leaning against people

roll on its back in response to a social challenge from a dog in a more dominant role, physically pinning a dog to the ground involves force and is more similar to what occurs in a dog fight than what happens in a ritualized social communicative display.

> *TECHNICIAN NOTE* Technicians should avoid recommending "scruff shakes" and "roll overs" and counsel dog owners about these dangers.

Technicians are encouraged to learn more about canine ethology by reading items from the Recommended Resources list, especially those by McConnell, Serpell (editor), and Coppinger.

Important Aspects of Social Behavior and Social Hierarchies in Cats

A mythology about cats wanting to be "dominant" over people has not developed the way it has in reference to dog-human relationships. The "don't pet me anymore" behavior of cats is the one most common problem attributed to a cat's attempt to "dominant" a person. In this behavior, the cat after permitting petting for a period of time will suddenly turn and bite or attempt to bite the person petting him. More commonly seen in males than females, this behavior is poorly understood, and there has been no observational research to support attributing this behavior to the order of the social hierarchy between a cat and a person.

Both the social behavior and domestication history of cats is quite different than that of dogs, resulting in significant differences in cats' social behaviors toward people as compared with those of dogs. Cat behavior scientists have speculated that the cat-person relationship is more analogous to kitten-mother, rather than peer to peer (conspecific), as is true for dogs and people (Bradshaw, 1992).

Cats' social hierarchies appear to be even more fluid than those of dogs. In a study of in-home pet cats, resource allocation was often time dependent rather than one individual always having priority access when in competition with another. For example, cat A might have priority access to the best window perch in the morning, but cat B would have priority in the afternoon (Bernstein and Strack, 1996). In studies of free-ranging cats, males were more likely to leave and avoid a confrontation the closer they were to the opponent's territory.

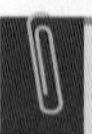

> *TECHNICIAN NOTE* Cats' social hierarchies can be quite fluid.

Cats do not seem to guard resources in the same way as dogs yet through subtle communication may be able to exclude other household cats from food dishes, litter boxes, and other necessities. Cats do not have ritualized play invitations or submissive behaviors in their social behavioral repertoire, so play "fights" can more easily escalate into real conflicts. Because many aggression problems between family cats are motivated by territoriality and defensiveness, many can be prevented through proper introductions. This is why it is so important for technicians to create wellness plans for new pet introductions, as explained later in the chapter.

Technicians are unlikely to find cats attempting to "dominate" them in the veterinary practice. The most common reason for a cat's aggression toward people in this setting is fear and defensiveness. Cats do not "scruff" other cats to assume and maintain social superiority, so this restraint technique does not mimic cats' behavior anymore than scruffing and pinning mimics dogs' behavior.

> *TECHNICIAN NOTE* Technicians are unlikely to find cats attempting to "dominate" them in the veterinary practice.

Technicians are encouraged to expand their knowledge of cats' behavior by reading several of the scientific books on cats' behavior contained in the Recommended Resources list at the end of this chapter. Technicians who will be working with horses and birds should also make use of the suggested readings about the social behavior of these species.

COMPONENTS OF A BEHAVIOR WELLNESS PROGRAM

DEFINING BEHAVIORALLY HEALTHY PETS

Technicians are taught how to recognize healthy animals according to certain criteria. These commonly include good condition of the skin and coat, clear eyes, a lack of external and internal parasites, proper weight, clean teeth, healthy gums, etc.

Criteria for behavioral health are often not considered. Behavioral health is more than the absence of behavior problems. As defined previously, it is the presence of normal and acceptable pets' conduct that enhances the human-animal bond and the pet's quality of life (Hetts, Heinke, Estep, 2004).

Specifying the criteria for normal and acceptable pets' conduct allows technicians to help pet owners set goals for promoting desirable behaviors, rather than just reacting when problems arise. Suggested criteria for behaviorally healthy cats and dogs are listed in Box 11-7. Technicians can use these as a basis for discussion with veterinarians and other co-workers to establish criteria within their hospitals. Criteria for other species can and should be established. The assessment of behavioral health by using these and other criteria is another component of behavior wellness care that will subsequently be discussed.

ESTABLISHING REALISTIC EXPECTATIONS AND HELPFUL ATTITUDES

Anthropomorphic explanations for and unrealistic expectations about pets' behavior contribute to relationship problems between owners and pets. Technicians can play a vital role in educating clients in these areas.

BOX 11-7 Criteria for Behaviorally Healthy Cats and Dogs

- Are affectionate, without being "needy."
- Are friendly toward or at least tolerant of people, including children, and other members of their own species.
- Enjoy or at least tolerate normal, everyday handling and interactions.
- Eliminate only in acceptable areas.
- Are not overly fearful of normal, everyday events or new things.
- Adapt to change with minimal problems.
- Play well with others by not becoming uncontrollable or rough.
- Are not nuisances or dangerous to the community.
- Can be left alone for reasonable time periods without becoming anxious or panicked or consistently misbehaving.
- Readily relinquish control of space, food, toys, and other objects.
- Vocalize (bark, meow) when appropriate, but not to excess.
- In addition, behaviorally healthy dogs:
  Reliably respond when told to sit, down, come, or stay.
- In addition, behaviorally healthy cats:
  Scratch only items provided for this purpose.

BOX 11-8 Anthropomorphic Interpretations and How to Reinterpret Them

1. Rather than having a moral sense of right and wrong, pets learn what behaviors, and in what circumstances, result in pleasant, unpleasant, or no consequences. Dogs do not learn that it is "wrong" to dig in the yard, and cats do not learn that it is "wrong" to scratch the stereo speakers. Instead, they learn that these are enjoyable behaviors (pleasant consequences) unless someone is present to discipline them for engaging in them. This is why pets learn to engage in certain behaviors only in the owners' absences.
2. Whereas for dogs, cats, and other species of animals, urine (and sometimes feces) has communicative value (to designate territory and to assess reproductive status), they do not perceive the products of elimination as vile and disgusting. Animals do not urinate or defecate in certain locations to "tell owners something" or to indicate their dislike of that person.
3. There is no scientific evidence that the behaviors of animals (with perhaps the exception of the nonhuman primates) are motivated by spite or revenge. Technicians should learn to apply the principle of parsimony when explaining behavior and choose the simplest explanation that explains the set of behavioral observations. For example, there would be no reason to claim that a dog or cat got into the trash because they were mad at the owner, when the behavior is easily accounted for as a foraging behavior.

Realistic Expectations

Technicians can routinely tell new pet owners to expect to lose something of value simply because they share their lives and their homes with an animal. To put it in terms pet owners will understand, clients will lose something of monetary or sentimental value (or both) when their pets chew up, tear up, eat, track mud on, shed on, relieve themselves on, and vomit or have diarrhea on their possessions. Most people expect some problem behaviors from puppies and kittens, but surprisingly many owners do not expect their 8- or 9-month-old cat or dog to still be prone to chewing and destructive play behaviors. Even well-behaved pets will inadvertently engage in behaviors that cause damage.

Clients who have recently acquired adult animals often make the erroneous assumption that their new pets are already "trained," and they will not have to worry about house training or chewing and other destructive behaviors. Adult animals new to the home, however, should be treated just like puppies or kittens for the first few weeks to prevent problems as a result of owners' expectations that are too high; adult pets often need training and supervision while they are making the adjustment to their new homes.

Reinterpreting Anthropomorphic Interpretations

Technicians can also help clients understand that their pets' behavior is not motivated by spite, revenge, rebelliousness, jealousy, or guilt. When owners realize that their pets are not vindictive or mean spirited, do not have a moral sense of right and wrong, or misbehave even though they "know better," they are usually more willing to work with their pets' behavior and to listen to possible solutions.

Technicians can tell people that animals do what works for them—to meet a need, cope with stress, or control their environment. Destructive behavior that occurs when a pet is left alone, for example, is not motivated by revenge. Alternative explanations are separation anxiety, playful behavior, or the pet's realization that unpleasant consequences do not occur in the owner's absence.

Technicians often have the opportunity to correct pet owners' misinterpretations that their pets "know better" and look "guilty" when evidence of their misbehavior is discovered. "Guilty looks" are submissive behaviors, such as the avoidance of eye contact, crouched body posture, flattening of the ears, and lowering of the tail when threatened by their owners. When owners discover evidence of misbehavior, they display behaviors, such as yelling, pointing fingers, and staring, that pets find intimidating and that in turn trigger submissive behaviors that are misinterpreted as guilt.

Other examples of how technicians can clarify misinterpretations can be found in Box 11-8.

PROVIDING PET-SELECTION INFORMATION

The most proactive behavior wellness service is the education of clients about pet selection. Unfortunately, few clients seek this service from the veterinary practice. Technicians can play a helpful role by regularly asking clients whether they are considering adding a new pet to the family and reminding them that the veterinary practice can assist them in selecting a pet that will best meet their expectations.

A closely related subject is helping owners introduce pets to one another. Better relationships between family pets could be created if introductions were better managed. Pet owners do not usually ask for help until relationship problems between pets have already begun so creating opportunities for early intervention will be up to the veterinary professional. How the new pet is getting along with resident pets should be a standard question put to clients when the newly acquired pet is brought in for its first veterinary appointment. A plan for introducing pets to one another that follows the Five-Step Plan for Positive Proaction (Hetts, Heinke, Estep, 2004), which will subsequently be discussed, should also be given to clients (see Box 11-14).

IMPORTANCE OF SOCIALIZATION

Most species of social animals have a sensitive period during which socialization to their own species, to humans, and to other animals occurs most easily. Socialization refers to the process by which an animal develops appropriate social behaviors toward members of its own and other species (Bateson, 1979). In dogs, this period is from 4 to 12 weeks of age (Scott and Fuller, 1965); in cats, it is from 3 to 7 weeks of age (Karsh and Turner, 1988); and in horses, it begins at birth (Waring 2003). There may also be sensitive periods for the acclimatization of animals to new places, situations, and things, which occur around the same ages; but the precise time of these is unknown.

The process of socialization requires providing the young animal pleasant experiences with people, situations, inanimate elements of the environment, and other animals. Adequate socialization helps the animal to adapt to change and not react with fear or aggression to common, everyday events.

Technicians should educate pet owners about how early socialization can prevent the development of many behavior problems, especially those caused by fearful behavior. Cats are typically undersocialized, as evidenced by the tendency of many to hide when visitors come, be afraid in unfamiliar environments, and not enjoy human handling.

A practical approach to socialization advice is that during its sensitive period, a young animal should be exposed to elements of its world that are relevant to its adult role. A foal should have positive experiences with the horse trailer, kittens should be introduced to friendly dogs, and puppies should interact with friendly, well-behaved children.

Veterinarians have historically been reluctant to recommend early socialization programs for kittens and puppies because of concern about disease transmission. If recent outbreaks of contagious disease have been rare in the local area and the percentage of vaccinated animals is high, early socialization may present little hazard.

Although the veterinarian will set practice policy regarding early socialization programs, as one prominent veterinary behaviorist wrote "... the risk of a dog dying because of infection with distemper or parvo disease is far less than the much higher risk of a dog dying (euthanasia) because of a behavior problem" (Anderson et al, 1999) that could have been prevented through early socialization and training. One finding from a study of puppies adopted from humane societies found that puppies were more likely to remain in their homes if their owners had attended puppy socialization classes with their puppies (Duxbury et al, 2003).

With proper training and the support of the veterinary practice, technicians can offer puppy and kitten socialization classes. This limits concern over disease transmission if all attendees are immunized patients of the veterinary practice. Resources to help technicians work with veterinarians to offer classes are available (e.g., Hetts and Estep, in prep, Landsberg, Hunthausen, Ackerman 2003).

FIVE-STEP POSITIVE PROACTION PLAN

The topic of preventing behavior problems is not a new one for technicians. However, a behavior wellness view focuses on promoting desirable behaviors, not just preventing problems.

This Five-Step Positive Proaction Plan (Hetts, Heinke, Estep, 2004) organizes information and provides a framework that technicians can use when they talk with pet owners about how they can create behavior patterns that define a behaviorally healthy pet. Having a means to organize information makes it easier to develop practical educational handouts about promoting healthy behaviors. The best time to at least introduce elements of this plan is the first veterinary visit or series of puppy and kitten visits after a new pet has been acquired. The plan can also be used during future appointments as a partial response to behavior concerns as they are discovered through behavior assessments and observations of the pet. The five steps in the plan follow, in client-friendly terms, with more technical phrases and terms in parentheses:

1. Catch your pet doing something right. (Elicit and reinforce appropriate behavior.)
2. Do not let bad habits develop. (Prevent or minimize inappropriate behavior.)
3. Meet your pet's behavioral and developmental needs.
4. Use the "take-away" method (negative punishment) to discourage inappropriate behavior.
5. Minimize "discipline" (positive punishment) and use it correctly when necessary.

Each of these steps will be discussed in some detail.

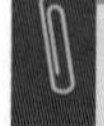
TECHNICIAN NOTE Animals need to be taught and encouraged to perform desirable behaviors.

Step One: Elicit and Reinforce Appropriate Behavior

This step is all about encouraging clients to more often positively reinforce their pets for good behavior *and* assisting them in finding ways to elicit good behavior that they can reward. Clients need specific instructions about how to proactively get their pet to do what they want, rather than reacting to unwanted behavior. For example, technicians can tell owners to have treats at the door for occasions when people are greeted and to encourage the dog to sit, rather than yelling and pushing the dog off when he jumps up (Figure 11-1).

In some situations eliciting good behavior is integrally connected to meeting the pet's behavioral needs, another step in the proactive plan. For example, establishing reliable litter-box behavior is primarily dependent on creating a litter box that meets the cat's behavioral preferences.

Technicians should also instruct owners to reward their pets when they catch them doing something right. It is easy to forget that behaviors that are rewarded are likely to be repeated. This is a powerful behavior modification method to which owners seldom devote enough effort. It is about providing animals sufficient feedback about their behaviors. Most pets are more likely to receive feedback when they misbehave, rather than when they are behaving appropriately.

Whenever the dog eliminates outside, the cat plays with its own toys, the foal nuzzles rather than nips at your hand, the puppy is lying down quietly, or the kitten is resting on a chair because owners expect these good behaviors, they are less likely to provide the animal feedback about them. Instead, good behavior is often passively accepted or ignored when owners should actively reinforce the behaviors they desire.

Reinforcement may consist of a tidbit, presentation of a new or favorite toy, petting, or any other event that the pet finds rewarding. Praise alone, especially when an owner is first establishing a relationship with a new pet, is often not adequate reinforcement. Praise usually first needs to be paired with petting, play, or food for a time to become sufficiently reinforcing.

Technicians may need to educate owners about the value of using food in training. Both food and toys are powerful ways to elicit and reinforce behavior when used correctly. The owner controls access to both, so the old adage that "a dog should work for me, not for food" is a useless argument. Pet owners may also resist the use of food to aid in establishing good behavior because they may believe this results in "he'll only do it when he knows I've got a treat." Although this can happen, it is due to training errors, rather than an inherent problem with using food. To overcome these errors suggest the following:

- Rather than using the food as a lure to elicit the behavior (the pet sees the food before performing the behavior), the pet must not see it until after the behavior has been performed (the food is used only to reward the behavior).

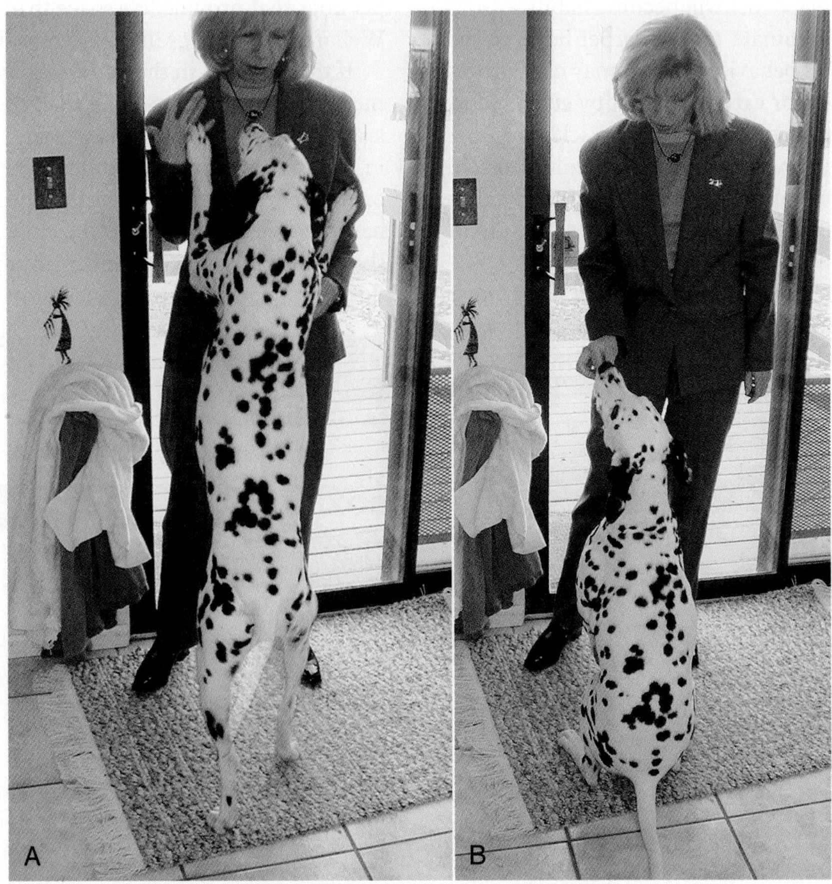

FIGURE 11-1 The lure-reward method of encouraging a dog to sit rather than jump on people.

- Until the behavior is well established, the food should be used to reinforce every occurrence of the correct behavior. Once the pet is responding well, the food should be given on an intermittent schedule (e.g., for some correct responses but not others) on an unpredictable basis (petting or praise should always be used). Intermittent reinforcement maintains correct responding better than continuous reinforcement.
- Because the pet must not know when food will be used to reward behavior and when it will not, all cues (e.g., a treat pouch, sound of food being removed from a container before behavior is performed, etc.) that the pet can use to predict whether food is available must be eliminated.

> TECHNICIAN NOTE The fewer opportunities animals are given to engage in undesirable behaviors, the less likely such behaviors are to become habits.

Certified Professional Dog Trainers (CPDT) should easily be able to help clients understand these procedures. Their website is listed in Box 11-3.

Step Two: Prevent or Minimize Inappropriate Behavior

When pets do not have the chance to make "mistakes," it is much easier to create good behaviors. The fewer opportunities an animal has to repeat or "practice" undesirable behaviors, the less likely such behaviors will become habits.

A cat that begins to eliminate on the carpet because the litter box does not meet its behavioral needs may quickly develop a surface preference for carpet. If a puppy gets used to pulling on the leash while walking, this can quickly become a habit, making loose leash walking more difficult to teach. Playing with a kitten with hands and feet rather than its toys can result in a cat that bites hands and considers human body parts to be playthings.

The technician should instruct owners that they must manage the pet's environment to prevent unwanted behaviors from occurring and developing into habits. Constant supervision of young animals and pets new to the household is an absolutely critical component of house training and also of teaching puppies and kittens to chew and scratch their own toys rather than household items.

Supervision can be accomplished in a number of ways, including crate training, use of baby gates to keep the pup in either a puppy-proof area or in the same room with the owner (Figure 11-2), or tethering the dog with a leash and collar to the owner or an object near the owner. Supervision of cats and kittens may mean closing doors to certain parts of the house.

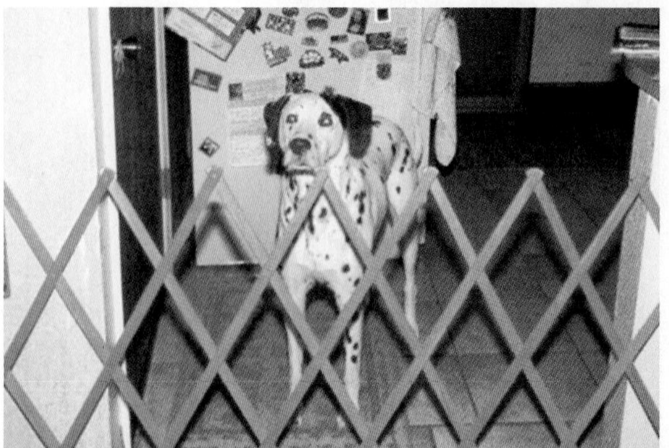

FIGURE 11-2 Environmental management with a baby gate to prevent opportunities for unwanted behavior.

Crate Training

A crate can be an extremely useful method of supervision, especially for puppies. Dog owners too often misuse or overuse crates because they are not given good information about their use. Technicians can play a vital role by giving dog owners accurate and complete information about crating to counteract the misinformation clients are likely to come across through other means, such as the Internet and television programs.

In the popular literature, crates are portrayed as analogous to dens. As the comparison points in Box 11-9 show, they are not. If technicians recommend crate training to pet owners, they should also cover the following topics:

Correct size of crate. Dogs need to be comfortable in their crates. This means sufficient room to stand up to full height, easily turn completely around, and lay down on a side, fully relaxed. Some dog-training books recommend crate sizes for pet dogs that provide less space than required by the Animal Welfare Act for dogs in research facilities.

If the dog soils in the crate, it is *not* appropriate to recommend a smaller crate. Soiling the crate does not mean it is too large; it means something is wrong. The dog may be confined in the crate for longer than he or she can control himself, he or she may be anxious and frightened, or he or she may even have a medical problem. The technician and the veterinarian should help the owner decipher why the dog is soiling, whether this means a medical work-up and/or a behavior consultation.

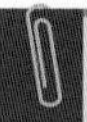

> TECHNICIAN NOTE If the dog soils in the crate, it is *not* appropriate to recommend a smaller crate.

BOX 11-9 A Comparison of Dens and Crates

1. Wild canids become familiar with dens starting at birth. Dogs are not introduced to crates until much later, sometimes not until adulthood.
2. Wild canids are seldom, if ever, left alone in dens. If the dam is gone, the pups are usually together as a litter. For dogs, being confined in the crate is usually synonymous with being left alone.
3. Wild canids can choose when to come and go from the den. Dogs confined to crates when home alone cannot.
4. Once mobile, older pups and adult wild canids spend little time in the den. Dogs can spend as much as 50 hr/wk or more confined in crates.

BOX 11-10 Basic Steps in Crate Training

Goal 1: The dog enters and exits the crate willingly, without reluctance, with the door open.
Goal 2: The dog can stay in the crate for brief times while relaxing with a chew toy with the owner in view, with the crate door closed for about 15 to 20 min.
Goal 3: The dog can stay in the crate for brief times while relaxing with a chew toy with the owner not in view, with the crate door closed for about 30 min and/or overnight.
Goal 4: The dog can stay in the crate with the owner gone for 1 hr.

How to acclimate the dog to the crate. Dogs do not automatically like being confined in crates. They must be introduced to them gradually by following steps similar to those listed in Box 11-10. This acclimation process may require just a day or two or as long as several weeks with dogs who have previously been anxious when crated.

How to acclimate the dog to being left alone in the crate. This step is frequently overlooked. Just because the dog is comfortable in the crate when someone is home does not mean he will be when left alone. Technicians need to educate owners about the importance of gradually acclimating the dog to being crated when alone. The first absence, for example, may need to be a maximum of 15 minutes. If the owner has any concern about how the dog is tolerating the crate when left alone, the technician can suggest that the client videotape or audiotape the dog.

How and when to make the transition to leaving the dog alone, free in the house. Crates should be a short-term management tool, not a way of life. The goal is for the dog to be unconfined in the home (perhaps with access to a backyard) when left alone. One study (Patronek et al, 1996) revealed that dogs that spent most of their day crated were at an increased risk for relinquishment. The explanation for this finding might be that crating merely manages a problem, such as house soiling or destructiveness. The continued existence of the behavior problem puts the dog at risk for surrender when management, for whatever reason, is no longer possible or effective.

Warning signs that a dog is not adjusting well to the crate. An important related subject that should be discussed is guidelines for when a crate should not be used, such as when separation anxiety problems exist or when the dog becomes panicked when it is confined (Box 11-11).

Step Three: Meet the Pet's Behavioral and Developmental Needs

Animals do things to get their needs met. Technicians can teach owners how to meet their pets' needs in ways that encourage and provide for desirable behaviors. This is much more effective than owners vainly trying to suppress normal behaviors, such as chewing, playing, or elimination. Instead, these behaviors should be directed onto appropriate targets, or steps should be taken to help the behaviors occur at appropriate times or locations.

BOX 11-11 Signs a Dog Is Not Tolerating the Crate

Even though a dog willingly enters a crate, this does not necessarily mean that he is relaxed there when left alone. The only way to determine this is to audiotape or videotape the dog.

- Reluctance to enter the crate
- Excessive whining, barking, or vocalizing
- Attempts to get out of the crate
- Soiling in the crate, even if crated for brief time periods
- Excessive salivation or drooling, as evidenced by the dog's wet fur on its chest and/or around its mouth
- The dog moving the crate, even slightly, through frantic movements, which are usually fear motivated.
- Any damage to the crate or injuries to the dog as a result of escape attempts

BOX 11-12 Behavioral Needs of Companion Animals

- Provision of a safe, comfortable place to rest and sleep
- Freedom from, or the ability to escape from, unnecessary pain, fear, and threats or discomfort
- Ability to control some aspects of the environment
- Opportunities to express species-typical behaviors, such as chewing, scratching, elimination, etc.
- Opportunities for exercise and play that are appropriate for that individual
- Opportunities for mental stimulation
- Opportunities for pleasant social contact with co-species and/or people to which the animals have been socialized and that are appropriate for that individual

Defining a list of widely accepted behavioral needs for pets, although difficult and controversial, has been proposed (Hetts, Heinke, Estep, 2004) and can be found in Box 11-12. This list presupposes that an animal's basic survival needs for food, water, and shelter have been addressed.

An Example of Meeting the Pet's Elimination Needs

Technicians can educate cat owners about cats' behavioral needs regarding a litter box based on the list in Box 11-13. Many litter-box problems develop because the areas the cat is soiling meet the cat's behavioral preferences for elimination better than the litter-box area.

Figure 11-3, for example, shows a litter box that is unacceptable in several ways, as follows:

- Dirty
- In an area, such as an unfinished basement, where the cat is unlikely to spend much time
- Next to noisy appliances
- On a cold cement floor
- Not easily accessible, such as a closet that has little space or the door to which can easily close unexpectedly

BOX 11-13 Litter Box Characteristics Associated With Meeting Cats' Behavioral Needs

- Type and number of boxes
- Size—average, smaller, larger
- Cover or not—start without unless a good reason to cover
- As many boxes as cats
- Litter
  Type—the finer the better
  Depth—1½ to 2 in generally
  Unscented preferred
- Liners or not
  Some cats may dislike
  Ease of cleaning may result in cleaner litter box
- Location
- Where in house
  Balance privacy with accessibility
  Avoid startling noises or other stimuli
- Where in room
  Ability to see and be protected
  Escape routes—more than one
  Access routes—easy to access, no obstacle courses
  Comfortable surface—soft and warm generally
- Multiple boxes not adjacent to one another
- Away from food, water, and resting places
- Cleaning
  Scoop at least daily
  Litter always appears dry and clean
  Wash with mild, odor-free cleaners—no dried urine or feces on box
  Self-cleaning litter boxes can be an option for some owners

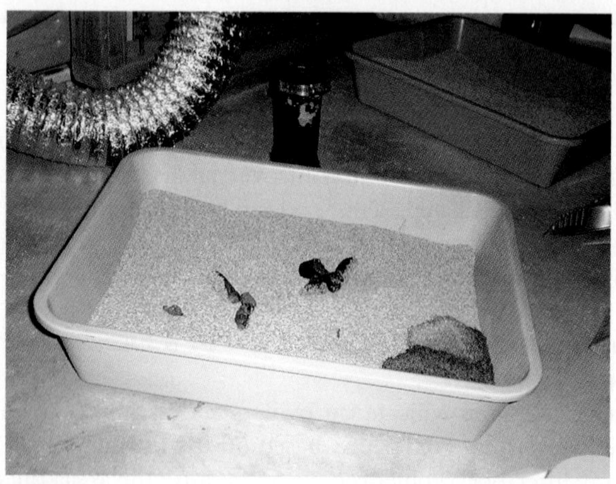

FIGURE 11-3 A litter box that will not meet the behavioral needs of most cats. See text for reasons.

Compare it with a clean litter box (Figure 11-4) located in a quiet, accessible, but private area. It is clear which box better meets the cat's behavioral needs and is therefore more likely to be used.

An Example of Meeting the Pet's Play Needs

Owners who do not realize that they must be prepared to devote time to playing with their pets may become frustrated with their pet's "hyperactivity" or pestering behavior that

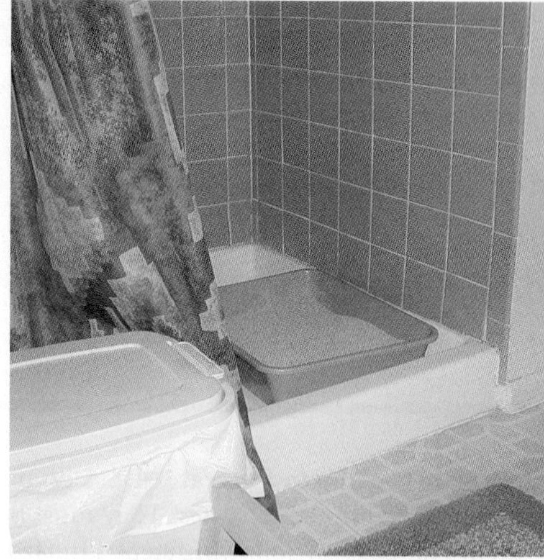

FIGURE 11-4 A cat-friendly litter box. See text for important characteristics.

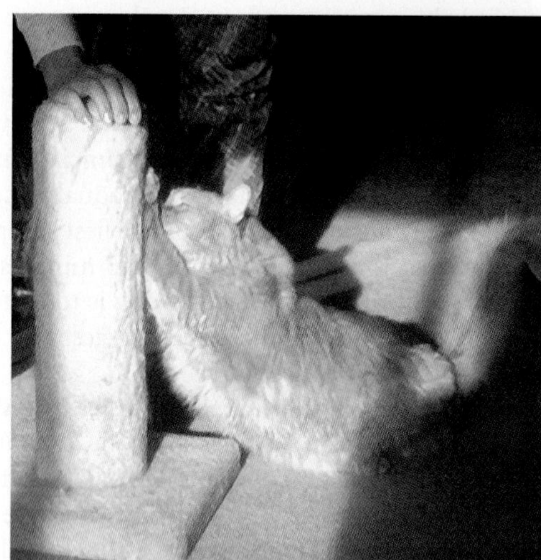

FIGURE 11-5 Cat with a preference for scratching vertical surfaces.

results when this need is not met. Other behavior problems that can result from a lack of physical activity and mental stimulation include self-injurious behaviors, destructive behaviors, excessive vocalizations, difficulties in basic training, and ignoring directions from the owner.

Pets need time for social play with their owners or other animals and for object play with toys. A variety of toys that allow for chewing, chasing, stalking (cats), and retrieving (dogs) should be provided.

Determine Individual Preferences

Technicians can explain to owners that sometimes it may be necessary to create choice situations so that they can determine their pet's preferences relative to various behavioral needs.

For example, cats need objects to scratch, but individual differences exist for what they prefer. Most cats tend to prefer a scratching post that is oriented vertically (Figure 11-5), although some prefer a horizontal scratching area (Figure 11-6). An owner can discover the specific preferences of a cat by giving the cat choices among vertical and horizontal

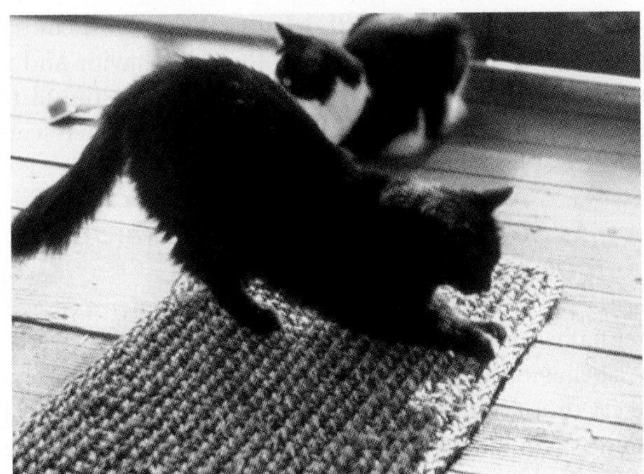

FIGURE 11-6 Cat with a preference for scratching horizontal surfaces.

TABLE 11-2 Examples of Choice Tests to Determine a Pet's Preferences

Preference of Interest	Choice 1	Choice 2
Litter material	Clay	Clumping
Location of pet bed	Adjacent to owner's bed	Bathroom
Cat toys	Puzzle box	Catnip mouse

scratching posts presented at the same time in the same location and then noting which one is most used. Similar choice "tests" can be used to determine what individual animals prefer in the way of toys, bedding, litter boxes, and surfaces for elimination. See Table 11-2 for examples of preferences that could be subjected to testing.

> *TECHNICIAN NOTE* Pet owners may need to set up choice situations to determine their pets' behavioral needs.

Step Four: Use the "Take-Away" Method (Negative Punishment) to Discourage Inappropriate Behavior

Parents may be familiar with the concept, but rarely think to use it with animals. As a reminder, the "take-away" method refers to negative punishment (see Box 11-4 and Table 11-1). To stop an unwanted behavior, technicians can tell owners how to take away something the animal wants. This is similar to taking away a child's television privileges as a consequence of bad grades.

If a puppy is playing too rough, rather than yelling, pushing, or slapping the pup, the owner can walk away and ignore the puppy. The puppy learns that rough play loses him his chance to play at all.

If a horse becomes "pushy" when the handler enters the stall with grain, the handler does not feed the grain to the horse and leaves the stall.

If a cat is meowing for attention, the owner can shut herself in another room for 5 or 10 minutes and not allow the cat to join her.

Negative punishment does not involve the application of aversive stimuli, so it is often preferred over what pet owners generally think of as "discipline" (yelling, hitting, pulling on the collar, squirting the pet with water, scruffing, or pinning), which is discussed in step five. However, if the owner cannot control the pet's access to the "good thing," negative punishment is not the right choice. Behavior that is internally reinforced because it makes the animal "feel better" will not be much affected by any kind of punishment. Barking and meowing, for example, may release tension as a result of fear or anxiety, so ignoring the behavior will not help decrease the frequency of these kinds of vocalizations.

> *TECHNICIAN NOTE* Behavior that is internally reinforced because it makes the animal "feel better" will not be much affected by any kind of punishment.

Examples of situations in which negative punishment can be applied instead of positive punishment are:

- Pet paws at person who is petting her—person stops petting and walks away
- Dog attempts to dash through door before being given permission—owner shuts door and walks away
- Bird screams for attention—owner covers the cage with a towel
- Dog will not release toy for owner to throw—owner walks away and refuses to play with dog
- When told to sit, dog lies down instead—owner withholds tidbit
- Cat A stalks family cat B—cat A is put in a small bathroom for 3 minutes

The last example is a timeout, a "take-away" technique. Technically, the term is "timeout from reinforcement." Practically a timeout means that as a consequence of unwanted behavior, the animal is immediately taken to a place where he does not want to be. A kitten that bites during play can be immediately placed in a small, dark room for a few minutes.

Although theoretically a quite useful technique, using a "timeout" effectively often presents some logistical difficulties. One is finding an appropriate timeout location. Putting a dog outside for a "timeout" if it plays too rough inside will stop the behavior at that moment, but will not have any value in preventing rough play in the future if the dog enjoys being outside.

After episodes of misbehavior, owners often confine their pets for hours in a garage, crate, or small room or ignore them for days, thinking prolonged periods of deprivation will be more effective than shorter ones. This is erroneous. Longer "timeouts" are not more effective than shorter ones. Technicians should actually recommend that owners set a clock to remind them to release the animal from its timeout after about 15 minutes.

Step Five: Minimize "Discipline" (Positive Punishment) and Use It Correctly When Necessary

When the other four steps are followed, discipline becomes less necessary.

For punishment to be used effectively and humanely, several criteria must be met. Some of the more important criteria for effective punishment are as follows.

Immediacy

Any punishment must be delivered within a few seconds after the undesirable behavior occurs. Any longer delay prevents the animal from associating the punishment with the unwanted behavior and increases the likelihood that the pet has performed another behavior before the punishment is delivered. Pet owners mistakenly believe that if a pet can be shown the results of its misbehavior, such as a puddle on the carpet, trash on the floor, or a damaged personal item, the animal will make the connection between past behavior and later attempts at "discipline" when delays of short or long duration separate one from the other.

This belief stems from owners' observations of what they label "guilty looks" when they attempt to deliver punishment after the fact. Such behaviors that dogs display are nothing more than submissive behaviors triggered by the owner's presence and/or her threatening behavior directed toward the dog. Rather than showing submissive behaviors, cats generally hide when they are intimidated.

Some pets learn to determine that when the owner comes home and there is a mess somewhere in the house (trash overturned, feces on the floor, a torn-up couch cushion), bad things will happen to them. If the owner comes home and there is no mess, nothing bad happens, and the pet displays normal greeting behaviors.

Consistency

All occurrences of the undesirable behavior must be punished for punishment to be most effective. If an owner catches the pet misbehaving some of the time but not all of the time, it is likely the behavior will continue because the pet continues to play the odds that it will not be punished. With most behaviors, it is unrealistic to expect owners to be available to immediately and consistently deliver a positive punishment. This is one reason that there are a limited number of situations and problems that can benefit from owner-delivered positive punishment.

Appropriate Intensity

Animals will learn to tolerate higher levels of aversive stimuli if they are presented with such stimuli in gradually increasing intensity rather than initially experiencing a moderately intense stimulus. For example, an owner might gently tell his or her dog "no," which is not sufficient to stop the misbehavior. The owner may say "no" in gradually increasing threatening tones until it is necessary to scream at the dog to get him to stop the behavior. In contrast, an owner who says "no" in a more firm, authoritative tone of voice initially is more likely to successfully stop the misbehavior and not have to scream. Unfortunately, many aversive stimuli that are intense enough to inhibit behaviors can also elicit fearful and aggressive responses.

Remote Punishment Is Usually Preferable to Interactive Punishment

Positive punishment that comes from the owner has several potentially undesirable outcomes. First, the pet often learns that a behavior will be punished only in the owner's presence. The cat thus scratches the stereo speaker or the dog lifts his leg on the couch only when the owner is at work. This leads owners to incorrectly and anthropomorphically conclude that the pet "knows better" because the behavior only occurs when the owner is not present. Second, owner-delivered punishment, especially if it is severe (scruff shakes, rollovers, hitting) or does not meet the other criteria, can result in the pet being afraid of or aggressive toward the owner and has a negative impact on the human-animal bond. Remote punishments or booby traps are more likely to be immediate and consistent. Examples of remote punishers are as follows:

- Citronella Anti-Bark Collar (Premier Pet Products) (Figure 11-7)
- Motion detector (SSSCAT, Premier Pet Products) (Figure 11-8)
- Scat Mat (Contech, Inc.) (Figure 11-9)
- Hand-held noisemaker, such as an air horn (Safety Sport) (Figure 11-10) or ultrasonic device
- DirectStop, a harmless spray of dilute citronella oil that nonetheless most pets find unpleasant because of its odor and startling delivery (Figure 11-11)

These last two products require activation by the owner, who must be able to covertly, immediately, and consistently activate them.

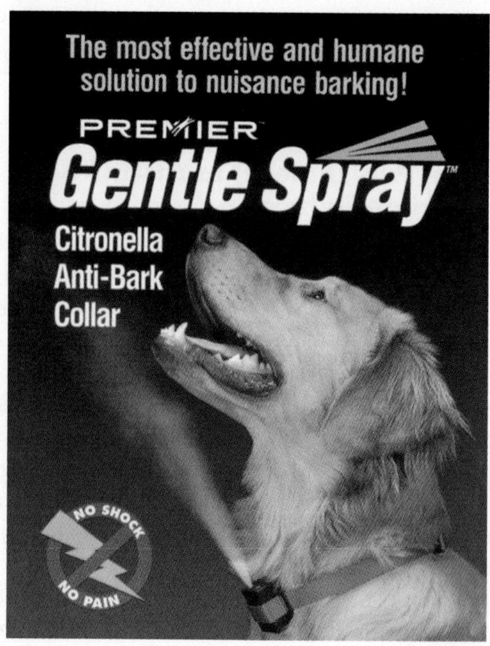

FIGURE 11-7 Citronella Anti-Bark Collar. (Premier Pet Products.)

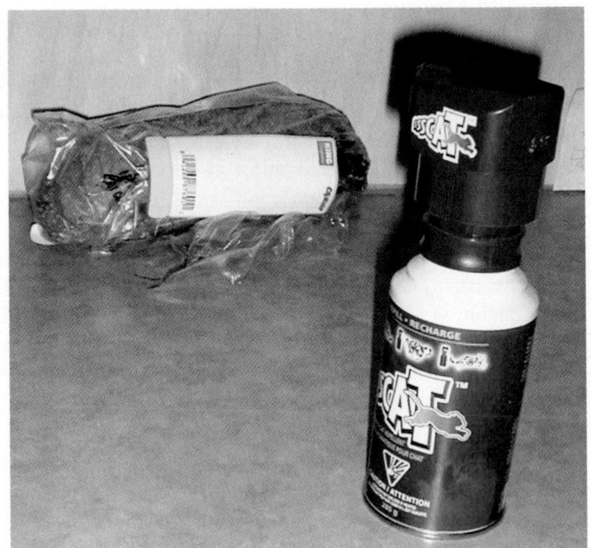

FIGURE 11-8 Motion detector. (SSSCAT, Premier Pet Products, Inc.)

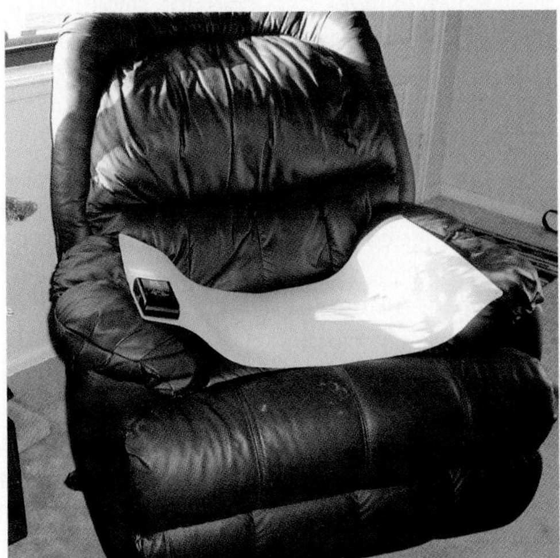

FIGURE 11-9 Scat Mat. (Contech, Inc.)

By definition, punishment decreases the frequency of the behavior it follows. If an owner has repeatedly attempted to punish a behavior but the pet is still showing the behavior at the same frequency, then the behavior has not really been punished.

A general guideline that technicians can give owners is that if positive punishment has not been successful after three to five applications, it probably will not be successful. Either this is not the best technique for the problem, or it is being implemented incorrectly.

> *TECHNICIAN NOTE* Technicians can tell owners that if positive punishment has not been successful after three to five applications, it probably will not be successful.

Even more importantly, technicians should encourage owners to shift their perspective from "how can I get my pet to stop a certain behavior?" which implies the need for some sort of aversive consequence, to "how can I get my pet to do what I want so I can reward it?" With this perspective, the first three steps of the five-step plan are usually the most important.

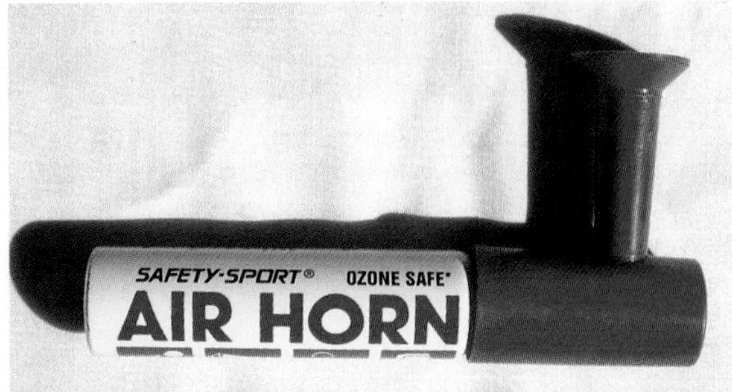

FIGURE 11-10 Hand-held noisemaker, such as an air horn. (Safety Sport.)

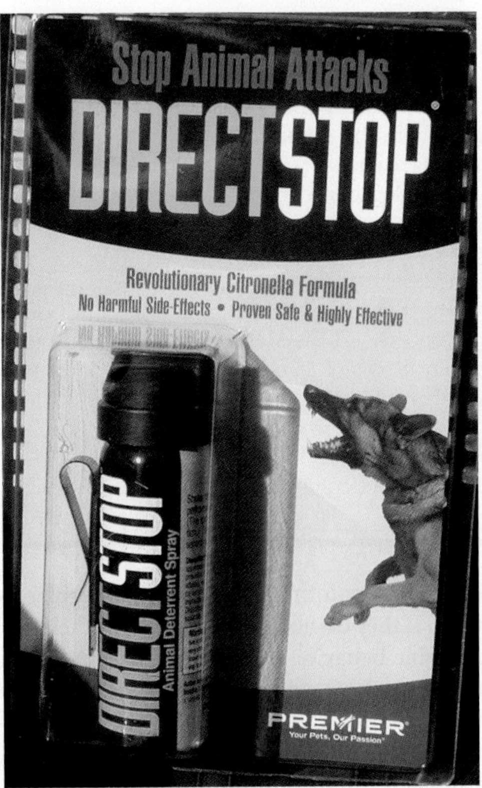

FIGURE 11-11 DirectStop, citronella deterrent spray. (Premier Pet Products.)

Examples of how the five-step plan can be applied to canine house training and to introducing pets to one another can be found in Box 11-14 and Box 11-15, respectively, and a list of behaviors and situations for which technicians should provide owners a five-step plan is provided in Box 11-15.

BEHAVIOR ASSESSMENTS

A recent study showed that as few as 25% of veterinarians routinely discuss behavior issues with clients, 17% never do, and only 11% of veterinarians thought it was their responsibility to initiate discussions about behavior problems with clients (Patronek and Dodman, 1999).

A behavior wellness approach requires that technicians and other veterinary professionals take the initiative during every wellness appointment and perhaps other

BOX 11-14 Using the Five-Step Positive Proaction Plan to Introduce Dogs to Cats

1. Catch the pets doing something right. Place towels impregnated with the other's scents under food bowls, in favorite resting locations, on the pet's bed, and in locations that have pleasant associations for both pets. Feed each pet on either side of a closed door to encourage calm, relaxed behavior in each other's presence.
2. Do not let bad habits develop. Keep the pets separated and allow them to only hear one another and smell one another's scent initially. Use confinement and restraint to safely and gradually allow visual and later physical contact and prevent fear or aggressive behaviors from either pet.
3. Meet the pet's behavioral needs. Provide the cat with hiding and other safe places to avoid or escape from the dog or, in rare cases, vice versa. Each pet should have sufficient play, exercise, and social time. The resident animal's routine should be disrupted as little as possible.
4. Use the "take-away" method to discourage unwanted behavior. A dog can be put on a leash and required to lie down and stay (he has his freedom taken away) should he begin to chase the cat.
5. Minimize "discipline" and use it correctly, when necessary. Punishment should not be a large part of introducing one pet to another. Owners, however, should be prepared to punish one animal *immediately* if they fear for the other's safety. For "discipline" to be used in a timely fashion, owners must be prepared to deliver it within the 3-sec time frame, if necessary. A dog, for example, could be sprayed with DirectStop, carried on the owner's belt, should it chase the cat.

nonemergency appointments to perform regular behavior assessments. If they do not, opportunities for helping owners create desirable behavior and for early detection and intervention when problems do arise will be lost.

Owners will resort to inquiring about behavior only at the crisis stage in which the pet's continued presence in the home is at risk. With the support of the veterinarian, trained technicians are best positioned to conduct behavior assessments before the start of the medical appointment.

Behavior assessments involve the following five major areas:

1. How well the animal meets the criteria for a behaviorally healthy pet
2. Family conditions or changes that put pets at risk for surrender
3. The pet's daily routine, lifestyle, and whether its behavioral needs are being met
4. Identification of early warning signs and problems
5. The pet's behavior observed at the veterinary hospital

How Well the Animal Meets the Criteria for a Behaviorally Healthy Pet

For each behavior listed in Box 11-16, owners can be asked to rate their pet's behaviors on a 5-point Likert scale (always, usually, sometimes, rarely, or never). Technicians can discuss in depth those behaviors that owners rank as "rarely" or "never." Certain behaviors may be sufficiently important to discuss, even if an owner rated them as "sometimes." A pet that is only "sometimes" friendly with people may have

BOX 11-15 Using the Five-Step Positive Proaction Plan to Facilitate Canine House Training

1. Catch the dog doing something right. Reward the dog with a treat, praise, and/or petting for eliminating outside. Go to the dog rather than waiting for the dog to return to the door. If the treat is given after the dog has returned to the door, that is the behavior that is rewarded. If the dog enjoys leash walks and eliminating terminates the walk, eliminating is being negatively punished (it ends the opportunity to continue walking).
2. Do not let bad habits develop. The dog should be constantly supervised (or crated when left alone during house training) so that he does not have an opportunity to house soil.
3. Meet the pet's behavioral needs. Provide the dog with sufficient opportunities for elimination and locations that meet its behavioral preferences. Many dogs prefer soft surfaces, such as grass, so a gravel-covered pen may not be acceptable. Provide an outside area that is protected from weather extremes (wet and cold for small, short-coated dogs or hot and humid for heavy-coated dogs). Accustom puppies to those surfaces that they will be expected to use for elimination as adults. For urban dogs, these may be city streets and curbs.
4. Use the "take-away" method to discourage unwanted behavior. This step is not directly applicable to house training. If the owner catches the dog soiling, the dog should merely be taken outside immediately. The owner should evaluate where the breakdown occurred that allowed the house soiling. Was the dog allowed too much freedom? Had too much time elapsed since his last chance to relieve himself?
5. Minimize "discipline" and use it correctly, when necessary. The process of house training is creating the correct preferences for where and on what the dog likes to eliminate and helping the dog learn that the entire house is his living area (or den) and should not be soiled. Discipline is not important in house training.

BOX 11-16 Behaviors and Situations for Which the Five-Step Plan Should Be Given to Clients

- Elimination behavior
- Play behaviors
- Normal destructive behaviors (play, investigation, chewing, or teething)
- Barking
- Introducing new pets to the family, especially children and resident pets
- Introducing new pets to resident family pets
- Acclimating dogs to being left alone
- Acclimating pets to being handled and examined

BOX 11-17 Behavior Assessment: Questions About Family Lifestyle Changes That Put Pets at Risk for Problems

- Are you planning a move to a different house?
- Will the composition of your family change in the near future (new baby, marriage, divorce, children moving home, etc.)?
- Will any infants or young children reach the crawling or walking stage in the near future?
- Will any family member's schedule undergo a significant change in the near future (e.g., resuming or leaving work, school, hours or shift change at work)?
- Will you be going on vacation? Different preparation may be needed for the pet if it is going with the family, left at home with a pet sitter, or will be boarded.
- Will you be doing any home improvement or construction?
- Will you be acquiring another pet, or have you recently lost a pet?

BOX 11-18 Behavior Assessment Questions Regarding Pet's Management, Lifestyle, and Provision for Behavior Needs

- Does your pet have free run of the house when you are gone, or is she kept crated; left outside, in the basement, or in the garage; or confined to a small part of the house on a regular basis? If the pet is confined, why?
- Where does your pet sleep at night?
- Is your cat allowed outside? When and for how long? Supervised, leashed, confined or not?
- Is your pet recently spending more time outside because its behavior inside the house has become more of a problem?
- How do you discipline your pet? What does your pet need to be disciplined for? What is the strongest discipline procedure you have ever used?
- How many hours does your pet spend alone?
- How much exercise and play time does your pet receive each day?
- What toys does your pet have? How does your pet like to play?

an aggression problem that requires immediate assistance. A checklist form of these behaviors can be downloaded for free from www.AnimalBehaviorAssociates.com.

Family Conditions or Changes That Put Pets at Risk for Surrender

A move, addition of a new baby, a change in a family member's schedule, vacation, remodeling, and the addition or loss of another family pet are all examples of changes that frequently trigger behavior problems. If impending changes are identified, additional behavioral services can be provided to pet owners to help them proactively prepare their pets and minimize the potential negative effects on the pet's behavior. Examples of questions to ask are provided in Box 11-17.

The Pet's Daily Routine, Lifestyle, and Whether Its Behavioral Needs Are Being Met

Recent research shows that where a pet spends its time during the day may be a risk factor for relinquishment. One study revealed that dogs who were confined in crates, left outside, or confined to a small part of the house on a routine basis were at a greater risk for surrender to a shelter than those who had free run of the house (Patronek et al, 1996a). Similarly, cats that were allowed outside were also at a greater risk (Patronek et al, 1996b). Thus it may be important to find out where the pet spends most of its time.

Problem behaviors can occur when an animal's behavioral needs are not being met or when the animal is getting its needs met by using inappropriate behaviors. Technicians can inquire about the pet's behavioral needs based on the categories in Box 11-12. Box 11-18 gives examples of questions regarding the pet's routines and whether the pet's behavioral needs are being met.

Identification of Early Warning Signs of Problems

Owners often do not interpret behaviors as early warning signs of potential problems, such as the following:

- The dog leaves the room and avoids an infant whenever the infant is placed on a blanket on the floor. The owner may not understand that this is an indication that the dog is fearful, a behavior that could escalate to growling and snapping when the infant reaches the crawling or toddler stage.
- The cat often urinates right next to the litter box. The owner tolerates and never mentions this behavior because it occurs on cement in the unfinished basement. The owner may not have the foresight to see that when he or she decides to finish the basement, this will likely result in the cat urinating on the new carpet.
- An owner who reports the adult dog that they just added to their home is "just fine" when meeting and greeting new people, but you observe the dog to be quite still, eyes wide and dilated, and without any evidence of friendly behavior when you approach him.
- A dog owner who is a teacher has been home all summer with a new puppy. She or he thinks it is cute that the puppy cries, paws, and becomes distressed at the door when the owner steps outside for a short time to get the mail or mow the yard. The owner does not view this behavior as an indication of a potential separation anxiety problem when she or he goes back to work in the fall.

The important point in these examples is that the owners would never think to discuss these behaviors with the technician because they do not see them as problems or potential problems. People surrendering their pets to a shelter

BOX 11-19 Behavior Assessment: Questions to Ask to Identify Early Warning Signs

- Is there anything you (or any other family member) are afraid or reluctant to do with or to your pet?
- What does your pet not like done?
- What things is your pet afraid of? How does she behave when afraid?
- What does your pet do when you do the following:
  - Clip nails
  - Brush her
  - Take food or toys away
  - Roll her over on her back
  - Touch her body in certain places
  - Discipline her
  - Pick her up
  - Pet her for awhile
  - Reach for her collar
  - Walk by or disturb her when she is resting
  - Tell her to move from the bed or furniture
  - Disturb her while she is asleep

had often experienced some lifestyle change that either prevented them from continuing to tolerate the problem or, as in these examples, resulted in the same behavior becoming less tolerable (DiGiacomo et al, 1998; Scarlett et al, 1999). A behavior assessment can be used to detect these situations and identify problems or potential problems earlier.

Box 11-19 gives examples of questions that technicians can ask owners for the purpose of identifying these warning signs. Things owners mention that the animal does not like and activities that elicit fearful, threatening, aggressive, or avoidance behaviors may later be associated with full-blown behavior problems.

The Pet's Behavior Observed at the Veterinary Hospital

Technicians should make note of the pet's demeanor at the veterinary hospital. This is important not only in assessing the pet's behavioral health, but in keeping the staff safe when handling the pet. Occurrences of fearful, threatening, or aggressive behavior should be put in the patient's record, shared with the staff, and discussed with the owner. It is a good idea to mark the front of a fractious or dangerous patient's file with a hard-to-miss symbol so that technicians are aware of the patient's behavioral history before attempting any interactions. In addition, technicians should receive clear instructions or protocols from the veterinarian as to what they should do differently when a patient identified in this way comes into the hospital.

When technicians observe dangerous or threatening behavior from a patient, they must discuss this with the veterinarian. The veterinarian must in turn share this information with the owner. Under the veterinarian's direction, technicians may be asked to discuss these problems with the owner. Veterinarians and technicians can prepare a script for the conversation with the owner. Examples of

BOX 11-20 Points for Discussion With the Owner When Behaviors of Concern Are Observed in the Veterinary Hospital

- We are concerned about the pet not receiving top-quality care.
- We are concerned about safety of the staff.
- Pet should be able to tolerate basic handling.
- Discuss the pet's behavior, rather than labeling the pet as a problem.
- We did everything we could to minimize his stress, yet he still became upset.
- Behavior was out of proportion to the situation.

discussion points are listed in Box 11-20. To gain a sense of the breadth of the problem, technicians should also ask the owner whether the pet has displayed similar behavior in other contexts.

> *TECHNICIAN NOTE* Veterinary professionals should make behavior assessments a routine part of every pet's ongoing health care.

Interpersonal Skills to Use During Behavior Assessment

Interviewing Skills: Asking Good Questions

Initiating discussions requires excellent interviewing skills. Such skills are important not only in behavioral wellness programs, but also during the process of taking a medical history. The first important interviewing skill is asking nonleading, open-ended questions. Good questions do not lead the client into a particular answer and require more than a yes or no answer. Questions such as "Is your pet showing any problem behavior?" or "Do you have any questions about setting up a litter box?" do not meet these criteria. A client could answer both questions "no" and yet have a 6-month-old dog who growls when people come too close to the food dish (the owner thinks this is normal and therefore not a problem), or the owner may have located a new kitten's litter box in the basement on a cement floor next to the furnace (the owner sees nothing wrong with this placement and thus has no questions). More productive questions might be: "What does your pet not like you to do with him?" and "Would you describe your kitten's litter box to me?" Follow-up questions may be necessary, and the technician may need to ask the same question in several ways to obtain concrete, detailed information.

Interviewing Skills: Interpersonal Communication

For owners to provide good information about their pets, they need to feel comfortable talking to the veterinary technician. Clients need to know that technicians are not just "going through the motions," but are genuinely interested in them, their pets, and what they have to say. Even on a busy day, a harried technician can make a good impression and encourage clients to open up, while at the same time keeping the conversation on track, by using a few simple communication skills.

Put clients at ease by sitting down. Conducting the behavioral interview sitting down puts the technician and client at the same level and also helps relieve any tension or nervousness. The technician who remains standing gives the impression of being in a hurry or less approachable. Having clients sit down helps to relax them and put them more at ease.

> *TECHNICIAN NOTE* When talking to clients, the technician should face them to communicate that they are the focus of attention.

Use active listening skills. A technician should face clients when talking to them to communicate that the clients are the focus of attention. If the technician's body is directed elsewhere, the message is that so is his or her attention. The technician can keep an open body posture by trying not to cross legs or arms, hold a clipboard or folder at chest or face level, or stand behind a barrier, such as an examination table. Doing so sends the message that the technician is not completely open to hearing the client. Maintaining casual eye contact by looking at the client from time to time, rather than burying one's face in papers, enhances communication. Looking up while still being able to take notes takes practice, but it is a skill worth developing. The technician can acknowledge what the client is saying by giving frequent feedback without interrupting; by nodding his or her head; by saying "OK," "Hmmm," or "I see"; or making other neutral, quick statements to let the client know that the technician is engaged in the conversation. A warm or neutral tone of voice, rather than an abrupt or abrasive one, should be used.

Obtain behavioral descriptions, not interpretations. Owners often describe their pets' behavior in relatively vague terms, such as "He goes crazy at the door!" Consider the following three examples of what this statement might actually mean. When the doorbell rings, the dog does the following:

- Barks, growls, runs to the door, and lunges at the people he sees outside
- Wildly jumps up, grabs his ball, races to the door, tail wagging, with a "happy face," and thrusts his wet, slimy ball into the visitor's hand
- Barks continuously, shies away from the door, hides behind the owner, and will not allow visitors to get near him

These are just three of many possible things that "He goes crazy at the door!" might mean. This illustrates the importance of obtaining behavioral descriptions, rather than interpretations. The technician can ask, "What does your pet do at the door? Describe the behaviors you see." The technician should continue to probe for additional information until he or she is certain what a client is attempting to describe. Repeated questioning may be necessary to obtain descriptions that provide a mental picture of the behavior in question. While probing for more information, the technician should use good communication skills so that clients understand that he or she is genuinely attempting to clarify information rather than harassing them with repeated questions. The technician can paraphrase a client's description of the pet's behavior by asking, "So when the doorbell rings, your dog barks and jumps on people—is that correct?" This question gives the client an opportunity to agree with the technician or provide additional information.

Using the Results of Behavior Assessments

The behavior assessment should be made a part of the pet's permanent record, and the technician should discuss the results with the veterinarian. An action plan could include a medical examination, an in-house behavior consultation, referral to a behavior consultant, referral to a dog trainer for obedience classes, dissemination of educational materials, or a recommendation for particular behavior-management products. The veterinarian may ask the technician to present or assist in presenting all or part of this action to the client. Technicians should be sure that they understand what role they play in delivering this information and avoid taking it upon themselves to develop any part of this action plan—including referrals—without approval from the veterinarian.

Follow-Up for Behavior Assessments

Once the veterinarian has created an action plan, technicians can be responsible for conducting behavioral follow-up telephone calls, just as many currently do for medical cases. After routine surgeries, suturing, or dental procedures, technicians are often given the responsibility of calling clients to inquire about the pet's status and progress. Behavior issues deserve the same type of follow-up. Technicians can call the client to determine whether the pet owner followed through with the suggested referral, implemented any training or behavior modification techniques that were suggested, or purchased behavior-management products that were recommended. Technicians can also help owners implement a behavior modification plan created by the veterinarian or outside behavior consultant. Few veterinary practices have routine procedures in place to follow up on behavioral problems in the same way they follow up on medical problems, so well-informed technicians have the opportunity to set important precedents.

> *TECHNICIAN NOTE* When behavioral concerns or issues are identified, a behavior wellness approach demands that these be addressed and not ignored. The practice should give pet owners specific recommendations or action plans.

MAKING THE VETERINARY PRACTICE A BEHAVIORALLY FRIENDLY PLACE

Visiting the veterinary practice is stressful for some pets and consequently for their owners. An animal that is stressed or fearful is more likely to injure a staff member. Animals in such states are more difficult to handle and consequently may not receive the best possible medical care. Each visit that results in stress and unpleasantness for the pet ensures that future visits will become more difficult.

One of the ways pet owners judge the quality of the veterinary hospital, the staff, and the services provided is by how their animals are treated. Using behaviorally friendly methods with patients is "walking the talk" of behavior wellness care. Clients will better understand the idea of behavior wellness care when they see technicians use positive and proactive techniques when handling their pets. It is to everyone's benefit to take a behavior wellness approach and help patients be more relaxed at the veterinary practice. Rather than having to calm down animals that arrive at the practice already stressed, a proactive behavior wellness approach seeks to create patients that have positive expectations when they arrive at the veterinary practice.

The first step in lowering patient stress is to understand species-typical behaviors when an animal feels threatened or challenged.

Understanding Social Conflict Behavior

When animals feel threatened or challenged in social interactions, they have a variety of choices as to how to respond. These choices are called agonistic behaviors. By understanding the choices animals may make in social conflict situations, technicians can often decrease conflict, more humanely handle and restrain animals with less use of force, and be safer themselves. The most common agonistic behaviors technicians are likely to see in a veterinary medical context are described in following sections.

> *TECHNICIAN NOTE* Technicians should understand the choices animals may make in social conflict situations.

Escape and Avoidance

Many animals initially try to avoid conflict. Animals may try to get away or struggle to avoid restraint. Sometimes it may be better to allow the animal to avoid conflict rather than escalating forceful restraint. Backing off, giving the animal a chance to calm down, and trying other techniques are safer choices for the technician and less stressful for the animal. Allowing avoidance to "work" for the animal is usually not as bad as forcing the issue and escalating the situation until the animal and possibly the technician are out of control.

An animal that is trying to escape and avoid conflict is *not* trying to "be dominant," a common misinterpretation of the situation. Although there is the rare patient that is offensively motivated in this way, if the technician pays close attention to the animal's body language, using the information given later in this chapter, it will be easy to recognize the difference.

Submissive Behavior

Dogs that show passive submissive behaviors (Figure 11-12) when threatened are not dangerous to handle. They are acquiescing, or "giving in." Technicians should handle and restrain such animals gently. Some submissive behaviors, such as lowered ears and tail and a crouched position, are also displayed when a dog is fearful (see Figure 11-24), so technicians may ease the dog's stress by changing their behaviors so as to appear less threatening.

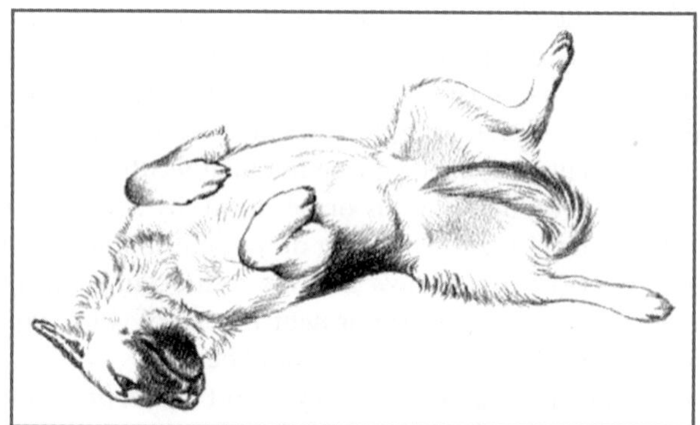

FIGURE 11-12 Submissive dog. Canine submissive postures and behaviors include rolling over or crouched body posture, avoidance of eye contact, low tail carriage, ears back, whining, and/or a submissive grin. (Copyright 2008. The American Society for the Prevention of Cruelty to Animals® [ASPCA®]. All Rights Reserved.)

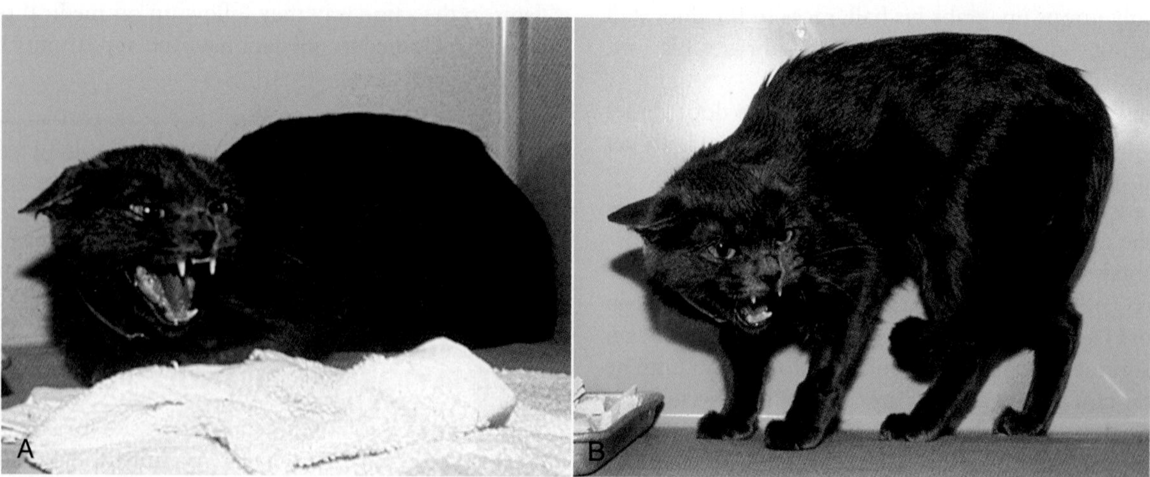

FIGURE 11-13 Defensively threatening cats. Feline defensive postures and behaviors include hissing, ears back or flattened to the side, baring teeth with an open mouth, rolling over or upright posture with arched back, tucked tail.

Cats and other species of animals that do not live in structured social groups typically do not show submissive behaviors. When cats cannot avoid conflict, they typically become defensively threatening or aggressive (Figure 11-13). Cats may sometimes be fearful without being threatening (Figure 11-14).

Threatening Behavior

The goal of threats is to warn, not to harm or hurt. Many behaviors that are commonly referred to as "aggression" are more accurately categorized as threats. These include baring teeth, growling or hissing, lunging, barking, scratching, and attempts to bite or inhibited bites. Animals that "air-snap" or bite without injury are being threatening. It is generally not true that a technician can avoid a bite by being quicker than the animal. Rather it is usually the case that the animal was never intent on biting, only on threatening. Threats can be either offensive or defensive. An offensive threat is accompanied by the body postures seen in Figures 11-15 and 11-16. Defensive dogs and cats are shown in Figures 11-13 and 11-17. Animals are much more likely to be defensive in a veterinary context. This means they are both fearful and threatening. Defensive animals do not take the initiative to charge their opponents and will not bite if left alone. Offensive animals can lunge, charge, and chase their targets.

Technicians should always assume that threatening behaviors can escalate into aggression at any moment.

Aggressive Behavior

Aggressive behavior harms the opponent. Threats and aggression can overlap. An animal may initially respond to a threat by showing threatening body postures, but may eventually bite or snap. Whereas a bite attempt that never touches the opponent is clearly a threat, a bite that leaves

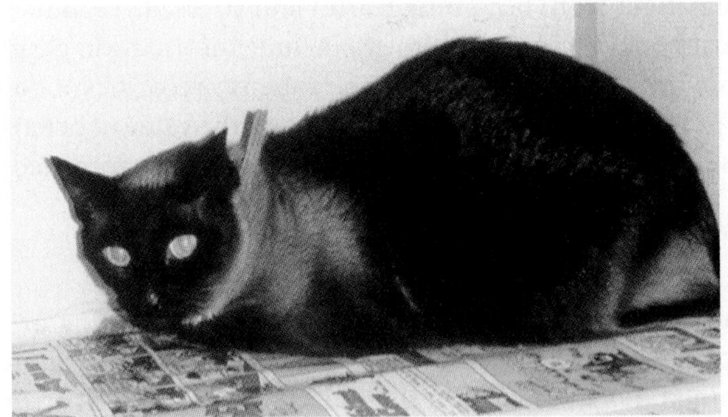

FIGURE 11-14 Fearful cat. Feline fearful postures include crouched body carriage, tail and feet tucked under body, and dilated pupils.

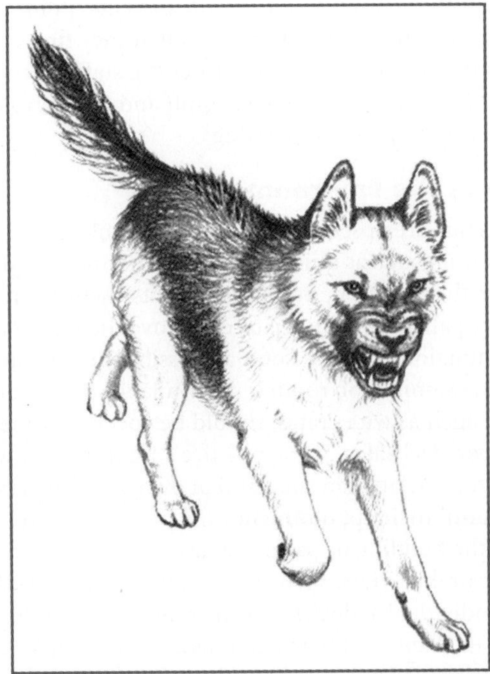

FIGURE 11-15 Offensively threatening dog. Canine offensive threats include upright ears, tail carried high, direct stare, piloerection, baring teeth with vertical lip retraction, stiff upright body carriage, and barking or growling. (Copyright 2008. The American Society for the Prevention of Cruelty to Animals® [ASPCA®]. All Rights Reserved.)

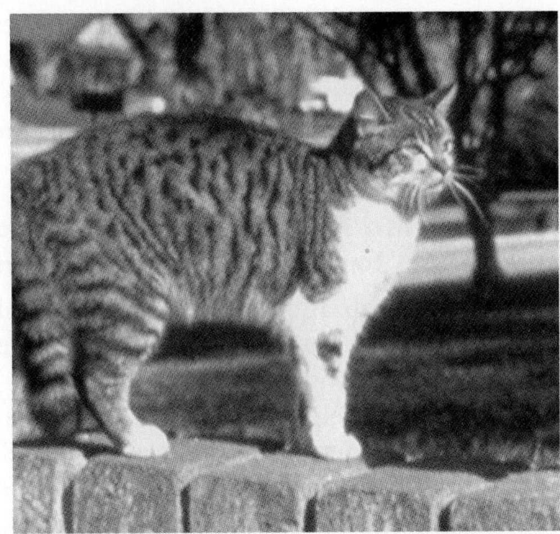

FIGURE 11-16 Offensively threatening cats. Feline offensive threats include a stiff upright posture, direct stare, ears upright, piloerection, tail stiff and held straight down. The tabby cat on the right has a slight arch to its back, indicating a small defensive component to its behavior.

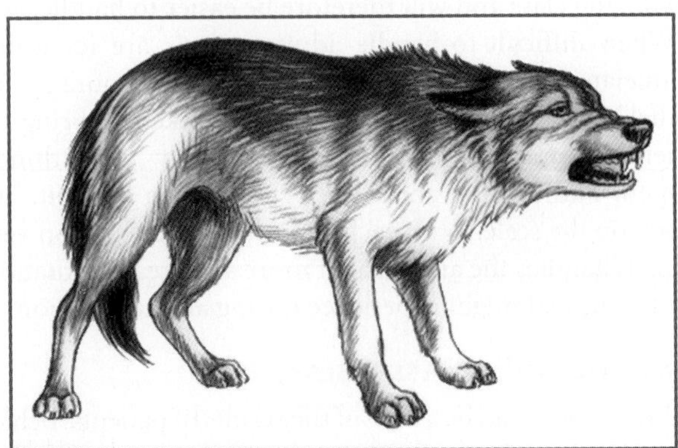

FIGURE 11-17 Defensively threatening dog. Canine defensive threats include avoidance of eye contact, crouched posture, ears back, tail down, teeth bared with horizontal retraction of the lips, barking or growling. (Copyright 2008. The American Society for the Prevention of Cruelty to Animals® [ASPCA®]. All Rights Reserved.)

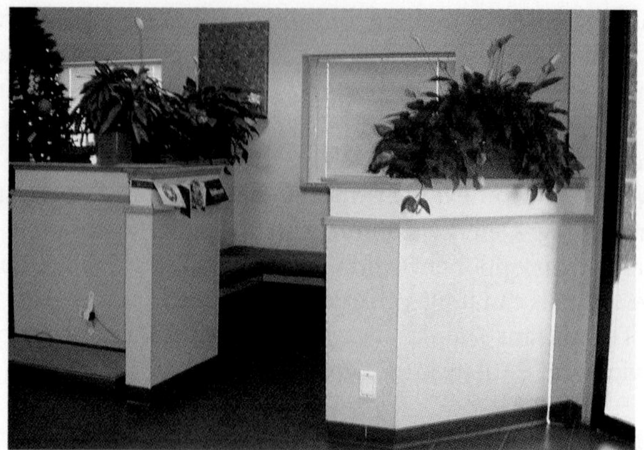

FIGURE 11-18 Cubicle in a veterinary practice reception area. The cubicle creates social distance between patients, creates a barrier from the entrance, and helps to keep patients' arousal levels low.

TABLE 11-3 Postures to Avoid When Approaching Fearful or Unfamiliar Dogs

Postures to Avoid	Appropriate Postures
Direct eye contact	Look at the floor, off to the side, or above the dog's head
Frontal approach	Turn the side of the body toward the dog or approach at a slight angle rather than head on
Reaching toward or over	Allow the dog to approach, let the dog sniff a hand held at the side of the body, pet the dog from under the chin
Leaning forward, over	Bend at the knees or stand straight up over the dog's body

a red mark, indentation, bruise, or other minor injury is in an area of transition between a threat and aggression. As with threats, most aggressive behavior that technicians will see in the veterinary context is likely defensive rather than offensive. This is why it is so important for technicians to use the proactive, nonthreatening techniques to be discussed to prevent patients from becoming fearful and feeling the need to defend themselves.

Using Puppy and Kitten Classes to Socialize Young Animals to the Veterinary Practice

Puppy and kitten socialization classes, which have already been mentioned, are one way to help create positive expectations and associations with the veterinary practice. These socialization classes can help young animals become familiar with the sights, sounds, and smells of the practice under enjoyable conditions. During class, young animals can be put on the scale and an examination table and subjected to brief handling procedures paired with treats and petting. This allows them to become somewhat familiar with the staff and with the physical environment. When they come for their next appointment, they will be entering a familiar environment, expecting the same sort of pleasant experiences they had during class and will therefore be easier to handle.

When difficult-to-handle adult animals are identified, technicians can suggest that veterinarians encourage "remedial" socialization visits. Owners are asked to bring the patient in for a brief visit during which only "good things" happen. Perhaps the animal is petted, given a tidbit, and placed on the scale. With each succeeding socialization visit, the staff handles the animal a bit more and creates situations that the animal might experience during an examination.

Using Behavior Assessments

Technicians should be aware of the results of patients' behavior assessments (Boxes 11-17 through 11-19) before handling them. By a forewarning about what a pet does not like, how the pet reacts to everyday handling, and whether the pet has shown aggressive or threatening behavior under certain circumstances, the technician can be better equipped to prevent the patient from becoming fearful and stressed. Technicians must be sure to take the time to include information gleaned from behavior assessments in the patient's record. Not doing so puts fellow staff members at risk, and the value of behavior assessments will be lost if the information is not recorded.

Establish a Positive Expectation in the Waiting Area

The emotional reactions patients have in the waiting or reception area will affect their arousal level when they are examined. If experiences in the waiting area increase patients' arousal, patients will be more difficult to handle. Such experiences, particularly with cats, are common triggers for aggression later redirected toward technicians. Technicians can assess the waiting area from the patients' point of view. What do the animals see and hear when they first enter the door to the veterinary practice? Does the staff approach too quickly? Is a dog close enough to sniff and frighten a cat in a carrier or to lunge at another dog?

Manage the Environment

Animals that are upset or overly excited should be moved out of the waiting area as quickly as possible. This not only helps to lower their arousal, but also prevents them from agitating other patients. Technicians can move these animals into an examination room as soon as possible or even an office area if an examination room is not available. See-through cat carriers, such as wire crates, should be covered immediately so that cats feel safer. If the practice's location and weather permit, technicians can suggest that owners leave patients in the car until their appointment time or take dogs for a walk around the building or parking area.

Structural barriers, such as half walls (Figure 11-18) that create individual cubicles, are helpful additions to reception areas. Plants or other inanimate objects can be used to block patients' views of one another. Chairs can be arranged to create more space between patients and placed back to back so that pets and their owners are not sitting across the room facing one another. Owners can be asked to position their pets or their carriers so that the animals are facing them (or a wall) rather than another patient. Ideally, cats and dogs should have separate entrances or at least be segregated into different sections of the waiting area.

Interactions With Staff: Greetings

Technicians must know how to approach patients in a nonthreatening way. The behaviors most people use to greet dogs are all, to the dog, offensive threats. These postures are listed in the left-hand column of Table 11-3 and illustrated in Figure 11-19. Cats also tend to perceive these postures as threatening.

Technicians must develop the habit of using nonthreatening behaviors when greeting patients. In general, these are the opposite of the behaviors described previously and are listed in the right-hand column of Table 11-3 and illustrated in Figure 11-20.

> *TECHNICIAN NOTE* Technicians must develop the habit of using nonthreatening behaviors when greeting patients.

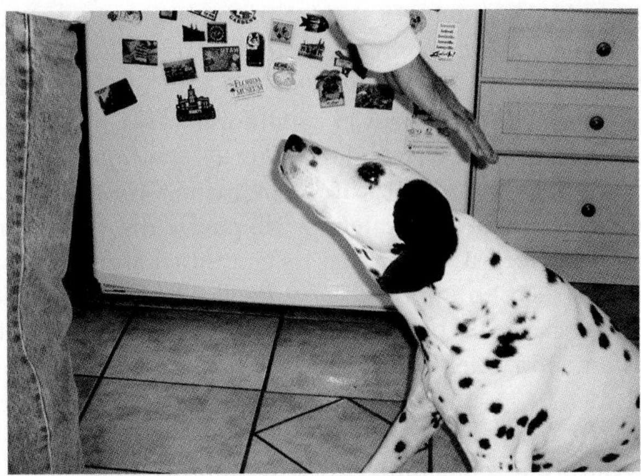

FIGURE 11-19 Threatening-appearing greeting. Person is reaching over dog's head, facing dog, and leaning over dog.

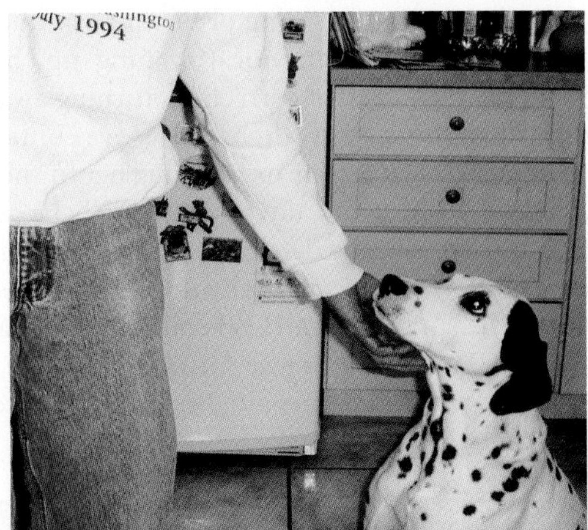

FIGURE 11-20 Nonthreatening greeting. Person has turned side of body toward dog, is not bending at the waist, and is petting dog under chin.

When possible, technicians can allow the pet to approach them rather than invading the animal's personal space. These nonthreatening behaviors make an immediate, significant, observable difference in patients' behaviors.

Before petting a cat, the technician should first allow the cat to sniff either a finger or an inanimate object, such as a pen (Figure 11-21). This mimics a typical friendly cat-to-cat greeting of sniffing noses (Figure 11-22). Many cats do not like to be stroked down their backs or patted on the head, particularly by an unfamiliar person. Instead, technicians can rub cats on their scent glands located on their cheeks and in front of their ears (Figure 11-23).

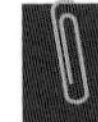

> *TECHNICIAN NOTE* Most cats do not like to be stroked and patted in the same way as dogs.

Because cats are extremely sensitive to odors, technicians should wash their hands before greeting a cat and consider spraying Feliway (Abbott Laboratories) on their hands. Feliway is a synthetic analog of the cat's facial pheromones and is said to have a calming effect on cats when they are in unfamiliar surroundings. Feliway can also be sprayed on an examination table or in a holding cage before the cat is placed in it. (This product has received mixed reviews and

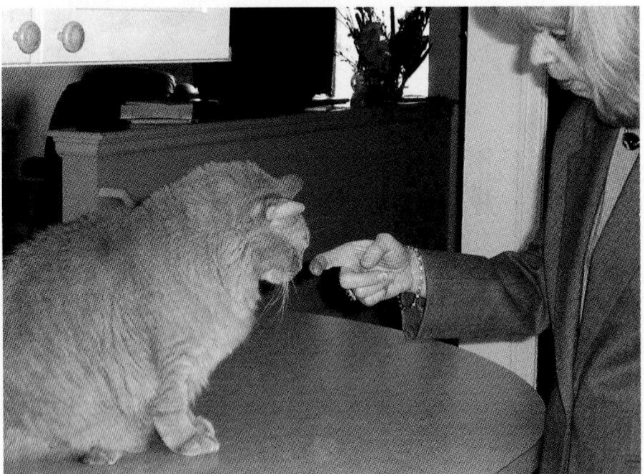

FIGURE 11-21 Friendly cat greeting person. Cat is sniffing the person's finger, similar to how it would sniff the nose of another cat.

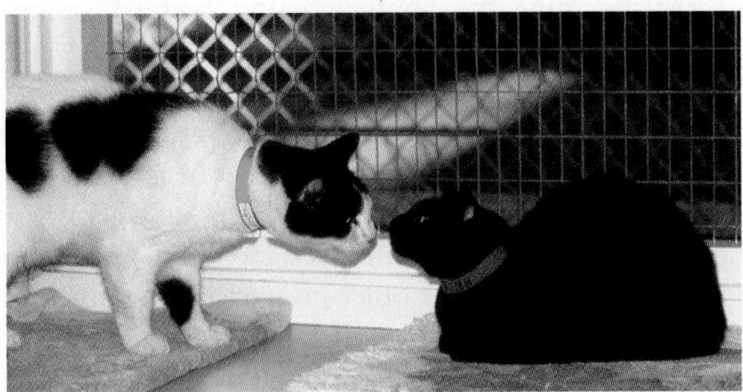

FIGURE 11-22 Friendly cat-to-cat greeting by sniffing noses.

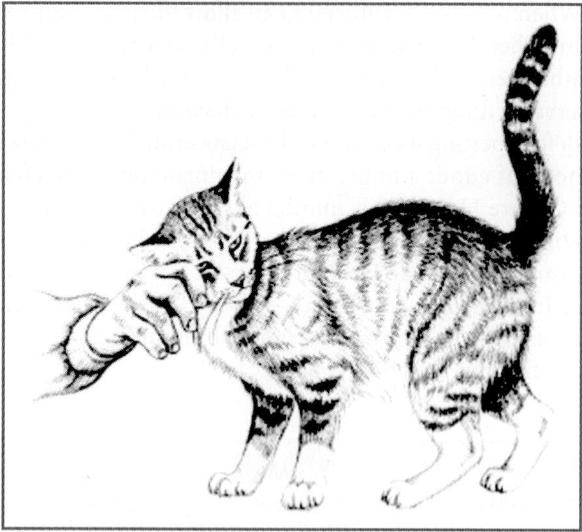

FIGURE 11-23 Recommended way to pet an unfamiliar cat. (Copyright 2008. The American Society for the Prevention of Cruelty to Animals® [ASPCA®]. All Rights Reserved.)

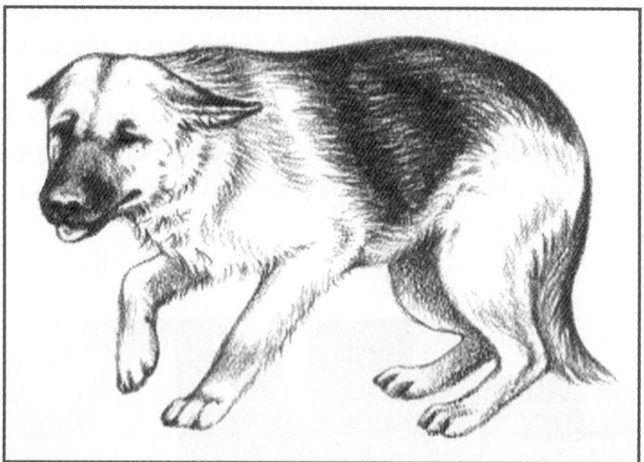

FIGURE 11-24 Fearful dog. Canine fearful postures overlap with submissive postures and can also include shaking, urination or defecation, shedding, panting, and dilated pupils. (Copyright 2008. The American Society for the Prevention of Cruelty to Animals® [ASPCA®]. All Rights Reserved.)

may work best to prevent the cat from becoming aroused, rather than to calm it once aroused.)

Interactions With Staff: Use of Food

Fearful or Threatening Animals

When patients are highly aroused and are displaying fearful, threatening, or aggressive behavior, technicians should try to decrease their emotional arousal. This may require more than just assuming the nonthreatening postures described previously. Technicians should also try offering the animal something that will elicit a more relaxed, friendly, or happy emotional reaction. For many animals, this means food or toys. Technicians and other staff members can offer patients small, highly palatable tidbits (assuming this will not interfere with the reason for the visit) from an open palm, not feeding from the fingers, while assuming other nonthreatening postures illustrated in Figure 11-20. An animal that refuses tidbits is likely stressed or anxious. This reaction should be noted and shared with other staff members who will be handling the patient.

BOX 11-21 How Classical Conditioning Works to Change Emotional States

Emotions are not amenable to reinforcements and punishments (operant conditioning). Thus reassuring a fearful animal does not make it more fearful (reward the fear). Consider the following example:

- Being cut off in traffic by another driver triggers an angry reaction.
- Whenever this occurs, your passenger gives you $10.
- After many repetitions, you are likely to be less angry about being cut off and may even look forward to the event, anticipating another $10.
- The $10 has made you less angry, not more.

Pairing the $10 (a pleasant event) with being cut off by another driver (an unpleasant event) is classical counterconditioning. In classical conditioning, an animal learns the association between two events, a phenomenon first illustrated by Ivan Pavlov.

If the animal attempts to avoid the technician (backs away, attempts to hide), displays fearful body postures (see Figures 11-14 and 11-24), or displays threatening behaviors (see Figures 11-13 and 11-15 to 11-17), the treat or toy should be dropped near the animal or into the carrier. Even when a pet will not eat the food, the sight and odor of the desirable tidbit may, through classical conditioning (see Box 11-20), still have a positive effect on the animal's emotional state.

Technicians need not worry that giving a treat to an animal that is fearful or threatening will reward these behaviors. Such behaviors are motivated by emotional arousal. Treats and toys serve to improve the animal's emotional reaction through classical conditioning. To better understand this phenomenon, refer to Box 11-21.

Unruly Dogs

For unruly dogs, a more assertive approach can be used (facing the dog, making eye contact), and the dog can be required to sit, lie down, or perform any trick it knows (e.g., shake hands) before receiving the tidbit. The tidbit can be used to lure the dog into a sitting or down position, if necessary. Any undesirable behavior (jumping up, barking) should be ignored (no verbal correction, turning away from the dog, moving out of its reach, breaking eye contact). Attempting to push the dog away or touching her to "help" her into the desired position (sit, down) will usually be counterproductive and can even be dangerous. If the dog jumps up, it is never appropriate to step on the dog's feet, squeeze the paws, or knee her in the chest. Head collars, such as a Snoot Loop or Gentle Leader (see Figure 11-27) work quite well to control such dogs. Head collars are discussed in more detail later in the chapter.

> *TECHNICIAN NOTE* Fearful or aggressive animals tend to respond better if they are allowed to approach a person, rather than the other way around.

BOX 11-22 Body Postures of Offensive Dogs and Cats

Offensively threatening dogs will usually show one or more of the following:

1. Standing up tall with a stiff body posture, oriented toward the subject of the threat
2. Weight distributed on all four legs or slightly more on front legs, leaning-forward appearance
3. Piloerection (erection of the hair) on the back
4. Tail held high, may be straight up in a vertical line, may be wagging slowly
5. Erect ears up and forward, floppy ears pricked forward
6. Direct eye contact or staring
7. Teeth bared with vertical retraction of the lips
8. Barking and/or growling
9. May lunge or move toward the target

Offensively threatening cats will show one or more of the following:

1. Standing, rear hips higher than front hips, tail down
2. Direct eye contact or staring
3. Ears up or rotated slightly outward
4. Growling, hissing, spitting

BOX 11-23 Body Postures of Defensive Dogs and Cats

Defensively threatening dogs will usually show one or more of the following:

1. Crouched body posture
2. Piloerection may occur
3. May or may not be directly oriented toward the subject of the threat
4. Tail usually down
5. Ears may be pinned back
6. Eyes not directly staring. May look away from subject of threat or alternate between staring and avoidance of contact
7. Teeth bared in horizontal retraction of lips
8. May be growling, barking, or whining and whimpering

Defensively aggressive cats will show:

1. Standing up, back arched, tail up or down (Halloween cat)
2. Lying down, rolled slightly to the side, feet and claws extended
3. Ears flat to the side or against the head
4. Eyes dilated, may avoid direct eye contact
5. Growling, hissing, spitting

Creating a Good First Impression in the Examination Room

Fearful and threatening patients respond better if they are allowed to approach a person, rather than the other way around. With dogs, the technician and/or the veterinarian should enter the examination room first so that the dog is coming into their space rather than vice versa. If the technician has already placed a problem dog in the examination room, one strategy might be for the technician to take the dog out of the room to the scale to be weighed. While the dog is gone, the veterinarian can enter the room and sit down. Fearful dogs may tolerate handling better if they are examined on the floor, rather than the table. Both dogs and cats may be more comfortable on a nonslip surface, so technicians can place a rug or mat on either the floor or the examination table to provide better traction.

> *TECHNICIAN NOTE* If the dog is intimidated and frightened by being on the examination table, the technician can try conducting the procedure on the floor.

Keeping Cats Calm

Before the cat and owner are brought to the examination room, Feliway can be applied to the examination table. Before attempting to take the cat out of the carrier, the technician should assess the cat's arousal level. What does the cat do if the carrier is moved, if the cat is touched with a pen or other harmless object (not a finger) through the wires or air holes of the carrier? Is the cat vocalizing? Does the cat appear relaxed, friendly, fearful, or defensive based on the illustrations of cat body postures in this chapter?

If the cat is significantly stressed or aroused, when possible, it may be better to delay handling and examinations until the cat is calmer. The carrier with its door left open can be put directly in a holding cage with a towel draped across the cage door, creating a quiet, dark hiding place for the cat.

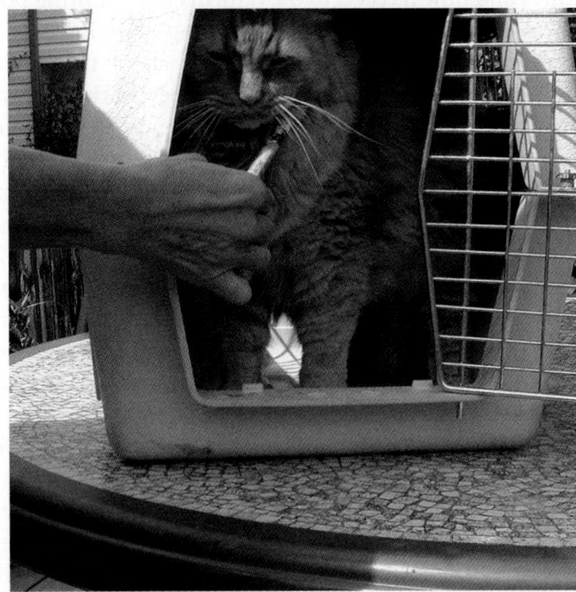

FIGURE 11-25 Allowing the cat time to exit the carrier rather than pulling him out.

Removing Cats from Carriers

If a cat is in a plastic carrier that can be separated into top and bottom halves, it is safer to remove the top half of the carrier rather than reaching into the crate. Some cats can be enticed out of their carriers using toys they can chase. Others may exit by following a small trail of tidbits. Taking a bit of extra time to allow the cat to exit the carrier on his own will go a long way toward keeping the cat's stress level down (Figure 11-25).

BOX 11-24 Warning Signs Stressed Cats May Display

- Twitching, swishing tail
- Head turns; intention movements
- Rapid change of ear carriage
- Freezing or moving little
- Tense body
- Paws, tail tucked in
- Hiding
- Dilated pupils
- No interest in food or toys
- Lack of friendly behaviors

Observe Body Postures Carefully

As mentioned previously, careful observation of an animal's body postures is the best way to assess its emotional state and its intentions. Even experienced technicians often get in a hurry and fail to take the time to watch the animal for a bit before attempting any interaction. This oversight contributes to bite injuries.

Before approaching or handling a pet in the examination room, technicians should carefully observe the animal's body postures and how it reacts to movements (e.g., shifting positions on the chair, reaching for something, standing up).

Technicians should be knowledgeable about the species-typical social behaviors of all the species they work with. At a minimum, for dogs and cats, technicians must be intimately familiar with the offensive and defensive postures illustrated in the accompanying pictures and summarized in Boxes 11-22 and 11-23. Technicians should also look for warning signs that indicate stress and/or arousal summarized in Boxes 11-24 and 11-25.

One category of warning signs is displacement behaviors. Displacement behaviors (yawning, grooming, lip licking, sneezing) are conflict behaviors. They are normal behaviors, but are displaced out of their expected context and indicate an animal is stressed and unsure about how to respond. If, for example, a cat is unsure of whether to bite or make a run for it, he may begin scratching or licking himself instead.

A lack of friendly behaviors is also a concern. This pattern easily goes unnoticed, or the significance of their absence is not realized. Technicians should be cautious of animals that stare or watch them closely without any other behavioral responses (e.g., no tail wags, no avoidance responses, no fearful or threatening behavior).

Be Proactive Rather than Reactive

Because initial friendliness is not always predictive of how an animal is going to react to restraint and handling, the technician should not assume an animal will be tolerant and should not move too quickly when initiating handling procedures. Erring on the side of caution is better than being bitten. To continue to help animals maintain relaxed, friendly attitudes about the upcoming examination, the technician can offer a tidbit with one hand (Figure 11-26) while doing one of the following:

- Touching the pet's collar
- Touching or reaching toward the pet's feet
- Touching an ear
- Running a hand down the patient's back

Pairing the touch of potentially sensitive areas with something positive for the patient can help decrease fear or anxiety. Although it could be argued that this requires additional staff time, it may require less time for one technician to conduct these proactive handling exercises than the extra time required when patients become unmanageable.

BOX 11-25 Warning Signs Stressed Dogs May Display

- Displacement behaviors, such as frequent yawning, licking of the lips, grooming, or sleeping (see text for explanation)
- Ambivalent behaviors—alternating between different motivational states, such as fear and friendliness or submission and defensive threat
- Redirected behaviors—behaviors directed at other animals or people not directly involved with the animal; redirected aggression is particularly dangerous for others in the area if a dog is aggressively motivated but cannot get to the original target
- Lack of friendly behaviors
- Frozen, moving little
- No interest in toys or food

For additional information on observing and interpreting canine and feline body postures, the videotape Canine Behavior: Body Postures, available from Animal Care Technologies, 2701 Hartlee Field Road, Denton, TX 76208, 800-357-3182, is an excellent resource.

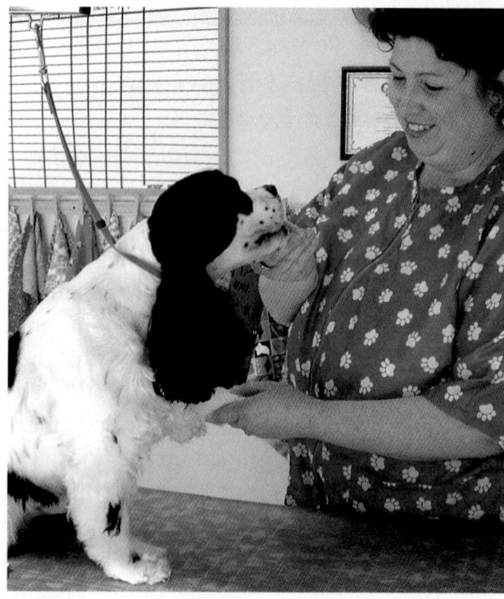

FIGURE 11-26 Pairing touching and holding paw with a treat for the dog.

Create a Protocol for Handling Exercises to Be Practiced at Home

For patients that, from past experience, are known to be threatening, aggressive, or generally difficult to handle, technicians can give clients a step-by-step plan to accustom their animals to basic handling procedures. Initial steps in this process would be similar to those listed in the previous section. As the pet begins to become more comfortable, owners can gradually do more, such as hold a paw rather than just touching it, squeeze the foot, and so on while pairing these procedures with something that the pet enjoys. Technicians can encourage veterinarians to partner with certified trainers, certified behaviorists, and others who can easily create these types of handling programs for clients.

Dealing With Threatening and Aggressive Animals

There are two issues in threatening situations: the technician's safety and well-being and the animal's safety and well-being. Good behavior skills should minimize the occurrence of those situations in which emergency restraint must be used for safety reasons.

When handling animals, it is best to assume an attitude of cautious calm (Hetts, 1999), as follows:

- Respect the animal and its ability to injure, without being overly fearful.
- Although knowledge of breed tendencies is helpful, be careful that breed biases do not result in approaching or handling the animal in a manner that could be counterproductive.
- Have confidence in your ability to accurately observe, interpret, and react accordingly to the animal's body postures and other communication signals without overconfidence or feeling invincible.
- Know what can be done to avoid being bitten or getting in a confrontation with the animal.
- Know when to back off (or use proper restraint) if you do not think you can accurately interpret the animal's intentions or when you realize the animal will bite if you persist. If the situation permits (e.g., if the procedure does not need to be performed immediately), it may be most helpful to put the animal in a cage, cover the front with a towel, and allow the pet to calm down.
- Avoid taking the animal's behavior personally and becoming angry, frustrated, and impatient. Another technician or staff member may be better able to handle the pet. Certain animals and certain people have personality conflicts, just as people do.

The minimal amount of physical restraint necessary for the technician's safety is the maximum that should be used. For example, if a dog or cat tries to bite, it is usually appropriate to stop and muzzle it rather than increasing the level of physical restraint. Additional information on animal restraint can be found in Chapter 7.

The goal of restraint and force is to keep personnel safe while they are performing necessary procedures. It is not to "teach the animal a lesson" or "show him who's boss." The technician should keep in mind that using physical force may allow one to do what needs to be done at the time, but the price may be creating an animal who becomes increasingly difficult or even impossible to handle during future visits.

In addition, the animal's behavior may be adversely affected in situations outside the veterinary hospital. Animals that have had a bad experience with restraint and handling have been known to become threatening or fearful toward people they are not familiar with, in reaction to quick arm or hand movements in their direction, and more difficult for their owners to restrain and groom.

These outcomes can occur after only *one* bad experience and become more and more likely with repeated ones. If owners observe an episode of what, to them, appears to be unnecessary roughness, it may also cost the practice clients.

The case of a veterinarian who was charged (and later acquitted on appeal) with cruelty to animals for hitting a dog in the face when it tried to bite him clearly illustrates that the issue of animal handling and restraint is an important one, not only to the veterinary profession but also to the public (Nolen, 2000). Rather than increasing the level of interactive, social restraint, technicians may want to use, and encourage veterinarians to use, appropriate equipment that can be less intimidating to the animal and safer for technicians and other staff members. Examples of such equipment are described in the following sections.

Muzzles

Rather than struggling to control a pet with increased force because of concern that the animal might bite, a muzzle can be applied (Figure 11-27). With a muzzle on the animal, the technician will be less concerned with the need for tight restraint, and the animal may calm down if it is less tightly restrained. Technicians can also educate owners on how to accustom their pets to tolerate a muzzle for short periods. The practice can consider selling muzzles to ensure clients' compliance. With this proactive approach, owners can muzzle their animals immediately before entering the veterinary hospital.

If using a nylon sleeve-type muzzle (see Figure 11-27, *B*), technicians may want to slit the side seams of the muzzle (an inch or so). The slit should not be so long as to allow the dog to open his mouth wide enough to bite, but sufficiently long to allow him to breathe and pant a little easier. Muzzles that do not allow this cause many dogs to panic, resulting in increased struggling, which is counterproductive.

Head Collars

The biggest advantage of a head collar is that it gives the technician control of the dog's head. Several brands of head collars are available, including the Gentle Leader (Figure 11-28). By exerting gentle but steady pressure directly upward on the leash (not horizontally, as seen in the figure) it is possible to raise the dog's head. By passing the leash through a ring attached to a wall at the level of a dog's head, it is possible to prevent the dog from turning its head to bite.

Although some dogs become somewhat panicked when first introduced to a head collar, based on personal experience, this is not as frequent with the Snoot Loop. To further

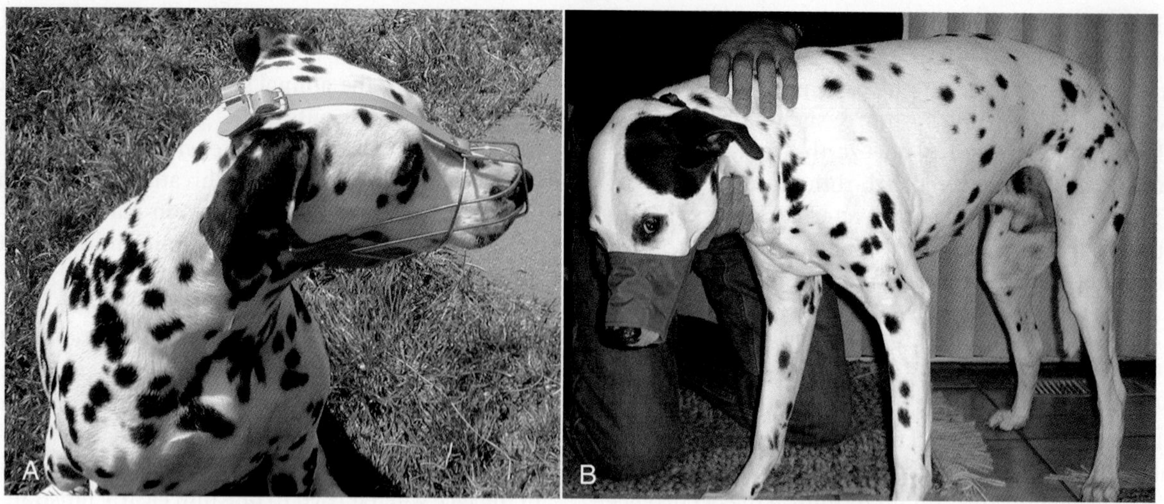

FIGURE 11-27 Dogs wearing wire basket **(A)** and nylon-sleeve **(B)** muzzles.

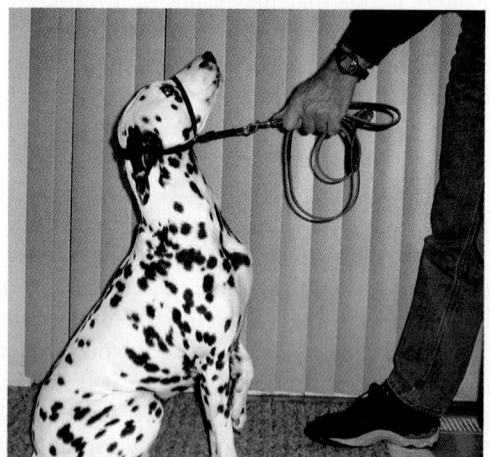

FIGURE 11-28 Control of the head with a Gentle Leader. (Premier Pet Products, Inc.)

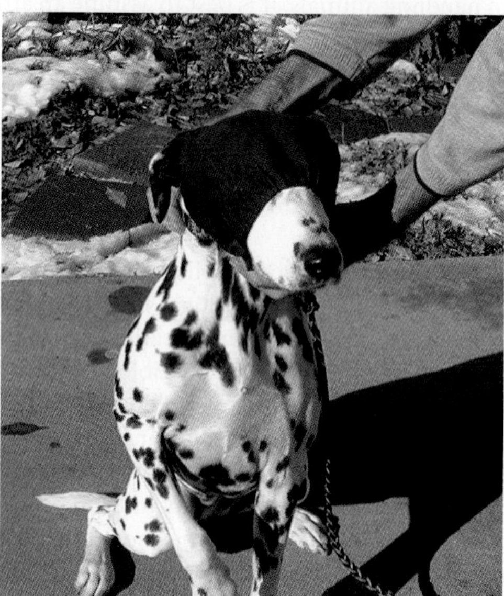

FIGURE 11-29 Dog wearing a Calming Cap.

reduce resistance to a head collar, technicians should encourage owners to use one as standard practice in place of choke chains or pinch collars. This recommendation can be made during puppy class or the dog's first wellness examination. When dogs are accustomed to a head collar, technicians can more easily use it to control dogs in the practice.

Calming Caps

Developed by a trainer to reduce a dog's reactivity when riding in a car, a Calming Cap is much like a hood used on horses (Figure 11-29). It "filters" the dog's vision and reduces the intensity of visual stimuli, thereby also reducing the intensity of the dog's response. The Calming Cap can be put on dogs that are quite reactive to various procedures, including nail trims, injections, examinations, or restraint in general. The dog can still see to move about and can be easily walked on a leash in the hospital.

Cat Bags

When possible, fractious cats should first be given a chance to calm down, as explained earlier. If the aggressive cat is still in a carrier, another option is to put the opening of the carrier directly into a large canvas cat bag. Some cats will crawl into the bag because it appears to be a darker, safer hiding place than the carrier. The cat can then be handled through the zippered opening of the bag. Some cat bags with frames (Figure 11-30) allow the cat to be put into the bag directly from a standard cage.

Plexiglas Shield

If the cat is in the larger cage, a Plexiglas shield (Figure 11-31) can be used to push and hold the cat to the rear of the cage if an injection is the only or first treatment that needs to be administered. This avoids having to handle the fractious cat at all until it is medicated. (Bag and shield are available from Animal Care Equipment and Services (ACES), 800-338-2237 or aces@gte.net; Boulder, Colo.)

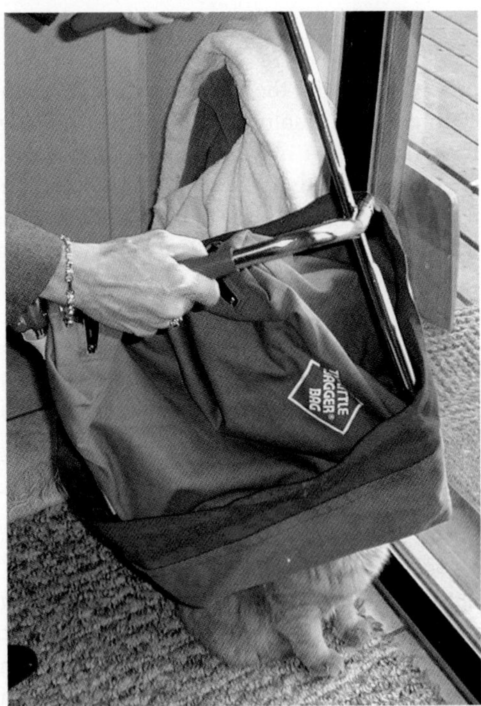

FIGURE 11-30 Cat Bagger (available from ACES, Inc.) with frame held over a cat.

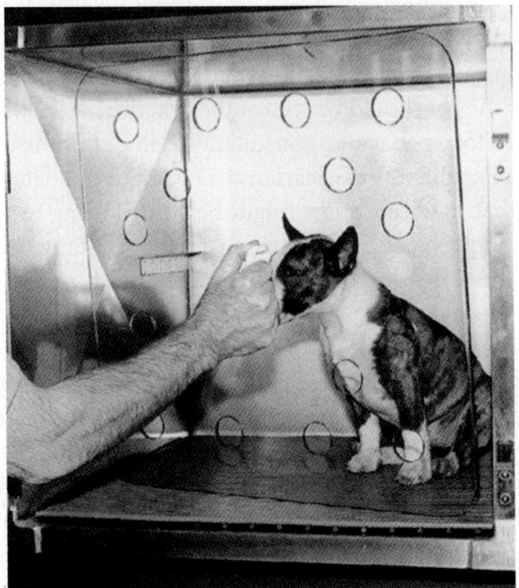

FIGURE 11-31 Plexiglas shield (available from ACES, Inc.) used to push a dog to the back of the cage. Injections can be given through holes in the shield.

Towels

One of the best and easiest tools to use when handling cats is simply a large, thick towel (Figure 11-32). Holding the towel high to partially block the cat's view of the technician's face makes the technician appear less threatening.

Setting Limits and Knowing When to Stop

Not all procedures are emergencies or must be done when initially scheduled. Nail trims and other routine procedures are not emergencies. Technicians should recognize when attempts to perform a procedure should be halted, both for their safety and the animal's well-being. Some veterinarians have set guidelines that if restraint requires more than two persons, other techniques will be used. This may include using the equipment already mentioned, sedating the animal, or sending the owner home with medication to be given before bringing the animal back.

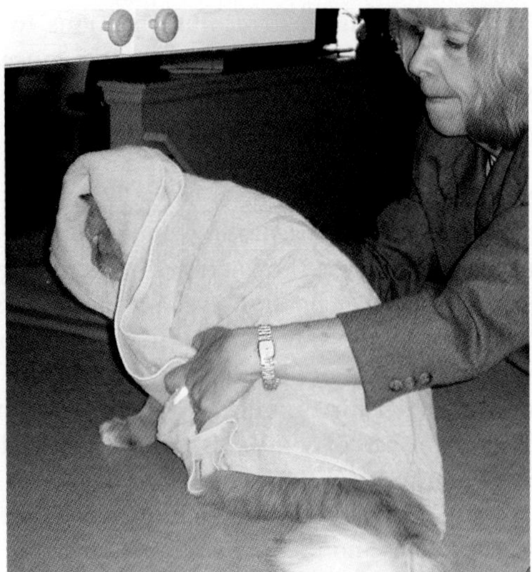

FIGURE 11-32 Using a towel to handle a cat.

PROBLEM-RESOLUTION COMPONENT

Problem resolution is not something to be taken lightly or attempted with an offhand, "try this, try that" approach. Behavioral problems should be approached in a systematic way: analysis of the behavior, creation of a behavior modification plan, and follow-up. Attempting to intervene with a behavioral problem without knowing the cause or motivation for the behavior can be just as disastrous as attempting to treat a medical condition without a diagnosis. For example, surgery would not be considered for a limping dog until it was determined why the dog was limping; similarly an antibark collar should not be recommended for a barking dog until the reason for the barking has been determined.

Technicians should always look to the veterinarian for guidelines regarding their role in providing problem-resolution information to clients. Owners often ask technicians questions about their pets' behavior even before they ask the veterinarian. Both veterinary technicians and veterinarians should be aware of the disadvantages to jumping into problem solving without adequate preparation.

Dangers of Problem Solving Without Adequate Preparation

Attempting to problem solve without being prepared is not helpful to the technician, the client, or the pet. Behavioral consulting requires knowledge about animal behavior and animal learning, having sufficient time to obtain a behavioral history and explain detailed recommendations to clients, and being available to follow up after the initial consultation. Attempting to problem solve without sufficient preparation can have the following unwanted consequences.

Owners' Frustration

Behavioral problems are frustrating, and many pet owners can quickly lose patience. If owners are investing their time to implement recommendations yet see no results, their frustration level may quickly increase. In one case, an owner was advised to confine her cat in a large crate with a litter box, food, and water for 1 month to "retrain" the cat to use the litter box. The cat, of course, used the box reliably while confined. When released from confinement, the cat walked over to the other side of the room and urinated on the carpet. Both the owner and the cat were frustrated, and the cat was surrendered to an animal shelter. What makes cases like this sad is that most litter-box problems can be resolved with proper intervention.

Technicians' and Practice's Credibility

If clients discover from other sources that the information the veterinary technician provided was not accurate, appropriate, or helpful, they may lose faith in the technician and the veterinary practice. Consider this example. An owner's dog was barking excessively when left home alone. The owner was told to sneak back and throw a can of coins at the dog to reprimand the barking. When the problem was later diagnosed as separation anxiety and the owner told that this approach would probably exacerbate the problem and increase the dog's anxiety, she no longer trusted the veterinarian who gave her inappropriate information and took her dog to another practice instead.

Liability for Injuries

A technician who advises a pet owner to handle his or her pet in a certain way that elicits an aggressive response from the animal may be legally liable for injuries that result. In one case, an owner was advised to give her dog a scruff shake when it did not obey her commands. When her dog failed to get off the bed when told, she grabbed the dog by the neck as instructed, and the dog promptly bit off her finger. The owner sued the trainer who had given this instruction, and the case was settled out of court in her favor.

Worsening Problems

A playful kitten was pouncing on its owner's ankles as he sat in a chair. He was told to grab the kitten by the scruff of the neck, throw her into a room by herself, and leave her there for several hours. The kitten did not learn to stop pouncing on the owner's ankles. Instead, she learned that whenever her owner reached for her, she needed to defend herself. She began to hiss, scratch, and bite whenever the owner tried to touch her. The problem had escalated from simple play-motivated aggression, which might well have resolved on its own, to a much more difficult, defensive-aggressive behavior problem.

Self-Assessment

As technicians work with the veterinarian to determine what their role in problem resolution will be, the self-assessment questions in Table 11-4 may help guide decisions. Can the technician correctly analyze the reason or motivation for the behavior by knowing what questions to ask in a thorough behavioral history? If the technician cannot answer yes to most of the questions in Table 11-4, then problem solving may not be an appropriate role at this time.

> *TECHNICIAN NOTE* Veterinarians will want to evaluate the possibility that medical causes might be contributing to the pet's behavioral problem before making a referral.

Referring Behavior Cases

When to Refer

Technicians are sometimes put in the role of referring clients to behavioral consultants or dog trainers without sufficient direction from the veterinarian. Veterinarians and technicians should work together to develop guidelines for when it is appropriate for a technician to make the referral. Technicians should not take it upon themselves to make the referral without these guidelines. For example, owners often call the veterinary practice for advice when a cat is urinating outside the litter box, a dog has bitten a neighborhood child, or a dog is lifting his leg on the furniture. It should be the veterinarian's decision whether the pet should be seen at the practice before the owner is referred for a behavioral consultation, either in-house or to an outside consultant. Veterinarians will want to evaluate the possibility that medical causes might be contributing to the pet's behavioral problem before making a referral. Many behavioral consultants will not accept a referral until this has been done.

Type of Referral

For dogs, the first decision that needs to be made is whether the referral should be for behavioral consulting or for obedience training. Obedience classes are helpful when dogs are unruly and not responsive to verbal directions from the owners. Jumping up, door dashing, pulling on the leash, and not coming when called are examples of undesirable behaviors that can be improved through a good obedience class. Obedience classes, however, do not resolve problems, such as separation anxiety, excessive barking, house soiling, destructive behavior, or aggression. These type of problems require behavioral consultations that include analysis and subsequent modification of the problem behavior. When the decision is made to refer a cat for a behavioral problem, obviously the owner should be referred to a behavioral consultant knowledgeable and experienced in cat behavior.

Evaluating Behavioral Consultants and Dog Trainers

Technicians can be helpful to the veterinary practice by assisting with the evaluation of behavioral consultants and dog trainers the practice may be considering for use as referral

TABLE 11-4 Self-Assessment Before Problem Solving

Question	Case Example
Can I take a behavioral history about this problem? Do I know what questions to ask to determine the type of problem that is causing the behavior? Can I obtain a behavioral symptom?	Excessive barking can be caused by separation anxiety and territorial behavior (among other things). Can I obtain a behavioral history that will distinguish between these two problems?
Will my recommendations for resolving the problem address the specific type of problem rather than merely treating the symptom? If not, is there a rationale that makes the symptomatic approach appropriate?	Constructing a higher fence to resolve an escaping problem is a symptomatic treatment. The reason for escaping is ignored. If the higher fence keeps the dog in the yard without additional problems, this may be sufficient. However, if the escaping is motivated by separation anxiety, other symptoms of the problem are likely to be seen. Can I determine when a symptomatic approach is appropriate and when it is not?
Am I familiar with a variety of possible problem resolution methods, only a few of which are based on aversive techniques?	One approach to destructive chewing is to give off-limits items with an unpleasant taste. Am I familiar not only with other ways of discouraging unacceptable chewing, but also with even more ways to *promote* acceptable chewing behavior?
Do I have the time to complete all the components of a behavior case that includes analysis (diagnosis), treatment (devising and explaining a plan), and following up?	Obtaining a history and explaining a treatment plan to an owner may require several hours, certainly more than 10 or 15 minutes. Follow-up contacts can occur over several months. Can I realistically expect to have sufficient time to handle the case properly?

From Hetts S: *Pet behavior protocols: what to say, what to do, when to refer*, Lakewood, Colo, 1999, AAHA Press.

resources. Veterinarians know that clients' experiences with referrals, both good and bad, will reflect directly back on the veterinary practice. Because there is such a great variation in the qualifications and methods of behavioral consultants and dog trainers, it is incumbent on the veterinary practice to evaluate the credentials and competency of the people to whom it refers clients. This can be a time-consuming process, but one that can benefit greatly from using the skills of trained technicians.

The technician who has been given the assignment of gathering information about individuals in the community who offer behavioral consulting services should know that anyone can use the professional titles of animal behaviorist, behavioral consultant, dog behaviorist, cat behaviorist, and so on, regardless of background and training. There are also no restrictions against nonveterinarians using the title behavior specialist. Although there is a veterinary board specialty in behavior and the Animal Behavior Society professionally certifies academically trained behaviorists who meet its criteria, relatively few individuals are certified in this manner, and it is likely that one is not located near a particular veterinary practice (for a complete listing of both Certified Applied Animal Behaviorists [CAAB] and Board Certified Veterinary Behaviorists [DACVB], refer to the respective websites listed in Box 11-3).

Because some CAABs provide behavioral consultations by telephone directly to the client and both CAABs and DACVBs will consult with veterinarians by telephone, access to one is always an option, regardless of the location of the veterinary practice. In addition, many people with a wide variety of backgrounds who are not certified offer behavioral consulting services, including veterinarians with a special interest in animal behavior, who are often members of the American Veterinary Society of Animal Behavior (AVSAB), and dog trainers. Obtaining information about the consultant's education and experience, and observing a consulting appointment are critical tasks that the veterinary practice can assign to the technician before agreeing to refer its clients to a noncertified consultant. Veterinarians can then make informed decisions about which professionals are best qualified to provide consulting services to the practice's clients.

The Certification Council of Professional Dog Trainers certifies trainers who have passed an examination and met other criteria. The Association of Pet Dog Trainers promotes the use of dog-friendly training methods, but certification is not a requirement for membership.

Technicians can be designated to observe several obedience classes and, ideally, participate in the class with a dog before the veterinary practice agrees to refer clients to any given trainer. Box 11-26 provides recommendations for assessing behavior consultants and trainers. Professional standards for dog trainers can be obtained from the Delta Society (see Box 11-3).

BOX 11-26 Guidelines for Evaluating a Dog Trainer or Behavioral Consultant

Finding and Working With Dog Trainers

Look for trainers who rely on teaching methods that use positive reinforcement for the right response rather than punishing the wrong one.

Observe an obedience class without your dog. Are the dogs and people having a good time? Talk with a few participants and see if they are comfortable with the trainer's methods. If someone will not let you sit in, do not enroll.

Do not allow trainers to work with your dog unless they tell you first exactly what they plan to do.

Do not be afraid to tell a trainer to stop if she or he is doing something to your dog that you do not like.

If a trainer tells you to do something that you do not feel good about, do not do it. Do not be intimidated, bullied, or shamed into doing something that you believe is not in your dog's best interest.

Avoid trainers who offer guarantees about results. They are either ignoring or do not understand the complexity of animal behavior.

Avoid trainers who object to using food as a training reward. Food is an acceptable positive reinforcement training tool.

Avoid trainers who use only choke chains. Head collars are humane alternatives to choke chains and pinch collars.

Look for trainers who treat people and dogs with respect, rather than an "I'm the boss" attitude.

Finding and Working With Behavioral Consultants

Look for academic training in the science of animal behavior and hands-on experience.

Certification by a professional organization tells you that the individual has met the requirements for education, experience, and professional ethics.

Look for people who recognize the importance of you working through the problem with your pet rather than sending it somewhere to be "fixed."

Membership in a professional organization suggests communication with colleagues and a means to keep current on new information.

Ask for professional references, such as former clients, colleagues, or veterinarians who refer cases.

Knowledge of positive reinforcement methods; behavior modification techniques, such as counterconditioning and desensitization; how to use food rewards appropriately; and humane products, such as head collars, is a must.

Look for people who treat you with respect and are not abrupt and abrasive.

Avoid people who guarantee problem resolution. Animals are complex, and no one knows everything there is to know about them.

Avoid quick fixes. This approach does not do justice to you, your pet, or the problem.

How to Make the Referral

If technicians will be making the referral to a dog trainer or behavioral consultant, such referrals must be conducted in a professional manner. A good guideline is to consider how a referral to a medical specialist is made. When a client is referred to a veterinary oncologist, technicians or veterinarians do not say, "Try calling these people and see if they can give you a few tips for dealing with your pet's cancer." This sounds ludicrous, but in reality, this is similar to what many clients are told when they are referred to a behavior consultant. When a referral is made to a behavior consultant, clients should first be told what to expect from the referral. From a previous evaluation of the consultant or trainer, the technician will know what kind of services are offered and what fees are charged. Provide the client with this information rather than referring the client for "tips" or "advice." It frustrates the client and the behavioral consultant if the client expects a "25-words-or-less" solution free of charge. How the technician makes the referral will have a significant impact on clients' perceptions of behavioral consulting and how likely they will be to follow through with an appointment. If clients get the impression that this is a trivial referral, they are also unlikely to take it seriously or believe that a behavioral consult can successfully help them change their pets' behavior. Similarly, clients will not take the importance of training classes seriously if the suggestion is made in an offhand manner, rather than emphasized as an important component of a behavior wellness program. A technician might say, "Your pet needs to see a behavior consultant because her problem requires more care than we can provide. Please call Dr. X at this number to set up an appointment. Dr. X will need to interview you at length and probably observe your pet as well. You can expect to pay for a fee for Dr. X's services. We know Dr. X and we recommend him highly. I'll call you in a week to see when your behavior consultation is scheduled."

SUMMARY

This chapter has discussed the important role that technicians can play in making behavior wellness care an integral part of the practice of veterinary medicine. A focus on behavior wellness rather than on resolving complex behavioral problems makes sense for technicians and the veterinary practice. It also fills a need for pets and their owners that is too often going unmet. More effective promotion of how to create desirable behavior patterns and early detection of problems when they do occur has a great potential to keep pets out of animal shelters and prevent euthanasia for behavioral problems. Behavior wellness programs can be applied to any species of companion animal by inserting species-typical behavioral information. It is hoped that this chapter can motivate technicians to seek additional continuing education in animal behavior so they can make greater contributions to behavior wellness. Technicians interested in behavior should join the Society of Veterinary Behavior Technicians.

LITERATURE CITED

Anderson RK, Line S, Jackson J: *Early learning for puppies—a program guide for humane societies and veterinary clinics*, Richmond, Va, 1999, Premier Pet Products.

Bateson P: How do sensitive periods arise and what are they for? *Anim Behav* 27:470-486, 1979.

Bernstein PL, Strack M: A game of cat and house: spatial patterns and behaviour of 14 cats *(felis catus)* in the home, *Anthrozoos* 9:24-39, 1996.

Bradshaw JWS: *The behaviour of the domestic cat*, Wallingford, Oxon, UK, 1992, CAB International.

DiGiacomo N, Arluke A, Patronek G: Surrendering pets to shelters: the relinquisher's perspective, *Anthrozoos* 11:41, 1998.

Duxbury MM, Jackson J, Line SW et al: Evaluation of association between retention in the home and attendance at puppy socialization classes, *JAVMA* 221(1):61-66, 2002.

Hetts S: *Pet behavior protocols: what to say, what to do, when to refer*, Lakewood, Colo, 1999, AAHA Press.

Hetts S, Estep D: *Pet behavior protocols: what to say, what to do, when to refer*, ed 2, Lakewood, Colo, AAHA Press, in prep.

Hetts S, Estep DQ: *Canine behavior: I. Body postures II. The behaviorally healthy dog*, Denton, Tex, 1999, Animal Care Training, Inc (videotapes).

Hetts S, Heinke ML, Estep DQ: Behavior wellness concepts for general veterinary practice, *JAVMA* 4:506-513, 2004.

Karsh EB, Turner DC: The human-cat relationship. In Turner DC, Bateson P, editors: *The domestic cat: the biology of its behaviour*, New York, 1988, Cambridge Univ Press.

Landsberg G, Hunthausen W, Ackerman L: *Handbook of behavior problems of the dog and cat*, ed 2, New York, 2003, W B Saunders.

New JC et al: Moving: characteristics of dogs and cats and those relinquishing them to 12 US animal shelters, *JAAWS* 2:83, 1999.

Nolen RS: New Jersey veterinarian acquitted of cruelty conviction, *JAVMA* 216:1888, 1894, 2000.

Patronek GJ, Dodman NH: Attitudes, procedures, and delivery of behavior services by veterinarians in small animal practice. *JAVMA* 215:1606, 1999.

Patronek GJ et al: Risk factors for relinquishment of dogs to an animal shelter, *JAVMA* 209:572, 1996a.

Patronek GJ, et al: Risk factors for relinquishment of cats to an animal shelter, *JAVMA* 209:582, 1996b.

Price G: President's message, *Newsletter Soc Vet Behav Technicians* 9:1, 2001.

Salman MD et al: Human and animal factors related to the relinquishment of dogs and cats in 12 selected animal shelters in the United States, *JAAWS* 1:207, 1998.

Scarlett JM et al: Reasons for relinquishment of companion animals in US animal shelters: selected health and personal issues, *JAAWS* 2:41, 1999.

Scott JP, Fuller JL: *Genetics and the social behavior of the dog*, Chicago, Ill, 1965, University of Chicago Press.

Waring GH: *Horse behavior*, ed 2, Norwich, NY, 2003, Noyes Publications.

Wood F: Boost your passive income, *Vet Econ* 38(8):56-62, 1997.

RECOMMENDED READINGS

Bradshaw JWS: *The behaviour of the domestic cat*, Wallingford, Oxon, UK, 1992, CAB International.

Coppinger R, Coppinger L: *Dogs: a startling new understanding of canine origin, behavior, and evolution*, New York, 2001, Scribner.

Leuscher AU: *Manual of parrot behavior*, Ames, Iowa, 2006, Blackwell Publishing.

McConnell PB: *For the love of a dog*, New York, 2006, Ballantine Books.

McConnell PB: *The other end of the leash*, New York, 2006, Ballantine Books.

Reid PJ: *Excel-erated learning: explaining how dogs learn and how best to teach them*, Berkeley, Calif, 1996, James and Kenneth Publishers.

Serpell J, editor: *The domestic dog: its evolution, behaviour and interactions with people*, Cambridge, 1995, Cambridge University Press.

Turner DC, Bateson P, editors: *The domestic cat: the biology of its behaviour*, ed 2, Cambridge, 2000, Cambridge University Press.

Waring GH: *Horse behavior*, ed 2, Norwich, NY, 2003, Noyes Publications.

Wright JC, Lashnits JW: *Ain't misbehaving*, Emmaus, Pa, 2001, Rodale Press.

12 Small Animal Nutrition

Mary Tefend Campbell

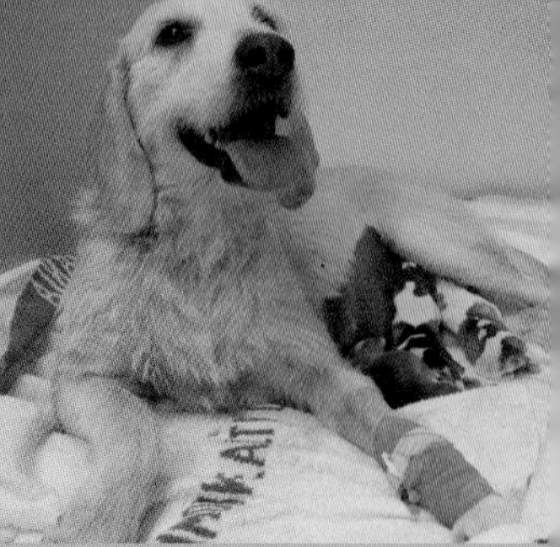

OUTLINE

LEARNING OBJECTIVES

When you have completed this chapter, you will be able to:

1. List the energy-producing and nonenergy-producing components of food.
2. List the classes of carbohydrates and describe the catabolism of carbohydrates.
3. Differentiate between lipids and fats and describe the general structure of triglycerides.
4. Describe the structure and functions of proteins.
5. Differentiate between essential and nonessential amino acids.
6. Explain the importance of water in metabolic reactions.
7. Differentiate between microminerals and macrominerals and give examples of each.
8. List the fat-soluble and water-soluble vitamins and explain the importance of vitamins in metabolism.
9. Define the following terms: nutrient, ingredient, formula, nutrient profile, calorie, and kilocalorie.
10. Differentiate between dry, semimoist, and moist food and describe the characteristics of each.
11. Describe considerations in evaluating home-prepared diets.
12. List the legal requirements of pet food labels and considerations in evaluating pet food label information.
13. Describe the components of a nutritional assessment for dogs and cats.
14. List special considerations in feeding adult, pediatric, geriatric, pregnant, lactating, injured, and ill dogs and cats.
15. List and describe routes and procedures for providing nutritional support to hospitalized patients.

KEY TERMS

Anorexia
Body condition scoring system
Calorie
Carbohydrates
Energy
Enteral tube feeding
Esophagostomy feeding tube
Fats
Gastrostomy feeding tube
Jejunostomy feeding tube
Kilocalorie
Malnutrition
Minerals
Nasogastric feeding tube
Nutrients
Obesity
Parenteral feeding
Proteins

INTRODUCTION

Nutrition plays a critical role in the health of companion animals. The responsibility of the veterinary technician to educate clients about proper nutrition is therefore key in promoting the quality and longevity of a pet's life. Communication between the technician and client should include a discussion of the diverse nutritional needs of healthy companion animals and simple instructions regarding the frequency of feedings and the type and amount of food to offer. When appropriate, indications for therapeutic diets in clinically ill animals should also be discussed. Veterinary technicians who provide this level of nutrition counseling increase the quality of care provided to patients, help establish a valuable personal and professional bond with clients, and increase profitability for the practice.

Research in nutrition, particularly during the past decade, has greatly enhanced our understanding of what companion animals require in a balanced diet. Commercial diets are now formulated to help prevent nutritional deficiencies, boost the immune system, improve cognitive health, and help slow the aging process. Because obesity is now commonplace among pets, the veterinary technician should also be prepared to discuss weight-management regimens and other nutrition-based wellness programs.

Nutritional support is particularly important in times of illness and injury. The technician should be able to assist in assessing the hospitalized patient's body condition, hydration, daily energy requirements, and help administer specialized feedings. Failure to recognize or address a patient's metabolic needs may have negative consequences and may adversely affect the patient's outcome.

NUTRITIONAL OBJECTIVES AND PRINCIPLES

The goal of feeding companion animals is to maximize the length and quality of the animal's life by reducing nutritional risk factors. For example, the veterinary professional will correlate diet with the life stage of the animal so that an adult dog is fed an adult maintenance food and not a food formulated to meet the needs of puppies. The nutritional goals for companion animals may differ sharply with those for food animals, where the goal in meat production is to encourage rapid weight gain and not necessarily longevity.

Energy is essential for sustaining life in all animals. It is derived from the components of food and food mixtures known as "the diet." These energy-producing components include carbohydrates, fats, and proteins. Water, vitamins, and minerals are also essential for life because they are important in many biochemical reactions. However, they cannot be broken down to produce energy directly. The components of food that produce energy are classified as carbohydrates, fats, and proteins; the components of food that do not produce energy, such as water, vitamins, and minerals, are all called **nutrients.** Nutrients can be defined as any substance that when ingested supports life (Figure 12-1). In summary, nutrients are divided into six categories: proteins, fats, carbohydrates (which are energy producing) and water, vitamins, and minerals (which are nonenergy producing).

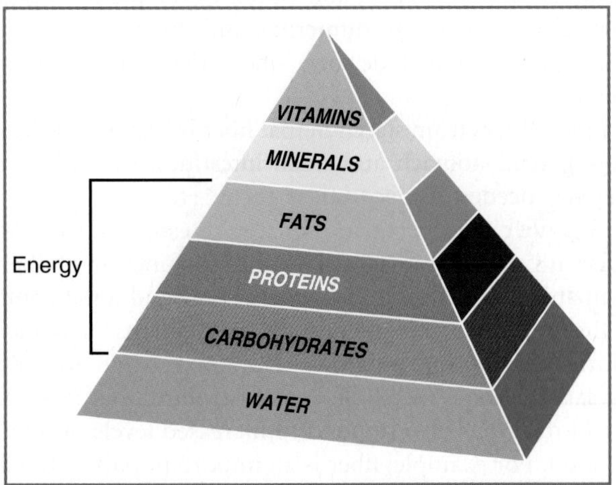

FIGURE 12-1 Six basic classes of nutrients are important for life sustenance. Carbohydrates, fats, and proteins may be used for energy, but also serve as structural components.

> *TECHNICIAN NOTE* Nutrients are divided into six categories: proteins, fats, carbohydrates (which are energy producing) and water, vitamins, and minerals (which are nonenergy producing).

NUTRIENT TERMS

The terms *nutrient, ingredient, formula,* and *nutrient profile* are easily confused and sometimes used interchangeably. Nutrients are fundamental energy and metabolic substrates classified as essential or nonessential. Ingredients are the raw materials used in food compounding. The formula selects and apportions ingredients for a particular diet. The nutrient profile describes the resulting quantitative distribution of the individual nutrients within the finished formula. These definitions are important to understand and distinguish from one another because clients easily confuse them.

Many pet food companies advertise their product as being "unique" or including fine ingredients. In this way, clients are led to believe that the product has a superior nutrient profile when compared with other brands. Although listing ingredients can be useful in evaluating a pet food, the nutritive value cannot be identified solely on an ingredient statement. An analysis of a particular food can give an indication of its nutrient content and the availability of a particular nutrient, but it is the *absorptive* capability of the nutrient (combined with availability) that lends nutritional value. In other words, digestibility of a food is a measure of the biologic availability. A balanced diet should supply all the key nutrients and energy needed to meet the daily requirements of the animal at its particular life stage.

Feeding a food with higher digestibility may allow animals to consume less of a particular food. Consequently, feeding highly digestible food may be more economical than feeding a less expensive food with lower digestibility. In addition, because more of the food is biologically usable, there is less waste to clean up in the yard. Digestibility of a food is determined by a mathematic equation comparing the amount of a nutrient in the food and the amount of the same nutrient in the feces (Box 12-1). Above-average digestibility can be defined as protein, fat, carbohydrate, and energy digestibility more than or equal to 85%, 90%, 90%, and 85%, respectively. Food higher in fiber will be lower in digestibility.

BOX 12-1 Food Digestibility

$$\frac{\text{Nutrient food} - \text{nutrient feces}}{\text{Nutrient food}} \times 100\% = \%\ \text{nutrient digestibility}$$

BOX 12-2 Palatability Factors

- Moisture
- Odor
- Fat and protein levels
- Temperature
- Texture
- Cats: shape (dry food)
- Acidity

Palatability of a food involves sensory factors, such as taste, smell, color, and even texture of food (Box 12-2). Palatability is an essential component of an animal's behavior toward a particular food, and first impressions are generally important. Sensory components, such as smell, can entice an anorectic patient to eat, particularly if the food is warm and strong smelling.

Additives are nonenergy, nonnutrient substances purposely added to food to enhance color, flavor, texture, and stability. Preservatives are defined as substances capable of inhibiting food-deteriorating microbes. Protection against microbes can also be achieved by both physical and chemical means, such as in dehydration (dry food), heat (moist and dry food), and chemical treatments (semimoist and some dry food). Many preservatives are organic acids, and their salts are added to retard oxidation, discoloration, or spoilage.

Humectants are preservative additives that bind to water to inhibit mold and fungal growth. Other chemical agents, such as antioxidants, can inhibit oxidation of fatty acids and fat-soluble vitamins, which protects them from becoming rancid and losing potency. Antioxidants, such as vitamins C and E, are natural preservatives.

> *TECHNICIAN NOTE* Additives are nonenergy, nonnutrient substances purposely added to food to enhance color, flavor, texture, and stability.

ENERGY-PRODUCING NUTRIENTS

Carbohydrates can be further broken down into simple sugars, fats into triglycerides, and proteins into amino acids. The digestion, assimilation, and metabolism of each of these nutrients produce chemical energy that is stored in the atomic bonds of "storage molecules," such as adenosine triphosphate (ATP). Storage molecules are portable and can be moved to any portion of the cell where energy is needed to complete an important job. In the case of ATP, the energy is stored in the bond that holds the last phosphate atom. When the phosphate atom breaks off, energy is released when the bond is broken. The energy can then be used to carry out a cellular process. Much of the energy that is gained from food is used to maintain and repair cell structures, such as the cell wall and the cytoskeleton. Animals that are growing, reproducing, exercising, or healing from an injury or combating a disease process have a higher degree of cellular activity than animals that are not engaged in these activities. These animals have higher energy (nutritional) demands. Oxygen synthesis and transport, heat production, muscle contraction, and the synthesis of new tissue are additional examples of cellular activity that requires energy.

As mentioned, **carbohydrates** provide the body with energy. The consumption of carbohydrates in excess of the body's immediate energy needs are stored as glycogen or converted to fat. Carbohydrates include sugars, starches, and fibers.

Sugars are numerous and include monosaccharides (simple sugars) and disaccharides (complicated sugars). Multiple sugars can bond and link to form complex sugar polymers. Polymerized sugars include starch and fiber. Simple sugars and complex sugars are broken down (catabolized) to provide energy, which is stored in the form of ATP. The type of polymer that is formed depends upon the sugar template and the type of polymer bonds in the molecule. Glycogen is an animal-specific starch and can quickly depolymerize into units of glucose. Stores of glycogen, therefore, provide a rapid supply of glucose to tissues when sugar is urgently needed. Most of the glycogen in the body is stored in the liver and in skeletal muscle tissue.

Digestion of carbohydrates and starch is a multifactorial process involving complex microbes and enzymes throughout the digestive tract. Dogs and cats lack certain salivary enzymes; consequently, digestion of starchy substances is not initiated in the mouth. Food is mixed with hydrochloric acids and other proteolytic enzymes in the stomach, where primarily protein is digested. Carbohydrates and starch are primarily digested and absorbed in the small intestine.

Insoluble fibers are referred to as complex carbohydrates, such as cellulose and lignin, and they make up the structural elements of grass, plants, and wood. In the plant kingdom, starches and fibers are numerous and diverse (Box 12-3). Sources of starch include corn, wheat, rice, barley, oats, and potatoes.

Fiber differs from starch in that fiber is indigestible by the monogastric stomach and small intestines, which lack the enzymes needed to decompose them. However, fermentation of fiber does occur in the large intestine of some animals with simple stomachs. The primary function of fiber in companion animals is to increase the bulk and water content of the intestine. This effect finds applications in reducing caloric density for weight-control food while maintaining satiety. Some metabolic and gastrointestinal (GI) tract transit disorders also respond to increased levels of fiber in the food. For example, fiber is an important part of the diet for dogs with diabetes mellitus because it helps to stabilize blood sugar levels by extending the time that nutrients are absorbed.

BOX 12-3 Carbohydrates

Soluble	Fiber
Starches	Pectin
Sugars	Lignin
	Cellulose
	Mucilage
	Gum

Fiber is digestible by bacteria and protozoan microbes in the rumen, cecum, and large intestine of grazing animals. Short-chain fatty acids result from fiber digestion, which in turn are transformed into glucose. Thus fiber serves as a major energy source for grazing animals. The role of fiber in the diet generally depends on the physiology of the animal's digestive tract, but in most species, fiber assists in regulating bowel function. In addition, the products of microbial fermentation (of fiber) play an important role in maintaining normal colonic function by decreasing pathogenic intestinal bacteria and may play a part in preventing intestinal cancer.

TECHNICIAN NOTE Cellulose, and other types of insoluble fiber, is a tough, structural component of grass, plants, and wood. Mammals do not have the digestive enzymes needed to break down fiber directly. However, horses, cattle, and other grass eaters house microbes and protozoa in their GI tracts (rumen, cecum, and large intestine) that break fiber down via fermentation.

Lipids and Fatty Acids

Lipids that are solid at room temperature are referred to as fats, whereas lipids that are liquid at room temperature are referred to as oils. The lipid is classified as dietary fat. Dietary fats are primarily made up of units called triglycerides, composed of three fatty acids held together by a molecule of glycerol. Fatty acids are the primary components of vegetable and animal fats.

The type of fatty acid primarily determines the structure and characteristic of fat. There are several families of fatty acids, named according to the position of the first double bond. Fatty acids with no double bonds in the primary hydrocarbon chain are referred to as saturated. Subsequently the fatty acid with one double bond is called monosaturated, and the one with more than one double bond is called polysaturated.

The type and distribution of constituent fatty acids determine the physical, nutritional, and biologic characteristics of the fat and oil. Lipids have one to three molecules of fatty acids, are highly digestible, and have twice the caloric density of a similar quantity of carbohydrates or protein.

TECHNICIAN NOTE Fats serve as primary sources of energy, supply essential fatty acids, facilitate digestion, and act as carriers for the fat-soluble vitamins (A, D, E, K).

Fat also facilitates digestion. The length of the carbon chain *backbone* identifies a fatty acid as *long-chain, medium-chain,* or *short-chain.* Short-chain fatty acids (one to eight carbon atoms in length) from rumen fluids and gases are important sources of energy for grazing animals. Long-chain fatty acids (12 to 20+ carbon units) are the most common components of dietary fats and oils in companion animals.

The primary function of fat and fatty acids is multifold. They serve as principal sources of energy, provide palatability and texture to food, and most importantly, supply essential fatty acids and act as carriers for the fat-soluble vitamins (A, D, E, K).

Essential fatty acids are polysaturated, long-chain fatty acids that are necessary for normal body function. Mammals cannot synthesize essential fatty acids; they must be obtained by the food. There are three known essential fatty acids, linoleic, α-linoleic, and arachidonic acids. Linoleic and α-linoleic are the parent compounds from which more complex essential fatty acids are made (Box 12-4).

The essential fatty acids serve many important functions. They are an integral part of kidney and reproductive function and key components to cell membrane formation and prostaglandin production. Deficiencies of essential fatty acids include alopecia, dull hair coat, anemia, and hepatic lipidosis. In the critical patient, essential fatty acid deficiency will increase susceptibility to an infection, weaken cutaneous capillaries, and illicit poor wound healing. Fatty acid deficiency is rapidly reversible if essential fatty acids are reintroduced orally or parenterally.

TECHNICIAN NOTE Lipids have one to three molecules of fatty acids, are highly digestible, and have twice the caloric density of a similar quantity of carbohydrates or protein.

Amino Acids and Protein

Amino acids are defined as any organic compound containing the amino and carboxyl group. Amino acids occur naturally in plant and animal tissue and are the chief constituents of protein. **Proteins** are long chains of amino acids held together by peptide bonds. There are roughly 22 known amino acid groups, but these can be arranged in a countless number

BOX 12-4 Essential Fatty Acids

Cats	Dogs
Linoleic	Linoleic
α-linolenic	α-linolenic
Arachidonic	

of ways, each having unique properties and characteristics. Amino acids are considered the building blocks for plant and animal protein.

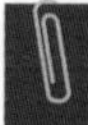

TECHNICIAN NOTE Amino acids are the building blocks for plant and animal protein.

Proteins are essential to all living cells. Functions include the regulation of metabolism, cell membrane construction, muscle fiber formation, and tissue growth and repair. Proteins are the principle structural component of all body organs and tissues, and serve as enzymes, hormones, and antibodies.

Amino acids are classified as either essential or nonessential. Essential amino acids (Box 12-5) are substances that cannot be synthesized in the body in adequate quantities and must be supplemented in the diet. Nonessential amino acids can be synthesized from other sources. Both are of equal importance in physiologic processes. Taurine is an essential amino acid in the cat because the feline liver has limited capacity to synthesize taurine. Taurine deficiency in the cat results in retinal degeneration, reproductive insufficiency, impaired immune function, and has been linked to dilated cardiomyopathy. Clinical signs of taurine deficiency occur only after prolonged periods of depletion (i.e., 6 months to 2 years). Pet owners typically report visual changes or poor depth perception ("miscalculating" jumps).

The quantity and distribution of essential amino acids in a protein are important features determining a protein's biologic quality. All proteins are not of equal worth, and an ideal protein contains the exact essential amino acid distribution profile to meet a specific requirement. In other words, the proportion in which it can be used for growth and maintenance of normal body systems measures the biologic value of a protein. Animal proteins generally have a higher biologic value than plant-based proteins.

Protein-containing ingredients are added to most commercial pet food to supply necessary amino acids; consequently, protein digestibility and amino acid composition must be considered in any dietary analysis. Digestibility is an important factor because the ease of digestion aids in easier absorption. Such digestible proteins are of high nutritional value; consequently, smaller amounts are added to the diet to meet an animal's amino acid requirement. As protein quality is increased, the amount of protein needed decreases. The quality of the protein is often the limiting factor in the amount that must be fed to meet daily requirements.

BOX 12-5 Essential Amino Acids

- Arginine
- Histidine
- Isoleucine
- Leucine
- Lysine
- Methionine
- Phenylalanine
- Threonine
- Tryptophan
- Valine
- Taurine (essential in cats only)

The improper balance of amino acids can decrease protein quality. Even if digestibility is high, the correct balance of amino acids must be present to classify a protein high in biologic value. Pet food companies will often mix animal and plant substances to provide multiple protein sources to improve the overall quality of the food by providing a wide amino acid profile. In addition, an individual amino acid may be added to the diet if the main protein source is limited to ensure a high biologic value. High-quality protein is especially needed during periods of growth, physical exertion, pregnancy, lactation, and for the repair of damaged tissues.

Amino acids are not stored in the body like fat and carbohydrates. If the animal is unable to consume the required levels of amino acids (e.g., during starvation), the breakdown of protein in the viscera and skeletal muscle will then occur. Skeletal muscle and visceral protein breakdown provide amino acids for energy. The breakdown of circulating and structural protein into glucose is called gluconeogenesis. Gluconeogenesis is initiated by the liver and the kidneys using glycerol, lactate, and glucogenic amino acids. Prolonged starvation or food deprivation in normal animals results in a reduction in metabolic rates to slow fat and muscle catabolism in an effort to survive long-term starvation. Eventually, muscle mass will decrease over time if protein needs are not met. Other signs of protein deficiency include weight loss, dull hair coat, **anorexia,** immunodeficiency, poor mentation, generalized edema, and death. Note that even a deficiency of a single essential amino acid can be detrimental.

Cats are specifically adapted to high-protein, low-carbohydrate diets and rely on gluconeogenetic amino acids as a major source of energy. Continuous protein catabolism limits the cat's ability to conserve protein, leading to higher requirements than found in the dog. Dentition patterns of the cat further demonstrate carnivorous eating behaviors, with curved and tapered teeth suitable for tearing the flesh of their prey. Animals subject to chronic anorexia or starvation are in a state of catabolism, which can be reversed by the slow reintroduction of a complete and balanced diet. Metabolic complications can occur if food is consumed or administered too rapidly. Termed "refeeding syndrome," electrolyte shifts occur from extracellular to intracellular compartments as amino acids are reintroduced. Clinical signs can include cardiac arrhythmias, muscle weakness, hemolytic anemia, and respiratory failure.

Dietary protein in excess of the body's requirement is converted to fat and stored as adipose tissue. Although the cat must consume twice the protein as the dog, feeding a food with proper levels of protein is essential. The metabolism of excess amino acids increases the liver and kidney workload by increasing the processing and excretory requirements for the urea and organic acid waste by-products.

Protein Requirements

Dietary protein must be consumed every day to replace amino acids lost to catabolism. Protein synthesis will be limited if certain amino acids are not present or available. In addition, pets with trauma, an infection, severe sepsis, or burns will increase protein turnover. Amino acids are not stored to the same degree that excess fat and carbohydrates are stored.

Clients often inquire about the best protein intake for animals. Crude protein quantity (on the label) is the usual concern, and clients assume that more is better. However, a high protein number is not always the defining criterion for food quality. Chemical analysis for crude protein measures only total nitrogen content. Unfortunately, the essential-to-nonessential amino acid profile, protein digestibility, and amino acid bioavailability may or may not be measured or stated on the label. It is best to contact the manufacturer directly to obtain this information. Lower quantities of a higher biologic-quality protein usually represent a higher-quality food, thus a more appropriate nutritional objective.

> *TECHNICIAN NOTE* The quality of the protein is often the limiting factor in the amount that must be fed to meet daily requirements.

NONENERGY-PRODUCING NUTRIENTS

Water

Although water does not produce energy, it is considered the most important nutrient. Water is essential for almost every chemical reaction, such as the digestion (hydrolysis) of carbohydrates, proteins, and fats. Other functions of water in the body include the transport of solutes and gases, temperature regulation, lubrication of joints and eyes, and electrolyte balance. Water is the largest and heaviest component of our body, making dehydration a common threat to sick patients unwilling or unable to eat and drink. In addition, the physiologic loss of water through diarrhea, vomiting, burns, an infection, etc., in the ill or injured animal will exacerbate anorexia and weakness.

Minerals

Minerals are inorganic chemicals that are an important part of a balanced diet. More than 18 mineral elements are believed to be essential for mammals. Minerals are divided into two groups: macrominerals and microminerals. Macrominerals are required in relatively large amounts, whereas microminerals are required in very small amounts and are therefore also known as "trace elements."

> *TECHNICIAN NOTE* Minerals are inorganic chemicals that are an important part of a balanced diet. More than 18 mineral elements are believed to be essential for mammals.

Macrominerals

Macrominerals include calcium, phosphorus, magnesium, sodium, potassium, chlorine, and sulfur (Table 12-1).

Calcium and phosphorus are constituents of bone and structural proteins. They sustain the structural rigidity of bones and teeth and participate as cofactors and catalysts in many biochemical reactions. Calcium is also a necessary ingredient in normal blood clotting, nerve transmission, and muscle function.

Phosphorus is also an important macromineral and is a major constituent of bone and muscle formation, energy production, and reproduction. Deficiencies impair growth and normal physiologic processes (Table 12-2). The ratio of calcium and phosphorus is of great clinical significance and should be maintained at 1:1. An imbalance of this ratio, such as an increase of phosphorus to calcium, can lead to serious bone malformation. However, nutritional excesses are far more common than deficiencies; excessive levels of calcium and phosphorus in commercial diets have recently been linked to excessive dental plaque formation.

Calcium deficiency results in nutritional secondary hyperparathyroidism, where there is increased bone resorption to restore circulating calcium levels. As a result, growing animals have skeletal deformities and lameness. Calcium deficiency frequently develops when inappropriate homemade food is prepared for dogs, cats, and reptiles. Conversely, high levels of calcium and phosphorus are also harmful. Developmental skeletal diseases, such as wobbler syndrome, hip dysplasia, and osteochondrosis, are thought to be associated with high calcium-phosphorus ratios. Feeding vitamin-mineral supplements, dairy products, and just overfeeding the growth or puppy diet may create a nutritional excess of calcium and/or phosphorus.

Concentrations of all macrominerals in the diet are of fundamental importance. Minerals circulate as cation (+ charge) or anion (− charge) electrolytes and play important roles in the osmotic fluid balance, nerve conduction, muscle contraction, blood clotting, blood pH buffering,

TABLE 12-1 Mineral Categories

Macrominerals*				Microminerals†	
Sodium and Chloride	NaCl	Zinc	Zn	Copper	Cu
Potassium	K^+	Selenium	Se	Iron	Fe
Phosphorus	P	Manganese	Mn	Boron	B
Magnesium	Mg^{2+}	Iodine	I	Molybdenum	Mo
Calcium	Ca^{2+}	Fluorine	F	Cobalt	Co
Sulfur	S	Chromium	Cr		

*Measured in %.
†Measured in ppm or mg/kg.

TABLE 12-2 Mineral Functions and Effects of Deficiency and Excess

Mineral	Function	Deficiency	Excess
Calcium	Constituent of bone and teeth, blood clotting, muscle function, nerve transmission, membrane permeability	Decreased growth, decreased appetite, decreased bone mineralization, lameness, spontaneous fractures, loose teeth, tetany, convulsions, rickets (osteomalacia: adults)	Decreased feed efficiency and intake, nephrosis, lameness, enlarged costochondral junctions, adverse effect on bone and cartilage maturation
Phosphours	Constituent of bone and teeth; muscle formation; fat, carbohydrates; and protein metabolism; phospholipid and energy production; reproduction	Decreased appetite, decreased feed efficiency, decreased growth, dull hair coat, decreased fertility, spontaneous fractures, rickets	Bone loss, urinary calculi, decreased weight gain, decreased feed intake, calcification of soft tissues, secondary hyperparathyroidism
Potassium	Muscle contraction, transmission of nerve impulses, acid-base imbalance, osmotic balance, enzyme cofactor (energy transfer)	Anorexia, decreased growth, lethargy, locomotive problems, hypokalemia, heart and kidney lesions, emaciation	Rare Paresis, bradycardia
Sodium Chloride	Osmotic pressure, acid-base balance, transmission of nerve impulses, nutrient uptake, waste excretion, water metabolism	Inability to maintain water balance, decreased growth, anorexia, fatigue, exhaustion, hair loss	Occurs only if there is inadequate good-quality water available; causes thirst, pruritus, constipation, seizures, and death; chronic amounts may complicate hypertension
Magnesium	Component of bone, intercellular fluids, neuromuscular transmission, active component of several enzymes, carbohydrate and lipid metabolism	Muscular weakness, hyper-irritability, convulsions, anorexia, vomiting, decreased mineralization of bone, decreased body weight, calcification of aorta	Urinary calculi
Iron	Enzyme constituent: activation of O_2 (oxidases, oxygenases), O_2 transport (hemoglobin, myoglobin)	Anemia, rough hair coat, listlessness, decreased growth	Anorexia, weight loss, decreased serum albumin concentrations, hepatic dysfunction, hemosiderosis
Zinc	Constituent or activator of 200 known enzymes (nucleic acid metabolism, protein synthesis, carbohydrate metabolism), skin and wound healing, immune response, fetal development, growth rate	Anorexia, decreased growth, alopecia, parakeratosis, impaired reproduction, vomiting, hair depigmentation, conjunctivitis	Relatively nontoxic Reported cases of Zn toxicity from consumption of die cast Zn nuts or pennies
Copper	Component of several enzymes (oxidases), catalyst in hemoglobin formation, cardiac function, cellular respiration, connective tissue development, pigmentation, one formation, myelin formation, immune function	Anemia, decreased growth, hair depigmentation, bone lesions, neuromuscular, enzootic ataxia, aortic rupture, reproductive failure	Hepatitis, increased liver enzyme activity
Manganese	Component and activation of enzymes (glycosyl transferases), lipid and carbohydrate metabolism, bone development (organic matrix), reproduction, cell membrane integrity (mitochondria)	Decreased growth (rare in dogs and cats), impaired reproduction	Relatively nontoxic
Selenium	Constituent of glutathione peroxidase and iodothyronine-5-deiodinase, immune function, reproduction	Muscular dystrophy, reproductive failure, decreased feed intake, subcutaneous edema, renal mineralization	Vomiting spasms, staggered gait, salivation, decreased appetite, dyspnea, "garlicky" breath, nail loss
Iodine	Constituent of thyroxine and triiodothyronine	Goiter, fetal resorption, rough hair coat, enlarged thyroid glands, alopecia, apathy, myxedema, lethargy	Similar to deficiency, decreased appetite, listlessness, rough hair coat, decreased immunity, decreased weight gain, goiter
Boron	Regulates parathyroid hormone, influences metabolism of Ca^{2+}, P, Mg^{2+}, and cholecalciferol	Decreased growth, decreased hematocrit, hemoglobin, and alkaline phosphate values	Similar to deficiency

From Hand MS et al, editors: *Small animal clinical nutrition*, et 4, Topeka, 2000, Mark Morris Institute.
Ca, Calcium; *P*, phosphorus; *Mg*, magnesium; *Zn*, zinc.

and numerous other physiologic processes (see Table 12-2). Examples of macrominerals include potassium, sodium, chloride, and magnesium. Deficiencies of macrominerals are uncommon in animals fed a standard commercial diet, but can occur in cases of anorexia, starvation, or dietary insufficiency. Excess macromineral intake can result from feeding large amounts of supplements, such as bone meal, or a diet limited to meat. The owner's supplementation leads to excess total intake when most commercial diets are already adequate in macrominerals. The technician most commonly encounters this situation among well-intentioned, but uninformed, purebred animal hobbyists.

Macrominerals are measured in the diet as a percentage (%), whereas microminerals are expressed in parts per million (ppm). When evaluating feed as a potential source of minerals, it is best to consider not only the amount of mineral contained in the food, but also on how much the mineral can be used by the animal. Mineral availability in the diet depends upon solubility, metabolic interactions with other nutrient compounds, the signalment of the animal, and the animal's ability to store the mineral. Animals consuming meat, for example, will consume much higher levels of minerals than animals consuming plant-derived food substances.

> *TECHNICIAN NOTE* Minerals are divided into two groups: macrominerals and microminerals. Macrominerals are required in relatively large amounts, whereas microminerals are required in very small amounts and therefore are also known as "trace elements."

Microminerals

Trace elements, or microminerals, are nutrients that are required in relatively small amounts, but are, nevertheless, essential for normal health in companion animals. Important microminerals include iron, manganese, copper, iodine, and selenium. Dietary requirements for these minerals are in ppm (mg/kg) instead of the percentage amounts for macrominerals (see Table 12-1).

The micromineral iron is a central component of the hemoglobin and myoglobin molecules, which carry oxygen in blood and muscle, respectively. Iron is also important in the enzymatic processes of cellular respiration. Because of the limited capacity of the body to excrete iron, homeostasis is obtained by iron absorption. Iron is stored primarily in the liver, bone marrow, and spleen. Because most commercial pet food has high concentrations of iron, as a result of the meat content, iron deficiency is not common among healthy animals fed standard commercial diets. Iron deficiency can be seen in animals with chronic blood loss, such as those with hookworm or other parasitic infestations. A hypochromic microcytic anemia results when iron stores become depleted. Nursing pediatric patients are particularly susceptible to anemia because milk is low in iron.

Other micromineral constituents are chromium, fluoride, nickel, molybdenum, silicon, vanadium, and arsenic. Such trace elements play roles in cell membrane function, teeth and bone development, and growth and reproduction. The amounts required in the diet are low, and deficiencies are rarely seen in animals fed a balanced diet. Dietary excesses of trace elements can be toxic. The proportion of microminerals ingested must be appropriate, or pathologic conditions can result.

Both microminerals and macrominerals can interact with one another. These interactions tend to be of two types, either antagonistic or synergistic. Antagonistic interactions are defined as the presence of one mineral reducing the transport or efficacy of the other. Synergistic interactions are two minerals acting in a complementary fashion by either enhancing biologic function or sparing the other mineral. Most mineral interactions are antagonistic and occur through a number of different mechanisms, such as during processing, digestion, storage, transport, or in the excretory pathway. Even a marginal deficiency of one vitamin can alter the efficacy of another.

> *TECHNICIAN NOTE* The micromineral iron is a central component of the hemoglobin and myoglobin molecules, which carry oxygen in blood and muscle, respectively.

Vitamins

Vitamins are organic compounds necessary for normal physiologic function. Most vitamins cannot be synthesized in the body and must be present in the diet. Vitamins are classified as either fat-soluble (vitamins A, D, E, K) or water-soluble (B-complex vitamins and vitamin C).

As a result of such differences in solubility, vitamins are absorbed in the body through a variety of means.

> *TECHNICIAN NOTE* Vitamins are classified as either fat-soluble (vitamins A, D, E, K) or water-soluble (B-complex vitamins and vitamin C).

Fat-soluble vitamins require bile salts and fat clusters for passive absorption through the wall of the duodenum and ileum. In contrast, water-soluble vitamins are absorbed via active transport. Water-soluble vitamins are poorly stored in the body, with excesses lost via the urinary tract. Consequently, frequent intake is critical. On the other hand, fat-soluble vitamins are stored in lipid deposits in all tissues and are required in smaller daily doses. As a result of such different absorptive and storage patterns, deficiencies and toxicities vary among fat- and water-soluble vitamins.

Vitamins are not energy nutrients, and not all types are essential for every species. In addition, an intake in excess of requirements does not improve performance. Oversupplementing fat-soluble vitamins may lead to toxic syndromes (Table 12-3). Conversely, water-soluble vitamins are depleted faster because of a limited storage capability, making toxicity less likely than deficiency.

TABLE 12-3 Vitamins

Vitamin	Function	Deficiency	Toxic Effects
Vitamin A	Component of visual proteins, differentiation of epithelial cells, spermatogenesis, immune function, bone resorption	Anorexia, retarded growth, poor hair coat, weakness, increased cerebrospinal fluid pressure, eye disorders, aspermatogenesis, fetal resorption	Cervical spondylosis (cat), retarded growth, anorexia, erythema, long-bone fractures
Vitamin D	Ca^{2+} and P homeostasis, bone mineralization and resorption, insulin synthesis, immune function	Rickets, osteoporosis, osteomalacia	Hypercalcemia, calcinosis, lameness, anorexia
Vitamin E	Biologic antioxidant, maintains membrane integrity	Sterility (males), steatitis, anorexia, dermatosis, immunodeficiency, myopathy	Minimally toxic, increased clotting time reversed with vitamin K
Vitamin K	Allows blood clotting protein formation	Prolonged clotting time, hemorrhage, hypoprothrombinemia	Minimally toxic, anemia (dogs), none described in cats
Vitamin B complex	Multiple metabolic reactions, component of energy-producing biochemical reactions that produce energy and allow proper function of tissues and organs	Retarded growth, diarrhea, emaciation, ataxia, anemia, dermatitis	Low toxicity, except niacin in the cat, which can cause convulsions and death
Vitamin C	Synthesized from D-glucose in dogs and cats; synthesis of collagen proteins and carnitine, biologic antioxidant	Deficiency symptoms have not been described in normal dogs and cats	None described in dogs and cats
Choline	Component of membranes, neurotransmitter	Fatty liver (puppies), thymus atrophy, decreased growth rate, anorexia	None described in cats and dogs
Carnitine (vitamin-like nutrient)	Transports long-chain fatty acids into the cell	Hyperlipidemia, cardiomyopathy, muscle asthenia	None described in cats and dogs

From Hand MS et al, editors: *Small animal clinical nutrition,* ed 4, Topeka, 2000, Mark Morris Institute.
Ca, Calcium; *P,* phosphorus.

All commercial pet food contains vitamins. However, patients can have vitamin deficiencies. For example, cats fed home-cooked diets rich in polyunsaturated fatty acids (found in fish) are at risk for developing a deficiency of vitamin E. The deficiency causes a painful inflammation of adipose tissue and is commonly known as "yellow fat disease" or pansteatitis.

Vitamin K deficiency is also clinically observed. Vitamin K plays a critical role in the coagulation of blood, and deficiencies result in clotting abnormalities and hemorrhage. Warfarin, found in rodent poison, interferes with the availability of vitamin K and causes fatal hemorrhaging in mice and rats. Pets that consume warfarin-poisoned rodents can become poisoned themselves and may slowly bleed to death without emergency supplementation of vitamin K.

> *TECHNICIAN NOTE* Vitamin K plays a critical role in the coagulation of blood, and deficiencies result in clotting abnormalities and hemorrhage.

Certain vitamins, such as vitamins C and E, are antioxidants and help free the body of the damaging effects of free radicals. The supplementation of these vitamins above the normal daily requirements can be beneficial. Antioxidants function as electron donors and oxygen and free radical scavengers. They also destroy invading organisms and help to restore damaged tissues. Nutritional antioxidants in canine food helps protect immune function and improve cognitive dysfunction in senior dogs.

Breakthrough research in the field of animal nutrition has also improved senior pet food by the addition of multiple antioxidant agents and omega-3 fatty acids to support cell membranes, protect against free radical damage, and help improve skin and coat condition. In addition, antioxidant additives in pet food may be a natural alternative to synthetic preservatives and improve palatability.

There are vitamin-like compounds that exhibit properties similar to those of vitamins, but are technically not classified as true vitamins. These include carnitine, carotenoids, and bioflavonoids. Their functions include: the metabolism of fatty acids, support of electron transport, and antioxidant capability.

An emerging area of food and food technology includes the clinical use of nutraceuticals. Nutraceuticals are defined in veterinary medicine as endogenous substances that may provide medical or health benefits. They are either specifically defined by the FDA or not defined or regulated. Nutraceuticals have grown in popularity over the past decade; currently, dietary supplements are sold in health food stores, supermarkets, pharmacies, and over the Internet. Clearly, there is a need for increased scientific research in the area of alternative medicine focusing on the mechanism of action, efficacy, and safety of nutraceuticals. Information should be sought directly from the manufacturer of any nutraceutical to advise clients on product selection and use. Examples of nutraceuticals include chondroitin sulfates and glucosamines, which may inhibit inflammatory mediators and promote joint stability, and omega-3 fatty acids, for modulating the immune response in patients with cancer.

PET FOOD EVALUATION

Many clients will ask for recommendations of the best food to feed their pet and will inquire about the many differences between commercial brand foods. Other owners will ask about the suitability of home cooking or about supplementing an existing diet with table food. Note that although various homemade food can be suitable for daily maintenance, most commercial pet food is superior in nutrient content, convenience, cost, and overall quality. Published homemade pet food recipes are generally imbalanced; energy and nutrient requirements for companion animals are not linear, and long-term use will result in nutrient deficiencies or excesses.

Nutritional terms commonly used in commercial pet food includes phrases such as complete and balanced. A complete diet contains nutrients with appropriate bioavailability, and a balanced diet provides the proper amount and nutrient ratio needed for a 24-hour period. In combining these two diets, the animal fulfills both its nutrient and energy requirements. If nonenergy nutrients are in proper concentration to the energy density of the food, the diet is also considered balanced. Complementary diets combine two or more food sources to improve outcome. For example, a small amount of a canned dog food mixed with dry food increases palatability for many dogs.

Other nutritional terms include: all purpose and special purpose. All-purpose food is marketed under the premise that one particular type of diet meets nutritional demands at every life stage. Such diets are typically found in grocery stores to target the uninformed consumer and are generally sold as off-brand or generic food. Formulated for the growth and lactation periods of companion animals, such diets are not appropriate for the other stages of life. In other words, all-purpose food provides nutrients in excess of what is required by the adult or geriatric animal.

> TECHNICIAN NOTE All-purpose food provides nutrients in excess of what is required by the adult or geriatric animal.

Special-purpose food provides specialized nutrition for individual needs. Special-purpose food is designed for animals with specific nutritional needs, such as the obese or obese-prone animal, the working dog, or the sick and injured pet. Special-purpose food is often sold in veterinary hospitals, where clients are educated about which diet is most beneficial for the individual needs of their pets. Many such special-purpose foods are designed to slow down progression of a disease process, such as heart or renal failure, and will require a veterinarian's approval for purchase.

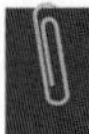

> TECHNICIAN NOTE The quality of a diet is not related to the percentage of moisture it contains.

NUTRIENT CONTENT AND FORMS OF PET FOOD

Commercial pet food is prepared with varying amounts of water. Three basic forms are available to the consumer: dry, semimoist, and moist. Dry food typically has 3% to 11% water. Semimoist food has 25% to 35%, and moist food, which is the most palatable to dogs and cats, contains 70% to 83% moisture. Nutrient profiles vary with each type of food so that both high- and low-quality food can be found in every form. Thus the quality of a diet is not related to the percentage of moisture it contains.

Dry food characteristically has lower proteins, fat, and minerals on a dry-matter basis than most moist food. In addition, dry food is produced with higher caloric density and typically costs less than most moist food. Dry food may also provide a dental hygiene benefit, although neither dry food nor hard-baked treats should replace regular dental prophylaxis.

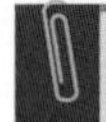

> TECHNICIAN NOTE Neither dry food nor hard-baked treats should replace regular dental prophylaxis.

When dry pet food is made, raw ingredients are mixed and moistened into dough. The dough is kneaded, cooked, and processed via extrusion. Extrusion uses high temperatures to fully cook and shape kibbles, which leads to digestibility and palatability. It is the most common method of making dry and semimoist diets, and it is important in killing the microorganisms that may be carried in the raw materials.

Although dry pet food is less palatable than moist forms, they have the advantage of having a lower *true cost* (Box 12-6). The true cost of feeding is the cost of feeding a pet per day or cost per year. This important concept needs to be explained to the pet owner because there are significant differences between dry and canned food. Evaluating both types of food on a cost-per-pound or a cost-per-calorie basis may result in an economically sound decision. For example, dry food costs approximately one third as much as moist food on a cost-per-calorie basis. In general, dry pet food is the major source of calories in North America. In addition to being cost-effective, dry food is convenient, easy to use, and allows the owner to leave food out for extended periods of time. In this way, pets may eat on an ad-lib basis. Access to unlimited dry food may contribute to obesity; annual health examinations should include body condition scoring and pet food consultation as the animal ages.

Water may be added to create a "gravy" that improves the acceptability of a dry pet food. In addition, palatability may also be improved by mixing dry food with canned food.

BOX 12-6 Cost of Feeding

The cost of feeding on a per-day basis is a better measure of value than the unit cost of the can or package.

Pet owners usually compare the cost of pet food on the price per unit (e.g., price per bag or price per can) rather than the true cost of feeding (cost per day or cost per year). It is easy to compare the price per unit when evaluating two different pet foods, but more difficult to compare the true cost of feeding. The following example demonstrates that veterinarians and their health care team members need to discuss the true cost of feeding with pet owners when clients are concerned about the price of a particular food.

Moist Cat Food

A 4.5-kg, 3-year-old neutered male cat is diagnosed with LUTD caused by struvite urolithiasis. A moist veterinary therapeutic food (food A) is recommended to help prevent further episodes of struvite urolithiasis. The cat's owner is concerned about the "high cost" of the veterinary therapeutic food, but would be willing to use food A if it costs the same as what she now feeds her cat (food B, a gourmet grocery brand). This calculation shows that the veterinary therapeutic food costs markedly less to feed than the cat's current food. By feeding a therapeutic food formulated to prevent FLUTD, recurrence may decrease and the owner may have additional savings in decreased veterinary bills.

	Food A	Food B
Cost/can	.99	.50
Size of container	156 g	100 g
Cost/g	.006	.005
Feeding amount (300 kcal)	285 g	350 g
Cost/day	$1.28	$1.75
Cost/year	$468	$639

Keep in mind, however, that if dry food is moistened with water and left outside in high temperatures, bacterial proliferation is possible.

Food-borne illnesses can be prevented by ensuring consumption of moist food within a few hours. Certain bacteria (e.g., *Bacillus cereus*) are found in soil, grains, cereal products, and other food. These bacteria may be found in small numbers in dry pet food and are normally of no health significance. However, they can rapidly increase in number when moisture levels are raised (e.g., adding water or moist food to dry pet food) at room temperature. These bacteria can produce a potent toxin that causes vomiting and diarrhea. Pet owners should be warned not to add water to dry pet food and leave them exposed to high ambient temperatures for prolonged periods. Dry pet food with added water or mixed with moist food are usually safe if consumed within a few hours.

TECHNICIAN NOTE Dry food moistened with water and left outside in high temperatures can cause bacterial proliferation and consequent food-borne illnesses. Ensure consumption of moist food within a few hours.

Semimoist and soft-dry food have a moisture content ranging from 25% to 40% and are composed of a meat and cereal mixture extruded into small, attractive shapes. Artificial flavors provide a sweet, savory flavor yielding high palatability. Humectant preservatives and cellophane wrapping provide a reasonable shelf life and convenience to the pet owner. Antimicrobial additives help prevent spoilage or bacterial proliferation. It is important to know that semimoist food has readily available soluble sugars and simple carbohydrate sources that are not recommended in the obese or diabetic animal or any other animal in which blood sugar needs to be regulated. Sodium concentrations may also be elevated in semimoist and soft-dry food and must be used with caution in the pet with cardiovascular disease.

Soft-dry food is the combined result of semimoist and dry products. Such hybrid mixes give the advantages of the dry food enhanced with the palatability found in the semimoist food.

TECHNICIAN NOTE Semimoist food has readily available soluble sugars and simple carbohydrate sources not recommended in the diabetic animal or any other animal in which blood sugar needs to be regulated.

Canned or moist food is typically 70% to 83% water and has three forms: a ration loaf, an all-meat appearance, or processed meats and flours bound into a jellied matrix by gums or alginates. The high palatability of canned food results from a high content of water, protein, fat, and the inherent flavor of animal-source tissue. Moist food requires portion-controlled feeding to prevent overconsumption because most pets prefer canned products to dry food. Most moist food in North America is sold as complete diets, with all nutrients present.

Moist food is preserved with heat sterilization and vacuum techniques to ensure an anaerobic environment. Enamel liners insulate the product and provide excellent nutrient stability. The shelf life ranges from 12 to 18 months, provided care is taken in storing at normal temperatures. Palatability may decrease toward the end of the shelf life.

Moist food has a low caloric density. Moist food is expensive on a per calorie basis because fresh and frozen meat by-product ingredients are more costly than equivalent meals and flours. In addition, higher packaging costs correspond to a higher daily feeding cost to the pet owner.

The use of moist food as a combination mixer with dry food is an acceptable practice to increase palatability and control cost. Note that as the ratio of moist food increases in a mix, the palatability and percentage of fat and protein calories usually increase.

TECHNICIAN NOTE The use of moist food as a combination mixer with dry food is an acceptable practice to increase palatability and control cost.

TABLE 12-4 Nutrient Characteristics of Human Snack Foods*

Food	Serving Size	kcal/Serving	kcal/g	Protein (g)	Fat (g)	Sodium†
Cow's milk (3.5%)	1 C = 244 g	150	0.6	8	8	122/81
Whole egg (boiled)	1 egg = 50 g	79	1.6	6.1	5.6	69/87
Ice cream (vanilla, 10% fat)	1 C = 133 g	266	2.0	4.8	14.3	116/43
American cheese	1 oz	93	3.3	5.6	7	337/362
Cottage cheese (low fat, 2%)	1 C = 226 g	203	0.9	31	4.4	918/452
Gelatin	1 C = 280 g	162	0.6	3.2	0	108/67
Hot dog	8/lb = 57 g	180	3.2	6.9	16.3	585/325
Bologna (beef)	1 slice = 23 g	72	3.1	2.8	6.6	226/313
Big Mac	1 sandwich = 200 g	570	2.9	24.6	35	979/172
Peanut butter (smooth)	2 T = 32 g	188	5.9	9	5.4	234/124
Popcorn (w/butter)	3 C = 37 g	192	5.2	2.8	11.5	273/142
Corn chips	1 oz	153	5.5	1.7	8.8	218/142
Potato chips	1 oz	148	5.3	1.8	10.1	133/90
Pretzels	1 oz	110	3.9	3.0	1.2	543/493

All values from Pennington JAT: *Food values of portions commonly used*, ed 15, New York, 1989, Harper & Row.
C, Cup; *T*, tablespoon.
*Metabolizable energy for humans.
†Sodium content per serving/sodium content per 100 kcal.

Treats are small food rewards that the pet owner may give as a training aid or to reinforce love or affection. Commercially prepared treats or snacks should not be given in excess because such practice could interfere with normal appetite, dietary balance, and may contribute to obesity (Tables 12-4 and 12-5). Chocolate is not recommended because it is toxic in high concentrations. Because treats may be a substantial source of calories and protein for some pets, it is important for the technician to inquire about the use of treats when completing the patient's history. This is particularly important if the pet suffers from diseases that require dietary restrictions, such as diabetes mellitus, urolithiasis, cardiac and renal insufficiency, and obesity. Commercial treats are not subject to testing as is pet food. Nutritional excesses are common in many commercial pet food treats.

The use of supplements should not be confused with treats. Whereas treats are nutritionally trivial when used in small amounts, the supplement is generally administered to correct a nutritional deficiency. The routine use of supplements is not necessary if the pet is provided with a balanced commercial pet food.

HOME-PREPARED DIETS

Many dog and cat owners prefer to prepare homemade food, despite the fact that most commercial food is easier to use, is less expensive, and provides better nutritional balance. Public interest in homemade diets has increased significantly as a result of the 2007 wheat gluten–related pet food recall. Homemade recipes may not be appropriate for individuals with unique physiologic requirements; consequently, close monitoring of the diet's efficacy is essential. This may include monitoring weight changes, fecal quality and consistency, food acceptance or refusal, pet activity level, water consumption, complete blood count and serum biochemical changes, and urinalysis changes.

Formulation of a home-prepared diet also requires detailed knowledge of the specific nutrient need, nutritional value of the ingredients, knowledge of any possible dietary interactions, possible deterioration of nutrients during cooking and storage, and consideration of the time and effort required in making such a diet. It is imperative that the owner follow a veterinarian-approved recipe so that a balanced diet is made. There are no human daily supplements that can be added to make a complete and balanced homemade pet diet. If human supplements for vitamins, minerals, and choline are used, splitting the capsules into proper proportions is risky and can easily lead to administration of toxic amounts.

Although it is possible to achieve the same nutrient balance with a homemade food as with a commercially prepared food, it is important for the client to understand that homemade recipes are not tested or evaluated as is commercial pet food. Pet owners interested in feeding a homemade diet should consult with a competent veterinarian or preferably a board certified veterinary nutritionist to obtain a balanced recipe. Veterinarians and technicians together should provide pet owners with recommendations or provide guidelines in assessing homemade food. In addition, the owner's compliance should be regulated by the veterinary professional and diets kept in conformity with the animal's needs.

> *TECHNICIAN NOTE* Pet owners interested in feeding a homemade diet should consult with a competent veterinarian or preferably a board certified veterinary nutritionist to obtain a balanced recipe.

Most homemade recipes have been crudely balanced using the average nutrient content of specific food and computer formulation. Unlike commercial food, few of the numerous published homemade recipes for dogs and cats

TABLE 12-5 Dog and Cat Treats

Treat	Manufacturer	Weight (g/treat)	Calories (kcal/ml)	Protein (g)	Fat (g)	Fiber (g)	Calcium (mg)	Phosphorus (mg)	Potassium (mg)	Sodium (mg)	Magnesium (mg)
Dog Treats											
Milkbone (small)	Nabisco	5	16	1.1	0.3	0.1	71	54	30	21	7
Beggin Strips Orginal Bacon Flavor	Purina	10.3	29	1.7	0.6	0.1	44	49	33	65	11
Bonz	Purina	20.4	66	3.1	1.3	0.3	241	155	86	53	24
Purina Biscuits (medium)	Purina	10.2	37	2.5	1.3	0.2	114	106	91	29	21
Meaty Bone (medium)	Heinz	18.2	64	2.3	1.8	0.4	8	55	71	116	20
100% Natural Treats	Heinz	7.6	26	1.3	0.5	0.1	17	49	48	41	15
Snausages (beef flavor)	Heinz	6.6	17	1.5	0.6	0.1	61	46	98	44	7
Pup-Peroni Jerky Snack Sticks	Heinz	6.6	21	1.8	1	0.1	55	44	59	73	7
Original Jerky Treats	Heinz	6.8	22	2	1.3	0.1	35	35	71	140	7
Fiber Formula Biscuits (medium)	Stewart	10.1	26	1.5	0.3	1.7	63	37	NA	7	NA
Science Diet (adult maintenance)	Hill's	5	17	1.1	0.5	0.2	29	29	29	11	4
Science Diet (light)	Hill's	5	15	0.8	0.3	0.6	29	29	38	11	7
Science Diet (senior)	Hill's	5	16	0.8	0.4	0.4	30	27	28	7	5
Prescription Diet	Hill's	5	15	0.8	0.3	0.8	28	21	36	5	6
Cat Treats											
Pounce (with tuna)	Heinz	1.5	3.7	0.32	0.13	0.01	13.5	11.3	1:1.2	9.2	1.2
Pounce Hairball Treatment	Heinz	1	2.9	1.7	0.4	0.2	2	6	7	5	0.6
Whisker Lickin's (Kluckers)	Purina	1.1	3	0.32	0.12	0.01	9	10.7	1:0.8	6.2	0.7

From Hand MS et al, editors: *Small animal clinical nutrition*, et 4, Topeka, 2000, Mark Morris Institute.
ME, Metabolizable energy; *NA*, not applicable.

have been tested to document performance over sustained periods, including tests for palatability, digestibility, and safety. Therefore veterinarians and veterinary technicians should encourage regular dietary histories and patient monitoring for pets fed homemade food. The pet owner must be committed to ensuring consistent, proper homemade food; home-cooked food is more expensive, inconvenient, and requires a major time investment. The purchase of new equipment (kitchen scales that weigh in grams, blender or food processors, etc.) may be required by the pet owner.

The veterinary technician should help evaluate the patient on a homemade diet by noting body weight, body condition score, activity level, and conducting a thorough physical examination. Veterinary technicians should be willing to assess an existing homemade food recipe, offer nutritionally adequate recipes, and make appropriate formula substitutions for clients. Taking the time to counsel clients on the different homemade diets will prevent common problems and increase the client's compliance.

It should be noted that many homemade diets contain excessive protein and are deficient in calories, calcium, vitamins, and minerals. Most formulations for dogs use staples such as carbohydrates and meat sources containing more phosphorus than calcium, often exceeding the animal's nutritional requirements. Homemade feline food often is deficient in fat and has low energy density. In addition, no single supplementation can be added to meet the mineral and vitamin requirements found in most commercially prepared food.

Home-Prepared Diet Analysis

Homemade formulations can be checked for nutritional adequacy and adjusted using the following "quick check" guidelines:

- **Do five food groups appear in the recipe?**
- A carbohydrate, fiber source from a cooked cereal grain or potato
- A protein source, (preferably of animal origin; if multisources of protein are used, at least one source should be of animal origin)
- A fat source
- A source of minerals, particularly calcium
- A multivitamin and trace mineral source
- **What is the type and quantity of the primary protein source?**
- The overall protein quality in a homemade food can generally be improved by using an animal-source protein. Skeletal muscle protein from different animal species has very similar amino acid profiles; therefore there is no great advantage to feeding one meat source over another. Note that any cooked animal protein source should provide most of the essential amino acid requirements.
- **Is the primary protein source lean or fatty?**
- The fat content of different cuts of meat varies. When the specified protein source is lean, an additional animal or vegetable fat source should compose 2% to 5% of the formula to ensure energy density requirements.
- **Is the carbohydrate source a cooked cereal or potato? Is it present in a higher or equal quantity than the meat source?**
- The carbohydrate/protein ratio should be approximately 1:1 to 2:1 for cat food and 2:1 to 3:1 for dog food.
- **Is a source of calcium and other minerals provided?**
- A homemade food is almost never balanced in minerals; most homemade food requires a specific calcium supplement.
- **Is a source of vitamins and other nutrients provided?**
- Supplements providing vitamins, microminerals, fatty acids, taurine, and other specific nutrients of concern for cats and dogs should be used in homemade recipes. Owners should consult their veterinarian for proper supplement ratios.

Specific instructions as to feeding and storing homemade food are of utmost importance. Most homemade food lacks preservative agents and is high in moisture content; consequently, such food is very susceptible to bacterial growth. Pet owners should be advised to refrigerate or freeze homemade food and monitor food for color and odor changes. Patients that eat homemade food should be brought in for regular veterinary examinations and nutritional reviews (at least two visits per year). The technician should ask the client to record and submit a 3- to 5-day food history as part of the evaluation.

> *TECHNICIAN NOTE* The veterinary technician should help evaluate the patient on a homemade diet by noting body weight, body condition score, activity level, and conducting a thorough physical examination.

Cooking techniques need to be reviewed in the homemade diet. Although cooking improves digestibility of starch in the carbohydrates, longer periods of cooking may depreciate vitamin concentration and cause protein denaturation of meat sources.

Increased digestibility and caloric density have an inverse relationship to the amount of feces produced in both homemade diets and commercially prepared food. Many owners may be concerned with the volume and firmness of feces excreted by their pet. Notice in Figure 12-2 that the quantity and texture characteristics of feces relate to the amount of dry matter eaten and its digestibility.

Ingredients for both homemade food and commercially prepared food are packaged to provide useful information, some of which is legally required. Labels should identify both the product and target species.

PET FOOD LABELS

Pet food regulation varies from country to country; the pet food label represents a contract between the manufacturer and the consumer. The Association of American Feed Control Officials (AAFCO) establishes standards for label information and the description of ingredients on pet food sold in the United States. The AAFCO ensures that adequate information is communicated to the consumer about the food product. The association is made up of representatives from a wide range of professional organizations, including: the American Veterinary Medical Association (AVMA), the American Animal Hospital Association (AAHA), and the Pet Food Institute (PFI). Pet food labels provide useful information that enables both the veterinarian and the pet owner to make decisions about what to feed and how frequently to feed it. It should be noted that in the United States, health claims on pet food labels or in accompanying literature are subject to FDA investigation. Pet food labels are required to state:

- Net weight
- Product designator (e.g., cat food)
- Name and address of the manufacturer or distributor
- Guaranteed analyses in percentages for crude protein, fat, fiber, and moisture
- A list of ingredients in descending order of preponderance by weight
- Nutritional adequacy statement
- Feeding guidelines

Many labels contain more information than what is listed previously. Feeding instructions, caloric content, and a statement that the diet is complete and balanced with respect to a particular life stage are all additional statements commonly found on pet food labels (Figure 12-3). The veterinary professional should counsel clients on how to read a pet food label (e.g., the consumer should consider whether there is a nutritional adequacy statement based on feeding trials and if there is a telephone number on the label for further inquiries).

The nutritional adequacy statements on pet food labels may vary. Nutritional adequacy statements may use terms such as *totally nutritious* or *complete and balanced.* By AAFCO regulations, the nutritional adequacy of a food only requires recommended levels of essential nutrients at two different life stages: growth and reproduction. A statement such as "formulated to meet the AAFCO dog food nutrient profile" (or similar wording) only indicates laboratory analysis for a minimal chemical content. Such testing is not an animal feeding performance trial and says nothing about adequacy, bioavailability, or excesses.

The AAFCO establishes minimal standards for testing new pet food products. These protocols are used by pet food manufacturers during feeding trials to substantiate the

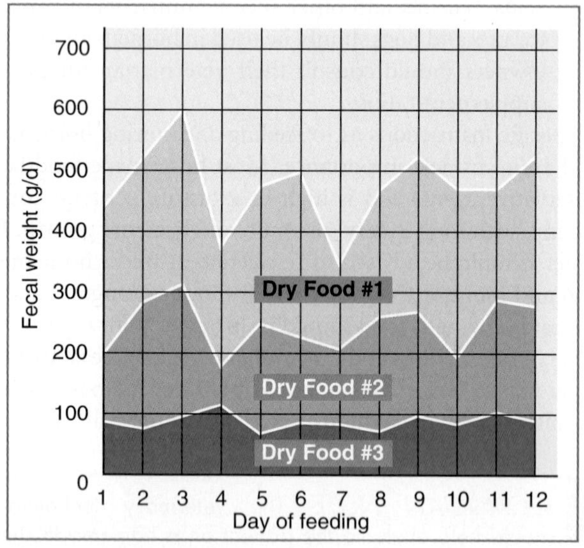

FIGURE 12-2 Increased digestibility and caloric density have an inverse relationship to fecal volume. Food 1 was a lower-energy food and produced voluminous stool volume with difficult cleanup characteristics. Food 3 featured high digestibility and was energy dense, and stool cleanup was quick and nonmessy.

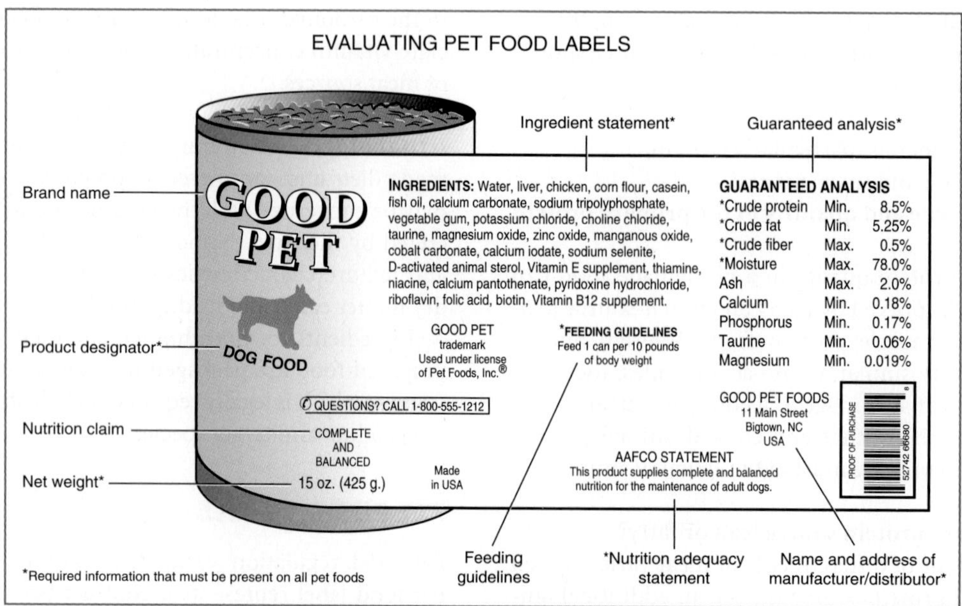

FIGURE 12-3 A pet food label is the contract between the manufacturer and the consumer. A label provides information required by law and may have optional information, such as a statement of calorie content, the Universal Product Code, batch information, or a freshness date.

nutritional adequacy of their product. The AAFCO animal feeding test statement (see Figure 12-3), which is required on pet food labels, lets the consumer know that the product was used in animal feeding tests and that it performed at acceptable levels. Consequently the veterinary technician should recommend feeds to clients that have the "feeding test" information on the label and not the food with the "formulated" statements, if given a choice. It is important to recognize that under current regulations, a pet food company does not have to run feeding trials on each individual product to be able to claim nutritional adequacy.

Nutritional adequacy statements are not needed on treats or snacks intended for intermittent feeding.

There are no government requirements in Canada for the substantiation of nutritional claims on pet food labels. Pet food that meets nutrient standards and passes digestibility feeding trials is given special seals of certification by the Canadian Veterinary Medical Association.

Evaluating Pet Food Labels

Although there is substantial information on pet food labels regarding food quality, there are also some pitfalls to be examined and considered. For example, percentages listed in the guaranteed analyses state only maximum and minimum levels and do not reflect the exact amounts of each nutrient. In addition, because feed labels are a legal contract between the manufacturer and consumer, the guaranteed nutrient levels are conservative and may be far different from the actual analysis. The manufacturer can often supply a more reliable source of data.

Finally the ingredients on labels are listed by weight, with the heaviest ingredients first and the lightest ones last. This often means that water-containing ingredients are listed before drier ingredients even though a dry ingredient may make up a larger portion of the food on a dry-matter basis. The guaranteed analysis, depending on the country, can also give information as to the average content of the food or at least the minimum and maximum values for key ingredients.

Ingredient Percentages

Percentage rules for listed ingredients are important to note when analyzing a diet for nutritional need. According to AAFCO rules, when a label statement identifies only one ingredient, at least 70% of the total product will consist of that named ingredient (e.g., beef). If any modifying words accompany the named ingredient, the amount of the named ingredient that must be present declines to 10% for moist food and 25% for dry food (chicken *dinner,* fish *entree,* liver *stew,* etc.). In addition, if a named ingredient is modified by the word *with* (e.g., with beef), the total portion of the named ingredient declines to 3%. Furthermore, if the term *flavor* is used (e.g., cheese flavor), the named flavor must be detectable only by the animal. The designator *food* (e.g., dog food) means that there are no rules regarding the minimum content of ingredients. Indirectly the technician may gather further quality information about a product through understanding these nuances of pet food labeling.

Percentage rules also apply to moisture content. In the United States, the maximum moisture content is 78%; pet food may exceed this amount if labeled as stew, gravy, juice, or containing a milk replacer.

> TECHNICIAN NOTE A patient's assessment and daily feeding performance analysis will provide greater insight into an animal's well-being than the most informative of pet food labels.

MARKET CATEGORIES

Understanding market objectives for a product may assist with some aspects of assessing a food's quality. Grocery brands are generally well-recognized pet food sold in grocery stores with large-scale advertisement and distribution. Most grocery brands are all-purpose food, balanced for the growth or lactation life stages (see Pet Food Evaluation). "Premium" grocery bands are specific-purpose food types with a more nutritional focus than traditional grocery brands. Other food types include "gourmet" food to sell the consumer on increased palatability for finicky pets.

Generic (white label) and private label (a grocery chain's own brand) food is made at contract feed mills using least-cost formulation methods. Private label brands are common in large supermarket settings and pet retail outlets. Markets emphasize low cost and high palatability and generally sell on anthropomorphic appeal. Flavor, shape, color, ingredients, and brand name proliferation characterize these products, allowing them to engage the largest amount of shelf space.

Specialty brand pet food is often sold in veterinary hospitals, pet superstores, and regular stores. Often called "premium" or "super premium" food, they generally stress better-quality ingredients with exceptional nutritional focus. Although differences in nutritional philosophy may be noted among different manufacturers, these brands are consistent in the *overall* objective of emphasizing a philosophy of optimal nutrition. This specialty brand food typically uses the life-stage and special-needs approach, with a general aim at disease prevention.

COMPANION ANIMAL NUTRITION

ENERGY REQUIREMENTS

An estimate of the energy requirement of an animal is needed to determine how much food to feed. If you recall from the Energy Producing Nutrients section of this chapter, the nutrients that provide energy include proteins, carbohydrates, and fats. When these nutrients are burned, they release energy in the form of heat. Each nutrient releases a different amount of heat, which is measured in kilocalories, or **Calories** (note the upper case "C"). A **kilocalorie** is the amount of heat (energy) needed to raise the temperature of 1 kg of water 1° C. With this in mind, the energy requirements (food) of an animal would be calculated and expressed in kilocalories.

Daily energy requirements are the number of calories needed to maintain an animal's weight. Obviously an increase in the animal's exercise, lactation, and growth would increase energy requirements, whereas a decrease in these activities would lower energy requirements. Increased energy demands over and above the needs for maintenance are called production energy requirements.

Predictive equations are useful in calculating nutrient requirements, but judging the body composition and condition of the animal is also important in determining the caloric needs of the animal. Body condition can be assessed by feeling the ribs with flat palms. Ideally the ribs should be felt, but not seen (Figure 12-4).

Body condition scoring gives the veterinary professional an estimate of an animal's body composition. The body condition score can subjectively assess a pet's fat stores and muscle mass. Note that the body condition scoring system was developed with regard to both age and species.

NUTRITIONAL ASSESSMENT

A thorough nutritional assessment consists of a patient's history and a physical examination including body weight, body condition scoring, and hydration status. The primary goal of nutritional assessment is to identify the dietary needs of the patient. In the course of a disease or treatment process, a patient's nutritional needs can change, and these changes need to be monitored regularly and discussed with the pet owner.

A baseline nutritional assessment should be made upon admission to the hospital and followed by serial assessments throughout the course of the hospitalization (see Clinical Nutrition). The veterinary technician is particularly well positioned to identify baseline data and ongoing changes in nutritional status because the technician typically spends the greatest amount of time with hospitalized patients. Nutritional intervention is crucial to recovery and survival, particularly with the critical patient, and appropriate consideration as to the type and route of nutrition should be given based

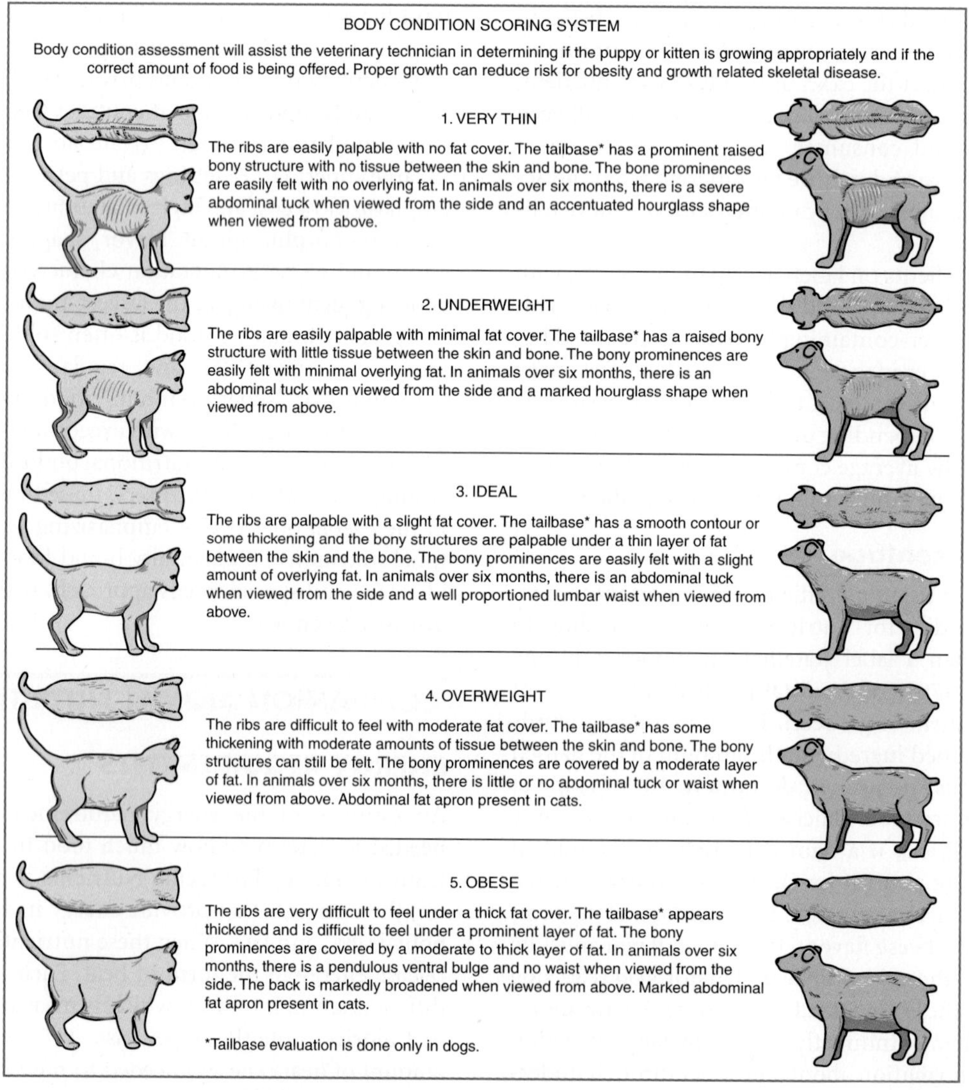

FIGURE 12-4 Body conditioning scoring system.

on the underlying disease process or diagnosis (see Routes of Feeding and Tube Selection).

> *TECHNICIAN NOTE* A thorough nutritional assessment consists of a patient's history and a physical examination including body weight, body condition scoring, and hydration status.

FEEDING DOGS

Dogs are typically omnivores and exhibit eating behaviors similar to their relatives the wolf *(Canis lupus)* and the coyote *(Canis latrans)*. Dogs are opportunistic eaters, predators, and scavengers and have developed anatomic and physiologic traits that allow for the digestion of a variety of food. Although dogs are omnivorous, pet food advertising emphasizes the carnivorous aspects of the canine diet ("meatier is better"). Many domesticated dogs eat vegetables, grains and pastas, meat, processed food, various dairy products, and fruit. Some pet owners complain that their dog eats grass and feces, though such behavior is natural. Cayenne pepper sauce on feces has been helpful in reducing their dog's objectionable behavior.

Because dogs range in size, age, and activity level, nutritional energy requirements are calculated based on the animal's metabolic body weight, or the weight of actively metabolizing tissue. Variations in body composition and breed are also considered. In addition, nutritional requirements should be based on the particular life stage to achieve biologic performance and overall good health (Table 12-6).

The amount of food needed to meet the nutritional requirements of healthy dogs is calculated from the energy value of the food (see Energy Producing Nutrients). Whereas most commercially prepared food contains the essential nutrients needed for a particular life stage, each companion animal should be evaluated individually because of differences in both activity and environment. Regular weighing and body condition scoring will enable the technician to provide general feeding recommendations. If treats or table scraps are added to the staple diet, their energy content must also be taken into account when calculating the amount of food to give.

The frequency of feeding normal dogs may vary. Most adult dogs in the maintenance life stage can obtain daily energy requirements by eating once a day, or two to three times a day to coincide with family meal times. Feeding dogs in the late evening should be avoided so that the owner is not inconvenienced by having to take the dog outside to eliminate in the middle of the night. In addition, large meals should be avoided before exercise, particularly in large-breed dogs, so that the possibility of gastric dilation and torsion is minimized.

TABLE 12-6 Nutrient Guidelines for Wellness*

	Energy	Protein	Fat	Fiber	Calcium	Phosphorus	Sodium
Life Stage	kcal ME/g	Dry Matter					
Dog							
Growth/reproduction	3.5-5.0	22-35	10-25	5 max	0.7-1.7	0.6-1.3	0.35-0.6
Large-breed growth	3.0-4.0	22-35	8-12	10 max	0.7-1.2	0.6-1.1	0.3-0.6
Adult maintenance	3.5-4.5	15-30	10-20	5 max	0.5-1.0	0.4-0.9	0.2-0.4
Obesity Prone	3.0-3.5	15-30	7-12	5-17	0.5-1.0	0.4-0.9	0.2-0.4
High energy	>4.5	22-34	26 min	5 max	0.5-1.0	0.4-0.9	0.2-0.5
Geriatric†	3.5-4.5	15-23	7-15	10 max	0.5-1.0	0.2-0.7	0.15-0.35
Cat							
Growth/reproduction	4.0-5.0	35-50	18-35	5 max	0.8-1.6	0.6-1.4	0.3-0.6
Adult maintenance	4.0-5.0	30-45	10-30	5 max	0.5-1.0	0.5-0.8	0.2-0.6
Obesity Prone	3.3-3.8	30-45	8-17	5-15	0.5-1.0	0.5-0.9	0.2-0.6
Geriatric†	3.5-4.5	30-45	10-25	10 max	0.6-1.0	0.5-0.7	0.2-0.5

Max, Maximum; *min*, minimum; *C*, cup.

*Nutrients are expressed as % dry matter. Energy is expressed as kcal metabolizable energy (ME) per gram dry matter.

†Older animals require frequent body condition scoring. Feed intake adjustment may be required to maintain an ideal body condition because some older individuals tend to be heavy and others tend to lose weigh.

Average Caloric Content of Pet Foods

Dog food (generic, private label, grocery)	
Dry	350 kcal/C
Soft-moist	275 kcal/C
Canned	500 kcal/14- to 15-oz can
Cat food (generic, private label, grocery)	
Dry	300 kcal/C
Soft-moist	250 kcal/C
Canned	180 kcal/5.5- to 6.5-oz can

> *TECHNICIAN NOTE* Large meals should be avoided before exercise, particularly in large-breed dogs, so that the possibility of gastric dilation and torsion is minimized.

Canine Pediatric Nutrition

Milk provides a complete food source for neonates, containing water, protein, fat, vitamins, and minerals. Colostrum is the key nutritional factor immediately after birth. Owners should ensure that the dam is producing colostrum and that the puppies are consuming it. This is particularly pertinent if the bitch delivered the puppies via cesarean section. Colostrum provides fluid for vital postpartum circulatory expansion and carries protective maternal antibodies that are absorbed through the intestine of the puppies. Colostrum is somewhat sticky and viscous, which can make nursing more difficult in the weaker puppy.

Most puppies are healthy and are capable of active nursing. Ensure that the mothers are lactating well and are attentive to the litter. In general, no assistance is needed from the technician or owner. Exceptions may include extremely small, toy-breed puppies for which frequent, assisted hand feedings may be needed to prevent hypothermia and hypoglycemia.

Technicians should advise clients to weigh their puppies if there is concern about poor milk production by the dam or an inadequate consumption of milk by the pups. The examination and expression of the mammary glands is also helpful when assessing milk production. Regular checks are important to ensure good milk flow and to make an early detection of mastitis or other mammary gland complications.

The normal growth rate for puppies is 2 to 4 g/day/kg of anticipated adult weight. Weight gain below this rate and accompanied by restless, hungry-seeming puppies is generally a sign that the puppies are not receiving adequate amounts of milk.

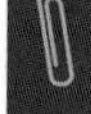

> *TECHNICIAN NOTE* The normal growth rate for puppies is 2 to 4 g/day/kg of anticipated adult weight.

Feeding Orphan Puppies

Neonatal puppies that are unable to nurse should be fed a canine milk replacement formula. Canine milk is higher in protein and lower in lactose than bovine milk; consequently, water should be used to mix the replacement formula and not cow's milk.

The orphan formula dose is initially 15% of the puppy's weight per day divided into several doses. The process of feeding puppies can be facilitated by using a syringe and a flexible, rubber feeding tube (Figure 12-5). If the animal has a strong suckling reflex, a small animal nursing bottle or doll's baby bottle may be used. The nipple may be pierced with a hot needle so that a drop forms over 1 to 2 seconds when the full bottle is tipped upside down. A syringe or eyedropper is not recommended, but can be used in an urgent situation where a bottle is not available. It is essential to deliver the liquid into the mouth slowly to prevent aspiration.

If a feeding tube is used, care must be taken not to place it in the trachea. The stomach capacity of the neonate is approximately 50 ml/kg. Initially, puppies are fed 10 ml q 4 to 6 hours, and kittens are fed 5 ml q 4 to 6 hours. The amount is gradually increased by 1 ml/feeding (dog) or 1 ml/day (cat) until the recommended guidelines are reached. Although feeding frequencies vary, generally the first 3 days of life are the most critical.

Typically the stomach is full from feeding when the belly is distended or the animal turns its head away from the nursing bottle and squirms. New formula should be made at each feeding and not stored reconstituted to prevent bacterial contamination. Food substances should be room temperature before administration. All equipment should be meticulously clean or sterile. Before the litter of puppies is

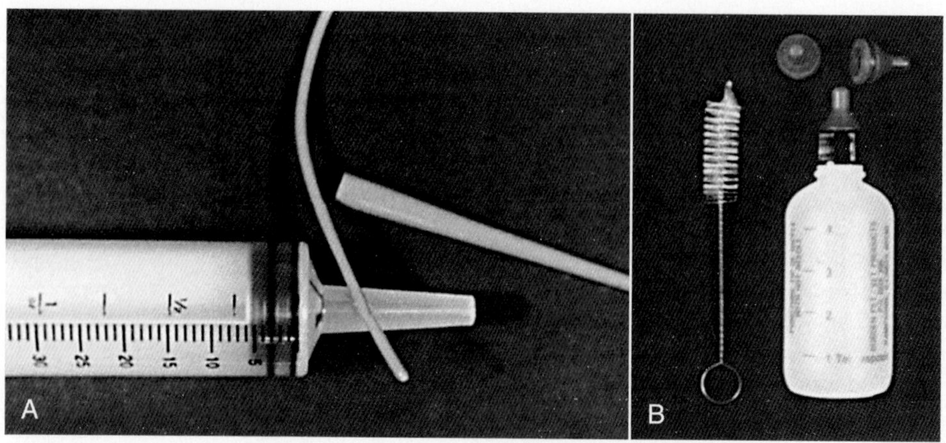

FIGURE 12-5 **A,** Orphan puppies and kittens are raised on species-specific milk replacement. Tube lavage with flexible feeding tube and a catheter-tip syringe is an easy and safe technique in neonatal puppies and kittens. **B,** Pet nursers are used in neonates with adequate sucking vigor. Always test the flow and temperature of formula in advance and sanitize equipment between uses.

discharged, the veterinary technician should pretest the flow rate from each of the nipples and give explicit instructions for keeping the system clean. When the puppy reaches 2 to 3 weeks of age, the food dose should approximate 25% of the body weight divided into four to six daily feedings. Monitoring weight gain by the use of a gram scale is a good way to evaluate food intake.

If the puppies are unable to consume formula or dam's milk on their own, a 5F or 8F infant feeding tube is typically used for gavage. Placement techniques include measuring from the tip of the nose to the last rib, marking the tube, and passing it down the left side of the mouth. A gag reflex is not present until 10 days, but easy passage to the premeasured distance usually indicates correct placement. After delivery of the fluid, kink the tube before withdrawal and withdraw it quickly to prevent aspiration. The animal should be burped after feeding by holding it at a 45-degree angle, massaging the stomach, and patting it gently on the back with fingertips only. The residual stomach volume should be measured by the gentle aspiration of stomach contents (which are then returned to the stomach) before each treatment or feeding to document that fluids are being absorbed and gastric motility is adequate.

When the puppies are able to eat solid food on their own, small amounts of food should be given incrementally until the puppies become content. Satiation is often indicated when the puppies become quiet and fall asleep.

Low birth weight is correlated with an increase in mortality. Puppies with low body weights are more prone to hypoglycemia, hypothermia, and sepsis. The bitch should also be monitored for behavior changes toward any particular pup because the bitch may shun hypothermic and ill puppies. Because body fat is generally low in puppies, the environment should be kept between 84° F and 90° F.

Eternal warming should always be provided if the neonate is separated from its mother. Warming protocols should include the use of circulating hot water blankets only; electric heating pads are not recommended. Other alternatives include warmed rice bags, hot water bottles, heat lamps, or Bair Hugger units, if hospitalized. A pan of water can increase the humidity in the environment. Neonatal incubators can be used to provide a temperature of 85° F to 90° F and a humidity of 55% to 65%.

Whichever heat source is used, the neonate should be able to crawl away from the heat source and the temperature monitored at least every 20 to 30 minutes on the recumbent patient. A thermometer should be placed near the neonate to check the ambient temperature. Hypothermia is common in neonates and is associated with shallow respirations, bradycardia, GI paralysis, and coma. Feeding is contraindicated if the animal is hypothermic (<94° F) because GI motility and digestive function can be impaired.

The neonatal body temperature should be increased slowly. The most effective method is the use of warm inspired air because it warms the core and the external shell (such as provided by the Bair Hugger units, if hospitalized) or an incubator or heated oxygen cage.

Constipation or diarrhea may occur with formula feeding. If diarrhea occurs, the formula should be diluted 1:2 with a balanced electrolyte solution until diarrhea resolves. During the administration of food substrates, the patient's response may not be typical because the gag reflex does not develop until 10 days of age. Consequently, care should be given for the proper placement of a feeding tube. A baseline birth weight should be recorded; healthy puppies are expected to gain 1 to 1.5 g daily for each pound of anticipated adult weight. Assist elimination every 2 to 4 hours (or after each feeding) for up to 4 weeks using cotton balls soaked in warm water to wipe the caudal abdomen and anogenital region. Wipe down the entire animal with a slightly damp, warm face cloth or soft nailbrush one to two times per day.

> *TECHNICIAN NOTE* The orphan formula dose is initially 15% of the puppy's body weight per day divided into several doses.

Weaning Puppies

Peak lactation occurs at 4 weeks, and weaning concludes at 6 to 8 weeks. Begin introducing puppies to semisolid gruel made from two parts of water to 1 part high-quality, dry, canine growth-lactation pet food. Three weeks of age is a suitable time to introduce a semisolid gruel, except for toy breeds and weak animals, which need more time before they are offered solid food. Gruel can be finely chopped or mashed and placed in a shallow bowl for easy consumption. This serves as an important transition food and acclimates puppies to eating solid food. At 5 weeks of age, puppies are reducing their intake of mother's milk and are consuming larger amounts of gruel. The ratio of water can be reduced as the puppies are slowly moved from semisolid to solid food. After weaning, the ability for the pup to digest lactose becomes less efficient. Consequently, it is important to avoid feeding weaned dogs large quantities of milk, which might cause diarrhea. In addition, puppies can exhibit competitive eating as early as 5 weeks of age; puppies should be supervised during feeding to ensure adequate and equal consumption.

Feeding Growing Dogs

Proper nutrition for growing dogs is essential for normal growth and development. An excessive intake, however, can lead to medical complications. Overfeeding, for example, can result in obesity in small breeds and rapid growth rates in large-breed dogs. Inciting stress on the juvenile skeleton by overfeeding in the large breeds can cause abnormalities, such as osteochondritis, hip dysplasia, panosteitis, and wobbler's syndrome. Nutritional requirements change rapidly during a puppy's growth, with growth rates varying between dog breeds. Nutrient guidelines for small- and medium-breed versus large- and giant-breed dogs are listed in Table 12-6. Supplements are generally not needed if the puppies are fed name-brand commercial diets.

Most growing puppies eat four or five times daily during the postweaning period, or until about 10 weeks of age. Meal frequency should be cut to three meals a day until they have reached approximately 50% of their adult body weight, or approximately 4 months of age. Technicians should advise pet owners to feed small meals several times a day and not allow the puppies continuous access to food because many puppies will overeat when fed ad lib.

Growing Concerns For Large-Breed Dogs

Research studies have documented that improper feeding during growth is associated with several skeletal disorders in large-breed dogs. About 22% of dogs less than 1 year of age are affected by developmental skeletal disorders, and more than 90% of these cases are influenced by nutritional factors. Such nutritional factors include free-choice feeding of a diet with excess calories and supplementing calcium during the growth phase. The onset of bone developmental disorders is usually associated with rapid growth of the long bones. As previously mentioned, the most common of these disorders are canine hip dysplasia, osteochondrosis, and hypertrophic osteodystrophy.

Calcium and dietary fat are, however, key nutrients for growing puppies. Unfortunately, some growth types of pet food contains excessive amounts of calcium, even at appropriate levels of dry-matter intake. A study of two populations of Labrador retriever puppies examined the effects of nutritional excess. One group ate ad lib, and the second group was limited to 75% of the ad-lib quantity. Serial pelvic radiography for 2 years showed significant reductions in hip laxity in the meal-limited group.

To help control the risk of abnormal orthopedic development in large- and giant-breed puppies, experts recommend that the caloric content for large-breed dogs should be less than that for smaller breeds and should contain no more than 12% fat on a dry-matter basis.

> *TECHNICIAN NOTE* The caloric content for large-breed dogs should be less than that for smaller breeds, and should contain no more than 12% fat on a dry-matter basis.

Feeding Adult Dogs

The primary objective in feeding the adult dog is to find the maintenance energy requirement and proper food dose to maintain the ideal body composition. Recommended nutrient guidelines for adult dogs are found in Table 12-6. Note that in the adult dog, ad-lib feeding is commonly associated with over consumption and obesity.

The amount of feed needed to meet energy requirements is based upon the energy value of the food. Activity levels also vary between dogs and should be taken into consideration when compiling a feeding protocol. Diverse canine breeds, specifically the variation in breed size, may reflect different metabolic rates and different growth rates. For example, small and toy breeds have a higher energy requirement per unit of body weight than the large and giant breeds because basal metabolic rate is related to total body surface area. Since the smaller breeds have a higher ratio of surface area to body weight than large breeds, they require more energy per unit of weight (lb or kg). In addition, the small breeds have relatively small stomachs, so their ability to consume food is somewhat limited. Consequently, small-breed diets should have a higher energy content and a more nutrient-dense matrix than diets designed for larger breeds. High digestibility is also an important consideration so that optimal nutrition can be provided in small meals. Small, kibble-size dry food should also be considered to aid in chewing and consumption.

Regular weighing and body condition scoring will allow both technician and owner to assess the adequacy of feeding. In addition, environment plays a key factor in energy expenditure. Note that by spaying an animal, energy requirements may decrease 10%; consequently, adjustments in diet may be necessary to prevent weight gain.

> *TECHNICIAN NOTE* An animal's energy requirements may decrease 10% after spaying; consequently, adjustments in diet may be necessary to prevent weight gain.

Feeding each pet separately is best, whenever possible. In the time-restricted method, feed each dog from one to three times daily with ad-lib consumption for 5 to 15 minutes. If the dog consistently leaves a little food in its dish and also maintains an ideal body condition, the conclusion must be that the animal is self-regulating its food intake at its energy requirement.

Time-restricted feeding works well for many dogs and their owners; however, some dogs ravenously overeat during the allotted time. In dogs that overeat, try volume-restricted meal feeding by serving a calculated food dose. To determine the daily volume, divide the energy requirement by the food's caloric density. Then feed one half to one third of the daily volume two or three times per day. An average caloric density guideline for pet food is listed in Table 12-6. Other aids for calculating how much food to feed are: the feeding instructions found on the pet food label, food dose calculators, and technical information from manufacturers. Maintenance pet food is recommended for the average house pet who is 1 to 7 years of age.

It is recommended that table food be eliminated or used in moderation (10% or less). Fat trimmings quickly unbalance a base diet and lead to finicky behavior and a predisposition to obesity. Avoid feeding animal bones because sharp fragments may wedge between teeth, lacerate the esophagus, or cause GI obstruction or constipation. Nylon bones and chew toys are safer substitutes for natural bones, but still cause problems in some individuals. Table 12-6 lists guidelines for assessing pet food used in life-stage feeding.

It is best for each dog to be fed individually; however, as a result of time and labor costs, this may be impractical in animal colonies and kennels. Problems associated with group

BOX 12-7 Feeding Dos and Don'ts

Dos

Provide fresh water.
Feed for control of calorie intake.
Feed for ideal weight and body condition.
Feel but do not see ribs.
Provide a consistent food and ritualize the time and place of feeding.
Use life-stage feeding concepts by correlating diet to pet's life stage.
Feed treats with nutrient profile and caloric density considerations.

Don'ts

Provide stagnant or frozen water.
Allow excess calorie consumption.
Feed obesity-prone dogs on an ad-lib or free-choice basis.
Rotate flavors or brands on a frequent basis.
Make rapid transitions.
Use growth-lactation food for adult maintenance.
Supplement a balanced, high-quality food.
Allow competitive eating.

feeding include anorexia in the timid animal and overconsumption in the aggressive or dominant dog. Group feeding may also result in competitive eating. Competitive eating can trigger quick consumption of food, initiating gastric distention from swallowing or quickly gulping air (aerophagia). In larger breeds, aerophagia may predispose the animal to gastric dilation and torsion. Box 12-7 lists general feeding guidelines.

It is common for the boarded animal to be stressed or compromised and as a result stop eating. The late detection of anorexia may lead to significant medical consequences for the animals not having an adequate intake. Technicians should frequently assess the appetite of boarding animals and feed on an individual basis.

TECHNICIAN NOTE Avoid feeding animal bones because sharp fragments may become wedged between teeth, lacerate the esophagus, or cause GI obstruction or constipation. Nylon bones and chew toys are safer substitutes for natural bones, but they may still cause problems in some individuals.

Feeding Adult Dogs With Increased Energy Needs

Increases in physical activity require extra energy to support increased muscular action. Diet and feeding protocols vary according to training schedules and the amount of work performed. Supplying extra energy to working dogs by using pet food with increased fat, caloric density, and digestibility will allow optimal performance. In addition, feeding diets with extra energy content allows dry-matter intake and gastric fill to remain at familiar, nonexcessive levels. Increasing the quantity or frequency of a regular food is a secondary option to increase performance.

The specific nutrient composition of diets for working dogs varies and depends upon the type of activity performed. In general, staples include fats and carbohydrates for intense muscular exercise. Note that in the sprinting or racing dog, short and intense bursts of energy are required, typically obtained by readily available muscle glycogen stores. Large quantities of carbohydrates may be useful because this may help maximize muscle glycogen reserves.

On the other hand, diets high in carbohydrates may be counterproductive in other working dogs and may even reduce athletic performance. High-carbohydrate diets may lead to lactic acid accumulation during *prolonged* exercise, resulting in muscle fatigue and/or damage. Endurance dogs therefore may benefit from higher fat diets because their muscle activity is powered primarily by aerobic fatty acid oxidation (approximately 70% to 90%).

Animals can be aerobically conditioned before extensive fieldwork. Aerobic training increases the efficiency of fatty acid metabolism in the muscles and the cardiovascular system. Such aerobic conditioning spares the rate of glycogen consumption in muscles and increases the capacity for work. At the start of aerobic conditioning, technicians can advise clients to slowly convert the dog to a more calorie-dense food and suggest feeding the majority of daily calories *after* the completion of training to help prevent hypoglycemia. This is particularly pertinent in hunting dogs.

Unfortunately, most clients feed the caloric-dense food before work or training. Subsequently, after the meals' digestion, insulin is released as a result of glucose absorption, allowing for a high rate of glucose transfer into the cells. If the animal simultaneously begins hard work, the combination of the two glucose-consuming activities may precipitate hypoglycemia. If working dogs show consistent signs of hypoglycemia, even after conditioning, they may be fed 10% to 15% of the daily calorie dose as a light feeding at 2-hour intervals during work. Clients should also be reminded of the importance of an adequate water intake throughout the work period.

Feeding During Pregnancy and Lactation

During lactation, a proper nutrient intake is directly linked to successful milk production. Technicians should recommend a growth-lactation formula to meet the increased requirements. Lactation markedly increases energy, protein, and mineral requirements; nutrient requirements during lactation are greater than at any other adult life stage. After whelping, the bitch returns to her regular body weight (Figure 12-6). Expect the food intake to rise rapidly by 50% the first week and by 200% to 400% by the fourth week of lactation. Free-choice food should be available to the bitch. The water intake should also be monitored because water is the most important nutrient during lactation. After whelping, energy requirements return to maintenance levels in approximately 8 weeks. Frequent physical examinations should be performed to maintain normal health and to assess the adequacy of the diet.

Key nutritional factors in the lactating bitch include highly digestible protein, increased concentrations of fat (in proportion with other nutrients), 10% to 20% soluble carbohydrates, and approximately two to five times more calcium than during the maintenance life stage (Table 12-7).

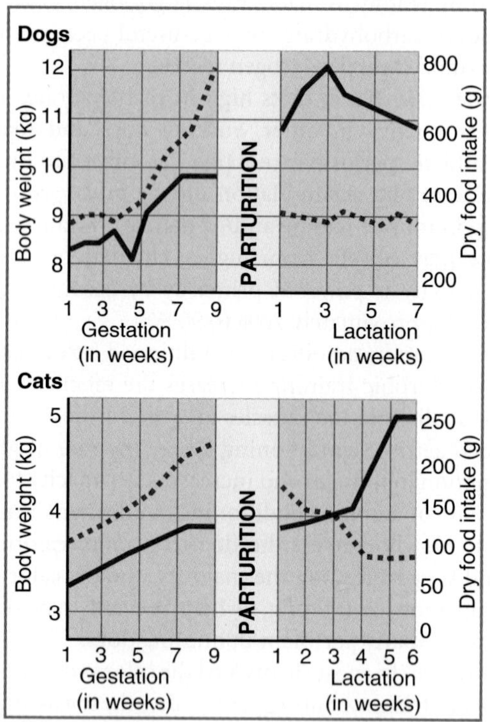

FIGURE 12-6 The pattern of normal weight gain during gestation and loss in the postpartum and lactation periods differs between cats and dogs. *Solid line* indicates food intake. *Dashed line* indicates body weight.

Supplements are generally *not* needed for normal animals when high-quality pet food is used.

> TECHNICIAN NOTE Expect the food intake to rise rapidly by 50% the first week and by 200% to 400% by the fourth week of lactation. Feeding the bitch free choice is recommended.

Feeding Methods During Weaning

The food intake should be terminated for 24 hours to help the bitch slow and stop her milk production. Restricting food will reduce nutrients needed for milk production, resulting in mammary gland reduction. Technicians should advise clients not to allow any puppies to nurse because such practices do not alleviate mammary gland engorgement and may stimulate milk production.

The food intake for the bitch can be resumed using maintenance food at one third of the customary maintenance level. On the second day, two thirds of the normal feeding dose is recommended, with a full intake on day three. As lactation quickly dries from acute calorie deprivation, the bitch will more readily reject the puppies' attempts to continue to nurse.

Obesity-Prone Animals

Definition, Causes, and Health Risks of Obesity

The incidence of obesity in companion animals is almost epidemic. Obesity is currently the most common nutritional disorder that occurs in companion animals in the United States. Surveys taken in 2007 have reported incidence rates

TABLE 12-7 Key Nutritional Factors for Reproduction

	Recommended Levels in Food (Dry Matter)	
Factors	Gestation/Lactation*	Lactation†
Energy density (kcal ME/g)‡	3.5-4.5	4.5-5.0
Energy density (kJ ME/g)‡	14.6-18.8	16.7-20.9
Crude protein (%)	22-32	25-35
Crude fat (%)	10-25	≥18
Soluble carbohydrates (%)	≥23	≥23
Calcium (%)	≤5	≤5
Phosphorus (%)	0.75-1.5	1.0-1.7
Ca/P ratio (%)	1:1-1.5:1	1:1-2:1
Sodium (%)	0.35-0.60	0.35-0.60
Chloride (%)	0.50-0.90	0.50-0.90
Digestibility	Above average	Above average

From Hand MS et al, editors: *Small animal clinical nutrition,* ed 4, Topeka, Kan, 2004, Mark Morris Institute.
*Gestation for all bitches and for lactation of bitches with four or fewer puppies.
†Lactation for bitches with litters of more than four puppies. Some giant-breed bitches may need this type of food during gestation to maintain body weight, particularly during late pregnancy.
‡If the caloric density of the food is different, the nutrient content in the dry matter must be adapted accordingly.

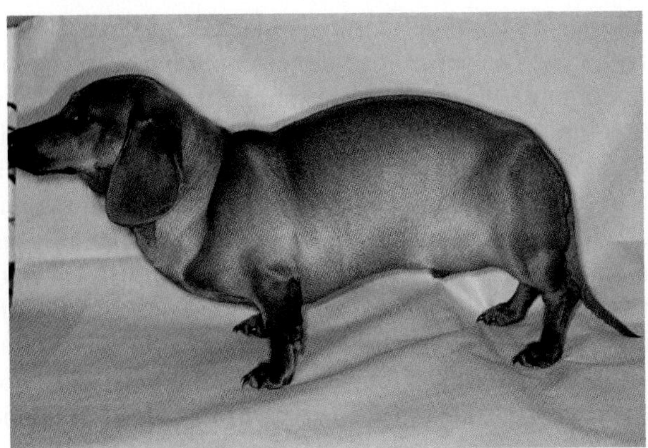

FIGURE 12-7 Once formed, fat cells are present for life, though they can shrink. Animals that eat too much as juveniles experience fat-cell division and are subsequently predisposed to excess weight gain throughout their lives.

of between 24% and 34% in adult dogs, and between 25% and 40% of the cats seen by veterinarians were considered to be overweight or obese.

Among dogs and cats, certain factors contribute to clinical obesity, including genetic background, high-calorie diets and snacks, physical inactivity, the presence of endocrine or neuroendocrine disorders, and gonadectomy. By definition, obesity means a body composition with a ratio of too much fat to lean tissue or body weight 15% to 20% greater than optimum (Figure 12-7).

The early detection of breeds that are prone to obesity is important in preventing and treating the condition. Veterinary technicians can play a vital role in recommending feeding regimens, exercise strategies, and educating the client on the health risks of obesity. Routine weighing, body condition scoring, and counseling clients during routine examinations can further benefit patients' health.

> *TECHNICIAN NOTE* Canine and feline obesity estimates are approximately 25% to 40% and can vary within age groups.

A primary cause for obesity is overfeeding during growth life stages. A positive calorie balance during juvenile growth may induce increased numbers of fat cells (hyperplasia). Once formed, these fat cells are present for life and have minimum volumes of triglyceride content below which they cannot shrink (Crane, 1991). Therefore a lifelong predisposition for excess weight develops. Adipocyte hyperplasia is prevented by using meal feeding for puppies, kittens, and foals.

Overeating during maintenance life stages is another factor contributing toward obesity. Consuming more energy than is expended can lead to excess body fat. In addition, feeding the picky eater table food and other diets high in fat contributes significantly to obesity. Excess dietary fat is typically stored as body fat, with storage capabilities almost limitless. Volume-restricted meals and the elimination of calorie-rich treats are recommended to prevent obesity. Adult pets can be fed high-fiber, low-fat treats if snacks are important to the pet owner.

BOX 12-8 Obesity-Prone Dog Breeds

- Beagle
- Labrador
- Sheltie
- Cocker spaniel
- Golden retriever
- Cairn terrier
- Scottish terrier
- Dachshund
- Basset hound
- Cavalier King Charles spaniel

A third cause of obesity is genetic predisposition. Evidence has linked genetic inheritance with resting metabolic rates (Crane, 1991). Breeds at greater risk include the Labrador retriever, cairn terriers, cocker spaniels, long-haired dachshunds, Shetland sheepdogs, basset hounds, and beagles (Box 12-8). Mixed-breed cats tend to be more overweight than purebred cats (McIntosh, 2000).

Another cause for obesity includes a declining lean body mass and declining activity level during normal aging processes. Decreases in energy requirements may be considered in a geriatric feeding program (Markham, Hodgkins, 1989). As pets become older and less active, lean body mass is reduced. Goals for maintaining optimal nutrition in the geriatric animal include avoiding food with excessive protein, phosphorus, and sodium chloride. Refer to the section in this chapter titled Feeding the Geriatric Pet.

Competitive eating may also provoke obesity. Multianimal households or other group-feeding situations may need volume-restricted feeding and separation of the competitive individuals during feeding.

Surgical neutering of males and females can also alter metabolism, deregulate satiety, and increase the desire to feed. The technician may recommend less calorically dense food concurrent with suture removal after neutering, particularly in the obesity-prone breed.

Health Risks of Obesity

The health risks of obesity are numerous. Among the most common include:

- Coronary heart disease
- Type 2 diabetes and insulin resistance
- Hypertension
- Pulmonary disorders
- Liver, kidney, and gallbladder disease
- Colon, ovarian, endometrial neoplasia
- Musculoskeletal diseases, including joint stress, hip dysplasia, and osteoarthritis
- Muscular injuries, including cranial cruciate ligament rupture

In addition, obese patients are anesthetic risks and are typically exercise and heat intolerant. Obese patients with ailments such as cardiovascular disease, asthma, elongated soft palates, or laryngeal paralysis are even further compromised and often have increased mortality. In addition, obesity is a predisposing factor for hepatic lipidosis in cats and is associated with some endocrine diseases, such as hyperadrenocorticism, hypothyroidism, and diabetes mellitus. Chemistry and endocrine profiles in the obese animal can be particularly important in identifying compounding disorders. Because obesity is such a common disease among pets, clients should be made aware of the many health risks associated with it. Obesity-related disorders can be prevented or delayed with proper feeding and exercise regimens.

> *TECHNICIAN NOTE* Obese patients are anesthetic risks and are often intolerant of exercise and high ambient temperatures.

Diagnosis and Treatment of Obesity

Assessing obesity among dogs and cats can be accomplished by examining the quantity of subcutaneous fat deposits both visually and by palpation over the ribs, groin, and tail head. Radiographs of the abdomen and thorax will also reveal fat accumulations. Weighing the animal indirectly measures body composition, but using ideal weight tables for purebred animals is useful. **Body condition scoring** (see Figure 12-4) is a visual and useful method for combining various assessment criteria into an opinion regarding the pet's body composition and relative fatness. The dietary history should always be included in the patient's history.

Obesity is best prevented, but can be treated by caloric restriction and exercise. Specific treatment requires teamwork among the owner, the veterinarian, and the technician. In general, dietary recommendations include feeding calorie-restricted, low-energy food. Certain food with increased dietary fiber provide satiety and aid in weight reduction. In addition, feeding a diet high in fiber can reduce total energy intake and improve blood glucose and lipid levels. Clients should be continually reminded of the benefits of weight control because the process can be both slow and frustrating. The veterinary technician can be a critical support person for the pet owner who is enforcing a pet weight-reduction program at home. The technician should recommend to the owner a realistic time frame for weight loss so that frustration is minimized, and the weight-reduction goal is more likely to be reached and maintained. An important part of a pet weight-reduction program is the restriction of supplemental calories in the form of treats, including both human snack food and commercial pet treats (see Tables 12-4 and 12-5). This concept must be especially stressed to the owner who is easily influenced by a begging pet with a plaintive expression.

Feeding Geriatric Dogs

The definition of geriatric as it pertains to the dog is not precise because of breed variability. In general, toy and small-sized breeds are geriatric at 7 years, medium-sized dogs at 6 years, and large and giant breeds as early as 5 years of age.

Geriatric pets undergo physiologic changes similar to elderly humans. Older animals, for example, have a higher incidence of multiple organ failure, benign and malignant tumor formation, osteoarthritis, dental disease, and loss of hearing and vision. Age-associated changes in physiologic function include reduced immune response, reduced digestive and renal function, reduced glucose tolerance, and smell and/or taste perception changes. Unfortunately, no specific diet or nutrient formula can delay the onset of disease or slow down the aging process. However, the dietary practices in the first three fourths of an animal's life can impact the nutritional consequences manifested in the last part of its life (Burkholder, 1999). Older pets become less active and have reduced lean body mass and have a reduced basal metabolic rate.

Nutritional recommendations for the geriatric pet should be influenced by the individual body condition and health history. The ideal goal in geriatric animals is the maintenance of optimum weight. Commercially available senior diets should be evaluated and only recommended based on the status of the animal. Dietary modifications should be considered if a particular disease state could be ameliorated by the absence or presence of a particular nutrient. Pet food specifically intended for seniors emphasizes moderate energy density with good palatability and reductions of some excess nutrients, as found in all-purpose pet food.

Senior food varies depending upon the manufacturer. Common nutritional factors to take into consideration when recommending a balanced senior diet in the healthy pet include reduced protein, reduced phosphorus and sodium, and increased fiber concentrations. Keep in mind that healthy older cats should not be fed a low-protein diet just because they are old; limiting protein in cats with normal renal and hepatic function can contribute to muscle loss.

Age-related behavioral changes, such as disorientation, owner interaction changes, disturbances in sleep, and loss of bladder or bowel control, may be ameliorated by diets enhanced with antioxidant formulations (Head, Zicker, 2001). Specific therapeutic diets are now available that may help combat the signs of brain aging and improve the learning ability of senior dogs. Exclusive blends of antioxidants and other nutrient formulations help protect against free radical damage, improve cell membrane health, and optimize senior health.

Calorie control may begin or be continued in some older animals. However, blanket feeding recommendations based solely on age are unwise without consideration of the individual. For example, though many geriatric animals have a propensity to put on weight, there are many that lose weight. Weight loss may be a symptom of systemic illness, dental or oral pain, a failing sense of smell, or heightened finicky tastes or fixed food addictions.

Renal Disease

As animals age, many of their organ systems function less efficiently. Chronic progressive renal disease, for example, is common in older dogs and cats. Unfortunately, there is no "quick fix" for chronic renal failure. However, dietary adjustments can slow down the progression of renal aging and prolong the life of a beloved pet.

There are a number of ways that diet can be used to improve a patient's quality of life and alleviate clinical signs of renal disease. The optimal diet for any given dog or cat will vary according to the stage of its disease, its body condition, if concurrent diseases exist, and practical considerations, such as palatability of the diet to the pet. The progressive loss of renal function can ultimately reduce the animal's ability to excrete phosphorus, urea, and other by-products of protein metabolism. Controlling excesses of intake during the geriatric periods does no harm, even in the absence of clinical signs of renal failure. Therefore the recommendation to avoid excessive protein, phosphorus, and sodium chloride seems medically prudent. In addition, cats with renal insufficiency have elevated potassium requirements. Commercial prescription diets are designed with these goals in mind and are readily available from a veterinarian. In addition, current research has indicated that feeding diets containing omega-3-fatty acids may be beneficial to the canine with renal insufficiency.

FEEDING CATS

Cats are not "small dogs" and are physically, physiologically, and behaviorally made to be solo-hunting, carnivorous predators. Protein metabolism is unique in cats; typically, cats require higher amounts of protein in their daily diet as compared with dogs (see Amino Acids and Protein).

Key nutritional factors for feeding cats include higher percentages of total dietary calories from an ideal protein source (biologic value of 100%) or approximately 8% in adult cats as opposed to roughly 4% in adult dogs. Carbohydrate metabolism is limited as a result of low liver glucokinase activity, making the feline liver unique in energy metabolism. In general, cats require high-protein, low-carbohydrate food. Feeding dog food to cats for convenience or economy is ill advised because of the different nutritional composition. Feeding a dog food will not specifically provide the required amount of fat and protein. To summarize, cats have obligate and daily needs for additional protein, specific requirements for certain amino acids (e.g., taurine, arginine), increased requirements for many B vitamins, and a reduced ability to digest, absorb, and metabolize carbohydrates.

Taurine is an eleventh essential amino acid in cats. AFFCO has determined that dry feline food must contain 1000 mg/kg of taurine and canned feline food must contain 2000 mg/kg of taurine to prevent diseases associated with deficiencies. Most feline food is now appropriately supplemented in taurine. Other feline-specific requirements include vitamin A, niacin, and pyridoxine. In addition, arachidonic (fatty) acids are not synthesized in the cat; consequently, arachidonic acids are required in the feline diet.

Although calculating energy requirements for cats in differing life stages can be useful, each pet should be examined individually, and nutritional recommendations should be made based on signalment, body condition score, activity level, hydration status, and medical and dietary history. It is important for the technician to consider the influence that diet has in oral health and the texture food can play in preventing dental disease. The palatability and acceptability of a particular food is often influenced by offering food at body temperature, particularly in the hospitalized or ill feline (see Clinical Nutrition).

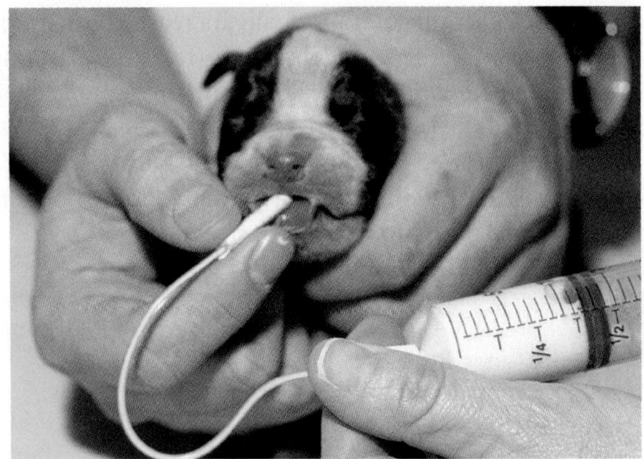

FIGURE 12-8 Tube feeding a neonate. Orphaned kittens can be given milk replacer by tube lavage.

Feline Pediatric Nutrition

An adequate colostrum intake for all kittens is critical and should be monitored immediately after birth. Like puppies, the orphaned kitten can be raised by tube lavage or pet nurser systems to administer milk replacement (Figure 12-8). It is important to ensure the correct placement of a gastric tube to prevent pulmonary aspiration. Stable environmental factors for pediatric felines are similar to pediatric canines; warm, dry bedding is paramount. Heating pads should cover only half the box for kittens and mother to crawl away from the heat source if it is too hot (see Feeding Orphaned Puppies). In addition, orphaned kittens may need assistance in urination and defecation, similar to orphaned puppies.

Kittens weigh between 85 and 120 g at birth and gain an average of approximately 100 g/week (McCune, 2003). Similar to canine pediatric care, the use of gram scales to monitor weight as an indicator for a proper nutrient intake is recommended. Caloric needs for most puppies and kittens are 22 to 26 kcal/100 g of body weight for the first 3 months of life. Feedings should be scheduled at least four times a day. In general, male kittens grow faster than females.

The formula should be warmed to about 100° F (37.8° C) before feeding. The initial feedings should have less volume (but not frequency) than those directed by the manufacturer. Over the next several days, gradually increase the volume of formula to the amount recommended by the manufacturer. Subsequent increases will be needed based on weight gain and satiation. The formula preparation should follow label instructions, and all feeding equipment must be cleaned immediately after use. The stomach capacity of the neonate is approximately 50 ml/kg. Initially, kittens are fed 5 ml every

4 to 6 hours. The amount is gradually increased by 1 ml/day until the recommended guidelines are reached. Although feeding frequencies vary, generally the first 3 days of life are the most critical.

Kittens are weaned later than puppies—generally at 7 to 9 weeks. Growth-sustaining kitten food are fed two or three times daily until the kitten is 10 months of age.

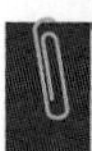

TECHNICIAN NOTE Kittens are weaned later than puppies—generally at 7 to 9 weeks.

Feeding Adult Cats

During the adult maintenance life stage, it is recommended to feed a consistent diet and employ a feeding schedule to eliminate finicky behavior and food aversion.

The technician may encounter owners that vary food types as a response to the large number of cat food flavors on supermarket shelves. Providing a variety of flavors is unnecessary, and a transient "newness" factor can temporarily increase food intake and can lead to weight fluctuations.

Most cat owners tend to feed ad lib. When allowed continuous access to food, cats usually eat small, frequent meals throughout the day. A common belief is that cats are better than dogs at maintaining their body condition. However, the latest epidemiologic studies no longer support this idea. When offered a highly palatable, high-fat diet, cats fed ad lib tend to overeat, especially if they are neutered or lead a sedentary lifestyle. A survey of 500 practitioners showed that although most clients were aware of the potential for weight gain in their sterilized cats, only 10% of the veterinarians recommended that the cats be switched to a low-fat diet (Biourge, 2001).

Commercial feline treats are usually nutritionally synonymous with dry cat food (see Table 12-5). As such, they are appropriate to be used as treats, but only if given in moderation. Some cat owners prefer "natural" treats, such as raw or cooked poultry necks, oxtails, or liver. Although little harm results from the use of these treats in moderation, finicky behavior and subsequent nutritional imbalance are potential hazards. Specifically, liver contains an inverted Ca/P ratio (1:17), and potentially toxic levels of vitamin A (hypervitaminosis A) can occur with long-term consumption.

Hairballs occur commonly in cats because of their meticulous grooming habits and the sharp barbs on their tongues, which increase the apprehension and consumption of hair. Hairballs are periodically regurgitated from the oropharynx or esophagus or vomited from the stomach. Occasionally, hairballs pass into the intestinal tract where they are voided in the feces. Owners may observe periodic gagging, retching, and regurgitation or vomiting of hair and mucus. Hairballs are often tubular and usually do not contain food or bile. Although hairballs do not usually cause significant clinical disease, they can be of concern to the owner. Many laxatives, lubricants, treats, and food are available for routine management of these problems. Laxatives and lubricants should be used intermittently because large daily doses may interfere with normal digestion and nutrient absorption. Several complete and balanced moderate-fiber food is now available for control of hairball problems in cats.

Feeding Cats During Pregnancy and Lactation

During the reproductive life stage, energy and nutrient requirements must support both queen and offspring during pregnancy, lactation, and milk production. At peak lactation, energy and nutrient requirements can be three to four times normal maintenance. Because ingesting larger amounts of food may not be feasible, owners can feed a diet that is more energy and nutrient dense, with increased digestibility to reduce bulk. It is important to advise clients that supplementation, with vitamins and minerals, is not necessary as long as the queen is fed a balanced diet.

There are significant differences in the food intake between the bitch and the queen during the initial stages of lactation (see Figure 12-6). As a solitary hunter, the queen hunts less during the early part of lactation and uses the body fat stored during gestation to support her milk production. The practical significance here is that clients may question a low food consumption in their new mother cat. Such clients can be advised that the queen will eat heavily, as expected, by the third week of lactation.

Feeding Geriatric Cats

An evaluation of the geriatric individual is crucial in determining an appropriate food that will maintain a proper body weight and still provide adequate nutrient levels. In selecting the optimal diet for an older cat, overall health must be considered. The food intake should be monitored in association with changes in weight. Hyperthyroidism, for example, is characterized by chronic weight loss despite a ravenous appetite. The water intake should be noted since an increased frequency of drinking and urination may also be symptomatic of disease.

No single food can meet the needs of every geriatric cat. Dietary modification can help to optimize health in the healthy cat and to modulate disease in cats as they age. Significant protein restriction is not recommended in the healthy geriatric cat because of the high protein requirements in felines (see Amino Acids and Proteins). A moderate restriction of protein is recommended for the cat with evidence of chronic renal failure (see Clinical Nutrition). Commercial diets are available with balanced nutrient contents for optimizing the health of the elderly cat. Oral hygiene is an important factor in feline geriatrics; routine dental examinations should be performed to ensure that there is no tooth pain and that food can be apprehended and chewed.

Similar to geriatric canine nutrition, certain dietary adjustments can help improve clinical signs or even slow progression of disease (see Feeding the Geriatric Animal). The best diet, however, should be based on the individual cat's clinical signs, body condition score, laboratory results, and stage of disease.

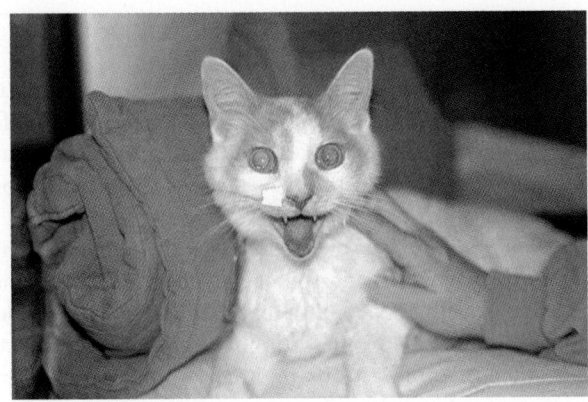

FIGURE 12-9 Fasting in obese cats has been associated with the accumulation of lipids in the liver, which in turn causes icterus.

Feline Obesity

Feline obesity, like canine obesity, is a common nutritional problem. One important role of the technician is to educate the client and to encourage participation in weight-reduction programs. A detailed dietary history is helpful when calculating the amount of food that will be offered during a caloric-restricted diet. Fasting in obese cats is not recommended because fasting has been associated with the accumulation of lipid in the liver. This can become pathologic over a 5- to 6-week period, and it mimics idiopathic feline hepatic lipidosis (Figure 12-9).

Obesity can be prevented if the veterinarian and the technician provide nutritional counseling during routine yearly examinations. In addition, the owners of felines that have a gonadectomy should also be counseled as to the amount of food given after surgery to prevent excessive weight gain. Dietary therapy should only be instituted after a complete physical examination, biochemical profiling, and compilation of medical history. It is important to instruct the client to gradually introduce a new food over a period of 7 days. Obese cats that are given a new diet all at once may become anorexic.

Statistics show that cats being fed high-fat (±20%) premium and superpremium diets are two to three times more likely to become overweight. Conversely, cats fed a diet containing around 10% fat are 50% less likely to be overweight. Dietary recommendations for feline obesity include feeding multiple small meals throughout the day to optimize digestive and absorptive energy expenditures. Traditionally, diets are composed of low-calorie, high-fiber substances. Recommendations for caloric restriction range from 50% to 80% of maintenance calories to achieve optimum weight (Burkholder, 2000). Commercial and prescription canned diets are now available that are tailored for the obese cat. Such canned food includes a low-carbohydrate, high-protein matrix. Cats fed some (50% is a good starting point) tailored canned food as part of their diet will reduce the carbohydrates and better control calories (dry food is very calorie dense) and will help increase the amount of water consumed daily. In addition, low-carbohydrate, high-protein formula have been clinically proven to alter a cat's metabolism for effective weight loss and may help prevent diabetes mellitus in the aging feline. The addition of L-carnitine also helps the feline patient lose weight while maintaining lean muscle mass and decreasing the accumulation of fat in liver cells.

Feline Urolithiasis and Lower Urinary Tract Diseases

The two most common calculi that occur in cats are struvite and calcium oxalate calculi, both of which can lead to lower urinary tract diseases. The amount and balance of mineral elements in the diet of a cat can have significant effects on the formation of urinary calculi. Other important factors in calculi formation include urinary pH, urine concentration, and high dietary magnesium. Although there are many factors that can contribute to the formation of uroliths that are related to diet, uroliths are rarely, if ever, the direct result of diet. The diet can, however, have an impact on the urinary concentration of calculogenic substances.

The water intake is a major factor in determining urine concentration and to some extent frequency of urination. Other factors that can affect urine concentration include the sodium, fat, and carbohydrate content because energy metabolism results in the production of metabolic water. The digestibility of the diet will also determine the amount of water lost in the stool and the quantity of minerals that are absorbed and ultimately excreted. Other aspects of diet that can influence the development of uroliths include the dietary content of minerals, quantity of diet consumed, and the influence of diet and eating frequency on urine pH because some uroliths are more or less soluble in certain pH ranges.

Certain feline diets are formulated to induce acidic urine because of the addition of acidifiers, such as methionine, ammonium chloride, and phosphoric acid. Struvite crystal formation is not possible at a urine pH below 6.5. Particular animal proteins and corn glutens found in feline diets can also promote acidic urine, as opposed to diets composed of vegetable proteins and mineral salts, such as calcium carbonate, which promote alkaline urine.

Urine acidification is not without potential toxicity. Excessive acidity can overpower the ability of the kidneys to excrete protons and induce uncompensated metabolic acidosis. Consequently, chronic acidosis in cats can increase urinary potassium losses and could potentially slow growth, increase urine calcium excretion, and promote bone demineralization.

Acidifiers also can be toxic. Acidifying diets are recommended to safely prevent and manage struvite-related lower urinary tract disease (LUTD). Technicians should refer to the veterinarian before recommending any acidifying diets. These diets are not recommended for kittens because they are not formulated for growth and may interfere with bone formation.

Acidifying diets may also be contraindicated in the older cat; older felines are at a higher risk for calcium oxalate urolith formation and renal insufficiency. No diet will promote the dissolution of calcium oxalate uroliths, but minimize the risk of crystal formation, diets for mature and older cats should be formulated to induce a higher urinary pH. Maintaining urine acidity (pH 6.2 to 6.4) and keeping the magnesium intake at nonexcessive levels are prudent risk-control measures for struvite crystalluria. Maintaining a more alkaline urine pH (6.4 to 6.8) while avoiding excess calcium, sodium, and magnesium are prudent risk-control measures for calcium oxalate crystalluria. It is also beneficial to increase the cat's water consumption. Feeding a canned food will decrease the cat's urine specific gravity and increase the overall volume of urine, thus decreasing the possibility of crystal formation.

Note that the main difference between canine and feline urolithiasis is that struvite uroliths are usually associated with urinary tract infections in the dog. Feline struvite uroliths are generally sterile. Bacteria, such as staphylococci and other urease-producing organisms, generally create an alkaline environment, which enhances the formation of struvite and other uroliths. Antibiotic therapy is therefore only recommended in patients with a positive urine culture.

> TECHNICIAN NOTE Important factors that influence calculi formation include urinary pH, urine concentration, and high dietary magnesium.

It is an oversimplification to state that controlling urine mineral concentrations or pH always controls feline lower urinary tract disease (FLUTD). FLUTD syndrome is multifactorial; not all causative agents or combinations of contributory factors are presently known. The term *idiopathic FLUTD* is used in cats where there is no known cause. Potential causes of idiopathic FLUTD include a viral infection, stress, and neurogenic inflammation. Idiopathic FLUTD is not well understood; however, water seems to be a key factor in controlling the recurrence of the disease. Canned and other high-moisture food increases total urine volume and are the preferred products for cats with idiopathic FLUTD.

FLUTD is typically caused by struvite uroliths or urethral plugs, calcium oxalate uroliths, or by a syndrome known as feline idiopathic cystitis (FIC). Clinical signs of FLUTD include urinating outside the litter box, frequency of urination, and/or straining to urinate. Prescription diets are now available that are formulated to provide nutritional management in feline patients with either struvite or calcium oxalate uroliths or FIC. Such diets contain controlled levels of magnesium, calcium, phosphorus, and oxalate to reduce building materials needed to construct potentially harmful crystals and uroliths. In addition, certain specialized prescription feline urinary diets contain limited sodium and high levels of omega-3 fatty acids that may inhibit the inflammatory cascade associated with FLUTD.

> TECHNICIAN NOTE The FLUTD syndrome is multifactorial, and not all causative agents or combinations of contributory factors are presently known.

CLINICAL NUTRITION

Nutritional support during times of stress, disease, or injury has provided the hospitalized animal a greater chance for recovery. The failure to consider nutrition as an important therapeutic strategy to improve health can have tremendous negative consequences.

Clinical nutrition is a veterinary medical subspecialty with the objective of modifying the cause, progression, or end-stage effects of illness by applying specific nutrient profiles. Numerous nutrient profiles support various prophylactic and therapeutic applications in small animal patients and are summarized in Table 12-8.

Table 12-8 provides a general guide for dietary therapy based on disease history.

NUTRITIONAL ASSESSMENT OF THE HOSPITALIZED PATIENT

The primary goal of a nutritional assessment is to identify which patient is at risk for malnutrition. Because altered nutritional status is associated with adverse clinical outcomes, it becomes paramount to address the nutritional needs early in *every* hospitalized patient, particularly the critically ill or injured. Although clinical status alone may dictate the need for nutritional intervention, a thorough nutritional assessment consists of evaluating both clinical and biochemical data, including the patient's history, and a thorough physical examination including body weight and body condition scoring. A baseline nutritional assessment should be followed by serial assessments throughout the course of hospitalization.

The veterinary technician is in a crucial position to identify baseline data and ongoing changes in nutritional status because it is the technician that spends most of the time with the patient. Baseline data includes such physical examination findings as weight, body condition score, hydration status, cardiopulmonary sounds, the body temperature, and a nutritional background on the patient. The owner or referring veterinarian must be questioned as to when the last complete meal or nutritional support was given because the intake is often impaired days before the initial visit to the veterinarian. Nutritional intervention is crucial to recovery and survival, and appropriate consideration as to the type and route of nutrition should be given based on the underlying disease process or diagnosis.

> TECHNICIAN NOTE A thorough nutritional assessment consists of evaluating both clinical and biochemical data, including the patient's history, and a thorough physical examination including body weight and body condition scoring, hydration status, and cardiopulmonary sounds.

PATIENTS AT RISK FOR MALNUTRITION

Any patient that is anorexic or NPO for 3 days or longer is a candidate for malnutrition. However, animals in danger of nutritional insufficiency include those with increased

TABLE 12-8 Summary of Small Animal Clinical Nutrition*

Disease	Objectives	Considerations	Product	Comments
Allergy, food				
Dog	Reduce antigen ingestion	Novel highly digestible protein source or protein hydrolysate Reduce total protein content Simplify food Distilled H_2O	Prescription Diet[†] Canine d/d or Canine z/d	8 to 10-wk trial period Avoid treats, snacks, access to other food sources,chewable medications, supplements
Cat		Same as dog except Control Mg^{2+} intake Provide taurine Control urine pH	Prescription Diet Feline d/d or Feline z/d	
Anemia	Support RBC production	↑ Iron, cobalt, and copper ↑ B complex vitamins ↑ Protein	Prescription Diet Canine p/d Feline p/d	
Anorexia	Prevent protein/caloric malnutrition Stimulate appetite	Establish fluid/electrolyte balance Acid-base balance ↑ Protein and fat ↑ Micronutrients	Prescription Diet Feline/Canine a/d Canine p/d Feline p/d	Cat foods are suitable for dogs in acute care settings
Ascites	Reduce fluid retention	Restrict sodium chloride	Prescription Diet Canine h/d, k/d Feline p/d	h/d = marked salt restriction k/d = moderate salt restriction
Bone loss and fracture healing	Correct deficiency of energy and protein	Maintain hydration ↑ Protein ↑ Energy Avoid supplementation	Prescription Diet Canine p/d Feline p/d	Extra dietary calcium does not increase rate of fracture healing
Cancer	Increase longevity and quality of life	↓ Soluble carbohydrate ↑ Fat and omega-3 fatty acids ↑ Arginine	Prescription Diet Canine n/d Canine/Feline a/d	Use in conjunction with chemotherapy or other forms of cancer therapy
Colitis	Normalize gastrointestinal motility Rebalance microflora Provide local healing factors	Feed small meals 3-6 times/day Control dietary antigens Vary levels of dietary fiber	Prescription Diet Canine w/d, l/d, d/d Feline w/d, d/d	
Constipation	Normalize gastrointestinal motility Maintain stool water Maintain stool bulk	>10% fiber	Prescription Diet Canine w/d Feline w/d	No table scraps or bones Increase exercise Encourage water intake Cats: keep litter box clean
Copper storage disease	Restrict copper intake	<1.2 mg copper/100 g dry diet	Prescription Diet Canine l/d	No table scraps or treats
Debilitation	Restore tissue, plasma, and nutrients	↑ Protein ↑ Fat ↑ Macronutrients and Micronutrients	Prescription Diet Canine/Feline a/d	Assist feed if needed
Developmental orthopedic disease	Reduce rapid growth	↓ Fat and energy density ↓ Calcium	Prescription Diet Canine p/d Large Breed	Avoid calcium-phosphorus supplements

*Nutrients in table are expressed on a dry weight basis.

Continued

TABLE 12-8 Summary of Small Animal Clinical Nutrition—cont'd

Disease	Objectives	Considerations	Product	Comments
Diabetes mellitus	Even rate of glucose absorption Consistent caloric intake	>10% fiber ↓ Soluble carbohydrates	Prescription Diet Canine w/d Feline w/d	Weigh animal frequently and note in medical record
Feline urolithiasis (struvite): Treatment	↑ Urine volume ↓ Urine pH (5.9-6.1) Restrict Mg^{2+}, Ca^{2+}, PO_4	↑ Caloric density ↓ P and Ca^{2+} Mg^{2+} >20 mg/100 Kcal ↑ Na^+ Urine pH (6.2-6.4)	Prescription Diet Feline s/d	Dissolution is complete 1 mo after negative radiographs Recurrence is high if prevention is not implemented
Prevention	Maintain physiologic levels of urinary solutes and urine pH ↑ Caloric density	Mg^{2+} >20 mg/100 Kcal (0.1% DMB) ↓ P Urine pH (6.2-6.4)	Prescription Diet Feline c/d-s	In obesity, use calorie-restricted diets that maintain urine pH 6.2-6.4 (Prescription Diet w/d is suggested)
Feline urolithiasis (calcium oxalate): Prevention	↑ Urine volume ↓ Urinary Ca^{2+}, oxalate ↑ Urine pH	↓ Protein ↑ Nonprotein calories ↓ P, Ca^{2+}, Na^+ Mg^{2+} <20 mg/100 Kcal	Prescription Diet Feline c/d-oxl	Monitor urinary crystalluria
Vomiting	Minimize gastric secretion Gastrointestinal rest	↑ Digestibility ↑ Caloric density	Prescription Diet Canine i/d Feline i/d	Frequent, small meals
Diarrhea, acute	Normalize gastrointestinal tract motility and secretion	Withhold food for 1-2 days Feed small amounts 3-6 times/day ↓ Fiber ↓ Sugar ↑ Digestibility	Prescription Diet Canine i/d Feline i/d	Electrolyte disturbances and dehydration are common
Eclampsia	Provide Ca/P in correct quantity and ratio prepartum	High digestibility of diet Balanced minerals/vitamins	Prescription Diet Canine p/d Feline p/d	Avoid supplementation
Flatulence	Decrease aerophagia Avoid food fermentation	Avoid milk or milk products Feed small meals 3-6 times/day ↑ Caloric density	Prescription Diet Canine i/d Feline i/d	Feed in a flat, open dish Avoid vitamin or fatty acid supplementation Separate competitive eaters
Gastric dilatation/bloat (postoperative)	Prevent gastric distention	Avoid exercise before and after feeding ↑ Digestibility of diet Small, frequent feedings	Prescription Diet Canine i/d	Diet form or type is NOT related to risk of occurrence or recurrence
Heart failure				
Dogs	Control Na^+ retention	↓ Na^+ intake Maintain energy and protein intake ↑ B complex vitamins ↓ Na^+ intake	Prescription Diet Canine h/d Canine k/d	Prescription Diet k/d has moderate Na^+ restriction

Cats		↑ Taurine Control Mg^{2+} levels	Prescription Diet Feline h/d Feline k/d	Avoid high Na^+ treats and water (see Table 12-5)
Hyperlipidemia	Control fat intake	↑ Fiber intake ↓ Fat intake	Prescription Diet Canine w/d Feline w/d	Common in schnauzers Consider fat in treats, table foods, and supplements
Hyperthyroidism (cats)	Support increased energy need	↑ Energy intake ↑ Vitamins and minerals ↑ Protein	Prescription Diet Feline a/d	Monitor for evidence of concurrent renal disease
Liver disease (fat tolerant)	Reduce protein metabolism Maintain liver glycogen Prevent ammonia toxicity	↑ Digestible energy Protein restriction High biologic value proteins Control Na^+ intake	Prescription Diet Canine l/d Feline l/d	May feed small meals (4-6 times/day)
Lymphangiectasia	Decrease dietary fat	↓ Intake of long-chain triglycerides Control protein levels Consider medium-chain triglycerides	Prescription Diet Canine w/d or r/d	Medium-chain triglyceride oils and powder can increase caloric density
Obesity	Maintain intake of all nutrients except energy	↓ Energy digestibility Replace digestible calories with indigestible fiber Increase bulk to control hunger Add carnitine	Prescription Diet Canine r/d Feline r/d	Requires professional advice and teamwork with veterinary technician and client
Oral disease: gingivitis (gum inflammation) periodontus (loss of tooth attachment)	Control accumulation of plaque, stains, and calculus Maintain gingival health	Food that promotes chewing and mechanical cleaning of teeth	Prescription Diet Canine t/d Feline t/d	Many treats make dental claims but are not effective
Pancreatics, acute (recovery phase)	Control pancreas secretions	↓ Fat ↑ Digestibility Feed small meals 3-6 times/day	Prescription Diet Canine i/d Feline i/d	Frequent, small meals
Pancreatic exocrine insufficiency	Reduce requirements for digestive enzymes	↓ Fiber ↓ Fat Highly digestible carbohydrates ↑ Caloric density	Prescription Diet Canine i/d Feline i/d	Pancreatic enzymes complement highly digestible food
Renal failure	Reduce signs of uremia Slow progression of disease	↓ Protein (↑ biologic value of protein) ↑ Nonprotein calories ↓ Phosphorus and sodium Increase B complex vitamins	Prescription Diet Canine k/d Canine g/d Canine u/d Prescription Diet Feline k/d Feline g/d	Small meals 4-6 times/day Conversion to a protein-restricted diet may take 7-10 days Water available at all times

Mg, Magnesium; *RBC*, red blood cell; *Ca*, calcium; *DMB*, dry matter basis; *Mg*, magnesium; *Na*, sodium; *NH_4*, ammonium; *P*, phosphorus; *PO*, phosphate; *RBC*, red blood cells.

†Other North American therapeutic brands with wide distribution include CNM (Purina), VMD, Medi-Cal, and IVD Select Care (Heinz), Eukanuba Veterinary Diets (Iams), and Waltham Veterinary Diets (Mars).

Continued

TABLE 12-8 Summary of Small Animal Clinical Nutrition—cont'd

Disease	Objectives	Considerations	Product	Comments
Canine urolithiasis (struvite): Treatment	↑ Urine volume ↓ Urine pH Restrict Mg^{2+}, NH_4^+, PO_4	↓ Protein ↓ PO_4, Mg^{2+} ↑ Na^+ ↓ Urine pH (5.9-6.1)	Prescription Diet Canine s/d	Evaluate and treat urinary tract infection Average duration of stone dissolution is 36 days; follow-up via radiography
Prevention	Maintain physiologic level of urinary solutes and urine pH	Control protein excess ↓ Ca^{2+}, P, Mg^{2+} ↓ Sodium mildly ↓ Urine pH (6.2-6.4)	Prescription Diet Canine c/d	Monitor urine sediment for crystalluria and infection
Canine urolithiasis (ammonium urate): Prevention		↓ Protein ↑ Nonprotein calories ↓ Nucleic acids ↓ Ca^{2+}, P, Mg^{2+}, Na^+ Urine pH (6.7-7.0)	Prescription Diet Canine u/d	Drugs plus diet may be successful treatment Monitor urinary crystalluria Prevention may require long-team drug treatment
Canine urolithiasis (calcium oxalate and cystine):	↓ Urinary concentration of calcium oxalate or cystine	↓ Protein ↑ Nonprotein calories	Prescription Diet Canine u/d	Treatment by surgical removal Prevention by dietary management with or without drugs
Prevention		↓ Ca^{2+}, P, Na^+, Mg^{2+} ↑ Urine pH (6.1-7.0)		

metabolic stress levels, including surgical patients, dehydrated patients, sepsis patients, burn victims, trauma patients, head injuries, patients with respiratory difficulties, and those with chronic vomiting or diarrhea.

In the healthy pet, short-term food deprivation results in quick adaptive mechanisms to maintain blood glucose levels. The body mobilizes its own tissue reserves to provide nutrients for basic physiologic processes while lowering the metabolic rate to reduce energy expenditure. Within a few days, fat becomes the major source of fuel. Unfortunately, not all cells can use fat stores; the brain, kidney, and red blood cells require a continuous supply of glucose for energy. Tissue proteins are used to provide amino acids for glucose conversion.

In the ill or injured animal, such adaptive mechanisms are altered. During the initial shock of injury or illness, tissue perfusion is provided by intravascular fluid shifts in a compensatory fashion to the severity of the patient. Often the initial metabolism is lowered as a result. After such fluid shifts are corrected and hemodynamic stability returns, the metabolism is accelerated to support healing and resistance to an infection.

Hypermetabolic states increase both the resting energy expenditure and the rate of oxygen consumption. Hypermetabolic states result from increased catecholamine releases to increase fuel production. Unfortunately, the increased metabolic rate and subsequent catabolism rapidly exacerbates weakness in patients without nutritional support. Even more serious is the loss of visceral proteins, such as serum proteins, immunoglobulins, and leukocytes, needed to maintain immunocompetence to fight an infection. The animal's nutritional requirements shift from an omnivore to an obligate carnivore requiring higher amounts of protein and fat. Chronically ill or injured patients not supported nutritionally can result in a cumulative tissue protein depletion state termed protein-energy malnutrition or PEM, which can have an adverse effect on recovery.

Undernourished patients are three times as likely as well-nourished patients to have major surgical complications.

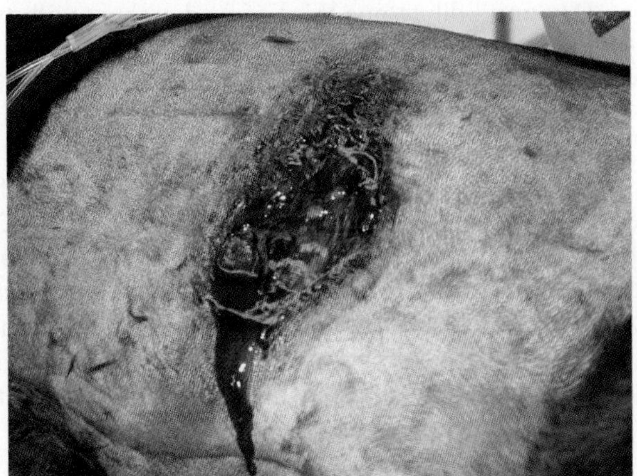

FIGURE 12-10 Undernourished patients are three times as likely to have major surgical complications, such as wound dehiscence (pictured here) and poor healing.

Wound dehiscence, decubital ulcers, sepsis, and pulmonary complications, such as pneumonia, are secondary to poor nutritional status (Figure 12-10). Pediatric patients are especially susceptible to malnutrition and often have dangerously low blood glucose levels. In addition, the technician must always remember to monitor the appetite of healthy patients in boarding kennels because they often become too stressed to eat and may go unnoticed until clinical signs are present.

Indications for nutritional support include recent weight loss of more than 10%, an absent or poor food intake for more than 2 days, acute illness or injury, acute muscle wasting, and heavy GI or urinary system losses of protein or electrolytes. In addition, specific nutritional support is indicated if physical changes are accompanied by hypoalbuminemia, a body condition score under an optimum value of 3, or surgical intervention or hospital procedures that may result in a reduction of the oral intake over 3 to 5 days.

> *TECHNICIAN NOTE* Monitor the appetite of patients in boarding kennels because they can become too stressed to eat and may go unnoticed until clinical signs are present.

FEEDING HOSPITALIZED SMALL ANIMAL PATIENTS

The technician frequently uses a subjective global assessment (SGA) to determine nutritional status. An SGA considers the dietary history, the body's condition scoring system (see Figure 12-4), and the current morbidity index of the illness or injury. Body scoring is done by physical examination, with 0 = cachexia and 5 = obesity. Albumin, total protein, blood urea nitrogen (BUN), and other markers for malnutrition decline with energy deprivation and protein-calorie malnutrition. However, these objective indicators change too slowly to be functional prognosticators, and the use sof an SGA permits functional, early clinical recognition of nutrient depletion and negative nitrogen balance. The most important outlook for the hospital is an awareness of the critical "need to feed" and the need to do so early. These steps reduce catabolism and improve responses to virtually all other therapy.

The technician assesses daily needs and progress in conversation with both the veterinarian and other technicians by both patient progress notes and patient rounds. The clinical signs, the patient's desire and ability to eat, and response to therapy can all rapidly change. Benefits of nutritional support in the debilitated animal can be reviewed in Box 12-9.

Routes of Feeding

Enteral Feeding

The enteral route is the preferred method of feeding, whenever possible, because this is the safest and least expensive route to provide nutrition. Enteral nutrition may be defined as the use of the upper alimentary tract (mouth, esophagus, stomach, and small intestine) for assisted feeding (Figures 12-11 to 12-13).

BOX 12-9 Benefits of Nutritional Support in the Debilitated Animal

Protein
Helps maintain lean body mass
Provides amino acids to support metabolism
Promotes wound healing
Enhances immune function
Provides a source of fuel for muscle

Fats
Primary source of energy
Provide essential fatty acids
Modulate immune function
Promote wound healing

Vitamins and Minerals
Enhance cellular and humoral immunity
Enhance the ability to taste and smell
Provide antioxidants

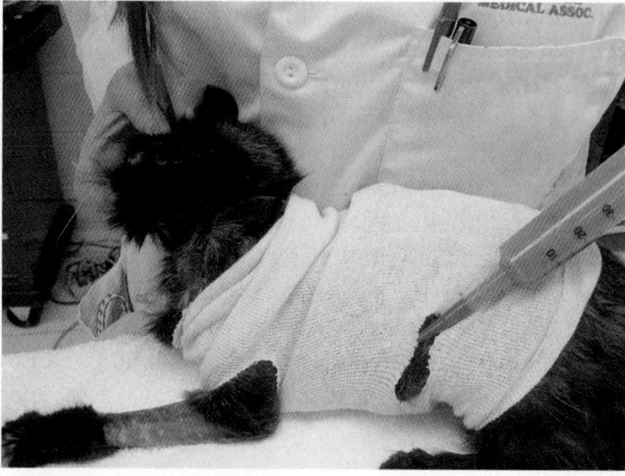

FIGURE 12-12 Gastronomy-tube feeding of an anorectic cat. A large range of diet formulations can be used because of the ease of administration, facilitated by large tube diameter.

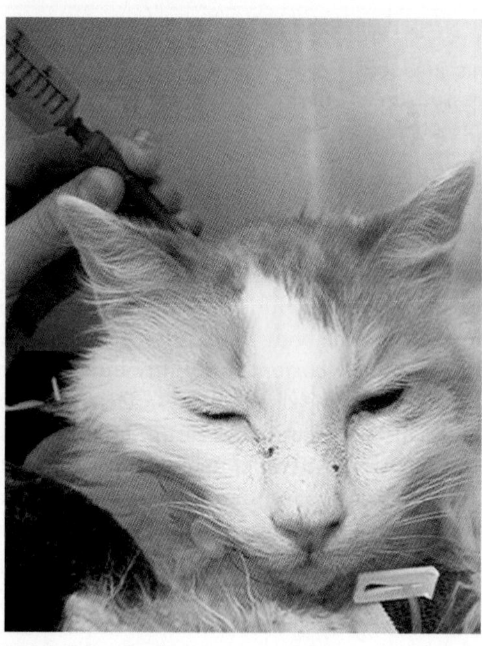

FIGURE 12-11 Feeding via an esophagostomy tube is well tolerated in cats.

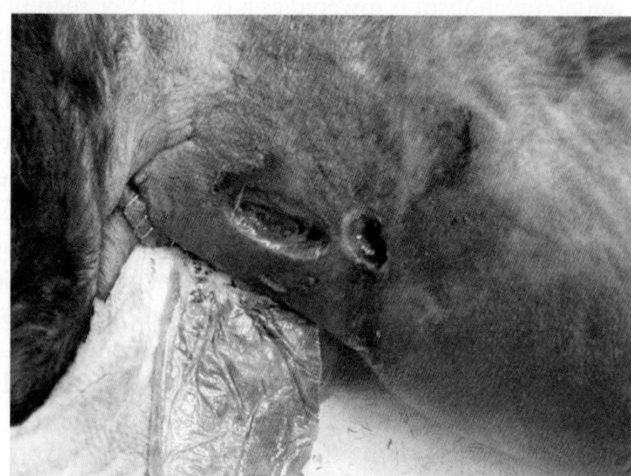

FIGURE 12-13 Tube migration of a J-tube.

There are four separate enteral feeding methods: coax feeding, appetite stimulation with drugs, forced oral feeding, and various tube administration te chniques. Options in enteral feeding are reviewed in Table 12-9 and Chapter 20.

Feeding schedules and enteral administration techniques. Proportions of fat, carbohydrates, and protein in food fed to hospitalized patients should be similar to that which the liver is estimated to be using from body stores. By the fifth day of food deprivation or longer, patients should receive the majority (greater than 50%) of their calculated resting energy requirement (RER) as fat. For dogs, use a food that provides protein of at least 4 to 6 g/100 kcal; for cats, use a food that provides at least 6 to 8 g/100 kcal.

In general, most food types are diluted in water, particularly if administered through a feeding tube. In addition, when using a feeding tube, using a blender and straining loaf products or adding water to moist, homogenized products will facilitate easier flow and will yield fewer complications with clogging. Box 12-10 reviews general enteral feeding guidelines. Feeding schedules are recommended as follows:

- **Day one**—dilute one third of food amount with two thirds water
- **Day two**—dilute two thirds of food with one third water
- **Day three**—full food amount

The amount fed should be divided into portions and fed every 4 to 8 hours or fed continuously by fluid pump. The patient's response to feeding is important to note. Initially the animal may feel slight discomfort with administration, but will adapt after several feedings. Food should be warmed to room temperature and should be fed slowly over several minutes. After feeding, the tube should be flushed with water to prevent obstruction.

The patient's response to feedings is important during administration. Patients that show signs of discomfort during feeding, such as restlessness, salivation, abdominal bloating, or vomiting, may have an improper tube

TABLE 12-9 Options in Enteral Feeding

Objectives	Techniques	Advantage	Disadvantage
Owner Hand Feeding			
Overcome partial anorexia	Hospital visit; bring favorite food	Familiarity with food preferences should be explored	No effect in full anorexia
Temptation			
Overcome partial anorexia	Use an unfamiliar food with strong odor	New odor may stimulate food exploration	No effect in full anorexia
Force Feeding Pet Food			
Overcome partial anorexia	Bolus of moist food; mouth held to force swallowing	Food is complete and balanced	High handling stress Probably limited calorie intake
Forced Feeding (Calorie Pastes)			
Overcome partial anorexia	Administer flavored pastes from tube	Moderate handling stress	Pastes not complete food Limited calorie intake Severe protein restriction
Assisted Feeding			
Achieve full caloric intake Overcome partial anorexia	Use oral syringe to give specific formula	User and patient friendly Moderate handling stress High calorie intake Food given at rate for comfortable swallowing	Learned aversion if nauseous
Orogastric			
Achieve full calorie intake	Intubate esophagus and stomach	Rapid administration No tube clogging Best for short-term use	High handling stress Intolerance to repeated feedings
Nasoesophageal			
Bypass oral cavity and swallowing Achieve full caloric intake	Indwell 6-10F tube in nostril	Ease of intermediate use	Sedation or topical anesthesia Liquid food only
Pharyngostomy			
Bypass oral cavity and swallowing Achieve full caloric intake	Indwell 16-28F tube in pharynx	None	General anesthesia required Mechanical interference with laryngeal function Possible gagging and vomiting Possible esophagitis
Esophagostomy			
Bypass oral cavity and swallowing Achieve full caloric intake	12-18F tube in left lateral cervical esophagus	Easy to maintain and install Easy to "eat around the tube" Minimal risk of esophageal stricture	General anesthesia required
Gastrostomy			
Bypass proximal GI tract for full or partial caloric intake	16-28F tube placement at laparotomy Percutaneous endoscopic placement Nonendoscopic placement	Well-tolerated long term Effective and efficient	General anesthesia required Gastrocutaneous fistula forms in 5 days Wait 24 hr to use
Gastroduodenostomy			
Bypass stomach	Duodenum cannulated via tube gastrostomy	Achieve full caloric intake	Loss of mechanical and chemical phases of gastric digestion May require endoscopic equipment
Jejunostomy			
Bypass stomach and duodenum	10F tube through submucosal tunnel Anchor bowel and tube to body wall	Achieve full or partial caloric intake Predigested food required to maximize nutrient delivery and minimize digestive work	Water transfer to gut lumen may cause cramping and diarrhea

BOX 12-10 General Guidelines For Enteral Nutrition

1. Do not use tube for 24 hours (unless nasogastric or naso-esophageal)
2. Begin by flushing tube with 5 ml/kg of warm water. Monitor patient response; discontinue if the patient coughs or shows signs of distress.
3. On the first day, feed ⅓ of daily caloric requirement divided into six feedings (every 4 hours).
4. Warm food to room temperature and administer slowly.
5. Aspirate tube before each feeding; if more than half of previous meal is aspirated, the feeding should be skipped—consider promotility drugs.
6. Always flush tube before and after feeding with 5-10 ml of warm water.
7. Increase feeding to ⅔ of requirement on day 2, and full feeding by day 3.
8. Keep the skin wound clean and change the bandage daily; monitor the tube for migration and signs of infection. Elizabethan collars may be necessary to prevent premature removal.

position. Other common but serious complications of tube feedings include pulmonary aspiration, diarrhea, constipation, tube occlusion, peritonitis from an improper tube position, and delayed gastric emptying. Such complications can be prevented by checking the tube placement before feeding, measuring gastric residue before each feeding, monitoring gastric tubes for migration during daily bandage changes, and evaluating both the type of diet and concurrent medications to determine the cause of the diarrhea or constipation. In general, slow "trickle" feeding via a fluid or enteral feeding pump is more tolerated by hospitalized patients and has a lower incidence of gastric bloating or vomiting than intermittent-bolus feedings. Box 12-11 outlines common complications and solutions to tube feedings.

Bacterial contamination can also occur during enteral tube use. It is important to use clean techniques during tube placement and handling, to keep opened containers of formula refrigerated and discarded after 48 hours, and to routinely change enteral bags and administration lines every 24 hours. If constant-rate infusions are required, the administration bag should contain only a few hours of solution at a time to ensure stability.

The technician must also carefully monitor all assisted-feeding methods for the stress associated with restraint and monitor all feeding tubes for mechanical blockage or kinking, particularly with small-bore tubes. Capping the tube prevents air from entering the catheterized viscus between uses. It is preferable for the same person to feed because this may allow quicker notation of flow and resistance changes in the tube.

Gastric motility should be monitored, and depending upon the type of tube used, the contents of the stomach should be aspirated before feeding. If greater than one third of the previous feeding remains in the stomach, I recommend

BOX 12-11 Tube Feeding Complications and Their Remedies

Vomiting
Aspirate stomach contents before feeding; do not feed if greater than one third of previous meal is present or aspirating large quantities of air.
Stop feeding and restart more slowly.
Consider constant rate infusion (CRI).

Diarrhea
Check diet composition with veterinarian.
Consider adding fiber (Metamucil).
Use CRI if animal cannot tolerate bolus feedings.

Tube Ejection
Prevent vomiting—antiemetics.
Consider E-collar.

Aspiration Pneumonia
Confirm tube placement and alveolar lung disease with radiographs.
Treat with antibiotics as recommended by veterinarian.

Clogged Tube
Always flush with warm water before and after feeding.
Avoid giving pills in tube.
Instill carbonated beverage or cranberry juice.

Cellulitis
Change bandage regularly.
Monitor site for redness, swelling, and discharge.
Keep site clean and dry.
Antibiotics may be necessary.

that the subsequent feeding be skipped. If two consecutive feedings are missed, pharmacologic agents may be instituted by the veterinarian to promote gastric motility. Feces should be analyzed for normal composition.

The stomach capacity of dogs and cats is varied. In general, the stomach volume of the dog is approximately 90 ml/kg. However, the amount fed typically should not exceed 50 ml/kg. In the cat, the general stomach capacity should never exceed 100 ml.

The tube placement should always be confirmed with a radiograph to prevent airway complications. In the sick or debilitated animal, coughing may not be present if a tube is inadvertently placed into the trachea. In this way, a "silent" aspiration may occur to critically ill or weak patients. The technician should monitor the patient for increased lung sounds, areas of dullness on auscultation of the lungs, coughing, and fever. If such clinical signs are present, feedings should be discontinued and oxygen supplied immediately. The patient may benefit from partial parenteral nutrition (PPN) or total parenteral nutrition (TPN) while recovering from aspiration pneumonia.

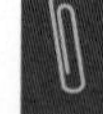

TECHNICIAN NOTE Upright feedings are recommended for patients at risk for aspiration.

ENTERAL FEEDING WORKSHEET

1. Calculate resting energy requirement (RER) RER = (70) 3 (kg)$^{0.75}$

70 3 [ ]$^{0.75}$ = [ ]
Body weight (kg) RER (kcal/day)

2. Choose a veterinary-specific critical care formula

3. Calculate volume of diet required

[ ] Name of diet chosen

[ ] 4 [ ] = [ ]
RER (kcal/day) kcal/ml ml formula/day

4. Number and volume of feedings

[ ] 4 [ ] = [ ]
ml formula/day Number feedings/day ml formula/feeding

FIGURE 12-14 Enteral feeding worksheet: Calculations for the daily food dose are done by dividing the patient's kcal requirement by the kcal/ml energy content of the food. The daily amount (ml) of food is usually divided into small portions that are given frequently.

Calculating nutrient requirements and food selection. (Figure 12-14) Consider physical form and other nutritional characteristics before selecting a feeding product. For example, oral calorie paste supplements are extremely deficient in protein, and meat baby food are neither complete nor balanced. In addition, 5% dextrose does not provide adequate calorie concentrations and is devoid of protein. Table 12-10 summarizes the nutrient profile of selected commercial enteral products used in small animal patients.

1. Calculate the RER as follows:
   RER = 30 × (body weight [BW] in kg) + 70
   For animals less than 2 kg or greater than 45 kg use: RER = 70 × (BW in kg)$^{0.75}$
2. Calculate the illness energy requirement (IER): IER = RER × illness factor
3. Calculate the amount of food required:
   Food amount (ml) = IER ÷ caloric density of selected food (kcal/ml)

Disease factors for determining energy requirements in dogs and cats are suggested as follows:

- Cage rest 1.1
- Surgery, trauma, cancer, sepsis 1.2-1.5
- Severe burns, head trauma, ventilator patients 1.7-2.0

Most hospitalized veterinary patients have metabolic rates very near their RER. Therefore initially feeding patients at their RER is a logical and safe recommendation. Regular nutritional assessment of the patient is strongly recommended to adjust initial feeding rates (see Nutritional Assessment of the Hospitalized Patient).

Parenteral nutrition (PN) refers to the delivery of nutrients intravenously (IV). Candidates for PN include patients who are unable to digest or absorb nutrients via the GI tract or have uncontrolled vomiting. Examples include patients with severe pancreatitis, inflammatory bowel disease, peritonitis, or postoperative intestinal surgery patients needing bowel rest.

PN is a compounded solution containing electrolytes, amino acids, and lipids in a standard crystalloid suspension. Calculations are based upon the patient's RER, disease history, protein levels, and hydration status. PN solutions can also be obtained from human hospitals and independent pharmaceutical companies, although concentrations of each nutrient must still be calculated.

PPN does not supply all of the patient's nutrient needs, but can provide short-term support for animals that are expected to recover soon. PPN solutions are usually given at a maintenance dose (60 ml/kg/day), and additional fluid needs are met with crystalloid solutions as described earlier. Procalamine (McGaw, Inc.) is a commercial product that contains 3% amino acids, 3% glycerol, and electrolytes. A "homemade" PPN solution can be made by adding 300 ml of 8.5% amino acid solution (Travenol, Baxter, Inc.) to 700 ml of lactated Ringer's solution with 5% dextrose. The addition of lipid emulsions is controversial. Although lipids are rich in caloric content, they have been associated with immunosuppression through the impairment of reticuloendothelial function and reduction in white blood cell phagocytosis.

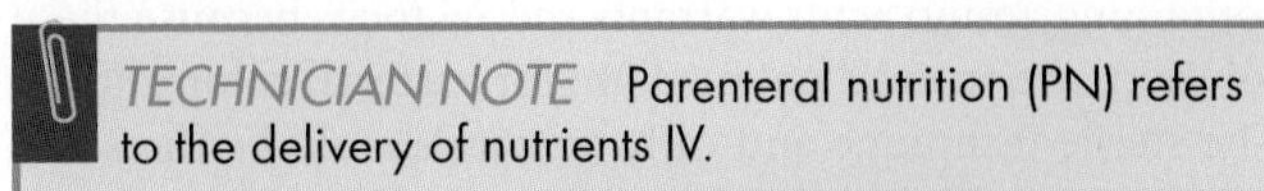
TECHNICIAN NOTE Parenteral nutrition (PN) refers to the delivery of nutrients IV.

The administration of PN is through a central, peripheral, intraosseous, or intraperitoneal catheter. However, the administration is typically through a central venous catheter because of the hypertonicity of the solution to prevent such common complications as phlebitis and an infection. In addition, if long-term parenteral support is anticipated, central venous catheters made of polyurethane are recommended because they need not be removed at a predetermined time.

TABLE 12-10 Composition of Commercial Enteral Diets

Product	Caloric Content (kcal/ml or g)	Protein Content (g/100 kcal)	(% Prot Cal)	Fat Content (% Fat/cal)	Carbohydrate Content (% CHO Cal)	Cost (cents/kcal)
Veterinary Polymeric						
CliniCare Canine powder*	0.9	6.0	24	64	12	2.5
CliniCare Canine liquid	0.9	5.5	25	59	16	3.5
Renal Care Canine	0.8	2.8	14	66	20	3.7
CliniCare Feline powder*	0.8	9.1	36	53	11	2.6
CliniCare Feline liquid	0.8	8.6	36	48	16	4.2
Renal Care Feline	0.8	5.6	25	60	15	4.0
Eukanuba Nutritional Recovery Diet	2.1	7.4	29	41	30	—
Prescription Diet a/d	1.3	8.8	36	51	13	0.5
Feline p/d†	0.9	9.3	37	56	7	0.2
Feline k/d†	0.9	4.4	21	67	13	0.2
Feline c/d†	0.6	8.9	33	52	15	0.2
Canine k/d‡	0.6	3.1	13	49	39	0.2
Canine u/d‡	0.7	1.9	8	48	45	0.2
Canine i/d‡	0.6	5.9	24	31	45	0.2
Waltham Instant Concentration Diet*	1.5	9.3	37	37	25	
Nutri-Cal	4.6	0.3	1	62	37	1.2
Human Polymeric						
Jevity	1.1	4.2	18	30	52	2.5
Pulmocare	1.5	4.3	17	55	28	2.5
Osmolite HN	1.1	4.4	17	30	53	2.5
Sustacal	1.0	6.8	24	21	55	2.5
Ensure HN	1.1	6.0	23	40	38	2.5
Baby food, turkey	1.0	14.6	58	42	0	1.0
Human Monomeric						
Peptamen	1.0	4.4	16	33	51	5.0

Reprinted by permission of Macintire DK: *Manual of small animal emergency and critical care medicine*, 2002, Lippincott Williams & Wilkins.
CHO, Carbohydrate.
*Diluted with water according to manufacturer's directions.
†In a blender mix ½ can (224 g) + ¾ cup (170 ml) water.
‡In a blender mix ½ can (224 g) + 1¼ cup (284 ml) water.

PN is expensive and requires a strict antiseptic technique in catheter placement (Figure 12-15). The nursing management of catheters carrying hyperosmolar solutions containing amino acids warrants special focus because these solutions are an excellent medium for bacterial colonization. The sterile technique and catheter care should be the same for *any* type of fluid administration, regardless of PN administration, but a sterile protocol should be strictly enforced for patients receiving PN.

Catheter care includes a strict sterile technique during insertion, including proper skin preparation, placement of a sterile underwrap over the insertion site, and a strict aseptic technique of IV tubing and administration bags. The IV lines should not be disconnected; if diagnostic testing or frequent walking is necessary, the IV lines and administration bags should accompany the patient. IV injections should follow the sterilization of the injection port. If a multilumen catheter is placed, proper identification to each port is necessary, with one line dedicated to the TPN solution only (usually the proximal port).

Laboratory analysis during PN use is important to monitor electrolytes, liver pathologic conditions, coagulopathies, and thrombocytopenia in addition to signs of an infection or patient compromise. Drug administration or drug additions into a parenteral solution are not recommended.

Maintaining enterocyte function is important to reduce PN complications, such as bowel atrophy and bacterial translocation. Combined enteral and parenteral feeding has been recently recommended to prevent intestinal mucosal deterioration, intestinal hypertrophy, and to facilitate healing by promoting intestinal growth. Therefore a small portion of enteral feeding to support the bowel during parenteral use is encouraged.

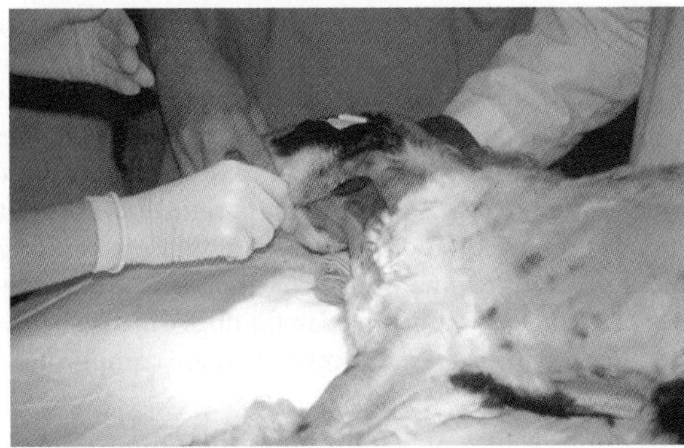

FIGURE 12-15 Central venous catheter preparation. Administration of PN is typically through a central venous catheter, which can remain in place for a prolonged period.

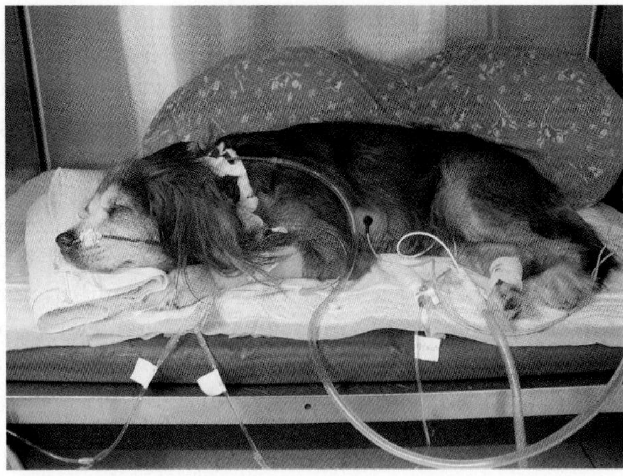

FIGURE 12-16 Critical patient with unexplained weakness. Note that various administration lines are clearly labeled.

Early enteral nutrition is also important to promote intestinal regeneration. A liquid diet (CliniCare) can be offered initially, or a gruel can be made with an easily digestible high-carbohydrate, low-fat diet. The addition of glutamine powder (0.5 g/kg divided q 12 hours) to drinking water may promote GI healing in dogs recovering from viral enteritis. Various veterinary recovery diets are available for care after hospitalization. The initial feeding should consist of small amounts of an easily digestible low-fat diet fed frequently. The normal diet is gradually reintroduced after the appetite and stool have returned to normal.

TECHNICIAN NOTE Candidates for PN include patients who are unable to digest or absorb nutrients via the GI tract or have uncontrolled vomiting.

NUTRITIONAL CONSIDERATIONS FOR THE CRITICAL PATIENT

Critical illness is associated with an increase in metabolism to provide energy for immune responses and healing. This hypermetabolic process is an effort by the body to mobilize its supply of circulating nutrient substrates, such as glucose and amino acids. Unfortunately, this mobilization occurs at the expense of body tissue and function at a time when protein synthesis demands are also high. The body becomes reliant on its protein stores to provide gluconeogenesis because glucose is desperately needed as a fuel source. The consequent loss of protein results in weight loss and alterations in protein homeostasis. The loss of lean body mass is associated with patient morbidity and mortality, and it is crucial to be able to recognize symptoms of nutritional insufficiency.

In the critically ill or injured patient, the hypermetabolic state continues as the body attempts to heal itself. As a result, a patient's resting energy expenditure and oxygen demands are increased (see Patients at Risk for Malnutrition). Clinical signs of such metabolic events include tachycardia, tachypnea, hyperglycemia, and the eventual net breakdown of skeletal muscle protein and the mobilization of body fat.

Unexplained weakness or dull mentation often accompanies the nutritionally starved critical patient (Figure 12-16). Dull mentation and weakness is often a reflection of the loss of skeletal muscle mass from altered protein homeostasis. Because patients are using protein reserves from multiple body organs, organ dysfunction is an eventuality without nutritional support. Obese and overweight critical patients can also develop malnutrition, in spite of excessive amounts of fat reserves. The overweight patient's nutritional needs may also be overlooked because the signs of muscle weakness and muscle wasting are less obvious. All critically ill patients, regardless of body weight, need the same degree of nutritional assessment and monitoring.

TECHNICIAN NOTE Dull mentation and weakness is often a reflection of the loss of skeletal muscle mass from altered protein homeostasis.

Respiratory function deteriorates as intercostals and diaphragmatic muscles waste as a result of poor nutritional support, exacerbating poor ventilation and hypoxia. Chronic hypoxia results in pneumonia and atelectasis. Increased respiratory efforts and increased respiratory rates are often present in the critical patient, requiring tremendous amounts of energy. In addition, the critical patient is often recumbent. Recumbent patients are at the greatest risk for respiratory insufficiency because the nutritional uptake is generally poor, with muscle fatigue and muscle wasting further complicating patient recovery. Recumbent patients with muscle wasting are prone to megaesophagus and aspiration pneumonia. Limb edema can also be present, suggesting hypoproteinemia.

Kidney function can also deteriorate because decreased urea concentration in the renal medulla reduces the kidney's ability to concentrate urine. Poor nutrition can cause decreased muscle function leading to decreased motility and malabsorption in the GI tract. Sadly, even cardiac muscle can become weak by the increased demand for oxygen consumption as a result of the hypermetabolic state from injury or illness.

In essence, no organ is spared during malnutrition of the critically ill patient. It is important to note that the interrelationships between organ function and nutrition are complex and delicate. Wherein no single parameter or observation can define the degree of nutritional insufficiency, an awareness of the nutritional need for the patient's maintenance is an important step in providing good patient care.

Routine laboratory tests can also provide additional evidence of nutritional insufficiency in the critical patient. Tests of immune function, such as a lymphocyte count, are important in addition to the hematocrit and reticulocyte count if anemia is present. In addition, serum albumin is important to measure in nutritionally challenged patients. It is important to note that any abnormal lab findings can also be from several underlying disease processes that are complicated by poor nutrition.

CASE PRESENTATION 12-1 EXOCRINE PANCREATIC INSUFFICIENCY

A 7-year old male named "Dash," a castrated whippet was seen for chronic diarrhea and weight loss over an 8-week period. On a physical examination, a BCS of one was observed, with a grade III/VI systolic heart murmur. Lab results showed a mild anemia (Hct of 35%, normal 37-55), lymphopenia (452, normal 1000-4000), panhypoproteinemia (albumin 1.8, normal 2.6-3.5, globulins 1.3, normal 3.6-5.0), and a possible UTI with rods identified on the urine sediment despite negative urine culture results. Chest radiographs showed mild to moderate left-sided heart enlargement. No significant findings were identified on abdominal radiographs or abdominal ultrasound. Bile acid results were unremarkable. Results are most consistent with a severe protein-losing enteropathy, with intestinal biopsies recommended to the owner, or other small-intestinal diseases, such as exocrine pancreatic insufficiency (EPI), small-intestinal bacterial overgrowth (SIBO), or lymphangiectasia. Pancreatic function tests (TLI) later revealed a diagnosis of **EPI.** Cardiac ultrasound revealed mitral insufficiency. The treatment included antibiotics, PN administration, enzyme replacement therapy, and a restricted diet on discharge from the hospital. Combined enteral and parenteral feeding was implemented to prevent intestinal mucosal deterioration, intestinal hypertrophy, and to facilitate healing by promoting intestinal growth

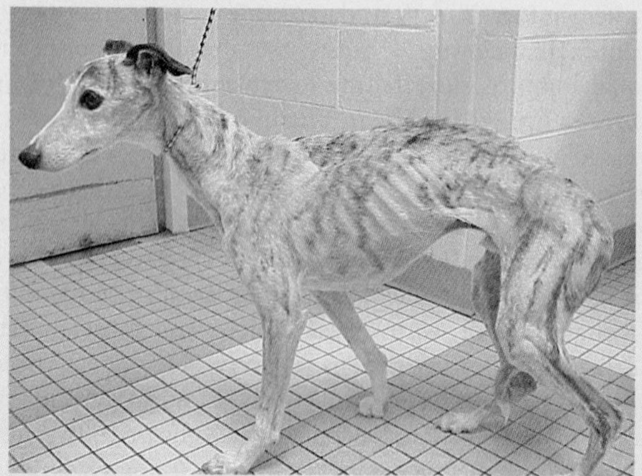

FIGURE 1 "Dash" a 7-year-old castrated male whippet had chronic diarrhea and weight loss.

Discussion

Restriction of dietary fat is recommended for such small-intestinal diseases as exocrine pancreatic insufficiency. Chronic diarrhea occurred as a result of interference of normal digestion and absorption of nutrients. Nutrients can be retained within the intestinal lumen, exerting an osmotic effect leading to the retention of water and diarrhea, often referred to as osmotic diarrhea. Although osmotic diarrhea is most commonly seen with nutritional overload, it is also associated with deficiencies of digestive enzymes, such as found in EPI. EPI is a disease of maldigestion as a result of a lack of digestive enzymes. Digestion of fat is significantly impaired.

Diet plays a fundamental role in the management of EPI. Recommended dietary treatment includes:

- ✓ Restriction of dietary fat
- ✓ Moderate to high quantities of good-quality protein
- ✓ Highly-digestible carbohydrates, such as rice
- ✓ Avoidance of dietary fiber
- ✓ Supplementation of water-soluble vitamins, such as B complexes and folate

Note that severe protein deficiency can further compromise a diseased intestinal tract. Protein-enriched food are critical in the management of such diseases. In addition, because protein plays a key role in dietary sensitivity (because most allergens are proteins), sources of dietary protein should be limited to one or two ingredients not normally associated with sensitivity reactions.

Carbohydrate digestion can be impaired with EPI; therefore highly-digestible carbohydrates are recommended in the diet. Simple sugars, such as lactose, should be avoided because the enzymes required for digestion may be insufficient.

Fiber is contraindicated in EPI because it may interfere with pancreatic enzyme activity. Although fiber may improve fecal consistency, it may interfere with digestion and absorption, thereby further compromising the patient. In addition, increased intestinal permeability may accompany low blood protein levels, as intestinal pore size becomes large and fluid filled, allowing proteins to escape, creating protein-losing enteropathies and diarrhea.

TECHNICIAN NOTE Poor nutrition can cause decreased muscle function leading to decreased motility and malabsorption in the GI tract.

NUTRITION OF BIRDS AND SMALL EXOTIC PETS

FEEDING PET BIRDS

Box 12-12 gives nutritional deficiencies of birds and the resulting conditions. Nutritional problems encountered in avian medicine include inadequate diets and poor feeding practices. Nutritional disease is common in pet birds. Box 12-13 lists human food that can add diversity to the diet of companion birds. Ill avian patients need nutritional support that may differ from their normal diet. An excessive or inadequate energy intake, supplementation imbalances, and the ingestion of toxic substances, such as heavy metals and inappropriate plant material, will create additional nutritional challenges to the veterinary professional.

Dietary-induced diseases frequently occur in psittacine and passerine bird species as a result of diverse nutrient requirements. Unfortunately, each species of bird means differences in nutritional demands, with little data to determine specific quantities or qualities of a diet. All-seed diets (particularly diets composed of only one type of seed, such as millet or sunflower) and diets supplemented with fruits, vegetables, and other human food are often thought to be complete food for birds. Such practices lead to feeding and nutritional disorders.

Small birds have high metabolic rates and high energy requirements; therefore a continuous supply of food should be available. However, most commercially available seeds are deficient in certain limiting nutrients (e.g., specific amino acids, vitamins, trace minerals, and macrominerals, such as calcium and sodium). In addition, seeds are not the primary or natural diet of most species of companion birds. Natural diets contain a wide variety of insects, fruits, and seeds; captive birds are commonly fed seed diets. In addition, seed diets are composed primarily of sunflower seeds high in fat but low in calcium and vitamin A, perpetuating obesity and/or nutritional deficiencies.

TECHNICIAN NOTE Small birds have high metabolic rates and high energy requirements; therefore a continuous supply of food should be available.

Perhaps the most common cause of dietary-induced diseases in companion birds is the practice of adding fruits and vegetables sold for human consumption to commercially prepared food or supplemented seed mixtures. The most readily available fruits and vegetables contain primarily water, carbohydrates, and fiber. They are severely deficient in protein, vitamins, and minerals when compared with the nutrient recommendations for psittacine and passerine birds.

BOX 12-12 Nutritional Deficiencies Typically Found in Companion Birds

- Vitamin A (squamous metaplasia, hyperkeratosis)
- Iodine (hypothyroidism)
- Vitamin E (encephalomalacia)
- Zinc (failure to thrive)
- Selenium (muscular dystrophy)

BOX 12-13 Feed Diversity for Companion Birds

- Cheerios
- Pellets, crumbles, crimps
- Cooked vegetables
- Bananas

Fruits and vegetables primarily dilute key nutrients present in nutritionally balanced commercially prepared food. Birds often preferentially eat fruits and vegetables because of their high water content instead of dry extruded or pelleted food and seed mixtures. Birds often select food items based on water content, texture, color, or taste rather than nutrient content, resulting in very imbalanced nutrient intakes.

Captive birds also develop nutritional deficiencies by habitually selecting specific food items from a variety of offerings. Because malnourished birds often tend to overeat the food items presented to them, it is unclear whether this is a cause or an effect of malnutrition. Unfortunately, such eating behavior leads to the popular misconception that birds are able to preferentially balance their diets.

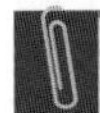

TECHNICIAN NOTE Each species of bird has its own unique nutritional requirement.

All birds do have similar nutritional requirements, including water, proteins and amino acids, carbohydrates, fats, vitamins, inorganic elements, and minerals. Different species require different amounts of these substances. The mineral required in the largest quantity is calcium, necessary for bone mineralization and eggshell calcification. The calcium requirement(s) for psittacine species have not been determined, but the maintenance requirement for chickens is 0.1% of the diet. Many of the seeds consumed by companion birds are less than 0.03% of the diet, suggesting that the requirement is larger than 0.05%. African gray parrots are particularly prone to hypocalcemic seizures. The pathophysiology is unknown. Hypocalcemia can be alleviated if birds eat at least half of their diet as pellets because vitamin D_3 is provided. Sunlight is needed to convert the inactive form of vitamin D to the active form, or it needs to be supplied in some food on a regular basis.

Proteins required by companion birds are composed of approximately 20 amino acids. Ten of these amino acids are essential: arginine, histidine, isoleucine, leucine, lysine, methionine, phenylalanine, threonine, tryptophan, and valine.

In the infant bird, glycine (or serine) and proline are of utmost importance. In the United States, methionine and lysine are often absent in the diet. Evidence suggests that increased protein may be needed during certain points in the reproductive cycle. In the wild, insects supply these increased needs. It is difficult for bird owners to meet these special needs by feeding only seed mixtures.

White worms (*Enchytraeus* larvae) are available commercially and can be kept for long periods, much like earthworms, in a cool, damp moss and leaf litter substrate. These worms are especially useful to provide when parent birds are brooding and feeding their young. Ant pupae, which bird fanciers have relied on heavily for their avian diets, are now available commercially in large outlets and by mail order. Water shrimp (*Daphnia* spp.) are relished by some species and greatly enhance red pigments in their plumage. Aphids that feed on members of the rose family concentrate the same pigments and may be more appropriate for small passerine birds. Moth larvae, commonly known as wax worms, and beetle larvae, called mealworms, supply extra protein and fat, especially at the onset of the breeding season. Care should be taken to restrict the intake of these insects, or birds will rapidly gain weight and become obese.

> TECHNICIAN NOTE Care should be taken to restrict the intake of certain insects, or birds will rapidly gain weight and become obese.

Food appropriately balanced with carbohydrates, protein, fats, vitamins, minerals, and water are essential for all birds. The stewardship of confined birds must address good nutrition at several levels: the daily satisfaction and health of the bird and the long-term contributions to growth, maturation, defense against disease, and reproductive health (the hallmark of good nutrition).

The major benefits of commercially prepared food are nutrient balance and convenience. Manufacturers commonly formulate commercial food using sound scientific principles following established nutrient recommendations. Although the adherence to these recommendations and ingredients' quality may vary among manufacturers, an extruded or pelleted diet supplies all the nutrients in one particle. Such formulations help prevent the alteration of nutrient balance by uninformed owners who feed imbalanced seeds or human food or by birds that consume different quantities of imbalanced food that are fed separately.

A potential disadvantage of feeding commercial food is that testing protocols for nutritional adequacy have not yet been established for avian food as they have been for commercial canine and feline food. Nevertheless, the probability of producing a nutritional imbalance by feeding a commercial avian food is significantly less than seeds or human food that are prepared by uninformed owners.

Although seeds are a popular, convenient, and inexpensive method of providing nutrients to companion birds (Figure 12-17), they are not necessarily the best or even the most natural food for pet birds. The types of seed present in most commercial mixes are not native to areas where most pet bird species originate.

> TECHNICIAN NOTE Although well-balanced seed mixtures supply essential nutrients, they are rarely sufficient to meet all of the nutritional needs of pet birds.

A well-balanced seed mixture can supply essential nutrients, such as fats, carbohydrates, and some minerals. However, seeds are rarely, if ever, an appropriate sole nutritional source because they provide inadequate levels of protein, vitamins, and minerals. Commercially available seed mixtures vary greatly in type and quality. Individual types of seed are also sold in most stores; thus formulating seed mixtures is a common practice. Unfortunately, the availability of individual types of seed promote nutrient imbalance when uninformed owners create a mixture based primarily on the price and physical appearance of the seeds. The creation or use of homemade seed mixtures should be discouraged.

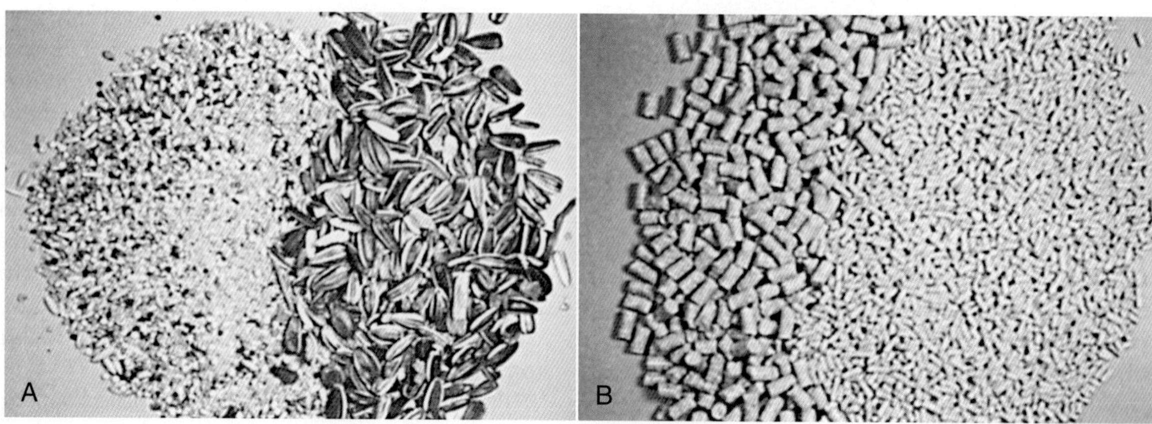

FIGURE 12-17 A, Seeds are an important part of many avian diets. However, high-oil seeds and nuts, such as sunflower seeds and peanuts, may cause addictions and nutritional imbalance. Oil seeds are deficient in proteins relative to calorie content and in calcium and micronutrients. **B,** Complete and balanced avian food are available as fortified seed mixtures and extruded and pelleted food.

TABLE 12-11 Suggested Diet for Maintenance of Adult Caged Birds

	Canary	Budgerigar	Cockatiel	Conure	Amazon/African Gray Parrot	Macaw/ Cockatoo
Offer Daily						
Whole-grain bread cubes or primate biscuit	¼ T	½ T	1 T	1½ T	2 T	4 T
Fresh dark green or yellow vegetables	½ T	1 T	2 T	4 T	3 T	½ C
Protein source (cheese, hard-cooked eggs, meat, mature legumes)	¼ Size of pea	½ Size of pea	Size of pea	¼ t	½ t	1 T
Dry seeds (two 15-min periods) (sunflower)	0	0	1 T	2 T	2 T	4 T
Small seeds (canary, niger, poppy, rape, millet, safflower, hemp)	Ad lib	Ad lib	Ad lib	Ad lib	Ad lib	Ad lib
2 to 3 Times Weekly						
Fruit (cantaloupe, apricot, apple)	⅛ t	⅛ t	1 t	1⁄12 Apple	1⁄12 Apple	⅙ Apple
Citrus fruit	0	0	0	1⁄12 Orange	1⁄12 Orange	⅙ Orange
Fresh corn on the cob	3 or 4 Kernels	⅛ Piece	½ Piece	½ Piece	½ Piece	1 Piece
Peanuts	0	0	0	1	2	4
Add Temporarily for New Birds						
Vitamin A (from 10,000 IU capsule)	1 Drop/wk	2 Drops/wk	3 Drops/wk	1 Drop/day	1-2 Drops/day	4 Drops/day
Yogurt	Drop	Few drops	¼ tsp	¼ tsp	½ tsp	1 tsp
Always Available						
Calcium and/or mineral supplements (cuttlebone, mineral treat block, oyster shell, calcium lactate)						

Modified from Harrison GI, Harrison LR: *Clinical avian medicine and surgery*, Philadelphia, 1986, WB Saunders.
C, Cup; *T*, tablespoon; *t*, teaspoon.

A wide variety of homemade mixed-food diets have been suggested as alternatives for birds that will not accept commercially prepared food or seed mixtures even with added fruits and vegetables. These diets can result in excellent feathering and an appropriate body mass for the species, with no discernible signs of nutritional deficiency, if prepared carefully from scientifically developed recipes. These diets often contain varying amounts of ingredients, such as seeds, nuts, cooked eggs, low-fat yogurt or cheese, vegetables, fruits, grains, bread, pasta, multigrain cereals, legumes, seed mixes, pelleted or extruded psittacine diets, vitamin supplements, and calcium supplements (Table 12-11). When converting birds to a new homemade diet, have the client offer a mixture containing all the ingredients at one time. This practice usually prevents preferential selection of certain ingredients. Although larger parrots have difficulty eating small seeds, such as milo or oat groats, a seed mixture containing 30% hulled safflower, 30% milo, 30% oats, and 10% peanuts works well for smaller birds.

Insoluble and soluble mineral grit are often given to birds as a dietary supplement. Insoluble grit (quartz or silica) remains in the gizzard, where it may facilitate mechanical digestion. Soluble grit (oyster shells or cuttlefish) is completely digested and supplies a source of such minerals as calcium and phosphorus. However, be advised that oversupplementing mineral grit can be harmful to caged birds and may lead to gizzard impaction.

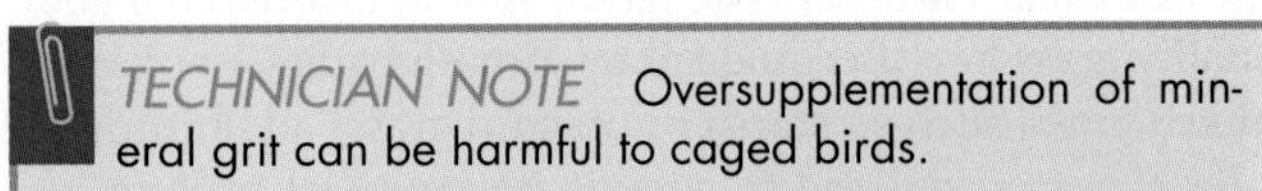
TECHNICIAN NOTE Oversupplementation of mineral grit can be harmful to caged birds.

Although homemade mixed-food diets may provide adequate nourishment, most companion bird owners are unwilling to devote the time necessary to adequately prepare these diets. In addition, owners must be willing to regularly observe which food components are being consumed to prevent birds from developing or reverting to preferential selection of specific ingredients.

Although feeding a well-balanced food is essential, it is easy to overlook the single most important dietary component: water. Water makes up more than 50% of a bird's body weight. Because birds have no sweat glands, the water intake plays an important role in thermoregulation. Breeding females may require increased amounts of water for egg production and for heat regulation while incubating eggs.

Although some food is high in water content, others require free water for efficient digestion and absorption. Some avian species are more physiologically adept at extracting water from their food. As a general rule, birds should never go for more than a few hours without access to fresh, clean water. Studies have shown that canaries will die within 48 hours if water is withheld.

Water should be provided in containers that are easily accessible, but not in a location that will allow feces, feathers, or food particles to accumulate. For this reason, water bowls should be attached to the wall of enclosures, near or above food bowls. In addition, large water bowls should be discouraged because they may invite bathing.

> TECHNICIAN NOTE Water should be provided in containers that are easily accessible, but not in a location that will allow feces, feathers, or food particles to accumulate.

RABBITS

The dietary requirements vary according to the age and use of a rabbit. For example, a balanced mixture of timothy grass, grass hay, and vegetables is the best diet for most pet rabbits, wherein show and production rabbits typically do better on a commercially produced alfalfa meal-based pellet. In general, however, rabbits are herbivores with high fiber requirements.

The best pet rabbit diet is an alfalfa-based pellet with a hay supplement given on a daily basis. Pellets are fed at the rate of 0.25 cup/2.27 kg (5 lb) body weight divided into two meals. During gestation and lactation, the amount of protein and available energy should be increased. This may require increasing the amount of pellets in the diet. Sugary treats should not be fed. "Treats" of fresh greens or other vegetable supplements are encouraged only as occasional rewards. Food recommended includes the carrot, small pieces of ripe banana, rice cakes, dry wheat bread, or dandelion leaves. It is important to remove any uneaten portion because spoilage can cause GI upset. The rabbit should be offered a good quality grass hay (Bermuda grass, timothy grass, oat hay, or mixed grass, such as marsh or orchard grass) ad libitum; alfalfa hay is considered to contain an excess of protein and calcium and thought by some to contribute to urinary calculi. Fresh, dark leafy greens should be fed at a rate of 1 cup/0.45 kg (1 lb) body weight.

Regular feeding schedules are important to the rabbit. Because rabbits are nocturnal in nature and consume most of their feed during the night, hay should be given in the morning and pellets with grains in the afternoon or evening. Adequate fresh water is essential to ensure a proper feed intake. Water delivery systems can be superior to water bowls that may tip or become contaminated with feces. The application of syrup or molasses to the tip of the waterspout may induce use and encourage water consumption.

> TECHNICIAN NOTE Rabbits are nocturnal and consume most of their feed during the night; hay should be given in the morning and pellets with grains in the afternoon or evening.

Other components of rabbit nutrition include vitamin supplementation. Vitamin A deficiency can result in infertility and other reproductive complications, central nervous system defects, and increased neonatal mortality. Most fresh alfalfa pellets contain adequate vitamin A to prevent such deficiencies; adding a supplement to a diet already rich in vitamin A can cause excesses with consequences just as harmful. Technicians should advise rabbit owners to buy fresh alfalfa pellets and monitor the rabbit's appetite.

All commercial feed should have a mill location and date of manufacture clearly printed on the bag; it is recommended to purchase feed within 90 days of production. Feed more than 6 months old have poor nutritional quality. In addition, feed that contains antibiotics is generally not recommended. Antibiotics may disrupt the intestinal floral balance, resulting in diarrhea, anorexia, or death.

Pellets high in calcium or excessive vitamin D can occasionally produce chalky-white or cream-colored urine. Termed dystrophic calcification, excess calcium causes urinary lithiasis or the excessive excretion of calcium "sand" and may even cause calculi to form in the kidney and ureter. Although rabbits have unusual calcium metabolism, dietary management to regulate the calcium intake includes feeding alfalfa-based diets without additional calcium supplementation. Normal urine color in the rabbit varies from straw to a reddish brown color.

> TECHNICIAN NOTE Dietary management to regulate the calcium intake includes feeding alfalfa-based diets without additional calcium supplementation.

GUINEA PIGS

Guinea pigs are notoriously fastidious eaters. They are herbivores with normal coprophagous behavior. Any abrupt changes in feed or feeding systems can result in a refusal to eat or drink for extended periods of time.

Recommended diets include types of food with increased fiber because insufficient levels can cause cecal impaction and fur chewing, resulting in the formation of hairballs. Diets should be composed of freshly milled guinea pig feed found in most pet or grocery stores, with a good quality hay to satisfy fiber requirements. As a result of specific nutrient and vitamin requirements, guinea pigs *should not* be fed rabbit or any other diet designed for another species. Guinea pigs should also be given access to hard-food diets that promote gnawing because malocclusion can prevent eating and drinking.

Guinea pigs lack an enzyme in glucose to the vitamin C pathway, thus requiring a daily dietary ascorbic acid supplement. Commercially prepared guinea pig diets generally contain minimum vitamin C concentrations, with depleted concentrations with a shelf life of more than 3 months. Fresh fruit can be used to supplement commercial diets; avoid abrupt changes in diet to prevent GI upset. Diets supplemented with produce high in ascorbic acid are recommended: spinach, kale, parsley, chicory, bell peppers, and oranges.

Absolute requirements of 10 mg/kg/day of ascorbic acid are recommended, with increases up to 30 mg/kg/day if pregnant (Puschinsky, 1995). If supplementation is not provided in the feed, 1g/L may be added to the water or one small handful of cabbage or kale or one fourth of an orange may be given daily. Clinical signs of vitamin C deficiency include alopecia, anorexia, dehydration, poor wound healing, with eventual periodontal disease including brown discoloration of teeth and temporomandibular joint (TMJ) inflammation.

Fresh water is essential to the guinea pig and should be provided daily. Water bottles or other water delivery systems are recommended to prevent water contamination or spillage. Note that the guinea pig has a propensity for chewing and gnawing; water valves should be located outside the cage to prevent destruction.

> *TECHNICIAN NOTE* Guinea pigs lack an enzyme in glucose to the vitamin C pathway, thus requiring a daily dietary ascorbic acid supplement.

HAMSTERS

Hamsters are omnivores and should be provided with hard-food diets, such as the occasional dog biscuit, to promote gnawing and chewing to prevent malocclusion and overgrowth of teeth. Dietary recommendations include pelleted diets or mixes designed for the hamster, supplemented with treat food, such as washed vegetables, seeds, fruits, crackers, and cooked meat. Food should be given at night because the hamster is typically nocturnal. Stale food should be removed from the cage because hoarding is a common social behavior.

Water should also be provided either in a heavy bowl or in a water delivery system to prevent contamination or spillage.

GERBILS

Gerbils are herbivorous or granivorous. In the wild, gerbils typically eat plants, seeds, and insects. Commercial pelleted food designed for the gerbil is available, although adult gerbils can be fed a good quality rat or mouse diet. Note that gerbils will preferentially eat sunflower seeds at the expense of other dietary ingredients, resulting in obesity and possible calcium deficiency. Technicians should advise gerbil owners to avoid mixes containing large amounts of sunflower seeds.

Gerbils typically eat frequent small meals, up to eight times a day. Weight loss will occur if food supplies are limited. Diets should be supplemented with green vegetables, fresh fruit, and hard food or pieces of wood to prevent tooth malocclusion.

Wherein gerbils can conserve water very efficiently, fresh water should be provided on a daily basis. Heavy water containers or water delivery systems are recommended to prevent contamination or spillage.

> *TECHNICIAN NOTE* Gerbils typically eat frequent small meals, up to eight times a day. Weight loss will occur if food supplies are limited.

Both rats and mice are omnivorous. Commercially available pellet-based diets supply most known nutritional requirements, although it is generally recommended to supplement diets with small amounts of apples, tomatoes, or biscuits. "Treats" may be given to encourage handling, but should be used sparingly to prevent obesity. Fresh water should be supplied in sipper bottles on a daily basis.

CHINCHILLAS

Chinchillas are hindgut fermenters, meaning they have complex digestive systems for fermenting fiber in the food. Inappropriate food (such as diets devoid of fiber) can cause diarrhea, constipation, bloat, or rectal prolapse. Recommended diets include mainly grasses and seeds, supplemented with small quantities of dried fruits, nuts, carrots, green vegetables, or green grass. Commercially prepared diets are available specifically for the chinchilla, although rabbit or guinea pig food is suitable. Hard food or pieces of wood should be available to prevent malocclusion.

Chinchillas should be provided with a dust bath for grooming needs. It is recommended to allow bathing for only short periods in the day; keeping dust baths in the cage may result in fecal contamination. Daily fresh water is also necessary, either in a heavy bowl or in a water delivery system.

FERRETS

Ferrets are typically carnivores, with general requirements of roughly 30% protein and 25% fat in a daily diet. High-fiber diets are not recommended. Pelleted commercial ferret diets are available, although high-quality dry cat food can be substituted. Commercial diets may occasionally be supplemented with mice or chicken heads to provide required protein. Small amounts of apples, cooked meat, or dried fruit can also be offered, although consistency in diet is generally recommended because the ferret may resent dietary changes. Body weight may have seasonal fluctuations with summer and autumn months having possible weight reduction. Fresh water should be provided on a daily basis.

FEEDING CAPTIVE REPTILES

Chelonians

Land tortoises are primarily herbivores, but will occasionally eat insects and small rodents. In captivity, diets should primarily be composed of vegetables (mainly dark leafy greens, grasses, and weeds), some fruits, and limited quantities of high-protein food. Typical tortoise diets include the following substrates:

- Eighty-five percent vegetables, such as collards, radish, turnip greens, dandelions, kale, cabbage, bok-choy, broccoli, cauliflower, and summer and winter squash
- Ten percent fruit, such as grapes, apples, oranges, pears, peaches, plums, dates, melons, strawberries, raspberries, mangos, and tomatoes
- Greater than 5% high-protein food, such as dry maintenance dog food, parrot chow, cereals, mice, scrambled eggs

Successfully caring for captive tortoises relies heavily on varying the diet. A shallow water dish should be provided to allow consumption, although caution should be taken not to overfill with water because the tortoise and box turtle cannot swim and will drown if submerged. The water should be changed daily because turtles may defecate in the water dish.

Sunlight or ultraviolet light should be provided to allow cholecalciferol (vitamin D) synthesis for shell formation and repair and to stimulate the appetite and basking behavior. Multivitamins containing vitamin D may be added to the diet every 1 to 2 weeks.

Aquatic turtles need a variety of food to achieve a balanced diet. The majority of the diet should be composed of whole animals, such as mice, earthworms, chopped goldfish or guppies, and slugs. Small amounts of insects, such as crickets, mealworms, flies, and grasshoppers, can also be offered. It is not recommended to feed such meats as hamburger or shellfish. Vegetables, such as dark leafy greens, cabbage, or romaine lettuce, can also be offered in small amounts. Commercial diets are available in floating stick forms, but keep in mind that supplementing with natural food, such as earthworms and small fish, is also recommended. Some tropical fish food can also be used to provide variation in diet. Note that aquatic turtles will only feed if they are in the water.

The most common nutritional deficiency in captive turtles is vitamin A deficiency. Clinical signs include respiratory infections, edematous eyes, urogenital tract obstructions, and beak overgrowths. Hypovitaminosis A can be prevented by providing the proper diet that supplies β-carotene, found in such food as earthworms, small fish, and green leafy vegetables. The most common clinical findings of sick turtles are due to anorexia and dehydration. Anorexia and dehydration are primarily husbandry related; causes include stress, a lack of food, an improper ambient temperature, improper diet, a parasitic infection, or metabolic disorders.

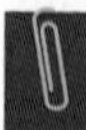

TECHNICIAN NOTE Successfully caring for captive tortoises relies heavily on varying the diet.

SNAKES

Snakes are carnivores and need to be fed a varied diet. Specific dietary needs depend on the species of snake, although staples generally include rodents. The size of the rodent fed should be about the same diameter as the snake's body and about one eighth of the length. Typical rodents used for snake food include the rabbit, rat, mouse, gerbil, chicken, lizard, or other snakes. It is usually prudent to feed frozen or freshly killed rodents to prevent injury or an infection caused by prey bites to the snake.

Most species of snake are fed once every 1 to 2 weeks, but the size of prey and frequency of feeding depends on both the time of year and the signalment of the snake. If the snake is fed more than once a week, the environment needs to be warm enough to facilitate digestion. The incidence of nutritional deficiency in the captive snake is rare because most are fed whole prey. Note that as snakes eat infrequently, inappetence or weight loss may go undetected. Periodic weighing is recommended to prevent nutritional deficiency. Although water requirements are low, it should be supplied on a daily basis.

LIZARDS

Most captive lizards are omnivorous, eating such food as mealworms, crickets, locusts, and silkworm larvae. Most insects are calcium deficient, however, and the insects themselves should be fed nutritional supplements to pass on to the lizard. Lizards in the wild are primarily carnivorous, eating invertebrate or vertebrate prey. In general, captive lizards require vitamin and mineral supplementation with an emphasis on a variety of food. Juvenile lizards should be fed one to two times a day, with adults requiring feeding two to three times per week. Most lizards are diurnal and require day feedings and time to bask in natural or ultraviolet light.

Herbivorous lizards, such as the green iguana, require a varied diet to ensure an adequate nutritional balance. Recommended diets for herbivores include leafy greens (romaine lettuce and collard greens), mustard greens, and clover. Vegetables are also adequate dietary substances, including green beans, okra, carrots, and squashes. It is important, however, to note that certain vegetables, such as spinach, cabbage, peas, and potatoes, contain substances that bind calcium and other trace minerals, inhibiting their absorption. Alfalfa rabbit pellets can also be fed to the common iguana.

Commercially prepared diets are available with additional supplementation unnecessary if the captive lizard is fed a diet based primarily on such purchased food. Homemade diets of vegetables and fruit should always be supplemented with appropriate vitamins and minerals. Technicians can advise lizard owners to purchase a quality reptile vitamin, containing vitamin D_3, administered one to two times a week if provided a good diet (Puchinsky, 1995).

TECHNICIAN NOTE Captive lizards require vitamin and mineral supplementation with an emphasis on a variety of food.

Common iguanas also require protein for normal growth and development. Juvenile iguanas in captivity generally need more protein and calcium than do adults. Common protein sources include dark green leafy vegetables such as collards, turnip greens, kale, bok choy, and broccoli with leaves. It was thought that meat-based protein was a requirement for iguanas, but that is no longer felt to be true.

Water should be provided in a bowl for bathing and drinking. Note that some lizards, such as the chameleon, will only drink water if it is on droplets on plants. Therefore it is important to spray or mist the tank several times a day. In addition, most lizards should be sprayed with water or allowed to bathe to prevent skin problems associated with low humidity.

AMPHIBIANS

Amphibians include such pets as frogs, toads, salamanders, and newts. Most adult amphibians are carnivores, eating live prey when not in a captive environment. Captive amphibians may adapt to eating dead prey or meat; raw meat must be supplemented with calcium at a recommended dose of 10 mg/g of meat (McCune, 2003). In general, captive amphibians should be fed two to three times a week.

Frogs and toads eat a diet based primarily on insects, such as crickets, mealworms, and fruit flies. Salamanders eat earthworms, slugs, and other insects. Note that with each individual species of amphibian, owners should be encouraged to replicate their natural environment to ensure food consumption and longevity.

ACKNOWLEDGMENT

The author and editors wish to acknowledge the exceptional contributions of Drs. Philip Roudebush; Stephen W. Crane; Susan Berryhill, RVT, VTS; and Sheila R. Grosdidier, RVT whose original contributions served as the foundation for the material appearing in this edition.

BIBLIOGRAPHY

Crane SW: Occurrence and management of obesity in companion animals, *J Small Anim Pract* 32:275, 1991.

Markham RW, Hodgkins EM: Geriatric nutrition, *Vet Clin North Am* 19:165, 1989.

McCune S: Nutrition. In *Veterinary nursing,* ed 3, 2003, Butterworth-Heinemann.

RECOMMENDED READING

Bonagura JD: *Current veterinary therapy XIII,* Philadelphia, 2000, WB Saunders.

Management of anorexia, pp 69-74.

Nutritional assessment of pet food labels, pp 74-80.

Parenteral nutrition products, pp 80-84.

Mechanical devices for percutaneous placement of gastrostomy tubes: use of Eld applicator, pp 87-94.

Refeeding syndrome, pp 87–89.

Microenteral nutrition, pp 136-140.

Hypoallergenic diets for dogs and cats, pp 530-536.

Essential fatty acids, pp 538-542.

Esophageal feeding tubes, pp 597-599.

Dietary sensitivity, pp 632-637.

Nutritional management of diarrheal diseases, pp 653-658.

Nutritional management of liver disease, pp 693-697.

Nutritional management of heart disease, pp 711-716.

Summary of dietary recommendations in urinary diseases, pp 841-846.

Hand MS, editors: *Small animal clinical nutrition,* ed 4, Topeka, Kan, 2000, Mark Morris Institute.

Small animal clinical nutrition: an iterative process, pp 1-19.

Nutrients, pp 21-107.

Introduction to commercial pet foods, pp 112-126.

Making commercial pet foods, pp 127-146.

Pet food labels, pp 147-161.

Making pet foods at home, pp 163-181.

Food safety, pp 183-198.

Health maintenance programs for dogs and cats, pp 201-211.

Normal dogs, pp 213-260.

Normal cats, pp 291-347.

Assisted feeding in hospitalized patients: enteral and parenteral nutrition, pp 351-399.

Obesity, pp 401-430.

Dental disease, pp 475-504.

Developmental orthopedic disease of dogs, pp 505-521.

Renal disease, pp 563-594.

Feline lower urinary tract disease, pp 689-718.

Feeding small exotic mammals, pp 943-960.

Feeding reptiles, pp 961-977.

Feeding passerine and psittacine birds, pp 979-991.

Neonatal, pediatric and orphaned puppy and kitten care, pp 1012-1019.

Comparative analysis of milks and milk replacers, pp 1064-1072.

Feeding orphaned and injured birds, mammals, amphibians and reptiles, pp 1101-1121.

Hawley B, Ritzman T, Edling TM: In Olsen GH, Orosz SE, editors: *Manual of avian medicine,* St Louis, 2000, Mosby.

Merton BD: Nutraceuticals: *Quality, safety and efficacy,* 2002, Proceedings ACVIM Forum.

Michel KE: *Dietary management of lower urinary tract disease,* 2002, Atlantic Coast Veterinary Conference.

Orosz SE: *Avian nutrition revisited: clinical perspectives,* 2005, AAV.

Quesenberry KE, Carpenter JW: *Ferrets, rabbits, and rodents, clinical medicine and surgery,* ed 2, St Louis, 2004, WB Saunders.

13 Large Animal Nutrition

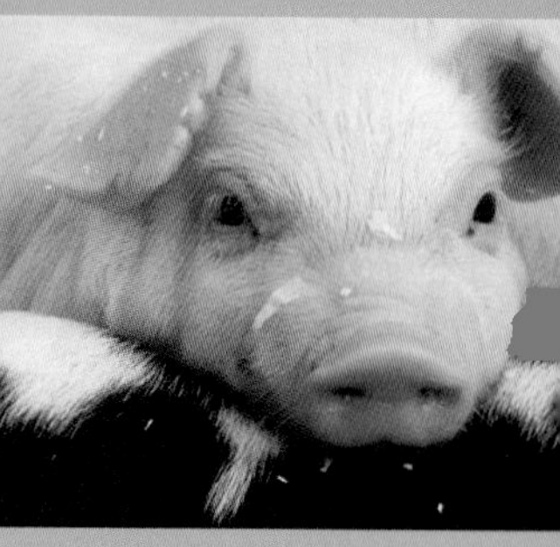

William D. Schoenherr

OUTLINE

KEY TERMS

Amino acids
Biologic value
Concentrates
Digestible energy
Digestion
Forage
Gross energy
Maintenance nutrient requirements (MNRS)
Net energy
Protein efficiency ratio
Total digestible nutrients (TDN)

LEARNING OBJECTIVES

When you have completed this chapter, you will be able to:

1. Explain the relationship between productivity and profitability in livestock production.
2. List the energy-producing and nonenergy-producing components of food.
3. Define the following terms: digestion, maintenance nutrient requirements, biologic value, protein efficiency ratio, total digestible nutrients, gross energy, digestible energy, metabolizable energy, and net energy.
4. List the variables affecting energy requirements of livestock and factors affecting the water intake of livestock.
5. Differentiate between essential and nonessential amino acids.
6. Explain the importance of water in metabolic reactions.
7. Differentiate between microminerals and macrominerals and give examples of each.
8. Describe the two commonly used feeding systems for dairy cattle.
9. Describe special considerations for feeding beef cattle, sheep, and swine for specific productive purposes (maintenance, growth, finishing, lactation, work, wool, or eggs).
10. List advantages and disadvantages of pasture feeding of livestock.

INTRODUCTION

Optimal nutrition has often been identified as the most expensive element in achieving full productivity and profitability in livestock (Ensminger, 1990). The veterinary technician must have a strong fundamental knowledge of nutrient needs and be able to identify the potential for problems and increase the client's understanding of essential feeding philosophies. The client who has the greatest need for this type of information is not the large, intensive livestock farmer who normally has feed professionally formulated for optimum production. Most often, the questions will be from clients who run small operations, have family members raising livestock for 4-H or children's clubs' (e.g., as Future Farmers of America) projects, or possess a "hobby farm." With these needs in mind, this chapter focuses on common nutritional problems and sound principles to help the veterinary technician provide meaningful, relevant information for livestock and horses.

Various nutritional disorders can be very similar to a vast array of diseases and may not be easily identified by the livestock producer or horse owner as a nutritional disorder until the problem becomes chronic and additional assistance is sought. It is essential to get a complete history, including a detailed feeding regimen, on any livestock or horse patient who is exhibiting signs of illness.

Dramatic enhancements have occurred in large animal nutrition, including studies that have increased understanding of the specific nutrient needs of livestock to maximize the genetic potential for efficient production, successful breeding, and the generation of high-quality, lean meat. Future research will continue to improve our understanding of animal physiology and lead to improvements in livestock production and equine nutrition (Table 13-1).

TABLE 13-1 Feeding Problems in Ruminants

Symptoms	Cause	Prevention	Comments
Bloat			
Distention of the left flank and then the right flank Hypersalivation Profuse burning ↑ Froth or gas accumulation in the rumen Respiratory distress Cyanosis Death	↑ Change in pasture with heavy fertilizer Genetics Bacterial overgrowth Overeating	Feed coarse grasses or dry forage before turnout to quick-growing pastures. Avoid straight pastures. Keep stock on pasture continuously rather than sporadically. Allow full access to water and salt.	Watch legume exposure for all ruminants.
Enterotoxemia (Overeating Disease)			
Death is often the first symptom Circling Progressive weakness Head butting Convulsions	Often occurs in faster-growing juveniles *Clostridium perfringens* Excess consumption of high-energy feed or lush pasture or heavy milk supply	Vaccinate with *Clostridium perfringens* type D for lambs and types C and D for breeding ewes.	Applies primarily in sheep and goats; sometimes cattle. If outbreak occurs, consider enterotoxemia antiserum for 21-day protection in lambs.
Fescue Toxicosis			
↓ +/− Lameness Necrosis of tail end Milk production Abortion	↑ Change in parasitized animal ↑ In malnourished animal Endophyte fungus *Acremonium coenophialum*	Avoid heavy parasitism and malnutrition. Use fungus-free fescue seed for planting.	Applies for cattle and sheep (fescue foot) mostly. Highest occurrence is in fall and winter in all fescue pasture.
Grass Tetany (Hypomagnesemia)			
Disorientation Paddling Convulsions Muscle twitching	Most common in cows 4 yr and older ↑ Occurrence during early lactation in heavy milking cows Pastures with ↓ Mg^{2+} and ↑ K^+ and ↓ Ca^+ availability	Start providing Mg^{2+} 30 days before high-risk times. ↑ Mg^{2+} in lactating and older cows and ewes. Highest risk is during spring, winter, and fall. Molasses supplement with Mg^{2+} may be required.	Stress from weather, movement, or environment increases risk.
Milk Fever (Parturition, Paresis, or Hypocalcemia)			
↓ Appetite Nervous behavior Collapse Wrenching of head toward back	Postcalving in high-producing cows ↓ Blood Ca^{2+}	Feed ↑ P, ↓ Ca^{2+} 14 days before parturition. Feed balanced Ca^{2+}/P rations. Vitamin D intake provided 1 wk before parturition. Avoid obesity.	Watch Ca^{2+} and P levels in dry periods.
Displaced Abomasum			
↓ Appetite ↓ Milk production Diarrhea, discolored feces	Pregnancy Lack of bulk in diet Sudden jarring of fresh cows Poor muscle tone Mycotoxin exposure	Avoid acidosis or alkalosis. Eliminate or reduce moldy or mycotoxin-laden feed.	Occurs most frequently in high-producing, heavily fed dairy cattle near parturition.
Ketosis			
Occurs: 14-50 days after parturition in cattle 2 wk before parturition in sheep ↓ Milk production ↓ Appetite	↑ Chances in multiple births with ewes and does Rapid loss of body fat and low availability of carbohydrates in diet	Maintain lean body condition and prevent excess fat. ↑ Energy intake before parturition and ↓ after parturition. Avoid sudden changes in the physical nature of the feed.	Ewes are at risk before lambing. Cows are typically at risk after calving.

Continued

TABLE 13-1 Feeding Problems in Ruminants—cont'd

Symptoms	Cause	Prevention	Comments
Ketosis—cont'd			
Sugary-acid breath ↓ Body weight Frequent urination Trembling Collapse			
Thiamine-Deficiency Polio			
Decreased vision Incoordination Acute death Excitable	Thiamine deficiency Overgrazing Feeding lambs in rich pasture	Cause not fully discovered. ↓ Grain intake while ↑ roughage quality, 1 wk before. ↑ Animals' intake of high-energy diets.	Occur primarily in feedlot and young cattle under 2 yr old. Goats may be affected while nursing young.
Rickets			
In young animals, enlarged joints Painful gait Leg bowing	Incorrect Ca^{2+}, P, vitamin intake	Provide balanced Ca^{2+}, P, and vitamin D diets.	
Urinary Calculi			
Difficult urination	↑ Increase in feedlots	Provide readily available water.	Males have ↑ risk.
Urolithiasis			
Bloody urine	High K^+ consumption, ↑ P, ↓ Ca^{2+}	Balance P/Ca^{2+} ratio.	
Water Belly			
Kicking at abdomen Rupture of bladder	Vitamin A deficiency Excess silicate intake	Prevent vitamin A deficiency. ↑ Salt availability. Balance ratios.	
White Muscle Disease			
Irregular gait Hunched-back appearance Heart irregularities Death	Se deficiency Geographic distribution: ↓ Se in many areas of United States and Canada	↑ Se in dietary intake in known deficient areas.	Most commonly occurs in most rapidly growing individuals in flock or herd.

From Naylor JM et al: *Large animal clinical nutrition,* St Louis, 1991, Mosby; McDonald P et al: *Animal nutrition,* New York, 1995, Longman Scientific and Technical; Maynard LA et al: *Animal nutrition,* ed 7, New York, 1979, McGraw-Hill; Ensminger ME et al: *Feeds and nutrition,* Clovis, Calif, 1990, Ensminger Publishing.

NUTRIENTS

Nutrients are ingested to support life. Livestock producers and horse owners want to obtain the most desirable results from the nutrients their animals consume at an economical rate and with an advantageous financial return. Ingested nutrients are either retained by the animal or excreted in the urine and feces. Retained nutrients are used for a wide array of body functions, such as homeostasis, replenishment and development of tissues, reproduction, and milk, wool, and meat production.

Maintenance nutrient requirements (MNRs) are the levels of nutrients needed to sustain body weight without gain or loss (Box 13-1). The MNR is the minimal level of dietary need; usually the vast percentage of published requirements is higher than this standard. As a general rule, one half of consumed and absorbed nutrients are used to fulfill MNRs. Individual variation results in fluctuation from this standard; be sure to evaluate need against all information to achieve the most accurate results.

Feeding standards are available listing the amounts of nutrients required by different species for specific productive purposes, such as maintenance, growth, finishing, lactation, work, wool, or eggs. The most widely used feeding standards in the United States are those published by the National Research Council (NRC), and they are established for beef cattle, dairy cattle, sheep, goats, swine, poultry, and horses (see Recommended Reading). Periodically the feeding standards are updated and published by a committee appointed by the NRC.

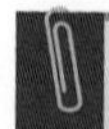

TECHNICIAN NOTE MNRs are the level of nutrients needed to sustain body weight without gain or loss.

Digestion (the process of protein, carbohydrate, and fat breakdown into absorbable nutrients) is accomplished by both chemical and physical methods. It is essential to remember that it is not the alfalfa hay, corn, or oats that

BOX 13-1 Elements That Influence Nutrient Requirements of Livestock

- Body size
- Health status
- Stress
- Environment
- Exercise
- Behavior
- Genetics
- Reproductive status
- Gender
- Breed

BOX 13-2 Relative Importance of Livestock Feed (% of Total Tonnage Fed)

- Pasture and grasslands 40.0%*
- Corn 23.3%
- Hay 12.2%
- Grains and high-protein feed 16.9%
- Silage and miscellaneous 7.6%

From the U.S. Department of Agriculture (USDA) Economic Research Service, 1983-1984.

*Varies significantly by season and pasture quality.

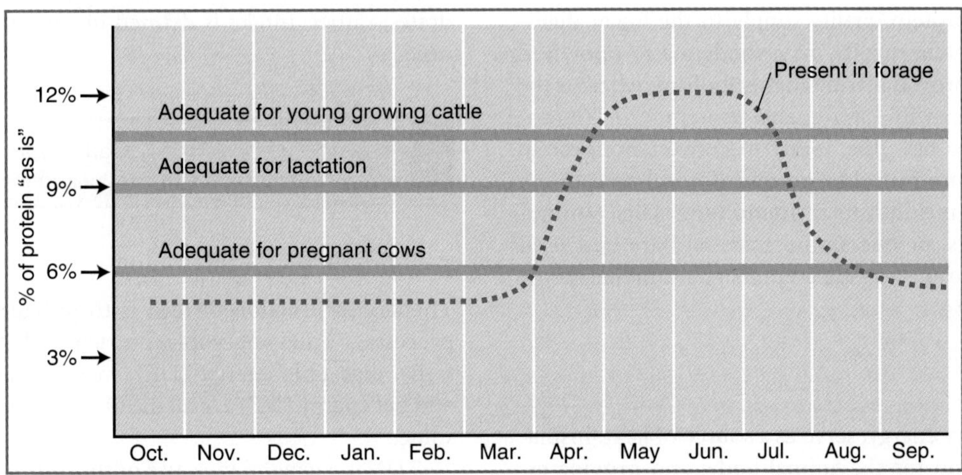

FIGURE 13-1 Nutrient content of forage varies with pasture quality and season.

is actually used by the cells of animals, but rather the digested and absorbed nutrients, such as amino acids, sugars, fatty acids, minerals, and vitamins, that present at the cellular level. The quality, quantity, and cost of nutrients that can be provided by the feedstuff are of primary importance when choosing ingredients for farm-animal feeding.

PROTEIN

Protein is the principal constituent of organs and soft tissues. It is constructed of building blocks called *amino acids* that are linked together in a chain. The arrangement of amino acids in the chain and the length of the chain are two factors that help to determine the composition of the protein. There are 10 essential and 12 nonessential amino acids. Essential amino acids must be supplied in the diet because the animal body cannot synthesize them fast enough to meet its requirement. Amino acids consist of nitrogen, carbon, oxygen, and sulfur. The deconstruction or deamination process releases these elements into the body's system and results in either their elimination from the body or their use as energy.

> *TECHNICIAN NOTE* Protein is a common component of plants, with the highest concentration in the seed and leafy portions.

Animal feed (Box 13-2) is identified often by crude protein content, but the measurement rarely illustrates the quality or use potential of the protein. A feed can possess a high protein content, yet the *biologic value* of that protein is low. Protein biologic value is the percentage of true absorbed protein that is available for productive body functions. Conceptually, it is the "amino acid grade card" because it defines the available amino acids. In general, proteins of animal origin have greater biologic value than do proteins of plant origin. The higher the biologic value, the better the protein used for productive purposes. Protein quality is also measured as the *protein efficiency ratio,* which is the number of grams of body weight gain per unit of protein consumed (McDonald, 1995).

Animal and plant proteins vary greatly in their distribution of amino acids and biologic value. When combined in correct proportions with other protein (e.g., animal protein), protein that individually has very poor biologic value (e.g., corn) may yield a biologic value similar to that of a single high-quality protein. The quality of protein depends on disallowing the overprocessing of feed, overheating in storage, and form of the feed (Nash, 1985) (Figure 13-1).

Use by Ruminants

Rumen digestion facilitated by microbes has the ability to convert most feed protein into peptides and amino acids, many of which are further degraded into ammonia, organic

BOX 13-3 Categories of Carbohydrates

- *Fiber-forage:* Structural carbohydrates, cellulose, hemicellulose
- *Sugars (molasses, growing plants):* Glucose, sucrose, fructose
- *Starches:* Stored carbohydrates, grains

BOX 13-4 Variables Affecting Energy Requirements

- Activity
- Environment
- Body size
- Life stage
- Reproductive status

acids, and carbon dioxide. The ammonia released on microbial degradation of feed protein will be removed from the rumen by absorption through the rumen wall or used by the microorganisms for synthesis of microbial protein. Microbial protein synthesis by the microorganisms results in a fairly constant protein quality supply to the lower digestive tract. The protein quality from moderate to poor feed will usually be improved by rumen metabolism, whereas the opposite may occur with high-quality protein feed. The rumen microbes also have the ability to convert nonprotein nitrogen sources into microbial protein. Typical nonprotein nitrogen sources include urea, ammonium salts, ammoniated by-products, or free amino acids and are best used judiciously because an excess or an imbalanced intake can be toxic (Church, 1984).

FATS

Fats provide dietary energy; serve as a source of heat, insulation, and protection for the animal body; and provide essential fatty acids. Fat has 2.25 times more energy per gram than protein or carbohydrates. Fats also aid the absorption of fat-soluble vitamins. Linoleic, linolenic, and arachidonic fatty acids are considered essential, even though linoleic acid is capable of being converted to arachidonic acid. However, the process to make these conversions is arduous and inefficient, and as such, arachidonic acid should be considered conditionally essential (McDonald, 1995).

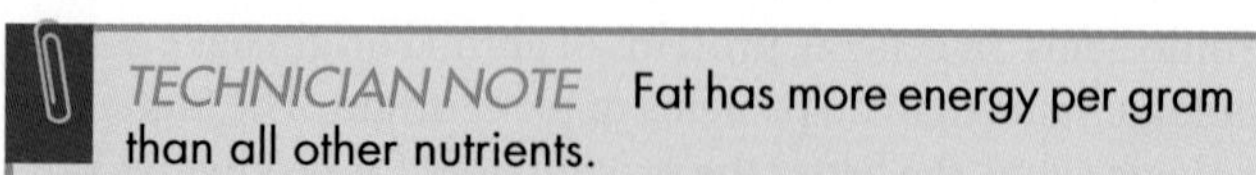

TECHNICIAN NOTE Fat has more energy per gram than all other nutrients.

CARBOHYDRATES

Carbohydrates (Box 13-3) are the primary energy source in livestock rations. They are less expensive and more readily available than protein or fat. Most feedstuffs of plant origin are high in carbohydrate content, especially cereal grains. Carbohydrates must be broken down into simple sugars for absorption from the digestive system. This requires digestive enzymes generated by the host or by microflora inhabiting the digestive system of the host. The carbohydrate-splitting enzymes are effective in splitting most complex carbohydrates into simple sugars except those with the beta linkage, as found in cellulose (fiber). Microflora in the rumen of ruminants and the cecum of some nonruminants, such as the horse or rabbit, produce an enzyme so that these species can use fiber for energy. Carbohydrates are commonly categorized into animal feed as concentrates (grains, high-starch compounds) and forage (grass, hays, legumes). There are no minimum or maximum requirements for carbohydrates; rather, intake is defined in conjunction with energy need.

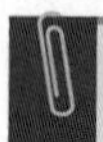

TECHNICIAN NOTE Carbohydrates are the primary energy source in livestock rations.

Feedstuff Energy

The largest function of feed is to provide energy for body processes. Total digestible nutrients (TDN), gross energy (GE), digestible energy (DE), metabolizable energy (ME), and net energy (NE) are all different measures of feed energy value.

TDN is a general measure of the nutritive value of a feed. Digestibility coefficients are used to compute the content of TDN. The usefulness of TDN as a measure of feed energy is limited in that it does not take into account energy losses in urine, combustible gases, and heat. The discrepancies can be large for forage-based feed because they tend to overestimate the energy available for productive purposes. TDN is expressed as a percentage of the ration or in units of weight and not as an actual caloric number.

Gross energy (GE) is the total energy (Box 13-4) potentially available in a feed consumed by an animal. All energy values used in the following scheme are expressed in kilocalories (kcal) or megacalories (Mcal) per unit of weight. During digestion and absorption, a portion of the GE escapes the body in the form of undigested food residue in the feces. Subtraction of the energy lost in the feces from the consumed GE accounts for energy that was digested and absorbed, or *digestible energy* (DE). The measurement of DE uses the same elements as TDN and gives similar energy values to feed. DE values and TDN are used extensively in horse feed. Energy that is digested and absorbed by the body is not used with 100% efficiency; a portion of the absorbed energy is lost in the urine and as combustible gases. Accounting for these energy losses leads to a step beyond DE or TDN, *metabolizable energy* (ME). The energy values for ME are used widely in the formulation of swine and poultry feed. One further refinement in this energy scheme is accounting for heat lost from the body during metabolism of the nutrients. *Net energy* (NE) represents the actual portion of energy available to the animal for use in maintaining body tissues or during pregnancy or lactation. NE values are used extensively in the beef, dairy, and sheep industry.

MINERALS AND VITAMINS

Minerals and vitamins are needed in small amounts compared with other nutrients, but play integral roles in many metabolic processes. Minerals are divided into two categories: microminerals and macrominerals (Box 13-5). The list of minerals and vitamins and their functions are given in Tables 13-2 to 13-4.

WATER

Water is the cheapest and most abundant nutrient. It makes up 65% to 85% of an animal's body weight at birth and 45% to 60% of body weight at maturity. Water is derived metabolically from the breakdown of organic nutrients in the animal tissues or drinking water or obtained from foodstuffs. Because water is the largest constituent of the animal, deprivation of water of only a few percentages of body weight is life threatening. Clean, fresh water should be readily available to maintain a zero water balance (Table 13-5).

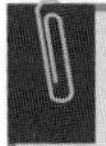

TECHNICIAN NOTE Water is the cheapest and most abundant nutrient.

DAIRY CATTLE

The dairy industry is successfully using many different production systems. Systems are based on geographic area and feedstuff availability. The traditional pasture system continues to be used in areas with readily available land, whereas dry-lot systems are more popular in urban and suburban areas (Figure 13-2).

Regardless of the dairy production system, two feeding programs are most frequently employed. Total mixed ration (TMR) is the practice of weighing and blending all feedstuffs into a complete ration. Each bite consumed by the cow contains all of the required levels of nutrients. The other program is a forage and grain diet fed separately. The animals are provided hay free choice at all times, silage is offered once or twice per day, and feed concentrates are fed twice daily.

Feeding, more than any other single factor, determines the productivity of lactating dairy cows. Feed represents about 50% of the total cost of milk production. Therefore a good feeding program is necessary for profitable milk production. Nutrient requirements for lactation are large and often several times the MNR (Figure 13-3 and Tables 13-6 to 13-8). Water is also important for dairy cows (Boxes 13-6 and 13-7).

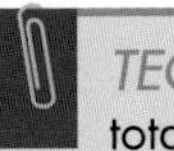

TECHNICIAN NOTE Feed represents 50% of the total costs of milk production.

BOX 13-5 Mineral Categories

Macrominerals*
Salt (sodium chloride; NaCl)
Potassium (K)
Phosphorus (P)
Magnesium (Mg)
Calcium (Ca)
Sulfur (S)

Microminerals†
Zinc (Zn)
Selenium (Se)
Manganese (Mn)
Iodine (I)
Fluorine (F)
Chromium (Cr)
Copper (Cu)
Iron (Fe)
Silicon (Si)
Molybdenum (Mo)
Cobalt (Co)

*Measured in kg.
†Measured in ppm or mg.

Energy

Carbohydrates (forage, concentrate) are the major energy source for lactation, followed by fats and proteins. Carbohydrates constitute 50% to 80% of energy on a dry-matter basis of much of the forage and many grains. Forage possesses a significant fiber content that is broken down by the microbial population in the rumen and used as energy.

Although the rumen capacity of the dairy cow is considerable, she cannot eat sufficient forage to meet her extensive nutrient needs during lactation. The estimated daily intake for forage is based on body weight and forage quality. A guide for estimating the consumption of forage (dry-matter basis) fed on a free-choice basis is in Box 13-8 and Table 13-9.

If cows are allowed to consume all the forage they want, they will not have sufficient rumen capacity to consume enough concentrate to meet the energy requirements for lactation. In general, most dairy farmers try to feed forage at a rate of 1.75% of body weight. The concentrate fed with the forage will vary with the kind of forage offered (a high-protein concentrate will be needed with a low-protein forage) and the availability and cost of the feedstuffs. The concentrate provides more energy and usually is higher in protein than the forage. Fat use varies with age, environment, and reproductive status. Fat intake during lactation can be 5% to 6% of the total energy intake. Excessive dietary fat intake can negatively affect rumen microbial activity, depressing fiber use (Shirley, 1986).

Protein

The restriction of protein or energy during lactation can lead to reduced milk production and increased reproductive problems. Protein is supplied by the forage or concentrate and should be added at levels to ensure that minimum

TABLE 13-2 Macrominerals for Livestock

Use	Toxicity	Deficiency	Sources
Calcium			
Nerve transmission Clotting cascade Cardiac function Muscle contraction Milk production	Calcium kidney stones ↑ Calcium deposition into soft tissue Osteomalacia ↑ Blood calcium level ↓ Absorption of Zn, Mg, Fe, Cu	↓ Quality of bone and teeth ↓ Milk production Fish by-products Osteoporosis Hypocalcemia (tetany) Rickets	Alfalfa Milk Soybean meal Bone meal Dicalcium phosphate supplement
Phosphorus			
Milk secretion Building muscle Teeth and bone development Acid-base balance Protein metabolism	↓ Absorption of Ca Urinary stones if Ca low	Similar to Ca Osteomalacia Rickets Hematuria Pica ↓ Breeding capability	Meat meals Soybean oil meal Wheat bran Bone meal Monosodium phosphate supplement
Sodium			
Muscle contraction Absorption of carbohydrates Part of sweat and bile Acid-base balance Water balance	↑ Toxicity with ↓ H_2O intake Staggering Blindness Hypertension Neurologic disorders	↓ Breeding capability Cravings: urine drinking ↓ Growth rate ↓ Milk production Weight loss ↓ Appetite	Molasses Meat by-products Salt and mineral blocks Monosodium glutamate Osmotic pressure supplement
Potassium			
Heart function Insulin secretion Acid-base balance Muscle development	↓ Heart rate ↓ Mg use Exaggerated when ↓ Mg and H_2O restricted	↓ Growth Excess NaCl depletes K Irregular gait Pica ↓ Weight	Molasses Forage Soy by-products Carrots Potassium gluconate supplement
Chlorine			
Water balance Osmotic pressure Acid-base balance HCl production in stomach	↑ When water is restricted Rare	↓ Appetite ↓ Growth Alkalosis ↓ Respiratory rate Muscle cramps Convulsions Alfalfa	Meat meals Molasses Salt blocks (NaCl) Potassium chloride supplement
Magnesium			
Cellular energy metabolism Alkalinizer Nerve impulse relaxant Bone and teeth	Rare	↑ Grass tetany ↑ Body temperature Respiratory rate Hypersalivation Death	Meat and bone meal Molasses Wheat bran Alfalfa supplements
Sulfur			
Carbohydrate metabolism Insulin production Hair and wool production	Hydrogen sulfide gas production	↓ Growth ↓ Hair and wool production	Meat meal Yeast Whey Supplements

TABLE 13-3 Microminerals for Livestock

Use	Toxicity	Deficiency	Sources
Zinc Skin Hair Bone maintenance Synthesis of protein Development of reproductive organs	↓ Growth Anemia Bone changes ↑ Appetite Stiff gait	↓ Growth ↓ Appetite Bone irregularities ↓ Wound healing Wool and hair loss Parakeratosis	Meat meal Corn gluten or germ meal Wheat by-products Supplements
Selenium Vitamin and sparing-tissue damage Fatty acid oxidation	Weight loss Blind staggers Lameness Anemia Paralysis	White muscle disease (sheep) Liver necrosis (pigs)	Poultry and fish meals Wheat by-products Cereals Oil-seed meals
Manganese Bone and cartilage growth Clotting cascade Metabolism of nutrients	Nontoxic	↓ Growth Lameness Reproductive disorders	Wheat Grass, alfalfa, hay Corn Sorghum supplements
Iodine Hormone production Influence growth Muscle tissue development Milk production Nutrient metabolism	*Horse:* Hyperparathyroidism Goiter ↓ Use of iodine	↓ Hair quality ↓ Growth Reproductive problems Abortion	Molasses Meat and bone meal Oats Wheat Iodized salt Soybean meal
Fluorine Bone Teeth	↓ Feed use ↓ Hair and wool quality Deformed teeth and bone	Rare	Fish meals Present in most foods
Chromium Synthesis of some fatty acids ↑ Insulin use Stabilizes DNA and RNA	Rare	Hyperglycemia glucosuria ↓ Fat metabolism	Wheat Potatoes Corn Vegetable oil Supplements
Copper Pigment of hair and wool Reproduction Skeletal structure Hemoglobin construction Absorption of iron	Although rare, sometimes seen in sheep ingestion of copper foot bath Gastroenteritis Hypersalivation ↓ Appetite Thirst	Swayback (lambs) ↓ Wool quality Lameness Anemia Diarrhea	Safflower oil Molasses Grass hays Cotton seeds Mineral mix
Iron Hemoglobin production Muscle oxygenation Enzyme activation	Irregularity in red blood cell production Reproductive disorders	Anemia Pica Diarrhea ↓ Hair coat quality ↓ Iron in milk	Fish and meat meals Safflower Alfalfa Corn gluten meal Supplements
Silicon Skeletal development	Calculi formation	Skeletal abnormalities	Meat by-products Grains

Continued

TABLE 13-3 Microminerals for Livestock—cont'd

Use	Toxicity	Deficiency	Sources
Molybdenum			
Metabolism of fats, carbohydrates, proteins Growth promotion Enamel production	Diarrhea Weight ↓ Hair quality ↓ Reproduction	Rare	Grass, alfalfa, hay Meat meal Corn Oats Wheat
Cobalt			
Formation of vitamin B_{12}	Rare	↓ Skin and hair coat quality Abortion ↓ Milk ↓ Appetite	Soybean meal Meat and poultry meal Corn Wheat Molasses

TABLE 13-4 Water-Soluble Vitamins for Livestock

Function	Toxicity	Deficiency	Sources
B Complex			
Biotin			
Metabolism of carbohydrates, fats, proteins Enzyme activities	No known toxicity	↓ Growth ↓ Hair quality Lameness ↓ Reproduction	Young grasses Safflower meal Soybean meal supplements
Thiamine (Vitamin B_1)			
Coenzyme of energy metabolism Peripheral nerve function Maintenance and assistance of appetite	No known toxicity	Heart irregularities ↓ Body temperature	Wheat Millet Oil-seed meals Oats Supplements
Pyridoxine (Vitamin B_6)			
Nitrogen metabolism Fat and carbohydrate metabolism	Nontoxic	Anorexia ↓ Growth Eye discharge Anemia	Green pastures Meat and fish meals Corn gluten meal Safflower meal Alfalfa
Cobalamin (Vitamin B_{12})			
Red blood cell formation Maintenance of nerve tissue DNA synthesis	Nontoxic	↓ Coordination (blackleg: pigs) ↓ Reproduction	Fish and meat meals Whey Brewer's yeast supplements
Niacin			
Growth ↓ Cholesterol levels Release of energy from fats, proteins, carbohydrates	Nontoxic	↓ Growth ↓ Appetite Diarrhea Unthriftiness	Wheat barley Yeast supplements
Folic Acid			
Construction of hemoglobin Manipulation of protein Choline synthesis	Nontoxic	Anemia Diarrhea ↓ Growth	Soybean meal Alfalfa Wheat Meat and fish meal Supplement
Pantothenic Acid			
Metabolism of fats, proteins, carbohydrates Hemoglobin production Maintenance of normal blood levels	Nontoxic	Neurologic disorder Goose stepping (swine) ↓ Hair quality Enteritis	Wheat bran Alfalfa Safflower meal Supplements

TABLE 13-4 Water-Soluble Vitamins for Livestock—cont'd

Function	Toxicity	Deficiency	Sources
Riboflavin (Vitamin B_2)			
Metabolism of amino acids and fatty acids Retinal pigment Adrenal function	Nontoxic	↓ Growth Moon blindness (horses) Anemia Unthriftiness ↓ Reproduction (swine)	Alfalfa Green pastures Sweet and white clover Supplements
Vitamin C			
Absorption of iron Metabolism of folic acid Antioxidant Teeth and bone integrity	Rare in food animals	↓ Wound healing Hemorrhage Enlarged joints Ulcerated gums	Green pastures Hay Potatoes

protein requirements are met (see Tables 13-6 to 13-8). Protein intake that exceeds the requirement is used as energy at a premium value. Protein is an expensive nutrient and is not an economic source of energy. Most cows are fed a high-protein legume hay, such as alfalfa, and grain, which should supply most or all the protein needs during lactation. Nonprotein nitrogen supplied as urea also can be an effective feedstuff to supply protein equivalents in dairy rations. The use of animal protein sources derived from ruminant species *is not allowed* in dairy rations to prevent the possible transmission of bovine spongiform encephalopathy (BSE).

Minerals and Vitamins

Milk is composed of 0.7% minerals on a dry-weight basis. The average cow will lactate 140 lb of mineral as a portion of the milk produced per year. A balanced mineral intake is essential; mineral requirements for lactation are given in Tables 13-6 to 13-8.

Rumen microorganisms can synthesize the water-soluble vitamins, whereas vitamin K is the only fat-soluble vitamin readily synthesized by microorganisms. The supplementation of water-soluble vitamins or vitamin K normally is not necessary in rations for ruminants.

Forage of good quality and properly harvested normally contains adequate levels of vitamin E and the precursor of vitamin A, carotene. Vitamin A is stored for extended periods in the body. Vitamin D is synthesized through ultraviolet radiation by the skin or added to a dairy ration as sun-cured forage or a vitamin supplement.

Although water-soluble vitamins are synthesized by the rumen microflora, some evidence indicates that supplemental thiamin, choline, and niacin may be beneficial in cows undergoing heavy stress or various disease states. Daily requirements for vitamins for lactating dairy cows are found in Table 13-8.

DAIRY CALVES

Newborn calves require the mother's colostrum within the first 72 hours of life to acquire energy and maternal immunity from disease. Peak benefits of colostrum intake are realized within the first 24 hours postpartum. Optimally the first milking colostrum should be given to the calf at 10% to 12% of the calf's weight with at least one half administered within 4 to 6 hours after birth. Colostrum can be successfully frozen and used at a later date and diluted equally with water should diarrhea occur because of the richness of the colostrum. The initial sucking of the calf will create a bypass of the rumen, allowing the milk to go directly into the abomasum. This ability will decrease as the calf ages and the rumen becomes functional. Calves normally start on milk replacers and then are offered calf starters within the first week of life. Calf-starter rations are commonly fed until about 3 months of age at a rate of 5 to 7 lb of calf starter per day. During the first week of life, a forage source should be added to the diet selection and free-choice water. Calves are typically weaned at 4 to 8 weeks of age and accustomed to solid food.

BEEF CATTLE

Feeding represents almost three fourths of the cost of production of beef cattle (Neumann, 1977). Beef producers control their profitability by obtaining optimal nutrient intake with the least-cost feed formulation. Profitability hinges on the ability to balance the use of resources, such as pasture and feedlot, with the production of high-quality finishing animals generated by the breeding herd. Beef production usually is divided into two primary areas: cow-calf production and finishing cattle.

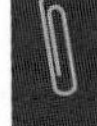

TECHNICIAN NOTE Feeding represents 75% of the cost of beef cattle production.

COW-CALF PRODUCTION

A live calf from each cow each year should be the goal of the profitable cow-calf producer. Nutrition has a large impact on the beef-breeding herd. Cows gaining weight just before and during the breeding season have a shorter period between calving and the first estrus period and typically have higher conception rates.

TABLE 13-5 Water Consumption Guidelines

Species	Weight (lb)	Consumption (gal/Day)
Swine		
Pigs	30-125	0.3-2.0
Feeder pigs	126-200	2.0-3.2
Finisher pigs	201-250	3.2-4.0
Sow and boar maintenance	150-400	1.3-3.5
	401-600	3.5-5.2
Sow: late gestation	250-400	4.5-5.0
	401-600	5.0-7.5
Sow: lactation	250-400	5.5-6.5
	401-600	6.5-9.8
Sheep		
Lambs	20-50	0.4-0.6
Feeder lambs	50-110	0.5-1.4
Finisher lambs	111-125	1.4-1.8
Ewes: grain and hay intake*		
Maintenance	150-300	0.3-1.2
Lactation	150-300	0.5-2.4
Rams: grain and hay intake	150-300	0.3-2.0
Cattle		
Calves	100-200	1.2-2.5
	201-400	2.5-4.9
Developing steers and heifers	401-600	4.5-6.2
	601-800	6.0-8.2
	801-1000	8.0-9.8
Finishing steers		
Pasture	1001-1200	8.5-10.2
Maintenance	800-1000	3.6-4.6
	1001-1200	4.4-7.2
	1201-1400	5.0-7.2
	1401-1600	6.0-9.0
Cows: late gestation	800-1000	4.4-5.5
	1001-1200	5.3-6.6
	1201-1400	6.4-7.9
	1401-1600	7.7-9.5
Beef cows: heifer lactation	800-1000	6.7-15.6
	1001-1200	8.3-18.8
	1201-1400	10.0-21.8
	1401-1600	11.7-25.0
Dairy cows: heifer peak lactation†	800-1000	14.8-20.6
	1001-1201	18.5-24.3
	1201-1400	22.5-28.8
	1401-1600	28.0-32.2
	1601-1800	30.5-36.0

*Intake is influenced dramatically by factors found in Box 14-6. Table is intended as a guideline.

†Dairy cattle intake varies on milk production more than beef cattle.

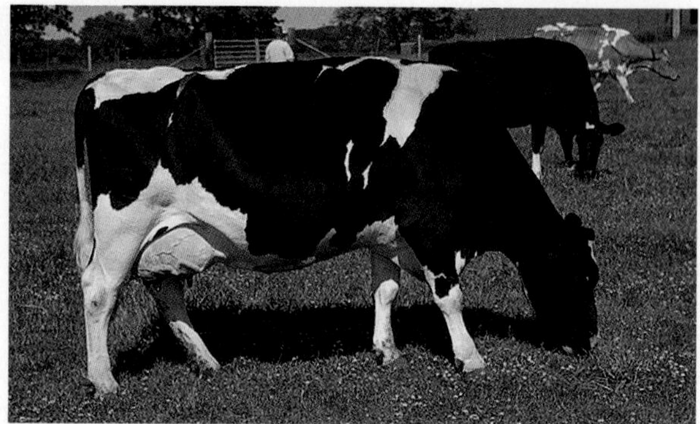

FIGURE 13-2 Holsteins are the predominant breed in the dairy industry.

Energy

Carbohydrates are the major energy source for beef cows, followed by proteins and fat. Forage commonly fed to beef cows possess a significant fiber content that is broken down by the microbial population in the rumen and used as energy.

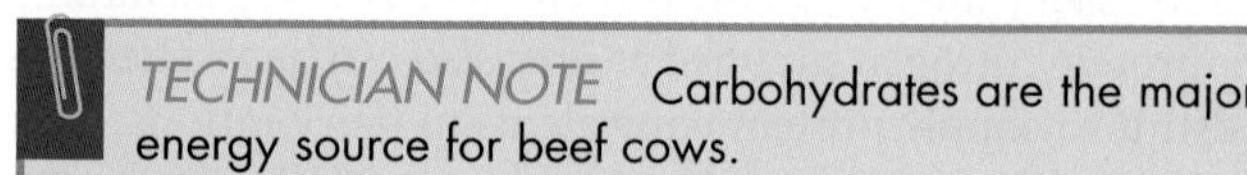

TECHNICIAN NOTE Carbohydrates are the major energy source for beef cows.

Feeding beef cows can be very economic because high-quality forage or pasture can supply all energy needs with no need for energy supplementation from grains or fats (Figure 13-4). In the summer, pasture normally will supply adequate energy for the cow. If pasture is inadequate, supplemental energy should be provided in the form of silage or hay. In the winter, pregnant cows are fed wintering rations (a combination of forage, grain, and a protein source supplemented with vitamins and minerals) to meet energy needs with minimal weight gain (Box 13-9). Cows in good condition are more tolerant to the stresses of winter and require less maintenance energy per unit of weight than do cows in poor condition.

Protein

Most pasture, silage, and forage contain adequate levels of protein to meet the needs of the breeding cow. If low-grade roughage (e.g., cobs, straw, stalks) are fed over extended periods of time, the ration must be supplemented daily with 1 to 1.5 lb of a 35% to 45% crude protein supplement. A review of deficiency and toxicity signs can be found in Boxes 13-10 and 13-11. The use of animal protein sources derived from ruminant species *is not allowed* in beef-breeding–herd rations. This is to prevent the possible transmission of BSE.

Minerals and Vitamins

Mineral supplementation will be necessary and is usually offered on a free-choice basis when animals are on pasture (Figure 13-5). Trace-mineral salt blocks and granular salt are popular methods of offering minerals and salt to animals on pasture. Good-quality pasture and roughage are adequate

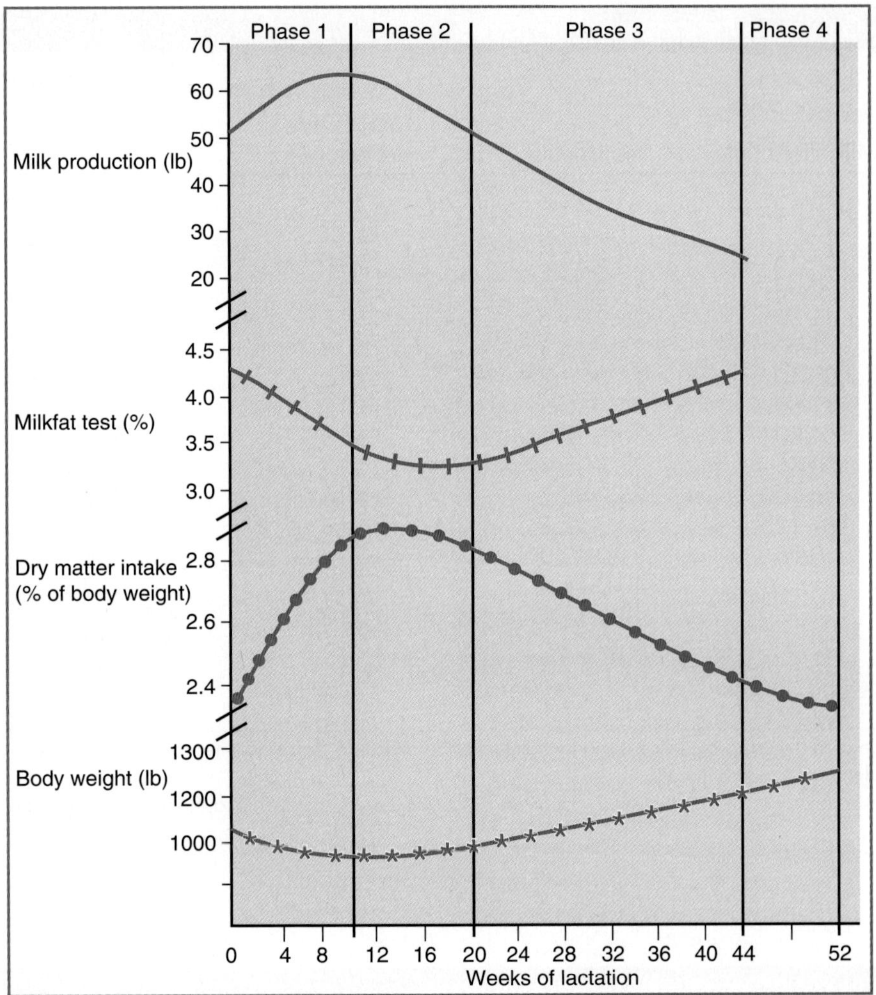

FIGURE 13-3 Milk production varies during a typical 52-week production phase. Disparity is also observed in milk fat content, dry-matter intake requirements, and body weight.

TABLE 13-6 Daily Feeding Considerations in Developing Female Dairy Cattle*

Weight (lb)	NE (Mcal)†	Total Crude Protein (%)	Minerals‡ Ca^{2+}	Minerals‡ P
200-399	6.4-11.5	16-18	15-18	9-15
400-599	11.5-15.4	12-16	18-23	13-15
600-799	15.4-19.5	12-14	23-24	15-17
800-999	19.5-23.9	12-14	24-26	17-18
1000-1199	23.9-28.4	12-14	26-28	18-19
1200-1399	28.4-33.8	12-14	28-30	19-21

*Ranges shown in table are to be used as guidelines, recognizing that variations can occur as a result of breed, milk production levels, butter fat content, rate of gain, and lactation cycle.

†Net energy (NE) expressed in megacalories (Mcal).

‡Ca^{2+}/phosphorus ratio needs to be maintained from 0.43%-0.66%; levels above 0.95%-100% can result in decreased performance and metabolic abnormalities.

TABLE 13-7 Daily Guidelines for Lactating Dairy Cows*

Weight (lb)	Milk Yield (lb)	NE (Mcal)†	Total Crude Protein (%)	Minerals‡	
				Ca^{2+}	P
800	15-45	13.1-21.6	12-16	40-77	25-49
	45-60	21.6-25.8	16-17	77-96	49-61
	61-75	25.8-34.0	16-18	96-115	61-78
1000	20-40	14.9-20.3	12-16	44-70	29-44
	41-70	20.3-25.6	16-18	70-114	44-73
	71-90	25.6-36.3	16-18	114-146	73-86
1200	20-40	17.0-23.7	12-16	50-81	33-52
	41-60	23.7-30.3	16-18	81-110	52-70
	61-80	30.3-37.0	16-18	110-139	70-87
1400	50-75	27.7-35.7	15-17	95-131	62-83
	76-100	35.7-43.7	16-18	131-165	83-104
	101-125	43.7-51.7	16-18	165-200	104-126
1600	60-90	31.0-40.0	15-17	108-146	69-92
	91-120	40.0-48.3	16-18	146-184	92-116
	121-150	48.3-57.0	16-18	184-221	116-137
1800	60-90	40.9-44.6	16-18	121-164	78-104
	91-120	44.6-54.4	16-18	164-207	104-131
	121-150	54.4-64.1	16-18	207-249	131-157

*This table is designed to be used only as a guideline. Feed to maintain body condition. Table assumes a 4% milk fat content of lactation.
†Net energy (NE) measured in megacalories (Mcal).
‡Mineral values assume that balance has been established. Variations occur with breed, lactation phase, milk yield, and age.

TABLE 13-8 Daily Nutrient Considerations for Dairy Cattle*

Weight (lb)	ME† (Mcal)	Total Crude Protein (g)	Minerals (g)‡		Vitamins (1000 IU)	
			Ca^{2+}	P	A	D
Females: 60 Days Before Gestation						
800-1000	13.8-16.4	850-925	24-30	16-18	30-35	12-14
1000-1200	16.4-19.2	925-1000	30-35	18-22	35-42	14-17
1200-1400	19.2-21.5	1000-1100	35-42	22-26	42-48	17-19
1400-1600	21.5-23.6	1100-1200	42-45	26-30	48-56	19-22
Dairy Bulls						
1000-1300	14.3-17.8	775-900	16-20	10-12	17.00-21.00	2.7-3.3
1301-1500	17.8-19.7	900-1000	20-24	12-15	21.00-25.25	3.3-3.9
1501-1700	19.7-21.6	1000-1125	24-28	15-18	25.25-29.50	3.9-4.6
1701-1900	21.6-23.5	1125-1225	28-32	18-20	29.50-33.75	4.6-5.3
1901-2100	23.5-25.3	1225-1325	32-36	20-22	33.75-38.00	5.3-5.9
2101-2300	25.3-27.0	1325-1425	36-40	22-25	38.00-42.50	5.9-6.6
2301-2500	27.0-28.8	1425-1520	40-44	25-28	42.50-46.60	6.6-7.3
2501-2700	28.0-30.4	1520-1610	44-48	28-30	46.60-50.90	7.3-7.9
2701-2900	30.4-32.1	1610-1700	48-52	30-32	50.90-55.10	7.9-8.6

*Ranges shown in table are to be used as guidelines, recognizing that variations can occur because of milk production levels, butter fat content, rate of gain, and lactation cycle.
†Metabolizable energy (ME) measured in megacalories (Mcal).
‡Ca^{2+}/phosphorus ratio needs to be maintained from 0.43%-0.66%; levels above 0.95%-100% can result in decreased performance and metabolic abnormalities.

BOX 13-6 Factors Affecting Water Intake

- Dry-matter intake
- Reproductive status
- Activity
- Type of feeding regimen
- Environment
- Weight
- Age
- Rate of gain

BOX 13-7 Importance of Water

- For digestion, absorption, and use of nutrients
- For production requirements
- Watering methods
- Free water always available
- Twice-daily watering
- Cleanliness
- Water heaters in winter to prevent freezing
- Troughs kept clean

BOX 13-8 Factors Affecting Dry-Matter Intake

- Stage of lactation
- Body condition
- Quality of feed
- Environment
- Size of cow
- Milk production
- Feeding regimen
- Age

TABLE 13-9 Forage Quality

Forage Quality	Daily Intake (% Body Weight)
Excellent	3.0
Good	2.5
Average	2.0
Fair	1.5
Poor	1.0

in vitamins A and E with ample levels to meet the needs of breeding cows. Supplemental vitamin A should be provided when low-grade roughage or long-stored hays are used as a major source of energy in wintering rations. There are mineral mixes that contain a stabilized form of vitamin A.

CALVES

The basic food for calves consists of the mother's milk (Box 13-12) plus access to pasture or forage fed to the cows. Many cow-calf producers offer calves a highly palatable creep feed to supply additional nutrients, leading to improved weaning weights and decreased weight loss by nursing cows. Creep-fed calves will weigh an extra 30 to 50 lb by weaning time. The greatest response to creep feeding is found when pasture is inadequate or the quality is poor. Beef calves generally are weaned at 7 to 8 months of age.

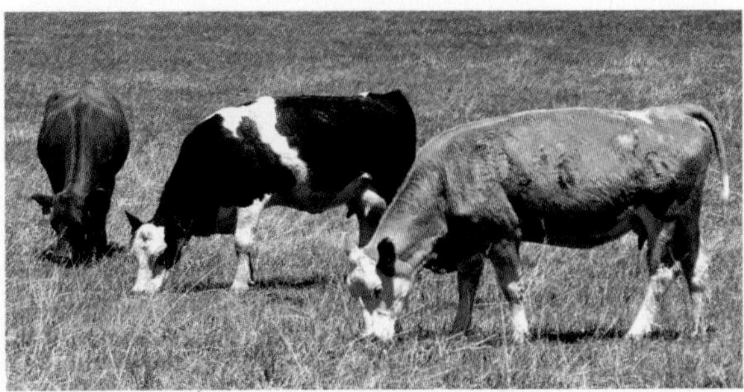

FIGURE 13-4 Beef cows are the majority used in pasture production systems. Good pasture rotation management ensures optimal nutrition for grazing animals.

BOX 13-9 Typical Grain: Nutritional Overview

- 20% (or less) protein
- 18% (or less) crude fiber
- Variable moisture
- 85% (or less) carbohydrate
- 6% (or less) fat
- 75%-80% TDN

BOX 13-10 Signs of Undernutrition

- ↓ Growth
- ↓ Hair and/or skin quality
- Skeletal irregularities
- ↓ Reproductive capabilities
- ↓ Immune function
- Death

BOX 13-11 Protein Deficiency and Toxicity in Cattle

- Deficiency
- ↓ Appetite
- Weight loss
- ↓ Growth
- ↓ Reproductive capability
- ↓ Milk production
- Toxicity
- Ammonia: Avoid >40% excess protein or nonprotein nitrogen (NPN) intake

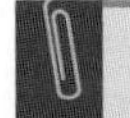

TECHNICIAN NOTE Creep-fed calves can weigh 30 to 50 lb more by weaning time.

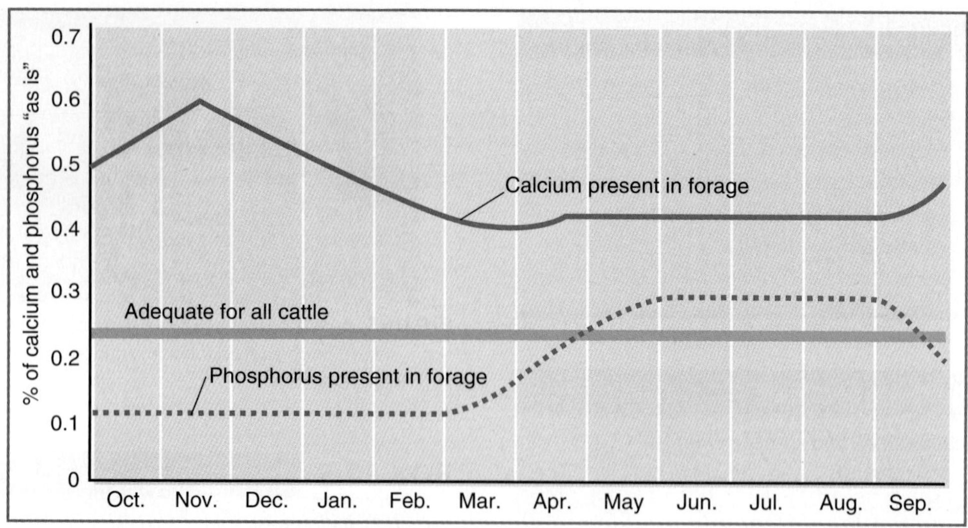

FIGURE 13-5 Calcium and phosphorus availability varies greatly during the seasons of the year and should be supplemented if inadequate amounts are present in livestock forage sources.

FINISHING CATTLE

The *finishing* of cattle refers to the time in the growth phase of growing cattle when they are fed to produce beef that is desirable to the food consumer. Most finished cattle are between 1 and 2 years of age and weigh more than 1000 lb. The goal of the finishing feeding program is to maintain a maximum feed intake and weight gain without causing digestive upsets (Table 13-10).

Energy

High-energy diets are used to increase weight gain, improve the carcass characteristics, and decrease the cost of energy compared with diets high in fiber. Total dry-feed intake commonly will be 2% to 3% of the animal's body weight. The feed contains high levels of grains to supply readily available energy (Figure 13-6). Cattle fed these rations are more prone to develop digestive upset (rumen acidosis), founder, or liver abscesses and require more attention and management to prevent these problems.

Protein

Protein requirements (9% to 14%) are greatly affected by age, size of animal, and growth rate. Young cattle require higher levels of protein (as a percentage of the diet) than do older cattle. Protein sources cost more than feed grains, but experienced finishing cattle producers know that a protein deficiency is more expensive than a slight protein excess in the ration. When protein is deficient, energy is not well used, and performance suffers.

Supplemental protein for finishing cattle can be provided by natural protein sources or nonprotein nitrogen (e.g., urea). Nonprotein nitrogen sources are used most efficiently by cattle consuming relatively high levels of grain. A normal range of urea intake for many finishing rations is 0.10 to 0.15 lb per animal per day. The use of animal protein sources derived from ruminant species *is not allowed* in finishing cattle rations to prevent the possible transmission of BSE.

BOX 13-12 Feeding Considerations for Calves

Dairy Calves

Days 1-3: Obtain colostrum from dam.

Days 4-7: Transition to milk replacer or other liquid feed; begin offering starter and free-choice water.

Days 5-84: Starter and free-choice water through weaning; begin offering forage.

Beef Calves

Ensure that calf nurses within 2 hr of birth to obtain vital colostrum.

Ensure that calf continues to thrive and that cow does not show signs of mastitis or decreased milk production.

Orphans

Can sometimes be grafted to another cow.

Ensure that colostrum has been administered.

Feed like dairy calves.

Minerals and Vitamins

Calcium is often added to the high-grain diets fed to finishing cattle. Generally, when forage (especially legumes) constitutes more than 25% of a finishing ration, additional calcium is not required. Grain contains adequate levels of phosphorus to meet the needs of finishing cattle. Finishing rations are balanced to contain a calcium/phosphorus ratio of 2:1 or higher. Salt is added to diets or fed on a free-choice basis to finishing cattle to meet the sodium requirement (Box 13-13). The less forage that is formulated into the diet, the more need there is for trace-mineral supplementation.

High-quality forage contains adequate amounts of vitamin A precursors and vitamin E. Generally, finishing rations are supplemented with 20,000 to 30,000 IU of vitamin A daily because they contain high levels of grain. Vitamins E and D are added to finishing rations when the feed ingredients are devoid of these vitamins or the production practices merit their inclusion (see Table 13-10).

TABLE 13-10 Daily Nutrient Considerations for Beef Cattle*

Weight (lb)	Net Energy (NE; Mcal)	Total Protein (lb)	Minerals (g)	
			Ca^{2+}	P
Growing/Finishing†				
300-400	3.0-3.6	0.75-1.5	10-42	6-8
401-500	3.7-4.4	0.90-1.9	11-40	8-18
501-600	4.4-5.0	1.0-2.0	12-38	9-19
601-700	5.0-5.6	1.1-2.1	13-36	11-19
701-800	5.6-6.2	1.3-2.1	14-34	12-20
801-900	6.2-6.8	1.4-2.2	15-33	14-20
901-1000	6.8-7.3	1.5-2.3	16-37	16-22
1001-1100	7.3-7.5	1.6-2.3	19-35	18-23
1101-1200	7.5-7.8	1.7-2.4	20-34	20-24
1201-1300	7.8-8.4	1.8-2.4	20-32	20-24
Yearling Heifers, Early to Late Gestation				
700-800	8.0-8.6	1.3-1.6	19-28	19-22
801-900	8.6-9.1	1.4-1.7	21-28	15-19
901-1000	9.1-9.8	1.5-1.7	20-23	14-20
1001-1100	9.8-10.3	1.5-1.7	23-25	18-20
1101-1200	10.3-10.8	1.6-1.8	25-27	20-21
1201-1300	10.8-11.4	1.6-1.8	26-28	21-23
1301-1400	11.4-12.0	1.8-2.0	26-28	23-24
Lactating Cow/Heifer				
800-900	10.0-14.0	2.0-2.4	23-35	19-20
901-1000	10.4-14.5	1.9-2.5	24-36	19-20
1001-1100	11.0-15.0	2.0-2.6	25-38	20-22
1101-1200	11.5-15.5	2.0-2.7	27-39	22-23
1201-1300	12.0-16.2	2.1-2.3	23-41	23-25
1301-1400	12.5-17.0	2.2-2.9	30-42	25-26
Breeding Bulls				
1300-1500	9.3-10.3	2.0-2.2	23-31	22-25
1501-1700	10.3-11.3	1.7-2.2	23-31	22-25
1701-1900	11.3-12.3	2.0-2.2	26-29	26-29
1901-2100	12.3-13.3	2.0-2.3	27-33	27-33

From National Research Council: *Nutrient requirements of beef cattle*, ed 8, Washington, DC, 1990, National Academic Press.
*Values represent guidelines, and individual variations dictate the constant appraisal of body condition to ensure desirable results.
†Assumes medium- to large-frame steers.

SHEEP

Feeding represents the single largest cost of production for all types of sheep operations. Sheep producers control their revenue by offering feed that supports optimal production, is cost-effective, and minimizes nutrition-related problems. Sheep production is divided into two principal areas: the breeding flock and lamb production.

BREEDING FLOCK

Ewes are the foundation of the sheep operation; they produce lambs and generate wool (Box 13-14). These two cash crops can be influenced greatly by feeding management. The mature ewe (3 to 8 years of age) needs only sufficient feed to maintain her normal weight from the time her lambs were weaned until 15 weeks (21-week gestation) into her next pregnancy, assuming not much weight was lost during lactation. Pasture is adequate to meet her nutrient needs during this period of production (see Figures 13-1 and 13-5 for reviews of the nutrient composition of pasture).

Energy

The energy requirements of the ewe largely depend on the stage of the reproductive cycle (Box 13-15). During the first two thirds of the pregnancy, energy requirements are close to those required for MNRs, and good pasture or hays can supply all the energy needs (Box 13-16). In the last trimester, energy requirements increase, and forage must be supplemented with grains. Poor care during the last trimester of pregnancy leads to lambing problems, lower wool output, and depressed milk production. A common problem attributed to poor nutrition in ewes is lambing paralysis or ketosis. Feeding inadequate forage with little or no grain can create a deficiency of usable carbohydrates during the last trimester of pregnancy in ewes carrying twins or triplets and can lead to paralysis and coma

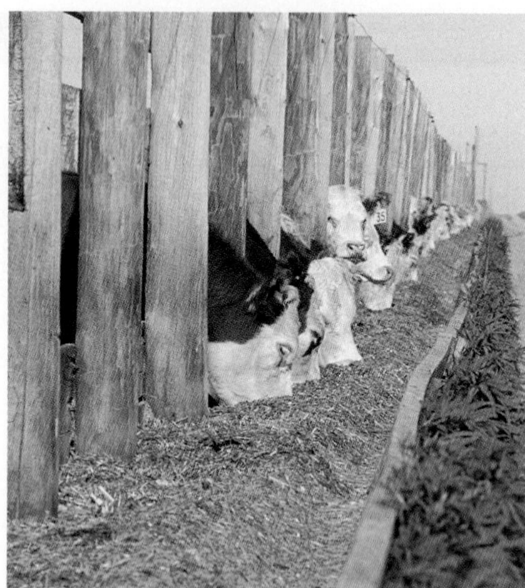

FIGURE 13-6 Large quantities of forage and grain are ingested by finishing cattle on a daily basis and are paramount to fulfillment of energy requirements.

BOX 13-13 Salt Use in Cattle

Rule 1: Supply
3-5 lb in each spring and summer mo
1-1.5 lb in each fall and winter mo

Rule 2: Availability
Make salt available at all times

Rule 3: Rotation
Continue to rotate salt
Mangers throughout pasture

in the mother. Prevention is the least expensive route to avoid pregnancy disease in the breeding flock. Energy requirements are highest during lactation and proportional to the number of lambs the ewe is nursing (Figure 13-7 and Table 13-11).

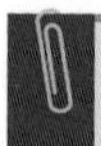

TECHNICIAN NOTE A common problem attributed to poor nutrition in ewes is lambing paralysis or ketosis.

Protein

An adequate protein intake ensures good wool production and reproductive function (Box 13-17 and Table 13-11). The most limiting amino acid for the maturation of wool is methionine; protein ingested by the breeding flock must contain adequate levels of this amino acid. Most pasture, silage, and forage contain adequate levels of protein and amino acids to meet the needs of the breeding flock. If low-grade roughage (e.g., cobs, straw, stalks) are fed over extended periods of time, the ration must be supplemented daily with a protein supplement or a nonprotein nitrogen source (Box 13-18). The use of animal protein sources derived from ruminant species *is not allowed* in ewe rations to prevent the possible transmission of BSE.

BOX 13-14 Common Sheep Breeds

Wool Breeds
Rambouillet
Merino
Debouillet
Columbia
Targhee

Meat Breeds
Suffolk
Dorset
Hampshire
Shropshire
Southdown
Oxford

Combination Breeds
Polypay
Texel
Tunis
Leicester
Cheviot

BOX 13-15 Energy Intake Variables in Sheep

- Breed size
- Gender
- Reproductive status
- Weaning age
- Multiple birth
- Age
- Environment
- Stress
- Shearing
- Forage quality

BOX 13-16 Advantages and Disadvantages of Pasture Feeding Livestock

Advantages
- Provides exercise
- Uses land unsuitable for other purposes
- Decreases diseases transmitted through close contact with other animals
- Decreases feed costs
- Good-quality pastures can provide quality feedstuffs

Disadvantages
- Depends on soil quality (deficiencies result in poorer quality pasture)
- Large acreage often needed to support animal's energy requirements
- Land may be made valuable for other uses

Minerals and Vitamins

Trace-mineral salt blocks and granular salt represent popular methods of offering minerals and salt to ewes on pasture. Sheep store copper quite well in various organs and

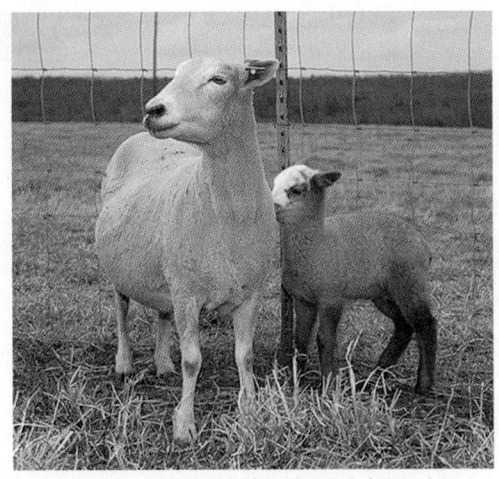

FIGURE 13-7 Ewes are the foundation of the sheep operation. Good feeding management ensures healthy lambs and first-class wool production.

tissues and develop toxicity symptoms to copper more rapidly than other livestock. Care should be taken to prevent exposing sheep to high levels of copper in their trace-mineral source.

Good-quality pasture and roughage are adequate in vitamins A and E with ample levels to meet the needs of the breeding flock. Supplemental vitamin A should be provided when low-grade roughage or long-stored hays are used as a major source of energy in wintering rations (see Table 13-11).

LAMBS

Lambs must be nursed with colostrum milk within the first hour after birth to improve survivability. Colostrum milk provides immunologic protection and energy for the newborn lamb. The lamb must consume at least 6 to 8 oz of colostrum to receive immunologic protection. Lambs are weaned successfully at 8 weeks of age or earlier.

TABLE 13-11 Daily Nutritional Considerations in Sheep

				Minerals (g)		Vitamins	
Weight (lb)	ME (Mcal)*	Daily Consumption (as fed) (lb/Day)	Total Crude Protein(lb/Day)	Ca^{2+}	P	A(1000 IU)	E(IU)
Weaned Lambs to Finishing							
20-40	1.3-2.6	1.2-2.9	0.35-0.45	4.9-6.5	2.2-2.9	0.47	12
41-60	2.6-3.2	2.9-3.4	0.45-0.48	6.5-7.2	2.9-3.4	0.95	24
61-80	3.2-3.8	3.4-3.7	0.48-0.51	7.2-8.6	3.4-4.3	1.40	21
81-100	3.8-4.0	3.7-4.1	0.51-0.53	8.6-9.4	4.3-4.8	2.30	25
101-Finish	4.0-4.2	3.8-4.1	0.53	8.2-9.4	4.5-4.8	2.80	25
Ewe Lambs							
Early							
80-100	2.9-3.0	3.4-3.7	0.35-0.36	5.2-5.5	2.7-2.8	3.0-3.1	21
101-120	3.0-3.1	3.7-3.9	0.35-0.36	5.2-5.5	2.8-3.0	3.1-3.4	22
121-140	3.1-3.2	3.7-3.9	0.35-0.36	5.5	3.0-3.3	3.4-3.7	24
141-160	3.1-3.3	3.9-4.1	0.35-0.36	5.5	3.3-3.4	3.4-3.7	26
Late							
80-101	5.0-5.4	3.7-3.9	0.41-0.44	6.4-7.8	5.0-5.4	3.1-3.9	22
101-120	5.4-5.8	3.0-4.1	0.44-0.45	7.8-8.1	5.4-5.8	3.9-4.3	24
121-140	5.8-6.2	4.1-4.4	0.45-0.48	8.1-8.2	5.8-6.2	4.3-4.7	26
141-160	6.2-6.3	4.4-4.7	0.46-0.48	8.1-8.2	6.2-6.3	4.3-4.7	27
Lactation							
80-100	2.9-3.0	5.1-5.7	0.67-0.71	8.4-8.7	5.6-6.0	4.0-5.0	32-34
101-120	3.0-3.1	5.7-6.1	0.71-0.74	8.7-9.0	6.0-6.4	5.0-6.0	34-36
121-140	3.1-3.2	6.1-6.7	0.74-0.77	9.0-9.3	6.4-6.9	6.0-7.0	36-38
Ewes: Maintenance to Early and Midgestation							
110-130	2.4-2.6	2.4-2.9	0.21-0.27	2.0-3.2	1.8-2.5	2.35-2.80	18-20
131-150	2.6-2.7	2.5-3.1	0.27-0.29	2.5-3.5	2.4-2.9	2.80-3.30	20-21
151-170	2.7-2.9	2.9-3.7	0.29-0.31	2.8-3.8	2.4-3.3	3.30-3.75	21-22
171-190	2.9-3.1	3.0-3.9	0.31-0.33	2.9-3.9	2.8-3.4	3.75-4.25	22-24
Ewes: Late Gestation (Last 30 Days) and Lactation							
100-130	4.0-6.0	4.1-5.9	0.43-0.45	5.6-6.9	4.8-5.2	4.25-5.10	24-27
131-150	4.2-6.6	4.4-6.1	0.45-0.47	6.9-9.1	5.2-6.6	5.10-5.95	26-28
151-170	4.4-7.0	4.7-6.3	0.47-0.49	7.6-9.5	6.6-7.4	5.95-6.80	28-30
171-190	4.7-7.5	4.9-6.6	0.49-0.51	8.5-9.6	6.8-7.8	6.80-7.65	30-33

*ME (metabolizable energy) is measured in megacalories (Mcal); 1 Mcal = 1000 kcal.

BOX 13-17 Variables in Protein Requirements of Sheep

- Breed size
- Reproductive status
- Age
- Body condition
- Ratio of protein to energy
- NPN availability

BOX 13-18 Feeding Guidelines for Nonprotein Nitrogen (NPN) Use in Sheep

- Balance NPN within total nutritional profile. Feed continuously after 3- to 6-wk transition.
- Avoid sporadic availability.
- Maintain nitrogen/sulfur ratio at not more than 10:1.
- Restrict use to not more than 1.0% dry matter, with one third of total nitrogen ration as NPN.
- Prevent excess intake and possible toxicity.
- Watch NPN levels when they coincide with high roughage intake.

From Ensminger ME et al: *Feeds and nutrition,* Clovis, Calif, 1990, Ensminger Publishing; Maynard LA et al: *Animal nutrition,* ed 7, New York, 1979, McGraw-Hill; McDonald P et al: *Animal nutrition,* New York, 1995, Longman Scientific and Technical; Naylor JM et al: *Large animal clinical nutrition,* St Louis, 1991, Mosby.

TECHNICIAN NOTE Lambs must receive colostrum within the first hour after birth to have immunologic protection.

Lambs also can be successfully weaned from their mother at 1 day of age and offered a milk replacer (Box 13-19). They should be weaned from the milk replacer at 3 to 4 weeks of age and transitioned to a high-quality, palatable solid feed. Postweaning rations (until lambs reach 50 lb) should be high-quality protein (16% to 20% crude protein), high energy, and well fortified with vitamins and minerals.

Grower (50 to 85 lb) and finisher (more than 85 lb) rations for lambs are normally formulated to contain 15% to 16% and 13% to 14% protein, respectively. A simple ration of shelled corn, long alfalfa hay, and supplement (protein, calcium, vitamins, trace minerals) can be fed to growing-finishing lambs (Figure 13-8). Research does not clearly indicate the need for vitamin additions to rations for early lambs, but it has become a common practice to fortify the rations with vitamins A, D, and E (see Table 13-11).

Large, fast-growing lambs are susceptible to overeating disease (enterotoxemia), which can cause death. This disease is caused by toxins produced by *Clostridium perfringens* and appears to be related to overeating by lambs of a ration high in grain. A vaccination with bacterin or toxoid can be used for lambs older than 2 months of age and will virtually eliminate symptoms of overeating disease.

BOX 13-19 Milk Replacement for Lambs

Optimal Requirement
25% to 30% fat
20% to 25% protein derived from milk product
<30% lactose derived from milk product

Feeding
Provide ration immediately.
Ration should be 20% to 24% protein, high in vitamins and minerals, well balanced, and ground fine.
NOTE: Avoid cow's milk (too high in lactose).

From Ensminger ME et al: *Feeds and nutrition,* Clovis, Calif, 1990, Ensminger Publishing; Maynard LA et al: *Animal nutrition,* ed 7, New York, 1979, McGraw-Hill; McDonald P et al: *Animal nutrition,* New York, 1995, Longman Scientific and Technical; Naylor JM et al: *Large animal clinical nutrition,* St Louis, 1991, Mosby.

SWINE

The swine industry has changed dramatically over the past 30 years. Most pigs are raised in confinement to reduce labor requirements for the owner and to improve the environment for the animal. The genetic base of the swine industry has changed to a more prolific breeding herd and better-muscled, faster-growing offspring. Feed still constitutes 60% to 70% of the cost of raising swine. Few swine are grazed on pasture; most are fed complete high-grain rations in self-feeders or are limit fed if in the breeding herd. The production of pigs normally is divided into three distinct areas: the breeding herd, starter pigs, and growing-finishing pigs.

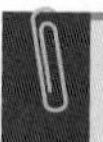

TECHNICIAN NOTE Feed constitutes 60% to 70% of the cost of raising swine.

BREEDING HERD

For profitable production of swine, the sows must be bred, gestate 114 days, nurse a litter for 21 to 35 days, rebreed within 10 days after weaning, and continue the cycle for five to seven litters. Nutrition plays a key role in allowing this to occur, especially during lactation (Table 13-12).

Energy

After breeding and for the first two thirds of gestation, the energy intake is limited to 6000 to 7000 kcal ME per day. The total amount of feed is increased during the last third of gestation, providing 9000 to 10,000 kcal ME per day, which contributes additional energy to the developing fetuses during this last stage of gestation. Overfeeding energy during gestation has a direct negative impact on the lactation feed intake, which can impair lactation performance.

In lactation, the goal of the swine producer is to encourage as much energy intake by the lactating female as possible (15,000 to 20,000 kcal ME per day). Sows are often fed twice per day to ensure fresh feed and improved energy intakes. Frequently, fat is added to the lactation ration to improve palatability and energy density. Sows peak in milk production between the second and third weeks of lactation, and they should be full fed to support the production of milk. A rule of thumb for feeding lactating sows is to offer 4 to 5 lb of the base ration plus 1 additional pound for every pig nursing (Figure 13-9).

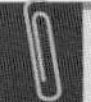

TECHNICIAN NOTE Sows are often fed twice daily to ensure an adequate energy intake.

Protein

The protein requirements during gestation are relatively low (11% to 12% crude protein, 0.5 lb of protein per day). The development of the fetuses and reproductive tissue requires small amounts of protein each day.

During lactation, sows require higher levels of protein intake to support milk production (2 to 3 lb of protein per day), which is accomplished by feeding a ration with a higher protein content at a greater intake level. Sows not fed adequate levels of protein or energy during lactation will support milk production with a loss of body tissue stores. Sows can lose more than 100 lb in weight during lactation if not fed proper amounts of energy or protein.

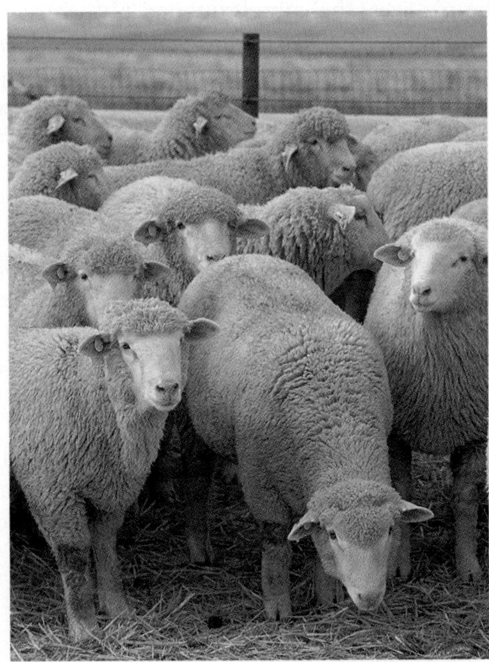

FIGURE 13-8 Optimal feed regimens in sheep will provide excellent results.

Minerals and Vitamins

Minerals and vitamins need to be supplemented throughout the life of pigs. The breeding herd is normally fed diets fortified with the minerals calcium, phosphorus, salt, zinc, iron, copper, iodine, selenium, and manganese. Calcium and phosphorus are kept in a balance of 1:1 to 2:1 for all stages of production. Low levels of calcium and phosphorus in the breeding-herd rations can lead to fractures and lameness in the female.

Sow's milk is virtually devoid of iron, and anemia of nursing pigs will occur unless they are supplemented with another source of iron (Box 13-20). The two most common ways to supply additional iron are as follows:

1. Injection of iron (150 to 200 mg) as iron dextran or other iron-carbohydrate complexes at 3 days of age
2. Oral iron solution given at 3 days of age or swabbed onto the dam's udder several times during lactation

The vitamins supplemented in breeding-herd diets are the fat-soluble vitamins A, D, E, and K and the water-soluble vitamins thiamin, riboflavin, niacin, pantothenic acid, B_6, B_{12}, choline, biotin, and folic acid. Adequate additions of these vitamins ensure proper development of the fetus in gestation and milk production in lactation (Box 13-21).

TECHNICIAN NOTE Sow's milk is devoid of iron, and nursing pigs will develop anemia unless they are supplemented with iron.

TABLE 13-12 Complete Feed Ration Considerations in Swine

	Complete Ration		
Stage Weight	Protein (%)	Fed (lb)	Comments
Weaning pigs (12-20 lb)	20-24	Free feed	Use if weaned early and transitioning to solid feed.
Starter pigs (up to 40 lb)	18-20	Free feed	
Feeder and finisher pigs (40 lb to 220-250 lb finishing weight)	13-18	Free feed*	May be limited in feed after 125 lb.
Gilts and sows			
Breeding and maintenance	11-14	4-6	Increase amount to maintain body condition and last mo of gestation through weaning.
Gestation	11-14	4-6	
Lactation	14-20	10-15	
Boars	14-16	4-7	Increase in breeding season.

*See text on feeding methods.

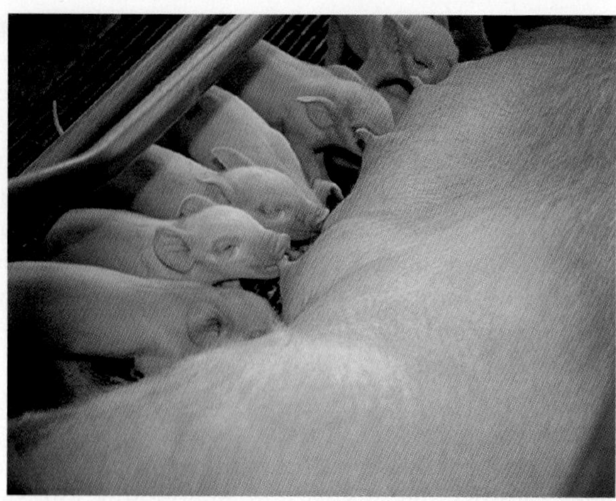

FIGURE 13-9 Sow nursing piglets in containment of farrowing pen.

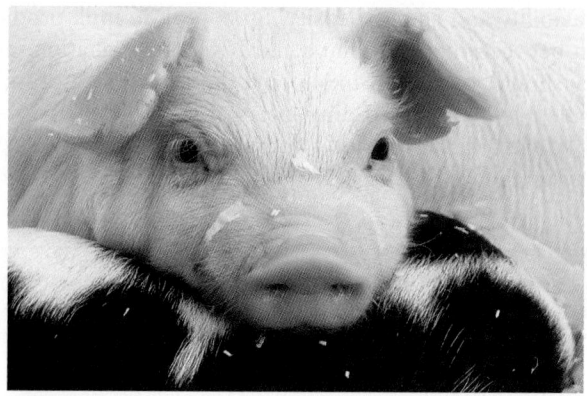

FIGURE 13-10 Young pigs need to be kept in a clean, dry, draft-free environment for optimal health and growth.

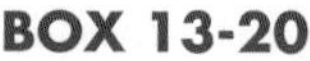

BOX 13-20 Prevention of Iron Deficiency Anemia in Baby Pigs

- Allow access to soil that has not been in contact with other pigs.
- Inject 100-200 mg iron before 72 hr of age.
- Paint sows' teats lightly with iron solution periodically.
- Encourage prestarter ration creep feeding early.
- Provide iron supplementation in creep feeder.

BOX 13-21 Orphan Piglet Feeding

Homemade Replacer

32 oz whole cow's milk
Water-soluble antibiotics
1 raw egg
16 oz half-and-half

Directions for Feeding Piglets

Give 2 oz per feeding per piglet every 3 hr.
Feed in a shallow, clean feeding pan.
Be sure that all piglets are eating.
Give iron supplementation as needed.
Start creep feeding at 7 days of age.

STARTER PIGS

Pigs are commonly weaned at 3 to 5 weeks of age and remain in the starter phase until they weigh 40 to 50 lb (Figure 13-10). The earlier the age at weaning, the more complex is the ration required to help in the transition from mother's milk to solid food. Starter diets (20% to 24% protein) are very complex and nutrient-dense complete feed and therefore often purchased from a commercial feed manufacturer. The highest-quality ingredients are used to make starter diets and include milk products, fish meal, spray-dried blood products, oats, corn, and fat. Vitamin and mineral supplementation levels are high in starter diets. This feed typically is pelleted and quite costly (see Table 13-12).

As the pig ages, the complexity and nutrient density of the starter ration decrease, leading to a lower-cost formula. In the last 2 or 3 weeks of the starter period, crude protein decreases to 18% to 20%, and the diet is often offered as a ground feed.

GROWING-FINISHING PIGS

Growing-finishing diets have been modified to complement the changes in the genetic base of modern swine. The leaner pigs require higher levels of protein and consume less energy than previous generations (see Table 13-12).

Energy

Complete grower-finisher rations are based on cereal grains and frequently have fat added to increase caloric intake. Fibrous feed ingredients often are not used or are used sparingly to prevent depressions in caloric intake. Corn, wheat, sorghum, and barley are the more popular cereal grains used to supply energy and comprise 60% to 85% of the ration.

Protein

Contemporary swine nutrition concentrates not on the protein content of feed, but on the amino acid levels. Lysine typically is the first limiting amino acid in swine formulas. Amino acid levels decrease as a percentage of the diet throughout the growing-finishing phase.

Amino acid levels are matched to muscle growth throughout the growth period to maximize lean tissue growth. Underfeeding of amino acids depresses muscle deposition, and overfeeding amino acids leads to excess, which is costly.

Typical protein sources in growing-finishing diets are soybean meal, meat and bone meal, and synthetic amino acids. When protein sources are expensive, synthetic amino acids can replace a portion of the protein source with no loss in performance. The most commonly available synthetic amino acids are lysine, methionine, threonine, and tryptophan (Figure 13-11).

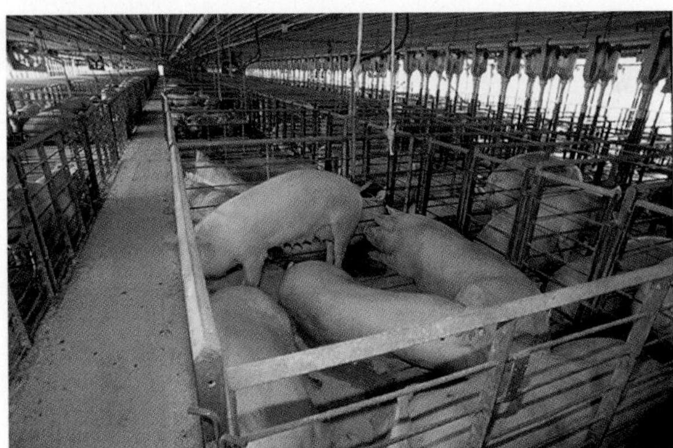

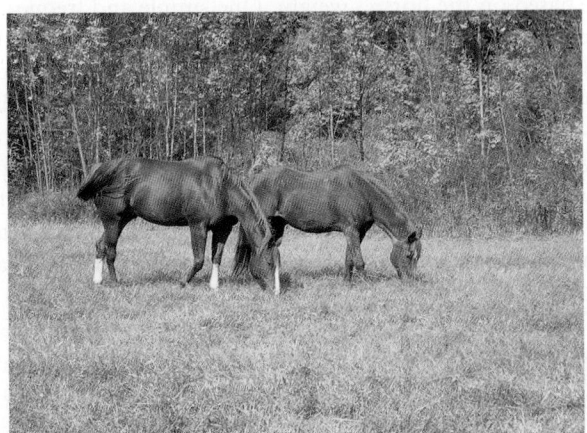

FIGURE 13-11 Grower-finisher pigs are fed large quantities of complete rations to obtain the most desirable carcass quality.

FIGURE 13-12 Horses evolved to forage on grasses and legumes. Good turnout and pasture may serve as the foundation for providing the nutrient needs to horses. (Courtesy J. Bassert.)

Minerals and Vitamins

Growing-finishing swine are fed diets fortified with the minerals calcium, phosphorus, salt, zinc, iron, copper, iodine, selenium, and manganese. Calcium and phosphorus are kept in a balance of 1:1 to 2:1 throughout this period. Deficiencies of phosphorus will depress growth performance as the animal grows.

Riboflavin, niacin, pantothenic acid, and vitamin B_{12} are the water-soluble vitamins most likely to be deficient in swine diets formulated with grains and plant protein. The fat-soluble vitamins A, D, E, and K also should be added to growing-finishing rations.

HORSES

Horses evolved eating grass and other range forage. Consequently, grass and hays serve well as a foundation for feeding all horses (Figure 13-12). Feed constitutes the greatest single cost in the horse business, but its economic significance varies more widely than with any other class of livestock. Most horses are kept for recreation, sport, or hobby purposes, whereas the vast majority of other large animal species are maintained for strictly business purposes: meat or milk production. Consequently, meeting the nutrient needs of horses is a major factor in determining their efficiency and years of service. As with other animals, the horse needs nutrients for maintenance, growth, reproduction, and production. But with horses, the production need is for work—mostly for recreation and sport. The work typically is irregular and often strenuous—characteristics which create a particular stress on the animal and make the job of feeding according to the nutritive needs very difficult. Horse production typically is divided into three areas: gestation and lactation, foals, and maintenance of adults.

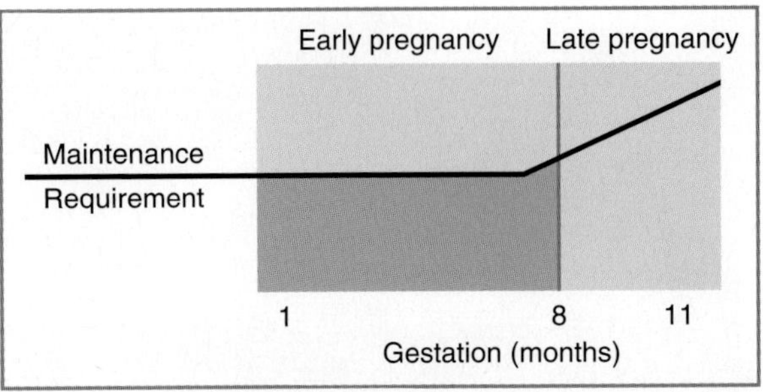

FIGURE 13-13 During early gestation, the mare should be fed for maintenance. However, in the last trimester of pregnancy, requirements for energy, protein, and minerals increase.

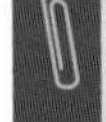

TECHNICIAN NOTE Good-quality grass and legume hay are crucial for the adult horse.

GESTATION AND LACTATION

Broodmares require good-quality, balanced rations, and their nutrient requirements change considerably as they advance from being open (not pregnant) through pregnancy and lactation (Figure 13-13).

Energy

In general, during the first 7 months of pregnancy, the energy requirements are very similar to those for maintenance at the time of breeding. However, from the eighth month of pregnancy, the requirements of the mare increase by 20% to 50%. During lactation, the mare requires even more energy, up to twice the amount that she was receiving at breeding time. It is estimated that 2 months following foaling, mares may produce 20 to 25 lb of milk daily (Figure 13-14).

Protein

Most high-quality forage contains adequate protein for the nutrient needs of the first two trimesters of gestation. Concurrent with the increased energy needs in the eighth month of pregnancy and beyond, protein requirements of the gestating broodmare increase by 20% to 25%. Restriction of protein during lactation can lead to reduced milk production and increased reproductive problems. Protein is supplied by the forage or concentrate and should be added

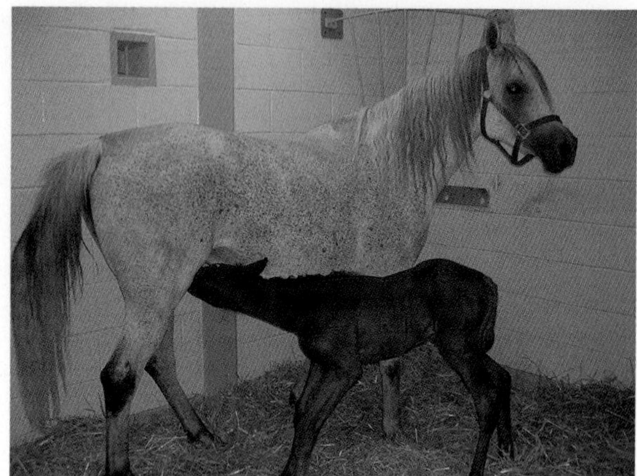

FIGURE 13-14 The mare's nutrient requirements double during lactation. It is estimated that 2 months following foaling, mares may produce 20 to 25 lb of milk daily. (Courtesy J. Bassert.)

at levels to ensure that minimum protein requirements are met. Most mares are fed a high-protein legume hay, such as alfalfa, and grain, which should supply most or all the protein needs during lactation.

Minerals and Vitamins

In general, it is important that the ration of the gestating-lactating mare supply sufficient calcium, phosphorus, vitamins A and D, and riboflavin.

FOALS

Peak lactation in the mare occurs at 6 to 8 weeks after foaling; and usually there is a drop in milk production after 3 months. It is at this time that consideration needs to be given to individual feeding or creep feeding of the foal. Foals will begin to nibble on grain and hay by 3 weeks of age. Creep feeding should be initiated at an early age and with small amounts of creep feed. A general rule of thumb is to offer 1 lb of creep feed per month of age per day up to a maximum of 6 lb. Foals typically are weaned at 6 months of age and then offered 1 to 1.5 lb of grain and 1.5 to 2.0 lb of hay daily per each 100 lb of live weight.

MAINTENANCE

Good-quality grass or legume hay, free-choice water, calcium, phosphorus as needed, and trace-mineralized salt are the only foods needed by the adult horse during the maintenance life stage.

Energy

In general, the energy requirements of the adult horse are related to the intensity of work they perform. The horse owner may base an individual horse's energy requirements on observation or by calculation. By simple observation, if the horse is too thin, increase the energy intake; if too fat, decrease energy intake. Equine food-offering calculations are based on the horse's weight. One simple and frequently used method is the calculation of the amount of feed per 100 lb of horse. A horse weight tape is a simple tool to measure girth circumference and estimate body weight (Table 13-13). Once the weight is estimated, the horse owner can use the recommendations in Figure 13-15 to estimate daily food offerings. Table 13-14 summarizes different dry-matter intake levels for various activity and physiologic states. Note that feedstuffs should still be weighed to ensure accurate proportions.

TABLE 13-13 Estimating Horse Weight

Girth Circumference		Body Weight	
(in)	(cm)	(lb)	(kg)
64.5	163.8	800	363.6
67.5	171.5	900	409.1
70.5	179.1	1000	454.5
73.0	185.4	1100	500.0
75.5	191.8	1200	545.5
77.5	196.9	1300	590.9

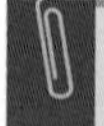

TECHNICIAN NOTE Routine body condition assessments should be included in all horses' examinations.

Protein

Most high-quality forage contains adequate protein for the nutrient needs of adulthood. The protein requirements for work are minimal and are not increased by workload; they are the same for maintenance, medium exercise, and intense exercise.

Minerals and Vitamins

Some forage or forage-grain combinations need calcium and phosphorus supplementation. Most commonly, a source of phosphorus is added only when good legume hay is the sole source of nutrition. Powdered mineral supplements are often mixed with hay or loose rock salt and provided as a part of the diet. Loose rock salt should be a 50:50 mix of dicalcium phosphate and salt.

FEEDING SICK HORSES

Hospitalized horses can develop protein-calorie deficits, hypermetabolic stress, or catabolic wasting states. These have negative clinical effects, and early interventional feeding is vital in equine critical care. Major gastrointestinal tract (colic) surgery is especially challenging in the perioperative period. The animal needs diets rich in protein, calories, and micronutrients despite **reduced gastrointestinal motility.** The veterinarian will focus closely as to when

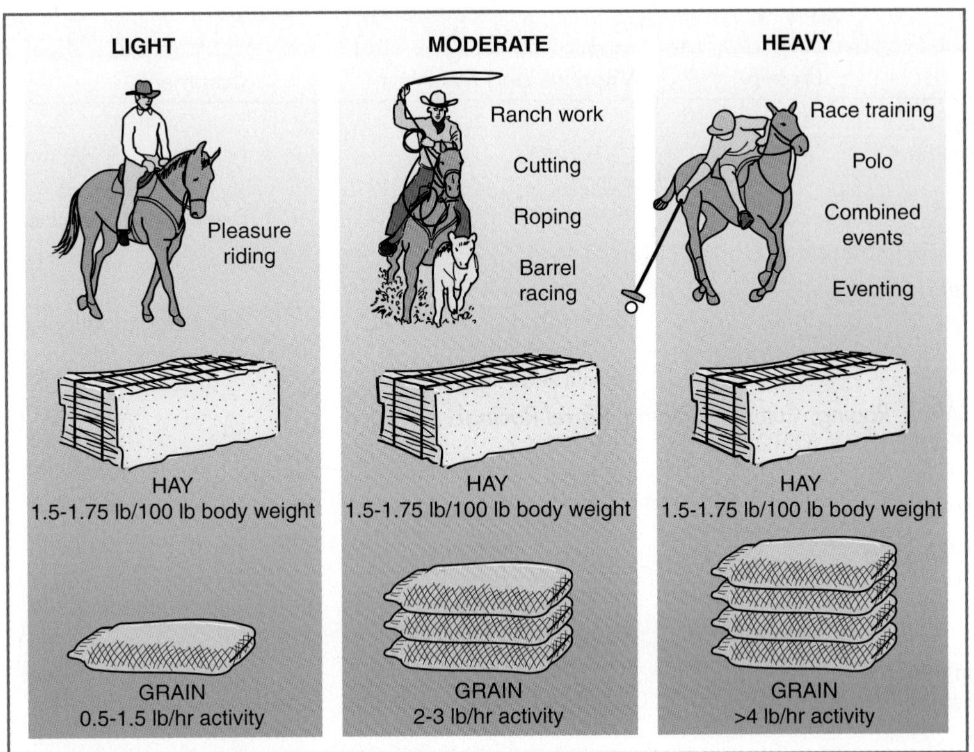

FIGURE 13-15 Adjusted feeding based on an activity level. Maintenance feed levels can be based per 100 lb of weight. Supplemental feeding over maintenance should be based on the level and duration of work.

TABLE 13-14 Nutrient Supply for Horses*

Energy	Protein	Vitamins and Minerals	Comments
Nursing Foals			
Supplement mare's milk	>16%	Ca^{2+} >0.85%	At 2-3 mo of age, begin 1 lb if foal is very thin; concentrate mixture/mo of age/day
		P >0.5%	Adequate Ca^{2+}, P, trace minerals in grain mix
		Cu >25 mg/kg	If creep feeding, mix 50:50 chopped hay to grain
		Vitamin A 50 IU/kg BW	Wean at 4 mo
Weaning			
Adequate to feel but not see the ribs	15%	Ca^{2+} 0.7%	Dry-matter intake = 3% of BW
		P 0.4%	Free-choice good roughage and trace-mineral salt
		Vitamin A 50 IU/kg BW	1 lb concentrate mix/mo of age/day: 7-9 lb mix
Yearling			
Adequate to feel but not see the ribs	13%	Ca^{2+} 0.5%	Dry-matter intake = 2.5% BW
		P 0.3%	Free-choice good roughage, trace-mineral salt
		Vitamin A 50 IU/kg BW	1lb concentrate mix/100 lb BW: 7-9 lb max
			Feed as mature horse at 90% of mature weight

Continued

TABLE 13-14 Nutrient Supply for Horses*—cont'd

Energy	Protein	Vitamins and Minerals	Comments
Adult Maintenance			
Adequate to feel but not see the ribs	8.5%	Ca^{2+} 0.3% P 0.2% Vitamin A 50 IU/kg BW	Dry matter = 1.5% BW ½-1½ lb roughage/100 lb BW Free-choice trace-mineral salt
Adult Working			
Light (Pleasure Ride)			
Add 0.5-1.5 lb of grain/hr of activity/day	8.5%	Ca^{2+} 0.3% P 0.2% Vitamin A 50 IU/kg BW	Amortize grain supplement over the wk
Moderate (Ranch Work, Roping, Cutting, Jumping, Barrel Racing)			
Add 2-3 lb grain/hr of activity/day	8.5%-10%	Ca^{2+} 0.3% P 0.2% Vitamin A 50 IU/kg BW	
Heavy (Race Training, Polo)			
Add 4 or more lb of grain/hr of activity/day	8.5%-10%	Ca^{2+} 0.3% P 0.2% Vitamin A 50 IU/kg BW	Dry matter = 1.75% BW
Adult Reproduction—Mares			
Feed at maintenance until late pregnancy	8.5%-10%		
Late Pregnancy			
Needs 20% more energy	11%	Ca^{2+} 0.5% P 0.35% Vitamin A 50 IU/kg BW	Feed 1½-1¾ lb grass hays/100 lb BW with addition of ½-¾ lb grain or concentrate mix/100 lb BW Free-choice trace-mineral salt–mineral Ca^{2+}/P mix
Last 3 Wk of Pregnancy			
Needs 30% more energy		Needs 100%, more Ca^{2+} and P Vitamin A 60 IU/kg BW	1¼-2 lb legume hay/100 lb BW Free-choice trace-mineral salt–mineral Ca^{2+}/P mix
Lactation			
Allow 75% energy increase at peak lactation	14%	Ca^{2+} 0.5% P 0.35% Vitamin A 60 IU/kg BW	Dry matter = 1.75%-2.0% BW free-choice grass hay Add 1½-2 lb/100 lb BW of concentrate Add Ca^{2+}/P mix and trace mineralized salt At weaning, stop concentrate; return to maintenance forage
Adult Reproduction—Stallions			
Feed for maintenance			

BW, Body weight; *Ca*, calcium; *Cu*, copper; *P*, phosphorus.
*Free-choice, potable water should be available at all times.

gastrointestinal motility returns to support the sick horse. Often, homogenized, moistened alfalfa pellet mashes are high-protein, high-energy, and nonirritating formulas designed for replenishing nutrients. Such diets may be given as slurries through nasogastric tubes and are often enriched with nutriment modules. Liquid enteral formulas based on mare's milk replacement and commercial equine critical care formulas are available and well tolerated. Formulas should be given in small, frequent feedings via indwelling nasogastric tubes.

REFERENCES

Church DC: *Livestock feeds and feeding.* Corvallis, Ore, 1984, O and B Books.

Ensminger ME: *Swine science.* Danville, Ill, 1990, Interstate Printers and Publishing.

Lewis LD: *Equine clinical nutrition, feeding and care.* Media, Pa, 1995, Williams & Wilkins.

McDonald P et al: *Animal nutrition.* ed 7, New York, 1995, Longman Scientific and Technical Publishing.

Miller ER et al: *Swine nutrition.* Boston, 1991, Butterworth-Heinemann.

Nash MJ: *Crop conservation and storage*, Oxford, England, 1985, Pergamon Press.
Neumann AL: *Beef cattle*, New York, 1977, John Wiley & Sons.
Shirley RL: *Nitrogen and energy nutrition of ruminants*, Orlando, 1986, Academic Press.

RECOMMENDED READING

Cunha TJ: *Swine feeding and nutrition*, New York, 1977 Academic Press, Inc.
Garmsworthy PC: *Nutrition and lactation in the dairy cow*, London, 1988, University Press.
Haresign DJ: *Recent developments of pig nutrition*, London, 1985, Butterworth.
Jones DH, Wilson AD: Nutritive quality of forage. In Hacker ED, editor: *The nutrition of herbivores*, Sydney, 1982, Academic Press.
Kruesi WK: *Sheep raiser's manual*, Charlotte, Vt, 1985, Williamson Publishing.
Linciciome DR: *Sheep: applied and basic research information*, Scottsdale, Ariz, 1983, International Goat and Sheep Research.
Lloyd LE, et al: *Fundamentals of nutrition*, ed 3, San Francisco, 1978, WH Freeman & Sons.
Machlin LJ: *Handbook of vitamins*, New York, 1984, Marcel Dekker.
Maynard LA, et al: *Animal nutrition*, ed 7, New York, 1979, McGraw-Hill.
Menzies CS: United States sheep and goat industry, Ames, Iowa, 1982, CAST Report.
National Research Council: *Nutrient requirements for beef cattle*, ed 7, Washington, DC, 2000, National Academic Press.
National Research Council: *Nutrient requirements for dairy cattle*, ed 7, Washington, DC, 2001, National Academy Press.
National Research Council: *Nutrient requirement of horses*, ed 6, Washington, DC, 2007, National Academy Press.
National Research Council: *Nutrient requirements for sheep*, ed 6, Washington, DC, 1985, National Academy Press.
National Research Council: *Nutrient requirements for swine*, ed 10, Washington, DC, 1998, National Academic Press.
Naylor JM, Ralston SL: *Large animal clinical nutrition*, St Louis, 1991, Mosby.
Pond WG: *Swine production and nutrition*, Westport, Conn, 1984, AVI Publishing.
Taylor RE: *Beef production and the beef industry*, Minneapolis, 1984, Burgess Publishing.
Tribble LG, Stansbury WF: *Swine report*, Dallas, 1985, Texas Technical University.
Webster J: *Calf husbandry: health and welfare*, London, 1984, Collins.

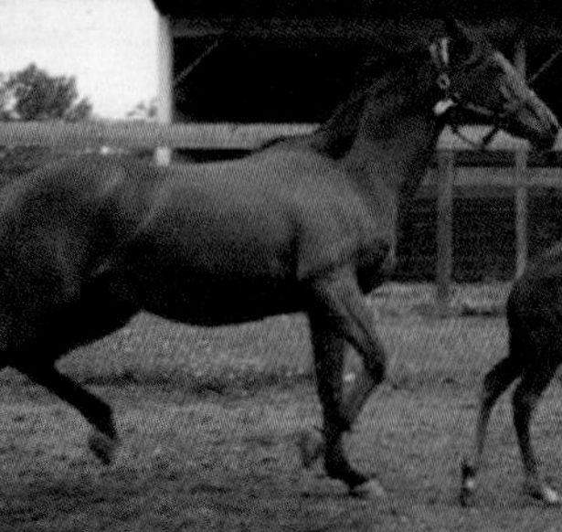

14 Animal Reproduction

Carlos R.F. Pinto, Bruce Edward Eilts, and Dale L. Paccamonti

OUTLINE

KEY TERMS

Allantois
Amnion
Artificial insemination (AI)
Chorioallantois
Chorion
Chromosomes
Colostrum
Corpus luteum (CL)
Cryptorchid
Embryo
Estrogen
Follicle
Gilt
Heifer
Luteinizing hormone (LH)
Oxytocin
Parturition
Placenta
Placentomes
Progesterone

LEARNING OBJECTIVES

When you have completed this chapter, you will be able to:

1. List the stages of the canine estrous cycle and describe the events that occur in each stage.
2. List the female reproductive hormones and describe their roles in the process of reproduction.
3. Describe the formation and structure of the placenta in domestic animals.
4. List and describe methods used to confirm pregnancy.
5. Describe the events that occur in each of the stages of whelping in the canine.
6. List clinical signs of pyometra, eclampsia, metritis, mastitis, and brucellosis in canines.
7. List the stages of the feline estrous cycle and describe the unique features of the feline reproductive process.
8. Differentiate between polyestrous, seasonally polyestrous, and induced ovulator reproductive cycles.
9. Describe the procedures and tests used for performing a breeding soundness examination in the mare.
10. Describe methods for synchronization of estrous in herd animals.

INTRODUCTION

The events that occur in the process of reproduction in domestic animals are elegant processes of checks and balances that ultimately result in the birth of a newborn, which carries the genes for the next generation. The birth of offspring is essential to produce the next generation of animals as commodities (meat, milk, and fiber production from cows, pigs, and sheep), as companions (dogs, cats, and horses) and for sport (horses). The production of food and fiber animals requires efficient reproduction to provide economical commodities to consumers and has been a cornerstone of many herd health programs. Reproduction in horses used as companions and for sport has had many advances recently. The interest in small animal reproduction has also blossomed in the last 10 to 20 years. Reproduction has many similarities between species and unique aspects within each species. A basic knowledge of hormones, hormone interaction, breeding, fertilization, pregnancy, and birth is needed to understand the normal aspects of reproduction in all species. When the normal aspects are understood, the problems that can occur when normal processes go awry are more easily comprehended. If normal and abnormal processes are learned for one species, transfer of that knowledge to other species may help solve problems or understand differences between species. This chapter provides a generic overview of female and male reproductive events, followed by more in-depth reviews of the most important aspects of reproduction in the canine, feline, equine, bovine, swine, ovine, caprine, and camelid species.

There are two embryologic tubular systems present in the early embryo that will become either the male genitalia or the female genitalia. If an animal has XY chromosomes, it will become a male, and one tubular system (Wolffian) will persist. In the male, the female tubular system regresses, and the Wolffian system becomes the epididymis and vas deferens. If an individual has an XX karyotype, the other tubular system (Müllerian) will persist and develop into a female reproductive system. In the female, the Müllerian system becomes the uterine tubes, uterus, cervix, and anterior vagina. Because there are two systems, many potential abnormalities can occur when sections of the systems fail to regress or fail to develop fully. An example of an embryonic malformation would be the hermaphrodite, which has developed both male and female gender organs.

In both the male and female, the brain is the initiator of the reproductive cycle. Neural input from higher brain centers results in the release of gonadotropin-releasing hormone (GnRH) from neurons in the hypothalamus into the hypophyseal-portal vessels. The GnRH then enters the anterior pituitary, causing release of the gonadotropins, follicle-stimulating hormone (FSH), and luteinizing hormone (LH).

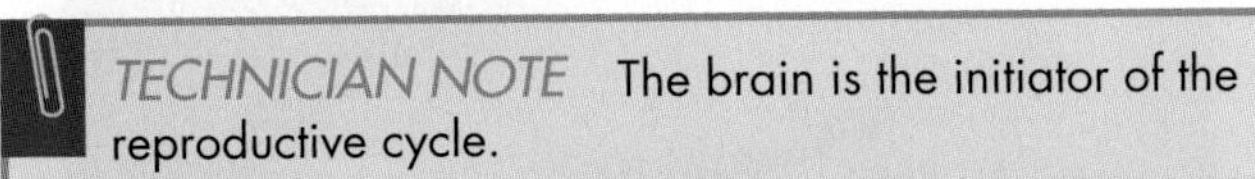

TECHNICIAN NOTE The brain is the initiator of the reproductive cycle.

Both FSH and LH are large, complex hormones that are stored within granules inside cells in the anterior pituitary. These hormones are glycoproteins, a complex of carbohydrates and proteins. Because the gonadotropins are extremely large and complex, they cannot be synthesized in the laboratory. The complexity and protein nature of the gonadotropins make them antigenic, and exogenous administration of these drugs derived from other species can induce antibody formation.

GENERAL FEMALE REPRODUCTION

THE ESTROUS CYCLE

The normal stages of reproduction are proestrus (the time leading to estrus), estrus (the time of mating), and diestrus (the time when pregnancy is being established). In most species, pregnancy is the normal event that ensures species survival. However, if pregnancy does not occur, the female will return to a sexually active state to entice mating with a male. If pregnancy is not established, the events will recur, thus forming a cycle of proestrus, estrus, diestrus, proestrus, estrus, diestrus, and so forth. The other normal events in the reproductive life of an animal are puberty (the time of first ovulation), pregnancy, and anestrus (time when the animal is not undergoing any reproductive events). The name given to these recurring events is the estrous cycle. (Note that estrus is spelled estrous when it is an adjective, as in estrous cycle.)

The beginning of an estrous cycle in most females starts with GnRH from the hypothalamus, causing the release of FSH from the anterior pituitary (Figure 14-1). The FSH is released into the bloodstream and is carried to the ovaries where it initiates its follicle-stimulating action, causing the growth of ovarian follicles. Ovarian follicles are structures on the ovary that contain the egg, or oocyte (Figure 14-2). All the oocytes that a female will ever have are present on the ovary at birth, and most of the follicles contain no fluid. Some follicles are selected to grow and start to develop fluid around them (an antrum) in a process that is independent from FSH stimulation. Once a follicle has reached the antral stage, the action of the FSH causes rapid growth of the

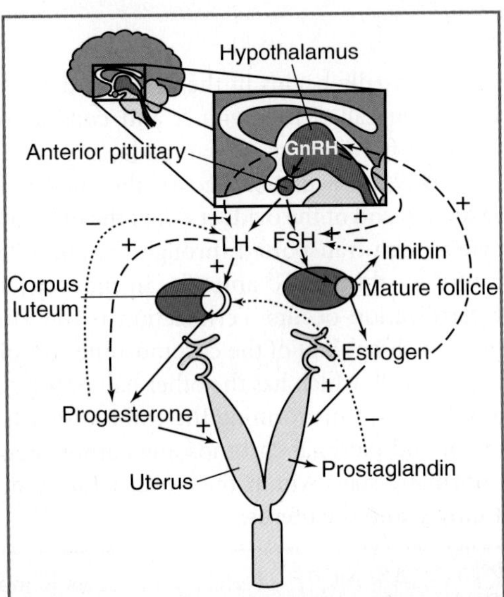

FIGURE 14-1 The general hormonal control of female reproduction: Pulsatile GnRH causes FSH to be released from the anterior pituitary. FSH causes follicular growth and maturation, where estrogen is produced. Inhibin from the follicle feeds back on the anterior pituitary and causes less FSH to be released. A surge of estrogen from the follicle causes GnRH release from the hypothalamus, which causes an LH surge. LH causes ovulation of the follicle and the formation of a CL, which produces progesterone. If a pregnancy signal is not secreted by the early embryo (bovine, equine, ovine, caprine), prostaglandin is released from the uterus, goes to the CL, and causes luteolysis (luteal death). The cycle then starts over with follicular growth.

follicle. The follicle wall is composed of two layers, the thecal cell layer and the granulosa cell layer. As the follicle grows, it produces the steroid hormone estrogen. Estrogen is the hormone that causes the characteristic behaviors and sexual receptivity when the female is in estrus. The oocyte within the follicle also begins to mature so that it will be ready for fertilization after ovulation. As the follicle grows and reaches maturity, the granulosa cells also produce a protein hormone called inhibin. Inhibin inhibits further FSH release so that only a species-specific number of follicles are chosen for final growth and maturation (depending on the species, this may be one or more).

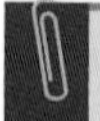

TECHNICIAN NOTE Estrogen causes the female to become sexually receptive to the male.

The estrogen surge produced by the developing follicle stimulates the release of GnRH from the hypothalamus, which causes release of LH from the anterior pituitary. At the ovary, LH causes the mature follicle to ovulate. Ovulation is the release of the oocyte into the oviduct. After ovulation, the follicle transforms into a corpus luteum (CL), or yellow body. The CL (Figures 14-2 and 14-3) has been transformed by the LH surge to produce only progesterone, the hormone that maintains pregnancy.

TECHNICIAN NOTE Progesterone is the hormone that maintains pregnancy.

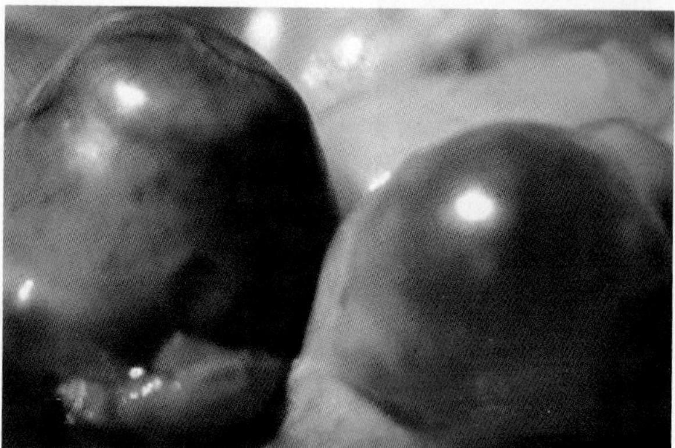

FIGURE 14-2 A bovine CL and follicle on the ovaries.

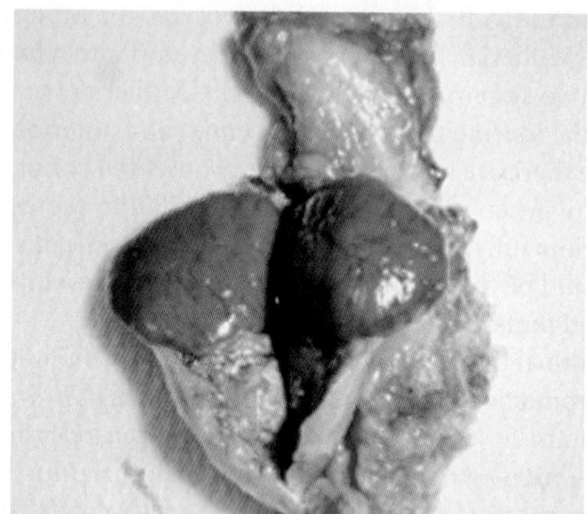

FIGURE 14-3 A cut section of a bovine CL.

Pregnancy actually begins in the uterine tube. The uterine tube is often called the oviduct and consists of three segments: the infundibulum, the ampulla, and the isthmus (Figure 14-4). When ovulation occurs, the oocyte is picked up by the dilated end of the oviduct called the infundibulum. The oocyte is then transported through the ampulla to the junction of the isthmus and ampulla. In most species, this is where fertilization occurs. Fertilization is the joining of the oocyte, which has half of the chromosome complement, with the sperm cell, which has the other half of the chromosome complement, thus forming the embryo that has both the maternal and paternal chromosome complements. The embryo normally stays within the oviduct for several days before it moves into the uterus.

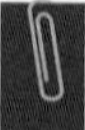

TECHNICIAN NOTE Fertilization occurs in the uterine tube (oviduct).

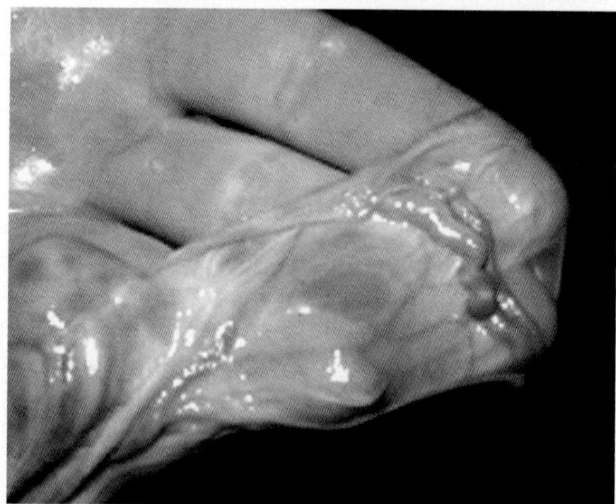

FIGURE 14-4 A bovine oviduct showing the fingers inserted in the infundibulum.

If the oocyte is not successfully fertilized, the CL still develops and maintains progesterone production for a time that is consistent within each species. This time of progesterone domination is called diestrus. It is the early embryo in most species that signals to the uterus and ovary that pregnancy has been established. If the signal for pregnancy is not received by the uterus, most species (not the dog and cat) will initiate an ending of diestrus so that the animal can return to estrus and have another chance to become pregnant. In most species, this occurs when the hormone prostaglandin is released from the uterus. Prostaglandin is a small molecule derived from arachidonic acid. When prostaglandin is released, it binds to receptors on the CL and lyses it. Because the CL is the source of progesterone, after the CL is destroyed by prostaglandin, the progesterone concentration in the blood falls. When progesterone is not present, there is a rise in FSH that allows new follicles to grow. This time of growing follicles after the death of the CL is called proestrus. As the animal enters proestrus, the follicles grow, estrus follows, the LH surge causes ovulation, and a CL forms. Therefore the animal has estrous cycles until pregnancy is established.

Once the embryo is in the uterus, it must establish itself as a viable pregnancy before prostaglandins destroy the CL. Different species have different mechanisms to do this. Each species appears to have a relatively unique substance produced by the early embryo that prevents the CL from being destroyed by prostaglandins released from the uterus. Dogs and cats appear rather unique in that their corpora lutea (plural for corpus luteum) appear to have preprogrammed life spans without any endogenous destruction by prostaglandins if they are not pregnant.

As pregnancy progresses, the early embryo changes from an embryonic disk to a more complex structure that includes the embryo or fetus and placenta. After all the bodily organs are formed, the embryo is called a fetus. The placenta forms from specialized cells on the embryo. These cells develop into the chorion and allantois. The amnion is a fluid-filled sac that immediately surrounds the fetus, whereas the chorion and allantois fuse to form the chorioallantois. The fetus has two fluid-filled sacs surrounding it (Figure 14-5). The chorion attaches to the uterus and has the function of transferring nutrients from the uterus to the fetus. The structure of the placenta varies from species to species (Figures 14-6 and 14-7). The ruminants have many individual attachment areas called placentomes. Dogs and cats have a zone of the placenta that attaches to the uterus. Horses and pigs have a more generalized attachment (diffuse) of the placenta to the uterus. In some species, such as the ewe and horse, the placenta produces the progesterone that maintains the pregnancy instead of the CL.

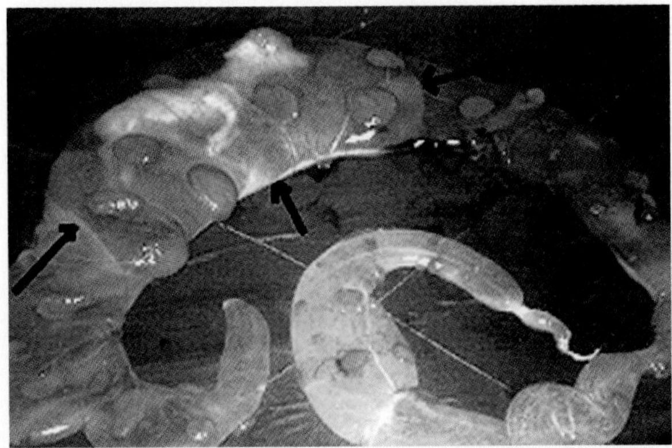

FIGURE 14-5 A bovine fetus within the amnion *(arrows)*, which is within the chorioallantois.

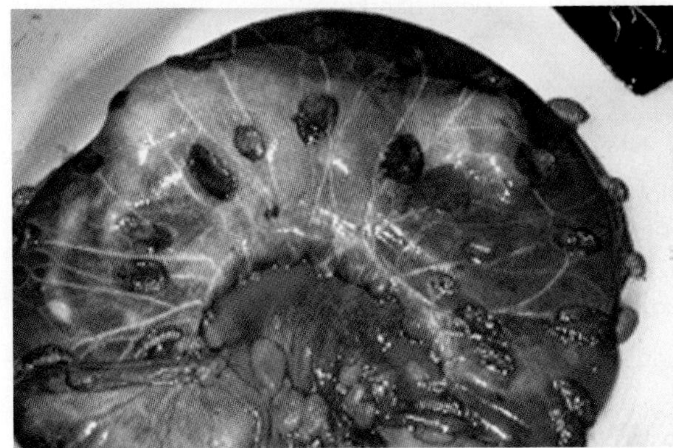

FIGURE 14-6 Cotyledons on the bovine chorioallantois.

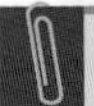

TECHNICIAN NOTE Parturition is the act of giving birth.

Parturition is the act of giving birth. The only domestic species in which the entire parturition mechanism is completely understood is sheep; other species are hypothesized to be similar. As gestation progresses, the fetal hypothalamus and pituitary mature enough to cause the fetal release of corticotropin-releasing hormone from the hypothalamus, which causes the fetal adrenal gland to produce high concentrations of cortisol. The high cortisol concentrations cause a change in placental production of progesterone to estrogen and a release of prostaglandins from the uterus. These hormones cause the cervix to dilate and the uterus to contract, thereby forcing the fetus out. Parturition is normally divided into three stages: I, II, and III. Stage I is the preparatory stage. Maternal pelvic ligaments relax and the cervix softens, preparing for delivery. Behaviorally the female becomes restless and prepares to give birth. The expulsion of the fetus is stage II (Figure 14-8). Stage III is the expulsion of the placenta. The timing of the events of parturition varies by species. A summary of the length of the estrous cycle and the length of gestation is found in Table 14-1.

CANINE REPRODUCTION

The estrous cycle of the bitch has four phases: proestrus (9 to 10 days average), estrus (9 to 10 days average), diestrus (57 to 58 days average), and anestrus (2 to 5 months average) (Figure 14-9). Interestrus consists of diestrus and anestrus combined and usually lasts 4 to 7 months. Interestrus periods of less than 4 months are associated with infertility.

During proestrus, the bitch is attractive to male dogs, but will not allow mating. The vulva appears swollen, and

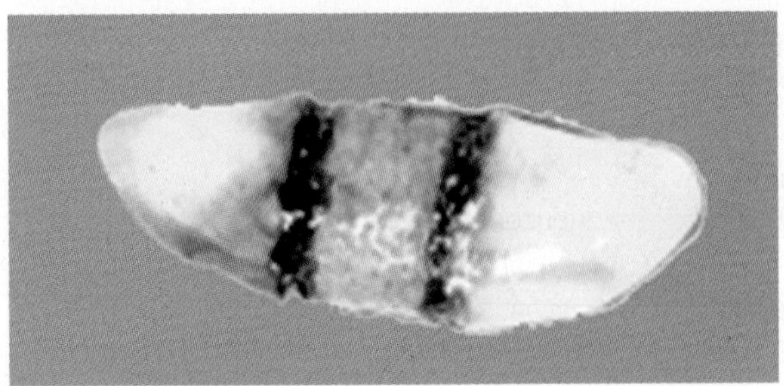

FIGURE 14-7 A canine puppy with the zonary placenta surrounding it.

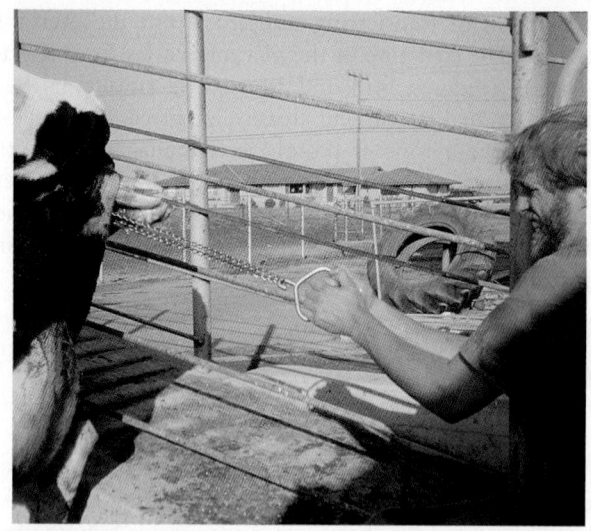

FIGURE 14-8 Chains placed around the legs of a bovine calf in a normal delivery position.

a serosanguineous discharge is present. Estrogen, which is rising during proestrus, causes the epithelial cells in the vagina to cornify. Vaginal cytology is a common tool used to follow a bitch's cycle. To prepare a vaginal cytology slide, moisten a long cotton swab and pass it through the vulva and vestibule (Figure 14-10). The canine vagina is nearly vertical at the entrance. To get a swab into the cranial vagina, once past the vulvar lips, direct the swab nearly vertical (toward the anus) until it will go no further. Redirect the swab horizontally and twirl it to obtain a sample. Roll the swab on a slide and stain the slide using a modified Wright's or Giemsa stain. Noncornified cells have a rounded cytoplasm and a large stippled nucleus. Cornified cells have a more angular-shaped cytoplasm, and the nucleus is either pyknotic or not apparent. The percentage of cornified cells increases approximately 10% per day, reaching 90% to 100% (full cornification) by the onset of estrus (Figure 14-11).

TABLE 14-1 Summary of the Lengths of the Estrous Cycle and Gestation Periods in Domestic Animals

Puberty	Estrous Cycle Length	Estrus Duration	Ovulation	Optimal Breeding (Fresh/Frozen)	Gestation
Canine (Dog or Bitch)					
6 mo	No true cycle (estrus is 2 times/yr)	9 days	2-4 days after onset of cytologic estrus	Days 3 and 5 or 4 and 6 after LH peak/day 5 or 6 after LH peak	57 days from first day of cytologic diestrus or 63 days from ovulation or 65 days from LH peak
Feline (Cat or Queen)					
6-12 mo	Seasonally polyestrous and depends on whether ovulation occurs	8 days	Induced ovulators after coitus	After third day of estrus and >2 hr apart for at least 3 breedings	65 days
Equine (Horse or Mare)					
18 mo	Seasonally polyestrous, 21 days (diestrus is consistently 15 days)	4-7 days	1-2 days before end of estrus	(Within 48 hr of ovulation) At ovulation	330 days, variable
Bovine (Cow)					
12 mo	21 days	12-18 hr	12-18 hr after end of estrus	12 hr after end of estrus	283 days
Caprine (Goat or Doe)					
6-9 mo	Seasonally polyestrous, 21 days	24-36 hr	24-30 hr after onset of estrus	18-24 hr after onset of estrus	150 days
Ovine (Sheep or Ewe)					
6-9 mo	Seasonally polyestrous, 17 days	24-48 hr	24-30 hr after onset of estrus	12-30 hr after onset of estrus	150 days
Porcine (Pig or Sow)					
5-6 mo	21 days	2 to 3 days	Day 2 of estrus	24 and 36 hr after onset of estrus (12 and 24 in gilts)	114 days
Llama					
10-12 mo	Induced ovulators	1-36 days (induced ovulators)	Induced ovulators	Induced ovulators	344 days
Alpaca					
10-12 mo	Induced ovulators	1-36 days (induced ovulators)	Induced ovulators	Induced ovulators	344 days

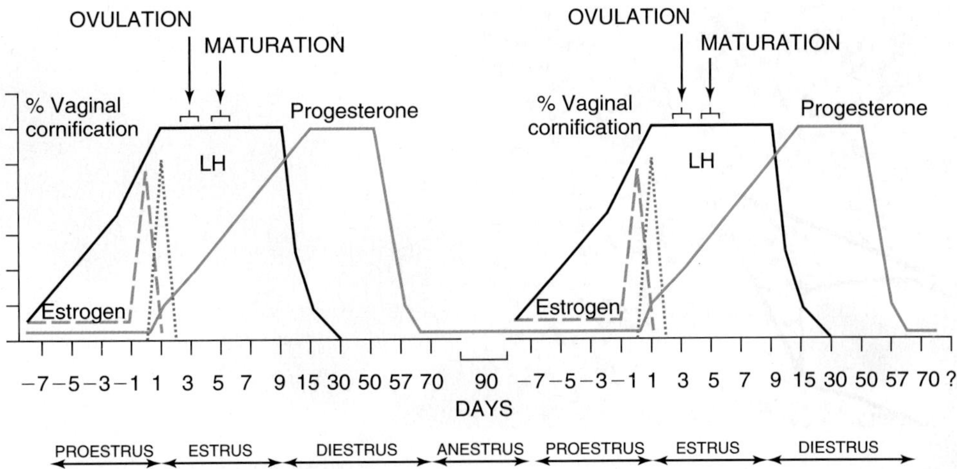

FIGURE 14-9 The canine estrous cycle. Proestrus lasts about 9 days. During proestrus, the vaginal cornification increases about 10% per day, and estrogen peaks at the end of proestrus. There is 100% vaginal cornification throughout a 9-day estrus. At the beginning of estrus, the LH peaks. At the same time the LH peaks, progesterone starts to rise. About 2 days after the LH peak, ovulation occurs, followed by a 2- to 3-day maturation of the oocytes. At the start of diestrus, the vaginal cornification abruptly declines to less than 50% cornified. Diestrus lasts about 57 days and is characterized by high progesterone. At the end of diestrus, progesterone declines, and the bitch enters a 90- to 150-day anestrus. The cycle then starts over again.

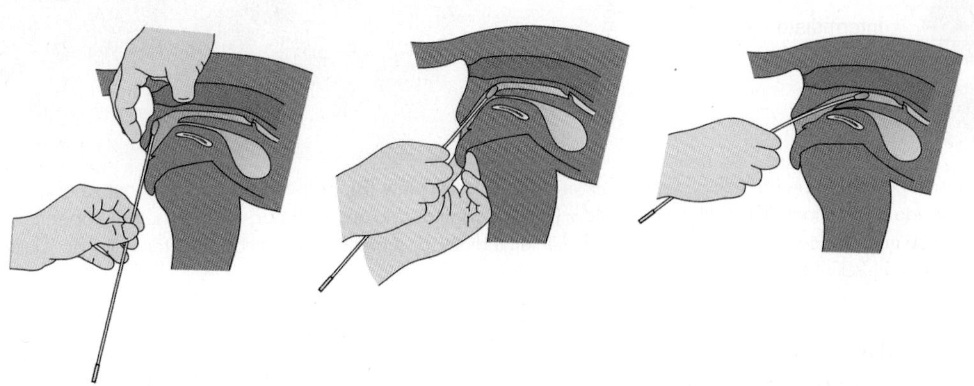

FIGURE 14-10 A diagram demonstrating cell collection for vaginal cytology preparation and examination. (From Eilts, BE: Determining estrous status, *NAVC Clinician's Brief* 5:40-41, 2007.)

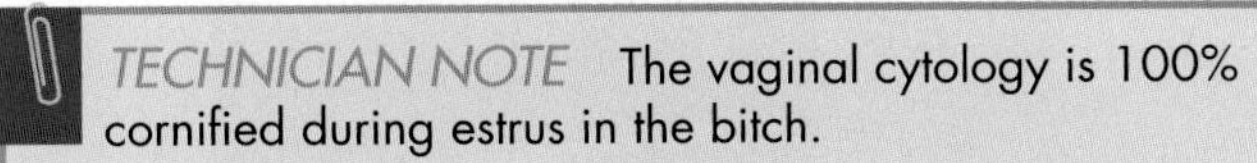
TECHNICIAN NOTE The vaginal cytology is 100% cornified during estrus in the bitch.

Estrus is the period of receptivity when the bitch will allow mating. During estrus, the vulvar swelling typically decreases slightly, and the bloody discharge changes to a straw color, although a bloody discharge may continue throughout estrus. Vaginal cytology is fully cornified, and the background of the slide is clear. No white blood cells should be present. Occasionally, bacteria may be seen on the slide.

The end of estrus, or the first day of diestrus, is typified by an abrupt decline in the percentage of cornified cells. This day is important to detect because whelping can be accurately predicted from day 1 (D1) of diestrus. D1 of diestrus also correlates well with the LH peak (8 days before D1) and ovulation (approximately 6 days before D1).

To maximize fertility, viable sperm must be present when the oocyte is ready to be fertilized. If the male is readily available, mating every other day is usually practiced. If performing artificial insemination (AI) and male availability is not limited, breeding three times per week (e.g., Monday, Wednesday, Friday) for as long as the vaginal cytology is fully cornified provides equally good results. However, when the number of breedings is reduced to one or two during a single estrus, such as with frozen or fresh cooled semen, timing insemination to coincide with ovulation becomes critical. Ovulation occurs approximately 2 days after the LH surge. The bitch ovulates immature oocytes that require 2 to 3 more days for maturation. Mature oocytes are then viable for another 2 to 3 days. Therefore the fertile period is 4 to 8 days after the LH surge, with peak fertility occurring 5 to 6 days after the LH surge.

TECHNICIAN NOTE The bitch ovulates immature oocytes that require 2 to 3 more days for maturation.

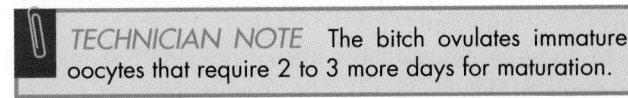

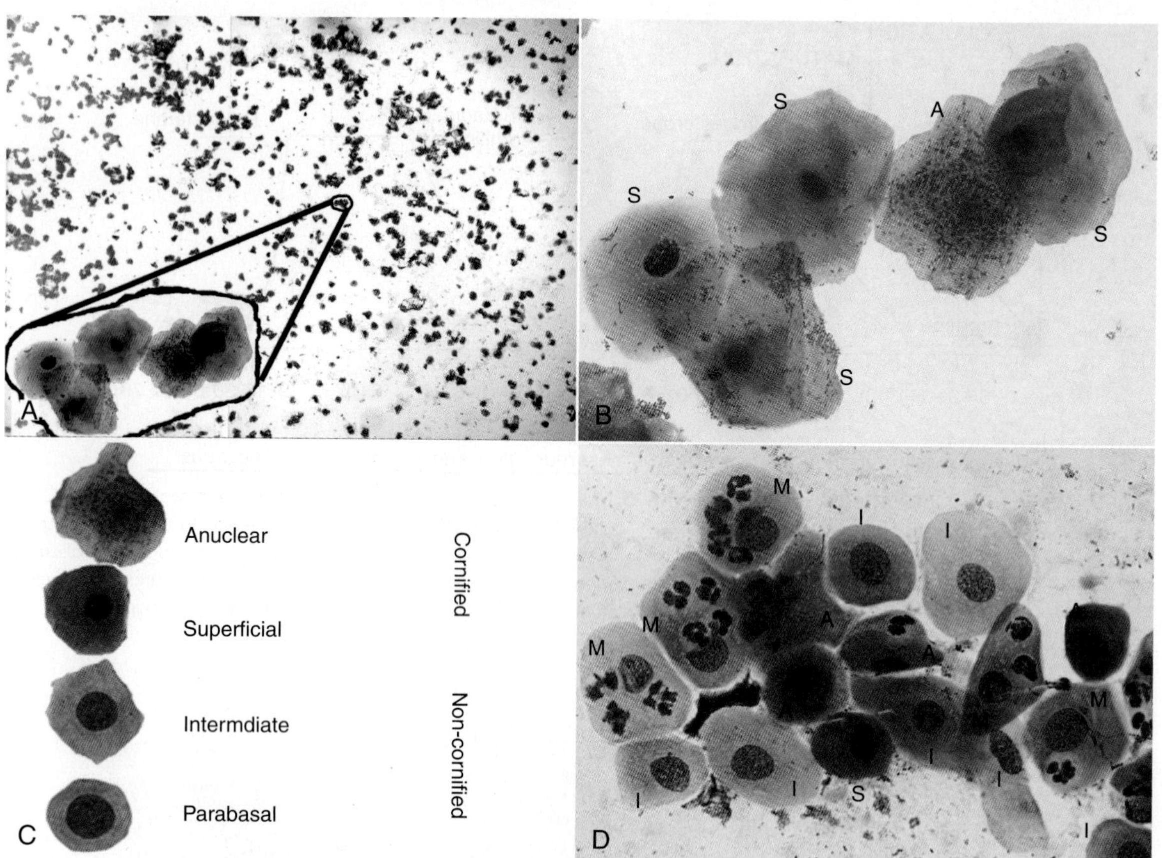

FIGURE 14-11 A low-power **(A)** and a high-power inset from the low-power view **(B)**, of a vaginal cytology sample of a dog in estrus. Cell types demonstrated in a canine vaginal cytology **(C)**. A high-power view **(D)** of a vaginal cytology of a dog in diestrus. The upper right and lower right cells are labeled with the cell type from the lower left (*M*, metestrum cell; *I*, intermediate; *S*, superficial; *A*, anuclear). (From Eilts, BE: Determining estrous status, *NAVC Clinicians Brief* 5:40-41, 2007.)

To best estimate the day of ovulation, hormone assays should be used. Vaginal cytology does not give a precise prediction of ovulation. The LH peak may occur anywhere from the same day of or up to 2 days after full cornification. Unlike most species, serum progesterone rises before ovulation in the bitch. Therefore progesterone is useful to predict the LH surge because the increase in serum progesterone is closely associated with the LH peak. Before the LH surge, serum progesterone is less than 1 ng/ml. On the day of the LH surge, serum progesterone rises to 1.5 to 2.0 ng/ml (2 ng progesterone = 3.18 nmol progesterone) and after that continues to rise during diestrus or pregnancy. By identifying this initial rise in progesterone, the day of the LH surge can be estimated and insemination performed during the period of peak fertility. Although LH can be measured semiquantitatively with in-house test kits (Figure 14-12), the peak only lasts 1 day, so serum must be tested daily. Progesterone assays provide some advantages because after the initial rise (on the same day as the LH surge), progesterone continues to rise, so the day of initial rise can be estimated even if a day is missed. Ovulation occurs 2 days after the LH rise and is associated with a progesterone concentration of 5 ng (15.90 nmol)/ml.

In-house, semiquantitative kits for progesterone analysis are available (Figure 14-13). The in-house tests are easy to perform, and results are available in about 20 minutes. Some aspects of the tests require attention to detail to achieve meaningful results. The kits need to be at room temperature before use, and the manufacturer's recommend that the kits be placed at room temperature for approximately 2 hours before use. If the test is run using a cold kit, results will be incorrect, often giving a false high progesterone. Blood should be allowed to clot at a cool temperature (in the refrigerator),

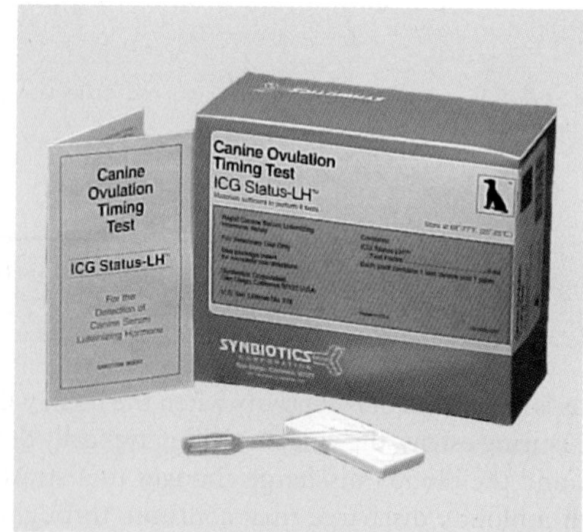

FIGURE 14-12 A commercially available kit to perform qualitative LH analysis.

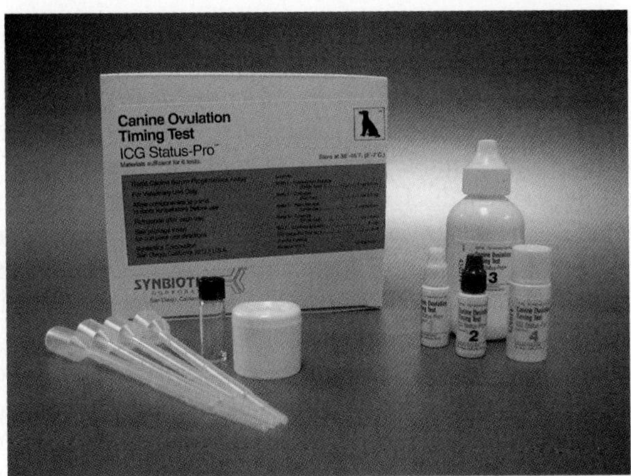

FIGURE 14-13 A commercially available kit to perform semiquantitative progesterone analysis.

and cells should be separated from serum or plasma as soon as possible (within 20 minutes of collection is the manufacturer's recommendation). If serum is allowed to remain in contact with the red blood cells, progesterone will be bound by them, and test results will be artificially low. Hemolyzed or lipemic samples may also cause erroneously low results. Serum samples may also be frozen for analysis later. If a laboratory is available that can give rapid turnaround time and provide quantitative results, this is preferable when breeding with frozen semen or any time breedings are limited.

If only two breedings are performed, such as with fresh cooled semen, insemination should be performed on either days 3 and 5 or days 4 and 6 after the LH peak or initial rise in progesterone, keeping in mind that the viability of fresh chilled semen is reduced, and the timing of insemination is more critical. The viability of frozen semen is reduced even further, and the timing is even more critical. When frozen semen is used, usually a single surgical insemination is conducted. Insemination with frozen semen should be performed on day 5 or 6 after the LH peak or initial rise in progesterone or 3 days after a progesterone level of 5 ng (15.90 nmol)/ml. Insemination with frozen semen is performed either surgically or by a transcervical endoscopic method. It is beneficial to continue to monitor vaginal cytology and identify D1 of diestrus, which usually occurs 8 days after the LH peak or 6 days after ovulation. Significant variations of the first day of diestrus from this expected time frame are associated with decreased fertility.

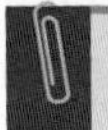

TECHNICIAN NOTE The fertile period is best identified using hormone assays for LH or progesterone.

VAGINAL CULTURES

Vaginal cultures can be taken from the bitch for various reasons, including prepubertal or postpubertal vaginitis, postparturient discharge, discharges during pregnancy, postabortion discharge, and prebreeding in normal or infertile bitches. Vaginal cultures are best performed with a guarded swab to prevent contamination as the culture swab is passed through the vestibule. If a culture is to be performed as part of a prebreeding examination and the client needs a negative culture before breeding, the performance and interpretation of the culture become critical. Bacteria, including mycoplasma, can be cultured from the vagina of the majority of fertile and infertile bitches. Once a culture has been obtained, it must be interpreted. If the culture was obtained as part of a work-up for a clinical problem, a pure culture is probably significant. However, a vaginal culture as part of a prebreeding examination in the absence of clinical signs often produces results of little significance.

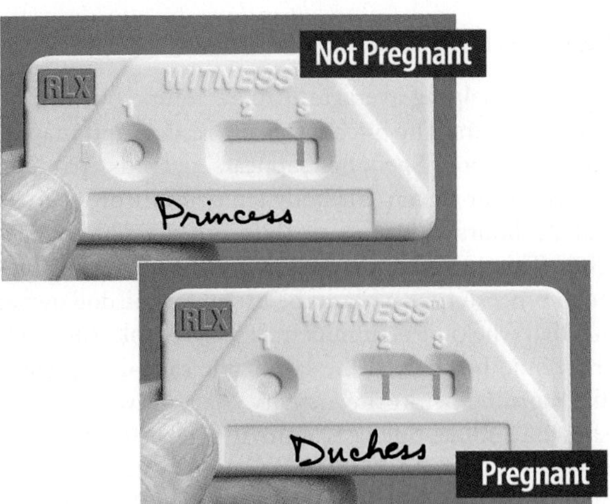

FIGURE 14-14 A commercially available kit to measure canine relaxin to determine pregnancy in a bitch.

CANINE PREGNANCY DIAGNOSIS

Pregnancy diagnosis can be performed by abdominal palpation, hormone assay, ultrasonography, or radiography. Palpation can be performed during a 7- to 10-day window beginning around day 21 after D1. After approximately day 30 post-D1, the embryonic vesicles become confluent and the ability to diagnose pregnancy by palpation is lost until late in gestation. Ultrasound can be used after approximately day 20 post-D1, possibly earlier, depending on the machine and probe used, until parturition. Radiography can be used after day 45 post-LH (day 37 post-D1). An in-house assay for relaxin is available and is reliable after about day 28 post-LH (day 20 post-D1) (Figure 14-14). When pregnancy testing, it is helpful to know the day of progesterone rise or D1 of diestrus to be able to estimate gestation length. Whereas gestation length seemingly can be as short as 55 days or as long as 70 days when timed from breeding, it is a reliable 57 to 58 days when timed from D1 of diestrus. Because a bitch is receptive to the male for 9 or 10 days, the timing from breeding is quite variable, resulting in errors (false-negative results) when examining for pregnancy or predicting whelping.

TECHNICIAN NOTE Pregnancy diagnosis can be performed by palpation, hormone assay, ultrasonography, or radiography.

PARTURITION AND DYSTOCIA

Stage I of whelping averages 6 to 12 hours, but can be as long as 36 hours. The bitch is usually restless and may show nesting behavior. She often appears nervous, pants, and may tremble or shiver. The body temperature drops to 99° F about 24 hours before stage II in approximately 85% of bitches. This temperature drop is related to the abrupt decline in progesterone and can be useful for the dog owner to signal that whelping is imminent. To be reliable, the temperature should be taken at the same time each day, preferably in the morning before any activity. Stage II, when the bitch pushes the puppies out, lasts approximately 20 to 60 minutes per puppy (Figure 14-15). However, no more than 2 hours should elapse between each delivery. Stage II usually lasts a total of 3 to 6 hours, but may be as long as 24 hours total. The presentation of the puppies is 60% anterior in the bitch. A blackish-green discharge is normal during parturition and comes from the site of placental attachment to the uterus.

Guidelines for recognizing dystocia (difficult birth) are strong continual contractions for 30 minutes without progress; weak, infrequent contractions for 2 hours without progress; or a prolonged interval between puppies. If any of these criteria are met, a veterinary examination is warranted. Ultrasound can be used to assess fetal viability, but radiography is the only reliable method to accurately determine the number of pups in utero, their relative size, and their position.

POSTPARTUM PROBLEMS

The bitch has the longest postpartum uterine involution period of the domestic species. A nonodorous hemorrhagic vulvar discharge is normal for 8 to 10 weeks after whelping and does not indicate metritis. Clients are often concerned when a bloody discharge persists for that length of time, but should be reassured that it is normal. When the discharge persists for a prolonged period, such as 12 weeks or more, the bitch is considered to have subinvolution of the placental sites (SIPS).

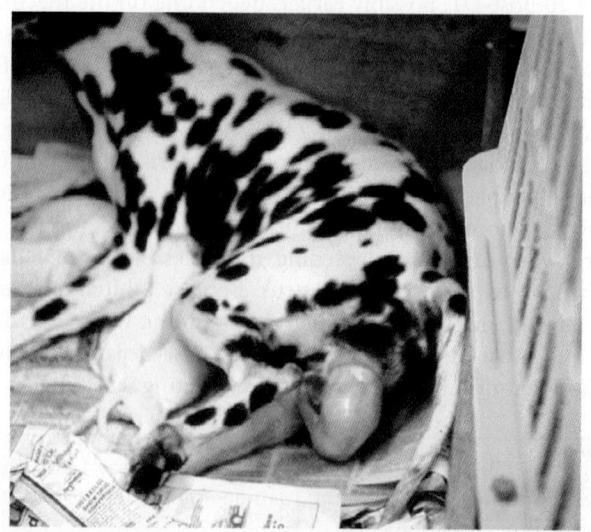

FIGURE 14-15 A puppy delivered during a normal canine parturition.

Treatment in these cases can be medical (ergonovine), surgical (ovariohysterectomy), or conservative (monitoring).

Indications that a bitch is suffering from postpartum problems include signs of discomfort, such as crying and whining, by the pups. Metritis is characterized by a foul-smelling vaginal discharge. Retained placenta results in a green discharge. Clinical signs of mastitis in the dam include fever, lethargy, and swollen mammary glands. The glands may be discolored. In many cases of metritis or mastitis, the pups will need to be hand fed or at least supplemented.

Eclampsia, or hypocalcemia, is characterized by tremors and excitation and is more common in smaller breeds. It most commonly occurs in the postpartum period. It is a true emergency. Hyperthermia and convulsions may require sedation or short-term anesthesia in addition to calcium treatment.

PSEUDOPREGNANCY

All bitches experience a 57- to 58-day period of elevated serum progesterone after estrus, whether pregnant or not. As progesterone declines at the end of a nonpregnant diestrus, many bitches, even if not pregnant, will experience mammary development, lactation, and maternal behavior. Clients may be concerned that the bitch is uncomfortable, or the behavioral changes may be unacceptable. With time, clinical signs will fade, and the bitch will return to normal. Alternatively, hormonal treatment with the prolactin inhibitor cabergoline or the androgen mibolerone can be used. Treatment with a progestogen, such as megestrol acetate, is contraindicated because signs of pseudopregnancy will return when therapy is halted.

Pyometra (uterine infection) can be a life-threatening situation in the bitch. It is progesterone related, usually occurring during diestrus, and may follow inappropriate estrogen therapy. The bitch may have a vaginal discharge depending on whether the cervix is open or closed. A bitch with pyometra is often lethargic, depressed, febrile, and exhibits polyuria and polydipsia. A leukocytosis is found on a complete blood count (CBC). Palpation or ultrasonography reveals an enlarged, fluid-filled uterus. If the breeding potential of the bitch is to be preserved, medical treatment with prostaglandins, cabergoline, and antibiotics is indicated; otherwise, surgical treatment (ovariohysterectomy) is usually recommended.

> *TECHNICIAN NOTE* A bitch with pyometra is often lethargic, depressed, and febrile and exhibits polyuria and polydipsia.

MISMATING

It is not unusual to have a client bring in a dog that has been bred accidentally or escaped while in estrus and request that she be "mismated" (aborted). In the past, few options were available other than estradiol cypionate (ECP), ovariohysterectomy, or allowing her to whelp. The use of ECP is not without risks. If given late in estrus or at the beginning of diestrus, there is a significant risk of pyometra. Another serious potential complication with the use of ECP is aplastic anemia. Further, many bitches seen for mismating may actually not have been bred or will not become pregnant. In one report, more than half of the bitches seen for pregnancy termination were not pregnant and would have been treated needlessly. For these reasons and the availability of suitable alternatives, the use of ECP for mismating is no longer recommended, and it is no longer manufactured in the United States. In many cases, the preferred method is to wait until such time as pregnancy diagnosis can be performed. If the bitch is pregnant, therapeutic options include prostaglandins, cabergoline, bromocriptine, or dexamethasone.

Prostaglandins effectively terminate pregnancy and are safe in dogs if used properly. Prostaglandins should be given subcutaneously, rather than intramuscularly. Further, a single dose will be ineffective in lysing the corpora lutea, so multiple small doses are used, usually two or three times per day for 5 to 7 days. Side effects include vomiting, diarrhea, and urination. An uncommon complication is cardiovascular collapse. Therefore an intravenous catheter is often recommended during the initial phases of treatment in case fluid therapy is necessary.

An alternative to prostaglandins is cabergoline (or a related compound, bromocriptine). Both are dopamine agonists, and administration will result in progesterone decline and pregnancy loss. Bromocriptine may be associated with vomiting, whereas cabergoline causes few side effects.

Dexamethasone is an attractive alternative to the previously mentioned drugs. It is administered orally, so it can be given at home. With any of these drugs, it is important to monitor pregnancy loss and continue therapy until abortion is complete. In addition, if the pregnancy is advanced when therapy is begun, it is important to inform the client that fetal discharge may be observed.

BRUCELLOSIS

Canine brucellosis, although typically thought of as a disease characterized by abortion and infertility, may manifest itself in a variety of ways. Although usually considered a venereal disease, *Brucella canis* is also spread through oronasal routes. Aborted fetuses and vaginal discharges are rich sources of *B. canis* organisms. Infected males shed the organism in their urine in addition to their semen. Transmission can occur between adult dogs in the absence of aborted material or sexual contact.

Because *B. canis* is an intracellular organism, the disease is extremely difficult to treat effectively, and cures are nearly impossible to achieve. No treatment has been found that is 100% effective in achieving a cure, although serum titers may decrease. Because of the nature of the disease and the potential for spread, euthanasia is commonly recommended for breeding animals in a kennel situation. A less drastic choice for pets is neutering and antibiotic therapy, although a persistent infection is still likely.

Because of the finality of neutering or euthanasia, a correct diagnosis is imperative. Unfortunately, many testing methods result in a high incidence of false-positive results and can be regarded as screening tests only. For example, antibodies against antigens of *Pseudomonas aeruginosa, Bordetella bronchiseptica,* and some *Staphylococcus spp.* can cause a false-positive result in a brucellosis test. Therefore a positive reaction on a screening test does not mean a dog is infected, but does suggest the need for a further, more definitive diagnosis.

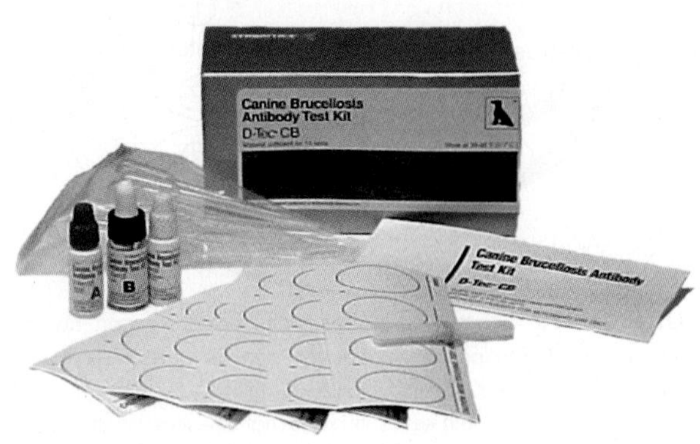

FIGURE 14-16 A commercially available kit to check for *B. canis.*

The in-house screening test (D-Tec CB, Synbiotics) is rapid and sensitive. False-positive results are common (20% to 50% of dogs with positive test results do not have brucellosis, and some breeds, such as English sheepdogs, have exceptionally high false-positive rates) (Figure 14-16). A negative result is highly accurate, provided the infection did not occur within 3 to 4 weeks before testing. Screening tests can give a false-negative result when a dog is infected for less than 4 weeks or is chronically infected and has recently received antibiotic treatment. If a dog has a positive result on the in-house test, samples should then be submitted to a diagnostic laboratory for further testing with a more specific test.

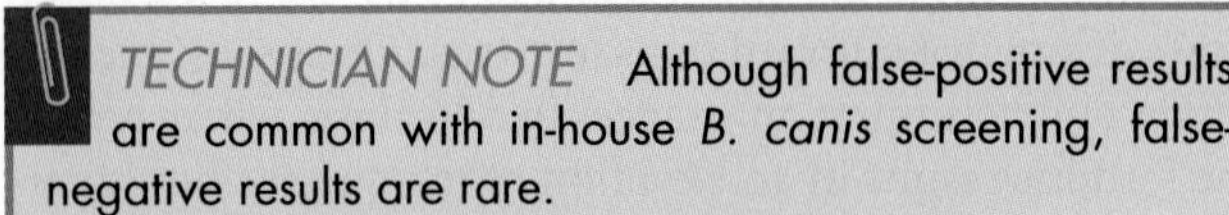
TECHNICIAN NOTE Although false-positive results are common with in-house *B. canis* screening, false-negative results are rare.

FELINE REPRODUCTION

Although most species have a spontaneous LH surge that causes ovulation during every estrous cycle, the queen must have vaginal stimulation to induce an LH surge. The queen is therefore an induced ovulator. Because the queen does not necessarily ovulate during each estrous cycle, there are unique aspects in the queen's estrous cycle that are not seen in other species. When a queen comes into estrus, there are three potential outcomes after estrus: the queen can ovulate and become pregnant, the queen can ovulate and not become pregnant, or the queen may not ovulate (Figure 14-17). Each of these outcomes results in a different series of subsequent events and time sequences for a return to estrus. The outcomes also depend on the season of the year because queens are seasonal breeders.

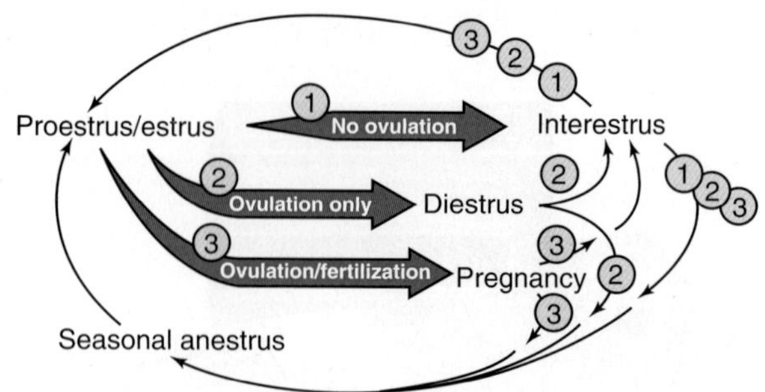

FIGURE 14-17 The feline estrous cycle. Depending on the season and whether ovulation occurs, the queen can do one of six things on entering an 8-day estrus. 1. If ovulation is not induced, the queen can go into a 2- to 14-day interestrus or seasonal anestrus. 2. If the queen ovulates but is not pregnant, a 36-day diestrus followed by either a 2- to 14-day interestrus or seasonal anestrus can occur. 3. If the queen ovulates and is pregnant, a 65-day pregnancy followed by either a 2- to 6-week interestrus or seasonal anestrus may occur.

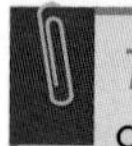
TECHNICIAN NOTE The queen is an induced ovulator.

SEASONALITY

Most queens have estrous cycles during the spring and are considered long-day breeders. This may be masked by the fact that most domestic cats are kept indoors under artificial lighting. The artificial lighting may be sufficient to stimulate estrous cycles all year long. The season and effect of artificial lighting must always be taken into account when discussing the queen's estrous cycle.

ESTROUS CYCLE

Proestrus in the queen is only 1 to 3 days long and may not be apparent. Estrus in the queen lasts 8 to 10 days, and the queen shows distinctive outward signs of estrus. These signs include rolling and assuming an exaggerated lordosis when petted. The lordosis results in an elevation of the queen's hindquarters. These signs are so intense that queens in estrus may be brought in for neurologic problems. Unlike other species that automatically enter a diestrus period of progesterone domination after estrus, the queen must have adequate vaginal stimulation to ovulate. The vaginal stimulation must come after the third day of estrus, and there must be multiple stimulations at least 2 to 3 hours apart to induce an LH rise of sufficient magnitude and duration to cause ovulation. Even if breeding does occur, vaginal stimulation will not necessarily be adequate to elicit a sufficient LH rise to cause ovulation.

If the queen ovulates and becomes pregnant, the gestation period is 63 to 66 days after mating. After parturition, the queen undergoes an anestrous period of variable duration. Anestrus is a time when nothing is happening on the ovaries, and the queen does not come into estrus. Postpartum anestrus may be as short as 2 weeks or as long as 6 weeks. Depending on the season and/or lighting conditions, the queen may return to proestrus or go into seasonal anestrus.

If a queen is bred, ovulates, but does not become pregnant, a diestrus (or pseudopregnancy) of approximately 40 days follows the estrus. During diestrus, the queen has a high concentration of progesterone in the blood that is produced by the corpora lutea on the ovaries that prevents the return to estrus. These corpora lutea apparently have a finite life span and cannot be lysed with exogenous prostaglandins, as in the bitch. After a nonpregnant diestrus, a short anestrus occurs. This anestrus is approximately 2 weeks long. Depending on the season and/or lighting conditions, the queen may return to proestrus or enter a seasonal anestrus.

If the queen is not bred or is bred and has insufficient stimulation to cause an LH surge, ovulation will not take place. If there is no ovulation, the follicles on the ovary regress. At this time, there are no structures on the ovaries (follicles or CLs), so this is called anestrus. This is a transitory anestrus, so a better term is interestrus. Depending on the season and/or lighting conditions, the interestrus may be 3 to 14 days or may extend into a long seasonal anestrus.

TECHNICIAN NOTE Pregnancy can be diagnosed in the queen from 16 to 30 days postcoitus by abdominal palpation, after 14 days postcoitus to term by ultrasound, and after 43 days by radiography.

Pregnancy can be diagnosed in the queen 16 to 30 days postcoitus by abdominal palpation, after 14 days postcoitus to term by ultrasound, and after 43 days postcoitus to term by radiography. Palpation must be done within a limited time frame because the gestational sacs are too small before day 16 and they become too confluent after day 30 to distinguish. Ultrasound can detect if the fetus is alive by seeing the fetal heartbeat, but it is difficult to count the number of fetuses and to estimate their size. Radiography is the best method to count the number of conceptuses and to estimate their size, but fetal mineralization of the skeleton must be adequate to detect them radiographically.

COMMON REPRODUCTIVE PROBLEMS

Queens are generally fertile and have few infertility problems. Because most pet queens have ovariohysterectomies performed at an early age, few of these queens are seen for reproductive problems.

The most common questions arise from the clinical signs that accompany estrus in the queen and irritate the owner. Queens that have not undergone an ovariohysterectomy may be seen for prolonged estrus. Although cystic ovaries do occur in queens, they are not often the cause of the prolonged estrus. More commonly a queen with persistent estrus is undergoing normal estrus, with a short 1- to 2-day interestrus, followed by another estrus. This makes it seem like the queen is in constant estrus, when there are normal periods of estrus and interestrus occurring. Treatment for this condition is either performing an ovariohysterectomy or induction of ovulation.

Ovulation can be induced by vaginal stimulation with a cotton swab, glass rod, or thermometer. The stimulations must meet the same criteria as breeding to be effective: the vaginal stimulation must come after the third day of estrus, and there must be multiple stimulations at least 2 to 3 hours apart to induce an LH rise sufficient to cause ovulation. An alternative to vaginal stimulation is the administration of GnRH or human chorionic gonadotropin (hCG). The GnRH will cause an endogenous release of LH from the anterior pituitary, thereby resulting in ovulation. The drug hCG has LH action and will directly cause ovulation. After ovulation induction, estrus will not be shortened; however, the queen will then enter diestrus and interestrus phases, so estrus will not recur for approximately 2 months. There are no drugs approved to control the estrous cycle in the queen.

Another common complaint is the queen that comes into estrus after an ovariohysterectomy. It is important to document the presence of extra ovarian tissue by hormone analysis. This is most easily done using the same techniques to induce ovulation. If the queen goes out of estrus and has high progesterone, then extra ovarian tissue must be sought surgically. If not, then the adrenal glands may be the source of the estrogen causing the signs of estrus.

Parturition in the queen (queening) can last as long as 36 hours. The following criteria can be used to diagnose dystocia (abnormal birth): 20 minutes of intense labor with no kitten, 10 minutes of intense labor when a kitten is present, acute depression, or the presence of fresh blood for more than 10 minutes. If any of these criteria are noted, it is advised that the queen be examined. Although most queens do not have problems queening, an examination and radiographs will help rule out if a cesarean delivery is required.

The normal postpartum discharge is a red-black, nonodorous fluid that can be seen as long as 3 weeks after queening. If the queen appears depressed or the kittens are dying, the queen should be examined for mastitis or metritis.

> *TECHNICIAN NOTE* The normal postpartum discharge is a red-black, nonodorous fluid that can be seen as long as 3 weeks after queening.

Pyometra in the queen has similar signs as seen in the bitch, including depression and vaginal discharge. Bitches with pyometra tend to be older, whereas queens can be any age.

EQUINE REPRODUCTION

Mares are seasonally polyestrous, meaning that during the breeding season they cycle repeatedly. The natural breeding season centers around the period of long day length. Under natural conditions, mares begin cycling in late March or early April and continue until September or October. Some mares may continue to cycle year round. In the northern hemisphere, many breed associations have designated Jan. 1 as the birth date for all horses born in a given year. This means that a horse born in January and a horse born in June will both be considered 1 year old the following January when they are actually 12 months and 7 months old, respectively. This is a large difference for horses competing as 2 year olds. Therefore there is a great deal of pressure to have foals born early in the season (January or February), but many mares are not cycling at this time. The most cost-effective method to stimulate earlier cyclicity is to "trick" the mare into perceiving that the days are lengthening by providing artificial lighting and mimicking a 16-hour daylight period. This should be started by December 1 to get the most benefit. A 200-watt bulb in a 12 × 12-foot stall is sufficient. For an outdoor situation, eight 1000-watt metal halide floodlights at a height of 20 feet will provide sufficient light for an 84 × 66-foot paddock. Artificial lighting should be added in the evening, rather than in the morning. Turning the lights on earlier in the morning is less effective than leaving them on later in the evening.

During the breeding season, the mare's estrous cycle averages 21 to 22 days in length. Diestrus, the period when a CL is present and producing progesterone, is a consistent 15 days in length based on hormone levels (Figure 14-18). During this time, the mare will tease "out," resisting the stallion's advances by kicking, squealing, pinning her ears back, and clamping her tail between her legs. Based on behavioral signs, diestrus is shorter (approximately 14 days) because she does not tease out until 1 day or so after ovulation. Estrus, or the period of receptivity, is shown by teasing "in." The mare squats, urinates, lifts her tail, and "winks" (everts her clitoris) on the approach of the stallion.

> *TECHNICIAN NOTE* Estrus, or the period of receptivity, is shown by teasing "in."

Between the noncycling period (anestrus) and the cycling period, a period called transition occurs. Transition varies in length and is characterized by irregular periods of estrous behavior, but without ovulation. A mare may exhibit estrous behavior for 2 or 3 days, then stop for a few days, and then begin again. Alternatively the mare may exhibit estrous behavior continuously without ovulation for 3 weeks or more. Although follicles may be present during these periods, they do not ovulate. The transitional period is a physiologically normal occurrence. Although cyclicity can be induced earlier in the year, a transitional period will still precede the onset of cyclicity. An awareness of this can help to reduce needless breedings and help mare owners understand this sometimes aggravating period. The administration of altrenogest, a synthetic progestogen, will stop the estrous behavior and is often used during transition.

During the breeding season, the duration of estrus is variable (4 to 7 days). Estrus tends to be shorter near the peak of the breeding season (June) and longer further away from June, such as March or September. Follicular development can be monitored by palpation per rectum and ultrasonography during estrus to decide optimal breeding time.

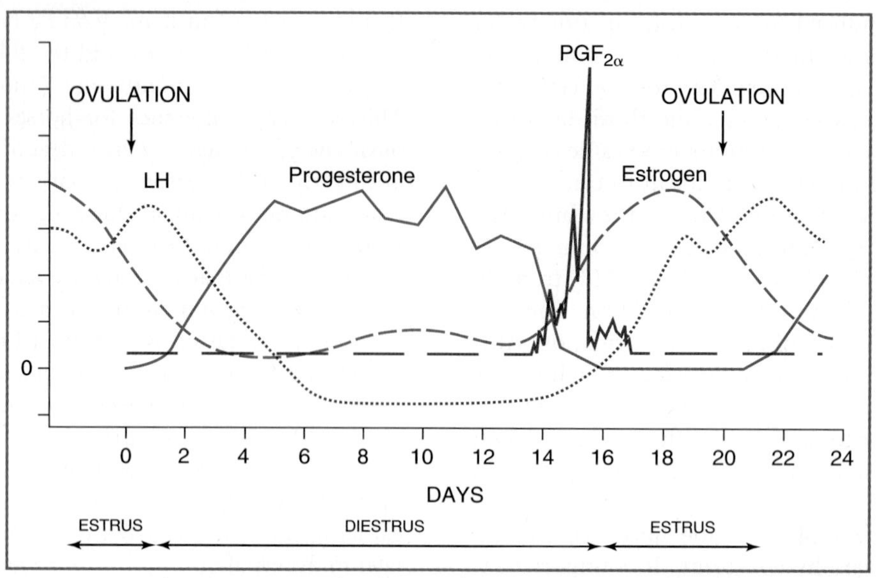

FIGURE 14-18 The equine estrous cycle. Estrus is 4 to 7 days long, and LH peaks after ovulation. Diestrus begins around 2 days after ovulation. Progesterone is high throughout a 14- to 15-day diestrus. If a pregnancy signal is not secreted by the early embryo by day 14 to 16, prostaglandin is released from the uterus, goes to the CL, and causes luteolysis (luteal death). The cycle then starts over.

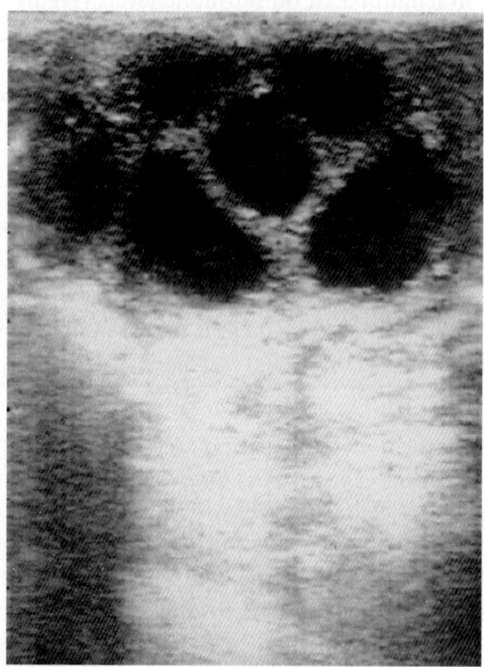

FIGURE 14-19 An ultrasound image of the black appearance of multiple follicles on an equine ovary.

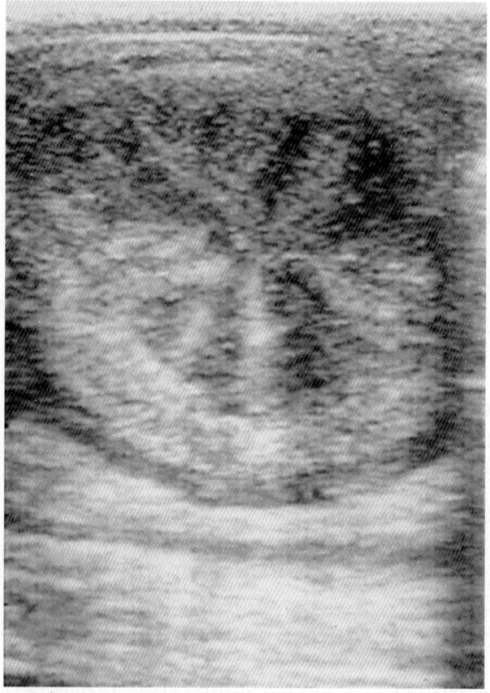

FIGURE 14-20 The "sliced-orange" ultrasonographic appearance of the uterus of a mare in estrus.

BREEDING SOUNDNESS EXAMINATION

Breeding soundness examinations are commonly performed at the sale or purchase of a mare or when a mare fails to become pregnant after breeding. A typical breeding soundness examination consists of palpation per rectum, ultrasonography, a vaginal speculum examination, uterine culture and cytology, and a uterine biopsy. During the ultrasonographic examination, structures on the ovaries and, more importantly, features of the uterus can be observed. Fluid-filled structures, such as follicles (Figure 14-19) and endometrial cysts will be black. Corpora lutea have a variable appearance, ranging from a rather homogeneous gray to a "spider web" trabecular pattern with a brighter thick-walled circumference. An important indication of the stage of the estrous cycle is the ultrasonographic appearance of the uterus. During diestrus, it has a homogeneous hyperechoic appearance, but in estrus it has a characteristic appearance caused by edema in the endometrial folds. It has been described as looking like the spokes of a cartwheel, a sliced orange, or pizza (Figure 14-20).

A vaginal speculum examination, uterine culture and cytology, and uterine biopsy are performed aseptically. First, wrap the tail with a clean tail wrap or gauze. Prepare a clean bucket with clean water and add small (approximately 10 cm × 10 cm) pieces of cotton. Rather than placing disinfectant in the bucket, it is preferable to place the soap on the cotton itself before scrubbing the vulva, thereby leaving clean water to rinse the vulva. Otherwise, disinfectant residues may remain on the vulva and be carried into the vagina, with a potential spermicidal or tissue-irritating effect. Cleansing of the perineal area should be done using the "clean hand-dirty hand" technique. One hand (the clean hand) is used to retrieve clean pieces of cotton from the bucket. The cotton is then transferred to the other hand (the dirty hand), which is then used to scrub the perineal area. This method keeps the bucket with clean water and cotton from being contaminated. The vulvar labia should be scrubbed in a manner similar to that for surgical preparation (i.e., from the center of the area being cleaned to the perimeter and repeated until clean). Check the inside of the labia during the procedure to be sure no feces have entered as a result of the palpation and ultrasonography procedures.

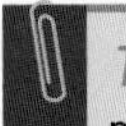

TECHNICIAN NOTE All vaginal procedures in mares should be performed aseptically.

A vaginal speculum examination can discern trauma to the cervix; discharge emanating from the uterus, cervix, or vagina; urine pooling in the cranial vagina; and other conditions associated with subfertility. After aseptically preparing the vulva, a small amount of sterile lubricant is placed on the end of a speculum, the labia are parted, and the speculum is placed into the vagina. A light source is then used to look through the speculum and examine the vagina and cervix (Figure 14-21).

The next procedure usually performed is a uterine culture and cytology. The importance of performing a cytologic examination in conjunction with the culture cannot be overstated. Without a cytologic specimen, it is impossible to differentiate between an infectious process and a contaminant resulting from improper sampling or mare preparation. When obtaining a culture and cytology specimen, only guarded swabs should be used. After aseptically preparing the vulva, a sterile sleeve is used to introduce the culture-cytology instrument into the vagina, through the cervix, and into the uterus. After the swab is withdrawn, the sample can be used to prepare a cytology specimen. Stain the cytology slide using a modified Wright's or Giemsa stain. The slide should contain numerous epithelial cells and be examined for inflammatory cells, primarily neutrophils. A positive cytology slide will contain numerous inflammatory cells, whereas a negative slide will not. Bacteria isolated from a culture with a negative cytology finding can be considered contaminants. An argument can be made to not submit the culture if the cytology slide is negative. However, if the cytology slide is positive, not only do culture results reveal the causative agent, but also sensitivity results aid in making a therapeutic choice. Excess lubricant used during the procedure can interfere with the interpretation by staining darkly and obscuring the field.

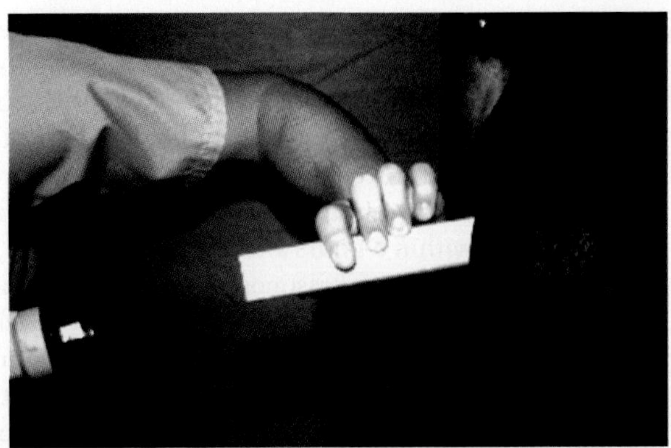

FIGURE 14-21 A vaginal speculum examination performed on a mare using a disposable speculum.

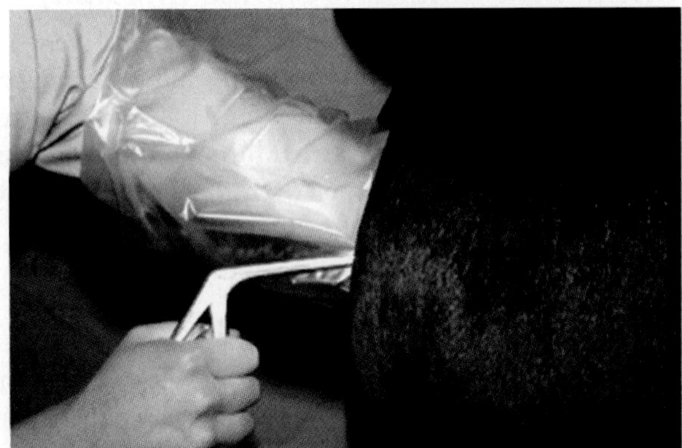

FIGURE 14-22 A uterine biopsy instrument inserted through the vagina and cervix into the uterus.

TECHNICIAN NOTE Endometrial cytology should always be performed in conjunction with an endometrial culture to aid in the interpretation of results.

The next, and often final, step in the breeding soundness examination is to obtain an endometrial biopsy. As with the previous procedures, it is done in an aseptic manner. The closed instrument is carried into the uterus, wearing a sterile sleeve (Figure 14-22). The instrument is held in the uterus while the hand is withdrawn and placed in the rectum. The instrument is then opened to permit endometrial tissue to enter the jaws and then closed to snip off a piece of endometrium. The tissue is next placed in a fixative and processed through a laboratory.

BREEDING MANAGEMENT

Monitoring follicular development by palpation and ultrasonography per rectum allows the mare to be inseminated close to ovulation. This has numerous benefits, including making sure that sperm are present when the oocyte is released, minimizing overuse of a stallion, and reducing the number of times a mare is bred during an estrus. Reducing the number of breedings per estrus becomes more important as a mare's fertility declines. When breeding a mare with fresh cooled or frozen semen, daily or even more frequent examinations are usually performed. With fresh cooled semen use, the semen is usually ordered after a follicle reaches 35 mm in diameter, and semen is shipped overnight to the mare's location. With frozen semen, the semen is stored in liquid nitrogen, and insemination must occur within 24 hours before to within 6 hours after ovulation.

After a mare is bred, an ultrasonographic examination is usually preformed the following day (possibly sooner or later depending on the mare and the particular situation) to confirm that ovulation has occurred and to examine the uterus for the presence of fluid. The failure of a mare to clear the fluid from the uterus after breeding has been associated with decreased fertility and is the reason for many postbreeding treatments.

Artificial Insemination (Uterine Infusion)

Breeding a mare by artificial insemination is a relatively simple procedure. It is an aseptic procedure, and the same procedure is used for uterine infusion as for AI. A sterile sleeve is donned and a sterile pipette carried through the vagina and cervix into the uterus. The semen or intrauterine medication is then deposited directly into the uterus.

Postbreeding Treatments

If fluid is detected in the uterus by ultrasonography 8 hours or more after breeding, a treatment to aid uterine clearance is indicated. Oxytocin or cloprostenol are the two most commonly used drugs to stimulate uterine clearance.

In addition to oxytocin or cloprostenol injections, common postbreeding treatments include intrauterine infusion of antibiotics and uterine lavage. Intrauterine infusion and lavage are performed in the same aseptic manner using sterile equipment as AI.

Uterine lavage is performed using a large-bore catheter with an inflatable cuff (Figure 14-23). The catheter is placed in the uterus, and the cuff is inflated and seated against the internal cervical os to provide a good seal. Sterile saline, usually 1 L at a time, is infused into the uterus and then retrieved. This is repeated until the saline retrieved is clear. This procedure helps to clear the uterus of debris.

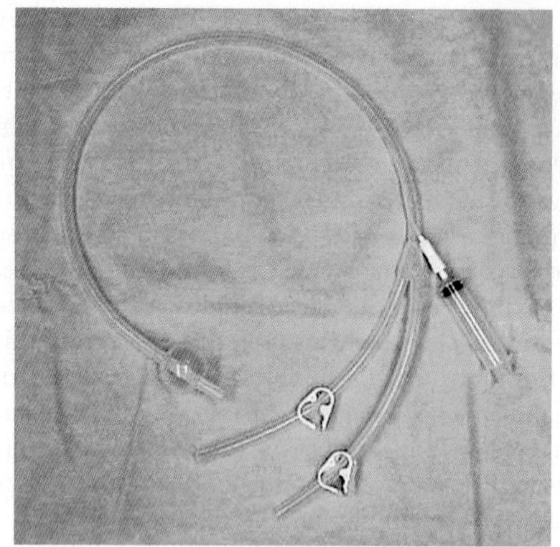

FIGURE 14-23 A large-bore catheter used to lavage a mare's uterus.

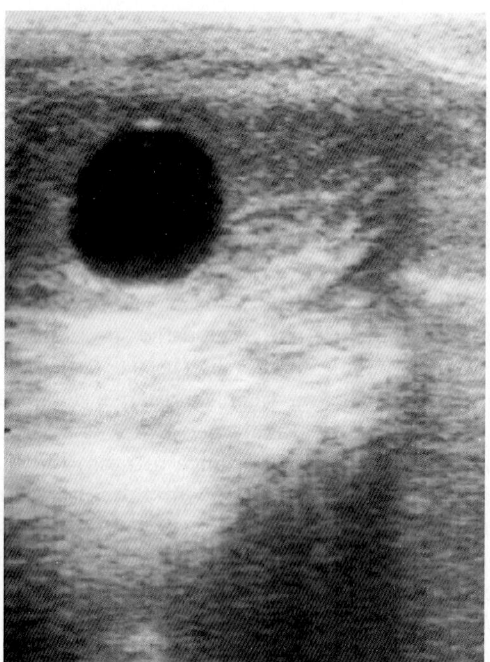

FIGURE 14-24 An ultrasound image of a 14-day pregnancy in an equine uterus.

EQUINE PREGNANCY DIAGNOSIS

Pregnancy diagnosis is usually done with the aid of ultrasonography 2 weeks after ovulation. With experience, the characteristic ultrasonographic appearance of the conceptus at various stages can be easily recognized and used to evaluate its growth and health (Figure 14-24). The term conceptus refers to everything derived from the fertilized ovum, including the fetal membranes and fluids the embryo or fetus. Fetal sexing is most commonly performed between 60 and 70 days by identifying the position of the genital tubercle.

> *TECHNICIAN NOTE* A pregnancy examination in the mare is usually performed 14 days after ovulation with the aid of ultrasonography.

Hormonal methods for pregnancy diagnosis exist. They can be useful in cases where palpation per rectum is not feasible, such as with small miniature horses or wild, fractious mares. Pregnant mares will have a positive result for equine chorionic gonadotropin (eCG), formerly called pregnant mare serum gonadotropin (PMSG), from 35 days until approximately 120 days of gestation. False-positive results happen if fetal death occurs during that period. Another hormone used for pregnancy testing is estrone sulfate. The benefit of estrone sulfate compared with eCG is that it is produced in high quantities by a viable feto-placental unit beginning around 60 days of gestation. If the pregnancy is lost, estrone sulfate drops off rapidly, so false-positive results are uncommon. Progesterone cannot be used to test for pregnancy because it is elevated during diestrus in nonpregnant mares and during gestation in pregnant mares.

VACCINATIONS

Equine herpesvirus can be a significant cause of abortion in horses. Vaccines are available, and a good program consists of vaccination at 5, 7, and 9 months of gestation. Either a killed-virus or modified live-virus vaccine may be used. Repeated vaccinations at these intervals are necessary each time a mare is pregnant to provide good protection. In addition, it is advisable to minimize stress, and it is important to keep pregnant mares separated from new additions to the herd or horses that have significant outside contact.

It is also recommended to give an annual booster for flu, encephalitis (Eastern, Western, West Nile), and tetanus at 10 months of gestation. This practice will help ensure good-quality colostrum and increase the protection level provided to the foal by passive transfer of antibodies through the colostrum. Additional information on preventive health programs is found in Chapter 9.

TECHNICIAN NOTE An annual booster vaccination given to the mare at 10 months gestation can improve the quality of the colostrum and enhance the foal's immunity.

Induction of Parturition

The gestation length in mares is generally quoted as 330 to 340 days. However, there is a wide variation in normal gestation length, ranging from 320 to 400 days. It is important to remember that the fetus determines the gestation length. For this reason, chemical induction of parturition based on the gestation length alone is risky and can result in the birth of premature foals. The decision to induce parturition is based on the following criteria:

1. Gestation length greater than 330 days
2. Relaxation of pelvic ligaments
3. Presence of colostrum in the udder
4. Relaxation or softening of the cervix
5. Most importantly, milk calcium more than 400 ppm with milk potassium higher than sodium

The electrolyte changes are well correlated with fetal maturity and are the best way to assess readiness for birth. Calcium can be measured with a water hardness test kit, but be sure to use one that measures only calcium, not just divalent cations. Magnesium, another divalent cation present in colostrum, rises slowly as parturition approaches and can interfere with the interpretation of the results. Milk calcium greater than 400 ppm and potassium less than sodium can occur in cases of placentitis or twins, so induction of parturition should not be considered unless potassium is greater than sodium, along with the increase in calcium.

PARTURITION

Parturition is a rapid process in horses. In the normal course of events as the mare begins labor (stage I), she will lie down, get up, roll, and so forth. During these maneuvers, the foal is getting into the correct position. Finally, at the end of stage I, the chorioallantois ruptures ("water breaks"), signaling the onset of stage II. Usually within 10 minutes, a bluish white membrane (amnion) appears at the vulvar opening. Within another 10 minutes, the feet will protrude through the vulva, still within the amnion. After another 10 minutes, the head protrudes, and delivery will be completed soon thereafter (Figure 14-25).

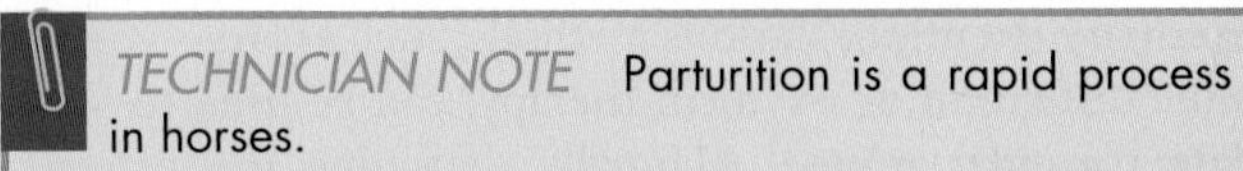

TECHNICIAN NOTE Parturition is a rapid process in horses.

A red membrane protruding from the vulva, the chorioallantois, is an indication of premature placental separation, or "red bag" (Figure 14-26). This is an emergency, and the chorioallantois must be ruptured manually and delivery assisted or the foal will quickly die.

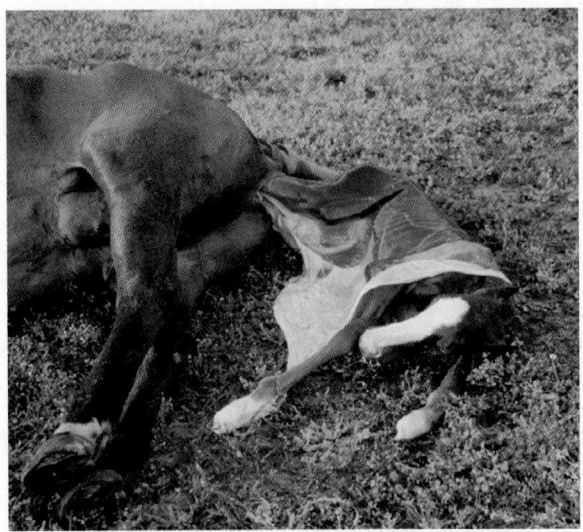

FIGURE 14-25 A foal delivered by a mare.

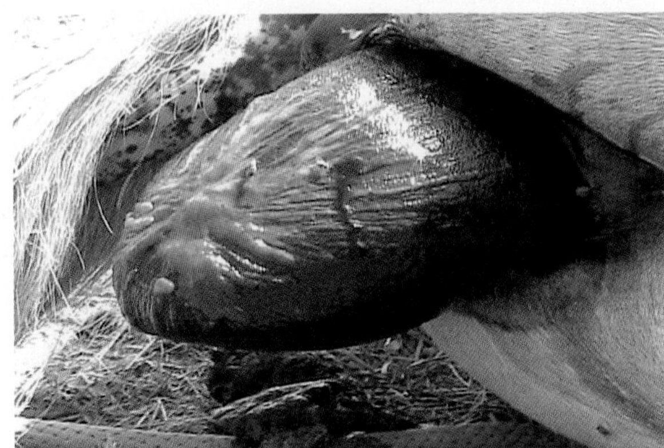

FIGURE 14-26 Premature placental separation ("red bag") during parturition in the mare. The chorioallantois is observed protruding through the vulvar opening.

If the guidelines for the time frame of delivery are not being met, an examination for possible dystocia is indicated. It is critical to perform any obstetric manipulations in as clean a manner as possible and with sufficient good-quality obstetric lubricant. The failure to adhere to guidelines of strict cleanliness and ample lubrication invites complications in the postpartum period and can compromise future fertility.

POSTPARTUM PROBLEMS

Mares do not experience postpartum problems as commonly as cows, but when they do, they can be life threatening. A retained placenta for more than 6 hours duration deserves veterinary attention. Various methods, such as large-volume saline distention or oxytocin therapy, can be used to stimulate placental release. Manually detaching the placenta should not be done because of the potential for causing damage to the uterus and hemorrhage. Systemic antibiotics, anti-inflammatories, and tetanus toxoid are usually administered in cases of placentas retained more than 6 hours.

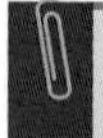

TECHNICIAN NOTE A retained placenta for more than 6 hours duration deserves veterinary attention.

A prolapsed uterus is a true emergency and must be dealt with as quickly as possible. Unfortunately, even with proper treatment, mortality can approach 50%. The mare should be restrained and the uterus protected from trauma until the veterinarian arrives.

The clinical signs of postpartum hemorrhage as a result of a ruptured uterine artery, usually either into the broad ligament or the abdomen, include signs of abdominal pain and pale mucous membranes. Mares exhibiting such signs in the postpartum period should be kept calm and quiet and be confined to a stall until examined by a veterinarian.

Postpartum metritis, often a sequela to retained placenta or contamination during obstetric procedures, can lead to septicemia and laminitis. As a result, treatment should not be delayed in a postpartum mare that has a foul-smelling vaginal discharge or is febrile or depressed.

HORMONE USE IN MARES

Prostaglandin

Prostaglandin F_{2a} and its analog cloprostenol can be used to lyse a CL and return a mare to estrus. It is effective beginning about 5 or 6 days after ovulation, when the CL has matured sufficiently to respond. Mares will return to estrus in 2 to 7 days after prostaglandin administration. Prostaglandins should not be used to induce parturition because of the high incidence of premature placental separation, dystocia, and fetal death.

Human Chorionic Gonadotropin

Human chorionic gonadotropin (hCG) is used to induce ovulation in mares that have a follicle 35 mm or larger. Doses commonly used range from 2000 to 3500 IU given intravenously, and ovulation can be expected to occur in 36 to 48 hours in approximately 80% of mares. Although concerns about antibody production have been expressed, no correlation between antibodies and the failure to induce ovulation has been shown. Nevertheless, some mares fail to ovulate after receiving HCG repeatedly.

Deslorelin

An alternative to hCG for ovulation induction is an analog of GnRH, deslorelin. Ovulation occurs within approximately the same time frame as with hCG. However, deslorelin appears to be more effective on slightly smaller (30-mm) follicles than hCG, and the failure of the mare to ovulate is reportedly less common.

Progestins

Altrenogest (Regu-Mate, Intervet) is a progesterone-like compound that is administered orally. It is used primarily for pregnancy maintenance and estrous cycle control. Its use for pregnancy maintenance is empiric in that true progesterone deficiency as a cause of pregnancy loss has not been documented. However, anecdotal reports of mares failing to maintain pregnancy unless supplemented with altrenogest are not uncommon. Because the fetoplacental unit eventually takes over progestogen production, altrenogest therapy can usually be discontinued at about 4 months of gestation.

The other reason to use altrenogest is estrous cycle control. Altrenogest mimics progesterone in the mare. Therefore mares given altrenogest act as if they are in diestrus. Altrenogest can be used for estrus synchronization in embryo transfer programs and to manipulate the estrous cycle to prevent or control the onset of estrus in performance mares. Altrenogest is also used in mares in late gestation when there is concern about possible impending abortion. Through its action, uterine motility is inhibited, thereby supporting maintenance of pregnancy.

Oxytocin

A common cause of infertility is persistent mating-induced endometritis. An inflammatory response to sperm cells normally occurs after breeding, whether by natural service or AI. This inflammatory response is necessary to remove excess semen and debris and to prepare the uterus for pregnancy. Uterine clearance mechanisms, such as uterine motility and lymphatic drainage, are critical in this process. Infertility results when uterine clearance mechanisms fail and fluid remains in the uterus after breeding. An ultrasound examination 12 hours or more after breeding should reveal no fluid in the uterus. If fluid is still present, oxytocin therapy (20 IU intravenously or intramuscularly) should be instituted. Oxytocin is effective in aiding uterine clearance and can be given as often as every 2 or 3 hours.

Oxytocin is also the only drug available to safely and reliably induce parturition. If the mare has met the criteria and is ready to give birth, a small dose (10 IU intravenously) of oxytocin is sufficient to initiate parturition. Lower doses result in a more natural process, whereas higher doses result in a faster and more forceful delivery.

Domperidone

Domperidone is a dopamine antagonist used to alleviate the effects of fescue toxicosis and stimulate lactation. It has also shown some promise to stimulate cyclicity in mares with lactational anestrus and may be beneficial in hastening the onset of cyclicity in the spring, but this has not yet been well documented.

BOVINE REPRODUCTION

The cow is a nonseasonal polyestrous species, meaning that cows have estrous cycles all year around. The entire estrous cycle averages 21 days long, but it can be as short as 18 days and as long as 24 days (Figure 14-27). Estrus lasts 18 to 20 hours, but may be shorter in hot, humid weather because of heat stress. Estrus is the time the cow is in "standing heat" and will stand with all four legs firmly braced to be mounted by a bull or another cow. Ovulation occurs 12 to 18 hours after the end of estrus. Estrus is followed by metestrus, which is 3 to 5 days long and is the time of luteal development. A bloody discharge from the vulva may be noticed in nearly half of all cows and heifers 1 or 2 days after they are in estrus. This bloody discharge is no indication of fertility or infertility, but merely a sign that the individual was in estrus 1 or 2 days earlier. During metestrus, a corpus hemorrhagicum (CH) is formed at the site of ovulation. This structure will develop into a CL over the next few days. However, during metestrus, the CL is not yet mature and not yet susceptible to the luteolytic action of prostaglandins. The next phase is called diestrus and lasts from day 5 or 6 until day 17 of the estrous cycle and is the time that the mature CL ("yellow body") is present and producing progesterone. During diestrus, there are waves of follicular growth that are important in understanding a cow's response to estrous cycle synchronization. At the end of diestrus, if an embryo is not present in the uterus to provide a pregnancy signal, the uterus releases a prostaglandin that lyses the CL, resulting in a decline of progesterone, and the cow returns to proestrus.

BOVINE PREGNANCY DIAGNOSIS

Various methods of pregnancy diagnosis exist, but the most commonly employed is palpation per rectum. An experienced person can diagnose pregnancy by 30 days of gestation. Ultrasonography is becoming more popular for pregnancy diagnosis. Machines have become more affordable, and accurate pregnancy diagnosis can be performed by 24 days or earlier in some cases. Fetal viability can be assessed, and fetal sexing is possible between 55 and 70 days.

> *TECHNICIAN NOTE* Various methods of pregnancy diagnosis exist, but the most commonly employed is palpation per rectum.

Progesterone tests should not be regarded as pregnancy tests. Although a progesterone test can detect the presence of a CL, many scenarios exist where a CL is present and progesterone is high, but the cow is not pregnant.

BREEDING/ARTIFICIAL INSEMINATION

Most dairy cattle, and increasing numbers of beef cattle, are bred by AI. There are numerous advantages to AI, with rapid genetic improvement being the primary one. However, the need for estrus detection to time insemination is a major drawback. Fortunately, cows, especially dairy cows, exhibit "standing heat" when in estrus, and observation of this

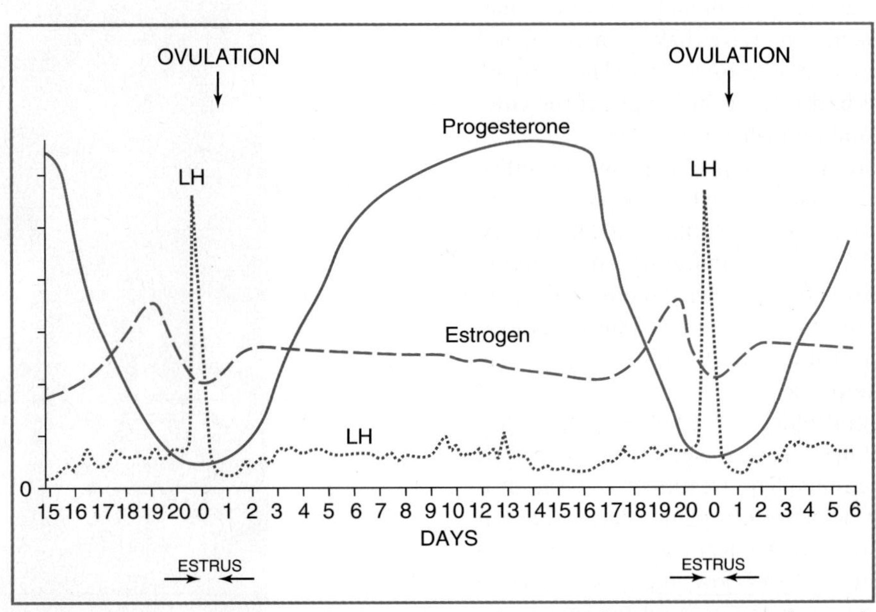

FIGURE 14-27 The bovine estrous cycle. Estrus is 12 to 18 hours long, and LH peaks during estrus. Diestrus lasts until about day 17, and progesterone is high throughout diestrus. If a pregnancy signal is not secreted by the early embryo by day 16 or 17, prostaglandin is released from the uterus, goes to the CL, and causes luteolysis (luteal death). The cycle then starts over.

behavior is the best method of estrus detection. "Teaser" bulls, bulls that have been surgically altered to prevent vaginal penetration with the penis and have had vasectomies to render them sterile, can be used to help with estrus detection.

Estrus synchronization, through the use of hormones, also helps improve estrus detection. Many schemes have been devised using prostaglandins to lyse the CL. Other schemes use progestogen to mimic the luteal phase and suppress follicular growth. An ear implant, Synchro-Mate B, containing the progestogen named norgestomet, has been successfully used for years in cattle, but it is no longer available in the United States as of the time of writing this chapter. Recently an intravaginal device has been approved for synchronization of estrus in dairy heifers and for synchronization of return to estrus in lactating dairy cattle. The product is called EAZI-BREED CIDR and contains 1.38 g of progesterone in silicone molded over a nylon spine. EAZI-BREED CIDR is the first and only approved source of progesterone for use in dairy cattle. EAZI-BREED CIDR can be used in association with prostaglandin F_{2a} (PGF_{2a}). Another popular method for synchronization of estrus involves an injection of GnRH at a random stage of the estrous cycle, followed by an injection of PGF_{2a} 7 days later, followed by a second injection of GnRH 48 hours later, and insemination 16 to 18 hours after that.

ABNORMALITIES OF THE ESTROUS CYCLE

Anestrus

The most common reason for the failure of a cow to show estrus is pregnancy, whether as a result of poor record keeping or an unknown visit by a neighboring bull. For this reason, it is always advisable to have a cow examined for pregnancy before attempting to "bring her into heat" with prostaglandins. After calving, a period of postpartum anestrus is common. This period is usually shorter for dairy cows (2 to 4 weeks depending on nutrition and environmental conditions) than for beef cows. Beef cows nursing calves have a longer period of postpartum anestrus, usually 45 to 90 days. The postpartum anestrus period in beef cattle is prolonged if the cows are not in good body condition when they calve.

Pathologic reasons for anestrus include pyometra, luteal cysts, and cystic ovarian disease (COD). Pyometra may be caused by a number of factors, including trichomoniasis, bovine viral diarrhea (BVD) virus, and postpartum uterine infection. It is characterized by a pus-filled uterus and a persistent CL. The treatment consists of simply administering a prostaglandin, although two injections 24 hours apart may be needed to improve response.

Luteal cysts arise from follicles that fail to ovulate, but do form luteal tissue. Progesterone is elevated, and a period of prolonged diestrus results. The treatment consists of a prostaglandin injection. COD results from follicles that fail to ovulate and do not form true luteal tissue. Progesterone secreted by thecal cells in the cyst is low, and although some cows may exhibit persistent or frequent estrus, anestrus is much more common. The treatment consists of GnRH or hCG administration.

ABNORMALITIES OF PREGNANCY

Uterine Prolapse

Uterine prolapse is easily recognized by the presence of the mucosal, or inner, surface of the uterus, with its characteristic caruncles, hanging from the vulva (Figure 14-28). It is more common in dairy than beef cattle. It occurs in the immediate postpartum period and is often associated with hypocalcemia or dystocia. Uterine prolapse should be considered an emergency, and the uterus should be replaced to its normal position as soon as possible. Uterine prolapse is not hereditary and is not considered likely to recur.

Vaginal Prolapse

Although seemingly similar to uterine prolapse, vaginal prolapse is actually quite different. This is a hereditary problem; therefore affected individuals should not be kept as breeding stock. It occurs under conditions associated with elevated estrogen, most commonly seen during late gestation, although it may also be associated with cystic follicular degeneration or the ingestion of certain plants. Typically the affected animal will be a beef cow or heifer in late gestation, and the vagina and possibly the cervix will be protruding from the vulva. Various methods have been described to treat the condition, but all consist of cleaning the exposed tissue, replacing it, and preventing recurrence. It must be remembered that in most cases,

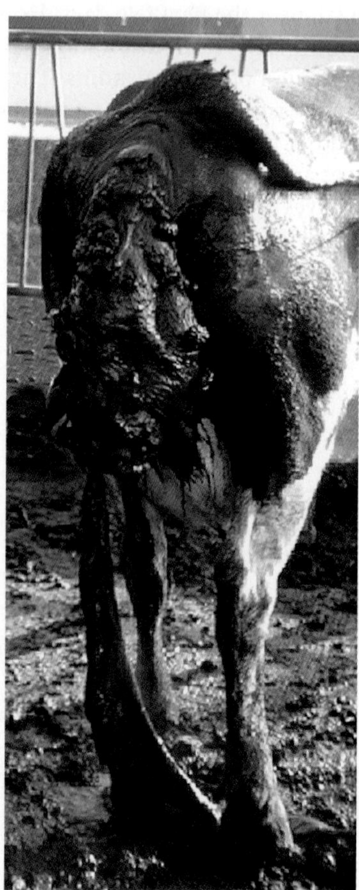

FIGURE 14-28 A bovine uterine prolapse. Note the caruncles on the exposed interior uterine surface.

the cow will not have calved yet, so care will need to be taken to monitor her to reduce the chance of dystocia and mortality.

Dystocia

Dystocia is much more common in cattle than in mares. It is most commonly caused by fetal-maternal disproportion in size. Uterine torsion is also a fairly common cause of dystocia. As with mares, cleanliness and lubrication are essential for successful management of dystocia.

Milk Fever

Milk fever, or parturient hypocalcemia, most commonly occurs during the postpartum period, although it may also occur during parturition. It is more common in dairy cattle than beef cattle. Milk fever is characterized by flaccid paralysis. The incidence is increased when cattle are fed high levels of calcium prepartum. This condition should be viewed as an emergency and is treated by a slow intravenous infusion of calcium gluconate or oral administration of a calcium-containing gel.

SWINE REPRODUCTION

PUBERTY

Gilts usually reach puberty at 4.5 to 6 months of age. Social environment and nutrition are important factors determining the onset of cyclicity in gilts. The onset of puberty is commonly seen in gilts weighing 82 kg or more. Direct contact between boars and gilts is important in swine reproduction. Boars have pheromone-secreting salivary glands that sexually stimulate female pigs. This "boar effect" (stimulating or detecting estrus) is even more evident if mature, experienced boars are used. Daily exposure of 5- to 6-month-old gilts to a mature boar will hasten the onset of cyclicity. Season probably influences the onset of puberty because gilts born in the fall start to cycle earlier than their spring-born counterparts. In addition, all factors that contribute to good management, such as number of gilts per pen, adequate physical space per gilt, ambient temperature, and health status (diseases, parasites) in general, will ensure that gilts reach puberty around 5 to 6 months of age.

Pharmacologic agents can also induce puberty. Fertile estrus and ovulation can be induced using exogenous gonadotropins. eCG in association with hCG is effective in inducing estrus in gilts. These two gonadotropins are marketed in a combination to induce estrus and ovulation. Estrogen administration is also effective, but does not yield as reliable results as the eCG-hCG combination. GnRH is effective, but it is expensive and needs to be delivered in a pulsatile fashion (every hour for 3 to 4 days), making this difficult to be done in a commercial unit.

ESTROUS CYCLE

Domestic pigs are nonseasonal polyestrous animals. Female pigs exhibit estrus at 21-day intervals after they reach puberty. Longer estrous cycles, such as 26 days, have been associated with early embryonic mortality.

During proestrus, follicular development intensifies as the corpora lutea in the nonpregnant pig start to regress around day 15 of the estrous cycle. Initial behavioral signs of estrus are not always easily recognized. They include increased restlessness, reduced appetite, mounting other animals, homosexual behavior (malelike sexual activity), and lordosis. The vulva swells and becomes more pink and moist. A cloudy mucous discharge may be present during this phase.

Estrus is the period when the female pig is responsive to the boar's approach. If a male and female are put together during this stage, they start to show a precopulatory behavior (foreplay) that includes sniffing each other and head-to-head contact; the male starts to compulsively follow the female pig and initiate mounting attempts. Courtship culminates with the female pig standing still and allowing the boar to mount. Estrus also can be detected by checking the female for lordosis. Lordosis occurs when pressure is applied on the pig's back by someone sitting on it and the female pig stands still, quiet, and passive, assuming a mating position. The duration of estrus can be variable among individuals of different breeds or age or during different times of the year (longest in summer and shorter in winter). Estrus lasts on average 40 to 60 hours (2 to 3 days), but it can vary from 1 to 4 days. Ovulation usually takes place during the second day of estrus (36 to 44 hours after the onset of estrus), and mated females reportedly ovulate 4 hours before unmated female pigs. Follicular rupture of all follicles present in the ovary (10 to 20) may take 1 to 9 hours.

Diestrus is behaviorally characterized by a lack of sexual receptivity and lasts for 18 days if the female pig is not pregnant. Anestrus is mainly seen when sows are lactating.

PREGNANCY

The deposition of semen in pigs is intracervical. The presence of cartilaginous rings in the sow's cervix in association with the fibroelastic spiral tip (corkscrew) of the boar's penis provides a natural and strong lock of the penis inside the cervix. Subsequently, during mating, strong contractions of the cervix are potentiated by oxytocin release in response to coitus. Several billion sperm cells are released during coitus in an average of 200 to 250 ml of semen. Uterine contractions allow a controlled number of sperm cells to reach the oviduct, where fertilization occurs. It seems that a minimum of four embryos must be present in the uterus to cause appropriate maternal recognition of pregnancy. The average length of gestation is 114 days (3 months + 3 weeks + 3 days). Piglets are born weighing on average 1.4 to 1.6 kg. A tail-first presentation is not abnormal. The interval time between piglets averages 10 to 15 minutes. Intervals greater than 20 minutes are associated with an increasing number of stillbirths. All fetal membranes should be delivered in 4 to 6 hours.

CONTROL OF FARROWING

Farrowing can occur at any time of the day or night. Each sow may take several hours to deliver all the piglets and fetal membranes. It is important to assist sows during delivery because the early detection and correction of potential problems during farrowing prevent piglet losses. Assistance during farrowing can be facilitated by pharmacologically inducing parturition. Accordingly, prostaglandin administration after day 112 of gestation will induce parturition in 20 to 30 hours. Combining a prostaglandin with oxytocin or xylazine will help to improve the precision of response to prostaglandin administration.

PHARMACOLOGIC CONTROL OF THE ESTROUS CYCLE

Exogenous hormones can be used to alter or manipulate the estrous cycle in pigs. Estrus and ovulation can be induced by different means either in cycling pigs or in early pregnant pigs to synchronize estrus (Table 14-2).

The preparation P.G. 600 contains 400 IU of eCG and 200 units of hCG. It can be used to induce estrus in prepubertal gilts or in sows showing anestrus after weaning. It can also be used in cycling sows after day 16 of the estrous cycle. Administering P.G. 600 will cause estrus and ovulation in 3 to 5 days following treatment. Estrus and ovulation can also be induced by administering ECG and HCG 2 days apart. Prostaglandins can be used to terminate pregnancy or diestrus only if given 12 days after ovulation. Before day 12, multiple injections (twice daily for 5 days) of prostaglandins are necessary to interrupt diestrus (short cycling) or to terminate pregnancy. Weaned sows usually show spontaneous signs of estrus in 11 to 12 days after weaning. Administering P.G. 600 on the day of weaning will also induce estrus in 3 to 5 days. Sows that do not come into estrus in 2 weeks after weaning will show signs of estrus if P.G. 600 is administered.

Artificial Insemination

AI with fresh or cooled semen is commonly performed in the swine industry. The boar is easily trained to mount a dummy and have semen manually collected. After collecting the sperm-rich portion of the ejaculate, semen is evaluated to determine its quality and how much extender to add. A sow should be inseminated with 3 to 4 billion sperm cells in a volume of 80 to 100 ml. The number of total insemination doses from an ejaculate will depend on the frequency of collection, age of boar, breed, and some individual variation. Farrowing rates from sows artificially inseminated are comparable with those observed in sows naturally mated. Artificially inseminating twice 12 to 24 hours apart is likely to improve pregnancy rates. In a commercial unit, heterospermic insemination (mixing semen from two or more boars) is sometimes used and reportedly increases pregnancy rates.

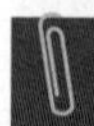

TECHNICIAN NOTE AI with fresh or cooled semen is commonly performed in the swine industry.

Swine Pregnancy Diagnosis

Ultrasonography procedures are used to diagnose pregnancy in pigs. Doppler and amplitude-depth ultrasound were the first methods to be employed and are accurate between 30 and 90 days of gestation. Real-time (B-mode) ultrasound is being used with more frequency in the swine industry as equipment cost decreases. Accuracy is greater than 90% if used after 20 days of gestation.

Postpartum Complications and Diseases

Retained placenta is not a common occurrence in pigs. Fetal membranes from all piglets are usually expelled after the last piglet is born. A manual examination of the birth canal is warranted if the placenta is not passed out after sows apparently deliver their last piglet.

Obstetric problems are also not common, and the great majority of sows and gilts deliver without any technical or veterinary assistance. Nevertheless, persistent and forceful abdominal contractions without delivery of a piglet for longer than 1 hour suggest potential complications. A problem will be even more evident if it is accompanied by vaginal discharge but not expulsion of a fetus. An increased time interval between deliveries is also suggestive of dystocia. The reason may be a primary absence of uterine contractions (primary inertia) or secondary to the presence of either an oversized, malpositioned, or malformed fetus. Oxytocin can be administered for primary uterine inertia. The removal of piglets is also helpful for stimulating progression of delivery. Occasionally a cesarean delivery is needed to deliver the piglets.

Prolapse of the uterus can occur during parturition or after all piglets have been delivered. Excessive straining or a large pelvic inlet may predispose to uterine prolapse. Uterine prolapse is likely fatal. Vaginal prolapse generally happens a few days before parturition. It requires veterinary

TABLE 14-2 Hormones Used in Swine Reproduction

Desired Effect	Drug	Regimen
Induction of puberty	P.G. 600	5 ml IM
	eCG/hCG	400-1000 IU/200-1000 U IM
Estrus/ovulation	P.G. 600	5 ml IM
	eCG/hCG	500-1000 IU/500-1000 U IM
	Regu-Mate	15 mg/gilt/day for 18 days orally
Abortion	$PGF_{2\alpha}$	10 mg Lutalyse or 500 mg Estrumate 12-45 days after breeding

eCG, Equine chorionic gonadotropin; *hCG*, human chorionic gonadotropin; *IM*, intramuscularly; *$PGF_{2\alpha}$*, prostaglandin.

intervention to reposition it, and sows should be watched for any problems during labor.

Metritis and mastitis are the main diseases of the postpartum period and consequently lead to a disturbance in milk production. Hypogalactia (low milk production) and agalactia (absence of milk production) are often associated with mastitis and metritis. Any signs of abnormal, fetid vaginal discharge or abnormal enlargement of the udder warrant veterinary assistance. Oxytocin can be used to stimulate milk let-down during treatment.

> *TECHNICIAN NOTE* Metritis and mastitis are the main diseases of the postpartum period and consequently lead to a disturbance in milk production.

OVINE AND CAPRINE REPRODUCTION

SEASONALITY

Sheep and goats are seasonally polyestrous, short-day breeders. Estrous cycles start to occur in the late summer and autumn. The photo period is the primary environmental cue controlling seasonal breeding in the ewe. Exposure of sheep and goats to increasing or long day length induces anestrus, whereas short or decreasing day length initiates estrous cycles. Perception of the day length by the eye is signaled to the pineal gland, which will cause melatonin release. Melatonin will induce the secretion of GnRH and LH, which initiates cyclicity. Low ambient temperature also cues small ruminants to start to cycle. Sheep and goats kept in tropical or subtropical areas do not display marked seasonality and can cycle almost year-round.

The geographic origin of a specific breed influences the length of the breeding season. For example, some breeds have a 2- to 4-month breeding season, and some cycle all year long. Suffolk and Suffolk crosses average 6 months of breeding season. Dorset and Finn sheep have an extended breeding season (8 months), whereas Merino ewes cycle almost year-round.

Dairy goats (Saanen, Toggenburg) cycle from August to February in the northern hemisphere. Most meat or crossbred-type goats have a more extended breeding season and undergo anestrus in late spring and summer.

ESTROUS CYCLE

Ewes cycle regularly every 17 (range 14 to 19) days and does every 21 (range 18 to 22) days during the breeding season. During proestrus, ewes and does are not sexually receptive, but attract the male's attention, and courtship is initiated.

Estrus lasts 24 to 48 hours in ewes and 24 to 36 hours in does. Estrogen causes the vulva to be edematous and moist. Does show overt signs of estrus more often than ewes. Accordingly, does may exhibit homosexual behavior, but ewes do not. Estrus detection is efficiently achieved using males that have undergone a vasectomy. Both species actively seek the male as they advance into estrus. Multiple copulations during the same estrus are correlated with higher pregnancy rates. A cloudy vaginal discharge may be seen at the end of estrus and should not be mistaken for an infectious vaginal discharge. Ovulation occurs 24 to 30 hours after the onset of estrus in both species. Diestrus lasts 15 to 17 days in ewes and 18 to 20 days in does.

BREEDING MANAGEMENT

Puberty of ewes occurs at 6 to 9 months, but it can be as late as 1 to 2 years of age depending on breed, nutrition, and the time of birth during the year (e.g., lambs and kids born in the fall come into puberty later than spring-born offspring). Pubertal ewes and does should be bred only if they have attained 65% of their mature body weight. The male/female ratio should be 1:50 in natural breeding situations or 1:10 for synchronized breeding. Fresh or frozen semen can be used for AI. The deposition of semen can be intravaginal, intracervical, or intrauterine (Table 14-3). Laparoscopic procedures have become common practice in the sheep and goat industry.

PREGNANCY

Gestation lasts approximately 150 days in both species. Ewes are dependent on luteal function only during the first 2 months of gestation. Because pregnancy maintenance in ewes is accomplished by placental hormones after day 50 of gestation, administration of prostaglandin after 2 months of gestation does not induce abortion or parturition. Does are dependent on luteal function throughout gestation, and prostaglandin administration interrupts pregnancy at any stage. Parturition can be safely induced by prostaglandin administration in goats after day 146 of gestation. Does go into labor an average of 28 to 36 hours after prostaglandin administration. Dexamethasone induces parturition in ewes within 36 to 48 hours if administered after day 144 of gestation. Twinning is common, and lambs and kids should be standing within 15 minutes and nursing within 1 hour after birth.

TABLE 14-3 Artificial Insemination (AI) Breeding in Ewes

Semen	Semen Dose (Number of Spermatozoa)	Lambing Rate (%)
Laparoscopic IU		
Fresh or frozen	20-40 × 10^6	40-100
Transcervical IU		
Fresh or frozen	50-100 × 10^6	30-80
Cervical		
Fresh only	200 × 10^6	40-80
Vaginal		
Fresh only	400 × 10^6	20-60

Modified from Youngquist RS, editor: Current therapy in large animal theriogenology, St Louis, 1997, WB Saunders.
IU, Intrauterine.

RAM/BUCK EFFECT

Male pheromones produced under androgenic stimulation dramatically influence cyclicity in ewes and does. The introduction of a new, mature, odoriferous male during the transition from the anestrus season into the breeding season will induce estrus in most females. Ewes ovulate in 3 to 6 days, but the CL of this first cycle is short lived. After the second ovulation, regular cyclicity is established. The buck effect is more efficient in does inasmuch as cyclicity is regularly initiated with the first ovulation.

> *TECHNICIAN NOTE* Male pheromones produced under androgenic stimulation dramatically influence cyclicity in ewes and does.

PHARMACOLOGIC CONTROL OF THE ESTROUS CYCLE

Intravaginal sponges delivering progestogen are used to synchronize estrus in ewes and does. Controlled intravaginal drug-releasing devices (CIDRs) are widely used internationally, but are not yet commercially available in the United States. Recently a vaginal sponge impregnated with flurogestone acetate (45 mg/sponge) has been approved by the Food and Drug Administration (FDA) for synchronizing estrus in cycling adult ewes during their normal breeding season. This vaginal sponge has not been approved for use in ewes that have not had lambs. Prostaglandins (extralabel use) are also used to synchronize estrus alone or in combination with progestogen.

OVINE AND CAPRINE PREGNANCY DIAGNOSIS

Pregnancy diagnosis can be performed by checking for returning to estrus, ballottement (palpation) of the fetus in the abdomen, or ultrasonography. The return to estrus can be observed by using a marking harness and crayon on the male (Figure 14-29). Doppler ultrasonography is 90% accurate after 75 days of gestation. Real-time (B-mode) ultrasonography using a 5-MHz probe is 100% accurate after 60 days.

PERIPARTURIENT PROBLEMS

Dystocia usually results from an abnormal fetal disposition or fetopelvic disproportion. It is important to recognize dystocia because the cervix will close after 2 to 3 hours of nonproductive labor. A cesarean delivery is the treatment of choice. Ringwomb refers to the failure of the cervix to dilate during parturition.

Pregnancy toxemia is a common problem seen in ewes in the last 6 weeks of gestation. It is associated with multiple fetuses and inadequate nutrition. Hypoglycemia in these cases may lead to neurologic signs and incoordination. Vaginal prolapse usually occurs in late gestation (3 to 6 weeks before parturition), and dystocia is likely to result in a cesarean delivery.

Hypocalcemia is a condition of pregnant ewes and does leading to cool extremities, failure of the cervix to dilate, and generalized weakness. The treatment is intravenous calcium administration. The hypocalcemic female should be examined 3 hours after calcium treatment. If no progress in delivery is observed, a cesarean delivery is indicated.

Pseudopregnancy is a common condition in goats. It is characterized by a collection of fluid inside the uterus without pregnancy (hydrometra). If not treated with prostaglandins, the natural expulsion of the fluid is called a cloudburst.

INFERTILITY

The natural absence of horns in goats is associated with abnormal sexual development. This condition is called polled (hornless) intersex. The polled condition is determined by an autosomal-dominant gene that is the same or closely linked to a recessive gene causing infertility. Homozygous polled genes cause sex reversal in the female. Affected animals may be genetically female, but exhibit male, female, or mixed characteristics and sexual behavior. The polled gene is dominant, but fortunately the intersex condition is seen only in homozygous animals. Therefore this condition can be prevented by having at least one horned parent.

> *TECHNICIAN NOTE* Camelids do not have regular estrous cycles. They are induced ovulators, similar to cats.

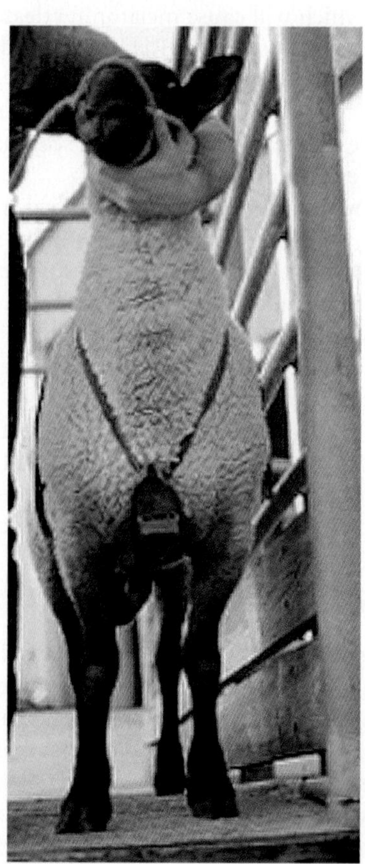

FIGURE 14-29 A ram fitted with a marking harness to detect estrus in ewes.

CAMELID REPRODUCTION

New world camelids include the llama, alpaca, vicuna, and guanaco. They developed from a common ancestor in South America before the arrival of Europeans. Many aspects of reproduction are similar, but there are differences that can be attributed to speciation.

ESTROUS CYCLES

Puberty occurs at 10 to 12 months of age when the animal reaches approximately 60% of the adult body weight. Although llamas have peak fertility during the summer, they cycle year-round. Environmental and endocrinologic factors responsible for the onset and cessation of sexual activity are not yet clearly defined.

Camelids do not have regular estrous cycles. They are induced ovulators, similar to cats. Sexual receptivity can vary from 1 to 36 days. Coitus lasts 5 to 50 minutes with an average of 18 minutes. One mating is sufficient to induce ovulation, which occurs 1 to 3 days later. Delayed ovulation occurs in 30% and absence of ovulation in 10% of females after a single copulation. Treatment with hCG (500 to 700 IU) or GnRH (800 mg) is effective to induce ovulation. The use of a male that has had a vasectomy is more effective to induce ovulation. The ovulatory follicle can be on either ovary, but the pregnancy is invariably in the left horn. Luteolysis is mediated by PGF_{2a}. The CL remains functional throughout gestation. Prostaglandin F_{2a} can be used to induce parturition.

The gestation length averages 344 days (range 331 to 347 days). Parturition lasts 1 to 2 hours, and few complications occur. Approximately 90% of crias (baby camelids) are born between 7:00 AM and 1:00 PM.

GENERAL MALE REPRODUCTION

The male differs greatly from the female in the production of gametes. Whereas in the female only 1 to 10 oocytes ovulate during an estrous cycle, males are continually producing and excreting millions of sperm cells. Testicular anatomy differs significantly from ovarian anatomy. The testis is made up of many tubules, each of which connects to a central collecting duct. Between the tubules are the interstitial cells, which continually produce testosterone (Figure 14-30). Each tubule is lined by primordial germ cells (immature sperm cell

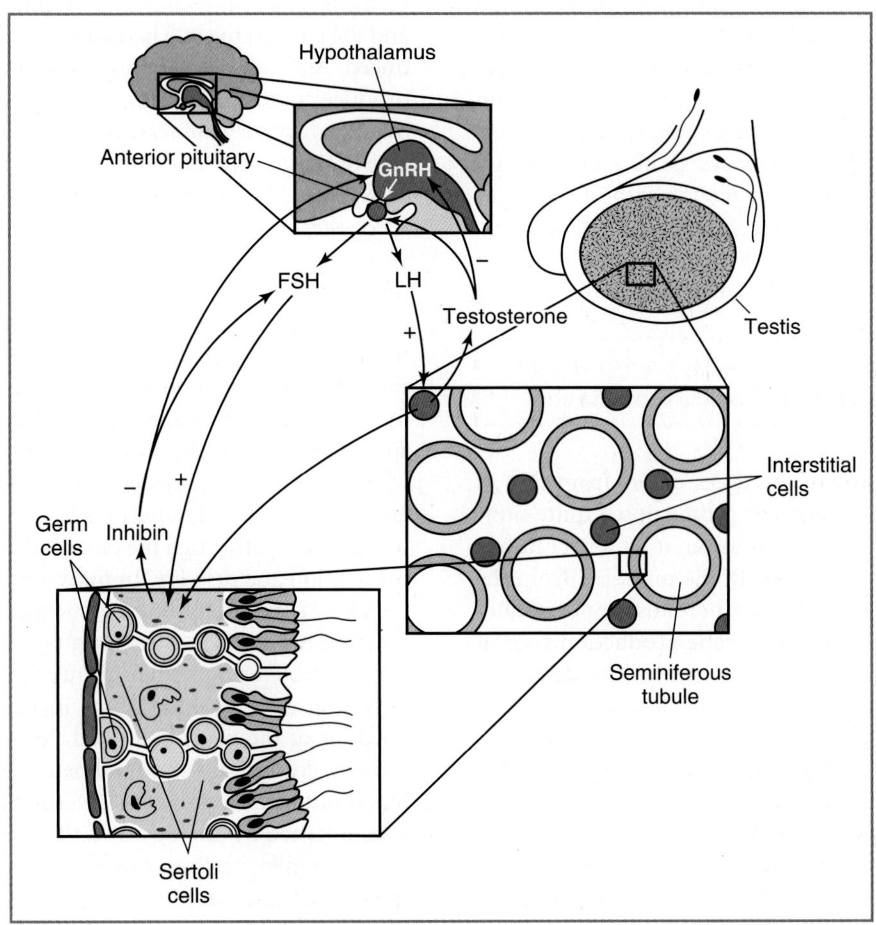

FIGURE 14-30 The general hormonal control of male reproduction: Pulsatile GnRH causes FSH to be released from the anterior pituitary. FSH causes increased sperm growth, maturation, and release. Inhibin from the Sertoli cells in the tubules feeds back on the anterior pituitary and causes less FSH to be released. GnRH secretion from the hypothalamus also results in LH release, which causes testosterone production by the interstitial cells of Leydig. The rise in testosterone causes less LH and GnRH to be released.

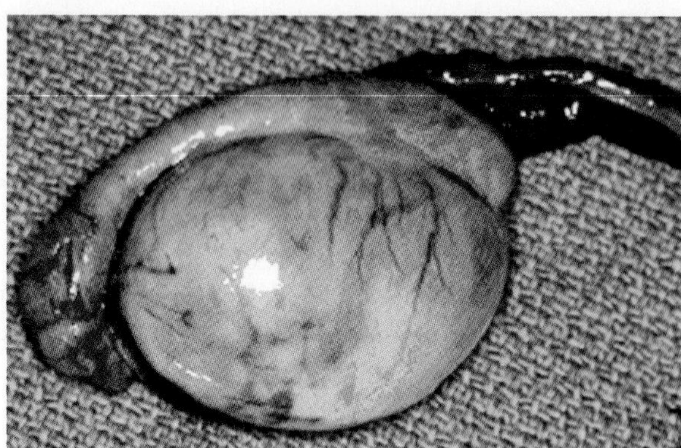

FIGURE 14-31 A canine testis showing the capsule surrounding the testicular tissue.

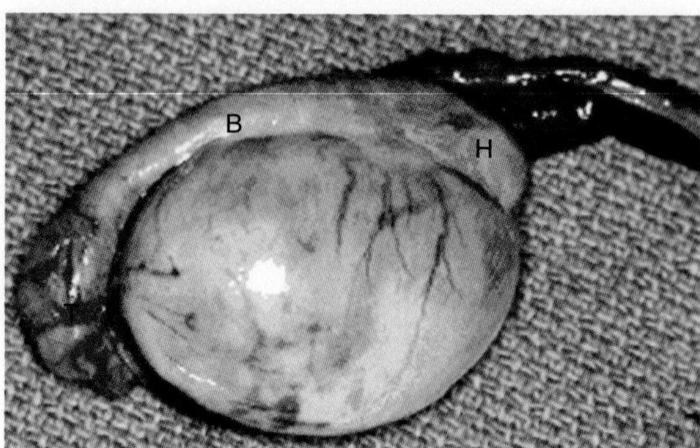

FIGURE 14-32 Lateral view of the right canine testis and epididymis with the head *(H)*, body *(B)*, and tail *(T)* of the epididymis.

precursors) and Sertoli cells. The Sertoli cells surround all the developing sperm cells, leaving them with no other contact to the body. This is critical in that the developing sperm are recognized as a foreign substance to the male and would be destroyed by the immune system if they were not protected. As the sperm cells mature, they leave their attachment to the Sertoli cell and are moved through the tubules.

The entire testis is covered by a tight capsule, the tunica albuginea (Figure 14-31). The paired testes are contained within the scrotum. The scrotum maintains the testes at a lower body temperature than the rest of the body. If the testes are not kept at a lower temperature, sperm cell production will cease. However, even though sperm cell production ceases, the interstitial cells still produce testosterone. A common example of these consequences is in a cryptorchid animal. A cryptorchid animal has one or both of the testes retained in the abdomen. If the testes are in the abdomen, the animal is sterile, but will still show masculine behavior because testosterone is still produced by the testes.

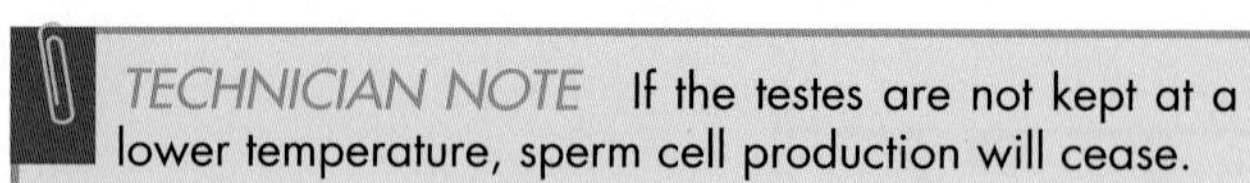

TECHNICIAN NOTE If the testes are not kept at a lower temperature, sperm cell production will cease.

Although the anatomy of the testes differs from that of the ovary, the control of sperm cell production is quite similar to that of oocyte production; however, it is more continuous and does not occur in cycles. In the male, LH from the anterior pituitary causes an increase in testosterone production (see Figure 14-30). As testosterone production rises, it causes a decrease in GnRH and LH release. The decreased GnRH and LH release causes less testosterone to be produced. As less testosterone is produced, it follows that more GnRH and LH are produced, thus resulting in a balanced feedback mechanism and a relatively constant testosterone production. Testosterone is essential for the production of sperm cells. If testosterone is not present, sperm cells will not be produced. The concentration of testosterone within the testis is 10 times that in the systemic circulation. The administration of testosterone decreases endogenous testosterone production because of the negative feedback on the anterior pituitary and hypothalamus. This will result in lower testosterone concentrations within the testis. Because testosterone is needed for sperm cell production, the exogenous testosterone will eventually decrease sperm cell production.

The other hormone involved in sperm cell production is FSH. Just as in the female, FSH release is triggered by GnRH from the hypothalamus. The FSH acts on the Sertoli cell to increase the division of primordial sperm cells and to release more sperm cells that are embedded in the Sertoli cells. As sperm cell production rises, the hormone inhibin feeds back on the hypothalamus and anterior pituitary to decrease GnRH and FSH, respectively. This causes fewer sperm cells to be produced. As fewer cells are produced, the FSH will increase to produce more sperm cells, thereby keeping sperm cell production relatively constant. In general, FSH causes production of the gamete (oocyte in the female and sperm cell in the male), and LH causes production of the dominant hormone (progesterone in the female and testosterone in the male).

After the sperm cells are released, they move through the tubules and into the head of the epididymis. Within the epididymis, the sperm cells attain motility and the ability to fertilize. The movement through the epididymis to the tail of the epididymis is relatively constant and cannot be increased by increasing the number or frequency of ejaculates. The sperm cells are finally stored in the tail of the epididymis, where they are either ejaculated or voided in the urine if they are not ejaculated (Figure 14-32).

Ejaculation through the penis is the final process in sperm production and delivery. In most domestic species, the penis comprises cavernous blood tissue surrounded by a firm covering, or tunic. An erection occurs when the male is sexually stimulated. During sexual stimulation, parasympathetic innervation causes a blood flow increase into the cavernous portions of the penis. As blood flow increases to the penis, muscles around the proximal penis also contract to prevent blood outflow. Because the cavernous portions of the penis are contained within the tunic, the pressure increases, resulting in a penile erection. Any disruption of the cavernous tissue or the tunic can result in an erection failure.

During an erection, the sperm cells in the tail of the epididymis are moved to the end of the ductus deferens into the ampullae in the process called emission. Once the sperm cells are present in the ampullae, the stimulation to the penis during mating causes ejaculation. Ejaculation is the forceful expulsion of the semen through the penis. The force comes from sympathetic nerves causing smooth muscle contractions in the urethra. During ejaculation, the sperm cells are mixed with fluid from the accessory sex glands. The accessory sex glands include the ampullae, prostate, vesicular glands, and bulbourethral glands. Each species has one or all of these glands, and different glands have different clinical problems in each species. When the sperm cells are mixed with the accessory sex gland fluid, the result is now termed semen. Secretions from the accessory sex gland fluid add various components to the ejaculate, increase the volume, and stabilize the sperm cell membrane. Once the sperm cells enter the female reproductive tract, the sperm cell membrane undergoes a physical and biochemical change called capacitation. Capacitation is required before the sperm cells are capable of fertilization. In the uterus, the sperm cells are quickly moved to the oviduct, where fertilization occurs. Sperm cells are moved to the oviduct by uterine contractions.

> TECHNICIAN NOTE Once the sperm cells enter the female reproductive tract, the sperm cell membrane undergoes a physical and biochemical change called capacitation.

CLINICAL EXAMINATION OF THE MALE

Depending on the species, an evaluation of the male as a sound potential breeder may employ different techniques to collect semen and evaluate sperm output. Although semen collection procedures may differ among species, analysis of the semen is quite similar.

SEMEN ANALYSIS

When evaluating semen, it is important to have all equipment at 37° C. Sperm cells are susceptible to cold shock and osmotic shock. Semen is best handled with a thin wooden stick because the wood is thermoneutral and will not cold shock the sperm cells. The first step in semen analysis is to examine the motility. The motility will decline with time because of changes in the semen temperature and pH. The gross motility is examined by placing a drop of semen on a warm slide and examining it at 100 times magnification (10 × objective). The light on the microscope needs to be reduced greatly to see the cells. The sample is only evaluated for movement; however, the concentration can be estimated to help prepare other samples.

After the gross motility is evaluated, the percent of progressively motile sperm is assessed. Individual motility slides are made by placing a drop of semen on the slide and then placing a coverslip over the sample. The sample should be evaluated at 400 times magnification (40 × objective). It is desirable to have approximately 10 cells per high-power field. If there are more cells, the motility cannot be estimated accurately. The motility is estimated by determining the percent of cells that move progressively across the field. Cells that move in tight circles are not progressively motile. If more than 10 cells are seen per high-power field, the sample can be diluted. Dilution can be done by placing a drop of warm saline on a slide and then placing a small amount of semen into the saline (concentrated bull and ram semen usually only requires a quick touch of the saline with a wooden stick dipped into the semen). If the cells were alive on the gross motility examination but are dead on the individual motility examination, the saline may be hypertonic. As saline remains opened, the water evaporates and increases the osmolarity of the solution. Replace the saline and repeat the motility evaluation.

> TECHNICIAN NOTE Sperm motility is the first parameter assessed because it can change quickly under adverse conditions.

Sperm morphology is generally examined after staining with an eosin-nigrosin stain (Lane Manufacturing). Slides are made by painting a line of the stain across one end of the slide. A small amount of semen is placed in the stain. A second slide is then used to push the stain across the length of the slide. The objective of making the slide is to have a dark background to highlight the cells. If there are lighter and darker areas on the slide, it may be easier to find a more suitable area to examine the cells. To examine the morphology slide, always use 1000 times magnification (100 × objective, oil). Lower magnification will not allow adequate assessment of the sperm cells. A total of 100 cells are counted, and they are classified as normal or abnormal. A spermiogram can be performed to differentiate the different type of sperm abnormalities, which include proximal droplets, distal droplets, kinked tails, coiled tails, acrosome abnormalities, midpiece abnormalities, and misshaped heads.

> TECHNICIAN NOTE Sperm morphology is assessed under high magnification (1000 × magnification or 100 × objective, oil).

Sperm concentration is also performed in situations where a physiologic ejaculate is obtained, such as with a stallion or dog. In those species in which the sperm cell output is estimated using scrotal circumference (SC), a sperm count is not done. The concentration of sperm is determined by diluting the sample 1:100 and then counting the diluted sample on a hemacytometer. The easiest way to make a 1:100 dilution is to prepare two tubes of 0.9-ml formal buffered saline. Add 0.1 ml of raw semen to the first tube and mix. Take 0.1 ml of diluted semen from the first tube and add it to the second tube. The second tube now has a 1:100 dilution. Place the 1:100 dilution on a hemacytometer and count all the sperm cells in the middle big square surrounded by triple lines (it has 25 smaller squares). The total number of sperm cells counted and multiplied by 10^6 gives the concentration per milliliter. The volume of the sample multiplied by the concentration gives the total number of sperm cells in the ejaculate.

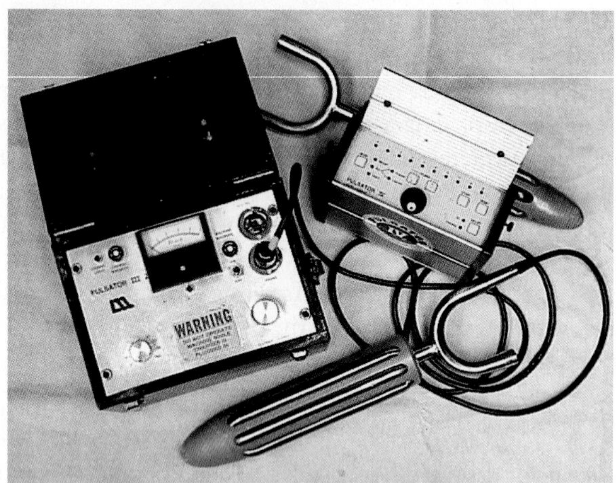

FIGURE 14-33 Two models of ruminant electroejaculators and two rectal probes.

BULL, RAM, AND BUCK

The bull, ram, and buck have a fibroelastic penis that has a low blood volume in the cavernous space, but there is high pressure within the penis. The stimulus for ejaculation in these species is temperature. When sensors on the penis encounter the correct temperature in the vagina, the male ejaculates. It is important to note that even though there is no pain response on the penis, the temperature sensors may still be able to signal ejaculation. However, it is also difficult to ascertain whether the temperature sensors are functional. To obtain a physiologic ejaculate, an artificial vagina (AV) needs to be used to collect the semen. Most AVs consist of a hard shell with a rubber liner inserted. Warm water is placed between the rubber liner and the shell. The temperature of the water is critical in inducing ejaculation.

The animal is allowed to become sexually stimulated and mount an estrual female, restrained male, or immobile object; the collector then diverts the penis into the AV. Because this is not easy to do and most ruminants are not trained to breed an AV, most semen collections in the field are performed using an electroejaculator (Figure 14-33). An electroejaculator consists of a probe inserted into the rectum. On the ventral side of the probe are electrodes that stimulate the sympathetic and parasympathetic nerves. The probe is connected to a control box. The box controls how much stimulation the animal receives. The stimulation is low at first and is gradually increased until the animal has an erection, protrudes the penis, and ejaculates. The ejaculate is then collected into a receptacle. Some machines have an automatic progression of power settings, whereas other machines have to be stepped up manually to control the power.

Although commonly used, electroejaculation may be a painful process for the animal. As long as the power is applied, that animal will produce fluid (from the accessory sex glands), so the "ejaculate" is not truly physiologic. Because the ejaculate is not physiologic, other estimates must be used to estimate sperm output. Sperm output is generally estimated by measuring the SC. When measuring the SC, the testes and epididymides are also palpated for size and consistency. A normal bull testis has the consistency of a flexed human bicep. Standards have been set for the desired SC of different ruminant species of different ages.

TECHNICIAN NOTE When measuring the SC, the testes and epididymides are also palpated for size and consistency.

In the ram, it is important to palpate the epididymides carefully because *B. ovis* causes infertility and epididymitis. In the bull, a rectal examination is performed to evaluate the vesicular glands. Other body systems to evaluate are vision, teeth, and locomotion. The animal must be able to see, eat, and move around to be a successful breeder. Guidelines have been set by the Society for Theriogenology regarding the minimal criteria needed for an animal to be acceptable for breeding. Breeding soundness evaluation forms and criteria are available for veterinarians from the Society for Theriogenology (Figure 14-34).

Bulls commonly get seminal vesiculitis, and white cells will be seen in the semen. Other common problems in bulls are penile hematomas and preputial injuries (Figure 14-35). A penile hematoma usually occurs when a bull is breeding and the penis bends. This increases the pressure in the penis and causes a rupture of the penile tunic. The rupture almost always happens at the distal sigmoid flexure, and a blood clot forms. Preputial injuries are common in *Bos indicus* bulls. These bulls have a redundant prepuce that often is everted or hangs out. When the prepuce is damaged, it swells, and the bull cannot retract it. Conservative therapy is common in these cases, but a reefing surgery or a circumcision may be needed.

STALLION

Semen is collected most commonly with an AV (Figure 14-36). The temperature and pressure of the AV are the criteria that contribute to the stallion ejaculating. A final temperature of 45° C to 48° C is generally needed, and the pressure must be adequate. Some stallions prefer hotter and some colder; some prefer more pressure, and some prefer less pressure. Once the AV is prepared, the stallion is teased with an estrual mare until attaining an erection. The penis should be washed with clean warm water, avoiding the use of disinfectants because they can disrupt the normal commensal organisms on the penis and are spermicidal. If a mare is used for a mount, the stallion is led to the side of the mare and allowed to mount. The stallion will then position himself on the mare. As the stallion begins to thrust, the penis is diverted into the AV, and the stallion is allowed to thrust and ejaculate into the AV. As the stallion dismounts, the AV is held vertical to prevent semen from draining out the open end. Immediately after the dismount, the water in the AV should be drained out to prevent heat shock to the cells and to allow the semen to drain into the collection bottle.

Bull Breeding Soundness Evaluation

Guidelines Established by Society for Theriogenology
530 Church Street, Suite 700 • Nashville, TN 37219
Phone 615/244-3060 • FAX 615/254-7047 • www.therio.org

OWNER	CASE NO.	DATE
ADDRESS	BULL NAME	BREED
ZIP	I.D. NO.	Brand ❑ Tattoo ❑ Ear tag ❑
TELEPHONE ( )	BIRTH DATE	AGE (MO.)
HISTORY: Previous BSE DATE	CASE NO.	CLASSIFICATION

PHYSICAL EXAMINATION		SEMEN EXAMINATION		
Body condition score ____ Thin ❑ Moderate ❑ Good ❑ Obese ❑ Beef 1, 2, 3, 4, 5, 6, 7, 8, 9 Pelvic Ht. ____ Width ____ Area ____ Dairy 1, 2, 3, 4, 5		Collection method: EE ❑ AV ❑ Massage ❑ Response: Erection ❑ Protrusion ❑ Ejaculation ❑		
Feet/legs	❑	Semen characteristics	Ejaculate 1	Ejaculate 2
Eyes	❑	Motility Gross (or) individual (%)		
Vesicular glands	❑			
Ampullae/prostate	❑	% Normal cells		
Inguinal rings	❑	% Primary abnormalities		
Penis/prepuce	❑	% Secondary abnormalities		
Testes/spermatic cord	❑	WBC, RBC, other		
Epididymides	❑			
Scrotum (shape)	❑			
Other				

SCROTAL CIRCUMFERENCE (CM) ________ . ________

This bull has been examined for physical soundness and quality of semen only. Unless otherwise noted, no diagnostic tests were undertaken for libido, mating ability or infectious disease status of this bull.

Remarks and interpretation (diagnosis, prognosis, recommendations)

CLASSIFICATION

Interpretation of data resulting from this examination would indicate that *on this date,* this bull is a:

❑ Satisfactory potential breeder

❑ Unsatisfactory potential breeder

❑ Classification deferred

Re-examination recommended on ________
DATE

Signed: ________
MEMBER—SOCIETY FOR THERIOGENOLOGY

Clinic:

FIGURE 14-34 Bull breeding soundness examination form. These forms are copyrighted and available from the Society for Theriogenology (Society for Theriogenology, PO Box 3007, Montgomery, AL 36109).

> *TECHNICIAN NOTE* Stallion semen often has a large gel fraction that must be removed before analysis can be performed.

Stallions can also be trained to mount dummies, or phantoms. A dummy allows the collection of a stallion's semen without an estrual mare present and is a safer way to collect semen. Stallion semen often has a large gel fraction that must be removed before an analysis can be performed. This is usually done with an in-line filter attached to the collection bottle. Alternatively the ejaculate can be filtered in the laboratory after collection. Motility and morphology assessments are performed the same as in other species. Stallion semen may be diluted and counted manually or using a densitometer. A densitometer measures the amount of light that passes through the semen sample. The higher the concentration of cells, the less light passes through, the less the percent transmittance. Commercially available machines are calibrated to read out the sperm cell concentration based on internal calculations made from the percent transmittance (Figure 14-37).

If semen is being collected as a part of a breeding soundness evaluation, two ejaculates are obtained 1 hour apart. If the second sample has about half of the number of sperm as the first ejaculate, the ejaculates can be considered representative. Stallions are also seasonal, and both sperm production and libido decrease in the winter when day length is short and increase in the summer.

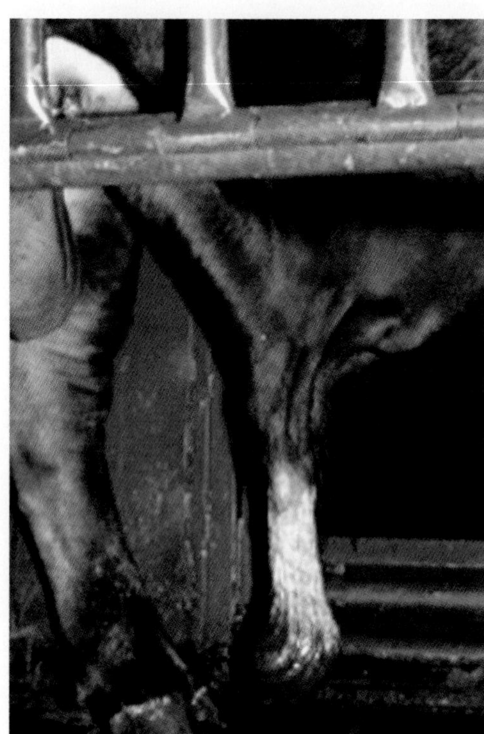

FIGURE 14-35 *Bos indicus* bull with a preputial prolapse.

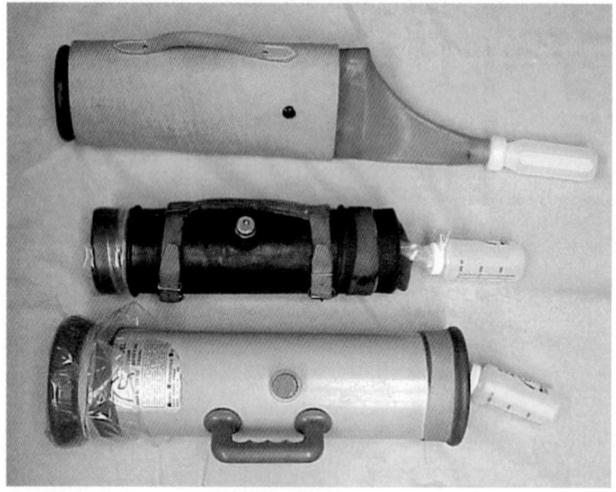

FIGURE 14-36 Three models of equine artificial vaginae. From the top, Missouri, Hannover, ARS/Colorado.

The transport of cooled stallion semen is becoming more and more popular with certain breeds. Commercially available shipping containers cool the extended semen at a specific rate and keep it cool for up to 48 hours. Extenders are liquids added to the semen to help the longevity of shipped semen. Most extenders are made from skim milk and glucose and have some antibiotics added. When extending stallion semen, the final concentrations should be between 25×10^6 and 50×10^6 cells/ml; however, the final dilution ratio should be at least four parts of extender to one part of semen. If the semen cannot be extended to that concentration and ratio, the semen must be centrifuged and the resulting pellet resuspended to the desired 25 to 50 million/ml concentration. Many stallions, despite having semen that appears good, do not have semen that withstands even the best cooling and shipping procedures.

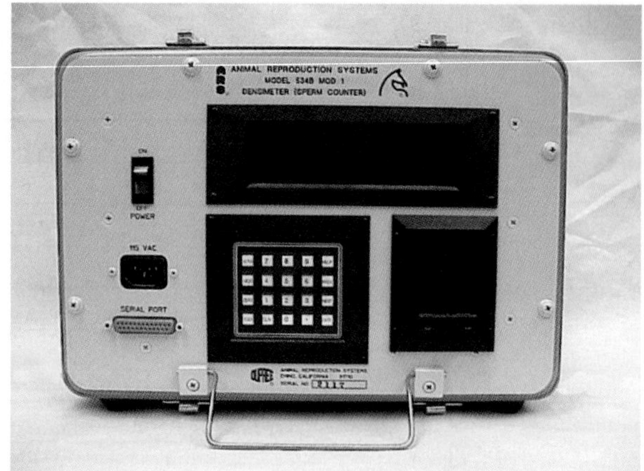

FIGURE 14-37 Densitometer used to measure the concentration of stallion semen.

Stallions may have problems with a decreased libido, hind limb lameness resulting in breeding difficulties, blood in the semen (hemospermia), or urine in the semen (urospermia). These may be challenging problems for the veterinarian to diagnose and treat. The most common breeding injury in the stallion is when the mare kicks the penis or scrotum. The sequel to a kick on the penis is often a hematoma. This is a large blood clot on the outside of the penile tunic, which results in paraphimosis (the penis will not go back into the sheath). If the scrotum is kicked, the testes can swell and be damaged by both the heat from the inflammation and pressure necrosis of the testicular parenchyma swelling within the confined testicular tunic. Conservative therapy for these conditions includes hydrotherapy and antiinflammatories.

CANINE

Canine semen evaluation is performed as in other species, which includes motility, morphology, and a semen count. The main difference is the way the semen is collected. Dog semen is collected by a manual massage of the penis. It is best to have an estrual bitch present when the collection is attempted. Once the dog is somewhat aroused, the prepuce is pushed caudal to the bulbus glandis with a rubber or plastic cone. Circumferential manual pressure is then applied proximal to the bulbus glandis. Pressure is applied while the dog ejaculates. The initial portion of the ejaculate is clear, followed by the sperm-rich fraction. The final portion of the ejaculate is the clear prostatic portion. Normally, it is not necessary to collect the prostatic fraction. It is common for the dog to step over the collector's hand during the collection process, thereby resulting in the male and female "tied" and facing opposite directions. The criteria for a dog to be a good potential breeder have been published by the Society for Theriogenology. The most common reproductive disorder in the dog is prostatitis. A dog with prostatitis will have white blood cells in the ejaculate and possibly show pain during ejaculation.

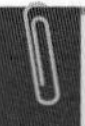

TECHNICIAN NOTE The most common reproductive disorder in the dog is prostatitis.

TOM

It is uncommon to collect semen from the tom. However, semen can be collected using a small AV or an electroejaculator. A tom must be extensively trained to use an AV and must be anesthetized to use an electroejaculator. This is why semen evaluations are rarely performed in the tom. One option is to use a vaginal swab to detect the presence of sperm cells in a queen that has just been bred. The tom will also have retrograde ejaculation into the bladder, so after breeding, a cystocentesis can be performed in an attempt to find sperm cells as another option. The most common causes of infertility in the tom are poor teeth (because the tom bites the queen's neck during breeding) and hair rings around the penis.

BOAR

Semen from the boar is collected by manual pressure of the distal penis. The boar is led to an estrual sow or can be trained to mount a dummy. As the boar mounts and extends the penis, the collector grasps the penis "backhand" such that the tip of the penis is grasped mainly with the little finger. It is the manual pressure on the penis that elicits ejaculation in the boar. The tip of the penis is diverted to an open container. The bottle should be covered with gauze or cheesecloth to filter out the gel fraction of the ejaculate. The boar takes approximately 10 to 20 minutes to ejaculate and will continue to ejaculate as long as pressure is applied to the penile tip (the collector's hand usually tires before the boar). The most common breeding problems in boars are bite wounds to the penis and infections of the preputial diverticulum.

CAMELID

Llamas and alpacas can have semen collected by electroejaculation or with an AV, or they can have semen recovered from the vagina of the female after natural mating. The AV is the best method to obtain a semen sample. The copulatory pattern of the llama is somewhat unique when compared with other domestic species. The female llama lies down, and the male llama will lie on top of the female during copulation. Copulation can take as long as 30 minutes, and the male may ejaculate several times. Semen is evaluated as with other species.

RECOMMENDED READING

Knottenbelt DC et al: *Equine stud farm medicine and surgery*, Edinburgh, 2003, WB Saunders.

Root Kustritz MV, editor: *Small animal theriogenology*, St Louis, 2003, Butterworth-Heinemann.

Samper JC, Pycock JF, McKinnon AO, editors: *Current therapy in equine reproduction*, St Louis, 2007, Saunders.

Younquist RS, editor: *Current therapy in large animal theriogenology*, ed 2, St Louis, 2007, Saunders.

15 Care of Birds, Reptiles, and Small Mammals

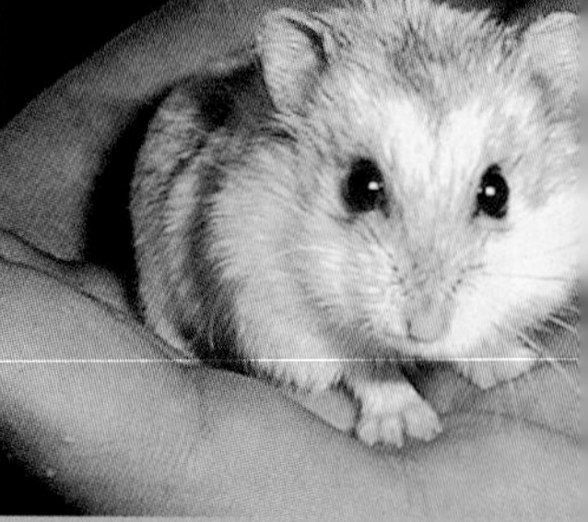

Thomas N. Tully Jr.

OUTLINE

KEY TERMS

Basilic vein
Capillaria
Chelonian
Cloaca
Colonic wash
Conjunctivitis
Crop
Giardia
Glottis
Heterophils
Medial metatarsal vein
Palpebral edema
Perineum

LEARNING OBJECTIVES

When you have completed this chapter, you will be able to:

1. List and describe the components of the clinical history for avian and reptile patients.
2. Describe physical examination considerations and sample collection procedures for avian and reptile patients.
3. Describe the indications for and procedures used to perform a cloacal swab, oral examination, and crop wash in avian patients.
4. Describe methods for the administration of medications, trimming of nails, and clipping of wing feathers in avian patients.
5. List and describe basic feeding guidelines for common pet bird and reptile species.
6. List the unique equipment required for care and treatment of reptiles.
7. Describe the indications for and procedures used to perform a colonic wash, bone marrow and urine sample collection, and stomach lavage in reptile patients.
8. Describe common diseases of ferrets and diagnostic procedures used for the diagnosis and treatment of ferrets, rabbits, and rodents,
9. Describe unique considerations related to the administration of anesthesia in small animals.
10. List and describe common zoonotic diseases of birds, reptiles, and small mammals.

INTRODUCTION

The veterinary field of exotic or nondomestic pet medicine is expanding in the areas of pet ownership and money owners are willing to spend on their animals (see Figure 15-1). Caged and aviary birds are now the third most common small animal pet. The 2007-2008 American Pet Products Manufacturers Association's (APPMA) National Pet Owners Survey reported that 6.4 million households owned a total of 16 million birds. Pet bird owners are using veterinary care for their animals according to the 2002 American Veterinary Medical Association's *U.S. Pet Ownership and Demographics Source Book* (Wise, 2002). This chapter discusses avian and nondomestic pet species, with particular attention paid to the individual requirements of birds, reptiles, and small mammals. It is important to note that approximately 85% of the problems seen in exotic pet medicine result from the lack of basic husbandry information among pet stores, pet owners, veterinarians, and veterinary technicians. With increased veterinary public education, all species covered in this chapter will have a greater chance of living long and healthy lives. For handling and restraint of the animals described in this chapter, see Chapter 7.

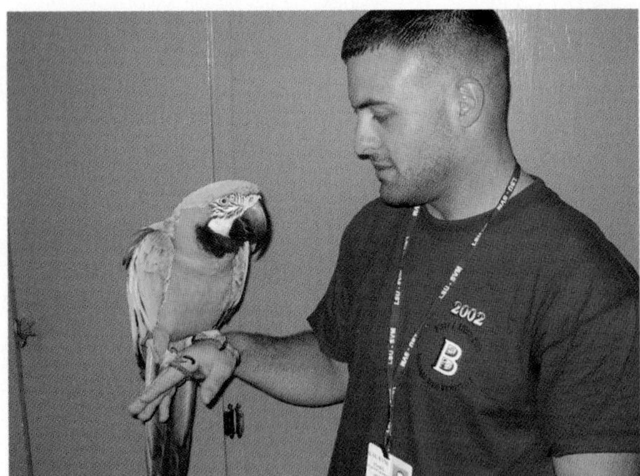
FIGURE 15-1 A bird is an attractive, popular companion.

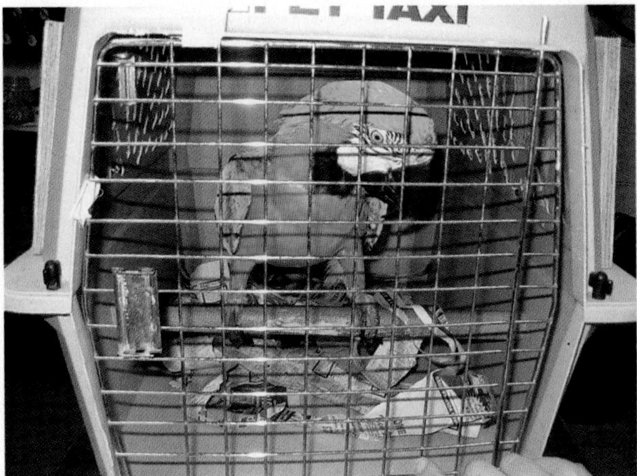
FIGURE 15-2 A pet carrier is recommended for transport of companion birds to the veterinary hospital.

> TECHNICIAN NOTE Approximately 85% of the problems seen in exotic pet medicine result from lack of information on the part of pet stores, pet owners, veterinarians, and veterinary technicians.

BIRDS

The veterinary technician may, on occasion, be involved in telephone communication with clients. When clients call regarding avian patients, it is important to instruct the owner in the following areas. Ask the owners to bring the bird in its own cage or carrier, if at all possible. If the bird is larger and the cage cannot be transported, then the bird should be transported in a plastic small animal carrier. Small animal carriers work well for birds, particularly the carriers with the door in the front. Newspaper or a towel can be used as material to cover the bottom, which is easily cleaned when removed. Wooden dowels can be placed in the carrier as perches and secured in place with screws and washers from the outside (Figure 15-2). Owners should always be advised never to bring their bird to the practice nonsecured; the bird should be in either a carrier or, if small, its cage. They should not clean the cage, except to empty the water dish to prevent it from spilling during the trip. A good evaluation of the bird's environment is helpful to the veterinarian, and clean papers and a clean cage do not provide that information.

BOX 15-1 Common Pet Birds

Psittacines
Budgerigar
Cockatiel
Amazon parrot
Macaw
Conure
Lovebird
African gray parrot

Passerines
Canary
Zebra finch
Java rice bird

> TECHNICIAN NOTE Owners should always be advised never to bring their bird to the practice nonsecured; the bird should be in either a carrier or, if small, its cage.

All grit should be removed because some birds tend to gorge themselves on grit, particularly when ill. The cage should be covered with a towel or blanket to protect it from the weather, and the owner should be instructed to bring along any medication and vitamin supplements the bird is taking and a sample of food. Most avian telephone inquiries should be considered emergencies because of most owners' inability to note early signs of illness, the bird's inherent ability to mask clinical problems, and the rapid speed with which avian species succumb to disease.

TAKING THE CLINICAL HISTORY

The following is a suggested list of questions to ask the client regarding avian patients:

- What is the chief complaint?
- Obtain the signalment (includes the species, gender, and age) (Box 15-1).
- Origin: Where was the bird obtained? How long has it been owned by the presenting party?
- Environment: What is the construction and design of the cage? Is it painted? If so, what type of paint has been used? What is the design and composition of the water and food bowls, substrate (newspaper, wood shavings, corncob, etc.), and perches? Where is the bird kept (indoors or outdoors)? In what room of the house is it kept (e.g., kitchen or garage where potential toxins may be located)? Is it close to a window? Are insecticides, household cleaners, or other chemicals used around the house in the vicinity of the cage? Is the bird allowed out of the cage? If so, is it allowed to fly freely, and how well is it supervised?

TABLE 15-1 Recommended Psittacine Diet

Food Group	What It Supplies	What It Lacks
Cereals and grains, 45%-50%	Proteins, fats, B vitamins	Vitamins A, D, and K and calcium (high phosphorus)
Vegetables, 45%-50%	Vitamins A and K, fiber, carbohydrates ± calcium	Protein, fats, vitamin D_3
Fruit, approximately 5%	Sugars, simple carbohydrates	Proteins, vitamins, minerals
Meats (in combination with dairy products), about 5%	Proteins, fats, calcium	

Mineral supplements (e.g., cuttlebone, oyster shell, mineral blocks, or avian vitamins) may be added to the above diets.
Commercial pelleted diets are primarily a cereal-and-grain-based diet with vitamin and mineral supplementation added.

- Diet: What is the bird being fed (e.g., seed, fruits, vegetables, grain)? How often is it fed? Are vitamins and minerals added to the food? How often is the water changed? How is the food prepared and stored? (Table 15-1)
- Appetite: Notes should be made regarding the bird's overall appetite and daily food consumption.
- Feces: Questions regarding the consistency, color, and number of droppings per day are all important. The client should be asked whether feces have been previously submitted for parasite evaluation.
- Cage mates: Are there other animals in the collection in the same cage or in the household? If so, how many, what species, and what degree of contact do they have with the patient? Does the owner maintain a quarantine policy?
- Molting cycle: When did the bird go through its last general molt, and are there any abnormalities in the feather coat or feather growth?
- Behavior: What is the overall attitude and behavior, including voice quality and changes in vocalization? Have there been behavior-related problems in the past (e.g., feather picking, screaming, or other abnormal behavior)?
- Previous medical history: Has the bird been ill before? Is there a history of disease in other pets in the house? If so, what illnesses have been diagnosed and treated in the past? Have they been to a veterinarian before?

BEHAVIOR CONSIDERATIONS DURING THE EXAMINATION PROCESS

As recommended, all birds should be brought to the practice in a carrier or cage (see Figure 15-2). Although a carrier may be recommended, there are avian patients that will arrive unrestrained. However a bird enters the room, there should be an understanding that the patient is in an unfamiliar, stressful environment. To reduce behavior complications that may arise as a result of the examination, certain considerations are recommended. Capture and restraint is necessary for an examination, but pain and stress should be reduced as much as possible. To achieve this goal, capture and restraint should be accomplished using a towel that covers the hand being used to grasp the bird. The bird should be in a standing position with the towel in full view as the hand approaches the patient's head. Most birds will allow the hand within the towel to grasp behind the neck with very little resistance if the towel is slowly advanced in full view. All diagnostic testing materials and medication should be ready before the bird is restrained. The examination, diagnostic sample collections, treatment, and procedures must be performed quickly to reduce the stress and adverse psychological effects of the hospital visit (Figure 15-3). Once the examination is completed, positive reinforcement of scratching the bird behind its head and communication will aid in transitioning the bird back to the owner.

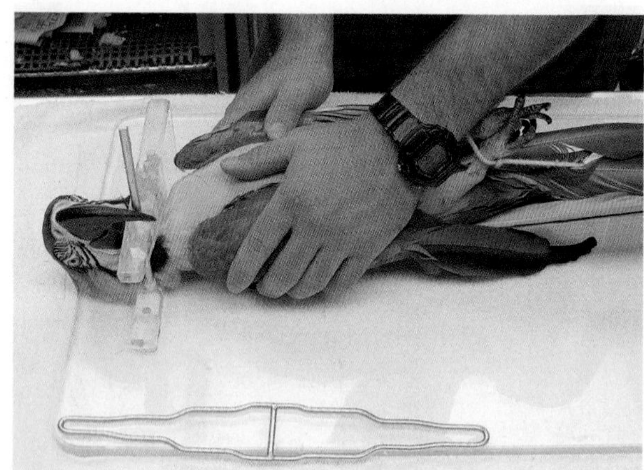

FIGURE 15-3 Once the bird is restrained, an avian examination board may be used to easily examine the patient and obtain diagnostic samples. Care should be made to prevent chest compression by the handler.

If the avian patient has to be hospitalized, placing the bird's cage within a hospital cage will help with accommodation to the unfamiliar surroundings. If the cage is too big to place in the hospital cage, familiar food and toys will help promote psychologic well-being. One point to emphasize to pet bird owners is that returning their bird to its familiar home surroundings as soon as possible will not only help the animal's psychologic comfort, but possibly aid in healing.

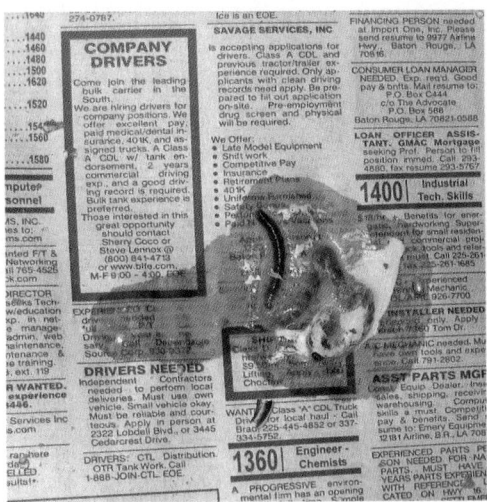

FIGURE 15-4 Normal psittacine stool. Note the dark solid feces, white solid urates, and liquid urine.

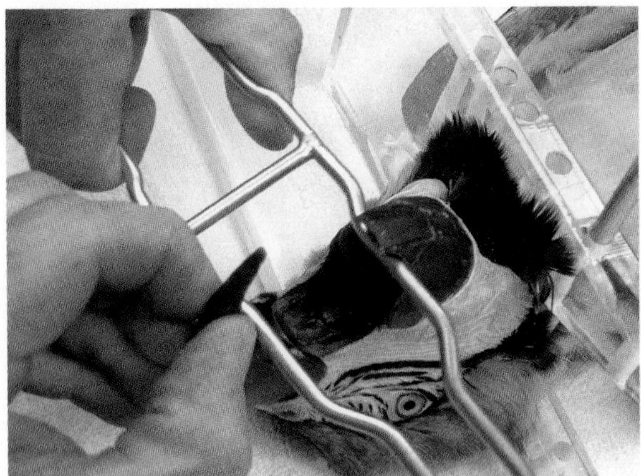

FIGURE 15-5 Oral examination demonstrating the use of a beak speculum on a macaw.

SAMPLE COLLECTIONS AND DIAGNOSTIC PROCEDURES COMMONLY USED IN BIRDS

Diagnostic plans in avian species are no different from the clinical approach to other domestic pets. The evaluation of the stool is an important first step. The technician should become familiar with normal stool presentation to determine differences between polyuria (excessive urine output) and diarrhea (change in the fecal consistency and amount) (Figure 15-4). Fecal parasites may be detected on fresh smears with saline and a coverslip. This is the best method to check for protozoa, such as *Giardia*. Fecal flotation will bring some parasite ova to the surface (e.g., ascarids and *Capillaria*). Fecal sedimentation is an important procedure for the diagnosis of flukes, which may be seen in wild avian species, including raptors. Fecal specimens that are Gram stained are useful to determine the bacterial flora of the digestive tract. Most cage-bird species have preponderantly gram-positive organisms inhabiting the digestive system. Fecal Gram stains are only a preliminary diagnostic test and should be followed up with a bacterial culture.

> TECHNICIAN NOTE Most cage-bird species have preponderantly gram-positive organisms inhabiting the digestive system.

Cloacal Swab

A cloacal swab is often done on a psittacine species to determine the bacterial flora of the lower gastrointestinal tract. A cotton swab is moistened, inserted into the cloaca, and gently rotated. Cloacal swabs are useful for cytologic evaluations and looking for inflammatory cells, such as heterophils. They may also be used for culture and sensitivity tests and *Chlamydia psittaci* or viral isolation.

Oral Examination and Crop Wash

The technician should become adept at assisting in the performance of an oral examination and crop wash by the veterinarian. Good restraint technique is essential (see Chapter 7). An avian beak speculum is placed in the bird's mouth parallel to the commissure and rotated to open the beak (Figure 15-5). A choanal culture should be taken when birds are exhibiting upper respiratory signs. The culturette is placed in the rostral area of the choana to prevent cross contamination with flora in the oral cavity (Figure 15-6).

Another important diagnostic technique is the crop wash. The crop wash permits the examination of the upper gastrointestinal tract. A sterile or clean tube is passed through the mouth into the crop or into the esophagus in those birds with an underdeveloped crop. A syringe of sterile saline is connected to the tube, and a simple flush is performed (Figure 15-7). Tubes may be made of plastic, rubber, or metal and have a ball tip (Figure 15-8). The crop wash is important for a direct microscopic examination to check for protozoans, such as *Trichomonas* spp. or yeast *(Candida albicans)*, using a wet mount technique. Slides may be prepared for cytologic examinations with Diff-Quik stains or Wright's stain, looking for inflammatory cells, such as heterophils. A Gram stain is often done on crop wash samples from psittacine species, or the sample may be submitted for culture and sensitivity (see Chapter 18). A culturette may be passed into a bird's crop for culture and sensitivity diagnostics. Care must be taken so the patient does not bite the culturette and swallow it. Young psittacine species readily accept culturettes into the crop through normal feeding responses.

Passing a tube into the crop of the psittacine bird is an important technique to learn because tube feeding is often necessary to administer medications and/or nutritional supplementation (see Figure 15-7). The tube should be passed over the trachea at the base of the tongue down the esophagus and palpated in the crop at the level of the thoracic inlet. Food that is administered using a feeding tube must have a lower temperature than the bird. Most psittacine species have a body temperature of 102° F to 104° F, so the food should

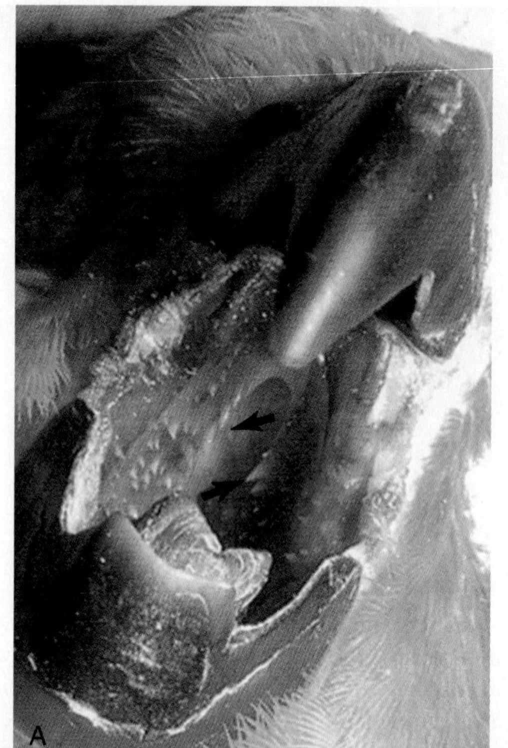

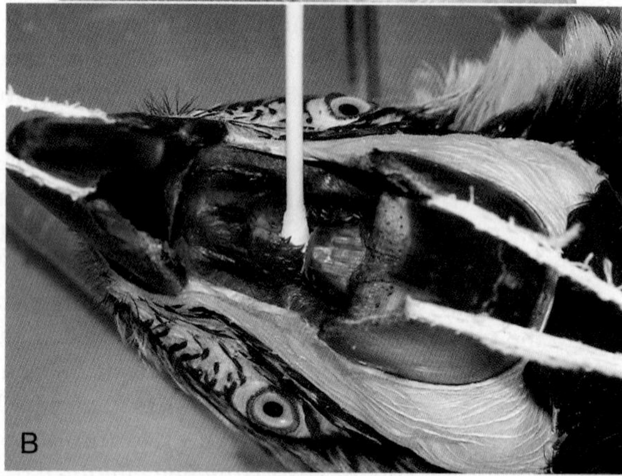

FIGURE 15-6 *A,* Arrow indicates correct placement of culturette. *B,* Culturette placement in the rostral aspect of the choana.

be between 98° F and 101° F. The feeding formula must be thoroughly mixed before uptake into the syringe. Many baby birds develop thermal burns from hot feeding formula (hotter than the birds body temperature), usually on the weight-dependent ventral surface area of the crop. This injury can be prevented by careful preparation of the food by the attending technician. The one rule of thumb to remember when using a tube for either feeding or a crop wash is to try to pick a tube with a diameter larger than the glottis.

> *TECHNICIAN NOTE* Thermal burns to the crop of young birds can be easily prevented by the proper preparation of food and feeding at the recommended temperatures.

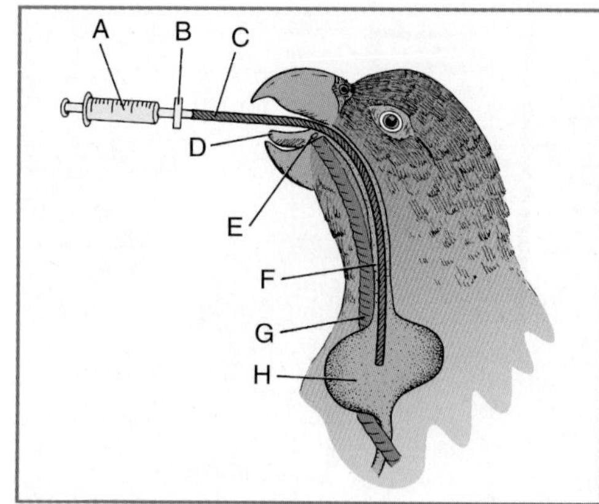

FIGURE 15-7 Proper tube placement for a crop wash or for tube feeding a bird. The bird's neck should be gently stretched. *A,* Syringe. *B,* Adapter, if necessary. *C,* Tube. *D,* Tongue. *E,* Tracheal opening. *F,* Proximal esophagus. *G,* Trachea. *H,* Crop.

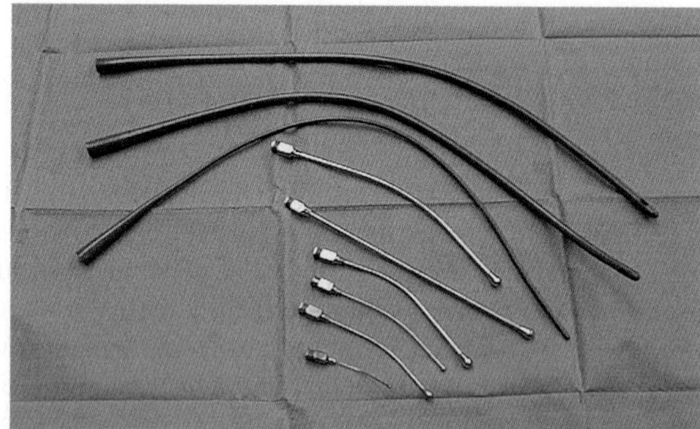

FIGURE 15-8 Various tubes used for tube feeding and crop washes.

The glottis of the bird is located at the base of the tongue and is easy to visualize. The tube may be passed into the crop easily by positioning the tube in the side of the bird's mouth (see Figure 15-8). The tube is easily palpated through the wall of the crop and the skin. While doing a crop wash or tube feeding, the handler should watch the back of the bird's mouth to ensure that food or water does not begin to accumulate. If the crop is overfilled, the bird may aspirate. If the crop overfills, put the bird down and let it attempt to clear its airway. The bird itself has a better chance of clearing its airway than does the technician or veterinarian using cotton-tipped applicators. Never handle a bird after placing oral medications into the crop or filling the crop unless the bird is experiencing respiratory difficulty.

> *TECHNICIAN NOTE* Never handle a bird after placing oral medication into the crop or filling the crop unless the bird is experiencing respiratory difficulty.

Hematology

Hematology is an important part of the diagnostic examination in avian species. Common venipuncture sites include the basilic vein, right jugular vein, and medial metatarsal vein, but other sites may be used depending on the avian species and experience of the phlebotomist. Each has its own advantages and disadvantages, and the veterinarian and technician will tend to develop their own sites of preference, but the right jugular vein is the recommended site for most, if not all, psittacine species.

The right jugular vein is large and easily found in most birds on the right dorsolateral aspect of the neck. However, it is highly mobile and therefore difficult to stabilize. In most birds, the right jugular vein is located in a featherless tract lateral to the trachea. With minimal practice and proper restraint, avian jugular venipuncture becomes an easy procedure to perform. An avian restraint board is recommended for blood collections from larger psittacine patients (see Chapter 7). Small psittacine and passerine patients can be handheld when blood is being drawn for diagnostic tests.

In general, the basilic vein is accessible but difficult to completely immobilize in the psittacine patient because of the tremendous strength of the pectoral muscles (Figures 15-9 and 15-10).

The medial metatarsal vein is easy to immobilize and secure, even on an awake, fractious patient. However, if large volumes of blood are to be collected, the medial metatarsal vein may not be a good choice in psittacine patients.

A toenail-clipping blood sample may be obtained, but it is painful to the patient and often causes lameness for several days following the procedure. It may result in a poor blood flow, low yield, and invalid results. Therefore blood obtained from toenail clipping is only recommended for DNA-based gender determination testing.

The blood may be collected in syringes, microhematocrit tubes, or blood collection tubes from the hub of the needle. A 3-ml syringe with a 26G needle should be used to collect blood in most avian patients. In extremely small psittacine and passerine patients, a 1-ml syringe with a 30G needle may be used. The technician should learn to proficiently perform a complete blood count (CBC) on avian blood.

Radiography

Radiography is an important diagnostic tool in avian patients. Typically, lateral and ventrodorsal views of the whole body or selected extremities may be taken (Figure 15-11). Technique charts must be developed based on the equipment available. Contrast films may be made with standard contrast agents, including iohexol and barium sulfate. Because good positioning and the absence of motion are important to high-quality radiographs, it is generally recommended that all avian patients be sedated or anesthetized, except those who may be too ill. Proper positioning is important, and an avian restraint board is essential (Figure 15-12). Other diagnostic procedures, such as laparoscopy, endoscopy, tracheal or air sac washes, biopsies, cytologic examinations, and bone marrow aspirates, may be performed on the patient. The technician's role may be to secure the animal with good restraint during these more sophisticated procedures.

HUSBANDRY AND TREATMENT IN THE HOSPITAL

Generally speaking, drugs administered in the food or water will not reach adequate therapeutic levels in the avian patient. This is an unreliable way to administer most medications because of the inconsistent intake of water by most birds. Direct oral absorption is inconsistent with tablets, but most liquid suspensions tend to work well. Injections of drugs into birds are best done in the large pectoral muscle mass. Drugs injected into the caudal half of the animal (e.g., the legs) may result in the agent's absorption into the bloodstream and shunted toward the kidneys by way of the renal portal system. Potentially nephrotoxic drugs, such as aminoglycosides, should never be administered by injection into the legs except in ostriches, emus, and rheas and only when the patients are adequately hydrated.

> TECHNICIAN NOTE Injections of drugs into birds are best done in the large pectoral muscle mass.

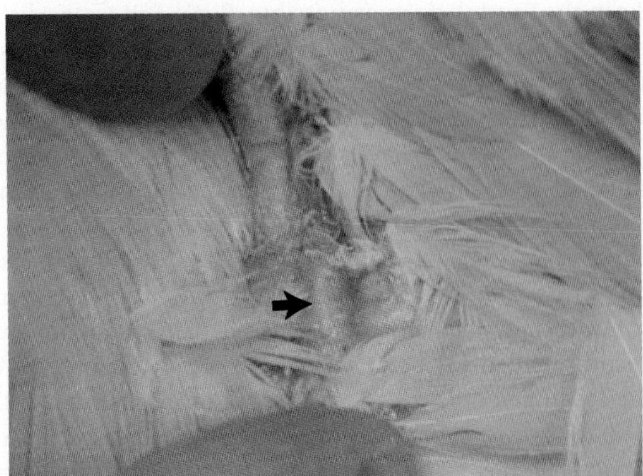

FIGURE 15-9 Location of the basilic vein *(black arrow)*. Ventral view of humerus, radius, and ulna.

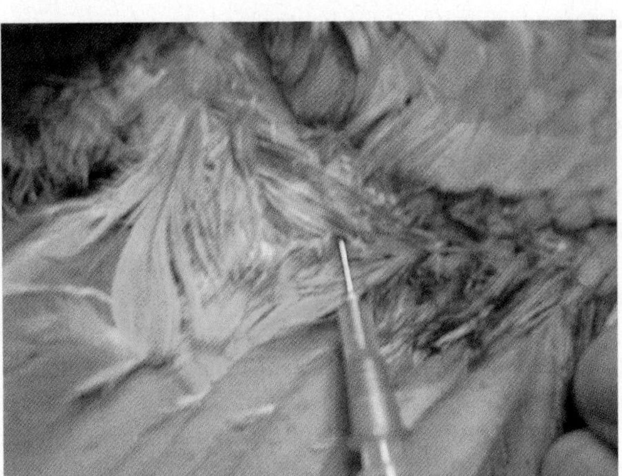

FIGURE 15-10 Intravenous injection using the basilic vein of a blue and gold macaw.

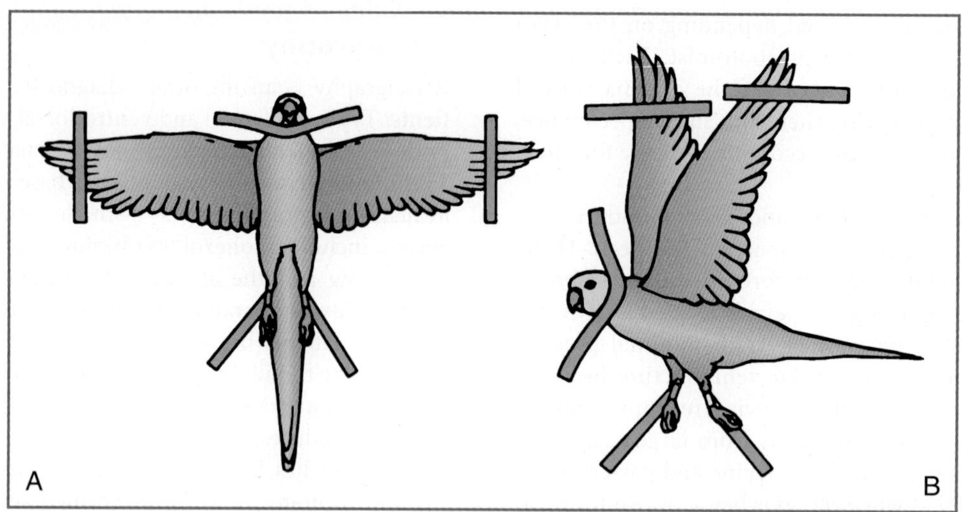

FIGURE 15-11 Positioning of a budgerigar for radiographs using masking tape. **A,** Ventrodorsal and **B,** Lateral positions.

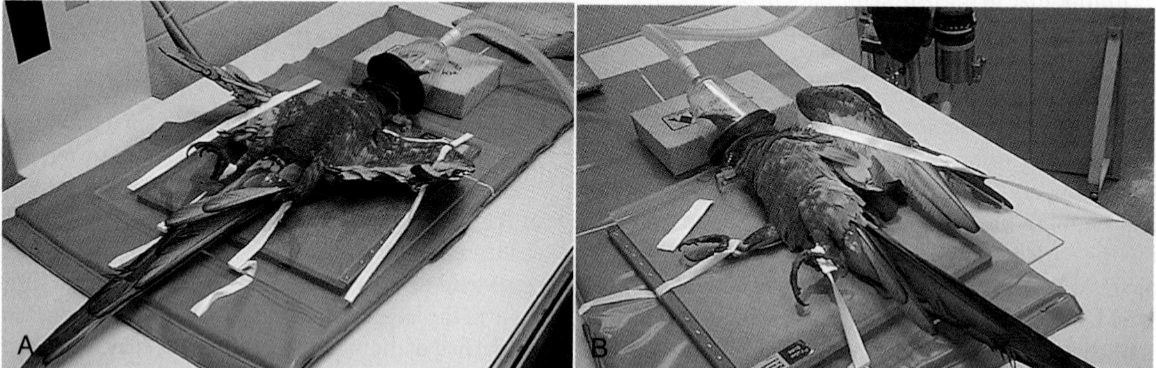

FIGURE 15-12 **A,** Ventrodorsal and **B,** Lateral positioning of a macaw with the use of adhesive tape. The bird is on a Plexiglas avian restraint board for uniform positioning of patients. A face mask is used for the administration of inhalant isoflurane anesthesia.

Common procedures that the veterinary technician often performs are nail trims and clipping of the wing feathers. Figure 15-13 illustrates one technique for clipping the flight feathers of pet birds. Both wings should be clipped for a symmetric effect, but there are many different feather-clip variations that owners request. Typically the primary flight feathers are cut for heavier birds and both the primary and secondary feathers for lighter birds to achieve maximal flight restriction. If only one wing is clipped, the bird cannot control its flight and will be prone to injury. Feather clipping is flight restriction, not prevention. Find out what the owner wants to achieve through the feather trim and how the owner wants the feathers clipped. No trim technique will prevent the bird from flight. In the end, both the owner and technician or veterinarian has to be happy with the look and flight restriction of the trim.

Trimming nails in larger psittacine species should be done with a Dremel Motor Tool (Dremel, Inc., Racine, Wis.). For small psittacine species and passerines, human nail clippers or an electrocautery unit can be used. Cautery units can be used on the nails of birds of all sizes, but work especially well on the smaller species (Figure 15-14). Grinding with a Dremel Motor Tool cauterizes as it reduces the length of the nails (Figure 15-15). Chemical cautery (as with silver nitrate sticks) should be available if bleeding occurs, especially in younger birds.

Dietary management and nutritional support are particularly important in the compromised avian patient. Table 15-1 provides the basic feeding guidelines for psittacine species and other seed-eating birds. It is important to remember to keep the cage as clean as possible. Food and water dishes should be cleaned at least daily and occasionally more often. Fresh fruits, vegetables, and meats should only be left in a food dish for short periods of time. Food consumption should be closely monitored. New food should be introduced gradually, especially the pelleted avian diets. Some food may provide the bird a source of activity while eating, such as peeling vegetables, fruits, and nuts. Tube feeding in psittacine birds is an important nursing procedure. Generally a commercially available cereal-based baby avian formula is recommended for hand raising young psittacine species. Tube feeding should begin with small amounts frequently, which are slowly increased in volume and decreased in time interval. The bird should be weighed one or two times per day to chart weight gain. The crop should be monitored for prompt emptying, and the stools should be examined for

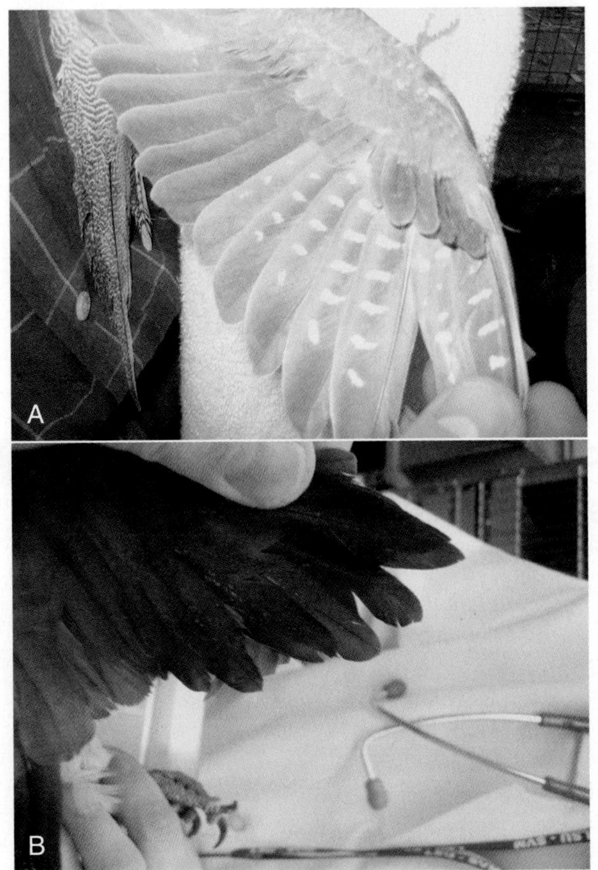

FIGURE 15-13 A, Ventral view of extended wing (when performing a proper feather trim, a symmetrical cut of the 10 outermost feathers is cut below the level of the dorsal coverts). **B,** Proper feather trim of wing on African gray parrot.

consistency. The basal metabolic rate (BMR) may be calculated as a rough approximation of energy requirements using the formula $K(W^{0.75})$. The normal K value for a nonpasserine species, such as parrots, is approximately 78, while W is the weight of the bird in kilograms. This should be doubled for an ill bird. For passerine species, 130 times the body weight raised to the power of 0.7 should be used. For carnivorous birds, such as raptors, a high-quality carnivore critical care diet (Lafeber Co., Ordell, Ill.) may be used to meet their energy requirements.

Hospital facilities must be appropriate for the species that are housed. Bird cages should be in a separate room, if possible, to minimize the stress of sounds and sights of other species. The isolation of birds also prevents the contamination of potentially pathogenic bacteria. For example, psittacine birds have a mostly gram-positive gut flora. Housing birds near animals with gram-negative gut flora, such as dogs, cats, reptiles, and carnivorous birds, could result in gram-negative enteric infections. A visual barrier should be provided for the hospitalized bird, such as a cage cover or hide box in the cage. Large parrots may do well in standard dog or cat cages if adequate perches and water and food bowls are provided. Alternatively, Plexiglas custom cages are an excellent alternative and easily cleaned. Perches should be disposable, simple to disinfect, and sized according to the individual patient. An isolation area is required for avian psittacosis suspects. Cleanliness is one of the most important details in the hospital.

Temperature control is important, particularly with sick birds. In general, birds will tolerate cold better than heat. Sudden changes in temperature and drafts should always be

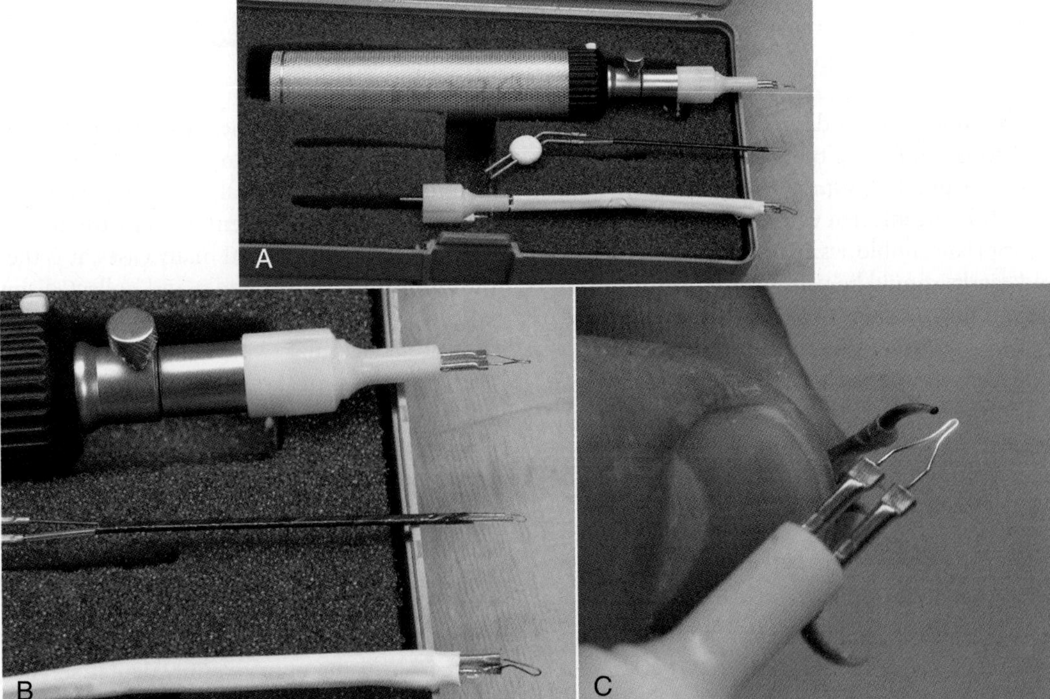

FIGURE 15-14 A, Electrocautery unit for trimming small birds' nails. **B,** Different electrocautery tips. **C,** Trimming bird nails with cautery unit.

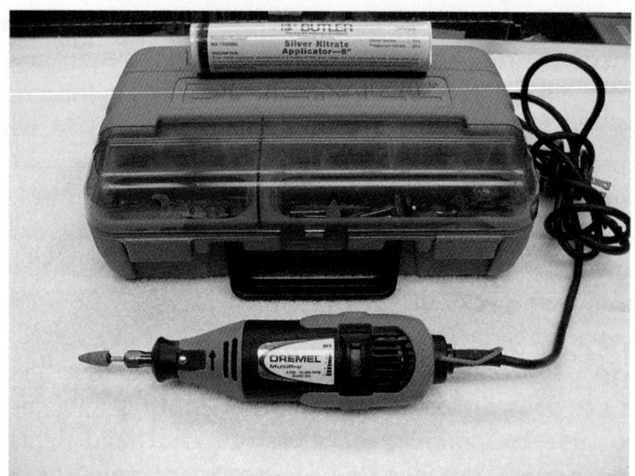

FIGURE 15-15 Motor tool for grinding larger birds' nails and grooming beaks.

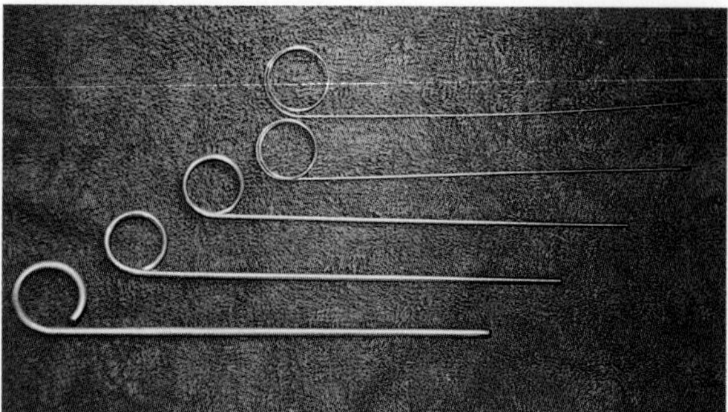

FIGURE 15-16 Snake cloacal probes for sexing.

prevented. Sick birds have difficulty maintaining and regulating their own body temperature, as do birds with poor feather coats, oil-damaged feathers, or plucked feathers. Therefore these birds should be kept warm, but not hot. Temperatures between 80° F and 90° F are best. The bird should be observed for signs of heat stress or shivering. Common signs of heat stress in avian patients are panting, wings extended, flushed (reddish) facial patches on macaws, and depression. An environmentally controlled cage or unit should be available for the intensive-care avian patients.

ZOONOSES AND COMMON CLINICAL PROBLEMS

Chlamydophila psittaci is commonly diagnosed in pet bird species. Avian chlamydiosis is considered a top differential diagnosis for a sick bird that has nonspecific clinical illness (e.g., signs of diarrhea, vomiting, or just not doing well). Patients that have recently been through quarantine or pet shops and exposed to other birds are most suspect.

Avian chlamydiosis is a disease transmissible to humans, caused by the bacterium *C. psittaci*. Those patients suspected of potentially being infected with *C. psittaci* should be treated with appropriate antibiotics. The bird should be isolated, gloves and masks should be used, and feces should be disposed of through the cleaning of the cage and bagging the disposable substrate. The transmission is primarily through respiratory inhalation of the infectious elementary body. Psittacosis is a potentially fatal disease in humans. Many wild birds may carry *C. psittaci* organisms without showing clinical signs. It is important that the veterinary technician working with birds become familiar with this disease.

REPTILES

It is estimated that there are 9 million pet reptiles in the United States according to the AAPMA 2003-2004 pet survey. Although the number of pet reptiles does not match dog and cat populations, there is a significant population of animals that require veterinary health services. The diversity of reptile species maintained in captivity requires owners' education in health, nutritional, and environmental management (Box 15-2). With excellent owner care, most reptile species live long, healthy lives. In many cases, it is the responsibility of the technician to handle and collect diagnostic samples and educate the owner about their captive reptile.

BOX 15-2 Reptiles Commonly Maintained as Pets

Snakes
Boa constrictor *(Boa constrictor)*
Ball python *(Python regius)*
Corn snake *(Elaphe guttata guttata)*
Burmese python *(Python molurus)*

Chelonia
Box turtle (*Terrapene* spp.)
Red-eared slider *(Trachemys scripta elegans)*
Mud turtle (*Kinosternon* spp.)

Lizards
Bearded dragon *(Pogona vitticeps)*
Common tegu *(Tupinambis teguixin)*
Green iguana *(Iguana iguana)*
Green anole *(Anolis carolinensis)*
Jackson's chameleon *(Chamaeleo jacksoni)*
Panther chameleon *(Chamaeleo pardalis)*
Leopard gecko *(Eublepharis macularius)*
Tokay gecko *(Gekko gecko)*
Savannah monitor *(Varanus exanthematicus)*
Water dragon *(Physignathus lesueurii)*

Once a veterinary hospital decides to treat reptiles, there are a few pieces of specialized equipment needed to provide an adequate hospital environment and aid the technician and veterinarian. Required medical equipment includes an electronic gram scale, an incubator, heating pad, tuberculin and microliter syringes, exotic animal formulary (see Recommended Reading), microhematocrit tubes, snake cloacal probes, and metal feeding tubes (Figures 15-16 to 15-18). Common material used on turtle-shell repair includes epoxy, resin, and fiberglas patches. There has been a move away from using epoxy resins, dental acrylics, and patches on turtle-shell repair and toward fracture fixation using cerclage wire and open wound healing. We have found that a

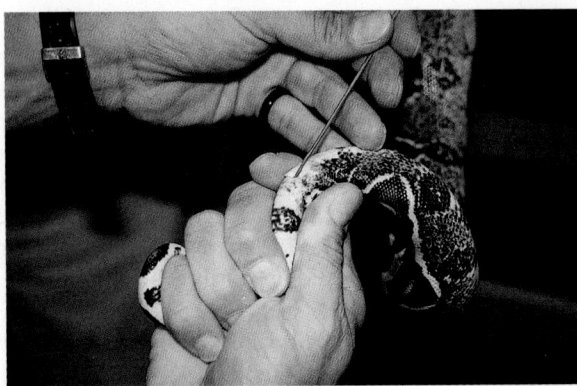

FIGURE 15-17 Snake sexed with cloacal probe.

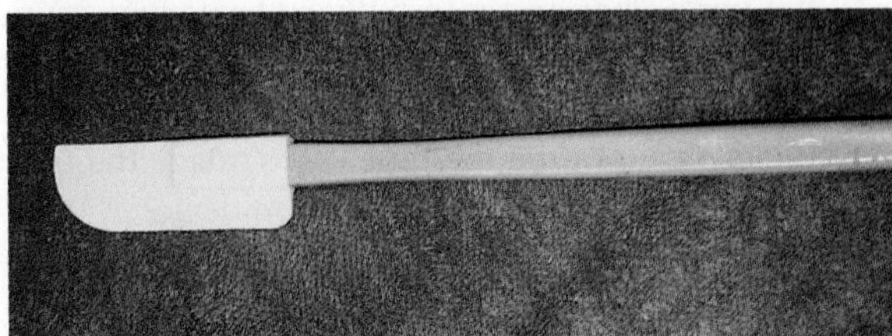

FIGURE 15-18 A spatula is often used as a reptile oral speculum.

combination of both the cerclage fixation of fragments and protection of the fracture site with epoxy resin lead to faster healing and release. Surgical equipment used for reptiles, but available in most exotic animal practices, includes a Dremel Motor Tool, stainless steel suture material, transparent surgical drapes, and a magnifying surgical headset.

Reptile housing equipment must be adaptable to the different species that may be hospitalized. Examples of hospital caging and equipment include fluorescent light tubes (regular and full spectrum), humidifier, fiberglas cages, small aquaria with secure ventilated tops, a heated room, or heat lamps and pads. To aid in capture and restraint, a snake hook, tongs, Plexiglas tubes, and pole snare should be available. As with other exotic species, proper restraint reduces stress to the client, animal, and health care personnel. Once a practice is properly equipped and personnel are trained, interesting patients and cases will begin to receive quality health care.

TAKING THE CLINICAL HISTORY

The following is a list of questions to ask clients regarding reptile patients:

- Chief complaint: Why does the owner want the pet examined?
- Signalment (including the species as specifically as possible): What is the age and gender of the animal, and how long has the client owned the animal?
- Origin: Where did the animal come from?
- Environment: Factors such as cage design, construction materials, substrates, perches, or branches are of critical importance in determining the health of these species. Temperature and humidity and photo period and exposure to sunlight or full spectrum artificial light may have a significant impact on the animal's health. The owner should be questioned as to where the cage is kept in the house, the type of heat source used, and the usual temperature gradient within the cage. For aquatic species, questions pertaining to water quality control, filter systems used, sources of water, and frequency of water change are important. Owners need to list types of cleaning agent and disinfectants used and the frequency of use.
- Food: How often is food offered? How much is consumed? What is the source of the food? How is the food stored, and how is it presented to the animal?
- Water: How often is the water cleaned or changed? How is it offered to the animal? If a water bowl is used, how large is it? For many species, it is important to offer water in a bowl large enough for the animals to completely submerge.
- Feces: How often does the animal defecate in relation to feeding? What are the color and consistency of the stool? Has the owner submitted a fecal sample previously for a parasite evaluation?
- Cage mates: Does the client have other animals in his or her collection or in the same cage? If so, what species are they, and where are they kept? Does the owner maintain a quarantine policy? If so, for how long?
- Behavior: What are the current attitude and behavior of the patient, and have there been any recent changes?
- Shedding: For lizards and snakes, how often does the animal shed? When was the last period of shedding, or ecdysis?
- Previous medical history: Has the animal been ill previously? If it has, it is important to get the owner to describe its illness and any treatments that were done. It is often helpful to include the attending veterinarian's name. Have other animals in the collection ever been ill?

SAMPLE COLLECTION AND DIAGNOSTIC PROCEDURES

Diagnostic approaches in reptiles are often similar to those of other small animal species. As with any diagnostic procedure, ability through experience and confidence determines who will collect the sample needed from the patient. Any of the procedures listed in this section can be mastered by the technician who has the proper sampling equipment and desire.

Colonic Wash

Fecal samples may be collected and examined for gastrointestinal parasites. A fresh sample should be examined under a wet mount, and fecal flotation and sedimentation should be evaluated. If a fecal sample is not available at the time of the examination, specimens may be collected by performing a colonic wash; this is done by passing a lubricated tube or catheter through the cloaca into the colon. A syringe of sterile saline is attached, and a typical flush is performed. The volume of saline is recommended at a volume of 1% or less of the animal's weight. Samples may then be examined for parasites or parasite eggs or prepared for cytology or culture and sensitivity tests.

Bone Marrow

Large lizards, crocodilians, and some other chelonians yield adequate diagnostic bone marrow specimens from their femoral cavities (Frye, 1995). Bone marrow from turtles and tortoises may also be obtained by drilling a hole between the outer and inner layers of the bony shell and using a biopsy needle (Vim-Silverman, Becton-Dickinson Primary Care Diagnostics) to obtain the sample (Frye, 1995). The hole should be patched with epoxy or acrylic resin (Frye, 1995). Snake diagnostic bone marrow specimens may be obtained from the marrow cavities in their ribs.

Stomach Lavage

To examine the upper gastrointestinal tract, especially for identification of cryptosporidiosis, a stomach wash is often performed. This procedure is well tolerated by most reptiles and is a quick and easy procedure to execute in the practice. A lubricated soft rubber catheter is advanced through the mouth into the stomach after premeasuring alongside the animal. The stomach area is in the midcranial body area, and this location should be used as a reference point for the tube placement length. A syringe containing sterile isotonic saline is attached to the catheter, and a simple flush is performed after agitating the stomach with external palpation. Samples obtained are used for a direct microscopic examination for parasites, to prepare slides for cytology, or to perform Gram stains for culture and sensitivities.

Urine Samples

Urine samples may be collected from those species that produce a large volume of urine. Many turtles and lizards have urinary bladders. All reptiles have a cloaca into which the reproductive, gastrointestinal, and urinary tracts empty. A routine urinalysis may be performed on fresh urine samples. A cystocentesis may be performed on turtles by advancing a needle cranial to the hind limb. Turtles will typically void when stressed; thus handling the patient may yield a urine sample. Green-stained solid urates rehydrated with saline may reveal amoebic cysts or fluke ova when examined under a microscope.

Blood Samples

Blood collection in reptiles varies considerably, depending on the species. Do not withdraw more blood than is necessary. If you are not sure of the volume needed, contact your diagnostic laboratory. Direct cardiocentesis and venipuncture can be done using the ventral and lateral caudal veins, jugular, brachial, popliteal, periorbital and pterygopalatine veins, and dorsal postoccipital sinuses depending on the species and size of the animal (Frye, 1995). Toenail clipping is not recommended for blood sample collection because of the inability to obtain reliable hematologic results from this site.

Venipuncture techniques in snakes depend on the experience of the handler. Sites that are often used include the caudal or coccygeal vein of the tail, cardiac puncture, and the ventral abdominal vein or palatine vessels. For blood collection at any site, good restraint of the reptile patient is necessary. For lizards, the caudal tail vein is often most accessible; however, cardiac puncture and the ventral abdominal vein may also be used (Figures 15-19 and 15-20). In turtles, large jugular veins are present and are easily used for venipuncture sites (Figure 15-21).

In large crocodilians, turtles, and tortoises, the occipital sinus or the caudal tail vein may be used. The site chosen will depend on the veterinarian and the technician and their experience with the particular species that is tested. In small lizards, the peribulbar and retrobulbar plexus may be used for blood samples by inserting a heparinized microhematocrit tube between the eyelids and directing it to the inner edge of the orbit. Rotating the tube will damage the plexus, yielding enough blood to fill the collection device.

RADIOGRAPHY

Radiography often is useful to aid in the diagnosis of reptile patients. For many species, radiographs may be taken on unsedated animals by restraining them in shallow boxes, acrylic tubes, or canvas bags. It is important to remember to take at least two views. With turtles, a third (frontal) view

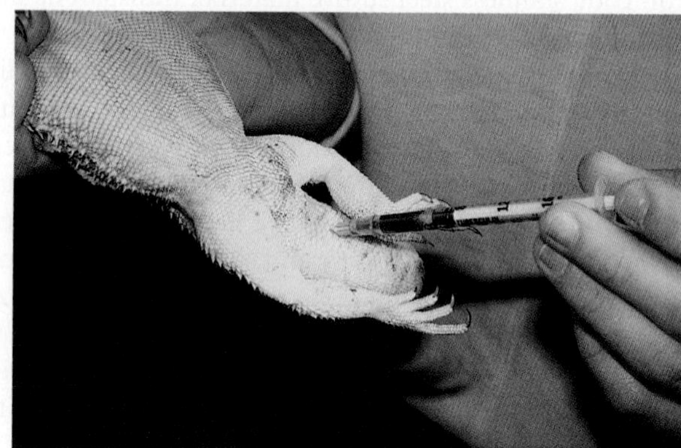

FIGURE 15-19 Restraint of a bearded dragon for venipuncture using the tail vein.

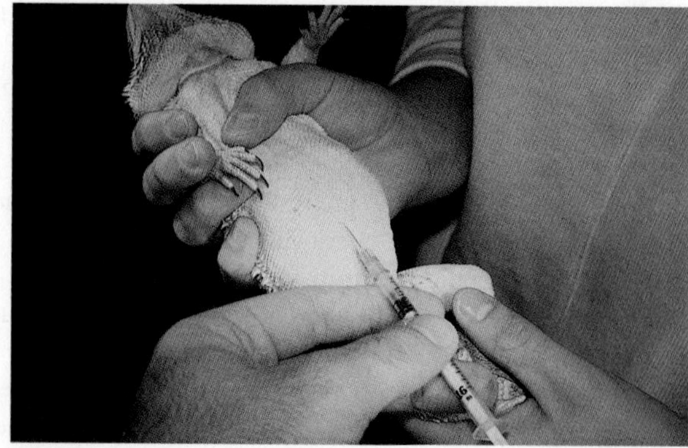

FIGURE 15-20 Venipuncture from the ventral abdominal vein.

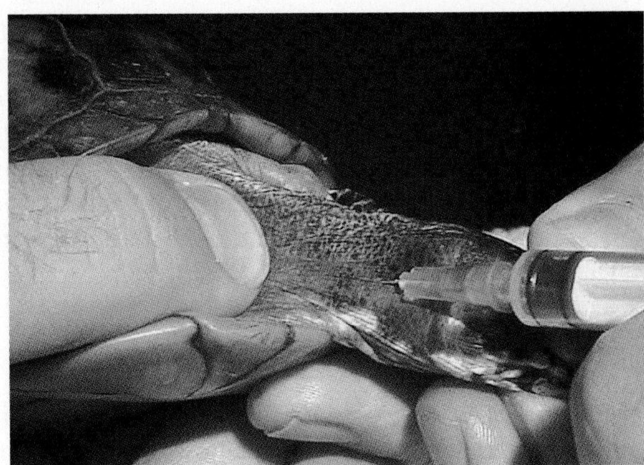

FIGURE 15-21 Jugular venipuncture in a box turtle. The jugular veins are located dorsally at the 10 o'clock and 2 o'clock positions.

should also be taken. Contrast studies may be done, and barium sulfate is easily administered; however, gastrointestinal transit times are long, and it may take 1 week to complete a gastrointestinal barium study. Various other diagnostic procedures may be used, according to the preference of the veterinarian. The technician's knowledge of restraint and reptile behavior will aid in any immobilization process.

HUSBANDRY IN THE HOSPITAL

Reptiles require a controlled microenvironment in a hospital setting. It is important to remember that the temperature and humidity are important because these animals are poikilothermic (i.e., they depend on their environment to regulate their body temperature). A temperature gradient should be provided, whenever possible, by using a thermostat at each end of the cage, resulting in a cooler end and a warmer end. For most species, temperatures should not exceed 32° C (90° F) or dip below 24° C (75° F). The humidity is the other important environmental consideration that is determined by species-specific requirements. In general, the majority of captive reptile species accommodate well in humidity ranges of 50% to 70%. The technician must remember that jungle species usually require a higher humidity, whereas desert species do better in lower humidity ranges.

TECHNICIAN NOTE In general, the majority of captive reptile species accommodate well in humidity ranges of 50% to 70%. The technician must remember that jungle species usually require a higher humidity, whereas desert species do better in lower humidity ranges.

It is important that hospitalized reptiles are maintained at the upper end of their temperature gradient during convalescence to aid in recovery. For many species, a variety of aquaria are sufficient for short-term hospitalization. Any substrate used should be one that is easily cleaned and disinfected or disposable, such as newspaper. It is important to house reptiles separately from psittacine birds, in particular, to prevent the contamination of birds from the normal gram-negative flora of most reptiles. Cages should be provided with hide boxes or areas of seclusion and perching for some species, such as iguanas and some snakes.

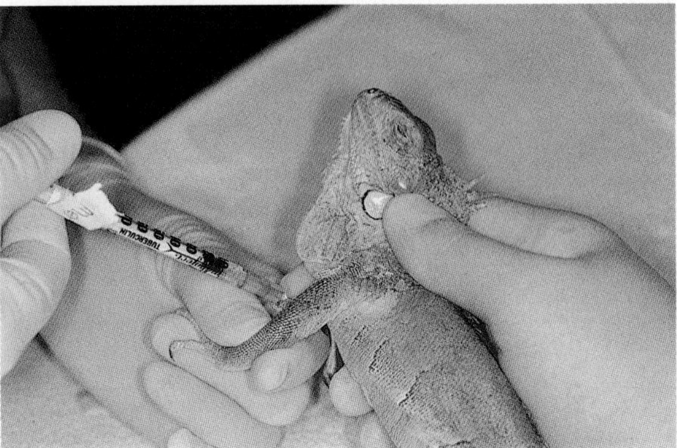

FIGURE 15-22 Injection into the forelimb of an iguana.

TECHNICIAN NOTE It is important that hospitalized reptiles are maintained at the upper end of their temperature gradient during convalescence to aid in recovery.

Tube feeding is an important technique for the veterinary technician to learn. Supplemental feed administration using a tube is easily accomplished, even by technicians without much experience with reptiles. A tube should be well lubricated and passed the distance necessary to place it in the stomach. The glottis of reptiles is adjacent to the base of the tongue and is easily avoided. The glottis of snakes may actually be extended by the animal outside the mouth to accommodate large prey items. The tube is gently passed all the way to the stomach, and food injected. Fluids may also be administered by this route. For patients that are anorectic, supplemental tube feeding may be accomplished by using a blended formula of food that is appropriate for the species. There are also commercial critical care supplements (Carnivore Critical Care, Lafeber Co., Ordell, Ill., Critical Care for Herbivores, Oxbow Pet Products, Murdock, Neb.) available that can be tube fed to herbivorous, carnivorous, and insectivorous species after reconstitution with water. Dietary references for reptile species are listed in Recommended Reading. It is imperative that the technician become familiar with proper reptile diets to maintain healthy animals and supplement sick patients.

Injections given to reptiles are usually performed on the cranial half of the animal's body, primarily the epaxial muscles and the muscles of the forelimbs (e.g., biceps brachii and long heads of the triceps brachii) (Figure 15-22). This is due to the renal portal system that routes blood from the caudal third of the body through a capillary network into the kidneys before returning it to the general circulation. It is important to refrain from giving nephrotoxic drugs in the caudal third of the reptile patient's body. Injection sites are easily found in all reptile species, either in the forelimbs or in the epaxial musculature of the snake. Oral medications are

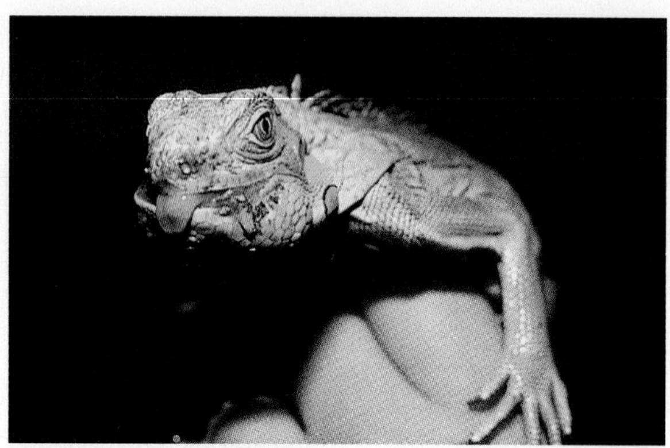

FIGURE 15-23 Metabolic bone disease in a lizard caused by an improper diet.

easily given using a stomach tube. Liquids are preferred over tablets, which are not consistently absorbed.

> TECHNICIAN NOTE It is important to refrain from giving nephrotoxic drugs in the caudal third of the reptile patient's body.

Dietary requirements vary tremendously from species to species and may be an important factor in the disease of the patient. Dietary deficiencies are not commonly seen in snakes, which eat a whole-animal diet; however, a variety of dietary deficiencies are commonly seen in lizards, turtles, and crocodilians. One of the most common is metabolic bone disease. Metabolic bone disease is caused by an inappropriately low calcium intake, low vitamin D_3 intake, or excessive phosphorus intake (Figure 15-23). This may be prevented by a suitable diet and exposing the animal to ultraviolet (UV) light, either naturally or artificially. It is essential that reptiles, especially lizards, have full-spectrum light available during normal daylight hours. Sunlight through glass does not provide the needed light supplementation because of the blocking ability of glass; direct sunlight or the appropriate artificial lighting is needed. Animals with metabolic bone disease must be treated very gently because their bones are subject to pathologic fractures. Vitamin A deficiency is commonly seen in turtles and tortoises and usually manifests itself by an overgrown beak, palpebral edema, and conjunctivitis. This underscores the importance of thoroughly researching the dietary history of the reptile patient.

> TECHNICIAN NOTE It is essential that reptiles, especially lizards, have full-spectrum light available during normal daylight hours.

SKIN

There are clinical dermatologic diseases noted in reptilian species, as in other animals. Proper diagnostic techniques are needed to identify the problem to implement the appropriate treatment.

Skin specimens may be cultured for bacterial and fungal organisms. For fungal identification, dermatophyte test medium (DTM), fungal growth medium, or Sabouraud culture medium may be used. Bacterial organisms may be isolated on blood agar or subcultured in a thioglycollate-containing medium. Samples for skin culture may be taken using cotton-tipped culturettes or by using pieces of the affected skin, scales, or dermal scutes.

FECES

Fecal material can be very useful in diagnosing parasite infestations, bacterial infections, pancreatic enzyme levels, and the presence of blood in the gastrointestinal tract. The fecal specimen should be as fresh as possible. If a fresh voided sample is not available, fecal material may be removed from the terminal alimentary tract by gentle palpation or by the insertion of a fecal extractor or cotton-tipped applicator stick through the cloacal vent (Boyer, 1998). The aid of a warm water enema may stimulate defecation in difficult cases. As with the colonic wash, an enema of 1% or less of the animal's body weight is recommend as the fluid volume to use for most captive reptile species.

SPUTUM

To obtain a sample of sputum, insert a cotton-tipped applicator into the discharge. Roll the sample applicator across a microscope slide, add a drop of coloring agent, apply a coverslip, and examine for parasite ova (Boyer, 1998). Common parasites diagnosed in sputum samples are *Rhabditis* spp., *Entomelas* spp., and *Strongyloides stercoralis.* When handling diagnostic samples, proper hygiene is essential because of the zoonotic potential of many animal diseases and parasites.

ZOONOSES AND COMMON CLINICAL PROBLEMS

The technician should be aware of common zoonotic infections and clinical problems associated with reptiles.

SMALL MAMMALS

FERRETS

Ferrets have been gaining in popularity as a companion animal. As ferrets gain popularity, they are also seen with increasing frequency in veterinarians' offices; thus it is imperative that technicians become familiar with these pets.

Ferrets do not have retractable claws, but they do have a vascular "quick" delineation that can be used as a point to trim. Small nail-trim scissors or human nail clips are recommended for ferret nail trims. If bleeding occurs after a nail trim, silver nitrate sticks can be used for chemical cautery. Ferret nails are sharp, and owners often request nail trims to blunt the claws.

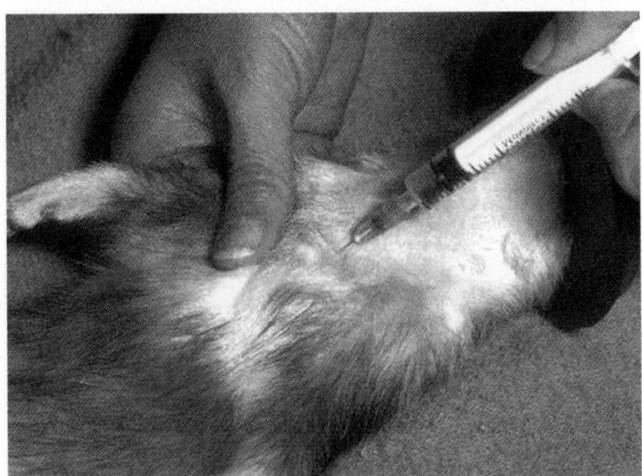

FIGURE 15-24 Cranial vena cava venipuncture of an anesthetized ferret with its head in an anesthetic mask.

When obtaining sample collections of blood, physical restraint alone is often inadequate. Chemical restraint is commonly employed. Blood samples are drawn from the jugular vein, the cranial vena cava, or the cephalic vein. To draw samples of blood from these sites, the animal's head must be securely restrained and grasped around the neck with thumb and fingers resting on the mandibles. To position an animal for jugular venipuncture, it is often best to stretch the animal out, using the other hand to grasp the hind limbs. The ferret's thick skin and subcutaneous fat make blood collection from the jugular vein difficult. To draw adequate blood samples, the cranial vena cava may be preferred (Figure 15-24).

> *TECHNICIAN NOTE* The ferret's thick skin and subcutaneous fat make blood collection from the jugular vein difficult. To collect adequate blood samples, the cranial vena cava may be preferred.

Ketamine hydrochloride or gas anesthetic agents, such as isoflurane or sevoflurane, may be used for chemical restraint. When using a gas anesthetic, an induction chamber is recommended for induction. The patient may be removed from this chamber as it loses the ability to right itself. The anesthetic may then be continued with the use of a face mask. Sample collection on the anesthetized animal is much easier, safer, and less stressful to the animal. Urine may be obtained by cystocentesis because the bladder is easily palpated. If desired, for prolonged anesthesia, ferrets are easily intubated with small standard endotracheal tubes or Cole tubes.

Strategies for treating ferrets in the practice revolve around the handler's ability to restrain the animal and perform the treatment in the most efficient and quickest manner possible. For giving drugs, Nutrical, dairy products, and sweets are useful in bribing animals and in hiding medications. Most ferrets will do almost anything for yogurt or ice cream. Liquid medications are much easier to administer than pills.

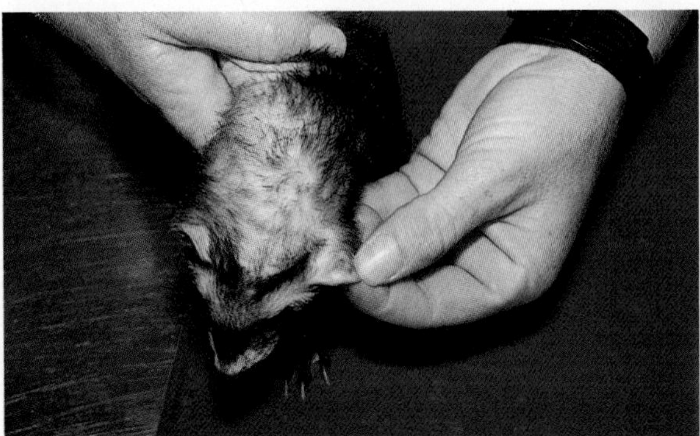

FIGURE 15-25 A tattooed dot indicates this is an early spayed or neutered, descented ferret.

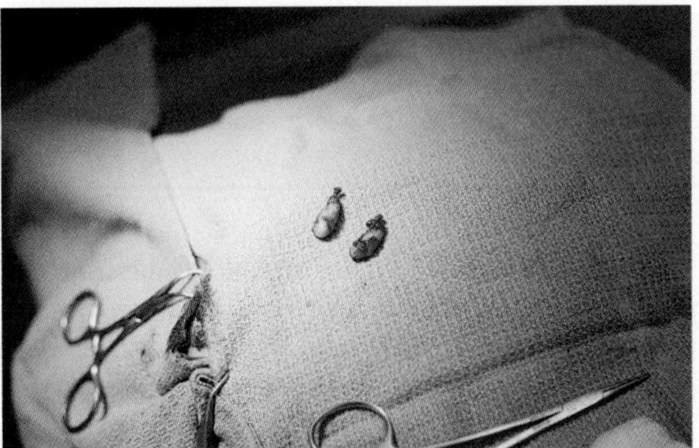

FIGURE 15-26 Anal sacs removed from a ferret.

A potentially fatal common clinical problem of the ferret is estrogen toxicity in females as a result of prolonged estrus. Female ferrets are induced ovulators and occasionally will not cycle out of heat unless bred. These animals become severely anemic and thrombocytopenic because of the toxic effects of estrogen on the bone marrow. Ferrets often are brought into the practice with signs of lethargy, dyspnea, petechial hemorrhages, vomiting, and diarrhea. This is best treated by prevention and education of the client. Female ferrets not intended for breeding should be spayed before their first heat. Since most ferrets in the United States have been spayed and descented before purchase, this is not a concern with most owners. Ferrets that have been spayed or neutered and descented by a breeding facility at an early age will have one or two tattooed blue dots on the surface of the pinna (Figure 15-25). When an owner talks of descenting a ferret, the procedure involves surgically removing the two anal scent glands of the animal. The two anal scent gland openings are located at the 4 and 8 o'clock position when the anal mucocutaneous junction is slightly everted (Figure 15-26). Most ferrets have had the anal scent glands removed before purchase (look for the ear tattoo), but still have a musky odor. Shampooing the ferret on a regular basis will reduce the musky smell, but not eliminate the odor. Ferret-specific shampoo and cologne products are recommended and can be purchased at most large retail pet outlets.

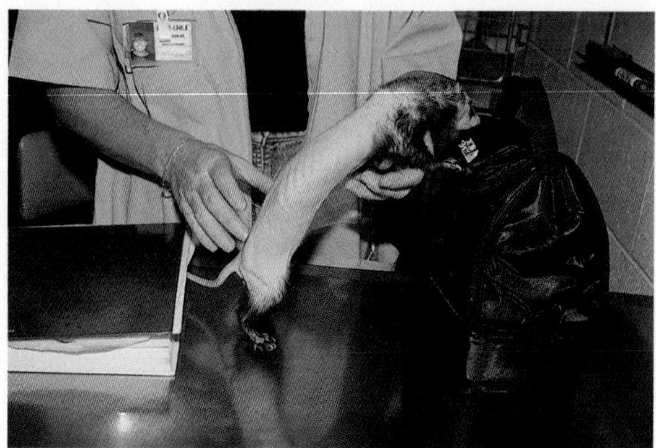

FIGURE 15-27 Hair loss in a ferret as a result of adrenal gland disease.

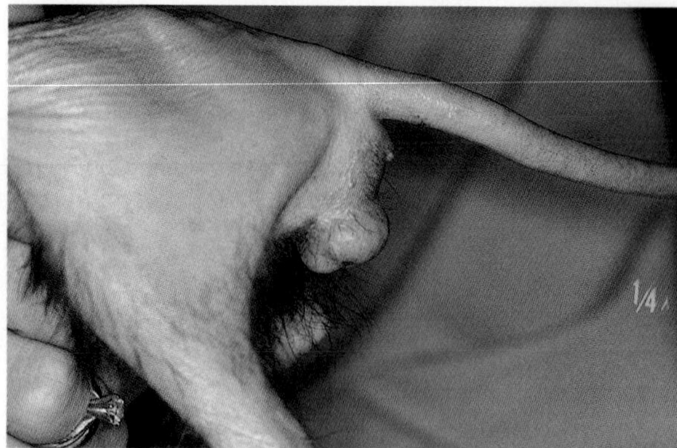

FIGURE 15-28 Swollen vulva in ferret as a result of adrenal gland disease.

> *TECHNICIAN NOTE* Ferrets that have been spayed or neutered and descented by a breeding facility at an early age will have one or two tattooed blue dots on the surface of the pinna.

Clinical signs similar to those of prolonged estrus include hair loss and a swollen vulva, which may be caused by adrenal hyperplasia (Figures 15-27 and 15-28). Female ferrets that have been spayed at an early age are extremely susceptible to this clinical condition. An adrenal hyperplasia work-up should be performed on an older spayed female ferret exhibiting signs of vulvar swelling. Adrenal hyperplasia can be treated by a partial adrenalectomy and/or the administration of therapeutic agents (e.g., leuprolide acetate). The response to therapy and surgery has been varied.

Ferrets are susceptible to human influenza, and clients should be counseled that when members of the family have influenza, the ferret should not be handled. Human influenza in a ferret must be differentiated from canine distemper and bacterial pneumonia, to which ferrets are also susceptible. Both have similar signs of respiratory disease: nasal and ocular discharges, coughing, and sneezing. The ferret with influenza will, in most cases, recover from the infection on its own in 5 to 10 days. A treatment protocol that includes antihistamines and decongestants may be of benefit. The nonvaccinated ferret will not survive a canine distemper infection, and signs usually progress to severe dyspnea, anorexia, and sometimes involvement of the central nervous system.

> *TECHNICIAN NOTE* A potentially fatal common clinical problem of the ferret is estrogen toxicity in females caused by prolonged estrus.

Parasites are a problem that must be understood by the ferret owner. Heartworm prevention is required in animals that are maintained in an outdoor enclosure where they are exposed to mosquitoes. Fleas commonly plague ferrets, even if maintained within a household setting. Feline flea control products are generally safe to use on flea-infested animals. Ear mite treatment and control and heartworm prevention are also important issues that need to be addressed with the owner (see Chapter 17).

Ferrets are also fond of chewing on objects, preferably soft rubbery toys, and should be watched closely for foreign body ingestion. A ferret that has signs of anorexia should be considered to have a potential gastrointestinal obstruction. Toys for ferrets should be limited to objects they cannot bite or "ferret tubes" in which they can crawl. Ferrets have very strong jaws and sharp teeth; there are few leather or rubber objects that they cannot bite and eventually swallow. There are also many reports of various neoplastic diseases in ferrets, including insulinomas, osteomas, lymphosarcomas, and fibrosarcomas. If a ferret is depressed or moribund, a blood serum glucose test should be performed because of common hypoglycemia.

Ferrets should be vaccinated for canine distemper using the PUREVAX ferret canine distemper vaccine (Merial, Duluth, Ga.) or the Galaxy-D vaccine. The American Ferret Association, Inc. (AFA) recommends that 1 ml of the vaccine be injected subcutaneously in healthy ferrets at 8, 11, and 14 weeks of age and then annually. If the ferrets are older than 14 weeks of age or with an unknown or outdated vaccine history, a series of two vaccines should be given 2 weeks apart then annually on the anniversary of the first booster. In cases where kits are exposed, the vaccine may be given as young as 6 weeks of age. Ferrets are not susceptible to feline panleukopenia and therefore should not be vaccinated. In many jurisdictions, ferrets are required to have a rabies vaccine and tag, although they are often not required to wear the tag. It is unlikely that an indoor ferret will be exposed to the rabies virus, but the IMRAB-3 rabies vaccine (Rhone Merieux, Inc., Athens, Ga.) will protect the ferret in the event of exposure and support its quarantine if a person is bitten. The AFA recommends that all ferrets be vaccinated against the rabies virus. Other preventive medicine measures regarding ferrets include good dental care and surveillance for gastrointestinal parasites. Ferrets are strict carnivores and should be fed a diet that meets their unique nutritional requirements. There are a number of commercially available diets that will provide the proper nutrition for the pet ferret. If the ferret diets are not available, a high-quality cat food may be used. Although a cat food diet may be slightly low in protein requirements for the pregnant or lactating ferret, few problems have been reported in ferrets eating high-quality cat food diets.

TECHNICIAN NOTE Ferrets should never be vaccinated against canine distemper using a vaccine of ferret cell origin.

The administration of fluids in a ferret that is less than 5% dehydrated may be administered per os or subcutaneously, whereas an indwelling intravenous catheter should be placed in any animal that is greater than 5% dehydrated. Subcutaneous fluids may be administered in the subcutaneous space between the shoulder blades. The cephalic and lateral saphenous veins are routine sites for intravenous catheter placement.

Fecal samples are often voluntarily given by patients before or during an examination. If a fecal sample needs to be obtained, a lubricated, small, feline fecal loop will often provide a sufficient sample for a test evaluation.

RABBITS

The rabbit is not a rodent, but rather a lagomorph of the family Leporidae. Rabbits may be housed indoors or outdoors and fed primarily a grass-based diet (Oxbow Enterprises, Murdock, Neb.) with supplemented grass-based pellets. Rabbits come in many sizes, ranging from the Flemish Giant (6 to 7.5 kg) to the Dutch and Polish breeds (1 to 2 kg). If proper husbandry practices are maintained, a pet rabbit should live a long, healthy life (5 to 6 years). Rabbits are sensitive to extreme hot and cold conditions, but primarily heat.

Rabbits defend themselves by using their long incisors to bite and by kicking with the hind legs. When kicking, their sharp claws can seriously injure the handler. Owners often inquire about "declawing" their rabbit, but this surgical procedure is strongly discouraged. To sex the rabbit, stretching the perineum while the animal is in dorsal recumbency will reveal the anogenital area. Males have a round urethral opening; females have a slit opening.

The rabbit that is a candidate for anesthesia should have food withheld for 8 to 12 hours and be free from respiratory disease. Some breeds of rabbits have atropinesterase, which inactivates atropine. Atropine may be given subcutaneously as a preanesthetic agent to decrease salivation. If a rabbit has atropinesterase, it may be necessary to increase the dose of atropine. Although recommended, rabbits are seldom intubated during anesthesia because they rarely regurgitate and are extremely difficult to intubate. Recommended endotracheal tubes in rabbits have inside diameters of 2 to 4 mm. A medium laryngoscope or rigid endoscope will aid in passing the tube into the rabbit's glottis to near the thoracic inlet. Do not use a topical anesthetic on rabbits to prevent laryngospasm.

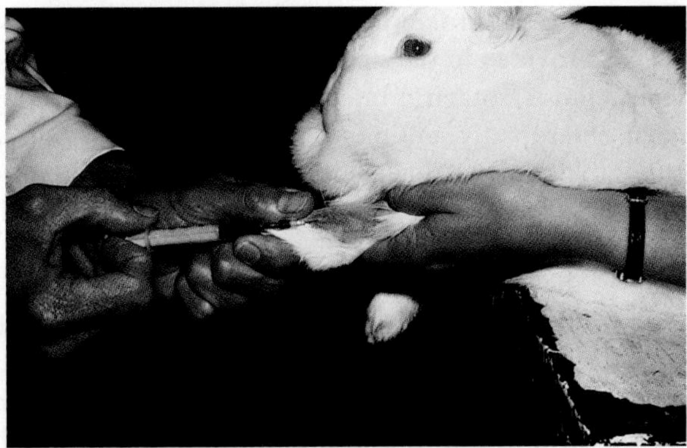

FIGURE 15-29 Blood collection from cephalic vein of rabbit.

TECHNICIAN NOTE Although recommended, rabbits are seldom intubated during anesthesia because they rarely regurgitate and are difficult to intubate.

Injectable anesthetic agents used in rabbits include ketamine, xylazine, and acepromazine; isoflurane is the inhalation anesthetic agent of choice. The movement of the nictitating membrane over approximately one third of the cornea, a respiratory rate of 18 to 24 respirations per minute, abdominal musculature relaxation, and the loss of the ear, mouth, toe pinch, and palpebral reflexes indicate a suitable plane of surgical anesthesia in the rabbit.

By placing a rabbit in dorsal recumbency and gently stroking its ventrum, one causes hypnosis to occur. Hypnosis is a good restraint for injections and radiographic procedures.

When giving intravenous injections to rabbits, the dorsal surface of the ear should be shaved to expose the marginal ear vein. Visibility of this vein will increase if alcohol is rubbed on the area. The central artery of the ear or the cephalic or lateral saphenous vein can also be used for bleeding (Figure 15-29). Cardiac puncture for blood collection should be used only under strict professional supervision and only as a last resort in the clinical setting. The lateral saphenous vein, which is located higher on the leg than in dogs, may be used to place an indwelling catheter.

Rabbits are affected by a number of infections and parasitic organisms. A pet rabbit may have hair loss caused by self-trauma; nutritional deficiencies; bacterial dermatitis (*Pasteurella multocida, Pseudomonas aeruginosa, Staphylococcus aureus,* and *Fusobacterium* spp.); parasites (ear mite *Psoroptes cuniculi* [Figures 15-30 and 15-31]); fur mites, *Cheyletiella parasitovorax;* and rabbit lice, *Haemodipsus ventricosus.* Flea prevention and control is also needed for rabbits, especially animals that are maintained outside (see Chapter 17). Ulcerative lesions on the ventral surface of the rear hocks are usually due to poor husbandry or environmental pressures. Fungal organisms that have been noted to cause dermatopathies in rabbits are *Microsporum gypseum* and *Trichophyton mentagrophytes.*

An anorexic pet should be examined for malocclusion, hairballs, trauma, dietary change, stress, dysbiosis, or poor feed. Heat stress (stroke) is common when adequate cooling is not provided in the summer. Diarrhea may be caused by colibacillosis, rotavirus infections, *Clostridium* infections, mucoid enteropathy, antibiotic intake, or Tyzzer's disease *(Bacillus piliformis)*. A high-fiber diet, which includes timothy hay, has been shown to improve digestive tract function and reduce incidence of hairballs.

One of the main disease problems in rabbits is *P. multocida* infection (snuffles). Clinical signs include nasal discharge, torticollis, abscesses, conjunctivitis, and respiratory distress. Venereal spirochetosis should always be considered when rabbits are exhibiting infertility. *Eimeria stieda* is a hepatic coccidium that may affect attitude and eating habits.

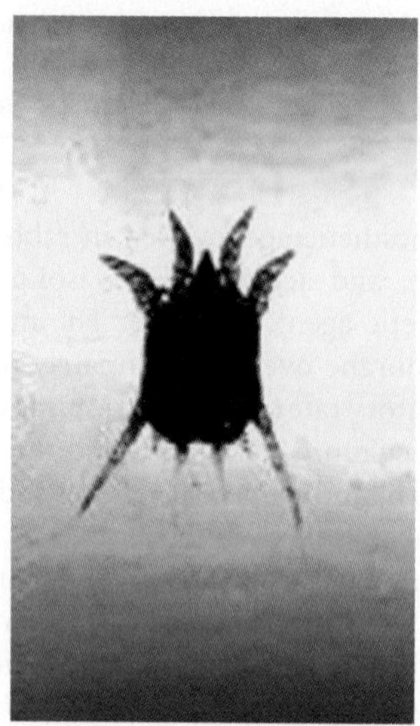

FIGURE 15-30 Microscopic view of *P. cuniculi*, the rabbit ear mite.

Rabbits are territorial and fight when sexual maturity is reached or a male is placed in a female's cage for breeding. Neutering or an ovariohysterectomy is recommended to prevent unwanted offspring.

Malocclusion often leads to elongated incisors and sharp enamel points on the molars. Rabbit-specific dental instruments should be used (Jorgensen Laboratories, Loveland, Colo.) to reduce teeth fracture and other complications associated with dental procedures (Figure 15-32). Most teeth-trimming procedures are done under general anesthesia, particularly when a Dremel Motor Tool is used. Gingival, lingual, and buccal lacerations are the primary complications when trimming molars. To access the oral cavity when trimming molars, a nose cone is used to maintain gas anesthesia, and buccal specula are recommended.

RODENTS

Rodent species commonly seen in the veterinary hospital include guinea pigs, hamsters, gerbils, rats, and, to a lesser extent, mice. Although all of these animals are rodents, each species has particular anatomic characteristics, dietary requirements, and diseases. Blood collection in most rodent species can be accomplished using the anterior vena cava with the patient placed under general anesthesia.

Antibiotic Therapy

Care must be taken when prescribing antibiotics to rodents. Guinea pigs, rabbits, and hamsters are extremely sensitive to the penicillin class of antibiotics, which may cause severe intestinal flora changes (dysbiosis); penicillins, streptomycin, and dihydrostreptomycin are drugs that may cause this problem. Tetracyclines work well in cases that require

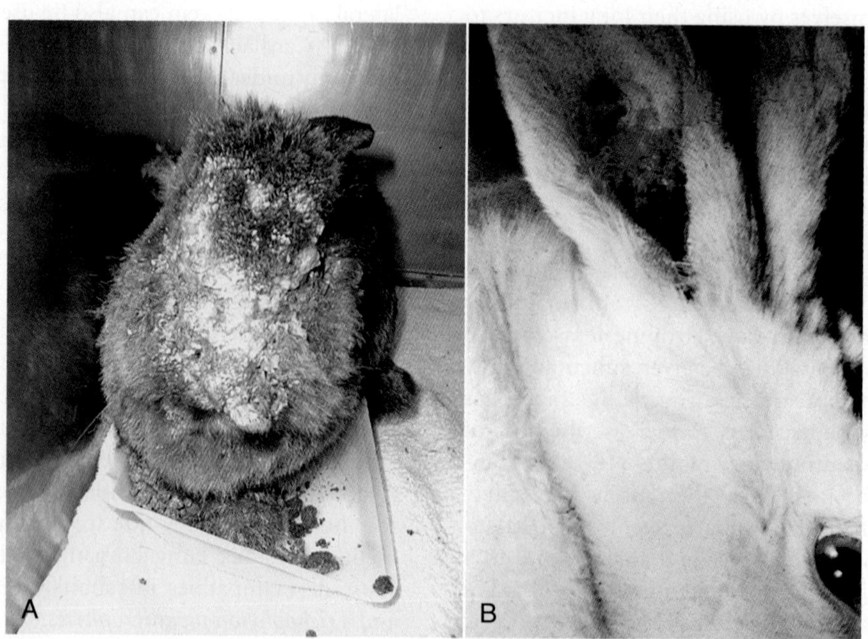

FIGURE 15-31 **A,** Rabbit exhibiting severe clinical signs of *P. cuniculi* infestation, extending to the face. **B,** *P. cuniculi* infestation in external ear canal of rabbit.

antibiotic therapy. An exotic animal formulary is essential to an exotic animal practice to obtain specific information and dosage.

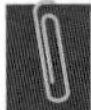

TECHNICIAN NOTE Guinea pigs, rabbits, and hamsters are extremely sensitive to penicillin antibiotics.

Anesthesia

Ketamine hydrochloride, pentobarbital sodium, and thiamylal sodium are injectable anesthetic agents that may be used in rodents. Isoflurane or sevoflurane are the anesthetic agents of choice, providing quick induction and recovery while providing an adequate plane of anesthesia. Chapter 27 discusses anesthesiology.

Antiparasitic Agents

Carbaryl powder, dichlorvos, and ivermectin can be used to treat ectoparasites. Dichlorvos, thiabendazole, and ivermectin are adequate to treat internal parasites. See Chapter 17 for additional information on parasitology.

GUINEA PIG

The cavy, or guinea pig, is a rodent related to porcupines and chinchillas. Guinea pigs have a long gestation that leads to the birth of large, precocious young. The most common guinea pig species kept as pets are the English or American, Abyssinian, and Peruvian long hair (Figures 15-33 and 15-34). The guinea pig has open-rooted teeth that may become maloccluded (Figure 15-35). The overgrown teeth will irritate the gingiva, causing excessive salivation. Although the female has only two mammary glands, it can successfully raise litters of three or more offspring.

A female guinea pig that is bred past 7 or 8 months of age may have trouble separating the pubic symphysis, causing a nondeliverable dystocia. Fat pads may also occlude the pelvic canal, complicating parturition. These problems usually lead to dystocia or death. If the sow is experiencing dystocia, a cesarean retrieval of the young can often save the babies. Food preferences are established within a few days after birth for the young. Hand rearing of the young requires regular stimulation of the anus for defecation and urethral opening for urination, as with most neonatal mammals. Females usually allow foster nursing of other young.

Guinea pigs rarely become excited or bite when handled. Through their gentle nature, they become conditioned to their surroundings. However, if a group is contained in an enclosure, subordinate animals may be traumatized (as by hair loss and bite wounds) by dominant cage mates.

Footpad dermatitis resulting in ulcers may develop on animals placed on wire (Figure 15-36). Metal, plastic, and glass make excellent cages for guinea pigs. The substrate may be paper (shredded), wood shavings, or hay. Chewing their substrate is a vice commonly associated when animals

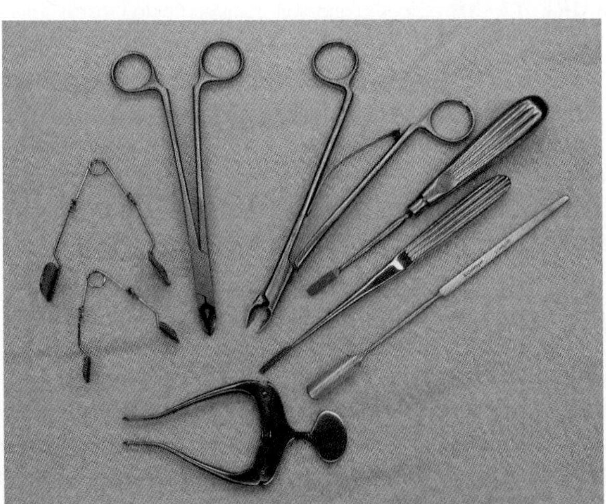

FIGURE 15-32 Rabbit dental instruments.

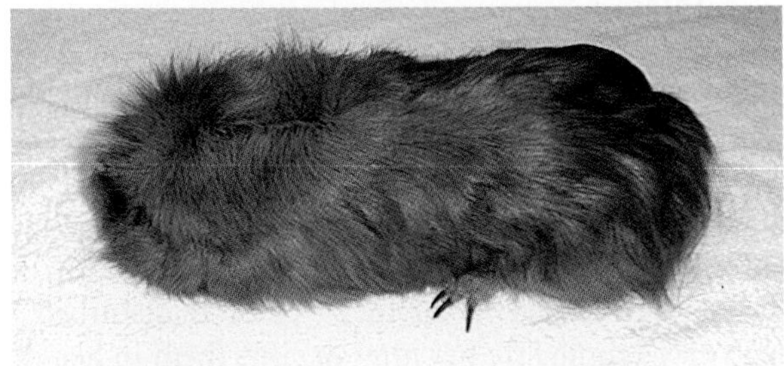

FIGURE 15-33 An Abyssinian guinea pig.

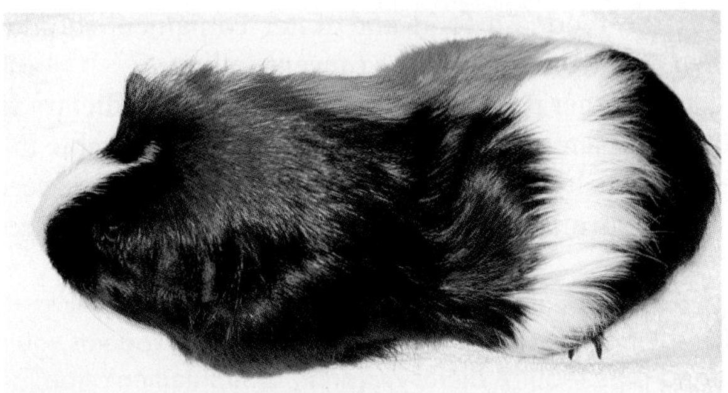

FIGURE 15-34 The English guinea pig, a common house pet.

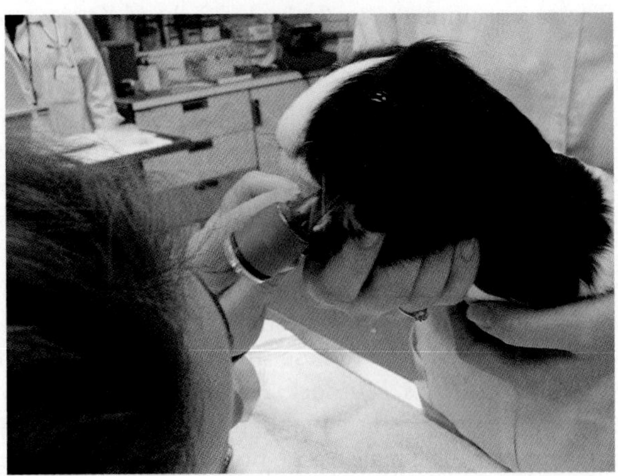

FIGURE 15-35 An otoscope with a disposable head may be used to examine a guinea pig's premolars and molars.

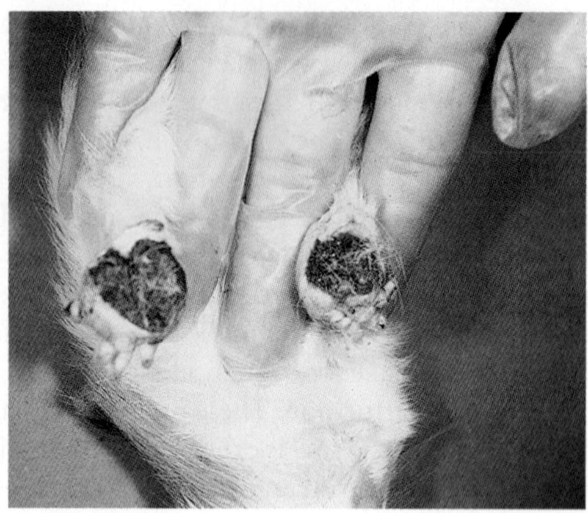

FIGURE 15-36 Footpad dermatitis is a common problem that affects guinea pigs.

develop submandibular abscesses. Hard fibrous splinters penetrate the oral mucosa, inoculating the tissue with bacteria (usually *Streptococcus zooepidemicus*) that develop into abscesses. Changes in the substrate may be indicated to stop this problem, although it may be difficult to find an adequate alternative substrate, which must have absorptive qualities for the opaque, pale yellow, crystalline urine.

The feed and water are best placed in bowls that cannot be chewed (e.g., stainless steel or ceramic crocks). A vitamin C supplementation may be added to the water, such as Tang (Kraft). The food should be a freshly milled, complete guinea pig ration. Storage in a freezer or refrigerator will extend the life of the food. All food and water containers should be placed above the substrate to prevent soiling.

Unlike other pet rodents, guinea pigs require dietary vitamin C supplementation. Vitamin C is highly unstable in the feed, especially when exposed to heat. The use of old feed is one of the primary reasons vitamin C deficiencies are seen.

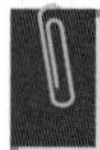

TECHNICIAN NOTE Unlike other pet rodents, guinea pigs require dietary vitamin C supplementation.

The cavy requires 0.5 mg/kg body weight of dietary ascorbic acid per day because it lacks L-gulonolactone oxidase. Published dosages of vitamin C for guinea pigs are 1 to 30 mg/kg intramuscularly twice daily or 200 to 400 mg/L in drinking water (freshly mixed daily). Guinea pigs must be fed species-specific food within 90 days of milling. Fruit and vegetable supplementation is discouraged because of the possibility of disturbing the normal gut bacterial flora. To ensure that the guinea pig is receiving adequate doses of vitamin C daily, oral supplementation in the form of specifically manufactured tablets for these animals is recommended (Oxbow Pet Products, Murdock, Neb.).

To sex a guinea pig, the handler must observe the urethral orifice and anus. The male has no break in the ridge between the openings, whereas the female has a shallow U-shaped break.

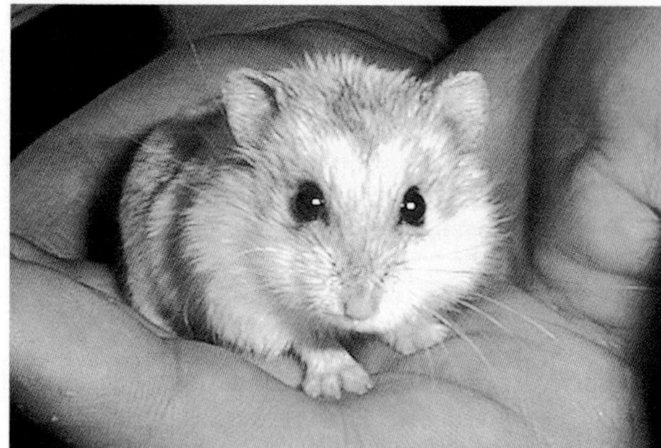

FIGURE 15-37 Siberian dwarf hamsters are popular pets.

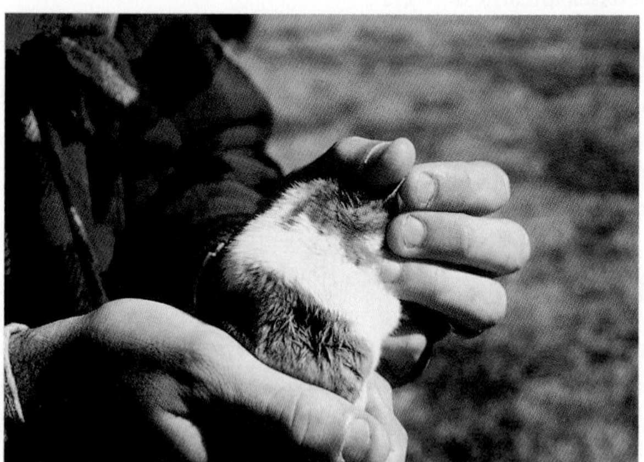

FIGURE 15-38 Flank glands on hamsters, noted in this figure by the moistened area in the caudodorsal region of the animal.

One boar will service up to 10 sows beginning at 8 weeks of age. The sow becomes sexually mature around 5 to 6 weeks of age. The gestation length is on average 63 to 68 days, with litter size ranging from one to six precocious offspring.

HAMSTER

The golden hamster is a native of Syria and comes in many different color varieties (Figure 15-37). Cheek pouches that extend along the head and neck to the proximal dorsum of the back serve as a food transportation device. Along the caudal lateral abdominal region lie the flank glands. A dark brown patch of skin on each side delineates these sebaceous glands that are used to mark territory and in mating rituals (Figure 15-38).

Hamsters have a tendency to bite and are good at chewing through cage material. To accommodate the animal's physical nature, an exercise wheel should be placed in the cage.

Female hamsters often attack newly introduced males and females. Hamsters live 18 to 24 months, have a gestation length of 16 days, and produce about five offspring. Young hamsters are weaned in 20 to 25 days. If disturbed, the female may cannibalize her litter or hide them in her cheek pouches. When the young are hidden in the cheek pouches, they may suffocate. Hamsters can be picked up by the nape skin at the base of the neck or by cupping the hands under the hind limbs.

> *TECHNICIAN NOTE* Hamsters live on average 18 to 24 months and have a gestation period of 16 days.

There are several commercially available hamster habitats. An aquarium with a mesh top may be used to house a hamster, with hardwood shavings as the substrate of choice. Aromatic shavings, such as cedar or pine, may cause ocular and respiratory irritation, severe dermatitis, and allergic reactions. Sipper bottles are perfect for water dispensing, and nonchewable bowls should be used for food containers, or food should be placed on the floor of the enclosure. All food and water access should be made available to the young.

Males have a greater anogenital distance than females. Hamsters may be mated monogamously or in a harem. It is important that females with young are not disturbed so that cannibalism and abandonment of the litter do not occur.

Wet tail is a general term to describe diarrhea in the hamster. Bacterial infections, cestodiasis, and antibiotic administration are a few causes of diarrhea in these rodents.

GERBIL

The Mongolian gerbil is a popular pet native to Mongolia and northeastern China. It is an active burrowing animal adapted to a desert environment.

> *TECHNICIAN NOTE* Under no circumstances should gerbils be grabbed by the tail. As a defense mechanism, the tail skin will deglove, necessitating a tail amputation.

The gerbil has a life span of 3.5 years, with a gestation length of 25 days without lactation and 24 to 48 days with lactation. The litter sizes average five offspring that wean in approximately 25 days (Figure 15-39). Certain gerbil lines are prone to epileptiform seizure activity. Gerbils are friendly rodents that may be housed in hamster units (Figure 15-40). These animals are good at escaping; therefore the cage should be designed to prevent chewing.

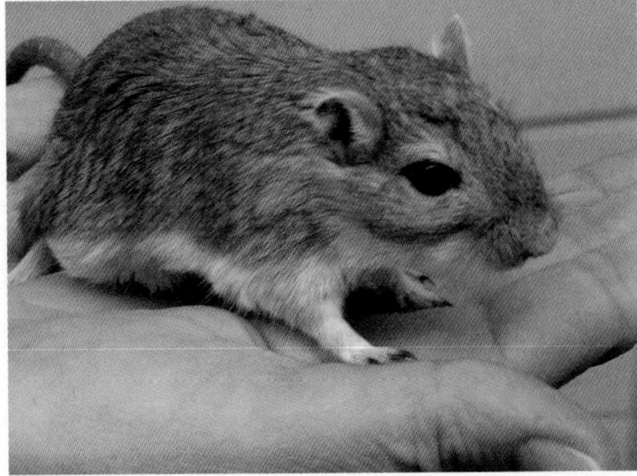

FIGURE 15-39 Rats make one of the best companion animals of all rodent species.

The gerbil's diet may be similar to that of the hamster, and water can be supplied in a sipper bottle. Sexing is accomplished by measuring the urogenital distance. The male has a much longer distance than the female. Males aid in the care of the young.

Gerbils commonly have a nasal dermatitis caused by a bacterial infection initiated by their burrowing activity. A topical antibiotic treatment is recommended for resolution of this infection.

Tyzzer's disease may be diagnosed in gerbils and is caused by *B. piliformis*. Dietary change and colibacillosis also cause diarrhea in these animals.

MOUSE

Mice are small rodents that are used most often in the research setting, but are maintained as pets. Mice are usually aggressive and bite. They are territorial animals and quickly develop a hierarchy when placed in groups (Figure 15-41). These small animals require small amounts of food and water, but are escape prone and may develop an unpleasant odor.

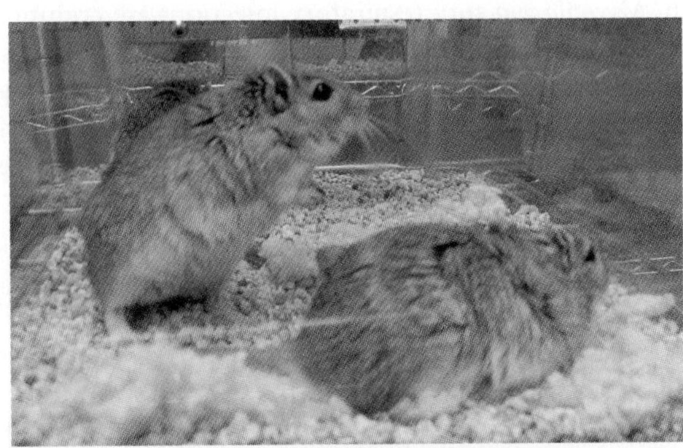

FIGURE 15-40 Young gerbil.

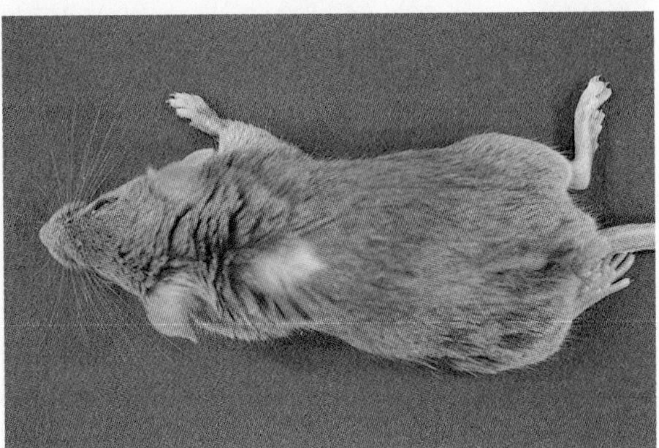

FIGURE 15-41 Trauma (cage mate–inflicted hair loss) on a mouse. This is commonly referred to as barbering.

Common clinical conditions affecting mice include ectoparasites, neoplasia, and trauma. Most mice have a life span of 2 years and are prone to geriatric disease conditions within a relatively short time of ownership. One of the most common geriatric disease conditions is neoplasia. Tumors of various types have been identified in mice, making the education of owners particularly important to aid in early detection and treatment.

Housing should be similar to that of gerbils and hamsters. Hardwood shavings or chips are recommended instead of the aromatic softwood chips (cedar and pine) because of potential liver damage and epithelial damage.

Housing should be cleaned regularly to prevent odor and health problems. Pelleted rodent feed and fresh water in sipper bottles are recommended to be supplied free choice.

Male mice have a greater urogenital distance than females. Female mice become sexually mature at 50 days of age and are best bred in the harem scheme, with one male combined with two to six females.

RAT

Rats are clean and unassuming and can be trained to be good pets (Figure 15-42). These animals may live up to 3 years or longer and become sexually mature at 1.5 to 2 months of age.

As with mice, rats are relatively short lived, predisposing them to geriatric diseases. Rats are also very susceptible to neoplasia, particularly mammary gland tumors. In addition, *Mycoplasma* spp. respiratory infections are commonly diagnosed and clinically may appear as dyspnea with signs of nasal discharge. The nasal discharge is commonly tinged with a red color as a result of the pigment of the harderian gland secretions. Enrofloxacin and tetracycline have been used to treat *Mycoplasma* spp. infections in rats.

> TECHNICIAN NOTE **Rats seldom bite, but caution must be used in a stressful situation.**

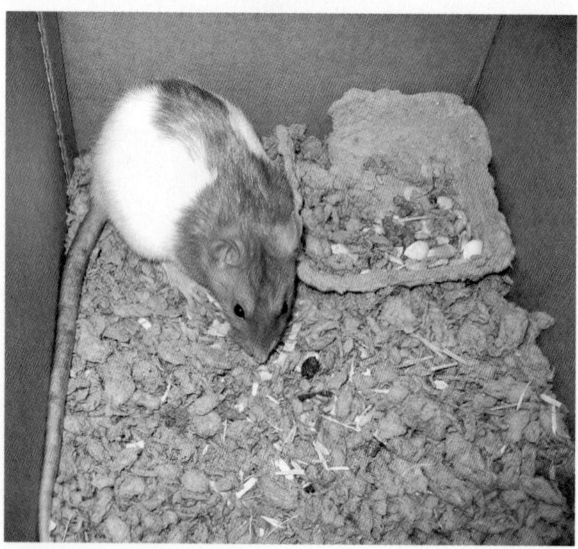

FIGURE 15-42 Typical small rodent cage containing gerbils.

Commercial rodent cages can be obtained for proper housing. The substrate should be similar to that of other rodents.

Males have a longer anogenital distance than females. The gestation length is 22 days, and nesting material should be provided before birth.

PRAIRIE DOGS

The black-tailed prairie dog *(Cynomys ludovicianus)* may be brought to a veterinary practice, even though it is illegal to keep wild North American species as pets. Wild prairie dogs may carry *Hantavirus*, rabies, ectoparasites, *Salmonella* spp., the plague bacteria, monkeypox, and other zoonotic agents (see Chapter 35). Some prairie dogs have been raised in captivity and are therefore less likely to carry dangerous zoonotic diseases. Nevertheless, it is recommended that all prairie dogs remain where they belong, in their natural habitat (Figure 15-43).

Prairie dogs may live up to 10 years and can survive on rodent chow and timothy grass hay. They are, however, susceptible to obesity, making it essential to monitor food intake, especially in adult animals. Digging and tunneling are important parts of their daily activity. The provision of deep bedding enables this type of exercise and allows them to hide and feel secure. Prairie dogs can be managed much like rats in regard to their management and care. The scrotal sac is the identifying characteristic of male prairie dogs when sex determination is required. Venipuncture is best accomplished using the lateral saphenous or cephalic vein. Jugular venipuncture or cranial vena cava collection should only be attempted when the patient is under general anesthesia.

Common disease problems identified in captive prairie dogs are obesity, respiratory disease, malocclusion, infectious pododermatitis, trauma, and neoplasia. The most difficult situation to overcome for most prairie dogs raised in

BOX 15-3 Recommended Daily Diet for Hedgehogs

- 3 tsp high-quality cat or kitten chow
- 1 tsp fruit-vegetable mix
- Four-eight small meal worms or two-three small crickets

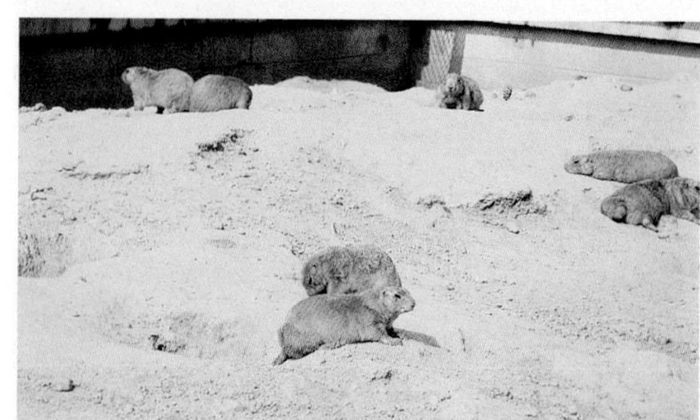

FIGURE 15-43 Sociable prairie dogs are not recommended as a companion animal.

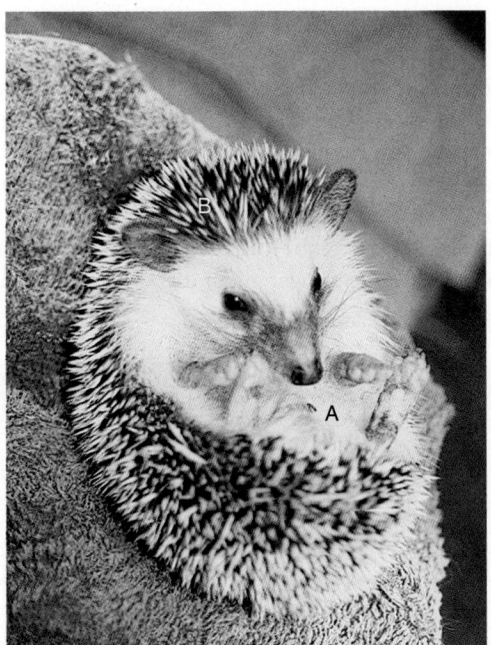

FIGURE 15-44 The ventral surface of hedgehogs is devoid of spines, but the dorsal aspect is covered with sharp spines.

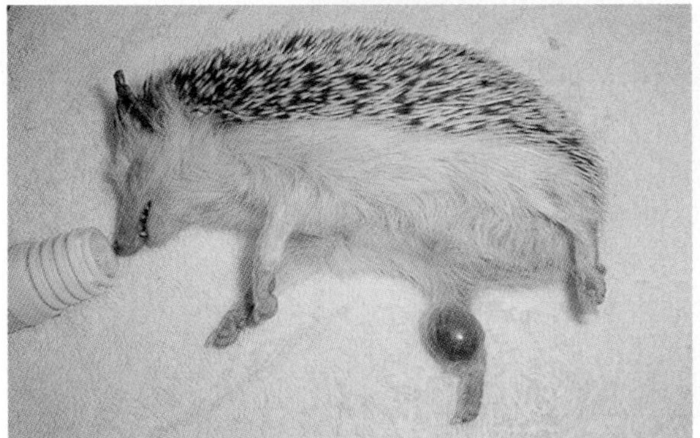

FIGURE 15-45 This hedgehog has a tumor on its rear leg. Tumors are common in hedgehogs.

captivity is obesity. Obesity usually complicates concurrent disease states, making it difficult at times to differentiate the primary disease problem from complications caused by excess body fat.

HEDGEHOGS

The African hedgehog *(Atelerix albiventris)* has become an increasingly popular pet in recent years. These nocturnal spinal animals often adapt best to captivity when left alone. Hedgehogs like to hide, like dark quite areas, and will burrow to escape. Hedgehogs may be maintained much like rodents. For example, enclosures that are 20 gal or larger and lined with an absorbable paper bedding make excellent habitats.

The life span of hedgehogs is 3 to 5 years. The most common disease conditions are neoplasia and external parasites. Yearly physical examinations are needed for teeth cleaning, nail trimming, and tumor checks. Hedgehogs are not rodents and rely on an insectivore-omnivore diet, such as the one listed in Box 15-3.

One feature of hedgehog medicine is that hedgehog patients must be anesthetized simply to be examined. The spines are very sharp, so caution must be taken during handling; gloves are necessary, particularly before anesthesia (Figure 15-44).

Blood collection sites are cranial vena cava, jugular vein, cephalic vein, and lateral saphenous vein, with the cranial vena cava as the site of choice. Common diseases diagnosed in hedgehogs are neoplasia, obesity, otitis externa, dermatitis, external parasites, and respiratory disease (Figure 15-45).

SUGAR GLIDERS

Sugar gliders are nocturnal marsupials from Australia (Figure 15-46). As with hedgehogs, they are unusual pets with unique qualities that should be considered carefully by a potential owner before a purchase is made. They are very social animals. If maintained as a single pet, a glider will

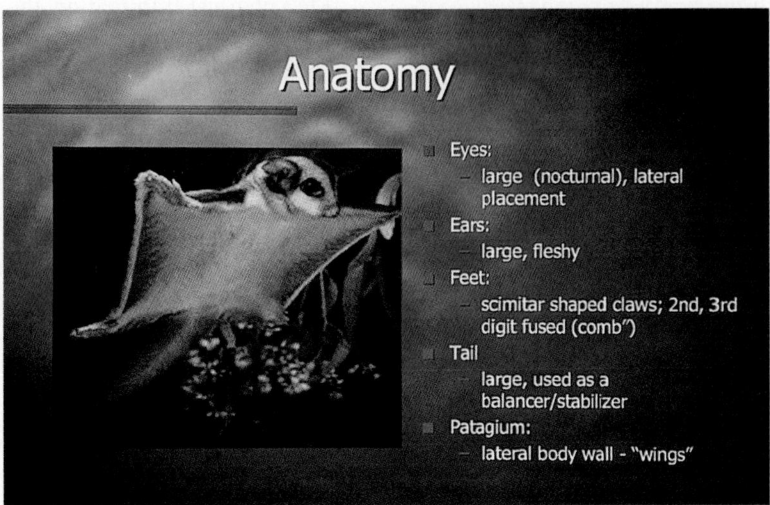

FIGURE 15-46 A sugar glider with its skin stretched out, giving it the ability to "fly" and also its name.

require additional attention from the owner to meet its psychologic needs. In addition, their nocturnal habits give rise to much activity throughout the night, which can be annoying to those who wish to sleep.

Housing needs to be a tall wire enclosure with fresh branches and places to hide, such as a bird box (Figure 15-47). The wire mesh should have spacing no more than 1-inch square to prevent escape. The bottom tray should be lined with shredded paper or pelleted paper products for easy cleaning and the optimal absorption of urine, food, and water.

Malnutrition (e.g., hypocalcemia, hypoglycemia) is one of the most common disease conditions diagnosed in sugar gliders. There are commercial pelleted glider diets available, but they are not actively marketed in most areas. One source of information worth exploring is the Internet. Websites that focus on these animals can be found via most search engines. An example of a complete sugar glider diet is listed in Box 15-4.

BOX 15-4 Daily Sugar Glider Diet

- Zoo-formula insectivore diet
- Equal amounts:
  - Chopped apple
  - Grapes
  - Carrot
- Sweet potato
- Hard-cooked egg yolk
- 10-12 small meal worms
- Dust food and insects with vitamin mineral powder

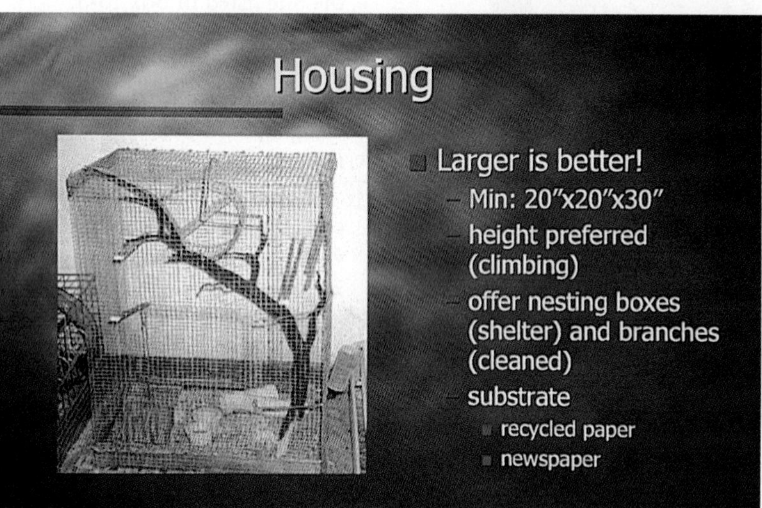

FIGURE 15-47 A typical sugar glider enclosure.

CASE PRESENTATION 15-1

"Dragontale," an 18-month-old bearded dragon *(Pogona vitticeps)*, came to the veterinary practice with a 3-4 week history of lethargy and anorexia (Figure 1). The bearded dragon had been owned for about 14 months and was maintained in a 10-gal glass aquarium with wood shavings as a substrate. The habitat was located on the floor and had a single 60-watt bulb as a heat source. When cleaned, the shavings were removed, the inside wiped down with a kitchen cleaner of unknown brand, and new substrate was placed in the bottom of the enclosure. The animal was fed lettuce, carrots, and crickets that had been dusted with a calcium-rich powder one time a day. Tap water was used as the water source and provided in a bowl. The owners had observed Dragontale becoming lethargic, nonmobile, sleeping more often, and anorexic. Another concern was that the tongue always seemed to be sticking out, and there was an apparent dark red lesion on the tip. The reluctance of their pet to eat had resulted in the owners force feeding crickets to the sick animal.

On a physical examination, the patient was responsive but depressed, exhibited very limited voluntary movement, and did not hold its head in a normal position. The lesion on the tip of the tongue was determined to be a slight irritation of the surface as a result of exposure from a reluctance to retract it into the oral cavity. Anatomic swellings were noted in several locations (e.g., tibia, carpus, pelvis, proximal dorsal tail), and the mandible was extremely flexible (Figures 2 and 3). Dehydration was estimated at 8% based on corneal moisture, the tackiness of oral mucous membranes, and skin tenting. Radiographs indicated a low bone density based on the radiolucent skeletal structure (Figure 4). There was also evidence of a fracture involving the proximal tail vertebra (Figure 5). Blood was collected from the ventral tail vein for a complete blood count and plasma chemistry panel (Figure 6). The only abnormality noted from the hematology results was an approximate 1:1 calcium/phosphorus ratio (7.9 mg/dl calcium, 7.1 mg/dl phosphorus). The normal calcium to

CASE PRESENTATION 15-1—cont'd

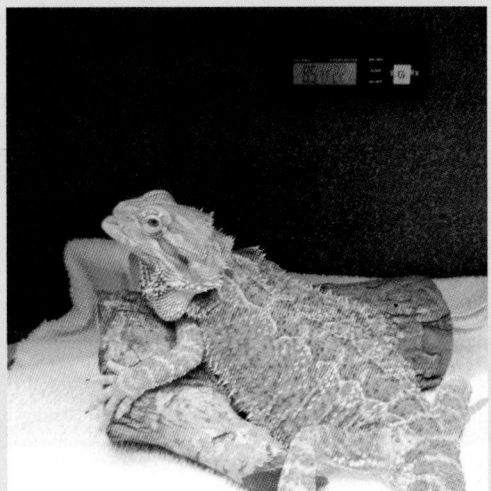

FIGURE 1 Dragontale, a bearded dragon that presented with a 3-4 wk history of lethargy and anorexia.

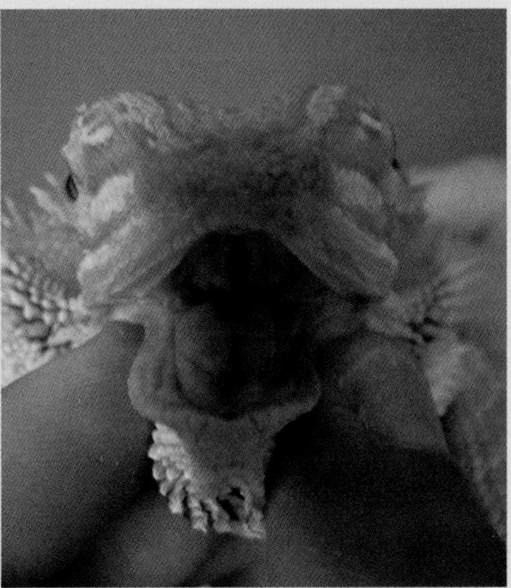

FIGURE 3 The mandible was extremely flexible upon examination.

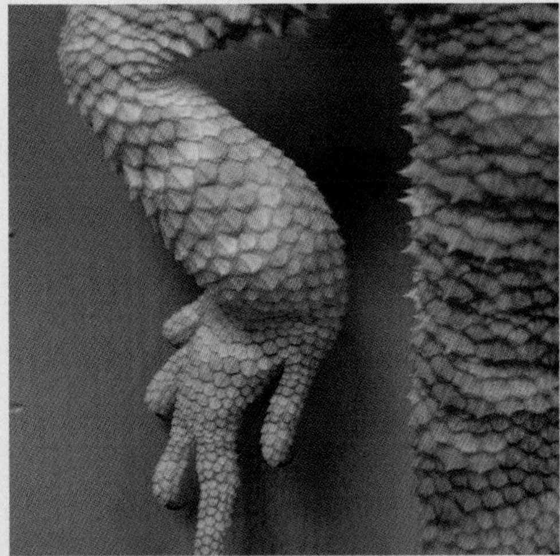

FIGURE 2 Swelling of tibia, a clinical sign linked to metabolic bone disease in lizard species.

phosphorus ratio in bearded dragons should average 2.2:1.[1] Based on the history, physical examination, and diagnostic test results, the top differential diagnosis was nutritional secondary hyperparathyroidism (NSHP) or "rubber jaw."

Nutritional secondary hyperparathyroidism is a form of metabolic bone disease (MBD). Metabolic bone disease is a descriptive term to describe a collection of medical disorders that affect the integrity and function of bones.[2] Husbandry effects, including chronic nutritional deficiencies of calcium and/or vitamin D_3, an imbalance of the calcium:phosphorus ratio (feeding crickets as a primary food source), or inadequate exposure to UV radiation in diurnal animals, will predispose reptiles to MBD. Although many reptile species are susceptible to NSHP, lizards and aquatic turtles seem to be most commonly affected.[2] If the animal is not receiving enough calcium in the diet or has an inability to absorb calcium from the gastrointestinal tract as a result

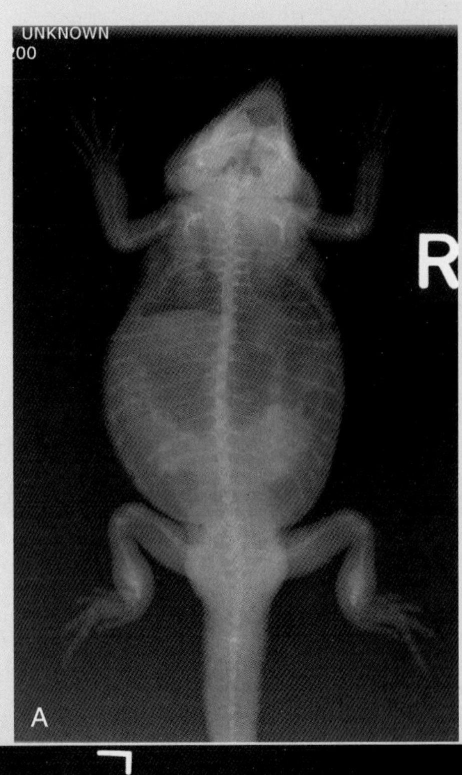

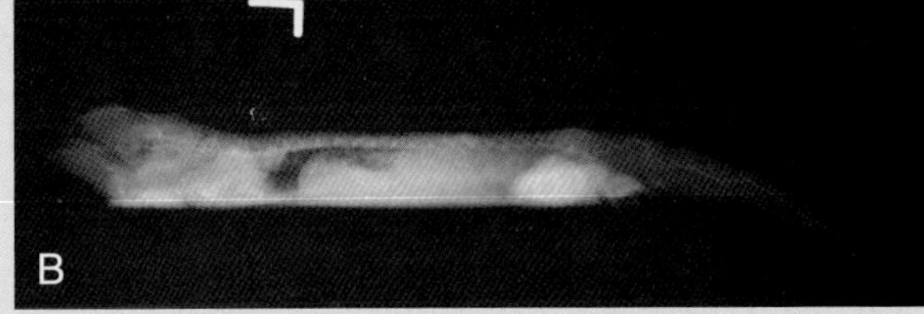

FIGURE 4 Dorsoventral **(A)** and lateral **(B)** radiographic images reveal a general lack of bone density.

Continued

CASE PRESENTATION 15-1—cont'd

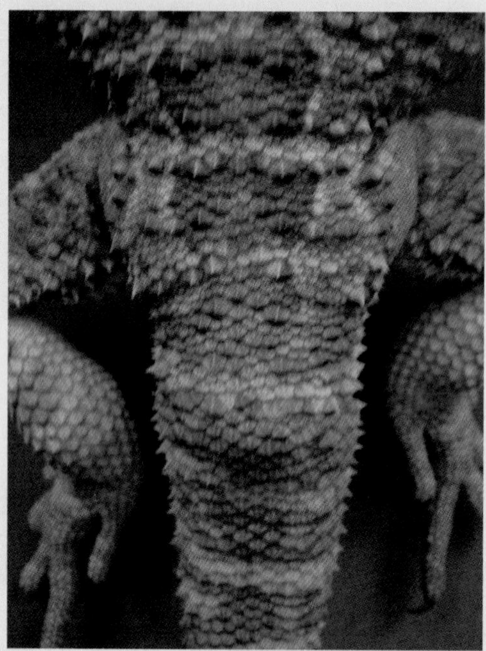

FIGURE 5 An elevated area at the proximal tail area that resulted from a fracture associated with a general lack of bone density.

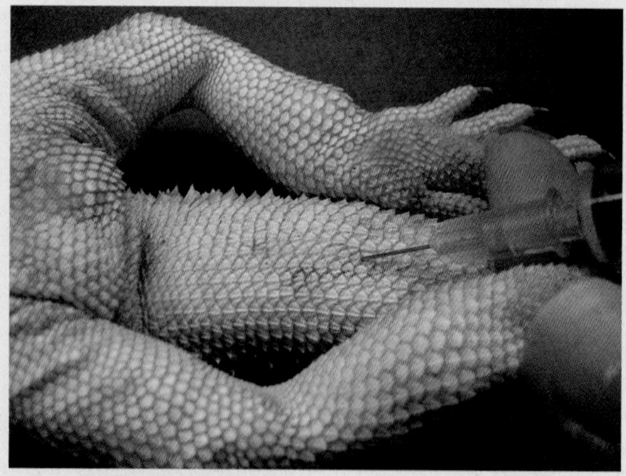

FIGURE 6 Blood collection from the ventral tail vein.

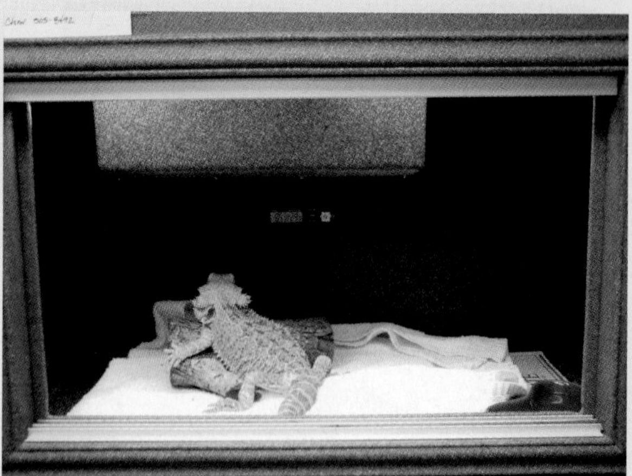

FIGURE 7 Proper hospital enclosure for reptiles with patient inside.

of the lack of vitamin D_3, the body will resorb calcium stores from the bone. Although the serum calcium levels remain within normal limits to maintain life, the bone become weaker with the loss of the stabilizing mineral. To compensate for the loss of calcium and subsequent bone instability, the affected skeletal structures stimulate immature bone cell development that increases the diameter of the bones. This gives the false impression of large "muscles." Instead of muscle tissue, the increased size of the extremities or jaw is actually underdeveloped bone.

In lizards that have a history of depression, anorexia, and a reluctance to move, as with Dragontale, NSHP should be considered a top differential diagnosis. Other signs of NSHP include an enlarged and/or "rubberlike" mandible, evidence of fractures, and enlargement of long bones. Radiographs of clinically affected animals will reveal thin bone cortices, pathologic fractures, or evidence of recently or partially healed fractures.[2]

The most important part of the treatment plan is communicating, informing, and educating the owner on proper nutritional and dietary requirements for the species. For bearded dragons, the diet should be supplemented with calcium and vitamin D_3, and the environment must have the proper temperature range with the animal's exposure to natural sunlight and UV light in the 290- to 320-nm wavelength. For bearded dragons, the preferred optimum temperature range (day 84° F to 88° F; night 68° F to 74° F, winter cool down 62° F to 69° F) with a 50- to 75-watt sun spotlight bulb and natural spectrum lighting required.[3] The artificial UV light and sunlight are needed to convert vitamin D in the body to vitamin D_3 (cholecalciferol), which is active and facilitates calcium uptake in the intestinal tract. Two commercially available lights, Vitalite (Durotest Corp, Lyndhurst, N.J.) and Colortone 50 (Westinghouse, Somerset, N.J.) are recommended for the proper UV wavelength exposure to reptile species.[2] To aid in UV ray exposure for lizard species, a black light bulb and natural sunlight are encouraged.

The treatment for Dragontale consisted of calcium supplementation with calcium gluconate 50 mg/kg subcutaneously, q 24 hours, once and repeated weekly for 4 to 6 weeks as needed, (American Pharmaceutical Partners, Schaumburg, Ill.); calcium glubionate 10 mg/kg orally, q 24 hours, until condition resolves (Calcionate Syrup, Rugby Laboratories, Inc., Duluth, Ga.); fluid therapy, replacement of dehydration deficit, and maintenance 25 ml/kg/day for 5 days then switch to oral administration until animal drinking on its own (Normasol, Hospira, Inc., Lake Forest, Ill.); vitamin A, D_3, and E 0.1 ml IM once, repeat in 1 week (Northwest Pharmacy and Compounding Center, Houston, Tex.); dietary supplementation 10% of body weight up to 5 cc orally q 24 hours (Carnivore Care, Oxbow Co, Murdock, Neb.); offer Critical Care for Herbivores (Oxbow Co., Murdock, Neb.), fresh vegetables with a calcium to phosphorus ratio of greater than 1.5:1 (e.g., watercress, kale, broccoli tops, carrots, oranges, cantaloupe, raisins), and a mealworm dusted with

CASE PRESENTATION 15-1—cont'd

calcium supplementation; and pain medication, meloxicam 0.2 mg/kg orally, q 24 hours, until pain is resolved (Metacam, Boehringer Ingelheim Vetmedica, Inc., St. Joseph, Mo). To supplement the therapeutic treatment regimen, the lizard was placed in a heated environment within its physiologic optimum temperature range, provided artificial UV light, and exposed daily to direct sunlight (Figure 7). Dragontale recovered from NSHP, and with a proper diet and husbandry, he has maintained excellent health.

REFERENCES

1. Eliman MM: Hematology and plasma chemistry of the inland bearded dragon, Pogona vitticepts, *Bull Assoc Reptile Amphibian Vet* 7(4):10-12, 1997.
2. Mader DR: Metabolic bone disease, In Mader DR, editor: *Reptile medicine and surgery,* ed 2, St Louis, Elsevier/Saunders, 2006.
3. Rossi JV: General husbandry and management. In Mader DR, editor: *Reptile medicine and surgery,* ed 2, St Louis, Elsevier/Saunders, 2006.

REFERENCES

Boyer TH: *Essentials of reptiles a guide for practitioners,* Lakewood, Colo, 1998, American Animal Hospital Association.

Frye FL: *Reptile clinician's handbook,* Malabar, Fla, 1995, Krieger.

Wise JK: *U.S. pet ownership and demographics sourcebook,* Schaumburg, Ill, 2002, American Veterinary Medicine Association.

RECOMMENDED READING

Campbell TW, Ellis CK: *Avian and exotic animal hematology & cytology,* Ames, Iowa, 2007, Blackwell Publishing Ltd.

Carpenter JW: *Exotic animal formulary,* ed 3, St Louis, 2005, Saunders.

Fox JG: *Biology and diseases of the ferret,* ed 2, Philadelphia, 1998, Lippincott, Williams & Wilkins.

Harcourt-Brown F: *Textbook of rabbit medicine,* Oxford, 2002, Butterworth-Heinemann.

Harkness JE, Wagner JE: *The biology and medicine of rabbits and rodents,* Philadelphia, 1995, Lea & Febiger.

Johnson CA, Harrison LR: *Exotic companion medicine handbook for veterinarians,* Lake Worth, Fla, 1996, Wingers Publishing.

J Avian Med Surg, Lawrence, Kan, Association of Avian Veterinarians, Allen Press (published quarterly).

J Herpetological Med Surg, Lawrence, Kan, Association of Reptilian and Amphibian Veterinarians, Allen Press (published quarterly).

J Zoo Wildl Med, Lawrence, Kan, American Association of Zoo Veterinarians (published quarterly).

Lewington JH: *Ferret husbandry, medicine and surgery,* Edinburgh, Butterworth-Heinemann.

Mader DR: *Reptile medicine and surgery,* ed 2, St Louis, 2006, WB Saunders.

Mitchell MA, Tully TN: *Manual of exotic pet practice,* St Louis, 2009, Saunders.

Quesenberry KE, Carpenter JW: *Ferrets, rabbits and rodents clinical medicine and surgery,* ed 2, St Louis, 2004, WB Saunders.

Spadafori G, Speer BL: *Birds for dummies,* Foster City, Calif, 1999, IDG Books.

Tully TN, Lawton MPC, Dorrestein GM: *Avian medicine,* Oxford, 2000, Butterworth-Heinemann.

Tully TN, Mitchell MA, editors: *Semin Avian Exotic Pet Med,* Philadelphia, Elsevier (published quarterly).

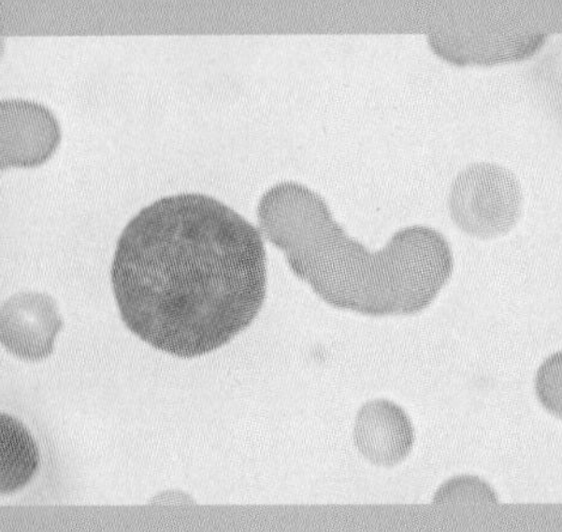

Clinical Sciences

PART THREE

Clinical Pathology

16

Jeffrey R. Sirninger and Jan L. VanSteenhouse

KEY TERMS

Agglutination
Anisocytosis
Anisokaryosis
Band or stab
Control solutions
Coombs' test
Degenerate left shift
Hemacytometer
Hematocrit (hct)
Heterophil
Hyposthenuric urine
Isosthenuric urine
Left shift
Mean corpuscular hemoglobin concentration (MCHC)
Mean corpuscular volume (MCV)
Mucin clot test
Nucleated RBCs (NRBCs)
Packed-cell volume (PCV)
Polychromatophils
Refractometer
Reticulocyte
Rouleaux
Spherocytes
Standard solutions
Toxic change

OUTLINE

LEARNING OBJECTIVES

When you have completed this chapter, you will be able to:

1. Describe proper handling of blood samples for hematology, coagulation, and clinical chemistry testing.
2. List the tests included in the complete blood count and the equipment needed to perform those tests.
3. Describe the procedure for counting white blood cells and platelets with the Unopette system.
4. Explain the procedures for the determination of the packed-cell volume and plasma protein concentration.
5. State the calculations for the determination of erythrocyte indices.
6. Describe the procedure for preparing and evaluating a differential blood cell film.
7. Describe normal blood cell morphology and list and describe common morphologic abnormalities of blood cells in a variety of species.
8. State the calculations for the determination of absolute values.
9. State the advantages, disadvantages, and limitations of automated cell counters and clinical chemistry analyzers.
10. List the indications for and the types of tests used in clinical chemistry testing.
11. Describe methods of collection and handling of urine samples.
12. List the test performed and describe the methods used for the evaluation of the physical properties and chemical composition of urine samples.
13. Describe methods for preparing urine samples for the microscopic examination of urine sediment.
14. List and describe the formed elements commonly found in urine sediment.
15. Describe the procedure for the collection of cytology samples by fine-needle aspiration and list the cytology tests performed on body fluids.

INTRODUCTION

Accurate clinical pathology data are invaluable components of the minimal database used in the diagnosis of diseases in all species. The repetition of selected test results also provides a means of monitoring and evaluating disease progression and the success of chosen treatment regimens. Erroneous data, however, may result in misdiagnoses and be a more serious disadvantage than a lack of data.

Each practice will be faced with the decision of whether laboratory data will be generated within the practice or be obtained from a reference laboratory. The practice's caseload, availability, and turnaround time of a qualified reference laboratory and experience of the technician are important criteria used to make this determination. Having clinical laboratory data available within 1 hour can be a great advantage to the veterinarian in determining the diagnosis, especially during life-threatening emergencies.

Whether samples are submitted to a reference laboratory or analyzed in the practice, the appropriately trained veterinary technician can be an invaluable asset in ensuring that valid, reliable data are obtained. In either case, knowledge of proper sampling techniques and proper sample handling is essential. The veterinary technician should be familiar with the type and amount of sample to submit for various tests, whether an anticoagulant should be used, and how the sample should be prepared, transported, and stored if it is not immediately analyzed.

It is the veterinary technician's responsibility to have a thorough working knowledge of any in-house analyzer, its sample requirements, its routine maintenance procedures, and basic quality control procedures to ensure accurate laboratory results. The technician should also be familiar with the care and maintenance of all supportive laboratory equipment necessary to keep instruments functioning properly.

Should it be decided that a reference laboratory is more time or cost efficient for an individual practice, the veterinary technician must communicate with the personnel of that laboratory. The laboratory should be consulted regarding appropriate sample submission for specific tests to prevent unnecessary delays and invalid results. Precautions must be taken to ensure that the samples are not damaged or destroyed during transport.

Accurate interpretation of test results requires a reference range of normal values specific to each species. Ideally, these ranges are generated by the laboratory that provides the test results. The use of veterinary-specific laboratories is recommended because different diagnostic criteria may be used by human laboratories (e.g., definition of a band neutrophil) in addition to assay methodologies, which may yield factitious results for nonhuman samples (e.g., use of reagents that inaccurately measure albumin). Ideally the most appropriate reference intervals would be generated from healthy animals that most closely matched the patient, but in practice, these can be difficult to obtain; more commonly, age-matched intervals may be available. In exotic species, reference intervals may not be available at all, and one may have to rely on a few reported values in the literature; alternatively the clinician may submit samples from the same species that they believe to be healthy and determine if the patient's values vary from their mean value by more than an arbitrary value, such as 30%.

This chapter addresses the more commonly used clinical laboratory techniques and procedures in veterinary hematology, urinalysis, clinical chemistry, and cytology. Techniques and methods are emphasized rather than interpretation. Although interpretive examples are given for commonly seen atypical findings, these examples are not meant to be exhaustive. The recommended reading list provides detailed reviews. Laboratory instrumentation and necessary quality control systems for clinical chemistry and hematology are reviewed and summarized. In addition, errors in sampling and sample handling and the consequence of misleading values, which complicate the interpretation of laboratory data, are discussed.

HEMATOLOGY

Although the microscopic evaluation of whole blood can occasionally provide direct diagnostic information on infectious and neoplastic blood-borne diseases, more frequently the clinician will indirectly deduce the presence of primary disease at distant tissue sites on the basis of common patterns of hematologic abnormalities.

The basic equipment necessary for hematologic analyses includes a microscope, microhematocrit centrifuge, refractometer, hemacytometer, clean slides, and a modified Wright's stain. The benefits of conscientious care and cleaning of these items cannot be overlooked. The complete blood count (CBC) provides the veterinarian with invaluable information regarding the patient's red blood cell (RBC or erythrocyte) mass, white blood cell (WBC or leukocyte) number and distribution, platelet number, and plasma protein. The CBC consists of a packed-cell volume (PCV) and/or hematocrit (Hct), WBC count, RBC count, hemoglobin determination,

RBC indices, platelet count or estimate, total plasma protein determination, and evaluation of the blood smear for RBC morphology and a WBC differential count. Hematologic procedures are performed on anticoagulated whole blood. The preferred anticoagulant is ethylenediaminetetraacetic acid (EDTA) because it does not interfere with blood cell morphology and staining. EDTA is commercially available in purple-top Vacutainer tubes in a variety of sizes. A Vacutainer is a sterile, glass tube that is sealed with a removable rubber stopper. There is a vacuum or negative pressure inside it that allows blood to flow freely into it from the intravenous needle without force. Many Vacutainer tubes contain substances, such as EDTA or heparin, to keep the blood from clotting. The color of the rubber stopper indicates the substance in the tube. For example, tubes that have lavender or purple colored stoppers contain EDTA whereas tubes with green stoppers contain heparin and "red-tops" do not contain any additive and are therefore referred to as "clot tubes" because the blood inside them is allowed to clot. Choosing the correct type and size of vacutainer is essential to obtaining accurate results because having a small amount of blood in a large tube will alter some of the values. The various types of sample tubes available and their appropriate uses are listed in Table 16-1.

The morphology of the normal and abnormal blood cells is briefly reviewed, but it is strongly recommended that the technician have on hand and consult the appropriate references listed at the end of this chapter. Table 16-2 contains sample reference intervals for normal hematology values in common domestic species.

TABLE 16-1 Recommended Sample Tubes

Color of Topw	Anticoagulant	Purpose
Purple	EDTA	CBC, platelet counts
Red	None	Chemistries
Tiger (red-black)	Separator gel	Chemistries
Green	Heparin	Electrolytes, Stats
Turquoise	Citrate	Coagulation assay

CBC, Complete blood count; *EDTA*, ethylenediaminetetraacetic acid.

EQUIPMENT

When a microscope is chosen, the laboratory's needs must first be assessed. The fewer "extras" that are included will reduce the requirements for maintenance, service, and repairs. A good-quality binocular microscope with a mechanical stage, an adjustable substage condenser, and good-quality objective lenses will accommodate the needs of any hematology laboratory. The most important aspect, and often the cost determinant, of a good laboratory microscope is the objective lens. Planachromatic lenses are recommended because they provide a flat field of vision with superior optical properties. The entire field will be in focus, resulting in reduced eyestrain and improved microscopic images. The basic laboratory microscope should have 10×, 40× (high dry), and 100× (oil immersion) objective lenses in addition to standard 10× ocular objectives. Many microscopists find an additional 50× oil-immersion objective lens useful for evaluation of both blood films and cytology specimens. The manufacturer's manual should provide directions for adjusting the light for optimal intensity (Köhler illumination), which enhances the clarity of the image. Proper adjustment of the substage condenser is necessary for optimal image quality; in general the condenser should be in a higher position for stained preparations, whereas dropping the condenser in combination with increasing light intensity is needed to visualize unstained wet preparations.

Proper care of the microscope is essential for providing accurate results for an extended period. Great care should be taken to follow the manufacturer's directions for proper use, cleaning, and maintenance. The oil-immersion lenses require a drop of special immersion oil on the blood film to achieve the appropriate optics. The immersion oil should be wiped from the objective after use to prevent damage to the lens. It is essential that all other objectives be kept free of oil.

TABLE 16-2 Hematology Values

	Canine	Feline	Equine	Bovine
PCV (%)	37-55	30-45	32-48	24-46
Hemoglobin (g/dl)	12-18	8-15	10-18	8-15
Reticulocytes (%)	0-1.5	0-1.0	0	0
WBCs (n/μl)	6000-17,000	5500-19,500	6000-12,000	4000-12,000
Segments	3000-11,400	2500-12,500	3000-6000	600-4000
Bands (n/μl)	0-300	0-300	0-100	0-120
Lymphocytes (n/μl)	1000-4800	1500-7000	1500-5000	2500-7500
Monocytes (n/μl)	150-1350	0-850	0-600	25-850
Eosinophils (n/μl)	100-750	0-750	0-800	0-2400
Basophils (n/μl)	Rare	Rare	0-300	0-200
TP (g/dl)	6.0-7.5	6.0-7.5	6.0-8.5	6.0-8.0
Fibrinogen (mg/dl)	150-300	150-300	100-400	100-600
Platelets (n/μl)	200,000-500,000	300,000-700,000	100,000-600,000	100,000-800,000

n, Number; *PCV*, packed-cell volume; *TP*, total protein; *WBCs*, white blood cells.

In practice, the 40× lens (high dry) is most easily dragged through oil while changing magnification, which in many multiuser environments will require constant cleaning or eventually lead to degradation of the lens as oil seeps through the lens seal. Lenses should be cleaned with lens paper only. A dust cover should be placed over the microscope when it is not in use to prevent collection of dust and hairs on the lenses and other surfaces.

> *TECHNICIAN NOTE* No laboratory equipment or instrument, regardless of cost, is any better than the care and maintenance it receives.

A microhematocrit centrifuge is required for the determination of the PCV. The force generated by the centrifuge separates the cellular components of blood from the plasma. The manufacturer's manual should be consulted for recommended speed settings for the sample being spun. As with all laboratory equipment, the accuracy and functional longevity of the centrifuge are directly related to proper care and use. For the purpose of safety, the centrifuge should not be operated unless the lid is closed and properly secured. Samples should always be balanced to ensure accurate separation and reduce wear on the motor. Periodic maintenance, such as lubricating the bearings and checking the commutator, should be scheduled according to the manufacturer's recommendations to extend the life of the centrifuge and ensure accurate results.

The refractometer is used to determine the plasma protein concentration by measuring the refractive index of the plasma. Careful cleaning of the sample surface is imperative to prolonging the accuracy and functional life of the refractometer. Several models are available, including one designed specifically for veterinary use (Figure 16-1). The veterinary model is less expensive, has a more shock-resistant casing, and is most appropriate for use in the veterinary determination of urine specific gravity (SG). Human calibrated refractometers will have the greatest degree of inaccuracy when reading feline urine SG, but even so the error is generally only a few thousandths higher than the actual value. The calibration of the zero setting should be checked periodically with distilled water and adjusted according to the instructions in the manufacturer's manual if necessary.

The Neubauer (recommended) hemacytometer is a small but valuable specialized counting chamber used for determining WBC and platelet counts per microliter of blood (Figure 16-2). With the 1:100 dilution Unopette system (Becton Dickinson Inc., Franklin Lakes, N.J.) for WBC and platelet counts, all nine of the large primary squares are counted for WBCs at 10×, and platelets are counted in all 25 squares within the center primary square at 40×. Appropriate calculations are provided with the system used to determine cells per microliter. The hemacytometer has a special weighted coverglass to prevent it from floating upon filling of the chamber because the calculation of the cellular concentration is dependent upon a set 0.1-mm distance between the counting chamber surface and coverglass; should it be damaged, a regular microscopic coverslip cannot be substituted because overestimation of cellular concentration will result if a greater volume of fluid than that corresponding to the expected 0.1-mm depth is present as a result of a floated coverslip. Both the hemacytometer and coverslip must be cleaned carefully to prevent scratching of the surfaces. One must realize that the hemacytometer method is notoriously inaccurate in comparison with many automated cell-counter methodologies. Inaccurate dilutions, high dilution factors, chamber overfilling, miscounting of debris, and the overall relatively low number of cells counted all factors into an erroneous determination of final cellular concentrations. Additionally, cells on two of the four edges must be designated as in the counting field, whereas cells on the other two edges are ignored.

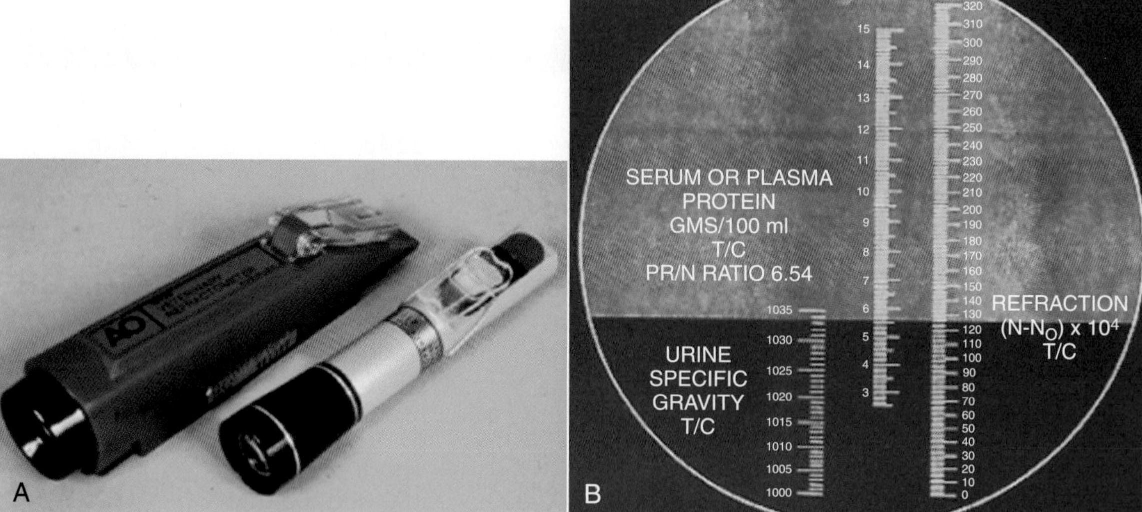

FIGURE 16-1 **A,** Veterinary *(red)* and human refractometers. **B,** The reading scale within the refractometer.

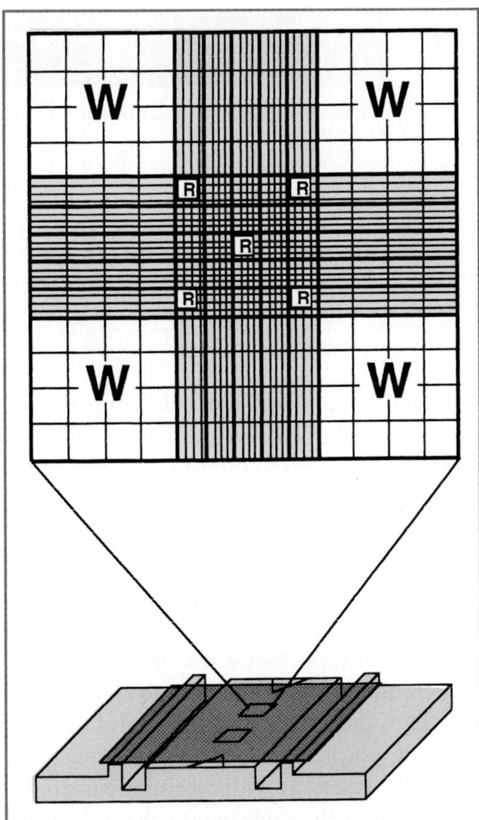

FIGURE 16-2 Neubauer hemacytometer. The large Ws indicate the squares that are counted for a total WBC count with the 1:20 dilution WBC Unopette system. The small Rs indicate the squares that are counted for an RBC count with the RBC Unopette system.

New, clean glass slides are essential for making usable blood films. Slides that are frosted on one end are preferred for labeling purposes. Attempts to save money by washing and reusing slides is discouraged because inferior smear preparations will result, thereby impeding accurate interpretation and resulting in the loss of material that can be archived.

SAMPLE HANDLING

In general, EDTA is the required anticoagulant for hematology. Be sure to use a tube of the appropriate size for the sample drawn. It is often difficult to obtain large samples from small dogs and cats; the 2-ml pediatric collection tube is best for a patient of this size. There are collection tubes for smaller volumes (0.5-ml Microtainer tubes, Becton Dickinson Inc., Franklin Lakes, N.J.). These tubes are excellent for samples from puppies, kittens, and small exotic animal species. Excess anticoagulant resulting from a small amount of blood in a too large tube can erroneously decrease the PCV and increase total protein values determined with a refractometer. Extended storage time in EDTA may lead to changes in the appearance of neutrophils. These changes may resemble those caused by disease processes and may lead to an erroneous diagnosis.

Anticoagulated blood samples should immediately be mixed by gentle inversion of the tube. Blood films should be made from well-mixed blood within 15 minutes of obtaining the sample to decrease in vitro morphologic changes in the blood cells. If the practice uses a reference laboratory, unstained blood films should be sent with the EDTA sample. If samples must be held overnight, refrigerate the whole blood but do not refrigerate the blood film. Water will condense on the surface of the blood film if it is placed in the refrigerator and cause lysis of the RBCs. The blood film and cytology slides should be protected from formalin vapors because formalin will interfere with cell preservation and staining. If samples are sent out, they should be packaged in separate bags.

> *TECHNICIAN NOTE* Blood films should always be made from fresh blood before refrigeration, regardless of whether the CBC will be performed in the practice or sent to a reference laboratory.

DETERMINATION OF ERYTHROCYTE NUMBERS

The determination of the PCV, the percentage of total blood volume accounted for by RBCs, is the easiest and most common means of evaluating the RBC mass. This is achieved by filling a plain microhematocrit capillary tube with anticoagulated blood, sealing one end of the tube with a specific type of clay, and spinning the sample in a microhematocrit centrifuge. During centrifugation, the red blood cells separate from the other components of blood and from a solid mass of tightly packed cells at the bottom of the hematocrit tube. The percentage of packed red blood cells relative to the total volume of blood can be deduced by holding the hematocrit tube against a special chart. This method provides a quick and accurate measurement if samples are spun for a standard length of time at a consistent speed. The specific time and speed depend on the particular centrifuge used. Accuracy also depends on the care and operation of the centrifuge. Blood samples from cattle, sheep, and goats may require centrifugation for a longer time because their smaller RBCs do not pack as well as dog and cat RBCs. The plasma portion at the top of the tube should be evaluated for color and clarity and will also be used for a determination of plasma protein values. The Hct provides basically the same information, but is obtained by calculation when an automated analyzer is used and thus may be slightly different from the measured PCV. This is most commonly seen in blood samples from collection tubes that have an inadequate volume of blood (less than 1 ml in a 5-ml tube or less than 0.5 ml in a 2-ml tube). The excess anticoagulant causes the RBCs to shrink, erroneously decreasing the PCV. When the blood is diluted by the electronic cell counter, the diluent reexpands the RBCs to their true size, providing the true value for the Hct.

The actual number of erythrocytes may be determined by using an automated cell counter, which is primarily available in reference laboratories. Erythrocyte counts may also be performed manually, but are too tedious and inaccurate to be of diagnostic value. RBC counts vary proportionately with the PCV and have little to no advantage over a PCV. The major advantage of automated cell counters is that they also measure hemoglobin and measure or calculate the RBC indices. Hemoglobin is the protein in RBCs that is responsible for carrying oxygen from the lungs to the tissues.

RED BLOOD CELL INDICES

RBC indices are commonly provided when automated analyzers are used; these indices include mean corpuscular volume (MCV), mean corpuscular hemoglobin (MCH), mean corpuscular hemoglobin concentration (MCHC), and red cell distribution width (RDW). The MCH is of little value, but the MCV and MCHC are useful in evaluating and determining the cause of anemias. MCH and MCHC values calculated with an electronic cell counter will be erroneous if the cells in the sample have ruptured (hemolyzed) during the blood draw or during rough handling. These values will also be affected if the patient is not fasted, and the blood is filled with lipid (lipemic) which is not uncommon in carnivores and omnivores after a meal. Samples with these properties cannot be used to determine MCH and MCHC.

$$\text{MCV (femtoliters)} = \frac{PCV \times 10}{\text{RBC } (10^6)}$$

$$\text{MCH (picograms)} = \frac{hemoglobin \times 100}{\text{RBC} \times (10^6)}$$

$$\text{MCHC (g/dl)} = \frac{hemoglobin \times 100}{\text{PCV}}$$

The RDW is the coefficient of variation of the RBC volumes and is a measure of anisocytosis. An increased RDW signifies that a greater variation in cell volumes are present, but does not imply their actual size (i.e., there may be smaller and/or larger RBCs present).

$$\text{RDW (\%)} = \frac{\text{standard deviation}_{\text{MCV}} \times 100}{\text{MCV}}$$

DETERMINATION OF LEUKOCYTE COUNTS

The total WBC count may be determined manually with the hemacytometer or an automated cell counter. Either way, it is important that the blood tube be well mixed before the sample is taken. The use of the Unopette dilution system is the most accepted method for performing manual WBC counts. Several Unopette systems are available for counting various cell types (Table 16-3), but the system preferred for counting leukocytes is also used for counting platelets and determining cell counts on samples such as synovial fluid. This system consists of a disposable reservoir containing diluent and an agent to lyse RBCs to accommodate the counting of leukocytes. Each Unopette system comes with detailed instructions for obtaining reliable results and a capillary pipette with which to draw a specific volume of blood. The interchangeable use of pipettes from another cell counting system, such as one for RBCs, to obtain WBC counts will result in significant errors and inappropriately decreased WBC counts.

TABLE 16-3 Unopette Systems for Counting Different Cell Types

Test	Pipette	Volume	Dilution	Diluent
Red cell count	<10 µl	<1:200	<0.85%	Saline
White cell count	20 µl	1:100	3%	Acetic acid
White cell count	25 µl	1:20	3%	Acetic acid
Platelet count	20 µl	1:100	1%	Ammonium oxalate
Eosinophil count	25 µl	1:32	—	Phloxine

The accuracy of a manual WBC count depends on adherence to the directions and the proper performance of each step. Care must be taken to accurately fill the capillary tube and wipe off any excess blood on the outside of the tube without touching the tip of the pipette and drawing any of the sample out of the pipette; residual blood will artifactually elevate the WBC count. The blood sample must be carefully transferred to the reservoir with careful mixing to ensure the complete delivery of the sample into the diluent. Blood left in the capillary tube or accidentally expelled from the top of the pipette during mixing will result in erroneous WBC counts. It will take practice and may require multiple attempts to completely and accurately fill the hemacytometer chamber. The chambers on both sides of the hemacytometer must be filled for accurate results. Counting both sides and comparing results also serve to check accuracy because the number of cells on one side should closely approximate the number of cells on the other side. Overfilling or underfilling the chamber will cause errors in the final cell count. After the hemacytometer chambers have been charged, the hemacytometer must be allowed to sit for several minutes to allow the cells to settle. WBCs will be counted with the use of the 10× objective; lowering the condenser on the microscope will increase the contrast, making the cells more prominent and easier to identify and count accurately.

Immature red blood cells that still contain nuclei may be released prematurely from the bone marrow during some conditions. These nucleated RBCs (NRBCs) may be erroneously counted along with WBCs by either manual or automated electronic counting methods, resulting in falsely elevated WBC counts. The number of NRBCs encountered on the blood film is counted while the differential count is performed on 100 leukocytes. The WBC count is then corrected by using the following formula:

$$\text{measured WBCs} \times 100/(100 + \text{number of NRBCs per 100 WBCs}) = \text{corrected WBC count}$$

For example, if 15 NRBCs are counted while the 100-cell differential count is performed and the initial WBC count is 30,000 cells/ml, the corrected count is then calculated as follows:

$$30{,}000 \times 100/(100 + 15) = 26{,}087 \text{ cells/ml}$$

Although this formula may be applied whenever NRBCs are noted, in practice, some laboratories do not perform corrections if there are less than 10 NRBCs per 100 WBCs since the degree of error is not clinically significant.

Increased WBCs are referred to as leukocytosis, whereas decreased WBCs are referred to as leukopenia. The diagnostic significance of either leukocytosis or leukopenia cannot be appreciated without the WBC differential count. The differential count is performed by examining the blood film (see the discussion of blood film evaluation). At least 100 leukocytes are identified and counted according to cell type (as neutrophils, bands, lymphocytes, monocytes, eosinophils, or basophils). The more cells that are counted, the more accurate the differential count will be. The percentages of each cell type counted are then multiplied by the total WBC count to provide absolute numbers of the cell types present. These numbers are the values used for interpreting changes in the leukogram.

Dramatic increases or decreases in the WBC count may also be noted by looking at the thickness of the buffy coat. The buffy coat is the white band of concentrated WBCs and platelets that is visible in the hematocrit tube between the layers of packed RBCs at the bottom and plasma at the top. Though the buffy coat does not give specific counts of the various WBC types, as does a differential, high numbers of concentrated WBCs on buffy coat smears allow for a rapid, general assessment. For example, infections, and neoplasia may be suspect if the buffy coat is thicker than normal. In addition, the blood-borne, swimming larva of heartworm, called microfilaria, may be seen by examining an intact microhematocrit tube under a microscope. In this way, a quick diagnosis of heartworm disease might be made.

AVIAN AND REPTILIAN LEUKOCYTE COUNTS

Unlike mammals, birds and reptiles have NRBCs (Figure 16-3), and this prevents a determination of their WBC counts by the methods described. However, the WBC counts of these nonmammalian species may be determined indirectly by using another Unopette system for an eosinophil determination. This special Unopette is filled with anticoagulated blood, mixed well, and allowed to incubate for approximately 5 minutes to allow uptake of the stain by the cells. If the sample is allowed to stand for a prolonged time, all the cells will take up the stain, and results will be erroneous. The hemacytometer is filled as for the manual WBC count described, and the red-staining cells are counted in all nine squares of the grid. With proper staining, only the eosinophils and heterophils (equivalent of neutrophils) will be stained. In contrast to the performance of the mammalian manual count, it is important to keep the microscope condenser up to decrease contrast. If the condenser is down, it will be more difficult to count the heterophils and eosinophils because of RBC interference. At the time of writing, this system has had limited availability, and many laboratories have had to make the staining solution themselves; a formula for an acceptable solution follows:

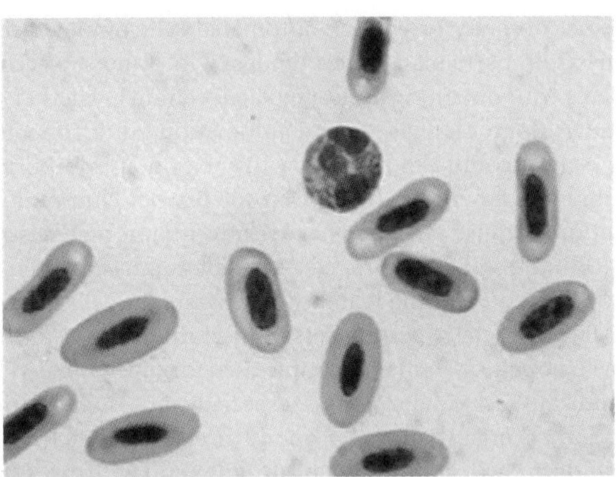

FIGURE 16-3 NRBCs and a heterophil from a cockatoo.

Mix in a 1-L volumetric flask: 1g phloxine + 500 ml propylene glycol, q.s. to 1 L with water.

Filter; protect from light; wrap flask in foil; use within 6 months.

Mix 0.8 ml stain with 25 μl blood in tube; incubate for 5 minutes; count on hemacytometer.

The number obtained does not represent the WBC count, but is used in conjunction with the differential count to calculate the WBC count. When the differential count is completed and the percentages of the various cell types present are known, the WBC count is calculated with the following formula:

$$\frac{\text{cells counted on hemacytometer} \times 32 \times 100}{\text{\% heterophils + eosinophil}} = \text{WBCs}/\mu\text{l}$$

The factor of 32 is a simplified mathematic combination of a variety of other factors. For example, if 282 cells are counted on one side of the hemacytometer and you have 70% heterophils and 5% eosinophils on the differential count, the total WBC count would be as follows:

$$\frac{282 \times 32 \times 100}{70 + 5} = 12{,}032 \text{ WBCs}/\mu\text{l}$$

PLATELET DETERMINATION

The determination of platelet numbers is important because platelets play an important role in clot formation. Several diseases cause decreased numbers of platelets (thrombocytopenia), and these can often be diagnosed and treated before a severe bleeding disorder develops; additionally, increased platelet numbers (thrombocytosis) are associated with certain conditions and as such represent useful diagnostic information. Like WBCs, platelets can be counted manually on a hemacytometer or with an automated cell counter. Feline platelets, in particular, have a tendency to clump, which interferes with obtaining accurate platelet counts; whether the count is done manually or by automation, an erroneously low platelet count can result. For this reason, it is important to always examine the blood film for platelet clumping. In addition, because cats often have relatively large platelets and cat RBCs are small, automated electronic counts are often inaccurate because of the inability to separate the cells by size.

Manual platelet counts can be performed by using the same Unopette system and sample used for the manual WBC count. This task can be tedious, especially if the hemacytometer and coverglass are not properly cared for. Scratches and small dust particles are difficult to differentiate from platelets. If platelet clumps are present, the resultant count will be inaccurate. It would be best to obtain another sample with special attention given to ensure a clean venipuncture and adequate mixing of the blood with the anticoagulant. Platelets are identified with the use of the 40× objective and will be easier to see if the condenser is lowered and the light intensity is moderate. The instructions that accompany the Unopette must be followed with regard to the squares of the grid that are counted and the method of determining the total count.

> *TECHNICIAN NOTE* The blood film should always be scanned for platelet clumps, especially for cats, to prevent reporting erroneously low platelet numbers.

When platelet counts are not available or when it is necessary to verify counts obtained manually or electronically, the number of platelets can be estimated from the blood film. During an examination of the appropriate area of the blood film in which RBCs are spaced in a uniform monolayer, the average number of platelets per 100× oil-immersion field in several fields (10 or more) is determined. This average number of platelets multiplied by a factor of 15,000 to 20,000 will provide an adequate estimation of the number of platelets per microliter.

Decreased platelet counts can have serious implications for the patient. Therefore before low platelet counts are reported, all technical problems must be considered. The feathered edge of the blood film must be checked for platelet clumping. The tube of blood from which the sample was taken should be checked for small clots, which could deplete platelets. Either or both of these problems may occur despite the use of an anticoagulant. If neither the blood film nor the tube reveals evidence of platelet aggregation, the low platelet count should be reported as determined. If platelet clumping or clots are found, another sample should be drawn, and the counts should be repeated.

BLOOD FILM EVALUATION

Examination of the morphology (appearance) of cells is one of the most valuable parts of the CBC, and its importance cannot be overstressed. Cells that appear too big or too small, for example, are indications of disease. The morphology of cells is best examined by spreading a very thin layer of blood over a glass microscope slide. The feather edge or tail of the smear, where the cells are spread at their thinnest, is often the best location for examination of the blood smear.

The blood smear or blood film evaluation not only reveals morphologic abnormalities or normalcy (as the case may be), but may also confirm or refute automated cell count figures. If there appears to be a discrepancy between what the technician sees on the film and the numbers reported by the automated instrument, the counts should be repeated with special attention given to determining what could be causing the difference. A common cause is that the blood tube was not adequately mixed before sampling for either the count or the blood film. Another common problem is seen with platelet clumping. Platelet clumps may be counted as WBCs in the impedance-based automated cell counting systems, resulting in falsely higher WBC counts made by these instruments, although many of the newer systems that use multiple methods to classify cell type do not have this problem. Small platelet clumps may erroneously increase the mean platelet volume (MPV) estimates when in fact the platelet volume is normal. Probably the most commonly encountered error caused by platelet clumping is a decrease in platelet concentration because the platelet clumps are not properly counted by machines. With time and experience, the technician will be able to scan the blood film and recognize the discrepancies between the number of leukocytes apparent on the film and the number of WBCs reported by the instrument. As a general rule, there should be approximately 20 leukocytes per 10× field in a normal canine blood sample.

There are a variety of ways to make quality blood films. New slides should always be used, and they should be handled only by the edges because the transfer of oils from fingers to the slide will result in poor-quality films. If the slides have inadvertently been exposed to dust and debris, it may be helpful to clean them with a nonabrasive tissue, such as Kimwipes. (The reader is referred to Recommended Reading for examples of the different techniques.) What is most important is to try several methods, find the one that is most comfortable, and practice repeatedly until quality films are consistently produced. Most commonly a small drop of blood is placed at one end of a slide, and the edge of a second slide is used to spread the drop. It is important to make the film in one even stroke and not use excessive downward pressure. Increased downward pressure on the spreader slide can cause the leukocytes to be carried to the feathered edge and may even cause the cells to rupture or become distorted. In either case, the accuracy of the differential count will be decreased. The thickness of the blood film can be altered to accommodate samples from severely anemic or dehydrated animals. Increasing the angle between the two slides will concentrate the cells when the PCV is low. Conversely, decreasing the angle will allow greater spreading of the cells in a concentrated sample (Figure 16-4). Alternatively, one can prepare highly reproducible blood smears by placing a small drop of blood between two coverslips, rotating one

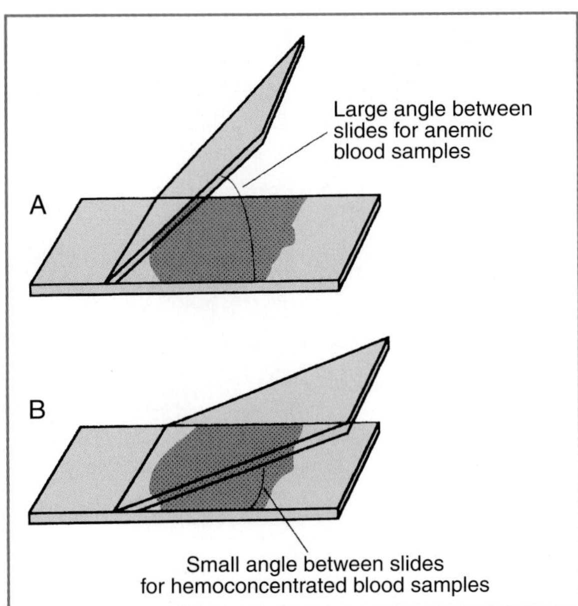

FIGURE 16-4 Difference in slide angle necessary for making blood films from anemic or hemoconcentrated blood. **A,** Large angle for anemic blood. **B,** Small angle for hemoconcentrated blood.

45-degrees in relation to the other, and then pulling one by a corner away from the other. These are then stained and mounted upon slides.

Manual staining methodologies with traditional Wright-Giemsa stains are labor intensive and require frequent filtering of the stains. More equipment, a source of distilled water, and critical timing are necessary. Several modifications of the traditional Wright's stain are available for the suitable staining of blood films for veterinary practices. Stat Stain (VWR Scientific, Philadelphia, Pa.), Diff-Quik (Baxter S/P, McGaw Park, Ill.), CAMCO Quik Stain (Baxter S/P), and Protocol Hema3 (Fischer, Waltham, Mass.) are commonly used. They are relatively economical, less time consuming, and technically easy to use and maintain. The components may be kept in individual Coplin jars. The lids should always be securely replaced after use, and the stains should be freshened or refilled as necessary. Stains should be replaced on a regular basis to prevent bacterial contamination and the accumulation of debris with repeated usage. The disadvantages of these stains are few. Polychromatophilic RBCs do not stain as obviously as they do with Wright-Giemsa stain, and some mast cell and eosinophil granules may be washed out leading to misdiagnosis. Conversely, distemper inclusions (clumps of distempter virus particles inside cells) may be more readily visualized with some of the rapid stains.

It is best to develop a routine for evaluating a blood film and follow the same approach each time to prevent oversights and mistakes. The blood film should first be examined under low power (10×). While scanning on 10×, one can get an impression of the general distribution of nucleated cells (clumped at the edges or spread evenly throughout), estimate the total WBC count (low versus normal versus high), and examine the feathered edge of the blood film for aggregates

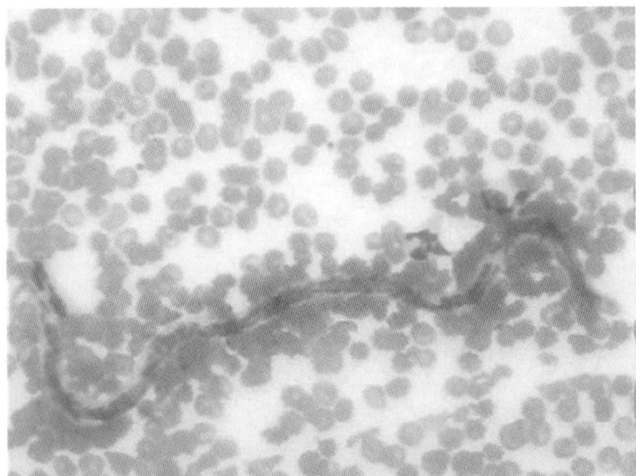

FIGURE 16-5 A microfilaria of *D. immitis* in a canine blood smear. The parasite is about the same width as an erythrocyte.

of platelets, the larger leukocytes, neoplastic cells, and microfilaria of *Dirofilaria immitis* or *Dipetalonema reconditum* (Figure 16-5). During the low-power examination, one may identify structures or areas that need a closer look. Last, on low power, one should identify the appropriate area in which RBCs are distributed in a uniform monolayer and the leukocytes are sufficiently spread so that morphologic identification on high power is possible. It is especially important to avoid going too far into the body of the blood film, where the WBCs are rounded and darkly stained. In this area, it is often difficult to differentiate the leukocytes.

The blood film is then studied under high power, generally under oil immersion (100×). The WBC differential count is performed at this power. Erythrocytes should be evaluated for morphologic changes and parasites, and platelets should be evaluated for morphology and counted to make the estimated count. These evaluations may be made before or after the differential count is performed, but they should be done consistently as part of the routine so that they are not overlooked. Platelets in mammals are cytoplasmic fragments, so they have no nuclei, whereas the platelet equivalents known as thrombocytes, which are found in avian and reptilian species, are nucleated; thrombocytes for a given species must be closely examined to differentiate them from relatively similar-appearing lymphocytes. They are generally round to oval or spindle shaped with purplish granules and multiple pointed projections (Figure 16-6). They may vary greatly in size, but increased numbers of large platelets may indicate an increased output from the bone marrow. After the platelets have been evaluated, the erythrocytes should be studied.

ERYTHROCYTE EVALUATION

The erythrocytes of most mammals are disk shaped and anuclear. They appear flat with a varying degree of central pallor (pale area in center of cell with less hemoglobin), depending on the size. The RBCs of different domestic species differ markedly in size, with those of the dog having the largest diameter (7 mm); followed by those of the horse, cow, and cat (5.8 mm); sheep (4.5 mm); and the goat (3.2 mm).

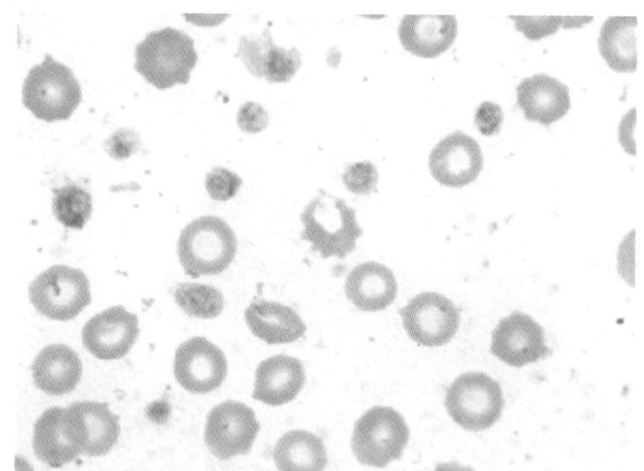

FIGURE 16-6 Canine blood smear showing hypochromic erythrocytes with increased central pallor as seen in iron deficiency anemia. Several platelets are also present between the erythrocytes.

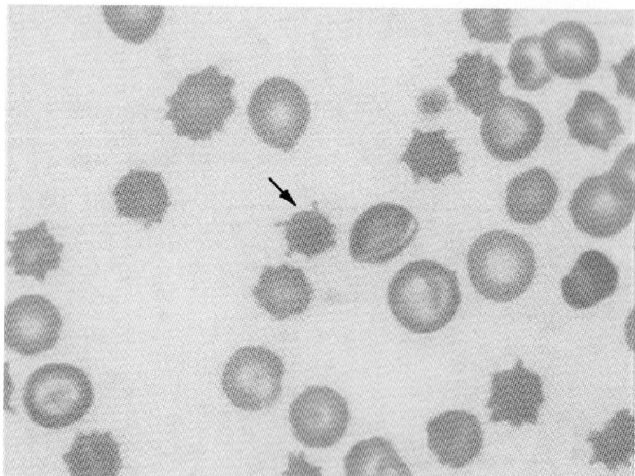

FIGURE 16-7 Canine blood film with acanthocyte.

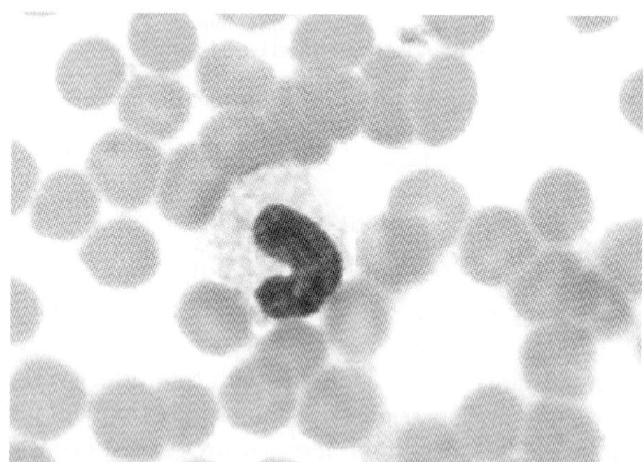

FIGURE 16-8 Feline erythrocytes. Note the lack of central pallor. There is also a toxic band neutrophil.

Some species have RBCs that vary in size, which is termed anisocytosis. Cows normally have more anisocytosis than do other species. In other species, extreme anisocytosis implies either that many of the RBCs are smaller (microcytic), which may indicate iron deficiency, or that many are larger (macrocytic), which may indicate increased production and release of immature RBCs from the bone marrow in response to anemia. An increase in MCV has been associated with feline leukemia virus (FeLV) infection frequently without an associated regenerative anemia. There are important species and breed variabilities that should not be mistaken as abnormalities. Some poodles have RBCs with increased MCVs as compared with other dogs. Some Akita dogs normally have smaller RBCs. These are genetic traits and do not indicate a change in RBC dynamics.

Poikilocytosis is the general term used to indicate changes in RBC shape. Leptocytes are RBCs with an increased surface area that makes them highly deformable. Target cells (codocytes) and cells with a transverse fold are two common forms of leptocytes. Acanthocytes are RBCs with a membrane abnormality that causes them to develop multiple, irregularly spaced, club-shaped projections from the cell surface (Figure 16-7). These must be differentiated from crenated cells, which have numerous rounded, evenly spaced projections. Crenation is most frequently an artifact resulting from high temperatures or slow drying of the blood film, but may also be seen secondary to certain drugs, hypophosphatemia, and in some cases of snake bite venom toxicity. Acanthocytes may be encountered in normal cattle, but in other species, they are often associated with some neoplasms (especially visceral hemangiosarcoma), disorders of lipid metabolism, and with liver dysfunction. Schistocytes are fragmented RBCs. They can be seen during a serious condition called disseminated intravascular coagulation (DIC). The disorder causes blood to clot in vessels leaving strands of fibrin criss-crossing through veins and arteries like a spider's web. As cells pass through the vessels, they are cleaved by the fibrin strands. DIC is such a grave condition, that it is sometimes referred to as "death is coming" and "dead in cage."After all of the clotting factors are used up, animals bleed uncontrollably in the terminal stages of DIC. Heartworm disease, and occasionally diseases of the spleen or liver that involve fibrin deposition within the vasculature of those organs, are conditions that can also cause schistocytes to form.

Spherocytes are RBCs that appear smaller than normal RBCs, exhibit no central pallor, but have MCVs comparable with normal RBCs as a result of the increased volume to surface area of a sphere (see Figure 16-6). Spherocytes are most commonly seen in immune-mediated hemolytic anemia (IMHA) and can also be seen after blood transfusions. One must be confident that spherocytes are actually present because many clinicians will start treatment for IMHA if they are reported because of the strong association with this disease process. They are more spherical because bits of their membrane have been removed, making them more rigid and unable to assume the discoid shape more typical of RBCs. They are most easily identified in canine blood because normal canine RBCs are larger and have a distinct zone of central pallor. In the other species with smaller RBCs, including the cat, which typically exhibit little or no central pallor, spherocytes are difficult to confirm (Figures 16-8 and 16-9).

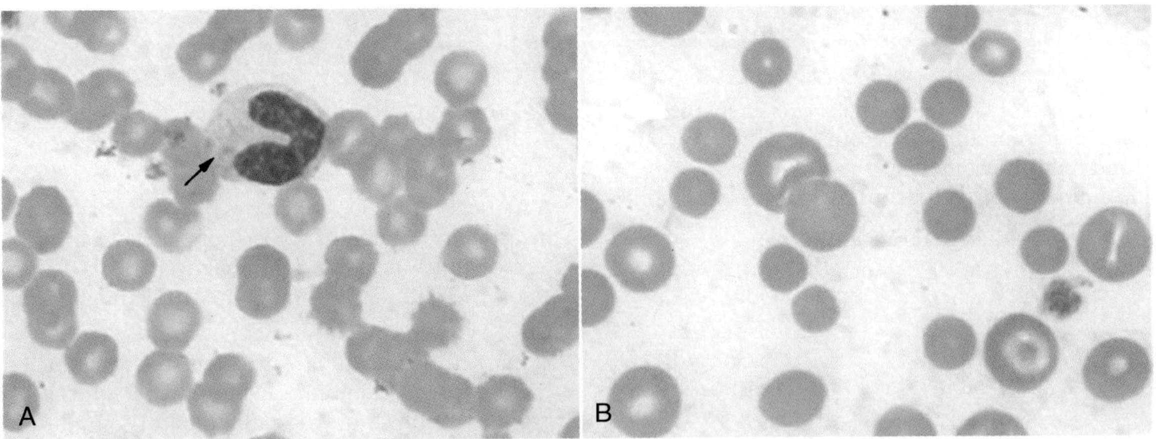

FIGURE 16-9 **A,** Normal canine RBCs. Note the distinct central pallor. There is also a toxic band with Döhle's bodies *(arrow)* in the cytoplasm. **B,** Blood from a dog with IMHA. Note the lack of central pallor in several smaller cells (spherocytes) and the large polychromatophilic cells.

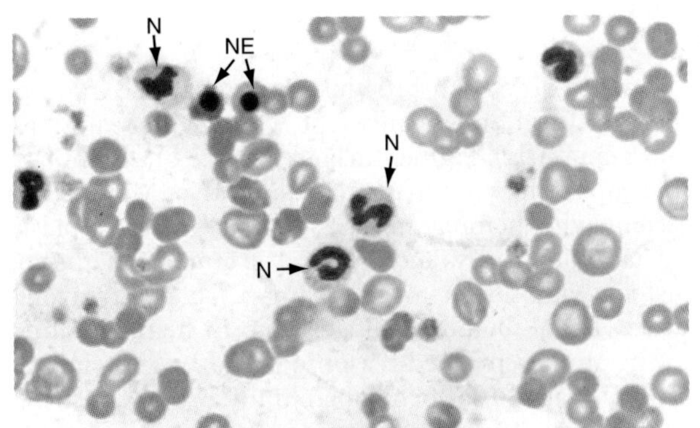

FIGURE 16-10 Canine blood film with several polychromatic erythrocytes, two nucleated erythrocytes *(NE)*, and neutrophils *(N)*.

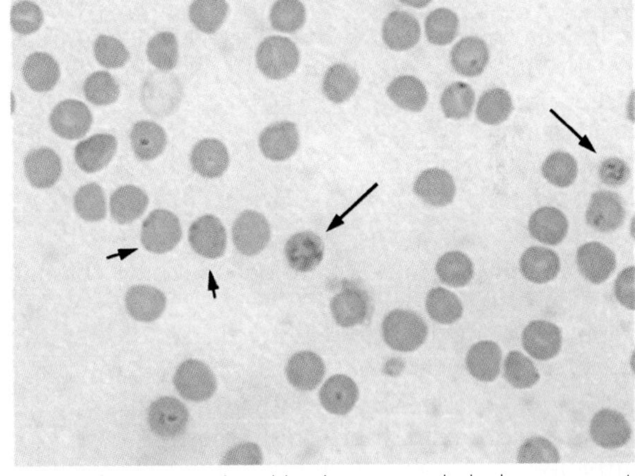

FIGURE 16-11 Feline blood smear with both punctate *(short arrows)* and aggregate reticulocytes *(long arrows)*.

NRBCs, or metarubricytes, may be seen in peripheral blood films. An occasional NRBC may be found in a normal animal, but increased numbers are a significant finding and should be reported as the number of NRBCs per 100 WBCs; NRBCs may be increased in cases of strongly regenerative anemias or may be representative of bone marrow pathologic conditions, as may be seen with toxins (such as lead) and neoplasia. Care must be taken to avoid confusing NRBCs with lymphocytes. NRBCs of a size similar to small lymphocytes will have more cytoplasm relative to nuclear size, and the cytoplasm will be faintly eosinophilic (reddish). Remember to correct the WBC count if more NRBCs are found (see previous discussion of determination of leukocyte counts).

The color of erythrocytes should be noted during the examination of the blood film. Polychromasia is the term used to describe a variation in the color of RBCs. Polychromatophilic RBCs (Figure 16-10) are bluish, although this is not as consistently evident with Diff-Quik stain as it is with Wright's stain. Some polychromasia may be seen in normal, healthy animals, but increased polychromasia in animals with anemia suggests that the anemia is regenerative (corresponding to an increase in reticulocytes); in other words, the bone marrow is responding to a need for RBCs and releasing immature RBCs. Little or no polychromasia detected on a blood film from an anemic animal suggests that the anemia is nonregenerative (i.e., the bone marrow is not responding appropriately). Although the presence of polychromasia may be suggestive of a bone marrow response to anemia, confirmation cannot be made without a reticulocyte count; because the reticulum of the immature RBCs are not being directly stained with Wright's staining procedures, they cannot be confirmed as reticulocytes, but instead appear as large bluish polychromatophils (these also may appear as leptocytes).

Polychromatophilic RBCs can be identified as reticulocytes (Figure 16-11) when the blood is stained with new methylene blue (NMB). Equal amounts of blood and stain (2 to 5 drops) are mixed in a small tube and left to stand for 5 to 10 minutes. Stain kits (ReticSet, Curtin Matheson Scientific, Houston) in which liquid stain is not used are available for reticulocyte counts. Instead, these kits include stain-coated plastic tubes into which 3 to 5 drops of whole blood are placed and then agitated. Whichever method is chosen, a blood film is made from the mixed sample.

CASE PRESENTATION 16-1 IMMUNE-MEDIATED HEMOLYTIC ANEMIA (IMHA) AND THROMBOCYTOPENIA (IMT)

Signalment: 2-year-old, spayed female, cocker spaniel
History: acute presentation of severe exercise intolerance, lethargy, and reddish urine
Physical Examination: pale mucous membranes, tachypnea

CBC:			Reference Interval
Hct	8	L	35-54 (%)
RDW	17	H	12-14 (%)
MCV	73	H	63-71 (fl)
MCHC	37	H	33-36 (g/dl)
Abs Retics	260	H	($\times 10^3$)
NRBC	7		

RBC morphology 2+ anisocytosis, 3+ polychromasia, 2+ spherocytes, agglutination noted (negative saline dispersion test)

Platelets	30	L	220-600 ($\times 10^3$)
MPV	7.0	L	8.0-12.5 (fl)
P. Protein	7.6		6.0-7.8 (g/dl)
Total WBC	32.0	H	8.0-14.5 ($\times 10^3$)
Neutrophils	28.4	H	3.0-11.5 ($\times 10^3$)
Bands	1.5	H	0-0.3 ($\times 10^3$)
Lymphocytes	0.3	L	1.0-4.8 ($\times 10^3$)
Monocytes	1.8	H	0.1-1.4 ($\times 10^3$)
Eosinophils	0.1		0.1-1.2 ($\times 10^3$)

WBC morphology 2+ Döhle's bodies, 2+ basophilia, 2+ vacuolation
P. appearance moderately hemolyzed (reddish)
Urinalysis (cystocentesis):

color	reddish-brownish (unspun), reddish-brownish (spun)
turbidity	clear
USG	1.025
pH	7.0
Protein	1+
Glucose	neg
Ketone	neg
Bilirubin	1+
Blood	3+
Sediment	occasional reddish casts

Interpretation

CBC, RBCs

A marked anemia is present, which is regenerative on the basis of the increased absolute reticulocyte count. Reticulocytosis is also supported by the other data, such as the increased MCV, measures of RBC size variation (RDW and morphologic assessment of anisocytosis), and the presence of polychromasia. Although reticulocytes typically have decreased MCHCs, in this case, the presence of free hemoglobin (supported by the reddish plasma) has artifactually increased the MCHC.

Primary IMHA can be deduced from the presence of agglutination and spherocytes, which are strongly associated with immune-mediated RBC destruction, and the lack of transfusion history.

Increased NRBC release in the face of a strongly regenerative anemia is appropriate and commonplace.

CBC, Platelets

A marked thrombocytopenia is present, which is assumed to be accurate because of the lack of platelet clumping. It is interesting to note at this point that decreased MPVs have been associated with IMT, but they are not pathognomonic for it.

CBC, WBCs

A marked neutrophilia with a left shift is defined as an inflammatory leukogram. Lymphopenia and monocytosis are commonly found in inflammatory conditions, either directly as a result of inflammation and/or secondary to a superimposed stress leukogram.

Toxic changes (Döhle's bodies, basophilia, and vacuolation) are present secondary to the intense inflammatory demand.

Urinalysis

The presence of reddish-brownish urine that does not clear upon centrifugation is consistent with pigmenturia (ruling out hematuria). Pigmenturia in the face of a hemolyzed plasma appearance and marked presumptive IMHA is most consistent with hemoglobinuria; the lack of clear plasma and a lack of history and physical examination findings consistent with severe muscle damage rule out myoglobinuria. The 3+ blood reading is due to hemoglobinuria given the aforementioned reasoning. The 1+ protein reading is likely also due to hemoglobinuria, but concurrent hemoglobinuric nephron damage cannot be ruled out; the protein reading is expected to be of a lesser degree than the blood reading in this case as a result of the relative insensitivity of the protein strip to hemoglobin. The reddish casts are most likely hemoglobin imbibed hyaline casts. The 1+ bilirubinuria may be related to hyperbilirubinemia associated with IMHA, but this could also be a normal finding in the dog; the lack of visible icteric plasma should not be surprising given that bilirubinuria precedes hyperbilirubinemia and the potential for it to be masked by the concurrent hemolyzed plasma appearance.

Summary

IMHA is primarily deduced by the presence of a marked anemia with agglutination, spherocytes, a hemolyzed plasma appearance, and findings most consistent with hemoglobinuria; it is important to note that IMHA may be also present in cases that do not have every one of the aforementioned findings. Additionally, IMHA commonly is associated with an inflammatory leukogram (sometimes with toxic neutrophils) and a strongly regenerative anemia (unless there is concurrent immune-mediated destruction of reticulocytes).

IMT may be associated with IMHA (known as Evans syndrome in human medicine), but other potential causes of thrombocytopenia need to be ruled out, especially DIC because of its strong association with primary IMHA.

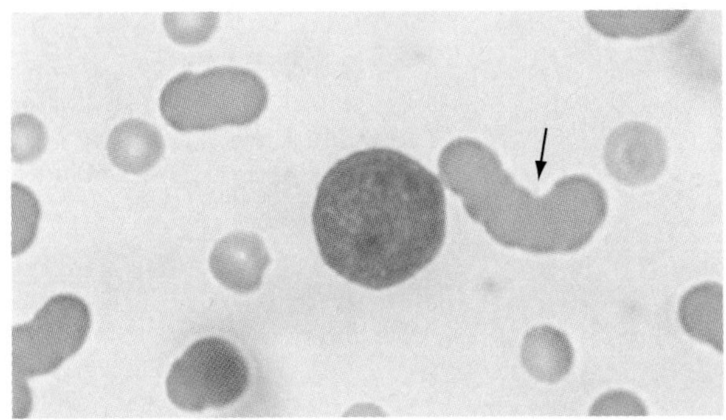

FIGURE 16-12 Feline blood film showing rouleaux formation *(arrow)*.

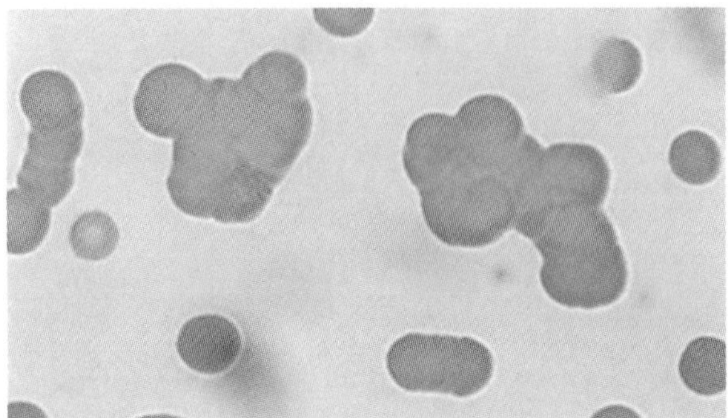

FIGURE 16-13 Feline blood film showing agglutination.

Normal RBCs appear yellowish green with NMB. The reticulocytes will be the same color, but will contain deeply basophilic (bluish) dots or strands. Cats have two types of reticulocytes, punctate and aggregate (see Figure 16-11). Only the reticulocytes that have prominent clumps of reticulum (aggregate reticulocytes) are counted. The RBCs with small single dots (punctate reticulocytes) are generally not included in the count, but their presence should be noted. A reticulocyte count is the number of reticulocytes noted in a count of 1000 RBCs expressed as a percentage. In dogs and cats, reticulocyte counts expressed as percentages should then be corrected to account for the patient's PCV or Hct (the corrected reticulocyte percentage [CRP]), or the absolute reticulocyte count per microliter can be reported by multiplying the percentage of reticulocytes by the RBC count.

% Reticulocytes = 40 reticulocytes counted in 1000 RBCs = 40/1000 or 4%

CRP = (% reticulocytes × patient's PCV)/45 (dog) or 37 (cat)

CRPs greater than 1% in the dog and greater than 0.4% in the cat and absolute reticulocyte counts greater than 80,000/μl and greater than 60,000/μl in the cat are supportive of a regenerative anemia, with the degree of response expected to be proportional to the severity of the anemia. Horses do not release immature RBCs from the bone marrow, even when they are severely anemic, so polychromasia and reticulocytosis are not seen in equine peripheral blood. Although an increased MCV is strongly supportive of a regenerative response in an anemic equid, an MCV within the reference interval does not exclude a regenerative response.

Hypochromic RBCs have an increased area of central pallor with a narrow, peripheral rim of hemoglobin resulting from an abnormally low amount of hemoglobin within the cell. The most common cause of hypochromasia is iron deficiency. Hypochromasia can be confirmed by a low MCHC provided by automated instruments. True hypochromic RBCs (see Figure 16-6) must be differentiated from "punched out" RBCs, which are normochromic, but have a more distinct central pallor with a thick dense rim of hemoglobinized cytoplasm. These cells are an artifact of blood film preparation, not a significant pathologic change. Hyperchromasia, or increased hemoglobin content, does not occur in RBCs, although increased MCHC values may be seen secondary to hemolysis, lipemia, icterus, and Heinz body formation. Because this elevation in MCHC is not a symptom of a diseased process but rather is a result of an error in collection, sample storage or patient preparation, it is referred to as an *artifact* and the MCHC is said to be "artifactually" elevated.

Rouleaux are groupings of RBCs that resemble stacked coins (Figure 16-12). Marked rouleaux formation is normal in horses and, to a lesser extent, in cats. In dogs, rouleaux formation may occur in inflammatory or neoplastic diseases. It is important to differentiate rouleaux from true agglutination (clumping) of RBCs. Agglutinated RBCs tend to appear as clumps rather than as stacked coins. The clumping is caused by strong attachments formed between antibodies on the surfaces of RBCs. This can be seen, for example, when an animal has a reaction during and after a blood transfusion. If the blood of the donor is not compatible with that of the recipient, the RBCs will form strong attachments to one another (Figure 16-13). Needless to say, this is a serious and life threatening complication. Blood types can be tested to see if cross-reactivity occurs by mixing the blood samples together in a glass tube or on a glass slide. If agglutination of RBCs occurs, it can often be seen grossly as clumps on the side of the blood tube and on the blood film. If there is some question about whether a blood sample is exhibiting rouleaux or true agglutination, a saline test can be performed. The blood cells are washed by adding 1 drop of blood to 5 ml of saline solution and centrifuging for 3 minutes. The supernatant is poured off, the RBCs are resuspended in saline solution, and a wet mount preparation is made. Rouleaux will disperse as a result of the dilution of the serum protein, but agglutinated RBCs will remain clumped because of their strong cross-linking.

A Coombs' test may be requested to confirm the presence of immune mediated hemolytic anemia (IMHA). In IMHA, an animal produces antibodies that attach to and ultimately leads to the destruction of its own RBCs. The Coombs' test is a species-specific test that detects the presence of these antibodies. Gross or microscopic RBC agglutination precludes the use of a Coombs' test because surface-bound antibodies are presumed to be present during agglutination. In

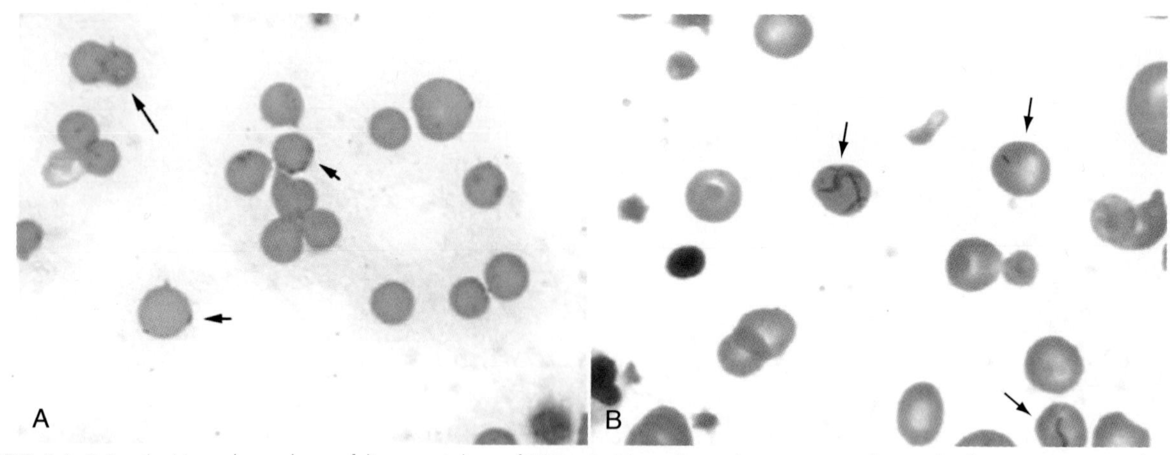

FIGURE 16-14 A, *Mycoplasma haemofelis* on periphery of RBCs. **B**, *Mycoplasma haemocanis* with strands of organisms across the surface.

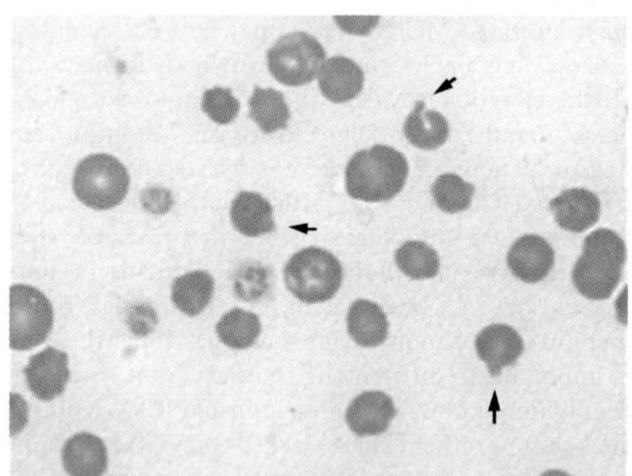

FIGURE 16-15 Feline blood film showing Heinz body formation. Note the RBCs with variably distinct, pale, rounded projections from their surface (Wright's stain, 100×).

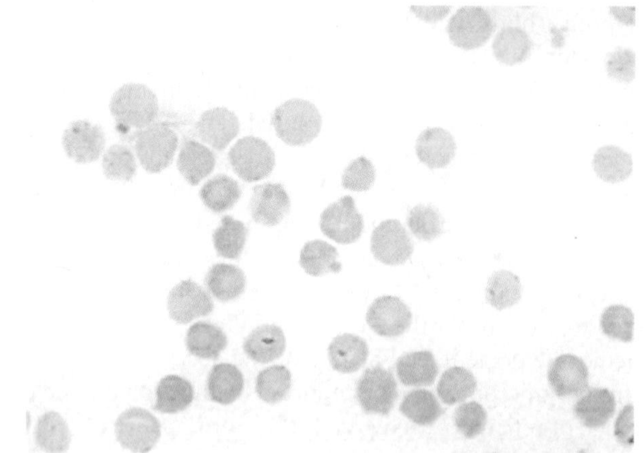

FIGURE 16-16 Distinctly basophilic, protruding Heinz bodies stained with NMB.

other words, if you see clumps of RBCs, don't bother doing a Coombs test, because you can assume it will be positive.

The evaluation of erythrocytes under oil immersion should also include a search for RBC parasites, particularly in cases of anemia. *Mycoplasma haemofelis* (formally known as *Haemobartonella felis*), the parasite responsible for feline infectious anemia, appears as small coccoid or rodlike structures on the surface of RBCs (Figure 16-14, *A*). A careful search for *M. haemofelis* organisms should be performed on any anemic cat. These parasites may be difficult to identify because they can be easily confused with protein and stain precipitates adhered to the cell surface. *Mycoplasma haemocanis* (formally known as *Haemobartonella canis*) is rarely seen, but is more readily identified (Figure 16-14, *B*). Other *Mycoplasma* spp., formally known as *Eperythrozoon* spp., which are found in cattle, sheep, and swine, may appear similar to *M. haemofelis* or may occur as ring forms on the RBCs. *Anaplasma marginale,* a parasite of bovine RBCs, appears as a small spherical body within the RBC, close to the cell margin. Another RBC parasite is *Babesia* spp. *Babesia* spp. are larger and lighter staining than the previously mentioned parasites, and they tend to occur as tear-shaped structures (often paired) within the RBCs. It is important to note that these parasites are diagnosed on standard Wright's-stained blood smears; one must take care to not misinterpret reticulum staining with potential parasites when using an NMB stain.

Other RBC morphologic abnormalities include Howell-Jolly bodies, basophilic stippling, Heinz bodies, and viral inclusions. Howell-Jolly bodies are small, often singular, deeply basophilic nuclear remnants that are occasionally seen on normal blood films. Increased numbers of Howell-Jolly bodies can be seen with regenerative anemias and in splenectomized animals. Basophilic stippling is due to staining of small amounts of cytoplasmic RNA in RBCs. These inclusions are multiple tiny, lightly basophilic dots in the RBC cytoplasm. They can be found in cases of markedly regenerative anemia in dogs and cats, but are found more commonly in cattle. Basophilic stippling may also be seen occasionally in cases of lead poisoning. The most consistent finding in lead poisoning is increased numbers of NRBCs with mild to no anemia. Heinz bodies are denatured hemoglobin that has fused to the RBC membrane and appear as hard to distinguish lightly eosinophilic, spherical inclusions (Figure 16-15). These inclusions are most readily seen when the reticulocyte (NMB) stain is applied. They appear as distinct, darkly staining inclusions frequently protruding from the cell surface (Figure 16-16). Distemper virus inclusions

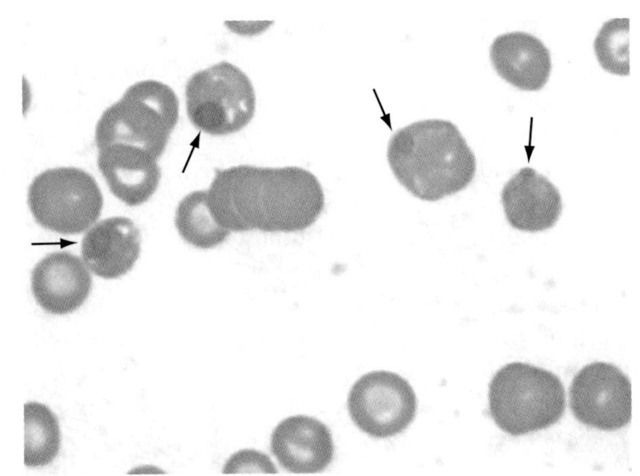

FIGURE 16-17 Canine blood film with viral (distemper) inclusions in RBCs (Wright's stain, 1000×).

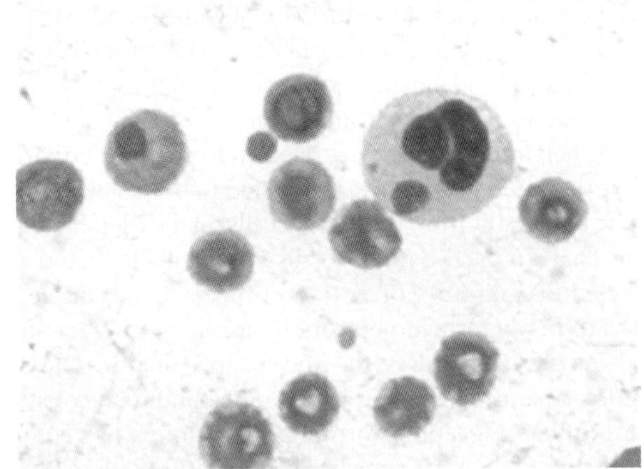

FIGURE 16-18 Canine blood smear with viral inclusions in RBCs and neutrophil (Diff-Quik stain).

may be seen in either RBCs or WBCs. These appear as distinct, spherical, eosinophilic to lightly basophilic inclusions and may sometimes be more readily appreciated with some of the rapid Wright's stains (Figures 16-17 and 16-18).

LEUKOCYTE EVALUATION

The WBCs also known as leukocytes (leuko = white) are categorized on the basis of nuclear segmentation and cytoplasmic granularity. Leukocytes may have distinct nuclear segmentation, such as neutrophils, eosinophils, and basophils, or may have round to oval nuclei, such as lymphocytes and monocytes; additionally, monocytes may display nuclear lobulation, but not segmentation. Leukocytes can also be characterized on the basis of the presence or absence of cytoplasmic granules, and further subdivided by granule coloration in addition to shape for some species that have similarly colored granules (heterophils and eosinophils). Eosinophil granules have eosinophilic (reddish-orange) coloration, basophil granules are basophilic (bluish-purple), and neutrophil granules are neutral (clear, but identifiable by dropping the substage condenser). The morphologic term heterophil is used to describe the appearance of obvious fine, reddish cytoplasmic granules normally found in neutrophil equivalents that are found in species such as elephants, rodents, avians, reptilians, amphibians, and nonhuman primates. Agranulocytes, such as monocytes and lymphocytes, typically do not display distinct cytoplasmic granulation, but a fine reddish-pinkish granularity may occasionally be seen in monocytes. Certain less commonly encountered subsets of lymphocytes can display focal accumulations of low numbers of small reddish granules (granular lymphocytes).

The evaluation of leukocyte numbers and morphology is important to define various disease states too broad in scope to detail herein, but often such information is used to differentiate potential systemic inflammatory conditions from other causes of neutrophilias, such as secondary to stress (mediated by glucocorticoids) and excitement (mediated by epinephrine). The interpretation of leukocyte responses should be based upon absolute cell concentrations ($10^3/\mu l$) instead of percentages.

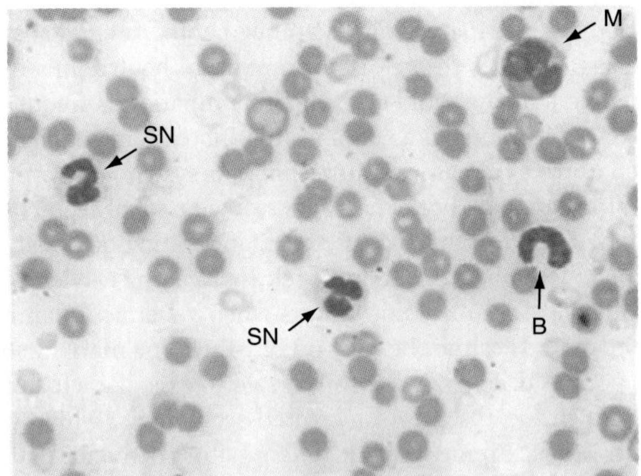

FIGURE 16-19 Canine blood film. Two segmented neutrophils *(SN)*, a band *(B)* to the right, and a monocyte *(M)* in upper right corner.

Neutrophils

In domestic species such as the dog, cat, and horse, the predominant WBC is the mature segmented neutrophil, referred to as a segmenter or seg (Figure 16-19); in contrast, the predominant leukocyte in cattle, sheep, and goats is the lymphocyte, and as such, a predominance of neutrophils (lymphocyte-neutrophil inversion or reversal) may be indicative of systemic inflammation. Pigs exhibit about equal numbers of lymphocytes and neutrophils. The average time spent by the neutrophil in the blood before entering tissue is only about 5 to 10 hours, so peripheral neutrophil numbers are used as one method of assessing recent systemic inflammatory reactions. Normal neutrophils have deeply staining, clumped, segmented nuclei (three to five lobes) with relatively clear cytoplasm. The degree of segmentation observed for a mature neutrophil varies with species and is important to recognize to prevent misclassification of lesser segmented immature forms.

> *TECHNICIAN NOTE* Extra care must be taken in differentiating monocytes from toxic band neutrophils, particularly in horses.

Charts that depict the maturation of white blood cells typically list the most immature form of the cell on the left hand side of the page and illustrate increasingly mature stages of the cells as the reader moves from the left to the right side of the page. When immature cells are released from the bone barrow before they are fully mature, this is said to be "a left shift" referring to the shift from the mature cells on the right hand side of the chart to the less mature cells toward the left hand side. A left shift is indicative of a disease process. For example, the nuclei of newly formed neutrophils are single circular structures. As the cell matures, the nucleus invaginates and bends forming a band (like a head band). The band then constricts in a number of locations forming thin isthmus-like connections between thicker segments. These mature cells are called segmenters and the immature cells are called bands. During a blood smear evaluation, an important morphologic change in neutrophils is the appearance of immature band-shaped nuclei. Because mature nuclei are segmented, a band shaped nucleus indicates the release of immature neutrophils from the bone marrow. Mild systemic inflammation is frequently reflected in the CBC as an absolute increase in segmenters also known as a mature neutrophilia. As systemic inflammation increases, the bone marrow's storage pool of segmenters cannot fully meet this increased demand for neutrophils, and increased numbers of bands are released leading to a left shift. In other words, a left shift occurs when systemic inflammatory demands cannot be fully met by the bone marrow storage pool. A degenerate left shift is said to exist if a left shift is present in the absence of increased segmenters, which may occur when extreme systemic inflammatory demands deplete the bone marrow's storage pool. A band nucleus is less segmented, and nuclear borders assume a more uniform parallel appearance (see Figures 16-8, 16-9, and 16-19). Even more immature cells, with bean-shaped or oval nuclei (metamyelocytes or myelocytes, respectively), may be seen in cases of extreme tissue demand for neutrophils. Neutrophils, mature or immature, may also show evidence of inflammatory disease as demonstrated by certain cytoplasmic characteristics known as toxic changes; these include any combination of Döhle's bodies, cytoplasmic vacuolation, cytoplasmic basophilia, and, rarely, retention of fine, reddish granules called toxic granulation. Notice that the band neutrofils in Figures 16-8 and 16-9 also show toxic changes. Toxic changes represent cytoplasmic defects in the maturation of blood neutrophils that develop secondary to intense granulopoiesis; this terminology must not be confused with degenerate changes, which represent nuclear dissolution in dying neutrophils found in tissue and fluids. Frequently, toxic changes are quantitated using scales that vary in scoring methodology between laboratories. Döhle's bodies are small, pale, bluish-gray, irregular cytoplasmic inclusions of RNA containing rough endoplasmic reticulum. Neutrophils from healthy cats may occasionally exhibit a few small Döhle's bodies, but greater numbers and/or larger ones are likely to be associated with systemic inflammatory disease. Generalized cytoplasmic basophilia is representative of increased amounts of RNA. Cytoplasmic vacuolation occurs secondary to organelle abnormalities. In contrast to these cytoplasmic changes, nuclear hypersegmentation (nuclei with five or more lobes) is a normal aging change that implies a nontoxic environment and prolonged circulation of neutrophils. They are most frequently seen in the presence of excessive steroids, in which neutrophils remain in circulation longer than normal.

An animal's gender may also be determined by the appearance of a small drumstick-appearing nuclear appendage called a Barr body. The Barr body represents an inactive X chromosome that is present in females. If these are reliably found on blood smears of an animal, it is likely to be a female; if Barr bodies are not found, one cannot determine the animal's gender.

Eosinophils

Eosinophils help to control allergic or anaphylactic hypersensitivity reactions. They are attracted to the sites of these reactions by substances released from sensitized mast cells; therefore eosinophils tend to occur where mast cells congregate. The eosinophil is characterized by a segmented nucleus, colorless to pale blue cytoplasm, and distinct eosinophilic (reddish-orange) staining granules in the cytoplasm.

The morphologic appearance of eosinophil granules varies from species to species, so they can be used to identify the origin of a blood sample. The eosinophils of cats contain numerous tiny rod-shaped granules that may obscure the nucleus. The eosinophil granules of dogs are less numerous and are usually round, but may vary considerably in size. Differences may be found between breeds; many Greyhounds have eosinophils that display clear nonstaining granules within a grayish cytoplasm and a relatively less segmented nucleus, which must not be mistaken for toxic bands. The eosinophil granules of horses are extremely distinctive; they are large and round and a much brighter orange than those of small animals. Bovine eosinophil granules are also bright orange, but are much smaller and more numerous than those of the horse and much more uniform in size than those of the dog. Figure 16-20 illustrates the diversity of eosinophil granules found in various domestic species.

Basophils

Basophils are relatively rare in blood films, but, when present, tend to occur in association with increased eosinophils. Classically, they have dark basophilic (blue) granules, but they also may vary considerably from species to species. Feline basophils tend to have light lavender to almost pink granules, rather than the dark purple granules seen in other species. Canine basophils may have few to no granules and must be differentiated from neutrophils on the basis of an elongated nucleus and a more basophilic cytoplasm (Figure 16-21). Equine and bovine basophils tend to have variable numbers of the more typical dark basophilic granules. Basophils are frequently confused with mast cells because of similar granules, but the basophil nucleus is segmented, and the mast cell nucleus is round or oval.

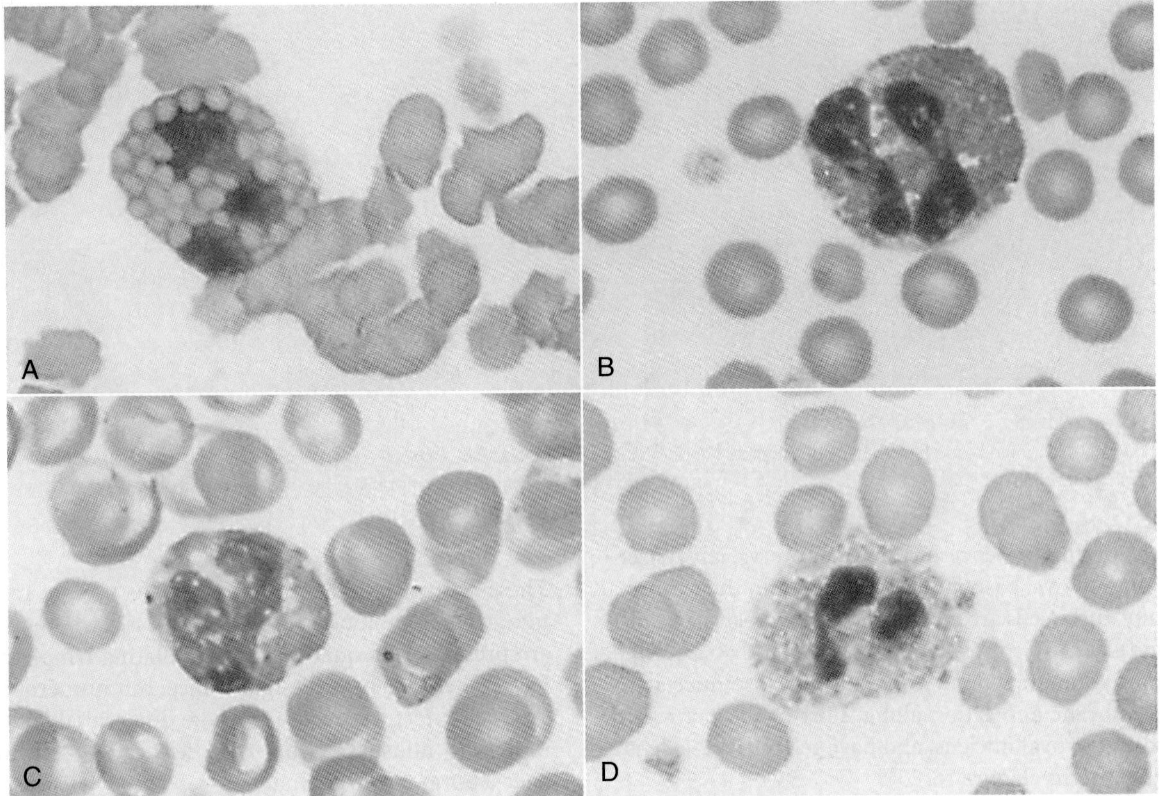

FIGURE 16-20 Species variation in eosinophil granules. **A,** Equine eosinophil. **B,** Bovine eosinophil. **C,** Canine eosinophil. **D,** Feline eosinophil.

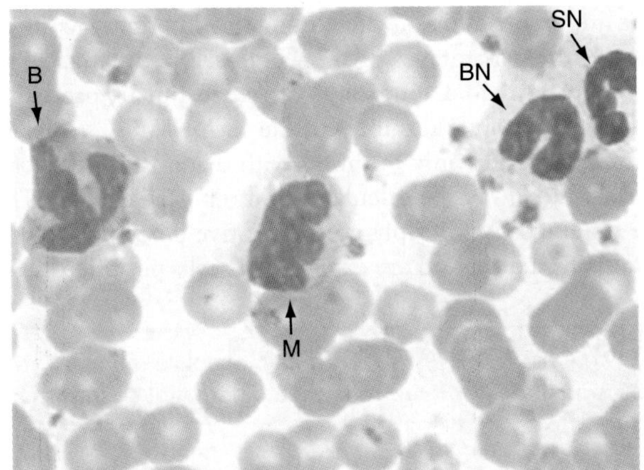

FIGURE 16-21 Canine blood film. From left, basophil *(B)*, monocyte *(M)*, band neutrophil *(BN)*, and segmented neutrophil *(SN)*. Note that the basophil has an elongated nucleus and darker cytoplasm, but no distinct granules. There are several platelets between the RBCs and few overlying RBCs.

FIGURE 16-22 Canine blood smear with mature lymphocytes with scant, basophilic cytoplasm. The number of cells is compatible with lymphocytic leukemia.

Lymphocytes

Lymphocytes are usually small- to medium-sized mononuclear cells. The nucleus of lymphocytes dominates the cell so that only a thin rim of light blue cytoplasm is visible surrounding the nucleus. Lymphocytes are therefore said to have a high nuclear to cytoplasmic ratio or N/C ratio (Figure 16-22). Intermediate- to large-sized lymphocytes may be present more frequently in large animals, but can also be present in most species secondary to antigenic stimulation. These cells have clear cytoplasm, moderate N/C ratios, centralized oval nuclei with a brushed chromatin pattern, and may display a focal accumulation of low numbers of small reddish granules. During periods of antigenic stimulation in all species, some of the lymphocytes in the blood film may have extremely basophilic cytoplasm with a small, pale, perinuclear zone (the site of the Golgi apparatus) and possibly azurophilic granules. These cells are referred to as reactive lymphocytes. Intermediate lymphocytes and reactive lymphocytes and monocytes must be differentiated from lymphoblasts (immature lyphocytes), which may be found circulating in cases of lymphoma and lymphoid leukemias. Lymphoblasts

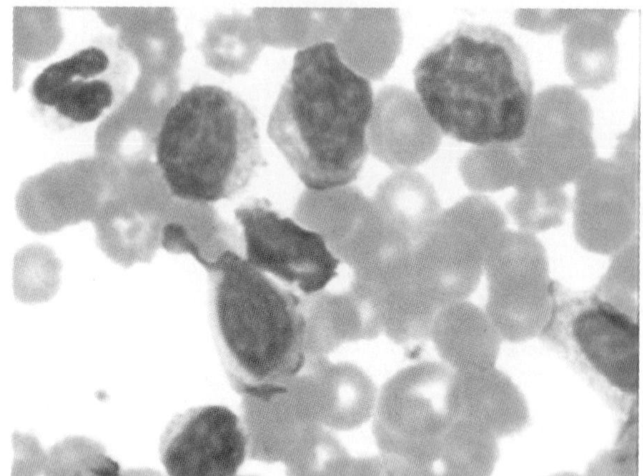

FIGURE 16-23 Canine blood film with large, atypical lymphocytes compatible with lymphoblastic leukemia.

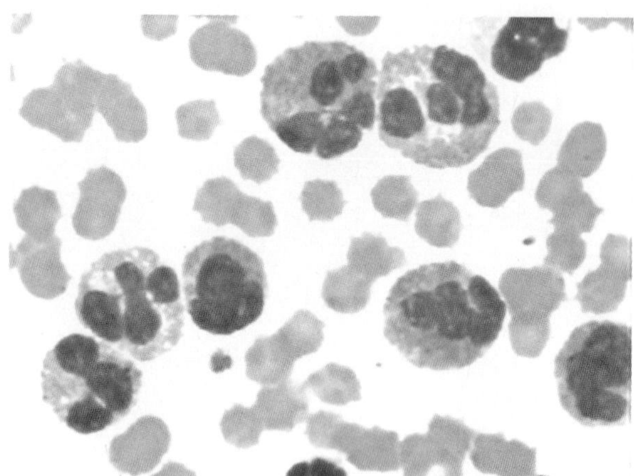

FIGURE 16-24 Feline blood smear. All of the nucleated cells in this smear are eosinophils. The large number of cells is indicative of eosinophilic leukemia.

are defined by the presence of one or more variably sized usually round to oval basophilic nucleoli within their nuclei; additionally, these cells are intermediate to large in size, with low to moderate N/C ratios, moderately to darkly basophilic cytoplasm, frequent apparent Golgi zones, close nuclear to plasma membrane apposition along most of the perimeter of their round to oval nucleus, and have relatively less dense chromatin patterns (Figure 16-23).

Monocytes

Monocytes (see Figures 16-19 and 16-21) are derived from the bone marrow and circulate in the blood briefly before entering the tissues in which they become macrophages. Macrophages phagocytize (ingest) large particles and cellular debris that neutrophils cannot handle. Monocytes have gray-blue cytoplasm that frequently has a fine, subtle, lightly eosinophilic granulation and may contain a few clear vacuoles and a variable-shaped nucleus. The nucleus can be round, oval, reniform, ameboid, or lobed. The monocyte is usually larger than the lymphocyte or neutrophil. The most common problem associated with the identification of monocytes is the tendency to confuse monocytes that have a lobate or reniform-shaped nucleus with a toxic band or metamyelocyte, respectively; nontoxic neutrophils have less basophilic cytoplasm and lack cytoplasmic vacuolation. Reactive monocytes may occasionally be seen (e.g., secondary to chemotherapy) that may be difficult to differentiate from lymphoblasts; these cells may have more darkly basophilic cytoplasm and perhaps apparent Golgi zones, but are not expected to display nucleoli.

Other Cells

Occasionally, the evaluation of the blood film reveals abnormal circulating cell types, such as mast cells, lymphoblasts, myeloblasts, and erythroblasts. The number and type of abnormal cells should be noted because they may indicate leukemia (see Figures 16-23 and 16-24) or systemic mastocytosis. Smudge (or basket) cells are swollen nuclear remnants from lysed cells that appear as pale, fibrillar, eosinophilic nuclear material lacking a cytoplasmic or nuclear membrane. These occur when excessive pressure is used in making the film, when old blood is used, and in cases where fragile cells are present (infrequently with circulating lymphoblasts). A few of these are of little significance, but numerous smudge cells can affect the accuracy of the differential count. Blood films with unusual or abnormal cells can be sent to a reference laboratory for evaluation.

ABSOLUTE VERSUS RELATIVE NUMBERS

The numbers obtained when doing the differential count are relative, or percentages of the whole cell population. These numbers have no diagnostic significance, but are used to calculate the absolute numbers of the various WBCs. Absolute numbers are the only numbers with diagnostic significance and should always be calculated and reported as such. These are obtained by multiplying the relative percentages by the total WBC count and are expressed as cells per microliter.

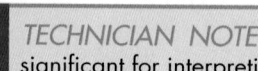

TECHNICIAN NOTE Only absolute numbers are significant for interpreting the differential count.

AUTOMATED CELL COUNTERS

A basic understanding of the principles of electronic cell counting is useful for the veterinary technician, regardless of whether the practice has an in-practice laboratory. Many practices find it convenient to use human reference or hospital laboratories, but these instruments must be specially calibrated for use with veterinary samples because of the wide variation in blood cell size among the different species. Several instruments have been designed specifically for veterinary medicine (e.g., Vet ABC-Diff Hematology Analyzer, Heska, Fort Collins, Colo. [Figure 16-25]) that are computer driven with species options and automatically change the instrument settings for multiple-species use. The major advantages of electronic cell counters are their speed, accuracy, and reproducibility. In addition to providing RBC, WBC,

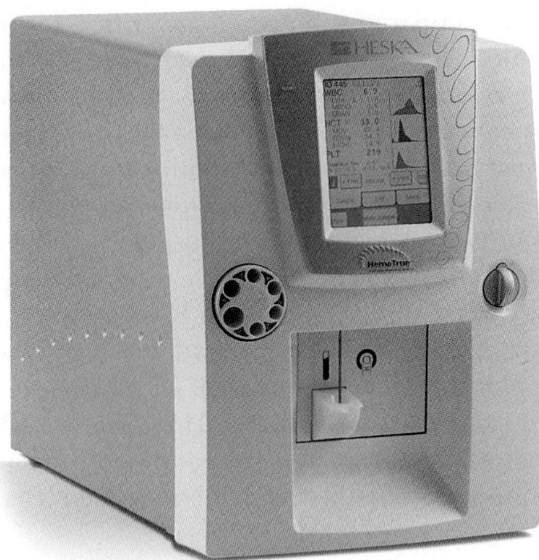

FIGURE 16-25 Heska Corporation's HemaTrue® Veterinary Hematology Analyzer provides an accurate CBC in only 55 seconds. (Courtesy Heska Corporation, Loveland, CO.)

and platelet counts, most cell counters will measure hemoglobin and calculate the RBC indices.

The disadvantage of electronic cell counters is the quality control and maintenance requirements. The veterinary technician must be able to recognize when the instruments are not functioning properly and determine the problem. The manufacturer should be willing to train the technician to perform quality control and calibration procedures, keep adequate quality control records, and handle minor adjustments. In addition, the manufacturer should be available for service calls, if needed. In some practices, consideration should be given to the purchase of a service contract; this should be discussed before investing in a major instrument.

The operating principle involved in electronic cell counting is based on a type of flow cytometry (the counting of particles as they flow past a detection device). This technology allows the instrument to count blood cells and measure the size. Most instruments use a simple orifice through which an electrical current passes. As particles (e.g., blood cells) move through the orifice, they disrupt the current by increasing the resistance (impedance) proportional to the size of the particle. The instrument is set to detect and count only particles that produce a signal that exceeds a specific resistance or threshold. The threshold settings will determine what particles are counted based on their size. This principle is important when an instrument is evaluated for use in veterinary medicine. Many instruments developed for human medicine do not accurately count RBCs with a volume of less than 55 femtoliters (fl). The RBCs of the cat, horse, cow, goat, and pig have mean cell volumes below this value. More advanced analyzers also attempt to determine cell type on the basis of differential staining patterns and other optical properties. Although veterinary-specific software exists for some of these machines, each laboratory needs to evaluate the validity of automated differential counts for the species in which they are interested; having said that, these results should never be considered absolutely accurate without a technologist's slide review.

WBCs from different species also have varying sizes after exposure to RBC lysing solutions. Total WBC counts on some instruments can be falsely decreased in the dog because of its small leukocytes. The reverse is true in the cat. The cat's platelets tend to form large clumps that are counted as leukocytes, thus falsely elevating the WBC count. A close inspection of the blood film will help the technician identify this problem.

Whole blood can be diluted for counting either before introduction of the sample into the machine (predilution) or by the instrument as part of the sampling cycle. In the newer instruments, whole blood is aspirated and diluted for the RBC count, and a portion of the sample is lysed to remove the RBCs and allow the WBCs to be counted. The lysed sample is often used for hemoglobin determination.

It is important to reiterate the limitations of these devices; differential counts obtained should not replace the blood film examination; the automated reticulocyte or platelet count should not be taken at face value. Blood cell morphology is important in evaluating the numbers obtained in the blood cell counts. The automated instruments cannot tell the technician whether band neutrophils, toxic neutrophils, polychromatophilic RBCs, RBC parasites, or NRBCs are present. Although clinicians may sometimes request manual platelet counts in cases of marked thrombocytopenias, automated are more accurate than manual platelet counts if platelet clumping has not been noted and associated quality control parameters are in order.

> *TECHNICIAN NOTE* The differential count provided by automated analyzers is not an adequate substitute for microscopic evaluation of the blood film.

PLASMA PROTEIN DETERMINATION

The determination of the plasma protein concentration is another standard component of the routine CBC. After plasma color and turbidity have been noted, the capillary tube used for measuring the PCV is broken at a point slightly above the buffy coat (cream-colored layer of WBCs and platelets just above the RBCs), and the plasma is allowed to run through the unbroken end onto the prism of a refractometer by capillary action. Lifting the cover and tapping the Hct tube on the prism may scratch the surface of the prism. Plasma protein values obtained with a refractometer are accurate as long as the plasma is clear. If the plasma is lipemic, hemolyzed, or otherwise cloudy, the refractive index will be increased and provide an erroneously high protein measurement. The lipemic samples often have an indistinct or unfocused line on the refractometer scale. In contrast to the dilution effect of a small blood sample in a large tube, excess anticoagulant will artifactually increase the plasma protein value obtained.

A semiquantitative determination of plasma fibrinogen levels may be useful in the detection of inflammatory processes, particularly in cattle and horses. Two capillary tubes of blood are centrifuged; one is used for the PCV and plasma protein determination, as described. The second tube is placed in a 56° C to 58° C water bath for 3 minutes to cause the precipitation of fibrinogen. The tube is then recentrifuged so the fibrinogen settles just above the buffy coat. The tube is broken above the fibrinogen, and the remaining plasma is placed on the refractometer for protein determination. The difference between the protein concentration of the first tube and the protein concentration of the second tube is the fibrinogen concentration.

Fibrinogen is usually expressed in milligrams per deciliter; therefore if the first tube had a protein concentration of 7.3 g/dl and the second tube has a protein concentration of 6.9 g/dl, the plasma fibrinogen concentration is 0.4 g/dl, or 400 mg/dl. Plasma from cattle with notably increased fibrinogen may completely coagulate during incubation; when the specimen is respun, the fibrinogen does not settle out, and a fibrinogen value cannot be determined.

COAGULATION TESTING

Animals will occasionally be seen with abnormal bleeding tendencies. The ability for blood to clot (hemostasis), depends on vascular integrity, adequate numbers and normal functioning of platelets, and a complete complement of coagulation factors. These are counterbalanced by several thrombolytic factors to prevent excessive thrombosis. When vascular injury is present, the platelets are exposed to collagen fibers normally secluded within the vessel wall. The platelets adhere to the periphery of the lesion and aggregate to form an initial plug to stem the immediate flow of blood. The formation of this initial plug is called primary hemostasis. Subsequently, a complicated cascade of biochemical reactions occurs that leads to the formation of a fibrin mesh that envelopes the plug of platelets and stabilizes it forming a strong clot. This latter stage of coagulation is called secondary hemostasis. Without a fibrin net, the platelets would lose their attachments to one another and the initial plug would break apart. Consequently, bleeding would begin again.

Hemostasis relies upon a wide range of proteins called clotting factors and cofactors such as calcium and vitamin K. These substances interact with one another, forming a cascade of biochemical reactions that ultimately transforms prothrombin into thrombin which in turn converts fibrinogen to fibrin. Each clotting factor is essential for the formation of fibrin. If any single factor is absent, the clotting cascade cannot be completed and a fibrin mesh cannot be manufactured. Basic coagulation testing therefore includes a platelet count and an evaluation of the two major pathways (intrinsic and extrinsic) that leads to the conversion of prothrombin to thrombin. The activated partial thromboplastin time (PTT) test evaluates the intrinsic pathway while the prothrombin time test evaluates the extrinsic pathway.

Most of these tests require special instrumentation and are submitted to a reference laboratory; however, careful sample collection and submission are critical for obtaining valid results. The venipuncture must be accurate to prevent tissue injury, which will invalidate coagulation assays. In addition to collection in an EDTA tube for the platelet count, blood must be collected in tubes with citrate anticoagulant (turquoise or blue top) for coagulation assays. The proper amount of blood must be drawn to maintain the 9:1 ratio of blood to anticoagulant for reliable results. Only plastic or siliconized glass should be used in handling these samples because contact with regular glass will invalidate the results. The samples should be centrifuged, and the plasma should be tested immediately or frozen. The reference laboratory should always be contacted for additional directions before samples are obtained and submitted for coagulation testing.

> *TECHNICIAN NOTE* Proper filling of the citrate collection tube for coagulation testing is essential for reliable results.

CLINICAL CHEMISTRY

The blood and urine of healthy animals contain biochemical substances such as enzymes, hormones, and electrolytes that remain stable within certain ranges. These ranges indicate that organs and tissues in the body are functioning normally. In the healthy state, the organs and tissues release specific amounts of these biochemicals into blood and urine. In the unhealthy state, these substances may increase or decrease beyond the normal ranges. Blood and urine is collected from unhealthy animals and evaluated to determine which organs and tissues are diseased. Numerous chemistry parameters can then be evaluated via specialized tests called assays. For example, there are specific enzymes that are produced or processed by the liver that can be analyzed to evaluate liver function. Aspartate aminotransferase (AST) and alanine aminotransferase (ALT) are intracellular enzymes that may be elevated as a result of damage to hepatocytes (liver cells). AST, in particular, may also be increased with muscle injury. Alkaline phosphatase and γ-glutamyltransferase are also produced in the liver, but are more often associated with bile duct (cholestatic) disease. They may also be increased because of steroid use. Abnormal blood levels of bilirubin and albumin may also be associated with liver disease, but may also be altered as a result of injury to other systems.

Two tests that can be used to evaluate kidney function are blood urea nitrogen (BUN) and creatinine. Concentrations of these compounds are used to differentiate simple dehydration from kidney (renal) dysfunction. The interpretation of concentrations of these two substances requires urine to be examined at the same time. An urinalysis and the specific gravity (SG) of urine must be performed at the same time the blood is analyzed.

Measurements of total protein (comprised of albumin, fibrinogen, and globulins) is generally included in the basic chemistry panel. Variations in these proteins may be indicative of a variety of disorders. Values may be increased with dehydration, inflammation, or autoimmune disease. Albumin values may be decreased in association with liver failure, gastrointestinal disorders, or renal glomerular disease.

Levels of serum sodium, potassium, chloride, calcium, and phosphorus, collectively referred to as electrolytes (ions that dissociate in water and have the capacity to conduct electricity; "-lyte" able to be dissolved), can also be affected by various disorders. They may reflect changes in fluid balance, gastrointestinal disorders (vomiting, diarrhea), acid-base disturbances, renal dysfunction, or metabolic and endocrine disorders. Calcium and phosphorus are intimately associated with bone growth, and levels may be higher in younger animals than in adults. Calcium circulates bound to albumin; therefore calcium levels may be low in cases of decreased albumin levels. Phosphorus levels are regulated in the kidney, so the phosphorus level often increases in cases relating to decreased urine production. Phosphorus is also present in RBCs, so if there is hemolysis or serum is allowed to remain on the cells, serum phosphorus results may be falsely elevated.

Several small, relatively inexpensive clinical chemistry instruments have been developed. As with all equipment, veterinary practices must have a demand for these and must be able to justify the expense. Two general types of chemistry analyzers are commonly used: liquid reagent chemistry and dry chemistry. Instruments that use liquid reagents require more technical expertise and time in preparing reagents and monitoring the performance. The dry chemistry instruments are simpler to use and provide consistent performance. The principles of operation differ significantly between the two types of instruments, as does the extent to which specimen quality affects the measurement. An important practical consideration in purchasing an instrument is the per test operating cost versus the relative ease of running individual tests; in general, large run wet reagent costs will have lower per test costs than individual dry reagent methodologies, but the latter may be more appropriate for less requested tests and for after-hours use.

EQUIPMENT

Regardless of whether an in-house chemistry analyzer is maintained and operated, veterinary practices will need a sample collection system consisting of either syringes and needles or Vacutainers plus clean plastic or glass tubes in which to store or transport samples. A centrifuge and pipettes will be necessary for the separation of the serum or plasma from the cells.

CLINICAL CHEMISTRY INSTRUMENTATION

The liquid reagent–based instruments use the principle of photometry (the measurement of light transmittance by a solution). Beer's law states that the concentration of a substance in a liquid is indirectly proportional to the amount of light that passes through the liquid. In other words, the higher the concentration of a substance in a liquid, the less light is able to pass through it. Most instruments have a spectrophotometer to measure the amount of light transmitted. A spectrophotometer consists of a light source directed through a specific path and a photosensitive detector that converts light into electrical energy. Each substance will transmit light at a specific wavelength. For the purpose of increasing the specificity of the measurement, filters are placed between the light source and the sample to allow only a specific wavelength to pass through the sample. The magnitude of the electrical current produced by the detector corresponds to the concentration of the substance measured.

The instruments that use dry reagents are becoming more popular for in-practice use. The major advantage of these instruments is the elimination of liquid reagents, which must be reconstituted or diluted before use. Dry chemistry instruments use reagent slides or cartridges. A specific amount of the patient's sample is added as directed, and the intensity of the color that develops is measured by the principle of reflectance. Light is transmitted to the analyte slide, and the reflected light is conducted to a photodetector. The density of the color formed by the chemical reaction is determined and is proportional to the concentration of the substance measured. There is less interference from lipemia or hemolysis because this method does not depend on reading light transmitted through a liquid as with the spectrophotometer-based instruments.

Several dry chemistry instruments (e.g., Heska SPOT-CHEM and i-STAT, Abaxis VetScan, IDEXX VetTest) that are designed specifically for use with veterinary samples are available (Figure 16-26). Available tests may vary from analyzer to analyzer, and new tests are often added. The primary advantage of using an instrument intended for veterinary testing is the availability of predetermined reference intervals, which can be used until the laboratory can establish its own values. In most cases with these instruments, little variation occurs from instrument to instrument or operator to operator. Veterinary samples can vary significantly from human samples in the concentration of particular substances. This can be problematic if an analyzer not specifically designed for

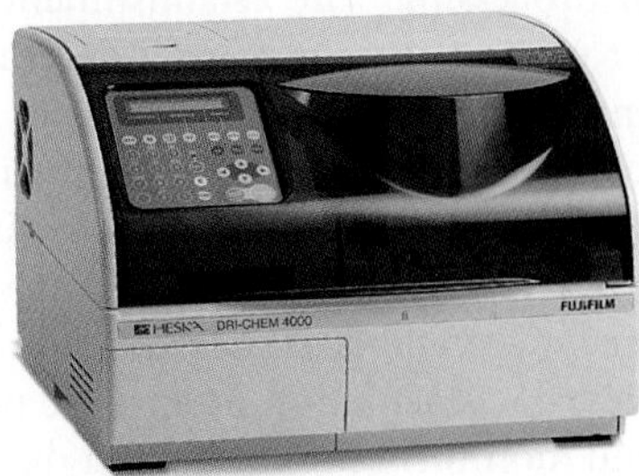

FIGURE 16-26 Heska Corporation's DRI-CHEM® Veterinary Chemistry Analyzer offers 22 tests including Electrolytes and Lipase. Take the guesswork out of making dilutions or calculating results with automated dilution. (Courtesy Heska Corporation, Loveland, CO.)

BOX 16-1 Common Causes for Inaccurate Results

- Poor-quality or outdated reagents
- Failure to calibrate or run controls
- Improper pipetting techniques
- Improper maintenance of instrument
- Lipemic or hemolyzed samples
- Allowing serum to sit on clot
- Use of inappropriate cuvettes
- Power surges or failure

veterinary samples is used, because the limits of the chemistry test (ranges established for humans) must be adhered to.

QUALITY CONTROL PROGRAMS

Any veterinary practice that decides to establish an in-house laboratory must make a commitment to quality control. Laboratory instruments will provide valid accurate results only if the samples are handled correctly, a well-maintained instrument is used, and the tests are performed correctly. The importance of routine maintenance and calibration procedures for all instruments cannot be overemphasized. However, even the most sophisticated, accurate, and well-maintained instrument cannot overcome errors in technique or poor sample quality. The technician should be familiar with the principles and limitations of all assays performed in the laboratory. Some of the more common causes for inaccurate results because of technical errors or sample quality are listed in Box 16-1. A quality control program consists of monitoring results of known control samples for identification of irregularities in reported values and following generally accepted laboratory procedures. Several textbooks on clinical chemistry and laboratory medicine (see Recommended Reading) provide excellent in-depth reviews of quality assurance programs. The following discussion deals primarily with the basics in monitoring an instrument to ensure the accuracy of reported data.

The three levels of quality control are preanalytic procedures, analytic procedures, and analytic quality monitoring procedures. The preanalytic procedures deal with how the patient is prepared (fasting versus nonfasting samples), patient and specimen identification, specimen acquisition, and specimen processing. The establishment of standard procedures for each of these steps will decrease the likelihood that samples will be misidentified or of poor quality (hemolyzed or lipemic). This aspect of quality control is important even in practices that send their clinical pathology samples to a reference laboratory. Analytic variables include the analytic method, standardization and calibration procedures, documentation of analytic protocols and procedures, and monitoring of equipment during use. This aspect of quality control is usually well defined by the manufacturer of the instrument and should be followed closely. The final level, the monitoring of analytic quality by using statistical methods and control charts, is the aspect that involves the use of control products and record keeping. This aspect is the responsibility of the technician performing the tests.

TECHNICIAN NOTE Despite sales claims, valid results cannot be ensured without the inclusion of appropriate control samples and proper calibration.

CONTROLS AND STANDARDS

Standard solutions are quality control products that contain the analyte of interest at a validated "true" concentration as determined by the manufacturer using "gold standard" methodologies; these are expected to accurately represent the stated concentration and as such can be relatively expensive. Control solutions are quality control products that may report a given expected concentration of the analyte of interest, or alternatively a laboratory may use a sample, possibly pooled, from representative animal(s) that has had its concentration repeatedly determined by the analyzer itself; although commercially available control solutions are expected to approximate the reported analyte concentration, they generally have not undergone the same level of rigorous validation and, as such, are generally less expensive than standard solutions. In general, quality control products should have an overall composition similar to the sample assayed, be stable, be available in premeasured amounts to prevent alterations caused by repeated freeze-thaw cycles, and have little vial-to-vial variation. Quality control products can be purchased from an independent source or from the company that makes the test kit or instrument. Most of these products are available as normal, high abnormal, and low abnormal values. The quality control products are analyzed in a manner identical to that used for patients' samples. The accuracy of an analyzer is judged upon how similar results of a measured standard solution are in comparison with the manufacturer's reported "true" concentration. The precision of an analyzer is judged upon the reproducibility of repeated measurements of a control solution. An analyzer can be precise and not accurate if the measured values are reproducible, but consistently higher or lower than the "true" value of a standard solution; although the establishment of a laboratory reference interval may allow for such data to still retain diagnostic utility, ideally the sources of the inaccuracy should be identified and resolved.

Many products are provided in a lyophilized (dehydrated) form that requires rehydration with distilled water or a diluent provided by the manufacturer. The solution must be diluted properly to ensure that the concentration of the analytes is correct. Imprecision in diluting the products will yield inaccurate values, even though the instrument is working properly. It is highly recommended that volumetric or other precise pipettes be used to dilute the control products (a graduated cylinder is not acceptable).

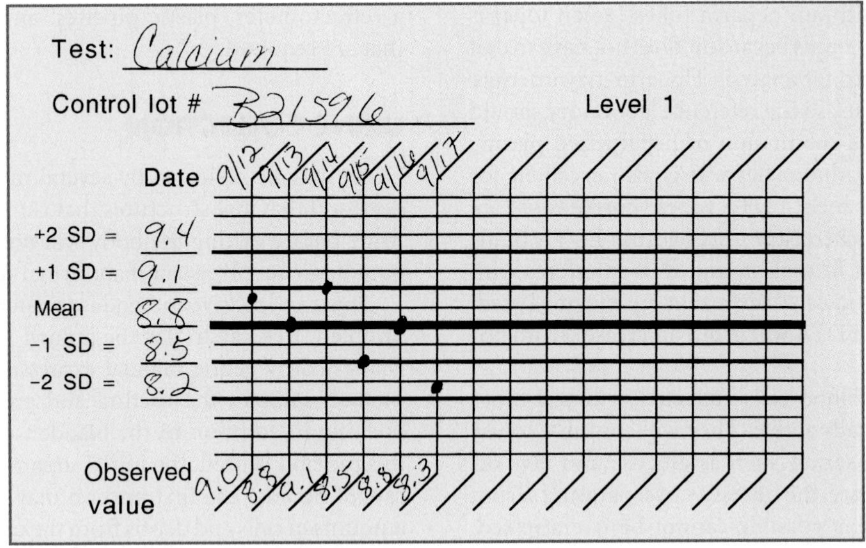

FIGURE 16-27 Levy-Jennings chart illustrating the common procedure used for following the performance of an individual test control serum.

The control values must fall within a specific acceptable interval, which usually encompasses the mean ±2 SD (standard deviations). This range is established by the manufacturer of the product by repeated assay of the solution. When the instrument reports a control value above or below the established interval, there is a problem with the procedure, and test results for that particular sample should not be reported until the problem is identified.

A separate log of the quality control results should be kept and reviewed periodically. A useful visual display of the instrument's performance for quick inspection and review is the Levy-Jennings chart. Figure 16-27 shows the use of the Levy-Jennings chart to keep track of quality control data. By inspection of control data over 1 month, a technician can see the control values gently drift upward or downward, indicating possible deterioration of the control product or a change in the light source intensity. A wide scatter of values outside the range on both the low and high ends indicates imprecision on the part of the instrument or technician. It is best to keep the chart close to the instrument, not hidden in a file drawer. Everyone who uses the instrument must be willing to run controls and chart the results. Other useful laboratory records include calibration logs, sample logs, and maintenance logs.

SAMPLE HANDLING

Sample handling is a critical step in obtaining accurate laboratory data. Several factors can interfere with the analysis of a sample. The most common problems in veterinary medicine are hemolysis and lipemia. Difficulty in performing the venipuncture or excess pressure applied to the syringe during collection can cause significant hemolysis. The most common cause of lipemia is collection of a sample after the patient has eaten. At times, both hemolysis and lipemia are unavoidable because they are the result of a disease process.

The effect hemolysis and lipemia will have on laboratory data is method dependent. There are no general rules to assist the interpretation of changes caused by sample quality. A good reference laboratory will provide information on how each of its tests is affected by these two changes. Manufacturers of the instruments and reagents should provide information on how interfering factors, such as hemolysis and lipemia, affect the methods used in their instrument. Hemolysis will commonly affect inorganic phosphorus resulting in artifactually increased or decreased values depending on the assay methodology. Lipemia will interfere with any method that depends on an optical density read on a spectrophotometer. Some chemistry instruments can compensate for this change. The reference laboratory should be able to indicate which tests are affected. Errors in processing the sample can also cause artifactual changes in laboratory data. It is important to use the appropriate collection tube for the test performed.

Samples collected for chemistry profiles can be collected in clot tubes (red tops), which contain no anticoagulant, or in lithium heparin tubes (green tops). Blood collected in clot tubes (tubes without anticoagulant) must be allowed to completely clot before the sample can be centrifuged and the serum removed; complete clot formation usually takes about 30 minutes. Clot tubes with activator gels (tiger tops) will promote clotting, thus decreasing the time required for complete clot formation and facilitating separation of the serum from the RBCs. The sample should not be refrigerated before complete clot formation because this inhibits good serum separation. In addition, a fibrin clot forms above the RBCs if the blood is centrifuged before complete clot formation or at too fast a speed.

TECHNICIAN NOTE Serum must be removed from the clot as soon as possible to prevent inaccurate results.

Blood collected in lithium heparin tubes (green tops) is excellent for emergency needs because it does not have to clot before it can be separated for analysis. Heparin may interfere with a few chemistry tests, so the reference laboratory should be consulted before the submission of heparinized plasma for chemistry panels. Lithium heparin is also excellent for emergency electrolyte panels. EDTA tubes (purple tops) are unacceptable for most chemistry tests because EDTA binds calcium to prevent clot formation and thus interferes with many of the assays, particularly those that are enzyme based. In addition, potassium EDTA will greatly increase serum potassium levels.

Keep in mind that blood cells collected in blood tubes are alive and metabolically active. They will continue to use up nutrients from the serum such as glucose and give off waste products. Therefore, the necessity of separating serum from the clot as soon as possible cannot be overstressed. Prolonged exposure of serum to the cells will erroneously decrease the glucose level; will increase the phosphorus level; may increase the potassium level, depending on species (especially in the horse); and may affect some enzyme activities. Do not depend on the reference laboratory courier service to get the sample to the laboratory in time to prevent these changes. It is best to take the time and responsibility to separate the serum and ensure the quality of the sample.

URINALYSIS

Urinalysis is one clinical laboratory procedure that should be performed as a part of any minimal database in all veterinary practices. A typical urinalysis consists of gross examination, a urine specific gravity (SG), chemical analysis, and sediment evaluation. Because the concentration of urine changes with the hydration status of a normal animal, a concurrent urine SG is necessary for the accurate evaluation of renal parameters (BUN and creatinine). In other words, if the BUN is elevated, is this due to kidney disease or dehydration? The hydration of the animal must be assessed via SG at the same time the blood is evaluated for abnormal elevations of substances. This is particularly important if fluid therapy has been initiated because the hydration status of the animal is changing. It is an important that urinalysis be performed on fresh urine, when possible, because protein and other substances that might be found in urine can degenerate with time. The techniques involved are simple and require no special instrumentation. Urine samples should be collected into clean glass or plastic containers. In general, no preservatives are necessary.

EQUIPMENT

The equipment necessary for performing the urinalysis is minimal. A supply of clean glass or plastic collection containers, a centrifuge and conical centrifuge tubes, chemical reagent strips, clean glass slides and coverslips, a refractometer, plastic pipettes, and a microscope are all that are required.

URINE COLLECTION

Urine may be collected by several methods. It must be understood that any structures that came into contact with the urine before exiting the body will potentially be a source of pathologic involvement if abnormal results are obtained.

The least invasive method is to catch a free-flow nonsterile sample ("free catch") as the animal voids spontaneously or is assisted by gentle manual expression. Unfortunately, this method samples the urethra and area around the external opening in addition to the bladder, ureters, and kidneys. If this method is used, the initial stream of urine should not be caught because the first portion may contain especially high amounts of cells and debris from the urethra and lower genital tract. It is better to collect a midstream sample, avoiding collection of the beginning or the end of a voided urine sample.

A second method that may be used to collect urine is cystocentesis. This procedure involves placing a needle (with a syringe attached) through the ventral abdominal wall into the lumen of the bladder and aspirating urine. Aseptic technique must be used. By performing cystocentesis, secretions and debris of the lower urogenital tract are avoided, and the interpretation of urinalysis findings is simplified. Hemorrhage induced through the collection process (iatrogenic hemorrhage) can occur during cystocentesis; therefore it is not unusual to have a widely varying number of RBCs in the sediment of samples obtained by this method.

Another method for collecting urine is by catheterization of the bladder. This procedure must be done as aseptically as possible to prevent the introduction of bacteria into the urinary tract. Urine collected in this manner frequently contains increased numbers of epithelial cells (including squamous cells), which may appear in sheets and clusters. A "traumatic catheterization" is sometimes purposely performed where the clinician tries to abrade a mass with the tip of the catheter to increase the yield of potentially neoplastic cells; this is a method of choice for sampling transitional cell carcinomas since needle aspiration of these masses has been associated with tumor spread along the needle track. Additional information on cystocentesis and catheterization can be found in Chapter 20.

Regardless of how the urine sample is collected, it should be analyzed as soon as possible. Many changes begin to occur immediately. Bacteria present in the urine will multiply, cells may degenerate, casts may dissolve (especially if the urine is alkaline), and bacteria that produce urease will convert urea to ammonia, causing the pH to increase. If there is to be any delay in performing the urinalysis, the sample should be refrigerated to slow these processes. However, refrigeration may cause a change in urine SG and interfere with some of the chemistry reactions on the chemistry reagent strip. Before a urinalysis is performed on refrigerated urine, the specimen should be allowed to come to room temperature.

EVALUATION OF PHYSICAL PROPERTIES

As with all laboratory procedures, it is wise to follow the same routine protocol with every urine sample analyzed. The physical properties evaluated in most routine urinalyses include color, appearance or turbidity, and SG. After making sure the sample is mixed well, the color (e.g., yellow, gold, red) and appearance (e.g., clear, hazy, flocculent) should be recorded.

COLOR

Normal urine is yellow to amber, depending on its concentration and constituents. Bright red urine indicates hematuria (RBCs in the urine) or hemoglobinuria (hemoglobin in the urine). Reddish-brown urine usually suggests hemoglobinuria or myoglobinuria (myoglobin in the urine); note that these two pigments cannot be distinguished from one another solely on the basis of color. High concentrations of bilirubin or urobilin cause yellowish brown urine that when shaken may produce yellowish foam. Whenever an unusual discoloration of the urine occurs, the history of any drug therapy should be evaluated because many drugs can produce abnormally colored urine. Urine that is notably discolored may make it difficult or impossible to interpret color changes when chemical reagent strips are evaluated.

TURBIDITY

Fresh urine is normally transparent at the animal's body temperature, but as it cools to an ambient temperature, some salts may precipitate, causing the urine to become cloudy. Except for equine urine which is normally cloudy, fresh urine that is cloudy is often pathologic, and it must be examined microscopically to identify the cause: pus, blood, mucus, bacteria, casts, or crystals. Fresh equine urine is normally cloudy because it contains mucus and calcium carbonate crystals. Even clear urine should be examined microscopically because some abnormal constituents may be present in small amounts that may not cause urine to be visually cloudy.

SPECIFIC GRAVITY

A healthy kidney can concentrate and dilute urine depending upon the hydration status of the animal. Therefore determining the SG is one of the most important parts of a urinalysis and gives key insight into hydration status of the patient. SG may be determined before or after centrifugation of the urine sample because the material that settles during centrifugation has little to no effect on SG. The SG value depends on the number and size of particles in the solution and is an indicator of the ability of the kidney to concentrate or dilute urine. The SG is most accurately determined with a refractometer, which is used for determining plasma protein and requires only 1 drop of urine. If the urine sample is turbid, the SG may be determined from the supernatant after centrifugation. Reagent strips are inaccurate for the determination of SG. Common terminology is to state the first two digits as "ten" and the last two digits as either "o" + 1 to 9 or as the number itself if greater than 9; for example 1.008 is stated as "ten-o-eight" whereas 1.035 is stated as "ten-thirty five."

There is no normal SG for urine, only appropriate SG values for a given hydration state. Animals are expected to concentrate their urine when dehydrated and dilute it when overhydrated. The minimum appropriate SG threshold for a dehydrated adult animal is as follows: cat 1.035, dog 1.030, and horse or cattle 1.025. Inability to achieve this threshold in a dehydrated animal points to renal dysfunction (actual physical damage and/or functional impairment) or postrenal involvement (obstruction and/or rupture of the ureters, urinary bladder or urethra). Dilute urine (SP <1.008) indicates that the kidneys are functioning by actively diluting the urine. The major determinant of urine SG is salt concentration because of the large number of particles involved. Protein, in contrast, has little influence on SG because they are relatively fewer in number. Glucose, likewise, has relatively little effect on SG. Both of these components, however, when found in large amounts in the urine will increase the SG by about 0.001 to 0.002. SG provides a good indication of how well the kidneys are able to function in maintaining the body's water and osmotic balance. In addition, SG is important in interpretation of other test results. For example, a 2+ protein in dilute urine (SG <1.012) suggests a greater loss of protein than a 2+ protein in concentrated urine (SG >1.030).

As blood enters the kidney, non-cellular components including small- to medium-sized molecules are filtered through glomeruli. The liquid produced from this filtering process is called glomerular filtrate. The specific gravity of glomerular filtrate is the same as plasma. Later, as the filtrate moves through the renal tubules the SG of the filtrate is adjusted depending upon the hydration status of the animal. Urine that has the same SG (1.008 to 1.012) as the glomerular filtrate is called isosthenuric. Isosthenuria indicates that the tubules have not attempted to concentrate or dilute urine. Isosthenuric urine is not abnormal in an adequately hydrated animal. However, if an animal is dehydrated, the renal tubules are expected to concentrate urine. Similarly, if the animal is overhydrated, the kidney is expected to dilute urine.

CHEMICAL EVALUATION

Reagent strip chemistries should be performed on unspun urine, unless the urine is turbid (cloudy). If it is turbid, the chemistry tests may be done after the sample has been centrifuged. Levels of protein, glucose, ketones, blood, and bilirubin in the urine are routinely determined in addition to urinary pH. The strips contain pads that are impregnated with reagents and result in a color change when the appropriate urine constituents are present. Although the strips are simple to use, proper technique and accurate timing for reading the results are critical. The key for evaluating the pad color reactions is commonly found on the bottle itself along with the proper time to read out the result. Automated strip analyzers are available and allow for a consistent and convenient strip analysis. The strips must be properly stored, the urine must be at room temperature and well mixed, and excess urine must be shaken from the strips to obtain valid results. Significantly discolored urine may interfere with the ability to discern colors and color changes on the reagent pads.

Some commercially available strips contain reagent pads for other components, such as leukocytes; the leukocyte strip is not valid for veterinary use.

> *TECHNICIAN NOTE* Refrigerated urine samples must be brought to room temperature before chemical analysis is performed.

pH

pH determines the acidity or alkalinity of a substance using a scale from 0 to 14 where 7 is neutral. A pH below 7 is acidic and a pH above 7 is alkalinic. The pH of a fluid decreases as the hydrogen ion concentration increases and vice versa. Small changes in pH represent large changes in hydrogen ion concentration. Physiologically neutral serum pH is generally 7.3 to 7.4 for most species. Readings in the serum above the pH reference interval are said to be alkalemic, and those below are academic. In the case or urine, pH is detected by reagent strips with chemical indicators. Unexpectedly high urinary pH is termed alkaluric, and those below are aciduric. In general, omnivores and carnivores (such as dogs and cats) tend to have more acidic urine than do herbivores (such as cattle, horses, and human vegetarians). A fresh sample must be used because as urine stands, it loses carbon dioxide (analogous to an acid), and bacteria that are present may produce ammonia, both of which result in increased alkalinity (raising the pH). A major function of the kidney is to metabolically compensate for serum pH abnormalities; as such, urine pH is expected to rise and fall in parallel with serum pH if the kidneys are functioning appropriately, but one cannot assume that urinary pH is always an accurate indicator of serum pH.

PROTEIN

Most commercial urine reagent strips include a test for protein. Urine normally contains a small amount of protein, which is due to normal leakage and secretion from the urinary tract lining. However, this normal amount of protein is not detected by routine methods. If the reagent pad shows a positive protein test, the reaction is usually graded trace to 1+ through 4+. As mentioned, a positive protein reaction in dilute urine implies a greater protein loss than the same level of reaction in a concentrated sample. As with most reagent strip chemistry tests, results are at best only semiquantitative and are subject to several types of error. The pH directly affects readings, with false-positive results occurring in alkaline urines (pH >8). The strips are more sensitive to albumin than to other proteins, such as globulins, hemoglobin, and myoglobi, which can result in false-negative or falsely low readings. Newer, more sensitive species-specific enzyme-linked immunosorbent assay (ELISA)-based strip tests (E.R.D., Heska Corp., Fort Collins, Colo.) are now available for the dog and cat that can detect low levels of proteinuria normally undetectable by traditional strips that in theory could aid in the detection of early renal disease; studies are ongoing to determine the clinical utility of this test.

Renal protein loss can occur at the level of the glomerulus and/or the renal tubules. Protein loss into urine can actually result in hypoproteinemia if glomerular dysfunction is severe enough; the degree of protein loss with pure tubular dysfunction is low and will not result in hypoproteinemia. One can make a subjective evaluation of the amount lost by comparing the results with the SG, as previously mentioned; however, a more exact method is to collect all urine produced in a 24-hour period and calculate its total protein content. The collection of 24 hours of urine output generally requires a metabolism cage and is not practical. The urine protein to urine creatinine ratio (UPC) in any single sample is a good index of protein loss in the urine. Both urinary protein and creatinine concentrations increase with an increasing urine concentration, because neither protein nor creatinine is secreted nor resorbed by the tubules. A UPC of less than 1.0 (some state 0.5) is considered normal; a ratio greater than 3.0 (some say 2.0) supports significant glomerular protein loss; and a ratio between these values supports tubular and/or early glomerular protein loss. A urine sample with an active sediment (increased WBCs and/or high numbers of RBCs) is not suitable for the determination of the UPC because the protein present may be secondary to inflammation, tissue damage, and/or hemorrhage and as such is not necessarily indicative of renal loss. For example, an increased UPC in urine from cystocentesis with an active sediment could simply be present secondary to a cystitis (bladder infection). Additionally, prerenal causes of proteinuria must be ruled out before a UPC can be performed; small proteins, such as free hemoglobin (pathologic from hemolysis), myoglobin (pathologic from massive muscle damage), light immunoglobulin chains (pathologic from plasma cell tumors), or postcolostral ingestion, can overload the tubules' ability to resorb them and result in proteinuria. The pathologic prerenal overflow-overload causes of proteinuria are not directly indicative of renal dysfunction, but may actually lead to renal damage if severe and/or chronic enough. UPCs are usually done at a reference laboratory because they require a sensitive protein determination. There are a few extrarenal factors that may temporarily alter glomerular permeability to protein and result in proteinuria; they include fever, strenuous exercise, shock, and cardiac or central nervous system disease.

When excessive hemorrhage into the urinary tract occurs, the result of the test for urine protein will be positive, and erythrocytes will be seen in the sediment. Possible causes of urinary tract hemorrhage include trauma, neoplasia, and inflammation. It should be noted that free hemoglobin or myoglobin in the urine will cause a positive protein test result and a positive blood test result. In either of these cases although the urine will appear reddish, intact RBCs are not a significant part of the sediment, and centrifugation of the urine will not clear the urine of reddish discoloration.

GLUCOSE

In addition to urine protein, a common reagent strip test for urine is the test for glucose. The reagent strips are quite specific for glucose. However, as with all reagent strip tests, they are not quantitative. Tablets that detect glucose, which are somewhat more quantitative, but not specific, are available.

Normally, urine contains no detectable glucose. Glucose is filtered by the glomerulus, but the body preserves this energy source by reabsorbing it in the proximal renal tubules. This resorption ability is exceeded once the blood glucose level rises above the renal threshold, which is 180 mg/dl in the dog, 280 mg/dl in the cat, or above 100 mg/dl in the cow or horse. The primary cause for glucosuria therefore is hyperglycemia. For confirmation of hyperglycemia as the cause, the blood glucose level should be determined at the same time as the urine glucose level; it should be noted that because urine may sit in the bladder for an indefinite amount of time, glucose may still be present from a previous hyperglycemic event that exceeded the renal threshold and not represent that degree of hyperglycemia in a concurrent serum glucose. Diabetes mellitus is a common cause of hyperglycemia and glucosuria.

KETONES

A test for urine ketones is included on many reagent strips; tablets are also available. Ketones will appear in the urine before they build up to a detectable level in the bloodstream, so ketonuria may occur before a detectable ketonemia occurs. Ketonuria indicates excessive fat metabolism, a deficiency in carbohydrate metabolism, or both, but is most commonly seen in conjunction with glucosuria as a complication of diabetes mellitus.

BILIRUBIN

There are reagent strips and tablets for detecting bilirubinuria, both of which use a similar reaction (diazotization), but the tablets are less subject to interference by urine color than are the strips. The tablets are also highly sensitive, so a 1+ reading, especially in concentrated urine, may not be significant. Bilirubin may be oxidized on exposure to light, so if there is much delay between obtaining the urine sample and performing the urinalysis, the sample should be protected from light to prevent false-negative results. Normal dogs may exhibit low levels of bilirubinuria in concentrated urine because the renal tubular cells can conjugate bilirubin. Bilirubinuria frequently precedes hyperbilirubinemia in most species.

BLOOD

The designation "blood" is somewhat misleading because this test actually detects intact RBCs, hemoglobin, and myoglobin. If the urine is red and erythrocytes are present in the sediment, hematuria is the reason for the positive blood reaction.

Hemoglobinuria (hemoglobin pigment in the urine) results in red to brown urine with a positive urine blood reaction and no erythrocytes in the sediment. A positive urine protein test result may also be apparent, but the degree of positivity will be less than the blood strip since the former is less sensitive to hemoglobin or myoglobin. In contrast to hematuria, hemoglobinuria will be accompanied by hemoglobinemia, imparting a pink to reddish discoloration to the serum or plasma.

Myoglobinuria (myoglobin pigment in the urine) will similarly result in red to brown urine with no erythrocytes in the sediment, a positive urine blood reaction, and a positive urine protein test result. However, during myoglobinuria, the blood serum or plasma generally remains clear. Myoglobin, which is derived from muscles, is a smaller molecule than hemoglobin and does not bind to serum protein; thus it is rapidly excreted into the urine before reaching levels sufficiently high to produce discoloration of the serum. Animals with myoglobinuria generally do not show evidence of anemia, but have some type of muscle disease, such as exertional myopathy in horses ("tying up" syndrome), trauma, electrical shock, or pressure necrosis from prolonged recumbency.

MICROSCOPIC EXAMINATION

The sediment should be prepared for microscopic examination. A urine sediment examination may reveal extremely useful diagnostic information and be crucial for the correct interpretation of the chemical analyses. A few cells and a few casts may be found in normal urine, but increased numbers of various elements indicate certain diseases. A reference is provided for assistance with the sediment evaluation.

Sample Preparation

Pour a standard volume (10 ml is recommended) of urine into a conical-tip centrifuge tube. If the sample available is less than 10 ml, use all that is left after the reagent strip chemistries and SG determinations have been completed. Centrifuge the urine at a slow speed (1500 rpm) for 5 minutes. Higher speeds for centrifugation may disrupt the cells and casts that are present. Decant the supernatant, leaving the sediment in the bottom. Gently tap the tube to resuspend the sediment in the small amount of urine remaining on the sides and in the bottom of the tube. With a small pipette, transfer a drop of suspended sediment to a glass slide and place a coverslip on it. Commercial stains (e.g., SediStain, Clay Adams, Parsippany, N.J.) are available for evaluating urine sediments, but with practice and experience, they are not necessary.

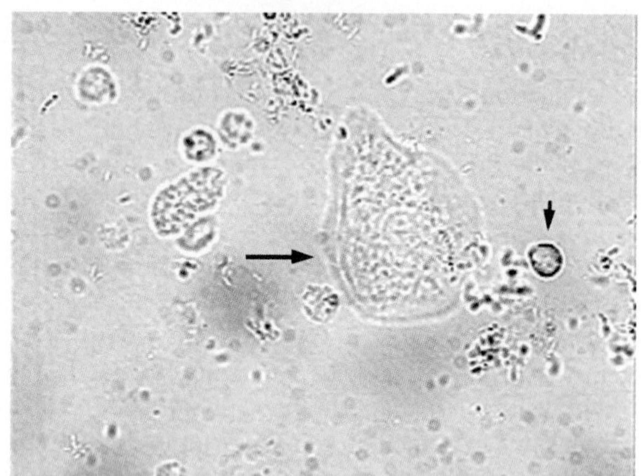

FIGURE 16-28 Urine sediment with a large squamous epithelial cell *(long arrow)*, crenated RBCs *(short arrows)*, and bacteria in the background.

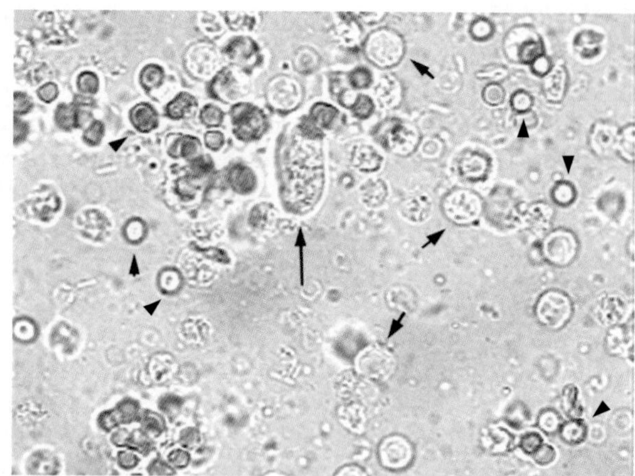

FIGURE 16-29 Urine sediment with a cast *(long arrow)* and several RBCs *(arrowheads)* and WBCs *(short arrows)*.

To examine unstained urine sediment, lower the condenser of the light microscope and reduce the intensity of the light. The slide should first be examined at 10× magnification to obtain an overall impression of how much and what type of sediment is present. The 40× or 45× power (high dry) is then used to make the final identification and count of various components. At least 10 microscopic fields must be evaluated, and the average numbers of various cells and casts per high-power field are reported. The presence and relative amounts of other components are also noted.

Epithelial Cells

Three types of epithelial cells can be found in urine sediment: squamous, transitional, and renal tubular. Squamous epithelial cells (Figure 16-28) are large, with angular borders and small nuclei. The cells originate from the lining of the distal urethra and vagina or prepuce and are not generally indicative of disease. Transitional epithelial cells are medium sized and oval, spindled, or caudate cells found lining the proximal urethra, bladder, ureters, and renal pelvis. They may occur in groups, especially if the urine was obtained by catheterization. If transitional epithelial cells are large and variable, basophilic, or found in large clusters, they should be further evaluated for possible neoplasia. Renal tubular epithelial cells are small, round cells and may indicate tubular degeneration.

Blood Cells

Erythrocytes in unstained sediment appear colorless or yellowish and are round and slightly refractile with no internal structure. They may be confused with fat droplets, but erythrocytes are fairly uniform in size and do not float in and out of planes of focus as do fat droplets. If there is doubt, a drop of diluted acetic acid will lyse erythrocytes, helping to differentiate them from fat droplets. In concentrated urine, erythrocytes may lose fluid and become crenated (shrunken and spiked). In dilute urine, water may enter the cell causing it to swell or even lyse. Leukocytes in urine sediment are round and granular and larger than erythrocytes, but smaller than epithelial cells (Figure 16-29). The presence of more than five to eight WBCs per high-power field indicates inflammation of the urinary or urogenital tract, depending on the method of collection. When this occurs, a careful check for bacteria should be made.

Casts

Casts are another prominent feature of urine sediment. They are elongated structures composed of protein from plasma and mucoprotein from the renal tubules. In general, they form in the distal tubules, in which the urine is more concentrated and acidic. Any structures that happen to be in the tubules at the time the casts form (erythrocytes, leukocytes, or epithelial cells) become embedded in the casts. The presence of increased numbers of casts helps to localize the renal disease to the tubules, but the numbers do not necessarily correlate with the severity of disease. For instance, severe chronic nephritis may be accompanied by just a few casts.

The five main types of casts are as follows:

1. Hyaline casts are colorless, homogeneous, and semitransparent. These may be difficult to see unless the light is reduced. The casts occur in health and also in association with mild glomerular leakage.
2. Cellular casts contain recognizable cells embedded in the protein matrix. Cellular casts may be epithelial cell casts that contain sloughed tubular epithelial cells, erythrocyte casts that indicate renal hemorrhage, or leukocyte casts that indicate renal inflammation or pyelonephritis.
3. Granular casts are derived from degenerating cells or cellular casts. Granular casts are characterized by a nonspecific granular matrix and are designated as either coarsely or finely granular depending on the degree of degeneration. This is probably the most common type of cast found in animals.
4. Waxy casts are wide and homogeneous, usually with distinct blunt or squared ends. These indicate a more chronic renal lesion.
5. Fatty casts contain fat globules from degenerating tubular epithelial cells and are most common in cats because of the high lipid content of feline tubular epithelium.

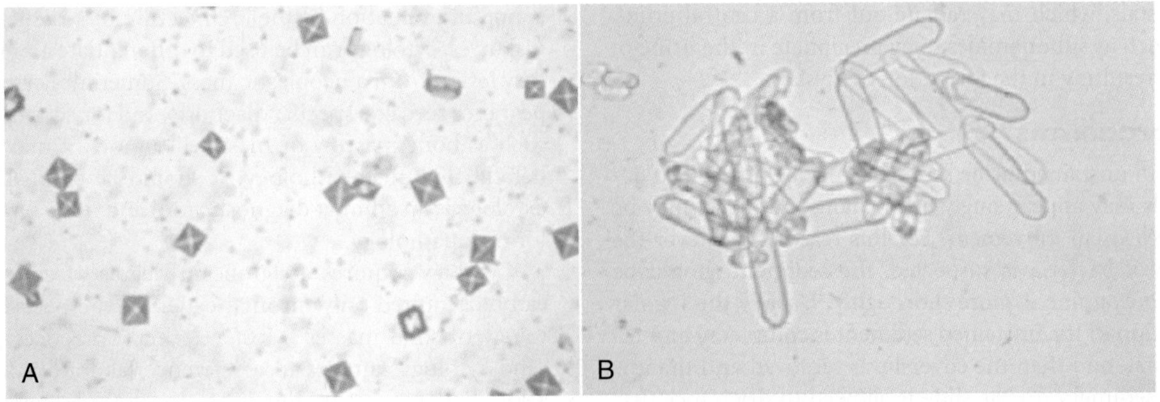

FIGURE 16-30 Canine urine sediment showing the two forms of calcium oxalate crystals. **A,** Dihydrate form. **B,** Monohydrate form.

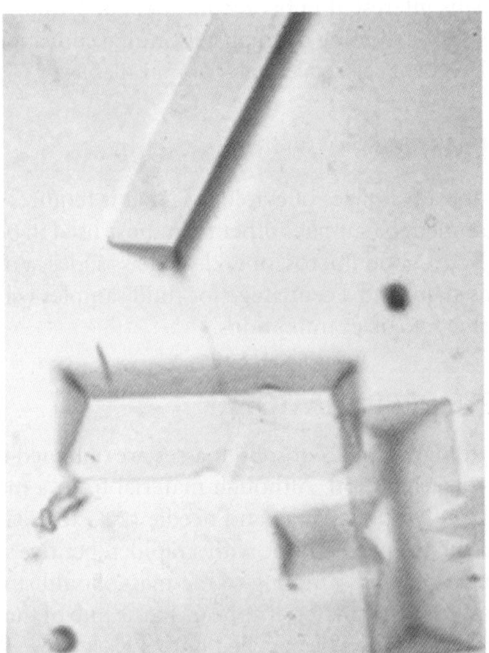

FIGURE 16-31 Urine sediment with triple phosphate crystals.

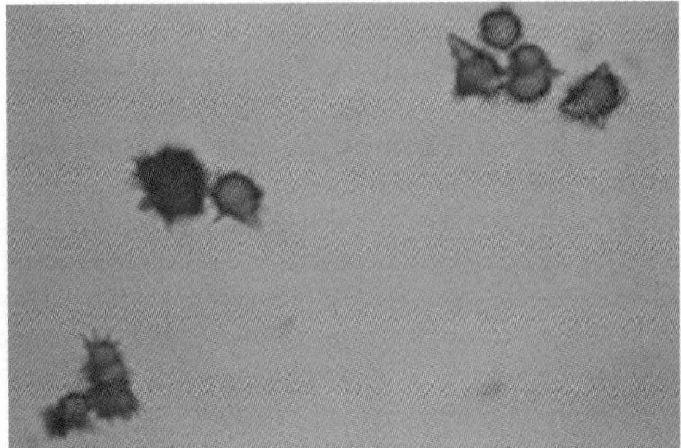

FIGURE 16-32 Urine sediment with ammonium biurate crystals.

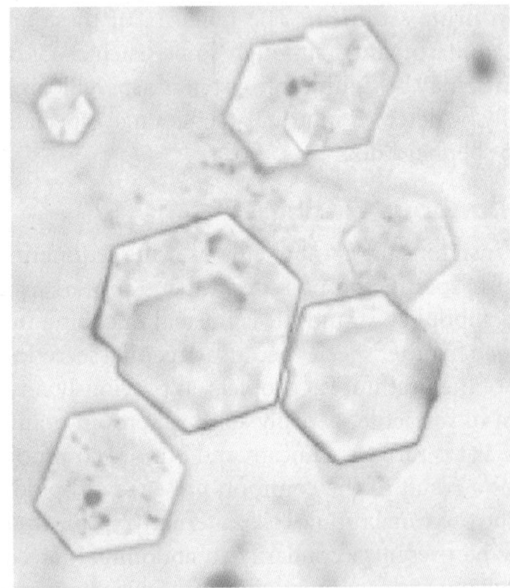

FIGURE 16-33 Urine sediment with cystine crystals.

Crystals

Crystals are another major component of urine sediment. The precipitation and presence of crystals depend on the urine pH and the solubility and concentration of the substance forming them. Urine crystals that accompany pathologic conditions include ammonium biurate, monohydrate calcium oxalate, bilirubin, triple phosphate (struvite, ammonium, magnesium phosphate), and cystine crystals. Dihydrate calcium oxalate crystals can be found in normal urine, but appear distinctly different from the monohydrate calcium oxalate crystals found with ethylene glycol (antifreeze) toxicity. Figure 16-30 shows these two types of calcium oxalate crystals. Bilirubin crystals generally occur in conjunction with bilirubinuria with little to no additional significance. Triple phosphate crystals (Figure 16-31) are often found in alkaline urine when urease-producing bacteria, associated with lower urinary tract disease, are present. Ammonium biurate crystals (Figure 16-32) are dark with distinct, multiple, irregular protrusions and are often associated with portal caval shunts, a specific liver disorder. Cystine crystals (Figure 16-33), although sometimes seen in the urine of healthy dogs, are also found in the urine of dogs with a congenital defect of cystine metabolism that leads to cystinuria. Brushite or calcium phosphate crystals may be found in the acidic urine of healthy dogs and appear as long, relatively thin, rectangular, clear crystals, which may radiate out from a central point. Drugs, such as sulfonamides, may precipitate in the urine of animals, resulting in the formation of crystals.

Microorganisms

Bacteria in unstained urine sediment may be difficult to detect. Rods may appear singly or in chains, but cocci may be lost in brownian movement. For this reason, whenever the presence of bacteria is suspected, the sediment should be stained to examine it more thoroughly. Usually the regular examination of the unstained sediment is completed and recorded first, and then the coverslip is removed and the underlying sediment on the slide is allowed to dry. Once dry, the slide can be stained with Gram stain or one of the modified Wright's stains, and any bacteria present can be identified. On Gram stain, the gram-negative, rod-shaped bacteria may be difficult to see among all the pink-staining cellular debris. With Wright's stain, all bacteria stain dark purple and are relatively easy to find.

Bacteria in a voided sample are often not significant because they may be normal flora from the distal urogenital tract, especially from the prepuce or vagina. Bacteria are significant if they occur in catheterized or cystocentesis samples. The presence of bacteria is most often correlated with leukocytes in urine because bacteria with no leukocyte response should raise suspicion of contamination of the sample, but urine from diabetic patients may sometimes be an exception. If bacteria are present in a urine sample, they can multiply as time passes, so this should be taken into consideration when the sample is being analyzed. Rarely, fungal organisms are found in urine sediment. The majority of these are insignificant contaminants, although some, such as *Blastomyces* organisms, may be significant; systemic aspergillosis may occasionally be detected in urinary sediments, especially in the German shepherd dog.

Miscellaneous Findings

Usually insignificant components of urine sediment include mucus, fat, sperm, and parasites. Mucus appears as narrow, twisted, ribbonlike strands. It is normal in equine urine and can be seen in other species because of genital secretions or irritation of the urethra. Fat droplets, as previously noted, take the form of refractile, variably sized spheres in many planes of focus. Fat is rarely significant and is more commonly seen in cats as a result of the common presence of lipid droplets within the proximal tubule cells; alternatively, the lipid droplets may be present secondarily to abdominal fat contamination during cystocentesis collection. Sperm are commonly seen in male canine urine samples. Parasites that can occur in urine include the ova of *Stephanurus dentatus, Dioctophyme renale,* and *Capillaria plica* and microfilaria of *D. immitis.*

CYTOLOGY

Cytology is the study of cells, specifically involving the microscopic examination of individual cells that have exfoliated from a tissue or structure. Unlike histopathology, cytology is not an evaluation of the architecture of a tissue. In most instances, cytology can be used to differentiate an inflammatory lesion from a neoplastic mass. Sometimes cytologic appearance reveals a specific diagnosis, and for certain samples, such as bone marrow or mast cell tumors, it may be more helpful than histopathology. It should be emphasized that cytology is an adjunct diagnostic tool and not a replacement for histopathology.

Cytology requires a significant degree of expertise that can be acquired only through experience, especially for cytology of solid masses. Most veterinary practices prefer to send cytology samples to a reference laboratory for evaluation. For this reason, the discussion on cytology is limited to the preparation of samples from solid tissues for submission to a reference laboratory and fluid analysis. Veterinary technicians interested in becoming adept at cytology should obtain specific training through continuing education workshops. Excellent reference material is available.

EQUIPMENT

One of the advantages of cytology is that it requires no special equipment or supplies other than those used in performing a CBC. A good microscope, clean glass slides, a modified Wright's stain, and a centrifuge for fluid samples will suffice for most cytologic examinations.

SAMPLE PREPARATION

Most cytology samples of solid masses are obtained through fine-needle aspiration. Although material from a mass may be aspirated with a syringe and needle (22G to 25G), some prefer using the needle alone with a rapid, repetitive stabbing motion. In general, sampling of the mass should stop when blood and/or other material appears in the hub of the needle. The sample can then be expelled onto a glass slide. The material is then spread by placing a second slide on top of the first and without applying downward pressure, slowly sliding it across the first, ideally creating a flame-shaped smear. A gentle compression of the slides before sliding can be done to help spread out thick material. Cells are often fragile, so gentle smear preparation is needed to prevent distortion or damaging the cells, which may make identification difficult, if not impossible.

When handling excised pieces of tissue for cytologic study, keep them wrapped in gauze and slightly moistened with saline solution so they do not dry out. Do not allow the sample or the prepared slides to be exposed to formalin or formalin fumes until after the cytologic slides have been stained. Excised solid masses should be blotted with absorbent paper to remove blood and tissue fluid and gently touched to a slide to make an impression slide. If the mass is of a dense consistency that does not exfoliate cells easily, it may be necessary to scrape it with a scalpel blade and then spread the material gently and thinly onto the slide. An alternative method is to crosshatch cut the surface of the tissue with the scalpel blade and make an imprint preparation. The crosshatching method

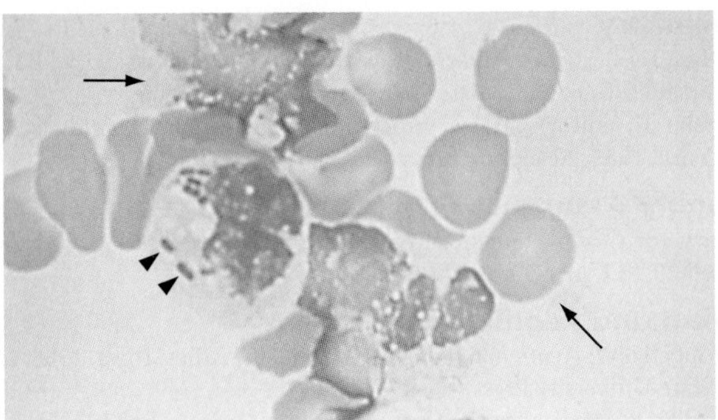

FIGURE 16-34 Equine abdominal fluid showing a degenerate neutrophil with intracellular rod-shaped bacteria *(short arrows)*. Two smudge cells are also present *(long arrows)*.

is often gentler than the scraping method and preserves the cells better. Always make impressions of the cut surface unless otherwise specified by the surgeon; impression smears of superficial surfaces are likely to yield mesothelial-lining cells unrelated to the material comprising the mass.

If the slides are to be sent to a reference laboratory, the use of flat slide mailers should be avoided because many slides will arrive shattered. Most reference laboratories prefer unstained slides, which can be stained at the laboratory by means of their standard stain protocol. If a slide has been stained and there are questions pertaining to that slide, it is a good idea to include that slide for comparison purposes.

FLUID ANALYSIS

For fluid analysis, a refractometer and a cell-counting method (e.g., Unopettes and a hemacytometer) are also needed. Once a sample for cytology has been obtained, slides should be made as soon as possible before the cells degenerate in the fluid. This is especially true of low-protein fluids, such as cerebrospinal fluid and tracheal washings. Many fluid samples can be prepared in the same manner as a blood film, leaving a feathered edge where the largest cells tend to migrate. If the fluid has few cells, as is the case with cerebrospinal fluid, a direct preparation may not provide a sufficient number of cells for a thorough examination. A routine fluid analysis of samples, such as abdominal, thoracic, or synovial fluid, usually includes a WBC count, which is more appropriately referred to as a total nucleated cell count, because some of the cells (mesothelial cells, synovial cells, etc.) may not be derived directly from blood. The total nucleated cell count can be performed in the same manner as a WBC count. If there are numerous cells present, these can be counted on an automated instrument, but lower cell counts will require the use of a hemacytometer as for a manual WBC count but with no dilution.

Total protein is another helpful parameter in fluid analysis and can be done by refractometer, generally with the supernatant portion of a centrifuged fluid sample. Total erythrocyte (RBC) count is often included in the fluid analysis if done on an automated instrument, but the RBC count alone is rarely helpful in evaluating fluid because of the frequency of peripheral blood contamination of samples. It is more important to check for erythrophagocytosis (phagocytosis of RBCs by macrophages) during the cytologic examination because erythrophagocytosis generally implies that the RBCs were present in the fluid before sampling rather than as contaminants.

Fluid samples that have neutrophils as the predominate cell type should be closely evaluated for the presence of bacteria. Bacteria should be present within cells (intracellular) to be considered significant (Figure 16-34). If the bacteria are only extracellular, the possibility of contamination of the sample should be considered. If no bacteria are found, it should not be assumed that they are absent. Bacteria may be present in low numbers and difficult to find. The degree of preservation of the neutrophils needs to be noted because dying or "degenerate" neutrophils may be associated with infectious causes even if organisms were not seen.

Fluid color and clarity should always be noted.

SYNOVIAL FLUID

The analysis of certain fluids includes specific tests that may add more information than routine tests. For instance, the mucin clot test is done on synovial (joint) fluid by mixing a diluted acetic acid solution (0.1 ml of 7N acetic acid in 4 ml of distilled water) and adding 1 ml of synovial fluid; EDTA anticoagulated samples cannot be used for this test. Normal synovial fluid contains mucin, which forms a tight white clot in the acetic acid; if the mucin has been digested by bacterial or cellular enzymes and/or diluted by effusion, the clot will be less distinct or may not form at all, leaving only hazy or cloudy fluid. Therefore good mucin clot formation usually accompanies normal or noninflamed joints, whereas a poor or absent mucin clot is commonly associated with inflammation and/or effusion. The WBC Unopette system cannot be used to obtain nucleated cell counts from synovial fluid because it contains acetic acid as the diluent in the reservoir, which would cause similar clotting of mucin. Total nucleated cell counts of joint fluid samples should be done with the Unopette system for both WBCs and platelets. The reservoir in this system contains ammonium oxalate, which will not precipitate mucin.

> *TECHNICIAN NOTE* Good mucin clot formation usually accompanies normal or noninflamed joints, whereas a poor or absent mucin clot is commonly associated with inflammation and/or effusion.

Although only semiquantitative, the mucin clot test is the least subjective of tests of joint fluid viscosity; the "string test" and direct microscopic examination of joint fluid also can yield valuable, albeit even less quantitative, information on viscosity. The string test is a simple test where a stick is placed into the joint fluid and then withdrawn; a string of greater than 2 to 3 cm in length is considered adequate. A microscopic assessment of viscosity is the least quantitative and relies upon the subjective assessment of the density of typical finely granular eosinophilic background material; whereas joints with decreased viscosity still have high amounts of this material, it is of a lower density than that from normal joints, which have an uninterrupted carpet of pink material that wells up upon the cell edges.

RECOMMENDED READING

General

Duncan JR, Prasse KW: *Veterinary laboratory medicine/clinical pathology*, Ames, Iowa, 1994, Iowa State University Press.

Stockham SL, Scott MA: *Fundamentals of veterinary clinical pathology*, Ames, Iowa, 2002, Iowa State University Press.

Laboratory Equipment

Tietz NW: *Fundamentals of clinical chemistry*, ed 4, Philadelphia, 1995, WB Saunders.

Hematology

Harvey JW: *Atlas of veterinary hematology: blood and bone marrow of domestic animals*, Philadelphia, 2001, WB Saunders.

Jain NC: *Essentials of veterinary hematology*, Philadelphia, 1993, Lea & Febiger.

Reagan WL, et al: *Veterinary hematology: atlas of common domestic species*, Ames, Iowa, 1998, Iowa State University Press.

Urinalysis

Graff L: *A handbook of routine urinalysis*, Philadelphia, 1983, JB Lippincott.

Osborne CA, Finco DR: *Canine and feline nephrology and urology*, Philadelphia, 1995, Lea & Febiger.

Chemistry

Coffman JR: *Equine clinical chemistry and pathophysiology*, Bonner Springs, Kan, 1981, Veterinary Medicine Publishing.

Kaneko JJ, editor: Clinical biochemistry of domestic animals, New York, 1989, Academic Press.

Quality Assurance Programs

Henry JB: *Clinical diagnosis and management by laboratory methods*, ed 20, St Louis, 2001, WB Saunders.

Avian and Reptilian Hematology

Campbell TW: *Avian hematology and cytology*, Ames, Iowa, 1988, Iowa State University Press.

Frye FL: *Biomedical and surgical aspects of captive reptile husbandry*, Edwardsville, Kan, 1981, Veterinary Medicine Publishing.

Cytology

Baker R, Lumsden JH: *Color atlas of cytology of the dog and cat*, St Louis, 2000, Mosby.

Cowell RL, et al: *Diagnostic cytology and hematology of the dog and cat*, ed 3, St Louis, 2008, Mosby.

Cowell RL, et al: *Diagnostic cytology and hematology of the horse*, ed 2, St Louis, 2002, Mosby.

Menard M, Papageorges M: Fine-needle biopsies: how to increase diagnostic yield, *Compend Cont Educ Pract Vet* 19:738, 1997.

Raskin RE, Meyer DJ: *Atlas of canine and feline cytology*, Philadelphia, 2001, WB Saunders.

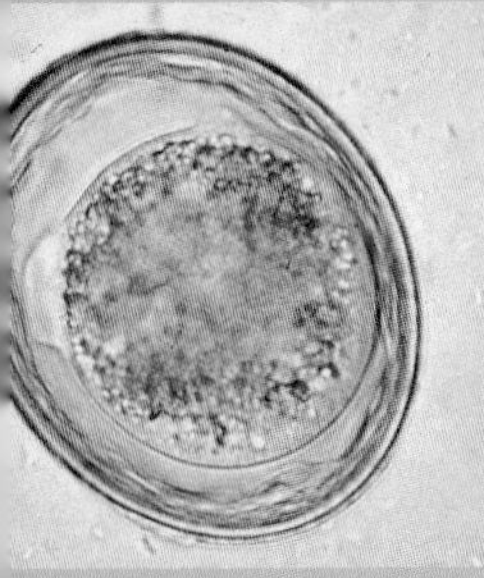

Parasitology

17

Charles M. Hendrix

KEY TERMS

Ascarid
Cestode
Definitive host
Ectoparasite
Endoparasite
Intermediate host
Life cycle
Microfilaria
Myiasis
Nematode
Obligatory parasite
Parasitism
Paratenic (or transport) host
Protozoan
Reservoir host
Trematode
Vector
Zoonosis

OUTLINE

LEARNING OBJECTIVES

When you have completed this chapter, you will be able to:

1. Define the following terms: intermediate host, definitive host, reservoir host.
2. State the scientific and common names for the nematode, cestode, trematode, and protozoal parasites commonly encountered in small and large animal practice.
3. List the definitive and intermediate hosts for the nematode, cestode, trematode, and protozoal parasites commonly encountered in small and large animal practice.
4. Describe the collection and handling of fecal samples from small and large animals.
5. Describe the procedures for the gross examination and direct examination of fecal samples and state the advantages and limitations of the procedure.
6. List the methods commonly used to concentrate parasitic material in fecal samples.
7. Describe the procedure for performing standard fecal flotation and centrifugal flotation.
8. List and describe the procedures for the identification of blood parasites.
9. List the scientific and common names for ectoparasites commonly encountered in small and large animal practice.
10. List and describe the procedures for the collection of samples and the identification of ectoparasites.

INTRODUCTION

Most parasites are capable of causing significant damage to the host. This potential damage may be a function of the number of parasites present, location within the host, production of toxins, or interference with the host's normal physiologic processes. Clinical signs associated with parasitism may include life-threatening anemia, hypoproteinemia, diarrhea, vomiting, and intestinal obstruction; however, the damage from most parasites is often more insidious, such as interference with normal weight gain or milk production. Parasitism is most severe in animals younger than 1 year, but it may affect animals of any age.

Parasites are divided into two large groups: endoparasites (internal parasites), which include: nematodes, cestodes, trematodes, protozoa, and acanthocephalans, and ectoparasites (external parasites), which include: fleas, lice, ticks, mites, chiggers, biting flies, and myiasis-inducing flies. There are endoparasites and ectoparasites on or in all animals and in every tissue and organ system. Some parasites are host specific, whereas other parasites are capable of infecting a broad range of species. Modes of transmission vary considerably from direct transmission to an extremely complex life cycle involving the use of intermediate hosts or transport hosts. In all modes of parasite transmission, specific environmental conditions play a key role.

There have been entire textbooks written about veterinary parasitology, and it would be impossible to cover all of the parasites that affect animals in a single chapter. Therefore this chapter will focus on identification of the most commonly found parasites in North America. The veterinary technician should become familiar with both the common and scientific names of the common parasites and should be proficient in the diagnostic tests that lead to a specific diagnosis.

ENDOPARASITES OF DOMESTICATED ANIMALS

Endoparasites live within an animal. They derive their nutrition and protection at the expense of the infected animal, which is called the host. The various internal parasites have many different life cycles. Each parasite's life cycle is distinctive and is composed of various developmental stages, all of which may occur within the same host or separately within sequential hosts.

The host that harbors the adult (sexually mature) stage of a parasite is called the definitive host. The dog, for example, is the definitive host for *Dirofilaria immitis;* adult male and female heartworms are found in the right ventricle and pulmonary arteries of the dog's heart. The host that harbors the immature (asexual) stages of a parasite is called the intermediate host. For example, the mosquito is the intermediate host for *D. immitis* because first, second, and third larval stages of *D. immitis* are found within this insect.

The life cycle of most parasites has at least one stage at which the parasite may be passed from one host to the next. Diagnostic procedures frequently detect this stage, and it is therefore called the diagnostic stage. The microfilarial stage is the diagnostic stage of *D. immitis* because a concentrated blood sample will frequently show the presence of *D. immitis* in the blood. The diagnostic stage of a parasite may leave the host in many ways; through excreta, such as feces or urine, or through the bloodstream when an arthropod, such as a mosquito, takes a blood meal. In the case of *D. immitis,* the female mosquito ingests microfilariae during a blood meal and transports it to the definitive host (the dog) when it later feeds on the dog.

CLASSIFICATION OF ENDOPARASITES

Nematodes (Roundworms)

Nematodes often are referred to as roundworms and are one of the most important groups of parasites in veterinary parasitology. They may be found in almost any tissue of domestic animals, including the intestines, skin, lungs, kidneys, urinary bladder, nervous tissue, musculature, and blood. As a group, nematodes have diverse, complicated life cycles. They have separate sexes (male nematodes and female nematodes). Their eggs or larvae are most commonly recovered from the feces, but some species that inhabit the urinary bladder and kidney may shed their eggs in the urine. Examples of intestinal nematodes found in dogs include ascarids *(Toxocara canis, Toxascaris leonina),* hookworms *(Ancylostoma caninum, Uncinaria stenocephala),* and whipworms *(Trichuris vulpis).* Roundworms found in the urinary system include canine kidney worms *(Dioctophyma renale).* Those found in the respiratory system include the lungworms of cattle and sheep *(Dictyocaulus* spp. and *Muellerius capillaris).* Nematodes of the blood vasculature are a special group, of which the heartworm of dogs *(D. immitis)* is an example. Adult female heartworms give birth to small, wormlike prelarval (embryonic) stages called microfilariae. The microfilariae may be observed in a peripheral blood smear and are approximately 310 μm long. Mosquitoes acquire the microfilariae from a blood meal, and within the mosquito, the microfilariae develop into infective third-stage larvae, which are subsequently transmitted to other animals by the infected mosquitoes.

Cestodes (Tapeworms)

Cestodes (tapeworms) are long, flat, segmented worms that resemble strips of white ribbon. They are hermaphroditic, meaning that they possess both male and female sex organs and can reproduce alone. The long ribbonlike body is divided into proglottids, which are segments connected like train cars behind a scolex or "head." The scolex allows the tapeworm to attach to the wall of the host's intestine. Most tapeworms release proglottids from the terminal end into the lumen of the gut where they emerge from the animal during defecation and can be found in the feces. A few tapeworms release eggs rather than proglottid segments directly into the gastrointestinal tract of the host.

Proglottids can be observed with the naked eye. Because the proglottid segments have muscles that enable them to move about, it is not unusual for the owners of infected animals to see "little white worms" crawling on the pet's feces, hair coat, or bedding. Fresh proglottids are said to resemble "cucumber seeds," whereas dried ones resemble uncooked grains of rice.

Tapeworm proglottids often contain eggs when they are passed into the feces. Each egg contains a hexacanth embryos that contaminate the vegetation where the host has defecated.

An intermediate host, such as a rabbit, ingests these hexacanth embryos as it feeds on ground dwelling vegetation and seeds. The hexacanth embryo grows within the tissues of the intermediate host to a "bladderworm" stage, which is a fluid-filled larval stage. The definitive host, such as a cat or dog, becomes infected by ingesting the intermediate host (e.g., rabbit), which contains the bladderworm larval stage. Examples of tapeworms that develop into the bladderworm stage in the intermediate host are the canine taeniid tapeworm *(Taenia pisiformis)* and the coenurus tapeworm *(Multiceps multiceps)*. In some tapeworms *(Echinococcus granulosus, Echinococcus multilocularis)*, the larval stage within the intermediate host forms a large, fluid-filled cyst called a hydatid cyst, which forms in internal organs, such as the lung, liver, kidney, spleen, and brain of the animal (or human).

When the intermediate host is an arthropod, such as a flea or a grain mite, the hexacanth embryo develops into a microscopic larval stage known as a cysticercoid. The cysticercoid stage is tiny and contains a small fluid-filled space. The definitive host becomes infected by ingesting the intermediate host, which contains the cysticercoid larval stage. The cysticercoid stage is associated with the fringed tapeworm of cattle *(Thysanosoma actinoides)* and the double-pore tapeworm *(Dipylidium caninum)* of dogs and cats.

Trematodes (Flukes)

The trematodes are leaf-shaped, flatworms with unsegmented bodies. Adults are hermaphroditic, and in domestic animals in the United States are found primarily in the intestinal tract, but some species have also been found in the liver and lungs. Flukes of veterinary importance include the liver flukes of cattle and sheep *(Fasciola hepatica, Fascioloides magna, Dicrocoelium dendriticum)* and the lung fluke of dogs and cats *(Paragonimus kellicotti)*.

Adult flukes lay eggs that are passed in the feces. The end portion of many fluke eggs has a small cap or lid called an operculum, and this is easily identifiable under a microscopic examination.

Within each fluke egg is a larval stage known as a miracidium, which hatches and exits the egg through the operculum. This stage penetrates the first intermediate host, which is usually a snail. Within the snail, the miracidium develops into a sporocyst, which then produces many tiny internal structures called rediae. Each redia may produce many internal cercariae. The cercariae exit the snail and may take one of three pathways before entering the definitive host: it may be ingested by a second intermediate host and become encysted as the metacercarial stage within the second intermediate host (which is subsequently ingested by the definitive host); it may encyst on vegetation, which is subsequently ingested by the definitive host; or cercariae may directly penetrate the skin of the definitive host.

Protozoa (Unicellular Organisms)

Protozoa are unicellular, or single-celled organisms, some of which may be parasitic in domestic animals and can infect a variety of tissue sites within the definitive host. The most common sites for their detection are in blood samples and in fecal samples. If they inhabit blood, they are called blood protozoa, and if they inhabit the gastrointestinal system, they are called intestinal protozoa. The protozoan's life cycle may be simple or complex.

Most hemoprotozoa seen in the United States are found in red blood cells (RBCs) during an examination of a stained blood smear. Ticks usually serve as intermediate hosts and transmit the hemoprotozoa from one animal to the next while feeding on multiple hosts. *Babesia bigemina* is a tear-shaped hemoprotozoan found within the RBCs of infected cattle. It is transmitted by the tick, *Boophilus annulatus*.

Trypanosomes are another group of hemoprotozoans occasionally found in the United States. Rather than being found within RBCs, trypanosomes are extracellular and "swim" within the blood. They are 3 to 10 times as long as an RBC is wide and are banana shaped. They have a lateral undulating membrane and a thin, whiplike "lash" (flagellum) that is used for swimming. These parasites are also transmitted by blood-feeding arthropods.

Acanthocephalans (Thorny-Headed Worms)

Acanthocephalans (thorny-headed worms) are uncommon parasites with complicated life cycles. Like the nematodes, they have separate sexes. On the cranial end of these helminths is a spiny proboscis, which is used to attach to the lining of the intestinal wall. Thorny-headed worms do not have a true gut; they absorb nutrients through their body wall. Acanthocephalans usually are recovered at necropsy.

A famous acanthocephalan is *Macracanthorhynchus hirudinaceus,* a parasite of pigs. This parasite has the dubious honor of possessing the longest scientific name among the parasites of domestic animals. *Oncicola canis* is an acanthocephalan found in the small intestine of dogs.

ENDOPARASITES OF DOGS AND CATS

The Gastrointestinal System

Nematodes (Roundworms)

Esophageal worms. *Spirocerca lupi,* the esophageal worm, is a nematode that often forms nodules in the esophageal wall of dogs and cats. Occasionally, it may be found in gastric nodules in cats. Adult worms reside deep within these nodules and expel their eggs through tunnel-like openings in the nodule. Eggs are passed through the host animal's intestine and out in the feces. The thick-shelled eggs contain a larva when they are laid; these eggs have a unique "paper clip" shape. Figure 17-1 shows the characteristic ovum of *S. lupi*. Eggs can usually be observed on fecal flotation and can be recovered when vomitus has been subjected to a standard fecal flotation procedure. A radiographic or endoscopic examination may also reveal characteristic granulomas within the esophagus or within the stomach.

Stomach worms. *Physaloptera* spp. are stomach worms of dogs and cats. Although they are occasionally found in the lumen of the stomach or small intestine, *Physaloptera* spp. are usually firmly attached to the mucosal surface of the

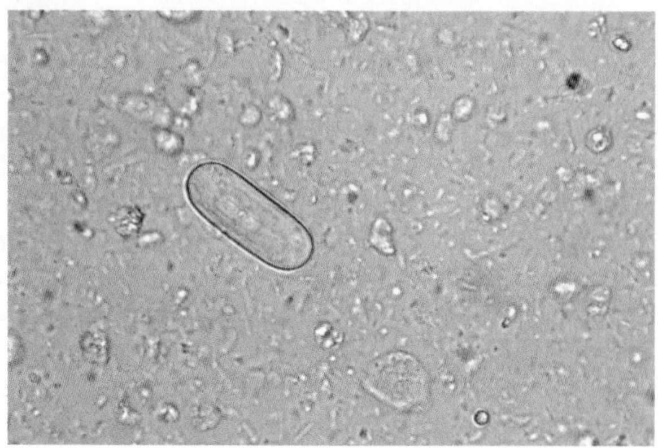

FIGURE 17-1 Characteristic ovum of *S. lupi.* The thick-shelled eggs contain larvae and measure 30 to 38 μm by 11 to 15 μm. Eggs usually may be observed on fecal flotation and may be recovered when vomitus has been subjected to a standard fecal flotation procedure.

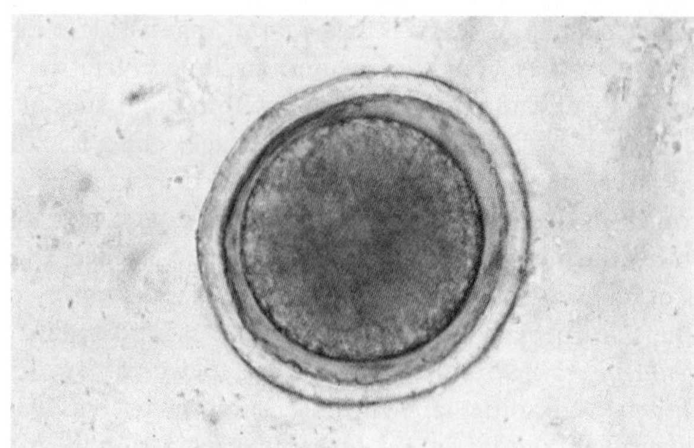

FIGURE 17-3 Characteristic ovum of *T. cati.* These eggs are smaller than those of *T. canis,* measuring only 65 to 75 mm in diameter.

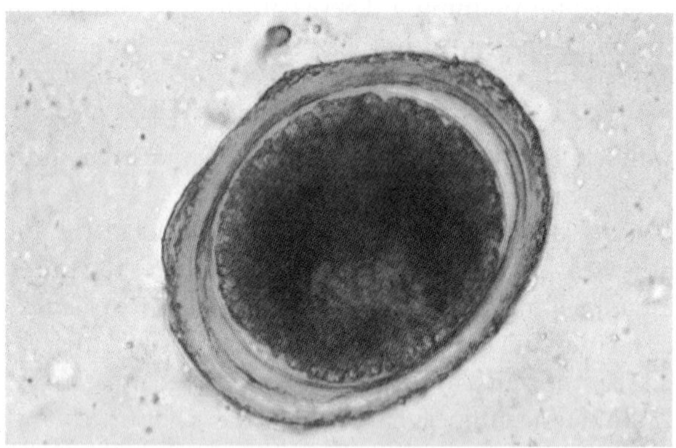

FIGURE 17-2 Characteristic ovum of *Toxocara canis.* These eggs are spherical, with a deeply pigmented center and a rough, pitted outer shell. Eggs of *T. canis* are 75 to 90 μm in diameter.

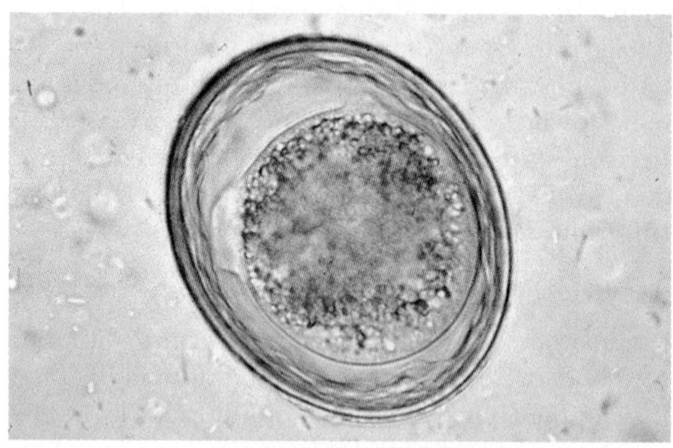

FIGURE 17-4 Characteristic ovum of *Toxascaris leonina.* These eggs are spherical to ovoid, with dimensions of 75 by 85 μm. They have a smooth outer shell and a hyaline or "ground glass" central portion.

stomach, where they suck blood. At this site, it is possible to view these nematodes using an endoscope. Their diet consists of blood and tissue derived from the host's gastric mucosa. Their attachment sites continue to bleed after the parasite detaches. Vomiting; anorexia; and dark, tarry stools may be observed in affected animals.

The adult worms are creamy white, sometimes tightly coiled, and 1.3 to 4.8 cm long. They are often recovered in the pet's vomitus and can easily be confused with the ascarids (roundworms). A quick way to differentiate these two parasites is to break open an adult specimen and (if that specimen happens to be female) examine the egg type microscopically. The eggs of *Physaloptera* spp. are small, smooth, thick-shelled, and contain a larva when passed in the feces. Eggs can usually be recovered on a standard fecal flotation, using solutions with a specific gravity above 1.25. If a vomiting dog is suspected of harboring *Physaloptera* spp., a fecal flotation can be performed on the vomitus to determine if the characteristic eggs are present.

Ollulanus tricuspis, "the feline trichostrongyle" is usually associated with vomiting in cats. This nematode is most commonly identified by examining the cat's vomitus with a dissecting or compound microscope. Feline vomitus can also be examined using a standard fecal flotation procedure. The best flotation solution for detection is a modified Sheather's flotation solution. Adult female *O. tricuspis* are 0.8 to 1.0 mm long and have three major tail cusps (i.e., toothlike projections [hence, the epithet *tricuspis*]). Adult males are 0.7 to 0.8 mm long and have a copulatory bursa. The female worms are larviparous (they bear live larvae). These larvae mature to the infective third-stage larvae, and they complete development to the adult stage in the cat's stomach. Free-living stages in the external environment are not required for the completion of the life cycle. Transmission occurs through the ingestion of vomitus from infected cats.

Ascarids. *Toxocara canis, T. cati,* and *Toxascaris leonina* are ascarids of dogs and cats. They are large, robust, white to cream-colored nematodes. Mature specimens measure about 3.5 to 5 cm (males) and 10 to 15 cm (females). Eggs of the *Toxocara* spp. are large, round to oval, and dark colored with thick, rough shells (Figures 17-2 and 17-3) *T. leonina* eggs are lighter in color and more egg shaped and have thick, smooth shells (Figure 17-4). All three species of ascarids are common in most geographic regions of the United States. The larval stage develops within the eggs; it will develop to the second stage larva, the infective stage for this parasite. Ascarid eggs are highly resistant to adverse conditions and in ideal environmental conditions become infective in about 2 weeks. Once ingested, *Toxocara* spp. hatch in the small intestine, penetrate the mucosa, migrate through the liver, pass through the heart, and go into the lungs, in which they develop within a short period. Larvae are coughed up and swallowed, and they mature to the adult stage in the small intestine within 4 to 6 weeks.

> *TECHNICIAN NOTE* In dogs and cats, all three species of ascarids, *T. canis, T. cati,* and *T. leonina,* are common in most geographic regions of the United States.

T. canis eggs hatch in the small intestine, and the larvae penetrate the intestinal mucosa to develop for about 2 to 3 months and then return to the intestinal lumen as adults. In dogs older than 3 months, most of the larvae leave the circulation and are stored in the somatic organs until the dog becomes pregnant. Between the 42 and 56 days of gestation, these larvae leave the somatic tissues, cross the placenta, enter the fetal lungs, and remain there until birth. The larvae then complete the cycle already described. Consequently a high percentage of dogs are infected via the prenatal or transplacental route. In pregnant dogs and cats, some of the activated *Toxocara* larvae migrate to the mammary glands. These larvae are ingested by puppies and kittens when they start to nurse. Transmammary infections are more common in cats than in dogs. The eggs of all three ascarids can be ingested by other animals (e.g., mice, chickens) and remain infective in their tissue until these animals are eaten by an appropriate canine or feline host. All three species are readily identified by several techniques, and they are amenable to treatment with several anthelmintics. Control is difficult because the eggs are resistant; control measures include thorough cleansing of kennels, runs, yards, and so forth. It is important that these eggs containing the infective larvae be removed from the premises. If these eggs are ingested by a human (e.g., a small child), the larvae will hatch from the eggs and undergo a migration through the liver and lungs or the eyes of the child. This condition is a zoonotic condition and is called *visceral larva migrans.*

Hookworms. Hookworms are a type of nematode found throughout the world and are common in tropical and subtropical areas of North America. A hookworm infection, which can produce severe anemia in young kittens and puppies, can be a serious problem in kennels and catteries. The prepatent period depends on the species of hookworm and the route of infection.

Ancylostoma caninum, the canine hookworm, is found in the small intestine of dogs, foxes, coyotes, wolves, raccoons, and badgers; *Ancylostoma braziliense* is found in dogs and cats; *Uncinaria stenocephala* occurs in dogs, cats, foxes, coyotes, and wolves; *Ancylostoma tubaeformis* is found in cats and wild Felidae. Hookworms are all short, thick parasites; adult males measure 6 to 12 mm, and females measure 6 to 20 mm. Hookworms produce strongyle-type eggs (Figure 17-5). *Ancylostoma* spp. are generally found in coastal areas of high rainfall, whereas *U. stenocephala* is found in the northern portions of North America. All hookworm species have a similar life cycle. Undeveloped eggs pass into the environment, develop and hatch, releasing first-stage larvae that undergo a free-living existence until they develop into infective third-stage larvae. Hookworms are capable of establishing themselves in the host after ingestion, but the normal mode of infection is skin penetration. After larvae penetrate, they enter the venous circulation, going ultimately to the lungs, in which they develop for a short period. They are then coughed up and swallowed, and they enter the small intestine and mature. This generally occurs within 4 to 6 weeks.

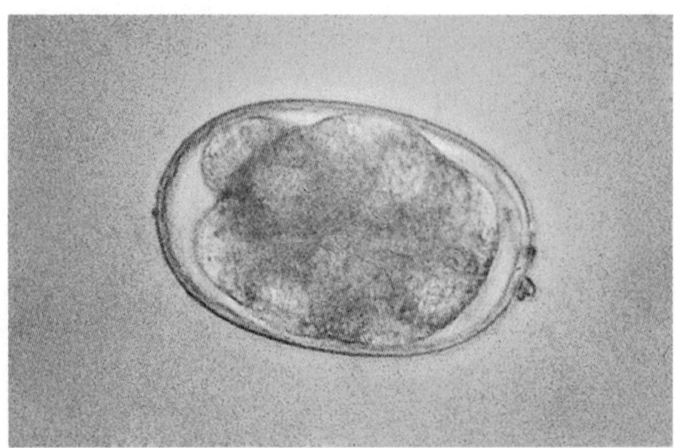

FIGURE 17-5 Characteristic hookworm ovum. The eggs of *A. caninum* are 56 to 75 μm by 34 to 47 μm, those of *A. tubaeformis* are 55 to 75 μm by 34.4 to 44.7 μm, those of *A. braziliense* are 75 μm by 45 μm, and those of *U. stenocephala* are 65 to 80 μm by 40 to 50 μm.

A. caninum has developed the additional modes of transplacental and transmammary infection. Third-stage larvae penetrate the skin and circulate in the pregnant female host, ultimately crossing the placenta. The larvae are also stored in somatic tissues until the female host becomes pregnant. In dogs, most of the somatic larvae activated at the time of pregnancy migrate to the mammary glands of the bitch and are passed on to nursing puppies. The diagnosis can be made by the identification of the eggs with a number of techniques, and these species are amenable to treatment with a number of anthelmintics. Control is difficult, especially in warm, humid geographic regions, necessitating regular thorough cleansing of yards, kennels, and other areas.

If the infective third stage hookworm larvae penetrate the skin of a human being (particularly children as they play in the sand or dirt), these larvae will migrate through the skin, producing a red, itchy, winding tunnel in the skin. This condition is a zoonotic condition and is called *cutaneous larva migrans.*

Intestinal threadworms. *Strongyloides stercoralis* is a nematode that is a tiny parasite that is found in the small intestinal mucosa of dogs, cats, foxes, humans, primates, and possibly other wild carnivores. Only the female nematode is

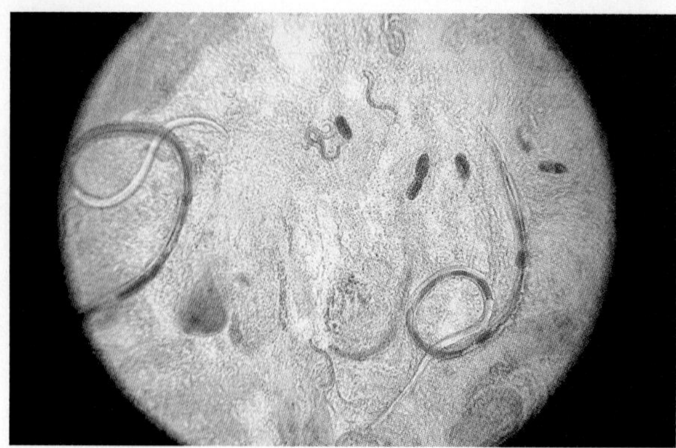

FIGURE 17-6 Parasitic adult females, eggs, and first-stage larvae of *Strongyloides* spp. These larvae are 280 to 310 μm long and have a rhabditiform esophagus, with a club-shaped cranial corpus, a narrow median isthmus, and a caudal bulb.

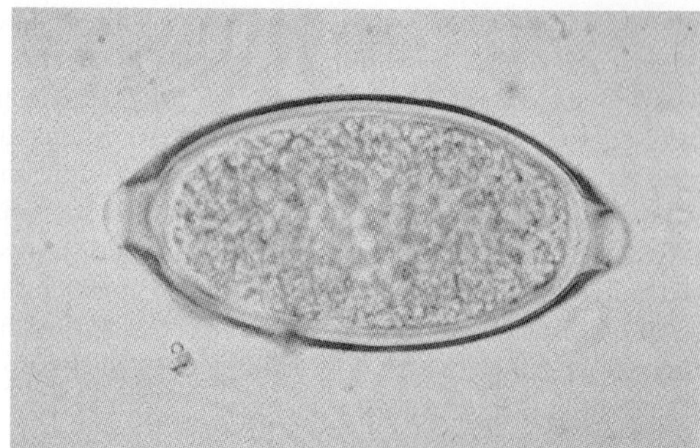

FIGURE 17-7 Characteristic ovum of *Trichuris vulpis*. Eggs of *T. vulpis* are 70 to 89 μm by 37 to 40 μm.

parasitic; there are no parasitic males. The females reproduce by parthenogenesis (reproduction without fertilization from a male). The eggs develop in utero, and nematodes give birth to eggs that will hatch into first-stage larvae (Figure 17-6) while they are within the host. The chromosome number of the larvae determines whether they will develop into a parasitic generation that must develop to an infective third-stage larvae that must infect a new host or whether they will become a free-living male or female stage that will breed and produce eggs that will eventually develop into third-stage infective larvae that must infect a new host.

The infective larvae are capable of establishing an infection by oral ingestion, after which they penetrate the small intestine and develop there. However, the primary mode of infection is skin penetration. If the larvae penetrate the skin, they then penetrate the venous circulation, going ultimately to the lungs to develop for a short period. Larvae are then coughed up and swallowed and penetrate the mucosa of the small intestine. In immunologically compromised animals, infections may be severe. *S. stercoralis* is widespread in tropical and subtropical regions and in kennels and pet shops in which environmental conditions are suitable. The diagnosis is not difficult. Frequently a direct smear of fresh feces is suitable for the identification of eggs containing first-stage larvae. The treatment is not always satisfactory, and alternative anthelmintics should be considered. Control necessitates thorough cleaning of facilities and allowing the facilities to dry.

Whipworms. *Trichuris vulpis* occurs in the cecum of the dog, fox, and coyote. Like all whipworms, *T. vulpis* has a slender anterior end with its mouth at the tip and a thickened posterior extremity, resulting in its unique whiplike appearance. Male and female worms are about the same length, measuring 45 to 75 mm. The symmetrical eggs are distinctive, possessing thick, brown-yellow shells with a clear polar plug at each end (Figure 17-7). *T. vulpis* is widespread in temperate zones, and the incidence of infection is frequently high. The life cycle is simple and direct. The larvae develop within the eggs to the infective second stage. When the eggs are ingested, the larvae are released in the intestine, which they penetrate. Larvae develop within 8 to 10 days, return to the lumen of the intestine, migrate to the cecum, and bury their anterior ends into the mucosa of the cecum. They mature to the adult stage in an additional 60 to 80 days. The diagnosis can be effectively accomplished by a number of procedures, but eggs are quite heavy, and an interpretation of the severity of the infection based on the number of eggs present is not possible. Several treatments are available. Control is difficult because eggs are highly resistant to environmental conditions. Sanitation, as applied for ascarids, is the best approach.

Whipworm infections are quite rare in cats and wild Felidae in the United States; however, *Trichuris campanula* has been reported to occur in the United States. Whipworm eggs can be confused with the eggs of *Aonchotheca putorii*, the gastric capillarid of cats. Occasionally, eggs of *Capillaria* spp. have been found in feces of both dogs and cats. The eggs of *Capillaria* spp. are similar, but not as dark in color, and on average, the eggs are somewhat smaller than those of whipworms. Frequently the eggs of trichurids or capillarids parasitize the prey of outdoor cats, such as mice, rabbits, or birds. The eggs of these nonfeline trichurids or capillarids may pass unaltered through the cat's gastrointestinal system, remaining intact and unembryonated, thus appearing to infect the feline host. Veterinary technicians should be careful not to be fooled by these pseudoparasites when examining a cat's feces.

TECHNICIAN NOTE Frequently the eggs of trichurids or capillarids parasitize the prey of outdoor cats, such as mice, rabbits, or birds. The eggs of these nonfeline trichurids or capillarids may pass unaltered through the cat's gastrointestinal system, remaining intact and unembryonated, thus appearing to infect the feline host. Veterinary technicians should be careful not to be fooled by these pseudoparasites when examining a cat's feces.

Pinworms. *Enterobius vermicularis* is the human pinworm and does not parasitize dogs or cats. Nevertheless, the family pet is often falsely incriminated by physicians, family practitioners, or pediatricians as a source of pinworm infection in young children. The veterinary technician should remember this rule: pinworms are parasites of omnivores (mice, rats, monkeys, people) and herbivores (rabbits, horses), but never are parasites of carnivores (dogs, cats).

Cestodes (Tapeworms)

True tapeworms. Dogs, cats, the wild Canidae, and some of the wild Felidae are susceptible to infection by a number of adult tapeworms. The most commonly found tapeworm species are *Dipylidium caninum, Taenia hydatigena, T. pisiformis, Taenia ovis, Taenia krabbei, Multiceps serialis, Echinococcus granulosus,* and *E. multilocularis.* Cats, and some of the wild Felidae, are generally infected with *Taenia taeniaeformis* and *D. caninum.* The species of tapeworms found in dogs and cats depends on the pet's geographic location and the amount of free-ranging activity the animals are allowed to pursue.

Some tapeworms use an intermediate host in which the larval stage (a microscopic cysticercoid stage) develops. *D. caninum,* the double-pored or cucumber seed tapeworm, uses a flea as its intermediate host; the flea contains this larval infective cysticercoid stage. *T. hydatigena, T. ovis,* and *T. krabbei* use ruminants, usually sheep, deer, elk, and moose, as intermediate hosts. In these hosts, the larval infective stage (a fluid-filled bladderworm or cysticercus) develops in the body cavity *(T. hydatigena)* or muscles *(T. ovis* and *T. krabbei).* The fluid-filled bladderworms or cysticerci of *T. pisiformis* develop in the body cavities of rabbits. *M. serialis* develops in subcutaneous areas or in the muscles (as a fluid-filled coenurus) of rabbits; this larval infective stage is known as *Coenurus serialis.* The larval infective stage of *T. taeniaeformis* (a strobilocercus) develops in the livers of mice, rats, and other small rodents. *E. granulosus* uses ruminants, such as sheep, deer and elk, and humans, as intermediate hosts. This tapeworm's larval infective stage is a rather large, fluid-filled bladder called a unilocular hydatid cyst that is easily recognized by its large size (25 to 100 mm in diameter). This hydatid cyst is typified by the presence of numerous small pieces of larval tapeworms (brood capsules lined with thousands of protoscolices) on its inner lining surface and the presence of compartments within the body of the cyst in which daughter cysts have grown and fused together. *E. multilocularis* uses rodents, such as rats, mice, and voles, as intermediate hosts. This tapeworm's infective larval stage is a fluid-filled bladder called a multilocular hydatid cyst that is easily recognized by its many compartments and invasive nature. This hydatid cyst also contains numerous small pieces of larval tapeworms (brood capsules with thousands of protoscolices) on the inner lining surface. In all instances of tapeworm life cycles, the canine or feline host becomes infected by ingesting the respective tissues containing these assorted larval infective stages.

The diagnosis of *Taenia* spp. and *D. caninum* infections in the dog or cat is normally made by finding the proglottids (tapeworm body segments), or chain of proglottids, around the host's anal region or on its hocks. Although the eggs of these tapeworms will float in a standard fecal flotation, they are usually not released to mix with the feces. Proglottids of *Taenia* spp. have one genital lateral opening or pore per proglottid, whereas proglottids of *D. caninum* have two, one on either lateral side of the proglottid (Figure 17-8). The further identification of *Taenia* spp. beyond the genus designation is extremely difficult, requiring morphologic study of the intact parasite, most specifically the anterior end or scolex with its unique double row of hooklets.

Gravid proglottids of *D. caninum* are filled with thousands of egg packets. Each egg packet may contain up to 30 hexacanth embryos. Dried proglottids of *D. caninum* resemble uncooked grains of rice. When water is added, the proglottids assume their natural form (Figure 17-9).

The eggs of *Taenia* spp. contain a single oncosphere with three pair of internal hooks. The oncosphere is often called a hexacanth embryo. The eggs of *Taenia* spp. are similar to those of *Echinococcus* and *Multiceps* spp. (Figure 17-10). These eggs are often referred to as "typical taeniid-type eggs."

E. granulosus eggs frequently mix with the feces (unlike *Taenia* spp.), but the eggs are typical *Taenia*-type eggs, possessing thick, striated egg shells and containing a six-toothed (hexacanth) embryo. *D. caninum* eggs, if seen in feces, occur in packets or groups of 20 to 30 embryos contained within a thin-walled membrane. Several treatments are available.

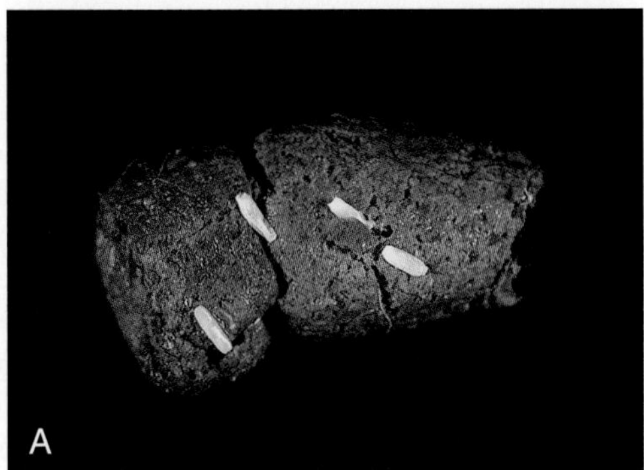

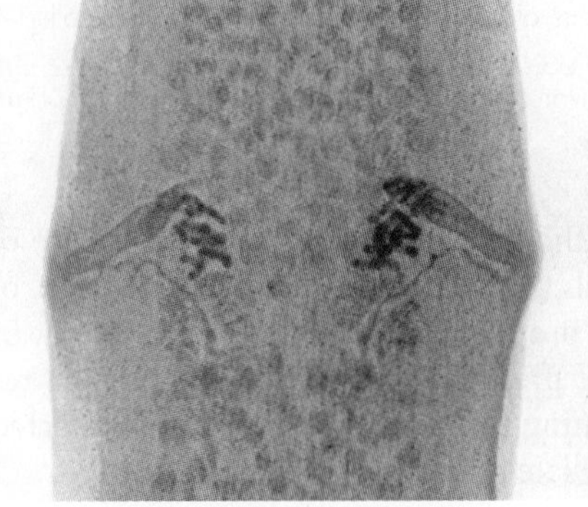

FIGURE 17-8 **A,** Characteristic motile, terminal, gravid proglottids of *D. caninum* on canine feces. In the fresh state, these proglottids resemble cucumber seeds; hence, the common name, the "cucumber seed" tapeworm. **B,** These proglottids of *D. caninum* have a lateral pore along the midpoint of each long edge, thus the second common name, double-pored tapeworm.

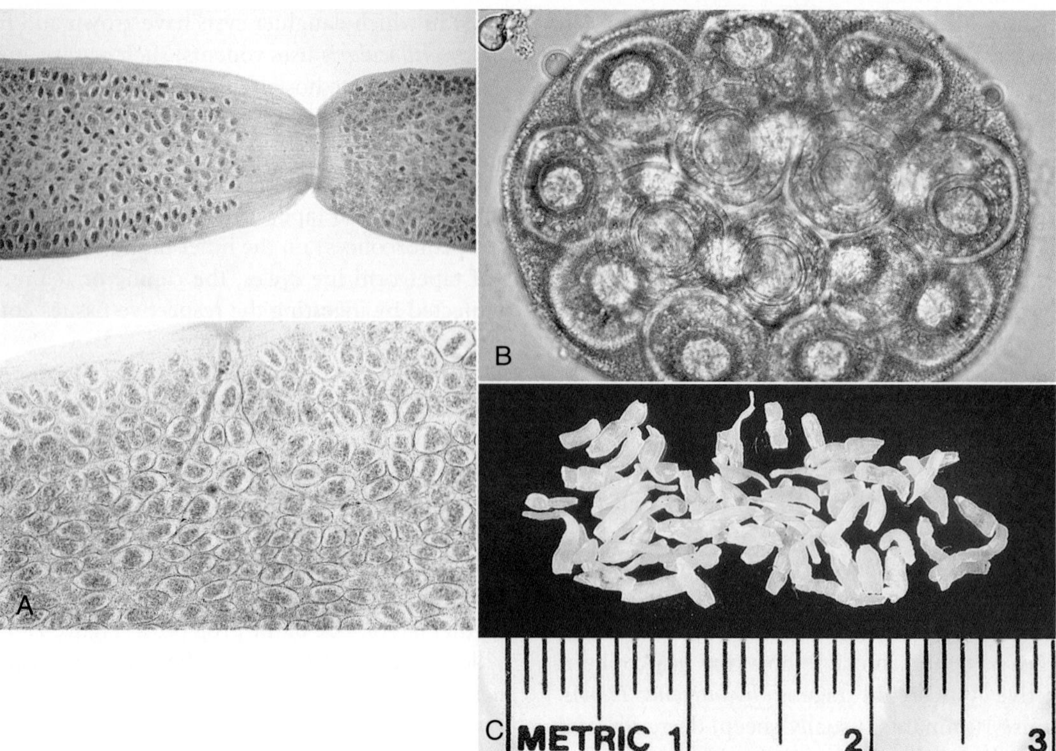

FIGURE 17-9 **A,** Gravid proglottids of *D. caninum* are filled with thousands of egg packets. **B,** Characteristic egg packet of *D. caninum.* **C,** Dried proglottids of *D. caninum* resemble uncooked grains of rice.

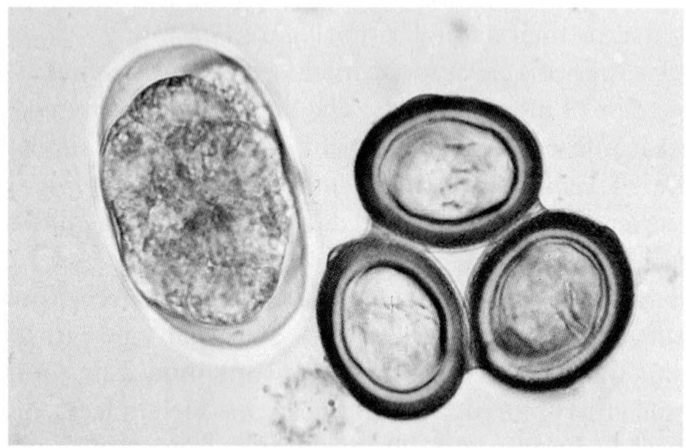

FIGURE 17-10 Characteristic ova of the taeniid tapeworms are slightly oval and 43 to 53 μm by 43 to 49 μm in diameter *(T. pisiformis),* 36 to 39 μm by 31 to 35 μm in diameter *(T. hydatigena),* and 19 to 31 μm by 24 to 26 μm *(T. ovis).* Eggs of *Taenia* spp. contain a single oncosphere with three pairs of hooks. The oncosphere is often called a hexacanth embryo. The eggs are similar to those of *Echinococcus* and *Multiceps* spp. The dissimilar ovum is that of *A. caninum,* the hookworm.

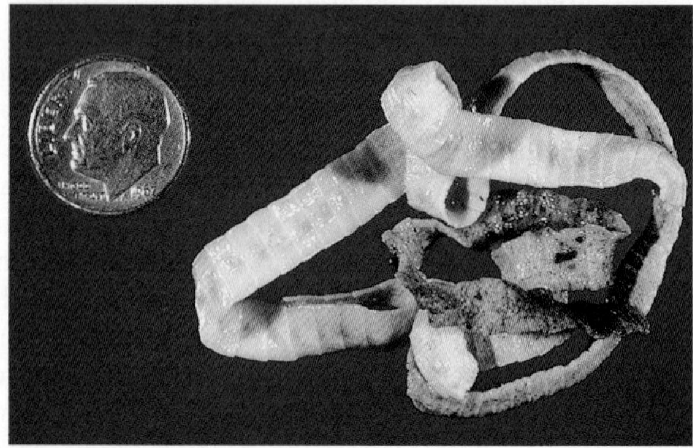

FIGURE 17-11 Spent proglottids of *S. mansonoides,* the "zipper tapeworm."

Control depends on the tapeworm species. The presence of *D. caninum* obviously necessitates the implementation of rigorous flea control programs. When *Taenia, Multiceps,* or *Echinococcus* spp. are present, dogs and cats should be restricted from consuming the flesh or viscera of the infected mammalian intermediate hosts.

Pseudotapeworms. *Spirometra* spp., "zipper tapeworms" or sparganum tapeworms (Figure 17-11), are often found in the small intestine of dogs and cats in Florida and along the Gulf Coast of North America. Gravid segments usually are not discharged into the pet's feces. While the adult tapeworm is attached to the host's jejunum, the mature proglottids will often separate along the longitudinal axis for a short distance along its length; the tapeworm appears to "unzip." This "zipped" and "unzipped" appearance gives the tapeworm its common name, the "zipper tapeworm." The egg of *Spirometra* spp. resembles that of a fluke, or digenetic trematode (Figure 17-12). This egg has a distinct operculum at one end of the pole of the shell. The eggs are oval and yellowish brown and are unembryonated when passed in the feces.

Diphyllobothrium latum often referred to as "broad fish tapeworms," may be 2 to 12 m long; however, it probably does not grow as large as 12 m in dogs and cats. These tapeworms continually release operculated eggs until they exhaust their uterine contents. The terminal proglottids become senile rather than gravid and detach in chains rather than individually. The egg of *Diphyllobothrium latum* also resembles that of a fluke (digenetic trematode). The egg is oval and light brown and possesses a distinct operculum at one end of the shell. The eggs are unembryonated when passed in the feces.

Trematodes (Flukes)

Platynosomum fastosum is the "lizard poisoning fluke" of cats (Figure 17-13). The adult flukes inhabit the liver, gall bladder, bile ducts, and less commonly the small intestine. The brownish, operculated eggs are 34 to 50 μm by 20 to 35 μm.

Nanophyetus salmincola is the "salmon poisoning fluke" of dogs in the Pacific Northwest region of North America. The adult fluke inhabits the small intestine and serves as a vector for rickettsial agents, which produce "salmon poisoning" and "Elokomin fluke fever" in dogs. The eggs are unembryonated when laid and measure 52 to 82 μm by 32 to 56 μm (Figure 17-14). The eggs have an indistinct operculum and a small, blunt point at the end opposite the operculum.

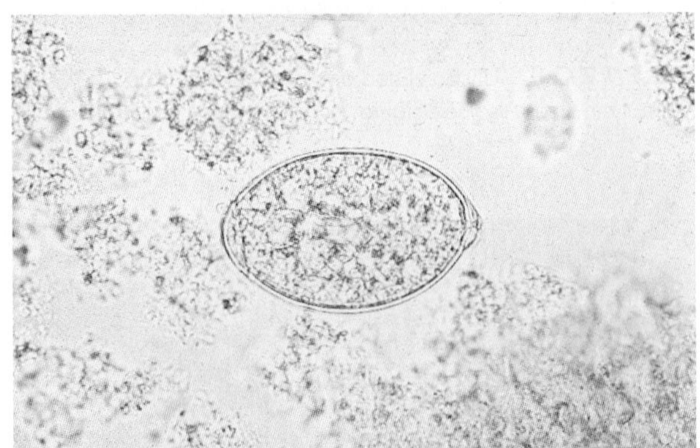

FIGURE 17-12 Characteristic ovum of *S. mansonoides*. The egg of *Spirometra* spp. resembles that of a fluke (digenetic trematode). The eggs average 60 by 36 mm and have an asymmetric appearance. These eggs tend to be rather pointed at one end.

Alaria spp. are intestinal flukes of dogs and cats and are found throughout the northern half of North America. Their ova are large, golden brown, and operculated (Figure 17-15). They are 98 to 134 μm by 62 to 68 μm.

Protozoa (Unicellular Organisms)

Giardia spp. are common protozoan parasites of dogs and cats in the United States. A higher incidence of infection occurs in dogs, cats, humans, and beavers than in other animals, such as deer, sheep, moose, and antelope. There are two forms of *Giardia*. The motile form (the trophozoite), which is approximately 12 to 17 μm long and 7 to 10 μm wide, is found in the small intestine (Figure 17-16). The cyst form (the infective stage) is approximately 9 to 13 μm long (Figure 17-17). When the cyst form is ingested, the cyst wall is digested away in the small intestine releasing the trophozoite, which immediately divides into two organisms. These organisms attach to the epithelial cells lining the small intestine and continue to multiply by binary fusion over the next 6 to 10 days until a large population exists. At that time, diarrhea develops and *Giardia* spp. begin to produce cysts. The diagnosis can be accomplished by means of the direct fecal-saline smear or, more effectively, with the zinc sulfate centrifugal flotation technique. A treatment is available. *Giardia* infection is more commonly found among young dogs and cats crowded into kennels and animal shelters. The most effective control procedure is cleanliness and disinfection with quaternary ammonium compounds.

Coccidia. Dogs and cats are hosts for many species of *Isospora, Cryptosporidium,* and *Sarcocystis,* and the cat is the definitive host for *Toxoplasma gondii.* The incidence and severity of coccidial infection depend on the host's age and immune status, conditions in which the hosts are housed, and the diet and quality of drinking water.

The species of *Isospora* have a direct life cycle. The life cycle begins with an oocyst in the feces (Figure 17-18). This oocyst must sporulate (develop into its infective form) (Figure 17-19); it does so in less than a week, given optimal conditions of warmth and moisture. Once infective, the oocyst encloses two sporocysts, each of which encloses four small, banana-shaped, infective forms called sporozoites for a total of eight infective forms in each oocyst. When ingested, the

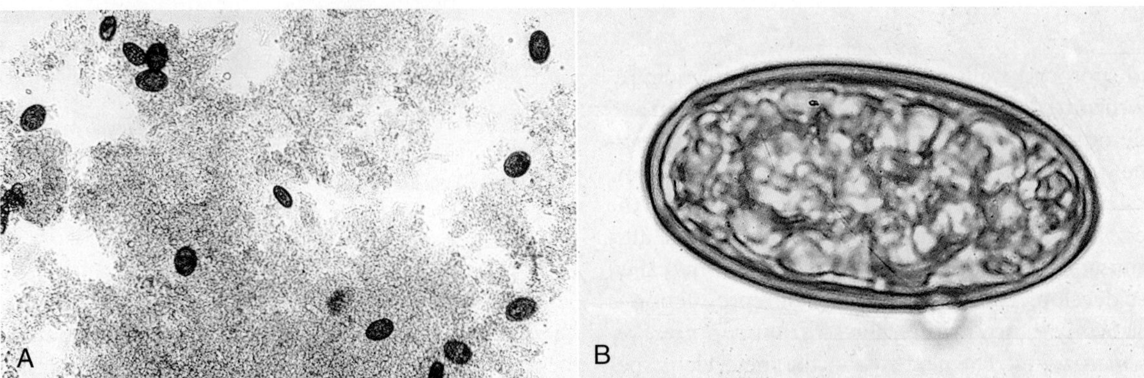

FIGURE 17-13 **A,** Characteristic ova of *P. fastosum*, the "lizard poisoning fluke" of cats. **B,** The brownish, operculated eggs are 34 to 50 μm by 20 to 35 μm.

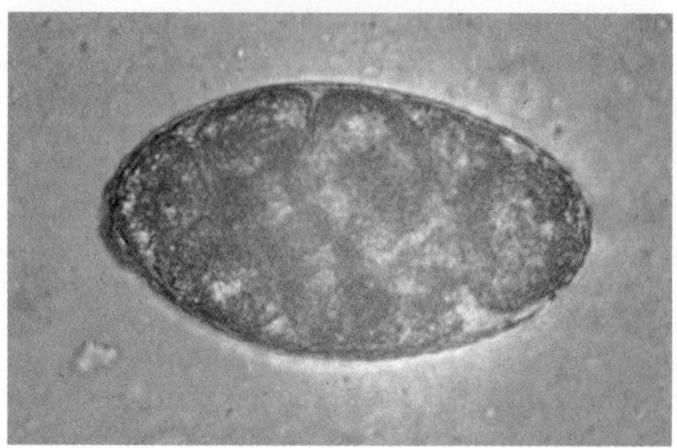

FIGURE 17-14 Characteristic ovum of *Nanophyetus salmincola.*

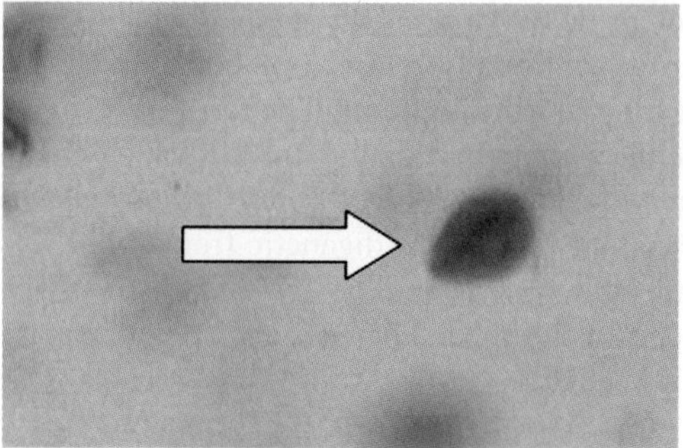

FIGURE 17-17 Cysts of *Giardia* spp. The mature cysts are oval and measure 8 to 10 μm by 7 to 10 μm. These have a refractile wall and four nuclei. Immature cysts, which represent recently encysted motile forms, contain only two nuclei.

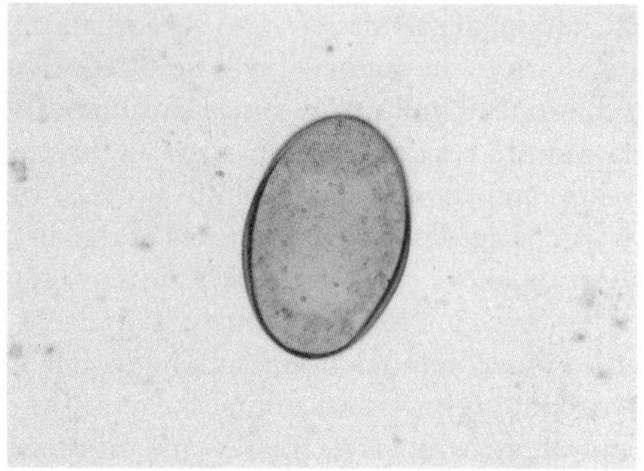

FIGURE 17-15 Characteristic ovum of *Alaria* spp., the intestinal flukes of dogs and cats.

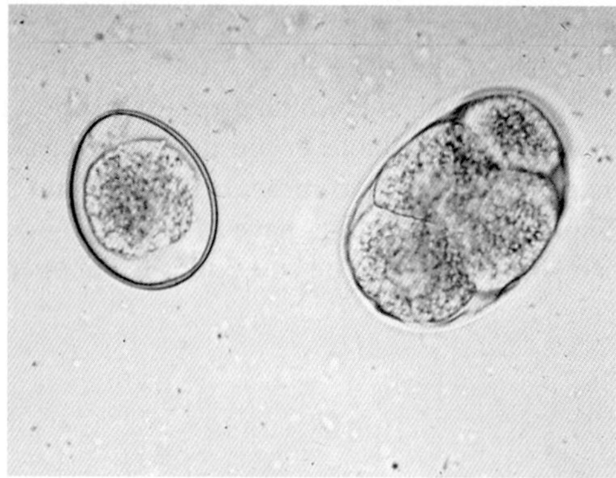

FIGURE 17-18 Unsporulated oocyst of *Isospora* spp. *(left).* Oocysts vary greatly in size. Also see Figure 17-19, *A. caninum (right).*

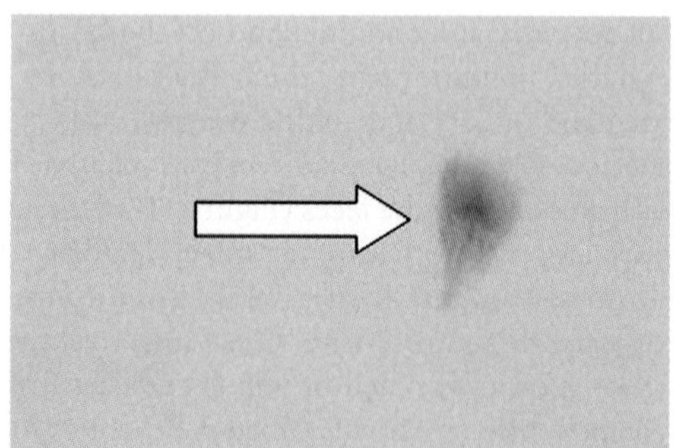

FIGURE 17-16 Motile trophozoite of *Giardia* spp.

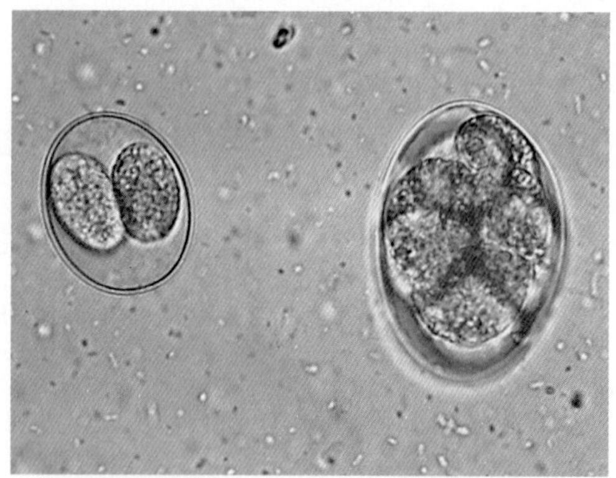

FIGURE 17-19 Sporulated oocyst of *Isospora* spp. The canine coccidians and their measurements are *I. canis,* 34 to 40 μm by 28 to 32 μm; *Isospora ohioensis,* 20 to 27 μm by 15 to 24 μm; and *Isopora wallacei,* 10 to 14 μm by 7.5 to 9.0 μm. The feline coccidians and their measurements are *I. felis,* 38 to 51 μm by 27 to 29 μm, and *Isospora rivolta,* 21 to 28 μm by 17 to 23 μm. *A. caninum (right).*

oocyst and sporocyst walls are digested in the intestine, releasing sporozoites to penetrate the intestinal epithelium and enter a cell for subsequent development. Within the intestinal cell, the sporozoites become spherical and begin to grow to a large size, the schizont, a large structure filled with the merozoites. The nucleus replicates several times, and ultimately, thousands of small, banana-shaped organisms called merozoites develop. This asexual process of reproduction is called schizogony. Once mature, the schizont ruptures, releasing its merozoites. The next step in the life cycle is species dependent, but usually the merozoites move farther down the intestine, penetrate a cell, and repeat the asexual process, but with smaller schizonts containing fewer merozoites. When released, the merozoites penetrate a cell, and some become macrogametes (ova), and some become microgametes (sperm). Once fertilization occurs, the oocyst is produced and passes in the feces to begin the life cycle again.

Although the life cycle is finite (e.g., only a given number of oocysts can be produced from a single oocyst infection), the reproductive potential is great for some species.

Species of *Cryptosporidium* have essentially the same type of life cycle. *Cryptosporidium* organisms inhabit the respiratory and intestinal epithelia of many hosts, including birds, mammals, reptiles, and fish. Dogs and cats develop an intestinal tract infection almost exclusively. Enteroepithelial (intestinal epithelial) development is limited to the luminal enterocytes; extraintestinal tissue cysts do not develop. The enteroepithelial life cycle begins with the ingestion of sporulated oocysts by a suitable host (Figure 17-20). After the ingestion of oocysts, eight sporozoites are released from each oocyst that penetrates intestinal epithelial cells. Asexual reproduction at the intestinal surface occurs with the production of merozoites that are released and penetrate other cells. Gametogony and sporogony occur, resulting in the production of thin-walled and thick-walled oocysts. Sporulated thick-walled oocysts are shed in the feces of an infected host and are immediately infective to a susceptible host. Thin-walled oocysts passed into the intestinal lumen rupture, releasing the sporozoites, which penetrate additional host cells and reinitiate the developmental cycle.

Species of *Sarcocystis* have essentially the same type of life cycle, except that carnivores act as hosts for the sexual stages (oocyst and sporocyst), and omnivores and herbivores act as hosts for the asexual (schizogony) stage. Infected carnivores pass a thin-walled oocyst, which will eventually rupture; the oocyst contains two small, thick-walled sporocysts in which four sporozoites have already developed and are immediately infective to the alternate host. Once ingested, the sporozoites are released and penetrate the epithelial tissue of the intestine. Generally, the sporozoites enter the circulatory system and begin the first asexual (schizogony) phase in the kidneys. The first schizont releases its small, spindle-shaped organisms, which then enter cardiac or smooth muscle, in which they develop into rather large schizonts called sarcocysts. When sarcocysts are ingested by a specific carnivore, and most species are specific for each carnivore-herbivore, the small, spindle-shaped organisms penetrate superficial epithelial cells of the intestine and immediately begin the sexual phase, terminating as a thin-walled oocyst about 11 to 14 days after the ingestion of the infected flesh.

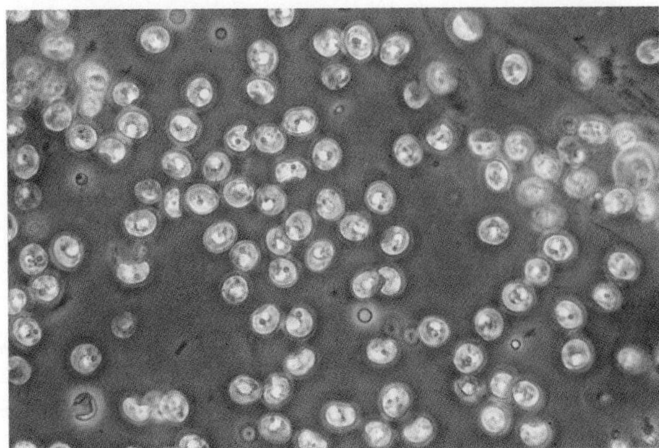

FIGURE 17-20 Oocysts of *Cryptosporidium* spp.

The life cycle of *Toxoplasma gondii* is similar to that of *Sarcocystis* spp. except that most animals are suitable hosts for the development of the asexual (schizogony) stages, but only the cat is suitable as a host for the sexual stages. The typical life cycle occurs when a cat ingests the small sporulated oocyst. In the intestine, the parasite goes through two asexual stages and then into the sexual phase, producing oocysts. If, for example, a mouse should eat the oocyst, the first asexual phase occurs in this animal. When a cat eats these schizonts, the parasite goes into one asexual cycle, in the cat's intestine, followed by the sexual cycle. If the first mouse is eaten by another mouse, *Toxoplasma* goes into the second asexual cycle in this mouse. When the second mouse is eaten by a cat, the parasites go directly into the sexual phase. The asexual cycle can go on indefinitely as animals eat the flesh of infected animals.

The diagnosis of an *Isospora, Cryptosporidium, Sarcocystis,* and *Toxoplasma* infection is based on recovery of the oocyst or sporocyst (for *Sarcocystis*) by a number of diagnostic procedures. A treatment is seldom administered for a *Sarcocystis* or *Cryptosporidium* infection, but when clinical disease occurs, a treatment is recommended for *Isospora* and *Toxoplasma* spp. infection. Control of *Isospora* and *Cryptosporidium* infections requires cleanliness, removal of the animal to clean premises, or both; however, the oocysts are extremely resistant to environmental conditions. Control of a *Sarcocystis* infection is generally not practiced for the carnivore host because it is considered nonpathogenic. If control is exercised, the best approach is to prevent the consumption of raw flesh from any source, including ground beef. The best control for *Toxoplasma* in cats is to prevent the consumption of raw flesh or carrion and to limit contact with feces of infected cats. Both *Toxoplasma* and *Cryptosporidium* spp. are zoonotic. *Toxoplasma* can cause birth defects in humans, and *Cryptosporidium* can produce a severe diarrhea, especially in immunocompromised individuals.

TECHNICIAN NOTE Both *Toxoplasma* and *Cryptosporidium* spp. are zoonotic. *Toxoplasma* can cause birth defects in humans, and *Cryptosporidium* can produce a severe diarrhea, especially in immunocompromised individuals.

The Integumentary System

Rhabditis strongyloides is a free-living saprophytic nematode that normally lives in moist soil and is considered to be a facultative parasite. These nematodes are normally free living in soil mixed with moist organic debris; however, under certain circumstances, they can invade mammalian skin and develop into a parasitic existence. The females produce eggs that hatch into first-stage larvae. These larvae invade the superficial layers of damaged or scarified skin, producing mild dermatitis. Dogs become infested by lying on contaminated soil. The skin may become reddened, denuded, and covered with a crusty material on the ventrum or medial (inner) surface of the limbs.

Adult *Dipetalonema (Acanthocheilonema) reconditum* is a nonpathogenic nematode that resides in the subcutaneous tissues of the dog. It may also be found within the body cavity. Occasional subcutaneous abscesses and ulcerated areas have been associated with this parasite. The intermediate host for this parasite is the flea, *Ctenocephalides felis*. Because this parasite is found in enzootic areas where *D. immitis* is present, it is often necessary to differentiate the microfilariae of these two parasites from each other Adults of *D. reconditum* rarely are recovered from their subcutaneous sites. Microfilariae may be recovered rarely in deep skin scrapings that draw blood. When subjected to the modified Knott procedure, the microfilariae of *D. reconditum* average about 285 μm long, with a buttonhook tail and a blunt (broom handle–shape) cranial end.

The Circulatory System

Nematodes (Roundworms)

Dirofilaria immitis, the canine heartworm, is a nematode and normally resides in the right ventricle and pulmonary arteries of its definitive host, the dog. Adult heartworms also may occur aberrantly and may be found in a variety of extravascular sites, including cystic spaces in the subcutaneous sites (Figure 17-21). When adult heartworms are found aberrantly, they are usually single, immature, isolated worms. Any female heartworms found within the cyst have not been fertilized by a male heartworm. Therefore such females are not gravid and do not produce microfilariae.

D. immitis and *D. reconditum* are the two filarial nematodes found commonly in dogs and the wild Canidae in the United States. *D. immitis* infections may also occur in cats and the wild Felidae, but not as commonly found as in dogs. The heartworm, *D. immitis,* is found primarily in the right ventricle and pulmonary arteries of the host, whereas *D. reconditum* is not found in the heart or pulmonary arteries, but instead is found in the subcutaneous tissues. Both nematodes produce a larval form called a microfilaria, which circulates in the blood (Figures 17-22 and 17-23). These filarial nematodes are found commonly in areas of the United States where the intermediate hosts (mosquitoes for *Dirofilaria* and fleas for *Dipetalonema*) occur; however, the heartworm is becoming more widespread as infected dogs and cats are brought into areas where the parasite is not normally found.

D. immitis males measure 12 to 20 cm, and the females are 25 to 31 cm long, whereas *D. reconditum* males are 9 to 17 mm long, and the females are 20 to 32 mm long. Both nematodes need an intermediate host to complete the life cycle. *D. immitis* uses several different species of mosquito, and *D. reconditum* uses the common dog and cat flea. Microfilariae when ingested by the intermediate host undergo reorganization and development to the infective third-stage infective larvae. Once infective, they go into the mouthparts of the arthropod and remain there until the arthropod feeds on the susceptible host. *D. immitis* infective larvae enter the tissue for 85 to 120 days and develop into young adults. The larvae then go to the heart and reach sexual maturity in

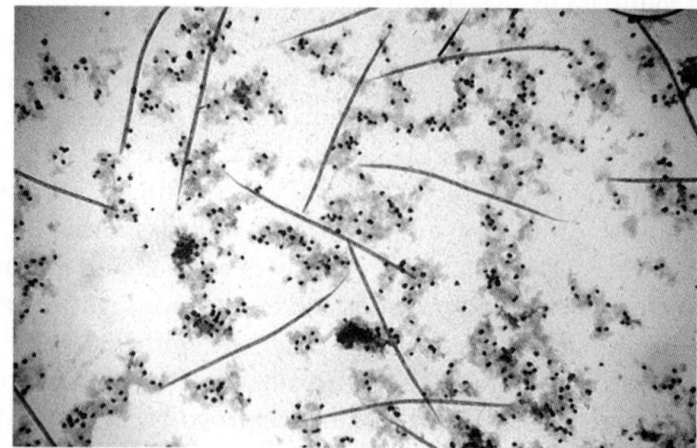

FIGURE 17-22 Microfilariae of *D. immitis* from a peripheral blood sample subjected to the modified Knott test. The microfilariae of *D. immitis* average 310 μm long. In contrast, the microfilariae of *D. reconditum* average 285 μm long.

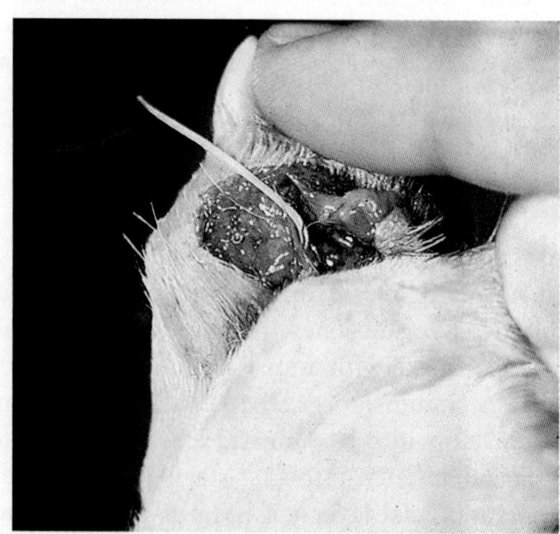

FIGURE 17-21 Aberrant adult *D. immitis* heartworm in a subcutaneous interdigital cyst in a dog.

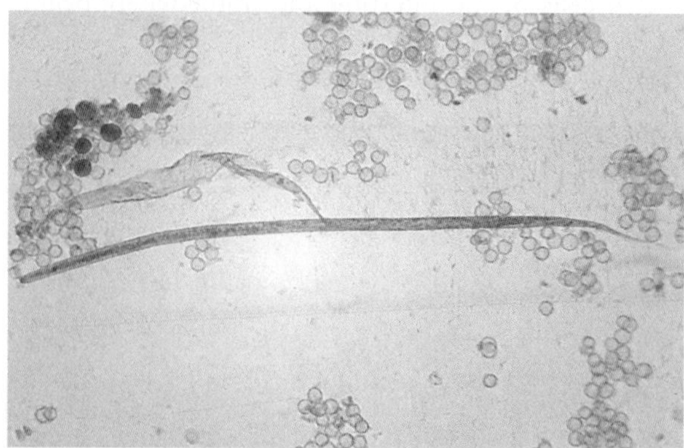

FIGURE 17-23 An individual microfilaria of *D. immitis* from a peripheral blood sample subjected to the modified Knott test. Note the tapered cranial end and straight tail. Microfilariae of *D. reconditum* have a blunt (rounded) cranial end and may exhibit a shepherd's crook (hooked) tail.

another 60 to 70 days, for a total of 145 to 190 days. Heartworms can also be aberrant or erratic parasites, getting "off course" en route to the heart and locating in sites other than the right ventricle and pulmonary arteries, such as the anterior chamber of the eye or in subcutaneous cysts in the skin. *D. reconditum* apparently goes directly into the subcutaneous tissues to develop to sexual maturity.

> TECHNICIAN NOTE The heartworm, *D. immitis,* is found primarily in the right ventricle and pulmonary arteries of the host, whereas *D. reconditum* is not found in the heart or pulmonary arteries, but instead is found in the subcutaneous tissues. Both nematodes produce a larval form called a microfilaria, which circulates in the blood.

A microfilaria of *D. immitis* is 295 to 325 μm long (average = 313 μm) and 6 to 7 μm in diameter (average = 6.9 μm), whereas a microfilaria of *D. reconditum* is somewhat shorter and more slender, measuring 250 to 288 μm in length (average = 276 μm) and 4.5 to 5.5 μm in diameter (average = 4.6 μm).

The diagnosis of heartworm disease in the dog is usually based on the identification of microfilariae in the peripheral circulation. Various techniques have been used to detect microfilariae, including the fresh blood-saline preparation; the capillary hematocrit tube test; and modified Knott test (or the filtration concentration) test. Fresh blood-saline preparations are helpful in differentiating *D. immitis* and *D. reconditum* microfilariae. *D. immitis* microfilariae move in place without directional motion, whereas *D. reconditum* microfilariae have a directional movement across the microscopic viewing field. Concentration tests are best used for the detection of *D. immitis* microfilariae because they are much more accurate than fresh blood-saline preparations or capillary hematocrit tube tests. Occult heartworm infections (adult heartworms without circulating microfilariae) occur in approximately 25% of dogs and 90% of cats. Several serologic tests are available in commercial kits to test sera of dogs and cats for occult infection; these commercial kits use the ELISA as the basis for diagnosis. The treatment of a *D. reconditum* infection is unimportant because these parasites are nonpathogenic. The treatment for a *D. immitis* infection requires the use of an agent effective against adult heartworms, followed by a microfilaricide. Control of *D. immitis* necessitates daily or monthly heartworm preventive therapy and mosquito control in enzootic areas.

Trematodes (Flukes)

Heterobilharzia americana, the canine schistosome, is a blood fluke that parasitizes the mesenteric veins of the small and large intestines and the portal veins of the dog (Figure 17-24). The blood flukes, or schistosomes, are unique flukes in that they are not hermaphroditic (most flukes are hermaphroditic). Among the blood flukes, there are separate sexes; therefore there are male schistosomes and female schistosomes. Because these flukes reside in the fine branches of the mesenteric veins, it is only natural that they should be long and slender. Females may be as long as 9 mm, and males are about 6.5 mm in length. This fluke is enzootic in the mud flats of the Mississippi delta and the coastal swampland of Louisiana. Although *H. americana* inhabits the blood vasculature, it manifests its presence by a bloody diarrhea. Infected dogs also exhibit emaciation and anorexia. The diagnosis is by the identification of the thin-shelled egg, about 80 by 50 μm, which contains a miracidium.

The Respiratory System

Nematodes (Roundworms)

Aelurostrongylus abstrusus is the feline lungworm. The adults live in the terminal respiratory bronchioles and alveolar ducts, where they form small egg nests or nodules. The eggs of this parasite are forced into the lung tissue, where they hatch to form characteristic first-stage larvae, approximately 360 μm long. Each larva has a tail with an S-shape bend and a dorsal spine (Figure 17-25). Characteristic larvae on fecal flotation or the Baermann technique can determine their presence. Recovering the larvae on tracheal washing is also possible.

Filaroides (Oslerus) osleri, Filaroides hirthi, and *Filaroides milksi,* the canine "lungworms," are found in the trachea, the

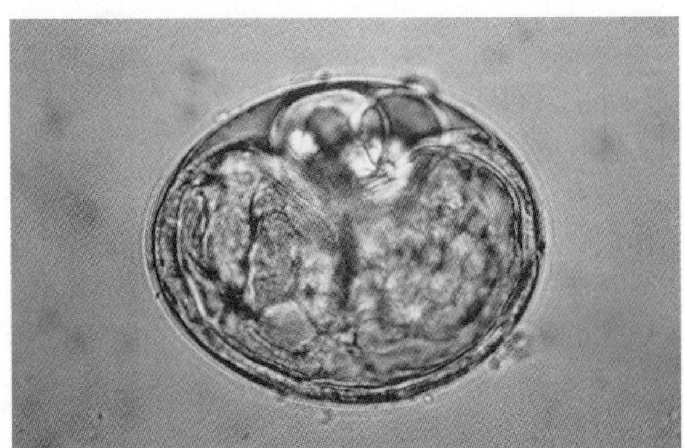

FIGURE 17-24 Characteristic thin-shell ovum of *H. americanum.* These ova are approximately 80 by 50 μm and contain a miracidium.

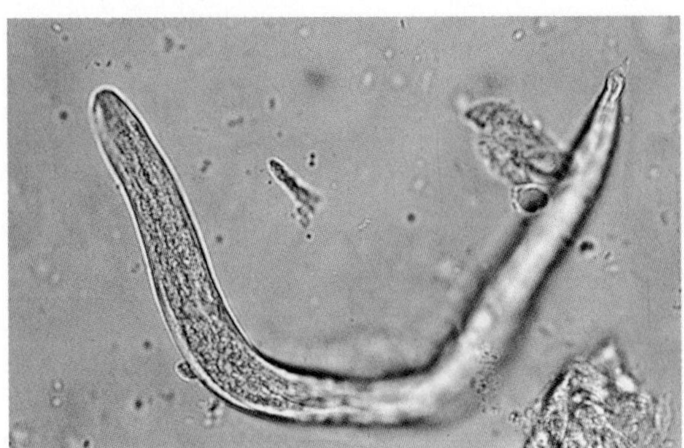

FIGURE 17-25 Characteristic first-stage larva of *A. abstrusus,* the feline lungworm. The diagnosis is accomplished by finding these characteristic larvae on fecal flotation or by using the Baermann technique.

lung parenchyma, and the bronchioles of canids, respectively. The larva is 232 to 266 μm long and has a short, S-shape tail. *Filaroides* spp. are unique among the nematodes in that their first-stage larvae are immediately infective for the canine definitive host. No period of development is required outside the host. The diagnosis is by finding these characteristic larvae on fecal flotation or by using the Baermann technique. Figure 17-26 shows the unique infective larvae of *F. osleri*. Nodules of *F. osleri* are usually found at the bifurcation of the trachea, where they can be observed via an endoscopic examination.

Eucoleus aerophilus (Capillaria aerophila) is a capillarid nematode found in the trachea and bronchi of both dogs and cats. The prepatent period is approximately 40 days. In standard fecal flotations, eggs of *Eucoleus* spp. are often confused with those of *Trichuris* spp. (whipworms). Eggs of *E. aerophilus* are smaller than whipworm eggs (59 to 80 μm by 30 to 40 μm), more broadly barrel shape, and lighter in color. The egg also has a rough outer surface with a netted appearance.

Trematodes (Flukes)

Adult *Paragonimus kellicotti* are flukes found in cystic spaces within the lung parenchyma of both dogs and cats. These cystic spaces connect to the terminal bronchioles. The eggs are found in sputum or feces. Adult flukes are thick, brownish-red flukes measuring up to 16 mm long by 8 mm wide. Eggs are yellowish brown, with a rather distinct operculum. The eggs are 75 to 117 μm by 42 to 67 μm; the shell at the pole opposite the operculum is somewhat thickened. See Figure 17-27 for the operculated ovum of *P. kellicotti*. These fluke eggs can be recovered using fecal sedimentation techniques; however, the eggs of *P. kellicotti* are usually recovered using standard fecal flotation solutions. The eggs of *P. kellicotti* can also be recovered in the sputum via tracheal washing. Cystic spaces in the lung parenchyma can also be observed via thoracic radiography.

The Urogenital System

Dioctophyma renale is the "giant kidney worm" of dogs. This largest of parasitic nematodes frequently infects the right kidney of dogs and gradually ingests the renal parenchyma, leaving only the capsule of the kidney. Eggs may be recovered by centrifugation and the examination of the urine sediment. They are characteristically barrel shape, bipolar, and yellow brown. The egg's shell has a pitted appearance. Eggs measure 71 to 84 μm by 46 to 52 μm. *D. renale* also may occur freely within the peritoneal cavity. When it is in this location, eggs are not passed to the external environment. The prepatent period is approximately 17 weeks.

Capillaria plica and *C. (Personema) feliscati* are nematodes of the urinary bladder of dogs and cats, respectively. The eggs may be found in urine or in feces contaminated with urine. Eggs are clear to yellow in color, measure 63 to 68 μm by 24 to 27 μm, and have flattened bipolar end plugs. Their outer surface is roughened. These eggs may be confused with those of the respiratory and gastric capillarids and with those of the whipworms.

The Eye and Adnexa

Thelazia californiensis is the "eyeworm" of dogs and cats. Adult parasites can be recovered from the conjunctival sac and lachrymal duct. An examination of the lachrymal secretions may reveal eggs or first-stage larvae. As mentioned previously, *D. immitis* may be recovered from a variety of aberrant sites, such as the anterior chamber of the eye.

The Musculoskeletal System

In the United States, canine hepatozoonosis, a protozoan, is most commonly diagnosed by a muscle biopsy rather than by the examination of peripheral blood smears for infected leukocytes. Muscle lesions consist of large cysts, pyogranulomas, and myositis. The cysts produced are round to ovoid and range from 250 to 500 μm in diameter. The center of the cyst demonstrates a basophilic nucleus surrounded by small basophilic bodies. Surrounding the nucleus and the basophilic bodies are concentric layers of fine multilaminated membranes, giving an "onion-skin" appearance. In most cases, no inflammatory response is associated with the cyst.

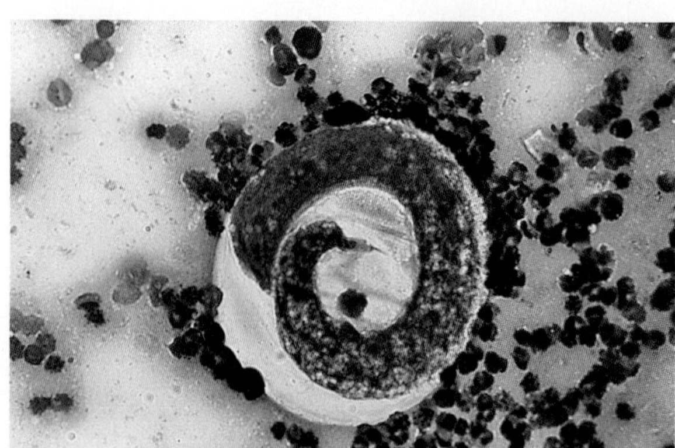

FIGURE 17-26 Characteristic infective first-stage larva of *F. osleri*, a canine lungworm.

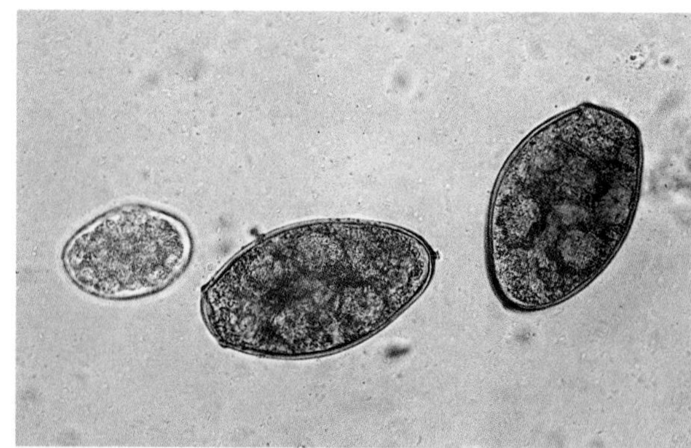

FIGURE 17-27 Characteristic ovum of *P. kellicotti*, the lung fluke of dogs recovered by standard fecal flotation. The eggs may be found in either sputum or feces, but often are recovered on fecal flotation. The yellowish-brown, operculated eggs measure 75 to 118 μm by 42 to 67 μm. *A. caninum* egg *(left)*.

ENDOPARASITES OF HORSES

The Gastrointestinal System

Horse Bots (Gasterophilus species)

Gasterophilus spp. is a common parasite of horses. However, it is unusual because the adult form of the parasite (a fly) is an ectoparasite and the larval form (bots) is an endoparasite. Larval *Gasterophilus* spp. parasitize the stomach of horses. Because these stages are larval or immature stages of the adult flies, no demonstrable egg stage may be recovered from horse feces; however, adult flies do deposit eggs on the hairs on the legs of horses (Figure 17-28). The larval stage exits the gastrointestinal tract via the feces; therefore this stage may be recovered from the feces. The brown larvae are up to 20 mm in length and have dense spines on the cranial border of each segment. A pair of distinct mouth hooks is found on the cranial end of the first segment and a spiracular plate on the caudal end. The veterinary technician should be able to grossly identify horse bots as *Gasterophilus* spp. (Figure 17-29).

Nematodes (Roundworms)

Stomach worms. *Habronema* and *Draschia* spp. are nematodes that are found in the stomach of horses. *Habronema microstoma* and *Habronema muscae* occur on the stomach mucosa, just beneath a thick layer of mucus; *Draschia megastoma* is often associated with large, thickened, fibrous nodules within the stomach mucosa. Larvae of both genera may parasitize skin lesions, causing a condition known as "summer sores." The prepatent period for these nematodes is approximately 60 days. Larvated eggs or larvae may be recovered on standard fecal flotation. The eggs of both genera are elongated, have thin walls, and measure 40 to 50 μm by 10 to 12 μm.

Ascarids. The ascarid of horses (*Parascaris equorum*) has a creamy white color. Male ascarids measure about 28 cm, whereas females are about 50 cm in length. The female ascarids produce dark brown, thick-shelled oval to spherical eggs that are resistant to environmental conditions. The eggs measure 90 to 100 μm in diameter (Figure 17-30). The equine ascarid is common throughout the United States, and the incidence of infection, especially among younger horses, is frequently high. The larval stage develops within the eggs and develops to the infective second-stage larva within the egg. This development to the infective stage requires about 2 weeks. When the eggs are ingested by the horse, the larvae are released in the intestine, penetrate the intestinal mucosa, enter the circulatory system, and pass through to the liver, heart, and ultimately the lungs, in which they develop for a short period. Subsequently, larvae pass up the bronchial tree, enter the mouth, and are swallowed. They are passed into the small intestine and mature. This entire life cycle requires 10 to 12 weeks. The diagnosis is readily made by using a number of techniques, and these parasites are amenable to treatment by several anthelmintics. Control is difficult because eggs are extremely resistant to environmental conditions, and the coprophagous habits of foals tend to ensure infection.

The large and small strongyles. *Strongylus vulgaris, Strongylus equinus,* and *Strongylus edentatus* are the three species of "large strongyles," along with 40 species of "small strongyles" of horses. The 40 or more species of small strongyles, of which there are several different genera, are bloodsucking nematodes. Strongyles vary in length from less than 12 mm (small strongyles) to 38 to 47 mm (large strongyles). However, some small strongyles, such as *Triodontophorus* spp., are nearly as large as *S. vulgaris,* the smallest of the large strongyles. All of the strongyles produce similar thin-walled eggs, each of which contains 4 to 16 brownish-colored cells when deposited (Figure 17-31). Regardless of whether these endoparasites are small strongyles or large strongyles, their eggs are virtually identical. Identification to the species level is accomplished by fecal culture and the identification of larvae. Strongyle eggs are most often observed in a standard fecal flotation. They measure approximately 70 to 90 μm by 40 to 50 μm. When these characteristic eggs are found on fecal flotation, the observation is recorded as "strongyle-type" ova, rather than as a particular species of strongyle.

All of the equine strongyles are common in horses throughout the United States, and the incidence of infection is generally high. The small strongyles that have been studied have a simple, direct life cycle. The eggs pass in feces, and first-stage larvae develop within the eggs. Once developed,

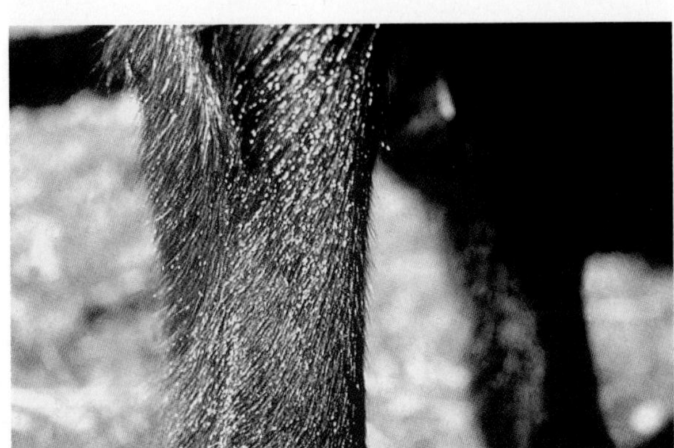

FIGURE 17-28 Numerous eggs cemented to forelimb of a horse.

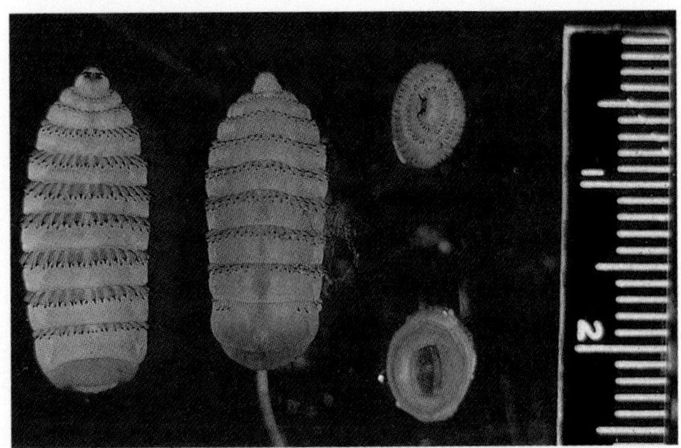

FIGURE 17-29 Final larval stage of *Gasterophilus* species within feces of host.

the larvae hatch and undergo a free-living existence, developing and molting to second-stage free-living larvae. They then develop to third-stage larvae that do not feed and await ingestion. In ideal environmental conditions, development from the egg stage to the infective larval stage will occur in less than 1 week. Once small strongyles have been ingested, the larvae go to the cecum, penetrate the cecal mucosa, and develop for 1 to 2 weeks. The larvae return to the mucosal surface and mature in an additional 1 to 2 weeks. The species in the genus *Strongylus* all have very complex life cycles.

The development of the larval stages for large strongyles in the environment is the same as that for the small strongyles, and once ingested, large strongyles also penetrate the mucosa of the cecum and develop in a short period. *S. vulgaris,* the most important of the large strongyles, leaves the mucosa and migrates through the cranial mesenteric artery and its branches and develops in the lumen of the arteries over the next 6 months, becoming a young adult. It then returns to the cecum and matures; the entire prepatent period (the period after ingestion and before eggs pass in feces) requires about 180 to 200 days. *S. equinus* leaves the cecal mucosa and enters the peritoneal cavity. It then goes to the liver and develops into a young adult. The route taken back to the cecum is incompletely understood, but it may enter the pancreas. The entire prepatent period may be as long as 265 days.

S. edentatus leaves the mucosa and enters the subperitoneal tissue, particularly in the right dorsal flank. Eventually, it enters the venous circulation and goes to the liver. It leaves the liver and about 2 months later migrates in the mesenteries to the perirenal fat for an additional 3 months. It again migrates in the mesenteries to the large intestine, which it penetrates, and develops to maturity in the lumen of the cecum. The entire prepatent period requires 300 to 322 days. The identification of the strongyles can be accomplished by a number of techniques, and strongyles are amenable to treatment by several anthelmintics. Control is difficult because the parasites are prolific egg producers, and development of the larvae occurs rapidly. Control is best achieved by regular anthelmintic treatment and management regimen based on environmental conditions and by limiting the number of horses on the pasture.

> TECHNICIAN NOTE *S. vulgaris, S. equinus,* and *S. edentatus* are the three species of "large strongyles," along with 40 species of "small strongyles" of horses. The 40 or more species of small strongyles, of which there are several different genera, are bloodsucking nematodes.

Intestinal threadworms. *Strongyloides westeri* is a common parasite of horses, principally of foals 2 weeks to 6 months of age, and is widespread across the United States. These nematodes are unique; only a parthenogenetic female (one that can lay eggs without copulating with a male) is parasitic in the host. Parasitic males do not exist. The life cycle is essentially the same as that of *S. stercoralis* of the dog, except that the parthenogenetic female produces thin-walled eggs containing first-stage larvae when deposited. These larvated eggs measure 40 to 52 μm by 32 to 40 μm. The diagnosis can be made by a number of techniques; however, fresh feces must be used because the eggs will hatch in older feces. Control requires good hygiene together with treatment because the parasite can be transmitted by the transmammary route. The prepatent period is 5 to 7 days.

Pinworms. The pinworm of horses, *Oxyuris equi,* is a white to slate gray-colored nematode with a slender, sharply pointed tail. Males are small, measuring less than 12 mm, and females are 75 to 150 mm long. The eggs are slender and somewhat flattened along one side (Figure 17-32). Frequently, the eggs contain first-stage larvae when deposited. The eggs are 90 by 40 μm, with a smooth, thick shell. Pinworms are common in horses in the United States. The life cycle is simple and direct. Female parasites living in the cecum pass out though the anal sphincter and deposit masses of eggs on the perineum. Eggs are cemented into masses with a gelatinous material. Eggs drop off, either singly or in masses, landing on the ground or feed and become infective in 3 to 5 days. Once ingested, the larvae are released in the small intestine, penetrate the intestinal mucosa, and develop for several days. Larvae then return to the mucosal surface, move to the large intestine, and reach maturity about 50 days after the initial ingestion of the eggs. A diagnosis can be made effectively only by the cellophane tape

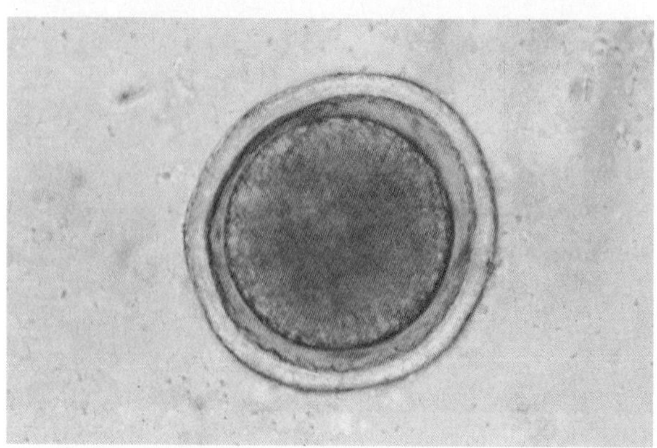

FIGURE 17-30 *Parascaris equorum* (equine roundworm).

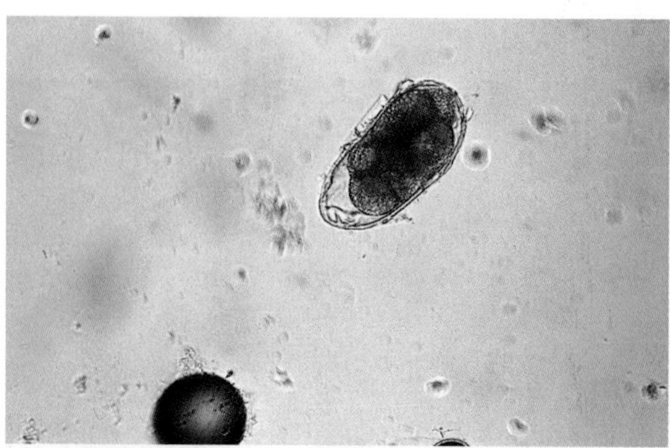

FIGURE 17-31 Strongyle-type ovum of horses. These eggs contain an 8- to 16-cell morula and measure approximately 70 to 90 μm by 40 to 50 μm.

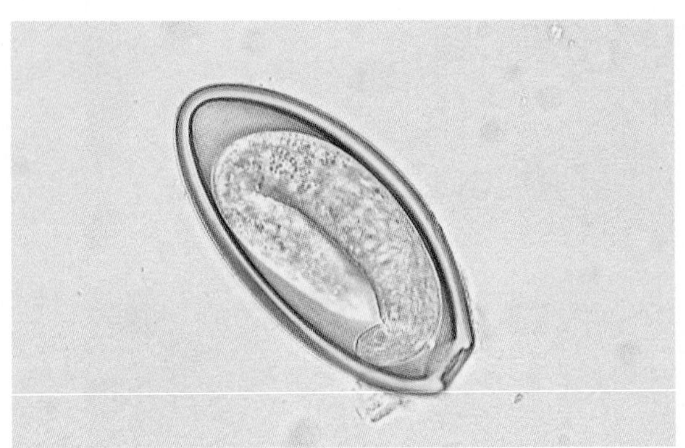

FIGURE 17-32 Characteristic ovum of *O. equi*, the pinworm of horses.

technique. Pinworms are amenable to treatment with several anthelmintics. Control is difficult because of the coprophagous habits of foals. The prepatent period is approximately 4 to 5 months. The diagnosis is by finding the characteristic eggs on a microscopic examination of cellophane tape impressions or by scraping the surface of the anus.

Cestodes (Tapeworms)

Anoplocephala perfoliata, Anoplocephala magna, and *Paranoplocephala mamillana* are the equine tapeworms. *A. perfoliata* is found in the small and large intestine and cecum. *A. magna* is found in the small intestine and occasionally the stomach. *P. mamillana* also is found in the small intestine and occasionally the stomach. They are broad, thick, and white and vary in length from about 2.5 cm *(A. perfoliata)* to about 75 cm *(A. magna)*. *P. mamillana,* the dwarf tapeworm, is only 4 to 6 mm in length. The eggs of *A. perfoliata* have thick walls, with one or more flattened sides, and measure 65 to 80 μm in diameter. Those of *A. magna* are similar, but slightly smaller, measuring 50 to 60 μm. The eggs of *P. mamillana* are oval and have thin walls, measuring 51 to 37 μm. Eggs of all three species have a trilayer egg shell, with the innermost lining called the pyriform apparatus. The life cycles of all three species are similar in that the eggs are ingested by a free-living mite for further development. Within the mite, a microscopic larval form, the cysticercoid, develops to the infective form in 2 to 4 months. Once ingested by the horse, the larval form is released from the mite and develops to an adult tapeworm in 6 to 10 weeks. A treatment or control is seldom practiced.

Protozoans (Unicellular Organisms)

Eimeria leuckarti is a coccidian found in the small intestine of horses. This protozoan demonstrates unique, large oocysts (80 to 87 μm by 55 to 60 μm) with a thick wall, a distinct micropyle, and a dark brown color. These oocysts can be recovered on fecal flotation and are the largest coccidian oocysts. They are frequently observed on a histopathologic examination. The prepatent period ranges from 15 to 33 days.

Protozoans (unicellular organisms) of the circulatory system. *Babesia equi* and *Babesia caballi* are intracellular parasites found within the RBCs of horses. These are also referred to as the "equine piroplasms." The diagnosis is by observing basophilic, pear-shape trophozoites in RBCs on stained blood smears. Trophozoites of *B. equi* may be round, amoeboid, or pyriform. Four organisms may be joined, giving the effect of a Maltese cross. Individual organisms are 2 to 3 μm long. Trophozoites of *B. caballi* are pyriform, round, or oval and 2 to 4 μm long. These occur characteristically in pairs at acute angles to each other.

The Respiratory System

Dictyocaulus arnfieldi, the "equine lungworm," is found in the bronchi and bronchioles of horses, mules, and donkeys. Its eggs are ellipsoid and embryonated, measuring approximately 80 to 100 μm by 50 to 60 μm. Eggs can be recovered on fecal flotation of fresh (less than 24 hours old) feces. Larvae hatch from the eggs within a few hours after feces are passed. The prepatent period for the equine lungworm is 42 to 56 days.

The Eye and Adnexa

Thelazia lacrymalis is the "eyeworm" of horses throughout the world. Adult parasites may be recovered from the conjunctival sac and lacrimal duct. An examination of the lacrimal secretions may reveal eggs or first-stage larvae. Also in the eye of horses, the unsheathed microfilariae of *Onchocerca cervicalis* have been incriminated as causing periodic ophthalmia and blindness. These may be detected by an ophthalmic examination.

The Abdominal Cavity

Setaria equina is the "abdominal worm" of horses. Adults are found free within the peritoneal cavity. The sheathed microfilariae are 240 to 256 μm long. The diagnosis is by demonstration of microfilariae in blood smears.

ENDOPARASITES OF RUMINANTS

The Gastrointestinal Tract

Nematodes (Roundworms)

The trichostrongyles. The bovine trichostrongyles comprise several genera of nematodes within the abomasum and small and large intestine of cattle and other ruminants. Genera that produce "trichostrongyle-type eggs" are *Bunostomum, Cooperia, Chabertia, Haemonchus, Oesophagostomum, Ostertagia,* and *Trichostrongylus* spp. These seven genera (and others) produce oval, thin-shell eggs. The eggs contain four or more cells and are 70 to 120 μm long. Some of these ova may be identified to their respective genera; however, the identification is usually difficult because mixed infections of bovine trichostrongyles are quite common in ruminants (Figure 17-33).

Nematodirus spp. and *Marshallagia* spp. are also "bovine trichostrongyles"; however, the eggs are much larger than those of the genera mentioned previously. These eggs are the largest in the trichostrongyle family. Figure 17-34 shows the large eggs of *Nematodirus* spp. In a standard fecal flotation, the eggs of *Nematodirus* spp. are large (150 to 230 μm

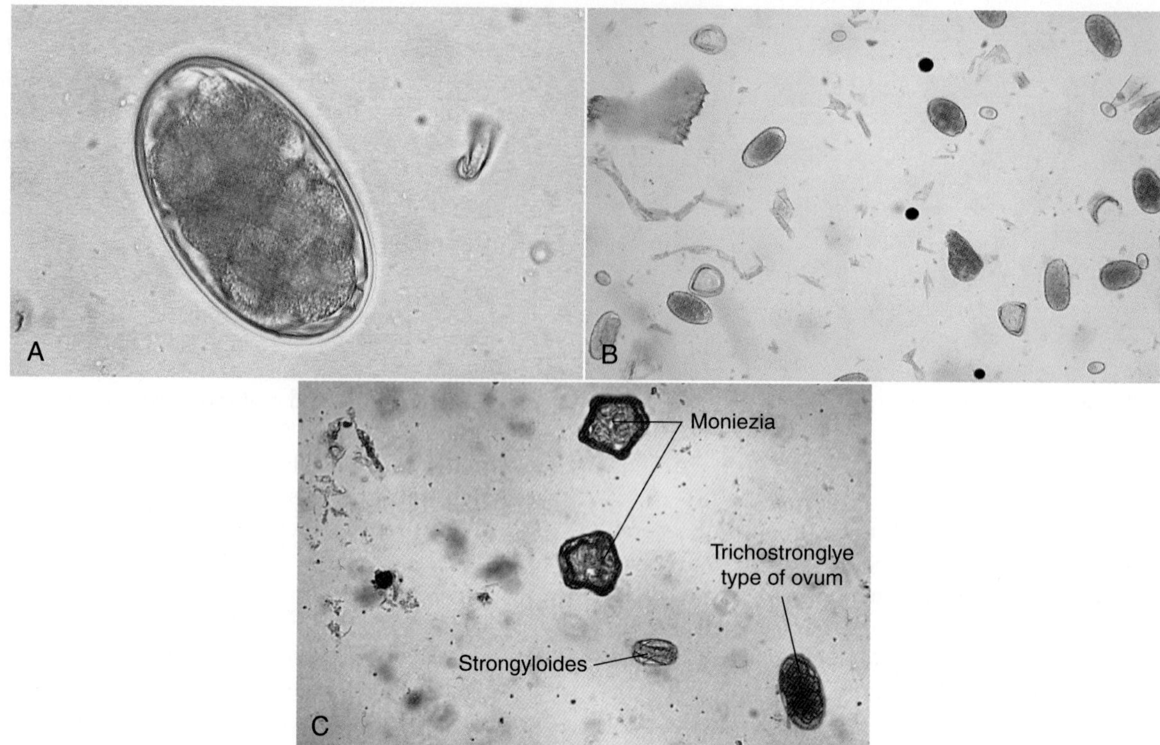

FIGURE 17-33 Characteristic trichostrongylus-type ova of the bovine trichostrongyles.

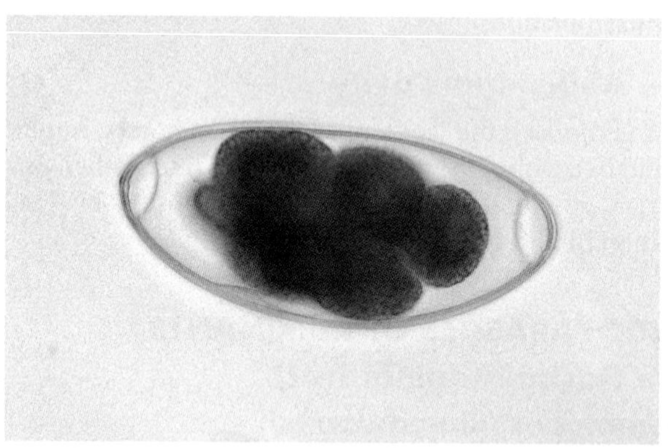

FIGURE 17-34 Characteristic large ova of *Nematodirus* spp.

by 80 to 100 μm) and have tapering ends and four to eight cells. The eggs of *Marshallagia* spp. also are large (160 to 200 μm by 75 to 100 μm), have parallel sides and rounded ends, and contain 16 to 32 cells.

The life cycles, though somewhat variable among these species of bovine trichostrongyles, are similar. The first-stage larvae develop within the eggs and hatch to undergo a free-living existence. The larvae develop within the eggs and grow and molt to the third-stage infective form in less than 2 weeks. Once ingested by the host, the larvae generally penetrate the mucosa in the site that they normally inhabit (stomach, small intestine, large intestine) and develop in a short period, then return to the surface of the mucosa and mature.

The bovine trichostrongyles are widely distributed throughout the United States, but the incidence depends on their ability to develop in the external environment. Some, such as *Haemonchus* spp., need considerable warmth and moisture; whereas others, such as *Ostertagia*, *Trichostrongylus*, and *Nematodirus* spp., will withstand colder, drier climates.

A diagnosis can be effectively made with most techniques. Upon the identification of the characteristic eggs, the veterinary technician should record the finding as "trichostrongyle-type egg." They should never be recorded by their individual genus names. The identification to genus and species usually can only be performed by fecal culture and larval identification.

Several treatments are available. Control is best achieved by a combination of treatment and pasture management in areas where there is an abundance of warmth and moisture to promote survival of the larval stages.

> *TECHNICIAN NOTE* The bovine trichostrongyles are widely distributed throughout the United States, but the incidence depends on their ability to develop in the external environment. Some, such as *Haemonchus* spp., need considerable warmth and moisture; whereas others, such as *Ostertagia*, *Trichostrongylus*, and *Nematodirus* spp., will withstand colder, drier climates.

Intestinal threadworms. *Strongyloides papillosus* is often referred to as the "intestinal threadworm." These nematodes are unique in that only a parthenogenetic female (a female nematode that lays eggs without copulating with a male) is parasitic in the host. Parasitic males do not exist. These females produce larvated eggs measuring 40 to 60 µm by 20 to 25 µm. Eggs usually are recovered in flotation of fresh feces. The prepatent period is 5 to 7 days.

Whipworms. *Trichuris ovis* is commonly called the "whipworm," infecting the cecum and colon of ruminants. The section on nematode parasites of the gastrointestinal tract of dogs and cats contains details regarding the unique gross morphology of adult whipworms. The egg of the whipworm is described as trichinelloid or trichuroid. It has a thick, yellow-brown, symmetric shell with plugs at both ends. The eggs are unembryonated (not larvated) when laid. Eggs of ruminant whipworms measure 50 to 60 µm by 21 to 25 µm.

Cestodes (Tapeworms)

Moniezia spp. are tapeworms found in the small intestine of cattle, sheep, and goats, and can reach lengths of 4 m. These tapeworms produce eggs with a characteristic cuboidal or pyramidal shape; under the compound microscope, these eggs appear to be square or triangular in silhouette. Two species are common, *Moniezia benedini* in cattle and *Moniezia expansa* in cattle, sheep, and goats. The eggs of both species can be easily differentiated using standard fecal flotation procedures. Figure 17-35 shows representative eggs of *Moniezia* spp. with the distinct pyriform apparatus as compared with a bovine trichostrongyle-type egg. The eggs of *M. expansa* appear triangular and measure 56 to 67 µm in diameter. The eggs of *M. benedini* appear square and are approximately 75 µm in diameter. The prepatent period for these tapeworms is approximately 40 days.

Thysanosoma actinoides is the "fringed tapeworm," found in the bile ducts, pancreatic ducts, and small intestine of ruminants in the western regions of the United States. *T. actinoides* is generally 25 to 30 cm long. Its life cycle is not known. Eggs of this tapeworm measure 19 by 27 µm. The diagnosis of a *T. actinioides* infection can be accomplished only by the observation of the pearly white bell-shaped proglottid with a prominent fringe on its posterior margin.

Trematodes (Flukes)

"Rumen flukes" are composed of two genera, *Paramphistomum* and *Cotylophoron*. These adult flukes reside in the rumen and reticulum of cattle, sheep, goats, and many other ruminants. The eggs of *Paramphistomum* spp. measure 114 to 176 µm by 73 to 100 µm, whereas the eggs of *Cotylophoron* spp. measure 125 to 135 µm by 61 to 68 µm. The prepatent period of *Paramphistomum* spp. is 80 to 95 days.

The common liver flukes of cattle and sheep are *Fasciola hepatica* and *Fascioloides magna*. Both trematodes are gray, flat, and leaflike in shape. *F. hepatica* is about 25 mm long, and *F. magna* is about 50 to 75 mm long. The eggs of both trematodes are similar and are large and yellow brown with an operculum or "lid" at one end (Figure 17-36). *F. hepatica* and *F. magna* are widespread throughout the United States, but only in wet, swampy, or subirrigated areas that will support substantial populations of the snail intermediate hosts. The natural hosts for *F. hepatica* are cattle and sheep, but the natural hosts for *F. magna* are members of the deer family. *F. magna* cannot complete its life cycle (by passing eggs into the environment) in cattle and sheep.

The life cycles of both trematodes are similar and quite complex. Eggs passing in the feces must land in water to develop. Inside each egg, a small, ciliated miracidium develops; the miracidium leaves the egg and penetrates the tissue of an aquatic snail, in which it undergoes asexual replication through larval stages called sporocysts and rediae, ultimately developing into cercariae. The cercariae leave the snail to encyst on vegetation to become metacercariae and await ingestion by the host. Once ingested, the juvenile fluke goes into the intestine, penetrates through to the body cavity, and penetrates the surface of the liver in which it wanders for several weeks. *F. hepatica* eventually enters the bile ducts, whereas *F. magna* will form a cyst wall around itself with an opening into a bile duct if it infects members of the deer family. In cattle, a calcite cyst is found, whereas in sheep, the parasite continues to wander throughout the liver. The eggs are heavy and will not float; consequently a sedimentation procedure is used for the diagnosis. An effective treatment

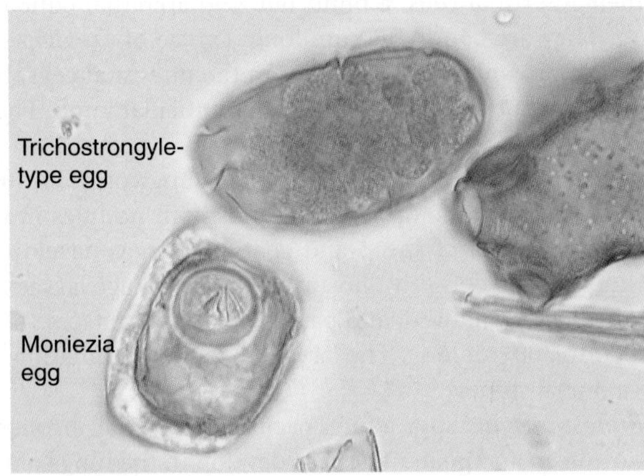

FIGURE 17-35 Characteristic ova of *Moniezia* spp.

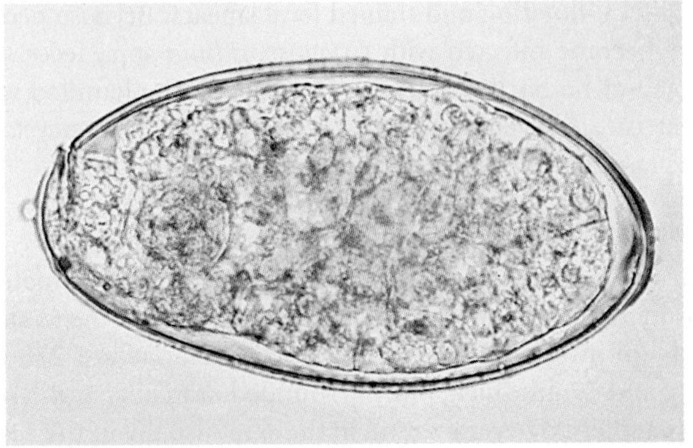

FIGURE 17-36 *Fasciola hepatica* (ruminant liver fluke).

is available. Control necessitates draining and drying wet, swampy pastures to prevent an overabundance of snails.

Dicrocoelium dendriticum is the "lancet fluke" of sheep, goats, and oxen. These tiny flukes reside within the fine branches of the bile ducts. The brown eggs have an indistinct operculum and measure 36 to 45 µm by 20 to 30 µm. Eggs may be recovered from feces using fecal sedimentation or a commercially available fluke egg recovery test.

Protozoans (Unicellular Organisms)

Several species of coccidia infect cattle and sheep, and all belong to the genus *Eimeria*. Coccidia are common throughout the United States, and most animals are infected with at least one of the *Eimeria* spp. The severity of the infection depends on environmental conditions (warmth, moisture), stocking intensity, age, and previous exposure. Oocysts of the *Eimeria* spp. sporulate in the environment and reach the infective stage in the same manner as do *Isospora* spp. *Eimeria* spp., however, develop four sporocysts, each of which contains two sporozoites, for a total of eight infective forms per oocyst. The life cycle of *Eimeria* spp. is almost identical to that of *Isospora* spp. The diagnosis may be accomplished effectively by a number of techniques. Several treatments are available for the clinical disease. Control is difficult because oocysts are highly resistant. The proper management for coccidiosis includes the prevention of overcrowding, prevention of contamination of feed and water, and the use of dry bedding.

Ruminants serve as host to many species of coccidia belonging to the genus *Eimeria*. It is often difficult to identify the individual species of coccidia because their oocysts are so similar in size and shape. The two most common species of coccidia in cattle, *Eimeria bovis* and *Eimeria zuernii*, can be differentiated on a standard fecal flotation. Oocysts of *E. bovis* are oval, have a micropyle, and measure 20 by 28 µm, whereas those of *E. zuernii* are spherical, lack the micropyle, and measure 15 to 22 µm by 13 to 18 µm. When oocysts are recovered on fecal flotation, the observation is usually recorded as "coccidia."

Cryptosporidium spp. is another coccidian parasite that parasitizes the small intestine of a variety of animals, including cattle, sheep, and goats. The sporulated oocysts in the feces are colorless and transparent and are extremely tiny, only 4.5 to 5.0 µm in diameter. The diagnosis is by standard fecal flotation and stained fecal smears. Because people may become infected with *Cryptosporidium* spp., feces suspected of harboring this protozoan should be handled with great care (see Figure 17-20 for features of the oocysts of *Cryptosporidium* spp.).

The Circulatory System

Elaeophora schneideri, the "arterial worm," is a nematode found in the common carotid arteries of sheep in the western and southwestern United States. Microfilariae are 270 µm long and 17 µm thick, bluntly rounded cranially, and tapering caudally. They are found in the skin, usually in the capillaries of the forehead and face. Filarial dermatitis is seen on the face, poll region, and feet of sheep. The diagnosis is by the observation of characteristic lesions and the identification of microfilariae in the skin. The most satisfactory means of diagnosis is to macerate a piece of skin in warm saline and examine the material for microfilariae after about 2 hours. In sheep, microfilariae are rare and may not be found in the skin of infected animals. A postmortem examination may be necessary to confirm the diagnosis. The prepatent period is 18 weeks or longer.

Protozoans (Unicellular Parasites)

Babesia bigemina is an intracellular parasite found within the RBCs of cattle. This parasite is a large piroplasm, 4 to 5 µm long by about 2 µm wide. It is characteristically pear shape and occurs in pairs, forming an acute angle within the erythrocyte. The intermediate host for this protozoan parasite is the tick, *Boophilus annulatus,* a tick that is reportable to the United States Department of Agriculture.

The Respiratory System

Dictyocaulus spp. are lungworms of cattle *(Dictyocaulus viviparus)*, sheep, and goats *(Dictyocaulus filaria)*. They are slender, white nematodes; males are 3 to 8 cm long, and females are 3 to 10 cm long. Females produce eggs containing first-stage larvae that hatch in the lungs. The first-stage larvae pass up the bronchial tree and are swallowed, passing with the feces. Lungworms occur in animals throughout the United States, but their distribution is discontinuous because the larval stages require a certain amount of warmth and moisture to survive. The life cycle is simple and direct. The first-stage larvae live on stored food granules, developing to the third-stage infective form within less than a week in optimal environmental conditions. Once ingested, the larvae enter the intestine, penetrate the intestinal mucosa, enter the lymphatic vessels, and develop for a short period in lymph nodes. They then go to the heart, enter the circulatory system, and then into the lungs to mature in a total of 25 to 30 days. Control is best achieved by proper management, ensuring that cattle and sheep do not occupy wet, swampy pastures. The prepatent period varies with the species, but is approximately 28 days.

The diagnosis is best made by use of the Baermann funnel technique. Larvae of *D. filaria* have brownish food granules in their intestinal cells, a blunt tail, and a cranial cuticular knob. They are 550 to 580 µm long. Larvae of *D. viviparus* also have brownish food granules in the intestinal cells, but have a straight tail; they lack the cranial cuticular knob. These larvae are 300 to 360 µm in length.

M. capillaris often is called the "hair lungworm." Adults are found within the bronchioles, mostly in nodules in the lung parenchyma of sheep and goats. The eggs develop in the lungs of the definitive host, and the first-stage larvae are coughed up, swallowed, and passed out with the feces. They are 230 to 300 µm long. The larval tail has an undulating tip and a dorsal spine.

Protostrongylus spp. adults occur in the small bronchioles of sheep and goats. The eggs develop in the lungs of the definitive host, and the first-stage larvae are coughed up, swallowed, and passed out with the feces. These larvae are 250 to 320 μm long. This nematode's larval tail has an undulating tip, but lacks the dorsal spine. The Baermann technique is used to diagnose a lungworm infection in ruminants.

The Urogenital System

Tritrichomonas foetus is a common protozoan parasite of cattle. This small, flagellated protozoan is equipped with three anterior flagella, an undulating membrane, and a trailing flagellum. Generally, *T. foetus* is a slender, pear-shaped organism. The bull acts as a carrier, with the parasite living on the surface of the penis or in the prepuce. When transmitted by coitus to the cow, the organism develops in the vagina and uterus, causing an abortion or fetal resorption. *T. foetus* multiples by binary fission; consequently, large populations can be generated in a short period. The cows, given a rest through two or three estrous cycles, will usually develop partial immunity. The diagnosis and treatment are performed on the bull. The diagnosis is difficult and complex. Control necessitates resting the cows and allowing immunity to develop, the treatment or elimination of infected bulls, and the purchase of virgin bulls for breeding.

The Eye and Adnexa

Thelazia rhodesii and *Thelazia gulosa* called the "eyeworms" are nematodes that parasitize the eyes of cattle, sheep, and goats. Adult parasites may be recovered from the conjunctival sac and lacrimal duct. The examination of the lacrimal secretions may reveal eggs or first-stage larvae.

The Abdominal Cavity

Setaria cervi is a nematode called the "abdominal worm" of cattle. Adults are found free within the peritoneal cavity. Their sheathed microfilariae are approximately 250 by 7 μm. The diagnosis is by the demonstration of microfilariae in blood smears.

Cysticercus tenuicollis is the metacestode or larval tapeworm of *T. hydatigena* and may be found attached to the greater omentum within the abdominal cavity of many ruminants. These cysticerci are usually diagnosed on a postmortem examination.

The Musculoskeletal System

Another metacestode is *Cysticercus bovis*, the bladderworm of *Taenia saginata*, the beef tapeworm of humans. It may be found within the musculature of the cattle that serves as the intermediate host. These cysticerci are colloquially referred to as "beef measles" and are usually diagnosed during a postmortem meat inspection. Humans become infected with the adult tapeworm by eating poorly cooked beef.

ENDOPARASITES OF SWINE

The Gastrointestinal System

Ascarops strongylina and *Physocephalus sexalatus* are nematodes known as the "thick stomach worms" of the porcine stomach. Both of these nematodes produce thick-wall, larvated eggs that may be recovered on fecal flotation. The eggs of both species are similar. The eggs of *A. strongylina* are 34 to 39 μm by 20 μm and have thick shells surrounded by a thin membrane that produces an irregular outline. The eggs of *P. sexalatus* are 34 to 39 μm by 15 to 17 μm. The prepatent period for both species is approximately 42 days. *Ascarops* and *Physocephalus* spp. use beetles as their intermediate hosts and rarely cause problems in swine.

Hyostrongylus rubidus is referred to as the "red stomach worm" of swine. The eggs are "trichostrongyle type"; (i.e., they are oval, thin-shell eggs). They contain four or more cells and measure 71 to 78 μm by 35 to 42 μm. These eggs may be recovered on fecal flotation. As with bovine trichostrongyles, a definitive diagnosis can be made only by fecal culture and larval identification. These eggs can be confused with the eggs of *Oesophagostomum*. The prepatent period is approximately 20 days.

Ascaris suum, the "swine ascarid" or the "large intestinal roundworm," is the largest nematode found within the small intestine of pigs. The eggs may be recovered on standard fecal flotation. They are oval and golden brown, with a thick albuminous shell bearing prominent projections. These eggs measure 70 to 89 μm by 37 to 40 μm (Figure 17-37).

Strongyloides ransomi, the "intestinal threadworm" of pigs, is found within the small intestine of pigs. This parasite is unique in that only a parthenogenetic female is parasitic in the host. Parasitic males do not exist. These females produce larvated eggs measuring 45 to 55 μm by 26 to 35 μm. Eggs are usually recovered in flotation of fresh feces. The prepatent period is 3 to 7 days (see Figure 17-6).

Trichinella spiralis occurs in the small intestine of many hosts, most notably the pig. Swine become infected with *T. spiralis* when they ingest infective larval stages (juveniles) in undercooked meat. The larvae mature into adults in the host's small intestine in a few weeks, and the female worms give birth to larvae. (The males die after fertilizing the females, and the females die after producing larvae.) The larvae enter the bloodstream of the host and eventually end up in the pig's musculature. See Swine Parasites of the Musculoskeletal System.

Oesophagostomum dentatum, the "nodular worm of swine," is found in the large intestine of swine. The prepatent period is 50 days. The eggs are "trichostrongyle type"; (i.e., they are oval, thin-shell eggs). They contain 4 to 16 cells and measure 40 by 70 μm. These eggs may be recovered on a standard fecal flotation. These eggs can be confused with the eggs of *Hyostrongylus*. As with bovine trichostrongyles, a definitive diagnosis may be made only by fecal culture and larval identification.

> TECHNICIAN NOTE *T. spiralis* occurs in the small intestine of many hosts, most notably the pig. Swine become infected with *T. spiralis* when they ingest infective larval stages (juveniles) in undercooked meat. *T. spiralis* is found in many species of carnivores and omnivores, but is often associated in humans with eating raw or undercooked pork.

Trichuris suis is commonly called the "whipworm," infecting the cecum and colon of swine. (See the section on nematode parasites of the gastrointestinal tract of dogs and cats for details on the gross morphology of adult worms.) The egg of the whipworm is described as trichinelloid or trichuroid. It has a thick, brown, barrel-shape shell with plugs at both ends. The eggs are unembryonated (not larvated) when laid. Eggs of porcine whipworms measure 50 to 60 μm by 21 to 25 μm. The prepatent period is 42 to 49 days.

Macracanthorhynchus hirudinaceus is the "thorny-headed worm" or acanthocephalan of the small intestine of swine. It is called "thorny-headed" because of its spiny proboscis, which it embeds as an anchor into the small intestinal mucosa of the host. The eggs have a triple-layer shell, are oval, and measure 67 to 100 μm by 40 to 65 μm. The eggs may be recovered on a standard fecal flotation. The prepatent period is 60 to 90 days.

Balantidium coli is the "ciliated protozoan" found in the large intestine of swine. Although commonly observed during a microscopic examination of fresh diarrheal feces, it is generally considered to be nonpathogenic. Two morphologic stages may be found in feces: the "cyst" stage and the motile "trophozoite" stage. Both stages may vary in size. This is a large protozoan parasite. The trophozoites may be 150 by 120 μm, with a sausage- to kidney-shape macronucleus. It is covered with numerous rows of cilia and moves about the microscopic field with lively motility. The cyst is spherical to ovoid and 40 to 60 μm in diameter, with a slight greenish-yellow color. Both of these stages may be easily recognized by a microscopic examination of the intestinal contents or fresh, diarrheal feces. Figure 17-38 shows the trophozoite stage of *B. coli* in histopathologic section.

Cryptosporidium is another coccidian parasite that parasitizes the small intestine of a wide variety of animals, including swine. The sporulated oocysts in the feces are colorless and transparent and measure only 4.5 to 5.0 μm. The diagnosis is by standard fecal flotation and stained fecal smears. Because people may become infected with *Cryptosporidium* spp., feces suspected of harboring this protozoan should be handled with great care (see Figure 17-20).

Isospora suis is the coccidian that parasitizes the small intestine of swine, especially young piglets. Oocysts are usually found on flotation of fresh feces. They are subspherical, lack a micropyle, and measure 18 to 21 μm (Figure 17-39). A postmortem diagnosis in piglets exhibiting clinical signs, but not shedding oocysts, can be achieved by a direct smear of the jejunum stained with Diff-Quik. The diagnosis is by the observation of the banana-shape merozoites. The prepatent period is 4 to 8 days.

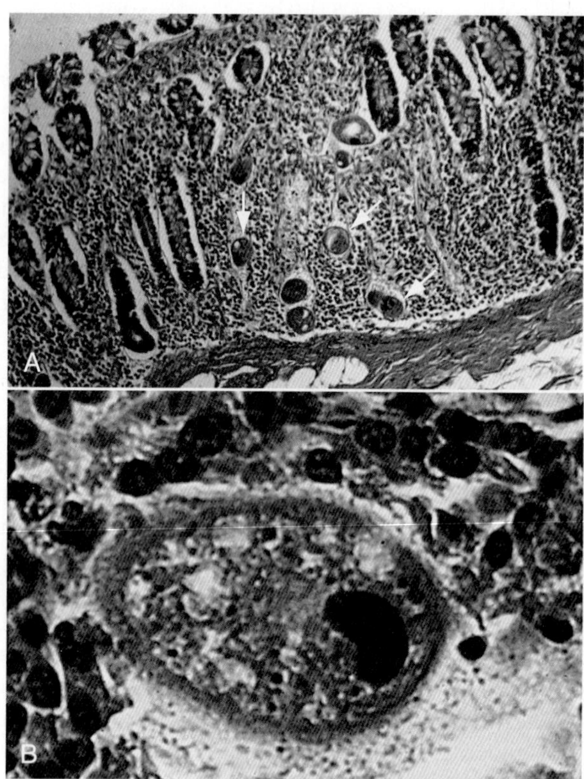

FIGURE 17-38 A, *B. coli* of swine in histopathologic section. This photomicrograph was taken at low magnification. Note that *B. coli* is quite large and easily visible *(arrows)*. B, *B. coli* of swine in histopathologic section. This photomicrograph was taken at higher magnification than A.

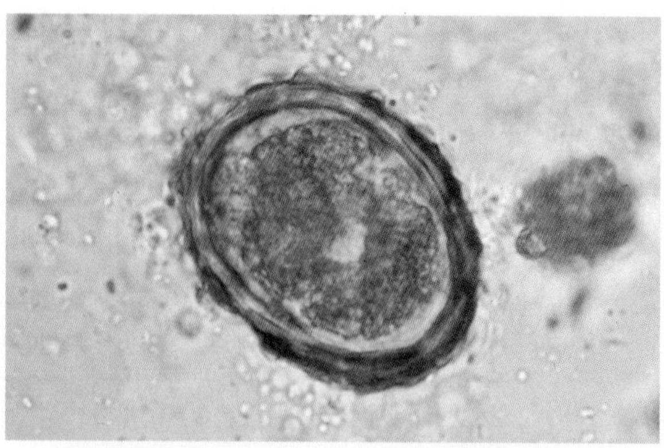

FIGURE 17-37 *Ascaris suum* (swine roundworm).

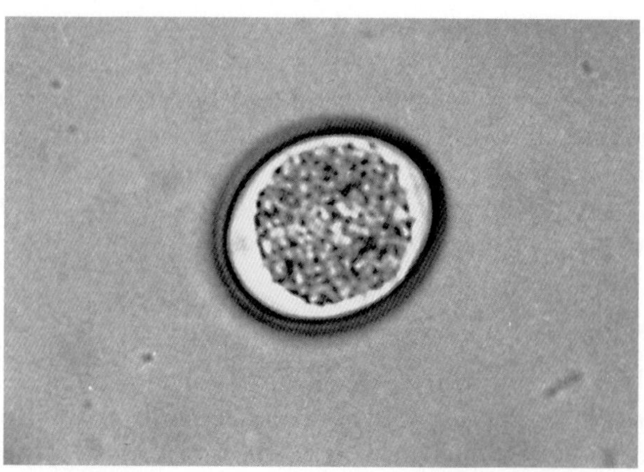

FIGURE 17-39 Oocyst of *I. suis* (swine coccidia).

Parasites of the Respiratory System

Metastrongylus apri, the "swine lungworm," is found within the bronchi and bronchioles of pigs. The oval, thick-wall eggs measure 60 by 40 µm and contain larvae. Eggs can be recovered on fecal flotation using a flotation medium with a specific gravity above 1.25 or by using the fecal sedimentation technique. The prepatent period is approximately 24 days.

The Urinary System

Stephanurus dentatus, the "swine kidney worm," is found in the kidney, ureters, and perirenal tissues of pigs. The eggs are "strongylus-type"; (i.e., they are oval, thin-shell eggs, containing 4 to 16 cells, and measuring 90 to 120 µm by 43 to 70 µm). Eggs may be recovered from the urine using urine sedimentation. The prepatent period is extremely long, approximately 9 to 24 months.

The Musculoskeletal System

T. spiralis is found in many species of carnivores and omnivores, but is often associated with raw or undercooked pork. Animals (including humans) become infected with *T. spiralis* when they ingest infective larval stages (juveniles) in meat. The larvae mature into adults in the host's small intestine in a few weeks, and the female worms give birth to larvae. (The males die after fertilizing the females, and the females die after producing larvae.) The larvae enter the bloodstream of the host and eventually migrate to the pig's musculature. Within the muscles, the larvae mature into infective encysted larvae. The next host becomes infected when it eats these larvae. Trichinosis is probably best known as a parasite that humans contract from eating raw or undercooked pork. It is usually diagnosed through proper meat inspection. Most recent outbreaks of trichinosis in the United States have been traced to pork products from pigs that have not been inspected and that have been slaughtered privately.

Cysticercus cellulosae, the bladderworm (larval or metacestode stage) of *Taenia solium,* the pork tapeworm of humans, may be found within the musculature of the porcine intermediate host. These cysticerci are colloquially referred to as "pork measles" and are usually diagnosed during a postmortem meat inspection. Humans become infected with the adult tapeworm *T. solium* by eating poorly cooked pork containing cysticerci. Humans may become infected with *C. cellulosae* in the muscles or within nervous tissue, such as the brain or the eye, by ingesting the eggs of *T. solium.*

DIAGNOSIS OF ENDOPARASITISM

Parasites can infect the oral cavity, esophagus, stomach, small and large intestines, and other internal organs of domesticated animals. The detection of the presence of these parasites involves the collection and microscopic examination of feces. The diagnosis is usually by finding life cycle stages of the parasite within the feces. These stages include eggs, oocysts, larvae, segments (tapeworms), and adult organisms. Veterinary technicians may perform the following procedures to detect parasitic infections.

COLLECTION OF FECAL SAMPLES

Fecal samples collected for routine examination should be as fresh as possible. Specimens that cannot be examined within a few hours of excretion should be refrigerated or mixed with equal parts of 10% formalin. The need for fresh feces stems from the fact that eggs, oocysts, and other life-cycle stages may be altered by their further development, making diagnosis extremely difficult.

Small Animal Fecal Samples

Several methods are used for collecting feces from companion animals. An owner may collect a fecal sample immediately after the animal has defecated. The feces may be stored in any type of container, such as a zippered plastic bag or a clean, small jar with a tight cap. Veterinary hospitals may dispense containers to their clients for this purpose. In either case, only a small amount of feces (1 tsp) is required for a proper examination by the technician. All specimens should be properly identified with the owner's name, animal's name, and species of animal.

Fecal samples also may be collected directly from the animal at the veterinary hospital, using a gloved finger or fecal loop. If a glove is used, the feces may remain in the glove, with the glove turned inside out, tied, and labeled. Samples collected with a fecal loop should be used for direct examination only because the amount collected is relatively small.

Large Animal Fecal Samples

Fecal specimens collected from livestock may be obtained either directly from an individual animal's rectum or from a number of animals to make up a pooled sample. Samples collected directly from an individual animal using a gloved hand can remain in the glove, with the glove turned inside out, tied, and labeled.

Pooled samples are collected from a number of animals housed together and then co-mingled in a single container. These samples are used to get an impression of the degree of infection within the group. Pooled samples can be collected in any type of container as long as it is clean and can be tightly sealed. These samples should be labeled with the species, pen or group number, owner, and time of collection.

EXAMINATION OF FECAL SAMPLES

Several precautions should be taken during fecal examination:

- Fecal samples are handled with care. The feces may contain parasites, bacteria, or viruses that are zoonotic (i.e., animal diseases that may be transmitted to humans). Appropriate clothing, such as a clean laboratory coat or jacket and latex gloves, should be worn during the laboratory examination. If gloves are not worn, hands should be frequently washed with soap and water. No food or drink should be allowed in the examination area. Likewise, workers should refrain from applying makeup or adjusting contact lenses. Laboratory coats should never be worn outside of the veterinary practice; this reduces the chances of spreading any infections.

- The laboratory area is cleaned thoroughly after the fecal examinations are completed. Spilled materials create a hazardous area in which to work and could pose a serious threat to staff members' health.
- Accurate and thorough records are maintained. Records should contain the date, owner's name, and any parasites found in the sample. If the sample's test results are negative, it should be recorded as such.

Gross Examination of Feces

Several characteristics of the feces also should be recorded and reported to the veterinarian. They are as follows:

- Consistency: Fresh feces should be somewhat formed, depending on the species of animal. Diarrhea or constipation could be the result of a parasitic infection.
- Color: Fecal color may be affected by the food an animal eats. Also malabsorption or a parasitic infection may alter the color of feces.
- Blood: Blood may impart a dark reddish-brown color to feces or it may appear as bright red streaks in the feces. In either case, blood may indicate a severe parasitic infection or other serious intestinal diseases. Blood in the feces is an important clinical finding and should be brought to the attention of the veterinarian. Digested blood has a dark, tarry appearance.
- Mucus: Mucus in the feces can be a result of digestive disorders or a parasitic infection. In either case, its presence should be reported to the veterinarian.
- Gross parasites: Adult parasites or tapeworm segments can be found in the feces. Adult roundworms resemble strings of spaghetti, whereas tapeworm segments look more like grains of cooked rice. Tapeworm segments may be identified by a microscopic examination. The segments of two common tapeworms infecting dogs and cats are shown in Figure 17-40.

Figure 17-41 shows common tapeworm segments, *Anoplocephala* spp. found in horse feces, and *Moniezia* spp., found in cattle feces.

Occasionally a client may submit a dried tapeworm segment to be identified. To identify the tapeworm species, the dried segments must be soaked in saline for 1 to 4 hours to rehydrate them. Once the segments are rehydrated, these may be identified by their unique size, shape, morphologic features, and the eggs contained within.

Segments of some tapeworm species do not contain eggs, and some segments may have expelled their eggs before the examination was conducted. In either case, a tapeworm segment may be identified as such by finding small mineral deposits (calcareous bodies) within the segment (Figure 17-42). This is done by crushing the tapewormlike segment

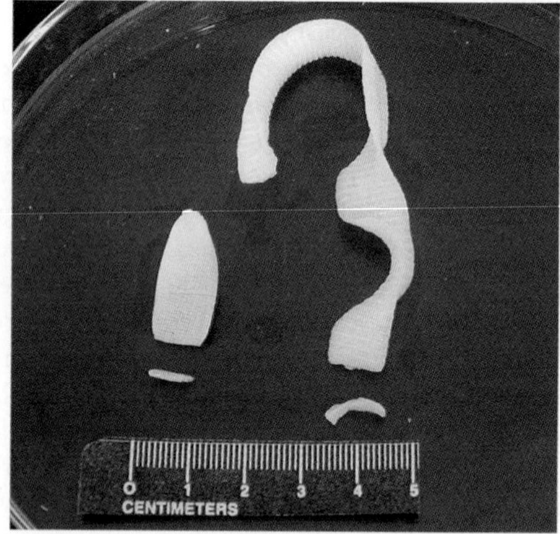

FIGURE 17-41 Chains and individually mature segments of tapeworms of horses, *Anoplocephala (left)*, and cattle, *Moniezia (right)*.

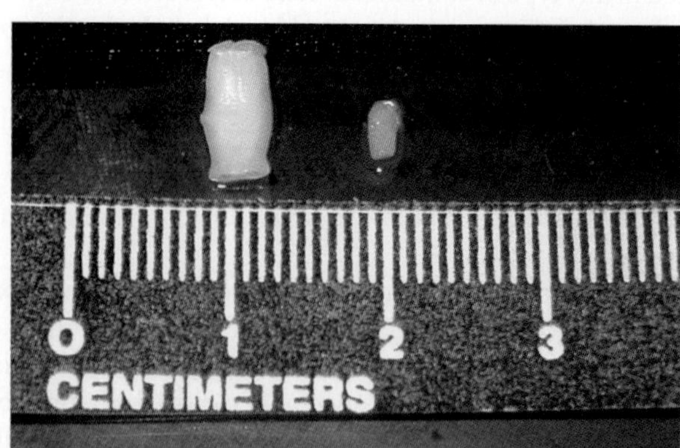

FIGURE 17-40 Mature segments of the most common tapeworms of dogs and cats. *Left, Taenia* spp. *Right, D. caninum.*

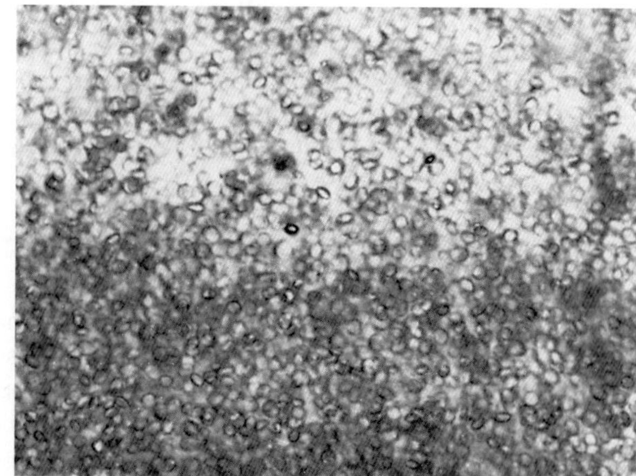

FIGURE 17-42 Microscopic calcium deposits (calcareous bodies) in tapeworm tissue.

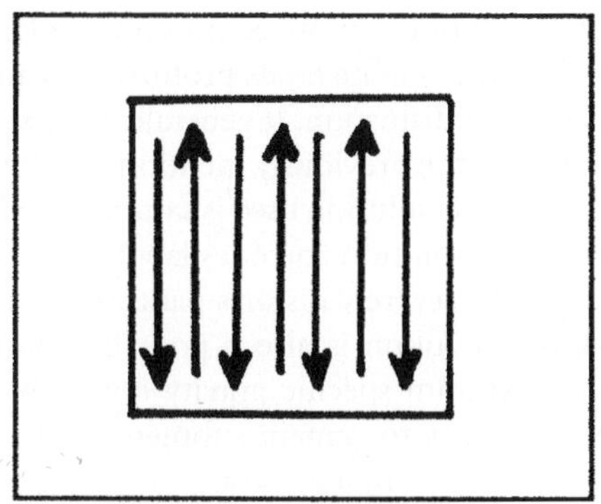

FIGURE 17-43 A scheme of movement of the microscopic field to examine the area under the coverslip thoroughly.

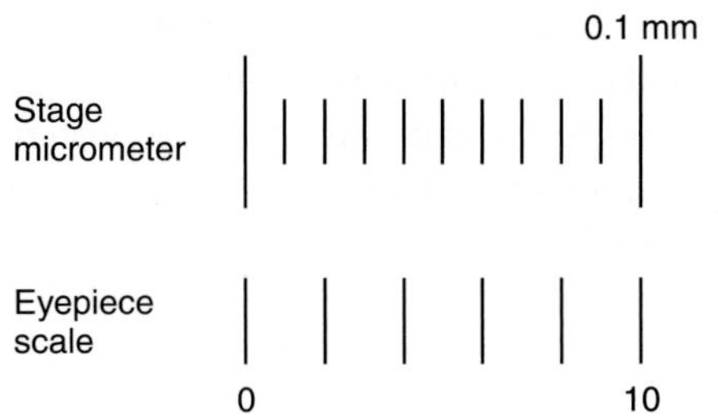

FIGURE 17-44 Stage micrometer *(upper scale)* and eyepiece scale *(lower scale)* used to calibrate the microscope.

between two glass slides and examining the material with a microscope.

Microscopic Examination of Feces

The microscopic examination of feces is the most reliable method to detect parasitic infections. A compound microscope with 4×, 10×, and 40× objectives is required for the proper examination of a fecal specimen. A mechanical stage is a necessity. An ocular micrometer is also recommended, but is not required.

Fecal specimens should be examined routinely using the 10× objective. The examination should begin at one corner of the slide and end at the opposite corner, moving over the slide in a systematic pattern (Figure 17-43).The microscope should be focused continually with the fine-tuning knob during the examination. The initial plane of focus should be that of air bubbles because most helminth eggs are found in this plane. Any material found during the initial scan, including parasite eggs, may be more closely examined using the more powerful objectives.

Calibration of the Microscope

The size of the various stages of many parasites is often important for correct identification. Some examples are *Trichuris* versus *Capillaria* eggs and *Dipetalonema* versus *Dirofilaria* microfilariae. Accurate measurements are obtained easily with the use of a calibrated eyepiece on the microscope. Calibration must be performed on every microscope to be used. Each objective (lens) of the microscope must be individually calibrated.

The stage micrometer is a microscope slide etched with a 2-mm line marked in 0.01-mm (10-μm) divisions (Figure 17-44). The veterinary technician should remember that 1 micron (μm) = 0.001 mm.

The eyepiece scale is a glass disk that fits into and remains in one of the microscope eyepieces. This disk is etched with 30 hash marks spaced at equal intervals. The number of hash marks on the disk may vary with different manufacturers, but the calibration procedure is the same for all.

The stage micrometer is used to determine the distance in microns between the hash marks on the eyepiece scale for each objective lens of the microscope being calibrated. This information is recorded and labeled on the microscope for future reference.

To begin the calibration procedure, the veterinary technician should start on low power (10×) and focus on the 2-mm line of the stage micrometer. Therefore 2 mm = 2000 μm.

The eyepiece is rotated so that the hash-mark scale is horizontal and parallel to the stage micrometer scale. The zero (0) point is aligned on both scales.

The point on the stage micrometer aligned with the "10" hash mark is determined on the eyepiece scale. For example, the 0.125-mm mark might align with the "10" hash mark.

This number is multiplied by 100. In the above example,

$$0.125 \times 100 = 12.5\ \mu m$$

This means that at this power (10×), the distance between each hash mark on the eyepiece scale is 12.5 μm.

These steps are repeated at each magnification (10×, 40×, 100×). The information is recorded on a label and attached to the calibrated microscope. For example:

Objective	Distance Between Hash Marks (μm)
10×	12.5
40×	2.5
100×	1.0

To measure an object, such as a parasite egg, one end of the egg is placed on the zero mark of the ocular scale, and the number of divisions to the other end of the egg is counted. The number of divisions counted is multiplied by the calibration factor for the objective used. For example, a trichostrongylus egg is 24 divisions long and 13.5 divisions wide when measured with the 40× objective. The calibration factor for the 40× objective is 2.5. Therefore the egg is:

$$24 \times 2.5 = 60\ \mu m \text{ long}$$

and

$$13.5 \times 2.5 = 33.75\ \mu m \text{ wide}$$

To measure a microfilaria, the head (the anterior end) is aligned with the zero mark of the ocular scale, and the number of divisions to the end of the tail (the posterior end) is counted. To measure round parasite eggs, the technician should measure through the middle of the egg at its greatest diameter. For more accurate measurements, the higher objective is used (40× instead of 10×).

Examination of Direct Smears

A direct smear of feces is used to rapidly estimate an animal's parasite burden. This procedure also is used to detect some of the motile protozoa found in feces.

Advantages of direct smears include short preparation time and minimal equipment required to run the procedure. Disadvantages include the small amount of feces examined, which may not be sufficient enough to detect a low parasite burden, and the amount of extraneous fecal debris on the slide, which could be confused with parasitic material.

A fecal sample for a direct smear preparation may be obtained from an animal using a fecal loop or a rectal thermometer (after measuring the animal's temperature). Either way, only a small amount of feces is needed.

Concentration Methods for Fecal Examination

The following methods are used to concentrate parasitic material in feces. A concentration technique makes it possible to examine a large amount of feces in a relatively short time. A low parasite burden can easily be identified. Two types of procedures are most often used in veterinary hospitals: flotation and sedimentation.

Fecal flotation methods are based on the specific gravity of parasitic material and fecal debris. Specific gravity refers to the weight of an object as compared with the weight of an equal volume of water. The specific gravity of most parasite eggs is between 1.100 and 1.200 g/ml, whereas the specific gravity of water is 1.000.

To allow for flotation of parasite eggs, oocysts, and other life-cycle stages, the flotation solution must have a higher specific gravity than that of the parasitic material. Several salt and sugar solutions work well for flotation. Most have a specific gravity of 1.200 to 1.250. In this range, heavy fecal debris sinks to the bottom of the container, and parasitic material rises to the top of the solution.

Sodium nitrate solution is the most common fecal flotation solution used in veterinary hospitals today. This solution is efficient for floating parasite eggs, oocysts, and larvae. It may be purchased with commercial diagnostic test kits or in individual aliquots. The major disadvantage of using sodium nitrate is the expense. Sodium nitrate also forms crystals and distorts eggs if allowed to sit longer than 20 minutes.

Another solution commonly used for flotation is saturated sugar solution. Sugar solution is inexpensive and does not crystallize or distort eggs. Sugar solution may be made anywhere and has a long shelf life. Although sticky to work with, spilled sugar solution may be removed with warm, soapy water.

Zinc sulfate solution is more commonly used in diagnostic laboratories. Zinc sulfate floats protozoal organisms with the least amount of distortion. It generally is used in combination with one of the previously mentioned solutions.

The least desirable solution used is saturated sodium chloride solution. This solution corrodes laboratory equipment, forms crystals, and severely distorts parasite eggs. Saturated sodium chloride solution is also a poor flotation medium because the maximum specific gravity obtainable is 1.200, allowing heavier eggs to remain submerged. A number of choices in flotation techniques exist.

> TECHNICIAN NOTE If testing multiple samples, the veterinary technician may want to use a numbering system to keep the samples in order. A number is assigned to the patient, and that number is written on the corresponding centrifuge tube with a marking pen. This minimizes the chances of error.

Standard fecal flotation. The standard or simple fecal flotation is one of the most common flotation techniques used in veterinary hospitals. This technique uses a test tube or vial, in which feces and flotation solution are mixed (Figure 17-45). A coverslip or microscope slide is placed on top of the test tube, and the unit is allowed to sit undisturbed. Any parasite eggs in the feces float to the top and adhere to the underside of the coverslip or microscope slide. The coverslip or slide is then removed and microscopically examined for parasitic material. Although the standard flotation technique is easy to perform, it is less efficient at floating parasitic material than the centrifugal technique, described later in this chapter.

Commercial flotation kits use the same principle as the standard flotation technique. These kits contain a vial with a filter; some also include prepared flotation solution. Examples of commercial flotation kits include Fecalyzer (EVSCO Pharmaceuticals, Buena, N.J.), Ovassay Plus (Synbiotics, San Diego), and Ovatector (BGS Medical Products, Venice, Fla.) (Figure 17-46). These kits are simple to use, but expensive when compared with the simple flotation technique. Some

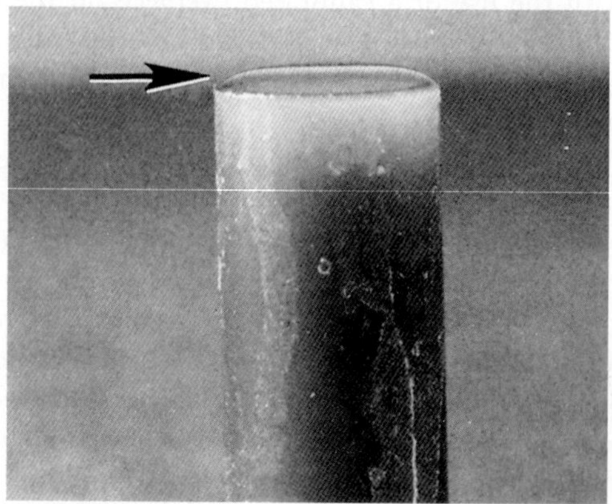

FIGURE 17-45 Vial filled with flotation solution, showing appearance of the meniscus.

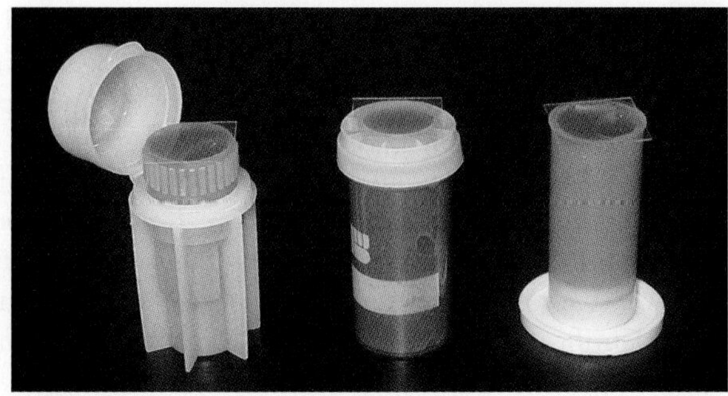

FIGURE 17-46 Three examples of commercial fecal flotation kits. *From left to right,* Fecalyzer, Ovassay, and Ovatector.

practices reduce the expense by washing and reusing the vials and filters; this practice should be discouraged.

Centrifugal flotation. Centrifugal flotation for parasite eggs, oocysts, and other parasitic material is the most efficient method available. It requires less time to perform than the standard flotation method. The only drawback to this procedure is that it requires a centrifuge with a horizontal (nonfixed) rotor that can hold 15-ml centrifuge tubes. If such a centrifuge is available, centrifugal flotation is preferred because it is easy to perform and samples can be run individually or in batches.

If testing multiple samples, the veterinary technician may want to use a numbering system to keep the samples in order. A number is assigned to the patient, and that number is written on the corresponding centrifuge tube with a marking pen. This minimizes the chances of error.

Fecal sedimentation. Fecal sedimentation concentrates parasite eggs, oocysts, and other parasitic material by allowing them to settle to the bottom of a tube of liquid, usually water. A disadvantage of this technique is that the amount of fecal debris that mixes with the parasitic material makes a microscopic examination somewhat difficult.

This procedure is used to detect heavy eggs that would not float in flotation solution or eggs that would become distorted by the flotation solution. Trematode (fluke) eggs are often considered too heavy for flotation and often found using fecal sedimentation. Although some flotation solutions can be adjusted to a specific gravity of 1.300 to float these eggs, such solutions are not routinely used because some distortion may occur.

Quantitative Fecal Examination

Quantitative procedures are used to determine the number of eggs or oocysts present in each gram of feces. These procedures are used as a rough indication of the number of parasites present within a host. Their usefulness is limited, however, by the fact that the various parasite species produce different numbers of eggs. Egg production by the parasites may be sporadic, and the number of eggs may not correlate with the number of parasites present. The last item is the most significant disadvantage because, in most cases, clinical signs of disease are caused by immature parasites that have not yet begun producing eggs or larvae.

Several quantitative procedures can be performed in veterinary hospitals. These include the Stoll egg count technique, the modified Wisconsin double centrifugation technique, and the McMaster technique. These procedures are fairly easy to perform; each requires its own specialized equipment.

Examination of Feces for Protozoa

All of the previously described procedures may be used to detect protozoal cysts. However, some protozoans do not form cysts and pass out of the host in the trophozoite form. Trophozoites are one-cell, motile organisms that lack the rigid wall of a cyst, making flotation without distortion or death of the trophozoite impossible. Therefore the direct smear technique, using saline and a stain, is the preferred procedure for the examination of a fecal sample for protozoal organisms.

In a direct smear, a trophozoite may be recognized by its movement. *B. coli,* a protozoan parasite found in the feces of pigs, is bean shape and covered with tiny hairs or cilia. It moves in a slow, tumbling fashion. *Giardia* spp. are tear shaped and have five to eight flagella. They move with a jerky motion. Trichomonads are pear-shaped organisms with multiple anterior flagella, which produce jerky movements. Amoebae move with a flowing motion, extending a part of the body (pseudopod) and moving the rest of the body after it.

Stains also may be used to recognize certain structural characteristics of trophozoites and cysts. Lugol's iodine and new methylene blue are common stains used with the direct smear procedure. These stains do not preserve the slide, but do facilitate the examination of the specimen, making identification easier.

If a protozoal parasite cannot be identified on direct smears, fecal smears containing protozoal trophozoites can be dried, stained with Diff-Quik, Wright, or Giemsa stain, and sent to a diagnostic laboratory. Many other procedures are used for staining and preserving protozoal trophozoites. Most of these procedures are used in diagnostic laboratories and are not explained here.

Special staining for coccidian parasites. Several coccidian parasites require special staining techniques for identification. Two procedures are discussed in this chapter.

The acid-fast staining technique is used to identify *Cryptosporidium* spp. in the feces. *Cryptosporidium* is a parasite of the gastrointestinal tract of many animals, including humans. The oocysts are 2 to 8 μm in diameter and are almost undetectable in flotation solution to the inexperienced eye. Acid-fast staining can aid detection of the oocysts in a fecal smear.

The second procedure uses Diff-Quik stain for the identification of *Isospora* spp. *Isospora* spp. are coccidia found in the gastrointestinal tract (especially the jejunum) of many animals, but they are of most concern in pigs. This parasite can cause the death of many piglets before any oocysts are found in the feces using conventional flotation methods. Therefore an intestinal mucosal scraping must be stained and examined for other diagnostic stages (schizonts, merozoites) of this parasite. This procedure involves scraping the mucosa of the jejunum and smearing the scrapings onto microscope slides. After the slides are air-dried, they are stained with Diff-Quik and examined with the oil-immersion objective.

For accurate results with either of these procedures, several samples should be examined. If such an examination is not possible, feces or intestines may be sent to a diagnostic laboratory. The collection and shipping of parasitic specimens are described later in this chapter.

Antigen tests. Antigen tests for *Giardia* and *Cryptosporidium* are available and may be used for the detection of these species.

Sample Collection at Necropsy

Necropsy (postmortem examination) is an important method of diagnosing many diseases, including parasitism. The types of lesions produced by immature parasites, any adult parasites found in the body cavity and tissues, and a histopathologic examination of infected tissues are used in diagnosis. Veterinary technicians are responsible for the samples collected, making sure they are contained, preserved, labeled, and shipped properly. Refer to Chapter 40 for more information about necropsy techniques.

Two methods may be used to recover parasites from the digestive tract at necropsy: the decanting method and the sieving method. With either method, the veterinary technician must separate the different parts of the digestive tract and work with the contents of each individually.

Parasites recovered from the digestive tract may be preserved in 70% alcohol or 10% neutral buffered formalin for later identification. Occasionally, bladderworms or cysticerci may be found attached to the viscera of domestic animals. A bladderworm is a fluid-filled, balloonlike structure that is actually a larval tapeworm. These should be handled with care because the fluid within the bladder can be allergenic and may also be zoonotic. To identify the parasites recovered, the veterinary technician should consult the references listed at the end of this chapter. If an in-hospital diagnosis is not possible, the samples may be preserved as previously described and sent to a diagnostic laboratory for identification.

Shipping Parasitologic Specimens

Any parasitologic specimen shipped to a diagnostic laboratory should be preserved with alcohol or formalin, unless otherwise directed by laboratory personnel. Specimens should be packaged in a leakproof container and sealed with Parafilm (American National Can, Greenwich, Conn.) or tape. If specimen containers are found leaking, the shipment will not be delivered. Feces can be sent fresh or mixed at a ratio of 1:3 with 10% formalin. Whole parasites or segments can be preserved in alcohol or formalin and placed in a leakproof container (clean small jar, medicine vial, clot tube).

All specimen containers should be labeled as to the site from which the specimen was obtained, the owner's name, the animal's species, name, or identification number, and the referring veterinarian (including telephone number and address). The labeled specimen container should be placed in a shockproof shipping container to prevent breakage during shipping. Styrofoam containers filled with shredded newspaper work well for shipping parasitologic specimens.

A cover letter should be included with the specimen and should contain a brief history of the animal, findings upon necropsy, and the reason for submitting the samples to the laboratory (e.g., fecal examination, special staining, and species identification). Without this background information, the diagnostic laboratory is unlikely to provide accurate results.

TECHNICIAN NOTE Any parasitologic specimen shipped to a diagnostic laboratory should be preserved with alcohol or formalin, unless otherwise directed by laboratory personnel. Specimens should be packaged in a leakproof container and sealed with Parafilm (American National Can, Greenwich, Conn.) or tape. If specimen containers are found leaking, the shipment will not be delivered.

Miscellaneous Procedures for Detection of Endoparasites

Cellophane Tape Technique

The cellophane tape technique is used to detect the equine pinworm, *O. equi*. Pinworms are nematodes found in horses, rodents and rabbits, and primates including people. They live in the colon and, as adults, migrate out the rectum to lay eggs on the skin around the anus. The eggs are contained within a sticky substance and fall off as the substance hardens or as the animal scratches. For this reason, pinworm eggs usually are not seen in a routine fecal examination.

Baermann Technique

The Baermann technique is used to recover nematode larvae from feces, tissues, or soil. This technique uses warm water to stimulate larvae to move about. As the larvae do so, they sink to the bottom of the funnel for collection and identification.

This technique is performed with a Baermann apparatus (Figure 17-47). The apparatus consists of a ring stand and ring holder, a glass funnel with a piece of rubber tubing on the end, a clamp, and a wire net or cheesecloth. The sample is placed on the wire screen or cheesecloth, and warm water is added to barely cover the sample. All air bubbles are allowed to flow from the tube of the funnel by releasing the clamp. The apparatus is allowed to sit undisturbed for 12 to 24 hours.

A drop of fluid from the bottom of the funnel is removed (usually the first drop) and placed on a microscope slide. If any larvae are found swimming on the slide, the slide is carefully heated with a match to render them immobile.

Larvae recovered from fresh large animal feces are almost always those of lungworms. Larvae from *S. stercoralis* can be found in fresh canine feces. If the feces are not fresh, all sorts of parasitic and nonparasitic larvae and adults may be seen. For more detailed information on the descriptions of larvae, consult the reference by Bowman.

EXAMINATION OF BLOOD SAMPLES

D. immitis, the canine heartworm, is the most important parasite of the vascular system in domestic animals in the United States. For this reason, in-hospital blood examinations are commonly performed to detect heartworms.

The following procedures can be performed by veterinary technicians to identify *D. immitis*. As mentioned earlier, a clean environment and proper handling of samples are vital to quality control in any laboratory. Any sample handled improperly may result in inaccurate results.

Direct Blood Smear

A direct examination of the blood for microfilariae is the simplest procedure to perform. This procedure detects movement of microfilariae and other parasites among the RBCs. As with a direct examination of feces, a direct examination of blood requires only a small sample. However, unless parasites are present in large numbers, they may be missed. For this reason, the direct smear is not a good diagnostic technique for diagnosing microfilariae.

Microfilariae of primary interest are those of *D. immitis,* the canine heartworm, and *D. reconditum,* a subcutaneous parasite of dogs. Differentiation between the two is extremely important because the treatment for heartworms is expensive, somewhat stressful, and involves the use of arsenical compounds.

In a direct blood smear, microfilariae of *D. immitis* spp. coil and uncoil, whereas those of *Dipetalonema* spp. may glide smoothly across the slide. However, this is not always the case. The number of *Dirofilaria* spp. microfilariae in a sample is usually greater than that of *Dipetalonema* spp. This is not always the case. A direct examination of the blood is only used to determine the presence of microfilariae, not the type. For this, a concentration technique, which "relaxes" and stains microfilariae, is used. These procedures are discussed later in this chapter.

Microfilariae can also be found in large animals. *Setaria* spp. are long, white nematodes found in the serous membranes of cattle and horses. Adults are most often seen during abdominal surgery or necropsy, and microfilariae are found during a differential white blood cell count.

Thin Blood Smear

The thin blood smear is prepared and stained in exactly the same way as a blood smear for a differential white blood cell count. When doing a differential white blood cell count on an animal, the veterinary technician should note any parasitic organisms seen. Occasionally, microfilariae may be found. Because of their size, microfilariae usually are found along the feathered edge. Because differentiation of the microfilariae is not possible in a thin blood smear, other procedures must be performed for identification. Trypanosomes, protozoans, and rickettsiae also may be found among or within cells. As with the direct smear procedure, a small blood sample is used, and mild parasitic infections may be missed.

Thick Blood Smear

A thick blood smear examines a slightly greater volume of blood than does a thin blood smear. Microfilariae may be seen, but they cannot be easily differentiated using this method.

Concentration Techniques

Buffy Coat Method

The buffy coat method is a concentration technique used on a small volume of blood. When blood is placed in a microhematocrit tube and centrifuged for determining the packed-cell volume (PCV), it separates into three layers: plasma, white blood cell layer (buffy coat), and RBC layer (Figure 17-48). Microfilariae can be found on the surface of the buffy coat layer. This technique is quick and may be performed in conjunction with a PCV and total protein evaluation. However, differentiation of microfilariae is not possible.

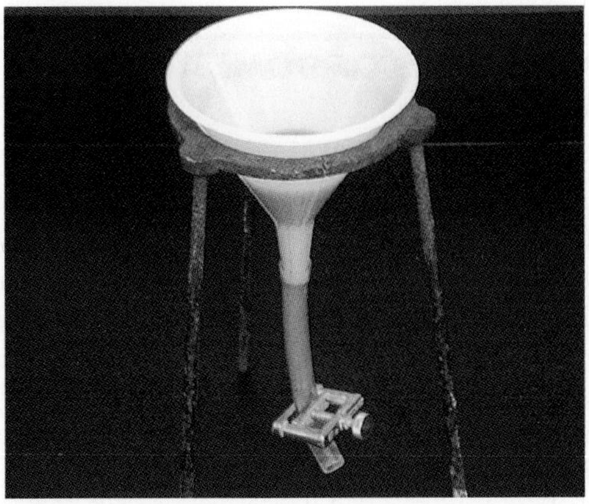

FIGURE 17-47 Baermann apparatus is used to recover larvae of roundworms from feces, soil, or animal tissues. This apparatus is most useful in recovering larvae of lungworms.

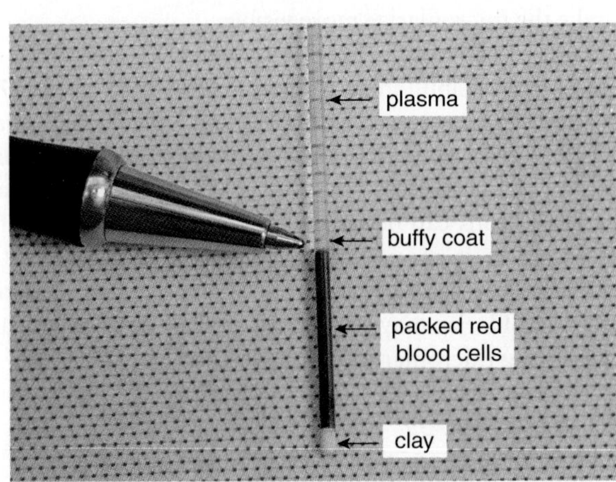

FIGURE 17-48 Buffy coat in a hematocrit tube lies between the plasma above and packed red blood cells below. A plug of clay prevents the blood from escaping the tube during centrifugation.

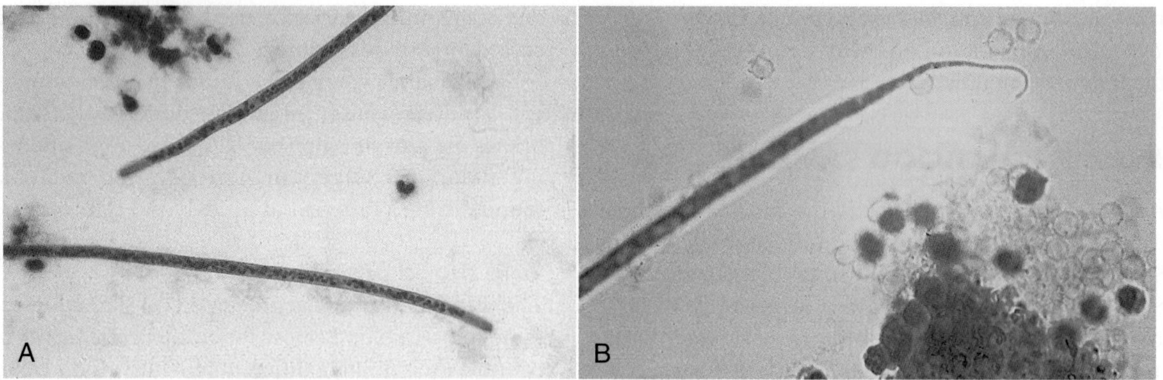

FIGURE 17-49 Cranial **(A)** and caudal **(B)** ends of a *D. reconditum* microfilaria.

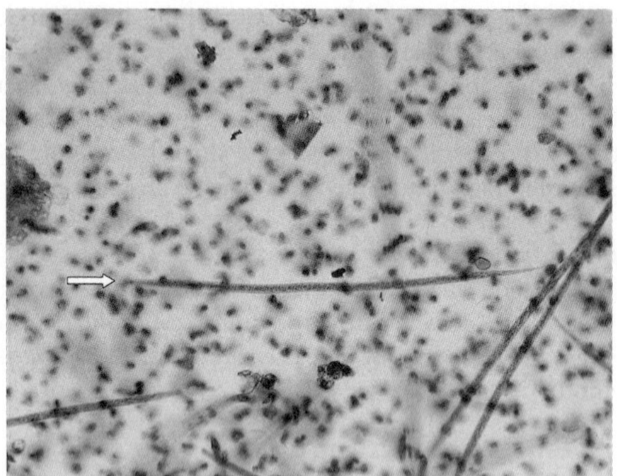

FIGURE 17-50 Microfilariae of *D. immitis* using the Difil-Test.

The following concentration techniques may be used for differentiating *D. immitis* from *D. reconditum.*

Modified Knott Technique

The modified Knott technique is a simple procedure that allows differentiation of microfilariae. This technique concentrates, "relaxes," and stains microfilariae while lysing RBCs to make the microfilariae more visible.

Figures 17-49 of *D. reconditum* and Figure 17-50 of *D. immitis* are helpful in identifying microfilariae. Table 17-1 shows the characteristics that may be used when differentiating these two microfilariae. The veterinary technician should always examine as many microfilariae as possible because mixed infections can occur. The most accurate method for differentiation is measuring the length and width of the body. However, with some practice, general characteristics of the microfilariae may be used for identification if a means of measuring microfilariae is not available.

TABLE 17-1 Differentiation of Microfilariae Using the Modified Knott Technique

	Dirofilaria immitis	*Dipetalonema reconditum*
Body length	310 μm	290 μm
Midbody width	6 μm	6 μm
Head	Tapered	Blunt
Tail	Straight	Hooked*

From Hendrix CM, Sirois M: *Laboratory procedures for veterinary technicians,* ed 5, St Louis, 2007, Mosby.
*Artifact of formalin fixation.

Filter Techniques

Filter techniques are the most common method used in veterinary practices for the detection of microfilariae in the blood. An excellent diagnostic kit is available for this procedure, the Difil-Test kit (EVSCO Pharmaceuticals, Buena, N.J.). These kits come complete with filters, lysing solution, stain, and directions for use.

Most kits require 1 ml of whole blood to test for heartworms. The blood is mixed with nine parts of lysing solution and passed through a filter. The filter is rinsed, removed, and placed on a slide. A drop of stain is added, a coverslip is applied, and the filter is microscopically examined for microfilariae. Differentiation of microfilariae is possible but difficult using the filter technique. If microfilariae are present, it is best to perform other diagnostic procedures for identification purposes.

ECTOPARASITES OF DOMESTICATED ANIMALS

The ectoparasites of domesticated animals usually belong to the phylum Arthropoda. The arthropodan ectoparasites include: bugs, lice, bloodsucking flies, myiasis-inducing flies, fleas, ticks, and mites. In addition, there are a few nematodes that inhabit skin lesions and bloodsucking leeches, which belong to the phylum Annelida that may also serve as ectoparasites.

Some arthropod ectoparasites are host specific, whereas others infect any number of animal species. The diagnosis is generally based on size and the appearance of external morphologic features, with the use of taxonomic keys. Control is often difficult, sometimes necessitating the treatment of the premises and prevention by prohibiting interaction with infested animals (e.g., other companion animals with fleas, ticks, or lice within the same environment).

TRUE BUGS

Whereas some adult hemipterans (true bugs) are wingless, most adult true bugs have two pair of wings. The posterior pair of wings is membranous in appearance. The anterior pair of wings has a leathery basal portion with a membranous apical portion, which gives the appearance of a "half wing," hence, the origin of the ordinal name: hemi-, meaning half, and -ptera, meaning wing. Two groups of true bugs are of veterinary importance: Reduviid bugs (kissing bugs) and bedbugs. Reduviid bugs (kissing bugs) are periodic parasites, making frequent visits to the host to obtain a blood meal. Kissing bugs serve as intermediate hosts for *Trypanosoma cruzi,* a protozoan parasite that can produce a rare disease in humans and dogs called Chagas' disease. This disease also is called South American trypanosomiasis and rarely occurs in dogs and other animals in the United States. Kissing bugs take blood meals from an infected host and transmit the parasite as they defecate.

Bedbugs are dorsoventrally flattened, wingless true bugs that often infest homes. They are periodic parasites, making frequent visits to the host to obtain a blood meal. Although bedbugs are human parasites, they also may be found in rabbit colonies, poultry houses, and pigeon colonies. Bedbugs are not capable of naturally transmitting any human or animal pathogen.

> *TECHNICIAN NOTE* Lice are some of the most prolific ectoparasites of domestic animals and usually are transmitted by direct contact. However, all life stages may be transmitted by fomites and are easily transmitted among young, old, and malnourished animals. It is often puzzling why certain animals in a flock or herd are heavily infested, whereas others have only a few lice.

LICE

Lice are some of the most prolific ectoparasites of domestic animals. Two orders of lice exist: the Mallophaga (chewing or biting lice) and the Anoplura (sucking lice). Lice are dorsoventrally flattened, wingless insects. They have three body divisions: the head, with its mouthparts and antennae; the thorax, with its three pairs of legs and its lack of wings; and the abdomen, the portion that bears the reproductive organs. These body divisions and their relationship to each other are important in diagnostic veterinary parasitology.

Members of the order Mallophaga, or chewing or biting lice, are smaller than sucking lice. They are usually yellow and have a large, round head. The mouthparts are mandibulate and are adapted for chewing or biting the host. Characteristically the head of every chewing louse is wider than the widest portion of the thorax. On the thorax are three pairs of legs, which may be adapted for clasping or for moving rapidly among feathers or hairs. Chewing or biting lice may parasitize birds, dogs, cats, cattle, sheep, goats, and horses (Figure 17-51).

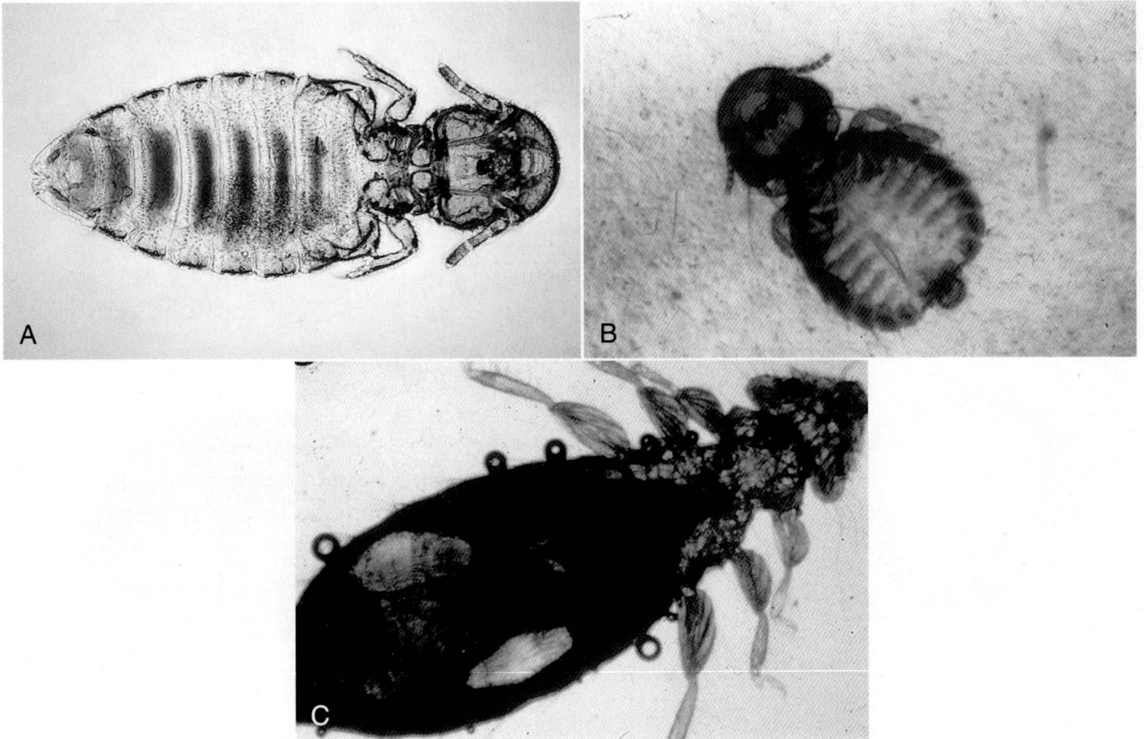

FIGURE 17-51 Assorted chewing lice of goats and fowl. **A,** *Damalinia caprae.* **B,** *Goniodes dissimilis.* **C,** *Goniodes gallinae.*

Members of the order Anoplura (sucking lice) are larger than members of the order Mallophaga (chewing lice). These lice are red to gray; their color usually depends on the amount of blood ingested from the host. In contrast to the wide head of the mallophagans, anoplurans' heads are narrower than the widest part of the thorax. Their mouthparts are piercing and are adapted for sucking blood. Their pincerlike claws are adapted for clinging to the host's hairs. They are found on many species of domestic animals (Figure 17-52).

Anoplurans and mallophagans have the same type of life cycle. This life cycle has only three developmental stages: the egg, nymphal, and adult stages.

The egg stage is also called a "nit." The nit is tiny, approximately 0.5 to 1.0 mm in length. It is oval, white, and usually found cemented to the hair or feather shaft of the host (Figure 17-53). Figure 17-54 shows a gravid female sucking louse and an associated nit collected from a dog. Nits hatch about 5 to 14 days after they are laid by the adult female louse.

The nymphal stage is similar in appearance to the adult. However, it is smaller and lacks functioning reproductive organs and genital openings. The three nymphal stages are each progressively larger than its predecessor. The nymphal stage lasts from 2 to 3 weeks.

The adult stage is similar in appearance to the nymphal stage, but larger. It has functional reproductive organs. Male and female lice copulate; the female lays eggs, cementing the eggs to the hair or feather; and the life cycle begins again. It takes 3 to 4 weeks to complete the cycle. Nymphal and adult stages live no longer than 7 days if removed from the host. Eggs hatch within 2 to 3 weeks during warm weather, but seldom hatch off the host.

Lice usually are transmitted by direct contact, but all life stages may be transmitted by fomites (inanimate objects, such as blankets, brushes, and other grooming equipment). Lice are easily transmitted among young, old, and malnourished animals. Veterinarians often cannot understand why certain animals in a flock or herd are heavily infested, whereas others have only a few lice. Lice are species specific (i.e., they will only parasitize their specific hosts). For example, dog lice parasitize dogs. They may temporarily reside on another species of animal, but they will not set up housekeeping on that animal.

Infestation by lice (whether mallophagan or anopluran) is referred to as pediculosis. Sucking lice can ingest blood to such a degree that they produce severe anemia; fatalities can occur, especially in young animals. The PCV can drop as much as 10% to 20%. Severely infested animals may harbor as many as one million lice. Infested animals become more susceptible to other diseases and parasites and may succumb to stresses not ordinarily pathologic to uninfested animals. When animals are poorly fed and kept in overcrowded conditions, they often become severely infested with lice and quickly become anemic and unthrifty.

A careful examination of the hair coat or feathers of infested animals easily reveals lice and the accompanying nits. Hair clippings also serve as a good source for lice. Infestation of animals with a thick hair coat may be easily overlooked. A hand-held magnifying lens or a binocular headband magnifier may aid the observation of adult or nymphal lice

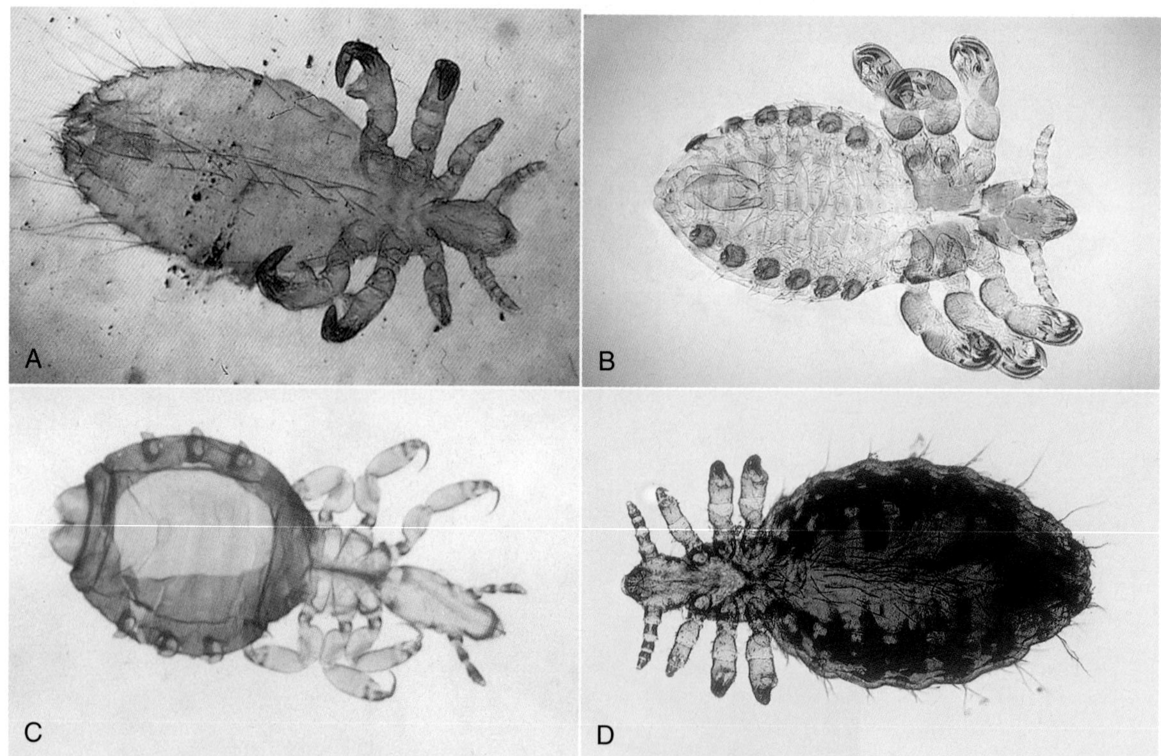

FIGURE 17-52 Assorted sucking lice. **A,** *Solenopotes capillatus* (sheep). **B,** *Pedicinus obtusus* (monkey). **C,** *Pedicinus obtusus* (monkey). **D,** *Linognathus setosus* (dog).

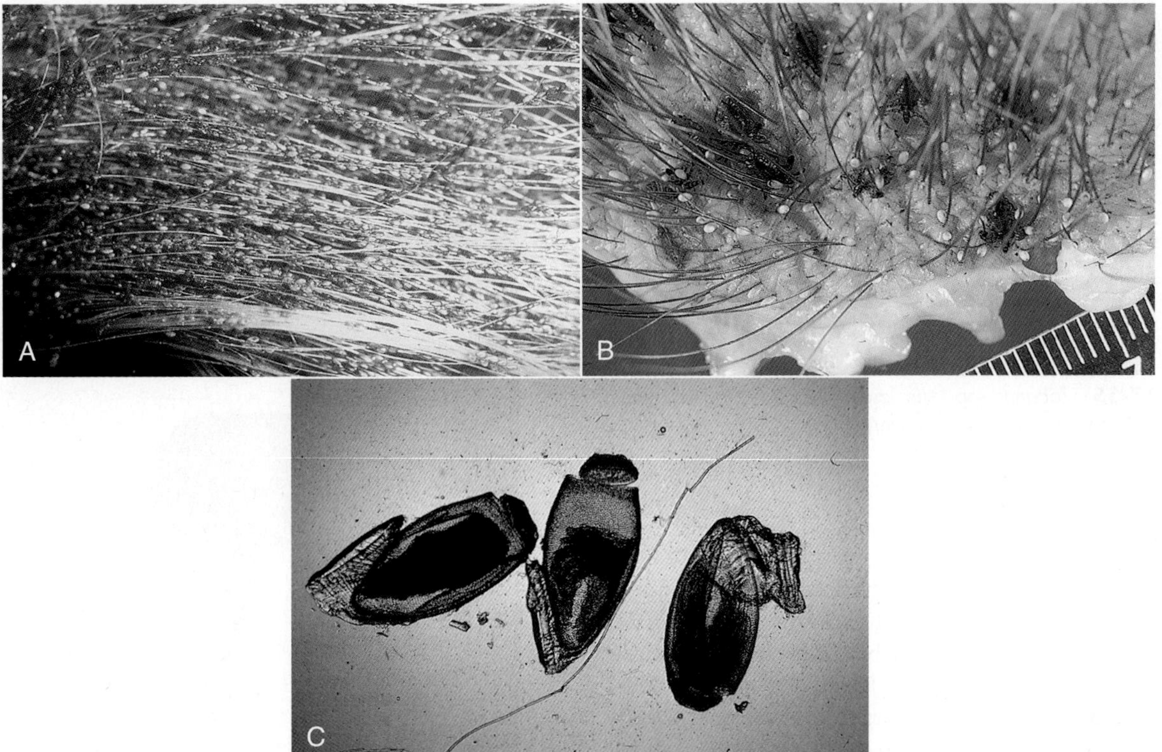

FIGURE 17-53 **A,** Thousands of nits can be cemented by female lice to the hair coat of domesticated animals. This calf's tail contains thousands of nits. **B,** Pediculosis can be defined as infestation by either chewing or sucking lice, in this case, *Haematopinus suis* infestation in a pig. **C,** Appearance of operculated nits viewed by compound microscope.

crawling through or clinging to hair or feathers or tiny nits cemented to individual hairs.

Any lice and/or their nits observed may be collected with thumb forceps and placed in a drop of mineral oil on a glass microscope slide. A coverslip should be placed over the specimen and the slide examined using the 4× or 10× objectives.

The identification of a louse as to genus and specific epithet is difficult and best left to a trained specialist. Veterinary technicians should be able to identify the specimen as anopluran (sucking) or mallophagan (chewing or biting) by a visual examination of the head size in relation to the width of the thorax.

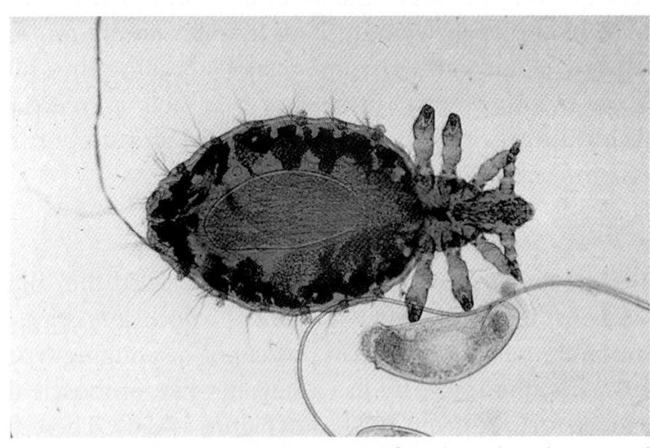

FIGURE 17-54 *L. setosus,* a gravid female sucking louse, and associated nit collected from a dog.

FLIES

Dipterans (two-winged flies) produce two contrasting pathologic scenarios. As adults, they may feed intermittently on vertebrate blood, saliva, tears, or mucus. As larvae, they may develop in the subcutaneous tissues or within internal organs. Adult dipterans that make frequent visits to the vertebrate host to intermittently feed on blood are referred to as periodic parasites. When dipteran larvae develop in the tissue or organs of vertebrate hosts, they produce a condition known as myiasis.

As periodic parasites, blood-feeding dipterans may be classified as to which sex feeds on vertebrate blood and as to food preference. In certain dipteran groups, only the females feed on vertebrate blood; these female flies require vertebrate blood for laying their eggs. In this group are the biting gnats (e.g., *Simulium, Lutzomyia,* and *Culicoides* spp.), the mosquitoes (e.g., *Anopheles, Aedes,* and *Culex* spp.), the horseflies (e.g., *Tabanus* spp.), and the deerflies (e.g., *Chrysops* spp.).

In the second group of blood-feeding dipterans, both male and female flies require a vertebrate blood meal. These species include the stable fly *Stomoxys calcitrans,* the horn fly *Haematobia irritans,* and the sheep ked *Melophagus ovinus.*

This section will discuss only those dipterans that may be seen by the direct observation of either large or small animals.

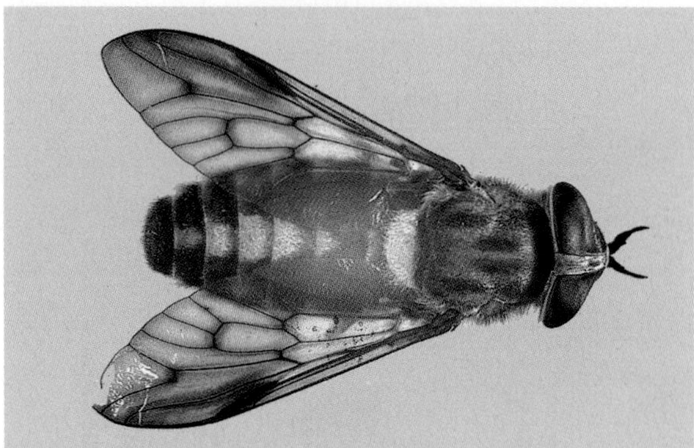

FIGURE 17-55 *Tabanus* spp., the largest blood-feeding dipteran. This tabanid is approximately 2.5 cm in length.

Horseflies/Deerflies

Chrysops spp. and *Tabanus* spp. are large (up to 3.5 cm long), heavy-bodied, robust dipterans with powerful wings. Horseflies and deerflies are the largest blood-feeding dipterans. Figure 17-55 shows *Tabanus* spp., the largest of the blood-feeding dipterans. Horseflies are larger than deerflies. Deerflies have a dark band passing from the cranial to the caudal margins of the wings.

Horseflies and deerflies feed a number of times at multiple feeding sites before they stop feeding. When disturbed by the animal's swatting tail or by the panniculus reflex (skin twitching), the flies leave the host, but blood continues to ooze from the open wound; these fly bites are painful. Affected horses and cattle become restless. Because they often feed on multiple hosts, these flies may acts as mechanical transmitters of anthrax, anaplasmosis, and the virus of equine infectious anemia.

Stable Fly

The stable fly, *Stomoxys calcitrans*, is often called the "biting housefly." It is approximately the size of *Musca domestica*, the common housefly. Rather than possessing a sponging type of mouthparts, the stable fly has a bayonet-like proboscis that protrudes forward from the head (Figure 17-56). These flies are found worldwide. In the United States, they are found in the central and southeastern states, where cattle are raised. Both male and female flies are avid blood feeders, feeding on any domestic animal. They usually attack the legs and ventral abdomen and may also bite the ears. These flies also feed on the tips of the ears of dogs with pointed ears, especially the German shepherd. These dogs' ears often demonstrate a loss of hair and the presence of dried, crusty blood on the ear tips.

This fly feeds on both horses and cattle, with horses the preferred host. The fly usually lands on the host with its head pointed upward. It is a sedentary fly, not moving on the host. The flies inflict painful bites that puncture the skin and bleed freely. Stable flies stay on the host for short periods, during which they obtain the blood meals. This is an outdoor fly; however, in the late fall and during rainy weather, it may enter barns.

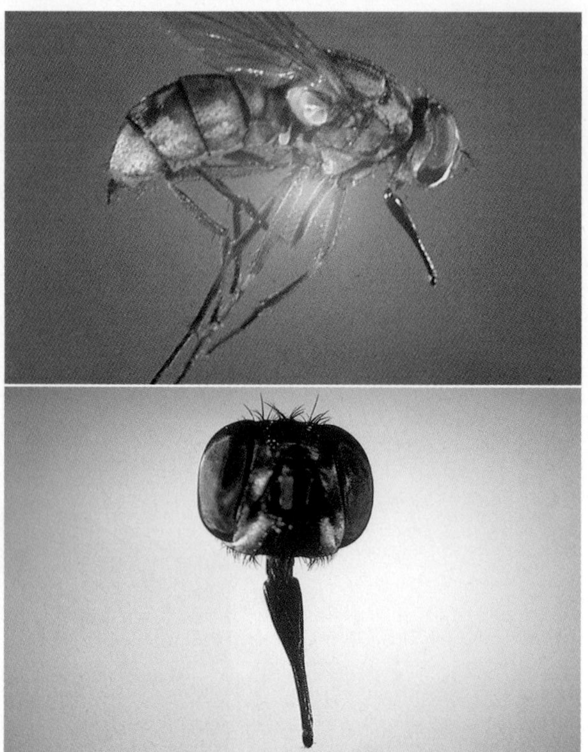

FIGURE 17-56 *Stomoxys calcitrans,* the stable fly. Note the bayonet-like proboscis that protrudes forward from the head. The stable fly is approximately the same size as a housefly.

Stable flies are mechanical vectors of anthrax in cattle and equine infectious anemia. They are the intermediate host for *Habronema muscae,* a nematode found in the stomach of horses. When large numbers of stable flies attack dairy cattle, milk production can fall. Beef cattle may refuse to graze in the daytime when they are attacked by large numbers of flies; as a result, these cattle do not gain the usual amount of weight.

Haematobia

Haematobia irritans is often called the horn fly. This dark-colored fly is approximately 3 to 6 mm in length, approximately half of the size of *S. calcitrans,* the biting housefly. Like the stable fly, the horn fly has a bayonet-like proboscis that protrudes forward from the head. These flies are found almost exclusively on cattle throughout North America.

When the air temperature is below 70° F, horn flies cluster around the base of the horns; this is the origin of the name horn fly. In warmer climates, thousands of flies often cluster on the hosts' shoulders, backs, and side; these areas are least disturbed by tail switching. On hot, sunny days, horn flies congregate on the ventral abdomen.

Adult horn flies spend most of their life on cattle and leave the host only to deposit eggs in fresh cow manure. Using tiny bayonet mouthparts, they feed frequently, sucking blood and other fluids, and cause considerable irritation. Female flies are more aggressive than males. Harassment by the flies and loss of blood often reduces weight gain and milk production in cattle. Horn flies probably cause greater losses in cattle in the United States than any other bloodsucking fly. Adult horn flies also cause focal midline dermatitis on the ventral abdomen of horses. These flies also serve as the intermediate host for *Stephanofilaria stilesi,* a filarial parasite that produces ventral, plaquelike lesions on the ventral abdomen of cattle.

Sheep Ked

Melophagus ovinus is often called the sheep ked. Members of the order Diptera usually have one pair of wings (two wings). Keds are an exception to that rule; they are wingless dipterans. Keds are hairy, leathery, and 4 to 7 mm in length. The head is short and broad, the thorax brown, and the abdomen broad and grayish brown. The legs are strong and armed with stout claws (Figure 17-57). Some observers say that keds have a "louselike" appearance, but they are not related to lice.

Keds are permanent ectoparasites of sheep and goats. Their pupal stages are often found attached to the wool or hair of the host. Keds are avid blood feeders. Heavy infestations can reduce the condition of the host considerably and even cause anemia. Their bites cause pruritus over much of the host's body; infested sheep often bite, scratch, and rub themselves, damaging the wool. Ked feces often stain the wool and do not wash out readily. Keds are most numerous in the cold temperatures of the fall and winter months. Their numbers decline as temperatures warm in the spring and summer months.

Louse Flies

Lynchia and *Pseudolynchia* spp. are often called louse flies, and like the keds, they are not related to lice. These dipterans are closely related to the wingless sheep keds, but they are found to parasitize a wide variety of birds—from songbirds to pigeons to raptors. They are found in among the feathers of these birds; however, they enjoy sucking from areas of the skin that are sparsely covered with feathers. These winged dipterans are dark brown in color, hairy, and leathery in appearance. These flies are from 4 to 6 mm in length with legs armed with stout, fierce claws. Louse flies are swift fliers and move about quickly—even attempting to get into a human's hair.

Face Fly

The final periodic parasite among the dipteran flies is one that is not a blood feeder, but instead feeds on the mucus, tears, and saliva of large animals, particularly cattle. Face flies, *Musca autumnalis* (Figure 17-58), are so named because they gather around the eyes and muzzle of livestock, particularly cattle. They also may be found on the withers, neck, brisket, and sides. Face flies feed mostly on liquid media—saliva, tears, and mucus. They usually are not considered blood feeders because their mouthparts are not piercing or bayonet-like. Instead, their mouthparts are adapted for sponging up saliva, tears, and mucus. They follow blood-feeding flies, disturb them during their feeding process, and then lap up the blood and body fluids that accumulate on the host's skin. Face flies are found on animals outdoors; they usually do not follow animals into barns.

Face flies produce considerable annoyance to the host. The irritation around the host's eyes stimulates the flow of tears, which attracts even more flies. This harassment ultimately interferes with the host's productivity. Face flies may be involved in the transmission of *Moraxella bovis,* a bacterium associated with infectious keratoconjunctivitis or pinkeye in cattle.

Files of the genus *Hippelates* feed on the mucus, tears, and saliva of large animals, particularly cattle. These tiny, fragile dipterans are nonbiting gnats with sponging mouthparts that are similar to the mouthparts of the common housefly. These tiny gnats are often found around a dog's penis (hence, they are often referred to by the common name of, "dog penis gnats." Because they have sponging type of mouthparts, these dipterans are not capable of biting the host, but often feed on liquid secretions from the host. Frequently, these nonbiting gnats are found around the teats of dairy cattle. They have been known to serve as mechanical vectors of a variety of bacteria.

Myiasis-Inducing Flies

The larvae or maggots of dipterans may develop in the subcutaneous tissues of many domestic animals and produce a condition known as myiasis.

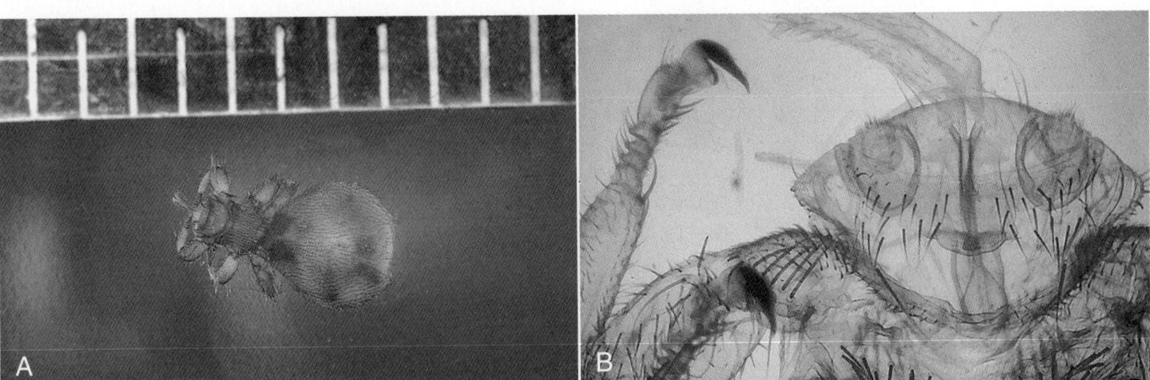

FIGURE 17-57 *Melophagus ovinus,* the sheep ked. Keds are hairy, leathery, and 4 to 7 mm in length. The head is short and broad. The thorax is brown, and the abdomen broad and grayish brown. The legs are strong and armed with stout claws.

Rabbit Bots and Fox Maggots

Cuterebra is known as the rabbit bot and *Wohlfahrtia* is known as the fox maggot. These species occasionally infest dogs, cats, rodents, rabbits, and other wildlife. *Cuterebra* flies usually deposit eggs around rodent burrows or runs. Eggs hatch, and the larvae penetrate the skin of the host, developing to the third stage in subcutaneous tissues without migrating in the host. The larvae then emerge from a hole in the host's skin (Figure 17-59) and pupate in the soil. The *Cuterebra* larvae are known for their aberrant or erratic migrations, having been found in a variety of extracutaneous sites, the cranial vault, the eye, and the pharyngeal regions. Clinical signs vary with the site of infection or infestation. Female *Wohlfahrtia* deposit larvae directly on the skin of the host, which is usually a young animal. The larvae penetrate the skin and develop in the subcutaneous tissues with limited migration. When they become third-stage larvae, they drop out and pupate in the soil. The treatment consists of surgical removal of the larvae and supportive wound treatment.

Horse Botflies

Gasterophilus intestinalis, Gasterophilus nasalis, and *Gasterophilus hemorrhoidalis*—the botflies of horses—are widespread and common wherever horses are found; but *G. intestinalis* is the most common species. The adult fly cements eggs to the hair of the horse (see Figure 17-28). The eggs either hatch by themselves and the larvae crawl into the horse's mouth or the eggs are stimulated to hatch by the horse licking them. Once in the mouth, the larvae penetrate the mucosa and move down the esophagus to the stomach, where they attach. These larvae develop into the third-stage larvae (see Figure 17-29). They usually spend about 10 months as larvae. Ultimately the larvae pass out with the feces, burrow into the soil, pupate, and later emerge as adult flies, usually in late summer. The diagnosis is based on the type of egg and means of attachment of the spines on each segment (single row, *G. nasalis;* double row, *G. intestinalis;* double row, smaller spines, *G. hemorrhoidalis*). The treatment is generally applied in the fall with a combination of insecticides and anthelmintics or a broad-spectrum compound. Control is difficult.

Heel Flies/Cattle Grubs/Ox Warbles

The heel flies of cattle, *Hypoderma lineatum* and *Hypoderma bovis,* whose larval stages are called grubs or warbles, are widely distributed wherever cattle are found. Emergence of these flies depends on environmental conditions. For example, they are active in early January in southern Texas and in early August in Montana. When both species are present, *H. bovis* emerges about 1 month later than *H. lineatum*. After emergence, H. bovis lays single eggs attached to hair, and *H. lineatum* lays a row of eggs just above the hooves. The

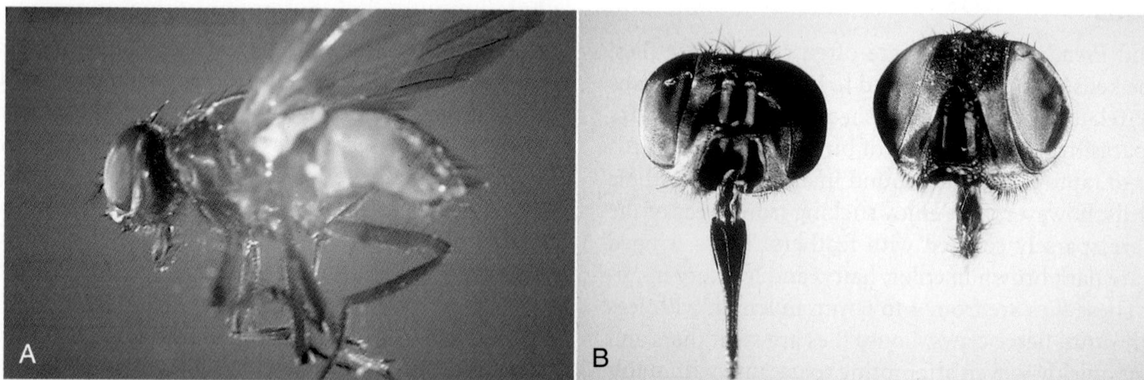

FIGURE 17-58 **A,** *Musca autumnalis*, the face fly. Its mouthparts are adapted for sponging saliva, tears, and mucus. **B,** *Stomoxys calcitrans* head (left) and *M. autumnalis* (right).

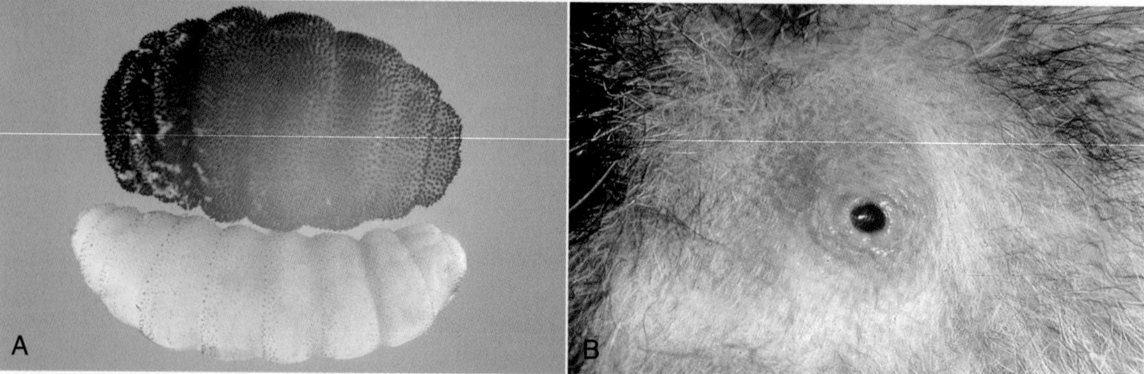

FIGURE 17-59 **A,** Different developmental stages of *Cuterebra* spp. Larval *Cuterebra* are either sparsely or thickly covered with tiny black spines. **B,** Larval *Cuterebra* spp. are usually found in swollen, cystlike subcutaneous sites, with a fistula (pore, or hole) communicating to the outside environment.

larvae hatch from the eggs, penetrate the skin, and wander in the subcutaneous tissue for 4 to 5 months. *H. lineatum* then goes to the esophagus for 2 months, and *H. bovis* goes to the epidural fat of the spinal cord for 2 months. Both then go to the subcutaneous tissue along the back for about 2 months (Figure 17-60). The larvae develop and drop out and burrow in the soil, in which they pupate for 1 month to 3 months. The diagnosis is generally based on the presence of warbles on the backs of cattle; however, the species can be identified on the basis of the morphologic appearance of the larvae. Several treatments are available, but they must be applied at a specific time of year.

Sheep Nasal Botflies

The sheep nasal botfly, *Oestrus ovis,* is common wherever sheep are found. Flies emerge from spring through fall and deposit first-stage larvae around the nasal opening. Larvae then enter the nasal cavity for 2 weeks to 9 months and migrate to the paranasal sinuses for a short period to complete development. The larvae leave through the nose and pupate in the soil for 15 to 60 days. The life cycle may be completed in 2 to 11 months, depending on environmental conditions. The diagnosis is based on the presence of these larvae in the nose or sinuses. There is no preferred treatment available.

> TECHNICIAN NOTE Economically the primary screwworm is the most important fly that may attack livestock in the southwestern and southern United States, but it may also be found in a small animal clinical situation, primarily in animals returning from foreign locales.

Primary Screwworms

Only one fly in North America, *Cochliomyia hominivorax,* is a primary invader of fresh, uncontaminated skin wounds of all domestic animals. These larvae must not be confused with the larvae of the more common facultative myiasis-producing flies described previously. *C. hominivorax* is often referred to as the "screwworm fly" because its third larval stage resembles a wood screw and because this same larval stage burrows deep into the host tissues. Economically, it is the most important fly that may attack livestock in the southwestern and southern United States, but it may also be found in a small animal clinical situation, primarily in animals returning from foreign locales.

Adult female flies are attracted to fresh skin wounds on any warm-blooded animal, where they lay batches of 15 to 500 eggs in a shinglelike pattern at the edge of wounds. The female lays several thousand cream-color, elongated eggs during her lifetime. They hatch within 24 hours. Larvae enter the wound, where they feed for 4 to 7 days before developing into third-stage (fully-grown) larvae. They may be as long as 1.5 cm in length. When fully mature, the larvae drop from the host to the ground and pupate for about a week, after which the adult flies emerge. The adult male and female fly mate only once during their lifetime, a fact that is used to control these flies biologically, a program known as the "sterile male release technique."

Adult flies are shiny and greenish blue, with a reddish-orange head and eyes, and are 8 to 15 mm long. Larvae often are identified by their wood-screw shape and by the deeply pigmented tracheal tubes on the posterior one third of the dorsal aspect of the caudal ends. Because of the obligatory nature of the screwworm with regard to breeding in the fresh wounds of any warmblooded animal, the veterinarian must report any screwworm infestations to both state and federal authorities. *C. hominivorax* has been eradicated from the United States, but occasionally surreptitiously enters the country in imported animals. The presence of this fly larva within U.S. borders must be reported to both state and federal authorities.

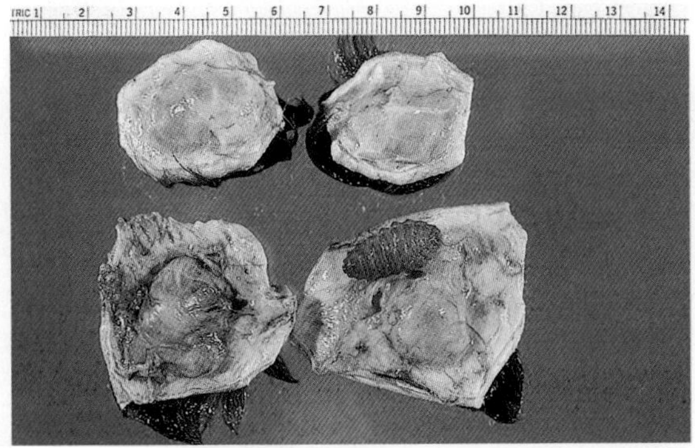

FIGURE 17-60 Mature larvae of *Hypoderma* spp. are 25 to 30 mm long, cream to dark brown in color, and covered with small spines. Lesions consist of large, cystlike swellings on the back, with a central breathing pore.

Secondary Myiasis (Fly Strike)

This group of flies includes *Musca domestica* (housefly) and *Calliphora, Phaenicia, Lucilia, Phormia* (blowfly, bottle flies), and *Sarcophaga* (flesh fly) spp. The adults of these fly species are colloquially known as "filth flies" because of their propensity to fly from feces to food. The adults of these flies are "vomit drop feeders," disgorging their stomach contents with the associated liquefaction enzymes and then lapping up the resulting liquid food. These adult flies are frequently seen in kennel situations, alighting on feces that have not been removed from dog runs.

Dipteran larvae that produce fly strike myiasis include the housefly, *M. domestic;* the blowflies or bottle flies *Calliphora, Phaenicia, Lucilia,* and *Phormia* spp.; and the flesh fly *Sarcophaga* spp. Larval stages of these flies usually are associated with skin wounds contaminated with bacteria or with a matted hair coat contaminated with feces or urine.

Under their "normal" living conditions, adult flies of these genera lay eggs in decaying animal carcasses or in feces. In "fly strike myiasis," the adult flies are attracted to an animal's moist wound, skin lesion, or soiled hair coat. These sites provide the adult fly with a moist medium on which it feeds. As adult female flies feed in these sites, they lay eggs. These eggs hatch, producing larvae (maggots) that move independently about the wound surface, ingesting dead cells, exudate, secretions, and debris, but not live tissue. These larvae irritate, injure, and kill successive layers of skin and produce exudates.

Maggots can tunnel through the thin epidermal layer into the subcutis. This process produces tissue cavities in the skin that measure up to several centimeters in diameter. Unless the process is halted by appropriate therapy, the infested animal may die from shock, intoxication, histolysis, or an infection. A peculiar, distinct, pungent odor permeates the infested tissues and the affected animal. Advanced lesions may contain thousands of maggots.

As adults, these flies can be pestiferous flies in a veterinary clinical setting. These flies are "vomit drop" feeders and fly from feces to food, spreading bacteria on their feet and their disgorged stomach contents. A veterinary practice with outdoor kennels is especially susceptible to the "assault" of these pestiferous adult flies.

A tentative diagnosis of maggot infestation in any domestic animal can easily be made by a veterinary technician because maggots can be observed in an existing wound or among the soiled, matted hair coat. When facultative myiasis has been diagnosed, the veterinarian must rule out the possibility of myiasis caused by the primary screwworm, *C. hominivorax.*

FLEAS

The most common flea of both dogs and cats is *Ctenocephalides felis,* the cat flea (Figure 17-61). Fleas are not host specific and will attack and may infest other animals and humans. Fleas are widely distributed, but are much more common in warm, humid environments. When environmental conditions are favorable, fleas have a great reproductive potential. Fleas thrive at low altitudes in temperature ranges of 65° F to 80° F (18.2° C to 26.6° C). Under these conditions, the flea life cycle can be completed, from hatching of an egg to the laying of the next generation of eggs, in as few as 16 days. See Figure 17-62 for a pictorial representation of the four life stages.

The female flea, *C. felis,* lays its eggs in the fur of dogs and cats. These flea eggs are not sticky and tend to fall out of the fur and survive in the protected places where the dog or cat sleeps or plays (Figure 17-63). The eggs will hatch into small maggotlike larvae, which are sparsely covered with fine hairs (Figure 17-64). These larvae feed on organic debris, especially the dried blood droppings (flea frass or flea dirt) defecated by adult fleas (Figure 17-65). The egg and larval stages of the flea are often recovered from the pet's environment and brought to the practice to be identified;

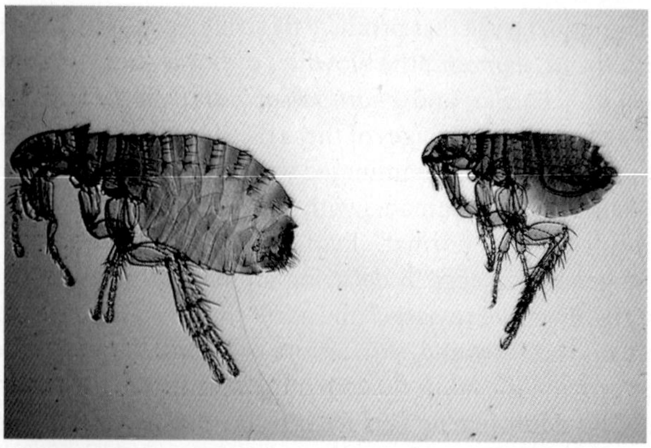

FIGURE 17-61 Morphologic details of the adult female and male *Ctenocephalides felis,* the cat flea.

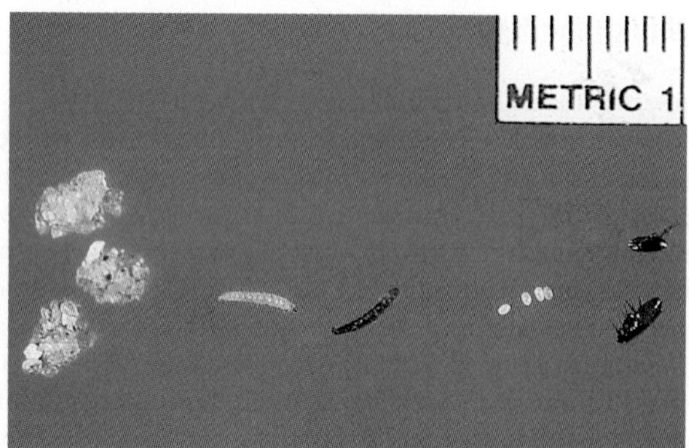

FIGURE 17-62 Life stages of *Ctenocephalides felis,* the cat flea. *Left to right,* Pupae, larvae, eggs, adult male *(top),* and female *(bottom).*

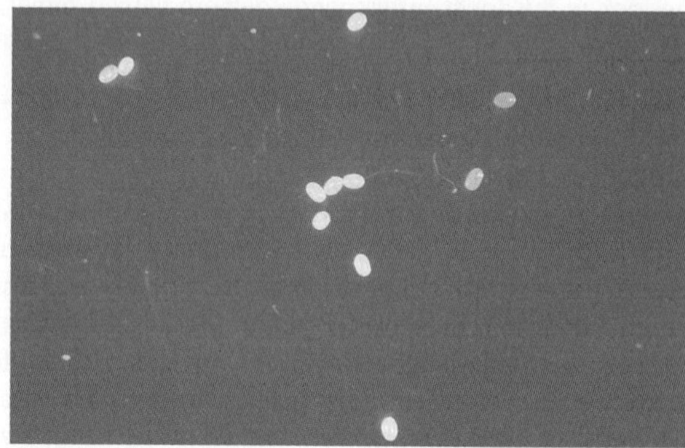
FIGURE 17-63 Eggs of *Ctenocephalides felis,* the cat flea.

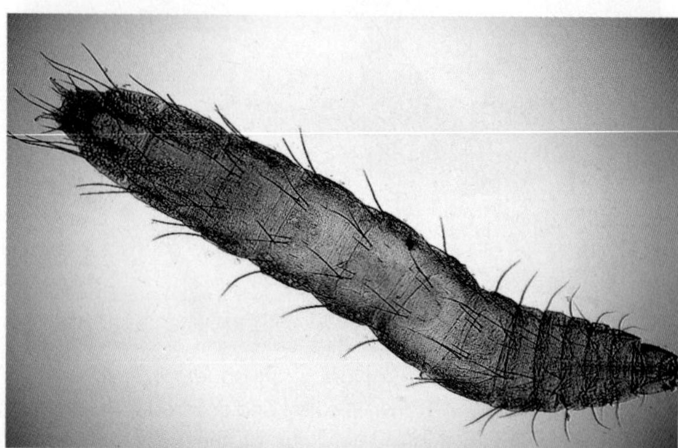
FIGURE 17-64 Larva of *Ctenocephalides felis,* the cat flea.

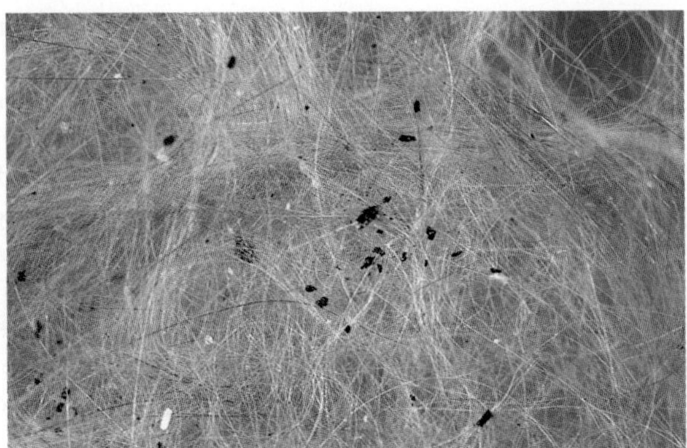

FIGURE 17-65 Flea dirt, flea feces, or flea frass of *Ctenocephalides felis,* the cat flea.

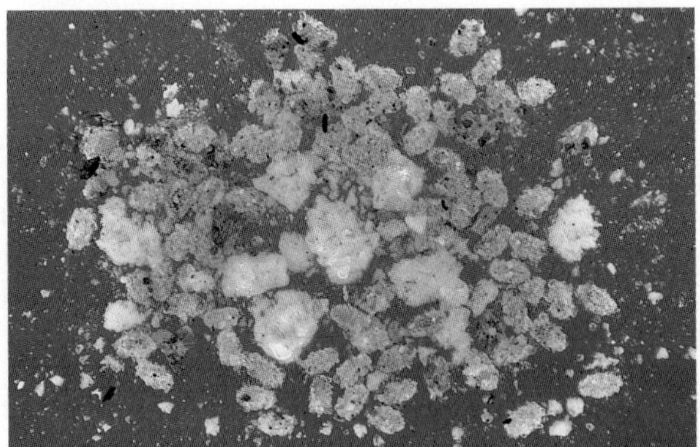

FIGURE 17-66 Sand-covered pupae of *Ctenocephalides felis,* the cat flea.

it behooves the veterinary technician to be able to identify these morphologic stages for the client. The flea larvae molt and form pupae that spin sticky, loose cocoons, to which sand and other environmental debris will adhere (Figure 17-66). The fleas will emerge as young and hungry adults in about 3 weeks. An important source of fleas to a dog and cat is these newly "hatched out" young fleas.

Once fleas have had a chance to establish the life cycle in a home or outdoor environment, no program that does not emphasize environmental control will be successful. Mechanical cleaning of the home and yard environment should precede any application of insecticides. In general, the same environmental control methods may be used in households with young dogs and cats as in those with adult animals. Care should always be taken that animals and people are not directly exposed to insecticides used in household extermination. All effective in-house programs should take advantage of new technologies in flea control. There are new insecticides that have truly long residuals (synthetic pyrethroids or microencapsulated products), and there are insect growth regulators (methoprene and fenoxycarb) marketed for preadult flea control.

Advances in outdoor environmental flea control have been less remarkable. At present, the use of insecticides (compounds that contain chlorpyrifos, malathion, or diazinon as their active ingredient) labeled for outdoor flea control is still the best and most economical approach. Such programs must incorporate repeated applications at 2-week intervals throughout the flea season where temperature and humidity are favorable for flea reproduction.

All topical insecticides should be used exactly according to label directions because it is not legally permissible to use or recommend the use of insecticide products beyond the label restrictions. In general, the use of organophosphate preparations on puppies younger than 16 weeks or on kittens younger than 6 months should be avoided. Any product containing lufenuron, fipronil, or imidacloprid as its active ingredient should never be administered to or used on nursing animals. Pyrethrin-based products are generally safe for frequent application; the most effective products are synergized pyrethrin sprays or foams. Very small animals and nursing animals sprayed with alcohol-based or other volatile organic solvents may be severely chilled as the solvent evaporates. Water-based sprays are preferable, and small animals and nursing animals should never be thoroughly saturated with a spray. The safest effective products are sprays and foams with microencapsulated pyrethrins. Flea collars that are safe for use on puppies or kittens are not effective in most environments. Topical treatments should be coordinated with in-home environmental flea control.

MITES

The first group of parasitic mites may be classified together as "sarcoptiform" mites. Sarcoptiform mites have several key characteristics or features in common. These mites may produce severe dermatologic problems in a variety of domestic animals. This dermatitis usually is accompanied by a severe pruritus. Sarcoptiform mites are small, barely visible to the naked eye, and approximately the size of a grain of salt. Their bodies have a round to oval shape. Sarcoptiform mites have legs with pedicels or stalks at the tip. The pedicels may be long or short. If the pedicel is long, it may be straight (unjointed) or jointed. At the tip of each pedicel, there may be a tiny sucker. Veterinarians and veterinary technicians should use the description of the pedicel (long or short, jointed or unjointed) to identify these sarcoptiform mites.

Sarcoptiform mites may be divided into two basic families: Sarcoptidae, which burrow or tunnel within the epidermis, and Psoroptidae, which reside on the surface of the skin or within the external ear canal.

TECHNICIAN NOTE Scabies is extremely contagious. These mites are spread by direct contact and can affect all dogs in a household or kennel. The dog owner can also become infested with this mite, but the infestation in humans is self-limiting. The mites burrow into human skin, producing a papulelike lesion, but they do not establish a full-blown infestation in humans.

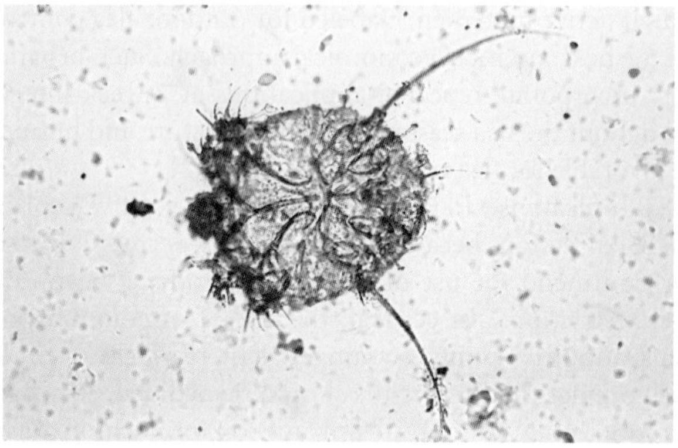

FIGURE 17-67 Adult *S. scabiei* mite. Note the long, unjointed pedicels (stalks), with suckers on the ends.

Sarcoptidae

Sarcoptic mites burrow or tunnel within the epidermis of the infested definitive host. The entire four-stage life cycle is spent on the host. Male and female mites breed on the skin surface. Female mites penetrate the keratinized layers of the skin and burrow or tunnel through the epidermis. Over a 10- to 15-day period, the female deposits 40 to 50 eggs within the tunnel. After egg deposition, the female dies. Larvae emerge from the eggs in 3 to 10 days and exit the tunnel to wander on the skin surface. These larvae molt to the nymphal stage within minute pockets in the epidermis. Nymphs become sexually active adults in 12 to 17 days, and the life cycle begins again.

The disease caused by *Sarcoptes scabiei* is called sarcoptic acariasis (Figure 17-67). This mite causes an extremely pruritic skin condition. Certain varieties of *Sarcoptes* mites infest specific hosts. For example, *S. scabiei* variety *canis* infests only dogs, and *S. scabiei* variety *suis* infests only pigs. Almost every species of domestic animal has its own distinct variety of this mite.

Scabies in dogs is caused by *S. scabiei* variety *canis,* which produces an erythematous, papular rash. Scaling, crusting, and excoriation are common. The ears, lateral elbows, and ventral abdomen are most likely to harbor mites. However, the host's entire body may be infested, whereas some dogs may be asymptomatic carriers. Scabies is extremely contagious. The mites are spread by direct contact and can affect all dogs in a household or kennel. The dog owner can also become infested with this mite, but the infestation in humans is self-limiting. The mites burrow into human skin, producing a papulelike lesion, but they do not establish a full-blown infestation in people. Nevertheless, this mite is considered to be zoonotic. *S. scabiei* variety *felis,* which causes scabies in cats, is an extremely rare mite.

Among large animals, pigs most commonly are affected by scabies mites. Lesions caused by *S. scabiei* variety *suis* include small, red papules, alopecia, and crusts, most commonly on the trunk and ears. The mite is rare in cattle (*S. scabiei* variety *bovis*). The main infested areas are the head, neck, and shoulders. *S. scabiei* variety *equi* of horses is even more rare. The main infested area is the neck. *S. scabiei* variety *ovis* does not infest the fleece of sheep and goats; the face and muzzle are the main areas affected.

Areas with an erythematous, papular rash and crust should be scraped, especially the areas most associated with sarcoptic infestation (ears, lateral elbows, and ventral abdomen of dogs). Repeated scrapings (as many as six scrapings) may be necessary to detect mites. Adult sarcoptic mites are oval and 200 to 400 μm in diameter and have eight legs. The key morphologic feature used to identify this species is the long, unjointed pedicel with a sucker on the end of some of the legs. The anus is located on the caudal end of the body. The eggs of *Sarcoptes* mites are oval.

Notoedres cati infests mainly cats; but on occasion it can parasitize rabbits. This sarcoptiform mite is found chiefly on the ears, back of the neck, face, feet, and, in extreme cases, on the entire body. The life cycle is like that of *S. scabiei,* with the mite burrowing or tunneling in the superficial layers of the epidermis. The characteristic lesion of notoedric acariasis is a yellowing crust in the region of the ears, face, or neck.

Notoedric mites are easier to demonstrate in cats than sarcoptic mites in dogs. Likely infestation sites should be scraped. Like *Sarcoptes* spp., *Notoedres* mites have a long, unjointed pedicel with a sucker on the end of some of the legs. Adult notoedric mites are similar to sarcoptic mites, but are smaller, with a dorsal anus. The eggs of notoedric mites are oval.

Knemidokoptes pilae causes "scaly leg" in budgerigars or parakeets. This mite tunnels in the superficial layers of the epidermis of the pads and shanks of the feet. In severe cases, the beak and cere also may be affected. The mite characteristically produces a yellow to gray-white mass that resembles a honeycomb. This condition may be disfiguring to the parakeet. The parasites pierce the skin underlying the scales, causing an inflammation with exudate that hardens on the surface and displaces the scales superficially. This process causes the thickened, scaly nature of the skin. A related species, *Knemidokoptes mutans,* produces scaly leg in chickens and turkeys.

Infested sites should be scraped. Great care should be taken in handling infested birds because parakeets are fragile creatures. The eight-legged, globular mites are about 500 μm in diameter. Adult female mites have short legs and no suckers on the end of their legs. Adult males have longer legs and a long, unjointed pedicel with suckers on the end of some of the legs.

Psoroptidae

Members of the family Psoroptidae reside on the surface of the skin or within the external ear canal. The entire five-stage life cycle (egg, larva, protonymph, deutonymph or pubescent female, adult egg-laying female) is spent on the host. Adult male and female mites breed on the skin surface (Figure 17-68). The female produces 14 to 24 elliptic, opaque, shiny, white eggs that hatch within 1 to 3 days. The six-legged nymphs are small, oval, soft, and grayish brown. The eight-legged nymphs are slightly larger than larvae. Larval and nymphal stages may last 7 to 10 days. The life cycle is completed in 10 to 18 days. Under favorable conditions,

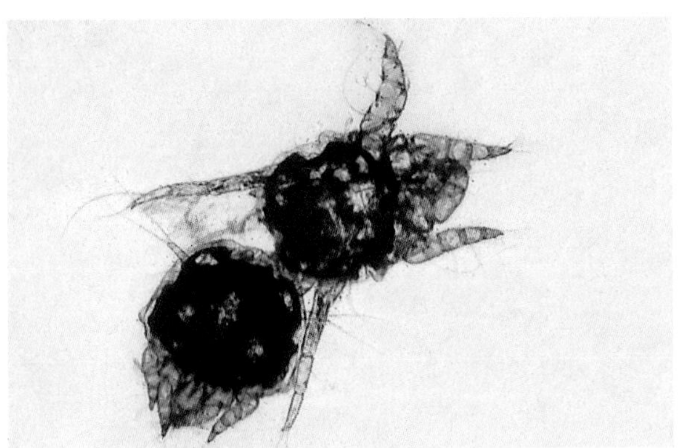

FIGURE 17-68 Adult *P. cuniculi* mites.

psoroptic mites can live off of the host for 2 to 3 weeks or longer. Under optimal conditions, mite eggs may remain viable for 2 to 4 weeks.

Psoroptes cuniculi occurs most commonly in the external ear canal of rabbits, but also has been found in horses, goats, and sheep. These mites live on the surface of the skin and feed on the rabbit host by puncturing the epidermis to obtain tissue fluids. Within the external ear canal of the infested host are the characteristic dried crusts of coagulated serum. The rabbit's ears appear to be packed with dried cornflakes. Affected animals shake their head and scratch their ears. Lesions sometimes occur on the head and legs. Severely infested animals may become debilitated. Loss of equilibrium may occur, with head tilt.

The mites within the crusty debris inside the ear can be easily isolated. The brownish-white female is large, up to 750 μm long. The mites exhibit characteristic long, jointed pedicels with suckers on the ends of some of the legs. The anus is in a terminal slit.

Psoroptes ovis, Psoroptes bovis, and *Psoroptes equi* are the scab mites of large animals, residing on sheep, cattle, and horses, respectively. These mites are host specific and reside within the thick-hair or long-wool areas of the animal. The mites are surface dwellers and feed by puncturing the epidermis to feed on lymphatic fluid. Serum exudes through the puncture site. After the serum coagulates and forms a crust, wool is lost. The feeding site is extremely pruritic, and the animal excoriates itself, producing further wool loss. The mites then migrate to adjacent undamaged skin. As the mites proliferate, tags of wool are pulled out, and the fleece becomes matted. Finally, patches of skin are exposed, and the skin becomes parchmentlike, thickened, and cracked. The skin may bleed easily. Infested sheep constantly rub against fences, posts, farm equipment, and anything else that might serve as a scratching post. The disease is spread by direct contact or infested premises.

P. bovis in cattle produces lesions on the withers, neck, and rump. These consist of papules, crusts, and wrinkled, thickened skin. *P. equi* in horses is rare and affects the base of the mane and the tail. Because of the intense pruritus and the highly contagious nature of the infestation, the occurrence of *Psoroptes* spp. in large animals should be reported to state and federal authorities and the United States Department of Agriculture.

These mites are host specific. Adults are up to 600 μm long. Psoroptic mites exhibit characteristic long, jointed pedicels with suckers on the ends of some of the legs.

Chorioptes equi, Chorioptes bovis, Chorioptes caprae, and *Chorioptes ovis* are the foot and tail mites of large animals, residing on horses, cattle, goats, and sheep, respectively. These mites are found on the skin surface on the distal (lower) part of the hind legs, but may spread to the flank and shoulder area. On cattle, they are frequently found in the tail region, especially in the area of the escutcheon. These mites do not spread rapidly or extensively. The mites puncture the skin, causing serum to exude. Thin crusts of coagulated serum form on the skin surface. The skin eventually wrinkles and thickens, although pruritus is not severe.

Infested horses stamp, bite, and kick, especially at night. Mites typically infest the pasterns, especially those of the hind legs.

The characteristic mites can be identified from skin scrapings of infested areas. Chorioptic mites have short, unjointed pedicels, with suckers on the ends of some of the legs. The female mites are about 400 μm long.

Ear mites, *Otodectes cynotis,* are a common cause of otitis externa in dogs, cats, and ferrets. Although they occur primarily in the external ear canal, ear mites may be found on any area of the body. A common infestation site is the tail and head region. As dogs and cats curl up to sleep, the head (and ears) are often in close proximity to the base of the tail. These mites are spread by direct contact and are highly transmissible both among and between the canine and feline species.

Ear mites are found within the external ear canal, where they feed on epidermal debris and produce intense irritation. The infection is usually bilateral. The host responds to the mite infestation by shaking its head and scratching its ears. Severe infestations may cause otitis media, with head tilt, circling, and convulsions. Auricular hematomas may develop.

Mites usually are identified by using an otoscope; through an otoscope, the mites appear as white, motile objects. The brown exudate collected by swabbing the ear may be placed in mineral oil on a glass slide and the mites observed with a low-power microscopic objective. These mites are fairly large, approximately 400 μm; they also may be easily seen with a magnifying glass or even the unaided eye. The mites exhibit characteristic short, unjointed pedicels, with suckers on the ends of some of the legs (Figure 17-69). The anus is terminal.

Demodex

Mites of the genus *Demodex* reside in the hair follicles and sebaceous glands of most domesticated animals and people. In many species, they are considered normal, nonpathogenic fauna of the skin. These mites are host specific and are not transmissible from one host species to another. The clinical disease, caused by an increased number of these mites, is called demodicosis.

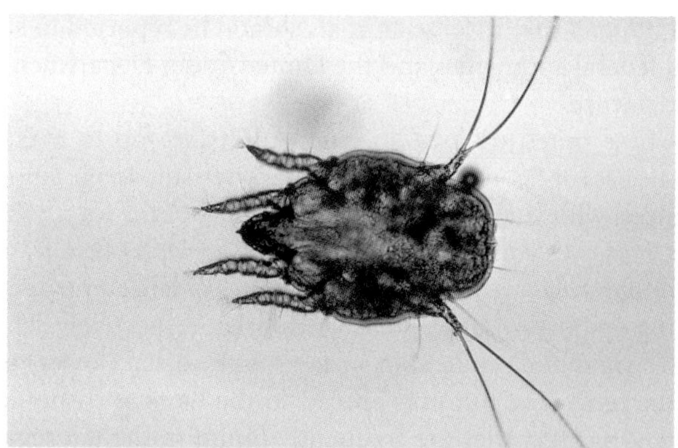

FIGURE 17-69 Adult female *Otodectes cynotis* mite.

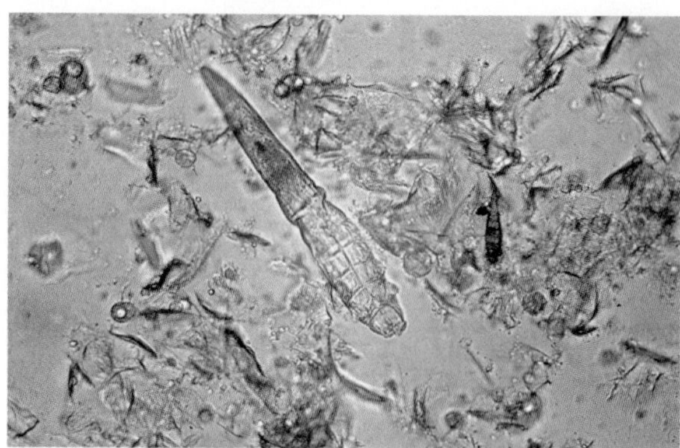

FIGURE 17-70 Adult *Demodex canis* mite.

Demodex mites resemble "eight-legged alligators." These are elongated mites with short, stubby legs on the anterior half of the body. Adult and nymphal stages have eight legs, whereas the larvae have six. Adult *Demodex* mites are approximately 250 μm long (Figure 17-70). The eggs are spindle shaped or tapered at each end.

The life cycle of *Demodex* spp. has five stages: egg, larva, protonymph, deutonymph, and adult. The developmental periods of these various life-cycle stages are not well known.

Of all the domestic animals infested with *Demodex* spp., the dog is the most commonly and most seriously infested. Small numbers of these mites are considered part of the normal skin flora of all dogs. In dogs with immunodeficiencies, however, these mites proliferate and cause skin disease.

Demodicosis occurs in two forms in dogs: localized demodicosis and generalized demodicosis. The preponderant clinical sign of the localized form is patchy alopecia, especially of the muzzle, face, and forelimbs. The mites presumably are acquired during intimate contact when the dam nurses the puppy. As a result of that close contact, localized demodicosis often develops in the region of the face. Generalized demodicosis is characterized by diffuse alopecia, erythema, and secondary bacterial contamination over the entire body surface of the dog. An inherited defect in the dog's immune system is thought to be an important factor in the development of generalized demodicosis.

> *TECHNICIAN NOTE* Of all the domestic animals infested with *Demodex* spp., the dog is the most commonly and most seriously infested. Small numbers of these mites are considered part of the normal skin flora of all dogs. In dogs with immunodeficiencies, however, these mites proliferate and cause skin disease.

Cats are infested by two species of demodectic mites: *Demodex cati* and an unnamed species. *D. cati* is an elongated mite, similar to *Demodex canis*. The unnamed species has a broad, blunted abdomen as compared with the elongated one of *D. cati*. The presence of either species on the skin of cats is rare. In localized feline demodicosis are patchy areas of alopecia, erythema, and occasionally crusting on the head (especially around the eyes), ears, and neck. In generalized feline demodicosis, the alopecia, erythema, and crusting usually involve the entire body. Demodicosis also has been associated with ceruminous otitis externa.

Demodectic mites reside in the hair follicles of other species of domestic animals, but rarely produce clinical disease. Cattle and goats are most commonly infested, but then only rarely. In cattle, *Demodex bovis* causes large nodules (abscesses) on the shoulders, trunk, and lateral aspects of the neck. In goats, *Demodex capri* occurs in small, papular or nodular lesions on the shoulders, trunk, and lateral aspect of the neck. In sheep, *Demodex ovis* rarely causes pustules and crusting around the coronet, nose, ear tips, and periorbital areas. In pigs, *Demodex phylloides* rarely produces pustules and nodules on the face, abdomen, and ventral neck. In horses, *Demodex equi* occurs around the face and eyes and rarely produces clinical disease.

Skin areas with altered pigmentation, obstructed hair follicles, erythema, or alopecia should always be scraped. In localized demodicosis, the areas most commonly affected are the forelegs, perioral region, and periorbital regions. In generalized demodicosis, the entire body may be affected; however, the face and feet usually are the most severely involved. In dogs, areas of apparently normal skin also should be scraped to determine if the disease is generalized. The areas should be clipped and a fold of skin gently squeezed just before scraping. Gentile scraping of affected areas should be continued until capillary blood oozing is observed because these mites live deep in the hair follicles and sebaceous glands (Figure 17-71).

Nodular lesions in large animals should be incised with a scalpel and the caseous material within smeared on a slide with mineral oil, covered with a coverslip, and examined microscopically for mites.

The mites on the slide should be counted and the live: dead ratio determined. The presence of any larval or nymphal stages or eggs should be noted. During therapy for *Demodex* spp., a decrease in the number of eggs and live mites is a good prognostic indicator.

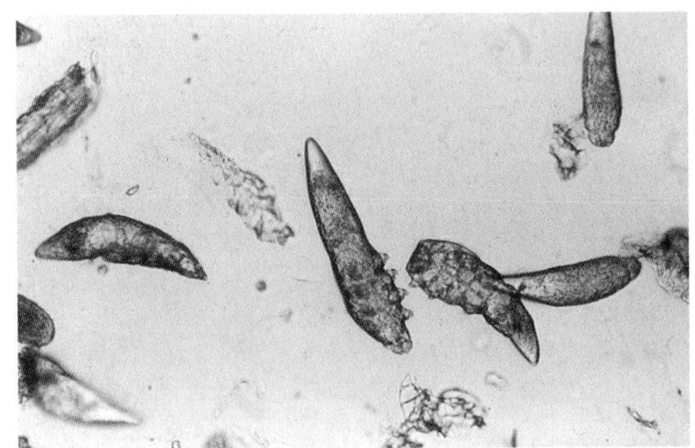

FIGURE 17-71 A deep skin scraping produces numerous mites of *D. canis.*

Cheyletiella

Mites of the genus *Cheyletiella* are surface dwelling (nonburrowing), residing in the keratin layer of the skin and in the hair coat of the definitive host, which may be a dog, cat, or rabbit. These mites ingest keratin debris and tissue fluids. *Cheyletiella* mites are sometimes referred to as "walking dandruff" because the mites resemble large, mobile flakes of dandruff. Cheyletid mites have distinct key morphologic features. They are large (386 by 266 μm) and visible to the naked eye. With the compound microscope, the most characteristic key morphologic feature may easily be seen: the enormous hooklike accessory mouthparts (palpi). These palpi assist the mite in attaching to the host as it feeds on tissue fluids. The mite also has comblike structures at the tip of each leg. Members of the genus also are known for a characteristic body shape resembling a shield, a bell pepper, an oak acorn, or a western horse saddle when viewed from above. Eggs are 235 to 245 μm long and 115 to 135 μm wide (smaller than louse nits) and supported by cocoonlike structures bound to the host's hair shaft by strands of fibers. Two or three eggs may be bound together on one hair shaft.

The key feature of *Cheyletiella* spp. infestation is often the moving white "dandruff" flakes along the dorsal midline and head of the host. A hand-held magnifying lens or Optivisor (binocular headband magnifier) often are used to view questionable dandruff flakes or hairs; these are perhaps the quickest methods of diagnosing cheyletiellosis. A fine-tooth flea comb may be used to collect mites; combing dandruff-like debris onto black paper often facilitates the visualization of these highly mobile mites. Using clear cellophane tape to entrap mites collected from the hair coat often simplifies viewing with the compound microscope.

TICKS

Ticks have dorsoventrally compressed, leathery bodies. The tick's head, or capitulum, serves as an organ of cutting and attachment. It is made of a penetrating anchorlike sucking organ, the hypostome, and four accessory appendages, two chelicerae and two pedipalps, which act as sensors and supports when the tick fastens to the host's body. The tick's body may be partially or entirely covered by a hard, chitinous plate, the scutum. Mouthparts may be concealed under the tick's body or may extend from the cranial border. Most ticks are inornate (i.e., reddish or mahogany, without markings). Some species are ornate (i.e., they have distinctive white patterns on the dark scutum background). Adult ticks have eight legs, with claws on the ends of the legs.

Ticks are important parasites because of a voracious blood-feeding activity. Ticks are important also because they can transmit many parasitic, bacterial, viral, and other diseases, such as borreliosis (Lyme disease), among animals and from animals to humans. These pathogenic organisms may be transmitted passively, or the tick may serve as an obligatory intermediate host.

The salivary secretions of some female ticks are toxic and can produce a syndrome known as "tick paralysis" in people and animals. Tick species commonly associated with tick paralysis are *Dermacentor andersoni* (the Rocky Mountain spotted fever tick), *Dermacentor occidentalis* (the Pacific Coast tick), *Ixodes holocyclus* (the paralysis tick of Australia), and *Dermacentor variabilis* (the wood tick).

Ticks of veterinary importance may be divided into two families: the argasid, or soft, ticks and the Ixodid, or hard, ticks. Argasid ticks lack a scutum, or hard, chitinous plate. The mouthparts of the adults cannot be seen when viewed from the dorsal aspect. Ixodid ticks have a hard, chitinous scutum that covers all of the male tick's dorsum and about one third or less of the female's dorsum. Depending on the degree of engorgement, male ticks are much smaller than female ticks.

Two species of argasid ticks are important: *Otobius megnini* (the spinous ear tick) and *Argas persicus* (the fowl tick). Thirteen economically important tick species are in the Ixodid family. These include *Rhipicephalus sanguineus, Ixodes scapularis, Dermacentor* spp., and *Amblyomma* spp. Of these species, only *R. sanguineus* infests buildings; the remaining ticks attack their hosts outdoors.

The specific identification of ticks is difficult and should be performed by a veterinary parasitologist or a trained arthropodologist. Ticks usually are identified by the shape and length of the capitulum, the shape and color of the body, and the shape and markings on the scutum. Male and unengorged female ticks are easier to identify than engorged females. Determining the species of larval or nymphal ticks is most difficult. Common species may be identified by size, shape, color, body markings, host, and the location on the host.

Four major stages exist in the life cycle of ticks: egg, larva, nymph, and adult. After engorgement on the host, female ticks drop off the host and seek protected places, such as within cracks and crevices or under leaves and branches, to lay eggs (Figure 17-72). The six-legged larvae, or seed ticks, hatch from the eggs and feed on a host (Figure 17-73). The larva molts to the eight-legged nymphal stage, which resembles the adult stage, but lacks the functioning reproductive organs of the adult stage. After one or two blood

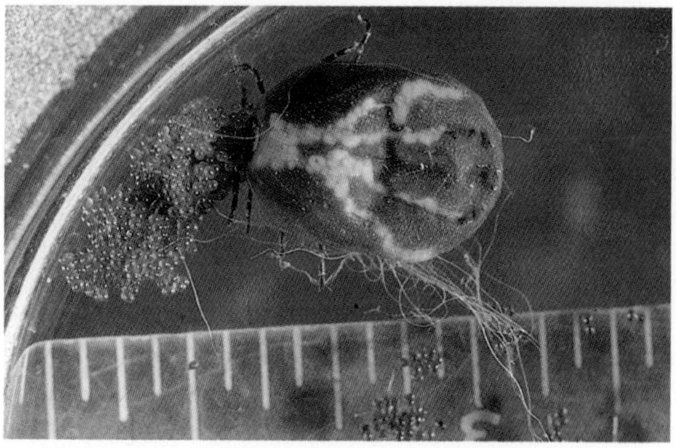

FIGURE 17-72 Adult female *Dermacentor variabilis* tick laying hundreds of eggs.

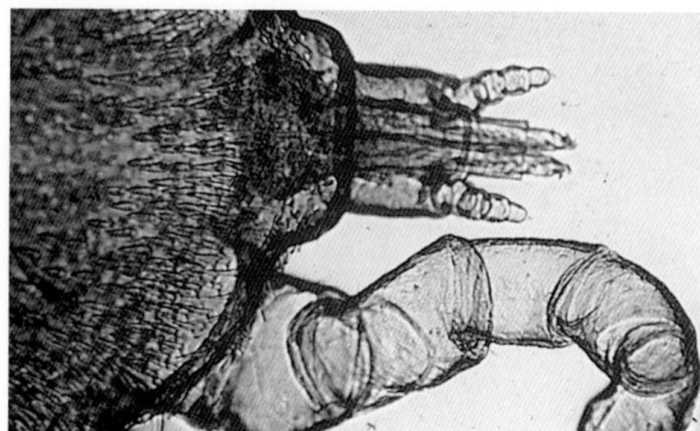

FIGURE 17-74 *Otobius megnini,* the spinous ear tick, is an unusual soft tick in that only the larval and nymphal stages are parasitic. The mouthparts may not be visible when viewed from the dorsal aspect.

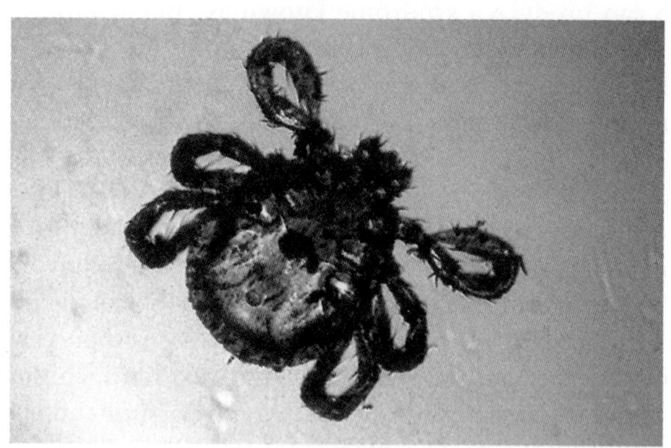

FIGURE 17-73 Six-legged larval *Rhipicephalus sanguineus.*

meals, the nymph matures and molts to the adult stage. During the larval, nymphal, and adult stages, ticks may infest one to three or even many different host species. This ability to feed on several hosts during the life cycle plays an important role in the transmission of disease pathogens among hosts. Any infestation of domestic animals by mites or ticks is referred to as acariasis.

Most ticks do not tolerate direct sunlight, dryness, or excessive rainfall. They can survive as long as 2 to 3 years without a blood meal, but females require blood before egg fertilization and deposition. Tick activity is restricted during the cold winter months.

Soft Ticks (Argasid)

Otobius megnini, the spinous ear tick, is an unusual soft tick in that only the larval and nymphal stages are parasitic. The adult stages are not parasitic, but are free living, found in the environment of the definitive host, usually in dry, protected places, in cracks and crevices, under logs, and on fence posts. The larval and nymphal stages feed on horses, cattle, sheep, goats, and dogs. These ticks usually are associated with the semiarid or arid areas of the southwestern United States. With widespread interstate movement of animals, this soft tick may occur throughout North America. As with most soft ticks, the mouthparts may not be visible when viewed from the dorsal aspect (Figure 17-74). The nymphal stage is widest in the middle, almost violin shape. It is covered with tiny, backward-projecting spines, which is the origin of the name spinous. Larvae and nymphs usually are found within the ears of the definitive host, which is the origin of the name ear tick.

Spinous ear ticks are extremely irritating to the definitive host. They often occur in large numbers, deep within the external ear canal. These ticks imbibe large amounts of host blood; however, because they are soft ticks, they do not enlarge with feeding. Large numbers may produce ulceration deep within the ear. The ears become highly sensitive, and the animals may shake their head. The pinnae may become excoriated by the animal's shaking and rubbing its head.

The ticks may be visualized in the ear with an otoscope. Any waxy exudate should be examined for larval and nymphal spinous ear ticks.

Hard Ticks (Ixodid)

Rhipicephalus sanguineus, the brown dog tick, is an unusual hard tick; it may invade both kennel and household environments. This tick is distributed throughout North America. It has an inornate, uniformly reddish-brown scutum, and it feeds almost exclusively on dogs. *R. sanguineus* also has a distinguishing morphologic feature. Its basis capitulum has prominent lateral extensions that give this structure a decidedly hexagonal appearance (Figure 17-75). The engorged female is often slate gray. In southern climates, the tick is found outdoors, but in northern climates, it becomes a serious household pest, breeding indoors.

The bites of this tick can irritate dogs. Severe infestations may cause heavy blood loss. This tick is also an intermediate host for *B. canis,* the agent that causes piroplasmosis in dogs.

This tick may be identified by its inornate brown color and characteristic lateral projections of the basis capitulum. These ticks are unique; they may be found in indoor or kennel environments.

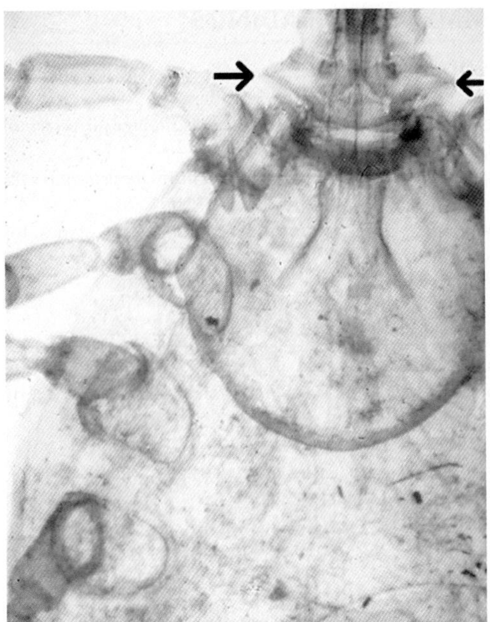

FIGURE 17-75 Lateral expansion of the basis capitulum (base of the head) *(arrows)* of an adult *R. sanguineus*. This key morphologic feature is used to identify this parasite, which can breed in the host's environment.

Dermacentor variabilis

Dermacentor variabilis, the American dog tick or wood tick, is found primarily in the eastern two thirds of the United States; however, with the increased mobility of American households, the tick may occur throughout the country. Unlike *R. sanguineus,* this tick only inhabits grassy, scrub brush areas, especially roadsides and pathways. This three-host tick initially feeds on small mammals and rodents; however, dogs (and people) can serve as hosts for this ubiquitous tick. This tick is a seasonal annoyance to people and domestic animals. It can serve as a vector of Rocky Mountain spotted fever, tularemia, and other diseases and may also produce tick paralysis in animals and people. This tick has a dark brown, ornate scutum with white striping. Unfed adults are approximately 6 mm long, whereas adult engorged females are about 12 mm long and blue gray (Figure 17-76).

This tick may be identified by its morphologic features. It has a rectangular base of the capitulum and characteristic white markings on the dorsal shield.

> TECHNICIAN NOTE *D. variabilis,* the American dog tick or wood tick, is found primarily in the eastern two thirds of the United States. It can serve as a vector of Rocky Mountain spotted fever, tularemia, and other zoonotic diseases and may also produce tick paralysis in animals and people.

Amblyomma americanum

Amblyomma americanum, the Lone Star tick, gets its common name from a characteristic white spot on the apex of its scutum. The spot is more conspicuous on male ticks than on female ticks. This tick is distributed throughout the southern

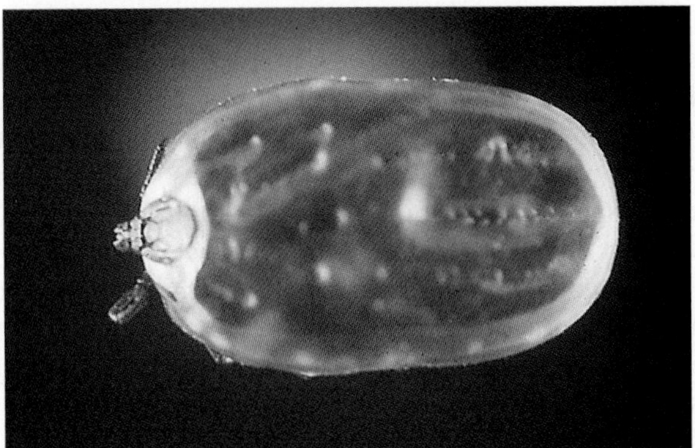

FIGURE 17-76 Adult female *Dermacentor variabilis*. Unfed adults are approximately 6 mm long, whereas engorged adult females are about 12 mm long and a blue-gray color.

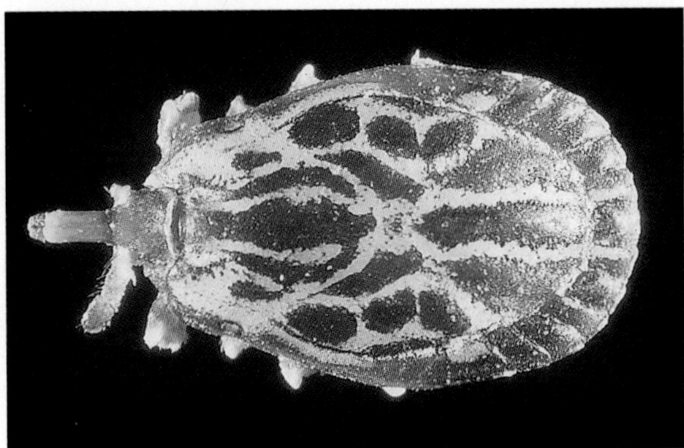

FIGURE 17-77 Ornate adult male *Amblyomma maculatum*.

United States, but is found also in the Midwest and on the Atlantic coast.

This three-host tick is found most often in the spring and summer months, parasitizing the head, belly, and flanks of wild and domestic animal hosts. It also feeds on people and is said to have a painful bite. It can produce anemia and has been incriminated as a vector of tularemia and Rocky Mountain spotted fever. *A. americanum* is easily identified by a characteristic white spot on the apex of the scutum.

Amblyomma maculatum, the Gulf Coast tick, is a three-host tick found in the ears of cattle, horses, sheep, dogs, and people. It occurs in areas of high humidity on the Atlantic and Gulf coasts. It produces severe bites and painful swellings and also is associated with tick paralysis. This tick has silvery markings on its scutum. Larval and nymphal stages occur on ground birds throughout the year. The number of adult ticks on cattle decreases during the winter and spring and increases in the summer and fall. When the ear canals of cattle and horses are infested, the pinna may droop and become deformed. *A. maculatum* is easily identified by the silvery markings on its scutum (Figure 17-77).

Boophilus annulatus

Boophilus annulatus is often called the Texas cattle fever tick or the North American tick. This one-host tick has historical significance in that it is the first arthropod shown to serve as an intermediate host for a protozoan parasite, *B. bigemina* of cattle, a discovery milestone in veterinary parasitology. This tick has been completely eradicated from the United States; however, any *Boophilus* spp. infestation should be reported to the proper regulatory agencies. The tick should be identified by a specialist and control methods applied. *B. annulatus* frequently enters the United States from Mexico.

The engorged female tick is 10 to 12 mm long and the male 3 to 4 mm. The mouthparts are short, and no festoons are on the caudal aspect of the abdomen. Because this is a one-host tick, larvae, nymphs, and adult ticks may be found on the same animal. They do not have to leave the host to complete the life cycle. Animals with heavy infestations are restless and irritated. In an attempt to rid themselves of ticks, they rub, lick, bite, and scratch themselves. Irritated areas may become raw and secondarily infected. Heavily infested cattle may become anemic. Suspect ticks from an enzootic area or from animals originating from the Texas-Mexico border should be submitted to a laboratory recommended by regulatory agencies.

RECOMMENDED READINGS*

Bowman DD, Lynn RC, Eberhard ML: *Georgi's parasitology for veterinarians,* ed 9, St Louis, 2009, Saunders.

Hendrix CM, Robinson E: *Diagnostic parasitology for veterinary technicians,* ed 3, St Louis, 2006, Mosby.

Hendrix CM, Sirous M: *Laboratory procedures for veterinary technicians,* ed 5, St Louis, 2007, Mosby.

Sloss MW et al: *Veterinary clinical parasitology,* ed 6, Ames, Iowa, 1994, Iowa State University.

*All figures in this chapter are originally from Hendrix CM, Robinson E: *Diagnostic parasitology for veterinary technicians,* ed 3, St Louis, 2006, Mosby.

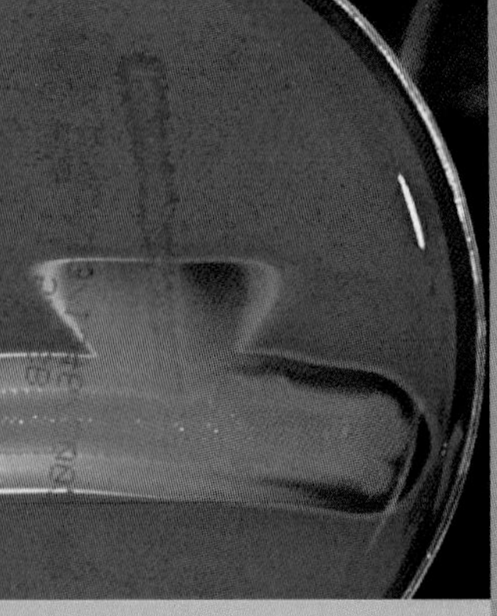

Clinical Microbiology

18

Robert L. Jones

KEY TERMS

Abscess
Acid-fast stain
Aerobe
Anaerobe
Antibiogram
Antigen
Antimicrobial susceptibility test
Catalase
Coagulase
Dermatophyte
Differential medium
Enrichment medium
Fastidious
Gram stain
Hemolysis
Immunoglobulins
Microflora
Minimum inhibitory concentration
Mycosis
Nosocomial infection
Oxidase
Selective medium
Serology
Transport medium
Yeast

OUTLINE

LEARNING OBJECTIVES

When you have completed this chapter, you will be able to:

1. Describe methods for collection and handling of samples for microbiology testing.
2. List the steps of the Gram stain procedure.
3. Describe the procedure for inoculation of agar plates, broth, and slant tube media and explain proper incubation methods for bacterial cultures.
4. List types of culture media commonly used for primary isolation of microorganisms and explain the specific use of each.
5. List and describe the characteristics of bacterial colonies that are evaluated on primary isolates.
6. Describe common staining procedures and biochemical tests used for identification of bacteria.
7. Describe the procedures for performing blood and urine cultures.
8. List common bacterial species encountered in small and large animal practices.
9. Describe the procedure for performing antimicrobial susceptibility testing.
10. List the common fungal organisms encountered in veterinary practice and describe the procedures for sample collection and identification of these organisms.
11. Describe the general principles of serologic analysis for bacterial and viral antigens.
12. Define nosocomial infection and explain methods for control of nosocomial infections.

INTRODUCTION

The purpose of the clinical microbiology laboratory is to rapidly and accurately provide the veterinarian with information that assists in establishing a diagnosis of infectious disease, formulating specific treatment and preventive programs, and predicting the prognosis and possible complications of the disease. The veterinary technician may have a direct impact on the quality of patient care through a variety of activities, ranging from collection of specimens to performance of laboratory assays. The sophistication of diagnostic microbiology that is undertaken in a local practice laboratory depends on the size and type of practice, cost of performing tests, and availability of a technician with appropriate diagnostic microbiology knowledge and skills compared with the services available through referral laboratories and their turnaround time for results. Many practices find it cost effective to operate a limited microbiology laboratory that is capable of processing routine bacterial cultures and performing a limited number of diagnostic tests with readily available test kits.

This chapter provides veterinary technicians with a broad overview of clinical microbiology and introduces some of the more common laboratory diagnostic procedures that may be performed. Common procedures that will be discussed include collection and handling of specimens, processing specimens for staining and microscopic examination, bacterial and fungal cultural procedures for isolation and presumptive identification of possible pathogens, antimicrobial susceptibility testing, use of packaged diagnostic kits for detection of microbial antigens and antibody responses, and immunoglobulin quantitation. Emphasis will be placed on those procedures that can be performed in the laboratories of most veterinary practices. For more advanced procedures, the focus will be on applications and interpretations rather than methods. The problems of nosocomial infections and hospital infectious disease control will be introduced because technicians have a critical role in identifying and solving these problems. This chapter introduces technicians to a variety of diagnostic microbiology activities, but it is not designed to serve as a substitute for detailed technical manuals that should be part of equipping a laboratory. Technician note reference manuals for the identification of bacterial and fungal pathogens are listed at the end of this chapter. These manuals provide detailed descriptions and complete identification characteristics of agents.

DIAGNOSTIC METHODS

The choice of methods for examining a specimen in the microbiology laboratory depends on the type of specimen and the pathogen sought. Traditionally, microbiologists have attempted to *isolate agents* in various types of culture systems and then use various identification schemes to characterize them. This is still the most frequently used method in bacteriology. However, there are times when the organism may be difficult to cultivate or may not be viable in the specimen presented to the laboratory. In these cases, demonstration of *specific microbial antigens* or *nucleic acid* in the specimen may be more rapid and cost effective. Immunohistochemical assays that have been introduced into veterinary diagnostics include enzyme immunoassays, latex particle agglutination, and protein A coagglutination procedures. In some diseases, such as botulism and mycotoxicoses, establishing the presence of a *microbial toxin* is necessary, rather than identifying the organism that produces it. Sometimes, a specific *immunologic response* by the patient to an infectious agent can establish the diagnosis. Serum can be tested for the presence of specific antibodies, or skin tests can be performed. Another diagnostic method is *direct examination* of exudates and tissue biopsy specimens. Some microorganisms present such unique morphologic characteristics, host inflammatory responses, and lesions that a preliminary diagnosis can be established without the need for further laboratory testing.

Recent developments in biotechnology are providing new methods for direct detection of infectious agents. Direct *nucleic acid hybridization probe* and *gene amplification* protocols have tremendous potential for detecting microbial pathogens. These procedures are highly specific and can be extremely sensitive. Because they detect the genes (or portions of genes) of organisms and can differentiate closely related organisms based on the presence of a unique genetic sequence, the identified strains are frequently described as genotypes. DNA probe assays are particularly well suited for in situ hybridization in tissue in which the location and distribution of the organisms must be determined, identification of slow-growing or difficult-to-isolate organisms, and for identification of toxicogenic strains of bacteria that cannot be differentiated from nontoxicogenic strains through the use of conventional methods. Nucleic acid amplification assays use primers and *polymerase chain reaction* (PCR) to provide specificity and sensitivity to detect as few as one organism or 1 to 10 copies of the specific gene sequence. Because of this exquisite sensitivity, specimen collection and handling procedures are critical. Cross-contamination of samples with as little as a single copy of a microbial gene carried on gloves, laboratory bench tops, or aerosolized droplets may result in false-positive test results.

> *TECHNICIAN NOTE* Reference laboratories should be consulted for preferred methods of specimen collection and handling for nucleic acid detection methods to avoid false-positive results from minute contamination of samples.

Ultimately, the goal of these molecular techniques is the direct determination of identities and antimicrobial susceptibility patterns of microorganisms in clinical specimens. As the technology for nucleic acid amplification currently stands, application of the procedure is limited to large referral laboratories and research laboratories. Partial or full automation and improved technology will begin to reduce costs and increase access to these assays. Despite their sensitivity, molecular detection procedures will not totally replace conventional culture and serologic procedures because the results of nucleic acid amplification procedures and the results of culture or serology mean different things. Nucleic acid amplification procedures are used to determine whether DNA or RNA from a particular organism is present in the specimen; they reveal nothing about the viability of the organism (because they can detect DNA from dead organisms) or whether the organism is involved in an infectious process. Culture, on the other hand, clearly demonstrates the viability of the organism, whereas a rise in titer of antibody to a specific organism strongly suggests infection.

COLLECTION OF SPECIMENS

A tremendous diversity of microbial agents, specimen sources, and samples are routinely considered in the microbiology laboratory. Specimen selection, collection, and transport requirements may also vary significantly, depending on the agent to be detected and the assay to be performed. Therefore it is important that technicians be alert to the potential of receiving and implementing specific instructions about specimen collection and handling for each patient rather than anticipating generic procedures.

PROPER SPECIMEN COLLECTION

The goal of specimen collection is to obtain a sample from the patient that is representative of the disease process. Therefore the culture specimen must be from the actual *infection site* (Figure 18-1). It must be collected with a minimum of contamination from adjacent tissues or secretions. Material swabbed from superficial body surfaces (skin or mucous membranes) will usually yield a mixed growth of bacteria, often making it difficult to identify a significant pathogen. Culture specimens recovered from body orifices and draining tracts are frequently contaminated with normal flora. The most useful specimens are those aspirated from normally sterile, closed body compartments after the surface has been aseptically prepared.

Optimal times and *sites* for specimen collection must be observed. Infections by some viruses and mycoplasmas are acute processes that are followed by secondary invasion by opportunistic bacteria; therefore sampling must be performed early in the course of a disease. When viruses and bacteria localize in specific tissues, collection should target such sites. Specimens obtained at necropsy for culture should be collected as soon as possible after the death of the animal (see Chapter 39).

Whenever possible, culture specimens should be obtained before the administration of antimicrobials, especially if the suspected pathogen may be susceptible to the antimicrobial or the antimicrobial may be concentrated at the site of infection. However, the administration of antimicrobials does not necessarily preclude the usefulness of cultures. The antimicrobial drug may be diluted to an ineffective level in culture medium, thereby allowing the pathogen to grow. Antimicrobial-resistant or superinfecting bacteria may still be recovered. In addition, the effectiveness of therapy can be evaluated by determining the relative numbers of bacteria present.

An *adequate quantity* of material should be obtained for complete examination. Aliquots of body fluids (>1 ml), exudates, or pieces of tissue (>3 cm^3) are always more useful than a swab. Smears can be prepared for direct examination, and multiple culture media can be inoculated when adequate material is submitted. Quantitative results can also be obtained if needed.

Appropriate collection devices and specimen handling must be used to ensure optimal survival and recovery of significant microorganisms (Figure 18-2). Sterile swabs are acceptable for transferring most samples from the patient to culture media. If the culture medium is not immediately inoculated, the swab must be placed in a swab transport system (CultureSwab, BD Diagnostic Systems; Copan Transport Swabs, Copan Diagnostics, Inc.) or into a transport medium. *Transport media* are designed to maintain optimal conditions for survival of the suspected pathogen without allowing overgrowth by contaminating saprophytes. Semisolid transport media, such as Amies transport medium with charcoal for *aerobic bacteria* (growth in the presence of oxygen) or the Port-A-Cul Anaerobic Transport System (BD Diagnostic Systems) for *anaerobic bacteria* (requires absence of oxygen), can preserve specimens on swabs for several days. Swabs should not be placed in nutritive broths before inoculation of isolation media because an insignificant nonpathogen may overgrow and prevent recovery of the pathogen. Specimens can be collected in various sterile containers that do not contain preservatives or anticoagulants for transport. If tissues are collected for culture, each piece must be packaged separately in a leak-proof, sterile container.

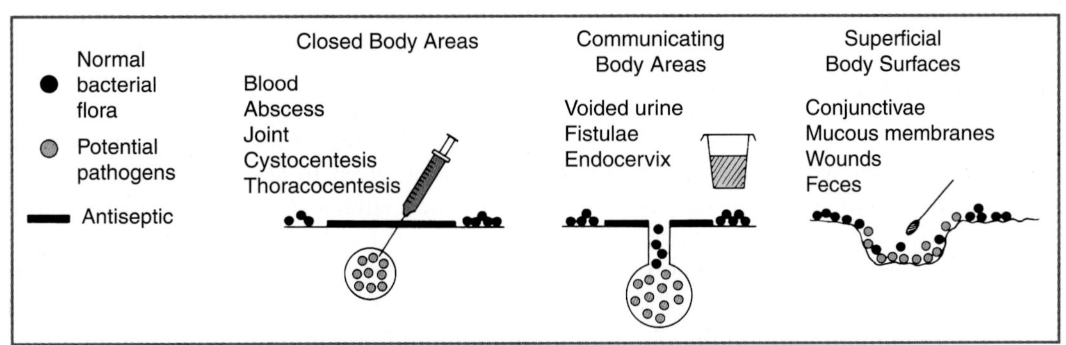

FIGURE 18-1 Methods used to collect bacterial culture specimens and probable sources of contamination.

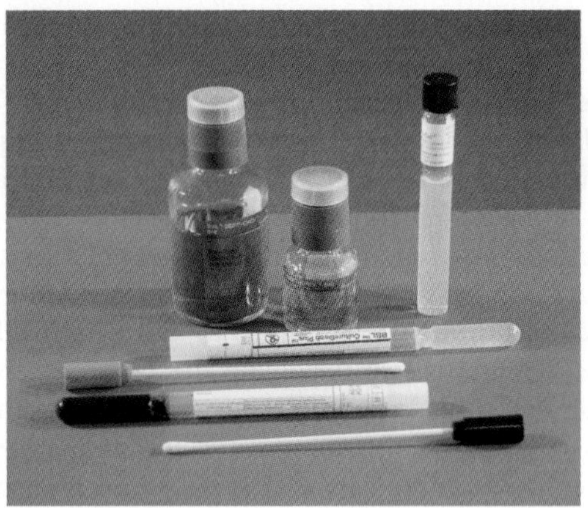

FIGURE 18-2 Culturette swab transport systems with transport media (black medium is Amies transport medium with charcoal), Port-A-Cul Anaerobic Transport Tube (BD Diagnostic Systems), and blood culture bottles. Swabs are used to collect culture inoculum and placed into transport systems or tube of medium for preservation of the viability of bacteria during transportation to the laboratory for culture. Blood culture bottles are inoculated with blood to prevent coagulation and contamination during transport to the laboratory for incubation.

> *TECHNICIAN NOTE* Transport media can serve as excellent vehicles for submitting a bacterial isolate to a reference laboratory for further characterization. A heavily inoculated swab of the pure culture should be placed in the appropriate medium for shipping rather than being submitted in an inoculated growth medium (plate or tube).

Each culture specimen container must be *properly labeled.* Identification of the patient by name, species, case number, or owner, as appropriate, should be legibly indicated. If more than one veterinarian works in the practice, the one in charge of the case should be identified so that questions about history and preliminary reports can be communicated efficiently. The source of the specimen should also be included on the label. As discussed later, the source of the specimen will be a significant factor in deciding how to set up the culture, which bacteria to identify, and how to interpret the results. If the culture specimen is to be sent to a referral laboratory, additional clinical history should be included. Results of previous culture attempts, other laboratory tests, and antimicrobial treatments should be reported, as well as the major clinical manifestations and duration of illness, so that laboratory personnel will be able to recognize and identify significant findings.

SPECIAL COLLECTION AND HANDLING PROCEDURES

Some groups of microorganisms require special collection and handling for optimal isolation. Anaerobic bacteria must be kept away from oxygen. Often, a sterile syringe with a fine-gauge needle (22- to 23-gauge) is the best collection device for aspirating exudates from an infected site. The specimen can be transported to the laboratory in the syringe: if air is expressed, the needle is removed to prevent injuries, and the syringe is capped to prevent leakage. Otherwise, the specimen should be transferred to an appropriate anaerobic transport device. Survival and subsequent isolation of anaerobes are enhanced by keeping them in the reduced microenvironment in which they are found. Therefore, as stated previously, exudate and pieces of tissue are better specimens than swabs. If a swab is collected, it must be placed in an appropriate anaerobic transport device. Handling a specimen as if it contains anaerobes will not jeopardize the viability of aerobic bacteria. Exudates, biopsy material, and tissue should be submitted as quickly as possible to the microbiology laboratory.

For attempts to isolate fungi and mycobacteria, swabs are usually not the best specimens. These agents tend to cause chronic infections, often with small numbers of organisms present. Too few organisms may be present on a swab, or in the case of mycobacteria, they may adhere to the swab, and culture results will be negative.

The more fastidious groups of microorganisms (e.g., *Mycoplasma*, *Chlamydia*, and *Rickettsia* and viruses) require special selective transport media. These media are usually formulated to contain antimicrobials that will inhibit the growth of other microorganisms while preserving the viability of the desired agent. Specific transport media and instructions for proper use should be obtained from a referral laboratory that is capable of providing the desired culture service.

> *TECHNICIAN NOTE* Selective transport media differ from anaerobic transport systems because they usually contain antimicrobial agents. Anaerobic systems only reduce the availability of oxygen to maintain viability of the anaerobes, but the lack of oxygen is not detrimental to other microorganisms during transport.

PROCESSING SPECIMENS

Processing of specimens should be performed in a dedicated laboratory work area to reduce the risk of transmission of infectious agents to patients and staff. Laboratory work should not be performed in areas such as hallways where personnel could accidently become contaminated while walking by. Care also must be taken to avoid cross-contamination of specimens by aerosol or transfer of agents on the laboratory bench surface. Unnecessary traffic and excessive air currents can easily contribute to the creation of aerosols, cross-contamination, and environmental contamination of culture media, thus resulting in spurious culture results.

Each specimen received in the microbiology laboratory should be carefully and individually evaluated, with consideration given to anatomic source and condition of the specimen, animal family of the patient, clinical history, and special requests from the veterinarian. Each pathogen has a preferred habitat in which it will grow and specific mechanisms for causing disease. Therefore, for a particular manifestation of disease, there will be a limited number of agents that should be considered as likely pathogens. Table 18-1 lists

TABLE 18-1 Common Bacterial Species Associated With Infections

Canine	Feline	Equine	Porcine	Ruminants
Dogs	*Cats*	*Horses*	*Swine*	*Ruminants*
Conjunctivitis				
Staphylococcus *Streptococcus* *Pseudomonas*	*Staphylococcus* *Pasteurella* *Chlamydophila*	*Streptococcus* *Staphylococcus*	*Streptococcus* *Staphylococcus*	*Moraxella bovis* *Branhamella* *Streptococcus* *Staphylococcus* *Mycoplasma* *Escherichia coli*
Central Nervous System				
Rare	Rare	*Streptococcus* *Actinobacillus* *Escherichia coli*	*Streptococcus* *Escherichia coli*	*Histophilus somni* *Listeria monocytogenes* *Escherichia coli* *Pasteurella trehalosi*
Gastroenteritis				
Salmonella *Clostridium perfringens* *Campylobacter* *Clostridium difficile*	*Salmonella*	*Salmonella* *Escherichia coli* *Actinobacillus* *Rhodococcus equi*	*Salmonella* *Escherichia coli* *Brachyspira* *Clostridium perfringens*	*Salmonella* *Escherichia coli* *Clostridium perfringens* *Mycobacterium paratuberculosis*
Genital Tract				
Brucella canis *Escherichia coli* *Streptococcus* *Staphylococcus* *Mycoplasma*	*Streptococcus* *Pasteurella* *Escherichia coli*	*Streptococcus* *Escherichia coli* *Klebsiella* *Pseudomonas*	*Brucella suis* *Streptococcus* *Leptospira*	*Brucella* *Listeria monocytogenes* *Arcanobacterium pyogenes* *Campylobacter* *Mycoplasma*
Mastitis				
Staphylococcus	*Staphylococcus*	*Streptococcus*	*Streptococcus* *Staphylococcus* *Escherichia coli* *Actinobacillus* *Arcanobacterium pyogenes*	*Streptococcus* *Staphylococcus* *Arcanobacterium pyogenes* *Mycoplasma* *Mycobacterium* *Escherichia coli* *Klebsiella* *Nocardia*
Musculoskeletal				
Staphylococcus *Escherichia coli* *Pseudomonas* *Brucella canis* Anaerobes	Rare	*Streptococcus* *Actinobacillus* *Escherichia coli* *Rhodococcus equi* *Staphylococcus* *Clostridium*	*Streptococcus* *Mycoplasma* *Escherichia coli* *Erysipelothrix* *Arcanobacterium pyogenes*	*Clostridium* *Arcanobacterium pyogenes* *Escherichia coli* *Streptococcus* *Erysipelothrix* *Histophilus somni* *Mycoplasma*
Otitis				
Staphylococcus *Pseudomonas* *Streptococcus* *Clostridium perfringens*	Rare	Rare	Rare *Streptococcus*	Rare *Streptococcus* *Pasteurella* *Arcanobacterium pyogenes* *Mycoplasma*
Upper Respiratory Tract				
Bordetella bronchiseptica	*Pasteurella multocida*	*Streptococcus equi*	*Bordetella bronchiseptica* *Pasteurella multocida*	*Histophilus somni* *Arcanobacterium pyogenes* *Fusobacterium*

Continued

TABLE 18-1 Common Bacterial Species Associated With Infections—cont'd

Canine	Feline	Equine	Porcine	Ruminants
Dogs	*Cats*	*Horses*	*Swine*	*Ruminants*
Pneumonia				
Bordetella bronchiseptica *Pasteurella* *Klebsiella* *Escherichia coli* *Mycoplasma* *Streptococcus* *Staphylococcus*	Rare *Pasteurella* *Chlamydia* *Bordetella*	*Streptococcus* *Actinobacillus* *Rhodococcus equi* *Pasteurella* *Staphylococcus* *Klebsiella* *Pseudomonas* *Bordetella bronchiseptica*	*Bordetella bronchiseptica* *Pasteurella multocida* *Mycoplasma* *Haemophilus parasuis* *Actinobacillus pleuropneumoniae* *Streptococcus*	*Histophilus somni* *Arcanobacterium pyogenes* *Mannheimia haemolytica* *Pasteurella multocida* *Arcanobacterium pyogenes* *Fusobacterium* *Mycoplasma*
Pleuritis				
Fusobacterium *Prevotella* *Porphyromonas* *Actinomyces*	*Prevotella* *Porphyromonas* *Fusobacterium* *Pasteurella* *Nocardia*	*Streptococcus* *Anaerobes*	*Actinobacillus*	*Mannheimia* *Pasteurella* *Arcanobacterium pyogenes*
Skin Wounds, Abscesses				
Staphylococcus *Streptococcus* *Pseudomonas* *Nocardia* *Actinomyces* *Fusobacterium*	*Pasteurella multocida* *Streptococcus* *Staphylococcus* *Anaerobes*	*Streptococcus* *Corynebacterium pseudotuberculosis* *Pseudomonas* *Dermatophilus* *Staphylococcus*	*Streptococcus* *Staphylococcus* *Arcanobacterium pyogenes*	*Arcanobacterium pyogenes* *Dermatophilus* *Actinomyces* *Actinobacillus* *Staphylococcus* *Corynebacterium pseudotuberculosis*
Urinary Tract				
Escherichia coli *Proteus* *Staphylococcus* *Streptococcus* *Klebsiella* *Pseudomonas* *Mycoplasma*	*Staphylococcus* *Escherichia coli*	*Streptococcus* *Escherichia coli*	*Actinobaculum suis* *Streptococcus*	*Corynebacterium renale* *Arcanobacterium pyogenes*

the most common bacterial species associated with infections of various sites in animals. If the technician can focus the search for pathogens on these most likely agents, results will often be obtained much more rapidly and with less expense.

CONDITION OF THE SPECIMEN

If there is evidence that the specimen has become grossly contaminated or dried out, if it is of insufficient quantity, if there has been excessive delay in receipt, or if any other evidence of mishandling is present, an attempt should be made to obtain a second sample. Specimens should be processed the same day they are collected, or they should be kept refrigerated if a delay is anticipated.

DIRECT MICROSCOPIC EXAMINATION

Direct microscopic examination of exudates, impression smears from tissues, or infected body fluids is the most important laboratory procedure that can be used for microbiologic diagnosis. It provides immediate information on the types and numbers of microorganisms present and the type of host cellular inflammatory response. The likelihood of infection can be determined, as can the probable type of agent (i.e., virus, bacterium, or fungus), which in turn determines the nature of the diagnostic assays needed. The most likely pathogen (or predominant organism) may tentatively be identified. This information may be used to provide guidance in selection of optimal culture conditions and as the basis for the interpretation of the significance of subsequent culture results. In some cases it may be all the information the veterinarian needs.

In many situations, application of Gram stain is the procedure of choice because it allows differentiation of gram-positive and gram-negative bacteria. However, some bacteria do not stain well with Gram stain. Gram-negative bacteria may not be well differentiated from the background in exudates and tissue impression smears.

Other tissue stains (i.e., Giemsa and Wright stains or methylene blue wet mounts) may be more useful for detecting all microorganisms present in the smear. Although these stains are more efficient in demonstrating the presence and morphology of bacteria, they do not provide differentiation of gram-positive and gram-negative bacteria. Careful direct examination may be sufficient for diagnosis without cultures, or it can narrow the diagnostic likelihood to a few bacterial species. This information helps in the selection of optimal culture conditions for identification of suspected pathogens.

> *TECHNICIAN NOTE* Microscopic examination of urine for bacteria should not be used as a substitute for urine culture. Caution must be exercised in the examination of unstained preparations of urine sediment to avoid interpreting artifacts as bacteria. Cocci are difficult to detect without staining, whereas rod-shaped bacteria may be more readily detected. Significant bacteruria is rarely present in the absence of an inflammatory response, and the detection of bacteria within the cytoplasm of phagocytes suggests phagocytosis rather than contamination of the sample.

Gram Stain Procedure and Interpretation

The technique for preparing a gram-stained slide is as follows:

1. Prepare a thin smear from tissue exudates or bacterial suspension on a clean slide and allow smear to air dry.
2. Fix material to the slide so that it does not wash off during the staining procedure by passing the slide, right side up, through a flame three or four times.
3. Flood smear with crystal violet solution, and let stand for 1 minute.
4. Wash smear briefly with tap water.
5. Flood smear with Gram iodine solution, and let stand for 1 minute.
6. Wash with tap water, and decolorize until solvent flows colorlessly from the slide. This usually requires 5 to 10 seconds.
7. Wash briefly with tap water, and flood the slide with safranin counterstain for 30 to 60 seconds.
8. Wash briefly with tap water, blot and air dry, and examine.

The stained smear is best examined by using the 100× (oil immersion) objective of the microscope. Gram-positive bacteria retain the crystal violet iodine complex and appear dark blue or purple. Gram-negative bacteria lose the primary complex, take up the secondary dye safranin, and appear red. Fungi (yeasts) appear gram-positive. Inflammatory cells appear gram-negative, and epithelial cells may appear gram-positive or gram-negative, depending on the thickness of the smear. Backgrounds usually appear gram-negative but may appear gram-positive if they are thick and inadequately washed. Fibrin, mucus, and erythrocytes often stain gram-negative and may mask detection of gram-negative bacteria.

BACTERIAL ISOLATION AND IDENTIFICATION PROCEDURES

The equipment and supplies required for the performance of basic diagnostic bacteriology tests depend on the scope of services to be provided. Some of the more common items are as follows: binocular microscope, incubator, anaerobic culture system, staining reagents or kits, specimen collection devices, swabs, transport media, isolation and identification media (Table 18-2), packaged identification systems (Boxes 18-1 and 18-2), and miscellaneous instruments, supplies, and appropriate reagents for the diagnostic procedures to be performed.

The most expensive item is a good-quality binocular light microscope with a 100× oil immersion objective. Dark-field and phase-contrast options are useful but not essential. Small countertop incubators are available. Important characteristics of a quality incubator include (1) insulated walls to maintain a constant temperature; (2) an adequate seal to maintain a humid atmosphere; (3) a capacity for plates, tubes, and candle jars; (4) a thermometer to check the temperature, which should not fluctuate more than ±2° C; and (5) an adjustable, thermostatically controlled heating element.

CULTURE MEDIA

Several formulations of media are needed in the bacteriology laboratory for isolation of various microbial agents and for identification of these microorganisms. Both dehydrated and prepared media are readily available today. It is usually much more convenient for small laboratories to purchase prepared media than to prepare their own. In addition, the quality of purchased media will be much more consistent, and these media will usually be quality tested before they are distributed. There are numerous distributors of prepared media throughout the United States. A few national and regional distributors are listed in Box 18-2. Names and addresses of other suppliers can be obtained from local hospitals and by searching the World Wide Web. Some microbiology supply distributors have a full line of prepared plates and tubes of media available, and ancillary biochemical reagents, stains, and miscellaneous supplies.

Purpose of Specific Media

Solid media in plates are used for primary isolation of bacteria from clinical specimens. This type of medium allows distribution of the specimen in such a way that *isolated colonies* develop, each representing a single bacterial cell. Some primary isolation media contain inhibitory ingredients that allow them to be *selective* for specific groups of bacteria. MacConkey agar is selective for bacteria that can grow in the presence of bile salts, which is similar to the environment found in the intestines. A *differential* medium contains an indicator system that can distinguish different bacteria, even though both types may grow. The lactose-fermenting ability of bacteria on MacConkey agar is a differential reaction. Table 18-2 lists some of the more commonly used culture media, the indicated use of the media, and selective and differential characteristics.

> *TECHNICIAN NOTE* Common laboratory media are optimized to support growth of many, but not all pathogens. Occasionally, strains of common organisms such as *Staphylococcus*, *Streptococcus*, and *Clostridium* spp. that mostly grow poorly, if at all, in the laboratory are observed.

TABLE 18-2 Bacteriologic Plate and Tube Media for the Practitioner's Laboratory

Purpose and Inoculation	Reactions and Interpretations
Blood Agar Plate (Trypticase Soy Agar With 5% Sheep Blood)	
Primary isolation medium for all specimens in which pathogenic bacteria are suspected. Always streak for colony isolation.	Observe growth rates, colony morphologic characteristics, hemolysis. Test selected colonies for Gram reaction, catalase, and oxidase. Inoculate differential tests and antimicrobial susceptibility tests from well-isolated colonies.
MacConkey Agar	
A primary isolation and differential plating medium for selection and recovery of *Enterobacteriaceae* and related gram-negative bacteria. Inoculate by streaking for colony isolation.	Growth is usually gram-negative. Pink to red colonies (with increased redness of the medium) are lactose fermenters (e.g., species of *Escherichia*, *Klebsiella*, and *Enterobacter*). Colorless colonies (often with a slight change of the medium to yellow) are nonlactose fermenters.
Hektoen Enteric Agar	
A direct plating medium for fecal specimens that is highly selective for *Salmonella*. Inoculate by streaking for colony isolation.	Disaccharide fermenters are moderately inhibited and produce bright orange to yellow to salmon to pink colonies. *Salmonella* colonies are blue-green, typically with back centers from hydrogen sulfide. *Proteus* colonies may resemble *Salmonella*.
Selenite Broth or Tetrathionate Broth	
Enrichment broth for the selective enhancement of growth by *Salmonella* from specimens containing heavy concentrations of mixed bacteria, such as feces. Inoculate relatively heavily, and incubate 18-24 hr.	Subculture to MacConkey agar and Hektoen enteric agar for isolation of *Salmonella*.
Triple Sugar Iron (TSI) Agar Slant	
A differential medium for detection of carbohydrate (glucose, lactose, sucrose) fermentation and production of hydrogen sulfide. Inoculate by the butt once with an inoculating needle and by streaking the slant. Incubate with a loose cap.	Yellow color change indicates acidification caused by carbohydrate fermentation. In the butt, glucose stabbing fermentation is detected; in the slant, lactose and sucrose fermentation is detected (includes glucose fermentation as an intermediate product). Red color change indicates alkalinization caused by lack of carbohydrate fermentation. Black color indicates hydrogen sulfide production. Results are recorded as slant/butt; A = acid (yellow), K = alkaline (red), or NC = no change.
Christensen's Urea Agar Slant	
A differential medium for detection of urease production by an organism. Inoculate by streaking heavily over the slant.	Urease-positive bacteria produce a pink-red color change in the slant and sometimes throughout the butt. Urease-negative bacteria allow the medium to remain the original yellow color.
Motility Media*	
A test medium for determining if an organism is motile or nonmotile. Inoculate by stabbing the center of the tube with an inoculating needle. Incubate at 35° C for most organisms; incubate at room temperature if *Listeria* is suspected.	Motile organisms migrate from the stab line, flaring out to cause turbidity in the medium. Nonmotile organisms grow only along the stab line; the surrounding medium remains clear.
Indole Test Media*	
A test medium for detecting the ability of bacteria to produce indole as one of the degradation products of tryptophan metabolism. Inoculate, incubate 24-48 hr, then add Kovac's reagent to detect indole.	Development of a red color at the interface of the reagent and the broth within seconds after adding the reagent indicates a positive test result.

*Combination media that provide for several tests in the same tube, such as SIM (sulfide-indole-motility), MIO (motility indole ornithine), or MIL (motility indole lysine), can be purchased.

Inoculation of Media

Before media are inoculated, each tube or plate should be labeled with a distinct identification and the date of inoculation. Plates should be labeled on the bottom with a waterproof marker. The swabs used for collection of most clinical specimens can be used for direct inoculation of primary isolation media. In the laboratory, a sterile swab can also be used to transfer inoculum material from liquid and tissue specimens to isolation media. The same swab can be used for inoculation of several media if the least inhibitory medium is inoculated first and the most inhibitory medium is inoculated last; for example, blood agar can be inoculated first, and then MacConkey agar can be inoculated.

Between one fourth and one third of the surface of the agar plates should be inoculated with the specimen. The inoculum is then progressively diluted across the agar by successive steps

BOX 18-1 Commercial Kit Systems for Identification of Microorganisms

Enterobacteriaceae
API 20E (bioMérieux, Inc.)
Enterotube II (BD Diagnostic Systems)
MicroID (Remel)
Staphylococcus
API Staph (bioMérieux, Inc.)
Streptococcus
API 20 Strep (bioMérieux, Inc.)
SMALL GRAM-POSITIVE BACILLI
API Coryne (bioMérieux, Inc.)
OTHER GRAM-NEGATIVE BACTERIA
API 20E (bioMérieux, Inc.)
Oxi/Ferm Tube II (BD Diagnostic Systems)
Yeast
API 20C AUX (bioMérieux, Inc.)
Anaerobic Bacteria
API 20A (bioMérieux, Inc.)

See Box 18-2 for addresses of product manufacturers and distributors.

BOX 18-2 Commercial Sources of Microbiology Laboratory Supplies

This is a partial list of manufacturers and distributors of various microbiology laboratory supplies, such as prepared plate and tube media, stains and reagents, susceptibility test supplies, loops, slides, swabs, incubators, microscopes, anaerobic systems, and diagnostic kits. Through consultation with other local microbiology laboratories (e.g., hospitals) and searching the World Wide Web, other local or regional suppliers may be discovered.

- Anaerobe Systems, 15906 Concord Circle, Morgan Hill, CA 95037, (408) 782-7557
- Bacti-Lab, Inc., PO Box 1179, Mountain View, CA 94042, (800) 227-7300
- BD Diagnostic Systems, 7 Loveton Circle, Sparks, MD 21152, (800) 675-0908
- BD, 1 Becton Drive, Franklin Lakes, NJ 07417, (888) 237-2762
- bioMérieux, Inc., 595 Anglum Drive, Hazelwood, MO 63042, (800) 634-7656
- Copan Diagnostics, Inc., 2175 Sampson Avenue, Suite 124, Corona, CA 92879, (800) 216-4016
- Heska Corp., 3760 Rocky Mountain Avenue, Loveland, CO 80538, (800) 464-3752
- IDEXX Laboratories, Inc., One Idexx Drive, Westbrook, ME 04092, (800) 248-2483
- ImmuCell Corp., 56 Evergreen Drive, Portland, ME 04103, (800) 466-8235
- Midland BioProducts Corp., 800 Snedden Drive, PO Box 309, Boone, IA 50036, (800) 370-6367
- Remel, Inc., 12076 Sante Fe Drive, Lenexa, KS 66215, (800) 255-6730
- Synbiotics Corp., 11011 Via Frontera, San Diego, CA 92127, (800) 228-4305
- VMRD, Inc., PO Box 502, Pullman, WA 99163, (800) 222-8673

of streaking with a bacteriologic loop (Figure 18-3). There are several different streaking technique modifications, and any method that yields isolated colonies is satisfactory. With the practice of a light touch to avoid tearing the agar and experience in anticipating the amount of bacterial growth that will occur, slight modifications can be made in technique from one specimen to the next to achieve the best isolation of colonies.

Media dispensed in tubes may be a broth or semisolid agar, or media may be poured as a slant. Broth media can be inoculated with a loop or an inoculating wire by touching the side of the tube just below the surface of the medium. Depending on the purpose of the slant medium, it may require inoculation by stabbing the deep (or butt) portion of the agar (e.g., triple sugar iron [TSI] slants); the slant surface is then streaked from bottom to top (Figure 18-4). When a semisolid medium for motility testing is inoculated (Figure 18-5), it is important for the inoculating wire to be inserted and removed along the same tract within the medium.

INCUBATION CONDITIONS

Inoculated plates are incubated in an inverted position to prevent condensation of water on the lid. If water drops to the agar surface, it can mix the bacterial growth rather than

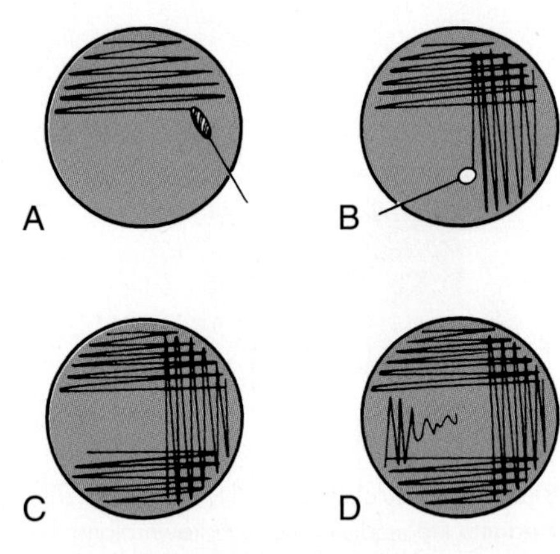

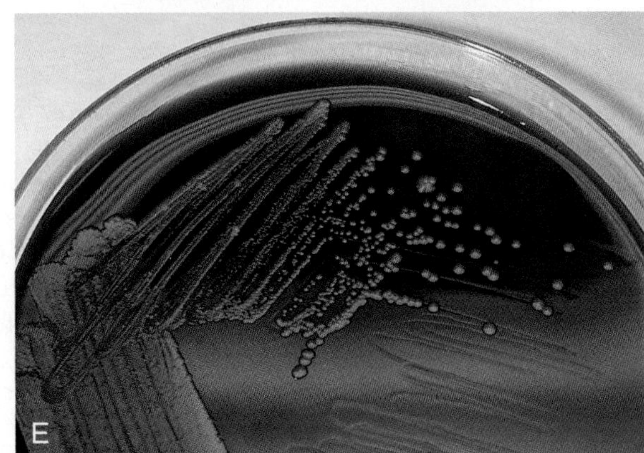

FIGURE 18-3 Plate inoculation and streaking method for isolation of bacterial colonies. **A,** Inoculate with swab, covering one fourth to one third of plate. **B,** Streak lightly, overlapping previous area. **C,** Flame loop, allow it to cool, and streak next area. **D,** Repeat as in C. The photo illustrates well isolated colonies.

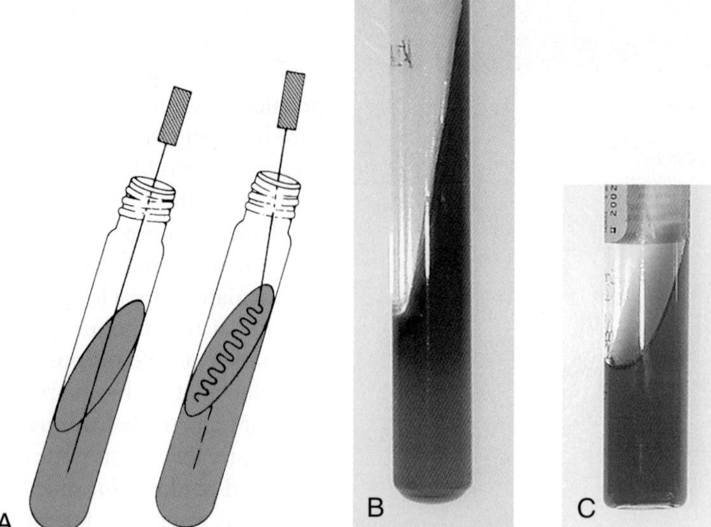

FIGURE 18-4 Inoculation procedure for agar tube media. **A,** Inoculation of agar slant and butt, such as triple sugar iron (TSI). The inoculation needle is first stabbed into the butt and then removed and streaked over the agar slant surface in a back-and-forth motion. **B,** Alkaline slant and acid butt reaction (K/A) in TSI. **C,** Positive urease reaction after slant inoculation.

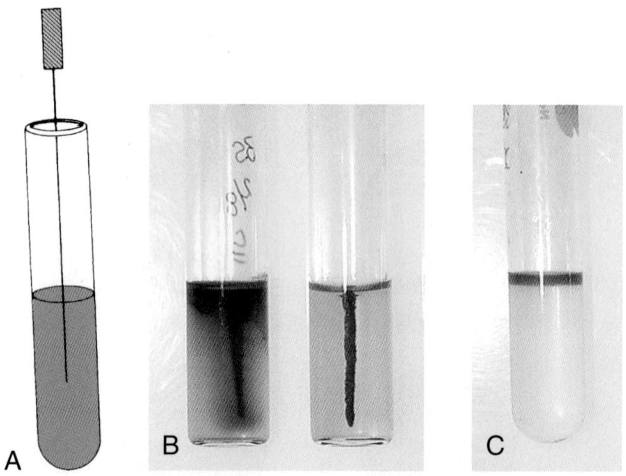

FIGURE 18-5 **A,** Inoculation of motility test media. The inoculation needle is stabbed into the medium and withdrawn along the same tract. **B,** Motile bacterial growth in the left tube and nonmotile growth in the

allowing it to develop as isolated colonies. If tube media have screw tops, they should be left loose during incubation.

Cultures should be placed in incubation at an optimal temperature as quickly as possible. The majority of cultures for isolation of pathogenic bacteria are incubated at 35° C. Although optimal growth may occur at other temperatures, in most cases, alternate temperatures are more important for differentiation of bacteria than for primary isolation.

Atmosphere

Most common pathogenic bacteria are aerobes or facultative anaerobes and will grow well in an atmosphere of room air. However, oxygen is toxic to obligate anaerobic bacteria, requiring that a special culture container from which all oxygen has been removed be used for incubation. Two excellent anaerobic systems for the small laboratory are the BioBag Type A environmental chamber and the BBL Gas-Pak anaerobic system (BD Diagnostic Systems, Sparks, MD). Each system consists of a hydrogen generator, a catalyst to facilitate the depletion of oxygen from the atmosphere by combining with the hydrogen, and a sealable container to hold these components and the culture plates. Certain bacteria—such as *Campylobacter*, *Brucella*, *Haemophilus*, and *Mycoplasma*—have specialized atmospheric and nutritional requirements so that specimens to be cultured for these agents are best forwarded to reference laboratories.

Time

All inoculated plates should be examined after 15 to 24 hours of incubation (overnight). Most cultures will have sufficient growth for evaluation and identification at this time. Culture specimens that contained bacteria on direct microscopic examination but yield negative results after this time or specimens that may be expected to contain slow-growing bacteria should be incubated for up to 3 days before a final negative report is issued. Incubation of primary isolation plates beyond 3 days is rarely indicated unless there is reason to suspect the presence of an unusually slow-growing pathogen.

ROUTINE CULTURE SYSTEM

The majority of specimens for culture in the veterinary microbiology laboratory can be processed in a routine manner with a minimum of media. The approach presented in this section is not represented as a comprehensive culture system that will successfully isolate and identify all potentially pathogenic bacteria; rather, it is meant as a basic guideline for the veterinary technician who has the opportunity to provide a diagnostic bacteriology service within a private veterinary practice. The system is designed to be cost effective when used for routine aerobic cultures, which will usually account for 80% to 90% of culture requests. Often, the veterinarian's immediate objective is for the laboratory to characterize the isolate sufficiently to guide antimicrobial selection or to perform an antimicrobial susceptibility test rather than to pursue definitive identification. The challenge for the technician is to discern when it is better to refer a specimen to another laboratory for more sophisticated diagnostic evaluation.

Primary Isolation Media

Blood agar, containing 5% sheep blood, is the most widely used primary isolation medium because of its ability to support growth of most pathogenic bacteria. It is also a standard medium used extensively for describing colony morphologic characteristics and hemolytic patterns. MacConkey agar is also commonly used as a primary isolation medium. Although use of MacConkey agar is not always essential, it often provides significant information about bacteria and may provide presumptive identification, or at least group classification, of the isolate. If MacConkey agar is inoculated as a primary isolation medium, rather than used as a differential medium for subcultures, the identification process is often moved forward by 1 day.

In many laboratories, it is customary to include an *enrichment broth* as part of the primary isolation medium. One of the most common broth media used for this purpose is thioglycolate. This medium can support growth of many anaerobic or facultative anaerobic bacteria that might not be recovered on primary plates incubated aerobically.

> *TECHNICIAN NOTE* Enrichment media are formulated to facilitate cultivation of microorganisms that may be present in the specimen in very low numbers or have special growth requirements.

Primary growth in a broth medium is frequently difficult to interpret. It must always be compared with a direct microscopic examination because contaminating bacteria from the environment or indigenous flora may overgrow a pathogen in the specimen. Specimens should never be cultured solely in a broth medium for primary isolation. Further discussion of the interpretation of broth subcultures is presented later.

When specific pathogens are sought in specimens, modifications of the basic culture setup can be incorporated into the laboratory routines. Procedures that may enhance the likelihood of recovering specific pathogens are discussed later in this chapter.

Preliminary Evaluation of Cultures

Efficient evaluation of primary cultures requires considerable skill, which is acquired through experience in the microbiology laboratory. Decisions that must be made about isolated bacteria include their possible significance as pathogens, which bacteria require further identification, and what additional tests are needed. As the veterinary technician gains experience in the laboratory and becomes acquainted with common bacterial pathogens, these decisions will become less challenging. Clinically useful results usually only require that identification of bacteria is usually carried to the presumptive level by a few key characteristics rather than to a definitive identification. Only isolates considered to be clinically significant need to be identified. Identification of bacterial growth that results from environmental contamination or indigenous microflora is wasted effort.

From the initial examination of primary cultures, considerable information can be obtained to help distinguish which bacteria should be characterized in further detail. The important characteristics of primary cultures to be noted include (1) the number of different types of bacteria isolated, (2) the relative number of each type, (3) the colony morphologic characteristics of the various isolates, and (4) the changes in the media surrounding the colonies. While making the preliminary evaluation of primary cultures, the technician must keep in mind the source of the specimen. If it was obtained from a normally sterile body site (e.g., joint fluid) and was properly handled, any growth is likely to be significant. If the specimen is from a site normally colonized by microflora (e.g., intestinal tract), interpretation becomes much more difficult. In general, if there is scant aerobic growth of three or more bacteria, the result probably reflects normal flora. Most bacterial infections, other than mixed anaerobic infections, are usually caused by only one or two agents. When a specimen from an infectious process is carefully collected, growth of a single organism in nearly pure culture will often be observed. Therefore the most abundant colony type is usually the most important.

Some general guidelines for selection of significant isolates can be derived from colony morphologic characteristics, although exceptions will always occur. Usually circular, smooth, raised or convex, opaque to gray colonies with an entire edge are more likely to be significant. Large, rough, granular, irregular, spreading, or heavily pigmented colonies

> *TECHNICIAN NOTE* Some bacterial species characteristically produce hemolysins that can be demonstrated when the bacteria are cultured on blood agar plates, and their hemolysis affects the red blood cells (RBCs) in the zone surrounding the hemolytic colony. The following types of hemolytic activity may be observed:
>
> - *Complete hemolysis:* Complete lysis of RBCs in the medium resulting in a clear, colorless zone surrounding the colony. For *Streptococcus* spp., this is referred to as β-hemolysis.
> - *Incomplete hemolysis:* Partial destruction of RBCs with some loss of hemoglobin. Because of streptococcal action on hemoglobin, a zone of greenish discoloration of the agar appears and is known as α-hemolysis.
> - *Nonhemolytic:* No apparent lysis of RBCs, although there may be some discoloration of media. For *Streptococcus* spp., this is sometimes referred to as γ-hemolysis.

are likely to be insignificant unless large numbers are recovered in nearly pure culture.

Changes in the media should be carefully noted. *Hemolysis* in blood agar is often a good indication of a possible pathogen. Sometimes the hemolytic pattern provides adequate identification (Figure 18-6), such as the double zone of hemolysis produced by many coagulase-positive isolates of *Staphylococcus* spp. Pigment production can be an important characteristic to note on primary cultures. The differential features of MacConkey agar (i.e., ability to grow, lactose fermentation) are important bits of information that can aid in the identification of an isolate. Odors produced by bacteria are difficult to describe adequately but, after experience is gained, become another useful identifying characteristic.

The novice microbiologist may be required to rely on several differential tests for the identification of isolates. As experience is gained and confidence develops, more isolates will be recognized on the primary plates. Knowledge of the more common bacterial species to expect from a specimen (see Table 18-1) will provide a differential list of bacteria to consider so that it is not necessary to face each culture as a complete unknown.

Recording, Interpreting, and Reporting Results

Although it is impossible to devise rigid rules that provide for adequate processing of all specimens, some routines are helpful for observing and recording results of cultures. A laboratory worksheet should be developed for recording all observations. These records should contain sufficient detail so that anyone who works in the laboratory can take over and complete the culture without a special briefing. A worksheet that provides adequate room for a flow chart type of illustration of culture processing and observation is easy to follow (Figure 18-7). These work records may become part of the medical record, so care should be taken to ensure that they are complete and accurate (see Chapter 5).

As an aid to interpreting culture results, the relative abundance of growth of each type of colony should be recorded. A convenient system of recording is a scale of 1+ to 4+, in which each step on the scale represents the number of quadrants of the primary culture plate in which the colony is growing. For example, if the only colonies are in the initial streak lines in which the specimen was inoculated on the plate, growth would be rated 1+. If growth is so abundant that colonies are found in the fourth quadrant (the final streak lines), growth is rated 4+. Any bacterium isolated from broth subculture, but not on primary inoculated plates, is rated 1+, regardless of the abundance of growth on the subculture plate. Bacterial cultures should not be evaluated empirically as positive or negative because this semiquantitative method helps the clinician to interpret the significance of the results. Specimens from most acute bacterial infections that have not been treated with antimicrobials will yield 3+ to 4+ growth. However, because of poor collection technique, mishandling the specimen, presampling antimicrobial therapy, or chronic infections, a smaller number of bacteria may be recovered. The clinician must decide whether these smaller numbers of bacteria are significant. If the culture is from a normally sterile body site, these culture results are often significant.

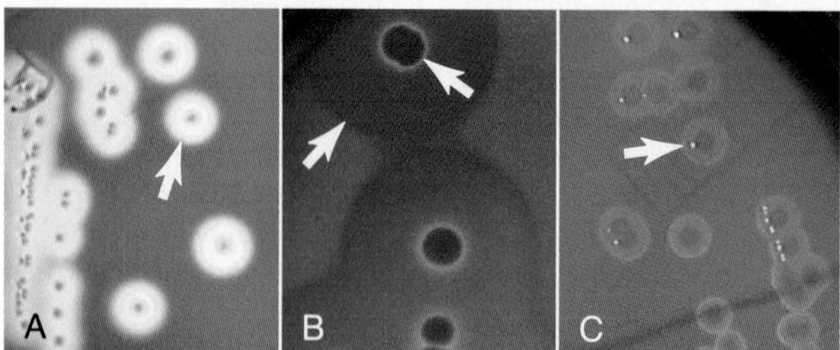

FIGURE 18-6 Types of hemolysis observed in blood agar plates: **A,** Complete hemolysis also named β-hemolysis if organism is *Streptococcus*. **B,** Double-zone hemolysis as produced by *Staphylococcus intermedius*. **C,** Alpha-hemolysis produced by some strains of *Streptococcus*.

> *TECHNICIAN NOTE* With the advances in molecular taxonomy, names of many bacterial species have recently been changed, and more changes are expected. A useful source of information for updates in nomenclature and cross-references to synonyms can be found on the Web at *http://www.dsmz.de/bactnom/bactname.htm* or *http://www.bacterio.cict.fr/*.

Indigenous Flora

Specimens cultured from sites populated with indigenous bacterial flora (often described as normal flora) are more difficult to interpret. Usually these cultures are insignificant if they result in scant growth, especially if it is a mixture of bacteria. To avoid wasting time precisely identifying the microflora, the technician should become familiar with the organisms normally found at various body sites (Table 18-3). Many of these bacteria are potential pathogens. If they are identified because of common recognition and are specifically reported while other, less familiar bacteria are overlooked, the report may mislead the clinician by implying undue significance.

Reporting results of cultures from sites with indigenous flora can be a perplexing problem. Often, it is better to specify which specific pathogens have been *excluded* by careful cultural examination, such as "no *Salmonella* isolated." Between the extremes of trying to identify everything and reporting "normal flora," the technician and clinician must agree regarding the most useful information expected from a given specimen. Perhaps certain potential pathogens that may be considered significant for the specimen should be carefully sought. In other situations a predominant bacterium can be identified or groups of organisms reported (e.g., coliforms, diphtheroids).

DIAGNOSTIC MICROBIOLOGY WORKSHEET

Date *Oct. 14, 2008* Lab No. *1036*
Patient ID *# 3053 Heidi*
Owner *Smith*
Veterinarian
Animal species *Canine*
Specimen *urine – cystocentesis*

Procedures requested:
✓ Aerobic cult
___ Anaerobic cult
___ Fungal cult
✓ Susceptibility
___ Acid-fast stain
___ Other:

Direct exam: *>10 gram – neg. rods per field*

Daily log of laboratory activities and observations:

10 – 14 Inoculate BA 10⁻² 10⁻³ MAC

10 – 15 TNTC >100 cfu hemolytic smooth colony → Micro – ID #23431; Susceptibility test. MAC: Strong lactose – fermenter

10 – 16 Record susceptibility

SUMMARY OF FINDINGS:
1. *E. Coli >10⁵ cfu/ml (hemolytic)*
2.
3.

Reported by *JS* Date reported *10 – 16 – 08*

KEY REACTIONS						
Isolate:	*E. Coli*					
Hrs:	24	48	24	48	24	48
Hemolysis	+					
Gram reaction	–					
MacConkey growth	+					
Oxidase	–					
Catalase						
Coagulase						
TSI						
Urea						
Motility						
Indol						
H_2S						

SUSCEPTIBILITY							
ANTIBIOTIC	Code	mm	Int	mm	Int	mm	Int
Amikacin	AN	24	S				
Amox / Clav	AmC	20	S				
Ampicillin	AM	0	R				
Cefotaxime	CTX						
Ceftiofur							
Cephalothin	CF	14	R				
Chloramphenicol	C	0	R				
Clindamycin	CC						
Enrofloxacin	ENO	26	S				
Erythromycin	E						
Gentamicin	GM	24	S				
Kanamycin	K						
Oxacillin	OX						
Penicillin G	P						
Pirlimycin							
Rifampin							
Tetracycline	TE	0	R				
Tilmicosin							
Tobramycin	NN						
Trimeth/Sulfa	SXT	18	S				
Triple Sulfa	SSS	0	R				

FIGURE 18-7 Example of a laboratory worksheet for recording results of various laboratory procedures, including microbial identification and susceptibility tests.

Identification Procedures

Identification of clinically significant bacteria is best accomplished by means of a few rapid tests that can presumptively differentiate organisms. To one who is experienced, such characteristics as colony morphology, hemolysis, growth on MacConkey agar, and odor may be adequate for presumptive identification. Often, additional differential tests are needed for more precise identification. Figure 18-8 presents a useful approach to identification of unknown isolates when needed.

Gram Reaction

The first differential characteristic to be considered is the reaction to Gram stain. Staining with *Gram stain* can be performed on thin smears of bacteria from a single colony (see Gram Stain Procedure and Interpretation). Potassium hydroxide, 3%, may be used as an alternate and more rapid test for Gram reaction of isolated colonies. A small drop of 3% potassium hydroxide (no larger than a colony) is dispensed on a slide, and a colony of bacteria is picked from the blood agar plate with a bacteriologic loop and mixed into the 3% potassium hydroxide. The loop is slowly and gently lifted at 5-second intervals to see whether a viscous gel is sticking to the loop. The formation of any sticky strand that can be lifted with the loop indicates a gram-negative bacterium. The reaction should appear within 20 to 30 seconds. Gram-positive organisms will diffusely mix in the 3% potassium hydroxide. Cellular morphologic characteristics of the gram-positive bacteria are important differential characteristics that require careful examination of a stained smear.

TECHNICIAN NOTE Luxuriant growth on a MacConkey agar plate is presumptive evidence of a gram-negative organism and usually does not need to be confirmed by Gram stain.

TABLE 18-3 Indigenous Bacterial Flora

Aerobes	Anaerobes
Skin, Ear	
Staphylococcus, *Micrococcus*, diphtheroids, and transient environmental and fecal contaminants	
Mouth, Nasopharynx	
Micrococcus, *Staphylococcus*, *Streptococcus* (alpha and beta), *Bacillus*, coliforms, *Proteus*, *Pasteurella*, *Actinobacillus*, *Haemophilus*, and *Mycoplasma*	*Bacteroides*, *Prevotella*, *Porphyromonas*, *Fusobacterium*, *Actinomyces*, spirochetes, and others
Trachea, Bronchi, Lungs	
No residents, only transient contaminants	
Stomach, Small Intestine	
Small numbers of α-*Streptococcus*	*Lactobacillus*
Large Intestine	
Streptococcus, *Escherichia coli*, *Klebsiella*, *Enterobacter*, *Proteus*, *Enterococcus*, and others	*Clostridium*, *Fusobacterium*, *Bacteroides*, *Porphyromonas*, *Prevotella*, spirochetes, *Lactobacillus*
Vulva, Prepuce	
Diphtheroids, *Micrococcus*, *Staphylococcus*, and fecal organisms	
Conjunctiva, Uterus, Mammary Glands	
These areas may occasionally contain small numbers of insignificant bacteria.	

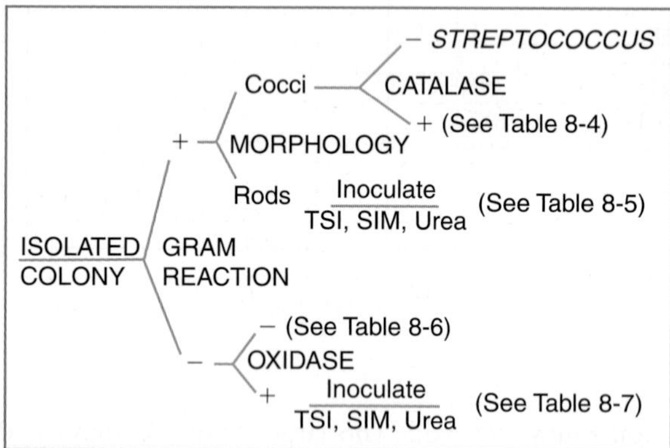

FIGURE 18-8 General flow chart for identification of common aerobic veterinary bacterial pathogens. *TSI*, Triple sugar iron; *SIM*, sulfide-indole-motility.

Catalase Test

Catalase activity is an important and rapid test for differentiating *Staphylococcus* from *Streptococcus* spp. and *Erysipelothrix* spp. and *Arcanobacterium pyogenes* from other small gram-positive rods. Hydrogen peroxide (3%) is the only reagent needed and can be readily purchased from any drugstore. It should be stored in a dark bottle in the refrigerator. The *slide catalase test* is performed by picking bacteria from the center of a colony with a needle or loop and smearing the bacteria on a clean, dry slide. A drop of hydrogen peroxide is added over the bacteria and immediately observed for bubbles of oxygen that will be released if catalase is present (Figure 18-9). Lack of bubbles is a negative test result. The order of the test procedure must not be reversed, or false-positive results may be obtained. If any blood agar is introduced into the test, it can also cause a false-positive result.

Oxidase Test

Cytochrome oxidase activity should be determined for all gram-negative bacteria except strong lactose fermenters, which will be negative. Commercial cytochrome oxidase test reagents are readily available (Figure 18-10). The reaction is supposed to be clearly visible within a few seconds, but with some reagents, the reaction may be delayed for up to 2 minutes for *Pasteurella* and *Actinobacillus* spp. A heavy inoculum must be used for accurate testing. A wooden stick or platinum loop should be used to pick colonies for testing because trace amounts of iron from other loops can cause false-positive results.

Presumptive Identification

When Gram reaction, cellular morphologic characteristics, and catalase and oxidase results have been determined, the bacteria can be tentatively grouped, and differential tests can be selected as indicated in Figure 18-8 for identification.

Isolates of *Streptococcus* are usually characterized by the type of hemolysis (see Figure 18-6) they produce. β-hemolytic *Streptococcus* isolates are usually considered to be potential pathogens. α-Hemolytic and nonhemolytic *Streptococcus* isolates usually originate from normal flora of skin and mucous membranes and are not considered significant unless they are obtained from normally sterile sites.

Isolates of *Staphylococcus* should be differentiated from those of *Micrococcus* (Table 18-4), which are considered to be nonpathogenic. Glucose-fermenting ability, determined in TSI agar slants, can be used for differentiation of these genera. If a double zone of hemolysis (see Figure 18-6) is observed on the blood agar plate, the bacterium can be identified as a coagulase-positive *Staphylococcus* without need for further testing. All other *Staphylococcus* isolates should be tested for coagulase activity because coagulase activity correlates with pathogenicity. Speciation of coagulase-positive and coagulase-negative *Staphylococcus* spp. may be attempted in special cases, if desired, by using a range of tests or commercial identification kits.

The small gram-positive rods can be differentiated by inoculating TSI, urea, and sulfide-indole-motility (SIM) medium. The results of these tests, and colony morphology and catalase activity, can identify the isolate (Table 18-5). Individual characteristics of the important pathogens in this group will be discussed later.

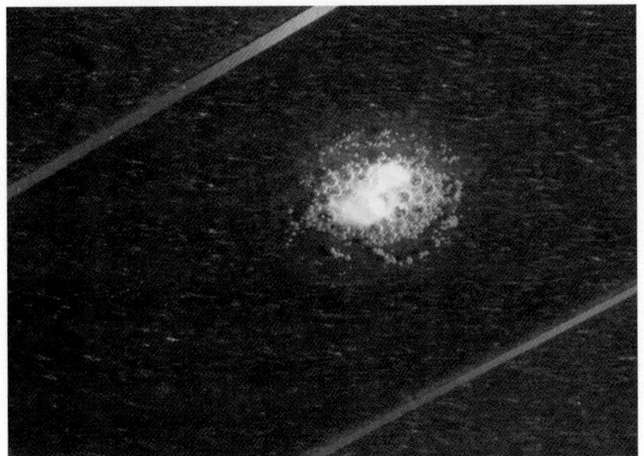

FIGURE 18-9 Positive slide catalase test demonstrating release of bubbles of oxygen.

Most gram-negative, oxidase-negative bacteria are members of the Enterobacteriaceae family. These bacteria are reactive in biochemical tests and can be identified by one of several different systems. The most rapid and economical methods for differentiating the Enterobacteriaceae family members are the commercially available packaged multitest systems. These systems are discussed later. A few other organisms that are oxidase-negative may be isolated infrequently. The most common reason for nonenteric oxidase-negative results is a false-negative oxidase test result. When such results are suspected, further differentiation of oxidase-negative bacteria, as shown in Table 18-6, is necessary.

The most frequently isolated oxidase-positive, gram-negative bacteria of veterinary importance can be differentiated by using three tubes of media (TSI, urea, SIM) as shown in Table 18-7.

Definitive Identification

The identification procedures discussed in this chapter are presumptive methods. Definitive identification of some isolates may require extensive testing. The cost of such identification in time, media, and specialized techniques is usually not justifiable in a small practice laboratory. Unusual isolates should be forwarded to a referral laboratory for further identification. The isolate should be subcultured to an agar slant medium that does not contain a fermentable carbohydrate, or it should be heavily inoculated onto a swab. The swab can be transported in a transport medium, such as Amies transport medium. Do not attempt to ship agar plates. Invariably, they become contaminated and overgrown, dehydrated, or broken.

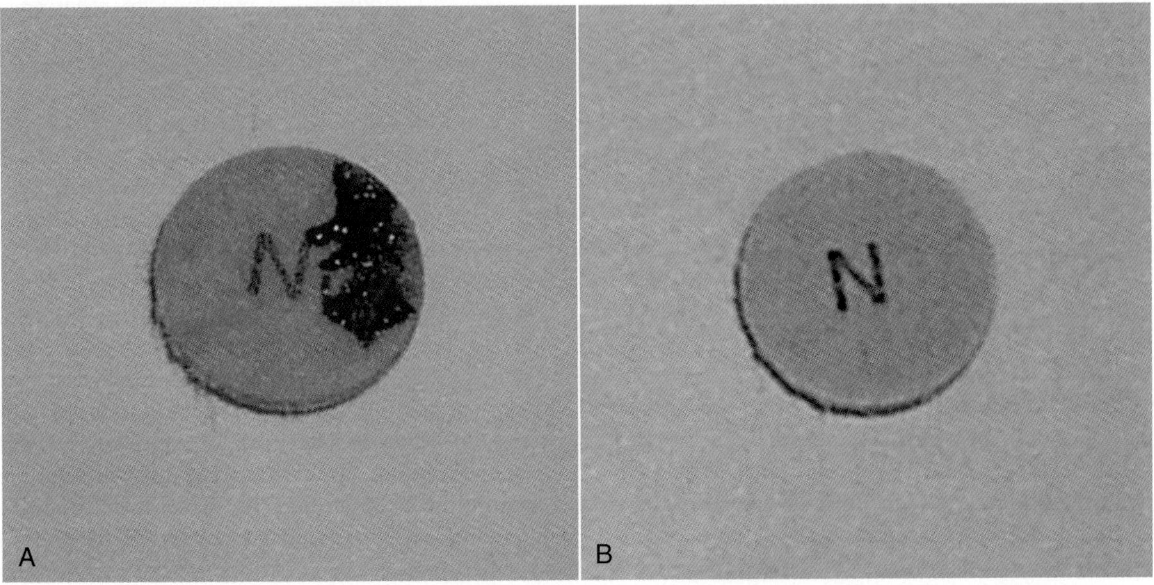

FIGURE 18-10 Positive and negative oxidase reactions using Taxo-N discs (BD Diagnostic Systems).

TABLE 18-4 Differentiation of Gram-Positive, Catalase-Positive Cocci

Organism	Hemolysis	Hyaluronidase	Glucose Fermentation	Coagulase
Staphylococcus aureus	+*	+	+	+
Staphylococcus intermedius†	+*	–	+	+
Staphylococcus (coagulase-negative spp.)	±		+	–
Micrococcus	–		–	–

*Double zones of complete and incomplete hemolysis are frequently observed.
†*S. intermedius* is positive for pyrrolidonyl arylamidase activity when PYR disks are used; this quickly differentiates it from *S. aureus*.

TABLE 18-5 Differentiation of Small, Non–Spore-Forming Gram-Positive Rods

Organism	Motility (22° C)	Catalase	Hydrogen Sulfide in TSI	Urease	Hemolysis	Colony Morphologic Characteristics
Listeria monocytogenes	+	+	–	–	Complete	Very small
Erysipelothrix rhusiopathiae	–	–	+	–	Slow, greenish	Very small
Arcanobacterium pyogenes	–	–	–	–	Complete	Very small
Corynebacterium renale	–	+	–	+	V	Medium size, entire
Coryebacterium pseudotuberculosis	–	+	–	+ (w)	V	Dry, grainy white
Rhodococcus equi	–	+	–	+ (d)	–	Large, mucoid, pink
Other diphtheroids	–	+	–	V	V	V

d, Delayed, may require up to 2 weeks; *TSI*, triple sugar iron (agar); *V*, variable results; *w*,weak.

TABLE 18-6 Differentiation of Gram-Negative, Oxidase-Negative Bacteria

	Growth on MacConkey	TSI	Motility	Identification Method
Enterobacteriaceae	+	A/A, K/A	+*	MicroID (Remel) or API 20E (Bio Mérieux, Inc.)
Pasteurelle, Actinobacillus, Mannheimia	–	A/A, A/NC	–	See Table 8-4†
Pseudomonas	+	K/NC	+	
Acinetobacter	+ (w)	K/NC	–	

A, Acid; K, alkaline; *NC*, no change; *TSI*, total sugar iron (agar); *w*, weak.
*Klebsiella is a nonmotile.
†Negative oxidase results are caused by very weak reactions.

Commercial Identification Kits

Commercial development of kit systems for identification of bacteria has been one of the most important advances in clinical bacteriology. These systems provide a cost-effective method for identification of bacteria in low-volume laboratories. Most kits consist of a number of test compartments arranged in a compact unit. The systems generally involve the use of microtechnique tests in various types of media systems. They may include compartments of solid agar, dehydrated broth, substrate or reagent disks, and supplementary conventional tests. All compartments are inoculated with organisms from an isolated colony or colonies. After the specified period of incubation and the addition of required reagents, the results are recorded as positive or negative for

TABLE 18-7 Differentiation of Gram-Negative, Oxidase-Positive Bacteria

Organism	Glucose Fermentation in TSI Agar	Growth on MacConkey Agar	Motility	Hemolysis	Urease	Indole
Aeromonas spp.	+	+	+	+	−	+
Actinobacillus spp.	+	±	−	+*	−	−
Mannheimia haemolytica	+	±	−	+*	−	−
Pasteurella multocida	+	−	−	−	−	+
Pasteurella spp.	+	−	−	−	±	−
Pseudomonas aeruginosa	−	+	+	+	±	−
Pseudomonas spp.	−	+	+	V	V	−
Bordetella bronchiseptica	−	+ (w)	+	−	+	−
Moraxella bovis	−	−	−	±	−	−
Brucella canis	−	−	−	−	+	−

TSI, Total sugar iron; *V*, variable; *w*, weak.
*Hemolysis under the colony.

each test. For many of the systems, these reactions have variously weighted values so that the positive results will produce a unique profile number for each combination of positive and negative results. Most systems provide profile directories or registers for identification of the isolate most likely to produce the set of observed reactions.

The low-volume laboratory may find these systems to be more cost effective than attempting to maintain a large inventory of conventional media. They have a reasonable shelf life (6 to 18 months) and require minimum storage space because of the compact construction. Accuracy is better than that achieved with conventional media in most small laboratories because most reactions are easy to interpret and results can be decoded more rapidly compared with sorting through conventional identification tables. Finally, depending on the specific system, most bacteria can be identified within 4 to 24 hours after isolation.

The manufacturer's directions and precautions must be carefully observed or misidentification will occur. If the system is limited to oxidase-negative enteric bacteria, only those organisms should be inoculated. Other organisms can still yield a profile number, which will result in an incorrect identification. Problems can also arise from inoculation with an older culture, improper concentration of inoculum, or mixed cultures. As experience is gained, accuracy will be increased.

> *TECHNICIAN NOTE* Identification kits can only correctly identify organisms listed in their database. New or rare organisms are likely to be either incorrectly identified or not identified at all.

When one of these systems is selected, factors to consider include the ease of inoculation, manipulations required to add reagents, the availability of interpretive charts or numeric coding devices, and the database used in development of profile registers. Often, it is difficult to discover whether significant numbers of veterinary pathogens are included in the databases for there to be a reasonable probability of correct identification of unique veterinary pathogens. The most beneficial use of these systems is the identification of members of the Enterobacteriaceae family (see Box 18-1). All enteric identification systems have essentially the same degree of accuracy and reliability of performance. The systems that seem to have gained widest acceptance in veterinary bacteriology include API 20E (bioMérieux, Inc., Hazelwood, MO), MicroID (Remel, Lenexa, KS), and Enterotube II (BD Diagnostic Systems, Sparks, MD). They provide excellent results.

Several packaged kit systems are marketed for identification of bacteria other than Enterobacteriaceae (see Box 18-1). Although these systems may provide more definitive identifications of some organisms, they have limited usefulness in small veterinary laboratories. Presumptive identification methods outlined in this chapter are frequently adequate.

The identification kits for yeast and anaerobes are useful for large-volume laboratories, but usually, the need for them in the small laboratory is not adequate to be cost effective.

SPECIAL CULTURE PROCEDURES

Blood Cultures

The detection of viable bacteria in an animal's blood has considerable diagnostic and prognostic importance. Blood cultures are indicated for fever of unknown origin; suspected bacteremia associated with endocarditis, arthritis, or meningitis; and neonatal septicemias. Blood cultures should be obtained from dogs that have antibodies to *Brucella canis* to aid in confirmation of the diagnosis.

> *TECHNICIAN NOTE* Special care must be taken to avoid contaminating blood cultures with skin microflora because some of these same organisms are frequently associated with significant bacteremia (usually <10 bacteria/ml of blood). Blood culture systems are not designed to differentiate small numbers of contaminants from bacteremia.

Special care must be taken to prevent contamination of blood cultures with skin microflora. The venipuncture site should be decontaminated by using surgical scrubbing procedures (see Chapter 28) and should not be palpated after preparation unless a sterile glove is used. Blood can be obtained by using a syringe and needle or a closed-vacuum bottle system. Often the concentration of bacteria in blood is too low to detect by direct inoculation of plate media. Therefore inoculation of commercially available blood culture media bottles is recommended. Ideally, a sample of 5 to 10 ml of blood should be obtained for culture. Blood samples in anticoagulants, such as heparin and ethylenediaminetetraacetic acid (EDTA), are not acceptable for culture because of the poor survival of some bacteria in the presence of these anticoagulants.

Blood culture bottles should be incubated at 35° C to 37° C for at least 7 days and examined daily for macroscopic evidence of growth. Positive cultures can be recognized by one or more of the following characteristics: turbidity, gas bubbles, fluffy or compact colonies, and hemolysis of the blood. When growth is observed, gram-stained smears and subcultures on plate media should be prepared for examination and identification of the organism. Negative-appearing blood culture broths should be subcultured in blinded fashion before being discarded and reported as negative. Blood cultures in which attempts to isolate *Brucella* spp. have been made should be incubated for 2 to 4 weeks before being discarded as negative.

Urine Cultures

Urine is an excellent growth medium for many bacteria because it contains electrolytes, water-soluble vitamins, residual amounts of glucose, and various nitrogenous compounds. Therefore careful attention must be given to proper collection and handling of urine for culture, or a small and insignificant number of bacteria can rapidly multiply to significant numbers. Urine specimens for culturing can be collected in three ways: free catch, catheterization, or cystocentesis (see Chapter 28). The distal urethra and genitalia are colonized with microflora that contaminate free-catch and catheterization specimens. If the skin has been adequately prepared for cystocentesis and the needle does not come in contact with any abdominal organ other than the bladder, any bacteria isolated from the specimen should be significant. Cultures should be set up within 2 hours of collection to reduce overgrowth with insignificant bacteria that may contaminate urine specimens. If cultures cannot be established within 2 hours, the sample must be refrigerated to slow the bacterial growth. Refrigeration begins to fail after 18 to 24 hours. Therefore the best method for identifying urinary tract infections is to establish cultures as soon as possible.

The use of blood agar and MacConkey agar as selective and differential isolation media is recommended for the culture of all urine specimens. There is no need for broth medium for enrichment. The bacteriologic examination of urine specimens collected by methods other than cystocentesis should provide an estimate of the number of microorganisms per milliliter of urine as an aid to interpreting the results. This can be accomplished by inoculating the blood agar plate with a standard dilution loop calibrated to deliver approximately 0.001 ml (Figure 18-11). Each colony that grows represents 10^3 organisms/ml in the specimen; therefore the number of colonies is multiplied by 1000 to obtain the concentration of organisms in the specimen. The number of bacteria can also be estimated through direct microscopic examination of a gram-stained smear of uncentrifuged urine. If one or more bacteria per oil immersion field are observed, usually more than 10^5 organisms/ml should be present in cultures. If more than two types of bacteria are isolated, a second specimen

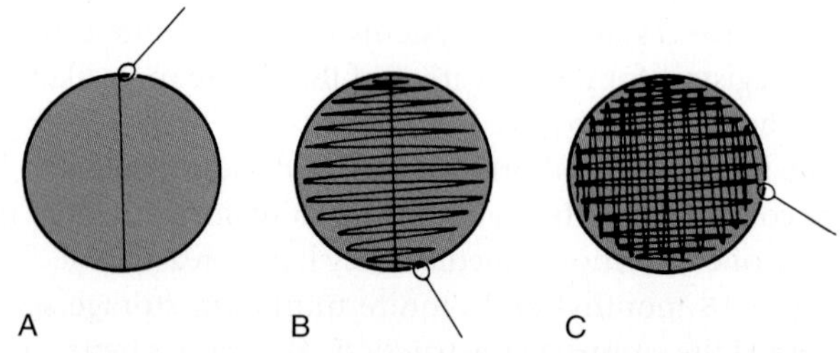

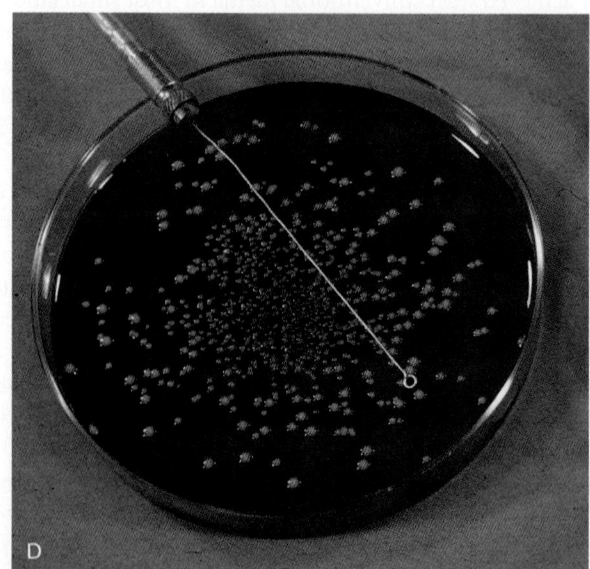

FIGURE 18-11 Procedure for inoculating media for semiquantitative bacterial colony counts when culturing urine. **A,** Primary inoculation with calibrated loop. **B,** Streak at right angles to primary inoculation. **C,** Streak at right angles to previous streak. **D,** Photo illustrates a plate with >100 colonies resulting from inoculation with a 1 μl loop indicating >10^5 bacteria/ml of urine.

should be collected and cultured to distinguish a mixed infection from contamination or mishandling of the specimen. Bacterial counts can be low because of improper handling of the specimen, dilution from forced fluid therapy, or cystocentesis samples from patients with urethritis that has not become established as a concomitant cystitis.

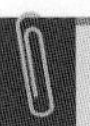

TECHNICIAN NOTE The following guidelines can be used for interpretation of urine cultures:

- For a single species, more than 10^5 bacteria/ml indicates significant bacteria.
- Between 10^3 and 10^5 bacteria/ml suggests infection if the urine has been properly collected and neutrophils are present.
- Fewer than 10^3 bacteria/ml suggests contamination or mishandling of the specimen. If there is doubt about interpretation of a colony count, the culture should be repeated with a second specimen.

COMMON BACTERIAL SPECIES

The bacterial pathogens frequently associated with many infectious processes are listed in Table 18-1. Some of the colony morphologic, growth, and identifying characteristics of these bacteria are listed in Table 18-8. Additional details are given in the following discussion of special isolation and identification techniques. Clinically important characteristics are noted.

GRAM-POSITIVE COCCI

Staphylococcus Species

Staphylococcus spp. are catalase-positive cocci that occur in grapelike clusters. They are frequently isolated from pyogenic lesions, such as wounds, dermatitis, otitis, mastitis, cystitis, and osteomyelitis. They are usually divided into coagulase-positive and coagulase-negative groups. The coagulase-positive species, *S. aureus* and *S. intermedius*, are more important pathogens, and the others are usually considered to be less pathogenic. One of the most important identifying characteristics that should be noted is the development of a double zone of hemolysis (an inner zone of complete hemolysis and a second zone of incomplete hemolysis, see Figure 18-6). This is a common identifying characteristic of most coagulase-positive isolates from animals. Mannitol fermentation is not a reliable correlate of coagulase activity in staphylococcal isolates from animals. Because of a high incidence of acquired antimicrobial resistance, these organisms should be tested for antimicrobial susceptibility.

Streptococcus Species

Streptococcus spp. are catalase-negative cocci that occur singly, in pairs, or in short chains. Chain formation is more easily demonstrated in broth cultures. *Streptococcus* is the most common bacterial pathogen of the horse and can be found to cause pyogenic infections and mastitis in all species of animals. However, each species tends to be rather host specific. Therefore the streptococcal pathogens of humans rarely cause infections in animals, and animals are usually not reservoirs of human pathogens. Some species cause specific diseases. *Streptococcus equi* ssp. *equi* is the cause of strangles in horses. *Streptococcus agalactiae* is an important cause of bovine mastitis. It can be identified by the CAMP test (Figure 18-12). Definitive biochemical and serologic (Lancefield typing) testing is usually not clinically important. For clinical interpretation, it is important to evaluate the hemolysis produced on blood agar (see Figure 18-6). β-hemolysis (complete clearing) usually correlates well with potential pathogenicity; α-hemolysis (incomplete greenish discoloring) and γ-hemolysis (nonhemolytic) are usually indications of normal flora of skin and mucous membranes. However, when isolated in nearly pure culture from normally sterile body sites, these organisms can be considered to be clinically significant. Susceptibility to antimicrobials is usually predictable, which means antimicrobial susceptibility testing may be an unnecessary expense.

The enteric group D streptococci have been renamed as *Enterococcus* spp. Urinary tract infections are the most common presentation of these organisms; and *Enterococcus* spp. occasionally infect wounds and cause bacteremia. They are emerging as significant nosocomial agents and are particularly troublesome because they are likely to be resistant to many antimicrobials.

TECHNICIAN NOTE *Streptococcus agalactiae* is an obligate parasite of the bovine udder and should be differentiated from other *Streptococcus* spp. that are of environmental origin when causing mastitis. *S. agalactiae* is the only species that produces a positive CAMP test.

ANAEROBIC COCCI

Most anaerobic cocci belong to the genus *Peptostreptococcus*. When isolated, these agents are usually associated with mixed anaerobic infections.

GRAM-POSITIVE RODS

Spore Formers

Bacillus spp. are common contaminants isolated in the laboratory. They are ubiquitous in soil, water, air, and dust. They are large spore-forming rods that usually grow as large, rough, granular, or spreading colonies. They are usually hemolytic. Occasionally, strains of *Bacillus* will be isolated that react as if they are gram-negative and oxidase-positive. However, they can be identified by the presence of spores in stained smears. *Bacillus anthracis* (the agent that causes anthrax) is the important pathogenic species. It is extremely virulent for humans. *Do not attempt to culture it.*

Clostridium spp. are large, spore-forming anaerobic rods. The pathogenic species are noted for their potent toxins and extensive destruction of tissue. Infections may be

TABLE 18-8 Identifying Characteristics of Common Veterinary Bacterial Pathogens

	Blood Agar	MacConkey Agar	Other Characteristics
Gram-Positive			
Staphylococcus	Smooth, glistening, white to yellow pigmented colonies	No growth	Catalase-positive glucose fermenter; double-zone hemolysis usually indicates coagulase positive; coagulase activity is a useful differential test
Streptococcus	Small, glistening colonies; hemolysis	No growth except some enterococci	Catalase-negative, usually identified by type of hemolysis; beta-hemolytic strains more likely to be pathogens; other are often part of flora; streptococcus agalactiae CAMP-positive
Arcanobacterium pyogenes	Small, hemolytic, streplike colonies	No growth	Catalase negative; slow growth, often requiring 48 hr for distinct colonies; growth enhanced in candle jar
Corynebacterium pseudotuberculosis	Slow-growing, opaque, dry crumbly colonies; usually hemolytic	No growth	Catalase positive; weak urease positive
Corynebacterium renale	Small, smooth, glistening colonies (24 hr); become opaque and dry later	No growth	Catalase positive; urease positive
Rhodococcus equi	Small, moist, white (24 hr); become large, pink colonies; no hemolysis	No growth	Catalase positive; delayed urease positive
Listeria monocytogenes	Small, hemolytic, glistening colonies	No growth	Catalase positive; motile at room temperature
Erysipelothrix rhusiopathiae	Small colonies after 48 hr; greenish (alpha) hemolysis	No growth	Catalase negative; hydrogen sulfide positive
Nocardia	Slow-growing, small dry, granular, white to orange colonies	No growth	Partially acid fast; colonies tenaciously adhere to media
Actinomyces	Slow growing, small, rough, nodular white colonies	No growth	Require increase carbon dioxide or anaerobic incubation; not acid fast
Clostridium	Variable, round, ill-defined, irregular colonies; usually hemolytic	No growth	Obligate anaerobes
Bacillus	Variable, large, rough, dry or mucoid colonies	No growth	Usually hemolytic; large rods with endospores
Gram-Negative			
Escherichia coli	Large, gray, smooth, mucoid colonies; hemolysis variable	Hot pink to red colonies; red cloudiness in media	Hemolysis frequently associated with virulence
Klebsiella pneumoniae	Large, mucoid, sticky, whitish colonies; not hemolytic	Large, mucoid, pink colonies	Nonmotile; require biochemical tests to differentiate from Enterobacter
Proteus	Frequently swarming without distinct colonies	Colorless; limited swarming	
Other enterics	Gray to white, smooth, mucoid colonies	Colorless colonies	Biochemical tests for identification; serotyping indicated for Salmonella
Pseudomonas	Irregular, spreading, grayish colonies; variable hemolysis; may show a metallic sheen	Colorless, irregular colonies	Oxidase positive; fruity odor; may produce yellow greenish soluble pigment in clear media
Bordetella bronchiseptica	Very small, circular dew-drop colonies; variable hemolysis	Small, colorless colonies	May require 48 hr for distinct colonies; oxidase positive; rapid urease positive; citrate positive

TABLE 18-8 Identifying Characteristics of Common Veterinary Bacterial Pathogens—cont'd

	Blood Agar	MacConkey Agar	Other Characteristics
Brucella canis	Very small, circular, pin-point colonies after 48-72 hr, not hemolytic	No growth	Oxidase positive; catalase positive; urease positive
Moraxella	Round, translucent, grayish white colonies; variable hemolysis	No growth	Oxidase and catalase positive; often nonreactive in routine biochemical tests; colonies may pit media
Actinobacillus	Round, translucent colonies; variable hemolysis	Variable growth; colorless colonies	Glucose fermenter, non-motile; urease positive; sticky colonies
Mannheimia haemolytica	Round, gray, smooth colonies; hemolysis under the colony	Variable growth; colorless colonies	Glucose fermenter in TSI; weak oxidase positive
Pasteruella multocida	Gray, mucoid, round to coalescing colonies; no hemolysis	No growth	Glucose fermenter in TSI; weak oxidase and indole positive

TSI, Triple sugar iron (agar).

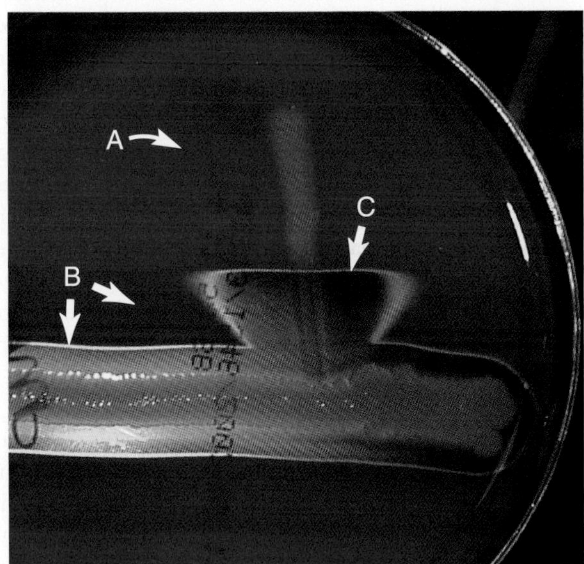

FIGURE 18-12 CAMP test for *Streptococcus agalactiae*. The isolate *(A)* to be tested is inoculated perpendicular to a stock strain of double-zone hemolytic *Staphylococcus (B)*, producing a synergistic triangle of hemolysis *(C)* as a positive CAMP test.

accompanied by an accumulation of gas (emphysema) in the tissues. Laboratory diagnosis of the toxic diseases (tetanus, botulism, enterotoxemia) and differentiation of the infectious diseases (blackleg, malignant edema, bacillary hemoglobinuria, etc.) require the assistance of reference diagnostic laboratories. Often a gram-stained smear is useful for ruling out clostridial disease or indicating it as a possibility. *Clostridium perfringens* is occasionally isolated from deep wounds with extensive tissue necrosis, such as compound fractures. The bacterium requires an anaerobic atmosphere for growth and frequently produces a double zone of hemolysis.

C. perfringens is also associated with enteritis and diarrhea in dogs. In some cases, the presence of enterotoxigenic strains of *C. perfringens* can be presumptively identified in fecal smears by evaluating the smears for the presence of increased bacterial spores because sporulation is associated with the release of enterotoxin. Spores appear as unstained, small, oval structures and are usually surrounded by a halo of stained bacterial cellular debris unless a specific spore stain is applied (Figure 18-13).

Small Rods

Corynebacterium spp. are small, club-shaped rods that tend to occur in palisades or in an angular arrangement because of their "snapping" division. Colonies are usually quite small at 24 hours, but continue to enlarge and vary greatly by species. Most species are catalase-positive. *Arcanobacterium pyogenes* (previously called *Actinomyces pyogenes*) produces a small pinpoint colony, hemolysis, and a catalase-negative reaction. Cellular morphologic characteristics must be evaluated carefully to differentiate it from *Streptococcus* spp. It is the most common pyogenic agent in ruminants. *Rhodococcus equi* is a cause of pneumonia and abscesses in foals. Morphologically, individual cells are coccobacillary and larger than other *Corynebacterium* organisms. *Corynebacterium pseudotuberculosis* causes chronic abscesses in goats and sheep, and it has recently reemerged in the western United States as the cause of abscesses in horses known as pigeon breast disease. The *Corynebacterium renale* group causes pyelonephritis and cystitis in cows. There are many other *Corynebacterium* spp. that are nonpathogenic commensals of the skin; they are frequently referred to collectively as diphtheroids.

Listeria monocytogenes is a small, non–spore-forming rod that is catalase-positive. It is the only small gram-positive rod that is motile at room temperature. It is an infrequent cause of abortion in large animals and septicemia in young animals. In ruminants, it causes an encephalitis known as *circling disease*. The bacteria localize in the pons and medulla (brainstem). Cultures from other parts of the brain may be negative. Isolation may require specific selective and enrichment techniques available in reference laboratories.

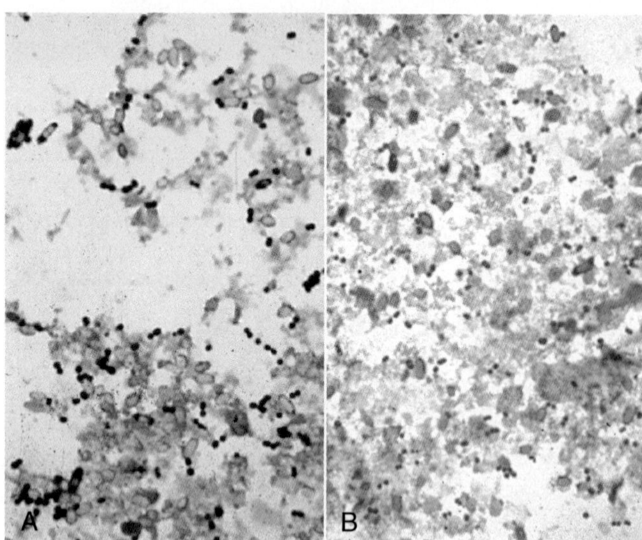

FIGURE 18-13 Stained fecal smears with abundant spores typical of *Clostridium perfringens*. **A,** Spores are not stained by modified Wright stain. **B,** Spores stained with malachite green.

Erysipelothrix rhusiopathiae is a pleomorphic rod that is usually slender and small. The colony is small, and an incomplete, greenish hemolysis (alpha like) is produced. The cellular morphologic characteristics must be carefully evaluated to differentiate it from *Streptococcus* spp. because both are catalase-negative. A definitive characteristic that differentiates it from other gram-positive rods is the production of hydrogen sulfide. *E. rhusiopathiae* is most commonly encountered as a cause of septicemic or arthritic disease of pigs, but it is occasionally a cause of endocarditis in dogs.

Filamentous Rods

The Actinomycetaceae family contains several clinically important bacteria that are distinguished by forming branching, filamentous gram-positive rods. Most *Actinomyces* spp. are anaerobic bacteria that may tolerate low levels of oxygen. Therefore some species can be isolated in a candle jar, but the most efficient isolation can be achieved with an anaerobic system. *Actinomyces* spp. colonies are slow to develop, requiring up to 5 days, and are usually raised and irregular in shape. When isolated, they are usually recovered from pyogranulomatous lesions of soft tissue, pyothoraces, or osteomyelitis. *Nocardia* spp. are partially acid-fast, which means a modified staining procedure must be used to differentiate them from *Actinomyces* spp. In place of the acid-alcohol decolorizer, only an acid decolorizer is used to demonstrate acid-fastness. *Nocardia* spp. are aerobic bacteria with colonies usually appearing after 2 to 5 days of incubation. The colonies are rough and have a dry, granular texture. They adhere tenaciously to the media. *Nocardia* spp. are occasionally isolated from pyothoraces and wounds. They may be serious mastitis pathogens in some dairy herds. *Dermatophilus congolensis* is another branching, filamentous bacterium. It often has a beaded appearance with transverse and longitudinal divisions. It is an uncommon cause of skin infections of horses and ruminants. The organism can be demonstrated in smears of pus from under the elevated scabs containing tufts of hair. *Streptomyces* spp. are aerobic, filamentous bacteria that are not acid-fast. They are abundant in soil and may be isolated as contaminants.

Anaerobes

Anaerobic, gram-positive, non–spore-forming rods belong to the genera *Bifidobacterium*, *Eubacterium*, and *Propionibacterium*. If definitive identification of these organisms is needed, culture specimens should be sent to a reference diagnostic laboratory. They are usually isolated in mixed cultures from pyogenic lesions.

ACID-FAST BACTERIA

Mycobacteria are mostly small, short rods but are occasionally pleomorphic. They stain poorly with Gram stain but are acid-fast. These bacteria are rarely isolated in veterinary practice laboratories because special procedures and media are usually required. However, preparation of an acid-fast stained impression smear can be a useful diagnostic procedure for making a presumptive diagnosis of mycobacterial infection. Positive findings are significant; however, negative findings have limited predictive value. *Mycobacterium avium* ssp. *paratuberculosis* may be demonstrated in acid-fast stained smears prepared from intestinal mucosa or mesenteric lymph nodes of ruminants. *Mycobacterium avium* infection of birds can frequently be confirmed by examination of acid-fast smears prepared from the liver or intestinal mucosa. Occasionally, abundant acid-fast organisms can be demonstrated in the feces.

Isolation of the zoonotic agents of tuberculosis, *Mycobacterium bovis* and *Mycobacterium tuberculosis*, should not be attempted in a practice laboratory. Infrequently, a rapid-growing *Mycobacterium* sp. may be isolated from a case of bovine mastitis. The colonies will usually appear after 3 to 5 days of incubation. These organisms should be forwarded to a reference laboratory for definitive identification.

GRAM-NEGATIVE BACTERIA

The Enterobacteriaceae family of bacteria is the largest group of potential pathogens and the most frequently isolated bacteria. The normal habitat of these organisms is the digestive tract and soil; therefore they will usually grow on MacConkey agar and are frequently insignificant contaminants of specimens. They are small gram-negative rods, with some pleomorphism. Some of the common identifying characteristics include oxidase negativity, glucose fermentation, and motility (except *Klebsiella* spp.). Genus and species identification requires numerous biochemical tests, and serotyping and genotyping are frequently necessary to identify pathogenic strains. Acquired antimicrobial resistance from R-factors (plasmids) is common in this family of bacteria, making antimicrobial susceptibility testing a necessary clinical evaluation of isolates.

Most non-Enterobacteriaceae, gram-negative bacteria are oxidase-positive, and growth on MacConkey agar is variable.

Coliforms

Escherichia coli can frequently be presumptively identified by the strong lactose fermentation reaction it produces on MacConkey agar. Strains causing tissue infections and cystitis are frequently hemolytic. *E. coli* is frequently associated with diarrhea in neonates (especially pigs, calves, and lambs). The pathogenic strains causing diarrhea are best identified by genotyping and other specialized laboratory testing, such as use of the *Escherichia coli* Antigen Test (K99 Pilitest, VMRD, Inc., Pullman, WA). However, presumptive evidence of *E. coli* involvement in diarrhea (scours) can be obtained by gram-staining a smear taken from small intestinal mucosa shortly after the death of the animal. If a large number (>25) of gram-negative rods are observed in each oil immersion field, it is a strong indication that *E. coli* is a cause of diarrhea. *Klebsiella* spp. and *Enterobacter* spp. are occasionally involved in infections of the respiratory and urinary tracts and in mastitis. They are becoming more important in veterinary medicine as superinfecting agents after antimicrobial therapy.

Salmonella Species

Salmonella spp. can cause diarrhea and septicemia in all animals and in humans. When feces are to be cultured, selective and enrichment media should be used to increase the probability of successful isolation of *Salmonella*. Hektoen enteric agar and selenite enrichment broth (see Table 18-2) are recommended (brilliant green agar and XLD agar are also commonly used selective media). The enrichment broth should be subcultured to both MacConkey and Hektoen enteric agar. Nonlactose-fermenting colonies can rapidly be screened with *Salmonella* polyvalent O antiserum to identify them. For the purpose of defining the epidemiology of salmonellosis outbreaks, the isolates should be forwarded to a reference laboratory for serotyping.

Proteus Species

Proteus spp. are frequently isolated as specimen contaminants or secondary invaders. They are important pathogens of the urinary tract. Related genera of bacteria that do not swarm on blood agar are *Morganella* and *Providencia*, and they can be readily identified by using kits. The swarming *Proteus* spp. sometimes interfere with isolation of other organisms. This problem can be solved by using phenylethyl alcohol (PEA) blood agar plates. *Proteus* and other gram-negative organisms will be inhibited, providing easier isolation of gram-positive organisms.

Other Enteric Organisms

There are many other members of the Enterobacteriaceae family—including *Serratia*, *Citrobacter*, *Edwardsiella*, *Enterobacter*, *Pantoea*, and *Hafnia* spp.—which are infrequently isolated. Careful clinical evaluation is necessary to determine their significance. Often a repeated culture helps confirm the significance of isolation.

Aeromonas Species

Aeromonas spp. are oxidase-positive rods that grow on MacConkey agar. They are commonly found in soil, water, and sewage and frequently infect aquatic animals. They are infrequently a cause of septicemia in terrestrial animals.

Actinobacillus

Actinobacillus spp. are oxidase-positive, small rods that usually grow on MacConkey agar. The colony morphologic characteristics are similar to those of *Pasteurella* spp. *Actinobacillus equuli* is the most frequently isolated species. It produces a sticky colony. It is frequently the cause of septicemic infections in foals. It can be isolated from most horses as part of the mucosal flora, but is generally only an opportunistic pathogen in older horses.

Pasteurella Species

Pasteurella spp. are usually associated with respiratory tract infections in most animals. In cats, they are frequently recovered from abscesses. They are small, oxidase-positive coccobacilli. *Pasteurella multocida* produces a characteristic musty odor. Identification can be aided by noting the typically weak glucose fermentation reaction in a TSI tube. *Pasteurella* spp. tend to be nonreactive in most commercial identification kit systems and may be misidentified. Hemolytic strains, previously known as *P. haemolytica*, have been renamed *Mannheimia haemolytica* for bovine respiratory isolates, and some ovine strains are now called *P. trehalosi*. Antimicrobial resistance is a growing problem in isolates from food animals, indicating a need to perform susceptibility tests.

Haemophilus Species

Haemophilus spp. are often part of the normal flora of mucous membranes. A few species are important pathogens, usually of the respiratory system. They are small coccobacilli that require specially enriched media for growth. They may grow as satellite colonies around *Staphylococcus* spp. on blood agar. In addition to the nutritional growth requirements, an increased concentration of carbon dioxide is necessary. These bacteria are susceptible to antibiotics and environmental stress factors, such as drying; therefore specimens must be collected and handled carefully or isolation will be unsuccessful.

Pseudomonas Species

Pseudomonas spp. are common soil and water bacteria. They are usually considered to be opportunistic pathogens of wounds and otitis. Infrequently, they are isolated from the respiratory and urinary tracts. There are many species, but *Pseudomonas aeruginosa* is the most common pathogen. It produces water-soluble yellow-green pigments that diffuse into the medium, and it has a distinctive odor that aids in recognition. Most isolates are quite resistant to antimicrobials and should routinely be tested for susceptibility.

Bordetella bronchiseptica is a small coccobacillus that is frequently recovered from respiratory tract infections of dogs and is emerging as an important respiratory pathogen of cats. It is associated with atrophic rhinitis in pigs and is infrequently isolated from respiratory tract infections of other animals. Colonies are slow to develop and may only be pinpointed after 48 hours. Growth occurs on MacConkey agar. It is oxidase-positive, urease-positive (often within 4 hours), and citrate-positive.

Brucella Species

Brucella spp. are small coccobacilli that are usually associated with reproductive failure: abortion and infertility. Some species require increased carbon dioxide for growth; however, *Brucella canis* can be isolated in an aerobic atmosphere. Growth is slow, often requiring 3 to 7 days for colonies to be detectable. Suspected *Brucella* isolates should be sent to a reference laboratory for definitive identification because of the regulatory and zoonotic importance of these agents.

Other Gram-Negative Rods

Many gram-negative bacteria have limited or undetermined clinical importance. Included are bacteria such as *Moraxella*, *Acinetobacter*, and *Branhamella* spp. and related pleomorphic coccobacilli. These organisms are commonly found as part of the flora of mucous membranes and are usually secondary, opportunistic pathogens. They are relatively nonreactive in most conventional biochemical tests. Thus identification is usually difficult, even for reference diagnostic laboratories.

Anaerobes

The gram-negative anaerobes (*Bacteroides*, *Porphyromonas*, *Prevotella*, *Fusobacterium* spp.) are frequently involved in mixed infections in abscesses and necrotic tissue. *Porphyromonas* spp. have recently been associated with canine periodontal disease. The obligate anaerobes are normally found in the digestive tract, so infections resulting from contamination of tissues with mucous membrane flora or intestinal contents frequently contain these organisms. If obligate anaerobes are isolated, evaluation of the cellular morphologic characteristics provides adequate clinical information. Species identification is rarely important. Taxonomic advances have resulted in the reclassification of some former *Bacteroides* spp. into the genera *Dichelobacter*, *Porphyromonas*, and *Prevotella*.

> TECHNICIAN NOTE Observation of bacteria that do not grow aerobically in gram-stained exudate from a pyonecrotic lesion is often a significant indication that obligately anaerobic bacteria are present.

SPIROCHETES AND CURVED BACTERIA

Leptospira spp. cause febrile infections, often followed by abortion and infertility. These spirochetes are difficult to isolate and usually die within a few hours while being transported to a laboratory. Dark-field examination of urine may aid in establishing a diagnosis. Most diagnoses are made by serologic testing or PCR assay.

Borrelia burgdorferi is a tick-transmitted spirochete that causes Lyme disease in humans and arthritis and lameness in dogs. Canine borreliosis may be accompanied by high rectal temperature and lymphadenopathy. Detection of serum antibodies to *B. burgdorferi* is the diagnostic test of choice in dogs. Isolation of *Borrelia* by culture is difficult and often nonproductive. Borreliosis is of importance in the United States in dogs and other animals only within areas infested by ticks carrying this agent.

Brachyspira hyodysenteriae is a spirochete that causes dysentery in pigs. Cultural isolation is beyond the capability of most laboratories. Diagnosis of this infection may be made by examining smears of colonic mucosa for numerous large spirochetes.

Campylobacter spp. cause two different types of disease conditions. One group contains important reproductive pathogens, causing abortion and infertility. Because of special needs for enrichment and selective media and a microaerophilic atmosphere, specimens for isolation of *Campylobacter* spp. should be sent to veterinary diagnostic laboratories specially equipped for *Campylobacter* culture. The second group includes important zoonotic enteric pathogens. Most public health and hospital laboratories are equipped to isolate this group. *Campylobacter* spp. are curved gram-negative rods. They can be recognized by dark-field or phase-contrast microscopy by their darting motility.

Helicobacter spp. are helical or curved gram-negative bacteria that colonize the gastric mucosa of humans, dogs, and cats and the intestinal tracts of some rodents, birds, and swine. Some species have been associated with gastritis and peptic ulceration, whereas other species are considered to be nonpathogenic flora of the gastric mucosa of animals. They can be detected and identified in histologic sections, by culture in reference laboratories, and by association with strong urease activity in gastric mucus.

MYCOPLASMA SPECIES

Mycoplasma spp. are small bacteria that lack cell walls and, as a result, are not easily stained and observed in exudates. Arthritis and pneumonia are the most common mycoplasmal diseases. The role of *Mycoplasma* spp. in urogenital infections is not well characterized. Occasionally, strains can be isolated on blood agar plates inoculated with urine from dogs with cystitis. Special media and techniques are required for isolation and identification of most *Mycoplasma* spp. Therefore arrangements should be made with a reference laboratory for *Mycoplasma* transport media and specimen shipping instructions.

The agent of feline infectious anemia (formerly *Haemobartonella felis*) has recently been renamed *Mycoplasma haemofelis*. Examination of a stained blood smear frequently results in identification of clinical cases. Molecular detection assays are also available.

OTHER FASTIDIOUS BACTERIA

Diagnosis of several fastidious bacterial infections is best accomplished by using molecular detection systems specific for gene sequences of nucleic acids or serology. Some of the agents most amenable to molecular detection include *Bartonella, Rickettsia, Neorickettsia, Chlamydophila, Chlamydia, Ehrlichia, Mycoplasma,* and *Mycobacterium* spp.

ANTIMICROBIAL SUSCEPTIBILITY TESTING

One of the most important functions of the clinical microbiology laboratory is to provide information that can assist in the selection of appropriate therapy for infectious diseases. All antimicrobial agents have limitations in their spectra of activity. Therefore a universal antimicrobial for all infections is not available. Some organisms are intrinsically resistant to an antimicrobial, whereas others acquire resistance. The most common mechanism for acquired resistance is the acquisition of extrachromosomal pieces of DNA, such as plasmids (R-factors) and bacteriophages. As a result, the bacteria are able to produce enzymes that modify or inactivate the antimicrobial, enable the cell to resist accumulation of the drug, or alter target sites and reduce the activity of the drug. Because the acquired resistance traits are not static, the antimicrobial susceptibility pattern *(antibiogram)* is not predictable for many organisms. Therefore susceptibility tests are necessary.

> *TECHNICIAN NOTE* Antimicrobial susceptibility testing by means of standardized test systems is indicated for clinically significant bacterial isolates with unpredictable (changing) patterns of susceptibility.

INDICATIONS FOR SUSCEPTIBILITY TESTING

Susceptibility testing is indicated for most rapidly growing, aerobic and facultative anaerobic, clinically significant bacteria. Testing should be avoided for isolates representing normal flora and for those bacteria with predictable susceptibility to the antimicrobial of choice. Gram-positive bacteria other than *Staphylococcus* spp. have rather predictable antibiograms; therefore routine testing is not needed. However, susceptibility testing may be indicated if the antimicrobial of choice cannot be safely and economically administered to the patient. Unpredictable resistance patterns are frequently observed with the gram-negative bacteria, thus requiring testing. Most slow-growing and anaerobic bacteria have rather predictable antibiograms, so testing is not necessary. If acquired resistance is found to be a problem in these organisms, special methods will be necessary for testing them.

In most cases the veterinarian will have started antimicrobial therapy before the laboratory results are available. When the test results become available, therapy can be altered or modified to provide safe, effective, least-cost therapy. In some situations the culture specimen will be from a moribund or dead animal. Susceptibility testing may still be important because it can establish patterns of antimicrobial susceptibility for the organism when encountered in other animals in the herd or region.

SUSCEPTIBILITY TEST METHODS

The simplest type of susceptibility test is one that determines the presence of an enzyme that can inactivate an antimicrobial. Penicillin resistance in *Staphylococcus* spp. is acquired by gaining the ability to produce β-lactamase, an enzyme that inactivates most penicillin derivatives. Sensitive and rapid tests, such as Cefinase (BD Diagnostic Systems), are available for detection of this enzyme. If the test result is negative, penicillin or a penicillin derivative is usually the drug of choice, and no further testing is needed. If the isolate is producing β-lactamase, further antimicrobial susceptibility testing will be needed to select an alternative therapy. A β-lactamase test can be a useful part of a mastitis culture procedure to rapidly evaluate the appropriateness of penicillin therapy because penicillin is one of the most frequently administered antimicrobials.

In most cases, tests for antimicrobial-inactivating enzymes are not available. Therefore most routine susceptibility tests measure the degree of susceptibility of the isolate to each of several antimicrobials. The broth dilution susceptibility test system is the most precise method and is considered the reference method. This test is performed by introducing a standardized inoculum of an organism into a series of tubes (or wells in a microculture plate) containing serial dilutions of an antimicrobial in medium (Figure 18-14). The lowest concentration of antimicrobial that macroscopically inhibits growth of the organism is the *minimal inhibitory concentration (MIC)*. The MIC of an antimicrobial for a given isolate represents the degree of susceptibility to the drug. If the antimicrobial is going to be used in therapy, the MIC must be achieved at the site of infection to effectively inhibit bacterial growth.

The most commonly used method of antimicrobial susceptibility testing in small laboratories is the agar diffusion test in which antimicrobial-impregnated paper disks are applied to the surface of agar that has been streaked with a standardized inoculum. As the antimicrobial is absorbed from the disk into the agar, it begins diffusing in a radial pattern (Figure 18-15). As the antimicrobial diffuses, it becomes more dilute, thereby creating a gradient effect of decreasing concentrations. The bacterial inoculum on the agar begins to grow in all areas except the places in which the antimicrobial concentration exceeds the MIC of the isolate. Zones of inhibition of growth can be observed around the disks. In carefully controlled studies, the diameters of the zones of inhibition have been correlated with MIC values. The results of the diffusion test can then be semiquantitatively interpreted, usually as susceptible, intermediate, or resistant.

The diffusion test is easy to set up, but it requires careful attention to detail to ensure that the results are accurate.

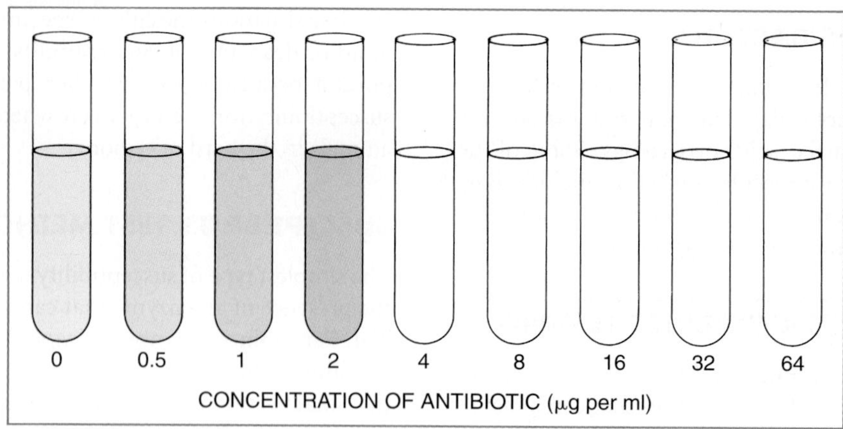

FIGURE 18-14 Broth dilution susceptibility test. The organism grew in broth containing antibiotic in the amounts of 0.5, 1, and 2 μg/ml, but growth was inhibited in the tube containing 4 μg/ml. Therefore the minimal inhibitory concentration is 4 μg/ml.

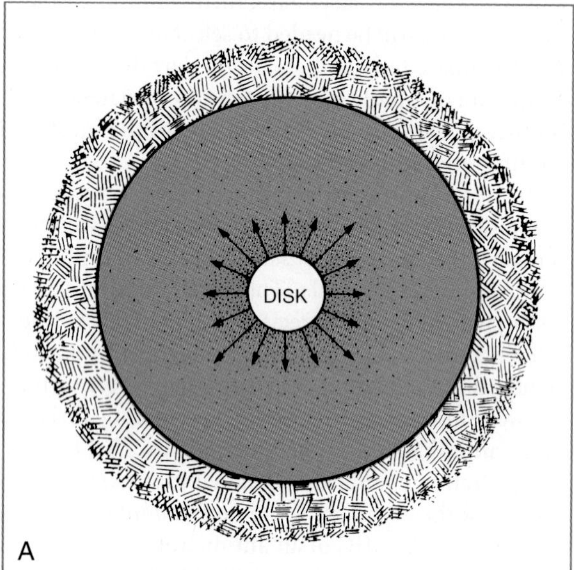

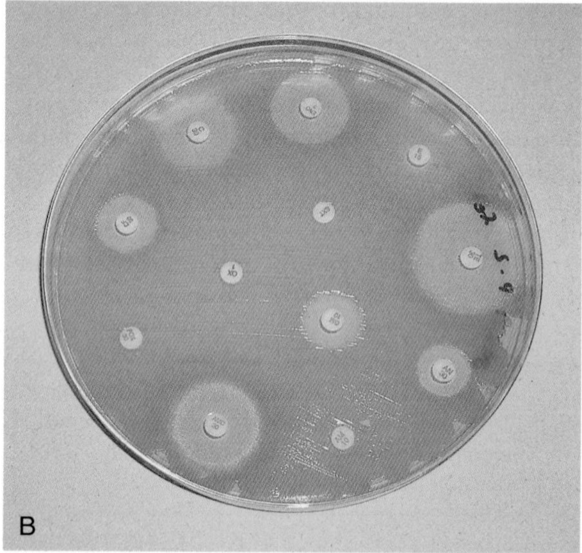

FIGURE 18-15 Antibiotic diffusion susceptibility test. **A,** As antibiotic diffuses from the disk, the concentration of antibiotic is highest near the disk and logarithmically diluted as it diffuses radially into a larger area. At some point, the antibiotic is diluted below the minimal inhibitory concentration for the test organism, which allows the organism to grow. **B,** The resulting zones of inhibition are measured and interpreted with the use of Table 18-9.

Mueller-Hinton agar has been selected as the standard culture medium so that the composition of the agar can be more uniformly controlled. However, this medium will not support growth of some fastidious pathogens, such as *Streptococcus*, *Listeria*, *Corynebacterium*, *Erysipelothrix*, and *Pasteurella* spp. and some other gram-negative bacteria. For these bacteria, serum or blood enrichment is necessary. Therefore it may be more practical to use blood agar plates for susceptibility tests in low-volume laboratories. Results are usually comparable to those obtained with Mueller-Hinton agar; however, false-resistant results will often be obtained on the blood agar during testing of trimethoprim and sulfonamide activity. Fresh plates with the proper depth of agar must be used to avoid altering the kinetics of antimicrobial diffusion in a shallow or dehydrated plate.

Inoculum density should be standardized to prevent significant variations in zone sizes and misinterpretations. Susceptibility tests should always be performed with a pure culture of bacteria. Bacteria in mixed cultures can inhibit growth of slower-growing or fastidious organisms. Therefore if mixed cultures are tested, antimicrobial resistance of a pathogen may not be detected. Direct susceptibility testing of clinical specimens is discouraged, and, if performed, the results should always be verified by testing isolates in pure culture.

Standard antimicrobial disks should be purchased rather than attempting to prepare them from therapeutic drug solutions. It is important to make certain that the disks contain the same amount of antimicrobial as is listed in the interpretation chart (Table 18-9). Otherwise the results will not correlate with the desired MIC values. All cartridges of disks not in current use should be stored in a −20° C freezer; those currently in use should be kept in the refrigerator to prevent deterioration of the antimicrobials.

TABLE 18-9 Zone Diameter (Measured in Millimeters) Interpretive Standards for Susceptibility Tests

Antimicrobial Agent	Disk Content	Susceptible	Intermediate	Resistant
Amikacin	30 µg	≥17	15-16	≤14
Amoxicillin/clavulanic acid (staphylococci)	20/10 µg	≥20		≤19
Amoxicillin/clavulanic acid (other organisms)	20/10 µg	≥18	14-17	≤13
Ampicillin* (gram-negative enteric organisms)	10 µg	≥17	14-16	≤13
Ampicillin* (staphylococci)	10 µg	≥29		≤28
Ampicillin* (enterococci)	10 µg	≥17		≤16
Ampicillin* (streptococci)	10 µg	≥26	19-25	≤18
Cefazolin	30 µg	≥18	15-17	≤14
Ceftiofur (respiratory pathogens only)	30 µg	≥21	18-20	≤17
Cephalothin†	30 µg	≥18	15-17	≤14
Chloramphenicol	30 µg	≥18	13-17	≤12
Clindamycin‡	2 µg	≥21	15-20	≤14
Enrofloxacin	5 µg	≥23	17-22	≤16
Erythromycin	15 µg	≥23	14-22	≤13
Florfenicol	30 µg	≥19	15-18	≤14
Gentamicin	10 µg	≥15	13-14	≤12
Kanamycin	30 µg	≥18	14-17	≤13
Oxacillin§ (staphylococci)	1 µg	≥13	11-12	≤10
Penicillin G (staphylococci)	10 units	≥29		≤28
Penicillin G (enterococci)	10 units	≥15		≤14
Penicillin G (streptococci)	10 units	≥28	20-27	≤19
Penicillin/novobiocin‖	10 units/30 µg	≥18	15-17	≤14
Pirlimycin‖	2 µg	≥13		≤12
Rifampin	2 µg	≥20	17-19	≤16
Sulfonamides	250 or 300 µg	≥17	13-16	≤12
Tetracycline¶	30 µg	≥19	15-18	≤14
Ticarcillin (*Pseudomonas aeruginosa*)	75 µg	≥15		≤14
Ticarcillin (gram-negative enteric organisms)	75 µg	≥20	15-19	≤14
Timicosin	15 µg	≥14	11-13	≤10
Trimethoprim/sulfamethoxazole#	1.25/23.75 µg	≥16	11-15	≤10

*Modified from National Committee for Clinical Laboratory Standards document M31-A2, Table 2, pp. 55-59, 2002.
Ampicillin is used to test for susceptibility ot amoxicillin and hetacillin.
†Cephalothin is used to test all first-generation cephalosporins, such as cephapirin and cefadroxil. Cefazolin should be tested separately with the gram-negative enteric organisms.
‡Clindamycin is used to test for susceptibility to clindamycin and lincomycin.
§Oxacillin is used to test for susceptibility to methicillin, nafcillin, and cloxacillin.
‖Available as an infusion product for treatment of bovine mastitis during lactation.
¶Tetracycline is used to test for susceptibility to chlortetracycline, oxytetracycline, minocycline, and doxycycline.
#Trimethoprim/sulfamethoxazole is used to test for succeptibility to trimethoprim/sulfadiazine and ormetoprim/sulfadimethoxine.

DIFFUSION TEST PROCEDURE

Inoculum

Select four or five well-isolated colonies of the same morphologic type from an agar plate culture. Touch the top of each colony with a wire loop, and transfer the growth to a tube containing 0.5 to 1 ml of saline solution or broth. The turbidity of the bacterial suspension should be equivalent to a MacFarland No. 0.5 standard, which is just turbid enough that a slight change in optical density of the tube is macroscopically visible. Within 15 minutes after preparing the inoculum suspension, dip a sterile nontoxic cotton swab into the suspension, and rotate the swab several times with firm pressure on the inside wall of the tube to remove excess inoculum from the swab. Then inoculate the agar plate by streaking the swab over the entire agar surface. Repeat the streaking procedure two or more times, rotating the plate approximately 60 degrees each time to ensure an even distribution of inoculum.

Test Procedure

Place the appropriate antimicrobial-impregnated disks, selected from the list in Table 18-9, on the surface of the agar. Note that some disks serve as class disks for a group of related antimicrobials, thereby reducing the need for testing each drug individually. The disks should be distributed evenly on the surface of the agar so that they are no closer than 24 mm from center to center. This is best accomplished with a dispensing apparatus. Using a sterile forceps or needle tip, gently press each disk to the agar to ensure complete contact. Because some of the drug begins to diffuse immediately, a disk should not be moved once it has come in contact with the agar. Finally, invert the plates, and place them in the incubator. The inoculated test plate is incubated in an aerobic atmosphere at 35° C for 18 hours.

Measuring Zones of Inhibition

After 16 to 18 hours of incubation of a properly inoculated plate, zones of inhibition around the disks should be uniformly circular with a uniformly confluent or almost completely confluent lawn of growth between zones. If only isolated colonies grow, the inoculum was too light, and the test should be repeated. The zone diameters should be carefully measured, including the diameter of the disk, and recorded to the nearest millimeter. The endpoint should be taken as the area showing no obvious visible growth (not including faint growth of any colonies that can be detected only with difficulty at the edge of the zone of inhibited growth). Large colonies growing within a clear zone of inhibition should be subcultured, reidentified, and retested. Strains of *Proteus mirabilis* and *Proteus vulgaris* may swarm into areas of inhibited growth around certain antimicrobials. The zones of inhibition are usually clearly outlined, and the veil of swarming growth is ignored. With the sulfonamides, organisms may grow through several generations before they are inhibited. Slight growth (80% or more inhibition) with sulfonamides is therefore disregarded, and the margin of heavy growth is measured to determine the zone diameter.

Results

Interpret the sizes of the zones of inhibition by referring to Table 18-9, and report results for the organism as susceptible, intermediate, or resistant to each antimicrobial.

INTERPRETATION AND LIMITATIONS

Antimicrobial susceptibility is not an all-or-none phenomenon. Instead, bacteria have a *degree of susceptibility* as defined by the MIC value. Therefore interpretation of diffusion test results as "zone or no zone" is unacceptable. Small zones may represent organisms that can tolerate higher levels of the antimicrobial (high MIC) than can be achieved at the site of infection. The measured diameter of the inhibition zone must be compared with the standards in Table 18-9 to determine whether the degree of susceptibility is comparable to the therapeutic level of the antimicrobial. The classification of "susceptible versus resistant" is a practical simplification of the various susceptibilities of organisms in terms of expected clinical response to standard dose therapy.

Although the diffusion test has been accepted as a standard test and is used in most veterinary microbiology laboratories, some limitations should be kept in mind. This test system is not applicable to slow-growing isolates or for use in special atmospheres. In many cases the interpretative criteria (see Table 18-9) are based on assumptions derived from knowledge of pharmacodynamics of antimicrobials in humans and efficacy in treating human pathogens. Dosages, absorption, and distribution of antimicrobials may be significantly different in the various species of animals. Levels of drug in tissues may significantly differ from levels in serum, such as low levels in cerebrospinal fluid. From the chart, a test result may be interpreted as susceptible, but the drug may not be able to penetrate to the site of infection. Conversely, ampicillin, for example, is concentrated several fold in the urine and may exceed the MIC value for an organism that has a small zone of inhibition. Therefore susceptibility test results are not absolute rules for antimicrobial therapy. They should be used as guidelines in selecting therapy in addition to clinical judgment and knowledge of the pharmacokinetics and pharmacodynamics of the antimicrobials.

Some veterinary microbiology laboratories are using microdilution tests to determine the MIC of clinical isolates. The MIC value can be compared with the levels of drug that can be obtained in the animal for final interpretation.

> TECHNICIAN NOTE *Susceptible* implies that infection caused by the strain may be appropriately treated with the standard dosage of antimicrobial recommended for that type of infection and infecting species, unless otherwise contraindicated.

Intermediate indicates infection caused by a strain with antimicrobial agent MICs that approach usually attainable blood and tissue levels for which response rates may be lower than for susceptible isolates. This category implies clinical applicability in body sites in which the drugs are physiologically concentrated (e.g., quinolones and lactams in urine) or when a high dose of drug can be used (e.g., lactams).

Resistant strains are not inhibited by the usually achievable systemic concentrations of the antimicrobial when normal dosage schedules are used, and/or they may have MICs that fall within the range in which specific microbial resistance mechanisms are likely and clinical efficacy has not been reliable in treatment studies.

MYCOLOGY

The fungal agents that technicians will most likely be expected to identify in a clinical laboratory are *dermatophytes* and some *yeasts*. Dermatophytes can be readily cultured and identified in local laboratories. The invasive *systemic mycoses* are usually encountered less frequently and require specialized laboratory facilities and procedures for identification.

DERMATOPHYTES

The dermatophytes are keratinophilic (keratin-seeking) fungi that invade hair, nails, and the superficial layers of the skin but not living tissue. They may cause chronic, mild inflammation rather than intense inflammation. Lesions are usually characterized by spreading areas of pruritus and accumulating crusty debris. Lesions can be single or multifocal, and hair loss is variable. Because of the peripherally expanding nature of the lesion, it is also referred to as *ringworm*. Lesions can be notably different in various species of animals, from a dry, minimally inflamed lesion without hair loss on cats to a large, wartlike crusty lesion on ruminants.

Specimen Collection

Representative bits of hair, scale, or crust should be collected from the area of suspected dermatophyte lesions. Care must be exercised to prevent heavy contamination with saprophytic fungi or bacteria, which can overgrow the culture of the desired pathogen. If the lesion is likely to be contaminated, it should be cleansed gently with 70% alcohol before samples are collected. Various dermatophytes are best recovered from unique parts of the lesion, and so samples of scale, crust, and hair should be selected. Pluck broken, frayed, or distorted stubs of hair within the lesion area. Do not cut off hair to use as a specimen for culture. Brush-sampling is the preferred method for obtaining a dermatophyte culture specimen from asymptomatic cats. Use a sterilized (or new) toothbrush to vigorously brush suspected lesions or brush the entire animal for 2 to 3 minutes as if grooming. Then lightly press the brush against the surface of the culture medium several times for inoculation. Avoid pressing too firmly because the agar may tear and subsurface inoculum will not grow well. Crush and separate large pieces of debris when inoculating media. To culture nails suspected of having dermatophytic invasion, make fine shavings with a scalpel. Scatter the specimen over the entire surface of the culture medium. Press the hair and scale onto the agar, but do not bury them in the medium. If samples are not placed directly on culture media, they should be placed in a clean, dry envelope. Do not seal them in a tube or place in transport media. When moisture is allowed to accumulate, bacteria and yeast may overgrow.

Direct Examination

All specimens for fungal culture should be evaluated by direct microscopic examination. Direct mounts can be prepared by mixing a small portion of the material in two or three drops of 10% potassium hydroxide on a microscope slide. Addition of black India ink to the potassium hydroxide solution will facilitate observation of fungal elements in the specimen. Add a coverslip over the wet mount, and examine for the presence of delicate hyphae in skin scales or for the accumulation of spores on the surface of an infected hair (ectothrix).

Culture Procedure

Sabouraud dextrose agar is the standard medium for isolation of fungi and can be used for the successful isolation of dermatophytes. Selective media, such as Mycosel (BD Diagnostic Systems, Sparks, MD), are modified with antibiotics to inhibit bacteria and saprophytic fungi. A selective and differential medium (DTM [dermatophyte test medium]) is the most convenient medium available (Synbiotics Corp., San Diego, CA; BactiLab, Inc., Mountain View, CA). The medium contains a phenol red indicator, which turns red as a dermatophyte grows and produces alkaline metabolic products. Occasionally, dermatophytes do not sporulate as well on DTM as on Sabouraud medium, which can hinder identification. This problem can be overcome by using a supplemental medium, such as Rapid Sporulation Medium (BactiLab, Inc., Mountain View, CA), to enhance sporulation and identification of dermatophytes.

After the agar is inoculated, the cap should be replaced but left loose so that air exchange can occur. The culture is allowed to incubate at room temperature (22° C to 25° C). Placement on an open shelf or counter allows daily observation for up to 2 weeks for growth and color change in the medium. Dermatophytes are identified on the basis of both their gross colony characteristics and microscopic morphologic characteristics. Rate of growth, texture, pattern of growth, color of the colony, and pigmentation of the reverse of the colony should be noted. Most dermatophyte colonies are white or light shades of apricot, yellow, or cream to tan. Darkly colored brown or black fungi are likely to be contaminants. The dermatophytes rapidly change the color of the DTM agar to red, even before a colony is apparent. The red color may appear as early as 3 to 5 days after inoculation and rapidly spreads to most of the agar. Nonpathogenic fungi that grow on the medium do not produce an early color change, although the medium may become red after it is heavily overgrown.

Definitive identification of a dermatophyte and speciation require microscopic examination of wet tape mounts prepared in lactophenol cotton blue stain. The slide is examined for microconidia, macroconidia, hypha structures, and other identifying characteristics. The distinguishing morphologic features of the common dermatophytes are illustrated in most clinical microbiology textbooks.

> *TECHNICIAN NOTE* Morphologic features of fungi serve as the basis for identification, much like identification of plants. Although fungi can be identified by using dichotomous keys, most clinical microbiologists prefer to compare structures with photomicrographs published in atlases.

SYSTEMIC MYCOSES

The three most important systemic mycoses are coccidioidomycosis, histoplasmosis, and blastomycosis. They are serious zoonotic agents; therefore the small laboratory should not attempt to isolate them in culture systems. All culture work must be carried out in an approved biohazard safety hood. The small laboratory is limited to direct microscopic examination of clinical material. Stained smears and wet mounts are useful diagnostic tools. The size and structural characteristics of these agents in the tissue or yeast phase can serve as specific identifying criteria. If cultures are desired, the clinical material should be inoculated onto isolation media, and the inoculated tubes should be shipped to a reference laboratory. Delays in inoculation of isolation media will result in loss of viability and overgrowth of the sample by contaminating bacteria.

Sporotrichosis is a chronic infection characterized by nodular lesions of the skin or subcutaneous tissues. *Sporothrix schenckii* usually gains entrance by traumatic implantation into the tissue. Therefore there is little danger of contagion except from cats that frequently harbor large numbers of yeast cells in lesions. The agent can be observed in direct examinations of tissue and exudates or isolated and identified by routine methods.

YEASTS

There are only a few clinical situations in which yeasts are significant veterinary pathogens. In general, animals seem to be much more resistant to yeast infections than humans. If yeasts are suspected, a direct smear of exudate should be stained for microscopic examination. The best approach to the isolation of yeast is to inoculate blood agar and Sabouraud dextrose agar. The blood agar is incubated at 35° C, and the Sabouraud agar at room temperature. Media should be held at least 2 weeks before discarding them as negative. Therefore agar slants in tubes are preferable to plates because they do not dehydrate as rapidly. Culture and identifying methods for the most common pathogenic yeasts are described.

Malassezia pachydermatis

Malassezia pachydermatis is frequently found in cases of external otitis and is emerging as a cause of seborrheic and hypersensitivity reactions associated with dermatitis. It is readily observed in smears of exudate stained with Gram stain as an oval, bottle-shaped, monopolar budding yeast (Figure 18-16). Isolation in cultures can be difficult, but is best attempted by inoculating Sabouraud dextrose agar and incubating it at 35° C in a carbon dioxide incubator.

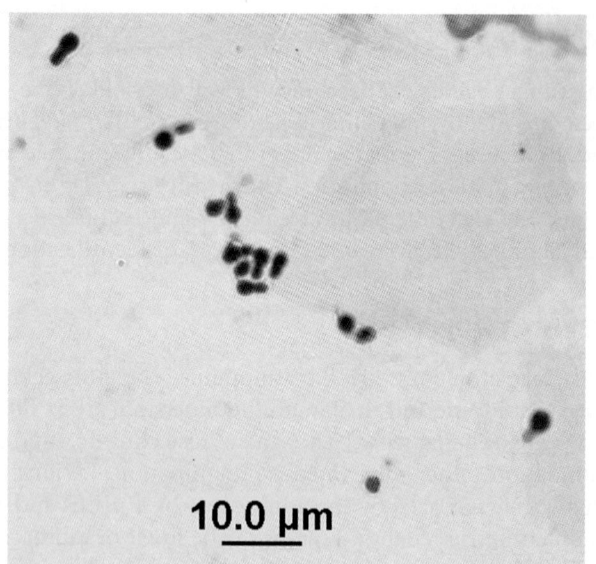

FIGURE 18-16 Gram stain of *Malassezia* spp. in a smear prepared from canine external ear canal swab.

Cryptococcus neoformans

In direct smears, *Cryptococcus neoformans* may be presumptively identified by its abundant capsular material. Negative staining with India ink provides a black background that outlines the clear capsule for easier observation. It can be isolated on Sabouraud dextrose agar or blood agar. *Cryptococcus neoformans* can be differentiated from other nonpathogenic yeasts because it will grow at 35° C to 37° C and is urease-positive. The urease test is performed by inoculating the same urea agar slant that is used for differentiating bacteria.

Candida albicans

Candida albicans is a frequently encountered opportunistic fungal pathogen. Infections usually involve mucous membranes. In direct microscopic examinations of wet mounts, unicellular budding yeasts without a capsule are observed. Limited hypha development may also be observed. *Candida albicans* is readily isolated on Sabouraud dextrose agar or blood agar. Definitive identification can be made by demonstration of germ tube (pseudohypha) development after 3 to 4 hours of incubation in rabbit serum.

Other Yeasts

Other yeasts are isolated much less frequently. It is usually not feasible for small laboratories to attempt to identify these rare isolates. They should be forwarded to a reference laboratory for definitive identification.

VIROLOGY

Laboratory diagnosis of viral diseases depends on the examination of appropriate specimens for evidence of viral infection and then attempting to correlate infection with disease. Because of the nature of viruses and the special laboratory procedures required, most clinical laboratories perform only limited viral diagnostic procedures. Viruses are obligate intracellular parasites. Therefore they are best recovered from living tissue. Isolation of viruses in dead tissues is reduced in direct proportion to the length of time since death and the extent of autolysis.

> *TECHNICIAN NOTE* Rapid detection of viral infection usually depends on some form of molecular diagnostics, such as antigen detection or nucleic acid detection.

VIRUS ISOLATION

Isolation and identification of viruses depend on the inoculation of susceptible living cells for cultivation of the virus. The major methods of providing these living cells include monolayer cell cultures, embryonated hen eggs, and laboratory animal inoculation. These techniques require special laboratory facilities and up to 2 weeks for recovery of a virus. Special care must be taken to ensure that a viable virus is delivered to the laboratory for isolation attempts. Therefore specimens should be collected early in the course of infection when viruses are most numerous. At death, virus numbers in the tissues are usually reduced, and extensive postmortem bacterial growth is often present. The presence of bacteria in the sample can be damaging to the cells that are being used as recovery hosts for the virus. Therefore specimens should be carefully collected, refrigerated, and promptly delivered to the diagnostic laboratory. Special arrangements should be made with laboratory personnel so that they can be prepared to process the sample when it arrives. Transport media containing antibiotics and virus-stabilizing agents are often available from viral diagnostic laboratories.

MICROSCOPIC EVALUATION

In some cases, viral infection can be identified by microscopic examination of infected tissues for the presence of pathognomonic changes or of body fluids for the presence of viral particles. Some viral infections produce distinct changes in host cells, such as the intranuclear inclusions of infectious canine hepatitis, which can provide a definitive diagnosis. Electron microscopic examination of body fluids and washings allows the direct visualization of viral particles. This procedure is often used for diagnosis of respiratory and enteric viral infections because it is rapid and can detect mixed viral infections. The procedure does not require viable viruses, as long as they have retained their structural integrity. Direct electron microscopic examination is limited to cell-free viruses, such as those found in body fluids, rather than examination of infected tissue. Most diagnostic laboratories perform negative-contrast staining; therefore virus identification is limited to morphologic identification. If immunoelectron microscopy procedures are available, the type of virus within a group can be identified.

ANTIGEN DETECTION

Antigen detection methods are the most frequently used viral diagnostic procedures. Advantages of antigen detection compared with viral isolation include rapid results, less expense, less technically demanding procedures, and less dependence on the presence of viable virus in the sample because most viral antigens remain intact after death of the virus. The most common methods of antigen detection are immunohistochemical staining, hemagglutination, and solid-phase immunoassays. Hemagglutination assays are not easily standardized for use in clinical laboratories.

Immunohistochemical Staining

Examination of selected clinical specimens by using a specific antibody labeled with a marker as a probe to identify viral antigen is a rapid and highly reliable diagnostic method. Markers on the antibody can include fluorescent compounds, enzymes, or colloidal gold. The two most important limitations of these procedures are the need for specific antibodies to the viral antigens and a system for detecting the marker. For immunofluorescence, a microscope with an ultraviolet (UV) light source is required.

In the *immunoperoxidase method assay*, the specific antibody is labeled with an enzyme (usually horseradish peroxidase) instead of a fluorescent label. Attachment of the antibody to tissue sections or smears is detected by using a chromogenic substrate that is deposited at the site of the enzyme-antibody attachment and produces a slide similar to other differential stains. The slide can then be examined by light microscopy. Several of these assays have been developed by using monoclonal antibodies to detect viral antigens in tissue, including examination of formalin-fixed specimens.

Solid-Phase Immunoassays

The use of enzyme immunoassays is based on the excellent ability of this method to be adapted to kits that meet practical needs, such as minimizing reagent cost, reducing technician time required to perform the assay, and simplifying the test protocol. These test systems are frequently referred to by the acronym ELISA (enzyme-linked immunosorbent assay). As a result, several kit systems are available for the detection of antigens from viruses and other infectious agents (Figure 18-17) and for detection of antibodies specific for infectious agents. Three typical configurations of ELISAs are illustrated in Figure 18-18. At present, there are several different solid phases commonly used in these assays. The most common solid phase for multiple tests is the microtiter well, but for individual clinical tests, dipstick, immunofiltration, immunomigration, and immunochromatographic formats are more efficient. Immunoassay diagnostic kit manufacturers usually offer technical assistance to kit users. If you have questions about a protocol or test result or are experiencing difficulty in conducting a test after carefully reading and following the manufacturer's instructions, call the company's technical services department and ask for assistance. Most companies provide a toll-free telephone number to facilitate this and will welcome an opportunity to assist you in using their products.

Assays that have been successfully developed for detection of viral antigen include feline leukemia virus (FeLV) in blood (Assure FeLV and Witness FeLV, Synbiotics Corp.; SNAP FeLV Antigen Test, IDEXX Laboratories, Inc., Westbrook, ME), FeLV in saliva (Assure FeLV), canine parvovirus in feces

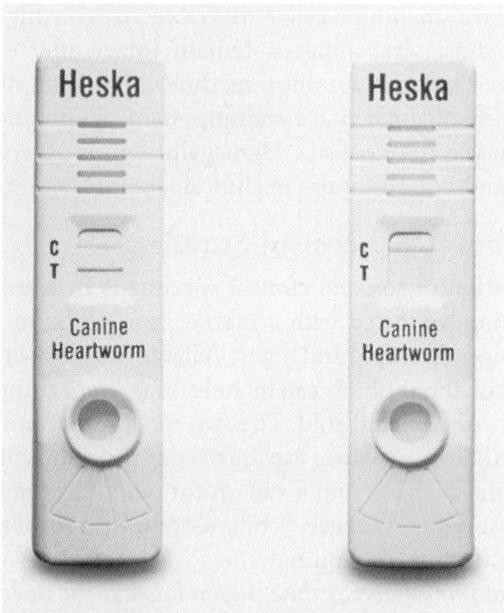

FIGURE 18-17 Solo Step CH (Heska Corp.) lateral flow immunoassay cassette for the detection of antigens produced by canine heartworms in serum. A positive test result has developed in the left cassette, and a negative test result is shown in the cassette on the right.

(Assure Parvo, Synbiotics Corp., San Diego, CA; SNAP Parvo Antigen Test, IDEXX Laboratories, Inc., Westbrook, ME), and influenza virus in respiratory tract specimens (Directigen Flu A, BD Diagnostic Systems, Sparks, MD). Kits are also available to detect bacterial antigens (*Escherichia coli* Antigen Test [K99 Pilitest], VMRD, Inc., Pullman, WA) and heartworm antigens (Solo Step CH, Heska Corp., Loveland, CO; SNAP Heartworm Antigen Test, IDEXX Laboratories, Inc., Westbrook, ME; Witness HW, Synbiotics Corp., San Diego, CA).

SEROLOGY

Serologic testing is an important tool in the diagnosis of infectious diseases. Serology is used extensively in the diagnosis of viral infections and in disease surveillance programs. Serologic tests for detecting a specific antibody have been developed for nearly every infectious agent. However, this indirect approach to diagnosing infection on the basis of a host immune response after exposure to an infectious agent has limitations. Serologic tests may vary in their sensitivity and specificity because of the type of test, immunogenicity and cross-reactivity of the antigen, and biologic variation of immune responses by individual animals. Nevertheless, serologic tests often remain the best diagnostic test available. In veterinary medicine, serologic tests are often required by regulatory agencies to prove an animal is not infected or a carrier of a particular infectious agent.

ANTIBODY RESPONSE TO INFECTION

The chronology of exposure to an infectious agent and subsequent development of an antibody response are illustrated in Figure 18-19. After exposure, there is a variable period of incubation, followed by clinical illness. During the time of clinical illness, the animal may be febrile, and this is when the greatest number of microorganisms are present. Therefore it is more likely to transmit the infectious agent, and the best samples can be obtained for recovery of the agent at this time. After a variable period from onset of clinical signs (usually after 5 to 10 days), the animal begins to produce antibodies to the agent. Continued production of antibodies after the animal is no longer ill, referred to as the convalescent phase, will cause the titer (serum antibody level) to rise for 1 month or longer.

INTERPRETATION OF SEROLOGIC TEST RESULTS

The presence of antibodies to a particular organism in an animal serum sample is not always a simple and absolute diagnosis of current or recent clinical illness caused by the organism. Sources of antibody in the serum of an animal include convalescent antibody after clinical disease or persistent infection, antibody response caused by exposure to an organism without clinical disease occurring, active immune response to vaccination, and passive transfer of maternal antibodies to the neonate. Therefore detection of antibodies in a single serum sample often has limited importance unless the finding can be correlated with other clinical indications of the disease. In most situations, it is necessary to collect two samples—the first one early in the course of the illness *(acute)* and the second one *(convalescent)* at a later time—to demonstrate a change in antibody titer that would indicate recent antigenic stimulation. The change must be at least two dilution increments (usually fourfold), such as an increase from 1:4 to 1:16 or greater, to be considered diagnostically significant. This change in titer is known as a *seroconversion*.

The presence of antibody in serum may be reported quantitatively as a titer or qualitatively as positive or negative. Qualitative tests have less diagnostic value than those tests that report titers, unless the result is negative, in which case the test can exclude some agents from the differential diagnosis unless the serum was collected early in the course of a disease. Most qualitative tests, such as immunodiffusion for equine infectious anemia (Coggins test) and bovine leukosis, are surveillance tests to identify animals that have been exposed and are possible carriers. Occasionally, a single, high-titered serum can aid in establishing a diagnosis, but it always leaves some question of whether the titer increased in association with clinical disease or is a stable, convalescent high titer.

When an animal is exposed to an infectious agent, the first antibodies produced are usually of the immunoglobulin (Ig) M class, with later antibody production being IgG. Some tests are designed to differentiate these antibody class responses, which can be helpful in confirming a diagnosis. If the antibody response to a virus is of the IgM type, the animal has recently been exposed. If the response is mostly IgG, it was probably exposed several weeks to months previously.

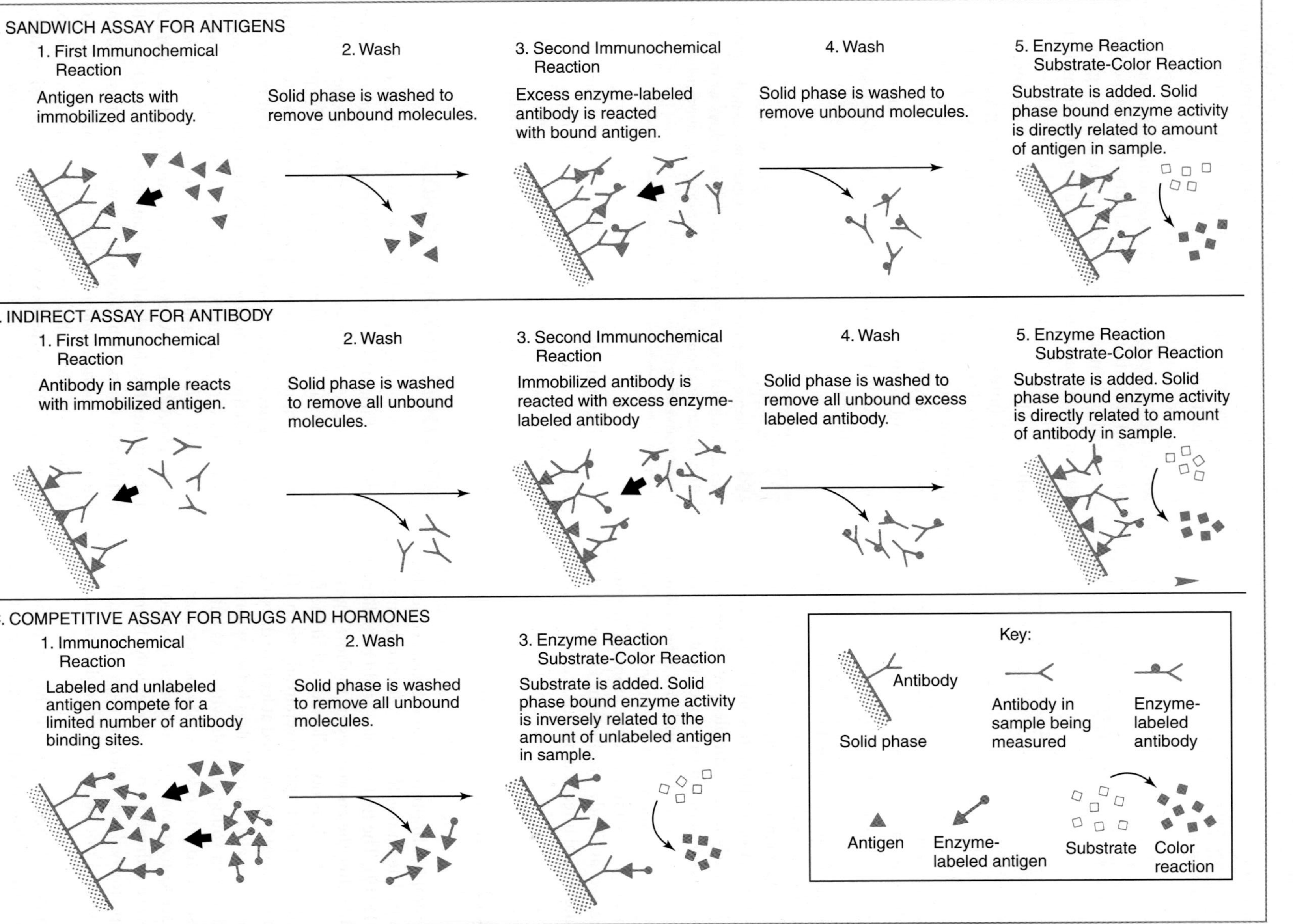
A. SANDWICH ASSAY FOR ANTIGENS
1. First Immunochemical Reaction
Antigen reacts with immobilized antibody.
2. Wash
Solid phase is washed to remove unbound molecules.
3. Second Immunochemical Reaction
Excess enzyme-labeled antibody is reacted with bound antigen.
4. Wash
Solid phase is washed to remove unbound molecules.
5. Enzyme Reaction Substrate-Color Reaction
Substrate is added. Solid phase bound enzyme activity is directly related to amount of antigen in sample.
B. INDIRECT ASSAY FOR ANTIBODY
1. First Immunochemical Reaction
Antibody in sample reacts with immobilized antigen.
2. Wash
Solid phase is washed to remove all unbound molecules.
3. Second Immunochemical Reaction
Immobilized antibody is reacted with excess enzyme-labeled antibody
4. Wash
Solid phase is washed to remove all unbound excess labeled antibody.
5. Enzyme Reaction Substrate-Color Reaction
Substrate is added. Solid phase bound enzyme activity is directly related to amount of antibody in sample.
C. COMPETITIVE ASSAY FOR DRUGS AND HORMONES
1. Immunochemical Reaction
Labeled and unlabeled antigen compete for a limited number of antibody binding sites.
2. Wash
Solid phase is washed to remove all unbound molecules.
3. Enzyme Reaction Substrate-Color Reaction
Substrate is added. Solid phase bound enzyme activity is inversely related to the amount of unlabeled antigen in sample.
Key:
Antibody
Solid phase
Antibody in sample being measured
Enzyme-labeled antibody
Antigen
Enzyme-labeled antigen
Substrate
Color reaction

FIGURE 18-18 Enzyme immunoassay configurations and major steps in assay procedures. (Courtesy E.S. Bean and E.T. Maggio, San Diego.)

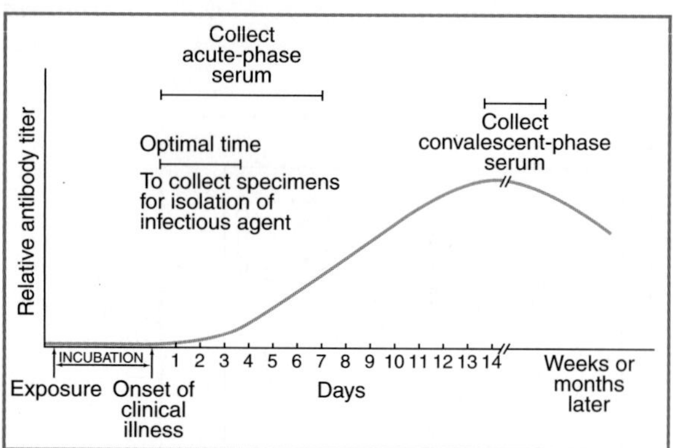

FIGURE 18-19 Antibody response to an infectious disease and optimal times for specimen collection.

Often IgM antibodies are less specific than IgG and may cross-react, resulting in false-positive test results. The test can be modified to exclude IgM reactions to prevent this from happening.

Serologic tests are frequently relied on as the only diagnostic procedures for abortion cases. Results are often difficult to interpret for two reasons. First, by the time abortion occurs because of infection of the fetus and its subsequent death, the dam is already in the convalescent phase of antibody production, so a seroconversion cannot be demonstrated. Second, the stress of abortion or other clinical illness may trigger reactivation of a latent viral infection. This provides an antigenic stimulus to the animal's immune system and increased antibody production. However, it is specific for the latent viral infection, not the current clinical illness.

COLLECTION OF SERUM

Technicians will frequently be responsible for collecting and handling serum samples. Improper methods can reduce the value of test results. The timing of serum collection is important (see Figure 18-19). The first sample should be collected as soon as possible after the animal begins to show signs of clinical illness. If the sample is not collected within the first 5 to 7 days, antibody titers might have already risen. The convalescent sample should be collected at least 10 days after the acute sample. Generally, 14 to 21 days between samples is recommended, but in young animals with a less efficient immune response, up to 4 to 6 weeks may be necessary to demonstrate a seroconversion. The technical procedures of serologic tests are difficult to duplicate exactly; therefore results of tests performed on different days or in different laboratories should not be compared to demonstrate a seroconversion.

Blood should be collected aseptically by venipuncture (see Chapter 28) with a new needle and syringe or evacuated clot tube (Vacutainer tubes and SST Sterile Serum Separation Tubes, BD). Do not use recycled, washed needles, syringes, or tubes. Residual detergent may cause hemolysis or may be toxic to cell cultures used in the test systems. Blood should be allowed to stand at room temperature until a clot has formed; the serum should then be removed from the clot and placed in a new, sterile tube. It may be necessary to separate the serum from the clot by centrifugation to prevent transferring cellular components of the blood. Anticoagulants should not be used to collect plasma because they can be toxic in some test systems. Avoid freezing the whole blood because that will cause hemolysis. The transfer of serum from the original blood tube must be performed aseptically. Contaminating microorganisms can grow rapidly in serum and alter the immunoglobulin molecules. Therefore serum samples (separated from the clot and cells) should be refrigerated until testing is commenced, if within 72 hours. For longer periods of storage, serum may be preserved in a freezer (−20° C). Frozen serum samples should be packaged and shipped with adequate insulation and ice to prevent thawing before arrival at the laboratory. If a second sample will be collected, the first sample should be held until both can be sent to the laboratory together for valid paired testing.

> *TECHNICIAN NOTE* The technical procedures of serologic tests are difficult to duplicate exactly; therefore results of tests performed on different days or in other laboratories should not be compared to demonstrate a seroconversion.

For shipment, the tubes of serum must be carefully labeled and packed so that they will not leak or break. When environmental temperatures are high, refrigerant and insulating materials should be used to preserve samples during transport.

SEROLOGIC TEST PROCEDURES

Only a few serologic tests have been standardized and packaged for efficient use in veterinary practice laboratories. When kits are used, it is important that the directions be followed carefully because modification of any part of the procedure can cause spurious results. A positive (or known titer) serum and a negative serum should be kept on hand (if not already included in the kit) and included in the test each time it is performed to verify accuracy of the results. Serology (antibody-detecting) kits are available for feline immunodeficiency virus (SNAP FIV Antibody/FeLV Antigen Test, IDEXX Laboratories, Inc., Loveland, CO), canine brucellosis (D-Tec CB, Synbiotics Corp., San Diego, CA), paratuberculosis (*Mycobacterium paratuberculosis* Antibody Test, ImmuCell Corp., Portland, ME), feline heartworm (Solo Step FH, Heska Corp., Loveland, CO), and canine borreliosis and ehrlichiosis (Canine SNAP 3Dx Test, IDEXX Laboratories, Inc., Westbrook, ME). The most frequent mistakes made in performance of serologic tests include the use of dirty or contaminated equipment, failure to adhere to instructions (especially incubation times), and unfamiliarity with interpreting results.

CLINICAL IMMUNOLOGY

PURPOSE OF EVALUATING IMMUNE SYSTEM FUNCTION

As the function and complexity of the immune system have been elucidated, an increasing need for laboratory diagnosis of dysfunction of the immune system has been recognized. Clinical immunologic laboratory support has become a well-established part of the diagnostic services and patient care procedures in human medicine. Similar assays are becoming available in veterinary medicine, but few tests are readily available for use in practice laboratories.

Several types of diagnostic problems present the need for laboratory evaluation of possible immunologic disorders. These disorders can be classified into four types: allergies, autoimmune diseases, immunodeficiencies, and immunoproliferative diseases. In young animals, disorders of the immune system may be observed as developmental defects (sometimes inherited) or may be caused by a failure of passive transfer of maternal antibodies. However, immune function abnormalities can be observed in animals of all ages because of effects of aging, various drugs, or environmental exposure to immunomodulating toxins. A few simple procedures will be discussed in this section. The Recommended Reading list should be consulted for detailed and theoretic discussions of other immune system function assays.

LABORATORY TESTS FOR IMMUNOLOGIC DISORDERS

Allergies are usually diagnosed by physical examination, history, and response to intradermal inoculation of test antigens.

Autoimmune disorders can be diagnosed more efficiently by evaluating lesions obtained by biopsy. Morphologic evaluation, combined with various immunohistochemical staining procedures, provides the most definitive diagnosis. It is best to consult referral laboratories to learn which specimens they are able to analyze and how the sample should be submitted.

Immunoproliferative diseases may result in the production of abnormal amounts or unusual types of immunoglobulin proteins, referred to as *gammopathies*. The techniques of electrophoresis (usually on cellulose acetate) and immunoelectrophoresis are the laboratory tests most frequently used to diagnose these disorders. Abnormalities of routine laboratory tests, such as total protein in serum or urine and albumin/globulin (A/G) ratios, frequently indicate a need for these specialized tests. Because of the infrequent demand for these tests and the cost of electrophoresis equipment, most practices request these services from referral laboratories.

Immunodeficiency or immunosuppressive disorders are the most frequently encountered immune system dysfunctions. Most assays of immune cell function require specialized equipment and procedures that are usually available in only a few reference laboratories. Some cellular function assays require submission of viable cells for evaluation. Recently developed assays are used to detect and quantify receptors on the surface of cells, such as CD18 deficiency in Holstein calves. Assays are being developed in research laboratories for genetic analysis of lymphocytes to detect both immunodeficiency and immunoproliferative dysfunctions. Determination of immunoglobulin levels, as an indication of B-lymphocyte function or passive transfer status, is a readily available laboratory test that will be discussed.

FAILURE OF PASSIVE TRANSFER

The newborns of most domestic animals depend on absorption of maternal antibodies from colostrum for protection from infectious diseases. Failure of the neonatal animal to obtain and absorb adequate colostral immunoglobulins is frequently associated with increased morbidity and mortality from bacteremia and common neonatal diseases. Determination of the passive transfer status of foals and calves is an important evaluation that can modify patient care. Although total serum protein levels can indicate relative levels of immunoglobulins, this indirect measurement is subject to considerable variability. The reference method for quantitating serum immunoglobulins is the radial immunodiffusion (RID) test. The RID test consists of agar containing antisera specific for a particular antigen. In this case, the antigen is a particular immunoglobulin class, such as IgG. Each test requires that quantitated standards be tested at the same time for comparison. Therefore if single samples are being tested, the cost per sample will be more, and it might be more cost effective to send samples to a referral laboratory. (Commercially produced RID kits for canine, feline, bovine, and equine immunoglobulins are available from VMRD, Inc.)

Passive transfer status of neonates can be evaluated rapidly and inexpensively in the practice laboratory. Field test kits that quickly assay plasma or blood concentrations of IgG are available for detecting failure of passive transfer in calves, foals, and llamas (VMRD, Inc., Midland BioProducts Corp., and IDEXX Laboratories, Inc.).

> TECHNICIAN NOTE Failure of passive transfer is the most common condition leading to infectious diseases and subsequent death in neonatal animals.

NOSOCOMIAL INFECTIONS

An infection that results from exposure to an infectious agent while the patient is in the hospital is considered to be *nosocomial* (hospital acquired). The nosocomial infection may become clinically apparent during hospitalization or after discharge from the hospital. Infections that are incubating at the time of admission are defined as *community acquired*, even though they become clinically apparent only during hospitalization. In veterinary practices, in addition to nosocomial infections of patients, zoonotic infections transmitted to the staff and clients can be considered part of the biosafety problem.

The incidence of nosocomial infections in veterinary hospitals is not well documented, but it is probably similar to the incidence in human hospitals, which ranges from 3% to 5% of hospitalized patients. The incidence is known to vary with the size and type of hospital and the sophistication of infection control programs. The highest incidence rates are observed in large referral or teaching institutions. The most important institutional risk factors appear to be an increased number of personnel having contact with the patient and an increased mean number of hospital days per patient. Therefore these infections are becoming an increasingly significant problem in teaching hospitals and large group practices in which intensive medical and surgical care is available through a large staff. These institutions also tend to care for patients with more critical and chronic diseases. Because these patients have increased susceptibility to opportunistic infection, the occurrence of a nosocomial infection does not necessarily indicate negligence by the hospital staff.

The stressed condition of hospitalized animals often makes them more susceptible to infections than the general population. Factors that predispose an individual animal to nosocomial infection may include extremes of age (old age or neonatal period); debilitating disease; diagnostic or medical procedures, such as urethral catheterization or immunosuppressive therapy (corticosteroids or cytotoxic drugs); long periods of hospitalization; antimicrobial therapy; presence of other infections; and presence of surgical hardware and drains. For some of the infectious diseases, such as canine distemper, the immunization status of the patient will determine its susceptibility.

Many nosocomial infections are caused by opportunistic microorganisms that infrequently cause infections in healthy animals. However, when the high-risk patient (increased susceptibility) is exposed, the agent can cause disease. Other highly virulent organisms, such as canine parvovirus and *Salmonella* spp., may cause disease in otherwise healthy patients. The greatest impact on the incidence of nosocomial infections can be made by understanding the sources of exposure and spread of these infectious agents. Microorganisms enter the hospital in or on people, animals, inanimate objects, air currents, and occasionally insects. Within the hospital, they are maintained in or on a variety of reservoirs, including patients with infections, healthy carriers, inanimate surfaces, solutions, food, staff, and insects. From these reservoirs, the potential pathogens may be disseminated by contact or by air to hospital personnel and patients.

The most important vehicles for the spread of nosocomial agents are the hands of hospital personnel. Therefore proper and frequent hand washing is the most important strategy for reducing the rate of nosocomial and zoonotic infections.

AGENTS OF NOSOCOMIAL INFECTIONS

Bacteria are the most frequent infectious agents involved in nosocomial infections, but viruses, fungi, and protozoa can also be involved. The commonly involved bacteria tend to be somewhat environmentally resistant, and the increasing use of antibiotic therapy has led to an increased level of antibiotic resistance by nosocomial agents. In the presence of limited antibiotic use, penicillin-susceptible, gram-positive cocci of the genera *Streptococcus* and *Staphylococcus* are the most common agents. With increased antibiotic use, penicillin-resistant *Staphylococcus* is frequently detected. Currently, the major problems are with multiple antibiotic-resistant, gram-negative bacilli, such as *Escherichia coli* and *Salmonella*, *Klebsiella*, *Enterobacter*, *Serratia*, and *Pseudomonas* spp. Methicillin-resistant *Staphylococcus aureus* (MRSA) and vancomycin-resistant enterococci are beginning to emerge as the next wave of serious nosocomial agents. Colonization (growth and establishment) of the body surfaces of the patient by these nosocomial bacterial pathogens is usually a prerequisite to infection. Therefore the patient becomes its own major reservoir of these agents once the organisms are transferred to it during hospitalization. Common reservoir sites are the lower intestinal tract and the naso-oropharyngeal area. Antimicrobial chemotherapy is the most important predisposing factor that allows the patient to become colonized because the antimicrobial suppresses normal flora and selects for resistant organisms. The most frequent locations of nosocomial bacterial infections are the urinary and respiratory systems and surgical wounds. Occasionally, infections become bacteremic. Clostridial enterocolitis in dogs has been identified as a nosocomial problem in several large teaching hospitals.

Viral infections are the second most frequent group of nosocomial infections in hospitalized patients, but are probably the most important nosocomial infections of outpatients. This is because some of these agents are easily transmitted and are highly infectious to susceptible but otherwise healthy animals. Diseases in this group include canine distemper, canine parvovirus, feline panleukopenia, and respiratory viral diseases of all animals (feline viral rhinotracheitis, equine influenza, infectious bovine rhinotracheitis, canine tracheobronchitis, etc.).

Other viral diseases that are not as contagious can be transmitted to susceptible patients at a veterinary hospital if adequate preventive measures are not followed. The resulting disease would be classified as a nosocomial infection. Examples include transmission of viruses of feline leukemia and equine infectious anemia by blood transfusions.

Fungi have rarely been recognized as nosocomial agents in veterinary medicine. As the awareness level of this problem increases, no doubt more fungal infections will be identified, especially with improved intensive care of immunocompromised patients. Yeasts, such as *Candida albicans*, have occasionally been identified. The dermatophytes do not cause life-threatening infections and are usually overlooked, but they can also be transmitted as nosocomial agents to both patients and hospital staff.

Infection of animals by protozoan pathogens can be acquired in the veterinary hospital. *Cryptosporidium* spp. are relatively resistant to disinfectants and have been the cause of nosocomial enteritis. If litter pans are not properly cleaned, other animals and hospital staff could be exposed to toxoplasmosis. Hemotropic parasites (*Mycoplasma haemofelis*, *Anaplasma*, *Ehrlichia*, and *Babesia*) can be transmitted to other patients by blood transfusions or surgical instruments that have not been adequately washed and disinfected.

RECOGNITION AND CONTROL OF NOSOCOMIAL INFECTIONS

Technicians frequently have the opportunity to be the first persons to recognize a nosocomial infection problem by taking note of an unusual number of isolations of a single pathogen or the appearance of an unusual antibiogram. Excellent diagnostic microbiology laboratory support for accurate identification and antimicrobial susceptibility testing of infectious agents is an essential tool for defining the scope of the nosocomial infection problem.

Measures that can help reduce or control nosocomial infections include sterilization of equipment and supplies, aseptic treatment techniques, isolation practices, judicious use of antimicrobial drugs, diligent hand washing between examining patients, disposal of trash, and establishment of sound housekeeping protocols. These protocols should provide for adequate cleaning, disinfection, and maintenance of patient-care equipment and environmental surfaces, such as cages, tables, floors, and walls.

> TECHNICIAN NOTE The hands of hospital personnel are consistently found to be the most important vectors of nosocomial bacterial infections. Diligent attention to hand washing after every contact with a patient and the use of exam gloves are essential to avoid contaminating the hospital environment and transmitting these agents.

The control measures that would be necessary to prevent all nosocomial infections are impractical and not economically feasible. Hospitals contain patients with increased susceptibility to infection, and short of total isolation in a controlled environment, few measures are biologically guaranteed. The risk for each patient of acquiring an infection must be individually evaluated. If the risk is sufficiently great, reverse isolation procedures may be indicated to prevent the patient from being exposed to potential pathogens. If active or passive immunizing products are available, their use should be encouraged. Routine immunization programs can effectively prevent many of the viral infections that have been discussed.

ANTISEPTICS, DISINFECTANTS, AND STERILIZATION

The effective use of antiseptics, disinfectants, and sterilization procedures is an important factor in preventing nosocomial infections. Microorganisms vary widely in their susceptibility to germicidal treatments. Bacterial endospores are the most resistant type. In descending order of relative resistance after bacterial spores are mycobacteria, fungal spores, nonenveloped viruses, vegetative fungi, enveloped viruses, and vegetative bacterial cells. The differences in chemical resistance of various vegetative bacteria are relatively minor, except for the mycobacteria, which are relatively resistant to many disinfectants. Other factors that may have a significant effect on the results of disinfection are concentration of the chemical, length of exposure to the chemical, amount of organic matter (soil, blood, feces) present, type and condition (porosity, cracks, etc.) of the material to be disinfected, ambient temperature, and the nature and number of contaminating microorganisms. Good physical cleaning will allow better penetration of crevices and porous material. Generally, the higher the concentration of the chemical agent or the longer a process is continued, the greater its effectiveness. For temperature-based procedures, increasing temperatures will usually increase efficacy.

Veterinary practices and hospitals should select disinfectants that are registered by the U.S. Environmental Protection Agency (EPA) and labeled as one-step cleaner-disinfectants for use in hospitals. The label should indicate that these products are effective in hard water up to 400 ppm hardness and in the presence of 5% serum. Most nonporous surfaces can be efficiently cleaned and disinfected with the newer combinations of twin-chain quaternary ammonium compounds (C_8/C_{10} dimethylammonium chloride) and alkyldimethylbenzylammonium chloride. Product labels must always be consulted for proper mixing and diluting instructions and intended applications. Chemical incompatibilities may occur if products are mixed. Therefore do not attempt to combine germicides or alter treatment procedures from the manufacturer's specifications.

BIOLOGIC SAFETY

Potential hazards in the veterinary hospital may be associated with infectious or chemical materials, physical facilities, and animal handling. Management should develop a comprehensive safety program that includes consideration of these dangers and preparedness for fire, accidents, and other disasters. This discussion will deal primarily with biologic hazards related to infectious agents in the laboratory and hospital.

Each individual has responsibility for protecting himself or herself and others from accidental infection. Laboratory coats should be worn to prevent contamination of street clothes and dissemination of pathogens to homes and families. Disposable examination gloves should be worn when handling heavily contaminated materials. Good hand-washing procedures should become a habit in the laboratory—between procedures if there is a chance of contamination and always before leaving the laboratory. Mouth pipetting should be prohibited in laboratories handling infectious material. Automatic or bulb pipetting devices should be used. Syringes and needles are poor substitutes for pipettes because they tend to favor creation of aerosols that may be inhaled. There is also the inherent danger of self-inoculation when handling syringes and needles. Self-inoculation must be guarded against, both in the laboratory and when inoculating animals. Centrifuge accidents, which may produce infectious aerosols, should be prevented by selecting compatible tubes, performing proper balancing, and not exceeding recommended centrifugal forces.

Good housekeeping procedures that will maintain a neat, uncluttered work area should be adopted. Eating, drinking, and smoking should not be allowed in work areas, even during break periods when there is no laboratory activity.

Immunization of personnel is recommended when they are at increased risk of infection. A minimal prophylactic immunization for all personnel employed in veterinary hospitals and laboratories should include rabies vaccine and tetanus toxoid. Other immunization products may be recommended in areas in which there is an unusually high risk of exposure to a particular infectious agent.

Primary containment equipment and laboratory design features are important factors in biologic safety. Directional airflow should be from clean areas to areas of contamination and should then be exhausted from the building without recirculation. Small veterinary laboratories and hospitals usually cannot justify the cost of biologic safety cabinets for diagnostic procedures. However, some infectious agents are of sufficient hazard that they must be handled only in laboratories with special design features, including biohazard cabinets. Zoonotic pathogens that small laboratories should not attempt to isolate include the agents of anthrax, brucellosis, plague, tuberculosis, tularemia, and systemic mycoses.

The clinical laboratory has a responsibility to decontaminate potentially infectious materials and wastes before they are discarded. Many states have adopted statutes and regulations that stipulate how hazardous waste materials must be handled. Clinical veterinary laboratories are required to comply with these rules and EPA and U.S. Occupational Safety and Health Administration (OSHA) requirements (see Chapter 6). All diagnostic specimens (swabs), inoculated media, viable cultures, glassware, instruments, and equipment should be considered to be contaminated. Decontamination methods should be applied before waste materials are discarded or reusable products are cleansed. The most practical decontamination procedure for most infectious wastes is use of the steam autoclave. Other methods include physical procedures (incineration, boiling, irradiation) and chemical agents (phenolics, hypochlorites, formaldehyde).

RECOMMENDED READING

Anonymous: *Difco & BBL manual,* Sparks, Md, 2007, BD Diagnostic Systems.

Clinical and Laboratory Standards Institute: *Performance standards for antimicrobial disk and dilution susceptibility tests for bacteria isolated from animals;* Approved Standard, ed 2, CLSI Document M31-A2,Wayne, Pa, 2002, Clinical and Laboratory Standards Institute.

Detrick B, et al: *Manual of molecular and clinical laboratory immunology,* ed 7, Washington, DC, 2006, American Society for Microbiology.

Greene CE: *Infectious diseases of the dog and cat,* ed 3, Philadelphia, 2006, Saunders Elsevier.

Hirsch DC, et al: *Veterinary microbiology,* Ames, Iowa, 2004, Blackwell Pub.

Larone DH: *Medically important fungi: a guide to identification,* ed 4, Washington, DC, 2002, American Society for Microbiology.

Murray PR, et al: *Manual of clinical microbiology,* ed 9, Washington, DC, 2007, American Society for Microbiology.

Research Committee of the National Mastitis Council: *Laboratory handbook on bovine mastitis,* Madison, Wis, 1999, National Mastitis Council.

Winn WC, et al: *Color atlas and textbook of diagnostic microbiology,* ed 6, Philadelphia, 2006, Lippincott Williams & Wilkins.

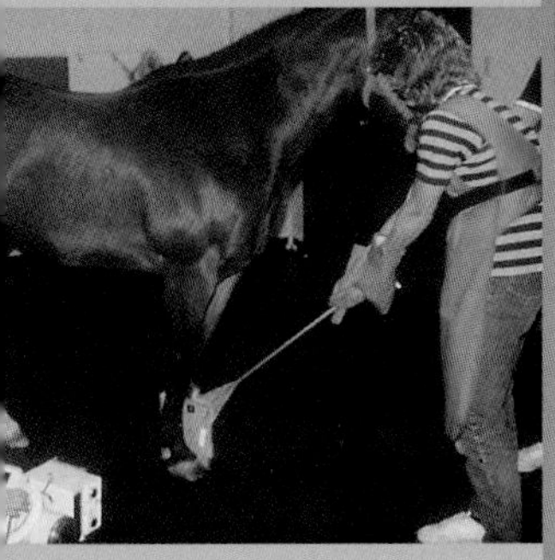

Diagnostic Imaging

19

Beth Paugh Partington and Lorrie Gaschen

KEY TERMS

Anechoic
A-mode
Anode
B-mode
Cathode
Computed radiography
DICOM
Digital radiography
Fluoroscopy
Grid
Heel effect
Hyperechoic
Hz
Ionizing radiation
Isoechoic
Kilovoltage
M-mode
Milliamperage
PACS
Rad
Rem
Rotating anode
Stationary anode
Teleradiology
X-rays

OUTLINE

LEARNING OBJECTIVES

When you have completed this chapter, you will be able to:

1. List and describe methods for labeling of radiographic films.
2. Describe the parts of the x-ray machine and explain the production of x-rays.
3. Differentiate between computed tomography, diagnostic ultrasound, nuclear medicine, magnetic resonance imaging, digital radiography, and computed radiography.
4. List advantages and disadvantages of digital radiography.
5. Define DICOM and explain its use in the veterinary practice.
6. Explain the procedure for developing a radiographic technique chart.
7. Describe the components of the x-ray intensifying screen and list the unique properties of rare earth intensifying screens.
8. Differentiate between screen and nonscreen x-ray film.
9. Explain the purpose and construction of the grid in radiology and differentiate between focused and nonfocused grids.
10. Describe use, care, and maintenance concerns related to x-ray film processing.
11. Differentiate between radiographic contrast and density, and explain how kilovoltage and milliamperage affect contrast and density of the radiograph.
12. List common artifacts encountered on radiographic images and methods for minimizing these problems.
13. List and describe safety issues related to radiography and methods for reducing exposure to radiology hazards.
14. List commonly used types of radiographic contrast agents and give examples of each.
15. State general considerations in positioning of patients for radiography.
16. Describe the preparation of a patient for ultrasound imaging and explain the importance of each step.
17. Identify basic ultrasound artifacts and describe their cause.
18. List tissues in order from most to least echogenic and identify basic anatomic structures on ultrasound images.

INTRODUCTION

Radiology and ultrasonography are the primary diagnostic imaging techniques available to the veterinarian. However, for the veterinarian to arrive at the correct diagnosis on the basis of a radiographic or ultrasound examination, images of high quality must be available. The responsibility to provide useful diagnostic images usually falls to the veterinary technician.

This chapter deals with the basic but essential information needed to produce x-ray films and sonograms of diagnostic quality. It is not the intent of this chapter to offer a course in radiation physics, ultrasound physics, and proper positioning of animals for examination. Excellent textbooks on these subjects have been written and should provide the veterinary technician with the detailed information needed; see Curry et al (1990), Douglas et al (1987), Han et al (2005), Lavin (2005), Morgan (1993), and Ticer (1984). These books should be consulted when the need arises. This chapter discusses the basic information needed to support and assist the veterinary technician in the area of radiology and diagnostic ultrasonography. A short introduction to the use of nuclear imaging, computed tomography, digital radiography, computed radiography, and magnetic resonance imaging is included. Every effort is made to simplify the radiation and ultrasound physics.

RADIOLOGY

LEGAL RECORDS AND FILM IDENTIFICATION

Radiographs are part of the medical record and should be clearly labeled as to which animal has been examined. The identification should include the name of the patient and owner or patient identification number, date of the examination, and name of the practice.

> *TECHNICIAN NOTE* Radiographs are part of the legal medical record and must be correctly identified and carefully labeled.

Several methods of film labeling are available. In one method, leaded numbers and letters are placed on the cassette at the time of exposure (Figure 19-1, *A*). These show up as white markings on a finished radiograph. Also available is a special graphite-impregnated tape on which the desired information can be written or typed and placed on the cassette, or the information can be taped on a special filter at the time of exposure (Figure 19-1, *B*). One of the better film identification methods is a light flasher system (Figure 19-2). It is simple and inexpensive. The required information is typed on a card that is placed in the imprinter. This system requires placement of a small, leaded blocker in the upper left-hand corner of the film cassette, which will prevent exposure to that part of the film. The card is placed in the light flasher in the darkroom. The unexposed, left-hand corner of the

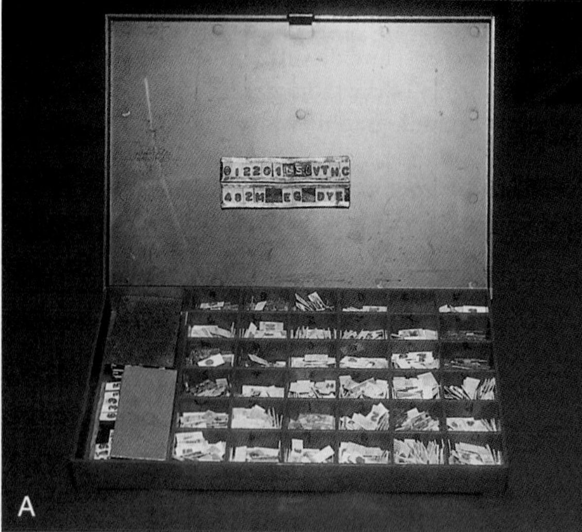

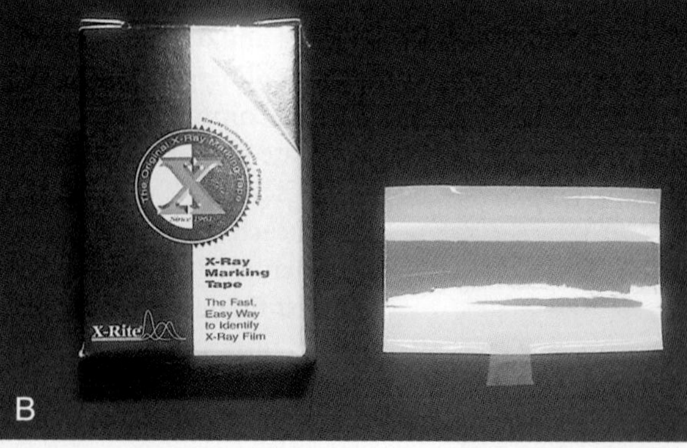

FIGURE 19-1 Film labeling. **A,** Leaded letters and numbers placed on the cassette at the time of exposure. **B,** Radiographic label tape.

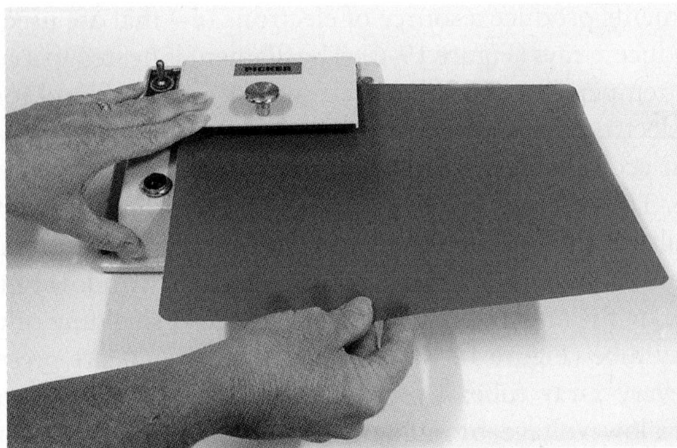

FIGURE 19-2 Light flasher. Patient information is printed onto a radiograph with an identification printer.

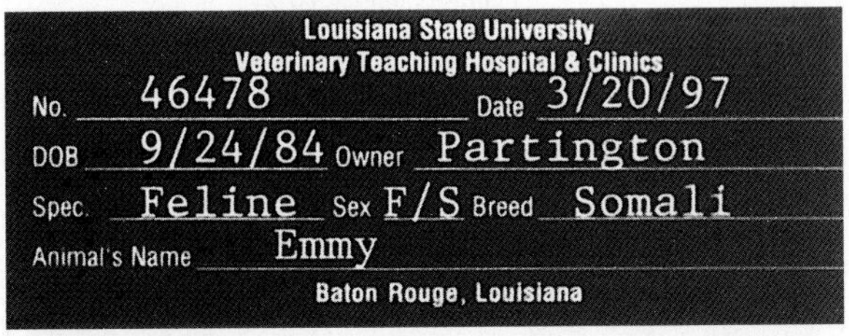

Louisiana State University
Veterinary Teaching Hospital & Clinics
No. 46478 Date 3/20/97
DOB 9/24/84 Owner Partington
Spec. Feline Sex F/S Breed Somali
Animal's Name Emmy
Baton Rouge, Louisiana

FIGURE 19-3 Film identification as it appears on a radiograph. The identification is flashed onto the film after x-ray exposure with a light flasher system or film identification camera.

exposed radiograph is placed underneath the card, and the light is flashed through the card. The information recorded on the card is transferred to the x-ray film and will be developed when the radiograph is processed (Figure 19-3).

One final identification method requires both a film identification camera and special windowed film cassettes. This method allows an individual to type the required information on a 3- × 5-inch card and to place the card into the ID camera. The windowed corner of the cassette is then automatically opened and "flashed" by the camera, and the information is exposed on the x-ray film. The benefits of this system are that the camera will automatically identify the date and time of the examination; it can be done in daylight, and the area on the film in which the identification information is placed is constant (Figure 19-4).

In addition to the legal identification imprinted on the film, it is necessary to identify the part x-rayed at the time of exposure. Leaded right and left markers should be placed on the cassette at the time of exposure to identify the extremity being examined or the side on which the animal is positioned for examination (i.e., right or left lateral recumbency). Additional specialty film markers include Mitchell markers, each of which consists of a plastic bubble containing two to four tiny lead balls that fall toward gravity. These are primarily used in standing radiography of the equine head to assist in identifying fluid levels in paranasal sinuses. Timing markers are used in contrast studies, such as upper gastrointestinal studies and excretory urography, to indicate when the film was obtained in relation to when the contrast medium was administered (Figure 19-5). Front leg versus hind leg and medial versus lateral side identification markers are

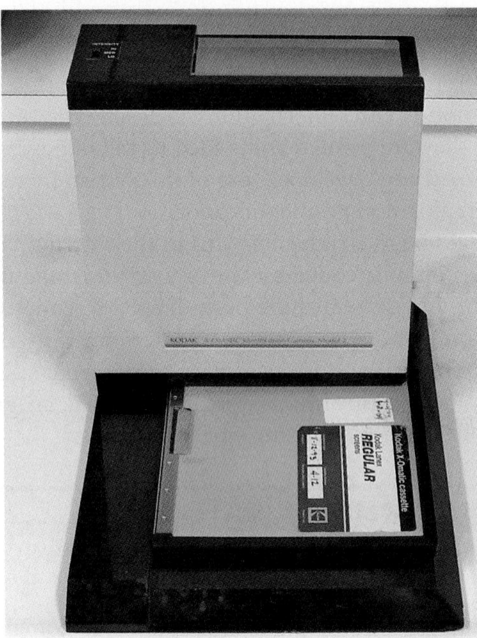

FIGURE 19-4 Film identification camera and special windowed x-ray cassette. Patient information is typed onto a 3- × 5-inch card and inserted into the top of the camera. The special cassette slides into the camera, which opens the window and flashes the identification onto the film.

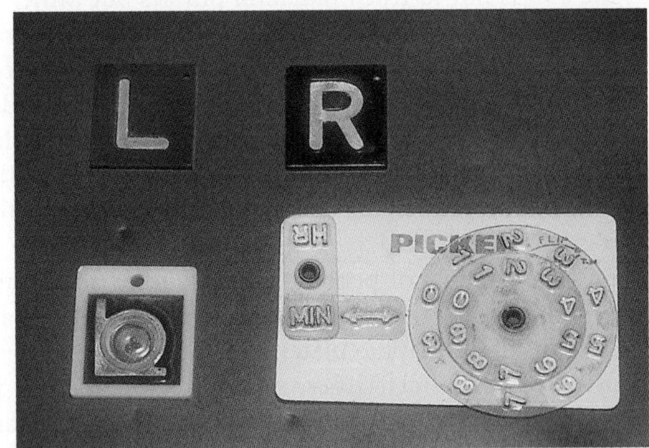

FIGURE 19-5 Leaded letters for film labeling. Left and right markers are used to label extremities and side of recumbency. The Mitchell marker *(lower left)* is used to identify gravitational direction, and the timer marker *(lower right)* is used with contrast studies to identify length of time since contrast medium administration.

critical for proper interpretation of equine lower-extremity radiographs.

FILING OF THE RADIOGRAPH

Because a radiograph is part of the medical record, one must be able to retrieve it when needed. The radiographs of each examination should be placed in an x-ray envelope and filed according to the filing system used for other hospital records (i.e., by last name or case number). The following information should be recorded on the envelope: owner's address, animal identification, date, and type of examination. In addition, the radiographic technique used for the examination can be recorded on the envelope to provide an easy reference for follow-up studies. Many of the veterinary practice software programs have radiograph and film folder labels automatically available for printing when the patient information is entered. The film labels are convenient, but because they are printed and added to the radiograph after it is exposed and developed, use of this system increases the risk for radiograph misidentification.

It would be most advantageous to the veterinarian if the envelope could be coded for use as a self-teaching file. Several color tape systems have been devised to code cases for specific purposes. The system could be refined to include a combination of color to identify species, breed, system examined, and so on. Morgan (1993) outlined an excellent color-coded system for x-ray retrieval purposes.

PRODUCTION OF X-RAYS

BASIC PRINCIPLES

A basic understanding of x-ray production, radiologic image formation, interactions of radiation with tissue, and radiation protection is essential. For those with little knowledge of physics or mathematics, the idea of having to learn basic radiation physics may seem like a large undertaking. However, the aim is not to teach radiation physics but rather to present basic concepts that are useful for those who use x-ray equipment. X-rays can be defined as nonluminous electromagnetic radiation that is similar to visible light and to radio and television signals but are of much shorter wavelengths. The shorter the wavelengths, the greater is the energy of the x-ray beam. The greater the energy of the x-ray beam, the greater is its penetration.

X-rays are capable of penetrating opaque or solid substances, ionizing gases, and tissues through which they pass and affecting photographic plates and fluorescent screens. Because of these characteristics, x-rays are widely used in medicine for the study, diagnosis, and treatment of certain organic disorders, especially those of internal structures of the body.

Unfortunately, because of their short wavelengths, x-rays are not visible. As a consequence, many veterinarians, physicians, x-ray technologists, and veterinary technicians tend to become careless in the day-to-day use of x-rays by neglecting to use protective equipment or apply basic radiation safety rules.

THE X-RAY TUBE

Filament and Focusing Cup

The source of x-rays used in diagnostic radiology is the x-ray tube. The generators and transformers used in radiology exist only for the purpose of providing and controlling the amount of electricity reaching the x-ray tube. The x-ray tube is composed of an anode (+) and a cathode (−) enclosed in a vacuum within a glass envelope surrounded by a lead housing. The cathode contains one or two coiled wire filaments within hollowed-out wells or focusing cups. The filaments produce a source of electrons (e-) that are used to produce x-rays (Figure 19-6). The filament is heated to a critical temperature, and the electrons are boiled off and form an electron cloud within the focusing cup. The electrons are then accelerated rapidly toward the positively charged anode. The collision of the speeding electrons into the anode results in the production of heat and x-rays. The x-rays are directed downward or vertically through the window of the tube by the angle of the anode and the lead shielding of the x-ray tube (Figure 19-7). Two electrical circuits are present in every x-ray tube: a high-voltage, or kilovoltage, circuit and a low-voltage, or milliamperage, circuit. The kilovoltage circuit controls the electrical potential between the anode

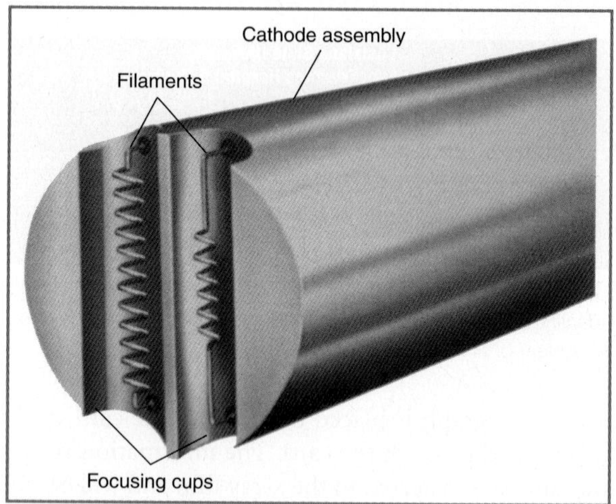

FIGURE 19-6 Cathode assembly showing focusing cups and filaments of two different sizes. Their arrangements produce electron beams that are focused onto narrow rectangles on the target. The smaller filament produces an electron stream of a smaller cross-sectional area and therefore a smaller focal spot. (From Eastman Kodak Co.: The fundamentals of radiography, ed 12, Rochester, NY, 1980, Eastman Kodak Co., Radiographic Markets Division.)

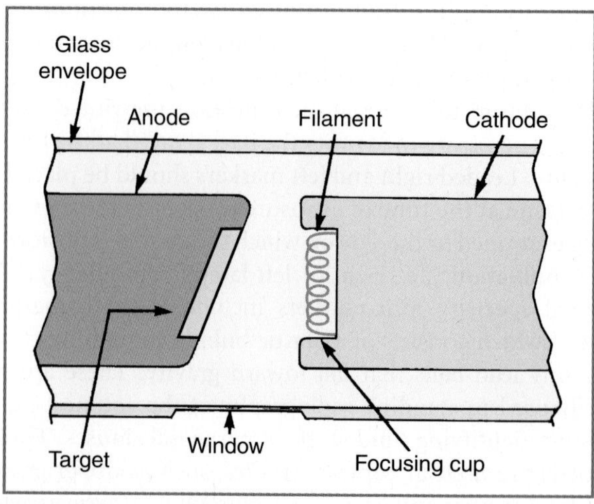

FIGURE 19-7 Stationary-anode x-ray tube. Diagram shows the relation of the anode and cathode. (From Eastman Kodak Co.: The fundamentals of radiography, ed 12, Rochester, NY, 1980, Eastman Kodak Co., Radiographic Markets Division.)

and cathode. This controls the speed of the electron acceleration and the energy level or penetrability of the resulting x-ray beam. The milliamperage circuit controls the electrical potential across the filament and affects the volume of electrons created and thus the number or volume of x-rays created. The filament must produce electrons without melting. To this effect, an alloy of tungsten is used because it is less brittle and more efficient than pure tungsten for the production of electrons. This alloy has a high melting point and is used for the manufacture of most x-ray tube filaments. The larger filament contains more tungsten than the small one and therefore can produce more electrons. As a result, the electron beam produced is larger and does not produce as sharp an x-ray picture as the smaller filament. Unfortunately, because of its size, the small filament may melt more rapidly than the larger one, if an excess load is placed on it. As a result, the veterinarian and veterinary technician must always be aware of the limits and capabilities of the equipment when selecting which filament (focal spot) to use for a given procedure.

Focal Spot

The smaller filament provides a small target region or focal spot for electrons at the anode. In general, the small filament is used to obtain images of higher quality. However, because of the limited number of electrons provided by a small filament, its use is generally restricted to lower mAs (milliamperage × time in seconds) settings used primarily in tabletop (nongrid) extremity radiography. When higher tube current and shorter exposure time are desired, the larger filament must be used, although there will be a loss of detail because the focal spot will be larger.

The size of the focal spot is determined by the size of the electron beam that is accelerated within the tube when high-voltage potentials are applied between the anode and cathode. Thus electrons traveling at an extremely high speed in the vacuum tube are suddenly stopped on the "target" area of the anode. As previously mentioned, the anode target is usually composed of an alloy of tungsten. Tungsten is used because it has the following special properties as a target material:

- High atomic number for the efficient production of x-rays
- High melting point to withstand the large amount of heat generated by the electron beam
- High capacity to transfer heat from the area in which electrons are absorbed
- High density to absorb the electron beam in a small surface area
- Low vapor pressure to maintain the vacuum inside the x-ray tube
- Relatively easy machinability into the appropriate shape at a reasonable cost

Stationary Anode

In early x-ray equipment, stationary anodes were used in most x-ray tubes. This type of x-ray tube is still prevalent in some veterinary practices in which older equipment is used, in dental equipment, and in small portable units used extensively in large animal extremity radiology.

In x-ray tubes with stationary anodes, the target area is a small tungsten block about 3.18 mm thick embedded in a large block of copper. The copper is used to absorb and diffuse the tremendous amount of heat generated by the interaction of the electron beam with the target areas. This type of tube is popular and effective in radiography of the extremities of horses and dogs. However, it has limited application for the abdomen and thorax. The stationary anode x-ray tube cannot produce a sufficiently powerful x-ray beam to penetrate thicker body parts. It is also limited in its ability to produce a rapid x-ray exposure of sufficient strength for chest radiography to eliminate respiratory motion artifact (see Figure 19-7).

Rotating Anode

Rotating anodes became popular with the advent of more powerful x-ray machines and the requirement for radiologists to obtain x-ray images of higher quality. Rotating anode tubes can use much higher tube currents, shorter exposure times, and focal spots as small as 0.1 mm because the electrons deposit their energy over a larger target region as the anode rotates (Figure 19-8).

The target of a rotating anode is a tungsten alloy bonded to molybdenum or graphite to help diffuse the tremendous heat generated by a high-powered x-ray machine. Rotating anodes are 7.5 to 12.5 cm in diameter. These tubes must dissipate enormous amounts of heat. The apparatus used to rotate the anode and dissipate the heat must be of the highest

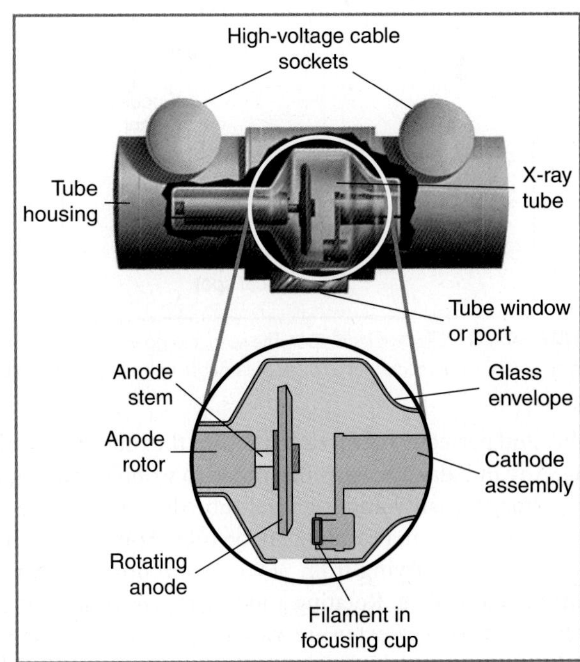

FIGURE 19-8 Modern rotating-anode radiographic tube. Exploded schematic view demonstrates the relationship of the filament to the rotating target. (From Eastman Kodak Co.: *The fundamentals of radiography,* ed 12, Rochester, NY, 1980, Eastman Kodak Co., Radiographic Markets Division.)

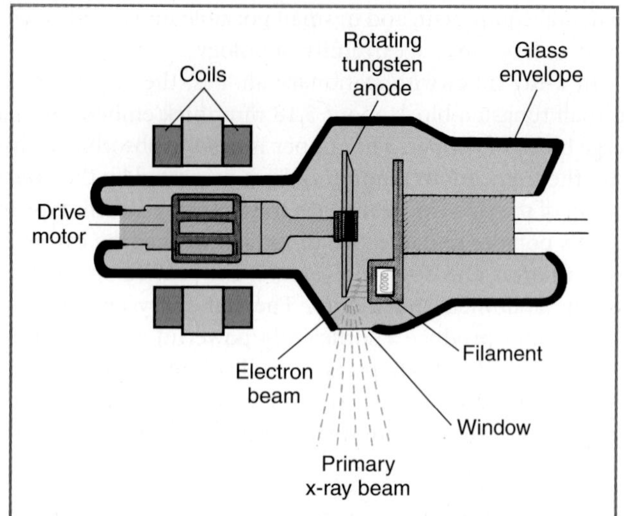

FIGURE 19-9 Rotating-anode tube. Heat is better dissipated by placing the target material at the circumference of a high-speed rotating disk.

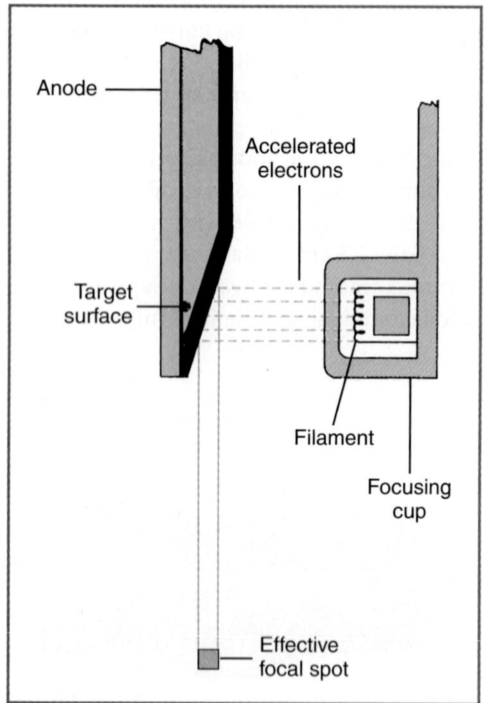

FIGURE 19-10 Effective focal spot. The surface area is decreased when the target area is constructed at a 20-degree angle to the electron beam.

quality and perfectly balanced to prevent the tube from wobbling. Any imbalance causes the anode to wobble, leading to loss of image quality and eventual tube destruction. Figure 19-9 is a diagram of a rotating anode tube. Some tubes may rotate at speeds varying from 3600 revolutions per minute (rpm) to 10,000 rpm. Rotating anode x-ray machines generally have a two-step exposure switch. The first step of the switch starts the anode rotating, and the second step of the switch activates the high-voltage circuit, resulting in x-ray production. The anode is angled for two reasons. One, the angle directs the x-ray beam vertically to exit the tube window; and two, it creates a smaller, more compact effective

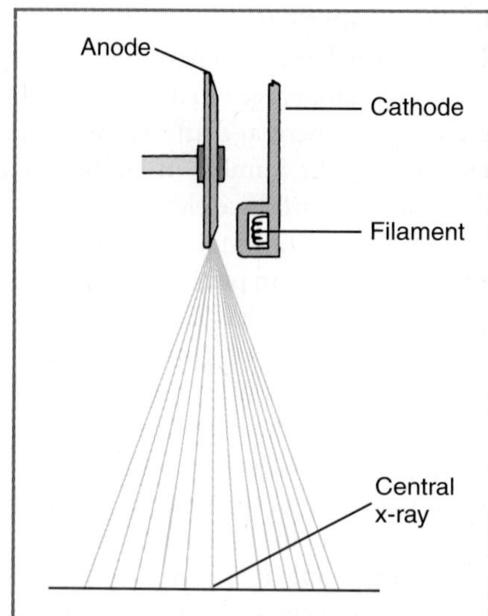

FIGURE 19-11 Heel effect, which is produced by the uneven intensity of the primary beam. The intensity decreases rapidly toward the anode.

focal spot to create better resolution and produce a higher-quality radiograph. The actual focal spot is the target on the anode. The effective focal spot is the tightly packed focused primary x-ray beam that exits the tube window. The actual focal spot is always larger than the effective focal spot (Figure 19-10).

Heel Effect

When an x-ray beam leaves the tube, it has an uneven x-ray photon distribution. This phenomenon is related to the angle of the target areas and the absorption by the anode and target material. As a result of this engineering feature, the x-ray beam is more intense at the side of the cathode than in the center of the beam or on the anode side. This phenomenon is called the heel effect (Figure 19-11).

This feature can be used to great advantage in veterinary radiology when x-raying parts of uneven thickness, a common problem in thoracic and abdominal radiography of deep-chested dogs. By placing the thickest part of the patient toward the cathode side of the x-ray tube, a more uniform density can be obtained on the radiograph.

> *TECHNICIAN NOTE* Always place the thickest part of the area being x-rayed toward the cathode side of the x-ray tube.

Tube Rating Chart

A rating chart is provided by all manufacturers of x-ray tubes. The tube rating chart provides important information on the maximum safe exposure time that can be used with specific milliamperage and kilovoltage settings. If longer-than-designated exposure times are used, tube damage may occur. The size of the anode focal spot determines the rating of the tube because size controls the amount of energy it can absorb and convert into x-rays and heat.

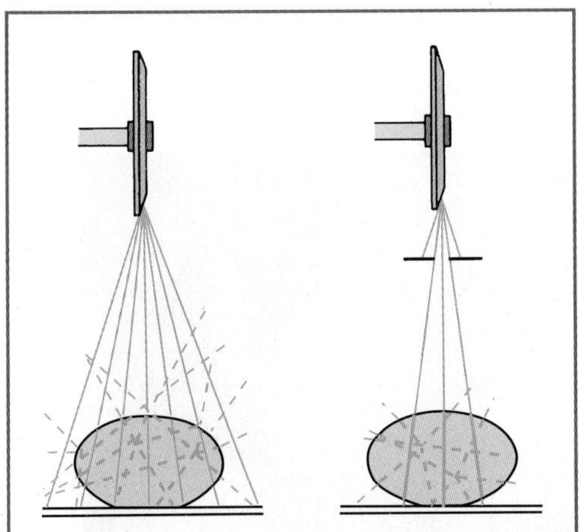

FIGURE 19-12 Scatter radiations. **A,** Scatter radiations are produced when the primary beam is redirected after interacting with structures in the patient's body. **B,** Reduction in the amount of radiation produced when the primary beam is restricted by a diaphragm or collimator.

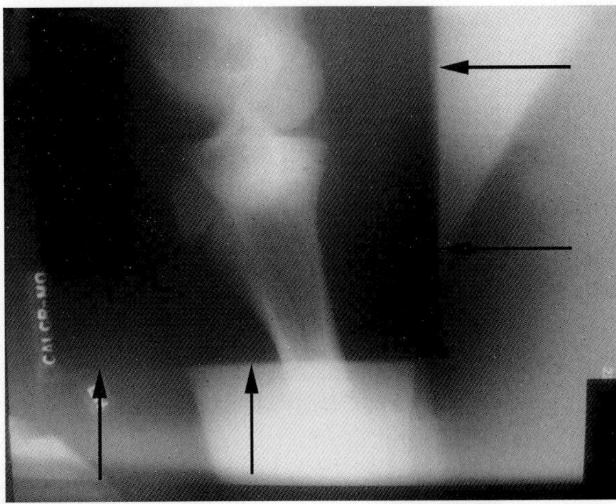

FIGURE 19-13 Lateral radiograph of an equine stifle. Note the close collimation on the joint *(arrows)* and that the scatter radiation from this area was of sufficient strength to penetrate the rest of the horse's leg and create an underexposed image of the leg on the rest of the radiograph.

THE PHYSICS OF X-RAY PRODUCTION

X-rays are produced when all the energy packed in extremely rapidly moving electrons comes to an abrupt stop on encountering the target in the x-ray tube. Most of the energy of the electrons is not converted into x-rays but is dissipated as heat. In fact, more than 99% of the energy dissipated in the target is lost as heat, and less than 1% is converted to x-ray energy. This explains the elaborate system of heat dissipation built into the x-ray tube described in the previous section.

Two events may occur when electrons approach the atoms of the target: (1) the electrons may miss the atom and its orbital electrons and go through the entire target and eventually be absorbed by the backing material of the target or the lead shielding of the x-ray tube, or (2) the incoming electrons may interact with the electron cloud of the atoms in the target material and produce x-rays by transferring their energy to these atoms. Both of these events produce x-ray photons, the majority produced by the slowing of the electrons as they are absorbed into the target. The faster the electrons travel, the greater is their energy and, therefore, the greater is the energy and penetrating power of the resulting x-ray beam.

SCATTER RADIATIONS

In passing through a patient, an x-ray beam becomes attenuated; in other words, its energy decreases gradually. Scatter radiations are lower-energy x-ray photons that have undergone a change in direction after interacting with structures in the patient's body (Figure 19-12).

Scatter radiation is of concern because it decreases film quality and increases radiation exposure to the person taking the radiograph. Most scatter radiations contribute to the overall film blackness or radiographic density, but do not contribute to the useful image. This results in reduced subject contrast. Scatter radiations are also the primary source of radiation exposure to technicians manually restraining patients. Scatter radiations are directly increased with increases in the following three factors: kilovoltage, thickness of the part being x-rayed, and size of the field (Figure 19-13).

Careful collimation with beam-limiting devices and close attention to technical factors to avoid the need for retakes are the best ways to decrease radiation exposure from scatter radiations. Several techniques are used to reduce scatter radiations and their effect on the radiograph. Beam-limiting devices, correct kilovolt peak (kVp) settings, compression radiography, and grids are a few devices that can be used to control scatter radiations. They are discussed later in this chapter.

> *TECHNICIAN NOTE* Scatter radiations coming from the area of the patient that is exposed during radiography are the main source of radiation exposure to the veterinary technician.

X-RAY EQUIPMENT

The kind of x-ray unit encountered in a veterinary practice will vary according to the caseload and type of practice. Because one may be working with a large or small animal practitioner, in a large corporate practice, or in a veterinary teaching hospital, it is necessary to be familiar with the several types of x-ray units found in such practices.

Regardless of type and model, most x-ray machines share many features. For small animal radiology, an x-ray machine must have a table on which the animal can be positioned (Figure 19-14). For larger animals, hand-held or stationary cassette holders are most often used (Figure 19-15). All x-ray machines must have a control panel to select kilovoltage, milliamperage, and time of exposure. An x-ray machine may have numerous auxiliary meters, buttons, dials, or switches; but kilovoltage, milliamperage, and time of exposure are the three primary factors of x-ray production (Figures 19-16

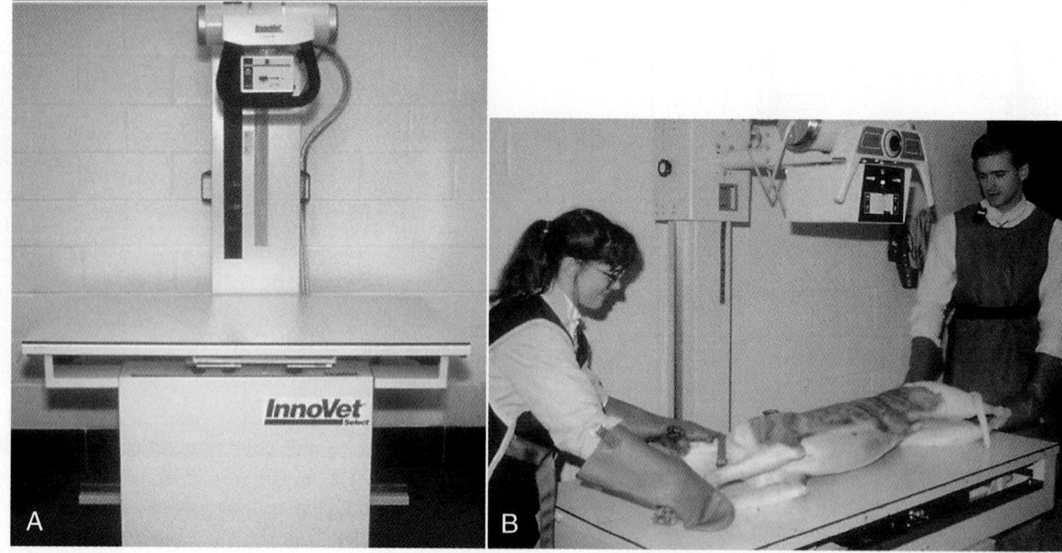

FIGURE 19-14 **A,** 300-mA x-ray machine commonly used in small animal practice. **B,** Canine patient correctly positioned on an x-ray table for a lateral thoracic radiograph.

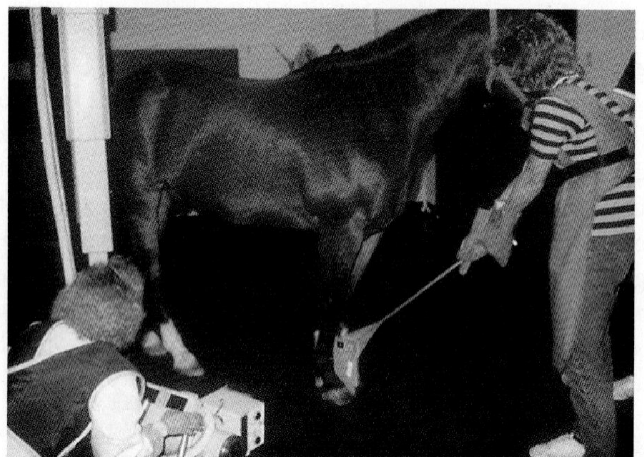

FIGURE 19-15 Large animal radiography unit with special film cassette holders for equine extremities.

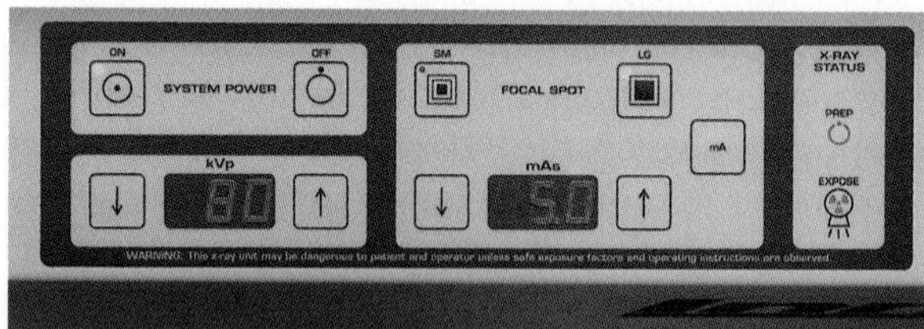

FIGURE 19-16 Typical instrument panel of an x-ray machine used by veterinarians showing digital panels with buttons for selection of milliamperage, time, and kilovolt peak (kVp).

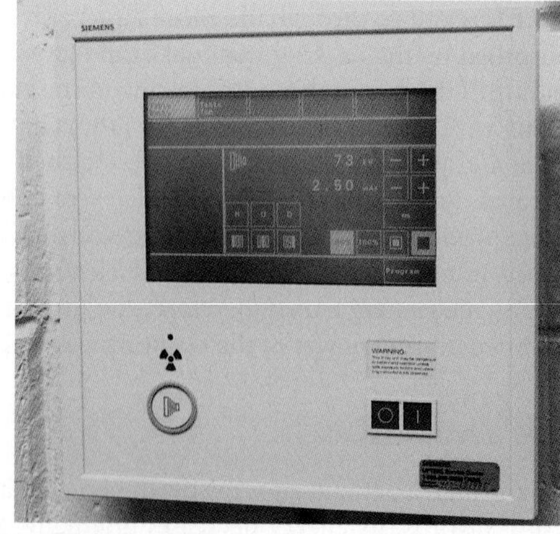

FIGURE 19-17 Wall-mounted operator control console used in some of the larger veterinary clinics and several veterinary teaching hospitals.

and 19-17). Many x-ray machines have a common selector control for milliamperage and time of exposure. This mAs dial or setting automatically sets the highest milliamperage station and fastest time to provide the requested mAs. Milliamperage ∞ time in seconds (mAs) controls the volume or number of x-ray photons produced. In older machines, milliamperage and time (in fractions of a second) must be set manually to produce a given mAs. The amperage (A) in mAs is always capitalized because it refers to Andre M. Ampere, the physicist credited with discovery of electric currents.

There are basically three types of x-ray machines used in veterinary practice: portable units, mobile units, and stationary units. Please refer to Chapter 32 for a discussion of dental radiographic units.

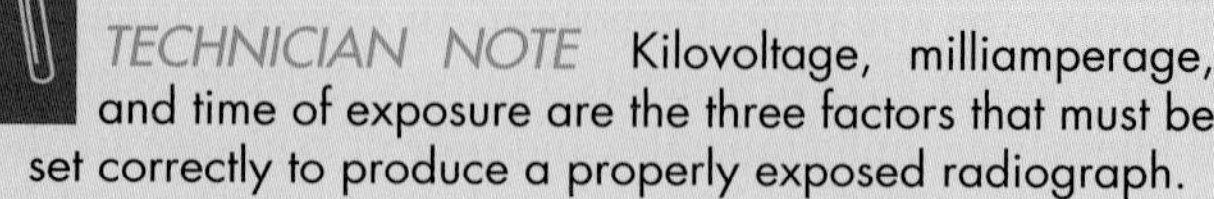

TECHNICIAN NOTE Kilovoltage, milliamperage, and time of exposure are the three factors that must be set correctly to produce a properly exposed radiograph.

PORTABLE UNIT

As the name implies, portable units can be carried "easily" from one location to another. Weight varies from 6.75 to 20.25 kg or more. They are generally used on blocks or custom-made stands. From a safety perspective, these units should never be handheld. This recommendation applies especially to lighter models that have less shielding. Hand holding an x-ray machine not only places the operator close to the x-ray tube but also decreases film quality because of tube motion during exposure.

Common characteristics of portable units include the following:

- A single focal spot of about 1.2 mm, stationary anode tube, and single filament, although a few models have two filaments and focal spot sizes
- Collimation varying from lead adapter plate to adapt to film size to lighted collimator with adjustable field size
- Tube output varying up to 90 kVp at 10 mA, usually with settings at 10, 20, and 30 mA and at 70, 80, or 90 kVp
- Electronic timer ranging from 0.01 to 10 seconds
- Electrical input of 110 V with an adapter to 220 V

Some models may use 12 DC (direct current) or operate on an automobile battery with converter (Figure 19-18).

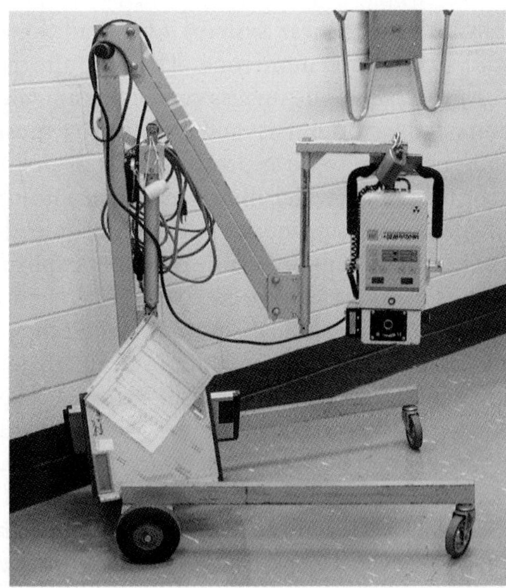

FIGURE 19-18 Portable x-ray unit. Such units are commonly used in large animal practices, mostly for the examination of extremities. This particular unit has a lighted collimator and a mobile operating stand.

MOBILE UNIT

Mobile units are medium-powered, wheel-mounted units that can be moved around the hospital. In many small animal practices, these units are used as fixed units and remain in one room. They are also popular in a mixed practice, in which the same unit can be used for both large and small animals.

These units are powered by 220-V or 110-V outlets. The 220-V units require more extensive electrical wiring, especially if the same units must be used at several locations. These units are equipped with a long, heavy power cord that can be a problem when working with large animals. The 110-V units are usually lighter and therefore easier to move around, and the power cord is smaller, which can be an advantage when taking x-rays of equine extremities. However, these units are usually less powerful than the 220-V units.

STATIONARY UNIT

Stationary units are more powerful and are found in most small and large animal hospitals. A typical stationary small animal unit is shown in Figure 19-14. Custom large animal units and radiography/fluorography rooms are common in all veterinary teaching hospitals. Some of these units are among the most powerful diagnostic x-ray units installed in the United States. They vary in size from 300 mA, 100 kVp up to 2000 mA, 150 kVp. They can be powered by single-phase or three-phase generators. The x-ray tube may be suspended from the ceiling or attached to a floor-stand support. The tube can rotate 90 degrees in all directions and usually has a heavy-duty collimator (Figure 19-19).

Stationary units commonly seen in small animal veterinary practices are of the 300 to 500 mA type with an exposure time of $\frac{1}{60}$ second to $\frac{1}{120}$ second. All these units can hold a cassette tray under the table with or without a Potter-Bucky grid. Some units have an image intensifier unit for fluoroscopic study or a fixed fluoroscopic screen.

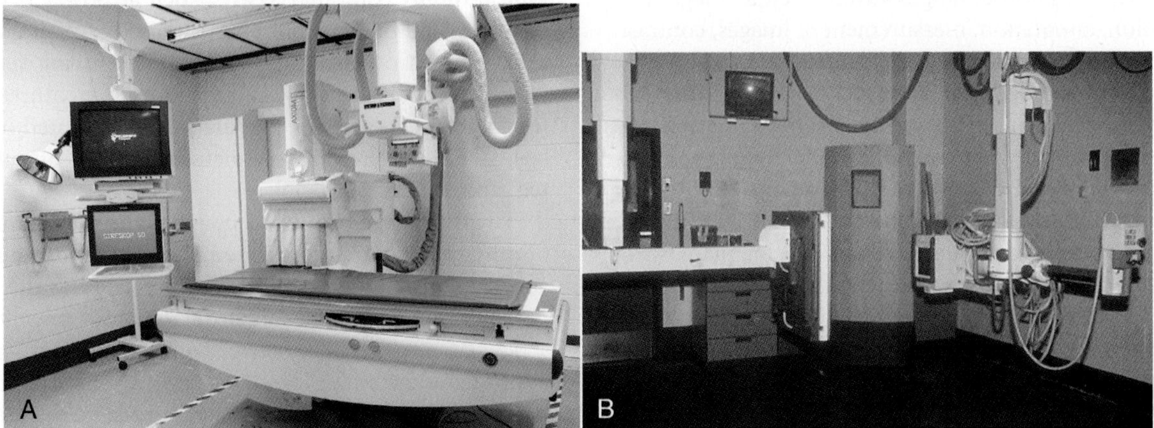

FIGURE 19-19 Stationary units. **A,** Radiography/fluorography used for special procedures, such as angiography, in a few large and small animal hospitals and all veterinary teaching hospitals. **B,** High-powered stationary large animal unit that includes a ceiling-suspended x-ray unit and a Potter-Bucky suspension system. The two units can be interlocked when needed for a fixed focal spot-film distance.

FLUOROSCOPY

Fluoroscopic units are more suited to the study of moving structures and dynamic processes than are x-ray films. Although films exposed close together in time provide some information about these structures and processes, an image that is continuous in time is required for maximum information. The presentation of a continuous image is called fluoroscopy, and it involves directing the x-ray beam through the patient and onto an image intensifier. The image intensifier amplifies the x-ray coming through the patient, thus reducing the amount of radiation needed for the continuous exposure. The resulting images can be videotaped for analysis, and the tapes can be stored as part of the permanent medical record. The use of fluoroscopy is usually confined to gastrointestinal studies and myelography and is essential to heart and vascular studies. A fluoroscopic unit can be a useful piece of equipment, but it is rarely used in veterinary medicine for economic reasons. For a more extensive discussion of fluoroscopy, review the chapters that cover this subject in Curry et al (1990), Douglas et al (1987), Eastman Kodak Co. (1980), Lavin (2005), and Morgan (1993).

DIGITAL RADIOGRAPHY

Medical imaging is currently undergoing rapid and revolutionary changes. With the advent of high-performance computers and high-resolution high-luminance monitors, digital radiography (DR) has been developed. Digital imaging techniques are applied to computed tomography (CT), diagnostic ultrasound, nuclear medicine, magnetic resonance imaging (MRI), DR, and digital fluoroscopy (DF). Computed radiography (CR) and DR are different. In DR, an x-ray tube coupled to a specialized receiver that changes x-rays into electrical signals is used. The analogue image is digitalized and displayed on the integrated computer screen (Figure 19-20). Creating an image in this manner allows postproduction digital enhancement. This enhancement can allow the operator to alter the image using software that has functions similar to conventional image-processing software such as magnification, rotation, annotation, measurement of images, contrast, brightness, and zoom. The main advantage to this ability to alter the image is a decrease in retakes that saves time and reduces the technician's exposure to harmful radiation. CR uses very similar equipment to conventional radiography except that in place of a film to create the image, an imaging plate is used. In this manner, all chemical exposure, expense, and darkroom time is eliminated as the imaging plate is run through a computer scanner to read and digitize the image. Both CR and DR images can be printed on a dry laser camera and will closely resemble typical radiographs, or they can be printed on a variety of imaging printers that process digital data. In most practices, the images are read on the computer screen, and the data are downloaded onto digital videodiscs (DVDs), compact discs (CDs), or magnetic optical disks (MODs) for permanent storage.

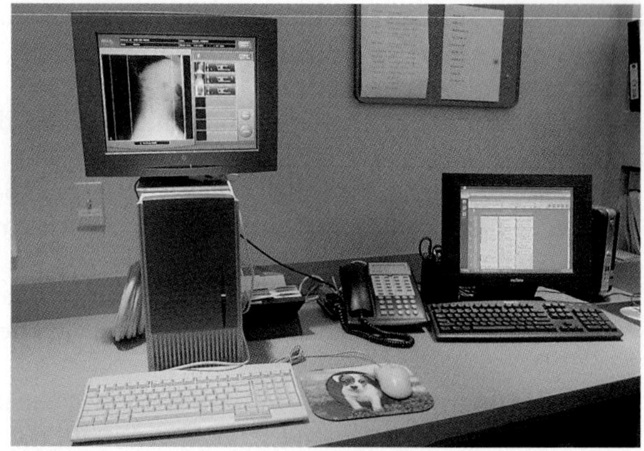

FIGURE 19-20 Digital radiology control system. Computer on the left is the digital radiography work station where images are viewed, optimized, and then stored or printed. Computer on the right is an RIS, or radiology information system, used to couple patient data to the images.

The advantages of these systems over traditional film/screen radiographs are numerous. They require no film, screens, or processing. The images can be manipulated after acquisition to adjust brightness and contrast so exposure parameters do not have to be as precise. Portions of an image can often be magnified, which improves visualization of small parts and enhances image interpretation in orthopedics and imaging of exotic animals. In equine practices, exposures can be repeated as many times as needed. This is a major advantage in field work as the study is not limited by the number of cassettes, the image can be seen almost immediately. This prevents having to return to the farm to repeat exposures and making trips to the hospital to develop films. Because 50 to 100 images can be downloaded on a single CD, DVD, or MOD much less physical storage space is required for archiving. Another major advantage is that because the data are digitalized, one can send these images via phone, DSL, and cable lines to other specialists or referral centers almost instantly for a second opinion and not have to wait for the mail or courier services to transport the radiographs. Disadvantages include increased initial equipment cost, problems typical of any computer system such as power failures and lost data, and the possibility of increased radiation exposure as a result of overuse. Although film archiving space is no longer needed, hard drive storage units are required to store the large sized data files that are being generated on a daily basis. This is referred to as a picture archival computing system and is discussed below.

The dynamic range of an image is the number of shades of gray that can be represented. The maximum number of shades of gray in a digital system is related to the numeric range of each pixel. The larger the dynamic range, the more shades of gray there are between white and black, providing a more gradual scale. The dynamic range of the x-ray beam is 2^{10}. It is impossible to appreciate this large dynamic range as the human eye can only see 2^5 or 32 shades of gray from white to black. However, a computer can display a much broader dynamic range. The dynamic range of a digital system is a function of the computer and software capacity. They range from 2^8 (0-255), 2^{10} (0-1023) to 2^{12} (0-4095). Images with low dynamic range have high contrast but only in some portions of the image. High dynamic range allows for wider image latitude.

Poor spatial resolution is a main disadvantage of digital radiography compared with film radiography. Conventional screen-film systems can image 100 μm-sized images, whereas DR is typically limited to 500 μm. Resolution is controlled by the design of the detector array.

COMPUTED RADIOGRAPHY

Computed radiography (CR) is similar to DR except that an x-ray receiver similar to a cassette is used and must be processed in a special machine (Figure 19-21). The special cassette contains a photostimulable phosphor that changes x-ray photons into a latent electronic image that is "read" by the processor and transferred to the computer. After that, the image data have all the advantages and disadvantages of DR. CR is primarily used in large human hospitals that have several x-ray machines in various departments and want a portable method to have digitized images from all of them. CR will probably not be as popular as the DR system in veterinary medicine, except at large teaching hospitals or specialty practices with several x-ray machines currently in use, because of the need for the special cassettes and latent image reader. There is some confusion about DR and CR in the veterinary marketplace, with some DR systems calling themselves "computed radiography." The question to ask is whether the x-ray receiver directly digitizes the image (true digital radiography) or whether a separate cassette and reader are needed to digitize the image (CR).

DICOM, PACS, RIS, AND TELERADIOLOGY

Medical imaging dissemination and archiving has been revolutionized since the introduction of the DICOM (digital imaging and communications in medicine) standard and transition from analog to digital imaging. Although DICOM is accepted as a universal image format, connectivity between workstations, modalities (ultrasound [US], MRI, CT, radiography, etc.) can still be difficult since vendors sometimes use proprietary methods that other systems cannot read. DICOM 3.0 is the current standard and is universally accepted. Images produced from equipment working with this standard can communicate with another vendor's software. This makes teleradiology possible. Images can be sent electronically from one hospital's workstation to another even though they don't possess the same imaging equipment or software.

Each DICOM image file contains image information and patient identification, modality used (CT, US, MRI, etc.), date and time of the examination, and display formats. Common DICOM files include images from CT, digital or computed radiography, MRI, US, or SC (secondary capture such as from a film scanner). DICOM functionality allows storage, query and/or retrieve, image display, and manipulation. The DICOM service objects are any images produced from any modality. DICOM roles are sender and receiver functions. A service class provider (SCP) and service class users (SCU) allow DICOM communications to happen.

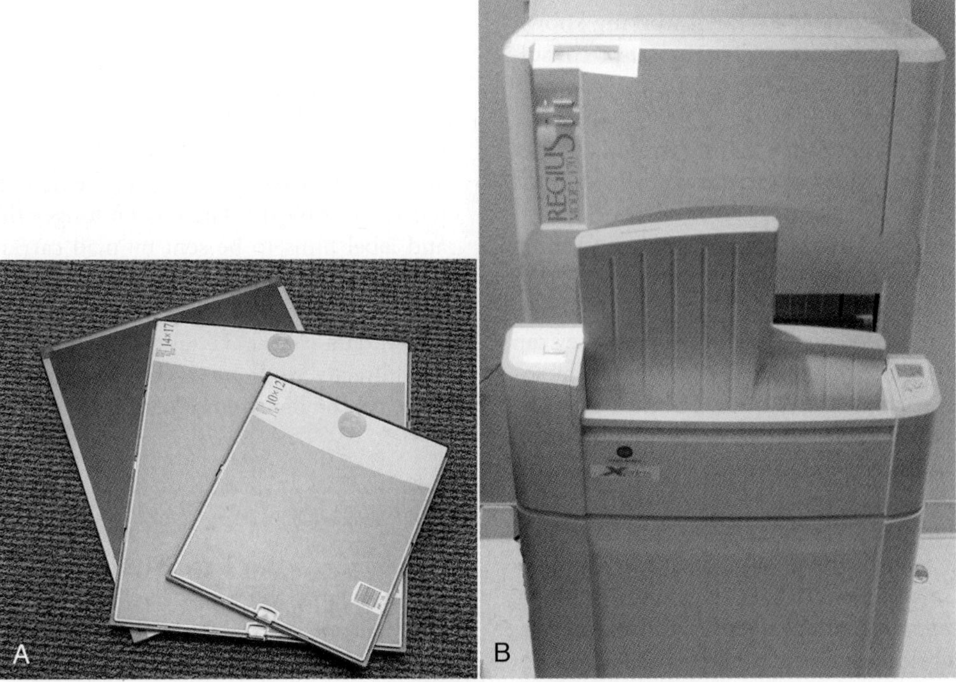

FIGURE 19-21 Computed radiology. **A**, Special cassettes containing a photostimulable phosphor instead of film to capture the latent x-ray image. **B**, The computed radiology reader that takes the specialized cassette and downloads the latent image into a computer.

DICOM service classes specify types of communications, such as store, print, send, and retrieve.

When images are performed from any modality, DICOM standard arranges them in images, studies, and series. Each patient has a number of images that are part of a study. Each study may consist of one or more series of images. A series can be a single image or several images. The imaging software reads the tags of each image so that it recognizes which images belong to which series and study. Therefore, when a patient's record is pulled up with the hospital's software, the images are organized automatically into groups according to date, modality, study, and series. DICOM functions also allow generation of a work list and print functions. A work list can communicate with the HIS (hospital information system) or RIS (radiology information system) so that the images become part of that patient's digital hospital record. DICOM print allows digital images to be printed out onto a medium. This is often done on film produced from a dry laser printer.

PACS

PACS are "picture archival computing systems" and are used to move images around to several computer work stations within a single hospital or between hospitals and as a method of storing imaging data permanently. They use DICOM standard. Benefits of the PACS are: eliminate need to generate and store film hard copies, improved communication between other veterinarians for information dissemination, tracking down lost films is no longer an issue and multiple users can view the images at the same time. With any computer system, however, there are inherent disadvantages. When computer systems go down, become blocked, or lose connectivity, decreased productivity may occur and data can also become lost (like a film radiograph). Furthermore, users need to have good and preferably excellent working knowledge of computer systems or have a department or consultant of the hospital that can troubleshoot and maintain the PACS at all times.

A PACS consists of various imaging modalities, a server for archiving images, and viewing stations connected to the LAN (local area network). Each imaging modality is "told" where to send the DICOM image information by introducing an IP address, AE title (application entry), and port number of the recipient of the images. In turn, the archive server has the same information of the modality so they can communicate. The AE title will be assigned by the technologist and is a name, such as "Ultrasound Room One." The port is the electronic route that the information will travel and the IP address is the computer's individual address, like a street address.

Three components of the PACS that the technologist may work with are the server, workstation, and monitor. The server receives the images and catalogs them into a database. The imaging software searches this database using either the patient name, identification number, date, modality, doctor's name, etc. The workstation consists of a computer with imaging software to display the DICOM information as an image (radiographic, ultrasound, CT, MRI, etc.). The workstation allows the images to be sent (exported) and received, manipulated (contrast, brightness, magnification, etc.), measurements to be made (length, width, circumference, angle, etc.), viewed on dual monitors, printed, and copied onto a CD-Rom with a DICOM viewer imbedded. Monitors are critical to image quality. There exist numerous combinations of monitor size, resolution, luminosity, graphics card quality, type (liquid crystal vs. cathode ray tube), and cost. A high quality graphics card is necessary for viewing cine-loops such as with ultrasound studies. Ultrasound, CT, MRI, and NM (nuclear medicine) images are of inherently low resolution and do not require high resolution monitors to view them adequately. Digital radiographic images, however, do require high resolution monitors. Minimally, monitors should have 1024 × 768 at 32 bit resolution for all digital imaging viewing.

RIS

RIS systems are "radiology information systems" and are computer software programs that allow all the patient data to be available and coupled to the digital imaging data. The advantage of the RIS is that when patient identification information or results of a test is entered by any individual in the hospital it is "coordinated" with all the other hospital's forms and records. For instance, when the patient's identification and details are entered into the digital file, that information will be automatically transferred to radiology forms, for example. There is no need for redundant entering of patient ID's by each secretary, technologist, or doctor. These systems are fairly new and are just now being integrated into the veterinary marketplace. For more information on computerized medical records, please read Chapter 4, Computer Applications in Veterinary Practice.

Teleradiology

Teleradiology allows the transmission of digital data across telephone, cable, and ISDN lines from private practices to referral centers around the world. Specialists can receive images almost instantly, interpret them, and send back a written report quickly. There is no longer the need to package and label films to be sent by mail carriers, which also delays the response time. This has improved patient care and continuing education for the practitioner dramatically. Any digital data (MRI, CT, ultrasound, digital, and CR) can be sent directly, and analog data (regular radiographs and lab data) can be digitized or scanned into a computer and sent as well.

EXPOSURE FACTORS

The veterinary technician is responsible for selecting an x-ray technique that will provide a diagnostic radiograph. The factors that must be selected are time of exposure, milliamperage, and kilovoltage. As previously mentioned, most recent x-ray machines have a common dial for time of exposure and milliamperage, called the mAs setting. The selection of each factor is based on an accurate technique chart. Preparation of a technique chart is discussed later in this chapter.

Other factors that enter into the production of a diagnostic radiograph are focal-film distance, type of intensifying screen, type of x-ray film, and tabletop versus grid technique. All of these variables are discussed in greater detail.

MILLIAMPERAGE

The milliamperage setting controls the quantity of electrons boiled off the filament in the x-ray tube. It is a quantity factor because it controls the amount of x-rays that will be produced at the target area. Most diagnostic units used in small animal radiology are operated at settings from 50 to 300 mA. The smallest portable x-ray unit commonly used in large animal practices may use current flow as low as 10 or 20 mA, whereas the larger units used in small animal hospitals and veterinary teaching hospitals may have a current flow of 2000 mA.

Adjustments of the milliamperage setting control on an x-ray machine will control the amount of x-rays produced. When one increases the milliamperage setting, radiographic density, or film blackness, increases; conversely, when one decreases the milliamperage setting, a reduction in radiographic density, or a lighter film, results.

EXPOSURE TIME

The exposure time is the time in fractions of a second during which the anode is positively charged. The longer the exposure time, the greater is the number of electrons that flow from the cathode to the anode and the greater is the number of x-ray photons. Because both exposure time and milliamperage affect the number of photons created and because you want the shortest exposure time possible to decrease patient motion blur, you should always use the highest milliamperage setting and the lowest time setting to arrive at the desired mAs. By using the highest milliamperage setting, you are maximizing the number of electrons in the focusing cup so you only have to charge the anode for a short period (exposure time) to get the number of electrons needed to the anode to create the desired number of x-ray photons.

> *TECHNICIAN NOTE* Always use the highest milliamperage setting and the lowest time setting to arrive at a particular mAs. This will decrease motion blur on the radiograph.

As an example to illustrate this concept, an exposure made at 100 mA and $\frac{1}{10}$ second should produce a film of equivalent density to an exposure made at 200 mA and $\frac{1}{20}$ second. In both cases the mAs factor (milliamperage X time) is the same and is equal to 10 mAs. Shorter exposure times reduce the problem of motion, which may result in loss of detail. For this reason, a thoracic radiograph on a dog or cat should be taken at $\frac{1}{20}$ to $\frac{1}{60}$ second to prevent blurring of the radiograph as a result of respiratory motion.

KILOVOLTAGE

Kilovoltage is a quality factor that regulates the energy of the x-ray beam. This setting regulates the voltage differential applied between the anode and cathode in the x-ray tube. The higher the voltage, the faster the electrons are accelerated and the greater is the energy of the x-ray beam. The greater the energy, the greater is the amount of patient tissue that can be penetrated. Increasing the kilovoltage will also increase radiographic density, or film blackness, because of increased x-ray photons passing through the patient. The kilovoltage setting most often used in diagnostic radiology varies from 40,000 to 150,000 V (40 to 150 kV).

The kilovoltage setting affects the scale of contrast on a radiograph. The scale of contrast refers to the number of shades of gray that can be seen. In general, the higher the kVp, the greater is the scale of contrast, and the quality of the x-ray film is improved because small differences in soft tissue density are more visible. Higher kilovoltage, lower mAs settings are used for soft tissue examination, such as thoracic examinations with low inherent contrast. Lower kilovoltage, higher mAs settings are used for bone structures with high inherent contrast.

The kVp setting must be high enough to penetrate the patient. If the radiograph is too light from exposure problems and mAs is increased with no increase in film density or blackness, there may be insufficient x-ray photon energy (too low a kVp) to penetrate the patient.

> *TECHNICIAN NOTE* You can increase radiographic density or film blackness by either increasing the energy level of the x-ray photons (kVp) or the total number of x-ray photons (mAs).

FOCAL-FILM DISTANCE

The focal-film distance refers to the distance between the target in the x-ray tube and the surface of the x-ray cassette. This factor is normally kept constant from one exposure to another. It is usually kept at a distance of 70 to 85 cm for large animal radiology and 90 to 105 cm for small animal radiology.

It is important to keep the focal-film distance constant from one exposure to the next because it has a significant influence on exposure factors. An increase in distance decreases the number of x-rays reaching the film. This is not a linear relationship. If you double the focal-film distance, the number of x-rays reaching the film will be reduced by a factor of four. This is often referred to as the inverse square law, which states that the intensity of the x-ray beam at a given point is inversely proportional to the square of the distance from the x-ray source.

> *TECHNICIAN NOTE* If you double the film distance from the x-ray source, you will decrease the x-ray beam intensity to one fourth of the original strength. Small changes in focal-film distance can result in big changes in radiographic density.

It is sometimes necessary to change the focal-film distance to obtain proper positioning. The following simple calculation will help you choose the new mAs setting when the distance is changed:

$$\frac{\text{Old mAs} \times \text{New distance F2}}{\text{Old distance F2}} = \text{New mAs setting}$$

For example, if an x-ray taken at 10 mAs at 100 cm must be taken at 50 cm, by using the formula given, the new mAs setting can be calculated as follows:

$$\frac{10 \text{ mAs} \times 50 \text{ F2}}{100 \text{ F2}} = 2.5 \text{ mAs}$$

This new mAs setting should produce an x-ray of similar radiographic density to the original setting of 10 mAs.

TECHNIQUE CHART

A technique chart is an essential component for obtaining diagnostic x-ray examinations in a consistent way. A technique chart must be formulated for each x-ray machine because there are differences in output with each machine (even those made by the same manufacturer). Therefore you should never use an x-ray chart formulated for another x-ray machine without making appropriate changes. If you select exposure factors from a good technique chart, consistent radiographic examinations of diagnostic quality will be obtained. In addition, there will be a savings on x-ray film because waste from repeated exposures will be avoided.

Several types of technique charts can be formulated. Each type must be formulated with the goal of using the maximum potential of a particular x-ray machine. Perhaps the most popular type of technique chart used by veterinarians is a variable kilovoltage chart. A variable mAs chart is probably more appropriate for the most powerful x-ray machines. However, a combination of variable kilovoltage and mAs technique charts is best. Such charts take into consideration the need to adapt a technique chart for different body systems, such as a thoracic and abdominal study, and examinations involving the musculoskeletal system.

This chapter cannot discuss appropriately every type of technique chart. The principle of how to prepare a variable kilovoltage technique chart, along with an example of such a chart (Table 19-1), is given. For a more extensive discussion of how to prepare different technique charts with examples of each, please refer to the discussions of this topic by Han and Hurd (2005), Lavin (2005), Morgan (1993), and Ticer (1984).

TABLE 19-1 Variable kV Technique Chart for an X-Ray Machine of 300 mA, 125 kV, 1/120-Second Timer with FFD of 40 inches

Thickness (cm)	kV	mA	Seconds	mAs	Grid a:1
4	48	300	1/120	2.5	No
5	50	300	1/120	2.5	No
6	52	300	1/120	2.5	No
7	54	300	1/120	2.5	No
8	56	300	1/120	2.5	No
9	58	300	1/120	2.5	No
10	63	300	1/60	5	Yes
11	65	300	1/60	5	Yes
12	67	300	1/60	5	Yes
13	69	300	1/60	5	Yes
14	71	300	1/60	5	Yes
15	73	300	1/60	5	Yes
16	75	300	1/60	5	Yes
17	77	300	1/60	5	Yes
18	79	300	1/60	5	Yes
19	81	300	1/60	5	Yes
20	84	300	1/60	5	Yes
21	87	300	1/60	5	Yes
22	90	300	1/60	5	Yes
23	93	300	1/60	5	Yes
24	96	300	1/60	5	Yes
25	99	300	1/60	5	Yes
26	102	300	1/60	5	Yes
27	105	300	1/60	5	Yes
28	99	300	1/30	10	Yes
29	102	300	1/30	10	Yes
30	105	300	1/30	10	Yes

FFD, Focal-film distance; *kV*, kilovolts; *mA*, milliamperes; *mAs*, milliamperes per second.
Radiographs were taken with Kodak Lanex Regular screens and Kodak TML x-ray film.

Formulation of a Technique Chart

A technique chart is formulated by a series of trial-and-error exposures. It is necessary, however, to standardize as many variable factors as possible before starting trial exposures. Factors such as the type of cassette and intensifying screen, type of x-ray film, and the focal-film distance must be constant, and a grid should be used if available. The darkroom procedures must be standardized to include fresh solution and developing time recommended by the manufacturer based on the temperature of the solution. All of these factors should be constant because the technique chart will be valid only under the conditions of formulation. If, for example, cassettes and intensifying screens in a veterinary practice are of different age or speed, the film density for a given technique will be different from one study to the next, even though the same factors are used.

To begin making our variable kVp chart for the abdomen we must begin with an initial technique. For trial exposure, a normal dog with a lateral abdominal measurement (measuring over the liver) of approximately 15 cm should be selected. A trial exposure at a setting of 80 kVp at 7.5 mAs is suggested. Two exposures are made at this setting. In selecting the mAs setting, the shortest possible time of exposure for a given mAs setting is selected. The two films are then developed according to standard technique and are examined for proper "diagnostic" density. If the films are either overexposed or underexposed, a second series of exposures is made. Use the 15% rule for kVp. If the radiograph is too dark then decrease the kVp by 15%. If the radiograph is too light then increase the kVp by 15%. Once you are close to a properly exposed radiograph using the 15% rule keep increasing and decreasing the kVp in 5% increments until your exposure is just right. All films should be examined and compared with each other for consistent density between exposures. Once the best film is selected you can begin formulating the technique chart. Start with the factors that produced the "diagnostic" film. Then, subtract 2 kVp dor each cm decrease from the original measurement. Then add 2 kVp to the original kVp for each cm increase from the original measurement up to 80 kVp. Add 3 kVp for each cm increase when the kVp is above 80 until you get to 100 kVp. Add 4 kVp for each cm increase when the kVp is above 100 kVp until you get to a maximum of 125 kVp.

Because there is an increase in scatter radiation with an increase in thickness of a part to be x-rayed, it is recommended that a grid be used for thicknesses greater than 10 cm. If you are creating a technique chart for extremities or areas under 10 cm a grid will not figure into your technique formula.

Table 19-1 shows a variable kilovoltage technique chart formulated for an x-ray machine of 300 mA, 125 kV, and $\frac{1}{120}$ second minimum time of exposure. Remember, however, that this is only an illustration of how to formulate a technique chart and should not be used with any one x-ray machine without adaptation to that particular machine.

> *TECHNICIAN NOTE* Technique charts are developed for a specific focal-film distance, film, cassette screen, and development process. If you change any one of these factors within your practice, the technique chart will need to be updated.

IMAGE FORMATION

When an x-ray beam penetrates a body system and reaches an x-ray film, a latent image is produced that will be revealed when the film is processed chemically. Several factors are involved in the formation of a high-quality latent image. This section discusses the factors that enter into the formation of an x-ray image.

X-RAY CASSETTE

Cassettes (film holders) used in veterinary medicine are of two types. The nonscreen type is a direct-exposure cassette in which the film is placed in a cardboard cassette or a plastic film holder (Figure 19-22). This nonrigid system must be light-proof and is used when great detail is needed for an examination. The disadvantage of this type of cassette is that it will require an exposure time in excess of 26 times the normal exposure time of a regular par screen cassette system. Nonscreen exposures should be used only when the animal is under general anesthetic or heavy sedation to stop motion and when no personnel are required for restraint in the radiology room. Nonscreen exposures are used primarily for intraoral occlusal studies of the nasal cavity and dental arches.

The second type is the more conventional image intensifying screen, which is placed in a rigid cassette (Figure 19-23). It is important that the hinges of the cassette be of the highest quality to ensure excellent and uniform contact between the x-ray film and the intensifying screen and to prevent light leakage that could fog or darken the film. Various materials are used in the manufacture of x-ray cassettes. Most cassettes have a solid front made of either plastic or light metal. Recently, carbon fiber (mostly graphite) has also been used. Such cassettes are excellent and may reduce the amount of x-rays needed to make an exposure by as much as 20%. The cassette back may be made of steel and can sustain moderate patient weight without being damaged. Sometimes a small area of about 7 × 3 cm is shielded from the primary beam for the purpose of film identification (see Figure 19-4).

Cassettes are expensive and should be handled with care. When dropped, they may warp, or if the cover is forced, the hinges may be damaged, resulting in a cassette that does not close properly. If the film contact is not perfect along the surface of the cassette, distortion of the x-ray image will occur.

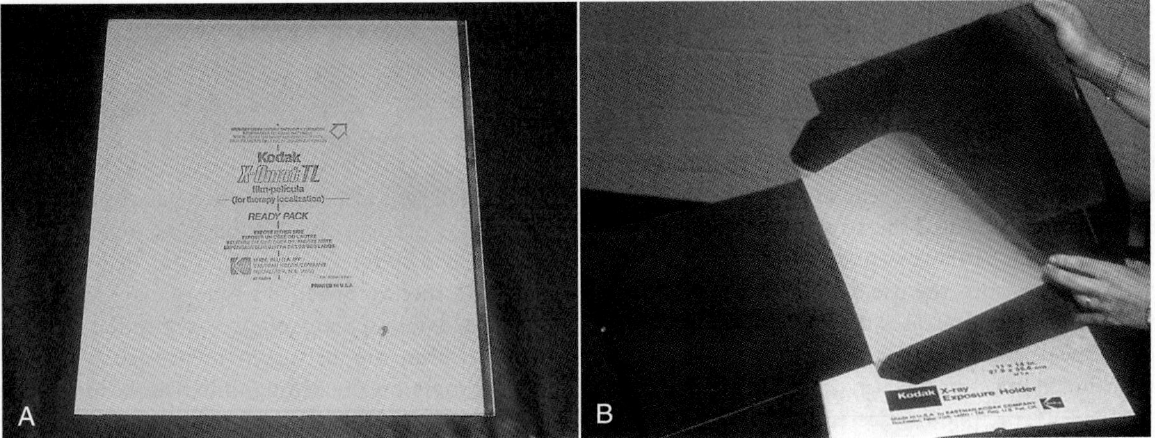

FIGURE 19-22 Nonscreen film. **A,** Ready pack film with a special emulsion for direct exposure. **B,** X-ray exposure holder for regular screen film. Such a soft cassette necessitates exposure time in excess of 26 times the normal exposure time of a regular par screen cassette system. (From Eastman Kodak Co.: The fundamentals of radiography, ed 12, Rochester, NY, 1980, Eastman Kodak Co., Radiographic Markets Division.)

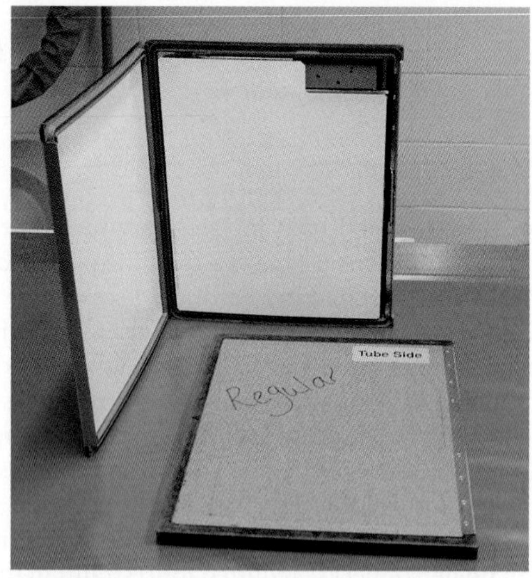

FIGURE 19-23 Open and closed rigid film cassette with image intensifying screens.

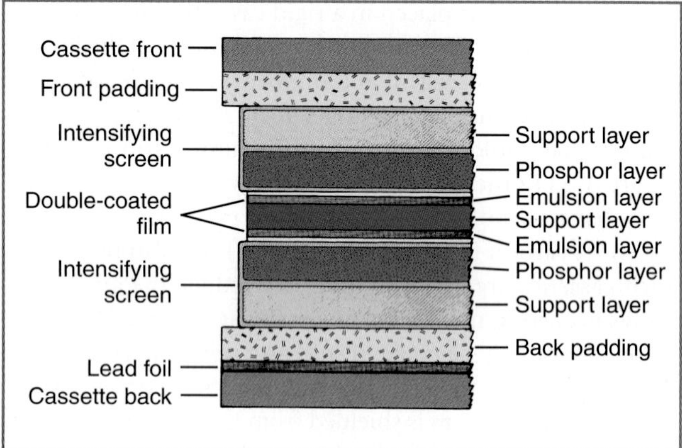

FIGURE 19-24 Cross section of a cassette intensifying screen system.

The surface of the cassette should be kept clean at all times to prevent the creation of film artifacts.

INTENSIFYING SCREENS

Intensifying screens are the smooth shiny white inner surfaces of the film cassette. They are made of layers of tiny crystals bonded together on a plastic support and covered with a protective coating. These crystals fluoresce, or emit light, after exposure to x-rays. The screens are placed in the inner surfaces of the cassette, and the x-ray film is sandwiched between. Because film is more sensitive to light exposure than to radiation exposure, the use of fluorescent intensifying screens dramatically decreases the amount of radiation needed to produce a film of diagnostic radiographic density. Screens allow much lower mAs settings, which decrease loss of detail as a result of motion, decrease patient radiation exposure, and help to prolong the life of the x-ray tube. In addition, intensifying screens increase radiographic contrast and therefore improve radiographic detail.

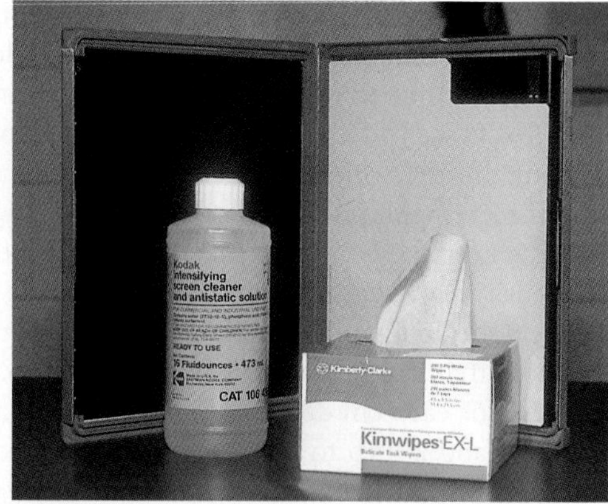

FIGURE 19-25 Open film cassette with a single intensifying screen (shiny white surface), used for detail extremity radiography. Screens should be handled carefully and cleaned regularly with approved solutions.

Intensifying screens are mounted in pairs in an x-ray cassette (Figure 19-24). They are made of the following four components:

1. A backing of cardboard or plastic, most commonly a Mylar material
2. Reflecting layers, such as titanium dioxide, that reflect light from the active layer back toward the x-ray film
3. An active layer of light-emitting phosphor, such as calcium tungstate or rare earth material, that produces the fluorescence that exposes the film after absorption of x-rays
4. A plastic coating that reduces static electricity and provides a protective covering that can be cleaned

The screens must be cleaned on a regular basis—at least monthly or whenever screen artifacts are noted on a radiograph. It is best to use a cleaning product recommended by the manufacturer for this purpose. If such a product is not available, a 70% alcohol solution will work (Figure 19-25). The surface of the screen must be thoroughly dry before an x-ray film is inserted or the cassette is closed; otherwise, the film will stick to the screens and permanently ruin them. Any stain on the surface of the screen will interfere with transmission of light from the screen to the film and cause an artifact. The technician must be careful not to spill or splash darkroom chemicals onto the surface of the screens, or they may be ruined. For this reason, emphasis is placed on the maintenance and cleanliness of screens.

SCREEN SPEED

The speed of a screen pertains to its ability to convert absorbed x-ray energy into visible light. Screen speed is a relative term that refers to the amount of radiation required by that screen to produce a film of diagnostic radiographic density. A fast screen requires less radiation than a regular, medium, or par screen to produce the same degree of blackness on the radiograph. The faster the screen, the poorer is the radiographic detail or resolution. Fast screens have a thicker phosphor layer and larger crystals to increase x-ray absorption and light production. Slower or detail screens have smaller crystals and are less efficient at light conversion but produce a radiograph of greater detail and resolution. Detail screens are also called fine screens and generally require four times the amount of radiation as a medium or par screen. These are best for obtaining radiographs of birds and small exotic animals. Regular screens are intermediate in speed between par or medium and fast screens.

The original phosphor used in intensifying screens was calcium tungstate. This phosphor produces light in the blue spectrum and is commonly found in veterinary hospitals that have acquired used cassettes and screens from local human hospitals. Improved rare earth phosphors introduced in 1975 emit light in the green spectrum and are able to produce the same degree of radiographic detail as calcium tungstate screens with less radiation exposure. Table 19-2 shows the relative speed of various calcium tungstate and rare earth screens. Rare earth screens are more efficient because they absorb more x-ray photons per crystal and produce more light per absorbed photon. These properties of rare earth screens have definite advantages in veterinary medicine and include the following:

- Reduced exposure time
- Reduced motion artifacts
- Decreased tube voltage, resulting in improved contrast
- Decreased tube current, which prolongs the life of the tube
- Reduced production of heat in the x-ray tube
- Reduced patient radiation dose

TABLE 19-2 Relative Speed of Calcium Tungstate* and Rare Earth† Screens

Screen Type	ASA Film Speed
Fine-detail calcium tungstate	30
Par calcium tungstate	100
Fine-detail rare earth	150
Regular calcium tungstate	200
Fast calcium tungstate	250
Medium rare earth	300
Regular rare earth	400
Fast rare earth	600

*Kodak X-O MAT with X-O MAT RP film.
†Kodak Lanex with T MAT L film.

TECHNICIAN NOTE Rare earth screens are advantageous for veterinary radiography because they require fewer x-rays to produce a diagnostic radiograph. Lower exposures mean lower radiation doses to the patient and technician, fewer retakes because of patient motion, and longer x-ray tube life.

The main disadvantage of rare earth screens at this time is their cost, which is much greater than that of regular calcium tungstate screens. They have a definite place in large animal radiology because of their speed. This is an important factor when they are used with the smaller, low-capacity portable x-ray units. Table 19-3 presents an example of a technique chart that can be used with a small, portable x-ray unit in combination with the rare earth screen.

There is a misconception in veterinary medicine that intensifying screens last forever. This is not true. Screens have a predictable lifetime and gradually wear out with repeated use. Most rare earth screens are worn out after 10 to 12 years of regular use. The radiograph produced with an old screen will have a white speckled pattern, most notable in the black areas on the film. This artifact is called screen craze. Most screens have a company name and screen number printed on the edge. By calling the manufacturer, the technician can find out the age of the screen and the best type of film to use with that particular screen.

X-RAY FILM

Because the recording medium for most x-ray examinations is photographic film, some basic principles of photography must be understood.

An x-ray film is prepared from a suspension of light and x-ray-sensitive granules embedded in a gelatin emulsion coated over a polyester base. The sensitive granules are

TABLE 19-3 Technique Chart for Portable X-Ray Unit of 10 mA at 90-kV, 15 mA at 80-kV, and 20 mA at 70-kV Capacity Kodak Cassette When Rare Earth Screen of Regular Speed* Is Used

Examination	Size	View	kVp	Time (sec)	Distance (cm)
Fetlock	Foal	DP or obliques	80	0.02	60
	Large adult		80	0.04	70
Carpus	Foal	DP or obliques	80	0.02	70
	Large adult		80	0.04	70
Tarsus	Foal	Lat	80	0.02	70
		DP	80	0.04	70
	Adult	Lat	80	0.04	70
		DP	80	0.08	70
Stifle	Adult	Lat	80	0.1	70
		CdCa	90	0.25	70

DP, Dorsoplantar or dorsopalmar; *kV*, kilovolts; *mA*, milliamperes; *kVp*, kilovolt peak; *Lat*, lateral; *CdCa*, caudocranial.
*For a more complete treatment of cassette and image-intensifying screens, refer to Douglas et al (1987) and Morgan (1993). Both have excellent discussions of all types of screens available on the market today.

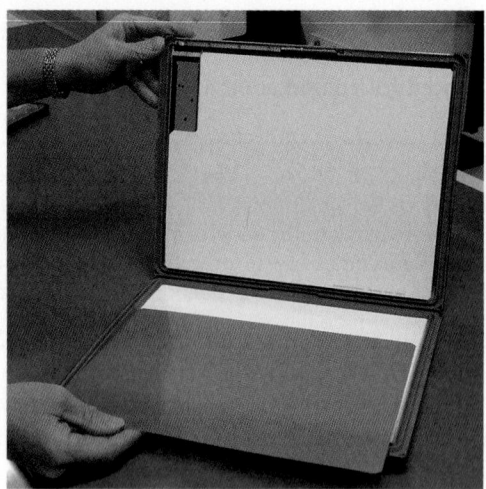

FIGURE 19-26 Screen film manufactured for the special purpose of being used with image-intensifying screens. Such film, when used with the proper combination of screen, will drastically reduce x-ray exposure time.

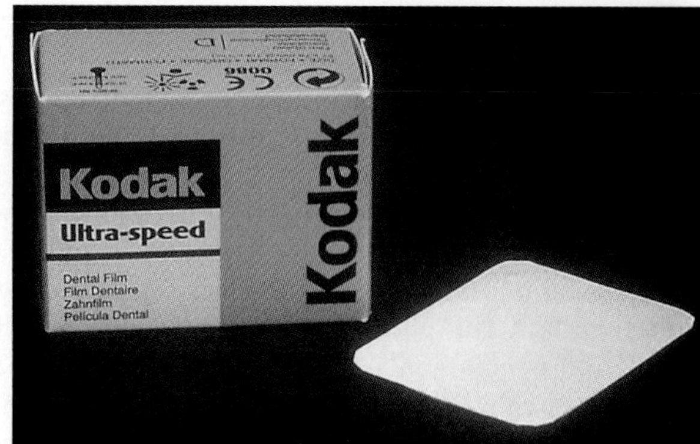

FIGURE 19-27 Prepackaged nonscreen film that can be used for dental and occlusal intraoral radiographic examinations. This type of film requires long exposure times because of the lack of intensifying screens. Patients should be under general anesthetic, and the technician should make the exposure from outside the room or behind a radiation safety barrier.

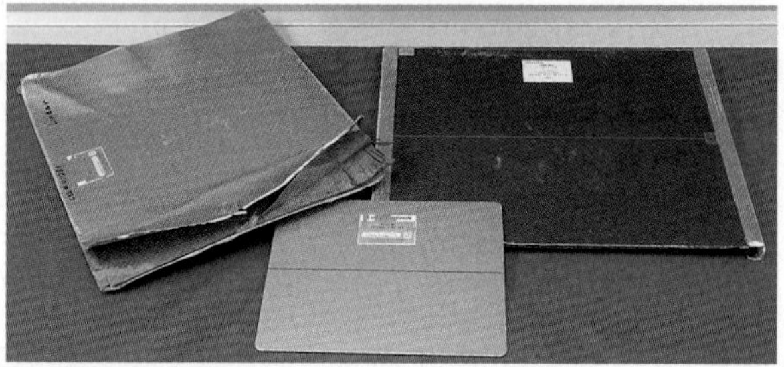

FIGURE 19-28 Three grids commonly used in veterinary radiology of large and small animals. The upper left grid has been damaged and opened, allowing you to see the hundreds of thin layers of metallic strips used to stop scatter radiation.

usually silver bromide crystals of different sizes. The gelatin matrix is protected by a thin covering called the T coat. Just like the image-intensifying screens, the sensitive crystals come in various sizes. Images of exceptional detail can be recorded on films containing fine crystals. In faster films, the crystals are larger, which results in a loss of detail, which is compensated for, however, by possible shorter time of exposure. Because of the shorter time of exposure, faster films may sometimes provide better image detail because the images contain fewer motion artifacts.

X-ray film can be separated into two categories: screen film (Figure 19-26) and nonscreen film. Screen film is sensitive primarily to the wavelengths of light emitted from intensifying screens. Nonscreen films are designed for direct exposure to x-rays and are relatively insensitive to visible light from screens. Nonscreen films provide superb detail and are especially good for intraoral examination of the nasal cavity, dental studies, and bony extremities. Because this type of x-ray film is exposed by x-rays only, it has the disadvantage of needing long exposure times to obtain necessary film density (Figure 19-27). Patients should be under general anesthetic and no personnel should be in the room during nonscreen film exposures.

Screen type of films are less sensitive to direct ionizing radiation, but are sensitive to visible light. This type of film requires less exposure to produce a radiograph because of its sensitivity to the fluorescence emitted by the intensifying screens. Remember that screens produce a specific color or spectrum of light. The film used should be matched in sensitivity to the light spectrum of the screen.

Rare earth screens do need special x-ray films to produce an optimal radiograph. Every x-ray film manufacturer produces a rare earth type of x-ray film. There is great confusion because of the endless names and types of combinations of x-ray film and image-intensifying screens available on the market. Again, please refer to (Douglas et al, 1987) and (Morgan, 1993) for a more elaborate discussion of this important topic.

TECHNICIAN NOTE Be sure the x-ray film you are using is maximally sensitive to the spectrum of light your screens are emitting.

GRIDS

When x-rays enter a patient, some pass straight through to the film cassette, but a great many are scattered or redirected along a different path before exiting the patient. The purpose of a grid is to control the scatter radiation before it reaches the x-ray cassette. A grid is constructed of a sheet of lead strips interfaced with radiolucent spacers made of plastic or aluminum. These strips are encased in an aluminum protective cover for durability. Grids come in various sizes, similar to x-ray cassettes, and are placed directly over the cassette between the animal and the cassette, or more commonly, in a special tray just under the x-ray table above the cassette tray (Figure 19-28).

The purpose of a grid is to allow only the primary x-ray beam to pass through and prevent scatter radiation from reaching the film. The grid is constructed in such a way as to absorb all radiation that does not pass between the lead strips. This arrangement may absorb most scatter radiation if grids of high ratios are used. However, it has the disadvantage of absorbing part of the primary x-ray beam and therefore requires greater exposure time to obtain a given film

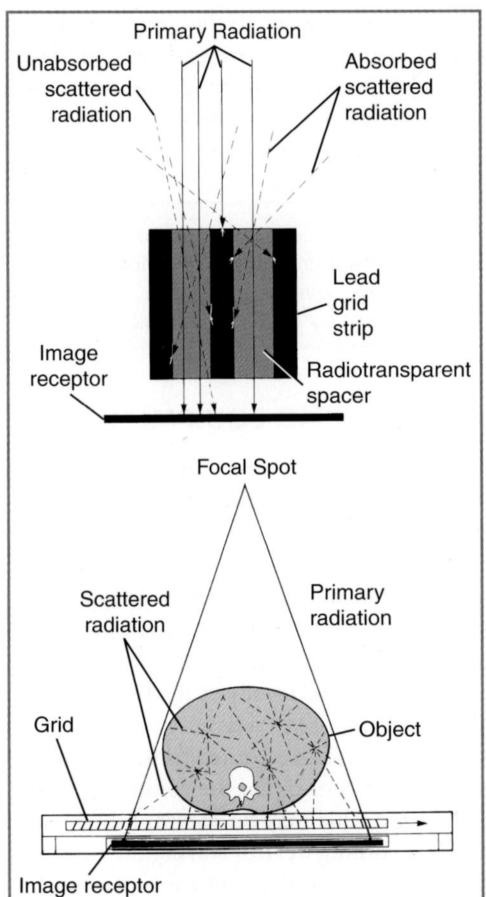

FIGURE 19-29 Cross section of a grid. **A,** Diagram of a small section of a grid showing how a large proportion of the scatter radiation is absorbed and image-forming primary radiation passes through to the image detector. **B,** Diagram of focused Potter-Bucky diaphragm being moved toward the right. (Modified from Eastman Kodak Co.: The fundamentals of radiography, ed 12, Rochester, NY, 1980, Eastman Kodak Co., Radiographic Markets Division.)

density. Figure 19-29 shows how a grid absorbs scatter and secondary radiation and prevents it from reaching the film.

Grids are made of different ratios and number of strips per 2.5 cm. The ratio varies from 5:1 to 16:1 and from 60 lines (strips) per 2.5 cm to 120 lines per 2.5 cm. The higher the ratio and the number of lines per 2.5 cm, the more radiation is absorbed by the grid. The ratio of a grid refers to the relation between the height of the lead strips and the width of the radiolucent spaces. For example, if the height of the lead strip is 12 times greater than the thickness of the space, the grid ratio will be 12:1, and if it is 10 times greater, the ratio will be 10:1. The greater the ratio, the more efficiently the grid absorbs scattered radiation. Figure 19-29, *A*, shows the ratio of a 5:1 grid. For veterinary work, a grid with a ratio of 8:1 at 103 lines per 2.5 cm is recommended.

The grid is most useful when x-raying parts of the body in which scattering is considerable, which in practice includes all thick parts of the body (e.g., thorax, abdomen, skull) and those joints and bones in excess of 10 cm thickness. The grid lines are visible on the resulting film, but this is made up for by the increased resolution of the image on the radiograph.

Grids may be parallel or focused. A parallel grid is one constructed with strips parallel to each other. A focused grid is one in which the lead strips and spacers are gradually angulated from the center to the periphery of the grid. The distance from the point of convergence, or focal point, is referred to as its focal distance, or radius. The advantage of a focused grid is that it allows unobstructed amounts of radiation to pass through it at the center and at the edge of the grid as long as the radiation is parallel to the axis of the lead strips. Such grids can be used only at a specific focal-film distance specified by the manufacturer. If distances above or below the focal-film distance are used, grid cutoff will occur, which means that part of the primary beam will be absorbed by the grid. With grid cutoff, large areas that are incompletely exposed will be found on the resulting radiograph.

Potter-Bucky Diaphragm

One other type of grid encountered in veterinary hospitals is the Potter-Bucky diaphragm. This is simply a movable grid. The movement of the diaphragm is timed to suit a particular exposure, and the grid moves across the film during the exposure so that the grid lines are not shown on the resulting film. When a movable grid is used, the exposure time must be increased by a factor of four, or the kilovoltage must be increased by about 20%. Usually, Potter-Bucky diaphragms are positioned under the table and electronically linked to the timer of the x-ray machine (Figure 19-29, *B*).

Another method of reducing scatter radiation is the air gap technique. It is a simple technique that consists of increasing the distance between the patient and the surface of the cassette. With this technique, the amount of scatter radiations produced is not reduced, but less scatter radiations reach the film because of the increased distance between patient and film. With the air gap technique, it is not necessary to increase the exposure factors, as must be done with a grid. However, this technique will decrease the sharpness of the image because of increased subject-to-film distance. It is also less effective at high kilovoltage settings because the higher-energy scatter occurs in a forward direction. This technique is used most commonly in veterinary radiology for magnification purposes.

> *TECHNICIAN NOTE* Always use a grid between the patient and the film cassette when the body part being x-rayed is greater than 10 cm thick.

THE DARKROOM

The importance of the darkroom in radiography cannot be overemphasized. Radiography unquestionably begins and ends in the darkroom, in which films are loaded into cassettes ready for exposure and returned for processing into a finished radiograph. Most mistakes made in veterinary radiography are related to the processing of radiographs. It is necessary to keep the darkroom clean and light proof. It is also essential for the technician to have a thorough knowledge of x-ray darkroom technique and of conventional or automatic processing. The chemicals should be changed, replenished, maintained, and mixed according to the strict directions of the manufacturer.

EQUIPMENT

A darkroom need not be spacious. For most veterinary practices, a small room of about 240 × 240 cm is adequate. However, it is essential that this room be made totally dark. If there is a window in the room, there is no reason not to open it for ventilation when the darkroom is not in use; however, the window should be light proof when closed. One can easily determine whether a darkroom is light proof by turning off all lights, including the safelight, closing the door tightly, and slowly turning around in the center of the darkroom, looking for any light leaking into the room. It is also important that a lock or light-proof cylindrical entrance be placed on the door to prevent its being opened while films are being processed. A darkroom need not be completely dark because a safelight can be used during film processing. A safelight is a light bulb shielded by a plastic filter that stops any light to which the film is sensitive from penetrating the filter and entering the room. It is important, however, that the safelight bulb not exceed the wattage recommended for the type of filter used; otherwise, the exposed films will be "fogged," or partially exposed, and the quality of the radiographs will be compromised. The proper type of light filter must be used in the darkroom. Orange, red, or yellow filters may be used with most x-ray films; but with the rare earth type of x-ray film, a special red filter must be used (Figure 19-30). No films should be exposed to the safelight any longer than necessary. It is important to work rapidly but carefully when processing x-ray films and loading and unloading films in the cassettes.

There should be a worktable in the darkroom for loading and unloading cassettes, located as far away from the processing tanks as possible so that liquid or dry chemicals will not be spilled on it. Above or below the bench, there should be shelves to store film hangers and unexposed films and cassettes. X-ray film must be kept in a cool, dry place protected from extraneous x-rays.

> *TECHNICIAN NOTE* Remember that all film and safelights are not created equal. Make sure the wavelength or color of light to which your film is sensitive is completely blocked by your safelight filter.

HAND PROCESSING EQUIPMENT

The processing equipment should include a developing tank, rinsing tank, and fixer tank. The tanks should be big enough to accommodate several 35-cm ∞ 42.5-cm films at the same time. Running water in the rinsing tank is ideal. If it is not available, the water should be changed frequently. Development and fixer solutions should be changed every 90 days, regardless of use, and more frequently if radiograph volume is high. The tanks should ideally be made of stainless steel for ease of cleaning (Figure 19-31).

In certain areas of the United States, it will be necessary to heat up or cool down the solutions during certain times of the year. This may be accomplished with an electric heater or a cooling device. During the heat of the summer, it may be necessary to add ice to the washing water to keep the solutions at the proper temperature. An inexpensive way to keep the solution temperature constant in processing tanks is by installing a good-quality shower-bath mixer valve. This type of valve is sufficient and economical enough to maintain the solution at a constant temperature in a low-volume practice. It is also important to have separate stirring rods made of stainless steel, plastic, or rubber and to mix the solutions thoroughly every day before starting the processing of films. Good ventilation is necessary to keep the room dry and prevent accumulation of volatile chemicals.

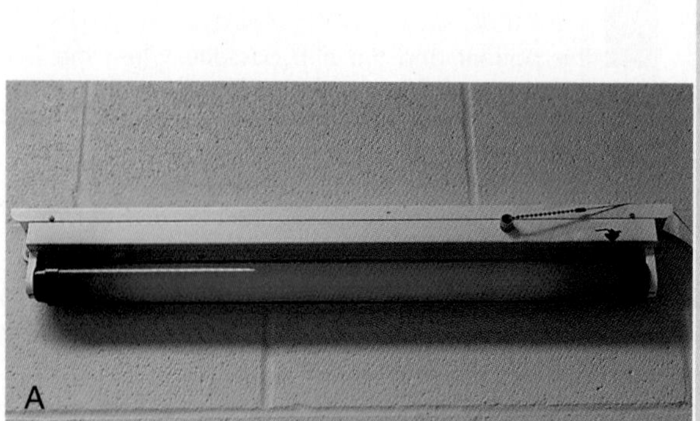

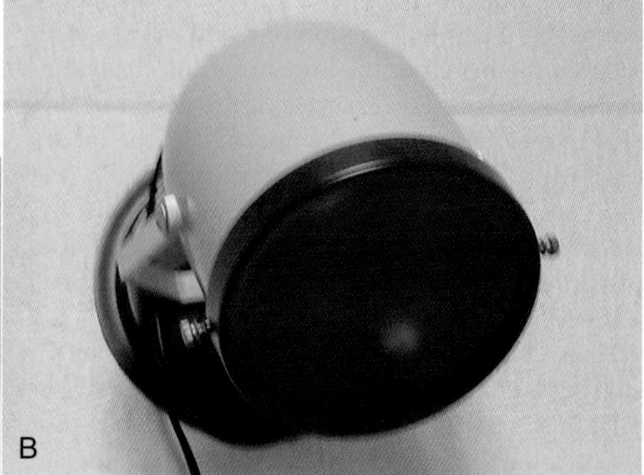

FIGURE 19-30 A and B, Two examples of darkroom safelights. The filters must be matched to the light sensitivity of the film being used in the darkroom and must not be cracked or incompletely sealed by the filter holder.

AUTOMATIC FILM PROCESSORS

There are several makes and sizes of automatic processors on the market. In recent years, many veterinary hospitals have invested in automatic processing systems. There are small-capacity, 90-second processor units that can be installed in most darkrooms without remodeling. The larger processor units necessitate some remodeling because the input tray must be in the darkroom and the output side must be out of the darkroom. This usually requires some structural and plumbing modifications (Figure 19-32).

As with manual processing tanks, it is necessary to maintain fresh solution and ensure that the solutions are flowing properly within the processor. Automatic processors may speed up and standardize film processing but require similar, if not more, maintenance compared with manual processing tanks. It is important to provide ventilation in the darkroom when automatic processors are used. Usually, a good-quality, light-tight exhaust fan installed in the ceiling is adequate.

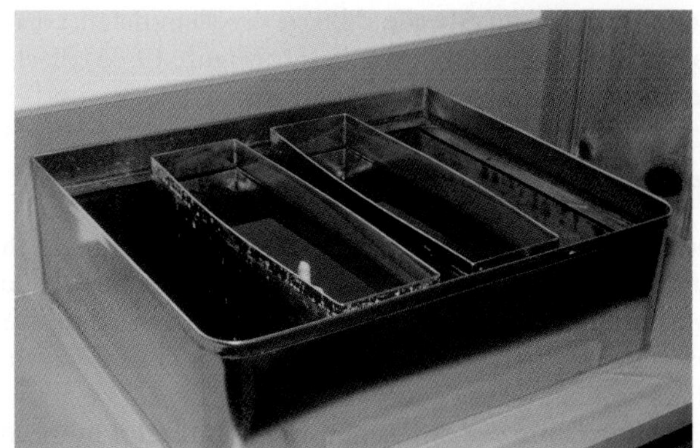

FIGURE 19-31 Processing tanks holding the developer *(left)*, two central fresh water tanks to wash the films *(middle)*, and fixer *(right)*.

FILM STORAGE

X-ray films must be handled and stored properly for maximum usefulness. The film must be protected from light, x-radiation, gamma radiation, heat, moisture, and pressure. All these hazards may result in film fogging and decreased radiograph quality. As previously mentioned, the darkroom can fulfill this function if the room is kept clean and free of moisture. It may be helpful if the x-ray films are kept in their original boxes and placed in a cabinet. Special bins to store x-ray films can be purchased, but they are an unnecessary expense if proper care is used in storage (Figure 19-33).

CASSETTE LOADING AND UNLOADING

Care must be taken when transferring x-ray film from its box to the x-ray cassette to prevent static electricity, bending, creasing, or scratching. The film should be handled carefully, held only by the corners, and pulled from the box in a continuous and slow motion manner (Figure 19-34). The film should be carefully placed in the cassette, and the edges should not extend over the edge of the film cassette. Great care should also be taken in removing x-ray film from the cassette to prevent damage or soiling of the intensifying screen.

HANGING X-RAY FILM

When exposed films are placed on a film hanger or automatic processor tray, they must be handled carefully. X-ray film is more sensitive after exposure and before development than at any other time. The films should be handled only by the corners and attached to the stationary bottom clip first and then to the flexible top clip. It is most important to have dry hands when handling exposed, nonprocessed films. Any developer or fixer solution touching the film will create an artifact on the processed film.

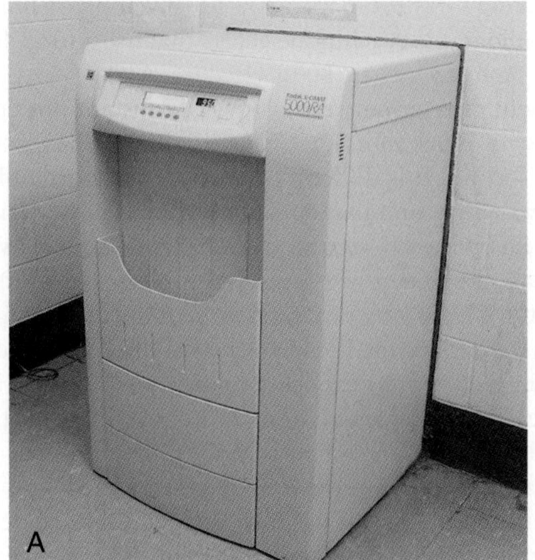

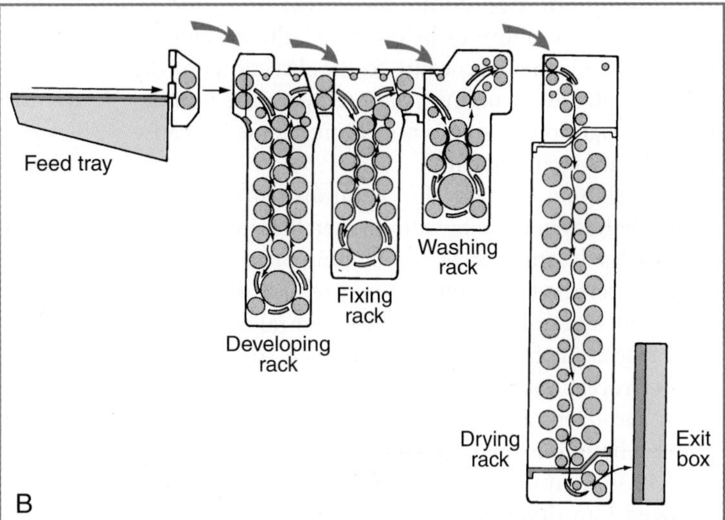

FIGURE 19-32 Automatic processor. **A**, Kodak X-OMAT processor (a 90-second processor). **B**, Diagram of a typical automatic x-ray processor.

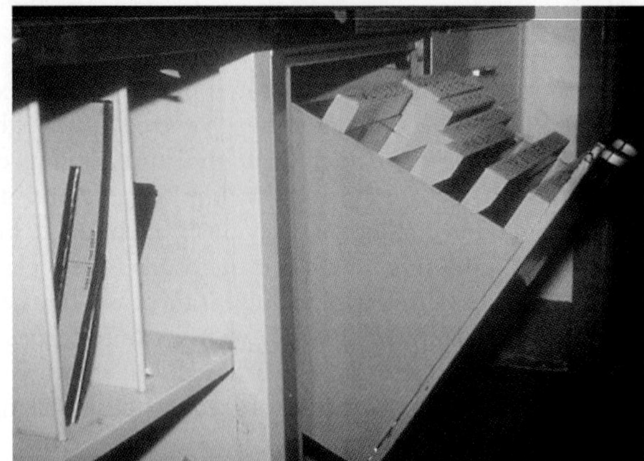

FIGURE 19-33 Film storage bin commonly used in darkrooms; it is designed to store open x-ray box films to load x-ray cassettes. This bin is wired to a switch that will automatically turn off the darkroom lights when opened.

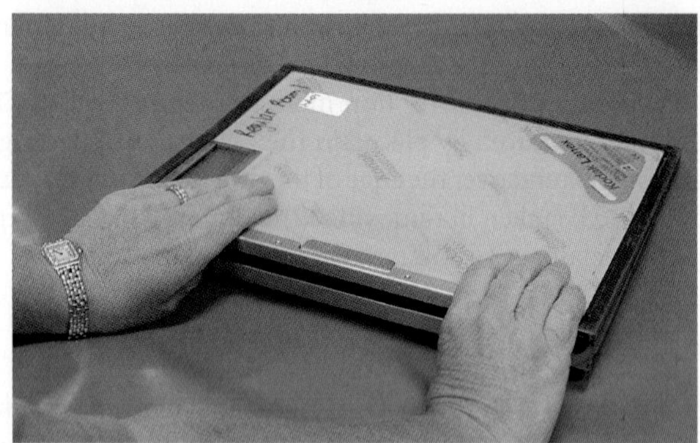

FIGURE 19-34 When loading a cassette, use both hands to prevent kink marks, and carefully place the film into the cassette. The cassette must be closed and latched gently.

DEVELOPING X-RAY FILM

As previously mentioned, processing solutions (developer and fixer) should be stirred before the film is inserted. When the film is placed in the developer, it should be agitated up and down a few times to remove air bubbles from its surface. The film should be developed for 5 minutes at 20° C (68° F). If the temperature is above or below 20° C, the developing time should be adjusted according to the directions of the manufacturer. Rapid (3-minute), high-temperature film development or sight processing is not recommended because of decreased radiograph quality.

In the developing solution, the chemicals reduce the exposed silver halides in the x-ray film to metallic silver, which is black. Gradually, through the developing process, the latent image is revealed. The film is then removed from the developer tank and quickly rinsed in the central water bath. It is then placed in the fixer solution, which stops the development process and preserves the film. The film should remain in the fixer for approximately twice the development time. The film is then placed in the central rinse tank for about 15 to 20 minutes. Films can be dried in a special air-circulated film dryer box or allowed to hang until dry in a well-ventilated, dust-free area. For a more complete discussion of the chemistry of x-ray processing, please refer to the Eastman Kodak publication The Fundamentals of Radiography (1980).

SILVER RECOVERY

In larger veterinary practices, the silver contained within the x-ray film emulsion may be removed and recovered. Most of the silver that is not exposed to x-rays is not converted to metallic silver and accumulates within the fixer solution. Silver recovery units can be attached to the fixer solution to remove the silver by an electrolytic process. This, however, is only economical for the larger-volume veterinary hospital. The silver can also be recovered from exposed and nonexposed x-ray film. A few companies specialize in recycling x-ray film for silver recovery. This could be the source of a small bonus at the time an x-ray file is purged from the old cases on file.

RADIOGRAPHIC FILM QUALITY

It is of utmost importance to produce radiographs of excellent quality to arrive at a radiographic diagnosis. A film of good diagnostic quality should have excellent detail, correct scale of contrast, and optimal density (Figure 19-35). Each of these film characteristics is briefly discussed.

DETAIL

Radiographic detail refers to the degree of sharpness that defines the edge of an anatomic structure. It is the best possible reproduction of an organ. Detail is influenced by every possible factor, but some factors are more influential than others.

The focal-film distance is one important factor in the loss of detail. If the focal spot is too close to the part x-rayed, there will be magnification and lack of distinction at the margins of the structures. Therefore it is important to keep the focal-film distance as long as possible without significantly reducing x-ray beam intensity. Most veterinary hospitals have radiographic technique charts that use a focal-film distance of 36 to 48 inches (80 to 110 cm).

Movement in veterinary radiology is a constant problem, especially with older units that have a minimum exposure time of $\frac{1}{10}$ second. It is difficult to produce diagnostic films of the thorax with a unit that does not have a minimum time of exposure of at least $\frac{1}{30}$ second and ideally $\frac{1}{120}$ second. With large animals, movement is a constant problem with a small, portable unit. This is why rare earth screens are becoming so popular in veterinary medicine; they have the advantage of requiring a much shorter exposure time.

The size of the focal spot is another important factor that regulates detail. The larger the focal spot, the poorer is the detail. Because most equipment in veterinary medicine has a rather large focal spot of 0.8 mm or more, loss of detail may be significant, especially with older units that have focal spots of 1.2 to 2 mm. Therefore it is important to place

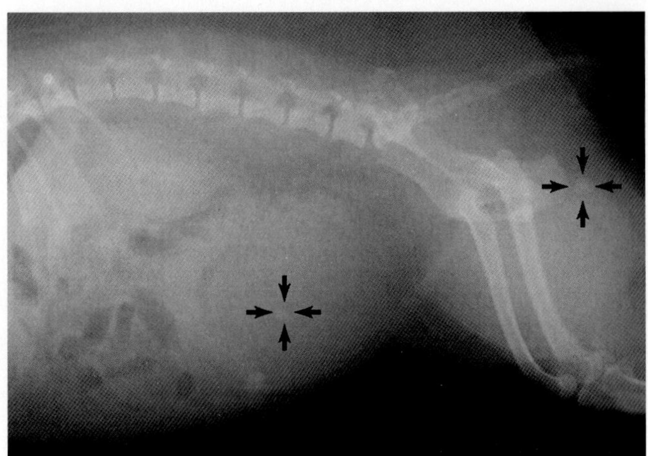

FIGURE 19-35 Lateral radiograph showing good radiographic detail and contrast. There are round, mineral opaque structures (uroliths) within the urinary bladder *(arrows)*. The urinary bladder is large due to obstruction by another stone within the urethra *(open arrow)*.

the part to be x-rayed as close as possible to the x-ray film. If the part is too far from the film, there will be magnification and distortion, resulting in a loss of detail. This is especially important in large animal radiology.

Other exposure factors that affect detail are poor film-screen contact and overexposed or underexposed radiographs that often result from an improper technique chart or carelessness. Poor radiographic processing causes more ruined radiographs than all other factors combined. All processing errors affect detail. It is therefore important to standardize the developing process by following exactly the instructions of the manufacturer.

RADIOGRAPHIC CONTRAST

Radiographic contrast refers to the density or opacity difference between two areas on a radiograph. High contrast means the opacity differences are large and there are fewer shades of gray. High-contrast radiographs are very black and white. Latitude refers to the range of different opacities on the radiograph. Long-latitude radiographs have a much larger number of shades of gray, but the difference or contrast between each shade is small. High-contrast radiographs are preferred for spine and extremity films. Long-latitude, low-contrast radiographs are preferred for thoracic films.

Kilovoltage is the exposure factor that has the greatest influence on radiographic contrast. The higher the kilovoltage, the greater the latitude and therefore the greater the number of shades of black, gray, and white. The absorption of the x-ray beam at high kilovoltage is more uniform among the various tissues in the body, resulting in less contrast. Therefore for thoracic examinations, a high-kilovoltage technique is recommended. For skeletal studies, a lower-kilovoltage technique is recommended.

Other factors reducing contrast are scatter radiation (which can be greatly improved by the use of a grid), light leakage, and rapid, high-temperature processing techniques.

RADIOGRAPHIC DENSITY

Radiographic density refers to the degree of blackness of the film. It is the result of the amount of light that was transmitted to the x-ray film after interaction of the crystals in the intensifying screens with the x-ray beam. When a film is properly exposed, the anatomic part x-rayed will have good contrast with good differential absorption of the x-ray beam by the various tissue densities. Therefore the part should be clearly seen but should not be so dark as to overexpose the anatomic structures to the degree that they are difficult to differentiate from the background film density. The thickness and density of the anatomic part x-rayed do affect density. The thickest part will absorb more radiation, sometimes as much as denser tissues of lesser thickness.

The primary factor affecting density is the mAs setting. As discussed previously, the mAs factor is a quantity factor that regulates the amount of x-rays produced. If more x-rays reach the film, more light will be emitted by the screens, and the film will be darker. Therefore it can be stated that high mAs settings will increase film density and low mAs settings will reduce film density.

Another factor that affects film density is the kilovoltage setting. At a higher kilovoltage, the x-ray tube is more efficient in producing x-rays and therefore increases the energy level of x-rays produced. If all other exposure and development factors are kept constant, increasing the kilovoltage will increase the radiographic density. This effect is more apparent at lower-kilovoltage settings for a given part than at higher-kilovoltage settings.

The distance from the focal spot to the surface of the film is another important factor in film density. If everything remains constant but the distance, a given examination could be substantially overexposed if the distance is reduced, or it could be underexposed if the distance is increased. This effect can be dramatic because the intensity of the radiation is reduced or increased as the square of the distance is changed. This effect is discussed in the section regarding inverse square law. It does emphasize the need for consistency and accurate measurement of the focal-film distance.

MAGNIFICATION

Magnification is a technique rarely used in veterinary practices, but it is popular in veterinary teaching hospitals. Magnification is based on the principle that a larger image of an anatomic structure can be obtained if the distance between the object and the film is increased. Generally, the object to be magnified is placed halfway between the film cassette and the focal spot of the x-ray tube. This results in an x-ray image twice as large as the actual anatomic structure. However, to obtain diagnostic films, it is necessary to have a small focal spot. A focal spot of 0.3 mm or smaller is needed for radiographic magnification. If larger focal spots are used, the advantage of direct magnification is lost because of the blurring at the margin of an organ produced by the larger focal spot. This technique would be useful to veterinarians, especially for studies of extremities in small dogs and cats and for studies of the skull.

TECHNICAL ERRORS AND ARTIFACTS

Several errors can be made in handling x-ray films or in setting up a technique for an examination. In general, these errors will reduce the quality of the radiograph and in certain cases may nullify its diagnostic value. Boxes 19-1, 19-2, and 19-3 are intended to help the technician identify the cause of errors and take corrective measures. Box 19-1 deals with technical errors other than those occurring as a result of film processing. Boxes 19-2 and 19-3 deal with errors caused by poor film processing.

The advent of automatic processing equipment has helped tremendously in eliminating many errors made in hand tank processing techniques. It has standardized film processing and made it easier to trace the cause of processing mistakes, which are usually mechanically related. Even with automatic processors, many mistakes can be made and must be recognized and corrected to obtain the best possible radiographs.

Several other mechanical failures may occur with automatic processors. It is important to keep the processor clean at all times. It is especially important to wash the roller assembly thoroughly at least once each week. Processors are sophisticated machines that must be serviced regularly by professionals. It is unreasonable and cost ineffective for a veterinarian to expect the technician to service the processor. However, it is the responsibility of the technician to be able to recognize processor problems and correct them when possible. It is also the technician's responsibility to keep the processor clean at all times and to ensure that fresh developer and fixer solutions are provided as needed.

RADIATION SAFETY

Since 1970 there has been a tremendous growth in the use of x-ray equipment by veterinarians. There are few diagnoses in medicine or surgery that cannot be aided by the use of diagnostic radiology. It therefore behooves technicians to be aware of the hazard of using x-rays or any other type of ionizing radiation.

It is the responsibility of the veterinarian to ensure that proper radiation safety measures are observed in the hospital. It is also the veterinarian's responsibility to instruct the technician in the proper use of the equipment and to ensure that the design of the x-ray room meets state regulations.

All animal tissues are sensitive to radiation; that is, absorption of radiation doses above a certain minimum roentgen value will change or alter the tissue. The following tissues (not in order of sensitivity) are most readily affected by ionizing radiation: skin, lymphatics, hemopoietic and leukopoietic (blood-forming) tissues, breast, thyroid, bone (especially the epiphysis or growing centers), and the germinal epithelium or gonads. These tissues are sensitive to all forms of ionizing radiation. All animal species are affected, including humans, even though there are different degrees of sensitivity among species. The more rapidly dividing tissues are affected most by radiation.

BOX 19-1 Technical Errors

Increased Film Density
Too high mAs or kV settings
Too short focal-film distance
Wrong measurement of anatomic part
Equipment malfunction
Speed of intensifying screen too fast

Decreased Film Density
Too low mAs or kV settings
Too long focal-film distance
Wrong measurement of anatomic part
Speed of intensifying screen too slow

Black Marks or Artifacts
Film scratches
Crescent mark from rough handling
Static electricity (linear dots or tree pattern)
Top of film black, resulting from exposure to light while still in box
Defective cassette that does not close properly, exposing margins of film to light

White Marks (Artifacts)
Dirt or debris between the film and screen
Defect or crack in screen
Contrast medium on tabletop, skin, or cassette

Gray Film
Film accidentally exposed to radiation (scatter, secondary, or direct)
Lack of grid for examination of a thick part
Outdated film
Film stored in too hot or too humid place

Distorted or Blurred Radiograph
Motion: patient, cassette, or machine
Too great focal-film distance, causing magnification and distortion
Poor film-screen contact
Poor centering of primary x-ray beam

Linear Artifacts
Gridlines
Grid out of focal range
Primary beam not centered
Grid upside down
Grid damage, causing distorted gridlines

Miscellaneous Artifacts
Cone cut, causing underexposed margins
Target damage, resulting in inconsistent film density: requires tube replacement
Double exposure
Blank film: faulty equipment, nonexposed film processed

kV, Kilovolts; *mAs*, milliamperes times seconds.

Technicians should remember that one of the best means of protection at their disposal is the ability to avoid retakes. Careful attention to patient positioning, thickness measurements, setting techniques, and film processing will decrease the need for radiograph retakes and reduce technician and patient radiation exposure. See Chapter 6 for additional radiation safety information.

BOX 19-2 Film Processing Mistakes in Wet Tanks

Increased Film Density
Film overdeveloped
Temperature of solution too high
Wrong concentration of developer
Defective thermometer

Decreased Film Density
Film underdeveloped
Temperature of solution too low
Exhausted developer
Contamination of developer
Developer too diluted or improperly mixed
Failure to add replenisher solution as needed
Defective thermometer

Fogged Films
Light leakage in darkroom from defective safelight, door, windows; light leakage around processor pipes; or turning lights on in darkroom before film is cleared
Film exposed to radiation from any source: through wall if storage room adjacent to x-ray room, cassette left in x-ray room while exposure made
Overdeveloped film
Contaminated developer

Yellow Radiograph
Fixation time too short
Exhausted fixer solution

White Spots
Defective screens: pitted, scratched
Dust or grit on surface of film
Fixer on film before processing

Black Spots
Drops of developer solution on film before processing
Films stacked together in fixer

Air Bubbles
Film not agitated when placed in developer; air bubbles form on surface of film

Reticulation
Solutions have uneven temperature from bottom to top of tanks
Need to stir up solution to even up temperature in tanks
Weak fixer or lack of hardening solution

Brittle Radiographs
Drying temperature too high
Drying time too long

Miscellaneous Mistakes
Film wet: too short drying time
Grit on films: dirty tanks and solutions
Corner marks: wet or dirty fingers on hangers
Sticky film: film washed or dried improperly
Static electricity: low humidity and rough or too fast handling of films
Scratches: careless handling

RADIATION FILTRATION

The x-ray beam is a composite or spectrum of x-ray photons of various energy levels. The kVp setting is the highest energy level within the beam, but there are photons of all levels from the kVp on down. The useful portion of the x-ray beam (the portion that passes through the patient to interact with the film and screens) is the upper two thirds of the energy levels. The lower third of the x-ray beam energies is too weak to pass through the patient. This radiation is called soft radiation. It is of no use for image formation and only causes increased radiation exposure of the patient. Aluminum has a marked effect on filtration of softer (lower energy level) x-rays. Insertion of 1 or 2 mm of an aluminum filter into the path of the primary beam at the portal of the x-ray tube is essential to filter out or absorb the soft x-rays that are a component of all x-ray beams in the diagnostic range. By absorbing this soft radiation, the filter reduces the amount of radiation absorbed by the patient. Increased aluminum filtration also generally improves latitude and detail by improving the quality of the x-ray beam.

BOX 19-3 Common Technical Errors With Automatic Processors

Increased Density
Temperature of developer too high
Overreplenishment
Light leak from cover or in darkroom
Speed too slow
Faulty thermostat

Decreased Density
Temperature of developer too low
Underreplenishment
Exhausted developer, necessitating thorough cleaning of tanks every 6 months
Faulty thermostat

Processing Streaks
Crossover rollers dirty
Dirty wash water
Air tubes need cleaning

Scratches on Film
Guide shoes misaligned or dirty
Dryer air tubes mispositioned

Wet or Damp Film
Thermostat malfunction
Dryer temperatures too low
Insufficient air venting
Film not hardened sufficiently

Film Overlap
Film fed too rapidly into processor
Tension on rollers too high

RADIATION MEASUREMENT

To understand radiation safety and radiation dose units of measurement, it is necessary to define a few terms commonly used in the measurement of radiation exposure.

Roentgen

The roentgen (R) is defined as a unit of radiation exposure that will liberate a charge of 2.58×10^{-4} coulombs per kilogram of air. Roentgens are a measure of radiation exposure or x-ray machine output and are generally evaluated with an ionization chamber placed below the primary x-ray beam. As an example, 1 R is the approximate exposure to the body surface for an anteroposterior radiograph of the abdomen for an average adult human.

Rad

The unit of absorbed dose of ionizing radiation is called a rad. It is the energy imparted by ionizing radiation to a unit mass of irradiated material and is equal to 100 ergs/g of tissue. The number of rads deposited in tissue per roentgen of radiation exposure varies with the energy of the x-ray beam and with the composition of the absorber.

Rem

Rem is an abbreviation for rad equivalent man; it is the product of the dose in rads and the relative biologic effectiveness of the radiation used. This unit of measurement makes allowance for the fact that the effect of radiation on different tissue varies with the type of radiation or relative biologic effectiveness. A rem is equal to the absorbed radiation dose in rads multiplied by a quality factor:

$$\text{Rem} = \text{Rads} \times \text{Quality factor}$$

Because the quality factor for diagnostic radiation is 1, for all practical purposes in veterinary practice, 1 rem = 1 rad. For larger particles of radiation, such as neutrons, protons, and alpha particles, the quality factor increases from 3 to 20. These larger, more dangerous particles of radiation are not emitted from diagnostic x-ray machines.

The old units rad, roentgen (R), and rem have been replaced with SI units. The following is a list of conversions to the new units of gray (Gy), coulomb/kg (C/kg) and sieverts (Sv):

The rad (rad) is replaced by the gray (Gy) 1 kilorad (krad) = 10 gray (Gy) 1 rad (rad) = 10 milligray (mGy) 1 millirad (mrad) = 10 microgray (μGy) 1 microrad (μrad) = 10 nanogray (nGy)

The gray (Gy) replaces the rad (rad) 1 gray (Gy) = 100 rad (rad) 1 milligray (mGy) = 100 millirad (mrad) 1 microgray (μGy) = 100 microrad (μrad) 1 nanogray (nGy) = 100 nanorad (nrad)

The roentgen (R) is replaced by coulomb/kg (C/kg) 1 kiloroentgen (kR) ~ 258 millicoulomb/kg (mC/kg) 1 roentgen (R) ~ 258 microcoulomb/kg (μC/kg) 1 milliroentgen (mR) ~ 258 nanocoulomb/kg (nC/kg) 1 microroentgen (μR) ~ 258 picocoulomb/kg (pC/kg)

Coulomb/kg (C/kg) replaces the roentgen (R) 1 coulomb/kg (C/kg) ~ 3876 roentgen (R) 1 millicoulomb/kg (mC/kg) ~ 3876 milliroentgen (mR) 1 microcoulomb/kg (μC/kg) ~ 3876 microroentgen (μR) 1 nanocoulomb/kg (nC/kg) ~ 3876 nanoroentgen (nR)

The rem (rem) is replaced by the sievert (Sv) 1 kilorem (krem) = 10 sievert (Sv) 1 rem (rem) = 10 millisievert (mSv) 1 millirem (mrem) = 10 microsievert (μSv) 1 microrem (μrem) = 10 nanosievert (nSv)

The sievert (Sv) replaces the rem (rem) 1 sievert (Sv) = 100 rem (rem) 1 millisievert (mSv) = 100 millirem (mrem) 1 microsievert (μSv) = 100 microrem (μrem) 1 nanosievert (nSv) = 100 nanorem (nrem)

Maximum Permissible Dose

The maximum permissible dose (MPD) should be of great interest to the veterinary technician because it is the maximum dose of radiation a person is allowed to receive during occupational exposure over a certain time. This dose is 0.1 rem for an average weekly dose or 3 rem over 13 weeks, 5 rem per year, and a maximum accumulated dose of 1(N − 18) rem, where N is age in years. The N − 18 indicates that an individual should not have occupational exposure to radiation before the age of 18. The technician should remember that the MPD is the dose that the U.S. Nuclear Regulatory Commission has determined should not harm the person receiving it during her or his lifetime. The MPD is maximum occupational exposure allowed by law; technicians should try to keep radiation exposure as low as possible by carefully following radiation safety practices.

Personal Monitoring

To protect the staff from overexposure, the radiation that each person receives can be measured on a film badge. A film badge is a container that holds a special film designed to record a wide range of exposures. The film holder incorporates several different types of metal filters that permit differentiation of the type of ionizing radiation exposures. This badge should be worn outside the apron on the collar at the level of the thyroid gland (Figure 19-36). Film badges can be exposed by heat, pressure, and chemical fumes. The film badge should be taken care of and stored outside the radiology area so that the amount of radiation it detects is actually the amount to which the person is occupationally exposed.

Radiation monitoring badges come in several forms: rings, clips, and wrist badges. Several companies offer a badge service. These badges are mailed back to the company and analyzed on a monthly or quarterly basis.

Film badge readings are reported in millirem (mrem), or $^1\!/_{1000}$ rem. The annual MPD equals 5000 mrem. Technicians using x-ray machines should insist that the veterinarian for whom they work provide them with a radiation monitoring device.

PROTECTION OFFICER

Every veterinary hospital should have an employee who is in charge of radiation safety. His or her responsibilities should include maintaining badges, ensuring the x-ray machine is properly calibrated, and maintaining a good exposure control system that includes an updated technique chart system. Low-exposure techniques that provide quality diagnostic radiographs should be the ultimate goal. Safe reliable radiography equipment that is clean (and in the case of digital equipment: calibrated correctly), has software that is regularly updated, and has a server that can handle

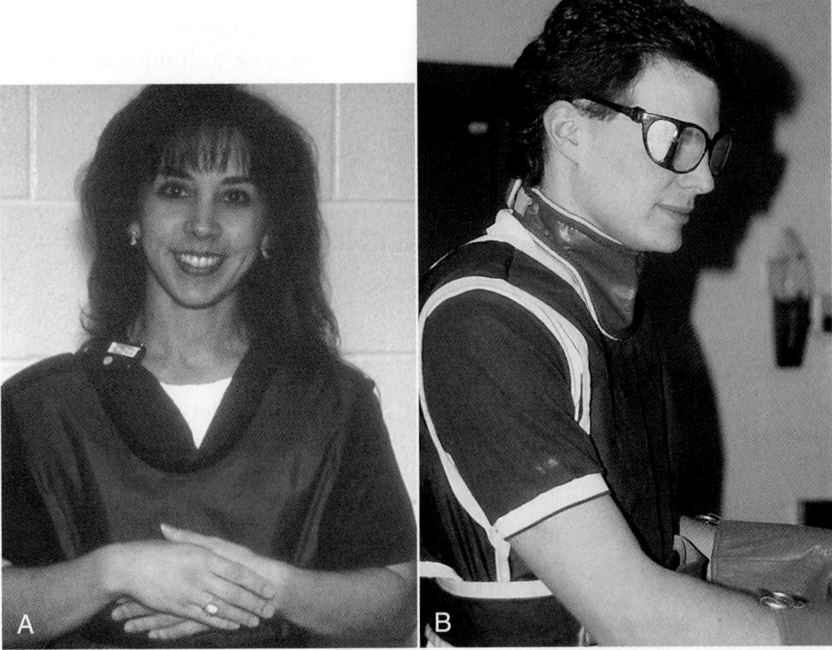

FIGURE 19-36 Each technician working in radiology should have a film badge to measure occupational radiation exposure. A, The film badge should be worn outside the lead apron at the level of the upper neck. This technician also wears a ring badge inside her lead gloves to measure the dose to the hands. B, This technician who works in a busy radiology department wears leaded glasses and a thyroid shield in addition to gloves and an apron.

the amount of data necessary to efficiently operate the veterinary practice are all imperative. A reliable shielding program *requiring* all staff to follow the ALARA (as low as reasonably achievable) principle whenever they are creating an image is equally important. The employee in charge of this essential part of the veterinary practice must also ensure that compliance with all government regulations is a priority.

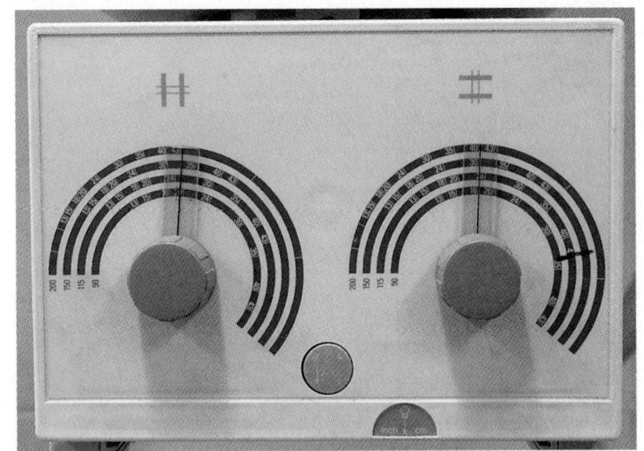

FIGURE 19-37 A collimator is used to limit the size of the x-ray beam to the part to be examined. By coning down on the area of interest, the amount of scatter and secondary radiation can be drastically reduced, improving image quality and decreasing technician exposure.

PROTECTION PRACTICES

- Always use a collimator and always use the smallest possible aperture that will cover the anatomic area of interest (Figure 19-37).
- Make sure there is an aluminum filter at the portal of the x-ray tube. This is to protect the patient, not the technician.
- Make sure the proper exposure factors are used to prevent the need for retakes.
- Make sure the animal is positioned properly the first time—again to prevent the need for retakes.
- Never permit any part of your body to be in the path of the primary x-ray beam even if it is covered by lead shielding. The protective equipment is designed to protect your body from scatter radiation. It is of no use if the body part is placed in the primary beam.
- Protection includes use of your well-maintained lead gloves, apron, thyroid shield, and lead glasses, if your practice provides them. If this basic safety equipment is not provided, you have three choices: purchase your own, ask the practice managers to make the purchase, or change jobs!
- Always wear an apron, thyroid shield, and gloves when holding an animal or if you must be in the room when an exposure is made. The apron, gloves, and thyroid shield should have 0.5-mm lead equivalent minimum to ensure good protection from secondary and scatter radiation. Lead eyewear is becoming commonplace in veterinary practice as more technicians and veterinarians become aware of the damage long-term radiation exposure can cause to the lens of their eyes (Figures 19-38 and 19-39).
- Use accessory equipment designed to reduce radiation exposure, such as cassette holders, restraining devices, and positioning devices (Figures 19-40 and 19-41).

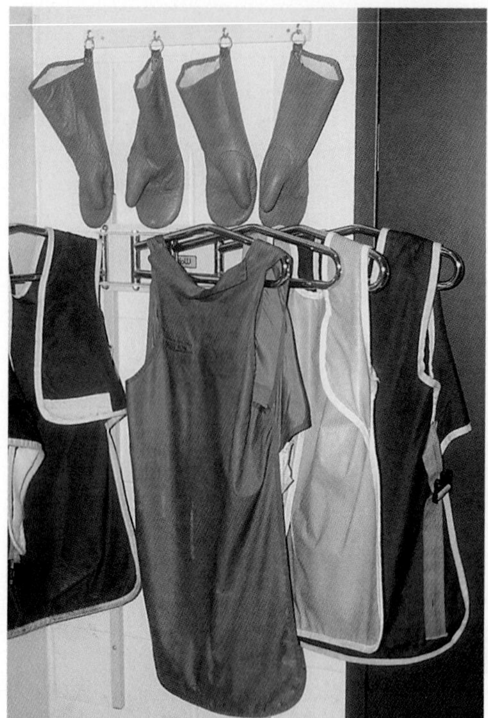

FIGURE 19-38 Aprons and gloves on a stand. It is important to keep the apron on a stand and the gloves well aerated when not in use to increase the useful life of the apron and gloves. The apron should have a minimum of 0.5 mm of lead equivalent.

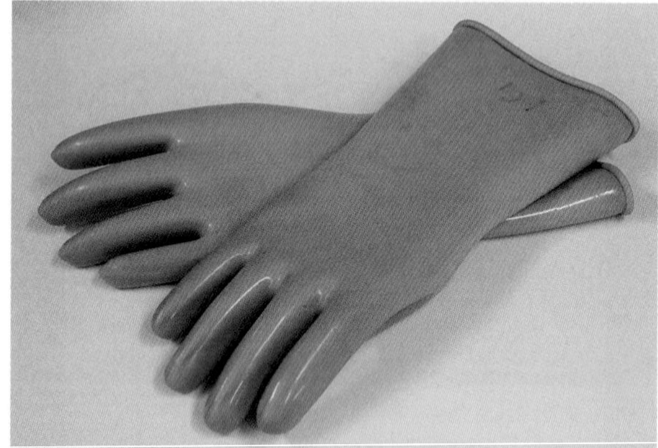

FIGURE 19-39 Lead gloves should have a minimum of 0.5 mm of lead equivalent; 1 mm of lead equivalent is ideal. They should always be worn when restraint is needed for examination.

- Anesthesia or tranquilization of the patient should be used every time an animal cannot be controlled easily and adequately for a given examination.
- Only required personnel should be in the examining room at the time of exposure. A pregnant woman should not be in the room, nor should anyone younger than 18 years.
- If you have to restrain manually, and you are therefore unable to leave the room, *always look away* and lean back as far as possible from the x-ray table when you are firing the machine.
- "Dose creep" is a term used in digital radiography to describe the incremental increases made in technique in an attempt to reduce the amount of "noise" affecting the quality of the image. Technicians should never increase technique and therefore personal and patient exposure to potentially harmful radiation in an effort to cut down on noise.
- Use good, fast screens to reduce the milliamperage settings as much as possible.

> TECHNICIAN NOTE When working in radiology, always remember the "big three" of radiation safety: time, distance, and shielding.

Radiation safety is a frame of mind. It is a habit, and it requires awareness of the danger of radiation. It is easy to become careless with radiation because it is invisible, tasteless, and odorless and produces no external stimulation at diagnostic levels. Technicians should always remember that although invisible, radiation is dangerous to one's health. X-ray effects are cumulative. The ionization that results from continued exposure to x-rays and other high-energy rays constitutes the cumulative effect. These rays can destroy all living tissue if the absorbed doses are high enough. Secondary radiation is less harmful than primary radiation, but is still extremely harmful. Therefore carelessness has no place in radiology. Remember the big three methods of radiation protection: time, distance, and shielding. Time means avoiding retakes; do it right the first time. Lower the time of exposure; keep the mAs as low as possible to still produce diagnostic radiographs. Distance means staying as far away as possible from the patient and x-ray beam. Shielding means always wearing an apron and gloves. It is important to take care of your apron and gloves. Hang them carefully after use, and do not allow the apron to be folded. Careless use causes creases and cracks to develop in the gloves and aprons and reduces their effectiveness.

RADIOGRAPHIC CONTRAST AGENTS

In radiology, contrast means density difference. In many radiographic examinations, there is insufficient natural or inherent contrast of the anatomy to make a diagnosis; this is especially true in gastrointestinal, urogenital, and spinal cord disease. The addition of positive or negative contrast medium can increase the radiographic density difference between anatomic structures and increase the likelihood of correct image interpretation. In veterinary medicine, the following four types of contrast media are used (Figure 19-42):

1. Radiolucent gases: air, nitrous oxide, carbon dioxide
2. Insoluble inert radiopaque medium: barium sulfate
3. Soluble ionic radiopaque medium: iothalamate, diatrizoate
4. Soluble nonionic radiopaque medium: iohexol, iopamidol

Radiolucent gases absorb small amounts of radiation, resulting in images of greatly reduced radiographic opacity. These agents are used primarily in double-contrast gastrograms, double-contrast cystograms, and rarely, pneumoperitoneography. Contraindications for their use are primarily

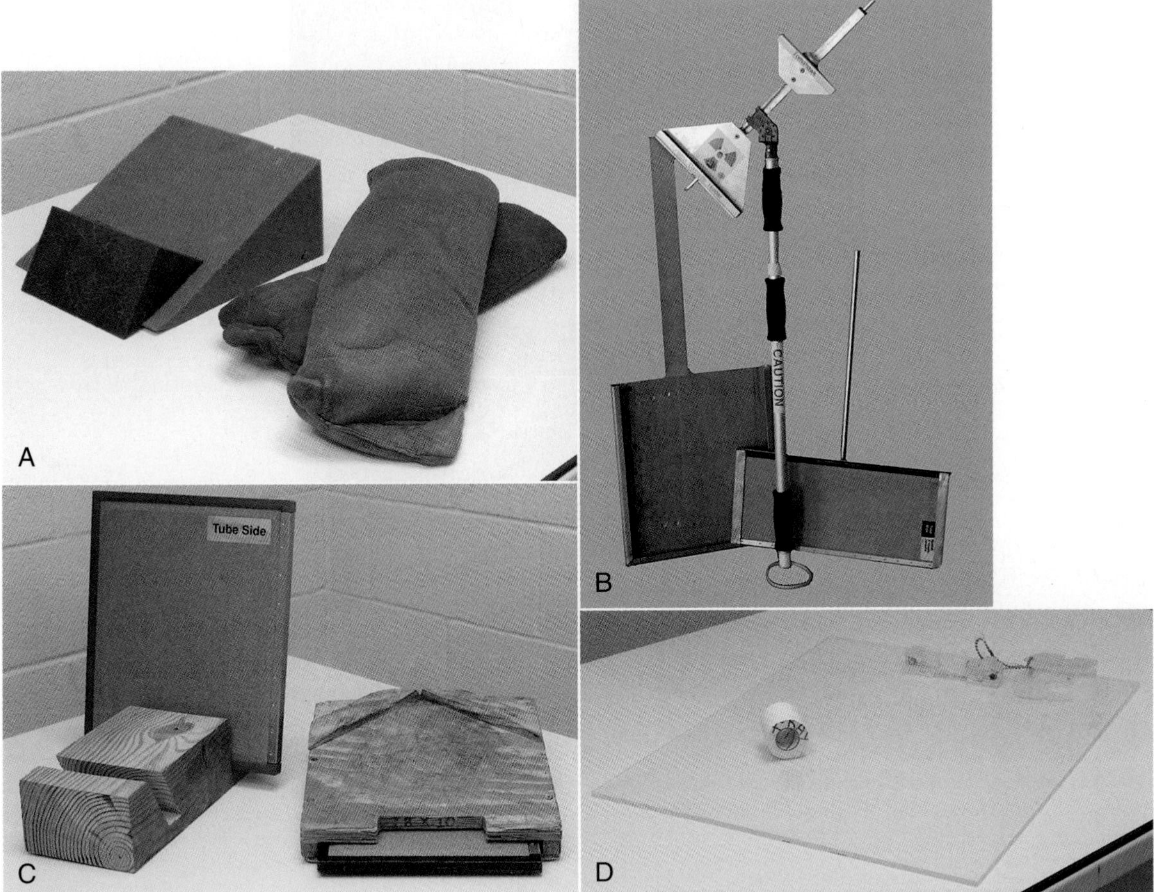

FIGURE 19-40 A number of commercially available positioning devices can be used to help position animals and reduce the time needed to perform the examination. **A,** Various foam wedges and sand bags used to position small animals. **B,** Cassette holder for large animal examinations. **C,** Wood blocks for examination of large animal feet. **D,** Lucite tray with neck restraint holder for avian radiology. Porous tape is used to position wings on anesthetized birds.

in patients with severe hemorrhagic cystitis, in which there is an increased likelihood for gas absorption into the circulation. Nitrous oxide and carbon dioxide are considered safer than room air because their increased solubility is less likely to cause serious air embolization.

Barium sulfate has a high atomic number and absorbs a large amount of radiation, resulting in greatly increased radiographic opacity. It is used almost exclusively for upper and lower gastrointestinal examinations. Barium sulfate is inert, nonabsorbed, and fairly soothing to the gastrointestinal tract. It coats the gastrointestinal mucosa better than organic iodides, improving visualization of the luminal surface. Barium sulfate is available in powder, paste, or liquid form. Micropulverized, solubilized barium sulfate solutions are vastly superior to powdered barium sulfate products because of the increased uniformity in mucosal coating. Contraindications for use include patients with severe constipation or upper or lower bowel perforations. As with all oral contrast media, care should be used in patients with known aspiration pneumonia or a high likelihood of aspiration.

Soluble radiopaque ionic contrast media include iothalamate and diatrizoate. The negatively charged iothalamate and diatrizoate are benzoic acid derivatives with three iodine molecules. They are coupled with positively charged sodium or meglumine to form a soluble salt. The high atomic number of iodine increases radiation absorption and increases radiographic opacity. These products can be used orally for gastrointestinal examinations; intravascularly for venous or arterial studies and excretory urography and in the peritoneal tract, bladder, and urethra; and intraarticularly and in draining wounds for fistulography and in salivary ducts for sialography. Ionic organic iodides should not be used in the respiratory tract or intrathecally for myelography. Because ionic iodides are essentially a hyperosmolar salt solution, they can result in an increase in intravascular fluid volume when used intravascularly followed by an osmotic diuresis. The hyperosmolarity can cause diarrhea when ionic iodides are administered orally. Because of these properties, these agents are contraindicated in dehydrated patients and patients with a known iodine sensitivity.

The newest class of positive contrast agents includes the nonionic organic iodides, represented by iohexol, iopamidol, iotolan, and, historically, metrizamide. These agents can be used like ionic organic iodides but have the advantage of not dissociating into positively and negatively charged ions in solution. This allows the agents to be used intrathecally (in the cerebrospinal fluid space around the spinal cord) for myelography and everywhere ionic iodides can be used. These contrast agents are still hyperosmolar but much less so

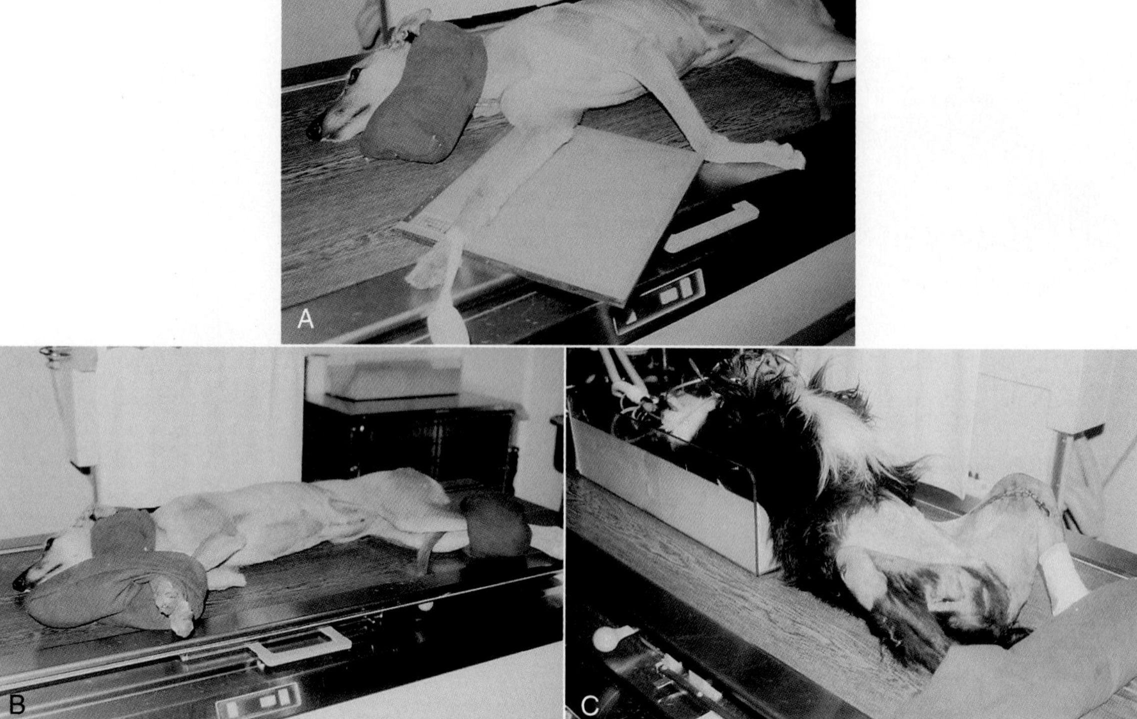

FIGURE 19-41 **A,** Sand bags and porous tape can help position tranquilized patients for some extremity radiographs. **B,** Sand bags can take the place of manual restraint for thoracic and abdominal lateral radiographs. **C,** Lucite positioning trays and sand bags can often take the place of technical restraint in postoperative radiography.

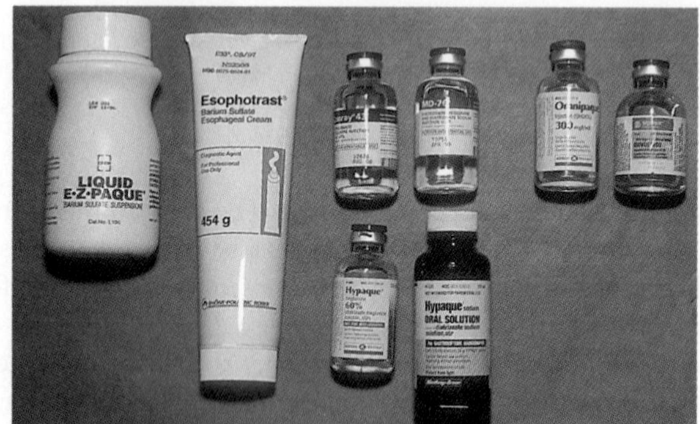

FIGURE 19-42 Positive contrast medium used in veterinary radiology. The first two containers are barium to be used orally or rectally only. The next four are ionic iodinated contrast, and the last two on the right are nonionic iodinated contrast.

than the ionic organic iodides. They appear to have a lower incidence of adverse effects and contrast reactions but have the disadvantage of increased cost.

Organic iodides (both ionic and nonionic) may cause serious contrast reactions, or adverse effects, when given intravenously, intraarterially, or intrathecally. These reactions are much less likely when the agents are used orally. Contrast reactions include nausea and vomiting, hypotension, cardiac arrest, and anaphylaxis. These reactions occur infrequently, but it is advised to have a catheter in place when these agents are used and rapid access to fluids, oxygen, endotracheal tubes, and cardiovascular arrest resuscitation drugs during organic iodide contrast procedures. Do not leave these patients unattended after contrast administration. For a thorough discussion of contrast media and contrast procedures, see Douglas et al (1987), Han and Hurd (2005), Lavin (2005), Morgan (1993), and Thrall (2007).

COMMON CONTRAST MEDIA AND APPLICATIONS

Esophagus

Contrast Agents

Barium sulfate, weight/volume (wt/vol) suspension 100%, is used alone and diluted to evaluate an enlarged esophagus or as a thick paste if the esophagus is not enlarged. Barium mixed with food may be more appropriate for diagnosis of esophageal strictures. Oral organic iodides (ionic or nonionic) are used when perforation of the esophagus is suspected.

Procedure

No special preparation is needed. Ideally, the study is done by using fluoroscopy. If this is not available, the exposure must be made when the animal swallows. The barium is administered with a syringe into the buccal pouch.

Stomach and Small Bowel (Upper Gastrointestinal Studies)

Contrast Agents

Three kinds of contrast agents are used for upper gastrointestinal studies: barium sulfate 25% to 30% wt/vol, oral iodides, and negative contrast, including air, carbon dioxide, and nitrous oxide. Barium sulfate is the most commonly used agent for upper gastrointestinal studies when perforation is not suspected. Negative contrast media are used in combination with barium sulfate for double-contrast studies. Oral iodinated products are given when perforation is suspected because barium sulfate will not be resorbed once it leaks into a body cavity.

Procedure

Food should be withheld for 24 hours, and warm water enemas should be administered about 2 to 3 hours before the gastrointestinal study. Acepromazine can be used without adverse effects on gastrointestinal motility.

Dosage

The dosage for barium sulfate is 10 ml/kg and for oral Hypaque or Gastrografin, 3 ml/kg.

Film Sequence

The survey film consists of a ventrodorsal and a lateral view. Immediately after administration of contrast medium, four films should be taken to completely evaluate the stomach: a ventrodorsal view, a dorsoventral view, and both a right and left lateral view. At 15, 30, and 60 minutes, the film sequence consists of ventrodorsal and right lateral views. These same views are taken at various intervals until contrast reaches the large bowel. The timing sequence will vary with the patient and the suspected disease process.

Large Bowel (Lower Gastrointestinal Study, Barium Enema)

Contrast Agents

Barium sulfate 10% to 15% (wt/vol) or iodinated preparations, such as Gastrografin or oral Hypaque, are used for the lower gastrointestinal studies.

Precautions

Barium sulfate should not be used when a perforation is suspected. A barium enema should not be performed for 48 hours after a biopsy specimen of the colon or rectum has been obtained.

Preparation

The patient is fasting for 24 to 48 hours and may be given a gastrointestinal cleansing agent such as Golytely (Braintree Labs). Warm water enemas must be given before the examination because it is essential that the entire large bowel be cleansed before a barium enema is performed. A Bardex (French; Bard Hospital Division, C.R. Bard) catheter and barium container are needed for the study.

Procedure

The animal should be anesthetized. The balloon-tipped catheter is inserted into the rectum, and the cuff is inflated to form a firm seal against the colonic wall. The barium or iodine is placed in the colon by gravitational flow. A 15% wt/vol barium sulfate solution is used for barium enemas. The dose is 5 to 10 ml/0.45 kg of body weight. Ideally, the study is done by using fluoroscopy. Radiographic views needed are lateral, ventrodorsal, and right and left ventrodorsal oblique views. After completion, the barium is evacuated, and air is injected to obtain a double-contrast study of the large bowel.

Urinary Tract

Contrast Agents

Several kinds of contrast studies are available for evaluation of the kidneys. However, because the intravenous pyelogram (IVP) is the one most used in practice, this discussion is limited to it.

An IVP, or excretory urogram, is performed by injecting contrast medium intravenously. Ionic organic iodide products are most commonly used. A meglumine diatrizoate and sodium diatrizoate preparation is probably the most popular contrast product used for IVP examinations. The standard dose of contrast is 800 mg of iodine per kilogram, which may be increased by 50% in patients with poor renal function.

Complications

The most common complications encountered with an IVP are vomiting, anaphylactoid reactions, and hypotension. Vomiting is a transient reaction of short duration and is not serious in nature. Care should be taken that the animal does not aspirate during the procedure. Anaphylactoid reactions are rare but must be attended to immediately. It is necessary to have epinephrine available for immediate administration whenever an IVP is done. Hypotension is rare, but when it occurs, it can be life threatening and may lead to renal failure.

Contraindications

The only serious contraindication is dehydration or iodine sensitivity.

Procedure

The animal should be fasting for 24 hours, but water should be available to prevent dehydration. Enemas should be given when needed, at least 2 to 3 hours before the IVP. Ventrodorsal and lateral films should be taken before the examinations. Films should be taken in the ventrodorsal and lateral positions immediately after injection of the contrast medium and at 5 and 15 minutes after injection. When needed, follow-up studies at 20 or 25 minutes after injection may be performed.

> TECHNICIAN NOTE The intravenous pyelogram (IVP) is the most commonly used contrast study of the kidneys.

Urinary Bladder

Contrast Agents

Ionic organic iodide contrast materials are most desirable for retrograde cystography. Nonopaque contrast materials, such as air, carbon dioxide, and nitrous oxide, are used in addition to organic iodides for double-contrast cystography. Do not use barium sulfate.

Procedure

The colon should be cleansed. Depending on the breed and size of the animal, different catheters may be used. A Foley catheter, tomcat catheter, or soft flexible male catheter may be needed. In addition, a syringe and three-way valve are needed. Two types of cystography are commonly performed in veterinary practice: positive-contrast cystography and double-contrast cystography. Positive-contrast cystography is used to detect leaks or rupture of the lower urinary tract after trauma. Ionic organic iodide contrast at concentrations of 10% to 15% is injected retrograde into the urinary bladder at 5 to 15 ml/kg of body weight. Double-contrast cystography is used to detect all other forms of urinary bladder disease. A catheter is placed into the urinary bladder, and all urine is removed. Next, 3 to 10 ml of organic iodide contrast is injected, followed by carbon dioxide or room air at 5 to 15 ml/kg of body weight. Because of the variability of urinary bladder volume, it is best to fill the bladder to palpable turgidity. Lateral and oblique ventrodorsal radiographic views are most helpful.

Urethrography

Contrast Agents

Ionic organic iodide compounds at 20% concentration are best for urethrography.

Procedure

A balloon-tipped catheter (Foley type) is placed into the distal urethra. The cuff is inflated for a snug fit to prevent contrast from leaking around the catheter. Contrast, 10 to 20 ml, is hand-injected rapidly. The x-ray is taken during injections of the last few milliliters. A lateral view and two oblique views should be taken during the separate injections of the contrast material.

Spinal Cord

Myelography is the contrast examination most frequently performed to localize and characterize spinal cord lesions. Myelograms are always performed with the animal under general anesthetic. Nonionic iodinated contrast medium is injected into the subarachnoid space (cerebrospinal fluid space) at the cisterna magna (skull-C1 space) or in the caudal lumbar spine area (L4-L6). Myelography is most commonly performed before surgical intervention.

Contrast Agents

Two nonionic contrast agents are currently in wide use in veterinary medicine: iopamidol (Isovue, Bracco Diagnostics) and iohexol (Omnipaque, Sanofi Winthrop). The dose of contrast medium ranges from 0.25 ml/kg for cervical evaluation with a cisternal injection to 0.45 ml/kg for cervical evaluation from a lumbar injection. The concentration of iodine should be between 240 and 300 mg/ml, and injection volume should not exceed 15 ml.

Contraindications

Contraindications for myelography include infection of the spinal cord and meninges. If the veterinarian chooses to treat spinal disease medically rather than surgically, myelography would be contraindicated.

Procedure

Survey films should be taken first. The site of injection should be aseptically prepared. Spinal needles of 20 to 22 gauge and 3.75 to 8.75 cm should be available because the size of the animal may vary considerably and some dogs may be so obese that even an 8.75-cm needle is short. Carefully collimated films are taken in the ventrodorsal and lateral positions immediately after administration of the contrast medium.

POSITIONING

Proper positioning is essential to obtain diagnostic radiographs. It is again the responsibility of the veterinary technician to properly position the animal. It is not the intent of this chapter to discuss positioning at length. Please refer to the excellent treatment of this topic by Butler et al (2000), Douglas et al (1987), Han et al (2005), Lavin (2005), Morgan (1993), and Ticer (1984).

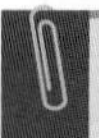

TECHNICIAN NOTE Proper positioning is essential to obtain diagnostic radiographs.

PRINCIPLES OF POSITIONING

To achieve proper positioning, the technician should remember that two views at right angles are necessary to obtain a diagnostic study. This principle applies to all examinations in small animals and to extremities in large animals. The exceptions to this rule are thoracic examinations and spinal examinations in the horse and examinations in cases of trauma or in debilitated animals when only lateral views can be taken without causing undue stress to the animals.

Another principle to remember is the importance of centering the primary beam on the lesion itself, when known. This is especially important in orthopedic cases in both small and large animals. For example, fracture healing may look different when the x-ray beam is centered over the fracture line as opposed to a short distance away from it. Costly errors have been made by veterinarians who removed supporting devices before the correct time. These errors occurred because fractures may have appeared healed when the primary beam was centered away from the fracture line itself.

It is also important when performing a radiographic examination to use an x-ray film that is sufficiently large to completely cover the system to be examined. When x-raying large dogs, it may be necessary to use two films for the abdomen: one for the cranial abdomen and one for the caudal abdomen, which is generally taken at a lower kilovoltage peak. For extremities, the primary beam should be directed at the lesion. It is good to have a radiograph large enough to include the proximal and distal portions of the joint to obtain a good spatial anatomic relationship of the lesion.

These principles are basic but essential. Proper positioning is achieved through practice. These topics are well illustrated and discussed in the references mentioned. A positioning reference textbook should be available in the radiology room of every veterinary practice.

RESTRAINT

The importance of restraint to achieve proper positioning cannot be overemphasized. It is part of radiation safety. Without proper restraint, many examinations should not be undertaken. In some cases, attempting to make examinations without restraint would be life threatening with large animals and dangerous with certain small animals.

There are many types of restraint; some are mechanical or manual, and some are chemical. For the purpose of radiation safety, manual restraint should be avoided as a routine procedure. When it is essential to be in the room with the animal, a protective lead apron, thyroid shield, gloves, and preferably lead glasses, should be worn, and the x-ray beam should be limited to the system to be examined by coning devices or by adjustment of the collimator.

Mechanical restraint comes in various forms. A number of commercial devices designed for animal positioning are available, varying in price from a few dollars to several hundred dollars. One of the most useful and inexpensive devices for use with dogs is a simple muzzle, which often has a calming effect on an animal (see Chapter 7). Sandbags and sponges can also be used to obtain excellent positioning. When the animal is positioned properly, it is most important to take the radiograph rapidly because one can hope for only a few seconds of restraint before the animal moves.

Chemical restraint can be achieved with tranquilizers, analgesics, or anesthetic (see Chapters 26 and 27). Chemical restraint has contributed greatly to the progress made in radiology by allowing positioning that would otherwise be impossible to achieve. For example, complete examination of the skull should not be attempted without anesthesia. Every time total immobility or relaxation is required for proper positioning, anesthesia should be used. Most spinal examinations will prove nondiagnostic unless the examination is done with the animal under anesthesia. In several circumstances, tranquilization is adequate to control most animals. Tranquilizers are excellent for control of frightened or aggressive dogs and cats. They are also most useful for controlling large animals.

> *TECHNICIAN NOTE* Chemical restraint has contributed greatly to the progress made in radiology by allowing positioning that would otherwise be impossible to achieve.

Again, good positioning is essential in producing diagnostic x-ray films. It takes time to learn and become proficient in achieving every position needed for a variety of examinations in large and small animals. However, most organs can be x-rayed with proper techniques, equipment, and accessory devices and the use of mechanical or chemical restraint or both.

Ultrasound imaging is becoming an essential diagnostic tool in veterinary practice. It is portable; does not require the use of ionizing radiation; and is noninvasive, well tolerated by patients, and accepted by clients. As ultrasound equipment becomes affordable, the only problem with its introduction into practice is the long learning curve associated with its use. Recent veterinary graduates are more familiar with the uses and indications for ultrasonography because veterinary schools have integrated ultrasonography into the curriculum. All new veterinary technicians are encouraged to familiarize themselves with the basics of diagnostic ultrasonography, but remember that ultrasonography is user dependent. The image and interpretation are only as good as the person doing the examination.

ULTRASONOGRAPHY

ULTRASONOGRAPHY BASICS

Sound is a mechanical pressure wave made up of a series of compressions and rarefactions transmitted through a medium. Sound waves are characterized by their wavelength or distance between compressions, their frequency in cycles per second, and their velocity or speed of transmission (Figure 19-43). These characteristics are integrated by the following formula:

$$\text{Velocity} = \text{Wavelength} \times \text{Frequency}$$

For simplicity, assume that the speed of sound in the body is 1540 m/sec. Therefore as the frequency of sound increases, the wavelength decreases. Shorter sound waves produce increased image resolution but decreased patient penetration. The frequencies used in veterinary diagnostic ultrasound examination generally range from 2.5 to 12 megahertz (MHz). A hertz (Hz) is 1 cycle per second. Therefore typical ultrasound frequencies will range from 2 million to 12 million cycles/sec, or 2.5 to 12 MHz. Audible sound will range from 20 to 20,000 Hz.

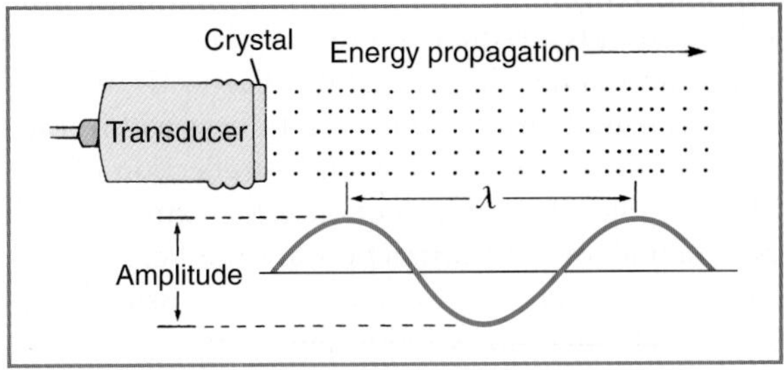

FIGURE 19-43 Sound wave with a wavelength = λ. Closely spaced dots, compressions; widely spaced dots, rarefactions. The amplitude is proportional to the loudness.

Real-time, gray-scale ultrasonography is based on the pulse-echo principle. A short pulse of sound, usually 2 or 3 cycles long, is produced from the transducer and transmitted into the patient. The sound wave strikes an echogenic surface in the patient and returns some of the sound to the transducer. The strength of the returning sound wave determines the brightness of the image, and the time it takes for the sound to travel into the patient and back to the transducer determines where the echo will be seen on the screen. Remember that the time it takes for a sound wave to traverse a distance and be reflected back is a function of the distance between the sender and reflector and the speed of the sound wave in that medium. For all practical purposes, the speed of sound in small animal tissues is constant at 1540 m/sec.

Ultrasound production and reception are based on the piezoelectric effect. A piezoelectric crystal will change shape or thickness when subjected to a voltage pulse. Rapid pulses of electrical energy are transformed into mechanical energy or sound waves by the vibrating crystal. Returning sound waves cause the crystal to vibrate, and that mechanical energy is transmitted into electrical energy by the transducer. This electrical signal is transformed into the gray-scale image on the screen. The transducer acts as both the sound transmitter and the receiver. The operating frequency of the transducer is partially determined by the thickness of the piezoelectric crystal. The thinner the crystal, the higher the transducer frequency. The transducer transmits sound 0.01% of the time. It receives returning sound waves 99.9% of the time.

TECHNICIAN NOTE Ultrasound production and reception are based on the piezoelectric effect. A piezoelectric crystal will change shape or thickness when subjected to a voltage pulse.

ULTRASOUND-TISSUE INTERACTION

To better understand the ultrasound image, it is important to understand the interaction of ultrasound within tissue. As the sound wave proceeds through the body, it is progressively attenuated or weakened. This attenuation limits the depth of penetration of the sound wave and therefore limits the depth of structures that can be effectively imaged. The ultrasound beam is attenuated or weakened by absorption, reflection, scattering, refraction, and diffraction. Reflection is a redirection of the sound beam back to the transducer and is the basis of the diagnostic image. Absorption is sound energy converted to heat within the tissues. Scattering is the intertissue microreflection of sound, which is responsible for much of the echo texture of various organs. Refraction and diffraction are the bending of the sound beam as it crosses areas of differing tissue densities. Refraction attenuation is important in the generation of several ultrasound artifacts.

Sound reflection or echo production forms the basis of the ultrasound image. An echo is produced whenever the ultrasound beam crosses an acoustic interface. An acoustic interface is the boundary between two tissues of differing acoustic impedances, or Z. See the following equation:

$$\text{Acoustic impedance (Z)} = \text{Density (P)} \times \text{Speed of sound transmission (C)}$$

or $Z = P \times C$

If we assume the speed of sound in soft tissue to be constant at 1540 m/sec, then the main factor that influences acoustic impedance is the density or composition of tissue. Thus the more different two adjacent tissues are, the greater will be the echo reflection between them. This is why homogeneous populations of cells (lymphoma, lymph nodes, regenerative liver nodules) produce few echoes and are generally hypoechoic (darker). If the acoustic interface difference is small, only a small percentage of sound will be reflected. If the difference is large, a large portion of sound will be reflected. Most soft tissues have a Z, or acoustic impedance, within 1% to 2% of liver.

Interface	% Reflection
Fat-muscle	0.94
Fat-bone	49.00
Tissue-air	100.00

By looking at this list, one can see the acoustic impedance (Z) between fat and muscle is low, whereas the acoustic impedance between fat and bone and between soft tissue and air is high. This property is why ultrasound cannot be used to image through bone or gas. Too much of the sound beam is reflected back from bone and gas interfaces because of the large change in tissue density.

PATIENT PREPARATION

Patient preparation is important because 100% of the sound is reflected when the ultrasound beam intersects air. Hair traps air, which is how it insulates the animal, but if one tries to pass an ultrasound beam through hair, the majority of the beam is reflected before it ever enters the animal. A careful close clip of the area to be examined, and removal of dirt and scales, will improve the ultrasound image. A generous volume of ultrasound gel is also beneficial to displace air and couple the transducer to the skin (Figure 19-44). Small animals are placed in a padded V-trough table on their backs or in lateral recumbency for abdominal examination and in lateral or sternal recumbency for cardiac examination. Most small animals tolerate abdominal and cardiac examinations well and rarely require tranquilization. A special cardiac table with large and small holes in it is helpful for echocardiography. The animal is placed in lateral recumbency with the chest area over the appropriate-size hole, which allows for better ultrasound transducer access (Figure 19-45). Large animal examinations are done in the standing tranquilized animal. Again, close clipping, especially for tendon examinations, is critical for an optimal examination.

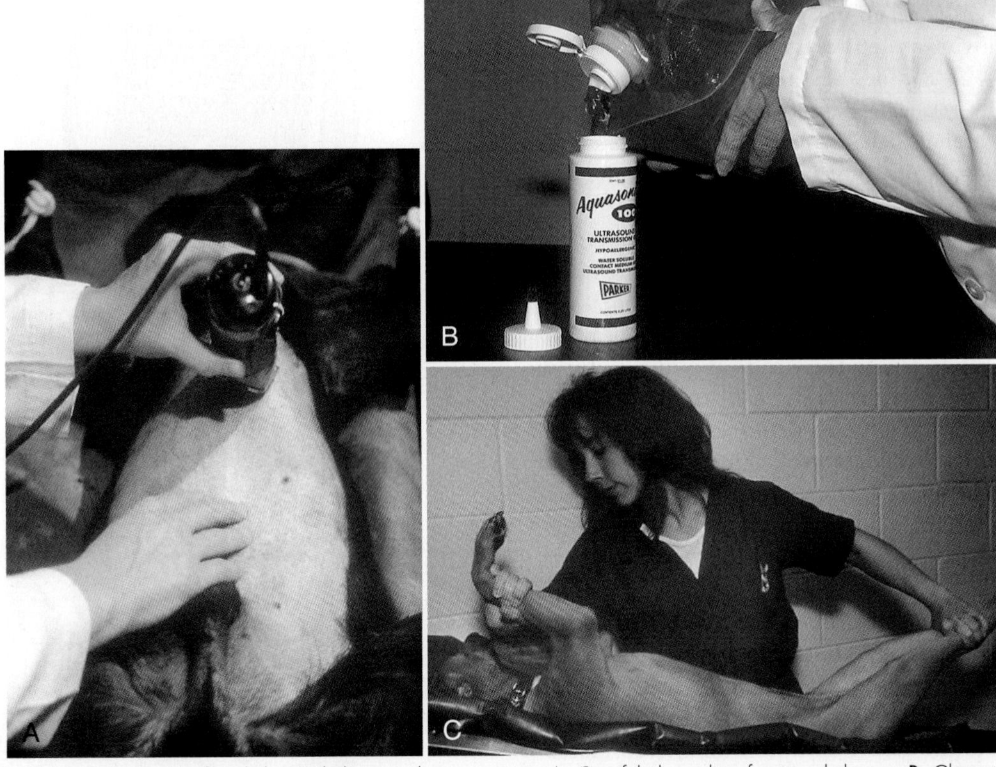

FIGURE 19-44 Patient preparation for abdominal ultrasound examination. **A,** Careful close clip of entire abdomen. **B,** Clean the skin surface, and use a generous volume of coupling gel. **C,** Place the animal in dorsal recumbency on a padded V-trough, and gently restrain during the examination.

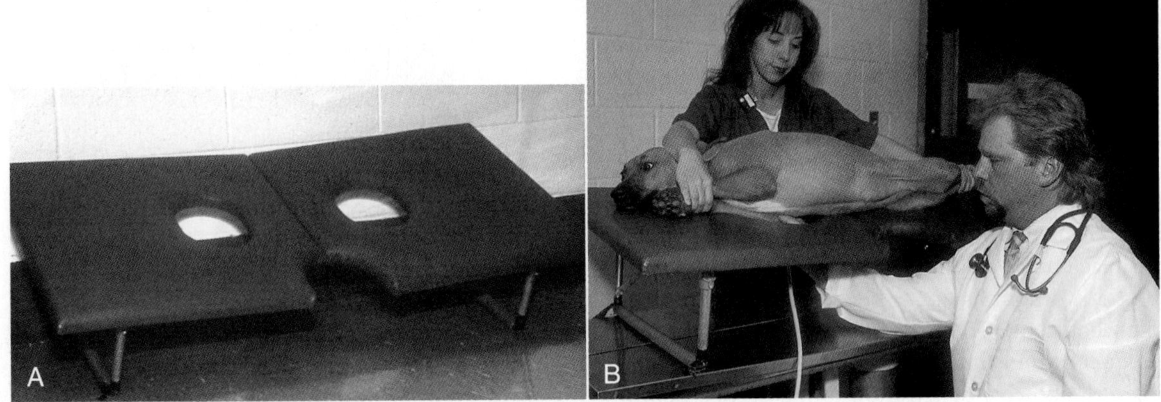

FIGURE 19-45 **A,** Small animal cardiac ultrasound table. **B,** Patient properly positioned and restrained for echocardiography. The dog's cardiac notch is placed over the table hole so the sonographer can access the chest from beneath the table.

TECHNICIAN NOTE Hair traps air, which is how it insulates the animal, but if one tries to pass an ultrasound beam through hair, the majority of the beam is reflected before it ever enters the animal. This is why good patient preparation is so critical.

ULTRASOUND DISPLAY MODES

The returning echo can be displayed in several ways. A-mode, or amplitude mode, displays the returning echoes as spikes from a baseline. The echo depth is determined by its location along the baseline. The echo intensity is displayed by the height of the spike. A-mode ultrasound machines are used predominantly in ophthalmology and have little value in veterinary practice.

B-mode, or brightness mode, forms the basis for two-dimensional imaging. The returning echoes are displayed as dots on the image screen. The brightness of the dot is a function of the strength of the returning echo. The placement of the dot is a function of the time it took for the echo to return to the transducer. The cross-sectional image is formed through data storage. The sound beam is automatically swept across the patient while the transducer is held steady and moved slowly over the area of interest. The rapid collection of images is called real time. This permits direct observation of moving structures, such as a beating heart or puppy motion. With B-mode real-time equipment, images are displayed in gray scale. Gray scale is a technique in which the various echo strengths are displayed in numerous shades of gray from black to white, similar to a black and white television picture.

M-mode, or time-motion (TM) mode, is produced by passing a narrow sound beam across a body part. Each echo interface is presented as a dot. The motion of the body part is displayed by sweeping the image across the screen or image recorder. M-mode can be thought of as a thin sector of B-mode displayed as a function of time. M-mode is primarily used for echocardiography. Ideal ultrasound equipment for veterinary practice would be a real-time B-mode scanner with M-mode capabilities (Figure 19-46).

The selection of appropriate transducers is critical when ultrasound equipment is purchased. Transducers vary in type, size, style, shape, and frequency. Linear array transducers are made with several piezoelectric crystals stacked side by side. The crystals are fired in rapid sequence to produce a rectangular cross-sectional image. The major drawback for older linear array transducers is their large footprint or contact area. It is difficult to use these transducers for intercostal cardiac studies and for subcostal studies in the cranioabdominal area in small animals. Linear array transducers are primarily used for transrectal reproductive examinations in cattle and horses. Newer microcase, small footprint linear array transducers are used effectively for small animal imaging.

Sector scanners produce a triangular field. The crystal is swept across the area by mechanical or electronic means, and the transducer generally has a small contact area. Newer, more expensive transducers may incorporate annular array and dynamic focusing technology. These transducers form the ultrasound beam by adding together many small beams from an array of small crystals. Dynamic focusing allows the operator to place any portion within the beam into maximum resolution without having to change transducers.

Deciding what frequency of transducer to use is easy. Use as high a frequency transducer as possible to maximize resolution while still allowing penetration to the needed depth. Remember that the higher the frequency of the transducer, the shorter will be the sound wavelength and the better will be the resolution. However, as the frequency increases, the depth of sound beam penetration decreases. For abdominal ultrasonography in small dogs (15 kg or less) and cats, a 7.5-MHz transducer is ideal. For middle-size to large-breed dogs, a 5-MHz transducer works well. A guide for selecting a transducer is as follows:

High frequency: Increases resolution
Increases attenuation
Decreases penetration
Low frequency: Decreases resolution
Decreases attenuation
Increases penetration

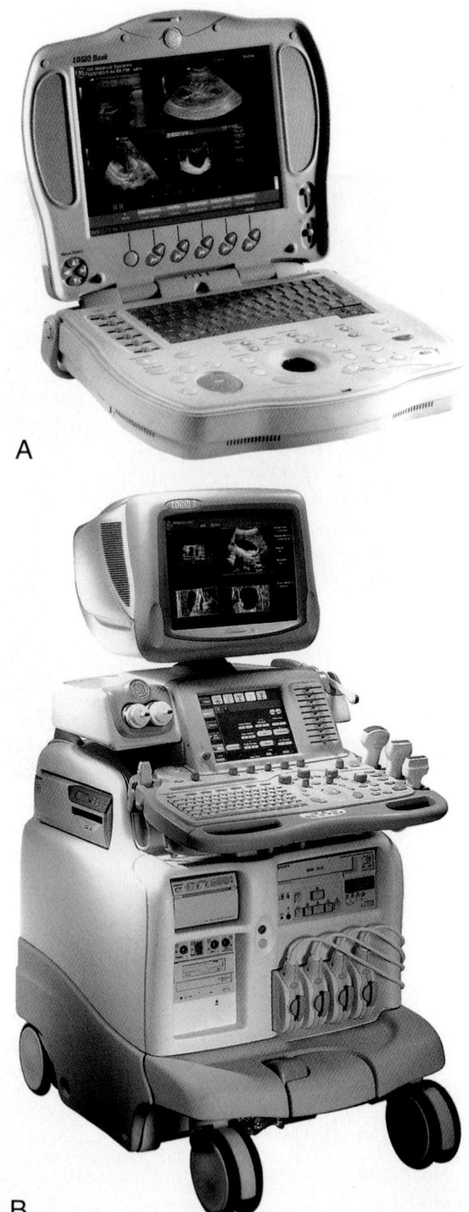

FIGURE 19-46 **A,** Portable notebook-style, real-time B-mode, M-mode, and color Doppler dedicated veterinary ultrasound unit that can be used on both large and small animals. **B,** Larger mobile veterinary ultrasound unit most commonly used in small animal practices. (Courtesy Sound Technologies, Inc, Carlsbad. Calif.)

TECHNICIAN NOTE Use as high a frequency transducer as possible to maximize resolution while allowing penetration to the necessary depth.

The ultrasound equipment controls vary from machine to machine, but the concept of time-gain compensation (TGC) is fairly universal. The echoes coming from acoustic interfaces close to the transducer are stronger than the echoes returning from farther away from the transducer. Time-gain amplification compensates for the progressive attenuation with depth in the ultrasound beam. TGC is operator dependent and is set for the best-looking uniform image. TGC controls are most often a series of slide pods on the front of the machine. The top pod is the near field of the image, and the lowest pod is the far field, or bottom, of the image.

THE ULTRASOUND IMAGE

As one begins using ultrasound, the need to restudy anatomy increases. The ultrasound image is a thin cross-sectional slice through the body in a new or different orientation. It will help to use a standard image orientation, which places the head or front of the animal on the left in the sagittal or longitudinal view and the animal's right on the left of the screen on the transverse or axial view.

Ultrasound terminology is easy to remember. Echogenicity refers to the strength or amplitude of the returning echoes. A structure that is sonodense or echogenic (bright) produces echoes. A structure that is anechoic or sonolucent (dark) produces few or no echoes. A structure is hyperechoic (brighter than) if it produces more echoes than adjacent structures. A structure is hypoechoic (darker than) if it produces fewer echoes than surrounding structures. An isoechoic (same as) structure has a level of echogenicity similar to that of adjacent structures. Remember that echogenicity is a relative term. Any structure can be made bright by adjusting machine control settings. Compare organs at the same depth and control settings to prevent misinterpretation of relative echogenicities.

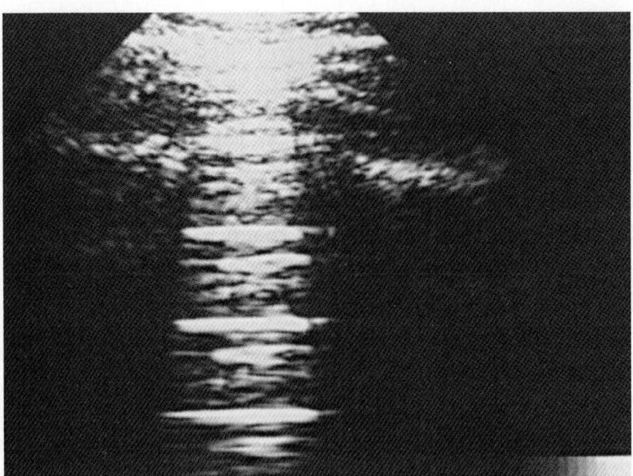

FIGURE 19-47 Reverberation artifact from the air-filled lung of a normal horse. The parallel, evenly spaced echogenic bands represent reverberation between the transducer and pleural surface.

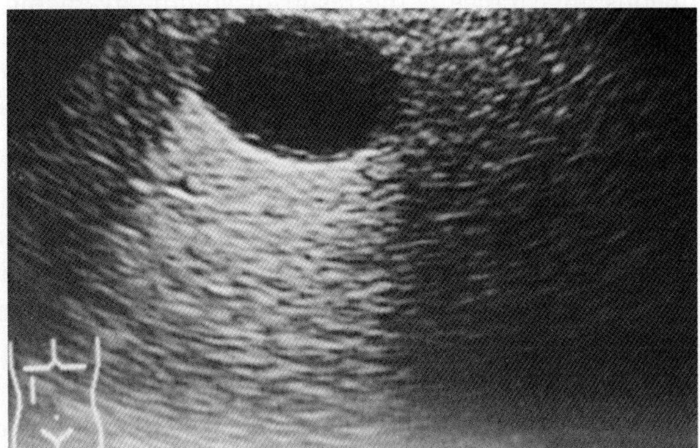

FIGURE 19-48 Bright echogenic band beneath the gallbladder represents acoustic enhancement. The ultrasound beam is not attenuated as much as it traverses the fluid-filled gallbladder as it is in the surrounding liver.

ULTRASOUND ARTIFACTS

Most people fail to take the time to fully understand ultrasound artifacts. They ignore artifacts because, by definition, an artifact does not contribute useful image information. This is not true of ultrasound artifacts. Ultrasound artifacts provide accurate clues to what makes up the ultrasound image.

REVERBERATION ARTIFACT

A reverberation artifact occurs when the ultrasound beam hits gas or air. Because of the large drop in acoustic impedance (soft tissue/air interface), all of the ultrasound beam is reflected back to the transducer. A portion of the reflected beam bounces off the transducer surface and reenters the patient. It hits the air interface a second time, and the same thing happens again. This occurs repeatedly and appears on the screen as a set of bright parallel lines that are the same distance from each other. Each parallel line represents the distance between the transducer and the gas interface. Reverberation artifacts can also be referred to as dirty shadowing or comet tails (Figure 19-47).

SHADOWING

A shadowing artifact occurs because of inadequate sound beam penetration through a highly reflective or sound-absorptive substance. Acoustic shadowing is an area of darkness or hypoechogenicity that occurs deep to dense material, such as bone, calcium, or calculi. Small objects cast an acoustic shadow only if they are within the focal zone or narrow portion of the ultrasound beam.

ACOUSTIC ENHANCEMENT

If the ultrasound beam passes through an area with few tissue interfaces (low attenuation region), the emerging ultrasound beam will have more intensity than would be expected and will be brighter or more echogenic distal to the nonattenuating structure. The best example of this is the normal gallbladder surrounded by the hepatic parenchyma. The liver tissue distal or deep to the gallbladder appears brighter than adjacent hepatic tissue (Figure 19-48). This artifact is seen deep to fluid-filled structures and is also referred to as through transmission.

REFRACTION, OR EDGE ARTIFACT

Refraction is a hypoechoic band or stripe at the margin of a curved structure caused by the refraction or bending of the sound beam. The sound beam is deflected from its true path and never returns, with an effect similar to shadowing. An edge artifact is helpful in identifying smooth round structures, such as early pregnancy vesicles.

MIRROR-IMAGE ARTIFACT

The ultrasound machine places the returning echo on the viewing screen as a function of the time it took the echo to return. If the sound wave reverberates within a highly echogenic structure before returning to the transducer, the image will be duplicated on the screen distal to the original image. This is most commonly seen as a duplication of the gallbladder in mirror image on the other side of the diaphragm.

SLICE-THICKNESS ARTIFACT

If the width of the ultrasound beam cuts through both the edge of a cystic structure and solid tissue, the solid tissue may look as if it is layered within the cyst. This artifact is responsible for the erroneous appearance of debris within the urinary bladder and gallbladder, although no debris are present. The erroneous appearance is the result of volume averaging of tissue by the ultrasound machine.

THE ULTRASOUND EXAMINATION

A complete ultrasound examination requires at least 20 to 30 minutes to perform. When ultrasound is used for a quick answer to a question such as pregnancy versus pyometra, the examination will be shorter. When ultrasound is used for abdominal disease diagnosis, a complete examination should be performed every time.

It is important to have a thorough understanding of the normal appearance of the various abdominal organs before trying to identify the abnormalities associated with disease. The ranking of small animal abdominal organs from least echogenic (darkest) to most echogenic (brightest) is as follows:

Least echogenic	Renal medulla
Liver	
Renal cortex	
Spleen	
Prostate	
Most echogenic	Renal sinus fat

Remember that echogenicity is a relative term, and one must compare organs at similar control settings and similar depths to avoid misinterpretation.

> *TECHNICIAN NOTE* It is important to have a thorough understanding of the normal appearance of the various abdominal organs before trying to identify the abnormalities associated with disease.

CLINICAL USE

The clinical application of ultrasound in veterinary medicine has exploded during the past 10 years. Equipment designed for use in humans is readily adaptable for use in veterinary medicine, and several companies are producing dedicated veterinary ultrasound machines. Both 5- and 7.5-MHz transducers are popular for small animal and nonreproductive large animal imaging. The 3- and 5-MHz linear array transducers are extensively used for transrectal large animal reproductive ultrasonography. Traditional cardiac and solid abdominal organ examinations remain the mainstay, but ultrasound is used to answer hundreds of clinical questions in a wide variety of species. The following section lists common ultrasound applications in both large and small animals.

USES OF ULTRASOUND IN LARGE AND SMALL ANIMALS

- Tendon injury evaluation and response to surgery or therapy
- Diagnosis of tendon sheath infections, adhesions, and foreign bodies
- Evaluation of joint effusions, intraarticular injury, osteomyelitis, and neoplasms
- Congenital and acquired cardiac disease and response to therapy
- Pleural effusion, pleuritis, and pleuropneumonia
- Soft tissue, neck, thyroid, parathyroid, tongue, and mediastinal disease
- Hepatic, renal, splenic, adrenal, urinary bladder, gallbladder, and biliary disease
- Abdominal and peripheral vascular malformations
- Peritoneal and pleural fluid assessment and sampling
- Abdominal masses of unknown origin
- Intestinal foreign bodies, intussusceptions, infiltrative disease, and neoplasia
- Testicular and prostate evaluation and location of retained testicles
- Pregnancy diagnosis, fetal evaluation, twin removal, and complete fertility evaluations
- Soft tissue neoplasia, granulomas, abscesses, and foreign bodies
- Umbilical infections and persistent and patent urachus
- Ocular and orbital evaluation
- Vascular thrombosis and catheter foreign body evaluation
- Guidance for fine-needle aspiration, drain placement, biopsy, and culture

NUCLEAR MEDICINE

ALTERNATIVE IMAGING MODALITIES

Many veterinary schools and several progressive specialized veterinary practices have nuclear medicine capabilities. Nuclear medicine can be divided into therapeutic and diagnostic procedures. Currently, veterinary therapeutic nuclear medicine involves the administration of radioactive iodine (^{131}I) for the treatment of hyperthyroidism and thyroid tumors. Diagnostic nuclear medicine involves the administration of radionuclides to the animal and detection of the electromagnetic radiation emitted from the animal with a gamma scintillation camera. Radionuclides are atoms with unstable nuclei that undergo radioactive decay. Radioactive decay is the transformation or disintegration of an unstable nucleus by spontaneous emission of electromagnetic radiation. Electromagnetic radiation that is of nuclear origin is termed gamma rays, in contrast to diagnostic radiation (x-rays), which originates from the electron cloud that surrounds the nucleus.

> *TECHNICIAN NOTE* Currently, veterinary therapeutic nuclear medicine involves the administration of radioactive iodine (^{131}I) for the treatment of hyperthyroidism and thyroid tumors.

Diagnostic nuclear medicine does not generate visual images equivalent to those of diagnostic radiology, but detects functional or physiologic, pharmacologic, and kinetic data from the patient in image or numeric data form. Figure 19-49 shows a standard gamma scintillation camera, control panel, and nuclear medicine computer. Common clinical uses of veterinary nuclear medicine include bone scanning for detection of tumor metastasis to bone and radiographically undetectable bone injury or infection, lung scanning for detection of pulmonary embolism and as a pulmonary function test, renal scans for assessment of kidney perfusion and function, and thyroid scans for the characterization of hyperthyroidism and the detection of metastasis. Other, less common nuclear medicine studies include hepatobiliary scanning, brain scans, labeled white blood cell scans for the detection of occult infection, lymphoscintigraphy, nuclear angiography, and scans for detection of an unknown focus of blood loss.

The most commonly used radionuclide is technetium 99m (^{99m}Tc). This agent is commercially available from a disposable technetium generator. Technetium is administered in an ionic form as $^{99m}TcO_4$ (pertechnetate) or bound to a specific organ-localizing pharmaceutical agent before administration. Technetium is the radiopharmaceutical of choice because it has a 6-hour physical half-life and emits a 140-keV gamma ray, which is appropriate for most imaging studies. The radioactive or physical half-life of a radionuclide is the time required for the number of radioactive atoms to decrease by 50%.

Radiation safety practices are important with nuclear medicine. When working in a practice that uses nuclear medicine, one should insist on receiving comprehensive instruction in radiation principles and safety. This chapter is meant only as an introduction.

The primary route of radionuclide administration to veterinary patients is intravenous. Latex examination gloves should be worn, and careful injection techniques should be used to ensure that the entire dose is delivered intravenously and not perivascularly. This is especially important in equine bone scans for which a large dose of radionuclide is administered. Please refer to Chapter 31 for additional information on nuclear scintigraphy in horses. The routes of excretion of the radioactive imaging agents vary with the agent used. Technetium is primarily excreted in urine, with a lesser amount in the feces. Animals should be housed in a separate restricted area of the hospital, and their stool and urine should be carefully collected and held for decay until the levels are below exempt quantities. Always wear latex examination gloves, and limit contact with patients to only that necessary for their care. Never eat or bring eating utensils (coffee cups, spoons, etc.) into a nuclear medicine area. The dose of radiation to the patient is small, but repeated physical contact or accidental ingestion of radionuclides

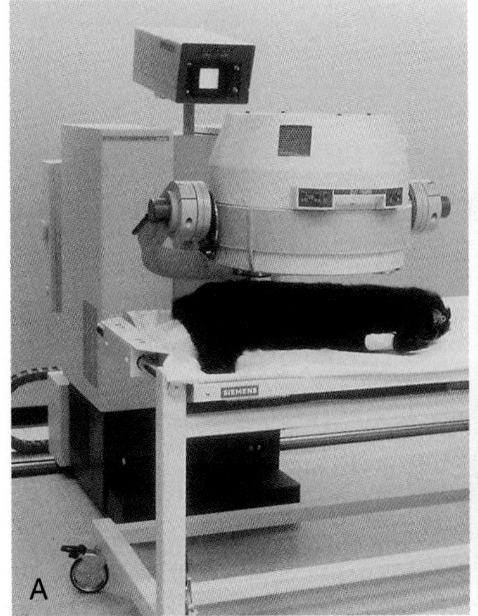

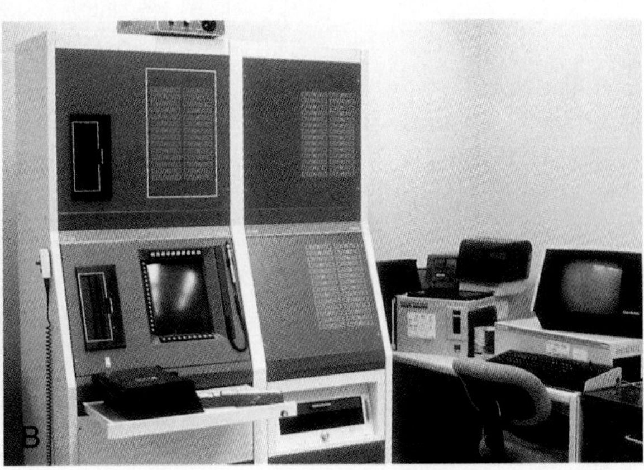

FIGURE 19-49 A, Gamma scintillation camera in position over a dog during a whole-body bone scan to check for metastatic neoplasia. **B,** Control panel monitor, nuclear medicine computer, and matrix camera.

may be harmful to the nuclear medicine technologist. Animals should be held in the restricted area until they pose no radiation threat to their owners or the population at large. This is generally 3 to 10 physical half-lives of the radiopharmaceutical, depending on specific state regulations.

> *TECHNICIAN NOTE* The primary route of radionuclide administration to veterinary patients is intravenous. Latex examination gloves should be worn, and careful injection techniques should be used to ensure that the entire dose is delivered intravenously and not perivascularly.

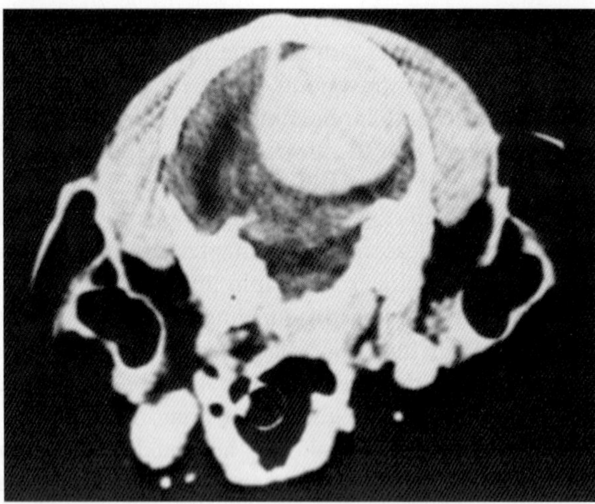

FIGURE 19-50 Computed tomogram of a dog brain showing a large contrast-enhancing brain tumor (meningioma) in the central cerebrum.

COMPUTED TOMOGRAPHY

In the past 15 years, there has been an expansion of the diagnostic imaging techniques available to veterinary patients. Most veterinary schools and several specialty practices have access to CT scanning. A CT scan is obtained by passing a thin x-ray beam transaxially through the patient and measuring the x-ray attenuation at multiple sites in a thin slice of the patient's anatomy. The computer then reconstructs the transmitted x-ray data into a cross-sectional image on a video monitor. The image can then be captured on film or videotape or stored on magnetic tape for later use. The advantage of CT over standard radiography is the greatly improved radiographic contrast, spatial resolution, and cross-sectional anatomic presentation. The most common use of CT in veterinary medicine is head and spinal examinations for neurologic disease. CT allows the veterinarian a noninvasive look inside the patient's skull (Figure 19-50).

When a CT scan is performed, the patient is placed in the ventrodorsal or dorsoventral position on the long, narrow, movable CT table. The table then moves the patient through the circular gantry that houses the x-ray tube and detectors (Figure 19-51). The table moves in a measured stepwise fashion. During each table step, the CT scanner obtains a single cross-sectional slice of data. The patient must be heavily sedated or under general anesthetic to prevent any motion and must be positioned perfectly straight. Most studies are performed twice on the same animal. The first study is performed without contrast, and the second is performed after intravenous administration of iodinated contrast. Urographic contrast agents are commonly administered at a dose of 800 mg of iodine per kilogram of body weight. Contrast will

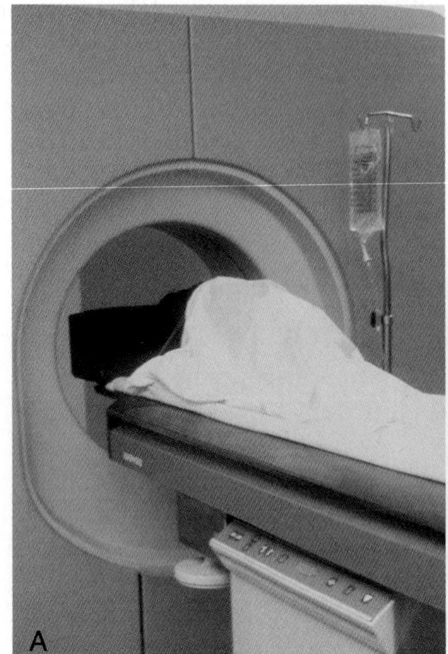

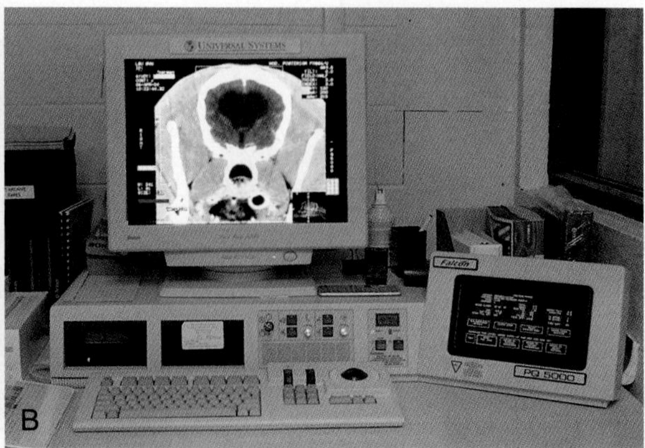

FIGURE 19-51 **A,** Dog in position for a brain computed tomogram. The large circular gantry houses the x-ray tube and detectors. The table moves the patient through the gantry in precise, measured, incremental steps. **B,** Computed tomography (CT) control panel located outside the shielded CT room.

highlight vascular structures, and some neoplasms will have a characteristic contrast enhancement pattern. In addition to examination of the brain, CT can be used to identify and characterize musculoskeletal, thoracic, and abdominal disorders.

> *TECHNICIAN NOTE* When performing CT studies, you use the same contrast agents you use for radiographic contrast procedures; you just use much less concentrated contrast medium because CT is much more contrast sensitive.

MAGNETIC RESONANCE IMAGING

The newest imaging modality to be used in veterinary medicine is magnetic resonance imaging (MRI). MRI is similar to CT in that the image is a thin slice of cross-sectional anatomy made up of a matrix of volume elements. MRI differs from CT in that it uses no ionizing radiation to create the image. Instead, the MRI represents the intensity of a radio wave signal from tissue in which hydrogen nuclei have been disturbed by a characteristic radiofrequency pulse. MRI is superior to CT in image resolution, anatomic definition, and sensitivity to tissue composition differences. Because of this, MRI is vastly superior to CT for imaging of the brain and spinal cord and is currently used primarily for head and spine evaluation. Figure 19-52 is a sagittal canine brain magnetic resonance image of a patient with a large contrast-enhancing pituitary tumor.

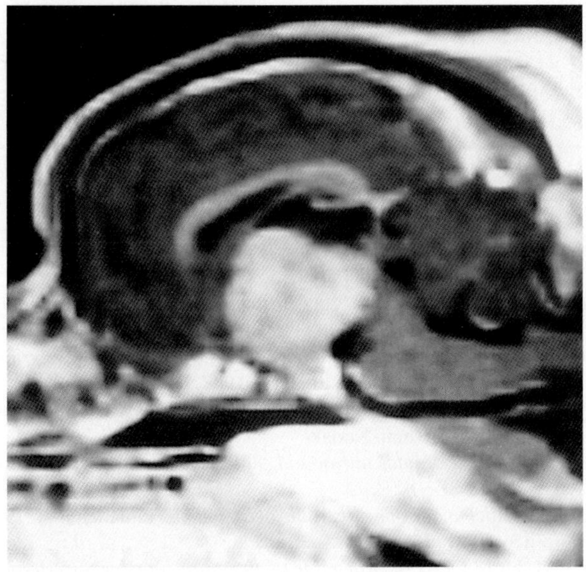

FIGURE 19-52 Sagittal T1 postgadolinium contrast magnetic resonance image of a dog with a large enhancing pituitary macroadenoma.

> *TECHNICIAN NOTE* MRI differs from CT in that it uses no ionizing radiation to create the image. MRI is superior to CT in image resolution, anatomic definition, and sensitivity to tissue composition differences. Because of this, MRI is vastly superior to CT for imaging of the brain and spinal cord and is currently used primarily for head and spine evaluation.

Two general types of MRI units (also called magnets) are used in veterinary imaging: low field strength open magnets (Figure 19-53, *A*) and high field strength, or superconductive, magnets (Figure 19-53, *B*). Magnetic field strength is measured in tesla (T). Low field strength magnets are 0.4T or less, and high field strength magnets are 0.6T and above. The most typical superconducting magnet has a field strength of 1 or 1.5 T. Regardless of the type of magnet used, the technician needs to be aware of several safety measures and patient management concerns peculiar to MRI.

About half of the veterinary teaching hospitals have in-house MRI units. In most private veterinary practices, CT and MRI are often done off the practice premises in an imaging center; a mobile, truck-based MRI unit; or a human hospital. Therefore everything needed to anesthetize, resuscitate, and recover a patient needs to be taken to the imaging site. Most practices that perform off-site imaging have a large tackle box or physician's bag filled with all necessary drugs, fluids,

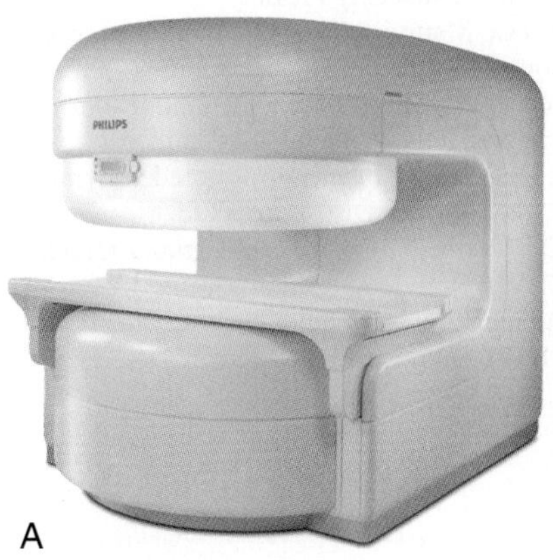

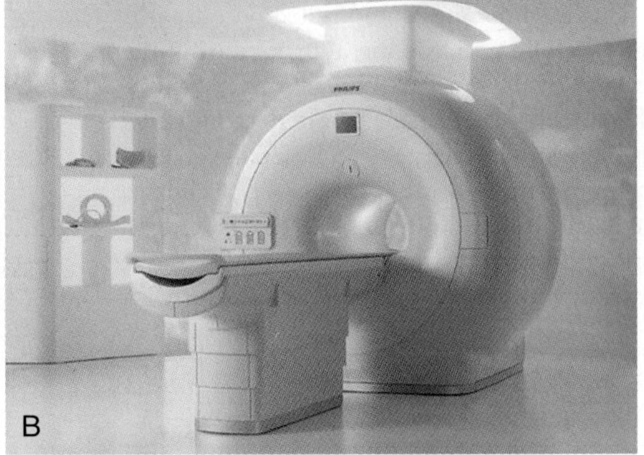

FIGURE 19-53 **A,** An open or low field strength magnetic resonance imaging (MRI) scanner. These machines make it easier to position and monitor the patient but may require longer scan times. **B,** Superconductive or high field strength MRI scanner. The circular closed MRI gantry can make patient positioning difficult.

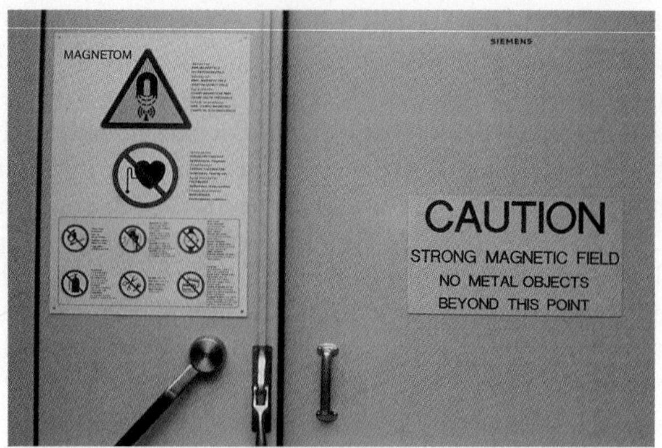

FIGURE 19-54 Warning signs positioned at the entrance to a magnetic resonance imaging (MRI) scanner. The technician must realize that the MRI magnet is always turned on and the high magnetic field may extend beyond the scanner room door. Never bring anything metallic into the MRI suite.

catheters, intravenous access lines, syringes, needles, tape, gauze, and endotracheal tubes. It often helps to do a mock run or pretend case before a clinical case to ensure that everything is correctly packed. Imaging centers and hospitals appreciate clean, odor-free, and flea- and tick-free veterinary patients. It is a good idea to bathe the patient within 24 hours before the examination if possible and to ensure that the patient's bowel and bladder have been evacuated before the patient enters the hospital or imaging center.

A serious problem with MRI is the strong magnetic field (Figure 19-54). One cannot use anything made of ferromagnetic metal in or around the magnet. The magnetic field will rapidly and forcefully pull these objects into the magnet, potentially injuring anyone in its path. Such objects include the gas anesthetic machine, oxygen tank, intravenous poles, clipboards, ink pens, leashes, collars, and beepers. There are nonmagnetic products available for use during MRI, but they are generally prohibitively expensive for most veterinary hospitals. The exception is an aluminum oxygen tank. Because of this limitation, anesthesia is generally performed with injectable drugs and heavy tranquilization. Patients must be absolutely still for MRI; any motion will severely degrade the image, so they must be under fairly deep injectable anesthetic. This is sometimes complicated because it is often difficult to carefully monitor the animals during the examination because of the narrow tubular shape of some magnets and the inability to use mechanized monitoring devices. Patients that cannot tolerate deep injectable general anesthetic with minimal monitoring are not good candidates for out-of-clinic MRI. MRI examinations generally take 45 to 60 minutes to perform and are done with and without intravenous contrast, similar to CT examinations, but with a paramagnetic contrast agent (usually gadolinium pentetic acid). Organic iodide contrast will not work for MRI examinations.

In addition to the anesthesia and monitoring difficulties created by the high magnetic field, personal safety is a concern, and precautions must be taken. It is important to remember that even though no images are being produced and the MRI technician is not at the controls, the magnet is still on at full power at all times. Credit cards and watches may be permanently damaged if carried too close to the high magnetic field. Any device that delivers a radiofrequency signal cannot be close to an MRI unit; these include but are not limited to televisions, radios, and pager transmitters. In addition, technicians with cardiac pacemakers, aneurysm or intracranial hemoclips, neural stimulators, metallic fragments within the orbits, or hearing aids should not be in charge of patient care during an MRI. If you ever have any questions regarding what can and cannot be brought into the MRI room, ask the MRI technician in charge before entering.

> TECHNICIAN NOTE The high magnetic field in an MRI unit is always on. It is never safe to bring anything made of a ferromagnetic metal close to the machine.

RECOMMENDED READING

Butler JA et al: *Clinical radiology of the horse,* ed 2, Oxford, England, 2000, Blackwell Scientific Publications.

Curry TS, Dowdey JE, Murry RC: *Christensen's introduction to the physics of diagnostic radiology,* ed 4, Philadelphia, 1990, Lea & Febiger.

Douglas SW, Herrtage ME, Williamson HD: *Principles of veterinary radiology,* ed 4, East Sussex, England, 1987, Bailliere Tindall.

Eastman Kodak Co.: *The fundamentals of radiography,* ed 12, Rochester, NY, 1980, Eastman Kodak.

Green RW: *Small animal ultrasound,* Philadelphia, 1996, Lippincott-Raven.

Hall EJ: *Radiobiology for the radiologist,* ed 4, Philadelphia, 1993, Lippincott-Raven.

Han CM, Hurd CD: *Practical guide to diagnostic imaging for veterinary technicians,* ed 3, St Louis, 2005, Mosby.

Lavin LM: *Radiography in veterinary technology,* ed 4, St Louis, 2005, WB Saunders.

Morgan JR: *Techniques of veterinary radiography,* ed 5, Ames, 1993, Iowa State University Press.

Nyland TG, Mattoon JS: *Small animal diagnostic ultrasound,* ed 2, St Louis, 2002, WB Saunders.

Rantanen NW, McKinnon AD: *Equine diagnostic ultrasonography,* Baltimore, 1998, Williams & Wilkins.

Stashak TS: *Adam's lameness in horses,* ed 5, Plymouth, United Kingdom, 2002, Plymbridge Distributors Ltd.

Thrall DE: *Textbook of veterinary diagnostic radiology,* ed 5, Philadelphia, 2007, WB Saunders.

Ticer JA: *Radiographic technique in veterinary practice,* ed 2, Philadelphia, 1984, WB Saunders.

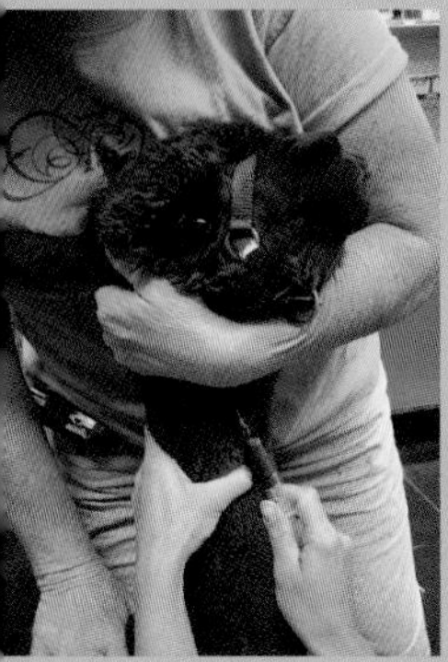

Diagnostic Sampling and Therapeutic Techniques

20

Harold Davis, Darlene L. Riel, Marika Pappagianis, and Kristin Miguel

KEY TERMS

Abdominocentesis
Anorexia
Arthrocentesis
Coupage
Cystocentesis
Diagnostic peritoneal lavage
Extravasation
Foley catheter
Gastrostomy
Hematoma
Hemolysis
Inflammation
Intraosseous
Leukocytosis
Neutropenia
Osmolality
Pancytopenia
Percutaneous
Phlebitis
Pleural effusion
Pneumothorax
Polymerase chain reaction (PCR)
Rumen
Stoma
Thoracentesis
Thrombocytopenia
Thrombosis
Vasodilation

OUTLINE

LEARNING OBJECTIVES

When you have completed this chapter, you will be able to:

1. List and describe general principles for the collection of samples for laboratory testing.
2. Describe the patient's preparation, positioning, and procedures for blood collection from peripheral veins and capillary beds in small and large animals.
3. Describe indications and procedures for collection of arterial blood samples in small and large animals.
4. List and describe procedures for collection of urine samples from small and large animals and give advantages and limitations of each method.
5. Describe the indications and procedures for performing thoracocentesis, abdominocentesis, arthrocentesis, fine-needle aspiration, bronchoalveolar lavage, and collection of vaginal cytology samples in small and large animals.
6. Describe the indications and procedures for performing diagnostic peritoneal lavage.
7. Describe the two methods for performing a transtracheal wash and give advantages and disadvantages for each method.
8. Describe procedures for obtaining cerebrospinal fluid (CSF) and bone marrow aspirate samples and list indications, contraindications, and potential complications of the procedure.
9. List the routes used for administration of medications in small and large animals and describe procedures for administration of medications by each route.
10. Describe the procedure for placement and care of a peripheral intravenous (IV) catheter.
11. Describe the indications and procedure for placement and care of a jugular catheter.

12. List requirements for monitoring of patients with IV catheters.
13. Describe indications and methods for administration of oral medication of enteral feeding of small and large animals.
14. Describe procedures for collection and evaluation of milk samples from dairy animals.
15. Describe procedures for collection of rumen fluid in large animals.

INTRODUCTION

The veterinary technician plays a vital role in the preparation, collection, and submission of diagnostic samples. Following diagnosis, therapeutic interventions may be required of the veterinary technician. For this reason, this chapter discusses sample collection first, followed by the administration of medication. Small and large animal techniques are discussed separately in keeping with the common delineation made between companion animal and large animal clinical practices. Given the advances in veterinary nursing, it is incumbent on the veterinary technician to have the knowledge, skills, and ability to collect diagnostic samples and perform therapeutic techniques. When performing or assisting in performing procedures, veterinary technicians should be aware of the indications, equipment needed, procedure technique, complications, and postprocedure nursing care. Technicians should have expertise in many basic and advanced procedures, such as blood and urine sample collection, IV and arterial catheter placement, and fluid and medication administration. These procedures and others will be addressed in this chapter.

BASIC GUIDELINES

Pretreatment blood and urine samples should be obtained before the administration of fluids and/or medications. The administration of fluids and the recent ingestion of a high-fat or high-protein meal may alter blood or urine laboratory values.

TECHNICIAN NOTE Pretreatment blood and urine samples should be obtained before the administration of fluids or medications.

All supplies needed for the collection of samples and for therapeutic procedures should be gathered ahead of time. Samples should be collected and stored in appropriate containers with the patient's name and hospital identification number printed on each label.

Whenever a needle is inserted through the skin as a part of a treatment (e.g., subcutaneous injection) or a sampling procedure (e.g., bone marrow aspirate), the skin should be properly prepared and free from obvious inflammation and infection. Microbes and other contaminants present on the skin surface may be introduced into the underlying tissue when the needle is inserted. Needles and IV catheters from which the protective coverings have been removed should remain sterile and should only be handled at the hub (e.g., the shaft should not be touched or set down on a nonsterile surface).

The knowledge of potential risk or complications will place the veterinary technician in a position to be proactive rather than reactive to problems. The technician should be able to assess the patient and recognize when problems are occurring and have a "game plan" in mind for addressing the problems. For example, a technician knowledgeable in IV catheter complications is performing IV catheter care and notices that the catheter insertion site is erythematous, swollen, painful, and warm to the touch. The veterinary technician assesses the problem as thrombophlebitis, determines that a new catheter is needed, and removes the old one.

SMALL ANIMAL SAMPLING AND THERAPEUTIC TECHNIQUES

BLOOD SAMPLE COLLECTION

Veterinary technicians perform venipuncture on a routine basis, either to collect blood samples for laboratory tests or to inject a drug or medication. Proper animal restraint is as important as the venipuncture technique (Chapter 7). Blood samples must be collected with minimal trauma to the vessel and minimal stress and discomfort to the patient (Box 20-1). Patients' stress can affect several laboratory tests (e.g., leukogram, cortisol and glucose concentrations).

A venipuncture is performed with either a needle and syringe or a Vacutainer collection system. The Vacutainer system consists of a double-pointed needle, plastic holder, and collection tubes with and without anticoagulants (Figure 20-1). The method and needle gauge selected depend on the vessel size, amount of blood required, intended use of the sample, and technician's preference.

The majority of venipunctures in cats and small dogs are performed with 22-gauge needles. Larger-gauge needles, such as 20- and 18-gauge, may be used in large-breed dogs and in most farm animals. For any venipuncture technique,

BOX 20-1 Venous Blood Collection

- Attach a 20- to 25-gauge needle to a 1- to 6-ml syringe.
- Occlude the vein with a tourniquet or digital pressure.
- Wipe the skin and hair on top of the vein with an alcohol-soaked cotton ball to help identify the vein.
- Insert the needle with the bevel facing up through the skin and into the vein at a 25-degree angle.
- Slowly retract the syringe plunger and collect a blood sample.
- Release the pressure on the vein and release the syringe plunger when a sufficient volume of blood has been collected.
- Remove the needle from the vein.
- Apply digital pressure to the venipuncture site as soon as the needle is removed until hemostasis occurs.

the needle should always be inserted into the vein with the bevel facing upward.

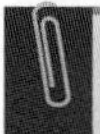

TECHNICIAN NOTE For venipuncture, the needle should be inserted with the bevel facing upward.

Blood collected for coagulation profiles (i.e., activated clotting time, prothrombin time, activated partial thromboplastin time) should be collected carefully with minimal tissue trauma and venous stasis. The needle should ideally penetrate the vessel on the first attempt to minimize the amount of tissue fluid that enters the sample; tissue fluid (thromboplastin) may initiate the clotting cascade.

Smaller, 25- to 28-gauge needles are used with smaller vessels, fragile vessels, or multiple venipunctures. Frequent sampling to establish a blood glucose curve is a situation in which the use of a small-gauge needle is appropriate. The amount of negative pressure applied to aspirate the blood into the syringe must not be excessive. Forceful retraction of the syringe plunger may result in hemolysis of the red blood cells as they pass through the needle, yielding erroneous laboratory values. The application of excessive negative pressure may also cause the vein to collapse.

Just before a venipuncture, the hair and skin over the vessel are wiped with a cotton ball saturated with 70% isopropyl alcohol. This helps to remove some superficial skin contaminants, causes vasodilation, and improves visualization of the vein. In animals with dense hair coats, the vessel may be easier to identify if the hair over the vessel is parted with the use of an alcohol-soaked cotton ball or shaved with a clipper. When blood is drawn for a bacterial culture, the region on top of the vein is shaved and aseptically prepared. Sterile gloves are worn when blood is collected for a culture.

The most important aspects of any venipuncture technique are the proper restraint of the animal and proper distention and immobilization of the vessel. These objectives are most easily accomplished when the procedure is done as a two-person project. The veterinary technician should only attempt the venipuncture when the vessel can be clearly

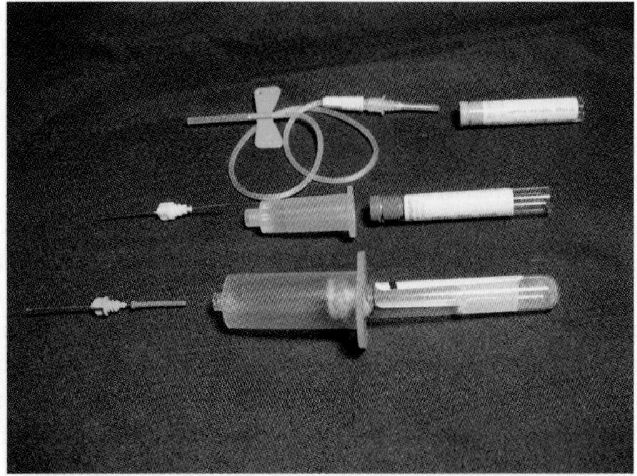

FIGURE 20-1 The Vacutainer blood collection system is used to collect blood samples directly into the collection tunes. The system consists of a needle, holder, and collection tubes. (From Hendrix CM, Sirois M, editors: *Laboratory procedures for the veterinary technician*, ed 5, St Louis, 2007, Mosby Elsevier.)

delineated. Blind venipuncture attempts are doomed to failure and unnecessary patient's discomfort. If the technician is unable to locate the vessel (by visual inspection or digital palpation), the manner in which the vessel is distended and immobilized must be changed.

TECHNICIAN NOTE The most important aspects of any venipuncture technique are the proper restraint of the animal and proper distention and immobilization of the vessel.

When collecting blood, excessive restraint should be avoided since it may incite more resistance from the animal than the venipuncture procedure itself.

To collect blood from a peripheral vein, introduce the needle into the occluded vessel as far distally as possible. If the initial venipuncture attempt is unsuccessful, reinsert the needle more proximal to the previous entry site. For a jugular venipuncture, the initial attempt is made in the caudal region of the jugular vein. Subsequent venipuncture attempts can be made in a more cranial region. If the vessel is damaged in the distal portion of the vein, a more proximal region is still patent and usable for blood collection.

After blood is collected, the needle is detached from the syringe, and the stopper is removed from the collection tube before the blood is transferred into the tube. This reduces the amount of hemolysis that may occur if blood is forcefully ejected through the narrow lumen of a needle. If blood is transferred into a tube containing an anticoagulant, such as lavender-topped ethylenediaminetetraacetic (EDTA) tubes, the stopper is quickly replaced, and the tube is gently inverted a few times to mix the blood with the anticoagulant. Vigorous shaking can cause hemolysis. The tube containing the anticoagulant should be at least half filled with blood to achieve the appropriate blood/anticoagulant ratio.

The most frequently used sites for canine blood collection are the cephalic, jugular, and lateral saphenous veins. The cephalic, jugular, femoral, and medial saphenous veins are used for feline venipunctures.

Cephalic Venipuncture

The patient may be positioned in sternal or lateral recumbency. The restrainer leans over the top of the animal and grasps the leg of interest at the elbow. The other hand and arm can be used to restrain the animal's head if the animal is awake to prevent an aggressive response to the skin puncture. If the animal is in sternal recumbency, the restrainer should lean on his or her elbow to help prevent the animal from withdrawing its leg at some critical time during the procedure. A tourniquet or thumb or forefinger is wrapped around the forearm at the level of the elbow. Pressure at this point occludes the cephalic vein. The skin is then rotated outward to roll the vein to the top (anterior) of the forearm.

The veterinary technician grasps the leg with one hand at the level of the metacarpus and further extends the leg. In "loose-skinned" animals, it may be necessary to flex the carpus. The objective is to tether the vein between the two points of traction (at the elbow and at the carpus) so that the vein is both distended and does not roll from side to side.

The needle is directed, as much as possible, along the longitudinal axis of the vein. The needle is inserted through the skin with the bevel facing up. The skin puncture is the painful part, and animals will often move in response to it. Once the animal has settled down, the needle can be directed into the vein. If blood does not spontaneously flow into the hub of the needle, gently aspirate to determine if the needle is or is not in the vein. If not, the needle should be advanced a bit farther and the process repeated. The needle can be advanced to its full length. If at this point the venipuncture has not been successful, the needle will have to be withdrawn to its subcutaneous (SQ) position (do not remove it entirely since another skin puncture will then be necessary). It is most important to withdraw the needle slowly, while gently aspirating. The deep wall of the vein may have been inadvertently penetrated, and the lumen will thereby be found as the needle is withdrawn.

Once the blood sample is taken or the drug is administered, the needle is withdrawn from the vein and digital pressure applied over the venipuncture site for at least 30 seconds. The site should be monitored for bleeding or hematoma formation for an additional several minutes.

Jugular Venipuncture

The patient may be positioned in sternal or lateral recumbency. Some large-breed dogs prefer to remain seated on the floor (Figure 20-2). Alternatively the patient is restrained on a table in sternal recumbency (Figure 20-3). One hand grasps the legs at the carpel joint and stretches the legs over the edge of the table. In any position, the head will need to be extended. Either the restrainer or the veterinary technician occludes the vein by applying occlusive pressure at the thoracic inlet. Care must be taken not to compress the trachea or impair breathing. Vein distention and immobilization can be maximized by pressing into the thoracic inlet in a caudal direction and by further extension of the head. Extensive longitudinal traction, however, can collapse the vein. With optimal positioning, the vein is easy to palpate (or visualize) and does not roll much from side to side. In sternal positioning, the venipuncture is usually done in a cephalad direction; in lateral positioning, the venipuncture is generally done in a caudal direction. The venipuncture is performed as previously described.

Lateral Saphenous Venipuncture

The patient is usually positioned in lateral recumbency (Figure 20-4). The restrainer grasps the upper leg at the stifle. The other hand and arm can be used to restrain the animal's forelegs and head if the animal is awake. Circumferential pressure is applied at the stifle to occlude and distend the vein. The veterinary technician grasps the leg with one hand at the level of the metatarsus. It should not be necessary for the veterinary technician to use his or her thumb to help immobilize the vein. The venipuncture is performed as previously described.

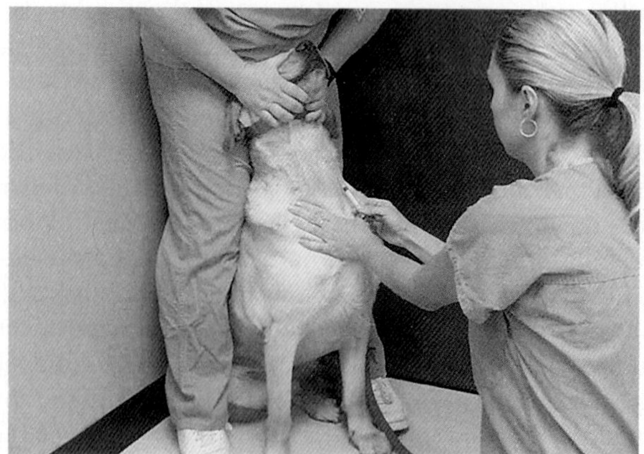

FIGURE 20-2 Dog positioned for jugular vein venipuncture by backing it into a corner. (From Ettinger SJ, Feldmen E, editors: *Textbook of veterinary internal medicine*, ed 6, Philadelphia, 2005, Elsevier Saunders.)

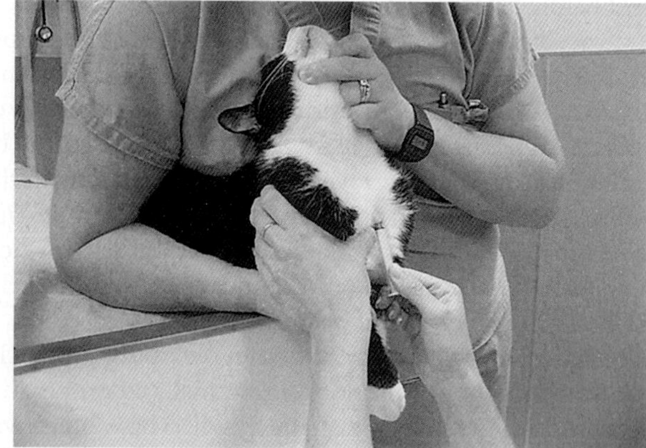

FIGURE 20-3 Cat positioned for jugular vein venipuncture. (From Ettinger SJ, Feldmen E, editors: *Textbook of veterinary internal medicine*, ed 6, Philadelphia, 2005, Elsevier Saunders.)

Medial Saphenous or Femoral Venipuncture

The medial saphenous or femoral vein is used to collect small volumes of blood. The patient is usually positioned in lateral recumbency. The restrainer grasps the lower leg at the stifle while reflecting the upper leg caudally with the forearm. The other hand and arm can be used to restrain the animal's forelegs and head if the animal is awake. Circumferential pressure is applied at the stifle to occlude and distend the vein. Alternatively, in the cat, grasp it by the scruff of the neck and place in lateral recumbency (Figure 20-5). The upper hind leg is abducted and flexed to expose the medial surface of the bottom leg. Applying pressure with the edge of the hand that abducts and extends the upper leg distends the vein. The veterinary technician grasps the leg with one hand at the level of the metatarsus. The venipuncture is performed as previously described.

Marginal Ear Venipuncture

On occasion, the technician will collect blood from a peripheral capillary bed to check for erythroparasitic organisms, such as *Babesia* spp. or *Haemobartonella* spp. The collection of a small drop of capillary blood is also used by clients who monitor their diabetic pets' blood glucose levels at home. A peripheral capillary blood sample can be obtained by clipping the quick of a toenail or lacerating the buccal mucosa. A more desirable, less painful alternative is to collect a sample from the marginal ear vein, which is most easily visualized as it courses around the periphery of the dorsal aspect of the pinna.

When a capillary sample is collected, the pinna of the ear is first warmed with a heated cloth, light source, or the technician's hands to help vasodilate the marginal ear vein and then wiped with a small amount of alcohol. A 25-gauge needle or lancet is used to nick the vein, and the pinna is massaged until a sufficient drop of blood is obtained (Figure 20-6). When a sample must be examined for erythroparasites, blood is collected into a heparinized capillary tube and is later smeared onto slides for a microscopic examination. If blood is collected to measure blood glucose, a Glucometer test strip is placed alongside the drop of blood on the pinna, and the blood is wicked directly onto the test strip. The test strip should be designed to measure a capillary, not venous, blood sample. The technician must make certain that the patient does not move its head or flick its ear, or the blood sample may be lost. After the blood sample has been obtained, firm pressure should be applied to the puncture site for approximately 15 seconds.

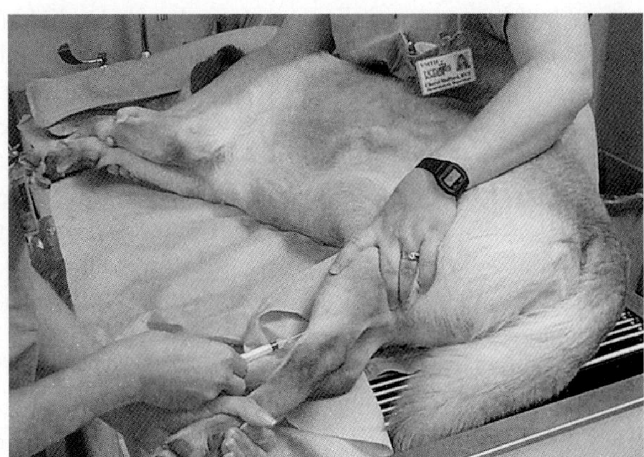

FIGURE 20-4 Dog positioned for venipuncture of the lateral saphenous vein. (From Ettinger SJ, Feldmen E, editors: *Textbook of veterinary internal medicine*, ed 6, Philadelphia, 2005, Elsevier Saunders.)

ARTERIAL BLOOD SAMPLE

One of the best ways to assess pulmonary function is through arterial blood gases. Blood gases tell us about the patient's ability to ventilate and oxygenate. Blood gases measure the partial pressure of carbon dioxide ($PaCO_2$—ventilation) and oxygen (PaO_2—oxygenation) in the blood. Blood gas measurements are performed on a pH and blood gas analyzer. In the last few years, new inexpensive point-of-care instruments have been developed to measure pH and arterial blood gases. These analyzers are cost-effective and easy to use.

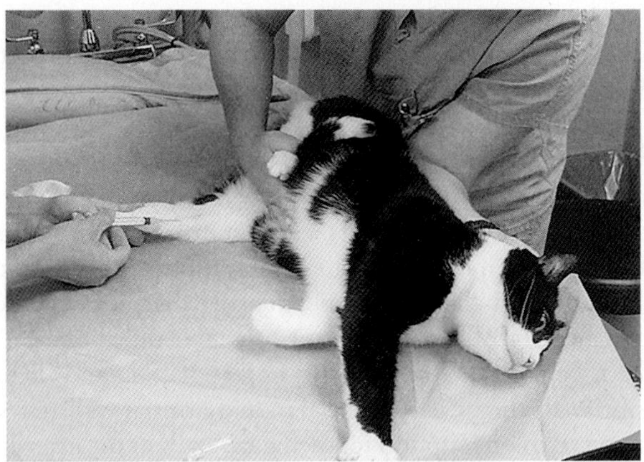

FIGURE 20-5 Cat positioned for venipuncture of the medial saphenous vein. (From Ettinger SJ, Feldmen E, editors: *Textbook of veterinary internal medicine*, ed 6, Philadelphia, 2005, Elsevier Saunders.)

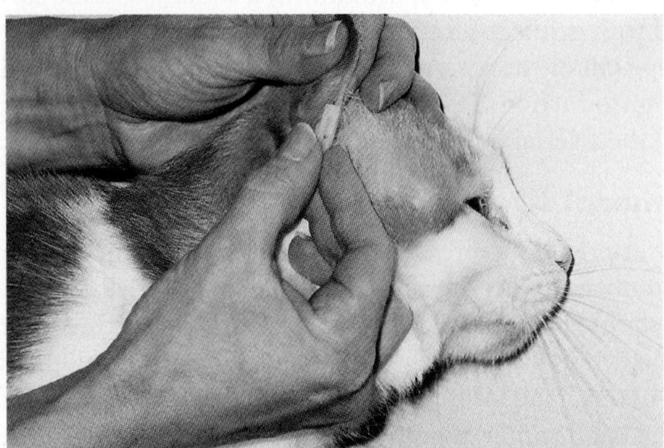

FIGURE 20-6 Collection of a peripheral capillary blood sample from the marginal ear vein of the cat with a lancet.

> TECHNICIAN NOTE One of the best ways to assess pulmonary function is through the measurement of arterial blood gases.

The collection of a blood sample for blood gas analysis entails a percutaneous puncture of an artery, such as the dorsal metatarsal or femoral artery. In the unconscious or anesthetized patient, the sublingual artery may be used. The dorsal metatarsal artery is smaller, but the interstitial connective tissues around it are "tighter" (compared with the femoral artery), which facilitates vessel positioning and minimizes postpuncture hematoma formation. The dead space of a 1- or 3-ml syringe (with a 25-gauge needle) is coated with lithium or sodium heparin (1000 U/ml); excess heparin is expelled from the syringe. In addition, a Vacutainer tube cork, alcohol swab, and a thermometer will be needed. When collecting the sample, care should be taken not to introduce air or apply excessive negative pressure, both of which can affect your PaO_2 measurement. Once the sample collection is complete, withdraw the needle and apply digital pressure over the puncture site for at least 1 minute and monitor for bleeding or hematoma formation for another 4 minutes. Air is expelled from the syringe, and the syringe is capped with the cork and placed in an ice water bath if the lab test cannot be performed immediately. Blood gas samples may stay in an ice water bath for several hours before metabolism alters the pH or blood gas values.

Dorsal Metatarsal Artery Sample

An arterial puncture is usually done with the animal in lateral recumbency; however, it can be accomplished when the animal is standing if it resents the lateral recumbent positioning. If the patient is in lateral recumbency with the hock extended, it may be helpful to tape the paw to a table or sandbag. The pulse is palpated with one or two fingers of one hand (Figure 20-7). With the bevel up, the skin and arterial wall may be punctured in one motion following the path of the artery, or a two-step fashion: skin first then artery. Watch for a back flash of blood in the needle hub and then gently aspirate a 1- to 1.5-ml sample. If the arterial puncture is unsuccessful, the needle can be inserted a bit farther. As for a venipuncture, when the needle is withdrawn, it should be done slowly and with gentle aspiration applied to the plunger in case the deep wall of the artery was inadvertently punctured during the introduction. The needle is withdrawn to its SQ position, and the arterial puncture is reattempted.

Femoral Artery Sample

The arterial puncture is performed with the animal in lateral recumbency with the down leg extended caudally. The top leg should be positioned so that it is out of the way. After the puncture site is properly prepared, the first and middle finger of one hand locates the artery, and the leading edge of the same hand can be used to slide the skin and underlying SQ tissues toward the inguinal region. The femoral artery must be immobilized properly to prevent it from rolling away from the needle. The syringe is held at a 45-degree angle over the site where the pulse is strongest. The needle is advanced through the skin as previously described and the sample collected.

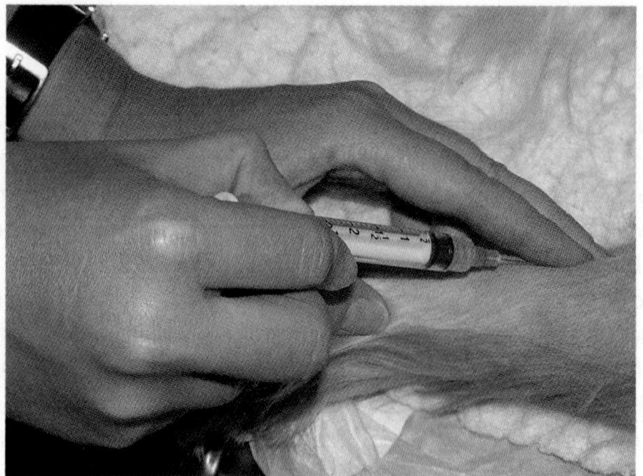

FIGURE 20-7 Palpating the dorsal metatarsal artery for arterial blood sampling.

Arterial Catheter Placement

Arterial catheters are inserted for the continuous measurement of direct arterial blood pressure and for the collection of multiple arterial blood samples. The most common artery selected for catheterization is the dorsal metatarsal artery. The dorsal metatarsal has many advantages over the femoral artery. The cylindrical nature of the tarsus allows the catheter to be taped rather than sutured. There is less risk of hematoma formation and hemorrhage because of the tight SQ tissues. It is easier to maintain the catheter position because the catheter does not move and kink in the SQ tissues.

A 20- or 22-gauge over-the-needle (OTN) catheter may be placed in the dorsal metatarsal artery. The patient is placed in lateral recumbency with the hock extended, it may be helpful to tape the paw to a table or sandbag. The insertion site is clipped and aseptically prepared. The catheter is flushed with heparinized saline. The artery to be catheterized is palpated with one or two fingers of one hand. A relief hole is made completely through the dermis with the beveled edge of the needle (without entering the artery). The catheter is positioned SQ above the artery with the bevel up. The needle tip and artery are palpated simultaneously with the finger(s) of the opposite hand. The catheter is inserted into the artery steeply at first just so that the tip of the needle penetrates the upper wall of the artery and then flat against the skin surface and parallel with the longitudinal axis of the artery so that the bevel of the needle and the end of the catheter lie in the lumen of the artery. A "flash back" of blood should be seen in the hub of the needle; the catheter is gently advanced into the artery to its full length. The needle is replaced with a T-connector and stopcock. The catheter is taped in place and flushed with heparinized saline. See the section in this chapter on securing the peripheral catheter.

The catheter is either attached to a continuous flush system or flushed with heparinized saline every 2 hours. The toes should be checked for warmth every 2 to 4 hours. If the toes are cool, the catheter will need to be removed. Catheter care is performed every 48 hours.

URINE SAMPLE COLLECTION

A urine sample may be obtained by several methods. The veterinary technician should be familiar with the various techniques. Urine is most often collected for a gross and microscopic analysis and a culture if indicated. Common collection techniques include obtaining urine from the patient as it voids, from manual expression of the bladder, from catheterization of the bladder, and by cystocentesis. Most references advocate a volume of 7 to 10 ml for a quantitative urinalysis; however, for example, smaller samples are sufficient for a culture or spot assays for ketones or glucose.

Urine collected is stored in clean, dry containers. Urine that is collected and to be cultured is collected and submitted in sterile containers. Samples that are not analyzed within 30 minutes of collection are refrigerated in secured sealed containers. Urine samples are returned to room temperature before the analysis.

VOIDED COLLECTION

A naturally voided sample is easy to collect. It is most commonly obtained from canine patients by walking the dog outdoors and catching a midstream sample. These samples are adequate for a routine urine analysis. They are not acceptable samples for a culture because these free-catch samples contain bacteria, cells, and debris from skin, hair, and the genitourinary tract. The initial void of urine contains the greatest concentration of contaminants and should be excluded from collection. Innovative collection devices can be easily made to catch the urine of a voiding dog because most dogs stop urinating if a person gets too close. Examples are devices made of a log rod or a straightened clothes hanger with a loop at one end holding a disposable cup or container.

> *TECHNICIAN NOTE* Urine is most easily obtained from a dog by walking it outdoors and catching a voided midstream sample.

Hospitalized patients can be elevated on a raised grate in a clean cage. The urine is collected from the cage floor with a syringe after the animal urinates.

Fresh voided urine samples of cats are obtained from litter boxes that are clean and empty. Lining the litter box with a plastic bag or clear plastic food wrap aids in collecting the sample. For cats that prefer litter in the boxes, shredded wax paper or specialty nonabsorbent litter made of plastic beads, such as NOSORB (Catco, Inc., Cape Coral, Fla.) are options. After the cat urinates in the litter pan, the urine is collected by a syringe or poured into a clean container.

MANUAL BLADDER EXPRESSION

Urine collected by manual expression of the bladder can be used for a routine urinalysis, but should not be used for a culture because the urine obtained by this method will contain contaminants from the lower urinary tract, skin, and hair. Bladder expression can be difficult to accomplish in some patients because the transabdominal compression causes the pressure inside the bladder to increase, but the urethral sphincter may not relax simultaneously. Manual expression of the urinary bladder is warranted in patients with neurologic impairments when the animal cannot initiate voluntary urination or does not have the ability to completely empty the bladder.

To perform manual expression of the urinary bladder, place a hand on either side of the caudal abdomen of a patient that is standing or in lateral recumbency. Isolate the bladder between the palmar surfaces of the fingers, and apply firm and steady pressure until urine is produced. In small-breed dogs and in cats, it is possible to use only one hand.

If urine cannot be produced by manual expression with moderate compression, an alternate method of emptying the bladder or obtaining a sample must be employed. Do not overexert pressure. Extreme caution is exercised in patients with an overly distended bladder in the presence of urethral obstruction, such as seen in obstructed male cats. Urethral or vesicular rupture may occur in these patients.

CATHETERIZATION

Indications for urinary catheterization include a urine sample collection, to empty the bladder, to relieve a urethral obstruction, to allow access to the urinary tract for radiographic studies, and for conditions in which an indwelling urinary catheter is indicated. Complications of urinary catheterization include a urinary tract infection, particularly with indwelling catheters or in patients with immunosuppression. Even though aseptic techniques are employed while placing the catheter, it may induce urethral inflammation and a bacterial urinary tract infection. Furthermore, urethra and bladder irritation and trauma can be other complications. Trauma from catheterization may cause increases in the red blood cell count, protein, and the number of transition epithelial cells in the sample. Urine samples may also contain contaminants from the genital region and urethra. Urine obtained by catheterization is, however, acceptable for a bacterial culture if a sample cannot be obtained by cystocentesis.

Indwelling urinary catheters are placed in patients at risk for urethral obstruction, such as male cats who have recently had urethral calculi removed, and also in patients with neurologic impairment or traumatic conditions that interfere with normal urination. Catheterization is also an important part of quantizing urinary output.

The prepuce or vulva is gently rinsed with a warm antimicrobial solution and water twice and then dried. Sterile gloves are worn to detach or connect the catheter to extension tubing or a collection system. A closed system is created by connecting the catheter to IV extension tubing that is connected to a sterile collection bag. Commercial urinary collection bags are available on the market, or an empty sterile fluid bag can be used. The collection bag serves as a urine reservoir. Its contents must be measured and emptied periodically.

Indwelling urinary catheters should be inspected for occlusion. The patient is also monitored for adequate urine output. A normotensive, normovolemic patient with intact renal function should produce 1 to 2 ml of urine per kilogram of body weight per hour. If there is not adequate urine in the reservoir bag, the patient's urinary bladder should be palpated for distention. The urinary catheter should be inspected for obstructions or kinks. The bladder can be gently compressed to determine whether urine will flow through the catheter. A small volume of sterile 0.9% saline solution can be flushed through the catheter as an attempt to relieve an obstruction.

Indwelling urinary catheters should be removed as soon as possible to reduce the inflammation of the urinary tract and catheter-induced infections. If catheterization is required long term, a new catheter should be placed every 4 to 5 days.

Urinary catheters are available in French sizes. See Table 20-1 of general guidelines for catheter selection. Note the length of available urinary catheters on the market. Many catheters that are manufactured for the human market do not possess the length for large breed canine male anatomy. Likewise, long-length catheters should be premeasured externally on the patient and excessive lengths not advanced in smaller patients because the catheter can tie itself in a knot within the urinary bladder, making withdrawal impossible without surgical intervention. Measurement therefore is made to the caudal portion of the bladder.

Male Dog

The placement of a urinary catheter in a male dog is not difficult unless a urethral obstruction exists. Polypropylene urinary catheters are rigid and easy to pass into the urinary bladder for a sample collection or to empty the bladder. If the catheter is to remain indwelling, a softer, flexible feeding tube or silicone self-retaining Foley catheter is more desirable and comfortable for the patient.

The dog is placed in lateral recumbency with the upper leg abducted. Carefully clip any long hairs around the preputial orifice. Flush the prepuce with a dilute antiseptic solution and rinse with warm sterile saline solution or water. An assistant retracts the prepuce so that the tip of the penis is exposed and maintains this position. The tip of the penis is gently washed with an antiseptic solution and rinsed with warm saline solution or water. Sterile gloves are donned. The catheter is taken aseptically out of the packaging, and the distal tip of the catheter is lubricated with a sterile water-soluble lubricant or sterile lidocaine ointment. If sterile gloves are not worn, the catheter should be kept wrapped so that it can be handled aseptically as it is advanced through the urethra. Sterile scissors can be used to cut a movable "butterfly" tab at the end of the packaging. The tab is then used to feed the catheter into the bladder and allows the operator to avoid touching the sterile catheter (Figure 20-8).

Insert and advance the catheter into the urethra. The catheter should never be forced. If the catheter cannot be passed, a smaller catheter should be used. It is common to feel some resistance at the level of the os penis, the portion of the urethra that curves around the ischial arch, and at the level of the prostate gland in older intact males. Steady gentle pressure should overcome this slight resistance. The catheter can be guided around the curvature at the ischial arch by applying digital pressure on the perineum externally or by pressing the catheter with an index finger placed in the rectum.

Urine should flow into the catheter as it enters the neck of the bladder. The catheter is then advanced 1 cm farther or to the predetermined measurement. A sterile syringe is attached to the catheter, and urine is slowly aspirated from the bladder. The first few milliliters of urine suctioned from the catheter should be discarded because it may contain contaminants and should not be submitted for a urinalysis or culture.

The catheter may be withdrawn from the bladder when the desired procedure is completed. If the catheter is to remain in

TABLE 20-1 Sizing Chart for Urethral Catheter Selection

General Guidelines for Selection of Urethral Catheters

Animal	Sex	Weight	Urethral Catheter Size
Canine	Male	<9 kg	3.5F
	Male	9-23 kg	5F or 8F
	Male	>23 kg	10F or 12F
	Female	<9 kg	5F
	Female	9-23 kg	8F or 10F
	Female	>23 kg	10F or 12F
Feline	Male	All weights	3.5F
	Female	All weights	3.5F

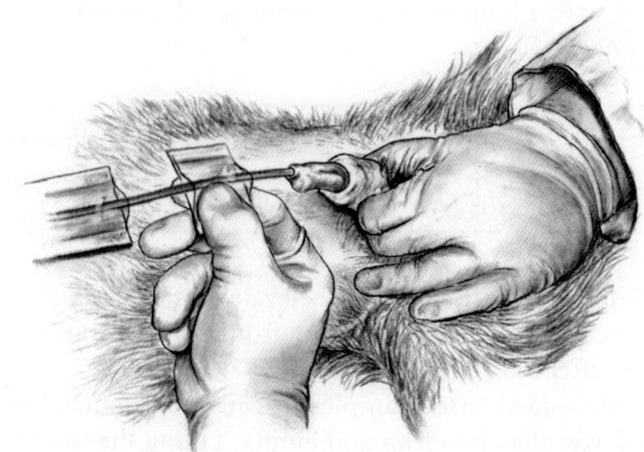

FIGURE 20-8 Urinary catheterization of a male dog. A butterfly tab is used to aseptically advance the catheter through the urethra. (From Ettinger SJ, Feldmen E, editors: *Textbook of veterinary internal medicine*, ed 6, Philadelphia, 2005, Elsevier Saunders.)

the bladder, it must be secured. If the catheter is a self-retaining Foley catheter, the appropriate volume of sterile saline or water is injected into its distal balloon cuff via the one-way valve at the proximal end of the catheter. The catheter must be secured in the following fashion (optional for a Foley catheter): Two stay-suture loops are made through the skin on two sides of the distal prepuce with 3-0 or 4-0 nylon suture material. An adhesive tape "butterfly" tab is folded around the catheter and over on itself at the location where the catheter exits the penis. A suture is then passed through one side of the tape and then through the nylon loop in the prepuce. This is repeated on the other side of the tape and the other nylon loop in the prepuce. This secures the catheter to the prepuce so that it remains in place. The stay-suture loops remain in place in the prepuce and allow catheter adjustments or changes without having to pass another needle through the prepuce.

Female Dog

Urinary catheterization is more challenging in the female dog than in the male. Catheterization can be accomplished with the patient in a standing position, in lateral recumbency, or sternal recumbency with the hind legs dangling from the end of the table. On a conscious dog, it is preferred that the dog stand with its hindquarters positioned at the end of an examination table. The assistant should support the patient under the abdomen to prevent lowering of the hindquarters during catheterization. Excessive long hairs are clipped from the vulvar area. The vulva and perineal areas are gently washed with a dilute, warm antiseptic solution and rinsed with sterile saline solution or water. The ventral vaginal floor is instilled with 1.0 ml of sterile 2% lidocaine jelly. The two techniques to pass the catheter are by visualization with the use of a speculum and a light source or a blind technique using a digit to palpate and guide the catheter. A sterile speculum is used for a visualization of the urethral orifice. Examples of a speculum include a lighted vaginal speculum, a Killian nasal speculum, an otoscope fitted with a large-diameter speculum, and a laryngoscope blade. The speculum of choice is gently inserted into the vagina. Exercise caution to avoid the clitoral fossa. After donning sterile gloves, insert the speculum vertically and straighten to horizontal when the pelvic canal is entered. With the aid of a light, locate the urethral papilla and urethral opening and insert a lubricated catheter. The papilla and urethral orifice can be found 2 to 4 cm into the vagina in most dogs (Figure 20-9). Advance the catheter until urine is obtained or at the premeasured length. If a speculum is not available, the blind technique can be performed. Wearing sterile gloves, the technician places a lubricated finger into the vagina and slides it 2 to 5 cm along the ventral floor until the papilla and external urethral orifice is located. The catheter is introduced into the vagina and guided into the urethral orifice by the finger in the vestibule. The technician will acknowledge the proper placement by palpating the catheter within the urethral orifice and not in the cranial vestibule (Figure 20-10). The catheter is advanced until urine is obtained or at the premeasured length. A sterile syringe is attached to the catheter, and gentle negative pressure is applied for the desired sample. If the catheter is to remain in place, it is ideal to select a self-retaining Foley catheter. Once the catheter is placed in the bladder, the balloon cuff is inflated with the appropriate volume of sterile saline or water to prevent the catheter from slipping out of the bladder. The catheter is then taped to the tail to prevent the dog from stepping on it. A closed collection system is placed on the free end of the Foley catheter.

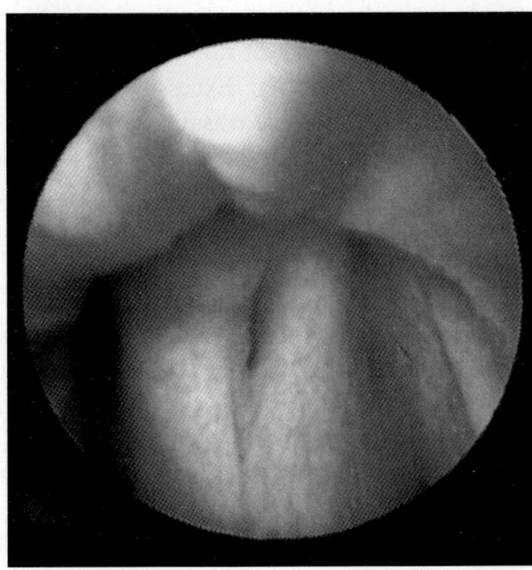

FIGURE 20-9 Urethral orifice on the ventral floor of the vagina in a female dog. (From Ettinger SJ, Feldmen E, editors: *Textbook of veterinary internal medicine,* ed 6, Philadelphia, 2005, Elsevier Saunders.)

> *TECHNICIAN NOTE* The most common reason for catheterizing a male cat is to relieve a urethral obstruction.

Male Cat

Routine catheterization of male cats for a urine collection is rare. The most common reason for catheterizing a male cat is to relieve a urethral obstruction. Catheterization of male cats will often warrant the use of sedation or a general anesthetic. Exercise extreme caution when sedating obstructed cats. Cats that have been obstructed long term are often obtunded and hyperkalemic and should therefore be

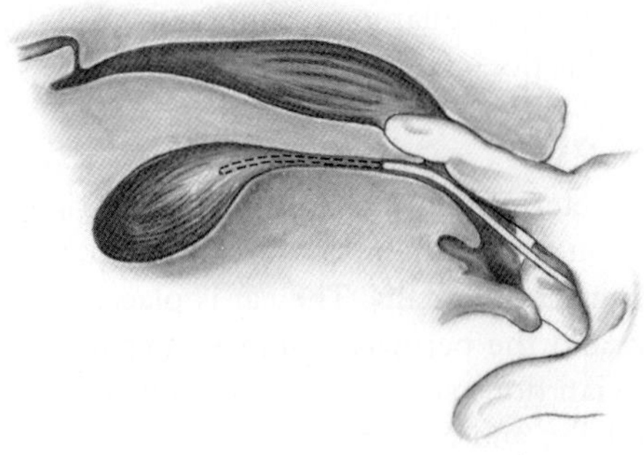

FIGURE 20-10 Urinary catheterization of a female dog. The finger in the vestibule over the urethral orifice guides the urinary catheter ventrally into the urethra. (From Ettinger SJ, Feldmen E, editors: *Textbook of veterinary internal medicine,* ed 6, Philadelphia, 2005, Elsevier Saunders.)

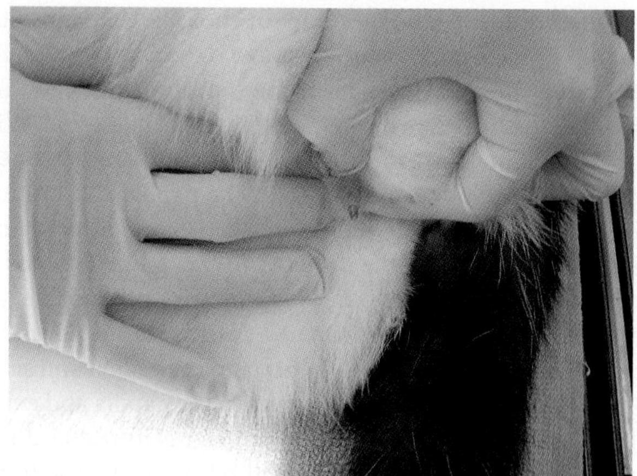

FIGURE 20-11 Retraction of the prepuce to expose the penis for feline urinary catheterization.

carefully evaluated and monitored before the administration of anesthetic agents. The cat is placed in lateral or dorsal recumbency with his hind legs drawn cranially. The prepuce is retracted to expose the glans of the penis (Figure 20-11). The perineum is prepared aseptically as described for the male canine catheterization, and the penis is extended dorsally so that the urethra is parallel to the vertebral column. An evaluation of the tip of the penis of an obstructed cat should be done at this time. Wearing gloves, first palpate the tip of the penis to check for the presence of a distal urethral plug or calculus. If an obstruction is present in the tip of the penis, gently massage the penis between the thumb and forefinger to attempt to dislodge the plug. If this is unsuccessful, proceed with catheterization. With sterile gloves, lubricate a 3.5F polypropylene or silicone tomcat catheter and pass it into the urethra. If resistance is met, the catheter is slightly withdrawn and slightly rotated as it is readvanced. If the catheter cannot be easily advanced, a small volume of sterile saline or water is injected through the catheter. Extreme care must be exercised when attempting retropulsion of a urethral calculus. Avoid excessive force or volume of fluid that could result in significant urethral trauma or rupture of the urinary bladder. Once the catheter is placed and there is good urine flow, secure the catheter in place in the same fashion described for the male dog. The cat should be fitted with an Elizabethan collar to prevent removal of the catheter and urine collection system.

Female Cat

Routine catheterization of female cats for a urine collection is also rare. Just as in the male cats, this is due to difficulty and sedation requirements. The cat is placed in sternal recumbency, and the perineal region is prepared aseptically. The technician dons sterile gloves, the lips of the vulva are pulled caudally, and a sterile 3.5F catheter is inserted into the vagina. Keeping midline, the catheter is advanced. The urethra papilla is located about 0.7 to 1.0 cm within the vagina. The catheter should pass into the urethra with little resistance. When urine flows out of the catheter, attach a syringe. Discard the first 1 to 2 ml of urine that flows and obtain a second sample for an analysis. Remove the catheter or secure the catheter in place and attach a closed urine collection system as previously described.

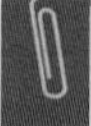

TECHNICIAN NOTE Cystocentesis is the percutaneous aspiration of urine from the bladder.

CYSTOCENTESIS

Cystocentesis is the percutaneous aspiration of urine from the bladder. A cystocentesis procedure is indicated to obtain a sterile urine sample for analysis and/or culture and sensitivity testing. The sample is free of bacteria, cells, and debris from the lower urinary tract. It also minimizes iatrogenic urinary tract infections caused by catheterization, especially in patients with preexisting diseases of the urethra and/or urinary bladder. Cystocentesis sampling can also aid in the localization of hematuria, pyuria, and bacteriuria. Cystocentesis is used as a last resort to empty an overly distended bladder when a urethral obstruction prevents urinary catheterization. The common contraindication for cystocentesis is an attempt to perform the procedure when there is inadequate urine in the bladder or when the patient resists restraint and abdominal palpation. It is recommended to wait until there is sufficient urine in the bladder or seek ultrasound guidance along with proper physical and chemical restraint, if necessary. Although statistically rare, laceration of the bladder and laceration of the bowel resulting in peritonitis add to the complication list. Patients having recent abdominal surgery or trauma, suspected bleeding disorders, pyometra, or suspected caudal abdominal or bladder tumors should not undergo cystocentesis procedures.

Supplies needed to perform a cystocentesis in canine and feline patients include a 22-gauge, 1- to 1.5-inch needle attached to a 12-ml or larger syringe. The patient can be standing, in lateral recumbency, or ventral recumbency. The site is ventral or ventrolateral insertion into the bladder wall, depending on the patient's positioning. When cystocentesis is performed, most but not all of the urine should be removed from the bladder. Excessive pressure from a full bladder might lead to extravasation of urine from the puncture site when the needle is withdrawn. On the other hand, the removal of the entire volume of urine increases the risk of contact between the needle and the bladder wall, which may result in damage to the bladder. Thus it is ideal to insert the needle a short distance cranial to the trigone region of the bladder. Having the needle a short distance cranial to the junction of the bladder with the urethra rather than the vertex of the bladder, permits the removal of urine and decompression of the bladder without the need for reinsertion of the needle into the bladder lumen. If the needle is placed in or adjacent to the vertex of the bladder, it may not remain in the bladder lumen because the bladder progressively decreases in size following the aspiration of urine. Furthermore, the technician should position the needle at a 45-degree angle through the bladder wall, creating an

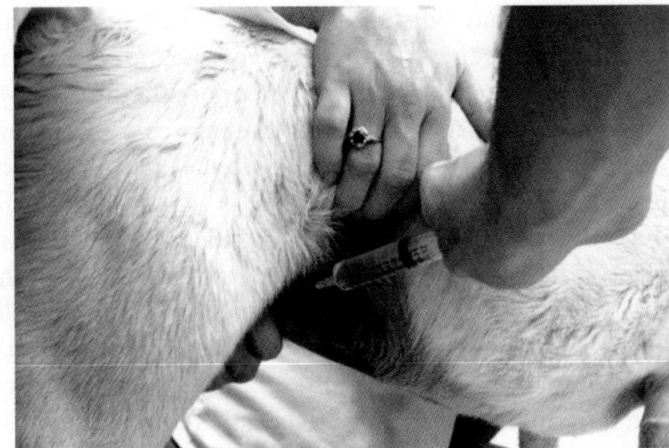

FIGURE 20-12 Performing a cystocentesis using a ventrolateral approach.

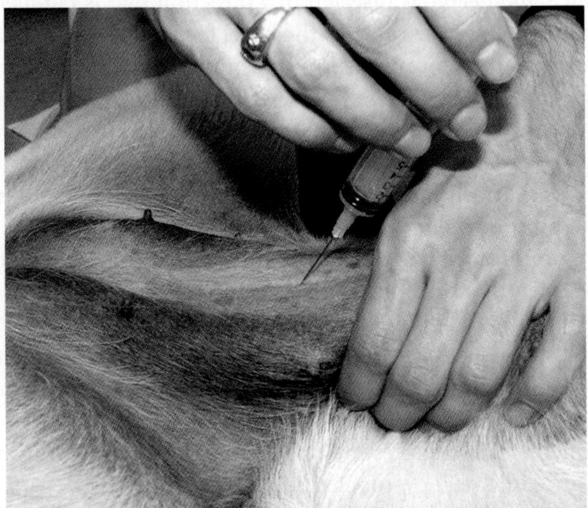

FIGURE 20-13 Performing a cystocentesis with the patient in ventral recumbency.

oblique needle tract. By directing the needle in this fashion, the elasticity of the vesicle musculature and the interlacing arrangement of the individual muscle fibers will provide a better seal of the small pathway created by the needle when it is removed. Procedures for ventrolateral (Figure 20-12) and ventral cystocentesis (Figure 20-13) procedures are outlined in Box 20-2. Note that in male dogs the prepuce and penis are diverted laterally, and the needle is inserted on the ventral midline or slightly paramedian. If blood enters the needle, another cystocentesis attempt is made with a different needle and syringe. The needle should never be redirected once it is in the abdominal cavity because accidental laceration of viscera may occur. Lastly the technician needs to remember to always release negative aspiration pressure on the plunger of the syringe before withdrawing the needle and syringe apparatus.

TECHNICIAN NOTE Remove negative aspiration pressure on the plunger of the syringe before withdrawing the needle when performing any paracentesis procedure, such as a cystocentesis.

BOX 20-2 Procedure for Cystocentesis

Procedure: Ventrolateral Cystocentesis

Patient is placed in either lateral recumbency or standing.

Palpate abdomen to determine size and location of bladder.

Hold the syringe with needle in one hand and stabilize the bladder from below with the free hand. The bladder should be pressed dorsally and caudally to immobilize it against the pelvis.

Wipe area of insertion with alcohol.

Insert the needle into the abdominal cavity and bladder, angling caudomedially at a 45-degree angle to the bladder wall and toward the trigonal region, as previously described.

Aspirate urine in the syringe. After the desired sample volume is obtained, stop aspiration or release negative pressure on the plunger of the syringe before withdrawing the needle from the bladder and abdominal cavity.

Procedure: Ventral Cystocentesis

Patient is placed in dorsal recumbency. This may take two assistants to accomplish this, especially in large-breed or deep-chested dogs.

Palpate abdomen to determine size and location of bladder.

Wipe the area of insertion with alcohol. Stabilize the bladder against the pelvis with one hand.

Insert the needle into the abdomen, staying on midline, into the bladder. The needle angle should be positioned at a 45-degree angle and directed caudally.

Aspirate desired sample. Release negative pressure on syringe plunger before withdrawing the needle.

FECES SAMPLE COLLECTION

Fecal samples are commonly collected from the ground, floor, cage bottom, or litter box after the animal defecates. Alternative methods include a lubricated fecal loop or a gloved finger inserted into the rectum to remove feces. Gross and microscopic examinations of feces for mucus, blood, intestinal parasites, and ova are commonly performed in veterinary practices. Fresh fecal samples are placed in a sealed container or bag. If the samples are to be checked for parasites but are not examined for several hours, the samples should be refrigerated. Refer to Chapter 17 for more information about a sample collection for a parasitologic examination.

THORACOCENTESIS

Thoracocentesis is a procedure, which may be used to diagnose or treat pleural filling defects (pneumothorax or pleural effusion). Air and fluid, which may compress the lungs within the pleural cavity, can be removed via thoracocentesis allowing the lungs to reexpand. Pleural filling defects should be considered when the patient has tachypnea; short, shallow breaths; respiratory distress; open-mouth breathing; and cyanosis. Chest auscultation may reveal diminished or absent breath sounds and muffled heart sounds. If a pneumothorax or pleural effusion is suspected, oxygen should be administered, and a thoracocentesis should be performed to

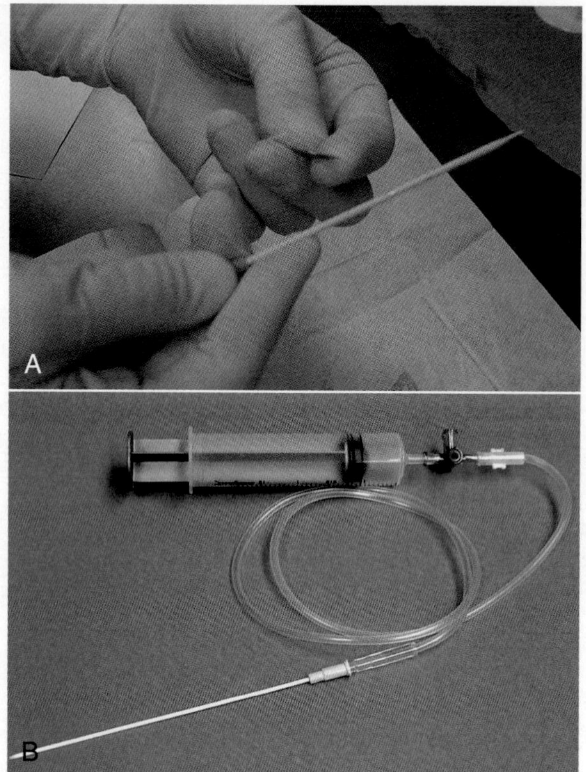

FIGURE 20-14 A, Using a blade to place two to three fenestrations in an OTN catheter. B, The setup for a thoracocentesis using a syringe, stopcock, extension tubing, and OTN catheter.

stabilize the patient before stressing the patient while taking radiographs.

> *TECHNICIAN NOTE* Pleural filling defects should be considered when the patient has tachypnea; short, shallow breaths; respiratory distress; open-mouth breathing; diminished breath sounds; and cyanosis.

The veterinary technician sets up for thoracocentesis by gathering sterile gloves, a 2-(5.08 cm) to 5-inch (12.7 cm) OTN catheter, IV extension tubing, three-way stopcock, syringe, #15 scalpel blade, 2% lidocaine, clippers, antiseptic scrub and solution, and lab tubes (EDTA and clot tubes and culture transport media). The thoracocentesis is performed at the seventh to eighth intercostal space. An area several inches in diameter is clipped and surgically prepared. It is best to prep an area on the thorax dorsally for the collection of air and ventrally for fluid. Lidocaine (1 to 2 ml) is injected into and around the intended insertion site.

After putting on surgeon's gloves, assemble the equipment. It is helpful to add two or three small fenestrations to the catheter with the scalpel blade. Attach the stopcock to the syringe, and attach the extension tubing to the stopcock (Figure 20-14). An additional extension tube can be added to the free port of the stopcock and the end of the tube placed in a bowl or graduated cylinder to collect the pleural fluid.

The patient may be standing or placed in either sternal or lateral recumbency. Intercostal vessels and nerves run along the caudal aspect of the rib, therefore the catheter will be inserted in the caudal aspect of the intercostal space and cranial to the anterior edge of rib. With the catheter perpendicular to the chest wall, the catheter is advanced gradually through the chest wall until a flash of fluid is seen in the hub or a pop is felt. The angle on the catheter is changed so that it is in the direction parallel to the long axis of the rib. The catheter is advanced a few millimeters so that the tip of the needle does not extend beyond the catheter; the needle and catheter are directed ventrally. The catheter is advanced off of the needle; the catheter is quickly attached to the extension tubing (Figure 20-15). In cats, a butterfly catheter can be used instead of extension tubing and catheter. In this instance, the needle is inserted in a direction that is parallel to the long axis of the rib with the bevel facing the thoracic cavity. If the thoracocentesis is nonproductive, it may be necessary to withdraw a few millimeters and redirect the catheter or needle. Using gentle pressure, aspirate until you achieve a slight negative pressure or until the patient's condition improves. Ultrasound can also be useful for determining the endpoint for the procedure.

Complications include: pneumothorax, lung laceration, and laceration of an intercostal vessel or internal thoracic artery leading to hypovolemia secondary to hemothorax.

Postthoracentesis nursing care includes close observation, respiratory rate measurement, auscultation of lung sounds, and measurement of oxygen saturation with a pulse oximeter. Lab samples may be submitted for cell count, total protein, cytology, biochemical analysis (e.g., triglycerides, glucose, and lactate), and culture and sensitivity.

ABDOMINOCENTESIS

Abdominocentesis is the aspiration of fluid from the abdominal cavity. The procedure is considered diagnostic and therapeutic. It can aid in the diagnosis of hemoabdomen or uroabdomen, peritonitis, or ascites (from cardiac or hepatic causes). It is not indicated when the patient has suffered a penetrating abdominal injury or is suspected of having a pyometra.

The veterinary technician sets up for the procedure by gathering sterile gloves, two to four 20- or 22-gauge needles, syringe, clippers, antiseptic scrub and solution, and lab tubes (EDTA and clot tubes and culture transport media). The abdominocentesis is performed at the right, midabdominal region so as to avoid the liver, spleen, and urinary bladder. An area several inches in diameter is clipped and surgically prepped. A local anesthetic is not usually necessary. The patient may be standing or placed in either sternal or lateral recumbency. Using aseptic technique, the needle is gently introduced into the peritoneal cavity. Gently aspirate or allow fluid to flow from the hub into the test tubes. Rotation of the needle or the placement of a second needle into the abdomen 2 cm from the first can stimulate fluid flow. If no fluid is retrieved, the procedure should be repeated in one or two

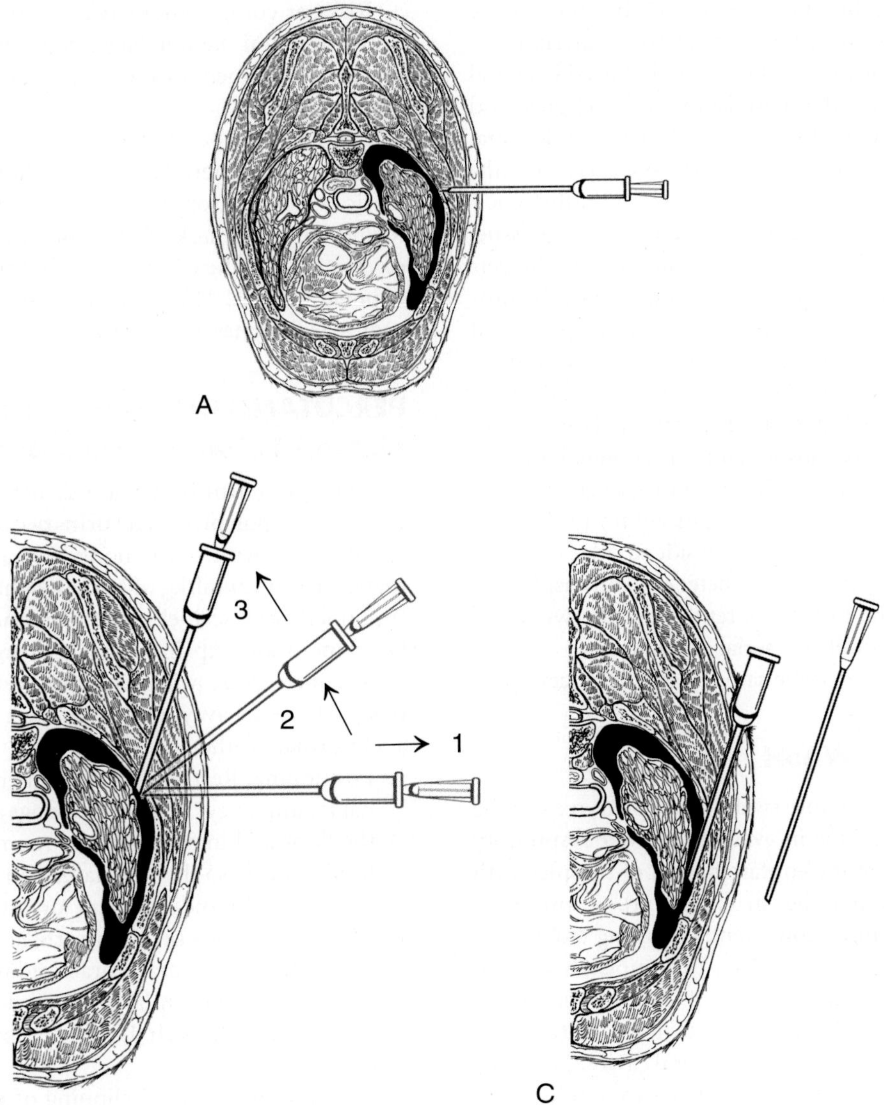

FIGURE 20-15 An OTN catheter is used to perform a thoracocentesis. **A,** The catheter is perpendicular to the chest wall and is advanced through the chest wall gradually. **B,** The needle is withdrawn slightly and the angle of the catheter changed so that it is parallel to the long axis of the rib. **C,** The catheter is advanced into the pleural space, and the catheter is attached to the extension tube, and gentle aspiration is applied. (From King LG: *Textbook of respiratory disease in dogs and cats*, St Louis, 2003, Saunders.)

other locations. As an alternative, the abdominocentesis can be performed with an 18- to 20-gauge OTN catheter.

This procedure has a high incidence of false-negative results. Large volumes (5 to 7 ml/kg) of peritoneal fluid are necessary for detection by this method. The use of a syringe can increase the likelihood of false-negative results as a result of the occlusion of the needle with omentum or viscera. If the abdominocentesis result is negative, a diagnostic peritoneal lavage may be indicated.

Postprocedure nursing care includes monitoring of vital signs, observing for pain, abdominal distention, and continued bleeding or bruising of the centesis site. Lab samples may be submitted for cell count, packed-cell volume, total protein, cytology, biochemical analysis (e.g., creatinine, potassium, bilirubin, and lactate), and culture and sensitivity.

DIAGNOSTIC PERITONEAL LAVAGE

Diagnostic peritoneal lavage (DPL) is the infusion of fluid into the abdominal and then the retrieval of the fluid for laboratory analysis. It has a higher diagnostic accuracy than abdominocentesis. The indications are the same as abdominocentesis or when the abdominocentesis result is negative. DPL has the same contraindications as abdominocentesis and is also not indicated when there is historical, physical, or radiographic evidence for the need for an exploratory laparotomy. Caution should be exercised in those patients with respiratory distress because the instilled fluid will place pressure on the diaphragm and potentially impair ventilation.

The veterinary technician sets up for the procedure by gathering a peritoneal lavage catheter or a long OTN catheter, IV administration set, isotonic crystalloid, basic surgical set, sterile gloves, lab tubes (EDTA and clot tubes and culture transport media), lidocaine, and surgical prep materials.

The bladder is emptied, and the patient is placed in lateral recumbency. The skin of the ventral abdomen is clipped and prepared caudal to the umbilicus. The skin and abdominal wall are infiltrated with lidocaine. If a peritoneal lavage catheter is used, the veterinarian may make a small midline incision just caudal to the umbilicus through the skin, SQ tissue, and superficial abdominal fascia. As an alternative, the veterinarian may make the incision just to the right of the umbilicus so as to minimize the risk of trauma to the spleen and descending colon. If an OTN catheter is used, the veterinarian will make a stab incision. The catheter is inserted through the incision and directed caudally and dorsally. The catheter is gently aspirated; if a diagnostic sample is obtained, there is no need to perform the lavage. If not, approximately 20 ml/kg of warmed crystalloid solution is infused into the abdomen. The patient is gently rocked from side to side. The fluid is allowed to flow freely from the catheter or gently aspirated. If the fluid is clear, the catheter is removed; otherwise, it is sutured in place temporally for serial evaluations.

Post-DPL nursing care is the same as abdominocentesis.

TRANSTRACHEAL WASH

It has been proven that culture swabs of the pharynx and the tonsil region are unreliable in evaluating lower respiratory tract disease because of the contamination of samples with oral flora (*Bordetella* may be an exception). Appropriate sampling is obtained more consistently by using techniques that bypass the mouth and oropharynx completely. Transtracheal lavage and aspiration provide a means to obtaining material from the tracheobronchial tree for a culture and cytology that is uncontaminated by the oral cavity. The technique is simple, clinically useful, and can be accomplished in a relatively short time period.

The veterinarian makes the decision to perform a transtracheal lavage based on clinical, radiographic, and hematologic findings. Specific examples for indications include: acute bronchopneumonia for a culture and cytology of the provocative agent; identifying the presence of inflammation and whether likely infectious or noninfectious; identification of the cells involved in inflammation (eosinophils, neutrophils, etc.); identification of parasitic eggs or larvae; identification of infectious agents (bacteria, fungi); and the identification of abnormal tracheobronchial cells (chronic inflammatory changes, neoplastic cells). The patient most likely will have a chronic productive cough. Patients may elicit a cough upon a physical examination by external palpation of the laryngeal area.

Patients who are not ideal candidates for a transtracheal lavage procedure are those with severe respiratory distress and are compromised when manipulated. Patients with coagulopathy conditions may require plasma transfusions before the procedure or may be best suited for a tracheal lavage procedure through a sterile endotracheal tube (see endotracheal lavage).

Risks or complications relative to the procedure include postprocedural hemorrhage, SQ emphysema, acute dyspnea, pneumomediastinum, pneumothorax, and iatrogenic infection.

Note that it is best to have the patient awake with a cough reflex present. Therefore heavy sedation or a general anesthetic is not advised for the procedure. An oxygen source, including a facemask, should be at hand at all times. Preoxygenation of the patient via a facemask is advised, even in eupneic animals. The following describes the common procedure techniques and approaches to tracheal lavages.

PERCUTANEOUS TECHNIQUE

Method 1: Two Catheter System

Equipment: A firm 16-gauge × 2-inch indwelling OTN catheter, a 3.5 Fr polypropylene urinary catheter, 20-ml or 35-ml syringe filled with sterile nonbacteriostatic saline (approximately 0.5 to 1.0 ml/kg of body weight), three-way stopcock (optional), #11 scalpel blade (optional), sterile gloves, 2% lidocaine drawn up in a syringe, bandage material (sterile 2- × 2-inch gauze with antiseptic gel, plus gauze roll and tape). Alternatively, you can also use a 14-gauge catheter and a 5 Fr urinary catheter. Technique:

1. Positioning. Restrain the animal either in sitting or sternal recumbency. Large-breed dogs are managed better on the floor and in a corner of a room. Extend the animal's head dorsally so that the nares point toward the ceiling.
2. Site. Cricothyroid ligament or intertracheal membrane (through trachea between cartilage rings). For the latter approach, it is generally practiced to use a lower site near the thoracic inlet in large-breed dogs to ensure that the catheter tip will reach the tracheal bifurcation (dependent on catheter length).
3. Preparation. Standard clipping of hair and surgical prep over area. Infiltrate with 2% lidocaine to level of ligament.
4. Incision. Stab incision 2 to 3 mm is optional. No suturing required. Alternatively, tenting of the skin and introduction of catheter through the skin before positioning and advancing through cricothyroid ligament or intertracheal membrane is advised.
5. Placement of catheters. Rigid 16-gauge indwelling catheter with stylet in place is placed through SQ tissues to level of the ligament. Steady the trachea with one hand, and with the other hand hold the catheter. With firm action then pass through ligament and into lumen of trachea. The catheter angle should be at 45 degrees once in the tracheal lumen, pointing down toward the tracheal bifurcation. Advance the catheter over the stylet and remove stylet. Keep a hand on the hub of the catheter at all times. Next, verify placement by attaching a syringe to the catheter in place in the trachea. Air should be easily aspirated. Pass the urinary catheter through the indwelling catheter to a predetermined level (measure from larynx to caudal border of the scapula to approximate distance to tracheal bifurcation) (Figure 20-16).

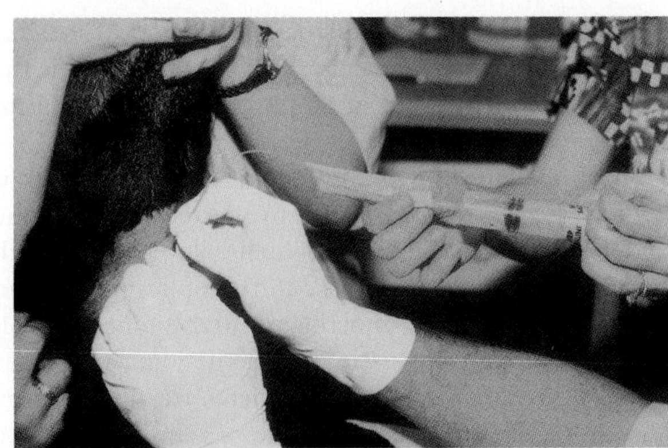

FIGURE 20-16 Percutaneous transtracheal lavage in a dog using a two-catheter system.

6. Obtaining sample. Attach a sterile 20-ml or 35-ml syringe containing no more than 10 ml of nonbacteriostatic saline to the urinary catheter. Rapidly infuse the saline and aspirate while slightly moving the urinary catheter back and forth in the trachea gently. It may be helpful to coupage the animal's chest at this time because the greatest amount of material will be aspirated if suction is applied while the animal coughs. Repeat this procedure until the fluid in the syringe is cloudy or contains visible clumps of mucus. The presence of the optional stopcock allows air to be evacuated from the syringe without disrupting the assembly. If desired, repeat aspiration procedure with a new syringe for two samples: one for a culture and one for cytology. When the procedure is complete, cap the syringe containing the lab samples with a new needle. Note: Do not expect to retrieve all of the saline infused through the catheter. A yield of 20% to 25% is common.
7. Patient monitoring. Monitor the patient closely during the sample collection. Oxygen can be delivered directly through the catheter or by facemask, if necessary.
8. Removal of catheters. Remove urinary catheter first, then the indwelling catheter. This will prevent contamination of soft tissues with the catheter tip.
9. Bandage placement. A light pressure wrap with a sterile 2- × 2-inch gauze square with antiseptic dressing applied on the entry site is sufficient. This may prevent excessive bleeding or SQ emphysema.

Method 2: Through-the-Needle Catheter

Equipment: Through-the-needle catheter, 19-gauge × 12 inches, 20-ml syringe filled with 10 ml of nonbacteriostatic saline, three-way stopcock, #11 scalpel blade (optional), sterile gloves, 2% lidocaine drawn up in a syringe, bandage material (sterile 2- × 2-inch gauze with antiseptic gel, plus gauze roll and tape). Technique:

1. Positioning, site, preparation, and incision (steps 1 to 4) are the same as in method 1.
2. Placement of catheter. The trachea is stabilized with one hand while holding the catheter with the other hand. The needle of the catheter is placed through the SQ tissues until it contacts the ligament. The angle of the needle is perpendicular to the trachea with the bevel pointing down. With a firm action, introduce the needle through the ligament, and then change the angle of the needle to 45 degrees, pointing downward toward the tracheal bifurcation. Advance the catheter through the needle, sliding the catheter down the enclosed plastic housing. Make sure the needle is pointing down toward the bifurcation. If not, the catheter may feed back up through the larynx and cause the animal to chew or gag. After advancing the catheter to its full length, withdraw the needle from the trachea and skin, leaving the catheter in place. If the needle is left in the trachea and the animal begins to move, the catheter may be severed off by the needle tip, leaving the catheter as a foreign body in the trachea. The needle guard provided with the catheter should be placed over the needle at this point to prevent injury to the animal or cutting of the catheter with the exposed sharp tip.
3. Obtain the sample and monitor the patient the same way as described in method 1 (steps 6 to 7).
4. Withdraw the catheter. Remove the catheter from the trachea and skin, making sure not to cut the catheter with the needle.
5. Bandage placement. Same as described in method 1 (step 9).

Method 3: Sterile Endotracheal Tube

Equipment: A sterile endotracheal tube suitable for the patient's size. A 5F or larger polypropylene urinary catheter, 20-ml syringe filled with sterile nonbacteriostatic saline, three-way stopcock, sterile gloves, 2% lidocaine (for feline patients to facilitate intubation and reduce laryngeal spasms), laryngoscope, gauze roll to secure endotracheal tube, anesthetic agents necessary to achieve intubation with endotracheal tube.

Technique:

1. An anesthetic plan should be established for the patient. It is necessary to induce anesthesia in the animal just to the depth necessary to cleanly place a sterile endotracheal tube. Care should be taken not to contaminate the tip of the endotracheal tube in the oral cavity. Laryngeal spasms may be reduced, especially in the feline patient, with the use of a few drops of 2% lidocaine placed on the arytenoids before intubation. Common anesthetic agents used are ketamine hydrochloride and diazepam, propofol, and thiopentathal. Monitor the animal closely. Apnea is a common finding with propofol and barbiturate induction agents. Once the endotracheal tube is placed and secured with roll gauze, the animal can be allowed to recover from the induction dose to a lighter plane of anesthesia so that a cough response is elicited when the procedure is performed. It is necessary to hold the head of the patient in case the animal begins to chew the endotracheal tube. It is ideal to position the patient in ventral recumbency.
2. Placement of catheter. With sterile gloves, advance the polypropylene urinary catheter to a predetermined

distance to the tracheal bifurcation (measure from larynx to caudal border of the scapula to approximate distance to tracheal bifurcation).

3. Obtain the sample as described in method 1, step 6.
4. Remove the polypropylene catheter.
5. Monitor and recover the patient. Provide supplemental oxygenation through the endotracheal tube as needed. Monitor patient's respiratory effort and signs for distress. Thickened mucus secretions may occlude airway. Suction endotracheal tube with an aspiration catheter, if necessary. Remove endotracheal tube when patient regains swallowing reflex and no longer tolerates the tube in place. Continue to monitor patient until ambulatory.

SAMPLE HANDLING

Tracheal lavage samples are commonly submitted for both a culture and cytologic examination. Aerobic and anaerobic cultures are often requested by the clinician. If a reference laboratory is used, check with the laboratory for their protocols on sample handling. They may provide transport media for your samples. If samples are submitted in a syringe, the needle should be sealed with a rubber stopper, the sample refrigerated, and cultured within 12 hours. If smears for cytology are made before shipment, make smears from both the supernatant and sediment after centrifugation. Be sure to make monolayer smears and air-dry. Smears may then be packaged in a protective container for shipment. If an on-site cytology examination is preferred, suitable stains are Romanovsky's or Giemsa-type stains.

CYTOLOGIC SAMPLE INTERPRETATION

The material obtained from deep transtracheal lavage procedures will include cellular elements normally lining the tracheobronchial tree; cells infiltrated from inflammatory, hemorrhagic, congestive, neoplastic, or other pathologic processes; and background material derived from mucus, proteinaceous exudate, or cellular fragments. Etiologic agents may be observed including bacteria, fungi, and parasites.

ARTHROCENTESIS

Arthrocentesis is the aspiration of fluid from a joint. The disorders involving joints are etiologically diverse, ranging from congenital, developmental, and acquired disorders to various infections and immunologic diseases. Depending on the specific disorder, joint disease may be a primary or secondary symptom. For the veterinarian to establish and differentiate the diagnosis of joint disease in the dog and cat, a synovial fluid analysis is essential.

Indications for a joint fluid analysis include persistent or cyclic fever, especially a fever of unknown origin (FUO). Indications also include patients that have generalized stiffness or limb lameness, especially associated with systemic signs of illness, fever, leukocytosis, neutrophilia, hyperfibrinogenemia, malaise, and anorexia. Arthrocentesis may be indicated in patients with a definite lameness. Palpation of localized pain and/or joint swelling may be detected along with a change in stability or range of motion involving the affected joint or joints.

Contraindications for joint fluid collection include those patients with moderate to severe pyoderma or lick granuloma. The risk is too great for potentially inoculating the joint from the infected skin. Risks and complications include trauma with or without hemorrhage into the joint, especially when degenerative changes involving the joint are present making access difficult, and when patients are uncooperative and are not immobilized. Iatrogenic contamination or inoculation of the joint is a complication prevented with good aseptic techniques.

PROCEDURE: JOINT FLUID COLLECTION OF DISTAL JOINTS IN THE DOG AND CAT

The equipment needed for arthrocentesis is: ¾-inch or 1-inch, 25-gauge needles and 3-ml syringes; 1-inch or 1½-inch, 22-gauge needles and 3-ml syringes; clean microscope slides and coverslips; sterile gloves; clippers; and aseptic surgical preparation supplies.

Patient restraint is essential. Joint fluid can sometimes be obtained from the distal joints without sedation or any type of anesthetic if the patient is not painful. However, sedation or light tranquilization and the use of analgesics are necessary for uncooperative and/or patients experiencing pain.

The patient's preparation includes placing the animal in lateral recumbency. Prepare the sites by clipping the animal's hair and proceeding with an aseptic surgical preparation.

With sterile gloves donned, palpate the joint space to be entered with the index finger. Introduce the needle attached to the syringe. Hold the syringe in such a manner that you can easily aspirate back on the plunger and you do not have to reposition your hands on the syringe. A steady hand is essential to minimize joint trauma and to produce a noncontaminated (bloody) sample (Figure 20-17). A slight negative pressure is applied to the syringe upon entry into the joint.

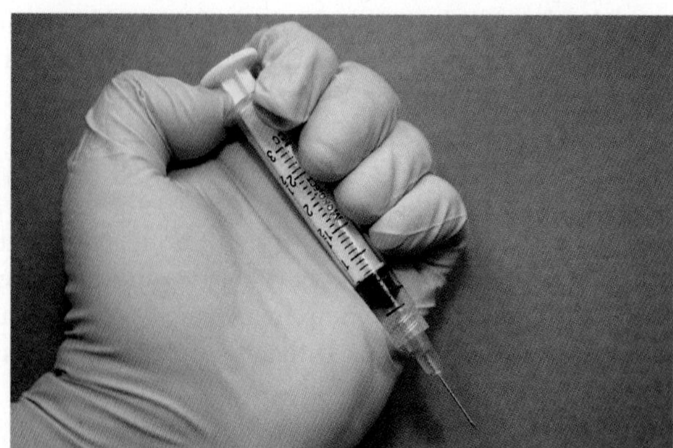

FIGURE 20-17 Hold the syringe in such a manner that you can easily aspirate back on the plunger and you do not have to reposition your hands. The shown "dart" technique is favorable with many clinicians and technicians.

The suction should always be released before withdrawing the needle. This will prevent contamination (blood) from the skin, SQ tissues, and synovium. An adequate sample is often just enough fluid to fill the needle hub.

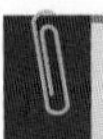

TECHNICIAN NOTE A steady hand is essential to perform arthrocentesis.

Common sites for arthrocentesis in the dog and cat include the distal joints, including the carpus, tarsus, and stifle (Figure 20-18). Techniques for these sites are as follows:

Carpus: The joint is held in flexion. The needle can be inserted in any palpable intercarpal space. The medial radiocarpal joint is most commonly used. This is to avoid the cephalic vein that courses over the carpal joint. The needle is inserted perpendicular to the skin to avoid the articulating surfaces.

Tarsus: The jock is held in partial flexion: 90 degrees with metatarsals and tibia. The joint may be approached either medially or laterally. During a lateral approach, care must be taken to avoid the caudal branch of the saphenous vein. The needle is inserted just caudal to the lateral malleolus and dorsal to the tibial tarsal bone. The needle is directed under the lateral malleolus where it forms a lip over the fibular tarsal bone. Keep the syringe and needle parallel (flat) with the metatarsal bones, heading in the direction of the animal's toes. The insertion of a ¾-inch, 25-gauge needle is often advanced to its full length before obtaining fluid in a medium-to large size dog.

Stifle: The stifle joint is partially flexed during the procedure. The patella, straight patellar ligament, tibial tuberosity, and the lateral condyle of the femur provide landmarks for tapping the stifle. These landmarks form a triangle that aid in entering the joint space. The needle is inserted just lateral to the straight patellar ligament. The needle is directed medially (approximately 35-degree to 45-degree angle) and slightly upward into the origin of the cruciate ligaments between the femoral condyles. A longer 1-inch to 1½-inch needle is usually necessary for tapping the stifle.

JOINT FLUID ANALYSIS

A single drop of synovial fluid is sufficient for gross and histologic appearance. The synovial joint analysis is complete with an additional drop of synovial fluid for a bacterial culture (aerobic, anaerobic, and *Mycoplasma*). If samples are submitted to a reference laboratory, synovial fluid can be placed in a small EDTA tube. When synovial fluid is minimal, excess EDTA should be decanted from the EDTA collection tube to minimize a diluting effect.

Gross appearance: A normal synovial fluid sample is a small volume of about 0.05 to 0.3 ml. It is colorless, clear, and viscous. An increased volume in synovial fluid can be observed in both noninflammatory and inflammatory joint diseases. A bloody tap as a result of trauma during the collection procedure can usually be distinguished from hemarthrosis because blood is incompletely mixed with the synovial fluid. Blood can be aspirated from inflamed (septic; acutely traumatized, coagulation defects) joints. A yellow-tinged fluid is a result of previous hemorrhage with release of hemoglobin pigments into the joint fluid (inflammatory, degenerative, and traumatic joint disease). If either red blood cells (RBCs) or white blood cells (WBCs) or both are in excess, an increase in turbidity or lack or clarity is observed. The viscosity can be subjectively evaluated by observing the fluid exiting the needle and onto a microscope slide. A normal joint sample will form a long string between the needle and slide. In addition, the drop on the slide should remain global rather than dispersing over the slide. A thin, runny consistency is a frequent, consistent finding in inflammatory disorders. Occasionally, poor viscosity is observed in degenerative or traumatized joints.

Culture: Aerobic, anaerobic, and *Mycoplasma* cultures are most often negative in polyarthritis. A negative culture therefore supports a noninfectious inflammatory polyarthritis disorder.

Histologic appearance: Normal values are noted in Box 20-3. Absolute cell counts can be done with a hemocytometer. Often joint fluid samples are small, and cell counts are estimated. Estimated counts are more often practiced in a clinical setting. This can be accomplished by recording the number of nucleated cells per microscopic field and comparing the counts with a peripheral blood smear of known concentration of nucleated blood cells.

Examples:

1. Blood smear = 6 WBC/high-power field (hpf) from a blood sample containing 18,000 WBC/μl
   Synovial fluid smear = 0 to 1 WBC/hpf
   Estimated count = 0 to 3000/mm^3
   The estimated count and zero to an occasional WBC observed suggest a normal joint.
2. Blood smear = 6 WBC/hpf from a blood sample containing 20,000 WBC/μl
   Synovial fluid smear = 12 WBC/hpf
   Estimated count = 40,000 mm^3

The estimated count and frequent appearance of WBCs on the smear suggest a markedly elevated nucleated cell count.

Differential: Mononuclear cells. Normal synovial fluid contains a mixture of small and large mononuclear cells. The absolute number of mononuclear cells varies considerably. Therefore the subclassification and absolute count of mononuclear cells provide limited diagnostic information. Elevations tend to occur with traumatized or degenerative joints, chronically inflamed joints, and joints with osteochondrosis.

Polymorphonuclear neutrophils (PMNs): They are generally absent or, if present, should account for less than 10% of the nucleated cell count. An increase in the relative (normal cell count) or absolute number of PMNs indicates inflammation of the synovial joint lining. Generally the more severely inflamed joints will contain a greater concentration of WBCs with a greater percentage of PMNs.

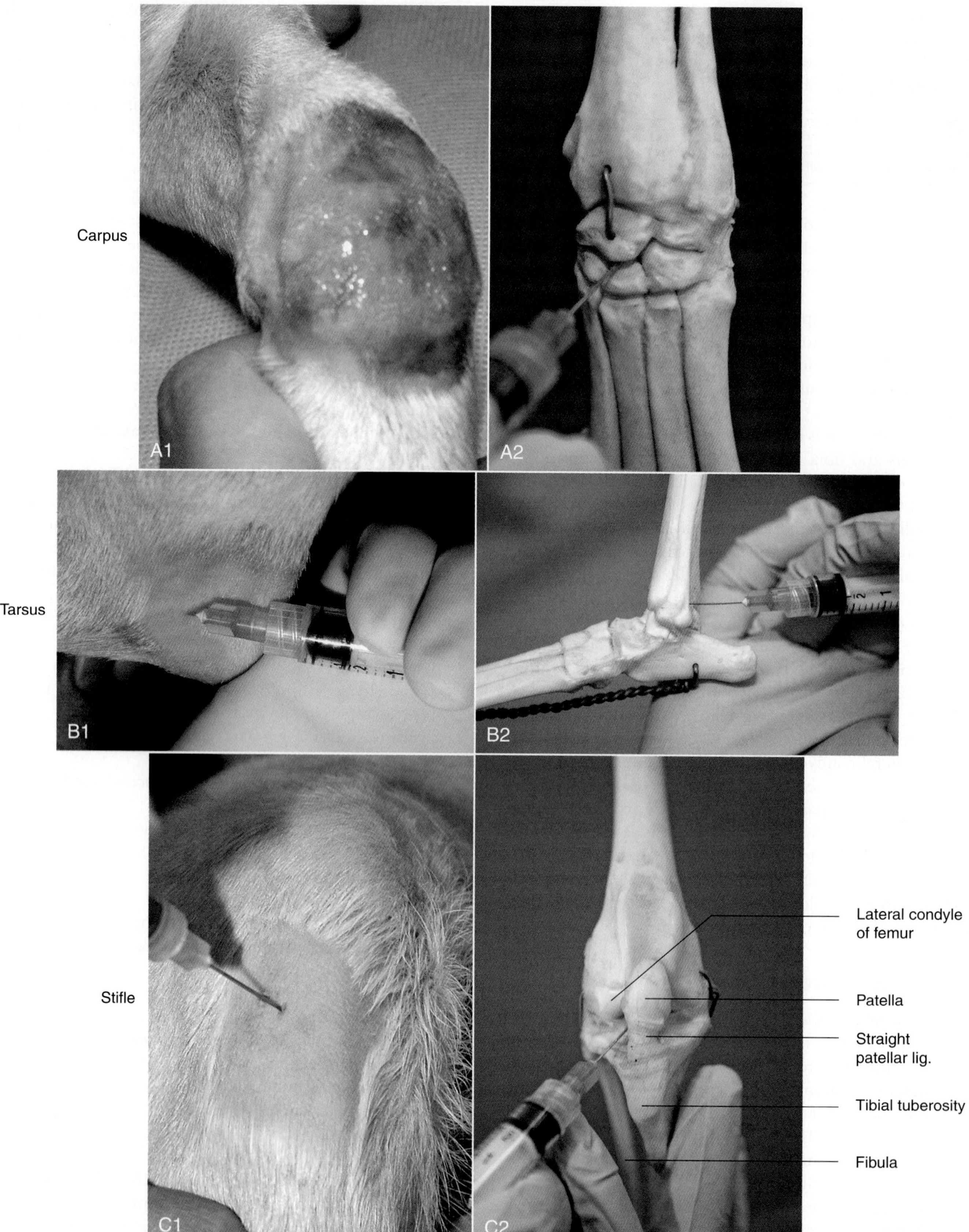

FIGURE 20-18 The carpus (**A1** and **A2**), tarsus (**B1** and **B2**), and stifle (**C1** and **C2**), are common sites for arthrocentesis in the dog and cat. Illustrations show the skeletal joint anatomy and a patient. The carpus can be approached perpendicular at any intercarpal space; **A1** and **A2**. The tarsus can be approached laterally with the needle directed caudal to lateral malleolus and keeping the syringe and needle parallel with the metatarsal bones; **B1** and **B2**. Reference landmarks for the stifle joint are the patella, straight patellar ligament, tibial tuberosity, and the lateral condyle of the femur **(C2)**.

BOX 20-3 Normal Values of Synovial Fluid

Normal Values of Synovial Fluid
Cell count
  Red blood cells—rare
  Nucleated cells/mm^3—250-3000
Differential for nucleated cells
  Mononuclear—94%-100%
  Neutrophils—0%-6%

TECHNICIAN NOTE Common sites for bone marrow aspiration include the iliac wing, femur, and humerus.

BONE MARROW ASPIRATION

Bone marrow aspiration is performed to evaluate the cells in the bone marrow. Bone marrow aspirations for cytology or a core biopsy are safe, easily performed techniques that may yield valuable information regarding the cause or pathogenesis of many disease processes.

Indications for bone marrow aspiration include patients with nonresponsive anemia, thrombocytopenia, neutropenia without suspicion of infection (i.e., sepsis), pancytopenia, suspected hematopoietic malignancies (i.e., myelogenous leukemia), polycythemia, and inappropriate RBC response, such as the presence of nucleated RBCs in peripheral blood without the presence of reticulocytes or without anemia. Patients that are suspected to have neoplasia, such as lymphoma or multiple myeloma, undergo bone marrow aspiration procedures. Clinical staging of lymphoma or mast cell tumors are also indications.

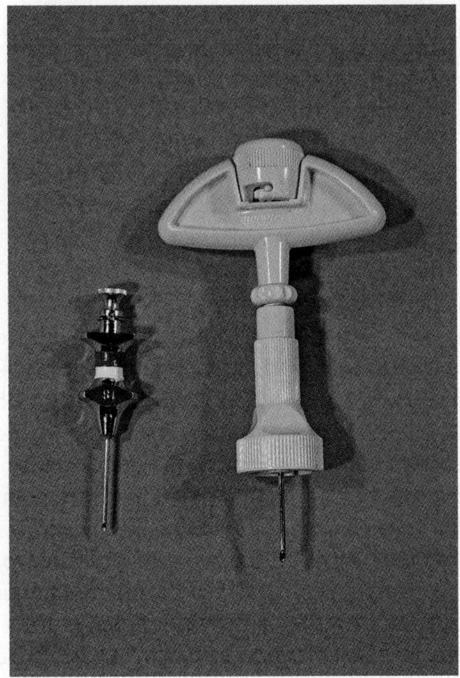

FIGURE 20-19 Bone marrow aspiration needles: 18-gauge stainless steel Rosenthal needle; 16-gauge Illinois-style needle with depth stop.

Contraindications include patients with clotting factor abnormalities and patients with severe thrombocytopenia. This is a relative contraindication and may require the administration of plasma or platelet-rich plasma before the procedure.

Complications include infection at the site if aseptic technique is not maintained, especially in leukopenic patients; damage to soft tissue structures; and hematoma formation if a coagulopathy or thrombocytopenia is present.

TECHNICIAN NOTE Stainless steel Rosenthal bone marrow aspirate needles are manufactured with a matched stylet. The stylet and needle both have a matching ID number that identifies them as a unit.

The supplies needed to perform a bone marrow aspiration procedure include a bone marrow aspiration needle. The needle may be purchased from a variety of manufacturers, but common types used in a small animal practice are 18-gauge, 1-inch Rosenthal needles with a matched stylet and 16-gauge, 15⁄16-inch Illinois needles with a matched stylet and depth stop (Figure 20-19). Other equipment required is: #11 scalpel blade, 12- or 20-ml syringe; sterile gloves; sterile drape; local anesthetic, such as 2% lidocaine in a syringe with a needle; clean glass slides; and EDTA collection tube. A complete blood count (CBC) with reticulocyte count is done within 24 hours before or after the aspirate so the peripheral and marrow cell populations can be composed. The bone marrow aspiration procedure is a very painful procedure. Heavy sedation with good analgesic agents in combination with a local infiltrate anesthetic or general anesthetic is warranted.

Bone marrow aspirations are most commonly performed in the ilium, humerus, and femur in small animal patients (Figure 20-20). The patient's size, age, and conformation determine which site is used. It is important to remember that aged patients' bone marrow is less active in long bones than flat bones, therefore in geriatric patients, a higher success rate for a cellular diagnostic sample is sought in a flat bone, such as the ilium. Bone marrow aspiration procedures are performed with strict aseptic technique. The hair over the site is clipped, and the skin is surgically prepared. Sterile gloves are worn by the person performing the aspiration. The patient's positioning for the dorsal iliac crest is sternal or lateral recumbency; lateral recumbency for the humeral head; and lateral recumbency for the intratrochanteric fossa of the femur.

ILIAC BONE MARROW ASPIRATION

The patient is placed in sternal or lateral recumbency with its legs drawn forward to better palpate the wings of the ilium. The hair is clipped from the procedure site, and the skin is prepared for aseptic surgery. Local infiltration of 2% lidocaine is done by injecting into the skin, SQ tissue, and periosteum of the bone. A stab relief incision is made into the skin over the

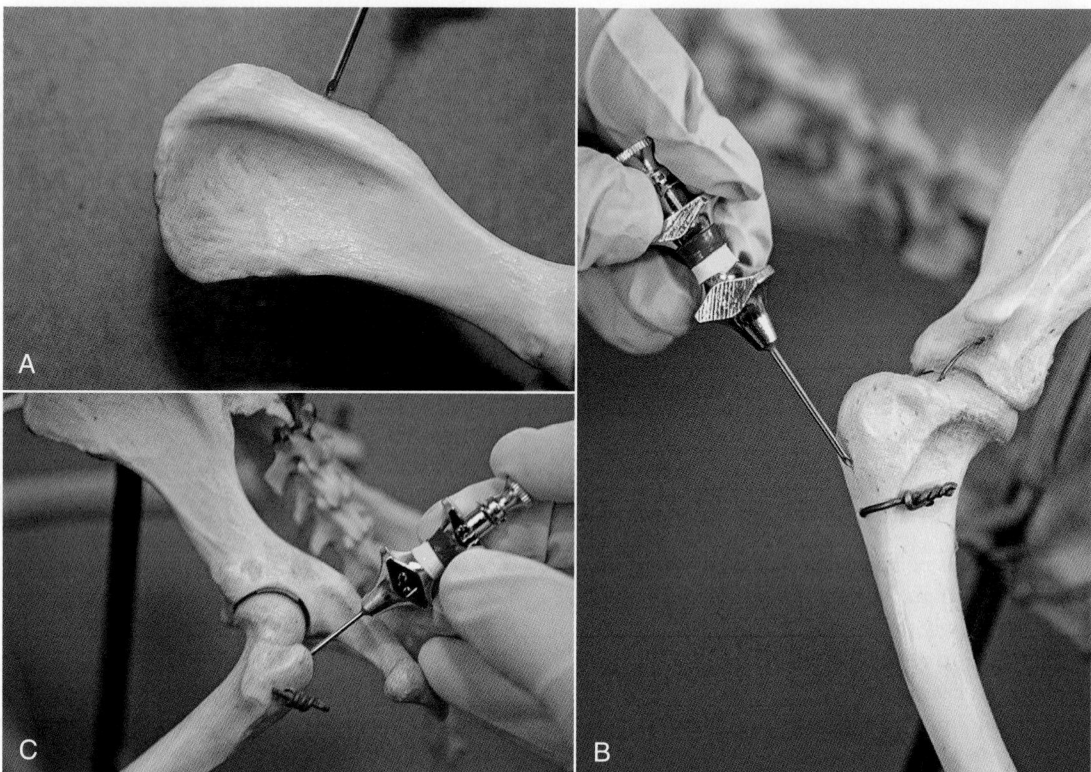

FIGURE 20-20 Common sites for bone marrow aspiration in the dog and cat patient: **A,** wing of the ilium, **B,** the greater tubercle of the proximal humerus, and **C,** the trochanteric fossa of the femur.

iliac crest with a #11 scalpel blade. The bone marrow needle's stylet is inspected, confirming that the stylet is perfectly occluding the distal tip and in place or the needle will become plugged with cortical bone. If a Rosenthal needle style is used, the operator must hold the needle in such a fashion that the stylet does not back out by placing counter pressure on the stylet with an index finger or palm of the hand. One hand is placed on the ilium to stabilize it. The bone marrow needle with its stylet in place is advanced through the skin incision and onto the bone. The needle is advanced into the bone by rotary motion, twisting the wrist only in a clockwise, counterclockwise motion. The goal is to keep a single axis and to avoid wobbling of the needle. This is accomplished by keeping the elbow immobilized and using wrist action only. Considerable force is typically required. The needle is advanced into the bone 1 to 1.5 cm or until the needle is well seated.

Once the needle is well seated and stabilized in the bone, the stylet is removed from the needle and placed on a sterile field. A 12- or 20-ml syringe is firmly attached to the bone marrow needle, and negative pressure is applied to the syringe plunger. The aspiration should be very quick and negative pressure immediately discontinued once 0.1 to 1.0 ml of sample is obtained. The actual aspiration of the marrow fluid is the most painful for the patient, and the conscious, sedated patients may show signs of discomfort. The restrainers of unanesthetized patients should be prepared for the patient to react with a yelp, cry, or movement.

Once the bone marrow enters into the syringe and negative pressure is released, the syringe is removed from the bone marrow needle. The sterile stylet is replaced into the needle. Immediately make six to eight fresh smears. This is accomplished by placing a drop of the sample on tilted microscope slides or by putting some of the sample into a Petri dish and tilting the dish so that the blood separates from the marrow particle. The bone marrow is usually more viscous than blood, contains bony spicules, is a deeper red, and contains fat globules (Figure 20-21). The bone marrow particles can be picked up with a tip of a hypodermic needle or microhematocrit tube and transferred to a microscope slide. A pull slide is made with each sample. A pull slide is made by placing a clean glass slide on top of the slide containing the sample and pulling the slides apart to create two slides for a cytologic analysis. The excess bone marrow sample should be immediately placed

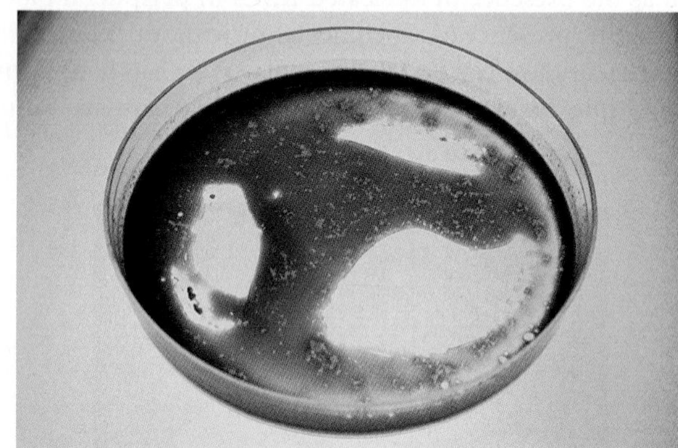

FIGURE 20-21 Bone marrow aspirate sample displayed in a Petri dish. Note the bone spicules.

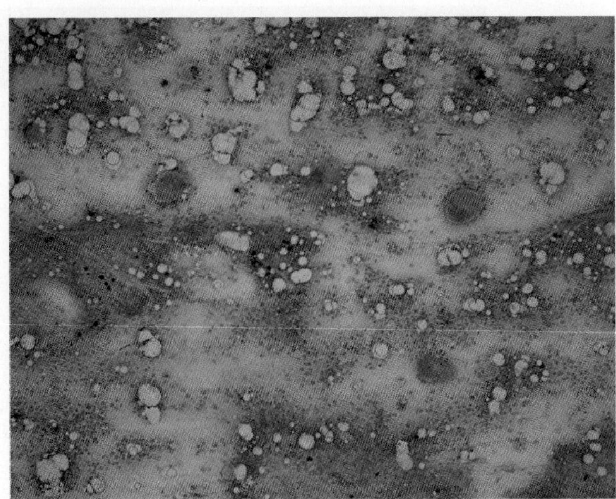

FIGURE 20-22 Microscopic view of a bone marrow aspirate under low 10x power stained with new methylene blue. Note nucleated precursor cells and large megakaryocytes.

in an EDTA collection tube. It is helpful to do this exercise simultaneously, having someone making slides and another pair of hands placing the excess sample into the anticoagulant EDTA collection tube. If this collaboration cannot be done, it is recommended to have the collection syringe precoated with an anticoagulant, such as 2.5% to 3.0% EDTA solution.

While the patient still has the bone marrow aspiration needle in place, quickly take one of the pull slides and examine it to determine if bone marrow elements are present (Figure 20-22). This screening can be done with a drop of new methylene blue stain and a coverslip. If the sample is not adequate, another sample can immediately be obtained. The patient will therefore not have to be rescheduled for another invasive procedure, and the veterinarian will not be delayed in getting a result and diagnosis.

Once the sample is determined to be adequate, the bone marrow needle is removed in the same fashion it was placed, by clockwise, counterclockwise motion, pulling out it. Once removed, pressure is held on the site until hemostasis occurs.

The dried unstained smears are packaged in a protective container for a reference laboratory along with the excess sample in the EDTA collection tube.

HUMERAL BONE MARROW ASPIRATION

The humerus is an excellent bone site for marrow aspiration. The craniolateral aspect of the greater tubercle of the proximal humerus is the insertion site. The advantage of this site is that it has less tissue, fat, and muscle overlying the bone. When a patient is heavily muscled or overweight, the dorsal iliac crest is difficult to palpate, and this site is always palpable and superficial in animals with this conformation. The humerus is also advantageous to use in animals with narrow iliac wings, such as small toy-breed dogs and cats.

The patient is placed in lateral recumbency, and the presenting proximal humerus is clipped, surgically prepped, and infiltrated with a local anesthetic. The bone marrow needle is placed perpendicular to the humeral shaft as the elbow is flexed, and the shoulder is rotated or abducted externally. The assistant holding the position of the limb should concentrate on using pressure points, such as the elbow and the blade of the scapula, as the operator advances the needle with constant pressure and force. Squeezing the soft tissues while trying to maintain the position of a limb often results in severe bruising in the thrombocytopenic patient. The techniques for site preparation, needle placement, bone marrow aspiration, and slide preparation are identical to those described for the iliac bone marrow aspiration.

FEMORAL BONE MARROW ASPIRATION

The femur can be used in small-breed dogs and cats for bone marrow aspiration. Site preparation, needle placement, marrow aspiration, and slide preparation procedures are identical to those described for bone marrow aspiration from the ilium.

The patient is placed in lateral recumbency, and the presenting hip region is surgically prepared over the palpable greater trochanter of the femur. The needle placement is within the trochanteric fossa of the femur on the medial aspect of the greater trochanter of the proximal femur. Once aseptically prepped, 2% lidocaine is injected into the skin, SQ tissue, and periosteum over the trochanteric fossa. A stab incision is made through the skin. The operator grasps the femur, and the hip is held in a flexed position. The bone marrow aspiration needle is introduced medial to the greater trochanter and parallel to the femoral shaft. Once the needle is well seated within the shaft of the femur, the sample is taken and processed as described previously.

FINE-NEEDLE ASPIRATION

Fine-needle aspiration is a quick procedure performed routinely in veterinary practices to acquire a sample of fluid or tissue cells from an accessible mass from the dermis, viscera, or a lymph node. These cytologic samples aid in differentiating between inflammation and hyperplasia of structures, such as lymph nodes or mammary glands. They also help to differentiate between inflammation, neoplasia, and hyperplasia of the skin, SQ, or other superficial masses. Complications of fine-needle aspiration procedures include minor hemorrhage, tissue damage, and infection.

Supplies needed to perform a fine-needle aspiration include 25- to 22-gauge needles. The needle lengths are determined by the depth of the mass to be sampled. Other supplies are 3- to 6-ml syringes, clean glass microscope slides, and surgical scrub or alcohol for skin preparation.

The animal is restrained so that the mass to be aspirated is accessible. The skin over the underlying mass is either surgically prepped (for visceral aspirates) or wiped with alcohol to remove superficial contaminants. Secure the mass with a free hand and introduce a 22-gauge needle into the mass with the other. In large masses, the needle is directed into the peripheral parts of the lesion to avoid the necrotic center. The needle is redirected within the tissue once or twice and is removed. A syringe containing at least 1 ml of air is attached to the needle. Depress the syringe plunger quickly because the expulsion should be rapid and forceful to remove all the material from the needle lumen onto a clean microscope slide. If the aspirated material is liquid, a push slide can be made; if the material is more viscous, a pull smear is made.

An alternate technique for performing fine-needle aspiration employs the use of a 3- to 12-ml syringe attached to the needle. After the needle is inserted into the mass, suction is applied to the syringe plunger to aspirate cells into the needle. During the process, the needle may be redirected once or twice; however, the negative pressure is released before withdrawing the needle from the mass. The needle is then detached from the syringe, and the operator aspirates 1 to 2 ml of air into the syringe and reattaches the air-filled syringe onto the needle. The syringe plunger is then forcefully depressed as described before, expelling the contents of the needle onto a clean microscope. Slides are made either by a push or pull technique.

VAGINAL CYTOLOGIC SAMPLING

The collection of vaginal cytology is a very quick and easy procedure to accomplish. Vaginal cytology is performed to determine the patient's present stage in the estrous cycle for breeding purposes or to collect samples to help determine the cause of vaginal disease. The patient is placed in a standing position with support under her abdomen so that she does not lower her hindquarters or in lateral recumbency. The vulva is gently wiped with warm water. The labia are separated with a gloved hand, and a cotton swab is carefully inserted and rolled against the vaginal wall. The cotton swab is removed from the vagina and is rolled onto a clean glass microscope slide for a cytologic examination.

ADMINISTRATION OF MEDICATION IN THE SMALL ANIMAL

Multiple routes exist for the administration of fluids and medication (Box 20-4). The route used depends on many factors, including, but not limited to, the patient's condition and temperament, type of medication or fluid, urgency involved in administering the fluid or medication, cost, ease of administration, and whether a systemic or local effect is desired.

INTRAVENOUS ADMINISTRATION

Many medications are administered directly into a vein. IV injection is used for drugs or fluids that must rapidly reach high blood levels or that would be irritating to tissue or insufficiently absorbed if given by another route (Box 20-5). Certain anesthetics, chemotherapeutic agents, anticonvulsant drugs, and drugs used in cardiopulmonary resuscitation are given IV. If an extremely rapid onset of action is required, the IV or intraosseous route is chosen.

BOX 20-4 Routes of Fluid or Medication Administration

- Intravenous
- Subcutaneous
- Intramuscular
- Intradermal
- Intranasal
- Intratracheal
- Intraosseous
- Intraperitoneal
- Topical ophthalmic
- Aural
- Transdermal
- Intrarectal
- Oral
- Per os
- Oroesophageal tube
- Orogastric tube
- Nasoesophageal tube
- Nasogastric tube
- Pharyngostomy tube
- Esophagostomy tube
- Gastrostomy tube
- Duodenostomy/jejunostomy tube
- Intramammary (primarily large animal)

BOX 20-5 Intravenous Injection

- Occlude the vessel with digital pressure or a tourniquet.
- Grasp the extremity and pull the skin tautly in a distal direction.
- Wipe an alcohol-soaked cotton ball over the hair and skin covering a distal section of a peripheral vein.
- Insert a 22- to 25-gauge needle attached to a syringe with the bevel facing up through the skin and into the vein.
- Aspirate a small volume of blood into the syringe to ensure that the needle is within the vein.
- Release the pressure from the vein.
- Inject the contents of the syringe into the vein.
- Remove the needle and apply digital pressure to the needle insertion site for 30 to 60 sec until hemostasis occurs.
- If a hematoma occurs when the needle is inserted, remove the needle and apply digital pressure over the hematoma until the bleeding subsides. Make another injection attempt either proximal to the initial site or in a different vein.

The most frequently used sites for IV injection in the dog are the cephalic and lateral saphenous veins. Cats are most often given IV injections in the cephalic, medial saphenous, and femoral veins. The jugular vein is used to administer injections in both large and small animals if an IV jugular catheter is in place.

When an IV injection is administered, the vessel is occluded with a tourniquet or digital pressure. Air bubbles are expelled from the syringe before the needle is inserted into the vein. The skin and hair over the vein is swabbed with

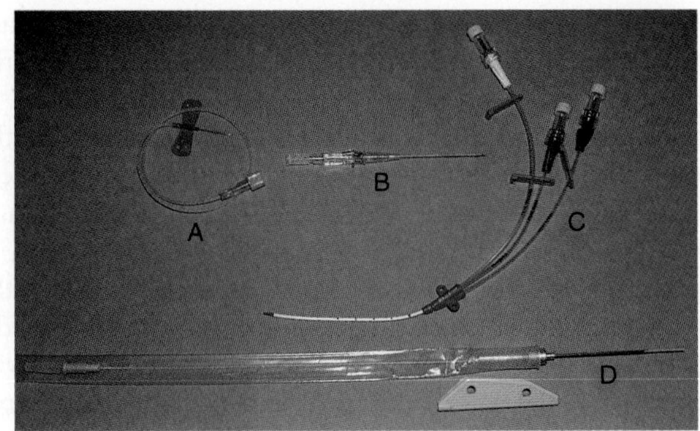

FIGURE 20-23 Examples of four types of IV catheters. Catheter *A* is a butterfly; catheter *B* is an OTN; catheter *C* is a multilumen (Triple-lumen); and catheter *D* is a through-the-needle.

alcohol, and the needle is inserted into the vein. Blood will appear in the needle hub when the needle penetrates the vein, but IV placement is confirmed by aspirating blood back into the syringe. Pressure is released from the vein, and the syringe contents are injected. The needle is withdrawn, and firm pressure is applied to the venipuncture site until hemostasis occurs.

Intravenous Catheter Placement

Patients often require temporary venous access for medications, fluid, and electrolyte replacement therapy or transfusion of blood products. Medications and fluids with osmolalities less than or equal to 600 mosm may be safely administered via a peripheral vein. Site selection depends on the available vessels, condition of the vessels and patient, expense, and the urgency of the situation. The veterinary technician should be familiar with the types of catheters, placement techniques, and catheter maintenance.

A variety of catheters are commercially available. The length and gauge (diameter) of the catheter to be used are dependent on the species and size of the patient and the veins available and their condition. There are four general categories of IV-access devices. They include the winged needle (butterfly), over-the-needle, through-the-needle, and the multilumen catheter (Figure 20-23).

The winged needle is for short-term use when the animal is not moving around very much. Applications might include blood collection or the administration of nonirritating medications. It is easy for the indwelling sharp needle to puncture the vessel wall, allowing for SQ infiltration of fluids or medications. The needles have plastic wings on the shaft to facilitate placement or taping in place. Plastic tubing of various lengths extends from the needle to the syringe connector port. The OTN catheter is the most common type of catheter used today. It is used primarily for peripheral vein catheterization. This type of catheter is fitted outside or over a steel needle. The needle point extends a millimeter or so beyond the catheter tip for entry into the vein. Catheters passed through the needle are called through-the-needle catheters. Through-the-needle catheters are usually longer than OTN catheters (8 inches to 12 inches) and are used primarily in the jugular vein. A plastic sleeve to prevent contamination protects the catheters. Once the catheter is placed and the needle withdrawn from the insertion site, a needle guard is placed. The needle guard protects the needle from sticking the animal and shearing the catheter, but can be fairly bulky in the small animal. Multilumen catheters have two to three separate lumens in one catheter. Multilumen catheters allow simultaneous infusions at one catheter site. Though one catheter is placed, the multilumen catheter provides the same functions as two to three separately introduced single-lumen catheters. The catheter placement is usually completed percutaneously with a guidewire. Multilumen catheters are more expensive than the commonly used IV catheters.

Although there might be slight variation, the setup for venous (peripheral and jugular) or arterial catheterization is essentially the same, no matter what type of catheter is being placed. The veterinary technician will gather a catheter (butterfly, OTN, through-the-needle, or multilumen); a syringe filled with heparinized saline flush; injection cap or T-connector; tape and/or nonabsorbable suture; bandage material; clippers; and antiseptic scrub and solutions.

Peripheral Vein Catheterization

Common peripheral insertion sites include the cephalic, medial (cat) and lateral (dog) saphenous veins. There is a tendency to insert a lateral saphenous catheter in the vessel as it traverses the hock; as an alternative, it might be preferable to insert the catheter in the lateral saphenous vein on the caudal surface of the leg because it is easier to secure in this location.

The area of the insertion site is generously shaved. A surgical preparation is performed with antiseptic scrub and solution. Aseptic technique is important to prevent indwelling catheter related infection. A facilitative incision or relief hole reduces the skin tension and friction against the catheter. The relief hole may be made with a #11 blade or a 20-gauge needle. A 0.5- to 1-mm incision is made directly over the vessel extending through the dermis.

> *TECHNICIAN NOTE* A facilitative incision or relief hole reduces the skin tension and friction against the catheter; it is indicated in severely dehydrated patients or patients with tough skin.

It is indicated in severely dehydrated patients or patients with tough skin. Care should be taken to avoid the vessel when making the relief incision. Local anesthetic blocks are rarely needed. The vein is occluded upstream of the insertion site by a tourniquet or an assistant. The distal portion of the leg is grasped in the palm of the hand of the veterinary technician, and the leg is extended to tense and immobilize the vein. It is not recommended to use the thumb to stabilize the vein since this compress and collapses the vein. Flexion of the carpus will increase the stretch on the vessel and improve the vessel immobilization in achondroplastic breeds. With the bevel up, the catheter is inserted through the skin or relief hole at approximately a 15-degree angle. The catheter is advanced into the vessel; when blood appears in the flash chamber (hub), the needle and catheter are advanced together as a unit for an additional 1 to 4 mm. This will ensure that the end of the catheter is entirely inside the lumen of the vessel. Then while holding the needle steady and maintaining the longitudinal tension on the leg, the catheter is then advanced off of the needle and into the vessel lumen. The catheter is capped with an injection cap or T-connector and flushed with heparinized saline. A ½-inch (1.3 cm) strip of adhesive tape is wrapped around the circumference of the hub of the catheter and leg to secure the catheter. A 2 × 2 gauze pad is placed over the insertion site. A 1-inch (2.54 cm) second piece of tape is placed sticky side down underneath the catheter and then wrapped around the leg. Roll gauze is wrapped around the catheter and leg proximal and distal to the insertion site. Finally, tape is applied to the top and bottom of the gauze where it interfaces with the skin.

Jugular Vein Catheterization

There are several advantages to the placement of a jugular catheter over a peripheral catheter: (1) Administration of fluids that have an osmolality greater than 600 mosm/L and constant rate infusions of drugs known to cause phlebitis, such as diazepam, pentobarbital, and mannitol; (2) measurement of central venous pressure (CVP); (3) facilitates frequent aspiration of blood samples; (4) necessary for the administration of total parenteral nutrition (TPN).

> *TECHNICIAN NOTE* Fluids or drugs that have an osmolality greater than 600 mosm/L should be administered through a jugular vein.

The key to a successful jugular catheter insertion is the patient's positioning and vessel immobilization. If the patient is not positioned properly, it can be difficult to visualize and immobilize the vein. Jugular catheters are placed antegrade with the tip of the catheter always directed toward the heart. The placement of the jugular catheter is best done with the patient in lateral recumbency. The patient's head is extended and its forelimbs positioned caudally by an assistant. Sedation of uncooperative patients is recommended. The placement of a bag of fluids, a sandbag, roll gauze, or rolled towels under the neck may be helpful (Figure 20-24). This flexes the neck and helps to make the vessel more accessible. The assistant should hold off the vein by pressing into the thoracic inlet, this should cause the vein to engorge and "stand up." The other end of the vein is immobilized by extending the head.

> *TECHNICIAN NOTE* The placement of a bag of fluids, a sandbag, or rolled towels under the neck helps to make the vessel more accessible for a jugular catheter placement.

The area of the insertion site is generously shaved. A surgical preparation is performed with antiseptic scrub and solution. To place a through-the-needle catheter, the catheter needle should be introduced SQ. The needle tip is positioned over the vein and aligned as close as possible to the longitudinal axis of the vein. The needle tip is inserted into the vein; it may be necessary to angle the needle somewhat to pick up the superficial vein wall. Once it is estimated that the entire needle tip is within the lumen of the vein, the needle is stabilized, and the catheter is threaded into the vein (Figure 20-25). Once the catheter is fully advanced into the vein, apply pressure over the venous puncture site and back the needle out. Once the bleeding has stopped, secure the needle guard around the needle. The plastic protective bag and stylet are removed; the catheter is aspirated to confirm its proper placement and to clear the catheter of air. It is then flushed with heparinized saline. The catheter should be capped with an injection cap or T-connector and again flushed with heparinized saline. The catheter is sutured or stapled close to the insertion site. The insertion site is then covered with a sterile 2- × 2-inch gauze pad and the catheter site is bandaged.

The Seldinger guidewire technique facilitates the placement of a multilumen catheter. The Seldinger technique uses a smaller introducing catheter, or trocar, and a guidewire to safely gain venous access. Before beginning the procedure, the required distance for catheter insertion is premeasured. The aim for a jugular catheter is to have the tip of the catheter lying within the thoracic cavity, just cranial to the right atrium. This distance is commonly estimated by measuring the distance

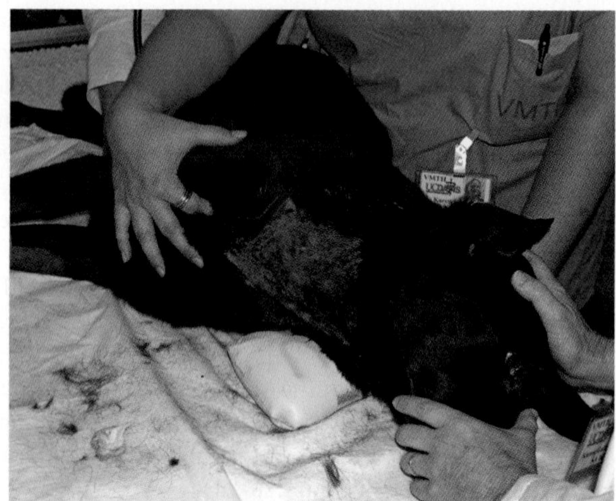

FIGURE 20-24 A sandbag placed under the neck facilitates jugular catheter placement by flexing the neck and providing better access to the vessel.

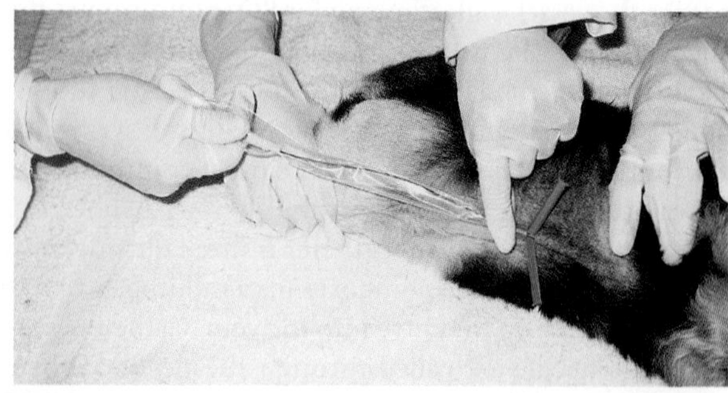

FIGURE 20-25 The catheter is threaded into the jugular vein through a protective sleeve.

from the intended insertion site to the caudal edge of the triceps muscle. The insertion site is widely clipped and surgically prepared in a routine manner. The infiltration of the intended insertion site with local anesthetic is recommended in awake animals. The technician wears sterile gloves; in some circumstances, a hat, mask, and sterile gown may also be appropriate. The distal port of the multilumen catheter is identified; this is the port that terminates at the very tip of the catheter and will be the one through which the guidewire is passed. All ports of the multilumen catheter are flushed with heparinized saline, and all ports with the exception of the distal port are capped. The insertion site is draped; this is important because the guidewire is long and flimsy and the risk for guidewire contamination is high if draping is not sufficient.

> *TECHNICIAN NOTE* The required distance for a jugular catheter insertion is estimated by measuring the distance from the intended insertion site to the caudal edge of the triceps muscle.

A small relief incision is made through the dermis with a scalpel blade at the site of the intended insertion. The introducing needle or short OTN catheter enters the skin through the relief incision and is inserted into the underlying vessel. The guidewire is threaded through the inserting needle or catheter into the vein (Figure 20-26). The distal end of the wire has a flexible J-tip to prevent puncturing through the vessel wall. In some instances when it is difficult to pass the J-tip along the vessel, it may be advantageous to use the straight end of the guidewire instead. To prevent embolism of the guidewire, the technician should retain a hold of the wire at all times. Once the guidewire is inserted approximately ⅔ to ¾ of its length into the vessel, the introducing needle or catheter is removed, and a vessel dilator is threaded over the wire, the skin entry site may need to be enlarged with a #11 blade to accommodate the dilator. The dilator is grasped near the distal tip, and using a forward twisting motion, the dilator is advance into the vessel (Figure 20-27). To minimize blood loss, pressure is applied over the insertion site with aseptic gauze pads as the dilator is removed leaving the guidewire in place. In the case of a sheath introducer, the dilator is incorporated in the sheath and is removed once the sheath is in place. The multilumen catheter is threaded over the guidewire until the proximal end of the guidewire protrudes from the hub of the catheter. If an excessive length of the guidewire was advanced into the vessel, it will be necessary to back the guidewire out of the vessel to achieve this. Finally, while holding the proximal end of the guidewire, the catheter is advanced into the vessel the desired distance as determined by a premeasurement (Figure 20-28). The wire is removed, and all ports are aspirated to remove any air and to ensure that blood is easily drawn through the catheter. If necessary, the catheter may be repositioned to allow the effective aspiration of blood; aseptic technique must be maintained throughout this time. All ports are then flushed with heparinized saline. The catheter is then sutured in place; the insertion site is covered by aseptic gauze and bandaged appropriately.

Intravenous Catheter Maintenance

IV catheter care should be performed every 48 hours or on an as-needed basis. The catheter dressing should be removed and the site inspected. The veterinary technician looks for signs of phlebitis, an infection, and/or thrombosis. Signs of phlebitis may include erythema, swelling, tenderness upon palpation, and an apparent increase in skin temperature over the vein. The signs of an infection include those seen with phlebitis and may include a purulent discharge. Thrombosis is characterized by a vein that "stands up" without being held off and a thick cordlike feeling to the vein. When signs of phlebitis or thrombosis are apparent, the catheter should be removed and a new one placed at a different site. While flushing the catheter with heparinized saline, the insertion site should be observed for leaking of fluid at the insertion site and pain upon injection. If either is observed, the catheter should be removed and replaced with a new one. If any portion of the catheter is exposed, it should not be reinserted, and it should be documented in the medical record. If the catheter site looks good, the site should be cleaned with an

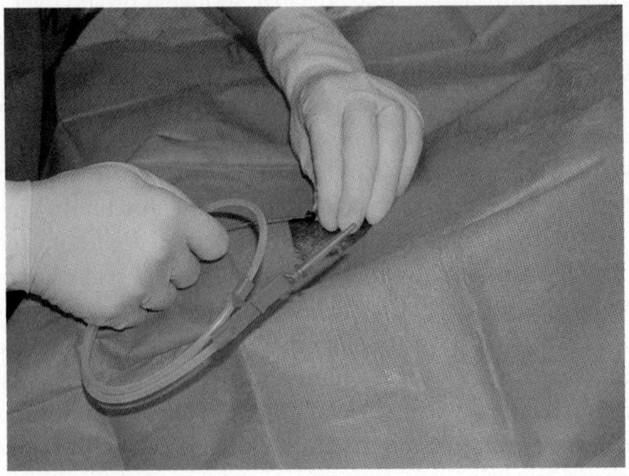

FIGURE 20-26 When using the Seldinger technique, the guidewire is threaded through the OTN catheter; care should be taken not to contaminate the flimsy wire.

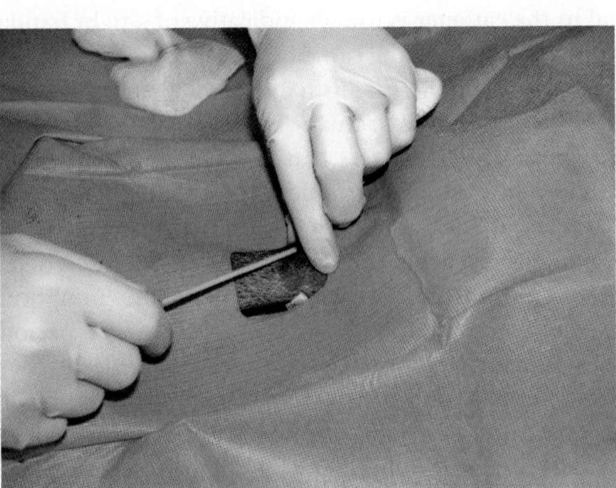

FIGURE 20-27 The dilator is used to enlarge the insertion site. The dilator is grasped near the distal tip, using a forward twisting motion, the dilator is advanced into the vessel.

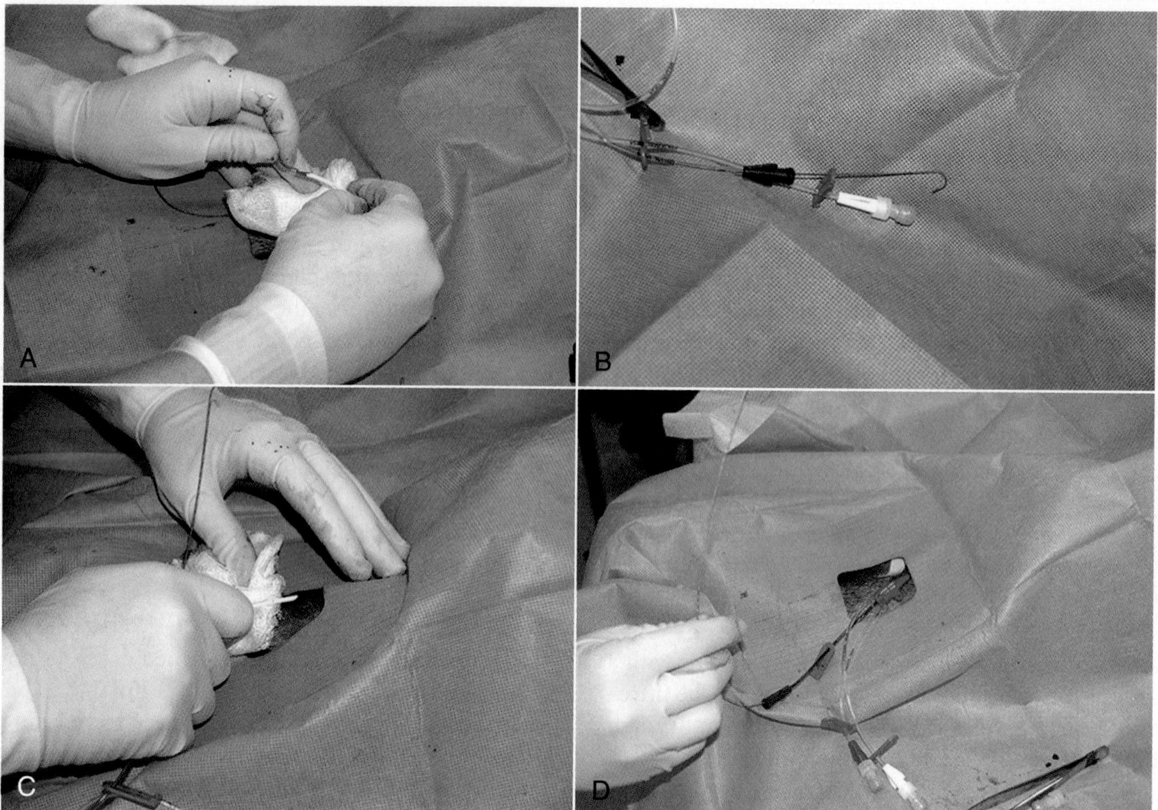

FIGURE 20-28 The proximal end of the guidewire is threaded up the catheter **(A)** until it comes out at the distal catheter hub **(B)**. The wire is then grasped and the catheter threaded into the vessel **(C)**. The wire is then removed from the catheter **(D)**.

iodophor or chlorhexidine solution. When the catheter site is dry, cover the insertion site with the sterile 2- × 2-inch pad. Then rebandage the catheter. Traditionally, it has been recommended not to leave a catheter in place any longer than 72 hours. These recommendations come from human medicine. It has been our experience that as long as routine catheter care is performed and the catheter removed when problems are first noticed, one can often exceed the 72-hour rule.

IV catheters should be observed several times a day. If the catheter bandage is found to be wet, the reason should be identified, and the bandage should be changed. Swelling distal to the catheter is usually indicative of a tight bandage. Swelling proximal to the catheter may be due to infiltration. If the patient is molesting its bandage, the reason should be investigated; there may actually be a problem with the catheter or bandage. Catheters that are not used continuously for fluid administration should be flushed with 4 U/ml of heparinized saline (1000 Units/250 ml normal saline) every 4 hours. Bags of heparinized saline should be discarded every 12 to 24 hours to minimize the risk of contamination. If a catheter is not going to be used for a prolonged period of time, a heparin lock should be considered. The dead space of the catheter is filled with 100 U/ml heparin every 12 hours. The concentrated heparin solution is never flushed into the patient; it is aspirated before the administration of medication or before renewing the heparin lock. The catheter should be clearly labeled so as to prevent inadvertent flushing of the concentrated heparin into the patient.

Intravenous Chemotherapy Administration

The use of chemotherapeutic agents to treat neoplasia is becoming more common in companion animal practices. The veterinary technician should be familiar with chemotherapy administration protocols and safety precautions (see Chapter 10). Because many chemotherapeutic agents are carcinogens, it is advisable to minimize exposure to the drugs during administration. Latex gloves, safety glasses, masks, and nonpermeable, long-sleeved, elastic-cuffed gowns should be worn. Materials used for chemotherapy administration should be discarded in leakproof hazardous waste containers. Drug aerosolization is decreased if an alcohol-soaked gauze sponge is placed over the catheter cap when the needle on the chemotherapy drug syringe is inserted into or removed from the catheter.

IV catheters are used to administer cytotoxic solutions, especially those that cause tissue irritation when injected extravascularly. Examples of such drugs, which are termed vesicants, include doxorubicin, vincristine, vinblastine, and actinomycin D.

IV chemotherapy catheters must be placed with extreme care. The catheter should be placed in a peripheral vein, and the vessel must be punctured only once during placement. If a "clean stick" is not achieved on the first placement attempt, a different vein should be used. This prevents tissue irritation caused by drug leakage from the previous puncture site. It is permissible, but not advisable, to place the catheter in the same vein in a more proximal site if the initial site has been given time to seal with a clot. Nonheparinized 0.9% sterile saline solution should be used to flush the catheter when specific chemotherapy drugs, such as doxorubicin, that precipitate when mixed with heparin are used.

Catheters used for drug administration should be frequently evaluated for patency. The area proximal to the catheter site should be freely visible so that extravasation may be observed. Signs that the chemotherapeutic agent has leaked out of the vein include the loss of catheter patency, redness or swelling at or proximal to the injection site, and vocalization or signs of discomfort by the patient.

If extravasation occurs, as much of the drug should be removed from the site as possible by aspirating 5 ml of blood back through the catheter. The tissue surrounding the site should be infused with saline solution, corticosteroids, or 2% lidocaine, and either warm or cold compresses should be applied, depending on the chemotherapy drug used.

When chemotherapy administration is complete, the catheter is flushed with several milliliters of sterile, nonheparinized 0.9% saline solution. An alcohol-soaked gauze sponge covers the catheter as it is removed from the vein. The skin puncture site is covered with an antibiotic-treated gauze pad and securely bandaged.

When less than 2 ml of a chemotherapeutic drug, such as vincristine, is injected IV, a 23- or 25-gauge butterfly catheter is often used. After the drug has been administered, the catheter is flushed with several milliliters of saline solution. The tubing is crimped to prevent fluid from leaking back out of the catheter, and the needle is removed from the vein. The needle is covered with an alcohol-soaked gauze pad as it is removed from the skin, and the venipuncture site is bandaged.

Subcutaneous Administration

The SQ injection is easily and frequently performed and is the most common route for vaccine administration. Although absorption may be slow in obese animals because of the relatively poor vascular supply in fat, SQ injections, in general, allow for relatively rapid absorption of the injected substance. However, the SQ route is not recommended in severely dehydrated or critically ill patients when immediate absorption is required. In an emergency situation, the IV or intraosseous route provides much faster absorption. The IV route is preferred when large volumes of fluid must be administered.

Moderate volumes of isotonic fluids can be injected under the skin to rehydrate animals if IV or intraosseous access is unavailable. Approximately 50 to 100 ml of body-temperature fluids can be injected per site, depending on the patient's size. Owners of patients that may require long-term fluid supplementation at home (e.g., those with chronic renal disease) can be instructed in how to administer SQ fluids.

The preferred site for most SQ injections is the dorsolateral region from the neck to the hips. The dorsal region of the neck and back should be avoided because of the difficulty in treating any abscesses or masses that may occur after an injection. When vaccinations are administered, especially to feline patients, the intrascapular region should be avoided because of the incidence of vaccine-induced tumors. Feline vaccinations should be administered in as distal a portion of an extremity as possible. The following sites are recommended for feline vaccination: right front leg, rhinotracheitis-calici-panleukopenia; right rear leg, rabies: left rear leg, feline leukemia. The intrascapular area should also be avoided for insulin injections because of the relatively poor absorption of insulin from that site and the fibrosis that may occur as a result of repeated injections. Insulin should be injected in alternating sites along the dorsolateral or ventrolateral aspect of the trunk.

When an SQ injection is administered, a fold of skin is tented, and the needle is inserted at the base of and parallel to the long axis of the fold. If the needle is inserted perpendicular to the long axis, the needle may penetrate both sides of the skin, and the syringe contents may be accidentally deposited on the patient's hair. The syringe plunger is retracted slightly, and the needle hub is checked for blood before injection. If blood appears in the hub, a vessel has been penetrated, and the needle should be removed and reinserted in another location. After the injection, the skin is briefly massaged to facilitate drug distribution. If multiple vaccinations or medications are administered, the injection sites should be a minimum of several centimeters apart.

INTRAMUSCULAR ADMINISTRATION

The intramuscular (IM) route is appropriate for the injection of small volumes of medication. Drugs are most often administered in the lumbosacral musculature lateral to the dorsal spinous processes or in the semimembranosus or semitendinosus muscles of the rear leg. Deep lumbar injections in the third to fifth lumbar region are used to administer heartworm treatment. The placement of the needle in the lumbosacral muscles is not recommended in very thin animals. When injections are made into the semimembranosus or semitendinosus muscles, the needle should enter the lateral aspect of the muscle and be directed caudally to prevent penetration of the sciatic nerve. Contact of the needle with the sciatic nerve may cause pain and lameness. Occasionally the triceps muscles on the caudal aspect of the front legs are used as injection sites. The neck is never used as a site for IM injections.

When an IM injection is performed, the muscle is isolated between the fingers and thumb, and a 22- to 25-gauge needle attached to a syringe is embedded in the muscle. As with SQ injections, the needle hub is checked for blood before the administration of medication to make certain a vessel is not inadvertently penetrated. If blood is observed, the needle is removed and inserted in another site. Once the placement within the muscle has been verified, the drug is slowly injected. The site is massaged for a few seconds after the injection to help distribute the substance.

INTRADERMAL ADMINISTRATION

Intradermal (ID) injections are performed to desensitize the skin with a local anesthetic or to perform allergy skin testing. Most animals will not tolerate skin testing unless they are sedated. The hair on the lateral aspect of the trunk is shaved with a #40 clipper blade. The skin is carefully wiped with a water-moistened gauze sponge. Vigorous scrubbing or the use of an antimicrobial cleaning solution is contraindicated because skin irritation that may occur interferes with testing. For an ID injection, a fold of skin is lifted, and a 25- to 27-gauge needle attached to a 1-ml syringe is inserted with the bevel up into the dermis. A 0.1-ml volume of allergen is injected. The injection site will look like a translucent lump if the injection is performed correctly. The skin is then examined for tissue reaction.

INTRANASAL ADMINISTRATION

Certain vaccines—such as those for feline infectious peritonitis, feline viral rhinotracheitis-calici-panleukopenia, and *Bordetella bronchiseptica*—are formulated for intranasal (and/or intraocular) administration. The patient's muzzle is held in one hand and elevated slightly. The tip of the vaccine dispenser is placed into the nostril, and the dispenser is compressed. Alternatively the patient's head can be tilted back, and the pipette containing the vaccine can be squeezed to dispense the liquid onto the plane of the nose. The vaccine runs into each nostril as the animal inhales. This method frequently results in less sneezing after the administration than when the dispenser tip is placed directly into the nostril.

Diazepam can be administered intranasally for the immediate treatment of status epilepticus if intravascular access cannot be obtained. Diazepam is absorbed more rapidly into the systemic circulation by the intranasal route than by the intrarectal route.

INTRATRACHEAL ADMINISTRATION

In an emergency situation, such as during cardiopulmonary resuscitation, drugs can be injected directly into the trachea of an unconscious animal. The absorption by this route is extremely rapid.

> TECHNICIAN NOTE In an emergency situation, such as during cardiopulmonary resuscitation, medications can be injected directly into the trachea because the absorption of the drug by this route is extremely rapid.

When an intratracheal injection is performed, a polypropylene urinary catheter or rubber feeding tube is inserted into the trachea, either directly or through an endotracheal tube. The drug contained in a syringe is forcefully injected through the urinary catheter or feeding tube. Approximately 10 ml of air or 3 to 10 ml of sterile saline solution is injected through the catheter or tube immediately afterward to disperse the drug. The acronym ALE (e.g., atropine, lidocaine, or epinephrine) is useful in helping to remember which drugs can be administered via the endotracheal tube. The intratracheal dosage is usually twice the IV dosage.

INTRAOSSEOUS ADMINISTRATION

Needles are placed directly into the bone marrow cavity to deliver fluids, drugs, and blood products when IV catheterization is not possible or cannot be performed rapidly. The intraosseous route is often overlooked and may be useful in emergency situations. Medications and fluids quickly enter the central circulation via the intramedullary vessels in the marrow cavity. The intraosseous placement of a needle or catheter allows rapid fluid delivery to neonates, small animals, and patients with circulatory collapse. Intraosseous needles are removed as soon as IV access can be established.

The placement of an intraosseous needle or catheter is contraindicated in patients with sepsis. Catheters are not placed in bones that are fractured or infected. Skin overlying the insertion site should be free of infection so that skin-surface pathogens are not introduced into the underlying tissue during an intraosseous needle placement. If the bone cortex is punctured multiple times during insertion attempts, a different bone should be used; fluid that is administered may leak from the bone into the SQ tissue.

Sites for intraosseous administration include the tibia, femur, humerus, and occasionally the iliac wing or ischium. The intraosseous catheter or needle should have a stylet that helps prevent the needle from bending or becoming occluded with a core of bone as it is inserted. Needles used include 15- to 18-gauge bone marrow needles specially designed for intraosseous access. If intraosseous access is needed in a neonate, an 18- to 22-gauge hypodermic needle can be used. If the hypodermic needle plugs with a core of bone, it can sometimes be flushed out with saline solution. A 22-gauge, 3.75-cm needle can be nested inside an 18-gauge, 2.5-cm needle to serve as a stylet during placement.

Needle placement for the purpose of delivering medications or fluids into the intraosseous space follows the protocol described for needle placement for bone marrow aspiration. When an intraosseous catheter or needle must be placed in the femur, the hip region is shaved and aseptically prepared. The patient is placed in lateral recumbency, and the technician stands at the dorsum of the patient. The trochanteric fossa of the femur of the upside leg is identified on the medial aspect of the greater trochanter of the proximal femur.

Approximately 0.5 to 1.0 ml of 2% lidocaine is injected into the skin, SQ tissue, and periosteum over the trochanteric fossa to provide local anesthesia. A stab incision is made through the skin. The femur is grasped, and the hip is held in a flexed position. The intraosseous needle is introduced medial to the greater trochanter and parallel to the femoral shaft. The needle is inserted through the skin incision and into the femur by using firm, steady pressure as the wrist is rotated back and forth. The insertion of the needle through a skin incision helps decrease the likelihood that skin contaminants will be carried into the bone. During a needle insertion, care is taken to prevent piercing the sciatic nerve, which is posteromedial to the greater trochanter of the femur. When the needle enters the marrow cavity, the needle will feel firmly embedded. The placement can be ascertained through aspiration of bone marrow into a syringe attached to the needle hub.

Once placed, the needle is secured by wrapping a "butterfly" tab of tape around it as it exits the skin. The tape is sutured to the skin. A povidone-iodine ointment-treated gauze pad is applied to the skin entry site. A bulky, gauze bandage is placed around the needle for further stabilization. The patency of the intraosseous needle is maintained by flushing every 6 hours with 1 to 2 ml of heparinized 0.9% saline solution. The needle may remain in place for up to 3 days, but is difficult to maintain in an ambulatory patient.

INTRAPERITONEAL ADMINISTRATION

The intraperitoneal (IP) route involves the placement of substances directly into the abdominal cavity. This route is occasionally used to administer noncaustic fluids, blood products, or medications. It may be used in neonates when intravascular or intraosseous access is difficult to obtain. Specific chemotherapy drugs, such as asparaginase, can be given IP. Body-temperature fluids may be infused into the abdominal cavity to lavage the abdomen in animals with peritonitis or pancreatitis. Warm or cool fluid IP lavage may be used to help treat patients with severe hypothermia or hyperthermia.

Substances injected into the peritoneal cavity are absorbed more rapidly than those administered SQ, but more slowly than those given by the intravascular or intraosseous route. When a drug or fluids must be administered into the peritoneal cavity, the ventral abdomen between the umbilicus and the bladder is shaved and aseptically prepared. An 18- to 22-gauge needle or catheter is inserted into the abdominal cavity on the ventral midline, a few centimeters caudal to the umbilicus. A syringe is attached and aspirated. If the needle is in the proper location in the peritoneal cavity, no blood or fluid will be aspirated into the syringe. If blood or fluid enters the syringe tip, the needle may have punctured a vessel or abdominal organ. The needle is removed, and a new needle is inserted in a different site. If the syringe remains empty when negative pressure is applied, the medication or fluids have been injected.

TOPICAL OPHTHALMIC ADMINISTRATION

If it is necessary to administer topical ophthalmic medications to treat ocular diseases or for specific vaccines, such as feline rhinotracheitis-calici-panleukopenia, there is a formulation designed for intranasal and/or intraocular administration. To successfully place a medication onto the surface of the eye, the technician must have good restraint of the patient. Control of the front limbs of the patient is essential, along with minimizing the movement of the animal, to prevent the medication from being inadvertently placed on the eyelids or face. The eye medication dispensed to a patient should only be used exclusively on that patient and no other patients to prevent transmitting ocular infections. The tip of the medication dispenser should not come into direct contact with any surface of the eye, including the cornea, to prevent contamination and scratching of the cornea. If an ophthalmic medication is a solution and it appears cloudy, contains particulate matter, or has a color change, it should not be used.

Ophthalmic medications should be administered slightly warm or at room temperature. The technician can take refrigerated medications and place them in the palm of his or her hand for 1 to 2 minutes before administration because this makes it more comfortable for the patient. The eyelids are held open with the thumb and index finger of one hand, and the hand holding the medication is rested on the patient's head as 1 drop of the medication is deposited onto the sclera (Figure 20-29). For medications that are ointments, the lids are held open with the thumb and index finger of one hand and a 3- to 5-mm strip of ointment is squeezed onto the upper sclera or lower palpebral border. The ointment dissipates across the cornea when the animal blinks.

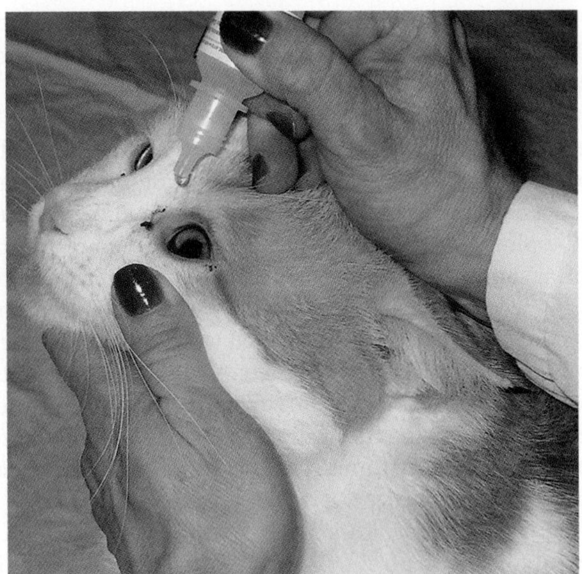

FIGURE 20-29 Ophthalmic drop is directed onto the sclera of a cat.

If the patient requires multiple topical ophthalmic medications in the same eye, these should be applied 3 to 5 minutes apart to allow for sufficient absorption. In the scenario of needing to administer both a solution and an ointment, the solution should be placed in the eye 3 to 5 minutes before the ointment. If the ointment is applied first, it may coat the cornea and interfere with the absorption of the solution.

AURAL ADMINISTRATION

The key to successfully medicating an ear is to have the medication in contact with the ear canals' epithelium to enhance the medication's absorption and effectiveness. Therefore the ear must be cleared of debris before the medication is applied.

When medication is placed in the ear canal, the pinna is grasped and pulled upward and slightly out laterally similar to the motion of introducing an otoscope cone for an otoscopic examination. This helps to straighten the vertical ear canal. The tip of the medication dispenser is then placed into the vertical ear canal, and the dispenser is squeezed. The base of the ear is massaged to distribute the medication.

TRANSDERMAL ADMINISTRATION

Certain medications applied topically to the skin have systemic and local effects. Many drugs commonly administered by the oral route, such as prednisone or methimazole, can be formulated into an ointment for transdermal application. Other medications, such as nitroglycerin, are manufactured as a cream to be applied directly on the skin.

Medications, such as nitroglycerin, may be absorbed by the individual making the application; therefore disposable gloves should be worn to prevent absorption. A small quantity of ointment is applied to a sparsely haired region, such as the pinna of the ear, the groin, or a shaved area on the ventral thorax. If gloves are unavailable, the ointment can be applied to a small piece of wax paper and wiped onto the skin. The treated area is covered with a light bandage so it will not be accidentally touched. A note is placed on the front of the patient's cage specifying the medication used, the site to which the medication has been applied, and the duration of time that must pass before the application site can be safely touched.

Many topical medications are dispensed in a liquid or aerosol form to control fleas, ticks, mites, heartworms, and intestinal parasites. Depending on the product, the medication is either sprayed on the hair on the entire body or applied to the skin between the shoulder blades. Manufacturer's directions regarding application should be followed closely. Gloves are worn during the application, and the site of administration should not be touched for a specified period after the application.

The transdermal application of analgesics is gaining popularity. One analgesic manufactured in a form specifically for transdermal application is fentanyl citrate. A fentanyl-impregnated self-adhesive patch is placed directly onto a shaved, dry region of skin. The technician should not touch the adhesive side of the patch containing the fentanyl because the medication is absorbed topically. Gentle pressure is applied with the palm of the hand over the patch application site for 1 minute to help the patch adhere to the skin. Each patch can only be applied once because it may not adhere to the skin and deliver the complete dose of fentanyl if it is removed and reapplied. The patch can be covered with tape on which the date and time of placement have been recorded.

It is important to place the fentanyl patch in a location from which the animal cannot remove it, such as on the intrascapular region. It should not be applied to skin that will be in contact with a heating pad, heat lamp, or other external heat source. The rate of drug delivery is increased when the skin beneath the patch warms and the cutaneous vessels vasodilate.

The topical application of creams (e.g., EMLA cream, lidocaine, and prilocaine) desensitizes the skin so that a venipuncture is more comfortable for the patient. This topical anesthetic must be in contact with the skin for at least several minutes (ideally 30 to 60 minutes) for it to reach its maximal effectiveness.

INTRARECTAL ADMINISTRATION

The mucosa of the large intestine is capable of absorbing medications delivered intrarectally. Medications delivered by this route may have both local and systemic effects. The absorption is most effective when the intestine is free of fecal material. Antiemetic tablets or suppositories can be administered intrarectally to vomiting patients that cannot be medicated orally. A gloved, lubricated finger is used to insert the tablet into the rectum a distance of at least 5 cm. The medication is then gradually absorbed.

Antiseizure drugs, such as diazepam, can be given intrarectally if an IV or intranasal administration is difficult to perform. A lubricated short rubber feeding tube or urinary catheter is inserted 8 to 10 cm into the rectum. The diazepam is placed into a syringe and injected through the catheter. Several milliliters of warm water are then flushed into the catheter to disperse the drug. Diazepam can also be injected directly into the rectum with a needleless syringe.

Enemas are also administered per rectum. A syringe containing the enema is lubricated and inserted into the rectum. After the enema is injected, the animal should be placed in an area where it can defecate, such as outdoors or near a litter box.

Warm-water enemas are administered through lubricated plastic tubing inserted through the rectum and into the large intestine. Water is funneled or injected into the end of the tube held in a raised position. The tube is moved back and forth and is slowly advanced up the intestinal tract as fecal material is expelled.

When a medication, such as lactulose, is added to the enema solution, it must be retained within the large intestine for a specified length of time. The solution is injected into a urinary catheter or feeding tube placed into the descending colon. The rectum is held closed with a gloved hand to prevent the enema from exiting. After the allotted time has passed, the catheter is removed and the intestine is evacuated.

ORAL ADMINISTRATION

The administration of medication by direct placement into the oral cavity is frequently and easily performed. Technicians should be adept at administering oral medications to animals and capable of demonstrating techniques to pet owners.

> *TECHNICIAN NOTE* Technicians should be adept at administering oral medications to animals and able to demonstrate techniques to pet owners.

Oral medications are usually administered in liquid, capsule, or tablet form. Liquids are easy to administer through a dropper or syringe. Pulverized tablets and the contents of capsules can be mixed with a small volume of food, water, or flavored liquid. When liquids must be administered with a syringe or dropper, the patient's lower lip is pulled out at the commissure. The tip of the syringe or dropper is placed between the cheek and the gums, and small volumes of liquid are injected. The muzzle should be held at a neutral angle and not elevated. Hyperextension of the neck or movement by the patient during administration may result in fluid aspiration into the trachea. If the patient struggles or coughs or if fluid spills out of the mouth, the patient should be allowed to rest before further administration attempts.

A tablet or capsule is most easily administered to a dog if it is hidden in meat, cheese, or a chunk of canned pet food. Cats rarely consume pills hidden in food. Cats will meticulously eat the food that surrounds the pill and leave the medication. If a patient has a diminished appetite, it may not consume the entire amount of medication-laced food and will not receive a sufficient dose of medication.

An animal that will not consume baited food is medicated by tilting the head back, prying open the jaws, and placing the pill far back on the base of the tongue (Figures 20-30 and 20-31). The tablet will be expelled if it is not placed far enough back in the pharynx. The technician holds the muzzle closed, rubs under the animal's chin, taps the tip of the nose, or blows air into the nostrils to stimulate the animal to swallow. When the animal licks its nose, it can be assumed that the tablet has been swallowed.

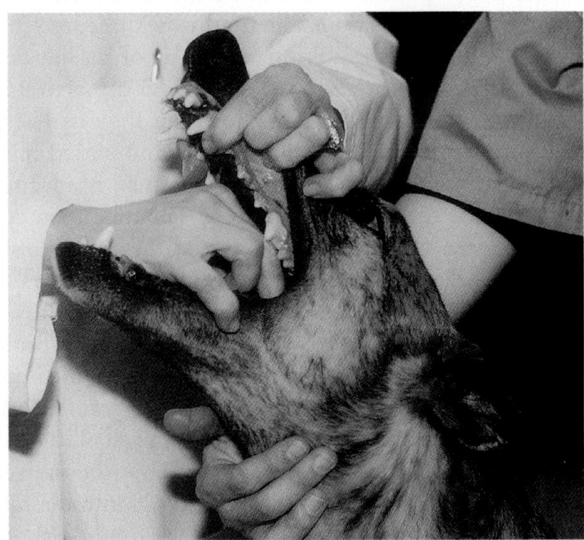

FIGURE 20-30 A dog's muzzle held open as a tablet is placed into the back of the mouth.

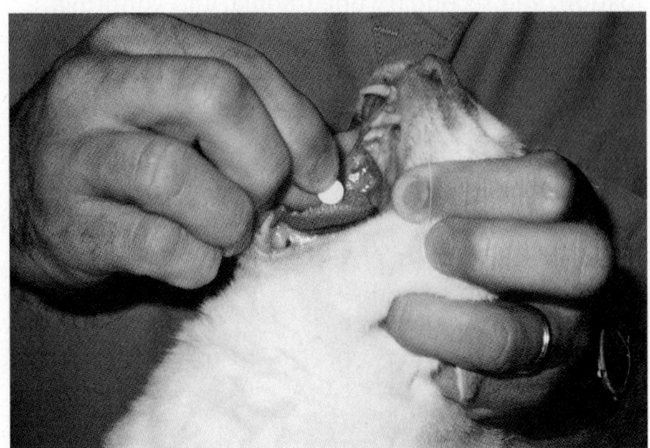

FIGURE 20-31 A cat's neck is hyperextended so its nose points toward the ceiling. The lower jaw is open as a tablet is placed in the back of its mouth.

A specially designed device is available to administer tablets to fractious cats and dogs. The tablet is secured in the tip of a plastic rod that is inserted into the back of the mouth. The rod plunger is quickly depressed, and the pill is propelled down the esophagus. Technicians can demonstrate the use of the "pill gun" to owners for the administration of medication at home.

OROGASTRIC INTUBATION

Sometimes it is necessary to administer medication, food, or fluids through a tube passed through the mouth and directly into the stomach. This technique is used to administer activated charcoal solutions or lavage the stomach to treat animals that have ingested toxins. Orphan or weak neonates who cannot nurse can be fed milk replacer via a tube passed through the mouth and into the distal esophagus or stomach. An orogastric tube (OGT) is also passed in an attempt to decompress a patient with gastric dilation (bloated stomach). Dogs usually permit an OGT placement with moderate resistance. Cats, with the exception of neonates, usually require sedation.

The length of 10 to 22F plastic or rubber tube required to extend from the tip of the nose to the thirteenth rib is measured and marked on the tube with tape or ink (Figure 20-32). If the tube is to be placed in the distal esophagus to feed an animal, the distance between the tip of the nose and the eighth rib is marked. Water-soluble gel is used to lubricate the tip of the tube. The animal is restrained in sternal recumbency or in a standing or seated position. A roll of tape, a plastic or wooden speculum with a hole in the middle, or a plastic syringe case with smooth ends is placed behind the canine teeth to hold the mouth open. The muzzle is kept in a normal position and held so the mouth speculum does not become dislodged.

The tube is slowly passed through the speculum (Figure 20-33). Swallowing will be noted as the tube passes over the base of the tongue and into the esophagus. If the animal coughs, the tube may have entered the trachea and should be

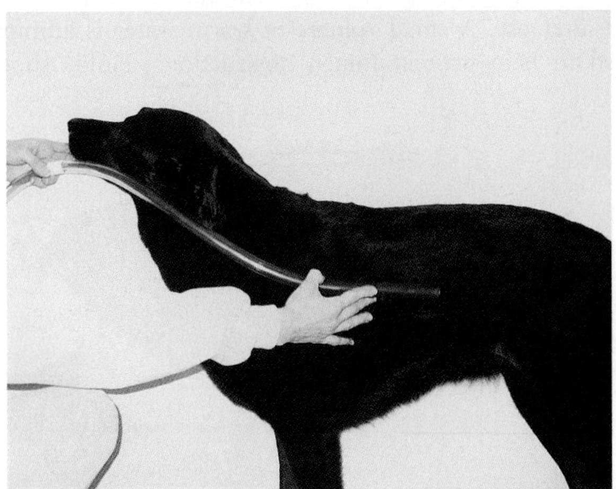

FIGURE 20-32 A length of stomach tube is measured from the nose to the thirteenth rib. It is marked with tape.

removed. Once the tube is in the esophagus, it is advanced the premeasured length until it enters the stomach.

The correct placement of the tube in the gastrointestinal tract should always be verified before the introduction of any medications or fluids. Refer to the discussion of nasoesophageal and nasogastric tubes (NGTs) for instruction on how to check the tube placement.

Fluid is added to the tube with a 60-ml syringe, metal drench pump, or funnel. After the fluid has been administered, the tube is bent to occlude it and then withdrawn in a downward direction. This technique prevents a backflow of fluid from entering the trachea.

Enteral Feeding Tubes

Enteral feeding has proved to be an excellent method for maintaining a normal nutritional status when oral intake is not possible. Indications for placing enteral feeding tubes include critically ill animals and patients with chronic disorders, such as renal impairment, that may not be able to normally consume enough calories for proper nutrition and therefore require nutritional support. If the gastrointestinal tract is capable of digestion and absorption, then food slurries, fluid, or medication can be administered through tubes placed directly into the esophagus, stomach, duodenum, or jejunum. The technician needs to be familiar with the technique that the veterinarian uses to place enteral feeding tubes and be knowledgeable about tube maintenance. The selection of the feeding tube device is dependent on many issues, including the duration of enteral support, aspiration risk, and the animal's temperament.

Nasoesophageal tubes are occasionally used for short-term feeding and the administration of medications. If a patient requires nutritional support beyond 10 days, the placement of an esophagostomy or gastrostomy tube is preferred (Figure 20-34). Esophagostomy and gastrostomy devices can remain long term (weeks to months), although occasional replacement may be necessary depending on the construction and wear of the tube. If the stomach must be bypassed completely, a duodenostomy or jejunostomy tube is surgically placed.

All enteral feeding tube types should be flushed before and after use. A small volume of warm water is administered to help prevent lumen obstructions. Fluids should always be injected slowly. Before the injection of fluid into a gastrostomy tube, the tube is aspirated with a syringe to make certain the stomach contents have emptied from the previous feeding. If the stomach is still full, the veterinarian should be consulted; the full volume of the next meal should not be instilled into the gastrostomy tube until the previous meal has passed from the stomach. The tube insertion site and tube position are inspected daily to make certain that the tube has not shifted and the skin is free from inflammation, redness, tenderness, and discharge.

Nasoesophageal Tubes

Nasoesophageal tubes are easy and inexpensive to place in an animal that requires short-term feeding, such as a severely anorexic cat. These tubes are contraindicated in patients that are vomiting or do not have a gag reflex. A 5 to 8 Fr pediatric feeding tube is held up to the animal to determine the appropriate length that is required. For nasoesophageal placement, the distance between the nares and distal esophagus at the eighth or ninth rib is marked on the tube with ink or tape. The patient is held in sternal recumbency, in a seated or standing position. The head is held securely with the neck slightly extended. From 0.5 to 1 ml of 2% lidocaine is infused into one nostril of the dog, and 5 drops of 0.5% proparacaine are placed into one nostril of the cat. The tip of the tube is coated with Xylocaine jelly and placed in the nostril dorsomedial to the alar fold. The tube is advanced into the nostril and directed ventrally. The tube then continues down the ventral meatus and into the nasopharynx. The animal will usually swallow when the tube enters the pharynx (Figure 20-35).

The tube is placed in the distal esophagus. The proper placement may be checked by injecting 5 to 10 ml of air into the tube and simultaneously auscultating the cranial abdomen. If gurgling sounds or borborygmi are present, the tube has been placed in the gastrointestinal tract. Alternatively, 5 ml of sterile saline solution may be injected into the tube; if the animal coughs, the tube is in the trachea and should be removed. A radiograph can also be taken to evaluate the tube placement. The most common complications of a nasoesophageal tube placement are epistaxis, rhinitis, tracheal intubation, and secondary pneumonia, and vomiting.

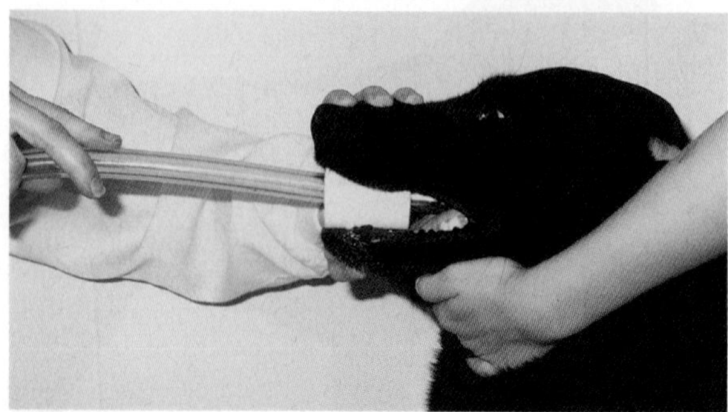

FIGURE 20-33 A roll of tape holds the mouth open as a stomach tube is passed through the roll and into the oral cavity.

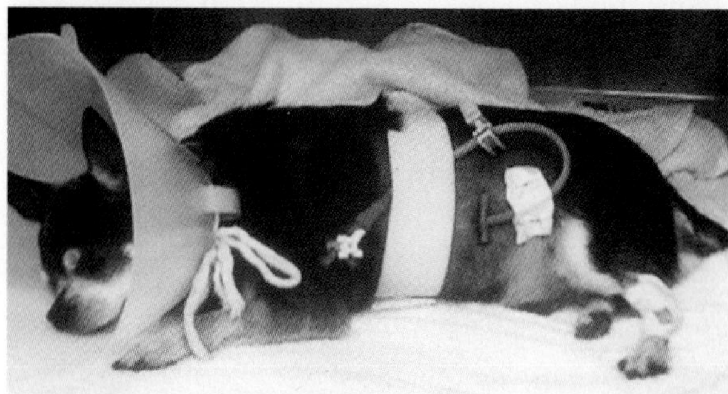

FIGURE 20-34 A gastrostomy tube is placed to feed a patient that has undergone esophageal surgery. The Elizabethan collar prevents chewing on the tube or IV lateral saphenous catheter.

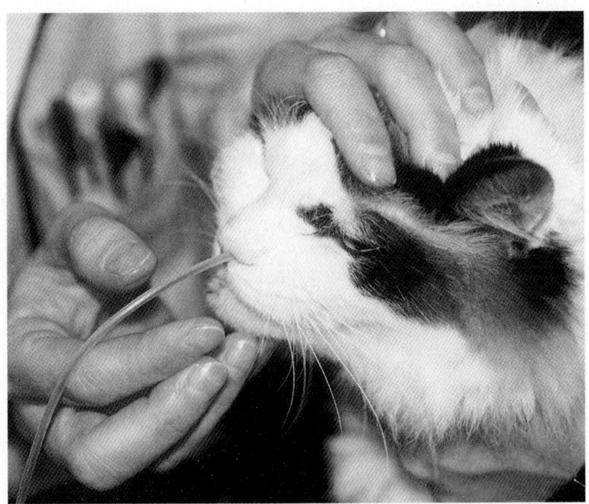

FIGURE 20-35 The tip of a nasoesophageal tube that has been lubricated is advanced into the nostril and directed ventrally. (From Ettinger SJ, Feldmen E, editors: *Textbook of veterinary internal medicine,* ed 6, Philadelphia, 2005, Elsevier Saunders.)

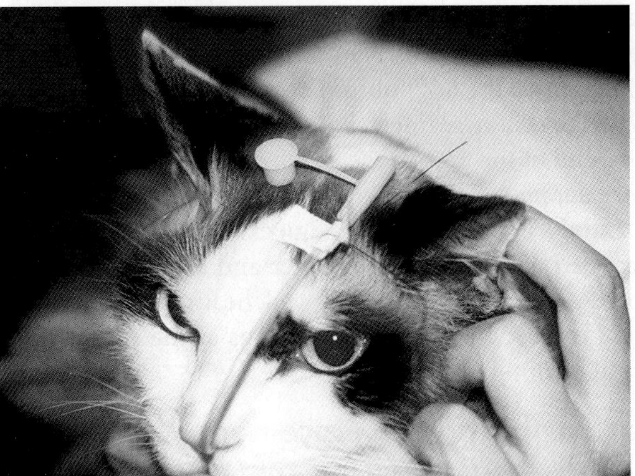

FIGURE 20-36 The nasoesophageal tube secured to the patient. The tube is sutured or glued close to the nostrils, on the bridge of the nose, and onto the forehead with "butterfly" tape. (From Ettinger SJ, Feldmen E, editors: *Textbook of veterinary internal medicine,* ed 6, Philadelphia, 2005, Elsevier Saunders.)

Suture material or tissue adhesive is used to secure the tube to the patient (Figure 20-36). The tube should be sutured or glued close to its entrance to the nostril, onto the bridge of the nose, and onto the forehead. The remainder of the tube should be taped to the dorsum of the neck, and the animal should be fitted with an Elizabethan collar to prevent chewing of the tube. A cap is placed on the end of the tube to prevent reflux.

Esophagostomy Tube Placement

The placement of a feeding tube directly into the esophagus to provide nutritional support has proved to be an effective technique. Esophagostomy tubes are preferred over pharyngostomy tubes because these cause less laryngeal irritation and obstruction and are less likely to induce vomiting and become dislodged. Esophagostomy tubes are easily inserted under a light general anesthesia plane, are minimally invasive, and no specialized equipment is required, such as an endoscope. There are, however, specially designed percutaneous kits available on the market: the ELD Tube Applicator (Jorgensen Laboratories, Inc.) and the Van Noort Oesophagostomy Tube Set (SurgiVet). Instruction sheets detailing the procedures involved in using these devices are available from the manufacturers. If a commercial kit is not used, the technique using right-angled forceps and a 14F to 20F red rubber feeding tube is commonly practiced.

> TECHNICIAN NOTE Patients tolerate esophagostomy tubes better than pharyngostomy tubes because these cause less laryngeal irritation and obstruction and are less likely to induce emesis and become dislodged.

An esophagostomy tube is placed in the midcervical esophagus on the left side of the neck (Figure 20-37). The animal is placed in right lateral recumbency, and the left cervical region is shaved and surgically prepared. The point of the shoulder and the angle of the mandible are used as guides to measure the distal and proximal limits of the cervical esophagus. The length of a red rubber feeding tube needed to extend from the skin of the midcervical region to the seventh rib is measured and marked on the tube with ink or tape. A pair of extra long curved forceps (such as Carmalt, Mixter, Schnidt, or Kantrowitz) is placed into the oral cavity and advanced to the left midcervical region of the esophagus. The forceps' tips should be palpable on the patient's neck. A stab incision is made with a scalpel blade through the skin and SQ tissue over the tips. The scalpel blade is used to carefully dissect the SQ tissue over the esophagus until the forceps are able to bluntly penetrate the esophagus. The tips of the hemostats are then brought to the exterior and opened just enough to grasp the fenestrated end of the feeding tube. The forceps with the attached feeding tube are withdrawn back through the skin and into the esophagus toward the

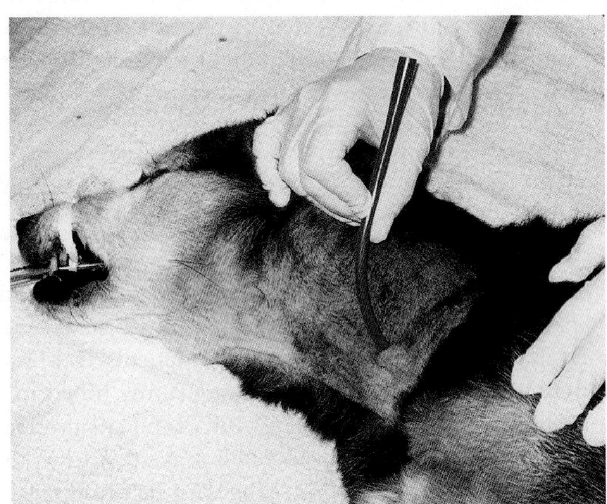

FIGURE 20-37 An esophagostomy tube for enteral feeding is placed into the midcervical esophagus on the left side of the neck.

oral cavity. Once the fenestrated end of the tube reaches the mouth, the tube is bent and redirected back down the esophagus to the level of the seventh rib. Retention sutures, such as the Chinese finger-knot suture, are used to secure the distal end of the tube to the skin. A povidone-iodine–treated gauze sponge is placed around the skin-tube interface, and a bandage is applied over the neck. The exposed tube end is capped with a catheter adapter and a catheter cap. Once esophagostomy tubes are removed, healing occurs by second intention. Stricture of the esophagus at the site of tube removal is minimal.

Gastrostomy Tube Placement

Gastrostomy tube feeding is recommended for long-term nutritional support and is especially suited for patients suffering from dysphagia; megaesophagus; and head, laryngeal, or esophageal trauma. Gastrostomy tubes are generally larger in diameter (18F to 24F). A gastrostomy tube placement for nutritional support is contradicted in patients that vomit frequently, have gastrointestinal obstruction, or are obtunded. Some animals require life-long gastrostomy tube feedings. This requires dedicated owners who are devoted to nursing their pets and ensuring that their animal receives daily nutritional requirements 365 days a year.

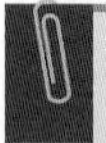

TECHNICIAN NOTE Percutaneous endoscopic gastrostomy (PEG) technique uses an endoscope.

Gastrostomy tubes can be placed percutaneously or during laparotomy. The placement is achieved with a PEG technique using an endoscope or a blind percutaneous technique. The percutaneous placement of a gastrostomy tube can be accomplished in 10 to 15 minutes. PEG tube kits are commercially available, but many hospitals make their own tube kits. Kits include a gastrostomy tube with its proximal end secured into a tapered plastic cannula or pipette to provide a sharp tapered guide, allowing the gastrostomy tube to be brought through the gastric and abdominal walls with minimal trauma. Also included are an external flange or stent, a clamp to anchor the external flange, a large clamp to prevent gastric contents from backing up into the proximal feeding tube, and a syringe adaptor to facilitate feeding.

Gastrostomy tube styles vary with the distal tip design. They may possess a Pezzer-style mushroom tip, or a rolled up "bumper," a round and flat disk, or a Foley balloon design (Figure 20-38).

Gastrostomy tubes are commonly made from either latex or silicone. The life of latex products is not long, usually up to 12 weeks. The volatile acidity of the stomach breaks down the latex, and the tube may dislodge as a result of the digestive disintegration of the tube. Furthermore, latex products can cause tissue irritation that can be observed at the stoma site. Latex gastrostomy tubes are soft and very pliable, and the long external feeding tube can be easily managed against the body wall. Latex gastrostomy tubes are inexpensive and are an excellent economical choice for short-term feeding. Silicone tubes can be more rigid and do not coil as easily against the body wall. They are, however, more tissue friendly, causing fewer tissue reactions. They are very sturdy in the gastric environment and are known to last 8 to 12 months, depending on the design of the tube. Silicone tubes with a Foley balloon design usually fail by 12 to 16 weeks because of balloon failure, but silicone tubes with a mushroom tip design will last many more months. Silicone tubes are, in general, more expensive than latex tubes, but are preferred for long-term feeding.

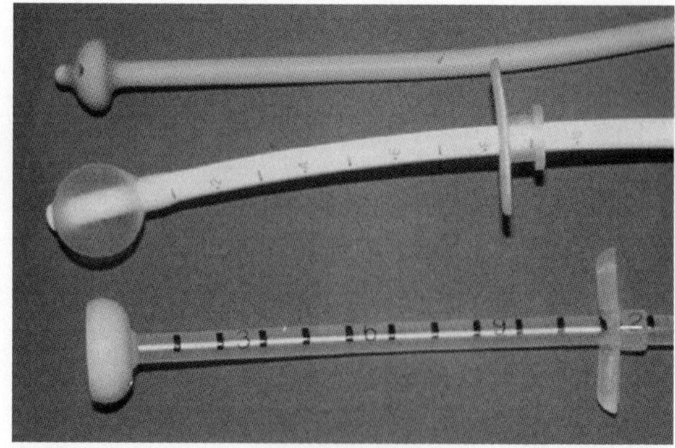

FIGURE 20-38 Examples of gastrostomy tube designs. From top to bottom: Pezzer or mushroom tip; Foley balloon; and bumper or disk style.

Endoscopic Placement Technique

Patients are placed in right lateral recumbency. Aseptic surgical preparation is done on the left paracostal area. A mouth gag is placed in the anesthetized animal, and a flexible gastroscope is inserted through the mouth and advanced into the stomach. The endoscopist fills the stomach with air until distention is obvious externally. Gastric distention is important because it will push the liver, spleen, and colon away from the gastrostomy site, leaving the gastric wall in direct contact with the left abdominal wall. Communication between the endoscopist and surgeon at the patient's side is necessary to confirm a good placement site by the surgeon poking with a gloved index finger just posterior to the thirteenth rib over the distended stomach. The endoscopist can visualize the gastric wall collapse around the finger of the surgeon. The endoscopist confirms the placement site location in the stomach, making certain that the site will be made in the body of the stomach or the greater curvature, outside the antrum. The surgeon then makes a small 3-mm incision with a scalpel blade at the desired site over the distended stomach. A needle or cannula is inserted through the skin incision and pushed through the abdominal and gastric walls. A strong nylon suture material is threaded through the needle or cannula into the stomach. The suture material is seen by the endoscopist who grasps the thread with an endoscopic snare or forceps. The suture thread is then brought out through the mouth along with the gastroscope. The needle or cannula is removed from the abdominal wall. A prepared PEG tube, attached in a tapered plastic cannula or pipette, is tied or attached to the suture exiting the oral cavity. The gastrostomy tube is well lubricated, and the surgeon places traction on the transabdominal suture, pulling the PEG tube through the animal's mouth, esophagus, and through the gastric and abdominal walls. The gastroscope is reintroduced, and the positioning of the gastrostomy tube is evaluated under direct vision. The surgeon applies traction on the gastrostomy tube until the gastric and abdominal walls are in contact. The contact should not be too tight because pressure necrosis can occur if the distal tip is too snug against the gastric mucosa. The endoscopist evaluates the gastric wall, making certain there are not any signs of mucosal blanching. The PEG tube is then fixed externally by a flange or stent, made of a small 3-cm piece of tubing with a hole cut in the center. The flange is simply passed over the PEG tube and placed in close contact with the abdominal wall. Care should be taken not to place the flange too snug. Allowance should be made for postoperative swelling. A plastic clip, a cable tie, or even tape should be placed around the PEG tube adjacent to the flange to anchor it in position. The flange helps to immobilize the tube and prevent inward and outward movement. A light dressing is placed around the gastrostomy tube site. The tube may be held in place against the body wall by a protective bandage or fishnet style stockinette (Figure 20-39).

Blind Percutaneous Placement Technique

There are several percutaneous placement kits commercially available. Each product varies with the manufacturer; however, all kits employ a rigid introduction tube, usually made of stainless steel. The patient is placed in right lateral recumbency and aseptically prepared, identical to the endoscopic technique preparation. The rigid introduction tube is passed through the mouth, esophagus, and into the stomach of an anesthetized patient. The rigid tube's distal tip is slightly angulated so that slight upward pressure on the tube presents to the surgeon the gastric wall against the prepared abdominal body wall. Suture material is introduced through the abdominal and gastric wall by a trocar blade mechanism inside the rigid introduction tube or a needle and wire passed from the exterior abdominal wall through the rigid insertion tube to the oral cavity. A prepared gastrostomy tube is attached to the suture or wire exiting the mouth. The gastrostomy tube is then advanced into the stomach by external traction by the surgeon, pulling the gastrostomy tube through the gastric and abdominal walls. The gastrostomy tube is then secured as described earlier.

Gastrostomy tubes should remain in place for 10 to 14 days, giving time for good stoma formation. If the patient removes the tube or tube failure occurs, resulting in undesirable removal of the gastrostomy tube, a new replacement tube should be inserted as soon as possible. Replacement gastrostomy tubes are available in various styles, just like the initial placement tubes. Foley balloon styles are the most common replacement tube type. Ideally, replacement gastrostomy tubes may be replaced through the existing stoma site, requiring little or no sedation of the patient. The new tube can be gently guided through the existing external stoma at the skin, through the adhered abdominal and gastric walls, into the stomach. The Foley balloon is inflated within the lumen of the stomach and retracted back against the gastric mucosa and secured by an external flange against the body wall.

Clients with pets that require long-term or lifelong gastrostomy tube feedings may want to consider a low-profile gastrostomy device. These devices set flush with the skin level, have a tube shaft the length of the patient's stoma, and possess a mushroom tip that sits snug against the gastric mucosa. A nice feature of most low-profile tubes is that they employ an antireflux valve at the mushroom tip, preventing gastric contents from leaking back through the tube. To replace an existing gastrostomy tube with a low-profile device, the stoma length must first be determined. Commercially available low-profile devices come with a measuring device. The stoma measuring device is inserted through the fistula into the stomach. The measuring device is retracted until the distal end of the device lies gently against the mucosa of the stomach. Depending on the manufacturer, the measuring device will have circumferential marks indicating depths from 1.5 to 4.4 cm. A gastrostomy device of an appropriate length is chosen on the basis of the length of the stoma, as determined by the distance from the distal tip of the stoma measuring device and the external surface at skin level. A technician can easily make his or her own measuring device with a simple Foley urinary catheter. Use a permanent marking pen to indicate incremental measurements from the inflated balloon. Design your measurements from commercially available lengths of low-profile devices. The low-profile gastrostomy device kits come with an obturator. The blunt-ended obturator is used to extend the mushroom at the distal tip of the tube. Placement of the obturator is never done through the shaft of the device because this will damage the integrity of the antireflux valve, but placed through the side holes of the mushroom tip. This elongates the mushroom tip, facilitating the placement through the stoma and into the stomach. Once the proximal end of the device is at skin level, the obturator is withdrawn, allowing the mushroom tip to regain its conformation. A plug or cap is placed in the tube opening. A connecting tube is attached to the gastrostomy device for feeding. Straight bolus feeding adaptors are preferred for veterinary medicine over angulated adaptors designed for enteral feeding pumps. A decompression tube is another accessory that penetrates through the gastrostomy device's antireflux valve. A syringe can be adapted to decompress the stomach in patients that accumulate excess trapped air and gas.

Low-profile devices available commercially are made from silicone, so they have higher tissue compatibility than latex tubes. Canine and feline patients tolerate the apparatus much better than the longer gastrostomy tubes. Owners of the patients are elated to "have their animal back," a pet that looks "normal," without a long tube, bandaging, or support device for the external tube. Owners have noted healthier stoma sites and appreciate the ease of feeding and care. Because of its snug low-profile fit, dislodgment of the tube does not occur as with the initial PEG tube. This is also a relief for the pet owner who may be accustomed to replacing gastrostomy tubes three to four times per year. A low-profile gastrostomy device can last up to 1 year (Figure 20-40).

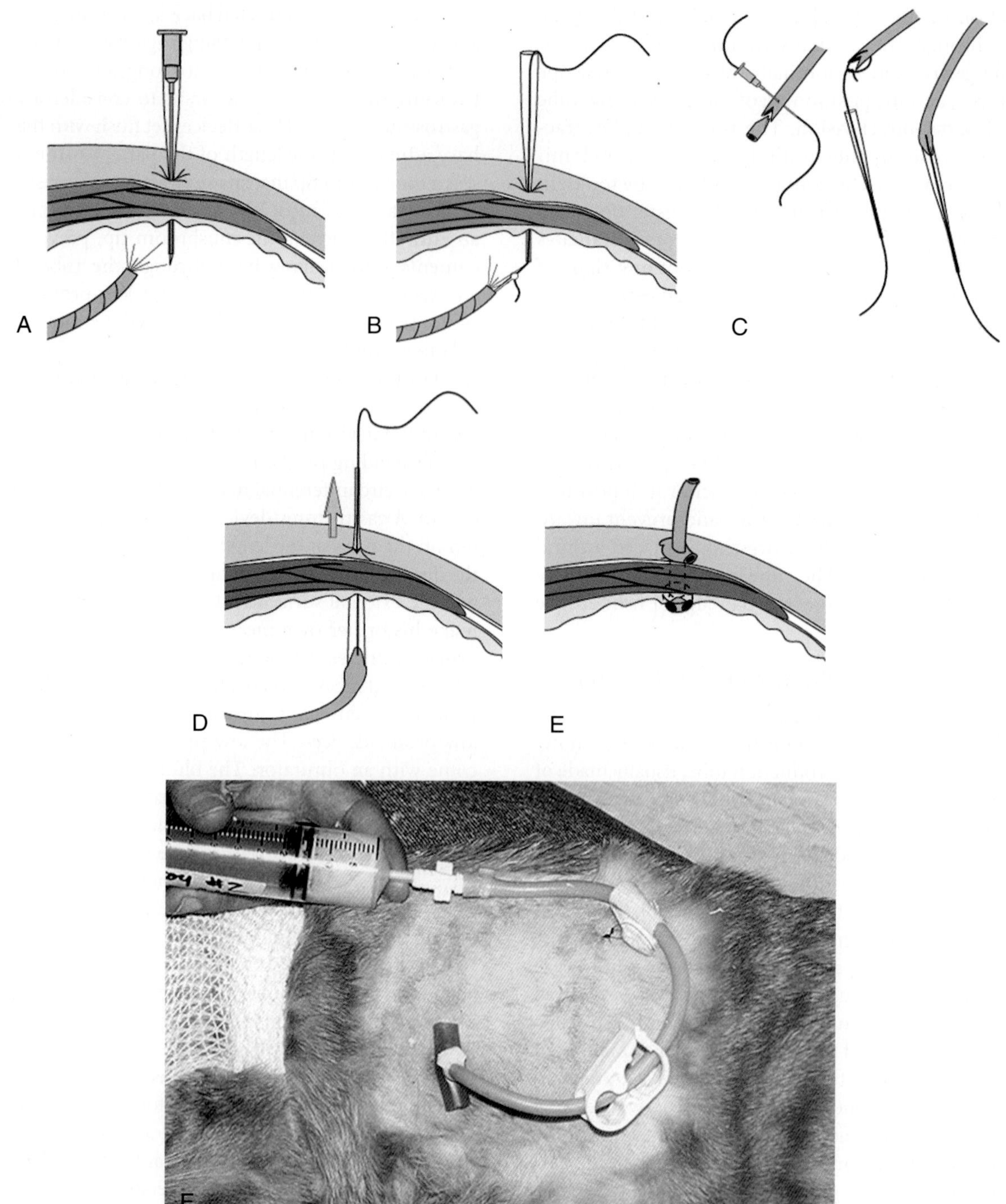

FIGURE 20-39 PEG technique. **A,** With the dog placed in right lateral recumbency, the gastroscope is introduced into the stomach. The lumen of the stomach is filled with air. A cannula with stylet is inserted through the skin and pushed through the abdominal and gastric walls. **B,** The stylet is removed from the cannula, and a nylon suture is advanced into the stomach. The endoscopist grasps the thread with an endoscopic snare or forceps. The suture is then brought out through the mouth along with the gastroscope. **C,** The prepared PEG tube, attached in a tapered plastic pipette, is tied or attached to the thread exiting the oral cavity. **D,** The gastrostomy tube is lubricated, and traction is placed on the transabdominal thread, pulling the gastrostomy tube through the animal's mouth, esophagus, and through the gastric and abdominal walls. The gastrostomy tube is advanced until its distal tip rests gently against the gastric mucosa. **E,** An external flange is fitted down the tube against the skin to prevent the tube from slipping into the stomach. **F,** Gastrostomy tube in place with clamp in open position for food administration. The stockinette dressing is pulled over the gastrostomy tube after feeding is complete. (From Ettinger SJ, Feldmen E, editors: *Textbook of veterinary internal medicine*, ed 6, Philadelphia, 2005, Elsevier Saunders.)

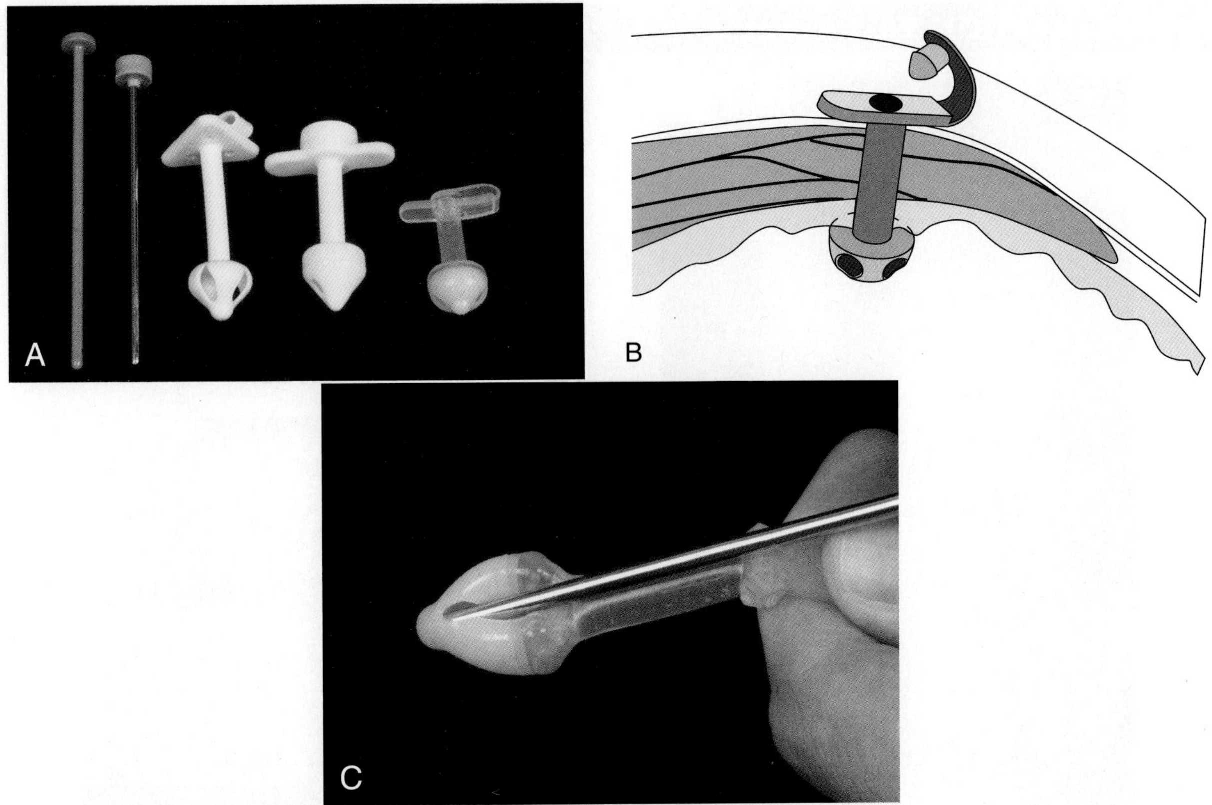

FIGURE 20-40 A, Low-profile gastrostomy devices and their obturators used to elongate the distal tip for placement. *Left to right:* The Ross Laboratories Stomate low-profile device, the Cook low-profile device, and the Bard "Button" low-profile device. B, The low-profile device placed in the stomach and its outer wings lying flush against the skin of the abdominal wall. The small cap is removed, and a feeding adapter with a syringe is connected to the low-profile device for administration of food. C, Correct technique to elongate the distal tip with the obturator before placement. Placement of the obturator is never done through the shaft of the device because this will damage the integrity of the antireflux valve located within the distal tip of the device. (From Ettinger SJ, Feldmen E, editors: *Textbook of veterinary internal medicine*, ed 6, Philadelphia, 2005, Elsevier Saunders.)

CASE PRESENTATION 20-1

Sandy is a 26.4 kg, 3-year-old, intact male Labrador cross. Sandy came to the hospital as a referral case from a local practice with the diagnosis of pyothorax. Two days earlier, the clients noticed sudden onset of dyspnea, difficulty breathing when lying down, panting excessively, and increased breathing effort.

Significant physical findings included: 5% dehydration, muffled heart sounds, absent breath sounds ventrally (bilateral) and present dorsally, and hyperpnea with increased abdominal component to the inspiratory phase. Sandy was placed in an oxygen cage with an FIO_2 (fractional inspired oxygen concentration) of 60% while the veterinary technician prepared for an IV catheter placement, thoracocentesis, and possible chest tube placement.

While on "flow by oxygen," an IV catheter was placed, and pretreatment blood samples were drawn for a CBC and chemistry profile; a urine sample was collected by free catch. The patient was started on lactated Ringer's solution with potassium supplementation. Following a surgical prep of the right chest wall, a thoracocentesis was performed with a 14-gauge OTN catheter. 1420 ml of purulent fluid was removed. A sample was submitted to the lab for cytology and a culture and sensitivity. It was decided to place a chest tube and initiate continuous chest drainage. Sandy was given Midazolam and butorphanol for sedation. Oxygen was administered by mask until he desaturated 10 minutes following sedation (SpO_2 decreased from 95% to 82%); at that point he was intubated and given 100% oxygen, the SpO_2 increased to 97%. The remainder of the procedure was uneventful, and radiographs were taken after chest tube placement (Figure 1). Sandy's chest tube was connected to a continuous chest drainage system (Figure 2), and Sandy was placed back in an oxygen cage.

Significant lab findings include: WBC 31,260 cells/μl (Normal 6000 to 13,000), metamyelocytes 1240 with moderate toxicity, bands 14,570 with moderate toxicity (Normal: rare), and neutrophils 8060 with slight toxicity (Normal 3000 to 10,500). The chemistry and urine analysis was unremarkable. Cytology revealed a total nucleated cell count of 193,560 with 88% neutrophils and 12% large mononuclear cells. The direct smear was noted to be markedly cellular and contained a small amount of blood. Nucleated cells consisted of a preponderant population of variably degenerate neutrophils. Mixed bacterial organisms (cocci and short and long thin rods) were occasionally seen within the cytoplasm of neutrophils. Lesser numbers of foamy activated macrophages were

Continued

CASE PRESENTATION 20-1—cont'd

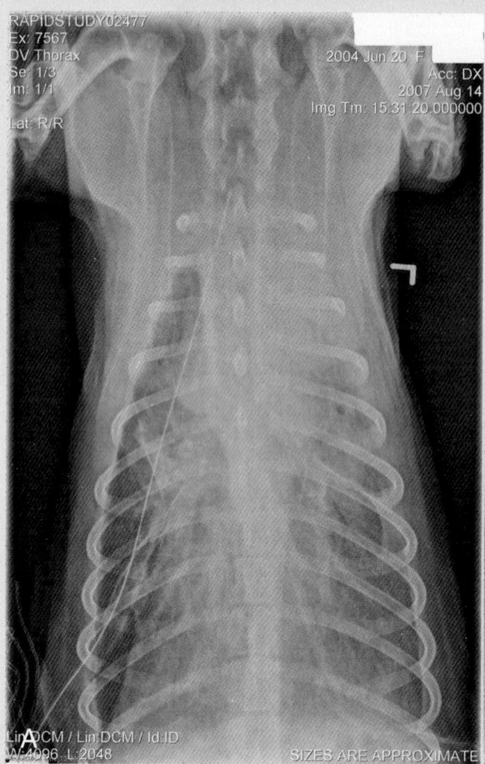

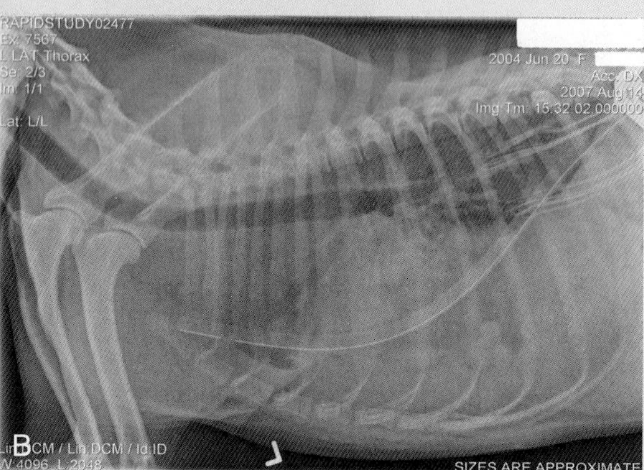

FIGURE 1 A and B, DV and lateral thoracic radiographs following chest tube placement. Bilateral pleural effusion is present.

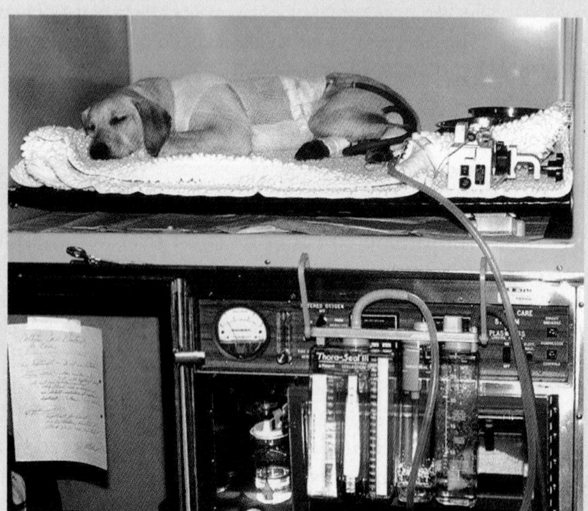

FIGURE 2 A, Patient (not Sandy) with a chest tube connected to a continuous chest drainage (Thora-Seal III) system.

seen. The cytology was interpreted as septic purulent exudate suspicious for a penetrating foreign body injury or migrating foxtail. Eventually the organisms identified from the culture were *Actinomyces* species and *Pasteurella multocida*.

Nursing concerns/plans included:

- Administer IV antibiotics (ampicillin and enrofloxacin). Care was given to administer at the proper rate and avoid administering with incompatible drugs.
- Continued monitoring of vital signs.
- Assess respiratory status by auscultation, respiratory rate and effort, oxygen saturation, and intermittent arterial blood gases.
- Monitor the chest drainage system and document the hourly chest drainage.
- Monitor body weight and ins and outs making adjustments in the fluid therapy plan to account for the abnormal fluid loss resulting from the pyothorax.
- Perform IV catheter and chest tube care per protocol.
- Ensure that the patient is eating and drinking.

On day 2 of the hospitalization, it was decided to try Sandy on room air and check an arterial blood gas. The blood gas results were: pH 7.42 (Normal 7.35 to 7.45), PCO_2 36 mm Hg (Normal 35 to 45), PO_2 64.6 mm Hg (Normal 80 to 120), HCO_3 22.5 mEq/L (Normal 18 to 24); the results confirmed hypoxemia (decreased PaO_2). Sandy was placed back on oxygen with an FIO_2 of 40%. His SpO_2 on room air was 90% and increased to 95% when on 40% oxygen.

The remainder of Sandy's hospitalization was uneventful; periodic samples of chest fluid were aseptically collected from the chest tube and submitted to the lab for an analysis. He was finally able to be placed on room air on day 6. The pyothorax resolved, and the chest tube was pulled on day 8. Sandy was discharged home on day 9 with orders to continue oral antibiotics and see the referring veterinarian in 1 week.

LARGE ANIMAL SAMPLING AND THERAPEUTIC TECHNIQUES

VENOUS BLOOD SAMPLE COLLECTION

Blood sampling is a routine and, in most cases, simple method to obtain a large amount of diagnostic data. The choice of blood collection tube (or syringe with anticoagulant added) will determine what laboratory parameters can be obtained. Some tests require serum (obtained after clotting of whole blood sample), some require plasma (the serum plus fibrinogen) obtained by using an anticoagulant, and some tests require whole blood for analysis. Blood sample tubes containing an anticoagulant should be filled to capacity to ensure the correct blood to anticoagulant ratio. Insufficient blood mixed with the anticoagulant may lead to erroneous laboratory results. Once collected, the sample should be gently inverted several times to ensure adequate mixing of the blood with the anticoagulant.

For all sites and species, the hair and/or skin should be cleaned with isopropyl alcohol to remove any obvious debris. In addition to providing antibacterial activity, the alcohol facilitates visualization of the vein and acts as a local vasodilator. If blood cultures are desired, a full sterile prep (as described earlier) is required.

> *TECHNICIAN NOTE* Cleaning the hair and/or skin with isopropyl alcohol provides antibacterial activity and facilitates visualization of the vein.

The choice of vein depends on the appearance of the vessels, the position of the animal, and the disposition of the animal. If repeated samples will be required, the technician should start first with a more distal venipuncture site, with subsequent samples taken progressively more proximal on the vein. The bevel-up position of the needle facilitates venipuncture and is less traumatic to the skin and vein on puncture. If the need to collect multiple samples is anticipated, placement of an IV catheter should be considered.

A syringe and needle may be used or Vacutainer needle and collection tube. When a needle and syringe are used, the needle may be inserted first and then the syringe attached, or in some cases, the needle may be attached to the syringe before insertion. The Vacutainer system can be used by inserting the long end of the double-ended needle into the vein and then slipping a blood collection tube over the exposed needle. Alternately the tube may be placed on the double-ended needle before injection by inserting the tube into the holder and pressing the rubber stopper against the metal end of the needle until the top of the rubber stopper is aligned with the circumferential score on the tube holder. Do not push it further until the needle is inserted into the lumen of the vein. Once in the lumen, the tube is pushed fully onto the needle. If the tube is pushed fully onto the needle before the other needle end is in the vein, the vacuum is broken, and the blood will not flow into the tube.

EQUINE VENIPUNCTURE

Common veins used for blood sampling in the adult equine include the jugular, the cephalic (located on the medial aspect of the forelimb), the transverse facial (runs transversely beneath the facial crest and above the transverse facial artery), and the lateral thoracic vein (located in the cranial ventral third of the thorax caudal to the point of elbow).

Additionally, for recumbent equine neonates, the saphenous vein (on the medial aspect of the hind limb) can be safely used.

Restrain the horse as necessary, depending on the behavior of the horse. A halter and lead rope may be the only restraint required, but additional restraint is necessary in some horses.

Jugular Vein

To occlude and distend the vein, pressure is placed on the jugular furrow in the lower third of the neck. Using an alcohol-soaked sponge or cotton ball, the ballottement of the vessel is performed (stroked several times in a downward direction). A 19- to 25-gauge × ⅝ to 1.5-inch needle is inserted into the lumen of the vessel, and blood is aspirated using a syringe or Vacutainer tube (Figures 20-41 and 20-42).

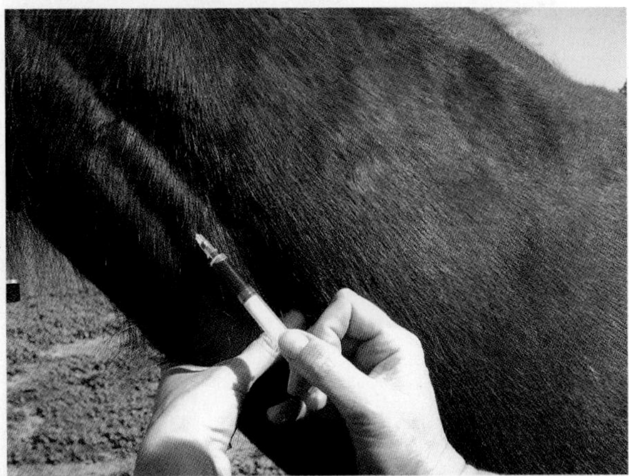

FIGURE 20-41 Venipuncture of equine jugular vein.

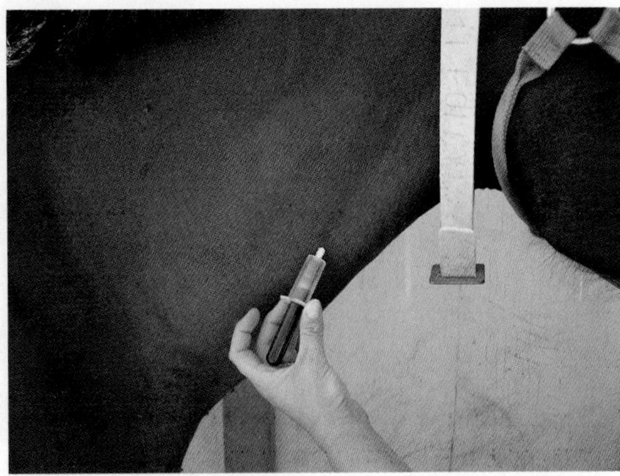

FIGURE 20-42 Blood collection from equine jugular vein using Vacutainer system.

Some animals object vehemently to the needle insertion. For these patients, if the needle is inserted first and the animal jumps, twitches, or otherwise moves, the needle is more apt to remain in place without the weight of the syringe. Once the animal settles, the syringe is attached. and the blood sample aspirated.

Transverse Facial Vein

This vein runs transversely beneath the facial crest and above the transverse facial artery and can be located midway between the medial canthus of the eye and the rostral end of the facial crest (Figure 20-43, *A*).

> TECHNICIAN NOTE To locate the site, the technician may place the thumb at the medial canthus and the index finger at the lateral canthus and draw an imaginary V shape diagonally down to the facial crest.

It is commonly used in nonfractious horses to collect small volumes of blood. There is no need to occlude the vein. A 22- to 25-gauge × ⅝- to 1-inch needle is inserted perpendicular to the skin beneath the facial crest and advanced until bone is felt. The syringe is then attached, and the needle is withdrawn slowly while aspirating. When blood enters the syringe, the placement is maintained until the collection is completed (see Figure 20-43, *B*). There is a very minimal risk for hematoma formation or bleeding from this site. Horses rarely object to the needle insertion at this site. Caution must be used when handling needles around the face of the horse because carelessness can lead to puncture of the eye. The hand that holds the needle should always be cupped, protecting the eye from the needle.

Cephalic Vein

The cephalic vein is located on the medial aspect of the forelimb and can be safely accessed in many horses. The site is cleaned with a wipe of rubbing alcohol, which also enhances

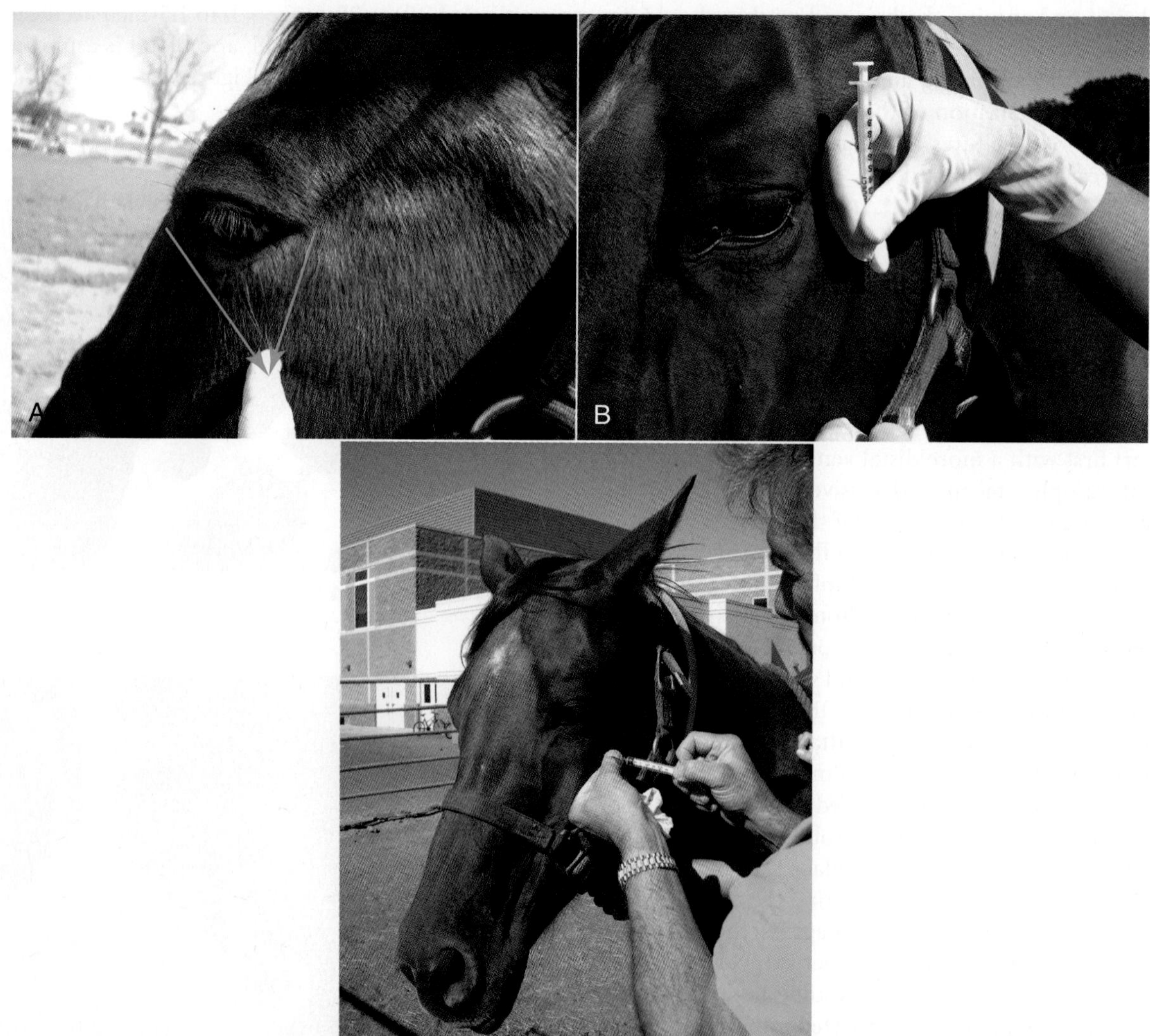

FIGURE 20-43 **A,** The needle insertion site for a transverse facial blood sample can be located by drawing imaginary lines from the medial canthus and lateral canthus, intersect them at the facial crest, and insert the needle just below the facial crest. **B,** Holding syringe to protect eye in case horse moves while preparing to insert needle. **C,** Blood collection from transverse facial vein.

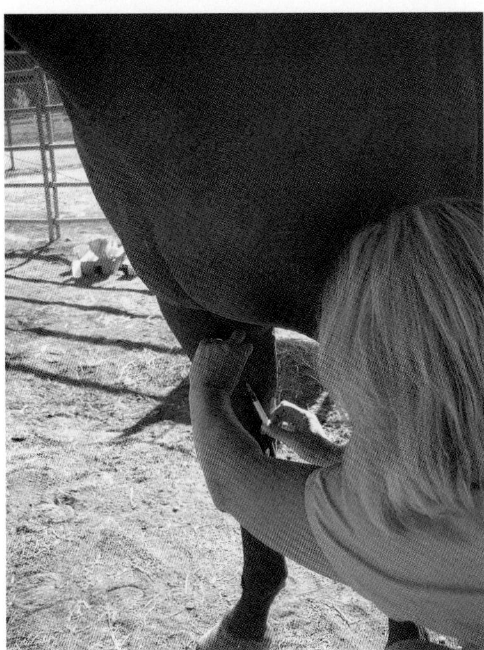
FIGURE 20-44 Venipuncture of equine cephalic vein.

the visibility of the vein. The vein is occluded above the needle insertion site (as with all veins, the blood flows back toward the heart). A 20- to 22-gauge × 1- to 1.5-inch needle is inserted (Figure 20-44). Horses may quickly lift up the foot when the needle is inserted, so it is beneficial to insert the needle first and then attach the syringe when the horse has placed the foot back on the ground to reduce the likelihood of the needle coming out of the horse when the foot is lifted. Since this site is low on the animal, the risk for hematoma formation is enhanced, so after removal of the needle, the technician must make a concerted effort to apply pressure to the site. If the technician is completing other work on the patient, a cotton ball may be placed on the site and adhesive tape wrapped around the limb, but this can only be left on very briefly because circulation can be compromised. The technician must remove the tape before leaving the patient.

Saphenous Vein

The saphenous vein is located on the medial aspect of the hind limb. It is unsafe for the technician to use this site in nonanesthetized adult horses. It can be used successfully in recumbent neonates. Care needs to be taken to apply sufficient digital pressure after the removal of the needle.

BOVINE VENIPUNCTURE

Jugular Vein

Restrain the animal with its head elevated slightly and tied securely. If necessary, nose tongs may be applied for additional restraint. Distend the jugular vein by placing pressure low in the jugular furrow. The bovine jugular vein is very large, and the palm of the hand should be used to occlude the vessel. Firmly wiping the jugular groove several times in a downward direction with an alcohol-soaked sponge aids in visualizing the vein. Thrust the needle (16- to 18-gauge × 1.5 inch) into the vein with the needle tip directed cranially at about a 45-degree angle (Figure 20-45). Maintain distention of the vein while collecting the blood and then apply digital pressure at the site when the needle is removed.

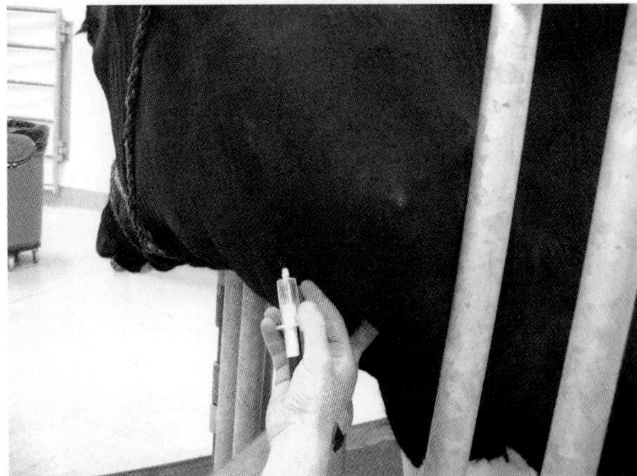
FIGURE 20-45 Blood collection from bovine jugular vein.

Coccygeal Vein (Tail Vein)

The tail vein is commonly used when bleeding a large number of cattle and when the individual's jugular vein is thrombosed or inaccessible. The animal is restrained in a chute or stanchion, and a tail jack is applied. The tail jack provides restraint and also places the tail in the best position for a venipuncture. With one hand, the tail is lifted up and toward the back of the animal until it is vertical. The ventral surface of the tail is cleaned with 70% isopropyl alcohol to remove dirt and fecal material. An 18- to 21-gauge × 1.5-inch needle is attached to a syringe. The diameter of the coccygeal vein is considerably smaller than the jugular vein, so larger needles are inappropriate. Locate the soft space between two vertebrae by palpating between two bony prominences. These are hemal processes, which are bony canals on the ventral aspect of the vertebral bodies that protect the artery and vein. Insert the needle perpendicular to the midline until bone is felt and then slowly back the needle out slightly from the bone while applying suction to the syringe. Blood should flow freely into the syringe. If preferred, a Vacutainer needle and tube can be used instead of the needle and syringe (Figure 20-46).

After the sample collection, withdraw the needle, lower the tail, and apply pressure to the site for approximately 15 seconds to discourage hematoma formation. The coccygeal artery lies in close proximity to the coccygeal vein and may be inadvertently punctured. If this is done, digital pressure should be applied to the site for at least 1 minute to prevent hematoma formation.

Subcutaneous Abdominal Venipuncture (Milk Vein)

The right and left milk veins are located along the ventrolateral body wall of the thorax and abdomen. These provide major venous drainage of the udder. Use of these veins for a venipuncture can result in life-threatening conditions for the cow. The milk veins are very large and are prone to prolonged

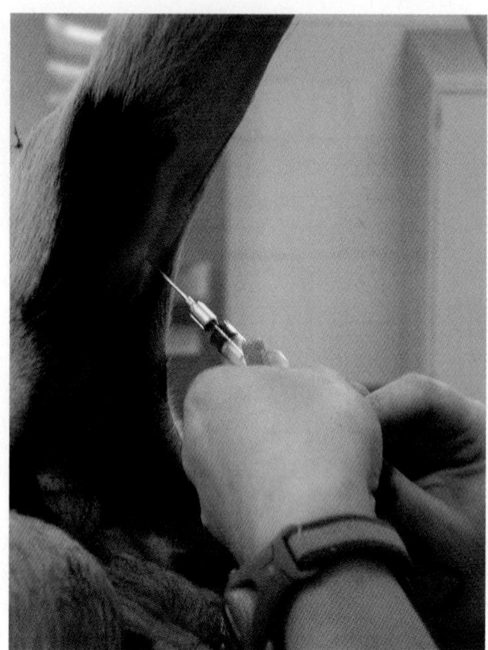

FIGURE 20-46 Venipuncture of bovine coccygeal vein.

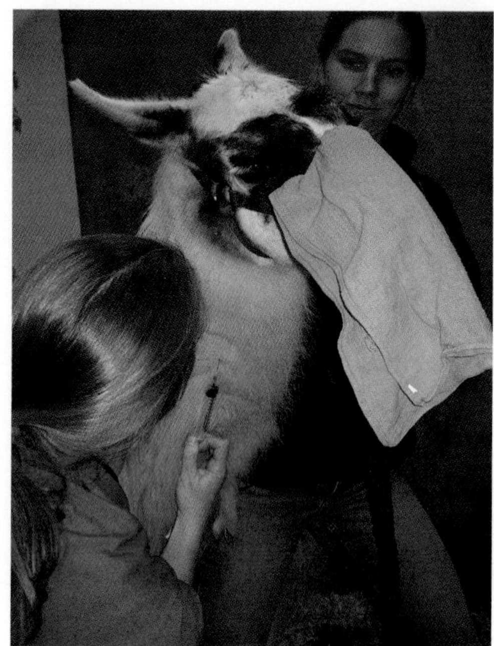

FIGURE 20-47 Blood collection from llama jugular vein. A towel can be draped loosely through the halter on bridge of nose to protect personnel from being spit upon if the animal objects to the procedure.

and pronounced bleeding, large hematoma formation, and are at great risk for an infection because they are easily contaminated by feces, dirt, and other material when the animal is recumbent. Thrombosis of the milk vein may lead to insufficient circulation to the udder, and collateral circulation is inadequate to overcome the problem. **It is recommended that these veins never be used for venipuncture.**

On very rare occasion and as a last resort, a veterinarian may direct the technician to collect a blood sample from the milk vein. In the event that no other vein is available for sampling and the veterinarian has deemed it necessary to collect a sample from the milk vein, the animal must be restrained adequately in a chute or stanchion with a tail jack or leg restraint applied. The technician should stand next to the shoulder of the cow facing the tail or stand close to the flank facing the head. Bend just enough to insert the needle while keeping your head up to avoid contact when the cow kicks (there is a strong likelihood that the animal will kick when the needle is inserted).

Select an accessible site. Clean with isopropyl alcohol, stabilize the vein with one hand, hold the skin taut, and insert the needle (18- to 22-gauge × 1.5-inch needle) in either direction (the blood flows cranially) with the syringe attached. Alternatively a Vacutainer collection needle may be inserted and a Vacutainer collection tube attached. After the needle is removed, prolonged digital pressure must be applied over the puncture site (for several minutes).

CAMELID VENIPUNCTURE (LLAMA, ALPACA, LAMOID, SOUTH AMERICAN CAMELID)

Jugular Venipuncture

Llamas and alpacas provide challenges to jugular venipuncture. In adult animals, visualization of the jugular vein is not possible. There is no visible jugular groove, the skin over the jugular vein is thick (in males it can be 1 cm thick), and they have long fiber. The transverse process of a cervical vertebra has a ventral projection that curves around the jugular furrow, and llamas and alpacas have valves in the jugular vein that function to keep the blood flowing toward the heart rather than allowing backflow when the head is lowered.

A jugular venipuncture can be performed in a high or low site. The high site can be located by creating an imaginary line along the ventral border of the mandible and dropping an imaginary line vertically down from just in front of the ear. The intersection of these two lines provides a guide for locating the vein. In some animals, a fluid wave may be visualized by occlusion and ballottement of the vein (stroking the vein toward the occluding hand). The skin is thickest at this point, but the jugular vein is separated here from the carotid artery by a muscle, making the likelihood of arterial penetration less at this site than the low neck site (Figure 20-47).

The low position is located by palpating the ventral projection of the transverse process of the sixth cervical vertebrae (this is close to the thorax and prominent) and occluding the vein just above the transverse process (Figure 20-48). As with the high neck site, ballottement of a fluid wave can help to identify the vein. The skin is thinner at this location, and movement of the head is less of a problem than with the high neck site, but the fiber is thicker. The carotid artery and jugular vein are in close proximity in this area, which increases the chance of arterial penetration.

Saphenous Venipuncture

The saphenous vein is superficial and on the medial aspect of the stifle. This vein can be used in recumbent animals. The vein lies in close proximity and cranial to the artery.

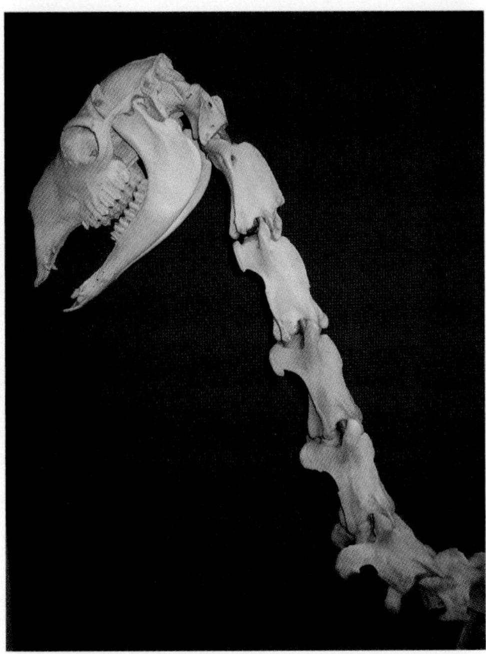

FIGURE 20-48 Cervical vertebrae of llama. The sixth cervical vertebra is used as a landmark for low neck venipuncture.

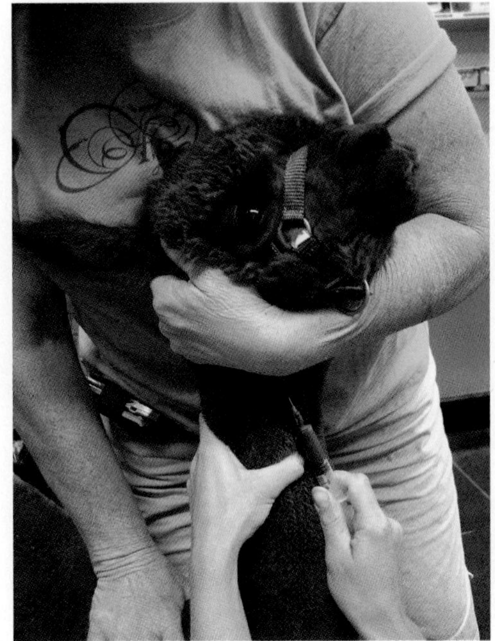

FIGURE 20-49 Blood collection from jugular vein in alpaca cria.

Auricular (Ear) Vein

The ear vein can yield small amounts of blood, sufficient for many laboratory tests. Digital pressure is usually sufficient to raise the vein, but if necessary, an elastic band can be wrapped temporarily around the base of the ear, as a tourniquet.

Middle Coccygeal Vein

Located as in cattle, but is more superficial in camelids, just under the skin.

Cephalic Vein

The cephalic vein lies similar in placement to that of dogs and can be accessed in adults when the animal is in sternal recumbency (Kushed position).

Neonatal Camelids (Crias)

The common veins used in neonates are the jugular, cephalic, saphenous, and occasionally the ear. The jugular vein is much easier to use in the neonate than the adult because the skin is thin and the jugular vein can be easily distended and visualized (Figure 20-49).

OVINE AND CAPRINE VENIPUNCTURE

The jugular, cephalic, and femoral veins are commonly used in sheep and goats. The ear also provides an accessible site for blood sampling.

Most sheep will be restrained in a "set up" position on their rumps with their back side leaning up against the handler (Figure 20-50). Jugular, cephalic, femoral, and ear samples can be taken from this position. Jugular, cephalic, and ear samples can be obtained from some sheep while they are standing, but having sheep "set up" on their rumps will drastically reduce the amount of effort required to carry out most procedures (Figures 20-51 through 20-54). The jugular, cephalic, and ear veins can be easily accessed in goats while they are standing. The handler can restrain the animal by backing it into a corner and by straddling the goat with the handler's legs tight

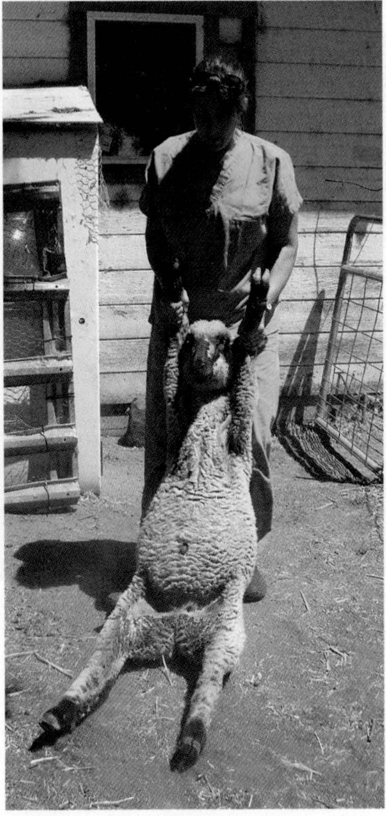

FIGURE 20-50 Setting sheep on the rump is an effective method of restraint for venipuncture and many other procedures.

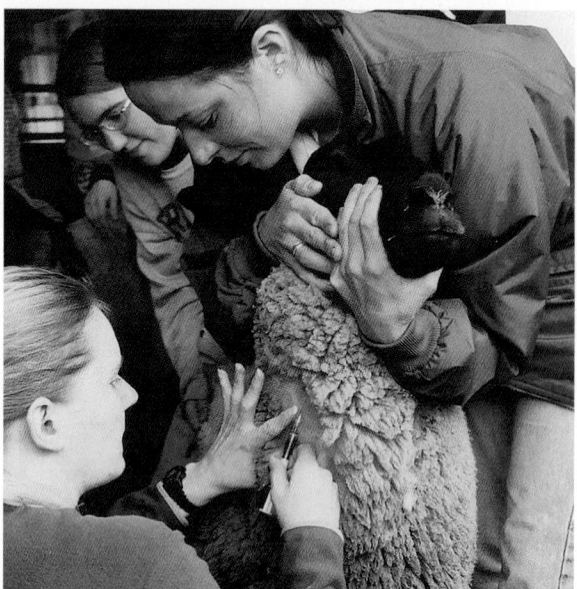

FIGURE 20-51 A technician crouches in front of a standing sheep to collect blood from the jugular vein. Note that the assistant at the rear of the sheep prevents the sheep from backing away from the technician.

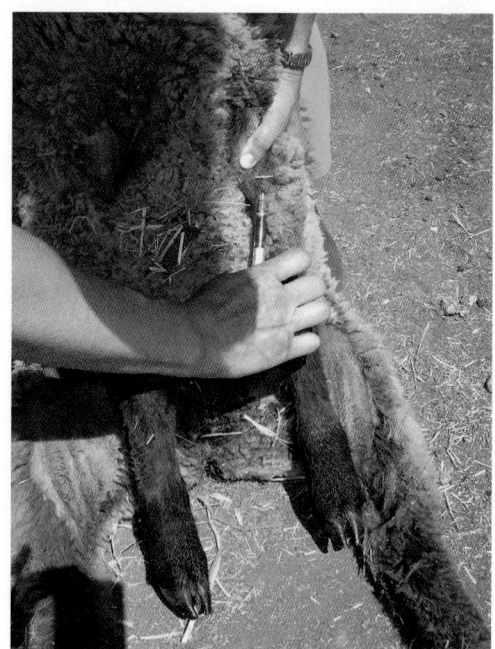

FIGURE 20-53 Collecting blood sample from cephalic vein while sheep set up on rump for restraint.

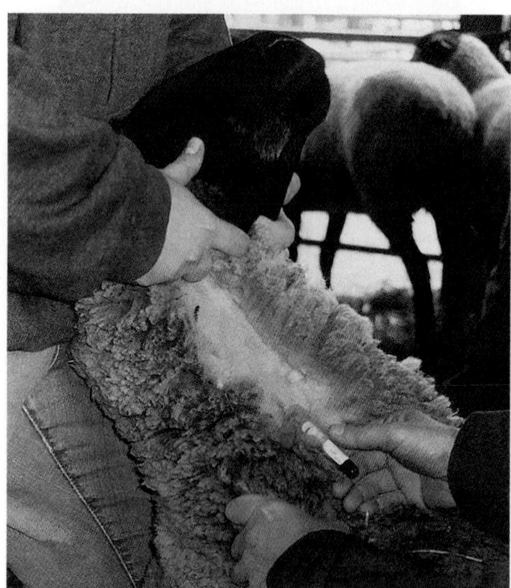

FIGURE 20-52 Sheep placed in a seated position to allow blood to be collected from the jugular vein.

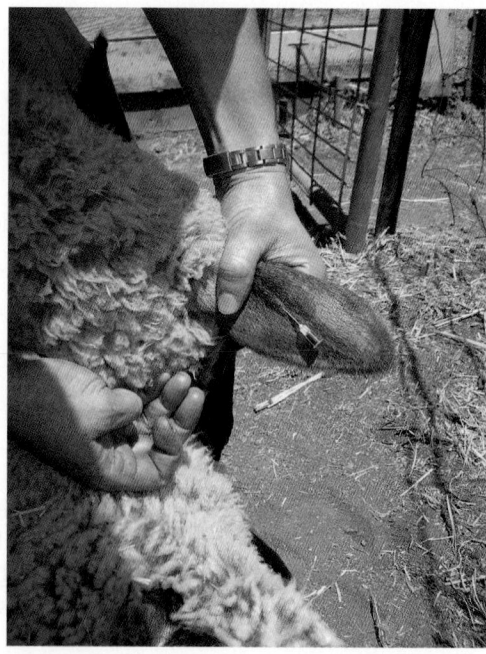

FIGURE 20-54 Blood samples can be obtained from auricular vein in sheep.

on either side of the neck or push the goat up against a wall. The femoral vein is accessible when the goat is in lateral recumbency.

PORCINE VENIPUNCTURE

Blood collection from swine is more difficult than in other large animals. They are challenging to restrain, have thick jowls, short legs, tough skin, and are fat. Sampling can be done with the animal restrained or with the animal under anesthetic. The technician should be aware that in addition to commercial hogs, many pigs that are receiving veterinary care are beloved pets, and the handling and restraint required for venipuncture and other procedures should be explained well to the owner.

The common veins used for venous blood collection in pigs include the cranial vena cava, jugular, auricular, cephalic, peripheral leg veins, and occasionally the orbital sinus or tail vein.

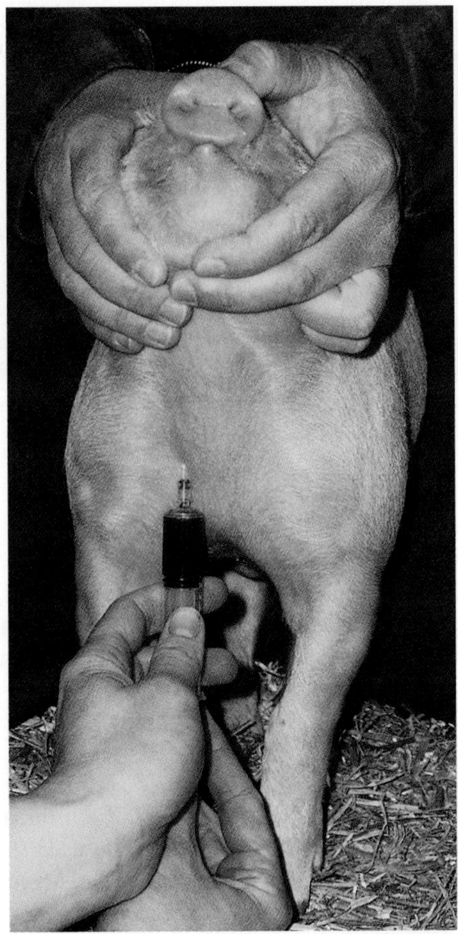

FIGURE 20-55 A blood sample from the right anterior vena cava is taken with the needle directed into the jugular fossa just lateral to the manubrium sterni.

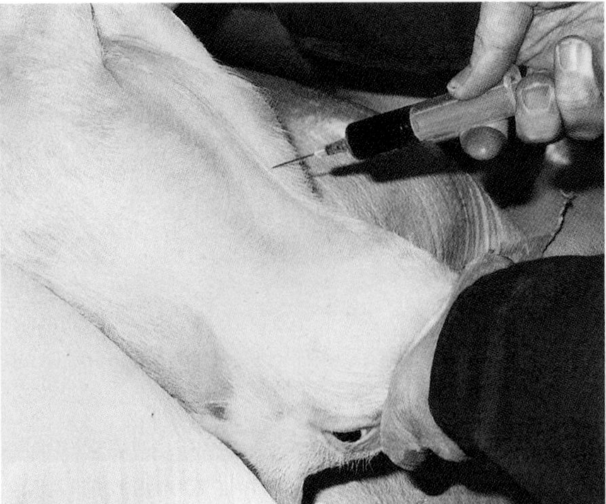

FIGURE 20-56 Venipuncture of right anterior vena cava in a small pig in dorsal recumbency.

Cranial Vena Cava

The cranial vena cava is located in the thoracic inlet between the first pair of ribs. The right side of the animal should be used to prevent damaging the phrenic nerve, which is anatomically more protected on the right side of the animal than the left. Hitting the phrenic nerve may alter the function of the diaphragm and can result in life-threatening cardiac or respiratory problems. For piglets, a 20-gauge × 1.5-inch needle is used. An 18- to 20-gauge × 1- to 1.5-inch needle is appropriate for small pigs (up to approximately 25 kg). For pigs weighing more than 25 kg an 18- to 20-gauge × 1.5- to 3.5-inch needle is used. Large adults require a 16- to 18-gauge × 4- to 4.5-inch needle.

To collect blood from a small pig, the animal is placed on its back (dorsal recumbency) on a 45-degree incline with the head lower than the hips. The head is extended and front legs pulled caudally. The jugular furrow is visualized, and the needle with a syringe attached is inserted in the furrow lateral to the manubrium of the sternum. The needle is pointed toward the caudal aspect of the top of the opposite shoulder blade (Figure 20-55). As the needle is inserted, the syringe plunger should be pulled slightly to maintain negative pressure. When blood enters the syringe, the needle is held in place while the desired amount of blood is aspirated.

Larger hogs are restrained with the use of a hog snare in a standing position with the head slightly elevated. The person with the syringe crouches in front of the right side of the pig facing the body of the pig or can crouch to the side of the right shoulder facing the neck. The needle is inserted into the right jugular furrow lateral to the manubrium (Figure 20-56), directed toward the shoulder. The cranial vena cava in large pigs is deep (4 inches may be required to reach the lumen).

Jugular Vein

The jugular vein can be used for a blood sample collection in pigs of any age. It is located in the jugular furrow. It is not as deep as the vena cava, so fewer potential complications are associated with its use. The jugular vein has a smaller diameter than the vena cava and is more difficult to access, especially in large or heavy pigs. The needle size selected depends on the size of the animal. A jugular venipuncture in piglets can be done with a 20-gauge × 1.5-inch needle. Large pigs may require 16-gauge × 3- to 3.5-inch needles. To prevent the puncture of the phrenic nerve, the right side of the animal should be used when possible. The needle should be inserted cranially to the manubrium where the jugular furrow appears deepest. The animal is restrained as for a vena cava venipuncture. An imaginary horizontal line that passes through the shoulders and manubrium sterni is visualized. A second line is visualized that extends from the manubrium sterni to the scapula at an angle of 45 degrees with the first line. The needle is inserted perpendicular to the skin at the intersection of the second line with the deepest part of the right jugular fossa. The needle is directed caudodorsally and should not be angled toward either scapula. Because the vein is superficial, the syringe plunger should be retracted slightly as soon as the needle penetrates the skin. The needle is advanced until blood is aspirated into the syringe. Once a sufficient volume of blood has been collected, the needle is removed.

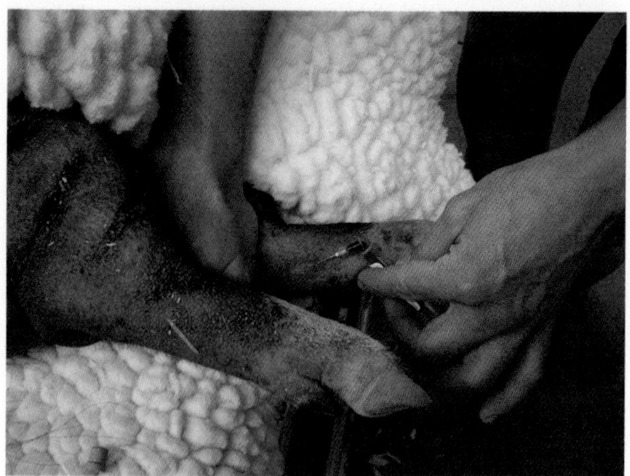

FIGURE 20-57 Collecting blood from peripheral leg vein in pig. Blood dripping from needle hub into collection tube prevents vein collapse.

The technician should be aware that fewer complications and a lower risk for incidental injury to the animal are associated with a venipuncture of the more distal veins listed below.

Auricular Vein

The auricular vein is located near the lateral border of the pinna of the ear. It is easily visualized on the dorsal side of the ear and can be seen even more clearly by placing digital pressure at the base of the lateral surface of the ear. The ear is held and digital pressure (or rubber-band tourniquet) applied at the base of the ear to distend the vein. A needle with a syringe attached can be inserted into the vein while gently pulling back on the plunger. To prevent the collapse of the vein with aspiration, some people prefer to insert the needle and allow the blood to drip from the needle hub directly into the uncapped collection tube. For most pigs, a 20-gauge × 1-inch needle is appropriate. For large adult pigs, an 18- to 19-gauge × 1-inch needle may be used. Vacutainer collection needles and tubes may also apply too much suction, and as in the case of excess pressure on the syringe plunger, these tend to cause the vein to collapse. When an adequate blood sample has been collected, pressure is released from the base of the ear, the needle removed, and pressure applied to the insertion site. For repeated sampling, the placement of an IV catheter should be considered.

Peripheral Leg Veins

The cephalic vein on the front leg, saphenous vein on the hind leg, and branches of veins located on the lower limbs are accessible in small pigs and can be used for venous sampling. The veins can be visualized and are readily accessible in anesthetized pigs. To prevent the collapse of the vein, the needle is inserted, and blood is allowed to drip from the hub of the needle into the open collection tube (Figure 20-57). The collection of blood from the standing and restrained pig can be done by placing hand pressure or a tourniquet above the collection site to distend the vein. A 20-gauge × 1- to 1.5-inch needle is inserted at approximately a 45-degree angle to the skin in the direction of the body.

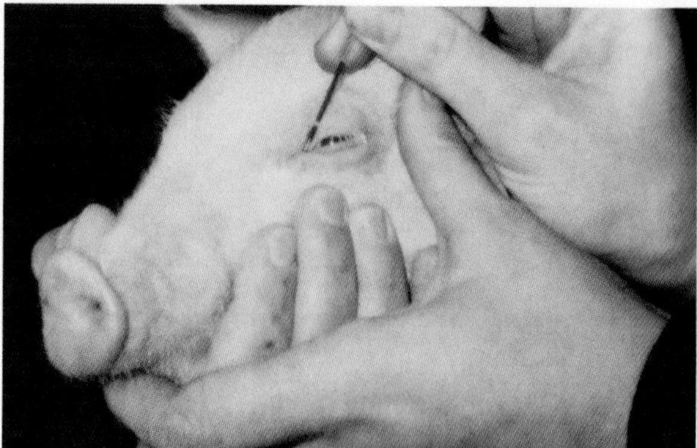

FIGURE 20-58 Small quantities of blood can be collected from the orbital sinus of the pig.

Coccygeal Vein

Though this site is not commonly used, it can be used for a venipuncture in adult pigs with intact (not docked) tails. A 20-gauge × 1-inch needle is inserted in the ventral midline of the tail perpendicular to the skin. Small blood samples can be obtained from this site.

Orbital Sinus (Medial Canthus of Eye)

The orbital sinus is adjacent to the medial canthus of the eye and can be used for the collection of small volumes of blood. A 20- to 22-gauge × 1 inch-needle can be used for piglets. Sampling on larger pigs may require a 16- to 18-gauge × 1.5-inch needle. The needle is inserted into the medial canthus deep into the third eyelid (nictitating membrane) and advanced at a 45-degree angle toward the opposite jaw until bone is felt. The needle is then rotated between the fingers until blood enters the hub. The syringe is attached and blood collected with gentle aspiration. When the collection is complete, the needle is removed and digital pressure applied over the medial canthus with the head elevated. A microcapillary tube with the end broken to form a rough point can be used in lieu of a needle (Figure 20-58).

ARTERIAL BLOOD SAMPLE COLLECTION

Arterial blood samples are commonly obtained for a blood gas analysis. This analysis usually provides information on the oxygen and carbon dioxide content, pH, base deficit, and bicarbonate in the sample. This information is used to evaluate respiratory status. If the data includes base deficit and bicarbonate, it is also used to assess the metabolic (acid-base) status. Arterial blood more accurately reflects the ventilation status of an animal than does venous blood because arteries carry freshly oxygenated blood from the heart to the body. Veins carry blood back to the heart for circulation to the lungs where the oxygen is replenished and carbon dioxide is released. Arterial blood gas samples are frequently performed intraoperatively on animals under a general anesthetic. Arterial catheters are commonly placed in anesthetized animals to facilitate sequential blood sampling. The values obtained from the sample analysis allow for close anesthesia monitoring.

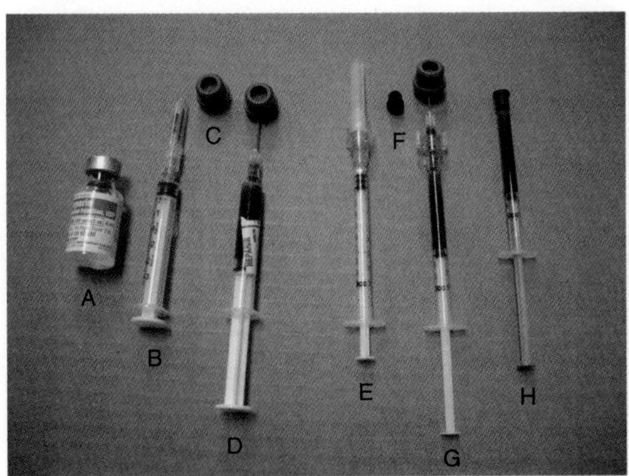

FIGURE 20-59 Syringes for blood gas sample collection. *A,* Sodium heparin (1000 U/ml). *B,* 3-ml syringe with barrel coated with heparin. *C,* Rubber stopper. *D,* Blood sample in syringe. *E,* Commercial preheparinized syringe (Micro A.B.G., Marquest). *F,* Stopper. *G,* Micro A.B.G. syringe with needle inserted into rubber stopper. *H,* Micro A.B.G. syringe with cap.

Arterial samples are routinely collected in nonanesthetized foals and crias, though less frequently in adult equines and camelids. Arterial sampling in cattle, sheep, goats, and pigs is rarely done on nonanesthetized animals.

The smallest gauge needle possible should be used to minimize trauma to the vessel. For most sample sites, a 25-gauge needle and 1- or 3-ml syringe are used. A very small amount of heparin (enough to fill the needle and appear in the hub) is aspirated into the needle and the plunger pulled back on the syringe to coat the syringe. The needle is removed, and a new 25-gauge needle is placed on the syringe, and then all of the heparin is expelled from the syringe and through the needle (this allows for the sharpest needle because the needle has not even punctured the stopper on a bottle of heparin). The heparin residue that remains is sufficient to prevent coagulation, but not enough to alter laboratory results. Some veterinarians prefer to use commercially prepared blood gas syringes containing powdered heparin (Figure 20-59).

Some veterinarians prefer to have sites for arterial puncture shaved before cleaning with alcohol (this is often the case with arterial samples on neonatal patients). The area is palpated to determine the location of the artery. Arteries pulsate, veins do not. The selected artery site is given a surgical prep or at least cleaned well with 70% isopropyl alcohol before insertion of the needle. It is not necessary to occlude arteries as is done with venous blood sampling. Depending on the patient's behavior and site selected, the needle may be inserted first and the syringe attached when blood comes from the hub or the needle may be inserted with a syringe attached. When the needle enters the artery, bright red blood pulses from the needle hub into the syringe. With most arterial samples, the blood will rapidly fill the syringe. Very little force is placed on the plunger of the syringe because the blood in the artery is under pressure and will spurt out. Do not expect blood to spurt from the needle as would be expected with a large-gauge needle. A minimum of 1 ml of blood should be collected into the syringe that has been prepared with liquid heparin to ensure results with diagnostic value. Smaller volumes can be taken using the commercial blood gas syringes because these syringes are designed to eliminate dilutional errors. When the needle is withdrawn, firm digital pressure should be applied immediately to the puncture site and should be maintained for several minutes. Arteries are far more susceptible to hematoma formation than veins. The technician must make sure to apply sufficient pressure long enough to stop bleeding and prevent formation of a hematoma. If care is taken with this step, the artery will be preserved and will be able to handle repeated sampling. If insufficient pressure and time is taken to hold off the collection site, the artery will become damaged, may become unusable for future sampling, and the related area may suffer from impaired circulation, thus compromising the condition of the patient.

> TECHNICIAN NOTE Following the collection of arterial blood samples, firm digital pressure should be applied immediately to the puncture site and maintained for several minutes.

Any bubbles present in the syringe are expelled, and the tip of the needle is inserted into a rubber stopper to occlude the needle tip and prevent air from entering the syringe. Samples for blood gas analysis must remain anaerobic (not contaminated by atmospheric air) because exposure to air will modify the oxygen and carbon dioxide values. The syringe should be rolled between the palms to ensure distribution of the anticoagulant throughout the sample. If the sample is not analyzed promptly, is should be placed in an ice water bath. Placing the sample in a freezer or on ice (with no water added) can damage the sample and affect the results of the analysis.

> TECHNICIAN NOTE Samples for a blood gas analysis must remain anaerobic (not contaminated by atmospheric air) because exposure to air will alter the laboratory values obtained.

EQUINE ARTERIAL SAMPLING

Arteries commonly used for blood sampling in horses include the facial (most often used in anesthetized animals), transverse facial, carotid, and metatarsal (in recumbent foals and anesthetized animals). In addition to those sites, arterial sampling on foals can include brachial and palmar (digital) arteries.

The facial artery is accessible in the area under the mandible to the facial crest. This site is commonly used for arterial catheterization in anesthetized animals (Figure 20-60, *A-D*).

The transverse facial artery lies caudal to the lateral canthus of the eye (Figure 20-61). Some people prefer to inject 0.25 ml of 2% lidocaine into the skin over the artery before a sample needle insertion, but often there is little or no objection from the horses when this site is used without a lidocaine block.

The carotid artery is accessible in the lower third of the neck, in the dorsal aspect of the jugular groove, and deeper

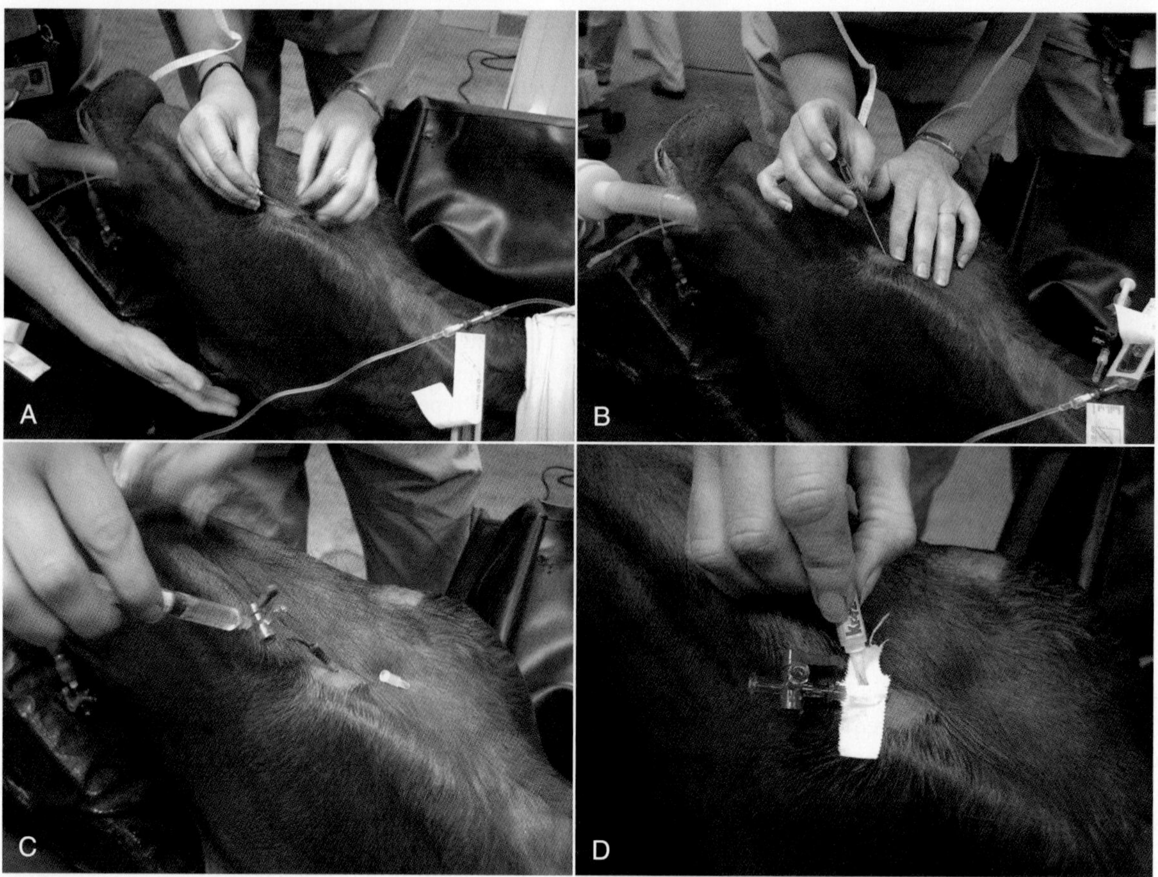

FIGURE 20-60 **A,** Nicking skin with needle to ease insertion for placing arterial catheter in facial artery. **B,** Inserting catheter. **C,** Placing stopcock on catheter. **D,** Securing arterial catheter with glue.

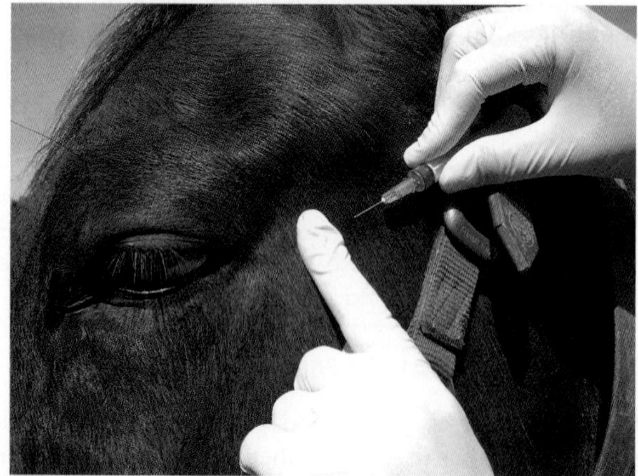

FIGURE 20-61 Collecting arterial sample from facial artery in awake equine.

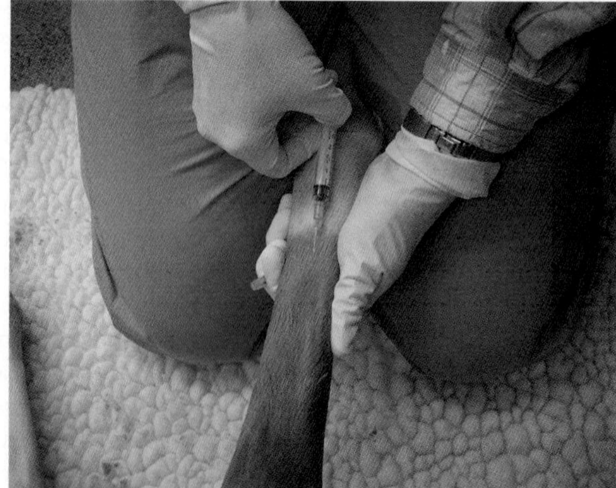

FIGURE 20-62 Restraining foal's hind leg between the technician's knees facilitates collection of arterial samples from the metatarsal artery in foals.

than the jugular vein. The artery feels like a cord, and a pulse is not usually palpable. An 18- to 19-gauge × 1.5-inch needle is directed into the artery at a 90-degree angle.

The dorsal metatarsal artery is located on the lateral aspect of the third metatarsal bone (cannon bone on hind limb) and is the preferred site in recumbent foals (Figure 20-62). A pulse is usually quite palpable. If a pulse is not obvious, the technician may put firm digital pressure proximal to the selected site, slowly release pressure, and feel for the pulse; this often enhances the pulse quality distally. In very sick neonates with poor blood pressure, the pulse may not be felt. In these patients, it is helpful to place a warm water bottle or compress over the artery to enhance the feel of local pulsation of the artery. The technician sits with the foal's hind hoof secured between the technician's knees. The artery is palpated with one hand and the needle inserted with the other hand. The foal's leg can be secured by holding it between the technician's legs (Figure 20-63). Some patients

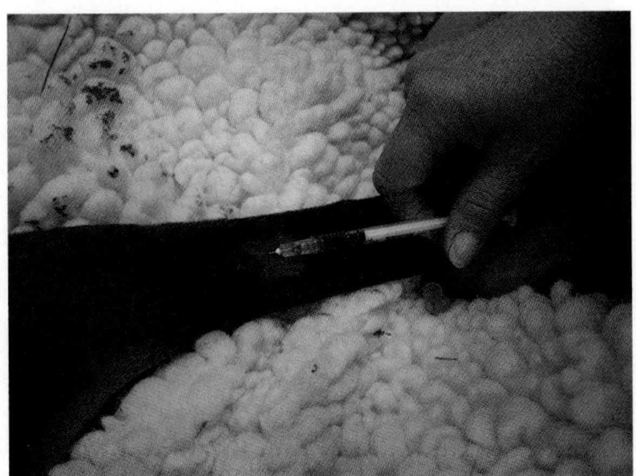

FIGURE 20-63 Collecting arterial sample from metatarsal artery in recumbent foal.

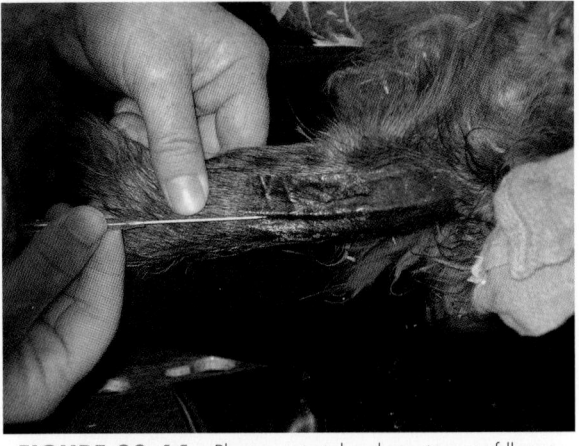

FIGURE 20-64 Placing arterial catheter in ear of llama.

require another handler restraining the foal, and the technician should make use of available help because procedures can be done quicker and with less stress to the patient and less risk for injury to the personnel when sufficient restraint is used. The behavior and condition of some foals allows the procedure to be done by the technician with no additional restraint. This will depend on the patient and the experience and skill of the technician. Many foals will accept this procedure if the needle is slowly and smoothly inserted into the skin. Some foals (even though very sick) will vehemently object to the needle insertion and jerk and kick the leg. In these foals, a quick insertion of the needle is done, and the syringe is attached after the foal's leg is again secured in place.

The palmar (digital) artery is palpable on the abaxial surface of the fetlock. This site is more difficult to access because the artery moves around quite a bit, so the location precludes restraining the foal's leg between the technician's legs.

The brachial artery may be palpated where it crosses the medial aspect of the proximal forearm and may yield a sample when attempts at other sites have been unsuccessful.

CAMELID ARTERIAL SAMPLING

The auricular (ear) artery is often used in llamas and alpacas for arterial sampling (Figure 20-64).

BOVINE, OVINE, AND CAPRINE ARTERIAL SAMPLING

Arteries used for sampling in these animals include the transverse facial, carotid, auricular, and dorsal metatarsal. As noted above, the collection of arterial samples from these animals is usually restricted to anesthetized individuals or neonatal patients.

ARTERIAL CATHETERIZATION

A short OTN catheter can be placed in the artery of an anesthetized patient.

Common arteries catheterized in the horse include the transverse facial and dorsal metatarsal. Common arteries catheterized in food animals include the transverse facial, dorsal metatarsal, and auricular.

URINE SAMPLE COLLECTION

Urine is collected from patients to screen for systemic (e.g., rhabdomyolysis, azoturia) or urinary tract disease. Urine is also routinely analyzed in race and performance horses for drug detection purposes. Urine can be collected for urinalysis from all large animal species in a free-catch midstream sample. Catheterization is recommended for samples that will be cultured, but as described later, bladder catheterization is not always possible. Cystocentesis is not practical in horses because of the inability to stabilize the bladder and the risk for intestinal perforation with a needle. It may be performed by some veterinarians on small ruminants.

For all urine samples, the sample should be collected in a dry, clean container (sterile if a culture is desired and catheterization is performed). A midstream sample should be collected because the initial stream contains more bacteria, mucus, and cell debris than the rest of the urine and does not as accurately reflect the actual content of the urine. Bacterial contamination in free-catch samples is significant. Urine samples degrade rapidly, so samples should be analyzed promptly (within 20 minutes) or refrigerated for no more than 2 days.

> *TECHNICIAN NOTE* Urine samples degrade rapidly, so they should be analyzed promptly or refrigerated for no more than 2 days.

Complications of urinary catheterization include infection of the urinary tract if sterile technique is not followed, mucosal irritation, slow and painful urination, and bacterial contamination of the sample.

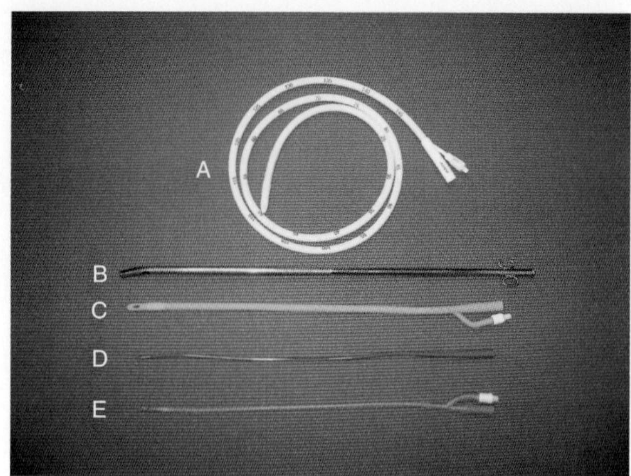

FIGURE 20-65 Urinary catheters. *A,* Stallion catheter. *B,* Mare Chambers catheter. *C,* 28F Foley catheter. *D,* 12 F Foley catheter. *E,* 12F red rubber feeding tube.

EQUINE URINE COLLECTION

Free-Catch Method

Urination may be encouraged by placing the horse in a freshly bedded stall. Sometimes standing the horse on a grassy area will encourage urination. Other suggestions include running water on cement and tickling the prepuce with a piece of straw. Some race and performance horses have been conditioned to urinate when whistled to. Recumbent neonates frequently will urinate when they are assisted to stand. The technician should be prepared by having a urine collection container within reach when helping a foal to rise or supporting it in a standing position.

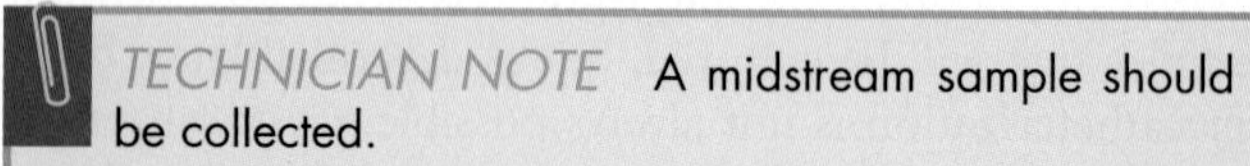

TECHNICIAN NOTE A midstream sample should be collected.

Cleansing of the external genital area is not necessary when collecting urine for drug testing.

Urinary Catheterization

Supplies needed:

Urinary catheter: use the tube with the smallest outer diameter as possible to minimize trauma to the urethra (Figure 20-65)
Adult males: Urinary (Foley) catheter 24F to 28F with 6- to 9-mm outer diameter and approximately 140 cm long
Colts: red rubber feeding catheter 12F
Adult females: Chambers catheter or Foley catheter 30F
Fillies: Foley catheter 12F
Sixty-milliliter catheter tip syringe
Sterile gloves
Gentle antimicrobial soap and 70% rubbing alcohol or other disinfectant cleanser (povidone-iodine solution and scrub)
Soft cotton
Sterile lubricant
Sterile collection containers (for urinalysis, cytology, and culture specimens)
Sedation

Male Horses

Sedation is usually required when catheterizing stallions and geldings for restraint and extension of the penis from the prepuce. The technician should be positioned cranially to avoid being kicked. Retract the prepuce, grasp the penis gently but firmly caudal to the glans penis (hold steady as the horse may attempt to retract the penis), and wash the penis with dilute antibacterial soap. Care must be taken to cleanse the urethral process and urethral diverticulum (a blind pouch located dorsal to the urethral opening) making sure to remove any smegma "bean" present in the diverticulum. It is then rinsed with water. This must be done to prevent the introduction into the bladder of bacteria that are present at the urethra and prepuce and to prevent bacterial contamination of the urine sample. Wearing sterile gloves, apply sterile water-soluble lubricant to the tip of a flexible urinary catheter. The penis is held with one hand, and the other hand is used to gently advance the catheter through the urethra and into the bladder. There is a curvature in the area of the ischial arch (just ventral to the anus), and slight force may be necessary to advance the catheter past this point. The horse will characteristically raise his tail when the catheter passes over the ischial arch just before it reaches the bladder.

If urine does not flow from the catheter, a syringe can be attached to gently aspirate the sample. Excessive negative pressure must not be used because it may cause minor hemorrhage and can alter the sample composition. A small volume of air can be injected into the catheter, or the catheter can be repositioned, if necessary, to encourage flow.

Female Horses

Wrap the tail and tie it out of the way to prevent hair from entering the vagina, touching the glove or catheter, and thus introducing contaminants.

Thoroughly clean the vulva and perineum. Using sterile gloves with sterile water-soluble lubricant locate the urethral orifice on the ventral aspect of the vaginal vault. The orifice is approximately 10 to 12 cm from the ventral commissure of the vulvar lips. A small Chambers catheter, stallion catheter, or Foley catheter can be used. Lubricate the catheter and using a finger, slide the catheter in and down into the urethral orifice and advance the catheter 5 to 10 cm (2 to 4 inches) until it enters the bladder (Figure 20-66, *A-D*). The flow of urine can be encouraged as described earlier.

CAMELID URINE COLLECTION

Free-Catch Method

Llamas and alpacas urinate and defecate on communal dung piles, so, if possible, the animal should be lead to a dung pile. Attaching a collection cup to the end of a broom or dowel facilitates collection without requiring personnel to be close enough to distract the animal. Both males and females urinate in a caudal direction while in a squatting position. Complete urination usually takes 30 to 60 seconds.

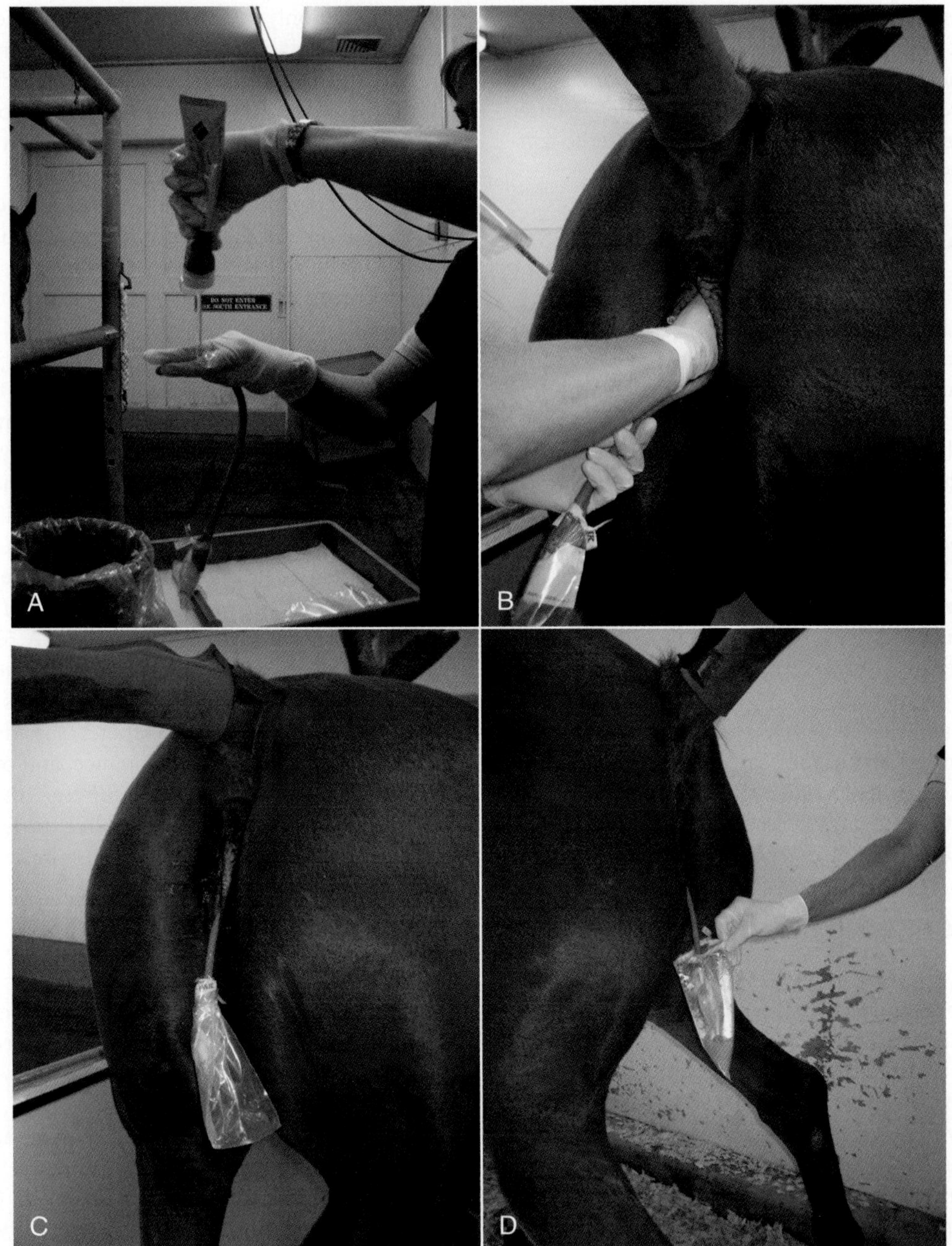

FIGURE 20-66 Urinary catheterization in mare. **A,** Applying sterile water-soluble lubricant to back of sterile gloved hand holding urinary catheter. **B,** Inserting urinary catheter. **C,** Urinary catheter with small plastic bag on end for sample collection. **D,** Collecting urine sample from catheter.

Urinary Catheterization of Llamas and Alpacas

In addition to the sigmoid shape of the penis, which makes passage of urinary catheters extremely difficult, male llamas and alpacas have a membranous flap at the ischial arch that prevents passage of urinary catheters into the bladder, so this procedure cannot be done in males.

Females

Supplies needed:

Sterile gloves
Sterile water-soluble lubricant
Sixty-milliliter catheter tip syringe
Red rubber tube or polypropylene catheter 5F
Gentle antimicrobial soap or other cleanser
Soft cotton
Sample collection containers (sterile if culture desired)
Sedation, if necessary

Restrain the llama or alpaca. Clean the lips of the vulva and dry the area. Wearing sterile gloves, place a small amount of lubricant on the glove. Insert a finger into the vulva and locate the external urethral orifice. This is felt as a groove on the floor of the vulva. When located, withdraw the finger slightly and slide the catheter along the dorsal aspect of the index finger into the orifice. Sliding the catheter along the finger in this manner avoids insertion into a blind ventral urethral diverticulum, which is located just caudal to the orifice of the urethra. Slowly advance the catheter. For most adult llamas or alpacas, the catheter is inserted about 25 cm from vulvar lips to enter the bladder. Collect a free-flowing sample into a sterile container or attach a syringe and gently aspirate the fluid.

BOVINE URINE COLLECTION

Free Catch

Place the animal in a chute or stanchion and allow the animal to relax. Urination in cows may be encouraged by lightly stroking the vulva tip and the skin beneath the vulva with fingers or straw. The technician may also try repeated parting of the lips of the vulva to elicit urination. Steers and bulls may oblige with urination if the prepuce is massaged and splashed with warm water. Urine is collected into a container or, depending on the required analysis, a urine dipstick (litmus paper test strip) can be held directly in the stream of urine. This technique is often used to monitor urine pH and ketones.

Urethral to bladder catheterization in male cattle is virtually impossible because of the anatomy and therefore is not performed by the technician.

Cows can be catheterized with a small-diameter (0.5 cm) catheter using similar techniques as used for mares. With sterile gloved and lubricated hand, a finger is inserted into the suburethral diverticulum, and the catheter tip is guided over the diverticulum and into the external urethral orifice.

OVINE AND CAPRINE URINE SAMPLES

Free Catch

Both ewes and does tend to urinate immediately after rising following a period of recumbency. The technician should be prepared to collect a urine sample when the animal rises. This is the easiest approach and causes the least stress to the animal.

Urination may be induced in ewes by occluding the nostrils for up to 45 seconds while the animal is standing. This causes stress to the animal. The animal will indicate discomfort by struggling, and as the nostrils are released and the animal allowed to breathe again, she will urinate. Two people are required for this procedure to go smoothly. One occludes the nostrils and restrains the ewe while the other catches the urine.

Holding the nostrils of does seldom results in urination. Sometimes urination may be encouraged by placing the animal in a new stall or pen.

Male ruminants may respond to manual stimulation of the prepuce, but the technician should be prepared with a collection container and make every effort to collect a sample when the animal obliges.

Urinary Catheterization

Males

As with male cattle, male sheep (rams) and male goats (bucks) have anatomic obstacles that make catheterization of the bladder extremely difficult, and the procedure is not commonly attempted. Catheterization of the urethra (not completely into the bladder) is commonly performed on blocked goats (urinary passage is blocked with urinary stones). The urethra opens 1 to 2 cm beyond the tip of the glans penis through the urethral process. It is difficult to enter this narrow structure with a catheter. The S-shaped curvature of the penis (sigmoid flexure) hinders the passage of a catheter beyond the flexure. There is also a urethral diverticulum (a blind sac) near the ischial arch that prevents the catheter from entering the bladder.

Females

Properly restrain the animal and hold or tie the tail out of the way during the procedure to prevent contamination. Cleanse the vulva. Wearing sterile gloves, apply sterile water-soluble lubricant to the fingers and pass the fingers into the vagina. The urethral opening is found midline on the ventral surface within 5 to 10 cm of the vulva (depending on the size of the animal). The vulvae of ewes and does are quite small. A small animal vaginal speculum may be helpful to allow visualization of the urethral opening. A 5F to 12F urinary catheter is inserted. Female ruminants have a small suburethral diverticulum (blind sac) that extends from the ventral aspect of the urethra. If the catheter is inadvertently fed into the diverticulum, it will not advance, and obvious resistance will be felt. If resistance is encountered, the catheter can be pulled out slightly and redirected in a more dorsal direction. Once in the bladder, urine may be collected by gravity flow or by aspirating with a sterile syringe.

PORCINE URINE COLLECTION

The technician should be ready with a collection cup because free-catch urine is necessary for a urinalysis in swine. It is common for adult swine to urinate two to three times a day.

Males should be confined and, if quiet and amenable, attempts to encourage urination can include stroking the prepuce with a warm, wet towel or soft brush. Male pigs cannot be catheterized because of the inaccessibility of the penis and the small diameter of the urethra.

Female pigs may respond when fingers, straw, or a soft brush are used to gently stroke the vulva. Females can be catheterized with the aid of a vaginal speculum and canine catheter, but the procedure is not routinely performed.

FECES SAMPLE COLLECTION

Fecal samples are collected for gross visual inspection; to check for the presence of mucus, sand, or blood (frank or occult); a microscopic examination to check for intestinal parasites; and for microbiologic culture or PCR assay. Occasionally, feces may be evaluated for osmolality and electrolyte concentration (to determine the presence of an osmotic diarrhea). The technician should be familiar with the normal character (content, consistency, color, and odor) and volume of feces for each species.

Feces contain a variety of bacteria that are normal and nonpathogenic. Fecal samples are cultured for specific microorganisms (such as *Salmonella*) by inoculating the feces into an enrichment medium that is designed to inhibit the growth of many normal bacteria while encouraging the growth of the specific bacterium to be identified. Some PCR assays that are now available are more sensitive and provide quicker results than a microbial culture for specific pathogens. If the animal is not producing feces, the technician may be asked to collect a rectal swab for a laboratory culture.

Fresh feces should be collected and placed in a clean container. Fresh feces will yield more accurate diagnostic information for parasite identification and an accurate culture result. Feces may be collected from the ground or from the rectum with a gloved hand.

> *TECHNICIAN NOTE* Fresh feces will yield more accurate diagnostic information for parasite identification and a culture.

If feces are to be collected directly from the rectum, the person must have their fingernails clipped short and should be wearing no rings or watches. The horse is restrained (preferably in stocks) and an obstetrical sleeve worn with generous amounts of lubrication gel applied to the sleeve. The person will stand slightly to the side of the horse, touch fingertips together, and slowly and gently insert the hand just far enough into the rectum to collect a handful of feces. The glove or sleeve can be turned inside out and tied in a knot to store the sample. The utmost care must be taken by the technician because rectal tears can occur and can be life threatening.

If sand colic is suspected in a horse, fecal sedimentation may be used as a diagnostic test. Feces can be mixed in the glove or sleeve with water and the sleeve hung up to allow the solid material to settle in the sleeve. Sandy material may be seen or felt through the fingers of the glove.

MILK SAMPLE COLLECTION

Milk samples are routinely collected from dairy animals to test for the presence of mastitis. Mastitis is an inflammation of the mammary gland and is commonly caused by a bacterial infection. Inflammation may be present without a bacterial component if the teat or udder has received a traumatic injury (kicked, stepped on, cut). Clinical mastitis refers to the presence of obvious clinical signs, including hard, hot udder; abnormal appearance or smell of the milk; and pain. Subclinical mastitis must be determined by diagnostic testing of the milk.

Colostrum samples are frequently collected from mares and tested to determine the quality of colostrum present.

STERILE MILK SAMPLE

Thoroughly wash and dry hands. Clean the teat end with an alcohol-soaked cotton swab. Repeat until the cotton is clean after rubbing the end of the teat. Allow the alcohol to dry. Using clean, dry hands, remove the top of a culture tube. Each quarter of the cow's udder (each half in small ruminants) is considered individually. If milk from more than one teat is collected, the teats nearest the milker should be sampled first to prevent contamination of the far-side teats by the arm of the milker. Hold the tube so that no dirt or debris will fall into the tube and do not allow anything to touch the opening of the tube. Discard the first few squirts of milk then squirt a stream of milk directly into the collection tube and replace the top. Refrigerate the sample for up to 24 hours before lab processing.

NONSTERILE MILK SAMPLE

Samples for California Mastitis Test

The California mastitis test (CMT) is commonly used to identify the presence of mastitis in cows (or does and ewes). The test involves the use of a white plastic test paddle with four cups labeled A to D and a reagent fluid (Figure 20-67).

The teats are cleaned and dried. It is not necessary to clean the entire udder. If washed completely, there is an increased risk of introducing contaminants from the udder into the teat orifice. Strip a small amount from one teat into one well of the paddle. Do the same for the remaining teats and note which teat was milked into each well (Figure 20-68). An equal volume of CMT reagent solution (one part milk to one part reagent solution) is added to each well, the paddle is gently moved to swirl the milk, and the resultant solution is graded based on gel formation.

0 = No gel
Trace = Precipitate that disappears with continued movement of the sample
1 = First visible precipitate does not disappear
2 = First visible gel—mixture moves toward the center of the cup, leaving the bottom of the outer edge of the cup exposed
3 = Egg yolk–type clot that sticks to the bottom of the plate
The number indicates the severity of inflammation.

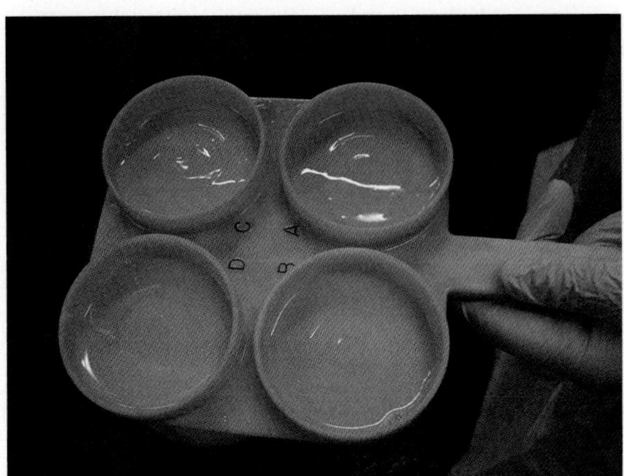

FIGURE 20-67 CMT (California mastitis test) paddle.

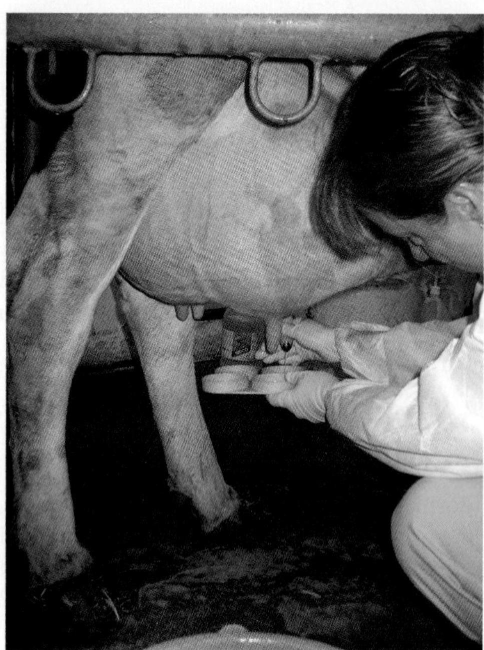

FIGURE 20-68 Collecting milk samples into CMT test paddle. Milk from each teat is collected separately into a cup on the paddle.

COLOSTRUM SAMPLE COLLECTION

Colostrometers provide a specific gravity assessment of the sample. Colostrum may also be submitted for a laboratory analysis, including immunoglobulin (Ig) (IgG) content and an antierythrocyte alloantibody determination. Sterile samples are not required.

The mare's udder should be washed well with soft cotton saturated with gentle soap and warm water and rinsed well before milking after foaling. The technician should be familiar with the use of a colostrometer and collect the appropriate volume (usually 5 to 10 ml) of colostrum. Samples can be milked directly into a collection tube or poured from another container into the necessary tubes.

RUMEN FLUID COLLECTION

Rumen fluid is collected for an analysis to aid in the diagnosis of diseases of the forestomachs (the reticulum, rumen, and omasum) in large and small ruminants. Characteristics of interest include the color, pH, odor, identification, and assessment of microbial organisms and numbers and electrolyte levels. Rumen fluid may also be collected for therapeutic purposes. When collected from a healthy animal, it may be used for transfaunation (inoculation of the sick animal's rumen with normal rumen flora needed to aid digestion).

ORAL GASTRIC TUBE (OROGASTRIC, ORORUMEN, STOMACH TUBE) METHOD

Tubes are inserted orally (through the mouth) in cattle. The nasal passages of cattle are a smaller diameter than horses, and this significantly limits the diameter of tube that can be placed nasally.

Equipment needed:

- Stomach tube—For adult cattle: medium to large diameter with internal diameter no less that 1.5 cm because smaller size is more likely to become obstructed with ingesta. For calves, sheep and goats, small and medium foal stomach tubes can be used
- Water-based lubricant
- Frick speculum (cattle)
- PVC pipe "speculum," block of wood with hole cut in center, roll of tape (sheep, goats)
- Dose syringe
- Sample collection container

TECHNICIAN NOTE A Frick speculum is commonly used on cattle to pass OGTs. For small ruminants, a short piece of polyvinyl chloride (PVC) pipe may be used as a mouth speculum.

BOVINE RUMEN FLUID COLLECTION

Restrain the animal to sufficiently limit movement of the head. Do not overly elevate the head during this procedure. Ruminants may regurgitate fluid around the tube and having the head overly elevated increases the likelihood of aspiration of the fluid.

Estimate the length of tube needed to reach the rumen by extending the tube outside the animal from the mouth to the rumen. The restrainer wraps one arm around the muzzle and places nose tongs (or places one finger into one of the animal's nostrils and a thumb into the other nostril and pulls the nose upward to open the mouth). Standing to the side of the animal, insert the speculum (to prevent biting of the tube) over the root of the tongue in the center of the mouth. A popping or "give" is felt as the speculum passes over the root of the tongue and into the pharynx.

Lubricate the tip of the tube with a water-soluble lubricant or with water. Insert the tube through the speculum. Resistance is usually felt when the tube reaches the back of the pharynx. As the animal swallows, the tube is advanced down the esophagus. If the tube is not easily advanced, it may be necessary to slightly withdraw and rotate the tube and try again. Blowing into the tube dilates the esophagus and may ease the passage of the tube. The proper placement of the tube in the esophagus is confirmed by palpating (the trachea and tube may be felt as two distinct tubular structures) or visualizing the tube in the esophagus and feeling mild resistance as it is passed. Coughing may indicate that the tube is in the trachea, and feeling air pass out of the tube upon exhalation may indicate the placement into the trachea (these are not always reliable).

The placement of the tube within the rumen can be confirmed by blowing into the tube and listening for gurgling from the end of the tube and by blowing into the tube with an assistant auscultating the abdomen with a stethoscope over the rumen (left paralumbar fossa) listening for gurgles. Air should be heard bubbling in the rumen. An additional confirmation of the placement is done by smelling the exposed end of the tube

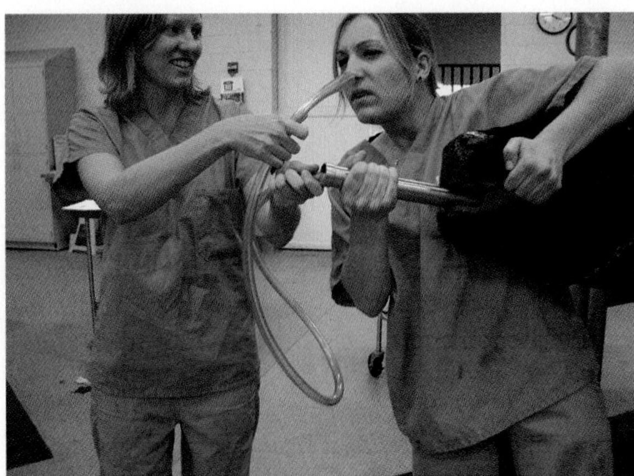

FIGURE 20-69 Checking for rumen smells to confirm placement of OGT in cow.

(Figure 20-69). The distinctive odor of fermented gas may be detected coming from the tube. The aspiration of rumen fluid (rumen juice) clearly confirms placement of the tube.

A dose syringe is used to collect the rumen fluid sample. The initial fluid is discarded because it often contains an excessive amount of saliva, which may erroneously elevate the pH of the fluid. When the process is complete, the tube is kinked and withdrawn with a smooth downward motion. This prevents the rumen contents from leaking out of the tube and entering the trachea as the tube is withdrawn. The pH of the sample should be measured immediately after the sample is obtained.

SMALL RUMINANTS RUMEN FLUID COLLECTION

Restrain as necessary. Sheep may be backed into a corner and straddled or "set up" on their rump; goats may be pushed against a wall or backed into a corner and straddled. A speculum is placed between the lower incisors and the dental pad. A short piece of PVC pipe may be used as a speculum or a block of wood with a hole in the center or even a roll of tape (Figure 20-70). Whatever is used must be long enough to reach the back of the mouth so that the tube is not deflected to the side where it can be bitten or chewed by the animal.

Select a suitable size and length tube (approximately ⅜- to ½-inch outside diameter) and estimate the necessary length as described for cattle and proceed with tube passage as described previously.

Rumenocentesis

This method is seldom done because of the ease and safety of the stomach tube method described earlier.

The ventral abdomen caudal to the xiphoid process and left of the ventral midline is clipped and surgically prepared. The veterinarian inserts a needle with a syringe attached (14-gauge needle for cattle, 16- to 18-gauge needle for small ruminants) through the skin and into the rumen. Rumen fluid is aspirated into the syringe.

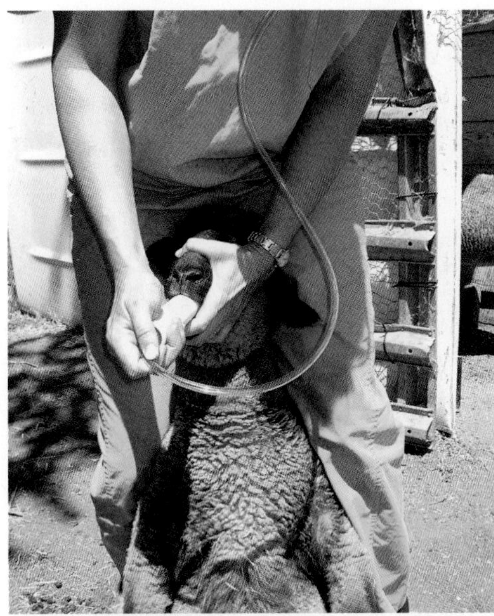

FIGURE 20-70 PVC pipe used as mouth speculum in sheep for OGT insertion. The speculum prevents the animal from biting the tube.

THORACOCENTESIS (THORACENTESIS, PLEUROCENTESIS, CHEST TAP, PLEURAL TAP)

Thoracocentesis is the aspiration of fluid from the thoracic cavity. It is performed in large animals to obtain pleural fluid samples for diagnostic purposes and therapeutically to drain fluid, air, or exudate from the pleural cavity. Pleural fluid is produced by the cells of the pleura, which line the pleural cavity and surface of the lungs. The fluid volume and character changes with the presence of disease in the pleural cavity or lungs. In the normal animal, little or no fluid is obtained from the thorax. When disease is present, large volumes of fluid may be obtained from the thorax. A gross analysis of the fluid includes the color, opacity, presence of fibrin material, pus, and odor. A laboratory analysis includes cytologic and microbiologic examinations and often pH, lactate, and glucose. Occasionally, a PCR analysis is done for the identification of certain pathogens.

This procedure is generally performed by the veterinarian, and the technician will be called upon to set up, prep, and assist with the procedure. If facilities allow, the technician may perform the laboratory analysis of the sample. When an indwelling chest drain is placed, the technician will be expected to maintain the drain and monitor the patient (Figure 20-71).

EQUINE AND BOVINE THORACOCENTESIS

Materials:

- Sterile gloves
- Ample collection tubes:
- EDTA (for cytology)
- Serum (for microbiology)

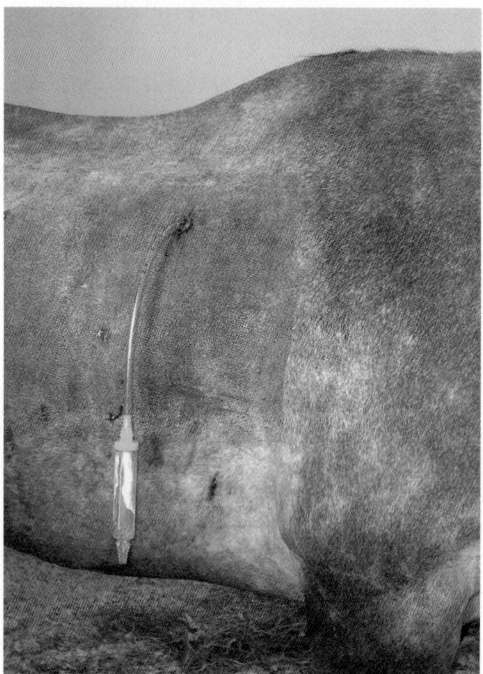

FIGURE 20-71 Indwelling chest drain with Heimlich valve.

- Heparin (for pH, lactate, and glucose) or fluoride (for pH and glucose), depending on specific laboratory analyzer requirements
- Instrument of veterinarian's choice:
- Needle (minimum 3 inches) with large gauge
  Or
- 14- to 16-gauge IV catheter
  Or
- Sharp trocar and cannula
  Or
- Teat cannula
  Or
- Bitch catheter
- Two percent lidocaine 3 to 5 ml
- Six-milliliter syringe with 20- to 22-gauge × 1-inch to 1.5-inch needle
- Scalpel blade #15
- Sterile 35- to 60-ml luer tip syringe
- Three-way stopcock
- IV extension tubing
- Suture material, needle drivers, and scissors
- Ultrasound machine, if available and requested by veterinarian

Restrain the horse and administer sedation, as needed. The veterinarian will select the appropriate site on the right or left lateral thorax and may use ultrasound to identify the most appropriate site. The patient may require thoracocentesis on both the left and right side. Each side of the thorax may yield different laboratory results because diseases of the plural cavity may cause blockage of the normal communication between the right and left side. It is possible that abnormal fluid may be present on one side while the other side remains essentially normal.

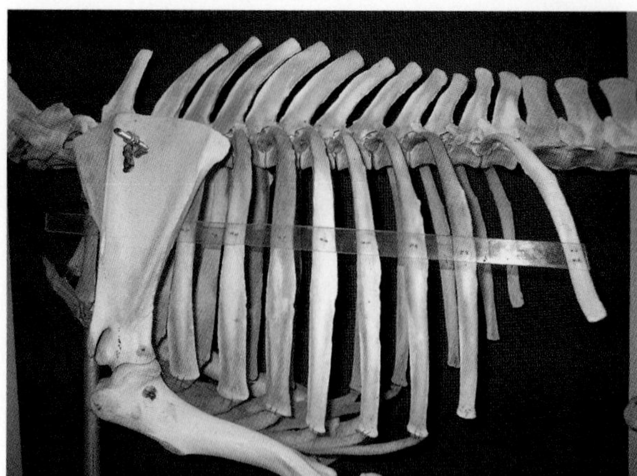

FIGURE 20-72 Side view of alpaca ribs.

TECHNICIAN NOTE A patient may require thoracocentesis on both the left and right side because each may yield different laboratory results.

Shave and aseptically prepare a large area from the olecranon back to the tenth intercostal space and from the point of the shoulder to well below the olecranon. The needle will be inserted in the ventral portion of the sixth and seventh intercostal (between the ribs) space 10 to 12 cm dorsal to the olecranon, above the lateral thoracic vein, and below the anticipated level of fluid. The site can also be determined with the use of ultrasonography, if indicated. Inject 5 ml of 2% lidocaine in the skin and SQ to make a bleb on the cranial aspect of the rib and deep enough into the intercostal muscles to include the parietal pleura. A stab incision is made into the anesthetized bleb with a scalpel blade. Avoid allowing the entrance of air during the procedure. A teat cannula (12- to 14-gauge × 3 inches) can be used to remove small volumes of air or fluid. A wider-bore sterile metal bitch catheter or human thoracic drainage cannula may be needed if there is a large volume of fluid or if the fluid is thick. The needle, catheter, or cannula with extension tubing and three-way stopcock attached is inserted cranial to the rib border and advanced through the parietal pleura. This approach is done to prevent damaging the intercostal vessels and nerves that run along the caudal border of the ribs. The heart, pericardial sac, and the lateral thoracic vein must be avoided. Once in the pleural cavity, a syringe is attached to the stopcock, and fluid is aspirated. When the fluid has been collected, the veterinarian may stitch a purse-string suture around the stab incision and tighten the suture as the cannula is removed.

CAMELID THORACOCENTESIS

The preferred site for thoracocentesis is at the sixth or seventh intercostal space 10 to 15 cm dorsal to the sternum (Figure 20-72). The area is clipped and surgically prepped. Any long fiber that may contaminate the shaved site should be taped back out of the way. Inject a local anesthetic as described for equines. A 14- to 16-gauge × 2-inch needle or teat cannula with a syringe attached is inserted near the cranial border of the rib. The pleural space is entered approximately 2 to 3 cm under the skin. The sample is aspirated into the syringe, and the needle is withdrawn and antibiotic ointment applied to the centesis site.

Thoracentesis in other large animals is similar to the procedures described for camelids and equines, with the cannula's size dependent on the animal's size.

Complications of thoracocentesis include pneumothorax, dyspnea, and iatrogenic infection.

Transtracheal Wash (Tracheal Wash, Trach Wash)

Transtracheal aspiration is the collection of fluid from the lower respiratory tract (bronchi, bronchioles, and alveoli) for a cytologic and microbiologic analysis and is performed to aid in the diagnosis of lower airway and lung disease. The fluid is a mixture of secretions and cellular material that has collected in the distal portion of the trachea.

EQUINE TRANSTRACHEAL ASPIRATION

The two methods used for this procedure are percutaneous and endoscopic.

Percutaneous Method

Restrain the horse appropriately and identify the location for the procedure. A horse may require mild sedation (heavy sedation should be avoided because it may suppress the cough reflex). Select a site on the midline of the neck directly over the trachea about one third of the way down the neck. Clip or shave an area approximately 4 inches × 4 inches, perform a sterile prep, and set up necessary materials.

> *TECHNICIAN NOTE* A horse may require mild sedation when a transtracheal wash is performed, but heavy sedation should be avoided because it may suppress the cough reflex.

Materials:
- Sterile gloves
- #20 to #30 surgical blade is used for adults, #15 to #20 for foals a few months old
- 12 Sixty-milliliter syringe containing 30 ml of 0.9% NaCl (do not use bacteriostatic saline). Place the syringe back into the case.
- Twelve- to 14-gauge Medicut IV cannula or 12- to 14-gauge needle
- Five to 6F polyvinyl canine urinary catheter placed on sterile field
- Twenty-five-gauge needle for capping the collection syringe after sample is obtained

Inject approximately 1 to 2 ml of 2% lidocaine ID and SQ over the selected site on the trachea and apply a final prep.

Wearing sterile gloves, tie the canine urinary catheter in a loose half hitch knot. This will allow the catheter to stay completely on the sterile field and makes it easier to control the distal tip to prevent contamination by accidentally touching it on something before or during the insertion. Using the scalpel blade, cut off the distal tip (approximately 1 inch) of the canine catheter and place it back on the sterile field. This step makes aspirating thick mucus possible.

Make a stab incision with the scalpel blade through the skin between the tracheal rings. Grasp the 12-gauge Medicut with one hand. Stabilize the trachea with the other hand, palm side up, use fingers and thumb placed on each side of the trachea and hold firmly. Insert the distal tip of the needle with bevel side down through the incision and advance it into the tracheal lumen. If resistance is felt, redirect the tip of the needle between the tracheal ring spaces, then advance into trachea. A burst of air will exit the needle when it penetrates the lumen of the trachea. A 3-ml syringe comes attached to the needle with the Medicut. The syringe can be kept attached to the needle and plunger pulled back to aspirate for the presence of air.

Remove the Medicut stylet. This prevents possible laceration and loss of the canine catheter tubing. Place on sterile field in case it is needed again. Insert the canine urinary catheter until it reaches the thoracic inlet. Attach the 60-ml syringe and retract the plunger. Air is aspirated if the catheter is within the tracheal lumen. If no air is aspirated, reposition the catheter because it may be bent or occluded against the tracheal wall. Once air is aspirated, infuse 30 ml of NaCl and immediately try to aspirate a 5-ml or greater fluid sample (only a small portion of the fluid that is instilled will be retrieved). A 5-ml sample should be sufficient for microbiology and cytology. Continue aspirating while slowly withdrawing the canine catheter. Stop withdrawing when fluid for aspiration is evident and collect as much as possible with a catheter at that location. Withdraw again as needed to continue the collection of fluid (do not reinsert the catheter). If fluid is not obtained, remove the canine catheter, insert a second sterile canine catheter, and infuse another 20 ml of NaCl and try again (Figure 20-73). The total volume of saline infused (first and second attempt) should not exceed 50 ml. Some horses will cough while the saline is infused, which may have the positive effect of increasing the yield of mucopurulent material. Unfortunately, coughing may also cause the catheter to kink cranially, which may prevent the collection of any sample. With a sample syringe, remove the 5F catheter while keeping the Medicut in place (this helps to prevent an SQ infection). Remove the Medicut, apply pressure to the site, control any bleeding, and place a 4 inch × 4 inch gauze with antiseptic ointment over the incision for 24 hours. Use a sterile needle to cap the syringe containing the sample for transport to the laboratory.

An alternate to using a Medicut catheter is to use a 12- to 14-gauge needle and insert the canine catheter through the needle. The needle is removed after the canine catheter

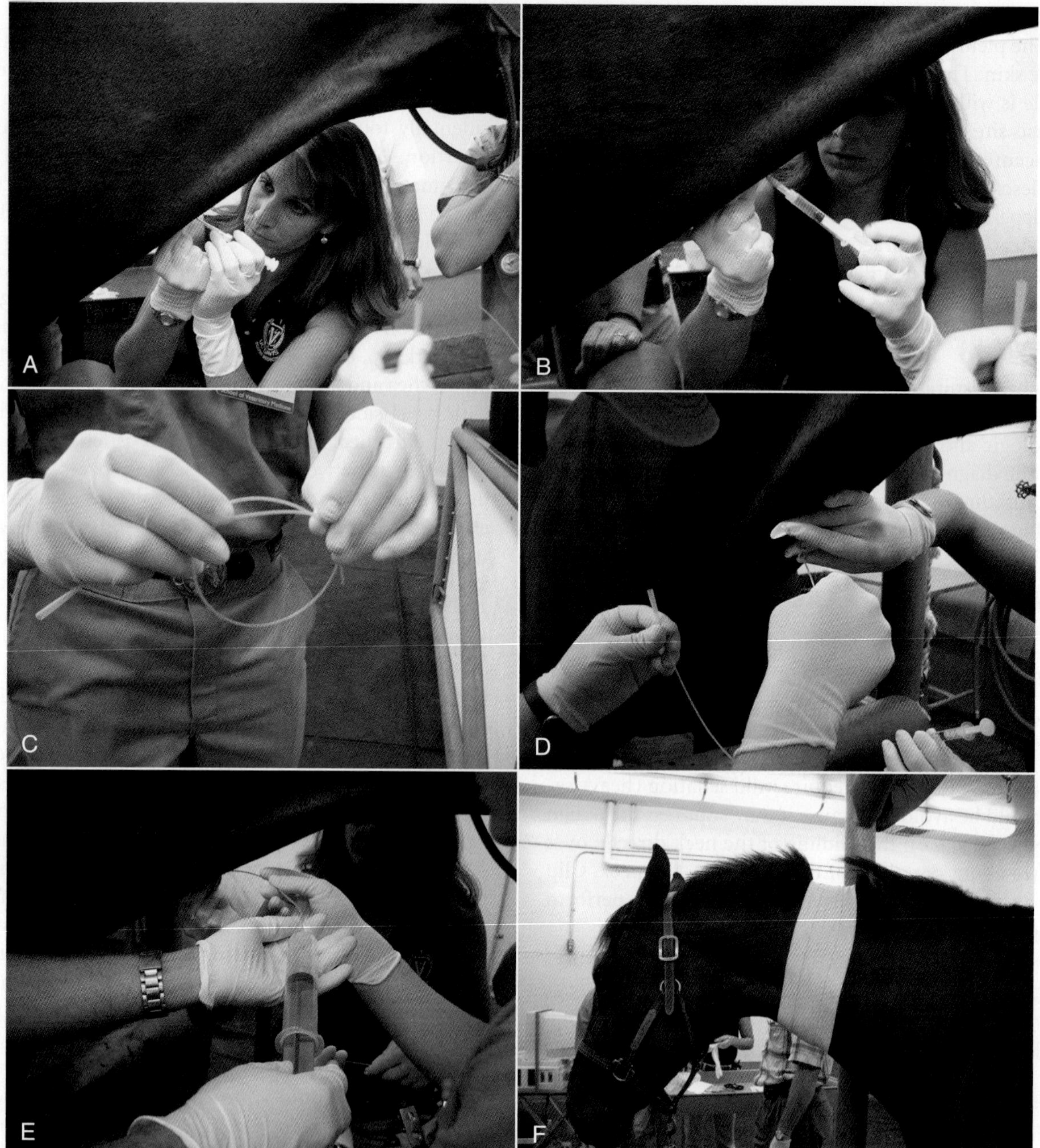

FIGURE 20-73 Transtracheal aspiration of equine patient. **A,** Insertion of Medicut needle. **B,** Aspirating air to confirm placement in tracheal lumen. **C,** Coiling catheter to keep sterile and easily controlled. **D,** Inserting catheter into trachea. **E,** Aspirating sample. **F,** Following completion of procedure, neck is wrapped to keep puncture site clean and dry.

is inserted into the tracheal lumen. Using the needle alone rather than an insertion catheter (Medicut) makes laceration of the canine catheter more likely and increases the likelihood of SQ contamination of the insertion site because the contaminated canine catheter will be in direct contact with the tissue at the insertion site when removed.

Cellulitis or SQ abscessation at the tracheal puncture site is the most common complication. If swelling occurs, warm compresses are applied. Other complications include SQ emphysema around the trachea, pulmonary foreign body as a result of the presence of a catheter piece in the airway, acute dyspnea, tracheal laceration, minor SQ hemorrhage, and iatrogenic infection.

Endoscopic Method

The use of an endoscope is considered noninvasive and allows for the visual examination of the upper airways, trachea, carina, and primary and secondary bronchi, but the presence of the endoscope leads to the questionable accuracy of the microbial samples recovered with this technique. An endoscope is inserted through the nasal cavity to the tracheal lumen. Special tubing (polyethylene tubing or endoscopic microbiology aspiration catheter) is placed through the biopsy channel of the endoscope and fluid injected and aspirated to collect the sample. The use of these specialized sample collection items decreases the likelihood of contamination from the pharynx or the endoscope that would otherwise

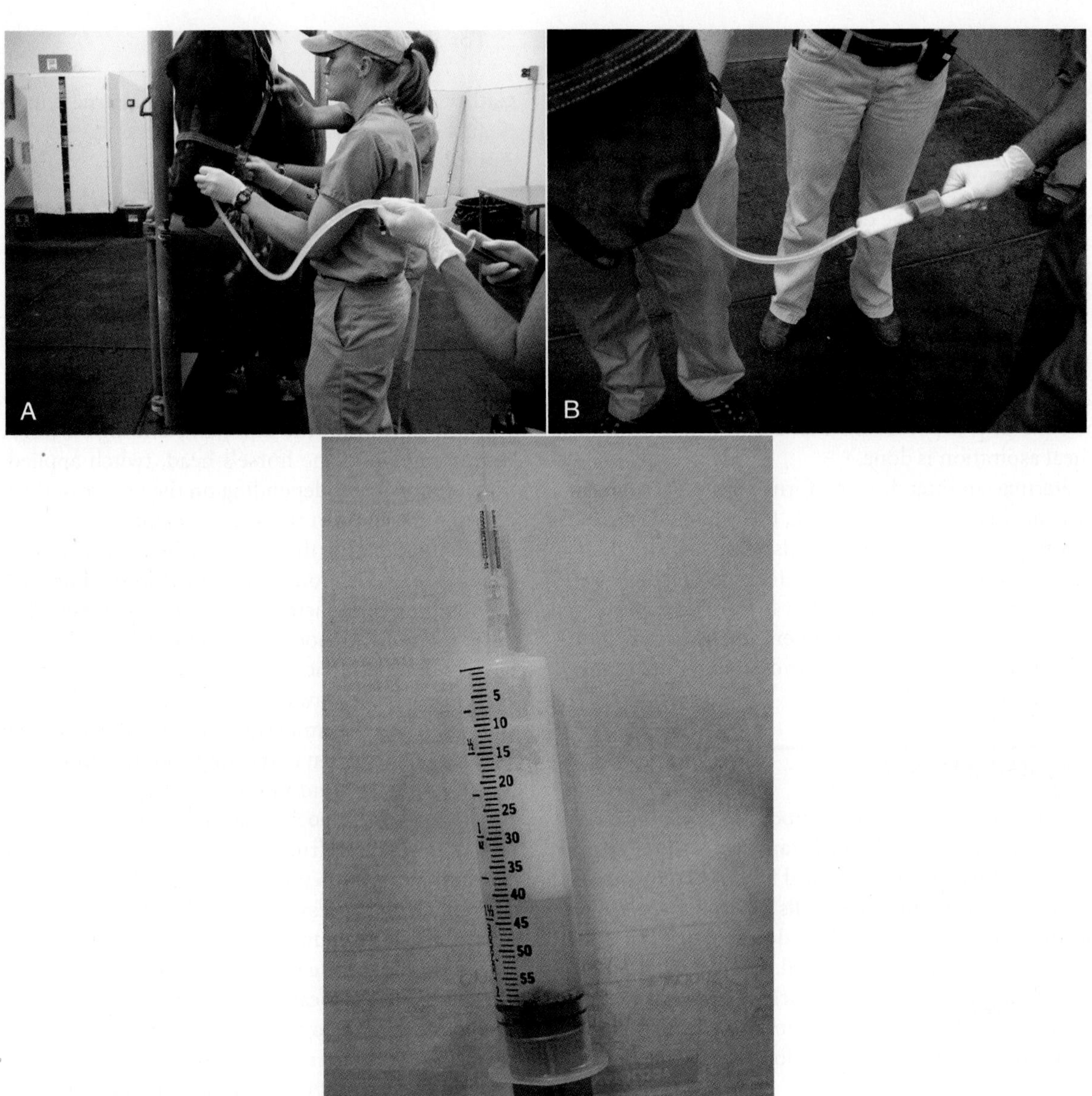

FIGURE 20-74 BAL of equine patient. A, Inserting BAL tubing with syringe containing lidocaine attached to end of tube. B, Collecting BAL sample. C, Syringe containing BAL sample is capped before transport to the lab.

occur with the endoscopic approach. It is usually necessary to infuse saline, as described for the percutaneous approach, to aspirate a fluid sample from the trachea.

BOVINE, CAPRINE, OVINE, AND CAMELID TRANSTRACHEAL ASPIRATION

Use methods as described for equines.

Bronchoalveolar Lavage (BAL)

Bronchoalveolar lavage is a procedure done to collect fluid samples from the lower airway. BAL provides fluid samples that are better for a cytologic assessment than samples obtained by transtracheal aspiration, but the fluid samples are representative of only a limited area of the lung and are subject to contamination from passing the tube through the nares. The BAL is done by the insertion of sterile tubing through the nares and down the trachea as far as possible. To prepare for the procedure, the technician should have sterile BAL tubing, a syringe containing 50 ml of 2% lidocaine, and three syringes each containing 60 ml of sterile saline (not bacteriostatic saline). The veterinarian may choose to use more or less saline, so the technician should check before the procedure to be sure of the desired amount of saline to have ready in syringes.

The horse should be sufficiently restrained and may require sedation. While the tube is passed into the trachea, 2% lidocaine is injected into the tube whenever the horse coughs. This acts as a local anesthetic to the bronchi and is done to decrease the cough reflex. It is not uncommon to use the entire 50 ml of lidocaine before the procedure is complete. Sterile saline (previously drawn up into three separate 60-ml syringes) is injected and aspirated (as is done with the transtracheal aspiration procedure) (Figure 20-74).

> *TECHNICIAN NOTE* While the BAL tubing is passed into the trachea, 2% lidocaine may be injected into the tube whenever the horse coughs to decrease the cough reflex.

The procedure can also be done with the use of an endoscope, with sterile tubing passed through the biopsy channel of the scope so that saline can be injected and fluid samples aspirated. This method is the preferred method for a sample collection when bronchial and/or alveolar disease is suspected. The use of the endoscope allows for sampling from specific areas of the lung, but a limited sample is obtained rather than the pooled secretions that are obtained when a transtracheal aspiration is done.

If the veterinarian intends to perform both a percutaneous transtracheal aspiration and a BAL, the transtracheal aspiration should be performed first. This will allow the fluid samples to be obtained before any contamination that may be introduced with the passage of the BAL tubing (or endoscope). Often the cough reflex is intentionally suppressed for the BAL, whereas a cough may be desirable during the transtracheal aspiration procedure.

ABDOMINOCENTESIS

Peritoneal fluid obtained by abdominocentesis (abdominal tap, peritoneal tap, paracentesis, belly tap) can provide valuable diagnostic information. Peritoneal fluid is produced by the cells of the peritoneum. These cells line the abdominal cavity and the outer surfaces of the abdominal organs. The composition of this fluid is determined by the condition of the abdominal organs. An analysis includes gross appearance, laboratory results, and the volume of fluid present. The accumulation of fluid in the abdominal cavity is abnormal.

> *TECHNICIAN NOTE* The composition of peritoneal fluid is determined by the condition of the abdominal organs.

Abdominocentesis is commonly performed on horses, camelids, cattle, sheep, and goats. The veterinary technician may be asked to prepare for and assist with the procedure or to perform the procedure. There are several variations on the procedure, and the technician will be directed by the veterinarian as to which approach is preferred. With any of the techniques, consideration should be made to ensure that the sample is not contaminated, that no contaminants are introduced into the patient, that as little trauma as possible is inflicted upon the patient, and that personnel are not injured while obtaining the sample.

Some indications for abdominocentesis include colic, suspected peritonitis, weight loss, abdominal distention, chronic diarrhea, signs of internal hemorrhage, abnormal ultrasound findings, and an FUO.

For all species:

Gather all required supplies (include alternate in case use of first-choice instrument is unsuccessful)
Appropriately restrain patient
Clip or shave the area chosen
Perform sterile prep
Wear sterile gloves and maintain sterility throughout procedure

EQUINE ABDOMINOCENTESIS

Many horses require minimal restraint for the procedure. If possible, restrain the horse in standing stocks. A handler should remain at the horse's head, twitch applied or sedation administered, depending on the nature of the horse and degree of discomfort the horse is exhibiting.

When preparing the site and when performing the procedure, the person should squat next to the horse adjacent to the forelimbs and facing the rear of the horse. This position reduces the likelihood of the person being kicked with the horse's hind leg. The person should take care to keep their head up and safely away from the belly and legs of the horse and be prepared to move quickly back if necessary to remain safe. If the technician is assisting with the procedure and will be collecting the fluid into tubes, they should be positioned similarly on the opposite side of the animal (if space permits) or wait until the instrument has been inserted and then squat or bend over next to the veterinarian (being prepared to step back quickly, if necessary) and with outstretched hand, place the collection tube under the needle or cannula.

Determine the site for the tap. Locate the lowest portion of the abdomen and locate the ventral midline. This is usually 2 to 4 inches caudal to the xyphoid. Abdominocentesis can be performed on the ventral midline, but a paramedian site 1 to 2 inches to the right of the midline reduces the likelihood of tapping the spleen (in horses) or the rumen (in ruminants). Abdominocentesis should not be performed through skin abrasions or surgical lesions and whenever possible, tapping through edema should be avoided. The clinician may perform ultrasonography to assist in determining the most desirable site for abdominocentesis and to prevent penetrating organs.

> *TECHNICIAN NOTE* Abdominocentesis can be performed on the ventral midline, but a paramedian site to the right of the midline reduces the likelihood of tapping the spleen (in horses) or the rumen (in ruminants).

Teat Cannula or Female Canine Urinary Catheter (Bitch Catheter) Method

Using a blunt-tipped bovine teat cannula or stainless steel female canine urinary catheter reduces the risk of bowel penetration, therefore this method may be chosen over the needle method for animals with abdominal distention or bowel distention (as identified with a rectal examination by veterinarian). This method requires the use of a local anesthetic.

Shave an area approximately 2 inches square. Perform a sterile prep. Aspirate 2 ml of 2% lidocaine into a 3-ml syringe. Perform local anesthesia by infusing the skin and SQ tissue with approximately 1 ml of the lidocaine using a 25-gauge needle. Insert the needle into the center of the shaved area (avoid any obvious cutaneous vasculature), aspirate to check for blood, and then infuse the lidocaine. Remove the 25-gauge needle and place a 19-gauge × 1.5-inch needle directly into the center of the SQ bleb. Insert the needle completely to the hub and inject the remaining 1 ml of lidocaine while slowly removing the needle from the patient. This is to block the parietal peritoneum.

Complete the sterile prep with a final swab of Betadine solution (or alternate antiseptic).

Assemble the equipment:

Four-inch teat cannula or bitch catheter
#15 scalpel blade
Two-milliliter EDTA tube
Three-milliliter serum tube
Heparin tube or syringe (depending on lab capabilities)
Sterile 4-inch × 4-inch gauze sponges
(Figure 20-75)

Create a sterile field by opening a pair of sterile gloves and placing the teat cannula (or bitch catheter or needle), scalpel blade, and sterile gauze 4 inches × 4 inches on the field (Figure 20-76).

Put on sterile gloves.

Puncture the center of one gauze 4-inch × 4-inch sponge with the scalpel blade and put the teat cannula through the gauze. This will help prevent contamination of the sample with blood or dust.

Using the scalpel blade, make a stab incision through the skin. Hold the blade with about ⅜ inch exposed. Using the back of the gloved hand, gently touch the horse's belly then insert the scalpel blade straight in the bleb and then pull it straight out. Avoid cutting the musculature. Slowly but firmly insert the teat cannula through the incision perpendicular to the musculature. The muscle will feel "gritty," and a slight "pop" will be felt when the peritoneum is punctured. A decrease in resistance is felt when the abdomen has been entered. If firm resistance is felt at this point, it may indicate contact with an organ, and care must be taken if further manipulation on the cannula is required. Once the cannula is in, expect to wait while the horse takes a few breaths before fluid begins to flow from the cannula. If fluid does not immediately flow, the cannula can be gently "flicked" with a finger in an effort to encourage the flow, and the cannula can be moved around slightly, rotated, or redirected. If necessary, a syringe may be attached to the cannula and aspiration may be attempted (Figure 20-77).

The first few drops of fluid may contain contaminants, so these drops should not be included in the sample. Collect the sample by gravity flow into collection tubes. The EDTA tube should be collected first since most of the desired laboratory tests will require this sample. The tube should be filled as much as possible to ensure the correct ratio of EDTA to abdominal fluid. If less than 1 ml of abdominal fluid is collected, the results of the laboratory analysis may be inaccurate. A common practice is to remove the rubber stopper from the EDTA tube and shake the tube to remove a bit of the EDTA before collecting the fluid sample. This is useful when a small sample volume is obtained. When refractometry is performed, excessive EDTA in relation to sample size will falsely elevate the protein reading. EDTA samples are used for cytologic analysis, protein measurement, and PCV (if fluid appears bloody). A serum (plain, clot) tube should be collected for bacterial culture (as little as 1 drop of fluid is sufficient for this purpose). Some facilities have the capability to perform pH, gas, lactate, and glucose analyses. The technician should be familiar with the laboratory capabilities and be familiar with the appropriate anticoagulant requirements. For many analyzers that perform these additional tests, heparin is the choice of anticoagulant. Some facilities will require a sodium fluoride tube for glucose and lactate measurements.

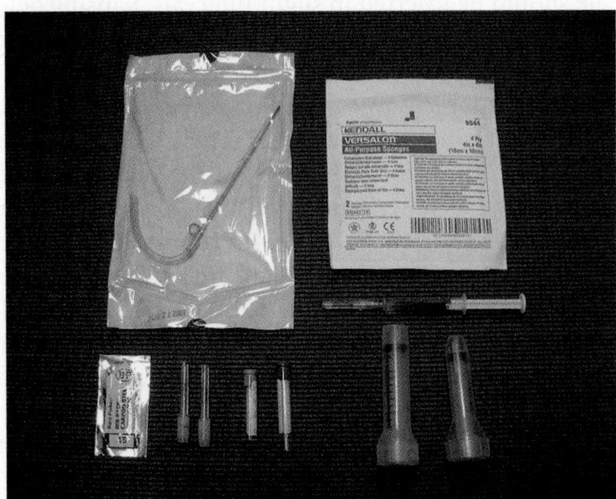

FIGURE 20-75 Supplies for abdominocentesis. Bitch catheter, 4-inch × 4-inch sterile gauze sponges, #15 scalpel blade, 19-gauge × 1.5-inch needles, 2-ml EDTA tube, 3-ml plain tube, 3-ml syringe with 25-gauge × 1-inch needle containing 2% lidocaine, 12-ml syringe, 6-ml syringe.

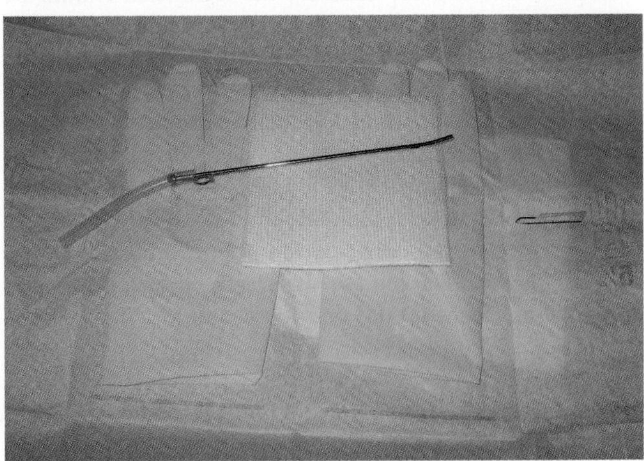

FIGURE 20-76 Sterile field with sterile supplies for abdominocentesis.

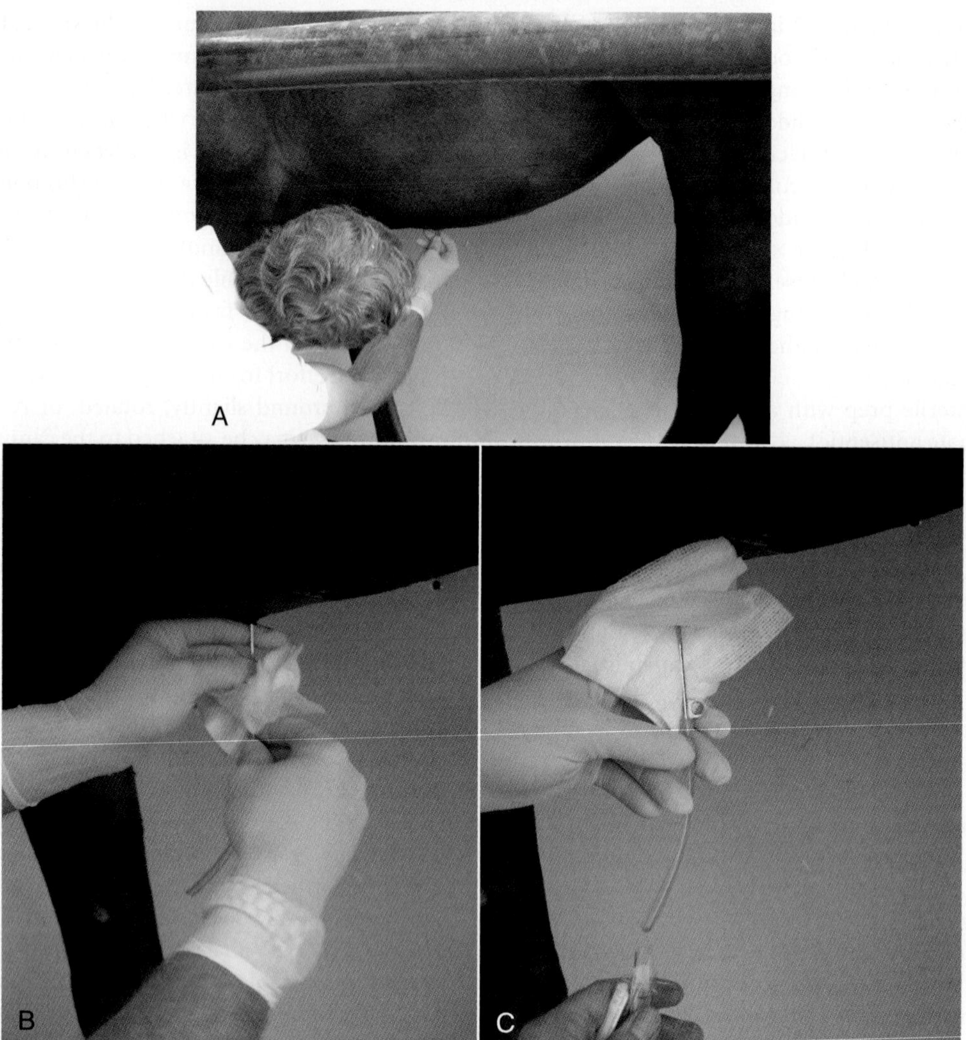

FIGURE 20-77 A, Incision on prepped and blocked ventral midline area for equine abdominal tap. B, Insertion of bitch catheter through incision. C, Collection of abdominal fluid through bitch catheter into collection tubes.

> *TECHNICIAN NOTE* The technician should be familiar with the laboratory capabilities and be knowledgeable about the appropriate anticoagulant requirements.

When removing the cannula, the technician should be aware that some omentum may have attached to the cannula and can follow the cannula out when the cannula is pulled from the site. To prevent it from being exteriorized, care should be taken to use fingers to guard close to the site when removing the cannula. As a result of the incidental perforation of skin vessels, slight bleeding is common after the removal of the cannula. Manual pressure applied to the site usually stops the bleeding. If necessary, the veterinarian will suture or staple the site. The centesis site can be cleaned gently and antibiotic ointment applied daily for a couple of days.

18- to 22-Gauge, 1.5-Inch Needle Method

A local anesthetic is usually not required for this method, but that will vary depending on the horse.

The needle is held midway between the thumb and forefinger and inserted through the skin while avoiding superficial veins. The fingers are then moved slightly to grasp the hub of the needle for gradual advancement. The needle should be inserted in slight intervals, pausing before each interval of advancement to notice (by feel) if a scratching sensation is present. The scratching sensation indicates that bowel is rubbing over the tip of the needle. The fingers should be removed from the needle periodically to watch for rotary or "flicking" movement of the needle, which is also indicative of bowel contact. Periodic back and forth movement of the needle in time with respiration is normal. The needle is advanced slowly to the hub if no bowel is encountered or until fluid is obtained. If abdominal fluid is not seen in the needle hub, the needle can be repositioned and rotated, and a syringe may be used to try and aspirate a sample. If fluid is not obtained, 1 to 2 ml of air (in a sterile syringe) may be injected in an effort to dislodge any material that might be occluding the needle. Another option to encourage the flow of fluid is to insert a second or third needle a few centimeters from the first (while leaving the first needle in place) to release the negative pressure in the abdomen.

> *TECHNICIAN NOTE* Periodic back and forth movement of the needle in time with the animal's respiration is normal.

18-Gauge, 3.5-Inch Spinal Needle Method

This long needle may be required in very large horses, draft horses, and obese individuals. Some clinicians report that this long needle is also useful in Arabian horses to facilitate penetration beyond the abdominal wall and subperitoneal fat layer.

A local anesthetic is not usually necessary for this method, but that will vary depending on the horse.

With the stylet in place, the needle is inserted to a depth of approximately ¼ inch. The stylet is removed before further advancement and the procedure continued as is done with a standard needle.

EQUINE ABDOMINOCENTESIS (FOAL)

Sedation is usually indicated. The procedure is safer for the patient and personnel if sufficient human assistance is used for physical restraint and positioning of the foal.

For neonates less than 1 month old or actively colicky foals, abdominocentesis can be done with the sedated foal restrained in lateral recumbency. A 20-gauge × 1- to 1.5-inch needle is inserted caudal to the xyphoid midline or right paramedian (off center but near the midline). Foal intestine is thin and fragile, and care must be taken to avoid contacting the bowel. A blunt-ended, small-diameter teat cannula or canine bitch catheter can be used and poses less risk for intestinal laceration than a needle, but a local anesthetic and stab incision are needed before the insertion of the cannula. The lack of subperitoneal fat in foals increases the risk for laceration of the bowel with a scalpel blade when a stab incision is made. The blade must be held with the fingers up near the tip of the blade to maintain control and ensure that it is not inserted too deeply. For foals older than 1 month of age, an 18- to 20-gauge × 1.5-inch needle, a teat cannula, or bitch catheter would be appropriate and the procedure performed as for younger foals.

> *TECHNICIAN NOTE* Foal intestine is thin and fragile, and care must be taken to avoid contacting the bowel.

CAMELID ABDOMINOCENTESIS (ADULT)

There are two common sites for abdominocentesis in camelids: a ventral midline site and a right paracostal (near the ribs) site. The paracostal site is easier to tap because camelids will frequently choose to drop to sternal recumbency ("kushed" position) when they object to a procedure, making the ventral midline site unavailable. The midline site is also complicated by a thick subperitoneal fat layer on either side of the linea alba, and the visualization may be obscured by a long-fiber coat hanging from the sides of the animal.

Provide appropriate restraint by using a camelid chute or having a handler push the left side of the animal up against a wall or fence. Chemical sedation may be required for some animals.

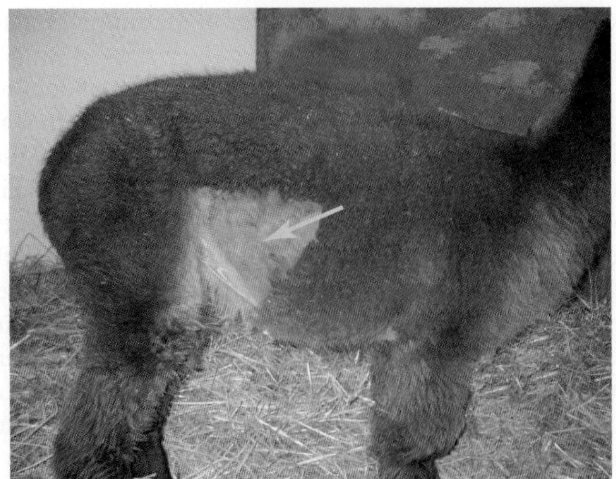

FIGURE 20-78 Paracostal site on alpaca for abdominocentesis.

The paracostal abdominal tap site is located on the right side of the animal about 4 inches behind the caudal most curve of the ribs (approximated by placing the palm of the hand behind the last rib) about one third of the way up between the ventral abdomen and the spine (Figure 20-78). Clip or shave a 3- to 4-inch square area. It is helpful to keep long fiber in the surrounding area clear of the site by taping it back.

Perform a sterile prep. Using a 22- to 25-gauge needle inject 1 to 3 ml of 2% lidocaine into the skin and SQ tissue. Perform a final sterile prep of the site. Using a #11 or #15 scalpel blade, make a stab incision. Using a quick, controlled thrust, insert a 4-inch blunt-ended teat cannula perpendicular to the abdomen. Advance it slowly into the abdomen. If fluid does not flow, the tip of the cannula can be gently repositioned, a syringe may be attached, and negative pressure applied or a few milliliters of air can be injected into the abdominal cavity.

For the ventral midline approach, select the lowest site, which is just caudal to the umbilicus. To avoid the retroperitoneal fat pads on either side of the linea alba (which will obstruct the cannula and prevent a sample collection), the site chosen should be directly on the linea alba. Clip a 3- to 4-inch area, perform a sterile prep, and inject a small amount of local anesthetic (as listed for method described earlier). Using a scalpel blade, create a small stab incision and insert a teat cannula as described for an equine abdominal tap.

CAMELID ABDOMINOCENTESIS (NEONATAL)

The cria (neonatal llama or alpaca) can be mildly sedated, as needed and should be restrained in lateral recumbency. A teat cannula or 20-gauge × 1-inch needle may be used in the same site as for the standing adult camelid.

BOVINE ABDOMINOCENTESIS (ADULT)

The animal is placed in a head gate, stocks or chute that will allow access to the right side of the animal. A tail jack restraint may be sufficient but chemical sedation may be necessary depending on the behavior of the animal and site used.

An 18-gauge, 1.5-inch needle is sufficient for abdominocentesis in most adult cattle, although some very large individuals may require a 3-inch needle. A teat cannula can be used instead of a needle. If "hardware disease" (traumatic reticulitis from the ingestion of heavy foreign objects) is suspected, the site selected should be just caudal to the xyphoid and to the right of the midline as described for horses. The person performing the tap should stand by the animal's forelimbs facing backward and be aware of the risk of being kicked. If general effusion or widespread disease is suspected, alternate sites can be the flank fold on the right side of the animal or the ventral abdomen at the lowest point approximately 2 to 4 inches to the right of the umbilicus. Tapping the abdomen through the flank fold can be done successfully without a local anesthetic.

BOVINE ABDOMINOCENTESIS (NEONATAL)

Abdominal taps on calves can be done with the animal standing or in left lateral recumbency. Appropriate restraint is necessary, and sedation may be necessary to keep the animal still. A ventral midline site about 4 cm (approximately 1.5 inches) cranial to the umbilicus or a paramedian site approximately 4 cm to the right of the umbilicus can be used. As described earlier, a needle or teat cannula can be used for the centesis.

OVINE AND CAPRINE ABDOMINOCENTESIS

Abdominocentesis in sheep and goats may be used to investigate abdominal distention, poor forestomach motility, and suspected uroabdomen (caused by urinary tract obstruction or ruptured bladder). A ruptured bladder is common in male goats (bucks) secondary to obstructive urolithiasis and leads to the accumulation of urine in the abdominal cavity.

> TECHNICIAN NOTE A ruptured bladder is common in male goats secondary to urolithiasis and leads to the accumulation of urine in the abdominal cavity.

Manually restrain the animal and sedate it, if necessary. A local anesthetic may be indicated, even if a needle is used for abdominocentesis. The procedure can be done with the animal standing.

Select a site at the lowest point of the abdomen 2 to 4 cm to the right of the ventral midline (to prevent tapping the rumen). Avoid the mammary veins (milk veins or SQ abdominal veins) of females and the penis and prepuce in males. An 18- to 20-gauge × 1.5-inch needle or teat cannula can be used. A local anesthetic is necessary for the stab incision required with the use of a teat cannula and may also be desirable, even if a needle is used. If peritonitis is suspected, the veterinarian may choose to tap multiple sites to increase the chances of a diagnosis. The additional sites include caudal to the xyphoid, medial to the right and left milk veins, and slightly cranial to the mammary gland on the right and left of the midline.

The most common complication associated with abdominocentesis is a failure to obtain a sample and slight skin hemorrhage. The protrusion of omentum through the site of puncture through the abdominal wall can also occur. More serious complications of abdominocentesis in large animals include penetration of the bowel, penetration of the spleen, damage to the xyphoid process if the centesis site is too cranial, and the introduction of bacteria leading to peritonitis or cellulitis. SQ abscessation and cellulitis are uncommon when an unremarkable abdominocentesis procedure is performed, but the risk for these complications increases markedly when the intestine has been punctured, if abdominocentesis is done through edematous tissue, and in animals that have septic peritonitis.

CEREBROSPINAL FLUID COLLECTION (SPINAL TAP, CSF TAP)

Cerebrospinal fluid may be collected from patients when central nervous system disease is suspected. A CSF fluid analysis includes the gross visualization of color, clarity, and presence of particulate matter. Total protein, cytology, and chemistry are performed on the fluid. The technician will be expected to prepare the site, restrain the patient, or assist the veterinarian while the veterinarian performs the procedure.

EQUINE

Atlanto-Occipital Site (AO Tap)

This site is located on the dorsal midline just caudal to the poll. Collecting spinal fluid from this site requires a general anesthetic. With the animal anesthetized, it is placed in lateral recumbency. The area is clipped, shaved, and a complete sterile prep performed. When all preparations have been made, the nose is directed down toward the front feet to flex the head. The head should be at a right angle to the neck. The veterinarian will insert an 18-gauge × 3-inch spinal needle into the atlanto-occipital space (about 5 to 7 cm depth) and once in, will remove the trocar (stylet) and place it on a sterile field. A sterile syringe is attached to the needle and a sample gently aspirated. Alternately the fluid may be collected directly into a tube by free flow. If the fluid is blood tinged, aspirate a few milliliters and then attach a new syringe. The technician should be prepared with additional syringes in case multiple samples can be obtained. The trocar (still sterile) is replaced in the needle, and the needle is withdrawn. Following the removal of the needle, any blood present can be cleaned from the site, and a Betadine-soaked gauze sponge can be placed on the site.

The AO tap in neonates is done with a 20-gauge × 1.5-inch needle directed at the mandible. Fluid should drip from the needle hub. Normally, 3 to 6 ml of fluid is obtained.

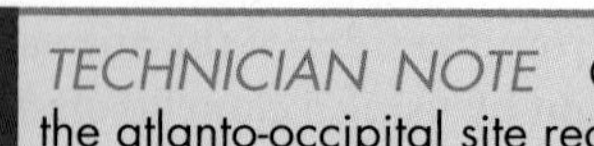

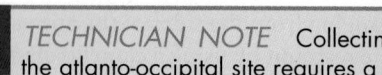

> TECHNICIAN NOTE Collecting spinal fluid from the atlanto-occipital site requires a general anesthetic.

Lumbosacral Site (LS Tap)

This site can be located by making an imaginary line across from the caudal edge of each tuber coxae and another line on the dorsal midline. A slight depression can be palpated using firm pressure at the intersection of these imaginary lines, just caudal to the sixth lumbar spinal process (L6). A large area is clipped, shaved, and a sterile prep performed. Sedation is required, and the use of a twitch for restraint is indicated because the animal must remain very still for the procedure. The horse should be placed in stocks. A local anesthetic is injected into the skin and SQ. The patient should be standing as squarely as possible (the best that its condition will allow) because an asymmetric stance makes collection more difficult (Figure 20-79, *A-F*). If sufficient personnel are available, it is helpful to have someone standing behind the horse to comment to the veterinarian as to the placement of the needle so that small errors in the direction of insertion can be noted and corrected. The veterinarian will insert a 6-inch (15 cm) × 18-gauge spinal needle perpendicular to the midline (about 11 to 15 cm, or 4.5 to 6 inches). For some draft horses and warmblooded animals, longer needles (up to 8 inches) may be needed. When the needle reaches the subarachnoid space, the patient may respond with movement. The trocar is removed from the needle and placed on a sterile field. The technician will place a sterile syringe in the veterinarian's still sterile, gloved hands. The initial sample may be contaminated with blood, so a second or third syringe may be collected if sufficient fluid is aspirated. The veterinarian may instruct assistants to occlude both jugular veins in an attempt to increase the intracranial pressure. The trocar (still sterile) is replaced into the needle and the needle removed.

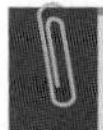

TECHNICIAN NOTE The patient should stand as squarely as possible for an LS tap.

The lumbosacral CSF tap in neonates can be done with the foal standing, in sternal recumbency, or in lateral recumbency using a 3-inch × 20-gauge spinal needle.

Complications that may result from CSF taps include trauma to the spinal cord during needle placement, herniation of the cerebellum (can occur with high intracranial pressure or from aggressive aspiration), and infection of the meninges. These can result in the death of the patient. The chances of these complications occurring are minimized by having the patient sufficiently restrained to remain still and by following strict sterile technique throughout the procedure.

Camelids

A CSF fluid collection from llamas and alpacas follows the same procedure guidelines as described for horses.

The atlanto-occipital site is located midline as it intersects the wings of the atlas. In adults, a 20-gauge × 2.5-inch spinal needle is used with the subarachnoid space usually reached at a depth of 4 cm.

The lumbosacral site is midline about 2 cm caudal to the dorsal spinal process of the seventh lumbar vertebra. The landmarks used to locate the site are the tuber sacrale of the pelvis and dorsal spinal process of the last lumbar vertebra. The site is cranial to the tuber sacrale. An 18- or 19-gauge × 3.5-inch spinal needle is appropriate for most adult llamas and alpacas.

TREATMENT TECHNIQUES IN LARGE ANIMALS

INTRAVENOUS ADMINISTRATION

IV injections are commonly performed on large animal patients. Drugs administered via the IV route are very rapidly absorbed. Some medications are quite caustic and injecting them into the vein dilutes the drug, making it less caustic than it would be if it were administered IM or SQ.

Equine

With most horses, minimal restraint (halter and lead rope) can be employed to successfully administer medication using this route. If the patient is uncooperative, aggressive, or sensitive to needles, placing the animal in the stocks or using a second person and a twitch may make the procedure easier and reduce the likelihood of injury to personnel and complications with misdirected puncture.

Jugular Vein

The jugular vein is the most common site used in equine patients for IV administration.

The right or left jugular vein is chosen, using the most cranial half of the neck. This is preferred because of the muscle layer that lies in the upper half of the neck that protects the underlying carotid artery from a potential puncture. The preference is the right jugular vein because in most horses, the esophagus lies within the left jugular furrow and could potentially be tapped with an aggressive venipuncture. The site is then wiped down with alcohol, and digital pressure is applied to the jugular furrow below the intended puncture site to distend the vein. For adult horses, a 1.5-inch needle is used (18-, 19-, or 20-gauge is adequate). Using the free hand, the needle is inserted into the vein in an upward direction (toward the head). Once blood drips from the hub of the needle, advance the needle all the way until just the hub is visible. It is critical to identify that the needle is in a vein and not an artery since the accidental injection of medication into the artery goes directly to the brain and can result in a serious, violent reaction and may even prove fatal. Certain substances that are injected perivascularly can cause severe necrosis to the tissue it comes in contact with (e.g., phenylbutazone). When a large-bore needle is inserted, arterial blood will forcibly pulse out of the hub of the needle and tends to be bright red, whereas venous blood will steadily drip from the hub of the needle and tends to be darker red.

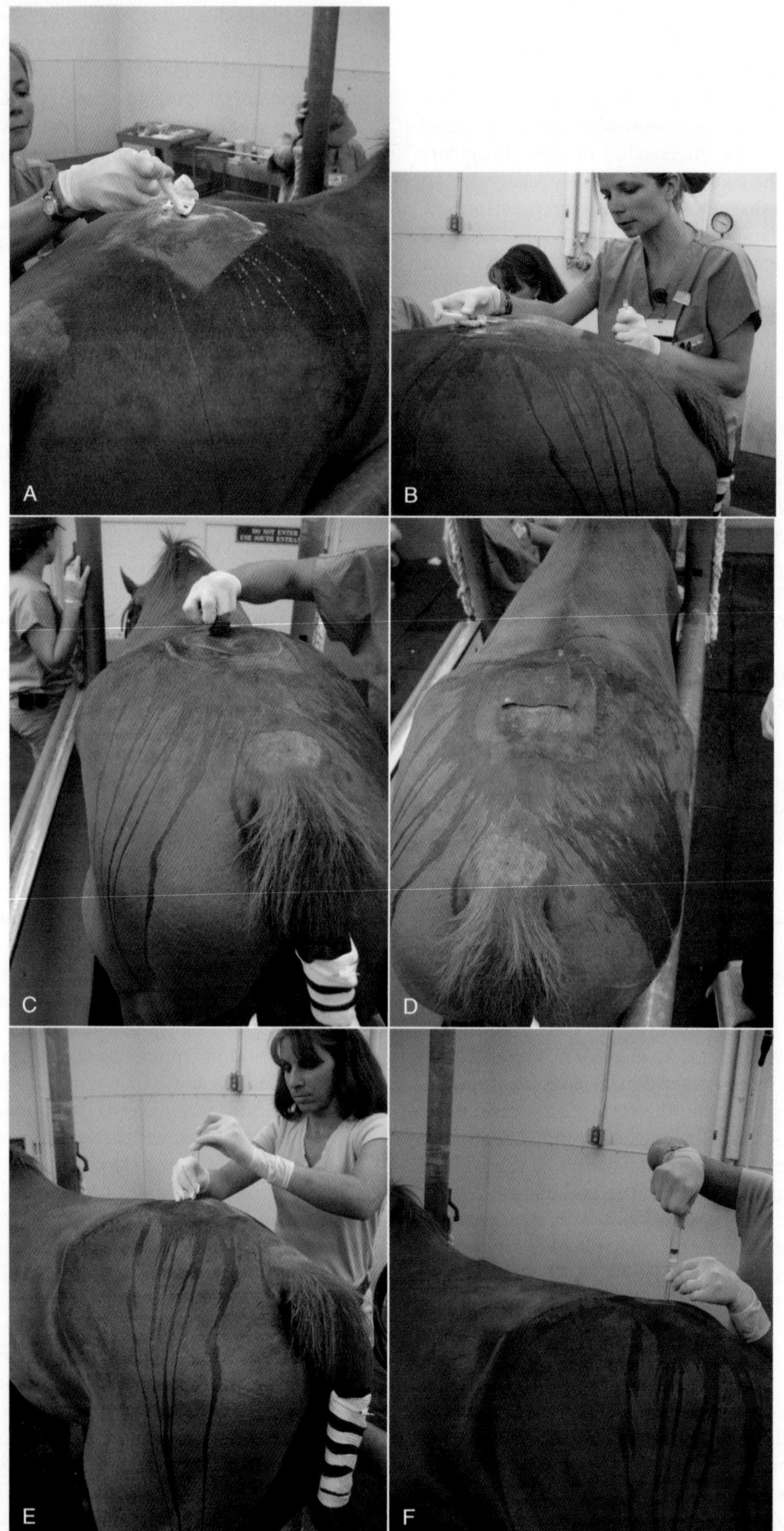

FIGURE 20-79 A, Shaving area for lumbosacral spinal tap. B, Injecting 2% lidocaine for local anesthetic block. C, Prepping site with Betadine solution. D, Site covered with Betadine-soaked gauze. E, Inserting spinal needle. F, Aspirating spinal fluid sample.

> *TECHNICIAN NOTE* Arterial blood will forcibly pulse out of the hub of the needle and tends to be bright red, whereas venous blood will steadily drip from the hub of the needle and tends to be darker red.

The syringe with medication can now be attached to the needle making sure not to inadvertently move the needle perivascularly. Before injecting any substance, confirmation of the placement needs to be reestablished. Gently aspirate the plunger of the syringe to confirm that blood enters the syringe and that it is not bright red in nature (indicating arterial puncture). Remove digital pressure from the jugular furrow and administer the medication in a slow and continuous fashion. Once all medication is administered, remove the needle and syringe and apply digital pressure over the site for a couple of minutes to reduce potential hematoma formation.

IV injection of a medication may result in an anaphylactic reaction (mild to severe). A reaction may include sweating, urticaria (hives), anxiety, agitation, difficulty breathing, and even collapse. If the technician notes any of these responses, the remainder of the drug in the syringe should not be given, the technician should move safely away from the animal, and the veterinarian notified of the situation. An injection of epinephrine may be necessary, and the technician should have prior arrangements with the veterinarian as to the amount to administer in the event that an anaphylactic emergency occurs when the veterinarian is not immediately present.

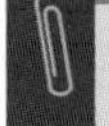

> *TECHNICIAN NOTE* The administration of a drug by any route can result in an anaphylactic reaction.

Other sites for IV injections include the cephalic vein and the lateral thoracic vein, but these sites are usually reserved for a catheter placement instead of routine injections of medications because they are more awkward to access on the patient.

Equine IV Catheterization

For repeated IV drug injections or when large volumes of IV fluids are required, an indwelling catheter should be placed in the jugular vein. If either jugular vein is not accessible as a result of thrombosis or trauma or if the horse pesters the jugular catheter, it may be necessary to catheterize the cephalic vein or the lateral thoracic vein. There are many different options for catheters, and the choice should be made based on the length of time the catheter will be in place and the number of ports that may be necessary. For adult equine patients, when using OTN catheters, 14 gauge × 5.25 inches is sufficient, but for neonates, small ponies, or miniature horses, 16 gauge × 3.25 inches may be preferred. Miniature horse neonates may require a smaller catheter, and an 18- to 20-gauge × 3-inch catheter may be used, with the realization that the size of the catheter will dictate the fluid administration rates that can be achieved.

> *TECHNICIAN NOTE* Polyurethane and Silastic catheters are less thrombogenic than catheters made of Teflon and can be maintained in veins for longer periods.

The site chosen is shaved and surgically scrubbed to remove all debris. A final wipe with Betadine solution over the area is then added and left on to dry. A "bleb" of lidocaine (ID administration using a 25-gauge needle and approximately 2 ml of lidocaine) should be administered over the intended injection site, including above the site, to desensitize an area for suturing the catheter in place. A sterile field is created by opening up a package of sterile gloves and aseptically laying the desired catheter on the gloves. All necessary items need to be either placed on the sterile field or readily accessible nearby.

Wearing sterile gloves, the technician grasps the catheter with the dominant hand and uses the other gloved hand to apply digital pressure to the jugular furrow. The catheter is inserted through the skin (into the "bleb") at approximately a 45-degree angle and should be inserted toward the heart, with the direction of blood flow. Once the lumen of the vein has been accessed (identified by the "flash" of blood at the hub of the catheter), the catheter is aligned more perpendicular to the vein and advanced 1 cm more. If the catheter is still in the vein (as indicated by flash back blood coming from catheter), the hand applying the digital pressure releases and then grasps the top of the stylet portion of the catheter. The catheter is then slid all the way into the vessel, removing the stylet at the same time. Recheck to make sure that the vein is still catheterized by applying digital pressure yet again (below the tip of the catheter) and watch for blood to drip from the hub. Once this has been identified, attach a PRN or T-port and suture the catheter into place (Figure 20-80, *A-E*).

> *TECHNICIAN NOTE* Once the stylet has been withdrawn from the catheter, it should not be reintroduced because the sharp tip may cut through the catheter causing a small piece to be dislodged into the vein or may make a very jagged edge on the catheter.

If the carotid artery is catheterized, bright red blood will forcibly pulse out of the catheter. If this should occur, immediately remove the catheter and apply digital pressure over the sight for a minimum of 5 minutes to prevent the formation of a hematoma. Neck wraps or stents can be placed over catheters to stabilize them and to prevent the patient from rubbing them out. A common practice is to apply a small amount of antibacterial ointment before placing a wrap over the catheter. If the catheter remains in place long term, the ointment used can be alternated (e.g., Nolvasan, Betadine, triple antibiotic) in an attempt to reduce the chances of a resistant staphylococcus infection taking hold. Foals and adult horses that spend a considerable amount of time in recumbency should have wraps placed over the

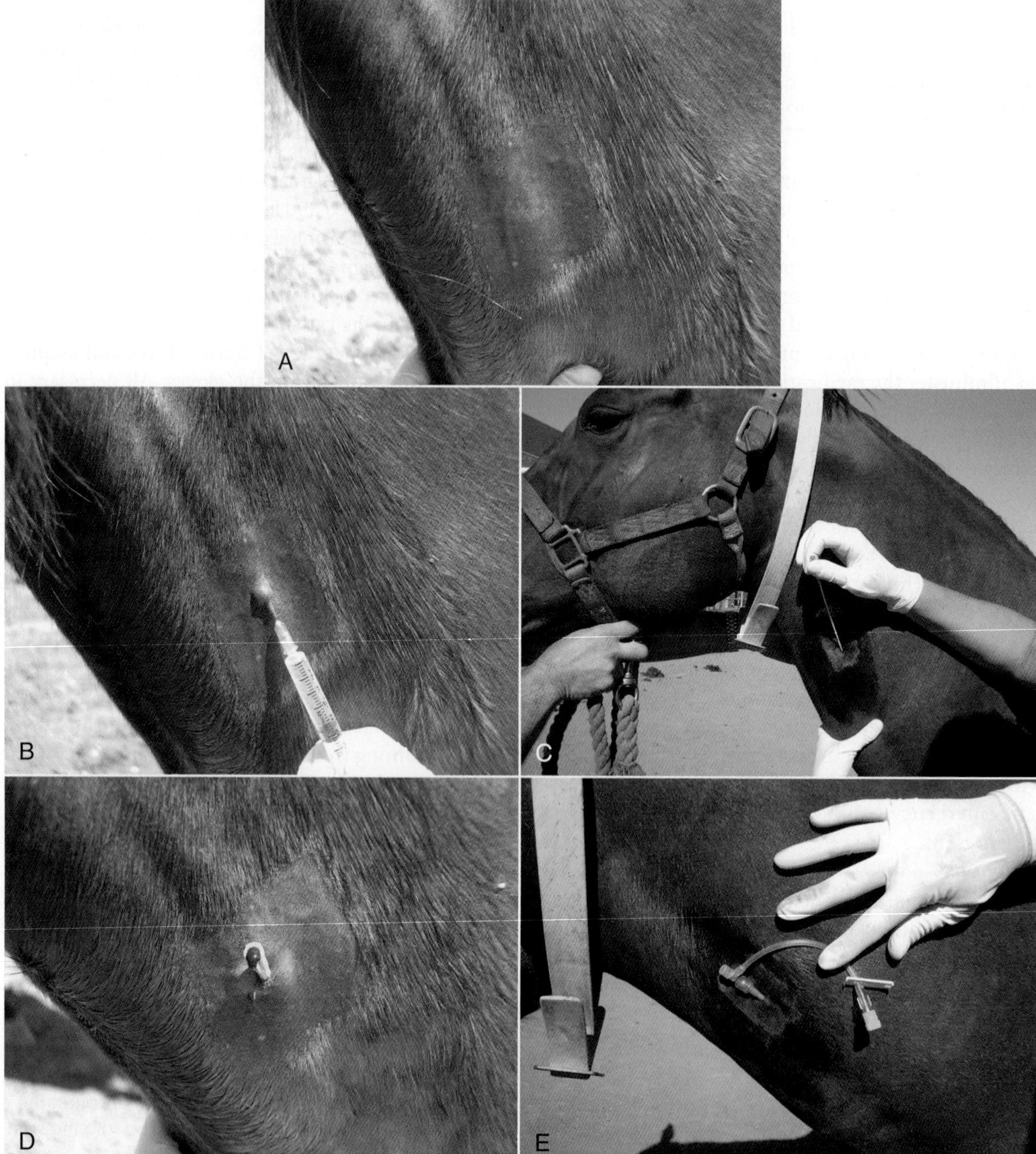

FIGURE 20-80 A, Distending the vein by placing pressure on the vein for IV catheter placement in equine jugular vein. B, Injecting ID lidocaine as local anesthetic. C, Inserting catheter. D, Catheter in vein, blood dripping from catheter confirms placement in the vein. E, T-port attached to catheter.

catheter to protect the site from bedding, urine, and manure. When placing IV catheters in recumbent neonatal foals, it is helpful to place a rolled-up towel under the neck to enhance the view of the jugular vein and stretch the skin. Making a small nick in the skin at the insertion site with a needle or blade will facilitate the insertion of the catheter. It is also helpful to have an assistant stretch the skin while applying digital pressure and thus maintaining distention while the catheter is advanced.

When administering fluids or medications into an IV catheter, the technician should always first clean the injection port with isopropyl alcohol to prevent bacterial contamination.

If the technician wishes to use a guidewire-type catheter, the same steps for preparing and placing the catheter are used, but the guidewire-type catheters entail a few extra steps (refer to Seldinger guidewire technique described for small animals or read directions on individual packages). The most important thing to remember when placing these types of catheters is to NEVER let go of the guidewire until the catheter is successfully placed and the guidewire is fully removed.

Cephalic Vein

For IV catheterization of the cephalic vein (Figure 20-81), the standard preparation is made and the catheter inserted proximal to the carpus and upward. A 14- to 16-gauge × 3.25- to 5.25-inch catheter is an appropriate choice for an adult equine. The placement of a T-port is beneficial and in some cases, a piece of IV extension tubing is connected to the catheter so that IV infusions can be made without disturbing the catheter wrap. The catheter can be covered with sterile gauze and elastic wrap.

Lateral Thoracic Vein

The site is shaved, and standard preparation is done. The IV catheter is inserted in a cranial direction (toward the front of the horse). This is a large diameter vein and can accommodate a large-bore catheter, if necessary. The vein is deeper than the other veins used for IV catheterization. A wrap is placed over the catheter and wrapped around the body of the horse.

Bovine

Jugular Vein

To administer IV medication or fluids to a bovine patient, the jugular vein is the most feasible route to use. Proper restraint of the animal is critical to the safety of the animal and the staff. For adult bovines, the head should be haltered, and ideally the animal should be placed into a head gate or stanchion. The head is slightly lifted and pulled away from the side to be used and tied with a quick-release knot. This will give the technician a good visual of the area and prevent the animal from knocking its head into the technician. Calves may be restrained standing with the handler holding the calf up against their body or in recumbency. Once the animal is sufficiently restrained, the site chosen is cleaned with 70% isopropyl alcohol until all organic material and debris are removed. Using fingers or a fist placed into the jugular groove, the technician occludes the vessel with one hand and performs a venipuncture with the other. Ballottement of the vessel (stroking with a finger over the vein in a downward direction) will help to make the vein more prominent and assist with visualization. For the jugular vein, a 16- to 18-gauge × 1½-inch needle should be used. The technician will introduce the needle into the skin at a 45-degree angle, using strong committed motion since the skin of cattle is relatively tough. Once the vein is accessed, blood should exit the needle hub. Confirmation of the placement in the vein and not an artery is made, and the needle is inserted all the way to the hub. At this time, the syringe containing the medication to be administered can be attached to the needle. By aspirating back, the technician can reconfirm that the needle is still in the vein. If no blood is obtained, the needle should be redirected without completely removing it from the skin. Once in the vein, pressure applied to the jugular groove for occlusion can be removed, and the medication can be administered. After the entire amount is administered, the needle and syringe are removed, and digital pressure is applied over the access site to prevent hematoma formation.

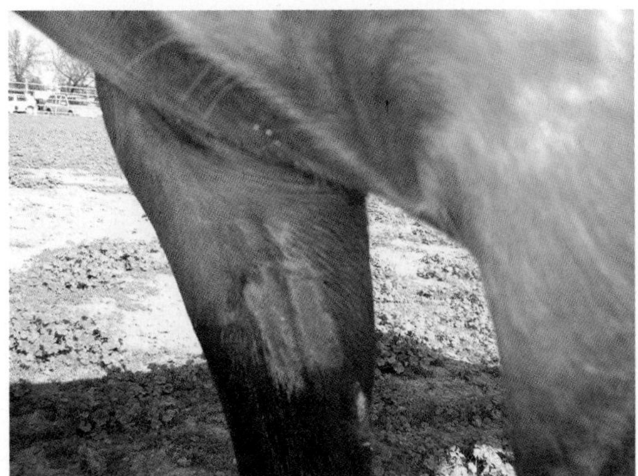

FIGURE 20-81 Site shaved for IV catheterization of equine cephalic vein.

Coccygeal Vein

For small volumes (up to approximately 5 ml) of nonirritating (xylazine, acepromazine, oxytocin) medication, the coccygeal vein can be used.

> *TECHNICIAN NOTE* Administering irritating drugs into the coccygeal vein can cause thrombosis of the vein and sloughing of the tail.

Dairy cows are fairly accepting of tail vein injections because holding the tail up vertically to access the vein also provides restraint ("tail jack"). Beef cattle may need to be placed in a chute for the safety of the personnel. An 18- to 20-gauge × 1.5-inch needle is appropriate for tail vein injections. Palpate the midline of the ventral surface of the tail, to determine the location of the second or third coccygeal vertebra. The site is cleaned with 70% isopropyl alcohol. The needle is inserted and the syringe attached (the needle may be inserted independent of the syringe or with a syringe attached) and plunger withdrawn slightly to check for placement in the vein. Once in the vein, the medication is injected (Figure 20-82).

Subcutaneous Abdominal Vein

The SQ abdominal (milk or mammary) vein is occasionally used to administer IV injections, but use of this vein is strongly discouraged, as noted in the section on blood sample collection. It is hazardous to the animal and dangerous for the technician.

Auricular Vein

This vein can be used for IV injections of very small amounts of medications. The animal's head is secured. Nose tongs may be helpful in preventing movement of the head.

Bovine IV Catheter

When administering large volumes of fluids or repeated IV administrations, a catheter should be placed in the jugular vein to perform these tasks successfully and without the potential for causing problems or damage to the vessels. To place an IV catheter, the same restraint techniques should be employed as outlined previously. The site that is chosen needs to be clipped and surgically prepared, and an antiseptic, such as Betadine solution, is wiped onto the site and left to dry. Because of the skin thickness of cattle, a cutdown using a #15 scalpel blade or a puncture with the same size needle as the catheter will allow for easier insertion of the catheter. If a blade is used to cut the skin before the catheter insertion, a local anesthetic bleb should be placed. A 12- to 16-gauge × 5¼-inch catheter is used on adult cattle, but a smaller size, such as 15- or 18-gauge × 3¼-inch, can be used for calves (Figure 20-83).

The cephalic vein can also be used to place a catheter if the jugular veins are inaccessible. The caudal auricular vein (ear vein) may be used for small-gauge catheters, but these are hard to maintain because it is difficult to stabilize the catheter and prevent the animal from rubbing the catheter (Box 20-6).

Camelid

Although the jugular vein is the most common site for IV injections for llamas and alpacas, it is not as easily accessed as the other large animal species. Injections can be given either high on the neck or low on the neck, but each has potential complications (see previous section of chapter). The high neck position is identified by landmarks as described earlier in the chapter for venous blood sampling. Using the same technique employed with all IV injections, the needle should be detached from the syringe and inserted to make sure that the vein has been punctured and not the artery. Once identified that you have successfully accessed the vein, the syringe is attached, aspirate back, and then gently administer the medication.

The same process is followed for the administration of the low neck site. The landmarks for jugular access on the lower neck are the space between the fifth and sixth cervical vertebrae. Locate the enlarged transverse process of the sixth cervical vertebra, and the jugular vein lies just medially to it. The advantage to choosing the low neck site is the thinner skin, better visualization, and fewer problems with the animal moving or flinching away from the needle and technician.

Camelid IV Catheterization

Camelids have very thick skin (up to 1 cm in adult males), and the large transverse processes of the cervical vertebrae help to protect the underlying vein. To place a catheter in the jugular vein, the lower third of the neck should be used. Fourteen gauge × 5¼ inches is acceptable for adults, and a 16- to 20-gauge × 3¼-inch catheter can be used for crias. The same process as outlined earlier should be used to place a catheter. In adult animals, it is beneficial to make a cut in the skin where the catheter will be inserted. The cephalic vein can also be used, but the placement and maintenance may be difficult because of the camelid's propensity to lie down in sternal recumbency ("kushed").

BOX 20-6 Materials Needed for Catheter Placement

- Catheter of choice
- Heparinized saline (flush) with syringe and needle
- T-port
- PRN adapter (intermittent infusion plug)
- Razor
- Surgical soap
- Suture material
- Sterile gloves
- Betadine-soaked gauze
- Alcohol-soaked gauze
- Wrap materials (antibiotic ointment, Elastikon, gauze)

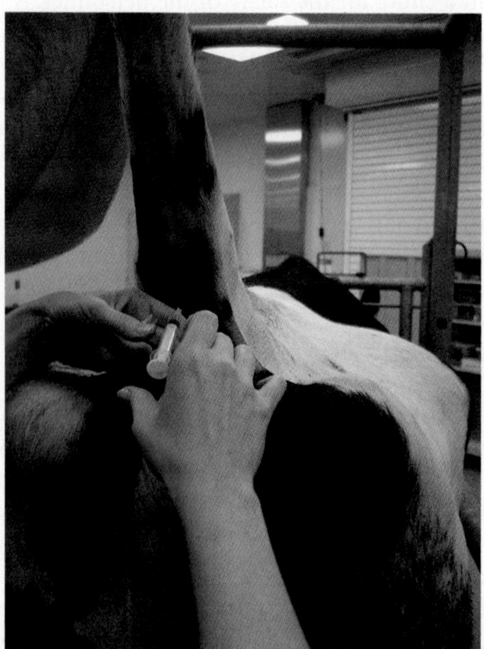

FIGURE 20-82 IV injection into coccygeal vein of cow.

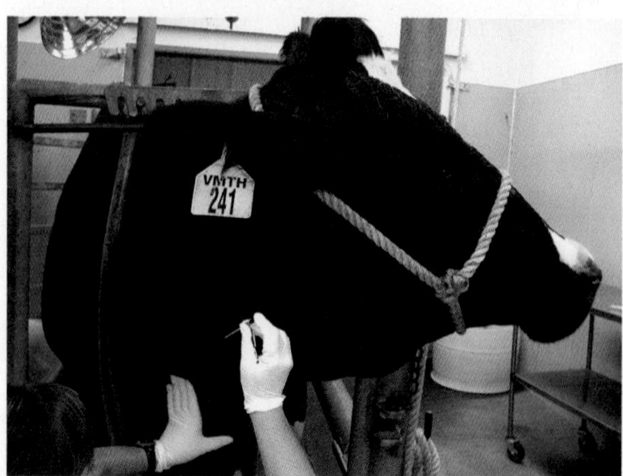

FIGURE 20-83 Jugular catheter placement in adult bovine.

> *TECHNICIAN NOTE* The thick skin and large transverse processes of the cervical spine help to protect these animals from exsanguination caused by bites from fighting males.

Ovine and Caprine

As with the other large animal species listed above, the most common route for IV administration in the goat or sheep is the jugular vein. Proper restraint is essential to administer the medication efficiently and effectively. It is possible to perform the procedure with one person, but having additional help will make the procedure smoother. For both sheep and goats, backing the animal up against a wall, the technician then straddles the patient over the shoulders facing the head and gently grasps under the mandible and lifts the head up and away from the vein to be punctured. For sheep, the wool should be parted for the visualization of the skin. Sheep can be set up on their rump and veins accessed as described for blood collection. The area is to be wiped down with isopropyl alcohol, digital pressure applied in the jugular furrow to distend the vein, and then a needle is inserted into the vessel (20-gauge × 1 inch for adults; 22-gauge × 1 inch for kids and lambs). Once the vein has been punctured and it is established that it is venous blood, the syringe with medication can be attached, aspirate back for confirmation, then slowly inject substance. After all medication is delivered, remove the needle, and apply digital pressure for a couple of minutes to prevent hematoma formation.

Ovine and Caprine IV Catheterization

The jugular vein is the most suitable site for placing a catheter, but the cephalic vein can also be used if jugular access is not an option. The procedure for placing a catheter in the goat or sheep is the same as described previously. For adults, 14- to 18-gauge × 3.5- to 5.25-inch catheters are appropriate, and for lambs and kids, 18- to 22-gauge × 1.5- to 3.25-inch catheters are used. It is helpful to nick the skin at the insertion site with a needle to ease the insertion of the catheter through the skin.

Porcine

IV administration to pigs is accomplished using the auricular veins, located on the dorsal aspect of the pinna. There are three veins, and the most common one for injection is the lateral vein. The pig should be restrained by using a snare or chute, or if small enough, an assistant can hold the animal against their body. Pigs have very sharp teeth and strong jaws. Without sufficient restraint, a bite is a serous possibility. The ear should be cleaned with alcohol-soaked gauze and the base of the ear occluded with digital pressure. A small-gauge needle is inserted into the vessel at a very shallow angle. The needle should be attached to the syringe at the time of insertion because of the very fragile nature of these vessels. Aspirate very gently to confirm venous placement, release occlusion, and then inject the substance with steady pressure. Remove needle and syringe and apply digital pressure. The cephalic vein can also be used, but in small piglets, the jugular vein should be used because of the small diameter and difficultly accessing the cephalic and ear veins at that age.

Porcine IV Catheterization

To catheterize the ear vein, a 19- or 21-gauge butterfly catheter or 18-gauge OTN catheter is used. The base of the ear is occluded with digital pressure or by using a rubber-band tourniquet, and the dorsal aspect of the pinna is surgically prepared. The catheter is then inserted toward the base of the ear into the vein as described previously for injecting into the vein, and the tourniquet or pressure is released. The catheter is then capped with a PRN and secured to the ear using glue. The pinna is supported by placing a roll of gauze or roll of tape on the inside of the pinna, and the margins of the ear are gently folded over and secured with strips of adhesive tape (Figure 20-84).

Complications of IV catheterization include phlebitis, thrombophlebitis, and local cellulitis. Septicemia may result if a venipuncture is made through dirt or fecal material. These can occur in veins that have been injected or catheterized, and thrombophlebitis can result in life-threatening conditions for the animal. Animals that are very compromised may develop these conditions, even when excellent cleanliness and technique are used. If veins are rendered unusable, it may become impossible to administer fluids and medications needed. The technician should be attentive to any changes in the appearance of the vein, including such things as swelling, heat, pus, a thick-corded feel to the vein, or the appearance of fluid from the catheter site, and promptly inform the veterinarian when any of these are noticed.

INTRAMUSCULAR ADMINISTRATION (IM)

Drugs that are administered directly into the muscle are absorbed relatively quickly. The IM route provides more rapid drug absorption than the SQ route and slower absorption than the IV route. The standard procedure for IM injections is to restrain the animal as needed based on its size and temperament and clean the injection site with 70% isopropyl alcohol or other appropriate disinfectant until dirt and debris are removed. Selection of the needle size is determined by the viscosity of the drug, the size of the muscle, and the volume to be administered. The needle is inserted into the muscle all the way to the hub, making sure to touch only the hub rather than the shaft. Inserting the needle without the syringe attached is useful so that if the animal moves, the needle is likely to remain in place. If the needle is inserted with the syringe attached, the added weight of the syringe may cause the needle to come out of the muscle if the animal moves. Attach the syringe containing the drug to be delivered and gently aspirate back to identify that you are in a muscle and have not hit a vessel. If you have punctured a vessel, remove the needle, start with a new needle, and repeat the process.

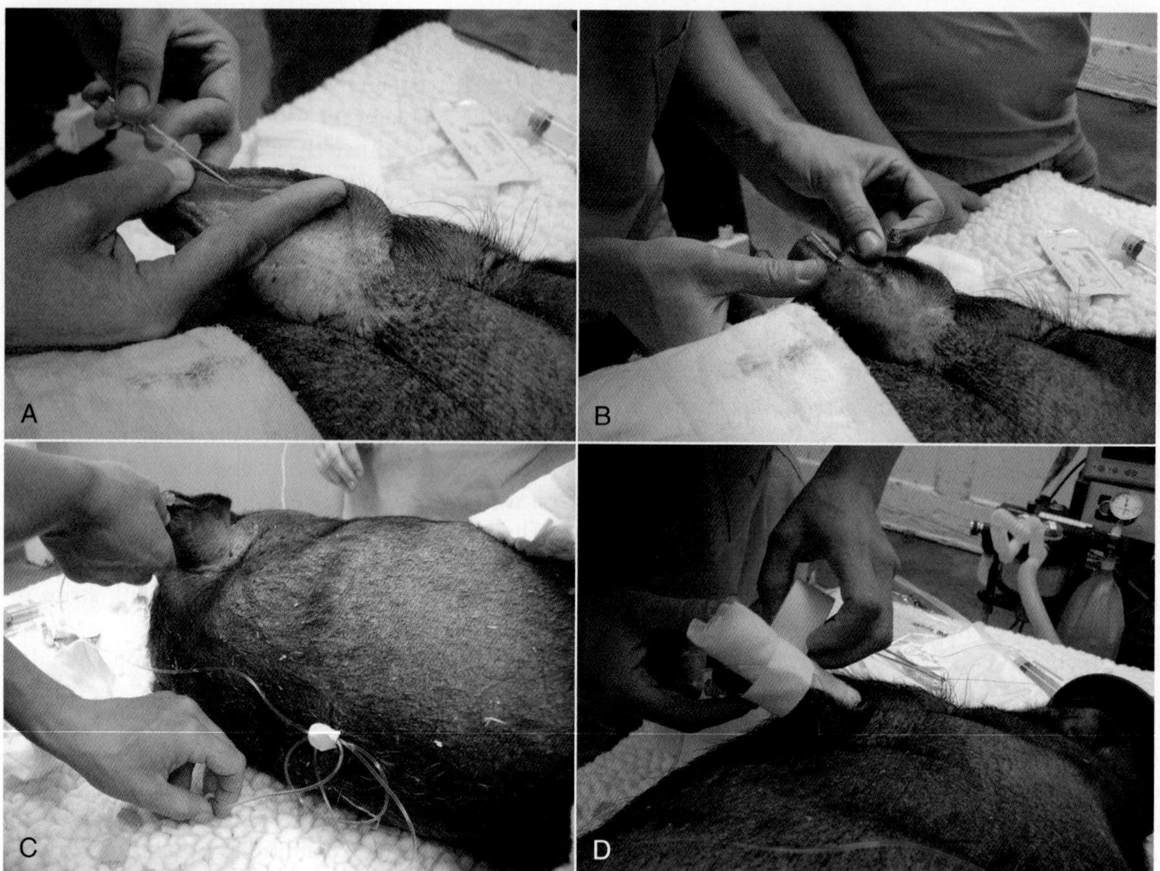

FIGURE 20-84 **A,** Inserting an IV catheter in the auricular vein of a pig. **B,** Removing stylet. **C,** Attaching IV line to back of pig. **D,** Wrapping the ear with gauze and tape to secure catheter.

> *TECHNICIAN NOTE* If the technician uses the same needle that hit a vessel on the first attempt, when aspirating back on the second attempt, residual blood will travel into the syringe causing the technician to believe that yet again a vessel has been struck.

Once you have confirmed that the needle is in the muscle, inject the substance with steady pressure. Do not aggressively force the solution into the muscle because the pressure may make the syringe detach from the needle, causing medicine to spray everywhere. The technician would be unable to determine the exact amount of drug actually delivered to the patient. Some substances that are injected can prove harmful to personnel if they come in contact with mucous membranes (eyes, mouth, etc.). Once the medication is delivered, remove the syringe and needle. Apply pressure if any blood comes from the injection site and massage the area gently.

If repeated IM injections are required on a patient, various sites should be used in an attempt to minimize muscle damage and pain.

Equine IM Administration

There are several locations that can be used on the equine patient for the IM administration of therapeutics. These sites include the lateral cervical (neck), semimembranosus and semitendinosus, and pectoral and gluteal muscles on both the left and right side of the animal. When choosing the location for IM injections, the technician should consider: the volume to be delivered, the viscosity of the solution, the potential injury to personnel, and the potential for complications in the muscle chosen. Restraint must be employed whenever giving an injection, with a halter and lead rope as the minimum. Placing a horse in stocks will greatly reduce the likelihood of the animal moving once the needle is introduced and will also prevent injury to personnel, although it can be detrimental to a patient that has a reaction to the medication given if they get caught in the stocks. Individual horses respond differently to needles. Some respond only slightly or not obviously at all. Others can respond violently. A method for desensitizing the injection site just before a needle insertion is to rub the site very firmly and rapidly back and forth 100 times using an alcohol-soaked cotton swab or piece of gauze and then immediately insert the needle. Some people like to tap the horse firmly with the edge of the fist just before inserting a needle into the muscle. This is also thought to desensitize the area before the insertion of the needle. Other people are convinced that tapping in this manner before a needle insertion simply lets the horse know what is about to happen. The technician should use whatever method proves to be a good approach for him or her.

Lateral Cervical (Neck) Muscles

IM injections into the neck allow for the safety of personnel. Small volumes should be delivered (less than 10 ml in an adult horse) into the lateral aspect of the neck. Choose a spot in the triangular space that is bordered dorsally by the nuchal ligament, ventrally by the cervical vertebrae, and caudad about 1 hand width in front of the cranial border of the scapula (Figure 20-85). An 18- to 22-gauge needle is appropriate for most horses. The needle is inserted with a quick thrust directly into the muscle. Some technicians make a point of grasping the skin next to the injection site between the fingers and pulling up. The injection is administered and the skin released back into place. This method results in the needle hole in the skin a few inches away from the needle hole in the muscle. When the skin is released, it acts as a barrier, preventing leakage of the drug. The neck muscles are not recommended for IM injections in foals because the soreness caused by the injections may make them reluctant to position themselves for nursing.

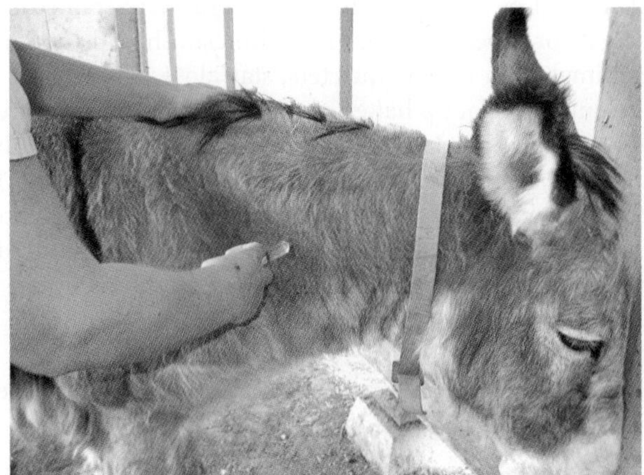

FIGURE 20-85 IM injection in neck of donkey. Needle is placed in an imaginary triangular area of the lateral neck to avoid the cervical vertebrae, the scapula, and the ligamentum nuchae.

Semimembranosus/Semitendinosus Muscles

Semimembranosus and semitendinosus muscles are located on the caudal aspect of the hind limb between the point of the buttock and the hock. These muscles are often used with minimal complications. Particular attention needs to be paid to the sciatic nerve that runs down the lateral aspect of the leg because an inadvertent injection into the nerve can cause paralysis. The technician should stand facing toward the tail end of the animal with his or her body next to the hip of the horse. Positioned with the body closely pressed into the horse's hip will lessen the impact if the animal chooses to kick. If the technician is tall enough, he or she can reach across the horse and insert the needle into the opposite leg (Figure 20-86, *A, B*). This reduces the chance of being kicked since a horse that kicks in response to the insertion of the needle will usually kick with the leg that has received the needle.

An 18- or 19-gauge × 1.5-inch needle should be inserted with swift action into this muscle group. Once the animal has stopped moving, attach the syringe and proceed as described previously. If injecting large volumes of medication, it is preferential to detach the syringe from the needle after 15 ml has been administered, withdraw the needle slightly, and redirect the needle within the muscle. There is no need to remove the needle completely, but care should be taken to avoid side-to-side movement because moving the needle

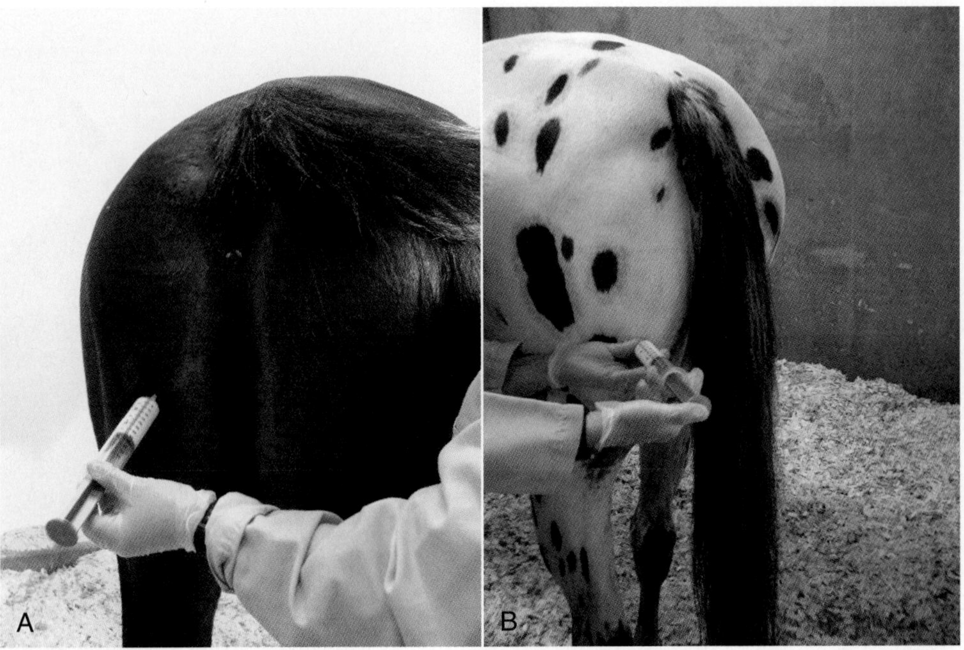

FIGURE 20-86 **A,** Technician positioned on opposite side from injection for an IM injection into semitendinosus muscle group of horse. **B,** Technician positioned on same side as injection.

can cause trauma to the tissue. Once the needle has been redirected, reattach the syringe, aspirate, and inject as described earlier. Continue this process until all of the solution has been administered.

Excessive distention by injecting large volumes of medication can result in necrosis of the tissue. When doing repeated injections into these muscle groups, it is advisable to rotate between the right and left sides to minimize muscle soreness and decrease the likelihood of puncturing a vessel. Because of the large size of the muscles in this area, it is a good choice for IM injections in foals. It can be used with the foal standing and restrained or when recumbent. Repeated IM injections in the hind legs may cause soreness that appears as lameness. It usually lasts for only a few days following the last injection. Repeated injections may also lead to increased vascularization in the area, making it more difficult to insert the needle without encountering blood.

Pectoral muscles. The pectoral muscles are located between the front legs. As with the hind end, safety needs to be considered when choosing this site. A needle insertion at this site usually elicits less of a reaction than an injection into the hind legs, but the technician should assess the temperament of the animal and be prepared for the horse to move forward, jump to the side, strike, or rear. The technician should stand next to the shoulder of the horse facing the head. Reaching around with the hand farthest from the horse, insert the needle all the way to the hub. An 18- to 20-gauge × 1- to 1.5-inch needle is appropriate (Figure 20-87). The pectoral muscles are relatively small, and repeated IM injections in this site may cause pain and swelling. The resultant edema that may be seen following an IM injection at this site can be temporarily unsightly and may be of consideration, depending on the planned use of the horse.

Gluteal Muscles

The gluteus, or rump, of the horse is the largest muscle mass on the hindquarters. It is located high on the rear limb, lateral to the spine, and caudal to the point of the hip (Figure 20-88). It can accommodate large volumes and repeated injections, but is not often chosen as the site for IM injections because it is difficult to detect inflammation caused by IM injections in the gluteus, and if an abscess forms, adequate drainage from this area can be very difficult. If the gluteus is used, the technician should stand close to the hip of the horse and insert the needle with a quick thrust, as for other IM sites.

Bovine IM Administration

Because most cattle are eventually consumed, IM injections are highly discouraged to prevent muscle damage. If it is absolutely necessary to give an IM injection, the muscles of the neck should be used. The animal should be restrained in a head gate or squeeze chute. The technician should approach the animal from the forequarters, stay close, and leaning in to the animal, place a halter on the head and tie it securely to the side. The borders are the same as described for equine patients (the spine, nuchal ligament, and the scapula). The needle should be inserted with a quick thrust into the muscle. Following beef quality assurance guidelines, the needle must be clean and sharp, the injection smooth so as not to cause too much muscle damage, and no more than 10 ml of substance is to be administered at any one time.

The semitendinosus, semimembranosus, and gluteal muscles should not be used for IM injections in cattle.

Ovine and Caprine IM Administration

Sheep and goats have small muscle masses. The most common muscle groups used for IM injections are the semitendinosus and semimembranosus muscles (Figure 20-89). The

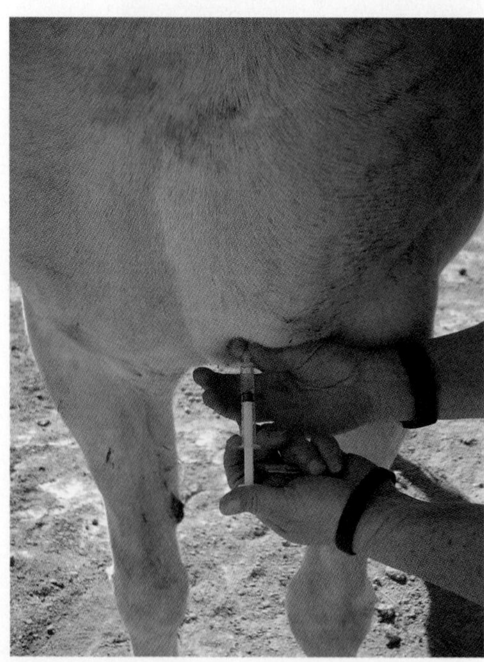

FIGURE 20-87 IM injection into pectoral muscles of horse.

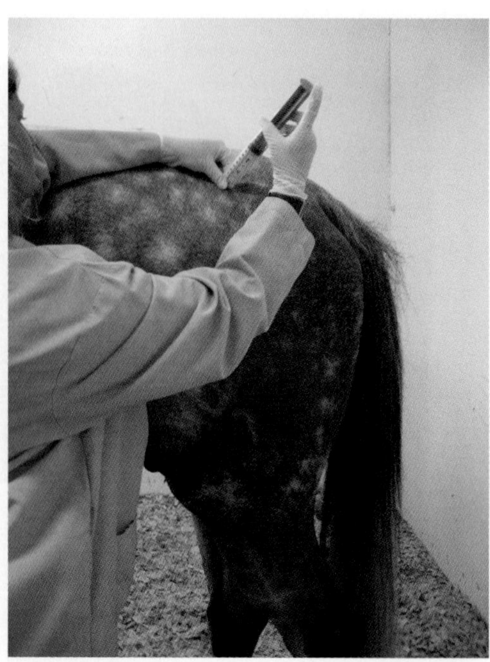

FIGURE 20-88 IM injection into equine gluteals.

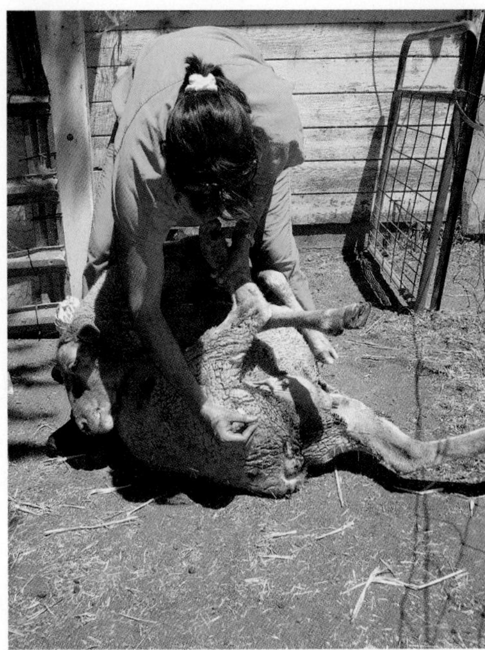

FIGURE 20-89 Technician administering IM injection to sheep.

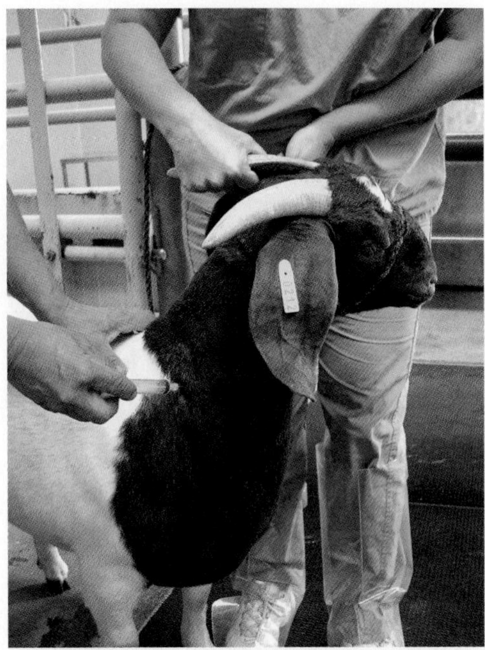

FIGURE 20-90 Site for IM injection in neck of goat.

technician must avoid the sciatic nerve, which runs down the caudomedial aspect of the hind legs. The neck, gluteals, and triceps can be used, but only for very small volumes (Figure 20-90). IM injections into the neck may cause significant soreness, and the animal may be reluctant to raise its head. This can be particularly problematic in kids and lambs because they may become too sore to nurse. Once the muscle to be used is identified, the standard procedure described for large animals is followed. For adult sheep and goats, an 18- to 20-gauge × 1-inch needle should be used. A 20- to 22-gauge × 1-inch needle is appropriate for lambs and kids.

Porcine IM Administration

IM injections in pigs can prove complicated because of the thickness of the skin, the tendency to store a thick layer of SQ body fat, the difficulty in restraining them, and potential damage to muscle (meat). Generally the cervical neck muscles are used just caudal and ventral to the ear. In adults, a maximum volume of 5 to 10 ml per site is recommended. Piglets can receive 1 to 2 ml per site. For adults, a long needle (at least 1.5 inches) should be used to avoid the fat because injecting into the fat will delay drug absorption. Depending on the size of the animal, the needle gauge can be anywhere from 20 gauge for piglets to 16 gauge for larger stock. Drug residues in various muscles will reduce the market value of the animal. The gluteal, semimembranosus, and semitendinosus muscles can be used, but not in animals destined to be used for meat. Following the same meat quality assurance guidelines as identified for cattle, the technician will grasp the skin in this area and pull cranially. With a firm motion, insert the needle at a perpendicular angle to the skin. Once the needle is in, attach the syringe, aspirate back, and inject the medication.

Camelid IM Administration

IM injection sites for llamas and alpacas are generally the same as in other large animal species. They do not have a large muscle mass in any one place, so SQ is the preferred route for the administration of large volumes or potentially irritating substances. The neck should not be used because of the potential for causing soreness in the area. The semimembranosus and semitendinosus muscles are good choices for IM injections in these animals (Figure 20-91). For adults an 18- to 20-gauge × 1-inch needle is appropriate. Twenty-gauge to 22-gauge × 1-inch needles are recommended for crias.

Subcutaneous Administration (SQ, Subq, SC)

In all species, SQ injections can be given anywhere that the skin is able to be lifted and tented. Medications that are administered SQ are absorbed less rapidly than IV or IM injections, but more rapidly than oral or intradermal (ID) administration. Therapeutic agents that are administered SQ include, vaccines, local anesthetics, and small volumes of other medications. Fluid therapy may also be administered via an SQ route for some large animal patients. SQ injections may be desired for use in show animals because there is less likelihood of a noticeable adverse reaction at the injection site with SQ versus IM injections. The meat animal production industry recommends that drugs be administered SQ in an effort to reduce any tissue damage (damage to the meat) that can occur with IM injections. There are strict regulatory requirements for the administration of pharmaceuticals to cattle, the medications must be administered per label, and most medications for use in cattle are labeled for SQ administration.

SQ injections are done by inserting a needle between the skin and the body of the animal. The site selected should have loose skin that is easily grasped. It is wiped with 70%

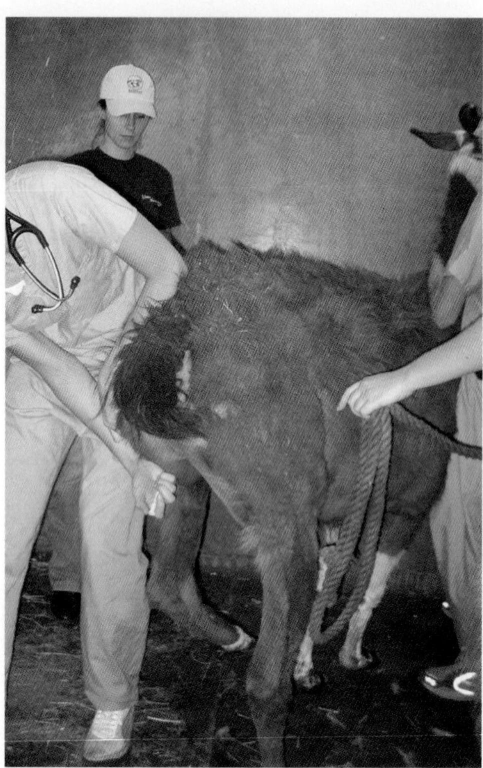

FIGURE 20-91 Llama receiving IM injection into semitendinosus.

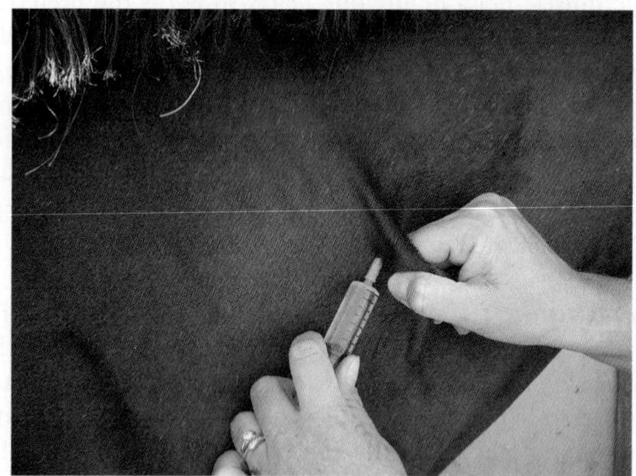

FIGURE 20-92 SQ injection into loose skin on lateral neck of horse.

isopropyl alcohol, the skin grasped and pulled away from the body of the animal, and then the needle inserted into the base of the tented skin. The needle size used will depend on the viscosity of the substance to be administered, the size of the animal, and the thickness of its skin. A 20- to 25-gauge needle no longer than 1 inch should be used for SQ injections in horses. An 18- to 22-gauge × 1.5-inch needle is a common choice for calves, sheep, goats, and pigs. Adult cattle may require a 16- to 18-gauge needle. Before injecting the substance from the syringe, aspirate back to make sure that the vessels have not been punctured. Once confirmation of the needle placement in the SQ space has been established, gently inject the medication. The solution should easily be

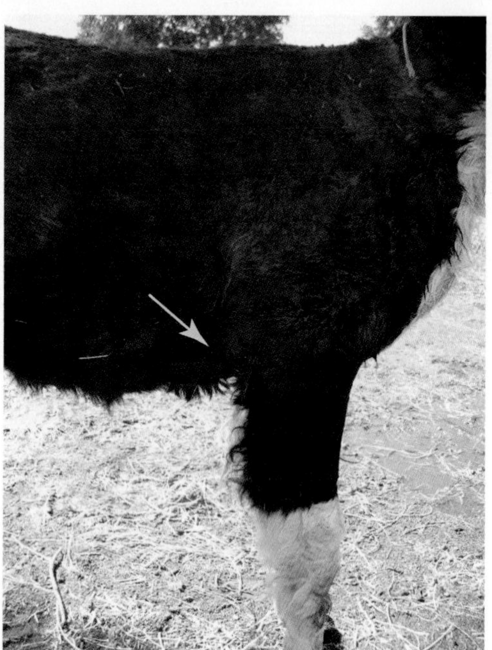

FIGURE 20-93 Loose skin located behind the elbow in llamas can be a site for SQ injections.

ejected from the syringe and a bleb, or bump, is often visible under the skin. A slow flow of solution may indicate that the needle is ID rather than SQ. If this resistance is felt, the needle should be repositioned before proceeding with the injection. After removing the needle and syringe, the injection area should be gently rubbed to lessen the bump that has been created and to increase circulation in the area, which promotes absorption of the medication. If an SQ injection is made into edematous tissue, a bump is not likely to be observed.

For equines, the loose skin on the side and at the base of the neck is the easiest spot for this type of SQ injection (Figure 20-92).

For bovines, the loose skin of the neck region is most easily used as the site for SQ injections. Large volumes of drugs may be injected SQ behind the elbow. Another site for SQ injections in cattle is in the loose skin on either side of the ischiorectal fossa. This site is used by veterinarians for the administration of leptospirosis vaccines in cattle that are restrained in lockup stanchions. The technician should not tent the skin when injecting *Brucellosis* vaccines. This is to make certain that there is no accidental injection of the drug into the person administering the drug.

For llamas, a common site for SQ injection is just behind the elbow (Figure 20-93).

In goats, injection sites for SQ administration include just behind the elbow (Figure 20-94), which can be done with the goat restrained in a standing position, and the axillary region where the forearm meets the body, which can be easily reached by lifting a front leg and the lateral chest, caudal to the shoulder (Figure 20-95).

For sheep, the sites chosen should be free of wool. SQ injections can be done with the animal restrained in a standing

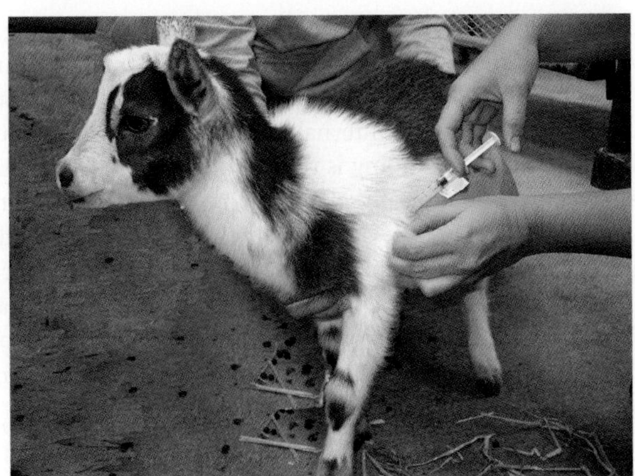

FIGURE 20-94 Goat kid receiving SQ injection behind the elbow.

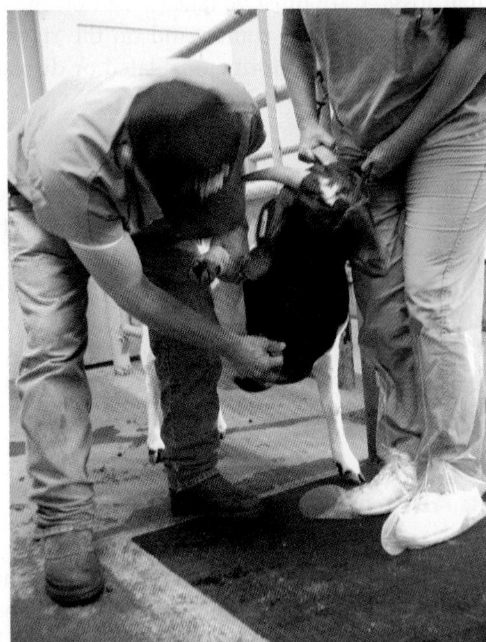

FIGURE 20-95 Lifting a front leg of goat provides access to axillary area for SQ injections.

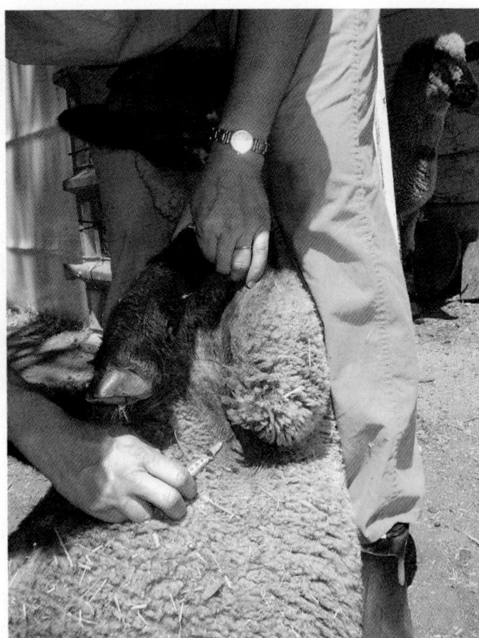

FIGURE 20-96 Technician administering SQ injection in axillary area of sheep while restraining in set up position.

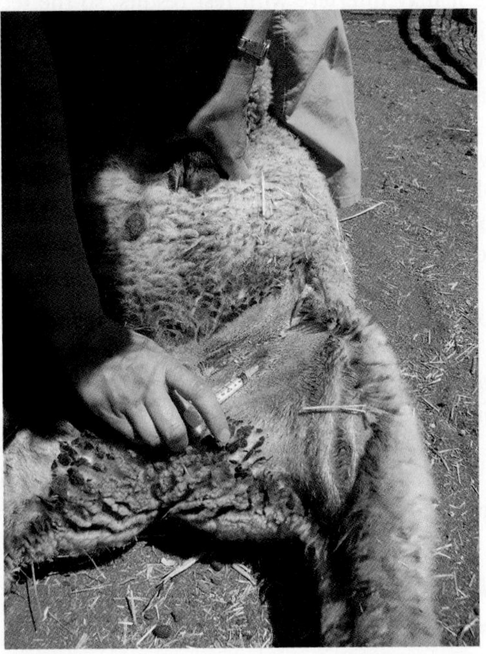

FIGURE 20-97 Administration of SQ injection in inguinal area of sheep.

position, but are facilitated by restraining the sheep set up on its rump. This provides easy access to the most wool-free site, including the axillary area where the forearm meets the body and the inguinal area and flank fold (Figures 20-96 and 20-97).

In pigs, it is challenging to find loose skin. Possible SQ injection sites include the axillary and inguinal regions and the skin caudal to the base of the ear. The size of the animal will determine where the injection can be given. For piglets, holding them up by the hind legs will expose an injection site on the inside of the flank along the abdominal wall. Grasp the skin and pull dorsally and make sure the injection is shallow. The needle should be inserted at an approximately 10-degree angle. Larger pigs should be restrained using a hog snare or chute to access the loose skin just caudal to the ear.

INTRADERMAL ADMINISTRATION (ID)

Intradermal administration is the injection of a substance between the dermis and epidermis (skin layers). This route results in very slow absorption. ID injections are made primarily for the purpose of skin testing, allergen identification, and to provide local anesthesia. Cattle, goats, and sheep are tested for tuberculosis by means of an ID injection into the

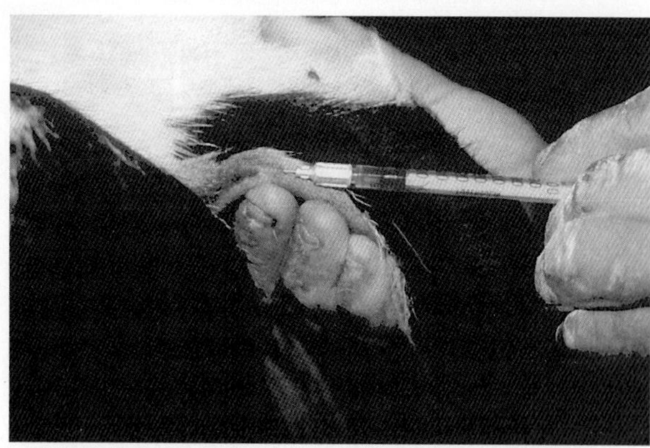

FIGURE 20-98 ID injection is made into the caudal skinfold to test for tuberculosis in the cow.

caudal tail fold (Figure 20-98). ID injections in swine can be given at the base of the ear. For allergy testing in horses, the side of the neck is commonly used. ID injections are also used to treat nodular skin lesions and sarcoids (a common tumor affecting the skin of horses).

For horses, the selected site should be clipped, cleaned, and allowed to dry. Depending on the purpose of the injection, the use of an antiseptic agent may be contraindicated because it may interfere with test results, so the technician preparing for the procedure should be clear on the intent of the veterinarian. The skin is grasped between the thumb and forefinger and pulled up from the body. A small needle (25 to 27 gauge × ⅝ inch) is placed parallel to the site with the bevel directed up and inserted at a slight angle. The syringe plunger is withdrawn slightly to aspirate and make sure that no vessels have been penetrated. The solution is slowly injected. Resistance should be felt if the needle is correctly placed in the dermis. A noticeable bleb should appear as the injection is made. If no bleb is visible, the needle has been placed too deep. Massaging the site (as is suggested with SQ injections) is not done following ID injections because the solution is intended to remain localized.

For goats, sheep, and swine, a 25- to 22-gauge × ⅕- to 1-inch needle is used. Cattle have very thick skin, and a 20- to 22-gauge × 1.5-inch needle is more appropriate.

INTRAPERITONEAL ADMINISTRATION

Equine Administration

In the equine patient, intraperitoneal (IP) administration of fluids and medication is usually accomplished through an abdominal lavage system. The drain system is inserted surgically by the veterinarian either during abdominal surgery or in a standing position when peritonitis is suspected and general anesthesia is not necessary. The technician will not be involved with the surgical procedure, but will be responsible for the care and maintenance afterward. To lavage the abdomen, latex tubing is attached to the desired fluids and connected to the drain system using a 5 in 1 connector. The desired amount of fluid (routinely 10 L for an adult equine patient, adjusted for smaller patients) is administered along with any medication (heparin, antibiotics, etc.), the latex tubing is clamped off, and the patient walked. This is done to attempt to distribute the fluid and medication throughout the abdominal cavity, washing internal organs, and breaking up any adhesions. The latex tubing is then unclamped, and the fluid is allowed to drain out of the abdomen back into the original fluid bag (Figure 20-99, *A-C*). Ideally the amount returned is equal to the amount originally administered. This process can be repeated several times per day. When handling the drain system, gloves should be worn, and the technician should pay careful attention to keeping the system clean and not introducing any contaminants during the administration.

Bovine Administration

IP injections may be indicated if IV administration is not possible and for treatment of peritonitis. If an IP injection is administered in cattle, the site selected is usually in the paralumbar fossa. Care must be taken when on the left side to prevent puncturing the rumen and on the right side to prevent puncturing the intestine or dilated or displaced internal organs.

Caprine and Ovine Administration

IP injections are usually reserved for neonatal kids and lambs with umbilical infections or hypoglycemia. The neonate is lifted by its front legs, and using a 20-gauge needle attached to the syringe filled with medication, the technician inserts it just to the left of the umbilicus up to a depth of 1 cm. Aspirate back to verify that you have not hit a vessel or internal organ. Once placement is confirmed, inject medication into the peritoneal cavity. Remove the needle and syringe.

Porcine Administration

In neonatal pigs, fluids are generally administered IP because of the impracticality of placing IV catheters and administering fluids using that route. Fluids should be body temperature, nonirritating, and isotonic. The site used needs to be prepared using aseptic technique to ensure that contaminants are not introduced. The piglet is held up by the rear legs, and an 18-gauge × ¾- to 1-inch needle is inserted paramedially between the midline and flank. The needle is stabilized to prevent damage to internal organs. To do this procedure in a mature, standing pig, follow the preparation guidelines and use a 16- to 18-gauge × 3-inch needle inserted through the paralumbar fossa.

Complications from IP administration include peritonitis, abscess, and injury to internal organs.

INTRANASAL ADMINISTRATION

Certain vaccines and local anesthetics are administered intranasally. Intranasal anesthetics may be used before performing other procedures involving the nasal cavity. The head of the patient needs to be secured. Small piglets can be held, whereas a hog snare should be used for restraining larger pigs. A halter and lead rope (and head gate for adult cattle)

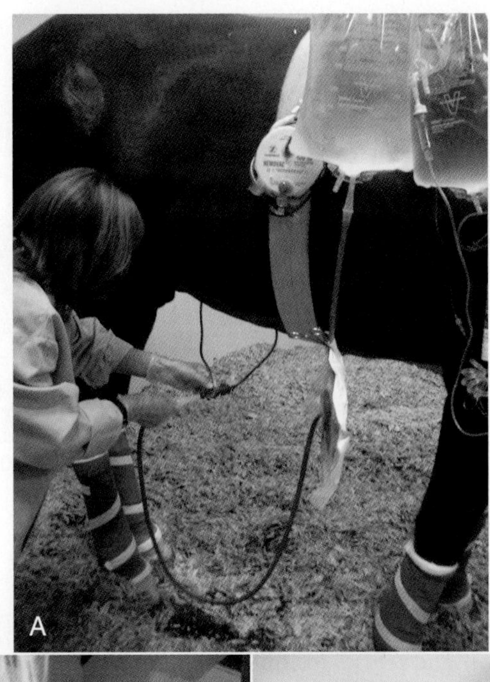

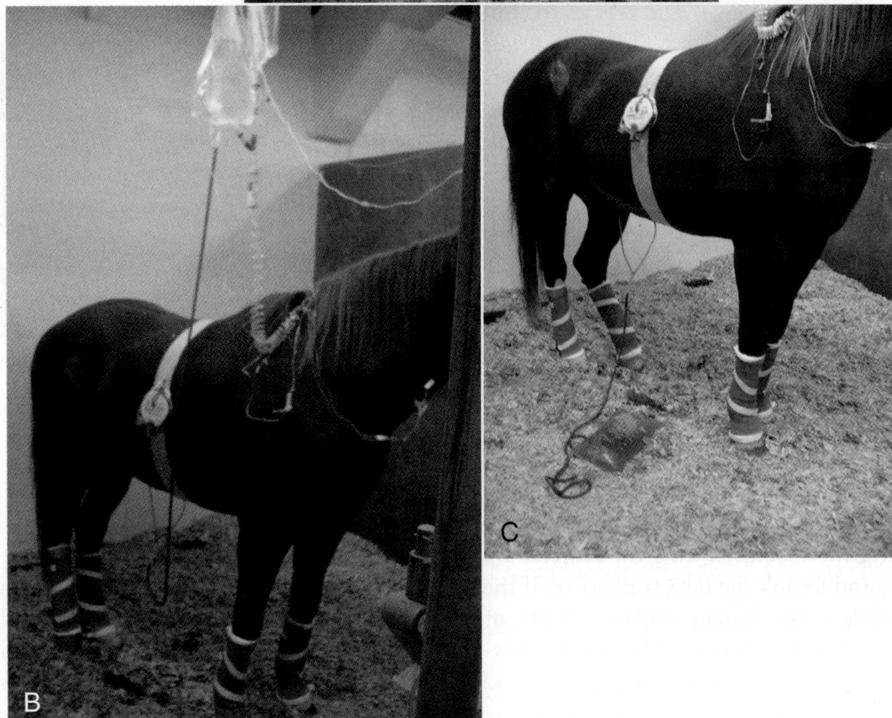

FIGURE 20-99 A, Technician attaches latex tubing from IV fluid bag to abdominal drain tubing from animal for equine abdominal lavage. B, Fluid bag is raised to allow fluid to flow through tubing and into abdominal cavity. C, The empty fluid bag is lowered to the ground to retrieve peritoneal fluid from the abdominal cavity.

may provide sufficient restraint for most large animals. The technician uses his or her free hand to steady the head. An easy method is to bring the free arm under the mandible and reach around placing the hand on top of the muzzle area. Any nasal discharge should be wiped away from the nares using damp gauze sponges. While slightly lifting the head, a needleless syringe containing the medication is introduced into the nostril, and the substance is injected, preferably when the animal inspires. The patient may sneeze afterward, causing the medication to spray. The technician should take precautions to prevent having his or her own mucous membranes sprayed from the sneeze.

Oxygen can be administered intranasally to help with certain conditions, such as pneumonia or hypoxic ischemic encephalopathy. Oxygen may be administered to preparturient females that are considered to have a high-risk pregnancy in an attempt to increase the oxygen content of the circulating blood in both the dam and fetus.

Using a commercially available product (AirLife O_2 catheter) or small rubber feeding tube, identify the distance from the medial canthus of the eye to the entrance of the nostril. This will be how far the catheter is to be inserted into the nostril. Gently insert the catheter ventrally into the nasal passage to the point that was measured. To maintain the catheter in the nostril for the long term, it is beneficial to first wrap adhesive tape (Elastikon works very well) loosely around the muzzle. Then the catheter, with a piece of butterflied 1-inch adhesive tape attached, can be secured using suture material to connect the butterfly to the Elastikon. The end can be hooked up to an oxygen source providing the desired oxygen flow in liters per minute.

ORAL ADMINISTRATION

Medications to be administered orally (per os, PO) come in a variety of forms, including tablets, capsules, powders, pastes, and liquids.

The simplest way to administer oral medications to all large animal species is in food or water. For a variety of reasons, this route may not always be feasible (patient is NPO, detects bitter substance in food or water and refuses to consume, decreased appetite associated with illness, multiple animals housed and fed communally). It is also extremely unreliable since it is hard to determine the amount that is actually ingested. The oral route provides for slower absorption than IV or IM administration, but in many instances is the only route for certain medications.

Oral medications are administered in a variety of methods, including syringes, drenching, balling guns, and nasogastric and orogastric intubation.

Syringes

Many commercially available products come in a paste form in premeasured dosing syringes, which make accurate dosing and administration easy. Other oral medications come in tablet form that need to be both crushed and mixed with water or simply dissolved in water over time. The easiest way to do this is by placing the tablets in a 60-ml catheter tip syringe, adding water, and letting the tablets dissolve. If the medication is unpalatable to the patient, molasses, Karo, or maple syrup or thin applesauce can be added to the mixture. To use the syringe method, proper restraint of the head should be used, with the free arm cradling the head, reaching around so that the hand is up over the muzzle. The technician then inserts the syringe into the mouth at the commissure of the lips near the interdental space, between the cheeks and teeth, and advances it as far back into the mouth as possible (Figure 20-100). With firm pressure, the medication is given, and the syringe can be withdrawn. Lifting the head slightly may encourage the animal to swallow instead of spit the medication out. The medication should not be injected too rapidly because it may be lost from the other side of the mouth or may be aspirated. The technician should be conscious of the probability of the patient spitting the material out and getting it on the skin or mucous membranes of the personnel. Always wash hands and skin that has been in contact with the medication.

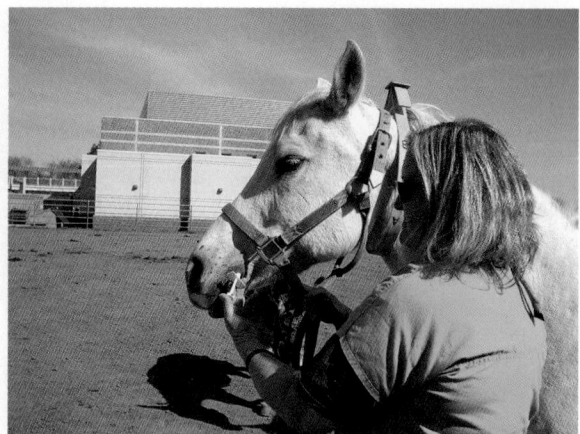

FIGURE 20-100 Administering oral medication via syringe to an adult.

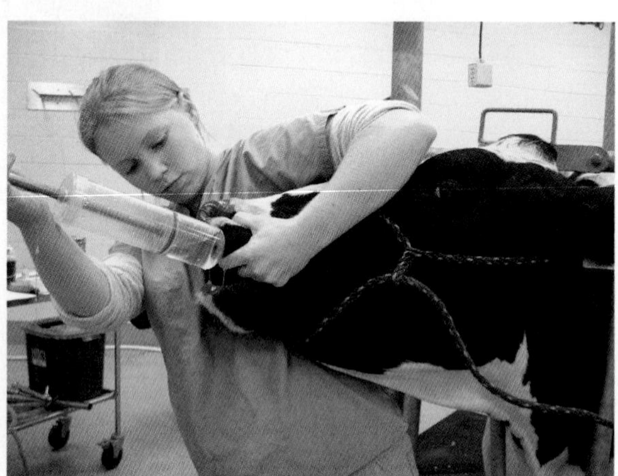

FIGURE 20-101 Bovine drench with dose syringe.

Drench (Dose Syringe)

Liquid medication or small volumes of fluid can be administered using a dose syringe. For calves, sheep, and goats, a catheter tip syringe can be used, whereas a large dose syringe is appropriate for adult cattle. Drenching in sheep and goats should be limited to small volumes of fluid (no greater than 30 ml). Holding the animal with the nose slightly elevated and pulled toward the handler, the tip of the dose syringe is inserted into the interdental space, and the fluid is slowly dribbled onto the tongue (Figure 20-101).

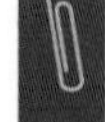

TECHNICIAN NOTE Mineral oil should never be given via drench. Inhalation of mineral oil can be fatal.

Balling Guns (Pilling)

For cattle, sheep, and goats, balling guns are commonly used to accomplish oral tablet administration. There are several sizes available, and the appropriate size should be picked in accordance with the size of your patient. Using a large balling gun on a small calf, goat, or sheep can result in a splitting of the soft palate and rupture of the pharynx. The balling gun should have a smooth end, preferably made of rubber to limit the trauma that can be caused to the back of the mouth, including the soft palate, pharynx, and esophagus. It should be inspected before each use to make sure that no sharp edges have formed. All food should be removed from the patient's mouth before dosing. For cattle, placing the patient in a head gate will help restrain the animal for the procedure. The technician should stand next to the animal's head facing the same direction as the animal. The arm nearest the animal reaches over and grasps the mouth at the interdental space and pressing on the hard palate, opens the animal's mouth. Alternately, placing a finger in one nostril and the thumb in the other and then pulling the nose dorsally will encourage cattle to open their mouth making insertion of the gun easier. The balling gun is inserted into the mouth and gently worked back to the pharynx. Once the thumb rings of the gun are at the commissure of the lips, the plunger is depressed (Figure 20-102). The animal's head should be kept down to prevent the loss of the medication. Cattle will lick their nostrils once they swallow the pill.

For sheep and goats, back them up to a wall and straddle the shoulders as stated before. Insert a hand into the interdental space at the commissure of the lips, open the mouth, and insert the balling gun to the back of the throat before depressing the plunger. If the balling gun is not inserted far enough, the medication may be chewed by the animal and spit out. If the balling gun is inserted too far, there is a risk for serious damage to the pharynx and larynx. To decrease the chance of aspiration of the medication, the head of the animal should not be overly elevated and the neck should not be overextended.

> *TECHNICIAN NOTE* Read labels carefully because certain medications can cause severe complications to the staff if they are mishandled. For example, chloramphenicol tablets should not be crushed because inhaling the powder has been shown to increase the risk to humans of developing fatal aplastic anemia.

Nasogastric and Orogastric Intubation

When large volumes of an oral medication need to be given (mineral oil, fluids, bismuth), oral fluid therapy or enteral feedings for extended periods of time are required, passage of an OGT (cattle, sheep, goats, pigs, and camelids) or an NGT (horses, cattle, adult sheep and goats, neonatal camelids) should be used.

Nasogastric intubation is a commonly used procedure in equine patients. Cattle, sheep, goats, and camelids have small nasal passages and although nasogastric intubation (with small diameter tubes) can be done (Figure 20-103), the usual method for these species is to place an OGT.

Nasogastric

There are many different sizes of tubes that can be used, and choosing one is dependent on the size of the patient and the thickness of the solution that needs to be given (or retrieved, if that is the intent of the procedure). An estimation should be made of the length of the tube required from the entrance of the nostril to the point of the stomach or rumen. For horses, it is helpful to mark the tube at a point where the tube should reach the pharynx (Figure 20-104). This is helpful because the tube can be rotated upward when it reaches the pharynx to deflect it into the esophagus rather than down the trachea. If the tube is cold, soaking it in warm water will make it more pliable for insertion. The tube should also be lubricated with water-soluble lubricant or warm water to aid in easy passage. The patient is restrained as outlined earlier, and with a hand over the muzzle and thumb placed into the nostril, the tube is passed in a ventral manner through the ventral nasal meatus and nasopharynx. Resistance is felt when the tube passes into the esophagus. Once the tube has passed into the esophagus and traveled down to the rumen or stomach, check the premeasured mark that you made with the tube, and then confirm you are in the rumen or stomach and not the trachea. Most patients will cough if the tube is placed in the trachea, but there are times when a cough will not be elicited

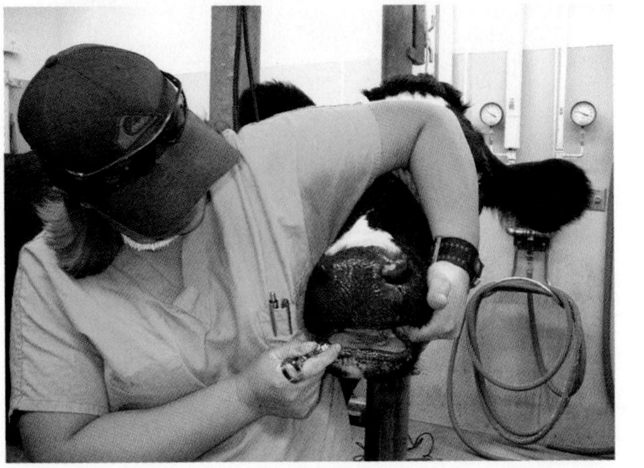

FIGURE 20-102 Using balling gun to administer medication in pill form to cow.

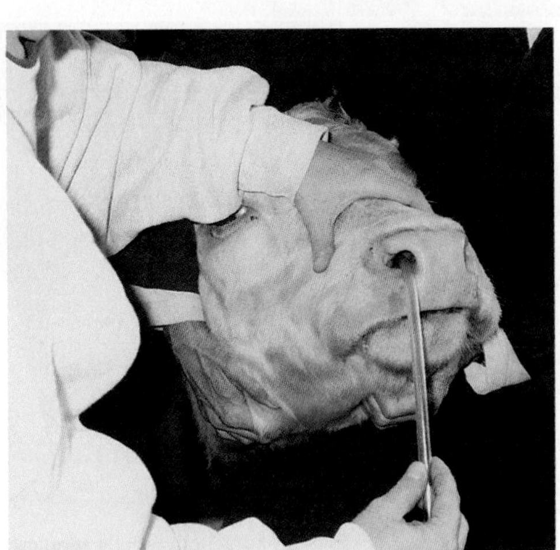

FIGURE 20-103 Nasogastric intubation of bovine with a foal stomach tube.

(small-diameter tubes; flexible, soft tubes used in neonates; comatose patients that are lacking cough reflex, etc.), and therefore it is essential that proper placement is confirmed before medication is administered. When the tube is passing through the esophagus, it is often possible to visualize the tube advancement and feel the tube. This view can be enhanced by moving the tube in and out a bit and looking at the neck for the movement. For all patients, blowing into the tube should elicit gurgles from the tube, rumen or stomach fluid smell, and if an assistant places a stethoscope over the area of the rumen or stomach, he or she should be able to hear bubbling as air passes over the fluid. Aspirating on the tube should reveal negative pressure (but this should not be the only check because the opening of the tube may be up against tissue). Placing one's mouth on the distal end of the tube and sucking back may result in an unpleasant mouthful of gastric fluid, and this has the potential for causing illness in the person if enteric bacteria is present. Once the position of the tube is verified, the patient is checked for gastric reflux. If no abnormal amount of gastric fluid is noted, the medication, fluids, etc. can be administered using a stomach pump, dose syringe, or gravity flow (Figure 20-105). For neonates, a 60-ml syringe is placed on the end of the tube and aspirated to check for reflux. For some patients requiring repeated administration of medications or food, the NGT should be left in place. This can be accomplished in adult equines by coiling and then taping the tube to the halter of the patient (Figure 20-106). A syringe case, tube cap, or other adaptor should be placed on the end of the tube. In neonatal patients, the tubes can be secured into place by using elastic tape around the muzzle of the patient and then coiling the tube off to the side of the mouth (make sure it does not interfere with the action of the mouth). A 1-inch piece of butterflied tape can be secured to the tube at the base of the nostril, and then using suture material, the tape can be affixed to the elastic tape around the muzzle (Figure 20-107, *A, B*). This method of securing the tube is preferred over suturing the tube directly to the nostril because that is irritating to the patient, causing it to rub at the tube and pull it out.

> *TECHNICIAN NOTE* When placing "stay" tape around the muzzle of a neonate, care must be taken to keep the tape loose enough to allow for opening of the mouth and secured well above the nostrils to prevent occlusion of the nostrils.

Once the process is complete, the pump is removed from the end of the tube, and the tube is held up above the patient's head to deliver any remaining medication from the tube into the stomach/rumen. A small amount of water or air can be pumped into the tube to clear the tube. Care should be taken not to aggressively or forcibly pump it in. The end of the tube is then covered with the technician's thumb, kinked, and in gentle, long motions, the tube is pulled out. Complications from the removal of the tube can include nosebleed

FIGURE 20-104 **A,** Estimating the length of tube required to reach the pharynx of horse. **B,** Inserting NGT in horse. Technician stands to side of horse for safe positioning.

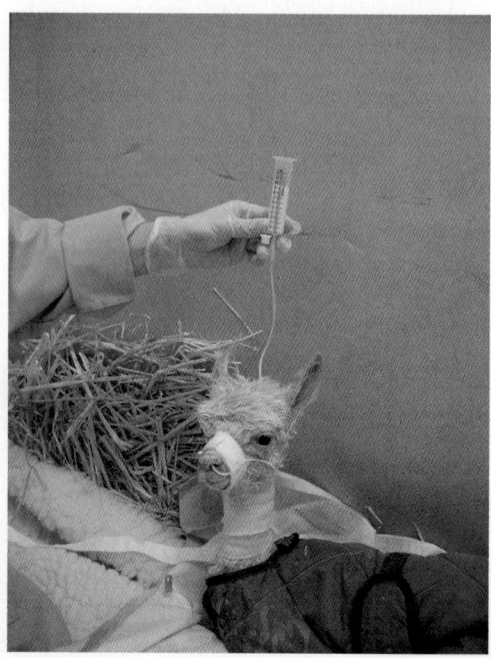

FIGURE 20-105 Technician administering enteral feeding via gravity flow into NGT in alpaca cria.

or aspiration of any residual fluid or medication. The patient should be closely monitored after delivering medication in this fashion for colic symptoms, bloat, or respiratory problems.

NGTs are routinely passed in horses to relieve gastric distention. The tube is passed as described earlier, and once placement in the stomach has been established, a known amount of water is pumped into the tube, causing a siphon, and gastric fluid and content is collected back from the tube into a bucket. The tube is manipulated as needed, and the procedure repeated while fluid is collected. If significant gastric fluid is retrieved, the tube can be secured in place by coiling it and taping it to the halter. This is less stressful to the patient than repeated passing of the tube and more time efficient for the staff. If a syringe casing is placed in the end of the tube, the gastric reflux can be very accurately quantified. If a large amount of gas is present, the veterinarian may decide it is prudent to leave the tube in place with no cap so as to provide continuous decompression and relief to the patient.

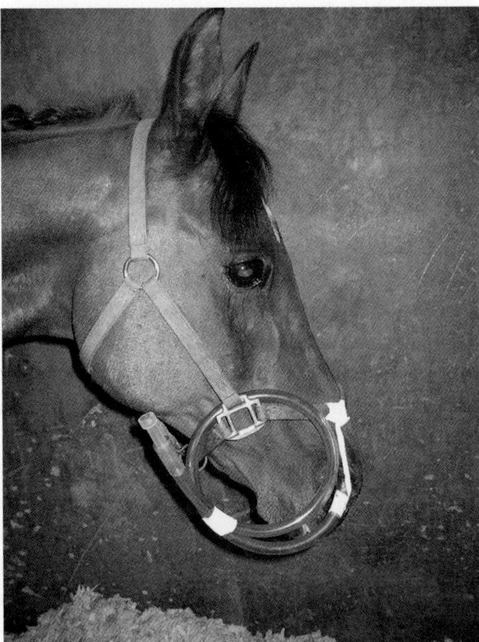

FIGURE 20-106 NGT secured to halter of horse for repeated NGT procedures.

NGTs may also be inserted to provide gastric lavage. This may be helpful in relieving feed impactions. Water is pumped into the tube and gastric contents collected as described earlier. As long as the water that is inserted is being retrieved, more water can be inserted and so on to attempt to dilute the impacted material.

Orogastric

As a result of small nasal passages, OGT is the routine choice for food animals and camelids (Figure 20-108). Medications and oral fluids can be administered, transfaunation of rumen contents can be accomplished, enteral feeding administered, and some bloats can be relieved. Using the same restraint techniques as described earlier, an OGT can be passed into a large animal patient. OGTs can be passed in sheep restrained set up on their rumps. Piglets can be lifted by the back of the head and neck. A ⅝- to 1-inch diameter tube can be passed in adult cattle, whereas a 9.54-mm diameter tube is appropriate for adult sheep and goats. Small-diameter 10F to 18F tubes are useful for neonatal kids, lambs, and crias. The technician should hold the tube next to the animal and place a mark at the point estimated to reach the rumen (from mouth to last rib). A speculum should be used in the animal's mouth to prevent the patient from biting down on the tub, although neonatal kids, lambs, and crias do not require the use of a speculum. A wide assortment of items can be used as speculums ranging from a roll of tape for small patients to PVC pipe or a piece of garden hose to a metal Frick speculum for cattle. The speculum needs to be inserted over the tongue root in the middle of the mouth. In cattle, a "popping" or "give" will be felt when the speculum passes into the pharynx. At this point, the tube is passed through the speculum and down the esophagus into the rumen. Slight resistance should be felt when the tube enters the esophagus. It is essential to make sure that you are in the rumen and not the trachea before any medication is

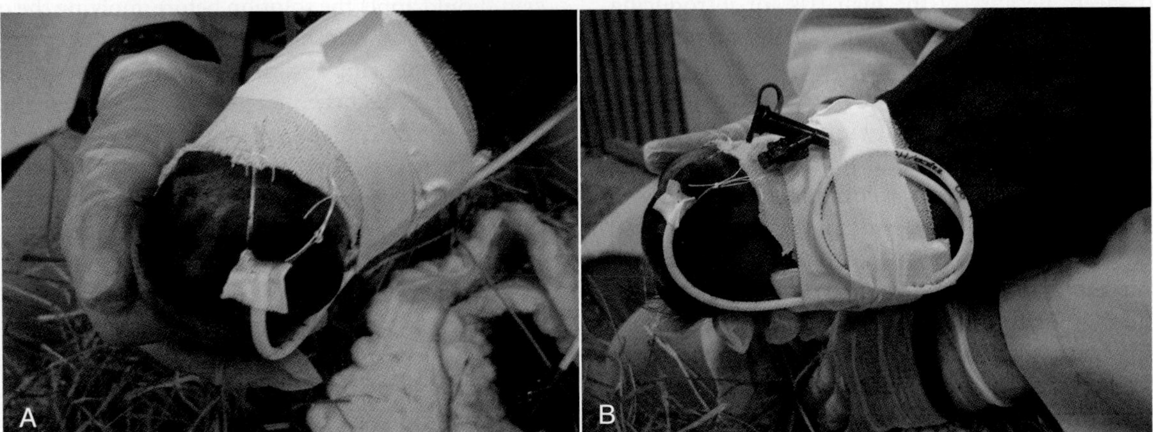

FIGURE 20-107 A, Placing suture loops in tape that is adhered to the muzzle of a foal allows for securing the tube without causing irritation to the nares that occurs when sutures are placed directly through the skin. **B,** NGT well secured to foal, easily accessible and very likely to stay in place, even with movement of foal.

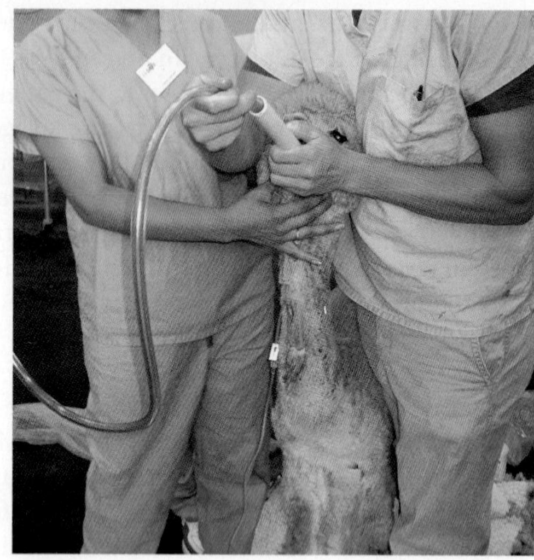

FIGURE 20-108 Passing OGT in alpaca patient.

administered. This can be done by blowing on the end of the tube and listening for gas crackles, feeling negative pressure, and the smell of rumen fluid. In ruminants, placing a tube into the rumen may stimulate regurgitation through and around the tube.

Once the placement is identified, the medication can be pumped into the patient or gravity flow used for smaller patients and neonates. Do not forcibly pump or administer medications to prevent rupture of the rumen or damage to the esophagus. When finished, the end of the tube is covered with the technician's finger and kinked, then pulled out using gentle motions.

> TECHNICIAN NOTE Occluding the end of the tube and kinking it prevents any residual fluid from entering the trachea when the tube is removed from the patient.

INTRAMAMMARY ADMINISTRATION

Intramammary infusion of antibiotics is used routinely to treat or control mastitis in cows and is also performed on goats and sheep. Because of the high risk for introducing contaminants during this process (organic debris, yeast, or other opportunistic organisms), the procedure must be performed aseptically. Minimal restraint is usually required, but a tail jack restraint may be necessary for some cows.

The udder is completely milked out and manually stripped. Residual milk present will dilute the medication. The teats are cleaned with a teat dip and then thoroughly dried using a separate cloth for each teat. Each teat is then wiped with an alcohol-soaked sponge and air-dried. The teats on the far side from the technician are cleaned before those on the near side. This will prevent transmitting contaminants from the dirty teats to the clean teats.

Teats on the near side are infused first. The teat is grasped at the base, and a sterile teat cannula or disposable mammary infusion cannula on an antibiotic syringe is partially inserted into the teat (up to 4 mm), and the antibiotic is injected slowly into the canal. For goats and sheep with a very small teat orifice, a sterile tomcat catheter can be used. Proceed to the next teat with the new cannula and syringe and then move to the teats on the far side and repeat. It is recommended that the end of the teat be occluded and the teat and udder gently massaged to distribute the medication. After the teats have been infused, teat dip is reapplied and left to dry. In very cold (0° C) conditions, chapping and frostbite can occur, so the animal should not be moved outside while the udder is wet.

> TECHNICIAN NOTE Partial insertion of the cannula into the teat canal delivers fewer contaminants to the udder than would occur with full insertion.

TOPICAL OPHTHALMIC ADMINISTRATION

To treat ocular diseases or conditions (ulcers, abrasions, lacerations, keratitis), topical ophthalmic ointment and solutions are routinely administered. When in an ointment form, a small amount is applied directly into the eye. To deliver the intended amount successfully into large animal patients (both adults and neonates), proper restraint of the head must be employed. Hands should be well cleaned or gloved. The lower eyelid of the particular eye that needs medicating is pulled down slightly, and the ointment is applied without touching the surface of the eye. The lid is then let go, and the blinking action will distribute the medication. Another method of ointment application is to wear sterile gloves and place a small ribbon of ointment on a gloved finger. The ointment on the finger is then touched directly to the eye. This eliminates the risk of scratching the eye with the end of the ointment tube.

Opthalmic solution can be applied by gently pulling the lower eyelid out slightly and placing drops into the lower conjunctival sac. Drops may come directly from a plastic bottle with dispenser or may be administered using a small sterile syringe—with no needle attached.

When applying both ointment and solution, the technician should apply the solution before applying the ointment. This will prevent the solution from running over the ointment without being absorbed directly on the eye.

Most patients become resentful of repeated applications into the eye, and many eye conditions are quite painful, so it may be necessary to place a long-term lavage system to properly treat the disease or condition.

> TECHNICIAN NOTE Eye conditions may require aggressive treatment with the administration of ophthalmic medication as often as every hour.

There are two types of lavage systems that will supply medication. The subpalpebral lavage system is inserted through incisions made into the upper or lower eyelids (Figure 20-109). The narrow rubber tubing is inserted through the incision(s) of the eyelid to open directly in the

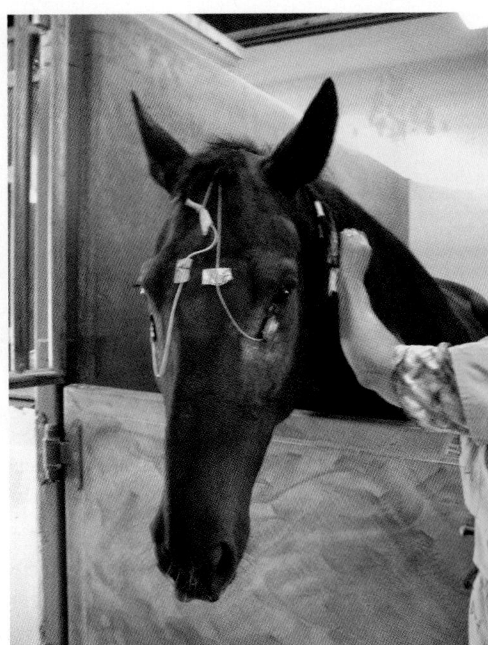

FIGURE 20-109 Subpalpebral lavage system in equine patient.

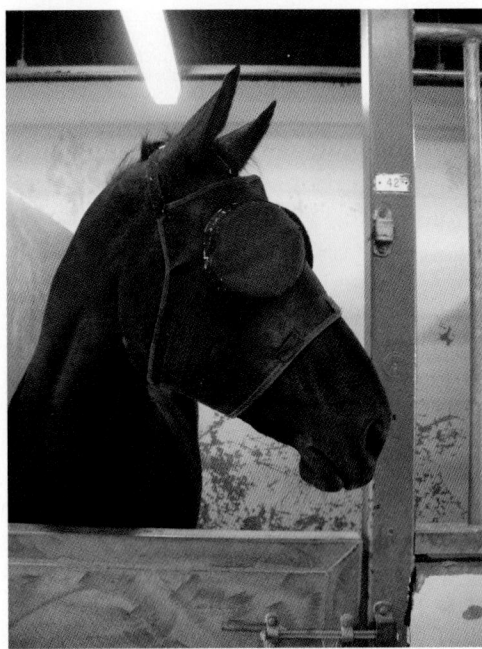

FIGURE 20-110 Guardian Mask (Guardian Mask Co.) placed on head to provide protection to eyes of horse.

conjunctival sac and away from the cornea. Since the tubing is very narrow, liquid solutions are delivered through the system instead of ointments. Once the tubing is placed, the system is secured to the skin above the eye and extended over the poll (IV extension tubing is attached to make the appropriate length to extend up and over the head). A PRN (intermittent infusion plug) is attached to the end of the system and should be changed every 24 hours or more often if it becomes friable from repeated injections. The medication to be delivered should be warm enough so as not to cause discomfort to the patient, and the lines should be cleared after the administration using either a saline flush or air. The injections should be made very slowly. If resistance is felt when injecting solution into the lavage system, the veterinarian should be notified so that the tube can be cleared of any debris. If air is used, the patient may startle when the air hits the eye, so the technician should be prepared for any adverse reactions.

The second type of lavage system is placed through the nasolacrimal duct (tear duct). The tubing is inserted into the nasal punctum, and a small stab incision through the nostril is created to pass the tubing through and attach to the skin. This will prevent the tubing from moving inside the nostril and prevent the patient from rubbing it out. The same method of medication delivery as described previously is used. This approach requires a greater volume of medication than the subpalpebral lavage method.

The veterinarian may choose to provide protection to the eye in the form of protective eye cups or hoods (Eye-Saver, JorVet; Guardian Mask, Guardian Mask Co.) (Figure 20-110). These provide protection from sunlight and provide a mechanical barrier, preventing the horse from rubbing the eye and keeping it free from debris.

EPIDURAL ADMINISTRATION

Epidural administration deposits drugs into the epidural space. The procedure may be done to provide anesthesia or for pain control. The epidural injection of analgesics or local anesthetics provides complete analgesia and muscle relaxation caudal to the block. For all species, proper restrain is required for the success and safety of this procedure. There are two locations for epidural administration. The cranial epidural is located at the lumbosacral junction (between L6 and S1), and the caudal epidural is located between S5 and C1 or C1 and C2. The veterinarian will choose the location for the epidural, depending on the effect that he or she wishes to achieve.

Equine Epidural Administration

The horse should be restrained in stocks and a twitch applied. Some horses will require the administration of a sedative. The technician will clip, shave, and aseptically prepare a 3-inch square (approximately) area over the first and second coccygeal vertebrae. This site can be determined by lifting the tail up and down with one hand while feeling for the vertebral space with the other hand (Figure 20-111). This area is usually close to where the coarse tail hairs originate. An SQ bleb of local anesthetic is placed. The technician should attempt to have the horse stand still and squarely upon its legs. If the animal is not standing squarely, there will be an uneven distribution of the drug because more will run into one side of the epidural space.

The technician should prepare the supplies necessary, including sterile gloves, local anesthetic, a sterile 12-ml syringe, 19-gauge × 1.5-inch needle (3.5 inches for very large horses), or an 18-gauge epidural catheter with stylet.

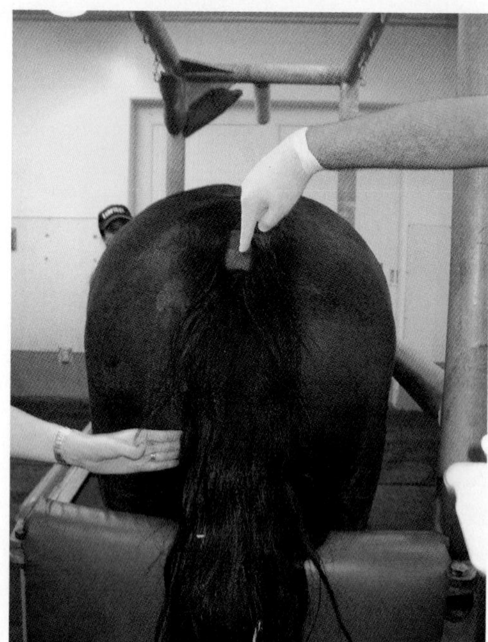

FIGURE 20-111 Locating site for equine epidural injection.

> *TECHNICIAN NOTE* To hand the sterile syringe to the veterinarian, open the plastic syringe casing and gently slide the syringe into the sterile gloved hand of the veterinarian without touching the outer casing to the glove. To provide him or her with a sterile needle, remove the needle cap and while holding the needle cover tightly, point the hub toward the veterinarian so that he or she may use sterile gloved fingers to pull the needle from the cover.

Directing the needle slightly cranially and ventrally into the epidural space at an approximately 45-degree angle to the rump, an 18- to 19-gauge × 1.5-inch needle is inserted about 1 inch in adult horses. When the needle enters the epidural space, a slight "pop" is felt, and there is a loss of resistance to the passage of the needle. The drug is injected, and the needle may be left in place to facilitate an additional injection. An epidural catheter may be placed and secured to the skin to facilitate repeated drug administration. When the needle or catheter is removed, antibiotic ointment is applied to the site.

The technician should be aware that hind leg instability may occur following epidural anesthesia. Lidocaine, Carbocaine, xylazine, and morphine are commonly administered as epidurals.

Bovine Epidural Administration

The technician must first ensure that the animal is sufficiently restrained. To locate the site, the tail is moved up and down using one hand while the other hand feels the top of the vertebrae to find the first moveable joint (S1 and S2). Clip, shave, and aseptically prep a 3 inch × 3 inch area (approximately). An 18-gauge × 1.5 to 3-inch needle is inserted perpendicular to the spine and into the vertebral space between S1 and S2 (Figure 20-112). A "pop" is felt when the space is entered. The epidural space is a relative vacuum compared with atmospheric conditions, and the medication will be sucked into the space. (A drop from the syringe into the hub of the needle should quickly be drawn into the needle.) Three milliliters of 2% lidocaine is commonly used for bovine epidurals.

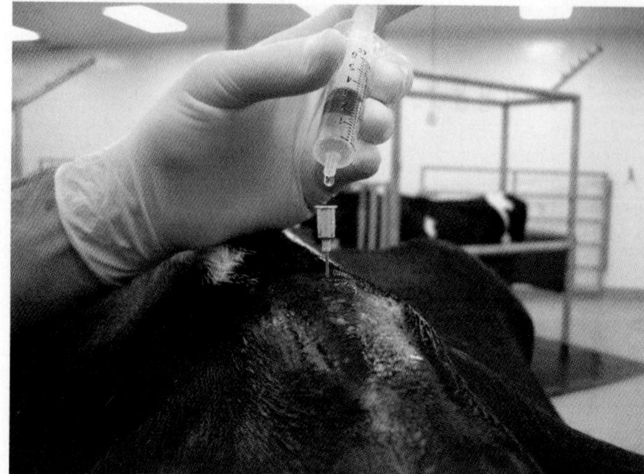

FIGURE 20-112 Technician performing epidural injection in bovine patient.

Camelid Epidural Administration

The site is clipped and surgically prepared. Owners may object to the clipping of the fiber, so efforts should be made to shave only a small site and secure the surrounding fibers away from the site with adhesive tape. The tail is moved up and down to locate the intervertebral space between S5 and C1. In most llamas and alpacas, this will be the first moveable joint because the five sacral vertebrae are usually fused. A 20-gauge × 1.5-inch needle is inserted. The veterinarian will determine a successful insertion as described for other large animals.

Ovine and Caprine Epidural Administration

Following the procedure guidelines for cattle, an 18- to 21-gauge × 1 to 1.5-inch needle is inserted at a 45-degree angle. Sheep and goats are very sensitive to local anesthetics.

Porcine Epidural Administration

The site for epidural injections in pigs varies from the site described earlier for other large animal species. The lumbosacral junction (between L6 and S1) is accessible for porcine epidurals. This is considered a cranial epidural, whereas the common sites described for other species are caudal epidurals. To locate the site, an imaginary line is drawn vertically up from the patella to the back and a dorsal midline site clipped and surgically prepared. An 18- to 20-gauge spinal needle may be used, with the length determined by the size of the animal.

TRANSDERMAL ADMINISTRATION (CUTANEOUS, TOPICAL)

The application of medications through the skin comes primarily in the form of an impregnated patch that is applied directly to the skin and left on to be absorbed. Fentanyl, scopolamine, nitroglycerin, and estrogen are all common medications that can be delivered in this fashion. When applying any type of impregnated patch to the skin, gloves should be worn so that the technician does not medicate himself or herself. The location that is chosen to place the patch should be shaved and the area cleaned with alcohol-soaked gauze. After the area has dried, the patch can be applied.

When it is time to remove or replace the patch, gloves need to be worn in case there is any residual medication left on the patch. The patch should then be disposed of according to local guidelines (fentanyl has strict legal disposal requirements). The area should then be wiped with a gauze sponge to remove any excess product.

Caution needs to be applied when using any product that is to be administered transdermally so that the technician or other personnel do not come in contact with the substance and absorb it through their own skin.

Many other ointments, solutions, and creams may be applied topically without the need for bandaging the area. With these, gentle application of the desired medication on gauze sponges, swabs, or directly from the gloved hand to the affected area will be effective. Before the application, the area should be cleared of any debris. In some instances, such as severe burns or wounds, the outer perimeter will first be débrided. The technician should wear gloves at all times when using topical or transdermal applications to limit the potential for contaminants to be added to the medication and for personal safety (to prevent inadvertent absorption of the substance).

INTRASYNOVIAL ADMINISTRATION

Patients may require the administration of medication, such as antibiotics or anesthetic agents, directly into a joint. Intrasynovial administration affords high drug levels localized in the joint compared with the levels that would be present from systemic drug administration. Veterinarians commonly perform intrasynovial injections on equine patients, but the procedure may be performed on other large animal species. Although the technician usually does not perform the injection, he or she may be asked to prepare the joint that will be infused and assist with the procedure.

The site that is to be injected needs to be surgically scrubbed and cleaned to minimize the chance of introducing a contaminant into the joint. The technician will lay out the appropriate size sterile gloves, several needles of the requested gauge and length (18- or 19-gauge × 1.5 inches is common for adult horses), and the syringe with the solution to be injected. All of these items must be handled in an aseptic fashion.

Proper restraint of the patient is necessary to ensure the safety of personnel and the patient. Using a twitch in addition to a halter and lead rope will lessen the likelihood of movement during the procedure. In addition, chemical sedation should be used to prevent movement and subsequent trauma while introducing the needle into the joint.

Once the injection is complete, the needle and syringe are withdrawn, and pressure can be applied to the site to prevent any seepage. The patient should be monitored for pain, heat, or swelling over the joint.

Joint flushing (joint irrigation, joint lavage) is commonly performed with the animal given a general anesthetic, but is also performed on young animals who have received injectable anesthetics or very heavy sedation (because of the risk involved, heavy sedation is not commonly used). Two needles are placed at different sites on the affected joint capsule, and sterile flush forced through one needle exits through the other. Joint lavage may be followed with an intrasynovial injection of antibiotics after removing the exit needle.

RECTAL ADMINISTRATION

Rectal administration of therapeutics in large animals is used as a method of delivering medication to a patient that cannot tolerate oral medication as a result of ileus or regurgitation or to deliver an enema to a constipated patient.

Rectal Medications

To deliver medication per rectum, the appropriate size tube should be selected based on the size of the patient. A Harris enema tube (24F) or fenestrated tube (multiple holes along the distal end) are appropriate for adult animals, foals, and calves, whereas smaller-diameter soft rubber tubes can be used for lambs, kids, and crias. The fenestrated tube may provide better distribution of the medication, but the fenestrations on some tubes may be rough and may cause irritation to the rectal mucosa. The technician should always check the tube for any rough edges before using and avoid using anything that is not smooth. The distal end of the tube is lubricated with a water-soluble solution (such as KY jelly), and the tube is inserted from 1 to 12 inches into the rectum. This distance is determined by the size of the patient. Appropriate restraint is used, tailored to the individual species and age of the animal. For standing animals, the technician should take precautions to stand to the side of the animal so as not to get kicked. Medications are dissolved in a small amount of water (or at the veterinarian's request, in another solution, such as DMSO) and injected gently via a catheter tip syringe into the tube followed by a small "chaser" of water (or air) to ensure that all of the medication is administered and none remains in the tube. The tube is then gently removed. It may be necessary to remove feces from the rectum before the administration of medications. The technician must clarify this with the veterinarian in advance because it may or may not be necessary, and there is an increased risk for injury to the animal when a hand is inserted into the rectum. Rectal tears can be fatal. If instructed to do so, the technician must have fingernails clipped short and wear no rings or watches. With a well-lubricated rectal sleeve, the technician will gently insert the hand a short distance into the rectum and gently remove obvious feces present before the insertion of the tube.

The veterinarian may administer 2% lidocaine per rectum to facilitate performance of a rectal examination by reducing

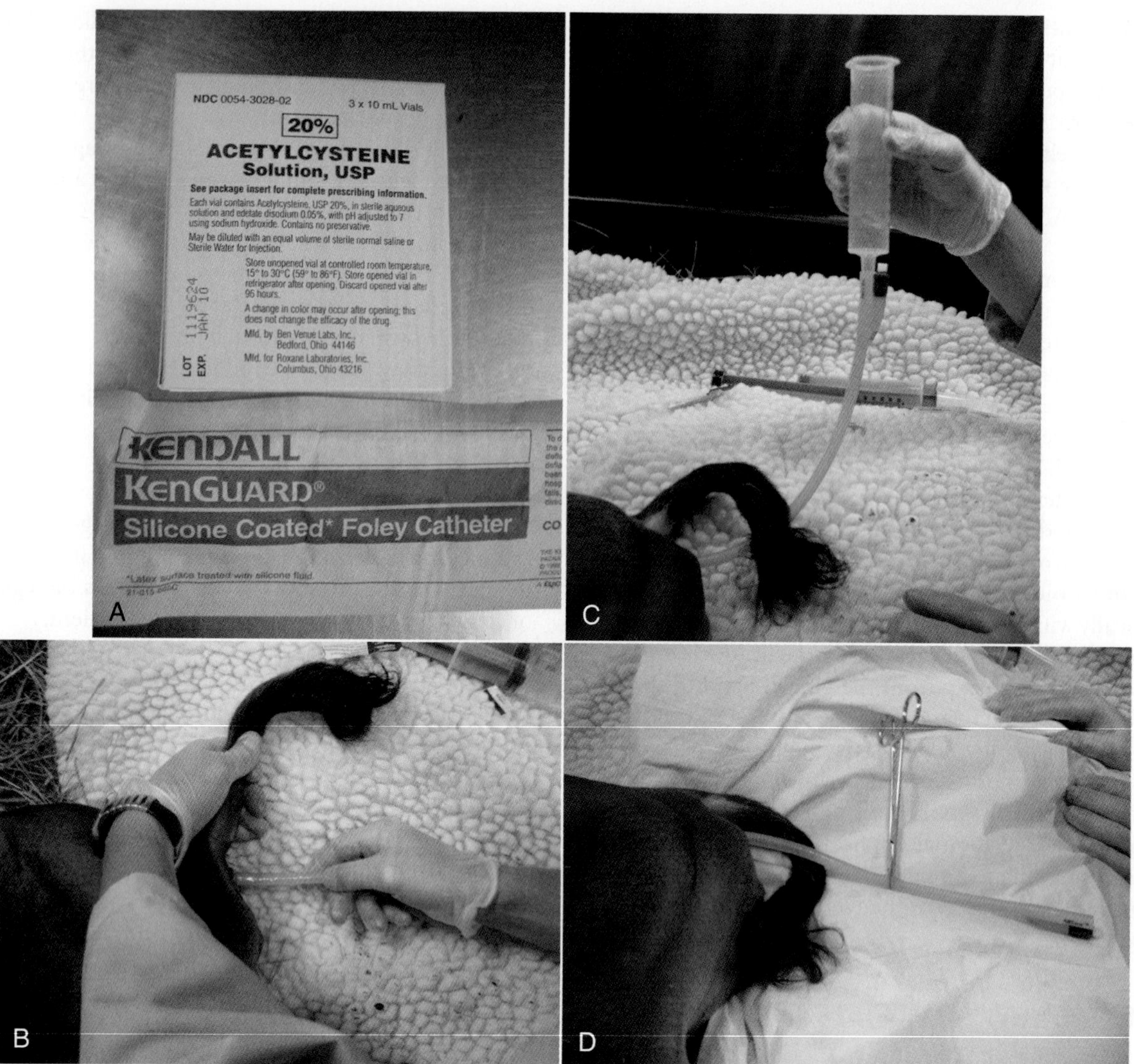

FIGURE 20-113 **A,** Acetylcysteine and Foley catheter for retention enema in equine neonate. **B,** Inserting well-lubricated Foley catheter into rectum. **C,** Administering enema solution via gravity flow. **D,** Foley catheter is clamped off to allow for retention of enema.

the straining of the patient. A 60-ml syringe containing lidocaine is attached to rubber tubing or IV extension tubing that is inserted into the rectum and the drug injected. Sedation may also be given via the epidural route for patients that are straining to prevent potential problems, such as rectal tears, during the examination.

Enema Administration

Enemas are administered to constipated animals to encourage defecation. They can be administered to animals of any age or species. The tube used, volume, and composition of fluid administered will vary with the size and condition of the animal. Fluids should be nonirritating and warmed to room temperature, but not above body temperature.

> *TECHNICIAN NOTE* The administration of cold enema solutions can lead to hypothermia in young patients.

Neonates

A common practice by many horse owners is to routinely administer a prepackaged human enema to newborn foals to encourage passage of meconium (fetal feces). Warm-water enemas and enemas containing other agents, such as gentle soap, mineral oil, or other lubricants, are administered using a tube and gravity flow. Retention enemas are routinely used in hospitalized neonatal patients. An excessive enema volume and repeated enemas can be damaging to the patient. The technician must be aware of the individual variation in the patients' size. The standard 120 to 180 ml of fluid delivered for an equine neonate would be far too much for a cria.

The tip of the tube is well lubricated with a water-soluble lubricant, and the tube is gently advanced into the rectum. Once the tube is inserted to the desired distance in the rectum, a 60-ml catheter tip syringe, funnel, or enema bucket can be attached to the end and the desired amount of solution delivered. Gravity flow is preferred to pumping fluid in because it is possible to tear the rectum. If a syringe is used, gentle pressure is applied until all of the enema solution has been delivered. After all of the solution has been administered, cap off the end of the tube with the thumb and gently remove the entire length of the tubing.

Retention Enemas

Retention enemas involve the insertion into the rectum of a well-lubricated Foley catheter with balloon. The tube is inserted a few inches (usually 2 to 4) into the rectum, and the balloon is inflated using a syringe containing air or water. The enema solution (often Mucomyst, acetylcysteine) is infused. The catheter is then clamped off using a hemostat and the tube left in place for at least 15 minutes. After that time, the hemostat is removed, the balloon deflated, and the catheter removed (Figure 20-113).

Enema Administration to Adult Animals

Enemas can be administered to adult animals. With the animal properly restrained, the technician stands to the side of the patient, inserts a well-lubricated tube (an NGT can be used for enema administration to large animals) and enema solution delivered. The technician administering the enema may find benefit from preparing in advance of the procedure by cutting one hole in the center of the bottom of a large plastic trash bag (for head) and cutting a hole on either side of the bottom of the bag (for arms). Wearing it as a protective covering may be desirable because the result of some enemas may be a rapid projectile expulsion of fluid and feces.

ACKNOWLEDGMENTS

The authors wish to acknowledge the faculty, residents, technical staff, and students at the William R. Pritchard Veterinary Medical Teaching Hospital of the University of California, Davis. Particular appreciation goes to Dr. Monica Aleman MVZ, PhD; Dr. Lisle George DVM, PhD; Fred Librach, Equine Clinical Instructor; Mike Reis, Food Animal Clinical Instructor; Sarah Hayes, RVT; and Teri Joseph, RVT.

RECOMMENDED READING

Bowden C, Masters J, editors: *Textbook of veterinary medical nursing,* London, 2003, Butterworth Heinemann.

Busch SJ, editor: *Small animal surgical nursing,* St Louis, 2006, Mosby Elsevier.

Colville T, Bassert JM, editors: *Clinical anatomy and physiology for veterinary technicians,* St Louis, 2002, Mosby.

Ettinger SJ, Feldmen E, editors: *Textbook of veterinary internal medicine,* ed 6, Philadelphia, 2005, Elsevier Saunders.

Fowler ME: *Medicine and surgery of South American camelids,* Ames, Iowa, 1998, Iowa State University Press.

Frandson RD, Wilke WL, Fails AD: *Anatomy and physiology of farm animals,* Baltimore, 2003, Lippincott Williams & Wilkins.

Hanie EA: *Large animal clinical procedures for veterinary technicians,* St Louis, 2006, Mosby.

Hendrix CM, Sirois M, editors: *Laboratory procedures for the veterinary technician,* ed 5, St Louis, 2007, Mosby Elsevier.

House JK, Smith BP, Van Metre DC, et al: Ancillary tests for assessment of the ruminant digestive system, *Vet Clin North Am Large Anim Pract* 8:203-232, 1992.

Jaffe TJ: Diagnostic sampling and therapeutic techniques, In McCurnin DM, Bassert JM, editors: *Clinical textbook for veterinary technicians,* ed 6, St Louis, 2006, Saunders.

Kopcha M, Schultze AE: Peritoneal fluid. II. Abdominocentesis in cattle and interpretation of nonneoplastic samples, *Compend Contin Educ Pract Vet* 13:703-710, 1991.

Lawhorn B: A new approach for obtaining blood samples from pigs, *J Am Vet Med Assoc* 192:781-782, 1988.

Macintire DK, Drobatz KJ, Haskins SC, et al: *Manual of small animal emergency and critical care medicine,* Baltimore, 2005, Lippincott Williams & Wilkins.

McKenzie EC: Abdominocentesis in large animals: methods and interpretation of results, *Proc 25th Forum ACVIM* pp 27-30, 2007.

Orsini JA, Divers TJ: *Manual of equine emergencies,* ed 3, St Louis, 2008, Saunders.

Sirois M, editor: *Principles and practice of veterinary technology,* ed 2, St Louis, 2004, Mosby.

Radostits OM, Gay CC, Blood DC, et al, editors: *Veterinary medicine, a textbook of the diseases of cattle, sheep, pigs, goats and horses,* ed 10, Oxford, 2007, WB Saunders.

Rockett J, Bosted S: *Veterinary clinical procedures in large animal practice,* Clifton Park, NY, 2007, Thomson Delmar Learning.

Rose RF, Hodgson DR: *Manual of equine practice,* ed 2, Philadelphia, 2000, WB Saunders.

Smith BP, editor: *Large animal internal medicine,* ed 4, St Louis, 2009, Mosby.

Smith MC, Sherman DM, editors: *Goat medicine,* Philadelphia, 1994, Lea & Febiger.

Taylor FGR, Hillyer MH, editors: *Diagnostic techniques in equine medicine,* Philadelphia, 1997, WB Saunders.

Terry C, Rashmir-Raven A, Linford RL: Placing an intravenous catheter in horses, *Vet Tech* 4:207-212, 2000.

Williams CSF: Routine sheep and goat procedures, *Vet Clin North Am Large Anim Pract* 6:737-758, 1990.

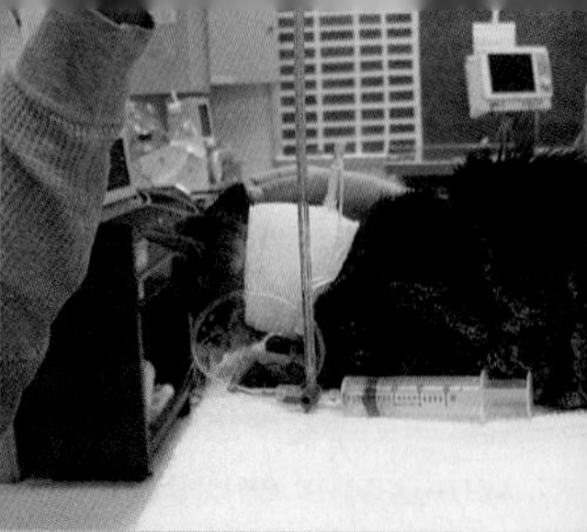

21 Small Animal Medical Nursing

Susan M. Eddlestone

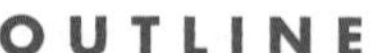

OUTLINE

LEARNING OBJECTIVES

When you have completed this chapter, you will be able to:

1. Describe general care of small animal patients, including bathing, grooming, ear cleaning, and nail trimming procedures.
2. Explain the special considerations in the care of recumbent, geriatric, and pediatric patients.
3. Describe the procedures for obtaining body temperature, blood pressure, pulse rate character, and respiratory rate.
4. Differentiate between sensible and insensible fluid losses and explain methods used to determine patient hydration status and calculate fluid requirements for rehydration of patients.
5. List routes of administration of fluid therapy treatments and describe monitoring procedures used for fluid therapy patients.
6. Describe the indications for and procedures used in blood transfusion and oxygen therapies.
7. List the canine and feline blood groups and describe procedures for blood typing and cross-matching.
8. List and describe the five methods of physical therapy used in small animal practice.
9. Describe the indications for and procedures used in respiratory and topical therapies in small animal practice.
10. List and describe common diseases of dogs and cats and provide an overview of small animal vaccines and vaccination protocols.
11. Define zoonosis and identify common zoonotic conditions and methods of control of zoonotic diseases.
12. List common diseases of the eyes and describe methods of diagnosis and treatment.
13. List and describe common cardiac and endocrine disorders of dogs and cats and describe methods of diagnosis and treatment.
14. List and describe common urogenital and gastrointestinal disorders of dogs and cats and describe methods of diagnosis and treatment.
15. List and describe common orthopedic disorders encountered in small animal practice.

KEY TERMS

Anaphylactic
Arrhythmia
Arterial blood gases
Atrophy
Capillary refill time
Central venous pressure
Cyanosis
Diastolic blood pressure
Dyspnea
Echocardiography
Electrocardiography
Epithelialization
Fomite
Gastric gavage
Glucocorticoid
Hemoglobin saturation
Hyperpnea
Hypoxia
Manometer
Peritonitis
Pulmonary thromboembolism
Septicemia
Systolic blood pressure
Tachypnea
Vasoconstriction

INTRODUCTION

Small animal nursing has changed over the last few decades from attending to the basic needs of the patient, such as feeding, walking, and cleaning to a more proactive role in the total needs of the medical patient. Problem solving is the basic skill needed to work with medical patients. This learned skill can be applied to almost every situation the medical nurse will encounter. Problem solving can be divided into several components:

data collection, data interpretation, implementation of a plan, and evaluation of the response to the plan.

Data collection for the technician begins with observation. This is the single most important tool needed to successfully manage a medical patient. If change in a patient's condition is to be recognized, careful, detailed, and systemic observation is required. Also, needed is an understanding that clinical problems are dynamic and can change at any time for better or for worse. The technician will usually notice these changes more so than the veterinarian because of the longer period of time he or she will spend with the patient. To monitor a patient, there needs to be an established baseline for the parameters being serially monitored. The precise system and nature of patient monitoring will vary depending on the specific clinical situation; however, the evaluation of all patients should take place according to a regular and reliable schedule.

> *TECHNICIAN NOTE* An integral aspect of any method of observation is the technician's ability to establish an accurate baseline for the parameter to be serially monitored.

Data interpretation by the veterinary technician consists of recognizing and correctly interpreting the observations that have been made. Stated differently, the technician must recognize and define the clinical problems. A clinical problem is anything that interferes with the well-being of the patient or anything that requires treatment or further diagnostic evaluation. Examples of clinical problems that might be recognized by the technician include diarrhea, vomiting, anorexia, and respiratory distress.

Once a problem is documented, a diagnostic or therapeutic plan is made. This may consist of repeating a clinical parameter such as a blood pressure reading or the patient's temperature before a more extensive plan is made. Once a clinical problem is positively identified, the attending veterinarian is consulted, and a diagnostic or therapeutic plan is implemented. For nursing to be optimally effective, a mechanism should exist for the ready exchange of information between technician and veterinarian. A team approach to animal health care is the ultimate goal, with veterinarian and technician each contributing their unique skills and abilities to the task of returning the patient to health. After a change of plan or treatment, continued observation of the patient is needed. The new plan or treatment may need to be altered again because of a changing clinical situation.

When implementing any diagnostic or therapeutic plan, it is important to remember that the quantity and nature of nursing care should always be individualized. One patient may readily accept a specific procedure, whereas another will resist to the point that the intended benefit is lost. Although excessive intervention may be detrimental to certain animals, this should not be construed as an excuse for medical neglect. The fundamental principle is that if a patient is not meeting a requirement for survival, the technician must promptly intervene. Certain animals require tremendous amounts of attention and affection from the technician simply to maintain the will to live during periods of separation from the owner.

Each technician and the head of every animal hospital should establish and maintain consistent standards of nursing care. Veterinary technicians have a professional and moral obligation to every patient to provide the following basic necessities:

- Clean, comfortable environment, as free of stress as possible
- Fresh food and clean water at all times unless restricted for medical reasons
- Adequate exercise and grooming care unless restricted for medical reasons
- Prompt and humane relief of suffering and pain
- Humane treatment of every patient with dignity at all times

GENERAL CARE

Grooming and bathing are aspects of the general care of the animal patient that are important for several reasons. First, a clean and well-groomed animal has an enhanced sense of well-being and potentially will recover from an illness more rapidly. Second, a clean animal is much less likely to develop severe contact dermatitis from urine scalding and fecal soiling of the skin, which, if it does occur, becomes another clinical problem to manage. Third, grooming and medicated baths are recommended for the prevention or treatment of many dermatologic problems. Bathing with shampoo that contains an insecticide is a useful adjunct in the control of ectoparasites. Finally, the cleanliness of the patient at the time of discharge is an indication to the owner of the overall quality of the health care provided.

Every animal hospital should have an adequate collection of grooming and bathing equipment and supplies (i.e., combs, brushes, scissors, towels for drying, electrical dryers, and a selection of shampoos appropriate for different situations). Care must be taken to prevent the spread of infections, such as dermatomycosis, from one animal to another via grooming instruments. These instruments should be thoroughly cleansed in an appropriate disinfectant solution after each use.

When clipping or removing hair from an animal for medical reasons, it is important to obtain the owner's permission, whenever possible. This is particularly important in animals used for show purposes. In certain breeds, such as the Afghan hound, regrowth of hair is extremely slow.

BATHING

The basic technique for bathing dogs and cats is to thoroughly wet the coat and then apply small amounts of shampoo starting at the head and working back to the tail. Rubbing the shampoo into the coat until a lather is produced, again starting from the head and working back to the tail is a generally accepted bathing method. The eyes should be protected from chemical injury by instilling a drop of mineral oil or a small amount of boric acid ophthalmic ointment in each eye before the bath. Care should be taken to prevent water from entering the external ear canal; this can be accomplished by placing a small piece of cotton in each ear. Remember to remove the cotton when the bath has been completed. Thermal injury from excessively hot water can be prevented by constantly monitoring the water temperature. Thorough rinsing with clean water prevents irritation of the skin from residual shampoo. The axillary and scrotal regions of long-haired dogs are particularly vulnerable to residual shampoo irritation. If a cage dryer is used, caution must be exercised to prevent overheating (hyperthermia). Shampoos containing insecticides should be used only with the approval of the attending veterinarian because of the possibility of cumulative toxicity or drug interactions with medications or other topically applied insecticides. If insecticidal dips are used, correct dilutions are necessary to prevent toxic reactions. If a complete immersion bath is contraindicated, localized soiling of the animal may be handled with a sponge bath. Orthopedic or neurologic patients may not be able to stand steady in the bath tub, and therefore a rubber mat should be placed in the tub to help reduce the risk of injury.

EXERCISE

Moderate exercise is beneficial for the general care of the animal patient. Exercise should take place in a secure, controlled, and safe environment so that injury or loss of the animal does not occur. Contraindications to exercise include many, but not all, respiratory, cardiovascular, and musculoskeletal problems. The decision whether to restrict exercise should be made after consultation with the attending veterinarian. Moderate exercise consists of taking the patient for a walk and can be considered the simplest and most basic form of physical therapy. It can be a useful means of reducing peripheral edema and improving muscle tone and strength.

> *TECHNICIAN NOTE* Moderate exercise consists of taking the patient for a walk and can be considered the simplest and most basic form of physical therapy.

FEEDING

The animal health technician plays a particularly pivotal role in ensuring that each patient remains in a positive energy balance, in which caloric intake exceeds metabolic requirements. The technician is in an excellent position to observe complete or partial anorexia and to take appropriate action to correct the situation. As long as the patient is not vomiting or the suppressed appetite is not due to a gastrointestinal problem, such as an ulcer or pancreatitis, there are a few things that should be tried to encourage the patient to eat. Substituting a more palatable food or texture such as canned food may solve the problem. Familiarity with the home feeding regimen will aid in the selection of palatable alternative diets. In certain instances, it may be advisable for the owner to prepare food at home and bring it to the hospital, such as chicken or hamburger and rice. It is helpful to stock a variety of types of food, such as canned, semimoist, and dry, in a variety of flavors to satisfy even the most discriminating patient. Personal attention at feeding time, such as talking to the patient and hand feeding the patient may work in some animals. Cats particularly may have an aversion to eating because they have lost the taste of food because of prolonged anorexia. Putting a small amount of canned food on the tongue or letting them lick it off the finger usually stimulates taste and interest in eating again. Force feeding, although not highly recommended, can be done in selected cases. This is done by mixing canned food with water for a slurry consistency and then administering the food with a syringe applied to the back of the animals mouth to stimulate the swallowing reflex. Care must be taken to avoid giving too much food at one time and to be sure that the animal is swallowing after each food bolus to prevent the patient from choking and/or aspirating food into the lungs causing life-threatening aspiration pneumonia. High-calorie density supplements, such as Nutrical (Evsco), may help to meet the caloric needs of the patient but by no means will meet the animal's daily requirement by themselves. Gastric gavage (stomach tubing) can be done in patients requiring force feedings for an extended period of time because it is less stressful to the patient and the technician. (The technique is discussed in Chapter 20.) More commonly, other methods of enteral feeding are being used with increasing frequency and include placement of nasoesophageal, esophagostomy, gastrostomy, and jejunostomy tubes. Specially tailored complete diets may be administered through these enteral tubes. All but the nasoesophageal tubes have large enough diameters to allow the use of commercially prepared prescription canned diets blended with water and strained to be easily administered through the tube. Only liquids (CliniCare diet, Abbott Laboratories) can pass through the nasoesophageal tube. Being able to use these complete diets ensures adequate nutritional requirements are being met in a variety of disease states, such as hepatic lipidosis in cats, and renal failure. Total or partial parenteral nutrition (TPN/PPN) may also be chosen and consists of administering a sterile liquid that contains a complete or partial nutritionally balanced diet and is given intravenously through a fresh and aseptically placed jugular catheter. Aseptic technique is needed for every feeding. This feeding option is very labor intensive and introduces the risk of sepsis to the patient if not administered properly. It is usually chosen for the most critically ill patients when other feeding options are not possible. Giving appetite stimulants to cats (does not work in the dog) is usually done when trying to get a cat to eat that has been off feed for quite a while and has no current illness, such as GI disease or nausea, from a metabolic disease to prevent them from eating. These drugs will increase interest in eating, but will not ensure adequate calorie intake by the patient.

TECHNICIAN NOTE Cats particularly may have an aversion to eating because they have lost the taste of food as a result of prolonged anorexia.

NAIL TRIMMING

Nail trimming (pedicure) is an important general care technique. Excessive nail length results in altered gait and the potential accentuation of lameness problems. Excessively long nails are more likely to split or to be traumatically avulsed. Finally, untrimmed nails can become ingrown (usually into the footpads), resulting in cellulites or abscess formation.

There are two common types of nail trimmers available (Whites and Resco; Figure 21-1). To avoid cutting pigmented (black) nails too short in the dog, the cutting surface of the nail trimmer should be held parallel to the palmar or plantar surface of the digital footpads, and the nail cut in this plane. In cats, the nails can be exposed by grasping the paw between the thumb and index finger and sliding the skin on the dorsum of the paw away from the nails (Figure 21-2). Once exposed, the nails can be trimmed as described for the dog. It should be noted that nails that have not been trimmed regularly have a "quick" or nail vein that extends further out into the claw than that of regularly trimmed nails. In this situation, one should be conservative with regard to how much nail is trimmed. The center of the nail takes on a fleshy, shining appearance in the region next to the quick (Figure 21-3). This is an indicator to trim no further. Because some animals vehemently resent handling of their feet for nail trimming, it is a good practice to routinely give a pedicure to any animal anesthetized or tranquilized for any procedure. If the blood vessel in the nail is inadvertently severed (the "quick" is cut), silver nitrate sticks can be used to stop the hemorrhage by means of chemical cautery. Other products available for chemical cautery include styptic powder and blood-stop powder, which are available from numerous companies. Owners can be instructed on the proper technique of nail trimming so that this routine task can be performed at home.

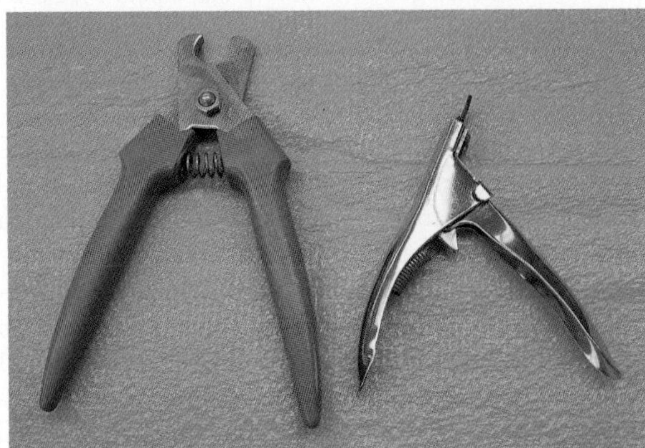

FIGURE 21-1 The two common types of nail trimmers, Whites *(left)* and Resco *(right)*. The Whites nail trimmer is useful for very long nails that have curled back toward the footpad.

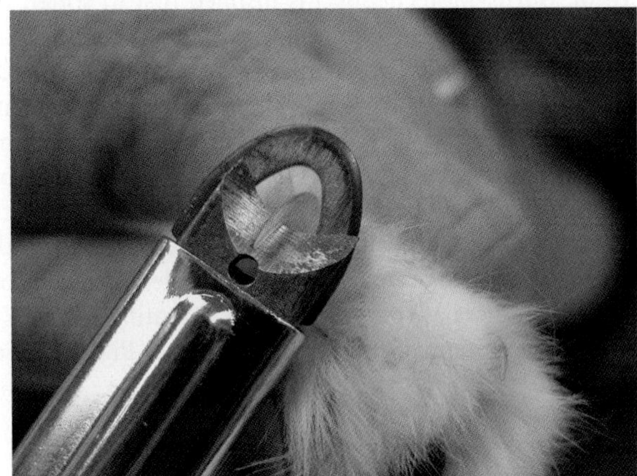

FIGURE 21-2 To trim the nails in cats, extend the claw by compressing the caudal part of the nail just in front of the footpad with the thumb and forefinger. At this point, one can visualize the vein or "quick" (pink area in claw), and the nail trimmer can be placed in front of the vein for trimming.

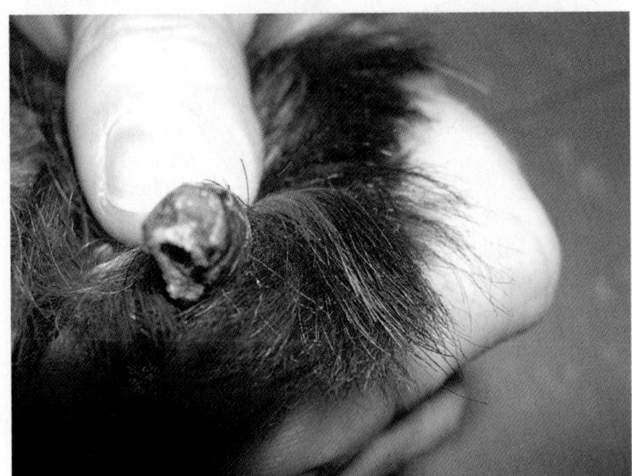

FIGURE 21-3 When trimming black nails, always trim a small amount at a time. Once you get close to the quick, you will note that the center of the nail begins to have a shiny, fleshy appearance. Once you see this, no further trimming is necessary.

EAR CLEANING

The external ear canal may accumulate cerumen, exudate, or cellular debris as a sequela to otitis externa or a foreign body (e.g., grass awn), which then requires cleaning. Certain breeds, notably poodles and terriers, may also accumulate excessive hair in the external ear canal. The initial and essential step in the treatment of any external ear problem is complete and thorough cleaning of the entire ear canal (Figure 21-4). Frequently, it is necessary to administer a short-acting general anesthetic or tranquilizer to properly clean the ears of patients that have painful ears and for patients that strongly resist ear cleanings. In some patients, it may be necessary to remove hair from the ear canals, whereas in others it may be left alone. This will depend on the severity of the ear infection, with the more severe inflamed ears responding to hair removal. A hemostat can be used to pull the hairs out, grabbing a small amount at a time. Excessive wax can be removed more easily if a ceruminolytic agent (i.e., dioctyl sodium succinate [Cerusol, Burns-Biotech labs]) is instilled first to soften the wax. Caution should be used before instilling ceruminolytics and certain ear cleaners that contain chlorhexidine when the integrity of the tympanic membrane is not known. Normal saline can be used for the initial cleaning agent until a proper ear canal examination can be performed to assess the tympanum. Using a soft rubber bulb syringe or a Luer-tipped catheter, excessive wax and debris can then be removed from the ear canals by gentle lavage with the chosen cleaning solution. Some practitioners advocate the use of pulsating streams of water from a dental hygiene apparatus (Water Pik, Teledyne Inc.) to clean the external ear canal. Approximately 5 ml of povidone-iodine (Betadine, Purdue-Frederick) or chlorhexidine solution (Nolvasan, Fort Dodge Laboratories) is added to approximately 236 to 384 ml of warm water. The stream of water should be applied in a rotating motion and directed parallel to the external ear canal. The excess water and debris can be collected in an ear irrigation basin or similar vessel. Avoid use of this method if the tympanum is not intact. Regardless of the irrigation system used, balls of cotton and cotton applicator sticks can then be used to gently wipe the wax from the external ear canal. It is important to remove only debris that is visible in the vertical canal so that debris is not pushed deep into the horizontal canal (Figure 21-4). Cleaning of the horizontal ear canal should be done only in the well-restrained patient and with caution to prevent damage to the tympanic membrane or the packing of debris deep into the horizontal canal (see Figure 21-4). A second otoscopic examination should be performed after the ear canals are cleaned to evaluate the completeness of the ear cleaning. Once the ear canal is sufficiently clean, the canal should be carefully dried with clean cotton swabs, and the initial dose of prescribed otic preparation instilled into each canal.

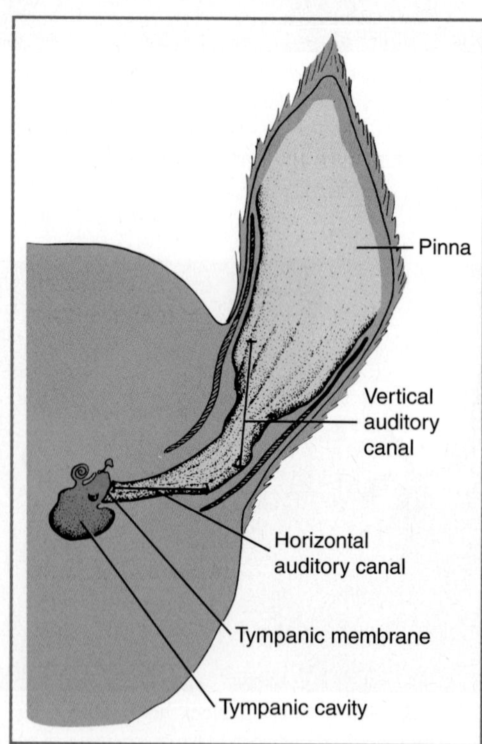

FIGURE 21-4 Schematic diagram of the anatomy of the canine ear.

Before cleaning, some of the debris should be mixed in mineral oil and smeared on a microscope slide to be examined under low-power magnification for the presence of *Otodectes* (ear mites). A small amount of the debris should also be smeared on a dry microscope slide and stained with Diff-Quik solution for examination under high-power magnification for overgrowth of bacteria and yeast. If the ear canal contains purulent debris, a sample should be obtained for cytologic evaluation (smear), bacterial culture, and antibiotic sensitivity testing (sterile Culturette) before inserting instruments or cleaning solutions. Based on the cytology (yeast, bacteria) and mineral oil slides (mites), appropriate therapy can be initiated and then adjusted if necessary based on bacterial culture and sensitivity results when available in a few days.

> *TECHNICIAN NOTE* Ceruminolytics and disinfecting solutions containing chlorhexidine should be used with caution if the integrity of the tympanic membrane is not known. Cleansing with warm normal saline should be attempted first.

ANAL SACS

The anal sacs are reservoirs for the secretions produced by the anal glands. The anal glands line the walls of the anal sacs and produce a foul-smelling fluid that varies from serous to pasty in consistency and is brown to off-white. The anal sacs are paired structures, approximately 1 cm in diameter, that lie between the internal and external anal sphincter muscles on either side of the anal canal. Each sac opens into the lateral margin of the anus by a single duct, at approximately the 4 and 8 o'clock positions of the anus (Figure 21-5).

Clinical signs associated with impacted anal sacs include excessive licking of the perineum; "scooting" or dragging the

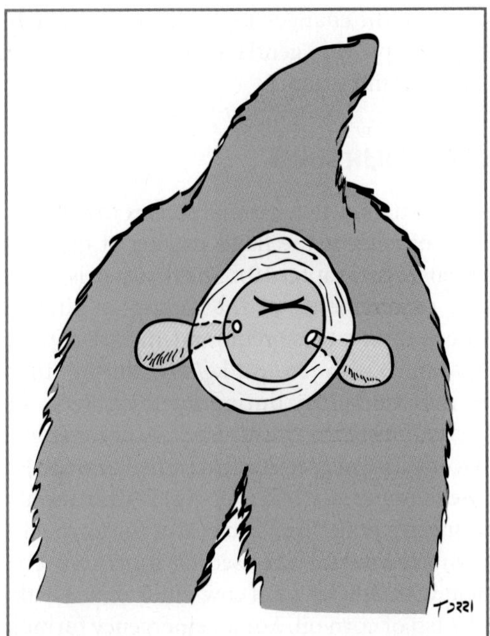

FIGURE 21-5 Schematic diagram of the anatomy of the canine anal sacs located approximately at the 4 o'clock and 8 o'clock positions.

perineum on the floor; abnormal carriage of the tail; and vague indications of pain or discomfort in the perineal region.

The anal sacs are best emptied, or "expressed," using the internal technique of inserting a lubricated, gloved forefinger into the rectum. The distended sacs are immobilized between the forefinger and thumb, which remains external to the anus. The sacs are generally found in a ventrolateral location. Gentle pressure is applied until the secretions are forced through the ducts. Because the ducts and the sac are occasionally compressed with this technique, if the sac cannot be expressed with gentle pressure, the finger and thumb are repositioned and pressure is reapplied. Paper towels, gauze, or cotton balls can be placed over the anus to collect the extremely unpleasant liquid from soiling the patient, environment, and the technician. External expression of the anal sacs is a technique that requires squeezing of the anal glands from the external anal sphincter. This technique is not recommended because of the frequent occluding of the ducts, inability to completely empty the sacs, and excessive pain it may cause the patient.

BEDDING

The optimal means of keeping an ambulatory dog clean is by the appropriate use of bedding and exercise runs. Several types of bedding are routinely used in small animal practice; they include newspaper, other types of paper products, blankets, towels, and lamb's wool products. It is important that the bedding material selected be either disposable or readily and effectively cleaned between uses. Because occasionally dogs will ingest their bedding, it is also important that the material be safe and nontoxic. Most dogs are extremely reluctant to urinate or defecate in their cage; therefore keeping the cage and patient clean is facilitated by the regular use of walks outside or use of an exercise run to allow them to urinate and defecate. Specifically, dogs should be walked or placed in the runs several times daily for an adequate period of time.

Generally, cats are easier to keep clean than dogs during periods of hospitalization. Cats will use litter pans and groom and clean themselves unless they are seriously ill. Litter should be changed daily, and pans or trays should be either disposable or constructed of materials that will allow thorough cleaning and disinfection between uses. To prevent litter from getting into open wounds or surgical incisions, newspaper shredded into long strips can be used in the litter pan in place of gravel litter. It is unnecessary to walk or place cats in exercise runs unless the hospital stay is unusually long.

DECUBITAL SORES

Prevention and management of decubital sores (bedsores) and urine scald are extremely important aspects of the care of recumbent patients. Animals with various neurologic or orthopedic problems can be recumbent for prolonged periods and require special care. Urine and fecal soiling can cause serious problems that can complicate recovery from the underlying condition. Scalding from urine or diarrhea can be prevented by a light topical application of a protective compound, such as Aquaphor (Beiersdorf, Inc.) or petrolatum (e.g., Vaseline) to susceptible perineal or inguinal areas.

Decubital sores not only complicate recovery, but can also be a source of sepsis, which can lead to the demise of the patient. The best treatment for decubital sores is prevention. Decubital sores develop over bony prominences as the result of continuous pressure and damage to the overlying skin. Various types of bedding have been advocated to reduce the frequency and severity of decubital sores; they include the use of air or water mattresses, foam padding, synthetic fleece, grids or grates, and straw. The material should either be disposable or have an impermeable surface that does not retain moisture or microorganisms and can be thoroughly cleaned. A potential problem with impermeable surfaces is that urine and moisture tend to remain in contact with the skin and can exacerbate the problem. Therefore care should be taken to keep the skin surface as dry as possible. This is why, for long-term management, straw is beneficial since adequate cushioning is available for the animal and urine drains through the straw and away from the patient.

Other routine measures that help to prevent decubital sores include frequent turning of the patient from side to side, intermittent use of slings or carts to prevent continuous pressure over the bony prominences, and frequent baths to keep the skin clean.

Once decubital sores have developed, they should be thoroughly cleaned with a surgical scrub. Surgical débridement of necrotic tissue may be necessary. After cleaning, the area should be completely dried. Soaking the affected area two to four times daily with a mild astringent will aid in keeping the decubital sore dry. A 1:40 astringent solution of aluminum acetate (Burow solution) may be made by dissolving one packet (Domeboro solution, Dome Laboratories) per pint of warm water. Ideally, the area of the decubital sore should be padded to prevent further pressure injury; however, the sore itself should remain exposed to the air to prevent retention of moisture. One way of accomplishing this is to fashion a "doughnut" from foam rubber and to fix this to the skin by means of adhesive tape. Unfortunately, it is difficult to maintain these pads in the proper location for long periods of time. Topical antimicrobial agents should be applied judiciously because many contain ointment or cream bases that form an occlusive dressing that will retain moisture. Further, it is questionable how beneficial they are in controlling an infected decubital sore.

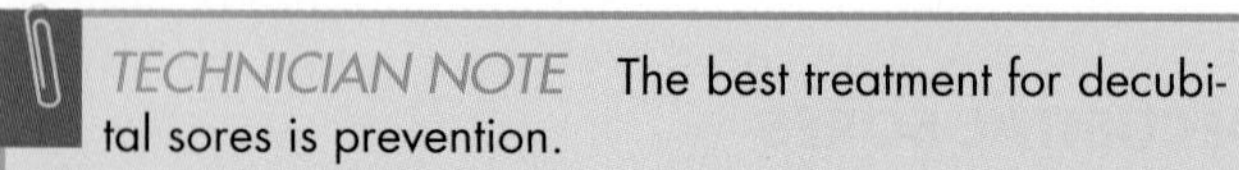
TECHNICIAN NOTE The best treatment for decubital sores is prevention.

GERIATRIC NURSING

With improved veterinary care, pets are enjoying an increased life span; consequently, the number of geriatric patients seen in small animal practices is increasing. The geriatric patient can be presented with a number of problems that directly influence the nursing process. These problems are generally related to or are secondary to degenerative diseases and other geriatric changes, such as arthritis, deafness, and blindness (see Chapter 37).

Dogs with arthritis or other degenerative diseases of the musculoskeletal system may be suffering from chronic pain. These animals are likely to react aggressively when an affected body part is touched or manipulated. Gentle handling when lifting or moving these patients and taking care to walk them at a slower pace than younger dogs is needed to prevent pain and fear in these patients. Dogs suffering from central nervous system disorders (e.g., a brain tumor or cerebral infarction) may also display aggressive behavior.

Deafness is another disorder that frequently accompanies old age. It is easy to surprise or startle a deaf, older dog, and certain dogs will instinctively respond by biting. When approaching a deaf dog, it is important that the patient is able to see you before you attempt to handle it or perform a procedure.

Blindness can occur in older dogs from cataracts, retinal degeneration, glaucoma, and other diseases. As is the case with deaf dogs, blind dogs should be approached cautiously. It is best to move slowly and speak while approaching the dog. Generally, elderly dogs and cats show less response to external stimuli. They appear to be less interested in their surroundings and frequently remain inactive for prolonged periods. In fact, they tend to resent any interference and react aggressively when disturbed. Some dogs forget previous training and may fail to respond to basic commands. Finally, the geriatric dog or cat is resistant to changes in daily routine. The stress of hospitalization alone can sometimes cause rapid deterioration. Obviously, it is impossible to correct or reverse many of the changes associated with aging; however, a willingness to provide gentle, compassionate nursing care is of paramount importance.

PEDIATRIC NURSING

The clinical situation that best illustrates the skills required in pediatric nursing is the hand rearing of orphaned puppies or kittens (see Chapter 10). The first step is to determine the caloric requirements of the puppy or kitten. During the first week of life, these requirements are approximately 27 cal/kg/day, 32 to 36 cal/kg/day during the second week, 36 to 41 cal/kg/day during the third week, and 41 to 45 cal/kg/day during the fourth week. A number of artificial milk replacers (Esbilac, Pet-Ag; Just Burn, Farnham) are available for use in puppies. KMR (Pet-Ag) is an artificial replacement for queen's milk. (See Table 21-1 for formula dosage.) The following formula can be used as a short-term emergency supplement in puppies: 8 oz of cow's milk mixed with two egg yolks and 1 tsp of corn oil. For an emergency formula in kittens, 4 oz of cow's milk can be mixed with two egg yolks and one drop of multivitamins. Once the total daily requirement has been calculated, this amount can be divided into four equal feedings. Frequent feedings are necessary to prevent overdistention of the stomach and subsequent emesis and aspiration pneumonia. Generally, it is faster and easier to use gavage via an orogastric tube than to bottle feed.

The technique for gavage is to use a soft rubber feeding tube (Fr 8 to 16). The tube is marked with a marking pen or tape at a point equal to the distance between the tip of the nose and the eighth rib. The tube is advanced into the pharynx and down the esophagus to the level of the midthorax. A syringe can be used to inject the artificial milk replacer slowly. The stomach capacity of puppies and kittens can be calculated by using the following formula: body weight in grams times 5% equals the capacity of the stomach in milliliters. This milliliter amount should not be in a single feeding.

If the puppies or kittens are vigorous nursers, an alternative technique would be to use Pet Nursettes (Peg-Ag) or human premature baby bottle nipples. This technique is slower but may satisfy the pups and kittens more, so the incidence of litter mates nursing on each other will be reduced.

The neonatal puppy is essentially poikilothermic (body temperature varies with ambient temperature); therefore it is imperative that the ambient temperature of the whelping box be maintained between 30° C and 33° C. If hypothermia

TABLE 21-1 Orphan Formula Dosage for Puppies and Kittens

Age (wk)	Dosage* (ml/100 g Body wt/Day)
1	13
2	17
3†	20
4	22

*Divide and feed four times daily.
†Begin to feed solid food.

occurs, it will reduce feeding by the neonate and may enhance the pathogenicity of certain viruses, such as canine herpes. To detect hypothermia in neonates, it is desirable to use a low-reading clinical rectal thermometer.

A highly effective monitoring technique during the neonatal period is to weigh the neonates frequently. Newborn puppies and kittens should be weighed daily. Puppies should gain approximately 10% to 20% of their birth weight daily for the first week of life. Postage or food scales should be used to weigh each animal two or three times daily, especially during the first 2 weeks of life. Weight loss or failure to gain weight each day may be the first sign of illness. Puppies and kittens less than 2 weeks of age often do not defecate or urinate on their own. The mother stimulates these functions by gently licking the genitals and anus. This can be simulated by using a warm, wet cloth to gently wipe the genital and anal area a few times daily.

> *TECHNICIAN NOTE* A highly effective monitoring technique during the neonatal period is to weigh the neonates frequently.

PRACTICAL NURSING PROCEDURES

In many veterinary practices, it is the responsibility of the veterinary technician to monitor the patient's vital signs (i.e., temperature, pulse, respirations).

TEMPERATURE

One routine method for determining the body temperature of a small animal is to use a standard mercury-in-glass clinical rectal thermometer. Veterinary thermometers differ from those used in humans in that the storage reservoir for the mercury is short and spherical rather than elongated. Human thermometers can be used in dogs and cats without difficulty. Thermometers can be calibrated in Fahrenheit or Celsius degrees. A Fahrenheit reading can be converted to Celsius by using the following formula: degrees C = (degrees F − 32) × 5/9.

When taking the patient's temperature, one should first shake the thermometer so that the mercury is below the constriction in the glass tube. The thermometer is well lubricated with petrolatum, mineral oil, or a mild soap and inserted into the rectum with a gentle twisting motion. The thermometer is advanced into the rectum beyond the bulb and is held in place for the minimum period of time stated on the thermometer. The patient is restrained to prevent the thermometer from being broken. The thermometer is withdrawn, and the bulb and stem are wiped clean with an alcohol-soaked cotton swab. The thermometer is held horizontally and rotated until the magnified scale is clearly visible. Because of the constriction in the glass tube, the level of the mercury does not fall until it is shaken down. Finally, the thermometer should be stored in an antiseptic solution (e.g., benzalkonium chloride). Hot water should not be used for cleaning thermometers.

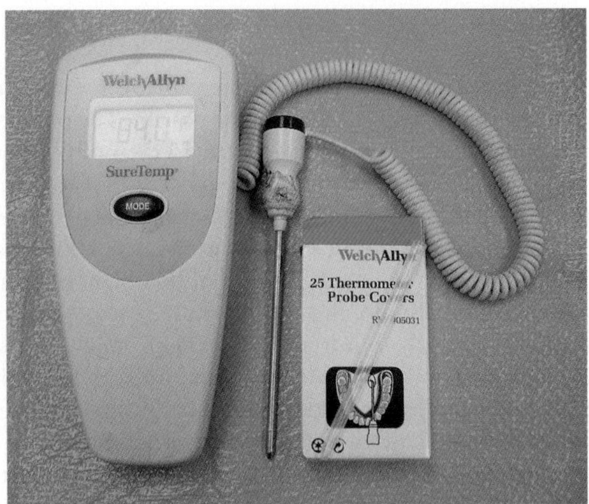

FIGURE 21-6 Digital electronic thermometer by Welch Allyn with removable and disposable plastic sheaths. These are very accurate and quick for the measurement of rectal temperature.

The more common and quicker method of obtaining a body temperature is with the use of digital thermometers (Figure 21-6). There are many brands available, and with most an auditory beep alerts the technicians when the reading is final.

Certain diseases that produce fever display a diurnal pattern (i.e., the temperature fluctuates) during the day. If the patient's temperature is taken just once per day, the periods of fever may not be recognized. If this situation is suspected, a temperature chart may be kept by taking and recording the temperature at regular intervals, for example, every 4 hours.

The normal rectal temperature in the dog is 101.0° F to 102.5° F. The normal rectal temperature in the cat is 100.5° F to 102.5° F. Excitement or activity can elevate the temperature above these limits. In rare clinical situations (i.e., rectal laceration, rectal prolapse), it may not be possible to measure the rectal temperature. In these situations, the temperature may be taken in either the axilla or the external ear canal. The temperature recorded in these sites will be significantly lower than the simultaneous rectal temperature. In general, 1° F can be added to an axillary or ear canal temperature to approximate rectal temperature. These alternative techniques for determining the body temperature are useful when the same site is used serially in an individual patient, and the results are compared. The temperature is taken by placing the bulb of the thermometer deep in the axilla or ear canal for several minutes.

Recently, infrared thermometers have been developed that record accurate body core temperatures by focusing the infrared beam on the tympanic membrane. This thermometer is helpful in those patients with very low rectal temperatures or in those for which taking a rectal temperature is contraindicated (Ototemp Veterinary, Exergen Corp.).

> *TECHNICIAN NOTE* The normal rectal temperature in the dog is 101.0° F to 102.5° F. The normal rectal temperature in the cat is 100.5° F to 102.5° F.

PULSE

The rate and character of the pulse are valuable means of assessing the cardiovascular status of the patient. The pulse can be palpated in any artery located close to the body surface. Using an index finger to palpate the pulse is best for sensitivity with the thumb being the least sensitive. The pulse is most commonly felt in the femoral artery. The femoral artery is palpated on the medial aspect of the thigh, proximal to the stifle. Palpation of the femoral pulse requires practice and can be difficult in a trembling patient or in a patient with short, heavily muscled legs. Alternative sites for taking the pulse are the palmar aspect of the carpus and the ventral aspect of the base of the tail. The normal pulse rate in adult dogs is 60 to 160 beats/min, up to 180 beats/min in toy breeds, and 220 beats/min for puppies. The maximum rate in cats is 240 beats/min.

The heart rate can be counted by palpation or auscultation at the point of maximal intensity of the heartbeat. The point of maximal intensity is located at the costochondral junction between the left fourth and sixth intercostal spaces. If the pulse rate is taken at the same time as the heart rate and the pulse rate is less, this is called a pulse deficit. A pulse deficit generally indicates an abnormal heart rhythm.

The dog can have heart and pulse rates that are "regularly irregular." Characteristically, the heart and pulse rates increase with inspiration and decrease with expiration. This normal variation is called sinus arrhythmia.

In addition to taking the pulse rate, it is beneficial to evaluate the pulse pressure and character of the pulse. Decreased pulse pressure may indicate systemic hypotension (drop in blood pressure) secondary to a process such as hypovolemic shock. Instrumentation has been developed for the noninvasive measurement of blood pressure in the dog and cat using the ultrasound Doppler method (Dinamap 8300, Critikon [Figure 21-7]; Parks 811-B, Parks Medical Electronics, Inc. [Figure 21-8]). Blood pressure readings are taken when the dog or cat has acclimated to the hospital environment to prevent falsely high readings. A neonatal cuff that has a width that is 40% the size of the limb circumference is placed over the medial tibial artery, which is found midway between the carpus and elbow or in the tibial area on a back leg. A small area is clipped free of hair distal to the cuff and transducer gel applied. The transducer is placed on top of the gel. Seven readings are taken for systolic and diastolic blood pressures. The highest and lowest values are omitted, and the remaining 5 values are averaged for the final value. The systolic readings are much more reliable than the diastolic readings with the Dinamap. The Parks ultrasound Doppler gives a more reliable reading in the cat. In the dog and cat, the normal systolic blood pressure is less than 160 mm Hg and normal diastolic blood pressure is less than 120 mm Hg.

> *TECHNICIAN NOTE* In the dog and cat, the normal systolic blood pressure is less than 160 mm Hg and normal diastolic blood pressure is less than 120 mm Hg.

RESPIRATION

The respiratory rate should be counted when the animal is at rest but not sleeping. Respiration involves both an inspiratory and expiratory phase. When counting the respiratory rate, it is necessary to count either inspirations or expirations but not both. The normal rate in the dog is between 15 and 30 breaths/min. Smaller breeds tend to have a more rapid rate of respiration than larger breeds. The rate in cats is between 20 and 30 breaths/min. In addition to determining the rate, it is important to characterize the respiratory status of the patient by inspection.

Several terms are used to describe respiratory function. Tachypnea refers to very rapid breathing. Hyperpnea indicates a condition in which the respiration is deeper and more rapid than normal. Depth of respiration indicates the volume of air inspired with each breath. Increased depth of respiration indicates a greater demand for oxygen. Shallow respiration can be caused by either metabolic derangement (e.g., acidosis) or mechanical injuries (e.g., fractured ribs). Dyspnea is a term used to indicate the subjective impression of increased difficulty or distress in breathing. Labored breathing is also used to describe difficulty in breathing and

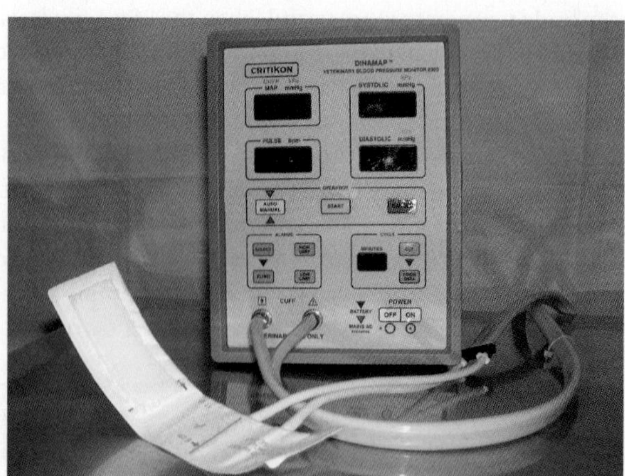

FIGURE 21-7 Dinamap 8300 (Citricon) instrument for noninvasive measurement of blood pressure.

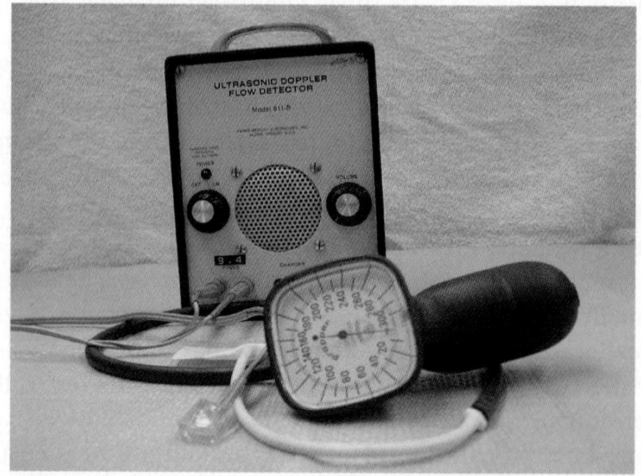

FIGURE 21-8 Parks 811-B (Parks Medical Electronics, Inc.) instrument for noninvasive measurement of blood pressure.

may include abdominal movements that occur simultaneously indicating the degree of increased effort to breathe by using abdominal muscles. Hyperventilation is seen as shallow, rapid breathing and occurs in severe metabolic acidosis and sometimes in severe respiratory disease.

All hospitalized patients should have their vital signs monitored at least once per day. Depending on the underlying problem and the status of the patient, it may be necessary to monitor the patient more frequently. The temperature, pulse, and respiration rate should be recorded in the medical record every time they are taken. This will facilitate recognition of abnormalities as early as possible. Further, serial observations will permit recognition of clinical trends.

ADMINISTRATION OF MEDICATIONS

It is important for the animal health technician to be familiar with several basic principles of clinical pharmacology. These principles are important when considering the route of administration of various drugs. Drugs can be administered parenterally (e.g., by injection), orally, or topically. The parenteral techniques routinely used in veterinary medicine include the intravenous, intramuscular, and subcutaneous routes. The specific techniques used to administer drugs by these various routes are discussed in Chapter 20. The discussion in this chapter is concerned with the selection of an appropriate route in various clinical situations.

In choosing the route of administration, a variety of factors must be considered. First, the pharmacologic properties of the drug should be considered. Certain drugs are not adequately absorbed when given by a certain route (e.g., gentamicin is poorly absorbed from the gastrointestinal tract). Similarly, insulin must be given by injection because it is destroyed in the gastrointestinal tract. Other drugs cannot be given by a certain route because they produce severe tissue reactions (e.g., thiamylal sodium causes sloughing of the skin if it is given subcutaneously). Another pharmacologic factor to consider is the rate of absorption. If an animal is critically ill, the route of administration that will provide the earliest onset of action is preferred. For example, an animal with a severe, overwhelming infection should receive an antibiotic intravenously rather than orally.

It is also important to consider the patient when considering the route of administration. For example, it is generally inadvisable to administer oral medications to a vomiting patient or to an animal with severe respiratory compromise or distress. The temperament of the patient should also be considered. In a fractious animal, it may be impossible to administer drugs topically, orally, or intravenously. Subcutaneous or intramuscular injections may be the only feasible routes of administration. Finally, convenience and compliance of the client will influence therapeutic decision. Obviously, the topical and oral routes are preferred for treatment at home.

The principal advantages of the oral route are convenience and reduced risk of infection or abscess caused by faulty injection technique. Disadvantages of the oral route include the potential for aspiration of liquid medications and the potential for animals to spit out the medication, so the prescribed dose is not absorbed.

> *TECHNICIAN NOTE* The principal advantages of the oral route are convenience and reduced risk of infection or abscess caused by faulty injection technique.

Advantages of parenteral injections include, in general, more rapid absorption and greater assurance that the prescribed dose is accurately delivered.

The major advantage to topical medication is that systemic effects are reduced and safety is thus increased. The major disadvantage is that most systemic illnesses do not respond to topical medication alone.

Whenever any drug is administered, it is essential to record the treatment (drug, dose, time) and route of administration completely and accurately in the medical record. The notation should be made immediately after administering the medication. If this procedure is consistently followed, patient care will improve because it is less likely that treatments will be omitted or inadvertently repeated. In addition to improving the level of patient care, it should be remembered that this policy is important because the medical record is a legal document, and every treatment should be recorded in case of subsequent litigation.

It is also of utmost importance that all medications, either those used in the hospital or those dispensed for use at home, be labeled correctly (see Chapter 25). The dispensing label information should include the complete name of the drug, size or concentration of the drug, number of tablets or capsules or milliliters of drug dispensed, dose and frequency of administration, name of the client, and name of the hospital. If potentially toxic drugs are dispensed, childproof containers should be used, as determined by state and federal regulations.

FLUID THERAPY

The veterinary technician generally will not be called on to formulate a fluid order in a hospitalized patient without supervision of the attending veterinarian. However, familiarity with certain fundamental points will allow the technician to participate actively in this essential process.

The total volume of fluid required to treat an animal can be approximated by considering the volume of fluid needed to rehydrate the patient, volume of fluid needed for maintenance requirements, and volume of fluid needed to correct ongoing losses.

Sensible losses are roughly equivalent to urine output. Insensible losses represent the fluid lost in the feces and during respiration. These losses are considered as part of the daily maintenance requirements. Contemporary losses are due to ongoing problems (i.e., vomiting, diarrhea).

The hydration status, and thus the rehydration requirement, can be assessed by the following physical examination criteria: skin turgor, dryness of the mucous membranes, capillary refill time, and degree of sinkage of the eyes into the bony orbit. Several laboratory criteria are beneficial, particularly if they are followed serially; these include the hematocrit, total protein determination, and urine specific gravity (SG). Finally, serial body weights can be valuable in determining changes in hydration status. One pound of body weight is equivalent to 1 pt or 480 ml of fluid.

By using the physical examination findings mentioned, the degree of dehydration is estimated as a percentage of body weight (Table 21-2). Thus an animal that shows only a slight alteration in skin turgor is approximately 5% to 6% dehydrated. Skin turgor is evaluated by pinching a fold of the skin and subjectively assessing the rate at which it returns to its normal position. This is not a valid test in older animals or animals that have recently lost weight because of the increased skin turgor that develops due to decreased fat in the subcutaneous space. An animal that is 10% to 12% dehydrated will display pronounced changes in skin turgor; dry, tacky mucous membranes; prolonged capillary refill time; and eyes that are sunken into the orbits. The physical alterations associated with dehydration are a continuum, so an animal that is 8% dehydrated should have abnormalities midway between the end points described. It should be stressed that physical examination findings are at best very crude indicators of the degree of dehydration. The quantitative value of these parameters is improved if they are carefully and critically assessed over time.

The laboratory criteria used to assess the degree of dehydration evaluate the extent of hemoconcentration. Thus the higher the hematocrit and the total protein determination, the more hemoconcentrated and thus dehydrated is the patient. These laboratory tests are useful in detecting relative changes and do not necessarily measure the absolute hydration status of the patient. If the concentrating ability of the kidneys is normal, a urine SG of more than 1.035 in the dog and 1.040 in the cat provides further evidence that the patient may be dehydrated.

Because changes in body weight over short periods are caused by changes in fluid balance rather than by the loss or gain of body mass, an accurate daily weight can also be helpful in assessing changes in the hydration status of the patient.

Once the degree of dehydration has been estimated, it can be used in calculating the volume of fluid needed to rehydrate the patient. The percent dehydration is multiplied by the body weight in kilograms and then by 1000. This is the number of milliliters needed to rehydrate the patient.

TABLE 21-2 Diagnosis of Dehydration: Physical Examination Findings

Dehydration (%)	Clinical Signs
<5	Undetectable
5-6	Skin slightly doughy, inelastic consistency
6-8	Skin definitely inelastic; eyes very slightly sunken in orbits
10-12	Increased skin turgor; eyes sunken in orbits, prolonged refill time, dry mucous membranes
12-15	Shock and imminent death

In addition to the volume required for rehydration, the maintenance requirement must be incorporated in the calculation of the daily fluid order. The maintenance requirement consists of estimates of both sensible and insensible losses.

As mentioned, sensible losses refer to the urine output. Insensible losses represent the fluid lost from the body via the gastrointestinal and respiratory tracts. Although sensible and insensible losses will vary somewhat depending on the clinical setting, a useful clinical approximation is 60 ml/kg/day (30 ml/lb/day). If the animal is not taking any liquid by mouth, a volume equivalent to the sensible and insensible losses (e.g., the maintenance requirement) should be included in the daily fluid order.

Most animals with problems that require fluid therapy do not have these problems resolve immediately on initiation of fluid therapy. Therefore contemporary or ongoing losses must also be considered in determining the daily fluid order. For example, if a patient has gastroenteritis, the volume of fluid lost with each episode of vomiting and diarrhea should be estimated and added to the rehydration and maintenance volumes. The volume of diarrhea and vomitus is frequently underestimated; therefore it has been recommended that the visual estimate be doubled to more accurately reflect the actual volume lost. Generally, the volume required to rehydrate the animal is not replaced immediately. Usually, the total volume is administered over the first 24 hours. Once rehydrated, maintenance requirement and ongoing losses are combined to calculate the fluid requirement for the next 24 hours and given over 24 hours (Box 21-1).

> *TECHNICIAN NOTES* An accurate daily weight can be helpful in assessing changes in the hydration status of the patient.

ROUTES OF FLUID ADMINISTRATION

Oral fluid administration is the preferred method because of reduced expense, ease of administration, and safety. Contraindications to oral fluid administration include vomiting and severe, life-threatening fluid imbalances that require immediate correction.

Many conditions respond well to subcutaneous administration of fluids. Fluids given subcutaneously should be

BOX 21-1 Calculation of Fluid Requirements

Body weight (kg) × % dehydration × 1000 = ml fluid deficit*
(60 to 80 ml/kg) × Body weight (kg) = ml of daily fluid requirement*
Estimation of ongoing losses × 2 = ml of ongoing losses*
Example: 20 kg dog, 8% dehydrated, 100 ml vomitus
20 kg × 0.08 1000 = 1600 ml
(20 kg) × (60 mg/kg) = 1200 ml
100 ml × 2 = 200 ml
Total volume = 3000 ml/24 = 125 ml/hr

*Add together for total volume to be replaced in milliliters over 24 hours. Divide total volume by 24 hours to get hourly fluid rate needed for digital pump administration of continuous fluids.

warmed to body temperature and must be isotonic with extracellular fluid. Isotonic fluids have an osmotic pressure approximately equal to that of extracellular fluid. Never give subcutaneously dextrose solutions with a concentration of more than 2.5%; sloughing of skin and abscess formation are common sequelae. The volume and rate of subcutaneous fluid that can be given will vary from patient to patient. A rough guideline for total daily volume is approximately 60 ml/kg (30 ml/lb). Absorption of subcutaneous fluid will occur over 6 to 8 hours; therefore this total daily dose can be divided and given every 6 to 8 hours. It is necessary and desirable to administer this divided dose in as many sites as possible. Subcutaneous fluid administration is safe and easy; however, it is not the recommended route of administration when prompt correction of severe deficits is required. Intravenous fluid administration is indicated when a patient is severely compromised with dehydration, hypovolemia, electrolyte imbalances, hypoglycemia, and so forth. The intravenous route is the most common way to give fluid in the hospital and is indicated particularly for serious, life-threatening illness and vomiting patients. Aseptic technique is required to place an intravenous catheter into the cephalic vein, saphenous vein, or jugular vein. The catheter and the fluid drip set must be kept sterile and free of blood clots to allow long-term use (3 to 5 days maximum) of the intravenous line. Heparinized saline or sterile saline may be used to periodically flush the catheter to prevent blood clots from forming in the catheter. Intravenous fluid can be given at a continuous rate using a digital fluid pump, or they can be given intermittently using the free-flowing drip method (Box 21-2).

The intraperitoneal route is not a routine method of fluid administration because peritonitis and intraabdominal abscess formation may result from this form of fluid therapy. The rate of absorption of intraperitoneal fluids is roughly equivalent to the rate of absorption of subcutaneous fluid and therefore the intraperitoneal route is not adequate when prompt correction is needed. The exception to this is the use of intraperitoneal fluid administration in the neonate and wildlife neonate, where this route may be very effective.

Signs of volume overload include restlessness, hyperpnea (increased respiratory rate), serous (watery) nasal discharge, chemosis (edema of the ocular conjunctiva), and pitting edema. Volume overload can be caused by either an excessive total volume or an excessive rate of fluid administration. Decreased cardiac function or decreased plasma protein can predispose to a volume overload state. If volume overload is suspected, the lungs should be auscultated for evidence of pulmonary edema, and the central venous pressure should be determined. Before the development of pulmonary edema or elevated central venous pressure, weight gain may be seen. Therefore it is advisable to weigh the animal three times daily while intravenous fluid therapy is being used, especially in those patients who are less able to handle a fluid load (e.g., patients with cardiac or renal disease). The placement of an indwelling urinary catheter (Foley) and urinary outflow collection system will allow quantitation of urine production. This will allow a more accurate assessment of how much fluid is coming out and how much intravenous fluid the patient actually needs to prevent overzealous fluid therapy.

BOX 21-2 Free Drip Calculations

$$\text{Drops per minute} = \frac{\text{Total infusion volume} \times \text{drops/ml}}{\text{Total infusion time (min)}}$$

For example, to administer 3000 ml over 24 hours using a 10 drop/ml drip set:

$$\frac{3000 \times 10 \text{ drops/ml}}{1440 \text{ min}} = 20 \text{ drops/min}$$

> *TECHNICIAN NOTE* Signs of volume overload include restlessness, hyperpnea (increased respiratory rate), serous (watery) nasal discharge, chemosis (edema of the ocular conjunctiva), and pitting edema.

Fluid therapy is a dynamic process that must be reassessed at frequent intervals and adjusted to obtain the maximum results. The technician's role in clinically assessing the patient is important in making appropriate adjustments. The chance of inadvertent fluid overload can be reduced by using indwelling intravenous catheters and administering fluid over prolonged periods of time rather than using rapid bolus techniques. In addition, Minidrip (Travenol Laboratories, Inc.) and Buretrol (Travenol Laboratories, Inc.) administration sets can be used in cats and small dogs. Also, syringe pumps are useful in administering fluid to cats and very small dogs (Medfusion 2010 [Medex, Inc.] Syringe Pump; Figure 21-9).

Several basic types of fluid are routinely used in small animal practice. They include physiologic (0.9%) saline, 5% dextrose in water, and extracellular fluid replacement solutions, such as lactated Ringer's solution or Ringer's solution. Combinations of these basic fluid types are also used. These basic parenteral fluid types can be supplemented with concentrated solutions of electrolytes and dextrose to produce the desired fluid composition appropriate for the specific clinical situation (Table 21-3).

Frequently, antimicrobials are added to intravenous fluid for administration. A number of the commonly used antimicrobials are incompatible with certain fluid (Table 21-4). The physical incompatibilities include precipitation of the drug out of solution and chemical inactivation. In addition to these incompatibilities, it has been noted that when certain drugs are mixed in infusion solutions, inactivation occurs. For example, when carbenicillin is added to a solution containing gentamicin, the gentamicin is inactivated. As a general rule, it is undesirable to mix multiple drugs in a syringe or intravenous fluid. Frequently, the interaction is visible on mixing, but other times it will not be observed before administration.

CENTRAL VENOUS PRESSURE

The measurement of central venous pressure is a useful aid in evaluating the fluid status of a patient. When used and interpreted properly, it can substantially reduce the likelihood

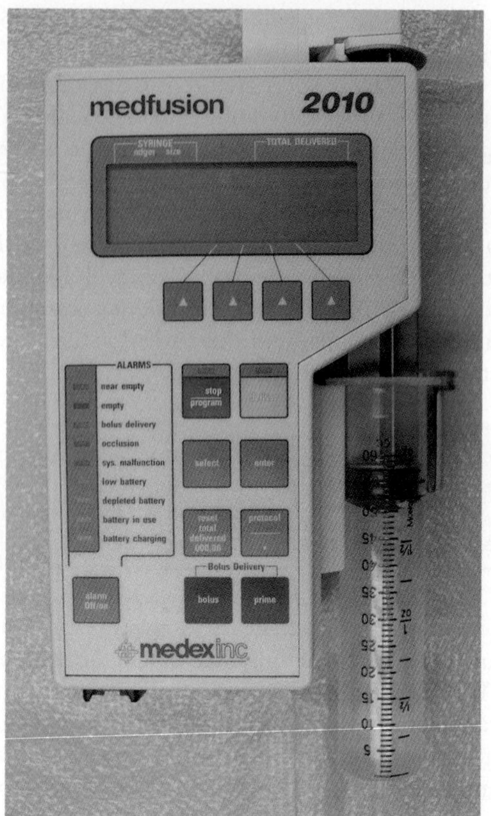

FIGURE 21-9 Medfusion 2010 (Medex, Inc.) Syringe Pump used for the administration of small volumes and slow rates of fluid to the cat and small dog.

of excessive fluid administration. Measurement of the central venous pressure is a simple technique that can be performed in all veterinary practices.

To measure the central venous pressure, an indwelling intravenous catheter is placed in the cranial vena cava via the external jugular vein. It is very important that the catheter tip be located in the cranial vena cava. If the intravenous catheter is properly placed, a 2- to 5-mm fluctuation in central venous pressure will be noted with each respiration.

Next, a sterile three-way stopcock is attached to the intravenous catheter. The open line of the three-way stopcock is connected to the intravenous fluid source. The intravenous fluid is used to prime the manometer; that is, the manometer is filled to overflowing with the intravenous fluid. With the patient in lateral recumbency, the zero point of the manometer is positioned at the level of the sternum (Figure 21-10). The central venous pressure is equal to the level of intravenous fluid in the manometer once equilibrium has been established. To improve accuracy, this determination should be repeated a total of three times. If the pressure is high, prevent blood from entering the manometer because a blood clot may alter the measurements.

The following points are important considerations when measuring and interpreting central venous pressure measurements. Serial measurements should be performed with the same zero point and the patient in the same position. If the catheter is obstructed because of blood clots or kinking, the central venous pressure will be falsely elevated. Obstruction

TABLE 21-3 Basic Fluids

	Fluid Composition per Liter					
Fluid Type	Na^+	Cl^-	K^+	Ca^{2+}	Lactate	kcal
Lactated Ringer's solution	130	109	4	3	28	9
Ringer's solution	147	156	4	5	0	0
0.9% Saline	154	154	0	0	0	0
2.5% Dextrose in ½ normal saline	77	77	0	0	0	85
5% Dextrose in lactated Ringer's solution	130	109	4	3	28	179
5% Dextrose in water	0	0	0	0	0	179
Normosol-R	140	98	5	0	0	18
Normosol-M in 5% dextrose Glucose 50	40	40	13	0	0	175

TABLE 21-4 Physical Incompatibilities of Antimicrobials in Intravenous Solutions

Antimicrobial	Incompatible With
Amphotericin B	Normal saline
Cephalothin sodium	Lactated Ringer's solution, calcium gluconate, calcium chloride
Chloramphenicol sodium	Vitamin B complex with vitamin C succinate
Chlortetracycline hydrochloride, hydrochloride, tetracycline hydrochloride	Lactated Ringer's solution, oxytetracycline sodium bicarbonate, calcium chloride
Penicillins	Dextrose-containing solutions with pH >8 (i.e., added sodium bicarbonate)
Penicillin G potassium	Vitamin B complex with vitamin C

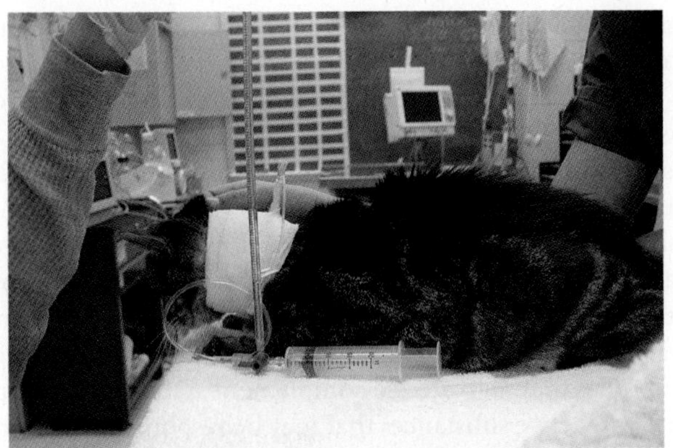

FIGURE 21-10 Use of a manometer to measure central venous pressure in a cat.

should be suspected if the level of the manometer does not fluctuate with respiration. Because continuous recording is not possible, pressure measurements are made intermittently. If intravenous fluid is not being administered between central venous pressure measurements, the catheter should be flushed with heparinized saline. Heparinized saline is prepared by adding 5 U of heparin per milliliter of saline. When evaluating the central venous pressure, it is better to evaluate trends rather than single measurements. Usually, changes of less than 3 cm of water are not significant. Using the sternum as the zero point, normal central venous pressure in the dog and cat varies between 0 and 5 cm of intravenous fluid. If the central venous pressure is consistently more than 8 to 10 cm of intravenous fluid, volume overload is suspected and fluid administration should be slowed or stopped.

> *TECHNICIAN NOTE* Heparinized saline can be prepared by adding 5 U of heparin per milliliter of saline. For example, add 500 U of heparin to a 100-ml bag of saline.

BLOOD TRANSFUSION

See Emergency Nursing, Chapter 33, for transfusion therapy.

Blood Collection

The donor may be sedated if necessary but in most dogs this is not necessary once they are use to the routine. A surgical aseptic preparation of the collection site is performed. The collection site in the dog and cat is the jugular vein. Blood collection should be performed rapidly and without interruption, using a single venipuncture of the vein to prevent excessive activation of the clotting cascade and damage to the RBCs. If acid citrate dextrose (ACD Evacuated Blood Collection Bottle, Diamond Laboratories, Inc.) is being used, a separate collection set should be used. If citrate phosphate dextrose (CPD) plastic blood pack units (with Integral Donor Tube, Fenwall Laboratories, Inc.) are used, the attached needle should be used. If vacuum bottles are used, care should be taken not to lose the vacuum at the time of venipuncture. Use of glass bottle blood collection systems should be avoided since they are not closed systems and allow the blood to be exposed to room air. Glass bottles also cause platelet inactivation and clumping on contact with the glass surface.

In the cat, a 19-gauge butterfly needle (Travenol Laboratories) and a large syringe containing the desired anticoagulant can be used.

Several anticoagulants are available for routine collection of blood. Blood drawn in heparin or sodium citrate must be used within 24 to 48 hours because of the lack of an RBC preservative, which results in a major increase in pH and the subsequent decrease in red cell adenosine triphosphate. These chemical changes result in rigid red cells that do not deform and thus are rapidly removed from the recipient's circulation.

If blood is to be stored for longer than 48 hours, either acid citrate dextrose (ACD Evacuated Blood Collection Bottle) or citrate phosphate dextrose (CPD Blood Pack Units with Integral Donor Tube) must be used as the anticoagulant and the blood stored at 1° C to 6° C. The temperature cannot vary by more than 2° C, and if the blood is out of refrigeration long enough to warm to 10° C (approximately 30 minutes), it must be used immediately. During storage, the blood should be gently mixed periodically. When collected and stored as described, blood drawn in ACD has an effective storage life of approximately 14 days, and blood drawn in CPD has an effective storage life of approximately 21 days. Blood stored in CPDA-1, with the added RBC preservative adenosine, has an effective storage life of approximately 35 to 45 days.

Blood should be gradually warmed to approximately 37° C or room temperature before administration. Refrigerated blood can be warmed by placing the bag in a 40° C water bath. Care should be exercised to prevent excessive warming (more than 50° C). Excessive warming will cause hemolysis.

It is essential that strict asepsis be maintained during collection, storage, and administration of blood and blood products. Once a blood storage container has been entered, the stored blood should be used within 24 hours. Blood should be administered through a sterile blood administration kit (Blood Administration Set, Diamond Laboratories, Inc.). A micropore filter is suggested to reduce the transfusion of microemboli found in stored blood. Administration of blood and blood products can be given by the intravenous (the most common route), intraperitoneal, or interosseous routes (into the bone marrow). The intraperitoneal and intraosseous routes are used more in the neonate.

> *TECHNICIAN NOTE* It is essential that strict asepsis be maintained during collection, storage, and administration of blood and blood products.

If the practice has a frequent demand for transfusion therapy, it is desirable to make optimal use of the available donors by separating blood into its components and administering only the needed component. Packed red cells can be produced by either centrifugation or by sedimentation of whole blood. Sedimented packed red cells are separated from plasma by gravity. The recovery of plasma is less efficient by this method;

however, a centrifuge is not necessary. If collected in glass vacuum bottles, approximately 25% to 30% of the blood volume separates into plasma by 7 to 9 days, and 45% of the blood volume is available as plasma after 14 to 16 days. Plasma is harvested from the glass collection bottles with a sterile 17.5-cm needle and a sterile syringe. Blood in plastic packs separates more rapidly than blood in glass bottles. Plasma can be collected from plastic packs by means of either a sterile needle and syringe or a plasma transfer pack (Plasma Transfer Sets, Fenwall Laboratories) and a plasma extractor (Plasma Extractor, Fenwall Laboratories). The plasma transfer packs have attached tubing, adaptors, and sealable entry ports. Thus the plasma can be collected in a closed, sterile system. If the plasma is to be stored at refrigerator temperatures (18° C to 68° C) for longer than 24 hours, a closed system is essential. Plasma frozen at less than −208° C has a storage life of longer than 1 year. If frozen plasma is to be used to treat bleeding disorders, it should be frozen within a few hours of collection.

If the major indication for transfusion is decreased oxygen-carrying capability, the patient should receive packed red cells. Packed red cells can be administered rapidly with less risk of creating volume overload in a patient with compromised cardiovascular function. The use of packed red cells will also reduce the frequency of transfusion reactions caused by plasma protein incompatibility.

Plasma transfusions are used primarily to expand the extracellular fluid volume. Plasma is also used for its transient benefit in the management of hypoproteinemia. Fresh frozen plasma is a source of coagulation factors for the treatment of warfarin toxicity, DIC, and inherited coagulation factor deficiencies.

An alternative to packed RBCs is bovine hemoglobin solution (Oxyglobin, Biopure, Inc.) also referred to as an acellular oxygen-carrying replacement fluid. The advantages of bovine hemoglobin are no need for blood typing and cross-matching, no transfusion reactions and the convenience of having the product stored on the shelf up to 3 years. Caution is necessary in the cat because of possible pulmonary edema when given rapidly. Bovine plasma is an active colloid solution and can cause volume overload if given to a patient with heart failure or renal failure or to any patient if given rapidly or in large amount. Discoloration of serum, urine, and mucous membranes to a yellowish-brown is seen with bovine hemoglobin. Also, certain laboratory tests are affected by bovine hemoglobin in the serum.

Transfusion Reactions

Complications of blood transfusion can be both immunologic and nonimmunologic in origin. Immunologic reactions can result from the transfusion of incompatible blood. Incompatible RBCs in a previously unsensitized recipient will be destroyed 7 to 10 days after transfusion. If the recipient is subsequently exposed to incompatible blood, a more acute hemolytic reaction may occur. Clinical consequences of hemolytic transfusion reactions include the rapid development of tachycardia, hypotension, vomiting, salivation, and muscle tremors. Laboratory changes associated with significant acute hemolysis include hemoglobinemia, hemoglobinuria, and possible acquired coagulation disorders.

Delayed hemolytic reactions will sometimes occur following multiple transfusions. Delayed hemolysis should be suspected if the PCV drops unexpectedly 2 to 21 days after transfusion. The clinical and laboratory signs of acute hemolysis mentioned may not be detected in delayed hemolytic reactions. Transfusion reactions may also be caused by immunologic reactions caused by leukocyte, platelet, or plasma protein incompatibilities. Reactions between antigens and antibodies may activate the complement system and thus release vasoactive substances that may be responsible for trembling, vomiting, and urticaria (hives). Prior transfusion is not required for these reactions to occur. The use of antihistamines (diphenhydramine hydrochloride) approximately 30 minutes before transfusion may reduce these reactions.

Transfusion-induced fever is due to the response of the donor to foreign proteins. The initial step in controlling transfusion-induced fever is to slow the rate of transfusion. If no response is noted when the rate is reduced, the transfusion should be discontinued, and the patient observed closely for more severe signs of reaction. Bacterial contamination of the transfused blood will also produce fever and should be considered. Starting another transfusion after a period of time may eliminate the problem.

Nonimmunologic transfusion reactions are principally due to vascular overload. Signs of vascular overload include coughing, increased respiratory rate, respiratory distress, and vomiting. If there is evidence of preexisting cardiac dysfunction, the rate of administration of blood should be reduced to approximately 1 ml/kg/hr. Because vomiting is a potential adverse reaction to transfusion, food and water should be withheld from the patient during the transfusion and any medications scheduled to be given during this time.

TECHNICIAN NOTE Since vomiting is a potential adverse reaction to transfusions, if the situation allows, the patient should have food and water withheld and avoid the administration of medications during the transfusion.

PHYSICAL THERAPY

See rehabilitation and physical therapy, Chapter 24.

OXYGEN THERAPY

The primary indication for oxygen therapy is hypoxia, which refers to a deficiency of oxygen at the tissue level. Tissue hypoxia may be caused by a reduction in perfusion (reduced blood flow) or a reduction in oxygen content of the blood. Hypoxia is probably more common than is recognized in veterinary medicine since a caged animal at rest will not show signs until the oxygen content of the blood is severely reduced.

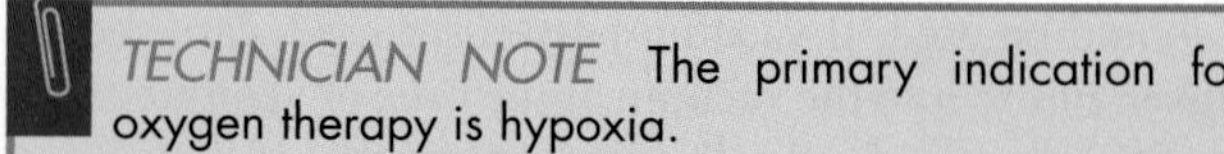

TECHNICIAN NOTE The primary indication for oxygen therapy is hypoxia.

Hypoxia can be manifested in a variety of ways, and the veterinary technician must be alert to identify these changes. Abnormalities that may be noted in the cardiovascular system include tachycardia or arrhythmias. An increased respiratory rate, open-mouthed breathing, and dyspnea may also be noted. Dyspnea is the term used to indicate subjective difficulty or distress in breathing. With severe hypoxia, central nervous system changes may be noted and include drowsiness, altered motor abilities, or increased excitability. Finally, cold extremities may indicate an inadequate supply of oxygen at the tissue level. Cyanosis is not a reliable indicator of hypoxia, especially if the animal is anemic. Cyanosis refers to dark bluish or purplish discoloration of the skin and mucous membranes.

Although the basic defect in hypoxia is decreased oxygen availability at the tissue level, it can occur by a variety of mechanisms. For example, it can result from lung disease, decreased cardiac output, or severe anemia.

In small animal practice, oxygen therapy is used primarily in the following clinical situations: pulmonary edema, severe bronchopneumonia, upper airway disease in brachycephalic breeds such as English bulldog and Boston terrier, pulmonary trauma, collapse of lung lobes, and shock. Measurement of hemoglobin saturation is performed with pulse oximetry (Figure 21-11). A pulse oximeter is used by applying a clip to nonpigmented skin or mucous membrane, such as the lip, tongue, pinnae, vulva, or prepuce to allow reading of hemoglobin saturation in the peripheral blood vessels. Hemoglobin saturation is an indirect way to monitor whether a patient has adequate peripheral arterial blood circulation. It is also a good indicator of hypoxemia due to decreased ventilation of air to the lungs. Direct measurement of oxygenation of arterial blood is monitored with the more invasive arterial blood gas. Arterial blood gas analysis determines the partial pressure of oxygen available in the bloodstream, which is a direct indicator of whether a patient can oxygenate blood in the lungs normally. An arterial blood sample is taken from the femoral artery to measure the arterial blood gas. Be careful not to incorporate air bubbles into the sample, and an immediate reading of the sample by a blood gas analyzer is imperative. A pulse oximeter reading less than 70% is considered decreased and an arterial blood gas PO_2 less than 95 mm Hg is considered decreased.

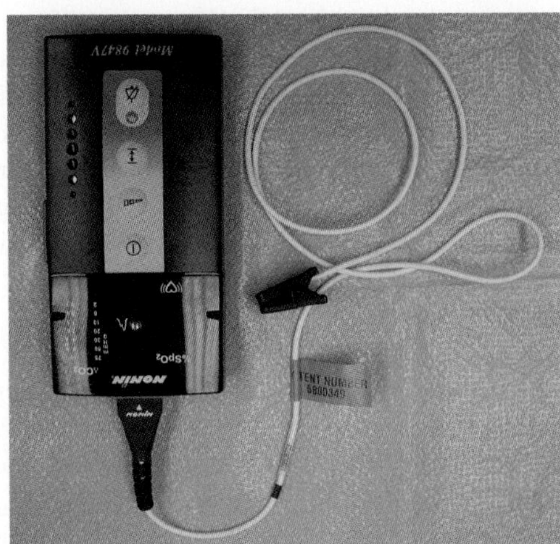

FIGURE 21-11 Pulse oximeter (Nonin 9847V) measures oxygen saturation.

Methods of oxygen therapy include oxygen cages, human pediatric incubators, masks, nasal catheters, endotracheal tubes, and intratracheal catheters.

Oxygen Cage

Oxygen cages for veterinary use are sold commercially. These cages permit control of not only the oxygen concentration but also temperature and humidity (Figure 21-12). These cages are useful in animals able to ventilate without assistance. However, they are expensive and consume large amounts of oxygen. Surplus human pediatric incubators are a less expensive means of providing similar therapy to small dogs, cats, or exotic animals. Oxygen cages and incubators should be flushed (filled) with oxygen after they have been opened. Some units are equipped with entry ports that allow access to the patient without excessive loss of oxygen.

An inspired oxygen concentration of 30% to 40% is adequate for animals requiring oxygen therapy. Excessively high oxygen concentrations can result in oxygen toxicity. Neonatal kittens appear to be particularly susceptible to retinal changes induced by oxygen toxicity.

Mask Induction

In certain circumstances, masks can be used to administer oxygen. Masks are available in a variety of sizes and shapes suitable for use in dogs and cats. If an oxygen mask is used, it is important to provide a high oxygen flow rate to prevent excessive accumulation of carbon dioxide. Administration of oxygen via a mask is suitable for short periods of time only and only in selected patients. Some patients will resist the use of an oxygen mask, and the resultant stress will negate any beneficial effect of the oxygen.

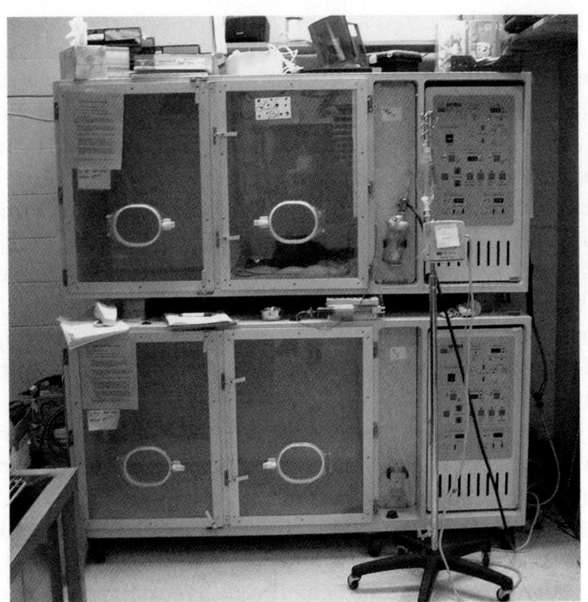
FIGURE 21-12 Small animal oxygen cage.

Intratracheal Catheter Induction

An alternative means of oxygen administration that is both inexpensive and effective is the intratracheal catheter. This technique is reserved for critically ill patients. The skin is aseptically prepared, and a local anesthetic is administered over the trachea in the midcervical area. An intravenous catheter (14, 16, or 18 gauge) is introduced into the trachea and advanced to a point craniad to the bifurcation of the trachea. The delivered oxygen should be humidified and administered at a flow rate of 0.5 to 4 L/min. The flow rate should be adjusted, depending on the size of the animal.

Nasal Catheter Induction

Nasal catheters can also be used to administer oxygen for brief periods to severely depressed animals. In this technique, a small (5 to 8 Fr) soft rubber feeding tube or urinary catheter is inserted through the external nares to the level of the caudal nasopharynx. The catheter can be coated with a topical anesthetic cream, or topical anesthetic drops can be instilled in the nostril to facilitate passage. Adhesive tape is attached to the catheter, and the tape is sutured to the forehead. An Elizabethan collar is used to prevent the patient from dislodging the catheter.

RESPIRATORY PHYSICAL THERAPY

Physical therapy of the respiratory system is a valuable adjunct to other forms of therapy for diseases of the lungs and airways. Appropriate physical therapy is also useful as a preventive measure in patients at high risk for the development of pulmonary disease. Secondary bronchopneumonia is a common complication in patients with lung lobe collapse. Stimulation of the cough reflex by compressing the trachea will expand the lungs maximally and help prevent lung collapse. Regular turning of recumbent patients will enhance drainage and circulation and thus prevent hypostatic congestion.

Percussion (coupage), also known as tapping or clapping, is a technique of striking the animal's chest to loosen bronchial secretion and thus facilitate drainage. The chest is struck with the hand held slightly cupped with fingers and thumb closed so that a cushion of air is trapped between the technician's hand and the chest wall. Best results come from using both hands alternately in rapid sequence for several seconds, moving from ventral to dorsal on the lung fields. When done properly, this is a noisy procedure; however, it is not painful to the patient. If the animal is ambulatory, a brief walk after coupage will aid in mobilization of respiratory secretions.

Whenever possible, animals with pulmonary problems should be maintained in an upright position (i.e., sternal recumbency). If necessary, slings or supports should be used to maintain this posture. When this is not practical, alternating sides of recumbency by turning the patient from one side to the other, every 2 hours, can prevent hypostatic congestion from developing.

> *TECHNICIAN NOTE* Coupage, also known as tapping or clapping, is a technique used to loosen bronchial secretions and facilitate drainage in patients with pneumonia.

TOPICAL THERAPY

Topical therapy plays an important role in the treatment of dermatologic disease. It can be used to treat a specific disease, such as sarcoptic mange. More frequently, however, topical therapy is used either in conjunction with systemic medications or as a form of symptomatic therapy when the diagnosis is unknown.

Plain tap water is one of the most effective topical agents. Depending on how water is used, it can either hydrate or dehydrate the skin. Frequent wetting of the skin will stimulate evaporation from the skin and thus cause dehydration. This approach can be useful in managing any acute moist dermatitis ("hot spot"). In contrast, if a film of oil (e.g., Alpha Keri, Westwood Pharmaceuticals, Inc.) is applied immediately after soaking with water, evaporation is slowed or stopped, and the skin remains moist.

Soaks

Soaks are an effective means of handling localized acute eruptions. Soaks can be applied with moist towels or by placing the animal in a water-filled basin or tub. Soaks for local acute dermatosis should be applied for 10 to 15 minutes three or more times daily. The involved area should be kept constantly moist, and the warm temperature of the soak should be maintained by adding hot water as needed. Some of the solutions commonly used for soaks in veterinary medicine include water, aluminum acetate (Burow's solution, Domeboro solution, Dome Laboratories), and magnesium sulfate or Epsom salts (1:65 solution in water, 1 tablespoonful per 1000 ml of water).

Astringents

Astringents precipitate proteins on the surface of an area of acute damage and form a beneficial covering. These agents do not penetrate deeply. Aluminum acetate is an excellent mild astringent. Another effective astringent is tannic acid. Tannic acid is combined with salicylic acid and alcohol in several products to form a potent astringent. These combination products are especially useful as part of the management of localized acute moist dermatitis; however, astringents should be applied only once to an involved area.

Baths

Cleansing baths are an important part of topical dermatologic therapy. Baths aid in the removal of dirt, debris, and scale. A variety of effective mild cleansing soaps or detergents are available. Mild dishwashing detergents or soaps (e.g., Joy, Palmolive Liquid) are effective and inexpensive. If a milder, less irritating product is desired, a balanced pH soap, such as Johnson's Baby Shampoo (Johnson & Johnson), can be used. If an even milder product is needed, vegetable oil soaps (coconut oil) are the most bland. Regardless of how mild the soap or detergent, it should always be thoroughly rinsed out of the coat with copious volumes of clean water.

A medicated bath can be applied as a shampoo or as a rinse applied to the animal after a routine cleansing bath. Medicated baths contain ingredients that enhance the actions of routine cleansing shampoos. Medicated shampoos should be lathered into the coat for 10 to 15 minutes. This allows the medicated component of the shampoo time for effect or limited absorption. Types of medicated baths used in small animal practice include colloidal oatmeal, tar-sulfur, sulfur-salicylic, and benzoyl peroxide products. Colloidal oatmeal (Aveeno, Cooper Care, Inc.; Epi-Soothe cream rinse, Allerderm, Inc.) baths are used for their soothing and antipruritic properties. Tar-sulfur shampoos (Lytar, Dermatologics for Veterinary Medicine, Inc.; Allerseb-T, Allerderm, Inc.) are used in the management of oily, flaky seborrheic conditions. Sulfur and salicylic shampoos (Sebalyte, Dermatologics for Veterinary Medicine, Inc.; Sebolux, Allerderm, Inc.) are used in the management of dry, flaky seborrheic conditions, and benzoyl peroxide shampoos (Oxydex, Dermatologics for Veterinary Medicine, Inc.; Pyoben, Allerderm, Inc.) are useful in the treatment of superficial pyoderma (bacterial skin infection), excessive crusting and debris problems, and oily seborrheic conditions. The underlying condition and the individual response to the medicated bath determine the required frequency of application.

Dips and Rinses

Dips or rinses use water as a means of delivering various antifungal or antiparasitic agents to the skin. Although applied to the skin, some of these agents have the potential to cause systemic toxicities. Clipping the hair and using cleansing baths help to obtain greater penetration in animals with excessive scale or crust. Dips that are useful in the treatment of dermatophytosis (ringworm) include dilute sodium hypochlorite solution, dilute Nolvasan solution (Fort Dodge Laboratories), dilute iodine solutions, or lime-sulfur solutions. Antiparasitic products used as dips or rinses include chlorpyrifos (Dursban), pyrethrins, pyrethroids, organophosphates (malathion), and carbamates. Amitraz (Mitaban, Upjohn Co.) is useful in the treatment of generalized demodectic mange.

Before using any topical agent the label should be checked to be sure it is safe to use in dogs, cats, puppies, and kittens. The age of young animals should be noted because some products are not recommended in the very young.

> *TECHNICIAN NOTE* Before using any topical agent the label should be checked to be sure it is safe to use in dogs, cats, puppies, and kittens.

Powders

Powders are occasionally used in veterinary medicine as drying agents and vehicles for parasiticides and to reduce friction and irritation. When used as a drying agent, powders may be in the form of true powders, shake lotions, or pastes. Components that improve the drying action of various powdered products include talc, zinc oxide, cornstarch, and tannic acid. Carbaryl powders are a valuable part of flea control programs in the dog and cat. Labels should be checked carefully to be certain that the specific product is safe for dogs and cats. The powder must be worked down into the hair coat to increase the parasiticidal effect. This can be accomplished by rubbing the hair coat against the grain as the powder is applied. The powder should be applied to the entire body, excluding the face. Fractious or frightened cats can be treated by wrapping them in a thick bath towel and medicating small sections until the entire animal has been covered. Flea sprays can be used similarly.

Creams and Ointments

Creams and ointments are also used in the topical treatment of dermatologic problems. The area of treatment should be clipped, if not hairless, and protected from immediate removal by licking. For practical and economic reasons, the area to be treated should be relatively small. Ointments are thicker than creams and leave a greasy feeling when applied to the skin. Ointments and creams soften, lubricate, and protect the skin and aid in the removal of scale and crusts. Ointments and creams form an occlusive covering and therefore are not indicated for moist or oozing skin lesions.

Topical creams and ointments can be used to treat localized dermatophytosis (ringworm). They can be used as the sole type of therapy or as an adjunct to oral therapy or topical rinses. Creams and ointments must be restricted to small lesions because of expense and convenience. Effective topical fungicidal products used in veterinary medicine contain miconazole and thiabendazole. Because the use of ointments and creams alone is often insufficient to clear the infection or prevent reinfection, rinses or dips are important.

Otic Preparations

Most topical otic preparations contain various combinations of antibiotic, antiinflammatory, fungicidal, and parasiticidal agents. Topical antimicrobial agents are indicated whenever infection is present. Chloramphenicol, neomycin, polymyxin, and gentamicin are the commonly used antibiotics in these combination otic preparations. Neomycin and gentamicin have been reported to cause ototoxicity when used for prolonged periods in dogs with ruptured eardrums. (Gentamicin is inactivated by purulent exudate; therefore the ears must be thoroughly cleaned before use.)

Corticosteroids are used in these combination products because they decrease inflammation and the buildup of discharge and, consequently, decrease self-trauma by the animal. The antifungals are useful in treating dermatophytes and yeast organisms such as *Malassezia pachydermatis* (Pityrosporon). Thiabendazole and miconazole are effective topical antifungal agents.

Certain drugs owe their efficacy to their ability to alter the pH in the ear canal. Acetic acid (dilute vinegar solution) and Domeboro Otic (Dome Laboratories) are specific examples.

Products that contain rotenone in oil or thiabendazole are used to treat ear mites. It is essential that treatment for ear mites be continued for at least 3 weeks and that all animals in the household be treated. Otic instillation of ivermectin, as a one-time application (on occasion, two to four treatments may be needed), has also been shown to be effective in the treatment of ear mites.

INFECTIOUS DISEASES

This section will discuss a number of common medical problems of dogs and cats. It is not intended to be a comprehensive review of internal medicine; rather, several specific problems have been selected that illustrate or emphasize important aspects of medical nursing.

CANINE RESPIRATORY DISEASE COMPLEX

Synonyms for canine upper respiratory disease complex include kennel cough and infectious tracheobronchitis. This complex is composed of a number of different disease processes. Causative factors include viral and bacterial agents, and predisposing environmental factors. These factors may occur singly or in combination. Fever, coughing, ocular and nasal discharge, vomiting, diarrhea, lethargy, and depressed appetite may occur for 24 to 48 hours. The clinical signs are usually gone after 48 hours, except for a dry, hacking cough, which can linger up to 2 weeks. The diagnosis of this complex is usually based on historical and physical examination findings rather than on laboratory tests. This problem is most often self-limiting, and the duration of signs generally is no more than 2 weeks.

> *TECHNICIAN NOTE* Kennel Cough (Infectious Tracheobronchitis) is most often self-limiting, and the duration of signs generally is no more than 2 weeks.

Treatment involves nursing care and the correction of any environmental factors that may have predisposed to the illness. The dog should be kept in a warm space that is well ventilated and free of drafts and should be fed a highly palatable diet. Appetite will be enhanced if eyes and nose are kept free of accumulated discharge. If appetite is suppressed, the patient should be encouraged to eat canned dog food or even selected table food, such as chicken and rice, for increased palatability. Intravenous or subcutaneous fluid therapy is occasionally necessary. Steam or vaporizer therapy may provide symptomatic relief of the dry cough. Steam therapy can be performed by placing the dog in a steam-filled bathroom several times per day. Alternatively, cold-mist vaporizers can be used several times daily.

The decision to use antitussive (cough suppressant) therapy should be based on the frequency of coughing and how prolonged the episodes are. If codeine-derivative cough suppressants are used to excess, depression and anorexia will result.

Treatment with antibiotics usually is not indicated unless there is evidence of lower respiratory or systemic involvement, for example, fever. The presence of a green- or yellow-colored nasal discharge may also warrant antibiotic therapy. If antibiotic therapy is instituted, a complete regimen of 10 to 14 days at full therapeutic doses should be completed. The selection of an antibiotic would ideally be based on the results of culture and sensitivity testing of a transtracheal wash. If these are not available, chloramphenicol, β-lactam penicillins, first-generation cephalosporins, or fluorinated quinolones are usually effective. The use of systemic products containing both antibiotics and corticosteroids is not indicated. Likewise, the intratracheal injection of any product is inappropriate therapy.

Because of the highly contagious nature of the causative organisms, an infected dog should be isolated from other hospitalized patients. If possible, hospitalization should be avoided. Once an outbreak occurs in a kennel or veterinary hospital, control is difficult. Ideally, the area should be kept vacant for approximately 2 weeks, and appropriate preventive measures should be instituted, consisting of the implementation of an effective vaccination protocol for every hospitalized patient. All dogs should preferably be vaccinated at least 10 days before exposure. At least every 3 years revaccination for the respiratory viruses of all patients over 1 year of age should be a consistent hospital policy. Vaccination with the intranasal vaccine for *Bordetella bronchiseptica* every 6 months is recommended for animals at high risk of exposure to the causative agents of infectious tracheobronchitis (e.g., frequent boarding or dog shows). The commonly used disinfectants, such as chlorhexidine (Novalsan) and benzalkonium (Roccal), effectively kill the causative bacteria and viruses.

> *TECHNICIAN NOTE* Because of the highly contagious nature of the causative organisms, an infected dog should be isolated from other hospitalized patients. If possible, hospitalization should be avoided.

FELINE RESPIRATORY DISEASE COMPLEX

The principal components of the feline respiratory disease complex are feline viral rhinotracheitis (herpesvirus) and feline calicivirus. Less frequently incriminated agents include feline pneumonitis *(Chlamydia psittaci)*, *Mycoplasma*, and *Bordetella bronchiseptica*.

Clinical signs of this complex include fever, cough, paroxysms of sneezing, and hypersalivation. As the infection progresses, mucopurulent ocular and nasal discharge, lacrimation, and open-mouthed breathing can be seen. Ulceration of the tongue, hard palate, and nasal pad has been reported with feline calicivirus. The severity of signs and the mortality are greatest in young (less than 1 year of age), nonvaccinated cats and kittens. The severity of the clinical signs will vary widely from patient to patient. The variability results from a number of interacting factors, which include the virulence of the virus, infecting dose of virus, and general health and immune status of the infected cat.

Diagnosis is based primarily on history and clinical signs rather than on laboratory findings. Occasionally, laboratory confirmation of the diagnosis by means of virus isolation or the demonstration of serum antibodies is indicated. The additional expense of laboratory confirmation is justified only when dealing with groups of cats having a chronic history of feline respiratory disease complex.

Treatment will vary, depending on the severity of signs. Some cats will show only mild, transient signs, and they require no treatment. Secondary bacterial infection will occasionally be a sequelae to the feline respiratory disease complex, and therefore a broad-spectrum antibiotic may be indicated in the very young kitten (<12 weeks of age).

General nursing care is of much greater importance than antibiotics in typical cases. Whenever possible, infected cats should be treated at home rather than in the hospital.

A vital part of nursing care is to gently clean away accumulated ocular and nasal discharge. If the nostrils are kept patent, the cat is more likely to continue eating because of the cat's reliance on smell to encourage appetite. To ensure that this happens, the owner should indulge the pet and provide highly palatable food. Strongly flavored or odorous food (fish flavored) is more likely to stimulate the appetite of an anorectic cat. Steam therapy is frequently useful and can be achieved by placing the cat in a steam-filled bathroom or by using a vaporizer.

In cats that become completely anorectic, subcutaneous or intravenous fluid may be required until the appetite returns to normal. Repeated syringe feeding may be attempted; however, in certain cats, the associated stress may negate any beneficial effect. Alternatives that appear to be better tolerated include nasoesophageal or pharyngostomy tubes. These procedures should be reserved for severely cachectic cats.

The virus is usually transmitted through direct contact with an infected cat. Sneezing with subsequent aerosolization of the virus will spread the virus a distance of approximately 15 to 20 cm. Fomite transmission via hands, clothing, letterboxes, and food and water dishes is a more significant means of transmission than aerosolization in veterinary hospitals. The agents responsible for the feline respiratory disease complex are sensitive to hypochlorite disinfection.

> *TECHNICIAN NOTE* Fomite transmission via hands, clothing, letterboxes, and food and water dishes is a more significant means of transmission than aerosolization in veterinary hospitals.

The best way to prevent outbreaks of feline respiratory disease complex in hospitalized cats is to have an effective immunization protocol that requires vaccination of the respiratory viruses at least every 3 years in cats over 1 year of age. Adequate ventilation will reduce the likelihood that infection will spread within the hospital. The humidity should be maintained between 30% and 50%. Disposable food trays and litter pans and autoclavable water dishes should be used. Cats should not be moved from one cage to another unless absolutely necessary during an outbreak. Cages should be thoroughly cleansed with a dilute hypochlorite solution. Finally, because the infection can be spread via hands and clothing, meticulous hygiene on the part of all hospital personnel is essential. It is important to understand that up to 80% of the cats that develop this respiratory complex remain lifelong carriers of the organism or organisms. They can pose a risk to other cats or can experience a recrudescence of the complex in stressful situations.

CANINE DISTEMPER

Canine distemper is an important viral disease of dogs because of the ubiquitous nature of the virus and the mortality associated with infection. The severity of signs will vary from a transient, subclinical infection to a severe fatal disease that involves several different organ systems. This variability is due to the differing virulence of various virus strains and differences in host immunity.

The initial phase of the infection is associated with fever, transient anorexia, lethargy, and a mild serous ocular discharge after an approximate 9- to 14-day incubation period. Obviously, these signs are not specific for canine distemper. Later, as the virus spreads to the respiratory and gastrointestinal systems, mucopurulent ocular and nasal discharge, coughing, diarrhea, and, occasionally, vomiting are noted. Many dogs are anorectic at this point and become severely dehydrated. Involvement of the central nervous system may occur and can be the only signs manifested by some dogs. These dogs may develop seizures or other evidence of neurologic disease. Some dogs will seemingly recover from the severe respiratory and gastrointestinal signs, but weeks or months later they develop neurologic signs that either are fatal or require euthanasia because of their severity.

Although the virus may survive in the environment for weeks at near-freezing temperatures, it is susceptible to heat, drying, and ultraviolet light. Routine disinfection is usually effective in destroying the virus in a hospital or kennel. Patients suspected to have distemper should be housed separate from the rest of the hospital patients. An isolation ward or cat ward would be acceptable to prevent the spread of the virus to susceptible canine patients. Diligent washing of hands and preventing fomite transmission after handling distemper suspects is also necessary to prevent spread of the virus.

> *TECHNICIAN NOTE* Patients suspected to have distemper should be housed separate from the rest of the hospital patients.

FELINE PANLEUKOPENIA

Feline panleukopenia is a potentially severe, highly contagious parvoviral disease of cats. Synonyms are feline distemper and infectious enteritis.

The typical clinical signs associated with feline panleukopenia include lethargy, anorexia, vomiting, and diarrhea after a 7-day incubation period. Characteristically, the feces are yellowish and semiformed to fluid in consistency; they may be blood tinged. Severe dehydration may be present. The temperature may be elevated or subnormal. Feline panleukopenia can be an acute disease. Rarely, development of signs is so rapid that the owner may suspect malicious poisoning. Kittens and young cats appear to be more severely affected.

Diagnosis of feline panleukopenia is based on the presence of the clinical signs described above in the presence of a low total leukocyte count (less than 2000 WBCs/mm^3). The low total count is primarily due to low numbers of neutrophils. The diagnosis of feline panleukopenia can be confirmed by virus isolation and serologic and histopathologic characteristics.

Treatment is primarily supportive because specific antiviral drugs are not available. The cornerstone of successful therapy is the correction of fluid and electrolyte imbalances and prevention of sepsis by the use of broad-spectrum antibiotics. Symptomatic control of vomiting and diarrhea is usually indicated. Another complication the technician should be aware of is the development of hypoglycemia. This may be manifested by the development of extreme weakness, seizure activity, or both.

The prognosis for recovery is good if the cat survives the initial 3 to 6 days of severe clinical signs. The prognosis for kittens and young cats is guarded. A rising WBC count indicates a more favorable prognosis. During the recovery phase, the WBC count may exceed 50,000/mm^3 and reveal a significant leftward shift. This should not be confused with the development of another infection because this can be a normal response.

If the queen is infected during pregnancy, fetal death or congenital defects in the kitten may result. The fetus is susceptible to the virus because most tissues have high cell-proliferation rates. If the fetus is infected just before or immediately after birth, the development of the cerebellum may be affected and hypocerebellum can occur. These kittens show balance and coordination problems beginning at about 3 to 4 weeks of age.

Fortunately, because of the availability of excellent vaccines, feline panleukopenia is currently an infrequent clinical problem.

FELINE LEUKEMIA VIRUS AND FELINE IMMUNODEFICIENCY VIRUS INFECTION

These two distinct retroviral infections in cats may cause similar clinical signs. Feline leukemia virus (FeLV) has been recognized for many years and may cause immunosuppression, neoplasia, or both. Lymphosarcoma and bone marrow disorders are the more common disorders associated with FeLV. The virus is transmitted between cats by direct contact through grooming, sharing food dishes, and fighting. The virus is easily killed in the environment, and isolation of an infected cat is adequate to prevent transmission to susceptible cats. Although most cats that are exposed to the virus successfully eliminate the infection, 1% to 3% of cats in single-cat households and up to 30% of cats in multiple-cat households will become persistently infected with the virus. These infected cats are then at risk for the development of the plethora of FeLV-related diseases. FeLV infection can be identified by an in-hospital test that detects viral antigen. There are many such in-hospital tests on the market and available to the practicing veterinarian. There are several vaccines available for the prevention of FeLV. These vaccines are not completely protective but do protect up to 70% of the vaccinated cat population.

Feline immunodeficiency virus (FIV), also called T-lymphotrophic T cell lentivirus (FTLV), is another virus that causes immunosuppression in the cat. Common clinical signs of infection with this virus include gingivitis, chronic diarrhea, generalized lymphadenopathy, fever, conjunctivitis, rhinitis, and dermatitis. It is notable that all these signs may be seen in cats infected with FeLV. FIV is found nationwide and, indeed, worldwide. Most cats infected with this virus will not become immune, which differs from FeLV infection. The disease is spread by inoculation of the virus through cat bites which allow blood transmission. Transmission of the virus by direct contact through grooming, sharing of food dishes, and close contact is less than that seen with FeLV. No treatment is available for this disease. Commercial kits detecting antibodies to this virus are available for in-hospital testing. A vaccine is currently available; however, the efficacy has not been established. Also, this vaccine will cause a positive FIV antibody test, complicating the ability to clearly document FIV infection in vaccinated cats.

TECHNICIAN NOTE FeLV infection is spread by direct and repeated close contact, such as grooming or sharing of food and water dishes, whereas FIV infection is transmitted by inoculation of the virus through cat bites.

ROUTINE IMMUNIZATION PROGRAM FOR DOGS AND CATS

One of the greatest areas of advancement in veterinary medicine in the past 50 years is in the prevention of infectious diseases. The purpose of any vaccination program is to prevent clinical disease by preventing or limiting infection. The vaccination program can also be the foundation of a complete well-animal health maintenance program. At the time of vaccination, owners should be counseled regarding nutrition, parasite control, and matters regarding reproduction. Chapter 9 provides a complete overview of canine and feline preventive health programs and vaccination recommendations.

A physical examination by the veterinarian at the time of vaccination is extremely important because a number of conditions will potentially influence the immunization procedure, such as pregnancy, debilitation, and fever.

Numerous factors influence the patient's ability to respond to vaccination. Factors that are of practical significance include colostral (maternal) antibodies, vaccine type, route of administration, age of the patient, nutritional status of the patient, and concurrent infection or drug therapy.

Colostral Antibodies

In puppies and kittens, approximately 95% of the circulating immunoglobulins come from absorption of colostrum (first milk) shortly after birth. These circulating immunoglobulins provide essential temporary protection, but they also have the ability to interfere with more permanent protection. Interference occurs because the vaccine does not reach the appropriate cells to stimulate the active immunity process. Consequently, it is necessary for the level of circulating immunoglobulins derived from the colostrum to be reduced before successful vaccination is possible. In puppies born to bitches that have received vaccinations against canine distemper and infectious canine hepatitis, this period of uncertain response to vaccination may extend to 14 weeks of age. Thus the last dose of vaccine should be administered at 14 to 16 weeks of age to optimize the success of the vaccination program. Colostral immunoglobulins to canine parvovirus may persist for at least 16 weeks in puppies; therefore the last dose of vaccine for parvovirus should be given no earlier than 16 weeks of age. In the Rottweiler and Doberman breeds, it is suggested that the last dose of parvovirus vaccine be given at 18 weeks of age.

An alternative technique to prevent or reduce the blocking effect of colostral antibodies on canine distemper vaccination is to use measles virus vaccine. Approximately 50% of puppies at 6 weeks of age will not respond to canine distemper virus vaccination, whereas the vast majority will respond to measles virus vaccine. The measles virus stimulates resistance against canine distemper in puppies regardless of circulating antibodies that the pup has acquired from the colostrum. Measles virus vaccine prevents clinical disease but does not prevent infection. Measles virus vaccine should be considered a temporary method of preventing canine distemper until the dog can respond to the canine distemper vaccine. There is no reason to use vaccines containing measles virus in dogs older than 16 weeks of age. There are no known public health dangers associated with the use of measles virus-containing vaccines. Measles virus vaccine does not provide protection against infectious canine hepatitis.

Methods of overcoming the effects of colostral (maternal) antibodies are not absolute. Therefore research is continuing in this area. Although colostral antibodies interfere with the immunization process, colostrum is extremely important for the protection of the neonate against a number of potentially harmful microorganisms. Puppies and kittens should never be deliberately deprived of colostrum.

Type of Vaccine

The type of vaccine is very important in formulating a successful vaccination program. Viral vaccines can be either inactivated or modified live virus vaccines. Because live virus vaccines depend on viral replication in the recipient animal to provide protection, the vaccine must be handled strictly according to the instructions supplied by the manufacturer. Inactivated vaccines are less labile; however, in general they must be administered several times to get an adequate protective response. It is impossible to state that one type of vaccine is categorically better than another; in the future, both inactivated and modified live virus types of vaccine will continue to be used.

To achieve the optimal response, the entire dose of vaccine should be given as recommended; the dose should not be split and given to more than one animal. Different vaccine products should not be mixed in the same syringe before administration. Frequently, vaccines contain preservatives that will interfere with another vaccine.

Route of Administration

The route of administration specified in the manufacturer's instructions should be followed. With certain viruses, significant differences in response occur, depending on the route of administration. For example, with measles virus and some rabies virus vaccines, the intramuscular route is much more effective than the subcutaneous route. The manufacturer's recommendations must be understood and followed for all vaccines.

With certain viruses (e.g., feline viral rhinotracheitis, calicivirus, feline infectious peritonitis) vaccines that produce local immunity have been developed. These vaccines are given by the intranasal and intraocular routes. An example of a bacterial disease for which an intranasal vaccine has been developed is *Bordetella bronchiseptica*. The basis for this approach is the concept that if the vaccine is administered by the same route that natural infection takes, greater local protection will be achieved. Unfortunately, these vaccines can produce mild clinical disease.

Because of the concern of development of feline sarcomas secondary to vaccination procedures, specific guidelines have been developed for vaccinating cats. Sarcomas have been associated more with rabies and feline leukemia virus vaccines than others. The suspected incidence of vaccine-induced sarcomas is approximately 1 in 1000 to 10,000 cases per year.

The suggested route of administration of rabies and feline leukemia vaccines is to give the rabies in the right rear leg (over the tibia) and the feline leukemia vaccine over the left tibia by the subcutaneous route. In this way, if a sarcoma does develop, amputation of the limb can be done to save the cat's life.

Age of Patient

The age of the animal is important, not only because of the persistence of colostral antibodies but also because of the relative immaturity of the immune response in the puppy and kitten during the first 2 weeks of life. This phenomenon is at least partially due to the hypothermia that exists during this period. Optimal functioning of the cells of the immune system depends on a normal body temperature. A puppy given vaccination at 8, 12, and 16 weeks and a kitten given vaccination at

9 and 12 weeks should be revaccinated at 1 year of age to ensure adequate response of the immune system to the vaccine.

Nutritional Status

An animal in poor nutritional condition may not respond adequately to vaccination. Generally, caution should be exercised in giving modified live virus vaccines to debilitated animals. However, a debilitated animal should be vaccinated if it is to be hospitalized. Although there is a chance the animal may not respond to the vaccination, it is also possible that the animal will be protected from infection with a virulent organism. If a debilitated dog or cat is vaccinated, vaccination should be repeated when the patient's nutritional status has improved so that immunity is more certain.

Concurrent Disease or Therapy

Occasionally, dogs and cats presented for vaccination are incubating an infectious disease. A detailed history of possible exposure to infected animals and a complete physical examination may suggest this situation. However, it is impossible to definitively diagnose most infections in the incubation stage. If there is a history of exposure to an infected animal, the owner should be informed that there is a risk of their animal developing disease despite vaccination.

Certain infections and diseases may be associated with alteration of the immune system and may interfere with successful response to vaccination; examples include dogs infected with demodectic mange and cats infected with feline leukemia virus or feline immunodeficiency virus.

It has been suggested that certain virus vaccines may increase the susceptibility of the recipient animal to the development of the disease for which one is vaccinating against, if the animal is incubating or infected with another virus simultaneously. For example, dogs infected with the canine parvovirus that are subsequently vaccinated with a modified live distemper vaccine may be prone to develop distemper encephalitis because of infection with the parvovirus.

Modified live virus vaccines are not recommended in dogs and cats receiving immunosuppressive agents. Drugs that suppress the immune system are frequently given to animals with cancer or autoimmune diseases, such as immune-mediated hemolytic anemia. Commonly used immunosuppressive agents include cyclophosphamide, azathioprine, methotrexate, and corticosteroids. When corticosteroids are used at antiinflammatory dose levels (less than 2 mg/kg of body weight), the response to virus vaccines is not altered.

> *TECHNICIAN NOTE* Modified live virus vaccines are not recommended in dogs and cats receiving immunosuppressive agents.

Program Guidelines

When all the clinical factors discussed are considered, along with economic factors, it is safe to conclude that there is no single perfect vaccination program. Nonetheless, certain general guidelines are possible. Every veterinary hospital should establish a specific vaccination policy and protocol and adhere to it at all times. This will prevent errors of omission that could result if the vaccination policy is not clearly defined. Usually, the first vaccination should be administered when the animal is between 6 and 8 weeks of age. Animals should be revaccinated at 10 to 12 and 16 to 18 weeks of age. New vaccine guidelines recommend that revaccination should occur at 1 year of age or 1 year after the last puppy or kitten vaccine. Annual revaccination is unnecessary for most viral diseases, but for others it is of critical importance. Every 3 years vaccination is recommended for dogs and cats over 1 year of age that were properly vaccinated as puppies and kittens. Rabies vaccination could be given every 3 years as well, but must be given based on the local county regulations, which can be as often as yearly.

Vaccine Reactions

Anaphylactic reactions to vaccines can occur after vaccinations are given. Typically it will occur on the second or third vaccination in the puppy or kitten series. Severe anaphylactic reactions occur immediately and up to 30 minutes after the injection. Severe reactions cause cardiovascular shock and respiratory arrest that can lead to death if not treated immediately with intravenous (IV) corticosteroids, epinephrine, and fluids. Vomiting, diarrhea, and urticaria are early signs of a reaction and should be treated immediately with IV fluids and corticosteroids. Milder reactions of vomiting and diarrhea should be noted in the medical record as a possible vaccine reaction. In severe life-threatening reactions, the animal should never be vaccinated again. In milder cases, the animal should be premedicated with an antihistamine (diphenhydramine hydrochloride) 20 minutes before the vaccination and monitored for at least 30 minutes after the vaccination before leaving the clinic. Many puppies and kittens will be lethargic or sleep more than usual the day after their vaccinations, and this is normal. Neurologic signs such as seizure may occur in dogs within a few weeks after vaccinations and may be due to the distemper vaccine. This form of vaccine-related distemper is rarely fatal and usually resolves with treatment. Polyarthritis in cats may occur within weeks after vaccination and may be due to the calicivirus vaccine. Owners may notice a lump or hard nodule at the vaccination site, which may last for a few weeks. If it is present longer than 3 weeks, a biopsy should be taken to identify whether it is neoplasia or just a tissue inflammatory reaction.

> *TECHNICIAN NOTE* Severe reactions cause cardiovascular shock and respiratory arrest that can lead to death if not treated immediately with intravenous corticosteroids, epinephrine, and fluids.

PET-ASSOCIATED ZOONOSES

A zoonosis is a disease of animals that is transmissible to humans under natural conditions. The technician is frequently questioned by clients about the public health significance of animal diseases. Hospitalized animals may represent potential sources of zoonotic infection; thus these infections may be considered occupational diseases.

It is beyond the scope of this section to discuss all the pet-associated zoonoses, but several of the more important infections are described. It is important to stress that when questions about human medical care arise, a physician should be consulted.

Canine brucellosis rarely occurs in humans. Transmission from an infected dog to a human can occur by contact with blood, urine, semen, milk, and infected tissues. Vaginal discharges, aborted fetuses, and placental material after abortion contain large numbers of bacteria. Infection in humans can be an insidious, chronic disease that resembles infection with other strains of *Brucella,* or it can result in relatively mild flulike symptoms.

Toxoplasmosis can be acquired by human exposure to cat feces containing infective oocysts. Cats are an obligate host in the life cycle of *Toxoplasma. Toxoplasma* oocysts can remain viable in the environment for as long as 6 months under ideal conditions. The following recommendations to reduce the exposure hazard from toxoplasmosis-infected cats should be followed.

- Plastic gloves should be worn when cleaning litter pans or handling potentially contaminated soil.
- Children's sandboxes should be covered, and basic principles of sanitation should be followed.
- Immunodeficient people and women of child-bearing age should exercise extreme caution to reduce the risk of exposure.
- Women contemplating pregnancy should have their antibody status determined by a physician.

Those with a significant titer against toxoplasmosis are probably protected from reinfection. Antibody titers in cats are of little value because they indicate exposure to the organism and do not indicate that the cat is currently infected or is actively shedding infective oocysts. An enzyme-linked immunosorbent assay (ELISA), currently available through the University of Georgia and Colorado State University veterinary schools, identifies immunoglobulin M (IgM) and immunoglobulin G (IgG) antibodies in a cat's serum and may provide evidence for an acute or a recent infection in a cat. It should be stressed to the concerned client that eating raw or improperly cooked meat probably is the most common source of human toxoplasmosis.

Campylobacter and *Salmonella* are bacteria that can produce pet-associated zoonoses. Pets appear to be relatively infrequent sources of *Campylobacter*. When pets are incriminated, it is usually a stray or recently adopted puppy or kitten that has had recent diarrhea. The incidence of *Salmonella* infection acquired from pets is unknown. Animals can be asymptomatic shedders of this organism for an average of 6 weeks. Because the route of transmission is the fecal-oral route, good sanitation is important.

Reports of human leptospirosis attributed to vaccinated pets have appeared in medical literature. The *Leptospira* bacteria that are used for routine immunization may not protect against subclinical infection and shedding of the organisms in the urine. Because transmission is via infected urine, good sanitation is essential.

Visceral larva migrans and cutaneous larva migrans are caused by the migration of animal parasite larvae in human hosts. The technician plays an important role in prevention by educating clients about the risks posed by pets infected with intestinal parasites. Treatment of infected animals and reducing environmental contamination will reduce the incidence of these problems.

Plague *(Yersinia pestis)* is an infectious disease of animals that is transmitted to humans by the bite of an infected ectoparasite, usually the flea. Although the majority of cases in humans result from exposure to infected wild rodents, domestic cats have been associated with a number of infections in humans. Infections have been reported in persons employed in veterinary hospitals. Cats with suppurative lymphadenitis (infected draining lymph nodes) should be considered plague suspects, and caution should be exercised by the veterinary technician when handling exudates or treating draining wounds.

Cat-scratch disease is a disease of humans that usually is associated with cat scratches or close contact with cats. Rarely, exposure to cats has not occurred, and other injuries are incriminated, such as splinters, thorns, or dog scratches. The causative agent is *Bartonella henselae*. It is presumed that cats simply act as vectors for the disease because they are not ill. Multiple cases in the same household have occurred over a period of months or even years. In immunocompromised patients (e.g., humans infected with the human immunodeficiency virus), the disease can cause severe problems and therefore may pose a significant risk to these individuals. Usually, the disease in humans is a mild, self-limited problem.

Rabies is an acute, fatal viral disease of the central nervous system that affects all mammals. Rabies is transmitted by infected secretions, usually saliva. In the United States, the skunk and bat are the most important sources of human exposure. However, raccoons, foxes, and unimmunized dogs and cats may also represent a hazard. In most areas of the world, the dog is the most important vector of rabies.

If human exposure to rabies is suspected, a physician or public health official should be consulted immediately. Technicians should be familiar with local laws governing the handling of animals who have bitten humans. Veterinarians and technicians that have a high exposure to rabid animals should be vaccinated for rabies virus with the human vaccine and have their serum titers checked periodically to ensure adequate protection.

> *TECHNICIAN NOTE* Technicians should be familiar with local laws governing the handling of animals who have bitten humans.

Animal bites can cause serious infectious complications, including cellulitis, lymphangitis, soft tissue abscesses, osteomyelitis, meningitis, and bacteremia. Humans who have undergone splenectomy are at particular risk of bacteremia and possibly death if the organism known as DF-2, isolated from the nasal and oral secretions of healthy dogs, is inoculated into tissues by a bite. Animal bites in the veterinary hospital should be washed thoroughly with a disinfectant solution (chlorhexidine) and examined by a physician for a prescription of antibiotics.

OPHTHALMOLOGY

GLAUCOMA

Glaucoma is defined as an increase in intraocular pressure. Glaucoma may cause blindness, and there are certain breeds predisposed to primary glaucoma (Box 21-3).

The signs in early glaucoma are often subtle and can be variable. Acute glaucoma is a painful process; signs include tearing, sensitivity to bright light, and pawing at the eye. Inspection of the eye may reveal congested episcleral blood vessels, a dilated nonresponsive pupil, and a cloudy cornea. In chronic glaucoma, the major finding is an enlarged globe.

The diagnosis is made by documenting an increased intraocular pressure. Several methods are used to measure intraocular pressure. Tonometers are the most accurate, but some are expensive. The Schiotz tonometer is useful and costs approximately $300 to $400, which is well within the means of most veterinary practices (Figure 21-13). Tonopens are less cumbersome to use but can be cost prohibitive in smaller practices, costing approximately $1200.00 each (Figure 21-14).

Glaucoma is considered a medical emergency because delay in treatment may result in permanent damage to the eye. Several drugs are available to treat glaucoma, all of which work by either reducing aqueous production or increasing the opening at the drainage angle.

BOX 21-3 Breeds Predisposed to Development of Glaucoma

- Afghan
- American cocker spaniel
- Basset hound
- Beagle
- Bedlington terrier
- Brittany spaniel
- Dachshund
- Dalmatian
- English cocker spaniel
- English springer spaniel
- Fox terriers
- Great Dane
- Malamute
- Norwegian elkhound
- Saluki
- Samoyed
- Sealyham terrier
- Siberian husky
- Toy and miniature poodles

TECHNICIAN NOTE Glaucoma is considered a medical emergency because delay in treatment may result in permanent damage to the eye.

CATARACTS

A cataract is a focal or diffuse opacity within the lens and its capsule. Cataracts may be hereditary or nonhereditary. They should be differentiated from nuclear sclerosis, which is a

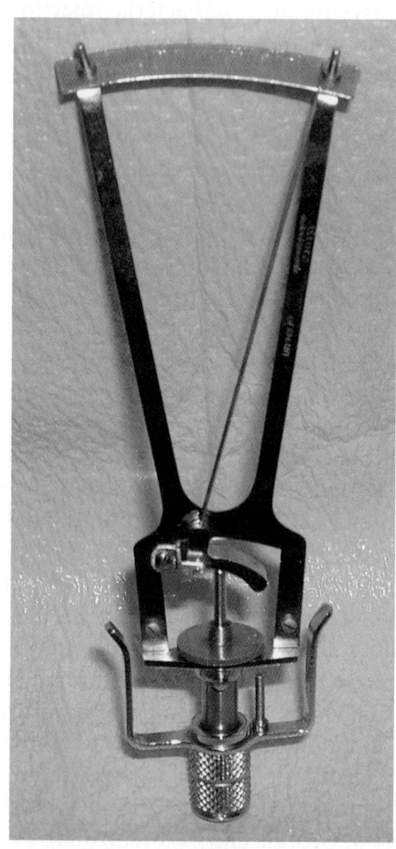

FIGURE 21-13 Tonometer (Schiotz Tonometer) used for measurement of intraocular pressure. The tonometer is placed on the cornea to obtain the pressure reading.

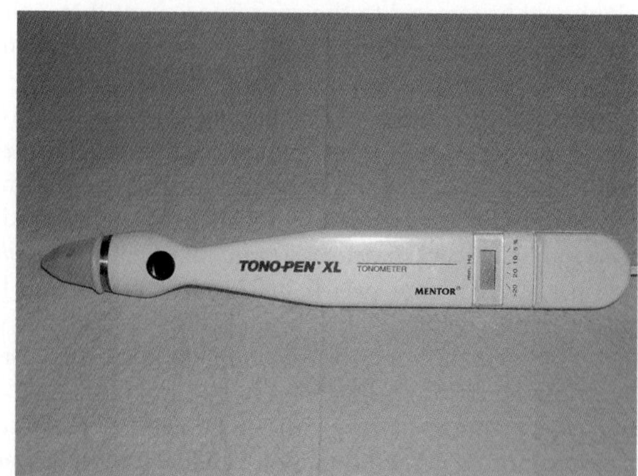

FIGURE 21-14 Tono-pen XL (Mentor) used for measure of intraocular pressure. Improved tonometer that is less cumbersome to use.

normal aging change that decreases the clarity of the nucleus of the lens.

Inherited cataracts occur in many breeds and may be associated with other eye abnormalities. Different modes of inheritance have been reported in different breeds. Breeds reported to have inherited cataracts include the beagle, German shepherd, golden retriever, Labrador retriever, Afghan hound, American cocker spaniel, Boston terrier, poodle, and miniature schnauzer. Inherited cataracts have not been reported in the cat.

Cataracts can be the result of metabolic abnormalities, such as diabetes mellitus, inflammation, or trauma. Inflammatory diseases associated with cataracts include feline infectious peritonitis, feline leukemia virus, leptospirosis, and systemic mycoses.

There is no successful medical treatment for cataracts, but any associated inflammation should be treated. Medications that dilate the pupil may be helpful in improving vision in cases of immature or hypermature cataracts. Currently, the only effective therapy for cataracts is surgical removal of the lens.

> *TECHNICIAN NOTE* Cataracts can be the result of metabolic abnormalities, such as diabetes mellitus, inflammation, or trauma.

CORNEAL ULCERS

Superficial corneal ulcers may result from trauma, decreased tear production (keratoconjunctivitis sicca), aberrant eyelashes (distichiasis, districhiasis), inward rolling of the eyelid (entropion), and inability to blink. Animals with superficial corneal ulcers experience a significant amount of pain. This pain is manifested as excessive tearing, sensitivity to bright light, and squinting (blepharospasm). Corneal ulcers are diagnosed by using fluorescein dye. Fluorescein is a water-soluble dye that will not stain the epithelial layer, but stains the underlying layers if the superficial epithelial layer is damaged.

Treatment should be directed first toward correcting the underlying cause. Once this has been accomplished, epithelialization of the ulcerated area is rapid and usually uncomplicated. Broad-spectrum antibiotics are generally used to eliminate infection. Antibiotic solutions and ointments that contain a corticosteroid should never be used with a corneal ulcer. Corticosteroids cause decreased healing with resultant deepening of the ulcer and possible corneal rupture. It has been shown that ointments may retard healing more than solutions; however, the difference in healing may not be clinically significant. One advantage to solutions is that the dose can be more easily controlled. Ophthalmic drops are applied by opening the upper and lower eyelid with one hand, tilting the patient's head slightly back, and then squeezing 1 to 2 drops of the solution into the eye with the other hand. Ophthalmic ointments are applied by the same restraint technique and then squeezing ⅛ inch of the ointment onto the cornea of the eye and then closing the eyelids shut for a moment to spread the medication. Systemic medications usually are not necessary with corneal ulcers. Occasionally, a surgical flap over the cornea or a special contact lens is necessary until epithelialization is complete.

> *TECHNICIAN NOTE* Animals with superficial corneal ulcers experience a significant amount of pain, which is manifested as excessive tearing, sensitivity to bright light, and squinting (blepharospasm).

DERMATOLOGY

Veterinary dermatology is an important part of small animal practice. Veterinary dermatology is a challenging discipline; although there are many causes of skin disease, there are only a limited number of ways in which the skin can react. Consequently, in many cases a specific etiologic diagnosis can be difficult to make.

It is beyond the scope of this chapter to consider all the common dermatologic diseases of dogs and cats.

CARDIOLOGY

CONGESTIVE HEART FAILURE

Congestive heart failure is a clinical term used to describe the state when the heart is unable to maintain adequate cardiac output. Because of decreased cardiac output, the body's tissues do not receive sufficient blood supply for normal function. The decreased cardiac output and the resultant increase in pressure within the vessels entering the heart stimulate complex compensatory mechanisms that contribute to the clinical signs of congestive heart failure. The term congestive heart failure does not indicate a specific cause.

Tachycardia and cardiomegaly (heart enlargement) are general signs associated with congestive heart failure. However, depending on the principal site of involvement, signs of left or right ventricular failure will predominate.

Left ventricular failure results from dysfunction of the left atrioventricular valve (mitral valve), ventricle, or both. Clinical signs associated with left ventricular failure include cough, exertional dyspnea, orthopnea, and at times syncope. Characteristically, early in left ventricular failure, the cough occurs in paroxysms and at night or in the early morning. The cough in left ventricular failure is usually secondary to the development of pulmonary edema or occurs because the left atrium has enlarged and compressed the left main-stem bronchus. Exertional dyspnea refers to labored breathing associated with increased activity. This may be manifested as decreased exercise tolerance or reluctance to exercise. Orthopnea means difficult or labored breathing in the recumbent position. Pulmonary edema refers to the accumulation of abnormal fluid in the interstitial spaces and alveoli of the lungs. It can be detected by auscultating rales (crackles) in the lungs or by observing the characteristic pattern on chest radiographs. Syncope, or fainting, results from decreased cardiac output to the brain.

Right ventricular failure results from a pathologic condition of the right atrioventricular valve (tricuspid valve), right ventricle, or both. Clinical signs associated with right ventricular failure include hepatic enlargement, ascites, pleural effusion, and subcutaneous edema. Increased pressure in the abdominal veins results in congestion and enlargement of the liver. Increased hydrostatic pressure in capillaries results in leakage of fluid and the subsequent development of ascites, pleural effusion, and subcutaneous edema. Subcutaneous edema is a relatively rare sign in the dog and is seen late in the course of the condition. (Box 21-4 provides a list of signs seen with left and right ventricular failure.)

Certain cardiovascular problems result in both left and right ventricular failure. Obviously, the signs described are not specific for heart disease. Consequently, when evaluating a patient for cough or ascites, the conditions to rule out should include noncardiac problems.

> *TECHNICIAN NOTE* Tachycardia and cardiomegaly (heart enlargement) are general signs associated with congestive heart failure.

MITRAL INSUFFICIENCY

Mitral insufficiency resulting from chronic mitral (left atrioventricular) valvular fibrosis is the most frequently diagnosed form of heart disease in the dog. It is followed in prevalence by chronic tricuspid (right atrioventricular) valvular fibrosis, which causes tricuspid insufficiency. Valvular insufficiency is a term used to indicate functional incompetence (leakage) of the valve with subsequent regurgitation (backward flow) of blood from the ventricle into the atrium during ventricular systole.

The signs associated with chronic mitral insufficiency are those of left ventricular failure (e.g., cough, exertional dyspnea, pulmonary edema). The specific cause of mitral valvular fibrosis is unknown; however, it appears to be associated with aging. Certain breeds appear to be predisposed, the majority of these being small breeds of dogs (e.g., miniature poodles). Mitral insufficiency as a cause of left ventricular failure is much less common in the cat. The diagnosis of chronic mitral insufficiency is based on the clinical history, auscultation of the heart and lungs, thoracic radiography, and electrocardiography. Although the traditional treatment for this condition has included the use of cardiac glycosides (e.g., digoxin), recent evidence indicates that cardiac contractility is normal to increased in the majority of these dogs, and therefore digoxin is not indicated until late in the course of the failure state.

Initially, the use of diuretics such as furosemide (Lasix), a sodium-restricted diet, and exercise restriction are the primary mode of therapy. Treatment with vasodilators, such as hydralazine (Apresoline), captopril (Capoten), and enalapril (Enacard), is also beneficial. These drugs work by decreasing the resistance against which the heart has to pump.

BOX 21-4 Clinical Signs of Left and Right Ventricular Failure

Left Congestive Signs

- Pulmonary congestion and edema resulting in cough, tachypnea, dyspnea, orthopnea, pulmonary crackles, tiring, hemoptysis, cyanosis
- Secondary right ventricular failure
- Cardiac arrhythmias

Right Congestive Signs

- Systemic venous congestion: high central venous pressure (CVP), jugular vein distention
- Liver and spleen enlargement
- Fluid in chest cavity (pleural effusion) causing dyspnea, orthopnea, and cyanosis
- Fluid in abdominal cavity (ascites)
- Subcutaneous edema
- Fluid in pericardial sac (pericardial effusion)

HEARTWORM DISEASE

Information on the life cycle and diagnostic procedures can be found in Chapter 17, Parasitology.

The treatment of heartworm disease can be divided into three phases. The first phase is to kill the adult heartworms (adulticidal therapy) that are present in the heart and blood vessels. The next phase is to eradicate the circulating microfilariae (microfilaricidal therapy). Finally, preventive medication (prophylactic therapy) is administered to those dogs at risk of developing heartworm disease. This would include any dog residing in or traveling to an endemic area.

Adulticide therapy consists of administering melarsomine dihydrochloride (Immiticide, Merial). It is an arsenical compound given by intramuscular injection into the epaxial muscles in the lumbar region. Two treatments are given 24 hours apart. If needed, a second treatment can be given 4 months later. In the clinically ill dogs, treatment to stabilize the disease is given, and then at a later date, the patient is treated with adulticide in two stages. One injection is given and then 1 month later two injections are given 24 hours apart. This allows a slower kill of heartworms with less chance of pulmonary reaction to dying worms.

The adult heartworms will die slowly over a 2- to 3-week period. Fever, coughing, and, in more severe cases, dyspnea and hemoptysis (coughing up blood) are the signs observed as the worms die and pass to the lungs (pulmonary thromboembolism). Prednisone therapy (1 mg/kg) is the accepted therapy for pulmonary thromboembolism. Administration of aspirin therapy (5 mg/kg once daily) is recommended in dogs with moderate to severe heart-worm disease to reduce thromboembolism. It may be started 1 week before treatment and continued for 4 to 6 weeks after treatment.

To minimize the development of clinical pulmonary thromboembolism, it is important to restrict exercise for 3 to 4 weeks after completion of adulticide therapy. If the signs associated with pulmonary thromboembolism are severe, hospitalization and the administration of bronchodilators, antiinflammatory drugs, and antibiotics are recommended. DIC may occur in dogs with severe clinical signs. Treatment of advanced DIC is usually unsuccessful.

Microfilaricidal therapy is begun 3 weeks after adulticide therapy. Ivermectin (Ivomec), 50 mg/kg orally once, is the current accepted method of treatment for microfilaria, even though it is not approved by the U.S. Food and Drug Administration (FDA) for this function.

Heartworm disease may be prevented with the use of one of several products. Some of these also have protective activity against some endoparasites. Table 21-5 lists the products currently available for heartworm prevention in the dog.

TABLE 21-5 Currently Available Heartworm Preventives

Ingredients	Company	Antiparasitic activity
Heartgard		
Ivermectin	Merial	Heartworm prevention
Heartgard-30 Plus		
Ivermectin Pyrantel pamoate	Merial	Heartworm prevention Roundworms Hookworms
Heartgard for Cats		
Ivermectin	Merial	Heartworm prevention Hookworms
Interceptor		
Milbemycin oxime	Novartis	Heartworm prevention Roundworms Hookworms Whipworms
ProHeart 6*		
Moxidection	Fort Dodge	Heartworm prevention Hookworms
Sentinel		
Milbemycin oxime Lufenuron	Novartis	Heartworm prevention Fleas Roundworms Hookworms Whipworms
Revolution (Dogs and Cats)		
Selamectin (topical)	Pfizer	Heartworm prevention Fleas *Otodectes cynotis* Ticks Roundworms Hookworms Sarcoptic mange
Advantix Multi (Dogs and Cats)		
Imidacloprid Moxidectin		Heartworm prevention Fleas *Otodectes cynotis* Roundworms Hookworms Whipworms (dogs)

*Injection given every 6 months.

Feline heartworm disease is far less common than canine heartworm disease due to dogs being the natural host for heartworms. In endemic areas, occasionally cats are infected with heartworms. Clinical signs differ from the dog with mild reactions causing occasional vomiting. Severe reactions cause severe respiratory distress because of pulmonary thromboembolism. Most cats with the severe form do not survive. If they do survive, they are treated with corticosteroids for pulmonary thromboembolism and oxygen, and then put on feline heartworm prevention to prevent further infections in the future (see Table 21-5). Currently, there are no safe and effective treatments to eliminate heartworms in the cat. Because the cat is not the natural host, the worms die over a 2- to 3-year period as compared with a 5- to 7-year period in the dog. Preventing further infection during this time may allow the cat to become heartworm free. Diagnosing heartworm infections in the cat is much more difficult than in the dog because of the lower number of worms infecting the cat. In-house antigen tests used in the dog are usually not sensitive enough to pick up antigen in the cat. Thoracic radiographs, angiography, positive antibody titer, and clinical signs are used to diagnose feline heartworm disease.

CARDIOMYOPATHY

Cardiomyopathy is a general term that merely indicates that the basic pathologic lesion involves the heart muscle. Cardiomyopathies can be primary or secondary. Primary cardiomyopathies indicate that the myocardial disease is not due to any recurrent or preexisting cardiovascular or systemic disease. Primary cardiomyopathies in cats are further subdivided into hypertrophic, dilated, and restrictive forms. Secondary cardiomyopathies in dogs and cats are less frequent and are the result of diseases such as infection, metabolic disorders (e.g., uremia), endocrine problems (e.g., hyperthyroidism), and infiltrative processes (e.g., neoplasia).

Feline Cardiomyopathy

Hypertrophic cardiomyopathy is characterized by increased thickness of the myocardium and a small left ventricular lumen. Clinical signs are seen in middle-aged cats of all breeds. The most prominent sign is the sudden development of respiratory distress secondary to pulmonary edema. Hind-limb paresis (weakness) and severe pain may also be present. These hind-limb signs are caused by aortic thromboembolism (blood clots) disrupting the blood supply to the hind limbs. This problem can usually be diagnosed easily if femoral pulses are found to be poor or absent. Diagnosis of cardiomyopathy is based on history, physical examination, radiography, electrocardiography, and echocardiography. If echocardiography is not available, nonselective angiocardiography may be necessary for diagnosis. The basic initial therapeutic approach may include diuretics (e.g., Lasix, Hoechst-Roussel Pharmaceuticals), cage rest, oxygen therapy, β-adrenergic blockers such as propranolol (Inderal,

Ayerst Laboratories), and calcium channel blockers such as diltiazem hydrochloride (Cardizem, Marion Merrell Dow). Long-term management consists of diuretics, beta blockers, calcium channel blockers, a sodium-restricted diet (feline H/D, Hill's), aspirin, and restricted activity. Aspirin is used to reduce the likelihood of aortic thromboembolism.

> *TECHNICIAN NOTE* Hypertrophic cardiomyopathy is characterized by increased thickness of the myocardium and a small left ventricular lumen.

Dilated cardiomyopathy is characterized by extreme ventricular dilation and moderate atrial enlargement. This results in impaired pump function of the ventricle. This type of cardiomyopathy is also known as congestive cardiomyopathy. Signs of right ventricular failure usually predominate. In addition, cats may show a gradual onset of lethargy and anorexia and at times may be brought in dehydrated, hypothermic, and in cardiovascular shock. Respiratory distress secondary to pleural effusion and aortic thromboembolism resulting in hind-limb paresis is also occasionally seen. The basic therapeutic approach is to mechanically remove as much fluid as possible from the pleural cavity (thoracocentesis), administer digitalis (digoxin therapy), and administer diuretics. Aspirin is used as a preventive measure against aortic thromboembolism. Vasodilators, such as nitroglycerin ointment (Nitrol ointment, Kremers-Urban Co.), may have a role in the management of dilated cardiomyopathy.

Some cats with dilated cardiomyopathy have low plasma taurine levels, and cardiac function will increase with oral taurine supplementation of 250 to 500 mg daily. Cardiac function usually improves over a period of months, and if cats are placed on a diet containing ample taurine, cardiac drugs and taurine supplementation may eventually be discontinued. It should be stated that because this association of low taurine levels and cardiomyopathy in the cat has been made, almost all commercial and prescription diets have adequate levels of taurine, so low-taurine dilated cardiomyopathy is much less common than it used to be.

Restrictive cardiomyopathy is the least common form of primary feline cardiomyopathy. A synonym is endomyocardial fibrosis. Respiratory distress is the most common clinical sign. Diagnosis is similar to the other forms of primary cardiomyopathy. Response to therapy is generally poor.

Canine Cardiomyopathy

Primary cardiomyopathies in the dog are categorized as dilated (congestive), boxer cardiomyopathy, Doberman pinscher cardiomyopathy, and hypertrophic cardiomyopathy.

Dilated cardiomyopathy is most common in large and giant breed male dogs aged 4 to 6 years; however, English and American cocker spaniels are smaller-breed dogs that may be affected. Presenting signs often include weakness, lethargy, respiratory distress, cough, anorexia, weight loss, and possibly ascites and syncope. The left ventricle and atrium are dilated with decreased contractility. Diagnosis is confirmed by physical examination, radiography, electrocardiography, and echocardiography. Treatment consists of diuretics, a low sodium diet, arteriolar dilators, and positive inotropes, such as cardiac glycosides (digitalis, digoxin). The long-term prognosis is guarded in that most dogs with the dilated form of cardiomyopathy have an average life span of 6 to 8 months after the diagnosis has been made.

> *TECHNICIAN NOTE* Dilated cardiomyopathy is primarily a disease of large and giant purebred dogs, although medium-sized breeds, such as English and American cocker spaniels, are being diagnosed with increasing frequency with this acquired heart disease.

A specific cardiomyopathy occurs in boxers. These dogs may be asymptomatic or have syncope and episodic weakness. Arrhythmias are common and may cause sudden death. Diagnosis is confirmed by the same methods as those used in dogs with dilated cardiomyopathy. Treatment with diuretics and antiarrhythmics, such as propranolol, may be useful; however, prognosis is still poor.

Doberman pinschers may have a primary cardiomyopathy that is similar to congestive or dilated cardiomyopathy. Ventricular contractility is often severely compromised, and atrial arrhythmias are common. These dogs are often in fulminant congestive heart failure and require supportive care with oxygen, diuretics, positive inotropes, and vasodilators. Prognosis is poor.

Hypertrophic cardiomyopathy is the most uncommon primary cardiomyopathy in the dog. It is most often seen in German shepherd dogs and other large breeds. Presenting signs are referable to cardiac disease, and sudden death may occur. Treatment with diuretics and propranolol may improve cardiac output and clinical signs.

ENDOCRINOLOGY

Canine hyperadrenocorticism (Cushing syndrome) is a disorder that results from the excessive production of cortisol by the adrenal cortex. The clinical signs of canine hyperadrenocorticism include polyuria, polydipsia, abdominal distention, polyphagia, muscular weakness, dermatologic changes, and reproductive problems (anestrus, testicular atrophy). Cushing syndrome can result from excessive production of adrenocorticotropic hormone (ACTH) by the pituitary gland (pituitary-dependent hyperadrenocorticism) or from a functional tumor of the adrenal cortex. Pituitary-dependent hyperadrenocorticism is by far the most common, comprising approximately 80% of the cases. Diagnosis is based on measurements of the plasma cortisol levels after stimulation with ACTH or suppression with dexamethasone. Treatment is different for these two conditions. If a functional adrenal tumor is present, the recommended treatment is surgical removal. The drug used to treat Cushing syndrome caused by excessive ACTH production is mitotane (Lysodren, Bristol Laboratories). Side effects associated with the use of mitotane include anorexia, lethargy, vomiting, and depression.

Hyperadrenocorticism is rare in the cat and usually is suspected because of the secondary consequences of the disease such as insulin resistance in a cat being treated for diabetes mellitus. Although there is much less known about this disease in the cat, diagnosis is similar to the dog. Treatment at this time is surgical removal of the adrenal glands. Medical therapy has not been as effective in the cat.

Canine hypoadrenocorticism (Addison's disease) is caused by a lack of glucocorticoid and/or mineralocorticoid levels and activity. It is generally seen in the middle-aged female, and the most common signs are gastrointestinal (vomiting, anorexia), weakness, depression, and collapse. These signs may have a waxing-waning course.

In an acute crisis these patients may present in acute collapse and in hypovolemic shock. The classic laboratory abnormalities are a low serum sodium (Na^+) level and a high serum potassium (K^+) level, resulting in a low Na^+/K^+ ratio (usually less than 25:1). These patients may also be azotemic and have a low urine specific gravity, which could be confused with renal failure.

The most accurate means of diagnosis is to perform an ACTH stimulation test and show that the patient has a very poor response to this drug because cortisol levels will not increase following ACTH administration.

The treatment consists of aggressive isotonic saline fluid therapy and supplementation with glucocorticoid and mineralocorticoid therapy. Prednisolone sodium succinate and desoxycorticosterone are the glucocorticoid and mineralocorticoid used to treat this disease. Addison's disease in the cat has not been reported.

HYPOGLYCEMIA

Canine hypoglycemia is a clinical problem associated with a variety of diseases rather than a specific diagnosis itself. The signs associated with hypoglycemia include weakness of the rear legs, generalized weakness, focal or diffuse muscle twitching, incoordination, blindness, generalized seizures, and behavioral changes. These behavioral changes include aggressive behavior and anxiety as evidenced by incessant running, barking, and loss of bowel and bladder control. These signs tend to be episodic, regardless of the cause of hypoglycemia. Hypoglycemia should be considered a differential diagnosis in any dog that is having seizures or is comatose.

The first step in evaluating a patient with suspected hypoglycemia is to verify or document that hypoglycemia exists. Improper handling of blood samples may result in falsely low blood glucose levels. The blood glucose level can be lowered if the serum is not removed from the clot or if the specimen is stored at room temperature for a prolonged period. It is preferable to remove serum from the clot within 10 to 15 minutes of drawing the blood sample. If this cannot be done, use of sodium fluoride tubes may be helpful.

Once hypoglycemia has been verified, the signalment, history, clinical findings, and further laboratory tests may be needed to reduce the long and rather diverse list of conditions that may cause hypoglycemia. Functional β-cell tumors (insulinomas of the pancreas), nonpancreatic tumors, hypoglycemia-ketonemia in pregnant bitches, glycogen storage diseases, septic shock, liver failure, juvenile and neonatal hypoglycemia, canine parvoviral diarrhea, and excessive insulin administration in diabetic patients are all examples of diseases that can cause hypoglycemia.

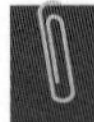

TECHNICIAN NOTE Improper handling of blood samples may result in falsely low blood glucose levels.

HYPOTHYROIDISM AND HYPERTHYROIDISM

Hypothyroidism is one of the most common endocrine disorders in the dog, but it is rare in the cat. Some of the common clinical signs include oily seborrhea, alopecia, thickened skin, weight gain, constipation, lethargy, and cold intolerance. There are some breeds with an apparent increased incidence of hypothyroidism (Box 21-5). The thyroid-stimulating hormone (TSH) stimulation test used to be the most accurate diagnostic test. TSH is no longer readily available; therefore a combination of three tests (total T_4, free T_4, and TSH levels) is used to diagnose the routine hypothyroid patient. Treatment of hypothyroidism consists of supplementation with thyroxine (T_4).

Hyperthyroidism is the most common endocrinopathy affecting cats older than 5 years of age, but it is rare in the dog. The most common clinical signs of hyperthyroidism are weight loss despite a good appetite, restlessness, hyperactivity, and diarrhea. In many cases, a thyroid nodule can be palpated in the ventrocervical region of the neck. The diagnosis can usually be confirmed by documenting an elevated serum T_4 level. Treatment may consist of medical therapy with

BOX 21-5 Breeds With an Apparent Increased Incidence of Hypothyroidism

- Afghan hound
- Airedale
- Beagle
- Boxer
- Brittany spaniel
- Chow chow
- Cocker spaniel
- Dachshund
- Doberman pinscher
- English bulldog
- Golden retriever
- Great Dane
- Irish setter
- Irish wolfhound
- Malamute
- Miniature schnauzer
- Newfoundland
- Pomeranian
- Poodle
- Shetland sheepdog

methimazole (Tapazole, Eli Lilly and Co.), surgical removal of the thyroid nodule, and/or radioactive iodine (^{131}I).

> *TECHNICIAN NOTE* Hyperthyroidism is the most common endocrinopathy affecting cats older than 5 years of age, but it is rare in the dog.

DIABETES MELLITUS

Diabetes mellitus is seen in the older dog and cat, and it is more common in the female dog and the male cat. Common clinical signs include excessive water intake (polydipsia), large volumes of urine (polyuria), weight loss in spite of a good appetite, and rapidly developing lens opacities (cataracts) in the dog. If the dog or cat is ketoacidotic, then weakness, vomiting, depression, and, possibly, coma may develop. The diagnosis of diabetes mellitus is made by documenting hyperglycemia, glucosuria, and, if the animal is ketoacidotic, ketonuria or ketonemia.

The technician's role in the treatment of patients with this endocrinopathy is twofold: (1) management of the ill ketoacidotic diabetic animal in the hospital and (2) education of clients concerning home management and treatment of their pets.

The ketoacidotic diabetic patient represents a true challenge for the veterinarian and technician alike, and it is important that they work in unison so that optimal patient care is achieved. The technician's role involves close monitoring of vital signs, ensuring fluids are given at the proper rate, frequent blood glucose determinations, and administering short-acting (regular/crystalline) insulin (see Table 21-6 for types of insulin). Because the ketoacidotic patient requires such close monitoring, the technician plays a major role in the minute-to-minute and hour-to-hour evaluation of the patient, so minor changes in the patient's condition can be recognized early and the veterinarian be informed. Because of the complexity of the ketoacidotic diabetic patient, all these functions should be done under the direct supervision of a veterinarian.

The second aspect of diabetic management involves the instruction of the client concerning home management of the pet. This can be a time-consuming function, and the technician who has a good understanding of diabetes management can be a tremendous asset to the veterinarian. Examples of areas in which the client should be instructed and/or shown include how to mix the insulin, read the syringes, draw up the insulin into the syringe, give the subcutaneous injection, and read urine test strips for urine glucose measurement. Having the owner practice giving injections to the pet by drawing up sterile saline in the syringe and giving saline injections is extremely helpful to the hesitant owner. In addition, the client needs to be instructed (1) about the type of diet to be fed and how much and when to feed, (2) not to give the insulin if the pet does not eat in the morning, and (3) to give the animal Karo syrup orally and call the hospital immediately if the pet has a seizure. All these items can be compiled into a handout that the technician can develop with the aid of the veterinarian. This handout can then be given to the client, who can refer to it as needed at home.

TABLE 21-6 Types of Insulin Used in Dogs and Cats

Route of Administration	Onset of Effect	Duration of Effect
Regular Crystalline		
IV	Immediate	1-4 hr (d&c)
IM	10-30 min	3-8 hr (d&c)
SC	10-30 min	4-10 hr (d&c)
NPH		
SC	30 min-2 hr	6-18 hr (d); 4-12 hr (c)
Vetsulin		
SC	4 hr, 11 hr	14-24 hr (d)
Glargine		
SC	1-4 hr	10-16 hr (c)

THERIOGENOLOGY

POSTPARTUM DISORDERS IN THE BITCH

The postpartum bitch may be brought to an animal hospital for a variety of serious problems after whelping. These problems include mastitis, metritis, and eclampsia. Mastitis refers to inflammation of one or more mammary glands. In severe cases, affected glands are hot and painful, and the patient is systemically ill. Bitches with septic mastitis are depressed, anorectic, and reluctant to care for the puppies. In less severe cases, the bitch may not be symptomatic; however, the puppies may fail to gain weight or may show signs of septicemia. Systemic antibiotics are used to treat mastitis. Because the affected glands produce abnormal milk, and the antibiotics excreted in the milk may be harmful to the puppies, it is recommended that the puppies be hand fed.

Severe mastitis may progress to abscess formation or gangrenous mastitis. Surgical drainage and treatment may be required in these cases.

Stasis of milk in the mammary glands can occasionally result in enlarged, painful mammary glands. Galactostasis may be observed during pseudopregnancy or at the time of weaning when the body is attempting to resorb milk. Unlike mastitis, dogs with galactostasis are not systemically ill. Treatment consists of application of cool towels and compresses to decrease inflammation. Care should be taken not to massage the glands because this can stimulate additional milk letdown.

Metritis is a uterine disease of the immediate postpartum period. Signs usually develop within the first week of whelping. Metritis is associated with retained placentae, retained fetuses, and dystocia. Clinical signs suggestive of metritis include fever, depression, and reduced interest in the puppies. A foul-smelling, brown or reddish-brown vaginal discharge may be present; the normal discharge after whelping is nonodorous and greenish. The diagnosis is based on history, clinical findings, and laboratory results. Laboratory tests that are useful include vaginal cytologic studies, CBCs, and bacterial cultures.

Initial therapy consists of replacing fluid deficits, treating shock, if present, and initiating antibiotic therapy after cultures have been obtained. Medical drainage of the uterus can be attempted in valuable breeding bitches. In severe cases, ovariohysterectomy may be indicated to save the bitch's life.

Hypocalcemia (eclampsia) usually occurs 2 to 3 weeks postpartum in small bitches with large litters but occasionally can occur before birth. Presenting signs include weakness and trembling and may proceed to tonic convulsions. The temperature is usually elevated during convulsions.

Diagnosis is based on clinical signs in a lactating female and low serum calcium levels. Treatment includes preventing the puppies from nursing on the dam, giving the dam intravenous 10% calcium gluconate, and ensuring the dam receives oral calcium lactate or calcium gluconate and vitamin D at home. The puppies are hand fed with nursing bottles and milk replacer until 4 weeks old. It is highly recommended that the dam have an ovariohysterectomy because of the high recurrence rate of eclampsia. See Chapter 14 for additional information on animal reproduction.

> *TECHNICIAN NOTE* The diagnosis of eclampsia is based on clinical signs in a lactating female and low serum calcium levels.

CANINE BRUCELLOSIS

Canine brucellosis is primarily an infection of the reproductive tract, although other organ systems may be involved. *Brucella canis* also has been isolated from dogs with discospondylitis and chronic recurrent fever. Brucellosis is a frequent cause of infertility and other reproductive problems in both males and females.

Definitive diagnosis requires demonstration of the organism by a culture of blood or body fluid. Serologic tests can be diagnostic as well. The rapid slide agglutination test is an easy, readily available test; however, false-positive results occur. The rapid slide agglutination can be used as a screen, with positive tests being confirmed using an alternative technique (e.g., agar gel immunodiffusion).

The mode of transmission is venereal. However, infection can also result from the ingestion of infected material, for example, aborted fetuses, placentae, and vaginal discharge. Because of these means of spread, brucellosis can quickly become a kennelwide problem.

Although a variety of antibiotic combinations have been recommended, therapeutic success cannot be guaranteed. After antibiotic therapy, some dogs will continue to harbor the organism and represent a risk to other dogs. Canine brucellosis is considered a possible zoonotic disease. For these reasons, some experts advocate removal of all infected dogs from the premises. Other experts feel that this position is extreme and instead recommend castration or ovariohysterectomy and antibiotic therapy for infected pet dogs.

Because treatment is not always successful, prevention is emphasized. All dogs should be tested before breeding or before introduction into a kennel.

PYOMETRITIS (PYOMETRA)

Pyometritis is a uterine disease that occurs during the luteal (approximately 1 to 2 months after estrus) phase of the reproductive cycle. It occurs in both bitches and queens. Pyometritis may be part of a complex that initially starts with cystic changes in the endometrium and endometrial hyperplasia. Prior estrogen therapy may predispose to pyometritis (see also Chapter 14).

Clinical signs are variable. A vaginal discharge may or may not be present, but, if present, the color of the discharge can be green, yellow, or reddish brown. Bitches with pyometritis frequently will be polydipsic and polyuric. Affected animals can be severely depressed and septic or clinically normal.

An enlarged uterus on radiographs and leukocytosis with a left shift are considered diagnostic. Fluid therapy to correct fluid and electrolyte deficits followed by emergency ovariohysterectomy is the treatment of choice in nonbreeding animals. In valuable breeding bitches, medical treatment with prostaglandin F_{2a} has been advocated to preserve the breeding life of the patient. Treatment with prostaglandin F_{2a} is expensive and potentially dangerous; therefore it should be strictly reserved for dogs of significant breeding value.

CANINE PROSTATIC DISEASE

Prostatic disease is occasionally seen in older intact male dogs. Clinical signs include straining to urinate (stranguria), painful urination (dysuria), blood in the urine (hematuria), and/or difficulty in defecation. The conditions that affect the prostate include benign prostatic hyperplasia, bacterial prostatitis, prostatic abscess, prostatic cyst, and prostatic neoplasia.

The following noninvasive techniques are used to evaluate the prostate: rectal palpation, routine radiology, sonography (ultrasound), urethrography, cytologic studies, and bacterial cultures of prostatic washes or the prostatic fraction of the ejaculate. Frequently it is difficult to differentiate neoplasia, infection, and hyperplasia with these noninvasive techniques. Consequently, surgical exploration and biopsy may be required to establish a definitive diagnosis.

Treatment varies, depending on the specific process. Dogs with benign prostatic hyperplasia respond to castration. Although estrogen therapy reduces the size of the prostate in benign prostatic hyperplasia, it is not recommended because of possible adverse reactions. Finasteride (Proscar, Merck & Co., Inc.) has been shown to be an effective medical treatment for reduction of prostatomegaly secondary to benign prostatic hyperplasia. Prostatic abscesses and cysts require surgical drainage. Bacterial prostatitis and prostatic abscesses are treated with antibiotics. Prostatic neoplasia is generally highly malignant, and treatment is directed toward palliation rather than cure. Some dogs with prostatic cancer may benefit from castration because the tumors possess testosterone receptors.

GASTROENTEROLOGY

ACUTE GASTROENTERITIS

Acute gastroenteritis is one of the more common problems seen in canine practice. Some examples of conditions that may cause this problem include dietary indiscretion, viral gastroenteritis, bacterial gastroenteritis, gastrointestinal foreign bodies, gastrointestinal parasites, intussusception, ingestion of toxins, acute pancreatitis, and hypoadrenocorticism. The clinical history, signalment, and physical examination may suggest the diagnosis. Frequently, response to symptomatic therapy is used to assess whether further diagnostic study is warranted. The intensity and degree of symptomatic and supportive care are determined by the severity of clinical signs.

> *TECHNICIAN NOTE* Acute gastroenteritis is one of the more common problems seen in canine practice.

The fundamental decision of whether to hospitalize the patient is based on a number of factors; they include the hydration status of the dog, severity and frequency of vomiting and diarrhea, presence or absence of blood in the vomitus or stool, and presence of fever or profound lethargy. Non–patient-related factors to be considered include the client's ability to provide adequate care for the patient at home and ability of the client to pay for hospitalized care.

Clinical management of outpatients consists primarily of dietary restriction, administration of locally acting gastrointestinal medications, and use of fluid therapy when indicated. Dietary restriction is the most important aspect of the symptomatic care of acute gastroenteritis. The objective is to rest the gastrointestinal tract. This is accomplished by withholding all food for 12 to 24 hours, depending on the details of the case. If vomiting is severe, water is also withheld. If diarrhea is present and vomiting has not occurred, warm electrolyte-containing solutions can be given by mouth. During this period of symptomatic therapy, it is imperative that the patient be observed closely to prevent ingestion of foreign material and detect any worsening of clinical signs.

After food has been withheld for the prescribed period, small, frequent, bland meals should be offered. These meals should be low in fat, low in fiber, and easily digested and absorbed. These criteria are met by prescription diets, such as Prescription Diet I-D (Hill's), and by homemade diets, such as cottage cheese and boiled rice. These diets should be warmed before feeding. These frequent, small, bland meals should be continued for 2 to 3 days. If the patient is doing well, the regular diet and feeding schedule can be gradually reintroduced over the next 3 to 5 days. If clinical signs recur during this process, the dog should be reevaluated. Further diagnosis, evaluation, and more intensive supportive therapy may be warranted.

Although a vast number of locally acting preparations are available for the treatment of acute gastroenteritis, most have not been proved effective in controlled clinical trials. An over-the-counter preparation containing bismuth subsalicylate (Pepto-Bismol) has been shown to shorten the duration of symptoms in humans with experimental viral enteritis. It is theorized that the beneficial response is not due to the coating action of the product but rather to the salicylate inhibiting prostaglandin synthesis. Prostaglandins play a role in diarrhea by affecting both motility and secretory activity of the gastrointestinal tract. The technician should be aware that Pepto-Bismol may cause the stool to be dark to black, giving the false impression that melena is present when it is not.

> *TECHNICIAN NOTE* Pepto-Bismol causes the stool to be colored black and therefore should not be confused with melena.

In animals that are slightly to mildly dehydrated, some form of fluid therapy is appropriate. Fluids can be administered by mouth if the patient is not vomiting. Commercial water and electrolyte solutions, such as Gatorade, can be used to restore hydration and correct electrolyte imbalances. Alternatively, a homemade solution can be prepared inexpensively. One formula that has been recommended consists of 3.5 g of sodium chloride, 2.5 g of sodium bicarbonate, 1.5 g of potassium chloride, and 20 g of glucose added to 1 L of water. Approximately 13.6 ml/kg/day of this solution will meet the maintenance requirements of the patient.

If the dog is mildly to moderately dehydrated or is vomiting, subcutaneous fluid is indicated. Lactated Ringer's solution or Normosol are the fluid of choice. If signs have been prolonged, the lactated Ringer's solution can be supplemented with potassium chloride. Generally, the dose of subcutaneous fluid is 4.5 to 9.0 ml/kg of body weight administered at multiple sites. This can be repeated if necessary.

Client education is an essential part of the symptomatic care for acute gastroenteritis. The client should be informed that a definitive diagnosis has not been established and that merely the symptoms are being treated. If the animal is getting worse or if the signs persist longer than 36 to 48 hours, the animal should be reevaluated. The technician should have a concerned, caring attitude during the outpatient visit so that if signs persist, the client will not hesitate to return or call for additional help. In many practices, it is standard procedure to telephone the client to receive follow-up progress reports. This ensures close client contact and thus improves the chances of successful management of the problem.

> *TECHNICIAN NOTE* Client education is an essential part of the symptomatic care for acute gastroenteritis.

If initial clinical signs are severe or there is no response to symptomatic therapy, hospitalization is necessary. A major indication for hospitalization is the need for intravenous fluid therapy. Details about intravenous fluid therapy have been discussed.

Medications that alter the motility of the gastrointestinal tract may be indicated in cases of severe gastroenteritis. Improved understanding of the pathophysiology of intestinal motility has resulted in the more rational use of medications that are used to symptomatically treat vomiting and diarrhea. Anticholinergics cause hypomotility of the intestines and thus are of questionable efficacy in treating diarrhea. Antispasmodics are of minimal benefit as well.

Narcotics and narcotic-like drugs increase the rhythmic segmental contractions of the bowel, slow the passage of ingesta, and thus help to control diarrhea. These drugs should be used cautiously because of potential problems. Generally, they are reserved for more chronic or severe cases that are unresponsive to conservative therapy. A major disadvantage of the narcotic derivatives is that they can cause central nervous system depression. The decreased ingesta flow rate may result in increased absorption of toxins and altered bacterial flora in the gut. These compounds are contraindicated in the presence of intestinal obstruction.

Drugs used for the treatment of acute vomiting can be divided into several categories (Box 21-6).

Drugs used to decrease gastric acidity include antihistamines or H_2 blockers, such as cimetidine (Tagamet, SK&F Lab Co.), ranitidine (Zantac,) and famotidine (Pepcid AC). Antacids do not decrease the secretion of acid; however, they neutralize the acid that is produced. Antacids must be given frequently because their duration of action is brief. Paradoxically, if antacids are not given frequently, total daily acid secretion increases. Antacids administered according to a schedule of two or three times per day are probably of no value and may, in fact, be harmful. In most practices, more frequent administration is not practical. Antidopaminergic drugs such as metoclopramide (Reglan) inhibit vomiting at the vomiting center in the central nervous system. Metoclopramide is contraindicated in intestinal obstruction because of its prokinetic or motility-stimulating activity. Phenothiazine-derivative tranquilizers, such as chlorpromazine, also work on the vomiting center of the central nervous system. These drugs are effective at controlling vomiting at much lower doses than the usual tranquilizer doses. These agents should be used with caution in dehydrated patients because of their blood pressure-lowering effects. Other antihistamines such as Dramamine act by inhibiting a neural center involved in vomiting called the chemoreceptor trigger zone. Vomiting induced by certain drugs, such as digoxin, is mediated by this center. Vomiting caused by motion sickness or vertigo may also respond to drugs in this group. Box 21-7 lists drugs used commonly for acute gastrointestinal disease.

When the patient has improved, oral fluid and frequent, small, bland meals can be instituted. After discharge from the hospital, the dog can be treated as already described under outpatient management.

CANINE VIRAL ENTERITIS

The most important cause of viral enteritis in the dog is canine parvovirus. Other viral agents can occasionally produce gastroenteritis; they include canine distemper and canine rotavirus.

Clinical signs vary from subtle lethargy and anorexia to severe, rapidly fatal hemorrhagic gastroenteritis. Dogs of any age can be affected; however, the more severe cases typically occur between 6 and 20 weeks of age. On physical examination, the pups are usually febrile, depressed, and dehydrated. Vomiting or diarrhea may be observed. The stool may be

BOX 21-6 Drugs Used for Acute Vomiting

Dopamine Antagonists
Metoclopramide (Reglan)
Domperidone

Serotonin Antagonists
Ondansetron (Zofran)
Dolasetron (Anzemet)

Neurokinin Receptor Antagonist
Maropitant (Cerenia)

Phenothiazines
Chlorpromazine (Thorazine)
Prochlorperazine
Darbazine (prochlorperazine, isopropamide)
Tigan (trimethobenzamide)

Antihistamines
Cyclizine hydrochloride
Diphenhydramine hydrochloride (Benadryl)
Dimenhydrinate (Dramamine)
Meclizine hydrochloride (Bonine)
Trifluoperazine

BOX 21-7 Commonly Used Drugs for Acute Gastroenteritis

Narcotics
Diphenoxylate and atropine (Lomotil)
Loperamide (Imodium)
Parepectolin (paregoric, pectin, kaolin)

Anticholinergics
Atropine
Scopolamine
Methscopolamine
Glycopyrrolate (Robinul-V)
Aminopentamide hydrogen sulfate (Centrine)
Prochlorperazine, isopropamide (Darbazine)

Locally Active Agents
Kaopectate (kaolin, pectin)
Kao-forte (kaolin, pectin)
Pepto-Bismol (bismuth subsalicylate)

Antihistamines
H_2 Blockers: Tagamet (cimetidine), Zantac (ranitidine), Pepcid AC (famotidine)

watery, watery with flecks of blood, or severely hemorrhagic. Occasionally, infected dogs will display abdominal tenderness or pain. The presence of fever is more commonly associated with parvovirus than with other enteric viruses. A history of vaccination does not rule out viral enteritis because maternal antibodies may have prevented a protective immune response to the vaccination.

Hemograms are usually normal with coronavirus enteritis but may be abnormal with parvovirus enteritis. Transient leukopenia is present in roughly one third to one half of dogs with parvovirus infections. Severely leukopenic patients may develop secondary infections because of a compromised immune system.

Plain abdominal radiographs do not reveal specific changes. Gastrointestinal contrast study changes may mimic small bowel obstruction. Abnormalities include dilated loops of bowel, tremendously prolonged passage time, and gas-capped fluid lines.

Definitive diagnosis is possible by several techniques. The viruses may be detected in the stool by electron microscopy. An ELISA performed on the feces can detect parvoviral antigen and can be used to demonstrate the virus in the feces during the period of active viral shedding. This period corresponds to the clinical illness. An easy-to-perform in-house test is available to check for parvovirus antigen in the stool (Probe-Canine Parvovirus Antigen test kit, Idexx Labs).

It should be stressed that the treatment of canine viral gastroenteritis is supportive because there are no effective antiviral agents. Treatment includes aggressive intravenous fluid therapy, antibiotics, injectable antiemetics, and keeping the animal clean and comfortable. One other complication seen with parvovirus infection, to which the technician should be alert, is the development of hypoglycemia. If profound weakness and/or seizures develop, a blood glucose level should be determined.

A myocardial form of canine parvovirus has been described in young pups. This form of the disease is characterized by sudden death in otherwise healthy pups; however, it is becoming less common. This may be because most pups have maternal antibodies at the critical period when they are susceptible to the myocardial form.

Canine parvovirus is highly contagious. The major route of the infection is fecal-oral. Dogs showing clinical signs will shed large numbers of viral particles for 1 to 2 weeks. The canine parvovirus is hardy; therefore once the environment is contaminated, infective virus will survive for prolonged periods. The virus has been shown to remain infectious in dog feces held at room temperature for longer than 6 months.

Good sanitation will reduce the numbers of infective virus in the hospital environment. Keeping infected patients isolated from other patients and wearing disposable gloves, gowns, and shoe covers every time the patient is handled will prevent spread of the virus within the hospital. Dilute hypochlorite (chlorine bleach and water, diluted to a ratio of 1:32) solutions have significant viricidal properties. However, because the virus is ubiquitous, the best means of prevention is an appropriate immunization program.

> *TECHNICIAN NOTE* Dilute hypochlorite (chlorine bleach and water, diluted to a ratio of 1:32) solutions have significant viricidal properties.

NEPHROLOGY AND UROLOGY

CANINE UROLITHS

A urolith is a pathologic stone formed from mineral salts found in the urinary tract. Clinical signs depend on location, number, size, shape, and whether there is concurrent urinary tract infection. Urolith classification is generally based on the predominant mineral component, such as phosphate or urate. In the dog, more than 90% of uroliths are located in the bladder and urethra and fewer than 10% are located in the kidneys. Although uroliths can occur in any breed, some breeds suspected to be at greater risk include the miniature schnauzer, Dalmatian, dachshund, pug, English bulldog, Welsh corgi, basset hound, Pekingese, and Scottish terrier.

> *TECHNICIAN NOTE* In the dog, more than 90% of uroliths are located in the bladder and urethra and fewer than 10% are located in the kidneys.

If the urolith is located in the bladder, there may be no clinical signs, but more commonly stranguria, increased frequency of urination (pollakiuria), and hematuria will be seen. If the urolith is in the urethra, there may be frequent attempts to urinate and dribbling of urine. If the urethra is completely obstructed by the stone or stones, abdominal distention, pain, anorexia, depression, and vomiting will be observed.

Laboratory findings generally are not specific for uroliths. Radiology, including contrast studies such as cystograms and pneumocystograms or ultrasound, may be necessary to establish the diagnosis. Generally speaking, uroliths are managed surgically. A prescription diet (S/D, Hill's) has been advocated as a means of medically treating phosphate uroliths. The diet is high in sodium and low in protein and phosphorus and has an acidifying effect on urine. Dissolution of the uroliths occurs over a period of weeks. Unfortunately, this medical approach has several important limitations. A prescription S/D diet is effective in the dissolution of only phosphate calculi and is not recommended as a long-term maintenance diet.

The overall recurrence rate for bladder stones is high, approximately 25%. Therefore efforts to reduce the chance of recurrence are very important. The first step is to analyze the mineral composition of the stone because different stone types are managed differently. It is also important to determine whether infection is present and, if so, which antibiotics are most likely to be effective.

Several preventive measures are appropriate regardless of the stone type. These include elimination of any infection and stimulation of increased urine output. The urine output can be increased by salting the diet and thereby increasing water intake.

Depending on the specific stone type, it may also be desirable to initiate dietary therapy and modify the urine pH. Ammonium chloride is commonly used to acidify the urine, and sodium bicarbonate is used to alkalinize it.

Because the recurrence rate for uroliths is high, client education is extremely important. First, long-term therapeutic compliance will be achieved only if the importance of these measures is stressed to the client. Second, the owner should be aware of signs that indicate recurrence of the problem.

FELINE LOWER URINARY TRACT DISEASE

Feline lower urinary tract disease (FLUTD) is the term used to describe a condition of unknown etiology in cats characterized by dysuria, hematuria, pollakiuria, urinating in uncommon places, and occasionally urethral obstruction. Urethral obstruction, if it occurs, is potentially fatal because of the associated severe metabolic derangements. The emergency treatment of feline urethral obstruction is covered in Chapter 33.

Because recurrence of the urethral obstruction is frequent, some clinicians prefer to routinely use indwelling urethral catheters for a brief period of time after relief of the obstruction. The justification for the use of indwelling catheters is to maintain urine flow without the trauma associated with recatheterization and manual compression of the bladder. Indwelling urethral catheters should be used judiciously because of the risk of ascending urinary tract infection and catheter-induced injury to the bladder or urethra. Complications associated with the use of indwelling catheters can be minimized if an appropriate catheter is selected. Commercially manufactured polypropylene catheters (Sovereign tomcat catheters and open-end tomcat catheters, Sherwood Medical Industries) can be either too short or too long. Therefore care should be taken to select a catheter with an appropriate length. Soft, flexible polyvinyl catheters, such as the Sovereign sterile disposable feeding tube and urethral catheter, are preferred because of decreased damage to the urethral and bladder mucosa. To pass these catheters, they are kept frozen until immediately before use. This will make the catheter sufficiently rigid to allow passage in a male cat. The catheter should be well lubricated before passage.

> *TECHNICIAN NOTE* Urethral obstruction, if it occurs, is potentially fatal because of the associated severe metabolic derangements.

Indwelling urethral catheters are generally secured by suturing the catheter to the prepuce. Adhesive tape is attached longitudinally and transversely to the end of the catheter. If the catheter is wet when the tape is applied, it may not stick. Two simple interrupted sutures on either side of the prepuce penetrate the tape and thus prevent movement of the catheter. If analgesia is required to place the sutures, the prepuce can be numbed by applying an ice cube for 1 or 2 minutes. When the catheter is sutured in place, it should be done in such a way that there is no chance of kinking. An Elizabethan collar should be used to prevent the cat from removing the indwelling catheter.

To prevent ascending urinary tract infection, sterile technique is required when placing and maintaining the indwelling catheter. The collection apparatus should be a closed, sterile system. The entire system—catheter, plastic tubing, and collection bottle—must be sterile initially and must be kept sealed to prevent bacterial contamination. Povidone-iodine ointment should be applied several times daily at the point at which the catheter exits the urethra.

Indwelling urethral catheters should be used for as brief a time as possible. The prophylactic use of antimicrobials does not reduce infection. If infection does develop, it is frequently caused by an organism resistant to the prophylactic antimicrobial.

Because the recurrence rate for feline urologic syndrome is high, preventive measures are an important aspect of its medical management. Unfortunately, because the etiology of feline urologic syndrome is unknown, preventive measures are largely empirical. The most frequently recommended preventive measures include providing an ample supply of fresh, potable water, cleaning the litter pan frequently, and lightly salting the food to increase water intake and thus urine volume. The most common urinary crystals and stones are magnesium ammonia phosphate (struvite) and calcium oxalate. To prevent struvite crystals/stones, exclusive feeding of diets that contain 20 mg of magnesium per 100 kcal or less and that maintain a urine pH of 6.4 or less is the most important preventive measure. Certain diets, such as C/D or Feline Maintenance (Hill's), meet this requirement. Although urinary acidification with ammonium chloride has been recommended, it should be emphasized that some diets, such as the ones mentioned above, cause urinary acidification, and additional acidifiers are contraindicated. The basis of acidifying the urine is to increase the solubility of this crystalline material, which is incriminated as the cause of feline urologic syndrome.

> *TECHNICIAN NOTE* Because the recurrence rate for feline urologic syndrome is high, preventive measures are an important aspect of its medical management.

If ammonium chloride is used with a nonacidifying diet, it should be thoroughly mixed with the food to improve palatability. It should also be administered with every meal. Any change in diet or introduction of a food additive, such as ammonium chloride or salt, should be done gradually over several days. This will reduce the chances of the cat rejecting the new or altered food. Enteric-coated ammonium chloride tablets are not effective in the cat.

In recent years, calcium oxalate bladder stones have become recognized in the cat as a new cause of FLUTD. Calcium oxalate stones are more likely to form in an acid urine, and therefore cats that eat an acidifying diet may be at risk for the formation of calcium oxalate stones. Cats at risk for forming both struvite and calcium oxalate stones can be managed on C/D Multicare (Hill's) diet.

In addition, some cats with FLUTD have no definable cause but may benefit from drugs, such as amitriptyline (Elavil) or glycosaminoglycans (Adequan).

CHRONIC RENAL FAILURE

Animals in renal failure should be fed diets containing reduced quantities of high-quality protein and adequate nonprotein calories. This can be accomplished by using prescription diets such as K/D (Hill's) or NF (Purina). These are moderate protein-restricted diets available for dogs in canned, semimoist, and dry forms. Feline K/D and NF canned and dry are products suitable for use in uremic cats.

If desired, homemade diets can be used. The following is a recipe for a moderately low protein diet for dogs:

¼ lb regular ground beef
1 hard-boiled egg, finely chopped
2 cups cooked rice without salt
3 slices white bread, crumbled
1 tsp calcium carbonate
Balanced vitamin and mineral supplement

The meat should be braised, retaining the fat, and thoroughly mixed with the other ingredients. This recipe will meet the daily requirements of a 13.5-kg dog.

The following is an example of a homemade protein-restricted diet for cats:

¼ lb liver
2 large hard-boiled eggs
2 cups cooked rice without salt
1 tbsp vegetable oil
1 tsp calcium carbonate
Balanced vitamin and mineral supplement

Dice and braise the liver, retaining fat. This recipe provides a total of 635 kcal/lb.

Many animals with renal failure are anorectic because of nausea and vomiting. Small, frequent meals are recommended to reduce the nausea. If the animal can tolerate food orally but is not eating, feeding by means of an orogastric tube is recommended. The diets described can be administered through a stomach tube if the ingredients are thoroughly mixed with water in a kitchen blender.

Supportive therapy for chronic renal failure includes the use of phosphorous binders, anabolic steroids, sodium bicarbonate, sodium chloride, calcium, and vitamin D metabolites. The use of these treatments should be based on documented abnormalities because the inappropriate or incorrect use of these agents can do more harm than good. Administration of subcutaneous fluid as a form of diuresis can be taught to the owner for use every other day or daily in advanced kidney failure. Surgically implanted subcutaneous catheters that do not require needle puncture for administration of fluid are a newer option for owners. Cats generally tolerate these catheters very well, and the owners can safely administer the fluid in a much shorter period of time because of the multiple fenestrations of the catheter allowing rapid fluid distribution without pocketing under the skin. This is also a less painful procedure for the patient.

> *TECHNICIAN NOTE* Administration of subcutaneous fluid as a form of diuresis can be taught to the owner for use every other day or daily in advanced kidney failure.

ORTHOPEDICS

CANINE HIP DYSPLASIA

Hip dysplasia refers to a developmental problem of the canine coxofemoral joint. Subluxation of the femoral head leads to abnormal wear and eventual degenerative joint disease. The acetabulum is more shallow than normal, and the femoral head is flattened.

The cause of hip dysplasia is multifactorial. Genetics and environmental factors such as nutrition appear to be important. Hip dysplasia is seen in most large breeds and is inherited by a polygenic mode of inheritance. This means that many genes are responsible for its development. It is also quantitative in its expression. In other words, affected dogs can show slight or severe changes. As is characteristic for traits with a polygenic mode of inheritance, hip dysplasia is modified by environmental factors. For example, it has been suggested that dogs fed a high-calorie diet during growth have an increased incidence, whereas dogs fed a low-calorie diet have a decreased incidence.

> *TECHNICIAN NOTE* Hip dysplasia is seen in most large breeds and is inherited by a polygenic mode of inheritance.

The Orthopedic Foundation of America in Columbia, Mo., is an organization established to evaluate the hip radiographs of potential breeding dogs. Radiologists identify those dogs with radiographically normal hip joints. Unfortunately, because of the factors mentioned, breeding two radiographically normal dogs does not ensure normal progeny. It is better to evaluate entire families (siblings and progeny) when selecting dogs to be included in a breeding program to decrease the incidence of hip dysplasia. It is also important to recognize that good hip joints should not be the sole criterion for selection. Other traits, such as disposition, working ability, and conformation, should also be considered.

The clinical signs of hip dysplasia vary tremendously from occasional slight discomfort to a severe disabling disease. It should be remembered that the clinical signs of hip dysplasia do not always correlate with the severity of hip dysplasia detected radiographically.

Dogs with hip dysplasia will respond differently to varying levels of exercise. Some dogs are most comfortable with minimal activity, yet others do best with a regular regimen of moderate exercise. Swimming is an excellent form of exercise, since muscle tone is increased with the hip joints in a non–weight-bearing position. Any exercise program should be instituted gradually. Forced sudden activity, such as ball playing or rough play, should be discouraged. Severely affected dogs should be treated symptomatically with analgesics and antiinflammatory drugs.

Several surgical procedures have been advocated for the treatment of hip dysplasia. They include procedures such as pectineal myotomy, pelvic osteotomy, excision arthroplasty, and total hip prosthesis. A discussion of these surgical procedures is beyond the scope of this chapter.

INTERVERTEBRAL DISK DISEASE

Intervertebral disk disease is a relatively common problem affecting the spinal cord of chondrodystrophoid and other breeds. Breeds commonly affected include dachshunds, Pekingese, cocker spaniels, poodles, pugs, and beagles. The chondrodystrophoid breeds tend to develop signs at an earlier age than the nonchondrodystrophoid breeds.

The intervertebral disks are structures located between the vertebrae and function as a shock-absorbing system. The disk itself is composed of two parts: the firm fibrous outer annulus and the softer inner nucleus. In intervertebral disk disease, the annulus undergoes degeneration, and the nuclear material protrudes or is completely extruded. The result is compression of the spinal cord with the subsequent development of neurologic signs. These signs vary from simple pain to complete paralysis.

Intervertebral disk disease can be managed either conservatively with strict cage confinement and antiinflammatory drugs or more aggressively with neurosurgery. Management decisions are based on the history, neurologic signs, and wishes of the owner.

If conservative therapy is elected, the technician plays a vital role. Extreme care should be taken in handling the patient because movement may result in the extrusion of additional disk material and worsening of signs. To reduce handling, these patients should be placed in lower cages whenever possible. Because these patients are frequently in severe pain, gentle, compassionate care is essential. Many cases will benefit from some of the physical therapy techniques described earlier.

Dogs with intervertebral disk disease receiving antiinflammatory drugs, such as dexamethasone, may develop secondary problems, such as gastrointestinal hemorrhage or acute pancreatitis. Consequently, these patients should be observed closely for fever, anorexia, abdominal pain, hemorrhagic vomiting, and diarrhea.

Additional information regarding orthopedics is found in Chapter 30.

CASE PRESENTATION 21-1

An 8-month-old, male, castrated, Rottweiler is brought in for not eating, vomiting, and having bloody diarrhea for 2 days. The dog had never been to a veterinarian before today. Abnormal physical examination findings are severe tenting of the skin and dry mucous membranes. Diarrhea is evident on the hind legs of the dog and the odor has a metallic smell. The dog is very depressed and lethargic. Given this dog's age and lack of vaccine history, a parvovirus ELISA test is performed on the feces right away because this is a very contagious disease and if positive, the dog would require isolation so that the virus is not spread through the hospital. Other differential diagnoses to consider are gastrointestinal foreign body, intestinal parasites, hemorrhagic gastroenteritis (HGE), ingested toxin, and Addison's disease. The parvoviral test is positive. The dog is admitted into the hospital in the isolation ward away from other hospitalized patients. An intravenous catheter is inserted into the cephalic vein to allow the administration of intravenous fluid to address the patient's severe dehydration. Intravenous broad-spectrum antibiotics are given to prevent sepsis. Because the parvovirus kills mucosal cells that line the intestinal tract, the internal wall of the gut sloughs and bleeds, exposing capillaries to the feces in the bowel. In addition, the weakened intestinal wall becomes a less effective barrier between the bowel's lumen and the surrounding, sterile peritoneal cavity. The migration of bacteria from the lumen to the blood supply and across the degraded bowel wall into the peritoneal cavity are dangerous possible sequelae. Thus, a broad spectrum antibiotic is administered to help guard against septicemia (a generalized infection) and/or peritonitis. In addition, antiemetics are given to prevent vomiting. Potassium and glucose blood levels are monitored twice daily because they tend to be low in parvoviral patients and are supplemented in the intravenous fluid. The patient needs to be kept clean from the vomitus and diarrhea with frequent cage cleanings because the patient should never leave the isolation ward to urinate and/or defecate. All used and dirty materials must be disposed of in garbage bags separate from the regular hospital garbage and not brought to other areas of the hospital. The veterinarian and veterinary technician must wear protective gowns, gloves, and shoe coverings when handling this very infectious patient so that other patients in the hospital do not contract the disease via fomites (contaminated objects and clothing). A bleach bath solution in a pan (1 part bleach; 20 parts water) for shoes must be available to dip the bottoms of shoes in before leaving the area. All thermometers, stethoscopes, and materials used to administer treatment must remain in the isolation area for this patient only and thoroughly cleaned with bleach solution or disposed of after the patient is discharged. Parvovirus is treated with aggressive supportive intravenous care. When treated promptly the patient has a good prognosis. Recovery occurs over the next 5 to 7 days. Parvovirus vaccination is essential at discharge as the patient is not immune to the disease after recovery. Client education is imperative at discharge with instructions for the owner to clean all of the dog's environment with a bleach solution including food bowls, blankets, beddings, and outdoor environment to prevent infection of other dogs. An area that has housed a parvoviral dog should be vacant for 1 month after cleaning before introducing a new dog.

RECOMMENDED READING

Feldman EC, Nelson RW: *Canine and feline endocrinology and reproduction,* ed 3, St Louis, 2004, WB Saunders.

Bonagura JD, Twedt D: *Kirk's current veterinary therapy XIV,* Philadelphia, 2009, WB Saunders.

Greene C: *Infectious diseases of the dog and cat,* ed 3, St Louis, 2006, WB Saunders.

Hand MS et al: *Small animal clinical nutrition,* ed 4, Marceline, Mo, 2002, Wadsworth Publishing.

Nelson R, Couto G: *Small animal internal medicine,* ed 4, St Louis, 2009, Mosby.

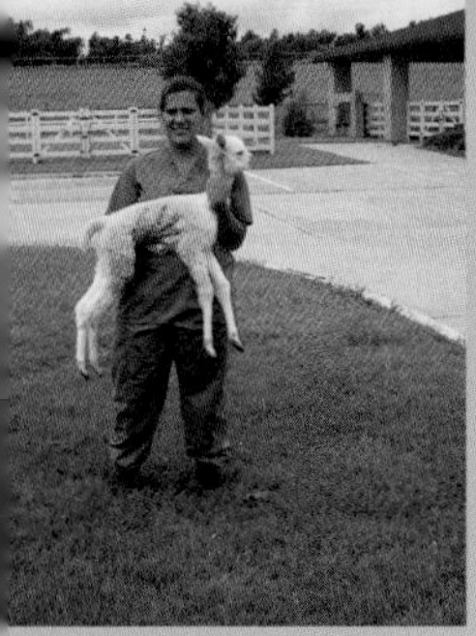

Large Animal Medical Nursing

22

Amy I. Bentz and Marjorie S. Gill

KEY TERMS

Anestrus
Azotemia
Catarrhal
Dystocia
Endotoxemia
Epistaxis
Epizootic
Keratoconjunctivitis
Ketosis, or acetonemia
Myositis
Pneumothorax
Proprioceptive
Pseudopregnancy
Septicemia
Serosanguineous
Serous
Strabismus
Strangury
Urolithiasis
Visceral
Xyphoid

OUTLINE

LEARNING OBJECTIVES

When you have completed this chapter, you will be able to:

1. List the common diseases and disorders of horses and describe the causes, symptoms, treatment, and control.
2. List the physiologic parameters used to monitor hospitalized equine patients.
3. Describe unique requirements for care of hospitalized recumbent and infectious equine patients.
4. Describe concerns related to the placement and care of intravenous (IV) catheters in horses.
5. List common medications used on equine patients and describe their indications.
6. Describe routine laboratory studies performed on equine patients.
7. List the common diseases and disorders of food animals and describe the causes, symptoms, treatment, and control.
8. List the common diseases and disorders of small ruminants and describe the causes, symptoms, treatment, and control.
9. List the common diseases and disorders of swine and describe the causes, symptoms, treatment, and control.
10. List the common diseases and disorders of camelids and describe the causes, symptoms, treatment, and control.

INTRODUCTION

In equine and food animal practices, the veterinary technician is a vital member of the veterinary health care team in providing efficient, quality medical care. A skilled veterinary technician monitors patients, administers treatments, provides nursing care, and educates clients. Treating horses and food animals for medical conditions requires knowledge of restraint and animal behavior. These topics are covered in Chapters 7 and 11, respectively. Whereas many principles of veterinary nursing are universal, techniques must be adjusted to compensate for the large body size of both horses and food animal species. In addition, unlike treating cats and dogs, technicians who work with large animals must be familiar with the behaviors and instincts particular to prey species. Large animals, for example, respond to body language and instinctively react to danger by running away. A quiet, calm voice and slow movement are essential to reassure large animal patients. However, animals are unpredictable, and large animals because of their size can be particularly dangerous. Therefore be practical and alert when nursing large animals. Dress appropriately and be sure to wear protective leather boots so that your feet are not injured under the weight of a large and heavy hoof.

This chapter is an overview of the common medical conditions encountered in equine and food animal species.

THE IMPORTANCE OF PHYSICAL EXAMINATION

A thorough physical examination is an integral part of the diagnostic assessment and monitoring of large animals. Because veterinary technicians play an important role in the day-to-day monitoring of hospitalized patients, learning to perform a thorough physical examination is vital. Refer to Chapter 8 for a detailed description of how to complete a physical examination on large animal species. Review the normal parameters for a horse in Box 22-1. It is crucial to record all observations and findings of the physical examination in the medical record. The medical record provides the only record of the patient's progress or deterioration and is a legal document. Refer to examples of medical records designed for the large animal patients in Chapter 5.

EQUINE MEDICINE

COMMON DISEASES AND CONDITIONS IN HORSES

RESPIRATORY DISEASES

Strangles

Strangles is a common, highly contagious respiratory disease of horses caused by the bacterial pathogen *Streptococcus equi equi*. Strangles typically produces swelling and abscesses of the submandibular and retropharyngeal lymph nodes. Affected horses have fever, depression, poor appetite, and painful swellings under the mandible. The abscesses under the mandible enlarge, rupture, and drain purulent exudate. Horses may develop abscesses within the guttural pouch, thorax, abdomen, and central nervous system (CNS). The development of an abscess in abnormal locations is termed bastard strangles. These cases are particularly difficult to treat successfully. Horses with complicated cases of strangles should be treated with antibiotics, and *S. equi equi* is typically sensitive to penicillin. Horses with strangles should be maintained under a strict isolation protocol. Recovered horses remain contagious and represent a threat to susceptible horses for approximately 6 weeks after recovering from clinical disease.

Immunization against *S. equi* can be helpful. The recently developed modified live virus intranasal vaccine induces mucosal immunity, providing better protection and fewer side effects, but it should not be given to pregnant mares and young foals. This attenuated vaccine will not completely prevent infection in horses, but minimizes clinical signs.

BOX 22-1 Normal TPR Parameters for an Adult Horse at Rest

T	99-101.5° F
P	28-44 beats/min (bpm)
R	8-20 breaths/min (bpm)

Guttural Pouch Empyema and Mycosis

The guttural pouches are two large symmetric dilations of the eustachian tube that are present in all Equidae. They are located just above the pharynx and larynx and can be accessed during an endoscopic examination through small openings in the dorsal lateral nasopharynx. The internal and external carotid arteries and several cranial nerves travel superficially under the surface of the guttural pouch lining and are vulnerable to damage from pathologic conditions. The purpose of the guttural pouches may be to lower the temperature of the blood to the brain (internal and external carotid arteries) during exercise. A bacterial infection of the guttural pouch is termed guttural pouch empyema and is often associated with strangles. A fungal infection of the guttural pouch is termed guttural pouch mycosis, and the causative agent is often *Aspergillus* spp.

A bacterial infection of the guttural pouch (empyema) usually is a sequela to strangles or retropharyngeal lymph node abscesses. Clinical signs include swelling in the throatlatch region and bilateral mucopurulent nasal discharge. Horses with guttural pouch empyema can be treated conservatively with antimicrobials and guttural pouch lavage; this may be effective in many horses that are treated early in the course of the disease. However, in more chronic cases, the mucopurulent material becomes inspissated and forms gelatinous concretions (chondroids) that lie in the floor of the guttural pouches. A resolution of empyema requires removal of the chondroids. Long-term effective drainage can usually only be achieved with surgical drainage.

During guttural pouch mycosis, fungal plaque usually forms over the internal carotid artery, adjacent to nerves that control swallowing. Horses may have a life-threatening blood loss from rupture of the internal carotid artery or dysphagia from damage to the nerves.

The accumulation of air in guttural pouches (guttural pouch tympany) occurs in foals and weanlings and is usually associated with an abnormality of the opening to the pouches. It can occur unilaterally or bilaterally and is characterized by a fluctuant, nonpainful swelling in the throatlatch region.

Influenza

Influenza is a highly contagious viral respiratory disease in horses characterized by an increased body temperature, e.g., 40.8° C (104.8° F), cough, and depression. The incubation period is short (2 to 3 days), and horses remain ill for 3 to 4 days. The equine influenza virus is transmitted through a herd via aerosolization of virus during coughing. The virus damages the clearance mechanisms in the lung and predisposes horses to bacterial pneumonia. Horses should be rested for a minimum of 3 weeks after recovery from viral respiratory disease.

Immunization against influenza is recommended. The intramuscular influenza vaccines do not provide consistent protection from an influenza virus challenge, but vaccination programs do reduce the incidence of disease within the herd and the severity and duration of disease in individual horses. On the other hand, intranasal influenza vaccine closely resembles the protective immunity achieved with natural infection. Sedentary adult horses not exposed to other horses are at a low risk for contracting influenza and may be vaccinated only once or twice per year. Young horses and horses engaged in performance activities (racing, showing, training) are at high risk for contracting influenza because of the exposure to other horses and should be vaccinated every 3 to 4 months or 3 to 4 weeks before exposure to other horses. Broodmares should be vaccinated with the injectable vaccine against influenza in the tenth month of pregnancy to ensure adequate colostral transfer of antibodies against influenza for the foal. Some horses may suffer a transient systemic reaction characterized by fever, inappetence, and depression several days after influenza vaccination.

Herpes

Equine herpesvirus (the causative agent of rhinopneumonitis) is a contagious virus that produces respiratory disease, abortion, and neonatal and neurologic disease (ascending paralysis) in horses. It is a reportable disease in some states. The clinical signs of respiratory disease caused by equine herpesvirus are milder, but hardly distinguishable from equine influenza. The incubation period is longer (2 to 10 days), and horses may remain ill for 4 to 5 days. Equine herpesvirus is transmitted through the herd by aerosol transmission, respiratory secretions, and fomite transmission. Protection against respiratory disease following equine herpesvirus vaccination is inconsistent and relatively short lived. Abortion secondary to equine herpesvirus occurs in the seventh to eleventh month of gestation and the mare does not appear sick at the time of abortion. Vaccination is recommended for performance horses and broodmares. Neurologic disease caused by equine herpesvirus is not common; however, there have been a few large outbreaks in the United States over the last few years with high morbidity and mortality. Affected horses demonstrate signs of incoordination, inability to urinate, and poor tail tone. The recovery from neurologic diseases is prolonged (2 to 3 months), and horses may not return to completely normal neurologic function. Standard quarantine protocols (e.g., quarantine all new horses for 30 days) and using individual equipment with proper disinfecting techniques are important to minimize disease transmission.

Protection against respiratory disease following equine herpesvirus vaccination is inconsistent and relatively short lived. None of the currently available vaccines claims to provide protection against the neurologic form of herpesvirus in horses. Sedentary adult horses not exposed to other horses may not be vaccinated or vaccinated only once or twice per year, whereas young horses and horses engaged in performance activities should be vaccinated every 3 to 4 months. Inactivated univalent vaccines should be administered to broodmares during the third, fifth, seventh, and ninth months of pregnancy to prevent abortion. Although 100% protection against abortion is not achieved, the incidence of abortion caused by equine herpesvirus is significantly decreased by adherence to a proper vaccination program.

Viral Arteritis

Equine viral arteritis is a contagious viral disease that produces limb swelling, conjunctivitis, abortion, and respiratory disease in horses. Limb swelling is painful and results from vasculitis (inflammation of blood vessels). Stallions infected after puberty develop a persistent infection in the accessory sex glands (ampullae) and transmit the viral infection to mares during breeding. Abortion can occur at any point during gestation and results from viral damage to the blood vessels of the placenta. The vaccine for equine viral arteritis is approved for use in stallions and nonpregnant mares under the supervision of the United States Department of Agriculture (USDA). Pregnant mares should not be vaccinated against equine viral arteritis. Vaccination induces seropositivity and may interfere with testing requirements for export. Therefore a negative status should be confirmed before vaccination.

Heaves

Heaves or recurrent airway obstruction (RAO) is an allergic airway disease caused by airway inflammation, narrowing of small airways (bronchoconstriction), and excessive mucus production. The clinical signs of heaves are cough, nasal discharge, flared nostrils, increased respiratory rate, increased expiratory effort, and wheezing. The severity of clinical signs may range from exercise intolerance to severe respiratory distress (dyspnea) at rest. Most affected horses are allergic to dust and molds present in hay and straw. Management, such as changing the environment to remove offending allergens, is the most important intervention to treat these cases. Ideally, horses should be maintained at pasture and not fed hay to minimize dust. Horses cannot be "cured" of heaves, but can often be controlled with appropriate management practices. Medical therapy of horses with heaves may be intermittently necessary in moderate to severely affected horses. Corticosteroids to reduce inflammation and bronchodilator therapy to relax small airways are used. They may be administered systemically (IV, IM, PO) or by inhalation using a special mask (e.g., Aeromask®).

CARDIOVASCULAR DISEASE

Equine Infectious Anemia

Equine infectious anemia (EIA) is a persistent viral disease of horses causing anemia, fever, and weight loss; however, some horses may appear healthy, but are inapparent carriers. The virus is transmitted from infected horses by large biting flies (tabanids). Once infected, horses become permanently infected and become carriers of the virus for the rest of their lives. Infected horses produce antibodies to the virus, so they will have a positive test result in the agar gel immunodiffusion test (Coggin's test) or the enzyme-linked immunosorbent assay (ELISA) for EIA virus. Horses must have a negative (Coggin's) test result for EIA within 6 months for the issuance of health certificates for interstate travel, international travel and show, and sale. A USDA-accredited veterinarian must draw blood for testing and provide a detailed description of the horse on specified forms. The health certificate for interstate travel cannot be issued until the negative test result is returned from a state or federally recognized laboratory. Horses not traveling or sold should still be tested on a yearly basis. If a positive test result is obtained, the entire herd is quarantined until all horses on the premises are tested (usually 60 days). Only the state veterinarian can release the quarantine. Because horses that have a positive test result for EIA are persistent carriers, they are a reservoir of the virus. Therefore infected horses must be quarantined for life (within a distance greater than 200 yards from other horses) or euthanized.

GASTROINTESTINAL DISEASE

Colic

See Colic section of Chapter 33, Emergency Nursing and Abdominal Surgery section of Chapter 31.

Gastric and Colonic Ulceration

Young horses are particularly prone to the development of gastric ulceration. Stress, a high-grain diet, musculoskeletal pain, and the administration of nonsteroidal antiinflammatory drugs (NSAIDs) are common predisposing factors. Clinical signs of gastric ulceration are bruxism (grinding teeth), hypersalivation, and abdominal pain after eating. Foals with gastric ulceration will often lie still in dorsal recumbency with their forelimbs over their head or extended out straight. Human antiulcer medications, such as histamine H_2 blockers, intestinal protectants, and hydrogen-ion pump blockers, are used to treat gastric ulceration in horses.

Phenylbutazone (NSAID) toxicosis in horses can produce renal insufficiency and oral, gastric, and colonic ulceration in horses. The colonic ulcers occur in the right dorsal colon and are difficult to treat. Colonic ulcers secondary to phenylbutazone toxicity can produce abdominal pain, marked protein loss, melena (blood in manure), peritonitis, colonic stricture, or colonic rupture. Dehydration and excessive dosages are the most important predisposing factors for development of phenylbutazone toxicosis.

Colitis

Colitis in horses can result in a rapid, life-threatening fluid loss (hypovolemia), shock, toxemia, electrolyte loss, and acid-base imbalance as a result of diarrhea. Some horses may develop hypovolemic shock and electrolyte imbalance before the appearance of diarrhea. In addition to diarrhea, clinical signs of colitis include depression, inappetence, abdominal pain, tachycardia (increased heart rate), injected (brick red) mucous membranes, and prolonged capillary refill time. Etiologic agents that produce life-threatening diarrhea in horses include *Salmonella* spp., *Clostridium* spp., and *Ehrlichia risticii*. Horses with diarrhea should be considered contagious and maintained under an isolation protocol. IV fluid therapy is crucial to support the cardiovascular system, replace fluid losses, and correct electrolyte and acid-base imbalance. Complications of colitis include laminitis (founder), cardiovascular collapse, cardiac arrhythmias, and thrombophlebitis.

> *TECHNICIAN NOTE* Choke refers to obstruction of the esophagus, usually as a result of impacted food in the esophagus.

Choke

Choke indicates obstruction of the esophagus. Chronic dental disease and retained deciduous caps are common predisposing conditions for the development of choke. Horses in overcrowded environments may eat feed too quickly and choke. Removing the competition usually alleviates this behavior. The esophagus is usually obstructed by grain or hay. Many horses will continue to attempt to eat despite their inability to swallow. Clinical signs include anxiety, gagging, excessive salivation, and feed and saliva coming from the nostrils. The obstruction can be visualized via an endoscopic examination (Figure 22-1) and in most instances can be relieved by sedation and time. Occasionally, manipulation and hydropulsion using a nasogastric tube is required. Horses must be heavily sedated to lower their head during manipulation of the nasogastric tube to prevent water and feed from entering the trachea. Aspiration pneumonia is a significant complication, therefore a preventative treatment is warranted. An esophageal stricture or rupture is a less common complication and occurs in horses with circumferential damage to the esophageal mucosa.

Potomac Horse Fever

Potomac horse fever is caused by *E. risticii* and produces diarrhea, fever, abortion, and laminitis. The mode of transmission is not completely elucidated, but it is suspected

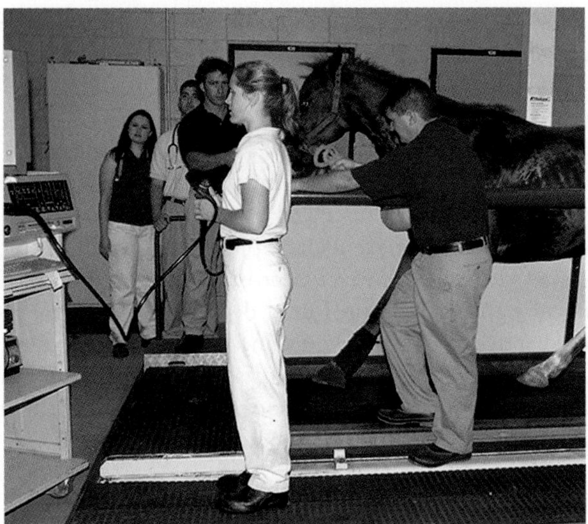

FIGURE 22-1 Use of dynamic endoscopy to evaluate the upper airway of a horse during exercise.

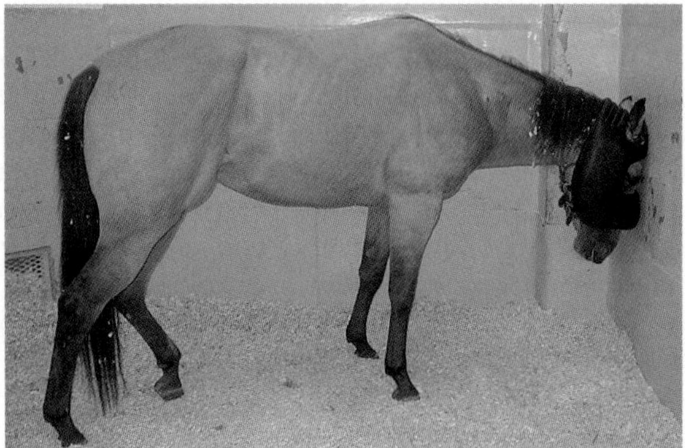

FIGURE 22-2 Horse head pressing as a sign of cerebral dysfunction.

to involve an arthropod vector. Geographically, clinical disease is observed preponderantly in states east of the Mississippi. Two inactivated bacterins are commercially available. Although the vaccine is not effective, horses living in affected areas may be vaccinated. Vaccination should precede the months of peak disease incidence (June through October).

NEUROLOGIC DISEASE

Brain and Brainstem Disorders

The four most common disorders of the brain and brainstem in horses are rabies, equine viral encephalitis (*Alphaviruses*: eastern, western, Venezuelan; *Flavivirus:* West Nile), leukoencephalomalacia (moldy corn toxicity), and head trauma. Damage to the cerebrum may produce altered mentation, altered states of consciousness, head pressing, and seizures (Figure 22-2). Damage to the brainstem may potentially damage the cranial nerves, which control the muscles of facial expression, facial sensation, mastication, swallowing, balance, vision, taste, and ocular position (Figure 22-3). Brainstem lesions also lead to incoordination of the limbs and altered breathing patterns. Diagnostic aids for the evaluation of horses with cerebral or brainstem dysfunction include cerebrospinal fluid (CSF) analysis and skull radiographs.

Rabies

Rabies is a zoonotic infection and is universally fatal. Horses usually acquire the infection by a bite wound from a wild animal. Skunks, foxes, raccoons, and bats are the most common reservoirs in North America. Clinical signs are highly variable, but often begin as fever, hind limb ataxia, and hyperesthesia (hyperresponsiveness to touch). Neurologic signs rapidly progress to involve the brain and brainstem. The duration of neurologic signs before death is relatively short, varying from 3 to 10 days.

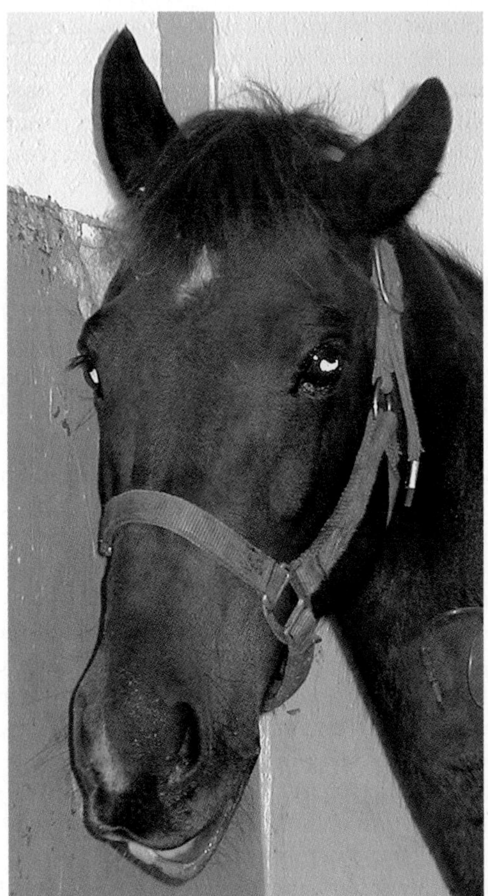

FIGURE 22-3 Horse with facial nerve paralysis (flaccid facial musculature, droopy ear and eyelid on the affected side) as signs of brainstem dysfunction.

Horses should be vaccinated against rabies on an annual basis. Vaccinated horses that have been exposed to a rabid animal should be revaccinated promptly and observed for 90 days. Unvaccinated horses with a known rabies exposure should be observed for 6 months and should not be vaccinated.

There is no accurate antemortem test for rabies; it is important to be cautious when handling horses with suspected rabies. The diagnosis of rabies is confirmed by fluorescent antibody stain of brain tissue. People handling potentially rabid horses should avoid contact with saliva, wear gloves, protective eyewear, disposable outerwear, wash hands thoroughly, and avoid contact with CSF. A list of individuals that had contact with the potentially rabid horse must be kept, and these individuals must be informed of the result of the test (generally 24 to 48 hours). A postexposure rabies vaccination should be administered to humans in contact with rabid animals. Individuals with occupational exposure to livestock and wildlife should undergo a prophylactic rabies vaccination series.

Viral Equine Encephalitis

There are four main types of viral equine encephalitis: Eastern, Western, Venezuelan, and West Nile. The viral equine encephalitides produce rapidly progressive, highly fatal neurologic disease in horses. Mosquitoes transmit the infection to horses; therefore disease incidence is seasonal in most geographic regions. Clinical signs of Eastern, Western, and Venezuelan encephalitis are practically indistinguishable and include profound depression, fever, ataxia, head pressing, dementia, and multiple cranial nerve abnormalities. The clinical signs of West Nile encephalitis include weakness, ataxia, muscle fasciculations, and cranial nerve deficits (such as droopy lip). Hyperesthesia (extreme sensitivity to touch) around the head and neck is a common clinical sign. The mortality rate is extremely high with Eastern Equine encephalitis (75% to 100%), moderate with Venezuelan (40% to 80%), and lower with western (30% to 50%) and West Nile (36% to 44%). The treatment consists of supportive care to provide hydration; nutrition; and a clean, dry environment. The prognosis is poor with eastern equine encephalitis and guarded with Western, Venezuelan, and West Nile encephalitides. The diagnosis is confirmed by serologic test (a high titer or a fourfold increase in antibodies to Eastern, Western, and Venezuelan viruses identified by complement-fixation, neutralization, or hemagglutination-inhibition assays or a positive IgM-capture ELISA for West Nile and Venezuelan). Fluorescent antibody or virus isolation in brain tissue is used to make a diagnosis from postmortem samples. The viral encephalitides can be prevented by vaccination 1 month before mosquito season. In southern regions of the United States, vaccinations should be administered two or three times per year.

Vaccines for Eastern and Western equine encephalitis are highly efficacious, and clinical disease in vaccinated horses is rare. A vaccine for West Nile has been available since 2001, and it appears to be efficacious. Horses in the United States should be vaccinated against eastern and western equine and West Nile encephalomyelitis viruses before the mosquito season in the spring. Horses living in southern states with a year-round mosquito season should be vaccinated in the fall in addition to the spring vaccination. Broodmares should receive a booster of their vaccination in the tenth month of gestation (use only killed-virus vaccines in pregnant animals) to ensure adequate colostral antibody protection for the foal. Vaccination against Venezuelan equine encephalomyelitis is not routinely recommended because the disease has not been reported recently in the United States and does not currently pose a threat to the U.S. horse population except those near the Mexican border.

Leukoencephalomalacia

Equine leukoencephalomalacia (moldy corn toxicity) is caused by the ingestion of a fungal toxin produced by *Fusarium moniliforme*. This mold has a predilection for corn, and affected kernels are usually pink to brown. The fungal toxin produces liquefactive necrosis of the cerebral cortex. Clinical signs include profound depression, head pressing, altered states of consciousness, incoordination, and aimless wandering. The treatment consists of supportive care, and the prognosis for recovery is poor. Horses often die within 24 hours of manifesting neurologic signs.

Head Trauma

Horses acquire two types of skull fractures depending on the nature of the traumatic injury. Horses that suffer a frontal impact with a solid object develop depression fractures of the frontal and parietal bones. The common neurologic signs observed in horses with this type of fracture are due to cerebral damage and include depression, seizure, stupor, and aimless wandering. Horses that flip over backward develop fractures of the petrous temporal bone and the junction of the basisphenoid and basioccipital bone. Neurologic signs associated with these fractures include abnormalities of balance, incoordination of limbs, nystagmus (rhythmic eye movement), abnormal respiratory patterns, and coma. The diagnosis is confirmed by a radiographic examination of the skull. The treatment consists of supportive care and antiinflammatory therapy (corticosteroids, dimethyl sulfoxide [DMSO]). Surgical decompression of frontal and parietal fractures may improve the neurologic status of some horses.

Spinal Cord Disorders

The five most common disorders of the spinal cord are cervical vertebral malformation caused by stenotic or dynamic compression of the spinal cord (wobbler syndome), equine protozoal myelitis, equine herpesvirus myeloencephalopathy (rhinopneumonitis), equine degenerative myeloencephalopathy, and vertebral fracture. Damage to the spinal cord causes spinal ataxia (incoordination of the limbs without abnormalities of the brain and brainstem), which may progress to dog sitting and recumbency (Figure 22-4). Muscle atrophy from a lower motor neuron disorder can also indicate a spinal cord disorder (Figure 22-5). Diagnostic aids to differentiate these diseases include a neurologic examination, cervical radiographic examination, myelographic examination, and CSF analysis. CSF can be obtained at the lumbosacral space in standing, sedated horses and at the atlantooccipital space in anesthetized horses. The CSF travels from the cranial area in a caudal direction. Typically, a CSF collection is performed at the lumbosacral space in a standing horse. A CSF collection can also be performed at the atlantooccipital space in horses while using a general anesthetic. Because some neurologic infectious diseases have zoonotic potential, most notably rabies, barrier precautions (e.g., face mask,

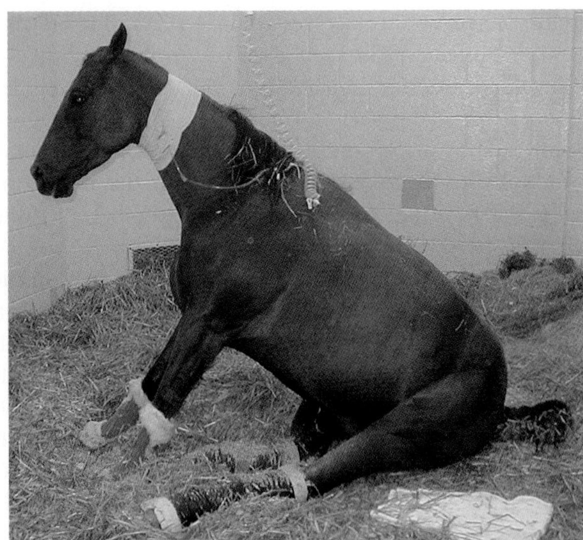

FIGURE 22-4 Horse in dog-sitting position as a result of a spinal cord dysfunction.

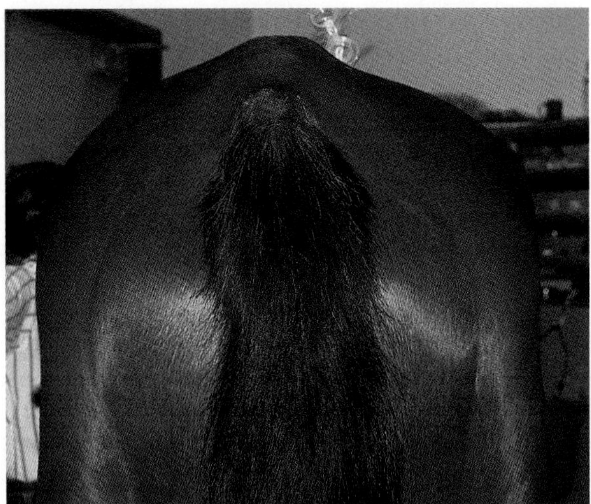

FIGURE 22-5 Asymmetrical gluteal muscle atrophy in a horse with spinal cord dysfunction involving a lower motor neuron.

double gloves) must be taken when collecting and handling CSF samples from horses with neurologic signs to minimize exposure to the infectious agent.

Wobbler Syndrome

Cervical vertebral malformation is a manifestation of developmental orthopedic disease characterized by compression of the cervical spinal cord by malformed or unstable cervical vertebrae. Males are affected four times more frequently than females, and Thoroughbreds appear to be predisposed. Clinical signs of symmetric incoordination usually begin between 6 months and 3 years of age. The hind limbs are usually more severely affected than the forelimbs. The likelihood of disease is determined by the evaluation of plain film cervical radiographs, and the diagnosis is confirmed by a myelographic examination. Surgical stabilization improves the neurologic status of some patients.

Equine Protozoal Myelitis

Equine protozoal myelitis (EPM) causes ataxia in horses. Horses are dead-end, aberrant hosts of the protozoan parasites. *Sarcocystis neurona* is the most common protozoan parasite that causes spinal cord disease in horses; opossums are the primary hosts of this parasite, and horses are likely infected via fecal-oral transmission. Birds are the secondary hosts and do not appear to be infectious for horses. The clinical signs of EPM are directly referable to the location of the organism in the CNS. Therefore EPM should be considered in a horse demonstrating neurologic signs. Most horses with EPM (85%) demonstrate signs such as ataxia, weakness, and muscle atrophy as a result of spinal cord damage. Clinical signs are often asymmetrical. Other signs such as cranial nerve deficits may occur. The diagnosis is confirmed by the identification of antibodies to the organism in CSF. The treatment of EPM consists of the administration of antiprotozoal drugs; the most common treatment for EPM is ponazuril. Another treatment is a combination of two antibiotics that inhibit folic acid metabolism: sulfadiazine and pyrimethamine, treating for an average of approximately 90 to 120 days.

Herpes

Equine herpesvirus can produce respiratory disease, abortion, and neonatal and neurologic disease in horses. The neurologic form is characterized by ascending paralysis with hind limbs more severely affected than forelimbs. Horses often demonstrate urinary incontinence, poor tail tone, and penile prolapse. The diagnosis is confirmed by a cytologic analysis of CSF. The administration of corticosteroids may improve recovery if administered early in the disease process. The prognosis for return to normal neurologic function is approximately 80%. Recently, there have been a number of outbreaks in the United States with a higher mortality than in the past. Cases are now considered reportable to the state veterinarian.

Equine Degenerative Myelopathy

Equine degenerative myelopathy results in symmetric spinal ataxia with both the forelimbs and hind limbs equally affected. Clinical signs appear between 6 months and 2 years of age. The disease appears to be familial in some breeds. There is no definitive antemortem diagnostic test, and the diagnosis is usually made on the basis of the neurologic examination, CSF analysis, cervical radiographs, and myelographic examination. Dietary supplementation with vitamin E may prevent the progression of disease and may result in improvement in clinical signs in some instances. The prognosis for return to normal neurologic function is poor.

Vertebral Fracture

The cervical vertebrae, caudal thoracic vertebrae, and thoracolumbar junction are the most common sites of vertebral fracture. A cervical vertebral fracture results in tetraparesis (weakness of all four limbs), whereas fracture of the thoracic and lumbar vertebrae produces paraparesis (weakness of hind limbs) or paraplegia (paralysis of hind limbs). The diagnosis is confirmed by radiography. If the fracture is nondisplaced, nuclear scintigraphy may aid in the identification of the fracture site. Surgical correction may be attempted for fractures of the cervical vertebrae, but the repair of thoracic or lumbar vertebrae is not attempted. The most consistent clinical sign associated with vertebral fracture is pain.

Tetanus

Tetanus is a highly fatal neurologic disease in horses characterized by a stiff, stilted gait; hyperexcitability; seizure; and coma. The causative organism is commonly present in the environment. The most common portals of entry for disease in horses include a subsolar abscess, penetrating wound, or infected intramuscular injection site. Tetanus toxoid (inactivated) is a safe and efficacious vaccine for preventing clinical disease. Healthy horses without risk factors should be vaccinated for tetanus annually. Unvaccinated horses at high risk for the development of tetanus (wounds, subsolar abscess, surgery) should receive tetanus antitoxin in addition to tetanus toxoid to provide immediate protection against disease. Tetanus antitoxin is associated with fatal serum hepatitis, and its administration should be limited to cases at a high risk for disease.

> *TECHNICIAN NOTE* Different neurologic diseases can have similar clinical signs in horses. It is important to take proper precautions, such as gloves and eye protection, when working with these cases. Rabies is a zoonotic infection (infectious to humans) and is fatal.

Botulism

Botulism is a rapidly progressive, often fatal neurologic disease in horses characterized by profound weakness, muscle fasciculations, and dysphagia (inability to swallow). The causal organism produces a neurotoxin that may gain entry to the body by colonizing the intestinal tract (foals), infected wounds, or contaminating feedstuff (Figure 22-6). Colonization of the intestinal tract in foals occurs in particular geographic regions of the United States, especially Pennsylvania, Ohio, and Kentucky (Figure 22-7). This is a preventable disease, and it is imperative to vaccinate for botulism in affected areas. The vaccine is effective, and unvaccinated horses can die quickly after an infection. The initial series is administered monthly for 3 months, then once a year.

DERMATOLOGIC DISEASE

Ringworm

Equine dermatophytosis (ringworm) is a fungal infection of the superficial layer of skin. The fungi commonly involved are *Trichophyton* and *Microsporum* spp. The transmission of the fungal infection is by direct contact between affected animals. Younger animals (less than 4 years old) are more likely to be affected. Infected areas of skin have a bull's-eye appearance with circular patches of hair loss with a circle of inflammation at the periphery of the lesion. The diagnosis is confirmed by a fungal culture on commercially available dermatophyte culture medium. Although the infection is usually self-limiting, the application of topical antifungal drugs will speed recovery.

Dermatophilosis (rain scald, rain rot) is a common bacterial infection caused by *Dermatophilus congolensis* that produces crusting lesions. The crusts can be pulled out with a tuft of hair, and the remaining lesion is a glistening yellow crater. The organisms readily colonize wet, macerated skin; therefore the disease is common in the winter and spring. An impression smear of the tuft should be stained with Wright stain. Organisms are identified as a double chain of cocci with a "railroad track" appearance. The organisms are usually easily cultured and form an applesauce-like colony on specialized growth medium. Affected horses should be bathed with an iodine-based or chlorhexidine shampoo and placed in a dry environment. The administration of penicillin will speed recovery in severely affected horses.

Culicoides Hypersensitivity

Culicoides hypersensitivity is a syndrome characterized by mane and tail rubbing whereby affected horses develop an allergic pruritic skin condition secondary to the bite of

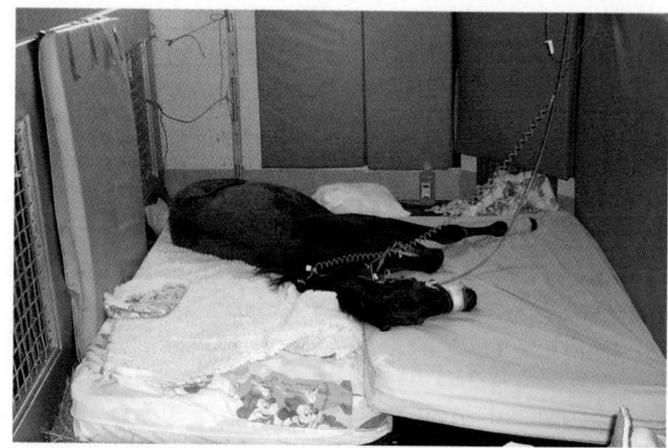

FIGURE 22-6 Recumbent foal with botulism.

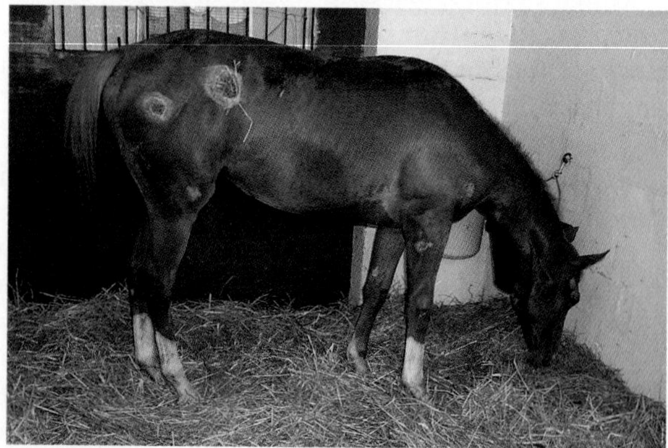

FIGURE 22-7 Recovered botulism patient with decubital ulcers.

Culicoides flies. The classic body regions affected include the face, ears, mane, withers, rump, base of the tail, and ventral abdomen. The dermatitis usually begins as a seasonal condition, but its severity and duration increase as the horse ages. Pruritus usually is noted during the fly season, but will vary in length depending on geographic location. The condition is diagnosed by correlating the time of year with physical evidence of self-mutilation, especially in the mane and tail areas. Intradermal skin testing can be useful in confirming the diagnosis. The treatment involves reducing insect exposure and concomitant use of antiinflammatory medication. Because *Culicoides* breeds in stagnant waters, affected horses should be moved away from ponds, lakes, or irrigation canals. Water troughs and barrels should be cleaned frequently and the water kept fresh to prevent use as breeding sites by the flies. Because *Culicoides* feeds primarily at dusk, night, and dawn, horses should be kept stabled during these times. Stabling is most effective if the doors and windows can be closed and if the stall is lined with a fine-mesh screen. Frequent application of insecticide to the screen may also be useful. Fans are helpful to reduce exposure because *Culicoides* cannot fly well in brisk breezes. The application of insecticides and repellents is a necessary part of disease control. The most effective products are those containing pyrethrins with synergists and repellents. Frequent bathing not only decreases scale and crust, but also seems to decrease pruritus. Corticosteroid therapy is often necessary in these cases to control the pruritus.

Sarcoid

Equine sarcoid is a benign, locally invasive tumor of skin and is the most common tumor in horses. These tumors produce either raised, hairless lesions with a corrugated surface that often bleed when traumatized, known as fibroblastic sarcoids, or a flattened form known as verrucous sarcoids. The cause of sarcoid is unknown, but a viral agent is suspected. Surgical resection, cryotherapy (freezing), laser therapy, immunotherapy (intralesional mycobacterial cell wall extract), radiotherapy (iridium 191), and chemotherapy (intralesional cisplatin) are accepted treatment modalities with variable success. It is difficult to predict the response to a given treatment modality, and combination therapy is often necessary.

Melanomas

Melanomas are relatively common skin tumors, particularly in gray horses. They occur most commonly in the perineal region, but can occur on other areas of the body. Melanomas appear as darkly pigmented nodules in the skin. They are usually benign, but tend to enlarge, causing mechanical problems, such as interfering with defecation. Most clinicians believe it is better not to attempt surgical removal unless they are located in an area that interferes with tack or they are so large that they interfere with normal body functions. The administration of cimetidine has been reported to be effective in many horses to reduce the size of melanomas. Once cimetidine is discontinued, the tumors usually enlarge. Autologous vaccines (making a vaccine from the horse's tumor) have also been used with some success.

OPHTHALMOLOGIC DISEASE

Equine Recurrent Uveitis

Equine recurrent uveitis (moon blindness) is the most common cause of blindness in horses. It is an immune-mediated condition, and many factors have been implicated (heredity, parasites, leptospirosis); however, the inciting cause is often unknown. Affected horses experience episodes of intraocular inflammation characterized by swelling of the eyelids, corneal edema, and hypopyon (inflammatory cellular exudate in the anterior chamber). Over time, the episodes become more frequent, severe, and produce permanent ocular damage, including retinal degeneration, cataracts, and synechiae (adhesions of the iris to either the lens or the anterior chamber). One or both eyes may be affected. Recurrent uveitis cannot be cured, but can often be controlled with long-term antiinflammatory therapy, including atropine and aspirin. Acute episodes are treated with ophthalmic preparations containing atropine and corticosteroids if there is no corneal ulceration. Systemic antiinflammatory therapy is beneficial (e.g., flunixin meglumine). Horses with end-stage uveitis are blind and have small, collapsed, ocular globes *(phthisis bulbi)*. If a corneal ulcer is present, antimicrobials and NSAIDs are used. Once the ulcer completely resolves, a topical steroid may be used. These cases require diligent observation and chronic treatment.

Corneal Ulceration

Corneal ulceration commonly results from ocular trauma. Fluorescein stain is used to detect corneal abrasions because it adheres to abnormal cornea (Figure 22-8). Defects in the corneal surface will stain an apple-green color. Corneal ulceration in most horses responds readily without complications to the administration of ophthalmic antibacterial ointment (bacitracin, neomycin, polymyxin B). In some instances, the ulcer will be colonized by fungus (e.g., *Pseudomonas* or *Aspergillus* spp.). These organisms produce collagenase, which destroys the cornea and creates a "melting" corneal

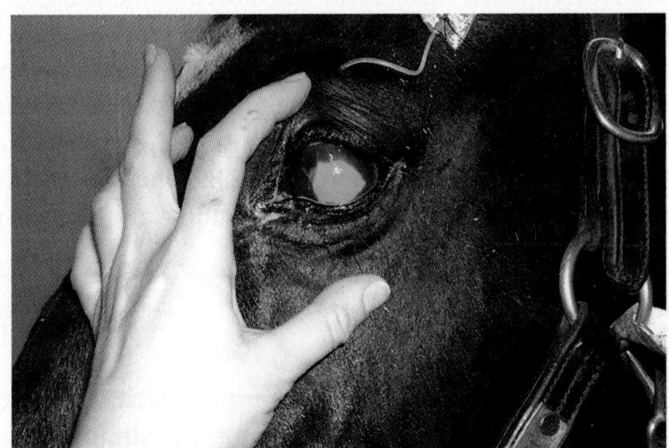

FIGURE 22-8 Patient with corneal ulceration stained with fluorescein.

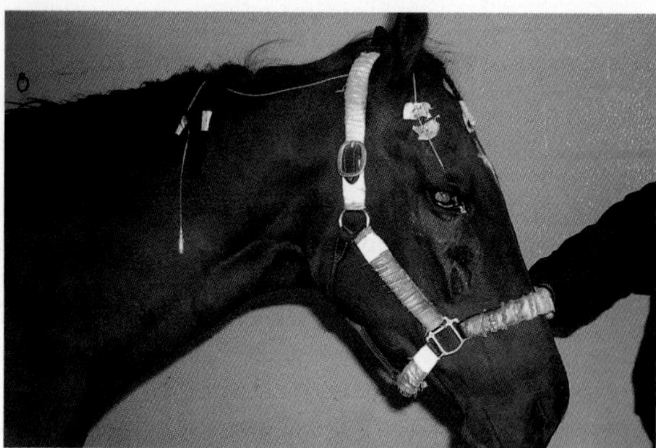

FIGURE 22-9 Subpalpebral catheter placement used to administer topical ocular medication.

ulcer. These ulcers are rapidly progressive, and the eye is prone to rupturing. Frequent antimicrobial dosage regimens may require the placement of a subpalpebral lavage system (Figure 22-9) to allow frequent medication administration for a painful eye. Aggressive topical antimicrobial therapy may be successful, but suturing a conjunctival pedicle flap to provide blood supply to the affected area may be necessary to save the globe in some instances. Deep, melting corneal ulcers often heal with a fibrous scar that may impair vision in the future.

> *TECHNICIAN NOTE* Recurrent uveitis (moon blindness, periodic ophthalmia) is the most common cause of blindness in horses.

MUSCULOSKELETAL DISEASE

Exertional rhabdomyolysis (myositis, tying up, azoturia, Monday morning sickness) is an acute inflammatory disease of muscle. It can be caused by exertion or a change in diet or exercise. It is characterized by a stiff, stilted gait with firm or hard muscles. The most commonly affected muscles are the hind limbs and back. Severely affected horses may be reluctant to move. Some may become recumbent and unable to rise. Affected horses are often anxious, sweat excessively, and have increased heart and respiratory rates and body temperature. Horses often have dark, discolored urine secondary to myoglobinuria from muscle damage. The confirmation of this disease is often based on increased serum muscle enzyme (creatine phosphokinase, aspartate aminotransferase) concentrations. The treatment involves exercise restriction, diet modification, IV fluid therapy, NSAIDs (phenylbutazone, flunixin meglumine), muscle relaxants, and tranquilization.

CARE OF THE HOSPITALIZED EQUINE PATIENT

In the equine hospital setting, veterinary technicians are responsible for primary patient monitoring, administration of medications, general daily care of horses, and supervision of lay technical support. This section provides an overview of the daily management of equine patients in the hospital setting.

PATIENT MONITORING

The level of patient monitoring required for a hospitalized horse depends on the severity and nature of the disease. Horses with infectious disease require frequent patient monitoring (e.g., every 6 hours). Any critically ill patients need constant IV fluid administration and intensive care monitoring. Most will be monitored frequently for signs of discomfort, heart rate, respiratory rate, hydration, capillary refill time, abdominal pain, respiratory distress, shock, laminitis, and gastrointestinal motility. An increased heart rate (tachycardia) is indicative of pain. 60 beats per minute (bpm) or greater indicates serious pain in an adult horse.

Patient monitoring forms are designed to identify trends in physical signs. Patient treatment forms coordinate treatment periods when several individuals may be responsible for administering medications. Treatment sheets and monitoring forms may be combined for low-maintenance, elective patients. However, for intensive care patients, monitoring should be more detailed, and many hospitals use a flow sheet. It is important to recognize that monitoring and treatment forms are a permanent part of the medical record, which represents a legal document to record all events during hospitalization.

Horses with contagious diseases should be hospitalized in isolation facilities. The most common diseases that require an isolation protocol are colitis (Salmonellosis) and strangles *(S. equi equi)*. Personnel wear disposable gloves, boots, and body suits while attending to isolation cases. A disinfectant foot dip should be used when entering and exiting each stall. Protective boots, gloves, and suits should be discarded when exiting the isolation area. Horses in isolation should not be walked in areas where other horses are grazing. Waste from the stall should be disposed of in an inaccessible area. If possible, personnel attending to isolation cases should not attend to foals or immunocompromised patients.

Recumbent horses are a particular challenge to manage effectively in a hospital setting. Neurologic and musculoskeletal diseases are the most common problems resulting in recumbency in horses. Recumbent horses and foals will quickly develop pressure sores (decubital ulcers) over the pelvis (tuber coxae), elbows, and head if not properly managed (see Figure 22-7). Manure- and urine-soaked bedding must be removed frequently because the horse will develop irritated skin and sores. Pressure sores rapidly become deep and may infect underlying bony structures. In addition, recumbent horses may have decreased intestinal motility and fail to void urine. Therefore soft feed, such as fresh grass, should be offered to recumbent horses to facilitate fecal evacuation and prevent impaction. Horses unable to defecate should have feces manually removed twice daily. The placement of an indwelling urinary catheter or periodic catheterization of the urinary bladder is often necessary when managing recumbent patients. Recumbent horses should be deeply bedded on straw, placed on a padded mat, or placed on a mattress to prevent the development of pressure sores (see Figure 22-6). The horse's position should be changed every 6 hours; multiple attendants are required to move an adult recumbent horse. A sling can only be used in horses that can support their own weight but are not able to stand on their own (Figure 22-10, *A, B, C,* and *D*). Horses cannot be supported solely by a sling because of the constriction of breathing and development of sling-induced pressure sores. Recumbent adult horses can rarely be managed for more than 1 or 2 weeks without the development of life-threatening complications (pneumonia, urinary tract infection, colic, pressure sores).

> *TECHNICIAN NOTE* Horses with infectious, contagious diseases should be hospitalized in isolation facilities. The most common infectious diseases requiring isolation are colitis (Salmonellosis) and strangles *(S. equi equi)*.

FEEDING

Whenever possible, hospitalized patients should be offered feed similar to what they are fed at home. Sudden changes in diet predispose horses to colic or diarrhea. When a horse is admitted to the veterinary hospital, it is imperative to ask the owner or trainer for details on the horse's typical diet. In some instances, feeding must be specialized to accommodate the patient's disease. After the medical resolution of colic, horses should be offered soft feed, such as bran mash, fresh grass, and small amounts of good-quality hay. Feed should be offered frequently in small quantities to horses with gastrointestinal tract disease rather than offering two large daily meals. Horses with heaves (recurrent airway obstruction) should be offered water-soaked hay and a dust-free complete pelleted diet. Inappetent horses should be offered highly palatable, calorie-dense feed to increase energy intake.

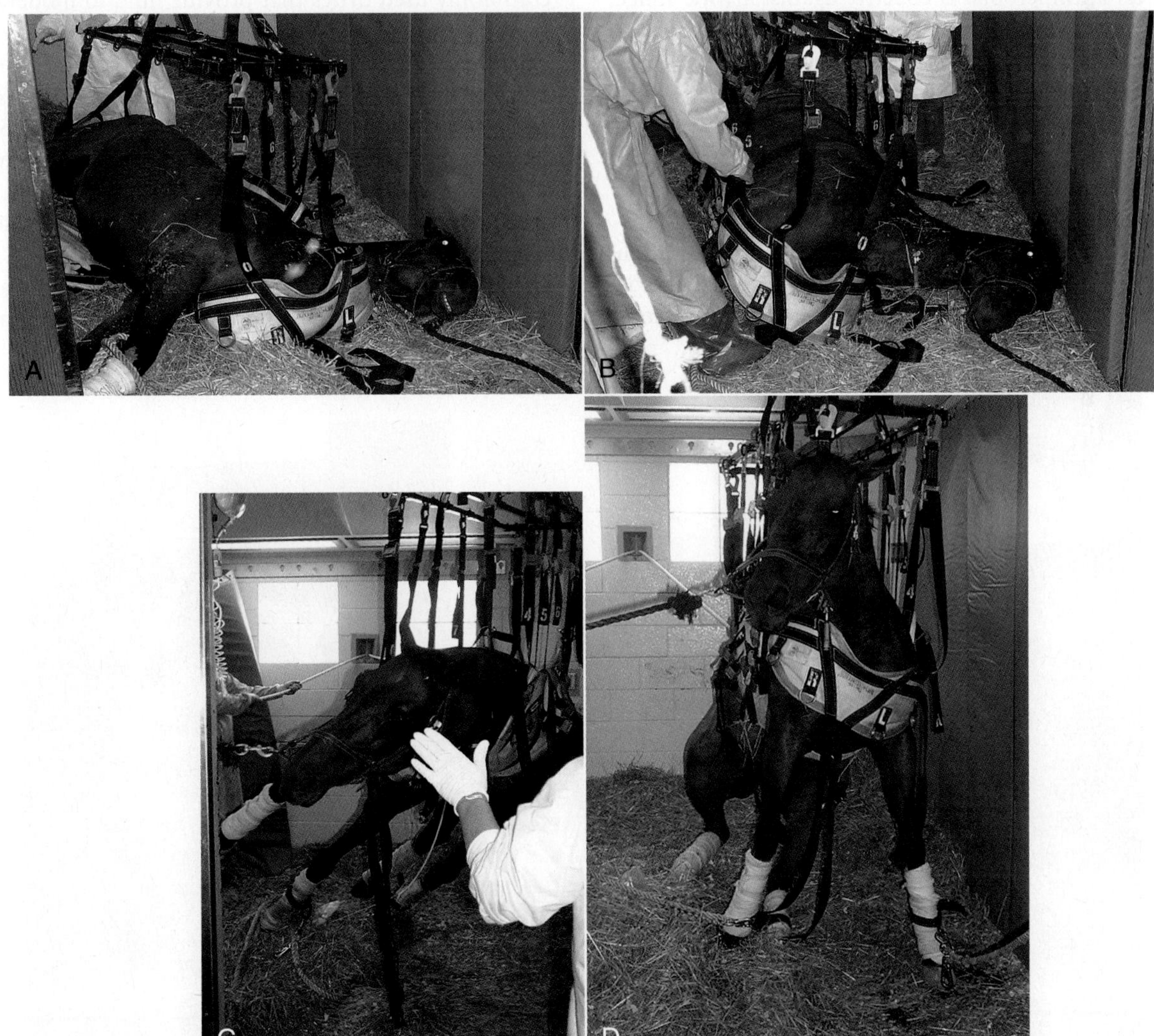

FIGURE 22-10 A, Placing sling over horse's head. B, Securing sling on recumbent horse. C, Slowly lifting recumbent horse in a sling using a mechanized pulley system. D, Recumbent horse is brought to a standing position.

THERAPEUTICS

An IV catheter can be placed for repeated administration of medications or continuous fluid infusion. IV catheters are usually placed in the jugular vein. Alternate sites include cephalic and lateral thoracic veins (Figures 22-11 and 22-12). Catheters should be placed aseptically and sutured appropriately to prevent dislodgment. Teflon catheters are relatively irritating and should be replaced every 3 days. Silastic catheters can remain in the vein as long these are patent and show no signs of infection. Central venous catheterization using a wire-guided polyurethane catheter is often used in critically ill patients. Polyurethane catheters are less traumatic, less thrombogenic, and ideal in peripheral veins, such as lateral thoracic and cephalic veins. IV catheters should be flushed with heparinized saline flush (2 to 10 U/ml) every 6 hours and monitored twice daily for heat, swelling, and pain. Infection at the catheter site may occur in the subcutaneous tissue or in the vein (septic thrombophlebitis). Septic thrombophlebitis can be life threatening in horses.

The ideal antimicrobial is effective against a wide range of bacterial organisms (broad spectrum), easy to administer, and nontoxic. Penicillin has good efficacy against common gram-positive pathogens in the horse *(Streptococcus zooepidemicus, S. equi equi)* and is relatively safe. It is frequently administered intramuscularly (procaine penicillin) and IV (potassium penicillin). Procaine penicillin should never be administered IV. Life-threatening anaphylactic reactions are reported with procaine penicillin administration and should be treated with epinephrine. Aminoglycoside antimicrobials (gentamicin, amikacin sulfate) are efficacious against gram-negative pathogens and can be administered intramuscularly or IV. These antimicrobials are nephrotoxic, so renal function should be monitored during therapy. Trimethoprim-sulfa antimicrobials have a moderate gram-positive and gram-negative spectrum and are administered orally or IV. Ceftiofur sodium has a good gram-positive and gram-negative spectrum and may be administered intramuscularly or IV. Metronidazole is administered orally or *per rectum* to treat anaerobic bacterial infections. There are specific indications for the administration of other antimicrobials, but some are not widely used because of the risk of antimicrobial-induced colitis. Chloramphenicol is used sparingly in horses because of the human health risk for idiosyncratic, fatal aplastic anemia from exposure during patient administration.

There are many analgesic medications available for horses. Phenylbutazone, ketoprofen, and flunixin meglumine are NSAIDs that provide mild to moderate pain relief. NSAIDs also reduce fever (antipyretic) and inflammation. Phenylbutazone is most effective for the treatment of musculoskeletal pain. Ketoprofen, meclofenamic acid, and naproxen are less commonly used drugs that provide mild to moderate analgesia for musculoskeletal pain. Flunixin meglumine is more effective for soft tissue and visceral (abdominal) pain. In addition, flunixin meglumine may combat the effects of toxemia in horses with gastrointestinal tract disease. Sedatives that also provide analgesia include xylazine and detomidine (alpha$_2$ agonists). Xylazine provides approximately 20 minutes of sedation and analgesia. Detomidine provides up to 1 hour of sedation and analgesia. Butorphanol is a narcotic agonist that provides up to 1 hour of sedation and analgesia for moderate to severe pain. Acepromazine has no analgesic

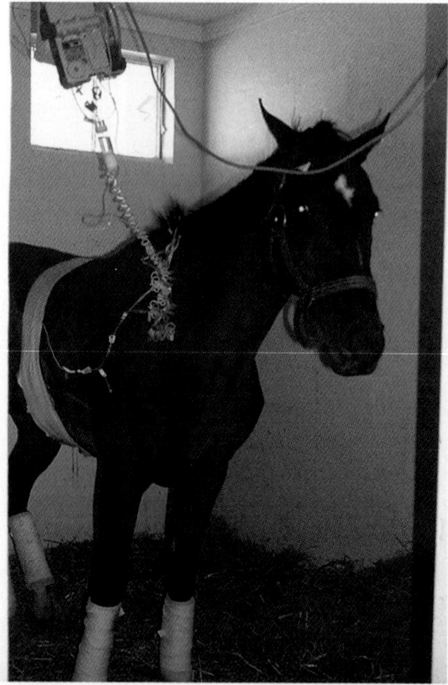

FIGURE 22-11 Patient with an IV catheter in the right lateral thoracic vein.

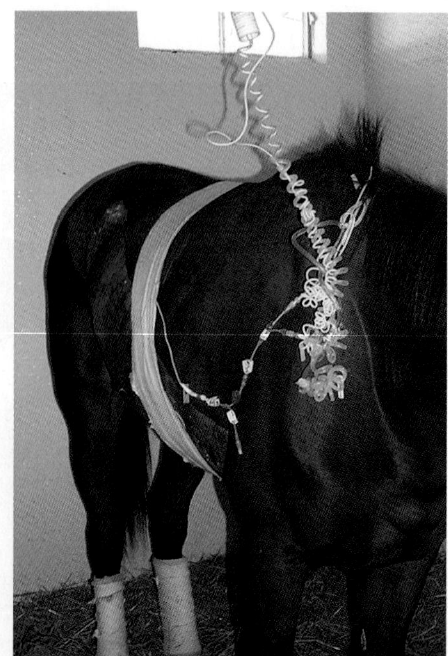

FIGURE 22-12 Close-up view of IV catheter in the right lateral thoracic vein.

properties and only provides moderate tranquilization. Acepromazine also causes hypotension and can cause persistent paraphimosis in stallions.

Corticosteroids have potent antiinflammatory properties and are administered for allergic airway disease, allergic skin conditions, immune-mediated disease, and joint inflammation. Corticosteroids are administered topically, orally, parenterally (IV or intramuscularly), and intraarticularly. Adverse effects of corticosteroid administration include immunosuppression, polyuria or polydipsia, poor hair coat, muscle wasting, poor wound healing, laminitis, and progression of degenerative joint disease. Therefore corticosteroids are administered with caution and only when specifically indicated.

DMSO is an antiinflammatory drug occasionally used in horses to relieve swelling and edema associated with CNS trauma, traumatic musculoskeletal injuries, laminitis, and myositis. DMSO may be administered topically, orally, or IV (diluted in crystalloid fluids as a 10% to 20% solution). Nitrile gloves are used while handling the product, because it can be absorbed wearing latex gloves. Rapid IV administration may result in hemolysis, hematuria, and sweating in horses.

> *TECHNICIAN NOTE* The veterinary technician plays a pivotal role in the day-to-day monitoring and caring for hospitalized patients; therefore the ability to be observant and to perform a thorough physical examination is vital.

LABORATORY STUDIES

Clinicopathologic testing provides important information for the veterinarian to identify an impairment of an organ system, confirm a clinical diagnosis, assess the response to therapy, and formulate a prognosis. The normal values of many clinicopathologic tests vary among species. In addition, there are species-specific characteristics associated with diseases and the significance of abnormal findings. This section concentrates solely on equine-specific alterations in clinicopathologic values in health and disease.

Hematology

A complete blood count (CBC) provides information pertaining to the red blood cell (RBC) count, RBC morphology, total white blood cell (WBC) count, WBC differential (including neutrophils, lymphocytes, eosinophils, monocytes), WBC morphology, and fibrinogen concentration. Samples for a CBC should be submitted in a tube with ethylenediaminetetraacetic acid (EDTA) anticoagulant (purple-top tube). The RBCs are most easily estimated using the packed-cell volume (PCV); low PCV (less than 30%) is indicative of anemia. Horses have a large muscular spleen that normally contains up to one third of the circulating RBC volume. With excitement and exercise, the PCV in horses can increase by as much as 50% secondary to splenic contraction. Therefore the resting PCV is highly variable and must be serially evaluated in excitable patients. In addition, the response of the spleen to massive hemorrhage precludes the use of the PCV to estimate the magnitude of blood loss for at least 24 hours. The normal range of the PCV depends on the breed, but generally is between 32% and 45%. Hot-blooded breeds (Thoroughbreds, Arabians, Quarter horses) have higher resting RBC counts compared with ponies and draft horses.

An evaluation of the total and differential WBC count is important to identify the presence of infection. In most instances, a bacterial infection will manifest as an increase in WBC count (leukocytosis) characterized by an increase in the number of mature neutrophils (mature neutrophilia). Fibrinogen is a coagulation factor and an acute-phase protein in horses, produced by the liver in response to inflammation. Fibrinogen concentrations remain increased until the infection is resolved.

Horses are particularly sensitive to circulating endotoxins released from the cell wall of gram-negative bacteria. Endotoxins cause margination and sequestration of WBCs. Therefore a profoundly low WBC count (leukopenia) characterized by low neutrophil count (neutropenia) and immature band neutrophils (left shift) is indicative of gram-negative septicemia or gastrointestinal disease with inflammation allowing mucosal absorption of gram-negative bacteria. High eosinophil counts (eosinophilia) are indicative of a massive parasite infestation or possibly allergic diseases. Low lymphocyte counts (lymphopenia) may be observed in horses with early viral infections.

Serum Chemistry

A serum chemistry panel provides specific information pertaining to the liver, kidney, muscle, and serum electrolyte concentrations. The serum sample should be drawn into a tube without anticoagulant (red-top tube) and submitted to the laboratory. Some laboratories can perform chemistry profiles in heparinized blood samples (green top). If there will be more than a 1-hour delay in submission, the tube should be centrifuged, serum or plasma removed, and stored in the refrigerator. Delayed sample submission without centrifuging produces artificially low serum glucose and high serum potassium concentrations. Horses normally have a yellow tint to the serum as a result of increased serum bilirubin levels because horses do not have gallbladders. Serum bilirubin concentrations will increase dramatically if feed is withheld for more than 24 hours as a result of a normal physiologic response and does not indicate liver disease. Most species develop low serum albumin levels with chronic liver disease because of decreased production; however, horses maintain production of albumin even with a marked impairment of liver function. Reliable indicators of liver dysfunction in horses are high serum γ-glutamyltransferase (GGT) activity, high serum sorbitol dehydrogenase (SDH) activity, high serum bile acid concentrations, low blood urea nitrogen (BUN) concentrations, and increased ammonia levels.

In most species, renal failure produces low serum calcium and high serum phosphorus concentrations. Horses are obligate calcium excreters, and chronic renal failure often produces a marked increase in the serum calcium concentration. Reliable indicators of renal failure in horses include high serum creatinine and BUN and electrolyte abnormalities, including low sodium and chloride and high potassium and calcium levels. The large colon of horses exchanges a vast amount of electrolytes and fluids on a daily basis. Horses with colonic inflammation may develop marked electrolyte abnormalities before the development of diarrhea. Low serum sodium, chloride, and potassium levels in horses with abdominal pain or depression often indicate a loss of electrolytes into the lumen of the colon and impending diarrhea.

Serum creatine phosphokinase (CK) is an indicator of muscle damage in all species. Horses have large muscle masses in comparison with ruminants and small animals. Moderate increases in serum CK levels (two to four times normal) readily occur in horses following prolonged transport, prolonged recumbency, exercise in an unconditioned horse, or rolling from abdominal pain. Moderate increases do not usually indicate primary muscle disease. Horses with primary muscle disease, such as exertional rhabdomyolysis (tying up, azoturia, Monday morning sickness) have increases in serum CK activity of up to 200 times normal values.

Urinalysis

A urinalysis is essential for evaluation of primary renal disease. Urine can be collected as a voided sample or after catheterization of the bladder. Urinary catheterization is performed in the standing horse. Females should have the perineum washed with 1% iodine and water. A sterile gloved hand is inserted into the vagina approximately 10 cm. The sterile catheter is gently inserted into the urethral orifice on the floor of the vagina to obtain urine. Males need to be sedated, and the penis is then grasped, gently extruded, and washed thoroughly with 1% iodine and water. While wearing sterile gloves, a sterile flexible stallion catheter is inserted into the urethral orifice and advanced until urine flows from the catheter. If no urine is spontaneously voided, slight negative pressure from a syringe attached to the catheter may produce a sample.

Normal horse urine is usually alkaline (pH 7 to 9) and contains many calcium carbonate crystals. Alkaline urine usually produces a false-positive reaction for protein on urine dipsticks. Horses have a large number of mucous glands located within the renal pelvis; therefore normal horse urine may appear thick and mucoid. Red urine is abnormal and results from the presence of frank blood (primary urinary tract disease), hemoglobin (hemolytic anemia), or myoglobin (myositis). The differentiation of these sources of red urine requires special testing of urine and serum samples. Urine specific gravity and urinary electrolyte excretion ratios should be obtained to investigate primary renal function. Urine specific gravity indicates the ability of the kidney to concentrate urine, and normal values in resting horses should be greater than 1.030. Urinary electrolyte excretion ratios indicate the ability of the kidney to conserve electrolytes. The identification of WBCs and numerous bacteria indicate a urinary tract infection. Protein in the urine (proteinuria), glucose in the urine (glucosuria), and casts indicate renal disease.

Evaluation of Body Fluids

The evaluation of cerebrospinal, synovial (joint), and abdominal cavity fluid provides important information pertaining to inflammation, an infection, or neoplasia within that particular body cavity. These body fluids are analyzed for total protein, total cell count, differential cell count, and bacterial culture.

Some neurologic diseases in horses require a CSF analysis for diagnosis. Because some neurologic diseases, such as rabies, have zoonotic potential, CSF must be collected and handled with caution (e.g., protective eyewear or face shields, lab coats, and gloves) to prevent exposure to the infectious agent. CSF is collected in standing, sedated horses with spinal cord disease from the lumbosacral space using a 6-inch 18-gauge spinal needle. In horses with brain and brainstem disease, CSF is collected in anesthetized horses from the atlantooccipital space using a 3-inch, 18-gauge spinal needle. Normal nucleated cell counts are less than five cells per microliter (predominately lymphocytes). The normal total protein concentration is variable depending on the laboratory, but is usually less than 80 mg/dl (higher than in other species). Abnormalities in protein and cell counts can identify an inflammatory, infectious, or neoplastic process, but CSF analyses are often nonspecific. Antibodies to the agents of several equine neurologic diseases (rabies, protozoal myelitis, herpes myeloencephalopathy, equine encephalomyelitis) can be detected in CSF, which provides specific information regarding the cause of neurologic signs. Complications associated with a CSF tap include iatrogenic (operator-induced) spinal cord trauma and the introduction of bacteria into the CNS.

Abdominal pain, an abnormal rectal examination, abdominal distention, and fever of unknown origin are indications for abdominocentesis in horses. Abdominal fluid is obtained by placing an 18-gauge, 1.5-inch needle into the peritoneal space of the ventral abdomen. The needle should be placed one hand's breadth behind the sternum, off the midline to the right of the horse (to avoid the spleen). If a 1.5-inch needle is insufficient to reach the peritoneal cavity, a teat cannula may be used. The use of a teat cannula is more invasive and increases the risk of traumatic bowel rupture. The normal abdominal fluid total protein is less than 2.5 mg/dl, and the normal total nucleated cell count is less than 5000/ml (50% neutrophils). The analysis of abdominal fluid can identify devitalized bowel in horses with acute abdominal pain (colic), an abdominal abscess, a tumor in horses with a mass in the abdomen identified via rectal palpation, and a ruptured bladder in foals with abdominal distention. Complications of abdominocentesis include traumatic bowel rupture, intraabdominal hemorrhage from trauma to the spleen, and iatrogenic septic peritonitis.

Bacterial Culture and Susceptibility Testing

The veterinary technician often plays an important role in the bacteriologic testing of specimens collected from patients with infectious diseases. Specimens (blood, joint fluid, abdominal fluid, urine, wound exudate, infected bone, etc.) are frequently collected from horses with infectious diseases for culture. Following proper procedures during the collection and transport of these specimens to the laboratory for culture and susceptibility testing improves the chances of growing the causative organism. There are specific guidelines followed for the collection and transport of different types of specimens. For example, blood is usually placed in a special enhancement medium immediately after collection for transport to the laboratory. There are also special methods for the collection and transport of samples submitted for aerobic and anaerobic culture. Identifying the causative agent in an infectious process and determining its in vitro susceptibility pattern to antibiotics are often critical in choosing the appropriate antibiotic regimen. Fecal samples are often submitted for *Salmonella* spp. or *Clostridium* spp. cultures from horses with diarrhea. Fecal samples for *Salmonella* spp. culture should be submitted daily for 5 consecutive days. If culture results are negative for these five samples, the horses are not shedding *Salmonella* organisms. Fecal samples may be tested for *Clostridium* toxins and *Clostridium* spp. culture; samples should be submitted daily for 3 consecutive days. Fecal samples may be submitted to other diagnostic tests, such as ELISA for rotavirus.

> TECHNICIAN NOTE Horses normally have yellow serum as a result of a high serum bilirubin level compared with other species because they do not have gallbladders. Serum bilirubin concentrations will increase dramatically if feed is withheld for more than 24 hours. This condition, fasting hyperbilirubinemia, is a normal physiologic response in horses and does not indicate liver disease.

Delivering exceptional medical care to the equine patient requires a team approach, and the veterinary technician plays a vital role in the diagnosis and treatment of these patients. Carefully monitoring hospitalized cases for potential complications is another important role for the veterinary technician. These horses often respond well to the treatment, and it is rewarding to see the horse recover with proper care.

FOOD ANIMAL MEDICINE

With fewer veterinarians choosing food animal practice, practice owners have been finding it increasingly difficult to hire an associate. For these individuals, optimizing the use of veterinary technicians is of great importance. Capitalization of technician skills can help meet client needs and improve practice productivity and efficiency. As a part of the professional team, the veterinary technician can assist in the restraint and handling of animals for an examination, sample collection, diagnosis, and treatment. Technicians can also prepare equipment, supplies, and animals for surgery and assist during the surgical procedure.

Other tasks performed by veterinary technicians in food animal practice include performing laboratory procedures and diagnostic tests, patient care, diagnostic imaging, anesthesia, preparation of pharmacologic and biologic agents, administration of injections and other treatments, ration balancing, body condition scoring in cattle and small ruminants, metabolic profiling of herds or flocks, monitoring records of postparturient cows, and planning herd consultation visits. Technicians are also valuable in educating clients. For example, instructing producers about the proper technique for the placement of growth implants in feedlot cattle and explanation of proper injection techniques based on meat quality assurance guidelines.

Veterinary technicians can also perform necropsies and collect tissue specimens. They record their findings and take digital pictures of the necropsy for subsequent review by the veterinarian. Technicians may also possess special talents or training, such as expertise in artificial insemination or corrective foot work, that could be offered as a service to clients. A cognizant, well-trained, and knowledgeable technician can anticipate the needs of the veterinarian and producer thereby enhancing the productivity of the professional team.

Finally, with current concerns of bioterrorism and foreign animal diseases in the United States (currently bovine spongiform encephalopathy and foot and mouth disease), the food animal veterinary technician might play a key role in the dissemination of information when handling public questions and concerns.

> TECHNICIAN NOTE Capitalization of veterinary technician skills in food animal practice can help meet client needs and improve practice productivity, efficiency, and revenue.

COMMON DISEASES AND CONDITIONS OF CATTLE

CARE OF THE NEONATE AND NEONATAL DISEASES

Food animal veterinarians are often asked to assist cows and heifers having difficulty calving. Often calves that are born via forced fetal extraction or cesarean section (C-section) are compromised. While the veterinarian attends to the mother, especially in the case of a C-section, the veterinary technician can provide intensive care to the neonate, if necessary. The most important step is to make sure the calf is breathing. All mucus should be cleared from the nose, mouth, and upper airway. There are several ways to achieve this. The calf may be hung upside down with the head off the ground to allow drainage of these fluids. A bulb syringe also works well to remove mucus from the nose and mouth, and it also provides nasal stimulus to breathe. A piece of straw or hay can also be used to tickle the nose and stimulate respiration. If all else fails, a technique known as gin chung, placing a small-gauge needle in the nasal septum, is often a successful respiratory stimulus. If these techniques fail, artificial respiration can be provided by mouth-to-nose resuscitation or by raising and lowering the uppermost forelimb while simultaneously pressing and releasing the rib cage. For difficult cases, a small amount of doxapram hydrochloride, a respiratory stimulant, may be injected under the tongue to induce respiration. Once the calf is breathing, it should be vigorously rubbed dry with a towel and the umbilical cord dipped in strong (7%) iodine.

Colostrum ingestion soon after birth is an important part of neonatal survival and prevention of infectious disease. Cattle and other ruminants (including sheep and goats) have a thick syndesmochorial placentation that prevents in utero transfer of high-molecular-weight immunoglobulins. These species are essentially agammaglobulinemic at birth and rely on the ingestion and absorption of colostrum-rich antibodies and nonantibody immune factors.

The transfer of immunity can be compromised by colostrum deficiencies, ingestion failure, or absorption failure. Immunoglobulins are absorbed by pinocytosis by specialized epithelial cells in the jejunum and ileum. These cells are replaced soon after birth by normal intestinal epithelium, and absorption terminates. Therefore it is important that the neonate receives colostrum within the first 6 to 8 hours of life. The calf should receive colostrum at the rate of 10% of its body weight within the first 12 hours (4.5 L/45 kg of body weight in 12 hours).

Several tests are available for the detection of failure of passive transfer (FPT), including single radial immunodiffusion (SRID), sodium sulfite precipitation, zinc sulfate turbidity, and serum protein analysis. The serum concentration of IgG using SRID should be greater than 1600 mg/dl. Serum protein can be measured using a refractometer. A serum protein concentration greater than 5 mg/dl in the absence of dehydration is indicative of successful passive transfer; values less than 4.5 mg/dl are consistent with FPT. For valuable calves, the treatment may be achieved by plasma transfusion at the rate of 20 to 40 ml/kg body weight.

Partial or total FPT can make a calf susceptible to a variety of disease conditions. Compromised calves are more likely to develop umbilical infections (omphalophlebitis), which may lead to any combination of the following problems: septicemia, septic arthritis, anterior uveitis, meningitis, vegetative endocarditis, pneumonia, and diarrhea. Calves experiencing these problems should immediately be given broad-spectrum antimicrobial agents, supportive therapy, such as fluids with dextrose and electrolytes, and other treatments specific to the problems encountered. If omphalophlebitis is present and does not respond to antimicrobial therapy, surgical removal of infected umbilical remnants should be considered if the patient is a good surgical candidate. Anterior uveitis and hypopyon often respond to the application of ophthalmic preparations of antibiotics and atropine. Septic arthritis may be treated with IV regional antibiotic perfusion or implantation of antibiotic-impregnated polymethylmethacrylate (PMMA) beads near affected joints.

> *TECHNICIAN NOTE* Colostrum ingestion soon after birth is an important part of the prevention of infectious diseases in neonates.

Diarrhea, a common problem in young dairy and beef calves, has multiple infectious and noninfectious causes. Viral causes include rotavirus, coronavirus, and bovine diarrhea virus (BVD). Bacterial enteritis may result if the calf is infected with *Escherichia coli*, *Salmonella* spp., or clostridial and protozoal diseases, such as cryptosporidiosis and coccidiosis, may also cause calf diarrhea. In addition, a variety of management conditions, including stress, poor nutrition, and improper sanitation, may cause or contribute to the development of diarrhea. Regardless of cause, affected calves often develop watery diarrhea, rapidly leading to severe dehydration, metabolic acidosis, hypoglycemia, shock, and hypothermia. The treatment is aimed at quick replacement of lost fluids and correction of acidosis and electrolyte abnormalities. Sick calves should be started on warm IV fluids, such as Normosol (Abbott Laboratories) supplemented with dextrose and bicarbonate as indicated. Milk and milk products should be withheld during the treatment of diarrhea, but for no longer than 48 hours total. In herds in which calf diarrhea is a persistent problem, it may be necessary to vaccinate cows and heifers before calving. Many polyvalent vaccines are available, and the product(s) used can be tailored to the needs of the individual herd.

Calves should be fed whole milk or quality calf milk replacer. Although milk replacers are never as complete as whole milk, the product chosen should be of good quality and meet the following standards: protein level 20% to 22%, and all protein must be milk derived (dried skimmed milk, dried whey, whey protein, casein, etc.), crude fat 18% to 20%, and fiber less than 10%. In general, calves are fed 10% of their body weight divided twice daily. This amount may need to be adjusted based on individual needs. It is important to carefully follow label directions when mixing milk replacers since a solution that is too concentrated or too dilute can cause problems, such as nutritional diarrhea. Well-informed veterinary technicians can question clients concerning the quality of their milk replacers, the method of mixing the milk replacer, and the technique of calf feeding and can then make appropriate recommendations to owners.

CONDITIONS OF THE DIGESTIVE SYSTEM

Actinomycosis and Actinobacillosis

Two common conditions of the head in cattle include actinobacillosis (woody tongue) and actinomycosis (lumpy jaw). Woody tongue is caused by a gram-negative bacterium,

Actinobacillus lignieresii, which is a normal inhabitant of the mouth of cattle. The organism may gain entry into the soft tissues of the mouth through wounds caused by weed or plant awns resulting in a granulomatous abscess, usually of the tongue. The tongue becomes hard with a diffuse nodular swelling. Clinical signs include excessive salivation and the inability of the animal to prehend food normally causing anorexia and weight loss. The tongue may become so swollen that it protrudes from the mouth (Figure 22-13). The diagnosis is usually based on clinical signs and an examination of the tongue; however, a biopsy and culture of the organism confirms the diagnosis. The successful treatment of this disease involves using sodium iodide and antibiotics. Sodium iodide is administered IV, and care must be taken during administration because perivascular injection may result in tissue sloughing. Woody tongue typically responds to treatment within a few days, but occasionally, repeated doses of sodium iodide may be necessary until signs of iodism occur (lacrimation, anorexia, dandruff, coughing). Prevention includes reduced exposure of the cattle to scabrous feed and plant awns (foxtails, horse nettles, pigweed) by keeping pastures as clean as possible.

Lumpy jaw is the common name for the disease caused by *Actinomyces bovis.* This organism is gram positive and also a normal inhabitant of the mouth of ruminants. This bacteria gains entry through wounds in the mouth and the infection results in osteomyelitis of the mandible and less commonly the maxilla. Affected cattle have a hard, immovable, nonpainful bony mass of the mandible or maxilla (Figure 22-14). If the mass becomes large enough or involves tooth roots, it may result in pain, an inability to masticate, and subsequent anorexia with weight loss. The treatment of lumpy jaw is the same as described for woody tongue; however, this disease is much less responsive to treatment. Repeated doses of sodium iodide are often necessary just to arrest the growth of the lesion. A more radical treatment involves surgical débridement and curettage of fibrous tissue and infected bone. The surgery is not without risk because these patients often lose significant amounts of blood and may require blood transfusions during the surgical procedure. However, surgical treatment followed by medical treatment offers the best long-term prognosis for valuable animals.

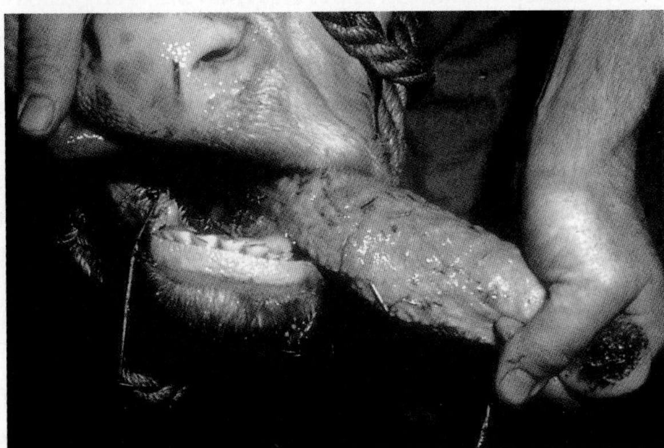

FIGURE 22-13 Bull with actinobacillosis (woody tongue). The tongue is enlarged and nodular in appearance.

Pharyngeal Trauma and Abscessation

Pharyngeal trauma occurs relatively frequently in cattle and may result in cellulitis, abscess, or hematoma formation. It is almost always caused by trauma associated with the improper use of a balling gun, long dose syringe, speculum, paste dewormer gun, or a rigid stomach tube. Less commonly, a foreign body (sharp stick or wire) may penetrate the pharynx.

Clinical signs include anorexia, salivation, malodorous breath, extension of the head and neck, feed coming from the nares, and mild bloat. In more severe cases, fever, obvious pharyngeal swelling, dysphagia, coughing, and aspiration pneumonia may occur. Careful digital palpation of the pharynx per os is often diagnostic. Always wear gloves during palpation of the mouth or pharynx in cattle because of the concern of rabies. Endoscopy and radiography may be of great benefit in diagnosing the site of the lesion, extent of the cellulitis, and the presence of a foreign body.

The treatment requires the aggressive use of antimicrobial drugs for 10 to 14 days. NSAIDs may help reduce the inflammation in the early stages of the disease. Supportive therapy is also important, especially if the animal cannot eat or drink. Feed and water may be forced with the use of a soft stomach tube or via a temporary rumenostomy. If a retropharyngeal abscess develops, it is best to drain the abscess into the pharynx by manually enlarging the original laceration.

The best way to prevent this condition is to exercise caution when using balling guns, dose syringes, and stomach tubes and make sure restraint is adequate to prevent excessive movement of the animal and subsequent injury. The veterinary technician can play an important role in educating the client-producer concerning the proper use of this equipment.

> *TECHNICIAN NOTE* Pharyngeal trauma in cattle can be prevented by the careful use of oral dosing equipment.

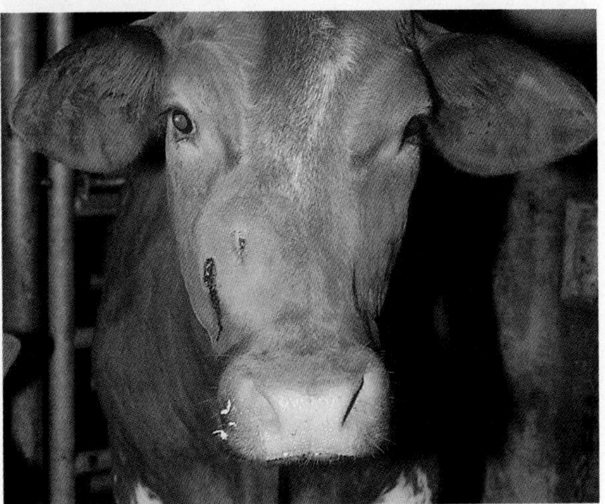

FIGURE 22-14 A bony mass on the maxilla of a cow with actinomycosis (lumpy jaw).

Grain Overload (Carbohydrate Engorgement, Lactic Acidosis)

Grain overload in ruminants results from the consumption of excessive amounts of highly fermentable carbohydrate feed with the production of large quantities of lactic acid in the rumen. Cattle with grain overload rapidly develop clinical signs of depression, anorexia, bloat, diarrhea with large amounts of grain, dehydration, incoordination, and recumbency leading to death.

Excess carbohydrate ingestion leads to an increased production of volatile fatty acids in the rumen, which lowers rumen pH and decreases rumen motility. *S. bovis* organisms then multiply producing lactic acid, which further lowers rumen pH (4.0 to 5.0). The acid-resistant *Lactobacillus* spp. then proliferate, producing more lactic acid. With the increased osmolarity of the rumen fluid, body water is drawn into the rumen creating a "splashy rumen" and leading to a loss of body water with severe dehydration and metabolic acidosis. Thus affected animals if not treated early may develop severe metabolic acidosis leading to shock and acute death. Animals that do not die from the acute acidosis may subsequently develop secondary problems, such as rumenitis with liver abscesses, laminitis (founder), and/or polioencephalomalacia.

The diagnosis is based on a history of sudden exposure to large amounts of grain, typical clinical signs, and a rumen pH of less than 5.0. Ruminal fluid analysis can be a valuable tool in the diagnosis of this and other rumen abnormalities.

Medical treatment involves removal of the rumen contents with a large-bore stomach tube (Kingman tube), which is accomplished by repeated flushing of water into the rumen followed by the outflow of rumen contents (lavage) (Figure 22-15). In addition, animals are given oral antacids, antibiotics (usually penicillin), NSAIDs when rehydrated, and thiamine, which all help prevent liver abscesses, polioencephalomalacia, and laminitis. In more severe cases,

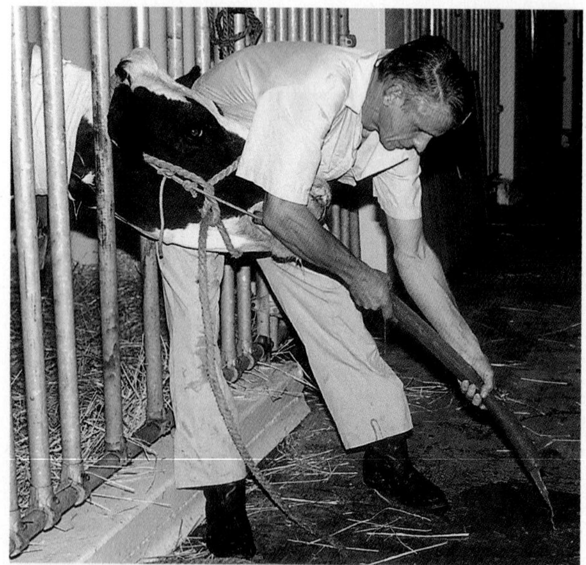

FIGURE 22-15 Rumen lavage or flushing using a large-bore stomach tube (Kingman tube).

IV fluids with sodium bicarbonate should be administered to correct dehydration and acidosis. It may be necessary in some cases to perform a rumenotomy to remove all rumen contents (see Chapter 31). Whether an animal is treated medically or surgically, rumen transfaunation is often helpful to reestablish normal rumen microflora and improve appetite during the convalescent period. Prevention of grain overload involves making dietary changes gradually. Rumen adaptation to dietary changes may take as long as 6 weeks. The veterinary technician can be instrumental in helping owners understand nutrition and the importance of making slow dietary adjustments in ruminants.

The analysis of rumen fluid is useful to establish the cause of indigestion from abnormal fermentation, such as occurs with the previously described grain overload. These are diagnostic tests that can be performed relatively quickly by a veterinary technician, providing the veterinarian with diagnostic information as to the cause of the indigestion and a treatment appropriate to the condition. Samples may be collected by using a 2- to 3-m–long × 1-cm-inner–diameter (ID) stomach tube. Nasogastric passage of the tube prevents continuous struggling during sample collection and reduces the amount of saliva (no mouth device) that can contaminate the sample and falsely elevate its pH. Samples may also be obtained via centesis of the left paralumbar area using an 18-gauge, 12- to 15-cm needle.

The evaluation of the fluid sample includes the assessment of color, consistency, odor, pH, sedimentation velocity, microscopic examination, rumen chloride, and redox potential. The normal color of rumen fluid is olive or brownish green. Grain overload results in fluid that is milky gray, whereas prolonged stasis or decomposition in the rumen changes the color to dark green or black. The consistency of normal rumen fluid is slightly viscous, and salivary contamination increases viscosity. The odor of normal rumen fluid is aromatic and strong, but it develops an acid smell with grain overload, a putrid odor with stasis and decomposition, and an ammonia scent with urea toxicity.

The pH of rumen fluid is normally 6.5 to 6.8 (5.5 to 6.5 with high grain diets). In general, anorexia will usually result in an elevation of rumen pH. Values below 5.5 and above 7.0 can cause anorexia because of an alteration in the normal microbial population. A pH less than 5.5 is suggestive of grain overload, whereas a pH greater than 7.5 may indicate the overzealous use of antacids or urea toxicity.

An evaluation of sedimentation velocity should be performed soon after sampling and serves as a crude evaluation of microbial activity. The sample is placed in a tube and observed for the time it takes for sedimentation to occur. Fine particles sink, and coarse particles float, buoyed by gas bubbles of fermentation. Normal sedimentation takes 4 to 8 minutes. Grossly inactive fluid shows rapid sedimentation, and frothy ingesta may show no sedimentation.

A microscopic examination is performed to assess the type of bacteria present and protozoal activity. The observation of protozoa requires no stain, and they can be easily seen at 40× to 100× magnification. Normally, ciliate and flagellate forms of various sizes and shapes are present and active. The importance of protozoa is their sensitivity to abnormalities in rumen fluid; the larger species are more sensitive to change, and all protozoa die at a pH less than 5. In the normal animal, gram-negative bacteria are predominate in the rumen. Grain overload results in mostly gram-positive bacteria (*Streptococcus* spp. and *Lactobacillus* spp.).

The rumen chloride concentration is normally less than 25 mEq/L and may be elevated in cases of vagus indigestion (failure of pyloric outflow and reflux of chloride back into the rumen). The redox potential test uses a new methylene blue (NMB) test to evaluate anaerobic fermentation. To perform the test, 1 ml of 0.03% NMB is mixed with 20 ml rumen fluid (control sample is untreated rumen fluid). The microflora, if active, reduce NMB, and it loses its color, and this usually takes about 3 minutes (1 to 3 minutes if on a grain diet, 3 to 6 minutes if on a hay diet). Animals with prolonged anorexia, after grain overload, or those receiving indigestible roughage may have a redox potential greater than15 minutes.

> *TECHNICIAN NOTE* To prevent grain overload and other indigestion in cattle, dietary changes should be made gradually over at least a 6-week period.

Rumen Tympany (Bloat)

Gas production is a normal occurrence during rumen fermentation, and healthy animals are capable of eructating far more gas than the rumen produces. However, in some cases, abnormal distention of the rumen with gas may occur resulting in bloat. Bloat is classified as either primary where eructation is normal but the gas cannot be expelled or secondary that is due to a failure of eructation. Primary bloat occurs when large amounts of legumes or grain are ingested resulting in development of froth in the rumen. A failure of eructation or secondary bloat may be associated with esophageal foreign bodies (choke); motor function abnormalities of the rumen, such as vagus indigestion; body position (lateral recumbency); hypocalcemia; or pharyngitis. Bloat is also described as free gas bloat or frothy bloat depending on the cause.

Clinical signs include distention of the left paralumbar fossa, discomfort (grunting, colic), dyspnea with open-mouth breathing, anorexia, salivation, anxiety, depression terminally, and sudden death.

The treatment of free-gas bloat involves passing a stomach tube either via the nasogastric or orogastric route. If bloat is due to the animal's position, the animal should be helped into sternal recumbency or a standing position. If hypocalcemia is the underlying problem, administration of calcium is therapeutic. Forced exercise also stimulates rumen motility and eructation. In addition, rumen stimulants improve motility and normal belching. If an animal is critically bloated and passing a stomach tube is too stressful, an emergency procedure called rumen trocarization should be performed using a large-bore trocar to enter the rumen through the left paralumbar fossa. The surgical treatment of chronic bloat is covered in Chapter 31.

Frothy bloat requires a different treatment in that the froth must first be consolidated into larger pockets of gas before it can be expelled. To reduce surface tension, several products may be used, including poloxalene, household detergent (Tide, 2 to 3 oz), mineral oil, or dioctyl sodium sulfosuccinate (DSS). Once the frothy bloat becomes a free gas bloat, it can be eructated or relieved via a tube. Nutritional management, such as preventing excessive exposure to grain or legumes, is important to prevent bloat in ruminants.

Traumatic Reticuloperitonitis

Traumatic reticuloperitonitis (TRP), or hardware disease, which results from the penetration of the reticulum by a foreign body, is one of the most common gastrointestinal problems affecting the forestomach compartments of mature dairy cattle. The indiscriminate eating habits of cattle, in contrast to small ruminants, can lead to the accidental ingestion of foreign materials that settle in the reticulum (Figure 22-16). The foreign bodies ingested by cattle are most often wires and nails, but also include steel objects. Most foreign bodies are ferromagnetic. Subsequent to ingestion of a foreign body, four outcomes are possible:

1. Attachment of the object to a magnet without further disease problems
2. Penetration of the reticular wall with acute inflammation and mild clinical disease if there is not penetration into the peritoneal cavity
3. Perforation of the reticular wall into the peritoneal cavity with acute localized TRP
4. Migration of the foreign body with penetration into the peritoneal or thoracic cavity and resulting abscessation (thoracic, reticular, hepatic), vagal indigestion, pericarditis, myocarditis, or other secondary problems

Acute cases of TRP result in anorexia, a sharp decrease in milk production, reluctance to rise or move, cranial abdominal pain, and kyphosis. Uncomplicated cases may improve in 3 to 5 days, but progression of the severity of signs may indicate either a failure to contain a localized peritonitis or extension of the infection to other organs. A heart rate

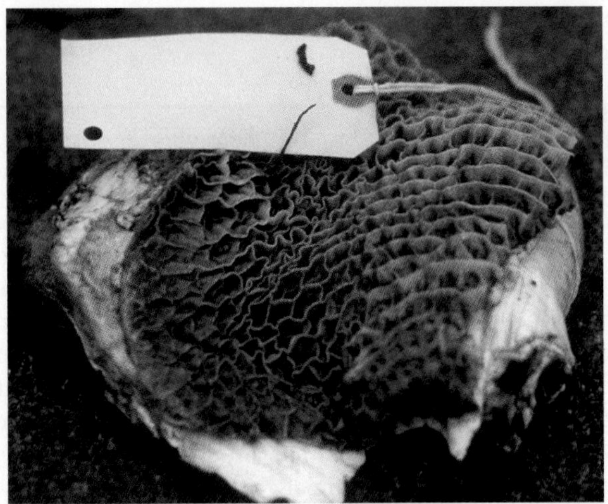

FIGURE 22-16 Metallic foreign body (wire) found in the reticulum of a cow with traumatic reticuloperitonitis (hardware disease).

greater than 90 bpm or a fever greater than 40° C generally indicates more severe disease, such as diffuse peritonitis or pericarditis. A heart rate less than 64 bpm is suggestive of vagus indigestion syndrome.

A differential white blood cell count (WBC) is a more reliable indicator of inflammation than is a total WBC. A neutrophilia (greater than 4000 cells/μl) with a left shift can be expected in acute cases, but in chronic cases, these changes are less consistent. A high plasma fibrinogen concentration (greater than 1000 mg/dl) usually occurs in both acute and chronic cases of TRP.

A peritoneal fluid analysis may be helpful in the diagnosis of TRP, especially in chronic cases when WBC changes are infrequently observed. It may be necessary to sample multiple sites because of the size of the rumen and that cattle are capable of localizing an infection by the formation of a large amount of fibrin. Failure to obtain a fluid sample does not rule out TRP. A relatively accurate diagnosis of peritonitis can be made if the nucleated cell count is greater than 6000 cells/μl and the total protein is greater than 3 g/dl (a more accurate diagnosis can be made if a differential is performed, and neutrophils account for greater than 40% of the cells and eosinophils for less than 10%).

Reticular or cranioventral abdominal radiography or ultrasonography can offer valuable assistance in the diagnosis and treatment of TRP.

Medical treatment of TRP is often successful. Even if a foreign body has perforated the reticular wall, in approximately half of the cases, it will return to the lumen. Medical treatment is geared toward treating reticulitis and/or peritonitis and preventing further perforation of the reticulum by the use of broad-spectrum antimicrobials and the oral administration of a magnet.

Surgical intervention may be necessary if TRP fails to respond to conservative treatment (see Chapter 31 for surgical details). Most abscesses that form secondary to TRP are located on the medial wall of the reticulum and are usually tightly adhered. These abscesses are the most common causes of vagal indigestion associated with TRP. These tightly adhered abscesses can be lanced and drained into the reticulum or omasum and then explored for the presence of a foreign body.

> *TECHNICIAN NOTE* TRP (hardware disease) may lead to peritonitis, liver or reticular abscesses, pericarditis, vagal indigestion, or other secondary problems.

Indications for performing paracentesis or abdominocentesis include an evaluation of accumulated abdominal fluid and diagnosis of abdominal diseases, such as TRP, peritonitis, abomasal ulcers (perforating), abomasal rupture, ruptured bladder or ureters, abdominal neoplasia (lymphosarcoma, mesothelioma), or intestinal obstruction or rupture. In monogastric animals, the most ventral aspect of the abdomen on the midline is the usual site for abdominocentesis; however, in cattle, centesis on the midline usually results in puncture of the rumen. Because bovine abdominal disorders are often localized (or effectively walled off), centesis of a single site might not reflect disease elsewhere in the abdomen. Centesis of four sites on the ventrolateral abdomen may be most productive. These areas represent four abdominal quadrants: left cranial, left caudal, right cranial, and right caudal.

Sampling should begin where the problem is suspected, such as start with the left cranial quadrant if hardware disease is likely. The animal should be standing and properly restrained. The area of centesis is surgically clipped and prepared. To approach the left cranial quadrant, palpate the foramen of the subcutaneous abdominal vein. The site to tap is one hand's breadth cranial and one hand's breadth (6 cm) medial to the foramen, or halfway between the xyphoid and umbilicus and half way between the midline and milk vein. The right cranial quadrant has the same landmarks as the left cranial quadrant only on the right side. This site would be most useful if abomasal disease is suspected. The left caudal quadrant can be located directly anterior to the attachment of the udder to the body (comparable location in the male) in the paramedian area. The right caudal quadrant has the same landmarks as the left caudal quadrant only on the right side. These sites are sampled using an 18-gauge, 3.8-cm needle and collecting any fluid in EDTA and serum tubes. Each quadrant sample should be individually analyzed if several sites are tapped unless it is necessary to combine samples because of small volumes. A sterile teat cannula may be used instead of a needle, but this requires some local analgesia and a small skin incision.

The sample is evaluated and classified as a transudate, which is a serous fluid accumulation as a result of an alteration in pressure, or an exudate, which may be a result of an abdominal infection. Transudates are clear, colorless, odorless, have a protein less than 2.5 g/dl and cell counts less than 5000/μl, and may be due to hypoproteinemia or hypoalbuminemia. Exudates are usually turbid and have a protein greater than 3 g/dl and cell counts greater than 10,000 cells/μl. The evaluation of peritoneal fluid in cattle includes the assessment of volume, color, turbidity, total protein, chemical analysis (urea nitrogen, creatinine), cell count, and cytology. In clinically normal animals, the ratio of neutrophils to mononuclear cells (eosinophils) is 1:1 with the exception of normal cows less than 2 weeks postpartum that may have total nucleated cell counts greater than 10,000 cells/μl, and neutrophils or eosinophils are predominant.

To evaluate cytology, a direct smear may be prepared or the sample may need to be centrifuged if cellularity is low. Hematologic stains, such as Wrights stain, NMB, or Diff-Quik, (Baxter S/P) can be used to examine neutrophil morphology (degenerative changes, bacteria). The classification of inflammatory fluids (exudates) is as follows:

1. Acute inflammation with 80% to 85% neutrophils (the rest of the cells are lymphocytes, eosinophils, macrophages), which may be nondegenerate as with a noninfectious irritant or degenerate as may occur with sepsis

2. Chronic active (subacute) inflammation with 50% to 70% nondegenerate neutrophils and 20% to 50% monocytes or macrophages
3. Chronic inflammation with greater than 50% monocytes and macrophages

> *TECHNICIAN NOTE* Abdominocentesis with an evaluation of accumulated abdominal fluid may aid in the diagnosis of abdominal diseases, such as TRP, peritonitis, abomasal ulcers (perforating), abomasal rupture, ruptured bladder or ureters, abdominal neoplasia (lymphosarcoma, mesothelioma), or intestinal obstruction or rupture.

Diarrhea in the Adult

Common causes of acute diarrhea in adults include coccidiosis, dietary gastroenteritis, acute salmonellosis, acute bovine virus diarrhea (BVD), and winter dysentery. Chronic diarrhea in the adult may be due to gastrointestinal (GI) parasites, Johne's disease, chronic BVD, chronic salmonellosis, bovine leukemia virus (BLV) , chronic renal disease, or chronic liver disease.

Winter dysentery, believed to be caused by a coronavirus, is an acute, contagious diarrheal disease of adult cattle. It is seen more commonly in dairy herds in the winter, and it is considered an epizootic disease since it spreads rapidly through infected herds. Morbidity is high, but mortality rare. The disease has a rapid onset of explosive diarrhea, mild depression, partial anorexia, and a decreased milk production in affected animals. The disease can spread through an entire herd in 2 weeks, and those individuals affected first usually recover within 1 week. The greatest economic loss to the producer is a loss of milk production as a result of body water loss secondary to severe diarrhea. No treatment is available, and most animals recover spontaneously; however, sick cows can be treated symptomatically with intestinal astringents, protectants, and absorbents. The provision of fresh drinking water and free-choice salt is also beneficial.

The most frequent cause of chronic diarrhea in cattle is parasitic infection, especially by *Ostertagia ostertagi* and *Nematodirus*. In adult cattle, the most common clinical parasitic disease is type II or pre-type II ostertagiasis.

In pre-type II disease, the fourth-stage *Ostertagia* larvae burrow into the abomasal wall and encyst instead of maturing into adults. This occurs in the fall in the northern United States and in the spring in the south. During encystment, the acid-secreting parietal cells of the abomasum are destroyed causing an increase in the pH of the abomasum. With the pH above 5, pepsinogen is no longer converted to pepsin, resulting in impaired protein digestion.

Type II ostertagiasis occurs in the spring in the northern United States and in the late summer, early fall in the south when large numbers of encysted larvae emerge into the lumen of the abomasum and mature. Much more damage occurs to the abomasal glands during emergence than during dormancy. Because of the extensive damage, clinical signs often persist long after the parasites are removed by effective anthelmintics.

Clinical signs include unthriftiness, weight loss, pale mucous membranes, diarrhea, and dependent edema in severe cases. Severe parasitism and associated clinical cases are more likely to occur when conditions are crowded, nutrition is marginal, and deworming programs are inadequate.

Parasite eggs may be absent in some cases of type II ostertagiasis. An increased serum pepsinogen concentration may be helpful in the diagnosis in cases of type II ostertagiasis (excessive amounts of pepsinogen are in the GI tract as a result of mucosal damage or decreased conversion to pepsin; the pepsinogen leaks into the bloodstream). For the treatment of these parasitic conditions, please refer to Chapter 17.

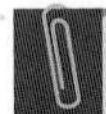

> *TECHNICIAN NOTE* The most frequent cause of chronic diarrhea in cattle is parasitic infection.

Johne's disease, characterized by chronic diarrhea and weight loss, is caused by *Mycobacterium paratuberculosis,* a slow-growing, acid-fast organism. The bacterium is transmitted from infected cows to their calves via the fecal-oral route, with calves less than 6 months the most susceptible to infection. Once the organisms have been ingested by the calf, these are taken up from the intestinal lumen by cells covering the Peyer's patches, particularly in the distal ileum, and are phagocytized by macrophages. The organisms reside and grow within macrophages eventually causing a severe granulomatous reaction with thickening of the intestinal wall. This leads to protein malabsorption and a protein-losing enteropathy so that even though these animals have good appetites, they continue to experience diarrhea and weight loss (Figure 22-17). Although the infection occurs early in life, clinical signs do not usually develop until the animal is at least 2 years of age.

Johne's disease is a terminal disease with no effective treatment. It can be difficult to diagnose because of a lack of reliable tests. There are several serologic tests available that may

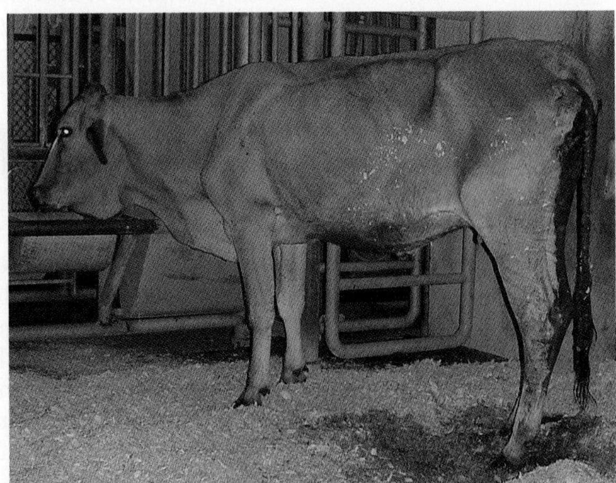

FIGURE 22-17 Severe emaciation, intermandibular edema, and chronic diarrhea in a cow with Johne's disease.

help diagnose this disease; however, most tests are clouded by false-positive and false-negative reactions. A deoxyribonucleic acid (DNA) test has recently become available, but it is relatively expensive and not 100% reliable. Once clinical signs are advanced, a rectal mucosal biopsy may be beneficial to achieve a quick diagnosis. Often the diagnosis is made based on history, clinical signs, and a lack of response to conventional treatments, such as antimicrobial and anthelmintic therapy (for both nematodes and trematodes) (Case Presentation 22-1).

Control programs have been outlined for producers who wish to eliminate the disease from their herd. These programs involve the use of repeated serologic testing, fecal cultures, culling of positive animals and clinically ill animals, and maintenance of separate disease-free and infected herds. These programs are costly and labor intensive, so most producers choose to live with the disease, culling clinically affected cows and the exposed offspring. A vaccine, the use of which is state controlled, is available and is used to control the development of clinical disease in herds with a high incidence of Johne's disease.

Salmonellosis typically manifests as an acute diarrhea, but in rare cases, individuals become chronically infected and have recurring bouts of diarrhea with or without fever, anorexia, and dehydration. Chronically infected cattle usually lose weight and become unthrifty. Salmonellosis is often associated with leukopenia, hyponatremia, hypokalemia, and hypoproteinemia. The submission of multiple fecal samples of adequate volume (up to 60 ml) for culture is necessary to establish a diagnosis. A culture of a rectal biopsy may enhance recovery of the organism.

Salmonellosis should be suspected when chronic diarrhea is preceded by an outbreak of acute diarrhea in a herd, especially if the outbreak was associated with the introduction of new livestock, a feed change, a water change, or a flood.

Other clinical diseases caused by *Salmonella* include septicemia, especially in the neonate, and abortion in adults. Severe cases may progress to endotoxemia, shock, and subsequent death. Animals that survive may continue to carry and shed the organism, posing a threat to other animals. The treatment includes antimicrobial drugs, NSAIDs, and fluid therapy, particularly in young calves with septicemia and/or endotoxemia.

BVD is a common virus-induced gastroenteritis affecting all ages of cattle. BVD manifests as sudden onset of fever, depression, anorexia, oral and GI ulcers and erosions, and diarrhea (sometimes with blood and mucus). The disease may progress rapidly through a group of animals. BVD also plays an important role in respiratory tract diseases in cattle by causing immunosuppression and susceptibility to secondary bacterial pathogens causing pneumonia. The virus is also responsible for abortions, in utero infections, and birth defects. The exposure of pregnant cattle to the noncytopathic strain of BVD between days 80 and 125 of gestation may result in an infected fetus, which becomes immunotolerant to the virus. Later in life, the calf may be exposed to cytopathic strains of BVD, which results in acute mucosal disease (MD) or chronic diarrhea (chronic BVD or BVD-MD), which has a nearly 100% mortality rate; affected calves rarely live to 1 year of age. Clinical signs of BVD-MD include intermittent or persistent diarrhea, weight loss, anorexia, unthriftiness, crusty eyes or muzzle, blunting of oral papillae (Figure 22-18), and chronic coronary band lesions. These cattle are also leukopenic and anemic and have no titer to BVD when serology is performed.

The diagnosis of BVD is made on a physical examination, characteristic necropsy findings, including linear erosions in the esophagus, necrosis of the Peyer's patches, blunted papillae in the buccal mucosa, and epithelial erosions on the tongue and ruminal pillars, virus isolation from tissues or

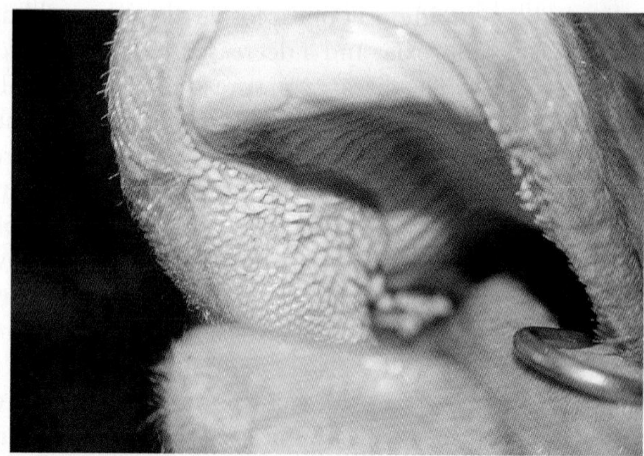

FIGURE 22-18 Blunted oral papilla seen in a calf with chronic BVD (BVD-MD).

CASE PRESENTATION 22-1

A 4-year-old crossbred beef cow was seen with a 4-month history of weight loss and diarrhea. She had been treated with LA200 (Liquamycin, Pfizer Animal Health, New York) every other day for three treatments, and she had been dewormed twice with IvomecPlus (ivermectin and clorsulon, Merial, Duluth, Ga.) at monthly intervals beginning 3 months before she was seen with no response. Clinical findings included emaciation (BCS of 2/9), submandibular edema, diarrhea, and good appetite. Differentials for chronic weight loss and diarrhea included Johne's disease, GI parasites, chronic salmonellosis, chronic renal disease, chronic liver disease, chronic BVD, and BLV. The clinical findings, chronicity of the disease, and failure to respond to conventional treatments made Johne's disease likely. A rectal mucosal biopsy was taken, and acid-fast organisms were found within the rectal mucosal cells. The cow was humanely euthanized and gross, and histopathologic findings resulted in a definitive diagnosis of Johne's disease. The owner was counseled to cull this cow's offspring, and education of the client concerning the disease impact on his herd was provided by the attending veterinary technician.

the buffy coat of whole blood samples, and serology (paired samples 2 to 4 weeks apart are most helpful).

There is no treatment for BVD, but antimicrobials are often used to prevent secondary bacterial infections. Vaccination of dairy and beef animals is important to help prevent the disease. Both killed virus and modified live virus vaccines are available. The use of the modified live virus vaccines should be avoided in pregnant cows, calves nursing pregnant cows, and immunosuppressed animals. Vaccination of calves experiencing chronic BVD using the modified live virus vaccine may result in the death of the animal.

> TECHNICIAN NOTE BVD may cause gastroenteritis, respiratory tract diseases, immunosuppression, abortions, in utero infection, and birth defects in cattle.

DISEASES OF THE RESPIRATORY SYSTEM

Bovine Respiratory Disease Syndrome

Bovine respiratory disease syndrome (BRDS) affects all ages of cattle, but particularly beef calves during the first 45 days in the feedlot and dairy calves younger than 6 months of age. The syndrome is caused by a complex interaction of respiratory viruses, bacteria, and stress. Transportation, cold weather, close confinement, stress with immunosuppression, and exposure to viral and bacterial pathogens predispose to the development of respiratory disease.

A number of viruses including infectious bovine rhinotracheitis (IBR), BVD, parainfluenza virus (PI3), bovine respiratory syncytial virus (BRSV), and respiratory coronavirus in addition to bacteria, such as *Mannheimia haemolytica* and *Histophilus somnus,* produce respiratory disease in susceptible, immunocompromised animals. Generally, infection with one or more of the respiratory viruses occurs first, followed by bacterial infection of the lower respiratory tract or bronchopneumonia. BRDS in feedlot cattle is often referred to as shipping fever.

Cattle with BRDS experience depression, standing with their heads lowered, anorexia, fever 40° C to 41.5° C (104° F to 107° F), mucopurulent ocular and nasal discharge, cough, and dyspnea (Figure 22-19). Morbidity and mortality within a group may be quite high.

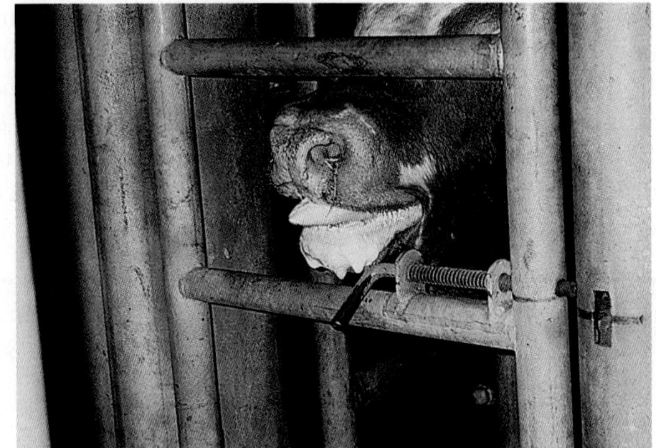

FIGURE 22-19 Severe dyspnea and open-mouth breathing in a calf with shipping fever.

The diagnosis of BRDS is based on a history of calves undergoing stress, typical clinical signs of pneumonia, and the presence of bronchopneumonia on necropsy. Samples from a transtracheal aspirate can be submitted for cytology, bacterial isolation, and antimicrobial sensitivity and virus isolation in cases of respiratory disease in cattle. A successful treatment of the disease hinges on early diagnosis and the institution of appropriate antimicrobial therapy. Individual sick animals should be isolated from the rest of the group and treated with broad-spectrum antimicrobial therapy for at least 5 days. Antimicrobial agents typically used for the treatment of shipping fever include ceftiofur sodium, ceftiofur hydrochloride, or ceftiofur crystalline free acid (Naxcel, ExcenelRTU, or Excede all produced by Pharmacia & Upjohn, Division of Pfizer Inc., New York), florfenicol (Nuflor, Schering-Plough, Union, N.J.), tilmicosin (Micotil, Elanco, Indianapolis, Ind.), tulathromycin (Draxxin, Pfizer Animal Health, New York), tetracycline (LA200, Liquamycin, Pfizer Animal Health, New York), and fluoroquinolone (Baytril, Bayer, Shawnee Mission, Kan.). When large numbers of animals are ill, antimicrobial agents may be added to the water to simplify the treatment. In addition, fresh water, hay, and adequate shelter should be provided. A procedure known as metaphylaxis is now commonly employed by feedlots and involves the treatment of cattle with long-acting antimicrobial agents, such as Micotil, upon arrival at the feedlot. Preconditioning (castration, dehorning, implanting, acclimation to feed and water, deworming, and vaccination) of calves before weaning and vaccination before transport from stocker to feeder operations decreases stress on the cattle during these transitions and may prevent the development or lessen the severity of disease. Vaccines typically used to prevent respiratory disease outbreaks include IBR, PI3, BVD, BRSV, *M. haemolytica,* and *H. somnus.*

> TECHNICIAN NOTE BRDS, which affects primarily feedlot calves and dairy calves younger than 6 months of age, is caused by a complex interaction of respiratory viruses, bacteria, and stress.

DISEASES OF THE MUSCULOSKELETAL SYSTEM

Lameness

Lameness is commonly encountered in cattle and is most often (88%) caused by lesions or problems in the foot. Upper leg problems, such as anterior cruciate ligament rupture, coxofemoral (hip) luxation, fractures, and arthritis, account for the remaining 12% of lameness. When foot problems occur, they are most often seen in the claws that bear the most weight, front medial and hind lateral claws.

Common foot conditions, especially in dairy cattle, include foot rot, laminitis, white-line abscess ("gravel"), sole ulcer, underrun heel and sole, and hairy heel warts. It is important to examine all foot problems early since many conditions can quickly lead to osteomyelitis and/or septic arthritis if not properly treated. Regardless of the cause of lameness, it can lead to a loss of production as a result of decreased milk production, weight loss, delayed breeding or anestrus, and culling. Intensive housing and feeding of large groups of animals has lead to an increased incidence of lameness.

> TECHNICIAN NOTE Lameness is commonly encountered in cattle and is most often (88%) caused by lesions or problems in the foot.

Interdigital Necrobacillosis

Interdigital necrobacillosis, or foot rot, in cattle is an infection of the interdigital skin and underlying tissues caused by the synergistic effects of *Fusobacterium necrophorum* and other anaerobic bacteria. The infection results in an ulcerated, foul-smelling area between the claws with resultant lameness (Figure 22-20). There may be swelling apparent above the coronary band, and in severe cases, cellulitis up to the carpus or hock may occur. The disease is particularly prevalent when cattle are kept in wet, muddy conditions. If left untreated, foot rot can invade the deeper tissues of the foot causing septic arthritis, osteomyelitis, and chronic lameness.

The treatment of foot rot in cattle can be successfully accomplished with aggressive topical treatment. In some cases, it may be necessary to débride necrotic tissue and even bandage the foot with antimicrobial agents to promote healing. In cases where cellulitis has occurred, it may be necessary to use parenteral antibiotics or the regional antibiotic perfusion technique. Foot rot usually has a low morbidity in any given herd, but in cases where there is a high incidence of foot rot, it may be necessary to initiate the use of a footbath containing zinc sulfate for the prevention or treatment of foot rot.

Papillomatous Digital Dermatitis

Papillomatous digital dermatitis (PDD), or hairy heel wart, has become an important cause of lameness in dairy cattle worldwide. Initially, PDD appears as a superficial inflammation of the skin of the bovine digit, but progresses to the typical mature lesions that are circumscribed, erosive, or proliferative and are usually located on the hind feet, adjacent to the interdigital ridge and heel bulbs (Figure 22-21). Granulation tissue develops with outgrowths of dermal tissue that grossly resemble hair, thus the common name, hairy heel wart. The disease seems to be contagious with a fairly high morbidity within any given herd.

At this time, the cause of PDD is still controversial; it is believed to be a multifactorial disease in which infectious agents are primarily involved. The economic impact includes a decreased milk production, impaired reproductive performance, an increased number of cows culled, and the cost of treatment and control. Antibiotics, such as oxytetracycline, lincomycin, or lincomycin-spectinomycin, have been used in addition to nonantibiotic products, such as triplex (solubilized copper, a peroxy compound and a cationic agent). The treatment is beneficial, but does not appear to be curative because disease outbreaks are common once a herd is infected.

Laminitis

Laminitis, or founder, is a diffuse, aseptic inflammation of the corium (sensitive lamina) of the feet. Acute laminitis occurs sporadically and may be due to sudden excess grain ingestion (see Grain Overload), or it may occur secondary to other diseases that occur during the postparturient period, such as retained placenta, metritis, mastitis, ketosis, or abomasal displacement. Chronic laminitis is more often associated with constant feeding of high-grain diets as occurs commonly in high-producing dairy cows, feedlot cattle, or show cattle.

Clinical signs include stiffness, pain, reluctance to walk, and difficulty in rising. Affected animals spend a lot of time lying down, and when they do stand, they may stand with their backs arched, front legs crossed, or kneeling on the front legs in an attempt to redistribute body weight because of the pain. Acute cases of laminitis are treated by correcting any existing underlying problem and the administration of NSAIDs. Laminitis often leads to serious sequelae, including sole ulcers, white-line disease, abnormal hoof growth with horizontal or vertical hoof-wall cracks (normal hoof growth is about 0.5 cm per month), underrun heel and sole, and

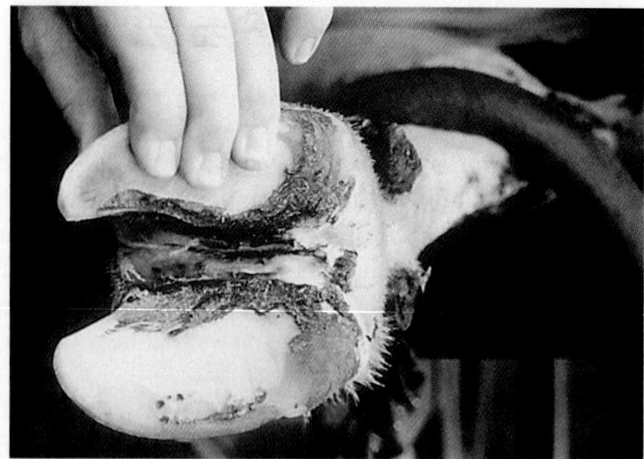

FIGURE 22-20 Interdigital necrobacillosis or foot rot in a cow.

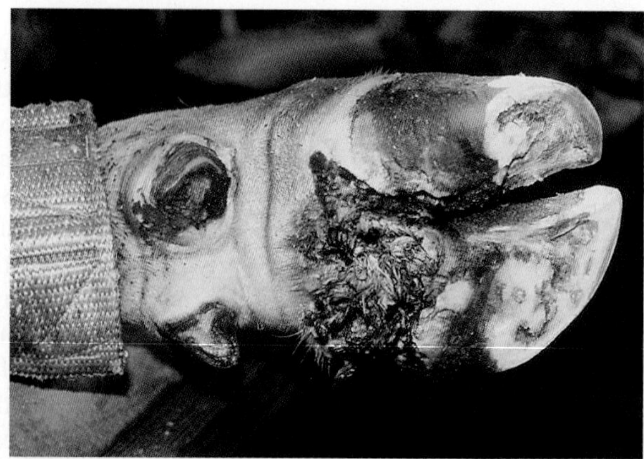

FIGURE 22-21 Papillomatous digital dermatitis or hairy heel warts of the hind feet cause severe lameness in affected dairy cattle.

even osteomyelitis or septic arthritis. Frequent foot trimming helps prevent the development of these problems.

> *TECHNICIAN NOTE* Acute laminitis may be due to sudden excess grain ingestion or may occur secondary to other diseases that occur during the postparturient period, such as retained placenta, metritis, mastitis, ketosis, or abomasal displacement.

Sole (Rusterholz) Ulcers

A sole ulcer is a circumscribed loss of sole that exposes the corium (sensitive lamina or "quick"). The typical location of the lesion is near the axial (inside) aspect of the hind lateral claws near the heel-sole junction. Lesions are usually bilateral involving both hind lateral claws. In some cases, sole loss is not evident, but there is a circular area of hemorrhage beneath the sole or the sole is yellow and soft; the ulcer becomes apparent when the undermined sole is trimmed away. Lameness usually is not severe until granulation tissue develops from the exposed corium and protrudes from the defect in the sole. This granulation tissue retards the development of new sole. These ulcers may become infected with extension of the infection into the deeper tissues (navicular bursa, coffin joint, and flexor tendons).

Sole ulcers are probably the direct result of laminitis. The higher incidence of ulcers in the lateral hind claws versus medial hind claws suggests an anatomic or mechanical difference, but it is not certain. The pressure on impact is greater at the heel-sole junction of the lateral claw. Localized ischemia from laminitis can lead to erosion of the sole.

Lameness can be severe and is worse when the granulation tissue protrudes or if deeper tissues are involved. The animal may abduct its leg slightly (an attempt to put more weight on the medial claw) or stand with the heel extending beyond the gutter. Since the condition is often bilateral, both hind feet should be checked, even though lameness may be apparent in only one leg (usually the lesion is more advanced in one foot than the other). The treatment is aimed at controlling granulation tissue and preventing extension of the infection into the deeper tissues. The treatment involves the excision of excessive granulation tissue, placement of a wooden or acrylic block on the medial claw to take weight bearing off the lateral claw, and use of a caustic substance, such as copper sulfate or phenol-formalin, with a bandage to control the granulation tissue. Prognosis is good if there is no deep infection; however, the treatment requires time and money.

White-Line Disease

The white line is the area of fibrous connective tissue that joins the rigid hoof wall to the more resilient sole. Since the white line is soft, it is more vulnerable to penetration by foreign material. Dirt-filled cracks and fissures in the white line are not uncommon in normal feet, but when abscesses develop under the sole, lameness follows. Factors predisposing to white-line disease are continuously wet feet and animals with previous bouts of laminitis, which result in poor horn quality and decreased white-line strength.

A serious sequela to white-line disease is an infection of the navicular bursa. Although the bursa is protected from direct penetration or infection by the flexor tendon, it is still vulnerable at the edges of the tendon. Occasionally, the infection extends up along the wall, forms an abscess in the navicular bursa, and drains above the abaxial coronet (called gravel).

White-line abscesses cause lameness. The animal may walk or stand with the heel slightly raised or the limb abducted (an attempt to shift weight to the medial claw). Hoof testers help localize the lesions that are not obvious. Black lines, cracks, and fissures should be followed and pared out. The opening of an abscess will often result in release of watery black exudate and gas. If the navicular bursa is involved, the heel will be swollen, hot, and painful. The sole should be pared to allow adequate opening and drainage of the abscess, and the lateral wall should be trimmed to prevent packing of dirt and manure back into the abscess hole.

Underrun Heel and Sole

This condition is also referred to as stable foot rot and occurs primarily in the hind feet. The erosive process begins at the heel bulb initially as pits or pockmarks, and then parallel horizontal grooves develop and fill with black necrotic material. The anaerobic bacteria *F. necrophorum* and *Bacteroides nodosus* have both been isolated from these cases. The sole can separate to form a flap that may extend to the toe with a new sole developing underneath (Figure 22-22). Debris can become packed between the sole layers causing lameness. Underrun heels may not cause lameness unless there is infection of deeper structures or a lot of debris gets packed between the sole layers.

This condition may result from chronic laminitis, which causes hoof overgrowth (especially at the toe) and shifting of the animal's weight to the area of the heel. The abnormal

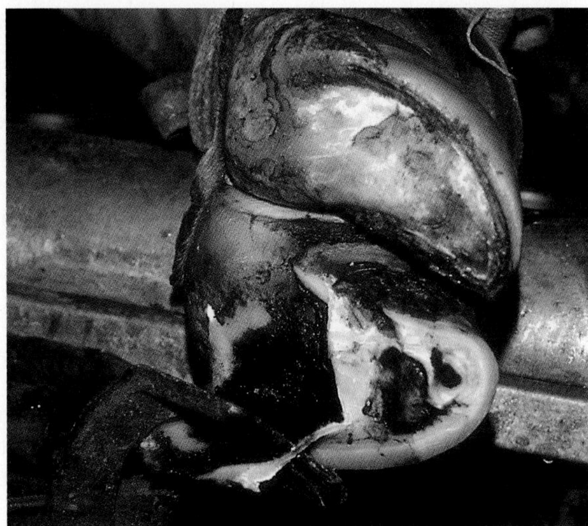

FIGURE 22-22 Debris packed between layers of sole causing lameness in a bull with underrun heel and sole.

and underrun sole should be removed to treat this condition. If sensitive lamina is exposed, the foot may need to be topically treated with antimicrobials and bandaged until the area becomes tough enough to bear weight. A wooden block on the opposite claw may be helpful during the healing process. Prevention includes regular hoof trimming to keep the animal from walking on its heels and the use of footbaths or regular topical treatment to control anaerobic bacterial infection in the area.

> *TECHNICIAN NOTE* Diseases of the foot may become so severe that they cannot be treated, thus necessitating the amputation of the affected digit.

Foot Block Application

Wooden or acrylic blocks or commercial rubber shoes may be glued to the bottom of healthy claws to reduce or eliminate weight bearing on a diseased or painful claw. These devices are adhered to the claw using an acrylic material (Technovit, Jorgensen Laboratories, Inc. or Equi-Thane Super Fast, Vettec Hoof Care Products). Wooden blocks may last as long as 6 weeks and may be allowed to wear off naturally unless they are wearing abnormally, in which case they may be manually removed earlier. Blocks or shoes help promote healing of affected claws and make the animal more comfortable when standing or moving.

Blackleg and Malignant Edema

Infections by *Clostridium chauvoei* (blackleg) and *Clostridium septicum* (malignant edema) are two important causes of lameness and sudden death in young cattle. These bacteria produce spores that enter the animal through either the digestive tract or skin wounds, producing a severe necrotizing myositis and cellulitis. Affected animals develop high fever and lameness as a result of severe muscle damage. The swollen muscle mass often contains gas pockets that are palpable subcutaneously as crepitus.

Animals with these infections are usually found dead. Those animals caught in the early stages of an infection may be treated with high doses of penicillin along with débridement and topical treatment of the wounds; however, the prognosis for recovery is poor. The best way to prevent these clostridial diseases and others is to vaccinate calves with a multivalent bacterin at 2 months of age followed by a booster 4 to 6 weeks later. Cows should be vaccinated before calving to provide colostral protection to the calves.

HEMOLYMPHATIC SYSTEM

Lymphosarcoma

The adult form of lymphosarcoma (LSA) is associated with BLV and is the most common neoplastic disease of cattle. Lymphosarcoma is mostly likely to affect cattle between the ages of 2 and 6 years. Although many cattle are exposed to BLV and any given herd may have a high incidence of cattle with titers to BLV, the actual number of cattle that develop neoplastic disease is small (less than 5%). Malignant tumors may develop in peripheral or deep lymph nodes, lymph tissue behind the eye or around the spinal cord, abomasum, heart, kidney, uterus, or other organs; therefore clinical signs may vary greatly depending on the organ(s) or system(s) involved. Occasionally a lymphocytosis with the presence of neoplastic lymphocytes is apparent when a CBC is performed. Diagnostic tests to help confirm lymphosarcoma may include a CBC, lymph node biopsy, paracentesis, thoracocentesis, a CSF centesis, or a BLV titer. A positive titer to BLV only suggests exposure to the virus, but does not confirm neoplastic disease. There is no treatment or vaccine available, and the disease is always fatal. Since BLV titers are so prevalent in cattle herds, it is unlikely that a test and cull program would ever be initiated. Because the virus is spread by infected lymphocytes, every effort should be made to prevent the transfer of blood between infected and noninfected animals (e.g., by changing needles and disinfecting surgery instruments between animals).

> *TECHNICIAN NOTE* Malignant tumors associated with LSA caused by BLV may develop in peripheral or deep lymph nodes, lymph tissue behind the eye, or around the spinal cord, abomasum, heart, kidney, uterus, or other organs; therefore clinical signs may vary greatly depending on the organ(s) or system(s) involved.

Anaplasmosis

Anaplasmosis, caused by the intraerythrocytic organism, *Anaplasma marginale,* is primarily a disease of adult cattle. RBCs infected with the organism are removed from the circulation by the liver and spleen and are subsequently destroyed resulting in a severe anemia. Resulting clinical signs from the development of acute anemia include pale mucous membranes, icterus, weakness, and depression or aggressive behavior as a result of anoxia to the brain. Anaplasmosis often causes sudden death without obvious clinical signs, and it must be differentiated from other causes of sudden death, such as anthrax, clostridial diseases, bloat, and lightning. The organism is sensitive to tetracycline, so this drug is used for the treatment and prevention of the disease. There is currently no commercial vaccine available for the prevention of anaplasmosis.

Anthrax

Bacillus anthracis is the etiologic agent of this acute disease causing sudden death in animals and humans. Anthrax is endemic in many areas of the southern United States. Since people can easily contract the disease, it is important not to perform a necropsy on any animal suspected of having anthrax. The exposure of anthrax bacilli to the air, as in the case of necropsy, results in spore formation by the organism and permanent contamination of the surrounding environment. If anthrax is strongly suspected as the cause of death, the area federal veterinarian should be notified immediately. Anthrax-contaminated carcasses should be buried in lime or incinerated. A live virus vaccine is available, and its use should be considered in high-risk areas. The organism is sensitive to penicillin, but in most cases, the treatment cannot be initiated quickly enough. In recent years, anthrax has become an important issue in cases of bioterrorism.

> TECHNICIAN NOTE Anaplasmosis, anthrax, clostridial diseases, lightning, and bloat are causes of sudden death in cattle.

REPRODUCTIVE SYSTEM/MAMMARY GLAND

Mastitis

Mastitis is inflammation of the mammary gland caused by the invasion of the streak canal of the teat by a variety of bacterial pathogens. Economically, mastitis is one of the most important diseases in the dairy industry, and it is the single most common disease syndrome in adult dairy cows. Anatomically the mammary gland is relatively resistant to infection, but severe environmental contamination of the teats, injury to the streak canal, or improperly functioning milking machine equipment may predispose the udder to infection.

Clinical signs of mastitis vary considerably based on the etiologic agent and may be seen as an asymptomatic subclinical infection to one in which the gland is markedly swollen and the milk is grossly abnormal. In general, mastitis can be subdivided into two broad but overlapping categories based on the source of the infection: contagious and environmental. Contagious mastitis is spread from an infected mammary gland to a healthy one via contaminated milking equipment, nursing calves, or by the milker's hands. *Streptococcus agalactiae* and *Staphylococcus aureus* are examples of bacteria causing contagious mastitis. Environmental mastitis results when bacteria within reservoirs in the environment gain access to the mammary gland and cause infection. Those organisms characteristically associated with environmental mastitis include the coliform bacteria. Other mastitis-causing organisms that fall between these two broad categories, maintaining alternate niches either in the host or in the environment, include *Streptococcus dysgalactiae* and *Streptococcus uberis.* Mastitis, depending on the cause, causes various abnormal secretions ranging from the presence of milk with flakes or clots to purulent material. The degree of inflammatory response varies also depending on the cause. Other classifications of mastitis include acute or toxic mastitis, usually caused by coliforms or *S. aureus,* chronic mastitis, caused by *S. aureus,* or acute gangrenous mastitis, the cause of which may be *S. aureus* or *Clostridium perfringens.* Cows with toxic mastitis are usually ill, have a watery or serous secretion from the affected gland(s), and have a low serum calcium level such that they may resemble a case of milk fever. Gangrenous mastitis causes gangrene of the gland with a distinct blue line of demarcation separating normal and affected tissues. Secretions from affected glands are watery and serosanguineous, the gangrenous portions will be cold to the touch, and these portions of the gland will eventually slough. Toxic and gangrenous mastitis may cause the death of the cow.

Mastitis is best diagnosed by a clinical examination of the udder and milk and the use of the California mastitis test (CMT). The CMT is performed by mixing equal parts of CMT reagent and milk. A plastic paddle with four separate compartments is provided with the test kit so that each quarter can be individually evaluated. The reagent reacts with leukocytes that are usually present in large numbers when mastitis is present. When this reaction occurs, the reagent-milk mixture thickens or gels in proportion to the number of white cells present and indicates the severity of the inflammation. The greater the reaction, the higher the CMT score. CMT scores are designated as negative, trace, 1, 2, and 3 with corresponding cell counts of 100,000, 300,000, 900,000, 2,700,000, and 8,100,000. The aseptic collection of a milk sample for culture and antimicrobial sensitivity often provides information on cause and appropriate drug therapy.

Depending on the etiologic agent, mastitis can be successfully treated if recognized early. The treatment of mastitis involves the use of appropriate antimicrobial therapy, systemic and/or intramammary. Frequent stripping of affected quarter(s) helps remove infected secretions and promotes quicker recovery. Cows with toxic mastitis may need intensive treatment with NSAIDs, IV fluid therapy, and calcium in those cows with hypocalcemia. Only antibiotics approved for use in dairy cows should be administered for the treatment of mastitis. In addition, antibiotic milk withdrawal times should be closely monitored. The veterinary technician should be familiar with these approved drugs and the withdrawal times and can serve as an important resource for education of the dairy farmer.

The prevention of mastitis is of paramount importance in the dairy industry. Control may be achieved by the implementation of the five-point plan for mastitis control, which includes:

1. Hygiene: premilking and postmilking teat dipping and efforts to keep cows clean and dry between milkings.
2. Use proper milking procedures with well-functioning equipment when milking.
3. Practice dry cow treatment of every quarter of every cow and develop a veterinary-prescribed therapeutic plan for clinical cases.
4. Cull cows as necessary based on economics.
5. Maintain good records on each cow concerning production, reproduction, milk quality, and clinical mastitis.

> TECHNICIAN NOTE Control of mastitis in cattle may be achieved by the implementation of the five-point plan for mastitis control.

Dystocia

Dystocia, or difficult calving, in cattle is relatively common, especially in first-calf heifers, and frequently requires veterinary assistance. Dystocia may result from fetal oversize, maternal undersize, or fetal malposition. To recognize if a problem exists, the veterinary technician should be familiar with the normal signs of impending parturition and the stages of parturition. When a cow or heifer is nearing parturition, relaxation of the pelvic ligaments, swelling of the vulva, and udder development occur. During stage I of labor, the cervix dilates and the chorioallantoic membrane ruptures, releasing a large volume of clear, yellow fluid. Stage II is marked by the appearance of fetal extremities at the vulva along with the amniotic membrane. Normally the cow or heifer will deliver the calf within 2 hours of this observation. If delivery takes longer than 2 hours or if the cow stops straining, the cow should be examined, and veterinary assistance may be indicated. Stage III involves the passage of the placenta.

When dystocia is suspected, the cow should be quickly and thoroughly examined to rule out hypocalcemia as a cause of uterine inertia. Before a vaginal examination, the vulva and perineal area should be thoroughly cleaned with a mild disinfectant. A sterile, nonirritating lubricant, such as carboxymethylcellulose, can be used to perform the vaginal examination, and it may be pumped into the uterus to facilitate manipulation, repositioning, and delivery of the calf. Once any malposition is corrected, obstetric chains can be placed on the legs of the calf to apply traction for delivery. The chains should be looped above the fetlocks and half hitched below the fetlocks to more evenly distribute the pulling forces on the legs. A single loop of the chain on each leg is much more likely to result in physeal fractures. If the calf's head is in normal position, a snare may be placed around the head to aid delivery. Excessive force should be avoided during forced fetal extraction to prevent nerve injury to the cow and fractures of the calf's legs. A mechanical calf extractor can be used carefully when manual traction is unavailable. If the calf cannot safely be delivered by this technique, then fetotomy or a C-section section should be considered.

Fetotomies are usually reserved for the removal of calves that are dead or emphysematous. It involves the use of specialized instruments to dissect the dead calf in utero to deliver it more easily. C-section for resolution of dystocia is covered in Chapter 31.

> *TECHNICIAN NOTE* During forced fetal extraction, obstetric chains should be looped above the calf's fetlocks and half hitched below the fetlocks to more evenly distribute the pulling forces on the legs to prevent physeal fractures.

Retained Placenta (Fetal Membranes)

After calving, the placenta is usually passed within 2 to 4 hours and is considered retained if it has not been expelled by 8 to 12 hours. Retained placenta is more common in dairy cows than beef cows. The cause is unknown, but it is more likely to occur following the birth of twins, following abortion during the last half of pregnancy, and in cases of dystocia. Selenium and vitamin A and E deficiencies have been suggested to cause an increased incidence of retained placentas.

The manual removal of the placenta should be avoided since this may result in endometrial damage and an infection with prolonged uterine involution and delayed breeding. Retained placenta and endometritis may be treated with intrauterine infusions of appropriate antibiotics. Although uterine infusion is controversial, most veterinarians agree that cows with signs of systemic illness as a result of retained placenta should receive parenteral antibiotic therapy.

If abortion is the cause of retained fetal membranes, vaccination of cows and heifers for diseases causing abortion should be considered. If nutrition is suspected as a predisposing factor, the ration should be evaluated making certain that it contains recommended levels and ratios of calcium, phosphorus, vitamins A and E, and selenium. An injection of vitamin E and selenium 1 month before calving may reduce the incidence of retained placenta in problem herds.

METABOLIC DISORDERS

Periparturient Hypocalcemia (Milk Fever)

Milk fever is a common metabolic problem in periparturient dairy cows usually occurring within 48 hours of calving. It is unlikely to occur in first-calf heifers, but the incidence of the condition increases with the age of the cow. It reportedly is more likely to occur in the Jersey breed. Milk fever is the result of a severe decline in the serum calcium level (normal, 10 mg/dl). Hypocalcemia results from feeding of diets high in calcium during the late dry period (the last 2 months of gestation), which causes a lack of response by the parathyroid gland and a decrease in vitamin D levels. As a result, the cow is slow to mobilize calcium reserves from the bone when there is a sudden demand for calcium at the beginning of lactation.

Cows with hypocalcemia develop muscle tremors, weakness, and a staggering gait eventually leading to recumbency. Cows with milk fever often lie in sternal recumbency with the head turned into their flank. Affected cows have a dry nose, rumen atony with bloat, and no urine or feces production. Some cows with milk fever may be found in lateral recumbency. The heart rate is increased and pupils dilated. Unless the cow is treated quickly, she may die of the effects of a low serum calcium level. It is important to get a down cow up as soon as possible since recumbency leads to the development of severe myositis of the muscles of the limbs and subsequent nerve damage resulting in a permanent "downer" cow.

The slow administration of calcium gluconate IV is the treatment of choice. Cows often respond rapidly to calcium therapy and will begin to lacrimate, eructate, urinate, and defecate. If the initial treatment helps but the cow does not stand, it may be necessary to administer additional calcium subcutaneously. If the cow does not respond to treatment, she should be reevaluated for persistent hypocalcemia or concurrent problems, such as mastitis, metritis, or musculoskeletal or nerve damage. Cows in the early stages of milk fever (before recumbency) often respond to the administration of oral calcium gel.

Prevention of milk fever is achieved by providing a well-balanced, low-calcium diet during the dry period. The total dietary intake of calcium should not exceed 20 g per head per day. It is important to keep dry cows separate from the rest of the herd so that they can be fed properly not only to prevent milk fever, but also to prevent overconditioning and fat liver syndrome.

> *TECHNICIAN NOTE* Milk fever is a common metabolic problem in periparturient dairy cows resulting from a severe decline in serum calcium level.

Ketosis (Acetonemia)

Ketosis occurs in high-producing dairy cows during the first few months of lactation if they are unable to meet the energy demands of lactation. To provide energy for milk production, the cow begins to mobilize fat, the breakdown of which results in the formation of ketone bodies that accumulate in the blood. Ketosis in dairy cows may result from a primary deficiency in energy intake, or it may occur secondary to a disease process, such as abomasal displacement, mastitis, or metritis, which can cause anorexia.

Ketones have a characteristic odor that can be detected in the breath, milk, and urine of affected cows. Excessive amounts of ketones and a low blood glucose level may cause the cow to display nervous symptoms known as nervous ketosis.

Ketosis responds to administration of energy sources, such as glucose IV, propylene glycol per os, or, where appropriate, systemic corticosteroids. It is important to determine the cause of ketosis and to correct the underlying problem. The cow's ration should be examined to make certain it contains adequate digestible energy to meet requirements for maintenance and lactation.

CARDIOVASCULAR SYSTEM

Vegetative or Valvular Endocarditis

Vegetative or ulcerative lesions may develop on the heart valves, in particular the right atrioventricular (AV) valve, as a result of septic emboli from other sites, such as omphalophlebitis or navel infection in calves. These lesions, if severe, may interfere with blood flow leading to congestive heart failure (CHF). The cause is bacterial, usually *Arcanobacterium pyogenes* or α-hemolytic streptococcus in cattle. Vegetative endocarditis in pigs is usually due to streptococcus or *Erysipelothrix.* If fragments detach from the heart valve, embolic endoarteritis and abscesses in showered organs may follow. Clinical signs in cattle include a history of an animal doing poorly, presence of a murmur or thrill, exercise intolerance, CHF with jugular vein distention and dependent edema in advanced cases, and fluctuating fever (Figure 22-23). Clinical pathology in acute cases may show leukocytosis (greater than 100,000 WBC) with a left shift, whereas chronic cases may have a normal CBC. Three serial blood cultures performed as the body temperature rises may yield bacterial growth.

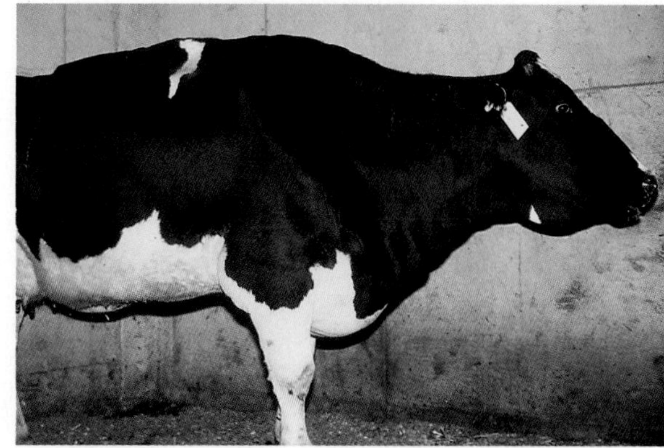

FIGURE 22-23 Ventral midline edema and jugular pulse in a cow with CHF.

On necropsy, the valve lesions may be large and cauliflower-like or small and wartlike. In chronic cases, valves may be shrunken and distorted or scarred. Treatment is not successful because of an inadequate penetration of the lesions with antibiotics and the presence of irreversible damage to the valves. Penicillin at high levels (44,000 IU/kg b.i.d.) for long periods of time (2 to 3 weeks) has given the best results, although cephalosporins may also prove beneficial and are commonly used to treat young calves. Echocardiography, when available, is quite useful for visualizing valve lesions.

Pericarditis

Pericarditis causes the inflammation of both the parietal and visceral surfaces of the pericardial cavity. True pericarditis is always infectious and nearly always exudative. It may be due to a blood-borne infection, but is usually due to traumatic pericarditis, an extension of traumatic reticuloperitonitis. Pericarditis develops after the penetration of the pericardial sac by a metallic foreign body (often occurs close to parturition). It results in a mixed bacterial infection that causes severe local inflammation. This inflammation causes deposition of fibrinous exudate leading to a friction rub (Figure 22-24). Effusion then develops creating splashing sounds around the heart, especially if the fluid is mixed with gas, or it may cause muffled heart sounds. Fluid accumulation compromises heart function and can lead to CHF. Clinical signs include pain as evidenced by kyphosis, abduction of the elbows, and shallow abdominal respirations. The temperature is slightly elevated, 103° F to 106° F. Pericardial friction sounds, fluid splashing sounds, or muffled heart sounds may be auscultated. Signs of CHF occur late in the course of the disease, and death is usually due to toxemia or CHF. Most cows die within 1 to 3 weeks, but a few persist with chronic pericarditis. These cows often have a leukocytosis (16,000 to 30,000 WBC). Pericardiocentesis can be performed at the four or fifth intercostal space at the level of the elbow on the left side to confirm the presence of pericarditis. Necropsy findings vary from hyperemia and fibrin deposition to the accumulation of purulent exudates, fibrin, and thickened pericardium and/or epicardium to adhesion of the pericardium to the epicardium as the condition progresses

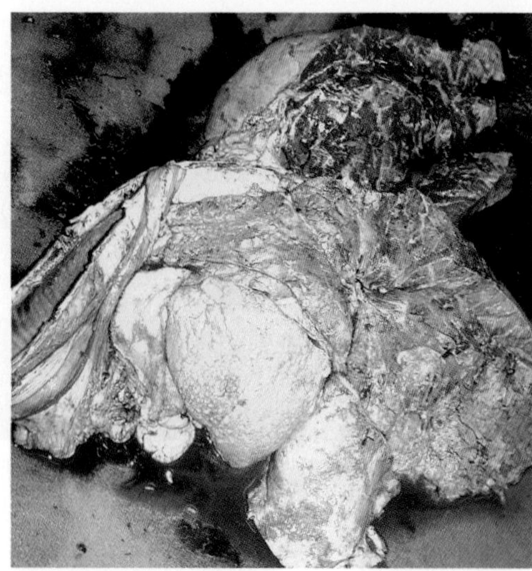

FIGURE 22-24 Severe fibrin formation with purulent exudate on the heart of a cow that died of pericarditis.

from acute to chronic. A metallic foreign body may also be present. No treatment is successful and requires long-term use of antibiotics. Pericardiocentesis provides only temporary relief, and pericardiotomy (fifth or sixth rib resection) for drainage and flushing purposes can be attempted, but is not highly successful.

> *TECHNICIAN NOTE* Pericarditis in cattle is usually due to the penetration of the pericardial sac by a metallic foreign body.

URINARY SYSTEM

Contagious Bovine Pyelonephritis

Contagious bovine pyelonephritis, caused by *Corynebacterium renale,* is an ascending urinary tract infection often affecting females because of the short, wide urethra. The infection occurs more often in the periparturient period when cows are more stressed and the urogenital tract is more susceptible to entry of bacteria.

Clinical findings include hematuria, pyuria, straining (strangury) and discomfort during urination, and frequent urination (pollakisuria). Affected cows may have a fluctuating fever, variable appetite, and decreased milk production. If the left kidney is affected, rectal palpation may reveal an enlarged, fluctuant, painful kidney.

The treatment is often unrewarding, but may be attempted using high doses of penicillin (44,000 U/kg b.i.d.) for long periods of time. In valuable animals in which only one kidney is affected, nephrectomy may be indicated.

NERVOUS SYSTEM

Rabies

Rabies is a fatal, viral, neurologic disease of warmblooded animals. Rabies is most often transmitted by the bite of an infected wild animal, with skunks, raccoons, and foxes being the greatest threat to domestic livestock. Two forms of rabies may occur: the furious form in which the affected animal demonstrates hyperexcitability, fear, or rage or the dumb form in which extreme depression, paresis, or paralysis manifest.

Clinical signs of rabies may include bloat, tenesmus, bellowing, aggressiveness, and increased sexual activity. Hydrophobia, the common name for rabies, stems from the inability of the animal to drink as a result of pharyngeal-laryngeal paralysis. Death occurs within 10 days of the onset of clinical signs. The definitive diagnosis is made by fluorescent antibody testing of the brain, the presence of Negri bodies (cytoplasmic inclusions in neurons) on histopathology, and mouse inoculation.

Several vaccines are available for use in cattle and sheep. Rabies poses a serious human health concern; therefore care should be taken when handling animals suspected of having rabies (i.e., gloves should be worn during an oral examination). Veterinary technicians who practices in areas where the rabies incidence is high should strongly consider a rabies vaccination for themselves.

> *TECHNICIAN NOTE* Rabies poses a serious human health concern; therefore gloves should always be worn during an oral examination of animals suspected of having rabies.

Polioencephalomalacia (Polio)

Polioencephalomalacia is a CNS disease that results from an underlying defect in thiamine metabolism. The disease may occur secondary to grain overload as previously discussed, or other sudden ration changes may precipitate its development. The coccidiostat, amprolium, administered at high doses or for long periods of time has induced polioencephalomalacia.

Affected animals show neurologic signs including blindness, ataxia, depression, opisthotonus, dorsomedial strabismus, convulsions, coma, and death. Polioencephalomalacia if treated early responds well to treatment with thiamine; however, the longer the animal has been affected, the longer it takes for recovery, and recovery may not be complete (i.e., blindness may persist). The addition of thiamine or brewer's yeast to the ration in high-risk situations may be beneficial in preventing disease.

Listeriosis

Listeria monocytogenes is responsible for three different clinical syndromes in ruminants: septicemia, abortion, and neurologic disease. Neurologic involvement produces fever, anorexia, depression, proprioceptive deficits, head tilt, and circling. Cranial nerve dysfunction causes unilateral drooping of the ear, eyelid, nose, and lips with excessive salivation. Although the ingestion of contaminated corn silage is blamed, the consumption of any rotting contaminated vegetation can serve as the source of infection.

The organism is sensitive to tetracycline or penicillin, but a treatment of listeriosis is often unrewarding. No vaccine is available for protection against this disease. The organism has zoonotic potential and poses a serious human health risk when contaminated milk, milk products, or meat have entered the food chain.

Thromboembolic Meningoencephalitis

Thromboembolic meningoencephalitis (TEME) is the result of septic emboli in the brain secondary to septicemia caused by *H. somnus*. Animals affected with TEME show neurologic signs that are consistent with the areas of the brain that are damage by the emboli. The organism is found primarily in the respiratory tract and usually causes pneumonia. It is not unusual for some individuals to develop neurologic disease after an outbreak of pneumonia in a group of feedlot cattle.

The diagnosis is made by finding the characteristic hemorrhagic lesions scattered throughout the brain. With confirmation of the disease, treatment of the herd with tetracycline may be beneficial in preventing more cases, and vaccination with *Histophilus* bacterin may be indicated.

DISEASES OF THE EYE

Infectious Bovine Keratoconjunctivitis

Infectious bovine keratoconjunctivitis (IBK), or pinkeye, is an infectious and contagious ocular disease of cattle characterized by conjunctivitis and keratitis with ulceration (Figure 22-25). Ultraviolet light and mechanical irritants, such as dust and weeds, may disrupt the corneal epithelium, allowing entry of *Moraxella bovis,* the etiologic agent of pinkeye. Flies have been shown to act as vectors for the bacteria.

Initial clinical signs include lacrimation, blepharospasm, and photophobia. Corneal inflammation followed by ulceration eventually develops. If ulceration becomes deep, the cornea may rupture, and vision will be lost.

The individual treatment of pinkeye involves a subconjunctival injection of antibiotics, usually procaine penicillin G (Figure 22-26). Eye patches may be applied to affected eyes to decrease photophobia and protect the eye from flies. More severe cases may require surgery, such as a third eyelid flap or tarsorrhaphy (suturing the lids closed) to protect deeper ulcers as they heal. In the case of herd outbreaks, it may be impractical to treat each animal with local therapy, so systemic antibiotics, such as long-acting tetracycline, can be administered to the group.

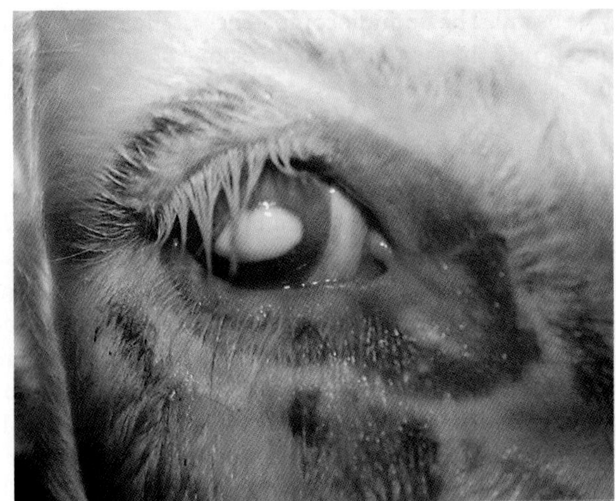

FIGURE 22-25 A large central corneal ulcer with abscess in a bull with IBK (pinkeye).

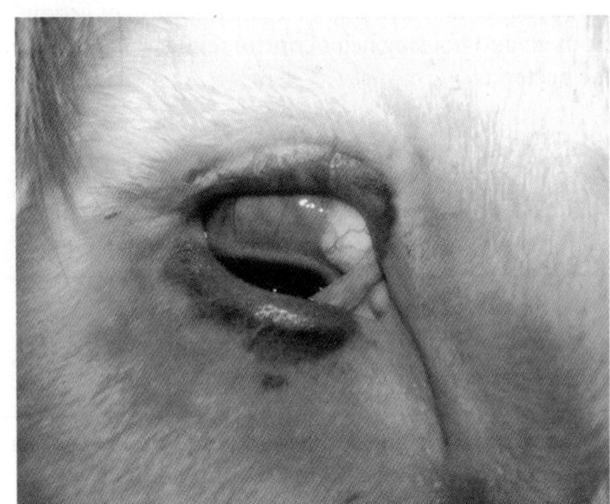

FIGURE 22-26 Procaine penicillin G injected subconjunctivally for treatment of IBK (pinkeye).

DISEASES OF THE SKIN

Cutaneous Papillomas (Warts)

Warts, a benign neoplasia caused by the papillomavirus, are common in young cattle. Warts appear as tan, white, or gray protruding masses with a dry, horny surface. Warts vary greatly in size and shape and can persist for 3 to 12 months at which time they often spontaneously regress.

Small warts may be crushed or surgically removed to help stimulate development of natural immunity and hasten healing. Cryosurgical treatment has also been successful. The use of autogenous and commercial vaccines has met with variable success. Since warts are usually self-limiting, no treatment may be necessary; however, in long-standing, severe, or nonresponsive cases, the immune status of the patient must be considered, and slaughter or euthanasia may be necessary.

Dermatophytosis (Ringworm)

Trichophyton verrucosum is the fungus responsible for ringworm in cattle. Ringworm is most likely to occur in calves housed in crowded conditions in the winter. Multiple circular lesions develop, particularly around the head and neck. The lesions, which are several centimeters in diameter, consist of an area of alopecia surrounding a slightly raised, whitish accumulation of dry, scaly skin. If left untreated, most lesions heal on their own in 2 to 3 months, especially if calves are turned out to pasture and exposed to the sunlight in the spring.

If treatment is desired, especially in the case of show animals, topical agents, such as iodine, bleach (1:10 in water), chlorhexidine, Captan, 5% lime sulfur, and thiabendazole may be useful. The immunocompetency of the animal hould be questioned in cases that do not respond spontaneously or with treatment.

Dermatophilosis (Streptotrichosis, Rain Scald)

Dermatophilosis is caused by the bacterium *Dermatophilus congolensis*. The bacteria invade the skin and produce crusts, which cause matting of the hair giving it a typical "paintbrush" appearance. The disease is more prevalent during periods of heavy rainfall or high humidity. Trauma, abrasions, concurrent disease, and poor nutrition make the skin more susceptible to infection. The disease may be transmitted by insect vector or direct contact with infected animals.

Treatment is accomplished by the removal of crusts by grooming followed by repeated iodine- or chlorhexidine-based shampoos. More severe cases may require systemic antimicrobials, such as penicillin or long-acting tetracycline. Exposure to the sunlight and disinfection of grooming equipment and housing helps control reinfection and spread of the bacteria.

> TECHNICIAN NOTE Dermatophilosis or rain scald, a common bacterial skin disease of cattle, is more prevalent during periods of heavy rainfall or high humidity.

BEHAVIOR

Since veterinary technicians are often responsible for the handling and restraint of cattle, it is important that they have a basic understanding of cattle behavior. Handling cattle can result in less stress to the cattle and increased safety for the handler if one has an understanding of the behavioral characteristics of the species. Minimizing excitement and stress is important since isolation, handling, and transportation stresses can lower the conception rate and suppress immune function. Nearly half of all bruises on livestock are due to rough handling with a cost of $46 million annually to the U.S. livestock industry.

Cattle have excellent wide-angle vision (greater than 300 degrees), but have difficulty with depth perception at ground level while moving along with their heads elevated. To see depth at ground level, the animal must lower its head, which may be one reason cattle stall when they see shadows. It is important to know that approaching an animal directly from the rear in its blind spot may result in the handler getting kicked if the animal is startled. Cattle are more sensitive to high-frequency noises than are people, and loud noises can cause distress in livestock.

When moving cattle in an open area or pasture, it is important to know that they will tend to follow fences. Shadows that fall across an alley or chute can cause cattle to stop moving; handlers should be careful about projecting moving shadows across the animal's line of vision. Cattle movement is facilitated by eliminating harsh contrasts of light and dark in loading ramps, chutes, and handling areas and sudden changes in floor level or texture. Cattle may also stop moving at puddles, drain grates, and bright spots of sunlight. Cattle have a tendency to move toward a more brightly illuminated area provided the light is not glaring in their eyes or causing a reflection off standing water on the ground. Care should be taken if leading halter-broken cattle from dim to bright light because they may unexpectedly run toward the light. It is sometimes difficult to move cattle under a roof or into a building for handling, but they will enter more readily if moved single file.

Cattle will tend to balk at the sound of clanking metal in chutes; rubber stops will help reduce the noise level. Moving or flapping objects (i.e., a coat hanging on a fence or a reflection from a truck bumper) will also cause cattle to stall. If cattle see people standing in front of the squeeze chute, they will frequently refuse to approach. However, a person in front of a squeeze chute containing an aggressive cow or bull may actually be advantageous to catching the head as the animal charges.

Movement of cattle in large pens is sometimes facilitated by a piece of cloth or plastic tied to a stick (commercial slapsticks are available). The noise and movement of these instruments causes the cattle to move away from the stimulus. Herding dogs should only be used in open areas where there is sufficient space for the cattle to move away. Electric prods should be used as sparingly as possible on cattle. Cattle quickly learn to associate the sound of the buzzer with receiving an electric shock and can often be moved by the noise alone. Cattle movement is more efficient if the working parts of the handling facility (squeeze chute) are oriented toward the "home" pasture or pen.

The flight zone of cattle is that space surrounding the animal that will elicit avoidance or escape when encroached upon. When a person enters an animal's flight zone, it will move away. If the handler penetrates the flight zone too deeply (gets too close to the animal), the animal will either bolt and run away or, if cornered, turn back and run past the person or charge the person. The best place for a handler to work animals is on the edge or perimeter of the flight zone. In this position, the animal will move away from the handler in an orderly manner (i.e., not show extreme flight behavior). The cattle will generally stop moving when the handler retreats from the flight zone.

The size of the flight zone depends on their relative degree of tameness. The flight zone of cattle raised on range may be many times greater than the flight zone of feedlot cattle. The "flight distance" can be roughly estimated by slowly walking toward the animal and noting how close the animal can be approached before it starts to move away. The flight distance can also be influenced by previous experience. Animals that have been handled gently and those that have been reared in close contact with people will have shorter flight distances than those handled roughly or with minimal human contact.

It is important not to invade the flight zone too deeply when moving cattle down an alley; if the animals attempt to turn back, the handler should retreat from the flight zone, which should terminate this escape behavior. Cattle sometimes rear up in a single-file chute or alley when the handler approaches too closely; backing up will allow the animal to settle down.

Cattle exhibit a strong tendency to follow and are highly motivated to maintain visual contact with each other. A single-file chute or alley should be long enough to take advantage of the animal's tendency to follow the leader. Cattle show visible signs of distress when isolated. This is especially true of Brahman-type cattle. An animal left alone in a crowding pen after the other animals have entered the alley or single-file chute may attempt to jump the fence to rejoin its herd mates. A lone steer or cow may become highly aroused and charge the handler. Many serious handler injuries have occurred when a steer or cow, separated from its herd mates, refuses to enter the single-file area. In this case, the handler should release the animal from the crowding pen and bring it back with another group of cattle.

Cattle should be able to see only one pathway of escape in the direction you want them to go and will move into a squeeze chute more easily if they can see other cattle ahead of them. Cattle can be driven most efficiently if the handler is situated at a 45-degree to 60-degree angle to the animal's shoulder. If the handler is behind the animal's shoulder ("point of balance"), the animal will move forward. If the handler is ahead of the animal's shoulder, forward movement will cease, and the animal will back up, if possible.

TECHNICIAN NOTE Handling and restraining cattle can result in less stress to the cattle and increased safety for the handler if one has an understanding of the behavioral characteristics of the species.

COMMON DISEASES AND CONDITIONS OF SMALL RUMINANTS

CARE OF THE NEONATE

One of the most important components of successful rearing of lambs is establishment of a strong ewe-lamb bond. Factors that may interfere with the bonding process include:

1. Lambing in a group housing situation
2. Conditions that prevent the ewe from licking the lamb immediately after birth
3. Separation of the lamb from the ewe during the first 24 hours for any reason

Sheep are gregarious and stay together as a group even during lambing, which may result in lamb "stealing" by late-pregnant ewes as a result of their maternal instinct. Lambing in individual pens (lambing jugs, 4 feet square and 30 inches high) helps prevent this from happening. Licking of amniotic fluid from the lamb by the ewe clears the airway and stimulates breathing and allows the ewe to identify that lamb as her own. Intervention during or right after parturition by the owner or veterinarian might confuse the ewe as to whether or not the lamb is hers. Ewes are capable of identifying their own lamb(s) after only a few hours of contact, whereas lambs require several days to identify their mothers. This is another reason for using individual lambing pens. The treatment of the lamb for hypoglycemia, chilling, or illness should be performed in the lambing pen if at all possible since separation of the lamb for more than 1 hour may result in rejection of the lamb by the ewe.

The first week of life is the most critical for the lamb; as much as 50% of lamb and kid mortality occurs during this time. The first 48 hours are the most critical. Two major problems that may occur are hypothermia and hypoglycemia. The relatively large body surface of a lamb (versus body mass) can serve as a significant drain of body heat and energy. A 55° F environmental temperature with a 12-mph breeze has an evaporative cooling effect equivalent to −25° F to a newborn; thus it is important to protect newborns from direct wind. Lambs and kids are born with minimal body fat stores; therefore hypoglycemia can develop if the newborns do not ingest colostrum (high in fat) within the first 12 to 24 hours. The dam's udder should be checked immediately postpartum to make sure it is functional. Ewes tend to have a thick wax plug that blocks the end of the teat before initial nursing. Occasionally the lamb is unable to remove the plug when it begins to nurse, which results in unsuccessful nursing. Another reason to examine the ewe's udder is for the presence of ovine progressive pneumonia (OPP) mastitis. The ewe's udder and milk will appear normal; however, the udder will feel firm when palpated as a result of the presence of fibrous connective tissue that occurs with OPP. Fibrous tissue development in the udder results in markedly decreased milk production. Lambs should be examined for congenital problems that might affect nursing, such as cleft palate, brachygnathism, prognathism, and tongue myopathies associated with vitamin E and/or selenium deficiency.

Hypothermia and hypoglycemia can usually be prevented with good management practices. Individual lambing pens work well to allow for bonding of the ewe and lamb, help keep the lamb warm, and allow the owner or veterinarian to check the ewe's milk supply and intervene if problems should arise. Pens should be built to prevent drafts and may even be designed with a supplemental heat source (heat lamp) for the lamb(s). It is helpful to have frozen sheep or goat colostrum available in case it is needed. Cow colostrum can be used; however, a small percentage of lambs have developed neonatal isoerythrolysis-type syndrome around 10 days after ingesting cow colostrum. Commercial lamb and kid milk replacers are available for orphan rearing or to supplement lambs or kids from poor-producing mothers. Lambs and kids need to be fed 10% to 15% of their body weight divided into three to four feedings during the first few days after birth. Later, twice-a-day feeding is adequate. They should be offered hay and starter rations early, but milk should be the major energy source until they are 5 to 6 weeks old. If a lamb or kid is hypoglycemic and hypothermic, it is best to rewarm the animal before any oral therapy. During a hypothermic crisis, the lower esophageal sphincter relaxes, and milk or oral supplements may be regurgitated and aspirated unless the animal is alert and sternal. Rewarming when the core body temperature is low is best achieved by immersing the neonate in warm water (100° F to 105° F) while supporting the head.

Sometimes lambs sustain "mama trauma" in the maternity pens, so it is important that the pens be of adequate size for large ewes. Lambs are sound sleepers, and it is instinctive for the ewe to roust the lamb(s) by pawing. Vigorous pawing in a small pen may result in fractured limbs, fractured ribs, and/or pneumothorax in the lamb. Signs of trauma include lethargy, lameness, inability to rise, dyspnea, or sudden death in the lamb(s). Securing a corner of the pen and providing a heat source in that area attracts the lamb(s) away from the ewe to rest and provides safety from the ewe's feet.

> *TECHNICIAN NOTE* The key to successful rearing of lambs is the establishment of a strong ewe-lamb bond; lambing in individual pens (lambing jugs) helps establish this bond.

GASTROINTESTINAL SYSTEM

Johne's Disease

Johne's disease in small ruminants has several unique features as compared with the disease in cattle. The most important difference is that Johne's disease in small ruminants is not characterized by diarrhea. Secondly, although Johne's disease is more infective to younger animals, exposed adults can develop clinical signs of the disease. A fecal culture, which is the "gold standard" in cattle, is unreliable and of no practical use in small ruminants because ovine strains, in particular, are difficult to grow. Agar gel immunodiffusion on a serum sample is fairly accurate and a good screening test to run.

Enterotoxemia

Enterotoxemia, caused by *C. perfringens,* is recognized worldwide as a common, frequently fatal disease of goats. Aspects of enterotoxemia peculiar to goats include a propensity for diarrhea to occur, severe enterocolitis at necropsy, and frequent failure of vaccination to protect from the development of clinical disease. The main cause of caprine enterotoxemia is *C. perfringens* type D, a gram-positive anaerobic rod that produces two main toxins, the most significant of which is epsilon toxin. Many outbreaks of caprine enterotoxemia involve dairy goats raised under intensive or semiintensive management conditions, whereas the greatest losses in sheep occur in lambs in feedlots receiving concentrate rations. Sudden feed changes have been associated with outbreaks of enterotoxemia, although outbreaks have occurred in situations where feeding practices were consistent. Specific feed changes include sudden accidental exposure to grain, turnout to lush pasture, feeding of bran or molasses mash to recently fresh does, feeding of bread or other bakery goods to goats, and feeding of garden greens to goats unaccustomed to green feed. Intestinal tapeworms are thought to predispose feedlot lambs to enterotoxemia by slowing GI transit time of grain rations allowing for more extensive proliferation of clostridia. In ruminant species, it is believed that commensal *C. perfringens* type D organisms reside in the gut without much damage, but sudden ingestion of readily fermentable carbohydrate-rich feed serves as a nutrient substrate for rapid proliferation of the organism. Excess carbohydrate intake may also reduce gut motility enhancing proliferation of *C. perfringens,* which increases the concentration and pathologic potential of the epsilon toxin. The toxin is necrotizing and neurotoxic. Death is due to damage of vital neurons, generalized toxemia, and shock. Clinically, lambs show lethargy, overt neurologic signs, minimal diarrhea, and death as opposed to kids, which show more prominent diarrhea and colic and fewer neurologic signs followed by death.

Glucosuria often occurs in goats affected with enterotoxemia, and soft or pulpy kidneys found on necropsy soon after death helps support the diagnosis. The most convincing evidence of enterotoxemia is the detection of epsilon toxin in diarrheal feces or intestinal contents (samples should be immediately refrigerated or frozen and sent to the lab). An ELISA test is available to identify the toxin.

The treatment includes balanced fluids with bicarbonate, NSAIDs, type C and D antitoxin (as much as 15 to 20 ml IV every 4 hours until stabilized), and antibiotics. In addition, cathartics and absorbents, such as activated charcoal, $MgSO_4$, and/or kaolin-pectin have been used. In the face of an outbreak, previously vaccinated goats should receive a booster vaccination, and unvaccinated animals should be vaccinated (to be repeated in 2 to 3 weeks) and given antitoxin. Any feeding of excessive carbohydrates should be immediately discontinued. Goats are considered highly susceptible to enterotoxemia and should be vaccinated at a maximum 6-month interval. In herds with a history of disease, 4-month vaccination intervals may be more appropriate. Initial vaccinations should be followed by booster vaccinations 3 to 4 weeks later; semiannual or triannual vaccinations should be followed by booster vaccinations 3 weeks before parturition for maximal benefit for the newborns. Kids should be vaccinated at 4 to 6 weeks of age and again at weaning. Vaccines with *C. perfringens* type C and D with or without tetanus are preferable to polyvalent clostridial vaccines available for cattle.

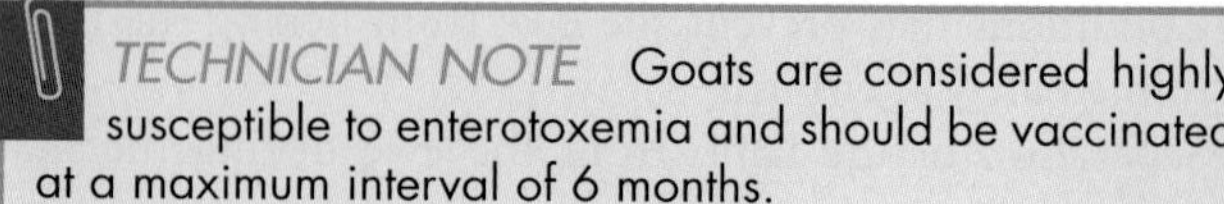

> *TECHNICIAN NOTE* Goats are considered highly susceptible to enterotoxemia and should be vaccinated at a maximum interval of 6 months.

RESPIRATORY SYSTEM

Pasteurella Pneumonia

Pasteurella multocida and *M. haemolytica* are both inhabitants of the pharynx of healthy animals, but may cause pneumonia in sheep and goats. Risk factors for development of pulmonary infection include initial infection with viral or mycoplasmal respiratory diseases, temperature extremes, overcrowding, respiratory tract irritants, transport, and other handling stresses. Clinical signs include bilateral nasal discharge, coughing, anorexia, and high fever. *M. haemolytica* causes an enzootic pneumonia with hemorrhagic bronchopneumonia as the primary lesion. The treatment includes the use of an antimicrobial to which the organism is sensitive. Drugs similar to those used for respiratory disease in cattle may be effective, but this use may be extralabel. Vaccines for pneumonic pasteurellosis are available, but are of questionable efficacy.

Ovine Progressive Pneumonia

OPP manifests as progressive respiratory failure, but also causes mastitis ("hard bag"), neurologic signs, and arthritis. The pulmonary form is predominant in the United States, and clinical signs include exercise intolerance, open-mouth breathing, exaggerated expiratory effort, and an occasional dry cough. In the later stages of the disease, weight loss occurs despite a good appetite. The disease causes an interstitial pneumonia, and affected animals usually die within 3 to 8 months of the onset of clinical signs. The diagnosis is based on clinical signs, necropsy, and serology using either AGID or ELISA (specificity of both is comparable, but ELISA is slightly more sensitive).

MUSCULOSKELETAL SYSTEM

Foot Rot

Lameness in multiple animals is usually due to contagious foot rot caused by *Dichelobacter nodosus* and *F. necrophorum.* Initial signs occur 10 to 20 days after exposure and include inflammation of the interdigital skin, followed by slight undermining of the sole at the heels. The undermining eventually progresses to the sole and wall. Some sheep are resistant to infection, some improve and clear the infection spontaneously, and others become chronic carriers of the disease. The usual source of bacteria is chronic carrier sheep or surfaces contaminated within the last 2 weeks by an infected animal. Infected feet have a characteristic foul odor.

The successful treatment involves thorough inspection of all animals and trimming and treatment of all affected animals. Animals should be divided into affected and unaffected groups and placed on clean pastures after treatment. As new cases develop in the unaffected group, these should be moved to the affected group. As cases in the affected group heal and respond to treatment, they should be placed in a third clean pasture. Footbaths are useful for treatment after trimming and may contain copper sulfate, zinc sulfate, or formalin. Zinc sulfate (10% to 20%) may be the best choice since it is less irritating than the other two. Copper sulfate poses a threat if sheep can drink the bath water, and formalin is a carcinogen and an environmental hazard. Once a treatment program has been initiated, all sheep should be checked weekly, trimmed if needed, and placed in the footbath. After 4 weeks of treatment, any animals with obvious hoof abnormalities or any that are still lame should be culled. The segregation of infected sheep and goats and culling of chronic carriers are essential for successful foot rot control. Vaccination can increase an animal's resistance to the organism, but it has little value in treating an active infection.

> *TECHNICIAN NOTE* The most common cause of lameness in sheep and goats is contagious foot rot caused by *D. nodosus.*

Tetanus

Spores of the bacterium *Clostridium tetani* may infect wounds resulting in tetanus. In an anaerobic environment, such as a wound, the organism produces several potent neurotoxins that are responsible for the typical clinical signs.

The disease commonly occurs following puncture wounds or surgical procedures, such as castration, tail docking, and dehorning. Animals with tetanus develop progressive muscle tetany characterized by stiff, erect ears; rigid extension of the limbs ("sawhorse" stance); and prolapse of the third eyelid (Figure 22-27). Affected animals are hyperresponsive to external stimuli, such as loud noises. Ultimately death is due to respiratory failure.

The treatment involves removal of the toxin-producing bacteria by cleaning, débriding, and disinfecting wounds or surgery sites. In addition, high doses of penicillin and tetanus antitoxin should be administered. Affected animals should be kept in a quiet environment and provided supportive care. Sedation may also be helpful.

Tetanus can be prevented by vaccination of pregnant ewes and does at least 1 month before parturition. Vaccination of kids and lambs should be initiated by 6 to 8 weeks of age. Tetanus toxoid and/or antitoxin should be given to small ruminants anytime a surgery is performed or an injury occurs.

> *TECHNICIAN NOTE* Small ruminants are extremely susceptible to tetanus; therefore tetanus toxoid and/or antitoxin should be given to small ruminants anytime a surgery is performed or an injury occurs.

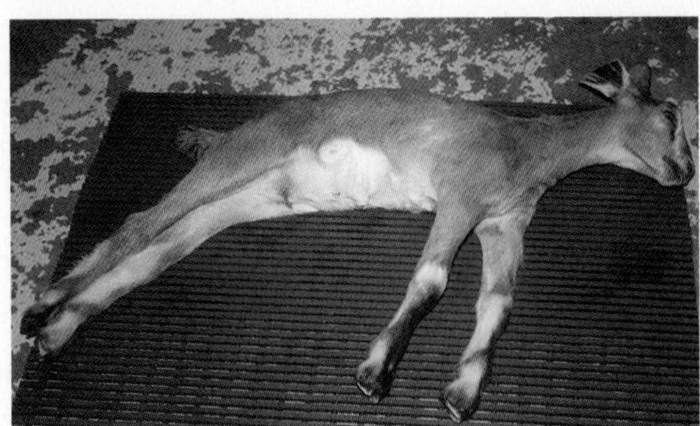

FIGURE 22-27 Severe extensor rigidity ("sawhorse" position) in a kid with tetanus.

White Muscle Disease

White muscle disease (WMD), also known as nutritional myodegeneration (NMD), occurs in young lambs, calves, kids, and pigs born to dams receiving diets deficient in selenium during gestation.

A dietary deficiency of selenium and/or vitamin E may cause degeneration of cardiac or skeletal muscle. If skeletal muscles are affected, muscular weakness or stiffness followed by eventual recumbency and death may occur. If the heart is primarily involved, sudden death can occur. On necropsy, the skeletal and cardiac muscles appear pale and may have the white streaks that give the disease its name.

Early cases of the skeletal form of WMD may respond to an injection of vitamin E and selenium. Prevention includes ensuring that the ration has adequate amounts of vitamin E and selenium and the injection of the dam before parturition in areas of the country where soil is deficient in selenium. Selenium can be toxic, so manufacturer's recommendations should be followed carefully.

HEMOLYMPHATIC SYSTEM

Caseous Lymphadenitis

Caseous lymphadenitis (CL) is the most common cause of lymph node abscess in small ruminants and is a major cause of carcass condemnation in sheep. The generalized or visceral form may cause chronic weight loss also known as thin ewe or thin doe syndrome. This highly contagious disease is caused by *Corynebacterium pseudotuberculosis.* The bacterium usually gains entry through broken skin, but the organism may also invade intact skin or enter the body via inhalation or ingestion. Once in the body, the organisms are carried in afferent lymph to regional lymph nodes where characteristic abscesses develop. The disease is readily spread from animal to animal by contact with contaminated materials (pus). The disease can become endemic in a herd or flock and is difficult to eradicate because of its poor response to therapeutics, its ability to persist in the environment for long periods (8 months in soil), and the lack of a reliable test to detect affected animals.

Abscessed lymph nodes have thick capsules and central cores of laminated, dry, green-white caseous material that may displace the remnants of the lymphoid tissue peripherally. Differentials for the visceral form (chronic wasting) include Johne's disease, chronic parasitism, caprine arthritis-encephalitis, and OPP in addition to other causes of chronic pneumonia. The presence of external abscesses is highly suggestive of CL, particularly in an endemic herd or flock, but a culture is needed to confirm the diagnosis.

In general, aggressive culling is recommended in herds or flocks with CL outbreaks since affected animals serve as reservoirs of infection. If a producer or owner is reluctant to cull infected animals, they should be encouraged to split the herd or flock into infected and clean groups and to manage each group separately. Kids and lambs should be separated from infected adults at birth and raised on pasteurized goat's (or cow's) milk and colostrum. Vaccinations may help limit the spread of CL in sheep flocks, but benefits have not been as apparent in goat herds, and there is a higher incidence of side effects in this species. Vaccination does not cure an infected animal; its primary benefit lies in its ability to prevent the establishment of infection in vaccinated animals if used before exposure to the organism. Treatment techniques include surgical removal of the unopened abscesses, lancing, draining, and flushing of opened abscesses, long-term antibiotic therapy (4 to 6 weeks), and intraabscess formalin injection. Control involves culling affected animals and practicing good hygiene during tail docking, castration, and shearing.

> TECHNICIAN NOTE CL, a highly contagious disease caused by *C. pseudotuberculosis,* is the most common cause of lymph node abscess in small ruminants.

Copper Toxicity

Sheep are the domestic animals most prone to development of copper toxicity, and young growing lambs are the most susceptible. Sheep absorb copper from the diet in proportion to the amount offered rather than according to the body's need. Copper accumulates in the liver causing liver damage that precedes the onset of clinical signs. Usually, stress, such as shipping, handling, traveling to shows, and feed changes, will trigger the release of copper from the liver. The sudden release of copper from the liver causes an acute hemolytic crisis.

Clinical signs are depression, anorexia, weakness, hemoglobinuria, hemoglobinemia, anemia, and icterus. The single toxic dose of copper for sheep is between 20 and 110 mg/kg. Chronic copper poisoning can occur after several months of a daily dose of 3.5 mg/kg. Sources of copper that have been responsible for toxicity in sheep include trace mineralized salt, rations containing greater than 20% chicken litter, pastures (and hay) fertilized with chicken litter or pig manure, forage from fruit orchard pastures that are contaminated with copper sulfate fungicides, parasiticides for GI helminths, copper sulfate footbaths, fungicide-treated fence posts, corroded overhead cables, copper-treated seed grains, and therapeutically administered copper salts.

Therapy, though usually not successful, includes diuresis with IV fluids (with caution), O_2 therapy, and blood transfusions, if necessary. Specific therapy for copper toxicity includes the use of D-penicillamine (Cuprimine, 52 mg/kg for 6 days) and oral administration of 100 mg ammonium molybdate and 1 g of anhydrous sodium sulfate per sheep. Ammonium tetrathiomolybdate (50 to 100 mg per adult sheep twice weekly) has shown some promise in the treatment of copper toxicity. Even if lambs live through the acute hemolytic crisis, often there is significant, irreversible renal damage as a result of the hemoglobinuria, which may result in death or necessitate humane euthanasia.

REPRODUCTIVE SYSTEM/MAMMARY GLAND

Pseudopregnancy

Pseudopregnancy is a common pathologic condition in goats that may develop in does with or without exposure to a buck. The condition is characterized by accumulation of fluid in the uterus and one or more corpora lutea (CLs) on the ovaries. The incidence of hydrometra is estimated to be 2% to 21%, and adult goats seem to be more prone to development of the condition than yearlings. Out-of-season breeding or delaying breeding until after the first or second estrous cycle during the fall breeding season appears to cause a higher incidence of pseudopregnancy. The treatment involves the use of luteolytic products, such as prostaglandin (PG) F_{2a} (5 mg, IM). Successful lysis results in uterine evacuation of fluid ("cloudburst"). However, in one study, hydrometra was found to recur immediately after induced cloudburst in 45% of does treated with a single dose of PGF_{2a}, and only 15% conceived from a breeding performed at the first estrus after treatment. By contrast, another group of does were injected twice with 5 mg of PGF_{2a} (at the time of diagnosis and 12 days after the cloudburst), and only 3% experienced recurrent hydrometra, and 48% conceived from a breeding performed at the estrus induced by the second injection. The examination for pregnancy should be performed 25 to 40 days after breeding (transrectal ultrasonography) or 40 to 70 days after breeding using the transabdominal method.

Mastitis

Mastitis in sheep and goats can be caused by a variety of bacteria including coliforms, *Staphylococcus* spp., *Pseudomonas* spp., *Streptococcus* spp., and *Pasteurella haemolytica*. Of much concern to sheep and goat producers is blue bag mastitis caused by *S. aureus* or *P. haemolytica*. *S. aureus,* which is most likely to be associated with the gangrenous form of mastitis, may progress rapidly and may be severe enough to cause death of the animal. A *P. haemolytica* infection may lead to abscess formation in the udder. The treatment of gangrenous mastitis includes antimicrobial therapy, NSAIDs, fluid therapy, and possible teat or udder amputation; however, therapy is often unrewarding.

> TECHNICIAN NOTE *S. aureus*, which is most likely to be associated with the gangrenous form of mastitis in sheep and goats (blue bag), may progress rapidly and cause death of the animal.

NERVOUS SYSTEM

Caprine Arthritis-Encephalitis

Caprine arthritis encephalitis most often affects dairy goats and causes a nonresponsive arthritis (usually carpi) in adults and an acute leukoencephalomyelitis in young goats. It may also cause chronic pneumonia (interstitial), chronic encephalomyelitis, chronic weight loss, and "hard udder." Clinical disease is less common than infection, and only about 15% of seropositive goats ever develop clinical disease. The primary mode of transmission is through infected colostrum and the milk of infected dams. Lactating goats housed together can seroconvert, but there is no evidence of nonlactating goats spreading the disease. There is also no evidence that the disease is spread during breeding. The arthritic form is seldom seen before 1 to 2 years of age. In general, the ELISA test developed for detecting caprine arthritis-encephalitis (CAE) virus infection is more sensitive than are the available agar gel immunodiffusion (AGID) tests. Positive tests in kids younger than 90 days old may reflect colostric transfer of antibodies; likewise, a negative serologic test result cannot be used to exclude a diagnosis of CAE because the time required for seroconversion is variable (some goats take months to years to seroconvert). A polymerase chain reaction (PCR) test for CAE is available and will detect positive goats sooner, but the test is labor intensive and expensive. Therefore serology will probably continue to be used more widely for eradication of CAE in individual herds.

Scrapie

Scrapie is a transmissible spongiform encephalopathy (prion protein) that manifests primarily as weight loss and since it generally takes years to develop the disease, weight loss is seen primarily in adults. Other clinical signs include pruritus with wool loss (Figure 22-28), ataxia, fine muscle tremors of the face, head pressing, abnormal gait, and disorientation. Scratching of the sheep's back will usually elicit nibbling or licking of the lips. An antemortem diagnosis may be attempted by immunohistochemistry on a biopsy of lymphoid tissue of the third eyelid, submandibular lymph node, and rectal mucosa. A postmortem confirmation can be achieved by histopathologic examination or immunohistochemistry of the brain. Scrapie is a reportable disease, and there is no known treatment. Genetic testing can be performed to predict the susceptibility of individual sheep to the scrapie prion. A scrapie eradication program is currently in place, and veterinary technicians play an important role in this regulatory work.

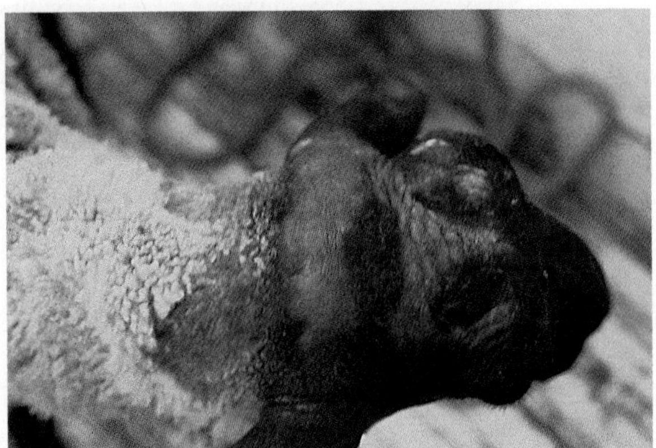

FIGURE 22-28 A ewe with scrapie exhibiting pruritus and wool loss over the poll.

Pregnancy Toxemia

Pregnancy toxemia is a metabolic disease that commonly affects pregnant ewes and does during late gestation. Clinical signs can occur in pregnant animals that are overconditioned, thin, or in normal body condition. Affected animals are generally pregnant with multiple fetuses and in the last month of gestation. The condition is typically limited to ewes or does in their second or subsequent pregnancies; it is uncommon in dams carrying a single fetus or yearlings bred for their first pregnancy. Clinical cases usually follow a period of negative energy balance resulting in hypoglycemia, increased fat catabolism, ketonemia, and ketonuria in susceptible animals. Traditionally, annual feed costs for the ewe flock account for 50% of yearly out-of-pocket expenses for producers; therefore this area of expenditure may be targeted for cost reduction to improve profitability resulting in an increased incidence of pregnancy toxemia in a flock.

A diagnosis of pregnancy toxemia should be considered whenever late-pregnant ewes or does exhibit neurologic signs or motor weakness leading to death within 3 to 10 days. Clinical signs include anorexia, hypoglycemia, ketonemia, ketonuria, weakness, depression, incoordination, mental dullness, and impaired vision, followed by recumbency and death. Urine can easily be checked for ketones using commercially available urine test strips. Recumbency is generally indicative of a poor prognosis. Characteristically, affected animals linger for several days to a week before dying. Differential diagnoses include hypocalcemia, listeriosis, polioencephalomalacia, hypomagnesemia, trauma, parasitism, and meningeal worm migration. Although treatment of the individual animal is often necessary, the owner should be reminded that prevention in the rest of the flock or herd is usually more important and cost-effective than is treatment of the individual animal. The treatment often includes propylene glycol (100 ml twice daily PO), IV dextrose or glucose at 5 to 7 g every 4 hours (e.g., 100 ml of 5% dextrose every 4 hours), 20 to 40 units of protamine zinc insulin every other day for 3 days, B vitamins, and calcium borogluconate if hypocalcemia is a problem. In addition, corticosteroids may be used to promote gluconeogenesis, increase appetite, induce parturition or abortion, and assist lung maturation in the fetuses. A recent report suggests that a single subcutaneous injection of 160 mg of a slow-release formulation of recombinant bovine somatotropin in combination with glucose and electrolyte treatments may show promise for increasing both ewe and lamb survival.

Body condition scoring of ewes or does 4 to 6 weeks before the expected date of parturition allows detection of problems and adequate time for correction of problems. Late gestation body condition scores (BCSs) should increase to a 3 to 3.5 level at parturition. Palpation of the lumbar epaxial musculature is a rapid and relatively simple means of evaluating the BCS in sheep (Box 22-2).

BOX 22-2 Body Condition Score for Sheep

0. Absence of lumbar musculature and subcutaneous fat, leaving a profound depression between the tips of the dorsal and transverse spinous processes
1. Moderate concavity between the dorsal and transverse spinous processes
2. Mild concavity between the dorsal and transverse spinous processes
3. No depression (straight line) between the dorsal and transverse spinous processes
4. Slight bulging (convexity) between dorsal and transverse spinous processes
5. Profound convexity between the dorsal and transverse spinous processes (cannot palpate spinous processes)

OPHTHALMIC SYSTEM

Pinkeye

Pinkeye, or infectious keratoconjunctivitis, is usually caused by *Chlamydia psittaci* in sheep and *Mycoplasma conjunctivae* in goats, although either organism can cause pinkeye in both species. Carrier animals and apparently uninfected animals in a herd or flock serve as an important source of infection. Both organisms may persist for months in ocular tissue and are spread by contact with infected ocular secretions. Clinical signs, regardless of the cause, include conjunctival hyperemia, epiphora, photophobia, blepharospasm, corneal edema, vascularization of the cornea, and ocular discharge. Severe cases may result in corneal ulceration or corneal abscessation. Both infections are self-limiting, and recovery can be expected in a few weeks; however, treatment with tetracycline systemically and/or topically is recommended to prevent spread of infection and development of severe eye lesions with loss of sight.

> TECHNICIAN NOTE Pinkeye, or infectious keratoconjunctivitis, usually caused by *C. psittaci* in sheep and *M. conjunctivae* in goats, is often treated with tetracycline in both species.

INTEGUMENTARY SYSTEM

Contagious Ecthyma

Contagious ecthyma (sore mouth, orf), a common viral disease of small ruminants, causes crusty, proliferative lesions around the mouth and nose of lambs and kids and similar lesions on the teats and udder of the ewes and does (Figure 22-29). The infection is self-limiting, taking 4 to 6 weeks to run its course. Since it is a viral disease, there is no treatment; however, antimicrobials may be given to prevent secondary bacterial infection. Supportive therapy may also be administered to those lambs and kids too painful to nurse. A live virus vaccine is available, but its use should be limited to those flocks or herds already experiencing a problem. The virus is zoonotic (transmissible to humans), so care should be taken when handling infected animals or administering the live virus vaccine (wear gloves).

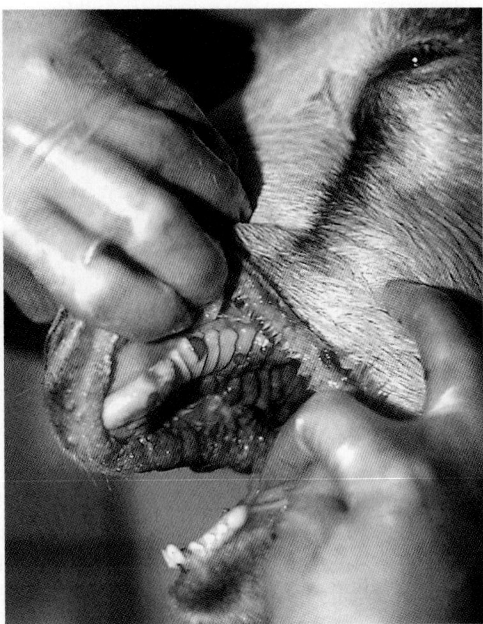

FIGURE 22-29 Ulcerative and proliferative lesions in and around the mouth of this doe are due to contagious ecthyma, or orf.

BEHAVIOR

Goats tend to flock together in extended family groups and have strong hierarchic structure in the herd. Both males and females will establish social dominance in their respective groups through head-to-head combat. Since goats use their horns to advantage during fighting, it is best if all goats in a group either be horned or dehorned to prevent excessive bullying by horned goats.

When goats are threatened or upset, they will turn to face an intruder or stranger and make a characteristic sneezing noise (sheep have a similar response). Goats will orally investigate everything in their environment, so destructible items should be kept out of reach. They are agile and are excellent climbers often found in trees, on rafters, or on top of vehicles (Figure 22-30). A rock pile or other elevated area within the pen or pasture will provide recreation and help control hoof overgrowth. Goats are notorious for learning to open gates and thus may escape the enclosure or may get into excessive amounts of stored feed (grain overload). Since goats can climb and get caught in fencing, electric fencing is recommended for their safety.

Goats are adaptable worldwide because of their efficient browsing ability and effective use of relatively poor quality roughage. Goats and sheep are seasonally polyestrous in temperate climates, breeding primarily in the fall. Bucks develop a stronger odor during breeding (rut) and may become quite aggressive during this time.

Sheep have wide-angle vision and can see behind themselves without turning their heads. Solid fencing should be used when moving sheep because they respect solid barriers and are less apt to be distracted or spooked. When moving sheep, it is important to know that they move toward light and will follow other sheep because of the flocking instinct.

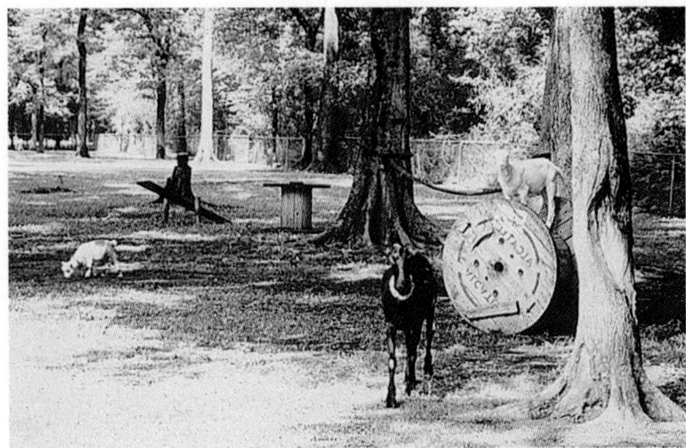

FIGURE 22-30 Goats are excellent climbers and should be provided with safe areas to climb and play for recreation.

> *TECHNICIAN NOTE* Contagious ecthyma (sore mouth, orf), a common viral disease of small ruminants, is zoonotic (transmissible to humans), so care should be taken when handling infected animals (wear gloves).

COMMON DISEASES AND CONDITIONS OF SWINE

CARE OF THE NEONATE

Neonatal pigs have little fat store and therefore require supplemental heat during the first few weeks of life. During the first week, the temperature of the sleeping area should be 92° F to 95° F, the second week 89° F to 92° F, and the third week 86° F to 89° F. Colostrum intake soon after birth is important in this species. Adequate nutrition is also important since hypoglycemia can quickly develop in the undernourished piglet. Hypoglycemia may lead to a weakened piglet that is susceptible to a variety of diseases or crushing by the dam when she lies down. Frequent observation of the sow or gilt and the pigs will help determine if nursing behavior is normal. Piglets that are hungry will circle the dam and squeal weakly. In this case, the sow or gilt should be examined to determine if she has mastitis or some other disease that requires immediate treatment. Baby pigs raised in confinement need iron dextran injections at 3 days of age (Figure 22-31). Needle teeth should also be clipped at this time to prevent injury to the dam's udder and to other piglets in the litter (Figure 22-32). Tails may also be docked at the same time to help prevent tail biting later, and castration may also be performed (Figure 22-33). These are common pig-processing techniques that are much less stressful to the pig if performed at a few days of age. If hypoglycemia develops, the piglet(s) may be treated with 5 to 10 cc of 5% dextrose injected by aseptic technique intraperitoneally. Pigs that are rejected, orphaned, or not receiving adequate nutrition by the mother may be supplemented with a milk replacer designed for pigs. Young pigs quickly learn to drink from shallow pans and therefore do not usually require bottle feeding, which can be labor intensive. These piglets can also be offered prestarter feed at an early age. Pigs are nosey by nature,

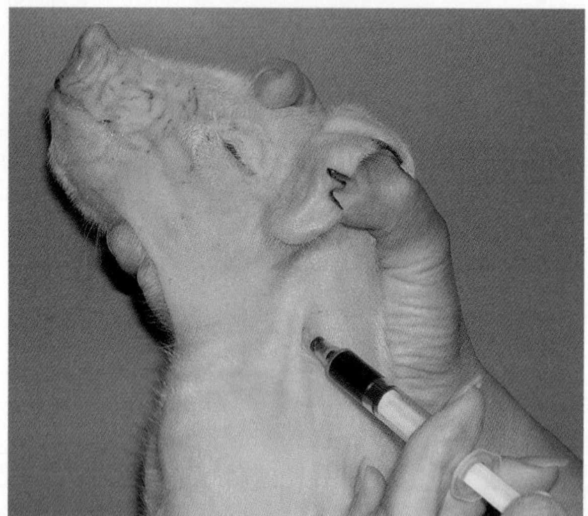

FIGURE 22-31 Baby pigs raised in confinement require iron dextran supplementation by 3 days of age.

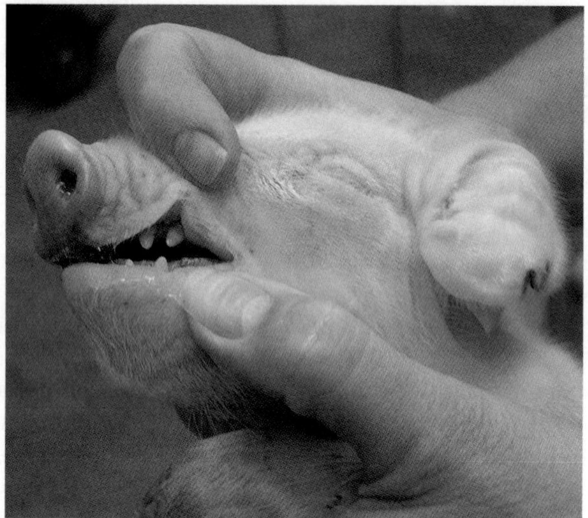

FIGURE 22-32 Needle teeth in neonatal pigs should be clipped to prevent bite injuries to the dam and littermates.

and through exploring their environment, they learn to eat solid feed quickly. A homemade milk replacer that can be used to raise piglets (more appropriate for potbellied pigs) consists of 1 qt of whole cow's milk, 1 oz of white corn syrup or honey, and 1 oz of cream or corn oil.

> *TECHNICIAN NOTE* Prevention of hypothermia and hypoglycemia in the neonatal period is important to successful pig rearing.

MULTISYSTEMIC DISEASES

Erysipelas

Erysipelas is caused by a bacterium that enters the body through lymphoid tissue, such as tonsillar or intestinal lymph tissue, or via breaks in the skin. Up to 50% of healthy swine may carry and shed the organism. Septicemia quickly

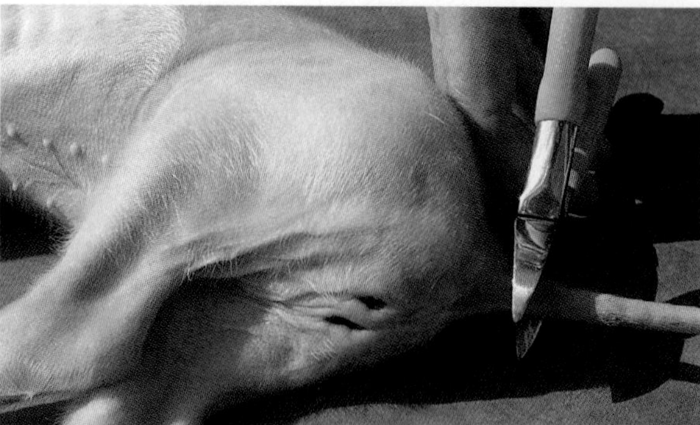

FIGURE 22-33 Tail docking is often performed at several days of age to prevent tail biting in pigs kept in confinement. Also note recent castration incisions.

develops after an infection, and the organisms tend to localize in the skin, heart, and joints. Infection causes a high fever and may produce characteristic diamond skin lesions. This form often results in death if not recognized early. The chronic form of the disease is more likely to result in vegetative endocarditis or chronic, nonsuppurative polyarthritis with lameness. The treatment of choice for the acute form is penicillin, but nothing is effective for treatment of the chronic form. Immunization against erysipelas is effective and inexpensive and should be provided at weaning and repeated every 6 months.

Pseudorabies Virus (Aujeszky's Disease, Mad Itch)

Swine are considered the natural host of pseudorabies virus (PRV), and although many other species are affected by this virus, most are dead-end hosts. An infection in baby pigs results in development of neurologic signs and in some cases vomiting and diarrhea. Mortality in this age group is high. Weaning and growing pigs exhibit fever, pneumonia, a dry, nonproductive cough, and flulike signs. Death loss can be high in nursery-age pigs, but fairly low in finishers. Infection in adults may cause reproductive problems, including early embryonic death, abortion, or stillbirths in pregnant sows or gilts. Serologic tests (ELISA) are used for screening herds for PRV. There is no treatment for PRV, and vaccination for the disease is closely regulated by state officials. There is currently a pseudorabies eradication program in place in the United States.

> *TECHNICIAN NOTE* PRV is responsible for development of neurologic signs in baby pigs, flulike signs in growing pigs, and embryonic death, abortion, or stillbirths in pregnant sows or gilts.

Porcine Reproductive and Respiratory Syndrome

Infection with the viral disease porcine reproductive and respiratory syndrome (PRRS) are prevalent in U.S. swine herds. The virus enters the body through the respiratory tract replicating in the pulmonary alveolar macrophage resulting in interstitial pneumonia. A viremia follows, and the virus may cross the placenta infecting embryos or fetuses. General clinical signs include fever, lethargy, inappetence, and cyanosis of the ears, vulva, tail, abdomen, and snout ("blue ear disease"). The respiratory syndrome is manifest by labored breathing, increased secondary respiratory infections, increased postweaning mortality, and decreased rate of gain and feed efficiency. The reproductive syndrome includes abortion, stillbirths, fetal mummies, and the birth of weak piglets. Diagnosis is based on clinical findings, histopathology, virus isolation, immunofluorescence, and/or PCR. Serology is also available, but since seroprevalence is high in U.S. swine herds, the presence of antibodies does not necessarily mean that the herd is experiencing clinical disease as a result of PRRS. There is no treatment for PRRS, but antimicrobials may be administered in the event of secondary bacterial infections. A modified live virus vaccine is available. Control measures are variable and dependent upon the current herd status and the goals of the producer.

GASTROINTESTINAL SYSTEM

Diarrhea in Young Pigs

Differentials for baby pig diarrhea include enterotoxigenic *E. coli* (ETEC) or colibacillosis, rotavirus, coronavirus or transmissible gastroenteritis (TGE), clostridial enteritis, coccidiosis, and parasites (*Strongyloides ransomi* or threadworms).

ETEC is the most important primary cause of diarrhea in piglets less than 5 days of age. Pathogenic strains are spread to susceptible pigs via the fecal-oral route. These strains of bacteria adhere to the lining of the small intestine via pili or fimbriae and produce enterotoxins. Dehydration and electrolyte abnormalities often result in death. Fecal pH is usually high (greater than 8) in pigs experiencing colibacillosis as a result of secretion of bicarbonate into the intestinal lumen. In contrast, malabsorptive diarrheas, such as those caused by viruses and protozoa, usually have a fecal pH of 7 or lower. Diarrheal stools are watery or pasty and yellowish. Definitive diagnosis is based on the isolation of large numbers of *E. coli* with appropriate virulence factors from the small intestine of affected pigs at necropsy. No villous atrophy occurs in the small intestine with colibacillosis. Treatment involves the use of antimicrobials to which the bacteria show sensitivity and supportive care, such as fluid and electrolyte therapy. Prefarrowing vaccination of the sow with a Köhler milk culture (oral vaccination of the sow with a live culture of the farm-specific strain of ETEC) or a commercial bacterin or subunit vaccine may be beneficial in preventing disease in the neonate.

TGE, caused by a coronavirus, occurs in an epizootic and enzootic form. The epizootic or acute form affects pigs of all ages. It causes vomiting, diarrhea, high morbidity, and high mortality in pigs less than 2 weeks of age and anorexia, vomiting, and diarrhea with low mortality in growers, finishers, and adults and usually occurs in the winter months. The enzootic or chronic form of TGE primarily affects pigs from 1 to 8 weeks of age and may occur year-round. With this form, diarrhea is usually not seen before 6 to 7 days and not after 2 weeks after weaning. Morbidity and mortality are much lower than with the epizootic form. The diagnosis is based on clinical signs, particularly in the epizootic form, presence of villous atrophy in the jejunum seen on histopathology, detection of viral antigen (ELISA, immunofluorescence, or electron microscopy), and a fecal pH of less than 7. Supportive care with fluid and electrolyte therapy and antimicrobials for prevention of secondary bacterial infections may reduce death losses. Vaccines, both injectable and oral, are available for sows and pigs for prevention of TGE.

Rotavirus is similar to enzootic TGE, though usually less severe. Diarrhea almost always occurs 3 to 4 days after pigs are weaned. Histopathology reveals villous atrophy in the small intestine, and the duodenum is not spared as in TGE. Treatment of rotavirus is as described for TGE. Vaccines are available for oral vaccination of pigs at 7 and 21 days of age.

Coccidiosis *(Isospora suis)* is responsible for diarrhea in 7- to 10-day-old piglets. Coccidiosis is more of a problem in production units with continuous farrowing operations and poor sanitation. Mixed infections, especially with *E. coli,* are common. Affected piglets have yellow to green watery feces without blood. The fecal pH in these cases is usually acidic.

The diagnosis is based on clinical findings, fecal flotation, and necropsy with histopathology and impression smears from the small intestine demonstrating merozoites. No coccidiostats are available for use in swine, so extralabel recommendations for treating baby pigs are oral amprolium or oral trimethoprim-sulfa. To reduce the chances of coccidiosis, all-in, all-out farrowing with cleaning and disinfection of premises is recommended.

C. perfringens type C causes enterotoxemia in 3- to 4-day-old pigs. Piglets consume the organism from carrier sows, and the bacteria attach to and invade the jejunal villi producing toxins that cause intestinal necrosis. Death results from secondary bacteremia, hypoglycemia, and toxemia. The peracute form may cause sudden death without prior clinical signs. The acute form has a 2- to 3-day course and causes a bloody diarrhea with shreds of necrotic mucosa. The subacute form had a longer duration with pigs that gradually waste away, whereas those pigs that have the chronic form become chronically stunted. Hemorrhagic diarrhea in nursing pigs is highly suggestive of clostridial enteritis. Characteristic gross lesions include bloody fluid and necrotic membranes in the jejunum, and large gram-positive rods may be apparent on histopathology. Any treatment is usually ineffective once clinical signs are obvious. The administration of type C antitoxin may benefit some cases. Vaccination of the sow prefarrowing with *C. perfringens* type C toxoid and improved sanitation are effective in prevention of this disease.

Despite the cause of diarrhea in young pigs, good nursing care is important to survival. Free-choice oral electrolyte solutions should be provided in shallow pans. Antimicrobials may be used if there is a risk of secondary bacterial infection. Finally, it is important to keep the piglets warm, at least 32.2° C (90° F), to prevent energy loss and rapid wasting.

> *TECHNICIAN NOTE* Baby pig diarrhea may be caused by ETEC or colibacillosis, rotavirus, coronavirus or TGE, clostridial enteritis, coccidiosis, and parasites (*S. ransomi* or threadworms).

Diarrhea in Grower and Finisher Pigs

Swine dysentery, salmonellosis, proliferative enteropathy (ileitis), and whipworms are all differential diagnoses for diarrhea in growing and finishing swine.

Swine dysentery is caused by a spirochete, *Brachyspira hyodysenteriae.* Morbidity with this disease in untreated herds may reach 90%. The disease is spread from pig to pig by the fecal-oral route. Once the bacteria are ingested, they attach to the colonic mucosa and produce virulence factors that cause a catarrhal colitis. The colon loses its reabsorptive capacity, leading to diarrhea and dehydration. Diarrhea begins with soft, yellow feces that progresses to diarrhea with large amounts of mucus and flecks of blood, then to a watery mixture of blood, mucus, and shreds of mucofibrinous exudate. Affected pigs become thin, weak, emaciated, and dehydrated. Most pigs recover in 2 weeks and may always do poorly, but up to one third may die. The diagnosis is based on clinical findings, gross lesions in the colon, observation of the organism by darkfield microscopy, examination of silver-stained histologic sections, culture, or PCR. Several drugs, including carbadox, lincomycin, tiamulin, and bacitracin methylene disalicylate, have helped in the treatment of swine dysentery. Prevention of this disease requires maintenance of a closed herd. Vaccination is not useful in control. Eradication of swine dysentery from an infected herd is possible and probably advisable from an economic standpoint. It may be accomplished without depopulation and involves culling, meticulous sanitation, and segregated early weaning.

Proliferative enteropathy (porcine proliferative enteritis, "garden-hose gut"), also transmitted through the feces, is caused by *Lawsonia intracellularis.* Clinical findings include intermittent diarrhea (hemorrhagic in older pigs), anorexia, weight loss, melena, and anemia. Gross lesions of thickened intestinal mucosa, or garden-hose gut, are usually limited to the distal third of the small intestine. Treatment is aimed at prevention by segregated early weaning; all-in, all-out pig production; stress reduction; and good sanitation.

RESPIRATORY SYSTEM

Atrophic Rhinitis

Atrophic rhinitis (AR) is a chronic, progressive disease of swine that results in atrophy of the nasal turbinates. Although AR is a multifactorial disease, *Bordetella bronchiseptica* and *P. multocida* are the primary infectious agents involved. The two pathogens together produce a more severe and persistent nasal atrophy than either agent alone. Environmental factors, such as high ammonia levels, stress, concurrent disease, and suboptimal nutrition, also play a role in development of AR. Piglets acquire the infectious agents from nose-to-nose contact with a chronically infected dam, and transmission may also occur among young pigs. Nationwide, probably 80% of swine herds are affected to some degree by turbinate atrophy. Early clinical signs include sneezing and mucopurulent nasal discharge in young pigs. Later, twisted or shortened snouts, excessive lacrimation, epistaxis, decreased growth rate, and decreased feed efficiency are apparent in grower and finisher pigs. Necropsy and slaughter checks can be used to assess the degree of turbinate atrophy and the prevalence of disease in a herd. At least 20 pigs should be evaluated by cross-sectioning the snout at the level of the second premolar. The severity of the lesion is evaluated by measuring in millimeters the space between the ventral turbinate and the floor of the nasal cavity and comparing it with an existing scoring scale. Treatment and control involves use of antimicrobial agents in the feed to maintain the rate of gain in pigs in the presence of AR. Vaccines are also available and are of greatest benefit when used in the dam prefarrowing. All-in, all-out farrowing; improved ventilation; control of concurrent diseases; farrowing older sows; and provision of adequate nutrition all help control the incidence of AR. Eradication may be achieved by depopulation and repopulation with AR-free swine. Other options for eradication include specific pathogen-free (SPF) programs and segregated early weaning.

B. bronchiseptica can also cause pneumonia in young pigs. Clinical signs include fever, anorexia, and coughing in nursing or recently weaned pigs. The disease causes an anteroventral hemorrhagic consolidation in the lung. Antimicrobials based on sensitivity should be administered to affected pigs, and vaccination of pigs with *Bordetella* bacterin aids in prevention.

> *TECHNICIAN NOTE* AAR, a chronic, progressive disease of swine, results in atrophy of the nasal turbinates, twisted or shortened snouts, excessive lacrimation, epistaxis, and decreased growth rate and feed efficiency in growing and finishing swine.

Swine Influenza

Swine influenza is a viral disease of swine that produces high fever, up to 108° F (42° C), anorexia, and a deep, dry "barking" cough. The disease is characterized by a high morbidity (nearly 100%) and low mortality. The clinical signs of the epizootic form of swine influenza are dramatic, distinctive, and highly suggestive of the disease, although diagnostic tests, such as FA, IHC, ELISA, PCR, serology, and virus isolation, are available for a definitive diagnosis. There is no specific treatment for swine influenza, but good nursing care and antimicrobial administration for prevention of secondary bacterial respiratory infections is suggested. Vaccines are available for protection against swine influenza. Though rare, swine influenza may be zoonotic and cause serious illness and even death in humans; therefore it is the veterinarian's responsibility to prevent infected animals from appearing at public exhibitions.

Mycoplasma Pneumonia

Mycoplasma hyopneumoniae is the most common cause of chronic pneumonia in swine, with most herds affected to some degree. The organism is spread by contact and aerosol, and disease may be mild, but other bacterial infections, such as *P. multocida, Streptococcus suis, Actinobacillus pleuropneumoniae,* and *Salmonella choleraesuis,* may occur as a result of compromised pulmonary defenses caused by *Mycoplasma.* The disease is usually not apparent until pigs are 3 to 6 months old when a chronic, nonproductive cough induced by exercise develops. The primary economic significance of the disease is the decreased growth rate experienced by affected pigs. Characteristic lung lesions are a purple to gray consolidation of the anteroventral lung. Several feed and water additives, such as lincomycin, tylosin, tetracycline, and tiamulin, have been shown to reduce the severity of pneumonia and improve feed efficiency. All-in, all-out rearing throughout the growing and finishing period is probably the most important management technique for control of pneumonia. Vaccines are also available and may reduce lesions and improve weight gain.

> TECHNICIAN NOTE *M. hyopneumoniae,* the most common cause of chronic pneumonia in swine, results in significant economic losses as a result of a decreased growth rate in affected pigs.

Pleuropneumonia

A. pleuropneumoniae, the cause of pleuropneumonia in swine, most frequently causes clinical disease in pigs from 12 to 16 weeks of age. The disease is spread among pigs by direct contact and aerosol transmission. Pigs may become susceptible when passive immunity from the sow wears off, and a high level of exposure can cause serious and often fatal disease. Recovered swine become carriers and can expose other susceptible animals to the disease. The peracute form causes sudden death without clinical signs. The acute form results in fever of up to 107° F (41.7° C), labored breathing, coughing, and often death within 36 hours. Pigs with the chronic form may display intermittent coughing, reduced appetite, and decreased weight gains. Lung lesions include pulmonary hemorrhage, edema and/or necrosis, usually more severe in the caudal lung lobes, with a fibrinous pleuritis. Chronic cases may develop abscesslike nodules and fibrinous pleuritis with adhesions. Acute cases may be treated with parenteral ceftiofur or high doses (10 times label dose) of procaine penicillin G. Administration of commercially available vaccines to pigs after weaning (twice, 2 to 4 weeks apart) can reduce the severity of the disease. Antimicrobials added to the feed or water may be effective in prophylaxis.

Pasteurella Pneumonia

P. multocida is the most common bacterial isolate from pneumonic swine lungs. The organism is a common inhabitant of the upper respiratory tract of swine and is an opportunistic pathogen. Other infections that impair pulmonary defense mechanisms (mycoplasma, ascarid migration, influenza) render the lung susceptible to *P. multocida* infection. Clinically, affected pigs have dyspnea; pyrexia, up to 107° F (41.7° C); moist, productive cough; and anorexia. The organism causes a purulent bronchopneumonia with an anteroventral distribution. Severe cases may develop fibrinous pleuritis and pericarditis. Affected animals should be treated parenterally with antimicrobial agents based on sensitivity. Since pasteurellosis is almost always a secondary infection, prevention of primary problems is important. Vaccination with *P. multocida* bacterins may offer some protection.

MUSCULOSKELETAL SYSTEM

Porcine stress syndrome (PSS) is also known as malignant hyperthermia (MH) or pale soft exudative pork (PSE). Susceptibility to PSS is caused by a single autosomal recessive gene, and disease is manifest only in pigs that are homozygous recessive for this gene. This defective gene is closely associated with desirable characteristics, such as good feed conversion and high percent lean. The gene for PSS has been identified in almost every breed of swine, but is especially prevalent in the Pietrain breed. Stress, halothane, and other anesthetics may precipitate the development of PSS. The severity of clinical signs is related to the degree of stress, and signs include muscle and tail tremors, dyspnea, alternating blanched and reddened areas of skin, elevated body temperature (hyperthermia), cyanosis, muscle rigidity, and death. At slaughter or on postmortem examination, the musculature is pale, soft, and watery. Susceptibility to stress can be diagnosed with a DNA probe test, which will identify both homozygous and heterozygous carriers. Once clinical signs develop, the affected animal may be treated by removing the stress, applying external cooling, and administration of dantrolene sodium, if available. It is more important to prevent this condition by genetic selection of breeding stock that is not stress susceptible.

REPRODUCTIVE SYSTEM

Agents responsible for abortion and reproductive failure in swine include PSR, brucellosis, PRRS, porcine parvovirus (PPV), and leptospirosis.

PPV is present in nearly 100% of swine herds worldwide. If the virus infects a male or nonpregnant female, the pig seroconverts and eliminates the virus with no clinical signs. If a pregnant female becomes infected, the virus crosses the placenta and infects rapidly dividing fetal cells. If the pregnancy is less than 30 days, the embryo is killed and resorbed by the dam. Between 30 and 70 days of gestation, the fetus is killed and mummified, and after 70 days of gestation, the fetus mounts an immune response and survives to term, although it may be born weak or dead. The only clinical signs of PPV are those of reproductive problems in pregnant sows or gilts. Mummies of different sizes, stillbirths, and live pigs may be present in the same litter. Abortions are not typical of parvovirus infection in swine. Since the virus is ubiquitous, a single positive titer is not useful in confirming a diagnosis of reproductive failure caused by PPV. Prevention may be achieved by natural exposure of gilts to sows before breeding. Natural infection usually results in lifelong immunity. Vaccines are available, but immunity only lasts 4 to 6 months, so vaccination must be repeated before each breeding. Vaccination may interfere with development of natural immunity.

Leptospira pomona and *Bratislava* are the primary serovars that are adapted to swine, although other serovars may incidentally infect pigs. The bacteria are shed through the urine and reproductive discharges of infected animals and enter susceptible animals through mucous membranes or broken skin. Once infected, a bacteremia develops, and the organism localizes and multiples in the kidney and in pregnant females may cross the placenta and infect and kill the fetuses. Aborted, weak, and stillborn pigs may be the only obvious clinical signs. Diagnostic tests include a demonstration of high antibody titers in the dam (interpret in light of vaccination status) or in fetal fluids, culture of the organism, darkfield microscopy of urine or fetal fluids, fluorescent antibody of fresh tissue, and PCR techniques. Treatment may be accomplished with the use of tetracycline in the feed or administration of parenteral tetracycline. Many monovalent and multivalent vaccines are available for the protection of breeding stock; however, the immunity is short lived, so animals should be vaccinated every 6 months at breeding.

> TECHNICIAN NOTE Pathogens responsible for abortion and reproductive failure in swine include PRV, brucellosis, PRRS, PPV, and leptospirosis.

NERVOUS SYSTEM

Salt poisoning, also known as sodium ion toxicosis or water deprivation, occurs in commercial and pet swine from an overconsumption of excess sodium (direct salt poisoning) or inadequate water intake (indirect salt poisoning) or possibly both. Water deprivation causes a hyperosmolarity of the CNS so that when water is consumed, the osmotic pressure draws water into the CNS causing cerebral edema. Affected pigs show signs of restlessness, pruritus, constipation, and thirst followed by depression, blindness, convulsions, and death. Salt toxicity is a well-recognized entity in commercial swine, but descriptions of medical treatment of affected animals is limited because it is usually not economically feasible to treat individual commercial pigs. Successful treatment of pet pigs has been reported. Treatment consists of slow rehydration with fluids that will gradually return sodium to a normal level. In one report, successful treatment of two potbellied pigs with salt toxicity was achieved using half-strength lactated Ringer's solution in 2.5% dextrose.

BEHAVIOR

The pig's normal response to fear is vocalization and attempts to escape. They are naturally curious and spend a great deal of time exploring their environment. The prehensile organ of the pig is the snout, and in general, they have a keen sense of smell. Pigs have poor eyesight, so with poor eyesight and a reliance on smell, pigs are reluctant to venture into areas with unusual odors and changes in light intensity. Once familiar with their surroundings, they begin to investigate by rooting with their snout, which may lead to destructive behavior. Co-mingling pigs, such as occurs at weaning, results in the reestablishment of hierarchy in newly mixed pigs. This reordering usually occurs within 12 to 24 hours with the dominant pig establishing itself first, followed by number two, three, and so on. Some changes of rank may occur within the middle members, but the top and bottom of the order remain fairly stable. The dominance hierarchy of swine is referred to as bidirectional, a subordinate pig sometimes directing antagonistic behavior toward a higher ranking pig; however, this does not affect the social status between individuals. In established hierarchies, the dominant pig assumes a recumbent position, and its belly is nuzzled by subordinates, possibly an allogrooming ritual. The best group size for socialization is not known for sure, but the order seems to become more complex when a group size is more than 20.

Abnormal behavior is more likely to develop because of stressful living conditions. An abnormal behavior may either be a new behavior or a normal behavior that has become misdirected or exaggerated. Abnormal behavior can be a valuable indicator of environmental (physical, climatic, or social) or managerial deficiencies. Tail biting begins as misdirected investigative behavior (harmless nibbling) at weaning that can escalate to vicious biting, an expression of predatory aggression, and appetite for blood. Tail biting can cause an ascending infection of the spinal cord or spinal abscesses and even hind limb paralysis and death. Contributing factors include stress of weaning (often begins at weaning), climatic stress, overcrowding, or an imbalanced diet. The behavior can be controlled by providing diversions, such as toys (bowling balls, inner tubes), for pigs to play within the pens. Commercial pigs in confinement have their tails docked to prevent this problem; however, tail docking may then lead to ear biting if the underlying problem is not corrected. Also, removing the "biter" often controls the problem within a group.

Ear biting and flank biting are different expressions of the same problem(s) that result in tail biting. In addition to the aforementioned reasons, ear biting may be initiated by fighting for social rank. Flank biting may begin by flank sucking that is misdirected nursing behavior (more likely to occur when piglets are weaned younger than 20 days) that escalates to varying levels of destructive behavior to the victim.

Aggression in the extreme may be an abnormal behavior. Some aggression in pigs is normal. In a group situation, such as within a litter, a pecking order is established by fighting. This begins as early as birth when a teat order is established. Since more milk is produced in the cranial mammary glands, the stronger, more assertive piglets will fight to claim these teats. This is the reason for trimming needle teeth shortly after birth to prevent serious injury to the piglets and to the sow's udder. Once teat preference is established, that order remains until weaning. In older groups of pigs, if groups are mixed or a pig is added or removed, the pecking order must be reestablished, usually by fighting. Mature boars have well-developed tusks for slashing and will bite each other as a part of normal aggressive behavior. If strange boars are mixed, they will fight and may seriously injure each other. Boars raised together undergo a dominance procedure, but typically do not violently fight each other. Sows and weaned pigs will also fight, and even though they do not have tusks, they will bite. Sows and young pigs will also ram their heads against an opponent's head or torso. Baby pigs are often observed play fighting in preparation for normal pecking order establishment later in life.

Pigs normally keep their sleeping and feeding areas clean from an early age. Poor manure habits or pen fouling may be indicative of environmental or management problems, such as overcrowding, a high ambient temperature, or inappropriate airflow pattern (resting area should be draft free). Lameness and diarrhea may contribute to the problem.

A dam's aggression toward piglets (hysteria) or savaging of baby pigs is usually exhibited by gilts. These same gilts may be normal during subsequent farrowings. Possible causes of hysteria include stress resulting from the inability of the gilt to make a "nest," human interference during farrowing, and perhaps genetic predisposition. Management of the condition includes removal of pigs as they are born and reintroducing the entire litter once parturition is complete because the initiation of nursing often calms the gilt.

POTBELLIED PIGS

Nutrition and Husbandry

Without proper knowledge of the potbellied pig's husbandry and nutritional needs, health and behavior problems are inevitable. According to one report, approximately 50% of potbellied pigs are abandoned or rehomed before they are 1 year of age. This occurs because of unrealistic expectations of the owners and their unwillingness or inability to provide for the pig's environmental needs. The most common misconception held by pet pig owners is that their potbellied pig will only weigh 40 to 50 lb when fully grown. Although a few pigs remain small, most of them will weigh closer to 120 lb when mature, and they do not reach full size until they are 2 to 3 years old. Breed standards set by the North American Potbellied Pig Association describe a pig weighing no more than 95 lb and having a maximum height of 18 inches at the shoulder at 1 year of age. The most common nutritional disease of potbellied pigs is obesity; however, many stunted and malnourished pigs are also seen owing to their owner's misguided attempt to keep them small. A number of companies have developed diets specifically for miniature pigs. Miniature pigs should never be fed commercial swine feed; feed for miniature swine are lower in protein and fat and have a higher fiber content than commercial swine rations. Miniature pig feed is generally classified as starter, grower, breeder, or maintenance. Starter rations are intended for newly weaned pigs. The most appropriate ration for the average potbellied pig is the maintenance ration, which contains 12% protein, 2% fat, and 12% to 15% fiber. Most potbellied pigs are adopted by owners at 6 to 8 weeks of age and are spayed or neutered in the first few months. They begin to lead sedentary lifestyles early, so maintenance rations are probably the best choice for these pigs. If the pig is not spayed or neutered and/or it leads an active life, grower rations may be a better choice. Some commercially available potbellied pig feed has urinary acidifiers to help prevent cystitis, so if this seems to be a problem, this specialty ration may be considered. Recommendations concerning the amount to feed potbellied pigs varies; some references suggest 2% to 2.5% of body weight, others suggest 1 cup of feed per 50 to 80 lb. These are general guidelines, and owners must be advised to feed their pets according to body composition.

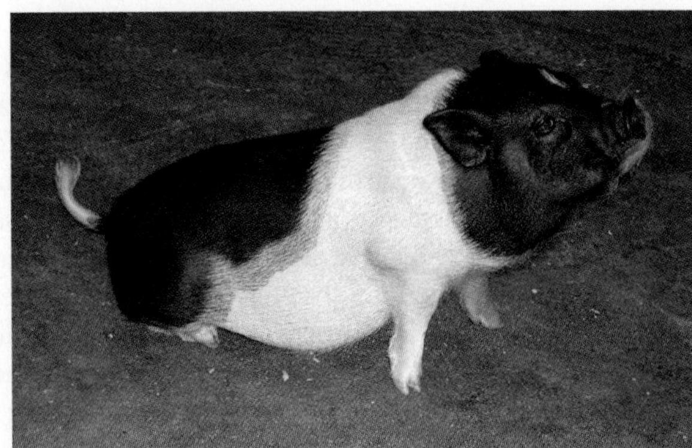

FIGURE 22-34 A healthy potbellied pig of appropriate size for its age.

Although the potbellied pig should have a rotund potbelly, they should never have turgid, fat-filled jowls or rolls of fat hanging over the hocks. They should have ribs that can be felt, but not seen (Figure 22-34). Appropriate treats for the pig include low-fat, low-salt (see salt poisoning under swine) snack food, such as popcorn (air popped without salt or butter), and small amounts of dried or fresh fruit. Requiring that the pig earn its treats is one way of continually reinforcing the pig's position as a subordinate member of the family. Obesity is likely to be the leading cause of health problems and decreased life span in pet pigs. Arthritis, heart disease, and kidney failure are just a few possible geriatric diseases that may be hastened by obesity. Sometimes entropion and corneal damage occur in morbidly obese pigs. Water intake in pigs is important for prevention of cystitis, urolithiasis, and salt poisoning. Pigs have a habit of alternating between eating and drinking and may make a mess at feeding time. Owners should be advised not to restrict water for this reason. Food and water should be provided in an easy-to-clean environment, such as a shower stall, or by placing the food and water in a large shallow pan to try to make cleanup easier. Pigs are also particular about the temperature of the drinking water, so the water should not be allowed to get too cold in the winter or too hot in the summer because this may restrict intake and cause problems. Pigs are foraging animals that normally spend much of the day either in search of food or at rest. When kept as a pet, pigs are fed two to three small meals a day and spend little time looking for food or eating. There are a variety of ways to extend mealtime, which increases the pig's exercise and makes them a more active participant in the acquisition of food. In good weather, the pig's ration may be broadcast over the grass in the yard. A rooting box can also be constructed out of wood or by using a plastic wading pool. The box is filled with large, smooth stones, and the food can be spread among the stones. This not only extends feeding time, but also allows the pig to fulfill its rooting needs in an acceptable place. Other useful techniques include the use of a Manna Ball or Buster cube, which allows the pig to slowly acquire its food while exercising at the same time.

> *TECHNICIAN NOTE* Obesity is the most common nutritional disease of potbellied pigs and is likely to be the leading cause of health problems and decreased life span in pet pigs.

COMMON DISEASES AND CONDITIONS OF CAMELIDS

In general, camelids are classified as either Old World or New World camelids. Old World camelids include dromedary, or one-humped camels, and Bactrian, or two-humped camels. The New World camelids, also called South American camelids (SACs), include the llama *(Lama glama)*, alpaca *(Lama pacos)*, guanaco *(Lama guanicoe)*, and vicuña *(Vicugna vicugna)*.

> *TECHNICIAN NOTE* The New World camelids, also called South American camelids (SACs), or camelids include the llama *(Lama glama)*, alpaca *(Lama pacos)*, guanaco *(Lama guanicoe)*, and vicuña *(Vicugna vicugna)*.

All SACs have 74 chromosomes and have therefore produced fertile hybrids. Camelids may live to be 15 to 20 years or more. The SACs became adapted to South American habitats and, in particular, the Andes; thus they became accustomed to dry climates and high altitudes. Camelids have a complex, three-compartment stomach with digestion similar to ruminants. Whereas llamas tend to browse, alpacas prefer to graze. Camelids regurgitate and rechew food as do ruminants, but they more efficiently extract protein and energy from poor-quality forage than do ruminants. SACs have pelleted feces and use communal dung piles (Figure 22-35). Their feces have been used for fuel and also as fertilizer. Llamas are typically used for meat, leather, fiber, and as pack animals, and alpacas are known for their superior fiber, but are also used as a source of meat and leather. Two breeds of alpacas, the huacaya and the suri, have gained popularity in the United States. The huacuya breed is the most common, and their fiber is crimped and shorter than that of the suri. The suri has a hair coat that consists of long fibers with no crimp that hangs from the body in ringlets.

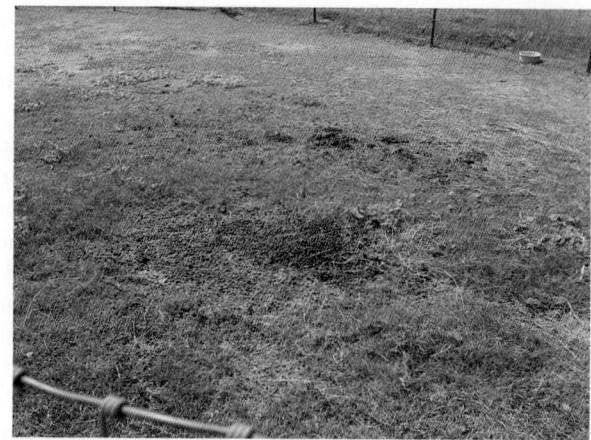

FIGURE 22-35 South American camelids have pelleted feces and use communal dung piles.

Llamas and alpacas are herd animals and therefore need to live with at least one other llama or alpaca. Gelded male llamas or adult female llamas can be used as guardians for sheep, goats, alpacas, cattle, or miniature horses.

> *TECHNICIAN NOTE* Llamas and alpacas are herd animals and therefore need to live with at least one other llama or alpaca. Gelded male llamas or adult female llamas can be used as guardians for sheep, goats, alpacas, cattle, or miniature horses.

CARE OF THE NEONATE AND NEONATAL DISEASES

Neonatal camelids are referred to as crias, and the newborn and its dam form a strong family bond (Figure 22-36). The newborn alpaca cria should weigh at least 12 lb at birth, and the normal llama cria should be greater than 15 lb; however, comparison with the average birth weight on any given farm may be of more significance. Crias are born with the eyelids open and the incisors erupted. The neonate is covered with an epidermal membrane that attaches at the mucocutaneous junctions, coronary bands, and the umbilicus. The camelid fetus is not surrounded by an amniotic membrane as occurs in other species, making the newborn much less likely to suffocate after birth. Camelid mothers do not lick the cria to dry it nor do they stimulate the baby to stand. The mother may nuzzle the cria and vocalize with a humming sound.

> *TECHNICIAN NOTE* The camelid fetus is not surrounded by an amniotic membrane as occurs in other species, making the newborn much less likely to suffocate after birth.

Following birth, crias should attempt to stand in 30 minutes and be successful by 60 minutes. Newborns should actively try to nurse the dam within the first hour and successfully nurse within 3 to 4 hours. If nursing has not occurred by 6 hours after birth, intervention is essential. Crias usually nurse three to four times per hour. During the first 3 days of life, the newborn may not gain any weight and may lose up to 1 lb; greater weight loss than this should be of concern. After the first few days, the cria should gain 0.5 lb per day for the first 2 weeks. Llama crias then continue to gain at the rate of 1 lb/day, and alpaca crias may gain 0.25 to 0.5 lb/day. The newborn should be alert and have clear eyes and erect ears. Typically, the body temperature is 101° F to 102° F; heart rate, 80 to 100 bpm; and respiratory rate, 10 to 30 breaths/min.

Camelids are obligate nasal breathers, so open-mouth breathing is considered abnormal and may be indicative of respiratory or congenital problems. As with other neonates, the newborn cria should be weighed, examined thoroughly, and the umbilicus dipped in disinfectant. Observation of nursing and assessment of passive transfer is also of great importance in neonatal care. It is not necessary to administer enemas to every neonate. Meconium should be passed within 18 to 24 hours after birth, and failure to do so, especially if the cria is straining, may warrant a gentle enema using 200 to 500 ml of warm water. Newborns should be carefully watched, especially during the first 48 hours of life. Crias that are considered "at risk" include premature crias, crias born to mothers with dystocia, newborns with congenital defects, crias that suffer excessive umbilical bleeding, crias born to the same mating that experienced problems in previous years, and crias that develop FPT. "At-risk" crias often show abnormalities in vital signs, labored respirations, weakness, depression, failure to nurse, failure to stand, and straining with failure to pass meconium.

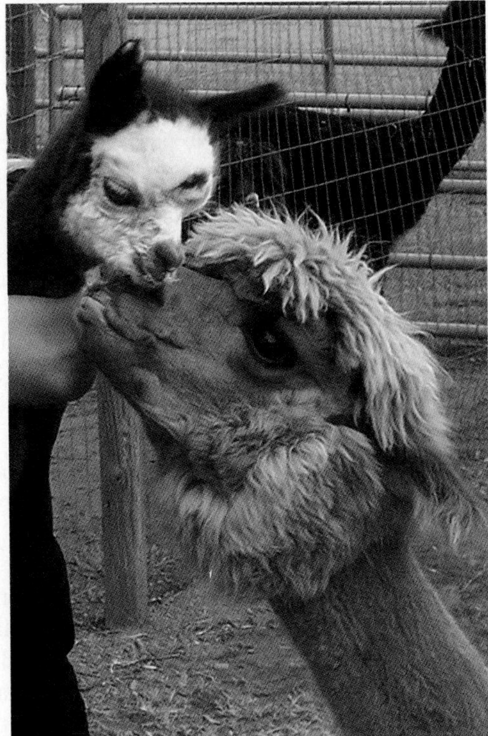

FIGURE 22-36 The neonatal camelid is referred to as a cria. The dam and cria form strong family bonds. (Courtesy of Ms. Vida Palmer.)

> *TECHNICIAN NOTE* Camelids are obligate nasal breathers, so open-mouth breathing is considered abnormal and may be indicative of respiratory or congenital problems.

There is considerable variation in gestation in alpacas and llamas (330 to 360 days), with some pregnancies lasting more than 1 year. This variation makes it difficult to determine prematurity based on length of gestation. In addition, in pasture breeding situations, undetected early embryonic death may be followed by another breeding several days later. Prematurity is not based entirely on gestational length. Signs of prematurity in the newborn are of more importance than time in utero. Low birth weight may be the most obvious sign, but premature crias also show signs, such as weakness and inability to stand or hold the head up to nurse. Affected crias also have excessive laxity of tendons and ligaments and may walk on their fetlocks. In addition, premature crias often have nonerect or curled ears as a result of immature cartilage in the ears (Figure 22-37), the hair coat is especially silky, and the rubbery covering of the toe persists for 1 to 2 days in premature babies (disappears in 6 to 12 hours in full-term crias). The incisors are not erupted in premature crias (Figure 22-38), and the mucous membranes are dark red from decreased oxygenation as a result of undeveloped lungs. Prematurity is life threatening and requires immediate and intensive therapy.

> *TECHNICIAN NOTE* There is considerable variation in gestation in alpacas and llamas (330 to 360 days), with some pregnancies lasting more than 1 year thus making it difficult to determine prematurity based on length of gestation.

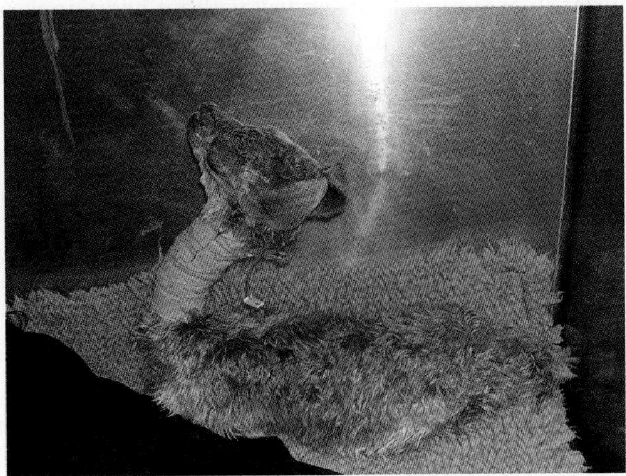

FIGURE 22-37 Premature crias often have nonerect or curled ears as a result of immature cartilage in the ears.

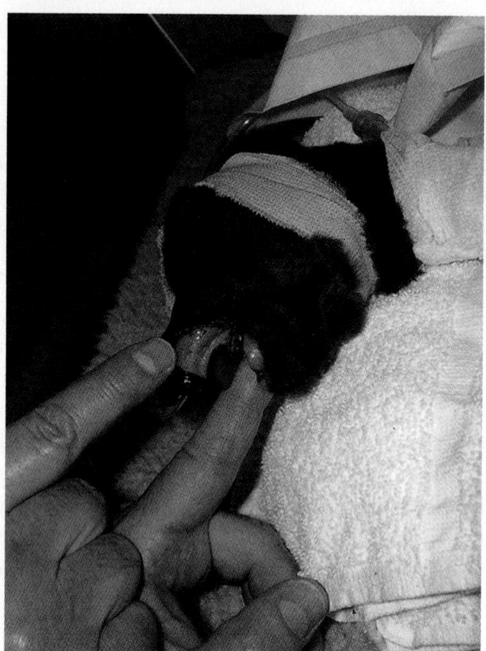

FIGURE 22-38 The incisors (bottom only) are not erupted in premature crias, and the mucous membranes appear dark red in color.

Once the condition of prematurity has been established, the cria should be provided supplemental heat and oxygen. Most premature crias are incapable of nursing the dam, so it is suggested that a warm plasma transfusion using camelid plasma (Triple J Farms, Redmond, Wash.) be administered. Following plasma transfusion, fluids, such as Normasol with 5% to 10% dextrose, can be given to meet any existing fluid deficits and prevent hypoglycemia. Premature crias are susceptible to infection, so administration of broad-spectrum antibiotics is usually initiated. In addition, thiamine and cimetidine are often given to promote neurologic development and prevent C3 ulcers, respectively. If the cria is strong enough to nurse, it should be fed milk at the rate of 10% to 12% of its body weight divided into four feedings a day. If the cria is incapable of nursing, tube feeding may be necessary via an orogastric tube (a stallion urinary catheter works well). Intensive care is continued until the cria matures appropriately or is capable of survival without additional support. Daily weights are helpful in assessing the health of the neonate and ensuring adequate oral nutrient intake.

> *TECHNICIAN NOTE* Most premature crias are incapable of nursing the dam, so it is suggested that a warm plasma transfusion using camelid plasma be administered.

Monitoring mucous membrane color, respiratory rate, and blood gases helps determine the point at which the cria can be weaned from oxygen supplementation. Other signs of maturation, such as eruption of the incisors and straightening of the ears, are important to assess. Any angular limb deformities may be addressed by application of light support splints; often these deformities improve as the neonate matures. The cria should be housed in close association or contact with the dam.

To prevent FPT, the newborn should be observed closely for the first 3 to 4 hours to make sure it nurses. It is desirable to get colostrum from the dam into the cria; however, if that is not possible, cow, goat, or sheep colostrum can be substituted. The cria should receive 20% of its body weight in colostrum in four to six feedings during the first 24 hours after birth. The use of commercial colostrum supplements or replacers should be avoided. It may be beneficial to feed colostrum to premature or sick crias for 3 to 4 days after birth. In the event the cria will not nurse, orogastric intubation should be performed to make certain that the cria receives adequate colostral immunity. Radial immunodiffusion is one of the most accurate tests used to check for passive transfer, but it is only useful if the cria received llama or alpaca colostrum, not cow, goat, or sheep colostrum. Sodium sulfite turbidity and total serum protein can be useful to access passive transfer status. These tests are most beneficial in crias that are from 24 hours to 7 days of age. If colostrum is not available, an IV plasma transfusion is strongly recommended. "At-risk" crias should be watched closely for any signs of septicemia for the first several months of life.

Orphaned crias may be bottle fed goat's milk, lamb milk replacer, kid milk replacer, or whole cow's milk. The cria should receive milk at 10% to 12% of its body weight per day. Initially, this amount can be divided into four to six feedings per day, but feedings can gradually be reduced to two to four feedings per day. Weighing the bottle-fed cria to document adequate weight gain is important. It is extremely important that orphans receive minimal human contact and are left with the herd at times other than feeding to prevent the development of "bezerk llama syndrome."

> *TECHNICIAN NOTE* It is extremely important that orphan crias receive minimal human contact and are left with the herd at times other than feeding to prevent the development of "bezerk llama syndrome."

Crias that do not nurse may need total parenteral nutrition (TPN). The recipe described for use in the foal (Smith) seems to work well for crias, and the TPN can be reduced incrementally as the cria begins to nurse on its own.

Congenital abnormalities are relatively common among camelids. This high prevalence is blamed on the narrow genetic pool available to breeders before importation of native South American camelids during the 1980s. Even with greater genetic diversity, congenital defects continue to plague breeders. Some common congenital defects include choanal atresia, atresia ani, wry face (maxillofacial dysgenesis), patent urachus, and cleft palate. Choanal atresia is the presence of a membranous or osseous separation of the nasal and pharyngeal cavities. Since camelids are obligate nasal breathers, the primary clinical sign in affected newborns is open-mouth breathing. Since this condition is probably hereditary and the prognosis for life is poor, euthanasia is recommended.

Diarrhea is an important cause of morbidity in neonatal camelids. Many factors may be involved in the cause of neonatal diarrhea, including management and nutritional factors and a variety of pathogens. The most common pathogens causing diarrhea in neonates are coronavirus, *E. coli*, *Cryptosporidium* spp., *Giardia* spp., and coccidia. If diarrhea in the young is not treated effectively, it may lead to the development of chronic diarrhea, which may ultimately result in chronic renal failure.

> TECHNICIAN NOTE Diarrhea is an important cause of morbidity in neonatal camelids and if not treated effectively, it may lead to the development of chronic diarrhea, which may ultimately result in chronic renal failure.

Coccidiosis is most frequently diagnosed in neonates and juveniles since adults are more resistant to infection as a result of their mature immune systems and prior exposure. Coccidiosis is typically associated with conditions of overcrowding and poor hygiene. The oocysts cause direct damage to the small intestinal epithelium resulting in diarrhea, enteritis, and sometimes straining. Chronic coccidiosis may cause nutrient malabsorption and subsequent poor growth in affected individuals. Sulfadimethoxine (Albon, Pfizer) dosed at 15 mg/kg orally twice daily for 5 days is an effective treatment for coccidiosis. Amprolium may also be used at the rate of 10 mg/kg orally once daily for 5 days. The correct dosing of amprolium is crucial because overdosing may produce clinical signs of polioencephalomalacia caused by thiamine deficiency. Ionophore antibiotics, such as monensin and salinomycin, which are commonly used to treat coccidiosis in cattle, are toxic to camelids and should therefore not be used in these species.

Diarrhea caused by *E. coli* often occurs in combination with neonatal septicemia secondary to FPT. Neonates are affected between 3 to 7 days of age and often exhibit profuse, watery diarrhea, lethargy, dehydration, and abdominal distention. Leukopenia with a degenerative left shift neutrophilia is often present in these crias. The treatment should include a good broad-spectrum antibiotic with gram-negative coverage along with fluid therapy. Sick camelids are often hypernatremic, so low-sodium IV fluids, such as 0.45% sodium chloride with 2.5% dextrose, are indicated.

Cryptosporidiosis *(Cryptosporidium parvum)* is a zoonotic disease that can cause severe and sometimes fatal diarrhea in neonates and immunocompromised individuals. The infection occurs by the fecal-oral route and may occur when contaminated feed or water are ingested. The diagnosis of cryptosporidiosis is accomplished by the examination of fecal smears using modified acid-fast stains. There is no specific treatment for cryptosporidiosis, so supportive therapy using IV fluids and/or TPN are important, especially since the disease results in malabsorption and maldigestion.

Giardiasis, also a zoonotic disease, primarily stems from contaminated water sources. The organism, which affects the small intestine causing villous atrophy, results in a malabsorptive diarrhea with dehydration and weight loss. Oral fenbendazole dosed at 50 mg/kg once daily for 5 days is an effective treatment for *Giardia*.

Salmonella spp. do not appear to be common causes of diarrhea in camelids.

Both rotavirus and coronavirus have been identified as causing diarrhea in neonatal camelids; however, of the two viruses, coronavirus appears to occur more commonly. Electron microscopy and fecal ELISA tests are the most useful for diagnosis of these viruses. There is no specific treatment for viral diarrhea, so supportive therapy, such as IV fluids, is useful. Monoclonal antibody vaccines, such as those available for oral use in calves and lambs, can be safely given to camelids on farms experiencing outbreaks of viral diarrhea, although the efficacy in these species is unknown.

Nematodes are capable of causing diarrhea in crias as young as 2 months of age because of the inherent lack of acquired resistance. Clinical signs include ill thrift, inappetence, anorexia, emaciation, and diarrhea. Fecal parasitology is useful in the diagnosis, and a 5-day course of oral fenbendazole at 20 mg/kg is usually effective.

Diarrhea in crias less than 7 days of age is likely due to nutritional factors in bottle-fed babies or gram-negative infections, especially in cases of inadequate colostrum ingestion. Viral diarrhea usually affects crias older than 7 days and is most often due to a coronavirus infection in the United States. *Cryptosporidium* and *Giardia* also tend to affect crias older than 7 days of age, and these infections are often due to overcrowding or sanitation problems on larger farms. Coccidiosis is unlikely to occur in crias less than 3 weeks of age, and it may be indicative of a herd problem. Diarrhea caused by GI parasites in crias less than 2 months of age is rare. It should be kept in mind that diarrhea may be multifactorial and can involve more than one pathogen. There are numerous diagnostic tests available to help determine the cause of neonatal diarrhea so that the clinician can initiate an appropriate treatment for affected individuals and control the spread of disease through the rest of the group.

> TECHNICIAN NOTE Diarrhea may be multifactorial and can involve more than one pathogen. Numerous diagnostic tests are available to help determine the cause of neonatal diarrhea so that the clinician can initiate an appropriate treatment for affected individuals and control the spread of disease through the rest of the herd.

RESTRAINT AND HANDLING OF CAMELIDS

Effective restraint requires knowledge of camelid behavior. Llamas and alpacas have been domesticated for thousands of years, and if they are accustomed to handling, they are docile and pleasant. Only rarely is an individual aggressive or a "spitter." Camelid ear and tail position expresses important information. The ears of a content, unaroused animal are in a vertical position and turned slightly forward. In an alarmed animal, the ears are pointed forward. Varying degrees of aggressiveness are manifest by ears that are positioned from barely behind the vertical to flattened on the neck. The tail position also reflects the emotional state of the animal. In an unaroused camelid, the tail lies flat against the perineum. With alarm, the tail position rises to horizontal or as much as 45 degrees above horizontal. Aggressive behavior is displayed by the tail in a completely vertical position. An accurate reading of body language is important to prevent injury to the handler and the animal.

Llamas and alpacas are usually calm, but the most common behavioral response to annoyance is spitting of regurgitated stomach contents. Once a spitter is restrained, the head can be turned away from handlers to redirect ingesta, or a towel or rag that covers the mouth can be tucked into the nosepiece of a halter to discourage continued spitting. A muzzle that hooks onto the halter can also be used to prevent spitting. Camelids may kick and generally "cowkick," although they can also kick directly backward. Biting is usually restricted to fighting between intact males, although llamas have been known to occasionally bite humans. Mature males have two upper and one lower canine teeth ("fighting teeth") on each side of the mouth that are sharp. These teeth occasionally need to be blunted or cut short for the safety of other animals and human handlers.

Dam-raised male camelids are usually no more difficult to handle than females (in contrast with bulls, stallions, bucks, and rams); however, bottle-fed orphan males or neonates that receive too much human contact may imprint on humans creating a dangerous behavioral problem. An imprinted male treats a human as if it is another male and can therefore become quite aggressive, especially when the male reaches puberty. A number of persons have been seriously injured as a result of this behavioral problem.

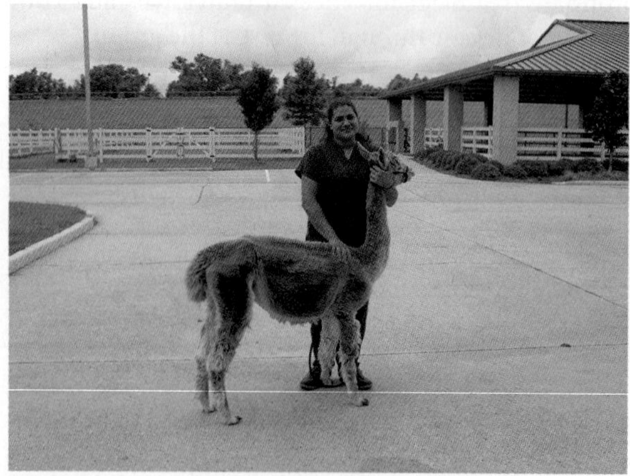

FIGURE 22-39 Restraint of the adult camelid is best accomplished by holding the head and neck close to the handler's chest while the other hand rests on the animal's shoulders with slight pressure.

> *TECHNICIAN NOTE* Llamas and alpacas are usually calm, but the most common behavioral response to annoyance is spitting of regurgitated stomach contents.

It is always desirable to use the least amount of restraint necessary to perform a procedure. Many alpacas have been halter broken and can be restrained with the use of the halter. Untrained individuals are best controlled by pulling the head and neck close to the handler's chest with one hand while the other hand rests on the top of the shoulders with slight pressure (Figure 22-39). As an alternative, the tail may be grasped and held upright by the second hand. Crias less than 20 kg (45 lb) may be lifted with one arm around the chest and the other arm supporting the abdomen in front of the rear legs, which has a calming influence on the cria and reduces struggling (Figure 22-40). Camelids can also be restrained in the kushed (sternal recumbency) position (Figure 22-41).

PHYSICAL EXAMINATION AND DIAGNOSTIC SAMPLING

The habitus of the animal should be evaluated before a complete physical examination. BCS should be completed (as described later under the hepatic lipidosis section) to access the overall nutritional state of the animal. The physical examination is similar to other ruminant species already described in this text. The normal temperature, heart rate, and respiratory rate for adult camelids are 99° F to 102.5° F, 60 to 90 bpm, and 10 to 30 breaths/min, respectively. The major fermentative process of camelid digestion takes place in compartment one (C-1) of the stomach. Since GI sounds are due to gas and liquid agitation, usually sounds are heard

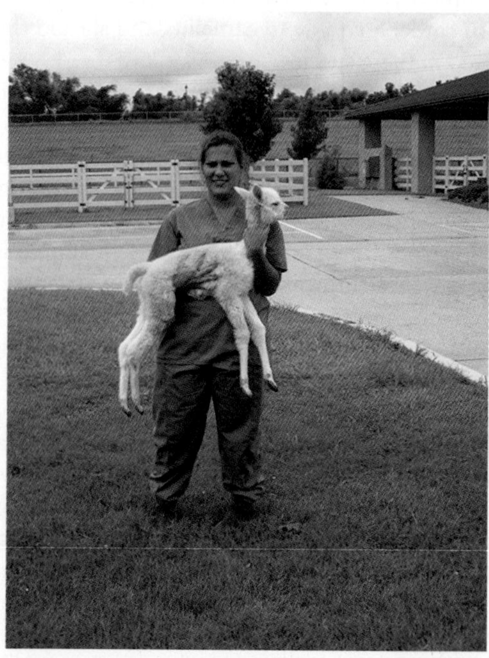

FIGURE 22-40 Crias may be held with one arm around the chest and the other arm supporting the abdomen in front of the rear legs.

only on the left side. Palpation of gastric motility is not possible as in the ruminant, so a stethoscope is necessary to hear the subdued sounds. The normal gastric motility rate is three to four sounds per minute. A fleece-free abdominal area is located just cranial to the thigh muscles of the hind limb. To expose the area for auscultation, it is necessary to reach under the fleece in what would be the flank area in other species and lift it up.

Blood analysis is often necessary for diagnosis of many different diseases in camelids. Venipuncture and blood collection is not as simple in camelids as in most other domestic species. Camelids have evolved protective mechanisms to prevent exsanguination from bite wounds inflicted when intact males fight. In all areas of the neck, one must be extremely careful not to accidentally cannulate the carotid artery when performing venipuncture. Two primary sites for jugular venipuncture are low on the neck near the thoracic inlet or high near the ramus of the mandible (Figure 22-42). There is no jugular furrow in camelids, and the skin of the neck is quite thick, especially in the high neck location. It is neither necessary nor desirable to clip fiber for collecting a blood sample. It may take 1 year to 18 months for the fiber to regrow, and owners are usually dissatisfied with clipping of the animal. The anatomy and location of the jugular vein in the two locations listed above should be reviewed before attempting venipuncture in camelids.

Gastric intubation is accomplished via the oral cavity. The nasal cavity is narrow and precludes passage of anything but a small tube. A speculum made from a piece of rubber garden hose slightly larger than the stomach tube or a polyvinyl chloride pipe padded with adhesive tape makes an excellent guide. Once the tip of the tube is in the oropharynx, it can be rotated to encourage the camelid to swallow. If properly located in the esophagus, the tube can be palpated as it traverses the left ventral cervical region. The tube may then be advanced into C-1; however, if the fluid or medication is intended to bypass C-1, the tube should be left in the esophagus. This is particularly important when force feeding neonates because milk deposited into C-1 may remain there and ferment rather than be digested normally in C-3.

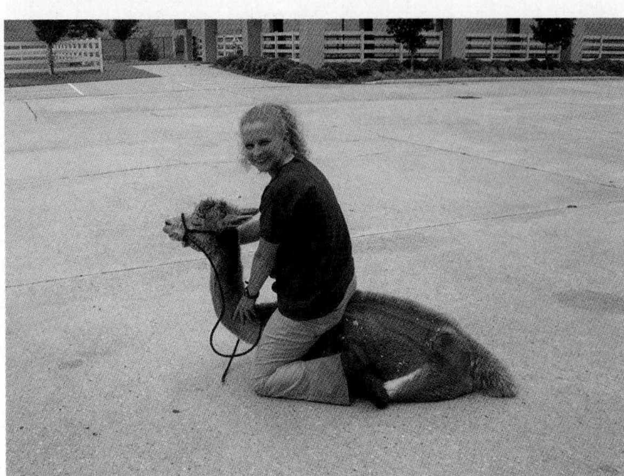

FIGURE 22-41 Adult camelids can also be safely restrained in sternal recumbency or the kushed position.

> *TECHNICIAN NOTE* Venipuncture and blood collection is not as simple in camelids as in most other domestic species since camelids have evolved protective mechanisms to prevent exsanguination from bite wounds inflicted when intact males fight.

HEALTH MAINTENANCE

Camelids are routinely vaccinated for *C. perfringens* C and D and tetanus. Vaccination for these diseases may be started as early as 2 to 3 days of age and repeated at 2 to 3 weeks of age. A booster vaccination is then suggested at 6 and 12 months of age. From that point, annual vaccination is recommended. Other vaccines that can be used in camelids include rabies, equine rhinovirus, equine influenza, equine herpesvirus, West Nile virus, leptospirosis, and *E. coli,* depending on the herd location and potential threat of these diseases within a given herd.

Camelids may acquire a great variety of internal and external parasites, some of which are common to sheep, goats, cattle, and horses. Parasite control programs are most effective if customized to the individual farm since recommendations from other farms or other areas of the country are of little use. Parasite control strategies should be developed through a local veterinarian with the aid of fecal parasite egg counts. The sugar flotation method is recommended for fecal egg counting because this method is more precise than traditional flotation methods. Fecal egg counts should be performed periodically and include all animals if there are fewer than 10 animals on the farm or 10% of the herd if there are more than 10 animals in the herd. Fecal egg counts performed approximately 2 weeks after deworming medication

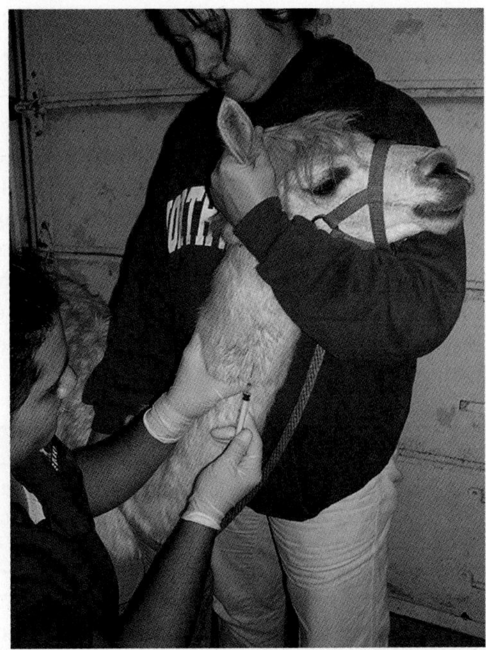

FIGURE 22-42 Jugular venipuncture may be achieved high on the neck near the ramus of the mandible.

has been administered are useful to evaluate the efficacy of the dewormer used and may aid in an evaluation of the development of anthelmintic resistance.

All camelids have canine teeth ("fighting teeth") that are particularly well developed in the intact male. There are two maxillary canine teeth on each side and one mandibular tooth on each side. It is a common practice in North America to blunt these teeth in some manner to prevent serious lacerations of the ears, throat, limbs, and scrotum when males fight. The teeth can be shortened using Gigli wire or a rotary tool.

Foot trimming is a routine part of health maintenance in camelids. The camelid foot is unique with two digits on each foot. The plantar surface is covered with a soft, cornified layer of epithelium similar to the heel bulb in small ruminants. This structure is called the slipper. A small, non–weight-bearing nail is located at the extremity of each digit and is closely attached to P3 via the corium or sensitive lamina. The nail may require periodic trimming.

> TECHNICIAN NOTE Parasite control strategies should be developed through a local veterinarian with the aid of fecal parasite egg counts.

NERVOUS SYSTEM

Meningeal Worm (Parelaphostrongylus tenuis)

One parasite that is of great importance to llama and alpaca producers is the meningeal worm, *Parelaphostrongylus tenuis*. The llama and alpaca and other animals, such as wild cervids and domestic small ruminants, are aberrant hosts of this parasite, whereas the white-tailed deer is the normal host. This parasite does not cause clinical disease in white-tailed deer, but in camelids, it causes high morbidity and mortality. The *P. tenuis* larvae migrate through the spinal cord of aberrant hosts causing neurologic deficits. Clinical signs appear around 45 to 53 days after infection. Most commonly, clinical signs reflect asymmetrical, focal spinal cord lesions, including hypermetria, ataxia, stiffness, muscular weakness, posterior paresis, paralysis, head tilt, arching neck, circling, blindness, gradual weight loss, apparent depression, seizures, and death. Clinical signs generally begin in the hind limbs and progress to the front limbs. The course of disease may be acute to chronic, ranging from death within days to ataxia that lasts months to years.

> TECHNICIAN NOTE *P. tenuis* larvae migrate through the spinal cord of aberrant hosts, such as the llama and alpaca, causing neurologic deficits that may be acute or chronic in nature.

Although consistent clinical signs and CSF eosinophilia are highly suggestive of a meningeal worm infection, the antemortem diagnosis of aberrant *P. tenuis* migration is often a diagnosis based on exclusion and response to therapy. The definitive diagnosis of a meningeal worm infection is made at necropsy. A confirmed diagnosis requires microscopic demonstration of the larvae within the brain or spinal cord.

A treatment regimen that has proven successful at Ohio State University involves fenbendazole (20 to 50 mg/kg body weight, PO, q 24 hours for 5 days) and flunixin meglumine (1 mg/kg, IV, IM, or SC, q 12 hours for 5 days) or dexamethasone in nonpregnant females and males (0.1 mg/kg, IV, IM, or SC, q 24 hours for 3 days). DMSO (1g/kg given in 500 ml of 5% dextrose solution, IV, q 24 hours) given to effect is useful in some cases, but may cause severe appetite suppression. DMSO should be discontinued if inappetence or anorexia occurs. Vitamin E, selenium, Vitamin B-complex, and Vitamin A are useful to assist healing of neural tissues.

Dexamethasone should not be administered to pregnant females because this drug may induce abortion. Alternatively, prednisolone sodium succinate (0.5 to 1.0 mg/kg, IV, IM, or SC, q 12 hours) has been used, but for no more than 3 days in pregnant females without subsequent abortion. Ivermectin is most effective against larval stages before the entrance into the spinal cord since it does not readily cross the blood-brain barrier; however, damage to nervous system tissues during larval migration may alter the permeability of the blood-brain barrier. The antiinflammatory drugs are critical to reduce the inflammation associated with the presence of the migrating larvae and the subsequent inflammatory response to the killed larvae. Use of antiinflammatory drugs is important to prevent the clinical signs from becoming more severe after instituting treatment.

In addition to drug therapy, supportive care and physical therapy are essential to aiding recovery. Using slings to support llamas that are unable to stand and performing physical therapy for muscles are beneficial (Figure 22-43). Hydroflotation therapy to facilitate recovery after prolonged recumbency may also help. A great deal of perseverance is required to care for severely affected camelids because recovery may take several weeks to months to years.

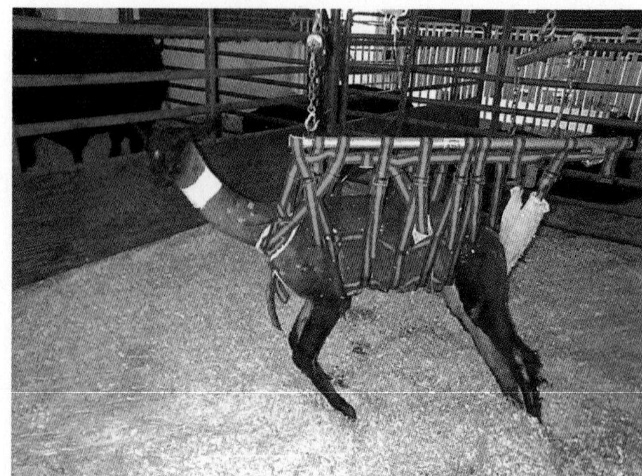

FIGURE 22-43 Camelids that are unable to stand may benefit from the use of slings and physical therapy. (Courtesy of Dr. Christine Navarre.)

The prognosis for survival depends upon how severe the clinical signs become. Clinical experience suggests that camelids that are unable to stand have a poor prognosis (10% to 20% recovery); those that are able to stand unaided have a fair to good prognosis (75% to 85% recovery). Animals that survive clinical disease do not seem to develop patent infections and are unlikely to pose a health risk to other animals. Many animals suffer permanent neurologic deficits. but may remain productive members of the herd for breeding and pets.

The prevention of a meningeal worm infection may be difficult. Ideally, llamas and alpacas should not graze the same pasture as white-tailed deer; however, in many areas of the United States, it may not be feasible to separate the two species. Placing a deerproof fence may offer some protection to prevent movement of deer. Additionally, thick ground cover can be removed to expose the environment to fluctuations in temperature, and vegetation-free buffer zones (i.e., gravel, limestone) can be placed around fence lines to reduce migration of snails and slugs into the pasture. Molluscicides may be considered to destroy snails and slugs that serve as intermediate hosts, thereby interrupting the life cycle of the meningeal worm and preventing infection in aberrant hosts. Drainage should be established in low-lying areas, and access to swampy areas may be restricted by fencing. These compounds present a potential environmental risk from contamination of ground water and may be toxic if consumed by camelids or other animals. The prophylactic treatment against migrating larvae may be achieved by administration of ivermectin (0.2 mg/kg) every 30 to 45 days during the high-risk periods or throughout the year in regions that have mild summers and winters. Anthelmintic resistance is unlikely to become a problem in the meningeal worm because these infections do not become patent. However, meningeal worm infection has occurred in some herds that maintain vigilant prophylaxis. These "breaks" in the prevention of larval migration may have been caused by insufficient dosing of anthelmintic, accidental failure to administer the anthelmintic, or some unknown mechanism.

> *TECHNICIAN NOTE* The prognosis for survival of the meningeal worm depends upon how severe the clinical signs become; camelids that are unable to stand have a poor prognosis, whereas those that are able to stand unaided have a fair to good prognosis for recovery.

METABOLIC CONDITIONS

Hepatic Lipidosis

When excessive fat accumulates in liver cells, the disease process is termed hepatic lipidosis, fatty infiltration, or fatty liver disease. This syndrome has been well defined in cats, cows, sheep, goats, ponies, and humans. Although there are differences in conditions that initiate hepatic lipidosis between these species, usually a period of inadequate energy intake (i.e., negative energy balance [NEB]) initiates body fat mobilization. Unfortunately, in camelids, the disease outcome is nearly always fatal if not recognized early and treated aggressively.

Although hepatic lipidosis in llamas and alpacas has not been frequently reported in the veterinary literature, it has commonly been recognized in cases of camelid illness and death. Veterinary diagnostic laboratories report some degree of fatty liver infiltration in the majority of llamas and alpacas submitted for necropsy; however, it may not always be clear whether hepatic lipidosis was the primary lesion causing the death of the animal or secondary to some other disease process.

One study at Oregon State University revealed a mostly middle-aged, pregnant, or lactating female population to be affected. In contrast to hepatic lipidosis in other species, males ranging from 5 months to 18 years accounted for 22.6% of the cases. The most common factor documented in histories from these affected camelids was a recent significant loss of appetite or severe weight loss varying from a couple of days to several weeks. Affected animals had a variety of BCSs (thin to obese). In some cases, there were other medical problems or changes in social or environmental conditions, such as uncharacteristically hot weather or movement of animals in or out of certain pastures or pens, evident around the time the condition developed. Some llamas were reported to be clinically normal less than 24 hours before they were found ill or dead. Most affected animals had elevations in enzymes that indicate liver disease. These are not, however, specific for hepatic lipidosis and may be increased with any cause of liver disease. A definitive diagnosis of hepatic lipidosis is only accomplished by microscopic or analytic measurement of fat content of liver biopsy specimens.

Since deficient energy intake is a hallmark factor in initiating hepatic lipidosis, therapy must be focused on increasing energy intake immediately. Offering a variety of browse and fresh grass clippings has been beneficial to stimulating feed intake. Blackberry leaves are particularly appealing to camelids. Injections of B-vitamins can be beneficial for appetite stimulation. If more aggressive oral supplementation is required, a liquid gruel can be administered via tube, if feasible. Soaking alfalfa pellets in hot water and mixing in calf electrolytes, calcium propionate, propylene glycol, and other ingredients can provide energy sources and fermentable material. Camelids are obligate nasal breathers, so indwelling nasogastric tubes are not practical. Rumen transfaunation can be used to repopulate the microbial fauna and restimulate fermentation. Collected rumen fluid from cattle, sheep, or goats can be used in llamas or alpacas.

In more severe cases, intensive supportive care and dietary management, including TPN, may be used. Since camelids may have insulin resistance, administration of an appropriate dose of insulin in conjunction with glucose therapy is warranted; never administer insulin without concurrent glucose therapy because this may result in hypoglycemia. The prognosis is always guarded in the more severe cases of hepatic lipidosis, even with aggressive nutritional support. All sick camelids should be considered at risk for developing hepatic lipidosis, especially those with anorexia or metabolic demands of pregnancy and lactation. Close monitoring of feed intake in sick animals is absolutely essential to prevent deaths.

> TECHNICIAN NOTE Deficient energy intake is a hallmark factor in initiating hepatic lipidosis, therefore therapy must be focused on increasing energy intake immediately.

The prevention of hepatic lipidosis is based on ensuring adequate energy and protein intake, especially in pregnant and lactating females, by feeding good-quality forage and appropriate supplementation. Forage testing is the only true way to know the quality of forage that is fed. Most cases of hepatic lipidosis are associated with the feeding of mature grass forage (less than 9% crude protein). The addition of some alfalfa or clover forage to grass forage will improve the quality of the diet. Grain supplements with some protein will be required to support lactation, though the amount and composition required will vary by production level and forage quality. Lactating dams have the highest nutrient requirements and should be fed the best-quality forage and potentially supplemented with a grain product containing energy and protein sources.

Given the strong association between significant weight loss and hepatic lipidosis, one can use routine (monthly or bimonthly) body weight determinations to assess potential risk. Body weight loss exceeding 15% over a short (1 to 2 weeks) period of time is a high-risk factor for this disease. Pregnant animals should gain approximately 10% to 15% of their body weight over the last 3 months of pregnancy to account for fetal growth. Lactating animals will be expected to lose body weight in support of lactation. This weight loss will vary by individuals and the amount of milk produced. A typical weight loss should be less than 10% of body weight following birthing. Excessive weight loss in early lactation is an indicator of inadequate dietary amounts or quality and can predispose to hepatic lipidosis problems. By far, the single best and simplest method of evaluating your nutritional program is body condition scoring. Body condition scoring is a method that subjectively grades animals by the amount of subcutaneous fat stores into defined "fatness" categories. A five-point system covering physical states of emaciated (1), thin (2), average (3), fat (4), and obese (5) has been developed. The ideal body condition is 3.0, having a moderate amount of body fat. Although some individuals will maintain a lower or higher BCS and remain healthy, this is just inherent individual differences in metabolism. BCSs 2.0 and below or 4.0 and above are considered abnormal and represent extremely thin or fat animals, respectively. Most animals other than those in late pregnancy or lactation should maintain a BCS between 2.5 and 3.25. Late-pregnant animals should have a slightly higher body condition (3.25 to 3.5) to have reserves to support impending lactation. Lactating animals will lose body condition rapidly as they produce milk. Lactating animals should not lose more than 0.5 to 0.75 condition scores. Important times to assess a BCS would be during early to mid pregnancy, early to mid lactation, and periodically (four to six times per year) for other animals of the herd to assess energy status.

> TECHNICIAN NOTE The best and easiest method of evaluating a camelid nutritional program is by body condition scoring using a five-point system defining the physical states of emaciated (1), thin (2), average (3), fat (4), and obese (5).

Heat Stress

Heat stress is a common occurrence for llamas and alpacas during the summer season. Since these animals originate from the Andes Mountains of South America, where high heat and humidity are not as common as in many areas of the United States, llamas and alpacas are not adapted to handle these conditions. It is critical to manage them in a way to protect them from heat stress because it can lead to illness and even death of the animal.

It is important to know when llamas and alpacas are most in danger for heat stress. Commonly used is the heat index, which is simply a formula to estimate the risk of heat stress. The heat index can be estimated by adding the temperature (F) and percent humidity (%). Typically a heat index of less than 120 is safe, 120 to 180 creates possible problems, and greater than 180 is the range where animals are in the most danger. During the warmer months of the year, there are many ways to keep animals cool. Shade is an easy way to keep them from getting too hot. The shade provided by trees is a great place for camelids to relax and stay cool during the heat of the day. If there are no trees available, artificial shade, such as tents, barns, and shelters, can be provided, keeping in mind that ventilation in these structures is important. Fans are an excellent way to keep the air moving and keep the animals cool. Tunnel ventilation barns are the most desirable because the "tunnel effect" maximizes cooling of the air. Fans placed in series (e.g., all facing the same direction) can create this effect and cool the barn. If available, having an air-conditioned room or area of the barn can help keep animals cool or be used as a place to move animals that begin to show signs of heat stress. Giving llamas and alpacas plenty of fresh water also helps prevent heat stress. There should be multiple sources of cool, clean water so that all the animals have a place to drink.

> TECHNICIAN NOTE The heat index can be used to determine when llamas and alpacas are at the most risk for developing heat stress, and the heat index can be estimated by adding the temperature (F) and percent humidity (%).

Shearing is one of the most important ways to help llamas and alpacas keep cool. Since the fibers work to trap the heat close to the animal's body, shearing helps the animal to lose

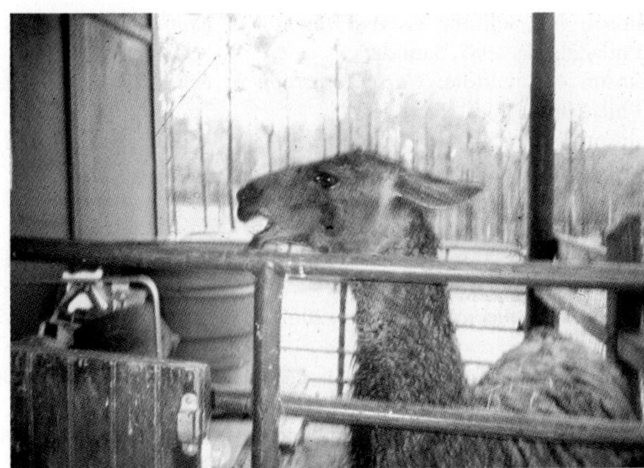

FIGURE 22-44 Monitoring of camelids during the hot summer months for signs of heat stress, such as open-mouth breathing is important. (Courtesy of Dr. David Pugh.)

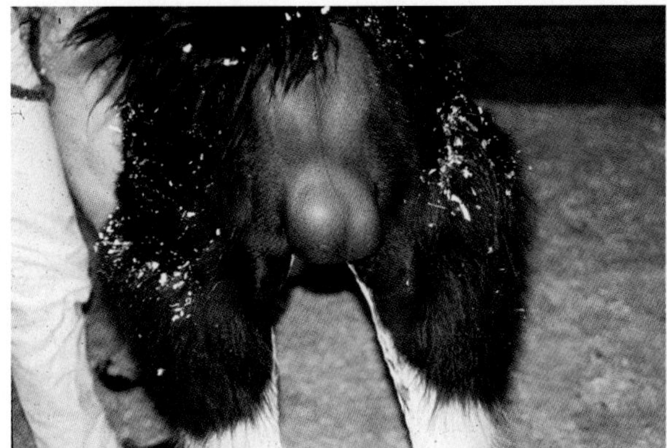

FIGURE 22-45 Another sign of heat stress in camelids is scrotal swelling in intact males. (Courtesy of Dr. David Pugh.)

heat through evaporation more effectively. If possible, shearing from head to toe (leaving about 1 to 3 inches of fiber on the body) is most effective, but barrel cuts (e.g., abdomen and thorax only) will also help. Differences are observed among the various camelids (e.g., llama, suri alpaca, huacuya alpaca, guanaco, vicuña) with respect to tolerance of hot and cold.

Proper management and husbandry can help prevent heat stress. For example, if the animals need to be worked or handled for any reason, it should be done early in the morning in the coolest part of the day. Breeding to have crias born in the spring is important since gestation and parturition can cause stress for the female and during the warmer months can cause considerable heat stress. Crias born in the warmer months are often born weak and can become dehydrated soon after birth. Weaning should also take place during the cooler months because it is a stressful time for both the cria and its mother.

The body condition of the animal also plays an important role in heat stress. Obese animals are more prone to the effects of the heat, so proper management of weight is a good way to help these animals cool themselves. On the other hand, emaciated animals also have increased susceptibility to extremes of environment. Proper nutrition of the animals is also important. In particular, providing adequate selenium,

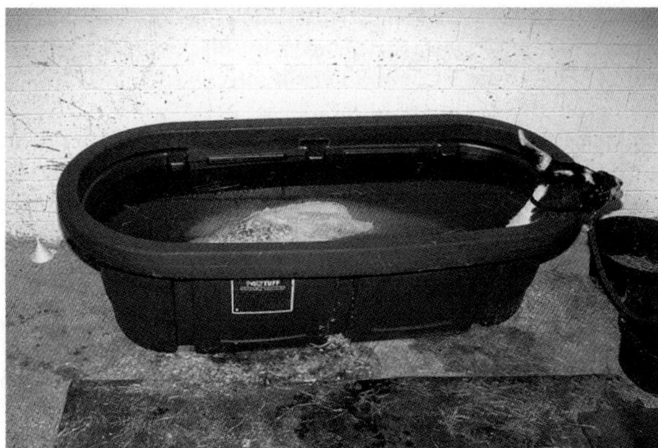

FIGURE 22-46 Animals that are recumbent as a result of heat stress may benefit from the use of water flotation tanks. (Courtesy of Dr. Christine Navarre.)

vitamin E, copper, zinc, and B vitamins, such as thiamine, can increase tolerance of environmental extremes. Monitoring the animals is important during the summer months so that any signs of heat stress can be caught early. Signs to watch for are nasal flaring, open-mouth breathing (Figure 22-44), tachypnea, dyspnea, drooling, depression or dullness, not eating feed, scrotal swelling in intact males (Figure 22-45), weakness, trembling, a rectal temperature greater than 104° F, a heart rate more than 90 bpm, or a respiratory rate more than 40 breaths/min. Taking temperatures often is a good way to learn what the normal temperatures of the animals are in the morning and afternoon so that abnormal temperatures are more easily recognized. Treatment of llamas and alpacas with heat stress should first be to cool the animal down using water or alcohol. Additional cooling with the use of a fan or air conditioner may be useful. If the animal has not been shorn, this may considered in the treatment regimen, but only if it does not cause further stress. Other therapies include cool IV fluids with electrolytes, steroids or NSAIDs, and good nursing care including lifting the animal periodically if it is unable to stand. Water flotation tanks are especially useful for this purpose (Figure 22-46). The most important aspect of heat stress is prevention.

> *TECHNICIAN NOTE* Shearing camelids before the onset of hot weather and careful monitoring of the animals during the summer months are important for the prevention of heat stress.

RECOMMENDED READING

Anderson DE, Rings DM: *Current veterinary therapy—food animal practice*, ed 5, St Louis, 2009, Saunders.

Cooper VL: Diagnosis of neonatal pig diarrhea, *Vet Clin North Am: Food Anim Pract* 16:117-133, 2000.

Cowart RP: *An outline of swine diseases,* ed 2, Ames, Iowa, 2001, Iowa State University, Blackwell Science.

Divers TJ, Peek SE: *Rebhun's diseases of dairy cattle,* ed 2, St Louis, 2008, Saunders.

Evans CN: *Alpaca field manual*, ed 2, Manhattan, Kan, 2005, Able Publishing and Ag Press.

Fowler ME: *Medicine and surgery of South American camelids,* ed 2, Ames, Iowa, 1998, Iowa State University, Blackwell Science.

Fubini SL, Ducharme NC: *Farm animal surgery,* ed 1, St Louis, 2004, Saunders.

Greenough PR: *Bovine laminitis and lameness—a hands on approach,* ed 1, Oxford, 2007, Saunders.

Hanie EA: *Large animal clinical procedures for veterinary technicians,* St Louis, 2006, Mosby.

Howard JL, Smith RA: *Current veterinary therapy—food animal practice,* ed 4, St Louis, 1999, Saunders.

Koterba AM, Drummond WH, Kosch PC, editors: *Equine clinical neonatology,* Philadelphia, 1990, Lea & Febiger.

Orsini JA, Divers TJ: *Manual of equine emergencies,* ed 3, St Louis, 2009, Saunders.

Pugh DG: *Sheep and goat medicine,* St Louis, 2002, Saunders.

Radostits OM, Gay CC, Hinchcliff KW et al: *Veterinary medicine,* ed 10, New York, 2007, Saunders.

Rebhun WC: *Diseases of dairy cattle,* Philadelphia, 1995, Lippincott Williams & Wilkins.

Reed S, Bailey W, Sellon D, editors: *Equine internal medicine,* ed 2, St Louis, 2003, Saunders.

Robinson NE, editors: *Current therapy in equine medicine,* ed 2, Philadelphia, 1987, Saunders.

Robinson NE, editors: *Current therapy in equine medicine,* ed 3, Philadelphia, 1991, Saunders.

Robinson NE, editors: *Current therapy in equine medicine,* ed 4, St Louis, 1997, Saunders.

Robinson NE, editors: *Current therapy in equine medicine,* ed 5, St Louis, 2003, Saunders.

Robinson NE, editors: *Current therapy in equine medicine,* ed 6, St Louis, 2009, Saunders.

Scott PR: *Sheep medicine,* London, 2007, Manson Publishing/The Veterinary Press.

Smith BP, editors: *Large animal internal medicine,* ed 4, St Louis, 2009, Mosby.

Tynes VV: Potbellied pig husbandry and nutrition, *Vet Clin North Am: Exotic Anim Pract* 2:193-207, 1999.

Tynes VV: Preventive health care for pet potbellied pigs, *Vet Clin North Am: Exotic Anim Pract* 2:495-510, 1999.

Wills RW: Diarrhea in growing-finishing swine, *Vet Clin North Am: Food Anim Pract* 16:135-161, 2000.

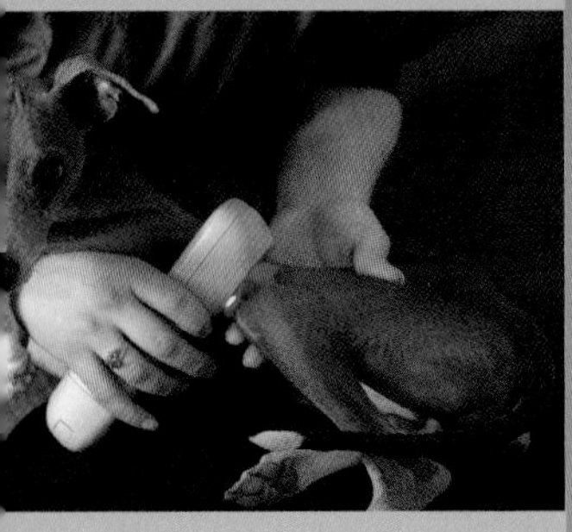

Nursing Concepts in Alternative Medicine

23

Laurie McCauley and Christine Jurek

KEY TERMS

Acupuncture
Applied kinesiology
Aroma therapy
Ayurvedic medicine
Chiropractic therapy
Glandular therapy
Holistic
Homeopathy
Myotherapy
Nutraceutical
Traditional Chinese medicine (TCM)

OUTLINE

LEARNING OBJECTIVES

When you have completed this chapter, you will be able to:

1. Describe considerations in the development of home-prepared diets for dogs and cats.
2. List the commonly used nutraceuticals and describe their therapeutic uses.
3. List the commonly used Western herbs and describe their therapeutic uses.
4. List the common ingredients found in Chinese herbal and ayurvedic herbal formulas.
5. Describe the principles of aromatherapy and list common aromatherapy oils and their uses.
6. Describe the basic principles of homeopathy and list forms of homeopathic preparations and considerations for storage and administration.
7. Describe the principles of flower essence therapy and list common flower essences and their uses.
8. Define applied kinesiology and list the techniques used for a patient's assessment and treatment.
9. List the theories that describe the principles of acupuncture and describe the role of the veterinary technician in acupuncture therapy.
10. List and describe the physical modalities used in alternative and complementary medicine.

INTRODUCTION

Complementary and alternative therapy can be an exciting and rewarding part of veterinary medicine. Whether you work at a completely nonconventional practice or a surgical referral center, you will have clients who seek a more natural approach to their pet's care than standard veterinary medicine provides. Quite often clients feel more comfortable speaking with a technician about less mainstream ideas than they do with a veterinarian.

The purpose of this chapter is to give you a basic knowledge and understanding of the most common complementary and alternative medicine modalities used in veterinary practice today. It is not meant to be a comprehensive explanation of each modality, nor is it intended as a "how to" guide. In addition to nutrition, the following modalities will be discussed: herbal medicine; homeopathy, homotoxicology, and flower essences; applied kinesiology (AK); acupuncture and TCM; and physical modalities, including chiropractic, massage, rehabilitation, and miscellaneous therapies. Case reports will illustrate the principles and practice of various therapies. For those interested in more information about alternative medicine, we have included a list of recommended reading and resources at the end of the chapter.

The term "holistic" refers to a "whole animal" approach to health care. It focuses on wellness as an ongoing, dynamic process with great variability in the state of health. On one end of the spectrum is perfect health, and on the other end is disease. Most patients fall somewhere in between. Holistic medicine seeks to bring the patient to an ever greater state of general health and well-being rather than the conventional approach of simply treating disease.

An animal in perfect health has bright eyes, a shiny coat, is muscular and fit, energetic, and robust. This animal is not only in balance internally, but it is also able to adapt to its environment in a much greater capacity. It is able to rebalance and heal easily after it receives an external insult, such as exposure to an infectious agent or trauma. Anything less than perfect health leaves room for improvement. The technician has a tremendous opportunity to contribute to holistic health care of the veterinary patient, both as an assistant and as a therapist under the supervision or direction of the veterinarian.

ALTERNATIVE CONCEPTS IN NUTRITION

One of the most commonly asked questions in veterinary practice is "what should I feed my pet?" Quite often, the technician is the staff member responsible for educating clients about nutrition. This is an important way that you can influence the health of your patients and become an outstanding part of the veterinary health care team. Basic nutrition is essential knowledge for every technician in every practice, with no exceptions. Even in a surgical referral practice, counseling clients on proper nutrition to optimize surgical recovery is an important aspect of providing the best and most complete health care. This section is meant to expand upon basic knowledge of animal nutrition and introduce some novel concepts in companion animal nutrition.

Nutrition becomes an even more commonly discussed issue in holistic practice because it is the foundation of achieving a state of ideal health. Many clients who seek alternative care for their pets are already educated about nutrition, sometimes even more than the staff. On the downside, misinformation and hype abounds, especially in the Internet age. It can be difficult to convince a client that a vegetarian diet is inappropriate for cats when the lady at the health food store swore it cured her Fluffy's cancer. It is therefore becoming an important issue in any practice because these clients need sound nutritional advice from an "expert" who is confident and well informed. Whether or not you or your veterinarians advocate a holistic approach to nutrition, it is imperative that you understand it and can justify your recommendations to these well-informed but sometimes misinformed clients.

A good holistic diet is based on using whole, natural ingredients in a balanced ration. For small animals, the most wholesome healthy diet is a *balanced,* home-prepared diet. In the case of herbivores, the best diet is pasture provided on a soil with balanced minerals, supplemented with hay and grain only when necessary. The term balanced is an important one because an improperly prepared or unbalanced diet can cause disease or at least be a hindrance to attaining ideal health. Balance can be achieved with each meal, as it is with commercial pet food, or it may be achieved on a daily to weekly basis, as our own diets do.

TECHNICIAN NOTE Not every client is willing or able to provide a balanced, home-prepared diet for his or her pet. There are many excellent nutritious and wholesome commercially prepared pet food that are easily accessible to the client.

It is also important to note that a healthy water source, such as spring water, is as significant to the patient's overall health. Water can be a source of healthy vitamins and minerals, or it can contain harmful toxins and additives. A good rule of thumb is if you would not drink your tap water, neither should your pet.

Some recommendations may simply be unattainable for our large animal patients, but we can do our best to optimize the resources that are available, such as proper pasture management and using sources of good-quality hay and grain, along with supplementation to balance the mineral and vitamin component of the diet. Soil testing and hay analysis for nutrient content is reasonably accessible and should be used regularly as food sources change.

We will now discuss home-prepared diets in a little more depth. Meat used in the home-prepared diet for carnivores may be raw or cooked, depending on the owner's preference and the pet's constitution. Raw diets are quite an area of controversy, and there is a great deal of information available on this topic. The theory behind raw diets is that a wild carnivore (feline or canine) catches prey and eats it; no cooking involved. Raw meat does contain more enzymes and is truly more "what nature intended." It is more highly digestible and contains more unspoiled nutrients than the cooked version (think about our vegetables). Although this is certainly undeniable, most people are unable to provide a fresh catch for their domestic cat or dog. Our raw meat is processed and packaged. This brings about the problem of bacterial contamination, which the carnivore is generally (but not always) well equipped to handle because of the more acidic pH of the stomach and intestines. The risk increases with ground meat, which has a higher surface area exposed to bacteria. Bacterial contamination is actually much more of a concern to the humans in the household who will be handling the food. Care must be taken to educate clients about the health risks posed to them and their families, especially when there are young, elderly, or immunocompromised members of the household. Basically the same procedures and precautions must be taken when handling raw meat that will be cooked: immediately clean and disinfect any surface that the raw food touches, including your hands.

Where raw bones are concerned, it is true that they do not splinter or break teeth as cooked bones do, but they are not without their dangers.

> TECHNICIAN NOTE Many dogs, when introduced to raw bones, are too enthusiastic about their new diet and consume large pieces, which can cause gastrointestinal (GI) obstruction. This is not as common an occurrence in cats, but it is not inconceivable. Bones must be introduced carefully, and if the pet is overzealous, the bones may be ground or a calcium powder must be substituted. This is not as ideal for dental health, but safety is more important.

On the subject of vegetables, these should be cooked (lightly steamed) and chopped or minced or grated because carnivores are less able to break down plant cell walls to obtain the nutritious substances inside. Generally, in the wild, the most substantial plant source is what is contained in the herbivorous prey's GI tract. This has already gone through part of the digestive process, and the nutrients are thus available for use by the carnivorous predator. There are now a variety of excellent, well-balanced commercially prepared raw diets. These come in both frozen and freeze-dried form and are becoming more readily available to pet owners. Some are even designed to be single-serving packages to minimize the need for directly handling the food. The bottom line on raw diets is that they can be a wonderful way to enhance an animal's health if properly prepared and balanced, but they are not indicated for every pet, nor are raw diets the cure for every disease or disorder.

Holistic-oriented commercial diets are also becoming more readily available. Many companies producing dry and canned food are including holistic product lines, and many smaller companies are focused solely on providing holistic diets for pets.

> TECHNICIAN NOTE It is important to realize that just because a company labels a diet "holistic" or "natural" does not mean that it is so. Careful research is important before deciding if a diet meets your standards. This includes not only inspection of the guaranteed analysis and ingredient list, but also information on the source of ingredients.

A recent contamination of grain imported from China resulted in numerous pet deaths, and many of the affected diets had an excellent mix of ingredients. Some of the recalled foods were considered to be high-quality, holistic diets. At this point, it may be best to steer clients to diets that obtain all ingredients from the United States, Canada, and New Zealand (which produces the majority of lamb for our pet food).

One newer trend in the pet food industry is the limited grain or grain-free diet. This mimics the nutrient profile of a raw diet without the concern for contamination. In addition, many of these diets are dry, which makes the convenience quite appealing. Some other dry diets are baked rather than extruded, providing a more natural nutrient profile with better digestibility.

Supplementation of the diet with probiotics and digestive enzymes may also be beneficial, particularly for those pets and breeds (such as the German Shepherd) that tend to have sensitive digestive systems. Addition of plain yogurt is a simple way to help balance the GI tract, but many commercially prepared products are also available.

Each patient must be assessed to find the best diet for him or her that is also feasible for the caretaker. An acceptable alternative to home-prepared meals may involve choosing several (three to four) commercial diets and rotating them to provide an overall balance in nutrients. For example, one diet may give an animal less than an ideal (although meeting *minimum* requirements) amount of a certain micronutrient. By rotating diets, this will likely balance out in the long run because another diet may have more of that nutrient (Case Presentation 23-1).

> TECHNICIAN NOTE Remember that holistic medicine is about treating each patient as an individual. With that in mind, there is no "best" diet for every animal. Each patient must be assessed to find the best diet for him or her that is also feasible for the caretaker.

NUTRACEUTICALS

The use of nutraceuticals is quickly becoming more mainstream in both human and veterinary medicine. The term refers to nutritional supplements that are not herbs and not approved for use as drugs, but are thought to convey therapeutic benefit to the patient. There are many types of nutraceuticals. They are *used to treat many conditions* and assist in maintaining the general health and well-being of the

CASE PRESENTATION 23-1 FELINE GASTROINTESTINAL DISEASE

Signalment: "Ivy," a 1-year-old spayed female domestic medium hair cat, 5½ lb

Chief Complaint: Soft stool and diarrhea of 6 weeks duration

Pertinent History: Ivy was rescued from an animal shelter 6 weeks before presentation and had always had soft stool. She had been vaccinated and dewormed three times while at the shelter. When she was spayed, she was found to have two mummified kittens in utero with a pyometra. She recovered nicely after surgery, but her stool became worse. The diarrhea was soft-serve consistency, foul-smelling, and voluminous. Fortunately, normal frequency without straining was evident, and she consistently used her litter box. A fecal examination was negative for parasites. Her diet initially consisted of dry and canned premium brand cat food. Although she ate voraciously in a large quantity for her size (½ cup dry plus 2 tbs canned b.i.d.), she had not gained weight since she had been rescued. A prescription diet (canned and dry, then canned only) for GI sensitivity had been tried for 3 days, but no improvement was noted, and Ivy began vomiting (partially digested food). Ivy had not been adopted to a permanent home because of her ongoing GI issues.

Significant Examination Findings: Ivy was quite thin (body condition score 3/10), and her hair coat was unthrifty (dull and brittle). Her intestines were palpably thickened. No further abnormalities were found.

Problem List:	Differential Diagnosis:
Chronic small intestinal diarrhea (localized based on volume, frequency)	Parasites, small intestinal bacterial overgrowth (SIBO), inflammatory bowel disease, food allergy, foreign body, infection, exocrine pancreatic insufficiency (EPI), neoplasia
Thickened intestinal walls	Parasites, inflammatory bowel disease, infection, neoplasia
Vomiting	Parasites, small intestinal bacterial overgrowth (SIBO), inflammatory bowel disease, food allergy, foreign body, infection, EPI, neoplasia
Thin body condition	Secondary to GI disease

Client Communication: Ivy's initial presentation made a definitive diagnosis difficult. A thorough work-up would be pursued, and a diet change and treatment would be initiated while results were pending. A fasting blood sample was drawn for a CBC and chemistry panel, with additional serum saved for further testing if indicated.

Initial Treatment Plan: Ivy was started on GI Encaps (*Thorne Research Inc.*—contains plantain, slippery elm, marshmallow, licorice), ½ capsule daily to soothe her GI tract, and Prozyme Plus (Prozyme products—contains rice starch, lipase, amylase, protease, cellulase, and lactase), ⅛ tsp added to each meal. Her diet was transitioned to a limited ingredient canned food with duck protein source over a period of 3 days.

Initial Diagnostic Plan and Results (in Order):

Fecal parasite examination: negative

CBC, comprehensive chemistry profile: within normal limits except borderline low albumin

Fecal culture: negative

Giardia titer: negative

TLI (Trypsinlike Immunoreactivity, a test for EPI): within normal limits

Cobolamin and folate levels: slightly low cobalamin, folate levels normal (diagnostic for SIBO)

Abdominal radiographs: within normal limits except for thickening in the walls of the small intestine

Working Diagnosis: SIBO of unknown cause

Progress and Revised Treatment Plan: Ivy responded favorably to her initial therapy (she stopped vomiting), but her stool remained soft, and she did not gain weight. Rather than pursue an immediate exploratory surgery with biopsies, we elected to transition Ivy to a raw diet. She was adopted to a home (mine) where her special dietary needs could be met consistently. Ivy was initially fed 2 tbs of raw chicken breast three times daily and monitored for adverse reactions (vomiting, worsening diarrhea). She was enthusiastic about her new diet and tolerated it well. Her stool started to become firmer after 3 days. At that point, chicken wings were introduced to try to transition her to whole food. This also was well tolerated. Since we would keep Ivy on a limited ingredient diet for several weeks, she was started on Thorne Feline Basic Nutrients Multivitamins (1 capsule daily), which she ate readily. GI Encaps were discontinued, but she remained on Prozyme Plus.

Two weeks later, Ivy had normal stool and had gained 1 lb. She regained a healthy weight within 2 more weeks and was transitioned to a more balanced diet including a small amount of pureed vegetables. After several months, an "accidental" trial of commercial dry cat food resulted in no adverse effects, and she currently maintains a healthy to generous weight on a dry food and raw chicken diet (fed at separate meals). Her diarrhea never recurred, and she has no health problems to date (6 years later).

Discussion: Ivy's GI issues likely were caused by a combination of a significant diet change (she was found as a stray on the streets of Milwaukee) and chronic infection (pyometra). Her work-up, like so many small animals with diarrhea, ruled out some problems, but never resulted in a definitive diagnosis. Although exploratory surgery with an intestinal biopsy would likely have yielded more information and possibly a definitive pathologic and histologic diagnosis, the cause would still likely be unknown. Traditional practice and therapy would have possibly included antibiotic therapy, metronidazole, or steroids and a limited or single-ingredient diet (food trial). Fortunately a simple diet change with a single, highly digestible protein was enough to help Ivy's body rebalance her GI tract and heal. Interestingly, cats, unlike dogs, are obligate carnivores, meaning they must have meat in their diet and can lead a healthy life without grains or even vegetables as long as vitamins and minerals are properly supplemented.

Whereas cooked, nonprocessed meat may have been a reasonable alternative, raw meat is more digestible. A part

CASE PRESENTATION 23-1 FELINE GASTROINTESTINAL DISEASE—cont'd

of my motivation to try a raw versus cooked diet with this cat was that my staff was quite skeptical about it at the time, and since she was kept at our clinic throughout this entire period, they were aware of the remarkable improvement in her health in a short amount of time after more conventional approaches had lead to more problems (vomiting). The most significant change and the one most indicative of a "cure" was that Ivy is now able to eat just about anything (including stolen strawberries and asparagus) and thrives on a diet now full of variety, including the dry food that she originally ate.

The technician's contribution to Ivy's care was significant and mainly conventional, including nursing care, blood collection and management, performing a fecal parasite examination, and taking radiographs. If Ivy had been adopted by a client, nutritional counseling and follow-up communication would have also been appropriate responsibilities. This is an excellent illustration of how holistic practice blends conventional and alternative care to help restore a patient's health.

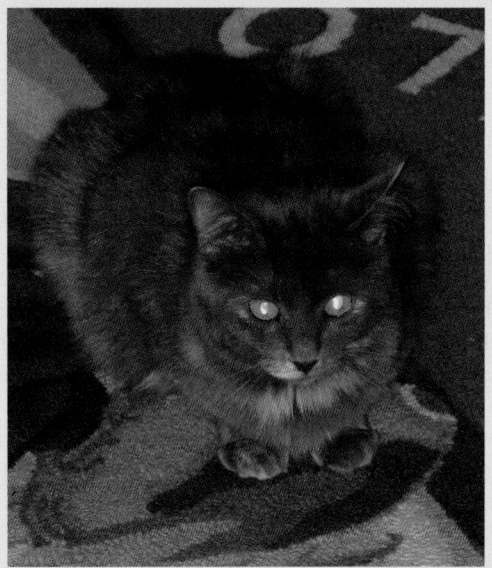

FIGURE 1 Ivy is now the picture of perfect health.

patient. The following is a brief list of the more commonly used nutraceuticals (Table 23-1).

GLANDULARS, CELL THERAPY, AND GLANDULAR-LIKE PRODUCTS

As the name implies, this type of supplement uses animal products to supply nutrients (steroids, enzymes, and raw materials of some organs, such as liver) to the patient. The theory behind use of glandulars is that by providing sources of whole tissue to a subject with a dysfunctional or suboptimally functioning organ or gland, the patient will receive the necessary substances to improve function and in some cases heal his or her own diseased tissue. A good example of this is to provide a product containing bovine thyroid gland for a patient with a low thyroid level.

Like any food ingredient, it is important to have a reputable source for these products because they are made from animal products. There are a handful of companies in the United States that use human grade ingredients in their products and have rigorously standardized and tested their products. These companies often provide guidelines for dosing and administration to animals. One company is now making products specifically for dogs and cats, using a powdered form that is quite palatable. This type of therapy is also sometimes a moral and ethical dilemma for holistic practitioners because of animal use, but the more reputable companies try to be as ethical and humane as possible in their formulations.

The technician should be familiar with the glandular-type and nutraceutical products used within the practice. He or she should be aware of the many types of diets that are appropriate and inappropriate for patients and should be able to explain the veterinarian's recommendations.

TABLE 23-1 Commonly Used Nutraceuticals

Nutrient	Primary Target Area(s)	Function
Glucosamine chondroitin, perna mussel, hyaluronate, cetyl myristoleate	Joints	Promote joint lubrication Reduce progression of or prevent arthritis Reduce pain and improve mobility
Shark and bovine cartilage	Joints	Reduce pain and improve mobility
	Cancer	Anticancer function (shark cartilage is significantly more potent)
MSM	Muscle	Supports muscle function and metabolism
SAM-E	Liver	Antioxidant
Coenzyme Q10	Heart, gingiva	Antioxidant: reduces free radical damage
Taurine	Heart, eye	Amino acids—used when deficiency occurs
L-Carnitine	Heart	Antioxidants/free radical scavengers
Superoxide dismutase		
Vitamin E/selenium		
Vitamin C		
Vitamin A		
Essential fatty acids (EPA, G)	Skin	Inhibit inflammation

HERBAL MEDICINE

Herbal or botanical medicine refers to the practice of using plant materials (including flowers, stems, leaves, bark, seeds, roots) to treat patients. Herbal medicine is the most ancient known medicine and the foundation of modern medicine. Using plants as medicine predated written communication, and evidence of the use of plants is widespread in ancient cultures. It is still a large practice in the world today, with an estimated 80% of the world's population using this form of therapy as a primary means of health care. Even today, about 20% of our drugs are derived from a plant source. The technician should become familiar with the herbal pharmacy, just as he or she knows about the drugs on the shelf.

Information about the medicinal use of herbs can be found in the *Materia Medica,* which is similar to a drug formulary.

> *TECHNICIAN NOTE* Herbs tend to be less toxic than drugs because the therapeutic substances are not as concentrated. Plants also contain other substances that can act synergistically with the active compound. Herbs are not, however, to be used carelessly. There are many herbs that are extremely safe at many times the therapeutic dose, but others, like some drugs, have a low margin of safety.

Many have not been proven safe in pregnancy, and some are toxic to cats. This is important to remember because many clients equate herbs with complete safety and need to be educated on their proper use and side effects, just as they should with any medication prescribed.

In the United States, herbs are regulated as a food. The FDA requires a rigorous testing procedure to approve a substance as a drug, at a cost to the manufacturer of more than $230 million. Because a natural substance cannot be patented, no pharmaceutical company would fund the research required for approval. Currently, we rely mainly on testing based in Europe and Asia to substantiate the effects of herbal therapy. Unfortunately, this does nothing to assure us of the quality or purity of the products because of the lack of FDA regulation. The herbal practitioner therefore must be cautious about the source of the prescribed herbs. This is another issue that must be emphasized to clients, who often do not understand the difference between the medication purchased at the practice versus the bottle they buy at the local supercenter.

If practicing with a veterinarian who uses therapeutic herbs, the technician should be familiar with commonly used preparations, just as he or she has knowledge of the commonly used drugs in the pharmacy. The technician may also be asked to assist in preparing and dispensing herbal products and explaining the proper use to the client.

WESTERN HERBS

Western herbal medicine is becoming a common practice in veterinary medicine. With the holistic movement in human medicine, most people are now familiar with products, such as echinacea, ginseng, and St. John's wort. Proper dosing and administration for animals have not been scientifically proven, but doses for the more commonly used herbs have been fairly well established.

The herbs come in many different forms (Figure 23-1), and each has advantages and disadvantages when used in animal species. Bulk herbs are the most commonly used preparation for herbivores. The product is often dried and prepared (chopped or powdered). Some of the tastier herbs are also administered to carnivores in this form. Capsules and tablets are often used for carnivores because they are more easily disguised. Teas are prepared by straining the herbs into water. They are fairly easy to prepare, but not always readily accepted by animals (depending on the patient and the herb). Extracts are made by concentrating the herb in alcohol or glycerin. A standardized extract is much like a drug, where a specific amount of active ingredient is measured rather than a measurement of the herb itself. Milk thistle, for example, is often sold as a standardized extract containing 70% silymarin. Poultices and compresses are used topically for short periods. These are made by soaking the herb or extract in hot water, then allowing it to cool. The product is then held in place manually or with gauze for a short period. Ointments are also used topically and are generally left in place. Essential oils may be used topically, and some can also be taken internally in extremely dilute form. They are concentrated and must be used cautiously.

Many herbs can be useful in combination. Some companies produce excellent and safe herbal combination products for animals. Beware, however, of combination formulas listed as "proprietary blend" because you do not know the exact dose of each herb in the formula, and patient safety could be at risk. Another precaution is using herbals and medications

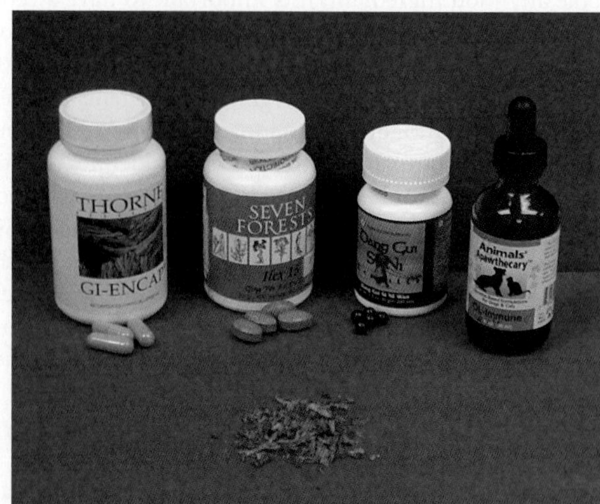

FIGURE 23-1 Commonly used herbal preparations: clockwise, left to right: capsules, tablets, tea pills, liquid, dried herbs (foreground).

with the same effect (i.e., antiinflammatory) because of the increased risk for adverse side effects.

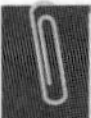

TECHNICIAN NOTE The use of herbs is not just limited to symptomatic treatment.

Herbs may also be used to support the general health of the patient (known as tonification). When used in this way, the herbs are taken over a long period of time. Ginkgo is often used in this way to support mental function in geriatric patients. Herbs may also be used in detoxification, such as the use of milk thistle to help protect and support the liver after steroid therapy (Table 23-2).

Administration of most herbs is generally best done on an empty stomach. For herbivores, this may be impossible. The next best way to administer herbs is with a small amount of water. Sometimes salt-free broth or clam juice works well for small animals. If food is the only way to get the herb to the patient, then try to avoid giving the herb with a full meal. It is also best to avoid any food with strong flavor, such as peppermint, near the time of administration.

CHINESE HERBAL MEDICINE

Chinese herbs actually consist of many substances, including minerals, and animal tissue. Individual botanical herbs may be used in the same way that Western herbs are. There is some overlap between Chinese and Western herbs. The main difference between the two is the use of traditional Chinese medicine (TCM) in a patient's diagnosis and treatment with Chinese herbs.

TCM is further discussed in the section on acupuncture. The Chinese herbal practitioner must have a clear TCM diagnosis when prescribing an herbal therapy. This involves a TCM examination, including tongue and pulse diagnosis. Herbal medicine is considered "stronger" than acupuncture. Practitioners often use the properties and taste of the herbs to choose the most appropriate herb or formula. Most TCM practitioners in China use acupuncture only in acute cases and prescribe herbs along with it to bring about a more thorough treatment. Often for more chronic conditions or to help patients maintain health, herbs alone are used. For example, the herb ma huang, or ephedra, is used to "disperse congestion in the Lung" and "release the exterior." In terms of TCM, the patient may be diagnosed with an exterior cold excess pattern of disease. In terms of our knowledge of pharmacology, this substance dries mucous membranes, and derivatives are used to treat the common cold, which is an exterior pathogen.

The formulas are named for their function or their main ingredients. Unlike Western herbs, each herbal formula is generally a combination of several products that work together to bring about an effect. It is a much more complex system than a Western approach. Certain herbs are found in many common formulas (Table 23-3). For this reason, the practitioner using Chinese herbs should undertake

TABLE 23-2 Commonly Used Western Herbs and Their Therapeutic Uses

Common Name	Scientific Name	Active Parts	Indications/Affinity
Aloe	*Aloe vera*	Gel layer of leaf	Skin irritation (topical)
Cranberry	*Vaccinium macrocarpon*	Fruit	Urinary tract infection
Dandelion	*Taraxacum officinale*	Root (whole plant)	Diuretic
Echinacea	*Echinacea purpurea*	Whole plant	Immune support
Eyebright	*Euphrasia officinalis*	Whole plant	Eye irritation (topical)
Ginkgo	*Ginkgo biloba*	Leaves	Promotes mental alertness
Hawthorn	*Crataegus laevigata*	Leaves, berries, blossoms	Supports heart function
Milk thistle	*Silybum marianum*	Seeds, fruit, leaves	Liver support, detoxification
Slippery elm	*Ulmus fulva*	Bark	Soothes the GI tract
Valerian	*Valerian officinalis*	Root	Anxiety, sleep disorders

TABLE 23-3 Common Ingredients in Chinese Herbal Preparations

Chinese Name	Common Name	Scientific Name	Indications TCM	Indications Western
Sheng jiang	Ginger	*Zingiber officianale*	Regulate stomach qi	Nausea
Ma huang	Ephedra	*Ephedra sinica*	Dispel wind cold	Bronchitis, asthma
Huang lian	Coptis	*Coptis japonica*	Clear damp heat	Inflammation
Sheng di huang	Rehmannia	*Rehmannia glutinosa*	Nourish yin	Adrenal, liver support
Chi shao	Red peony	*Paeonia rubra*	Invigorate blood	Pain
Tang kuei	Angelica	*Angelica sinensis*	Nourish blood	Itching
Wu rong	Maitake	*Grifola frondosa*	Enhance qi	Cancer (immune stimulation)
Yunnan paiyao	(Proprietary blend)		Stop bleeding	Hemorrhage

formal training. Forms are similar to Western preparation (see Figure 23-1), including tablets and pills, powders, granules, liquid teas and extracts, and topical preparations (ointments, plasters, and liniments). Many of the formulas come in tiny tablets known as tea pills. These are quite handy when treating cats, but large dogs may require 10 or more pills per dose.

As with Western herbs, and perhaps even more importantly, it is important that the herbs come from a reputable source that ensures quality control. The use of animal products in many formulations makes this a more serious concern. There are several companies in the United States that distribute products of uniform quality that are produced under the most ethical circumstances possible (e.g., some animal products from endangered species are substituted with a similar product from a related domestic animal). For some holistic practitioners, the use of animal products may result in a moral dilemma, and these veterinarians may choose to avoid these products in their pharmacy.

AYURVEDIC HERBS

Ayurveda means "the science of life." Similar to TCM, it emphasizes health and wellness, not just treatment of disease. It originated in India and is believed to predate TCM and even to have contributed to its foundation. It includes not only herbal prescriptions, but also diet, massage, exercise, and meditation as part of a patient's therapy. The goal of this system of medicine is to balance the three elements of nature, known as Doshas, which exist in every living organism.

Like Chinese herbs, ayurvedic herbs may be prescribed based on pharmacology (like Western herbs), according to the three Doshas (similar to TCM yin, yang, and qi), or based on taste and temperature. For example, licorice is considered a sweet herb. Sweet herbs are considered to be cold and wet and are used to nourish and soothe. In terms of pharmacology, licorice reduces the breakdown of prostaglandin, which protects the stomach from excess acid. Thus it is a treatment for stomach ulcers, which cause a burning sensation. Ayurvedic herbs also tend to come in formulations of multiple ingredients, and like Chinese herbs, some ingredients are commonly found in multiple formulations (Table 23-4).

> *TECHNICIAN NOTE* The technician who works with a practitioner who treats patients using the aforementioned herbal therapies should be familiar with the more commonly used herbs: indications, contraindications, precautions, and appropriate dosing. Awareness of common herb-drug interactions is also important.

The technician may be asked to prepare the herbal formula, to administer, to dispense, and to explain a prescribed formula to the client. This requires a thorough knowledge of the herbal pharmacy.

AROMATHERAPY

Aromatherapy is the therapeutic use of volatile essential oils to obtain a physiologic or psychological effect (Table 23-5). Oils are distilled or extracted from plants and are considered the "last possible and most sublime" parts of the plant. Flowers, buds, fruits, peels, leaves, bark, wood, roots, and seeds can be used. The oils can be applied topically by themselves or in a massage oil, ingested (not common), or administered by nebulization (the oil is made into a mist and inhaled). The effect of inhalation is most likely due to rapid absorption by both the nasal and lung mucosa. Plants or parts of the plants can also be burned and the smoke inhaled. Potential uses of aromatherapy include antibacterial and antifungal (tea tree oil and thyme oil), relaxation or sedation (lavender oil), behavior modification (positive or negative), conditioning (citronella bark collars), and medicinal.

> *TECHNICIAN NOTE* The technician's role in aromatherapy is to apply the oils at the recommendation of the veterinarian and to have a basic knowledge of their treatment purpose and be able to discuss their use and benefits.

> *TECHNICIAN NOTE* Lavender is the most widely used essential oil. It can be applied topically to the head for calming effects and on cuts, burns, insect bites, and abrasions to speed healing (see Table 23-5).

TABLE 23-4 Common Ingredients in Ayurvedic Herbal Formulae

Common Name	Scientific Name	Indications Ayurveda	Indications Western
Ashwagandha	*Withania somnifera*	Balance vata and kapha	Fatigue, skin disease
Boswellia	*Boswellia serrata*	Balance vata and kapha	Arthritis (antiinflammatory)
Cinnamon	*Cinnamomum zeylanicum*	Reduce vata and kapha	Digestive disorders
Licorice	*Glycyrrhiza glabra*	Pacify vata and pitta	Soothe urinary and GI tract
Neem	*Azadirachta indica*	Antiseptic	Wounds, rashes
Shatavari	*Asparagus racemosus*	Balance vata and pitta	Bladder infection
Turmeric	*Curcuma longa*	Reduce kapha	Arthritis, liver support

TABLE 23-5 Common Aroma Therapy Oils and Their Uses

How Applied	Action	Indications	Chemical Constituents	Contraindications
Basil				
Temples, navel and chest, insect stings and bites, inhale, or added to food	Antispasmodic, antiinfectious, antiviral, antiinflammatory, antibacterial, and decongestant	Gastroenteritis, lethargy, relax muscle, soothe insect bites, stimulate sense of smell, may help bronchitis	Methyl chavicol, linalool, terpene alcohol, terpene esters, phenols, ketones, camphor, oxides	Epilepsy, skin test for sensitivity
Birch				
Dilute with oil for massage, add to bath water	Analgesic, antispasmodic, antiinflammatory, liver stimulant, supports bone function	Arthritis, inflammation, muscular pain, tendinitis, hypertension, cramps, and cystitis	Esters, methyl salicylate	Topical use only, do not use in cats, skin test for sensitivity, epilepsy
Chamomile (German)				
Diffuse, topical, dietary supplement	Sedating, calming, antispasmodic, antiinflammatory, decongestant, supports digestive, liver, and gallbladder function, reduces scarring, relieves allergies	Insomnia, nervous tension, bursitis, tendinitis, dermatitis, liver and gallbladder disease, and inflammatory bowel disease	Sesquiterpenes, sesquiterpenols, sesquiterpene oxides, sesquiterpene lactones, coumarins, ethers	Nontoxic
Cinnamon				
Diffuse, topical, dietary supplement	Antimicrobial, antiinfectious antiviral, antifungal *(Candida)*, antibacterial, circulatory stimulant	External parasites, dental problems, and pneumonia	Ethers, eugenols, cinnamaldehyde	Repeated topical use can result in extreme contact sensitization, diffuse with caution because it may irritate the nasal membrane
Cypress				
Topical	Improves circulation, supports nerves and intestines, antiinfectious	Arthritis, bronchitis, intestinal parasites, pulmonary infections, spasms,	Monoterpenes, sesquiterpenols, diterpenols	Nontoxic
Lavender				
Diffuse, topical, dietary supplement	Antiseptic, analgesic, antitumoral, anticonvulsant, sedative, antiinflammatory	Burns, cuts and abrasions, allergies, seizures, insomnia, inflammatory skin lesions, depression, hives, insect bites, nervous tension	Monoterpenes, sesquiterpenes, esters, lavandula, ketones, sesquiterpenones, aldehydes, lactones	Nontoxic

Continued

TABLE 23-5 Common Aroma Therapy Oils and Their Uses—cont'd

How Applied	Action	Indications	Chemical Constituents	Contraindications
Lemon				
Diffuse or add a few drops to water and spray air, dietary supplement	Antiinfectious, disinfectant, antibacterial, antiseptic, antiviral, vitamin P–like action to improve microcirculation, enhance immune function	Anemia, asthma, promote leukocyte formation, digestive problems, respiratory infections, strengthens nails, insect repellent	Monoterpenes, sesquiterpenes, aldehydes	Very photosensitizing (avoid applying to skin that will be exposed to the sun)
Peppermint				
Diffuse, topical (massage on stomach for upset or temples for headache), dietary supplement	Anticarcinogenic, supports digestion, expels worms, decongestant, antiinfectious, antibacterial, antifungal, mucolytic, stimulant, stimulates gallbladder, expectorant, stimulates sense of taste	Gastroenteritis, colic, inflammatory bowel disease, diarrhea, fever, motion sickness, bronchitis, asthma, headaches when applied topically, cough	Monoterpenes, monoterpenols, monoterpenones, terpene oxides, terpene esters, coumarins	Avoid contact with the eyes, mucous membranes, or sensitive skin areas. Do not apply to a fresh wound or burn, Neurotoxic (respiratory depressant, convulsant), cardiac dysrhythmias
Rosemary				
Diffuse, topical, dietary supplement	Mucolytic, expectorant, antispasmodic, antibacterial, antiseptic, neurologic stimulant	Respiratory infections, bronchitis, nervous tension, cystitis, arthritis, dry or erythematous skin	Monoterpenes, sesquiterpenes, monoterpenols, terpene esters, terpene oxides, monoterpenones	Epilepsy
Thyme				
Dilute topical	Antimicrobial, antifungal, antiviral	Pneumonia, asthma, gastroenteritis, skin and oral infections	Monoterpenols, terpene esters	Dermal and mucous membrane irritant
Valerian				
Diffuse, topical, dietary supplement	Sedative to the central nervous system	Restlessness, sleep disturbances, nervousness, tension	Monoterpenes, sesquiterpenes, monoterpenols, terpene esters, sesquiterpenols, sesquiterpenones	Repeated use can result in contact sensitization

Note: If the animal is pregnant or nursing, oils should only be used with the veterinarian's consent. Many of these oils have not been tested on pregnant or nursing animals. Cats are more sensitive to most oils, and caution should be used when applying. Some oils that are therapeutic for dogs are toxic to cats.

HOMEOPATHY, HOMOTOXICOLOGY, AND FLOWER ESSENCES

Homeopathy is a system of medicine that is based on the principle that "like cures like." It involves treating each patient as an individual based on his or her group of symptoms. Practitioners use extremely diluted versions of herbs and other substances, which are called remedies, to treat patients. It is sometimes difficult to understand, but it can generate amazing results when used by a skillful practitioner. Homotoxicology and flower essence therapies are similar in practice, but can often be more easily used by a veterinarian with basic knowledge and understanding.

The technician should understand the basic principles of homeopathy and be able to properly administer and store remedies, and educate clients about their proper use and handling.

HISTORY AND PRINCIPLES

Samuel Hahnemann, a German physician, first used and developed homeopathy in the late 1700s. At the time, medications were given to patients without any ensuring safety. The scientific process as we know it did not exist, and trial and error determined which substances would be good medications. At the time, quinine was being used to treat patients with malaria, but often caused as much harm as good. This pioneering practitioner through diligent perseverance ultimately recognized that symptoms of disease were expressions of the body's attempt to restore homeostasis in response to an imbalance or insult.

The initial postulate was that giving a patient a medication that simulates the disease would stimulate the body's own defenses, and the patient would heal. This is similar to, though not completely the same as, the principle of vaccination. It is the reverse of allopathic (or Western or modern) medicine, which uses drugs to counteract symptoms, thereby suppressing them. For example, if you use cortisone to treat a rash, your symptoms will return if you do not repeat the dose for many days, sometimes even more severely than initially experienced. You may later show signs of a more serious disease, such as a stomach ulcer. Western medicine would consider the two conditions to be unrelated, but a homeopath considers them both to be signs of disorder in the body.

Hahnemann determined that the more he diluted medicine, the stronger the beneficial effects became, whereas the harmful effects diminished or disappeared altogether. Although important, this was not his most profound discovery. Whereas most physicians were concerned with treating one symptom, the "chief complaint" as we know it, Hahnemann astutely observed that these medications had many multiple effects on the body (some beneficial, some harmful, and some neither beneficial nor harmful). He decided to try his medications, which were then completely safe, on healthy patients. For example, if you were healthy and took cold medicine, you might experience a dry nose and throat in addition to drowsiness or even inability to sleep, depending on the drug combination. He recorded everything his patients told him about the effects the medicine had on them and observed every detail that he could, from physical signs to emotions that his patients experienced. This practice is known today as a "proving."

One of Hahnemann's beliefs was that the medication should match the symptoms more closely. He began collecting much more detailed information about his patients, and he was able to be more precise when choosing a medicine for each individual. A perfect example is the common cold: No two persons exhibit the same exact symptoms, even though they may have the same exact virus that caused the disease. Many people exhibit the same cold symptoms each time they are sick, regardless of the strain of the virus.

Because of the safety and efficacy of his medicine, others sought to learn how to treat patients in this manner. Hahnemann recorded his philosophy and findings in a book entitled *The Organon of Medicine*. Homeopathy is still widely practiced today in Europe, although less so in the United States. The earliest mention of veterinary homeopathy came from Hahnemann himself, when he stated in a lecture in the early 1800s that a similar approach was also applicable to animals. Today there are organizations and courses available worldwide for veterinarians who would like to practice homeopathic medicine.

PRACTICE

When a patient is seen by a homeopathic practitioner, a clear and detailed history is essential to a successful outcome. The owner is asked many questions, some of which may seem minute and unimportant. Any previous diagnostics and therapies (and responses) should be noted, even for minor problems. The patient is observed, and details about his or her physical status and personality and reactions to certain situations are noted and recorded. This should always include a thorough "Western" physical examination because these findings may lead to symptoms not discovered by the owner (such as a fast heart rate). The veterinarian may also note something of a serious nature that may need a "Western" approach before using homeopathy. For example, an older patient in congestive heart failure that comes to the hospital dyspneic and cyanotic needs to be stabilized first. Once out of a life-threatening situation, the patient can be evaluated, and a more long-term approach can be taken.

Minute details can be important when treating patients homeopathically. Even the way the patient greets the veterinarian can be important in finding the correct remedy. All of the details are recorded, and a list of remedies that are appropriate for each sign or symptom is compiled. This is called repertorizing. From this list, the most appropriate remedy is prescribed. In modern times, much of this work can be done by computer, although some practitioners still do all of their research by hand. The remedy is then dispensed to the owner with specific instructions on dosage and administration.

> *TECHNICIAN NOTE* It is important that the remedy be handled properly and that it is given exactly as directed.

Homeopathic remedies come in several strengths, called potencies. Potency is inversely proportional to dilution: the less actual substance present, the stronger the medicine. In general, it is best to use the lowest potency (or least dilute) necessary to bring about a cure. Sometimes the dose will be given only once, sometimes multiple times. The remedy should be discontinued when the symptoms cease or the patient shows improvement. Occasionally a patient will experience an exacerbation of symptoms, called an aggravation. This usually passes within a few hours and is not generally a concern. Usually, it indicates that the correct remedy was chosen, but if the patient becomes weaker, an "antidote" (another remedy) to the prescribed remedy can be given. Antidotes to each remedy are listed in the *Materia Medica*.

The remedies are fragile compared with Western medications. There are several forms (Figure 23-2). They should not be touched and should be administered away from food, whenever possible. The remedy is effective as soon as it gets into the mouth; as long as it touches the lips, gums, or tongue, it does not need to be swallowed. Remedies should never be returned to the bottle. They should be stored at room temperature away from moisture (keep container sealed) in a dark place, preferably in a cabinet away from strong herbs, Western medication, and magnetic fields (microwaves, computers, stereo speakers) (Table 23-6).

Homeopaths believe that things that suppress symptoms actually drive disease deeper into the body, or create more imbalance. Depending on how "deep" or serious the disorder is, it may take a succession of several remedies to restore a patient to health. Changes in symptoms are noted, and a new remedy is chosen until the patient is healthy.

> *TECHNICIAN NOTE* A disorder that may seem minor by traditional medicine may actually be quite serious from a homeopathic perspective. Similarly a patient may be considered healthy by Western standards, but may still be imbalanced and thus in need of further treatment when undergoing homeopathic treatment.

Homeopathy can be used at many levels. The least complex is the treatment of *acute* disease, which should quickly restore health to a vital, strong patient. An example of this is the use of *Arnica montana* to treat a patient with bruising from trauma. Several remedies are fairly easily used in acute situations, even without extensive training (Table 23-7). Next is treatment on a *constitutional* level, which takes into account the nature (physical traits, personality, emotions) of the patient and "disease" symptoms, past and present. The goal is to help the patient restore and maintain a state of health. The most complex is *miasmic* treatment, in which the ultimate goal of therapy is to prevent disease by addressing genetic weaknesses. This is quite challenging in the veterinary patient and is therefore not often undertaken.

Homeopathy can be further divided into *classical homeopathy,* in which the patient is treated with one remedy at a time, and modern homeopathy, in which the patient is given a combination of remedies to match his or her given set of symptoms. Homotoxicology is the most commonly used form of combination homeopathy in veterinary medicine. The remedies are compounded using the most commonly

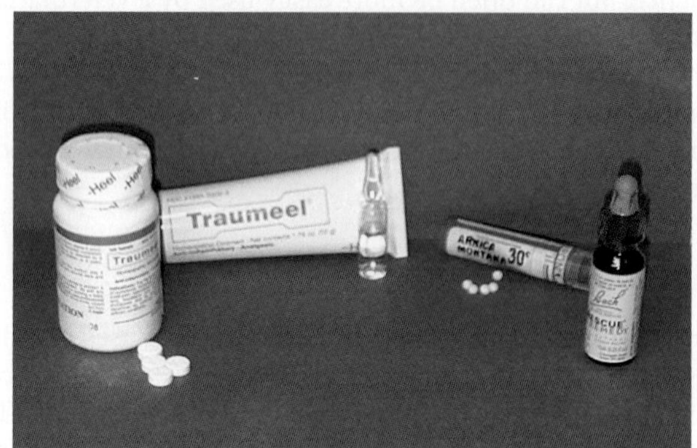

FIGURE 23-2 Homeopathic preparations: clockwise, left to right: tablets, ointment, injectable (foreground), pellets, liquid (flower essence).

TABLE 23-6 Homeopathic Preparations

Form	Administration
Pellets (sugar) or tablets	Use whole (dispense from cap into the patient's mouth, avoiding contaminating the cap) or crush between a folded sheet of paper Pour into patient's mouth or drop between the lips and gum Can also be dissolved in distilled or spring water and administered by dropper
Liquid	Use dropper and apply on tongue or between cheek and gums
Topical	Apply to affected area
Injections	May be used SQ, IM, intralesion Often used in acupuncture points

TABLE 23-7 Commonly Used Single Homeopathic Remedies for Acute Use

Remedy	Symptoms
Arnica	Bruising, bleeding
Calendula	Topical for skin irritation
Ledum	Hives, stings
Nux Vomica	Vomiting
Pulsatilla	Purulent discharge
Thuja	Vaccine reaction

indicated remedies used to treat a specific set of symptoms, such as low back pain. This therefore alleviates the need to repertorize and choose one remedy (Table 23-8).

The combination therapy can be used in a more "Western" approach. For example, Traumeel (see Figure 23-2) is a commonly used treatment for bruising, trauma, inflammation, and arthritis. It comes in several forms (oral tablets and liquid, injectable, and cream) and contains arnica, calendula, echinacea, and several other individual remedies that work together to provide the desired effect.

From a scientific standpoint, there has been much research on homeopathy. The individualized nature of the treatments can make it difficult to "prove" from a Western standpoint, but many double-blind placebo-controlled studies exist. Research on the biphasic nature of medication has assisted our understanding of how diluted forms of medication can have the opposite effect of the therapeutic dose of the same medicine on the body. For example, a clinical dose of atropine causes drying of mucous membranes, but a tiny dose has been shown to increase secretions of mucous membranes. Both in vitro and clinical studies have shown homeopathic remedies to be effective, but thus far we do not understand exactly *how* they work.

FLOWER ESSENCES

Flower essence therapy, developed by Edward Bach in the 1930s, uses an approach similar to homeopathy to treat patients. Bach believed that all substances used to treat patients should be completely nontoxic, even in undiluted form. He developed 37 essences derived from plants (flowers, bushes, trees) and one from water (rock water) for a total of 38 remedies (Table 23-9). These essences are not diluted to the extent that homeopathic remedies are.

The use of flower essences is based more on a psychologic or emotional than physical level. Bach himself described 12 pathologic emotional states that he believed would lead to physical disease if left untreated. For example, the remedy Aspen is used to treat patients with fear of the unknown, and holly is used to treat patients exhibiting jealousy or suspiciousness. Of course, the emotional nature of animals can be difficult to determine, but it is not unreasonable and can be quite rewarding. Flower essences may, like homeopathy, be used in acute situations in addition to treating patients on a constitutional basis.

The individual essences are all provided as a liquid. The most common remedy used is called Rescue Remedy (see Figure 23-2), and it is a combination of five flower essences (rock rose, cherry plum, star of Bethlehem, clematis, impatiens). The preparation may also be found in a cream. It is

TABLE 23-8 Commonly Used Homotoxicology Products and Their Indications

Product	Indications	Main Ingredients
Discus Compositum	Sciatica, hind limb weakness	Berberis, cimifuga, colocynthis
Spascupreel	Muscle spasm	Aconitum, colocynthis, atropinum
Traumeel	Inflammation, pain	Arnica, aconitum, belladonna
Vertigoheel	Vestibular issues	Cocculus, coneum
Zeel	Arthritis	Silicea, arnica, rhus tox

TABLE 23-9 Basic Flower Essences and Their Uses

Essence	Indications
Rescue Remedy	Shock, trauma, stress
Cherry plum	Panic, loss of control
Clematis	Lack of responsiveness
Impatiens	Impatience, irritability
Rock rose	Extreme fear
Star of Bethlehem	Shock, trauma
Agrimony	Prolonged grief, moping and withdrawing
Aspen	Fear of unknown things (strangers)
Beech	Intolerance, rigidness
Centaury	Submissiveness, timidness
Cerato	Indecisiveness (need constant reassurance)
Chestnut bud	Repetitive actions (helps break bad habits)
Chicory	Possessiveness (separation anxiety)
Crab apple	Detoxification
Elm	Overwhelming stress of (working, competing, travel)
Gentian	Depression
Gorse	Hopelessness
Heather	Attention-seeking behavior (constant barking, whining)
Holly	Jealousy, especially when aggressive or spiteful
Honeysuckle	Grief, homesickness
Hornbeam	Helps adjust to changes
Larch	Lack of confidence
Mimulus	Fear of known things (thunderstorms)
Mustard	Mood swings, depression, gloom
Oak	Workaholic (overworks to exhaustion)
Olive	Lack of energy, exhaustion
Pine	Excessive grief, rejection, guilt
Red chestnut	Worry, overprotectiveness
Rock water	Inflexibility
Scleranthus	Indecision with mood swings, motion sickness
Sweet chestnut	Extreme stress, mental anguish
Vervain	Excessive enthusiasm, hyperactivity
Vine	Aggression, dominance
Walnut	Stress as a result of change
Water violet	Aloofness, withdrawal
White chestnut	Restlessness, repetitive thoughts
Wild oat	Frustration, boredom, lack of concentration
Wild rose	Apathy, resignation
Willow	Resentment, sulkiness

used to treat animals in times of stress, anxiety, or trauma. For those interested in using flower essences, Rescue Remedy is an excellent starting point and can be used in such situations as trauma, surgery recovery, or even for the frightened and panic-stricken boarding patient. The remedies are administered like homeopathic remedies, but they are generally sold in stock bottles. The stock flower remedy should be diluted in spring water or a combination of water and alcohol (increases shelf life) to make a treatment bottle. Generally, 2 drops of each stock remedy (four if using Rescue Remedy) are placed in a 1-oz glass amber vial with a dropper. Up to five remedies may be combined in one treatment bottle (Rescue Remedy only counts as a single remedy). They are given by the dropper directly into the mouth. They may also be added to drinking water (from a few drops in a bowl for a cat to 15 drops per gallon for a horse). Another method is using the remedy in a spray bottle as a mist (usually into the environment), which is an effective and stress-free means of treating birds and small mammals. It can also be used topically. Administration is generally repeated at various intervals. In an acute situation, it may be as often as every 30 seconds. For a less urgent situation, it may be daily for several days or weeks. Flower essences should be stored like homeopathic remedies.

These flower remedies, like their homeopathic counterparts, are safe to use and can have a profound effect on a patient when the correct remedy is given. They are often used as an adjunct to other therapies that do not do as much to address the emotional aspect of healing. As you can imagine, the technician can be of great value to the veterinarian who practices homeopathy. By assisting in observation of the patient and clients' education, the technician can have a substantial impact on the success of the treatment.

APPLIED KINESIOLOGY

Applied kinesiology (AK) is an approach to health care that uses functional assessment measures, such as posture and gait analysis, manual muscle testing as a functional neurologic evaluation, range of motion, static palpation, and motion analysis to diagnose patients. These assessments are used in conjunction with standard methods of diagnosis, such as clinical history, physical examination findings, and laboratory tests to develop a clinical impression of the unique physiologic condition of each patient. Thousands of professionals belong to the International College of Applied Kinesiology (ICAK), including chiropractors, physicians, osteopaths, dentists, podiatrists, psychologists, and veterinarians. More than 2100 clinical research papers have been published by the ICAK. Veterinarians take a basic 100-hour certification course through the ICAK.

> *TECHNICIAN NOTE* AK is a diagnostic system using manual muscle testing to augment normal examination procedures.

George Goodheart, D.C., is recognized as the creator of the field of AK. As early as 1964, he recognized that dysfunction of the muscle and tendon receptors in a particular muscle could affect the strength of that muscle and have a negative effect on the stability of a related joint. Whereas most practitioners were treating musculoskeletal problems by addressing the hypertonic muscles, Dr. Goodheart saw that most of the time the problems were related to muscle paresis. He came to discover, and has since been supported by research, that muscle weakness could be caused by a large number of factors affecting output from the ventral horn. Dr. Goodheart investigated the effects of many different types of existing techniques on the efficiency of muscle function. These include the following techniques and relationships:

- Manipulative therapy
- Neurologic relationships
- Chapman's reflexes, which are known in AK as neurolymphatic reflexes
- Bennett's reflexes, which are known in AK as neurovascular reflexes
- Cranial sacral therapy
- Meridian therapy
- Nutritional and biochemical therapy
- Organ-muscle relationships
- Psychologic relationships
- Electrical and magnetic relationships

One of the tools in AK is manual muscle testing for functional neurologic assessment. It can be used to evaluate and correct functional imbalances in the structural, chemical, mental, and energetic systems of the patient. It is important to note that manual muscle testing is only a small part of AK, and these terms are not mutually interchangeable. In muscle testing, the professional places pressure against a certain muscle, and the patient tries to resist the motion caused by this pressure. For example, if one person held an arm out to their side parallel to the ground, the major muscle holding it there would be the deltoid muscle. If the professional put pressure downward and the deltoid muscle was weak, the arm would go down relatively easily. If the deltoid muscle was strong, it would take a much greater force to bring the arm down. The physician using AK finds a muscle that is unbalanced and attempts to determine why that muscle is not functioning properly. This may be due to improper facilitation or neuromuscular inhibition. On the basis of response to therapy, it appears that in some of these conditions, the primary dysfunction is due to deafferentation, the loss of normal sensory stimulation of neurons as a result of the functional interruption of afferent receptors. It may occur under many circumstances, but is best understood by the concept that with abnormal joint function (subluxation or fixation), the uncharacteristic movement causes improper stimulation of the local joint and muscle receptors. This changes the transmission from these receptors through the peripheral nerves to the spinal cord, brainstem, cerebellum, cortex, and then to the effectors from their normally expected stimulation. Symptoms of deafferentation arise from numerous levels, such as motor, sensory, autonomic, and consciousness, or from anywhere throughout the neuraxis. The physician works out the treatment that will best balance the patient's muscles. Treatments may involve specific joint manipulation or mobilization, various myofascial therapies, cranial techniques, meridian and acupuncture skills, clinical nutrition, dietary management, evaluating environmental irritants, and various reflex procedures. In human medicine, the application of AK diagnosis requires that the physician be competent in the testing of all accessible muscles of the body. In animal AK, the insertion of a surrogate tester reduces the number of muscles tested to one or two. It is hard to tell an animal to resist a given motion; this is where the veterinary technician plays a role. They are the missing link of the animal manual muscle test. The technician's role is to be a surrogate, adding another human being to the equation (Figure 23-3). When muscle testing adult humans, we test their muscles directly. It was discovered early on in AK that babies and quadriplegics could be tested indirectly by having a third person touch them while the physician tested the surrogate's muscle for changes in strength. The same tests or challenges are applied to the patient, but the muscle testing response is through the surrogate. This same principle has been applied with great success to animals. How surrogate testing works is not really known at this time. It is hypothesized that neurologic information, which is conveyed electrically, is transferred to the mostly salt and water surrogate by contact with the patient.

The technician is an important team member in a practice that uses AK. The involvement may include writing down examination findings and treated areas and assisting with restraint and communication with clients. The technician should have a basic knowledge of the procedure and what abbreviations or AK notations are used at the practice.

> *TECHNICIAN NOTE* In some cases, the examiner may test for environmental or food sensitivities by using a previously strong muscle to find what weakens it.

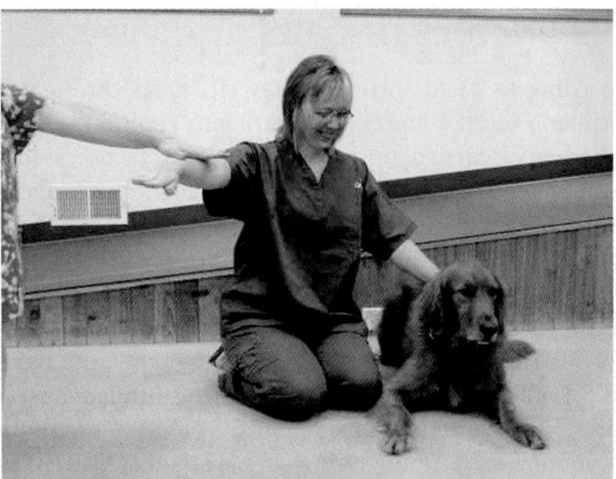

FIGURE 23-3 AK: a dog diagnosed with manual therapy.

ACUPUNCTURE

The term acupuncture comes from the Latin words acus, meaning "needle," and pungere, meaning, "to pierce." It is the technique of piercing the skin with a needle at specific, predetermined "acupuncture points." It is now known that these points can be stimulated by more than just needles; they can also be stimulated by injection of fluid, laser, ultrasound, surgically implanted material, and electrical stimulation.

Acupuncture has been used for more than 4000 years in the East as one medical method within TCM. TCM is a system of medicine that includes herbology, massage, and nutritional and lifestyle management. Early Chinese veterinary applications of acupuncture started with the domestication of animals. Veterinary acupuncture came to the United States in the early 1970s, and in 1974 the International Veterinary Acupuncture Society (IVAS) was organized with the aim of fully integrating acupuncture into Western veterinary science. Acupuncture is used to treat all species from ferrets and birds to dogs and cattle to elephants and killer whales.

In the United States, acupuncture is increasingly used as a modality in the treatment of musculoskeletal, neurologic, cardiovascular, respiratory, GI, reproductive, and dermatologic disorders. Although it has the ability to help many areas of the body, pain management is probably the most common use of acupuncture today.

TERMINOLOGY AND RECORD KEEPING

Acupuncture points are connected through pathways that are called meridians or channels. In TCM, it is believed that the body's vital energy or life force (bioelectricity) circulates in a cyclic predetermined course through the meridians. In most species, there are 14 classical meridians: 12 are associated with specific organ systems on which they have a primary influence, and two run on the midlines of the body. The paired organ-related meridians are named lung (LU), large intestine (LI), stomach (ST), spleen (SP), heart (HT), small intestine (SI), bladder (BL), kidney (KI), pericardium (PC), triple heater (TH), gallbladder (GB), and liver (LV). The unpaired channels are conception vessel (CV) that runs on the ventral midline and the governing vessel (GV) that runs on the dorsal midline. Individual acupuncture points are named and recorded by pairing the meridian and a number (e.g., LV3 is the third point on the liver meridian, and SP6 is the sixth point on the spleen meridian). In addition, there are "extra" points that do not lie on meridians and trigger points, which are temporary tender areas that can move on and off the meridians in episodes of pathologic conditions.

> *TECHNICIAN NOTE* Acupuncture points are connected through pathways that are called meridians or channels.

ACUPUNCTURE THEORIES

According to TCM theory, energy circulates through each meridian every 24 hours. The meridians run on the surface of the body, where acupuncture points can be accessed and manipulated. A blockage of energy circulation manifests as dysfunction or disease. Medical conditions that can be helped result from stagnant energy circulation or lack of sufficient energy to function optimally. Stagnant energy manifests as painful spasms or swelling, whereas deficient energy manifests as atrophy or weakness. To bring the body into balance and to facilitate healing, it is necessary to stimulate or sedate energy levels at acupuncture points. There are many theories about how acupuncture works. The most current acupuncture theories discussed in the human literature are as follows:

1. Gate theory
2. Endogenous opioid theory
3. Autonomic nervous system input theory
4. Humoral theory
5. Bioelectric theory

THE GATE THEORY

The gate theory explains the analgesic effects of acupuncture. It has been shown that different types of neurons transmit pain. When an acupuncture needle is inserted, thin myelinated nerve fibers carry a message to the spinal cord. The neurotransmitters are released and taken up by the interneurons. When the impulse from the unmyelinated pain nerve fibers causes the release of neurotransmitters, the receptors are full and the "gate" is closed to that signal with little to no message of pain reaching the brain.

ENDOGENOUS OPIOID THEORY

Opioids have been used for many years to combat pain (i.e., poppy, morphine, torbutrol). Depending on where the needles are placed, acupuncture has been shown to release β-endorphins, met-enkephalins, and leu-enkephalins in both the blood and cerebral spinal fluid. These endogenous opioids can be reversed with naloxone (an injectable agent used in veterinary medicine to reverse the effects of morphine). Opiates are also known to have systemic effects that can be produced by acupuncture. For example, opiate receptors in the gut are responsible for decreasing peristalsis and increasing segmental contractions, thus effectively controlling diarrhea.

AUTONOMIC NERVOUS SYSTEM THEORY

This theory looks at how needles inserted into the skin can have an effect on the muscles and organs of the body. Numerous viscerosomatic (relating the organs to the muscles) relationships have been studied, and it has been found that visceral and somatic fibers have adjacent tracts in the spinal cord and distribution in the dorsal gray matter. Examples of this relationship include muscle cramping seen secondary to inflammation of the intestines and the phenomenon of "referred pain," which is when there is pain felt in one part of the body but it is different from the part of the body that was stimulated.

HUMORAL THEORY

This theory was first postulated after studies showed that a transfer of blood, cerebrospinal fluid (CSF), or brain tissue from an animal under acupuncture analgesia to an animal not receiving acupuncture resulted in analgesia of the recipient. This analgesia was generalized and reversed by naloxone. β-endorphins are released by acupuncture and may contribute to analgesia, but it is not the only important component. Serotonin is also important and increases 30% to 40% in the systemic circulation after acupuncture. Acupuncture has also been shown to cause systemic increases in growth hormone, prolactin, oxytocin, luteinizing hormone, white blood cells, immunoglobulins, antibodies, and interferons, depending on which points are stimulated.

> *TECHNICIAN NOTE* The humoral theory was first postulated after studies showed that a transfer of blood, CSF, or brain tissue from an animal under acupuncture analgesia to an animal not receiving acupuncture resulted in analgesia of the recipient.

BIOELECTRIC THEORY

Becker and Reichmanis, in 1976, proposed a theory that the healing and analgesic properties of acupuncture are based on a direct current (DC) system. In this system, electric signals are generated and propagated by Schwann cells, satellite cells, and glial cells. Acupuncture points, like amplifiers, would boost the DC signal along the nerve pathways. The insertion of a metal acupuncture needle would, in effect, short-circuit the system and block pain perception. In this system, acupuncture points boost the DC signal along the meridian, comparable with an amplifier boosting electricity along a high-power tension wire.

TECHNIQUES

Dry needling is performed using stainless steel acupuncture needles (Figure 23-4). These needles are 25 to 36 gauge and range from ½ to 2 inches long when used with companion animals or up to 4 inches long when used with large animals. Large animal practitioners will often use hypodermic needles in their patients.

Moxibustion is the burning of dried leaves of the *Artemisia vulgaris* or mugwort plant. The moxa stick can be moved slowly over an acupuncture point or be placed on an inserted needle. This is often used for animals with degenerative changes that do better in warm dry climates than when it is cold or damp. In TCM, this adds energy to a deficient area.

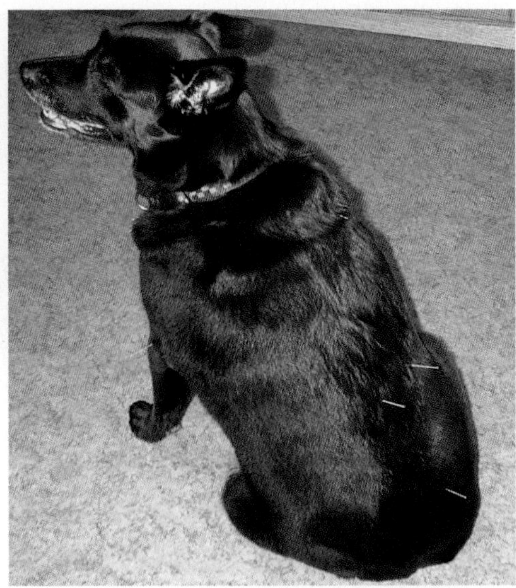

FIGURE 23-4 Acupuncture: Dakota has acupuncture treatment for spondylosis.

Aquapuncture is the injection of a solution into an acupuncture point. The most commonly used substance is vitamin B_{12}, although electrolyte solutions, saline, dimethyl sulfoxide (DMSO), vitamin C, antibiotics, herbal extracts, homeopathics, and local anesthetics can be used. It is thought that either the pressure on the point or the solution itself will stimulate the nerve fibers.

Electroacupuncture is the passing of electrical energy through acupuncture points. Stimulation is accomplished by connecting an electronic device to the inserted needles. Indications include paralysis or paresis, severe and chronic painful conditions, or conditions not responsive to dry needling.

To achieve a continuous stimulation of an acupuncture point, various materials may be surgically implanted at acupuncture points, called implantation. Though catgut, stainless steel, and silver can be used, the most common implant is gold in the form of solid beads or wires. This technique is most commonly used for young dogs with painful hip dysplasia, older dogs with coxofemoral arthritis, or epilepsy. This is considered a surgical procedure.

Low-intensity or "cold" lasers have been used to stimulate acupuncture points. Laser puncture is a noninvasive form of intense light therapy using various frequencies and wavelengths that promote positive physiologic changes within cells. It is used to (1) stimulate acupuncture points, (2) enhance healing of wounds and burns, and (3) treat acutely inflamed joints (Figure 23-5).

Ultrasound can be used to stimulate an acupuncture point, but it is not commonly done, perhaps because of the cost and also the necessity of shaving at each acupuncture point.

Microcurrent therapy is the use of a machine that generates a microcurrent of electricity that can be used on acupuncture points or directly over areas of pain or muscle spasm.

Acupuncture needles can be placed in the tissue perpendicularly or at an angle. When removing the needles, they should be gently pulled in the same direction that they went in. If there is resistance when removing the needle, tapping around the needle, rolling it back and forth, or gently holding down the skin on either side of the needle while pulling the needle gently will ease if from the tissue. Occasionally the needles will come out crooked, which is not unusual because they bend easily. All needles should be accounted for and placed into a sharps container.

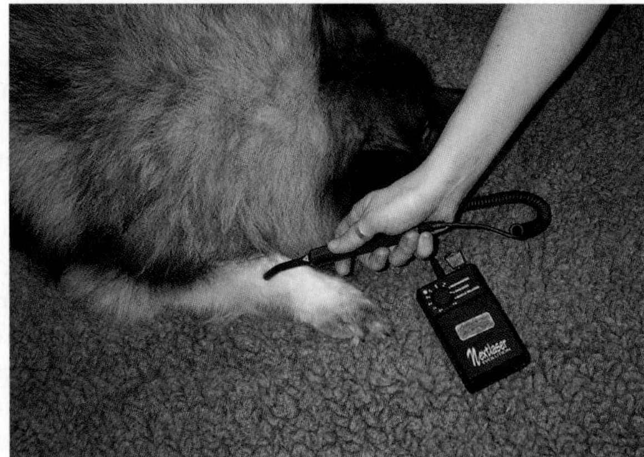

FIGURE 23-5 Laser acupuncture: Laser acupuncture can be used for painful or swollen areas or with animals that are sensitive to needling.

The technician's role in acupuncture includes having a general understanding of how and why acupuncture works to be able to discuss it with clients; charting the points in the record; aiding if patient restraint or diversion is needed; assisting in easing a patient's anxiety, if present; and removing and counting the needles.

> *TECHNICIAN NOTE* If there is resistance when removing the needle, tapping around the needle, rolling it back and forth, or gently holding down the skin on either side of the needle while pulling the needle gently will ease if from the tissue.

PHYSICAL MODAILITES

MASSAGE

Massage is defined as a systematic and scientific manipulation of the soft tissues of the body for the purpose of obtaining or maintaining health. Massage has been performed for thousands of years. There are more than 70 types of human massage philosophies, many of which can be applied to animals.

> *TECHNICIAN NOTE* The technician, if properly trained, can play the key role in massage therapy. Most massage certification courses are open to technicians, allowing them to be the primary massage therapist for animal patients. Training schools are listed at the end of this chapter.

Types

Shiatsu is a Japanese form of massage that literally means "finger pressure." Shiatsu practitioners use finger pressure on specific points in the body (correlating to acupuncture points) to increase circulation and stimulate the nervous system.

In trigger-point massage, or myotherapy, the therapist feels for taut bands or knots that have a point of maximal tenderness. Pressure on this point can cause local pain, referred pain, and muscle spasms in humans and animals. The manual technique for deactivating a trigger point is *ischemic compression*. By applying direct pressure over the point, the tissue becomes ischemic (blood is pushed out of the tissue), and when the pressure is removed, the tissue becomes hyperemic (blood quickly infiltrates the tissue). This will often relieve the tension, band, or knot, and the pain. This pressure is usually held for 8 to 15 seconds, and if a spasm is felt during the pressure, it should be maintained until the muscle stops firing.

Sports massage can be broken into event massage and maintenance massage. Event massage (relating to a massage done on an athlete before, during, or after competing) can be broken down into preevent, interevent, and postevent. The goal of preevent massage is to leave the animal relaxed and ready for the event. Interevent massage keeps the patient tuned up and ready for the next event, and postevent massage flushes out metabolic waste and reduces muscle spasms and soreness. The goal of maintenance massage is to help prevent injury and expedite the healing of injured tissue.

TTEAM is a system of massage for teaching physical awareness of the body. Originally designed for horses, and based on the human work of Dr. Feldenkrais, TTEAM is a form of massage that is devoted to nonhabitual motion to reeducate the nervous and musculoskeletal systems. It has an impact on an emotional level in addition to aiding focus, coordination, and balance. A major difference between TTEAM and other forms of massage is that whereas massage works on the deeper tissue, TTEAM manipulates only the skin. Although this was originally designed for horses, all species may benefit from this therapy.

Swedish massage is the most commonly used massage system in North America. These techniques began in the late 1700s and will be discussed for use on animals. Studies have shown that massage is beneficial in reducing stress, enhancing blood and lymph circulation, decreasing pain, promoting sleep, reducing swelling, enhancing relaxation, and increasing oxygen capacity of the blood.

Techniques

Effleurage is the most commonly used stroke in animals. It is a gliding stroke that follows the contour of the body. Hand over hand, thumb over thumb, or one hand on either side of the body are the most common variations. It is repeated several times at the beginning and end of the massage to evaluate the tissue and enhance blood flow (warm it up and then aid in flushing lactic acid). Animals usually prefer these stokes flowing with the hair. Although effleurage is often thought of as a light stroke, deeper strokes are used to lengthen muscles and aid in stretching.

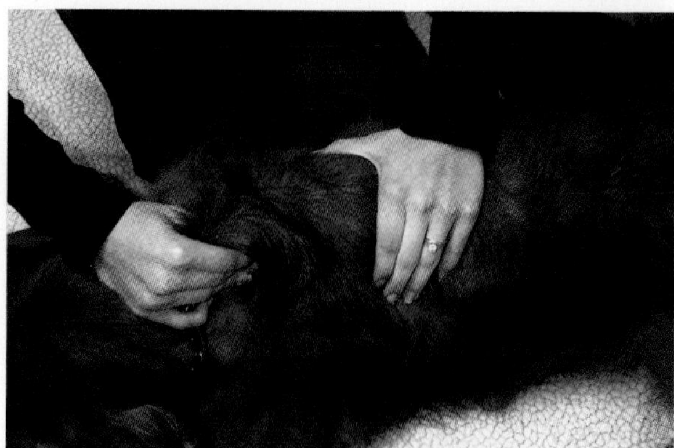

FIGURE 23-6 Pétrissage: Bandit receiving pétrissage, notice the "C" shape to the hands and the alternating pattern to the hands.

Pétrissage, or kneading, consists of rhythmic lifting, squeezing, and releasing the tissue. It assists in removing metabolic waste and increasing circulation. The hands form a C shape and can be alternated in a circular motion, can "roll" the skin, or can spread up and out to help widen or broaden the muscle (Figure 23-6).

Friction is the manipulation of tissue to increase circulation. It is commonly used over tendons when tendinitis is present, over knots and trigger points, and over joint capsules with excessive fibrous tissue. It is also used to break up skin adhesions and scar tissue (wait 3 to 4 weeks after injury or surgery before applying this technique). When applying this to deep tissue, one finger or thumb is placed on the skin and either rubs the skin or is attached to the skin and rubs the tissue underneath. This can be done longitudinally (with muscle fibers), cross fiber (perpendicular to the muscle fibers), circularly, diagonally, or in a J pattern.

Tapotement is a tapping motion of the hands or fingers. When done for a short time, it stimulates nerve endings (preevent sports massage or to tone atrophied muscles). When done longer, it has a more sedative effect. Coupage, which is used to loosen phlegm congestion in the lungs, is a form of tapotement. The hands are cupped, and the strokes start at the caudal aspect of the ribs and move forward. Proper positioning using wedges or pillows can help maximize the effectiveness of coupage. This stroke may be continued for 5 to 10 minutes on each side (Figure 23-7).

Vibration is a rapid shaking or slower rocking of the tissue. The speed of vibration will affect outcome: faster vibration will be stimulatory, whereas slower speeds will be inhibitory. It differs from tapotement in that the therapist's hands do not leave the patient's skin. It can aid in relaxing muscles, reducing trigger-point activity, and when used over a joint capsule in the proper position can act as a joint mobilization.

Swedish Massage

Swedish massage breaks down the massage into several elements. The elements include intention, touch, pressure and depth, excursion, speed, rhythm and continuity, duration,

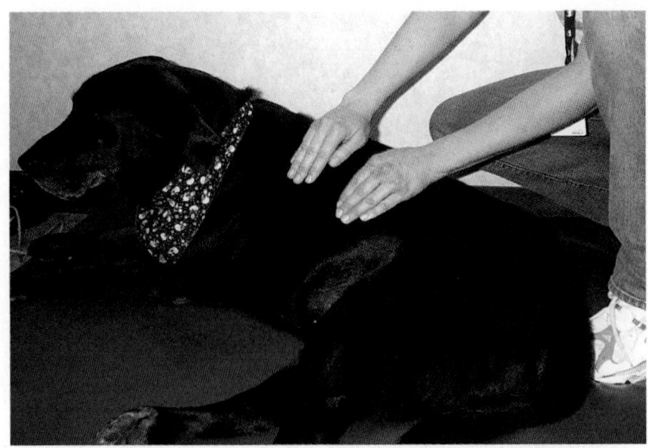

FIGURE 23-7 Tapotement: Coupage, a form of tapotement, is performed on Shadow. Note that the hands are cupped and alternating. The motion starts at the base of the ribs and moves forward.

and sequence. *Intention* is the consciously sought out goal of the therapist. Therefore the massage outcome is different if the therapist wants to create relaxation versus invigoration. *Touch* is the vehicle of massage and conveys the intention. *Pressure* is the force applied to the surface, usually through the therapist's hands. *Depth* is the distance traveled into the patient's tissue. The therapist controls the force, but the patient has more control over the depth. Often, applying less pressure slowly will increase depth, whereas fast, higher pressure will cause splinting (muscle contracting in a protective reflex) to occur. *Excursion* is the length of one massage stroke. In a cross-friction massage, meant to relieve tendinitis, the excursion may be only 1 to 2 cm, but in a beginning effleurage stroke, the excursion may be from the head all the way to the tip of the tail. *Speed* refers to how fast the hand moves over the patient. In an invigorating preevent sports massage, the speed will be much faster than if the therapist's goal is to achieve relaxation. The repetition or regularity of the stroke defines its rhythm, similar to music. The concept of *continuity* in massage refers to the uninterrupted flow of strokes and to the unbroken transition from one stroke to the next. It is hard for the patient to relax if the rhythm is not smooth or if the continuity is not fluid. *Duration* is the length of time devoted to one area. In humans, a relaxing massage does not usually last more then 1 hour without creating muscle soreness. The duration of a small animal massage is usually 30 minutes, and for a large animal, like the human, it is approximately 1 hour. A *sequence* is the arrangement of the massage strokes.

A typical example of a sequence would be:

- Start with effleurage on the face and head.
- Continue down the back and sides.
- Use pétrissage over the paraspinal muscles (including kneading, circles, or strokes going with or perpendicular to the muscle fibers).
- Apply ischemic compression on trigger points if found.
- Move on to one side of the neck.
- Carry on down the forelimb.
- Perform effleurage, with strokes running from the toes to the heart to flush toxins.
- Continue by using skin rolls along the body wall.
- Apply the same techniques you used in the forelimb to treat the rear limb.
- Gently flip the patient over if a canine or walk around to the other side if an equine.
- Repeat your techniques on the other side.
- Finish up with a final effleurage.

Signs of relaxation include sighing, yawning, licking the lips, hanging the head (equine), burping, or flatulence. Signs that the pressure is too great include increased respiratory rate, opening the eyes (if previously closed), fidgeting, and incessant licking (canine) or swishing the tail (equine).

Contraindication

There are several contraindications to massage, and there are also *endangerment sites*. Endangerment sites are areas of the body that are delicate and are relatively unprotected. Contraindications include massage over bacterially or virally infected lesions, over open wounds, over the area of an acute injury or inflammatory condition, over an area of hemorrhage, or following a recent high fever. Some endangerment sites include the throat, eyeballs, brachial plexus, abdomen (deep, near the aorta), and over the kidneys.

Precautions should be taken when massaging a patient with heart disease or over a neoplastic area.

> *TECHNICIAN NOTE* Effleurage is the most commonly used stroke in animals. It is a gliding stroke that follows the contour of the body.

VETERINARY CHIROPRACTIC

Chiropractic is perhaps one of the most familiar and most used complementary therapies that are used to treat veterinary patients. The term is derived from the Greek cheir ("hand") and praxis ("practice"). The purpose of chiropractic is to manually restore reduced motion in the spine and limbs, thereby improving patient mobility, comfort, and in many cases nervous system function. A. E. Homewood defined chiropractic as "that science and art which uses the inherent recuperative powers of the body and deals with the relationship between the nervous system and the spinal column, including its immediate articulations, and the role of this relationship in the restoration and maintenance of health."

The technician is an important team member in a practice that uses chiropractic. The involvement may include writing down examination findings and treated areas and assisting with restraint and communication with the client. The technician should have a basic understanding of the procedure, be able to properly stabilize an area to facilitate adjustment, and be familiar with what abbreviations or chiropractic notations are used at the practice.

The technician should have a basic knowledge of the procedure and what abbreviations or chiropractic notations are used at the practice.

History

Manipulation of the spine is an ancient practice. References were made to this form of treatment as early as 2700 BC in China. Even Hippocrates noted the effects of this type of therapy because he notes, "Look well to the spine for the cause of disease." Chiropractic began in the United States in 1895 with D. D. Palmer who began to treat the spine as a primary method of healing his patients. His son, B. J. Palmer, followed in his father's footsteps and further developed chiropractic into a system of medicine. He founded the first school of chiropractic in Davenport, Iowa. He claimed to have treated animal patients and people in his hospital at the school.

Chiropractic is becoming a more accepted and mainstream treatment in humans. Most major health insurance carriers now cover chiropractic care. This increased accessibility to people has contributed significantly to the increased demand for chiropractic care for veterinary patients. Also contributing to a wider acceptance is the growing amount of research that has been done on chiropractic in humans. Many of these same studies use animals as models for human disease, thus creating even more applicable research for veterinarians.

In most states, veterinary chiropractic adjustments must be performed by a trained professional (either a veterinarian or a chiropractor). Training leading to certification in veterinary chiropractic is available to both groups of professionals through postgraduate courses, but it is not yet a part of standard or elective coursework in either profession.

> TECHNICIAN NOTE Proper chiropractic technique requires a great deal of time and effort to learn. This is why human chiropractors go to school for 3 to 4 years before practicing. It is important that *only* a thoroughly trained professional adjust an animal patient. A weekend short course is a nice introduction, but it is not enough to prepare anyone to treat patients. Imagine a person taking a weekend course in veterinary nursing trying to take on the responsibilities that you have worked so hard to prepare for.

In the United States, certification is available to both groups of professionals through the American Veterinary Chiropractic Association (AVCA), which was founded in the 1980s. This involves approved coursework (consisting of at least 200 hours of lecture and hands-on labs), a certification examination (written and practical), and completion of several case reports. To remain certified, a veterinarian must complete 30 hours of continuing education every 3 years.

Philosophy and Theory

Chiropractic is much more than the stereotyped "bone out of place." A chiropractic problem, known as a subluxation or vertebral subluxation complex (VSC), involves an abnormal relationship between two adjacent vertebrae. This is an anatomically complex area known as the motor unit (Figure 23-8). It consists of muscles, ligaments, connective tissue, a spinal nerve and other smaller nerves, blood vessels, lymphatics, and CSF. The hallmark, or "triad" of signs that occur with a subluxation, includes altered mobility, pain on palpation, and abnormal tension in the surrounding (paraspinal) muscles.

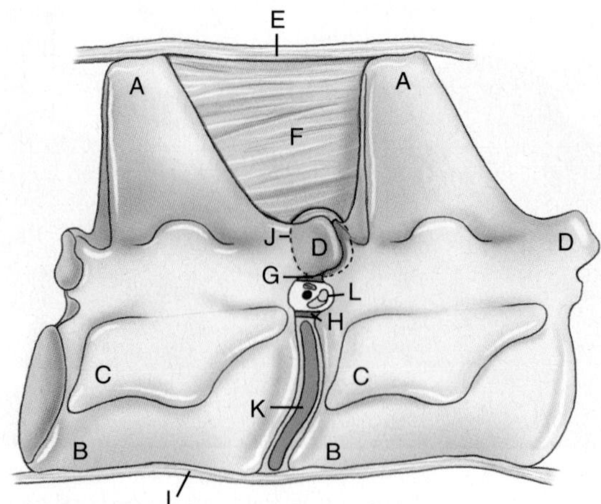

FIGURE 23-8 The motor unit is a complex anatomic and dynamic area that consists of two adjacent vertebrae and the tissues in between. *A,* Dorsal spinous process; *B,* vertebral body; *C,* transverse process; *D,* articular facet joint; *E,* supraspinous ligament; *F,* interspinous ligament; *G,* ligamentum flavum; *H,* dorsal longitudinal ligament; *I,* ventral longitudinal ligament; *J,* joint capsule; *K,* intervertebral disk; *L,* intervertebral foramen.

> TECHNICIAN NOTE A chiropractic subluxation is much more subtle than a partial luxation, or dislocation. It is more a description of function than anatomic position, and thus the disrelationship is not always apparent radiographically. Most often it is discovered by palpation.

There are many explanations about how subluxations occur that have been validated by scientific research. The causes of subluxation can vary from overt trauma to minute repetitive stress to the area, such as abnormal spinal movement secondary to left forelimb lameness. Clinical signs range from mild discomfort to reduced reflexes to serious organ dysfunction. By determining where abnormal motion exists and correcting reduced motion in the spine, we can restore normal biomechanics to the body and reset normal neurologic pathways, thus aiding proper nervous system function. In addition, restoration of full motion in the joints of the limbs can be equally important to maintain spinal health because the body functions as a whole, and all segments are connected.

The chiropractic appointment begins with a clear and detailed history. Hopefully the patient has previously received a thorough "Western" medical work-up before the chiropractic appointment, but this is not always the case. The examination proceeds with observation of posture and gait, palpation of the spinal column and the extremities (limbs and tail), neurologic evaluation, and review of diagnostic images and lab work. It is as detailed (or more so) than a typical general physical examination. Problem areas are recorded, usually using AVCA's notations. This creates a uniform way of communicating with other veterinarians who use chiropractic (much as abbreviations for a CBC or blood chemistry are universally understood).

Once the problem areas are identified, the veterinarian determines whether a chiropractic adjustment is an appropriate therapy for the patient at that time. Sometimes more diagnostics may be required, either in the future or before any adjustment is performed. For example, a horse may have neurologic deficits consistent with equine protozoal myelitis (EPM), and a spinal fluid analysis and EPM test may be indicated. A dog may be seen for lameness, and the veterinarian may find cranial drawer motion in the left stifle, indicating anterior cruciate ligament rupture. In both of these cases, chiropractic may help these patients and could be an appropriate therapy to perform at the initial visit, but other primary therapies are warranted. In some cases, such as when patients have acute paralysis secondary to intervertebral disk disease, it may be more appropriate to obtain further diagnostics (such as radiographs and a myelogram) before adjusting the patient to be sure that any areas of active disk disease are avoided.

The next step is for the veterinarian to adjust the patient. Although treatment principles are similar, each veterinarian has a unique technique that he or she has developed. The AVCA certifies veterinarians who are able to perform the basic techniques, but advanced techniques and variations may be learned. Often it is easiest to treat patients in a standing position (Figure 23-9). However, sometimes a sitting or sternal recumbent position may work better for small animal patients. Cats, in particular, are easier to treat while lying on the treatment table rather than being forced to stand. The best position for a patient is one that is comfortable for the patient.

The veterinarian will check the motion between two spinal segments by applying pressure aligned with the way the joint surface glides. If reduced mobility is found in a given area, the veterinarian takes the motion as far as it will go and applies a short, quick motion in the plane of motion of the joint. Sometimes a popping noise (like someone cracking a knuckle) will accompany the adjustment, although this is more common in people than in animals. The adjustment should generally be painless for the patient, although sometimes a problem area may present some momentary mild discomfort. If a seriously painful area is found, the veterinarian will likely avoid treating that area altogether, at least until further diagnostics have been done. It is important to keep the patient relaxed and make the treatment a positive experience (both for the patient and the client), so all of the problem area may not be corrected in one visit. Following the treatment, the veterinarian will instruct the client on aftercare and follow-up visits in addition to any additional recommendations. Usually, there will be some period of rest or reduced exercise recommended, and massage and stretching may need to be done at home.

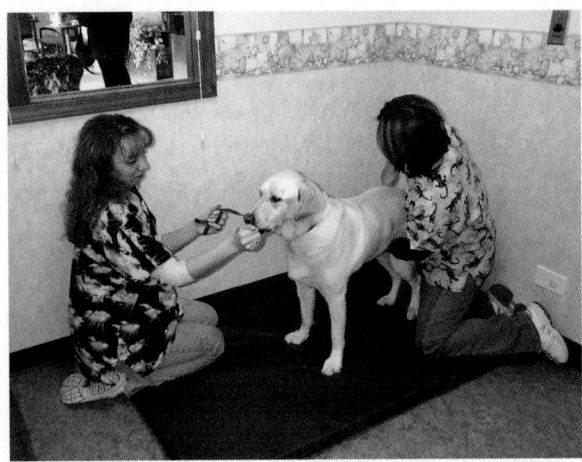

FIGURE 23-9 Chiropractic adjustment: A technician uses food to gently restrain a patient in a standing position while the veterinarian performs an adjustment.

The Technician's Role

Restraint is particularly important for the first-time patient because they are unsure about the process and may be nervous or frightened. Restraint can be simple, such as gentle petting, kind words, or a food distraction (see Figure 23-9). Often a patient may need to be repositioned so that the veterinarian is in the best position to perform the necessary adjustment. Most patients accept and enjoy the treatment, so generally, only gentle physical restraint is necessary. It may, however, be necessary to use more rigorous methods of restraint if the situation warrants. Some canine or feline patients may need to be muzzled (especially if they are regular patients at a general practice—they may be expecting a blood draw or a vaccine rather than a relaxing and comfortable treatment). Some horses will require twitching or hobbling, especially if they are not used to being routinely handled. In a large animal practice, sometimes the technician may be required to stabilize nearby segments so that an adjustment may be more effective or specific. Proper technique is required to provide the most effective treatment and for the assistant's safety. Occasionally, although most veterinarians avoid it, chemical restraint is necessary for some patients to relax enough to receive a safe and effective treatment. This is much more likely to happen early in the treatment program, and most patients will not need to be sedated more than once or twice. The technician should become comfortable with all anticipated restraint techniques before their use because any unfamiliarity or nervousness may contribute to patient anxiety, and it is important for the patient to be as relaxed aspossible. Practicing on the staff's pets is often a good method of developing proficiency in this important role.

In addition to restraining the patient, the technician may also be asked to stabilize certain areas of the spine for the veterinarian to effectively adjust a neighboring segment. This is especially true when assisting with large animals, such as horses. For example, when a veterinarian adjusts T6 in the horse, the technician must stand on the opposite side of the horse in a specific position (both body and hands) to stabilize T5 and T7.

CASE PRESENTATION 23-2 EQUINE HIND LIMB LAMENESS

Signalment: "Anna," a 6-year-old Trakehner thoroughbred mare in training as a hunter and jumper

Chief Complaint: Right hind limb lameness of 3 weeks duration

Pertinent History: Anna was purchased 3 months prior and had been completely sound until she came in from turnout. She was placed on stall rest for 1 week, with 10-minute hand walks twice daily. Initially, her lameness appeared to be in her left rear limb, then 5 days later it was noted in the right rear limb. A prior examination had resulted in no localization of the lameness. Current supplements included glucosamine and MSM.

Significant Examination Findings: Right rear limb lameness with a pronounced hip hike and somewhat shortened stride. Significant back pain with muscle tightness and tenderness in the lumbar spine. No pain was noted in the limb itself, and a thorough examination of her unshod foot revealed no pain or injury.

Problem List:

Right rear limb lameness

Back pain with muscle tightness and tenderness

Reduced spinal mobility particularly in the lumbar region and pelvis

Initial Therapy Plan: A chiropractic adjustment was performed to address the back pain and decreased mobility in the pelvis and lumbar spine, with follow-up pending response. No further treatments were done as a result of the inability to definitively localize the lameness.

Client Communication: The owner was instructed to hand walk Anna for 10 minutes after her adjustment to help loosen her muscles and stimulate her nervous system to "reset" her now improved posture and motion to "normal." She would be allowed short turnout (1 to 2 hours) in a small paddock for the 3 days following adjustment, and if sound at that point could do some walking and trotting on a loose rein for 20 minutes each day until her next visit 7 days later.

Progress: Anna responded favorably to her adjustment, showing significantly reduced lameness the following day. The lameness recurred 3 days later, so she was not ridden, but was still allowed turnout.

The following week, Anna's lameness remained unchanged, and no significant findings were noted in the limb itself. Her back was still a bit tender, but notably improved. Reduced mobility was still significant. Acupuncture was performed before chiropractic adjustment to try to alleviate some of the discomfort and loosen tight muscles. An aquapuncture technique using ½ ml of 50 mcg B_{12} inserted to a depth of ¾ inches at each tender-reactive point (local points around the pelvis: GBBDTC reactive and treated bilaterally; GB 27 and 28 reactive on the right, treated bilaterally; points along the back: BL 20 reactive on the right, treated bilaterally along with BL 21) was elected because of the ease of use and continued pain-reducing effects. Ting points (which are strong points in the feet at the ends of the channels that are used to unblock energy: BL 67 reactive on the right, treated bilaterally) were bled using a 25G ¾-inch hypodermic needle inserted to a depth of ¼ cm. After chiropractic adjustment (pelvis: RPI—Right side Posterior Inferior; lumbar spine: L7 Posterior, L6 Posterior, L4 Posterior Left; thoracic spine: T9 Posterior Left; cervical spine: C6 Body Left, APL—Atlas Posterior Left), the mare was still lame, but had a less pronounced hip hike. The same plan was followed for aftercare, with the understanding that further diagnostics (nerve blocks, possibly nuclear scan) would be indicated if Anna failed to respond favorably to combined therapy.

A follow-up report from the owner indicated that Anna was still sore the day following the treatment, but appeared completely sound on the third day. She maintained soundness all week so was lightly ridden at the end of the week with no relapse. On examination, she trotted soundly with an occasional short stride in the right rear limb, so the lameness was not completely resolved. Far fewer reactive acupuncture points were found (GBBDTC reactive on the right, treated bilaterally; BL 20 reactive on the right, treated bilaterally), and her spinal mobility was much improved. She exhibited minimal back pain, and her muscles were relaxed and supple. After chiropractic adjustment (RPI, L7P, L6P, L1PR, T8PL), she trotted off with excellent balance and symmetry. Her owner was instructed to increase the duration of exercise, with some collected activity at the walk and trot and canter work on a loose rein. She was also taught some stretching exercises to use before riding. Another treatment was scheduled the following week.

By week 3, Anna was working soundly under saddle as recommended. On examination, she walked and jogged without lameness and appeared nicely balanced. Her back was supple and pain free. No reactive acupuncture points were found. A chiropractic examination and adjustment was performed (L7P, L6PL, L3PR). At this point because her lameness had resolved completely, further exercises were recommended to help her maintain balance and strengthen her back (Cavaletti poles, leg yields).

Anna has maintained soundness since her second treatment. Her trainer remarked about how balanced and supple she had become, working much better after her treatments than before the lameness had appeared. She is now adjusted monthly to maintain mobility and help prevent injury and is competing successfully in hunters and equitation.

Discussion: Anna's rapid and complete response to acupuncture and chiropractic is fairly typical of a young horse without significant structural problems. Of greatest significance is that her lameness would have been quite a mystery if she were diagnosed and treated with a Western perspective: there was absolutely no sign of pain in the right rear limb itself. Antiinflammatory therapy may have resulted in temporary soundness, but prolonged use while she was in training could have resulted in permanent structural changes that would have caused further and more serious lameness over time. Early intervention with pain management and the restoration of joint mobility throughout her spine has given her not only relief from her lameness, but also better balance and symmetry than she had initially. This should lead to a longer career and reduced likelihood of injury as long as this mobility is maintained.

The technician's involvement in Anna's case was comprehensive and included assisting with the examination and restraint, preparation of acupuncture materials, segment stabilization for chiropractic adjustment, communication with the client, and demonstration of stretching techniques.

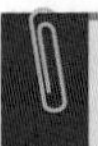

TECHNICIAN NOTE Thorough knowledge of skeletal anatomy is important for assistance with stabilization.

Immediately after the treatment, the technician may be asked to massage the patient, apply essential oils, or walk the patient for several minutes to help the patient "hold" the adjustment. The day after the treatment, the technician may be responsible for making a follow-up telephone call, so it is important to be familiar with expected results and the veterinarian's recommendations for aftercare. It is also helpful to be able to answer commonly asked questions about the examination, treatment, or aftercare. If there is a situation that deviates from the normal response, the veterinarian can be alerted, and the patient can be reevaluated in a timely fashion (Case Presentation 23-2).

PHYSICAL THERAPY AND REHABILITATION (SEE CHAPTER 24)

Physical therapy is a relatively new modality in both the human and animal realm. It has been used with horses and then companion animals for just more than 20 years, and although much has been learned, there is still much that we do not know. Physical therapy or rehabilitation is defined as the use of many modalities to relieve pain, build strength, and reeducate patients to walk in a balanced manner after an injury or illness. Many conditions benefit from physical rehabilitation. Passive range of motion, exercises, and cryotherapy and heat therapy will be touched on briefly, but will be discussed in more detail with all the other modalities of rehabilitation in Chapter 24.

PASSIVE RANGE OF MOTION

Passive range of motion (PROM) is the use of stretching to prevent the loss of normal range of motion, to return normal range of motion if absent, to increase cartilage nutrition in the joint, and to stimulate cartilage regeneration. Most of the nutrition received by the chondrocytes (cartilage cells) comes from the capillary-rich synovial capsule, which then bathes the cartilage via the synovial fluid. If the joint is stationary, the joint fluid is not circulated, and there is less nutrition available to the chondrocytes. In studies done in rabbits, after stabilizing a joint for 7 days, microscopic degenerative changes had already started in the cartilage.

If PROM is to be done postsurgically or in a joint with restricted motion, each joint that is stretched should be done separately. However, when PROM is performed on a patient with a neurologic disorder where it will be used to prevent loss of motion and increase cartilage nutrition and regeneration, each limb is done as a whole. The rules of PROM include:

1. It should never hurt.
2. If the patient is lying on his or her side, keep the limb that you are working on parallel to the ground to prevent torque of the joints.
3. Flex the most proximal joint first and work distally.
4. Do not let the stifle go under the rib cage.
5. Hold the limb flexed for 10 seconds, hold it in extension for 10 seconds (to the front, then 10 seconds to the back), and repeat this 10 times.
6. Massage the muscles you are stretching.
7. Guide the limb, do not pull it.
8. Do not hyperextend the carpus or tarsus because permanent tendon or ligament damage may occur. These joints are flexed and relaxed, unless there is a contracture issue involving these joints.
9. If it is postsurgical PROM, set up your hands on either side of the joint on which you are working (one joint is worked on at a time), and then move your eyes too and keep them on the surgery joint to prevent inadvertent motion of this joint.
10. The hip and shoulder joint have rotation and flexion and extension. Start with small circles and gradually increase the motion performing 10 rotations. Stabilize the distal joints.

The technician can take an active role in PROM, performing this modality under a veterinarian's direction. This can be used successfully in equine and canine patients.

Exercises

Exercises are used for strengthening specific muscles or muscle groups, building endurance, enhancing balance and proprioception, and reeducation of normal posture and gait. Examples of exercises and their purpose are in Table 23-10. Many of these exercises are custom made for the individual patient and condition (Figure 23-10).

It has been shown that a graded exercise program consisting of hand walking and using ultrasound returned horses to racing faster than either stall rest or putting out to pasture.

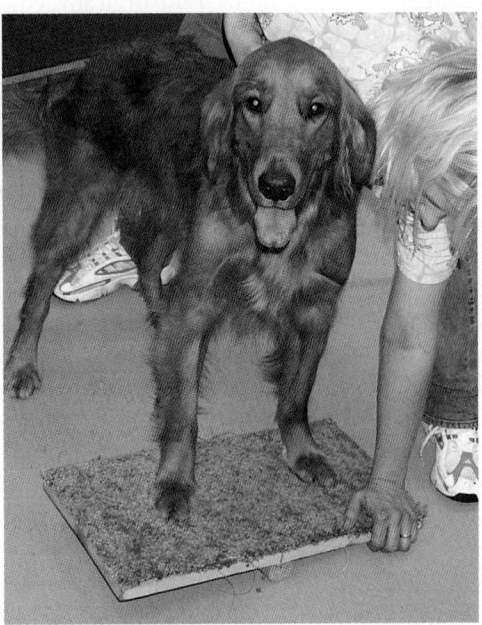

FIGURE 23-10 Exercises—rocker board: Rudy increases his forelimb balance and proprioception on the rocker board.

TABLE 23-10 Exercises

Exercises	Type	Used for
Sit to stand	Strengthening	Rear Limbs
Walking on a hill	Endurance	
Zigzag	Proprioception	Whole body
Parallel to top	Strengthening	Side closest to the top
Balance board	Balance	Limbs on the board
	Proprioception	Limb not on the board
	Strengthening	
Goosing (abdominal contractions)	Strengthening	Posture
Cavaletti poles	Proprioception	Gait training Flexing limbs
Flexing limbs	High-five/wave	Strengthening forelimb

The technician's role in exercises is to lead the patient in doing the exercises or to teach the owner to perform the exercises at home.

Cryotherapy and Heat Therapy

Cryotherapy, or cold therapy, when applied to the body, removes heat. Some of the actions are vasoconstriction, which reduces postsurgical bleeding and bruising (when the cooling agent is removed, there is a rebound vasodilation—red coloration may be seen in the skin); slowed nerve conduction (thereby decreasing pain sensation); and decreased enzyme activity (decreasing inflammation). The first 72 hours after an injury is the destructive phase of inflammation in which only cold and not heat therapy should be used. After that period, heat may be applied between cryotherapy sessions. An example would be 10 to 15 minutes of cold, 10 to 15 minutes of heat, and 10 to 15 minutes of cold up to three times daily. Small patients may require less time. Horses do not need more then 15 minutes of cryotherapy and heat therapy on their limbs. Postsurgically, cold can be applied by filling a Dixie cup three-fourths full and freezing it. The paper is unraveled, and gauze can be placed at the incision to prevent water from contaminating the incision. Commercial CoolPacks are easy to keep in the freezer. Frozen peas can also be used because they are moldable and hold the cold fairly well. A mixture of alcohol and water in a Ziploc freezer bag at a ratio of 2:1 stays cold and malleable. Double bagging is recommended. If the patient is shaved or short coated, wrapping the peas or alcohol bag in a towel may be required. In horses, running a cold hose over an injury is also effective. Therapeutic ice boots are also available for equine extremities. Sweat wraps in horses commonly contain DMSO, Furosin, and dexamethasone surrounded by plastic wrap and a quilted wrap. This is thought to decrease inflammation.

The actions of heat include increasing enzyme activity (beneficial 72 hours after the insult), increasing circulation, increasing muscle contractility, increasing collagen's ability to stretch, and decreasing pain. The recommended method is wet heat. A hand towel, for small areas, or bath towel, for larger areas, may be folded into thirds and rolled (to be unrolled around a joint) or accordion folded to be placed over a flat surface. Run the towel under warm to hot water and apply to the area. If you cannot keep your hand on the towel because it is too hot for you, then it is also too hot for the patient. A big, thick towel or plastic wrap may be placed over the wet towel to keep the heat in. Heat can be applied for 10 to 15 minutes between cryotherapy sessions, preceding exercises to warm up the muscles and joints, or if an area is cold to the touch on examination (signifying a chronic condition with decreased blood perfusion). Heat can also be used over an area of infection once the patient is taking antibiotics to enhance the drug's penetration into the area.

Contraindications

Do not use cryotherapy and heat therapy over areas that do not have sensory sensation because tissue damage may occur.

The technician's role in cryotherapy and heat therapy is to treat the patient and to instruct the clients on home care (Case Presentation 23-3).

MISCELLANOUS THERAPIES

LASER

Laser stands for light amplification by stimulated emission of radiation. Albert Einstein first introduced this concept in 1917. Low level laser therapy (LLLT) is the stimulation of tissue with low-energy lasers to achieve a therapeutic effect. LLLT's most common indications include treating acupuncture points (see Figure 23-5), trigger points, edema, wounds and ulcers, postoperative pain (seen commonly in human dentistry), stomatitis and gingivitis, and temporomandibular joint dysfunction. The lasers most commonly used in LLLT are the visible red helium-neon (HeNe), and the invisible infrared (IR) gallium-arsenide (GaAs) lasers and gallium-aluminum-arsenide (GaAlAs) lasers. Laser beams differ from conventional light because these are monochromic (one color creates a narrow spectrum) and coherent (the waves stay together and are consistent). Most lasers have polarized light (light waves oscillate in the same plane), have a small divergence (nearly parallel beam), and a high mean output power (MOP), indicating that many watts are put out. LLLT may be indicated for soft tissue trauma, wounds, tendinitis, and pain relief (Figure 23-11). Some of the biologic effects seen with LLLT include accelerated cell division, increased leukocyte phagocytosis, stimulation of fibroblasts and collagen formation, and the degranulation of mast cells (which may explain why it can be used in acupuncture because mast cell degranulation occurs when a needle is placed in an acupuncture point).

PRECAUTIONS

Lasers may induce retinal lesions and are therefore classified by their irradiation properties. Class I lasers have a 0.4-mW output (MOP) or less. Class II lasers have 0.5 to 1.0 mW

CASE PRESENTATION 23-3 CANINE INTERVERTEBRAL DISK DISEASE

Signalment: "Sebastian," a 7-year-old neutered male Beagle, 40 lb

Chief Complaint: Quadriplegia 5 days after ventral slot for IVDD at C5-C6

Pertinent History: Sebastian initially became painful 2 days before surgery. He cried when he lifted his head and was reluctant to move. He was examined by his regular veterinarian who took radiographs (which were unremarkable) and started him on prednisone (10 mg b.i.d. 3 days then s.i.d. 4 days). That evening he was more painful, so tramadol was prescribed (50 mg b.i.d.). The following morning, he was swaying while walking, so he was referred to the local emergency clinic, which monitored him over the weekend. Over the weekend, he lost voluntary motion. An MRI was performed by a neurologist, who found a compression at C5-C6. Sebastian was taken immediately to surgery and underwent a ventral slot procedure at the site of disk rupture with fenestration from C2 to C6. He was managed at the emergency clinic for 5 days, with pain control consisting of a fentanyl patch and tramadol 50 mg t.i.d. He was released for rehabilitation 5 days after surgery. His pain patch was removed before transfer. Additionally, he had undergone a femoral head ostectomy (FHO) on his right hip 3 months before presentation (as a result of hip dysplasia).

Significant Examination Findings: Contusion along ventral neck with heat and tight, tender, spastic muscles along the cervical spine; quadriplesia with no weight-bearing ability; crepitus at the right hip with moderate muscle atrophy in the right rear limb. Sebastian was able to maintain a sternal position when assisted to rise from lateral recumbency, but was unable to lift his head more than 2 inches off of the floor.

Problem List

Quadriplesia

Cervical pain post IVDD and decompressive surgery

Muscle spasm, tightness and tenderness along the cervical spine

Heat and inflammation along cervical spine

Contusion along incision line

Crepitus at the right hip secondary to previous FHO

Initial Therapy Plan	Purpose
Acupuncture daily for 3 days, then every other day for 1 week, tapering further as pain subsides with	Pain control, stimulation of healing and nervous system support
Spascupreel	Reduce muscle spasm
Cryotherapy two times daily	Reduce inflammation and pain
Massage 30 minutes daily	Relieve pain and tightness in the muscles, increase circulation to promote healing, stimulate nerve endings
Passive Range of Motion daily	Maintain range of motion, stimulate nerve endings

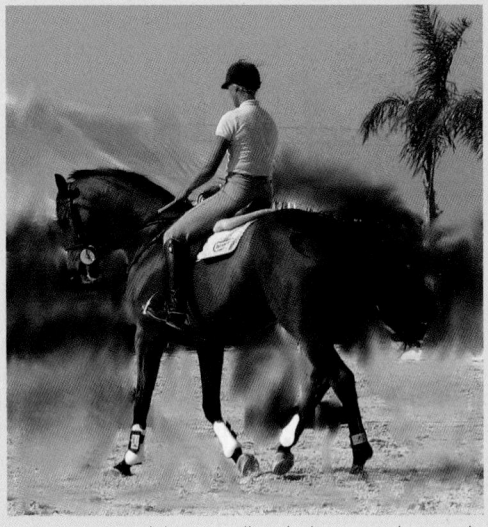

FIGURE 1 Anna exhibits excellent balance and strength with the help of regular chiropractic maintenance.

Initial Therapy Plan	Purpose
Neuromuscular electrical stimulation (NMES)—both triceps and supraspinatus muscles every other day	Promote muscle strengthening passively
Supplements:	
Vitamin C 250 mg b.i.d.	Antioxidant support
Vitamin E 400 IU/day	Antioxidant support
Vitamin B Complex 50 mg/day	Nervous system support
Traumeel 1 tab t.i.d.	Reduce bruising and pain
Discus Compositum 1 tab t.i.d.	Promote neurologic strengthening
Hako-Med electric current therapy daily for 3 days, then every other day for 1 week	Pain relief
Therapeutic exercises with weekly consultations to revise exercise plan	Neurologic stimulation, strengthening, reeducation of ambulation

Client Communication: The recommended therapy plan was presented to the client and immediately approved.

Treatment: Acupuncture was performed with a dry-needle technique (GV 14, Tip of Tail; BL 17, BL 27 to facilitate movement of qi down the governing vessel and bladder meridians that run through the spine; GB 20 and 39 to facilitate qi movement through the gallbladder meridian to the back legs; LI 10 and SI 3 to facilitate qi movement down the front legs) using Hwato needles (22G 1 inch) inserted to a maximum depth of ½ inch. Spascupreel (0.5 ml) was injected subcutaneously at gallbladder 21 bilaterally to reduce muscle spasms near the surgery site (lower cervical spine). Sebastian's urinary bladder was expressed manually until empty. He did not attempt or appear to be able to urinate on his own.

Continued

CASE PRESENTATION 23-3 CANINE INTERVERTEBRAL DISK DISEASE—cont'd

Progress

By the next morning, Sebastian was able to lift his head and support some weight in all four limbs for about 10 seconds. An exercise consultation was done with a physical therapist to determine what exercises would be appropriate for him. He still needed assistance to attain a sternal position from lateral recumbency, but did make an attempt. He needed assistance to attain and maintain a sitting and standing position. He continued to progress daily his first week and by the end of the week was able to move from a lateral to a sternal position unassisted, stand with only balance support for 1 minute, and was attempting to take steps with all four limbs (although he lacked coordination). Irritation at the pain patch site and at his incision was resolved, but his muscle spasms persisted, and his neck was sore at the end of the day. He had also started to urinate on his own, with excellent bladder awareness and control.

The following week, Sebastian continued to progress to increased weight-bearing activity, improved coordination to the point where ambulation training could be initiated, and comfort was improved, and muscle spasms had resolved. Pain management was greatly reduced (Tramadol, Traumeel, and Spascupreel were discontinued; Hako-Med therapy was also discontinued). After surgical staple removal, hydrotreadmill therapy was initiated with great success: Sebastian moved all four of his limbs independently with reasonable coordination.

At the beginning of week 3, Sebastian was able to transition from a down position to standing and could walk for several minutes with balance support. His right rear limb was the weakest partly as a result of his already present atrophy after his FHO surgery, so neuromuscular stimulation was changed to work on his right quadriceps, hamstrings, gluteals, and digital extensors. By the end of week 3, Sebastian was able to walk unassisted, negotiate a course of weave cones, small stairs, poles on the ground, and gentle hills.

Sebastian continued to progress, with ongoing acupuncture, hydrotreadmill therapy, and a home exercise program. Within 6 weeks after the initial injury, he was running and playing with no restrictions. After 3 months, he had regained enough strength in his right rear limb to be almost completely balanced and symmetrical.

Discussion

Sebastian's remarkable progress was largely due to compassionate holistic care. His response to therapy was dramatic and fairly rapid, but the treatments themselves only partly contributed to the speed of his recovery. He received intensive pain management and appropriate exercise to facilitate neurologic healing. He was kept in a nurturing environment where he received extra attention and got sufficient rest and a healthy diet. He was taken outside to eliminate at least four times daily and was encouraged with his favorite treats and toys. Sebastian was treated as an individual with specific needs that we strived to meet each day, and this holistic focus was what made the difference in his successful recovery.

In Sebastian's case, technicians played a fundamental role in his therapy and general care. In addition to assisting with the examination and acupuncture treatments, they took a primary role in performing cryotherapy, Hako-Med, massage, PROM, NMES, and exercises. They also were responsible for communication with the client and nursing care. This is an excellent example of how crucial technician care can be in returning a critically ill or injured patient to health and mobility.

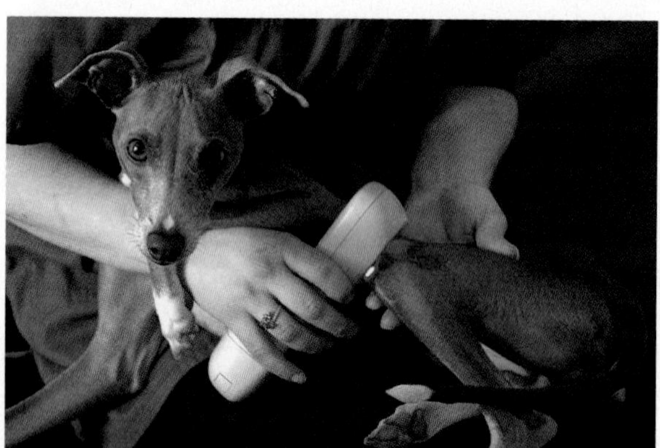

FIGURE 23-11 Laser Q-1000.

MOP, and if they shine in your eyes, a blink reflex is usually adequate to prevent retinal damage. A Class IIIa laser has 1 to 5 mW MOP, which means caution must be used near the eyes because retinal damage may occur if it is directed into the eye (even if the lid is closed). Class IIIb lasers have 5 to 500 mW MOP and are considered dangerous to the eyes. A class IV laser has greater then 500 mW MOP and is dangerous to the retina (special glasses must be worn at all times when the laser is in use) and a potential fire hazard. These are usually surgical lasers. Class III and above lasers are often only used by the veterinarian.

> *TECHNICIAN NOTE* Some of the biologic effects seen with LLLT include: accelerated cell division, increased leukocyte phagocytosis, stimulation of fibroblasts and collagen formation, and degranulation of mast cells.

MAGNETS

Magnets have been used for centuries in medicine. Magnetism can be separated into stationary magnets, which have a north and south pole, and electromagnetic therapy, which uses electricity of different frequencies along with magnets to create an electromagnetic field. The units of measurement for magnetism are gauss (G) and tesla (T). Most therapeutic magnets range from 1000 to 3000 G. Below 500 G has been deemed ineffective. The north and south poles of a magnet are reported to have different effects. The effects of using the north pole end of the magnet include pain relief, stimulation of bone healing, the enhancement of vasoconstriction, decreased blood pressure, and, by decreasing mitosis, slowing the growth rate of cancer cells and bacterial cells. The effects of using the south pole side of the magnet include strengthening and promoting growth by stimulating cell multiplication (therefore should not be used with bacterial or viral infections or close to tumors), enhancement of vasodilation, slowing bone healing, and increasing ascites, edema, and inflammation. Some therapeutic magnets have both north and south poles that may be held on a given area or wrapped over an area. Products are available that place magnets in horse blankets or leg wraps and dog and cat beds and collars.

In electromagnetic therapy, pulsating electromagnetic waves are produced by electrical charges undergoing acceleration. These waves can be generated with different frequencies and can create different physiologic changes in the body. For instance, it is known that there is an electrical field around each joint that plays a part in the continual regeneration of cartilage and connective tissue. There is a disturbance in this field if osteoarthritis or inflammatory joint disorders are present. Pulsed signal therapy (PST) is one type of pulsed electromagnetic field therapy (PEMF) (Figure 23-12). This allows reconstruction of the disturbed electrical field, which returns the natural regeneration capabilities and reactivates the chondrocytes (cartilage cells) and connective tissue to increase production of proteoglycan and collagen, which aids in repairing cartilage defects. Most of the research has been done in osteoarthritis, but there have also been significant improvements after treating many other conditions, including tendon and ligament injuries (this should not be used in partial cranial cruciate tears because the scar tissue is important in joint stabilization and this removes early scar tissue) and wound healing. PEMF has been used extensively in equine sports medicine for musculoskeletal and neurologic conditions. It has been used successfully to treat navicular disease, tendon injuries, arthroses, spavins, delayed wound healing, and diseases of the thoracolumbar spine. Artificial insemination centers also use PEMF on bulls that suffer from degenerative lumbosacral diseases to extend their productive capacity.

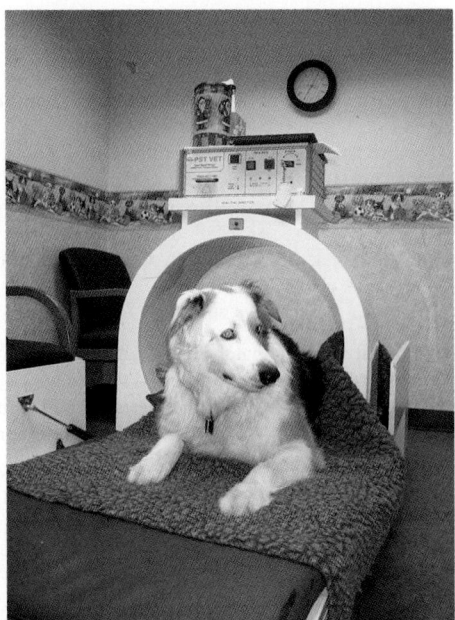

FIGURE 23-12 Dog in the PST: PST has an 80% to 85% success rate of treating osteoarthritis with good to excellent results. Since there is a 13-inch treatment area, often feet, hocks, stifles, hips, and lower back can be treated at the same time.

The technician's role in magnet therapy is to answer questions the clients may have, apply stationary magnets to the patients, and to position and sit with patients during PEMF therapy (see Figure 23-12).

> *TECHNICIAN NOTE* Most therapeutic magnets range from 1000 to 3000 G. Below 500 G has been deemed ineffective.

TTouch Wrap or Anxiety Wrap

TTouch is part of TTEAM, which is mentioned in the massage section (Figure 23-13). TTouch for small animals has various massage and other techniques to affect an animals well-being. A certification course is offered for both technicians and lay people. We will not review all of the techniques, but will discuss a method used for calming anxious dogs and helping dogs whose front and rear limbs seem like they are on two different dogs. Effects are usually seen within 5 to 10 minutes. An ace bandage is folded in half, and the halfway mark is applied to the chest. The ends are wrapped up over the chest, tied in a knot, wrapped around the abdomen, up and knotted over the back, and can be wrapped around the rear limbs (Figure 23-14). This technique can be applied before exercises, before working with anxious dogs, or to help dogs with separation or thunderstorm anxiety.

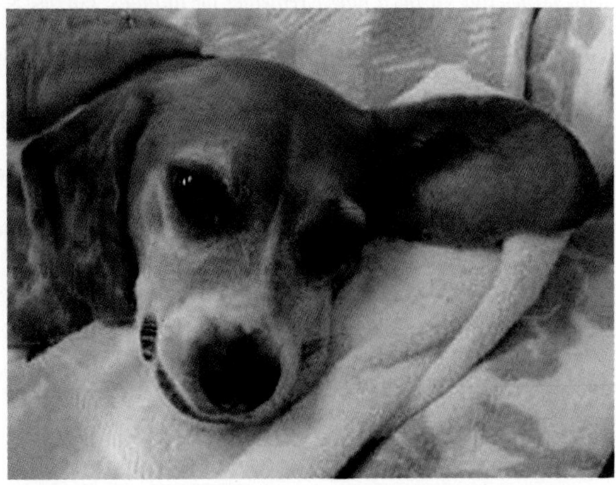

FIGURE 23-13 Sebastian: "the little Beagle that could."

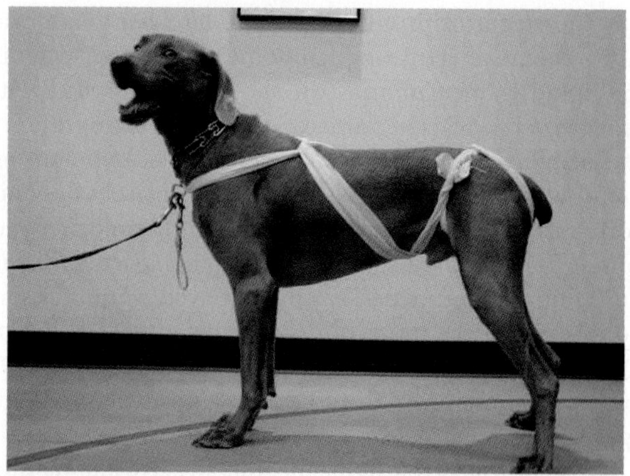

FIGURE 23-14 Dog wearing a TTouch wrap to assist calming.

CONCLUSION

Complementary and alternative veterinary medicine encompasses a vast amount of material. This chapter offers an overview of some of the more common modalities used today and not a comprehensive guide to alternative medicine. Many of the individual subjects discussed in this chapter have their own texts written on the subject and are taught in courses lasting months to years. The technician may become the "clinic expert" in many of these modalities (i.e., massage or flower essences) and can be a good source of information for the client in the other modalities (i.e., acupuncture and chiropractic therapy). As many clients are looking into alternative medicine for themselves, they are seeing the benefits and are looking into sharing the experience with their animals. There are numerous opportunities to be a part of the thrilling and gratifying fields of complementary and alternative medicine. Additionally, as more veterinarians are becoming certified in these areas, the employment opportunities will continue to grow.

RECOMMENDED READINGS AND REFERENCES

Books

Gersh MR: *Electrotherapy in rehabilitation*, Philadelphia, 1992, F.A. Davis.

Graham H, Vlamis G: *Bach flower remedies for animals*, Forres, Scotland, 1999, Findhorn Press.

Michlovitz SL: *Thermal agents in rehabilitation*, ed 3, Philadelphia, 1996, F.A. Davis.

PDR People's desk reference for essential oils, 1999, Essential Science Publishing.

Pitcairn R, Hubble Pitcairn S: *Dr. Pitcairn's complete guide to natural health for dogs and cats*, ed 2, St Martin's Press.

Pontinen PJ: *Low level laser therapy as a medical treatment modality*, Tampere, Finland, 1992, Art Urpo.

Salvo SG: *Massage therapy principles and practice*, St Louis, 2003, WB Saunders.

Schoen AM: *Veterinary acupuncture: ancient art to modern medicine*, St Louis, 1994, Mosby.

Schoen AM, Wynn SG: *Complementary and alternative veterinary medicine: principles and practice*, St Louis, 1998, Mosby.

Schwartz C: *Four paws five directions: a guide to Chinese medicine for cats and dogs*, Berkley, Calif, 1996, Celestial Arts Publishing.

Tisserand, Balacs: *Essential oil safety: a guide for health care professionals*, 1995.

Wynn SG, Marsden SM: *Manual of natural veterinary medicine: science and tradition*, St Louis, 2002, Mosby.

Wulff-Tilford M, Tilford G: *All you ever wanted to know about herbs for pets*, Irvine, Calif, 1999, Bowtie Press.

Journals

Haussler KK: Chiropractic evaluation and management, *Veterinary Clin North Am, Equine Pract* 15.1:195-207, 1999.

Videos

Schreiber M: *Sports massage for the equine athlete*, Equissage, telephone: 800-843-0224.

Vaughn L: *Body works for dogs*, Animal Healing, Pound Ridge, NY, telephone: 877-929-1515. Available at www.animalhealing.com.

Whalen-Shaw P: *Canine massage: an instructional guide*, Integrated Touch Therapy, telephone: 800-251-0007.

Contacts

Musculoskeletal Therapies for Animals, Madison, WI, telephone: 866-646-8684, www.MTAvet.com.

Hako-Med Systems: Contact person: Ken Becker, telephone: 843-572-0708, www.hako-med.com.

Professional Organizations

Academy of Veterinary Homeopathy: www.theavh.org

American Holistic Veterinary Medical Association: www.ahvma.org, telephone: 410-569-0795

American Veterinary Chiropractic Association: www.animalchiropractic.org, telephone: 918-784-2231

International Veterinary Acupuncture Society: www.ivas.org

Veterinary Botanical Medicine Association: www.vbma.org

International College of Applied Kinesiology: www.icak.com

Massage Schools

Equissage: Round Lake, Va, www.equissage.com, telephone: 800-843-0224

Healing Oasis: Sturtevant, Wis, www.thehealingoasis.com, telephone: 262-878-9549

Integrated Touch Therapy Inc: Circleville, Ohio, www.integratedtouchtherapy.com, telephone: 800-251-0007

TTEAM training USA, PO Box 3793 Santa Fe, NM, telephone: 800-854-TEAM

TTEAM training Canada, 5435 Rochdell, Vernon, British Columbia, Canada, telephone: 604-545-2336

Rehabilitation Training

Animal Rehab Institute, Loxahatchee, Fla and Aspen, Colo, www.caninerehabinstitute.com, telephone 561-792-6889

North East Seminars/University of Tennessee, www.NESeminars.com

The Healing Oasis, Sturtevant, Wis, www.thehealingoasis.com

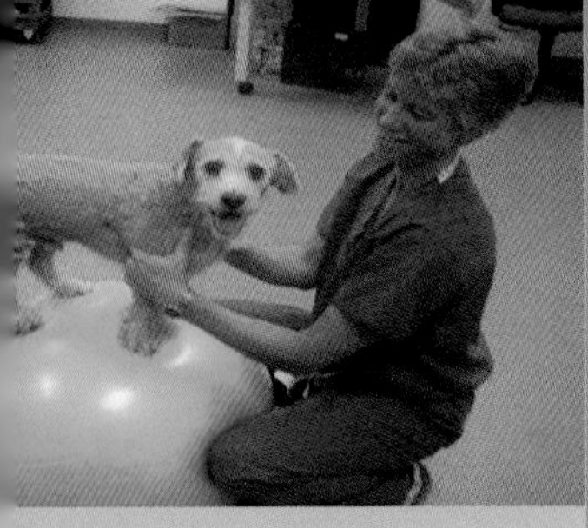

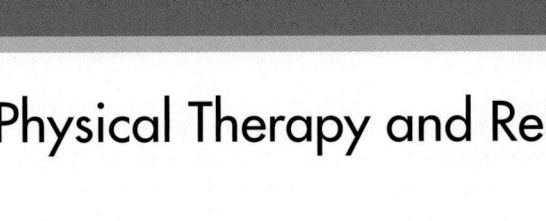

Physical Therapy and Rehabilitation 24

Caroline Adamson Adrian and Robert A. Taylor

KEY TERMS

Accessory motion
Active assisted range of motion
Active range of motion
Aquatic physical therapy
Bursae
Bursitis
Closed kinetic chain exercise
Cryotherapy
Electrical stimulation
Flexibility
Goniometer
Goniometry
Hydrotherapy
Hypermobile joint
Hypomobile joint
Joint mobilization
Ligament
Massage
Modality
Open kinetic chain exercise
Palpation
Passive range of motion
Proprioception
Range of motion
Sprain
Strain
Tendinitis
Tendon
Thermal agents
Ultrasound (therapeutic)

OUTLINE

LEARNING OBJECTIVES

When you have completed this chapter, you will be able to:

1. Differentiate between rehabilitation and physical therapy.
2. Describe the roles of the members of the animal rehabilitation team.
3. Describe the goals of and indications for use of physical therapy in animals.
4. List and describe the five elements of patient management in physical therapy.
5. Describe legal issues related to the practice of physical therapy.
6. List services commonly offered by physical therapists.
7. Differentiate between passive, active, and active-assistive exercise.
8. Describe the principles of hydrotherapy and explain methods to provide hydrotherapy to animal patients.
9. Define proprioception and give examples of proprioceptive activities performed with animal patients.
10. List supportive and assistive devices used with animal patients.
11. List and describe commonly used physical therapy modalities.
12. List common classifications of strokes used for myofascial manipulation.
13. Describe considerations in the design of training or conditioning programs for canine athletes.
14. Differentiate between orthotics and prosthetics.
15. Define common terms related to physical therapy and rehabilitation.

INTRODUCTION

The field of physical therapy (PT) in veterinary medicine is a rapidly expanding topic of interest. In 2007 , CareerBuilders named veterinary PT as one of the top 10 fastest growing professions in the United States.[1] This heightened interest within both the PT and veterinary medical professions is the result of client and consumer demand, increased longevity of our canine companions, and a higher level of surgical and medical sophistication. Patients with a pneumothorax, lymphoma, or neurologic condition all can benefit from PT. Of interest to many general practitioners is the large number of older, obese, and arthritic dogs. Many of these animals can benefit from muscle strengthening, improvement of joint range of motion, and weight control. PT can improve their quality of life and return them to the highest level of function after injury or disease.

This chapter is intended to introduce you to the field of PT and its application on animal patients. By no means is this a comprehensive chapter on the application of PT techniques nor is this a cookbook guiding the reader on the application of these techniques. For those interested in understanding more about the profession of PT, a reference and resource list is included at the end of this chapter.

HISTORY OF PHYSICAL THERAPY

The field of human PT has an extensive international history. If you travel back in time, different forms of PT were used centuries ago. Hippocrates was an advocate of massage, and Hector used aquatic therapy in 460 BC.[2] The first documented origin of PT as an established profession dates back to 1894 when the Chartered Society of Physiotherapy was formed in England.[3] PT began in the United States in 1914 in Portland, Ore., by a small group of female nurses with a physical education background. At this time, graduates of Reed College and the Walter Reed Hospital were called "reconstruction aides," a program that developed out of a need to manage the devastating injuries from World War I. Called the American Women's Physical Therapeutic Association, the first professional association was formed in 1921 with 274 members.[2] This was a landmark year because educational standards for university professional PT programs were instituted and programs became accredited by a national body. Scientific research and technology started to shape the profession.

By the end of the 1930s, membership grew to just under 1000, men were admitted, and the chapter changed its name to the American Physiotherapy Association. Ten years later, the official name changed to the American Physical Therapy Association (APTA) that opened its doors to their first office in New York City with a full-time staff.[2]

With the advent of World War II and a nationwide polio epidemic during the 1940s and 1950s, physical therapists were in greater demand than ever before. The Association's membership swelled to 8000, and the number of PT education programs across the United States increased from 16 to 39. The first two association sections, school and private practice, were created to promote and develop specific objectives within the profession.[2]

By the 1960s, membership in the APTA grew to 15,000, and education programs offered in the country expanded to 52. Today, headquartered in Alexandria, Va., APTA represents more than 75,000 physical therapists and physical therapist assistants nationwide. The goal of this association is to continue to foster advancements in PT practice, education, and research. There are currently 180 institutions that offer PT education programs, and 236 physical therapist assistant education programs are offered in the United States.[2]

THE PROFESSION OF PHYSICAL THERAPY

You may be familiar with the terms "rehabilitation" and "physical therapy." Rehabilitation is a more broad term that includes the processes of education and treatment for disabled individuals as a result of disease or injury that causes mental or physical impairments. PT is a more specialized term under the broader scope of rehabilitation. In the human realm, rehabilitation may include a variety of professionals, including a physiatrist (MD specializing in rehabilitation medicine), an occupational therapist, speech therapist, recreational therapist, and a physical therapist.

> TECHNICIAN NOTE *Rehabilitation* is a broad term that includes the processes of education and treatment for disabled individuals as a result of disease or injury that causes mental or physical impairments. *Physical therapy* is a more specialized term under the broader scope of rehabilitation.

AMERICAN PHYSICAL THERAPY ASSOCIATION

According to the APTA, PT is defined as "a dynamic profession with an established theoretical and scientific base and widespread clinical applications in the restoration, maintenance, and promotion of optimal physical function."[2] The terms physiotherapy and physiotherapist are synonymous with physical therapy and physical therapist, respectively.

Physical therapists started to move beyond hospital-based practice in the 1950s. However, the majority of them continued to practice in a hospital setting through the 1960s. Today, physical therapists practice in a wide variety of settings to include outpatient orthopedic clinics, public schools, geriatric settings, skilled nursing facilities, factories and the workplace, outpatient rehabilitation and medical centers, and hospitals.

Physical therapists provide their services to patients with impairments, disabilities, functional impairments, or those with "changes in physical function and health status resulting from injury, disease, or other causes."[2] Physical therapists also interact and collaborate with a variety of different professionals; assess risk factors that may negatively impact optimal functioning; prevent and promote health, fitness and wellness; educate and provide consulting services to other businesses or health facilities; engage in research; and supervise and direct PT services to include support personnel. Today, physical therapists continue to strive for scientific-based medicine, and key elements of the past remain the same focus in our profession today to include practice, teaching, and research.

Areas of expertise are designed to promote lifelong learning and professional development. APTA's special-interest sections were established to give members additional exposure to others who share their specific interests. Over the years, these specialties have continued to expand to a total of 18 special-interest sections, which include acute care; aquatic PT; cardiovascular and pulmonary; clinical electrophysiology and wound management; education; federal PT; geriatrics; hand rehabilitation; health, policy, and administration; home health; neurology; oncology; orthopedic; pediatrics; private practice; research; sports PT; and women's health.[2] Within each of these sections fall any number of special interest groups (SIGs) that focus on specific areas of PT practice. For example, within the neurology section of the APTA lie six SIGs: balance and falls, brain injury, degenerative diseases, spinal cord injury, stroke, and vestibular rehabilitation. Currently the animal physical therapist special interest group lies within the framework of the orthopedic section of the APTA.

THE PROFESSION OF PHYSICAL THERAPY FOR ANIMALS

In the past, there was little attention paid to postoperative care, and many animals were lost to follow-up following suture removal. This coupled with the notion that the animal would use the limb when it felt "good" and the reluctance on the part of veterinarians to urge early mobility were factors that limited the use and concept of PT. Despite recent advances, there are still veterinary surgeons that routinely immobilize their postoperative cranial cruciate repair patients for 4 to 6 weeks using casts, braces, or splints. Early motion has been shown to be efficacious in hastening recovery and limiting the effects of disuse on bone, cartilage, ligaments, and tendons.

Today's current challenge is to prove that PT is as meritorious in the dog as it is in the human. There are many new studies done in man demonstrating the value of PT on earlier recovery, resumption of a normal lifestyle, return to athleticism, and enhanced quality of life. However, there have been a few studies on animals. Some of the first and most notable are Johnson and Johnson's work on early use of electrostimulation[4]; Levine and Millis' work on goniometry,[5] and Steiss on ultrasound.[6] The recent interest will only stimulate new areas of investigation and research. One of the most recent articles was published in the *Journal of the American Veterinary Medical Association* in 2007 entitled "Treatment of Traumatic Cervical Myelopathy With Surgery, Prolonged Positive-Pressure Ventilation and Physical Therapy in a Dog."[7]

> TECHNICIAN NOTE *PT* is defined as a dynamic profession with an established theoretical and scientific base and widespread clinical applications in the restoration, maintenance, and promotion of optimal physical function.

GOALS OF PHYSICAL THERAPY

The goal of PT is to return the affected area and the animal back to its prior level of function. This may be accomplished by: (1) Reducing pain and accelerating healing of injured and inflamed neurologic and musculoskeletal tissues; (2) maintaining or restoring normal range of motion in affected joints of the forelimb, hind limb, or spine; (3) preventing fibrosis or soft tissue contractures in injured, weak, or paralyzed limbs; (4) preventing disuse atrophy (i.e., preserving muscle mass) of an affected limb during the healing phase of neurologic or musculoskeletal insults; (5) gaining strength and improving function in weak or paralyzed limbs; (6) providing a positive psychologic effect maximizing both the patient's and owner's well-being; (7) educating and providing the owner with individualized home-care programs to maximize the animal's functional mobility and preventing injury to the owner. Any one or a combination of these goals may be employed throughout the rehabilitation phase.

INDICATIONS FOR REFERRAL TO PHYSICAL THERAPY

Many veterinarians ask what type of patients may benefit from PT. Indications for referral to a physical therapist may be categorized by a specific pathologic condition or by a PT diagnosis (Box 24-1). Orthopedic cases may include those animals suffering from neurologic conditions or osteoarthritis, hip dysplasia, or tendinitis. Many are postoperative patients that have undergone a total hip replacement, bicipital tendon release or femoral head osteotomy, an arthrodesis or amputation, cruciate surgery (intracapsular or extracapsular procedures), or a fracture repair. General conditions may include delayed unions, geriatric support care or strengthening, and conditioning or weight loss programs. Wounds, such as degloving injuries, lick granulomas, and decubitus ulcers, are also rapidly resolved with rehabilitation. PT diagnoses focus more on a specific musculoskeletal problem. The list may include gait abnormalities or other movement dysfunction, pain and inflammation, decreased strength and endurance, joint stiffness, or loss of range of motion.

THE IMPORTANCE OF THE PHYSICAL THERAPIST EVALUATION

APTA's *Guide to Practice* (2001) describes the integration of five major elements in patient management. These elements include examination, evaluation, diagnosis, prognosis, and intervention.[8] Keeping these elements in mind, the ultimate goal of systematically carrying out these guidelines is to provide the best, most individualized, and effective quality of care for each patient. By conducting a comprehensive examination, the physical therapist is able to generate an accurate neuromusculoskeletal diagnosis. This allows the physical therapist to optimize the patient's outcome and choose the most appropriate plan of care to reach those outcome goals.

> TECHNICIAN NOTE The *neuromusculoskeletal evaluation* allows the physical therapist to optimize the patient's outcome and choose the most appropriate plan of care to reach those outcome goals.

BOX 24-1 Common Conditions Referred to Physical Therapy

Orthopedic Conditions
Geriatric support care
Tendinitis
Osteoarthritis
Patellar luxation
Osteochondritis dissecans

Postoperative
TPLO/TTA/extracapsular cruciate repairs
Arthrodesis
Fracture repair
Total hip replacement
Amputation
Femoral head osteotomy

Neurologic Conditions
Fibrocartilaginous embolism
Degenerative myelopathy
Chronic back or neck pain
Hemilaminectomy/laminectomy
Peripheral nerve disease
Lumbosacral disease
Increased tone, decreased conscious proprioception
Decreased voluntary motor function
Ataxia/uncoordinated gait
Balance/vestibular disorders

Other Conditions
Conditioning
Weight loss—diet and exercise
Wellness programs—injury prevention
Muscle strain and/or sprains
Patients in the critical care unit
Nonsurgical CCL rupture
Contractures
Fibrotic myopathy

Wound Care
Lick granulomas
Degloving injuries
Decubitus ulcers

Examination refers to the thorough screening of a patient and includes the history, tests, measures, and systems review.[8] *Evaluation* is the clinical judgments made by the PT diagnosis and is directed more at neuromusculoskeletal deficiencies rather than a specific medical condition or disorder.[8] For example, a veterinarian's diagnosis may be a ruptured cranial cruciate ligament, whereas the physical therapist's musculoskeletal diagnosis is muscle atrophy, movement dysfunction, pain, and inflammation. A *prognosis* is a prediction of the level of improvement and how long it will take to reach those levels.[8] Goals are established as part of the plan of care along with expected outcomes, level of predicted improvement, and interventions to be used, including duration and frequency. The *interventions* are the actual treatment techniques and procedures consistent with the diagnosis to improve a patient's condition.[8] A variety of physical therapy interventions will be discussed later in this chapter.

As with all evidence-based practice, it is the physical therapist's responsibility to provide appropriate, effective, and comprehensive quality of care to our animal patients and estimated prognoses for the clients. As mentioned, the proven effects of PT demonstrated in man are inferred when transferred to the dog. Much work needs to be done to prove that PT is as meritorious and beneficial in animals, and documentation is the key.

By measuring, assessing, and reevaluating, the physical therapist is able to determine how the animal is progressing or regressing and change the treatment plan as appropriate. Is the chosen intervention nearing the outcome goals? Do changes need to be made in the plan of care? This information is also vital when improving or changing protocols and justifies treatment and benefits for the owner. Documentation allows us to objectify our efforts, teach and/or perform research, chart progress or lack thereof, provide a continuity of care, prevent medicolegal issues, and show proof of success.

LEGAL ISSUES

You will notice the terms physical therapy and physical rehabilitation have been used interchangeably throughout this chapter. Inconsistent language stems from individual state practice acts that define physical therapy differently across the nation. Each state owns the right to legally define physical therapy and regulate its practice.

For example, in the state of Colorado, the term *physical therapy* is not a protected term. In other words, anyone providing this type of service may deem it physical therapy. However, calling oneself a *physical therapist* implies that you have gone through a rigorous training program in an accredited PT school and have passed the national licensure examination. Thus the term *physical therapist* may only be used by those holding a PT license. However, in California, both the terms *physical therapy* and *physical therapist* may only be used by those individuals possessing a license to practice PT. As a result of the nature of individual practice acts, the term physical rehabilitation will be used throughout the remainder of this chapter.

Laws, in general, are in place to protect the consumer and the patient. With the field of animal physical rehabilitation continuing to blossom, regulations and policies will continue to expand to ensure that providers of physical rehabilitation services are competent. In Colorado, the veterinarian is the gatekeeper for animal care and in the past, the one solely responsible for conducting and directing patient care and the ultimately legally responsible party. The veterinary practice act stated that anyone could work under the direction of and on-site premises of a veterinarian. The PT practice defined PT as the *examination, treatment, or instruction of human beings* to detect, assess, prevent, correct, alleviate, or limit physical disability, movement dysfunction, bodily malfunction, or pain from injury, disease, and other bodily conditions. As of July 1, 2007, the PT Practice Act, through 3 years of legislative lobbying efforts, was changed to read "clients and patient" in place of "human beings." With this change,

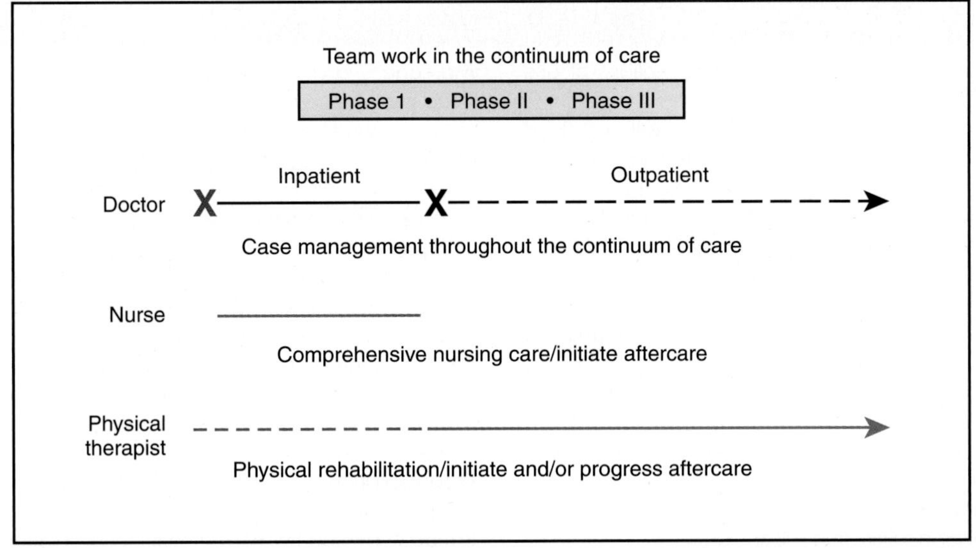

FIGURE 24-1 The ideal collaborative approach. (Courtesy Jackie Woelz, MS, PT University of California, Davis.)

comes the capability of a more comprehensive collaborative approach to patient care. With a veterinary medical clearance, instead of a referral, a physical therapist is now able to treat animal patients without direct supervision, in any environment desired, including home care. In addition, physical therapists are now responsible for half of the legal liability for treating offsite should a malpractice suit arise.

Under Colorado law, the veterinary technician must be under direct, on-site supervision of a veterinarian when performing tasks related to animal care. As a licensed or certified veterinary technician, you may not examine, evaluate, or develop a plan of care for an animal. In addition, most states require direct supervision of a technician by a veterinarian. Thus it is imperative that you are familiar with and abide by your state's physical therapy and veterinary medical practice acts before performing any type of physical rehabilitation.

TECHNICIAN NOTE It is imperative that you familiarize yourself with your respective state's physical therapy and veterinary medical practice acts before performing any type of physical rehabilitation.

TEAM APPROACH AND THE ROLE OF THE VETERINARY TECHNICIAN

A number of differently trained professionals may be involved in animal rehabilitation. They include veterinarians, physical therapists, veterinary technicians, and physical therapist assistants (PTAs). Ideally, animal rehabilitation is a collaborative effort between the veterinarian and the physical therapist, with additional assistance from the veterinary technician and the PTA. The degree of supervision and amount of autonomy for the veterinary technician and PTA will vary by state for each of these professionals according to state laws and regulations related to their individual practice.

BOX 24-2 Examples of a Physical Therapist Diagnosis or Neuromusculoskeletal Problem List

- Decreased range of motion and flexibility (soft tissue, joint)
- Decreased endurance and mobility (pneumothorax, obesity, osteoarthritis)
- Decreased strength
- Abnormal movement/gait patterns (ataxia, partial/non-weight bearing)
- Muscle atrophy (disuse, neurogenic)
- Contracture (prevention)
- Pain (acute or chronic)
- Inflammation
- Neurologic dysfunction
- Scar tissue (retard growth, break down)
- Muscle guarding and/or spasm
- Joint stiffness
- Depression

In the continuum of care (Figure 24-1), the veterinarian clears the animal of any zoonotic or concomitant disease and recommends PT. The veterinarian provides medical management and has the knowledge and expertise regarding the pathophysiology of the injury or problem. The role of the physical therapist is direct patient care. The physical therapist is responsible for performing the PT evaluation, predicting outcome goals, and delivers and progresses the rehabilitation according to an individualized care map, or protocol. The physical therapist interprets the results of the examination and uses the results as a guide to establish a PT diagnosis, or problem list (Box 24-2) and the patient's prognosis. This would also include developing realistic goals and a plan of care for that individual patient. Many aspects within the PT plan of care are delegated to the veterinary technician and PTA who serve to assist the physical therapist in the provision of PT. The degree of direction and supervision will depend upon the individual's education, experience, and

BOX 24-3 Key Terms in Physical Therapy

Accessory motion—the spin, roll, and gliding motions of one joint surface on another
Active assisted range of motion (AAROM)—patient is assisted manually or mechanically to achieve a normal range of motion when the prime muscle mover is weak or injured
Active range of motion (AROM)—ability of a patient to voluntarily move a limb through a range of motion
Aquatic physical therapy—specific treatment interventions using a water-filled pool
Bursae—fluid-filled sacs that decrease friction between structures
Bursitis—inflammation of bursae
Closed kinetic chain exercise—an exercise in which the distal limb segment is fixed
Cryotherapy—therapeutic techniques to decrease tissue temperature; cold therapy
Electrical stimulation—the use of electricity to stimulate soft tissues to facilitate healing and reduce pain
Flexibility—ability of a limb to move through a specific range of motion
Goniometer—tool used to measure joint range of motion
Goniometry—technique used to measure range of motion at a joint
Hydrotherapy—use of water for therapeutic effects
Hypermobile joint—excessive motion at a joint
Hypomobile joint—less than functional range of motion at a joint
Joint mobilization—specific passive movements applied to joint
Ligament—structure that connects bone to bone
Massage—varying types of manual strokes applied to the body to promote relaxation, decrease pain, or increase circulation to surrounding tissues
Modality—a wide group of agents that may include thermal, acoustic, radiant, mechanical, or electrical energy
Open kinetic chain exercise—an exercise in which the distal limb segment is free
Palpation—the sense of touch used to assess what structures lay below the skin and presence of potential injury to those structures
Passive range of motion (PROM)—that joint movement obtained by a therapist moving a limb with no assistance from the patient may include thermal, acoustic, radiant, mechanical, or electrical energy
Proprioception—awareness of body position and movement in space
Range of motion (ROM)—movement at a joint
Sprain—excessive stretching of a ligament
Strain—excessive stretch of a muscle that may cause tearing of the muscle fibers
Tendon—structures that connect muscle to bone
Tendinitis—inflammation of a tendon
Thermal agents—tools used to modify tissue temperature and change blood flow to surrounding tissues
Ultrasound (therapeutic)—tool used to modify tissue temperature and change blood flow to surrounding tissues through the application of high-frequency sound waves

responsibilities of the involved parties. Veterinary technicians and PTAs with additional education are competent to perform many delegated aspects of patient care, to include assessment, reassessment, and intervention techniques. With this combined effort, effective rehabilitation can get an animal "back on all fours" in no time.

LEARN TO TALK LIKE A PHYSICAL THERAPIST

As in any new professional endeaver, there arise differences in terminology. To help acquaint you with the PT profession, Box 24-3 lists many of the key terms used by physical therapists.

PHYSICAL THERAPY INTERVENTIONS

PT interventions include a variety of components. From admittance through discharge, the physical therapist is responsible for coordinating, communicating, and documenting the patient's physical rehabilitation needs to ensure appropriate, comprehensive, and effective quality care. Other interventions may involve client-related education, instruction, and procedural interventions. Procedural interventions may include therapeutic exercise, manual therapy techniques, supportive or assistive devices, airway clearance techniques, integumentary repair and protection techniques, physical

BOX 24-4 Common Services Offered in the Physical Therapy Department

Client education/individualized home-care programs
Custom orthotics and prosthetics
Cart fittings/assistive devices
DEXA scanner—body fat composition
Manual therapy
Myofascial manipulation
Neuromuscular reeducation
Computerized gait analysis—two- or three-dimensional
Pain management
Hydrotherapy
Wound care
Therapeutic exercise: spinal stabilization techniques, balance and coordination, strength, and appropriate progression of exercise plan
Modalities: low-intensity laser therapy, cold and heat modalities, ultrasound, electrical stimulation, extracorporeal shock-wave therapy of tissues

agents, and electrotherapeutic and mechanical modalities. See Box 24-4 for a more comprehensive list of services offered by physical therapists.

Education and *home-care programs* are necessary to provide the owner with a way to become involved in their

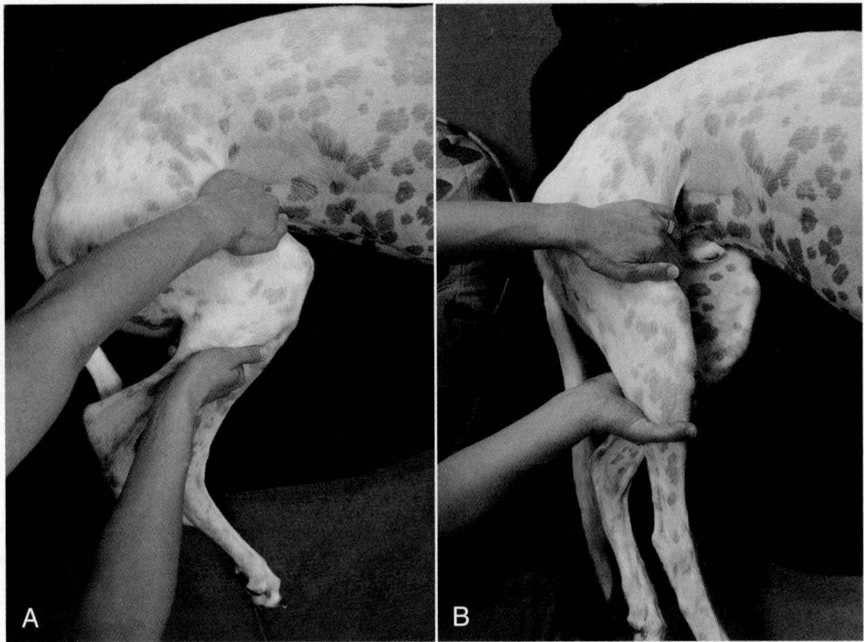

FIGURE 24-2 A, Passive range of motion exercise in flexion. B, Passive range of motion exercise in extension.

animal's rehabilitation phase. The program is individualized to each animal's needs and is progressed accordingly. Topics may include information on surgical procedures or pathologic conditions, specific therapeutic exercises, clients' education and/or recommendations on how to care for the animal without injury to the owner or further injury to the animal.

> *TECHNICIAN NOTE* Educating the client on surgical procedures or pathologic conditions, specific therapeutic exercises, and recommendations on how to care for the animal without further injury become important in daily physical rehabilitation routine.

Therapeutic exercise, limited only by one's imagination, plays a large role in rehabilitation and is the most cost efficient. Exercises may be structured according to the outcome desired, such as improving balance, coordination, endurance, strength, or flexibility. Exercise may be separated into passive, active-assistive, and active. **Passive** exercise mimics the normal muscle pumping action to improve blood flow and sensory awareness in affected limbs. It requires movement from an external force (e.g., gravity, a machine, or a person). There is no voluntary muscle contraction on the animal's part. Passive exercise may be used when an animal is unable or not supposed to actively stress a body segment, in the presence of inflammation, or when active range of motion is painful. It helps to maintain soft tissue and joint integrity, enhance synovial movement for cartilage nutrition and diffusion of joint materials, and minimizes the potential for contracture formation. When performing passive range of motion exercises, the joint in question must be supported from above and below (Figure 24-2).

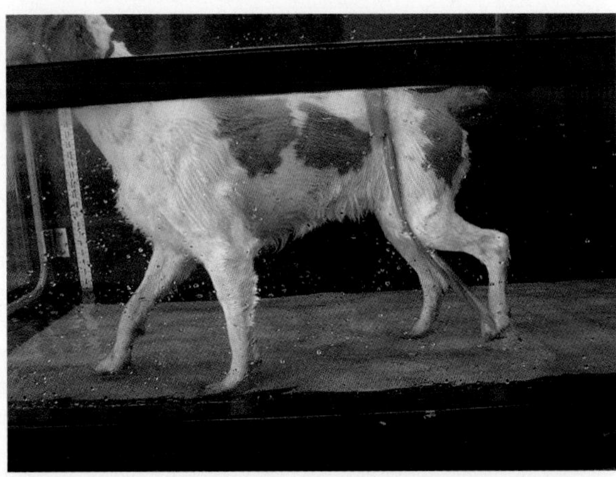

FIGURE 24-3 Use of Thera-Band to assist dorsiflexion and avoid knuckling of the right hind limb throughout the entire gait cycle.

Follow the joint through a comfortable range of motion by slowly and gently flexing and extending. Ten to 15 repetitions are typically sufficient for one treatment session and repeated three to four times per day. Passive range of motion is *not* a stretch, and range of motion should never be forced.

Active-assistive exercise requires an outside force to assist with the range of motion (Figure 24-3). Whether mechanical or manual, the outside force must assist the animal in achieving range of motion against gravity. Because of weakness or disease, the prime mover muscles require some degree of assistance to complete a full range of motion. This type of exercise is usually prescribed for gentle stretching or for a weak body part.

Active exercises produce movement by active muscle contractions (Figure 24-4). The patient is able to move its body part independently against gravity throughout a range

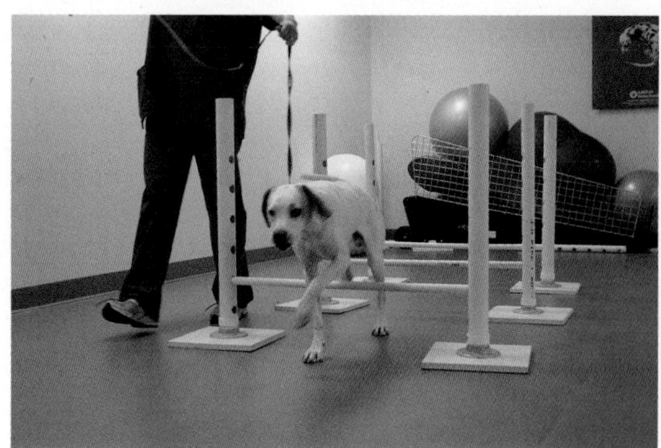

FIGURE 24-4 One example of active exercise using Cavaletti rails. Note the increased balance, coordination, strength, and flexibility this animal is demonstrating during this exercise.

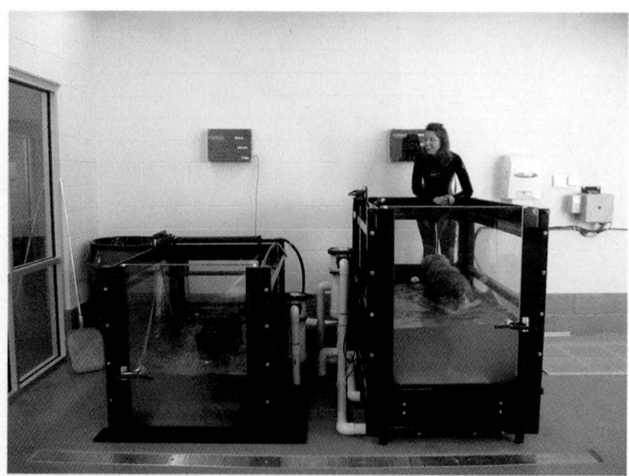

FIGURE 24-5 UTs used in physical rehabilitation.

of motion. Active exercise serves to increase muscle strength, cardiovascular function, and coordination. It maintains physiologic elasticity and contractility of involved muscles, provides sensory feedback from contracting muscles, and provides a stimulus for bone and joint integrity.

Hydrotherapy, via lakes or streams, an underwater treadmill (UT), pool, or whirlpool, is capable of reducing gravity, thus decreasing concussive forces on joints to allow earlier intervention and faster recovery times. Water provides resistance throughout the entire range of motion providing a closed chain exercise. The warm water assists in pain reduction and acceleration of the healing process. Older animals are capable of exercise effectively without undue stress. Water height is adjustable for the amount of desired weight bearing and capable of adjusting for different sized dogs.

> *TECHNICIAN NOTE* Hydrotherapy may be used not only for rehabilitation, but also for wellness, weight loss, conditioning, and recreation.

Hydrotherapy uses five inherent properties of water (thermal, buoyancy, hydrostatic pressure, cohesion, and turbulence) to help strengthen, improve lung capacity, and increase blood flow. Thermal properties are provided by heated units, most notably an indoor pool and UT. Temperature ranges from the low 80° F to the low 90° F. Thermal properties allow for superficial heating of the involved limbs, increasing circulation to help decrease pain, relax skeletal muscle, and increase flexibility. Buoyancy is the upward thrust of water that is created when a patient is submersed, producing a decrease in body weight. Buoyancy will counteract weight allowing for modified ambulation when weight bearing is contraindicated or limited. In addition, for neurologic patients, buoyancy helps the body regain a vertical position if a patient is tipped from the midline. While the animal is submersed, pressure is exerted by stationary fluid on the body. This phenomenon is called hydrostatic pressure. The amount of pressure will increase with depth, allowing increased circulation in the extremities and a reduction in edema. The cohesion property is explained by water molecules adhering to one another. The greater the cohesive forces, the greater the viscosity, in this case, water. A force is required to separate the molecules. This adds resistance to the limbs while the animal is moving through water. Finally, many of the hydrotherapy devices are equipped with jet systems. These jets provide a certain velocity of water at a given point that varies in magnitude and direction. When moving a body through water, turbulence is created causing a greater resistance during movement. The amount of turbulence may be increased by adding the jet system to the treatment session. Turbulence also offers a superficial massage to the area targeted by the jet system.

The most common forms of hydrotherapy in animal physical rehabilitation are UTs and pools. In the UT (Figure 24-5), dogs may walk comfortably on the treadmill without the "panic" of not being able to touch the bottom, as in a pool. Small dogs can even swim with adequate turning radius in an UT. UTs provide a more controlled, less erratic environment for more specific rehabilitation. However, should a dog exhibit an abnormal gait pattern, that pattern may be exacerbated and worsened by continued exercise in the UT if not addressed.

Most UTs have clear doors and windows for excellent viewing of an animal's gait pattern. A digital display shows speed, distance, and time, allowing for appropriate documentation during rehabilitation. These treadmills are typically large enough for one to two therapists and the canine patient in the water at the same time. This becomes important in the case of the neurologic patient that is unable to walk independently.

A pool (Figure 24-6) allows for a more erratic, less controlled environment, unless the activity is better controlled by a rehabilitation therapist entering the pool with the animal. Waders, wet suits, or even scrubs may be worn in a pool while providing assistance to the animal. Potential for increased injury to the animal exists if the patient is allowed to run around the side of or jump into the pool. The pool tends to be used later in the rehabilitation plan of care, as the animal is capable of higher levels of active exercise.

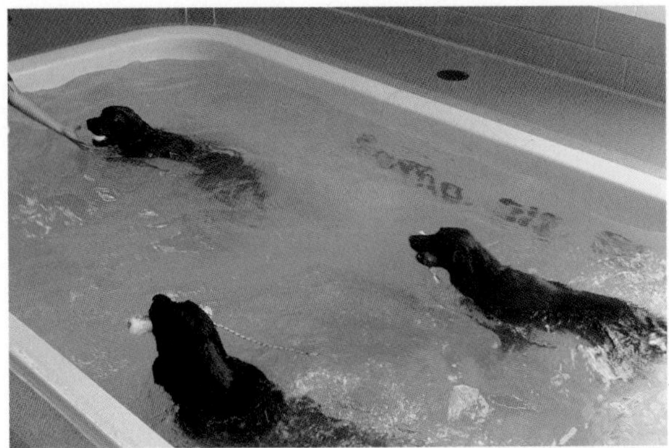

FIGURE 24-6 A pool may be used for recreation or rehabilitation.

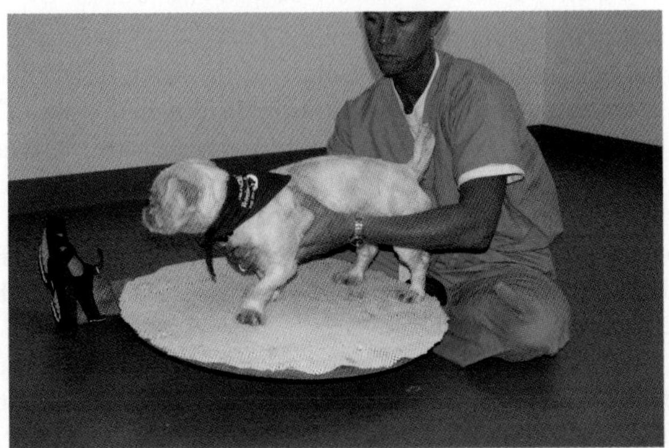

FIGURE 24-7 A balance board helps stimulate proprioceptive input.

Proprioceptive rehabilitation is a concept commonly overlooked in a patient. **Proprioception** refers to the conscious awareness of limb motion and position in space. Joint capsules, ligaments, synovium, and fat pads all contain a variety of highly specialized receptors that respond to varying types and degrees of sensory stimuli. Proprioceptive activities include exercises that facilitate rapid muscle contractions, focusing on closed kinetic chain exercises, and improve dynamic stability. Such examples may include a balance board, Theraball, figure eights, ambulating across couch cushions or different surfaces (Figures 24-7 and 24-8).

> *TECHNICIAN NOTE* Proprioception is conscious awareness of one's body position in space and is a concept commonly overlooked in rehabilitation for animals.

Manipulations and *mobilizations* may also be applied to decrease pain, restore pain-free functional range of motion, or increase flexibility in hypomobile joints. A manipulation is a passive motion of any kind as a form of treatment for musculoskeletal disorders. A manipulation pertains to all forms of passive movement, including mobilization. Manipulations are applied in a gentle fashion, with small changes in range of motion and are rarely forceful. A mobilization is

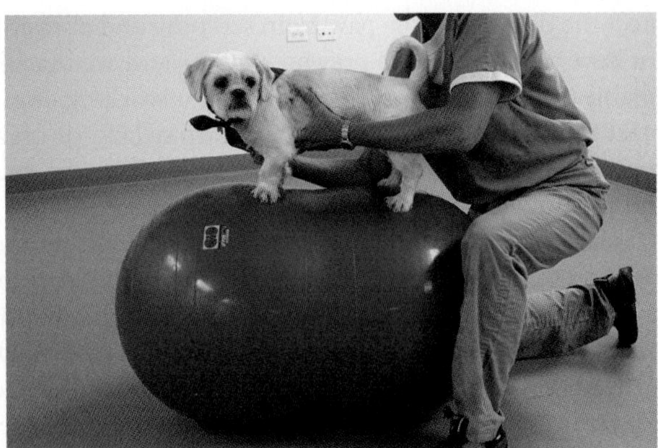

FIGURE 24-8 A therapy ball used to increase proprioception.

also a passive movement, typically an oscillatory movement that produces a sustained stretch on a particular joint.

A physiologic movement is a motion that a patient actively performs himself (flexion, extension, abduction, adduction). However, to have full physiologic range of motion, a joint must possess full accessory movements. Accessory motions are the movements of a joint that contain spins, rolls, and glides. Each type of joint possesses different combinations of accessory movement. Restrictions of accessory joint motion may limit normal physiologic movement and cause pain.

It is because of the complex nature of joints and the specific knowledge gained through extensive training in manual therapy that the application of manual techniques is limited to only licensed physical therapists. If done improperly, damage, in some cases severe, to the joint may be produced.

> *TECHNICIAN NOTE* Because of the complex nature of joints and the specific knowledge gained through extensive training in manual therapy, the application of manual techniques is limited to licensed physical therapists only.

Supportive and *assistive devices* can play an important role in the overall well-being of the animal patient with neurologic or orthopedic impairments. In addition to providing increased independence for the pet, these devices can provide additional autonomy for the owner. They provide support to a weak or nonfunctioning body part and may assist with rehabilitation. They can also help to prevent decubitus ulcers from forming, increase an animal's mobility, and prevent future complications in recumbent patients. Supportive devices may range from a single orthotic to protect an animal from knuckling to proper fitting for animals in need of a hind limb cart. These devices are available in a variety of forms: boots, slings, and two-wheeled and four-wheeled carts.

Boots

Boots are an ideal way to protect the feet when conscious proprioceptive deficits are present. Boots will act as a sock-like covering that is securely fashioned by a Velcro strap to protect the dorsum of the paw from scraping and abrasions. Most have a rubber sole to prevent slipping and are machine washable. These boots may also be used for working dogs to protect the feet from glass and other sharp debris, or on active dogs on long hikes, protecting them from jagged rocks and the elements.

It is important to remember to remove the boots periodically to preserve skin condition and it is advisable to remove boots before rehabilitation treatment. When performing therapeutic exercise, remove the boots to increase weight bearing and proprioception through the bottom of the pads. If not removed, these boots will decrease the amount of sensory input through the bottom of the paw in neurologically impaired patients. If not fitted properly, these boots can interrupt circulation, become cumbersome, and impede gait patterns or strides, potentially causing increased injury if the animal stumbles and falls. It is imperative that the proper size is ordered and appropriate instructions for skin care and rehabilitative exercises are communicated to the owner.

When choosing the proper boot, make sure that they are machine washable, waterproof, or water resistant. Be sure that they are manufactured out of durable material to prevent quick wear and tear and that they have a secure tread on the bottom to prevent slipping. Old socks may be considered for indoor use. However, exercise caution when securing the top with tape to prevent interrupting circulation.

Slings

Slings come in a variety of shapes, sizes, and manufacturers. Some may be wrapped around the belly or fitted around the forelimbs or hind limbs. They are equipped with long hand-held straps to prevent personal injury for the handler when supporting their pet. These devices aid the handler in transitioning a recumbent animal and assist with ambulation to prevent falls on slippery floors, especially after surgery to prevent further injury to the animal. Support slings are also available for forelimb assistance and patients with amputations or to reduce the weight on the front quarters after forelimb surgeries or injuries.

It is important to customize the size of the harness for the utmost safety and comfort of your patient. A wide variety of sizes are available, and they come conveniently designed for both male and female patients. With forelimb slings, the neckline should not obstruct respiration, and urine flow should not be compromised in the hind limb slings. A fleece or soft lining is recommended against the animal's skin to prevent skin breakdown. Be cautious that the sling is not too narrow in diameter, especially around the groin and belly region, to prevent occlusion of vital arteries and nerves in addition to rubbing and skin irritation. Should these devices become soiled, most can be machine washed.

Carts

At times, total body support is necessary and may be achieved through two- and four-wheeled carts, or canine wheelchairs (Figure 24-9). These carts provide additional support of either hind limbs or all four limbs, independence for both owner and animal, and prevention of the deleterious effects of a continual recumbent position in downed dogs. The frames are lightweight, and some harnesses are designed to distribute weight throughout the entire mass of the dog, rather than concentrated in one area of the body (such as over the scapulae). The pneumatic wheels make it easy for a dog to traverse a variety of terrains, such as small curbs, rocks, roots, and grass.

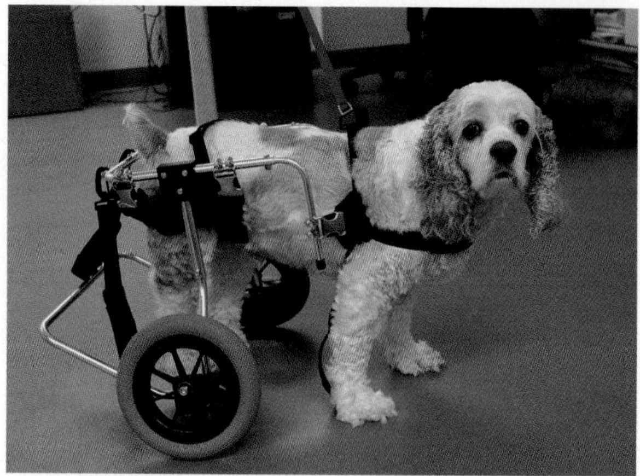

FIGURE 24-9 Dog fitted in a Doggon Wheels canine cart.

Carts are not intended to be used in place of a physical rehabilitation program. If fitted too early in the rehabilitation phase, the animal and owner may become too dependent on the cart's support and replace the rehabilitation program completely. The client must be encouraged to continue a home-care program to maximize neurologic return and maintain active movement as long as possible.

The transition into a cart should be a positive experience for the animal. Familiarize yourself with the cart and its parts before placing an animal in the device to prevent unnecessary stress on the animal. Animals should be supervised at all times when in a cart to avoid concern that they may fall out of the cart, tumble down a flight of stairs, or tip over or become stuck on a household or lawn object. Food bowls may need to be elevated; however, animals should have no problem eating in these carts. Frequent rest periods out of the cart are necessary, especially for larger dogs, because it is difficult for the animal to lie down and rest comfortably while placed in the cart.

MODALITIES

The term **modality** identifies a wide group of agents that may include thermal, acoustic, radiant, mechanical, or electrical energy. The goal of these modalities is to produce physiologic changes in tissues for therapeutic purposes. Modalities may include **cryotherapy** or heat therapy that act to decrease pain and inflammation, relax skeletal muscles, reduce muscle spasm, and decrease joint stiffness. **Ultrasound** may be used as a deep-heating agent that converts electrical energy into high-frequency sound waves. It is beneficial for problems such as muscle spasm and contractures and effective in accelerating wound healing, causing vasodilation and reducing pain. **Electrical stimulation** promotes muscle reeducation, slows muscle atrophy, and reduces pain and edema. Low-intensity laser therapy, in the form of infrared energy, acts to locally stimulate the production and release of nitric oxide concentrations. Nitric oxide has been shown to accelerate wound healing, decrease pain, retard scar tissue formation, and increase bone density. When documenting the use of a modality, the agent and the parameters used (intensity, duration, and frequency) must be included in the animal's medical record. In addition, treatment time, location of the body where the treatment was applied, and any other special notes or instructions must be documented. These may include whether the animal's fur is shaven or unshaven, any skin abnormalities, or any unusual reactions from prior treatments.

> TECHNICIAN NOTE When documenting the use of a *modality,* the agent and the parameters used (intensity, duration, and frequency) must be included in the animal's medical record.

Cryotherapy may be applied in a number of ways. Cold packs, ice massage, cold baths, and cold compression units are common cryotherapeutic modalities used to treat pain and inflammation. Cold transferred to the patient's skin, muscle, and tissue has several beneficial therapeutic effects. Vasoconstriction of the blood vessels in this localized area causes a decrease in the inflammation, thus reducing pain and swelling by anesthetizing the area, slowing nerve conduction velocities, and reducing the amount of painful chemical mediators. Cold also decreases hemorrhage (via vasoconstriction) and edema as a result of decreased histamine release. Muscle spasm caused or exacerbated by pain, ischemia, or muscle tension is also reduced by interrupting the pain cycle, and in neurologic patients, spasticity may be reduced. Cold application may be indicated in musculoskeletal trauma and in postsurgical cases.

Contraindications to the application of cold include frostbite, compromised circulation, improper thermoregulatory responses (in the very young and very old patient), and hypersensitivity to cold. Caution must be exercised when performing rapid exercises immediately after cold application because of the reduced speed of muscle contractions as a result of slower nerve conduction velocity.

Heat Therapy

Physical therapists may wrap a hot pack in several layers of towels and place them on the area in need of treatment. Hydrotherapy and ultrasound may also be used as a heating modality. The heat provided by these thermal agents causes vasodilation, or an increase in local circulation and metabolism. This causes an increase in permeability of capillaries and the lymphatic system to help reduce tissue swelling. Heat helps relax tight skeletal muscles, decreases pain, reduces muscle spasm, and decreases joint stiffness by increasing tissue extensibility.

Caution should be exercised over dermatologic conditions or infection, which may be exacerbated by moist heat.

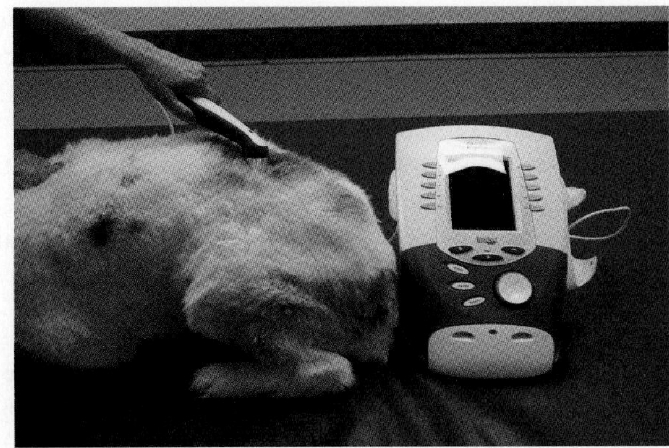

FIGURE 24-10 Ultrasound may be applied for thermal or nonthermal benefits.

Vascular insufficiency, lack of sensation, application over bony prominences, and dogs on long-term steroids (thinner skin, fragile capillaries) are also considerations to keep in mind when applying heat. Avoid laying the animal directly over a hot pack because this will increase the amount of pressure, thus increasing the amount of heat applied to one area and the potential for burns.

Ultrasound

Ultrasound is the use of high-frequency sound waves that are produced by vibration of a membrane (e.g., vocal cords). When a synthetic crystal vibrates at a certain frequency (as a result of its specific shape and geometry), the crystal contracts and expands when exposed to an alternating current. Ultrasound, at a frequency of 1 MHz, may penetrate tissues from a depth of 2 to 5 cm. At a frequency of 3 MHz, tissue penetration is 0.5 to 2 cm.

Ultrasound may be applied for thermal or nonthermal purposes (Figure 24-10). Thermal indications for ultrasound include an increase in metabolic rate, enzyme activity, circulation, and tissue extensibility and a decrease in pain. The biologic effects of ultrasound involve increasing joint range of motion (improve flexibility), tissue healing, collagen extensibility, decrease muscle spasm, joint adhesions, tendon repair, and retardation of scar tissue formation. Using the nonthermal parameters of ultrasound helps to reduce muscle spasm and pain, accelerate healing, aid in tissue regeneration and repair of soft tissue, and reduce swelling.

Ultrasound should never be applied over pacemakers, eyes, malignancy, infected wounds, areas of decreased circulation and sensation, thrombi, a pregnant uterus, carotid sinus, or exposed spinal cord (hemilaminectomy or laminectomy). Care should be taken when applying ultrasound over bony prominences, implants (including plastic), major nerves and arteries, and over epiphyseal plates in young animals.

When ultrasound is applied, parameters will be chosen by the physical therapist. The technician must ensure that the area to be treated is shaven, especially when applying thermal parameters. Protein in the hair coat may absorb the heat emitted from the ultrasound head and potentially produce burns. Be sure the skin is cleaned with alcohol. Use a water-soluble gel with the application of the sound head. Never apply ultrasound without a conducting medium. Immersing the sound head in water is an effective treatment method for uneven skin surfaces. Be sure to hold the transducer head ~0.5 cm away from the area to be treated. The treatment area should be no larger than twice the size of the transducer head.

> *TECHNICIAN NOTE* Ultrasound should never be applied without using a water-soluble get. Water immersion of the sound head may be used for uneven skin surfaces. Hold the transducer head ~0.5 cm away from the area to be treated.

Electrical stimulation

Electrical stimulation (ES) is the application of an electrical current to stimulate nerves, muscles, and soft tissue (Figure 24-11). ES comes in many forms: neuromuscular ES (NMES), functional ES (FES), and transcutaneous electrical nerve stimulation (TENS) are some of the more common types. Electrical stimulation is used to enhance muscle performance, retard muscle atrophy, increase strength and range of motion, accelerate wound healing, reduce pain and edema, and enhance transdermal administration of medications (called iontophoresis).

There are numerous electrotherapy devices sold on the market, making use and selection of these devices quite confusing. The physical therapist must have a clear understanding of the desired outcome from the ES device and an accurate and in-depth knowledge of the appropriate parameters to choose in regards to treatment intensity, frequency, voltage, and current type.

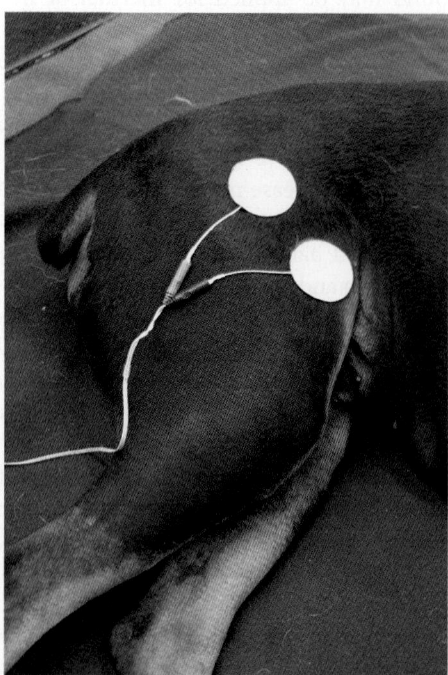

FIGURE 24-11 A dog receiving electrical stimulation to its quadriceps muscles.

When applying ES interventions, the physical therapist will choose the appropriate parameters. In preparation, fur or hair may need to be clipped to lower impedence. If the fur is short enough, simply wetting it down may be enough to achieve an adequate current. Skin should be cleaned to remove excess dirt and debris. ES requires constant supervision of the animal to prevent electrode migration. Parameters used with electrical stimulation intervention are defined below.

Frequency—pulses per second (PPS), Hertz (Hz) or pulse rate

Waveform—different current types (AC, DC, medium frequency, etc.); usually asymmetrical or biphasic

Pulse or phase duration—measured in microseconds; duration of a phase or pulse

Amplitude—intensity of the machine output

On-off time (duty cycle)—amount of time the stimulator is delivering a current versus rest time, usually measured in seconds

Ramp—(rise/decay time) allows current amplitude to build slowly (2 to 4 seconds)

Treatment time—15 minutes is an average treatment time, cycling through the duty cycle

Electrical stimulation should never be used over a neoplasm or infection site, skin lesion, carotid sinus, pacemaker, peripheral vascular disease, areas of analgesia, or an abdomen during pregnancy.

Low-Level Laser

The term, Equi-Light therapy, is synonymous with Anodyne. Equi-Light is used when referring to the application of a low-level laser on animals and Anodyne when applying this modality on human patients. Equi-Light is a low-intensity laser, or monochromatic infrared energy (MIRE) source, emitting a wavelength of 890 nm. At 890 nm, Equi-Light is capable of stimulating the local release of nitric oxide from hemoglobin. Nitric oxide has been shown to be beneficial in many capacities, notably one of the most natural vasodilators. It allows an increase in circulation to facilitate wound and soft tissue healing, increases lymphatic flow, decreases pain by stimulation of endorphin and enkephalin production, and retards and breaks down scar tissue.

This modality has shown promising results for human patients in treating decubitus ulcers, sprains, tendinitis, fasciitis, deep tissue bruising, rotator cuff injuries, fractures, and arthritic pain. It has been studied on horses for the treatment of wounds, pressure sores, and laminitis. Many promising results in dogs are proven to include the treatment of decubitus ulcers, lick granulomas, and delayed unions with other applications, such as generation of cartilage in osteoarthritic dogs, still being investigated in ongoing clinical trials.

Contraindications to Equi-Light therapy include its use over any active malignancy, over or near a pregnant uterus, or directly over a topical heating agent, such as BenGay (McNeil-PPC, Morris Plains, N.J.) or Icy Hot (Chattem, Inc.,

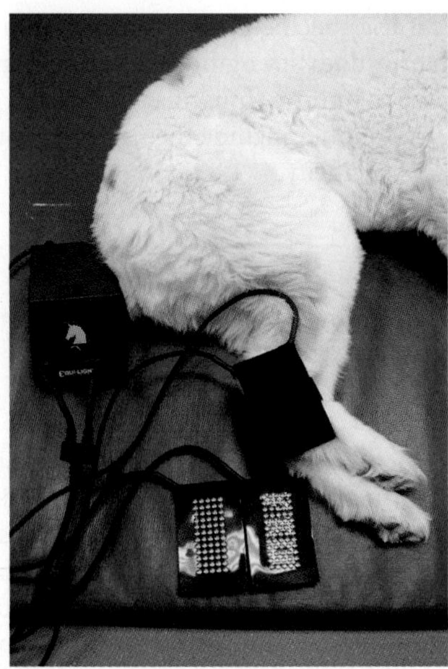

FIGURE 24-12 A patient demonstrating the use of Equi-Light to accelerate healing in open sores.

Chattanooga, Tenn.). Equi-Light may be used over metal implants, pins or screws, pacemakers, and defibrillators because of the absence of electrical current or deep heat with this device.

There are many devices on the market that employ a variety of wavelengths of photo energy. The term photo or light therapy must not be mistaken for monochromatic infrared energy. Photo or light therapy, is visible energy. Therapeutic monochromatic infrared energy sources are found just outside of the visible wavelengths on the light spectrum. At this specific wavelength (890 nm) of infrared light, photo dissociation of nitric oxide from hemoglobin has been proven. Currently, there is no evidence that other phototherapeutic devices affect serum nitric oxide levels in this manner.

Initially, Equi-Light was given FDA clearance for human use in 1994 to enhance circulation and reduce pain. The Equi-Light consists of a two- or four-pad flexible diode treatment pad configuration (Figure 24-12). Treatment times vary from 20 to 45 minutes, with constant monitoring of the animal treated to prevent pad migration.

MASSAGE

Touch is one of the most powerful forms of nonverbal communication. Myofascial manipulation, or **massage,** increases blood flow and lymphatic drainage to injured tissues. Specific techniques may be applied to stretch tendons and ligaments to decrease the potential for fibrosis and contractures.

> TECHNICIAN NOTE *Classifications of massage* contain several types that can be performed in a soothing or a stimulating manner, depending on the pressure and the rhythm applied.

Technique

When considering applying massage techniques, be sure to place the animal in a quiet room with minimal to no distractions. Place the animal on a soft blanket or pad and observe the temperament. Begin with gentle palpation of the dog's body. Do you feel muscle tightness (hypertonicity), increased or decreased tissue temperature, abnormal texture (warts, lumps, lipomas) or tenderness?

Begin with gentle, slow rhythmic strokes, preferably along the length of the muscles and following the direction of fur. Your speed of stroke will depend on the purpose or goal of the massage. Generally a massage will last 20 to 45 minutes, depending on the animal's tolerance.

During massage techniques, watch the animal for signs of discomfort, overstimulation, or pain. Should the dog attempt to move away, gently bring it back and begin again with less manual pressure. If a dog flinches during a technique, again reduce pressure and change the stroke.

Classification of Massage Strokes

Each class listed below contains several types of strokes, all requiring additional training, and each can be performed in either a soothing or a stimulating manner, depending upon the pressure and the rhythm applied. Many classifications occur with the most common listed below.

Effleurage is the most common stroke. It soothes and relaxes the nervous system, increases circulation, prepares the tissues for deeper work, and eliminates waste material from the tissues. Effleurage is a gliding movement that uses the palm of the entire hand following the contour of the body. Each hand is well molded, and at least one hand is in full contact with the body at all times.

Pétrissage is the foundation of a massage. The purpose of pétrissage is to also drain the tissues of waste material and increase circulation to the region massaged. Pétrissage contains a variety of strokes, such as shaking, vibration, muscle squeezing, skin rolling, chucking, kneading, and V-spread. Many of these techniques lift the muscles away from the underlying tissues and bone.

Shaking—skin is lifted and "shaken" over the underlying structures either using fingertips (small areas) or with the flat palm of the hand (large areas). The skin will move with your hands over the body parts.

Vibration is a quivering movement applied with fingertips or a flat hand. "Point vibration" uses only the thumb or fingertips for small, specific areas, and "flat-hand vibration" is used for larger areas.

Muscle squeezing uses one or two hands, palms only, to grasp and squeeze muscle; reduces muscle tension. Slow rhythm—to calm the nervous system; brisk rhythm—stimulates circulation and nervous system. Effective for the neck, legs, and tail.

Skin rolling uses both hands to grasp and lift superficial tissue with thumbs and fingers and rolls the tissues.

Chucking supports the foot with one hand while grasping tissue of the lower leg moving up and down along the length of the bone.

Kneading uses the surface of the middle three fingertips, providing overlapping movements, compressing against underlying bone structures, and pushing outward while maintaining contact at all times.

V-spread—place the thumbs together on the dog's body; move them up and out (away from each other) to form a "V."

Friction breaks down adhesions in muscles, tendons, ligaments, and fascia through circular or linear motion. This massage technique is often a heat-producing stroke. Use the tips of the thumb or middle three fingers for small areas or the heels of one or both hands for larger areas. Friction uses small, deep movements applied across the length or perpendicular to the muscle or fibrous tissue treated. This technique uses a fair amount of pressure that may be increased to tolerance.

Tapotement, or percussion, stimulates and energizes the body by increasing blood flow and lymph circulation and warms up muscle groups. Tapotement also assists with the toning of atrophied muscles. This technique applies a series of brisk blows, or repetitive striking movement in a rapid, alternating fashion. Hands are cupped, or the edges of hands are used for larger muscle groups and to penetrate into deeper tissues.

Certain behaviors elicited by the animal may indicate inappropriate massage techniques. All of the following behaviors may indicate that the masseuse needs to change his or her technique or apply less pressure: the animal's eyes are wide open; pupils are dilated; taking rapid, shallow breaths; pulling away from pressure; turning quickly to look at the masseuse; placing its muzzle over your hands or possibly licking the masseuse's hands; and attempting to rise and walk away.

MAXIMIZING PERFORMANCE OF THE CANINE ATHLETE

What is "performance?" What does "training" entail? There is much discussion surrounding these topics, and the "perfect" training program for our canine athletes remains a mystery. Of course, there are many components that may affect performance. In addition to proper training and conditioning, nutrition, the type of sporting event, and overall health of the animal must be considered. Before designing an optimal training or conditioning program for your four-legged athlete, a basic knowledge of tissue physiology is necessary. The focus of this section will include the necessary components to achieve maximal performance of your canine athlete. In addition, a better understanding of the optimal performance of involved tissues, including tendons, ligaments, muscles, bones, and cartilage, will be gained.

To maximize the function of each of these tissues, the "SAID" principle, "specific adaptation to imposed demands" is best applied.[9] Simply stated, exercises designed for a specific training program should mimic the anticipated function. For example, if the specific activity requires more muscular endurance than it does strength, then the training program should be geared to improve muscular endurance. Building an exercise program should include the necessary foundation—a framework of specificity.

> TECHNICIAN NOTE When considering an exercise program for the canine athlete, a *framework of specificity* is a necessary foundation.

It is this principle that applies to all body systems and is an extension of the theory that body systems will adapt over time to the stresses placed upon them, or Wolff's law.[10]

Improving cardiovascular endurance may be achieved by engaging in large muscle group activities, such as running, jogging, or swimming, at varying frequencies, durations, and intensities. Resistance training to enhance muscle strength, endurance and to maintain flexibility is equally as important.

Stretching is also a vital component to any training program. It improves joint range of motion and function, enhances muscle performance, and helps prevent musculoskeletal injuries. Pollock et al states that poor flexibility may lead to declining performance and subsequent injury. However, performance may be modified through flexibility training.[11]

The "warm-up" and "cool-down" phase of an exercise program is also a necessary component to achieving maximal performance. The purpose of a warm-up is to allow the body to make the physiologic adjustments necessary before the onset of activity. This allows the body to meet its physical requirements before physical activity. Following exercise, the cool-down period is necessary to prevent pooling of blood in the extremities and to enhance the recovery period by removing metabolic waste and replacing energy stores.

A basic understanding of the principles of exercise and a basic understanding of achieving maximal performance of important body tissues is a vital component when considering the development of an exercise plan. With these concepts, one is well on his or her way to developing an optimal training program for a canine athlete.

ORTHOTICS AND PROSTHETICS

Orthotic and prosthetic intervention has been a standard application in human PT to achieve mechanical and rehabilitative goals. An orthotic is defined as a device used to support an injured limb (see Figure 24-12). A prosthetic device is designed to replace a missing limb (Figure 24-13). Until recently the use of these assistive devices has been limited to the human realm of rehabilitation.

The goal of an orthosis includes: resting an injured limb, immobilizing or protecting a joint, controlling a limb, and/or to assist, prevent, or correct movement of an affected limb. If the physical therapist's goal is to rest a part of the body, the orthosis must be able to substitute for or assist with the action of the injured or weak muscles. On the other hand, an orthosis may be used to immobilize a limb to reduce pain or provide joint protection immediately following surgery or injury. In these types of cases, the orthosis must take over the role of intrinsic stability normally achieved by the bony, ligamentous, or muscular components of the animal.

> TECHNICIAN NOTE An orthotic is a device used to support an injured limb, and a prosthetic is designed to replace a missing limb.

Before consideration of a prosthetic device, rehabilitation goals must be met in a patient that has undergone a limb amputation (Figure 24-14). It is imperative for positive functional outcomes that the spared muscle groups are identified and the respective functions understood. Each of the remaining joints in the involved extremity must maintain full range of motion. Improvement of cardiovascular endurance and a decrease in pain and inflammation can be met using appropriate modalities. Finally, adhesion and scar management must be addressed to maintain mobility of the surrounding soft tissues. Once these goals have been met, the appropriateness of a prosthetic device may be evaluated. Treatment of the entire animal is necessary, especially evaluation of the uninvolved limb(s) because the concern for fatigue and overloading may often be present.

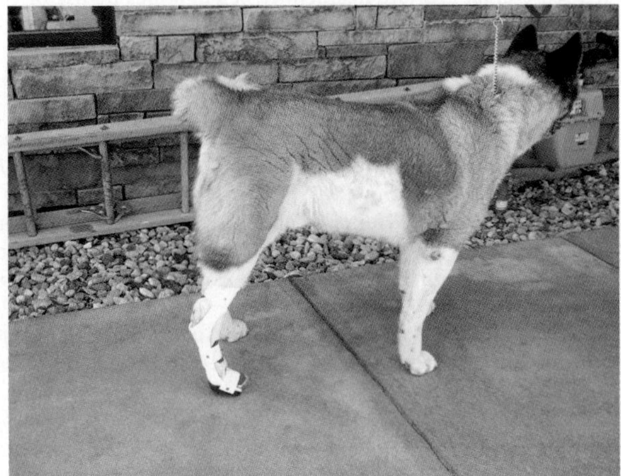

FIGURE 24-13 This Akita is donning a hind limb brace as an alternative to surgery to support an Achilles tendon rupture.

Many other considerations are also important for achieving a successful outcome when considering an orthosis or prosthesis. Proper healing at the site of the amputation and sensitivity of the distal stump must be known. The orthotic should not impact daily activities of the patient. The patient should be able to freely perform normal daily functional tasks, such as transitioning from sitting to standing, especially in patients with concomitant neurologic or musculoskeletal deficits.

PROTECT YOURSELF

In the animal world, when discussing safety and protection, most people think of avoiding dog bites and how to safely handle and restrain animals. In addition, you must consider that the field of animal rehabilitation is extremely physically demanding. You will find yourself lifting large neurologically impaired patients and crawling around on the floor more often than sitting in a chair. Besides slips and falls, back injuries are one of the most common injuries in the workplace. More than 50% of injuries are due to improper lifting. Six hundred

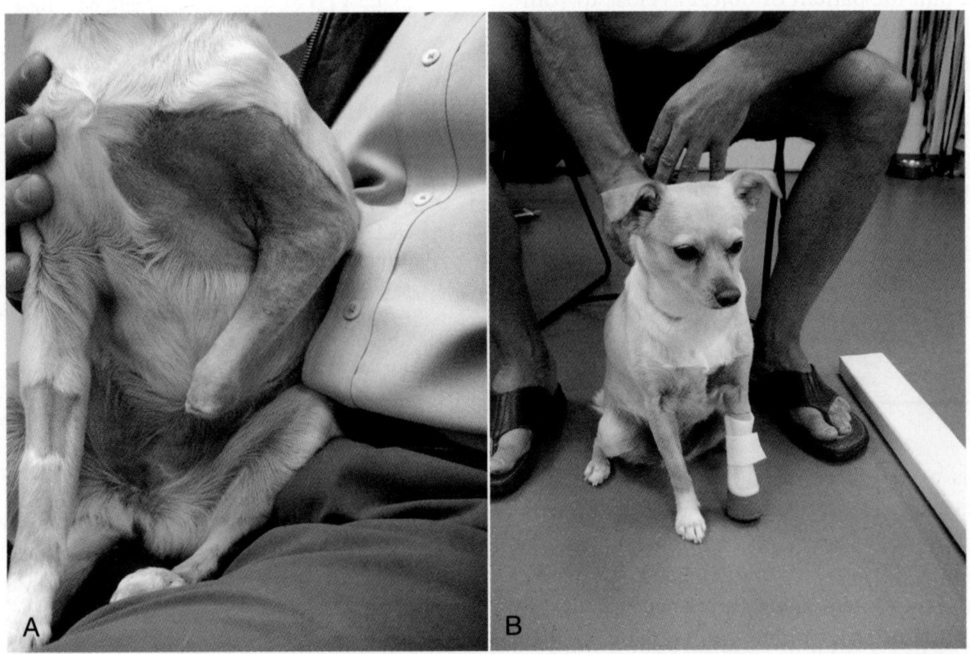

FIGURE 24-14 A, Rubi is a 6-year-old Chihuahua that suffered a left forelimb amputation caused by complications from a blood clot. B, Rubi donning her custom prosthetic. A gel liner lessens shear forces on her skin and provides a cushion to prevent constant irritation of her residual limb.

thousand back injuries per year are reported at a cost of $60 billion annually.

> TECHNICIAN NOTE The field of animal rehabilitation is extremely physically demanding. For this reason, understanding proper body mechanics will help to prevent back injuries.

Most back injuries are due to microtrauma of the nucleus pulposus and annulus fibrosis that occur gradually with a slow onset. It is difficult to trace any one single cause or injury. Macrotrauma typically occurs from improper lifting techniques in addition to the gradual damage from microtrauma and weakening of the muscles, ligaments, and disks surrounding the vertebrae.

Contributing factors to back injury may include reaching, bending, or twisting while lifting, pushing, or pulling heavy objects. Poor posture in standing or sitting in addition to weak abdominal musculature, poor physical condition, and strength also play a role in the gradual breakdown of the back structures. In addition, staying in one position for too long, incorrect lifting techniques, poor footing while lifting, fatigue, and repetitive lifting in awkward positions play a role in the potential for back injury. Dogs pulling on a leash, restraining animals on the floor, sudden jerks or movements by an animal to get away from pain or from fear, and bending over to pet, hold, or lift a patient are a few clinical examples of potential contributing factors to back injury.

When lifting properly, you should maintain a wide base of support on a dry surface. Bend your knees and keep your back straight while centering your body over your feet as much as possible. Tighten your abdominal muscles to support the spine and pull the patient or object as close to your body as possible. If you have to change direction, move your feet instead of twisting your spine. If you are unable to move your feet, put one foot in front of the other in the direction you want to move.

Correct sitting techniques include pulling the chair forward to allow your back to be supported against the back of the chair. Your chair should have an adequate lumbar (lordotic) support, and your feet should touch flat on the floor. Your hips should be equal to or higher than your knee level, and your computer should be in front of you at eye level.

SUMMARY

The field of PT is a well-established profession that encompasses a wide variety of applications. This chapter provides a small portion of the skill and techniques available to physical therapists. Physical therapists train for many years to establish these basics, with continued education throughout the remainder of their career. The veterinary technician may become a skilled assistant in physical rehabilitation, working side by side with physical therapists. As this newly defined career continues to expand, specialty certificates recognized by national organizations may develop along with numerous employment opportunities within the veterinary community. With the collaborative efforts of all professionals involved, animal patients will continue to benefit from this rapidly growing field, and physical rehabilitation therapy will become a standard of care in veterinary medicine.

REFERENCES

1. www.careerbuilders.com.
2. American Physical Therapy Association, Alexandria, Va, www.apta.org.
3. Chartered Society for Physiotherapy, London, www.csp.org.uk.
4. Johnson JM, Johnson AL: Rehabilitation of dogs with surgically treated cranial cruciate ligament-deficient stifles by use of electrical stimulation of muscles, *Am J Vet Res* 58(12):1473-1478, 1997.
5. Jaegger G, Marcellin-Little DJ, Levine D: Reliability of goniometry in Labrador Retrievers, *Am J Vet Res* 63(7):979-986, 2002.
6. Steiss JE, Adams CC: Effect of coat on rate of temperature increase in muscle during ultrasound treatment of dogs, *Am J Vet Res* 60(1):76-80, 1999.
7. Smarick SD, Rylander H, Burkitt JM, et al: Treatment of traumatic cervical myelopathy with surgery, prolonged positive-pressure ventilation, and physical therapy in a dog, *J Am Vet Med Assoc* 230(3):370-374, 2007.
8. American Physical Therapy Association: *Guide to physical therapist practice*, Alexandria, Va, 2001, American Physical Therapy Association.
9. McArdle WD, Latch FI, Katch VL: *Essentials of exercise physiology*, ed 2, Philadelphia, 2000, Lippincott Williams & Wilkins.
10. Kisner C, Colby LA: *Therapeutic exercise: foundations and techniques*, ed 4, Philadelphia, 2002, F.A. Davis.
11. Pollock ML, Gaesser GA, Butcher JD, et al: The recommended quantity and quality of exercise for developing and maintaining cardiorespiratory and muscular fitness, and flexibility in healthy adults, *Med Sci Sports Exercise* 975-991, 1998.

RECOMMENDED READINGS

Books

Kisner C, Colby LA: *Therapeutic exercise: foundations and techniques*, ed 4, Philadelphia, 2002, F.A. Davis.

Lippert L: *Clinical kinesiology for physical therapist assistants*, ed 3, Philadelphia, 2000, F.A. Davis.

McGowan C, Goff L, Stubbs N: *Animal physiotherapy: assessment, treatment and rehabilitation of animals*, Oxford, 2007, Blackwell Publishing.

Michlovitz SL: *Thermal agents in rehabilitation*, ed 3, Philadelphia, 1996, F.A. Davis.

Millis DL, Levine D, Taylor RA: *Canine rehabilitation & physical therapy*, Philadelphia, 2004, Elsevier.

Norkin CC, Levangie PK: *Joint structure and function: a comprehensive analysis*, ed 4, Philadelphia, 2005, F.A. Davis.

Snyder-Mackler L, Robinson AJ: *Clinical electrophysiology: electrotherapy and electrophysiologic testing*, Philadelphia, 1995, Lippincott Williams & Wilkins.

Journal Articles

Berry WL, Reyers L: Nursing care of the small animal neurological patient, *J S Afr Vet Assoc* 61(4):188-193, 1990.

Bocobo C, Fast A, Kingery W et al: The effect of ice on intra-articular temperature in the knee of the dog, *Am J Phys Med Rehab* 70(4): 181-185, 1991.

Jaegger G, Marcellin-Little DJ, Levine D: Reliability and goniometry of Labrador Retrievers, *Am J Vet Res* 63:979-986, 2002.

Jerrum RN, Hart RC, Schulz KS: Postoperative management of the canine spinal surgery patient, *Compendium* 19(2):147-161, 1997.

Johnson JM, Johnson AL, Pijanowski GJ et al: Rehabilitation of dogs with surgically treated cranial cruciate ligament-deficient stifles by use of electrical stimulation of muscles, *Am J Vet Res* 58(12): 1473-1477, 1997.

Millis DL, Levine D: The role of exercise and physical modalities in the treatment of osteoarthritis, *Vet Clin N Am* 27(4):913-930, 1997.

Steiss JE, Adams CC: Effect of coat on rate of temperature increase in muscle during ultrasound treatment of dogs, *Am J Vet Res* 60(1): 76-80, 1999.

Professional Organizations

American Physical Therapy Association, www.apta.org

American Veterinary Medical Association, www.avma.org

Physical Rehabilitation Training

Animal Rehabilitation Institute, Loxahatchee, Fla, 561-651-0760, www.animalrehabinstitute.com.

North East Seminars, University of Tennessee, 800-272-2044, www.neseminars.com.

Pharmacology and Anesthesia

PART FIVE

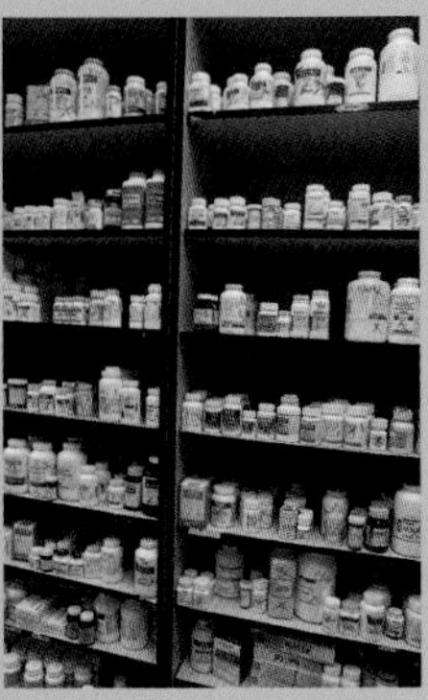

Pharmacology and Pharmacy 25

Marvene Augustus and Sonya Bremer Boss

KEY TERMS

Absorption
Analgesic
Anthelmintics
Anticholinergic agent
Antiinflammatory agent
Antimicrobial
Antipyretic
Cathartics
Cholinomimetic agents
Creatinine
Distribution
Diuretic
Emetics
Half-life
Neuromuscular blocker
Neurotransmitter
Opioids
Peak serum concentration
Pharmacodynamics
Reconstitute
Steady-state serum concentration
Therapeutic drug monitoring
Therapeutic window
Toxic dose

OUTLINE

LEARNING OBJECTIVES

When you have completed this chapter, you will be able to:

1. Define common terms related to pharmacology and pharmacy.
2. Describe the factors that affect the absorption and distribution of drugs and list mechanisms by which drugs may be biotransformed and eliminated.
3. List the dosage forms of medications, the routes by which medications may be administered, and factors that affect route selection.
4. Describe the classifications of drugs that affect the nervous, cardiovascular, and gastrointestinal (GI) systems and give examples of each.
5. List the classifications of agents used to treat common internal parasite infections of animals and name the parasite(s) that may be treated with each.
6. List the pharmacologic agents used in treatment and prevention of heartworm disease.
7. List the classes of compounds used to treat common external parasite infestations of animals.
8. List the classifications of antimicrobial agents used to treat animals and give examples of each.
9. List hormonal substances used in treatment of animals and describe indications for their use.
10. Describe legal issues and requirements related to purchasing, storing, dispensing, and administering pharmacologic agents.
11. Define compounding and explain legal issues related to compounding of medications.
12. Explain the purpose and uses of material safety data sheets.
13. Calculate quantities of medications in a variety of dosage forms for dispensing or administering to patients.
14. Define inventory turnover rate and explain its importance in managing pharmacy inventory.
15. Describe procedures for procuring, organizing, and pricing pharmacy inventory.

INTRODUCTION

In most practices, the technician shares the responsibility of administering drugs, which may range from the simplest chewable tablet to a gaseous anesthetic. As new drugs and strategies are applied to veterinary care, the role of the technician becomes increasingly sophisticated. The technician must have some knowledge regarding mechanisms of drug actions, therapeutic uses, and potential side effects. Verification that the drug and dosage are correct is a major responsibility of the technician. For this reason, the technician should be familiar with the dosage forms of drugs, able to recognize common medications, and translate drug dosages into the appropriate number of tablets or volume of drug for the individual patient. It is essential that the technician understand federal and state laws that regulate drug acquisition and distribution.

This chapter is intended to provide the technician with minimal knowledge of drug laws, inventory control, and calculation of dosages. The clinical chapters in this book will address drug classes with their pharmacology specifically. There are several good books written primarily for veterinary technicians dedicated entirely to the subject of drugs and they should prove helpful for those with greater interest in veterinary therapeutics.

PHARMACOLOGY

GENERAL PRINCIPLES

DEFINITIONS

A *drug* is defined as any chemical agent that affects living processes. These agents may be used to prevent, diagnose, or treat diseases. *Pharmacology* is a broad term defined as the study of drugs. Aspects of pharmacology include the history and source of drugs *(pharmacognosy);* physical and chemical properties of drugs and effects and actions of drugs on living organisms *(pharmacodynamics);* characteristic ability of living organisms to absorb, distribute, metabolize, and excrete drugs *(pharmacokinetics);* therapeutic uses of drugs *(pharmacotherapeutics);* and *toxicology,* the study of the symptoms, mechanisms, treatments, and detection of biologic poisoning. Toxicology has a set of related terms itself that need to be defined to better understand the study of pharmacology.

Therapeutic drug monitoring deals with the proper timing of blood samples drawn to determine the serum concentration of a drug. This value must be compared with accepted reported levels in consideration of the pharmacokinetic properties of the drug measured to ensure proper dosage and dose frequency.

Half-life is the time required for the serum concentration of a drug to decrease by 50%. It shows the intradose fluctuation of a drug and is useful in estimating the time a drug concentration should approach zero. Half-life is most helpful in determining optimal dosing schedules of oral agents and time required to reach steady state.

Steady-state serum concentrations are values that recur with each dose and represent a state of equilibrium between the amount of drug administered and the amount eliminated in a given time interval. It takes five half-lives to reach steady state after dosing has begun.

> *TECHNICIAN NOTE* Steady state is a state of equilibrium between the amounts of a drug administered and eliminated in a given time interval.

Peak serum concentration is the point of maximum concentration of drug on the time-versus-serum concentration curve.

Trough serum concentration is the minimum drug serum concentration (Figure 25-1) during a given dosing interval.

Therapeutic window (range) is a range of a drug serum concentration associated with a high degree of efficacy and a low risk of undesired dose-related adverse reactions. Correct timing is important for sample collection. Steady-state concentrations should be achieved because low readings may cause premature and erroneous dose increases.

Toxic dose is a dose greater than the upper limit of the therapeutic range (Figure 25-2) that causes poisonous or toxic symptoms.

Therapeutic index is the ratio between the toxic dose and therapeutic dose of a drug used as a measure of the relative safety of the drug for a particular treatment. A drug that has a narrow therapeutic index may cause toxic results with small changes in doses. These drugs require constant monitoring so that the dose of drug can be adjusted as necessary to ensure uniform and safe results. These ranges should only be used as guides for dosing because there are differences among patients in the manner in which drugs are distributed and are available at the receptor site. Some patients may achieve adequate relief of symptoms before the drug level is within therapeutic range and may experience toxic symptoms when the drug level is within the target range. Examples of drugs with narrow therapeutic windows and indices are digoxin, theophylline, warfarin, phenobarbital, and levothyroxine.

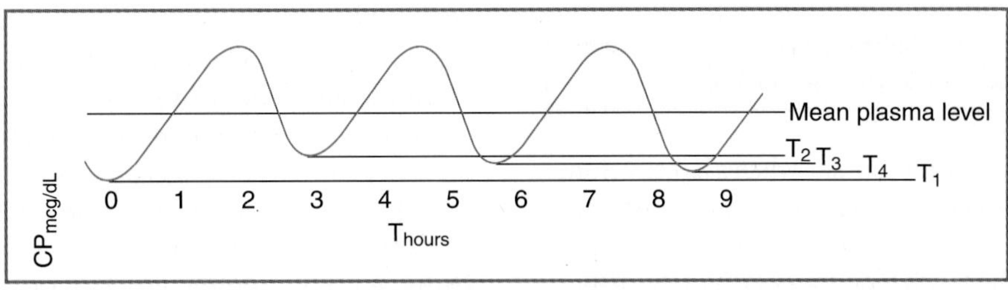

FIGURE 25-1 Illustration of trough levels after continuous doses of medications.

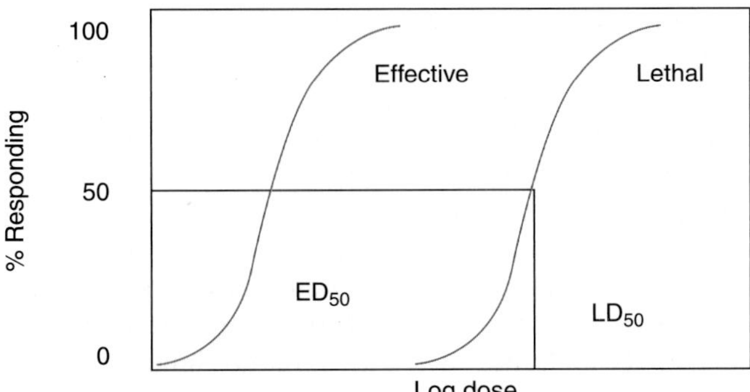

FIGURE 25-2 Illustration of toxic dose and therapeutic window.

LD_{50} is the dose of drug that kills 50% of the animals tested (LD = lethal dose). It is a standardized measure for expressing and comparing the toxicity of chemicals (see Figure 25-2).

ED_{50} is the minimum dose of drug required to cause the desired effect in 50% of the test subjects (ED = effective dose).

PRINCIPLES RELATING TO DRUG ACTIONS

The pharmacokinetic factors of a drug are absorption, distribution, metabolism, and excretion (ADME). These factors determine how the drug enters the body, reaches the site of action, and is removed from the body.

> *TECHNICIAN NOTE* Pharmacokinetic factors include absorption (how the drug enters the body), distribution (how the drug reaches the target tissue organs), metabolism (how the drug is chemically altered), and excretion (how the drug is removed from the body).

Drug Absorption

For drugs to exert an effect, they must reach their site of action (target tissue). For some drugs, a simple topical application accomplishes this. Most drugs, however, must cross several barriers of cell membranes to produce the desired action. Cell membranes also must be crossed for the subsequent deactivation and elimination of the drug from the body. *Absorption* is defined as the uptake of substances into or across tissues.

Drugs with systemic actions that are administered orally must cross the GI lining of the stomach or small intestine to be effective. Absorption of drugs from the GI tract will be influenced by several factors. To pass through the membrane lining of the GI tract, a drug must dissolve to some degree in oil (lipid soluble) because the membranes contain a high concentration of lipid (fat). Ionic (charged) forms of drugs do not easily pass through these membranes, whereas the nonionic forms of drugs pass more easily. Most drugs are weakly acidic or basic and have some lipid-soluble properties. The stomach is a highly acidic environment. The weakly basic drugs that are highly ionized (charged) in the acidic stomach will not be readily absorbed until they are farther down the digestive tract in the small intestine because it is basic in nature. In the small intestine, the weakly basic drugs exist in an unionized form, which permits easier transport across the lipid membrane. Drugs that are weak acids are unionized in the acidic stomach and diffuse more easily through the lipid membrane. They are rapidly absorbed from the stomach and therefore expected to exert their action more quickly than weakly basic drugs. Most drugs with poor lipid solubility cannot pass through cell membranes. Drugs, such as the antimicrobial aminoglycosides (e.g., gentamicin), have poor lipid solubility and therefore are inadequately absorbed and ineffective after oral administration.

Stomach contents may inactivate or trap certain drugs. The volume of stomach contents also may delay absorption, thus delaying action. In ruminants, one is confronted not only with slow absorption from dilution, but also with the effect of the action of the ruminal microorganisms on certain susceptible agents. Common drugs of plant origin, such as digoxin and atropine, are ineffective in the ruminant when administered orally because of digestive microorganisms.

Drugs that are administered by intradermal injection are deposited into the outer layer of the skin and are primarily used for diagnostic purposes, as in allergies and tuberculosis. The volume is less than 0.5 ml. The drug produces a local effect. Drugs that require injection subcutaneously or intramuscularly must be absorbed from the injection site to exert their action. The subcutaneous route is appropriate for small drug volumes (less than 1 ml) and drugs intended to be absorbed slowly. Because of limited blood flow, subcutaneous drug administration results in a more sporadic absorption compared with those drugs injected intramuscularly. Insulin and heparin are examples of drugs that are administered subcutaneously. In animals that are highly dehydrated, there is a restricted blood flow at body surfaces, so subcutaneous administration is not usually recommended.

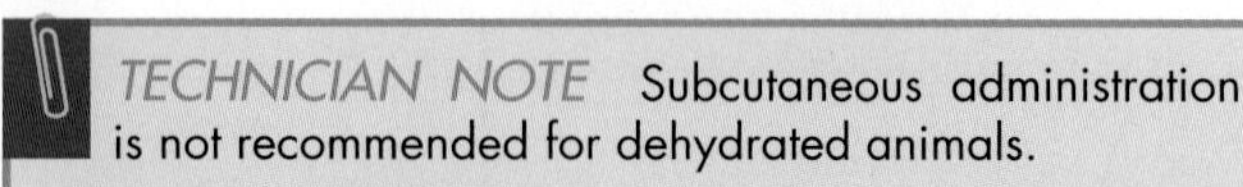

> *TECHNICIAN NOTE* Subcutaneous administration is not recommended for dehydrated animals.

Intramuscular injection is appropriate when a larger volume of drug must be administered. Absorption from the intramuscular site is faster than that from subcutaneous sites because muscles are better supplied with blood vessels than the skin.

Procaine penicillin is an example of a drug to be injected in the muscle.

Absorption from the subcutaneous or intramuscular site can be hastened by applying heat or massage to the site to accelerate blood flow. Applying ice packs at the injection site to decrease blood flow can slow absorption.

Drugs that are introduced into the vascular system (intravenous) will not go through an absorption phase. These drugs are placed directly into the plasma compartment and take effect immediately.

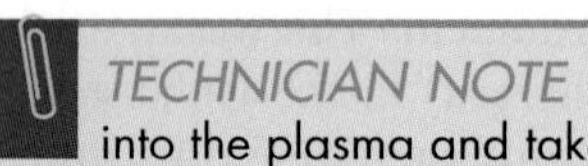

> *TECHNICIAN NOTE* Intravenous drugs go directly into the plasma and take effect immediately.

Drug Distribution

Drug distribution is the dispersion of the drug that is systemically available from the intravascular (within the vessels) space and extravascular (outside the vessels) fluid and tissues to the target receptor sites.

Figure 25-3 depicts the distribution of drugs after administration. Drug concentration is a dynamic process that continually varies at different sites until it is virtually all excreted. Generally, another dose of drug is administered before the complete removal of the previous dose, so the effective tissue levels (site of action) may be maintained. High lipid solubility and low protein binding are favorable characteristics indicative of the ability of a drug to diffuse through membranes. Drug transport into tissues involves passage through lipid-containing membranes. Diffusion is a difficult process for water-soluble compounds.

Most drugs in the bloodstream bind in varying degrees to plasma proteins, such as albumin. Only the unbound drug (free drug), which may be as little as 10%, is available to diffuse into tissues and produce biologic effects. As a rule, drugs bound to albumin or other proteins do not diffuse through capillary walls. Drug binding to albumin is a reversible process. Protein binding serves as a reservoir site because the drug becomes available as the plasma concentration of the free drug is reduced. Equilibrium is maintained at all times between protein-bound and free drug in the blood. A common form of drug interaction occurs when a second drug has a stronger affinity for the plasma protein. The first drug is replaced and becomes free to exert its effects in a greater concentration at its site of action.

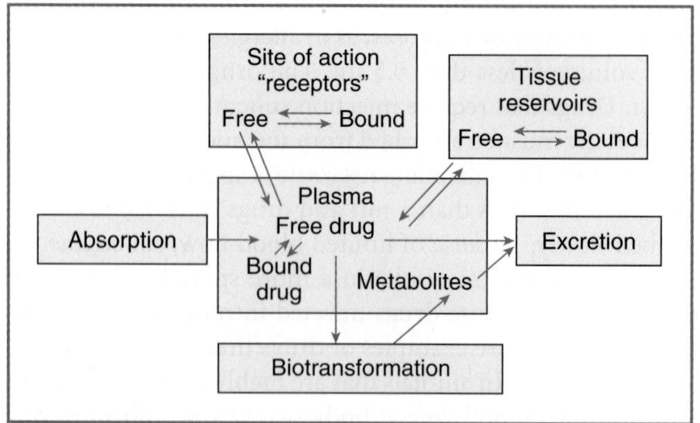

FIGURE 25-3 Schematic depicting fate of drug on administration.

Accumulation of drugs may occur in various body compartments, such as fat, muscle, and liver, prolonging the effects of the drug as it is released from these storage sites. The potential of a drug to accumulate at these different sites will vary greatly among drugs, depending on the physiochemical properties. For example, a highly lipid-soluble drug, such as thiopental, will accumulate in body fat. This accounts for the slow recovery of obese dogs from barbiturate anesthetics compared with leaner dogs, such as the greyhound.

Although all the aforementioned distribution sites of a drug are important, the amount of a drug reaching its site of action is of primary concern. The place at which a drug interacts with cellular components to exert its effect is called a receptor. There are numerous sites throughout the body. Some sites are specific for certain drugs, whereas others are general and may respond or interact with several types of drugs.

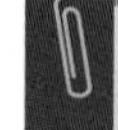

> *TECHNICIAN NOTE* A receptor is the place in the body at which a drug exerts its effect.

The ability of a drug to bind to a specific receptor determines the biologic activity of the drug. The interaction of a drug with a specific receptor is similar to a lock-and-key fit (Figure 25-4). Only a certain critical portion of the drug is usually involved in binding with the receptor. Drugs that have similar critical portions but differ in other parts of the biologic molecule might be expected to have similar biologic activity.

A drug, in interacting with its receptor, may mimic the action of a natural body substance (transmitter). For example, acetylcholine is a natural transmitter that is secreted at terminal nerve endings, causing muscle contraction. A drug, such as bethanechol chloride, that is chemically similar to acetylcholine produces similar effects. Such drugs that directly produce the normal function of the receptor are termed agonists.

Drug Metabolism

For free drugs to be removed (cleared) from the blood, they must be excreted directly without change or metabolized (biotransformed). Biotransformation is the ability of a living organism to modify the chemical structure of drugs so that

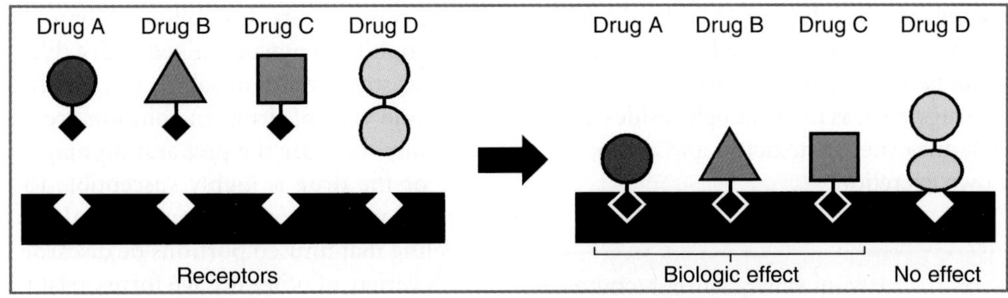

FIGURE 25-4 Lock-and-key fit between drugs and receptors through which they act.

they are no longer active (inactive metabolites). The liver is the principal organ responsible for biotransformation, but some of the activity may occur in the kidneys, brain, lungs, small intestine, and other organs.

TECHNICIAN NOTE The liver is the principle organ responsible for biotransformation.

Simple changes in the drug molecule, such as the removal or addition of certain atoms, may completely inactivate the drug. Through the mammalian enzyme system, potentially toxic compounds are changed into water-soluble compounds, which are more easily eliminated from the body by the kidneys. One means of removing many of the lipid-soluble drugs is through conjugation. This process involves the attachment of various endogenous substances to the drug. An example is the attachment of glucuronic acid to aspirin. After conjugation, the aspirin complex is much more water soluble, making it more readily excreted by the kidney. Cats are deficient in the enzymes required to conjugate drugs with glucuronic acid. This accounts for the relatively longer action of certain drugs in cats compared with most other mammalian species that do not have this deficiency.

Other common biotransformations of drugs by the liver include hydroxylation and acetylation. Biotransformation often inactivates drugs, but it does not always produce inactive products. Drugs, such as codeine, diazepam, and amitriptyline, are changed by the liver into metabolites that also exert a pharmacologic effect. These are called active metabolites.

In older animals or animals with hepatic disease, the ability of the liver to biotransform drugs may be impaired. Newborns less than 30 to 60 days of age are generally not capable of metabolizing many drugs because the liver enzyme system is not yet fully developed. To prevent drug toxicity, it might be necessary to reduce the drug dosage, increase the interval between doses, or switch to a drug that is not metabolized by the liver.

A few drugs are administered in an inactive form and do not become active until they are biotransformed by the liver; these are called prodrugs (i.e., angiotensin-converting enzyme [ACE] inhibitor enalapril must be converted by the liver to enalaprilat before it will exert any biologic activity).

Bacteria may carry out some biotransformation within the colon. This process may limit absorption of the drug from the bowel after oral administration, or it may help to eliminate drugs from the blood after parenteral administration.

Excretion

The kidneys eliminate (excrete) most drugs or the metabolites, although some may be removed via the bowel or lungs or in some other minor way in limited amounts. The removal of drugs from the blood by the kidney is somewhat complex and will vary from drug to drug. One route of elimination involves the liver and kidney. Biotransformation of drugs by the liver tends to form more polar compounds, which can be more efficiently excreted by the kidneys. For example, chloramphenicol (CHPC) is metabolized by the liver to chloramphenicol glucuronide. In this form, the drug cannot be reabsorbed via the kidney tubules from the urine back into the blood and therefore is excreted in the urine.

The pH of the urine will also influence excretion of drugs. Urine pH is normally basic, so drugs that are weakly acidic will exist in the ionized state and be more readily excreted. The weakly basic drugs will be in an unionized state and more apt to be reabsorbed back from the urine. For example, the elimination of aspirin, a weak acid, is enhanced in more basic urine. The reverse is true of weak bases in acidic urine. Ammonium chloride can be used to produce more acidic urine, and sodium bicarbonate can be used to produce basic urine.

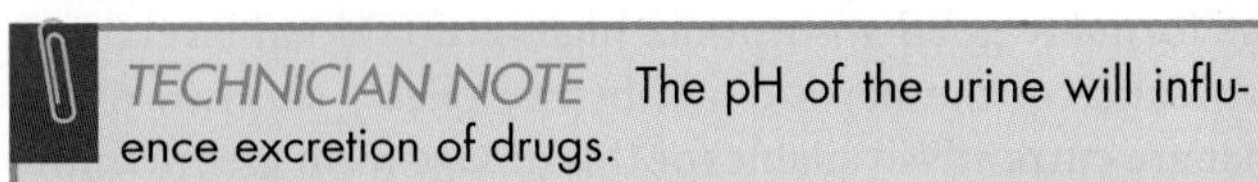

TECHNICIAN NOTE The pH of the urine will influence excretion of drugs.

Some drugs are not extensively metabolized by any organ in the body and are excreted unchanged in the urine. Some are excreted through passive diffusion into the glomerular fluid and are not reabsorbed to any significant degree and therefore enter the urine. Other drugs are actively secreted by specific systems in the renal tubules, which lead to more rapid drug elimination.

Drugs that are excreted by the kidney will accumulate in the body when there is a loss of kidney function. Creatinine (a natural waste product) levels in the blood are sometimes measured to determine the extent of renal damage so that the dose of various drugs can be adjusted accordingly. Kidney function declines with age, even in the healthy animal. Elderly animals may show a reduced ability to excrete drugs in the urine. Certain drugs, such as the aminoglycosides, may directly damage the kidney (nephrotoxicity) and ultimately interfere with their own excretion.

> *TECHNICIAN NOTE* Loss of kidney function causes drugs to accumulate in the body if the kidney excretes them.

Another route of drug excretion involves uptake by the liver, release into the bile, and elimination in the feces. Drugs in the bile enter the small intestine, in which they may be reabsorbed into the blood, returned to the liver, and secreted again into the bile. This process is called enterohepatic circulation. The drugs that are reabsorbed and resecreted will persist in the body much longer than the drugs that remain in the lumen of the intestine and pass out with the feces.

DOSAGE FORMS

To administer drugs through the various routes, manufacturers have produced products in different formulations to accomplish the desired effect. For oral administration, there are not only traditional tablets and capsules, but also chewable, flavored tablets to encourage animal acceptance and ease in owner administration. Care must be taken in dogs and cats with food allergies when considering the use of chewable flavor tablets. Many tablets are beef based and can cause adverse drug reactions in animals allergic to beef. Because of an undesirable flavor or high alcohol content, animals may not readily receive oral liquids developed for human use. Liquids specifically flavored and designed for dogs, cats, and exotic animals reduce stress for both client and patient during administration. Some cats are hard to orally administer drugs to. Compounding pharmacists can incorporate the drug into a gel that is placed on the outer or inner ear or a place with the least amount of hair. The advantages of using this dosage form are good absorption, high serum blood levels, and avoidance of the hepatic first-bypass effect. The two drugs that are currently available for this dosage form are methimazole and amitriptyline.

Equine owners often cannot administer many drugs to horses orally because of a disagreeable taste or odor and the amount to administer. Some crushed tablets and powders can be mixed with molasses or other suitable compounds then mixed with the animal's grain ration. Veterinary drug manufacturers have formulated granules and pellets for ease in oral administration. Oral paste forms, though somewhat more expensive, have gained popularity because of convenience to the owner and receptiveness of the animal.

Injectable drugs are frequently available in solutions or suspensions ready for use. Special buffers to maintain pH or absence of oxygen are required because of the instability of some components. Instability of some drugs may require a dry lyophilized powder mixed with a diluent (reconstituted), such as sterile water or saline, just before use.

Some vials of drugs in solution are designed for "single use only" because the preparation may not have a preservative or the drug is highly susceptible to oxygen in the air. Certain vaccines or intravenous products may advise on the labeling that unused portions be discarded.

A variety of other dosage forms exist for use in veterinary medicine, such as ophthalmic ointments, solutions, or suspensions; topical sprays, cream, ointments, and lotions; and otic drops. Most are designed for a local effect, although occasionally there may be sufficient absorption from the application site to produce some systemic side effect. Another dosage form that is gaining popularity is the transdermal system. A patch is designed for local application to produce systemic results. Duragesic (fentanyl) patches were introduced to veterinary medicine to control postsurgical pain. Compounding pharmacists are able to make a transdermal patch for any drug except antibiotics. The molecules of the antiotics are too large and will not pass through the lipid biolayer.

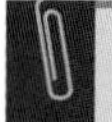

> *TECHNICIAN NOTE* A transdermal patch is designed to apply topically, but produce systemic results.

Intrauterine administration of some antibacterials is not uncommon in mares, cows, and other breeding stock. Antibiotics are also formulated for intramammary infusion for milk-producing animals. Some of these products are used to prevent (prophylactic) infections at the end of the milking period only. These agents are designated for use in dry cows and usually have a longer duration of action. Other mastitis preparations are for use in lactating cows to treat an infection during the milking period and for a time after the last treatment. The withdrawal time (usually 36 to 72 hours) will vary with the drug and formulation and is stated on the product label.

ROUTES OF ADMINISTRATION

Several methods are available for administering drugs to animals (Chapter 20). Each route of administration has advantages and disadvantages. The route selected will depend on a number of factors, including the patient's size, disease state, temperament, and unique species characteristics; the characteristics and commercial formulation of the drug; and the expertise and knowledge of the individual administering the drug. The cost of drugs should be a factor in the selection of a route of administration when all other clinical factors have been considered.

ORAL ADMINISTRATION

Oral administration is one of the most convenient methods used by clients and animal health personnel for giving drugs. Tablets and capsules are fairly economical and provide accurate and uniform doses. Oral liquids offer some convenience, but the amount of active ingredient administered may vary from dose to dose, depending on measurement or the animal's acceptance. Administration of oral liquids by force in cats usually results in an undesirable salivary gag reflex episode. Oral paste forms for horses and food-producing animals have gained popularity because of the ease of administration. The acceptance of oral granules and powders, although variable among animals, offers convenience for dosing larger species. Drugs formulated for mixing in the animal's drinking water are least desirable because water consumption is highly variable and unpredictable. However, when dealing with large numbers of sick animals in flocks or herds, the use of water mixes may be the only economical and feasible method of treatment. For small birds, medicated drinking water is sometimes used to prevent the stress that occurs with other methods.

Absorption of drugs administered orally depends on a number of factors. Even when accurate doses are given, the actual amount of drug absorbed may vary, altering the expected therapeutic response. Most medications that can be administered orally can also be administered via a feeding tube. It is preferred to give liquids by tube; however, some solid medications can be finely crushed and mixed with sufficient liquid to ensure complete passage of the drug into the stomach. Before administration of any drug via a tube, make sure that the tube is correctly placed and the drug can be crushed or mixed with aqueous solutions.

PARENTERAL ADMINISTRATION

Parenteral administration of drugs is usually accomplished by subcutaneous, intramuscular, intradermal (Figure 25-5), or intravenous injections. Parenteral administration of drugs requires sterile technique to reduce the possibility of introducing infection into the animal (see Chapter 20).

An intradermal injection is made just below the outer layer of skin (epidermis). This route of administration is used for allergy testing and giving local anesthetics. The volume of drug injected is small, usually less than 0.5 ml.

Subcutaneous injections are common in veterinary medicine because they are less painful to the animal than intravenous or intramuscular injections and are easily administered. Some drugs cannot be given in this way because tissue irritation or sloughing may occur. Many vaccines are given subcutaneously, but some require intramuscular injection to produce the desired immune response.

Increased risks are inherent in the intramuscular administration of drugs. One must ensure that the drug will not be injected into a vein or an artery by accident. The potential also exists for injecting the drug in or near a major nerve fiber, which could cause paralysis. One must have knowledge of the location of major nerves to prevent accidental damage.

When giving drugs subcutaneously or intramuscularly, only a limited amount can be administered at the injection site. Multiple sites may be used for some preparations, but the absorption may be more erratic.

The absorption from an intramuscular or a subcutaneous injection site is primarily through simple diffusion. A number of factors will influence the rate of diffusion from the site. Of primary importance is capillary circulation in the area. Because circulation is limited at subcutaneous sites, compared with intramuscular sites, one would expect a lower absorption and longer action for drugs given subcutaneously.

Label directions should be followed regarding route of administration when administering drugs by injection. There may be a few exceptions for preparations with which sufficient experience exists for administration by routes other than those stated on the label. In most cases, however, there is a definite reason why the recommended route is stated. For example, antibiotics given by subcutaneous injection may not produce adequate blood levels to destroy microorganisms.

For intravenous administration, one must not only know the location of the larger veins that are used, but also possess some skill in placement of the needle or catheter within these blood vessels. An immediate effect can be obtained from drugs administered intravenously without the delay of absorption encountered with other administrative routes. This route may also be used when larger volumes are required. Even certain irritating compounds can be given intravenously if they are given slowly, allowing adequate blood dilution.

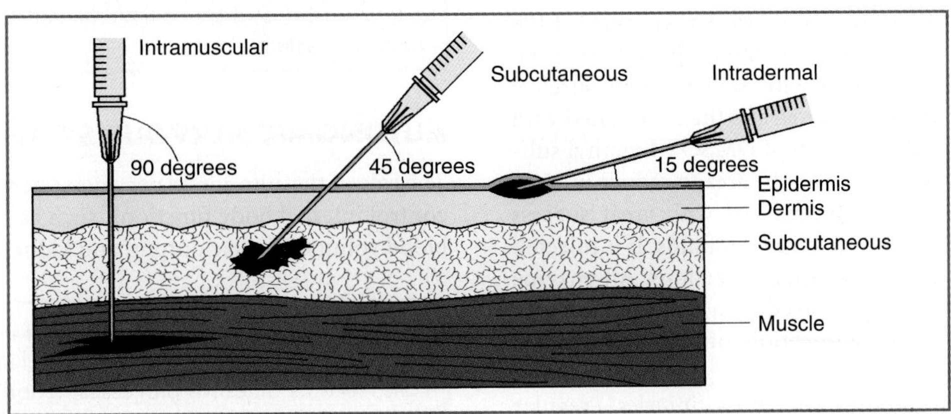

FIGURE 25-5 Comparison of angle of injection and location of medication deposit for IM, SQ, and ID injections.

Although intravenous administration has advantages, it also has risks. One major disadvantage is the immediate effect seen with an intravenous administration. In situations involving overdose or inappropriate drug selection, the response in an attempt to prevent major problems may not be successful. Highly irritating drugs, such as phenylbutazone, sodium thiopental, and triple sulfa, can severely damage blood vessels and surrounding tissue if injected outside the vein (perivascularly). Injecting certain drugs too rapidly may lead to untoward effects, including circulatory collapse and death. Some drugs may irritate vein walls, stimulate vasoconstriction, and raise the pressure inside a blood vessel until it ruptures. Drugs that leave the vein, leak into the soft tissue surrounding the vein, and cause tissue damage are vesicants. The leakage of intravenous drugs from the vein into the surrounding tissue is called extravasation. Once extravasation has occurred, damage can continue for months and can involve nerves, tendons, and joints. It may cause full thickness of skin loss above the area of injury and may require skin grafting. Delayed treatment to the area may result in the need for surgical débridement, skin grafting, and even amputation. Injury from extravasation can occur with any medication that is highly acid or basic, cytotoxic, or has a high osmolarity. Drug items noted for extravasation are cytotoxic agents (cancer drugs), intravenous nutrition, and solutions of calcium, potassium, bicarbonate, and 10% dextrose.

To prevent extravasation, great care must be taken to ensure that the veins are intact with a good blood flow since drugs may leak from sites of previous or recent punctures or occluded veins. The insertion site should not be distal to a recent venipuncture or an extremity with compromised circulation.

> *TECHNICIAN NOTE* Drugs noted for extravasation are cytotoxic agents, intravenous nutrition, and solutions of calcium, potassium, bicarbonate, and 10% dextrose. Highly irritating drugs can severely damage blood vessels or cause untoward effects, such as circulatory collapse and death.

The first line of treatment is to remove as much of the offending fluid as possible. One method reported has been to dilute the infiltrated fluid with saline. Small surgical incisions are made around the area and then suctioned with a liposuction device. Application of DMSO (dimethyl sulfoxide) has been used topically on the area to reduce inflammation. Hyaluronidase has been used with great success because it can work for a wide variety of fluids. It is injected into the area via a catheter or small injections. An enzyme degrades hyaluronic acid (involved with the inflammatory process), then enhances absorption of the extravasated fluid.

To treat tissue damage in most injuries, regular assessment of the site is all that is necessary. To facilitate healing of injuries leading to necrosis, follow wound care principles:

1. Remove necrotic tissue.
2. Eradicate infection.
3. Absorb excess exudates.
4. Obliterate damaged space.
5. Maintain a moist wound surface.
6. Insulate the wound.
7. Protect the wound from further trauma or bacteria.

NEUROPHARMACOLOGY

Many different classes of drugs affect the nervous system, even though they are used for a variety of therapeutic uses. Some drugs will cause a direct effect, and others will alter functions of the nervous system as a side effect. The central nervous system (CNS) includes the brain and spinal cord. Its function is to monitor, convey, and process signals from receptors throughout the body.

Neurons (nerve cells) relay information from the CNS to the rest of the body. They use neurotransmitters (NTs) to contact neurons and other cells. An NT, a chemical substance released from the axon terminal of a presynaptic neuron or excitation (stimulation), diffuses across the synaptic cleft to either excite or inhibit the target cell (receptor). Most neurons make only one kind of NT. The receptor recognizes only one specific NT and initiates a cellular response to it. The binding of the NT to its receptor is reversible. The stimulation of the cell is terminated when the NT is degraded or removed away from the receptor.

The nervous system is divided according to general function. The two primary divisions of the CNS are the autonomic nervous system, or involuntary system, and the somatic (motor) nervous system, or voluntary system. The somatic system initiates muscle contraction by both conscious and unconscious control. The autonomic system innervates involuntary activities of the body. Although both systems have efferent fibers leading from the CNS, the focus of this discussion is on those of the autonomic nervous system.

> *TECHNICIAN NOTE* The two primary divisions of the CNS are the autonomic nervous system, or involuntary system, and the somatic (motor) nervous system, or voluntary system.

AUTONOMIC NERVOUS SYSTEM

The role of the autonomic nervous system is to monitor and control internal body functions, such as digestive processes, blood volume, cardiac output, and kidney function.

> *TECHNICIAN NOTE* The role of the autonomic nervous system is to monitor and control interval body functions, such as digestive processes, blood volume, cardiac output, and kidney functions.

For impulse transmission to occur between nerves or between nerves and effector site (e.g., muscles, glands, organs), a small amount of NT must be released by the efferent nerve (Figure 25-6). Two major NTs exist in mammals: acetylcholine (ACh) and norepinephrine (NE). ACh is released into the synapse. ACh that diffuses into opposing membranes is degraded into acetate and choline by the membrane-bound enzyme acetylcholinesterase. ACh that diffuses into the blood is degraded by nonspecific cholinesterase in the blood and tissues. Enzymes deactivate NE, but reuptake of NE by the nerve that released it also occurs, and the NT is again stored in the granules.

The autonomic nervous system is subdivided into the sympathetic and parasympathetic nervous systems. Both divisions commonly act on a given organ, but they produce opposite responses. NE is the predominant NT in the sympathetic system, and ACh is the principal NT of the parasympathetic system. ACh is also the transmitter substance found at the ganglia and at the neuromuscular junction in the somatic nervous system.

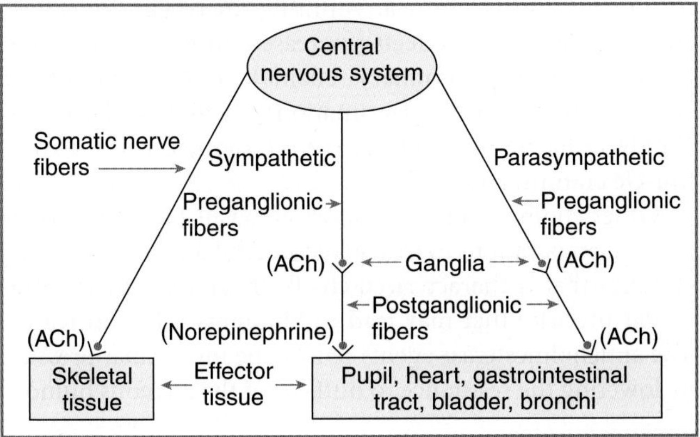

FIGURE 25-6 Schematic of efferent fibers showing sites of neurohumoral transmitters.

Within the sympathetic nervous system, at least three different types of receptors exist (α, β_1, and β_2) with others postulated. All these receptors may be found within the same effector tissue, and the response to the transmitter will vary, depending in large part on the type of receptor that is predominant at the site and on the amount of transmitter substance present. The general response of various effector tissues to normal sympathetic and parasympathetic stimulation are listed in Table 25-1.

This antagonism allows full control of organ function according to body requirements. It should be noted that sympathetic response is a fight-or-flight response in that the animal's heart rate increases, bronchioles are dilated for better ventilation, and blood vessels to the heart and skeletal muscle dilate to increase blood supply. In the parasympathetic rest-and-digest response, the heart rate slows, bronchioles constrict to restrict airways, and blood vessels constrict in the heart and skeletal muscle.

Drugs affecting the autonomic nervous system may mimic or block all or selected effects of the NT, or they may alter the synthesis, storage, release or degradation, and uptake of the transmitter. The classification of these drugs is difficult, not only because there are so many different types of action possible, but also because most drugs possess more than one specific action. Drugs are generally classified based on the primary or predominant action.

Cholinomimetic (cholinergic or parasympathomimetic) agents are drugs that mimic the stimulatory effects of ACh. Cholinomimetic drugs can be further divided into muscarinic and nicotinic agents. Receptor sites that are found to

TABLE 25-1 Partial Listing of General Responses Seen at Effector Sites

Effector Tissue	Sympathetic Stimulation (Dominant Receptor Type)	Parasympathetic Stimulation
Pupil	*Dilated*	*Constricted*
Glands		
Salivary	Scanty viscous secretion	Copious secretion (watery)
GI tract	—	Increased
Bronchioles	Dilated	Constricted
Heart		
Rate	Accelerated	Slowed
Contractile force	Increased	Decreased
Blood Vessels		
Muscle (skeletal)	Dilated	—
Heart	Dilated	—
Skin	Constricted	Dilated
GI Tract		
Muscle wall	↓ Peristalsis and tone	↑ Peristalsis and tone
Sphincter	↑ Tone	↓ Tone
Urinary bladder		
Wall	Relaxed	Contracted
Sphincter	Contracted	Relaxed

be postganglionic in the effector tissue may be stimulated by a naturally occurring alkaloid, muscarine. Most other ACh receptor sites, including end plates of muscle, may be stimulated by nicotine. Anticholinergic (cholinergic blocking or parasympatholytic) agents are those that are capable of blocking ACh effects. They can also be subdivided according to the site or sites blocked.

Sympathomimetic (adrenergic) agents and sympatholytic (adrenergic blocking) agents are those drugs that mimic or block, respectively, the effects of NE. These agents also are further classified by the particular receptor that they stimulate or block.

AUTONOMIC DRUGS

Cholinomimetic Agents

ACh is not effective systemically as a drug because it is rapidly hydrolyzed by the enzyme acetylcholinesterase at the receptor site. Only an ACh ophthalmic formulation is available for the immediate constriction of the pupil during eye surgery.

Bethanechol is similar in structure to ACh and mimics much of its pharmacologic action. Bethanechol is sufficiently different from ACh in that it can resist hydrolysis by the cholinesterase enzymes; therefore it is a fairly long-acting drug. It is used as a smooth muscle stimulant. When given orally, indications for bethanechol use include gastric atony or stasis and urine retention when there is no obstruction.

Adverse reactions to bethanechol in small animals are mild and may include vomiting, diarrhea, salivation, and anorexia. Arrhythmias, hypotension, and asthma are most likely to occur in overdosage.

Several drugs are able to bind with the cholinesterase enzyme, preventing it from breaking down ACh. This not only allows ACh to act longer, but also creates increased concentration, resulting in exaggerated effects. These agents are toxic (some related compounds were used as nerve gases in World War II), and the therapeutic usefulness is limited to a few unique medical problems. In veterinary medicine, the use of cholinesterase inhibitors is primarily for treatment of parasites—both internal and external.

Cholinesterase inhibitors (anticholinesterases) are divided into three groups on the basis of reversibility: truly reversible (short acting, 5 minutes), edrophonium chloride; reversible (long acting, 30 minutes to 4 hours), physostigmine, pyridostigmine, and neostigmine; and irreversible, organophosphates and echothiophate iodide.

Edrophonium chloride is a drug used to diagnose myasthenia gravis, a disease of the nerves and muscles that is characterized by weakness and a marked fatigue of skeletal muscles. Edrophonium chloride induces an immediate improvement, although it is of short duration. The longer-acting agents, physostigmine, pyridostigmine, and neostigmine, are used to treat the disease in humans. Myasthenia gravis is a disease with a poor prognosis. It is a condition that is expensive to treat; therefore treatment is rare in veterinary medicine.

A common veterinary use of injectable neostigmine is in the treatment of ruminal atony or gut stasis. Neostigmine is relatively short acting (2 to 4 hours), but its stimulatory effects may be beneficial in returning the rumen and GI tract to normal peristaltic activity after surgery. This agent is sometimes employed to treat urine retention because of its stimulatory effects on smooth muscle in the urinary bladder.

Neostigmine and physostigmine can also be used to treat atropine intoxication and to reverse the effects of certain neuromuscular blocking agents (e.g., tubocurarine, gallamine, pancuronium) used during surgery.

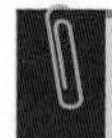

TECHNICIAN NOTE Neostigmine and physostigmine can be used to treat atropine intoxication.

Symptoms of overdose of the anticholinesterase agents include GI effects (nausea, vomiting, diarrhea), salivation, sweating, respiratory effects (increased bronchial secretions, bronchospasms, pulmonary edema), ophthalmic effects (miosis, blurred vision, lacrimation), cardiovascular effects (bradycardia or tachycardia, hypotension, cardiac arrest), muscle cramps, and weakness.

Other cholinesterase inhibitors are available only as ophthalmic preparations to treat glaucoma. Glaucoma is a disease complex that is characterized chiefly by an increase in intraocular pressure that may lead to blindness if left untreated. The anticholinesterase agents reduce the intraocular pressure by lowering the resistance to outflow of the aqueous humor.

Anticholinergics

As mentioned previously, nicotinic receptors are mainly at the end plates of skeletal muscle and autonomic ganglia. Muscarinic receptors are predominant in smooth muscle, heart, and glands. Some drugs have the capability of stimulating both types of receptors to varying degrees, whereas other drugs are capable of blocking both sites in varying degrees. Furthermore, some drugs may block the nicotinic effects at the skeletal muscle and not at the autonomic ganglia.

Drugs that inhibit the action of ACh at the muscarinic sites (antimuscarinic drugs) are used widely in veterinary medicine; the most popular drug in this class is atropine. Atropine is a belladonna alkaloid found in nature and commonly incriminated in plant poisoning. Other belladonna alkaloids, such as homatropine and scopolamine, are commercially available and have a slight difference in action.

Because anticholinergic drugs exhibit their usefulness in inhibiting the action of ACh by competing at a number of sites, their potential for correcting a disorder or altering a response is significant. One can rarely choose a single site for the therapeutic action without concomitant side effects occurring at other muscarinic sites. There have been numerous compounds synthesized in attempts to reduce certain unwanted actions and enhance desired effects. The success of such efforts has been limited, depending somewhat on the unique response of the individual patient.

The significant responses that are seen with therapeutic doses of atropine and related drugs are nearly the opposite of parasympathetic stimulation (see Table 25-1). The pharmacologic effects of atropine are dose related. Low doses will produce decreased salivation and bronchial secretions. Dilation of the pupil and increased intraocular pressure and heart rate are experienced with moderate systemic doses. High doses decrease motility and tone of the GI and urinary tracts.

The antimuscarinic drugs are frequently used before and during surgery in small animals to reduce or prevent secretions of the respiratory tract and to reduce bradycardia (decreased heart rate). Atropine and its analogs have been used in combination with other drugs to treat diarrhea (see later discussion of antidiarrheal agents).

Atropine is indicated in eye examinations and some ophthalmic surgery in which dilation of the pupil is desired. Atropine is long acting; therefore some of the shorter-acting mydriatics (dilating agents), such as tropicamide, are used. One of the most important uses of an antimuscarinic drug is to block spasms of the small ciliary eye muscles, thereby alleviating the associated pain.

Another significant use of atropine is as an antidote for organophosphates and other anticholinesterases found in many insecticides or parasiticides. Muscarine toxicity from poisonous mushrooms is also treated with atropine.

> *TECHNICIAN NOTE* Atropine is an antidote for organophosphates and other anticholinesterase poisoning. It is contraindicated in the horse except for life-threatening organophosphate toxicity.

Atropine must be used with caution because of potential side effects, which are merely extensions of the pharmacologic effects. Some clinicians believe atropine is contraindicated in the horse except for life-threatening organophosphate toxicity because the decreased peristaltic activity in the lengthy gut of the horse leads to gas and toxin complications. Atropine can increase ocular pressure and is therefore contraindicated in the treatment of animals with certain types of glaucoma.

Neuromuscular Blockers

Neuromuscular blockers (NMBs) act at the junction of the nerve and skeletal muscle to paralyze skeletal muscle. These compounds are classified according to the onset and duration of action. Older agents, such as d-tubocurarine, succinylcholine, gallamine, and pancuronium, are still available commercially. Newer agents, such as vecuronium and atracurium, are widely used in veterinary medicine.

Some NMBs have been used in darts to capture animals, but this use is dangerous because respiratory paralysis occurs. The main clinical use of NMBs is as an adjuvant in surgical anesthesia to obtain relaxation of skeletal muscle, particularly of the abdominal wall, and in orthopedic surgery. These agents are selectively used in veterinary medicine. Guaifenesin, another type of muscle relaxant, is commonly used in equine and bovine surgery to selectively depress transmission of nerve impulses at the internuncial neurons of the spinal cord, brainstem, and subcortical regions of the brain. Symptoms of NMB overdose include increased risk for hypotension, histamine release, and prolonged muscle blockade.

Sympathomimetics

The sympathetic nervous system is extensively involved in regulating a number of body functions, including heart rate, blood pressure, bronchial airway tone, body temperature, carbohydrate and fatty acid metabolism, and appetite. Although NE is the primary transmitter substance, epinephrine is released from the adrenal gland when an animal is stressed through physical, psychologic, or other stimulatory means.

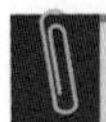

> *TECHNICIAN NOTE* Epinephrine is released from the adrenal gland when an animal is stressed.

Because the NE molecule can be modified extensively and still possess some type of stimulatory properties, numerous agents are commercially available. Manufacturers seek a molecule that produces a desired response and eliminates or reduces all the other adrenergic effects. NE possesses only alpha effects and has limited therapeutic use in the treatment of certain hypotensive shock conditions.

Epinephrine has several therapeutic applications in veterinary medicine, although the actual frequency of use is limited. Clinical applications include the following:

- Allergic reactions (often lifesaving in the face of shock)
- Bronchospasm (provides rapid relief)
- Cardiac effects (sometimes used in specific heart disorders)
- Local hemostasis (may be used in dilute solution [1:100,000 to 1:20,000] to control surgical bleeding in highly vascular tissue)
- Prolongation of the effects of local anesthetics (even though there may be undesirable systemic effects from epinephrine if overused)

Isoproterenol, which has few alpha effects, but powerful beta effects, is useful as a bronchodilator in respiratory disorders and as a cardiac stimulant in certain heart conditions. Isoproterenol is available in many preparations for humans that are designed for inhalation use or as tablets for under the tongue (sublingual). Only the short-acting injectable form has application in veterinary medicine.

Epinephrine and NE are not available in oral forms because both are destroyed by stomach acid. In addition, both drugs are relatively short acting when given by injection. Epinephrine and phenylephrine hydrochloride are also commercially available as ophthalmic preparations. They cause the pupil to dilate, but unlike atropine, they directly stimulate those muscles of the eye controlled by sympathetic nerves. This mydriatic effect is useful in selected cases of glaucoma and in ophthalmic examinations.

Symptoms of toxicity include arrhythmias, pulmonary edema, dyspnea, vomiting, headache, and sharp rises in systolic, diastolic, and venous blood pressures.

Sympatholytics

Many chemicals interfere with the function of the sympathetic nervous system. Some agents act by interfering with the synthesis, storage, and release of the transmitter substance. Others interfere with the ability of receptors to interact effectively with NTs. Some blocking agents are specific in their action (e.g., prazosin hydrochloride is specific in blocking the α receptors). Other agents (e.g., the phenothiazine tranquilizers, such as acepromazine) are nonselective in activity, blocking α and β_1 receptors (see Chapter 27 on information about preoperative drugs and drugs used in anesthetic emergencies).

α- and β-Adrenergic Blocking Agents

The α-adrenergic blocking agents, such as phenoxybenzamine, prazosin, and hydralazine, cause vasodilation and are used mainly in animals for lowering blood pressure or improving blood flow in certain vascular diseases.

Phentolamine, an expensive, injectable α-blocker, is used to diagnose adrenal gland tumors and during surgery to control abnormally high blood pressure. Adverse effects seen with use of α_1-adrenergic blocking agents include first-dose syncope, transient lethargy and dizziness, nausea, vomiting, diarrhea, and constipation.

> *TECHNICIAN NOTE* Phentolamine is used to diagnose adrenal gland tumors and during surgery to control abnormally high blood pressure.

β-Adrenergic blocking agents, such as propranolol and atenolol, are therapeutically useful as antihypertensive agents and in the treatment of certain heart arrhythmias.

Betaxolol and timolol are two β-adrenergic blocking agents that are widely used in veterinary ophthalmology. After topical application to the eye, each reduces both elevated and normal intraocular pressure with or without glaucoma. Overuse of β-adrenergic blocking agents results in symptoms of hypotension, bradycardia, bronchospasms, depressed consciousness to seizures, hypoglycemia, respiratory depression, and atrioventricular block.

Tranquilizers

Tranquilizers are drugs that act on the CNS to produce a calmness of mind or detached serenity without loss of consciousness or marked depression. The use in veterinary medicine is to modify the behavior of the animal to make it more manageable or less responsive to external stimulation.

Phenothiazines

Phenothiazine was originally used in veterinary medicine as an anthelmintic. Derivatives of the drug (chlorpromazine and acepromazine) have been synthesized to enhance the sedative effects of phenothiazine. Some of the derivatives are used as antihypertensive agents because they exhibit peripheral α-adrenergic blocking activity and cause vasodilation. The exact mechanism of action for sedation is unknown, but phenothiazines block postsynaptic dopamine receptors. These drugs have found usefulness as antihistamines, antiemetics, and antimotion sickness agents.

The phenothiazine tranquilizers are used as preanesthetics by "taking the edge off" the animal and enhancing or prolonging the effects of certain anesthetics. Some side effects to be aware of when administering the phenothiazines include a drop in blood pressure, paralysis of the retractor penis muscle in horses, and lowering of the seizure threshold in dogs.

> *TECHNICIAN NOTE* Phenothiazine tranquilizers are used to take "the edge off" the animal and to enhance the effects of some anesthetics.

α_2-Agonists

Although xylazine, detomidine, and medetomidine in the strictest sense may not be classified as tranquilizers, their sedative and analgesic properties are useful for chemical restraint, especially in the horse. Detomidine is approved for use only in the horse and has little application in other species. It appears to differ slightly from xylazine by producing greater analgesia and sedation. Although it is dose dependent, the duration of action of detomidine is longer than xylazine.

Both xylazine and detomidine are commonly used in combination with other sedatives, tranquilizers, and anesthetic agents. The effects of these drugs in combination are greatly potentiated and must be used with caution. Common side effects seen in the horse include muscle tremors, partial atrioventricular (AV) block, bradycardia, respiratory changes, sweating, penile prolapse, increased intracranial pressure, or decreased mucociliary clearance.

Xylazine has always been used widely in cattle. Only recently has the U.S. Food and Drug Administration (FDA) approved it for use in food-producing animals. The popularity in ruminants results from its excellent anesthetic properties. Ruminants are sensitive to xylazine, requiring approximately one tenth of the dose (based on body weight) used in horses. Adverse effects in cattle include ruminal atony, intestinal stasis, salivation, hypothermia, diarrhea, bloating, ataxia, and regurgitation with aspiration pneumonia.

Although xylazine is approved for the management of hyperexcitable behavior in the cat and dog, it is not widely used in these species. Vomiting is a common side effect seen in the dog and frequently in the cat soon after administration. A single episode usually occurs, but the use of antiemetics may delay this phenomenon. Xylazine is frequently used as an emetic when an emetic effect is desired (e.g., emptying stomach before surgery). Gaseous extension with use may occur in dogs, making radiographic interpretation difficult. Movement in response to sharp auditory stimuli may be observed. Increased urination may occur in cats following the use of xylazine.

Yohimbine is an α_2-adrenergic receptor antagonist that competitively blocks and antagonizes CNS depression or sedation and the bradycardia and respiratory depression caused by xylazine.

Atipamezole hydrochloride, a synthetic α_2-adrenergic antagonist, reverses the effects of medetomidine hydrochloride in dogs.

The use of propofol in veterinary medicine for induction of anesthesia in high-risk patients, such as those with compromised organ systems, is rapidly gaining popularity. It is used mainly for sedation and/or relaxation of 5 to 10 minutes in duration because it is rapidly metabolized. Because propofol can cause respiratory depression, its use should be restricted to situations where controlled intubation is available. Propofol may cause increased vasodilation and negative inotropy (weakening the force of muscular contraction) when used in conjunction with preanesthetic agents, such as acepromazine or opiates. Animals with preexisting cardiopulmonary disease, in shock, or suffering from trauma should be of particular concern. Propofol-induced bradycardia may be exacerbated in animals receiving opiate premedication, especially when anticholinergic agents are not given concurrently.

Drugs that inhibit the hepatic P-450 enzyme system and other basic lipophilic drugs may increase recovery times associated with propofol. Cats with liver disease as a preexisting condition may be susceptible to longer recovery time.

TECHNICIAN NOTE Propofol is useful for induction of anesthesia in high-risk patients. It should be used in situations with controlled intubation because of its ability to cause respiratory depression.

Anticonvulsants

Of the several different causes of seizures (convulsions) in dogs, only about two thirds can be controlled by the various anticonvulsant drugs. The benzodiazepine derivative diazepam may be the most popular injectable drug for use during seizures or in other emergency situations. This benzodiazepine agent depresses the subcortical levels of the CNS, thus exhibiting sedative, skeletal muscle relaxant, and anticonvulsant properties. Diazepam is relatively short acting (30 minutes to 2½ hours). Phenobarbital sodium, a barbiturate, is also available for injection when a longer effect (4 to 6 hours) is required.

Midazolam, an imidazobenzodiazepine, exhibits similar pharmacologic actions as other drugs in its class. The unique characteristic of lipid solubility at body pH gives it a rapid onset of action after injection. It is not used as an anticonvulsant, but finds use as a premedication before surgery, alone or in combination. When combined with potent analgesic and/or anesthetic drugs, such as ketamine or fentanyl, midazolam produces conscious sedation. Intracarotid artery injections must be avoided. Midazolam should be used cautiously in animals that are comatose, in shock, or have significant respiratory depression. Use in the first trimester of pregnancy should only occur when the benefits clearly outweigh the risks associated with the use. This drug should be used in an inpatient setting only or with direct professional supervision.

Adverse effects seen with benzodiazepine use include muscle fasciculations, weakness, and ataxia in the horse at sedative doses; irritability, possible development of hepatic failure, and aberrant demeanor in cats; and CNS excitement in the dog.

BARBITURATES

Phenobarbital is a barbiturate with CNS effects. The mechanism of action of this group of drugs is not quite understood, but they have been shown to inhibit the release of ACh, NE, and glutamate. Phenobarbital tends to depress motor activity without causing excessive sedation, which makes it a good anticonvulsant agent. One major side effect of this drug is dose-dependent respiratory depression.

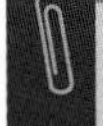

TECHNICIAN NOTE A major side effect of phenobarbital is dose-dependant respiratory depression.

An effective and inexpensive agent used to treat epilepsy (status epilepticus) and seizures caused by acute encephalitis or meningitis in dogs is oral phenobarbital. For some cases that are uncontrolled by phenobarbital, oral administration of potassium bromide has been effective. (Potassium bromide is not available in a commercial formulation. Authorization may be obtained from the FDA to compound preparations for treatment of refractory cases.) Compounding pharmacies may be a source for obtaining this product when its use is determined necessary.

Analgesics, Antipyretics, and Antiinflammatory Agents

Analgesics are agents that alleviate pain. Although local and general anesthetics inhibit the sensory perception of pain, analgesics are generally considered to increase the threshold of pain in the pain perception areas of the brain. Antiprostaglandins (e.g., aspirin, flunixin) inhibit the biosynthesis of these natural pain-producing substances and are also considered analgesics (see Chapter 26 for additional information on opioids).

Opioid Analgesics

The naturally occurring narcotics (e.g., morphine, codeine) and synthetic narcotics (e.g., hydrocodone, meperidine) are the most potent analgesics. These agents stimulate the μ-opioid receptor and are thought to have some activity at the δ-opioid receptor. Although these addictive agents are used for severe postsurgical or posttrauma pain in dogs and horses, their more common use is as an anesthetic or preanesthetic agent.

The pharmacologic effects differ somewhat among the various narcotics, but most will produce the following:

- CNS depression in the dog, monkey, and human
- CNS stimulation (excitement) in the cat and horse
- Cough sedation in the dog and human
- Respiratory depression (panting may initially be seen)
- Increased tone of intestinal smooth muscle, causing constipation
- The effects of these drugs are reversed by narcotic antagonists, such as naloxone

Unfortunately, narcotic analgesics are fairly short acting in the dog and the horse (2 to 4 hours). Gut stasis in the horse is a concern when considering opioid analgesics. The opioid analgesics have questionable efficacy in the ruminant.

The agonist activity of the synthetic opioid butorphanol is thought to be exerted at the κ- and σ-receptors. Butorphanol, a morphine congener, has shown promise in dogs as a longer-acting (4 to 8 hours) analgesic. Adverse effects seen in dogs include sedation (occasionally), ataxia, and anorexia or diarrhea (rarely). Transient ataxia and sedation may occur in the horse at usual doses. Butorphanol is used in horses as an effective analgesic, although its stimulatory effects must be suppressed by the concurrent use of depressant drugs, such as xylazine. Butorphanol is approved by the FDA for use as an antitussive and analgesic in dogs.

Gaining popularity in veterinary medicine for pain relating to surgery is fentanyl. Fentanyl shares the actions of the opioid agonists; the same precautions should apply. One advantage of using fentanyl is that it is marketed in a transdermal patch system for chronic pain management that delivers continual analgesia for about 72 hours. The patch is not recommended for use in management in postsurgical pain.

Hydrocodone bitartrate is a phenanthrene-derivative opioid agonist that exhibits the characteristics of other opiate agonists. It is used in veterinary medicine mainly as an antitussive agent. The mechanism is thought to be a result of direct suppression of the cough reflex on the cough center in the medulla. Hydrocodone is more sedating than codeine, but not as constipating.

Opioid Antagonists

The opioid antagonists reverse the pharmacologic effects of narcotics and have no analgesic activity. *Naloxone* appears to be the only true antagonist because it possesses no other apparent pharmacologic effect at usual doses. (It reverses the majority of effects associated with high-dose opiate administration—respiratory and CNS depression.)

> TECHNICIAN NOTE Effects of opioids may be reversed with the use of the narcotic antagonist naloxone.

Although narcotic antagonists are used commonly in human addicts to reverse overdoses of self-administered narcotics, the principal use in veterinary medicine is to reverse the sedative and quieting effects of analgesics used for temporary restraint. Dogs receiving narcotic sedation for minor procedures (e.g., radiographs, suture removal) are easily "reversed" with naloxone; the animal is almost immediately alert. The duration of action of naloxone is shorter than that of most narcotics, and generally the effects of the unmetabolized analgesic are inadequate to cause the animal to return to its sedated state.

Corticosteroids

Corticosteroids are extremely active compounds that have numerous pharmacologic effects on all organ systems. They have been used in an attempt to treat practically every malady that afflicts animals. They are valuable in the treatment of certain conditions; however, there are significant risks when one considers the potential adverse effects.

Because corticosteroids are naturally occurring body substances (cortisol is derived from the adrenal gland), one indication for the use of steroids would be replacement therapy to correct a deficiency. Such a deficiency is relatively rare. Most steroids used in veterinary medicine are given for the antiinflammatory effect; the mechanism for the antiinflammatory response is complex. They suppress the tissue swelling and pain that normally follow injury. Because inflammation is common in a variety of diseases, there is extensive use, perhaps overuse, of these agents.

Steroids also possess antiimmunologic effects, altering the immune response of the body. Therefore they are used in certain allergic diseases because they reduce the hypersensitive and allergic reactions of the patient. Immunizations generally should not be given during corticosteroid therapy because of the potential for inadequate immune responses.

> TECHNICIAN NOTE Immunizations should not be given during corticosteroid therapy because of the potential for inadequate immune responses.

Common side effects seen with the long-term use of steroids include GI bleeding; increased susceptibility to infections or wounds that will not heal; potassium loss, causing irregular heartbeats, muscle cramps, and weakness; sodium and water retention (edema or ascites); muscle weakness resulting from protein breakdown; and behavioral changes. The primary adverse effects associated with long-term administration, especially if given at high doses or on an alternate-day regimen, are generally manifested as symptoms of hyperadrenocorticism (Cushing's disease).

Dexamethasone is one of the most popular steroids used in veterinary medicine; it is fairly long acting (more than 48 hours). Prednisolone and prednisone are used interchangeably and are available in tablet form. Triamcinolone and betamethasone are also used extensively in veterinary medicine.

Steroids are found in various dosage forms, including ophthalmic, otic, topical, injection, and oral. It should be noted that long-term use of these steroids as ophthalmic or topical agents may lead to some of the systemic toxic effects previously mentioned.

Nonsteroidal Antiinflammatory Drugs

To prevent side effects inherent to steroids, other agents possessing antiinflammatory action have been synthesized. These are called nonsteroidal antiinflammatory agents (NSAIDs). NSAIDs exhibit antipyretic, analgesic, and antiinflammatory activity. The major mechanism of therapeutic effect is believed to be the result of inhibition of prostaglandin (PG) synthesis. Many inhibit both COX-1 and COX-2 isoenzymes. Phenylbutazone, one of the original members of this group of compounds, remains one of the most widely used agents in equine medicine. Phenylbutazone is not frequently used in small animals, although there is a label claim for use in dogs. Dogs metabolize phenylbutazone rapidly, which makes it difficult to maintain therapeutic levels of the drug. Cats metabolize the drug slowly and thus become prone to its toxic effects. Blood dyscrasias have been reported in several species receiving phenylbutazone. The drug has the potential for reducing the effects of other drugs metabolized by the liver because it increases the hepatic microsomal enzymes necessary to deactivate these drugs.

Flunixin has gained popularity not only for its antiinflammatory effects, but also for its ability to reduce GI pain in horses and ruminants. Although not approved for food-producing animals, flunixin appears to be the best analgesic available for ruminants, providing relatively long, effective relief.

Ketoprofen and carprofen are propionic acid derivatives structurally related to ibuprofen and naproxen. Ketoprofen has been approved for use in the horse to alleviate inflammation and pain associated with skeletal disorders. Carprofen has been approved for dogs only to relieve pain and inflammation associated with osteoarthritis.

Oral administration of the NSAIDs is apparently irritating to the GI tract and may cause ulceration in the mouth, stomach, or intestines. Newer generation NSAIDs (etodolac, meloxicam, deracoxib, and tepoxalin) are gaining in popularity because of once-a-day dosing and decreased adverse effects on the GI tract. Firocoxib is a new agent that has been recently marketed for use in equine medicine.

DIURETIC AND CARDIOVASCULAR DRUGS

Fluid and electrolyte imbalances and the treatment are discussed in Chapter 21. The function of the kidney and its role in maintaining proper fluid volume and electrolyte concentration are also mentioned. Blood is initially filtered in the kidney, and most of the filtrate is reabsorbed from the kidney tubules back into the blood. Most diuretic drugs affect the reabsorption process, preventing the reabsorption of some sodium and water from the filtrate. As a result, urine output and sodium excretion are increased.

DIURETICS

Diuretic drugs are used primarily to relieve edema (the presence and abnormally large amounts of fluid in the intercellular tissue spaces of the body) associated with diseases of the kidney, heart, or liver. Although there are numerous diuretic agents, furosemide appears to be the most routinely used diuretic in veterinary medicine. Furosemide is a loop diuretic that primarily inhibits reabsorption of sodium (Na^+) and chloride (Cl^-) in the kidney. It is commercially available in convenient forms for oral and injectable administration in small and large animals. Besides being potent and effective in most cases, furosemide is rapid acting and usually produces diuresis within 5 minutes when given intravenously.

Furosemide can cause a "wasting" of potassium, so serum potassium levels should be monitored for animals that take furosemide. Potassium supplementation may be indicated during furosemide therapy.

> *TECHNICIAN NOTE* Loop diuretics can cause "potassium wasting." Serum potassium levels should be monitored; potassium supplementation may be indicated.

Occasionally, when renal blood flow is inadequate because of trauma or shock, furosemide or similar diuretics are ineffective in altering tubular reabsorption. In such cases, an osmotic diuretic, such as mannitol, which is poorly absorbed from the glomerular filtrate, is used to produce diuresis. Animals that have been hit by cars may be likely candidates to receive mannitol. Crystallization may occur in solutions with concentrations greater than 15%. It is important to dissolve crystals before administering. Keeping the solution in a warm water bath prevents crystals from forming. The crystals can also be dissolved by running warm water on the bottle or rolling the bottle to and fro in the hands.

CARDIAC GLYCOSIDES

Cardiac (heart) drugs are probably the most potent and hazardous group of drugs used in medicine because of the effects on such a vital organ. Any carelessness in calculation, administration, or observation of the patient may lead to death. The dosage for these drugs should be individualized through frequent and careful monitoring to ensure the desired therapeutic response and prevent or minimize toxic effects.

The heart performs a relatively simple function (to circulate blood) and is essential to life. The heart consists primarily of myocardium (muscle), valves, and some specialized impulse-conducting nodes and fiber. Even though the heart has the ability to compensate for certain defects, disorders left untreated reduce the quality of life with severe disability, leading to premature death.

Significantly severe defects in the valves can only be treated surgically. Medical therapy is available for the treatment of a weakened myocardium and conductance disorders (arrhythmias).

The normal healthy heart can increase its output readily when demands, such as increased exercise, are placed on it. This increased cardiac output is a result of either an increased heart rate or an increase in the volume of blood pumped per beat (stroke volume), but usually, it is a combination of both. Heart muscle weakened with age does not contract as fully and therefore can lead to reduced output. Because the body cannot tolerate much decrease in cardiac output, the heart rate will increase slightly and the heart will become enlarged because the myocardium will thicken in an attempt to improve contractility. Congestive heart failure (CHF) is the condition of an enlarged heart with poor myocardium contractility.

Various glycosides found in the leaf of the digitalis plant have been found to be useful in the treatment of CHF. Digoxin is one of the glycosides that is commonly used in veterinary medicine. Digoxin is unique in that it not only improves the inotropic ability (contractility) of the myocardium, but also reduces the heart's demand for energy and oxygen. It also decreases the conduction of certain impulses within the heart and therefore decreases the heart rate. It is used for treatment of atrial fibrillation, an arrhythmic disorder of the heart.

Digoxin dosing is critical. Toxic effects of the cardiac glycosides are seen at doses close to the therapeutic dose (narrow therapeutic window) and therefore complicate its use. Owners should be aware of signs of toxicity, which include vomiting, diarrhea, loss of appetite, and depression. Associated with these symptoms are a decreased heart rate and drug-induced arrhythmias.

> *TECHNICIAN NOTE* Toxic effects of cardiac glycosides are seen at doses close to the therapeutic dose (narrow therapeutic window).

Further complications to digoxin therapy are animals with reduced liver or kidney function, as is common in the older animal. Good client compliance and close monitoring are essential in digoxin therapy because of the toxicity possibilities. The drug is available as an oral tablet, oral liquid, and injection.

Animals that are concurrently using a diuretic may have low serum potassium levels and are more susceptible to digoxin toxicity.

Although the cardiac glycosides are effective by injection in horses and cattle, and to some extent orally in horses, it is not feasible to use these drugs to treat CHF because of the long-term nature of the disease. These drugs are commonly used in dogs and cats. There is adequate absorption of digoxin from the GI tract in these species; however, it may differ somewhat among animals and can be influenced by feeding times.

ANTIARRHYTHMIA DRUGS

Arrhythmias of the heart fall into several categories and require skilled clinicians and electronic instrumentation for proper diagnosis and treatment. Some minor cardiac arrhythmias are likely to correct themselves and may be left untreated. The use of antiarrhythmic drugs in veterinary medicine is usually limited to treatment of those arrhythmias that are life threatening and require immediate attention.

Calcium channel blockers provide the veterinarian with an efficacious weapon in the treatment of certain cardiovascular disorders. This group of drugs has a low incidence of side effects. Of the numerous agents, diltiazem has surfaced as the most commonly used agent to treat supraventricular tachyarrhythmias in dogs and cats. It is used in the treatment of hypertrophic cardiomyopathy in cats. Diltiazem acts as an antihypertensive agent through arteriolar dilation, but the benefit of this action is not fully known.

Three older commonly used antiarrhythmic drugs are quinidine, procainamide, and lidocaine. The more ordinary uses are only mentioned because detailed discussion is beyond the scope of this chapter. Quinidine is used in horses and large dogs for the treatment of supraventricular and ventricular arrhythmias. Other uses include treatment of atrial fibrillation and atrial flutter. Procainamide is related chemically to procaine, and it is used in the treatment of ventricular extrasystoles and tachycardia, atrial arrhythmias, ectopic contraction and tachycardia, flutter, and fibrillation. Lidocaine, although used primarily as a local anesthetic, has therapeutic application in the treatment of ventricular tachyarrhythmias. Clinical monitoring and electronic evaluations should accompany the use of these drugs.

All antiarrhythmia drugs are toxic to the heart and may produce their own serious arrhythmias. In addition, in the horse, quinidine can produce urticarial wheals, GI disturbances (e.g., anorexia, colic, diarrhea), erythema, and edema of nasal mucosa with dyspnea and laminitis. Signs of quinidine toxicity in the dog include vomiting, depression, incoordination, and convulsions. Procainamide toxicities are exemplified in dogs by a loss of appetite, vomiting, and serious immunologic reactions with long-term use. A serious decrease in blood pressure may occur when procainamide is given intravenously. Lidocaine is not effective orally and has brief action when given intravenously. In large doses, lidocaine can produce a drop in blood pressure.

> *TECHNICIAN NOTE* All antiarrhythmia drugs are toxic to the heart and may produce their own serious arrhythmias.

ANGIOTENSIN-CONVERTING ENZYME INHIBITORS

Vasodilatory drugs, or angiotensin-converting enzyme (ACE) inhibitors, prevent the conversion of angiotensin I to angiotensin II (a potent vasoconstrictor). The drugs compete with angiotensin I for the active site of ACE. In veterinary medicine, this group of drugs is primarily used to treat canine CHF. Captopril was the first agent in this class to be commercially available. Treatment presented risks, such as renal failure. Other ACE inhibitors have been synthesized; they are prodrugs because they require a functioning liver to convert them to the active metabolite. Enalapril is commercially available with label indication for use in veterinary medicine. Other ACE inhibitors that are in use are human-labeled *benazepril hydrochloride* and *ramipril.*

> TECHNICIAN NOTE Hydralazine should be given with a diuretic because of water and sodium retention associated with its use.

The side effect profile of the second generation of ACE inhibitors has improved, and the dosing schedule is one or two times per day, which should help with client compliance.

Hydralazine is a phthalazine-derivative antihypertensive, vasodilating agent. The main use of hydralazine is an afterload reducer for the adjunctive treatment in CHF in small animals, particularly if the primary cause is mitral valve insufficiency. It is usually administered in cases where enalapril is not effective in clinically improving dogs with mitral valve insufficiency. Hydralazine should be given with a diuretic because of the sodium and water retention associated with its use.

Pimobendan is a benzimidazole-pyridazinone inodilator (positive inotrope-vasodilator) and is the newest drug introduced to treat CHF, dilated cardiomyopathy, and mitral regurgitation in the dog. It is a nonsympathetic, nonglycoside, positive inotrope (through myocardial calcium sensitization), and vasodilator. Pimobendan should not be used as a monotherapy, but in conjunction with an ACE inhibitor, furosemide, or digoxin.

> TECHNICIAN NOTE Pimobendan should not be used as monotherapy. It should be used as adjuvant therapy with an ACE inhibitor, furosemide, or digoxin.

AGENTS USED TO TREAT PARASITISM

TREATMENT OF INTERNAL PARASITISM

Anthelmintics (dewormers) are an extremely important group of drugs in veterinary medicine. The presence of internal parasites in an animal can shorten its life span or reduce the quality of life. It can contribute to considerable economic loss in food-producing animals. Although several different parasites are capable of infecting each species, most parasite infections can be effectively prevented or treated with proper care and medication. Current anthelmintics are much improved because they are more effective in eradicating the parasite and less toxic to the host. In addition, dosage forms, such as pastes or chewable tablets, are now available. These formulations are much more easily administered, which reduces stress to the animal and client.

There are a vast number of anthelmintics currently available; however, this discussion is limited to a select, popular few. Parasite treatment summary charts and specific parasite information are given in Chapter 17.

Benzimidazoles

Benzimidazoles are a large class of anthelmintics. They inhibit the enzyme fumarate reductase and thereby interfere with parasitic carbohydrate metabolism. Thiabendazole, oxibendazole, mebendazole, albendazole, parbendazole, fenbendazole, cambendazole, and oxfendazole are safe and effective agents against several GI parasites. They are formulated primarily for large animals to eradicate strongyli, pinworms, and ascarids in the horse and roundworms and several other parasites in cattle, sheep, swine, and goats. Albendazole shows activity against liver flukes. Fenbendazole and mebendazole are available for use in small animals to eradicate roundworms, hookworms, whipworms, and some tapeworms, although neither is effective for the common *Dipylidium* tapeworm. Adverse effects are not usually seen at recommended doses of benzimidazoles. Thiabendazole, parbendazole, and cambendazole are not commercially available in the United States.

Organophosphates

Trichlorfon, coumaphos, and dichlorvos are a group of agents that bind irreversibly to cholinesterase in the parasite, leading to ACh "poisoning" of the parasite. These drugs would also be toxic to the host, but they are selectively formulated to be poorly absorbed from the GI tract of the animal. Precautions must be taken so animals dewormed with organophosphates are not exposed to other organophosphates, cholinesterase inhibitors, pesticides, or muscle relaxants, such as succinylcholine, until a few days after treatment. There is potential danger to humans in administration of these agents.

Common toxic signs of organophosphate poisoning (e.g., widespread parasympathetic stimulation) include miosis, salivation, breathing difficulties, vomiting, defecation, and muscle fasciculation. Atropine is used as a specific treatment to block the muscarinic effects. Pralidoxime (2-PAM) is an expensive product for humans and may be used in severe cases of organophosphate poisoning to reactivate the cholinesterase enzyme.

> TECHNICIAN NOTE Pralidoxime (2-PAM) is used in severe cases of organophosphate poisoning to reactivate the cholinesterase enzyme.

The organophosphates are fairly effective in treatment of a number of principal parasites in horses, cattle, swine, sheep, dogs, and cats. With the potential toxicity of the organophosphates, many are being replaced with safer agents. The use of organophosphates is no longer professionally accepted; however, they are still obtainable.

Tetrahydropyrimidines

Pyrantel and morantel are two drugs in the tetrahydropyrimidine class. These drugs act as a cholinergic agonist and depolarize neuromuscular junctions. They are effective against the adult nematodes, but not active against larvae form.

Morantel is an analog of pyrantel that is safer and more effective in sheep and cattle than pyrantel. It is available only as a feed additive.

Pyrantel is widely used in horses for ascarids, strongyli, and pinworms. In dogs, pyrantel is used in the prevention and treatment of hookworms and ascarids. Tetrahydropyrimidine products are safe and nontoxic to all species at the recommended therapeutic doses. There is no contraindication for use of these agents with other cholinergic drugs.

Imidazothiazoles

Two popular drug agents, febantel and levamisole, are in the broad category of imidazothiazoles. Febantel is a prodrug that is metabolized in vivo to fenbendazole. It is approved by the FDA for use in a number of species against parasites. It has only been recognized to treat the most common equine parasites except bots and is reported to be safe in pregnant mares. Febantel is only commercially available in the combination product (Drontal Plus, Bayer).

Levamisole has broad anthelmintic activity in a large number of hosts, including sheep, cattle, pigs, horses, chickens, dogs, and cats. Use and FDA approval are limited primarily to food-producing animals. Although levamisole is relatively safe, some signs of toxicity occur similar to those of organophosphate poisoning. The toxic doses are only one or two times the therapeutic dose. Muzzle foam may be seen in ruminants after oral administration, but it usually disappears within a few hours. Transitory excitement has been seen in horses after treatment.

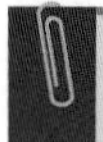

TECHNICIAN NOTE Toxic doses of levamisole are only one to two times the therapeutic dose.

Milbemycins

The milbemycins are macrocyclic lactones that act by interfering with the chloride-channel mediated neurotransmission in the parasite, thereby resulting in its paralysis and elimination.

Moxidectin is an oral dewormer and boticide for horses and ponies at least 4 months old. The label claims that one dose of the drug will suppress strongylus egg production through 84 days. Doramectin is an injectable drug marketed as a single dose for control of a wide range of roundworms and arthropod parasites in cattle and swine.

Ivermectins

The ivermectins enhance the release of gamma-aminobutyric acid (GABA), which paralyzes nematodes by blocking neurotransmission at excitatory motor neurons. Ivermectin has demonstrated effectiveness in a number of species against a wide variety of internal and external parasites. In cattle, swine, sheep, and goats, injectable ivermectin is used to treat infestations by numerous GI roundworms, lungworms, cattle grubs (cattle only), sucking lice, and mites. The paste and oral liquid forms of ivermectin have been approved for treatment of infestations by large and small strongyli, pinworms, and bots and for other equine parasite infestation. It is also approved for the treatment of ascaridiasis, although for some stages, it may be less effective than desirable.

Ivermectin has been approved for use in dogs and cats only for heartworm prevention; however, it has also been used at higher doses for treatment of other canine parasite infestations, including scabies. In certain dogs (most pure collie breeds) that are inherently sensitive to ivermectin, toxicities—sometimes fatal—have occurred with higher doses. Except for these unique toxicities, ivermectin has proved to be safe in other breeds and species when given at therapeutic doses. Overdose may manifest clinically as blindness, ataxia, and even death.

Agents Used In Heartworm Treatment and Prevention

There is considerable risk involved in the treatment of heartworms; therefore the American Veterinary Medicine Association (AVMA) Council on Veterinary Service established guidelines suggesting that first adult heartworms and then the microfilariae (the larvae forms of the filarial tissue) be eliminated. The adult worms usually stay in tissues, such as the heart, but the microfilariae migrate throughout the host. Heartworm disease is primarily seen in dogs; however, cats may also become infected. Dogs subject to infestation or reinfestation must be found free of microfilariae and adult heartworms before they are placed on a preventive heartworm regimen.

TECHNICIAN NOTE Dogs subject to infestation must be found free of microfilariae and adult heartworms before they are placed on a heartworm prevention program.

Melarsomine dihydrochloride is an arsenic agent used in treatment of heartworm disease caused by immature to adult infections. Dogs are at risk for posttreatment pulmonary thromboembolism; therefore they should be exercise restricted after treatment. The site of administration is critical for this drug, and it should be given only by deep intramuscular injection into the epaxial muscle. Adverse reactions observed with melarsomine dihydrochloride treatment include abdominal hemorrhage and pain, discolored urine, hematuria, tachypnea, disorientation, restlessness, and icterus. Melarsomine overdosage may show signs of arsenic toxicity. Dimercaprol (BAL) is an antidote for arsenic toxicity and may reduce signs of toxicity in overdoses. Coadministration of BAL may reduce the efficacy of melarsomine dihydrochloride.

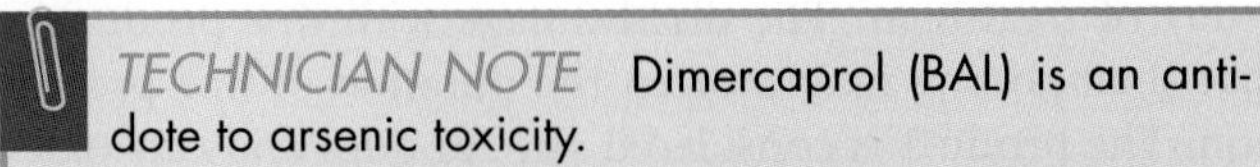
TECHNICIAN NOTE Dimercaprol (BAL) is an antidote to arsenic toxicity.

Microfilariae ingested by mosquitoes from infected animals molt in the mosquitoes and are then introduced back into other animals when another blood meal is taken. It is these reintroduced microfilariae that molt again into larvae and become adult heartworms. Drugs used for heartworm prevention, such as diethylcarbamazine (DEC), ivermectin, milbemycin, and moxidectin, act by killing the tissue-migrating larvae. To review the heartworm life cycle, see Chapter 17.

DEC should be administered daily at the beginning of mosquito season and continued for 2 months after the season is over. If ivermectin or milbemycin is used, it should be given within 1 month of the initial exposure and then once monthly. The final dose is given within 30 days of the last exposure. If more than 45 days elapse between doses, animals should be retested for heartworms before restoration of preventative therapy. In mild climates where mosquitoes prevail year round, prophylactic treatment must be administered for the lifetime of the dog.

Although relatively nontoxic at the low dose used for heartworm prevention, DEC is somewhat irritating to the gastric mucosa. Oral administration is therefore recommended immediately after a meal to reduce nausea and vomiting. These adverse effects are usually seen only with the higher doses of DEC that are sometimes used to treat ascarids.

Milbemycin and ivermectin are available as one-per-month heartworm preventatives. Milbemycin (Interceptor, Novartis) and ivermectin/pyrantel (Heartgard Plus, Merial Ltd.) have the added protection against adult hookworms caused by *Ancylostoma caninum*. Ivermectin toxicities (although rarely observed at the low-dose heartworm preventative level) unique to collie breeds are not seen with milbemycin.

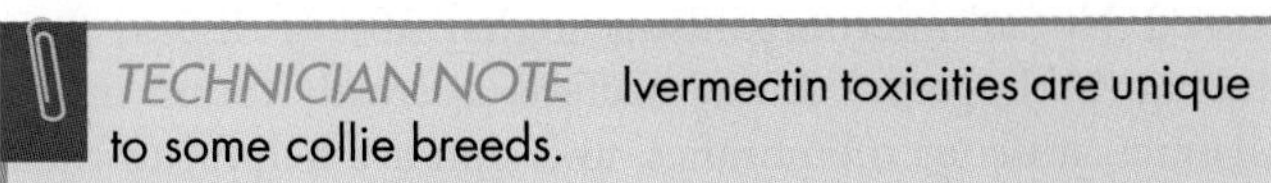
TECHNICIAN NOTE Ivermectin toxicities are unique to some collie breeds.

Moxidectin (ProHeart, Fort Dodge) activity results in paralysis and death of the affected parasites at the tissue larvae stage. Not only is moxidectin indicated for heartworm prevention use in dogs 6 months and older, but also treatment of existing larvae and adult hookworm infections. Moxidectin is the first antimicrofilaria that is injectable and provides 6 months of continuous protection in one dose. It should be administered by a Doctor of Veterinary Medicine (DVM). Professional administration avoids the need for the owner to remember when the dose is due.

Anticestodal Drugs

Anticestodal drugs kill and/or facilitate expulsion of tapeworms. The original drugs used were agents that temporarily paralyzed the tapeworms, causing them to lose their attachment to the GI tract. Even when these drugs contained purgative properties (causing the emptying, cleansing, or evacuation of the bowels) or were given with harsh laxatives, reattachment of a number of tapeworms was likely to occur. This treatment was stressful to the host because its ineffectiveness required repeated dosing. Newer drugs, although more expensive, kill the tapeworm and have replaced most other anticestodal drug on the market.

After oral administration, praziquantel is widely distributed throughout the body, which makes it unique in its effectiveness against various stages of tapeworm development, including the adult stage. In addition, it is nontoxic and has a wide margin of safety. It can also be given by injection.

Epsiprantel has proven to be safe and effective. Unlike praziquantel, only trace levels of it are absorbed after oral administrations, and it remains at the site of action within the GI tract. The exact mechanism of action has not been determined; however, this drug exerts its action directly on the tapeworm causing disruption of attachment to the host. The worm is vulnerable to digestion by the host animal.

Drugs Used To Treat Giardiasis

Giardia canis is a protozoan that may produce chronic diarrhea in dogs. Treatment with metronidazole is usually effective. In general, the toxicity is low; few adverse effects are reported during or after the 5-day treatment period.

Giardiasis is also found in cats, but clinically, it is usually not a problem (its diarrhea-producing role is not known). For treatment in the cat, metronidazole is given in a dosage regimen similar to that used in dogs. The margin of safety in cats is much narrower. Overdosing must be avoided because it may lead to death.

Investigations show that *Giardia* with presenting diarrhea may be successfully treated with an "alternating 7 days on-7 days off" regimen of fenbendazole. A label claim to this indication has not been made.

EXTERNAL PARASITE TREATMENT

Chlorinated Hydrocarbons

Various chlorinated hydrocarbon compounds (e.g., lindane and methoxychlor) were once popular and marketed in several different formulations for a variety of uses in a number of species. The compounds were effective and possess rapid knockdown capability, with some having residual effects for several days. The long-lasting residual properties posed a threat as an environmental hazard, and as a result, many of these types of products have been banned. Although the degree of toxicity will vary among the various chlorinated hydrocarbons, they should all be treated with caution and used as advised on the container label. Some diluted aqueous suspensions and powders may be applied directly to livestock. Signs of toxicity include vomiting, weakness, and other CNS effects, such as tremors, incoordination, convulsions, coma, and respiratory failure. Young, debilitated, or lean animals are more susceptible to the toxic effects. There is no specific antidote for chlorinated hydrocarbon toxicity. The animal should be removed from further exposure and given supportive treatment, such as barbiturates, to control seizures, if necessary.

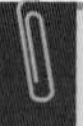

TECHNICIAN NOTE There is no specific antidote for chlorinated hydrocarbon toxicity.

Organophosphates

Organophosphates (ronnel, coumaphos, trichlorfon, malathion) are formulated specifically for the treatment of external parasites. As with chlorinated hydrocarbons, a number of preparations exist, such as sprays, dips, foggers, pour-ons, and pest strips. These compounds have good insect-killing ability, but residual effects are related to the vehicle used to apply the agent. Topical application of these preparations permits significant absorption through the skin to produce signs of toxicity. Signs and treatment of toxicity are the same as those mentioned in the discussion on internal parasitism treatment. Persons applying these agents should avoid getting them in their eyes or on their skin. The use of disposable gloves and eye protection is recommended. Prolonged breathing of spray mists should also be avoided.

Pyrethrins

Pyrethrum flowers (chrysanthemums) have been used as insecticides for centuries. Formulations for animal use are reported to be nontoxic to mammals in addition to having little effect on the environment. Some toxicity has occurred in cats.

Pyrethrins are marketed in numerous formulations for convenient use. Most have chemicals, such as piperonyl butoxide, added to potentiate their killing power. Also, microencapsulation has significantly increased the residual activity of these compounds that were known initially for their quick "knockdown" effect.

Permethrin, a synthetic pyrethroid, is formulated and used similarly to the natural pyrethrins.

Miscellaneous Agents

Several manufacturers have marketed new once-per-month flea control products. Lufenuron is a benzoyl-phenyl-urea derivative classified as an insect development inhibitor. The product does not kill adult fleas, but instead safely and effectively controls flea populations by breaking the life cycle at the egg stage. Preexisting flea populations may continue to develop and emerge after flea treatment, so noticeable control may not be seen for several weeks after dosing. Lufenuron is available in tablet formulation for dogs and oral liquid and injectable formulations for cats older than 6 weeks of age.

Imidacloprid is a flea adulticide formulated for topical application. It is classified as a nitroguanidine and acts as an NT blocker in the insect. Imidacloprid will kill fleas within 1 day of treatment. The disadvantage with this product is that shampooing may shorten the duration of flea protection. The product is considered safe for dogs and cats older than 4 months of age.

Fipronil is classified as a phenylpyrazole and acts as a GABA inhibitor. It is a topical formulation for control of fleas by killing adult fleas. There is a product label claim for killing all stages of brown dog ticks, American dog ticks, Lone Star ticks, and deer ticks. After an application, the animal can be handled immediately and shampooed the following day. Fipronil is safe for dogs and cats 8 weeks of age and older.

Moxidectin is an endectocide of the milbemycin class used to treat infections caused by internal and external parasites in cattle.

Selamectin, a member of the avermectin class, is a once-per-month topical treatment for dogs and cats 6 weeks of age and older. Selamectin kills adult fleas and prevents flea eggs from hatching for 1 month. It is indicated for the prevention and control of flea infestations, prevention of heartworm disease, treatment and control of ear mite infestation, treatment and control of sarcoptic mange, control of tick infestation in dogs, and treatment of intestinal hookworm and roundworm infection in cats.

ANTIMICROBIAL AGENTS

Initially, antibiotics (antimicrobials) were defined as substances produced by microorganisms, which in low concentrations destroy or inhibit growth of other species of microorganisms. Many of these substances may be produced totally or in part through chemical synthesis. Because antibiotics have the potential to cure life-threatening infections, they are one of the most popular and useful groups of drugs in veterinary medicine.

It is important to know the characteristics and uses of the various antibiotics and have a proper understanding of the principles of antibiotic therapy (chemotherapy). It is beyond the scope of this chapter to present a thorough discussion of chemotherapy; however, some basic principles are discussed. Not all microorganisms are harmful or disease producing (pathogenic). Many bacteria normally found in the GI tract, mucous membranes, and skin are helpful to their host. They compete with invading harmful pathogens and keep them from proliferating, thereby preventing progression to a disease state.

Each antibiotic is effective against specific groups of microorganisms. Some antibiotics are bactericidal (destroy bacteria), and some are bacteriostatic (inhibit growth); some may be both, depending on the concentration of the antibiotic (Box 25-1). The various species of bacteria that

BOX 25-1 Antibacterial Action at Usual Serum Concentrations

Bacteriostatic
CHPC
Tetracyclines
Erythromycin
Sulfonamides
Lincomycin

Bactericidal
Penicillin
Aminoglycosides
Cephalosporins
Trimethoprim-sulfa combinations
Quinolones

are affected by the antibiotic are known as the spectrum. Broad-spectrum antibiotics are those that are effective against a wide range of microorganisms, both gram-positive and gram-negative.

One method of classification of bacteria is to determine the tendency to absorb dye (gentian violet) into the cell wall. Those absorbing stain are referred to as gram-positive (dark blue cell walls), and those that do not absorb the stain are known as gram-negative (light pink cell walls) (Box 25-2).

BOX 25-2 Common Animal Pathogens

Gram-Positive Organisms
Streptococcus spp.
Staphylococcus spp.
Clostridium perfringens
Corynebacterium spp.

Gram-Negative Organisms
E. coli
Proteus spp.
Pseudomonas spp.
Klebsiella spp.
Salmonella spp.
Brucella
Vibrio
Pasteurella spp.

For an antibiotic to be effective, it must be able to reach the site of infection in a sufficient concentration to exert its effect on the microorganism. In addition, the antibiotic concentration must be maintained or reached frequently over a period of time to completely destroy all bacteria or inhibit bacterial growth and provide time for the natural defense mechanisms of the body to eradicate the pathogen.

> *TECHNICIAN NOTE* For an antibiotic to be effective, it must reach the site of infection in a sufficient concentration to exert an effect on the microorganism.

The length of antibiotic therapy may vary, depending on factors, such as the site of infection, the microorganism, and the duration of infection. When antibiotics are prescribed, the treatment is usually for a minimum of 5 days. Although improvement may be seen with inadequate antibiotic therapy, it is an unwise practice to stop treatment until the total regimen has been given. Microorganisms exposed to subtherapeutic antibiotic levels may develop resistance to that particular antibiotic, which will then be ineffective even when given at high doses. Bacteria not only can develop resistance to several antibiotics, but can also pass resistance on to other species of bacteria. Multiple antibiotic-resistant bacteria are also a serious problem if resistance is developed in a hospital or practice. Nosocomial (originating in clinical settings) infections from resistant bacteria can be treated with only the most potent and expensive antibiotics. Nosocomial infections are discussed in Chapter 18.

The choice of antibiotic is obviously critical to successful therapy. The microorganism must be sensitive to the antibiotic chosen. A sample from the site of infection (blood, urine, or tissue) should be collected for culture and antibiotic sensitivity testing to determine the causative organism and the effective antibiotics (see Chapter 18). This is not always economically or clinically feasible, so potentially effective antibiotics are frequently just chosen (empiric treatment). Empiric treatment usually includes agents effective against gram-positive, gram-negative, fungal, and viral infections. In selecting an antibiotic, one tries to choose an agent that is most likely to be effective against the pathogen and least likely to disturb normal, nonpathogenic bacteria. Even the narrow-spectrum antibiotics are effective against a number of types of bacteria, both pathogenic and nonpathogenic. Destruction of the nonharmful bacterial flora may allow a second pathogen to manifest and proliferate.

> *TECHNICIAN NOTE* Destruction of nonharmful bacterial flora may allow a second pathogen to proliferate.

Administered antibiotics that are not effective may actually worsen the disease by destroying nonpathogenic bacteria that are actively competing with the pathogen. Indiscriminate use of broad-spectrum antibiotics eventually leads to resistant strains, ineffective antibiotic use, and expensive, perplexing therapeutic problems.

PENICILLINS

The discovery of penicillin in 1920 has dramatically changed the outcome of many life-threatening infections. The basic penicillin molecule (Figure 25-7) has been continuously manipulated and changed to produce a number of improved penicillins with unique characteristics.

Penicillin G (benzylpenicillin), the first clinically used penicillin, is still used extensively in large animals in its procaine salt form. Procaine penicillin G is poorly soluble and is released slowly from its site of injection, providing adequate penicillin levels to allow once-daily dosing; however, twice-daily dosing is usually recommended. Penicillin G is effective when given orally, but high doses must be administered because only approximately one fourth of it is absorbed from the GI tract. Most of the antibiotic is destroyed by stomach acid, so it should not be given directly after feeding, when stomach acid is greatest.

Penicillin acts by blocking bacterial cell wall synthesis in the final stages of replication. Without a cell wall, the bacteria swell and cannot function properly, and some lysis (rupturing) may occur. New infections in a high-log growth phase are therefore most susceptible to penicillin. Penicillin has no direct effect on mammalian cells because they do not have cell walls.

TECHNICIAN NOTE Infections in the high-log phase are more susceptible to penicillin.

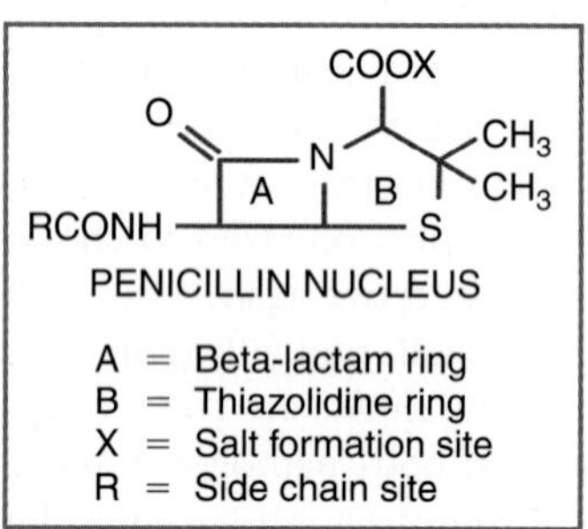

FIGURE 25-7 Penicillin nucleus.

Penicillin G is effective against most of the gram-positive microorganisms, including many of the streptococcal and staphylococcal species. Some staphylococcal species have the ability to produce penicillinase, an enzyme that hydrolyzes the lactam ring and thus renders the penicillin inactive. At high doses, penicillin G is effective against a few gram-negative species.

One alteration of the penicillin molecule was to make it more resistant to hydrolysis by stomach acid. For example, amoxicillin and potassium clavulanate, a specific β-lactamase inhibitor, is a combination product prepared to resist the action of penicillinase. Table 25-2 provides some comparison among various commercially available penicillins. From side-chain alteration of the molecule emerged penicillins that are effective against a wide variety of microorganisms. Some of the penicillins available for human use have a broad spectrum of activity and are the most important potent antibiotics for use against many gram-negative organisms that may be resistant to most other antibiotics.

There is documentation that some patients that are sensitive to the penicillins are also sensitive to another class of antibiotics: cephalosporins (cross-sensitivity). In general, the penicillins are safe. Allergic reactions, such as skin rashes, fever, urticaria, salivation, cutaneous edema, and other hypersensitivities, may occur and lead to justifiable concern.

AMINOGLYCOSIDES

Aminoglycosides (streptomycin, neomycin, kanamycin, amikacin, gentamicin) have a fairly broad spectrum, but are used primarily for the activity against gram-negative organisms. Aminoglycosides are not adequately absorbed when administered orally, but they may be used orally for intestinal tract infections or "sterilization" of the GI tract before

TABLE 25-2 Comparison of Penicillin Products

Product	Acid Stable	Resists Penicillinase Hydrolysis	Spectrum, Comments
Penicillin G	No	No	Mostly gram-positive
Penicillin V	Yes	No	Mostly gram-positive, less effective than penicillin G against some species
Procaine penicillin G	NA*	No	Same as penicillin G
Dicloxacillin, oxacillin	Yes	Yes	Mostly gram-positive
Ampicillin, hetacillin	Yes	No	Mostly gram-positive plus *Escherichia coli*, *Proteus mirabilis*, and a few other gram-negative organisms
Amoxicillin	Yes	No	Spectrum similar to ampicillin, better absorbed
Carbenicillin	Yes†	No	Gram-positive plus several gram-negative, including *P. aeruginosa* (oral form effective only in urinary tract infections)
Azlocillin, mezlocillin, piperacillin	NA	No	Broadest spectrum penicillins effective against most gram-negative organisms, including *Klebsiella* spp.

**NA*, Not applicable (no oral forms).
†Indanyl sodium salt for oral use.

surgery. Aminoglycosides exert their action by interfering with bacteria protein synthesis. Although toxicity may vary among agents, all are potentially ototoxic (affecting hearing balance) and nephrotoxic (renal toxicity). Neuromuscular blockage is also an adverse effect that is manifested by apnea and progressive paralysis of skeletal muscle. When aminoglycosides are administered to animals with preexisting renal damage, the patient must be closely monitored because potential for toxicity is much greater.

> TECHNICIAN NOTE All aminoglycosides are potentially ototoxic and nephrotoxic and may cause neuromuscular blockage.

Resistance, toxicity, and expense are major considerations in the selection of these agents. Resistance demonstrated by organisms may be to a particular aminoglycoside or commonly to several aminoglycosides within this class (cross-resistance).

Neomycin is nephrotoxic and therefore finds its use primarily in topical or ophthalmic preparations. Kanamycin, gentamicin, and amikacin are commercially available as veterinary products. Although expensive for humans, other aminoglycosides are finding use in veterinary medicine for highly resistant organisms that are not susceptible to other antibiotics.

Aminoglycosides are frequently used simultaneously with some of the newer penicillins or cephalosporins to treat stubborn gram-negative infections. Because the combinations are more effective than the use of either agent alone, the activity of the combination is called synergism. The use of aminoglycosides and CHPC together is contraindicated because it is an antagonistic combination, resulting in decreased antibacterial action.

CEPHALOSPORINS

Cephalosporins (cephalexin, cefadroxil, cephradine, cephapirin, cefuroxime, cefotaxime, ceftazidime, and ceftiofur) are somewhat chemically similar (Figure 25-8) to the penicillins and share a similar mechanism of action and spectrum. Cephalosporins are not destroyed by penicillinase-producing bacteria, although some resistance to them exists.

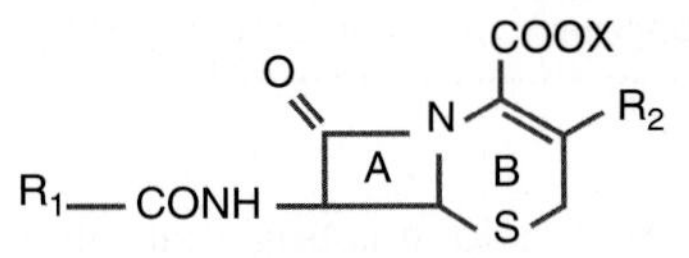

FIGURE 25-8 Cephalosporin nucleus.

The cephalosporins are subclassified primarily by spectrum into first, second, third, and fourth generations. Only minor differences exist in the spectrum of the first generation; all are effective against most gram-positive bacteria and several gram-negative species. The second generation has a somewhat broader spectrum, displaying activity against most clostridial species and adds more gram-negative coverage and less gram-positive coverage. Although *Pseudomonas aeruginosa* is not susceptible to the first- or second-generation cephalosporins, it may be treated with the third-generation cephalosporins. Severe infections, such as *Pseudomonas* infections, are usually treated with a combination of antibiotics to ensure eradication and limit the possibility of developing resistance. The fourth generation cephalosporin cefepime can be compared with the third generation, but is more resistant to some chromosomal β-lactams, such as those produced by *Enterobacter*.

The cost of the cephalosporins limits their use in veterinary medicine. Even with the availability of veterinary cephalosporin and generic products for humans, cost remains a major concern when considering second- and third-generation cephalosporins.

The cephalosporins have a low incidence of adverse effects. Long-term use of excessively large doses may lead to some complications similar to those of other antibiotics, including possible allergic reactions or overgrowth of nonsusceptible bacteria or fungi, leading to intestinal pain, bloating, and diarrhea.

QUINOLONES

Quinolones constitute a class of antibiotics finding extensive use in veterinary medicine for treatment of a wide variety of organisms, including *P. aeruginosa*. Enrofloxacin is approved primarily for urinary, skin, and respiratory infections in dogs and cats, but it is also being used to treat bone and other infections in several additional species. There is a subcutaneous injection approved for cattle not intended for food to treat bovine respiratory disease (BRD) associated with *Pasteurella haemolytica, Pasteurella multocida,* and *Haemophilus somnus*.

Enrofloxacin seems to be well tolerated, and few side effects have been noted in animals. It is contraindicated in puppies during the rapid growth phase because it can induce abnormal cartilage formation, leading to weakness or lameness. This potential adverse effect discourages the use of enrofloxacin in other young animals and in adult horses. Although bacterial resistance to enrofloxacin is not yet common, indiscriminate use to treat routine infections is likely to produce resistant strains, making this valuable drug worthless.

CHLORAMPHENICOL

Chloramphenicol use in humans is limited to a few specific infections because of a rare but potentially fatal occurrence of irreversible aplastic anemia. Personnel who handle and administer CHPC to animals should use care, avoiding direct contact with the drug. Although some blood dyscrasias have been seen in animals, particularly in neonates, the condition is usually reversible by withdrawal of the drug.

> TECHNICIAN NOTE CHPC causes reversible blood dyscrasias. Personnel who handle and/or administer CHPC should use care and avoid direct contact.

CHPC is an important antibiotic in veterinary equine medicine. Although CHPC is bacteriostatic, it has a fairly broad spectrum of activity. It is rapidly distributed to most body compartments and tissues in adequate therapeutic concentrations. A small amount of CHPC is excreted unchanged in the urine, but most undergo biotransformation in the liver to the inactive glucuronide conjugate.

Other adverse effects include anorexia, diarrhea, vomiting, and depression and other rare but severe effects. CHCP in combination with other antibiotics is usually contraindicated. It interacts with several specific drugs or groups of drugs, including anticonvulsants, penicillins, phenylbutazone, and lincomycin.

Florphenicol is a broad-spectrum, primarily bacteriostatic antibiotic with a range of activity similar to that of CHCP against many gram-negative and gram-positive organisms. It does not carry the risk of inducing blood dyscrasias.

TETRACYCLINES

Oxytetracycline and tetracycline are practically used interchangeably because of a similarity in spectrum and pharmacologic properties. One tetracycline, doxycycline, has gained acceptance for use in small animals. It requires less frequent dosing and penetrates the CNS better than other tetracyclines.

These bacteriostatic agents affect the vital protein synthesis of the microorganism. Although the tetracyclines possess a relatively broad spectrum of activity, the development of resistant organisms has been a factor that limits use. Through more judicious use of these agents, less-resistant strains are being encountered.

The absorption of tetracyclines from the GI tract is adequate, but is decreased in the presence of food, milk, or antacids. Some injectable preparations use propylene glycol as a solvent and are not recommended for intramuscular use because they are painful. When given intravenously, the tetracycline must be injected slowly because the solvent and drug may exert a blocking effect on the heart, causing the animal to temporarily collapse. Other injectable preparations contain povidone or similar agents, which reduce intramuscular irritation and eliminate the cardiac problem. The intramuscular product formulated for extended action must not be given intravenously.

Out-of-date or improperly stored tetracyclines should never be administered because they form nephrotoxic products.

> TECHNICIAN NOTE Tetracyclines form complexes with calcium in developing bones and teeth and should not be given to young animals.

Tetracyclines are relatively inexpensive and widely used, especially in food animals. The tetracyclines are also commonly used at low levels as a livestock feed additive to increase weight gain and decrease liver abscesses. This practice promotes the development of resistant strains of bacteria, rendering the tetracyclines useless for treatment even when given at therapeutic levels.

Although popular, the tetracyclines have toxicities. A common toxicity is the intestinal problems associated with disruption of the natural intestinal flora, including the possibility of superinfection by resistant organisms. Hypersensitivity reactions of rashes, fever, and liver damage may also occur with use of tetracyclines. The tetracyclines form complexes with calcium in developing bones and teeth; they should not be given to pregnant or young animals because tooth discoloration, increases in dental caries, and temporary suppression in bone growth may occur.

MISCELLANEOUS ANTIBIOTICS

Erythromycin and tilmicosin are classified as macrolide antibiotics because of their high molecular weight. The spectrum of activity is similar to that of penicillin; therefore they are commonly used instead of penicillin against penicillinase-producing microbes. Erythromycin does not alter intestinal flora extensively, but GI effects, such as vomiting and diarrhea, have been observed.

Tilmicosin is a macrolide used to treat bovine respiratory diseases, including those caused by *Mycoplasma*. A distinct advantage of tilmicosin is its long half-life, which allows a single-dose treatment. Tilmicosin must only be administered by subcutaneous or intramuscular injections because fatalities have been reported with intravenous dosage. Deaths have been reported after the use of tilmicosin in swine, horses, and nonhuman primates. The drug must be handled with extreme caution and administered in accordance with the detailed label instructions.

> TECHNICIAN NOTE Fatalities have been reported with IV use of tilmicosin; therefore it must be administered subcutaneously or intramuscularly only.

Azithromycin is a long-acting macrolide administered orally that is used to treat *Chlamydia* infections of the eye.

Lincomycin is in the class lincosamides. It has a spectrum of activity similar to erythromycin and is particularly effective against *Staphylococcus* and *Streptococcus* spp. It has been useful when resistant strains or hypersensitivities to other antibiotics exist. Favorable results have been reported in the treatment of bone infections and various skin disorders (pyoderma) with lincomycin. The drug is concentrated and excreted in the bile. Lincomycin causes severe intestinal flora disturbances in horses, hamsters, and rabbits, so it should be avoided in these species.

OTHER ANTIMICROBIAL AGENTS

In addition to the antibiotics discussed, other chemical agents exist that are effective against certain strains of microorganisms. The sulfa drugs were the first antimicrobial agents to be used systemically in the treatment of bacterial infections.

SULFONAMIDES

Numerous sulfonamides (sulfamethazine, sulfadiazine, sulfadimethoxine) have been formulated. Their value and use have declined with the discovery of newer antibiotics; however, a few sulfonamides remain useful for certain conditions. These agents are relatively inexpensive, which makes them attractive for use in large animals for herd or flock treatment. The sulfonamides are particularly useful in the treatment of various infections of the respiratory system and urinary tract, bacterial diarrhea, foot rot, and coccidial infections. Unfortunately, bacterial resistance to the sulfonamides limits their effectiveness. A toxicity seen with the original sulfonamides was crystalluria, a condition in which insoluble crystals formed in the urine, causing renal damage. Because the solubility of one sulfonamide is independent of other sulfonamides, the formulation of triple sulfa was developed to avert crystalluria. More soluble sulfonamides are also available, thereby further reducing concern. It is important that animals receiving sulfonamide have adequate water available.

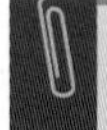

TECHNICIAN NOTE It is important that animals receiving sulfonamides have adequate water available.

The intravenous preparations of sulfonamides have a high (basic) pH and are therefore damaging to tissue when inadvertently given perivascularly (in spaces around blood vessels). In addition, the intravenous preparations should be given slowly to prevent acute toxicity demonstrated by CNS effects, such as salivation, vomiting, diarrhea, weakness, ataxia, and convulsions.

TRIMETHOPRIM-SULFONAMIDE COMBINATIONS

Effective antibacterials being used are combination products of one part trimethoprim and five parts sulfadiazine or sulfamethoxazole. Ormetoprim with sulfadimethoxine is a comparable combination with similar use and actions. These combinations block two essential sequential steps in the replication process of the bacteria, resulting in a synergistic antibacterial action. The combinations are effective against a wide range of organisms, but not *Pseudomonas*.

Undesirable side effects seen with these combinations are infrequent. Although vomiting may occur, diarrhea is seldom seen. Animals that are deficient in folic acid may be prone to develop blood disorders, as has been reported in humans.

NITROFURANS

The nitrofurans (nitrofurazone, nitrofurantoin, furazolidone) have been replaced to a great extent by newer, more effective, and safer antibacterials. These synthetic agents have a fairly broad spectrum of activity, but they are not effective against *Pseudomonas*.

Except for topical application, use in food-producing animals is strictly forbidden by the FDA because of carcinogenic properties.

Nitrofurantoin is sufficiently absorbed and has some use in small animals in the treatment of urinary tract infections. Nausea and vomiting, which are common adverse effects, can be reduced by administering nitrofurantoin with food or using the macrocrystal human preparations.

ANTIFUNGAL AGENTS

Numerous topical agents are available to treat fungal infections of the skin (dermatomycosis). Griseofulvin is administered orally; it has no antibacterial activity, but inhibits the growth of various skin fungi. It is an expensive product and is not usually the first-line choice unless the infection is widespread.

The treatment of systemic fungal infections (e.g., cryptococcosis, blastomycosis, histoplasmosis) is usually expensive, requiring lengthy treatment with limited success. Amphotericin B, an antibiotic used for various fungal infections, is toxic, causing kidney and liver damage, CNS abnormalities, and so on. A newer formulation of amphotericin B in a lipid complex suspension eliminates some toxic effects experienced with the original solution. Nystatin, another antibiotic, is relatively nontoxic, but has a narrow spectrum of activity. Nystatin has activity against a variety of fungal organisms, but is used systemically to treat oropharyngeal and GI *Candida* infections.

Ketoconazole, an expensive antifungal agent, has proven to be effective against a variety of fungal infections. Ketoconazole causes hepatotoxicity (liver damage), so liver enzymes should be monitored during therapy. Itraconazole is a newer agent that is efficacious against a variety of fungal infections and is less hepatotoxic than ketoconazole and more expensive.

TECHNICIAN NOTE Ketoconazole causes hepatotoxicity, and the liver functions should be monitored during use.

HORMONES AND SYNTHETIC SUBSTITUTES

Hormones that act on or are released by various organs are also used in treatment of specific diseases and disorders.

THYROID HORMONES

The thyroid gland is controlled primarily by the amount of thyroid-stimulating hormone released from the pituitary gland. When stimulated, the thyroid gland releases thyroid hormones consisting primarily of thyroxin. Because the thyroid hormones affect the metabolism of carbohydrates, protein, and fats, thyroid-deficient (hypothyroid) animals show signs of lethargy, reduced alertness, increased body weight, poor hair coat, and other related signs. Insufficient amounts of iodine in the diet can result in inadequate production of thyroid hormones. Such hormone deficiencies can be treated with desiccated thyroid because it is effective orally. Sodium levothyroxine may be the most popular agent for the treatment of hypothyroidism. Sodium liothyronine, the other active component of desiccated thyroid, is also available commercially.

Feline hyperthyroidism is treated with methimazole. It interferes with iodine incorporation into tyrosyl residues of thyroglobulin, thereby inhibiting the synthesis of thyroid hormones.

INSULIN

Insulin is normally produced and released by islet cells of the pancreas. This hormone is necessary to facilitate the use of food by the body, especially sugar. Insulin enhances the absorption of glucose in most cells of the body. Animals with inadequate insulin will have abnormally high blood glucose levels (hyperglycemia) and other associated metabolic disorders. Dog and cat insulin are thought to resemble more closely porcine than beef insulin. Insulin injection (regular Iletin) is a solution of dissolved insulin crystals, which accounts for its immediate action and short duration. There are other insulin preparations that are intermediate acting (approximately 24 hours) to long acting (approximately 36 hours). Isophane insulin suspension (NPH), an intermediate-acting insulin, tends to be widely used in small animal medicine.

Protamine zinc insulin (PZI) may take 1 to 4 hours for onset of action to occur. The effect of PZI peaks between 5 and 20 hours after dosing and may persist up to 30 hours. Dogs are generally controlled with once-a-day dosing. In cats, PZI insulin would begin to decrease blood sugar in about 1 to 3 hours and has its peak effect in 4 to 10 hours. The duration of action may be 12 to 30 hours. Nearly all cats require twice-daily dosing for good control.

With the emergence of recombinant products, it may be difficult to obtain insulin of animal origin. The newest product on the market, glargine insulin (Lantus), is another recombinant product that is being introduced in veterinary medicine. Glargine is a once-a-day recombinant product that peaks in about 12 hours. It was designed to prevent the highs and lows that the diabetic patient experiences with use of other insulin products. Animals that were originally administered insulin from animal sources may need to have dose adjustments if switched to recombinant products. Any change in insulin should be made cautiously and under the medical supervision of the veterinarian.

> *TECHNICIAN NOTE* Dose adjustments may be needed if animals are switched to recombinant products from insulin of animal origin.

Overdoses of insulin produce hypoglycemia, which, if severe, can lead to coma and death. Treatment of hypoglycemia consists of administration of intravenous dextrose or intramuscular injection of glucagon.

If an animal develops hypersensitivity (local or systemic reaction) or insulin resistance, a change in type or species of insulin should be tried.

OXYTOCIN

Oxytocin is a hormone released at the end of pregnancy to stimulate uterine contractions during parturition and induce milk letdown. The synthetically produced oxytocin is destroyed in the GI tract and must be administered parenterally. It is beneficial during delayed parturition, for aiding milk letdown, treatment of postpartum retained placenta, and metritis.

PROSTAGLANDINS

Prostaglandins are found in many mammalian tissues and have been shown to have a wide variety of effects on a number of body systems, including the CNS, cardiovascular, urinary, GI, and reproductive systems. Commercially available PGs, such as dinoprost and cloprostenol, are used because of the effects on the reproductive system.

In cattle, PGs can be used to regulate the heat cycle, so breeding and consequent calving times for a herd can be planned. PGs are approved by the FDA to abort feedlot heifers. For certain conditions in mares, PGs can effectively restore the normal heat cycle so that the animals can be bred.

Pregnant women should not handle these agents because they are abortifacients. Bronchospasm is another serious adverse effect in animals and humans that may occur as a result of contact with the product. Consequently, PGs should not be handled by asthmatics or used in animals with respiratory diseases.

> *TECHNICIAN NOTE* PGs are abortifacients and cause bronchospasms. They should not be handled by pregnant women or asthmatics or used in animals with respiratory disease.

GASTROINTESTINAL DRUGS

ANTIEMETICS

Certain species, such as horses, rabbits, and rodents, are unable to vomit, but protracted vomiting may become a problem in dogs, cats, and other species.

The vomiting reflex may be stimulated through at least four different pathways. For example, chemical substances in the blood (bacterial toxins or certain drugs) may mediate vomiting via the chemoreceptor trigger zone (CTZ) pathway (medulla of brain). Vomiting arising from movement of the head (motion sickness) is transmitted through another pathway (cortex of the brain). In selecting an antiemetic agent, it is desirable to know the underlying cause of vomiting and the pathway involved because some antiemetic drugs are specific in their site of action. Vomiting may be a symptom of a disease state, so initial attention should be directed to treatment of the primary disease.

Although independent of their antihistaminic activity, a few of the antihistamines (e.g., dimenhydrinate, cyclizine, clemastine, and meclizine) and scopolamine are effective in preventing vomiting induced by motion sickness. The principal side effect of the antihistamine is drowsiness, which may be desirable in pets that are traveling.

A number of phenothiazine tranquilizers (chlorpromazine, prochlorperazine, and triflupromazine) are classified as broad-spectrum antiemetics that control vomiting by blocking the CTZ at low doses and at the emetic center (in the medulla of the brain) at higher doses. Although these agents have the potential of producing a number of adverse effects, the risk of toxicity is low because of the low dose and short duration of therapy. Some potent broad-spectrum, human antiemetics (e.g., haloperidol and metoclopramide) are finding use in veterinary medicine.

Metoclopramide is a unique pharmacologic agent. Besides its potent antiemetic property, especially in drug-induced emesis (e.g., cancer chemotherapy), metoclopramide is also a peristaltic stimulant, increasing gut motility. It has been used for gastric stasis in a number of species, including horses and cattle. In addition, to facilitate radiologic examination of the stomach or small intestine, metoclopramide may be used to stimulate gastric emptying and intestinal transit of barium in cases where delayed emptying interferes. Reflux esophagitis in dogs and cats has also been treated with metoclopramide.

Cisapride is useful as an equine GI prokinetic agent (increases motility) in reflux conditions. Cisapride is no longer available commercially, but may be obtained from a compounding pharmacy.

Vomiting related to chemotherapy has been treated with ondansetron, granisetron, dolasetron, and butorphanol. Maropitant citrate (Cerenia, Pfizer) has been formulated specifically for targeting the mechanism that causes patients to vomit when undergoing chemotherapy.

EMETICS

Agents to induce vomiting are used clinically as a rapid means of eliminating certain poisons or to remove food from the stomach before induction of general anesthesia. A once common emetic used in veterinary medicine is apomorphine. Although still commercially available, it is extremely expensive and difficult to obtain. Apomorphine stimulates the CTZ and may be administered orally, intramuscularly, intravenously, or via the conjunctival sac of the eye. Because apomorphine depresses the emetic center, repeated dosage is not recommended when the initial dose is ineffective. Apomorphine should not be given to cats because it produces extreme excitement. Xylazine, a sedative analgesic, can be used as an emetic because of the routine vomiting it produces in the cat.

Ipecac, once used commonly in cats and occasionally in dogs, has the disadvantage of having to be administered via a stomach tube because of taste. In addition, its effects may be somewhat sporadic. Some toxic effects, including death, may be induced with ipecac in cats. However, ipecac syrup remains a popular, convenient emetic for children for the removal of accidentally ingested noncorrosive poison.

ANTIDIARRHEAL AGENTS

Diarrhea, like vomiting, may only be a symptom of an underlying problem. Ideally, it is best to identify the specific problem and correct it. Current trends are not to slow the gut, but to allow it to remain active to remove any present toxins or irritants. Most small animals with diarrhea recover regardless of therapy. Persistent diarrhea not only may be offensive to pet owners, but also may require supportive treatment, such as electrolyte and fluid replacement. Anticholinergics, such as the various belladonna alkaloids (atropine, homatropine, and scopolamine), have historically been used to treat diarrhea. Although peristalsis (propulsive intestinal contractions) is reduced, a minimal antidiarrheal effect results. The value of using anticholinergics is questionable because they have adverse effects, such as increased heart rate, dryness of mouth, and diarrhea from gut paralysis.

Opiates, including opium tincture, morphine, codeine, and similar derivatives, such as diphenoxylate, are unique in that they increase rhythmic segmentation contraction, which resists intestinal flow and decreases peristalsis. In addition, the opiates increase the tone of the various sphincters and valves in the GI tract, which further delays movement of the contents. The commercial product diphenoxylate hydrochloride with atropine sulfate is effective in treating diarrhea in dogs.

The use of antidiarrheal opiates in cats is controversial because this species may react with excitatory behavior. Opiate antidiarrheals should be used with caution in patients with head injuries or increased intracranial pressures and acute abdominal conditions, such as colic, because the opiates may obscure diagnosis or clinical course of the condition. Opiate antidiarrheals should be used with extreme caution in patients with hepatic disease and CNS symptoms of hepatic encephalopathy because hepatic coma may result.

The use of opiates in animals with acute diarrhea that may be bacterially induced may enhance bacterial proliferation, delay the disappearance of the microbe from the feces, and prolong the febrile state. Acute overdoses of the opiate antidiarrheals could result in central nervous, cardiovascular, or respiratory system toxicity.

Another over-the-counter (OTC) preparation that is extensively used in veterinary medicine is the human product loperamide. Loperamide is a synthetic piperidine derivative that slows intestinal motility through a direct effect on the nerve endings and/or intramural ganglia of the intestinal wall. In animals, loperamide does not have analgesic activity, even in extremely high doses. Loperamide is available in tablet, capsule, and oral liquid formulations.

Bismuth subsalicylate is thought to have weak antibacterial properties and is a protectant and antiendotoxic. Popular thought suggests that the compound is cleaved in the small intestine into bismuth carbonate and salicylate. The bismuth carbonate is responsible for the protective, antiendotoxic, and weak antibacterial properties. The salicylate component has antiprostaglandin activity, which may contribute to its effectiveness and reduce symptoms associated with secretory diarrhea. In humans, the preparation is used for other GI symptoms (e.g., indigestion, cramps, and gas pains) and in the treatment and prophylaxis of traveler's diarrhea.

CATHARTICS (LAXATIVES)

There are relatively few clinical reasons to use cathartics in veterinary medicine. Occasionally, an older animal may have constipation, but usually, alteration of the diet will correct the problem. Another indication might be for the treatment of hairballs in cats. After bowel or anal surgery, stool softeners may reduce stress at the surgery site until healing takes place. Cathartics and enemas may also be used before GI tract radiographic examinations, proctoscopy, or elective surgery. One of the most legitimate uses of cathartics is in treating food animals and horses suffering with overingestion of concentrated carbohydrates, such as grain. There are a few other unique circumstances in which the use of cathartics is appropriate; however, one is discouraged from overuse because it leads to dependence.

Cathartics increase the motility of the bowel by directly stimulating the smooth muscle or indirectly activating receptors through increased bulk. The irritant laxatives, which directly increase bowel motility, include (1) emodin, found in cascara sagrada, aloe, and senna; (2) sodium ricinoleate, a digestive end product of castor oil; and (3) danthron, a synthetic compound. Bulk-producing cathartics include (1) indigestible materials, such as psyllium seed, methyl cellulose, mineral oil, and white petrolatum, which not only increase bulk, but lubricate and soften fecal masses; (2) saline cathartics, such as magnesium sulfate, sodium sulfate, magnesium oxide, and phosphate salts, which draw water into the bowel; and (3) stool softeners, such as docusate sodium and dioctyl calcium sulfosuccinate. These are surface-active agents, such as soap, that increase bulk through water retention and lubricate and soften the fecal mass.

The cathartics as a group are relatively safe for short-term use, although some may be harsh and cause cramping and diarrhea. Chronic use of the petrolatum type of cathartics may lead to deficiencies in fat-soluble vitamins because of absorption interference.

ULCER MANAGEMENT DRUGS

Gastric ulceration and the subsequent blood loss appear to be related to acid damage commonly associated with high doses of corticosteroids or NSAIDs and to certain medical disorders. Several methods are currently available for treatment and prevention.

Antacids were initially used, but required around-the-clock administration every 2 to 3 hours to truly be effective. A major advancement in human medicine for ulcer management was the introduction of cimetidine, a histamine$_2$-receptor antagonist. Although these agents are not approved for veterinary use, cimetidine, ranitidine, and others are used to block the acid-producing effects of histamine on the gastric parietal cells.

Sucralfate in an acid environment forms an ulcer-adherent complex providing a protective, Band-Aid-like barrier for the damaged mucosa. Sucralfate also inhibits pepsin activity.

Omeprazole is an agent that acts directly on the parietal cell, blocking acid secretion. Omeprazole is formulated as an oral gel that is indicated for treatment and prevention of recurrence of gastric ulcers in horses and foals 4 weeks of age and older. Misoprostol not only blocks gastric acid secretion, but also appears to enhance natural gastromucosal defense mechanisms.

PHARMACY

DRUG LAWS

STATE LAWS

Most state pharmacy laws are primarily concerned with the distribution of drugs within the state. These laws specify who is authorized to prescribe and dispense legend drugs, the licensing of distributors, records required, and certain processing standards.

Because state laws are unique to each state, it is the responsibility of those practicing veterinary medicine to know the laws that apply to them. State laws work in conjunction with federal laws. Sometimes state laws are more restrictive than federal laws; in such cases, one should comply with the state law.

FEDERAL LAWS

Although the Food, Drug and Cosmetic Act of 1938 has been amended numerous times, it is still the basic federal law governing drugs in the United States. This law assures the public that drugs have been prepared through approved manufacturing standards and are safe and effective for the claims made. The Durham-Humphrey Amendment (1951) restricted the availability of certain drugs to prescription through licensed practitioners. This class of drugs, referred to as prescription drugs or legend drugs, is deemed unsafe for lay medication, even with clear and precise label directions.

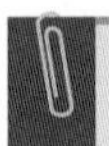

TECHNICIAN NOTE The FDA restricts legend drugs to prescription through a licensed practitioner.

Veterinary labeled prescription drugs bear the legend, "Caution: Federal law restricts this drug to use by or on the order of a licensed veterinarian." Human-labeled prescription drugs bear the legend, "Caution: Federal law prohibits dispensing without a prescription." Commercial packaging may elect to use the "*Rx*" symbol on the label copy to denote drug product status as a legend drug instead of the written caution.

The FDA has the responsibility for determining the marketing status of a drug, whether or not it is possible to prepare adequate directions for use under which a layperson can use the drug safely and effectively. Nonprescription or "*over-the-counter*" drugs may be sold directly to clients, but must bear extensive labeling, which includes warnings and instructions for proper use.

The AVMA has approved the following guidelines regarding the use and distribution of veterinary drugs: (1) A prescription drug can be dispensed only by or upon the lawful written order of a licensed veterinarian within the course of his or her professional practice where a valid veterinarian-client-patient relationship (VCPR) exists; and (2) all veterinary prescription drugs must be properly labeled when dispensed.

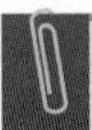

TECHNICIAN NOTE A prescription drug can be dispensed to a client only where a VCPR exists.

VETERINARIAN-CLIENT-PATIENT RELATIONSHIP

A VCPR exists when all of the following conditions have been met:

1. The veterinarian has assumed the responsibility for making clinical judgments regarding the health of the animal(s) and the need for medical treatment, and the client has agreed to follow the veterinarian's instructions.
2. The veterinarian has sufficient knowledge of the animal(s) to initiate at least a general or preliminary diagnosis of the medical condition of the animal(s).
3. The veterinarian is readily available for a follow-up evaluation or has arranged for emergency coverage in the event of adverse reactions or failure of the treatment regimen.

LABEL REQUIREMENTS

Labeling requirements vary between states, but may include:

- Name, address, and telephone number of practice
- Name of client
- Animal identification
- Species of animal
- Date
- Prescribing veterinarian
- Name of medication
- Quantity of medication dispensed
- Adequate directions for proper administration of medication
- Number of authorized refills
- Prescription transaction number (optional)

Auxiliary labels may also be required to caution or inform the client. Examples include "Shake well," "Keep refrigerated," "Do not use after (date)," "Poison," "External use only," and "For veterinary use only." It is the responsibility of the veterinarian to inform clients to whom prescription drugs are delivered or dispensed about appropriate handling and storage.

The ultimate responsibility for any medication dispensed through a veterinary practice lies with the authorizing veterinarian. In some states, the technician may be allowed to assist the veterinarian by typing labels, counting or pouring, attaching labels, and pricing. The technician *should not issue or refill medications without the veterinarian's approval.* For most medications, this would be in violation of the federal law.

Readily retrievable dispensing records may be required by some states to safeguard the public's health. Accidental ingestion of prescription drugs by animals and small children is not uncommon. Proper records can provide attending physicians with the name and the amount of medication dispensed so that appropriate treatment can be provided.

TECHNICIAN NOTE Readily retrievable dispensing records may be required to safeguard the public's health.

The Federal Poison Prevention Packaging Act passed in 1970 requires pharmacists and physicians to dispense medications intended for oral human use in childproof containers. The AVMA recommends that prescription drugs to companion animal owners be placed in child-resistant containers. Certain states mandate the use of such. Veterinary practices failing to use such a safeguard would be highly vulnerable to legal action in a case of accidental poisoning.

TABLE 25-3 Schedule of Controlled Substances

Schedule	Abuse Potential	Dispensing Limits	Distribution Restrictions	Schedule Examples	Comments
I	High	Research use only	DEA form C-222 required	LSD, heroin	No accepted medical use
II	High	Requires written prescription, no refills	DEA form C-222 required	Oxymorphone, sodium pentobarbital injection	Abuse may lead to severe dependence
III	Less than I and II	Oral or written, refills up to five times within 6 mo	DEA registration number	Hycodan, Tylenol with codeine, anabolic steroids	Abuse may lead to moderate dependence
IV	Low	Oral or written, refills up to five times within 6 mo	DEA registration number	Diazepam, phenobarbital	Abuse may lead to limited dependence
V	Low	No DEA limits	DEA registration number	Lomotil, Robitussin AC	Lowest potential for abuse

CONTROLLED SUBSTANCES

The Controlled Substances Act of 1970 reduced drug abuse by defining certain legal and illegal acts regarding substances of high abuse potential. It established and authorized the Drug Enforcement Administration (DEA) to enforce this law. The law is designed to provide an approved means for proper manufacture, distribution, dispensing, and use of controlled substances through licensing of legitimate handlers of these drugs. This "closed" system has been effective in reducing widespread diversion of these drugs into the illicit market. Controlled substances are classified into five classes (schedules) according to the use or abuse potential (Table 25-3).

TECHNICIAN NOTE The DEA enforces the law regarding substances of high abuse potential.

All veterinarians using these drugs in the course of their practice are required to have a DEA license number. Those who engage in administering or dispensing controlled substances in Schedules II, III, IV, and V are required to keep records of such transactions for 2 years. Receiving records for reports of controlled substances received must also be kept for 2 years.

TECHNICIAN NOTE All veterinarians using controlled drugs in the course of their practice are required to have a DEA license number.

In addition, practitioners who handle controlled substances are required to take an initial inventory at the opening of business of all controlled substances. Biannual inventories are required after the initial inventory. Records for receipts and dispensing of Schedule II substances must be kept separate from all other records. When records for Schedules III, IV, and V drugs are incorporated with other drugs, they should be identified with a red "C" in the lower right-hand corner of the record. All controlled substance records must be "readily retrievable." Each commercial container of a controlled substance shall have printed on the label the symbol designating the Schedule in which such is listed, (CII). The word "schedule" need not be used.

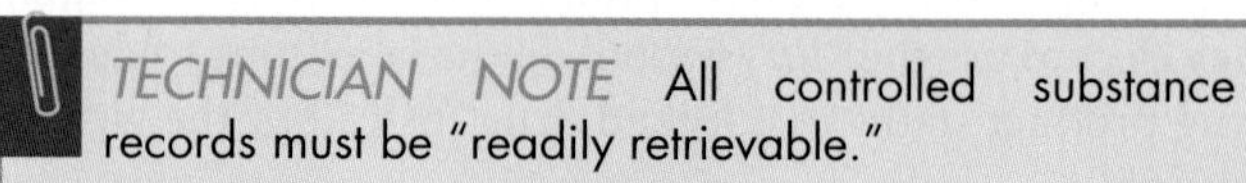

TECHNICIAN NOTE All controlled substance records must be "readily retrievable."

Acquisition and distribution of controlled substances should be monitored by maintenance of a perpetual inventory (Figure 25-9) for each product stored in the practice. Drugs in Schedule II must be ordered on a DEA Form C-222 and completed when drugs are received.

A perpetual inventory is a "checkbook" balance system that provides an up-to-date balance of each drug. It is easier to reconcile inventory when this system is used.

It is best that those persons responsible for handling controlled substances be familiar not only with federal laws governing them but also with state laws, which may be more strict. Agencies, such as the state boards of pharmacy or the local DEA office, are quite helpful in answering questions concerning compliance.

The law states that, "A practitioner who has controlled substances stored in his office or practice must keep these drugs in a securely locked, substantially constructed cabinet or safe." A secure area is usually interpreted as a double-locked container that cannot be picked up and moved. Examples would be a locked metal box stored inside a floor safe or an attached locked wall cabinet. The responsibility for access to controlled substances should be restricted to only one or two persons in the practice. Practitioners experiencing theft or a significant loss of controlled substances must report such a loss to the DEA regional office and the local police department when the loss is discovered.

TECHNICIAN NOTE Controlled substances should be stored in a securely locked, substantially constructed cabinet or safe.

CONTROLLED DRUG INVENTORY

Date	Dept. Rm No.	Vendor	Invoice No./ Control No.	Quantity Received	Quantity Issued	Balance on Hand	RPh	Date	Dept. Rm No.	Vendor	Invoice No./ Control No.	Quantity Received	Quantity Issued	Balance on Hand	RPh
			BEGINNING BALANCE →→→			20	MA								
1/2/04	SAICU		108221		1	19	MA								
1/7/04	SAICU		108236		1	18	SB								
1/9/04		M/D	9162710	25		43	MA								
1/10/04	63415		108376		1	42	MA								
1/13/04	64489		108389		1	41	SB								
1/15/04	64285		108401		1	42	MA								

FENTANYL TRANSDERMAL 75 MCG/HR (DURAGESIC)

FIGURE 25-9 Controlled drug inventory form.

A government publication entitled, *Physician's Manual: An Information Outline on the Controlled Substances Act of 1970* is an excellent guide for proper handling of controlled substances. This government manual may be obtained free by request from the following:

U.S. Department of Justice
Drug Enforcement Administration
1465 "I" Street, NW
Washington, DC 20537

COMPOUNDING

Compounding is the preparation of a drug product by mixing legally, obtainable ingredients and/or appropriate vehicles that have not been listed as an unapproved drug for animals by the regulatory action of the FDA, United States Department of Agriculture (USDA), or Environmental Protection Agency (EPA). When drug products are compounded, distributed, and used there is a possibility of harm to public health and animals if there is no adequate and well-controlled safety and effectiveness data and when there is no adherence to the good manufacturing practices (GMP). Death and adverse drug reactions may result from use of these compounded drugs.

Federal and state laws permit compounding because it sometimes provides value to patients. The practice of veterinary medicine continues to require medications to treat or prevent diseases and requires dosages for different animal species for which there are no commercially prepared, FDA-approved products currently available or efficacious. Concentrations, dosage forms, or combinations of medications that are unavailable can be compounded. Compounding can be used to prepare products that are hard to acquire or are temporarily unavailable from the manufacturer. Pharmacies require a written prescription specifying that the product can be compounded for a specific patient. Veterinarians may compound medicaments for their own patient use. Whether compounding is done at the local practice or in a pharmacy, a recipe is provided so that other pharmacists or veterinarians can provide refills of the same recipe.

Veterinarians, who compound themselves or make the decision to use a compounded product, must assume the responsibility for the safety of animals and wholesomeness of food of animal origin.

TECHNICIAN NOTE The veterinarian who prescribes a compounded product must assume the responsibility of safety to animals and wholesomeness of foods.

Both the pharmacist and veterinarian who compound must use professional judgment that is consistent with proper pharmaceutical and pharmacologic principles when compounding medications. The following points must be considered:

- The stability of the active ingredients
- The physical and chemical compatibility of the ingredients
- The pharmacodynamic compatibility of the ingredients
- The inactive ingredients and diluents must be of known compositions and not contaminated with harmful substances or agents or unapproved sources
- The prepared medication must be properly labeled before dispensing
- Compounded medications must not be advertised or displayed to the public

When compounded medications are used, appropriate records must be maintained. When compounded products are used in food-producing animals, appropriate residue tests, when available and practical, and other procedures for ensuring volatile residue avoidance should be instituted.

> *TECHNICIAN NOTE* Compounded products for food-producing animals require testing for volatile residues.

In the July 14, 2003, *Federal Register,* the FDA released a revised Compliance Policy Guide (CPG) section 608.400 entitled "Compounding of Drugs for Use in Animals" (61FR34840). The purpose of the guide is to ensure that the agency's enforcement policy regarding the compounding of drugs intended for use in animals is consistent, to the extent practical, with its policy regarding the compounding of drugs intended for use in humans. The FDA does not make a distinction between compounding and manufacturing or other processing of drugs for use in animals rather than in humans. It does acknowledge the use of compounding within certain areas of veterinary practice. Regulations specifically permit compounding of products from approved animal or human drugs under conditions set forth in 21CFR 530.13. The activity of compounding is not the subject of this guidance.

Veterinarians and pharmacies that are engaged in manufacturing and distributing unapproved new animal drugs in a manner that is clearly out of bounds of the traditional pharmacy or veterinary practice violate the act.

The three restrictions set for compounding by the FDA are:

- The drug product must not be identified by the FDA as a drug product that presents demonstrable difficulties for compounding in terms of safety or effectiveness.
- In states that have not entered into a "memorandum of understanding" with the FDA addressing the distribution of "inordinate amounts" of compounded drugs in interstate commerce, the pharmacy, pharmacist, or physician compounding the drug may not distribute compounded drugs out of state in quantities exceeding 5% of that entity's total prescription orders.
- The prescription must be "unsolicited," [section 353a(a)], and the pharmacy, licensed pharmacist, or licensed physician compounding the drug may "not advertise or promote the compounding of any particular drug, class of drug, or type of drug." The pharmacy, licensed pharmacist, or licensed physician may, however, "advertise and promote the compounding service" that they provide, [section 353a(c)]. *Thompson v. Western States Medical Center.*

Generally the FDA will defer to state authorities regarding the day-to-day regulation of compounding of animal and human drugs that are intended to be used in food-producing animals. When the scope and nature of activities raise concern associated with manufacturing resulting in significant violation of the new drug, adulteration, or misbranding provisions of the act, the FDA has determined it will seriously consider enforcement action. In determining whether or not to initiate such action, the agency will consider whether the veterinarian or pharmacist engages in any of the following acts:

- Compounding of drugs for use in a situation (a) where the health of the animal is not threatened and (b) where suffering or death of the animal is not likely to result from failure to treat.
- Compounding of drugs in anticipation of receiving prescriptions, except in limited quantities in relation to the amounts of drugs compounded after receiving prescriptions issued within the confines of a valid VCPR.
- Compounding of drugs that are prohibited for extra-label use in food-producing or non–food-producing animals under 21 CFR 530.41(a) and (b), respectively, because the drugs present a risk to the public health.
- Compounding finished drugs from human or animal drugs that are not the subject of an approved application or from bulk drug substances, other than those specifically addressed for regulatory discretion by the FDA, Center for Veterinary Medicine (e.g., antidotes). Inquiries about compounding from unapproved drugs or bulk drug substances should be directed to CVM, Division of Compliance, 240-276-9200.
- Compounding from approved human drugs for which the FDA has implemented a restricted distribution system.
- Using commercial scale manufacturing equipment for compounding drug products.
- Compounding drugs for third parties who resell to individual patients or offering compounded drug products at wholesale to other state licensed persons or commercial entities for resale.
- Failing to operate in conformance with applicable state law regulating the practice of pharmacy.
- Compounding of drugs for use in animals where an approved new animal drug or approved new human drug used as labeled or in conformity with 21 CFR Part 530 will, in the available dosage form and concentration, appropriately treat the condition diagnosed.

- Compounding from a human drug for use in food-producing animals if an approved animal drug can be used for the compounding.
- Instances where illegal residues occur in meat, milk, eggs, honey, aquaculture, or other food-producing animal products, and such residues were caused by the use of a compounded drug.
- Labeling a compounded drug with a withdrawal time established by the pharmacist instead of the prescribing veterinarian.
- Labeling of compounded drugs without sufficient information, such as withdrawal times for drugs for food-producing animals or other categories of information that are described in 21 DFR 530.12.

The foregoing list of factors is not intended to be all-inclusive. Other factors may be appropriate for consideration in a particular case.

Although many veterinarians say that in some cases the use of bulk drugs is medically necessary, the FDA regulations forbid the use of bulk drugs. The revised guide provides a list of bulk substances for compounding and subsequent use in animals that the FDA will not normally object to:

- Ammonium molybdate
- Ammonium tetrathiomolybdate
- Ferric ferrocyanide
- Methylene blue
- Picrotoxin
- Pilocarpine
- Sodium nitrite
- Sodium thiosulfate
- Tannic acid

REGULATION OF NUTRACEUTICALS

Chapter 23 provides detailed information on nutraceuticals. The use of nutraceuticals has plummeted, even though most are unproven and uncontrolled. Most do not meet USP *(United States Pharmacopeia)* standards. None requires the scrutiny of the FDA because it considers nutraceuticals as dietary supplements, not drugs. Pet products are regulated under the auspices of specific animal regulatory agencies.

Preparations of nutraceuticals do vary widely between manufacturers. There is no mechanism to establish the effectiveness of levels of products consumed or support label claims. There are no guarantees that the product is stable enough to withstand extreme temperatures or prolonged storage. There is no supportive documentation of stability of raw ingredients. In addition, some nutraceuticals are poorly manufactured. Some may be contaminated with bacteria or heavy metal. A number of side effects have been identified, but not passed on to the consumer.

There is truly a need for some level of government to regulate the safe use of nutraceuticals as effective dietary supplements for animals and accurate function claims. Before purchasing pet supplements, owners need to make sure that the products are truly helpful, safe, and effective. They need to make sure that the products have undergone many of the same scientific and clinical evaluations that are now required of human products.

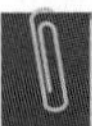

TECHNICIAN NOTE There are no government regulations on nutraceuticals.

EXPIRATION DATES AND DISPOSAL OF DRUGS

EXPIRATION DATES

The concept behind expiration dates is that the prescriber and consumer can be confident that the potency of the drug remains unaffected during the time of use. The expiration date guarantees if the drug is stored properly as instructed by the manufacturer, no toxic by-products will accumulate before completion of the drug regimen.

TECHNICIAN NOTE Expiration dates guarantee that no toxic by-products accumulate before completion of the drug regimen; potency of the drug remains unaffected during time of use.

Some manufacturers first began putting expiration dates on drugs in the 1960s. Although it was not required, the FDA began to mandate this practice in 1979 to set uniform testing and reporting guidelines.

The expiration date is set by the manufacturer after stability studies have been submitted to the FDA. This date is required in all labeling and should be clearly expressed as month, day, and year (i.e., 1/5/04 = January 5, 2004), and not as a code.

TECHNICIAN NOTE Expiration dates are set by the manufacturer and should be clearly expressed on labels as month, date, and year or month and year.

If this date is stated only in terms of month and year, according to the USP, the product becomes expired the last day of the stated month (i.e., 3/04 = March 31, 2004).

If a drug has not been stored properly and the integrity of the product has been compromised, the product's safety and effectiveness is questioned and should not be used. If a bottle of pills is wet or has been kept in a room with extremely high humidity and temperatures, the medication may go bad before its expiration date. Freezing temperatures may also ruin a drug's effectiveness. If capsules are sticking together or the shiny coat of a tablet is rubbing off in your hands, the drug may be degrading because it is stored in a place that is too moist. If a solution changes color or consistency, the product is light sensitive and has been stored under direct light. It should not be used even if the expiration date has not passed.

Drugs regulated by the *EPA* (i.e., Advantage, Bayer Animal Health) have no labeled expiration dates. The required shelf life is a minimum of 5 years.

Homeopathic medicine uses medication that works with your whole body to restore your health and are made from all natural substances. Unlike *synthetic* or man-made drugs, they never lose their potency or efficacy because all of the components are natural and not combined with any unnatural substances that will expire. If exposed to strong scents, left out in extreme heat or cold for a period of time, or contaminated by returning pills back to the bottle after they have been handled, they may be ineffective. If this happens, it is better to throw the product away. Do not reuse the bottle or send it to a recycling center. Homeopathic medicines are exempt from labeling laws that require expiration dates.

TECHNICIAN NOTE Homeopathic medicines are exempt from labeling laws that require expiration dates.

Commercially prepared products that are reconstituted (mixed with a diluent) before administration or repackaged must be labeled with an appropriate period limiting the time of use. If products are compounded, the compounder must establish an expiration date and appropriate withdrawal times for food-producing animals.

DISPOSAL OF DRUGS

Regardless of how well managed inventory control is, every facility will have drugs expire or unwanted drugs that need disposal. The EPA states that a drug product only becomes outdated when the decision is made to discard it. Whereas flushing was once, and in many instances still is, the most commonly used method of disposing leftover and expired medications, there are environmental concerns resulting from hormones and antibiotics contaminating drinking water supplies.

The Department of Environmental Quality (DEQ), EPA, FDA, and local boards of pharmacy have established guidelines to regulate drug disposal.

All drugs for discard are to be separated from usable stock and clearly marked as "outdated."

Medications that can be returned for credit are sent back to the manufacturer, distributor, or a *reverse distribution company* (RDC—a company that serves as a liaison between purchaser and vendor for credit). The purchaser will need to establish an account with the RDC of their choice before any drugs are sent to them.

When using an RDC, make sure it is understood which items were purchased or received using special programs so that problems will not be incurred in getting credit at the correct price. Understand that their fee for this service comes off the top, so your credit for returns will be less than the statement.

Items that are unacceptable for credit may also be discarded through the RDC on a "by the pound" basis. In most instances, this is determined after the medications reach the company. As an alternative, those items that are not accepted for credit may be destroyed through some waste disposal companies.

Open containers may be placed in the biologic waste collection containers for disposal. Prior arrangements must be made with the companies for destruction of medications.

The DEA regulates the disposal of controlled drugs. In no case should controlled drugs be forwarded to the DEA. The procedures established shall not be construed as altering, in any way, state laws or regulations for disposal of controlled substances.

The only approved method of disposal of controlled substances by the DEA is through the hire of an RDC. The registrant (practice) should complete a C-II request form (disposition and reporting form for expired Schedule II pharmaceuticals) from the RDC. This will list all C-II drugs that will need disposal, including partial containers. After completing the form and sending it back to the RDC, the registrant will receive the triplicate form C222 (U.S. Official Order Forms-Schedule I and II). The registrant now becomes the supplier and will keep the suppliers copy (now in brown color). The blue copy (purchaser's copy) and green copy (DEA copy) are included in the box of drugs to be sent to the RDC. The green copy is then forwarded to the DEA by the RDC.

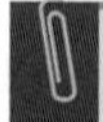

TECHNICIAN NOTE The DEA only approves disposal of controlled substances through use of an RDC.

An inventory should be taken of all controlled drugs in Schedules III to V. The registrant should submit a written or type written list of every item for disposal to the RDC. A copy of the list should be filed with the registrant.

After receipt and disposal of all drugs, the RDC will send the following records to the registrant as necessary:

1. C-II Manifest (DEA Form #41-Registrants Inventory of Drugs Surrendered)
2. Returnable Manifest (credit listed)
3. Nonreturnable Manifest (drugs destroyed)

All records pertaining to disposal of drugs should be kept for 2 years as required by the DEA.

Used drug containers should be disposed of properly to reduce the risk of environmental contamination with chemicals. Always use the manufacturer's label recommendation for disposal of empty or partial containers. Unused products should not be dumped down a drain, a toilet, or on the ground. Disinfectants should be added to unused portions of live virus or modified live virus vaccines to reduce accidental exposure to disease.

Disposal of medical wastes may be regulated by your state. Contact the agency in your state that oversees the disposal of medical waste. A list of agencies can be found at the following EPA website:

www.epa.gov/epahome/state.htm

MATERIAL SAFETY DATA SHEETS

The U.S. Occupational Safety and Health Administration (OSHA) under the authorization of the U.S. Department of Labor sets standards for current practice relations and requirements. The OSHA Act of 1970 was enacted to ensure the safe and healthful working conditions for working men and women. The law was based on the simple concept that every employee has the basic "right to know" the potential hazard of any substance in the workplace. Employees also need to know what protective measures are available to prevent adverse effects from occurring. Along with the federal government, the U.S. chemical industry developed a chemical identification system. It requires a paper document to accompany every chemical shipped, used, or stored. This paper document is called a *Material Safety Data Sheet* (MSDS) and is sent to users, such as industries, hospitals, universities, practices, and others when the chemicals are sent. The company that produces the chemicals writes the MSDS. Every drug and pharmaceutical aid has an MSDS. A file of these fact sheets must by maintained in the veterinary practice and be accessible to every employee.

> TECHNICIAN NOTE OSHA requires a file of MSDSs because every employee has a need and right to know the hazards and identities of the chemicals he or she is exposed to when working.

The essential parts to an MSDS are:

1. *Name, address,* and *telephone number* of the manufacturer or supplier.
2. *Chemical name* as it appears on the container's label: common name; scientific name: trade name or brand name that the manufacturer uses; synonyms for the mixture or chemicals.
3. For hazardous ingredients, the MSDS should list:
   a. The *permissible exposure level* (PEL)—amount of an air contaminant a worker can be exposed to for 40 hr/wk over a working lifetime (30 years) without suffering adverse drug reaction.
   b. The *threshold value* (TLV)—amount of a substance in the air nearly everyone can be exposed to daily without adverse drug reactions.
4. *Physical properties*: vapor pressure; specific gravity; appearance and odor; solubility; boiling point; melting point; freezing point; vapor density; evaporation rate.
5. *Potential for fire and explosion data*: flash point (when will a fire start and what should be done about it); flammability or explosive limit (lower and upper explosive limit) (LEL and UEL)—numbers used to describe the range in which a fire or explosion can occur; extinguishing media required to put out class A, B, C, and D fires.
6. *Health hazards:*
   a. Body entry by inhalation, ingestion, or transdermally.
   b. The short-term (acute) and long-term (chronic) harmful effects.
   c. Carcinogenicity *(cancer-producing)*, corrosive, or sensitizer *(an allergen or irritant that after an initial sensitizing exposure produced atopic or contact dermatitis)*, irritant, target organ effector.
7. *Reactivity:* conditions under which a chemical reaction will occur either by itself or with other materials; whether the chemical bonds are strong or weak and make the substance stable or unstable; incompatibility with other substances' storage compatibilities; if the substances will break down under conditions and release toxic or flammable vapor or gas; whether *hazardous polymerization* can occur (a chemical reaction that can cause a fire or explosion and possibly release hazardous gases).
8. *Spill or leak procedures:* Precautions for disposal of released substances should be taken during handling and storage.

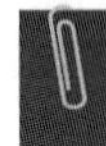

> TECHNICIAN NOTE Each MSDS shall provide methods of waste disposal.

9. *Special precautions:* Respiratory protection, ventilation, protective clothing and gear, and hygiene practices.
10. *Special precautions:* First aid in case of exposure.

MSDSs are written for:

- Employees who may by exposed to hazards at work
- Employers who need to know proper methods of storage, etc.
- Emergency responders, such as firefighters, hazardous material crews, emergency medical technicians, and emergency room personnel

MSDSs are not intended for consumers. It reflects the hazard of working with a material in an occupational fashion. Employees must have ready access to MSDSs while in the workplace. MSDSs must be on hand for every hazardous chemical known to be present in the workplace in such a manner that employees may by exposed under normal conditions for use or in a foreseeable emergency.

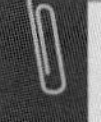

> TECHNICIAN NOTE MSDSs must be readily accessible.

CALCULATIONS

There is no need to fear calculations involved in dosing and compounding medications. Most are simple arithmetic. A methodical approach to each problem will simplify the concept and minimize the risk of error. Remember:

- If you are transferring data from a reference source, double-check what you have written down.
- Write down every step; expressing all quantities in the same system of units.
- Do not take short cuts; you are more likely to make a mistake.
- Try not to be totally dependent on your calculator. There is something to be said for "common sense."

Have an approximate idea of what the answer should be, and if you happen to hit the wrong button on the calculator, you are more likely to be aware that an error has been made.

- Finally, always double-check your calculations. There is frequently more than one way of doing a calculation, so if you get the same answer by two different methods, the chances are that your answer is correct. Alternatively, try working the problem in reverse to see if you get the starting numbers.

EXPRESSION OF CONCENTRATION

The metric system is the International System of Units (SI Units) for weight, volume, and length. The basic unit for weight is gram (g), and the basic unit for volume is the liter (L), and the basic unit of length is the meter (m). The prefix "milli" indicates one thousandth (10^{-3}) and "micro" one millionth (10^{-6}).

In some countries, the avoirdupois system (pounds and ounces) is still used in commerce and daily life. The apothecary system of volume (pints and gallons) is still a common system for commerce and household measurement. One should be aware of these systems to prevent serious errors in interpretation of prescriptions. It is important to be able to change between the systems (Box 25-3).

Example of unit conversions:

1. Express 70 grains in metric units (to 2 decimal places).
   You know: 1 grain (gr) = 64.8 mg
   Let Y = metric conversion

$$\text{Therefore:} \quad \frac{60\text{ mg}}{1\text{ grain}} = \frac{Y\text{ mg}}{70\text{ grains}}$$

$$Y = \frac{60\text{ mg}}{1\text{ grain}} \times 70\text{ grains}$$

$$Y = \mathbf{4200\text{ mg}}$$

To change the units to grams:
You know: 1 g = 1000 mg
Let X = Unknown number of grams.

$$\text{Therefore:} \quad \frac{1\text{g}}{1000\text{ mg}} = \frac{X\text{ g}}{4200\text{ mg}}$$

$$X = \frac{1\text{g}}{1000\text{ mg}} \times 4200\text{ mg}$$

$$X = \mathbf{4.20\,g}\text{ (to two decimal places)}$$

2. Sulfacetamide eyedrops contain 200 drops in a 10-ml bottle. Calculate the volume of 1 drop.
   You know that 200 drops = 10 ml (20 drops = 1 ml).
   Let y = volume of 1 drop.
   Therefore, *y* ml drop = 10 ml/200 drops = **0.05 ml.**

BOX 25-3 Mathematics Conversion Chart

Abbreviations

Weight
grain = grain
gram = g
kilogram = kg
milligram = mg
microgram = µg
pound = lb

Volume
cubic centimeter = cm^3
drop = gtt
gallon = gal
liter = L
milliliter = ml
ounce = oz
pint = pt
quart = qt
tablespoon = tbsp
teaspoon = tsp
unit = unit

Conversions

Weight Conversions
1 g = 1000 mg
1 mg = 1000 mg
1 g (mass) = 1 ml (volume)
1 kg (mass) = 1 L (volume)
1 lb = 16 oz
1 lb = 454 g
1 grain = 60 mg

Volume Conversions
1 L = 1000 ml
1 L = 32 oz
1 ml = 1 cm^3
1 drop = 0.05 ml
1 ml = 15-16 drops
1 tsp = 5 ml
1 tbsp = 15 ml
1 oz = 30 ml
1 gal = 3785 ml
1 pt = 473 ml
1 qt = 960 ml

EXPRESSION OF STRENGTH

Ratio is the relative magnitude of two like quantities.

Ratio strength is the expression of a concentration by means of a ratio (e.g., 1:10).

Percentage strength is a ratio of parts per hundred (e.g., 10%).

Thus 1:10 = 1 part in 10 parts total volume of solution.

If 1 ml of glucose is in 10 ml of solution, the ratio is 1:10. Therefore 10 ml of glucose is in 100 ml of solution. This can be expressed as a percentage, so it is equivalent to a 10% volume/volume (vol/vol) solution. The same concept applies whether the expression is % volume/volume (vol/vol), % weight/volume (wt/vol), or % weight/weight (wt/wt).

> TECHNICIAN NOTE 1:10 does not mean 1 ml of glucose and 10 ml of water. It means 1 ml of glucose and 9 ml water (1 ml of glucose in 10 ml total volume of solution).

1. Express 0.1% w/w as ratio strength.
   You know: 0.1% = 0.1 g/100 g
   Let Y = total parts.
   Therefore 0.1 g/100 g = 1 part/Y parts.
   Y = 100 × 1/0.1 = 1000.
   The ratio strength = 1:1000.
2. Express 1:2500 as percentage strength.
   You know: percentage is a ratio of parts/100 parts.
   Let Y = percentage strength.
   Therefore, 1 part/2500 parts = Y parts/100 parts.
   Y = 1 × 100/2500 = 0.04%.
3. Express 1 part per million (ppm) as percentage strength.
   You know that ppm is another expression of ratio strength (ppm = 1 part per million = 1:1,000,000).
   Let Y be the percentage strength.
   Therefore 1 part/1,000,000 parts = Y part/100 parts.
   Y = 1 × 100/1,000,000 = 0.0001% = 1×10^{-4}%.
   Percentage weight-in-weight (wt/wt) is the number of grams of an active ingredient in 100 g (solid or liquid)
4. How many grams of a drug should be used to prepare 200 g of a 5% wt/wt solution?
   You know: 5% = 5 g/100 g
   Let Y = the weight of the drug needed.
   Therefore Y/200 g = 5 g/100 g
   Y = 5 × 200/100 = 10 g.
   Percentage weight-in-volume (wt/vol) is the number of grams of an active ingredient in 100 ml of liquid.
5. If 6 g of iodine are in 240 ml of iodine tincture, calculate the percentage of iodine in the tincture.
   You know: % weight in volume is part (g)/100 ml.
   Let Y = percentage of iodine in the tincture.
   Therefore Y/100 ml = 6 g/240 ml.
   Y = 6 × 100/240 = 2.5% (wt/vol).
   Percentage volume-in-volume (vol/vol) indicates the number of milliliters (ml) of an active ingredient in 100 ml of liquid.
6. If 20 ml of Betadine are mixed with water to make 60 ml of solution, what is the percentage of Betadine in the solution? You know that % volume in volume is part (ml)/100 (ml). Let Y be the percentage of Betadine in the solution.
   Therefore, Y/100 ml = 20 ml/60 ml.
   Y = 20 × 100/60 = 33% (vol/vol).
7. Express 15 g of dextrose in 300 ml of solution as a percentage, indicating wt/wt, wt/vol, or vol/vol. You know that g (weight)/ml (volume) is expressed as % wt/vol.
   Let Y grams be the weight of dextrose in 100 ml.
   Therefore Y/100 ml = 15 g/300 ml
   Y = 15 × 100/300 ml = 5% wt/vol.
8. What is the percentage of sodium chloride in the following syrup?
   Sodium chloride 10 g
   Dextrose 420 g
   Water, q.s. ad 1000 ml
   You know: Percentage is the number of grams (w) of sodium chloride in 100 ml (v) of syrup.
   Therefore Y/100 ml = 10g/1000 ml.
   Y = 10 × 100/1000 = 1% wt/vol.

CALCULATING THE STRENGTH OF A DRUG SOLUTION

The following basic equation is used to calculate the concentration of a liquid dosage form:

Concentration (g/ml) = mass (g)/volume (ml)

If you know any two of these quantities, the third can be found.

Example 1: What is the strength of a 1-L solution containing 50 g of drug?

You know:

1. Volume of solution (1 L = 1000 ml)
2. Mass of drug (50 g)

Solution:

Substitute all known quantities in the equation. Solve for the unknown:

Concentration (g/ml) = 50 g/1000 ml = 5 g/100 ml × 100% = 5% solution.

Manipulation of this equation is frequently used for finding the quantity (mass) of a given volume of drug solution at a known concentration:

Mass (g) = volume (ml) × concentration (g/ml)

Example 2: How much drug is needed to prepare 4 oz of a 2% solution?

You know:

1. Volume of solution (4 oz = 120 ml)
2. Concentration of solution (2% = 2 g/100 ml)

Solution:

Substitute all known quantities in the equation. Solve for the unknown:

Mass (g) = 120 ml × 2 g/100 ml = 2.4 g

The original equation is also used to find out the total volume of drug solution that can be prepared at a desired concentration with a given quantity of drug:

Volume (ml) = mass (g)/concentration (g/ml)

Example 3: How much of a 10% solution can be prepared with 15 g of drug?

You know:

1. Concentration of desired solution (10% = 10 g/100 ml)
2. Mass of drug (15 g)

Solution:

Substitute all known quantities in the equation. Solve for the unknown:

Volume (ml) = 15 g/10 g/100 ml = 150 ml

CALCULATING THE STRENGTH OF DILUTED SOLUTIONS

A basic equation can be used to solve problems for dilution stock (concentrated) solutions. (A more concentrated [stronger] solution can never be made from a diluted [weaker] solution without adding pure drug.)

Concentration of desired solution × Volume of desired solution = Concentration of stock × Volume of stock

Knowing any three of these quantities, one can solve for the unknown.

Example 1: Prepare 2 qt of a 1:1000 solution from a 20% solution.

You know:

1. Concentration of desired solution (1:1000 = 1 g/1000 ml)
2. Volume of desired solution (2 qt = approximately 2000 ml)
3. Concentration of stock (20% = 20 g/100 ml)

Solution:

Substitute all known quantities in the equation. Solve for the unknown:

Volume of stock solution (ml) × 20 g/100 ml = 2000 ml × 1 g/1000 ml = 10 ml

Example 2: How much of a 1% solution can be prepared from 6 ml of a 5% solution?

You know:

1. Concentration of desired solution (1% = 1 g/100 ml)
2. Volume of stock (6 ml)
3. Concentration of stock (5% = 5 g/100 ml)

Solution:

Substitute all known quantities in the equation. Solve for the unknown:

Volume of desired solution (ml) × 1 g/100 ml = 5 g/100 ml × 6 ml = 30 ml

CALCULATING DRUG DOSAGES

A drug dosage is expressed as units or mass of drug per body weight (BW) of the patient. The usual dosage for human drugs is based on the ideal BW of 140 lb (70 kg). There is no ideal BW in veterinary medicine because of the variety of species and breeds of animals. The usual drug dose for animals is based on BW expressed in pounds or kilograms.

The following equation is used for calculating the quantity of drug to be administered based on BW:

$$\frac{BW \times dosage}{\text{Concentration of drug}} = \text{Volume of drug (dose)}$$

Example 1: An 88-lb dog is to receive a drug dosage of 25 mg/kg of BW. How many milliliters of the supplied drug at 50 mg/ml are required?

1. Drug dosage (25 ml/kg of BW)
2. Animal's BW (88 lb = 40 kg)
3. Concentration of drug solution (50 mg/ml)

TABLE 25-4 Conversion Tables for Weight (kg) to Body Surface Area (m^2)

Dogs				Cats	
kg	m^2	kg	m^2	kg	m^2
0.5	0.06	33	1.03	2.0	0.159
1	0.10	34	1.05	2.5	0.184
2	0.15	35	1.07	3.0	0.208
3	0.20	36	1.09	3.5	0.231
4	0.25	37	1.11	4.0	0.252
5	0.29	38	1.13	4.5	0.273
6	0.33	39	1.15	5.0	0.292
7	0.36	40	1.17	5.5	0.311
8	0.40	41	1.19	6.0	0.330
9	0.43	42	1.21	6.5	0.348
10	0.46	43	1.23	7.0	0.366
11	0.49	44	1.25	7.5	0.383
12	0.52	45	1.26	8.0	0.400
13	0.55	46	1.28	8.5	0.416
14	0.58	47	1.30	9.0	0.432
15	0.60	48	1.32	9.5	0.449
16	0.63	49	1.34	10	0.464
17	0.66	50	1.36		
18	0.69	52	1.41		
19	0.71	54	1.44		
20	0.74	56	1.48		
21	0.76	58	1.51		
22	0.78	60	1.55		
23	0.81	62	1.58		
24	0.83	64	1.62		
25	0.85	66	1.65		
26	0.88	68	1.68		
27	0.90	70	1.72		
28	0.92	72	1.75		
29	0.94	74	1.78		
30	0.96	76	1.81		
31	0.99	78	1.84		
32	1.01	80	1.88		

Solution:

Substitute all known quantities in the equation. Solve for the unknown:

Volume of drug = 40 kg × 25 mg/kg/50 ml/ml = 20 ml (dose)

The dosage of highly toxic drugs, such as *antineoplastic* (anticancer) agents, is calculated on the basis of body surface area (BSA). BSAs are difficult to calculate. Nomograms and charts (Table 25-4) have been constructed to help relate BW to BSA. BSA is expressed in square meters (m^2).

To determine dosage based on BSA, modification of the previous equation will enable this:

BSA (m^2) × drug dosage = volume of drug

Concentration of drug

Example 2: A 44-lb dog is to receive a dosage of 0.2 mg/m^2. What volume of a drug should be given at a concentration of 1 mg/ml?

You know:
1. BSA (44 lb = 20 kg = 0.74 m^2)
2. Drug dosage (0.2 ml/m^2)
3. Concentration of drug solution (1 mg/ml)

Solution: Substitute all known quantities in the equation. Solve for the unknown:

Volume of drug solution = 0.74 m^2 × 0.2 mg/m^2/1 mg/ml = 0.148 ml

CALCULATING INFUSION RATES

Many drugs must be administered intravenously by slow infusion rather than as a rapid bolus injection. Large volumes of fluids are also given by intravenous infusion. Disposable intravenous sets and infusion pumps are used to deliver intravenous fluids at a steady rate over a period of time.

Calculations of infusion rates can be found by using the following equations:

Rate (drops/min) = Total vol to be administered (ml)
Total time of infusion (hours) ×
conversion of hours to
minutes (1 hr/60 min) ×
calibrated IV set (drops/ml)

Example 1: If 500 ml of a solution is to be infused over 6 hours, what is the correct infusion rate (drops/min) if the set delivers 10 drops/ml?

You know:
1. Drops/min calibration of intravenous set (10 drops/ml)
2. Volume of solution to be infused (500 ml)
3. Hours of infusion (6 hours)
4. Conversion of hours to minutes (1 hr/60 min)

Solution:

Substitute all known quantities in the equation. Solve for the unknown.

Rate (drops/min) = 500 ml/6 hr × 1 hr/60 min × 10 drops/ml = 13.89 drops/min

Example 2: If a drug is to be infused at a dosage rate of 2 μg/kg/min into a 50-lb animal, what rate (ml/hr) should a pump be set on for a drug concentration of 400 mg in 250 ml of dextrose 5%?

You know:
1. Dosage rate = 2 μg/kg/min
2. Weight of patient = 50 lb (22.73 kg)
3. Concentration of drug solution 400 mg/250 ml = 1.60 mg/ml

Constant rate infusion (ml/hr) = Dosage rate (μg/kg/min) ×
weight (kg) ×
conversion of minutes
to hours (60 min/1 hr) ×
conversion of μg to mg
(1 mg/1000 μg)/
concentration (mg/ml)

Solution:

Substitute all known quantities in the equations. Solve for the unknown:

Constant rate infusion (ml/hr) = 2 μg/kg/min × 22.73 kg = 45.46 μg/min

45.46 μg × *60 min/hr* = 2727.6 μg/hr

2727.6 μg/hr × 1 mg/1000 μg = 2.72 mg/hr

2.72 mg/hr/1.60 mg/ml = 1.70 ml/hr

INVENTORY CONTROL

The maintenance of an active working inventory requires both planning and continuous monitoring. Failure to keep abreast of use and needs results in shortage, inefficient use of time, increased costs, and added stress. The time invested to maintain appropriate levels of stock is therefore beneficial to the overall operation of the practice.

Veterinary technicians who demonstrate interest in an active inventory may find themselves acquiring an increasing role in inventory control and maintenance. This additional responsibility not only increases employee value in the practice, but also adds to job satisfaction.

Ideally the quantities of each item stocked should be as small as possible without running out between reasonable ordering periods. Because it is worse to have a shortage of certain items than to have extra, most practices lean toward a higher inventory than actually required. *Inventory turnover* (the number of times per year an item is bought and sold) should be at least four to six times per year. Some items, such as pet food, may turn over 12 to 14 times per year. With the assistance of a computer, monitoring of daily usage, and keeping helpful records, the average turnover rate can usually be increased. The higher the turnover, the lower the investment in the item. Drug ordering can become a full-time duty if care is not given to organization and planning.

INVENTORY MAINTENANCE

The primary disadvantage of having a large inventory is the expense of having working capital tied up in drugs and supplies. A large inventory makes switching to equivalent products difficult, even at a cheaper price. There is great potential for product breakage, expiration, spoilage, and obsolescence when the inventory is large. Some states have an inventory tax that provides added incentive for keeping working stock to a minimum.

Occasionally, there is some justification for increasing the purchase of certain products. The "savings" claimed through many of the deals offered by vendors should be approached with caution. Unless one can accurately predict the use of certain products, quantity buying is difficult to justify. To participate in most marketing promotions, a significant financial commitment is usually required. Before entering into these agreements, one should truly determine whether the products offered are desirable and will be used within a reasonable period and whether the savings really merit the capital commitment.

Processing small orders is costly because the time commitment required to process the order is not much different from that of a larger order with several items. One is justified in increasing quantities on these small orders, especially if the items are inexpensive, to reduce ordering frequency and cost of acquisition. Some vendors charge handling fees if the total order is below a minimum required dollar amount or volume.

Availability of replacement goods is a factor that will affect the inventory turnover. With some items, one may be able to accurately predict monthly use and maintain a few weeks supply. Unfortunately the use of most items cannot be readily anticipated, which results in a larger inventory requirement, especially if delivery time cannot by predicted.

PROCUREMENT

Veterinary Suppliers

One may purchase supplies through veterinary wholesale suppliers (distributors) or directly from manufacturers. Distributors may specialize in one class of items, such as surgical supplies or bulk pharmaceuticals. Some wholesale suppliers may offer a complete line of products, ranging from buckets to gas machines.

One advantage in dealing with wholesalers is the ability to reduce the number of small orders that would be required in purchasing from several individual vendors. A few manufacturers only sell their products directly to veterinarians rather than distributors. The *Compendium of Veterinary Products* (see Recommended Reading) offers a complete reference to veterinary pharmaceutical companies and their product lines.

Veterinary Practices

It is an excellent idea to establish and maintain a good working relationship with another practice in the area. In a crisis, you can borrow items from that practice to see you through the emergency. Borrowing seldom-used items in an emergency is encouraged rather than stocking them. However, your practice is expected to order the item and return it. Thus inventory of seldom-used items should be maintained elsewhere, and record keeping is not necessary. Purchasing some items from another practice may be helpful, especially for expensive, short-dated items.

Several large buying groups have been established by some practices to increase their purchasing power and decrease costs.

Pharmacies and Drug Wholesalers

Using the services of a retail pharmacy is nearly essential to the practice of quality veterinary medicine. Veterinarians have a need for various human products that are not obtainable through veterinary suppliers. Retail pharmacies may not stock many injectable products, but they can help with most ophthalmic and oral products and some topical preparations. In some locations, a human drug wholesaler may deal directly with the small, individual practitioner. Most, however, do not welcome these small accounts and will serve only as a distributor for hospitals and pharmacies. The veterinary practitioner must make arrangements with pharmacists to obtain human products for practice or client use. Most pharmacists welcome this opportunity to serve the veterinarian.

Human Hospitals and Hospital Suppliers

A local human hospital may be a valuable resource for the veterinary practice. Federal laws restrict hospitals with special buying privileges from selling to anyone outside their institution. As a result, it may be difficult for veterinarians and their clients to obtain some of the more potent, expensive, or rarely used medical supplies, except in an emergency. Practicing veterinarians should make human hospital contacts to determine the local availability of human drugs and supplies. The hospital's library and clinical laboratory may also provide some welcome assistance.

Local hospital suppliers will stock items, such as syringes, needles, cotton balls, tongue depressors, and other disposable supplies. Although veterinarians do not routinely purchase from the local hospital, do not overlook them as an immediate source in times of shortages.

Other Sources of Suppliers

In addition to bulk chemicals, major chemical suppliers will stock glassware, balances, disposable beakers, brushes, carboys, and other laboratory and clinic supplies and equipment that would be useful in a veterinary practice. Most of these suppliers are located in metropolitan areas and have addresses and telephone numbers listed in the telephone directory.

Numerous mail order suppliers exist that provide not only pharmaceuticals, but also a wide variety of veterinary products and equipment. The quality of product and service may vary greatly among these outlets. Of major concern is the return policy for handling inferior or unacceptable items.

Feed stores and lay veterinary drug outlets can be used for an occasional urgently needed item. One may at times also want to take advantage of certain specials offered through these suppliers.

ORGANIZING THE PHARMACY

A comprehensive list of all activities conducted in the pharmacy should be prepared, whether planning a major hospital complex or rearranging a small portion of a hospital. Activities related to the pharmacy include storage (refrigeration, security), ordering, receiving, cleanup, dispensing, withdrawal and administration of medication, compounding and manufacturing, product information, and so forth. In the design, the location of each activity must be determined, and each activity should be coordinated with other areas when required. Although most areas will be multifunctional, some activities may be unique and have their own special requirements.

Regulating agencies require that refrigerators that store vaccines and biologics should be kept at 40° C. Minor fluctuations in temperature may occur. A daily temperature log must be maintained (Figure 25-10). Personal foodstuff should not be stored in the refrigerator designated for pharmacy use.

> *TECHNICIAN NOTE* Refrigerators should be kept at 40° C. Personal foodstuff should be stored separately.

A detailed list of functions pertaining specifically to the pharmacy inventory should include the following:

- *Ordering* requires a telephone, desk, file, and calculator.
- *Receiving* should be near an outside door and requires temporary counter or floor space.
- *Returns* require space for holding broken outdated, and damaged items.
- *Storage* areas must be adequate for working and backup stock. Refrigeration for perishable items and security for volatile hazardous bulk materials.
- *Pricing* involves the use of a computer or price book, markup schemes, record, and a collection of MSDSs for all products.

In addition, consideration should be given to the movement of items to areas of use for dispensing. Monitoring of inventory levels of all items is a much-needed function to ensure an adequate supply at demand without shortages.

REFRIGERATOR / FREEZER TEMPERATURE MONITORING CHART

Refrigerator Location: ______________ Month: ______________ Year: ________

Used for (÷ One): ❑ Medications ❑ Staff ❑ Nourishment ❑ Other: ______________

Freezer in Use: ❑ Yes ❑ No

Refrigerator Acceptable Range: 35-40 Degrees Fahrenheit or 2-8 Degrees Centigrade
Freezer Acceptable Range: Less than 0 Degrees Fahrenheit or Less than –18 Degrees Centigrade

** *IF THE TEMPERATURE FALLS OUTSIDE OF THE ACCEPTABLE RANGE, NOTIFY SUPERVISOR IMMEDIATELY AND RECORD ALL CORRECTIVE ACTION TAKEN ON THIS FORM.*

Date	Refrigerator	Freezer	Initials	Cleaned	Thawed	Corrective Action Taken	Initials
1							
2							
3							
4							
5							
6							
7							
8							
9							
10							
11							
12							
13							
14							
15							
16							
17							
18							
19							
20							
21							
22							
23							
24							
25							
26							
27							
28							
29							
30							
31							

PF-IC-1049 (Rev. 07/02)

FIGURE 25-10 Refrigerator-freezer temperature monitoring chart.

ARRANGEMENT OF INVENTORY

Working inventory should be placed on shelves in an organized fashion. One method is to arrange items by dosage form. Categories would include the following:

- Oral solids (tablets, capsules)
- Oral liquids
- Oral miscellaneous (boluses, powders, pastes)
- External liquids
- External miscellaneous (sprays, powders, ointments, creams)
- Ophthalmic drugs (ointments, suspensions, solutions)
- Small-volume injectables
- Large-volume injectables
- Mastitis preparations
- Miscellaneous, such as chemicals for compounding

Each section should be further arranged, perhaps by generic name, brand name, or the more common name used by individuals in the practice. One may wish to make exceptions for items that are popular, but they should be limited.

A different type of arrangement would be to group items by their most common therapeutic use. Classification would be similar to that in the discussion of drugs found in the first portion of this chapter:

- Anesthetics
- Tranquilizers
- Anticonvulsants
- Analgesics
- Antiinflammatory drugs
- Cardiovascular drugs
- Fluids and electrolytes
- Diuretics
- Parasiticides
- Antibiotics
- Other antibacterial drugs
- Antineoplastic agents
- Hormones and related substances
- GI drugs
- Vitamins

Each drug class could then be further divided into more specific uses, such as GI drugs divided into antiemetics, emetics, and antidiarrheals. Some classes may have only two or three items. Disadvantages of using this system are the poor use of shelf space and the possibility of gallon jugs ending up next to ampules.

Another arrangement is to group items by company or vendor. This method may be acceptable for backup stock because it is helpful when preparing orders. In an active inventory, there may be poor use of shelf space. Perhaps the greatest disadvantage is trying to recall the last supplier for rarely used items. Another disadvantage is purchasing generic items from multiple vendors, which may lead to multiple locations of the same item and duplicate stock.

Pharmacy organization is desirable and has advantages, primarily by assisting each individual in locating items. The best method of organizing stock is probably a combination of the various preceding arrangements. Each practice should design its own method. In addition to the methods listed, placement of selected items in areas where they are frequently used should be considered.

INTERNET PHARMACY

The Internet is rapidly transforming the way we live and shop in all sectors of the economy. In the area of health care, it permits individuals to obtain medical information to help them understand health issues and treatment options for themselves and their animals. The Internet allows consumers to shop online for health care products and get prescriptions filled.

There are great benefits and challenges that the Internet presents when consumers use it to shop. One of the greatest benefits of shopping online to fill prescriptions is the ease with which consumers can comparison shop. Many pharmacies offer price comparisons between their charges and that of other legitimate pharmacies, which helps to stretch the health care dollar. Some Internet pharmacies sell drugs for less than traditional "brick-and-mortar" pharmacies, which is most important for people who love their animals, but have limited income.

Legitimate online pharmacies offer valuable health care information in a searchable format. Drug prices and drug information are accessed by the website. It may be requested by e-mail. Consumers do not have to wait on the telephone for an answer or travel to the pharmacy to get it.

There is convenience and flexibility to ordering and receiving medications without leaving home, which is a tremendous timesaver. For the pet owner who has limited time, online prescriptions allow for the convenience of shopping 24 hours per day. This is especially valuable to homebound pet owners for whom a trip to the pharmacy may be difficult.

Online pharmacies provide more privacy than traditional pharmacies. Sometimes consumers are too embarrassed to purchase certain items or health care products from the local pharmacy. They may find greater anonymity by ordering online where staff may not be able to put "face to name."

CONCERNS ABOUT ONLINE SITES

As beneficial as computer technology is, the Internet also creates a new market place for illegal activity, such as the sale of unapproved new drugs and prescription drugs dispensed without a valid prescription. Consumers may encounter difficulties in identifying illegitimate sites.

One problem found with illegitimate online pharmacies is that they open and close on a daily basis. One company may have many URLs or web addresses, and they frequently sell customer links. Many customers are unable to contact the pharmacy because telephone lines are disconnected or there is no answer.

Often consumers experience nonreceipt of medications ordered, and they face credit card charges that these illegitimate pharmacies refuse to remove. Genuine risks exist when foreign drugs are dispensed.

Medications dispensed that are considered unsafe for laypersons to administer without monitoring by a licensed veterinarian are called *legend drugs* (they bear the word "caution," which restricts the use of the drug). For the veterinarian to write a prescription, he should have established a valid VCPR with the animal and its owner. This cannot be done online. Because online pharmacies only provide a questionnaire to be filled out, the PE (physical examination)—a requirement within a VCPR—cannot be done. When a VCPR is established without the PE, inappropriate medications can worsen an underlying, undiagnosed, serious disease state. When pharmacies do not employ licensed professionals, the animal's life may be threatened because the pharmacy may not sell the right drug.

Illegitimate online pharmacies use patient questionnaires and fee-based cyberspace consultations. They will sell legend drugs and controlled drugs without a consult. It is no longer legal to sell controlled drugs over the Internet.

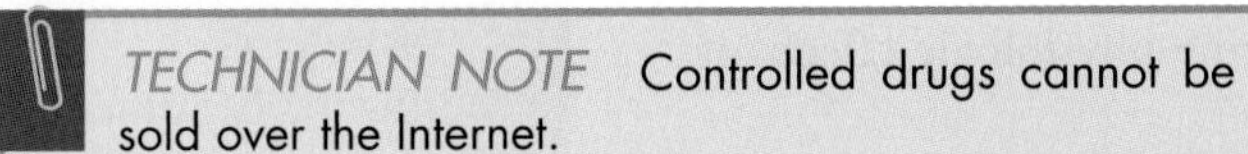

TECHNICIAN NOTE Controlled drugs cannot be sold over the Internet.

Many illegitimate sites will use drugs from foreign countries. The FDA generally prohibits the importation of foreign-made versions of prescription medications that are commercially available in the United States. Genuine risks exist when foreign drugs are dispensed. The safety and efficacy of these medications cannot be guaranteed. Online pharmacies may dispense expired, subpotent, contaminated, or counterfeit products; the wrong or contraindicated product; incorrect dose; or medications without adequate directions for use.

The prescription order should come directly from the prescriber to be valid—not the patient. Online sites that do not protect the integrity of the original prescription or do not verify the authenticity of the prescription may be in violation of the law.

REGULATIONS

The challenge for regulatory agencies concerning online prescriptions is to make sure that the protection for consumers is just as strong as that for consumers who purchase drugs at their corner pharmacy.

The FDA has actively engaged with a number of states in jointly pursuing illegal Internet sales. Regulation is primarily the jurisdiction of each state board of pharmacy with some federal oversight. Most states protect their citizens by licensing "out-of-state" pharmacies to ship medications in their jurisdiction. The National Association of Boards of Pharmacy (NABP) does not regulate online pharmacies.

The VIPPS is a voluntary certification to Verify Internet Pharmacy Practice Sites. The program offers an accompanying seal of approval that identifies to the public those online pharmacy sites that are appropriately licensed and are legitimately operating over the Internet. Those approved sites have successfully completed a rigorous review inspection.

The value of the VIPPS program is to provide members of the public a means to assure themselves that the Internet pharmacy they choose is a bona fide, fully licensed facility exercising competent Internet and interstate pharmacy practices. Regulations that apply to traditional "brick-and-mortar" mail-order pharmacies apply to online pharmacies.

VIPPS-certified pharmacies are required to offer customers free telephone consultations with a registered pharmacist and may offer free ask-a-pharmacist e-mail service.

VIPPS has a mechanism in place to report errors made by its certified pharmacies. They are to document, track, and analyze the types of errors to determine what went wrong and to make suggestions to prevent recurrences.

ADVICE FOR CONSUMERS

- Suspect the pharmacy if it will dispense medications without requiring a hard copy of the prescription to be mailed in.
- Suspect the pharmacy if it dispenses prescription medications and does not contact the prescriber to obtain a valid verbal prescription.
- Suspect the pharmacy if it will dispense medications solely based on a consumer questionnaire without a preexisting VCPR with a prescriber on-site.
- Suspect the pharmacy if it does not have a toll-free number and street address posted to the website.
- Suspect the site if the pharmacy merely has an e-mail feature as the sole communication between consumer and facility. Legitimate sites allow you to contact the pharmacist.
- Avoid the site if the site does not advertise the availability of a registered pharmacist for consultation.
- Avoid a pharmacy that does not have policies in place that address different issues.
- Always look for the VIPPS seal.

RECOMMENDED READING

Baumgartner K, Hoffman D, editors: *Controlled substances handbook,* Washington, DC, 1998, Government Information Services.

Bonagura JD, editor: *Kirk's current veterinary therapy 14: small animal practice,* St Louis, 2009, WB Saunders.

Compendium of veterinary products, ed 7, Port Huron, Mich, 2003, North American Compendium.

Hardarman JG et al: *The pharmacological basis of therapeutics,* ed 9, New York, 1995, McGraw-Hill.

Physician's desk reference, ed 57, Montvale, NJ, 2003, Medical Economics.

Plumb DC: *Veterinary drug handbook,* ed 4, White Bear Lake, Minn, 2002, PharmaVet Publishing.

USPDI: Drug information for the health care professional, ed 23, vol 1, Englewood, Colo, 2003, Micromedex.

Veterinary pharmaceutical and biologicals, ed 12, Lenexa, Kan, 2001, Veterinary Healthcare Communications.

26 Pain Management

Nancy Shaffran and Tamara Grubb

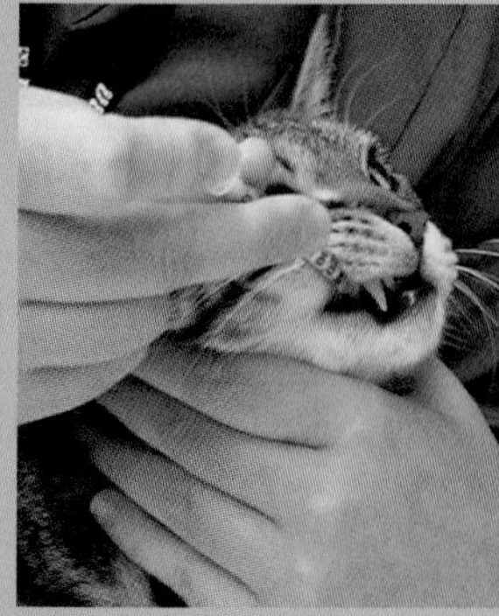

OUTLINE

KEY TERMS

Agonist
Allodynia
Antagonist
Dysphoria
Hyperalgesia
Modulation
Multimodal analgesia
Neurotransmitters
Nociception
Transduction
Transmission
Wind-up phenomenon

LEARNING OBJECTIVES

When you have completed this chapter, you will be able to:

1. Describe methods used to recognize pain and monitor response to analgesics in small and large animals.
2. Differentiate between dysphoria and pain response and describe physiologic effects of pain on body systems.
3. Differentiate between pain and nociception and describe the phases of nociception.
4. Define hyperalgesia and allodynia and explain their role in management of chronic pain.
5. Describe the concepts of pre-emptive analgesia and multimodal analgesia.
6. List the steps in calculating constant rate infusions.
7. List the classes of medications used in management of pain and give examples of each.
8. List the routes of administration of local and systemic anesthetics, analgesics, and sedatives.
9. List the types of adjunctive medications used in pain management.
10. List and describe non-pharmacologic options of treatment of pain.

INTRODUCTION

In recent years, the practice of pain management has become mainstream in veterinary medicine. The optimal use of analgesic drugs, combinations, methods of administration, and alternative therapies are still being developed as more is learned about the way animals feel and express pain. The search also continues for the most objective, scientific methods of measuring and assessing pain in nonverbal patients. Technicians continue to play a vital part in the field of pain management. Many veterinarians rely heavily on the veterinary technician's ability to recognize and report animal pain and use this input to guide decision making. This is not surprising given the huge role that nurses have played in pain management for nonverbal human patients. Human neonatal and pediatric nurses and veterinary technicians share the position of patient advocate, giving their patients a voice and attending to their needs. However, unlike in human medicine, veterinary technicians typically do this without the help of parents who play a large role in advocating for their hospitalized children.

The role of advocate for a nonverbal patient can be daunting. Veterinary technicians are responsible for the quality of patient care and the overall condition of their patients without the freedom to prescribe or initiate therapy. This can sometimes result in frustration while pursuing a positive response from veterinarians toward giving analgesia. Knowledge of the physiology of pain and pharmacology of analgesics is essential for good communication between veterinarians and veterinary technicians. Optimally the veterinarian regards the technician as an integral member of the pain management team. The skilled technician is a source of vital information required to choose and administer appropriate analgesics. He or she is a trusted caretaker for recovering patients. The success of this relationship is terribly important for all hospitalized patients and applies to elective, routine, and extraordinary cases.

THE ROLE OF THE VETERINARY TECHNICIAN AS A PATIENT ADVOCATE

COMMUNICATION

Technicians use their critical thinking, observation, and interpretation skills to make important pain management recommendations. Discussion about each case directly with the clinician might include the technician's particular concerns about a patient or a general approach to managing different types of pain. Based on his or her interaction with patients, the technician may offer suggestions for adjustments in analgesic regimens, changes or additions to drug protocols, or the possible addition of sedatives, if needed.

Veterinary technicians often complain that their requests for patient analgesia go unheeded. The actual method of communication plays a large part in achieving a positive outcome. For example, "Can I give Charlie something for pain" is inadequate to convey the situation and often results in the response "no." To be effective, technicians must present two sets of information; what is the patient doing that indicates painfulness and what has already been done that is considered inadequate. For example, "Dr. X … yesterday's cruciate repair, the black lab, Charlie, is not doing as well as I would like. Despite the fact that his bladder is empty and I have offered him food and water, he seems restless and has difficulty getting comfortable. He is panting excessively, although his temperature is normal. I checked the bandage, and it does not seem too tight. The record says he received morphine last night at midnight, which allowed him to sleep for 4 hours, but has not had any since. May I give him a repeat dose to see if it makes him more comfortable?" This approach delivers the necessary information to gain the veterinarian's confidence in the technician's assessment skills and knowledge of the case. He or she is much more likely to agree to administer pain medication under these circumstances.

Technicians can also play a vital role in the administration of preemptive medication, which is often overlooked in a busy hospital setting. For example, "I have noticed a difference in the recovery of the animals that are given a dose of NSAID before surgery. Would you like me to give an NSAID to this patient now?" This approach also applies to the placement of transdermal analgesic patches, starting constant rate infusions (CRIs), and performing local or regional nerve blocks. Technicians should provide as much feedback as possible as to which analgesic protocols are working well and which need to be improved to increase patient comfort.

PATIENT ASSESSMENT

Historically, animal pain has been recognized and treated only in those patients that display overt behavioral signs, such as vocalization. By waiting for signs, patients are forced to prove that they are in pain before they are given analgesics. In reality, dogs and cats instinctively hide pain just as they would in the wild to avoid becoming prey. Once animals display obvious signs of pain, the pain intensity they are experiencing is likely to be severe. Old or severely debilitated patients may be too ill or weak to display changes in behavior. Patients should never be required to prove that they are in pain. A sound approach to pain management favors anticipation of the severity and duration of pain that is likely to occur with any procedure, condition, or surgery. In many cases, animals do "appear" to tolerate pain better than humans. There may be several explanations for this. In contrast to pain detection threshold (the point at which pain nerve fibers are stimulated to send signals), pain tolerance (the greatest intensity of pain that is voluntarily tolerated) varies widely between species and individuals within a species. Like humans, animals tolerate pain to a certain point before they show changes in their behavior. Awareness that patients may exhibit a wide range of pain tolerance and a broad spectrum of behaviors can improve pain recognition and treatment. Recently, research in pain management has shifted toward identifying and even predicting known painful events. For example, severe pain is expected with cervical disk herniation, extensive inflammation, medical or surgical fracture repair, limb amputation, declawing, ear canal ablation, etc. Moderate to mild pain is expected with cruciate repair, laparotomy, mass removal, castration, dental procedures, etc. This approach encourages us to treat patients who undergo painful procedures or disease processes without requiring proof. It does not, however, consider the vast variation in pain tolerance in the individual. It seems reasonable to incorporate both concepts to develop a truly effective analgesic plan (i.e., to have direction given by what are known to be painful events and be prepared to provide adequate analgesia for the expected level of pain but also to look at the individual and tailor analgesic protocols accordingly). A more complete list of anticipated levels of pain associated with surgical procedures, illness, or injuries is available in *Veterinary Clinics of North America*, July, 2000.

Technicians observe patients closely for extended periods of time and are usually the first to notice changes in status. Familiarity with individual patients' personalities and usual reactions to stimuli gives insight into the meaning of behaviors. Experience establishes expectations of how particular patients may react to painful stimuli. This includes the differences in expression between dogs and cats, the young and old, and variations among certain breeds. For example, Siberian huskies and Dobermans that vocalize regularly are thought to be more "sensitive" to pain or possess a lower pain threshold than other breeds, whereas pit bulls and Labrador retrievers appear to remain stoic in the face of pain. The skilled technician factors this into his or her pain assessments.

> *TECHNICIAN NOTE* Companion animals retain survival instincts despite being bred into captivity. This includes a drive to hide pain from potential predators so that they do not appear to be weak compared with the rest of the pack. Much to their detriment in a setting without predators, dogs and cats attempt to hide pain from us. Because of this, many animals probably reach a high threshold of pain before showing changes in behavior. Conversely, some animals express more pain than expected. This may indicate an unusually low pain threshold and should be managed appropriately.

SIGNS OF PAIN

Diagnosis of pain in veterinary medicine is seldom made on the basis of a single observation or physiologic value. Because pain is an individual, subjective experience, assessment depends on a combination of good examination skills; familiarity with species, breed, and individual behavior; knowledge of the degree of pain associated with particular surgical procedures or illnesses; and recognition of the signs of stress and pain.

Signs of pain in animals can be categorized as physiologic or behavioral (Table 26-1). Physiologic pain signs may be obvious and include increased heart rate and blood pressure, increased respiratory rate, and vocalization. More subtle behavioral changes, such as general restlessness, decreased appetite, not sleeping, resenting handling, and not assuming a normal position, may be even more significant. Clinical signs of pain in dogs and cats most often reported include tachycardia, increased respiratory rate, restlessness, increased temperature, increased blood pressure, abnormal posturing, inappetence, aggression, frequent movement, facial expression, trembling, depression, and insomnia. Less frequently reported are: anxiety; nausea; pupillary enlargement; licking, chewing, and staring at the surgical site or wound; poor mucous membrane (MM) color; salivation; decreased CO_2; and head pressing.

The clinical manifestations may be quite different between species and even among different members of the same species. For dogs, standing or sitting for long periods or sleeping in an atypical position are considered pain signs. For cats, abnormal posture, hiding, and aggression are ranked as

TABLE 26-1 Behavioral Signs of Pain in Dogs and Cats

Posture	Temperament	Vocalization	Locomotion	Other
Dogs				
Tail between legs Arched or hunched back Twisted body to protect pain site Drooped head Prolonged sitting position Tucked abdomen Lying in flat, extended position	Aggressive Clawing Attacking, biting Escaping	Barking Howling Moaning Whimpering	Reluctance to move Carrying one leg Lameness Unusual gait Unable to walk Chewing painful areas	Unable to perform normal tasks Attacks other animals or people if pain site is touched (self-trauma) No interest in food or play
Cats				
Tucked limbs Arched or hunched head and neck or back Tucked abdomen Lying flat Slumped body Drooped head	Aggressive Biting Scratching Chewing Attacking Escaping Hiding	Crying Hissing Spitting Moaning Screaming Purring	Reluctance to move Carrying one leg Lameness Unusual gait Unable to walk Inactive	Attacks if pain site is touched Failure to groom Dilated pupils No interest in food or play

common pain signs. Because the signs of pain are so varied and diverse, any abnormal sign(s) in a veterinary patient that cannot be attributed to another cause is (are) suspected of indicating pain.

> *TECHNICIAN NOTE* Signs of pain vary among animals. Patients should assume normal positions (what you would expect to see at home) while caged in the hospital. Standing for long periods or sleeping in an abnormal position indicates discomfort. Normal posture and behavior is a good indication that the patient is comfortable.

All patients should be evaluated for pain upon admission and at regular intervals throughout the hospitalization period. The observer's subjective opinion and physiologic signs can be described using a pain scale, such as a visual analog scale (VAS). A VAS designed for use in nonverbal human patients uses pictorial rather than numerical rating systems. The most common scale for nonverbal humans has a series of faces with varied expressions. The main difference between a human and animal VAS is that in human medicine, the patient is the reporter of his or her pain level, whereas in veterinary medicine, VAS readings are most often provided by a veterinary technician who is always a second-party reporter. Veterinary VASs typically use subjective numerical ratings where 0 correlates with no pain, and the highest number is the worst pain imaginable for that particular procedure. A new pain scale for dogs and cats has recently been developed at Colorado State University (CSU) that uses numerical, pictorial, and descriptive assessments (Figure 26-1). In addition to the VAS score, a complete patient description including physiologic signs (temperature, pulse, respiration) and behavioral signs (vocalization, posturing, eating, and sleeping habits) should be documented in the medical record.

Pain assessments should be made at 4- to 6-hour intervals throughout hospitalization in the general patient population. During the immediate postoperative period and throughout the critical phase, patients should be monitored as often as every 30 minutes. Ideally, assessments on an individual patient are performed by the same person over time. Repeat recorded assessments allow for evaluation of the efficacy of analgesic protocols and make response to specific drugs easier to track.

Veterinary technicians are trained to recognize animal pain. By nature, technicians are quite skillful observers of behavioral changes in their patients, noticing the subtlest expressions of potential pain. Most experienced technicians also have an innate sense of how painful most procedures, conditions, and surgeries are likely to be based on repeated prolonged exposure to animals in the recovery phase. However, it is often difficult for even the most experienced technician to distinguish between pain and other stress. For example, postoperative patients frequently display aberrant behavior for several minutes up to hours after surgery. These behaviors may include vocalization, thrashing, rolling, self-mutilation, and tachypnea. When these behaviors are thought to be related to stress other than pain, they are often referred to as dysphoria (an emotional state characterized by anxiety, depression, or unease). Dysphoria is a general term that does not specify a cause. Abnormal postoperative behaviors are sometimes referred to as "emergence delirium" attributed to residual gas anesthetics. Some animals do in fact display this response upon awakening, but anesthetic-related behaviors should resolve within several minutes. Behaviors that persist beyond a few minutes require further investigation and attention. In any case, it can be difficult to discern between pain, dysphoria, and reaction to narcotics or general anesthetics. Differentiating between pain and dysphoria following drug administration or use of anesthetics is critical to provide appropriate treatment.

Most animals in pain will be able to be temporarily soothed by a technician speaking in low tones during a petting interaction, although painful behaviors normally resume when the technician leaves the cage. These patients appear to recognize that someone is with them and usually make eye contact. A patient who stops the abnormal behaviors in the presence of a calming person is likely to be in pain rather than having a drug reaction. Animals in pain will also respond when the suspected focus of pain is gently palpated. These two findings should confirm the suspicion of pain and prompt the administration of additional analgesics. Conversely, patients who appear delirious and cannot be "calmed" are more likely to be experiencing stress or a narcotic reaction and will more likely benefit from sedation. These patients typically do not seem to recognize that a human is with them, do not make eye contact, and do not necessarily respond to light palpation of painful sites. The practice of reversing analgesics is reserved for patients who do not respond to either of the above approaches and/or whose physiologic condition is of immediate medical concern.

> *TECHNICIAN NOTE* To differentiate pain from other types of stress: Carefully get into the cage with the patient speaking in a calm soothing tone. Stroke the patient and assess whether or not the patient responds favorably (stops abnormal behavior) and whether the patient makes eye contact. Gently palpate the region of suspected pain and assess for negative response (turns toward painful area or withdraws from touch). Patients who respond favorably to interaction and respond negatively to specific palpation are likely to be feeling pain, whereas those who do not respond or make eye contact are likely to be stressed or experiencing a drug reaction.

THE SCIENCE OF PAIN MANAGEMENT

PAIN IS BAD

Today in human medicine, preventing and treating pain are recognized as essential parts of overall patient management. Pain is considered to play such an important role in overall health and well-being that pain is now considered a fifth vital sign, ranking it of equal importance with temperature, pulse, respiration, and blood pressure. Not only do human health care providers view pain as a symptom of an underlying disease or condition, they view pain as an important syndrome in its own right. This is due to the vast array of negative physiologic events attributable to pain, regardless of the patient's underlying disease or condition.

Pain triggers a series of physiologic changes that increase stress. Although the nervous system is the main target of pain transmission and provides the means for the body to react to that information, the body's response to pain signals is not limited to the nervous system. Most, if not all, of the body's major systems are affected by inadequately controlled pain (Box 26-1). For example, increased cortisol levels that accompany pain may interfere with wound healing and reduce the immune system's ability to work effectively. In addition to suppressing the immune system, increased sympathetic nervous system activity associated with unrelieved pain may result in increased catabolism and metabolic rate, anorexia,

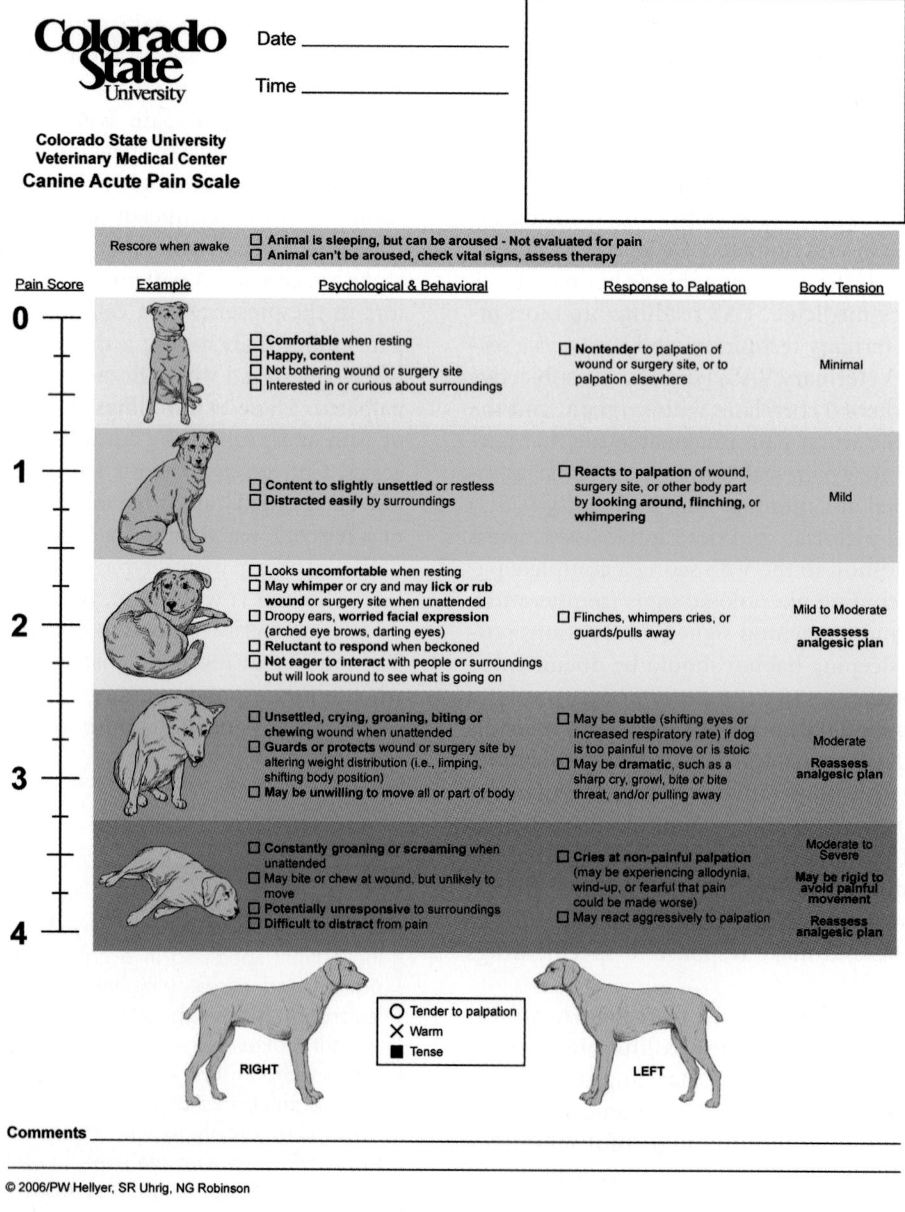

FIGURE 26-1 A and B, Colorado State University (CSU) pain scales. Acute animal pain scales developed by P. Hellyer et al at CSU for assessing pain in dogs and cats. Available at www.IVAPM.org.

Colorado State University

Date ____________

Time ____________

Colorado State University
Veterinary Medical Center
Feline Acute Pain Scale

Rescore when awake
☐ Animal is sleeping, but can be aroused - Not evaluated for pain
☐ Animal can't be aroused, check vital signs, assess therapy

Pain Score	Example	Psychological & Behavioral	Response to Palpation	Body Tension
0		☐ **Content and quiet** when unattended ☐ **Comfortable** when resting ☐ Interested in or **curious** about surroundings	☐ **Not bothered** by palpation of wound or surgery site, or to palpation elsewhere	Minimal
1		☐ **Signs are often subtle and not easily detected in the hospital setting**; more likely to be detected by the owner(s) at home ☐ Earliest signs at home may be withdrawal from surroundings or change in normal routine ☐ In the hospital, may be content or slightly unsettled ☐ **Less interested** in surroundings but will look around to see what is going on	☐ May or may not react to palpation of wound or surgery site	Mild
2		☐ Decreased responsiveness, **seeks solitude** ☐ **Quiet**, loss of brightness in eyes ☐ **Lays curled up or sits tucked up** (all four feet under body, shoulders hunched, head held slightly lower than shoulders, tail curled tightly around body) with eyes partially or mostly closed ☐ **Hair coat appears rough** or fluffed up ☐ May intensively groom an area that is painful or irritating ☐ Decreased appetite, **not interested in food**	☐ **Responds aggressively or tries to escape** if painful area is palpated or approached ☐ Tolerates attention, may even perk up when petted as long as painful area is avoided	Mild to Moderate **Reassess analgesic plan**
3		☐ Constantly **yowling, growling, or hissing** when unattended ☐ May bite or chew at wound, but **unlikely to move** if left alone	☐ **Growls or hisses at non-painful palpation** (may be experiencing allodynia, wind-up, or fearful that pain could be made worse) ☐ **Reacts aggressively** to palpation, **adamantly pulls away** to avoid any contact	Moderate **Reassess analgesic plan**
4		☐ Prostrate ☐ **Potentially unresponsive** to or unaware of surroundings, difficult to distract from pain ☐ **Receptive to care** (even mean or wild cats will be more tolerant of contact)	☐ **May not respond** to palpation ☐ **May be rigid to avoid painful movement**	Moderate to Severe **May be rigid to avoid painful movement** **Reassess analgesic plan**

RIGHT

○ Tender to palpation
X Warm
■ Tense

LEFT

Comments ____________

B

FIGURE 26-1, cont'd

ileus, and atelectasis. The cardiovascular system can also be adversely affected resulting in increased heart rate and blood pressure, irregular heart rhythms, and coagulopathies. Reducing or suppressing the stress response by managing pain can minimize adverse effects on the entire body. Given the potential consequences listed previously, it becomes obvious that, like humans, animals in pain require more intensive medical care than those in which pain is adequately managed. Recent changes to the American Animal Hospital Association's (AAHA) standards require a pain assessment in every patient, regardless of the presenting complaint. Other requirements include making repeat regular assessments throughout hospitalization and recording of those assessments in the medical record. A full listing of the AAHA pain management standards can be found on its website at www.aahanet.org/ (Box 26-2).

PHYSIOLOGY OF PAIN

Nociception and the Pain Pathway

From a physiologic standpoint, pain is processed identically in all mammals. Nociception, derived from the Latin word *nocere* (to injure), includes three distinct phases: transduction, transmission, and modulation. The pain pathway begins at the point of tissue trauma, site of inflammation, injury, or surgical incision, where nociceptors (pain receptors) are stimulated. These specialized nerve endings convert mechanical, chemical, and thermal energy into electrical

BOX 26-1 Negative Effects of Pain on All Mammals

Cardiovascular System
Arrhythmias

Gastrointestinal System
Nausea, vomiting

Pulmonary System
Tachypnea
Hypoxemia
Pulmonary edema
Pulmonary hypertension
Respiratory acid-base imbalance

Renal System
Renal hypertension

Metabolic System
Cachexia
Increased oxygen demand
Negative nitrogen balance

Immune Function
Hemorrhage

Sleep Pattern
Behavior changes

BOX 26-2 Summary of AAHA Pain Management Standards

- Pain assessment for every patient, regardless of presenting complaint
- Assessment recorded in the medical record
- Use of preemptive pain management
- Appropriate pain management for anticipated level and duration
- Pain management with ALL surgical procedures
- Reassessment for pain throughout procedures
- Medical and chronic pain is also treated
- Written protocols
- Teaching clients to recognize pain in their pets

impulses (transduction) once their threshold is exceeded. If the noxious stimulus is large enough to exceed the nociceptor's threshold, a nerve impulse is generated and transmitted along peripheral nerves to the spinal cord (transmission). These nerve fibers are highly specialized to carry pain information and are distinct from other nerve fibers that typically carry pleasant or neutral sensations. Once at the spinal cord, a nerve impulse is either projected upward to the thalamus and then to other parts of the brain or it may be transmitted to a nerve cell located entirely within the central nervous system (CNS) that activates sympathetic reflexes (Figure 26-2). In this way, the sensation of pain is dampened (modulation).

The fourth phase of the pain pathway is perception. Perception occurs in the conscious brain and is the awareness that "I hurt." Although the terms *pain* and *nociception* are often used interchangeably, these are not synonymous. What differentiates nociception from pain is consciousness. That means that patients under a general anesthetic (unconscious) do not perceive that they are in pain. However, nociception occurs even when an animal is in a state of unconsciousness.

> *TECHNICIAN NOTE* Without the benefits of analgesia, the nervous system is still activated to process pain signals, triggering negative physiologic effects, even though no pain-related behaviors are seen.

As anesthesia wears off and consciousness returns, postoperative pain perception occurs. This explains why many patients display pain signs immediately upon waking. Good pain management is designed to interrupt nociception, even if the patient is under a general anesthetic and should be initiated whenever pain is anticipated. When analgesia is provided to surgical patients, recovery is typically much more comfortable.

Wind-up Phenomenon

The CNS adapts adversely to bombardment by persistent pain impulses. This can cause a profound effect on the nervous system's architecture, altering pain processing. When spinal neurons are subjected to repeat or high-intensity nociceptive impulses, these neurons become progressively and increasingly excitable, even after the stimulus is removed. This condition is known as *central sensitization* or *wind-up phenomenon* and leads to nonresponsive or chronic intractable pain. Wind-up is the culmination of two distinct phases of change in the nervous system. First, pain-transmitting nerve fiber threshold is reset to a lower level. This resetting results in *hyperalgesia* where less and less stimulation is required to initiate pain. In the second phase, nerve fibers that normally carry pleasant or neutral information are recruited and become a part of the pain transmission process. This phase is termed *allodynia* and results in normally harmless sensations being interpreted as pain. The presence of hyperalgesia and allodynia collectively is considered wind-up phenomenon. This is apparent, for example, in the dachshund with vertebral disk disease that cries out in pain when any part of its body is touched or the cocker spaniel with a chronic ear infection that can no longer tolerate normal petting. People suffering from a migraine headache can attest to both the increase in pain sensitivity and the feeling that normally innocuous feelings (light touch, clothing, wind, etc.) have become unpleasant. Wind-up phenomenon highlights the need for effective analgesia to treat pain before it begins and at regular intervals once it occurs. Wind-up phenomenon is an important and newly understood concept in pain management. The vast majority of patients experiencing acute pain can be managed using common analgesics, such as nonsteroidal antiinflammatory drugs (NSAIDs). Patients experiencing wind-up require additional therapy just as the migraine sufferer would not likely be helped by taking two ibuprofen tablets, even though this approach would be adequate to treat a common headache. There are a variety of approaches to "unwind" the patient aimed at resetting neurologic processing so

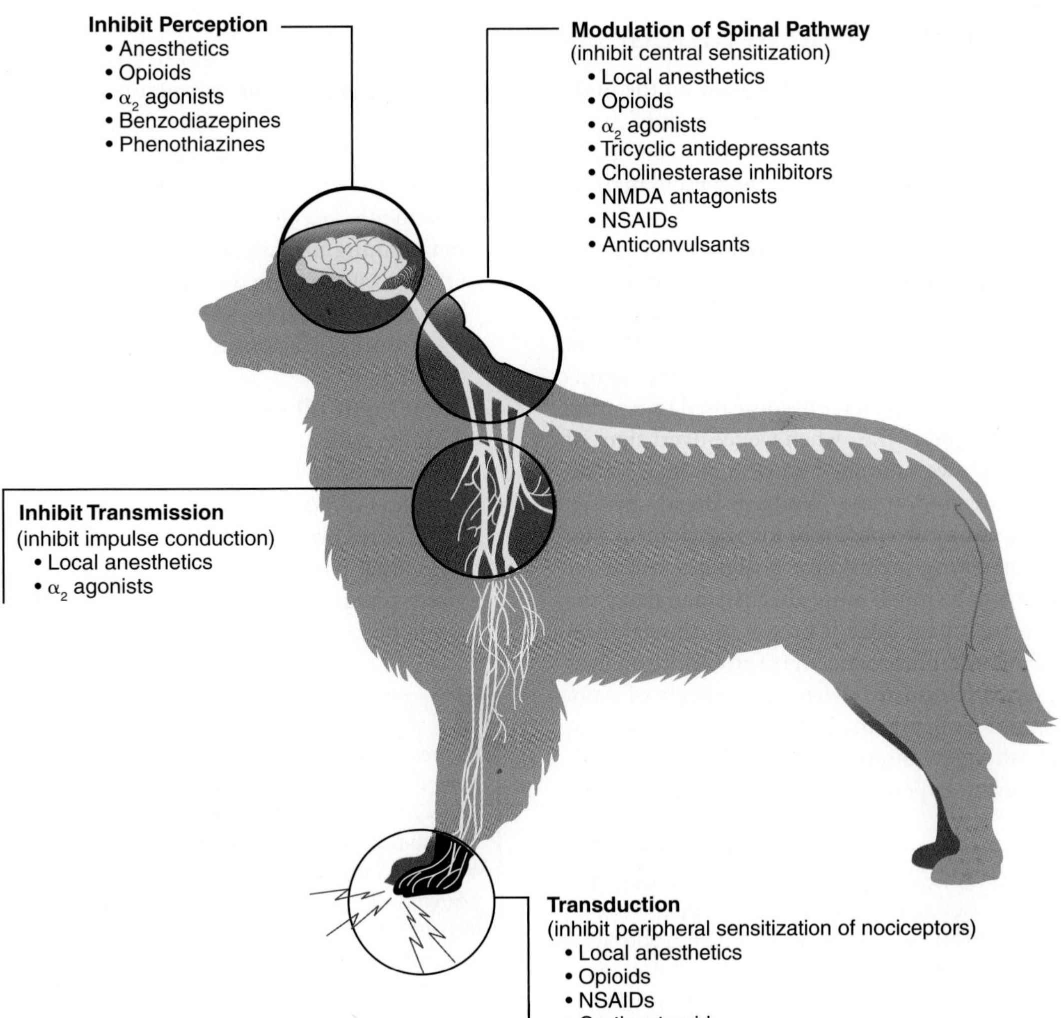

FIGURE 26-2 Nociception. Sites of analgesic action along the pain pathway. (From Tranquilli WJ, Grimm KA, Lamont LA: *Pain management for the small animal practitioner*, Jackson, Wyo, 2004, Teton NewMedia.)

that conventional medications will work again. These will be discussed in the analgesia section of this chapter.

TREATMENT OF PAIN IN SMALL ANIMALS

ENVIRONMENTAL AND EMOTIONAL CARE

Pain has both physical and psychologic components. Fear and anxiety can exacerbate pain and vice versa. Attending to an animal's physical and perceived emotional needs can reduce stress and consequently minimize pain levels. Environmental factors seem to affect the perception of pain in pets. The hospitalized patient in unfamiliar surroundings may be comforted by a favorite blanket or toy. Veterinary technicians must be adept at "reading" patients because the emotional needs of individual dogs and cats vary greatly. A comforting hand or a soothing voice can ease stress and make a pain assessment easier. Skilled technicians know when a visit by the owner would be therapeutic and when it would more likely create anxiety in the patient. Astute technicians can also sense which animals will recuperate better in a quiet environment and which patients are best distracted by exposure to a more active area of the hospital. The patient's comfort can be improved by minimizing painful procedures. Many nursing procedures, such as a venipuncture and injections, cause pain. Procedures should be coordinated to minimize the total number of painful events. Increased technical skill also reduces the intensity of related pain. Policies that protect patients, such as a "two stick rule" (any individual should stick the patient no more than two times) for invasive techniques (e.g., venipuncture and catheter placement), should be instituted. Environmental care, such as providing a clean cage of appropriate size, extra padding, and careful positioning to reduce pressure on painful areas, is important. Designate the patient's cage as a safe zone so that animals do not associate contact with an unpleasant experience. Any procedure that might be considered noxious should be performed outside of the cage, if possible. This allows the animal to feel comfortable and safe when in the cage. Nonpharmacologic actions can reduce pain by removing other stressors. However, tending to a patient's comfort needs should not be seen as a substitute for analgesia.

PRINCIPLES OF ADMINISTERING ANALGESIA

Improved understanding of the impact of pain on the body is shaping new philosophies in managing patients' pain. Several basic principles are used in the approach to designing analgesic protocols and are particularly important in managing pain effectively.

1. **The best way to treat pain is to prevent it.** This is the concept of **preemptive analgesia.** All research in human and veterinary medicine shows that preventing pain is unquestionably the best approach to treatment. It is an easy concept to grasp, but not so easy to remember to implement. That is because we have become used to treating animal pain on "request" (i.e., when we see overt signs of pain), even though we rationally know that once we see the signs, it is already too late. We have already missed the opportunity to most effectively manage pain in that patient. Administering preemptive analgesics whenever possible appears to be much more effective than using the same agent to treat pain once it occurs. Analgesia given before a noxious stimulus reduces postprocedure analgesia requirements, minimizes detrimental effects of pain, improves handling of patients, and potentially lowers sedation or anesthetic requirements. Reducing pain signaling helps to prevent hypersensitization at the spinal cord.

> *TECHNICIAN NOTE* Imagine that tomorrow at 5 PM you were going to have an excruciating headache, guaranteed. What would you do at 4:30? Probably, you thought, "I would take something," such as ibuprofen or another NSAID. You would make that choice because the looming headache is an example of a planned painful event. Knowing the pain is coming allows you the opportunity to stop that pain before it starts. Elective surgery is also a planned painful event. It makes sense to preempt the pain that is associated with *all* surgical procedures.

2. **Drug combinations often produce better pain relief than single agents.** The physiology of nociception gives rise to the concept of **multimodal analgesia.** Multimodal analgesia takes advantage of the synergistic effects obtained by combining two or more classes of analgesic drugs to alter more than one phase (transduction, transmission, modulation, and perception). Attacking pain from many angles is more effective than from one. Because the pain pathway has distinct phases, pain can be interrupted at various points. For example, in addition to preemptive NSAIDs (transduction), we may want to do a local block (transmission) and administrate opioids (modulation and perception). Using drugs from three different classes provides better pain control and has the added benefit of allowing use of lower doses of individual agents, thereby reducing side effects. Effective analgesia can also reduce the amount of gaseous anesthetic required for a procedure.
3. **Matching analgesics** (based on dosage and duration of action) to the degree of expected surgical pain rather than to the patient's ability to express pain in a recognizable way is a more effective way to ensure pain relief.
4. **Maintaining an analgesic plane once pain control is established.** This may include the use of epidurals, CRIs, or continued bolus dosing. Pain management is weaned off as patients are transitioned out of the ICU. Regimented treatment (i.e., dosing at regular intervals) is helpful in maintaining an analgesic plane. Otherwise, a roller coaster effect occurs leaving the patient in varying degrees of pain between treatments. Keeping a patient out of pain is always more efficacious than continually taking the patient out of pain.
5. **"Don't quit till the pain quits."** Send pain relief home with the patient. Many professionals agree that most soft tissue procedures, such as spaying or neutering, require 3 to 4 days of postoperative analgesia, whereas orthopedic procedures probably require a 1-week supply. Of course, individual patients may vary, and owners should be advised to request additional analgesia if they perceive their pet to be in pain beyond the anticipated period.

> *TECHNICIAN NOTE* Dispelling the pain myth that *pain is beneficial in limiting a recovering animal's activity* is critical to patient care. Although one of the mostly widely held myths about pain, studies demonstrate that animals in pain tend to be restless, change positions frequently, and bite and/or chew and/or lick at painful sites, whereas pain-managed animals tend to rest quietly. Aside from being morally questionable, allowing animals to remain in pain for the purpose of restraint is not medically sound. The type of pain produced by tissue injury, inflammation, or direct damage to the nervous system is never beneficial. The previously described negative effects of pain far outnumber any possible benefit, real or imagined. Providing effective analgesia reduces the pain-induced stress response, thereby enhancing patient comfort and recovery.

ADMINISTRATION OF ANALGESICS AND ANALGESIC TECHNIQUES

The basic principles of current pain management have just been described to include preemptive (preventive) analgesia, multimodal analgesia (using different classes of drugs simultaneously to interrupt the pain pathway at various points), and appropriate follow-up analgesia (postoperative and take-home). Using this strategy, an analgesic plan is designed for each patient that maximizes pain control, maintains patients on an analgesic plane, and reduces unwanted side effects (Table 26-2).

Choosing the correct analgesic therapy requires an understanding of both the pharmacokinetics of a wide range of drugs and the levels or type of pain associated with various conditions. The four categories of drugs, NSAIDs, local anesthetics, opioids, and α_2-agonists, are used in various combinations to inhibit the nociceptive process at more than one site. For this reason, combinations are more effective than single agents. Ultimately, pain relief, as assessed by the criteria

TABLE 26-2 Monitoring Patients on Analgesics

Adverse Effect	Monitoring
Opioids	
Sedation, low blood pressure, respiratory depression	Mentation, blood pressure, respiratory rate, and nature
Local Anesthetics	
None unless given by CRI. Then nausea, vomiting, neurologic signs, seizures	Observe regularly for muscle tremors and GI upset
NSAIDs	
GI disturbances, GI bleeding, renal disturbances	General observation, hydration status, stool quality, and urine production
α_2-Agonists	
Bradycardia, cardiac arrhythmias, hypertension, peripheral vasoconstriction	Palpate femoral pulse rate and quality, auscultate heart, blood pressure

previously described, is the only true measure of successful treatment. More recently, several classes of drugs have been added to the pain management regimen as adjunctive therapy in nonresponsive cases. This includes N-methyl-D-aspartate (NMDA)–receptor antagonists and anticonvulsants.

Anticipating pain level and duration provides a starting point for analgesic protocols. The initial approach is based on knowledge of the mechanisms of pain, drug dosages and expected duration, pain assessment, and the knowledge of the expected levels of pain for injuries, surgery, and diseases. Patients should be continually evaluated for breakthrough pain (exceeding usual protocol) or pain that persists beyond the expected period. Categorization of the expected severity (mild, moderate, severe) of pain is used to establish the initial type of analgesia and the duration of treatment. Later dosages can be adjusted according to individual patient response. For example, mild pain may be manageable with NSAIDs alone or in combination with a weak opioid, whereas moderate pain may require the addition of a stronger opioid. Severe pain might be best approached with an NSAID and a full opioid agonist or may require a CRI or additional therapies. Local and regional blocks can and should be added to the pain management plan, whenever feasible. When specific nerves cannot be identified for block, lidocaine can be administered by CRI for excellent systemic analgesia (Box 26-3).

> *TECHNICIAN NOTE* There are a variety of techniques for administering analgesics. Experienced veterinary technicians are able to deliver drugs by oral, transmucosal, subcutaneous, intramuscular (IM), intravenous (IV), transcutaneous, and epidural routes and by CRI.

BOX 26-3 Sound Approach to Developing an Individual Pain Management Protocol

The initial approach should be based on the following questions:

- How painful is the condition, procedure, or surgery expected to be?
- Are there any underlying factors, such as stress, anxiety, fear or preexisting chronic pain conditions, that could be causing an increased pain response?
- What is the normal behavior and disposition of the particular breed and for this animal in particular?
- Are there any contraindications to particular drugs or drug classes for this patient's condition?
- Does this animal have a history of drug sensitivities?

NSAIDs

Nonsteroidal antiinflammatory drugs (NSAIDs) provide analgesia by modifying the inflammatory response. The pharmacologic actions of NSAIDs include analgesia, antipyresis (fever reduction), and control of inflammation. Because they treat the underlying problem (inflammation) and pain is diminished as a result, NSAIDs are considered a therapeutic class of analgesia used. Since NSAIDs approved for use in dogs were introduced into the market, they have been universally accepted as the treatment of choice for osteoarthritis. NSAIDs remain the most widely used analgesics in the treatment of chronic pain. However, they are also extremely effective in reducing acute pain in the perioperative period (around surgery). Recent changes in understanding animal pain and the best ways to manage it and new FDA drug approvals have led to NSAIDs becoming one of the most widely used classes of veterinary analgesics in a variety of situations.

Research shows that pretreatment with NSAIDs greatly reduces intraoperative and postoperative pain from soft tissue or orthopedic procedures. Therefore patients undergoing everything from spaying to neutering to cruciate ligament repair potentially benefit from NSAID administration, especially when given preemptively. NSAIDs have been shown to have a synergistic effect when combined with other classes of drugs, such as opioids. Often, patients with severe acute pain can be weaned to NSAIDs alone as their pain diminishes. NSAIDs have an onset of action of 45 to 60 minutes. The duration of action is typically 24 hours in the dog and varies from 8 to 96 hours in the cat. NSAIDs are best suited for mild to moderate pain, whether acute or chronic in nature. In addition to controlling postsurgical pain, NSAIDs are extremely effective in controlling inflammatory pain associated with traumatic soft tissue injury, ophthalmic conditions, otitis, gingivitis, and some cancer pain.

Current commonly used veterinary NSAIDs include: Rimadyl (carprofen), Metacam (meloxicam), Deramaxx (deracoxib), Previcox (firocoxib), and Zubrin (tepoxalin). Regardless of the NSAID, patients should be normotensive (normal blood pressure), with normal renal and liver function, without bleeding abnormalities, and without evidence or concern for gastric ulceration. Patients that receive NSAIDs should not also be receiving other NSAIDs, corticosteroids, or aspirin.

> *TECHNICIAN NOTE* Cats can safely receive approved NSAIDs on a one-time basis because of their varying metabolic rate of excretion for this drug class (7 to 96 hours). Cats should *never* receive Tylenol (acetaminophen). Cats lack an enzyme required to metabolize acetaminophen, resulting in liver toxicity and an inability of the red blood cells to carry oxygen. One regular-strength tablet (325 mg) may be toxic to cats, and a second could be lethal. The most common abnormalities observed upon physical examination of cats are: increased respiratory rate; pale, muddy mucous membranes; hypothermia; and tachycardia. Other signs are CNS depression, anorexia, vomiting, swollen face and paws, salivation, diarrhea, coma, and death.

Take-Home Analgesia

The availability of NSAIDs has greatly improved outpatient pain management. These drugs are convenient to administer (once a day, chewable), relatively inexpensive, and provide long-lasting pain relief compared with other analgesics. The current anecdotal recommendation from pain management experts is that elective soft tissue procedures, such as spaying or castration, require 3 to 4 days of postoperative treatment with NSAIDs. Orthopedic procedures may require treatment for 1 week or more. Of course, each individual animal must be evaluated for presence of pain that persists beyond the expected time or that is of significant intensity as to require additional analgesics.

Local and Regional Anesthetics

Local anesthetics work by totally disrupting neural transmission of information. Blocking transmission of painful signals is one of the most effective ways of managing pain. Nerve blocks routinely performed by veterinary technicians include canine and feline dental blocks and feline declaw blocks. The use of lidocaine as a systemic blocking agent by CRI is also increasingly popular. There has been a great deal of work recently reviving the use of local or regional analgesia. Applying analgesia directly to the affected nerve endings can provide excellent pain control while reducing the need for systemic drugs.

Lidocaine, the most widely used local anesthetic, takes effect in 3 to 5 minutes and is effective for 60 to 90 minutes. The duration of lidocaine can be extended by combination with a 1:200,000 dilution of epinephrine. Epinephrine should *never* be used in circumferential limb blocks, such as feline declaw blocks. Marcaine (bupivacaine) takes longer to take effect (15 to 20 minutes), but its anesthetic and analgesic effects last 6 to 8 hours. Bupivacaine is not effective as a topical analgesic, but is an excellent choice for local infiltration.

Drugs, such as lidocaine and bupivacaine, are relatively safe if correctly administered. Most cases of toxicity in small animals occur as a result of accidental overdose or inadvertent IV administration. Signs of toxicity include seizures, coma, neurotoxicity, and cardiovascular collapse.

> *TECHNICIAN NOTE* If it ends in "caine," it blocks a nerve. All of the local anesthetics end in the suffix caine and block nerve transmission via the sodium channels. The difference between individual agents is in time to onset and duration of action. Most procedures in small animals are best performed using the longest-acting agent possible (bupivacaine), although mixing local anesthetics to get faster onset is not uncommon.

Routes of Administration

Topical. Application of topical analgesia to the surface skin or mucosa can reduce pain associated with minor procedures, such as wound suturing, venipuncture, arterial puncture, nasal cannulization, and urinary catheterization. Solutions of lidocaine, bupivacaine, tetracaine, and epinephrine can be used alone or in various combinations to provide desensitization at the application site. Gauze pads soaked with solutions can be applied directly to the site. Alternately, there are several commercially prepared topical anesthetic creams and jellies that can be applied as a thick paste. Regardless of application method, 20 to 30 minutes of direct contact time is required to ensure effective analgesia.

Local infiltration. Injection of lidocaine or bupivacaine into local tissue can reduce pain associated with various painful procedures. This technique is useful for small mass removal, digit amputation, arterial catheter placement, thoracocentesis, abdominocentesis, bone marrow sampling, etc. The entry area is infiltrated with small amounts of anesthetic before tissue penetration. An appropriate waiting time must be observed to ensure adequate desensitization of the area, as described earlier.

Circumferential ring block. This block is especially effective for use in feline declawing and involves subcutaneous (SQ) injections of bupivacaine or bupivacaine and lidocaine combination just above the carpal bend on the top of the paw and just above the accessory carpal pad on the underside (Figure 26-3). The dosage is 1 ml of 0.5% bupivacaine/10 lb

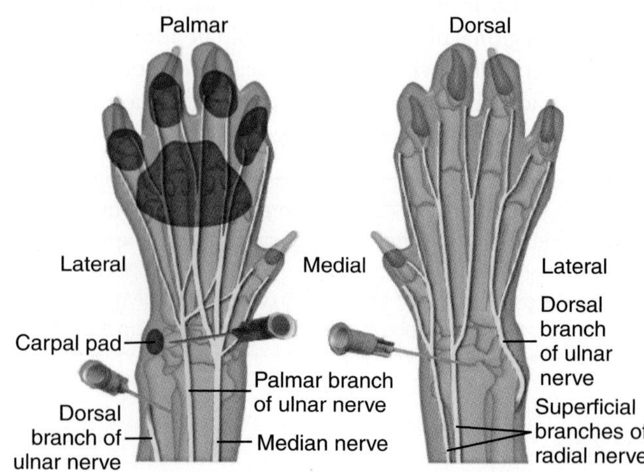

FIGURE 26-3 Circumferential block for feline declawing. The landmarks are shown indicating proper site for SQ injection of local anesthetic to provide block of the three major nerves in the feline forelimb.

of body weight divided among the injection sites. Sterile saline can be added to achieve sufficient coverage for smaller cats. The injections are made just above the carpal bend on the top side of the paw and just above the accessory carpal pad on the underside. The skin is tented horizontally, and the needle is fed under the skin. As the needle is withdrawn, the drug is injected slowly to leave behind a "line." When this is done on both surfaces, the lines will connect creating a bracelet or ring block around the limb. This four-injection technique provides regional nerve block sufficient to eliminate pain for up to 8 hours after surgery.

Dental nerve block. The entire muzzle can be anesthetized by blocking the infraorbital and mandibular foramen. This relatively simple technique is quite effective for dental extractions, oral mass removal, fracture repair, mandibulectomy, maxillectomy, and nasal biopsy (Figures 26-4 and 26-5). Lidocaine or bupivacaine can be used. Epinephrine can be added to reduce bleeding by coating the syringe with epinephrine before drawing up local anesthetic. Volume of administration is limited by the size of the foramen. Typically, about 0.5 ml per site is appropriate for a 50-lb dog, whereas about 0.1 ml per site is adequate in the cat.

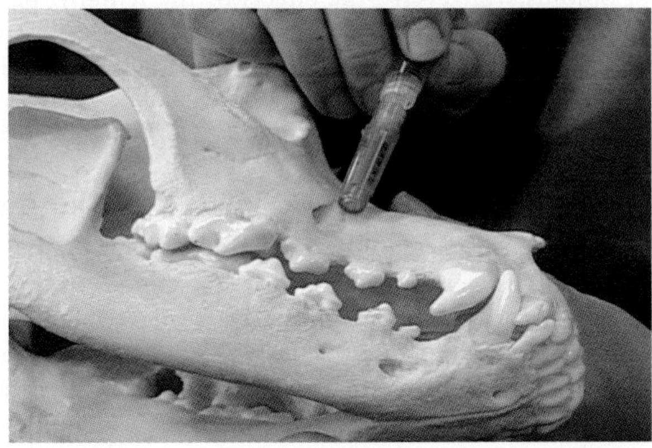

FIGURE 26-4 Location for blocking the infraorbital foramen in the dog. The infraorbital foramina are the sites for injection to provide nerve block to the entire maxilla. Left and right foramen can be located easily just above the third premolar and about midway up the gum line.

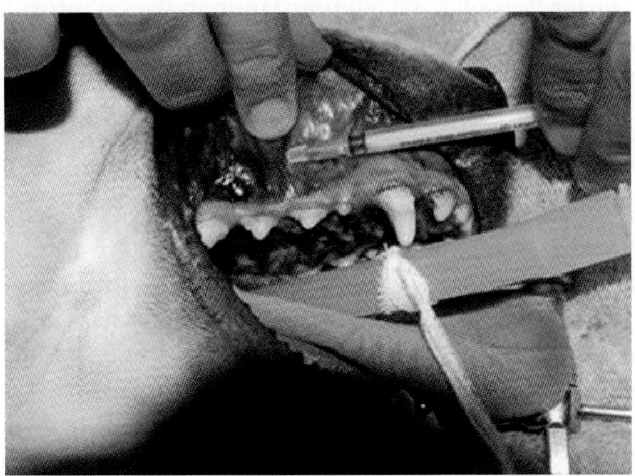

FIGURE 26-5 Blocking the foramen in the dog. Photo shows needle inserted into foramen to block the right maxilla. Care must be taken in shorter muzzled dogs not to overinsert the needle and enter the ocular orbit.

Intraarticular (joint space). Effective analgesia in preoperative and postoperative orthopedic cases has been achieved by injection of local anesthetics directly into the joint space, such as in cruciate ligament repair. Intraarticular morphine has also been shown to effectively reduce joint pain. The effectiveness of this technique when used preoperatively is evident in the smooth plane of anesthesia maintained when the joint capsule is incised. This is in sharp contrast to the spike in heart rate and "lightness" that is observed when the capsule is entered without anesthetic, indicating these responses are likely due to pain.

Pleural space. Interpleural bupivacaine infusion following thoracotomy surgery may have some analgesic benefit. Bupivacaine (1.5 to 2 mg/kg) is injected via an indwelling chest tube into the pleural space. Analgesia is thought to occur by direct blocking of the intercostal nerves. For maximum coverage, patients are held in sternal recumbency for 5 to 10 minutes after injection and gently rolled from side to side. Drug absorption through the pleural tissue should be considered.

Epidural nerve block. Injection of opioids (morphine, fentanyl) and/or local anesthetics (lidocaine, bupivacaine) directly into the epidural space have been used to provide analgesia to the caudal half of the body while minimizing sedative effects. This is a fairly simple and safe technique. Injection is generally made at the lumbosacral space. Epidural catheters can be inserted to allow long-term analgesic administration.

Transdermal. The lidocaine transdermal patch (Lidoderm) has recently gained widespread acceptance in human medicine for management of neuropathic pain associated with back injury or surgery. Work is underway to investigate the use of transdermal lidocaine patches in veterinary medicine for specific conditions and procedures.

Intravenous. IV administration of lidocaine by CRI is an effective technique for managing a variety of pain states. At the cardiac dose of 50 to 80 μg/kg/min, lidocaine provides excellent analgesia for visceral pain (e.g., pancreatitis, parvovirus) and in procedures with extensive nerve damage, such as limb amputation. Lidocaine by CRI can be administered as a sole agent or in conjunction with other analgesics.

> *TECHNICIAN NOTE* The addition of 0.1 ml of sodium bicarbonate per 10 ml of local blocking agents may reduce the stinging sensation and is advised when administering blocking agents to awake patients.

Opioids

Opioids are the most commonly used analgesics in hospitalized patients as a result of efficacy, rapid onset of action, and safety.

The efficacy of various opioids is determined by the specific receptors in the brain and spinal cord that they affect. The receptors are classified as mu, kappa, or sigma. Mu and kappa receptors are responsible for sedation, analgesia, and respiratory depression. Kappa receptors are responsible for analgesia and sedation. Sigma receptors are less clinically relevant and are thought to be responsible for the adverse effects of opioid administration, such as dysphoria, excitement, restlessness, and anxiety. Opioid drugs are classified as agonists (meaning that they stimulate the opioid receptors) or antagonists (meaning that they block particular opioid receptors). There are also mixed agonist-antagonist opioids that stimulate some receptors while blocking others and partial agonists with overall decreased effects at all receptor sites. In general, pure agonists are the most potent of the opioids, but also have the most severe adverse side effects. Mixed agonist-antagonist and partial agonist opioids can provide reasonably good analgesia without many of the deleterious side effects of pure agonists. Side effects may include vomiting, constipation, excitement, respiratory depression, bradycardia, and panting. The type of opioid is chosen based on the degree of analgesia required and the specific needs or limitations of the individual patient. The most commonly used pure agonists in the United States are morphine, hydromorphone, oxymorphone, and fentanyl.

> *TECHNICIAN NOTE* Emesis (vomiting) is a common side effect of some opioids, particularly morphine and hydromorphone. It occurs most frequently when an opioid is used as a premedication rather than when the opioid is administered as an analgesic to an animal already in pain.

Pure antagonists have the effect of reversing the narcotic properties of agonists. The availability of opioid antagonists makes opioid use extremely safe because the drug effects can be rapidly removed. Opioids are metabolized by the liver and excreted via the kidneys and should be used with caution in patients with renal or hepatic disease. Opioids are most effective when administered before the onset of pain. As a class, these drugs produce minimal side effects in animals. Virtually any animal patient experiencing pain is a candidate for opioid analgesia.

Opioids can be administered through numerous routes, ranging from IV, IM, transcutaneous, epidural, and oral routes and administration by CRI. Opioids can be administered concurrently with all other analgesics.

Severe Pain

Morphine sulfate (pure opioid agonist). Morphine is the gold standard for pure opioid agonists. All other drugs in this class are compared with morphine in terms of efficacy, duration of action, and cost. Morphine is commonly used to provide maximal analgesia and sedation. Its relatively low cost and similar efficacy makes it preferential over other opioids in some cases. However, morphine has additional side effects, particularly systemic hypotension and vomiting, that make it less desirable in many instances. Cats are particularly sensitive to morphine, therefore lower doses are used in the cat. Typical dosage for dogs is 1.0 to 1.5 mg/kg IV q 4 to 6 hours. The dosage in cats is 0.25 to 0.1 mg/kg SQ or IM every 4 to 6 hours.

Hydromorphone (pure opioid agonist). Hydromorphone has similar properties to morphine in terms of providing analgesia, but is thought to have fewer side effects. Specifically, hydromorphone is less likely to induce vomiting or hypotension than morphine. Elevated body temperature has been noted, especially in cats. Typical dosage in dogs is 0.1 to 0.2 mg/kg SQ or IM and 0.03 to 0.1 mg/kg IV. Cat dosage is 0.05 to 0.1 mg/kg SQ or IM and 0.01 to 0.025 mg/kg IV. The duration of action is 3 to 4 hours.

Fentanyl citrate (pure opioid agonist). Fentanyl is an extremely potent synthetic opioid with rapid onset, but short duration of action when administered IV or IM. It is most efficaciously used as a transdermal patch for long-term (3 days) analgesia. Fentanyl is contained in an adhesive patch of varying concentration to deliver 25, 75, or 100 μg/hr. Once applied to shaved, cleaned skin, the drug is continually absorbed. The onset of action is from 12 to 24 hours, therefore supplemental analgesia is recommended during the initial treatment period. Use of mixed agonist-antagonist opioids will reverse the effects of the fentanyl patch and should be avoided. Fentanyl can also be delivered as a CRI and its use in this manner will be described later in this chapter.

Moderate to Severe Pain

Buprenorphine (buprenex) (partial mu agonist). Buprenorphine is a partial mu agonist that is of a longer duration than morphine as a result of its slow dissociation from receptors, providing analgesia for approximately 6 to 8 hours. Partial agonists avidly bind and partially activate mu receptors. Buprenorphine use in veterinary medicine also is increasing primarily because its duration of analgesia is significantly longer in dogs. Buprenorphine is recommended for moderate pain in the dog and moderate to severe pain in the cat. Recent work has been done to demonstrate that buprenorphine is readily absorbed across mucous membranes in the feline as a result of the unique oral pH in this species. This allows for transmucosal administration in the cat, providing analgesia for up to 8 hours from a single dose. Transmucosal buprenorphine is the primary analgesic for take-home use in cats. It is extremely easy to administer by owners and provides long-lasting analgesia (Figure 26-6).

Mild Pain

Butorphanol tartrate (torbugesic) (mixed agonist/antagonist). Butorphanol is a kappa agonist and a mu antagonist. As a kappa agonist, it is a mild analgesic with marked sedative properties. Whereas the sedative effects of butorphanol may last for 2 or more hours, the effect of analgesia is only about 45 minutes, an important consideration when managing pain of any greater duration. As a mu antagonist, butorphanol can be used to reverse adverse events thought to be associated with mu opioid agonists, such as morphine. The dosage is 0.2 to 0.8 mg/kg SQ, IM, or IV.

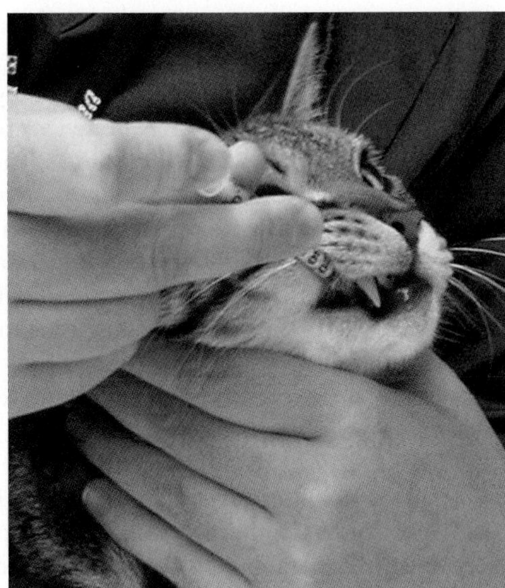

FIGURE 26-6 Administering transmucosal buprenorphine to cat. Transmucosal delivery of buprenorphine is extremely efficacious in the cat and provides up to 8 hours of pain relief in the hospital or at home.

> *TECHNICIAN NOTE* Butorphanol should not be used as the sole analgesic unless mild pain of short duration (less than 1 hour) is expected.

Opioid Reversal

Naloxone hydrochloride (pure opioid antagonist). One of the reasons that makes opioid use safe is the ability to rapidly reverse sedation and adverse side effects. Antagonists work by blocking opioid action at the receptors. Onset of reversal occurs within 1 to 2 minutes of IV administration and can last for 1 to 4 hours. Treatment may be repeated when reversing narcotics with a longer duration. Typical dosage is 2 μg/kg IV.

Butorphanol tartrate (torbugesic) (mu antagonist). See preceding comments.

Synthetic Opioid

Tramadol. Tramadol is a synthetic drug with opioid-like analgesic effects, but fewer side effects. Tramadol has opioid-like activity at the mu receptor and appears to be quite effective in controlling moderate pain, especially when used in conjunction with an NSAID. It is available in oral form making it suitable for long-term at-home management of postoperative, cancer, orthopedic, and other chronic pain. A wide variety of dosages have been tried and reported in both the dog and the cat. Current dosing recommendation is for 4 mg/kg PO b.i.d. to t.i.d. in the dog and cat. It is also unscheduled, an additional benefit. Tramadol may be effective in management of long-term cancer patients, problem osteoarthritis cases, or postoperative prolonged pain.

α_2-Agonists

Xylazine, medetomidine (Domitor), and dexmedetomidine (dexdomitor) are α_2-agonists widely used in veterinary medicine. Dexdomitor is the most potent and selective α_2-agonist and is playing an ever-increasing role in pain management and sedation. α_2-Agonists, which are nonnarcotic and nonscheduled agents, can be useful as adjuncts in a balanced analgesic protocol. The main effect is to produce significant sedation accompanied by visceral and somatic analgesia. There are a variety of new ways to use this drug class as a premedication, rough recovery rescue and ongoing management of in-hospital pain and anxiety. α_2-Agonist combinations are also extremely effective in cats for a variety of surgical and nonsurgical procedures.

α_2-Agonists inhibit release of the excitatory neurotransmitter norepinephrine to produce analgesia and sedation. α_2-Agonists are short-duration analgesics and can be rapidly reversed with α_2-antagonists. This characteristic makes these drugs suitable for procedures requiring short-term restraint and analgesia. α_2-Agonists may bind to the same receptors as opioids and act synergistically with them. The dosages of other analgesic and anesthetic agents can be significantly reduced if given concurrently with α_2-agonists. α_2-Agonists can have profound effects on the cardiovascular and nervous systems, but these adverse events can be minimized by using low dosages. Bradycardia and vomiting are the most common side effects with α_2-agonists.

> *TECHNICIAN NOTE* α_2-Agonists cause vasoconstriction and, like kinking a water hose, the narrowed vessels result in increased blood pressure or hypertension. Because heart rate normally goes up when blood pressure is low and down when pressure is high, slowed heart rate is expected. Bradycardia is considered a normal finding when using α_2-agonists.

Advantages of α_2-Agonists Over Other Sedatives

Other commonly used sedatives (e.g., acepromazine and diazepam) do not provide pain relief. The analgesia achieved with α_2-agonists is of moderate intensity and moderate duration. Even more importantly, α_2-agonists work synergistically with opioids (such as butorphanol or morphine) and improve both the intensity and the duration of pain relief. Other advantages are that the degree of sedation can be "tailored" or "titrated" by using different dosages and/or different drug combinations to provide mild to profound sedation and that α_2-agonists are reversible. Antisedan (atipamezole) is most commonly used to reverse Dexdomitor. Antisedan is the safest of all of the reversal agents because it works almost exclusively by simply displacing Dexdomitor from the α_2-receptors so that the nerve function can return to normal. After the administration of Antisedan, patients usually awaken in about 5 to 10 minutes and are able to stand or walk in less than 10 minutes. α_2-Agonists, are used in a variety of ways to provide patient comfort including as premedicant before surgery combined with an opioid, as a stand-alone sedative or analgesic for short procedures, such as x-rays, and as a rescue drug for patients experiencing rough recovery from anesthesia. The most common use of α_2-agonists in cats is in a combination called "kitty magic," which consists of an α_2-agonist, an opioid (most commonly buprenorphine), and ketamine. The addition of ketamine makes the combination a general anesthetic protocol rather than just a sedative protocol. Minor surgical procedures can be performed under kitty magic, or kitty magic can be used before a gas anesthetic for more advanced procedures. α_2-Agonist can also be administered as a CRI for patients with continual anxiety or pain.

> *TECHNICIAN NOTE* As with any sedative, α_2-agonists works best when it is administered to an animal that is not overly agitated. Agitated patients should be placed in a quiet place for 15 minutes after administration to allow the drug to take effect. Handling, loud noises, or any other sudden stimuli may cause a startled reaction, even if the animal is sedated. Caution should be used, especially when around the animal's head and neck.

Constant Rate Infusion (CRI)

Constant rate infusion allows continuous low-dose administration of various analgesics. Optimally, CRIs are established before tissue damage (i.e., preoperatively) and run for 6 to 12 hours postoperatively. CRI analgesia is also quite effective in management of hospitalized patients with preexisting or persistent medical pain. Many agents can be delivered, but this method most commonly uses local anesthetics (lidocaine), opioids (morphine or fentanyl), and NMDA antagonists (ketamine). These drugs can be used as single agents or in combination with one another. Technicians should be adept at calculating CRIs (Box 26-4).

Morphine

The main advantage of giving morphine as a CRI is preventing the peaks and valleys typically seen with opioid bolus dosing. A lower dose of morphine can be used in a CRI, which can reduce the unwanted side effects, such as dysphoria or panting. Morphine by CRI is useful to manage any severe pain and can be safely combined with ketamine and/or lidocaine. The CRI dose for morphine in dogs: 0.2 to 0.5 mg/kg SLOW IV loading bolus followed by 0.1 to 0.3 mg/kg/hr CRI. Cats: 0.05 to 0.1 mg/kg IV loading bolus followed by 0.025 to 0.2 mg/kg/hr CRI. **Fentanyl** is a full opioid agonist with similar properties to morphine. The main advantage of fentanyl over morphine is a rapid onset of action and short half-life, which allows for rapid cessation of unwanted side effects. The CRI dose for fentanyl is dog: 2 to 5 μg/kg IV loading dose followed by 5 to 20 μg/kg/hr CRI intraoperatively; cats: 1 to 2 μg/kg IV loading dose followed by 5 to 20 μg/kg/hr CRI.

Lidocaine is a local anesthetic that provides excellent systemic analgesia when delivered IV. Because it is safe for use in patients with GI disturbances, lidocaine is a good choice for analgesia in patients with gastric dilation volvulus (GDV) or other similar disorders. Lidocaine seems to also provide benefits for patients undergoing procedures with excessive nerve trauma, such as complicated back surgeries or limb amputations. IV lidocaine is extremely short acting and can be discontinued without residual effect almost immediately. Lidocaine CRI should be discontinued if the patient shows signs of toxicity, including muscle tremors, seizures, nausea, or vomiting. The CRI dose for lidocaine in the dog is 1 to 2 mg/kg IV followed by 30 to 50 μg/kg/min. There are reported lidocaine CRI dosages for cats, but typically, lidocaine is not recommended for use in cats because of potential for severe cardiotoxic effects.

Ketamine is a dissociative anesthetic and an NMDA antagonist. Stimulation of NMDA receptors in the spinal cord results in firing of neurons that transmit pain signals. Prolonged bombardment of these receptors, such as occurs with intense surgical pain or long-term chronic pain, results in wind-up phenomenon. "Wind-up" will be most evident in the postoperative period once the patient has regained consciousness. However, as an NMDA receptor antagonist, ketamine given as an intraoperative CRI binds at these CNS receptors and prevents "wind up." Because of its mechanism of action, ketamine is best used to manage neuropathic types of pain, particularly when the pain has been long standing and the patient has not responded well to other analgesics. Ketamine should always be given in combination with other analgesics and can be delivered in the same infusion. The CRI dosage for ketamine in the dog and cat is 0.5 mg/kg IV loading bolus followed by a 10 μg/kg/min CRI during surgery and 2 μg/kg/min for 24 hours following surgery.

BOX 26-4 Calculating Constant Rate Infusions

Step 1. Set up equation based on dosage μg/kg/min = μg to add to bag
Step 2. Replace hash marks with time signs μg × kg × min = μg to add to bag
Step 3. Enter known information dose and weight
Step 4. Solve for hours fluid bag size ÷ hourly rate = # hr bag will last
Step 5. Solve for minutes # hr above × 60 min/hr
Step 6. Solve equation μg × kg × min = μg to add to bag
Step 7. Convert μg to mg divide answer by 1000
Step 8. Calculate drug volume and add to bag desired mg ÷ concentration in mg/ml = ml

*A controlled rate infusion pump is required because the rate of drug delivery must be precisely controlled. This can be a syringe pump, cassette pump, or rotary pump.

Morphine-Lidocaine-Ketamine (MLK)

The MLK infusion combines an opioid (morphine), a local anesthetic (lidocaine), and ketamine to provide optimal analgesia and treat wind-up. The recipe for MLK is:

To a 500-ml bag of lactated Ringer's solution (LRS) add: Administer at 10 ml/kg/hr to provide

10 mg morphine (.66 ml)	morphine 0.2 mg/kg/hr
120 mg lidocaine (6 ml 2%)	lidocaine 2.5 mg/kg/hr
100 mg ketamine (1 ml)	ketamine 2 mg/kg/hr

Adjunctive Agents

The vast majority of patients experiencing acute pain can be managed with conventional analgesics, such as NSAIDs, opioids, and local anesthetics. Patients in which pain is unmanaged or that are in preexisting pain states may require additional therapy. In addition to the classic analgesic agents, medications with other indications can be used to help manage pain. These drugs are referred to as *adjunctive analgesics* and come from many separate classes of pharmacologic compounds. *Adjuvant analgesics* are agents that can enhance analgesic drugs when co-administered, but have few or no analgesic properties when given alone. Some examples of adjunctive and adjuvant analgesics are:

- **Tranquilizers** (phenothiazines, benzodiazepines), which alter an animal's response to pain and can relax muscles, are used in combination with true analgesics. These drugs also reduce anxiety and fear, which can exacerbate pain.
- **NMDA receptor antagonists,** such as CRI of ketamine or oral administration of amantadine, can enhance analgesia by blocking sensitization of neurons in the spinal cord and are especially useful for managing patients who have experienced wind-up phenomenon.
- **Anticonvulsants.** Gabapentin may play an important role in reducing neuropathic pain and central sensitization in chronic pain patients. Gabapentin is increasingly popular in both human and veterinary medicine as the first choice in patients whose pain does not respond to conventional therapies especially where neuropathic pain is suspected.
- **Corticosteroids** (prednisolone) have powerful antiinflammatory and immunosuppressive effects, "dampening the fires" of acute inflammation.
- **Tricyclic antidepressants** (amitriptyline, imipramine) are effective analgesics for chronic pain, especially neuropathic or cancer-related pain.

Nonpharmacologic Treatment Options*

When possible, multimodal therapy that includes both pharmacologic and nonpharmacologic modalities should be used to treat pain, regardless of whether the pain is acute or chronic. Nonpharmacologic options include thermotherapy, massage, therapeutic exercises, aquatic therapy, acupuncture, electrical stimulation, therapeutic ultrasound, extracorporeal shock-wave therapy, low-level laser, etc. Many of these modalities provide direct pain relief (e.g., acupuncture), whereas others are associated with pain relief secondary to improved function and strength (e.g., many therapeutic exercises).

- *Thermotherapy* includes the use of both heat and cold for treatment of pain, injuries, surgical incisions, etc.
- *Massage* decreases pain and accelerates recovery by relieving muscle tension, increasing blood flow to the painful muscles, and mobilizing adhesions.
- *Therapeutic exercises* are a part of physical therapy that is designed to improve active pain-free range of motion and flexibility, improve use of limbs and reduce lameness, improve muscle mass and muscle strength, improve daily function, and help prevent further injury. Forms of therapeutic exercises include passive exercises, proprioceptive training exercises, active exercises to improve limb use, and speed and strengthening exercises.
- *Aquatic therapy,* such as underwater treadmill exercises and swimming, may be used for rehabilitation after orthopedic surgery, rehabilitation after neurologic injury for muscle strengthening, and for improved joint function. Water is an excellent medium for therapy because the body bears less weight in water, which reduces the load on painful joints and allows the patient to exercise more comfortably and to do exercises that were not possible for the patient on land.
- *Electrical stimulation* indications include pain management (especially in arthritis, spondylosis, spondyloarthrosis, recovery from orthopedic surgery, and nerve regeneration), facilitation of fracture healing, relief of muscle tension, prevention of muscle atrophy from disuse, and muscle strengthening. Treatment modalities include neuromuscular electrical stimulation (NMES), transcutaneous electrical stimulation (TENS), and electrical muscle stimulation (EMS).
- *Acupuncture* has been used for thousands of years to treat pain, yet the mechanism of action is still not completely understood. The efficacy of acupuncture in relieving pain, especially chronic pain, is documented in the veterinary literature, and many veterinarians support its use.
- *Therapeutic ultrasound* has numerous applications, but seems to be especially effective in treating diseased and dysfunctional joints and joint components and certain muscle diseases. The goals of treatment are to reduce pain, improve the elasticity of fibrous structures, increase blood flow, and improve tissue nutrition.
- Indications for *extracorporeal shock-wave therapy* (ESWT) include joint disease (e.g., arthritis of the hip, knee, or elbow) and tendinopathies.
- *Low-level laser therapy* has many possible applications, including pain relief.

*Bockstahler B, Levine D, Millis D: *Essential facts of physiotherapy in dogs and cats: rehabilitation and pain management,* Germany, 2004, BE VetVerlag.

CASE PRESENTATION 26-1 FELINE ONYCHECTOMY (DECLAW)*

An 8-lb, 3-year-old spayed female Siamese is seen for destructive behavior at home, and the owners have elected declawing as an alternative to euthanasia. Pain is expected to be severe immediately following surgery and for 3 to 5 days postoperatively. How would you design an analgesic protocol that provides maximum preemptive, multimodal, and take-home analgesia for this cat?

Preemptive Pain Management

- Give one dose of NSAIDs SQ 1 to 2 hours before surgery.
- Administer 0.02 to 0.03 mg/kg buprenorphine IM with sedation 30 to 45 minutes before anesthesia.
- Perform circumferential ring block using 0.8 ml of 0.5% bupivacaine and allow 15 minutes to onset of action.

Postoperative Pain Management

- Administer subsequent doses of buprenorphine SQ or transmucosally every 6 to 8 hours until discharge.

Take-Home Pain Management

- Dispense buprenorphine to be given every 8 hours transmucosally by owners for 3 days.
- Reevaluate at day 4 and continue buprenorphine as needed. May repeat NSAID at this time if deemed necessary.

*Declawing is one of the most painful procedures performed electively in veterinary medicine. Maximum analgesia should be administered to every cat undergoing this procedure to minimize the associated pain.

CASE PRESENTATION 26-2 CANINE OVARIOHYSTERECTOMY (SPAY) AND TOOTH EXTRACTION

A 2-year-old golden retriever is being spayed, but physical examination reveals a fractured premolar tooth that needs to be removed while she is under a general anesthetic. What analgesia do you think would be appropriate for these two procedures?

Preemptive Pain Management

- Give NSAIDs SQ 1 to 2 hours before surgery.
- Administer a premedication combination of a strong opioid, such as morphine, combined with an α_2-agonist for sedation and analgesia about 15 minutes before induction.
- Perform an infraorbital nerve block on the affected maxillary side using approximately 0.5 ml of 0.5% bupivacaine. (Rinse syringe with epinephrine before drawing up bupivacaine to reduce bleeding from extraction.)

Postoperative Pain Management

- Administer additional doses of morphine every 4 to 6 hours for 12 to 24 hours.
- Can change to buprenorphine for its longer lasting effects (6 to 8 hours) in the evening if personnel are unavailable to assess during the night.

Take-Home Pain Management

- Continue once daily NSAIDs for 3 to 4 days postoperatively and longer, if indicated.

TREATMENT OF PAIN IN LARGE ANIMALS

INTRODUCTION

As poor as pain management can be in some small animal practices, sadly the situation in large animal medicine is generally even worse. Although we do not know exactly how many large animal patients receive analgesia in the United States, a survey of Canadian veterinarians sheds some insight on just how few horses, steers, and piglets actually receive analgesic drugs. For routine procedures, such as castrations in patients less than 6 months of age, only 0.001% of piglets, 6.9% of beef calves, and 18.7% of dairy calves received pain medication (Hewson, et al, 2007). Analgesia improved slightly in older patients where 19.9% of beef calves and 33.2% of dairy calves older than 6 months of age received some analgesic drugs. In horses, 95.8% of patients received analgesics for castration, and more than 90% of veterinarians used analgesic drugs for other equine surgeries, for cesarean sections in sows and cows, and for bovine claw amputations and omentopexies. However, even when analgesia was provided, it was often inadequate. In most cases, a sole agent was used to treat levels of pain that would have required multimodal analgesia for adequate pain control, and often that agent was a drug with a short duration of action.

IDENTIFYING AND ANTICIPATING PAIN

Why is large animal pain so grossly undertreated? Fortunately, some of the reasons are exactly the same in large animals as they are in small animals, so we can use our existing small animal knowledge to educate our large animal colleagues. However, there are also some species-specific treatment differences and differences in the economic perceptions of veterinarians and producers. Here are the main reasons that large animal pain is not addressed:

1. "Animals don't feel pain." As with pain in small animals, this is absolutely false. All mammals have the same pain pathway, so if a procedure or injury would be painful to you, it will be painful to other mammals—including large animals.
2. "Animals don't show pain." As occurs in small animals, this one is often true—but is absolutely no excuse for not treating pain. Unless an animal is in so much pain that it can no longer hide the pain, it is instinctual for them not to show pain. Remember, most farm animals are "prey," and in their world, the weakest member of the herd might be lunch for a "predator." It is in their best interest to be stoic. Thus each patient should be treated on the expected pain intensity and not forced to prove that it is in pain.

CASE PRESENTATION 26-3 HERNIATED DISK, SURGICAL REPAIR

A 9-year-old male castrated dachshund has acute lameness progressing to inability to walk within several hours. Owners report that the dog has been walking "funny" for several weeks. After an MRI confirms a herniated disk, surgery is scheduled ASAP. How do you think this dog's pain should be managed before, during, and after surgery?

Presurgery

- The dog is started on steroids immediately and therefore should *not* receive additional NSAIDs.
- Morphine, lidocaine, and ketamine CRI is started to treat existing pain and prevent wind-up phenomenon.
- Epidural block is performed using 0.5% bupivacaine and morphine.

During Surgery

- Continue MLK infusion throughout surgery.

Postoperative Pain Management

- MLK infusion is continued for 12 to 24 hours postoperatively.
- Steroids are continued.

Take-home Pain Management

- Send home on once daily NSAIDs for several weeks.
- Give tramadol as needed for multimodal pain control.
- After 2 weeks, the dog is able to walk and does not appear to be in pain, but is chewing persistently at his left hind toes. What could be added to treat this assumed nerve pain?
- Gabapentin is added, and signs resolve in 2 days.

3. "There are a limited number of analgesic drugs available for farm animals." This one is also often true—but absolutely no excuse for not treating pain. The analgesic drug classes that are available in small animal medicine (NSAIDs, opioids, local anesthetic agents, α_2-agonists, etc.) are available in large animal medicine. However, it is true that there are some species differences in how the patients respond to a drug (e.g., horses can get quite excited after opioid administration) and some species differences in how drugs are "handled" in the body (e.g., orally administered drugs may be inactivated in the rumen). However, there are effective drugs available for each species, and they are listed in the specific species discussions later in the chapter.
4. "Owners or producers won't pay for analgesia." This one may be true if we let it be true. It is definitely not true for most horses, and this is reflected by the large percentage of veterinarians in the Canadian study who provided at least some analgesia for their equine patients (Hewson et al, 2007). However, most farm animals have an absolute economic value (which is generally low), and the value to the producer is in the herd rather than in each individual animal; thus individual animal medicine is not a priority, and pain relief falls in the category of individual animal medicine. But to counter that argument, many of the analgesic drugs are quite inexpensive (e.g., lidocaine) and could be used without adding significant cost. Furthermore, the stress of pain causes decreased food intake, weight loss, decreased milk production, and other side effects, which can be expensive to the producer. There is more information on this topic under the "Cattle, Sheep and Goats" section of this chapter.

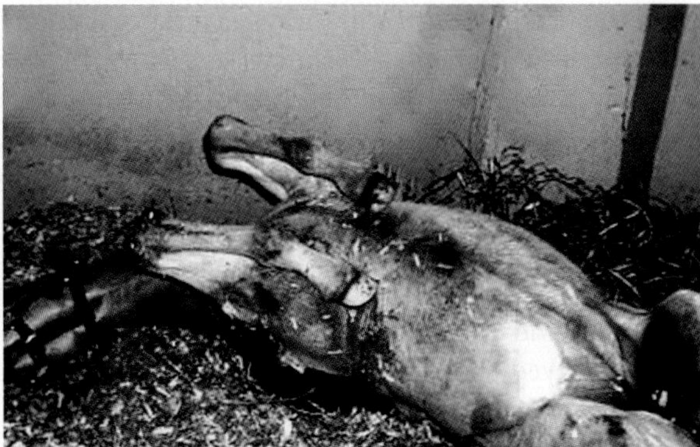

FIGURE 26-7 Painful horse rolling in the stall. Horses will occasionally roll in the pasture, presumably as a way to scratch an itchy back. However, horses that are rolling and thrashing violently and repeatedly are generally in pain, and the source of the pain is almost always from the GI tract. This degree of pain requires immediate attention.

As troubling as the situation seems, there are a few instances where the practice of large animal pain medicine might be slightly ahead of that practiced in small animals. For instance, equine practitioners are extremely comfortable with the use of NSAIDs for acute and chronic musculoskeletal pain and with the use of α_2-agonists for the control of acute abdominal pain (or colic). Of course, this perceived comfort level with analgesics sometimes stems from issues other than concern over the welfare of the patient. As an example, NSAIDs are administered because lame horses are not highly functional and certainly will not perform well if they are in competition. Colic pain is treated because severe GI pain can make horses become extremely violent and dangerous to humans. But for whatever reason that the analgesic agents are administered, the benefit to the patient is the same. However, veterinarians and veterinary technicians should continue to stress the message that large animals do indeed feel pain and that pain should be treated in all animals (Figure 26-7).

> *TECHNICIAN NOTE* All mammals, including large animals, have the same pain pathway and do experience pain, although they may not show signs of pain. Pain causes deleterious effects (e.g., hypertension, arrhythmias, GI ulceration, ileus, delayed healing, etc.) and should be treated based on what we expect the pain level to be following a given painful stimulus and not based on what the patient actually exhibits.

Identifying pain in large animals can be extremely difficult because these animals evolved in a prey-predator society, and all are in the "prey" group. This means that they instinctively hide weakness (and pain is a weakness) to survive. However, because the pain pathway is the same in all mammals, the phrase "if it hurts you, it hurts them" is appropriate to determine whether or not a patient might be in pain, regardless of whether or not the patient shows pain. Unfortunately, as with small animals, the negative effects of pain (see Box 26-1) occur any time pain occurs (whether the patient shows pain or not) and cause detrimental effects to the patient, including delayed healing. Treatment of pain is not just an ethical issue, but also a medical issue. Species-specific signs of pain are listed in Box 26-5.

Furthermore, because these animals often do not show pain until the pain is too severe to be hidden, the sequelae of pain may well be advanced by the time that a human realizes that the patient is in pain. The degree of pain that we expect the patient to be in should be anticipated and analgesia administered based on that expectation rather than on exhibited pain. Species-specific, commonly encountered painful conditions and surgical procedures and the degree of pain expected with each condition are listed in Tables 26-3 and 26-4.

BOX 26-5 Signs of Pain in Horses and Farm Animals

General Signs of Pain

Decreased interest in food to anorexia
Lethargy
Excitement, restlessness
Pawing
Vocalizing (especially cattle)
Bruxism
Reluctance to move
Lying down more frequently or for longer periods than usual
Any abnormal behavior

Additional Signs of GI Pain

Kicking or looking at abdomen
Violently trying to roll
Stretching out in abnormal posture (especially horses)
Standing with abdomen "tucked" (especially cattle)
Dog sitting (especially foals with GI pain)

Additional Signs of Musculoskeletal Pain

Lameness
Abnormal gait
Positive response to hoof testers or flexion tests

Other Signs of Pain (Horses Only)

Reluctance to be bridled (may be head or teeth pain)
Reluctance to be saddled (may be back pain)
Reluctance to be ridden (may be back pain, lameness, or general pain)

TREATING PAIN IN LARGE ANIMALS

All of the analgesic drug classes used to treat small animals can be used to treat large animals, but there are fewer FDA-approved drugs and, in general, less information about the use of these drugs in large animal species (Box 26-6). However, affordable and effective analgesic drugs are available for all species, and a "lack of drugs" is not a viable excuse not to treat pain.

As with small animals, the principles of pain management include the use of:

1. Preemptive analgesia (for surgical pain)
2. Multimodal analgesia (anytime pain is moderate to severe)
3. Analgesia of a duration that covers the entire painful period

Regardless of which analgesic drugs are chosen for the patient, these principles should be addressed every time an analgesic protocol is formulated. Drug classes that can be used in large animal analgesic protocols are listed in Tables 26-5 and 26-6 and include the following.

NSAIDs

NSAIDs are an ideal choice for most painful conditions because they are antiinflammatory and analgesic. Thus anytime pain is caused by inflammation, NSAIDs are treating

TABLE 26-3 Most Commonly Occurring Painful Conditions in Horses, Cattle, Sheep, Goats, and Camelids

Source of Pain	Signs/Severity	Treatment
Horses		
Musculoskeletal Pain: Conditions of the Foot		
Acute: sole abscess	Severe lameness of sudden onset	Treat source—remove abscess, treat with NSAIDs for 2-3 days to control inflammation.
Chronic: laminitis or navicular disease	Mild, moderate to severe lameness of long duration. May have bouts of severe lameness that must be treated more aggressively. These are extremely difficult conditions to treat.	Use NSAIDs to control inflammation, shoeing and hoof care are extremely important, local anesthetic blockade, opioids, other therapies (e.g., vasodilators), alternative care (e.g., acupuncture) all may be necessary.
Musculoskeletal: Joint Pain		
Acute: OCD	Moderate to severe lameness that occurs with exercise; joint effusion	Surgery is required for resolution of lesion. NSAIDs may be necessary long term. Joint supplements and chondroprotective agents may help.
Chronic: osteoarthritis	Mild to severe lameness that may decrease during exercise	NSAIDs long term, joint supplements and chondroprotective agents may help.

TABLE 26-3 Most Commonly Occurring Painful Conditions in Horses, Cattle, Sheep, Goats, and Camelids—cont'd

Source of Pain	Signs/Severity	Treatment
Soft Tissue Pain		
GI pain: colic	Moderate to severe pain, may have recurring episodes with chronic cases; restlessness; pawing; looking and/or kicking at abdomen; frequently lying down and rising; trying to roll; violent movements; bruxism; tachycardia; etc.	Requires treatment, may require surgery. For acute pain: NSAIDs, opioids, α_2-agonists, antispasmodic agents, CRIs, alternative therapy, etc., may all be included in the protocol. For chronic pain: depends on cause of colic.
Cattle		
Musculoskeletal Pain		
Foot (claw) and joint problems	Moderate to severe lameness; lying down more frequently than usual; anorexia; decreased milk production (dairy cattle)	NSAIDs, general foot care, may require antibiotics, local anesthetics for diagnostics, may need surgery.
Soft Tissue Pain		
GI pain: colic	Mild to severe pain; general restlessness; standing with abdomen "tucked"; bruxism	Requires treatment, may require surgery. For acute pain: NSAIDs, opioids, α_2-agonists, antispasmodic agents, CRIs, alternative therapy, etc., may all be included in the protocol. For chronic pain: depends on cause of colic.
Mastitis	Mild to severe depending on degree of inflammation; stilted gait, unwillingness to move, kicking at udder, redness and swelling of udder	NSAIDs, antibiotics, stripping of affected quarter.
Sheep and Goats		
Urolithiasis	Mild progressing to severe if urinary tract is blocked, spraying urine or inability to urinate, abdominal pain, restlessness moving to recumbency, anorexia	Requires treatment, may require surgery; NSAIDs, opioids, epidural analgesia.
Foot (claw) and joint pain	Moderate to severe lameness; lying down more frequently than usual; anorexia; decreased milk production (dairy cattle)	NSAIDs, general foot care, may require antibiotics, local anesthetics for diagnostics, may need surgery.
GI pain: colic	Moderate to severe lameness; lying down more frequently than usual; anorexia; decreased milk production (dairy cattle)	Requires treatment, may require surgery. For acute pain: NSAIDs, opioids, α_2-agonists, antispasmodic agents, CRIs, alternative therapy, etc., may all be included in the protocol. For chronic pain: depends on cause of colic.
Camelids		
Dental pain	Mild to severe depending on severity of disease; anorexia, lethargy, swelling on jaw, nasal discharge	Generally requires surgery, NSAIDs, antibiotics, opioids, and oral blockade with local anesthetics.
Dystocia	Can be severe during the actual dystocia, moderate to severe (depending on tissue trauma) following dystocia; signs of GI pain, lethargy, anorexia	Dystocia requires treatment and fetal manipulation, may require surgery; NSAIDs and epidural analgesia.
Foot and joint pain	Moderate to severe lameness; lying down more frequently than usual; anorexia; decreased milk production (dairy cattle)	NSAIDs, general foot care, may require antibiotics, local anesthetics for diagnostics, may need surgery.
GI pain: colic	Mild to severe pain; general restlessness; standing with abdomen "tucked"; bruxism	Requires treatment, may require surgery. For acute pain: NSAIDs, opioids, α_2-agonists, antispasmodic agents, CRIs, alternative therapy, etc., may all be included in the protocol. For chronic pain: depends on cause of colic.

TABLE 26-4 Most Commonly Occurring Painful Surgeries in Horses, Cattle, Sheep, Goats, and Camelids

Surgery	Pain Severity	Treatment
Horse		
Colic surgery	Severe	Opioids (morphine?), α_2-agonists, NSAIDs, CRIs
Joint surgery	Moderate to severe	Opioids, α_2-agonists, NSAIDs, intraarticular analgesia, epidural analgesia for rear limb pain
Sinus surgery	Moderate to severe	Opioids, α_2-agonists, NSAIDs
Castration	Mild to moderate	Butorphanol + α_2-agonist premedication, NSAIDs, testicular block?
Cattle		
GI or colic surgery	Severe	Opioids (morphine?), α_2-agonists, NSAIDs, CRIs
Abomasopexy	Moderate	Local anesthetics, NSAIDs
Claw removal	Moderate to severe	Local anesthetics, NSAIDs, opioids + α_2-agonists during surgery
Dehorning	Moderate to severe	Local anesthetics, NSAIDs
Teat surgery	Moderate to severe	Local anesthetics, NSAIDs, opioids + α_2-agonists during surgery
Castration	Moderate	Local anesthetic block? NSAIDs?
C-section	Moderate to severe	Local anesthetics, epidural? NSAIDs, opioids + α_2-agonists during surgery?
Sheep, Goats		
C-section	Moderate to severe	Local anesthetics, epidural? NSAIDs, opioids + α_2-agonists during surgery?
Perineal urethrostomy	Moderate to severe	Epidural analgesia, NSAIDs, opioids + α_2-agonists during surgery?
Castration	Moderate	Local anesthetic blockade, NSAIDs, opioids + α_2-agonists during surgery?
Dehorning (goats)	Moderate to severe	Local anesthetic blockade, NSAIDs, opioids + α_2-agonists during surgery
Claw removal	Severe	See comments under cattle
Camelids		
Dental surgery	Moderate to severe	NSAIDs, local anesthetic blockade, α_2-agonists and opioids during surgery
C-section	Moderate to severe	Epidural analgesia, NSAIDs, opioids and α_2-agonists during surgery

BOX 26-6 What FDA Approval Means

FDA approval for a drug in a particular species is gained only after a fair amount of research that proves that the drug is both safe and effective in that species. Thus FDA approval guarantees that the drug has been studied in the target species. However, many "off-label" or nonapproved FDA drugs are used when there is not an approved drug available for treatment or when nonapproved drugs may be more effective or safer than approved drugs. Approved drugs may also be used in a nonapproved way (e.g., medetomidine is approved for use in dogs, but not as a premedicant to anesthesia, yet it is commonly used this way) or at a nonapproved dose (e.g., the dose of butorphanol used clinically in horses is generally lower than the FDA-approved dose). Not all of the products mentioned in this chapter are FDA approved, but all are commonly used in veterinary practice, and all can be referenced in the veterinary literature.

the source of pain and the pain itself (Figure 26-8). They are also relatively safe, easy to administer, inexpensive, and long lasting (12 to 24 hours). Because of the long duration, NSAIDs are ideal to pair with more potent but short-acting drugs, such as the opioids and the α_2-agonists. Depending on which drug is chosen, NSAIDs can be used IV, IM, SQ, PO, or transdermally. The most commonly used NSAIDs in large animals are phenylbutazone ("bute") and flunixin meglumine ("Banamin"), but other NSAIDs are available (see Tables 26-5 and 26-6). The primary side effect of NSAIDs in large animals is GI ulceration.

TECHNICIAN NOTE **The most common side effect from NSAIDs in all species is GI upset and/or ulceration, with large animals more likely to experience ulceration. Patients with GI ulceration tend to stop eating and appear lethargic. Pain may cause the animals to stand with backs "hunched," (especially ruminants) or stretch out in abnormal postures (especially horses). Adult horses often grind their teeth when they are in pain, and foals may "dog sit" when they have stomach pain. Anorexia, lethargy, and/or abnormal behavior in any patient that is on therapy should prompt immediate evaluation of the patient and assessment for possible drug side effects.**

Opioids

Opioids are the most potent class of analgesic drugs and should be included in all moderate to severe cases of pain, especially acute pain. The opioid most commonly used in large animals is butorphanol, but morphine, buprenorphine, and fentanyl are also used. Opioids may cause excitement in large animal species, especially horses and pigs, so they are generally used with a sedative (e.g., xylazine, romifidine, or detomidine) in these species. Cattle, sheep, and goats

TABLE 26-5 Analgesic Drug Dosages for Horses

Drug Class/Drug	Dose (mg/kg Unless Stated)	Route	Dosing Interval	Comments
NSAIDs				
Phenylbutazone	2-4	PO, IV	q12 hr	FDA approved for use in horses; reduce dose to 2 mg/kg on second day; used most commonly for musculoskeletal pain.
Flunixin meglumine	1	PO, IV, IM	q 12 hr or 24 hr	FDA approved for use in horses. Used most commonly for GI pain and treatment of endotoxemia.
Ketoprofen	2-3	IV	q 24 hr	FDA approved for use in horses.
Firocoxib	0.1	PO	q 24 hr	FDA approved for use for up to 14 days for the control of pain and inflammation associated with equine osteoarthritis.
Diclofenac sodium	5-in ribbon of cream	Topical, over painful joint	q 12 hr	FDA approved for the treatment of joint pain and inflammation for up to 10 days.
Carprofen	0.7	IV	q 24 hr	Approved for horses in countries other than the U.S.
Meloxicam	0.6	IV	q 12 hr	Approved for horses in countries other than the U.S.
Opioids				
Morphine	0.1-0.3		q 3-4 hr	Inject slowly if administered IV; horses may have excitatory response.
	0.1-0.2	Epidural	q 24 hr	qs to 10-30 ml with sterile saline.
	0.1	Intraarticular	Once, intraoperative	
Butorphanol	0.02-0.1	IM, IV	q 2-3 hr	FDA approved for the relief of pain associated with colic at 0.1 mg/kg; ataxia associated with label dose and lower dosages are generally used clinically.
	23.7 μg/kg/min (0.013 mg/kg/hr)	IV	CRI	Loading dose 0.02 mg/kg.
Fentanyl	2 of the 100-μg patches/450 kg	Transdermal	Change patches at 48 hr	Can be used without sedation—no excitement noted.
Buprenorphine	0.004-0.006	IV, IM, SQ		
Tramadol	2	IV		Analgesic effects unknown.
α_2-Agonists				
Detomidine	0.01-0.02	IV	q 2-4 hr	FDA approved as a sedative-analgesic.
	0.02-0.04	IM		
	0.06	PO		
	0.15-0.3 μg/kg/min		CRI	Loading dose 6-10 μg/kg; adjust CRI to achieve desired sedation.
Romifidine	0.04-0.120	IM, IV	q 2-4 hr	FDA approved as sedative-analgesic and as a preanesthetic.
Xylazine	0.5-1.0	IV	q 2-4 hr	FDA approved as a sedative-analgesic.
	1.0-2.2	IM		
	0.17	Epidural		Generally added to lidocaine.
Medetomidine	0.005-0.007	IV	q 2-4 hr	
	3-5 μg/kg/hr	IV	CRI	Loading dose 5 μg/kg.
Local Anesthetic Agents				
Lidocaine	As needed for tissue infiltration; total dose <5 mg/kg	Tissue		
	50 μg/kg/hr	IV	CRI	Intraoperative or postoperative or for medical pain.
	0.35	Epidural		May be combined with morphine or xylazine.
	0.35	Intraarticular		

Continued

TABLE 26-5 Analgesic Drug Dosages for Horses—cont'd

Drug Class/Drug	Dose (mg/kg Unless Stated)	Route	Dosing Interval	Comments
Bupivicaine	As needed for tissue infiltration; total dose ≤2 mg/kg			Longer duration of action than lidocaine; can also be used for epidural and intraarticular administration.
Mepivicaine	2-15 ml 5-20 ml 10-15 ml	Tissue Epidural Intraarticular		FDA approved for use in horses; dosages are from label.
Joint Supplements and Chondroprotective Agents*				
Sodium hyaluronate	10-40 mg/joint	Intraarticular	Every 7 days	
Polysulfated GAGs	250 mg/joint 500 mg	Intraarticular IM	Every 7 days Every 5 days	
Other Agents				
Ketamine	40 µg/kg/min	IV	CRI	
Antispasmodic agents (Buscopan)	0.3	IV	One dose	FDA approved for one-time injection for spasmodic, flatulent, or impaction colic in horses. Administer slowly.

*There are numerous products in this category, and two examples are listed here. Use of these products should be governed by proven efficacy.

TABLE 26-6 Analgesic Drug Dosages for Farm Animals (Cattle, Sheep, Goats, and Pigs) and Camelids

Drug Class/Drug	Species	Dose (mg/kg Unless Stated)	Route	Dosing Interval	Comments
NSAIDs					
Phenylbutazone	All	4-6 2-4	PO IV	q 24-48 hr	Prohibited in dairy cattle older than 20 mo of age.
Flunixin meglumine	All	1	PO, IV, IM	q 12-24 hr	FDA approved in some species; withdrawal times are published.
Ketoprofen	All	2-3	PO, IV, IM, SQ	q 24 hr	
Aspirin	Cattle, sheep, goat	100	PO	q 12 hr	Widely used because of low cost, but absorption may be erratic.
Carprofen	All	0.7	IV	q 24-48 hr	
Meloxicam	Cattle Pig	0.5 mg/kg 0.4 mg/kg	SQ, IV IM	q 24 hr q 24 hr	
Opioids					
Morphine	All	0.05-0.1 0.1-0.4	IV IM	q 3-4 hr	Inject slowly if administered IV. May cause excitement, especially in pigs.
		0.1	Epidural		Commonly combined with local anesthetic agent.
	All	0.1-0.2	Epidural	q 6-12 hr	Dilute with 0.05 ml/kg sterile saline or combine with bupivicaine at 1.5 mg/kg.
	All	0.1	Intraarticular	Once, intraoperative	
Butorphanol	All Pigs	0.01-0.2 0.2 mg/kg	IM, IV IM, IV	q 2-3 hr q 2-3 hr	Camelids are extremely sensitive to sedative properties.

TABLE 26-6 Analgesic Drug Dosages for Farm Animals (Cattle, Sheep, Goats, and Pigs) and Camelids—cont'd

Drug Class/Drug	Species	Dose (mg/kg Unless Stated)	Route	Dosing Interval	Comments
Fentanyl	Sheep, goat Pig Camelid	50 μg/hr 50 μg/hr 150-225 μg/hr	Transdermal	48-72 hr	Dosage is for adult animals of the respective species.
Buprenorphine	Sheep, goat Pig Camelid	0.015 0.01 0.01	IV, IM IV, IM IV, IM		Rarely causes either sedation or excitement.
α_2-Agonists*					
Detomidine	Cattle, sheep, goat Pigs	0.003-0.01 0.1	IM, IV IM, IV	q 2-4 hr q 2-4 hr	
Romifidine	Cattle, sheep, goat Pig	0.003-0.005 0.1	IM, IV IM, IV	q 2-4 hr q 2-4 hr	
Xylazine	Cattle, sheep, goat Camelid Pigs	0.1-0.3 0.05-0.1 0.2-0.4 2.2-4.4	IM IV IV, IM IM Epidural	q 2-4 hr for all	Alpacas are more resistant than llamas and require a dose of 0.3-0.6 mg/kg IV or IM.
Medetomidine	Camelid Pig	0.01-0.03 0.08	IV, IM IV, IM	q 2-4 hr q 2-4 hr	
Local Anesthetic Agents					
Lidocaine	All	As needed for tissue infiltration; total dose ≤5 mg/kg	Tissue	q 1-3 hr	Goats sensitive to side effects—dose carefully.
	All	0.2-0.4	Epidural	q 1-3 hr	
	All	0.1	intraarticular	q 1-3 hr	
Bupivicaine	All	As needed for tissue infiltration; total dose ≤2 mg/kg	Tissue	q 4-6 hr	Goats sensitive to side effects—dose carefully; do not give IV.

*α_2-Agonists cause profound sedation in ruminants and camelids, but pigs are fairly insensitive to α_2-agonist–induced sedation.

generally become lightly sedated with opioids, but may have behavioral changes, such as restlessness and vocalization. Camelids are sensitive to the sedating properties of opioids. Opioids can be administered IV, IM, SQ, transdermally, epidurally, intraarticularly, and by CRI. Opioids are primarily used for acute medical or surgical pain. Other than butorphanol, opioid use in large animals has been fairly uncommon, but is increasing.

α_2-Agonists

α_2-Agonists, such as detomidine, xylazine, and romifidine, are used more commonly in large animals than in small animals and, although generally considered a sedative, actually provide moderate pain relief. α_2-Agonists are often combined with opioids (primarily butorphanol) for improved sedation and enhanced analgesia in patients that are experiencing acute pain (e.g., patients with colic) and patients that will undergo minor procedures (e.g., wound repair). The dosage of α_2-agonists is highly variable between species because the response to α_2-agonists is highly variable. Ataxia secondary to profound sedation is the most common side effect of this class of drugs in large animals. The heart rate drop that often follows α_2-agonist administration is rarely of concern because it is a normal physiologic response to increased blood pressure caused by α_2-agonist–mediated vasoconstriction.

TECHNICIAN NOTE There is a wide variation in species' response to the sedative effects of α_2-agonists. Pigs are the most resistant and require high dosages for sedation. Horses are next in sensitivity and require moderately high dosages. Cattle, sheep, and goats are the most sensitive, and all species require approximately one tenth of the horse dose. Camelids fall right in between horses and ruminants.

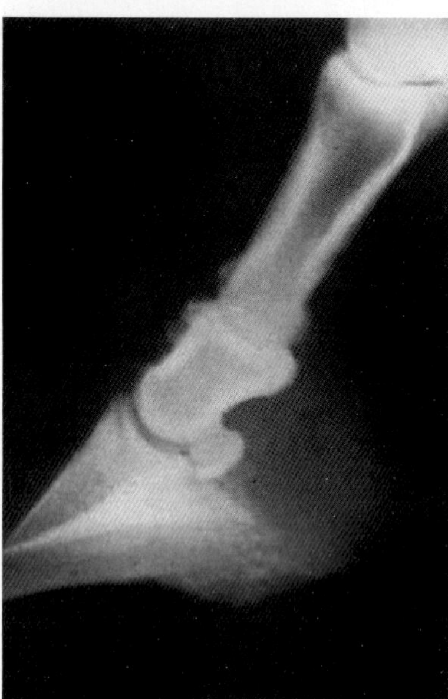

FIGURE 26-8 Radiograph of the pastern joint of a horse with "high ringbone." This is a slowly progressive disease that will cause a mild to severe lameness (depending on the degree of pathologic condition) that will limit the usefulness of the horse. Mild pain can generally be controlled with NSAIDs and light use, but more severe pain will require multimodal therapy.

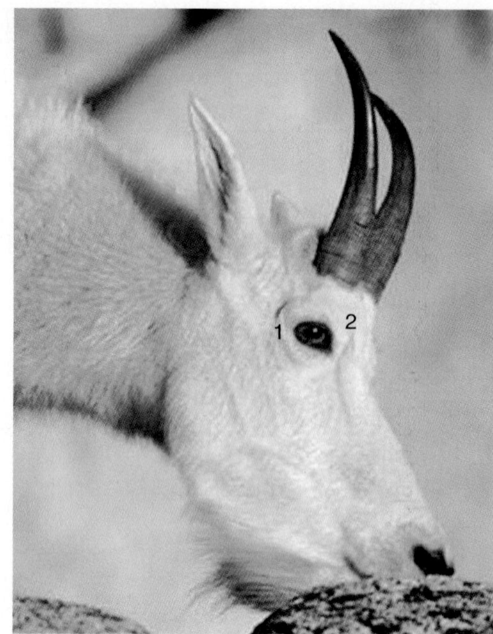

FIGURE 26-9 Locations for blocking the nerves supplying the horns in a goat. The number *1* indicates the location to block the cornual branch of the zygomaticotemporal nerve, and the number *2* indicates the location to block the cornual branch of the infratrochlear nerve. It is important to note that both nerves must be blocked in goats, as opposed to cattle in which only the cornual branch of the zygomaticotemporal nerve supplies the horns.

Local Anesthetic Agents

Local anesthetic agents are some of the most effective and least expensive (yet underused) analgesic drugs available. Local anesthetic agents are ideal for pain control in all species because they will block the transmission of painful impulses without causing systemic effects. Lidocaine, bupivacaine, and mepivacaine are all used locally in large animals, and lidocaine can be used IV as a CRI. Mepivacaine is often chosen for diagnostic nerve blocks because it has an intermediate duration of action between lidocaine and bupivacaine (Figure 26-9). For true analgesia (i.e., blocking nerves to control the pain of laminitis), longer-lasting drugs, such as bupivacaine, should be used. A lidocaine CRI is fairly commonly used to control intraoperative and postoperative pain, especially GI pain in horses.

Joint Supplements and Chondroprotective Agents

Joint supplements and chondroprotective agents, such as nutraceuticals, chondroitin sulfate, hyaluronic acid, and glycosaminoglycans (GAGs), are used more commonly in horses than in any other species, although they can be used in all of the species mentioned in this chapter. These products are generally not truly analgesic agents, but may help improve joint health and thereby decrease pain. Some, however, may have an antiinflammatory or other medical effect. These products are appropriate to add to a multimodal protocol (e.g., with NSAIDs) and are sometimes used alone for mild to moderate pain, especially in performing horses that cannot receive other pharmaceuticals because of drug administration rules. There are a large number of products in this category, and the choice of which one(s) to use should be based on proven efficacy of the product.

> *TECHNICIAN NOTE* Most nutraceuticals and other feed additives are not FDA regulated; thus research proving the efficacy and safety is not required by law. Reports of efficacy are generally anecdotal and not backed by research. Furthermore, the true content of the product is not regulated, and some products have been shown to have a lower percentage of active ingredients than the percentage listed on the label. However, this does not mean that these products do not work. It means that only products that are shown to be safe and effective and products that come from reputable companies should be used.

Miscellaneous Agents

Ketamine

Ketamine is an NMDA receptor antagonist that is used as a CRI to treat the pain of "wind-up" (see p. 866, general section in this chapter). Ketamine CRIs can be added to multimodal analgesic protocols in patients that are experiencing pain that is difficult to control. Ketamine CRIs have been shown to be useful in a variety of large animal species, including horses and llamas.

Antispasmodic Agents

Antispasmodic agents (e.g., Buscopan) are frequently administered as part of a multimodal plan in the initial treatment phases of colic in horses.

Alternative Therapy

Alternative therapy encompasses many modalities, including acupuncture, chiropractics, massage, low-level laser therapy, extracorporeal shock wave therapy, magnetic therapy, and many others (see "Nonpharmacologic Treatment Options" in the small animal section of this chapter). However, not all of the alternative modalities have scientific credibility, and all treatment modalities should be carefully researched before they are endorsed. These treatments may be used for acute pain, but are generally added to a multimodal protocol for chronic pain or used when pharmaceuticals are not allowed (e.g., in performance horses that will be drug tested).

Good Husbandry

Good husbandry and nursing care are always a major part of a good pain management program. This includes not only attention to comfort, as in small animals, but also attention to species-specific details, such as proper shoeing in horses with foot and limb pain and proper udder care in lactating dairy cattle.

More species-specific information on each drug class is available later in the species section and in Tables 26-5 and 26-6.

SPECIES-SPECIFIC INFORMATION

HORSES

Horses generally receive better analgesic treatment than other large animals for several reasons:

1. They are more likely to be treated as "companion animals," such as dogs and cats.
2. Horses are generally performance animals, and pain can affect their performance.
3. Horses may become violent and dangerous when in acute pain—especially with GI pain.
4. Most horses do not have an absolute economic value, such as cattle and pigs, and thus the owners are more likely to spend money on care.

More analgesic agents have been researched in the horse; thus we have more information about how to use the drugs in this species. The NSAIDs are the mainstay for both acute and chronic pain, and equine practitioners are often better at prescribing NSAIDs than small animal practitioners. Opioids are used more commonly in horses. Morphine is a potent analgesic agent that is used intraoperatively as an IV injection or used in the epidural or intraarticular space. When morphine is used parenterally in the horse, it is generally combined with an α_2-agonist to reduce the chance of an excitatory response. Butorphanol is commonly combined with an α_2-agonist to treat acute pain. Buprenorphine, albeit somewhat expensive in adult horses, has also been shown to provide analgesia and has a longer duration of analgesia than butorphanol. Fentanyl patches have been used in adult horses and foals for acute pain, and tramadol has been used in a few horses (with mixed success) for control of chronic pain. Other agents that are routinely used in horses include chondroprotective agents for joint pain and antispasmodic agents for GI pain. Ketamine and

CASE PRESENTATION 26-4 SEVERE COLIC

Lightning, a 4-yr-old quarter horse was found 1 hour ago kicking at his abdomen and trying to lie down and roll. His respiratory rate is 30 breaths/min, his heart rate is 60 beats/min, and his capillary refill time is 3 seconds. All other physiologic parameters are normal, but the horse is now pawing and aggressively trying to throw himself down to roll. On rectal palpation, the veterinarian discovers that there is a great deal of large intestine distention, and she decides to send the horse to a surgical referral center. How will you make the horse comfortable for the ride to the referral center?

ANSWER: Multimodal therapy is required for this degree of pain. Potent analgesic drugs that act quickly are the best choice. A combination of an α_2-agonist (xylazine, detomidine, and romifidine are all appropriate) and an opioid (most likely butorphanol) should be administered IV. NSAIDs do not work fast enough and are not potent enough to treat this horse's pain when used alone. However, they are long lasting and will become effective as the other drugs wear off, so an NSAID (most likely flunixin) should also be considered. An antispasmodic agent would also be a good addition.

CASE CONTINUED: The horse arrives at the referral center, and the surgeon determines that he needs to go to surgery immediately. What analgesic protocol will you recommend preoperatively and intraoperatively?

ANSWER: Preemptive, multimodal analgesia is required. Some analgesia is most likely still present from the α_2-agonist-opioid combination and the NSAID administered by the referring veterinarian. However, more α_2-agonist will be needed for induction of anesthesia, and the opioid will need to be repeated either at induction or just before the surgeon makes an incision. IV morphine just before the incision would be an excellent choice because it is a potent, long-lasting opioid. An NSAID should be administered if one was not administered before arrival at the referral center. A CRI of lidocaine with or without ketamine could be administered intraoperatively.

CASE CONTINUED: The horse had an obstructed bowel, which was corrected during surgery. He recovered well, but now, 6 hours after surgery, he seems a bit uncomfortable. What can be done postoperatively to control his pain?

ANSWER: Unless the horse is only mildly uncomfortable and would need only one dose of analgesic drugs, a CRI is the best choice. Lidocaine, ketamine, or butorphanol (or a combination of two or three of these drugs) can all be used. The best choice is probably lidocaine because it is inexpensive, not controlled, and causes neither sedation nor excitement (unless overdosed). Ideally, in our attempt to anticipate pain rather than force the patient to show pain, the CRI should have been started *before* the horse became uncomfortable. Multimodal analgesia will be required, so the horse should be continued on an NSAID (long duration and antiinflammatory properties). Flunixin is the most commonly used NSAID for colic pain.

lidocaine CRIs are used more and more commonly for intraoperative and postoperative pain and for medical pain (e.g., nonsurgical colic). Local and regional blockade (e.g., epidurals and intraarticular blocks) are becoming fairly standard.

> *TECHNICIAN NOTE* Do not be afraid to use potent opioids (e.g., morphine) in horses, especially for intraoperative and postoperative pain. These drugs are highly effective and extremely inexpensive. However, like cats, horses may exhibit excitement after receiving a potent opioid, so always administer a sedative (e.g., xylazine, romifidine, or detomidine) at the same time.

CATTLE, SHEEP, AND GOATS

Food-producing herd animals, such as cattle, sheep, and goats, are the least likely large animal patients to receive analgesia. Exceptions to the lack of treatment include animals kept as individual pets, valuable beef herd sires, and high-producing dairy cows. Problems specific to food-producing animals include that these animals often have an absolute economic value with a narrow profit margin, and pharmaceutical residue is not generally accepted in the food chain. The latter issue means that some drugs are totally prohibited in this group of patients, whereas other drugs have a withdrawal time that must be observed between the administration of the drug and the time that meat and/or milk can be used.

Economics

Although it is true that many farm animals have an absolute economic value with a low profit margin, it is also true that a number of the analgesic drugs are inexpensive (e.g., local anesthetic agents), and the side effects of pain (e.g., anorexia and weight loss) can be as or more costly than the analgesia. In many other countries of the world (e.g., the United Kingdom and several Scandinavian countries), analgesia is required by law for surgical procedures done on farm animals. The most common requirement is the use of local anesthetics, which will at least provide good analgesia for the duration of the block, have been shown to decrease the side effects associated with pain, and have minimal tissue uptake so that drug residues are of decreased concern. Analgesia may be difficult to regulate in the United States because many of the routine procedures (e.g., castration in calves, pigs, and lambs) are done by producers and not by veterinarians. However, as a profession, we should strive to ensure that all procedures done by a veterinarian are accompanied by analgesia. Unfortunately, even this seemingly simple step may be difficult, as evidenced by a few of the swine practitioners that participated in the Canadian study who were concerned about the loss of professional time and income while waiting for local anesthetics to take effect—a delay that is only 2 to 5 minutes in duration.

Drug Residues in Meat and Milk

Because drug residues in the human food chain could be harmful to human beings, there are strict regulations regarding the use of many pharmaceuticals in food-producing (meat and milk) animals. For instance, the use of phenylbutazone is completely prohibited in dairy cattle 20 months of age or older. On the other hand, some forms of flunixin (but not all brands) are approved for use in cattle and pigs, with withdrawal times of 72 hours for milk and 10 days for meat in cattle and 12 days withdrawal for meat in pigs. Because regulations change, people dealing with food-producing animals should routinely update the withdrawal information of the drugs that they are using. The best source for information is the Food Animal Residue Avoidance Databank (FARAD) at www.farad.org.

Finally, many food-producing animals are ruminants, and delivery of oral drugs into the rumen can inactivate them, slow their absorption, or otherwise alter the drug or the response to the drug. Fortunately, most oral drugs that are available to treat pain can be used in ruminants, and, of course, the IV, IM, SQ, transdermal, epidural, intraarticular, and local tissue infusion routes of administration can all be used.

> *TECHNICIAN NOTE* The latest guidelines for withdrawal times of drugs in food-producing animals can be obtained from the Food Animal Residue Avoidance Databank (FARAD) at www.farad.com.

All of the drug classes used in horses can be used in ruminants. The most commonly used NSAIDs are phenylbutazone, flunixin, and aspirin. α_2-Agonists are commonly used for acute pain, but this group of animals is extremely sensitive to the sedating effect of α_2-agonists, so low dosages

CASE PRESENTATION 26-5 OSTEOARTHRITIS

Rajah, an 11-year-old Arabian mare, has been diagnosed with osteoarthritis of the pastern joint ("high ringbone"). She has been a competitive endurance horse, but her owner is willing to retire her. However, she still wants a "performance" horse in that she would like to do some light trail riding with Rajah. What will you recommend to control chronic pain in this horse?

ANSWER: NSAIDs will be the mainstay of treatment because they will help to control both the pain and the inflammation associated with the disease. Phenylbutazone is the most likely choice. Nutraceuticals added to the feed, GAGs administered IM, or hyaluronic acid with or without steroids injected directly into the joint are all excellent additions to the NSAIDs. Proper shoeing will also greatly benefit Rajah. An increased dose of NSAIDs immediately before and the day after long rides may be needed to keep Rajah comfortable and able to enjoy the trail.

CASE PRESENTATION 26-6 DEHORNING

Bucky, a 6-month-old Spanish goat, comes to your practice for dehorning. How will you manage surgical pain?

ANSWER: For multimodal, preemptive analgesia, sedate Bucky with an α_2-agonist (xylazine or medetomidine would be good choices) combined with butorphanol. Use bupivacaine to block the nerves to the horn and give one dose of flunixin or ketoprofen IV.

CASE PRESENTATION 26-7 BONE FRACTURE

Willow, an 8-year-old adult female llama, has a fractured tibia that will be surgically repaired today. How will you handle the pain associated with this surgery?

ANSWER: For preemptive, multimodal analgesia, administer butorphanol and xylazine (or medetomidine) as a premedicant to anesthesia and give a dose of an NSAID IV. Once the patient is anesthetized, administer an epidural block of morphine and bupivacaine. For pain after the epidural wears off, there are three options: (1) place an epidural catheter (*easy* to do in large animals and my personal favorite for this case) and administer morphine b.i.d. for 2 to 3 days; (2) place a fentanyl patch for 72 hours of analgesia; (3) keep Willow on a lidocaine-ketamine CRI (this is probably the least practical because this patient will not likely be on fluids postoperatively). Whichever method is chosen, it should be combined with IV NSAIDs. Subsequently the patient should be discharged from the hospital on oral NSAIDs for 10 to 14 days.

should be used. Butorphanol is also commonly used for acute pain, and morphine is used occasionally. Fentanyl patches, buprenorphine, and both ketamine and lidocaine CRIs have been used to control pain in small ruminants (sheep and goats), but the use of these drugs and techniques are not as common in adult cattle simply because treatment of pain in this group is not as common. By far, the most commonly used analgesic drugs in ruminants are the local analgesic agents (primarily lidocaine and bupivacaine), and techniques include local field block (tissue block at the site of the surgery or injury), IV regional blocks, epidurals, paravertebral blocks, corneal blocks, etc. For a description of these blocks and how to perform them, see the chapter by Dr. Skarda (full reference in the Recommended Reading section of this chapter). Alternative techniques, such as acupuncture, are also appropriate for analgesia in ruminants.

TECHNICIAN NOTE Local anesthetic agents are an excellent choice for analgesia in all ruminants. However, keep in mind that sheep and goats are easily overdosed, so the drug dosage in these species must be calculated carefully.

CAMELIDS

Camelids (e.g., llamas and alpacas) are more likely to receive analgesic treatment than cattle, sheep, and goats (but not as likely as horses) because they are generally constrained neither by an absolute economic value nor by entry into the human food chain. These animals have a GI tract similar to that found in ruminants with a "third compartment" that functions like a rumen. Thus drug administration issues are the same in camelids as they are in ruminants, where orally administered drugs may be inactivated. All drugs used in other ruminant types of species can be used in camelids. NSAIDs are generally the first treatment for both acute and chronic pain. α_2-Agonists and butorphanol are used to treat acute pain, but these drugs cause fairly profound sedation in camelids, so they are used only when sedation is appropriate. Other treatment modalities include fentanyl patches, lidocaine CRIs, ketamine CRIs, local or regional blockade, and alternative therapies, such as acupuncture.

PIGS

The lack of good pain management in swine practice rivals the lack in cattle practice, but high-producing boars and sows along with pot bellied pigs kept as pets may receive better treatment. Like ruminants, pigs generally have an absolute economic value and are affected by their likely entry into the human food chain. All of the drugs discussed with the other species can be used in pigs.

SUMMARY

Providing effective pain management is not an individual endeavor. It requires a team approach involving everyone who participates in patient care. As true patient advocates, veterinary technicians constitute a vital force in this effort. A successful technician understands the goals of pain control and the analgesic options. Combining keen observation with good technical skills, the technician appropriately assesses pain and then requests and administers analgesics to his or her patients. Attention to environmental and emotional needs and differentiating other stress from pain is part of a technician's daily routine (Box 26-7). Veterinary technicians have played a vital role in bringing animal pain management to the forefront of veterinary practice. Through continued teaching and vigilant practice, technicians will no doubt be credited in large part with the continuing improvements in the practice of veterinary pain management. Much work is still to be done, particularly in the arena of large animal practice. Although it is true that large animals hide pain (often even better than small animals) and that there are some economic constraints and species-specific limitations in drug use or administration, it is not true that large animals do not feel pain. Pain management is often initiated at the technician's level because the technician is often the person who spends the most time with the patient and is the most likely to recognize pain in the patient.

BOX 26-7 Summary of Technician's Responsibilities

Technicians typically hold the responsibilities of:
- Patient assessment
- Identifying (or predicting) pain
- Providing nonpharmacologic comfort and care
- Differentiating pain from other stress
- Requesting appropriate analgesia and/or sedation
- Helping to develop appropriate protocols for pain management
- Administering medications, performing analgesic techniques
- Monitoring and treating drug effects
- Assessing patients postoperatively
- Communicating with clients
- Logging controlled substances

REFERENCES

Bockstahler B, Levine D, Millis D: *Essential facts of physiotherapy in dogs and cats: rehabilitation and pain management*, 2004, Germany, BE VetVerlag.

Hewson CJ, Dohoo IR, Lemke KA, et al: Canadian veterinarians' use of analgesics in cattle, pigs, and horses in 2004 and 2005, *Can Vet J* 48:155-164, 2007.

Skarda RT: Local and regional anesthetic and analgesic techniques. In Thurmon JC, Tranquilli WJ, Benson GJ, editors: *Lumb & Jones' veterinary anesthesia*, ed 3, Baltimore, 1996, Williams & Wilkins.

RECOMMENDED READING

Animal Welfare Act and Regulations. USDA website with other links. Available at www.nal.usda.gov/awic/legislat/usdalegl.htm.

Bath GF: Management of pain in production animals, *Appl Anim Behav Sci* 59:147-156, 1998.

Benson GJ, Rollin BE, editors: *The well-being of farm animals: challenges and solutions*, 2004, Blackwell Publishing.

Wildlife Information Network: Pain management in ruminants. Available at www.wildlifeinformation.org,

Valverde A, Gunkel CI: Pain management in horses and farm animals, *J Vet Emerg Crit Care* 15(4):295-307, 2005.

Mama K: Pain management and anesthesia, *Vet Clin North Am Eq Pract* April, 2002.

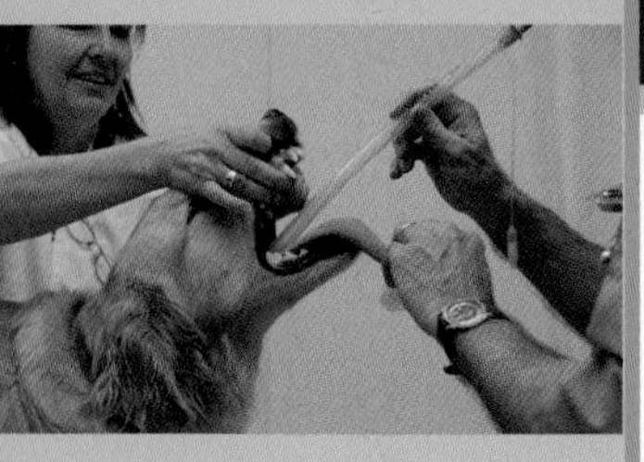

Veterinary Anesthesia

27

John A. Thomas and Phillip Lerche

KEY TERMS

Analgesia
Apnea
Atelectasis
Ayre's T-piece
Bain circuit
Cyanosis
Hypercarbia
Hypnotic
Hypothermia
Hypoventilation
Hypoxia
Miosis
Mydriasis
Nonrebreathing system
Oxygen saturation
Pneumothorax
Rebreathing system
Respiratory minute volume (RMV)
Tachycardia
Tachypnea
Tidal volume
Vasodilation

OUTLINE

LEARNING OBJECTIVES

When you have completed this chapter, you will be able to:

1. Define anesthesia and differentiate between general and local anesthesia.
2. Differentiate between sedation, tranquilization, and neuroleptanalgesia.
3. Explain the concept of balanced anesthesia and list the factors to consider in developing an anesthetic plan for a patient.
4. List the classes of injectable medications used in anesthetic protocols and give examples of each.
5. List and describe the features of the commonly used inhalant anesthetics.
6. List the parts of the anesthesia machine, describe the function of each part, and list procedures used for verifying proper operation.
7. Differentiate between nonrebreathing and rebreathing systems and explain the proper use, advantages, and disadvantages of each type of system.
8. List the reflexes used in monitoring of anesthetic depth and describe the relationship between vital signs, patient reflexes, and anesthetic depth.
9. List the stages and planes of anesthesia and describe changes in patient physiology and behavior in each stage.
10. Describe the equipment needed and procedures used for placement of an endotracheal tube.
11. Describe procedures used for IV, IM, mask, and chamber induction.
12. Describe general considerations for patient positioning, comfort, and safety during anesthesia.
13. Describe procedures used in monitoring patients during recovery from anesthesia.
14. Differentiate between manual and mechanical ventilation and explain indications, procedures, and complications of ventilation.
15. Describe common anesthetic problems and emergencies.

INTRODUCTION

Anesthesia is a unique discipline for several reasons. First, anesthetic procedures are performed not for their own sake, but to allow veterinary professionals to do other things that would otherwise not be possible. For instance, anesthesia enables surgery, dentistry, endoscopy, and other procedures that require patient immobility, unconsciousness, and pain control. It enables treatment, handling, and transport of exotic and feral animals. In some patients, it is necessary to perform procedures, such as nail trims, grooming, and radiographic studies, which—although not painful—evoke fear, cause discomfort, and are unwelcome. This wide range of indications makes anesthesia a constant presence in the professional life of the veterinary technician.

Second, the practice of anesthesia is much more than choosing machine settings, checking reflexes, or watching monitoring devices. It is an extremely complex discipline involving use of complicated equipment, administration of potentially dangerous drugs, and awareness of an intricate set of monitoring parameters that enable the anesthetist to assess the well-being of the patient.

General anesthesia is by nature high risk. Anesthetic drugs cause adverse physiologic changes in cardiac output, blood pressure, respiratory drive, and central nervous system (CNS) function that can be dangerous and even life threatening if not monitored and managed. Although a competent anesthetist is never controlled by fear, a healthy respect for the risks of anesthesia must be maintained at all times to keep the "edge" required for best performance.

Finally, changes in the status of anesthetized patients occur quickly and unexpectedly—often within minutes or even seconds. This urgency demands a high level of awareness and an ability to make critical decisions rapidly and effectively to ensure patient safety.

This unique combination of frequent use, complexity, high risk, and fast pace of veterinary anesthesia tests the knowledge and abilities of even the most experienced veterinary technician. Therefore the successful practice of anesthesia demands that the technician be prepared, skillful, alert, and attentive. The purpose of this chapter is to provide the reader with the information needed to reach this end.

WHAT IS ANESTHESIA?

Anesthesia is defined as an absence of sensation that affects either the whole body or an isolated part or region of the body. Tranquilization and sedation are by convention included in the study of anesthesia because these techniques are frequently used in conjunction with anesthesia. The effects appropriate for each patient vary depending on the procedure and may include light to heavy sedation, local anesthesia, general anesthesia, muscle relaxation, analgesia, or a combination thereof.

General anesthesia is characterized by unconsciousness and insensibility to feeling and pain induced by administration of anesthetic agents given alone or in combination. General anesthesia provides an environment in which general surgery or other painful procedures can be performed without the danger of patient movement or injury to personnel. Anesthetic induction is the process used to take the patient from a state of consciousness to general anesthesia. Anesthetic maintenance is the process used to keep the patient under general anesthesia until recovery.

In contrast, local anesthesia is the loss of sensation in a localized body part or region induced by the administration of a drug or other agent without the loss of consciousness. Local anesthesia is used for procedures that do not require the patient to be unconscious and for adjunct pain control. Administration of local anesthetic to remove a skin tumor, a nerve block performed on a horse to localize lameness, or an epidural used to provide analgesia for a patient undergoing an orthopedic procedure are all examples of local anesthesia.

Premedication refers to the administration of an agent or agents before induction of general anesthesia to calm and relax the patient, ease induction and recovery, minimize adverse effects, reduce the amount of general anesthetic needed, provide muscle relaxation, or provide pain control. A variety of tranquilizers, sedatives, anesthetics, and anticholinergics are used alone or in combination for this purpose. Premedication is also referred to as preanesthesia.

Sedation is a state of calm or drowsiness, whereas tranquilization is a state of relaxation and reduction of anxiety. Many tranquilizers also produce some degree of sedation. Consequently, these terms are often used interchangeably, even though they have somewhat different meanings.

Neuroleptanalgesia is a state of profound sedation and analgesia produced by simultaneous administration of an opioid and tranquilizer. Neuroleptanalgesia is commonly used to perform minor procedures, such as wound treatment or radiography, and to induce general anesthesia in sick patients.

The objectives of anesthesia are to produce a loss of sensation in the whole body or a body part or region and to provide muscle relaxation, analgesia, and alteration of consciousness appropriate to the procedure. In addition, patient safety must be preserved and adverse effects minimized, with special attention to respiratory and cardiovascular function. This can seldom be achieved with the use of only one drug. This is why the concurrent administration of two or more anesthetic drugs is commonplace. This use of drugs with complimentary effects, referred to as balanced anesthesia, enables the anesthetist to fulfill these diverse objectives. Although there are many commonly used protocols, premedication with acepromazine, anesthetic induction with a ketamine-diazepam mixture, anesthetic maintenance with sevoflurane gas, and administration of a morphine infusion for pain control is one example of balanced anesthesia.

PATIENT PREPARATION

The technician must accurately identify factors that can compromise a patient and must effectively communicate this information to the veterinarian before beginning any anesthetic procedure. Specifically, careful patient preparation is important for the following reasons:

- To minimize the likelihood of preventable complications, such as aspiration
- To allow treatment of any problems that may endanger the patient, such as dehydration, bleeding, organ dysfunction, or organ failure
- To allow the veterinarian to make anesthetic drug choices based on facts about the patient's condition
- To give the anesthetist awareness of potential problems that the patient may experience during the procedure

FASTING RECOMMENDATIONS

Swallowing reflexes become sluggish, lower esophageal sphincter tone decreases, and patients may experience nausea or vomiting during anesthetic procedures. This combination of factors may allow stomach contents to reflux into the esophagus and the pharynx resulting in a range of mild to devastating complications, including aspiration of stomach contents into the lungs, postanesthesia esophagitis, and esophageal stricture. Therefore it is vital to observe fasting recommendations before any anesthetic procedure in common domestic species. Although fasting recommendations vary widely from practice to practice, guidelines may be found in Table 27-1.

> *TECHNICIAN NOTE* Be certain that fasting instructions have been observed before admitting *any* patient for anesthesia.

GATHERING HISTORICAL INFORMATION

In addition to the usual historical information needed for any patient, such as vaccine status and the medical and surgical history, there are several additional pieces of information that must be determined before administering an anesthetic. The following is a list of questions that should be asked of a client at the time of patient drop-off:

- Has the patient been fasting for the recommended time?
- How is the patient feeling today?
- Are there any changes in the patient's condition since the procedure was scheduled?
- Is the patient up to date on routine preventive care?
- What is the patient in for today (including left or right side if the procedure involves a limb, eye, or ear; and including the location of tumors or other localized lesions)?
- Is the patient taking any medications?

Unless asked, a client may not reveal this information at the time of drop-off for a variety of reasons. For example, an owner who failed to observe fasting recommendations may be unwilling to admit a lack of willpower to withhold food, may not realize the importance of fasting, or may simply have forgotten to tell you. An owner may not think to inform you that the patient worsened or developed vomiting, coughing, or some other sign of significant illness. If the procedure is not verbally confirmed, the surgeon could mistakenly perform a procedure on the incorrect limb or the wrong surgery altogether. Thus any missing piece of information can make the difference between a successful and a potentially serious outcome.

TABLE 27-1 Fasting Recommendations

Species	Food Withholding Time (Hr)	Water Withholding Time (Hr)
Dogs and Cats	8-12*	2-4
Horses	8-12	0-2
Cattle	24-48	8-12
Small ruminants	12-18	8-12
Neonates (<8 wks old)	None	None

*Note that patients under 2 kg should be fasted for shorter lengths of time.

PHYSICAL ASSESSMENT

A physical assessment should be performed immediately before administering any anesthetic to uncover any problems that may increase patient risk or necessitate a change in patient management (see Box 27-1 for physical findings that should be reported to the veterinarian). The focus of this assessment should be on the nervous, cardiovascular, and pulmonary systems because the health status of these systems is closely associated with the outcome of any anesthetic procedure. Below is a list of important components of a preanesthetic physical assessment:

- Observe the patient's level of consciousness (e.g., bright, alert and responsive; alert but subdued; lethargic; stuporous; comatose).
- Observe the general body condition including body weight and hydration.
- Note weakness, abnormal gait, or recumbency.

BOX 27-1 Physical Findings That Should Be Reported to the Veterinarian

- Dehydration, obesity, or cachexia
- A change in consciousness or any other sign of neurologic disease (e.g., seizures, ataxia, abnormal pupil size)
- Pale mucous membranes or prolonged CRT
- Cyanosis or icterus
- An abnormal HR, rhythm, or heart murmur
- A weak or irregular pulse
- Increased respiratory effort or rate
- Abnormal lung sounds, such as wheezing or crackles
- Marked hypothermia or hyperthermia

- Look for parasites, wounds, tumors, or other external lesions.
- Examine body orifices for external signs of disease, such as diarrhea, nasal discharge, hematuria, or vaginal discharge.
- Determine vital signs (temperature, pulse, respiratory rate [RR]).
- Assess mucous membrane color and capillary refill time (CRT).
- Watch the patient breathe noting respiratory effort.
- Auscultate the lungs for abnormal respiratory sounds.
- Concurrently palpate the pulse and auscultate the heart.

DIAGNOSTIC TESTING

When preparing a patient for surgery, diagnostic tests are often needed to supplement the history and physical assessment. The purpose of these tests is to uncover abnormalities that may impair the patient's ability to compensate, that may lead to unanticipated complications, or that may impair the patient's ability to eliminate the anesthetics. Testing recommendations vary widely from practice to practice. Most diagnostic testing recommendations are based on the signalment and physical status class and may include blood work, urinalysis, thoracic radiographs, serology, electrocardiography, and other tests as indicated. In general, young, healthy patients receive relatively fewer tests, and patients that are older, sick, or have other risk factors receive more.

PATIENT STABILIZATION

Abnormalities identified during patient evaluation must be treated before administration of the anesthetic. This patient stabilization includes treatment or correction of dehydration, anemia, cardiac arrhythmias, respiratory compromise, major organ failure, electrolyte or acid-base imbalances and may involve administration of antibiotics, analgesics, fluids, blood, oxygen, or a wide variety of other agents. The veterinary technician will be intimately involved in this stabilization process and must be prepared to accurately calculate doses, place intravenous (IV) catheters, set fluid administration rates, and administer drugs, blood, and oxygen as ordered by the veterinarian.

PHYSICAL STATUS CLASSIFICATION

The information gleaned from the patient evaluation is used to determine a physical status classification. This system, developed by the American Society of Anesthesiologists (ASA), is a subjective rating of the patient's condition based on historical, physical, and laboratory findings that places the patient in one of five classes (Table 27-2). This system is a tool that can be used to guide the anesthetist in appropriate patient management because anesthetic protocols are often based on physical status classification. This classification is somewhat subjective, so use your best judgment based on the criteria listed. Any surgery that is an emergency, regardless of ASA class, is additionally assigned the letter "E."

ANESTHETIC AGENTS

Anesthetic agents used in veterinary patients may be classified in one of several ways. These may be grouped according to the route of delivery (topical, oral, injectable, or inhalant) or by primary use (preanesthetic, sedative, induction agent, or maintenance agent). Anesthetics may also be grouped into drug classes based on chemistry. Agents in any given class tend to have similar actions, properties, uses, and effects, so this system will be used to classify the anesthetic agents described.

TABLE 27-2 ASA Physical Status Classifications

Classification	Risk	Criteria	Representative Conditions
P1	Minimal	Normal, healthy patient	Patients undergoing elective procedures (OHE, castration, or declaw)
P2	Low	Patient with mild systemic disease	Neonatal, geriatric, or obese patients Mild dehydration Skin tumor removal
P3	Moderate	Patient with severe systemic disease	Anemia Moderate dehydration Compensated major organ disease
P4	High	Patient with severe systemic disease that is a constant threat to life	Ruptured bladder Internal hemorrhage Pneumothorax Pyometra
P5	Extreme	**Moribund** patient that is not expected to survive without the operation	Severe head trauma Pulmonary embolus Gastric dilation-volvulus End-stage major organ failure

Agonists, partial agonists, mixed agonist-antagonists and antagonists: Anesthetic drugs work by binding to specific receptors on or inside the cells of target tissues. In the case of many anesthetics, these target tissues are located in the central or peripheral nervous systems. Most anesthetic agents are agonists (drugs that bind to receptors and exert one or more effects). Some drug classes, such as the opioids and α_2-adrenergics, include drugs called antagonists that block or reverse the action of the corresponding agonist. These antagonists are referred to as reversal agents. In the opioid class, there are also agents that are classified as partial agonists and those classified as mixed agonist-antagonists. Partial agonists bind to receptors and exert a partial or milder effect, whereas mixed agonist-antagonists partially reverse the effects of pure agonists.

ANTICHOLINERGICS

Although not true anesthetic agents, anticholinergics are used to counteract effects of parasympathetic nervous system stimulation, such as bradycardia and excess salivation. Although many anesthetics cause these effects to some degree, the barbiturates and dissociatives have a notable tendency to cause excess salivation, and opioids and α_2-adrenergic agonists are especially likely to cause bradycardia. Atropine and glycopyrrolate are the most commonly used anticholinergics in veterinary patients.

Anticholinergics have many effects expected to result from a parasympathetic nervous system blockade, including increased heart rate (HR), bronchodilation, reduced tear secretions and salivation, reduced gastrointestinal (GI) activity, and dilation of the pupils, especially in cats. Protective ophthalmic ointment should be applied to patients receiving these agents to prevent drying of the corneas.

There are many potential adverse effects, including tachycardia, cardiac arrhythmias, bronchodilation, mydriasis, and ileus. The bronchodilation caused by these drugs can increase anatomic dead space, which increases the risk of hypoxemia. Mydriasis may render the pupillary light reflex unreliable. Anticholinergics may also cause a thickening of the mucus in the airways, especially in cats, which can result in blockage. Some anesthetists use anticholinergics routinely in small animal (SA) patients, whereas others do not.

In ruminants, copious salivary secretions become more viscid, pool in the pharynx, and may be aspirated, thus predisposing the patient to airway blockage. Horses may develop colic from GI stasis. For these reasons, anticholinergics are avoided in these species unless necessary to treat bradycardia.

Atropine is a rapid-acting agent that comes in SA and large animal (LA) strengths (0.54 mg/ml and 15 mg/ml, respectively). Glycopyrrolate is similar to atropine with the following differences: Glycopyrrolate has a slower onset and a longer duration. It is less likely to cause tachycardia, cardiac arrhythmias, and ileus and suppresses salivation more effectively. Unlike, atropine, it does not cross the placental barrier and will not adversely affect the fetuses if used for cesarean sections (C-sections). It also does not cross the blood-brain barrier and thus has less impact on vision than atropine.

> *TECHNICIAN NOTE* Anticholinergics are used to counteract bradycardia and hypersalivation. There are LA and SA concentrations of injectable atropine that differ in strength by a factor of almost 30. Do *not* mix them up.

Tranquilizers and sedatives are commonly used to provide patient restraint for minor procedures, such as grooming, diagnostic imaging, blood draws, nail trims, and wound treatment. They are used as premedications and also to produce specific effects, such as analgesia and muscle relaxation. Each of these drugs has unique properties and must be chosen based on the particular effects desired. For instance medetomidine (an α_2-adrenergic agonist) produces analgesia and muscle relaxation, whereas acepromazine minimizes vomiting and development of cardiac arrhythmias. Often tranquilizers and sedatives are used in combination or with other anesthetic agents to produce a combination of effects that cannot be achieved by using one drug alone.

PHENOTHIAZINE TRANQUILIZERS

Phenothiazine tranquilizers (also classified as major tranquilizers) are used to calm and sedate patients before general anesthesia. This helps improve the quality of anesthetic induction and recovery by reducing anxiety. The phenothiazine tranquilizer used most commonly for this purpose is acepromazine. In addition to its use alone, it is also often used in combination with other agents. Combinations include "RAT" (Rompun, generic name xylazine, acepromazine, and Torbugesic, generic name butorphanol) and "BAG" (butorphanol, acepromazine, and glycopyrrolate).

Acepromazine induces mild to moderate sedation and is antiemetic and antiarrhythmic. Unlike many other agents, it causes little respiratory or cardiac depression. It has a relatively long duration.

Acepromazine blocks α_1-adrenergic receptors in the sympathetic nervous system resulting in dose-dependent peripheral vasodilation. Consequently the main adverse effect of acepromazine is hypotension, which can lead to cardiovascular collapse. It also can cause hypothermia or hyperthermia, changes in the HR, prolapse of the third eyelid, and paradoxical excitement or aggression. Adverse effects specific to horses include excitement, sweating, tachypnea, and protrusion of the penis, which can lead to permanent injury. Therefore some clinicians will not use this drug in breeding stallions.

Give acepromazine IM at least 15 minutes before induction and allow the patient to remain in a quiet area because the tranquilizing effect may be overridden, especially in excited patients. Note that the commonly used dose of the injectable form of acepromazine is significantly less than the dose on the label. Use of higher doses will not increase the level of sedation, but will cause increased hypotension.

When administering acepromazine IV, give it slowly and avoid intraarterial injection. Boxers, greyhounds, and giant-breed dogs and debilitated, young, or geriatric patients may be sensitive to this drug, whereas terriers and cats are relatively resistant. Acepromazine should not be given to patients with seizure disorders because it may lower the seizure threshold. Inform owners to use caution when handling patients that have received this drug because personality changes may occur resulting in aggression.

> *TECHNICIAN NOTE* The commonly used dose of acepromazine (about 0.05 to 0.1 mg/kg in small animals with a maximum dose of 3 mg in dogs and 1 mg in cats; 0.03 to 0.05 mg/kg in horses) is significantly less than the labeled dose. Higher doses will increase hypotension, but not sedation.

BENZODIAZEPINE TRANQUILIZERS

Benzodiazepines (also classified as minor tranquilizers) are most often used in combination with other agents, such as opioids and dissociatives, to produce a range of effects from sedation to general anesthesia. Benzodiazepines are controlled substances. Diazepam, midazolam, and zolazepam are benzodiazepines commonly used in veterinary patients. Zolazepam is one of the two components in the product Telazol. The other component of this product is tiletamine (see Dissociatives for a discussion of this drug). Although benzodiazepine antagonists (flumazenil and sarmazenil) are available, they are seldom used because of the expense.

Effects of benzodiazepines include anxiety reduction and mild to moderate sedation, although young healthy dogs are resistant to these drugs, and sedation in cats is often unpredictable. Other effects include appetite stimulation in cats, skeletal muscle relaxation, and anticonvulsant activity. The effects generally last no more than a few hours.

Benzodiazepines are relatively safe and minimally affect the cardiopulmonary system, but can produce adverse effects that vary among species. Dogs tend to experience CNS excitement, anxiety, and fear, especially if young and healthy and may become more difficult to control. Aggressive animals may lose inhibition, prohibiting use in these patients. Horses may experience muscle fasciculations, weakness, and mild ataxia.

Following intramuscular (IM) injection, diazepam is erratically absorbed and causes pain. It can also cause bradycardia, apnea, hypotension, and pain if given rapidly intravenously as a result of the propylene glycol vehicle.

Do not store diazepam in syringes or IV bags because it is soluble in plastic and will lose potency. Diazepam is commonly mixed with ketamine (a dissociative anesthetic) in equal volumes and given intravenously to induce general anesthesia in small animals (see Boxes 27-7 and 27-8).

Midazolam is more potent than diazepam, but can be used with ketamine in place of diazepam for anesthetic induction. Midazolam is water soluble and is compatible with a variety of agents, unlike diazepam which is not water soluble and therefore cannot be mixed with other agents except ketamine.

> *TECHNICIAN NOTE* As a result of incompatibility with most other agents, injectable diazepam can only be mixed with ketamine. When administering diazepam by IV injection, give it slowly.

α_2-ADRENERGIC DRUGS

α_2-Adrenergic agonists are sedatives that are used alone or in combination with opioids, dissociatives, and other agents to produce a wide spectrum of effects from mild sedation to general anesthesia, including analgesia and muscle relaxation. Xylazine and medetomidine are α_2-agonists most commonly used in SA patients. Xylazine, detomidine, and romifidine are most commonly used in LA patients.

The main therapeutic effects of α_2-agonists are CNS depression, analgesia, muscle relaxation, and sedation. These agents may cause vomiting in dogs and cats. Effects on the cardiovascular system include an initial hypertension followed by prolonged hypotension. Bradycardia is common, and cardiac output decreases. At high doses, these drugs cause a decrease in both respiratory rate (RR) and depth. In horses, xylazine causes lowering of the head and relaxation of the facial muscles, leading to drooping of the ears and lower lip. Relaxation of limb muscles leads to ataxia and a wide-based stance.

α_2-Agonists can cause significant bradycardia, reduced cardiac output, heart block, cardiac arrhythmias, and hypotension. They can cause respiratory depression, especially when administered with other agents, and respiratory distress in brachycephalic dogs. Other adverse effects include pain upon IM injection, muscle tremors, and changes in body temperature. Dogs may bloat secondary to aerophagia, and horses may sweat. Ruminants may experience profound respiratory depression, hypersalivation, bloat, diarrhea, premature delivery, or abortion. Because sedated patients are sensitive to auditory stimuli, horses may kick, small animals may move, and aggressive patients may bite in response to loud noises.

The sedation produced by these drugs can be profound and prolonged, as can cardiovascular depression. Therefore give standard doses only to young, healthy patients and use cautiously in geriatric, diabetic, pregnant, pediatric, or sick patients. Most clinicians do not recommend routine use of anticholinergics with α_2-agonists because they can predispose the patient to development of arrhythmias and hypertension.

Xylazine is used in many domestic and exotic species as one component of anesthetic mixtures and is also used to induce vomiting in cats following ingestion of toxins. Xylazine comes in SA (2% or 20 mg/ml) and LA (10% or 100 mg/ml) concentrations. Ruminants are extremely sensitive to this drug, requiring about one tenth of the dose used for horses. Swine require a high dose, so xylazine is usually given in combination with other drugs in this species.

Medetomidine is used primarily in small and exotic animal species. When compared with xylazine, it is more potent and less likely to produce side effects. It can be used in equal volumes with the reversal agent atipamezole to sequentially sedate and awaken patients undergoing minor procedures. Sudden arousal has been reported in patients heavily sedated with medetomidine, resulting in bites.

Detomidine (Dormosedan) and romifidine (Sedivet) are α_2-agonists used in horses to produce sedation for procedures, such as dental work, and as a part of anesthetic combinations. Detomidine has a longer duration of action and provides more profound sedative and analgesic activity than xylazine. Romifidine generally causes less muscle relaxation than xylazine or detomidine.

> *TECHNICIAN NOTE* When giving α_2-agonists, monitor closely for hypotension, cardiac arrhythmias, bradycardia, and abnormal temperatures. Use special caution in geriatric, pediatric, and sick patients. There are LA and SA concentrations of xylazine—do *not* mix these up.

α_2-Adrenergic antagonists increase the HR, increase the blood pressure, and stimulate the CNS. These are used to "wake" patients following sedation or anesthesia and to reverse adverse effects of α_2-agonists. Unfortunately, these agents also reverse desirable effects, such as analgesia. Therefore an alternative analgesic must be administered if pain control is warranted. Adverse effects include apprehension as a result of rapid arousal, excitement, muscle tremors, and salivation.

Yohimbine is an α_2-antagonist used to reverse the effects of xylazine. Although it is labeled for use in dogs, it is used in other species. It should be used cautiously in patients with seizure disorders. Atipamezole (Antisedan) is used to reverse the effects of medetomidine (Domitor). Both the dose and concentration of this drug is five times that of medetomidine, so these two drugs are administered in equal volumes. Cats are more sensitive to this drug and are given a reduced dose. In addition to the general adverse effects of α_2-antagonists listed earlier, this drug can also cause vomiting or diarrhea. Atipamezole may also be used to reverse detomidine. Tolazoline is used to reverse the effects of α_2-agonists in a variety of species.

α_2-Antagonists may be given IM in all species. When given IV, α_2-antagonists should be given slowly to effect to avoid excitation and aggression that is sometimes seen with rapid reversal. Their IV use in cats may cause unwanted severe salivation and excitement and is thus contraindicated.

OPIOIDS

Opioids (also known as narcotics) are drugs related to morphine. Opioids are classified as agonists, partial agonists, mixed agonist-antagonists, and antagonists. Morphine, fentanyl, oxymorphone, and hydromorphone are examples of pure agonists. Buprenorphine is a partial agonist, butorphanol is a mixed agonist-antagonist, and naloxone is an antagonist. Opioids provide analgesia and sedation and are combined with tranquilizers to produce neuroleptanalgesia. With the exception of naloxone, most opioids commonly used in veterinary patients are controlled substances.

Opioids work by stimulating specific opioid receptors in the brain and spinal cord, each of which produces distinct effects. For instance, stimulation of the μ-opioid receptors produces analgesia, euphoria, dependence, miosis, hypothermia, and respiratory depression. κ-Receptor stimulation produces analgesia, miosis, and sedation. σ-Receptor stimulation produces dysphoria, hallucinations, respiratory and cardiac stimulation, and mydriasis. The effects of each opioid depend on its affinity for each of the various receptors.

Opioid agonists primarily stimulate the μ-receptors. They are used as sedatives, analgesics, and—when combined with tranquilizers—neuroleptanalgesics. The effects of opioid agonists vary according to the species. Cats and large animals tend to experience anxiety, excitement, hyperthermia, and mydriasis, whereas dogs and primates experience sedation, hypothermia, and miosis. High doses of opioid agonists can induce narcosis in dogs, a state in which the patient appears profoundly sedated, but can be aroused by loud noises or other stimulation. CNS effects may include euphoria and dysphoria. Euphoria is an exaggerated sense of well-being, whereas dysphoria is restlessness or discomfort. The opioid agonists are among the best analgesics available and are often used to control moderate to severe pain. Opioid agonists cause a variety of other effects, including cough suppression, respiratory depression, bradycardia, hypotension, and changes in urination and GI tract activity, which vary agent to agent.

There are many adverse effects of opioid agonists, including significant CNS and respiratory depression, which are of concern, especially when using morphine. Peristalsis initially increases then decreases in dogs, causing defecation followed by constipation. Dogs may pant, or—if not in pain—may whine or bark. Other adverse effects of opioids include vomiting, excessive salivation, and in horses sweating and increased locomotor activity. Special caution must be used in neonatal, geriatric, and debilitated patients; patients with head trauma or respiratory disease; or patients with a number of other major organ diseases. Rapid IV administration of morphine may cause histamine release and bronchoconstriction.

Morphine, hydromorphone, fentanyl, and many other pure agonists are class II controlled substances and consequently are subject to special record-keeping requirements. As a result of respiratory depression, monitor patients closely and be prepared to provide ventilatory support. Opioid agonists must be used with caution and in lower doses in cats and horses. GI activity should be monitored closely in horses receiving μ-agonist opioids because decreased motility may lead to colic.

Most opioid agonists have a duration of only a few hours necessitating administration by constant rate infusion for a sustained effect. When used for analgesia, morphine may also be administered by epidural injection, and fentanyl may be administered via transdermal patch (Duragesic). Oxymorphone and hydromorphone are used in a similar fashion to morphine.

Opioid partial agonists exert partial activity at the μ-receptors, but cannot stimulate the receptors to the same degree as a full or pure agonist, and thus cannot provide the same degree of analgesia. Buprenorphine, the drug example in this class, is available only as a solution for injection, but also can be given orally for pain control in cats. Buprenorphine must be given only every 8 to 12 hours because it has a long duration of action. At high doses, this drug can cause respiratory depression that is difficult to reverse with naloxone because buprenorphine binds tightly to the μ-receptors.

Opioid mixed agonist-antagonists exert agonist activity at the κ-receptors and antagonist activity at the μ-receptors. This results in many of the same effects as opioid agonists (sedation, analgesia, and cough suppression) but to a lesser degree. If given following a pure opioid agonist, they will partially reverse the effects of these agents including the analgesic effects. In other words, if given following a pure agonist, they will decrease the beneficial effects, not increase them.

Butorphanol, the representative drug in this class, is used as a premedicant, an analgesic for mild to moderate pain, an antitussive, and when given with tranquilizers, neuroleptanalgesia. In small animals, adverse effects of this agent are rare, but may include transient sedation and ataxia. Horses may also experience excitement at high doses. Because the analgesic effects of butorphanol last only about 1 to 2 hours, frequent administration is necessary for adequate pain control.

Butorphanol is available in oral and injectable forms. The injectable form is available in multiple strengths: 0.5 mg/ml, 2 mg/ml, or 10 mg/ml. It is important to be sure that you select the correct strength.

> *TECHNICIAN NOTE* Concurrent administration of opioid partial agonists or mixed agonist-antagonists (e.g., buprenorphine or butorphanol, respectively) and opioid agonists (e.g., morphine, hydromorphone, fentanyl) may decrease analgesia and other beneficial effects.

Opioid antagonists are used to "wake" patients following sedation with opioid agonists, partial agonists, or mixed agonist-antagonists and to reverse undesirable effects of these agents. Naloxone is the opioid antagonist most commonly used in veterinary patients. Adverse effects of this drug are uncommon. Naloxone may be administered by giving the calculated dose slowly intravenously to effect and the remainder by the subcutaneous route. The duration of effect is about 1 to 2 hours; so if the opioid you are reversing is of a longer duration than this, repeat doses may be needed. One to two drops under the tongue can be used to revive neonates delivered by C-section if the dam received opioids.

PROPOFOL

Propofol is a short-acting IV anesthetic used to induce general anesthesia in a variety of species. It may also be used to maintain general anesthesia by administering repeat boluses to effect or a constant rate infusion. Propofol is a phenolic compound that is chemically unlike any other anesthetic. It is not a controlled substance.

Following slow IV injection, it induces a state of general anesthesia in 30 to 60 seconds with a duration of approximately 2 to 5 minutes. The patient rapidly recovers when drug administration is stopped, will sit up within about 10 minutes, and stand within about 15 to 30 minutes. Propofol decreases intracranial and intraocular pressure, provides muscle relaxation, and exhibits antiemetic and anticonvulsant properties. It does not provide significant analgesia. Although propofol is safe when used as directed, it has a relatively narrow therapeutic index and so must be given with caution.

Respiratory depression including apnea may occur and can be severe following rapid injection or with high doses. Therefore it is important to monitor the RR and depth carefully, especially during the first 1 to 2 minutes following initial injection. Cardiac effects include bradycardia and decreased strength of contraction. It causes hypotension, which can be significant following rapid injection. Propofol should be given with caution to patients with preexisting hypotension.

Propofol can cause seizurelike symptoms following induction and allergic reactions in some patients. Transient excitement and muscle tremors may occur during induction if the drug is given slowly or if the patient is not premedicated. Cats can develop Heinz body anemia (a specific type of anemia induced by exposure to certain drugs or toxins), anorexia, lethargy, and diarrhea following repeat doses or use on a daily basis.

Unlike barbiturates, propofol is not cumulative and may be used in greyhounds and other sight hounds. It is available only as an IV injectable in the form of a milky emulsion containing soybean oil and egg lecithin and is an exception to the rule that cloudy liquids should never be administered IV.

Propofol will support bacterial growth. Therefore it is important to handle containers with strict aseptic technique. The manufacturer recommends discarding unused portions more than 6 hours old, although some clinicians believe that propofol can be kept in the refrigerator for up to 24 hours if sterile technique is observed. It must be well mixed before use. If the patient experiences apnea or is given an overdose, treat with supportive care (intubation, oxygen administration, manual or mechanical ventilation, fluid therapy, and diuresis) until vital signs normalize.

> *TECHNICIAN NOTE* For induction of general anesthesia, give about one fourth of the calculated dose of propofol every 30 seconds to effect. For maintenance, give boluses about every 3 to 5 minutes to effect or a constant rate infusion of about one tenth of the induction dose per minute. Monitor for respiratory depression or apnea.

DISSOCIATIVES

Dissociatives (also known as cyclohexamines) are a unique group of injectable anesthetic agents used alone to immobilize patients for minor or brief procedures. They are also used in combination with opioids and tranquilizers to induce and maintain anesthesia and to provide analgesia or other specific effects. Ketamine and tiletamine (one of two agents contained in Telazol) are the dissociatives most often used in veterinary patients. Both are controlled.

When used alone, dissociatives produce immobilization, but not surgical anesthesia. Ketamine and other dissociatives induce a state known as "catalepsy" or "dissociative anesthesia," in which the patient appears awake, but is immobilized and does not respond to its surroundings. Catalepsy is also characterized by open, central, and dilated eyes; nystagmus; increased muscle tone; increased sensitivity to light and sound; an exaggerated palpebral reflex; and intact pedal and laryngeal reflexes.

Dissociatives increase HR and blood pressure without the decrease in cardiac output characteristically seen with most other agents. Other effects include increased CSF pressure and intraocular pressure and superficial analgesia. They may also induce apneustic breathing, a pattern in which there is a prolonged pause following inspiration and a short pause following expiration.

Dissociatives can induce respiratory depression, cardiac arrhythmias, hypersalivation, vomiting, vocalization, prolonged recoveries, jerking movements, tremors, and pain upon IM injection. Increased salivation can be prevented by premedicating with a low dose of an anticholinergic. Dissociatives may induce seizurelike activity during recovery and should not be used in patients with seizure disorders. Ketamine may also cause behavioral changes that can in some cases last for days or weeks.

Tranquilizers or sedatives should be used with or before administration of dissociatives in dogs and horses to decrease adverse effects. Because the eyes remain open, use a corneal lubricant during dissociative anesthesia. Ketamine can be given at a rate of 100 mg/5 kg orally for restraint of fractious cats.

The product Telazol contains tiletamine in combination with zolazepam (a benzodiazepine) and when reconstituted, contains 50 mg of each drug/ml. Once reconstituted, Telazol is stable for 14 days if refrigerated. Telazol is used as an induction agent in healthy dogs and cats, especially if aggressive. Because it causes hypothermia, body temperature must be closely monitored.

A mixture of ketamine and diazepam (or midazolam) is commonly used to induce general anesthesia in dogs, cats, and horses. This combination has an onset of about 30 to 90 seconds and 5 to 10 minutes of working time. In small animals, the two drugs are mixed in a 1:1 volume ratio and given to effect at a rate of about 1 ml of the mixture/20 lb IV slowly over 30 to 90 seconds. Diazepam or midazolam (0.03 to 0.05 mg/kg) can be added to ketamine (2.2 mg/kg) for induction of anesthesia in horses.

Ketamine-α_2-adrenergic agonist mixtures are used to provide anesthesia in dogs, cats, horses, and exotics. These mixtures cause significant cardiovascular and respiratory depression and must be used cautiously. Other dissociative mixtures include TKX (Telazol-ketamine-xylazine) and TKD (Telazol-ketamine-Domitor).

> *TECHNICIAN NOTE* Unlike most other anesthetics, dissociative agents cause increased muscle tone, sensitivity to light and sound, intact or exaggerated reflexes, increased HR, and increased blood pressure.

BARBITURATES

Barbiturates, a class of drugs developed in the early 1900s, are used for a variety of purposes, including induction of general anesthesia, treatment of seizures, and euthanasia. All barbiturates are controlled. These agents are classified as ultrashort-, short-, intermediate-, and long-acting based on their duration of action.

The ultrashort-acting barbiturates, thiopental sodium and methohexital, are used in SA patients for induction of general anesthesia. The use of these drugs for induction of anesthesia in large animals is now rare, having largely been replaced by ketamine.

Thiopental sodium is rapidly absorbed into the brain, more slowly redistributed into muscle and fat, and later is metabolized and excreted. The patient recovers as the drug redistributes to the muscle and fat, thus decreasing the amount in the brain tissue. This results in rapid onset (30 to 60 seconds) and short duration (5 to 20 minutes) following a single dose. The effects of thiopental are cumulative if multiple doses are given, however, because the fat and muscle become saturated with the drug until it is metabolized and excreted. The result of this saturation is a prolonged recovery time. Because sight hounds have low body fat levels, saturation occurs more quickly, resulting in even longer recovery times than other animals.

Thiopental sodium causes a dose-dependent decrease in cardiac output, blood pressure, RR, and tidal volume ($\mathbf{V_T}$). It does not produce significant analgesia, however, and is a poor muscle relaxant. Adverse effects include hypotension, bradycardia, and arrhythmias, particularly ventricular premature contractions (VPCs) and bigeminy (alternating normal complexes and VPCs). It can also cause severe respiratory depression including a period of apnea following induction, which may require ventilatory support. Because neonates delivered by C-section also experience respiratory depression, this drug should not be used for this purpose.

Thiopental and other barbiturates cause swelling, pain, and tissue irritation if injected outside the vein. Treat perivascular injections by infusing the area with large volumes of normal saline with or without a local anesthetic.

If injected too slowly or without premedications, the patient may experience undue excitement during induction or recovery. The use of this drug alone in horses will induce ataxia and excitement and is not recommended. Other adverse effects include salivation, coughing, and laryngospasm, which can be decreased by concurrent use of anticholinergics. Thiopental should not be used in sight hounds because of the likelihood of prolonged recovery, in horses with leukopenia, or patients without suitable veins.

Barbiturates should be dosed based on lean body weight, patient condition, and concurrent administration of other preanesthetic and anesthetic drugs. Thiopental has a relatively narrow therapeutic index and must be administered cautiously. In healthy patients, give one half of the calculated dose intravenously as a bolus and the remainder to effect. Debilitated, hypothermic, geriatric patients or patients with major organ disease may require a much lower dose and may experience prolonged recoveries. Treat any overdose with supportive care.

Thiopental is packaged as a dry powder that must be reconstituted to a concentration ranging from 2% to 2.5% in small animals to 5% to 10% in large animals. The reconstituted solution has a shelf life of 7 days when refrigerated. Use the lowest concentration that is practical, and do not use thiopental if the solution is not clear.

Methohexital is an ultrashort-acting barbiturate used for induction and maintenance of anesthesia that has an onset of about 15 to 60 seconds and duration of about 5 to 10 minutes. This drug is reconstituted to a 1% solution and has a shelf life of 6 weeks at room temperature. It is considered safe in sight hounds because it is rapidly metabolized, and therefore repeat doses are not cumulative. Because it can cause excitement and seizures during induction or recovery, patients should be premedicated before administration.

Pentobarbital sodium is an intermediate-acting barbiturate that, although no longer used for routine anesthesia in clinical settings, is given intraperitoneally to induce general anesthesia in lab animals. It is also given intravenously to treat status epilepticus in small animals and is used in a concentrated form as a euthanasia agent.

> *TECHNICIAN NOTE* The ultrashort-acting barbiturate thiopental sodium is cumulative if multiple doses are given, should not be used in sight hounds, and must *not* be injected out of the vein.

IMIDAZOLE DERIVATIVES

Etomidate is a short-acting, injectable, imidazole-derivative sedative-hypnotic used for induction of anesthesia in dogs and cats. It is not a controlled substance. Etomidate causes minimal changes in cardiovascular and respiratory function and decreases both intracranial and intraocular pressure. It has a significantly wider therapeutic index than propofol and thiopental sodium. It is therefore the agent of choice for patients with severe heart disease or shock. Etomidate also produces good muscle relaxation, but no analgesia.

Although etomidate has a wide margin of safety, adverse effects include vomiting, muscle movements, sneezing, and excitement during induction and recovery. It also suppresses adrenocortical function. Premedication is recommended to reduce these adverse effects. IV injections may be painful and cause phlebitis, and rapid injection or repeat doses can cause hemolysis in cats. Administration through a running IV fluid line will decrease pain and hemolysis. Etomidate is not in common use because of its relative higher cost and adverse effects.

GUAIFENESIN

Guaifenesin, also known as "GG" or glyceryl guaiacolate, is an injectable muscle relaxant and sedative used in combination with other agents for short procedures or to improve the quality of induction and recovery in large animals. It is also used as an expectorant to treat respiratory conditions.

Adverse effects on the cardiovascular, respiratory, and GI systems are mild and of little consequence. If injected out of the vein, guaifenesin is irritating to the tissues. Solutions more than 7% in strength cause hemolysis in ruminants, whereas solutions more than 15% cause hemolysis in horses.

Guaifenesin is often administered as a 5% to 10% solution in dextrose by rapid IV infusion before ketamine or barbiturate induction to produce muscle relaxation in LA species. Several combinations are also commonly used. "Double drip" (ketamine and GG) is used for induction and/or maintenance of anesthesia in ruminants. "Triple drip" (xylazine, ketamine, and GG) is used for IV maintenance of anesthesia in horses.

INHALANT ANESTHETICS

Inhalant anesthetics are liquid agents that are vaporized in oxygen and administered via an anesthetic breathing system by endotracheal tube, mask, or chamber. Vapor pressure, blood-gas solubility coefficient, and minimum alveolar concentration measure properties of these agents that influence the way they are used. Therefore a basic knowledge of these concepts is necessary to use inhalant anesthetics effectively and safely.

Vapor pressure is a measurement of the tendency of a liquid to evaporate. Agents with a high vapor pressure evaporate readily, reaching dangerously high concentrations if not regulated and therefore must be administered using an agent-specific precision vaporizer. Conversely, low vapor pressure agents may be administered with a nonprecision vaporizer.

The blood-gas solubility coefficient is a measurement of the tendency of an agent to dissolve in blood. It is associated with the speed of induction, recovery, and change in anesthetic depth, each of which are faster when using agents with a low solubility coefficient and slower when using agents with a high solubility coefficient.

The minimum alveolar concentration (MAC) is the percent concentration of an agent required to prevent a response to surgical stimulation in 50% of patients and therefore is a measurement of the potency of an agent. An agent with a high MAC is less potent (more of the agent is required to attain surgical anesthesia) than an agent with a low MAC. Typically a dial setting of approximately 1.5 to 2 times the MAC is required to reach surgical anesthesia in a majority of patients.

HALOGENATED ANESTHETICS

These inhalant agents are used in a wide variety of species to induce and maintain general anesthesia. Isoflurane and sevoflurane are the halogenated anesthetics most commonly used in veterinary patients.

Halogenated anesthetics cause CNS depression, hypothermia, respiratory depression, hypotension, and muscle relaxation. Although they cause myocardial depression, cardiac function is maintained close to that of preanesthetic levels. These agents have little or no analgesic effect postoperatively.

Both isoflurane and sevoflurane have high vapor pressures (240 mm Hg and 160 mm Hg, respectively) and must be administered via a precision vaporizer. Both agents also have low solubility coefficients (1.4 and 0.6, respectively) resulting in relatively rapid inductions, recoveries, and changes in anesthetic depth.

Halogenated anesthetics induce a dose-dependent hypotension, which is more prominent with sevoflurane than isoflurane. They can also cause vomiting, nausea, and ileus in addition to a dose-dependent respiratory depression that can progress to apnea. Although the primary route of excretion for these agents is through the lungs, the amount that is metabolized by the liver and excreted by the kidneys varies agent to agent. About 3% of sevoflurane is metabolized, whereas only about 0.2% of isoflurane is metabolized, making it an excellent anesthetic choice for patients with kidney or liver disease.

There have been reports of fire or extreme heat production when sevoflurane is used with desiccated carbon dioxide (CO_2) absorbent. This problem is more common when using low oxygen flow over a long period of time. To prevent this complication, turn off the machine when not in use, replace absorbent granules regularly, avoid the use of low oxygen flow for protracted periods, and monitor the temperature of the absorbent canister. Sevoflurane also reacts with chemicals in CO_2 absorbent to produce compound A, a chemical that causes renal damage in rats. This effect has not been found to be clinically significant.

Although isoflurane and sevoflurane are similar, there are subtle differences in the way they are used. Because isoflurane is irritating to mucous membranes, patients may struggle and hold their breath during mask or chamber induction. In contrast, sevoflurane is not irritating, making it ideal for anesthetic inductions. One of the chief advantages of sevoflurane is the rapid inductions, recoveries, and changes in anesthetic depth associated with this agent. Therefore safe use of this agent requires subtle dial changes and vigilant monitoring on the part of the veterinary anesthetist.

> *TECHNICIAN NOTE* Although there is a perception that sevoflurane is safer than isoflurane, it causes more hypotension and must be monitored even more closely than isoflurane as a result of the more rapid response time.

Halothane was used extensively in veterinary anesthesia for many years, although use has gradually decreased as isoflurane and sevoflurane have gained wide acceptance. Halothane has a similar vapor pressure to isoflurane, necessitating use of a precision vaporizer. It can be used for mask or chamber induction, but has a higher solubility coefficient (2.4) than isoflurane. Consequently, inductions, recoveries, and changes in anesthetic depth take somewhat longer. Halothane has similar effects to isoflurane, but causes less respiratory depression, has a greater tendency to induce cardiac arrhythmias, and is a more potent cardiac depressant.

Methoxyflurane is currently off the market, but was used for many years to maintain anesthesia. Because of its low vapor pressure (23 mm Hg), methoxyflurane can be administered from a nonprecision vaporizer in-circle (VIC). It cannot be used for mask or chamber inductions, however, because of a high solubility coefficient (15). Methoxyflurane is 50% metabolized and has been linked to organ damage.

Desflurane is similar to isoflurane, but has an extremely high vapor pressure and low solubility coefficient. Because the boiling point of this agent is near room temperature, desflurane requires a special, expensive electronic vaporizer. Inductions and recoveries are even more rapid than with sevoflurane, producing what is sometimes referred to as "one-breath anesthesia." Desflurane is not arrhythmogenic, but causes a dose-related respiratory depression.

Enflurane has not found wide acceptance in veterinary medicine as a result of adverse effects.

NITROUS OXIDE

Nitrous oxide (N_2O), sometimes referred to as "laughing gas," is a gas at room temperature and is stored in compressed gas cylinders identified by a deep blue color. N_2O is administered along with oxygen through a gas-specific flowmeter that is blue in color.

N_2O is one of the oldest inhalant anesthetics, its use dating back to the mid-1800s. N_2O will not produce general anesthesia alone, but speeds the uptake of other agents into the bloodstream and allows lower doses to be used because it has analgesic properties. In the past, it was administered in conjunction with older halogenated agents, such as methoxyflurane. When used with newer agents, these benefits are of less clinical importance. It is therefore seldom used in practice.

Because N_2O displaces oxygen in the lungs and breathing circuit, it can cause hypoxemia during anesthesia or recovery. It also diffuses into air spaces, such as the chest cavity of patients with pneumothorax and the stomach of patients with gastric dilation-volvulus, thus worsening these conditions. Its use is contraindicated in ruminants and horses because of the large amount of air in the rumen and large intestine, respectively. Specific flow rates must be used to maintain oxygenation, and other precautions must be taken, which are detailed in most veterinary anesthesia textbooks.

ANESTHETIC EQUIPMENT

ENDOTRACHEAL TUBES

An endotracheal tube is a device that is placed inside the trachea of an unconscious patient, attached to a breathing circuit, and used to administer oxygen and inhalant anesthetics. Endotracheal tubes increase patient safety because they maintain an open airway; minimize the likelihood of pulmonary aspiration of blood, stomach contents, and other substances; facilitate administration of supplemental oxygen; and allow the anesthetist to ventilate the patient when necessary. Because of these benefits, many veterinarians prefer to place an endotracheal tube in all patients undergoing general anesthesia even if not receiving inhalant anesthetics.

Endotracheal tubes come in a variety of sizes, lengths, and types needed to accommodate the wide size variation of veterinary patients and may be made of red rubber (Figure 27-1, *D*), silicon rubber (Figure 27-1, *A*), or polyvinyl chloride (PVC) (Figure 27-1, *C* and *E*). Murphy tubes have a side hole called the Murphy eye (Figure 27-2, *J*) at the beveled end that permits airflow in the event of blockage of the tip. The patient end of a Cole tube is tapered and has no cuff (Figure 27-1, *B*). This type is used for small patients and birds, which do not have an expandable trachea.

An endotracheal tube consists of the following parts: The connector (Figure 27-2, *D*) is attached to the breathing circuit of the anesthetic machine or to an Ambu bag. The cuff (Figure 27-2, *H*) is a balloonlike part at the beveled patient end (Figure 27-2, *I*), which when inflated, creates a seal between the tube and the tracheal mucosa. This prevents mixing of room air and anesthetic gases and prevents aspiration of liquid or solid materials around the tube. The cuff is connected by a small tube to the pilot balloon (Figure 27-2, *B*) and a valve (Figure 27-2, *A*), which is used to inflate the cuff. The pilot balloon allows the anesthetist to monitor cuff inflation.

Although there are several different scales used to measure the diameter of an endotracheal tube, internal diameter (ID) is most common (Figure 27-2, *G*). Tubes for dogs and cats range in size from 3.0 to 14 mm ID. Small ruminants, swine, and foals require tubes between 6 and 18 mm ID. Small exotic animals may require tubes as small as 1.0 mm ID. Horses and mature cattle require sizes ranging from 16 to 30 mm ID.

LARYNGOSCOPES

Laryngoscopes are used to visualize the larynx while placing endotracheal tubes. A laryngoscope consists of a handle and a blade that is used to depress the tongue and includes a light-source to illuminate the throat (Figure 27-3). Common blade sizes range from 0 (small) to 5 (large), although longer blades are available for use in swine and some exotics. Miller blades are straight (Figure 27-3, *A* and *C*) and McIntosh blades are curved (Figure 27-3, *B* and *D*). Laryngoscopes are often used in small ruminants, camelids, and swine, may be helpful in dogs and cats, but are not used in adult cattle, which are intubated by digital palpation, and horses, which are intubated blindly.

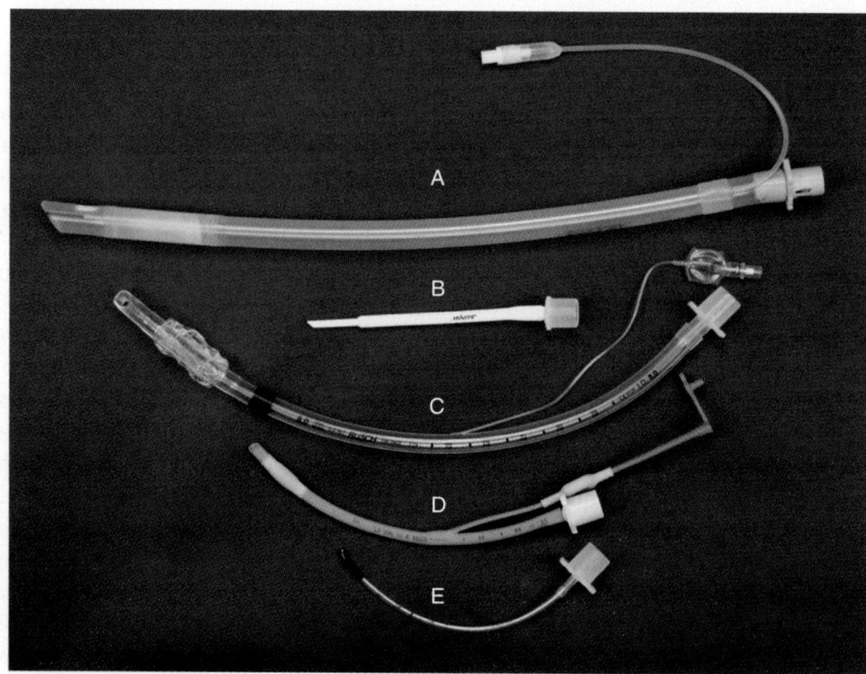

FIGURE 27-1 Endotracheal tube type, material, and size comparison. *A*, Cuffed 11-mm silicone rubber tube. *B*, 2.5-mm Cole tube. *C*, Cuffed 8-mm PVC tube. *D*, Cuffed 4-mm red rubber tube. *E*, Uncuffed 2-mm PVC tube.

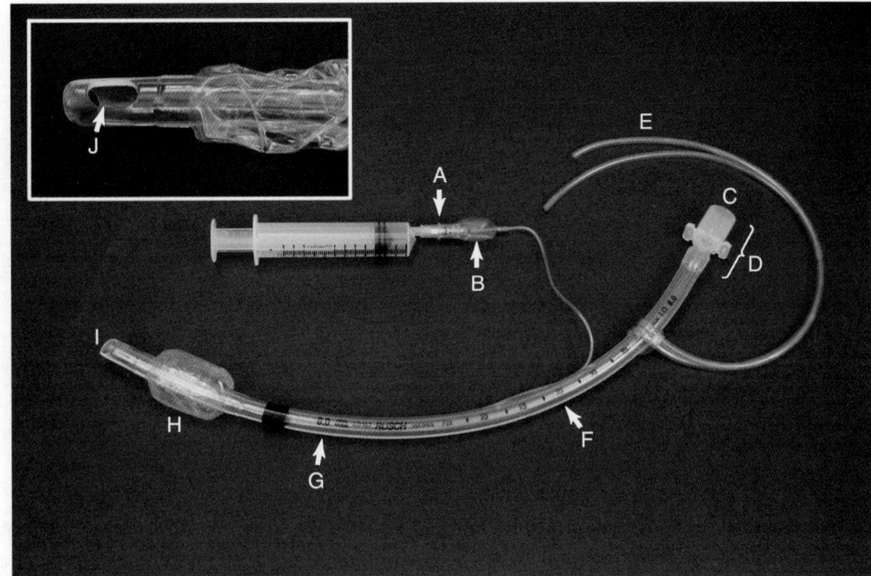

FIGURE 27-2 Endotracheal tube parts. *A,* Valve with syringe attached. *B,* Pilot balloon. *C,* Patient end. *D,* Connector. *E,* Tie. *F,* Measurement of length from the patient end (cm). *G,* Measurement of ID (mm). *H,* Inflated cuff. *I,* Patient end. *J,* Murphy eye.

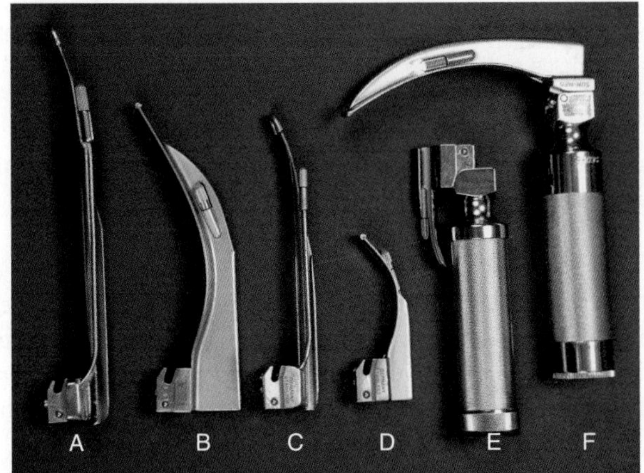

FIGURE 27-3 Laryngoscope handles and blades. *A,* Size-4 Miller blade. *B,* Size-4 McIntosh blade. *C,* Size-2 Miller blade. *D,* Size-1 McIntosh blade. *E,* Laryngoscope handle with size-00 Miller blade in unlocked position. *F,* Laryngoscope handle with size-3 McIntosh blade in locked position (note that the light turns on when the blade is locked).

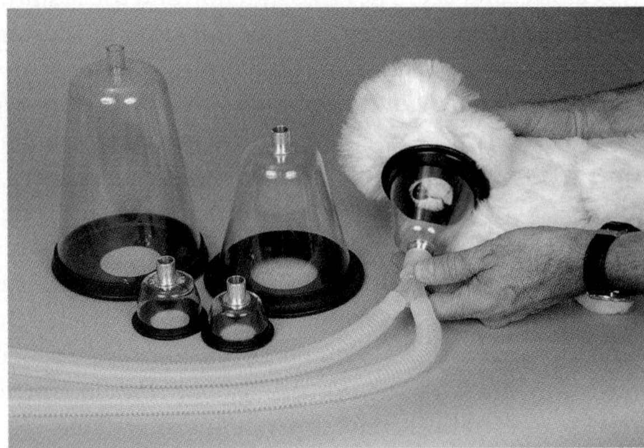

FIGURE 27-4 Anesthetic masks. Note the good fit around the patient's muzzle to minimize leakage.

MASKS

Masks are cone-shaped devices used to administer oxygen and anesthetic gases to patients that are not intubated (Figure 27-4). They are usually made of plastic or rubber, come in a variety of sizes, and have a rubber gasket designed to create a seal around the patient's muzzle. The smallest mask that comfortably fits the patient should be selected. Masks may be used to induce or maintain anesthesia. They are frequently used to administer anesthetic gases to small patients in which intubation is difficult. Masks may also be used to administer oxygen during the preanesthetic and postanesthetic periods. Masks do not maintain an open airway, do not protect against aspiration, nor do they afford the ability to ventilate the patient as does an endotracheal tube.

ANESTHETIC CHAMBERS

Anesthetic chambers are solid boxes used to induce general anesthesia in small patients that are feral, vicious, intractable, or cannot be handled without undue stress (Figure 27-5). Chambers are usually clear to allow the anesthetist to observe the patient. They have two ports, one of which is attached to a fresh gas source and the other that allows exit of waste gas. A common way to set up a chamber is to attach the inhalation tube and exhalation tube of a semiclosed rebreathing system to each port in place of the Y-piece. Chambers prevent close monitoring of the patient during induction, thus necessitating extreme care when anesthetizing patients using this method.

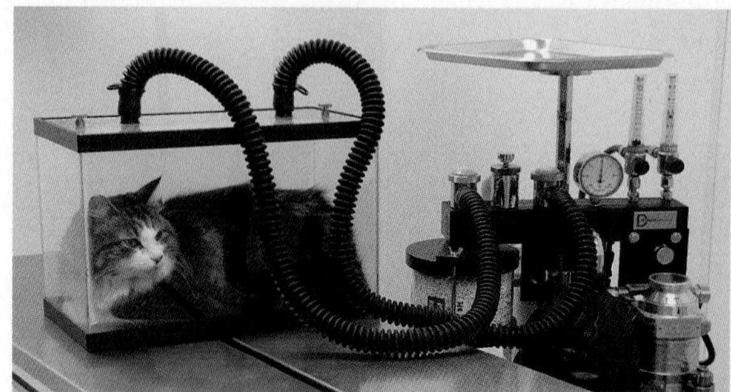

FIGURE 27-5 Anesthetic chamber attached to the corrugated breathing tubes of a semiclosed rebreathing circuit in place of the Y-piece.

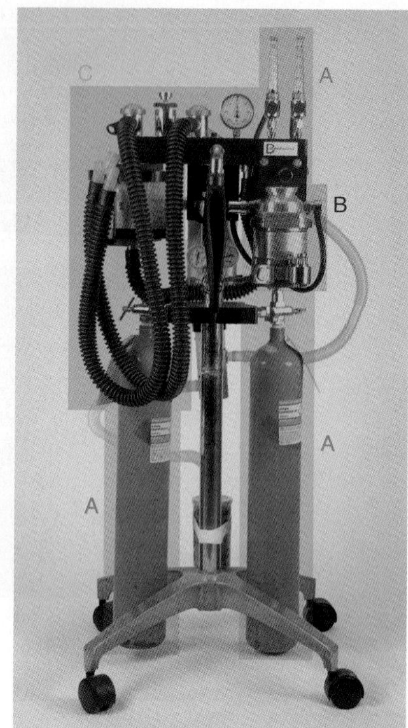

FIGURE 27-6 Anesthetic machine systems. *A,* Carrier gas supply: Note the two size-E compressed gas oxygen cylinders beside the "As" at the bottom of this image. *B,* Anesthetic vaporizer. *C,* Breathing circuit. Note that the scavenging system (see Figure 27-8) is not visible in this view.

THE ANESTHETIC MACHINE

Anesthetic machines are used to deliver inhalant anesthetics and oxygen to patients during general anesthesia. These machines are complex and have many specialized and distinct parts that must be properly used and maintained to ensure patient safety. Many different makes and models are in common use, ranging from state-of-the-art machines to those that have been in service for many years, so the veterinary technician may encounter a wide variety of machines in appearance, size, and age. The basic function and use is similar, however, and has not changed significantly over the past several decades. For this reason, a complete knowledge of anesthetic machine systems and associated equipment along with a review of the owner's manual will prepare the technician for operation of any machine he or she may encounter.

An anesthetic machine consists of the following general systems:

1. The carrier gas supply (Figure 27-6, *A*) delivers oxygen and other carrier gases to the patient at a controlled flow rate. Compressed gas cylinders, the pressure reducing valve, the tank and line pressure gauges, the flowmeters, and the oxygen flush valve are part of this system.
2. The anesthetic vaporizer (Figure 27-6, *B*) vaporizes a precise concentration of liquid inhalant anesthetic and mixes it with the carrier gases.
3. The breathing circuit (Figure 27-6, *C*) delivers the anesthetic and oxygen mixture to the patient via an endotracheal tube, mask, or chamber and conveys expired gases away from the patient. Breathing circuits are classified as either rebreathing systems (see Figure 27-6) or nonrebreathing systems (Figure 27-7).
4. The scavenging system disposes of waste and excess anesthetic gases (Figure 27-8).

PREPARING THE MACHINE

Box 27-2 highlights the steps required to prepare an anesthetic machine for use.

Machine Assembly

Before using any anesthetic machine, attach all necessary parts including the vaporizer inlet and outlet port hoses, the reservoir bag, the corrugated breathing tubes, the scavenging system hoses, and any other parts required for the machine that you are using.

Checking for Leaks

To check the low-pressure system of a nonrebreathing system for leaks, occlude the patient connector and the scavenging hose or pressure relief valve. Turn the oxygen on to fill the bag. When the bag is full, turn the flowmeter off. The system has no leaks if the bag remains inflated for at least 10 seconds.

To check the low-pressure system of a rebreathing system for leaks, assemble the machine and secure all connections. Close the pop-off valve completely. Place your thumb over the Y-piece, and use the oxygen flush valve and the oxygen flowmeter to fill the reservoir bag until the pressure manometer indicates a pressure of 30 cm of water. Turn off the flowmeter. No leaks are present if the pressure decreases no more than 5 cm of water (to the 25 cm of water mark) in 10 seconds. As an alternative, when the pressure in the system reaches 30 cm of water, you may turn the flowmeter back on just enough to maintain pressure. A leak is present if greater than 200 ml/min is necessary.

Setting the Pop-off Valve

When using a semiclosed rebreathing system, adjust the pop-off valve immediately after checking the low-pressure system for leaks. With the Y-piece occluded, turn the oxygen flow back on to the anticipated maximum for that procedure. A general rule of thumb is about 1 to 3 L/min for patients under 30 lb and about 3 to 5 L/min for patients more than

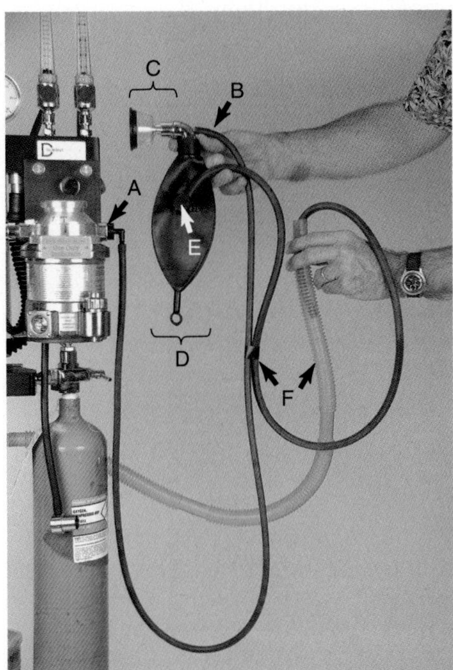

FIGURE 27-7 Parts of a nonrebreathing circuit. *A*, Outlet port of the vaporizer with keyed fitting. *B*, Fresh gas inlet. *C*, Connector with mask attached. *D*, Reservoir bag. *E*, Pressure relief valve. *F*, Scavenging hose.

30 lb. Then open the pop-off valve gradually until the pressure manometer indicates a pressure of 1½-2 cm of water.

THE CARRIER GAS SUPPLY

The gases into which the liquid inhalant anesthetic evaporates and that carry the vaporized anesthetic to the patient are referred to as carrier gases. Oxygen is the carrier gas used during all anesthetic procedures. Oxygen administration is necessary throughout anesthesia not only to carry the anesthetic, but also to compensate for the diminished RR, depth, and available oxygen that most patients experience during anesthesia. In some circumstances, N_2O may be used with oxygen, although in recent years, use of N_2O in veterinary patients has declined.

Compressed gas cylinders store carrier gases at high pressure (see Figure 27-6, *A*). They are attached to the yoke (Figure 27-9, *A*) of the anesthetic machine or alternatively may be stored in a remote location and connected to the machine via gas lines. An outlet valve is located on the top of all compressed gas cylinders (Figure 27-9, *C*). This valve must be opened when the cylinder is in use by turning the valve stem counterclockwise until it is fully open. When opened, gas will flow through the yoke and into the anesthetic machine. The valve is closed by turning it clockwise (see Figure 27-9, *right side*).

> TECHNICIAN NOTE The mnemonic "left-loose, right-tight" (loose meaning open and tight meaning closed) may be used to remember the proper direction to turn the compressed gas cylinder outlet valve, flowmeter dials, and the pop-off valve.

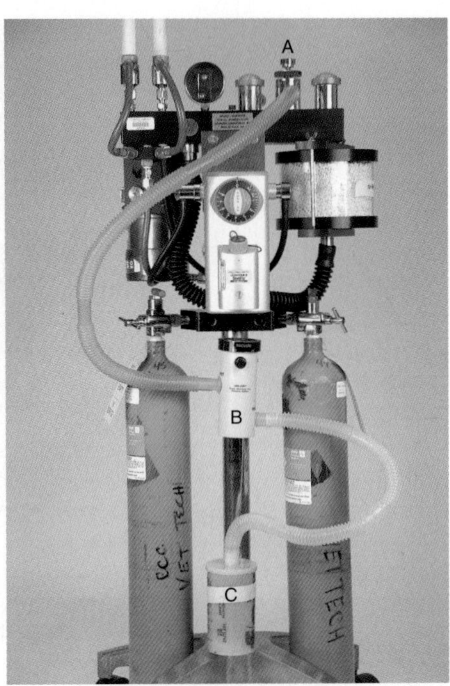

FIGURE 27-8 Scavenging system: The waste gas exits from the pop-off valve *(A)* of this rebreathing system (or the discharge hose of a nonrebreathing system), flows through the vacuum regulator *(B)*, and finally into either a charcoal canister *(C)* or alternatively into an outlet pipe in the ceiling or wall.

BOX 27-2 Preparing an Anesthetic Machine for Use

1. Check the amount of carrier gases in the compressed gas cylinders and replace them, if needed.
2. Check the level of inhalant anesthetic in the anesthetic vaporizer and refill it, if necessary.
3. Select a rebreathing system or nonrebreathing system based on patient size and requirements.
4. If using a rebreathing system, select an appropriately sized reservoir bag and breathing tubes.
5. Assemble the machine and check the low-pressure system for leaks.
6. Set the pop-off valve.
7. Assemble, turn on, and adjust the scavenging system.

Compressed gas cylinders are usually owned by a supplier that will pick up and refill them as needed. Always be sure that you have at least one spare full tank before commencing any anesthetic procedure. If the primary tank runs out, you will always have a second tank available.

Three holes are visible on the face of the outlet valve. The large hole is the valve port where the gas exits the cylinder (Figure 27-9, *D*). This port fits onto the nipple of the yoke (Figure 27-9, *F*) with a nylon washer in between (Figure 27-9, *H*). The two smaller holes (Figure 27-9, *E*) fit onto index pins (Figure 27-9, *G*), which hold the cylinder in place. These holes and pins are a specific distance apart for each gas, a feature that prevents a cylinder containing the wrong gas from being attached to the yoke.

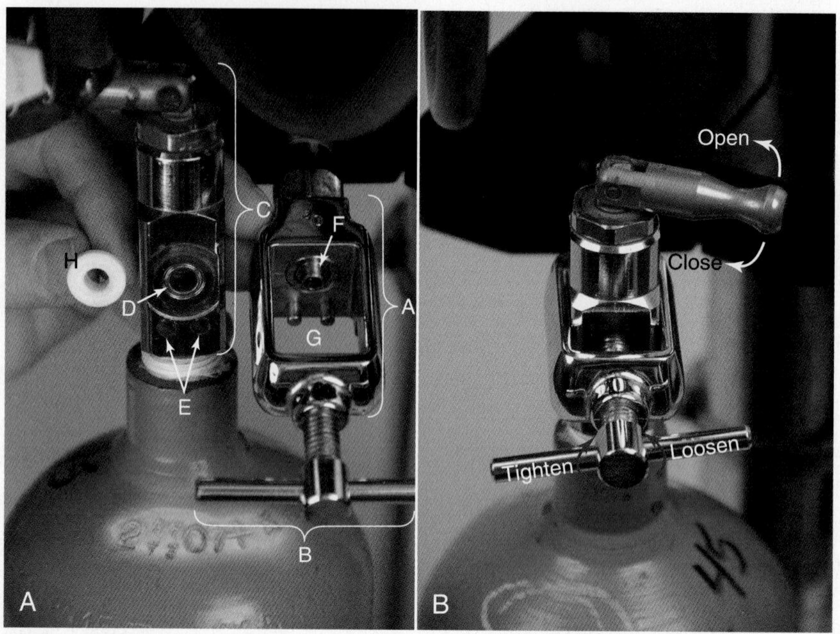

FIGURE 27-9 A *(right image)*, Parts of compressed gas cylinder and yoke. *A*, Yoke. *B*, Wing nut. *C*, Outlet valve. *D*, Valve port. *E*, Pin holes. *F*, Nipple of yoke. *G*, Index pins. *H*, Nylon washer. **B**, Opening-closing the outlet valve; loosening-tightening the wing nut.

When removing a cylinder from the machine, be sure the outlet valve is closed and the oxygen is evacuated ("bled off") from the system (see Tank Pressure Gauge for a review of this procedure). Support the cylinder, loosen the wing nut (Figure 27-9, *B*) and back the valve port off of the yoke. Carefully lower the tank until the valve clears the yoke. When attaching a full cylinder, first inspect the valve port for cleanliness then place a clean, undamaged nylon washer between the valve port and the nipple. Gently raise the tank into place, lining up the valve port and the pin holes with the corresponding structures on the yoke. Tighten the wing nut as securely as you are able to by hand. Open the valve slowly and listen for leaks. If there is a leak, recheck the holes for proper alignment, tighten the wing nut further, or use a new washer.

Compressed gas cylinders may contain different gases. To prevent confusion, cylinders are color coded as follows: Green (United States) or white (international) is oxygen; blue is N_2O. These cylinders come in two sizes called E tanks (see Figure 27-6, *A* at the bottom) and H tanks. E tanks are stored either on the yoke of the anesthetic machine or in a rack. H tanks are much larger and are stored on a movable cart or chained to the wall and are often used to feed centralized oxygen sources. A centralized oxygen source is one in which the oxygen from an H tank is piped to outlets at various points around the hospital. The outlets are then connected to anesthetic machines via quick-release connectors.

> *TECHNICIAN NOTE* The following rules must be observed when using compressed gas cylinders to prevent injury. Never leave an unattended compressed gas cylinder unsupported or lying on its side. Never attempt to remove the valve or index pins. When turning a tank on, keep skin and eyes clear of the valve port. Do not use oxygen near any source of ignition.

Some larger practices use a concentrator as a primary oxygen source. An oxygen concentrator is a machine that extracts oxygen from room air.

The tank pressure gauge (Figure 27-10, *B*) indicates the pressure in a compressed gas cylinder. When full, a cylinder contains oxygen at a pressure of approximately 2200 pounds per square inch (psi). As the oxygen is used, the cylinder pressure gradually decreases. Oxygen cylinders should be changed when the pressure reaches 100 to 200 psi or a level at which the tank does not contain enough gas to last the anticipated length of the procedure. It is important to check the pressure before and throughout the anesthetic period to be sure that there is enough oxygen to complete the procedure.

The volume of oxygen contained in an E tank (expressed in liters) can be estimated by multiplying the pressure in psi by a factor of 0.3. Therefore a full tank contains about 660 L of oxygen (2200 psi × 0.3 = 660). At a flow rate of 1 L/min, this will last about 660 minutes, or 11 hours. The volume of oxygen in an H tank in liters is about three times the pressure in psi. Therefore an H tank with a pressure of 1000 psi contains about 3000 L of oxygen. When a compressed gas cylinder is turned off, the tank pressure gauge will continue to register pressure until the system is evacuated or "bled off." This is accomplished by depressing the oxygen flush valve until the gauge reads 0 psi.

The pressure reducing valve (Figure 27-10, *C*) reduces the pressure of the gas exiting the compressed gas cylinder to 40 to 50 psi. This pressure is maintained regardless of the pressure in the cylinder. The line pressure gauge (Figure 27-10, *A*) indicates the pressure in the line connecting the pressure reducing valve and the flowmeter(s). When the oxygen is turned on, this gauge should read 40 to 50 psi. Both of these

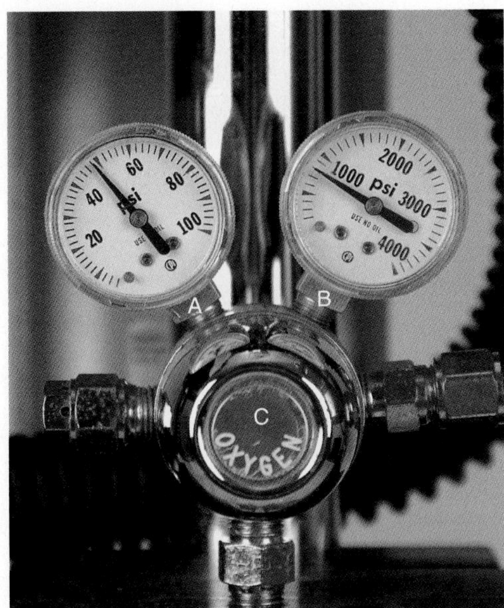

FIGURE 27-10 *A,* Line pressure gauge (registering 48 psi). *B,* Tank pressure gauge (registering 800 psi). *C,* Pressure reducing valve.

parts function passively and require no action on the part of the machine operator.

The flowmeter (Figure 27-11) controls the rate at which the carrier gas is delivered to the patient, and reduces the pressure from 40-50 psi to 15 psi. Carrier gas flow rates are expressed in liters per minute (L/min). Flowmeters are gas specific and color coded to match the compressed gas cylinders (green for oxygen and blue for N_2O). Therefore if using N_2O in addition to oxygen, there will be flowmeters to adjust the flow separately for each carrier gas. Some machines, such as the one pictured, have two oxygen flowmeters. The meter on the right is used for flow rates greater than 1 L/min, and the meter on the left is used for flow rates less than 1 L/min.

Turn on a flowmeter by turning the dial counterclockwise. All flowmeters have a ball or rotor indicator that rises to a height proportional to the flow of gas. Read the *center* of a ball indicator or the *top* of a rotor indicator. When turning off these meters, turn clockwise just until the ball or rotor drops to zero. Even though the knob can still be turned, do *not* turn it any further to prevent damage to the valve.

Oxygen flow rates must be carefully chosen to ensure patient safety, produce desired changes in anesthetic depth, and to conserve carrier and anesthetic gases. Although in some practices it is common practice to use a standard rate of 1 to 2 L/min for most SA patients, using specific rates will improve patient response, cost savings, and safety. Oxygen flow rates depend on the type of equipment and system used. When using a rebreathing system, higher rates should be used during induction, recovery, and when changing anesthetic depth. Lower rates may be used during maintenance (see Box 27-3 for recommended oxygen flow rates).

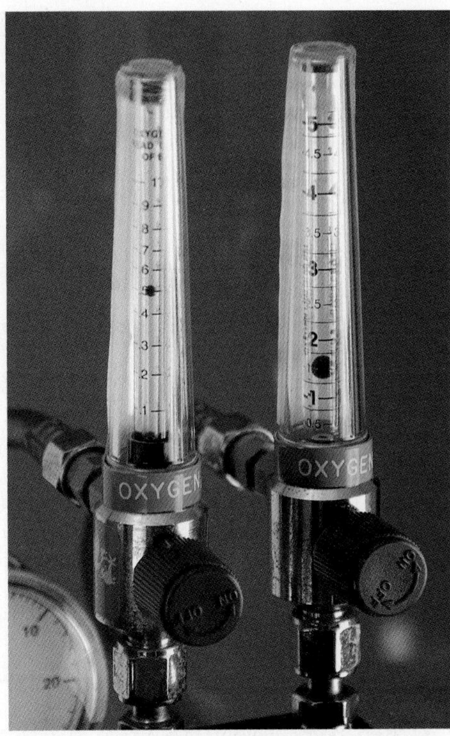

FIGURE 27-11 Oxygen flowmeters with ball indicators: The flowmeter on the left is adjusted to 0.5 L/min, and flowmeter on the right is adjusted to 1.5 L/min for a total oxygen flow of 2 L/min.

The oxygen flush valve (Figure 27-12, *F*) delivers pure oxygen at 35 to 75 L/min directly to the breathing circuit, bypassing the flowmeter and vaporizer. The oxygen flush valve is used to quickly fill an empty reservoir bag with fresh oxygen, but will dilute the concentration of inhalant anesthetic in the breathing circuit when it is used. It is also used to deliver fresh oxygen to a critically ill patient or to flush inhalant anesthetic out of the circuit during anesthetic recovery or during a crisis. To flush the circuit, turn off the vaporizer, force the gases out of the reservoir bag using gentle hand pressure, and press the valve to refill the bag with fresh oxygen. When using this valve, use only short bursts to avoid overfilling the bag and damaging the patient's lungs as a result of a buildup of pressure.

ANESTHETIC VAPORIZERS

The anesthetic vaporizer holds liquid inhalant anesthetic and adds controlled amounts of vaporized anesthetic to the carrier gas. Vaporizers may be classified as precision or as nonprecision.

Precision Vaporizers

The inhalant anesthetics isoflurane and sevoflurane require the use of a precision vaporizer designed and color coded specifically for the agent used (purple is isoflurane; yellow is sevoflurane) (see Figure 27-12). Turn on the vaporizer by disengaging the safety lock (Figure 27-12, *C*) and turning the dial to the desired percent concentration.

BOX 27-3 Oxygen Flow Rates

Oxygen Flow Rates for Small Animals, Foals, Calves, and Small Ruminants

Chamber and Mask Inductions:

Chamber induction: 5 L/min

Mask induction: *(300 ml/kg/min or 30 times the V_T)*

- 1-3 L/min for patients ≤10 kg
- 3-5 L/min for patients >10 kg

Rebreathing Systems:

Semiclosed system following induction, during a change in anesthetic depth, or during recovery: (200 ml/kg/min up to a maximum of 5 L/min. This is approximately equal to the respiratory minute volume.)

- **~1 L/5 kg body weight/min** up to a maximum of 5 L/min

Semiclosed system during maintenance: (20-40 ml/kg/min)

- **~0.1-0.2 L/5 kg body weight/min** with a minimum of 0.2 L/min regardless of patient size

(Note: The use of a maintenance rate of 0.1 L/5 kg/min is sometimes referred to as "low flow.")

Semiclosed system during maintenance with minimal rebreathing: (200 ml/kg/min)

- **~1 L/5 kg body weight/min** up to a maximum of 5 L/min

(Note: At this flow, the machine functions in a manner similar to a nonrebreathing system.)

Nonrebreathing Systems:

The following rate is used at all times when using these systems: *(200-300 ml/kg/min)*

- ~1-1.5 L/5 kg body weight/min

Oxygen Flow Rates for Large Animals

Rebreathing Systems:

(Note: Only rebreathing systems are used in LA patients.)

Induction and during a change in anesthetic depth: ~8-10 L/min

Maintenance: ~3-5 L/min

TECHNICIAN NOTE The level of the liquid anesthetic in the vaporizer should be noted before each procedure. To function properly, it must be between the upper and lower lines of the window (Figure 27-12, *D*). Refill as needed, but keep it at least one-half full at all times. Overfilling a vaporizer will result in anesthetic overdose, and underfilling will result in an inability to keep the patient anesthetized.

With the exception of some older models, the amount of inhalant anesthetic gas vaporized by a precision vaporizer is independent of variables such as ambient temperature, oxygen flow rate, RR, depth, and back pressure. This allows precise delivery of high vapor pressure inhalant agents, such as isoflurane and sevoflurane. Precision vaporizers are located out of the breathing circuit because of their high resistance to gas flow and are therefore known as vaporizer out-of-circle or VOC (Figure 27-13).

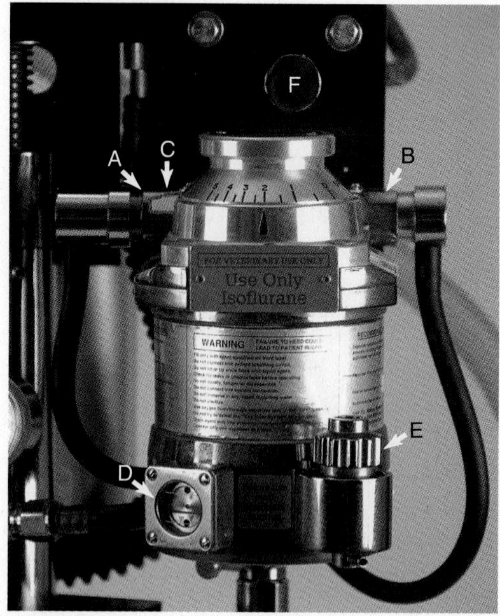

FIGURE 27-12 Precision anesthetic vaporizer for isoflurane set on 2%. *A*, Inlet port with keyed fitting leading from the flowmeters. *B*, Outlet port with keyed fitting leading to the fresh gas inlet. *C*, Safety lock. *D*, Indicator window. *E*, Fill port. *F*, Oxygen flush valve (part of the compressed gas supply).

All precision vaporizers will be somewhat affected by very high or very low carrier gas flow rates. Specifically, oxygen flows in excess of 10 L/min or lower than 500 ml/min may affect output. When flows are significantly less than the patient's respiratory minute volume (200 ml/kg/min), the output will decrease slightly as a result of a dilution effect by expired gases. Therefore higher dial settings may be needed under these circumstances.

Nonprecision Vaporizers

Nonprecision vaporizers are intended to be used only with low vapor pressure anesthetics, such as the discontinued agent methoxyflurane and, in contrast with precision vaporizers, are located in the breathing circuit (VIC) because they do not impede the flow of gases around the circuit as the patient breathes. These vaporizers do not measure a precise concentration and are affected by ambient temperature, oxygen flow rate, back pressure, and the patient RR and depth. Although infrequently used, these vaporizers may be used with high vapor pressure anesthetics, such as isoflurane, if specifically designed for this purpose.

Vaporizer Inlet Port, Outlet Port, and the Fresh Gas Inlet

The vaporizer inlet port (see Figure 27-12, *A*) is the point where oxygen and other carrier gases enter the vaporizer from the flowmeters. The vaporizer outlet port (see Figure 27-12, *B*) is the point where the oxygen, inhalant anesthetic, and other carrier gases exit the vaporizer. The point at which these gases enter the breathing circuit is referred to as the

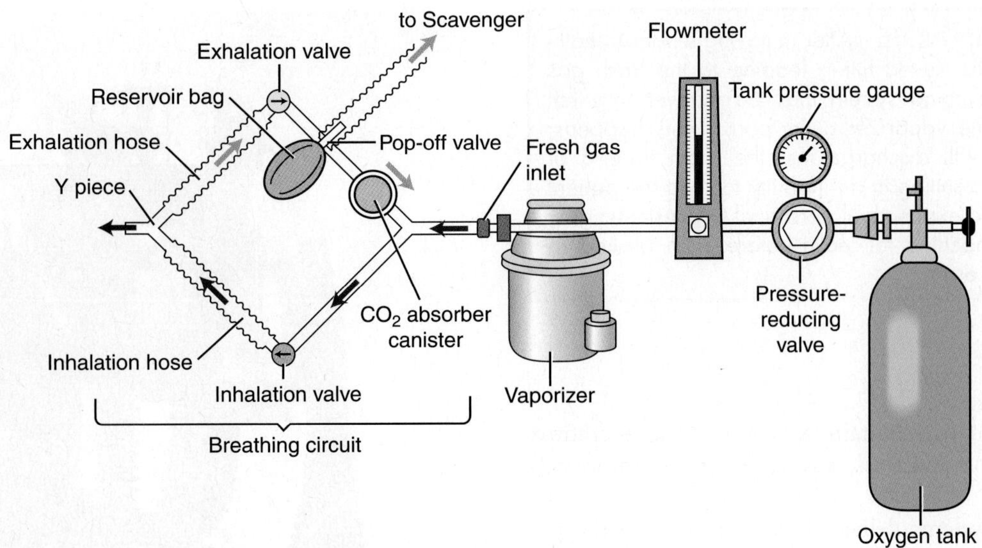

FIGURE 27-13 Diagram of an anesthetic machine with a rebreathing circuit and VOC. Note that the vaporizer is located outside of the breathing circuit.

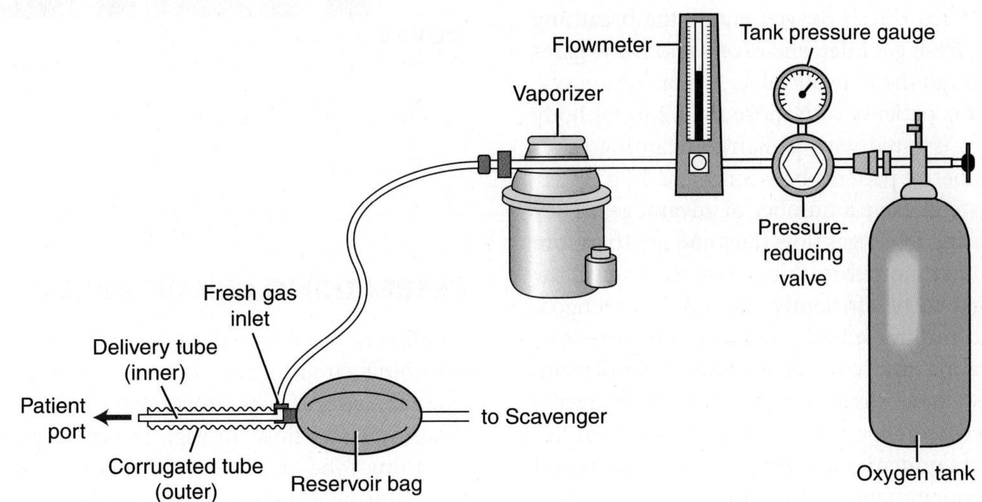

FIGURE 27-14 Diagram of an anesthetic machine with a nonrebreathing system attached to the vaporizer outlet port.

fresh gas inlet. The vaporizer outlet and inlet ports are connected to hoses with keyed fittings that prevent the operator from inadvertently attaching the wrong hose to the wrong vaporizer port.

BREATHING CIRCUITS

Breathing circuits circulate fresh gases to the patient and convey waste gases to the scavenging system. During inhalation and exhalation, the patient's lungs act like a bellows to move air through the breathing circuit. Nonrebreathing systems do not resist air movement and are generally used for smaller patients because they minimize the work required to breathe. In contrast, rebreathing systems resist air movement, thus impairing the ability of small patients to move the gases through the circuit.

The use of a nonrebreathing system (Figure 27-14) is recommended for patients under 7 kg in body weight. A nonrebreathing circuit is attached to the outlet port of the anesthetic vaporizer in place of the keyed fitting of a rebreathing circuit (see Figure 27-7, *A*). Fresh oxygen and inhalant anesthetic are delivered to the patient through a fresh gas inlet (see Figure 27-7, *B*) while exhaled gases pass into the scavenging system (see Figure 27-7, *F*), often after passing through a reservoir bag (see Figure 27-7, *D*). These systems flush out expired gases by use of a relatively high oxygen flow rate (200 to 300 ml/kg/min) and consequently do not require a CO_2 absorbent canister or unidirectional valves. Nonrebreathing circuits are available in a variety of configurations in which the position of some parts including the fresh gas inlet, the reservoir bag, and the scavenger outlet varies. The Ayre's T-piece; Mapleson A, D, E, or F circuits; and Magill, Jackson-Rees, and Bain circuits are names of some of the nonrebreathing circuits available.

Nonrebreathing systems have disadvantages. They do not conserve gases, moisture, or body heat, thus increasing the

> *TECHNICIAN NOTE* After removing a nonrebreathing circuit, the keyed fitting leading to the fresh gas inlet of a rebreathing system may be inadvertently left unattached to the vaporizer outlet port. If this happens, anesthetic gas will discharge into the room instead of into the circuit, resulting in an inability to keep the patient anesthetized and exposure of personnel to anesthetic gas. Checking the machine for leaks before each procedure will prevent this error.

vigilance required to maintain patient body temperature. Manual ventilation and waste gas scavenging are more difficult.

Rebreathing systems deliver anesthetic gases to the patient, remove CO_2, and recirculate carbon dioxide–free exhaled gases to the patient. These systems are also called "circle systems" because the gases move in a modified circular pattern (see Figure 27-13). Fresh oxygen enters the breathing circuit through the fresh gas inlet, and excess and waste gases exit the circuit through the pop-off valve. A rebreathing system may be used for patients with more than 2 kg of body weight providing it is fitted with pediatric breathing tubes when used to anesthetize patients between 2 and 7 kg.

Rebreathing systems have a number of advantages. They may be operated using lower gas flow rates and are therefore more economical than nonrebreathing systems. They allow waste anesthetic gas to be efficiently and easily scavenged. These systems also minimize body heat and moisture loss, and allow observation and control of patient ventilation. These systems also have disadvantages. Infectious agents may be transferred from patient to patient via microbe-laden moisture that condenses inside the machine parts and is inhaled by subsequent patients. Because the parts of these systems restrict air movement, they are not intended for use in small patients.

A semiclosed rebreathing system (partial rebreathing system) is a safe, practical, and economical system to use in general practice in all patients with a body weight greater than or equal to 2 kg. When using a semiclosed rebreathing system, the pop-off valve is partially open, the oxygen flow rate is higher than the metabolic needs of the patient (greater than 15 ml/kg/min), and waste gases exit through the pop-off valve.

A closed rebreathing system (total rebreathing system) is identical to the semiclosed system with two exceptions. The pop-off valve is nearly or entirely closed, and the oxygen flow rate is just enough to meet metabolic needs of the patient (7 to 15 ml/kg/min). In other words, in this system, approximately the same amount of fresh gas is added to the circuit as the patient consumes. With the exception of equine and bovine anesthesia, closed systems are infrequently used in practice because of the constant monitoring required, although most veterinary anesthesia texts include a detailed protocol for using these systems.

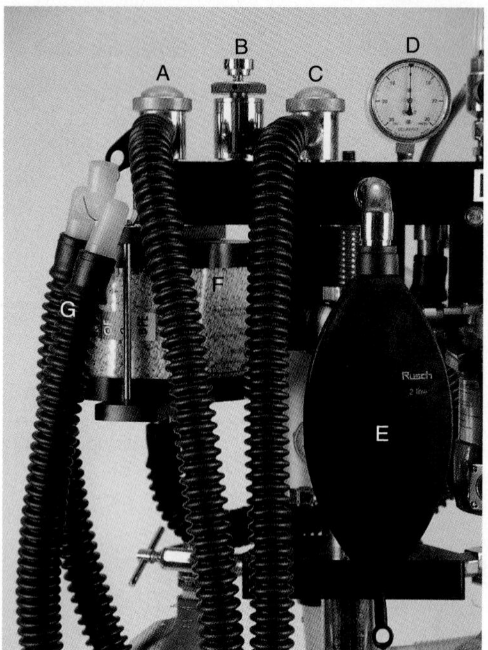

FIGURE 27-15 Parts of a rebreathing circuit. *A*, Exhalation unidirectional flow valve. *B*, Pop-off valve. *C*, Inhalation unidirectional flow valve. *D*, Pressure manometer. *E*, 2-L reservoir bag. *F*, CO_2 absorbent canister. *G*, SA corrugated breathing tubes.

REBREATHING CIRCUIT PARTS

Unidirectional flow valves keep the flow of gases in a rebreathing circuit going one way as the patient breathes. The inhalation (inspiratory) valve (Figure 27-15, *C*) opens to allow gas to flow through the corresponding corrugated breathing tube and into the patient's lungs during inspiration. During expiration, the exhalation (expiratory) valve (Figure 27-15, *A*) opens to allow expired gases to flow through the corresponding corrugated breathing tube into the CO_2 absorbent canister. Thus inhalation of expired gases containing CO_2 is prevented.

The reservoir bag or rebreathing bag (Figure 27-15, *E*) is a storage reservoir for anesthetic gases. It holds gases that will fill the patient's lungs during inspiration, receives gases breathed out by the patient during expiration, and therefore should deflate during inspiration and inflate during expiration. The reservoir bag also allows the anesthetist to visually observe patient respirations and to manually ventilate for the patient, when necessary. Reservoir bags come in a variety of sizes.

The bag should contain enough gas to fill the patient's lungs during an inhalation, but should not be so large as to prevent visualization of respiratory movements. The following rules of thumb can be used when selecting a bag: 500 ml for up to 5 kg; 1 L for 6 to 10 kg; 2 L for 11 to 25 kg; 3 L for 26 to 45 kg; 5 L for greater than 45 kg. Patients more than 200 kg or that are intubated with at least an 18-mm endotracheal tube require an LA anesthesia machine that uses 30-L bags.

> *TECHNICIAN NOTE* The V_T is the amount of air that passes in or out of the lungs during a normal breath. Normal V_T is about 10 to 15 ml/kg body weight. The size of the reservoir bag should be at least five times the patient's V_T.

When in use, the reservoir bag should be an average of three-fourths full. The amount of gas in the bag is influenced by a variety of factors, including oxygen flow, pop-off valve adjustment, and scavenging system adjustment. Low oxygen flows, a full-open pop-off valve, or a maladjusted scavenging system can cause the bag to empty. This will prevent the patient from filling its lungs with anesthetic gases during inspiration and will impair the ability to manually ventilate for the patient. In contrast, high oxygen flows, a closed pop-off valve, or malfunctioning scavenging system may result in an overfilled bag. This may impair the patient's ability to expire or cause a buildup of pressure within the lungs and will impair the ability to monitor respirations by sight.

The pop-off valve or pressure relief valve (Figure 27-15, *B*) allows excess gases to exit the breathing circuit, transfers these waste gases to the scavenging system, and prevents buildup of excess pressure within the circuit. The pop-off valve allows a range of settings from fully closed to fully open to maintain optimum volume in the reservoir bag. When fully open, it releases when the gas pressure in the circuit exceeds 0.5 to 1 cm of water. As the valve is tightened, more pressure is required for release. When using a semiclosed rebreathing system, the valve is kept partially open when the patient is spontaneously breathing. It is closed *only* when providing manual ventilation so that gases may be forced into the patient's lungs using hand pressure. Between each breath provided by manual ventilation, it must be opened again to allow the escape of gases and to prevent excess pressure in the chest, which can lead to decreased cardiac output and death.

The CO_2 absorbent canister (Figure 27-15, *F*) is connected to the exhalation valve and receives expired gases. The canister holds absorbent granules, such as calcium hydroxide, which passively remove CO_2 from the expired air. Be sure to purchase an absorbent intended specifically for the inhalant agent that you are using.

The absorbent granules in the canister must be fresh to prevent the patient from rebreathing toxic levels of CO_2. When saturated, the granules will no longer absorb the waste CO_2 and therefore should be changed after 6 to 8 hours of use or when one third to one half of the granules become saturated. Fresh absorbent granules are able to be crushed and are white in color, but when saturated, become hard and turn an off-white color that is visibly distinguishable from the original. Most absorbents also contain a pH indicator that will cause a color change to blue or violet when saturated. The color reaction does not always occur, however, and will dissipate after a few hours if not noted.

The pressure manometer (Figure 27-15, *D*) indicates pressure (expressed in centimeters of water) in the breathing circuit and the patient's lungs. This pressure is influenced primarily by oxygen flow and pop-off valve adjustment. The pressure manometer should read 0 to 2 cm of water when the patient is breathing spontaneously. It should read no more than 20 cm of water in small animals or 40 cm of water in large animals when providing manual or mechanical ventilation unless the chest cavity is open, in which case the pressure can be somewhat higher. Excessive pressure in the circuit can result in dyspnea, lung damage, pneumothorax, and decreased cardiac output. Therefore frequent monitoring of the pressure is critical during any anesthetic procedure.

The negative pressure relief valve admits room air into the breathing circuit if a vacuum is detected, thus preventing patient asphyxiation. A vacuum may occur if the scavenging system exerts excessive suction, if the oxygen flow is too low, or if the oxygen cylinder is empty.

The corrugated breathing tubes (Figure 27-15, *G*) complete the breathing circuit by carrying the anesthetic gases to and from the patient. The Y-piece connects the inhalation and exhalation corrugated breathing tubes together. The opposite ends of the breathing tubes attach to the unidirectional valves. The remaining port of the Y-piece is then connected to a mask or to an endotracheal tube. LA tubes are 50 mm in diameter. SA tubes (Figure 27-16, *A*) are 22 mm in diameter. Pediatric tubes (Figure 27-16, *B*), which are shorter and smaller than conventional SA tubes, decrease mechanical dead space and are intended for patients between 2 and 7 kg of body weight. The Universal F-circuit (Figure 27-16, *C*) is a type of SA breathing tube in which the inhalation tube is located within the exhalation tube. This arrangement is designed to conserve body heat. As the cold inspired gases travel through the inner turquoise tube, the warm expired gases travel through the outer, transparent tube, warming the inspired gases.

SCAVENGING SYSTEM

This system of hoses and pipes is connected to the pop-off valve (see Figure 27-8, *A*) or other breathing circuit outlet and transfers waste gas outside the building through a system of pipes. Active scavenging systems use a fan to remove waste gas, whereas passive scavenging systems work by gravitational flow. Some active scavenging systems have a vacuum regulator (see Figure 27-8, *B*) that can be adjusted to prevent inadequate or excessive vacuum.

All scavenging systems must be checked periodically to be sure that the tubes are not blocked and that the vacuum is properly adjusted. Excess vacuum from an active scavenging system will draw all the gas out of the breathing circuit. This may lead to asphyxiation and can be recognized by a collapsed reservoir bag. Obstruction of the scavenging system will have the same effect as a closed pop-off valve and is indicated by a full reservoir bag or pressure buildup in the circuit.

An activated charcoal cartridge (see Figure 27-8, *C*) is attached to the discharge hose of the scavenging system and may be used as an alternative when a conventional scavenging system is not available. The activated charcoal will absorb

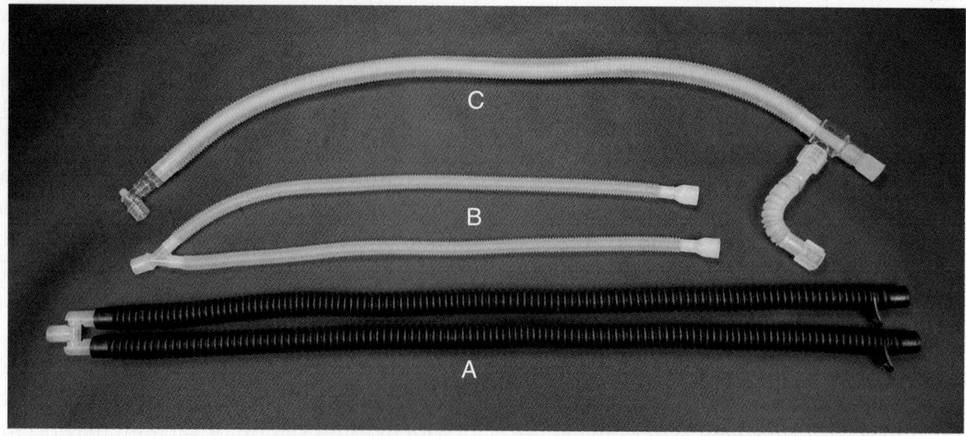

FIGURE 27-16 Corrugated breathing tubes. *A,* Standard 22-mm SA breathing tubes. *B,* 15-mm pediatric tubes. *C,* Universal F-circuit.

most commonly used inhalant anesthetics (except N_2O) as the waste gas is filtered through the cartridge. Activated charcoal cartridges should be weighed before use and must be replaced after a weight gain of 50 g.

ANESTHETIC MACHINE MAINTENANCE

All anesthetic machines require regular maintenance to keep them functioning properly. Whereas much of the maintenance of individual parts can be performed by the anesthetist as detailed later, the machine should be inspected and maintained by a repair professional at least once a year to ensure proper operation.

The tank pressure gauge, line pressure gauge, pressure reducing valve, flowmeters, oxygen flush valve, pop-off valve, negative pressure relief valve, and the pressure manometer do not require regular maintenance, but should be checked by a repair professional for proper function annually or when a problem is suspected. Corrugated breathing tubes, reservoir bags, and other detachable rubber parts should be cleaned periodically with a mild disinfectant, such as chlorhexidine, rinsed, dried, inspected for holes or defects, and replaced as necessary.

Unidirectional flow valves should be disassembled, cleaned with 70% isopropyl alcohol or mild disinfectant, dried, and inspected before reassembly to ensure that neither the valve nor valve seat is damaged or warped. An incompetent valve will allow rebreathing of expired CO_2—a serious and potentially fatal complication.

To change the CO_2 absorbent, disassemble the canister, dispose of the exhausted granules, check the gaskets for damage, and clean each part with mild soap and water. Rinse, dry, and reassemble the parts. Fill the canister loosely with fresh absorbent granules, leaving at least one half inch of air space at the top. Following reassembly, the canister must be airtight.

ANESTHETIC MONITORING

There is a common perception that modern anesthetic agents are safe. This belief can lead to the erroneous assumption that careful monitoring is not as important as it once was. Anesthetic monitoring is and always has been one of the cornerstones of the successful practice of anesthesia. Conditions that may lead to serious complications are often subtle, but must be recognized and corrected without delay. Serious anesthetic complications often develop rapidly and if not prevented, are devastating for the patient, the owner, and the anesthetist. Consequently the anesthetist must develop the ability to endure long periods of relative boredom in a state of readiness to manage periods of urgency and crisis. This requires that the anesthetist be knowledgeable, alert, and watchful for subtle changes in the condition of the patient.

During any general anesthetic procedure, the anesthetist must strike a delicate balance of sufficient depth of anesthesia to produce unconsciousness and insensitivity to pain without endangering the life of the patient by compromising cardiovascular and respiratory system function. Monitoring allows the anesthetist to achieve this balance through careful observation and precise regulation of the amount of anesthetic administered.

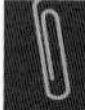

TECHNICIAN NOTE Principles of patient monitoring:
- Monitor patients frequently using your hands, eyes, and ears.
- Always check multiple parameters.
- Never depend on instrumentation alone.
- Do not attempt to judge anesthetic depth by drug doses or dial settings.

STAGES AND PLANES OF ANESTHESIA

In the early 1900s, a system of stages and planes of general anesthesia was developed to describe patient responses to diethyl ether, an early inhalant anesthetic that is no longer used in clinical practice. Changes in patient behavior, body movements, ocular signs, reflexes, and vital signs in response to the progression from consciousness to deep surgical anesthesia were observed and documented. Under this system, general anesthesia was divided into four stages (I to IV), and stage III was subdivided into four planes (1 to 4).

Stage I—The Period of Voluntary Movement

During this stage, the patient gradually loses consciousness. It is usually characterized by fear, excitement, and struggling. The HR increases, and the patient may hold its breath, urinate, or defecate. Near the end of stage I, the patient loses the ability to stand and becomes recumbent.

Stage II—The Period of Involuntary Movement

During this stage, also known as the excitement stage, the patient loses voluntary control and assumes a regular breathing pattern. It is usually characterized by involuntary reactions in the form of vocalizing, struggling, or paddling. The HR and RRs are often elevated, pupils are dilated, muscle tone is marked, and reflexes are present.

Stage III—The Period of Surgical Anesthesia

During this stage, the patient is unconscious and progresses gradually from light to deep surgical anesthesia. It is characterized by progressive muscle relaxation, decreasing heart and respiratory rates, and loss of reflexes. The pupils gradually dilate, tear production decreases, and the pupillary light reflex is lost. The increase in heart and respiratory rates seen in response to surgical stimulation during light anesthesia is gradually lost. Many authors now divide this stage into three planes corresponding to light (stage III, plane 1), medium (stage III, plane 2), and deep (stage III, plane 3) surgical anesthesia.

Stage IV—The Period of Anesthetic Overdose

During this stage, the nervous, cardiovascular, and respiratory systems are extremely depressed. Breathing stops, muscle tone is flaccid, pupils are widely dilated, and all reflexes are absent. The heart stops, and death follows quickly unless rapid action is taken.

PRINCIPLES OF MONITORING

Healthy patients (physical status class P1) should be monitored at least every 5 minutes during any general anesthetic procedure. Higher-risk patients (physical status classes P2 to P5) must be monitored more frequently and in some cases continuously. Ultimately the anesthetist must judge the frequency of monitoring that is appropriate for each patient. An anesthesia record should be used to document monitoring parameters, drug administration, and other information pertinent to the procedure (Figure 27-17).

At any given time during anesthesia, the patient should be somewhere between consciousness and deep surgical anesthesia (stage III, plane 3). Careful observation of the patient based on expected responses enables the anesthetist to determine the stage that the patient is in. For instance, unconsciousness, intact reflexes, eyes in a central position, marked jaw tone, and movement in response to stimulation are all expected responses from a patient in light surgical anesthesia (stage III, plane 1), a point inappropriate to perform surgery. In contrast, absent palpebral, pedal, and swallowing reflexes; moderate jaw tone; eyes in a ventromedial position; and an intact corneal reflex are all expected responses from a patient in medium surgical anesthesia (stage III, plane 2), an appropriate stage to begin.

There are many factors that influence progression through the stages of anesthesia and interpretation of physical signs. For instance, patients induced using IV agents often pass through stages I and II so quickly that they are minimally noticeable. In contrast, patients induced with an inhalant agent take longer to reach surgical anesthesia and may be difficult to control while passing though these stages. The administration of premedications generally decreases excitement seen during stages I and II and therefore eases passage into surgical anesthesia.

In addition, the anesthetic protocol will influence interpretation of physical signs. For example, a patient induced with an α_2-adrenergic agonist will often have a much lower HR than one induced with an inhalant agent. A patient may have dilated pupils if given a dissociative agent, but conversely may have constricted pupils if given an opioid. Consequently, physical signs must be interpreted in light of the agents administered.

After considering each of these factors, the anesthetist must ultimately answer two questions:

1. Is the patient safe or in danger?
2. Is the anesthetic depth inadequate, excessive, or appropriate for the procedure performed?

Monitoring parameters are the physical signs used to answer these questions. They are subdivided into vital signs, reflexes, and other indicators of anesthetic depth. Although all monitoring parameters are evaluated together, some are more useful for answering the first question, whereas others are more useful for answering the second.

VITAL SIGNS

Vital signs are used primarily to evaluate the cardiovascular and pulmonary systems. Vital signs include the HR and rhythm, RR and depth, mucous membrane color, CRT, blood pressure, and temperature. These parameters are used principally to answer the question: "Is the patient safe or in danger?" They are only loosely correlated with the depth of anesthesia. Specifically, patients in lighter planes of anesthesia tend to have higher HRs, RRs, and blood pressure; pinker mucous membranes; and more rapid CRT, whereas patients in deeper planes experience opposite effects (Table 27-3). However, other factors may change this association. For example, a patient in light surgical anesthesia given an opioid agonist may have a decreased HR. Conversely a patient in deep surgical anesthesia may have an elevated HR if in shock. Although vital signs are helpful in determining anesthetic depth, other parameters are better suited to this purpose.

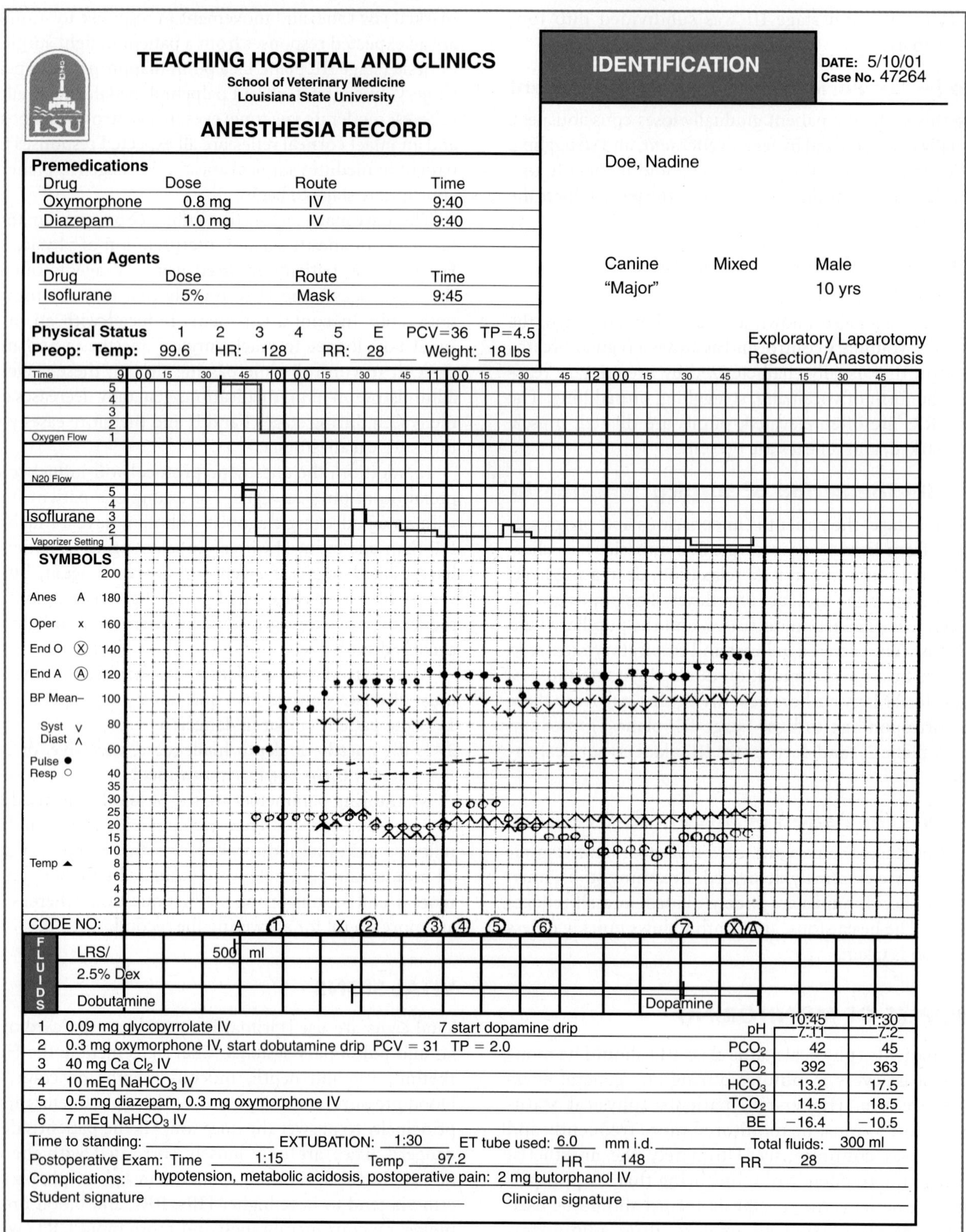
TEACHING HOSPITAL AND CLINICS
School of Veterinary Medicine
Louisiana State University

ANESTHESIA RECORD

IDENTIFICATION

DATE: 5/10/01
Case No. 47264

Doe, Nadine

Canine Mixed Male
"Major" 10 yrs

Exploratory Laparotomy
Resection/Anastomosis

Premedications

Drug	Dose	Route	Time
Oxymorphone	0.8 mg	IV	9:40
Diazepam	1.0 mg	IV	9:40

Induction Agents

Drug	Dose	Route	Time
Isoflurane	5%	Mask	9:45

Physical Status 1 2 3 4 5 E PCV=36 TP=4.5

Preop: Temp: 99.6 HR: 128 RR: 28 Weight: 18 lbs

FLUIDS	
LRS/	500 ml
2.5% Dex	
Dobutamine	Dopamine

			pH	10:45 7.11	11:30 7.2
1	0.09 mg glycopyrrolate IV	7 start dopamine drip			
2	0.3 mg oxymorphone IV, start dobutamine drip PCV = 31 TP = 2.0		PCO_2	42	45
3	40 mg $CaCl_2$ IV		PO_2	392	363
4	10 mEq $NaHCO_3$ IV		HCO_3	13.2	17.5
5	0.5 mg diazepam, 0.3 mg oxymorphone IV		TCO_2	14.5	18.5
6	7 mEq $NaHCO_3$ IV		BE	−16.4	−10.5

Time to standing: ______ EXTUBATION: 1:30 ET tube used: 6.0 mm i.d. ______ Total fluids: 300 ml

Postoperative Exam: Time 1:15 Temp 97.2 HR 148 RR 28

Complications: hypotension, metabolic acidosis, postoperative pain: 2 mg butorphanol IV

Student signature ______ Clinician signature ______

FIGURE 27-17 Anesthesia record: The form is used to document the anesthetic protocol, monitoring parameters, treatments, and other information pertinent to the procedure.

Heart rate measured in beats/min (bpm), and heart rhythm (Table 27-4) may be monitored by palpation of the chest wall, palpation of the pulse, auscultation, or use of monitoring equipment. The HR generally decreases gradually in response to increasing anesthetic depth because most anesthetic agents are cardiovascular depressants. This effect is extremely variable, however, and is influenced by the specific agents used, blood pressure, preexisting illness, and other factors. Although bradycardia is caused to some degree by most anesthetic agents, the opioids and α_2-adrenergic

TABLE 27-3 Relationship between Vital Signs and Anesthetic Depth

Vital Sign	Depth: Too Light	Depth: Surgical Anesthesia	Depth: Too Deep
HR	Usually elevated	Variable	Usually decreased
Respiration rate	Usually elevated	Variable	Usually decreased
Pulses	Strong	Palpable, but often less strong	Weak/nonpalpable
Mucous membrane color/CRT	Normal/normal	Normal but may be somewhat paler/normal	Pale/prolonged

TABLE 27-4 Normal and Abnormal Heart Rate and Rhythm

Species	Normal HR (bpm) (Awake/at Rest)	Normal HR (bpm) (Anesthetized)	*Report to the Veterinarian if:
Dog†	60-180	60-150	<60 (lg); <70 (sm); or >140 (lg); >160 (sm)
Cat	120-240	120-180	<100; or >200
Horse	30-45	28-40	<25; or >60
Cattle	60-80	50-80	<40; or >100

*In addition to the rates listed, any arrhythmia should be reported to the veterinarian.

†Because of the extreme variability of size, large dogs tend to have lower rates, whereas small dogs and puppies have higher rates.

agonists are particularly likely to have this effect. Conversely, dissociatives and anticholinergics may cause tachycardia.

During anesthesia, the normal heart rhythm is normal sinus rhythm (NSR) or sinus arrhythmia (SA) in dogs and NSR in cats. Large animals typically exhibit NSR, but SA may also be observed. Cardiac arrhythmias can be induced by anesthetic agents, particularly the α_2-adrenergic agonists, barbiturates, anticholinergics, and dissociatives, but can also be caused by other conditions, including hypoxia, gastric dilation-volvulus, hypercarbia, preexisting heart disease, and trauma.

Mucous membrane color (Table 27-5) is monitored by observing the color of the oral mucous membranes. Capillary refill time (Table 27-5) is the time it takes (in seconds) for the normal color to return following application of digital pressure to the gums near the base of a tooth. If the oral tissues are pigmented, the tongue, conjunctiva, or mucous membranes of the prepuce or vulva can be used as alternatives.

Pale mucous membranes indicate any cause of poor capillary perfusion or anemia. Prolonged CRT indicates poor capillary perfusion. Cyanosis indicates low oxygen saturation and is a medical emergency.

Blood pressure is monitored by indirect measurement using a Doppler or oscillometric monitor or by direct measurement via an arterial catheter. Pulse strength (see Table 27-5) as determined by palpation of a peripheral artery (such as the lingual, femoral, carotid, or dorsal pedal artery in small animals or the facial, auricular, digital, or dorsal pedal artery in large animals), gives the anesthetist a crude indication of blood pressure. A strong pulse is suggestive of normal blood pressure, and a weak one is suggestive of hypotension. The pulse strength varies widely among individuals, so the anesthetist should assess the pulse before anesthetic administration as a point of reference.

Respiratory rate measured in breaths/min (bpm), respiratory effort, and V_T (Table 27-6) are monitored by observing movement of the chest wall, expansion and contraction of the reservoir bag, or movement of the unidirectional flow valves or with monitoring equipment. Auscultation—an important tool for evaluating lung sounds—does not work well to monitor RR and depth. It is advisable to observe the patient's respiratory depth and quality while awake as a point of reference.

Since many anesthetic agents are respiratory system depressants, anesthetized patients will often experience a decrease in RR and about a 25% decrease in V_T directly related to anesthetic depth. This hypoventilation can lead to atelectasis. Atelectasis results in decreased gas exchange, which may lead to hypoxemia. This effect is common during anesthesia, particularly in the dependent lung (the one nearest the table). Many clinicians recommend gentle inflation of the lungs by periodic manual ventilation about every 5 minutes during anesthesia to prevent this complication. This technique is referred to as "bagging" or "sighing" the patient.

In addition to the effects of anesthetic agents, there are many other potential causes of hypoventilation, including postinduction apnea. As the name implies, postinduction apnea is a phenomenon that commonly occurs following anesthetic induction for the following reason. During

TABLE 27-5 Normal and Abnormal Mucous Membrane Color, CRT, and Pulse Strength

Vital Sign (All Species)	Normal (Awake/at Rest)	Normal (Anesthetized)	Report to the Veterinarian if:
Mucous membrane color	Pink (often described as "bubblegum pink")	Pink (may be somewhat paler than when awake)	Pale or blue
CRT	<2 sec	<2 sec	>2 sec
Pulse strength	Palpable with one pulse closely following each heartbeat	Often somewhat decreased in strength, but still palpable	Nonpalpable Irregular Excessively weak

TABLE 27-6 Normal and Abnormal Respiratory Rate, Effort, and Tidal Volume (V_T)

Species	Normal (Awake/At Rest)	Normal (Anesthetized)	Report to the Veterinarian if:
Dogs	10-30 (panting is normal)	8-20	<8 or >20
Cats	15-30	8-20	<8 or >20
Horses	8-20	6-12	<6 or >20
Cattle	8-20	6-12, although rapid, shallow breathing is common	<6 or >20
All species	Normal effort and V_T	Normal effort ~25% decrease in V_T	Increased effort >25% decrease in V_T

TABLE 27-7 Normal and Abnormal Body Temperatures

Species	Normal (Awake/At Rest)	Normal (Anesthetized)	Report to the Veterinarian if:
Dog and cat	100° F-102.5° F (37.8° C-39.2° C)	Variably decreased	>103.5° F (39.7° C) or <98° F (36.7° C)
Horse	99° F-100.5° F (37.2° C-38° C)	Variably decreased	>101.5° F (38.6° C) or <98° F (36.7° C)
Cattle	100° F-102.5° F (37.8° C-39.2° C)	Variably decreased	>103.5° F (39.7° C) or <98° F (36.7° C)

induction, all patients pass through lighter stages of anesthesia during which hyperventilation occurs for a period of time ranging from several seconds to as much as a few minutes. Hyperventilation of a sufficient length will cause the patient to expire excessive quantities of CO_2 resulting in a decreased concentration of CO_2 in the blood. In response to the decreased concentration, the patient then hypoventilates or stops breathing until a normal CO_2 level is reestablished.

Postinduction apnea can be frightening and dangerous if not understood and must be managed promptly with supportive care. Supportive care involves careful monitoring of other parameters, including oxygen saturation, and periodic manual ventilation about 2 to 4 times/min to maintain adequate oxygen levels until the patient begins to breathe spontaneously. When managing postinduction apnea, avoid ventilating too frequently so that the normal CO_2 level can be reestablished. The use of a capnograph allows precise measurement of CO_2 levels and so is a useful tool for managing this problem.

During anesthesia, the patient should exhibit normal respiratory effort. Dyspnea indicates a serious patient problem or machine malfunction that must be addressed promptly. Abdominal breathing is a unique breathing pattern associated with dangerously excessive anesthetic depth. It is characterized by a rocking motion of the abdomen and chest as a result of paralysis of the respiratory muscles and must be acted upon immediately.

Body temperature (Table 27-7) should be monitored about every 15 to 30 minutes with a rectal thermometer or probe. Although body temperature can be estimated by touching the skin of the paw or ear, it cannot be accurately determined this way. Hypothermia is experienced by most patients during anesthesia, but can lead to prolonged recovery and predisposition to anesthetic overdose if severe. Hypothermia usually occurs rapidly following induction and is often of a relatively large magnitude. Therefore the following steps should be taken to reduce heat loss during all anesthetic procedures:

- Do not allow the patient's body to contact stainless steel.
- Place a heat-retaining surface under the patient, such as a warm-water circulating blanket, blanket, towel, or lamb's wool.
- Warm IV fluids before administration.

- During preparation of the surgery site, avoid the use of alcohol as a rinsing agent or wetting the hair excessively.
- Avoid excessively low ambient temperatures in the surgical suite.

Malignant hyperthermia is a complication of general anesthesia in which the body temperature progressively rises to dangerous levels. Some animals, such as Pietrain, Landrace, and Poland China swine are genetically predisposed, but it may also be a reaction to certain drugs including the inhalant anesthetics. Malignant hyperthermia may occur in a variety of species, is a medical emergency, and must be promptly recognized, reported, and treated. Early signs include muscle rigidity and excessive production of CO_2, which leads to exhaustion of the CO_2 absorbent.

REFLEXES AND OTHER INDICATORS OF ANESTHETIC DEPTH (TABLE 27-8)

Reflexes are involuntary protective responses to stimuli (such as the "kick" response when your physician taps your knee with a neurologic hammer). Reflexes and other indicators of anesthetic depth are used to answer the question *"Is the anesthetic depth inadequate, excessive, or appropriate for the procedure being performed?"*

The palpebral reflex is induced by gently tapping the skin at the medial or lateral canthus of the eye with your finger. This reflex is present when the patient is too light, progressively diminishes with increasing depth, and is generally absent in surgical anesthesia in small animals, but may still be present in horses and ruminants until they are in a moderately deep plane of anesthesia.

The swallowing reflex is a normal reflex that occurs in response to the presence of saliva or food in the pharynx. It is detected by watching the throat for swallowing motions. The swallowing reflex is present when anesthetic depth is inadequate, but is absent in surgical and deeper stages of anesthesia and is therefore used to determine whether or not the patient is too light.

The pedal reflex is the withdrawal of a limb in response to a painful stimulus. To induce this reflex, place a limb in a relaxed position and vigorously pinch a toe. Withdrawal of the limb indicates inadequate depth of anesthesia.

The corneal reflex is induced by placing a drop of sterile artificial tears on the cornea. When the reflex is present, the eyeball will retract slightly within the orbit. When in lighter planes of anesthesia, a blink response may also occur. This response is difficult to interpret when the eyes are in a ventromedial position, but should be present during all planes of surgical anesthesia and therefore helps to determine if the anesthetic depth is excessive.

Muscle tone is most frequently determined in small animals by assessing jaw tone. Open the jaw with the fingers and feel for resistance. Muscle tone is high when the patient is too light, gradually diminishes with increasing anesthetic depth, and is described using the terms marked, moderate, loose, and flaccid. Muscle tone may alternatively be assessed by observing the size of the anal opening, which will be closed at lighter planes and progressively more open at deeper planes.

Eye position and pupil size are also useful in determining anesthetic depth. Eye position is central (straight forward) in light anesthesia, gradually shifts to a ventromedial position (toward the chin), and finally shifts back to a central position in deep anesthesia. In most patients, ventromedial deviation is common during surgical anesthesia. In some horses, eye position may change from ventromedial to central and back again. This is usually indicative of surgical anesthesia. The presence of nystagmus usually indicates a light plane of anesthesia in any patient.

Response to Surgical Stimulation

When stimulated by cutting or manipulation of viscera, the HR, RR, V_T, or blood pressure may increase. A sudden marked increase in any of these parameters indicates

TABLE 27-8 Interpretation of Reflexes and Other Indicators of Anesthetic Depth

Indicator	Inadequate Depth	Surgical Anesthesia	Excessive Depth
Palpebral reflex	Present	Absent*	Absent
Swallowing reflex	Present	Absent	Absent
Pedal reflex	Present	Absent	Absent
Corneal reflex	Present	Present	Absent
Muscle tone	Marked	Moderate or loose	Flaccid
Eye position	Central	Generally ventromedial	Central
Pupil size	Constricted	Gradually larger	Widely dilated
PLR	Present	Gradually nonresponsive	Absent
Lacrimal secretions	Present	Gradually decrease	Absent
Nystagmus†	Present	Absent	Absent
Response to surgical stimulation	Marked increase in HR, RR, or V_T	Mild or no increase in HR No increase in RR or V_T	No increase in HR, RR, or V_T

*Absent when using halogenated inhalant agents (small animals); may be sluggish when other agents are used to maintain anesthesia or in large animals.

†Nystagmus may be caused by severe hypoxia or hypercarbia in horses.

inadequate depth of anesthesia. Mild changes in HR may occur, however, even in surgical anesthesia. Realize that the appropriate depth for each patient may vary somewhat according to the degree of surgical stimulation and pain associated with the procedure.

MONITORING EQUIPMENT

Monitoring equipment is a useful addition to physical assessment, but should never be used alone. The main advantages of this equipment are to give early warning of impending problems before serious consequences develop and to provide a measurement of certain physical parameters, such as blood pressure, oxygen saturation, or expired CO_2, that is not possible with physical assessment. Monitoring equipment allows the anesthetist to assess the patient more precisely than would be otherwise possible. For instance, a pulse oximeter can detect hypoxemia long before cyanosis is visible. A capnograph can warn of inadequate or excessive ventilation accurately and rapidly, and an oscillometric monitor can detect subtle changes in blood pressure before a change in pulse strength is evident. In this section, the use of this equipment will be reviewed.

An esophageal stethoscope (Figure 27-18) is a device designed to amplify the sound of the heartbeat so that the anesthetist can monitor the heart from a distance. Although this device is not capable of determining the heart rhythm, changes in rate, irregularity, or interruption in the heart sounds can alert the anesthetist to a possible arrhythmia. Esophageal stethoscopes are inexpensive, easy to operate, and easily maintained.

Parts include esophageal catheters of various sizes, a sensor, and base unit, which amplifies and converts the heart sounds into an audible electronic signal. To use an esophageal stethoscope, lubricate the closed end of an appropriately sized catheter and insert it into the esophagus to the level of the heart (about the fifth rib). Attach the free end to the electronic base via the sensor. Adjust the position of the catheter and the volume until the signal is audible. Care is minimal. The base should be cleaned as needed and batteries must be changed periodically. Catheters should be washed with a disinfectant and dried following use. Avoid immersion or introducing water inside the catheter.

An electrocardiographic (ECG) monitor is used to monitor the HR and rhythm. Electrodes are attached to specific locations on the patient's skin, and the electrical activity of the heart and the HR are displayed on a screen in real time. These monitors generally require little care. When using an ECG monitor, realize that it is possible for the heart to stop beating and the electrical activity to continue for a time after the heart has stopped. Therefore never depend on this monitor alone as a guarantee of patient safety.

A pulse oximeter (Figure 27-19) is a device designed to detect changes in the oxygen saturation of hemoglobin. Red and infrared wavelength light is passed through or reflected off of a tissue bed, detected by a sensor, and analyzed. The sensor is sensitive to blood pulsation in the arteries, so it also determines the HR. The machine determines the percent oxygen saturation (%SpO_2) by calculating the difference between levels of oxygenated and deoxygenated hemoglobin. Both the HR and the oxygen saturation are digitally displayed.

Normally, when breathing pure oxygen, hemoglobin in the lungs is at least 97% saturated with oxygen. Therefore during oxygen administration, the oxygen saturation should be greater than 95%. Saturation between 90% and 95% indicates a problem that must be acted upon. Saturation less than 90% indicates hypoxemia. Saturation less than 85% for longer than 30 seconds is a medical emergency.

Parts include a computerized base unit and a variety of probes, each of which analyzes light either passed through or reflected off a tissue bed. Pulse oximeter probes are classified as transmission or reflective. Transmission probes are constructed in a clamplike configuration. One of the jaws houses a light source, and the other houses a sensor that detects the transmitted light. Transmission probes must be applied over a nonpigmented tissue bed that is thin enough to allow light transmission, such as the tongue, lip, ear, flank fold, prepuce, vulva, digital web, nasal septum, or foot of smaller patients. Although these probes are able to function through a thin hair coat, excessive hair will prevent operation. The lingual probe and the "C" probe are examples of transmission probes (see Figure 27-20 for examples of probe types and placement).

Reflective probes are often long and narrow. The light source and sensor are located next to each other on one side

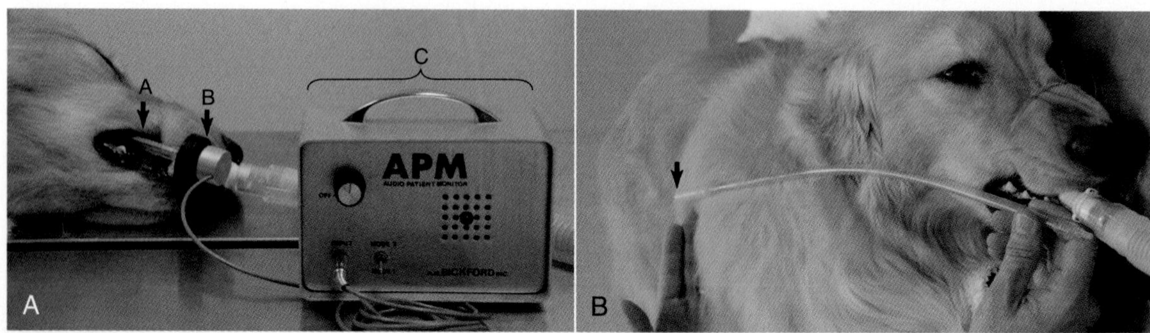

FIGURE 27-18 **A,** Esophageal stethoscope. *A,* Catheter. *B,* Sensor. *C,* Base unit. **B,** Measurement of the catheter to the level of the fifth rib or the caudal border of the scapula *(arrow).*

of the probe. These probes are placed inside a hollow organ, such as the esophagus or rectum, with the side housing the light source and sensor in contact with a tissue bed. When placing a reflective probe in the rectum, care must be taken to digitally displace the feces from the wall of the rectum and place the correct side of the probe against the tissue. A reflective probe may also be taped against the ventral surface of the tail (see Figure 27-20).

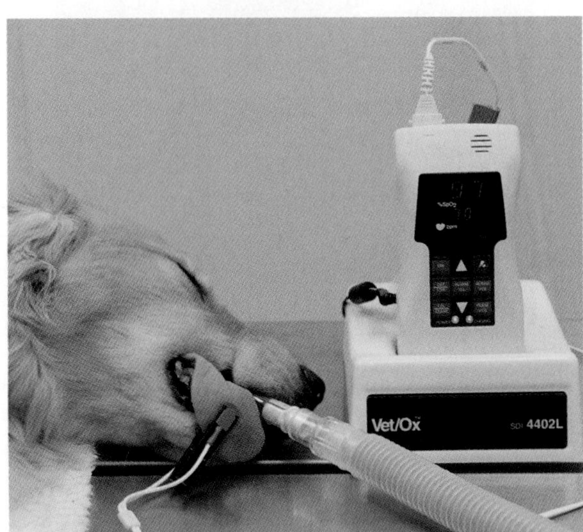

FIGURE 27-19 Pulse oximeter with transmission lingual probe: The upper number (97) represents the percent oxygen saturation (%SpO_2). The lower number (70) represents the HR in beats per minute.

Pulse oximeter probes can be frustrating to work with because of the high incidence of signal loss. When this happens, values will no longer appear on the display, the numbers will be incorrect, or an alarm may sound, and the probe must be readjusted or moved to a different location. Probe function is adversely affected by many factors, including tissue pigmentation, motion, excessive pressure, orientation in relation to ambient light, and patient conditions, such as anemia, icterus, vasoconstriction, or edema. Box 27-4 contains suggestions for trouble-shooting signal loss.

Pulse oximeters require little maintenance, but must be handled with care. Probes should be cleaned with alcohol or other mild disinfectant, but must not be immersed, scrubbed, or autoclaved.

An ultrasonic Doppler monitor (Figure 27-21) is a device that detects the flow of blood through small arteries and converts this motion into an audible signal. The blood flow is converted to a continuous sound similar to that of a heart murmur. Parts include an electronic base unit that processes the signal and a probe that emits and receives an ultrasonic wave. The hair overlying a small artery must be clipped and the skin cleaned and covered with a generous amount of ultrasonic gel. The probe is positioned over the artery, adjusted until an audible signal is detected, and then taped in place.

The placement of an ultrasonic Doppler probe requires patience and finesse. It must be oriented parallel to and precisely over the artery and must make firm, but not excessive contact. Sometimes subtle differences in position of only a millimeter or two can make the difference between success and failure in acquiring a signal.

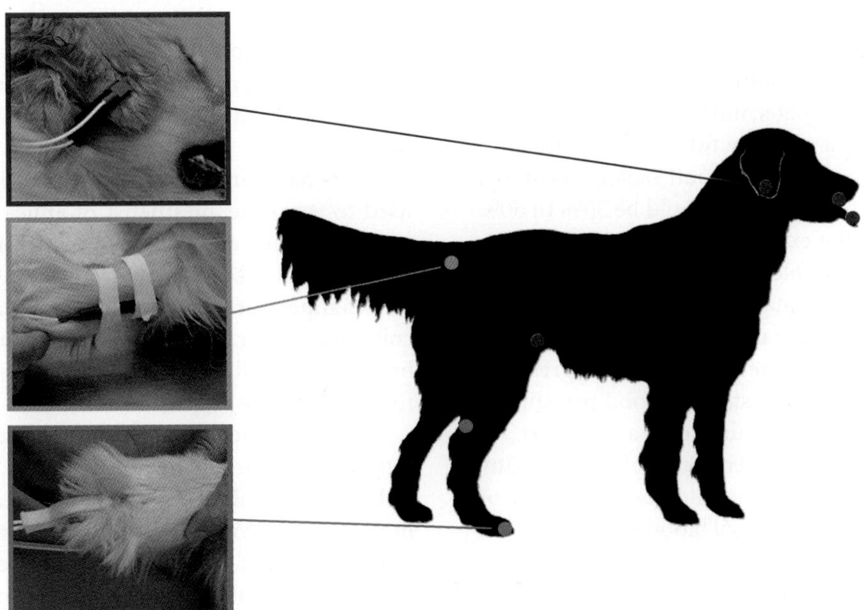

FIGURE 27-20 Examples of pulse oximeter probes and locations for placement. *Red,* Transmission probe on the ear flap. Additional red dots show alternate placement locations for this probe (tongue, lip, and flank fold). *Green,* Reflective probe taped to the ventral surface of the tail base. *Blue,* "C-probe" (a transmission probe) on the toe web. The other blue dot shows an alternate placement location for this probe (the skin fold between the Achilles tendon and the tibia).

BOX 27-4 Suggestions for Troubleshooting Pulse Oximeter Signal Loss

Transmission Probes

- Make sure the patient is safe by assessing vital signs.
- Remove and replace the probe.
- If the tongue is dry, rewet it.
- Be sure there is not excessive or inadequate pressure on the tissue.
- When possible, the jaw with the sensor should be oriented toward the ceiling to avoid interference from ambient light.
- Choose a different area that is not pigmented, covered with excessive hair, icteric, or edematous.
- If the area is heavily haired, clip and gently cleanse the area.

Reflective Probes

- Make sure the patient is safe by assessing vital signs.
- Be sure the side with the light source and sensor is oriented toward the tissue.
- Check for adequate tissue contact.
- When placed in the rectum, be sure that feces are not between the probe and the tissue.

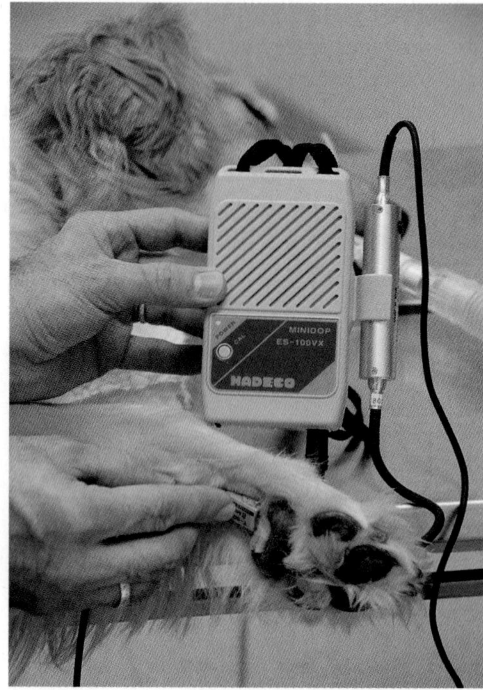

FIGURE 27-21 Doppler monitor: Base unit with the probe positioned over the ventral surface of the metacarpus proximal to the metacarpal pad.

Ultrasonic Doppler probes are delicate and expensive and must be handled carefully. They should be cleaned by wiping gently with a gauze sponge. Gentle cleaning with tap water is acceptable, but the probe must not be immersed, scrubbed, or autoclaved.

In SA patients, ultrasonic Doppler probes may be placed on the ventral surface of a paw proximal to the metacarpal or metatarsal pad, on the ventral surface of the tail base, on the dorsomedial surface of the hock, or on the medial surface of the thigh in patients less than 10 lb. In LA patients, the ventral tail is the most frequently used site (see Figure 27-22 for common locations to place the probe).

When used with a sphygmomanometer, the Doppler monitor can also be used to determine blood pressure (Figure 27-22, *top left*). Place a properly fitted cuff on the foreleg, metatarsus, or tail base with the cuff balloon centered over the artery. The width of the cuff should be 30% to 50% of the circumference of the extremity (Figure 27-23, *inset*). After establishing a good Doppler signal, inflate the cuff until the artery is occluded (the signal can no longer be heard). Gradually decrease the pressure until the audible signal can first be heard again. This represents the systolic pressure. These instruments tend to underestimate blood pressure in cats by about 15 mm Hg, but are fairly accurate in dogs. All indirect blood pressure measurements are subject to many inaccuracies, however, and must be interpreted in light of other signs (see Table 27-9 for normal blood pressure values during anesthesia).

An oscillometric blood pressure monitor (see Figure 27-23) is a device that is used to measure blood pressure and HR. Parts include a blood pressure cuff and a computerized base unit that inflates and deflates the cuff and analyzes the signals received by the cuff.

A cuff is placed around a leg or tail with the balloon centered over an artery, and the unit is turned on. The cuff is inflated and deflated automatically by the machine. The unit detects oscillations within the cuff bladder caused by pulsations of the arteries. Based on changes in the intracuff pressure, systolic, mean, and diastolic pressures are calculated. The cuff can be placed around the foreleg, metatarsus, metacarpus, or tail of small and large animal patients (see Figure 27-24 for example locations to place the cuff). For proper operation, the cuff should be at the same horizontal plane as the heart. This device is more accurate in patients more than 10 kg.

As its name implies, an apnea monitor (Figure 27-25) is used to warn the anesthetist of apnea. Parts include a base unit and a sensor. The sensor, which is placed between the endotracheal tube connector and the breathing circuit, detects temperature changes between the warm expired and cold inspired air. It emits an audible beep when the patient breathes and will sound an alarm when no breath is detected for a preset time period.

The sensor increases mechanical dead space, which can be significant, especially in small patients. For this reason, special endotracheal tube connectors are available that accommodate the sensor and minimize dead space. Although apnea monitors do not warn of inadequate respiratory depth, they may have difficulty detecting respirations if the patient's V_T is significantly decreased or the patient becomes hypothermic and will sound the apnea alarm. Consequently, as with any monitor, alarm signals must be confirmed by physical examination of the patient.

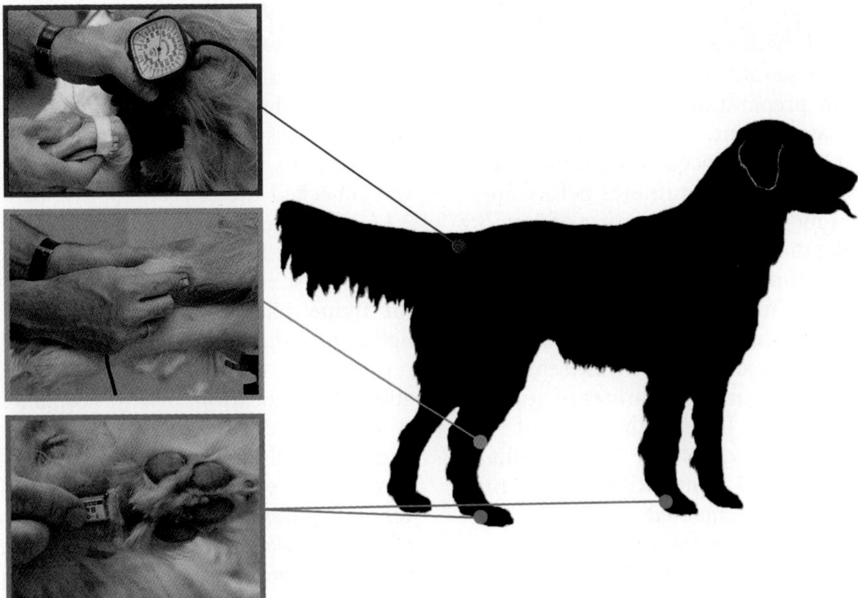

FIGURE 27-22 Locations for Doppler probe placement. *Red,* Determination of systolic blood pressure by use of a sphygmomanometer with the cuff placed around the tail base and the probe placed on the ventral surface of the tail distal to the cuff. *Green,* Probe over the dorsomedial surface of the hock. *Blue,* Probe proximal to the metatarsal pad or metacarpal pad.

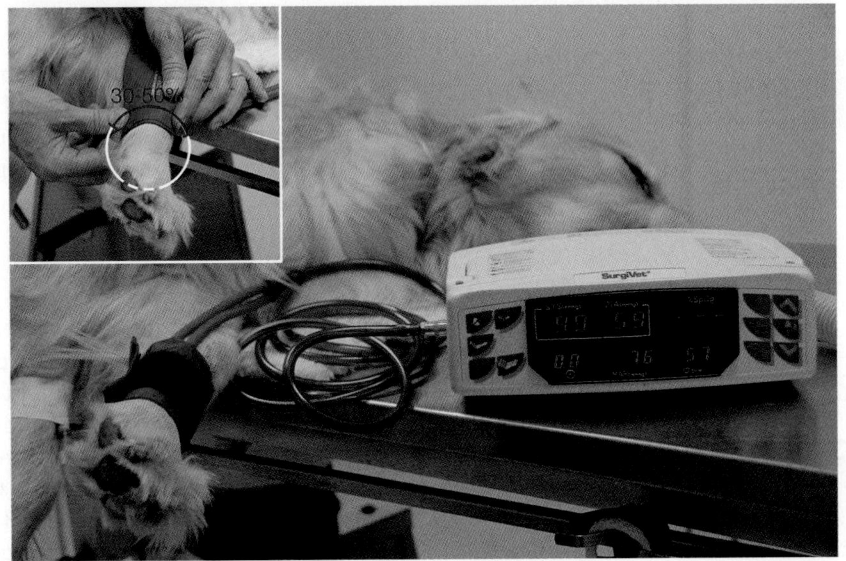

FIGURE 27-23 Oscillometric blood pressure monitor with a cuff placed on the metacarpus. The following measurements are indicated: Systolic BP: 99 mm Hg; diastolic BP: 59 mm Hg; mean arterial pressure (MAP): 76 mm Hg; HR: 57 bpm. *Inset,* Selecting an appropriately sized blood pressure cuff, the width of which should be 30% to 50% of the circumference of the extremity.

A capnograph, also known as an end-tidal CO_2 monitor (Figure 27-26), is a device that measures the level of CO_2 present in the inspired and expired air. Parts include a computerized base unit and a fitting that is placed between the endotracheal tube connector and the breathing circuit.

The capnograph enables the anesthetist to estimate the partial pressure of CO_2 in the patient's bloodstream and is one of the best indicators of adequate respiration. Because CO_2 is produced at the tissue level, carried by the vascular system, and eliminated by the lungs, abnormal readings may be caused by disease of the lungs, cardiovascular system, or tissues and equipment malfunctions.

In normal animals during inspiration, the level should be 0 mm Hg, and at the end of expiration, the level should rise to 35 to 40 mm Hg. Any change in the configuration of the curve can indicate a problem and should be explored. The interpretation of capnograph tracings is complex and beyond the scope of this chapter. The student is encouraged to explore the recommended readings for more information.

CASE PRESENTATION 27-1 ANESTHESIA OF A CANINE

Case Study: Cocoa, a 2-year-old, female, 15.2-kg spaniel mix, was anesthetized in preparation for a routine OHE. Based on preanesthetic assessment, she was classified as a physical status class P1 patient. Cocoa was premedicated with 0.1 mg/kg acepromazine IM 15 minutes before anesthetic induction and was induced with a mixture of 5 mg/kg ketamine and 0.25 mg/kg diazepam IV. After reaching surgical anesthesia, she was maintained with isoflurane at 2.5% and oxygen at a rate of 0.5 L/min. Pulse oximetry was used to monitor Cocoa via a transmission probe placed on the tongue. Following surgical preparation, she was transferred to the operating room. For the first 10 minutes of surgery, Cocoa's oxygen saturation (SpO_2) was in the range of 96% to 99%. Then over a 3-minute period, the SpO_2 gradually fell to 92%, although the HR (85 bpm), RR (8 bpm), mucous membrane color, and refill remained normal.

Normal SpO_2 for patients breathing oxygen is 95% or greater. Low SpO_2 can be caused by many factors, including preexisting disease, pulmonary edema, loss of signal, airway blockage, lack of adequate oxygen flow, and respiratory depression. When in this situation, the veterinary technician must rapidly determine whether the decrease is real or an artifact and then if real, must explore possible causes and correct the problem without delay.

The technician determined that the patient was in no immediate danger, based on assessment of the other vital signs. Preexisting disease was deemed unlikely based on this patient's medical history. She rapidly checked the airway, checked the oxygen supply, turned the oxygen up to 3 L/min and ruled out pulmonary edema based on normal lung sounds. Because pulse oximeter probe signals are frequently lost as a result of excess probe pressure, drying of the tissue, patient movement, interference from ambient light, and other factors, the technician removed the probe, rewetted the tongue, and replaced the probe with careful attention to location, orientation, and pressure.

Despite these measures, the SpO_2 remained between 90% and 93%. Although the RR was normal, careful observation revealed a V_T estimated to be less than 50% of normal. Manual ventilation was initiated with a maximum inspiratory pressure of 20 cm of water. Following the first breath, the SpO_2 rapidly returned to 96%. Intermittent positive pressure breaths were given about every 30 seconds for the first 2 minutes and then about every 5 minutes for the duration of the procedure. The oxygen saturation remained in the normal range. The case illustrates the importance of careful observation of respiratory depth during anesthesia, which in this patient was insufficient to maintain an adequate oxygen level.

TABLE 27-9 Normal Blood Pressure Values During Anesthesia

Blood Pressure Value (mm Hg)	Small Animal	Equine
Systolic	100-160	100-120
Mean	80-120	80-100
Diastolic	60-100	60-80
Minimum acceptable mean during anesthesia	60	70
Hypertension	Systolic >160	Systolic >140

PRINCIPLES OF ENDOTRACHEAL INTUBATION

Placement of an endotracheal tube offers several important advantages. It helps to maintain an open airway and allows inhalant anesthetics and oxygen to be administered precisely. It prevents pulmonary aspiration of stomach contents, blood, fluid, or other debris. It permits careful observation of RR and depth and gives the anesthetist the ability to ventilate the patient when needed. The following equipment is required to perform endotracheal intubation:

- Appropriately sized endotracheal tubes
- Hard roll gauze or IV tubing to secure the tube
- A gauze sponge to grasp the tongue
- A syringe to inflate the cuff (12 ml for small animals and 20 ml for large animals)
- A good examination light
- Some species require a laryngoscope with an appropriately sized blade
- Prepare a stylet if intubating small ruminants or swine, if using a narrow diameter tube, or if using any other tube that requires additional support
- Lidocaine to control laryngospasm (cats, small ruminants, and swine)

SELECTING A TUBE

Select a tube of appropriate diameter and length. Always prepare at least three tubes of different sizes so that you are prepared if your first choice does not fit the patient's trachea. The following rules of thumb may be used to select the diameter. Most cats require a 3- to 4.5-mm tube. The appropriate size for a dog is based on the patient's body weight. Prepare a 9-mm tube for a patient weighing 40 lb. Increase or decrease size 0.5 mm for each 5 lb body weight under or over 40 lb. In other words, prepare a 7.5-mm tube for a 25-lb patient or a 10-mm tube for a 50-lb patient. Be aware that usefulness of this rule of thumb depends on a variety of factors, including body condition and conformation, and may not apply to all patients, particularly brachycephalic breeds and small or obese animals.

Prepare a 7- to 12-mm tube for sheep and goats; a 6- to 14-mm tube for swine; a 9- to 16-mm tube for foals; a 9- to 18-mm tube for calves; and a 22- to 30-mm tube for adult horses and cattle.

Next determine if the tube is the appropriate length. The endotracheal tube should ideally extend from the tip of the nose to the thoracic inlet. If the tube is too long, one of two problems may occur. If inserted too far, the beveled end may inadvertently be advanced into only one

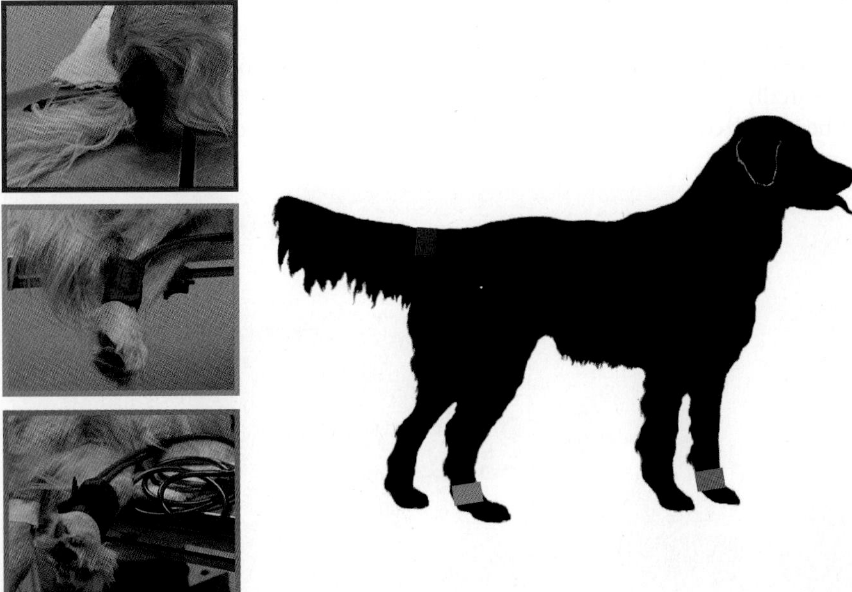

FIGURE 27-24 Locations for placement of a blood pressure cuff: *Red,* Base of the tail. *Green,* Metatarsus. *Blue,* Metacarpus.

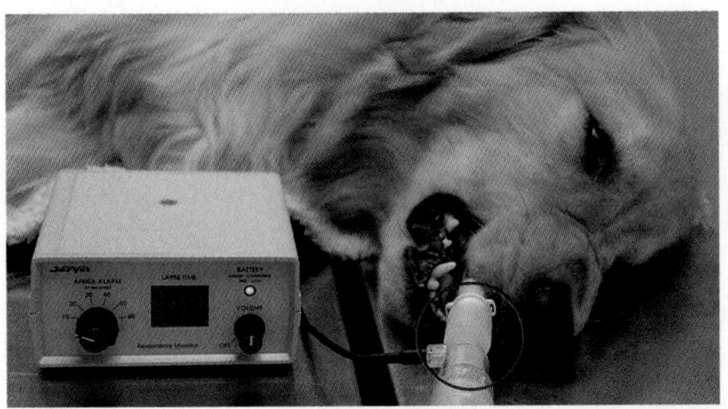

FIGURE 27-25 Apnea monitor. The probe *(circled)* is located between the breathing circuit and the endotracheal tube connector. The lapse time indicates the time in seconds since the previous breath. This alarm is set to sound if the interval between breaths exceeds 10 seconds.

main stem bronchus, thus only supplying one lung with oxygen and anesthetic. If inserted only to the thoracic inlet, the portion of the tube extending from the mouth will increase mechanical dead space. Either situation will predispose the patient to hypoventilation and hypoxia. If it is too short, it may not be long enough to reach the trachea.

Dead space is defined as the breathing passages and tubes that convey fresh oxygen to the alveoli but in which no gas exchange can occur. Increased dead space decreases the amount of fresh air that reaches the alveoli and is therefore available to the patient. Mechanical dead space is produced by the Y-piece, the portion of the endotracheal tube extending beyond the mouth, and anything placed between these structures, such as an apnea or capnograph monitor sensor, whereas anatomic dead space includes the mouth, nasal passages, pharynx, trachea, and bronchi. It is to the patient's advantage to decrease dead space as much as possible.

PREPARING THE TUBE

Check each tube for blockages, holes, or other damage. Check to be sure that the connector is securely attached and check the cuff by inflating it. If intact, the cuff should remain inflated after detaching the syringe from the valve. If the tube is soft or narrow, use a stylet that does *not* extend beyond the end of the tube to stiffen it during placement. The tube can be lubricated with a small amount of sterile water-soluble lubricant or with the patient's saliva immediately before placement.

> TECHNICIAN NOTE Before placing an endotracheal tube, check the length, diameter, and cuff. Be sure that the connector is not loose and the tube is not damaged or blocked with dried mucus.

Successful endotracheal tube placement requires knowledge of the anatomy of the pharynx and larynx including the glottis, epiglottis, vocal folds, and soft palate (Figure 27-27, *B* and *C*). Proper restraint, positioning, and visualization are also critical to success. The induction agent must be administered until the patient is in a state of readiness for intubation. Readiness for intubation is characterized by unconsciousness, a lack of voluntary movement, sufficient muscle relaxation to allow the mouth to be held open, and absent pedal and swallowing reflexes.

INTUBATION PROCEDURES

Intubation Procedure for Small Animals (see Figure 27-27)

- Place the patient in sternal recumbency.
- Have an assistant grasp the maxilla behind the canine teeth, extend the neck, and raise the head.
- Grasp the tongue with a gauze sponge and open the mouth fully by firmly pulling the tongue out and down.

- Adjust the light so that you have good illumination of the larynx.
- If necessary, use the tube or laryngoscope to gently displace the epiglottis ventrally or the soft palate dorsally until the glottis can be visualized (see Figure 27-27, *C*).
- Gently insert the tube past the vocal folds using a rotating motion. If the tube is too large to pass easily, change the tube for one of smaller diameter, but *never force the tube.*
- After the tube is placed, gently transfer the patient into lateral recumbency.

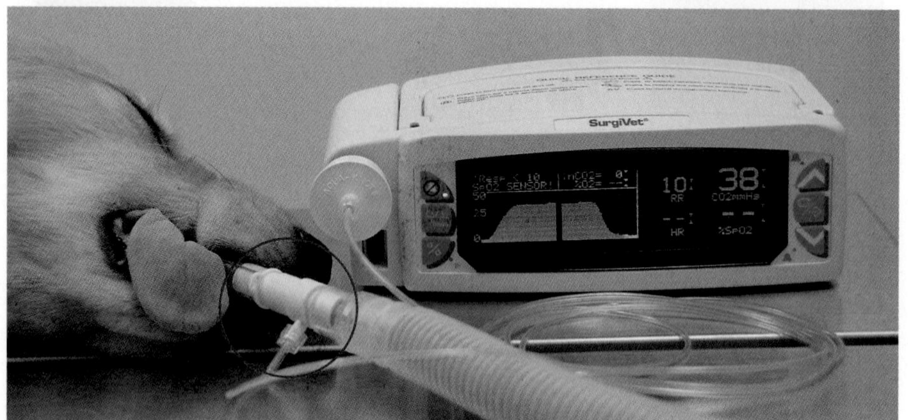

FIGURE 27-26 Capnograph registering an end-tidal CO_2 level of 38 mm Hg and a RR of 10 bpm *(upper right).* The sensor *(circled)* is located between the breathing circuit and the endotracheal tube connector. The graph indicates the CO_2 levels throughout the respiratory cycle, which in normal patients is 35 to 40 mm Hg during expiration and 0 mm Hg during inspiration.

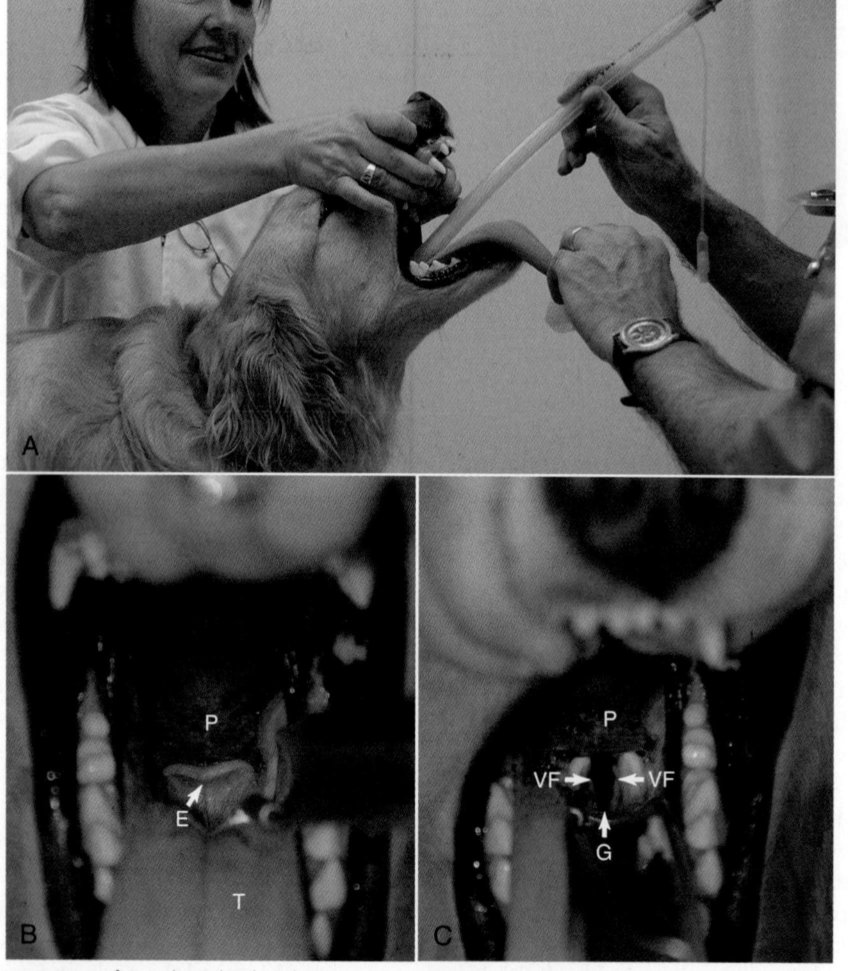

FIGURE 27-27 **A,** Proper position for endotracheal intubation in a small animal. **B,** The anatomy of the pharynx and larynx: *P,* palate; *T,* tongue; *E,* epiglottis, which in this view is covering the glottis. **C,** In this view, the epiglottis has been displaced ventrally with a laryngoscope. The glottis *(G)* is visible as the dark, oval opening between the vocal folds *(VF),* which move apart when the patient inspires and relax as the patient expires.

- Check the tube to ensure that it is in the appropriate distance and is oriented to match the natural curve of the trachea.
- Secure the tube with roll gauze or used IV tubing (over the nose for dolichocephalic dogs and behind the head for cats and brachycephalic dogs). Be sure that the tie is secure enough not to slip, but does not compress the tube.
- Connect the tube connector to the breathing circuit.
- Inflate the cuff and check for leaks.
- Ensure a patent airway by checking the position of the patient and tube. The neck and tube should assume a gentle natural curve.

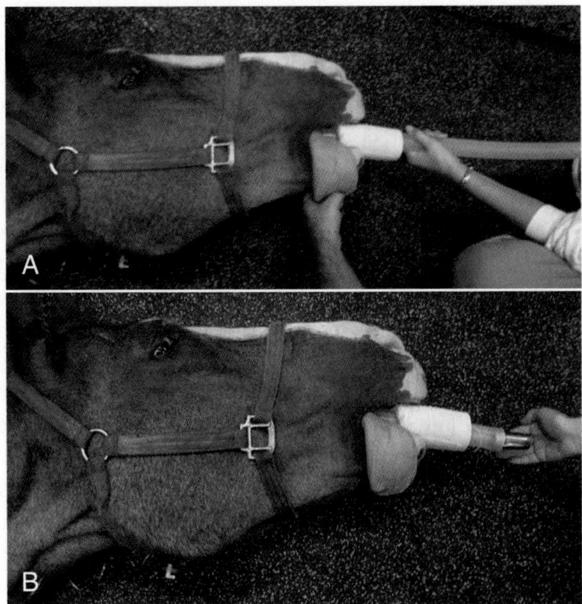

FIGURE 27-28 Equine intubation. **A,** The anesthetist advances the endotracheal tube blindly through a speculum in the mouth and into the larynx with the head extended. **B,** The anesthetist feels for movement of air when the horse breathes out to confirm correct placement of the tube in the trachea.

Intubation Procedure for Horses (Figure 27-28)

Endotracheal intubation is performed blindly in this species because the larynx is impossible to see.

- Extend the head to line up the mouth, oropharynx, and larynx.
- Place a speculum or mouth gag.
- Advance the tube over the tongue taking care to stay in the center of the oropharynx so that the molar teeth do not damage the cuff.
- During inspiration, advance the tube *gently.*
- If resistance is encountered, stop and pull the tube back 10 to 15 cm.
- Repeat if unsuccessful, each time rotating the tube 90 degrees.
- Once the tube passes easily into the larynx and trachea, check for correct replacement by feeling air passing out of the tube on expiration. If the horse is apneic, pressure on the thorax will produce the same effect.

It may be helpful to apply gentle pressure externally on the larynx (cricoid pressure) or to flex then reextend the head if intubation is difficult.

Intubation Procedure for Adult Cattle (Figure 27-29)

Endotracheal intubation is also performed blindly in this species.

- Place a speculum or mouth gag.
- Extend the head and neck.
- Insert your arm in the mouth.
- Palpate, then reflect the epiglottis forward.
- Remove your arm and grasp the endotracheal tube with the beveled end protected in your palm.
- Guide the tube into the larynx using the hand that is in the mouth while using your other hand to advance the tube into the trachea.

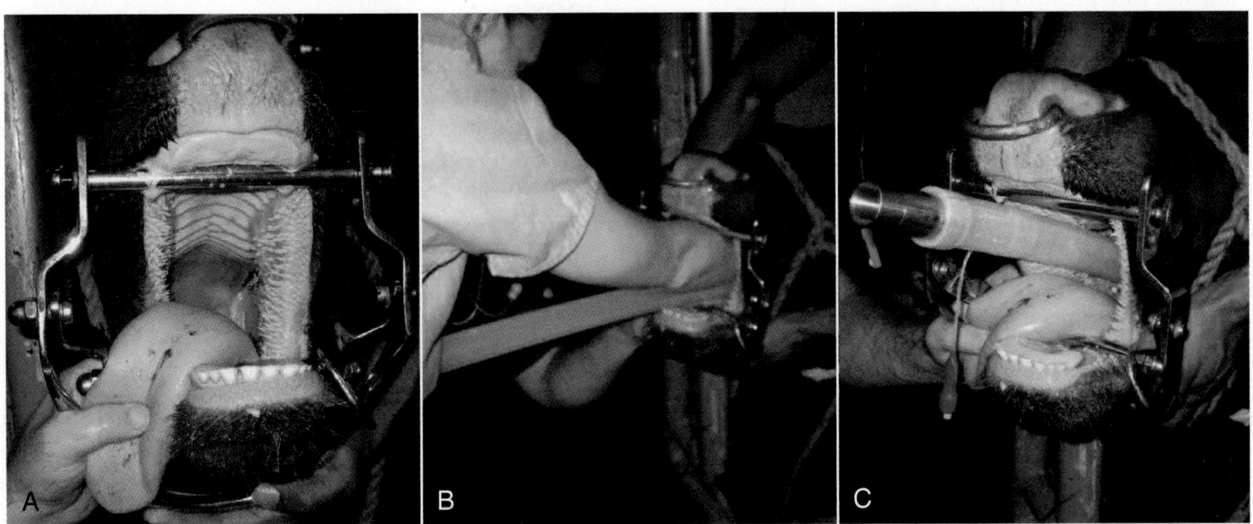

FIGURE 27-29 Bovine intubation. **A,** A mouth gag is placed and the head extended by an assistant. **B,** The anesthetist palpates the larynx with her fingers and directs the endotracheal tube into the trachea. **C,** With the tube in place, the cuff can be inflated and the mouth gag removed.

Intubation Procedure for Small Ruminants and Small or Young Cattle

These patients are intubated using a similar technique to SA patients. The oral cavity is long and narrow in these animals, so visualization of the larynx requires use of a laryngoscope with a long blade and a stylet.

- Extend the head and neck.
- Hold the mouth open.
- Gently pull the tongue down and out by grasping it with a gauze sponge.
- Insert a stylet that protrudes from the patient end of the endotracheal tube to facilitate intubation.
- Once the larynx is visualized, insert the stylet no more than 2 to 5 cm into the trachea.
- Holding the stylet firmly in position, pass the tube over the stylet into the larynx.

Because of limited space in the mouth, it may be necessary to remove the laryngoscope while passing the endotracheal tube. Goats may develop laryngospasm, so topical lidocaine may be used to desensitize the larynx before intubation. It is imperative to inflate the cuff as soon as the patient is intubated to prevent aspiration of regurgitated material or saliva.

CHECKING FOR PROPER PLACEMENT

An endotracheal tube can be easily misplaced in the esophagus and therefore may appear to be correctly placed when it is not. This will result in an inability to keep the patient anesthetized. Therefore confirmation of proper placement is essential. The following techniques may be used to confirm proper placement:

- Revisualize the larynx to confirm successful intubation (dogs, cats, and small ruminants).
- Watch for expansion and contraction of the reservoir bag as the animal breathes.
- Feel for air movement from the tube connector as the patient exhales.
- Check that the motion of the unidirectional valves coincides with breathing.
- Palpate the neck. The only naturally firm structure in the neck is the trachea. If the tube is properly placed, only one firm structure should be palpable. Palpation of two firm structures (the tube and the trachea) indicates placement of the tube inside the esophagus.
- If the patient can vocalize (whine or cry), it is not in the correct location (this most commonly applies to dogs).
- Although a cough reflex during intubation is indicative of proper placement, not all patients exhibit this sign.

CUFF INFLATION

The cuff of the endotracheal tube must be gently inflated until a seal is formed between the trachea and the cuff. This will prevent leakage of anesthetic gases and mixing with room air, which will result in a variety of complications, including contamination of the surgery suite with waste gases and difficulty keeping the patient asleep. To inflate the cuff, extend the patient's head to straighten the airway. Attach an air-filled syringe to the valve port. Have an assistant close the pop-off valve and gently compress the reservoir bag. Listen for gas leakage around the tube, which may sound like a soft hiss or gurgling. Slowly inflate the cuff until the leaking just ceases at pressures under 20 cm of water. Avoid overinflation of the cuff, which can result in a variety of mild to serious complications.

LARYNGOSPASM

Laryngospasm is a complication in which the glottis forcibly closes during intubation. This complication is most commonly encountered in cats, swine, and small ruminants. It is extremely difficult to place a tube in a patient experiencing laryngospasm because the glottis closes as soon as it is touched and cannot be safely forced open. Laryngospasm can lead to hypoxia and cyanosis in severe cases, but is prevented using one or more of the following strategies:

- Apply 2% injectable lidocaine via a syringe directly to the glottis before placement. Wait 30 to 60 seconds for the lidocaine to take effect before attempting intubation; 0.1 ml is appropriate for cats, whereas 1 to 2 ml can be used in sheep, goats, and pigs.
- Be sure that the patient is adequately anesthetized before attempting intubation because laryngospasm decreases with increasing depth of anesthesia.
- Prepare carefully, wait for the glottis to open before attempting placement, and try to get the tube in the first time. Repeat attempts worsen laryngospasm.
- *Do not force the tube.* This can lead to severe and potentially life-threatening complications, including tracheal rupture, pneumothorax, and pneumomediastinum.

COMPLICATIONS OF INTUBATION (BOX 27-5)

There are a number of hazards associated with endotracheal intubation. Most are associated with tracheal irritation, trauma, or failure to protect the airway. Although the larynx and trachea of mammals are relatively resilient structures, excessive force will result in damage, perforation, rupture, or irritation of the delicate mucosa. An endotracheal tube must therefore be chosen, maintained, placed, and monitored with care.

SMALL ANIMAL ANESTHESIA

A successful anesthetic procedure requires not only careful preparation, but also a good understanding of the sequence of events involved in taking a patient from consciousness to surgical anesthesia and back to consciousness. Box 27-6 summarizes these events when inducing an SA patient with injectable agents and maintaining with an inhalant agent.

BOX 27-5 Complications of Endotracheal Intubation

Cuff Not Inflated/Underinflated
- Inability to create a seal between the cuff and trachea
- Difficulty or inability to keep the patient anesthetized
- Aspiration of stomach contents
- Aspiration of foreign material and fluid during dental cleaning
- Pollution of the work space with anesthetic gas

Tube Diameter Too Small
- Inability to create a seal between the cuff and trachea leading to the same complications listed earlier
- Small tubes are more likely to block with mucus
- Increased resistance to breathing with increased respiratory effort

Cuff Overinflated/Tube Diameter Too Large
- Necrosis of the tracheal mucosa
- Possibility of tracheal rupture in extreme situations

Tube Too Long
- If placed past the thoracic inlet, intubation of only one main stem bronchus leading to hypoxia and difficulty in keeping the patient anesthetized
- If extending beyond the mouth, increased mechanical dead space leading to hypoventilation and hypoxia

Tube Too Short
- Inability to intubate the patient successfully
- Changes in patient position may dislodge the tube from the glottis

Overzealous Intubation
- Tracheal irritation leading to tracheitis and postoperative cough
- Trauma or tracheal rupture resulting in pneumomediastinum and/or pneumothorax

Tube Kinked or Obstructed
- Dyspnea and hypoxia
- Asphyxia and cardiac arrest if not corrected

Tube Not Removed Before Return to Consciousness
- Damage to the tube from chewing
- Blockage of the airway
- In extreme situations, a severed portion of the tube can be aspirated or swallowed

Tube Not Cleaned and Disinfected
- Transmission of infectious agents leading to tracheitis, bronchitis, or pneumonia
- Blockage of the tube with dried mucus or other foreign material

SELECTING A PROTOCOL

An anesthetic protocol is a list of the premedications and anesthetics for a particular patient including dosages, routes, and order of administration. Anesthetic protocols are commonly selected by the veterinarian in charge based on training and clinical experience. A suitable protocol takes into account the patient signalment, preexisting problems, the physical status class, and the procedure to be performed (see Box 27-7 for sample protocols used in physical status class P1 and P2 dogs and Box 27-8 for sample protocols used in physical status class P1 and P2 cats).

After the protocol is known, calculate all drug dosages, oxygen flow rates, and fluid administration rates and check them *carefully* because most anesthetic agents have narrow therapeutic indices and can easily be overdosed.

> *TECHNICIAN NOTE* The volume (in milliliters) of each injectable anesthetic drug to give must be calculated using extreme care. The general formula for most injectable anesthetics is as follows:
>
> **Volume** (ml) = **Drug dosage** (mg or μg/kg or lb body wt) ×
> **Patient body weight** (kg or lb) ÷
> **Drug concentration** (mg or μg/ml)

Note: When performing this calculation, drug dosage and body weight units must be the same (kg or lb) as must the drug dosage and drug concentration units (mg or μg).

Physical status class P3 to P5 patients require use of modified protocols based on the patient's primary condition (Table 27-10). Management of these cases can be quite challenging and requires customization of the anesthetic protocol by the veterinarian in charge.

EQUIPMENT PREPARATION

During a typical anesthetic induction, anesthetic agents are administered; the patient becomes unconscious and recumbent; the endotracheal tube is placed, secured, cuffed, and attached to the machine; the anesthetic gas level is adjusted; the patient is positioned and monitored; and adjustments are made as needed all within the first few minutes of the procedure. Because these events follow one another so rapidly, the technician has little to no time to leave the patient to locate necessary equipment. Consequently, all equipment must be carefully gathered, checked, and organized before commencing the procedure.

THE PREANESTHETIC PERIOD

The preanesthetic period is the time before induction of general anesthesia. During this period, a physical assessment is performed, the patient history and results of laboratory tests are reviewed, the patient is stabilized, an IV catheter is placed, and fluid administration is started. Premedications, including tranquilizers, α_2-agonists, opioids, dissociatives,

BOX 27-6 Sequence of Events for a Small Animal Anesthetic Procedure (Induction With an IV Agent and Maintenance With an Inhalant Agent)

1. Assess, prepare, and weigh the patient (see Part II: Patient Preparation for a discussion of patient assessment, preparation, and stabilization).
2. Determine the protocol (anesthetic agents including dosages, routes, and sequence of administration).
3. Calculate the volume of each agent to give, including fluid administration rates (preanesthetic, induction, maintenance, and analgesic agents).
4. Calculate the oxygen flow rates (see Box 27-3).
5. Prepare equipment required to administer drugs (scales, syringes, needles, agents, reversal agents, emergency cart, controlled substance log).
6. Prepare fluid administration equipment (clippers, antiseptic scrub, catheters, tape, heparinized saline, catheter cap, administration-extension set, fluids).
7. Prepare equipment for endotracheal intubation (see Part VI: Principles of Endotracheal Intubation for an equipment list).
8. Prepare monitoring equipment including anesthesia record, stethoscope, monitors, and probes (see Part V: Anesthetic Monitoring for a discussion of monitoring equipment).
9. Assemble and test the anesthetic machine (see Part IV: Anesthetic Equipment for a discussion of these procedures).
10. Administer premedications approximately 15-20 min IM or 5-10 min IV before anesthetic induction.
11. Place an IV catheter, attach the fluid administration set, and begin fluid administration.
12. Administer the induction agent.
13. Check the patient's readiness for intubation.
14. Place and secure the endotracheal tube (see Part VI: Principles of Endotracheal Intubation for a discussion of this procedure).
15. Turn on the oxygen and connect the endotracheal tube to the breathing circuit.
16. Check the patient's vital signs.
17. Turn on the inhalant anesthetic to the appropriate level.
18. Determine the patient's anesthetic depth and commence regular monitoring.
19. Position and secure the patient for the procedure with attention to padding, maintenance of an open airway, unrestricted blood flow, and unrestricted chest excursions.
20. Attach monitoring devices.
21. Continue to monitor and adjust the anesthetic and oxygen levels as needed until completion of the procedure.
22. Prepare the patient for recovery.
23. Discontinue the anesthetic and extubate the patient at the appropriate time.
24. Remove monitoring equipment, IV catheters, and any other equipment no longer needed.
25. Prepare the patient for continued hospitalization or discharge by applying bandages, administering medications, and performing any other procedures ordered by the veterinarian.

BOX 27-7 Protocols for Premedication, Sedation, and General Anesthesia in Physical Status Class P1 and P2 Dogs

Protocols for Mild to Moderate Sedation or for Premedication

1. Acepromazine: 0.05-0.1 mg/kg IM with a maximum dose of 3 mg (not for use in old or debilitated patients or in sensitive breeds).
2. Medetomidine: 0.003-0.005 mg/kg IM (equivalent to 3-5 μg/kg).
3. Midazolam 0.2 mg/kg IM and butorphanol 0.2 mg/kg IM. (Can add glycopyrrolate 0.01 mg/kg or atropine 0.04 mg/kg to this mixture. Halve the doses for IV administration.)

Protocols for Moderate to Heavy Sedation (for Minor Procedures, Such as Radiography or Grooming) or for Premedication

1. "BAG" (butorphanol 0.2 mg/kg, acepromazine 0.05 mg/kg, and glycopyrrolate 0.005 mg/kg mixed in one syringe and given IM or IV).
   (As an alternative, mix 1 ml acepromazine, 4 ml butorphanol (10 mg/ml), and 5 ml glycopyrrolate and give this mixture in a volume of 0.5 ml/10-20 lb of body weight.)
2. Medetomidine 0.01-0.02 mg/kg IM and butorphanol 0.2-0.4 mg/kg IM *(Note: Can use hydromorphone 0.1 mg/kg in place of butorphanol).*
3. Medetomidine 0.03 mg/kg IM and ketamine 3 mg/kg IM. *(Halve the doses for IV administration. Do not reverse the medetomidine until at least 40 min later.)*
4. Telazol 4 mg/kg IM or IV to effect (for aggressive patients).

Protocols for Anesthetic Induction

1. Ketamine 5 mg/kg IV and diazepam* 0.25 mg/kg IV mixed in the same syringe. (This is equivalent to 1 ml of the mixture/20 lb of body weight.) *Butorphanol at a dose of 0.1-0.2 mg/kg can be added for additional analgesia.*
   **Note: An equivalent volume of midazolam can be used in place of diazepam.*
2. Propofol 6-8 mg/kg IV to effect if not premedicated or 2-4 mg/kg IV following premedication.
3. Thiopental sodium 4-8 mg/kg IV to effect following premedication or 10-15 mg/kg if not premedicated *(note that administration without premedication is not recommended).*
4. Isoflurane 4%-5% or sevoflurane 6%-8% by mask or chamber.
5. Etomidate 1-3 mg/kg to effect.

Protocols for Anesthetic Maintenance

1. Isoflurane 1.5%-2.5% or sevoflurane 2.5%-4%
2. Propofol 0.2-0.4 mg/kg/min by constant rate infusion or by repeat boluses to effect every 3-5 min.

BOX 27-8 Protocols for Premedication, Sedation, and General Anesthesia in Physical Status Class P1 and P2 Cats

Protocols for Mild to Moderate Sedation or Premedication

1. Acepromazine 0.05-0.1 mg/kg IM up to a maximum dose of 1 mg
2. "BAG" *(same dose as for the dog)*
3. Medetomidine: 0.01-0.04 mg/kg IM

Protocols for Moderate to Heavy Sedation (for Minor Procedures, Such as Radiography or Grooming) or for Premedication

1. Medetomidine 0.01-0.05 mg/kg IM and ketamine 5 mg/kg IM
2. Medetomidine 0.01-0.02 mg/kg IM and butorphanol 0.2 mg/kg IM
3. Ketamine 10-20 mg/kg IM (causes immobilization with muscle rigidity)
4. Telazol 4 mg/kg IM or IV to effect (for aggressive patients)

Protocols for Anesthetic Induction

(Use the same protocols as for the dog.)

Protocols for Anesthetic Maintenance

(Use the same protocols as for the dog.)

Protocols for Injectable Anesthesia

1. Medetomidine 0.06 mg/kg with ketamine 5 mg/kg and butorphanol 0.2 mg/kg IM for elective surgeries
2. "TKX"—Add 4 ml of ketamine and 1 ml 10% (LA) xylazine to 1 vial of Telazol powder. Give at a dose of 0.015 ml/kg IM. Must dose accurately.
3. Add 2.5 ml butorphanol (10 mg/ml) and 2.5 ml medetomidine to 1 vial of Telazol powder. Give at a rate of 0.015 ml/kg IM for castration and 0.02 ml/kg IM for OHE.

TABLE 27-10 Recommendations for Physical Status Class P3-P5 Small Animal Patients

Primary Condition	Example Protocols and Other Considerations	Avoid These Agents/Circumstances
Cardiac disease	Premedicate with opioids and benzodiazepines Etomidate or propofol induction Ketamine/diazepam induction acceptable except in feline patients with hypertrophic cardiomyopathy Maintain with isoflurane or sevoflurane Maintain blood pressure in normal range	Acepromazine in patients with congestive heart failure α_2-Agonists Mask/chamber induction (as a result of stress) Ketamine/Telazol Thiopental sodium without premedication
Liver disease	No premedication or use opioids if needed Preoxygenation before induction Propofol or etomidate induction if mild to moderate Mask induction if severe Maintain with isoflurane or sevoflurane Maintain blood pressure and fluid balance	Acepromazine Barbiturates
C-section	Propofol or mask induction Maintain with isoflurane or sevoflurane Epidural analgesia is helpful to reduce the need for other analgesics Minimize anesthetic time If opioids used before delivery, administer 1-2 drops of naloxone sublingually to neonates If needed to stimulate breathing, administer 1 drop doxapram sublingually to neonates	Thiopental sodium and other barbiturates α_2-Agonists Opioids before delivery
Respiratory disease	Preoxygenate and minimize stress Premedicate with opioids and benzodiazepines Any induction agent that allows rapid control of the airway and ventilation Place endotracheal tube rapidly and be prepared to ventilate if needed Maintain with isoflurane or sevoflurane	α_2-Agonists N_2O
Kidney disease	Premedicate with opioids + or − benzodiazepines Mask or propofol induction Maintain with isoflurane or sevoflurane Maintain blood pressure and fluid balance	α_2-Agonists Ketamine in blocked cats

anticholinergics, or a combination thereof, are administered to calm and prepare the patient for anesthetic induction. Premedications are chosen to produce a specific set of desired effects, such as sedation, analgesia, and muscle relaxation. Most are given IM, although some may be administered IV. Following IM injection, place the patient in a quiet but observable location for about 15 to 20 minutes for the agents to take effect before proceeding; otherwise, the patient may partially override the beneficial effects.

ANESTHETIC INDUCTION

During anesthetic induction, the patient is taken from consciousness to unconsciousness. Agents commonly used for anesthetic induction in small animals include a ketamine and diazepam mixture, thiopental sodium, propofol, etomidate, neuroleptanalgesics, and inhalant anesthetics. Except for the inhalant anesthetics, these agents are most often given IV.

IV Induction

To induce general anesthesia by the IV route, draw up the calculated volume and administer it *to effect* until you are able to intubate the patient or until the patient is at an adequate plane of anesthesia to complete the planned procedure. The term "to effect" means that the drug is administered gradually in increments until the desired stage of anesthesia is reached. The entire calculated dose may or may not be given.

Immediately after giving the patient an initial dose, check the HR and RR to be sure that the patient is stable and breathing. Remove muzzles and other restraint devices. Make sure that the patient has passed through stage II and is deep enough to intubate. While giving the drug, there must be interplay between administration of the drug and monitoring the patient. Give the initial dose; then rapidly check the vital signs, pedal reflex, palpebral reflex, and jaw tone; give more if needed; check again, etc. If the patient is light and needs more or starts to wake up while being intubated, give a much smaller amount to effect (about one fifth to one tenth of the original volume) until the patient is in an adequate plane of anesthesia. Although all are given to effect, different induction agents are given at slightly different rates.

Propofol

Give one fourth of the calculated dose every 30 seconds to effect until at an adequate depth for endotracheal intubation. Be sure to give it rapidly enough to take the patient through stage II and into stage III.

Ketamine-Diazepam or Ketamine-Midazolam

Give slowly to effect over 30 to 90 seconds.

Thiopental Sodium

In healthy patients, give one half of the calculated dose over 10 to 15 seconds, then to effect. Old, ill, and debilitated patients may need much less and require that the drug be given much more cautiously and slowly.

IM Induction

To induce anesthesia by the IM route, draw up and administer the entire calculated volume. In general, the dosage for IM injection is generally about two to three times the corresponding IV dosage. When given IM, anesthetic agents have a slower onset and longer duration than when given IV. A typical induction will take 5 to 20 minutes. After peak effect, if the patient is still too light, administer additional drug or an inhalant agent with a mask until you are able to intubate the patient. Remember that some drugs, such as propofol, thiopental sodium, and etomidate *must not* be given IM.

Mask Induction

Mask induction requires the use of a rapid-acting inhalant anesthetic, such as isoflurane, sevoflurane, or desflurane. Once induced, an endotracheal tube can be placed to maintain the patient for the duration of the procedure. Mask induction is a special challenge for several reasons. Many patients struggle necessitating skillful restraint (enough to prevent operator and patient injury, but not so much as to restrict chest excursions or the airway). It is more challenging to monitor mucous membrane color and refill and ocular indicators of anesthetic depth because the mask partially obscures the eyes and muzzle. Therefore monitor carefully and do not be lulled into the belief that the monitoring requirements are less with this method of induction than with others.

To induce a patient by mask, first attach a well-fitted mask to the breathing circuit. Hold the mask over the patient's muzzle. Administer pure oxygen for 2 to 3 minutes at the recommended rate, and then turn on the vaporizer to 0.5% to 1% for about 30 seconds to allow the patient to become accustomed to the smell of the gas. Increase the setting to 4% to 5% if using isoflurane and 6% to 8% for sevoflurane. Some clinicians recommend a gradual increase over several minutes, which allows the patient time to become accustomed to the gas. Other anesthetists increase the vaporizer setting immediately, especially if the patient is difficult to handle when using the gradual method. If the patient struggles, monitor carefully for cyanosis or other problems and be ready to act quickly if the patient becomes compromised. As soon as the patient is laterally recumbent, assess readiness for intubation and adjust the anesthetic level as appropriate. From this point on, the patient is managed much the same as for IV induction. Mask induction is generally *not* appropriate for brachycephalic breeds.

Chamber Induction

Chamber induction may be used only for patients small enough to fit comfortably into the chamber. This technique is commonly used in place of a mask for small patients that are aggressive or difficult to handle. Once induced, an endotracheal tube can be placed to maintain the patient for the duration of the procedure.

To induce a patient using this method, place the patient in the chamber, close the lid, and attach the breathing tubes of a semiclosed rebreathing system to the ports. Deliver oxygen at 5 L/min and isoflurane at 5% or sevoflurane at 8%. As soon as the patient can no longer stand, shake the chamber gently to assess the patient's mobility. When the patient is immobile enough to allow it to be safely handled, remove it from the chamber, place a mask, and proceed as with mask induction.

Patients can get into trouble easily while inside a chamber from stress, trauma, vomiting, airway blockage, or other issues. Since it is impossible to accurately assess most monitoring parameters while inside a chamber, the anesthetist must be vigilant and prepared to act quickly if the patient shows signs of compromise.

> *TECHNICIAN NOTE* Patients must be restrained and watched *carefully* during both mask and chamber inductions because they can get into trouble suddenly and unexpectedly and cannot be monitored as closely under these circumstances.

MAINTENANCE OF ANESTHESIA

Following anesthetic induction and endotracheal intubation, the patient must be maintained with injectable anesthetics, inhalant anesthetics, or a combination thereof. The goal during maintenance is to administer enough anesthetic to keep the patient in the desired plane of surgical anesthesia. This requires that the anesthetist frequently evaluate the patient watching for subtle changes and adjust the amount of anesthetic administered based on this observation.

Most patients are light immediately following intubation and must be brought into surgical anesthesia. Because inhalant anesthetics are most commonly used to maintain anesthesia, this discussion will focus on maintenance using these agents. When maintaining with inhalant agents, there is a delay effect between the time the vaporizer dial setting is changed and the change in anesthetic depth because it takes time for the new concentration to fill the breathing circuit, reach the patient's lungs, and equilibrate with the blood and tissues. The time required is influenced by a number of factors, including the patient's respiratory drive, the agent used, the carrier gas flow rate, and the volume of the breathing circuit. For this reason, vaporizer setting adjustments must be anticipated as much as possible through close monitoring. In general, if a patient is significantly light or deep, larger dial changes are indicated, whereas if the patient is slightly too light or deep, more subtle changes are needed. Familiarity with appropriate dial changes is acquired through experience.

IV maintenance agents, such as propofol, may be used to maintain general anesthesia by administering repeat boluses every few minutes to effect or by constant infusion via a syringe pump. A syringe pump is a device that automatically delivers the drug through an IV line at a calculated infusion rate.

PATIENT POSITIONING, COMFORT, AND SAFETY

Below are some considerations that must be observed throughout both the anesthetic induction and maintenance periods.

- Prevent patient trauma by supporting the patient's body as consciousness is lost.
- When using an IV agent for induction: as soon as the patient is intubated, remove the needle and syringe to prevent accidental overdose.
- Following intubation, lay the patient in lateral recumbency and secure and cuff the tube.
- Before surgery begins, check the tube for proper placement and cuff inflation.
- Check the endotracheal tube for kinks or bends. An open airway must be maintained at all times.
- Temporarily disconnect the endotracheal tube from the breathing circuit while turning the patient to prevent trauma to the trachea caused by torsion of the tube.
- Support the corrugated breathing tubes so that they do not exert traction on the endotracheal tube.
- Place the patient in a position that is as normal as possible during the procedure without hyperflexion or hyperextension of the neck or limbs.
- Do not compress the chest with restraint devices or instruments.
- Place the patient on a heat-retaining surface, such as a warm-water circulating blanket. Do *not* use an electric heating pad, which can burn the patient.
- Do not restrict blood flow by overtightening leg restraint ropes.
- Place sterile lubricant in the eyes every 90 minutes.
- If one lung is diseased, place the normal side up to maximize oxygen exchange.
- Avoid more than a 15-degree elevation of the caudal aspect of the body to prevent pressure on the diaphragm.

ANESTHETIC RECOVERY

The recovery period is the period of time between discontinuation of the anesthetic and the time when the patient is able to walk without assistance. Many factors affect recovery including the length of the procedure, the anesthetic protocol, patient condition, body temperature, and patient signalment.

Preparation for Recovery

Upon completion of the procedure, transfer the patient to a recovery area where it can be extubated and monitored. Turn off the inhalant anesthetic, but continue oxygen administration at a rate of 200 ml/kg/min (1 L/5 kg body weight up to a maximum of 5 L/min) for 5 minutes after discontinuation of the anesthetic or until the animal swallows. If the patient is light and must be extubated, administer oxygen by mask or place an oxygen source close to the nose for 5 minutes. Remove all ties, catheters, monitoring devices, and other unnecessary equipment. Keep the patient warm. Turn the patient at least every 10 to 15 minutes.

Monitoring During Recovery

During recovery, the patient must be watched on a continual basis at close range. Put the patient in the cage in a position that allows observation of the mucous membranes and respirations, but never leave the patient in an open cage or on a table unattended because a recovering patient may fall and be injured. Monitor at least every 5 minutes paying particular attention to vital signs. Watch for and report unusual signs, such as vomiting or hemorrhage.

> *TECHNICIAN NOTE* Many anesthetic accidents occur during recovery. Monitor at close range and do not let down your guard. Never leave a patient unattended on a table or in an open cage because patients may awake rapidly, chew the tube, fall, or be injured.

Signs of Recovery

During recovery, gently comfort and reassure the patient. Recovery may be hastened through gentle stimulation by talking softly to the patient, rubbing or patting the chest, and by turning the patient. Gentle movement of the endotracheal tube will stimulate breathing.

As the patient recovers, it will progress back through the stages and planes of anesthesia. Passage through stage II during recovery may result in a variety of alarming signs, including excitement, vocalization, hyperventilation, and head thrashing. Be prepared to prevent self-trauma if the recovery is unusually violent or stormy.

Extubation

To prepare the patient for extubation, deflate the cuff by drawing out all the air until the pilot balloon is empty. Untie the tube to prepare for rapid removal. Both before and following removal, keep the neck in a natural but extended position to protect the airway. Remove the endotracheal tube gently when the swallowing reflex returns using a slow, steady motion. You may also remove it when signs of imminent arousal are present, such as voluntary movement of the limbs or head, movement of the tongue, or chewing. Delay extubation in brachycephalic dogs until the patient is able to lift its head unassisted.

The Postanesthetic Period

Following recovery, most SA patients should be given nothing by mouth for the first hour or two and no food for at least several hours. Upon discharge, instruct the client to reintroduce water gradually after arriving home and feed a small meal after several hours. Exceptions to these rules include small and neonatal patients, which require shorter withholding times. Monitor the patient for signs of pain and administer analgesics as prescribed.

EQUINE ANESTHESIA

All of the basic principles discussed under SA anesthesia apply to anesthesia of the horse. Additional challenges for the equine anesthetist include the temperament and physical size of the patient, the effects of inhalant anesthetics on cardiorespiratory physiology, and management of recovery. As with SA anesthesia, a successful anesthetic procedure requires careful preparation and a good understanding of the sequence of events involved in taking a horse from consciousness to surgical anesthesia and back to consciousness. Box 27-9 summarizes these events when inducing a horse with injectable agents and maintaining with an inhalant agent.

SELECTING A PROTOCOL

As for SA anesthesia, protocols are commonly selected by the veterinarian in charge. A suitable protocol takes into account the patient signalment, preexisting problems, the physical status class, and the procedure to be performed (see Box 27-10 for sample protocols used in physical status class P1 and P2 horses). After the protocol is known, calculate all drug dosages, oxygen flow rates, and fluid administration rates and check them *carefully*.

Physical status class P3 to P5 patients require use of modified protocols based on the primary condition (Table 27-11).

EQUIPMENT PREPARATION

It is critical in equine anesthesia to be prepared and check equipment before use, including any hoists and hydraulic tables that are to be used for lifting and positioning horses. Recovery pads, ropes, and other equipment, if used, should be organized before induction, if possible.

THE PREANESTHETIC PERIOD

The preanesthetic procedure in horses differs slightly from small animals. After appropriate patient assessment, the first step is placement of an IV catheter, almost always in one of the jugular veins. Some horses object to venipuncture and must be sedated first. Xylazine IV or IM is commonly used for this purpose. Once the horse is cooperative, a small bleb of local anesthetic is administered over the proposed site of catheterization to desensitize the skin.

Following catheterization, the horse's mouth should be rinsed out using a dose syringe placed between the cheek and teeth on each side of the mouth to flush out any feed material. This prevents aspiration of the material during intubation or in recovery. Feet should be cleaned before sedation, and then shoes should be removed or wrapped. Just before or immediately after premedication, the horse is positioned in an induction area or placed adjacent to a tilt table. Some horses startle easily in a strange environment,

BOX 27-9 Sequence of Events for an Equine Anesthetic Procedure (Induction With an IV Agent and Maintenance With an Inhalant Agent)

1. Assess, prepare, and weigh the patient (see Part II: Patient Preparation for a discussion of patient assessment, preparation, and stabilization).
2. Prepare equipment for and place IV catheter, which may require IM sedation in some horses (clippers, local anesthetic, antiseptic scrub, catheters, tape, heparinized saline, suture material, catheter cap, and/or extension line with three-way stopcock).
3. Rinse the horse's mouth, clean the hooves, and remove or wrap shoes when appropriate.
4. Determine the protocol (anesthetic agents including dosages, routes, and sequence of administration).
5. Calculate the volume of each agent to give including fluid administration rates (preanesthetic, induction, maintenance, and analgesic agents).
6. Review oxygen flow rates (see Box 27-3).
7. Prepare equipment required to administer drugs (scales, syringes, needles, agents, reversal agents, emergency cart, controlled substance log).
8. Prepare fluid administration equipment (fluids, administration-extension set, syringe pump, tape, heparinized saline).
9. Prepare equipment for endotracheal intubation (see Part VI: Principles of Endotracheal Intubation for an equipment list).
10. Prepare monitoring equipment including arterial catheterization materials, anesthesia record, monitors, and probes (see Part V: Anesthetic Monitoring for a discussion of monitoring equipment).
11. Assemble and test the anesthetic machine and ventilator (see Part IV: Anesthetic Equipment and Part X: Manual and Mechanical Ventilation for a discussion of these procedures).
12. Administer premedications approximately 20-30 min IM or 5-10 min IV before anesthetic induction.
13. If the horse is adequately sedate, administer the induction agent; otherwise, give additional sedation.
14. Check the patient's readiness for intubation.
15. Place and secure the endotracheal tube (see Part VI: Principles of Endotracheal Intubation for a discussion of this procedure).
16. Check the patient's vital signs.
17. Hoist, position, and secure the patient for the procedure with attention to padding of the face and lower limbs if the horse is in lateral recumbency, maintenance of an open airway, unrestricted blood flow, and unrestricted chest excursions.
18. Remove the halter.
19. Turn on the oxygen and connect the endotracheal tube to the breathing circuit.
20. Turn on the inhalant anesthetic to the appropriate level.
21. Determine the patient's anesthetic depth and commence regular monitoring.
22. Attach monitoring devices, including placement of an arterial catheter.
23. Continue to monitor and adjust the anesthetic and oxygen levels as needed until completion of the procedure.
24. Prepare the patient for recovery, including placement of a nasopharyngeal tube and removal of monitoring equipment, and ensure the recovery area has been prepared.
25. Discontinue the anesthetic and transfer the horse to the recovery area, paying attention to positioning.
26. Extubate the patient at the appropriate time and ensure the horse can breath through its nostrils without obstruction.
27. Assist the horse until it stands as directed by the veterinarian.
28. Prepare the patient for continued hospitalization or discharge by applying bandages, administering medications, and performing any other procedures ordered by the veterinarian.

BOX 27-10 Protocols for Premedication, Sedation, and General Anesthesia in Physical Status Class P1 and P2 Horses

Protocols for Mild to Moderate Sedation

1. Acepromazine: 0.03-0.05 mg/kg IV or IM (not for use in debilitated patients, or in breeding stallions)
2. Xylazine: 0.1-0.3 mg/kg IV
3. Detomidine: 0.005-0.01 mg/kg IV
4. Butorphanol: 0.02-0.05 mg/kg can be combined in the same syringe with any one of the sedatives listed above and given IV for additional sedation

Protocols for Moderate to Heavy Sedation (for Minor Procedures, Such as Wound Débridement, Radiography) or for Premedication

1. Xylazine: 1.1 mg/kg IV
2. Detomidine: 0.01-0.02 mg/kg IV
3. Romifidine: 0.05-0.1mg/kg IV
4. Butorphanol: 0.05-0.2 mg/kg IV can be added to any of the α_2-agonists listed previously to provide neuroleptanalgesia
5. Morphine: 0.05-0.1 mg/kg IV can be added to any of the α_2-agonists listed previously to provide neuroleptanalgesia

Protocols for Anesthetic Induction

1. Ketamine 2.2 mg/kg IV
2. Guaifenesin IV to effect followed by ketamine 2.2 mg/kg IV
3. Diazepam 0.03-0.05 mg/kg IV with ketamine 2.2 mg/kg IV *(midazolam can be used in place of diazepam)*
4. Guaifenesin IV to effect followed by thiopental 3.5 mg/kg *(postinduction apnea is common with thiopental)*

Protocols for Anesthetic Maintenance

1. Isoflurane 1.5%-2.5% or sevoflurane 2.5%-4%
2. "Triple drip" IV to effect: 500 mg ketamine and 250 mg xylazine are added to 500 ml of 5% guaifenesin. The mixture is then administered at 1-2 ml/kg/hr.

and some breeds (such as Arabians and thoroughbreds) have a higher drug tolerance. An excited horse should never be induced to anesthesia because this will increase the anesthetic maintenance requirement. This may result in difficulty keeping the patient anesthetized as a result of high levels of circulating catecholamines, requiring dangerously deep levels of anesthesia. Sedation is considered to be adequate when the horse's head (and lower lip) droops, the horse no longer pays attention to its surroundings, and the horse demonstrates a wide-based stance or reluctance to move (Figure 27-30).

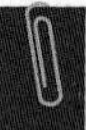

TECHNICIAN NOTE *Never* induce anesthesia in a horse that is not adequately sedated.

TABLE 27-11 Recommendations for Physical Status Class P3-P5 Equine Patients

Primary Condition	Example Protocols and Other Considerations	Avoid These Agents/ Circumstances
Colic	Premedicate with xylazine to effect Induce with a ketamine-based protocol Maintain blood pressure in normal range	Acepromazine Thiopental
C-section	Premedicate with xylazine to effect Induce with ketamine Maintain with isoflurane or sevoflurane Epidural analgesia is helpful to reduce the need for other analgesics Minimize anesthetic time Monitor oxygenation	Thiopental sodium Opioids before delivery

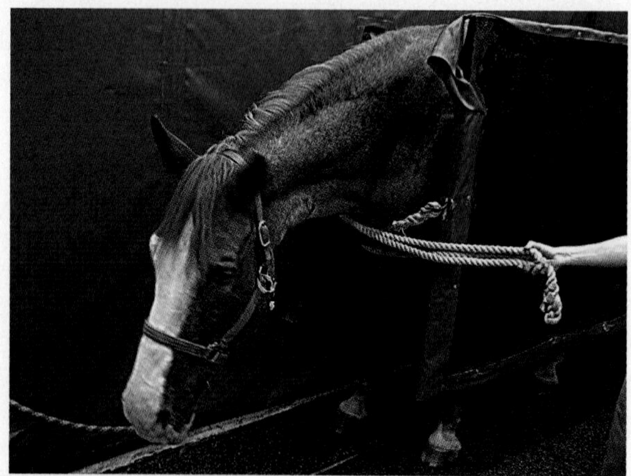

FIGURE 27-30 The horse is positioned behind a gate, which is secured to the fixed wall of the induction stall with a rope. Note the relatively wide-based stance and lowered head position. The horse is also not particularly interested in its surroundings. This indicates that the horse is adequately sedate before induction.

ANESTHETIC INDUCTION

Horses are generally induced to anesthesia by administering drugs intravenously.

IV Induction

Induction typically occurs in a special induction stall that has padded walls and often a padded floor. Induction may be done "free fall" or behind a gate that restrains the horse. Sometimes the induction stall is also used for recovery. In comparison with small animals where IV induction is given to effect, the goal of induction in horses is to rapidly take the horse from standing (sedated) to lateral recumbency (unconscious) so as to minimize excitement, which can lead to the horse injuring itself or personnel. All drugs are thus given as a bolus with the exception of the muscle relaxant guaifenesin, which is administered rapidly intravenously to effect by placing it in a pressure bag. Once the horse shows signs of ataxia, typically knuckling of the forelimbs at the fetlocks, the induction agent is given as a bolus.

Once the horse has been induced, the vital signs should be briefly checked. The horse is then intubated (see Figure 27-28, *A* and *B*).

In some practices, the floor of the induction stall forms part of the surgery table, but in many, the horse must be hoisted onto a table (Figure 27-31, *A*). It is important to understand how the hoist functions so that the horse can be transported safely and any problems can be resolved rapidly.

It is key to ensure that muscles and prominent nerves are protected when a horse is placed on a surgical table or surface (Figure 27-31, *B*). There are many table designs, and the anesthetist should make sure that muscle groups are well supported to prevent myopathy ("tying up") and that the facial and radial nerves are supported. Horses in lateral recumbency should have the forelimb closest to the table pulled forward, if possible, to decrease the pressure placed on it by the chest and opposite limb.

MAINTENANCE OF ANESTHESIA

Horses present the biggest challenge of all the domestic species to the anesthetist. Sudden unexpected movement can occur without any change in signs of depth. As a result of the large breathing circuit volume and patient size, response to changes in inhalant anesthetic and oxygen flow rates occur too slowly to return the patient to surgical anesthesia simply by altering machine settings. A syringe of thiopental or ketamine is typically drawn up before anesthesia and either attached to a three-way stopcock in the fluid administration line or kept close to the IV port for this purpose. Approximately one fifth of the IV induction dose is administered to the horse to return it to surgical anesthesia.

Compared with other species, horses are more likely to develop hypoxemia, hypoventilation, and hypotension during maintenance of anesthesia, particularly when using inhalant agents. To monitor blood pressure more accurately and to obtain arterial blood gas values, it is recommended that horses anesthetized with inhalants for procedures lasting more than 1 hour have an arterial catheter placed in a peripheral artery (facial, transverse facial, dorsal pedal) (Figure 27-32). Blood gas samples should be taken every 30 to 60 minutes or more frequently if the situation warrants.

Hypoventilation is so common in anesthetized horses, particularly those placed in dorsal recumbency, that a ventilator is often used to maintain normal ventilation. Hypotension (mean arterial blood pressure less than 70 mm Hg) has been shown to contribute to myopathy, so treatment with drugs is frequently indicated if increased IV fluid rate, decreased anesthetic depth, and surgical stimulation do not increase blood pressure. The most common drug used to support blood pressure is the positive inotrope dobutamine (commonly administered via a syringe pump). Dobutamine and many other positive inotropes may cause arrhythmias, so it is important to monitor the ECG closely when starting an infusion.

Hypoxemia can occur in any horse, regardless of the physical status class, but is more common in horses that are obese, pregnant, or have torsed intestines and those that are placed in dorsal recumbency. Hypoxemia has several possible causes, including hypoventilation, lung disease, and low cardiac output. Wherever possible, the cause should be investigated and corrected.

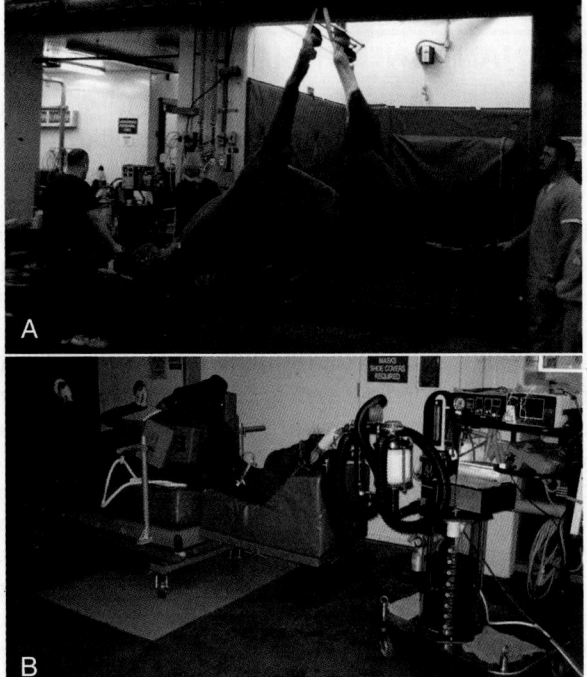

FIGURE 27-31 **A,** Once the horse is intubated and the anesthetist confirms that it is stable after induction, it is hoisted for placement on the surgery table. The anesthetist controls and supports the head while the patient is on the hoist. **B,** The horse is positioned on a thick foam pad to prevent muscle damage. Side paddles are used to keep the horse in dorsal recumbency on the table, and smaller foam pads support the large muscles of the upper forelimbs. Once the horse is positioned, it is connected to an LA anesthesia machine.

IV maintenance of anesthesia in horses is generally reserved for shorter procedures (less than 1 hour) in healthy patients and for procedures done away from a veterinary practice ("field anesthesia"). "Triple drip" is the mainstay of IV anesthesia in horses and is generally characterized by higher blood pressure, better breathing, and more active palpebral reflexes than inhalant anesthesia. Use of "triple drip" for short procedures is also associated with recoveries of good quality.

ANESTHETIC RECOVERY

Horses have an instinctive need to stand shortly after awakening from anesthesia, and it is this that makes recovery particularly dangerous. Some steps can be taken to minimize injury to the horse and anesthetist, but there is a high incidence of complications from anesthetic recovery in horses, and clients should be informed of the risks.

Preparation for Recovery

Replace the halter. Place a nasopharyngeal tube before movement if nasal edema is present (Figure 27-33, *A*). Upon completion of the procedure, turn off the inhalant anesthetic and transfer the horse to a padded recovery stall where it can be extubated and monitored. If possible and particularly if the horse was hypoxemic during anesthesia, provide oxygen support using a demand valve or insufflation (5 to 10 L/min delivered nasally or through the endotracheal tube via tubing that is connected to an oxygen flowmeter) until the horse is extubated or too light to tolerate an insufflation hose. If the recovery is assisted by ropes, a head rope should be attached to the halter and another rope tied to the tail (Figure 27-33, *B* and *C*).

Monitoring During Recovery

During recovery, it is ideal to watch the horse continuously so that it can be assisted or sedated, if necessary. While the horse is lying quietly, the anesthetist should watch respirations to make sure that the horse is breathing normally, take

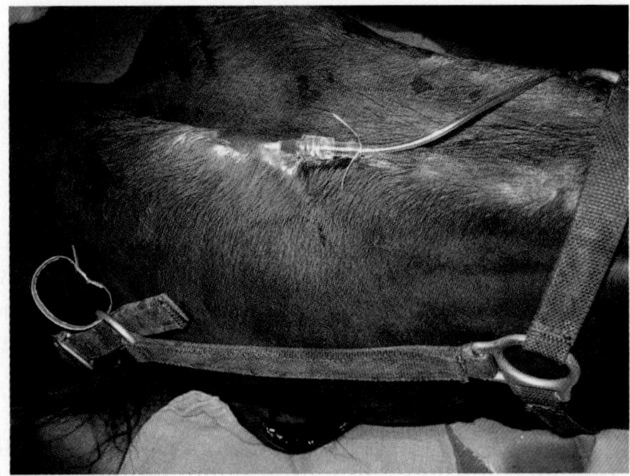

FIGURE 27-32 Placement of a catheter in the facial artery for monitoring blood pressure and taking blood samples for arterial blood gas analysis.

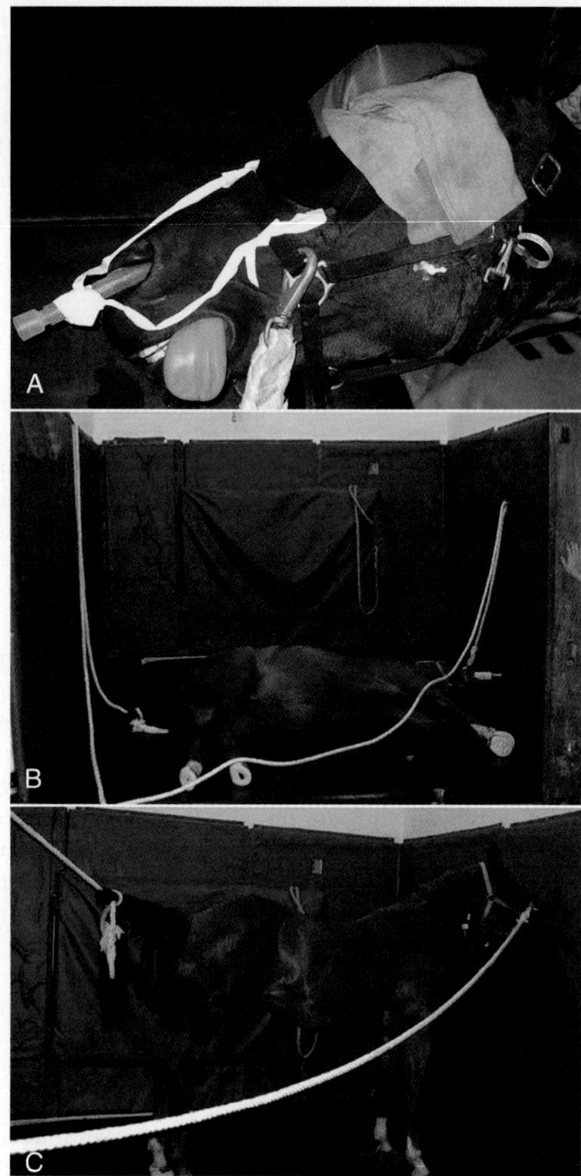

FIGURE 27-33 Recovery. **A,** A nasopharyngeal tube is placed and secured to the halter to ensure a patent airway. Note that the eye is covered to decrease stimulation during recovery. **B,** Placement of head and tail ropes for recovery. **C,** Recovered horse standing quietly. The nasopharyngeal tube stays in place until the horse is fully recovered.

the pulse (facial artery) occasionally, and assess the eye for depth of anesthesia.

Signs of Recovery

As the patient recovers, it will progress back through the stages and planes of anesthesia. Many horses develop nystagmus during recovery, and rapid nystagmus accompanied by "paddling" of the limbs generally means that a horse will try to get up too soon and have a "rough" recovery. In this event, it may be prudent to sedate the horse with 50 to 100 mg xylazine IV. Generally, maintaining control of the head by sitting on the neck or holding the head up off the floor will provide some control over the horse. However, once the horse is strong enough to lift an anesthetist off its neck, the anesthetist should retreat to a safe distance to observe the remainder of recovery.

Extubation

To prepare the patient for extubation, deflate the cuff by drawing out all of the air until the pilot balloon is empty. Both before and following removal, keep the neck in a natural but extended position to protect the airway. Remove the endotracheal tube gently when the swallowing reflex returns using a slow, steady motion. You may also remove it when signs of imminent arousal are present, such as voluntary movement of the limbs or head, movement of the tongue, or chewing. Check to make sure that the horse can breathe without obstruction. Horses can only breathe through their noses and will become distressed and compromised if they are unable to. If a nasopharyngeal tube has not been placed and the nasal passages are or become obstructed, one must be placed immediately. In the event that a nasopharyngeal tube does not alleviate the obstruction, a tracheostomy must be performed by the veterinarian, so materials for performing one must be close to the recovery stall at all times.

The Postanesthetic Period

Once the horse is standing and able to walk steadily, it can be returned to its stall. This can be assessed by walking the horse in a circle inside the recovery stall. Once back in its own stall, the horse should be muzzled for 1 to 3 hours, but should have free access to water.

RUMINANT ANESTHESIA

Ruminants do not pose quite the same challenge to the anesthetist as horses; however, an understanding of their unique digestive physiology is important where it impacts on the well-being of the patient under general anesthesia. Additionally, ruminants come for general anesthesia less frequently than small animals or horses do, so it takes longer to gain anesthetic experience. There are several reasons for this. Because of their relatively calm nature, ruminants require general anesthesia for relatively few procedures. Many surgeries can be conducted using local or regional anesthetic techniques. A discussion of local and regional anesthesia is beyond the scope of this chapter; this subject is covered in most veterinary anesthesia textbooks. Finally, administration of general anesthesia to production animals is often uneconomical.

The general principles discussed for other species also apply to ruminants, and careful preparation and planning is important to a successful anesthetic outcome. Box 27-11 summarizes the sequence of events when inducing a ruminant with injectable agents and maintaining with an inhalant agent.

SELECTING A PROTOCOL

As with other species, protocols are commonly selected by the veterinarian in charge. A suitable protocol takes into account the patient signalment, preexisting problems, the

BOX 27-11 Sequence of Events for a Ruminant Anesthetic Procedure (Induction With an IV Agent and Maintenance With an Inhalant Agent)

1. Assess, prepare, and weigh the patient (see Part II: Patient Preparation for a discussion of patient assessment, preparation, and stabilization).
2. Prepare equipment for and place IV catheter, which may require restraint in a chute with a head gate for larger or aggressive cattle (clippers, local anesthetic, antiseptic scrub, catheters, tape, heparinized saline, suture material, catheter cap, and/or extension line with three-way stopcock).
3. Determine the protocol (anesthetic agents including dosages, routes, and sequence of administration).
4. Calculate the volume of each agent to give, including fluid administration rates (preanesthetic, induction, maintenance, and analgesic agents).
5. Review the oxygen flow rates (see Box 27-3).
6. Prepare equipment required to administer drugs (scales, syringes, needles, agents, reversal agents, emergency cart, controlled substance log).
7. Prepare fluid administration equipment (fluids, administration-extension set, syringe pump, tape, heparinized saline).
8. Prepare equipment for endotracheal intubation. Have suction equipment assembled and turned on for small ruminants. Remove jewelry, watch, and ensure fingernails are trimmed short for digital intubation of adult cattle (see Part VI: Principles of Endotracheal Intubation for an equipment list).
9. Prepare monitoring equipment including arterial catheterization materials, anesthesia record, monitors, and probes (see Part V: Anesthetic Monitoring for a discussion of monitoring equipment).
10. Assemble and test the anesthetic machine and ventilator (see Part IV: Anesthetic Equipment and Part X: Manual and Mechanical Ventilation for a discussion of these procedures).
11. Administer premedications approximately 20-30 min IM or 5-10 min IV before anesthetic induction if this is considered necessary.
12. Administer the induction agent.
13. Check the patient's readiness for intubation.
14. Place and secure the endotracheal tube (see Part VI: Principles of Endotracheal Intubation for a discussion of this procedure).
15. Check the patient's vital signs.
16. Hoist or lift (as appropriate), position, and secure the patient for the procedure. It is imperative that the pharynx be positioned higher than the head, whenever possible.
17. Turn on the oxygen and connect the endotracheal tube to the breathing circuit.
18. Turn on the inhalant anesthetic to the appropriate level.
19. Determine the patient's anesthetic depth and commence regular monitoring.
20. Attach monitoring devices, including placement of an arterial catheter.
21. Continue to monitor and adjust the anesthetic and oxygen levels as needed until completion of the procedure.
22. Prepare the patient for recovery, including removal of monitoring equipment, and ensure the recovery area has been prepared.
23. Discontinue the anesthetic and transfer the patient to the recovery area.
24. Extubate the patient at the appropriate time with the cuff partially inflated. Place or prop the patient in sternal recumbency so that it can eructate.
25. Prepare the patient for continued hospitalization or discharge by applying bandages, administering medications, and performing any other procedures ordered by the veterinarian.

physical status class, and the procedure to be performed (see Box 27-12 for sample protocols used in physical status class P1 and P2 ruminants). After the protocol is known, calculate all drug dosages, oxygen flow rates, and fluid administration rates and check them *carefully*.

Physical status class P3 to P5 patients require use of modified protocols based on the primary condition (Table 27-12). Management of these cases can be quite challenging and requires customization of the anesthetic protocol by the veterinarian in charge.

EQUIPMENT PREPARATION

It is key to ensure that ruminants have been adequately fasted before anesthesia. Fasting reduces the size of the rumen and also decreases microbial activity. This in turn decreases gas production during anesthesia. Normally, ruminants eructate to expel the gas from the rumen; however, under anesthesia, this does not happen and can lead to bloating. A bloated rumen can put pressure on the diaphragm and large blood vessels (aorta, caudal vena cava) in the abdomen, resulting in respiratory and circulatory compromise. Once an anesthetized ruminant develops severe bloat, it can be difficult to treat and may lead to death if it goes unnoticed or untreated.

Any specialized equipment required for restraining or positioning anesthetized ruminants, such as head gates, transporters, and tilt tables, should be checked. In addition to the standard equipment, it is extremely helpful to have suction available for small ruminants to allow feed material, regurgitus, or saliva to be removed from the pharynx during intubation.

THE PREANESTHETIC PERIOD

Many ruminants are calm and tractable enough to allow IV catheterization and induction of anesthesia with minimal or no premedication and mild restraint. Adult cattle are typically restrained using the head gate of a transporter or chute. Premedication is often reserved for patients that are aggressive, excited, or stressed. Although many ruminants do not require sedation before anesthesia, premedication will

BOX 27-12 Protocols for Premedication, Sedation, and General Anesthesia in Physical Status Class P1 and P2 Ruminants

***Protocols for Mild to Moderate Sedation**

1. Acepromazine: 0.02-0.03 mg/kg IV *(may increase regurgitation)*
2. Xylazine: 0.01-0.05 mg/kg IV or IM *(unlikely to cause recumbency)*
3. Detomidine: 0.005-0.02 mg/kg IV

† Protocols for Moderate to Heavy Sedation (for Minor Procedures, Such as Radiography or Wound Assessment) or for Premedication

1. Acepromazine: 0.03-0.05 mg/kg IV
2. Xylazine: 0.05-0.1 mg/kg IV or 0.05-0.2 mg/kg IM *(likely to cause recumbency and potentially light anesthesia)*
3. Detomidine: 0.01-0.03 mg/kg IV
4. Midazolam 0.1 mg/kg plus butorphanol 0.1-0.2 mg/kg IV *(may produce ataxia, so recommended for small ruminants or restrained cattle)*

Protocols for Anesthetic Induction

1. Ketamine 2.5 mg/kg IV and diazepam* 0.12 mg/kg IV mixed in the same syringe. (This is equivalent to 1 ml of the mixture/20 kg of body weight and is given most commonly to small ruminants. Note the difference from SA dosage.) *Note: An equivalent volume of midazolam can be used in place of diazepam.
2. "Double drip" administered IV to effect (approximately 1-2 ml/kg). "Double drip" can be made by adding 500 mg ketamine to a 500-ml bag of 5% guaifenesin.
3. Telazol® 1-4 mg/kg IV or IM *(lower dose after xylazine premedication)*

Protocols for Anesthetic Maintenance

1. Isoflurane 1.5%-2.5% or sevoflurane 2.5%-4%
2. "Double drip" can be used to maintain anesthesia at 1-2 ml/kg/hr

*(Note that many ruminants require no sedation for standing procedures performed with local anesthetic.)
†(Note that many ruminants do not require premedication before anesthesia.)

TABLE 27-12 Recommendations for Physical Status Class P3-P5 Ruminant Patients

Primary Condition	Example Protocols and Other Considerations	Avoid These Agents/Circumstances
C-section requiring general anesthesia (live calf)	No premedication Induce with ketamine-based protocol Maintain with isoflurane or sevoflurane Epidural analgesia is helpful to reduce the need for other analgesics Minimize anesthetic time	Thiopental sodium and other barbiturates α_2-Agonists Acepromazine Opioids before delivery
C-section requiring general anesthesia (dead calf, septicemic cow)	No premedication or benzodiazepines Induce with ketamine-based protocol Maintain with isoflurane or sevoflurane Support blood pressure	Thiopental sodium and other barbiturates α_2-Agonists Acepromazine
Urethral obstruction	No premedication or premedicate with benzodiazepines (e.g., diazepam) Induce with "double-drip" or diazepam-ketamine Maintain with isoflurane or sevoflurane Monitor electrolytes preoperatively and intraoperatively Maintain blood pressure and fluid balance	Acepromazine α_2-Agonists

provide benefits, such as decreased dose of induction and maintenance drugs and muscle relaxation (Figure 27-34).

> *TECHNICIAN NOTE* Ruminants are sensitive to xylazine, requiring at most one tenth of the dose that horses do.

ANESTHETIC INDUCTION

IV Induction

Induction of large cattle may occur in a special induction stall that has padded walls and often a padded floor, in a transporter, or on a tilt table. Smaller ruminants can generally be induced next to the surgery table or if small or severely compromised, while lying on the surgery table. Although ruminants do not typically become excited during induction of anesthesia, the goal with larger patients is similar to that in horses: to rapidly produce unconsciousness and minimize injury of the patient or personnel. Drugs are thus given as an IV bolus, with the exception of "double drip," which is administered rapidly IV to effect. Smaller ruminants, particularly those that are compromised, can be given induction drugs IV to effect as for SA patients.

Once the patient is unconscious, it should be kept in sternal recumbency for intubation, whenever possible. It is important to be vigilant for regurgitation, which can occur at any point of the anesthetic procedure, but occurs most frequently when anesthesia is light or too deep. If regurgitation

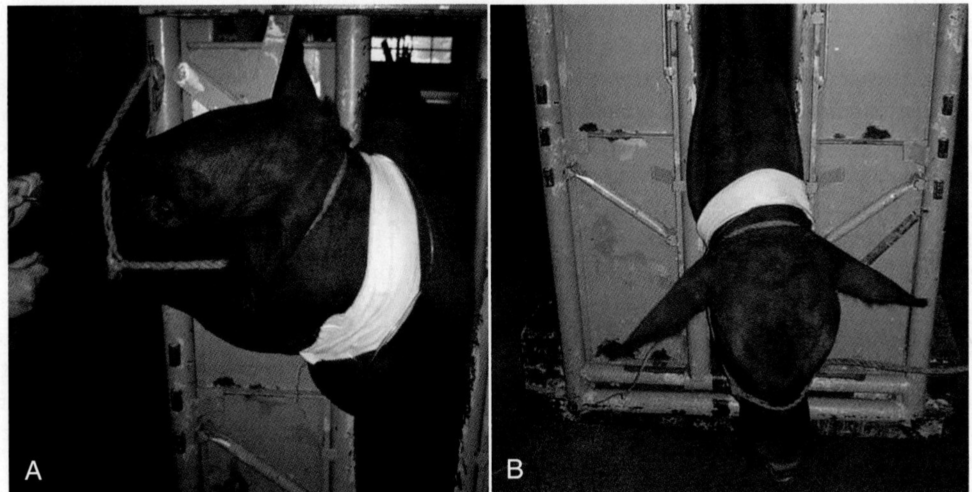

FIGURE 27-34 A, A 500-kg bull is restrained for jugular catheterization in a transporter with a head gate. B, The same bull after sedation with 25-mg xylazine IV.

occurs, the head should immediately be positioned so that it is lower than the body to prevent aspiration.

Once the patient has been induced, the vital signs should be briefly checked before intubation (see Figure 27-29).

All ruminants should be positioned for surgery with the mouth lower than the pharynx to allow drainage of saliva and any regurgitated material from the mouth, preventing buildup in the pharynx, which could lead to aspiration in recovery. Ruminants produce copious amounts of saliva each day, which is normally swallowed. Under anesthesia, this cannot occur, so it must be allowed to drain. Ruminants, even large cattle, are not predisposed to developing myopathy or neuropathy like horses; however, appropriate physical support and padding during anesthesia is prudent.

MAINTENANCE OF ANESTHESIA

Healthy ruminants typically have relatively few problems during the maintenance phase of anesthesia. Blood pressure is usually well maintained and is often much higher than that seen in SA and equine patients. Ruminants do, however, tend to hypoventilate and are often observed to breathe rapidly and shallowly, somewhat like a panting dog. This type of breathing pattern tends to lead to hypoxemia and difficulty keeping the patient anesthetized because of inadequate delivery of inhalant anesthetic to the lungs. Patients that demonstrate this breathing pattern should be placed on a ventilator.

Most ruminants have accessible arteries in their ears, and these are often catheterized so that blood pressure can be monitored directly and blood samples can be taken for blood gas analysis.

IV maintenance of anesthesia in ruminants is generally reserved for shorter procedures (less than 20 minutes) in healthy patients, although if the patient is intubated, the duration of anesthesia can be extended. "Double drip" is commonly used for this purpose.

ANESTHETIC RECOVERY

Unlike horses, ruminants are generally content to lie in sternal recumbency after they wake up from anesthesia. The development of complications from anesthetic recovery is generally limited to the residual effects of bloat. Ruminants rarely develop nasal edema during anesthesia and usually do not require nasal intubation.

Preparation for Recovery

Upon completion of the procedure, turn off the inhalant anesthetic and transfer the patient to a padded recovery stall where it can be extubated and monitored (large cattle) or a quiet, clean area on the floor (small ruminant). If possible, support or prop the patient in sternal recumbency.

Monitoring During Recovery

The patient should be monitored for signs of excessive bloating (visually large abdomen that feels tight to the touch).

Signs of Recovery

As the patient recovers, it will progress back through the stages and planes of anesthesia. Generally, this is not as dramatic in ruminants as it is in horses, even if the patient did not receive a premedication.

Extubation

In contrast to other species, the endotracheal tube cuff should either be kept inflated or only partially deflated to prevent aspiration of any material that may have become lodged in the pharynx during anesthesia. The anesthetist should wait for strong swallowing movements or coughing before extubation. Both before and following removal, keep the neck in a natural but extended position to protect the airway. Remove the endotracheal tube gently using a slow, steady motion. If there is difficulty removing the tube, remove some more air from the cuff and try again.

The Postanesthetic Period

Once a ruminant is lying in sternal recumbency without support and is no longer in danger of bloating, it can be left unattended. Many ruminants will lie quietly after anesthesia, only standing some time after the anesthetic period, unless they are stimulated to rise. It is not necessary to withhold food or water from ruminants postoperatively unless specifically instructed to do so.

MANUAL AND MECHANICAL VENTILATION

Ventilation is a process in which air or anesthetic gases are artificially forced into a patient's lungs. Although ventilatory support is necessary in patients with preexisting problems, such as lung disease, obesity, abdominal distention, or brain trauma, some ventilatory support is needed even in healthy patients to compensate for the respiratory depression that accompanies general anesthesia. This is especially true in healthy LA patients, and consequently, many practices will ventilate all horses and ruminants under general anesthesia.

Under certain circumstances, such as a loss of the normal vacuum in the chest cavity (e.g., thoracotomy for repair of diaphragmatic hernia, thoracic injuries, or pneumothorax) or paralysis of the respiratory muscles when neuromuscular blockers are used as a part of the anesthetic protocol, a patient may be unable to breathe. At these times, ventilation is mandatory throughout the procedure to keep the patient alive.

This support can be provided by the anesthetist by application of pressure to the reservoir bag with the pop-off valve fully or partially closed (manual ventilation) or by using a ventilator (mechanical ventilation).

MANUAL VENTILATION

Manual ventilation is used when a mechanical ventilator is not available, to provide ventilatory support to patients with temporary apnea or inadequate respiratory depth, or to prevent atelectasis in any patient. Depending on the need, manual ventilation may be either periodic or mandatory.

MECHANICAL VENTILATION

Mechanical ventilation is routinely used for large animals and at other times when mandatory ventilation is required. There are different types of ventilators that function in different ways. Pressure cycle ventilators force air into the lungs until a set pressure is reached. Volume cycle ventilators deliver a preset volume (usually 10 to 15 ml/kg). Time cycle ventilators force air into the lungs according to a set inspiratory time regardless of the volume delivered or pressure generated. Because of the wide variety of ventilators available, safe use requires a careful review of the operating instructions in the owner's manual.

To prepare for mechanical ventilation follow the procedure below:

- Connect the ventilator to an electrical supply, an oxygen source, and the scavenging system.
- Insert the pressure feedback sensor between expiratory valve and corrugated breathing tube.
- Remove the rebreathing bag from the anesthetic machine and attach in its place the tube that connects to the bellows of the ventilator.
- Close the pop-off valve.
- Check that the endotracheal tube cuff is inflated and the entire breathing circuit is airtight.
- Set the RR, maximum inspiratory pressure, V_T, and/or inspiratory time as indicated in the owner's manual.
- Turn on the ventilator and adjust the settings to achieve the target volume, pressure, and/or time.

PERIODIC VENTILATION

Periodic ventilation is used to support normal healthy patients and patients that are experiencing apnea or hypoventilation. To support healthy patients, many experts advise periodic manual ventilation of all SA patients once every 5 to 10 minutes. This technique used to prevent atelectasis is often referred to as "bagging" or "sighing" the patient. In contrast, hypoventilating or apneic patients may require breaths at 15-second to 5-minute intervals depending on the specific need as determined by observation of monitoring parameters and monitoring equipment. To provide periodic manual ventilation, first close the pop-off valve and gently squeeze the bag until the patient's chest rises as in a normal breath. Then immediately following each breath reopen the pop-off valve.

INTERMITTENT MANDATORY VENTILATION

Intermittent mandatory ventilation is used for the majority of LA patients, which are extremely prone to hypoventilation under inhalant anesthesia. It is also a necessity during procedures in which the thoracic cavity is exposed to the atmosphere and those in which neuromuscular blockers are used. To provide intermittent mandatory ventilation:

- Ventilate at a rate of 12 to 16 bpm (SA) or 6 to 10 bpm (LA) until spontaneous breathing ceases.
- Lower the rate to 8 to 12 bpm (SA) or 6 to 8 bpm (LA).
- For the duration of the procedure, adjust the rate based on data from blood gas analysis, capnography, pulse oximetry, and other monitoring parameters.
- When you are ready for the patient to resume spontaneous breathing, gradually reduce the rate to about 4 bpm (SA) or 2 bpm (LA).
- When the patient begins to spontaneously breathe, support the patient with periodic ventilation, as needed.
- Discontinue ventilation when the rate and V_T are normal.

COMPLICATIONS OF VENTILATION

There are risks of manual and mechanical ventilation. Positive pressure is generated in the chest during the inspiratory phase of normal ventilator cycling. This leads to a reduction in venous return to the heart and a temporary drop in blood pressure. Ventilation should therefore be used cautiously in the hypotensive patient.

If excess pressure is applied to the airways, alveoli can rupture, resulting in pneumothorax or pneumomediastinum. Additionally, high positive pressure in the thorax will decrease blood returning to the heart. This may lead to a life-threatening reduction in cardiac output. For these reasons, never allow the pressure in the breathing circuit to exceed 20 cm of water in small animals or 30 to 40 cm of water in large animals.

If the respiratory minute volume is excessive, respiratory alkalosis can occur as a result of a loss of CO_2. In contrast if respiratory minute volume is inadequate, the patient can develop hypercarbia and respiratory acidosis. For this reason, use of an appropriate RR and volume is critical to maintaining patient safety during ventilation. Capnography is the best noninvasive tool for judging the appropriateness of the rate and volume, with the gold standard as measurement of arterial CO_2 through blood gas analysis.

If using a nonprecision, VIC, anesthetic overdose is possible if the patient receives an excessive minute volume. Therefore careful monitoring of anesthetic depth is additionally important in these patients.

Finally, artificial ventilation is generally more efficient at delivering anesthetic gas, even from a precision VOC. A ventilator will thus deliver more inhalant anesthetic to the patient, which may lead to exacerbation of side effects, such as hypotension. Conversely, ventilators are often used in LA patients as anesthetic delivery devices to maintain a smoother plane of anesthesia than sometimes occurs with spontaneous breathing.

ANESTHETIC PROBLEMS AND EMERGENCIES

The majority of general anesthetic procedures are uneventful, but from time to time, problems develop that have the potential to cause transient or permanent harm to the patient. Most studies show that although as many as 1 out of 10 patients have complications of one sort or another, an average of only 1 or 2 out of 1000 healthy patients die as a result of anesthesia. Therefore it is likely that a technician will have experience with many successful anesthetic procedures before a serious complication ever occurs. This can easily lead to a false sense of security, which, unless tempered with increased watchfulness, may impair readiness to handle a crisis.

Although patients with preexisting conditions, such as major organ disease, are more likely to develop complications, healthy patients may also be at greater risk by reason of species, age, breed, reproductive status, body conformation, or a variety of other factors. For instance, brachycephalic dogs and geriatric, young (less than 8 weeks old), obese, and pregnant patients are at greater risk. Ruminants may bloat leading to cardiorespiratory compromise, and equine anesthetic recovery poses many risks, including myopathy and neuropathy. Therefore the anesthetist must approach any anesthetic procedure alert to problems that are likely to arise.

In addition, adverse drug reactions, equipment malfunctions, anesthetic overdose, complications of surgery, and human error are other possible causes of anesthetic problems and emergencies. Most can be managed successfully, however, if recognized early and acted upon before they reach crisis level. There are many indicators, which may be detected by careful and frequent observation throughout the procedure, that warn of developing problems. These indicators usually come from the machine (e.g., an overfilled reservoir bag or exhausted CO_2 granules), the patient (e.g., a patient that will not stay anesthetized or is experiencing a rough recovery), or monitoring devices (e.g., an SpO_2 below 95% or a cardiac arrhythmia).

The anesthetist may be able to manage some problems independently and quickly, whereas others require rapid and effective communication with the veterinarian in charge in addition to further exploration. For instance, mildly excessive or inadequate anesthetic depth can in most cases be managed by the anesthetist by simply adjusting the vaporizer setting and oxygen flow or altering the administration of injectable agents. On the other hand, problems such as hypotension or cardiac arrhythmias may require more complex action, such as changing the anesthetic protocol, treating blood loss, or interpreting data from a monitoring device. The remainder of this section highlights causes, solutions, and prevention of common anesthetic problems and emergencies.

A flowmeter or oxygen tank pressure gauge that registers zero indicates that the flowmeter is turned off or that the oxygen tank is empty or turned off. If the primary tank is empty, open the reserve tank. If it is impossible to solve the problem right away (there is no reserve tank on the machine and only one machine at your disposal), you should disconnect the endotracheal tube from the breathing system until the problem is rectified, although there is a risk that the patient may wake up or become hypoxemic in the interim.

Lack of movement of the reservoir bag or unidirectional valves when the patient breathes usually indicates that the endotracheal tube is not in the trachea, is disconnected, or is blocked. A disconnected or misplaced tube will result in difficulty keeping the patient anesthetized. A blocked tube will usually cause dyspnea and cyanosis. To manage this problem, first check that the tube is connected to the breathing circuit and is correctly placed. Next disconnect the tube and listen or feel for air flow when the patient breathes to rule out a blockage. If the tube is blocked or incorrectly placed, immediately remove the tube and reintubate the patient. If reintubation is not possible (e.g., no one to help you), administer oxygen and anesthetic via a mask until the tube can be replaced.

An overinflated reservoir bag or pressure manometer reading of more than 2 cm of water while the patient is breathing spontaneously occurs most commonly because the pop-off valve has inadvertently been left too far closed. Occlusions of the scavenging system, high oxygen flow, or overzealous use of the oxygen flush valve are other possible causes. If the pop-off valve is closed, open it immediately. If the pressure is dangerously high, (more than 20 cm of water) immediately disconnect the endotracheal tube from the breathing circuit and then correct the primary problem. If the pressure builds again when the tube is reconnected, check the scavenging system for a blockage. If high oxygen flow is causing the bag to overfill, the pressure in the circuit should not increase, but will remain less than 2 cm of water, even though the bag appears to be overinflated. In that case, gently press the bag to empty it as needed and—if safe to do so—decrease the oxygen flow.

An underinflated reservoir bag indicates inadequate oxygen flow, a leak in the system, a maladjusted scavenging system, or that the pop-off valve is too far open. If it is completely deflated, immediately increase the oxygen flow or use the oxygen flush valve to fill the bag one-half to three-fourths full. Then check the pop-off valve, machine assembly, and scavenging system adjustments. If the problem cannot be corrected quickly, change to another machine.

Violet or off-white, brittle absorbent granules indicate saturation of the CO_2 absorbent. The resulting increase in CO_2 in the breathing circuit will cause increased inspired and expired CO_2 levels on a capnograph and may also cause tachypnea or tachycardia. The solution to this problem is to change the granules as soon as the machine is no longer in use. For the duration of the procedure, change the patient to another machine. If you only have one machine, use high oxygen flow (1 L/5 kg body weight/min), continue close monitoring, and wake the patient as soon as possible, or if the patient is under 7 kg, change to a nonrebreathing system.

A PATIENT THAT WILL NOT STAY ASLEEP

Difficulty keeping a patient adequately anesthetized is most often related to problems with the machine and associated equipment. Check that the oxygen is on and flow is adequate, the vaporizer is not empty and is turned on, the machine is correctly assembled, there are no system leaks, and the endotracheal tube is properly placed and cuffed. Also check the RR and depth, which if decreased, may be insufficient to draw enough anesthetic into the lungs. If this is the case, bag the patient about every 5 to 10 seconds until in surgical anesthesia. If light, it may be necessary to prevent the patient from chewing the tube by applying gentle but firm pressure to the muzzle and to give additional injectable anesthetic until the source of the problem is identified and corrected.

Excessive anesthetic depth is usually due to excessively high vaporizer settings, equipment problems, or preexisting medical problems. Immediately inform the veterinarian, stop administration of all anesthetics, increase the flow of oxygen, and proceed as ordered by the veterinarian. Excessively deep patients may require bagging, IV fluid support, measures to increase body temperature, reversal agents or other drug therapy, and even resuscitation in extreme situations. If there is a suspicion of a vaporizer problem (overfilled, tipped over, out of calibration), change to another machine until the problem is corrected.

Cardiopulmonary arrest (CPA) most often follows uncorrected excessive anesthetic depth, but can happen at any time during anesthesia. Patients in physical status classes P2 to P5 are at especially high risk for CPA. A patient that has arrested has no heartbeat, pulse, or respirations and requires prompt initiation of cardiopulmonary-cerebral resuscitation (CPCR). The reader is directed to Chapter 33 for a complete discussion of CPCR.

Apnea or hypoventilation commonly occurs following any episode of hyperventilation as a result of a decrease in blood CO_2 levels. Apnea or hypoventilation is also common following induction with drugs that depress the respiratory system, but can also indicate excessive anesthetic depth and in some cases even respiratory arrest. To manage apnea, rapidly inform the veterinarian, check other vital signs, and then determine the anesthetic depth by assessing other monitoring parameters. If the patient is stable and at an appropriate depth, it may be necessary to "bag" the patient 2 to 10 times/min until normal respirations resume. Use the low end of this range if the apnea is secondary to hyperventilation to allow normalization of CO_2 levels.

Hypotension is a common anesthetic complication caused by preexisting conditions, blood loss, shock, cardiac arrhythmias, excessive anesthetic depth, and adverse effects of drugs. Hypotension is confirmed with Doppler, oscillometric, or direct monitoring, but may be suspected based on pale mucous membranes, increased CRT, and weak pulses. After informing the veterinarian, treat hypotension as ordered. Treatment often includes IV fluid therapy, reduction of the anesthetic, administration of additional oxygen, warming the patient, and drug therapy.

Cyanosis or low oxygen saturation indicate hypoxemia and can be caused by cardiopulmonary disease, ineffective respirations, airway blockage, or machine problems. Cyanosis is a medical emergency that requires immediate action. Dyspnea often accompanies or precedes cyanosis and must also be treated aggressively. Low oxygen saturation is defined as an SpO_2 of less than 95% on a pulse oximeter. Assuming the value is correct and is not due to a machine or probe problem, first inform the veterinarian and then check the oxygen flow, machine assembly, and the endotracheal tube for blockage. Also check that RR and depth is adequate.

Vomiting or regurgitation may occur at any time during an anesthetic procedure and can result in serious complications from pulmonary aspiration if the airway is not protected with a cuffed endotracheal tube. Vomiting is more common during induction and recovery, whereas regurgitation is more common during surgical anesthesia because of relaxation of the lower esophageal sphincter. Keep the tube cuffed at all times, and position the head level with or slightly higher than with the rest of the body during surgical anesthesia to decrease the likelihood of regurgitation. If the patient begins to retch or vomit at any time during general anesthesia, quickly position the patient's head lower than the body so that the vomitus flows out of the oral cavity and away from the pharynx. When the vomiting stops, carefully clean the oral cavity and pharynx with swabs, gauze, or suction.

Prolonged recovery may be seen in patients with preexisting disease or hypothermia, patients that have received barbiturates or dissociatives, or following prolonged procedures. These patients must be supported with IV fluids, good nursing care, measures to treat hypothermia, administration of reversal agents if indicated, and careful monitoring.

A rough or stormy recovery is one in which a patient thrashes, vocalizes, paddles, tries to bite, falls over, or exhibits any other uncontrolled behavior that can result in injury of the patient or personnel during the recovery period. Rough recoveries are more common in unpremedicated patients and may result from pain, fear, or disorientation. To manage a rough recovery, approach the patient with caution, administer sedatives or analgesics as ordered by the veterinarian, calm the patient, and use padding, restraint, and bandaging techniques to prevent self-trauma.

ACKNOWLEDGEMENTS

The authors would like to acknowledge the following individuals for production of the following photographs and graphics: Figures 27-1 through 27-27 (with the exception of 27-13, 27-14, and 27-17): Photography, photo editing, and photo illustration: Steven Ahern, AA, AAB; art direction and photography direction: William Fogarty, M.Ed.

RECOMMENDED READINGS AND REFERENCES

Blaze CA, Glowaski MM: *Veterinary anesthesia drug quick reference,* St Louis, 2004, Elsevier.

Greene SA: *Veterinary anesthesia and pain management secrets,* St Louis, 2002, Hanley & Belfus.

Love L, Harvey R: Arterial blood pressure measurement: physiology, tools, and techniques, *Compend Cont Educ Pract Vet* 28(6):450-462, 2006.

Marshall M: Capnography in dogs, *Compend Cont Educ Pract Vet* 26(10):761-778, 2004.

McKelvey D, Hollingshead KW: *Veterinary anesthesia and analgesia,* ed 3, St Louis, 2003, Mosby.

Muir WW et al: *Handbook of veterinary anesthesia,* ed 4, St Louis, 2007, Mosby.

Muir WW, Hubbell JAE: *Equine anesthesia,* St Louis, 1991, Mosby Year Book.

Thurmon JC et al: *Essentials of small animal anesthesia and analgesia,* Baltimore, 1999, Lippincott Williams & Wilkins.

Thurmon JC et al: *Lumb & Jones' veterinary anesthesia,* ed 3, Baltimore, 1996, Lippincott Williams & Wilkins.

Surgical Nursing

PART SIX

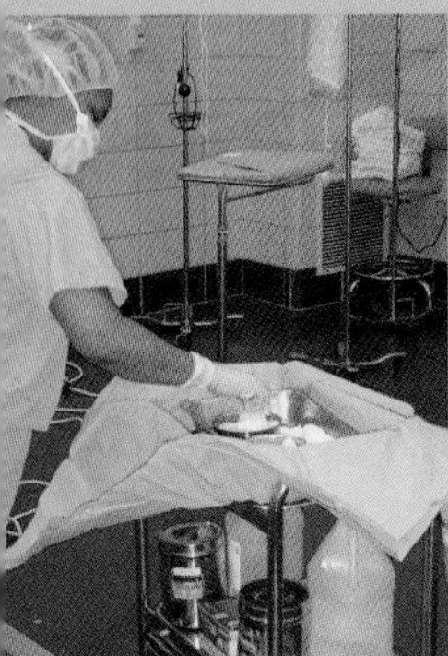

Surgical Instruments and Aseptic Technique

28

Jacqueline R. Davidson and Daniel J. Burba

KEY TERMS

Asepsis
Aseptic technique
Assisted gloving
Box lock
Closed gloving
Endogenous
Exogenous
Flash sterilization
Incise drape
Ingress port
Obturator
One-step prep
Open gloving
Osteochondral chip fragments
Prep
Prosthesis
Ratchet
Recumbency
Residual activity
Scrub in
Scrub suit
Sterile field
Sterile technique
Strike-through
Subchondral bone

OUTLINE

LEARNING OBJECTIVES

When you have completed this chapter, you will be able to:

1. Name and describe the commonly used surgical instruments.
2. State advantages of surgical stapling and list common surgical stapling devices.
3. List commonly used instruments and equipment for ophthalmic, orthopedic, and arthroscopic procedures.
4. List surgical instruments and supplies routinely included in general and emergency surgical packs for small and large animals.
5. Describe procedures for cleaning, packing, and sterilizing instruments.
6. Describe procedures for folding and packing cloth surgical drapes and gowns.
7. Differentiate between sterilization and disinfection.
8. List and describe physical and chemical methods of sterilization and methods of quality control of sterilization methods.
9. State safe storage times for sterile packs.
10. List and describe common antiseptic and disinfectant agents.
11. Describe requirements for preparation of the operating room and maintenance of operating room sterility.
12. Describe preparation requirements for patients, including skin preparation, patient positioning, and draping.
13. Describe preparation requirements for the surgical team and explain the procedures that may be used for hand scrubbing before surgery.
14. Describe the procedure for donning surgical attire.
15. Describe procedures for opening sterile items.

INTRODUCTION

The veterinary technician may need to assist the veterinarian with many aspects of surgery. The technician may need to prepare the patient for surgery, act as a circulating nurse in the operating room, and take responsibility for the care, cleaning, packing, and sterilization of the instruments. The technician is often responsible for ordering surgical instruments and implants, so familiarity with this equipment is essential. In addition, the principles of aseptic technique should be second nature. The technician may need to alert the veterinarian to potential problems with aseptic technique and may be required to "scrub in" to assist with surgical procedures. A surgical assistant can be of great value by anticipating which instruments the surgeon will need and by aiding in tissue retraction and hemostasis. The technician is an invaluable part of the surgical team and can greatly enhance the quality and efficiency of surgical procedures.

INSTRUMENTATION

Thousands of different surgical instruments are available, and new instruments are continually designed to increase the efficiency and ease of performing surgery. The surgical technician must know the purpose of each instrument to anticipate when it will be used and must understand how to handle and care for it.

> TECHNICIAN NOTE Each instrument is designed for a specific purpose, such as cutting, holding, clamping, or retracting.

GENERAL SURGERY INSTRUMENTS

SCALPEL

The scalpel is the best instrument for incising tissues with minimal trauma. A variety of disposable blades are designed to fit several different scalpel handles (Figure 28-1). The *Bard-Parker No. 3 handle* uses detachable blade Nos. 10, 11, 12, and 15 and is the most useful for small animal surgery. The *Bard-Parker No. 4 handle* is larger and uses detachable blade Nos. 20, 21, and 22. This handle is most commonly used for large animal surgery.

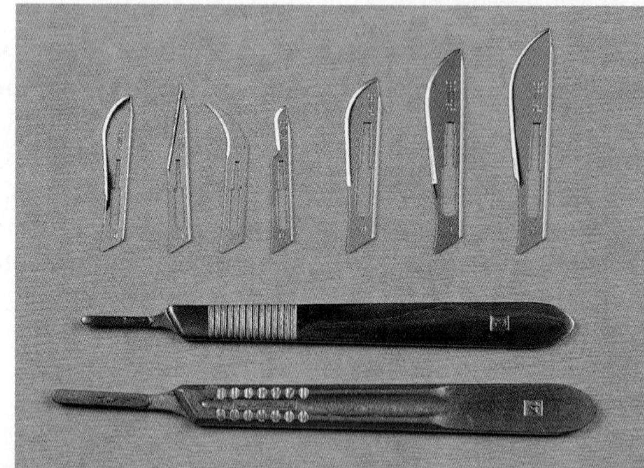

FIGURE 28-1 Scalpel handles and attachable surgical blades. Surgical blade Nos. 10, 11, 12, and 15 fit the Bard-Parker No. 3 scalpel handle, and surgical blade Nos. 20 to 22 fit the Bard-Parker No. 4 handle. The No. 3 handle and No. 10 blade are commonly used in small animal surgery. The No. 4 handle and No. 20 blade are commonly used in large animal surgery.

BIOMEDICAL LASERS

Surgical lasers may be used to cut or ablate (destroy) tissue. There are many different types of lasers. The most commonly used in veterinary medicine are carbon dioxide (CO_2) and neodymium:yttrium-aluminum-garnet (Nd:YAG) lasers. Advantages of incising tissue with a laser include some hemostasis and possibly less postoperative swelling and pain as compared with cutting with a scalpel blade. Disadvantages include delayed wound healing and safety issues associated with the use of lasers. Special glasses must be worn by everyone in the room, and care must be taken to prevent ignition of combustible materials. Smoke evacuators and laser-safe surgical masks should be used to reduce the amount of particulate debris inhaled from the smoke plume.

ELECTROSURGERY

Electroscalpels can be used to cut or coagulate tissue and help to minimize bleeding. They work by passing a high-frequency alternating electrical current through the tissue (Figure 28-2, *A*). Cutting or coagulation can be performed through the same handpiece, and the surgeon can activate it by a switch on the sterile handpiece or by a foot switch (Figure 28-2, *B*). However, the power level must be adjusted by a nonsterile technician. In *monopolar electrosurgery*, current passes from the handpiece (Figure 28-2, *C*) through the patient to a metal ground plate (Figure 28-2, *D*) that is placed under the patient. Poor contact between the patient's skin and the ground plate can burn the patient at the site of the ground plate. In *bipolar electrosurgery*, the current passes between two tips on the handpiece (Figure 28-2, *E*), which grasp the tissue. No ground plate is needed for bipolar electrosurgery.

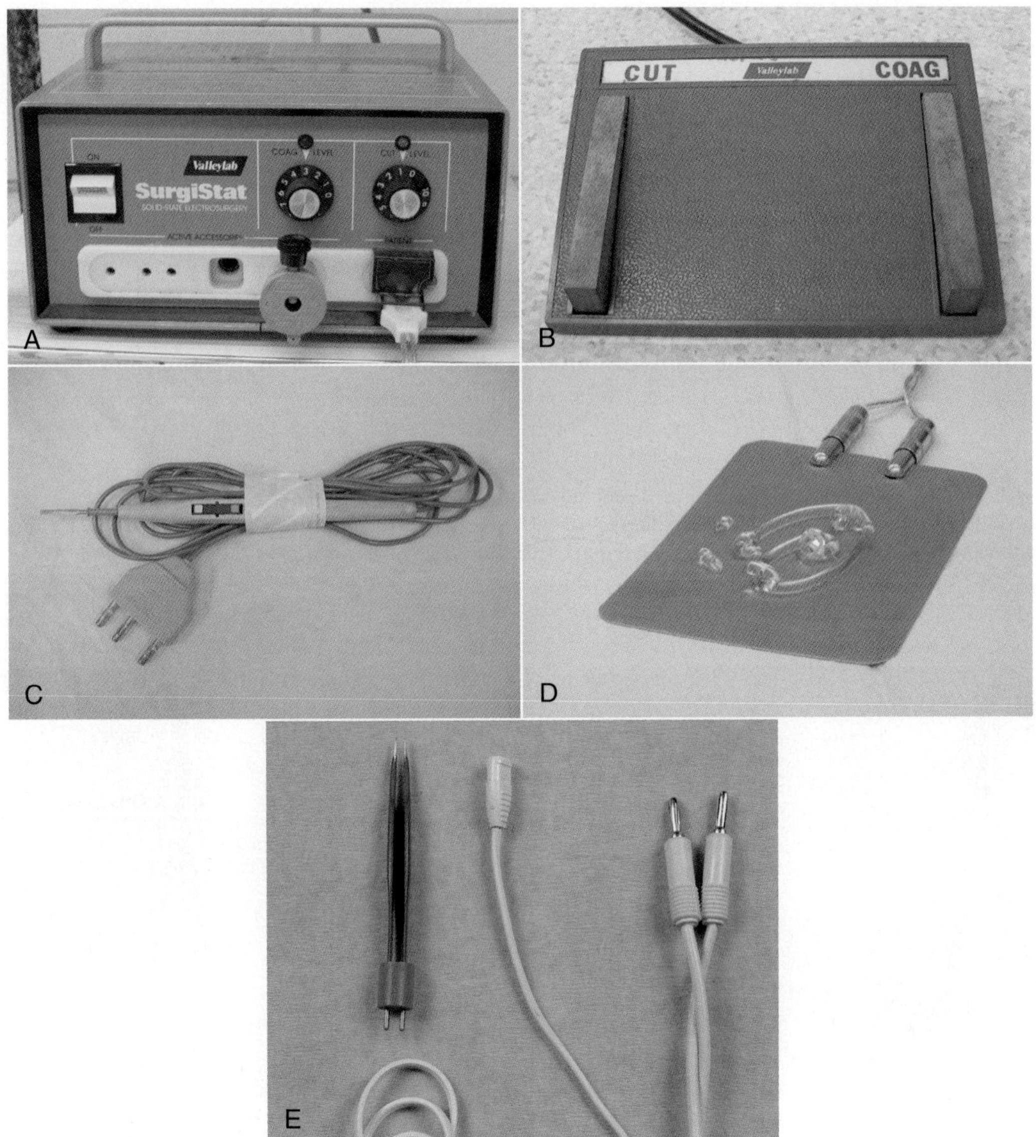

FIGURE 28-2 Electrosurgical equipment. **A,** Settings on electrosurgical unit are adjusted by nonsterile technician. **B,** Electrosurgical foot switch is placed near surgeon's foot. **C,** Monopolar electrosurgery handpiece. If the handpiece has a cutting-coagulation button, a foot switch is not needed. The handpiece is sterilized and given to the surgeon. The surgeon passes the end of the cord to a nonsterile assistant who plugs it into the electrosurgical unit. **D,** Ground plate on surgery table with gel to improve skin contact when the animal lies on it. Good contact is important for proper function. **E,** Bipolar handpiece is sterilized for use. A nonsterile foot switch is needed for activation.

SCISSORS

Specific scissors are designed to cut tissue, suture, wire, or bandage material (Figure 28-3). There are many types of dissecting scissors, made for precise cutting and dissection of tissue. *Operating scissors* vary by the type of blades (straight or curved), the type of points (blunt-blunt, blunt-sharp or sharp-sharp), and the cutting edge of the blades (plain or serrated). *Mayo dissecting scissors* are heavy scissors used for cutting tough tissue, such as heavy connective tissue. The blades may be straight or curved. *Metzenbaum dissecting scissors* are fine, curved scissors used for cutting delicate tissue, such as fat or thin muscle. Metzenbaum scissors are preferred for most soft tissue dissection. They should never be used for cutting suture because this dulls the edges and causes the blades to separate and lose effectiveness. Stitch scissors or *Littauer suture removal scissors* are used to cut all sutures except wire sutures. *Wire-suture–cutting scissors* can cut wire suture. *Lister bandage scissors* are available to cut bandage material. One blade of the Lister scissors has a blunt end to facilitate sliding under a bandage without poking the skin. To prolong the life of any scissors, it should be used only for its intended purpose.

> TECHNICIAN NOTE Scissors are specifically designed for many purposes, including tissue dissection and cutting suture or bandage materials.

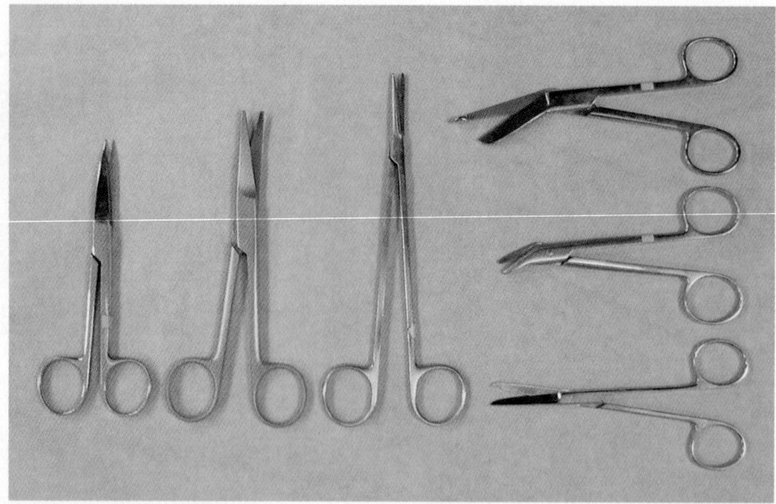

FIGURE 28-3 Scissors. *Left to right:* Sharp-sharp operating scissors, Mayo dissecting scissors, and Metzenbaum dissecting scissors. *At right, from top to bottom:* Lister bandage scissors, wire-suture cutting scissors, and Littauer suture removal scissors.

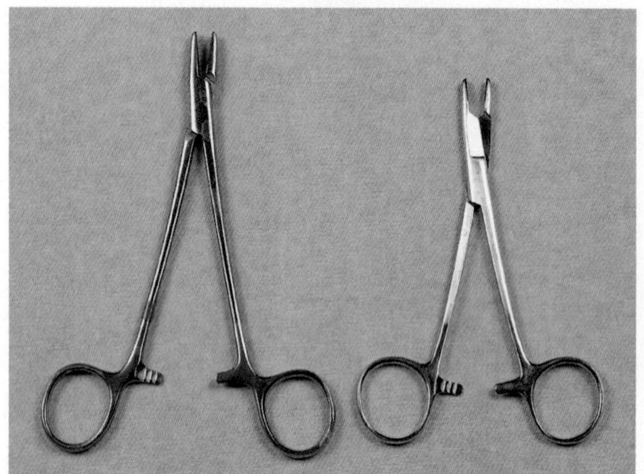

FIGURE 28-4 Needle holders. Mayo-Hegar needle holder *(left)*, Olsen-Hegar needle holder *(right)*.

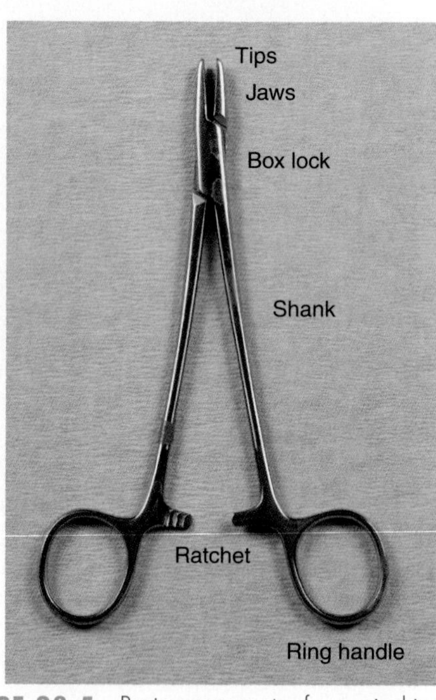

FIGURE 28-5 Basic components of a surgical instrument.

NEEDLE HOLDERS

Needle holders are designed for holding curved suture needles during suturing and for performing instrument suture ties. *Mayo-Hegar* and *Olsen-Hegar* needle holders are two commonly used needle holders (Figure 28-4). The Olsen-Hegar needle holder has built-in suture scissors, which negates the need for an assistant to cut suture. It allows the surgeon to work alone and cut suture without switching instruments. The potential disadvantage of this needle holder is that the suture may be accidentally cut during suture placement.

Needle holders consist of a set of jaws, a hinge or box lock, and handles with a ratcheted locking device (Figure 28-5). The size and design of these components vary greatly, depending on the intended use. The jaws commonly have tungsten carbide inserts that provide excellent grip. The tungsten carbide insert is hard, resistant to wear, and can be replaced when worn, thereby prolonging the life of the instrument. Worn inserts can result in improper closure of the jaws or sharp edges that inadvertently cut suture. Needle holders are available in different sizes, depending on the needle sizes they are designed to hold. Improper use of needle holders (such as using a needle holder that is too small for the size of the needle or using the needle holder to bend or twist wire) may not only damage the jaws, but may also spring the box lock and ratchet.

TECHNICIAN NOTE Needle holders are designed for handling the suture needle and performing instrument suture ties.

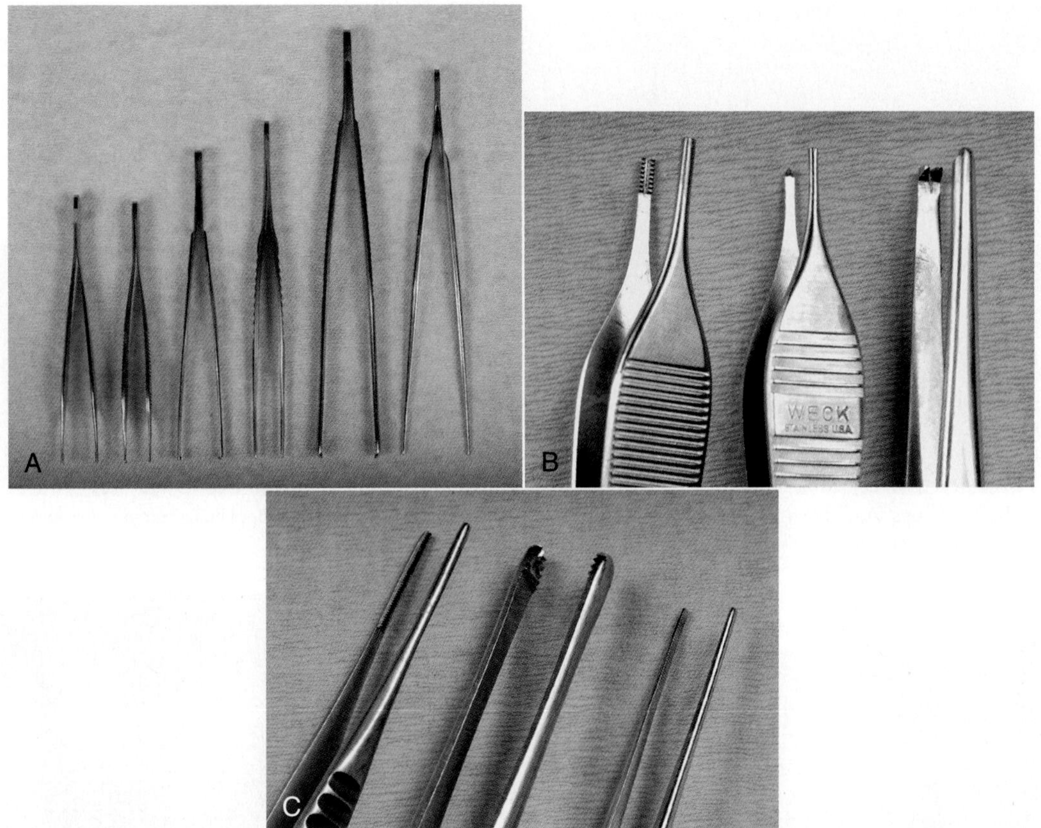

FIGURE 28-6 Thumb forceps. **A,** *Left to right:* Brown-Adson thumb forceps, Adson thumb forceps, rat-tooth thumb forceps, DeBakey vascular thumb forceps, Russian thumb forceps, dressing thumb forceps. **B,** Close-up of tips *(left to right):* Brown-Adson thumb forceps, Adson thumb forceps, rat-tooth thumb forceps. **C,** Close-up of tips *(left to right):* DeBakey vascular thumb forceps, Russian thumb forceps, dressing thumb forceps.

THUMB FORCEPS

Thumb forceps are special tissue forceps designed to hold and easily release tissue with a simple finger motion (similar to tweezers). They have a spring action, and the jaws are opposed by compressing the two metal handles together. Several different jaw surfaces are available and are designed for use with various tissues (Figure 28-6, *A* to *C*). *Brown-Adson thumb forceps* have multiple intermeshing teeth with a broad tip, providing good tissue and needle handling. They are commonly used during suturing and wound closure. *Rat-tooth thumb forceps* have large interdigitating teeth and are primarily used for skin or fascia. *Adson thumb forceps* have delicate intermeshing teeth ("rat toothed") that provide a good, atraumatic grasp of delicate tissues. They are commonly used during dissection. Cooley and *DeBakey thumb forceps* have long, narrow jaws with multiple delicate sets of teeth that are especially good for vascular surgery. *Russian thumb forceps* have a broad curved surface good for needle handling, but are traumatic when used to hold tissues. *Dressing thumb forceps* do not have teeth and are used for applying and removing dressings. They are not designed to grasp tissue and are undesirable for this use because the surgeon must squeeze hard and crush the tissue to grasp it. Thumb forceps are available in a variety of sizes, depending on the intended surgery. For example, thoracic forceps have long handles to enable the surgeon to reach tissues deep within the chest, but these same forceps would be too cumbersome and awkward to use on the skin.

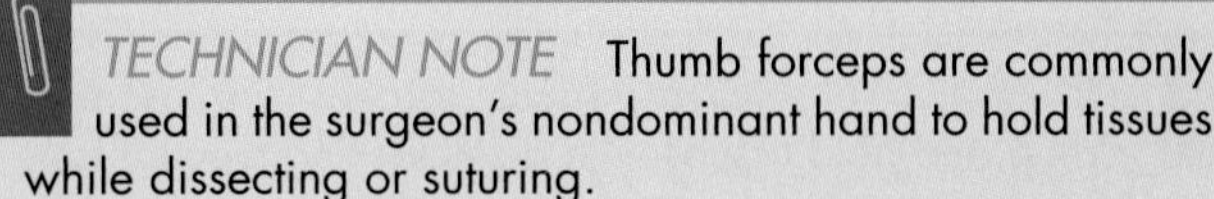

TECHNICIAN NOTE Thumb forceps are commonly used in the surgeon's nondominant hand to hold tissues while dissecting or suturing.

TISSUE FORCEPS

Tissue forceps are locking instruments that clamp tissues (Figure 28-7, *A*). Different teeth patterns allow them to grip various types of tissues without slipping. *Allis tissue forceps* securely grasp tissue, but also crush it (Figure 28-7, *B*). Therefore they are considered to be traumatic and should only be used on tissue that is being removed. *Babcock forceps* are shaped similarly to the Allis forceps, but are less traumatic because they have a smoother grasping surface and less tip compression (Figure 28-7, *B*). The Doyen intestinal tissue forceps (Figure 28-7, *A*) is a more delicate instrument used to occlude and hold intestine. The disadvantage of less traumatic tissue forceps is that they are less secure on the tissues.

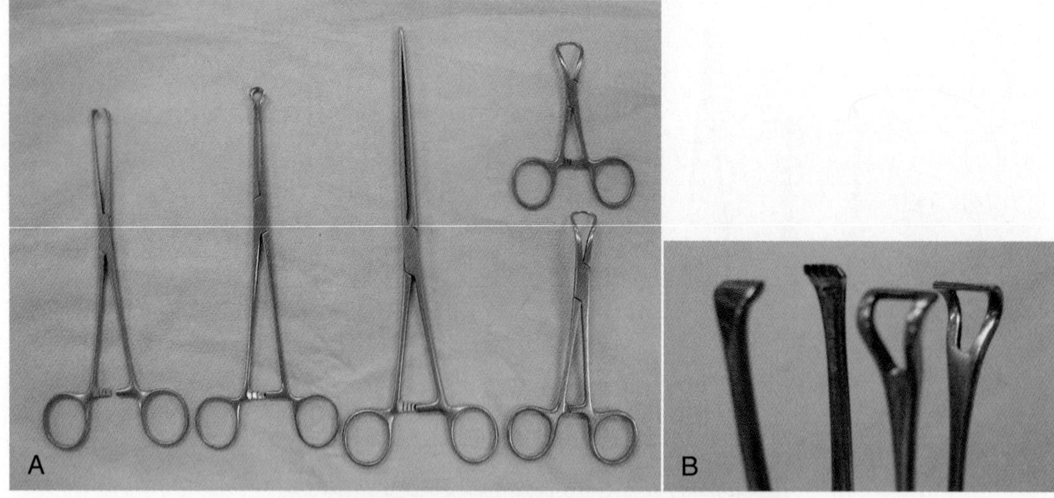

FIGURE 28-7 Tissue forceps. **A,** *Left to right:* Allis tissue forceps, Babcock tissue forceps, Doyen intestinal tissue forceps, Backhaus towel clamps (two sizes). **B,** Close-up of tips: Allis tissue forceps *(left)*, Babcock tissue forceps *(right)*.

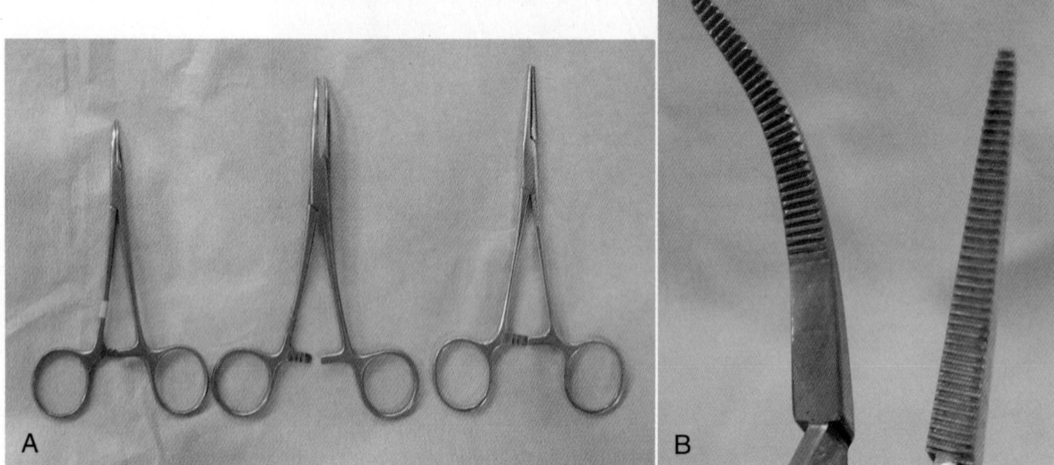

FIGURE 28-8 Hemostatic forceps. **A,** *Left to right:* Halsted mosquito hemostatic forceps, Kelly forceps, Crile forceps. **B,** Close-up of jaws: curved Kelly *(left)*, straight Crile *(right)*.

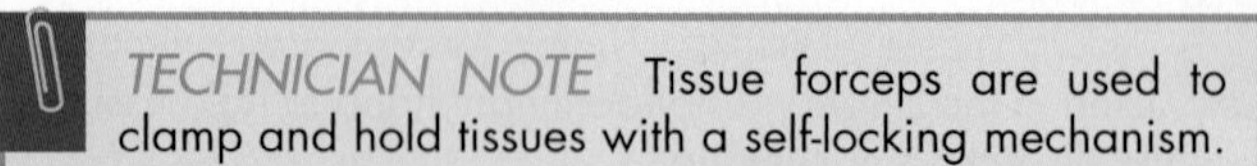

TECHNICIAN NOTE Tissue forceps are used to clamp and hold tissues with a self-locking mechanism.

Towel clamps are forceps used to attach towels and drapes to the patient. These forceps have pointed tips that curve and join like ice tongs. They are available in different sizes (see Figure 28-7, *A*). *Backhaus towel clamps* and *Roeder towel clamps* are two common designs. The Roeder towel clamp has a metal bead or ball stop attached to the jaws that prevents deep tissue penetration and prevents the towel from slipping toward the box lock of the forceps.

HEMOSTATIC FORCEPS

Hemostatic forceps are tissue forceps used to stop bleeding by crushing blood vessels (Figures 28-8 and 28-9). They are available in different sizes and may be straight or curved. Most hemostatic forceps have transverse grooves on the inside surface of the jaws to better grasp the tissue. *Halsted mosquito hemostats* are small and designed to occlude small vessels (see Figure 28-8, *A*). When using hemostatic forceps, the tips of the forceps should be used to grasp only as much tissue as necessary. *Crile forceps* and *Kelly forceps* (see Figure 28-8) are larger hemostatic forceps and are used on larger vessels. The jaws of the Crile forceps are transversely grooved for the entire length, but only the distal halves of the Kelly forceps are grooved. *Rochester-Péan forceps* are large, transversely grooved forceps that are used to clamp tissue bundles and large vessels (see Figure 28-9). *Rochester-Ochsner forceps* are similar to the Rochester-Péan forceps, but have interdigitating teeth at the tips (see Figure 28-9) that aid in grasping the tissue. Rochester-Ochsner forceps are used most commonly in orthopedic or large animal surgery. *Rochester-Carmalt forceps* are large crushing forceps with longitudinal grooves and cross-grooves at the tip to provide more traction (see Figure 28-9). These forceps are used for clamping across tissue containing vessels. The Rochester-Carmalt forceps are commonly used to crush the vessels of the ovarian pedicle or the body of the uterus during an ovariohysterectomy (spay)

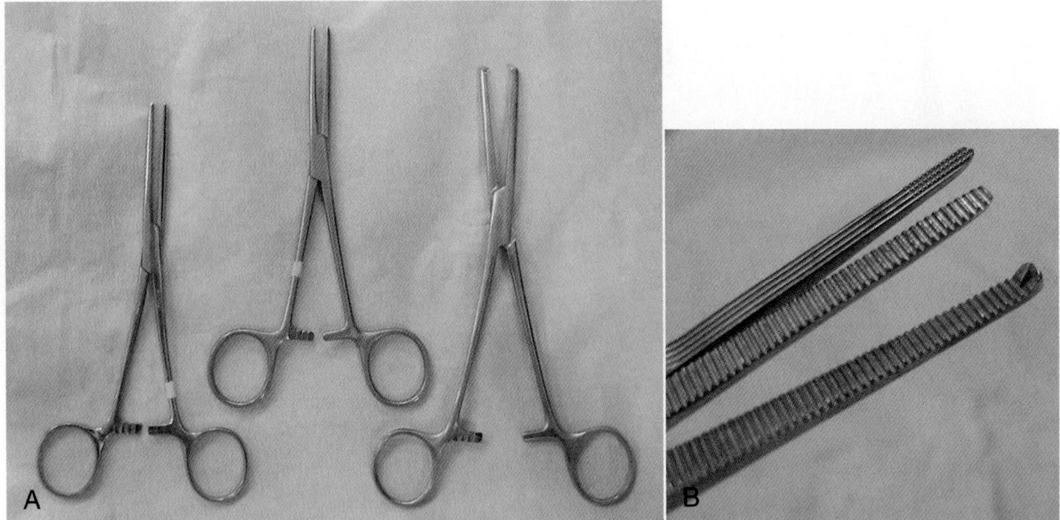

FIGURE 28-9 Hemostatic forceps. **A,** *Left to right:* Rochester-Carmalt forceps, Rochester-Péan forceps, Rochester-Ochsner forceps. **B,** Close-up of jaws *(left to right):* Rochester-Carmalt forceps, Rochester-Péan forceps, Rochester-Ochsner forceps.

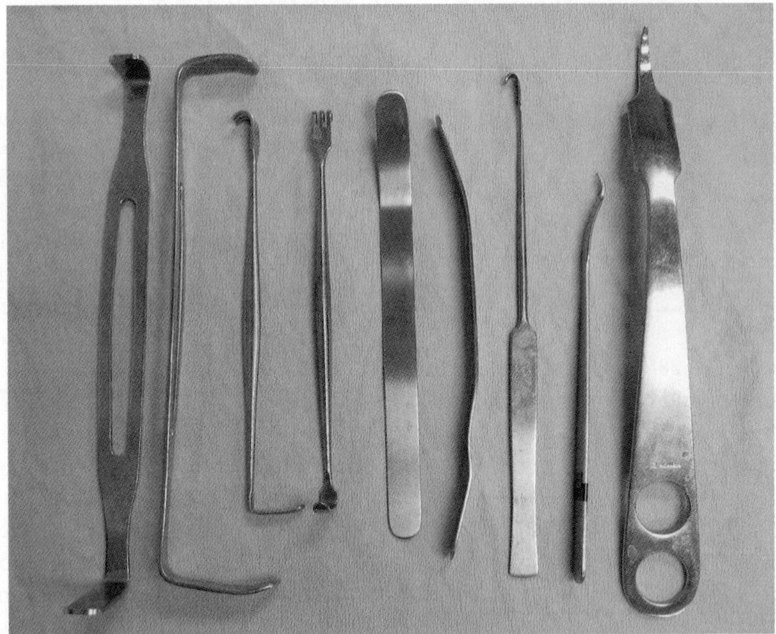

FIGURE 28-10 Hand-held retractors. *Left to right:* Two Army-Navy retractors, two Senn retractors, two small malleable retractors, Snook ovariohysterectomy hook (spay hook), two Hohman retractors (different sizes).

operation. When clamping across vessels, the forceps should be applied with the concave surface facing upward to facilitate tying the ligature. Refer to Chapter 29 for more information on the use of hemostatic forceps.

> *TECHNICIAN NOTE* Hemostatic forceps are used to clamp, crush, and hold blood vessels with a self-locking mechanism.

RETRACTORS

Properly placed retractors do not interfere with the surgery yet provide good visibility of the surgical site and allow more room for the surgeon to work. Retractors may be handheld or self-retaining. A surgical assistant is needed to maintain the position and tissue tension of a hand-held retractor. The *Army-Navy retractor* and the *Senn retractor* are double-ended hand-held retractors commonly used to retract skin, fat, or muscle (Figure 28-10). The Army-Navy retractor has smooth blades, whereas the Senn has one smooth blade and one blade with three sharp or blunt prongs. The *malleable retractor* is made of thin metal that is easily bent to the desired shape (Figure 28-10). It is commonly used to retract abdominal organs. The *Snook ovariohysterectomy hook* is a specialized type of hand-held retractor used to expose the horn of the uterus during an ovariohysterectomy (see Figure 28-10). The *Hohmann retractor* consists of a single blade and a handle that are used to lever tissues out of the

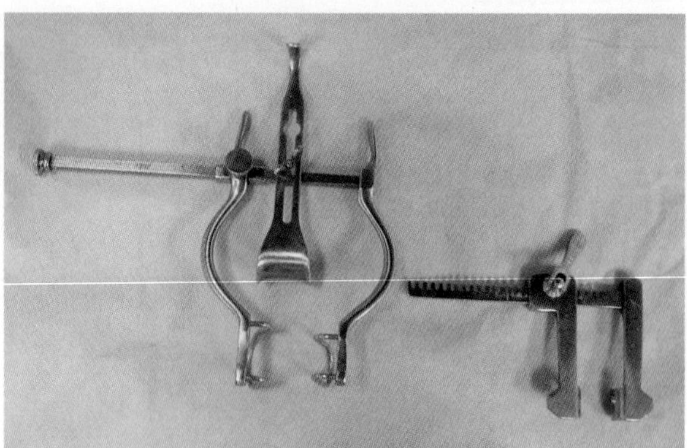

FIGURE 28-11 Self-retaining retractors. Balfour abdominal retractor *(left)*, Finochietto rib retractor *(right)*.

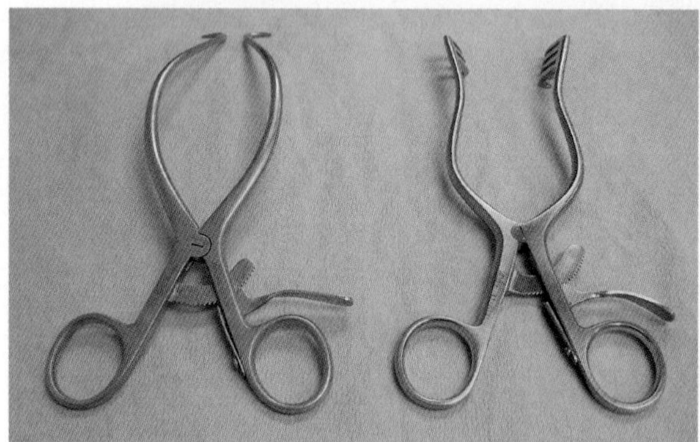

FIGURE 28-12 Self-retaining retractors. Gelpi retractor *(left)*, Weitlaner retractor *(right)*.

way for better visibility (see Figure 28-10). It is used almost exclusively in orthopedic surgery and can provide good visibility in certain joint surgeries.

> TECHNICIAN NOTE Retractors rather than hands are used to retract tissues and provide good visibility of the surgical site.

Self-retaining retractors are maintained in the desired position by some type of locking mechanism on the retractor handle. The advantage of the self-retaining retractors is that the surgeon and the assistant have their hands free for other tasks. The *Balfour retractor* provides increased exposure of the abdominal cavity (Figure 28-11). The two wirelike blades are used to distract the abdominal incision, and the solid spoonlike blade is hooked onto the sternum to distract it cranially. The *Finochietto rib spreader* retracts the ribs to expose the surgical field within the thoracic cavity (see Figure 28-11). The ratcheted part of the retractors is positioned at the dorsal aspect of the thoracic incision so that it does not interfere with the surgeon. *Gelpi retractors* and *Weitlaner retractors* (Figure 28-12) are self-retaining retractors commonly used for muscle retraction, especially in orthopedic and

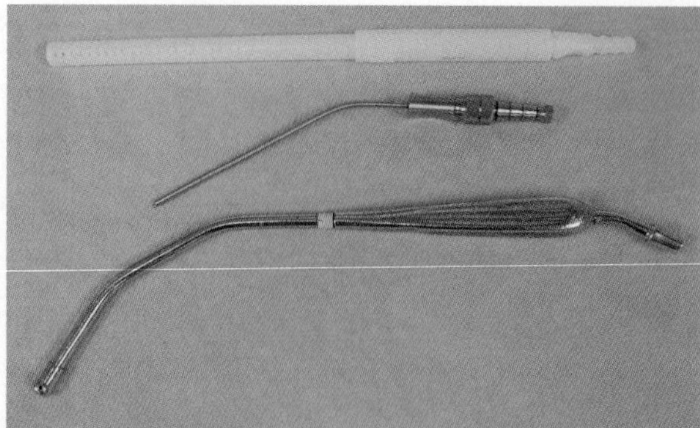

FIGURE 28-13 Suction tips. *Top to bottom:* Poole, Frazier, Yankauer. The suction tip is attached to a sterile hose. The surgeon hands the other end of the hose to a nonsterile assistant to plug it into the suction unit.

neurologic surgery. Refer to Chapter 29 for more information on retraction techniques.

SUCTION TIPS

Several different suction tips are commonly used (Figure 28-13). The *Poole tip* is used primarily in the abdominal or thoracic cavity because it has an outer sleeve with small holes to prevent tissue, such as fat, from becoming entrapped in the tip. The *Frazier tip* is most commonly used in orthopedic and neurologic surgery. The *Yankauer tip* is a general-purpose suction tip. The suction tip is attached to a long, sterile suction tube. The other end of the suction tube is connected to a nonsterile suction canister. Refer to Chapter 29 for more information on the use of suction.

STAPLING EQUIPMENT

Several different surgical stapling devices are available for an array of purposes (Figure 28-14). There are many advantages to using stapling devices in both large and small animal surgery. Stapling devices provide an easier and faster alternative to hand suturing. Some stapling devices also cut tissue after stapling. The staplers are named by an abbreviation of their designed function (Table 28-1). A number may be used after the name thoracoabdominal stapler (TA) or gastrointestinal stapler (GIA) to indicate the length of the row of staples (e.g., a TA 30 places two rows of staples 30 mm long).

MICHEL SKIN CLIPS

Drape material is often attached to the incised skin edge during surgical procedures to minimize contamination of the surgical field by the surrounding skin. The use of Michel skin clips is one method of attaching the drape to the wound edges (Figure 28-15). One end of the Michel clip-applying-and-removing forceps grips the clip. When the handles are squeezed, the clip bends to pinch the edges of the drape and the skin together. The other end of the forceps has jaws that remove the clip by bending it backward and disengaging it

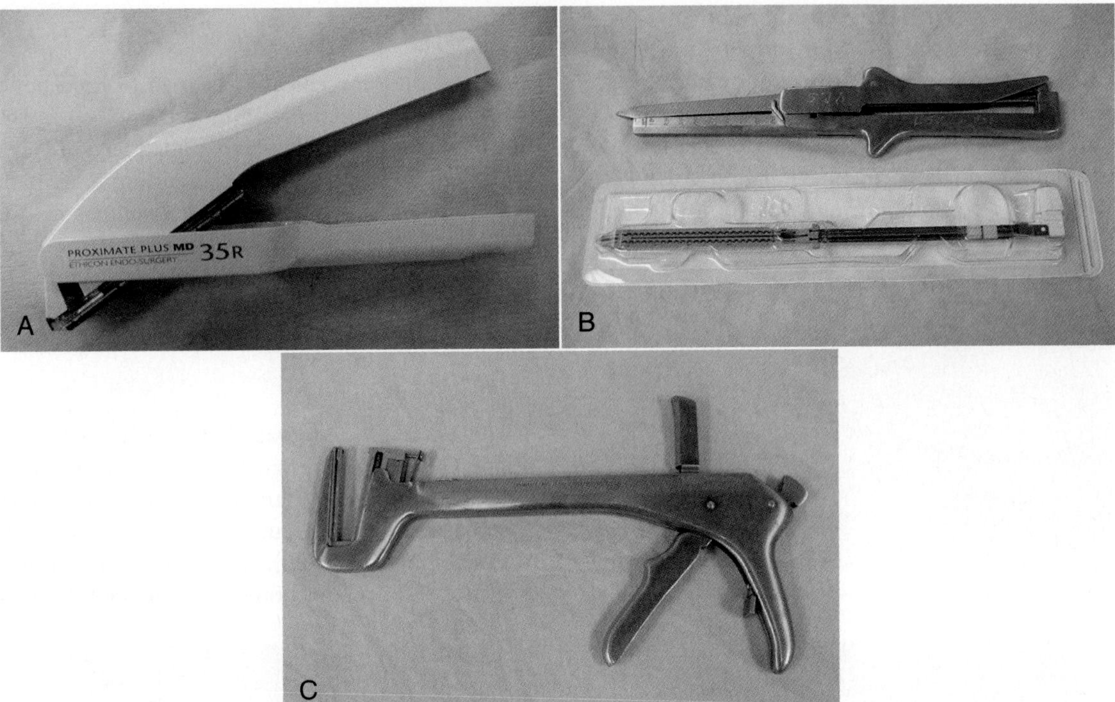

FIGURE 28-14 Surgical stapling equipment. **A,** Surgical skin stapler applies a single staple with each squeeze of the trigger (staple guns commonly hold 25 to 35 staples). **B,** Gastrointestinal stapler (GIA). Cartridge of staples are for one-time use and are purchased in presterilized package. **C,** Thoracoabdominal stapler (TA). Staple cartridges are purchased as for GIA. Shown here with staple cartridge in place.

TABLE 28-1 Stapling Equipment

Derivation of Name	Common Use	Comments
TA		
Thoracoabdominal	Lung resection	Places double or triple row of staples
GIA		
Gastrointestinal anastomosis	Gastrointestinal resection and anastomosis	Places four rows of staples and cuts between the middle two rows
EEA		
End-to-end anastomosis	Gastrointestinal anastomosis	Staples two intestinal segments together in a circular manner with a functional lumen
Skin and Fascial Stapler		
	Skin or fascia closures	Places a single staple
LDS		
Ligate-and-divide stapler	Blood vessel ligation	Places two staples on a vessel, and cuts between them

from the incision edge. There are alternatives to Michel clips, including the use of suture, "scalp clips," towel clamps, and adhesive drapes.

OPHTHALMIC INSTRUMENTS

Ophthalmic surgery requires the use of delicate instruments that must be handled carefully. Basic ophthalmic instruments include specialized scalpels, scissors, thumb forceps, needle holders, and retractors (Figure 28-16).

ORTHOPEDIC INSTRUMENTS

RONGEURS

Rongeurs have sharp cupped tips that are used to cut small pieces of dense tissue, such as bone, cartilage, or fibrous tissue (Figure 28-17, *A*). Rongeurs have a double-action or single-action mechanism (Figure 28-17, *B*). *Double-action rongeurs* have a smooth cutting action and are mechanically stronger than single-action rongeurs, but they are also larger.

Double-action rongeurs are preferred for removing large amounts of dense tissue. *Single-action rongeurs* are more commonly used in confined areas, as in removing bone to perform spinal surgery. *Kerrison rongeurs* have a gun-shaped appearance and are useful for spinal surgery. *Bone-cutting forceps* are similar to rongeurs, but have paired chisel-like tips. They are used for cutting bone and should not be mistaken for wire cutters (Figure 28-18).

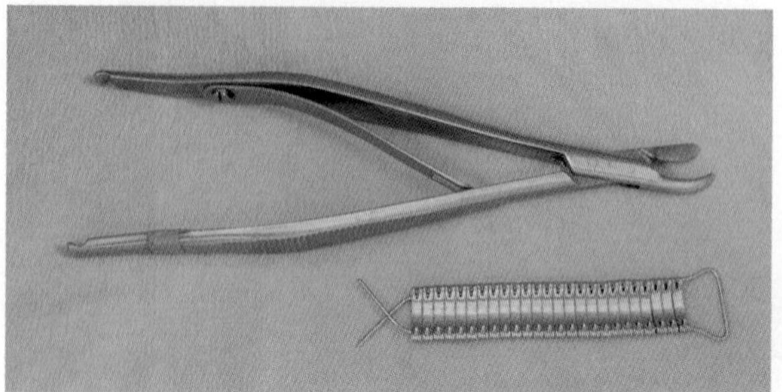

FIGURE 28-15 Michel skin clips and Michel clip forceps.

BONE-HOLDING FORCEPS

Bone-holding forceps are designed to hold bone and bone fragments in alignment while orthopedic implants (screws, pins, wires, or plates) are applied (Figure 28-19). Most bone-holding forceps are self-retaining. A *Kern bone-holding forceps* has a ratcheted handle that allows it to be clamped securely on the bone. The *self-retaining bone-holding forceps,* also known as *speed locks,* has a nut that tightens against one handle to squeeze the handles together.

CURETTES

Curettes are used to scrape hard tissue, such as bone or cartilage. Curettes are designed with a small cuplike structure at one or both ends of a handle (similar to an ice cream scoop). The cup has a sharp cutting edge and is available in various sizes (Figure 28-20). A common use of bone curettes is to retrieve cancellous bone from the medullary cavity (tibia,

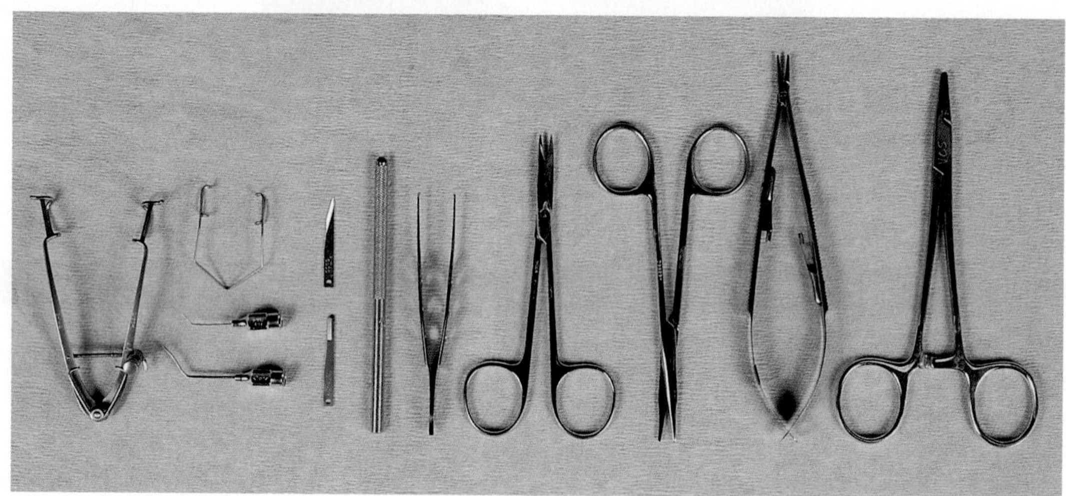

FIGURE 28-16 Common ophthalmic instruments. *Left to right:* Lid speculum, small lid speculum *(above)* and lacrimal cannulae *(below),* beaver blade handle with No. 64 and 65 surgical blades, Bishop-Harmon thumb forceps, iris scissors, tenotomy scissors, Castroviejo needle holder, and Derf needle holder.

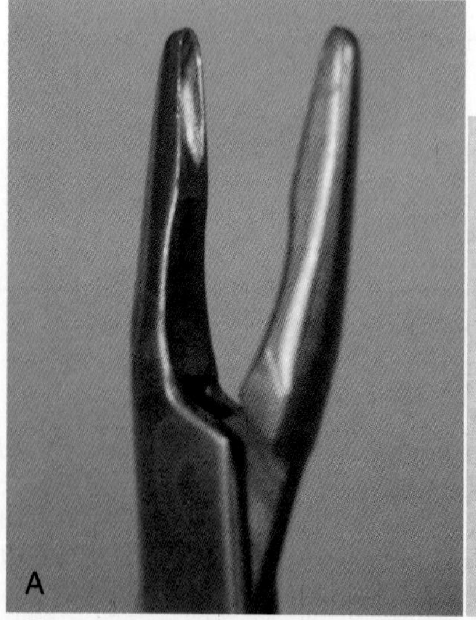

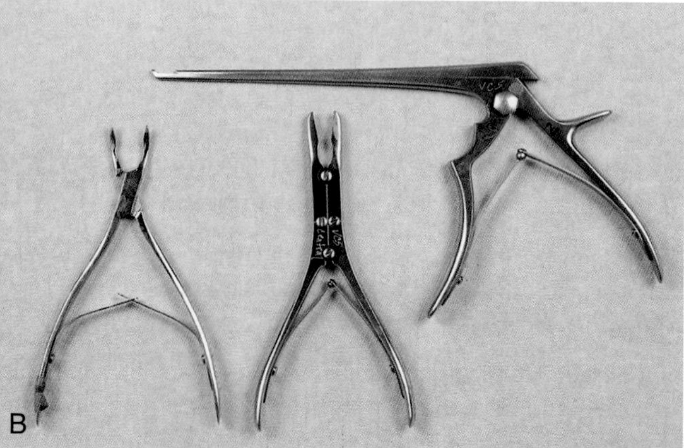

FIGURE 28-17 Rongeurs. **A,** Close-up of tips. **B,** *Left to right:* Single-action rongeur, double-action rongeur, Kerrison rongeur.

humerus, ilium) for use as a bone graft. Cancellous bone grafts are often used during fracture repair.

PERIOSTEAL ELEVATORS

Periosteal elevators are instruments that are used to pry periosteum or muscle from the bone surface. They have a bladelike structure at one or both ends of a handle. The blades have sharp or blunt edges and are available in various sizes (Figure 28-21).

OSTEOTOMES AND CHISELS

Osteotomes and chisels are used to cut bone. Osteotomes and chisels are used by pounding on the flared end of the handle with a mallet (Figure 28-22, *A*). The cutting edge of the osteotome is tapered on both sides, whereas the chisel is tapered only on one side (Figure 28-22, *B*).

GIGLI WIRE

Gigli wire is used to cut bone by placing the wire around the bone and drawing it back and forth in a sawing fashion. T-shaped handles hook onto the wire to give the surgeon a firm grasp of the wire.

TREPHINES

Trephines are T-shaped tubular instruments with a cylindrical cutting blade (Figure 28-23). Trephines are usually used to remove a core of bone for biopsy.

POWER EQUIPMENT

Some power equipment is commonly used in orthopedic and neurologic surgery. Although some drills are electric or battery powered (Figure 28-24, *A* and *B*), many orthopedic drills and saws are powered by nitrogen gas that is supplied via a sterile hose (Figure 28-24, *C*). The Hall air drill is a specialized high-speed bur that grinds bone (Figure 28-24, *D*). It is most commonly used for spinal surgery.

ORTHOPEDIC IMPLANTS

Orthopedic surgery sometimes involves the use of various products that are placed in or around the bone and left in place permanently or for an extended period of time. Metal implants are usually made of stainless steel alloy, cobalt-chromium alloys, or titanium. Of these three types, titanium is the most resistant to corrosion and has the best fatigue life. It is also the most expensive.

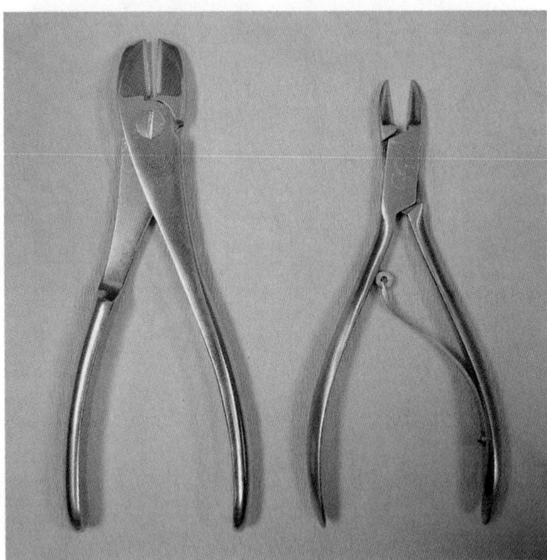

FIGURE 28-18 Wire cutters *(left)* and bone cutters *(right)*. They look similar, but should not be confused. Bone cutters have finer jaws.

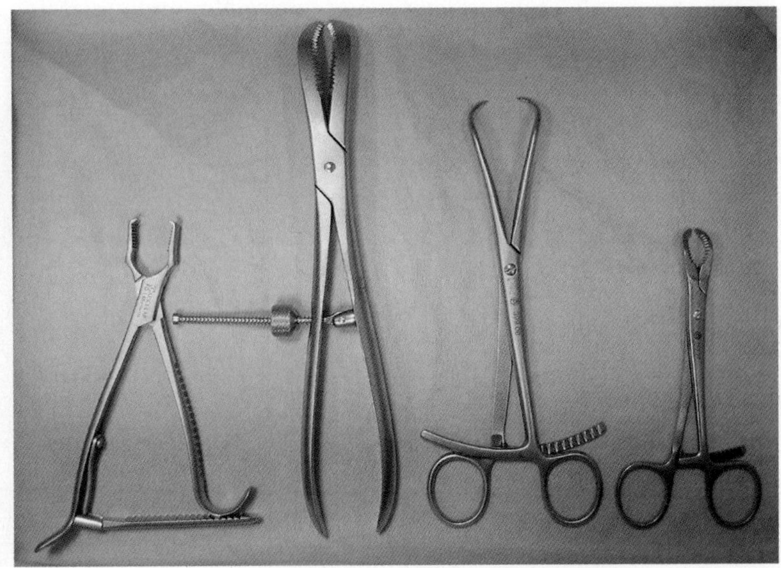

FIGURE 28-19 Bone-holding forceps. *Left to right:* Small Kern forceps, large speed-lock forceps, large point-to-point forceps, small clamshell forceps.

BONE PINS

Bone pins vary in diameter, length, and the type of points. *Steinmann pins* are smooth, stainless steel pins ranging in diameter from 1⁄16 to 1⁄4 inch. Three different types of pin points are available, including chisel, trocar, or threaded trocar. Some pins have threads, similar to a screw. A power drill or a Jacobs hand chuck is required to insert the pin into bone, and a pin cutter is necessary to cut it to the proper length (Figure 28-25). Steinmann pins may be called *intramedullary (IM) pins* because they are often placed in the medullary cavity of long bones for fracture fixation. *Kirschner wires (K-wires)* are similar to Steinmann pins, but are smaller and can be used to pin small bone fragments. The available sizes are 0.035-inch, 0.045-inch, and 0.062-inch in diameter.

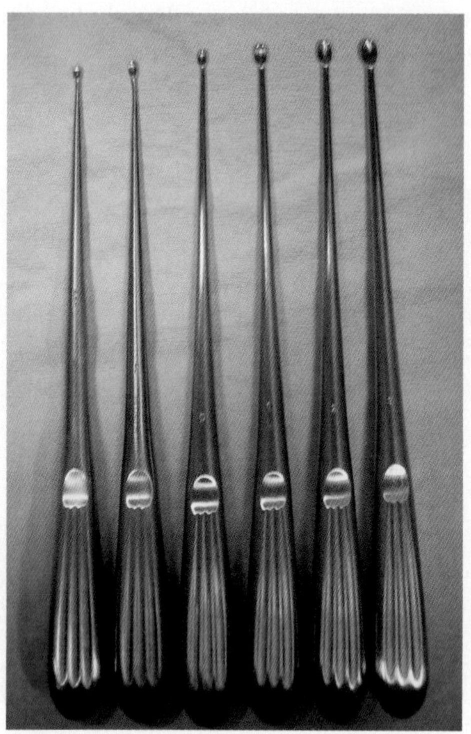

FIGURE 28-20 Bone curettes of various sizes.

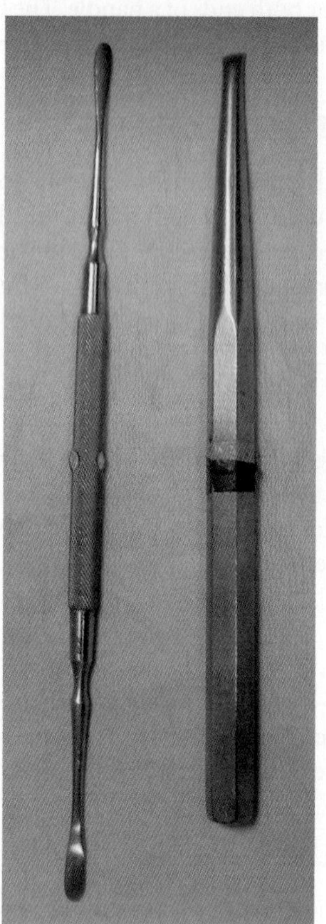

FIGURE 28-21 Periosteal elevators. Freer elevator and 1⁄4-inch Key elevator.

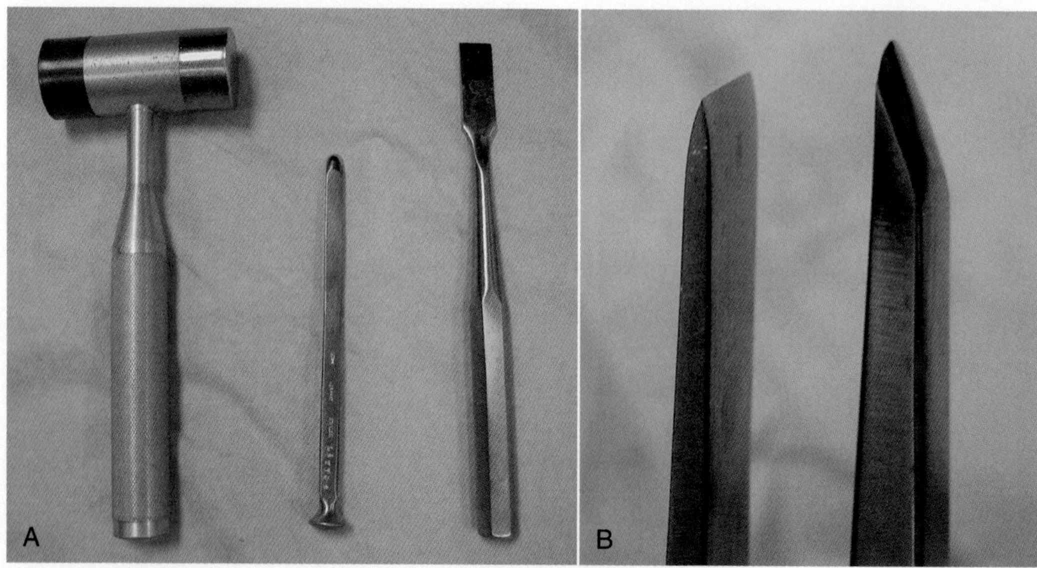

FIGURE 28-22 **A,** Mallet, chisel, and osteotome. **B,** Osteotome *(left)* and chisel *(right).*

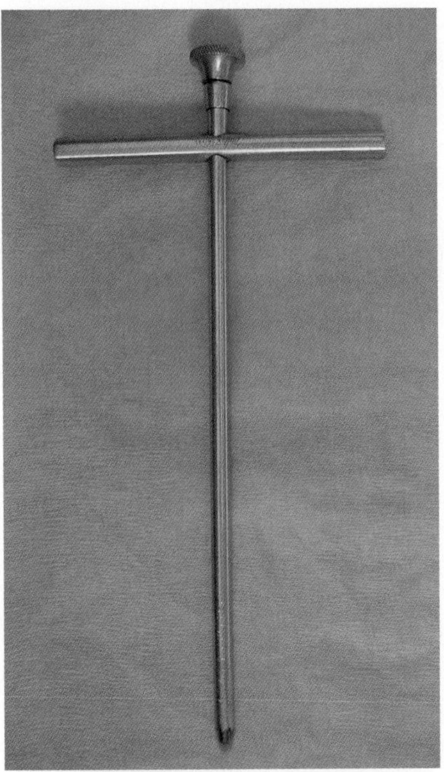

FIGURE 28-23 Michel trephine.

INTERLOCKING NAILS

Interlocking nails are similar to IM pins, but have preplaced holes through the pin that allow screw placement. Interlocking nails have more rigid fixation than IM pins. Equipment is similar to that required for pins, but specialized equipment is needed for screw placement.

ORTHOPEDIC WIRE

Stainless steel orthopedic wire is supplied on spools (Figure 28-26). The common sizes used in small animal surgery are 22 gauge, 20 gauge, and 18 gauge (Table 28-2). It is most commonly applied in a cerclage fashion by encircling the bone or bone fragments and twisting the ends in a "twist-tie" manner. Orthopedic wire is often used for fracture repair in combination with pins or bone plates.

EXTERNAL FIXATORS

External fixation is a means of stabilizing fractures using pins placed through the skin and bone. The pins are held rigid by a metal or acrylic connecting bar that is attached to the pins several centimeters from the skin (Figure 28-27). The metal apparatus uses special clamps to attach a metal connecting

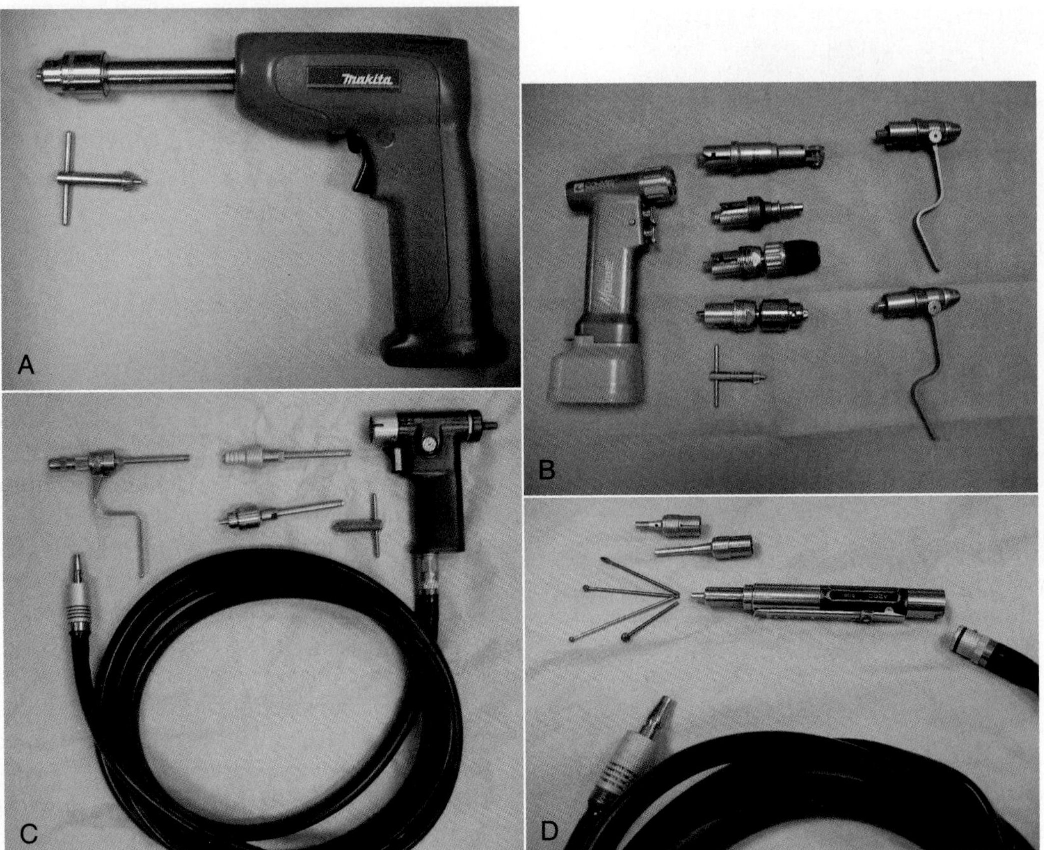

FIGURE 28-24 Power equipment. **A,** The Makita drill is an example of a battery-powered drill. **B,** ConMed Linvatec battery-powered handpiece *(left)*. Attachments shown are *(center, top to bottom)*: saw blade attachment, quick release for drill bit, keyless chuck, Jacobs chuck with key, and *(right)*: pin and wire drivers. **C,** The 3M Mini-driver is powered by a tank of pressurized nitrogen gas. It has an attachment for K-wires and quick-release or chuck attachments for drill bits. **D,** The Hall air drill has various sizes and shapes of burs, and two different length bur guards.

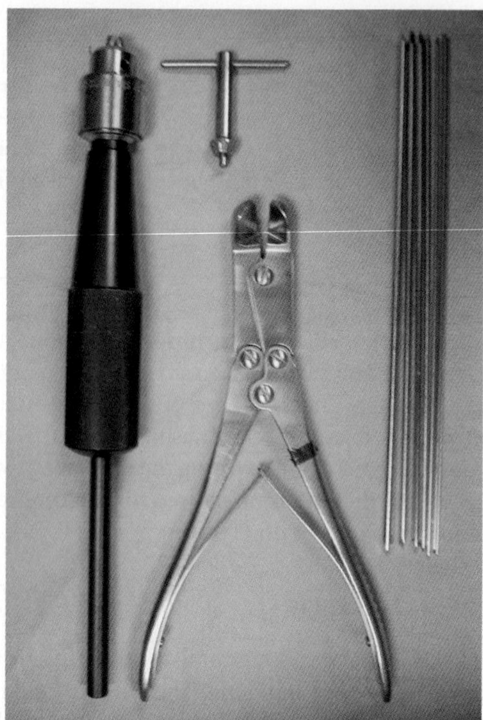

FIGURE 28-25 Jacobs hand chuck, key, pin cutter, and various sizes of Steinmann pins and K-wires.

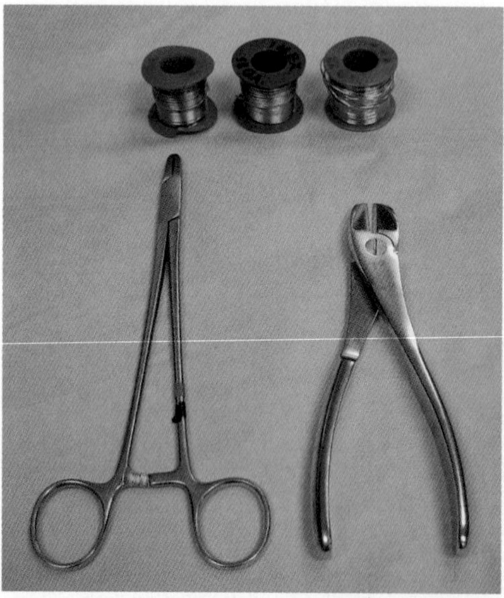

FIGURE 28-26 Orthopedic wire, wire twisters, wire cutters. Wire twisters look similar to needle holders, but are more rugged and designed to withstand higher forces.

bar to the pins. Acrylic (methyl methacrylate) connecting bars are often made from dental acrylics or hoof-wall–repair acrylics because they are less expensive than surgical grades of acrylic. The acrylic connecting bar is more versatile and lighter than the metal apparatus. Ring fixators use special wires instead of pins in the bone. Several metal rings encircle the limb and are fixed in alignment using rods. Each bone wire is clamped to one of the rings.

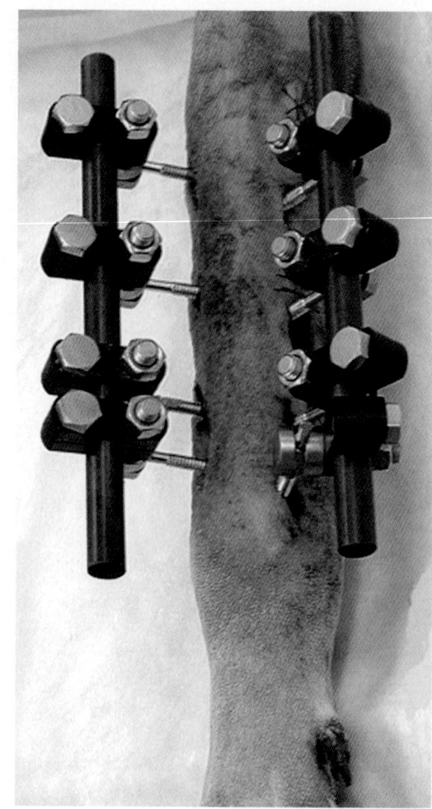

FIGURE 28-27 An external fixator on the radius of a dog. Pins that penetrate the skin and bone are fixed to bars using special clamps. (Courtesy Dr. James Toombs.)

TABLE 28-2 Commonly Used Orthopedic Wire Sizes

Gauge	Inches	Millimeters
22	0.025	0.64
20	0.032	0.81
18	0.040	1.02

BONE SCREWS

The two basic screw types are cortical and cancellous screws. Cortical screws are fully threaded screws that are designed for dense (cortical) bone. Cancellous screws are either partially threaded or fully threaded and are made with wider threads to have a better grip in the softer cancellous bone (Figure 28-28).

The general steps of screw placement include drilling a hole in the bone, measuring the hole with a depth gauge to determine the proper screw length, using a bone tap (a screwlike instrument with sharp threads) to cut a screw path in the bone, and inserting the screw with a specialized screwdriver. Bone screws may be used alone or in conjunction with a bone plate or interlocking nail.

Bone screws are named by both the screw length and thread diameter (in millimeters). Commonly used screws in small animal surgery are 2.7- and 3.5-mm diameter cortical screws and 4.0-mm diameter cancellous screws. All of these screws have hexagonal heads and are driven by the same hexagonal screwdriver. Smaller screws (1.5- and 2.0-mm diameter) have cruciate heads and require a small, cruciate screwdriver. Larger screws (4.5-, 5.5-, and 6.5-mm diameter) are used in large animal surgery. These screws use a large hexagonal screwdriver.

BONE PLATES

There are many different types of bone plates (Figure 28-29). Bone plates are named by the number of screw holes and by the screw diameter size that best fits the plate. For example, a seven-hole, 3.5-mm plate would use seven, 3.5-mm diameter screws. Bone plates must be bent to match the curve of the bone and fastened to it with bone screws. Instrumentation required to apply a bone plate is highly specialized and includes drills, drill bits, drill guides, depth gauges, bone taps, tap sleeves, screws, screwdrivers, and plate benders (Figure 28-30). Although bone plating is more complex than other types of orthopedic fixation, plate fixation is much more stable in most cases.

TOTAL HIP PROSTHESIS

Replacement of the hip joint with a prosthesis may be done in some dogs with severe arthritis. This procedure is done by highly trained veterinary surgeons and requires much specialized orthopedic equipment in addition to the prosthesis itself. The femoral prosthesis consists of a long stem that fits inside the proximal femur and a ball that replaces the femoral head. A special cup replaces the acetabulum.

ARTHROSCOPIC INSTRUMENTS AND EQUIPMENT

The arthroscope is used as a diagnostic and surgical tool in veterinary surgery. It is used mostly to examine various joints of the horse, including the scapulohumeral, humeroradial, carpal, fetlock, distal interphalangeal, coxofemoral (foals only), stifle, and tarsocrural. It is also used to examine various joints in the dog. Arthroscopy is used primarily to remove osteochondral chip fragments and osteochondritic lesions on the articular surface in joints of young horses and dogs. The arthroscope has been used to visualize intraarticular fractures for lag screw fixation, such as third carpal bone slab fractures in the carpus (knee) of horses and meniscal and cruciate injuries in dogs. The arthroscope has also been used to perform tenoscopy of the digital flexor tendon sheath and sinuscopy of the paranasal sinuses through trephined holes in the facial bones overlying the sinuses of horses. Most of the equipment used in veterinary arthroscopy has been adapted from human arthroscopy. New technology is constantly developed that will no doubt influence the veterinary field. This section is intended to allow the veterinary technician to become more familiar with the instruments and techniques of arthroscopy.

ARTHROSCOPE

There is a selection of different arthroscopes that have been developed with various diameters and viewing angles. For example, there is a 5-mm-outer-diameter (OD) arthroscope with either a 10-degree, 25-degree, or 70-degree lens angle; a 4-mm OD with a 10-degree, 30-degree, 70-degree, or 110-degree lens angle; a 2.7-mm OD with a 5-degree, 30-degree, or 70-degree lens angle; and a 1.9-mm OD with a 5-degree or 30-degree lens angle. A 4-mm OD, 25-degree or 30-degree angled lens scope is generally used by most equine surgeons (Figure 28-31), whereas a 2.7-mm OD, 30-degree angled lens scope is commonly used for canine arthroscopy. Most arthroscopes have a television camera permanently coupled to them, which allows the surgeon to view the joint on a television monitor (Figure 28-32). A television monitor has the advantage of a larger image. This greatly improves visualization of the intraarticular space compared with direct viewing through the eyepiece of the arthroscope. This method also provides better aseptic technique because the surgeon's face is not near the surgical field, and an assistant can operate the camera-scope unit, allowing the surgeon more freedom. A monitor also allows several persons to observe the procedure simultaneously, and a videotape record can be made for future replay.

ANCILLARY ARTHROSCOPIC EQUIPMENT

Along with the arthroscope come various instruments used to introduce the scope into the joint. Stab incisions are made in the skin over the joint space once the site is surgically prepared through which the arthroscope and hand instruments will be inserted once the animal is positioned for surgery.

Sharp Trocar and Sleeve

A pointed instrument called a *sharp trocar* is inserted inside a hollow, cannula type of instrument called the *sleeve* (Figure 28-33). The trocar and sleeve unit are used to penetrate the fibrous portion of the joint capsule through a stab incision.

Blunt Obturator

Once the sharp trocar has penetrated the fibrous joint capsule, the sharp trocar is replaced with a conical (blunt) obturator (Figure 28-34), which is used to penetrate the synovial membrane of the joint capsule and advance the sleeve into the joint space with less risk of damaging the articular cartilage. At this point, the obturator is withdrawn from the sleeve. The joint space is distended with a sterile, balanced electrolyte solution (fluids) before placement of the sleeve in the joint, so a rush of fluid through the barrel of the sleeve will occur as the obturator is removed. The obturator is replaced with the arthroscope (Figure 28-35), which is designed to lock onto the sleeve once it is slid into position in the sleeve.

Light Cable, Light Projector, and Television Camera

Once the arthroscope is positioned in the joint, a fiber-optic light cable (Figure 28-36) is attached directly to the optical light port on the arthroscope (Figure 28-37). A high-intensity light generated from a specially designed light projector is fed through the fiber-optic cable and through the arthroscope to illuminate the joint space (Figure 28-38).

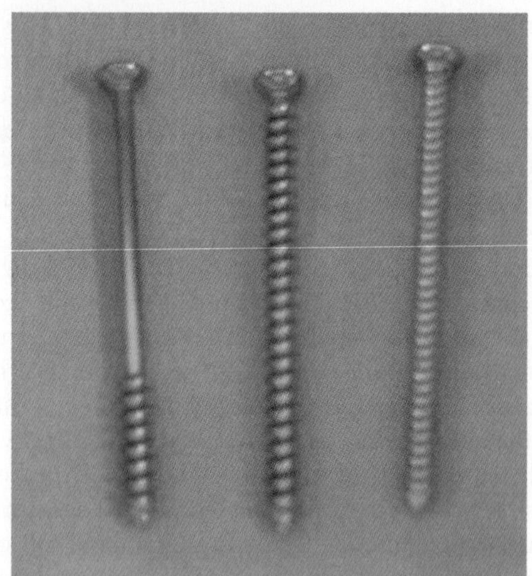

FIGURE 28-28 Bone screws. *Left to right:* Partially threaded cancellous screw, fully threaded cancellous screw, and fully threaded cortical screw.

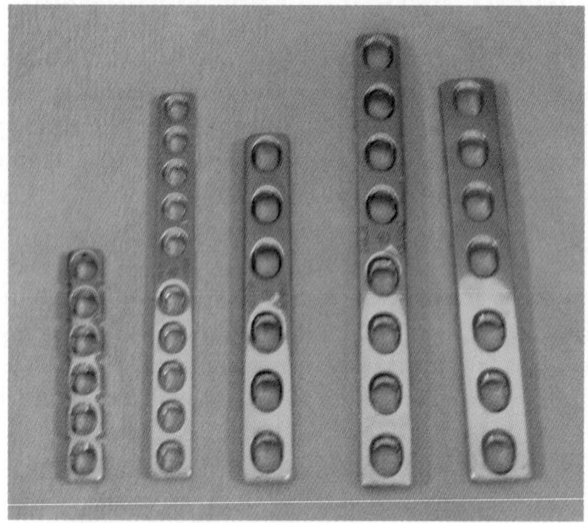

FIGURE 28-29 Various sizes of bone plates.

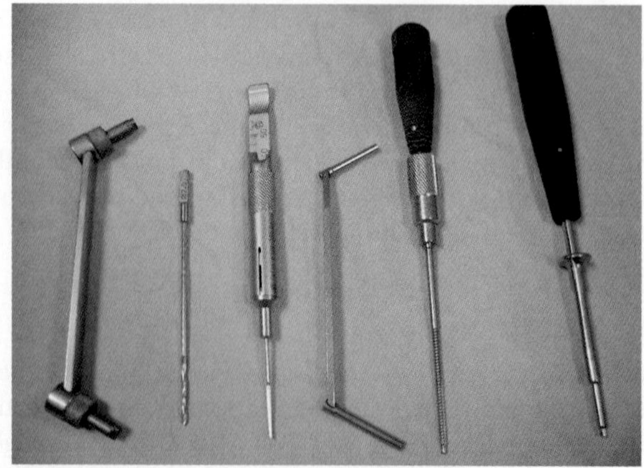

FIGURE 28-30 Bone plating equipment. *Left to right:* Drill guide, drill bit, depth gauge, tap sleeve (to prevent soft tissues from being caught on the bone tap), bone tap, and screwdriver.

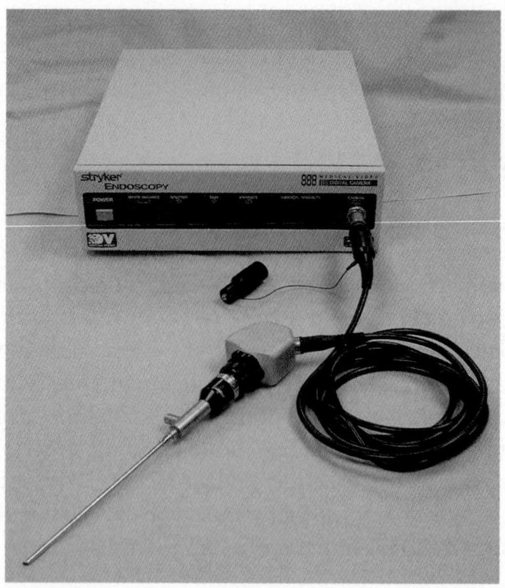

FIGURE 28-31 Television camera and 4-mm-OD arthroscope.

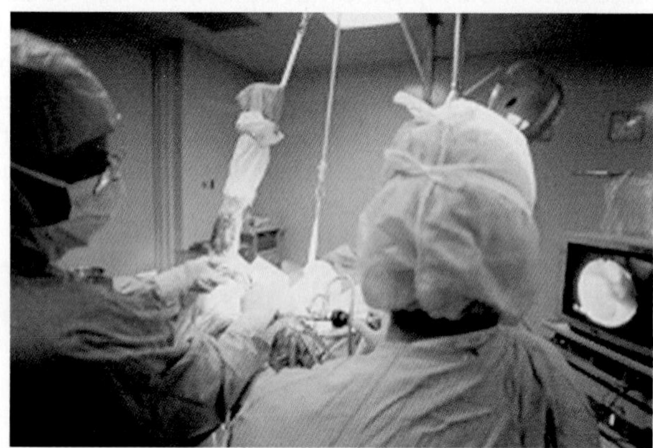

FIGURE 28-32 Most arthroscopic procedures are viewed on a monitor.

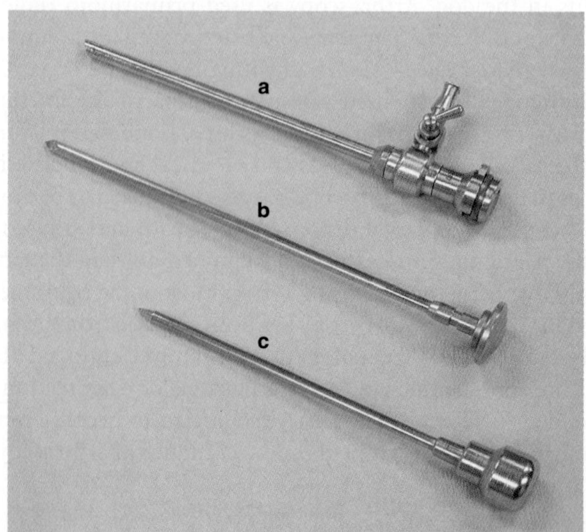

FIGURE 28-33 The sharp trocar *(b)* fits inside the arthroscope sleeve *(a)*. The unit is used to penetrate the fibrous joint capsule through a stab incision in the skin. The conical obturator *(c)* replaces the sharp trocar in the sleeve once the fibrous joint capsule is penetrated.

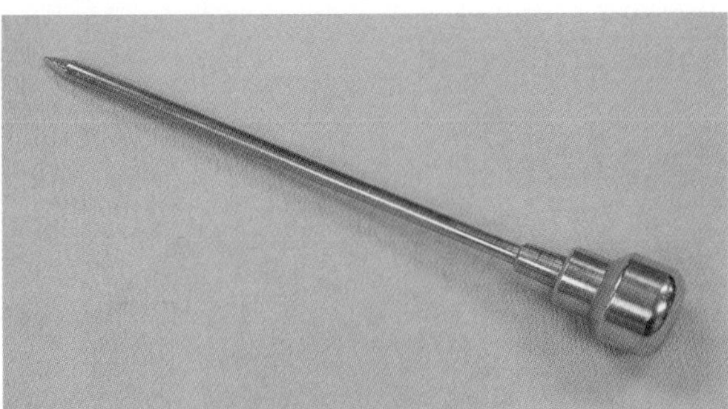

FIGURE 28-34 The conical obturator replaces the sharp trocar in the sleeve and is used to penetrate the synovial membrane portion of the joint capsule and advance the sleeve further into the joint.

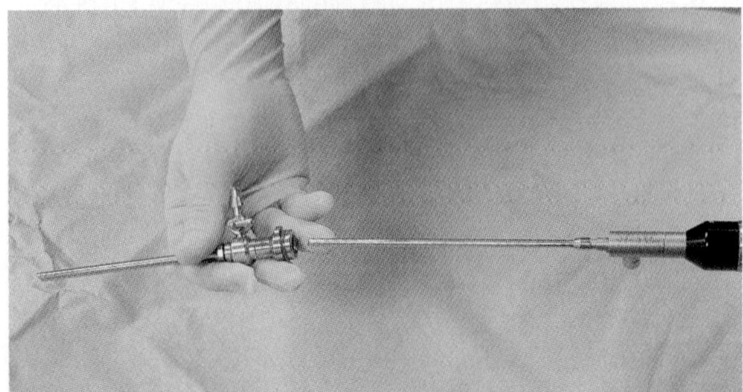

FIGURE 28-35 Once the sleeve is in position in the joint, the obturator is removed, and the arthroscope is placed into the sleeve.

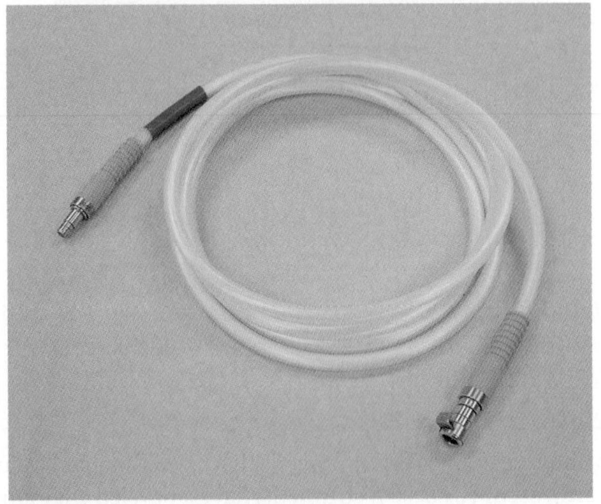

FIGURE 28-36 Fiber-optic light cable. It should be handled carefully to prevent damaging the optic fibers.

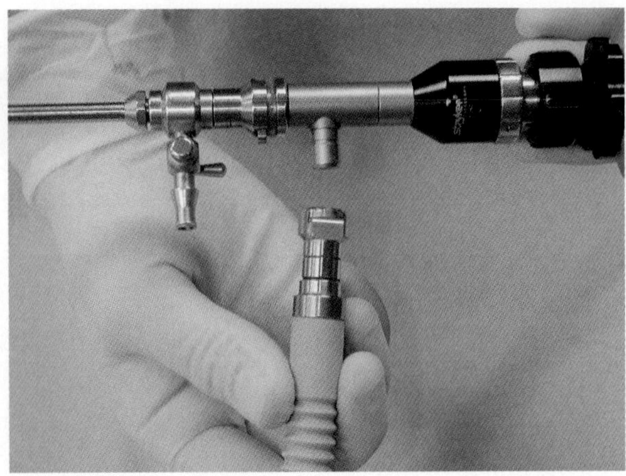

FIGURE 28-37 The fiber-optic light cable attaches to the light port of the arthroscope.

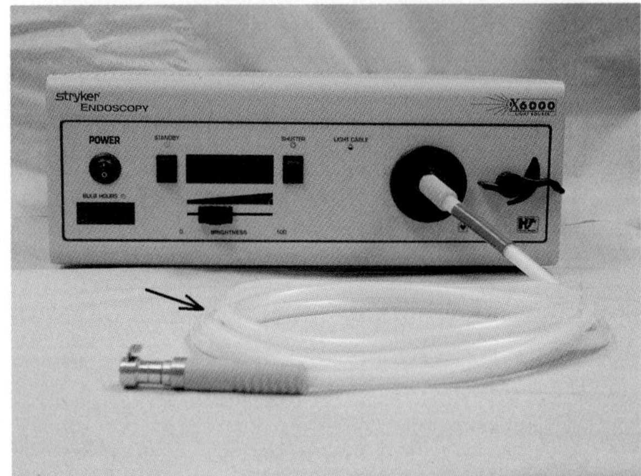

FIGURE 28-38 Light projector is designed to project light through a fiber-optic light cable *(arrow)* of the arthroscope.

FLUID DELIVERY SYSTEMS

Fluid, usually a balanced electrolyte solution, is infused into the joint under pressure to maintain distention of the joint capsule, which is essential for visualization of the intraarticular space. Gas insufflation, using CO_2 or nitrous oxide, has also been used as a method of distending the joint. However, a special system with a pressure-regulating device is required. One disadvantage of gas is that it does not allow for lavage of the joint space if osteochondral chip fragments become detached in the joint. The fluid is infused into the joint space through the sleeve, around the arthroscope. The sleeve has at least one stopcock that is used as an ingress port to connect a sterile fluid line (Figure 28-39).

Pressurized Bag System

Various systems are available to deliver fluid to the joint. One system is a pressurized bag design. A pneumatic pressure cuff is slipped around a bag containing sterile fluid. The cuff is inflated with air, which squeezes the fluid bag, thus pressurizing the fluid (Figure 28-40). The amount of pressure is regulated by the amount of cuff inflation.

Automated Pump System

Another type of system uses a motorized pump to regulate the fluid rate through the fluid lines connected to the arthroscope. One example of this type of system is the Hydroflex (Davol, Inc.) (Figure 28-41). The pressure and fluid volume going into the joint are automatically regulated within the fluid pump. This automated pressure-sensitive pump system regulates the pressure via a pressure feedback control. This allows the pump to maintain a preset pressure in the joint without the surgeon having to adjust the fluid pressure.

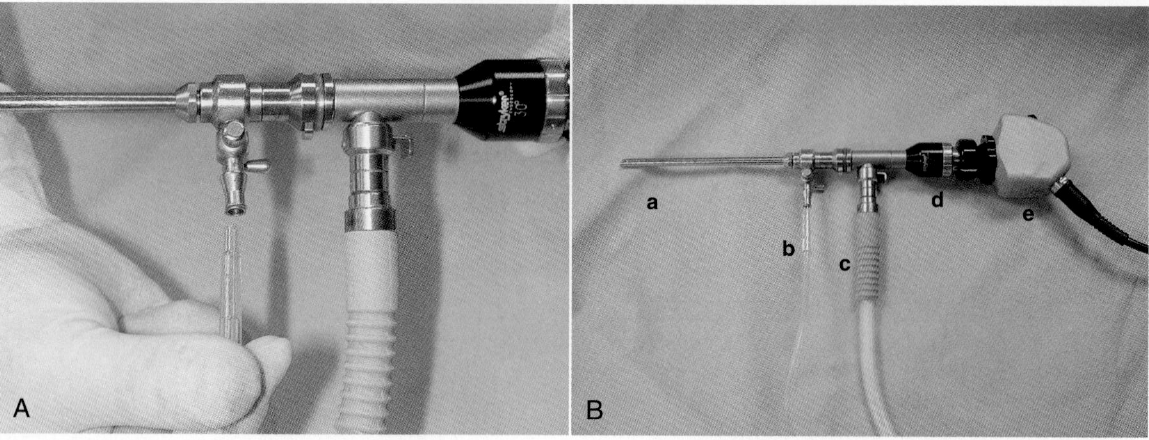

FIGURE 28-39 A, The fluid line is connected to the stopcock of the arthroscope. B, Arthroscopic sleeve *(a)*, fluid line *(b)*, light cable *(c)*, arthroscope *(d)*, and camera *(e)*.

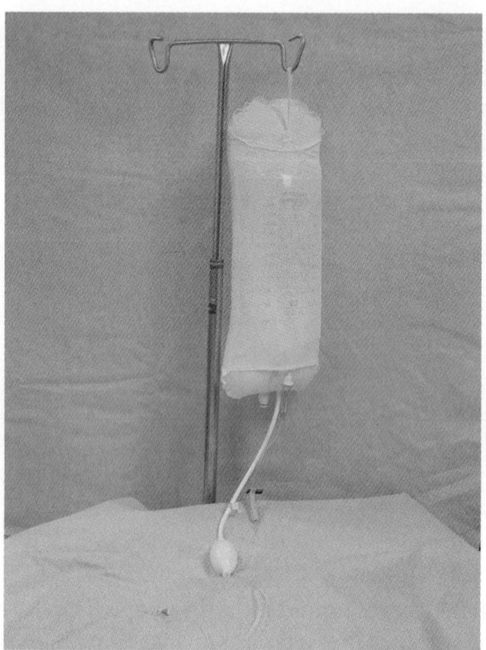

FIGURE 28-40 Pressurized bag of fluid can be used to distend a joint during arthroscopy.

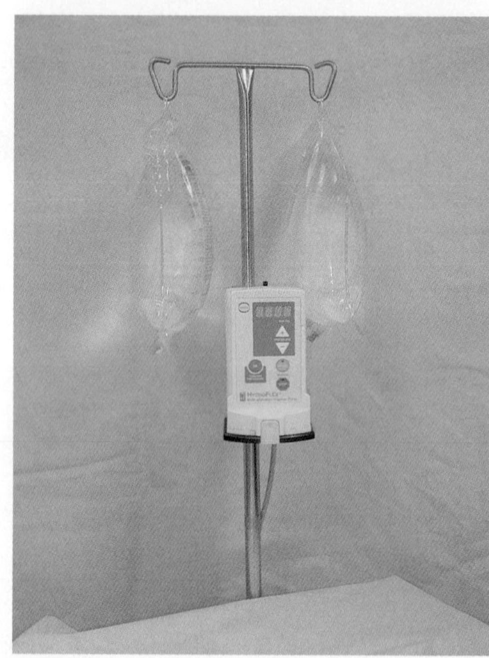

FIGURE 28-41 Automated fluid pressure pump can be used to infuse sterile fluid into a joint during arthroscopy. The pressure within the joint is automatically regulated by the pump.

HAND INSTRUMENTS FOR ARTHROSCOPIC SURGERY

Numerous hand instruments of various types are available or have been adapted for arthroscopy. They are used to remove or retrieve osteochondral chip fragments, débride articular cartilage or subchondral bone, or probe cartilage or cartilage lesions. The instruments are inserted into the joint through a separate stab incision, and the arthroscopic operation is performed via a technique called *triangulation*. Only the most commonly used instruments are discussed here.

Blunt Probe

The blunt probe is used to probe a site in the joint to determine such aspects as cartilage integrity or the extent of a cartilage lesion (Figure 28-42).

Rongeurs and Grasping Forceps

Various types and sizes of rongeurs have been adapted for use in arthroscopy. These instruments have a beveled edge along cupped jaws to cut the attachments of an osteochondral chip fragment as it is removed (Figure 28-43). Forceps are used to retrieve loosely attached fragments (see Figure 28-43).

Elevators and Osteotomes

These instruments have small beveled heads that are designed to cut or break down the attachments of an osteochondral chip fragment and elevate it from the parent subchondral bone bed (Figure 28-44).

Curettes

Curettes are inserted into the joint to débride a defect left in the articular cartilage or subchondral bone after removal of an osteochondral chip fragment or osteochondritic lesion (Figure 28-45).

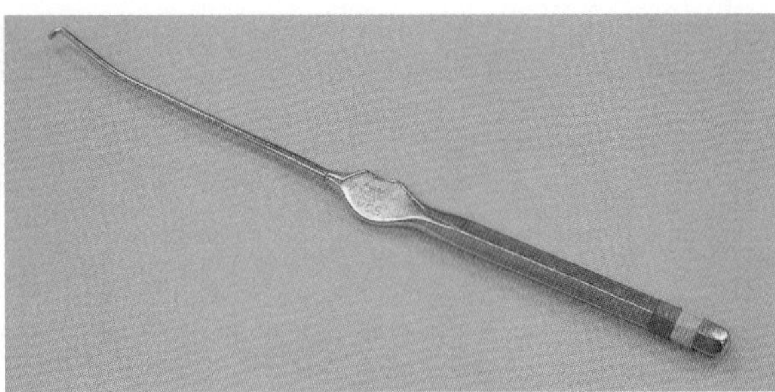

FIGURE 28-42 Blunt arthroscopy probe.

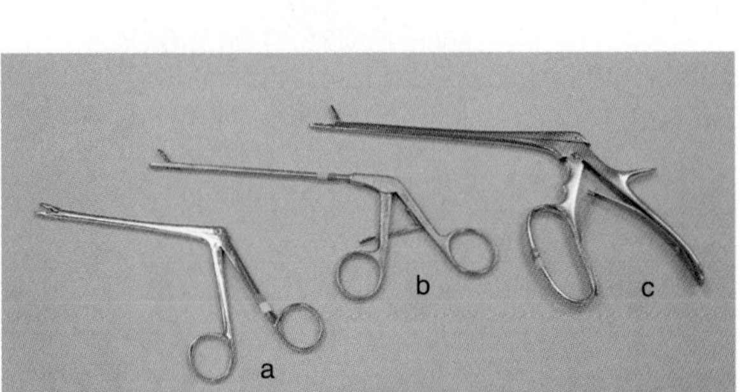

FIGURE 28-43 Rongeurs used in arthroscopy: Love-Gruenwald (a), grasping forceps (b), and Ferris-Smith (c).

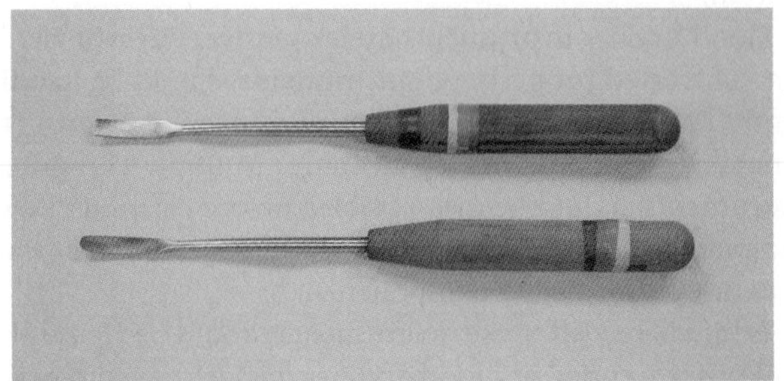

FIGURE 28-44 Elevator and osteotome used in arthroscopy.

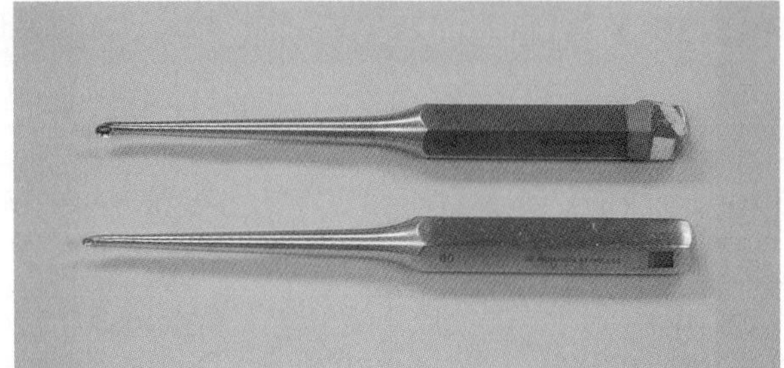

FIGURE 28-45 Small cupped bone curettes used in arthroscopy.

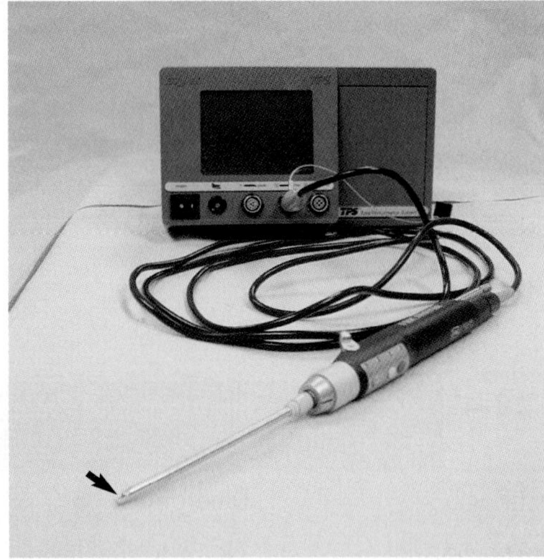

FIGURE 28-46 Motorized arthroplasty system with bur attachment (arrow).

Motorized Burs

Motorized burs are often referred to as a *motorized arthroplasty system*. The system consists of a small rounded bur attached to a power-driven shaft. The bur and shaft are enclosed in a sleeve, with a portion of the bur protected to prevent inadvertent damage to surrounding articular cartilage (Figure 28-46). This instrument is also used to débride a defect left in the articular cartilage or subchondral bone after removal of an osteochondral chip fragment or osteochondritic lesion. The speed of rotation of the bur can be adjusted, and the bur is usually operated at several thousand revolutions per minute. Most systems operate with an on-off foot-pedal switch for the surgeon.

INSTRUMENT PACKS

Most veterinary hospitals organize surgical instruments into several different instrument packs based on the type of surgical procedure. Surgical pack organization is dependent on the type of practice and surgeries performed, but some examples are as follows: general packs for soft tissue surgeries, bone packs for orthopedic surgeries, emergency packs for emergency and minor procedures, and neurologic packs for spinal surgeries (Tables 28-3 and 28-4). A pack system helps to organize the instruments so that the most commonly used instruments are readily available and infrequently used instruments are not contaminated and resterilized unnecessarily. For example, all commonly used instruments for spinal surgery are in one pack, so it is opened, used, cleaned, sterilized, and repacked only when necessary. Infrequently used instruments are typically wrapped individually. Large and bulky instruments are also packed separately. In addition, some commonly used instruments (e.g., scalpel handle, hemostats, thumb forceps, scissors, needle holders, sponges) may be wrapped individually to provide access to an additional instrument without having to open an entire instrument pack.

Each type of pack should be organized such that items are always placed in the same location on the tray (Figure 28-47). This makes it easier to inventory the instruments and facilitates finding the instruments quickly during surgery. Sponges may be counted at the beginning and end of each surgery to be sure that none has been left in the patient.

TABLE 28-3 Small Animal Instrument Packs

Soft Tissue/General Pack	Emergency Pack	Orthopedic
No. 3 scalpel handle	No. 3 scalpel handle	Army-Navy retractors
Brown-Adson thumb forceps	Brown-Adson thumb forceps	Senn retractors
Adson thumb forceps	Needle holder, Olsen-Hegar	Rongeurs
Needle holder, Mayo-Hegar	Mayo scissors, curved	Large Kern bone-holding forceps
Mayo scissors	Mosquito hemostats (3 curved, 3 straight)	Small Kern bone-holding forceps
Metzenbaum scissors	Crile or Kelly forceps (1 curved, 1 straight)	Bone curette
Wire-suture scissors	Allis forceps	Periosteal elevator
Mosquito hemostats (4 curved, 4 straight)	Towel clamps (4)	Steinmann pins (5/64, 3/32, 7/64, 1/8, 9/64, 5/32, 3/16, 1/4)
Carmalt forceps (2 curved)	Crile forceps (1 curved, 1 straight)	Wire (0.035, 0.045, 0.062)
Allis forceps (2)	Sponges (standard count)	Jacobs chuck and key
Ovariohysterectomy hook (Snook hook)	Sterilization indicator	Roll 18-gauge stainless
Towel clamps (8)		Roll 20-gauge stainless
Towels (6)		Roll 22-gauge stainless
Stainless steel bowl		Metal ruler
Sponges (standard count)		Michel clips and applicator
Lap sponges (2)		Sterilization indicator
Sterilization indicator		

TABLE 28-4 Large Animal Standard and Emergency Packs

Standard Pack	Emergency Pack
No. 3 scalpel handle	No. 3 scalpel handle
No. 4 scalpel handle	No. 4 scalpel handle
Rat-tooth thumb forceps (3)	Rat-tooth thumb forceps
Adson thumb forceps (3)	Brown-Adson thumb forceps
Needle holders (2)	Needle holder
Mayo scissors (1 curved, 1 straight)	Mayo scissors (1 curved, 1 straight)
Operating scissors (2 curved, 2 straight)	Mosquito hemostats (sharp-sharp)
Metzenbaum scissors (1 curved, 1 straight)	Allis tissue forceps (2)
Bandage scissors	Towel clamps (4)
Mosquito hemostats (4 straight, 4 curved)	Towel
Kelly or Crile forceps (2 straight, 2 curved)	Sponges (standard count)
Ochsner forceps, 15-cm (1 curved, 1 straight)	Sterilization indicator
Allis tissue forceps (2)	
Towel clamps (16)	
Towels (4)	
Saline bowl	
Sponges (standard count)	
Sterilization indicator	

INSTRUMENT CARE

Most surgical instruments are made of stainless steel, which is rust resistant and retains a sharp edge. The two common instrument finishes are polished or satin. The polished finish is durable, but tends to reflect light, which may impair the surgeon's vision. The satin or dull finish was developed to eliminate glare, but it is less resistant to spotting and discoloration.

Good quality instruments are expensive, but will last for years if treated properly. All instruments should be handled gently, and delicate instruments should be separated from the general instruments before cleaning. Multiple-component instruments should be disassembled before cleaning. Power equipment should be cleaned separately to ensure that water does not get inside the components.

Immediately after use, instruments should be rinsed with cold water to prevent blood and organic debris from drying in the serrations, hinges, box locks, or ratchets. Distilled or deionized water is preferable to tap water to prevent staining or corrosion of the instruments. If there will be a delay before final cleaning, the instruments can be immersed in water containing an instrument detergent. Each instrument is scrubbed with a soft brush in warm water using a neutral pH instrument detergent. Abrasive cleaning agents should never be used on surgical instruments. An ultrasonic (high-frequency sound) cleaner (Figure 28-48) is used after manual cleaning to remove tightly bound soil or clean areas that the brush cannot reach. Instruments should be placed in the ultrasound unit with the box locks open. Instruments of dissimilar metals (e.g., chrome and stainless steel) should not be put together in the ultrasound unit because this may result in pitting of the instruments. Instruments should be thoroughly rinsed and air-dried (wiping instruments may leave lint residue) before autoclaving to prevent rust spots.

Instruments with a working action, such as a hinge or box lock, should be treated with an instrument lubricant or instrument "milk" after each cleaning. The recommended lubricants are water soluble, so thorough cleaning will remove

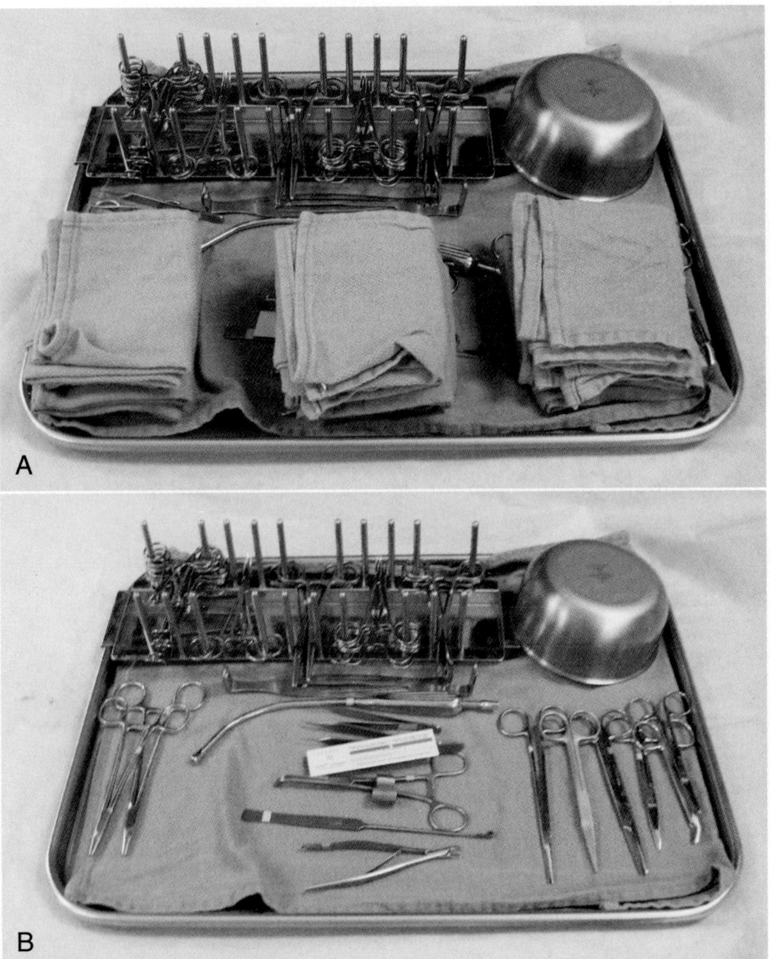

FIGURE 28-47 A, Properly organized instrument tray. B, Same tray, but towels have been removed.

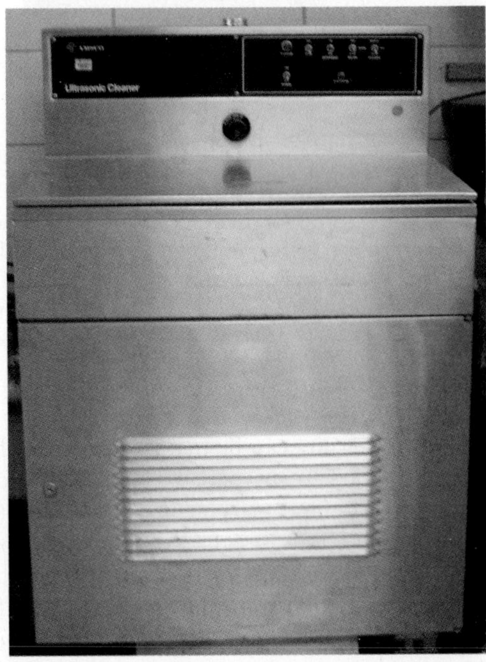

FIGURE 28-48 Ultrasonic cleaners are available in different sizes and models. Follow manufacturer's recommendations regarding use.

all the lubrication. Instrument lubricants are not oily or sticky, inhibit rust formation, and do not interfere with steam sterilization. Working components of power equipment should also be lubricated to maximize efficiency and to prolong the working lifetime of the equipment. Before instruments are repacked for sterilization, they should be thoroughly inspected for cleanliness, stiff or "frozen" hinges, improper jaw alignment, rust spots, and worn or broken parts. Defective instruments should be repaired or replaced.

DRAPES AND GOWNS

Surgical drapes and gowns may be paper or cloth. Paper drapes and gowns are designed to be disposable and should be used only once. They are bought prepackaged and sterilized for individual use. Cloth drapes and gowns are designed for repeated use, but they require washing after each use. Immediately soaking the cloth in cold water will prevent blood and other fluid from setting. All cloth drapes and gowns should be washed in a mild detergent and thoroughly dried before sterilization. They should also be inspected for holes or other signs of wear.

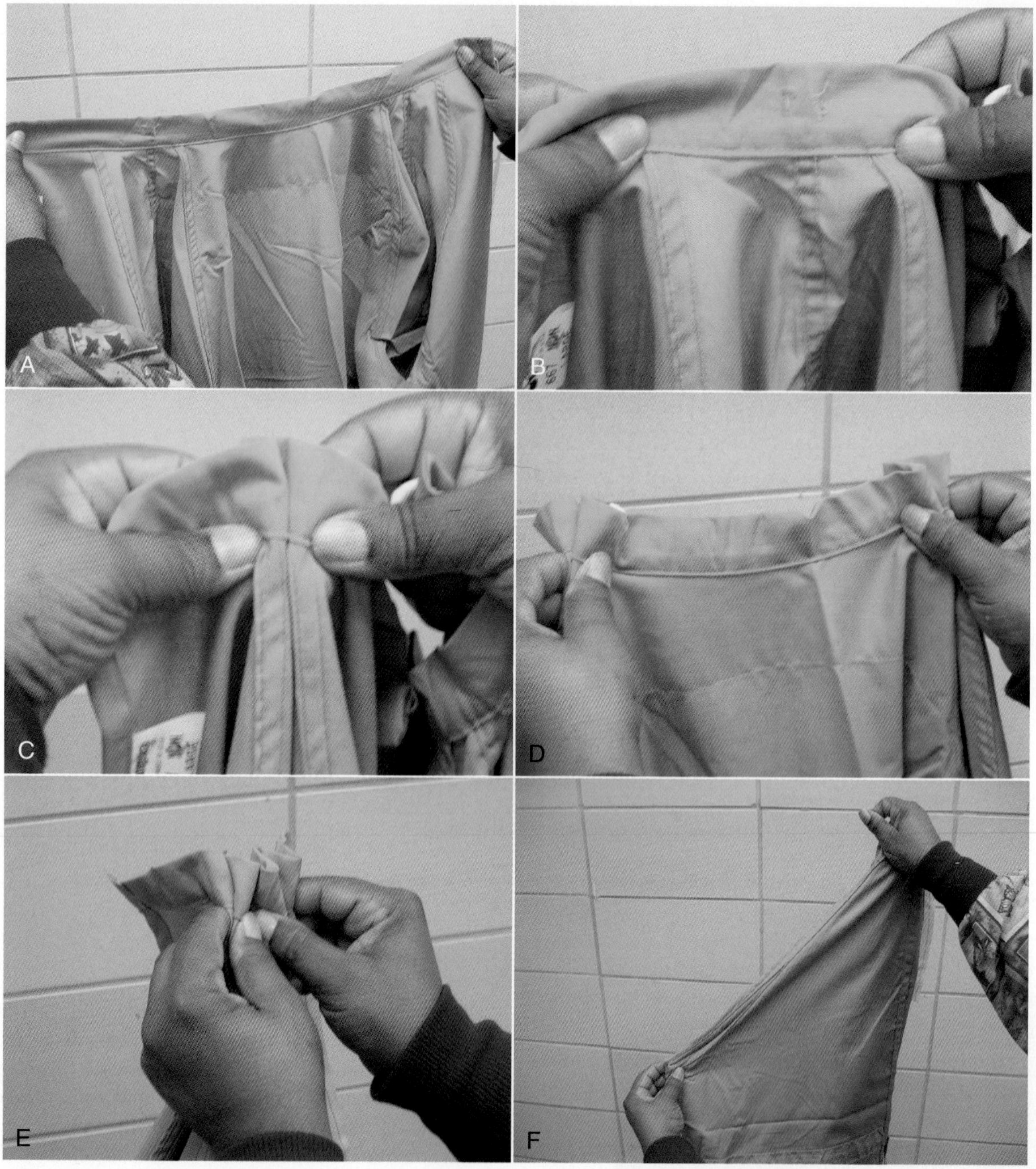

FIGURE 28-49 Method of folding a cloth surgical gown. **A,** The gown is held by the neck to see the shoulder seams on the inside of the gown. **B,** Close-up of the three seams of one shoulder. **C,** The gown is folded so the outer two seams of one shoulder are touching. **D,** The same fold is done with the other shoulder. **E,** The gown is folded so the seams of both shoulders are touching. **F,** The shoulders are held in one hand while the other hand aligns the armpit seams.

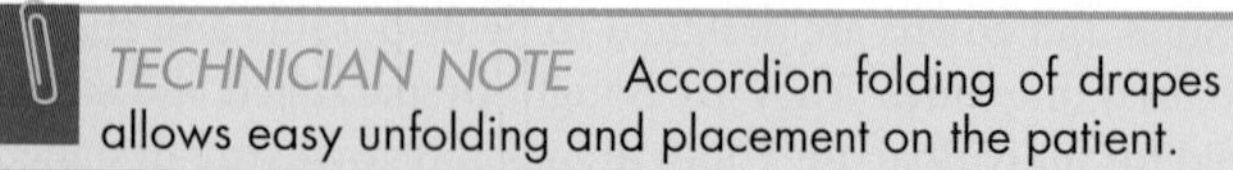
TECHNICIAN NOTE Accordion folding of drapes allows easy unfolding and placement on the patient.

Cloth gowns must always be folded and packed in the same manner (Figure 28-49). This technique allows the sterile gown to be unfolded and put on without contaminating the exterior surface. Cloth drapes must also be folded and packed such that sterility can be maintained while they are unfolded and applied to the patient. "Accordion folding" allows easy unfolding and placement of the drape (Figure 28-50). Many specifically designed drapes are also available, including adhesive drapes, transparent drapes, fenestrated drapes, stockinettes, and compressive wraps. After the drapes and gowns have been properly folded, they are usually double wrapped in muslin or a nonwoven barrier before sterilization (Figure 28-51).

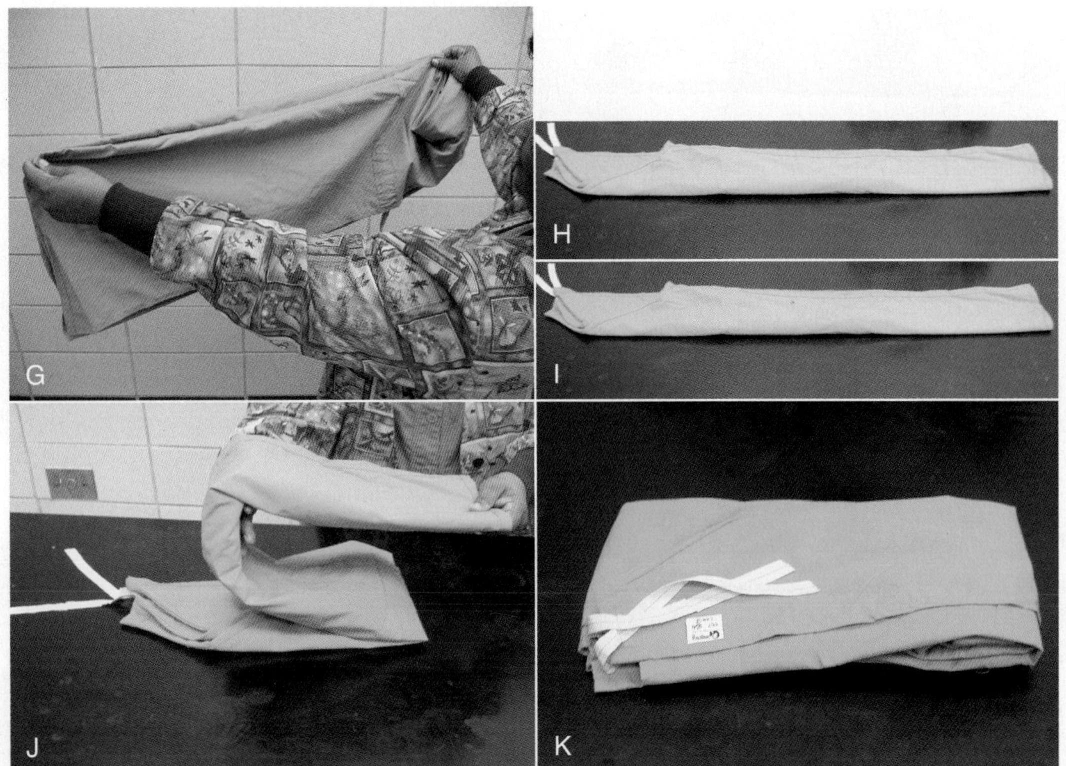

FIGURE 28-49, cont'd **G,** The shoulders and armpits are held in one hand while the other hand aligns the gown hem. **H,** The gown is laid flat on the table. (A tabletop method of folding is to first lay the gown open flat on the countertop with the outside of the gown facing up, sleeves on top. The side edges of the gown are each folded to meet near the middle, and then the gown is folded in half.) Only the inside surfaces of the gown are now exposed. **I,** The gown is folded in half lengthwise. **J,** The gown is folded in accordion fashion. **K,** The gown is laid on the table so the neck ties are uppermost. Proceed to Figure 28-51 to wrap the gown.

ASEPTIC TECHNIQUE

Asepsis is a condition of sterility, where no living organisms are present. Aseptic technique includes all steps taken to prevent contamination of the surgical site by infectious agents. A thorough understanding of aseptic technique is required to properly sterilize the surgical equipment and clean the operating room. Certain principles of aseptic technique must also be followed when scrubbing the surgical site and placing sterile drapes on the patient. The technician may need to act as a circulating nurse by getting the patient in the operating room and opening sterile equipment for the surgeon. Additionally the technician may be called upon to scrub in as a scrub nurse or surgical assistant to organize and pass instruments to the surgeon or to assist with the surgical procedure. A working knowledge of aseptic technique is necessary to perform these tasks correctly and also to monitor for inadvertent "breaks" in sterile technique.

Microorganisms must be introduced into the surgical site for infection to develop. The source of microorganisms includes exogenous and endogenous routes. Exogenous sources of contamination include the air, the surgical instruments and supplies, the patient's skin, and the surgical team. Endogenous contamination arises from within the patient and reaches the wound through the bloodstream. Examples of endogenous sources are bacteria from gingivitis or dermatitis.

During every surgery, some bacterial contamination occurs at the surgical site. Whether the contamination progresses to an infection depends on many factors, including the general health of the patient, the degree of tissue damage in the wound, the virulence of the infectious agent, and the number of infectious agents. The factor over which the surgical team has the most control is the number of infectious agents that are introduced into the wound by an exogenous route. Strict adherence to the principles of aseptic technique will minimize exogenous wound contamination and prevent many infections from developing.

All procedures do not require the same degree of vigilance regarding aseptic technique. For example, the débridement of a cutaneous abscess is considered to be a contaminated or dirty surgery, so aseptic technique would not be strictly followed. The wound would be scrubbed, but surgical instruments may be disinfected (cold sterilization) rather than sterilized (steam autoclave or gas sterilization), and the surgeon may wear sterile gloves, but forgo complete sterile surgical attire. It may be preferable for such a patient to remain outside the operating room to prevent contaminating it. In contrast, total hip replacement surgery involves the implantation of synthetic material, and infection can be devastating to the success of the surgery. In such cases, the surgical team adheres strictly to aseptic protocol. The surgeon will determine the degree to which the principles of asepsis are to be followed for each case.

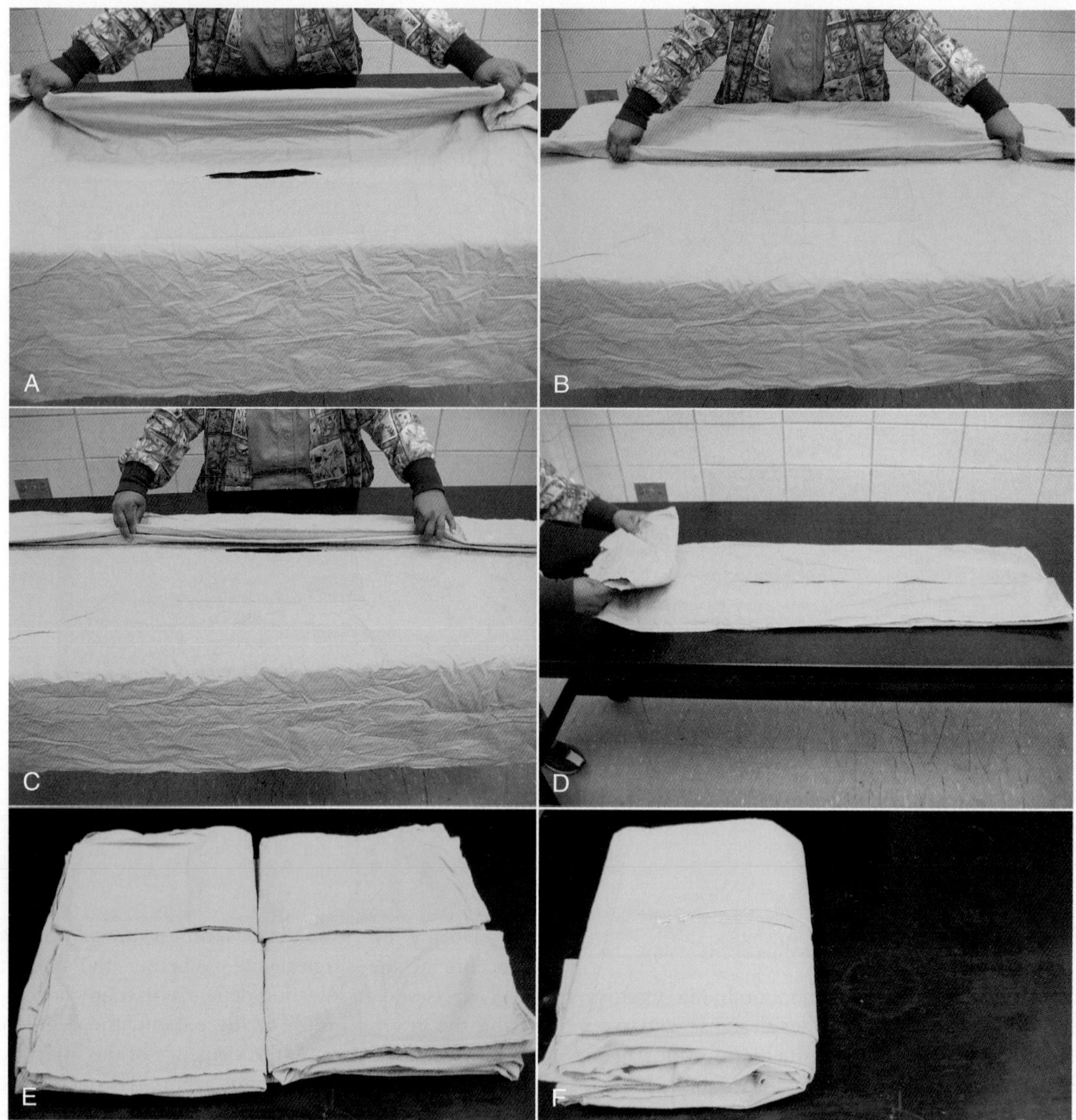

FIGURE 28-50 Cloth drapes are folded in accordion fashion so that they are easily unfolded onto the patient. **A, B,** A lengthwise fold is created in the drape (approximately 30 cm from the middle), and the folded edge is brought to the fenestration at the middle of the drape. **C,** This is repeated with a second fold, creating an accordion folding. Each section of folded drape is approximately 15 cm wide. **D,** The opposite side is folded in a similar manner. Then one end of the drape is folded to the center in accordion fashion. **E,** The opposite end is folded in the same manner. **F,** The drape is folded in half (half of the fenestration is visible), and it is ready to be wrapped as in Figure 28-51.

Sterilization is the destruction of all organisms and spores on an object. *Disinfection* is the destruction of the vegetative forms of bacteria but not the spores. Both sterilization and disinfection are used to prepare medical and surgical materials. The process used depends on the nature of the material and its intended use. Methods of sterilization and disinfection can be classified as either physical or chemical.

PHYSICAL METHODS OF STERILIZATION

The three general types of physical methods used for sterilization include filtration, radiation, and heat. Filtration and radiation are primarily used during the production and packaging of certain surgical products.

FILTRATION

Filtration is the use of a filter to separate particulate material from liquids or gases. Pharmaceuticals are commonly sterilized by filtration.

RADIATION

Some materials that would be damaged by other methods of sterilization can be safely sterilized by radiation. Radiation destroys microorganisms without causing any significant temperature elevation. Gloves and some suture materials are sterilized by radiation during the manufacturing process.

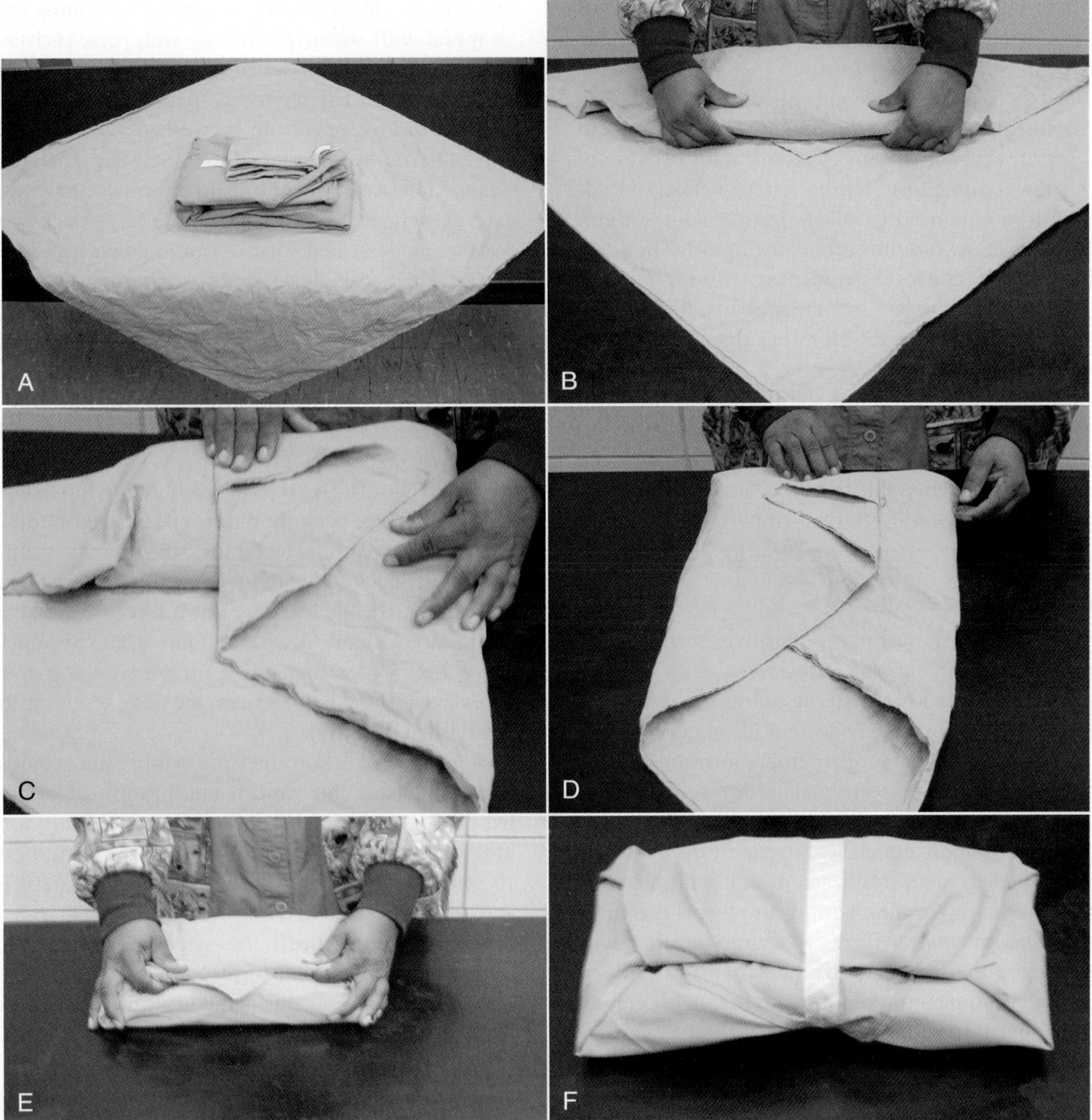

FIGURE 28-51 Wrapping a cloth drape or gown or an instrument pack. **A,** The gown along with an accordion-folded hand towel and sterilization indicator is placed diagonally onto the drapes. **B,** One corner is folded over the entire pack and tucked under it, leaving the tip visible. **C,** An adjacent corner is folded over the end of the pack, and the tip folded back so the drape is flat on top of the pack. **D,** The opposite corner is folded the same way. **E,** The pack is turned around, and the final corner is folded over the top of the pack and tucked under the folded drape edges, leaving the tip visible. **F,** The pack is then wrapped in a second layer in the same manner. The pack is secured with autoclave tape and is then labeled with contents, date, and the initials of the individual preparing the pack.

THERMAL ENERGY

The most common method used for sterilization is heat. The mechanism by which heat destroys microorganisms is not completely understood, but it is believed that death is the result of protein denaturation. This is probably a gradual process and may be reversible during the early stages of sterilization. The thermal susceptibility of microorganisms is influenced by several factors, including inherent resistance, individual variation, and age (young bacteria are more susceptible). There is no one temperature at which all microorganisms are killed instantly because death of bacteria and spores is a function of temperature and duration of heat.

The two basic types of heat sterilization are moist heat and dry heat. Dry heat is used to sterilize materials that cannot tolerate moist heat, but can withstand high temperatures. Oils, powders, and petroleum products are most effectively sterilized by dry heat, whereas rubber, fabrics, and some metals may be damaged by the high temperatures. An advantage of dry heat is that it will not rust or corrode needles or sharp instruments. Dry heat is more difficult to control than moist heat, and the sterilization time is longer.

Both dry and moist heat destroy bacteria through protein denaturation; however, dry heat kills by protein oxidation, whereas moist heat kills by coagulation of critical cellular protein. Moisture facilitates the coagulation of protein; thus moist heat kills bacteria and spores at lower temperatures and shorter exposures than dry heat.

Moist heat sterilization is accomplished by either boiling water or by steam under pressure. Boiling water at ambient pressures is not a reliable means of sterilization because of its relatively low temperature. The bactericidal effect of boiling water can be enhanced by alkalinization with sodium hydroxide (0.1 g/dl) or sodium carbonate (2 g/dl). The addition of these agents reduces instrument corrosion, but they cannot be used with glassware or rubber goods. Boiling water probably results in disinfection rather than sterilization and is rarely used.

The most common method of sterilization is saturated steam under pressure. Increased pressure causes steam to achieve a higher temperature. Materials to be sterilized in this manner must be penetrable by steam and not damaged by heat or moisture. Sterilizers that employ steam under pressure are called *autoclaves* (Figure 28-52).

Autoclave Sterilization

Autoclave sterilization is technique sensitive, so operating instructions accompanying the autoclave should be followed. An autoclave load is not sterile unless the steam has penetrated the packs completely so that all materials have been exposed to steam at the proper temperature and for the proper duration. Adequate steam penetration requires that the packs be properly prepared and loaded into the autoclave. The most common autoclaves are *gravity displacement* or downward displacement sterilizers, meaning the steam is introduced into the top of the chamber and forces the air to the bottom. In *prevacuum sterilizers,* a vacuum pump evacuates the air before the steam is introduced. This provides a more rapid and even penetration of steam than with gravity displacement, permitting higher temperatures and shorter time duration.

Proper pack preparation begins by checking that all materials are thoroughly clean and free from grease, oil, or protein residues. Complex instruments should be disassembled, and any box locks should be open. Packs must be properly wrapped with steam-permeable wrappers, such as double-thickness muslin (thread count of 140 threads per 6.45cm^2) or a nonwoven barrier (crepe paper or polypropylene fabric). Muslin wrappers can be washed and reused, but nonwoven barriers are designed for single use. Packs are usually wrapped in two layers of muslin or nonwoven wrappers. The external wraps are folded around a large pack in the same manner as described for drape and gown packs (see Figure 28-51). Heat-sealable paper or plastic or plastic peel pouches may be used for individual instruments (Figure 28-53). Each pack must be labeled identifying the pack contents, the person who prepared it, and the date it was sterilized.

Materials need to be packed as loosely as is practical to ensure good steam penetration. There should be 2.5 to 7.5 cm of space around each pack, and they should be arranged to allow steam to flow readily from top to bottom. For example, a large pack should not be placed on top of several small ones because it will block the flow of steam down to the smaller packs. Steam flow may be facilitated by positioning packs vertically (on edge). It is recommended that packs be no larger than 30 cm × 30 cm × 50 cm and weigh no more than 5.4 kg, depending on the type of material being autoclaved. In many practices, the pack size is limited by the size of the autoclave.

A number of minimum time-temperature standards have been established for routine sterilization of surgical packs. Exposure to saturated steam at 121° C (250° F) for 13 minutes is considered to be a safe minimum standard. Five to 10 minutes at 121° C will destroy most resistant microbes, and an additional 3 to 8 minutes provides a margin of safety. When the temperature in the exhaust line reaches the desired level, the entire content of the sterilizing chamber has been exposed to steam, so this is the beginning of exposure time.

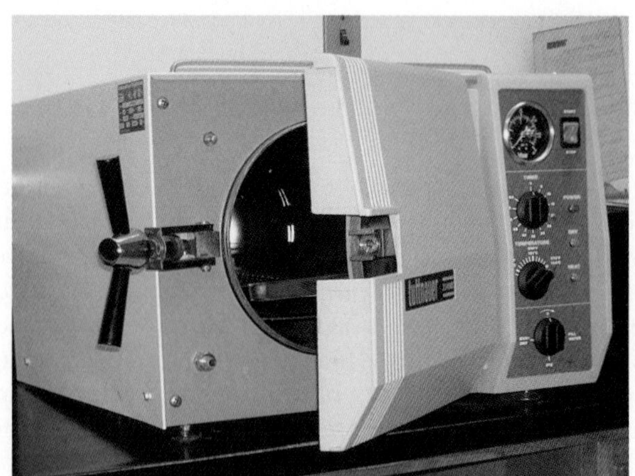

FIGURE 28-52 Autoclave. They are available in different sizes and models.

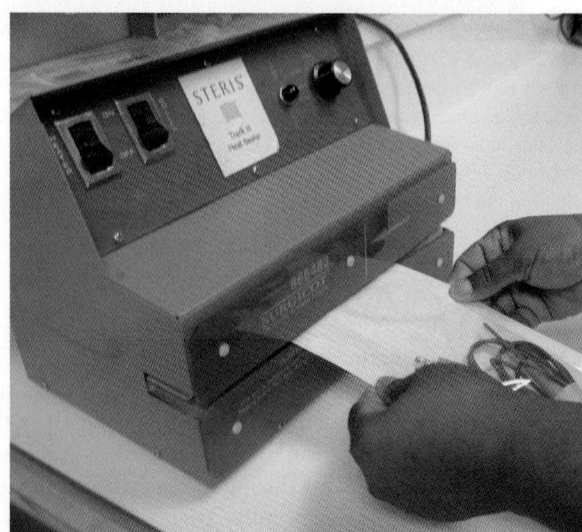

FIGURE 28-53 Individual instruments may be heat sealed in plastic or paper pouches in preparation for steam or chemical sterilization. The instrument should be positioned in the pouch so that the handle will be presented to the surgeon when the pouch is opened.

The time required to reach the sterilizing temperature is referred to as the *heat-up time* and is extremely short (about 1 minute) in prevacuum and pulsing type of sterilizers. Large linen packs require both a longer heat-up time and a longer exposure time. They should be saturated for 30 to 45 minutes at 121° C (250° F) in gravity displacement sterilizers and 4 minutes at 131° C (270° F) in prevacuum sterilizers.

> TECHNICIAN NOTE The safe minimum standard for autoclave sterilization is 121° C (250° F) for 13 minutes.

Emergency sterilization, also called *flash sterilization,* is usually performed in prevacuum sterilizers. The recommended exposure time is 3 minutes at 131° C (270° F). The unwrapped instruments are placed in a perforated metal tray for sterilization and then carried to the operating room using detachable handles.

After sterilization, the autoclave door is unlocked and "cracked" open. If the autoclave door is opened wide, the cool outside air will condense the steam in the materials, making them soggy and promoting corrosion of metal instruments. About 10 minutes after cracking the door, the remaining moisture will have vaporized and escaped, leaving the contents thoroughly dry. Paper-wrapped products should not be left in the autoclave more than 15 to 20 minutes after cracking the door. If left too long, the heat will dry the paper, making it brittle and likely to crack and split when handled.

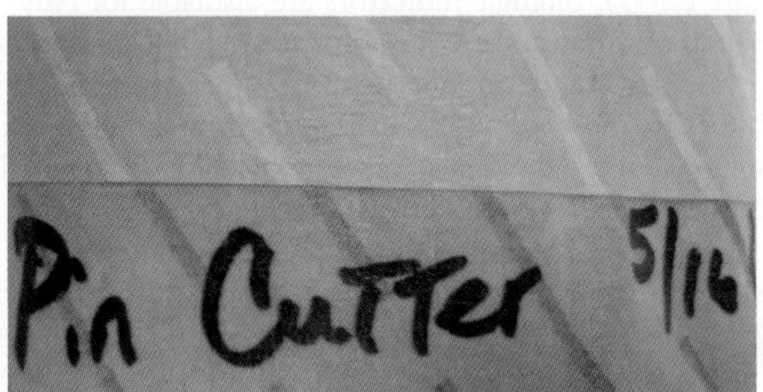

FIGURE 28-54 Autoclave tape before *(above)* and after *(below)* sterilization. Notice the appearance of the black stripes indicating exposure to steam.

Sterilization Quality Control

The only certainty that sterilization has been achieved is through proper technique and the use of dependable sterilization indicators. Indicators should always be checked before using the materials.

There are four types of sterilization indicators used in autoclaves: (1) autoclave tape, (2) fusible melting pellet glass, (3) culture tests, and (4) chemical sterilization indicators. These indicators are meant to be used in combination because no one test alone can provide quality assurance of sterility.

> TECHNICIAN NOTE The four types of sterilization indicators are (1) autoclave tape, (2) melting pellet glass, (3) culture tests, and (4) chemical sterilization indicators.

Autoclave tape is useful for identifying packs and articles that have been exposed to steam, but it does not indicate whether the proper requirements of time, temperature, and steam have been met (Figure 28-54). The fusible melting pellet glass type of indicator indicates that a temperature of approximately 118° C (244° F) was reached, but does not indicate whether proper time or steam saturation was achieved. Culture test indicators are strips that contain a controlled-count spore population of some particular strain of bacterium. This biologic challenge test is useful since it is the only test that proves microorganisms were killed. The disadvantages of this test are that the results are not immediately available and it does not assess steam penetration. Chemical sterilization indicators are available in many types, and they undergo color changes when subjected to saturated steam for adequate periods of time (Figure 28-55). Most practices will use a combination of autoclave tape on the outside of

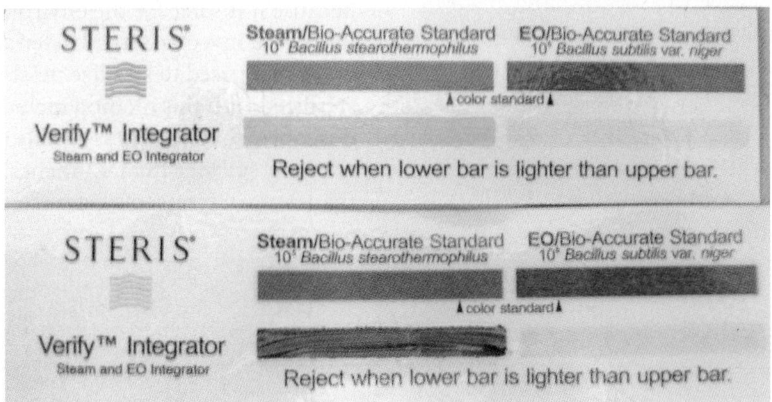

FIGURE 28-55 Chemical indicator strip to be placed inside pack. This strip can monitor steam *(left)* or gas *(right)* sterilization. Lower strip has been exposed to adequate steam, as indicated by the darkened bar.

the pack and a chemical sterilization indicator within the center of the pack to assess sterility.

In the prevacuum sterilizers, an air removal test can be run daily to ensure that air is sufficiently removed from the autoclave. In gravity displacement sterilizers, temperature graphs can be kept as a record of autoclave performance. Therefore quality assurance occurs at two levels, one to ensure that the pack runs through a sterilization cycle and another to ensure that the autoclave system is working properly. Quality control is essential for any surgical practice because failure to ensure proper sterilization can have far-reaching consequences.

Care and Handling of Sterile Packs

Sterile packs should be stored in a dust-free, dry, and well-ventilated area away from contaminated equipment. Closed cabinets provide a cleaner storage area than open shelving. Safe pack storage times are listed in Table 28-5. If a pack is dropped, the tape sealing the pack is broken, or the pack wrap becomes wet, punctured, or torn, the pack should be considered contaminated. If there is any doubt as to the sterility of an item, consider it to be nonsterile.

CHEMICAL METHODS OF STERILIZATION

Chemical sterilization is performed with certain liquids or gases. Liquid chemicals can be used for instrument sterilization. The most common agent used for liquid sterilization is glutaraldehyde. Gas sterilization is used for items that cannot tolerate the high temperatures or steam associated with autoclaving (some power equipment or plastic products). The most common agents used for gas sterilization are ethylene oxide and hydrogen peroxide gas plasma.

ETHYLENE OXIDE

Ethylene oxide is a colorless gas at room temperature. It is flammable, explosive, and toxic. It can cause skin burns, respiratory irritation, vomiting, headaches, and birth defects (see Chapter 6). The manufacturer's guidelines should be followed carefully to prevent injury to hospital personnel and patients. Ethylene oxide penetrates paper and plastic film packaging. The item to be gas sterilized is wrapped in plastic packaging (polyethylene, polycoated paper, and Mylar) and heat sealed before sterilization (see Figure 28-53).

TABLE 28-5 Safe Storage Times for Sterile Packs

Wrapper	Closed Cabinet	Open Cabinet
Single-wrapped muslin	1 wk	2 days
Double-wrapped muslin	7 wk	3 wk
Single-wrapped crepe paper	At least 8 wk	3 wk
Single-wrapped muslin sealed in 3-ml polyethylene		At least 9 mo
Heat-sealed paper and transparent plastic pouches		At least 1 yr

Ethylene oxide destroys metabolic pathways within the cells by alkylation, and it is capable of killing all microorganisms. Effective sterilization with ethylene oxide is dependent on the concentration of gas, exposure time, temperature, and relative humidity. Ethylene oxide activity is enhanced by increasing the temperature or the gas concentration. Ethylene oxide sterilizers usually operate at temperatures between 21° C and 60° C (70° F and 140° F). The activity of ethylene oxide approximately doubles with each 10° C increase in temperature. Doubling the ethylene oxide concentration decreases the sterilization time by approximately one half. Moisture is necessary for the lethal action of ethylene oxide, and optimum relative humidity for sterilization with ethylene oxide is 40%. Exposure time varies from 48 minutes to several hours, but 12 hours of exposure is commonly used when sterilizing at room temperature.

After ethylene oxide sterilization, materials should be quarantined in a well-ventilated area for a minimum of 7 days or in an aerator for 12 to 18 hours. Recommended aeration time varies with the type of material and other factors. Color-coded chemical sterilization indicators are commonly placed within the packs when using ethylene oxide sterilization (see Figure 28-55). Biologic indicators are available for ethylene oxide sterilization and are the only truly reliable test for sterility. Since results are unavailable for several days, biologic indicators are most commonly used to evaluate the sterilization system and not individual packs. External tape can be used to indicate exposure to gas sterilization (Figure 28-56).

> *TECHNICIAN NOTE* Because of the high toxicity of ethylene oxide, it is being replaced by hydrogen peroxide gas plasma sterilization.

HYDROGEN PEROXIDE GAS PLASMA

Gas plasma sterilization has been replacing ethylene oxide because it is safer for the environment and personnel. It can inactivate mycobacteria, bacterial spores, fungi, and viruses and can be used to sterilize most items. Items that cannot be sterilized with this method include linen, wood or paper, endoscopes, some plastics, liquids, and tubes or catheters that are long (greater than 12 inches) or of small diameter (less than 3 mm). Items to be sterilized are wrapped in nonwoven

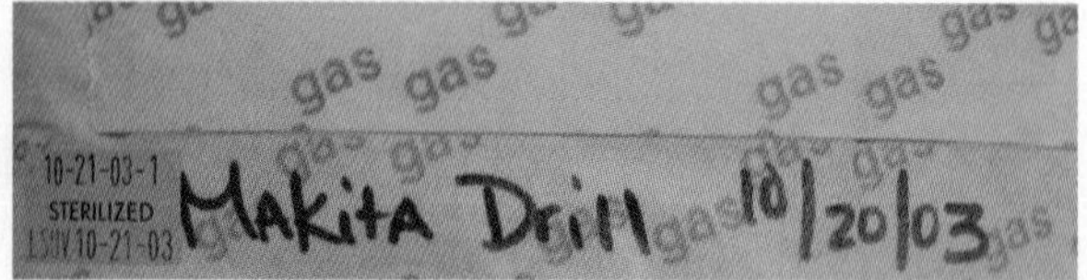

FIGURE 28-56 Gas tape before *(above)* and after *(below)* sterilization. Notice the change in color of the word *gas,* indicating exposure.

polypropylene fabric or plastic (Tyvek-Mylar) pouches and placed in the sterilization chamber. A vacuum is drawn, and hydrogen peroxide is injected and is vaporized. After 50 minutes, the pressure is lowered, and radio waves are applied to the chamber, creating a gas plasma. This creates free radicals, which kill the microorganisms. The process takes about an hour and requires no aeration. A biologic indicator is used to test for sterility, and a chemical indicator is used to show that hydrogen peroxide was present.

CHEMICAL DISINFECTION

A *disinfectant* is an agent that destroys bacteria or inactivates viruses. Disinfectants are chemical agents that are applied to inanimate objects to destroy the vegetative form of bacteria, but not necessarily the spore forms. Disinfectants that are capable of destroying vegetative bacteria plus spores, tubercle bacilli, and viruses may be used as chemical sterilizers.

Disinfection time is the time required for a particular agent to produce its maximal effect. It is influenced by many factors, including the nature of the material disinfected, the degree of soil and microbial contamination, and the concentration and germicidal potency of the disinfectant.

Antisepsis is the prevention of infection by inhibiting the growth of infectious agents. Antiseptic agents, such as iodine or chlorhexidine, are substances used on living tissue to effect antisepsis. A glossary of key terms used in describing aseptic technique may be found in Box 28-1.

ANTISEPTIC AND DISINFECTANT COMPOUNDS

Iodine

Iodine compounds are effective antimicrobial agents, but have limited activity against bacterial spores. Iodine solutions are used for surgical preparation, topical wound therapy, and joint and body cavity lavage. Iodine compounds are available as aqueous solutions, tinctures, and iodophors. *Aqueous solutions* contain higher levels of free iodine than iodophors and therefore have greater bactericidal activity. However, aqueous solutions are also cytotoxic and cannot be used in living tissue unless they are greatly diluted. Aqueous iodine also stains materials and is corrosive to instruments.

Tincture of iodine is a solution of 2% iodine in 50% ethyl alcohol and is intended for use on intact skin. It is not commonly used in veterinary practices.

Iodophors contain iodine complexed with surfactants or polymers, so free iodine is slowly released. The adverse properties of staining and irritation are reduced, and delivery of iodine to the tissues is enhanced. *Povidone-iodine* is the most commonly used iodophor and is available as scrubs or solutions. Dilution of stock solutions (common dilutions include 1:10, 1:50, and 1:100) increases the bactericidal activity and decreases the cytotoxicity. The residual bactericidal activity (i.e., continued action when left on the skin) of povidone-iodine is 4 to 6 hours, but this is greatly diminished in the presence of organic matter.

Povidone-iodine is one of the most common surgical scrubs used in veterinary hospitals. Although it is a relatively safe skin preparation, there are several considerations regarding its use. Alcohol, lavage solutions, or organic debris, such as blood, will destroy residual bactericidal activity. Povidone-iodine can cause skin irritation or acute contact dermatitis in up to 50% of canine patients, and it may be a problem for some hospital staff. Rarely, individuals who have repeated contact with iodine scrub solutions may develop systemic iodine toxicity, resulting in metabolic acidosis and thyroid dysfunction.

> *TECHNICIAN NOTE* The two most commonly used antiseptic agents are povidone-iodine and chlorhexidine.

Chlorhexidine

Chlorhexidine is an antiseptic agent that is available in aqueous, tincture, and detergent formulations. It is an effective antimicrobial agent with activity against bacteria, molds, yeasts, and viruses. Chlorhexidine has a rapid onset and a long residual activity that is not affected by alcohol, lavage solutions, or organic debris. It has become a popular surgical scrub because of its effectiveness and because it is nonirritating to the skin. In several human studies, chlorhexidine has been found to be superior to povidone-iodine as a surgical hand scrub. The effectiveness of povidone-iodine and chlorhexidine is similar when used as surgical scrubs for canine surgery.

> *TECHNICIAN NOTE* Chlorhexidine is an effective antimicrobial agent with rapid onset and long residual activity.

BOX 28-1 Glossary of Key Terms Associated With Aseptic Technique

Antiseptic—Agent capable of preventing infection by inhibiting the growth of infectious agents. This term is generally applied to living tissues.

Autoclave—Sterilizers that use saturated steam under pressure to achieve high temperatures for sterilization. Minimum exposure to saturated steam 13 min at 121° C (250° F).

Disinfectant—Agent that destroys or inhibits microorganisms. Typically refers to inanimate objects.

Ethylene oxide—Gas chemical sterilization agent used to sterilize objects that cannot withstand heat. A good exhaust system must be used.

Flash sterilization—Emergency sterilization in which object (instrument) is placed unwrapped in an autoclave and taken directly to the surgery following sterilization. Recommended exposure is 3 min at 131° C (270° F).

Sterilization—Destruction of all microorganisms. This term is generally applied to inanimate objects.

As a lavage solution for open wounds, chlorhexidine must be diluted 1:40 with sterile water or saline to produce a 0.05% solution. At this concentration, chlorhexidine has significant antibacterial activity with no cytotoxicity and is superior to povidone-iodine, saline, and other antiseptics. Higher concentrations can cause inflammation and cytotoxicity, so they are not recommended in open wounds. When chlorhexidine is mixed with electrolyte solutions (such as lactated Ringer's solution), it will precipitate, but this does not affect antimicrobial activity and the solution can still be used for wound lavage.

Alcohols

Alcohols are used as disinfectant and antiseptic agents. They are organic solvents that evaporate rapidly and leave no residue. Alcohols are bactericidal, but ineffective against spores and fungi. They have no residual effects and are inhibited by organic debris. Ethyl and isopropyl alcohols are more effective than methyl alcohol as disinfecting agents. Alcohols should never be used in open wounds because they are both painful and cytotoxic.

Phenols

Phenols (carbolic acid) have been used historically as both antiseptics and disinfectants, but phenols have been routinely replaced by newer, safer, and more effective agents. Hexachlorophene, a skin preparation, was one of the most popular phenols, but it has been replaced by povidone-iodine and chlorhexidine.

Quaternary Ammonium

Quaternary ammonium compounds are synthetic cationic detergents that act on cell membranes and are effective against bacteria, but not spores or some viruses. Bland and nontoxic, these agents are quite popular. Benzalkonium chloride is the most commonly used quaternary ammonium compound and is used as a disinfectant.

Chloride

Chloride compounds were among the first agents to be used as medical disinfectants and found popularity for wound treatment in World War I as Dakin's solution. Antimicrobial chlorine compounds, specifically the hypochlorites, have broad bactericidal and virucidal activity, but can be cytotoxic when improperly used on living tissues. Presently, sodium hypochlorite (bleach) is commonly used as a disinfectant in many hospitals.

Aldehyde

Formaldehyde and glutaraldehyde are the most commonly used aldehydes in veterinary medicine. They are both toxic and irritating, which restricts them from use on living tissues. They are effective antimicrobial agents, but may require several hours of exposure time. Formaldehyde is commonly used in the preservation of tissue specimens. Glutaraldehyde is commonly used for chemical sterilization in cold trays and for endoscopic equipment.

COLD STERILIZATION

Cold sterilization refers to soaking instruments in disinfecting solutions, such as chlorhexidine or glutaraldehyde. Metal trays used to soak instruments in disinfectant are called *cold trays* (Figure 28-57). Since sterility cannot be guaranteed, cold-sterilized instruments should be used only for minor procedures (superficial lacerations, dental procedures) or for equipment that cannot tolerate other forms of sterilization, such as endoscopic equipment. Exposure times should exceed 3 hours, and the equipment must be rinsed thoroughly before use.

STERILIZATION OF ARTHROSCOPIC EQUIPMENT

Most hand instruments and ancillary equipment can be steam sterilized. They can also be gas sterilized with ethylene oxide or cold sterilized using a glutaraldehyde-based solution (CidexPlus, Johnson & Johnson Medical Inc.). Cold sterilization affords the ability to use the equipment more than once in a single day, unlike steam and gas sterilization in most situations. The arthroscope, light cable, and camera can be gas sterilized or cold sterilized, but not steam sterilized.

> *TECHNICIAN NOTE* The arthroscope, fiberoptic light cable, and camera should never be steam sterilized.

With cold sterilization, the instruments are soaked for a minimum of 20 minutes in the Cidexplus just before surgery. The electrical plug of the camera cable is not submerged in the cold sterilization solution, which would damage it. The end is draped out over the top of the container with the Cidexplus. The surgeon or assistant double gloves and removes the instruments from the solution. The instruments are then placed in a sterile autoclave tray containing sterile water. Once the instruments have been submerged in the sterile water, each piece is gently agitated, individually removed

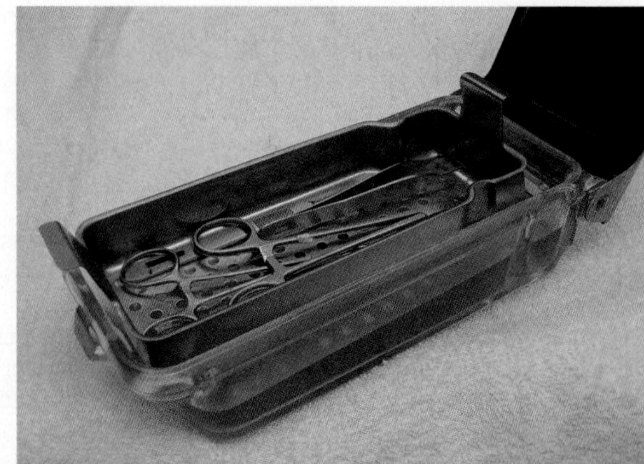

FIGURE 28-57 Cold sterilization tray. Instruments are kept submerged in disinfectant and retrieved by lifting the rack.

from the tray, rinsed with sterile water by a scrub nurse or other assistant, and transferred to the instrument table. The surgeon or assistant removes his or her outer gloves and dries the instruments. It is important that the Cidexplus be thoroughly rinsed from the instruments. Glutaraldehyde can cause a chemical synovitis and is injurious to chondrocytes. A double rinse further reduces the amount of glutaraldehyde residue remaining on the instruments.

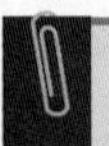

TECHNICIAN NOTE Glutaraldehyde causes a chemical synovitis and is injurious to chondrocytes.

OPERATING ROOM PREPARATION

Operating room design is important for ease of cleaning. The operating room should be simple and uncluttered. Commonly used equipment and materials should be readily available, but excess stock should not be stored in the operating room. When additional equipment is needed, it is brought to the operating room by the circulating nurse.

Operating room cleanliness is essential for proper aseptic technique. A routine daily and weekly cleaning schedule should be established to keep the operating room clean and dust free. The surgery table should be cleaned and disinfected, and soiled areas of the floor should be cleaned and disinfected by damp mopping immediately after each surgery. It is preferable to perform thorough daily cleaning at the end of each day because cleaning creates airborne dust that takes several hours to settle. Buckets should be emptied and cleaned. The operating table and all equipment should be cleaned and wiped with a disinfectant solution. (The operating room is never dry mopped or dusted because this produces excessive airborne dust.) The casters on equipment should be cleaned, and the entire floor should be mopped.

Once a week, the operating room should undergo a thorough cleaning in which movable equipment is removed and cleaned with a disinfectant solution. Permanent structures, such as walls, air vents, window sills, light fixtures, and the surgical table should also be wiped clean. Cabinets should be emptied, washed, and restocked. The operating room floor should be scrubbed and disinfected. Disinfectant can be applied with a mop, although this may actually spread dirt and microorganisms throughout the room. To prevent this, the mop head should be laundered daily and not stored in used disinfectant solution. The wet-vacuum method in which the clean floor is flooded with disinfectant solution and then vacuumed is superior to mopping. Cleaning equipment used in the operating room should be kept separate from all other cleaning equipment.

Daily cleaning of the surgical preparation room is also important because this room is subject to continual contamination. Sinks and plumbing fixtures should be scrubbed. Buckets and vacuum canisters should be emptied. Furniture and cabinets should be wiped clean and the floor scrubbed. If there are holding cages in the preparation room, they should be cleaned and disinfected. All surgical preparation solutions and supplies should be replenished.

TECHNICIAN NOTE Daily and weekly cleaning schedules should be established for the operating room.

SMALL ANIMAL PATIENT PREPARATION

SKIN PREPARATION—SURGICAL CLIP

The surgical site is usually prepared after the animal is anesthetized. The hair is first clipped in the same direction as the hair growth. Then it is clipped against the direction of growth to achieve the closest shave possible (using a No. 40 clipper blade). A wide region of skin is clipped around the proposed surgical incision. A general rule is to shave at least 2 to 4 cm in every direction from the proposed incision, depending on the size of the animal and location of the incision. For abdominal procedures, the clip should extend several centimeters cranial to the xyphoid, caudal to the pubis, and lateral to the nipples. For orthopedic procedures, the entire circumference of the limb is clipped from the foot up onto the body. Long hair growing near the periphery of the clipped area should be cut short enough that it cannot hang over the clipped area. Sterile, water-soluble lubricant may be placed in open wounds before clipping around them. The lubricant will collect hair, allowing it to be rinsed away before the surgical scrub. Areas that appear to be infected should be clipped last so that the clippers do not spread infected material. After clipping, a vacuum cleaner may be used to eliminate loose hairs on the skin. The surgical clip should be thorough but gentle. Unnecessary roughness will result in inflamed or traumatized skin, which can cause greater postoperative complications.

SKIN PREPARATION—SURGICAL SCRUB

Initial skin preparation is done in the preparation room to remove gross contamination. Before scrubbing the abdomen of a male dog, the prepuce should be flushed with an antiseptic solution. Examination gloves are worn to decrease contamination from the hands. The surgical scrub is performed by alternating an antiseptic scrub (such as povidone-iodine or chlorhexidine scrub) with alcohol or sterile saline. (Remember not to use alcohols or detergents in open wounds, eyes, or mucous membranes.) Scrubbing should begin over the proposed incision site and extend outward in a spiraling pattern, never going back toward the center with the same gauze sponge (Figure 28-58). The sponge is replaced with a clean one, and the process is repeated until no dirt is visible on the discarded sponges.

The sterile surgical scrub is done once the animal is properly positioned on the operating table. Sterile gloves should

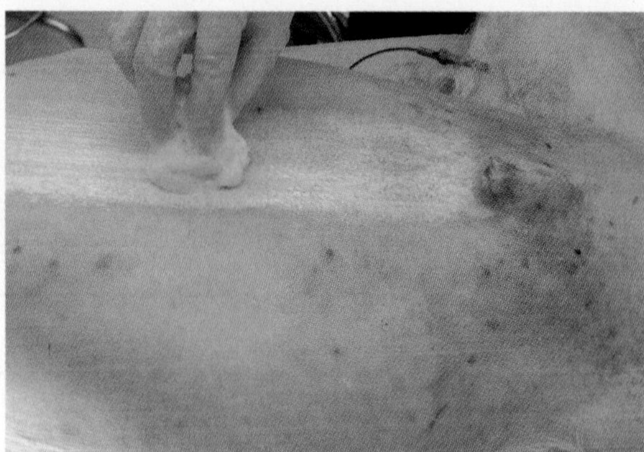

FIGURE 28-58 The surgical preparation should begin at the proposed incision site and should progress outward, never returning to the proposed incision line with the same gauze sponge. Gloves are worn during the preparation to decrease contamination from the hands.

be worn, and sterile sponges are used. If the sterile surgical scrub is performed by alternating povidone-iodine with alcohol, the total contact time of the povidone-iodine should be at least 5 minutes. After the final povidone-iodine scrub, a 10% povidone-iodine solution should be sprayed or painted on the skin. Alternatively the sterile surgical scrub may be performed by alternating chlorhexidine gluconate with either alcohol or sterile saline. Either chlorhexidine or sterile saline may be left on the skin at the end of preparation. Both povidone-iodine and chlorhexidine are effective scrub solutions, but the contact time for chlorhexidine is less critical than for povidone-iodine.

> TECHNICIAN NOTE It is generally recommended that the surgical site be scrubbed and rinsed at least three times. The sterile scrub should provide at least 5 minutes of contact time for povidone-iodine. An antiseptic solution is often applied to the skin following the scrubs.

Several skin preparations are now available that enable a "one-step prep" (Table 28-6). The solution is packaged in a small plastic bottle that is directly attached to an applicator sponge. After squeezing the bottle to activate solution flow, the sponge is used to "paint" a single uniform coat of the solution on the skin, starting at the incision site and working outward in a circular motion (Figure 28-59). It requires a 30-second application time and dries within 2 to 3 minutes, so the preparation time is much faster than the traditional alternating scrub described earlier. They contain isopropyl alcohol, which is a broad-spectrum antimicrobial with rapid onset of activity. The other substances in these preparations result in further antimicrobial action and the formation of a film that adheres strongly to the skin and provides long residual activity. These solutions should be applied to clean, dry skin. However the skin should *not* be scrubbed beforehand with Betadine or Hibiclens scrub because residues may prevent the one-step preparation from adhering appropriately. These one-step preparations should be applied to intact skin and are not appropriate for open wounds because of the high alcohol content (70% to 74%). These preparations enhance the skin adherence of incise drapes. The region will be flammable until it dries. Alcohol-free solutions are being developed.

> TECHNICIAN NOTE "One-step preps" are easy to apply, much faster than traditional scrubbing techniques, and effective for antimicrobial kill. They have a rapid onset and long residual effect.

There are many modifications to the surgical preparation technique. For example, in preparation for feline orchiectomy (castration), the scrotal hair is plucked rather than clipped. Feline onychectomy (declawing), tail docking, and dewclaw removal of neonatal puppies are commonly performed without clipping the hair. The surgical site is soaked or gently scrubbed with detergent and swabbed with alcohol or antiseptic solution. Bovine and porcine castrations are performed without clipping the hair, and an alcohol or antiseptic wash is usually used. Equine castrations may be prepared with three thorough washes using dilute chlorhexidine or povidone-iodine solution.

PATIENT POSITIONING

There are several common positions in which to place an animal for surgery. The position of the animal is described by the region of the body that contacts the table. For example, right lateral recumbency means the animal is lying on its right side, dorsal recumbency means the animal is on its back, and sternal recumbency means the animal is on its belly. Maintaining patient positioning is facilitated by the use of adjustable surgical tables, portable tabletop V troughs, sand bags, or vacuum-activated "beanbags."

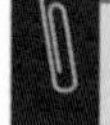

> TECHNICIAN NOTE The dorsal recumbent position is commonly used for abdominal surgical procedures.

In orthopedic surgery, the affected leg is often suspended from an overhead support or intravenous (IV) stand during skin preparation and initial surgical draping. The advantage of hanging the leg is that it allows aseptic preparation of the entire circumference of the limb, so the surgeon can manipulate it during surgery. To hang the leg, the distal limb is wrapped (using gauze or an examination glove covered with tape) to cover any unclipped areas, and strips of tape ("stirrups") are extended from the end of the foot. The leg is suspended by these stirrups (Figure 28-60). The entire limb circumference is clipped and scrubbed from the foot to the level of the inguinal or axillary region. The skin preparation usually extends to the dorsal and ventral midlines of the body.

TABLE 28-6 Common Antiseptic and Disinfectant Agents

Examples	Common Uses	Spectrum of Activity	Residual Activity
Povidone-Iodine Detergent			
Betadine scrub (Purdue Frederick) (brown sudsy solution)	Preoperative scrubs	Bacteria, viruses, fungi, protozoa, yeasts	4-6 hr, but inactivated by organic debris and alcohol
Povidone-Iodine Solution			
Betadine solution (Purdue Frederick) (brown solution)	Preoperative skin preparation; wound lavage when diluted 1:100	Bacteria, viruses, fungi, protozoa, yeasts	4-6 hr, but inactivated by organic debris and alcohol
Chlorhexidine Detergent			
Nolvasan scrub (Fort Dodge Laboratories) (blue solution), Hibiclens scrub (Stuart Pharmaceuticals) (pink solution)	Preoperative scrubs	Bacteria, viruses, fungi, yeasts	2 days; not inhibited by organic matter or alcohol; less skin irritation
Isopropyl Alcohol-Iodine Povacrylex			
DuraPrep (3M)	Preoperative skin preparation—one step Do not use in open wounds	Bacteria	Rapid onset; at least 1 day residual
Isopropyl Alcohol-Povidone-Iodine			
Prevail-Fx (Cardinal Health)	Preoperative skin preparation—one step Do not use in open wounds	Bacteria	Rapid onset; at least 1 day residual
Isopropyl Alcohol-Chlorhexidine Gluconate			
ChloraPrep (Cardinal Health)	Preoperative skin preparation—one step Do not use in open wounds	Bacteria	Rapid onset; 2 day residual; not inhibited by organic matter
Chlorhexidine			
Nolvasan solution (Fort Dodge Laboratories) (nonsudsy blue solution)	Preoperative skin preparation; wound lavage when diluted 1:40	Bacteria, viruses, fungi, yeasts	2 days; bactericidal, but solution not cytotoxic in open wounds at diluted concentrations
Alcohol, Isopropyl and Ethanol			
Many manufacturers	Surgical preparations; disinfection antisepsis; do not use in open wounds	Bacteria, some fungi	Rapid onset, but no residual activity
Ethyl Alcohol-Chlorhexidine Gluconate			
Avagard (3M)	Preoperative hand scrub—waterless	Bacteria	Rapid onset, with some residual activity
Phenol, Hexachlorophene			
pHisoHex scrub (Sanofi; Winthrop) (white)	Preoperative hand scrub	Bacteria (more effective against gram-positive than gram-negative species)	Up to 2 days
Phenol, Glutaraldehyde			
	Cold sterilization; not intended for living tissues	Bacteria, viruses, fungi, yeasts, spores	None; causes skin irritation

EQUINE PATIENT PREPARATION

PATIENT POSITIONING

Positioning of the equine patient for surgery can be quite an involved process. It requires more personnel compared with small animals. In most situations, the minimum number of persons required to position a horse on a surgery table is three. There are various ways in which a horse is moved or transported to the surgical suite and ultimately onto the surgical table. This is determined by the physical setup of the surgical facility. An overhead hoist system greatly facilitates the lifting and positioning of the horse onto the surgery table. As an example, the horse is walked into a padded induction room and anesthetized by using several persons pushing the horse against one of the walls during the induction of the anesthesia. As the animal becomes anesthetized, it is allowed to collapse to the floor and then roll into lateral recumbency. At that point, the horse is positioned in the center of the moveable floor that rolls into the surgical suite. Nylon leg bands

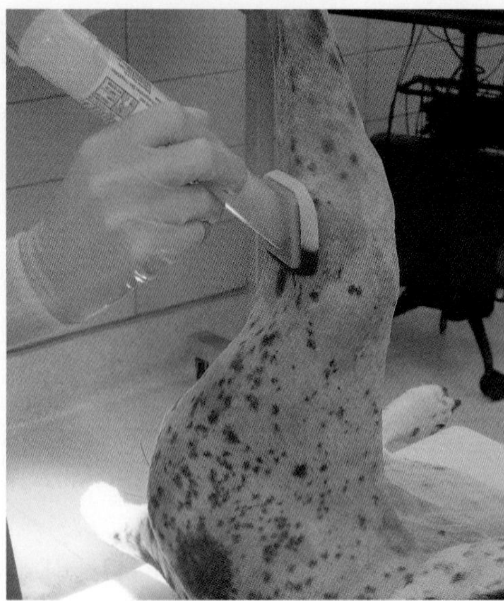

FIGURE 28-59 Skin preparation using a one-step prep method. In this case the planned incision will be along the lateral aspect of the femur. The applicator sponge is used to paint a single uniform coat of antiseptic solution on the skin, starting at the planned incision site and working outward in a circular pattern. (Photo courtesy Dr. Susanne Lauer.)

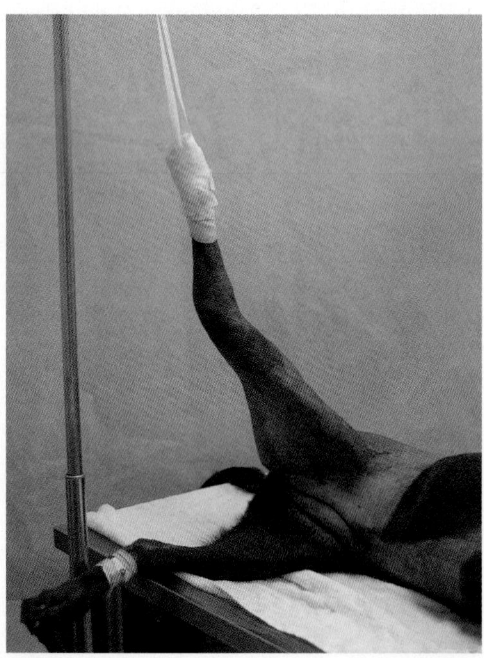

FIGURE 28-60 Hanging leg surgical preparation. This is commonly used for orthopedic surgeries of legs, including the shoulder and hip. The operated limb is suspended by tape stirrups that cover all distal leg hair. The surgical scrubs are started at the highest aspect of the clipped leg and worked downward with gravity in a circular fashion. Note the wide area of skin preparation on the body. At surgery, the taped foot is wrapped in a sterile towel, and the stirrups are cut.

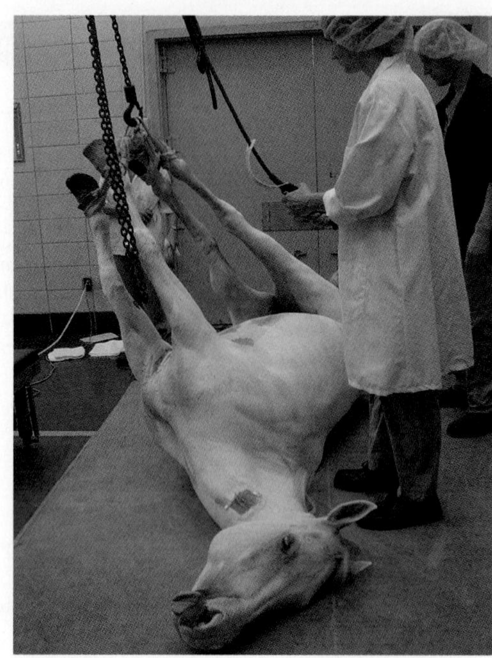

FIGURE 28-61 Nylon webbing leg bands are strapped to a horse's limbs at the pastern using double half-hitch loops. The leg bands are then attached to a chain hoist to transport the horse to the surgery table.

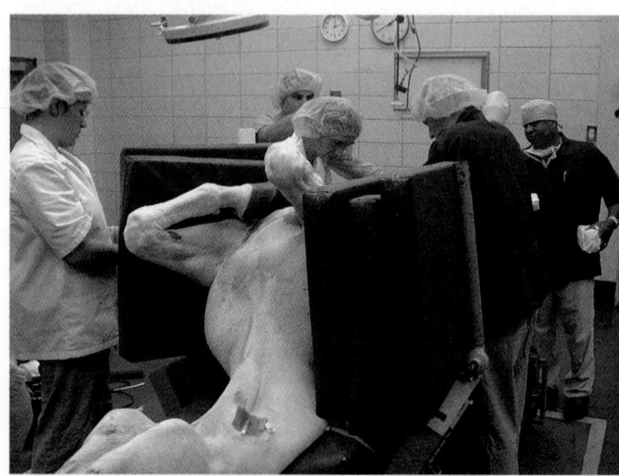

FIGURE 28-62 A horse maintained in dorsal recumbency for surgery, using side poles with pads wedged between the poles and the horse.

are strapped to the front and rear feet, and an overhead chain hoist is hooked to the bands (Figure 28-61). The horse is raised off the floor and moved onto the surgical table by way of a rail system that the chain hoist moves on. Once the animal is over the surgical table, it is gently lowered onto the table in the desired recumbency. If the horse is to be in dorsal recumbency, it is maintained in this position by the use of side poles with pads wedged between the poles and the horse (Figure 28-62). Once the horse is positioned on the table, the leg bands are removed, and the legs may be secured to the positioning poles or table to reduce shifting of the horse during surgery. The chain hoist is rolled away, and the rolling floor is pushed back into the padded induction room, and the surgical doors are closed. Large examination gloves or obstetrical (OB) sleeves are used to cover the feet of the horse to reduce contamination of the surgical suit (Figure 28-63).

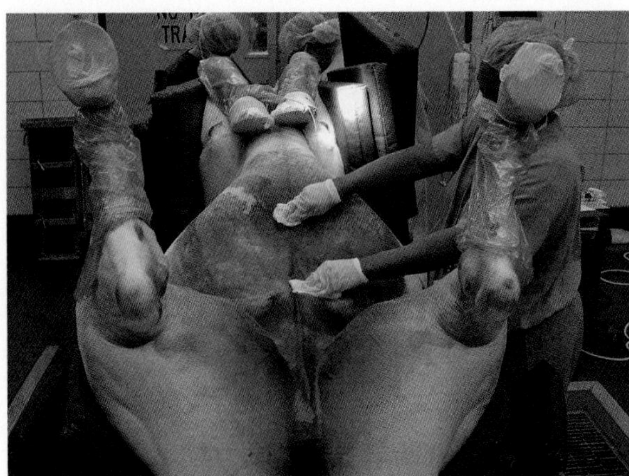

FIGURE 28-63 Large examination gloves or OB sleeves are used to cover the feet of the horse to reduce contamination of the surgical suite.

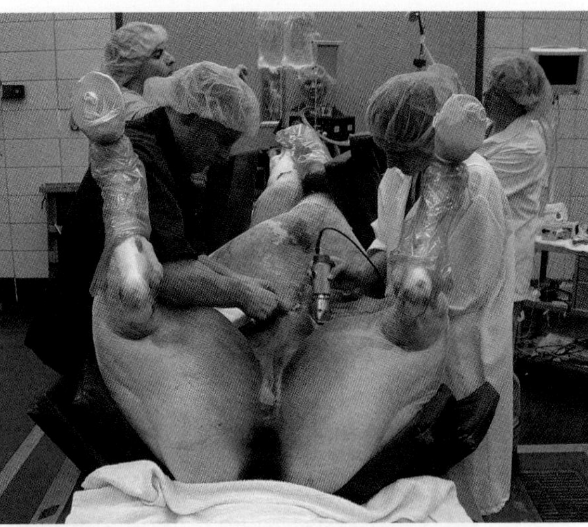

FIGURE 28-64 Surgical preparation of the ventral abdomen of a horse. A wide area of hair is removed with electric clippers.

As with proper technique, the personnel remaining in the surgical suite must wear proper surgical attire, including caps and masks. The surgical nurse should take charge to make sure that all personnel in the surgery suite are following protocol. During this preparation time, an anesthesiologist or anesthesiology technician is often placing arterial catheters in the hind limb or facial artery, attaching the ECG monitor, and attaching fluid lines to the IV catheters.

> *TECHNICIAN NOTE* The surgical nurse should take charge to make sure that all personnel in the surgery suite are following protocol.

SKIN PREPARATION

For some equine surgical procedures, particularly abdominal surgeries, it is difficult to clip the hair and perform an initial skin preparation before the horse is anesthetized. A wide area of hair at the intended surgical site is removed with electric clippers (Figure 28-64). An initial skin preparation is performed using chlorhexidine or povidone-iodine scrub with a rinse and wipe down of alcohol. During the initial preparation, the opening of a male horse's sheath (gelding or stallion) is packed with gauze sponges and sutured closed. This prevents urine and smegma from contaminating the surgical field (Figure 28-65). With female horses, it is imperative that the mammary area is cleaned thoroughly. Next a sterile skin preparation is performed with sterile gloves and sterile sponges (Figure 28-66). Three to five surgical scrubs alternating with the chlorhexidine and alcohol are performed, starting at the center of the surgical site and moving outward in a circular fashion (Figure 28-67). Preparation is complete when the sponges no longer collect visible dirt. Then the surgical area is sprayed with a chlorhexidine solution, which is left on the skin (Figure 28-68).

SURGICAL TEAM PREPARATION

ATTIRE

Proper surgical attire and proper scrubbing, gowning, and gloving procedures are important aspects of aseptic technique. Street clothing, especially shoes, are a major source of contamination and should not be worn into the operating room. Ideally, each person should have a pair of shoes designated for use only in the operating room. Disposable shoe covers may be worn in the operating room and discarded upon leaving the room. Lint-free scrub suits should be worn in the operating room. The shirt should be tucked into the pants to reduce the amount of skin debris dispersed into the room. Outside the operating room, scrub suits should be protected by a laboratory coat to reduce contamination.

During surgery, surgical caps and masks are worn by all persons who are in the room. The surgical cap covers the hair to reduce airborne contamination. Different types of surgical head covers are available to cover short hair, long hair, or beards (Figure 28-69). The mask protects the wound from saliva droplets, primarily by redirecting air flow out the sides of the mask. Masks are effective for relatively short periods and should be changed between procedures.

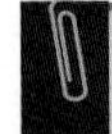

> *TECHNICIAN NOTE* Anyone entering the operating room should wear a cap, mask, and scrub suit.

HAND SCRUB

Scrubbing of the hands and arms, followed by gowning and gloving, is performed by all personnel who will be in close proximity to the surgical site. Surgical gloves may have tiny holes, so they cannot be solely relied upon to prevent contamination from the hands. The purpose of scrubbing the hands and arms is to remove dirt and decrease

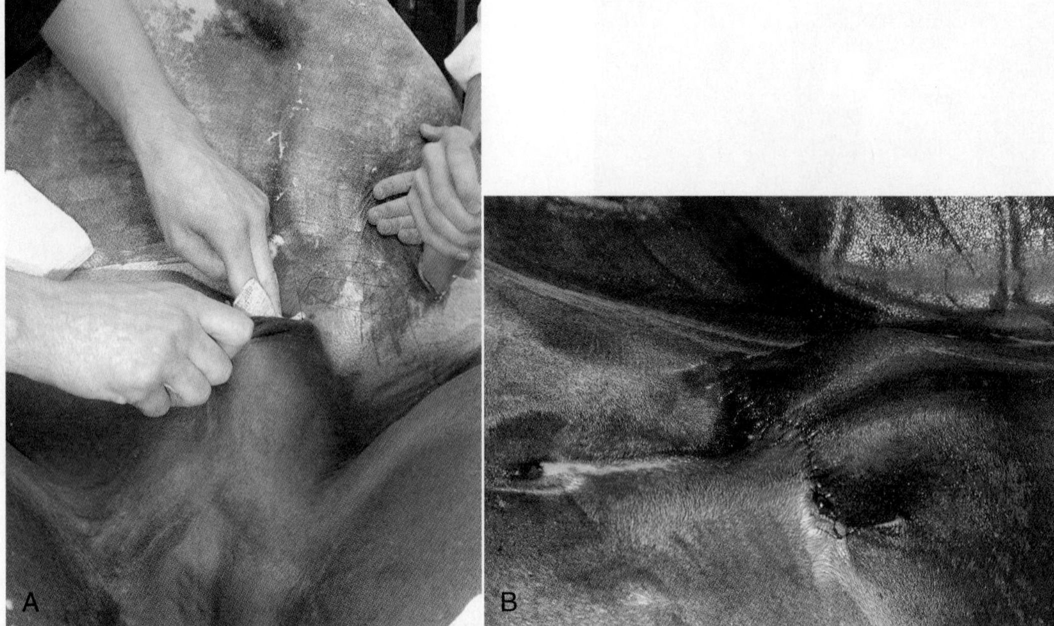

FIGURE 28-65 Surgical preparation of the ventral abdomen of a horse. **A,** During the initial preparation of the ventral abdomen of a horse for surgery, the opening of the male's sheath (gelding or stallion) is packed with gauze sponges. **B,** It is sutured closed to prevent urine and smegma from contaminating the surgical field.

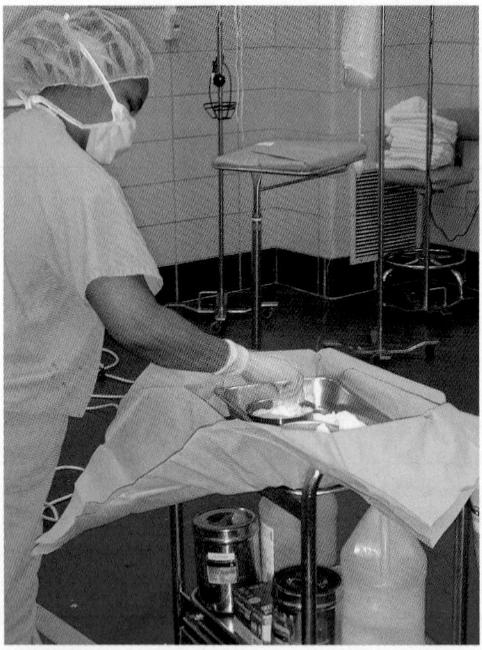

FIGURE 28-66 Sterile bowl and gauze sponges are used to do the final preparation of the surgical site on a horse. The inner sterile wrapping is opened with sterile gloves. The nurse should be wearing cap and mask.

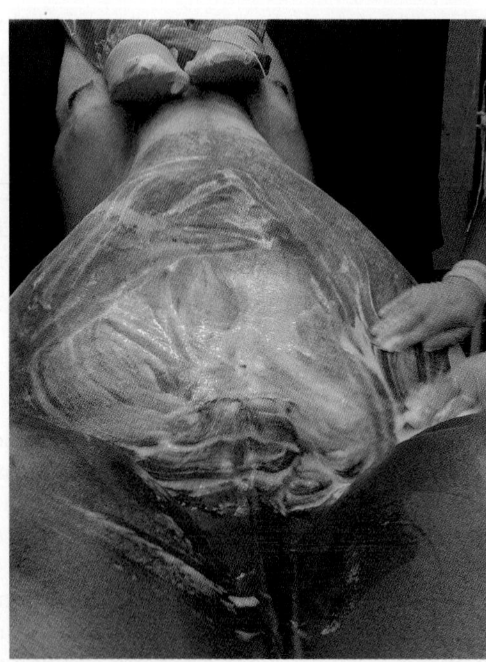

FIGURE 28-67 Surgical scrub on a horse. Three to five surgical scrubs, alternating with the chlorhexidine and alcohol are performed, starting at the center of the surgical site and spiraling outward.

the concentration of bacterial flora. The surgical cap and mask must be donned. The gown pack may be opened before scrubbing (Figure 28-70). All jewelry is removed from hands and arms before beginning the sterile hand scrub, and fingernails should be short and free of polish or artificial nails. Once the scrubbing has begun, the hands and arms should not touch nonsterile objects. If this occurs, the scrub is started over.

While scrubbing, the hands are always held above the level of the elbows so the water drains off the elbows. Soap is applied to a sterile brush, and a systematic scrub is begun. Scrub all four sides of each finger, with special attention to the fingernails (Figure 28-71, *A*). The back, both sides, and the palm of the hand are scrubbed. Next the wrist and forearm are scrubbed, working toward the elbow (Figure 28-71, *B*). After both hands and arms have been scrubbed, they are rinsed in running water (Figure 28-71, *C*). The entire scrub process is then repeated.

The two basic methods of surgical scrubs are the counted brush strokes and the timed. The counted brush strokes method is performed by counting the number of brush strokes used on each skin surface. Ten to 25 brush strokes are made on each surface of the fingers, hands, and arms before rinsing. This is performed four times. The timed method is more commonly used. This is done by repeatedly scrubbing and rinsing for a set period of time. The initial scrub of the day should last about 5 minutes. For subsequent scrubs during the day, 2 to 3 minutes is adequate.

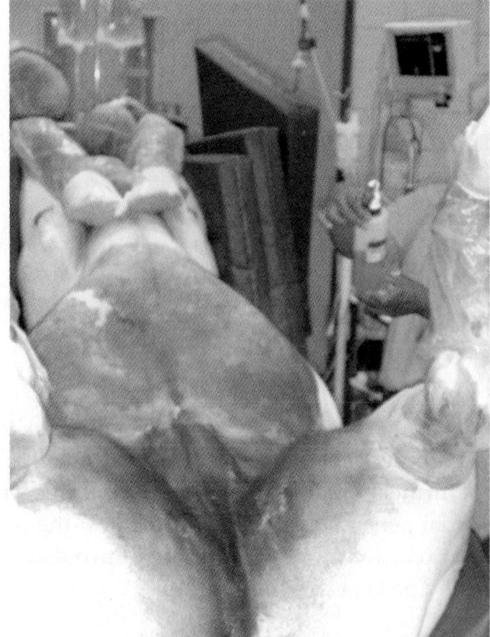

FIGURE 28-68 The surgical area is sprayed with a chlorhexidine solution, which is left on the skin once the final preparation is completed on a horse.

> *TECHNICIAN NOTE* The surgical hand scrub requires that all surfaces of the fingers, hand, and forearm be scrubbed. Skin-soap contact time should last 5 minutes.

Waterless hand antiseptics are now available that are at least as effective as the traditional hand-scrub technique described earlier and cause less skin trauma. These antiseptics contain an alcohol solution, which provides a rapid antimicrobial kill of a broad spectrum of microorganisms. They also contain a lotion to prevent drying of the skin. Hands must be clean and dry, but scrubbing is not necessary. The solution is rubbed briskly and evenly over one hand and forearm; a second application is applied to the other hand and forearm. A final application is applied to both hands and allowed to air-dry. The waterless antiseptics are fast, effective, easy to apply, and nonirritating.

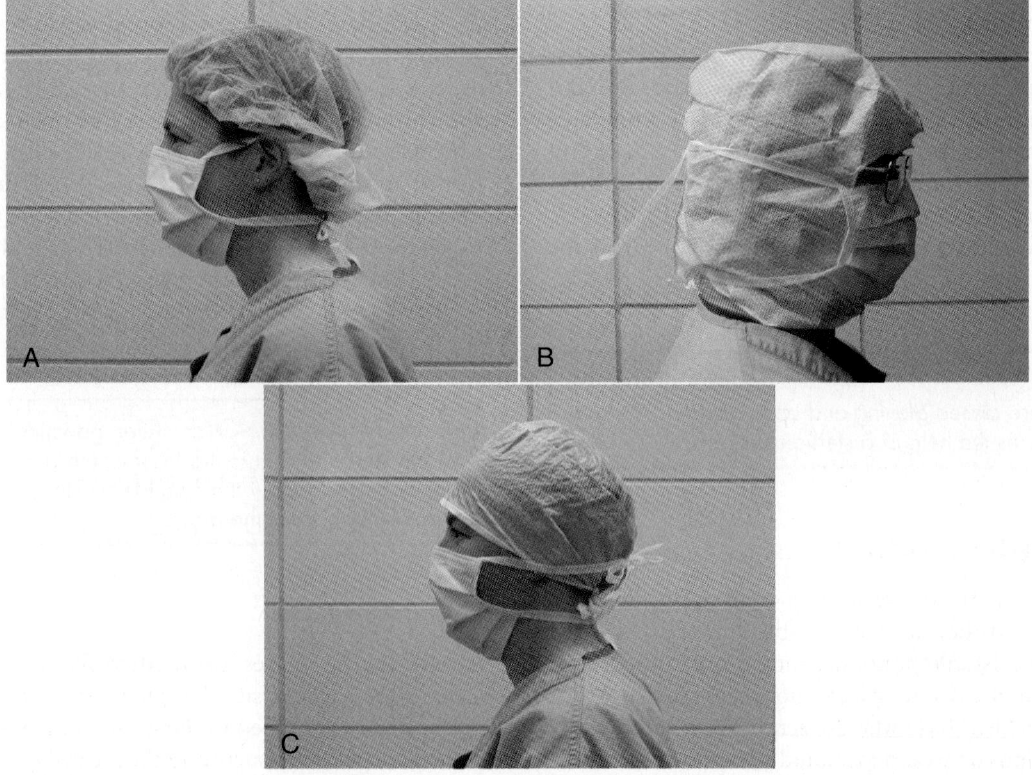

FIGURE 28-69 Surgical caps and masks. **A,** Bouffant head cover is used to cover long or short hair. **B,** Hoods are available for individuals with sideburns or a beard. **C,** A cap may be suitable to cover short hair.

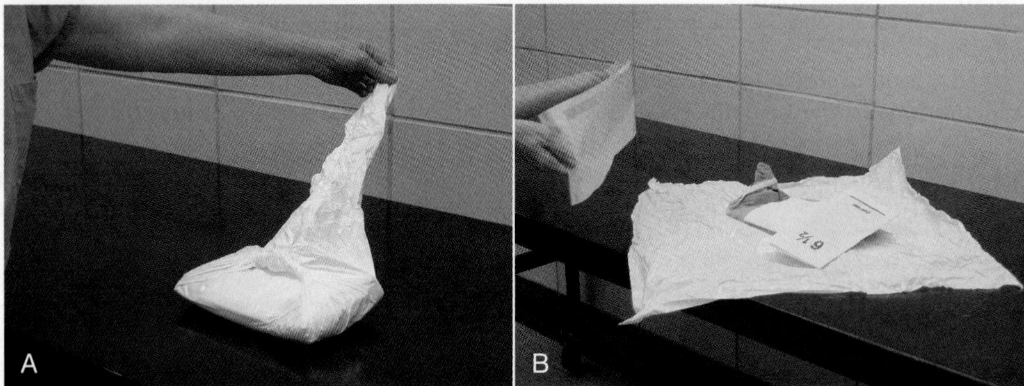

FIGURE 28-70 Open gown pack. **A,** The gown pack may be opened before scrubbing so that the hand towel is available. When opening a pack, always open the flap away from you first. Keep the arm off to the side, not directly over the pack. Then open the other three sides, touching only the corners of the wrap on the outside surface. **B,** The sterile gloves are opened onto the gown. With the package positioned at the edge of the sterile field, it is opened symmetrically. This gives the contents enough forward momentum to fall on the sterile field without having to reach over it.

> TECHNICIAN NOTE Waterless hand antiseptics are easy to apply, faster than traditional hand-scrubbing techniques, effective against microorganisms, and nonirritating to the skin.

GOWNING AND GLOVING

The hands and arms are thoroughly dried with a sterile towel (Figure 28-72) before gowning (Figure 28-73) and gloving.

The two methods for gloving yourself are *closed gloving* and *open gloving*. The risk of contamination is minimized with closed gloving (Figure 28-74) because the outside of the gloves never contacts skin. There is a much higher risk of contamination during open gloving (Figure 28-75), and it is generally reserved for minor procedures when a gown is not worn (e.g., sterile patient scrub, urinary catheterization). If it is necessary to replace gloves during surgery, it is preferable to have a nonsterile assistant remove the old gloves and simultaneously pull the gown sleeve so that the hands remain inside the sleeves (Figure 28-76). If the old gloves are removed in this manner, new gloves can be put on by the closed gloving method or by *assisted gloving* (Figure 28-77).

> TECHNICIAN NOTE The two methods of gloving yourself are *closed gloving* and *open gloving. Assisted gloving* requires the help of a sterile assistant.

MAINTAINING STERILITY

It is important for the entire surgical team to be conscious of sterility, even if they are not "scrubbed in" (i.e., gowned and gloved). Nonsterile personnel should only touch nonsterile items or areas and should not lean over or reach across sterile fields. Those who are scrubbed in should only touch sterile items or areas and should always face the sterile field. Only sterilized items can be placed on a sterile field. If anyone on the surgical team notices a potential source of contamination or "break" in sterile technique, it should be mentioned immediately so that steps can be taken to reduce the risk of further contamination. To reduce contamination, only essential personnel should be present in the operating room, and excessive movement should be avoided. Conversation should be kept to a minimum.

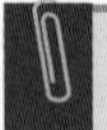

> TECHNICIAN NOTE Nonsterile personnel should not lean over or reach across sterile fields.

Scrubbed-In Personnel

The sterile area on a person is considered to be the front of the gown, from just below the shoulders (the neckline is not sterile) to the waist or the level of the table. The gown sleeves are also considered to be sterile. Note that the back of a gowned person is considered to be nonsterile, so it should not be turned to face any sterile field. Gloved hands may be rested on a sterile drape or clasped in front of the body in the zone between the shoulders and waist. The arms should not be folded across the chest because the armpit region is considered to be nonsterile, and the hands should not drop below waist level.

> TECHNICIAN NOTE After gowning and gloving, the sterile region is the front of the gown between the waist and just below the shoulders. The gown sleeves are also sterile, but not the back.

THE PATIENT

Sterile surgical drapes are used to maintain a sterile field around the surgical site. Draping is performed by personnel who have scrubbed in. First, four small towels (cloth or paper) are placed to surround the area where the surgical incision will be. These are called *quarter drapes* and they are secured to the skin using towel clamps. During this procedure,

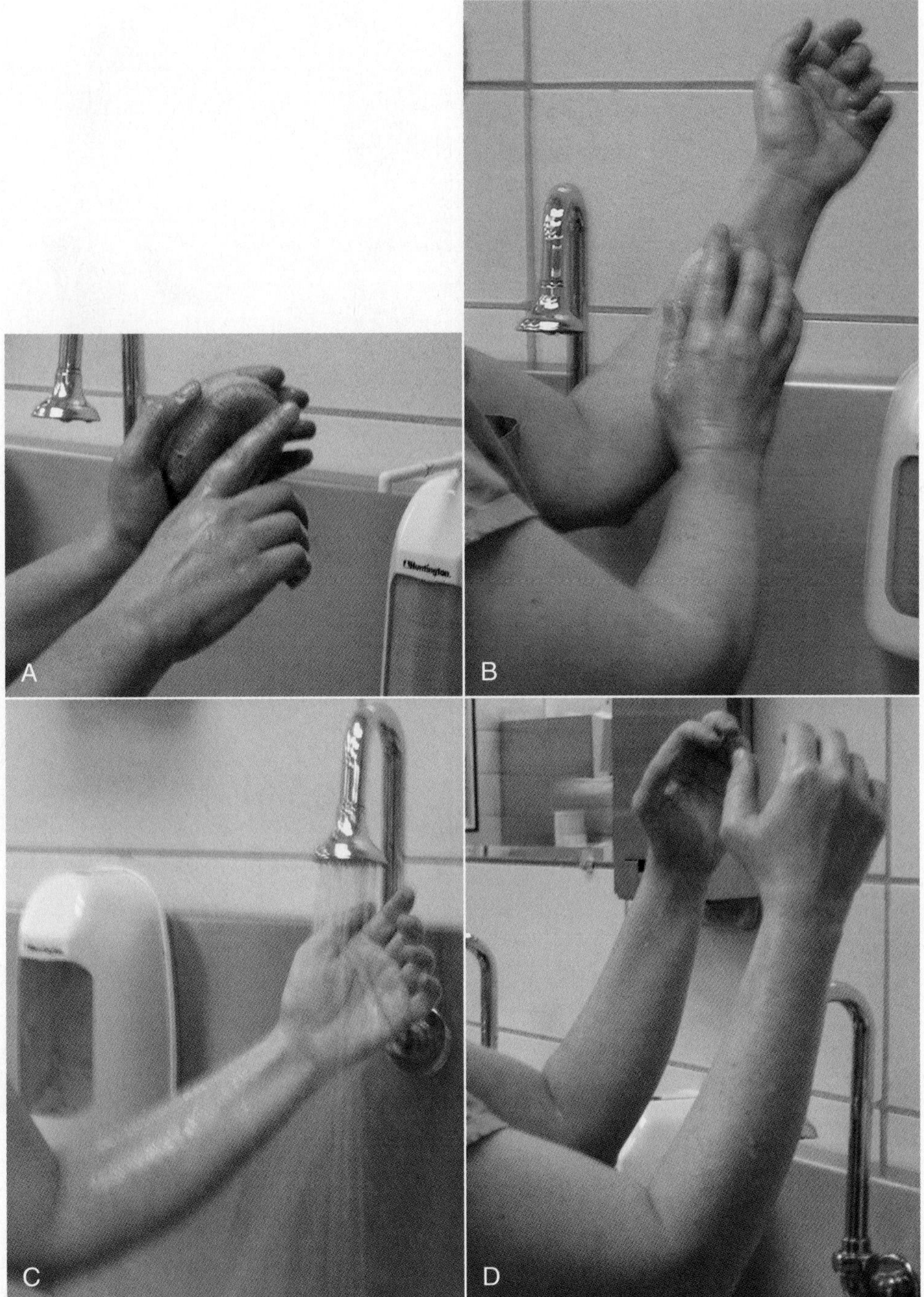

FIGURE 28-71 Surgical hand scrub. **A,** Imagine each finger as having a tip and four sides. Scrub each surface of each finger. Also scrub the palm, back, and sides of the hand. **B,** Imagine the forearm as having four sides and scrub each side. **C,** After scrubbing both hands and arms, rinse the brush, hands, and forearms. The hands are always kept above the elbows. **D,** After the last scrub, drop the brush, rinse, and let the excess water drip off the elbows.

one must be careful not to brush the front of the surgical gown against the surgical table. Then a large drape is placed over the animal, surgical table, and instrument stand to provide one continuous sterile field. Cloth drapes have an opening or "fenestration," which is positioned over the surgical site. If a disposable paper drape is used, the appropriately sized hole may be cut after the drape has been placed. Because skin preparations do not sterilize, but only disinfect, the skin, plastic incise drapes may be used to provide a sterile surface at the start of surgery. These are translucent, adherent plastic drapes that are used to completely cover any visible skin after the barrier drapes have been applied. Incise drapes are often impregnated with an antiseptic. The surgeon can cut through the incise drape simultaneously with the skin incision. Refer to Chapter 29 for more detail on draping procedures.

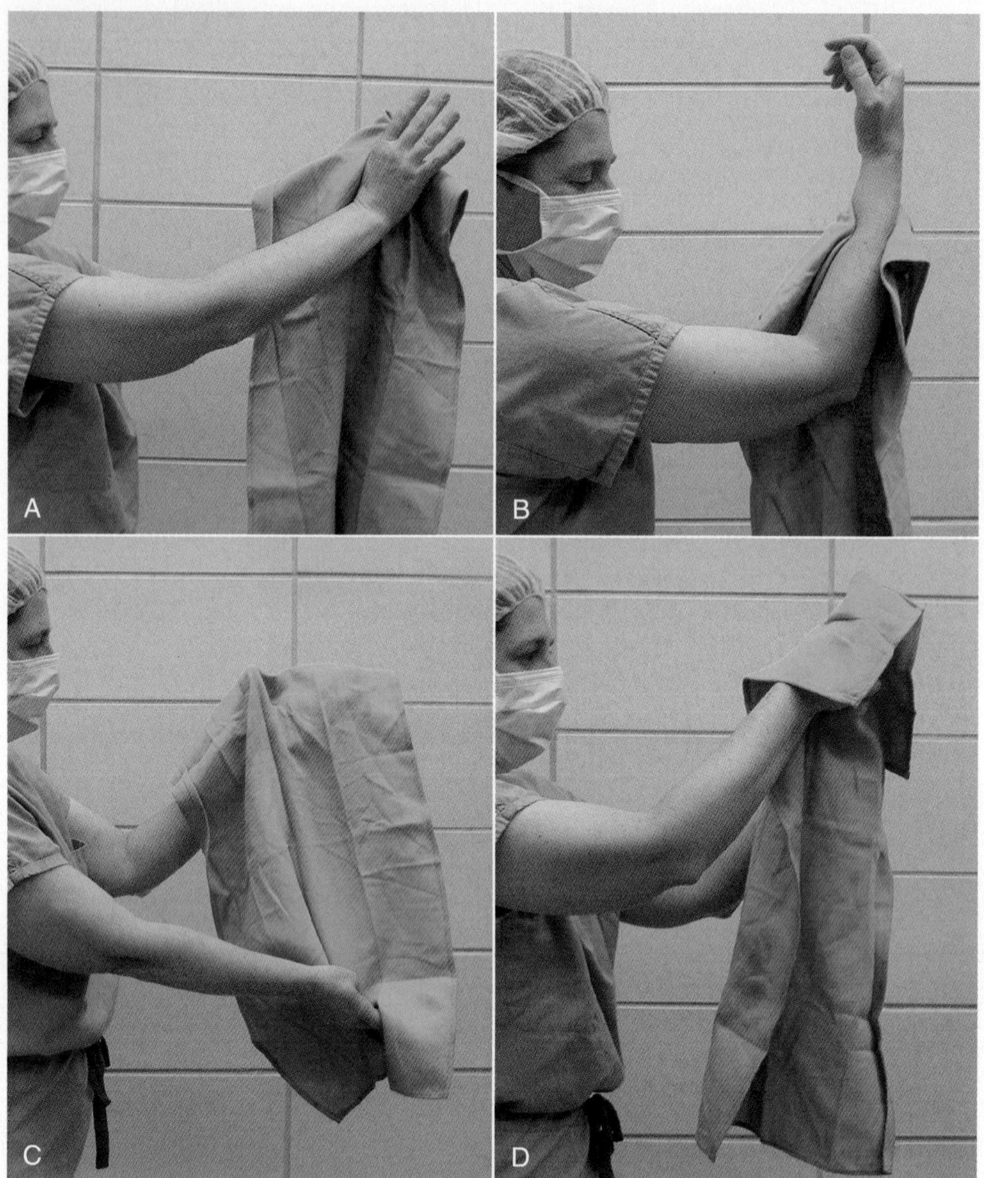

FIGURE 28-72 Towel dry. **A,** One hand is dried first, holding the towel away from the body. **B,** Move the towel down to dry the arm, using only the top end of the towel. **C,** The dry hand now grasps the dry end of the towel. **D,** The other hand and arm are dried. Note that the hands do not switch sides of the towel during the process.

If a limb has been suspended in preparation for an orthopedic procedure (as described under Patient Positioning), the quarter drapes are placed on the body, around the base of the limb. The distal limb is then held with a sterile wrap while a nonsterile assistant cuts the stirrups. The nonscrubbed, distal portion of the limb is covered with a sterile towel or sterile Vetrap. A sterile cotton stockinette or adhesive incise drape may be used to cover the entire leg. Finally the limb is passed through a hole in the large sterile drape that covers the entire animal.

> TECHNICIAN NOTE The *optimal* approach to draping includes isolating the surgical site with two layers of drapes: (1) four quarter drapes and (2) a large drape that covers the entire animal and the instrument table.

After draping is completed, sterile instrument packs, light handles, suture material, and other sterile equipment may be opened. Draped tables and instrument trays are considered to be sterile only on the top of the draped surface, so if part of a sterile item slips below the level of the tabletop, it is considered to be contaminated and should no longer be touched by the surgeons.

OPENING STERILE ITEMS

Nonsterile assistants must open all sterile items for the surgeons. Nonsterile assistants can only touch the outside of sterile packs and should never reach over a sterile field. Large or heavy packs, such as an instrument pack, may be set on a table to be opened. The four folded edges of the outer wrap are opened one at a time, while never extending the hand

and arm over the top of the pack (see Figure 28-70, *A*). If the pack can be placed on a Mayo instrument stand, this can be accomplished by moving around the stand and pulling each fold away from the center. The inner wrap may be opened by the surgeon or by a nonsterile assistant. Once the instrument tray is exposed, the surgeon can pick it up and set it on the draped instrument stand.

A smaller wrapped pack may be opened while holding it in one hand (Figure 28-78). As each corner of the pack is unfolded, it is grasped by the hand that is holding the pack. This prevents the edges of the wrap from contaminating the contents of the pack. The exposed item may be grasped by the surgeon or carefully set on the sterile field.

To open a plastic or paper pouch, scalpel blade, or suture package, the edges of the wrapper should be peeled back slowly and symmetrically, keeping the package opening directed away from the body. Some items may be dropped onto the sterile field; be careful not to lean or reach across the sterile field (see Figure 28-70, *B*). If the item is small or awkward to handle, the surgeon can grasp it with a gloved hand or sterile instrument. The item should not be allowed to touch the peeled edges of the pouch because the edges are considered contaminated.

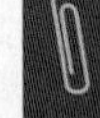

TECHNICIAN NOTE While opening a pack, make sure that the opening faces away from you.

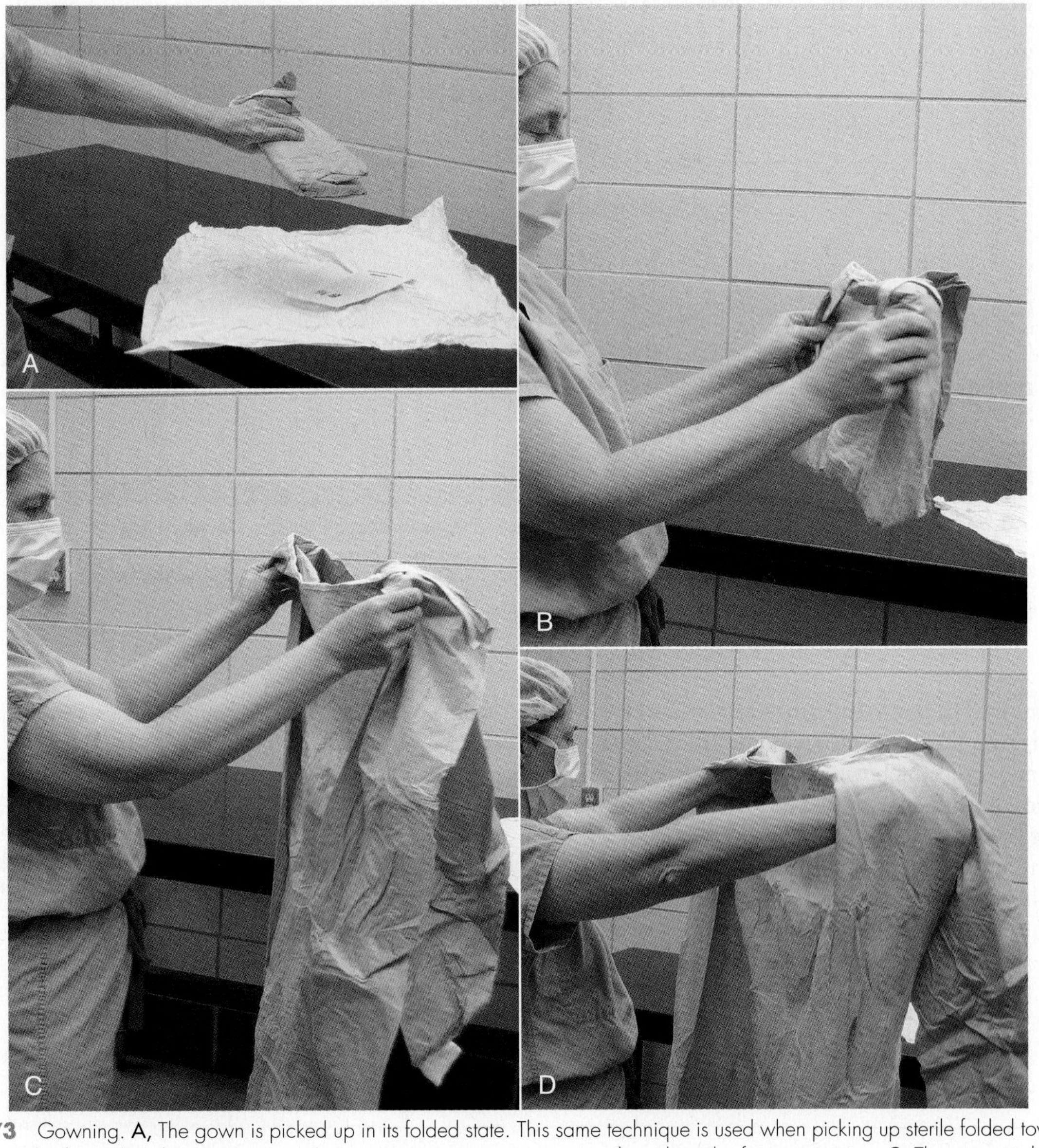

FIGURE 28-73 Gowning. **A,** The gown is picked up in its folded state. This same technique is used when picking up sterile folded towels or drapes. This reduces the risk of accidental contamination. **B,** Move to a spacious area to reduce the risk of contamination. **C,** The gown is held away from the body by the inside shoulder seams and allowed to unfold. **D,** The arms are slid into the sleeves, but the hands should not extend through the cuff openings.

Continued

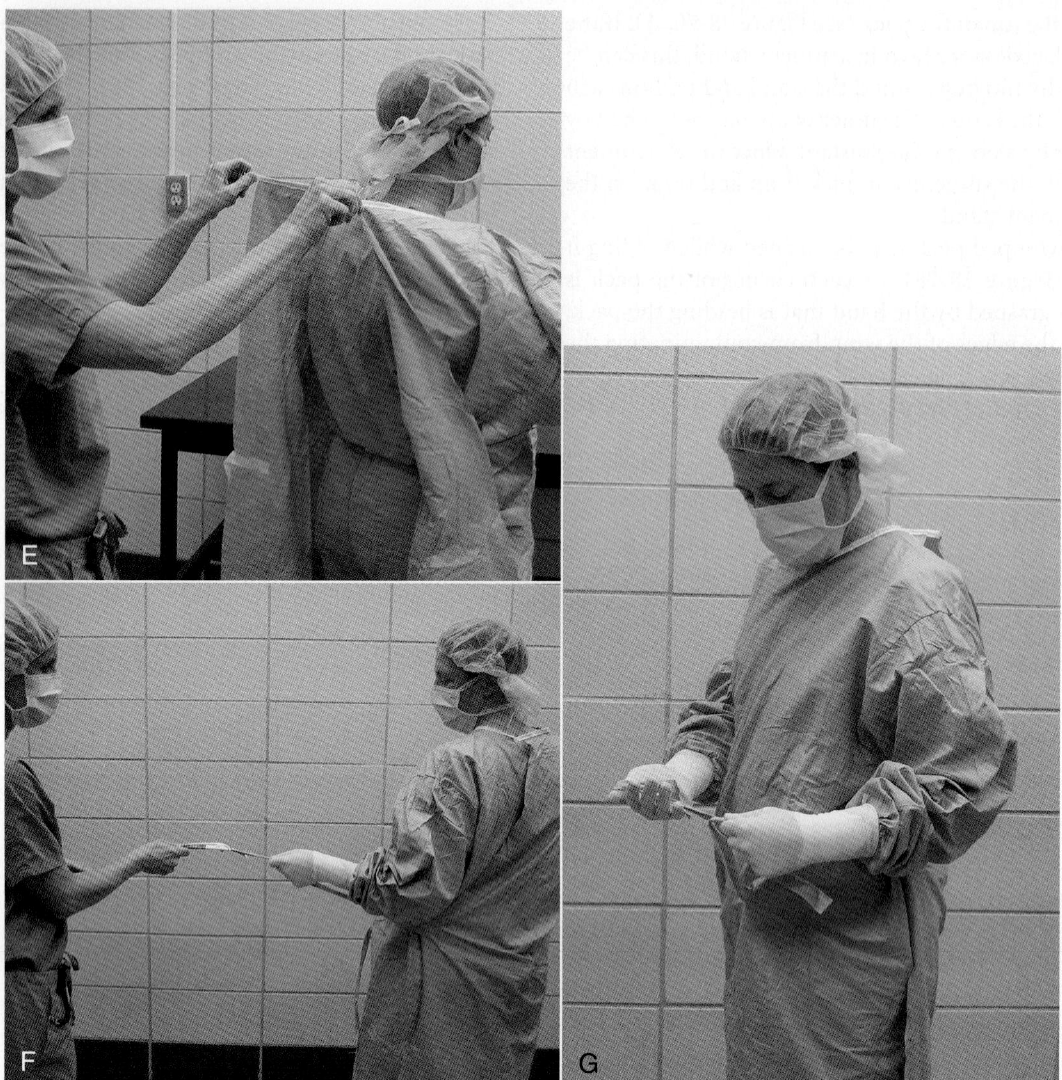

FIGURE 28-73, cont'd **E,** A nonsterile assistant pulls the gown over the shoulders and ties the back of the gown at the neck and waist. **F,** If the gown has a wraparound back, the last tie is performed after the surgeon has gloved. The surgeon hands the sterile tag to a nonsterile assistant. The assistant holds the end of the tag while the surgeon turns around, causing the gown to cover the surgeon's back. The surgeon takes the gown tie and pulls, releasing it from the tag that is still in the assistant's hand. **G,** The final tie is done in front by the surgeon.

Sterile saline may be poured into the sterile saline bowl. To avoid reaching over the sterile field with the saline container, the surgeon may hold the bowl away from the instrument tray or position it on the tray at the edge of the sterile field. The lip of the saline container should be a few inches above the rim of the bowl to reduce the risk of touching it, but not so high that the saline splashes as it is poured. If drapes or gowns (especially those made of cloth) become wet with saline or blood, they may no longer be impermeable to bacteria and are said to have "strike-through."

> *TECHNICIAN NOTE* If drapes or gowns (especially those made of cloth) become wet with saline or blood, they may no longer be impermeable to bacteria and are said to have "strike-through."

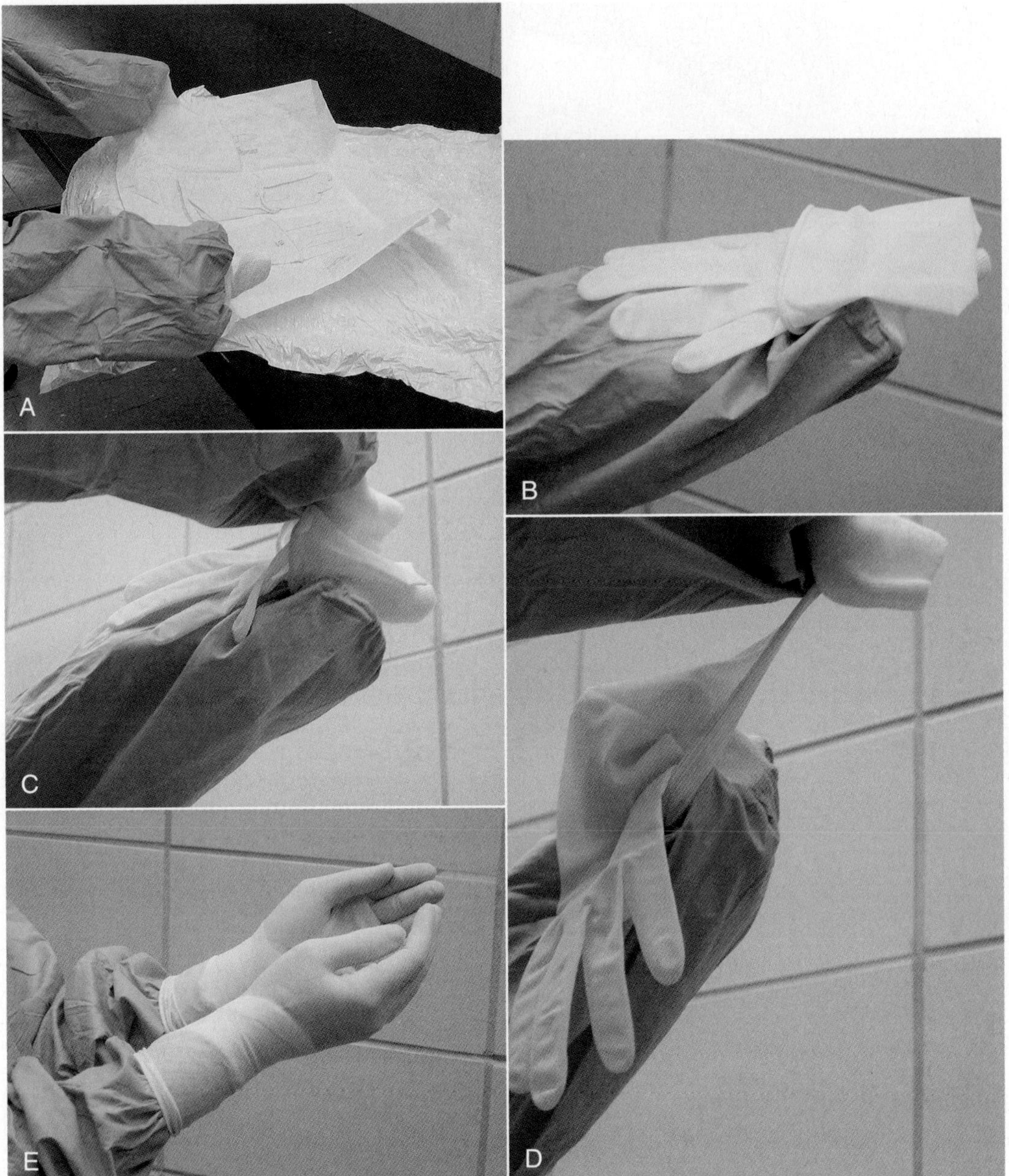

FIGURE 28-74 Closed gloving. **A,** The sterile pack is close to the table edge so that the surgeon can maintain some distance from the table to prevent contaminating the sterile gown. The sterile paper wrap containing the gloves is unfolded, and one glove is picked up. It is easiest for most people to glove their nondominant hand first. The fingers must be kept inside the sleeves at all times during closed gloving. **B,** The glove is laid on the hand to be gloved, with the glove fingers pointing toward the elbow and the glove thumb lying against the sleeve. The edge of the glove cuff is grasped through the gown sleeve. **C,** The opposite side of the cuff is grasped in the other hand. **D, E,** The glove is pulled over the hand. Now the gown and glove cuff may be grasped together to pull the glove completely onto the hand.

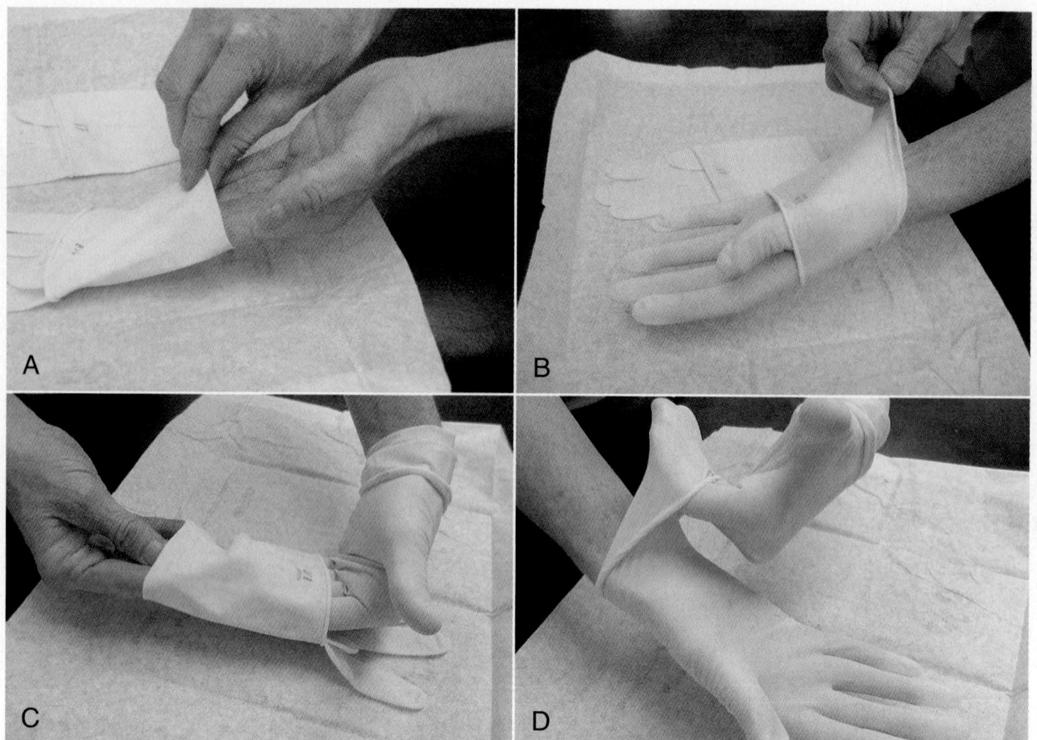

FIGURE 28-75 Open gloving. **A,** The glove pack is opened near the edge of a table. The hand is inserted into the glove opening, taking care not to touch the outside of the glove. The inside of the glove will not be sterile, so the cuff may be touched. **B,** The glove is pulled on by grasping the cuff fold with the other hand. The cuff will still be folded, but the glove is on well enough to allow use of the hand. **C,** The gloved hand is placed between the cuff and the palm of the glove to assist gloving the other hand. This protects the gloved hand from accidental contamination on the arm. **D,** The cuff can be unfolded. Now adjustments can be made to both gloves, taking care to touch only the sterile areas of the gloves.

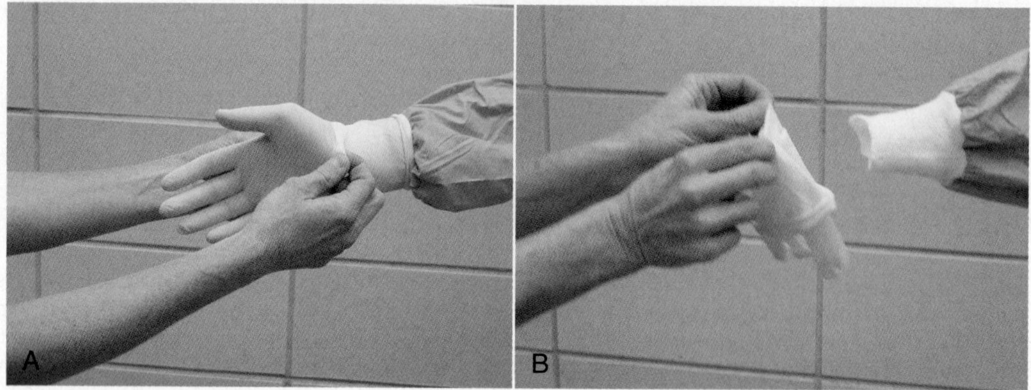

FIGURE 28-76 Removing gloves aseptically. **A,** A nonsterile assistant grasps the glove and gown cuff together without touching the gown sleeve. **B,** As the glove is removed, the gown is pulled over the fingers. The gown cuff is considered contaminated. The surgeon can reglove, taking care not to contaminate anything with the gown cuff. It may be preferable to perform an assisted gloving as shown in Figure 28-68.

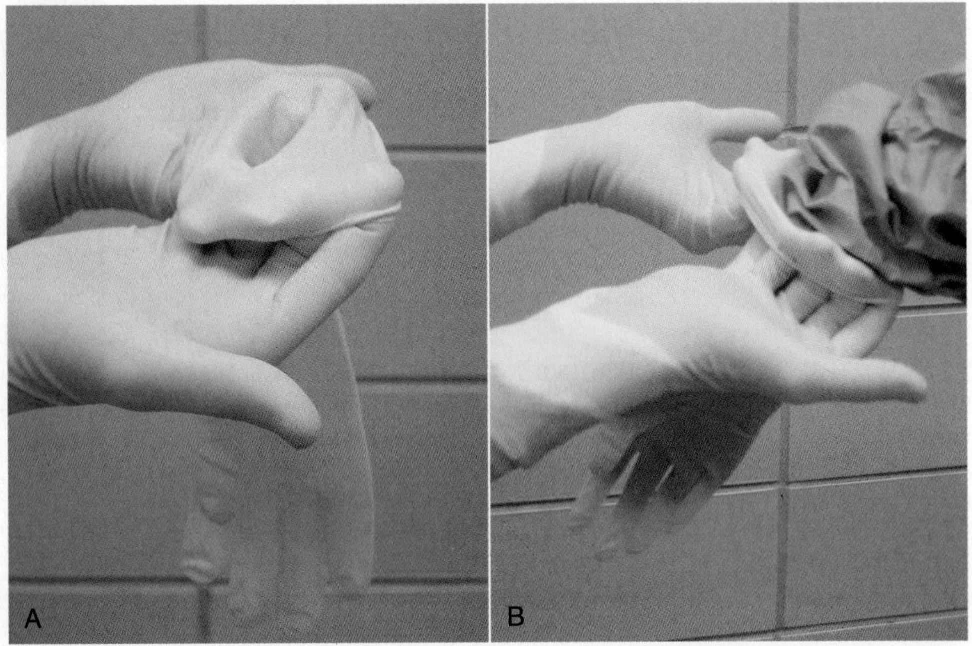

FIGURE 28-77 Assisted gloving. **A,** A sterile assistant picks up the appropriate sterile glove, holding it so the location of the glove thumb is apparent. The assistant hooks his or her fingers under the glove cuff and pulls to make the glove opening as large as possible. **B,** The surgeon slides his or her hand into the glove while the assistant pulls the glove cuff up to be sure it covers the gown cuff before releasing.

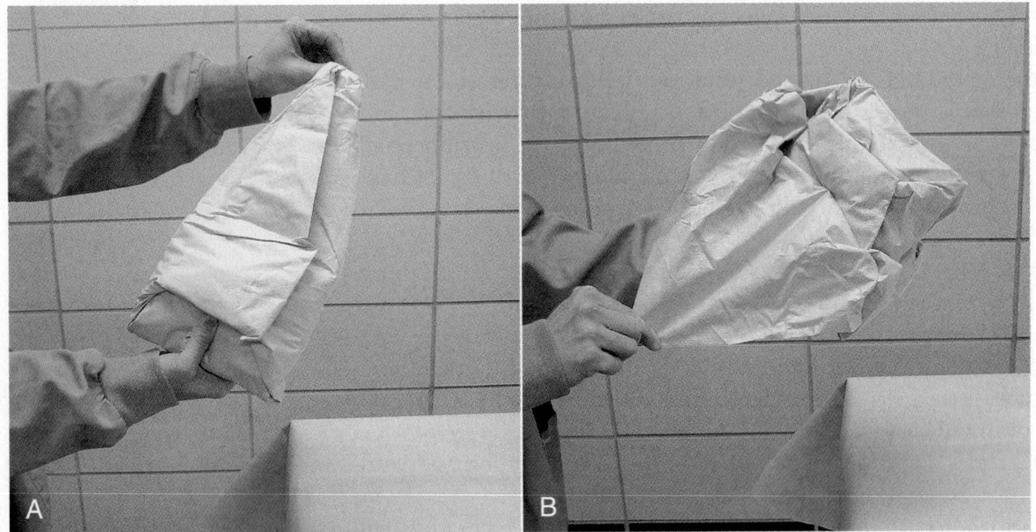

FIGURE 28-78 Opening a sterile pack that can be held in one hand. **A,** Open the first flap away from you. **B,** As each flap is opened, it is held together with the hand holding the pack. After the fourth flap is pulled back and secured, the inner package may be grasped by the surgeon. Move the wrap down and toward you as the surgeon lifts the contents up and toward them. Alternatively the package may be set on a sterile field near its edge to avoid reaching over the field.

RECOMMENDED READING

Beale BS et al: *Small animal arthroscopy,* St Louis, 2003, Saunders.

Busch S: *Small animal surgical nursing,* St Louis, 2005, Mosby.

Cockshutt J: Principles of surgical asepsis. In Slatter D, editor: *Textbook of small animal surgery,* ed 3, St Louis, 2003, Saunders.

Hobson HP: Surgical facilities and equipment. In Slatter D, editor: *Textbook of small animal surgery,* ed 3, St Louis, 1993, Saunders.

Lemarie RJ, Hosgood G: Antiseptics and disinfectants in small animal practice, *Compend Cont Educ Pract Vet* 17:1339-1352, 1996.

McIlwraith CW et al: *Diagnostic and surgical arthroscopy in the horse,* ed 3, Philadelphia, 2005, Mosby.

Mitchell SL, Berg J: Sterilization. In Slatter D, editor: *Textbook of small animal surgery,* ed 3, Philadelphia, 2003, WB Saunders.

Nieves MA, Wagner SD: Surgical instruments. In Slatter D, editor: *Textbook of small animal surgery,* ed 3, Philadelphia, 2003, Saunders.

Pavletic MM: Surgical stapling, *Vet Clin North Am* 24:225-429, 1994.

Shmon C: Assessment and preparation of the surgical patient and the operating team. In Slatter D, editor: *Textbook of small animal surgery,* ed 3, Philadelphia, 2003, WB Saunders.

Sonsthagen TF: *Veterinary instruments and equipment: a pocket guide,* St Louis, 2006, Mosby.

29 Surgical Assistance and Suture Material

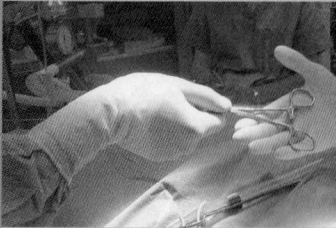

Susanne K. Lauer and Daniel J. Burba

KEY TERMS

Carpus
Laparotomy
Viscus

OUTLINE

LEARNING OBJECTIVES

When you have completed this chapter, you will be able to:

1. Describe the role of the veterinary technician in surgical assistance for large and small animal patients.
2. Describe the method of placing and securing surgical drapes on the patient and special requirements for surgical draping for orthopedic or neurologic surgeries.
3. Discuss considerations for placement of instruments on the instrument table and considerations for maintaining sterility of the gloved and gowned surgical team.
4. Describe proper handling of skin, hollow organs, muscle, and bone tissue during surgery.
5. Describe procedures and special considerations for retracting tissues during surgical procedures.
6. Describe indications for and complications of sponge hemostasis.
7. Differentiate between monopolar and bipolar electrosurgery modes and describe care, use, and safety issues related to electrosurgical units.
8. Describe commonly used hemostatic and cauterizing agents.
9. List the principles and procedures related to incision irrigation and lavage and surgical drains.
10. List and describe commonly used suture material and needles and methods for their preparation.

INTRODUCTION

The use of the veterinary technician in surgery has evolved over the past 20 years. The technician today is needed as a trained and skilled operating room (OR) assistant and circulating nurse. As technology and surgical equipment have increased in sophistication, the need for well-trained surgical assistants has become necessary in both companion animal and large animal surgery. The specific role of the veterinary technician as part of the surgical team is emphasized in this chapter.

GENERAL CONCEPTS WITH SMALL ANIMAL EMPHASIS

ROLE OF THE VETERINARY TECHNICIAN IN SURGICAL ASSISTANCE

The excellent support of a dedicated surgical technician can make a difference between successful surgical outcome and failure. The ideal surgical assistant "prethinks" and anticipates the surgeon's needs before the surgeon asks for it. Thus already on the day before surgery the surgical assistant generates a plan for the following day. As a rule of thumb, sterile surgeries are performed first and more contaminated surgeries later throughout the day with the intent to prevent surgical infections. The surgical assistant verifies that the required instruments, implants, surgical and diagnostic supplies, medications, anesthetic equipment, and OR are available and set up for surgery.

The surgical assistant supervises or performs preparation of the patient (see Chapter 28 for clipping, scrubbing, preoperative antibiotics) and positions the patient in an ideal secure position on the operating table according to the instructions of the surgeon. The surgical technician will then drape the patient for the surgeon and set up the instruments properly.

> *TECHNICIAN NOTE* The ideal surgical assistant anticipates the surgeon's needs before the surgeon asks for it and plans in advance.

Intrasurgical assistance includes improving the surgeon's visualization by providing retraction and hemostasis in the surgical field, familiarity with the objectives of the technique, and manipulating the instrumentation and tissues into position for completion of the surgical task. The second charge of the technician is to protect the patient from hazards of surgery, such as infection, by maintaining an aseptic surgical field and expediting surgical completion by anticipating needs for proper instruments and suture readiness. Because the surgeon is often concentrating on the surgical procedure, the technician must be constantly aware of the patient's anesthetic and cardiovascular status while assisting. After the surgery, the assistant will help with bandaging and anesthetic recovery of the patient.

PATIENT AND INSTRUMENT TABLES SETUP

POSITIONING OF PATIENT

Before sterile preparation is performed, the surgical patient is moved into the OR and secured to the table. The surgical site must be accessible for the surgeon and the assistant standing (sitting) in a neutral position to prevent long-term health problems secondary to abnormal posture. Depending on the surgical procedure performed, the patient is placed in the appropriate position and secured with V-shaped troughs, ropes, towels, sandbags, and vacuum-activated positioning devices (Figure 29-1). The patient is placed on prewarmed water-circulating heating pads and covered with warm-air circulating blankets (see Chapter 30). Many surgeons prefer the warm-air circulation to be only activated after the patient is draped to prevent potential blowing of particles into the sterile surgical field. If the surgeon plans to use monopolar electrosurgery, the ground plate must be positioned in direct contact with the patient under the animal. Care must be taken that the securing devices do not restrict respiratory function or apply excessive pressure on peripheral nerves, vessels, or muscles. When extremities with intravenous (IV) or arterial catheters or blood pressure monitoring devices are tied to the table, rope tension or position often have to be adjusted to allow for adequate flow of fluid and correct measurements.

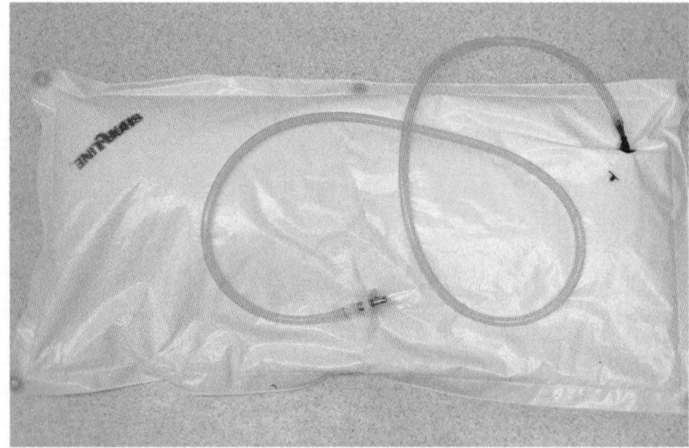

FIGURE 29-1 Vacuum-activated positioning device for accurate positioning of the patient on the table.

DRAPING

The function of draping is to separate the sterile surgical site from contaminated areas of the patient. Draping can only be performed by a sterile gloved and gowned member of the surgical team. Draping and instrument setup performed by the surgical assistant will speed up the procedure. Sterile quarter (field) drapes, Backhaus towel clamps, and large table-covering drapes are opened on a sterile table by a nonsterile assistant. The first field drape is unfolded and an edge folded under toward the patient. The corners of the drape are wrapped around the hands to protect these from contamination (Figure 29-2). The drape is floated above the patient and placed in the appropriate position without dragging the sterile drape along the patient's contaminated body. This is easier if the table is positioned relatively low considering the height of the draping person. When applying the drapes, keep in mind that the undraped surgical table is not sterile and cannot be touched by the person doing the draping. Therefore the draping assistant should stand at least 15 inches away from the table border and be constantly aware of his or her environment to prevent contamination of sterile hands and gown. The drape should only be adjusted

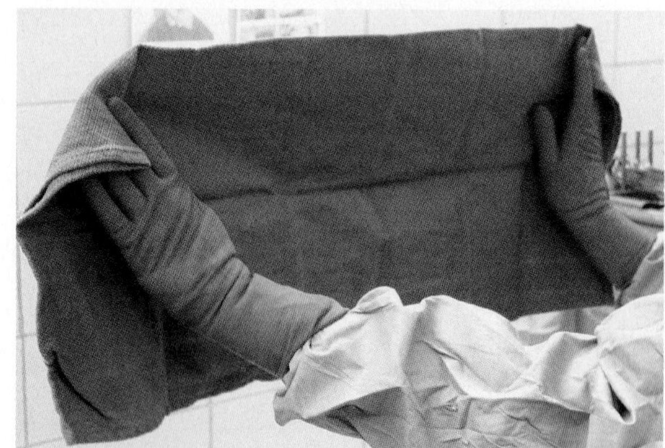

FIGURE 29-2 The drape is wrapped around the hands for protection of the sterile gloves.

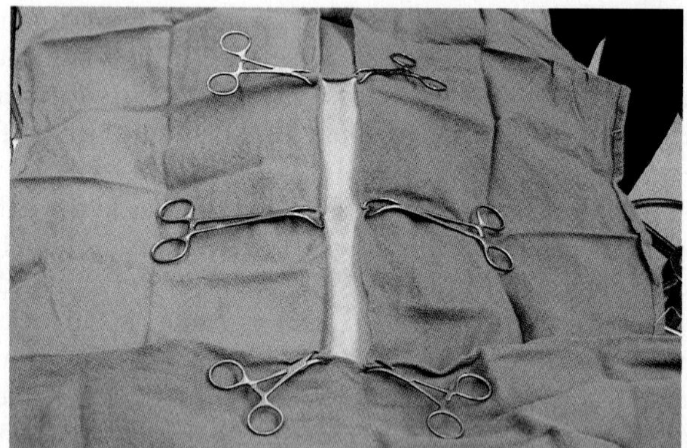

FIGURE 29-3 Four quarter drapes are secured with towel clamps approximate to the incision.

minimally once it has been laid onto the patient. If the drape needs to be adjusted, it should only be moved in a direction away from the sterile surgical site and never toward the sterile site. Four quarter drapes are secured to each other and to the patient's skin with Backhaus towel clamps around the incision site (Figure 29-3).

> *TECHNICIAN NOTE* If Backhaus towel clamps are positioned directly in the corners (of a four-toweled drape set) to attach the drapes to each other, the edges of the drapes will lie flat and not bulge up.

The Backhaus towel clamps are considered unsterile once they have penetrated the skin. If you need to remove towel clamps for readjustments, do not touch the contaminated tips; hand them off the table (to a nonsterile assistant) and use a new clamp. For final draping, a large fenestrated or unfenestrated drape is placed over the animal and the table (Figure 29-4). The fenestration is placed over the incision site, or a slit is cut into the unfenestrated drape at the incision site (Figure 29-5).

For orthopedic or neurologic surgeries (especially when implants are placed or if lengthy surgery is expected), exposed aseptic skin in the fenestrated area can be covered with additional adhesive drapes (Ioban, 3M Healthcare, St. Paul, Minn.) (Figure 29-6, *A* and *B*). Paint preparation of the surgical field with Iodine Povacrylex (3M DuraPrep, 3M Healthcare, St. Paul, Minn.) or even application of a spray adhesive to the skin augments the plastic's ability to remain in place throughout the surgery (Figure 29-6, *C* and Chapter 28).

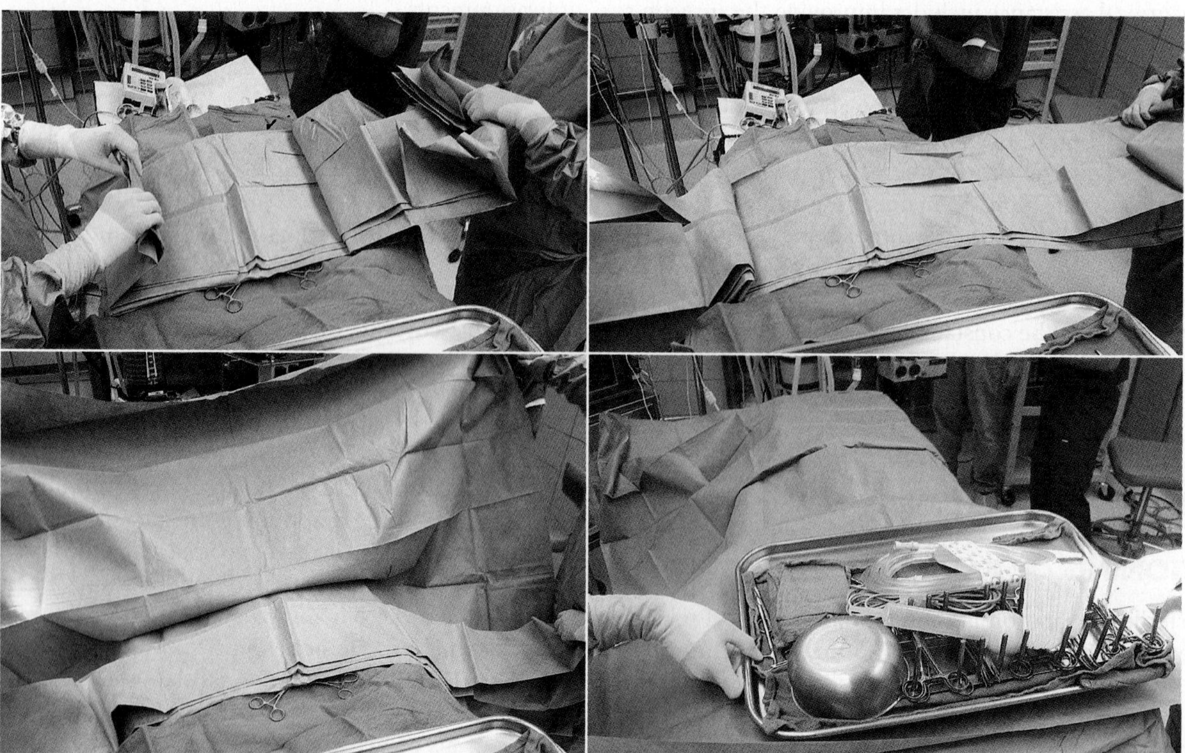

FIGURE 29-4 A large drape is placed over the four quarter drapes.

Alternatively, sterile towels or drapes may be applied to the margins of the skin incision to protect the deeper incision. These towels may be attached with additional towel clamps spaced every 5 to 10 cm along the incision, with Michel clips (Figure 29-7) or by suturing the rolled edge of the towel or drape to the subcutaneous tissue with a simple continuous pattern of a strong, inexpensive suture material.

For orthopedic surgery, the limb is often enclosed in a sterile nonpermeable stockinette (General Econopak, Inc., Philadelphia) to allow movement and manipulation and to limit exposed skin (Figure 29-8). The edges of the incised stockinette can be attached to the surgical incision as described above. The cut edge of the stockinette should be rolled under so that cut fragments of the stockinette material will not fall into the incision. The rolled-under stockinette is usually pulled over the skin edge and attached to the subcutaneous tissue to completely cover the cut skin edge. This will also control much of the minor hemorrhage that occurs following skin incision.

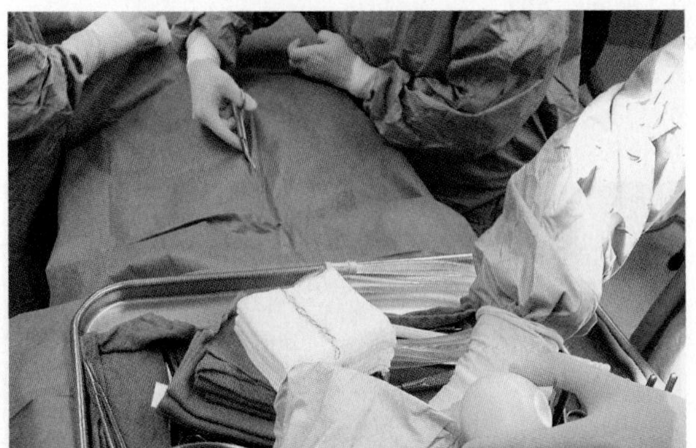

FIGURE 29-5 A fenestration is cut into the final drape to expose the incision site.

INSTRUMENT SETUP AND HANDLING

After the patient is draped, instrument packs are opened on an adjacent table with sterile cover. Depending on the surgical procedure and surgeon's preference, the cover of the instrument table is continuous with the surgical field or remains as an isolated sterile isle that can be independently moved. Cautery and suction tubing are attached approximate to the incision site with specialized nonpenetrating towel clamps (Lorna or Edna clamps) or with Allis tissue forceps to the drape (Figure 29-9). The assistant decides which instruments from the pack are required by the surgeon and the surgical assistant for the procedure and

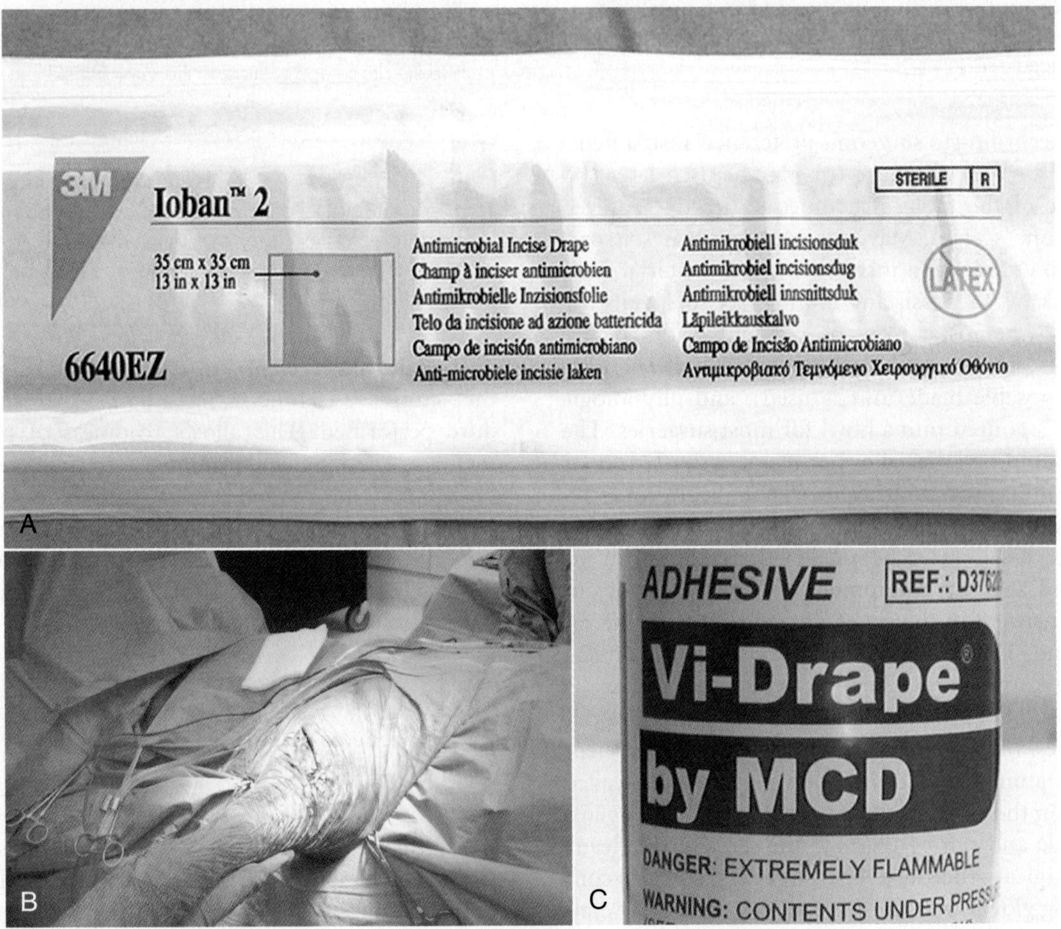

FIGURE 29-6 A, B, A sterile adherent plastic drape has been applied to the skin to minimize potential contamination. C, A spray adhesive is recommended to enhance adhesion of the plastic drape.

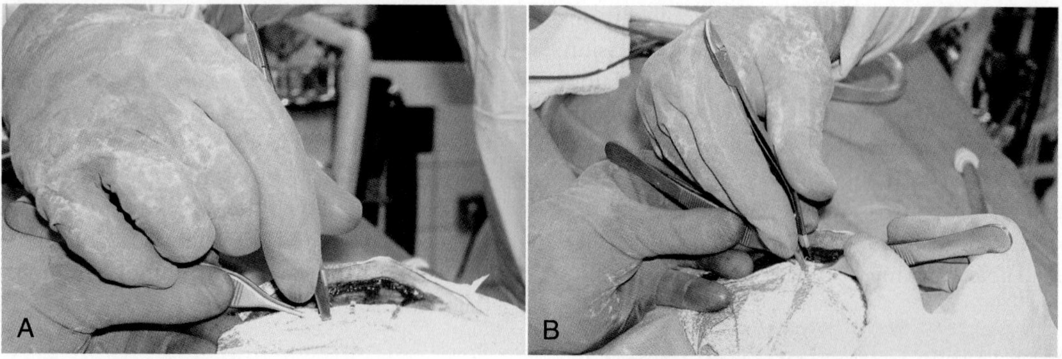

FIGURE 29-7 A, B, Towels or stockinettes can be attached to the skin with Michel clips.

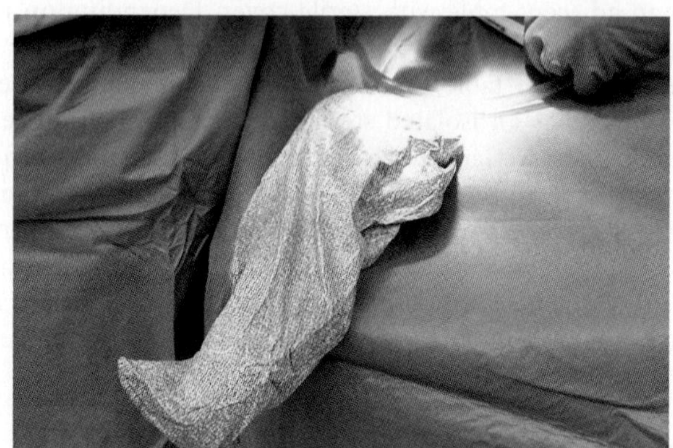

FIGURE 29-8 Nonpermeable stockinette to minimize contamination during orthopedic surgeries.

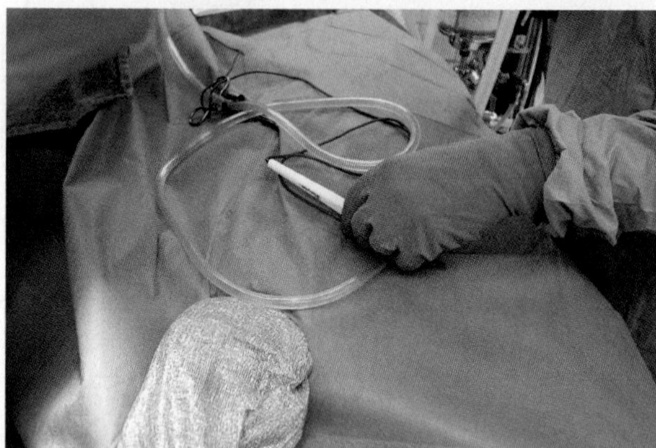

FIGURE 29-9 Cautery and suction are secured with Allis tissue forceps to the drape approximate to the surgical field.

places them according to surgeon's preference: instruments not required for the procedure (or may be used later) on the back side of the table, instruments directly required by the surgeon (scalpel, Mayo or Metzenbaum scissors) on the surgeon's side, and instruments and material typically handled by the assistant (suture scissors, sutures, needle holders, hemostats) on the assistant's side (Figure 29-10). Blades are attached to the surgical knife handles (unless a disposable blade unit is used), and physiologic sterile saline is poured into a bowl for most surgeries. The saline bowl should be placed either inside a sterile tray or on waterproof drapings to prevent wicking from underlying nonsterile surfaces. Although no specific organizational scheme is universally used because of the variation in instruments and specialty equipment, the surgical assistant should be consistent in the general arrangement of the instrument stand. This will save time and effort for the assistant and speed up the procedure.

Special precautions are taken for oncologic and contaminated surgeries. Instruments used for manipulation of neoplastic or contaminated tissues are only placed in a so-called dirty corner on the table. In this way, the other instruments are kept sterile and can be used for the remaining "clean" part of the surgical procedure. The surgeon might also consider changing gloves, suction devices, and potentially contaminated drapes and laboratory sponges during the course of surgery.

> *TECHNICIAN NOTE* Instruments that have been contaminated during the surgical procedure are placed only in a so-called dirty corner on the table. In this way, the other instruments are kept sterile and can be used for the remaining "clean" part of the surgical procedure.

To be truly efficient and effective as a surgical assistant, the veterinary technician must be familiar with the procedure performed. This allows readiness of proper instruments and supplies and minimizes the time spent explaining positioning and retraction. This may require maintenance of a card file detailing necessary equipment and a brief review of the operative technique for each procedure (Figure 29-11). Technicians should follow the progress of the procedure closely to anticipate the surgeon's needs.

> *TECHNICIAN NOTE* Card files about surgical procedures and surgeons' preferences allow more efficient setup of the OR.

When passing instruments, the assistant should firmly "snap" the handle or handles into the open palm of the surgeon (Figure 29-12). This keeps the instrument firmly under control and in position for use. When the surgeon has finished with an instrument, it should be quickly wiped clean

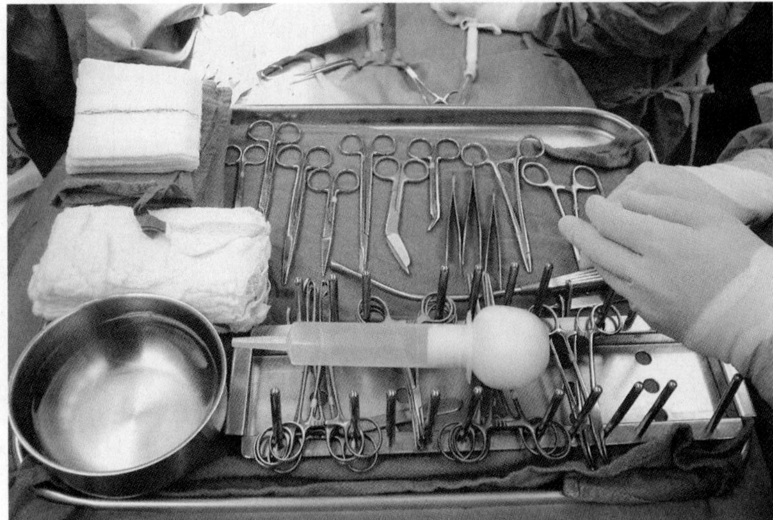

FIGURE 29-10 Example of a typical instrument arrangement.

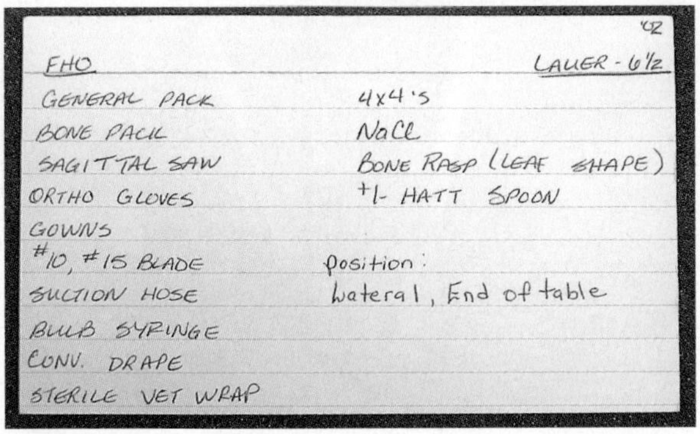

FHO	LAUER - 6½
GENERAL PACK	4x4's
BONE PACK	NaCl
SAGITTAL SAW	BONE RASP (LEAF SHAPE)
ORTHO GLOVES	+/- HATT SPOON
GOWNS	
#10, #15 BLADE	position:
SUCTION HOSE	Lateral, End of table
BULB SYRINGE	
CONV. DRAPE	
STERILE VET WRAP	

FIGURE 29-11 A technique card that is used to detail the necessary equipment for each surgical procedure.

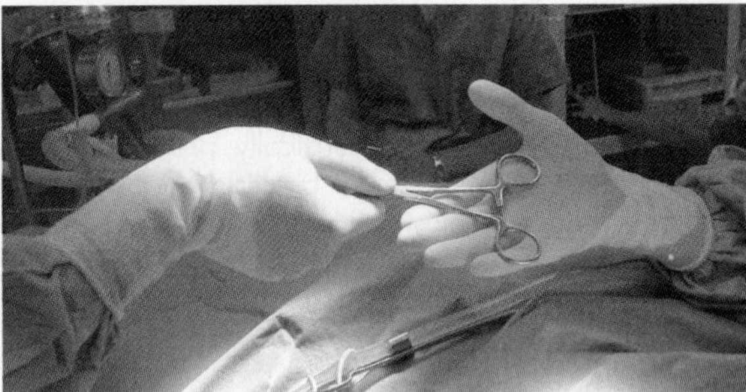

FIGURE 29-12 Instruments are passed, ready for use, into the open hand of the surgeon.

of blood and tissue and returned to its position on the instrument stand. Prolonged soaking of instruments in water (particularly saline) should be avoided because this ultimately causes corrosive damage to sharp cutting edges and hinges.

STERILITY IN THE OPERATING ROOM

Maintaining sterility during surgery is a demanding task and requires that the assistant be constantly aware of the OR environment. Especially in the beginning of surgery, when nonsterile assistants still move around to open instrument packs, to adjust the table height, or to adapt anesthetic equipment, communication is important, and position changes should be announced. The gowned and gloved sterile surgical team should primarily face the sterile field and must not touch or bend over nonsterile regions. The back of the surgical gown is always considered nonsterile, and only the front of the gown extending from below the shoulder level to the level of the surgical field is considered sterile. Therefore the assistant's hands must be positioned above the waist and below the shoulder. The sleeves of the gowns are considered sterile from 5 cm above the elbow to the level of the cuff (the stockinette cuff is not a bacterial barrier, and it is considered nonsterile and should be always covered by the gloves). Clasping of the hands in front of the body is recommended, or the hands can be simply rested approximate to the incision site ready to assist. Unnecessary traffic and visitors in the surgery suite should be avoided, not only during the procedure but at all times, to help control dust and aerial contamination of the facility.

PROPER TISSUE-HANDLING TECHNIQUES

Surgical manipulation of each tissue by hands and instruments results in trauma. If the technician understands the general surgical principles of each body tissue system, he or she can minimize iatrogenic tissue injuries by simple routine actions and measures (such as handling the gastrointestinal tract with saline-soaked sponges).

SKIN

The preparation of the patient's skin for surgery is described in Chapter 28. One must remember that preparation results in aseptic but not sterile skin. This means that the number of bacteria has been reduced below the number required to overwhelm the body's defense mechanism. However, with a depressed immune system or prolonged surgery, these

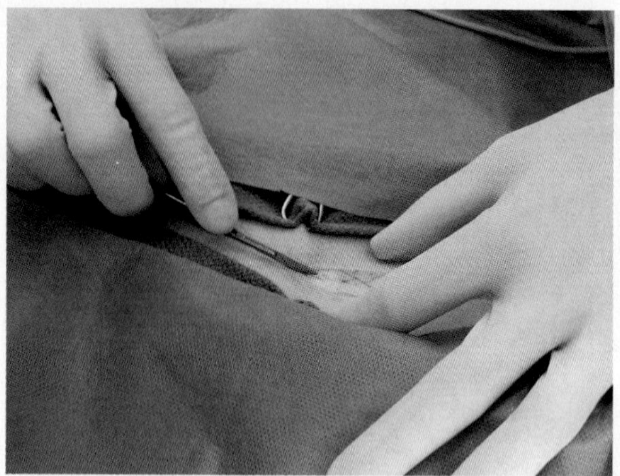

FIGURE 29-13 Skin incision with a scalpel blade results in rapid healing, with minimal trauma and scar formation.

resident bacteria can start to multiply and result in infection. Therefore the surgeon and assistant should avoid unnecessary direct handling of the skin.

> *TECHNICIAN NOTE* Surgically prepared skin is aseptic, and the number of bacteria on the skin has only been reduced below the number required to overwhelm the body's defense mechanism.

The skin incision itself should be performed with a sharp scalpel blade (Figure 29-13). A scissors will crush and shear skin as it cuts. Skin is generally sensitive to this form of injury and will commonly react with severe swelling and scar formation. The skin is relatively thick and elastic; therefore it will also tend to force or "spring" the blades of the scissors apart, damaging the instrument. A sharp incision with a scalpel blade results in the least trauma, most rapid healing, and the least amount of scar formation, but results in more hemorrhage compared with high-energy cutting incisions. Skin incision with high-energy cutting instruments (electrosurgical scalpel, plasma scalpel, and lasers) reduces resistance of wounds to infection and delays healing. Therefore after high-energy cutting, skin sutures or staples should remain in place 2 to 3 days longer compared with conventional scalpel incisions. The principles and use of the electroscalpel are discussed later under electrosurgery.

Skin edges can be controlled, rolled, and steadied with the thumb and index finger. Any instrument used to hold or manipulate skin should grip the tissue with teeth or hooks. Instruments that have smooth tips hold the tissue by pressure, which tends to crush skin and damage it in much the same way as scissors do. Traumatic surgical technique is known to contribute to postsurgical seroma formation.

HOLLOW ORGAN SURGERY

Surgery of the hollow organs (i.e., stomach, intestines, bladder, esophagus) requires both complete control of luminal contents to prevent contamination and gentle handling to prevent iatrogenic damage to these delicate tissues. The surgical site is isolated from the body cavity with saline-moistened laparotomy sponges (Figure 29-14). Doyen intestinal forceps have thin bowed jaws with longitudinal grooves that prevent luminal content leakage when performing enterotomies or intestinal resections (Figure 29-15). The jaw tips make tissue contact as soon as the ratchet's first teeth engage. Doyen intestinal forceps must not be overtightened or left in place too long because this might result in excessive tissue damage (Figure 29-16). Many surgeons prefer the assistant to occlude the intestinal lumen by using moistened gloved fingers (Figure 29-17).

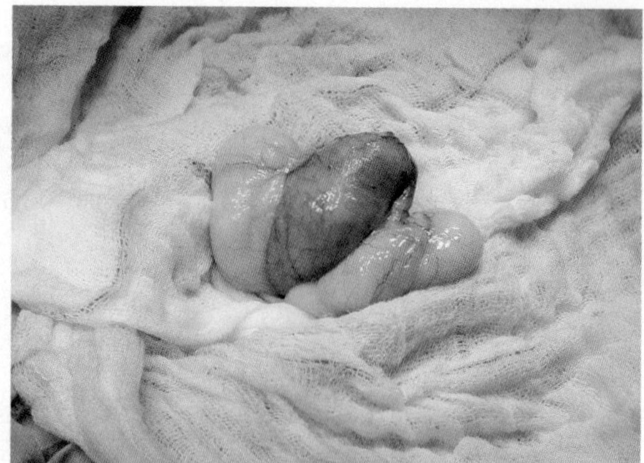

FIGURE 29-14 The bladder is isolated from the abdominal cavity with laboratory sponges before cystotomy.

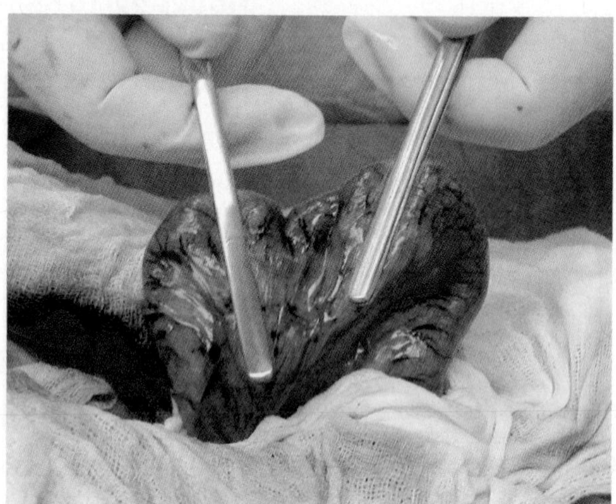

FIGURE 29-15 Use of Doyen intestinal forceps to prevent luminal content leakage during an enterotomy or a resection.

Large, hollow organs, such as the stomach or urinary bladder, often cannot be completely exteriorized. To prevent leakage of contaminated organ contents into the body cavity, the incisional region is elevated and stabilized with stay sutures. Stay sutures are simple loops of suture that pass through the holding layers of the viscus and are held together at the ends with a clamp (Figure 29-18). The surgical assistant applies controlled traction to the clamps to keep the incision in the desired location and elevated to prevent

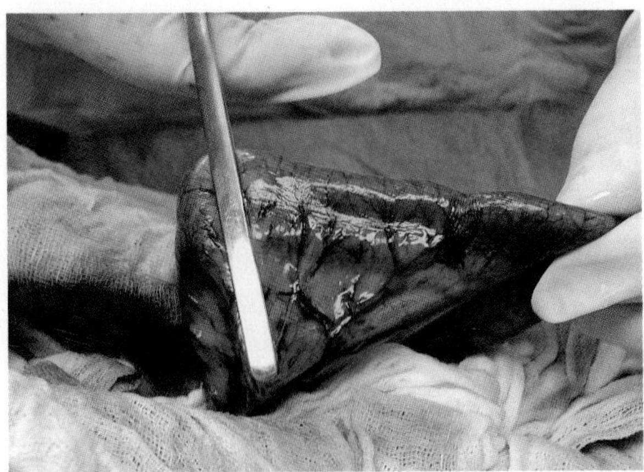

FIGURE 29-16 Area of intestinal damage from excessive tightening of a Doyen intestinal clamp.

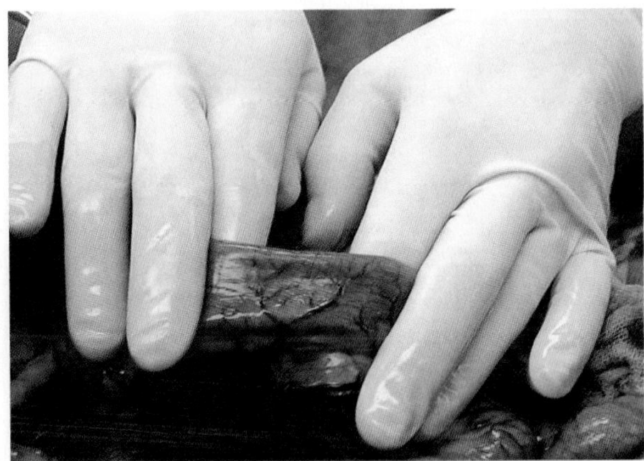

FIGURE 29-17 Use of moistened gloved fingers to occlude the intestinal lumen.

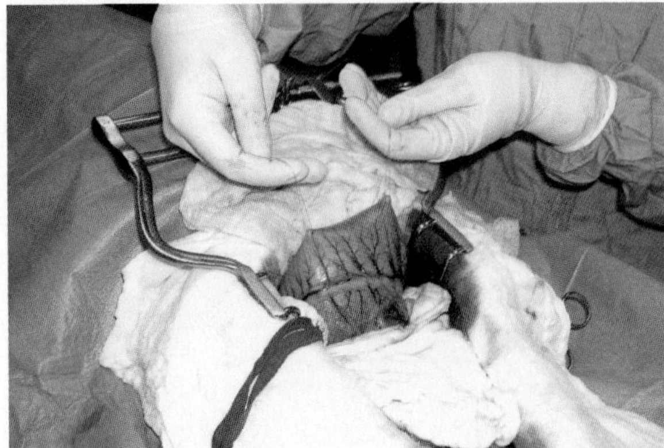

FIGURE 29-18 Stay sutures are passed through the outer layers of hollow organs. Both ends are held with a clamp. The assistant elevates the area of incision by applying traction to the stay sutures.

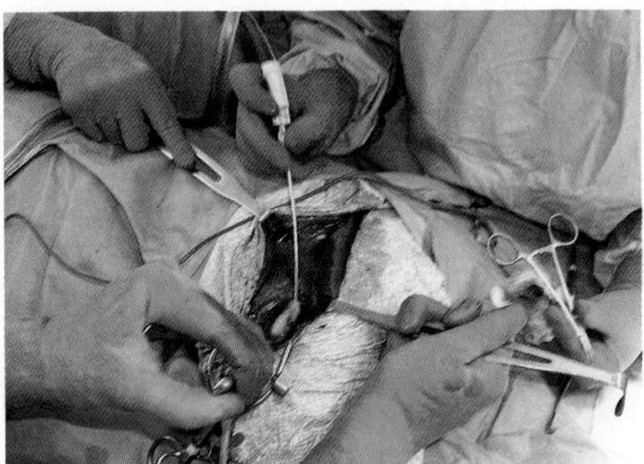

FIGURE 29-19 Exposure in the incision can be increased with hand retractors by the application of traction in one direction and countertraction in the opposite direction.

content leakage (Figure 29-19). Stay sutures are removed after the luminal incision has been closed.

MUSCULOSKELETAL SURGERY

Surgery of the musculoskeletal system often requires surgical assistance. Muscle itself is highly vascular and has great healing ability. The natural blood supply of bone is compromised after fractures, and healing only occurs if there is patent blood supply from the adjacent muscles. Consequently, all efforts should be made to preserve soft tissue attachment to the bone as the assistant retracts and manipulates fractures. The assistant must also be cognizant of adjacent nerves and vessels and protect them from damage by bony fragments or the surgeon. Specifically the radial, ulnar, and ischiadic nerves are often exposed during surgical approaches or course closely to commonly occurring fractures. The surgical assistant must be familiar with the anatomic location of these major structures.

> *TECHNICIAN NOTE* The surgical assistant must be familiar with vital structures to prevent injury during retraction of tissues during surgery.

RETRACTION TECHNIQUES

Retraction of tissues is used to increase visibility and ease of manipulation in the incision. This can be accomplished with handheld retractors by which the assistant provides traction in one direction with one retractor and countertraction in the opposite direction with a second retractor (see Figure 29-19). Retractors are available with various tips and blades to be used on different tissues (see Chapter 28). Care should be taken that retractors do not slide around or pull out of the incision because this causes significant tissue trauma. Consequently, sharp-tipped retractors that maintain a grip on the tissue (without crushing) are often preferable to blunt-tipped retractors, particularly for muscle and skin retraction (Figure 29-20). Self-retaining retractors are also used to free the assistant for other duties (Figure 29-21, *A* and *B*). Excessive retraction for prolonged periods must be avoided with self-retaining instruments to prevent pressure-induced tissue damage.

Manual traction on adjacent tissues is often used to increase visibility or expose organs.

Visualization of the liver and the diaphragm can be significantly improved if the assistant carefully pulls up the sternum (Figure 29-22). Deep structures of the right abdominal cavity can be clearly visualized by retracting the

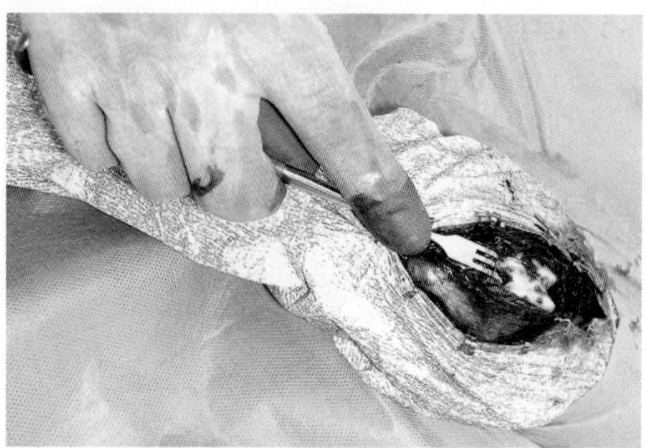

FIGURE 29-20 Use of a sharp-tipped, self-retaining retractor (Gelpi) to increase stifle joint exposure during an arthrotomy.

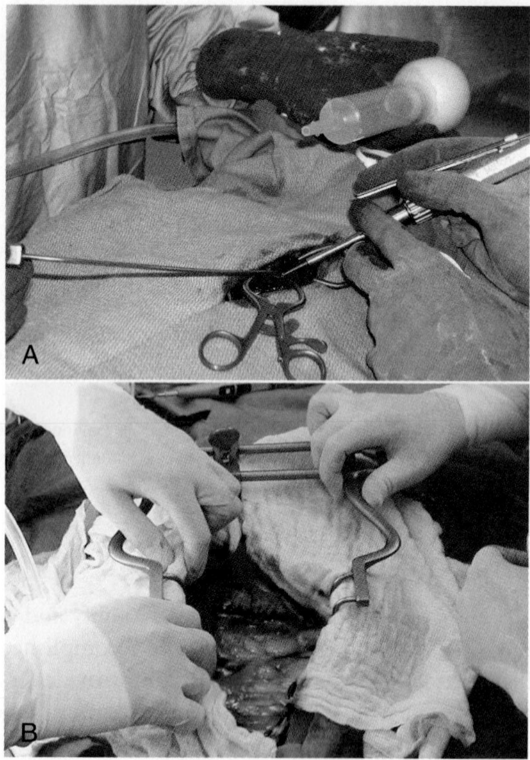

FIGURE 29-21 **A,** Self-retaining Gelpi retractors applied during a hemilaminectomy free up the hands of the assistant for suction and lavage while the surgeon removes bone with a drill. **B,** Placement of a blunt-tipped, self-retaining retractor (Balfour) in an abdominal incision verifying that abdominal organs are not entrapped.

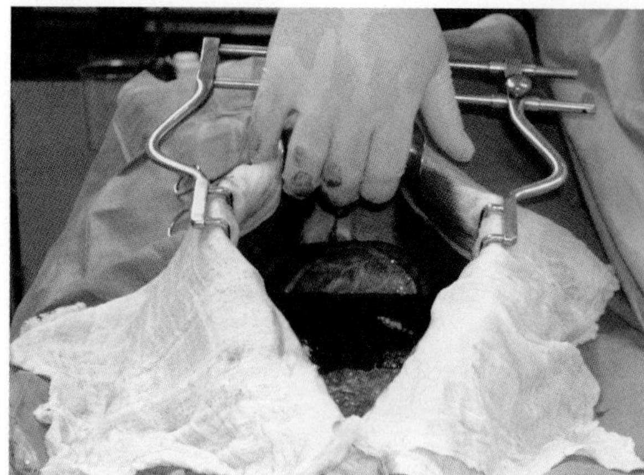

FIGURE 29-22 Gentle lifting of the sternum increases exposure of the diaphragm and liver during abdominal exploratory surgery.

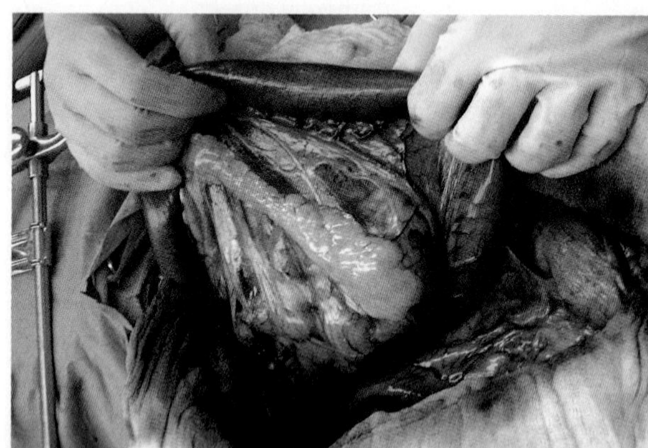

FIGURE 29-23 Retraction of the proximal duodenum and mesoduodenum to the left exposes the right adrenal gland, kidney, and ureter.

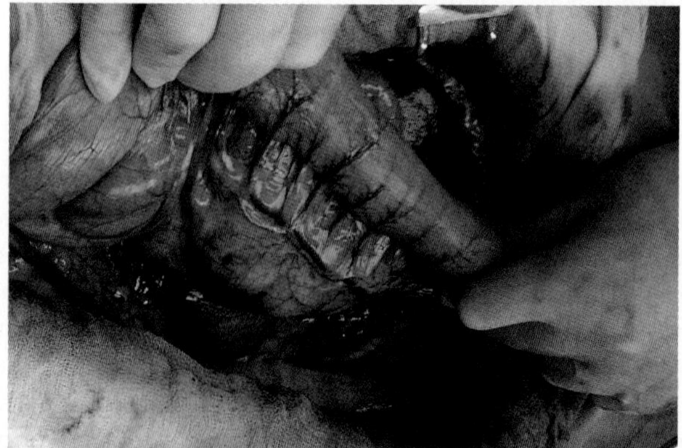

FIGURE 29-24 Retraction of the descending colon to the right exposes the left adrenal gland, kidney, and ureter.

proximal duodenum with mesoduodenum. If the abdominal viscera are positioned behind the mesoduodenum to the left, the right liver lobes, adrenal gland, kidney, and ureter are exposed (Figure 29-23). The left half of the abdominal cavity may likewise be visualized by retracting the abdominal viscera to the right, behind the mesocolon of the descending colon (Figure 29-24). The pancreas and portal vein are best exposed by gentle traction on the adjacent duodenum. As when using fingers for occluding the intestinal lumen, gloves should be moistened and excessive pressure avoided.

> *TECHNICIAN NOTE* Bleeders from the ovarian pedicles can be clearly visualized by retraction of abdominal viscera behind the mesoduodenum or mesocolon.

Nerves or large blood vessels are often retracted to improve visualization or to prevent potential damage. Careful blunt dissection is used to free the nerve or vessel from surrounding tissue. A broad, flat band, such as a Penrose drain

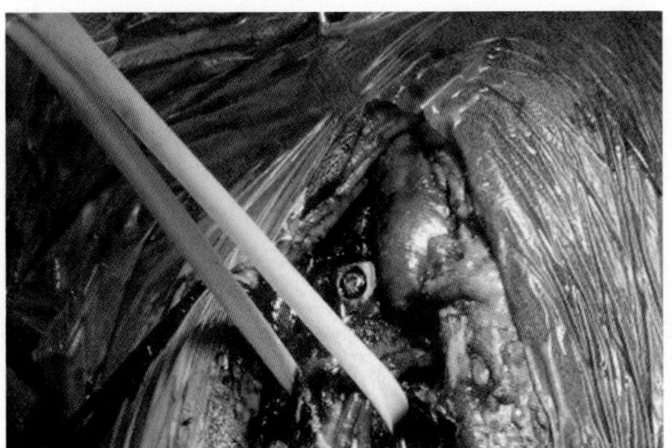

FIGURE 29-25 A Penrose drain is passed around the radial nerve and brachial muscle for atraumatic manipulation of the nerve during fracture repair with plate and screws.

or moistened umbilical tape, is passed around the structure (Figure 29-25), and the ends are clamped together, much like a stay suture. The assistant can gently retract the nerve or vessel to one side, carefully avoiding entanglement with other instruments or equipment.

HEMOSTASIS

Hemostasis is a physiologic response to arrest bleeding. Various surgical techniques can be used to augment this physiologic clotting process. The surgical assistant should be able to perform or to assist with routine hemostatic procedures.

Excellent hemostasis is vital (1) to obtain optimal visibility at the surgical site, (2) to limit the volume of blood loss, and (3) to decrease risk of infection (extravasated blood is an ideal medium for bacterial growth).

SPONGE HEMOSTASIS

Low-pressure bleeding from small vessels can be controlled by sustained pressure through gauze sponges or similar material. The sponge should be applied with a blotting type of motion. A wiping motion (especially if sponges are not moistened with saline) will irritate tissue and will often renew bleeding by pulling the forming blood clots out of incised capillaries. The pressure apparently stops hemorrhage by collapsing the vessels until clotting can occur. With persistent hemorrhage, pressure may need to be sustained for up to 5 minutes to allow adequate coagulation.

SPONGE COMPLICATIONS

Gauze sponges left in the body after closing of the incision will cause severe inflammatory reaction, adhesions, and drainage. The abdominal and thoracic cavities are particularly hazardous locations for sponges to become lost. Consequently, many surgical assistants count sponges in such areas to make sure all sponges have been removed. Before surgery begins, sterile sponges are counted out in piles on the Mayo stand. Usually, two or three piles of 10 sponges are used to start. The total number is recorded, and all other sponges (e.g., those used for skin preparation) are removed from the area. If additional sponges are required during surgery, they are supplied in packs of 10, and their number is added to the total. The used sponges are saved in a separate pile and are counted at the termination of the procedure before the incision is closed. The number of used sponges plus the remaining clean sponges must equal the total amount to account for all sponges. Additional precautions include use of sponges with radiopaque markers and never placing used or superfluous sponges approximate to the incision.

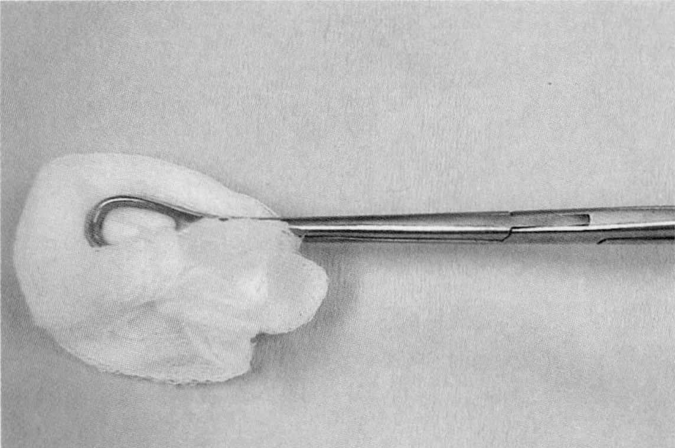

FIGURE 29-26 Gauze sponge held in a sponge forceps.

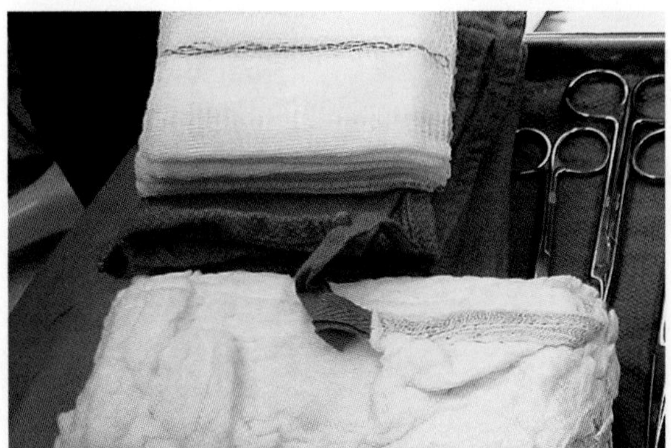

FIGURE 29-27 Laboratory sponges with tail and sponges with radiopaque markers can be used in deep incisions.

For particularly deep incisions, sponges may be held in a sponge forceps (Figure 29-26), or laboratory sponges can be used (Figure 29-27). The tape attached to the laboratory sponge is left extending out of the incision, and the sponge can be easily removed by pulling on it.

HEMOSTATIC FORCEPS

Hemorrhage from slightly larger vessels can be occluded by clamping with a hemostatic forceps. When the vessel wall is crushed with the hemostatic forceps, the bleeding stops temporarily, and the physiologic clotting mechanism is activated. The clamp should be applied perpendicular to the tissue surface and the bleeding vessel, with a minimal amount of adjacent tissue grasped in the tips of the clamp (Figure 29-28).

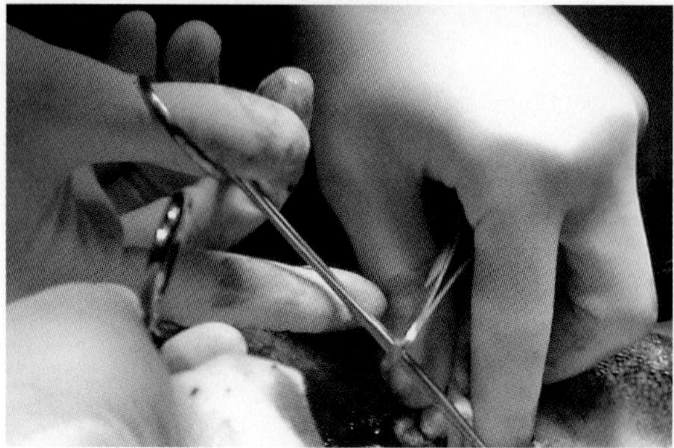

FIGURE 29-28 A hemostatic forceps is perpendicularly applied to the bleeding vessel with a minimal amount of adjacent tissue included.

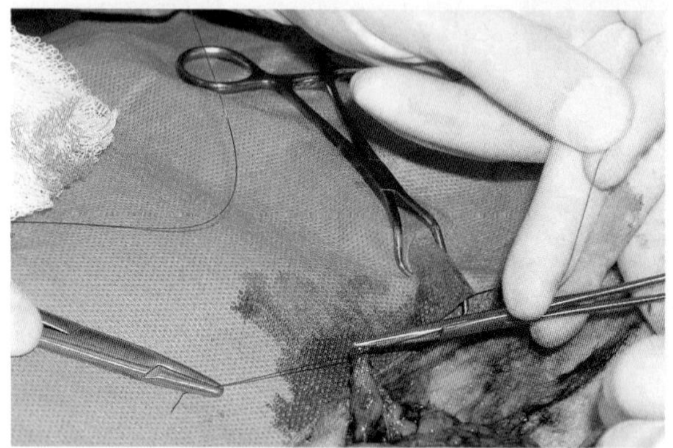

FIGURE 29-29 Lowering the handles of the hemostatic forceps raises the tips, forcing the ligation loop to form around the vessel.

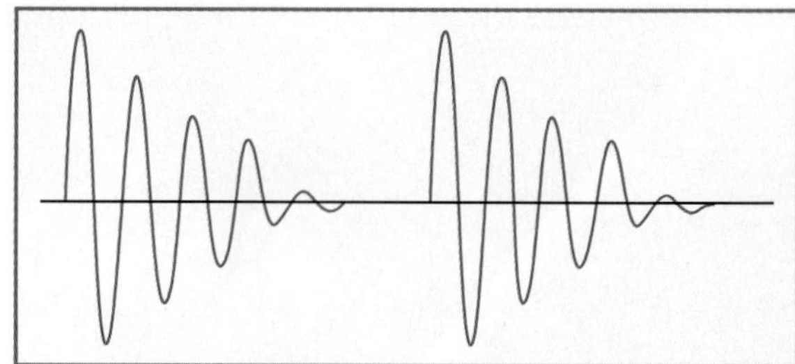

FIGURE 29-30 Diagram of the damped sine wave current, which causes coagulation.

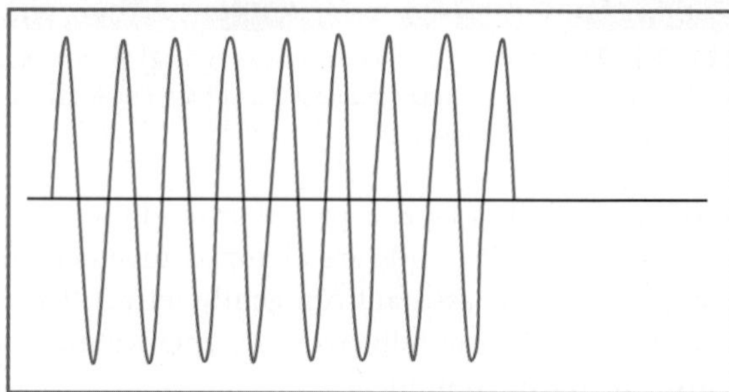

FIGURE 29-31 Diagram of the undamped sine wave current, which "cuts" tissues.

SUTURE LIGATION

A larger bleeding vessel that has been clamped can be ligated to achieve permanent hemostasis. After the suture material is passed around the vessel, the assistant lowers the handles of the clamp, which raises the tips (Figure 29-29). This causes the ligation loop to form around the vessel and not the instrument. As the first throw of the knot is pulled tight, the assistant releases the clamp. This allows the vessel to totally collapse, thus occluding the lumen. However, the assistant should return the vessel to its origin before releasing the clamp so that the knot is not snapped off the cut end of the vessel. After the surgeon finishes the knot, the assistant cuts off excessive suture, using the tips of the scissors. Care must be taken not to pull the ligature off the end of the vessel. Only enough material to secure the knot should be left. Arteries are commonly ligated twice, particularly if they are more than 2 mm in diameter.

ELECTROSURGERY

Electrocoagulation and Cutting Function

Electrosurgical units not only offer a means of stopping hemorrhage from an already cut vessel with electrocoagulation, but also allow prevention of hemorrhage with an electroscalpel that coagulates as it cuts a vessel. Most electrosurgical units allow both coagulation and cutting, depending on the waveform of the current selected.

Interrupted damped sine waves primarily result in coagulation, but they also allow for some cutting (Figure 29-30). The current causes protein coagulation of the blood elements within the blood vessel wall. Electrocoagulation should be used only on vessels smaller than 1.5 mm. As a rule of thumb, vessels with visible lumens should be ligated.

Continuous undamped sine waves primarily result in cutting associated with some minimal coagulation (Figure 29-31). Microcoagulation of the tissue protein occurs at a small point of contact.

Modulated pulsed sine waves allow simultaneous cutting and coagulation.

Monopolar and Bipolar Electrosurgical Modes

Most electrosurgical units allow both monopolar and bipolar modes of coagulation.

The monopolar mode is most commonly used in veterinary medicine and can be used for coagulation and/or cutting. The current flows from a small handpiece (active electrode) through the animal's body and returns to the current generator via a ground plate (indifferent electrode) that is necessary to complete the electrical circuit (Figure 29-32). Direct maximal contact between the patient and the ground plate is important to prevent burns approximate to the ground plate. For hemostasis, the current can be applied through a hemostatic forceps clamped on the vessel (Figure 29-33) or directly from the monopolar handpiece tip to the vessel. Monopolar electrocautery only works if all blood and fluid, which would dissipate the current, has been blotted away.

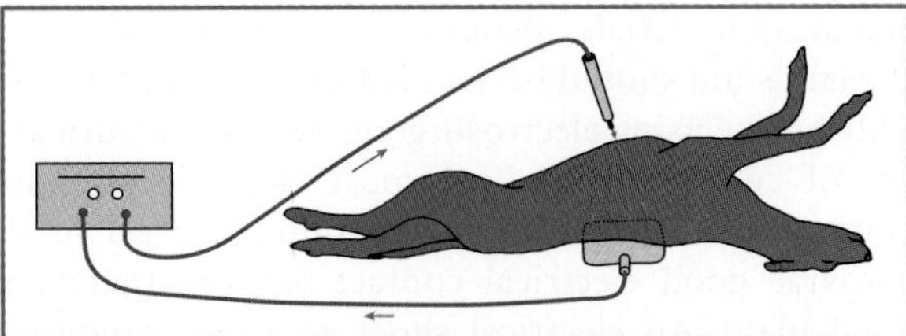

FIGURE 29-32 Diagram of electrical current passing from the handpiece, dispersing in the body, and returning to the generator via the ground plate.

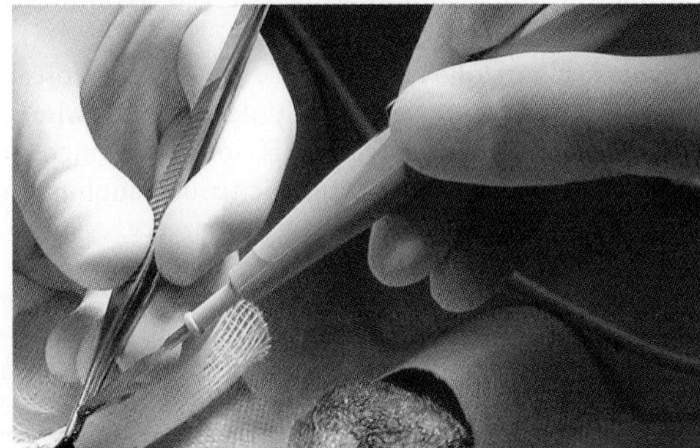

FIGURE 29-33 Application of current to a bleeding vessel by touching the handpiece to the Brown-Adson forceps.

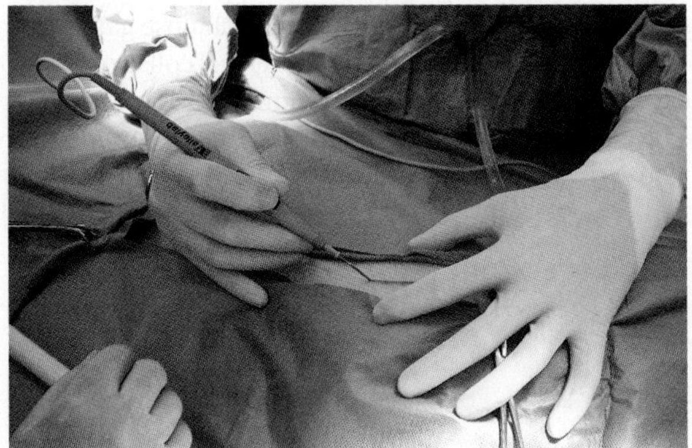

FIGURE 29-34 A bloodless incision can be obtained by blending, cutting, and coagulating currents.

For a truly bloodless incision (modulated pulsed sine wave mode), the handpiece is held in a modified pencil grip perpendicular to the tissue surface. Because the electrode cuts whatever tissue is contacted, continuous visualization is indispensable when the electrode is activated. To prevent lateral heat damage to adjacent tissues, it has been recommended to move the instrument slowly at a speed of 7 mm per second (Figure 29-34).

Bipolar electrocautery uses a thumb forcepslike handpiece as an active electrode (Figure 29-35). The vessel to be cauterized is grasped between the tips of the forceps, and the coagulating current runs from one blade to the other, not through the body (Figure 29-36). For effective use, a slight gap must remain between the tips when the tissue is grasped. Because the short current pathway results in minimal damage to adjacent tissues, this form of electrocoagulation is particularly useful in microvascular, ophthalmic, and neurosurgery. In contrast to the monopolar mode, bipolar coagulation is only used for coagulation, but it has the advantage to function in a wet surgical field.

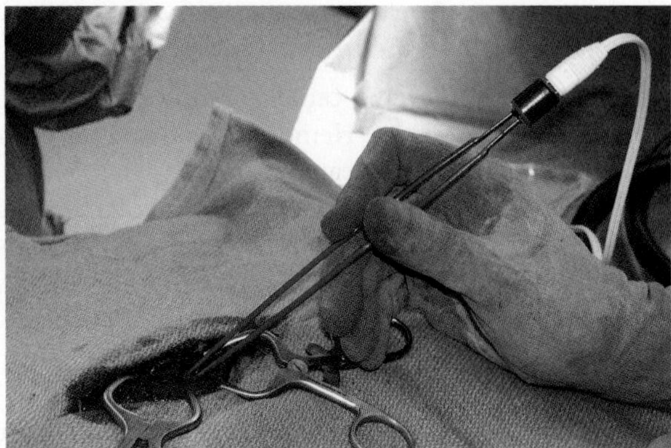

FIGURE 29-35 The thumb forcepslike handpiece used for bipolar cautery.

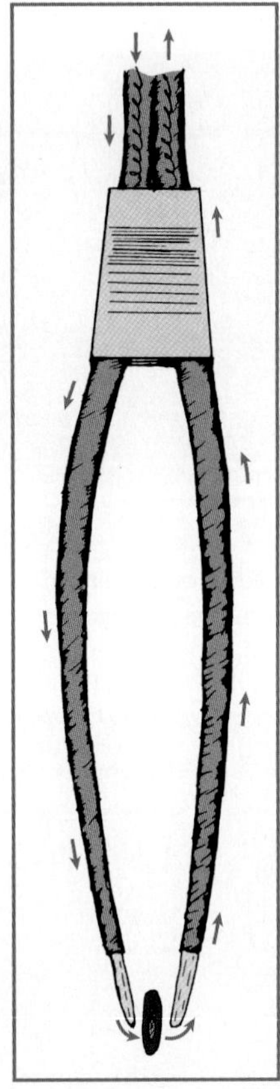

FIGURE 29-36 Diagram of the bipolar coagulation current as it passes from one tip of the handpiece to the other.

The monopolar setup allows for cutting and/or coagulation, but the bipolar setup only allows for coagulation.

TECHNICIAN NOTE Monopolar cautery only works in a dry surgical field, but bipolar coagulation also functions in a wet surgical environment.

Battery-Powered Cautery Units

Disposable battery-powered cautery units can be used for hemostasis of small vessels. Hemostasis is based on protein coagulation produced by a heated filament.

Carbon built up on the active tip of monopolar and bipolar handpieces should be periodically removed by the assistant, who scrapes it on a scratch pad (Figure 29-37) or with a hard metallic edge, such as the backside of a scalpel blade.

Safety With Electrosurgery

Electrosurgery will result in spark formation, and it should not be used when explosive anesthetics, such as ether and cyclopropane, are present. Likewise, some antiseptic preparation materials (alcohol based) and adhesive agents are volatile and should be avoided or allowed to dry thoroughly before using electrosurgery. To avoid a burn at the point of current grounding, most electrosurgical units require generous application of conductive gel or fluid to provide good electrical contact between patient and ground plate. An electrical shock to hands holding the clamp or electrosurgical handpiece is usually caused by a hole in the glove. Regloving should alleviate the problem. Continued shocking reflects poor grounding or an equipment malfunction that should be checked by a qualified service representative.

Tissue healing following the use of the electroscalpel has been shown to be significantly delayed. Likewise, the incidence of incisional infection is somewhat increased. Techniques of asepsis and atraumatic tissue handling must be strictly adhered to when using electrosurgery.

FIGURE 29-37 Buildup of protein on the handpiece tip, which prevents passage of current, can be removed with a scratch pad.

> *TECHNICIAN NOTE* Electrosurgery should not be used in the presence of explosive anesthetics (ether) or alcohol-based antiseptic materials.

HEMOSTATIC AGENTS

Absorbable hemostatic agents, such as gelatin sponges (Gelfoam, Upjohn), oxidized regenerated cellulose gauze (Surgicel, Johnson & Johnson), or bovine dermal collagen (INSTAT Collagen Absorbable Hemostat, Johnson & Johnson), can be used to achieve hemostasis on tissues that tend to continually ooze or to pack small bleeding cavities (Figure 29-38).

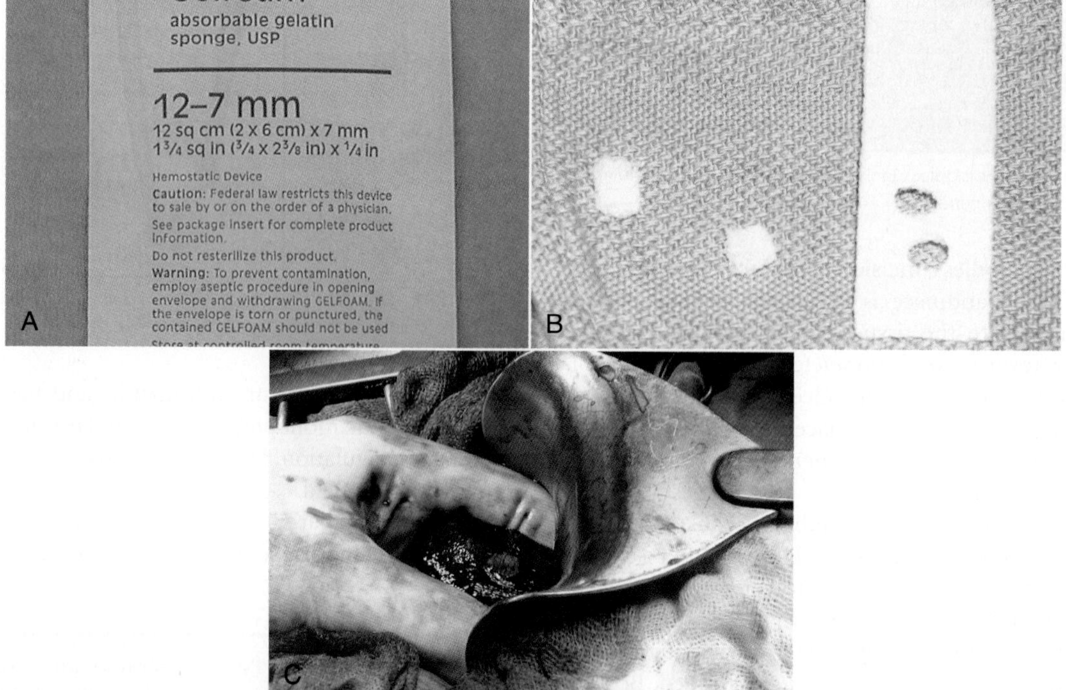

FIGURE 29-38 **A,** Biologic hemostatic agents, such as gelatin foam, promote coagulation and clot adherence. **B, C,** The foam is punched out of the sheet and placed in a bleeding liver biopsy site for hemostasis.

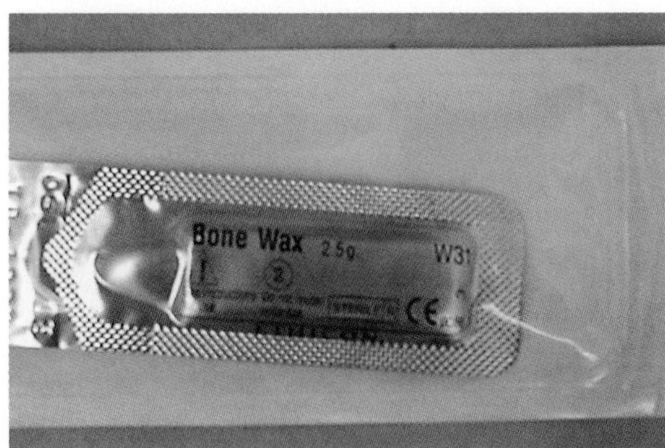

FIGURE 29-39 Bone wax is a nonabsorbable hemostatic agent used to control bleeding from exposed bone.

Gelatin sponges are applied dry, soak up blood, and provide a lattice for the forming clot to adhere to. They are normally absorbed in 4 to 6 weeks, but should not be used in infected areas.

Cellulose is a knitted material that only activates clotting of whole blood. Therefore it is not useful if oozing occurs in a serohemorrhagic environment.

Bovine collagen triggers clot formation via platelet aggregation and release of coagulation factors. Collagen's hemostatic capabilities are inactivated by autoclaving.

Bone wax is a nonabsorbable agent that is used during orthopedic (midfemoral amputation) and neurologic surgery to control bleeding from bone (Figure 29-39). Bone wax functions as a mechanical plug when pressed into bleeding bony surfaces. Keep in mind that it results in mild inflammation and should be used sparsely.

CHEMICAL CAUTERIZATION

Chemical cauterization by agents, such as phenol, ferric subsulfate, and silver nitrate, will achieve hemostasis by denaturing the protein of the tissues they contact, thus sealing small blood vessels. However, these agents are difficult to apply without contacting and damaging adjacent soft tissues. This usually precludes their use in general surgery. However, silver nitrate is commonly used to stop nail bleeding when the nail bed has been cut during routine nail trimming.

VASCULAR CLIPS

Metal clips made of noncorrosive materials (Hemoclip, Weck Closure Systems) and the specialized forceps to apply them are available in a variety of sizes and designs (Figure 29-40). They are effective and can be applied quickly to occlude vessels up to 5 mm in diameter in locations that are not accessible for ligation. Their use in veterinary surgery is becoming more widespread as the expense relative to convenience decreases. Vascular stapling devices that automatically occlude both sides of a vessel with small metallic staples in addition to dividing it are available (LDS, U.S. Surgical Corp.) and are commonly used in human surgery. Although the staple cartridges are expensive, the supplying company will often lease the application device.

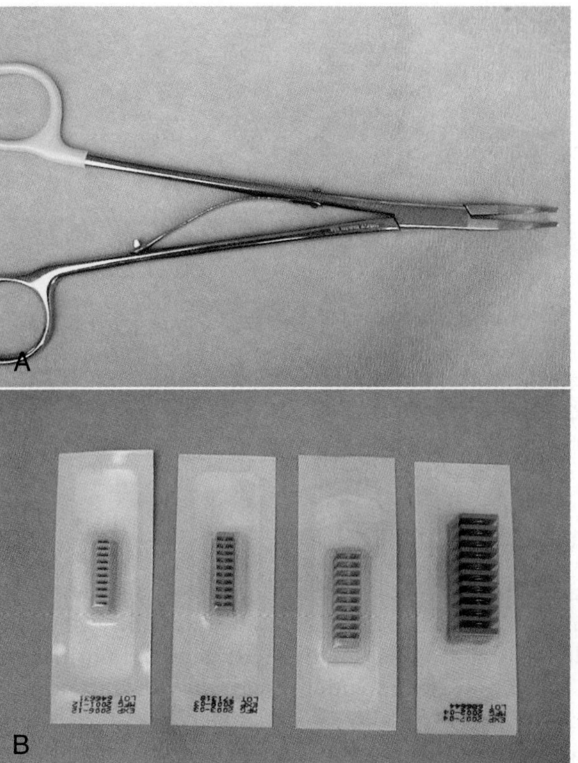

FIGURE 29-40 A, B, Metallic hemoclips with applicators are available in several sizes.

INCISION IRRIGATION AND SUCTION

Incision irrigation and suction (lavage) serve four main purposes. The first is to physically dilute and remove bacteria carried into the incision from the skin or the air or from spillage from incising a contaminated or infected structure, such as the intestine. The body has a tremendous ability to resist infection from low numbers of bacteria. Consequently, lavaging the site after the initial skin incision and periodically throughout the procedure to decrease bacterial numbers will dramatically reduce the incidence of infection. Second, irrigation and suction are used to remove hemorrhage, increasing visibility at the surgical site. This makes both hemostasis and surgical manipulations easier to accomplish. Third, lavage keeps the tissues moist, particularly during longer procedures. If the tissues desiccate (dry out), cell damage and death occur. This decreases the rate of healing and increases the incidence of infection by devitalizing the natural cellular defense mechanisms. There is an old surgical saying that "moist tissues are happy tissues." Finally, lavage is used to dilute and remove irritating and degenerative material, such as urine, bile, or bony fragments. Although these materials will not cause infection, they can cause undesirable biologic reactions and should be removed.

> *TECHNICIAN NOTE* Because any dry material is damaging to body tissues, slight moistening of sponges with saline before using them in the incision will reduce tissue trauma.

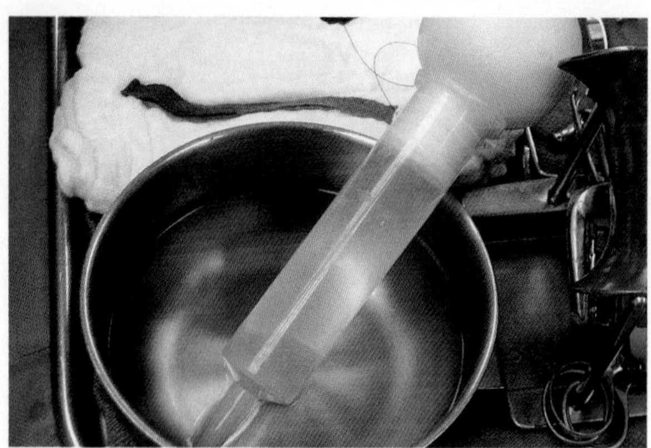

FIGURE 29-41 The saline bowl and bulb syringe are placed on a waterproof drape to prevent wick contamination after spillage.

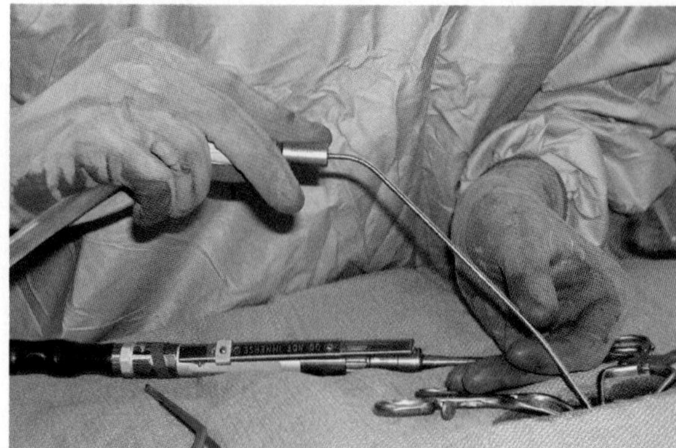

FIGURE 29-42 The single-orifice suction tip (Frazier) is used for precise control.

LAVAGE FLUID

Many different fluids are used for lavage, but they all have common characteristics. The fluid should be a physiologically neutral, isotonic solution (i.e., buffered normal saline or lactated Ringer's solution), meaning it has the same pH (acidity) and osmolality (mineral concentration) as serum. Excessively acidic or basic fluids can promote bacterial growth and cause cell damage. Hypotonic (less concentrated) solutions, such as distilled or tap water, will be imbibed by the tissues, resulting in significant edema. Hypertonic (more concentrated) solutions, such as hypertonic saline, will pull water out of tissues and result in dehydration. This reaction is occasionally used to reduce preexisting edema.

Antibiotic agents are rarely added to lavage solutions because systemic administration of IV antibiotics in general provides higher antibiotic tissue levels than topical application. Antibiotic solutions (e.g., tetracyclines) can be irritating to tissues when applied topically and result in chemical peritonitis or pleuritis. Antibiotic solutions should not be used with cancellous bone grafts because the antibiotic will diminish the graft's biologic activity.

Diluted antiseptics, such as povidone-iodine and chlorhexidine hydrochloride, have been used for lavage of wounds. Because these agents are irritating for synovium, pleura, and peritoneum, joints, thoracic cavity, and abdominal cavity are in general not lavaged with antiseptic solutions. The routine use of buffered normal saline is preferred.

LAVAGE TECHNIQUE

Irrigation solutions can be applied with a bulb syringe or a large syringe to obtain a hydraulic cleansing effect (Figure 29-41). They should be warmed to body temperature to prevent causing hypothermia. This is particularly important in small or debilitated patients. Cloth drapes should not become excessively damp during surgery because this will allow capillary movement of bacteria (wicking) from the underlying nonsterile area. Alternatively, waterproof draping materials, such as sterile baby crib sheets or diapers, may be used.

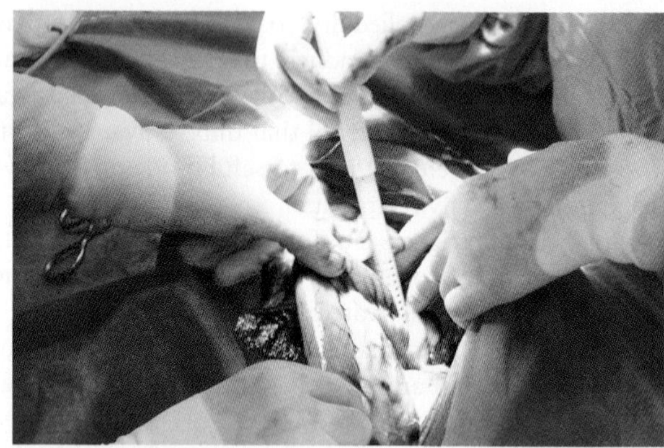

FIGURE 29-43 The multiple-fenestrated suction tip (Poole) is used to remove large volumes of fluids and to prevent omental occlusion.

Suction of the surgical incision requires a suction tip, tubing, and a suction bottle. The suction tip may have a single orifice or multiple fenestrations. The single-orifice tip (Yankauer or Frazier tip) is most useful in orthopedic surgery, neurosurgery, and general surgery in which the exposure is limited and relatively small amounts of liquid must be removed from precise areas (Figure 29-42). The surgical assistant controls the strength of suction by occluding the vent hole in the handle of the suction tip. If the tip becomes plugged, it can be cleared by passing a stylet made of slightly smaller stainless steel wire.

The multiple-fenestrated tips (Poole tip) are used in thoracic and abdominal procedures in which large volumes of fluid are removed (Figure 29-43). Fenestrated tips also reduce the incidence of plugging with movable soft tissue, such as omentum and mesentery. The assistant can also use his or her hands as a barrier between the omentum and the suction tip to prevent plugging. Periodic suction of clean irrigation solution during the surgical procedure will reduce the incidence of suction tube plugging and make cleaning of the tube much easier.

TECHNICIAN NOTE The assistant should remove all lavage fluid from the incision because remaining fluid might compromise phagocytosis and the bacterial defense mechanisms.

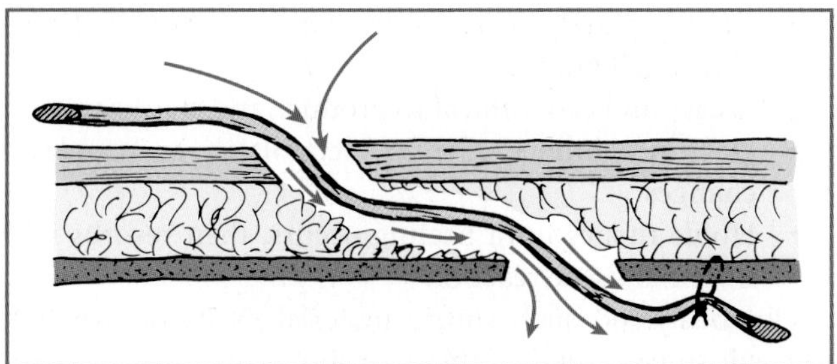

FIGURE 29-44 Diagram of discharge escaping around the outside of a Penrose drain.

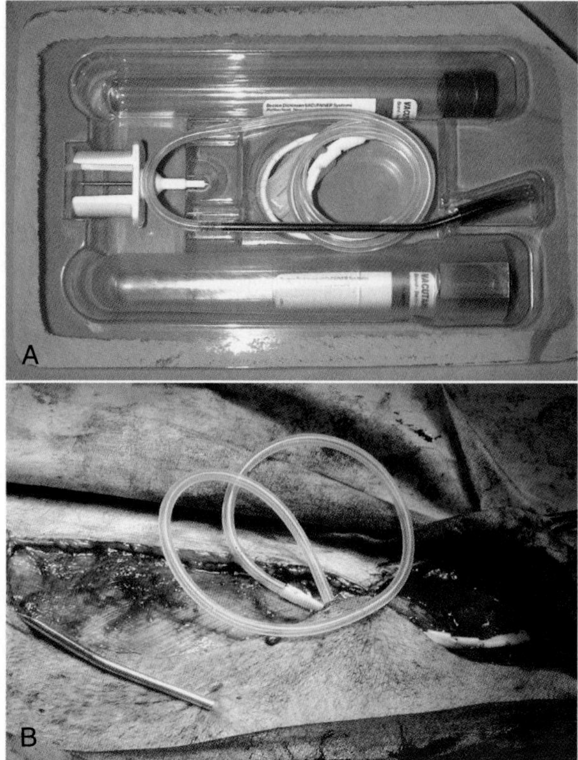

FIGURE 29-45 A, B, Multiple openings on the implanted end of a commercially available active suction drain (TLS) after mammary resection.

SURGICAL DRAINS

Postoperative drainage of the surgical area may be indicated for several different reasons. Any incision that is thought to be infected should be allowed to discharge. This can be accomplished by leaving the wound open or by inserting a drain. A drain is also indicated when soft tissues cannot be opposed to obliterate dead space. Serum tends to accumulate in such spaces, and seromas (serum pockets under the skin) can develop if a drainage route is not established. Drains commonly used in veterinary surgery are classified as passive and active drain devices. The draining effect of passive systems is based on gravity, whereas active systems produce negative pressure (suction) resulting in drainage.

PASSIVE DRAINS

Soft, thin-walled, collapsible, latex rubber tubes named Penrose drains are most commonly used as passive drains in veterinary medicine. Passive drains made of stiffer polypropylene, Silastic, or red rubber tubes are rarely used. Discharge escapes by moving along the outside of the drain (Figure 29-44). Therefore the holes in the tissues through which the drain runs must be kept spread open and clean for the drain to work properly. Cleanliness is particularly important because the hole and drain can act as an avenue for ascending infections.

ACTIVE DRAINS

Active (i.e., suction) drains are thick-walled tubes of rubber or Silastic. Suction is applied to the outside end of the drain, and discharges are pulled through the lumen of the tube. Multiple openings are present in the wall of the tube on the implanted end (Figure 29-45). Suction must be maintained for this type of drain to work. Negative-pressure activated devices are commercially available (Jackson Pratt, Allegiance) (Figure 29-46). A homemade device can be made from a large injection syringe, butterfly catheter, and a hypodermic needle (Figure 29-47).

Drains are foreign bodies and can be removed after 2 to 5 days when the discharge volume has decreased and becomes serosanguineous.

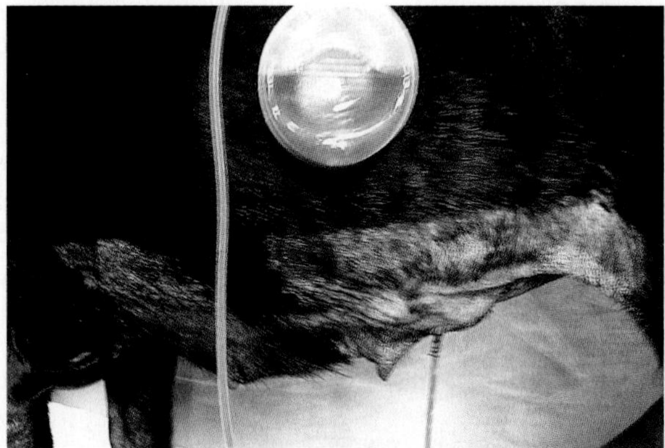

FIGURE 29-46 A commercially available negative-pressure activated, constant-suction device (Jackson Pratt drain).

> *TECHNICIAN NOTE* The exit point of the drain at the skin level should always be covered with a sterile dressing to minimize risk of infection along the drain. The dressing must be changed before strike-through occurs (Figure 29-48).

SUTURE MATERIAL

Suture is any material that holds tissues together until they heal. The use of suture has been documented since the first century AD. However, it was not until the advent of sterilization and aseptic technique that suture became commonly

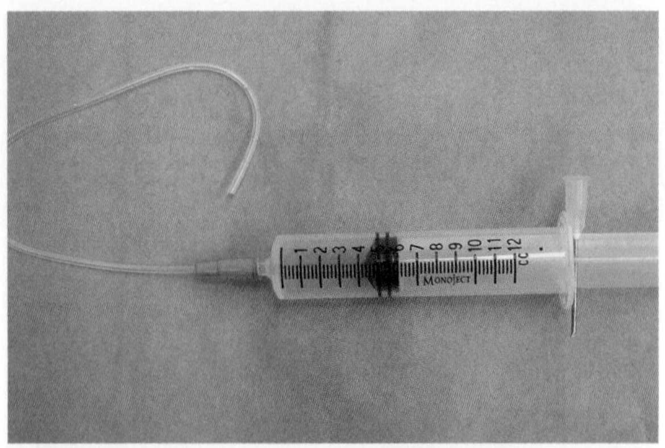

FIGURE 29-47 A homemade constant-suction device constructed from a large syringe, butterfly catheter, and hypodermic needle.

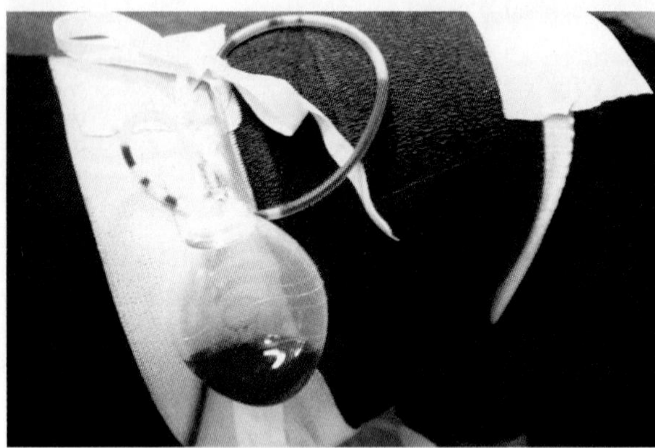

FIGURE 29-48 The exit point of the drain at the skin level should always be covered with a sterile dressing to minimize risk of infection along the drain. The dressing must be changed before strike-through occurs.

used. During the late 1800s and early 1900s, suture materials were derived mainly from natural sources. Synthetic suture materials first became available in the 1930s and are still being developed.

Some uses of suture include the following:

- Apposing the edges of an incision or wound
- Obliterating open space in which serum would tend to accumulate
- Tightening and stabilizing joints that have sustained ligament injury or have luxated
- Strengthening or replacing weakened tissues, as in hernias
- Ligating blood vessels or tissues that will be removed

QUALITIES OF THE IDEAL SUTURE MATERIAL

The ideal suture material would have the following qualities:

- Able to be used for any procedure with the same characteristics in all tissues
- Is easily handled and tied by the surgeon
- Causes minimal tissue reaction and does not support, spread, or sequester bacterial growth
- Has high tensile strength in a small diameter, yet not cut through tissues
- Knots securely with a minimum number of throws with small knot size
- Is easy and economical to produce and sterilize
- Does not induce allergic, electrolytic, or neoplastic changes
- Holds tissues until healing occurs, then resorbs with minimal tissue reaction

Obviously, no such suture material exists or probably ever will since several of these attributes are contradictory. Consequently, veterinary personnel must be aware of the advantages and disadvantages of all available sutures and choose the one most appropriate for the use at hand. The technician will need to become familiar with all sutures used by the surgeon.

SUTURE NOMENCLATURE

Suture material can be classified by a number of characteristics. Absorbable suture is broken down and resorbed by the body, resulting in a loss of tensile strength within 60 days. Consequently, it should be used in tissues that heal rapidly to adequate strength. Nonabsorbable suture does not significantly weaken with time. It is used in areas that heal slowly and are subject to disruptive stresses. Multifilament or braided suture material is made up of a number of small elements that are braided or twisted together to form the desired diameter (Figure 29-49). Multifilament suture tends to be relatively strong, handles well, and has good knot-holding abilities. However, many braided sutures induce significant tissue reaction and can harbor bacteria, leading to intractable suture tract infections if they become contaminated. Moreover, most braided suture will exhibit capillary or "wicking" characteristics in which fluid travels along the length of the suture between the filaments. Therefore multifilament suture should not be used in hollow organs or in the skin when part of the suture is exposed to a contaminated environment and the wicking fluid can carry bacteria into the body. Monofilament suture (Figure 29-50) prevents the capillary problem and consequently has a lower incidence of infection. It also has a low coefficient of surface friction, making it easy to generally pull through tissues. However, the low surface friction ("drag") results in poor knot security, necessitating many throws on each knot. Some monofilament suture also has a tendency to return to its original shape (called memory), resulting in poor handling characteristics (Figure 29-51).

> *TECHNICIAN NOTE* Suture material can be classified as absorbable or nonabsorbable and monofilament or multifilament.

ABSORBABLE SUTURE MATERIAL

Surgical gut is collagenous protein obtained from the submucosal layer of sheep small intestine. It was originally known as kit gut (meaning fiddle string because the material was used for stringed instruments). Over the years, the term

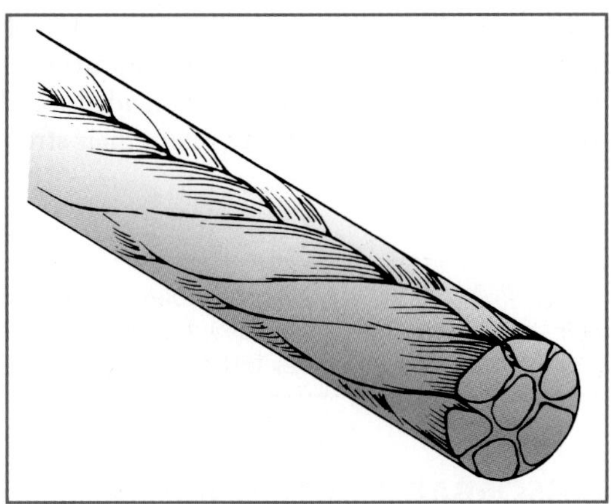

FIGURE 29-49 Constructed multifilament suture. (From Meeker MH, Rothrock JC: *Alexander's care of the patient in surgery*, ed 11, St Louis, 1999, Mosby.)

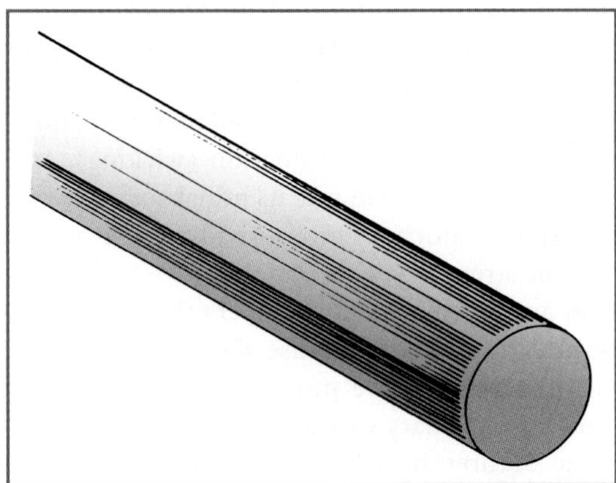

FIGURE 29-50 Monofilament suture. (From Meeker MH, Rothrock JC: *Alexander's care of the patient in surgery*, ed 11, St Louis, 1999, Mosby.)

kit was mistakenly changed to cat, resulting in the common misnomer catgut. When implanted in tissues, surgical gut incites an inflammatory reaction that ultimately resorbs the suture by phagocytosis. The severity of reaction, and consequently the rate at which the gut loses strength, can be decreased by tanning the material with chromic salts. Surgical gut has been classified into four groups: plain, mild, medium, and extrachromic and treated with resorption times of 10, 20, 30, and 40 days, respectively. Because surgical gut is broken down by phagocytosis, implantation in inflamed, highly vascular, or biologically active tissue will result in a faster rate of resorption. Medium chromic gut is relatively inexpensive and has predictable handling and knotting characteristics. However, its variability in rate of tensile strength loss, particularly in response to an inflammatory environment, should be considered and has led most surgeons away from its use for closure of support layers.

Other natural absorbable suture materials, such as collagen, kangaroo tendon, and fascia lata, have been developed, but have shown few distinct advantages over surgical gut.

Synthetic Absorbable Suture Material

Synthetic absorbable sutures are in general broken down by hydrolysis and have been developed to prevent the variation of resorptive rates in inflammatory environments. Synthetic absorbable sutures can be principally subdivided into sutures retaining strength for more than 21 days (Dexon, Vicryl, Maxon, PDS, and Polysorb) and sutures retaining strength for less than 21 days (MONOCRYL, BIOSYN).

Polyglycolic acid (Dexon, Kendall) is a synthetic polyester polymerized from hydroxyacetic acid. It is produced in fine filaments that are braided into sutures of various sizes. Consequently, it has excellent handling and knot-holding characteristics. Dexon is broken down in the body by enzymatic hydrolysis, which does not induce a

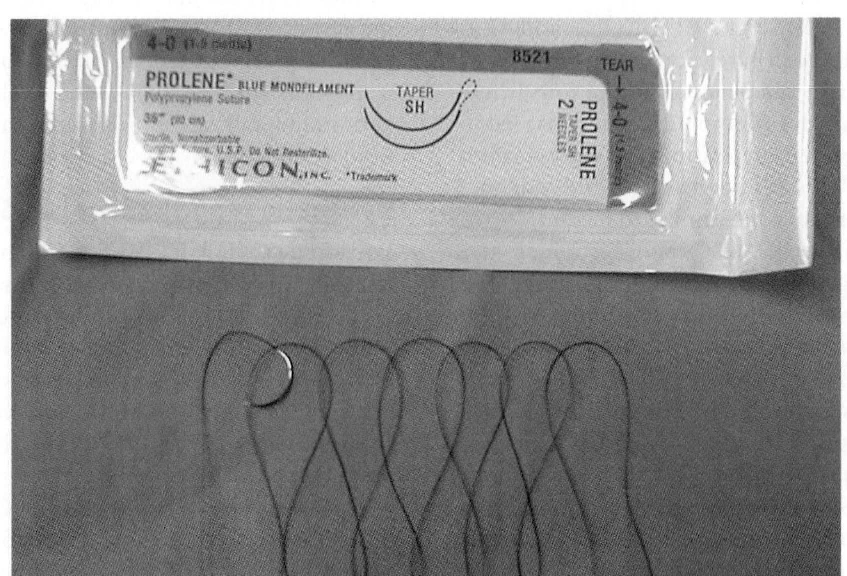

FIGURE 29-51 Memory is the tendency of suture to return to its package shape.

significant inflammatory reaction. Further, the rate of absorption is not affected by placement in an inflamed or infected environment. Dexon loses about 35% of its tensile strength in 14 days and 65% of its strength within 21 days. Some studies have shown that Dexon absorbs more rapidly in the presence of urine. Overall, it has a superior initial strength, but it loses its strength more rapidly than surgical gut.

Polyglactin 910 (Vicryl, ETHICON) is a coated multifilament suture consisting of a copolymer of lactic and glycolic acids. Its production and resorption processes are similar to those of Dexon. Vicryl also has a high initial strength that declines rapidly when implanted. Likewise, it has good handling qualities and knot security. Polyglactin 910 has become available with an antiseptic Triclosan coating (Vicryl Plus) to protect against bacterial colonization of the suture. Wound healing properties of Triclosan-coated polyglactin 910 and polyglactin 910 are similar.

Polydioxanone (PDS, ETHICON) and polyglyconate (Maxon, Kendall) are newer synthetic polyester materials that are pliable enough to be produced and used in monofilament form. Consequently, they have significantly less tissue drag in placement. However, they do possess some memory characteristics and must have multiple throws to gain a knot securely. The process of resorption is similar to that of the other synthetic absorbable materials. PDS retains 86% strength at 14 days and 69% strength at 42 days. Maxon retains 70% strength at 14 days and 45% at 21 days. Consequently, these are particularly useful in slow-healing tissues. Despite their absorbable classification, it takes about 180 days until PDS and Maxon are completely absorbed.

Polysorb (Kendall) is a multifilament glycoside-lactide copolymer with good knot-tying capabilities. Polysorb retains 80% strength at 14 days and 30% strength at 42 days. Although entirely absorbed at day 70, its bacterial wicking potential as a result of the braided characteristics should be considered.

Polyglecaprone (MONOCRYL, ETHICON) and Glycomer 631 (BIOSYN, Kendall) are more rapidly absorbed monofilament sutures that can be used in situations where healing occurs more quickly. Their predictability has led to their replacing gut for many applications. Monocryl is not as strong as and BIOSYN is as strong as PDS and Maxon.

Polyglecaprone absorbs at a rate similar to medium chromic gut. Polyglecaprone retains 60% to 70% strength at 7 days, 30% to 40% strength at 14 days, and 0% at day 21. The suture is absorbed between day 90 and 120. Similar to polyglactin 910, polyglecaprone is marketed with an antiseptic coating (MONOCRYL Plus, ETHICON) to inhibit bacterial colonization along the suture in high-risk patients (e.g., animals with diabetes, neoplastic diseases, FIV, FeLV, hypothyroidism, or immune suppression).

BIOSYN consists of 60% glycoside, 26% trimethylene carbonate, and 14% dioxanone. BIOSYN retains 75% strength at 14 days, 40% to 50% strength at 21 days, and 25% at 28 days. The suture is absorbed between day 90 and 120.

Vicryl and Dexon are more rapidly degraded in alkaline environments and dissolve faster in infected urine. Therefore PDS and Maxon have been recommended for closure of the bladder because these sutures retain their strength in urine.

> *TECHNICIAN NOTE* Absorbable sutures retain their tensile strength in tissues for several weeks, whereas nonabsorbable sutures last 60 days or more.

NONABSORBABLE SUTURE MATERIAL

Nonabsorbable suture retains its tensile strength for more than 60 days. It can be organic fiber, metallic, or synthetic and will be described according to origin.

Silk is one of the first and still most commonly used organic nonabsorbable materials. It is obtained from the cocoon of the silkworm and is braided or twisted into multifilament strands. It has excellent handling and knotting qualities and is commonly used in cardiovascular surgery. However, it can induce a severe soft tissue reaction, allow capillary migration of contamination (wicking), and serve as a nidus for infection. Despite its nonabsorbable classification, the inflammatory reaction usually results in complete loss of tensile strength within 6 months.

Cotton and linen are natural fibers that are also used to make suture. They both increase slightly in strength when wet, but otherwise behave much like silk. They have seen limited use in veterinary surgery.

Metallic sutures have been used since the fourteenth century, when the biologically nonreactive nature of gold was first described. Stainless steel is the major metallic suture in use today. It is biologically inert and will not support bacterial growth. Steel retains its high tensile strength when implanted. Consequently, it is particularly useful in infected wounds or tissues that are expected to be stressed while healing slowly. Stainless steel suture is available in monofilament and multifilament forms. The major disadvantage of steel is its poor handling quality and its tendency to kink. Silver, aluminum, and tantalum sutures have some limited use in human surgery.

Synthetic Nonabsorbable Suture Material

Polyamide (nylon, ETHICON) is a polymerized plastic that is available as suture in both monofilament and braided forms. It does not cause tissue reaction when implanted, but it gradually loses its tensile strength over several years. It is somewhat stiff and slippery, and it has significant memory, making handling and knot security exacting. Monofilament nylon is typically used for skin sutures that are removed.

Polypropylene (Prolene, ETHICON; Surgipro, Kendall) is a synthetic plastic that is similar to nylon. However, polypropylene does not weaken with time, making it useful when permanent suture support is needed.

TABLE 29-1 Limits on Suture Diameter

	Millimeters		Limits on Knot-Pull Tensile Strength	
Size	Minimum	Maximum	kg	lb
7-0	0.025	0.064	0.06	0.125
6-0	0.064	0.113	0.16	0.35
5-0	0.113	0.179	0.32	0.7
4-0	0.179	0.241	0.68	1.5
3-0	0.241	0.318	1.13	2.5
2-0	0.318	0.406	1.18	4.0
1-0	0.406	0.495	2.50	5.5
1	0.495	0.584	3.40	7.5
2	0.584	0.673	4.80	9.0
3	0.673	0.762	5.22	11.5

From US Pharmacopeial Convention: *United States pharmacopeia,* ed 16, Rockville, Md, 1960, The Convention.

Polybutester (NOVAFIL, Kendall) is a similar synthetic suture that is much more elastic. This means it can stretch and return to its original length without breaking, making it useful for repairing ligaments and other structures that must stretch under weighted motion.

Polyester fibers (MERSILENE, ETHICON; Ti-cron, Kendall) are braided to form a strong noncapillary suture. Handling quality is good, but five or six throws are required for good knot security. It also has significant tissue drag and induces just slightly less tissue reaction than silk. Some manufacturers coat the polyester fibers with Teflon (Tevdek and Polydek, Deknatel) or silicone (Ti-cron, Kendall) to reduce drag and reaction. However, chronic infection and draining fistulas remain common complications of polyester use.

Polymerized caprolactam (Supramid, S. Jackson; Braunamid, Vetcassette II, B. Braun Melsungen AG) is made of synthetic fibers coated with a smooth plasticlike material. It has high tensile strength and does not induce a significant tissue reaction. Because the outer sheath of these sutures often breaks, the underlying multifilament fibers allow bacterial migration. Therefore these sutures should not be used below the skin level because they predispose to fistulation and infection.

SUTURE SIZE AND STRENGTH

The size or diameter of suture has been classified by the *United States Pharmacopeia.* Table 29-1 lists the established limits of surgical gut from 7-0 (pronounced "seven ott" or "seven zero") to No. 3. Other suture materials use the same sizing limits and have extended down to an 11-0 nylon for microvascular anastomosis and up to No. 7 stainless steel for orthopedic use. The appropriate-sized suture for each procedure needs to be no stronger than the tissue on which it is used. Oversized sutures do not strengthen a wound and may lead to overtightening and strangulation of tissues. In addition to suture tensile strength, knot security should be considered when selecting suture size. Because the knot is the strength-limiting area of most suture and the relative knot security decreases as suture size increases, smaller suture offers a mechanical advantage. This is particularly true of the synthetic monofilament sutures, which have a low coefficient of friction (slippery). Besides untying, knotting decreases a suture's strength by converting the longitudinal tensile force into a shearing force that collects at the base of the knot, at which point strands cross and angle. The process of tying the knot also weakens suture by abrading its surface as strands cross. This is particularly true of surgical gut sutures and braided sutures. Excessive suture material should be cut off, leaving the ends just long enough to secure the knot on buried sutures. Of course, this length varies with surface friction and knot security. In general, multifilament and metallic sutures can be cut off quite close to the knot (about 2 mm). Monofilament sutures with memory and polyesters need to have 3 to 4 mm left to prevent knot untying (Figure 29-52). Skin sutures usually have about 0.5- to 1.0-cm tails to aid in easy removal.

TECHNICIAN NOTE Oversized sutures do not strengthen a wound and may lead to overtightening and strangulation of tissues.

SUTURE REACTION

As previously noted, some suture materials induce more tissue reaction than others. In descending order of reactiveness, surgical gut is most reactive, followed by multifilament natural fiber, synthetic multifilament suture, synthetic monofilament suture, and finally metallic suture. Recognizing a suture's reactivity becomes particularly important when suture reaction might affect function of the tissue, as in neurosurgery or cardiovascular surgery.

Tissue reaction also impedes healing of normal tissue. The presence of infection or contamination has a much

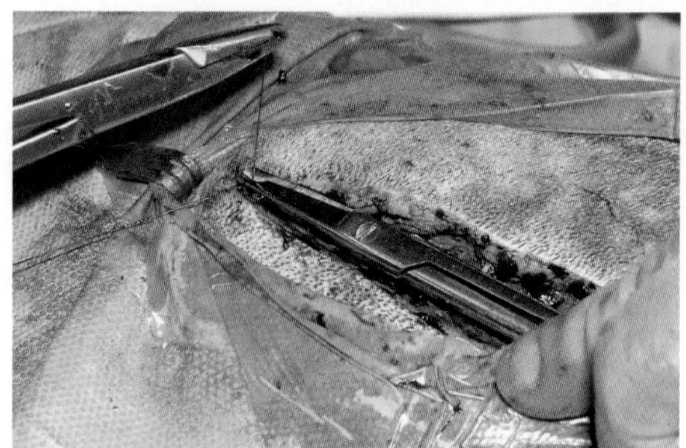

FIGURE 29-52 Monofilament sutures with memory and polyester sutures need to have 3 to 4 mm left to prevent knot untying.

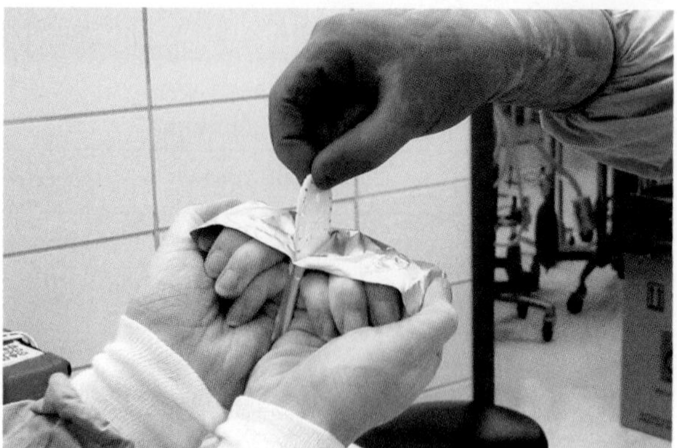

FIGURE 29-53 Peeling back the outer covering of a prepackaged suture material.

greater effect on the more reactive sutures. For example, the inflammatory process associated with infection will often phagocytose surgical gut at an increased rate, leading to resorption before healing and wound dehiscence. Likewise, the presence of silk has been shown to increase the incidence of infection 10,000-fold in contaminated incisions. Finally, nonabsorbable suture, such as silk or polyester, may cause ulceration of the gastrointestinal tract or serve as the nidus for stone formation in the urinary bladder or gallbladder if it penetrates the lumen of those hollow organs.

PREPARATION OF SUTURE MATERIAL

Several methods are used by suture producers to sterilize various suture materials. Many prepackaged sutures are sterilized by gamma irradiation. Ethylene oxide is used on those products that will not tolerate irradiation. Prepackaged suture material has a sterile shelf life that varies as denoted by the expiration date printed on the package. Consequently, expiration dates should be periodically checked and stock rotated when new supplies arrive. Steam sterilization (autoclaving) can be used on some materials, with variable damaging effects. The following describes the effects of autoclaving:

I. Severe damage, destroys tensile strength
   A. Surgical gut
   B. Polyglycolic acid (PDS)
   C. Polyglactin (Vicryl)
II. Mild damage, reduces tensile strength
   A. Silk
   B. Linen
   C. Cotton
III. Tolerates at least three autoclavings without loss of tensile strength
   A. Polyester
   B. Nylon
   C. Polypropylene
   D. Metallics

Sutures that can be steam sterilized are sometimes bought in bulk and are sterilized in the practice. When preparing such suture, an appropriate number of strand lengths (usually 30 to 60 cm) should be cut and coiled or loosely wound around a card or sponge. This will avoid repeated autoclaving, which will damage even the most steam-tolerant material.

Prepackaged suture material is opened (by a nonsterile assistant) onto the instrument tray by peeling back the outer packaging (Figure 29-53). The surgical assistant opens the inner pack by tearing off one end and grasping the suture end or swaged needle with needle holders as directed on the package. Before use, the suture should be stretched slightly to overcome memory, but not snapped because this commonly leads to contamination of the suture end. Any excessive preserving fluid should be wiped off. The tissue drag of many sutures (particularly the synthetic multifilaments) can be reduced by moistening with sterile saline. However, this will reduce the tensile strength of silk, and surgical gut will imbibe water to swell and soften. Multifilament suture strands tend to accumulate blood as they pass through tissue and should be wiped off with a moistened sponge between uses.

SUTURE NEEDLES

Suture needles vary considerably in shape, point design, method of attachment to the suture (eye), and size. The size and shape of the needle are determined by the thickness of the tissue sutured and the depth of the incision (Figure 29-54, *A*). Straight needles are usually used superficially in accessible locations where the needle can be manipulated with the fingers. Curved needle types are manipulated with needle holders. One-fourth (¼) circle needles are commonly used in ophthalmologic surgery, whereas three-eighths (⅜) and one-half (½) circle needles are most popular in general surgery.

The point design varies with the toughness of tissue being sutured (Figure 29-54, *B*). Skin, eye tissues, and some tough facial tissues are sutured with a cutting-edged needle. Cutting needles have two or three opposing cutting surfaces. Regular cutting needles have a third cutting surface on the inside curvature resulting in a "cutout" effect. Reverse cutting needles have the third cutting surface on the outside curvature, resulting in a more robust design with less

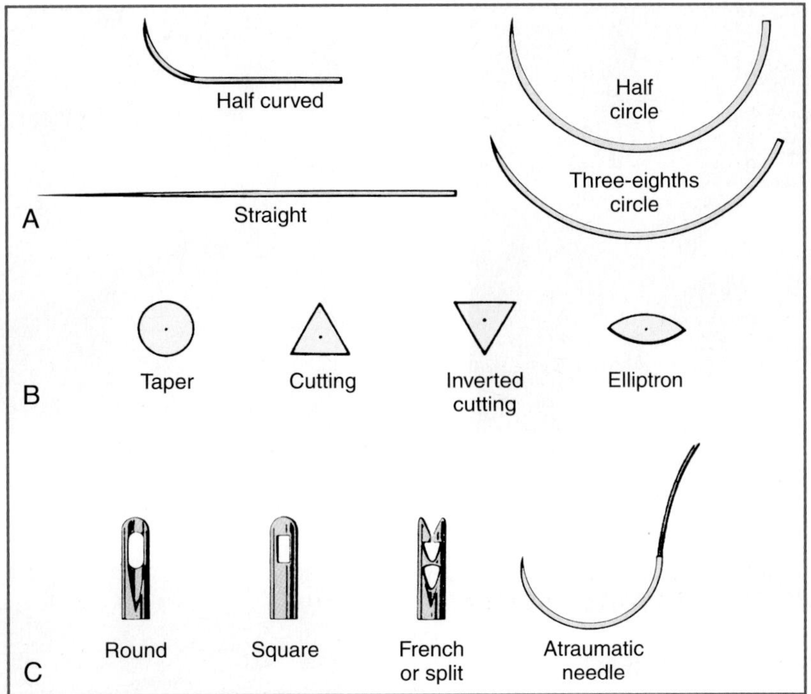

FIGURE 29-54 **A,** The size and shape of the needle are chosen according to the thickness of the tissue. **B,** The needle point design is determined according to the toughness of the tissue on which it is used. **C,** The needle is attached to the suture either by threading through an eye or by being swaged. (Courtesy Sherwood Davis & Geck, Milford, N.J.)

cut-out effect. Reverse-cutting needles (K needles) are therefore preferred by some surgeons because they do not bend or break as easily. The cutout effect makes passage of the needle and suture easier, but a true incision that can leak is created. Cutting-edged needles should not be used when an airtight or watertight suture line is required. Taper needles do not actually cut tissue, but spread it open around the needle and following suture. This spreading effect prevents hemorrhage and results in a sealed suture line. Taper needles and reverse-cutting needles are used in suturing most hollow organs.

> *TECHNICIAN NOTE* Cutting-edged needles should not be used when an airtight or watertight suture line is required (lung, urinary bladder, intestine, etc.).

The needle can be attached to the suture by three different methods (Figure 29-54, *C*). Single-eyed needles have one hole in the head of the needle. The eye should be single threaded because double threading leaves a large bulk of suture around the shank, which will cause excessive tissue drag and damage as the needle is passed. A curved needle is threaded from within the curve so that the short end of the suture falls away from the outside curve. About 10 cm of suture should be pulled through the eye. These steps will help to prevent the suture from pulling out of the eye during suturing. Spring or French-eyed needles have a complete eye and an incomplete "spring" eye. Suture is threaded through the complete eye and is forced back through the spring eye, which grips the suture end.

Eyeless or swaged needles are attached directly to the end of the suture by the factory. The surgeon draws a single strand through the tissue and automatically uses a new sharp needle with every strand. Therefore swaged needles are the most atraumatic and most popular surgical needles in veterinary practice.

EQUINE SURGICAL ASSISTANCE

ROLE OF THE VETERINARY TECHNICIAN IN SURGICAL ASSISTANCE WITH EQUINE PATIENTS

It is important, particularly with large animal surgeries, that the technician, whether as a scrub nurse or assistant, anticipates what is needed with regards to preparation of the equine patient and what will be needed during surgery (i.e., instrumentation) to reduce the anesthesia time. This will lessen the potential for any postanesthetic recovery complications. Surgeons rely instinctively on the technician in surgery to be prepared and have things moving in an efficient manner.

> *TECHNICIAN NOTE* To lesson postanesthetic recovery complications, it is important with large animal surgeries that the surgery nurse anticipates what is needed with regard to preparation of the animal and during surgery (i.e., instrumentation) to reduce the anesthesia time.

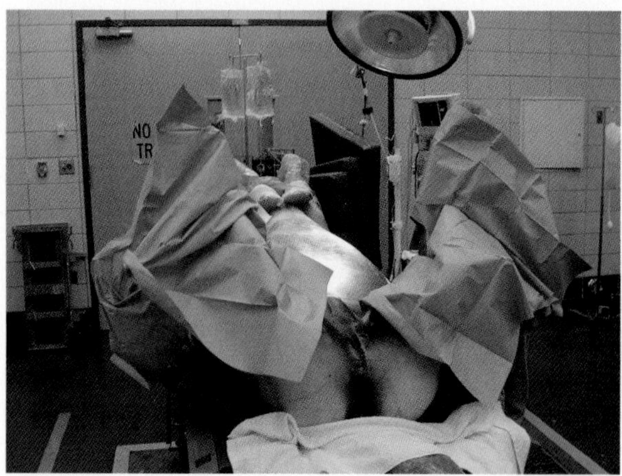

FIGURE 29-55 Draping of an equine surgery patient. Leg drapes are used to cover the rear limbs of the patient.

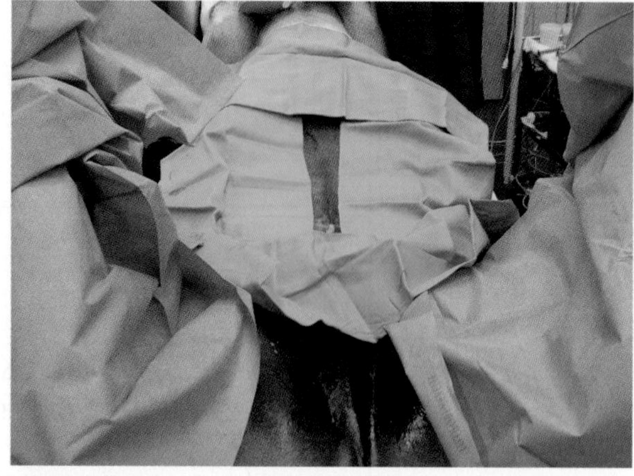

FIGURE 29-56 Draping the ventral abdomen of an equine surgery patient. Hand towels are placed in a four-quarter fashion around the incision site.

PATIENT AND INSTRUMENT TABLES SETUP

DRAPING OF THE EQUINE PATIENT

As with small animals, the function of draping is to separate the sterile surgical site from the rest of the contaminated area around the patient. Draping should only be performed by members of the surgical team who are aseptically gowned and gloved. In most cases, it takes at least two persons to correctly perform draping of a horse because of the size of the drapes. Abdominal surgery is one of the most common surgical procedures performed on a horse. Therefore draping of the ventral abdomen for abdominal surgery in the horse is described here as the example.

Once the animal has been surgically prepped, sterile stockinettes or leg drapes are placed individually over each hind limb (Figure 29-55). Next, the horse is draped in a similar manner as a small animal would be, with hand towels placed in a four-quarter fashion around the incision site (Figure 29-56). These are secured with several Backhaus towel clamps. Then a large laparotomy drape is placed with a person positioned on opposite sides of the patient carefully unfolding the large drape over the horse. The most effective way of doing this is first placing the drape over the center of the surgical site, on top of the already secured hand towels, and carefully unfolding the large drape with a backward step away from the horse. Then, in a coordinated fashion, the drape is unfolded longitudinally to cover the entire animal (Figure 29-57). If an equine laparotomy drape is used, these drapes are already fenestrated, so no cuts are needed to create the fenestration. Towel clamps are used to secure the laparotomy drape by clamping to the towel clamps underneath the drape (Figure 29-58, *A*). The exposed towel clamps are covered with a single 4 × 4 gauze, and an adhesive, impervious drape is placed directly over the incision site (Figure 29-58, *C*). An adhesive spray is necessary to get good contact (Figure 29-58, *B*). The gauze prevents the adhesive drape from sticking to the clamp. However, it is important that none of these gauze sponges fall into the abdominal cavity unnoticed. Serious life-threatening consequences could occur.

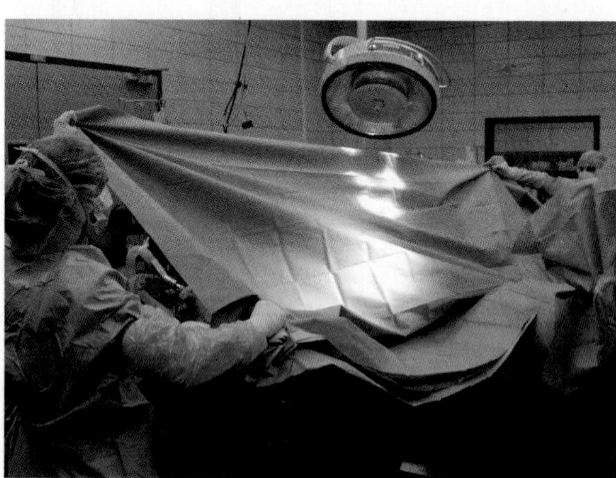

FIGURE 29-57 Draping of an equine surgery patient. Two persons are required to drape the patient.

> *TECHNICIAN NOTE* It is important that no gauze sponges fall into the abdominal cavity and not be retrieved.

INSTRUMENT SETUP AND HANDLING

If there is adequate surgical technical personnel, the surgical instrument packs are opened during the time that the surgical team personnel are draping the horse. This will reduce anesthesia time. There are some situations in which two tables are sterily draped, depending on the amount of instruments needed. This is often the case with orthopedic surgeries. Unlike small animal surgery setup, the instrument tray(s) are set up on a table separated from the patient table. The instrument table is draped by a nongowned assistant (Figure 29-59). The surgical instrument packs needed for the surgery are placed on a Mayo stand or similar type of table, and the outer wrap only is opened by the surgical nurse or technician that is not gloved and gowned (Figure 29-60). Then one of the surgical team personnel opens the inner wrap and removes the tray from the stand and moves it onto the instrument table.

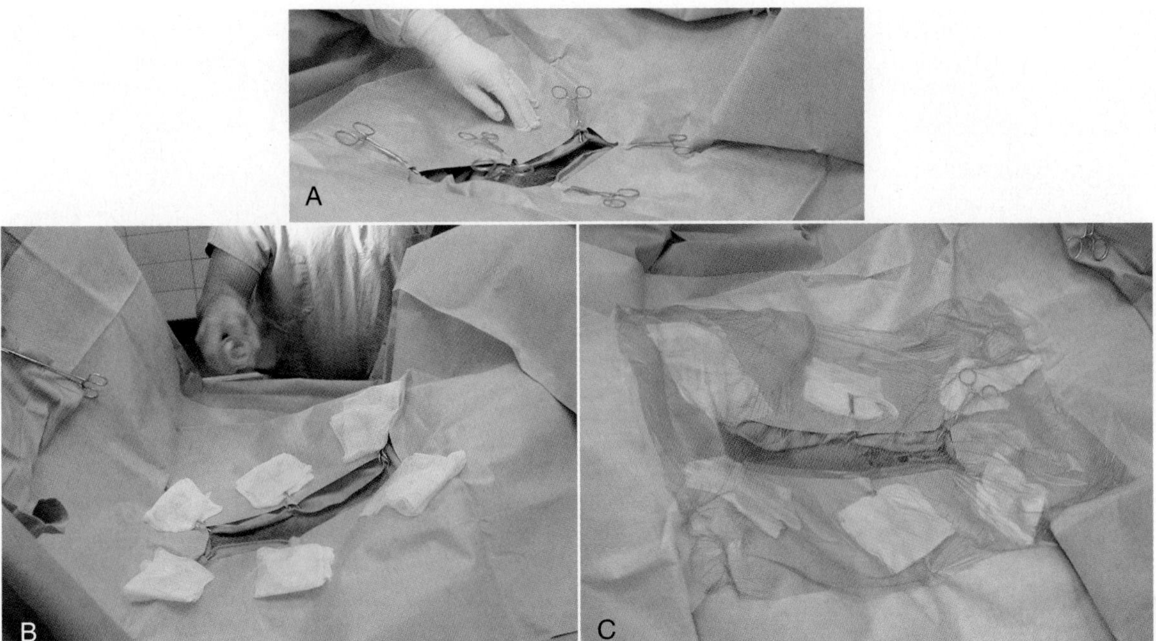

FIGURE 29-58 Draping the ventral abdomen of an equine surgery patient. Towel clamps are used to secure the laparotomy drape by clamping to the towel clamps underneath the drape. **A,** The exposed towel clamps are covered with a single 4 × 4 gauze, and an adhesive spray is used to improve the adhesiveness of the adhesive drape. **B,** An adhesive, impervious drape is placed directly over the incision site. **C,** The gauze prevents the adhesive drape from sticking to the clamp.

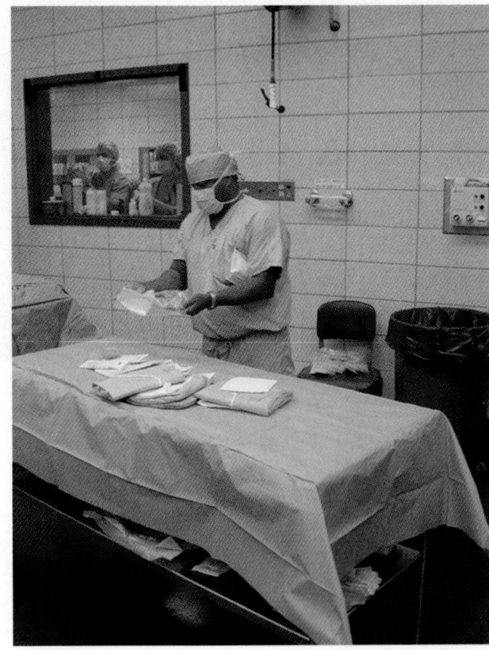

FIGURE 29-59 Instrument table is being set up for equine surgery. The surgical gowns were commercially packaged inside the drape.

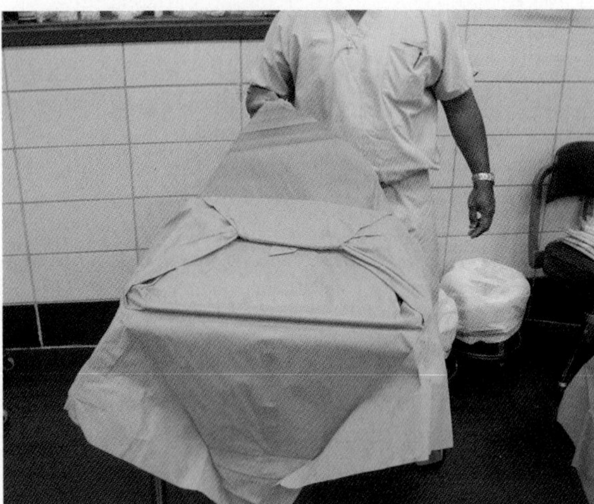

FIGURE 29-60 Preparing for equine surgery. The surgical nurse opens the outer wrap of the instrument pack. One member of the surgical team will aseptically open the inner wrap and move the pack onto the instrument table.

Setup of the surgery table includes the instrument tray, sterile light handles, suction hose, electrocautery, fluid bowl, and suture. During the positioning of the horse on the table, an electrocautery plate with contact gel is positioned under the animal and plugged into the unit at some point in time during the preparation of the animal. If the horse is draped for abdominal surgery, the surgeon and assistant create a pouch between the back legs of the horse by clamping a hand towel folded to the drape using a nonpenetrating instrument, such as Allis forceps (Figure 29-61). The suction hose and cautery line are run through the rings of these instruments to secure them to the table and held in this pouch. These are then run over the drapes between the legs of the horse and connected by the scrub nurse. A sterile IV fluid line may also be set up at this time. During this setup of the table, the surgeon's assistant should also be setting up the surgical instruments. The instrument tray is set to the back of the surgical table, a hand towel

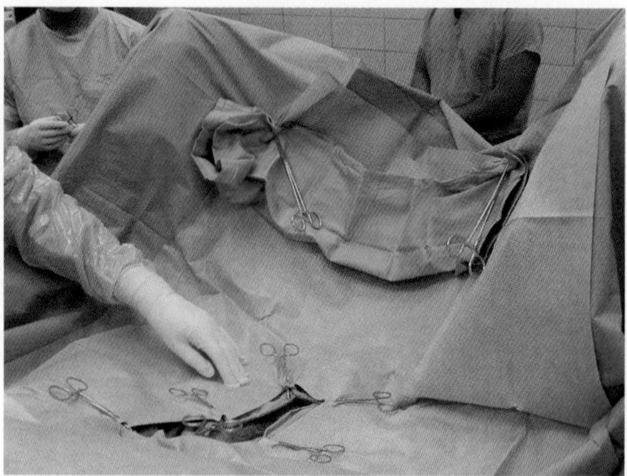

FIGURE 29-61 A pouch is made from a sterile folded hand towel and clamped to the surgery drape by nonpenetrating clamps between the horse's rear limbs to hold the suction hose and cautery line.

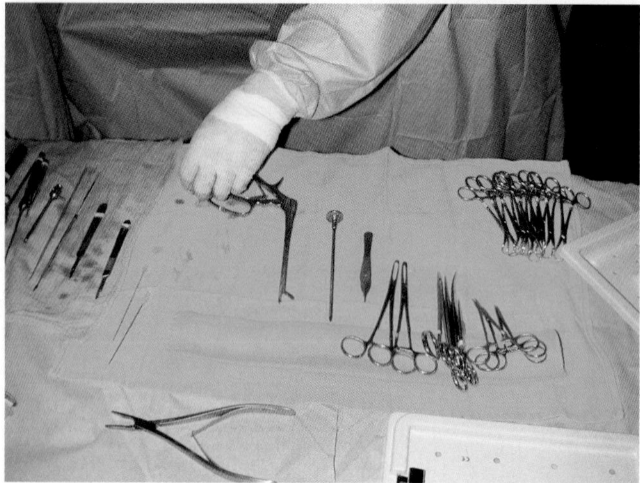

FIGURE 29-62 For efficiency in retrieving, the most frequently used instruments are placed in front of the instrument pack on a hand towel.

is placed in front of the tray, and the frequently used instruments are placed on the towel to allow for immediate access (Figure 29-62). The instruments include scissors, forceps, needle holders, and hemostats. The blades are attached at this time to the scalpel handles. The bowl is positioned on the edge of the table so that sterile saline can be poured into the bowl by a nongowned scrub nurse. It is important during the surgical procedure, particularly in horses, that the instruments be kept clean during the surgical procedure. This is done by taking a wet 4 × 4 towel and gently wiping the blood from the used surgical instrument and placing it back onto the instrument table. However, if an instrument becomes contaminated, such as opening a hollow viscus of the GI tract, this instrument is discarded from the surgical table. At any time in which a break in asepsis occurs whether a glove or a gown becomes contaminated, these need to be immediately discarded and replaced. It is important during the surgical procedure that the technical assistant be efficient and develop a thought process of anticipating the next move of the surgeon. This will create a more efficient surgical environment and reduce the anesthesia time.

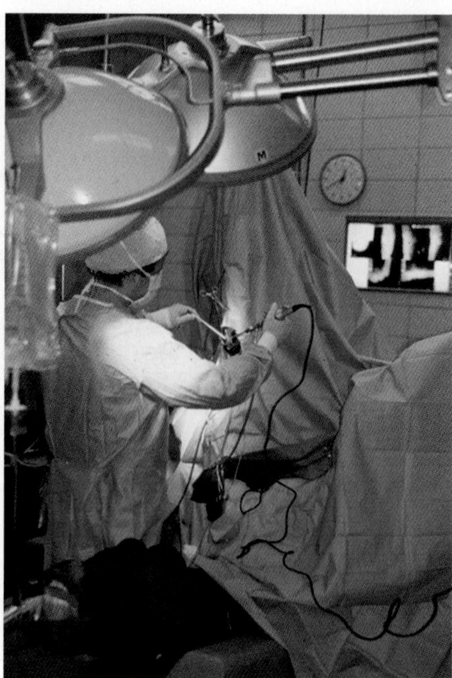

FIGURE 29-63 Arthroscopic surgery performed on the carpus of a horse.

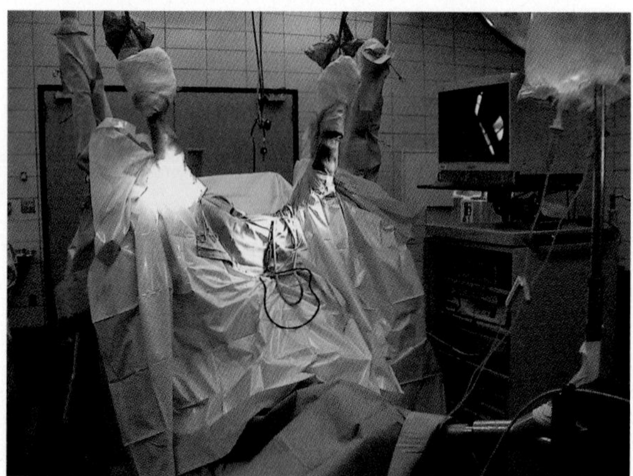

FIGURE 29-64 Horse draped for arthroscopic surgery of the carpi. Adhesive, impervious drapes are placed around the carpi to reduce surgical wound contamination from the skin.

> *TECHNICIAN NOTE* Any instrument that becomes contaminated during surgery is immediately discarded from the surgical table.

ORTHOPEDIC SURGERY

Positioning of a horse on the surgery table for orthopedic surgery greatly depends upon the location on the limb of the orthopedic problem and the procedure. Arthroscopic procedures in most cases are performed in dorsal recumbency (Figure 29-63). Impervious plastic drapes are used to reduce strike-through contamination and tearing. An adhesive, impervious type of drape is used directly over the surgical site (Figure 29-64).

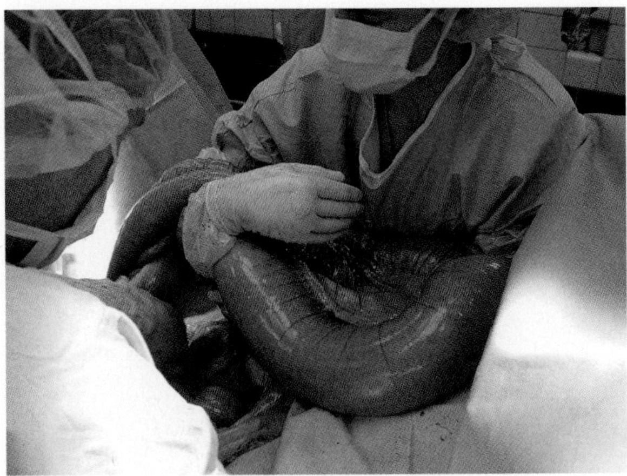

FIGURE 29-65 During abdominal surgery, the large intestines must be carefully handled during exploration of the abdominal cavity. In this photo, the large colon is being cradled by the assistant.

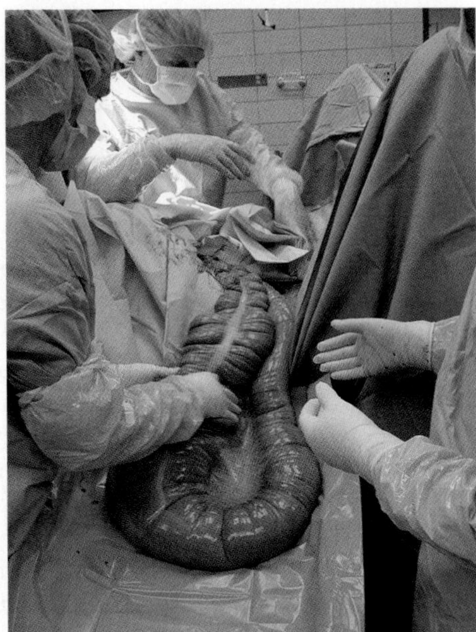

FIGURE 29-66 The large colon placed on the colon tray in preparation for an enterotomy and content evacuation. Notice that the opening of the abdominal cavity is being draped off.

As performed with small animal orthopedic surgery, a stockinette is usually not sutured around the incision site with horses.

PROPER TISSUE HANDLING TECHNIQUES IN THE EQUINE HOLLOW ORGAN SURGERY

Surgical manipulation of tissue in the horse is similar to small animal surgery. Refer to that section regarding this description. There are things that are different that will be expanded upon.

HOLLOW ORGAN SURGERY

Hollow organ surgery, especially intestinal, can be a quite involved procedure in the horse, mainly because of the size and length of the intestinal tract. The small intestine, for example, is more than 80 feet in length. Whereas the large intestine will contain several pounds of ingesta, which can create a problem when manipulating it. Because of the weight of the large colon in the horse, risk of tearing and ultimate contamination of the abdominal cavity is great. Thus as an assistant, careful handling of the large colon is important (Figure 29-65). If the contents from the large intestine is to be evacuated, this is done via a colon tray that is positioned along side of the horse and draped with sterile impervious drapes that allow the large colon to be placed onto the tray away from the abdominal opening. This allows the colon to be evacuated without the risk of contamination of the abdominal cavity (Figure 29-66). It is the responsibility of the assistant to maintain the large colon on the tray during the evacuation process so that it is not pulled back into the abdominal cavity until the enterotomy site is closed. If a small intestinal resection is performed in a horse, the segment of small intestine is isolated from the rest of the abdominal cavity as much as possible, using laparotomy sponges and impervious drapes. It becomes a coordinated effort between the surgeon and the assistant to ensure that the portion of the small intestine that is undergoing surgery be kept on the table and to keep the majority of the intestine in the abdominal cavity. It is important for the assistant to maintain proper orientation of the segments during reanastomosis and to maintain their proper positioning for the surgeon during this closure and suturing procedure. Any instruments that came in contact with the ingesta should be discarded from the surgical table and after the procedure is completed, a change of gloves may be in order before abdominal closure.

The intestinal tract can easily become dehydrated if the intestines are left out of the abdominal cavity for an extended period of time and ultimately can result in damage and possible risk of creating areas for adhesion formation. It is important that the assistant be aware of tissue dehydration during the entire surgical procedure and that the exposed intestinal segment is kept moist. This can be accomplished by several means, such as an IV drip set hooked to a pressurized fluid bag or a bulb syringe filled with irrigation saline (Figure 29-67).

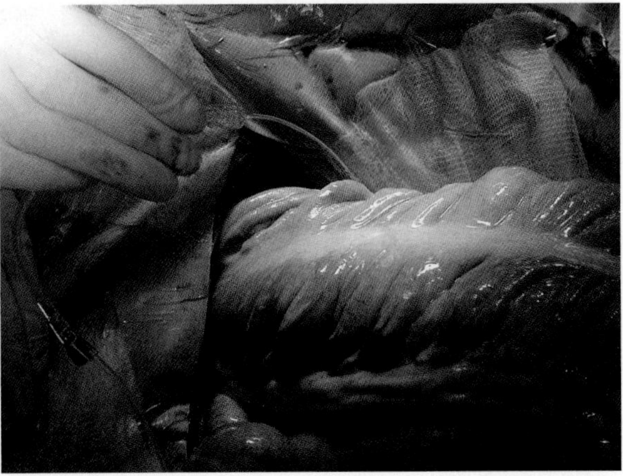

FIGURE 29-67 Photo of a segment of the large colon of a horse. It is imperative that the surface of the intestines be kept moist to prevent drying and subsequent tissue damage.

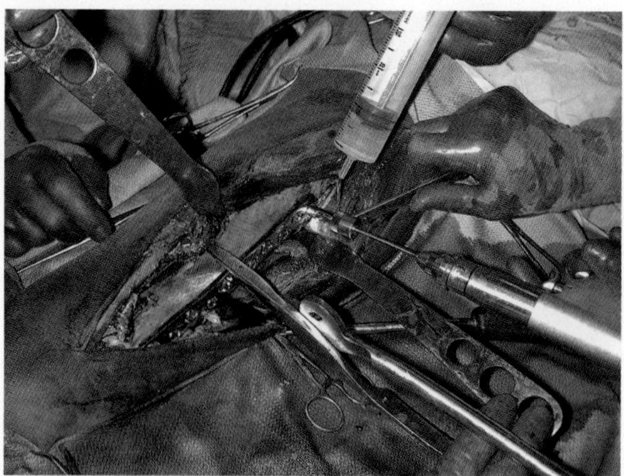

FIGURE 29-68 Repair of a radial fracture in a foal. Notice that the drill bit is bathed with sterile saline to reduce thermal damage of the bone.

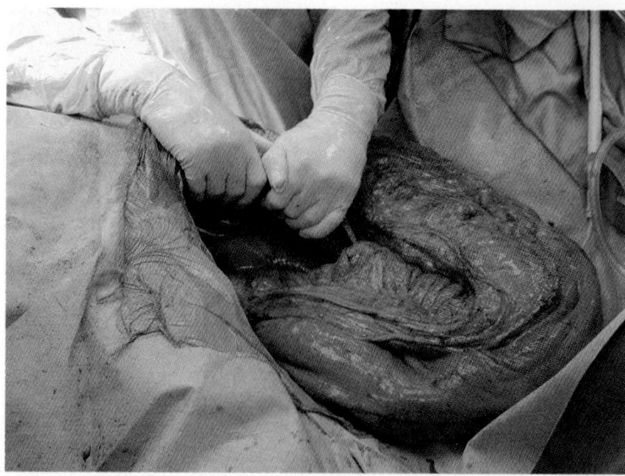

FIGURE 29-69 Abdominal exploration on a horse. Retraction of the ventral abdominal wall is performed by an assistant grasping it with their hands.

> *TECHNICIAN NOTE* It is imperative that a torn glove be replaced immediately during orthopedic surgery.

ORTHOPEDIC SURGERY

Aseptic technique is an absolute must. Instrument handling or sharp ends of fracture bones can result in glove tearing. It is imperative that torn gloves be replaced immediately. Frequent irrigation of the tissue is absolutely vital. Irrigation is an absolute must during bone drilling (Figure 29-68). Heat from the drilling process will cause thermal damage to the bone. Being proactive in keeping blood removed from the surgical field, via suction or blotting, will allow the surgeon to be more efficient and provide better visualization of the fracture during repair. Proper tissue retraction and fragment reduction during fracture repair are also important roles that an assistant plays in orthopedic surgery on the horse.

> *TECHNICIAN NOTE* Constant irrigation of the drill bit is necessary during bone drilling during fracture repair.

RETRACTION TECHNIQUES

Retraction techniques in equine surgery are, for the most part, quite similar as in small animals, with the exception of abdominal surgery. In these cases, it is difficult to maintain self-retaining retractors of any type within the abdominal incision to allow for exploration. Thus in some cases, the assistant retracts the abdominal wall with their hands (Figure 29-69). As with small animal orthopedics, retraction of muscle and tendon is necessary for visualization of fractures in horses. Hohmann retractors are effective hand-held retractors for deep tissue surrounding bone (see Figure 29-68).

HEMOSTASIS

Because of the size of the horse, loss of blood in most surgical procedures is not a major concern. It becomes a concern in surgeries, such as open sinusotomies, nasal septum resections, ovariectomies, castrations, or uterine trauma and cesarean sections (C-sections). Sponge hemostasis is avoided in abdominal surgery because of the potential for loss of a sponge within the abdominal cavity, which can be devastating and quite life threatening to the horse. The sponge will cause a severe inflammatory reaction resulting in peritonitis and adhesions that could significantly impair the normal function of the equine gastrointestinal tract. Thus in these cases, suction is used to evacuate fluids from the area. With actual cut arteries or large veins or a situation with large-vessel bleeding, these are clamped and ligated with suture material similarly described under the small animal section. With small-vessel bleeding, it is a common practice to use hemostats with a combination of electrocautery to fuse the vessel walls together (see Small Animal section).

SUTURE MATERIALS USED IN HORSES

Since the basic concept of suture types and use of suture material has already been covered in this chapter, it will not be discussed. However, because of the size of the horse, larger suture material is used compared with small animals. For closure of abdominal organs, in most cases, a 2-0 absorbable material is used. Closure of the ventral abdominal wall of a horse requires at least a No. 2 or a No. 3 absorbable suture material (Figure 29-70). PDS or Vicryl are commonly used suture material. For closure of the subcutaneous space, often a 0 absorbable suture material is used. Zero or 2-0 nonabsorbable material (nylon or Prolene) is used for

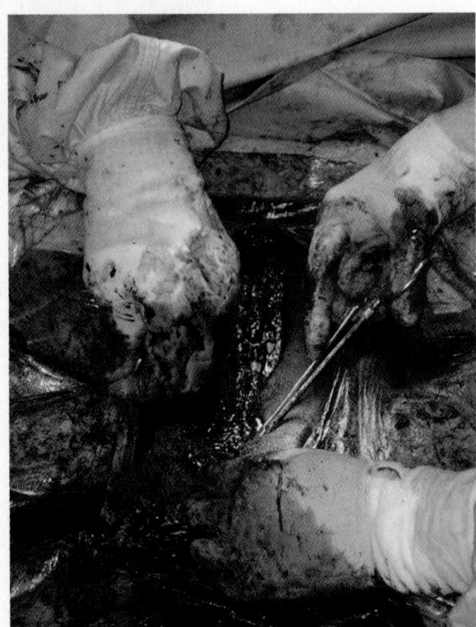

FIGURE 29-70 Closure of a ventral abdominal incision. Large suture material is needed to maintain closure.

apposition of the skin. In most cases, suture material with swaged needles are used. This saves time and improves efficiency. It is important for the surgical assistant to have the proper suture material readily available for the surgeon at the time it is needed. Often, the required sutures are discussed before surgery. It is a common practice for the surgical assistant to open the suture material and have it ready by arming a needle holder with suture just before the time it is requested.

ACKNOWLEDGMENT

The authors also wish to acknowledge the work of Erick L. Egger in editions one through five of this book.

RECOMMENDED READING

Evans HE, Christenson GC: *Miller's anatomy of the dog,* ed 3, Philadelphia, 1993, WB Saunders.

Slatter D: *Textbook of small animal surgery,* ed 3, Philadelphia, 2002, WB Saunders.

30 Small Animal Surgical Nursing

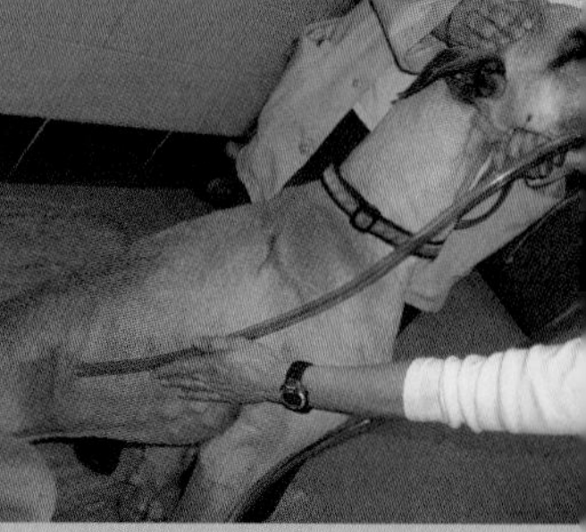

Loretta J. Bubenik

OUTLINE

KEY TERMS

Abdominocentesis
Anastomosis
Arthrodesis
Capillary refill time
Celiotomy
Cellulitis
Cystotomy
Dehiscence
Enterotomy
Evisceration
Gastrotomy
Hydrometra
Ileus
Intussusception
Mucometra
Onychectomy
Orchidectomy
Ostectomy
Osteochondrosis
Ovariohysterectomy
Pseudocyesis
Pyometra
Seroma
Splenectomy
Strangulation
Urethrostomy

LEARNING OBJECTIVES

When you have completed this chapter, you will be able to:

1. Describe the preoperative, intraoperative, and postoperative responsibilities of the veterinary technician in surgical assistance.
2. Describe indications and use of prophylactic antibiotics for surgical patients.
3. Describe signs of blood loss in the postoperative patient.
4. Discuss concerns related to hypothermia in anesthetized patients and describe methods for increasing patient body temperature intraoperatively and postoperatively.
5. Describe postoperative abnormalities that can occur in surgical incisions.
6. Describe the procedure for removal of skin sutures.
7. Discuss general considerations for care of bandages and drains.
8. List and describe indications, preoperative, intraoperative, and postoperative considerations for common elective procedures in dogs and cats.
9. List and describe indications, preoperative, intraoperative, and postoperative considerations for common nonelective procedures in dogs and cats.
10. List considerations related to client education for discharged surgical patients.

INTRODUCTION AND GENERAL PRINCIPLES

The veterinary technician's role in surgical assistance is an important part of hospital and patient management. Preoperative, intraoperative, and postoperative responsibilities should be considered for a successful outcome. The surgical candidate must undergo preoperative assessment, including examination and laboratory evaluation, the appropriate restraint, and adequate preparation for surgery. The technician's responsibility during surgery includes patient monitoring and surgeon assistance. In the postoperative period, patient monitoring and supportive care are also important. Duties of the veterinary technician include appropriate animal restraint; appropriate sample collection and diagnostic evaluation; administration of sedation, anesthesia, and pain medication; instrument preparation; operating room preparation; appropriate patient preparation and positioning for surgery; aseptic patient and instrument handling; patient monitoring; direct surgical assistance; patient recovery and securing of the operating room. Patient restraint, pain management, anesthesia, aseptic technique, instrumentation, and surgical assistance are discussed in Chapters 7, 26, 27, 28, and 29. This chapter will focus on familiarizing the technician with specific surgical procedures and highlighting technician responsibilities in the preoperative, intraoperative, and postoperative period.

Many operative procedures require the assistance of a veterinary technician. A working knowledge of common surgical procedures will ensure proficiency in surgical assistance. Proficiency will decrease surgery time, enhance the flow of surgery, and improve quality of care. Procedures that often require such assistance include orthopedic surgery (retraction, reduction, traction, countertraction), open chest procedures (artificial ventilation, retraction), and complicated abdominal procedures (diaphragmatic hernia repair, renal surgery, tumor resection). An understanding of aseptic technique, a familiarity with surgical instrumentation, and a working knowledge of the specific surgical procedure are prerequisites for proper intraoperative assistance.

Small animal surgical nursing is an important component of patient care. This chapter highlights important concepts involving preoperative evaluation, surgical preparation and assistance, and postoperative care. In addition, the more commonly performed small animal surgical procedures are discussed, with emphasis on the role of the veterinary technician.

PREOPERATIVE PATIENT ASSESSMENT

The veterinary surgical candidate should undergo a complete preoperative assessment. It is important to know what the primary problem is so that specific needs can be anticipated. Elective surgical procedures will not require the same demands that emergency or urgent surgical procedures will. Eating, drinking, urination, and defecation habits of the animal should be ascertained. An animal that has not been eating or drinking will likely require rehydration before anesthesia and surgery. Rehydration may then necessitate a blood or plasma transfusion because dilution of the blood cell volume occurs with rehydration. Fluids should not be withheld to prevent anemia. If the animal has eaten the day of scheduled surgery, the procedure will have to be delayed to decrease the risk of aspiration (inhalation of stomach contents into the trachea and lungs). The animal should not have food for at least 12 hours before anesthesia, but water should not be withheld. Emergency surgeries will have to be performed whether the animal has eaten or not, but owners should be warned of the increased risk of aspiration. Temperature, pulse rate and quality, respiration rate and character, capillary refill time, mucous membrane color, body weight, and demeanor should be assessed before surgery. Abnormalities should be brought to the attention of the surgeon.

Preanesthetic screening will depend on the animal's condition and reason for surgery. Specifics of this are covered in Chapter 27. From a nursing standpoint, it is important to discuss with the surgeon what diagnostics are appropriate before surgery and ensure that they are performed in a timely manner. Diagnostics might include blood work, such as packed-cell volume (PCV), total plasma protein (TP) concentration, blood urea nitrogen (BUN) concentration, blood glucose concentration, complete blood count (CBC), complete biochemical analysis, and heartworm test; blood gas analysis; electrocardiogram (ECG); radiographs; fine-needle mass aspiration; fecal analysis; and/or urinalysis. Abnormalities detected on the preanesthetic screen should be brought to the attention of the surgeon.

SURGICAL PREPARATION AND ANIMAL POSITIONING

It is the veterinary technician's responsibility to inquire about the surgical procedure to be performed and what instrumentation will be required. The technician should have all the necessary equipment readily accessible and prepared for use. The operating room should be clean and anesthesia equipment checked for functionality and ready for use. A heated circulating water blanket should be placed on the operating table, turned on, and covered with a towel so that it is warm by the time the animal is positioned on the table. A heated water blanket should also be set up in the recovery cage (or the warmed blanket from the operating table can be placed in the cage with the animal). Hair clippers and skin cleansing solutions should also be made available for use.

Inadequate animal preparation or inappropriate positioning can hinder surgical technique and will result in wasted time spent correcting deficiencies. Aseptic protocol should always be followed with animal preparation and draping and with surgical instrument handling. The hair should be liberally clipped around the surgical site and the skin cleansed appropriately (see Chapters 28 and 29). The veterinary technician should be familiar with the type of surgery performed so that animal preparation is consistent and adequate.

PERIOPERATIVE ANTIBIOTICS

Prophylactic antibiotics are used to decrease the risk of infection in clean or clean-contaminated surgeries, but their use will not entirely eliminate infections associated with a surgical procedure. Using antibiotics to treat active infection is a completely different process and will not be discussed here. Antibiotics should never be given indiscriminately to animals undergoing surgery. All antibiotics have potential side effects, and their use also increases surgery cost. More importantly, indiscriminant use of antibiotics contributes to the development of resistant strains of bacteria (hospital "superbugs") that are difficult to treat.

> *TECHNICIAN NOTE* Antibiotics should never be given indiscriminately to animals undergoing surgery because this contributes to the development of resistant strains of bacteria (hospital "superbugs") that are difficult to treat.

Indications for Prophylactic Antibiotics

- Operative time is more than 90 minutes. Open surgical wounds are constantly exposed to bacteria from the animal's skin, the operative team, and the air. The longer the wound is open, the higher the chance of infection. Prolonged anesthesia also increases the risk.
- The patient is at increased risk of infection. Things that might increase the risk of infection include immunosuppressive drugs (steroids), **Cushing's disease (hyperadrenocorticism),** some cancers, chemotherapy or radiation therapy, feline leukemia virus (FeLV) and/or feline immunodeficiency virus (FIV) positive, or any other immunosuppressive factor.
- A hollow **viscus** is to be entered (i.e., gastrointestinal [GI] tract, urinary bladder).
- The incision is to involve an area that is difficult to aseptically prepare (such as a toe or ear).
- Orthopedic implants are placed.
- Joint procedures that are long and aggressive or certain joint procedures that require multiple entrances into the joint (arthroscopy).
- Consequences of infection could be devastating, such as total hip replacement or spinal surgery of any kind.
- Prophylactic antibiotics are not recommended for short, clean surgical procedures, such as simple mass removal, osteochondritis cartilage flap removal, ovariohysterectomy, castration, and simple biopsy.

Therapeutic drug levels must be present in the wound fluid (serum) at the time of surgical incision or the antibiotics will not be effective. They should be given at least 20 minutes before the surgical incision is made. Antibiotics given 3 or more hours before the procedure select for resistant bacteria. Prophylactic antibiotics given more than 3 to 5 hours after the surgical incision has been made will likely not be effective in preventing infection. There is no advantage to continuing antibiotics beyond 6 to 24 hours after surgery unless it is necessary to treat an active infection or a break in sterile technique occurred during surgery. The appropriate antibiotic should be of narrow spectrum (but effective against the potential contaminant), achieve good tissue concentrations, and have minimal side effects. The veterinarian in charge should be questioned as to what antibiotic is appropriate for what surgical procedure and when antibiotic prophylaxis is needed. If a break in sterile technique occurred or the animal has an active infection, antibiotics are continued in the postoperative period according to the manufacturer's dosing recommendations and under the supervision of the veterinarian in charge. Continuing antibiotics for other reasons (i.e., you want to be on the safe side) is a misuse of prophylactic antibiotics.

MONITORING

Intraoperative and postoperative monitoring are critical to proper surgical nursing care. Chapter 27 covers anesthetic monitoring in detail, and the reader should refer to that chapter for further information. Some important components of patient monitoring as they pertain to surgery and recovery after surgery will be covered here.

During surgery, a surgical plane of anesthesia is crucial to appropriate surgical technique and animal well-being, and careful monitoring in the perioperative period might alert the observer to potential fatal complications. The postoperative phase is a critical transition period from general anesthesia to consciousness, and continual monitoring should be provided until the animal is safely extubated, normothermic, and in sternal recumbency. Surgery can result in several potential problems, including blood loss, hypothermia, pain, and cardiac and respiratory problems. The veterinary surgical technician must be prepared to deal with changes in animal status during and after surgery and address issues as the need arises. Monitoring should involve a series of evaluations and tests. Suspected complications during anesthesia and recovery are based on a group of signs consistent with a problem, not just one abnormality.

Patient monitoring does not stop once the animal has recovered from anesthesia. As long as the animal is hospitalized, vital signs, behavior, appetite, and the surgical incision should be evaluated. Depending on animal status, daily or more frequent observation of these parameters is performed. Abnormalities should be reported to the veterinarian in charge.

> *TECHNICIAN NOTE* One abnormal sign at one given time is not enough to diagnose a significant problem. All indicators (temperature, pulse, respiration, mucous membranes) should be evaluated serially to determine a trend in the animal's condition. It is this trend that will determine the severity of the postoperative problem and dictate the appropriate treatment.

BLOOD LOSS

Many procedures can result in substantial blood loss as a complication, or blood loss could be due to the inherent nature of the procedure. PCV and TP should always be assessed before surgery to obtain a baseline value. Preoperative anemia should be brought to the attention of the veterinarian in charge, and, if present, a CBC should be performed. If substantial blood loss occurred during surgery, the PCV and TP should also be assessed postoperatively. It can be difficult to determine if an animal is hemorrhaging or has lost a substantial amount of blood immediately postoperative because a painful, recovering animal can have similar clinical signs. Temperature, heart rate, pulse quality, respiration, and character of mucous membranes should be examined periodically during and after surgery. Animals with substantial blood loss may experience continued hypothermia or a drop in body temperature, rapid heart rate with weak peripheral pulses, rapid respiratory rate, and pale or white mucous membranes. Abnormalities should be promptly reported to the veterinarian in charge. Other signs include abdominal enlargement if intraabdominal hemorrhage occurs, incision swelling or oozing of blood, and dyspnea and decreased ventral lung sounds if intrathoracic hemorrhage occurs. Another important thing to remember is that changes in PCV and TP may not occur immediately with blood loss, and these tests may need to be repeated a few hours after the incident of blood loss to document abnormalities or to assess continued blood loss. It is not unusual for the PCV and TP to drop 10% just as a result of anesthesia and surgery, even when no major blood loss occurred.

Besides PCV and TP determination, abdominocentesis (aspiration of fluid from the abdomen), thoracocentesis (aspiration of fluid from the thoracic cavity), or fine-needle aspiration beneath the incision can be performed when the patient is suspected of having substantial bleeding. If the sampled fluid has a PCV nearly equal to the systemic PCV and clinical signs are consistent with hemorrhage, the index of suspicion should be high. Treatment strategies include crystalloid fluid bolus, colloidal fluid administration, blood transfusion, oxygen carrier fluid administration (Oxyglobin), pressure bandages, and/or reoperation with ligation of bleeding vessels. The treatment of choice depends on the animal's status and ability to maintain a stable condition. The reader should review the clinical signs and treatment strategies for various types of shock as discussed in Chapter 33.

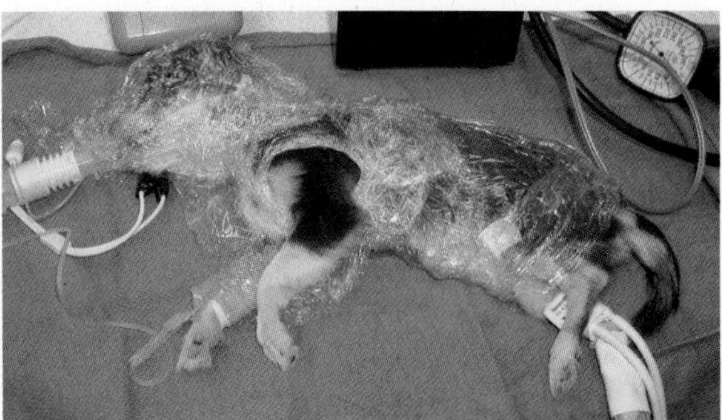

FIGURE 30-1 One method of heat retention during surgery is to wrap the animal in plastic. This works well for small dogs and cats.

HYPOTHERMIA

Hypothermia is defined as a subnormal body temperature. Once an animal is anesthetized, its body temperature begins to drop. It is important to monitor body temperature throughout general anesthesia and during recovery. All anesthetized animals should be placed on a heated circulating water blanket that is covered with a towel to help maintain body temperature, especially small dogs and all cats, during surgery. Although rare, if the body temperature rises above normal during the procedure, the heat source can be turned off. Small animals become hypothermic quickly when placed under general anesthesia, especially if a body cavity is opened. It is important to remember that the more surface area exposed (i.e., large incision exposing the abdominal organs), the faster and lower the body temperature is expected to drop. If the exposed area is moist, evaporative cooling occurs. Mechanisms to maintain body temperature during surgery include placing animals on heated circulating water blankets; wrapping paws and the body in plastic wrap to prevent heat loss (Figure 30-1); wrapping warm water bottles (or gloves filled with warm water) with a towel and placing them next to the animal; covering areas not involved in the surgical procedure with an insulated blanket; and using a warm air blanket (Bair Hugger, Arizant Healthcare, Inc.) on areas not involved in the surgical procedure. Heat lamps are not recommended because they can cause thermal burns, especially in an anesthetized animal that cannot respond to painful, concentrated heat. It must be remembered that electric heating pads should never be used to warm anesthetized animals. Electric heating pads concentrate heat and cause thermal burns (Figure 30-2). The veterinarian is liable for burns caused by electric heat units because it is a known cause of thermal skin injury during anesthesia.

After surgery, the animal is placed in a warm area to recover with a heated circulating water blanket. If the patient is severely hypothermic, a warm air blanket and/or warm water bath can be used to raise the temperature quickly (Figure 30-3). A warm water bath is made by filling a large, deep pan, big enough to place the entire animal in, three-fourths full with warm water, placing a thick garbage bag over the pan and water, and placing a towel over the garbage

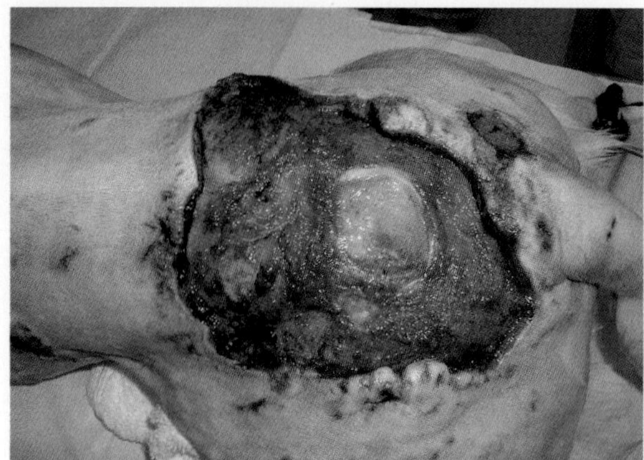

FIGURE 30-2 The area of denuded skin over the rump of this dog is a result of a thermal burn sustained from an electric heating pad used to maintain body temperature during ovariohysterectomy.

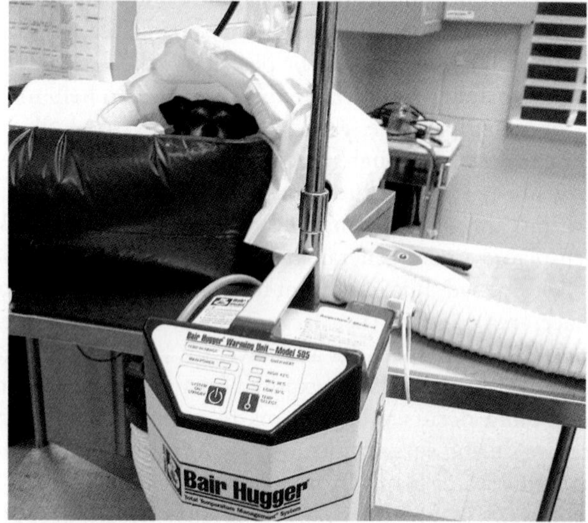

FIGURE 30-3 Blankets that blow warm air and warm water baths can be used to bring the body temperature up quickly. Notice the dog placed under the blue hot air blanket in a well-constructed water bath.

bag where the animal is to be placed (similar to a heated water bed). The animal is placed in the water bath allowing the warm water to "wrap" around the animal; the plastic prevents soaking. The animal must be monitored closely to prevent accidental puncture of the plastic and drowning (Figure 30-4). Only small dogs and cats can be warmed in this way.

Body temperature should show a steady rise as the animal recovers. When the animal's temperature approaches 100° F, heating sources can be discontinued, but the animal should be kept covered, and body temperature should be reevaluated periodically to ensure that it returns to and remains normal. If the temperature remains low or continues to fall, it may be an indication of a potential problem, and the veterinarian in charge should be alerted. Heat should be reapplied if the animal's body temperature begins to drop after heat sources are removed.

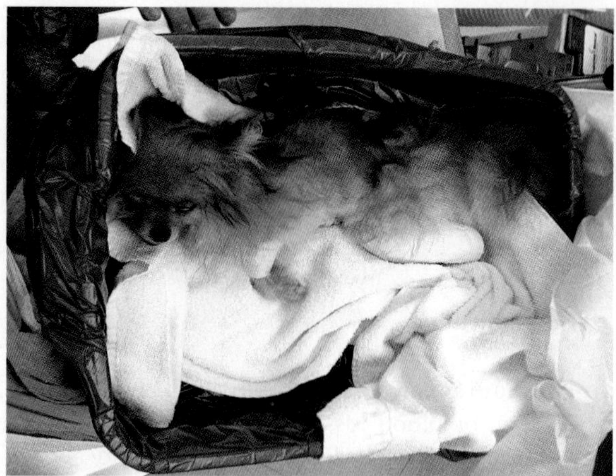

FIGURE 30-4 This is a close-up of a water bath. A large container is filled with warm water and covered with thick plastic and a towel. The dog or cat is placed on the towel in the container and is allowed to sink down into the warm water with the plastic preventing soaking. The animal must be monitored carefully to prevent accidental puncture of the plastic and drowning.

PAIN

Intraoperative and postoperative pain assessment is important for animal well-being and health. During surgery, increases in heart rate, respiratory rate, and blood pressure and lightening of the anesthetic plane can indicate that the animal is in pain. During recovery, animals that are in pain, among other things, may vocalize, have elevated heart and respiratory rates, thrash, bite or chew at the surgery site, and/or become aggressive. Other signs of pain include a disinterest in the environment, crying upon manipulation, insomnia, and lack of appetite (Figure 30-5). It should be remembered that changes in vital signs can mean numerous things (e.g., elevated heart rate could also signify substantial blood loss). The animal should be carefully evaluated by the technician and surgeon before drug administration. It is best not to allow the animal to experience pain before giving pain medication. If an incision was made, pain is going to be experienced by the animal. It is up to the veterinary technician and surgeon to decide how much pain a particular procedure might cause. Painful procedures include fracture repair, amputation, declaw, joint surgery, and any major abdominal procedure. Moderately painful procedures include minor abdominal procedures (spay, cystotomy) and simple body wall hernia repair. Mildly painful procedures might include simple mass removal or biopsy. It can be difficult to determine how much pain an animal is in because animals respond so differently to pain. Some animals may act as if in pain after spay, whereas others may not, even though they are both likely experiencing pain. When in doubt, it should be assumed that the animal is having some degree of postoperative discomfort.

Pain treatment is accomplished in several ways, and it depends on the animal, availability of pain medications, and the type of procedure that was performed as to what sort of

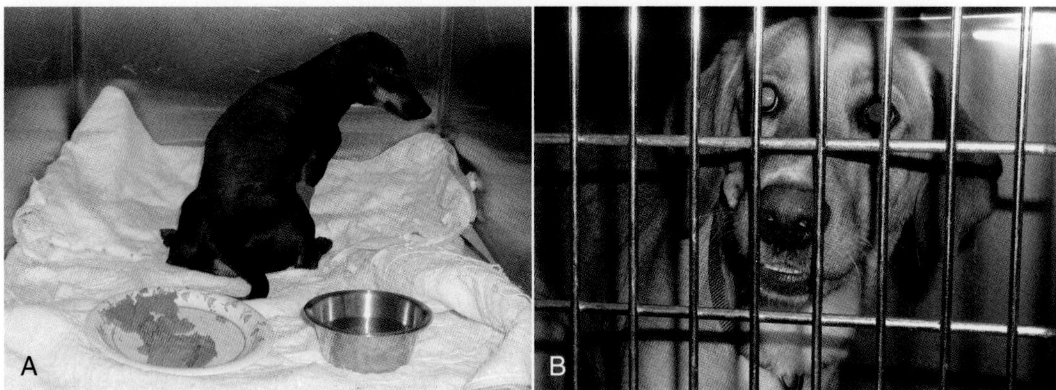

FIGURE 30-5 Note how the dog in **(A)** does not turn to face the door even when it is opened. Also note the full food dish in the front of the cage. This is a dog suffering from severe spinal pain and is uninterested in her environment. Comfortable animals are often interested in their surroundings and will come to the cage door to greet you. In spite of her tibia fracture, the dog in **(B)** is more than willing to interact with those around her.

regimen is chosen. Most soft tissue surgical pain will last 4 to 5 days after surgery. For bone and joint procedures, this should be extended another 4 to 5 days. It is best to preemptively manage pain rather than wait for the animal to show pain before administration of pain medication. If the animal is allowed to experience pain before administration of pain medication, then the pain is harder to treat and may not be relieved by the medication administered (see Chapter 26). Pain medication should be administered before surgery in the premedicants, and they should be continued throughout the surgical procedure and into the postoperative period according to the dosing regimen for the particular drug used. A wait-and-see attitude should never be adopted because this allows the animal to experience pain before treatment is given.

Another misconception is that animals will stay quiet and calm if they are in pain, so avoidance of pain medication is a form of treatment. You would never be treated that way in a hospital, and animals should not be treated that way. This is an ethical dilemma many veterinarians and technicians must face. An appropriately managed animal will likely sleep for several hours after surgery, should be comfortable when manipulated, should be alert and interested in its environment when aroused, and will likely be willing to eat and drink.

> *TECHNICIAN NOTE* The animal should not be allowed to be in pain before the medication is given. Pain medication should be administered at dosing intervals appropriate for the medication administered, not as needed.

INCISION EVALUATION

Visual and palpable inspection of the surgical wound should be made daily (see Chapter 34 for detailed information on wounds and healing). The surgical incision is usually left uncovered after surgery. Ointments and creams (even antibiotic topicals) should not be placed on the incision because this can cause irritation, and components of the ointment can delay wound healing. The incision can be covered with an adhesive or a wrap bandage for the first few days after surgery to keep the incision clean, prevent contact with the hospital environment, and absorb seepage.

Abnormalities that can occur in the early postoperative period (1 to 3 days) include redness, swelling, drainage, and dehiscence (wound breakdown). An incision should be evaluated with respect to the type of surgical procedure performed. Elective operations, such as ovariohysterectomy and castration, can be expected to produce mild redness and swelling with no drainage from the incision site (Figure 30-6). However, if the wound was contaminated (e.g., laceration, perianal wound) or if the surgical exposure was extensive, the incision is expected to be somewhat swollen, reddened, and warm to the touch and have mild to moderate drainage in the first 24 to 48 hours postoperatively (see Figure 30-6). Swelling secondary to surgical trauma will usually resolve within 3 to 7 days after surgery. However, seromas (serum accumulation under the incision) and hematomas (blood accumulation under the incision) may persist for weeks.

Surprisingly, most animals will not lick or chew at the surgical incision. Animals will usually lick or chew at the incision only if the character of the incision is irritating. Contributors to incision irritation include sutures placed too tight, traumatic tissue handling, suture reaction, tension on the suture line, clipper burn, prepping irritation, incision infection, and seroma formation. Only rarely will an animal chew the sutures because they are bored. Using appropriate suture technique will minimize incision self-trauma. However, if an animal begins to traumatize the incision via licking or scratching, an Elizabethan collar, bandage, neck brace, T-shirt, and/or chemical restraint should be used to protect the incision.

Seromas can form if extensive surgical dissection occurred beneath the incision, tissue planes could not be or were not adequately closed, or excessive motion occurs at the incision site. Seromas are recognized as localized areas of fluctuant swellings that are not usually painful or warm to the touch (Figure 30-7). Seromas will usually resolve without treatment. Warm compresses, hydrotherapy, and bandaging

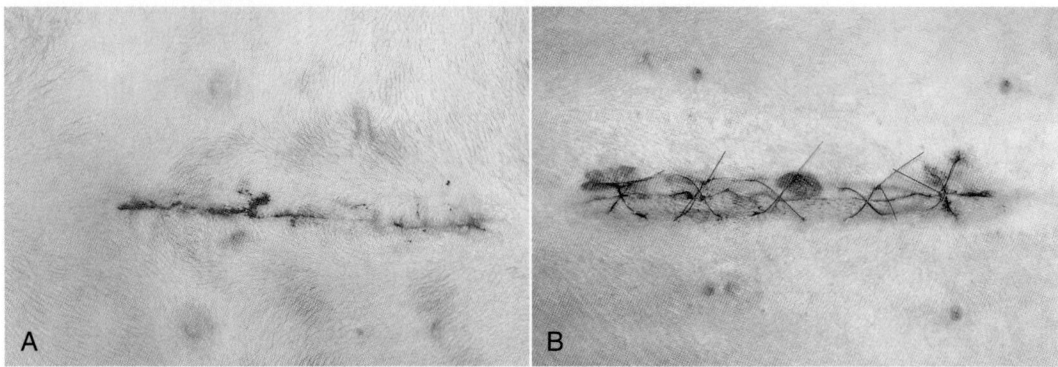

FIGURE 30-6 These photographs were taken 4 hours after surgery. **A** shows a celiotomy incision following routine ovariohysterectomy, whereas **B** shows a celiotomy incision following severe traction on the skin during surgery for exposure. Note the minimal redness, swelling, and drainage from incision **(A)** compared with incision **(B)**.

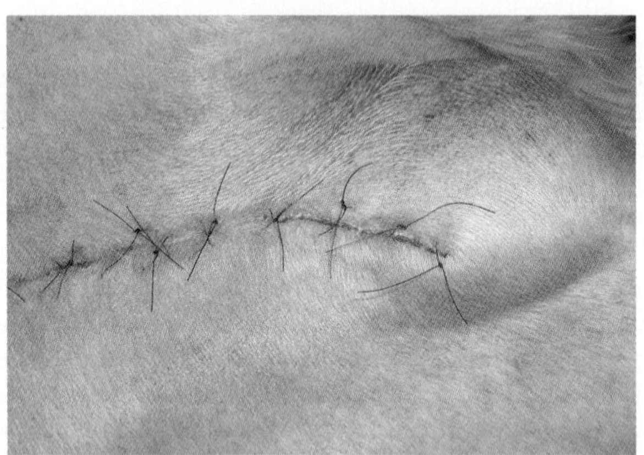

FIGURE 30-7 Note the swelling beneath the incision on cranial thigh of this dog. The swelling was nonpainful, and the dog's vital signs were normal. The swelling was diagnosed as a seroma.

may aid in resolution. If the seroma is large and/or is causing impairment, drainage is warranted. Drainage should be performed aseptically, and an active, closed drain should be placed. It is important to keep animals calm in the postoperative period to decrease the chance of seroma occurrence. Hematomas are treated the same way.

> *TECHNICIAN NOTE* Repeated aspiration of seromas can result in infection and should be avoided. If an area must be aspirated, it should be aseptically prepared before aspiration. Suspected abscesses should be aseptically aspirated for cytology and culture, but there is no reason to aspirate a suspected seroma unless for the purpose of treatment, which is rare.

If incision swelling occurs 4 to 6 days postoperative, is warm to the touch, or is associated with an elevated body temperature, reddened, and/or draining, the possibility of infection or cellulitis (infection along tissue planes) must be considered (Figure 30-8). Abscess or infection or cellulites must be treated by drainage, warm compresses, and systemic antibiotics. Some infected incisions can be flushed and managed with an active, closed suction drain, but others will require open wound management (see Chapter 35 for details on infected and open wound management).

Wound dehiscence is defined as the separation of all layers of an incision or wound. Early recognition is imperative in any wound, but especially in abdominal and thoracic incisions. Dehiscence is most often due to technical error in suture technique, but incision complications can also play a role. Things that will contribute to wound dehiscence include using inappropriate suture to close a wound, inappropriate suturing technique, tension on the incision line, incision infection, seroma formation, or disease and/or drug therapy leading to delayed wound healing. Rarely would an animal self-mutilate an incision and cause dehiscence (see previous discussion).

Early detection of surgical incision problems is of paramount importance to help prevent more serious complications. If dehiscence is suspected, the reason for dehiscence should be ascertained. If the external suture layer (skin) is dehiscing and it is only partial, conservative management may be possible. The open portion of the wound will heal by second intention. However, the open wound will likely need to be bandaged and the animal placed in an Elizabethan collar to prevent licking of the open wound and further dehiscence. If the phase of healing is early (first few days after surgery), cleansing and closure of the incision may be necessary depending on the degree of dehiscence. Dehiscence of deeper layers can be more serious and should be brought to the attention of the veterinarian in charge as soon as possible, especially if the incision involves the abdominal or thoracic cavity. Complete dehiscence of an abdominal wound can result in evisceration (exposure) of the abdominal organs, with subsequent contamination and infection (Figure 30-9). Complete dehiscence of a thoracic wound will result in a pneumothorax (air within the chest causing collapse of the lungs), a problem that may result in sudden death.

> *TECHNICIAN NOTE* Dehiscence of an abdominal wound or thoracic wall can result in life-threatening complications. The veterinarian should be alerted immediately of impending complications.

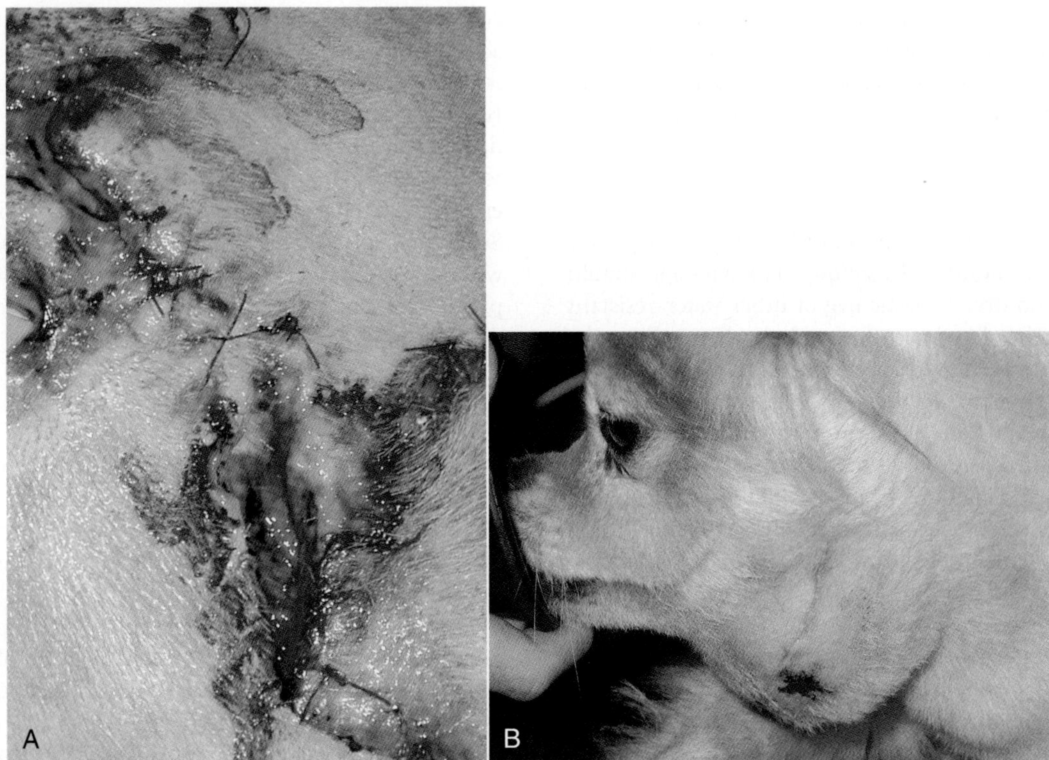

FIGURE 30-8 Incisional infection is recognized by drainage, redness, swelling, fever, dehiscence, and/or abscess formation. Notice the purulent discharge and partial dehiscence of the incision in **(A)**. **B** shows an abscess that recently ruptured.

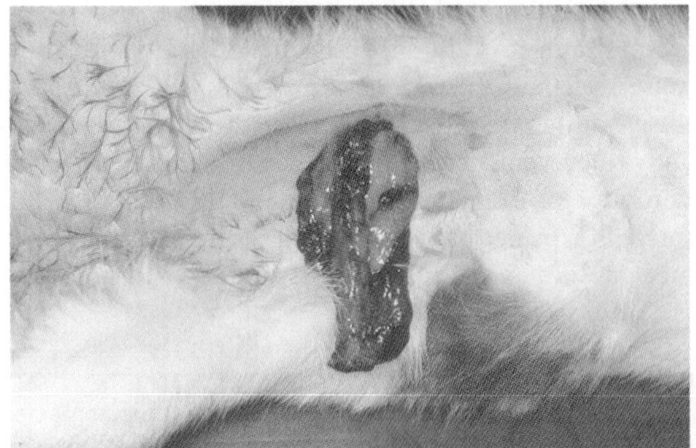

FIGURE 30-9 Complete dehiscence of an abdominal incision. Note the intraabdominal contents protruding through the incision.

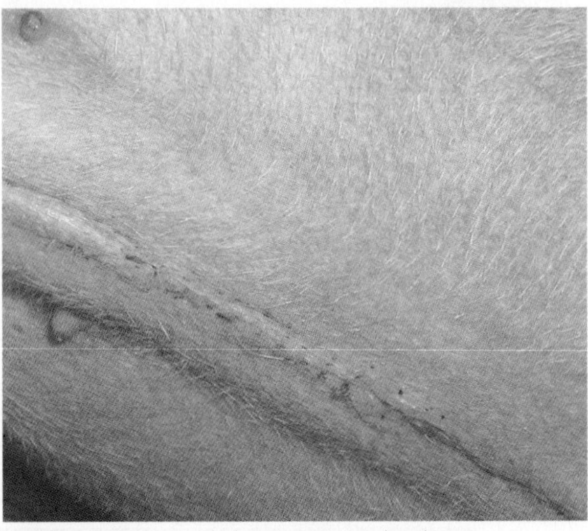

FIGURE 30-10 Healed incision. Note that the incision is not red, swollen, or draining. The skin edges are apposed, and the scar is slightly raised. This photo was taken 12 days after surgery.

SUTURE REMOVAL

Suture removal is commonly performed by the veterinary technician. The procedure is usually performed 10 to 14 days after surgery because this is the approximate time that the wound is beginning to strengthen (see Chapter 34). If internal sutures were placed in the dermis with the external skin sutures, external suture removal can be performed in 5 to 7 days because the internal suture layer will hold the incision closed while healing continues. The incision should be inspected carefully for adequate healing before removal. A healed incision is usually confluent, slightly raised, and whitish in color and has no gaps between skin edges (Figure 30-10). An appropriately healed incision should not be draining, severely reddened, or severely swollen. However, if complications were encountered, then some reddening, swelling, and excessive scarring is expected. Incisions that are swollen, draining, reddened, or have obvious separation should be inspected by the veterinarian in charge before suture removal.

Skin sutures are usually easy to remove in the calm animal. Suture scissors are simple to use and allow removal with minimal discomfort. The suture should be grasped with thumb forceps or your finger. Gentle traction is placed on the suture, and the suture is cut near the skin surface (Figure 30-11). The suture is manually pulled out of the skin after cutting. If metal staples were placed, a staple remover should be used to allow removal with minimal discomfort (Figure 30-12).

BANDAGE CARE

If a bandage was placed, the limb in which the bandage was placed should be monitored carefully. The bandage should be kept clean and dry. A plastic bag or other water-resistant covering should be placed over the bandage when walking the animal outside and removed once back inside. The plastic will prevent the bandage from getting wet, but it should not be left in place because moisture will accumulate under the plastic if left on for extended periods of time. The animal's toes should be checked twice daily for swelling or coldness as long as a limb bandage is in place. This is especially important immediately after placement. Swollen toes might be an indication the bandage is too tight. If the bandage gets wet, dirty, has an odor, or the toes become swollen or cold, it should be changed. A soiled, wet bandage can lead to sore formation and incision infection. Bandages placed too tight can result in vascular compromise to the skin with death and sloughing. Bandages are changed at intervals designated by the veterinarian in charge and depending on the reason for placement. Bandages covering open wounds will have to be changed daily. Some wounds drain excessively, causing serum to seep through the bandage and extend to the external environment. This is called strike-through (Figure 30-13). Strike-through must be prevented to help prevent wound infection. The bandage must be changed multiple times a day under such circumstances (see Chapter 34 for information on bandaging wounds).

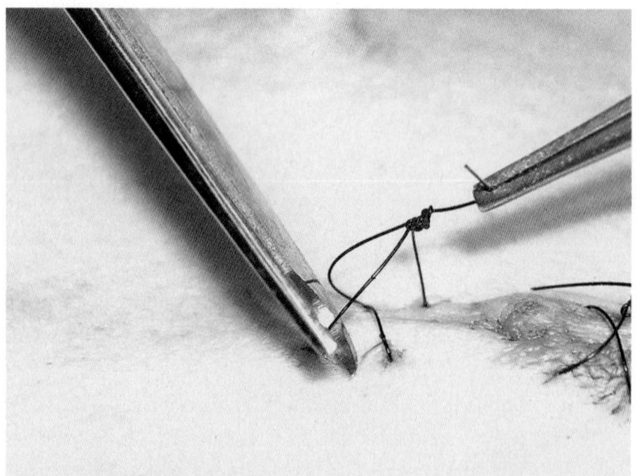

FIGURE 30-11 Suture removal. The suture is grasped with forceps or fingers and gently tensioned. It is cut with suture scissors near the skin and then pulled with slow, steady traction until it is completely removed.

DRAIN CARE

Drains are placed to collect fluid under a wound (surgical incision). They are often placed when large amounts of tissue are resected (mammary chains, amputation, large skin masses) or when a large amount of drainage is expected (a contaminated or infected wound). If a drain is placed, the drain exit site should be kept covered with a bandage. Additionally the animal should be placed in an Elizabethan collar to prevent premature removal or drain breakage by the animal. Active drains (drains that are sealed to the environment and actively collect fluid from the wound into a reservoir) should be emptied as needed (Figure 30-14). Passive drains (drains that provide an exit port for fluid to the external environment) should be avoided because of risk of ascending bacterial infection and difficult maintenance as a result of constant drainage of fluid through the drain exit site, though they are placed under some circumstances (see Figure 30-14). If passive drains are used, the bandage should be changed frequently to prevent strike-through. Drains are removed when the amount of drainage has substantially decreased. Some drainage is expected as long as a drain is in place as a result of tissue irritation by the drain, but it should be minimal.

> *TECHNICIAN NOTE* Some drainage is expected as long as a drain is in place as a result of tissue irritation by the drain, but it should be minimal.

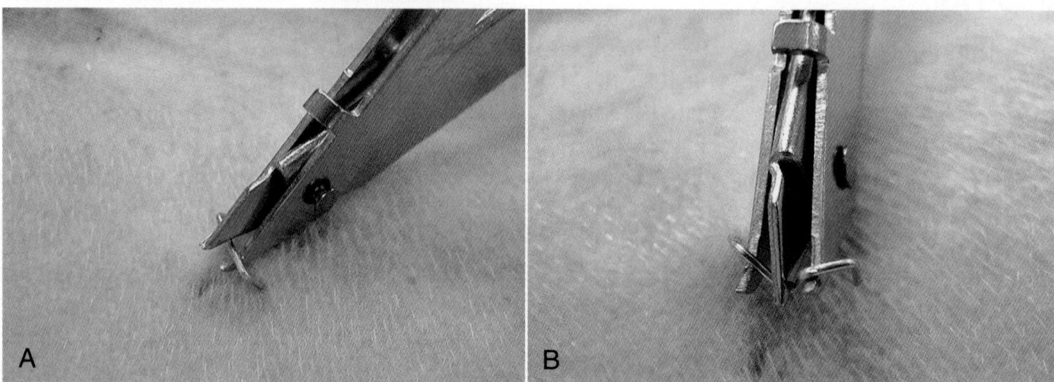

FIGURE 30-12 Staple removal. Staple remover is used. **A,** Staple remover is slipped under the staple. **B,** Staple remover is closed, causing the staple to be folded at its midsection and the teeth on either end of the staple to be dislodged from the skin.

RESTRAINT

Animal restraint is important for appropriate surgical technique. Naturally the animal will have to be manually restrained during the preoperative examination and sample collection; however, surgical restraint involves sedation and/or general anesthesia. The type of surgical procedure dictates whether simple sedation or general or local anesthesia will be required. The specifics of anesthetic drug administration are covered in Chapter 27 and should be reviewed. Appropriate protocol should be discussed with the surgeon before surgery so that preparation of the animal and the operating room can be initiated.

All animals should be well controlled after surgery to minimize complications. The length and severity of confinement depend on the type of procedure performed. Animals undergoing routine sterilization or simple mass removal usually require 10 to 14 days of restricted activity, whereas animals undergoing orthopedic surgery will likely require 6 to 8 weeks of confinement. No animal should be allowed to roam free immediately after surgery. Additionally, self-trauma should be prevented.

Besides crate, leash, and room confinement, chemical agents and mechanical devices can also be used for restraint.

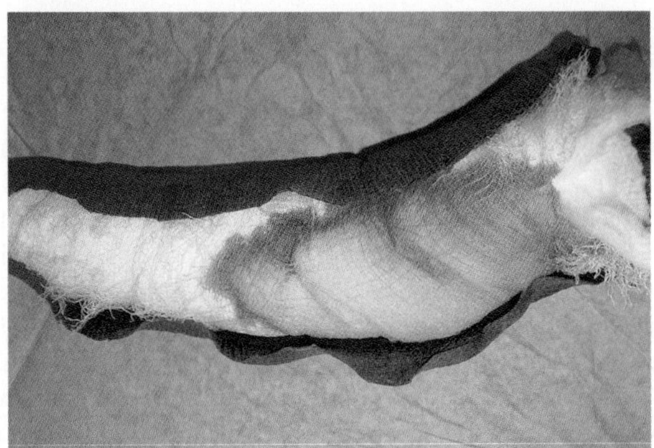

FIGURE 30-13 Strike-through. Notice red-tinged fluid seeping through the bandage from the wound bed.

Tranquilizers and noxious-tasting substances are commonly used chemical restraints. Tranquilizers must be used with caution because they can have undesirable side effects. They are not meant to be used long term. Phenothiazine derivatives (acepromazine) are commonly used tranquilizers in veterinary medicine, but α_2-adrenergic agonists, benzodiazepines, and cyclohexamines are also used (see Chapter 27 for more information on drugs used for sedation). Appropriate crate or room confinement usually will suffice without the addition of tranquilization.

Noxious-tasting agents are used to prevent animals from licking or chewing, and they must also be used with discretion. Some commonly used substances include Bandguard Cream (Schering-Plough), Bitter Apple (Grannick's), Tabasco, and various thumb-sucking preparations. The agent can be impregnated into bandage material, and some can be placed directly on the skin around the incision. These agents should never be placed directly on the incision because they can burn, irritate the incision, and have the potential to delay wound healing.

Mechanical restraint devices include the Elizabethan collar, the body brace, the side bar, hobbles, and various bandages. These devices are used to limit motion, prevent licking and chewing, and prevent weight bearing. The assembly, materials necessary, specific indications, contraindications, and complications have been adequately described elsewhere (see Chapter 34 and Recommended Reading) and are beyond the scope of this chapter. A properly selected, constructed, and applied device will be well tolerated by the animal and effective for its desired purpose.

COMMON SURGICAL PROCEDURES

The veterinary technician must have a working knowledge of common surgical procedures to properly prepare an animal preoperatively, act as an efficient surgical assistant, and manage the immediate and long-term postoperative care. The remainder of this chapter reviews common small animal surgical procedures performed in veterinary practice. A brief

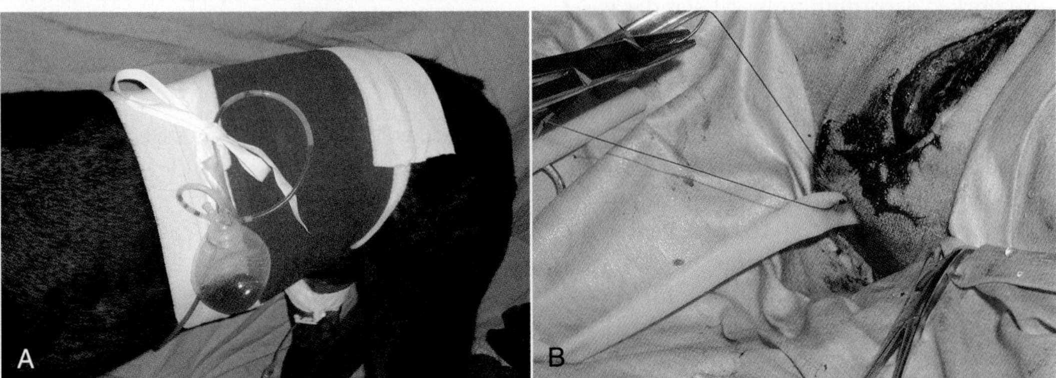

FIGURE 30-14 Drains. **A,** Active drains actively suck fluid from the wound bed into a sealed reservoir and are preferred over passive drains. **B,** Passive drains are placed under incisions and just provide surface area for fluid to drain from the wound with gravitational forces. They are more prone to ascending infection and are harder to manage. In photo **B** the wound is being closed over a rubber drain *(yellow)*. The incision and drain will be bandaged afterward.

description of the procedure, with emphasis on the role of the veterinary technician, will be given.

> *TECHNICIAN NOTE* The veterinary technician must have a working knowledge of common surgical procedures to properly prepare the animal for surgery, act as an efficient surgical assistant, and manage the immediate and long-term postoperative care.

ELECTIVE VERSUS NONELECTIVE SURGERY

Surgical procedures are divided into elective and nonelective. Elective procedures are performed at the veterinarian and owner's convenience, usually in healthy animals. Spay, castration, and declaw are examples of such procedures. Some procedures must be done to improve the animal's quality of life, but are not necessarily urgent, such as stifle stabilization for cranial cruciate ligament rupture, correction of patella luxation, and cancer resection. For these procedures, if animals are not ideal candidates for surgery at the time of presentation, surgery can be delayed. However, ideally, surgery would be performed at some point to alleviate the animal's clinical signs or to decrease the chance of tumor spread. Nonelective surgical procedures must be done urgently. These are usually emergency procedures performed on compromised animals.

TAIL DOCKING ON PUPPIES

DEFINITION

Tail docking refers to partial amputation (removal) of the tail.

INDICATIONS

Tail docking in young puppies is specifically performed for aesthetic reasons. Dog breeders have traditionally developed breed standards by alteration of the breed character with surgery. Tails are docked according to breed standards set forth by the American Kennel Club.

PREOPERATIVE CONSIDERATIONS

The dam can get upset as puppies are removed from her presence for the procedure. Some dams will even become aggressive. Care must be taken with removal and replacement of the puppies from the nest. If the dam becomes too upset, it may be necessary to place her in another room while the procedure is performed on the puppies. Alternatively, some dams are more comfortable in the same room with the puppies.

Tail docking should be performed during the first week of life (3 to 5 days of age). At this age, the procedure can be performed without general anesthesia and is minimally traumatic to the dam and puppies. It must be remembered that puppies of this age are immunogenetically naive. It is important to perform the procedure in an area where the puppies will not be exposed to a high concentration of infectious agents.

TECHNIQUE AND INTRAOPERATIVE CONSIDERATIONS

The puppy should be cradled in the palm of both hands with the hind limbs held between the index and middle fingers and the tail directed toward the surgeon. The surgical site is prepared using aseptic technique. The desired length of remaining tail is marked, and the skin of the tail is retracted craniad (toward the base of the tail). The tail is amputated with a pair of scissors, bleeding is controlled with electrocautery or pressure, and the skin is released, allowing it to retract over the exposed bone. One simple interrupted absorbable suture is placed to appose the skin edges, or the edges are glued with a tissue adhesive. If a surgical laser is used to remove the claws, the technician should ensure that the appropriate equipment and eye protection is available for the surgical team and that the surgery site is not prepared with alcohol. Furthermore, the technician must also be available to vacuum the emitted smoke from the laser because this smoke is harmful to people and animals.

POSTOPERATIVE CONSIDERATIONS

The puppies should be returned to the mother as soon as hemorrhage is controlled. The surgical site should be monitored for the first few hours for excessive bleeding. During the week following surgery, the tail should be monitored for drainage, redness, and swelling daily. The suture remains until it is absorbed or licked out by the mother. Complications are not expected following tail docking, but may include hemorrhage and infection. In some animals, too much skin is removed during the amputation. Those animals may have chronic wound healing problems and bone exposure at the amputation site. Revision of the surgery site may be necessary to correct the problem.

DEWCLAW REMOVAL ON PUPPIES

DEFINITION

The claws located on the medial aspect of the forelegs and hind limbs are known as dewclaws. Dewclaw removal is amputation of the claw.

INDICATIONS

Dewclaws are commonly removed from the forefeet and hind feet of purebred dogs for aesthetic reasons and from hunting dogs because they may be torn as the dog runs over terrain densely covered with shrubs. It should be remembered that in certain breeds (e.g., Great Pyrenees, Newfoundland) the presence of dewclaws is necessary for proper show quality.

PREOPERATIVE CONSIDERATIONS

The preoperative considerations are the same as those described earlier.

TECHNIQUE AND INTRAOPERATIVE CONSIDERATIONS

Dewclaws should be removed during the first week of life (3 to 5 days). Removal is generally performed at the same time as tail docking in most breeds. The surgical site is prepared aseptically. The puppy is cradled in the palm of one hand, and the extremity is extended with the other hand. Scissors are used to amputate the claw. Hemorrhage is controlled with electrocautery or pressure. The skin edges may be left to heal by second intention or apposed with one absorbable suture.

POSTOPERATIVE CONSIDERATIONS

The puppies are returned to the mother immediately. The surgical site should be monitored for the first few hours for excessive bleeding. During the week following surgery, the amputation site should be monitored for drainage, redness, and swelling daily. Complications are not expected following dewclaw removal, but may include hemorrhage and infection.

TAIL DOCKING AND DEWCLAW REMOVAL IN THE ADULT

Tail docking and dewclaw removal should ideally be done within the first week of life if it is performed for aesthetic purposes. In some instances, adult dogs are seen for one or both procedures.

INDICATIONS

Indications for tail docking or dewclaw removal in the adult dog include aesthetics, trauma, infection, and neoplasia.

PREOPERATIVE CONSIDERATIONS

One must consider the reason for tail or claw amputation before animal prepping and initiation of the procedure. If it is done to treat cancer, acceptable tumor-free margins should be taken with the removed tissue, and the appropriate amount of skin must be prepared before surgery. Removed tissues will have to be placed in formalin at a 1:10 ratio for eventual histopathologic evaluation. If trauma is the reason for the procedure, the animal may have to be stabilized before surgery can safely be performed. If amputation is performed as a treatment for infection, the veterinary technician should have culture swabs available so that the veterinarian can obtain appropriate cultures at the time of surgery.

TECHNIQUE AND INTRAOPERATIVE CONSIDERATIONS FOR DEWCLAW REMOVAL

The animal must be placed under general anesthesia. The surgical site is clipped and prepared using aseptic technique. The surgeon will make an elliptical incision at the base of the dewclaw. The dewclaw is dissected free and is transected at the carpometacarpal joint in the front paw or the tarsometatarsal joint in the hind paw. Hemorrhage is controlled with suture, electrocautery, laser, and/or direct pressure. If a surgical laser is used to remove the claws, the technician should ensure that the appropriate equipment and eye protection is available for the surgical team and that the surgery site is not prepared with alcohol. Furthermore, the technician must also be available to vacuum the emitted smoke from the laser because this smoke is harmful to people and animals. The skin edges are apposed with suture. The paw is usually bandaged to prevent swelling and self-trauma.

TECHNIQUE AND INTRAOPERATIVE CONSIDERATIONS FOR TAIL AMPUTATION

The tail should be clipped and hung from an intravenous stand. The skin should be prepared using aseptic technique. If the tail is to be amputated near the base, the rump adjacent to the tail base must also be clipped and aseptically prepared. A tourniquet may be placed at the base of the tail to help control hemorrhage and is placed before the animal is draped for surgery. The tail is amputated at the desired location by skin incision and disarticulation of the caudal vertebra at the appropriate site. The skin incision is made 1 or 2 cm distal to the expected amputation site to ensure adequate skin coverage of the stump. Blood vessels are identified and ligated. The skin edges are sutured over the remaining vertebrae, and the tourniquet is removed.

POSTOPERATIVE CONSIDERATIONS

The surgical sites should be monitored for hemorrhage, swelling, drainage, redness, evidence of self-trauma, and dehiscence. Elizabethan collars should be placed on those animals attempting to traumatize the surgical site. Bandages placed on the foot should be maintained as previously discussed. If placed, skin sutures are removed in 10 to 14 days. Pain medication is generally needed for 4 to 5 days following the procedure. Complications are rare for these procedures, even in adult animals.

FELINE ONYCHECTOMY

DEFINITION

Onychectomy (declawing) is removal of the claw and its associated third phalanx.

INDICATIONS

Onychectomy is an elective procedure to prevent scratching of owners and household items. Most veterinarians recommend declawing the front feet only. This does not significantly impair the cat's ability to climb trees or defend itself from intruders. Onychectomy is often performed at the same time as castration or ovariohysterectomy.

PREOPERATIVE CONSIDERATIONS

Onychectomy is a painful procedure. Preoperative analgesics should be administered.

TECHNIQUE AND INTRAOPERATIVE CONSIDERATIONS

The cat is placed under general anesthesia. The feet are surgically scrubbed, but need not be clipped unless the cat is a long-haired breed. If a laser is to be used during the procedure, alcohol should not be used to prepare the toes because it is flammable and likely to ignite when the laser beam strikes the soaked area. The nails are left long to aid in nail manipulation during the procedure (Figure 30-15). A tourniquet is usually placed to control hemorrhage during the procedure. It should be placed over the foot before aseptic preparation, but tightened when the surgeon is ready to perform the procedure. The tourniquet should always be placed distal to the elbow to prevent nerve damage (Figure 30-16). The radial nerve is more superficial just proximal to the elbow and can be permanently damaged if the tourniquet is tightened over that area (see Figure 30-16). The tourniquet should only remain in place for no more than 1.5 hours. The veterinarian should be alerted as that time approaches so the tourniquet can be removed.

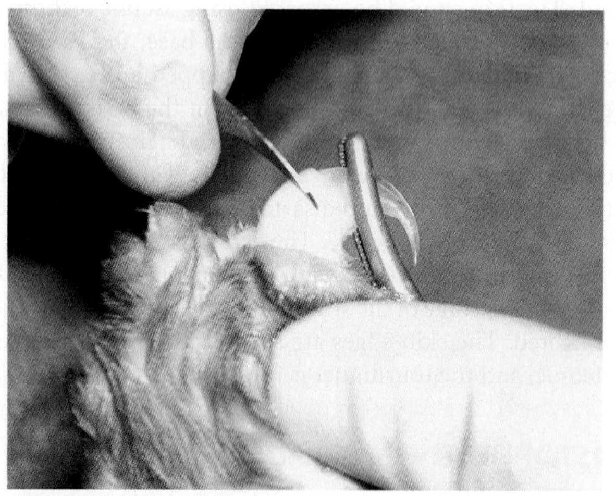

FIGURE 30-15 Declaw. The nail is not trimmed before surgery to aid in nail manipulation.

Three techniques can be used to remove the claws. The Rescoe (nail trimmer technique), scalpel blade, and the CO_2 laser techniques are all effective means to perform the procedure. For the Rescoe technique, a Rescoe nail trimmer is positioned snugly onto the dorsal surface of the toe between the second phalanx and third phalanx. During positioning of the nail trimmer, the claw should be pulled cranially. As little skin as possible should be excised. The cutting edge of the Rescoe nail trimmer is positioned at the cranial edge of the footpad. As the cutting edge is advanced, the pad is moved caudally while rotating the nail dorsally and caudally. The third phalanx is then excised by the Rescoe nail trimmer. Care is taken to prevent cutting the footpad. Each nail is amputated in a similar fashion. A portion of the third phalanx is usually left behind with this technique, but the entire germinal layer is removed to prevent regrowth of the nail. The blade technique amputates the entire third phalanx using a No. 12 scalpel blade. The phalanx is disarticulated dorsolaterally, first by cutting through the collateral ligaments, then the nail is cut away from the underlying tissue and digital pad. The pad is moved out of the way while the nail is removed to prevent inadvertent laceration.

The laser technique is similar to the blade technique except that it uses laser energy to dissect the third phalanx free from the second phalanx instead of a sharp edge. The surgical site usually does not bleed with the laser technique, so a tourniquet is not necessary. If a laser is used, the technician should ensure that plenty of saline-soaked sponges are available to cover the remainder of the cat's foot, instruments, and surgeon's fingers to absorb extraneous laser energy and prevent iatrogenic laser burns. It is best to use instruments approved for laser surgery to prevent reflected laser beams from inappropriately penetrating objects and tissues. Everyone in

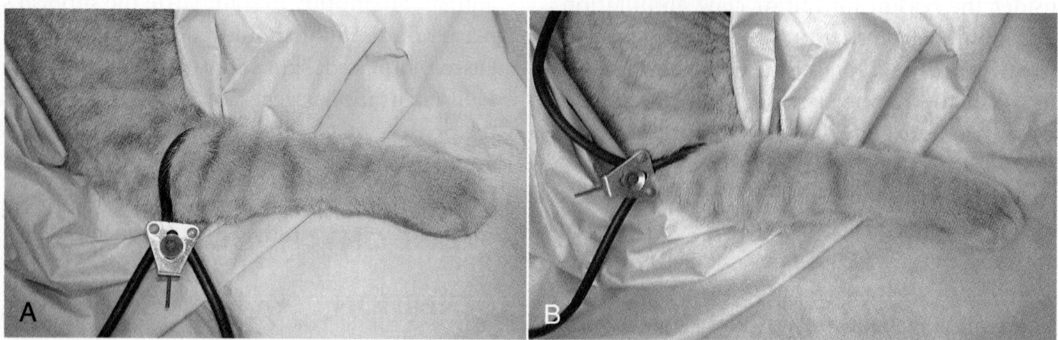

FIGURE 30-16 Declaw. A tourniquet should always be placed, distal to the elbow **(A)** rather than proximal to the elbow **(B)** to help prevent permanent radial nerve damage.

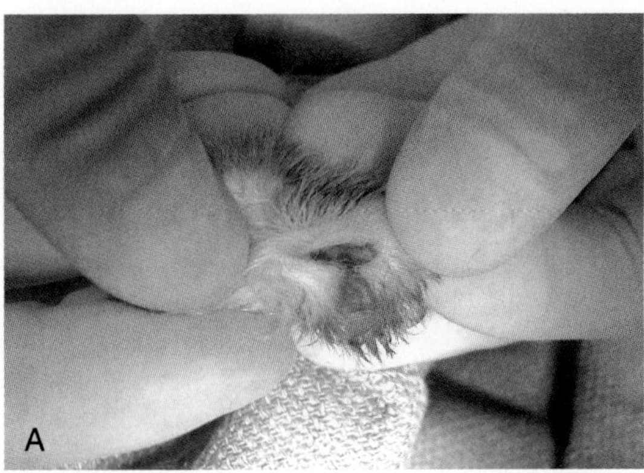

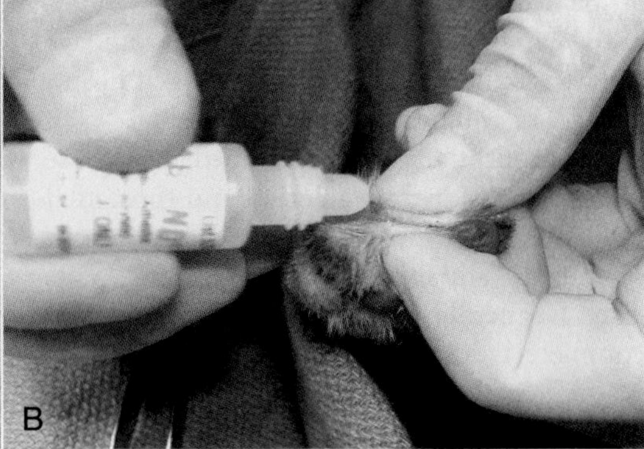

FIGURE 30-17 Declaw. **A,** When applying tissue adhesive to a wound, the glue should never be placed inside the wound created from removing the claw. **B,** The wound should be manually apposed and the glue placed along the skin edges.

the room should wear safety glasses to prevent inadvertent ocular damage, and the technician should be available to vacuum emitted smoke during the procedure. The technician should be familiar with laser safety before its use.

One to two sutures are often placed to appose the skin edges after nail removal. Surgical glue (cyanoacrylic tissue adhesive) is used instead of sutures in some instances. If surgical glue is used, it should never be placed on the exposed bone of the second phalanx or dropped inside the void (wound) created by removal of the third phalanx (Figure 30-17). Instead, the wound should be manually closed and a drop of glue placed only on the skin edges of the closed wound (see Figure 30-17). Dropping glue into the wound can cause chronic lameness and foreign body reaction. Some veterinarians do not appose the skin edges with anything other than a bandage.

> *TECHNICIAN NOTE* Do not place tissue glue into the open wound formed after a claw is removed. The wound should be manually apposed and the glue placed only on the skin edges. Placing surgical glue internally can result in chronic lameness and foreign body reaction.

After surgery, the paws are bandaged snugly with a gauze sponge and strips of tape. The sponge is placed over the ends of the digits. Strips of tape are placed longitudinally along the leg and distally around the paw. Tape is then placed circumferentially around the paw up to the elbow. Care is taken to lay tape on the leg and not to pull too tightly. Bandages placed too tight can result in vascular compromise to the foot with skin sloughing. The tourniquet is removed as soon as bandaging is complete.

POSTOPERATIVE CONSIDERATIONS

Onychectomy is painful. Pain medication should be administered to all cats in the postoperative period. It is appropriate to administer a pure opioid agonist for the first 24 hours after surgery (see Chapter 26 for details on the administration, advantages, and disadvantages of specific pain medications). A fentanyl patch can be placed the day before surgery to allow the fentanyl to take effect and can last up to 3 days postoperative, but pain control can be variable with the patch, and the cat should be monitored closely for continued pain in spite of having a patch in place. Alternatively, injectable pain medication can be given intermittently. Some nonsteroidal antiinflammatory drugs can also be used in cats; however, care must be taken to avoid overdosage. A wait-and-see attitude regarding pain medication for this procedure is not acceptable. Instead, medication should be given at the appropriate dosing intervals for at least 4 to 5 days postoperative.

The bandages are kept on for 24 hours, but no longer, and the cat should be hospitalized while the bandage is in place. After surgery, litter should consist of shredded paper or pellets to prevent accumulation of clay or sand in the surgical wounds with resultant irritation and infection. Normal litter should not be reintroduced until 10 days after surgery. The paws should be monitored for hemorrhage, swelling, drainage, and redness. Cats will be fairly sensitive on the front legs after surgery, but this should start improving within 2 weeks of surgery. If sutures were placed, suture removal is generally not necessary because the cats will remove them on their own, but if they are still present after 2½ weeks, the owner should have them removed by the veterinary staff.

> *TECHNICIAN NOTE* The bandage from an onychectomy should be removed within 24 hours. The cat should remain in the hospital until the bandages are removed.

Most cats allow removal of the bandages by carefully cutting the bandage apart longitudinally and gently peeling it off the leg. If the cat is intractable, the bandage may be cut and the cat returned to its cage. The cat will then remove the bandage on its own. If this technique is used; however, the cat will have to be monitored to ensure that bandage ingestion does not occur. In severely intractable patients, a light dose of a tranquilizer may be necessary to remove the bandages safely. Cats are monitored carefully for 8 to 12 hours after bandage removal for hemorrhage. Rebandage with prolonged hospitalization will be necessary if hemorrhage occurs.

Onychectomy complications can be divided into those that occur in the early postoperative period and those that occur in the late postoperative period. Early complications include loose bandages and postoperative bleeding. Cats should be checked frequently for evidence of loose, bloody bandages or complete bandage removal and severe hemorrhage. In the event of hemorrhage, the paws should be rebandaged snugly. Infection can also occur and generally becomes evident within the first 3 weeks of surgery. Infection requires antibiotic therapy and/or wound débridement. Late complications include regrowth of the claws, chronic lameness, or both. Claw regrowth requires reoperation and removal of remaining germinal epithelium. Chronic lameness without evidence of regrowth may be seen with incomplete removal of the phalanx or cut footpads. For this reason, it is essential that the pads be preserved during the operative procedure. Other complications include radial nerve damage secondary to tourniquet placement and skin sloughing secondary to tight, prolonged bandage placement.

CELIOTOMY

DEFINITION

Celiotomy (laparotomy) is a surgical incision into the abdominal cavity. There are several locations in which the incision can be made: ventral midline, paramedian, paracostal, parapreputial, and flank (Figure 30-18). The most commonly used incision site is ventral midline.

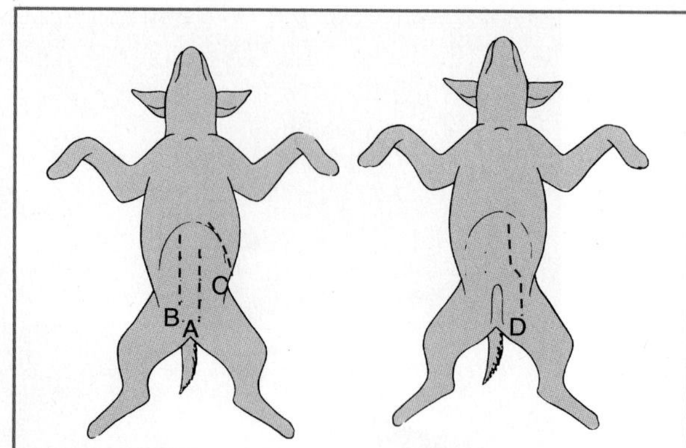

FIGURE 30-18 Locations for celiotomy incisions. *A*, Ventral midline. *B*, Paramedian. *C*, Paracostal. *D*, Parapreputial.

INDICATIONS

A celiotomy is performed for both elective and nonelective procedures. Some of the common elective procedures include ovariohysterectomy, organ biopsy, cystotomy, planned cesarean delivery, gastropexy, and retained abdominal testicles. Some common nonelective procedures include emergency cesarean delivery, gastric dilation-volvulus (GDV) (bloated, twisted stomach), intussusception, gastrointestinal foreign bodies, ruptured spleen, penetrating foreign bodies (e.g., knife wound, arrow wound, bullet wound), severe abdominal bleeding, and diaphragmatic hernia. In some instances, the animal is seen for an unknown abdominal problem. These patients may need elective or nonelective celiotomy, referred to as an exploratory celiotomy. Exploratory celiotomy is often performed for abdominal masses of unknown origin and to obtain biopsies for disease diagnosis.

PREOPERATIVE CONSIDERATIONS

Animals should always be clipped widely for abdominal incisions. At times, the incision must be extended, and an inappropriate prep will hinder surgical exposure. Animals undergoing abdominal incision because of illness or trauma may have to be stabilized before anesthesia is administered. If biopsies or cultures are to be taken, the veterinary technician should make sure that culture supplies and tissue sample cups with formalin are available.

TECHNIQUE AND INTRAOPERATIVE CONSIDERATIONS

For ventral midline celiotomy, the patient is placed in dorsal recumbency. Larger dogs should be placed in a V-trough to help stabilize them in that position (Figure 30-19). Smaller dogs and cats can be placed on moldable beanbags or between sandbags. The abdomen is widely clipped from 2 cm cranial to the xiphoid cartilage to 2 cm caudal to the pubis. The skin is aseptically prepared for surgery.

The various incisions (paramedian, paracostal, etc.) are all slight variations of the ventral midline incision and are less commonly used (see Figure 30-18). For this reason, emphasis will be given to the ventral midline incision.

The line of the incision is from the xiphoid process to the pubis. The length used varies with the type of procedure (see specific procedures). A surgical sponge count is performed before entry into the abdominal cavity. The incision is made with a scalpel blade or electrocautery in the cutting mode. The incision is carried through the subcutaneous tissue to the level of the linea alba, which is elevated with forceps to pull it away from the underlying abdominal viscera. This will prevent the inadvertent puncture of abdominal organs when entering the peritoneal cavity. A scalpel blade is used to penetrate the linea alba and enter the peritoneal cavity. The incision is extended the desired length with scissors or scalpel blade and forceps. Moistened laparotomy pads (sponges) are placed along the incision edges for protection during exploratory surgery. This is usually not necessary during ovariohysterectomy because the incision is small and manipulation is minimal. A Balfour self-retaining abdominal retractor can be introduced, if necessary, into the incision to facilitate visualization of abdominal structures (exploratory celiotomy). Surgical lights and air exposure

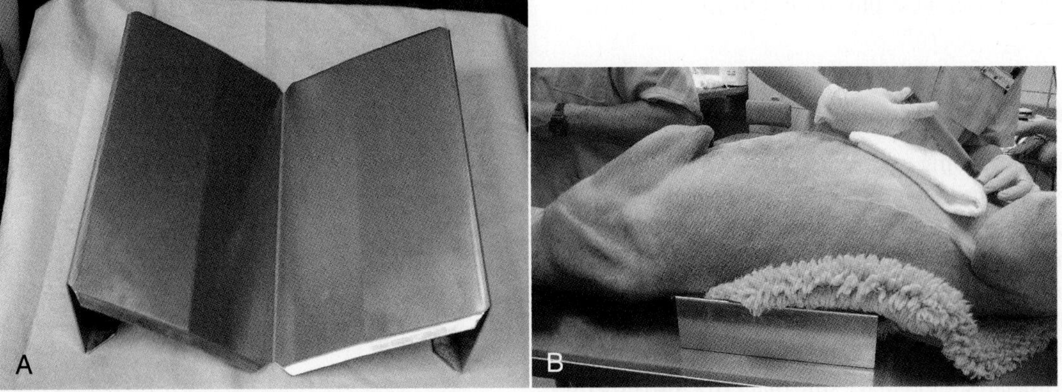

FIGURE 30-19 V-trough is used to stabilize large animals in dorsal recumbency for surgical preparation. **A,** Trough. **B,** Proper positioning.

of abdominal organs will quickly dry out abdominal structures. It is important for the surgical assistant to keep exposed tissues moist to prevent damage and decrease adhesion formation. The technician should pay special attention to viscera moved external to the abdominal cavity. Viscera temporarily moved outside of the abdominal cavity should be covered with warm, moist laparotomy pads. Abdominal viscera should be handled carefully and as little as possible. Whenever retraction or manipulation of structures is necessary, atraumatic technique is mandatory. Retract viscera with moistened laparotomy pads, manipulate viscera with moistened gloves, blot any excess hemorrhage with moistened sponges (do not wipe surfaces with sponges), and when using suction, be careful not to suck the walls of visceral structures against the suction orifice. A thorough inspection of the abdomen is performed. A postoperative sponge count should be made before closing the abdomen to ensure that all sponges are accounted for.

> *TECHNICIAN NOTE* Tissues exposed to the air during surgery should be kept moist to help prevent tissue desiccation with subsequent death or irritation.

> *TECHNICIAN NOTE* A thorough inspection of the abdomen should be made before closure to prevent leaving instruments or sponges in the abdominal cavity. A preoperative and postoperative sponge count is recommended.

The abdomen is sutured closed in three layers. The linea alba is the layer of strength and must be securely closed. The subcutaneous tissues are then sutured to decrease the amount of dead space. This helps reduce the frequency of postoperative hematoma or seroma formation. The skin is sutured to complete the celiotomy closure.

POSTOPERATIVE CONSIDERATIONS

During the first 24 hours, the skin incision should be examined carefully for swelling, drainage, excessive redness, dehiscence, and evidence of self-trauma. An Elizabethan collar should be considered if the animal appears to lick or chew the incision. Incision problems should be brought to the attention of the veterinarian. Incision monitoring should be continued for 2 weeks after surgery or until suture removal. Animals should be exercise restricted until the abdominal wound is healed. If there is evidence of dehiscence, the veterinary technician should notify the veterinarian immediately. Emergency closure may be necessary.

Some animals may be inappetent or vomit after celiotomy. Intestinal and pancreatic manipulation can lead to intestinal ileus (temporary loss of intestinal motility), nausea, and/or pancreatitis. One or two episodes of vomiting or lack of appetite for the first 24 to 48 hours after celiotomy is usually not concerning in and of itself. However, if the animal appears ill or vomiting and inappetence continues, further evaluation should be performed. Animals not eating or drinking after surgery should be supported with intravenous fluid therapy until oral alimentation is resumed.

GASTROINTESTINAL SURGERY

DEFINITION

Gastrotomy is incision (opening) into the stomach. Enterotomy is incision into the intestine. These are often done to obtain biopsies or to retrieve foreign material. Anastomosis is suturing portions of the gastrointestinal tract together to allow confluent ingesta flow. Anastomosis is performed after damaged tissue or tumor requires a segment of the gastrointestinal tract to be removed.

INDICATIONS

Gastrointestinal surgery has many indications. Gastrointestinal foreign body lodgment, neoplasia, biopsy for vomiting or diarrhea of unknown origin, GDV, gastrointestinal trauma, and gastrointestinal obstruction of unknown cause can all be reasons for abdominal exploration and gastrointestinal surgery.

PREOPERATIVE CONSIDERATIONS

Many animals undergoing gastrointestinal surgery have usually been recently vomiting or not eating for several days. The veterinary technician should stabilize the animal with appropriate fluid management to correct dehydration before surgery. The animal should be intubated as soon as possible with a cuffed endotracheal tube to help ward off aspiration of stomach contents should the animal vomit during induction. The veterinary technician should make sure that extra instruments are available in case the primary pack is contaminated with intestinal contents during the procedure. Prophylactic antibiotics are used if the gastrointestinal tract is to be entered.

> *TECHNICIAN NOTE* It is important to remember that gastrointestinal contents are not sterile. Materials that touch intestinal contents are considered contaminated and are removed from or kept in a separate place on the surgical field.

TECHNIQUE AND INTRAOPERATIVE CONSIDERATIONS

The animal is prepared for a full midline celiotomy (see Figure 30-18). An abdominal exploration is performed. Abnormalities are noted. Foreign bodies leading to gastrointestinal obstruction are removed via gastrotomy or enterotomy. The normal gastrointestinal tract is pink, has visible vasculature on the surface, and has active motility. In some instances, devitalized tissue must be removed via resection and anastomosis. Devitalized intestine is discolored and lacks blood supply. Purple and red discoloration does not necessarily imply devitalization; blood supply must be evaluated by direct visualization of cut sections, Doppler, or injection of vital stains. If the tissue is questionable, it should be resected (Figure 30-20).

Characteristics of intestinal devitalization are:

- Lack of motility
- Black discoloration
- Green discoloration
- Gray discoloration
- Severe thinning of the visceral wall
- Lack of bleeding on cut section
- Lack of fluorescein dye uptake
- Lack of Doppler blood flow

For biopsy or foreign body removal, the affected portion of the gastrointestinal track is isolated with laparotomy pads (Figure 30-21). Laparotomy pads are placed to prevent intestinal contents from leaking into the abdomen if accidental spillage occurs. Stay sutures are placed to steady the tissue on either side of the incision. Biopsy is performed by making a stab incision into the stomach or intestine between the stay sutures and removing a full-thickness portion of the tissue

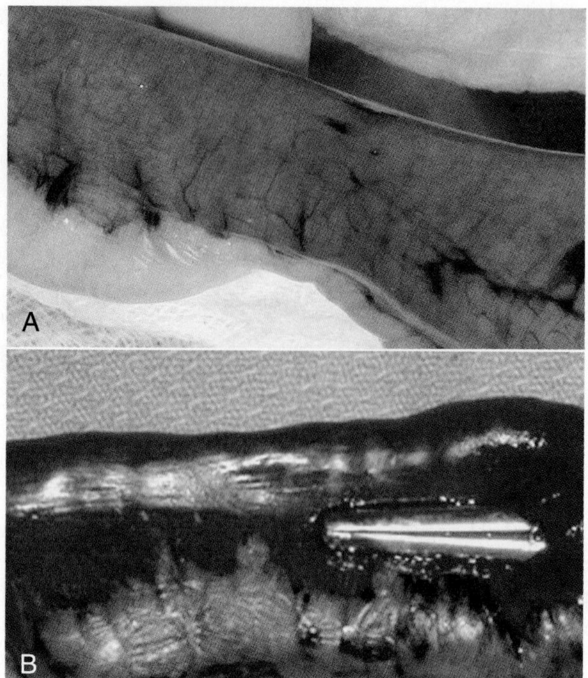

FIGURE 30-20 The normal intestine is pink with visible vessels and motility. Note the difference in color of the normal intestine **(A)** with the devitalized segment of bowel **(B)**.

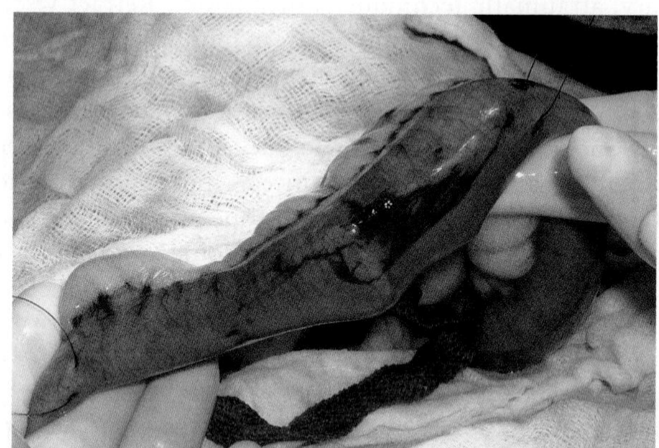

FIGURE 30-21 If a biopsy is to be performed on the gastrointestinal tract, the segment is packed off with laparotomy pads to prevent leaking ingesta from contaminating the abdominal cavity. Note the white pads surrounding the intestine. Ingesta is prevented from leaking from the cut surface of the intestine by placement of intestinal clamps or having an assistant gently pinch off the intestinal lumen on either side of the incision with fingers.

with a blade or scissors. If the incision is made simply to remove intraluminal material, the stab incision is extended enough to remove the material, and no tissue is removed for biopsy. The incision is closed in an interrupted pattern with absorbable, monofilament suture.

If a resection and anastomosis is to be performed, the vasculature to the portion of the intestine to be removed is ligated; the intestines are clamped with Doyen forceps, or the surgical assistant supports the intestines with fingers to prevent ingesta from leaking onto the surgical field (see Figure 30-21); the portion of the intestines to be removed is excised;

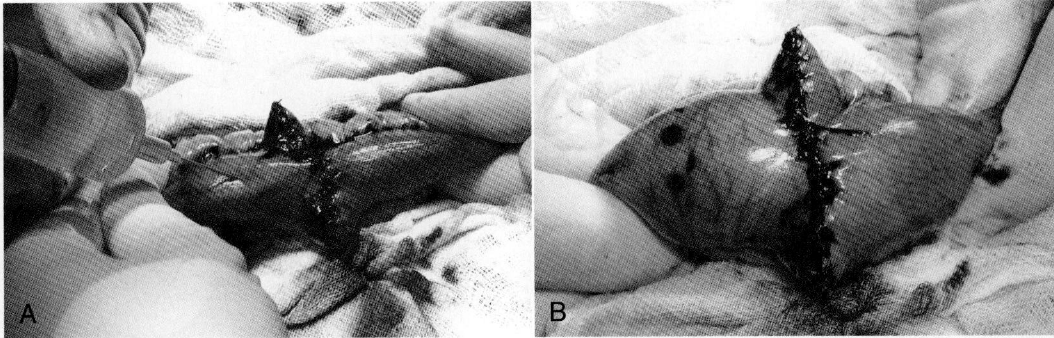

FIGURE 30-22 **A,** To check for leaks after intestinal anastomosis, the intestine is occluded on either side of the incision, and the occluded segment of intestine is filled with sterile saline. **B,** The incision is checked for leakage while the segment is filled with saline.

and the viable intestinal ends are sutured together in an interrupted pattern similar to a biopsy site. After completion of the anastomosis, the intestine is evaluated for leakage. This is accomplished by occluding the intestine on either side of the anastomosis site and filling the enclosed space with sterile saline using a syringe and small-gauge needle. The surgeon and assistant check for leaks along the incision. Leaks are sealed with additional suture (Figure 30-22). The intestine is flushed, and the laparotomy pads are removed from the abdomen and surgical field, being careful not to contaminate the rest of the abdomen or the surgical field with ingesta that might have leaked onto the pads. The technician should ensure that warm isotonic saline is available for flushing the abdominal cavity. Omentum is placed over the incision, and the abdomen is flushed. The celiotomy is closed routinely. Many surgeons will ask for a clean surgical pack, gloves, and drape to perform the celiotomy closure to prevent contamination of the celiotomy wound with ingesta from instruments used during the intestinal procedure.

POSTOPERATIVE CONSIDERATIONS

Careful patient monitoring is important following intestinal surgery. The main consideration is evaluation for intestinal leakage. If intestinal dehiscence or leakage occurs, septic peritonitis is likely to follow. Animals should be monitored for inappetence, vomiting, fever, painful abdomen, abdominal enlargement, incision drainage, and shock, which are all potential indicators of peritonitis. Most animals are willing to eat within 24 hours of intestinal surgery. Minor vomiting (one to two times) might be expected. However, protracted vomiting and inappetence should alert the technician to a potential impending problem with the intestinal surgery site. If intestinal leakage is suspected, abdominocentesis is performed. Material collected is evaluated for cell population and bacteria. If enough material is not obtained for evaluation from simple abdominocentesis, but leakage is still suspected, a diagnostic peritoneal lavage should be performed. A septic abdominal tap warrants abdominal exploration and correction of the problem.

Feeding animals after intestinal surgery is also a consideration. The gastrointestinal tract requires food for cellular health and proper function. Intestinal surgery can result in ileus and may cause inappetence, nausea, and vomiting. However, animals without complications are most often willing to eat within 24 hours. Unless the animal is vomiting, oral alimentation should be initiated as soon as the animal has an appetite. Animals should be introduced to water first. If no vomiting occurs after water intake, then food is introduced. A small amount of highly digestible, bland food should be fed initially (e.g., 1 to 2 tbsp of Hill's Science Diet I/D). If no vomiting occurs over 2 to 4 hours, another small amount can be fed. If vomiting does not occur, the amount fed can be gradually increased and frequency decreased. Animals are reintroduced to their normal or another maintenance diet gradually after recovery.

Monitoring as discussed for routine celiotomy should also be done.

GASTRIC DILATION-VOLVULUS

DEFINITION

Gastric dilation-volvulus is dilation of the stomach with ingesta and gas with rotation of the stomach into an abnormal position. This is a life-threatening condition that typically occurs in deep-chested, large, and giant-breed dogs. The cause is not specifically known, but genetics and chest/abdomen configuration play a role. Some animals have often eaten a large meal, drunk a large portion of water, and/or engaged in heavy exercise following either; however, others have not. Some animals develop the condition during times of stress, such as hospitalization or boarding. Vomiting, retching, and bloating (severe distention of the stomach) are classic clinical signs. Gastropexy is attachment of the stomach to the body wall with the goal of creating a permanent adhesion. It is performed to substantially decrease the chance of stomach rotation, but it does not prevent bloating. Partial gastrectomy is removal of part of the stomach. Splenectomy is removal of the spleen.

PREOPERATIVE CONSIDERATIONS

Animals suffering from GDV usually are in shock. If left untreated, these animals will die from cardiovascular collapse. The enlarged stomach compresses the caudal vena cava and

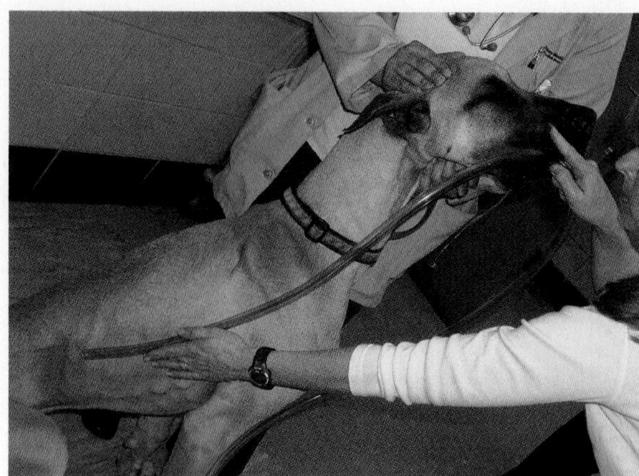

FIGURE 30-23 Before passing a stomach tube, the length of tube to be passed is marked by measuring from the nose to the last rib.

affects venous return to the heart. Hypovolemic shock results. Large-bore catheters should be placed immediately. It is important to place the catheters in the front legs or jugular vein because venous return from the caudal half of the body is impaired by the dilated stomach. These dogs are often large and require a substantial amount of fluid. It is best to place at least two catheters. Baseline blood work, ECG, and blood gas should be obtained. The veterinary technician should review treatment of hypovolemic shock (see Chapter 33).

> *TECHNICIAN NOTE* Intravenous catheters should be placed in the front half of an animal suffering from GDV. Venous return is compromised from the back half of the dog as a result of compression of the vena cava from the dilated stomach.

After fluids are started, the stomach must be decompressed to help stabilize the animal and decrease the chance of gastric wall necrosis secondary to vascular compromise from the severe distention. A stomach tube is measured from the nose to the last rib (Figure 30-23). Stomach tubes are large bore and thick. The mouth is held open with a roll of tape or a gag with a hole big enough to pass the tube. An assistant should hold the mouth closed with the gag in place while another person passes the tube (Figure 30-24). The tube is lubricated and gently passed down the esophagus to the stomach up to the premeasured mark. It is difficult to impossible to pass a tube of that size into the trachea, but if the animal begins to cough, the tube should be removed and repassed. It would not be possible to pass the entire measured length of the tube down the trachea without causing severe destruction of the trachea and lungs. Do not forcefully pass the tube if resistance is felt. Overinsertion of the tube may result in gastric rupture if the gastric wall is compromised as a result of vascular impairment. Gas is emptied from the stomach as the tube enters the stomach. Water can be pumped into the stomach to help break up ingesta. If the tube cannot be passed, the animal can be sedated with an opioid and benzodiazepam and another

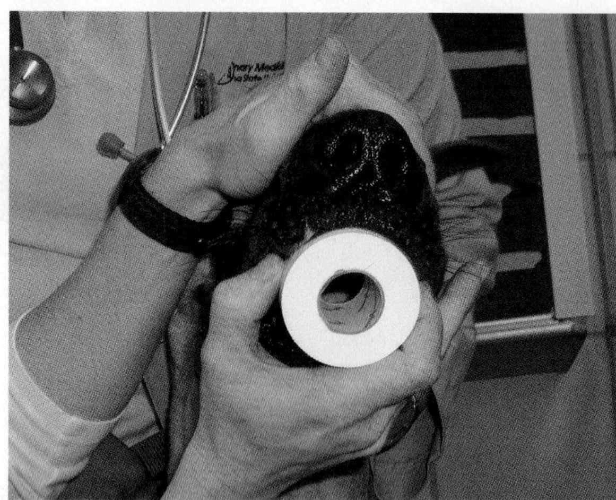

FIGURE 30-24 A roll of tape (pictured) or a mouth gag can be used to hold the mouth open while passing a stomach tube. The assistant should hold the mouth gag in place by holding the mouth shut around the gag.

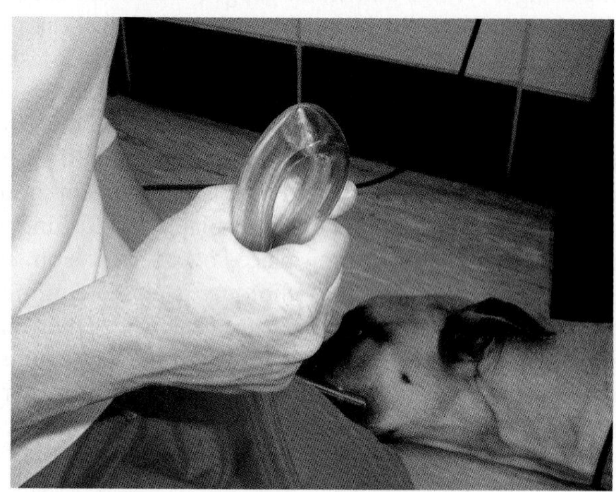

FIGURE 30-25 The assistant passing a stomach tube should pinch the tube off before removing the tube from the animal's stomach. This helps prevent aspiration of stomach contents into the lungs.

attempt made. The veterinary technician must always remember to pinch off the gastric tube before removing it from the stomach (Figure 30-25). If the tube is not pinched, material from the tube can leak down the trachea as the tube is removed, causing aspiration pneumonia.

> *TECHNICIAN NOTE* While removing a gastric tube from a dog, the tube lumen should be pinched or clamped off to prevent leakage of tube contents down the trachea during removal.

If the tube cannot be passed after sedation, the stomach should be decompressed by trocarization. The disadvantage of trocarization is the potential leakage of gastric contents into the abdominal cavity at the stomach puncture site or stomach rupture. For trocarization, the right side of the

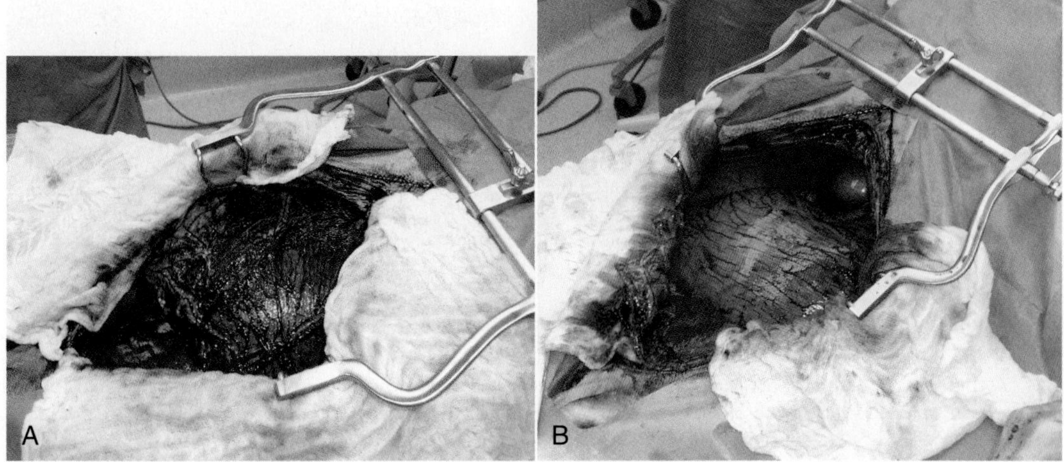

FIGURE 30-26 **A,** Note how the dilated, rotated stomach is pressed against the ventral abdominal wall and protrudes out of the abdomen. Inadvertent stomach puncture can occur if the abdomen is not entered carefully. **B,** The normally positioned stomach is still dilated, but recesses back away from the ventral incision and lies completely within the abdomen.

stomach is aseptically prepared behind the last rib. A large-bore needle is attached to a 60-ml syringe, a three-way stopcock is gently passed into the dilated stomach percutaneously, and air is aspirated until the stomach is decompressed enough to stabilize the dog.

After stabilization is under way and vital signs are improving, right lateral abdominal radiographs are obtained. This view is best for evaluating whether rotation of the stomach or simple bloat without rotation is present. Thoracic radiographs should also be performed because aspiration is a possibility. As a result of vascular compromise to the stomach wall, the animal should also be started on broad-spectrum antibiotics to help prevent septicemia should intestinal compromise lead to bacterial translocation from the gastrointestinal tract to the bloodstream. The animal is stabilized and prepared for emergency surgery.

Anesthesia can be challenging in these cases. Respiratory compromise is often present as a result of the gas-distended stomach compressing the diaphragm. Blood pressure is often low and difficult to maintain. If possible, an arterial access port should be established for continuous pressure and blood gas monitoring. Additionally, cardiac arrhythmias may also occur and may need to be treated. The veterinary technician should review Chapter 27 for specific anesthetic techniques and monitoring.

TECHNIQUE AND INTRAOPERATIVE CONSIDERATIONS

The dog is prepared for a full ventral midline celiotomy. The abdomen is opened carefully to prevent puncture of the stomach because gas distention pushes the stomach against the ventral aspect of the abdomen (Figure 30-26). If the stomach is substantially distended at the time of surgery, further decompression should be performed to make manipulation easier. The veterinary technician should make sure that a stomach tube, bucket, and pump are available in the operating room. The tube should be gently passed down the esophagus after lubrication while the veterinarian manipulates the tube into position within the stomach. The veterinarian can often gently express gas and fluid from the stomach through the tube. If decompression cannot be achieved in this manner, decompression can be performed with a syringe, three-way stopcock, and needle. The stomach must be handled with care. The tissue is often friable as a result of compromise of the tissues. Additionally the ingesta and fluid that accumulates in the stomach following GDV is heavy and can contribute to tissue tearing during manipulation of the stomach back into the normal position. Extreme care must be taken to prevent inadvertent damage. Once the stomach is in its normal position, it is evaluated for viability. The stomach is often discolored at the start of the procedure, but may improve as blood supply and venous drainage returns. A complete abdominal exploratory is performed while circulation is allowed to return to the stomach. The spleen is carefully evaluated. Vascular compromise to the spleen can occur with dilation and rotation of the stomach, or the spleen may rotate. If the spleen is discolored, the vascular pedicle is relieved of compromise, and the spleen is gently placed out of the abdomen and covered with moistened laparotomy pads while a gastropexy is performed. In most instances, the spleen will return to its normal character once blood supply is reestablished. After abdominal exploration, the stomach is reevaluated for viability. Partial resection is performed, if needed.

A gastropexy is then performed on the right ventrolateral aspect of the body wall near the last rib. There are many different techniques for performing gastropexy, and the discussion of each technique is beyond the scope of this chapter. Which technique is used depends on the comfort level and skill of the surgeon performing the procedure. Fixation of the stomach into the celiotomy incision at the time of closure is not recommended because future abdominal surgery can result in accidental perforation of the stomach when the abdominal cavity is entered. The surgical assistant is responsible for retraction of tissues and suture manipulation to keep the procedure running smoothly. It will often help the veterinary surgeon

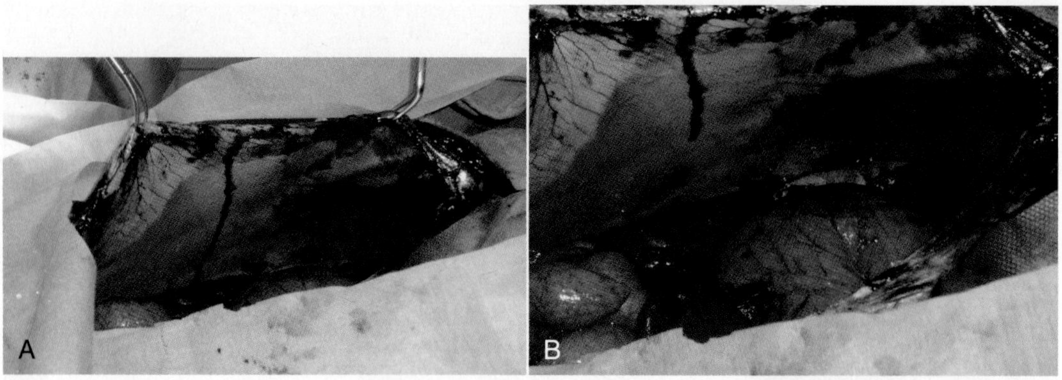

FIGURE 30-27 **A,** The surgical assistant can increase exposure for the surgeon during gastropexy by holding the abdominal wall up on the right side with towel clamps. **B,** Note how well this exposes the abdominal wall and the pylorus of the stomach.

if the assistant stands on the right side of the dog and holds the body wall up with towel clamps during the gastropexy. This will often expose the entire surgical field for the surgeon (Figure 30-27). After gastropexy, the spleen is reevaluated. If all or a portion of the spleen does not appear viable, all or part of the spleen is removed, respectively. The abdomen is flushed, and the celiotomy incision is closed routinely.

POSTOPERATIVE CONSIDERATIONS

Dogs suffering from GDV can have many postoperative complications. Arrhythmias can continue for 2 to 3 days postoperative. Treatment for the arrhythmias should be initiated if vascular compromise is present or is expected based on the abnormality. The veterinarian should be alerted as to the type of arrhythmia present. Hypotension and hypovolemia can continue postoperative and should be treated as needed. Urination should be monitored because prolonged hypotension under anesthesia can affect renal function. A urinary catheter should be placed if urine production is questionable. Some dogs will require a blood transfusion because of hemorrhage associated with tearing of blood vessels during bloating and rotation of the stomach and/or spleen. If a partial gastrectomy was performed, the dogs should be monitored for evidence of gastric wall dehiscence. Some of these dogs continue to develop gastric wall compromise after decompression and surgery. Fever, persistent inappetence, and vomiting may be an indication that this is occurring. Signs are similar to intestinal incision dehiscence as previously discussed. Antibiotics should be continued for at least 7 days postoperative. Immediately after surgery, antibiotics should be given intravenously to avoid oral administration. Gastrointestinal protectants, such as H_2 blockers, should also be administered for 3 to 5 days postoperative. Finally, gastric dilation can again occur in the postoperative period necessitating decompression. However, gastropexy should prevent rotation of the stomach.

Oral alimentation should be initiated slowly. Water is given in small amounts to start. If no vomiting occurs, food is gradually introduced. Feeding can start as soon as the animal is willing to eat; this is often within 24 hours of surgery. Some animals may require antiemetics in the perioperative period to help control nausea and vomiting. Long-term dietary management should be considered. When home, these dogs should be on a three- to four-times-a-day feeding schedule. If possible, a three-times-a-day feeding schedule should be continued for the rest of the dog's life. Water should always be available, but gulping of water should be avoided. Heavy activity should be avoided after feeding. Owners should be warned that bloating can still occur, even though gastropexy was performed, but surgery is likely to prevent gastric rotation, which is more life threatening. Stomach decompression may be needed if bloat is severe.

OVARIOHYSTERECTOMY IN THE DOG AND CAT

DEFINITION

Ovariohysterectomy (spay) is surgical removal of the uterus and ovaries.

INDICATIONS

The primary indication for ovariohysterectomy is prevention of pregnancy and subsequent production of unwanted puppies and kittens. Other indications for ovariohysterectomy include endocrine imbalances, infections, injuries, cysts, tumors, prevention of unwanted behavior, and congenital abnormalities. Endocrine disturbances are associated with varied clinical manifestations, such as sterility, skin lesions, mammary tumors, pseudocyesis (false pregnancy), and nymphomania. Ovariohysterectomy before the first estrus will greatly decrease the chance of mammary neoplasia in dogs. Uterine diseases that may require ovariohysterectomy include metritis, pyometra, uterine prolapse, endometrial hyperplasia, neoplasia, injury, neglected dystocia, and congenital abnormalities.

PREOPERATIVE CONSIDERATIONS

Ovariohysterectomy is usually performed between 5 and 6 months of age, but it can be performed at almost any age and during any phase of the reproductive cycle. Performing ovariohysterectomy around 6 months of age decreases anesthetic risk in younger animals and usually allows the procedure to be performed before the first estrus. If performed during estrus or pregnancy, increased vasculature may be encountered with potential for increased hemorrhage. This is more important for dogs than cats. The most favorable time to spay a mature dog is 3 to 4 months after estrus. After whelping, the operation should be done as soon as the puppies or kittens have been weaned and lactation has ceased, about 6 to 8 weeks following parturition.

TECHNIQUE AND INTRAOPERATIVE CONSIDERATIONS

The animal is clipped and aseptically prepared for a ventral midline celiotomy. The skin incision extends caudally 3 to 6 cm from the umbilicus in the dog and from 2 cm caudad to the umbilicus caudally 3 to 4 cm in the cat. When the abdominal cavity is entered, the uterine horns are located and exteriorized from the abdomen using a spay hook or digital manipulation. The ovarian arteries and veins (pedicles) are ligated with the appropriate-size absorbable suture material. The veterinarian or surgical assistant should check to ensure that both ovaries are completely removed after ligation and division of the ovarian pedicles. The uterine body is then exteriorized and ligated. The abdominal cavity is carefully examined for hemorrhage. The celiotomy incision is closed routinely.

Intraoperative complications include hemorrhage and anesthetic problems. If excessive intraabdominal blood is seen during surgery, both ovarian pedicles and the uterine stump should be evaluated before celiotomy closure. The abdominal incision will likely have to be extended. The left ovarian pedicle is evaluated by retraction of the descending colon to the right and viewing the pedicle just caudal to the left kidney. The right pedicle is evaluated by retraction of the descending duodenum to the left and viewing the pedicle just caudal to the right kidney. The uterine stump is visualized between the urinary bladder ventrally and the colon dorsally. Bleeding stumps are religated before abdominal closure.

POSTOPERATIVE CONSIDERATIONS

Postoperative, intraabdominal hemorrhage can also occur and can be fatal if not treated appropriately (see the section on monitoring blood loss). After ovariohysterectomy, the technician should monitor the animal carefully for the first 24 hours. Abnormalities should be promptly reported to the veterinarian in charge.

Incision complications can also occur after ovariohysterectomy. These include irritation, premature suture removal by the animal, seroma formation, infection, suture reaction, and dehiscence. Only rarely are these complications serious. The veterinarian should be alerted to impending incision complications.

Some animals experience renal dysfunction secondary to accidental ureteral ligation during surgery. Ligation typically occurs when overzealous attempts are made to alleviate hemorrhage from a bleeding stump with mass ligation of tissues and poor visualization. It is important to ensure that the ureters are visualized and are not in the mass of tissue to be ligated when controlling hemorrhage from bleeding ovarian or uterine stumps. Animals are unlikely to show signs of renal failure if only one ureter is ligated, but they may be seen for abdominal enlargement, abdominal pain, or signs consistent with renal infection at a later date. If both ureters are inadvertently ligated, the animal will begin to show signs within 24 hours and will die if steps are not taken to alleviate the obstruction of urine flow.

Body weight gain may occur as a late sequel to ovariohysterectomy. The reasons for this excessive weight gain are poorly understood, but may be partially caused by ovarian endocrine deficiency. In actuality, obesity can be controlled by proper diet and exercise. Other late complications include loss of stamina in working dogs (eunuchoid syndrome) and urinary incontinence. Although incompletely understood, urinary incontinence may be related to endocrine alteration following ovariohysterectomy or scar tissue formation around the urinary bladder and proximal urethra. These appear to be rare complications.

PYOMETRA

DEFINITION

Pyometra is a condition of the uterus in which endometrial hyperplasia has resulted in increased uterine secretions and accumulation of fluid in the uterus with secondary infection. Progesterone production from the ovaries during diestrus contributes to uterine gland hyperplasia and the disease process. The process typically occurs in middle-aged to older dogs 4 to 8 weeks following estrus. Mucometra or hydrometra is enlargement of the uterus with a sterile mucoid or serous fluid, respectively.

INDICATIONS

Ovariohysterectomy is the recommended treatment for pyometra. This is especially true for closed (nondraining) pyometra. Some owners will elect conservative management for open (draining) pyometras in valuable breeding dogs, but this should be discouraged because septicemia and/or endotoxemia is possible and the incidence of recurrence is high. Conservative management of closed pyometras is not recommended because of the risk of uterine rupture, septicemia and/or endotoxemia, and possible death.

PREOPERATIVE CONSIDERATIONS

An intact female dog with fever, lethargy, polyuria, polydipsia, vaginal discharge, abdominal pain, abdominal enlargement, inappetence, vomiting, and/or diarrhea should be evaluated carefully for pyometra. Animals with closed pyometra are more likely to have severe clinical signs. Baseline

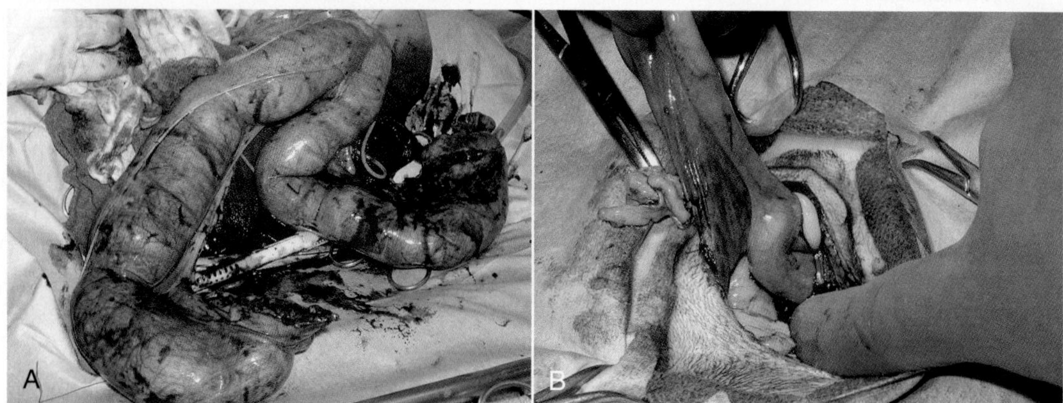

FIGURE 30-28 The uterus must be carefully handled in cases of pyometra because it is often large, friable, and heavy. Compare the pyometra uterus **(A)** with the normal uterus **(B)**.

biochemical values and blood cell counts should be obtained. Many of these animals are dehydrated, inappetent, and have metabolic and/or electrolyte abnormalities at the time of presentation (renal or hepatic dysfunction, glucose imbalances, etc.). They should be started on intravenous fluids and their metabolic/electrolyte abnormalities corrected, if possible, before surgery. If left untreated, pyometra can result in septicemia and/or endotoxemia and possible death. Additionally, uterine rupture and peritonitis is also possible. Palpation of the abdomen should be done with extreme care and cystocentesis to collect urine should be avoided in animals suspected of having pyometra. Broad-spectrum intravenous antibiotic therapy is initiated before surgery.

TECHNIQUE AND INTRAOPERATIVE CONSIDERATIONS

The animal is prepped for a ventral midline celiotomy. A routine ovariohysterectomy is performed with some exceptions. The uterus is usually large, heavy, and friable (Figure 30-28). It should be manipulated with extreme care during the procedure to prevent rupture and contamination of the abdomen. This means that the celiotomy incision should extend from the xiphoid to the pubis so that excessive tension is not placed on the uterus during manipulation. Vessels are usually prominent and may be increased in number, so care must be taken to ligate and separate vessels appropriately to prevent hemorrhage. The uterine contents should be cultured for aerobic and anaerobic bacteria and a bacterial sensitivity test performed after the uterus is removed from the surgical field. This is performed via aseptic aspiration of the fluid with a needle and syringe before the uterus is contaminated. The abdomen should be flushed before closure. The abdominal closure is routine.

POSTOPERATIVE CONSIDERATIONS

Animals should be monitored as for ovariohysterectomy. Special considerations include continued antibiotic therapy in the postoperative period. Antibiotics are given intravenously until the animal is stable and eating. Antibiotic therapy is continued for 7 to 10 days after surgery based on culture and sensitivity results. Electrolyte and metabolic abnormalities can continue postoperative, and monitoring for this is important. Abnormalities should be corrected. Intravenous fluids should be given until the animal is stable, eating, and drinking.

CANINE CASTRATION

DEFINITION

Orchidectomy (castration or neuter) is the removal of both testicles. Scrotal ablation is removal of the scrotum with the testicles at the time of castration.

INDICATIONS

There are numerous indications for canine castration; the most common is an elective procedure in the young male dog to help prevent roaming, aggressiveness, unwanted breeding, or a combination of these. Several medical problems may also be treated by castration, including prostate disorders, anal and perianal tumors, perineal hernias, and testicular tumors. Older dogs with a well-developed scrotum or animals with scrotal abnormalities should undergo scrotal ablation to prevent severe scrotal swelling, improve postoperative aesthetics, and/or treat disease.

PREOPERATIVE CONSIDERATIONS

There is not an optimal age for canine castration, but the procedure is often performed around 6 months of age. Performing castration before the development of unwanted male behavior—before sexual maturity—may help prevent this behavior from occurring. Castration after development of this behavior will often improve behavior, but may not eliminate it in all male dogs. Before surgery, a careful examination should be performed to ensure that both testicles lie within the scrotum.

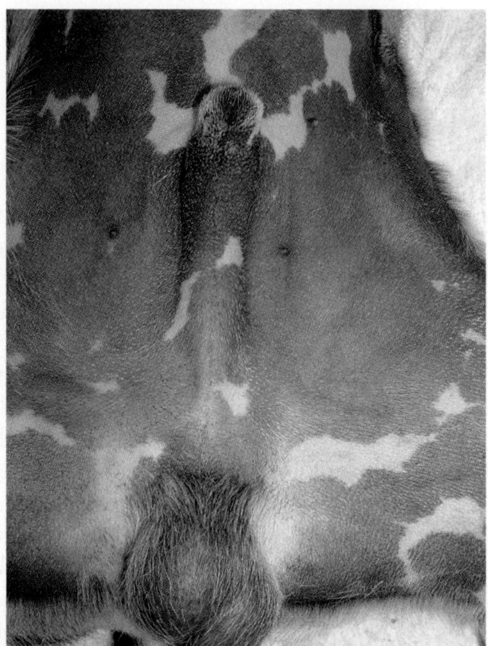

FIGURE 30-29 Proper positioning and preparation for canine castration. Note that the scrotum is not clipped.

TECHNIQUE AND INTRAOPERATIVE CONSIDERATIONS

The abdomen is clipped from the tip of the prepuce to the margin of abdominal skin and scrotal skin (Figure 30-29). The clipped area should extend widely into the inguinal region. The scrotum is typically not draped into the surgical field and is not normally clipped during surgical preparation. The scrotum has delicate, thin skin that is easily subject to clipper burn and laceration. If, however, there are long scrotal hairs protruding into the surgical field, they should be trimmed without touching the clippers to the scrotal skin. If scrotal ablation is to be performed, the scrotum is clipped and prepared aseptically along with the rest of the surgical field.

For simple castration, the dog is secured in dorsal recumbency, and a standard surgical preparation of the prescrotal skin (craniad to the scrotum) is performed. A testicle is pushed cranial beneath the prescrotal skin. A midline incision is made in the prescrotal skin centrally and over the cranially displaced testicle. With gentle pressure, the testicle is exteriorized through the incision by carefully incising over the common tunic (tissue that encases the testicle). The major vessels are then easily identified and ligated with two absorbable sutures. The remaining scrotal ligament is gently dissected from the testicle. The opposite testicle is handled in a similar fashion and is exteriorized through the same incision as the first. The incision is closed with a continuous subcuticular suture pattern.

For scrotal ablation, the incision is made circumferentially around the base of the scrotum. The subcutaneous tissue is bluntly dissected to expose the testicles and associated structures. Castration is carried out via ligation of these structures as for simple castration. The testicles and scrotum are removed and the incision closed. Care must be taken to avoid removal of too much skin around the scrotum to prevent excessive tension on the closure.

POSTOPERATIVE CONSIDERATIONS

Several postoperative complications can occur. If the presurgical preparation is not done carefully so as to preclude scrotal dermatitis (clipper burn, excessive scrubbing), the dog will lick aggressively at the scrotum and the incision. This often results in severe inflammation and swelling of the scrotal and prescrotal skin. If this problem is not detected early, the results can be premature suture removal and wound dehiscence. The best treatment is prevention. If scrotal dermatitis does occur, the dog should be placed in an Elizabethan collar.

Another less common complication is hemorrhage. When the testicles are removed from the scrotal sac, free space remains in the scrotum. If there is any hemorrhage, either from the subcutaneous tissue or common tunic, the space will fill with a considerable amount of blood before there is enough pressure to create hemostasis, resulting in a large hematoma within the scrotum. If a hematoma is detected early, before the scrotum is full, cold compresses can be applied with slight pressure to the scrotal area to encourage hemostasis. If the scrotum becomes excessively large, not only is it unsightly but trauma and skin sloughing may also occur. At this point, removal of the scrotum may be necessary.

A scrotal seroma is more likely to occur than hemorrhage and can also result in scrotal swelling. In older dogs with a well-developed scrotal tissue, fluid accumulation after castration can be excessive. Some advocate performing a scrotal ablation at the time of castration to help prevent this complication in older animals. Treatment is the same as for hematoma. It is important to restrict activity in these dogs to decrease the amount of fluid accumulation.

FELINE CASTRATION

DEFINITION

Feline orchidectomy (neuter) is the removal of both testicles.

INDICATIONS

The major indications for feline castration are to prevent fighting, roaming, and urine spraying and to decrease urine odor. Castration in the cat may provide a rapid response (2 to 4 weeks) to these objectionable characteristics, although complete resolution may not occur.

PREOPERATIVE CONSIDERATIONS

The cat is usually castrated around 6 months of age. Preanesthetic evaluation should include palpation of both testicles to confirm the gender of the cat and to detect retained testicles before surgery.

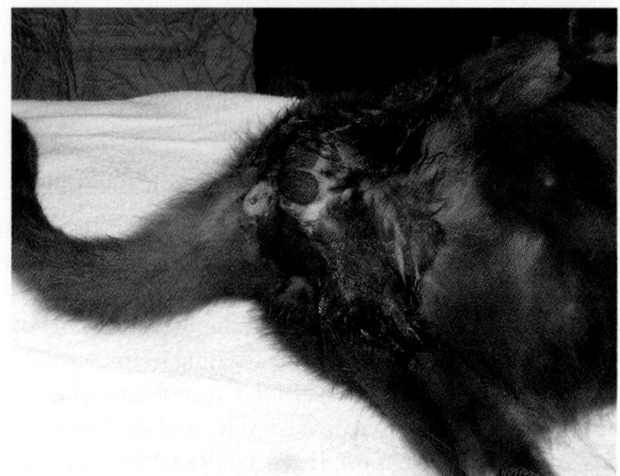

FIGURE 30-30 Proper positioning for feline castration. The legs are pulled forward, and the cat is in dorsal recumbency.

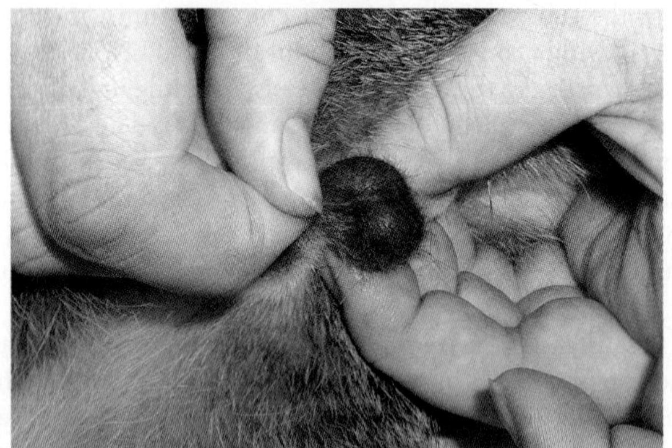

FIGURE 30-31 Technique for scrotal plucking to remove hair in preparation for surgery.

TECHNIQUE AND INTRAOPERATIVE CONSIDERATIONS

There are several acceptable techniques for feline castration. The patient is generally placed in dorsal recumbency with the legs tied craniad (Figure 30-30). Unlike the dog, the scrotum is the site of the primary incision and should be aseptically prepared for surgery. Scrotal dermatitis is not a major concern in the cat, although you should avoid putting alcohol on the scrotum during surgical preparation. Warmed sterile saline is a good substitute for alcohol. The scrotal hairs are gently plucked from the scrotum with the thumb and finger. This is easily accomplished by grasping the base of the scrotum by the thumb and index finger of one hand and gently pushing the testicles into the scrotum (Figure 30-31). With the other hand, the thumb and finger are used to gently strip the hair from the scrotal skin. The scrotum is then scrubbed and draped in an aseptic manner.

An incision is made directly through the scrotum. The testicle is protruded through the incision by gentle pressure with the thumb and index finger. The testicle and its spermatic cord (vessels) are exteriorized and may be ligated with suture, ligated with metal clips, or tied in a knot on itself, or the vessels can be separated from the vas deferens and tied in a square knot. The scrotum is left unsutured.

POSTOPERATIVE CONSIDERATIONS

Scrotal swelling and bleeding are the two most common complications of feline castration. Scrotal swelling is due primarily to traumatic surgical preparation and hair plucking. An Elizabethan collar may be necessary to control licking. If scrotal hemorrhage is noted after surgery, cold compresses on the scrotum for 5 to 7 minutes will help to encourage hemostasis. Severe hemorrhage can also occur and may actually occur intraabdominally. The veterinary technician should monitor these animals carefully (see discussion on blood loss) and bring clinical abnormalities to the attention of the veterinarian. Scrotal infection occurs rarely and should be treated with drainage (if not already draining), scrotal flushing and abscess drainage, Elizabethan collar, and appropriate antibiotics.

When the cat is sent home, the owner should be informed to change the litter from a gravel type of litter to a shredded or pelleted type of litter for the first 5 to 7 days. This will prevent pieces of litter from contaminating the surgical site.

CESAREAN DELIVERY

DEFINITION

Cesarean delivery derived its name from Caesar, allegedly the first to be born by such a technique. The procedure involves making an incision into the abdominal cavity and then into the uterus to deliver a neonate. It is usually performed on animals experiencing dystocia. Dystocia (Greek: dys, difficult + tokos, birth) literally translated means "difficult birth."

INDICATIONS

Cesarean delivery is indicated when a bitch or queen cannot deliver the pups or kits through the birth canal by normal uterine contractions because of either maternal or fetal abnormalities. Some breeders schedule planned cesarean deliveries in dog breeds that might typically have birthing problems, such as bulldogs. Some of the common causes of dystocia are seen in Figure 30-32. Normal stages of parturition are discussed in Chapter 14.

PREOPERATIVE CONSIDERATIONS

The aim of treatment should be the successful delivery of live and undamaged puppies or kittens without harm to the dam. Medical therapy to increase uterine contracture or to treat metabolic abnormalities in the dam should be considered before surgery; however, a diagnosis of the cause of dystocia must be made first. Medical therapy may do more harm than good when used in the wrong type of dystocia (e.g., giving a drug [oxytocin] that would increase uterine muscular contraction in a dam that has a uterine obstruction from a

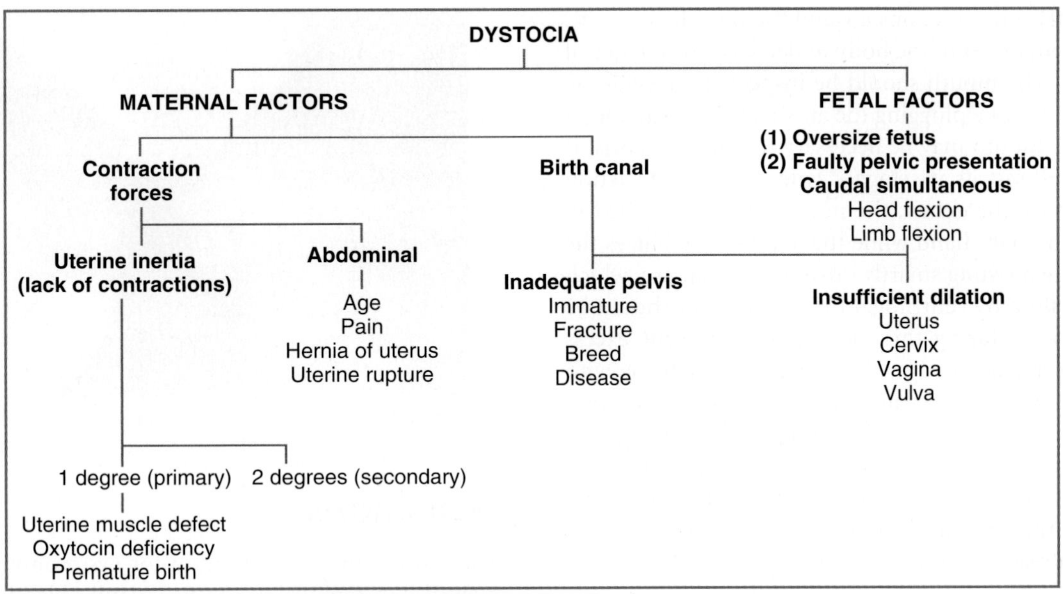

FIGURE 30-32 Common causes of dystocia.

malpositioned fetus or uterine torsion). When proper diagnosis of the type of dystocia is made and medical therapy is either contraindicated or not effective, the dam should be prepared for surgery. Metabolic alterations should be treated before or during anesthesia, if possible.

The anesthetic regimen is of prime importance when considering cesarean delivery. The dam that is dehydrated and exhausted with potential metabolic abnormalities from a prolonged attempted delivery is a poor anesthetic candidate. Anesthetic complications may be encountered. The selected agents should have minimal effects on the newborn. A detailed discussion of anesthetic regimens for the dystocia patient is given in Chapter 27.

TECHNIQUE AND INTRAOPERATIVE CONSIDERATIONS

The animal is clipped before anesthesia. After anesthetic induction and maintenance, the dam is placed in dorsal recumbency. It is important to remember that the increased weight of the gravid uterus on the diaphragm may compromise the normal breathing capacity of the dam, and intermittent manual respiration or a respirator should be considered.

A ventral midline celiotomy is performed (see Figure 30-18). The uterus is exteriorized and isolated with moistened surgical towels. Uterine isolation helps prevent the uterine contents from entering the abdominal cavity. An incision is made into the ventral aspect of the uterine body. Care is taken not to cut a fetus. A neonate and its associated fetal membranes are advanced through the uterine incision by applying gentle traction and pressure on the uterine wall. On presentation, the fetal membranes are removed, the umbilicus is clamped or ligated, and the neonate is handed to the assistant. The fetal membranes can be firmly attached to the uterus if the fetus was not full term. Severe hemorrhage can result if the membranes are pulled from the uterus under those circumstances. Each successive neonate is handled in a similar fashion until all are delivered. The birth canal is checked carefully before closure to ensure that a fetus is not wedged there. The uterine incision is closed in two layers. The abdominal cavity is flushed to remove any debris that might have leaked into it from the gravid uterus. The celiotomy incision is closed in a routine fashion. The skin should be closed internally with an absorbable suture to prevent premature removal by the puppies or kittens during nursing.

Some owners prefer that the dam be spayed at the time of cesarean delivery. This can be accomplished in two ways. An en bloc removal of the gravid uterus can be performed. This entails clamping both ovarian pedicles and the uterine body, cutting the gravid uterus out of the dam, then going back and ligating all the vasculature in the dam. The gravid uterus is given to an assistant, and the assistant cuts each neonate carefully from the uterus using sterile instruments and ligates or clamps the umbilicus. The neonates are then treated as previously described. The second method allows a formal cesarean delivery as already described followed by a routine ovariohysterectomy after uterine body closure. The technique chosen by the surgeon depends upon preference and assistance available to care for the neonates. There is not a proven benefit or downfall to either technique if performed appropriately. Removal of the uterus and ovaries at the time of neonate delivery does not affect milk production or motherly instincts. Alternatively the dam can be returned for ovariohysterectomy after the neonates are weaned.

POSTOPERATIVE CONSIDERATIONS FOR THE NEONATE

The assistant should be ready to grasp the neonate from the surgeon and immediately place it in a dry towel. The assistant can then massage the animal gently to stimulate respiration, dry any secretions around the mouth and nose, and dry the remainder of the body to decrease the chance of hypothermia. The mouth should be inspected for evidence of mucus that may be plugging the airway. Gentle suction of the nostrils or mouth may be necessary to remove debris. If the mouth and nostrils are clogged with mucus and suction does not remove the debris, the neonate can be cradled in the palm of the right hand while the left hand stabilizes the animal; it is then swung smartly downward in an arc, which removes any fluid by centrifugal force. The head should be firmly supported during this maneuver to prevent excess motion and cervical damage. Weak neonates or those with faint respirations may be stimulated by placing doxapram (a respiratory stimulant) under the tongue. A thorough examination for congenital defects is made, and the neonate is placed in an incubator or warm, padded area. Neonates stressed from the prolonged attempted delivery may not survive or may already be dead by the time cesarean delivery is attempted.

The neonates should be returned to the dam as soon as she has recovered from anesthesia. Care should be taken not to return them so early that the dam may unknowingly harm them by stepping or lying on them. The dam should be returned to her home environment as soon as possible so that she can begin caring for the neonates and to prevent transmission of hospital organisms to the immune-challenged neonates.

POSTOPERATIVE CONSIDERATIONS FOR THE DAM

The dam should be awakened from anesthesia as soon as possible so that the neonates can begin nursing. The mother and neonates should be monitored carefully as the two are introduced. Most dams will accept the young readily, but some may be aggressive. If the dam appears painful, pain medication should be considered. It must be remembered that all systemically administered pain medications will be delivered to the neonates through the milk; therefore dosing should be low. Epidural drug administration before surgery will minimize the need for pain medication and transmission of these drugs to the neonate (see anesthetic management of cesarean delivery, Chapter 27). Other considerations include the development of metritis secondary to retained fetal membranes or infection, excessive uterine hemorrhage from overzealous fetal membrane removal, and all the potential complications discussed for routine celiotomy or ovariohysterectomy, if that was performed at the same time. Some dogs may experience infertility after cesarean delivery as a result of scar tissue formation.

CYSTOTOMY

DEFINITION

Cystotomy means incision into the urinary bladder to expose the lumen or interior of the urinary bladder.

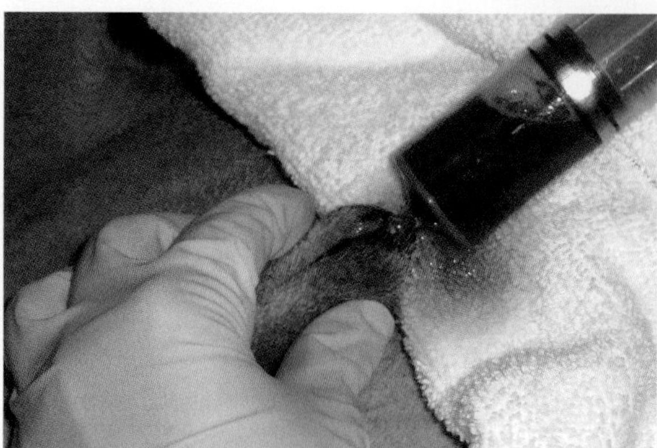

FIGURE 30-33 Proper technique for flushing the prepuce.

INDICATIONS

The most common indication for cystotomy in small animals is for removal of cystic calculi (bladder stones). A cystotomy is also indicated to remove tumors, to correct congenital defects, or to repair traumatic rupture of the urinary bladder. A final indication for cystotomy is placement of a cystostomy tube (a tube exiting the urinary bladder and abdominal wall) to provide an alternate outlet of urine in the case of tumor, calculi, or scar tissue causing obstruction of urine flow through the urethra.

PREOPERATIVE CONSIDERATIONS

Animals undergo cystotomy for various reasons. If urinary flow was obstructed, stabilization of the animal before anesthesia and surgery should be performed. Severe metabolic and/or electrolyte abnormalities might exist. Imaging studies may be necessary to identify the extent of disease and its exact location.

TECHNIQUE AND INTRAOPERATIVE CONSIDERATIONS

The abdomen is widely clipped from the xiphoid to the pubis. In male dogs, care is taken to clip the hair from the prepuce. The preputial orifice and penis are then gently flushed with a 1% povidone-iodine (Betadine) solution (Figure 30-33).

The animal is placed in dorsal recumbency and prepared for surgery with a standard skin preparation. For males, the abdominal skin incision will curve laterally to avoid the prepuce (see Figure 30-18, *D*). Care should be taken to thoroughly prepare this area aseptically. The prepuce is draped into the surgical field in the case of urinary calculi removal. This allows placement of a urinary catheter through the urethra for urethra flushing to aid in calculi removal. Although it is more common for urinary stones to lodge in the urethra of the male, a urethral catheter should also be passed in the female because urethral calculi have been reported to lodge there occasionally. The urinary catheter in the female dog should be placed aseptically before surgery. Care should be taken if bladder expression is attempted before celiotomy because an outflow obstruction from tumor, calculi, or scar tissue may result in inadvertent bladder rupture. Bladder expression should be avoided in those cases or when urinary bladder wall fragility is expected (e.g., urinary flow obstruction or tumor).

In the female, a standard caudal midline celiotomy is performed (see Figure 30-18, *A*). In the male, a caudal midline skin incision is made from the umbilicus to the sheath of the penis and is then extended lateral to the sheath. The caudal superficial epigastric artery and vein lateral to the prepuce are encountered. These are ligated and transected. The sheath is retracted laterally, and a ventral midline celiotomy is performed. The bladder is exteriorized and packed off with laparotomy pads to preclude urine spillage into the abdominal cavity. If a urinalysis and urine culture were not obtained before surgery, a syringe and needle are used to obtain a urine sample before cystotomy. An avascular area on the ventral aspect of the bladder is visualized and two stay sutures placed along the intended incision line. An incision is made along the proposed incision line between preplaced stay sutures. If cystic calculi are present, they are removed and submitted for stone analysis. If biopsies are taken for a suspected tumor, samples are placed in formalin and submitted for histologic analysis. Sample collection containers should be readily available; urinary calculi should not always be placed in formalin, and it is best to ask for appropriate sampling technique from the lab where they will be submitted.

Because calculi can lodge in the urethra, after removal, the entire lower urinary tract (bladder to urethra) is flushed with sterile physiologic saline solution until all calculi have been removed. The bladder wall is inspected for abnormalities and is then closed with a simple interrupted or inverting suture pattern. The laparotomy pads are removed, the abdomen is lavaged with sterile physiologic saline solution, and the incision is closed in a routine fashion. In the case of calculi, a postoperative imaging study may be necessary to determine if all the calculi were actually removed.

POSTOPERATIVE CONSIDERATIONS

The animal should be placed on intravenous fluids after cystotomy to help dilute blood clots and flush the urinary bladder. Urine production should be carefully monitored. If the incision was close to or involved the proximal urethra, postoperative swelling can obstruct urine flow. The veterinarian in charge should be alerted if the animal is straining to urinate and does not produce a urine stream or has not produced urine in 12 hours. Some straining to urinate can be expected following cystotomy as a result of swelling and bladder irritation, but a urine stream should accompany the straining, and the bladder should be nearly empty afterwards. During the first 48 to 72 hours postoperative, a mild hematuria (bloody urine) with or without blood clots and frequent urination can be expected. Owners should be informed of this if the animal is released during this time.

> *TECHNICIAN NOTE* During the first 48 to 72 hours following a cystotomy, a mild hematuria with or without blood clots and frequent urination can be expected.

Treatment ultimately depends on urinalysis, urine culture, and the type of disease present (type of calculi, type of tumor, type of congenital defect). If cystic calculi were removed, stone analysis must be performed before an appropriate treatment regimen can be initiated. Therapy will likely involve dietary alterations and/or antibiotics. The owners should be informed that calculi recurrence is a possibility and that dietary recommendations should be followed strictly to help decrease that chance.

Postoperative complications are rare following cystotomy. They include urinary outflow obstruction as a result of swelling, celiotomy incision complications, uroabdomen secondary to urine leakage through the cystotomy incision, and recurrence of the primary problem. If the animal is unable to urinate following cystotomy, a temporary urinary catheter may have to be placed to keep the bladder decompressed until the surgical swelling decreases. This is not done routinely because catheter placement can cause further irritation to the healing cystotomy incision and because it increases the chance of infection. If the animal is not producing urine or is producing minimal urine and abdominal distention is detected, a complete biochemistry panel, CBC, and paracentesis should be performed. Fluid taken from the abdomen should be spun for PCV determination and should undergo creatinine and BUN determination. Values higher than serum values indicate a problem and should be reported to the veterinarian in charge. Urine leakage through a cystotomy incision is treated with an indwelling urinary catheter or reoperation and appropriate urinary bladder incision closure.

URETHROSTOMY

DEFINITION

Perineal urethrostomy is the process of making an external opening in the urethra in the area of the perineum that is large enough for passage of urine, mucus, crystals, and small calculi without obstruction. It bypasses the narrow penile urethra where obstruction often occurs. The procedure is performed in male cats with recurrent urethral obstruction secondary to feline urologic syndrome. Urethrostomy is also performed in other locations and are named by their location (scrotal urethrostomy, prescrotal urethrostomy, antepubic urethrostomy, etc.). Scrotal urethrostomy rather than perineal urethrostomy is performed in male dogs prone to calculi obstruction or with penile scar tissue preventing normal urination because this location provides the best functional outcome. The general technique is the same.

INDICATIONS

The primary indication for a perineal urethrostomy is multiple episodes of obstruction in association with feline urologic syndrome. Other less common indications include rupture of the penile urethra secondary to traumatic catheterization or blunt trauma (e.g., hit by car, abdominal kick), stricture of the penile urethra, or obstruction secondary to cancer.

PREOPERATIVE CONSIDERATIONS

A cat with feline urologic syndrome can come in for examination with an array of clinical findings, as can dogs with urethral obstruction. The presentation often depends on the duration and completeness of the urinary obstruction. A common factor is straining to urinate. If the animal is brought for examination early, there is little chance that other organ systems are affected. If the animal is brought in 12 to 24 hours after a complete obstruction, severe electrolyte abnormalities, cardiac arrhythmias, kidney dysfunction, and shock can be present. These animals must have the obstruction removed and be stabilized with establishment of improved or normal renal function before surgery. Obstruction of urine flow is an emergency situation in both cats and dogs.

Depending on the suspected cause and location of the obstruction, preoperative imaging studies will be necessary to determine the exact location and extent of the problem.

TECHNIQUE AND INTRAOPERATIVE CONSIDERATIONS

The hair on the perineum and external genitalia is clipped. For perineal urethrostomy, the cat is placed in ventral recumbency with the perineum elevated approximately 30 degrees (Figure 30-34). The tail is extended directly over the dorsal midline and immobilized with tape. A purse-string suture is placed in the anus to eliminate fecal contamination of the surgical field. Standard skin preparation is performed. For scrotal urethrostomy in male dogs, the animal is placed in dorsal recumbency, and the area is prepped as for castration and scrotal ablation.

For perineal urethrostomy, an elliptical skin incision is made around the scrotum and prepuce. The testicles are removed if the cat is intact. The penis is dissected free from its pelvic attachments. A catheter is placed in the urethra, and a longitudinal incision is made through the penile urethra extending craniad to the level of the pelvic urethra. The diameter of the pelvic urethra is approximately two times that of the penile urethra. This allows normal urination in the face of crystalluria (sandlike material in the urine) and mucous plugs. The urethral mucosa is sutured to the skin. The remaining portion of the penis is amputated during urethra suturing, and the urinary catheter is removed. This results in a new, permanent opening that will accommodate the excess mucus and crystals. The bladder should be expressed at completion of the procedure to ensure that a good urine stream is obtained (Figure 30-35). Scrotal urethrostomy in male dogs is performed the same way except that the penis is not amputated. A skin incision is made in the area of the scrotum (castration with scrotal ablation is performed in intact dogs), followed by a urethral incision over a presurgically placed urethral catheter and then suturing of the urethral mucosa to the skin as for perineal urethrostomy.

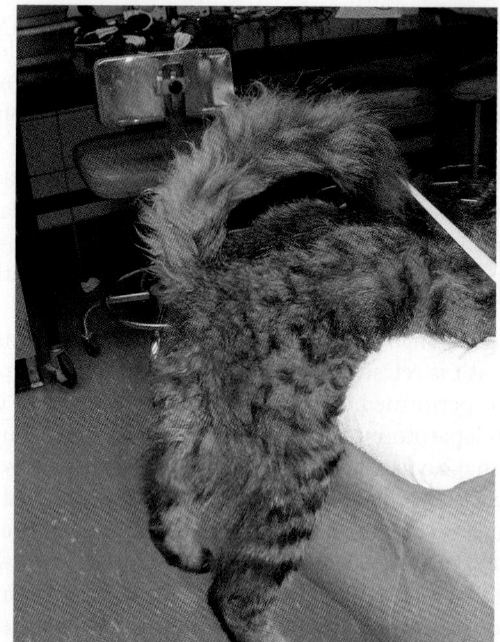

FIGURE 30-34 The perineal position can be used in the dog or cat.

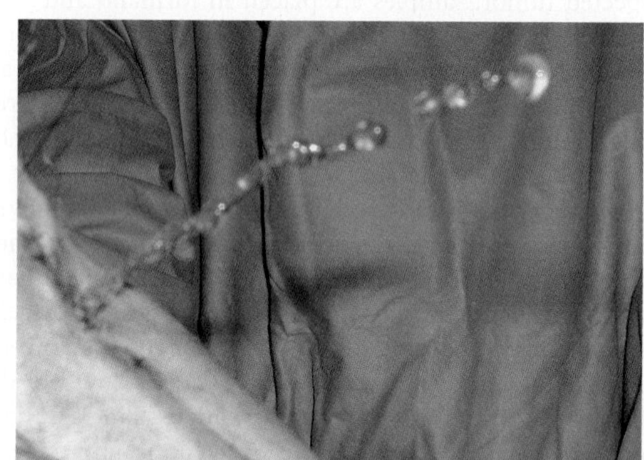

FIGURE 30-35 After urethrostomy in cats, the bladder should be gently expressed to ensure easy urine passage.

POSTOPERATIVE CONSIDERATIONS

The purse-string suture is removed. Immediate postoperative care includes placement of an Elizabethan collar and examination of the surgical site for evidence of hemorrhage. The Elizabethan collar is essential to keep the animal from licking the sutures. Mild hemorrhage during urination is expected for the first 24 to 72 hours after surgery (this may even continue for 2 weeks postoperative, especially in intact animals undergoing urethrostomy). This is usually of no consequence and will resolve on its own. Rarely is the bleeding severe enough to require additional surgery or transfusion. Animals should be placed on intravenous fluids for at least 24 hours after surgery, especially if urinary outflow obstruction was encountered, to maintain normal renal function and flush the urinary bladder and urethra.

The animal should be monitored carefully for normal urination in the early postoperative period. If no urine is produced for 12 hours after surgery, the bladder should be manually expressed until normal urination is seen. Postoperative catheters are discouraged because of the increased incidence of strictures at the surgery site. The urethrostomy site should be manipulated as little as possible. Ointments and warm cleansings are also discouraged. This may delay healing or aggravate hemorrhage. For cats, the use of shredded paper or pellets in the litter box is recommended for the first 7 to 10 days. Dietary alterations will likely be necessary depending on the composition of the mucous plug, grit, or calculi causing the obstruction and the presence or absence of a urinary tract infection. Owners will have to be counseled on the importance of dietary modification.

The most common late postoperative complication is stricture. This is generally manifested by chronic stranguria (straining to urinate). Complete obstruction of urine flow may also be noted. Stricture requires reoperation.

HERNIAS

The strict definition of hernia is protrusion of tissue from its normal cavity (generally the abdominal cavity) through a congenital or acquired defect in the wall of that cavity. Some common hernias in the dog and cat are umbilical hernias, inguinal hernias, and diaphragmatic hernias.

UMBILICAL HERNIA

DEFINITION

An umbilical hernia is one in which bowel or, more commonly, omentum and intraabdominal fat protrudes through a defect in the abdominal wall under the skin at the umbilicus. This hernia is most commonly congenital, and it is recognized on physical examination by the presence of a swelling at the umbilicus (Figure 30-36).

PREOPERATIVE CONSIDERATIONS

Most umbilical hernias are not life threatening and are surgically repaired at the time of ovariohysterectomy or castration. Small hernias in young dogs (2 to 4 months of age) may be self-limiting. Larger hernias or those in older dogs (6 to 9 months of age) generally require surgical repair. Large umbilical hernias can result in intestinal entrapment (incarceration) within the confines of the hernia with resultant strangulation (loss of intestinal blood supply with devitalization and possible intestinal perforation). If intestinal strangulation occurs, surgical repair becomes an emergency.

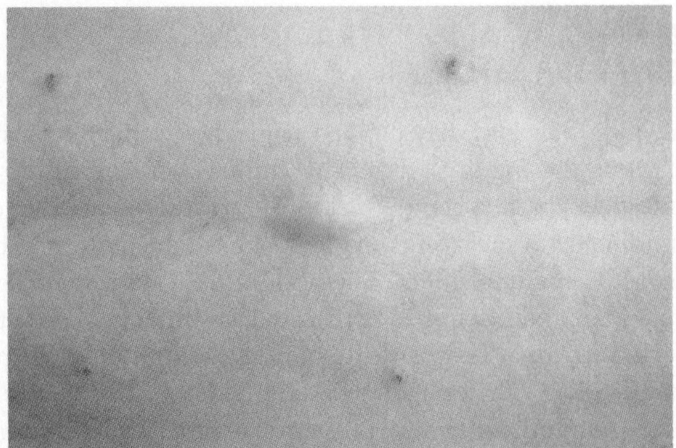

FIGURE 30-36 Note the raised lesion in the region of the umbilicus (umbilical hernia) on the ventral abdomen.

TECHNIQUE AND INTRAOPERATIVE CONSIDERATIONS

The abdomen is widely clipped from xiphoid to pubis. The patient is placed in dorsal recumbency, and a standard skin preparation is performed. A ventral midline incision is made directly over the hernia, being careful not to perforate the hernia contents. The skin is dissected away from the hernial sac; the contents are then exposed and are either replaced into the abdominal cavity (intestine) or excised (falciform or omental fat). The edges of the hernial ring are trimmed to ensure healing of the defect. The abdomen is closed in a routine fashion as for the celiotomy incision.

POSTOPERATIVE CONSIDERATIONS

Postoperative care is similar to that for any celiotomy incision. Recurrence is a rare complication of repair, and reoperation is necessary for correction.

INGUINAL HERNIA

DEFINITION

An inguinal hernia is one in which intestine, uterus, broad ligament, intraabdominal fat, and/or another abdominal organ protrudes through the inguinal canal as a result of a defect in the constraints of the canal. This is more common in the bitch than in the male dog. An inguinal hernia is diagnosed on physical examination by the presence of a soft, doughy, nonpainful mass in the inguinal region. Inguinal hernias can develop early or late in life. It does not spontaneously regress, and surgical correction is necessary.

PREOPERATIVE CONSIDERATIONS

The opposite inguinal ring should be carefully palpated for weakness. Owners should be told that hernias can develop bilaterally, even if a hernia is not present on the opposite side at the time of presentation. Owners should also be told that recurrence is rare, but possible.

TECHNIQUE AND INTRAOPERATIVE CONSIDERATIONS

The abdomen is widely clipped from the umbilicus to and including the inguinal area. The animal is placed in dorsal recumbency, and a standard skin preparation is performed. A midline skin incision is made in the caudal abdomen between the inguinal folds. The abdominal cavity is not entered. Lateral dissection is performed carefully to expose the affected inguinal ring with its hernial sac and external pudendal vessels. The hernial sac is emptied of its contents with gentle manipulation and pressure toward the abdominal cavity. The empty sac is then excised and sutured along with the margin of the inguinal ring. Care is taken during closure to avoid the external pudendal vessels that exit from the caudal medial aspect of the ring. The skin incision is closed as for celiotomy.

POSTOPERATIVE CONSIDERATIONS

The incision is monitored as any abdominal incision. The owner should monitor for recurrence or occurrence on the opposite side.

DIAPHRAGMATIC HERNIA

DEFINITION

A diaphragmatic hernia exists when abdominal contents protrude through an opening in the diaphragm into the thoracic cavity. Diaphragmatic hernias may be congenital or traumatic.

PREOPERATIVE CONSIDERATIONS

Any animal with a history of trauma or suspected trauma should be examined for presence of a diaphragmatic hernia. Diaphragmatic hernias can be life threatening or insidious and difficult to identify. Signs can also be masked by other problems. Presumptive diagnosis is based on a thorough physical examination. The classic signs of diaphragmatic hernia are a "tucked-up" abdomen (thin, empty abdomen), intestinal sounds in the chest, muffled heart and lung sounds, and dyspnea. However, some animals only have decreased lung sounds over the area of the hernia and mild exercise intolerance, if that. The diagnosis is confirmed by a thoracic radiograph.

> *TECHNICIAN NOTE* Animals with a diaphragmatic hernia should have oxygen and cage confinement to allow maximal oxygenation, minimal stress, and constant monitoring for respiratory insufficiency before surgery.

An animal with a massive hernia will have a diminished intrathoracic space as a result of the presence of abdominal contents within the thoracic cavity. The resultant space occupying mass does not allow the lungs to expand normally and compromises oxygen delivery to the blood. These animals can have life-threatening respiratory compromise and should be treated appropriately. Any animal with respiratory compromise should be stabilized. This includes minimal stress, oxygen cage or nasal oxygen insufflation, confinement, sternal recumbency, and constant monitoring for respiratory insufficiency or arrest. Sometimes holding the animal gently and with the head up and the rear legs hanging down will allow some abdominal contents to shift back into the abdomen. Along the same lines, the animal can be propped up such that the front half of the chest and shoulders are higher than the hindquarters. Intravenous access should be established in case of an emergency so long as the stress of catheter placement does not cause further respiratory embarrassment. Thoracic radiographs will be necessary for diagnosis and to assess for other pathologic conditions, but the animal should be stabilized as best as possible beforehand. Rarely is diaphragmatic hernia repair an emergency. Mortality is actually higher in those animals operated on acutely for the problem. Only in cases of massive hernia with severe respiratory distress or severe gas distention of a herniated viscus (stomach) is immediate operation necessary.

> *TECHNICIAN NOTE* Positioning an animal with a diaphragmatic hernia in sternal recumbency with the shoulders higher than the pelvis or gently raising the animal up from the front end may help reduce abdominal structures back into the abdomen from the thoracic cavity and improve respiration.

TECHNIQUE AND INTRAOPERATIVE CONSIDERATIONS

One of the most critical time periods for an animal with a diaphragmatic hernia is anesthetic induction. It is important to be thoroughly familiar with induction procedures and resuscitative techniques in the event of respiratory or cardiac arrest. The animal is placed in dorsal recumbency on an incline, with the head slightly higher than the hindquarters. It is important to remember that severe respiratory compromise may result when the animal is placed in dorsal recumbency, and the technician should be prepared to breathe for the animal. Mechanical ventilation or intermittent manual respiration will be necessary throughout the procedure.

The skin is widely clipped from about 3 inches cranial to the xiphoid to the pubis. The lateral thoracic wall on at least one side, preferably the side of the hernia, should be clipped and aseptically prepared for potential chest tube placement. A ventral midline celiotomy from xiphoid to umbilicus is performed. The edges of the incision are protected with laparotomy pads, and a Balfour self-retaining abdominal retractor is placed to enhance visualization. The diaphragmatic defect is inspected, and any herniated contents are gently reduced into the abdominal cavity. If the herniated contents do not reduce easily, the diaphragmatic defect is enlarged slightly to allow easy reduction. A thorough inspection of abdominal and thoracic viscera is made to rule out organ rupture or vascular compromise.

Diaphragmatic hernia repair requires working in a deep cavity. Gentle retraction of viscera to expose the defect during repair is necessary to preclude damage to abdominal organs to allow adequate visualization by the surgeon. The diaphragmatic defect is sutured with a nonabsorbable suture material in a simple continuous suture pattern. This will affect an airtight and watertight seal. Air is evacuated from the chest by thoracocentesis through the diaphragm or with chest tube placement. The celiotomy is closed in a routine fashion. After celiotomy closure, the chest cavity is once again aspirated from the lateral thoracic wall. If a chest tube was placed, evacuation of the thoracic cavity occurs through the chest tube.

POSTOPERATIVE CONSIDERATIONS

The animal should be monitored carefully for signs of respiratory distress. It is best to waken these animals with oxygen supplementation either through placement in an oxygen cage or through nasal insufflation. If a pulse oximeter is available, oxygen saturation should be checked frequently, especially as an attempt is made to wean the animal off oxygen. If dyspnea occurs or the animal cannot maintain normal oxygen saturation, the chest should be evacuated with a hypodermic needle, three-way stopcock, and a large syringe or through the chest tube. A rapid return to normal negative thoracic pressure and normal lung capacity should occur with evacuation of air and fluid.

If an indwelling chest tube was placed, periodic aspiration using positional changes (right lateral recumbency, left lateral recumbency, standing on hind legs, standing on front legs) will afford maximal removal of air and fluid. It is of utmost importance to keep the animal from chewing a hole in the drain or removing it from the chest cavity, and those involved in tube management should be informed on how the tube should be handled. An Elizabethan collar may be necessary, and the chest tube should be covered with a bandage. It is also imperative to keep all connections on the chest drain airtight. A security clamp should be placed on the tube to keep air from leaking into the chest if the free end of the tube is inadvertently opened. Premature removal, puncture, or inappropriate management (leaving the three-way stopcock open to the atmosphere) can result in acute animal death secondary to pneumothorax and resultant pulmonary dysfunction. Proper management of a chest tube requires full-time patient monitoring. A chart quantitating the amount of air and fluid removed during a given period of time (12 to 24 hours) will help to determine when the tube should be removed. Most chest tubes are removed immediately following surgery once negative intrathoracic pressure is obtained or within 12 hours of hernia repair. Otherwise, the tube can safely be removed as the amount of air and fluid decreases toward zero.

> *TECHNICIAN NOTE* The animal with a chest tube should be handled carefully to prevent inadvertent introduction of air around the lungs and potential death of the animal. Make sure the tube is airtight, all connections to the environment are closed, and that it is equipped with a protective clamp.

LUMPECTOMY

DEFINITION

Lumpectomy refers to local surgical resection of a mass. The term often refers to cutaneous or subcutaneous masses.

INDICATIONS

Indications for lumpectomy include masses of cancerous origin, rapidly growing masses or masses that appear to be changing, ulcerative masses, nonhealing wounds, or masses that are impairing function.

PREOPERATIVE CONSIDERATIONS

Some masses are related to biochemical or blood cell alterations. Blood work should be performed to evaluate for these abnormalities. Abnormalities should be corrected before anesthesia, if possible. Additionally, many animals undergoing surgery for mass resection are older and may have organ system failure, which should be evaluated before anesthesia. After a mass is diagnosed, fine-needle aspiration of the mass is performed. If the mass is considered benign (i.e., lipoma), resection can proceed or the owner can monitor the mass. If changes in the mass are noted, resection should be considered. If the mass appears cancerous, further work-up for detection of metastasis should be considered, and resection is strongly recommended. All surgically resected masses should be submitted for histologic evaluation. Removed masses are placed in formalin at a 1:10 ratio of mass to fluid.

TECHNIQUE AND INTRAOPERATIVE CONSIDERATIONS

The skin around the area to be resected is prepared for surgery. It should be remembered that a generous clip needs to be performed because normal margins will need to be removed with the mass. Additionally, large mass resections will require that normal skin around the mass be pulled into the surgical field during closure. If this skin was not prepared aseptically before surgery, it will contaminate the surgical field. Masses should be manipulated as little as possible before surgery. A sterile marker is used to draw an elliptical pattern around the mass to be removed. One to 3 cm of normal tissue is included in the resection plane with large margins reserved for cancerous lesions. The mass is removed and the wound closed in three layers with absorbable suture placed internally.

The mass is marked with ink or suture to note cranial and lateral margins. This will help future surgical planning if the mass was found to be incompletely resected according to histologic evaluation.

POSTOPERATIVE CONSIDERATIONS

The surgical wound should be monitored as any other surgical procedure. Large resections will result in tension on the incision line, making dehiscence more likely. Animals should be exercise-restricted until the wound is healed and sutures are removed. Owners should be told that further steps for treatment may need to be taken once a diagnosis is obtained (future surgery if complete resection was not obtained, chemotherapy, radiation therapy, etc.).

REMOVAL OF MAMMARY NEOPLASIA

DEFINITION

Mammary neoplasia is cancer of the mammary gland. It is the most frequently occurring neoplasm in the female dog and the third most frequently found tumor in the female cat. Mastectomy is removal of a mammary gland. Radical mastectomy is removal of a chain of mammary glands on one or both sides of the animal. Lumpectomy is removal of a mammary tumor with approximately 1 cm of normal marginal tissue, not the entire mammary gland.

GENERAL INFORMATION AND INDICATIONS

In dogs, there is a significantly higher incidence of mammary gland tumors in nonspayed females or females that are spayed after their first estrus. Spaying before the first estrus cycle provides a definite protective factor against mammary tumor development.

In the initial stages, the tumor will usually appear as a small, pea-shaped, firm mass in one or more of the glands of the mammary chain. Long-standing or fast-growing tumors may present a sizeable mass with ulceration and drainage. Early diagnosis and therapy is best when dealing with mammary neoplasia.

Before surgery is considered, an examination for possible metastasis of the tumor is done. Malignant tumors will generally metastasize to the lymph nodes and lungs. Chest radiographs may detect pulmonary metastases, and abdominal radiographs may show iliac lymph node enlargement suggestive of metastasis. About 50% of mammary tumors in dogs are malignant, and about 80% to 90% of mammary tumors in cats are malignant. Surgical resection of tumors that have already metastasized does not improve prognosis. At the time of surgery, biopsy of regional lymph nodes should always be performed.

Surgery is currently considered the most effective therapy. The primary objective of surgical treatment is to remove completely the tumor tissue for potential cure and to obtain a histologic diagnosis of type of tumor and behavior.

TECHNIQUE AND INTRAOPERATIVE CONSIDERATIONS

Two techniques are available for tumor resection. In dogs, there appears to be no advantage to radical gland resection versus lumpectomy unless the tumor is incompletely excised. Lumpectomy affords the same long-term outcome as varying forms of mastectomy as long as the tumor is freely movable, small, and on the periphery of the gland. If the tumor is centralized within a gland, multiple tumors are present within a gland or a chain of glands, or the tumor is large and/or fixed, a more radical excision is warranted. In cats, unlike in dogs, recurrence is decreased if a unilateral mastectomy is performed rather than local excision of the mass. If bilateral radical mastectomy is necessary, the procedure must be staged (removal of one side at a time) to allow less tension on the skin closure. The skin is clipped widely to include all affected mammary glands. The animal is placed in dorsal recumbency, and a standard skin preparation is performed. An elliptical incision is made, attempting to include a 1-cm margin around the tumor. The skin and tumor, with or without the mammary gland, are gently undermined and removed. The skin incision is often gaping after tumor excision if an entire gland is removed, requiring a meticulous subcutaneous closure. Subcutaneous tissues are closed with a simple interrupted pattern using absorbable suture material. An active drain may be placed if a large amount of tissue is removed to help prevent fluid accumulation under the skin. The skin is closed in a routine fashion. The excised mammary masses are placed in formalin and sent to a laboratory for histopathologic evaluation.

POSTOPERATIVE CONSIDERATIONS

Major complications that can occur postoperatively are generally related to the tension placed on the skin to adequately close the wound when large amounts of tissue are removed. Seroma formation is common, especially if a drain was not placed at the time of surgery and the resection was large. It is best to bandage these animals for 48 to 72 hours postoperative to help prevent large amounts of fluid from accumulating under the incision and to make the animal more comfortable. Warm compresses may be needed after seroma development. Dehiscence is not common, but the incision should be examined daily for evidence of separation, especially if a large amount of tissue is removed. Bruising along the incision edges is common and should be expected. Immediate postoperative hemorrhage can occur. In the event of oozing blood, an abdominal bandage should be applied with gentle pressure. If a drain was placed, a bandage should be placed over the drain. The drain is emptied several times a day and is removed when minimal drainage is noted. If the animal irritates the incision by licking, an Elizabethan collar should be applied until suture removal. An Elizabethan collar should be applied as long as a drain is in place to prevent self-inflicted pulling or breaking of the drain. The animal should be exercise restricted, especially if a large incision under tension is present, to help prevent dehiscence and seroma formation. Radical mastectomy is a painful procedure, and pain management should be continued for at least 5 days postoperative.

AMPUTATION

DEFINITION

Amputation refers to partial or complete removal of a body part, such as a limb or a toe. This section covers limb amputation.

INDICATIONS

Indications for amputation include appendicular cancer not amenable to local excision or other treatment modality (amputation may be curative or may be done as palliative therapy in some instances); severe neurologic dysfunction resulting in repeated trauma of a limb; nonunion fractures that will not result in limb function with orthopedic repair; irresolvable osteomyelitis; vascular disease of the limb, such as thrombosis or arteriovenous fistulae; and congenital deformity resulting in a nonfunctional limb not amenable to orthopedic repair. Simple limb fracture is not an indication for amputation, although some veterinarians may perform the procedure for that problem.

PREOPERATIVE CONSIDERATIONS

Amputation can involve considerable blood loss. It is important to perform presurgical blood work to determine PCV and TP. Transfusion should be given or anticipated depending on the animal's preoperative values. Additionally, coagulation times should be assessed. A thorough orthopedic examination should be done to evaluate concurrent orthopedic problems. The owner needs to be aware of other orthopedic conditions that are diagnosed and how they may affect function following amputation. Orthopedic problems in other limbs can make ambulation after amputation difficult, depending on the severity and type of problem. The owner should also be made aware of neurologic problems affecting other limbs. This too can lead to difficult ambulation after amputation. When amputation is done because of neoplasia, the animal should be screened appropriately for metastasis. The amputation must be planned such that adequate margins of normal tissue are obtained if cancer is involved. Amputation is a painful procedure, and analgesics are best initiated before surgery and continued without interruption in the postoperative period.

For rear limb amputations with disarticulation of the coxofemoral joint in intact male dogs, scrotal swelling is a major concern. Seroma formation after amputation is common, and fluid tends to accumulate in the scrotum. Scrotal swelling can become so severe that ablation is necessary. Additionally the scrotum is more visible after amputation and may not be aesthetically pleasing to some owners. It is best to perform a scrotal ablation and castration at the time of amputation in these dogs.

TECHNIQUE AND PERIOPERATIVE CONSIDERATIONS

The limb is suspended from an intravenous fluid stand as for an orthopedic procedure. The limb is clipped and aseptically prepared for surgery. The clip should be generous and include the skin around the base of the limb to prevent contamination during closure. In general, a skin incision is made around the limb in the area to be amputated. Subcutaneous and muscle tissue are dissected and transected to remove the limb. Vessels are ligated and transected, and nerves are blocked with local anesthetic and then transected. Depending on the site of amputation, the limb may need to be disarticulated or the bone severed to remove the limb. The remaining muscle and subcutaneous tissue are closed over the bone and/or wound bed. The skin is closed in three layers. If a large amount of dead space is present at the time of closure, a closed, active drain can be placed.

Thoracic limb amputation can be done by removing the scapula and the entire forelimb (forequarter amputation), disarticulation of the scapulohumeral joint, or by ostectomy (cutting of the bone) at the level of the proximal humerus. Forequarter amputation offers the advantages that the major vessels and nerves are well visualized, sectioning the bone is not required, and the prominent scapular spine will not be present as the scapular muscle mass atrophies. It is also indicated in neoplastic diseases of the humerus (especially proximal) or of the scapula. Disarticulation leaves a more full appearance to the thorax and requires less extensive dissection, but muscle atrophy over the scapula can be unsightly in some cases. If disarticulation is performed, the acromion process should be excised to improve appearance. Proximal humeral amputation may be faster for some.

Pelvic limb amputation can be accomplished by disarticulation of the coxofemoral joint or proximal femoral osteotomy. Proximal femoral osteotomy yields a more cosmetic result, particularly in an intact male dog. It is also faster and easier than disarticulation. However, the remaining stump will move as the animal ambulates, and the owners must be made aware of this. Neoplastic diseases of the femur will require disarticulation to obtain a normal margin of tissue.

POSTOPERATIVE CONSIDERATIONS

Postoperative complications are not a major concern, but should not be ignored. Animals undergoing amputation are painful, and analgesics must be given. It is best to give analgesics as schedule doses rather than on an "as needed" basis. Analgesics will likely be required for 4 to 5 days after surgery.

Seroma formation is common. The area can be cold compressed for the first 24 hours after surgery, and if a seroma forms, warm compresses can be initiated. The limb should be bandaged for the first 24 to 48 hours, if possible. This will provide some comfort for the animal and help minimize seroma formation. The animal should be exercise restricted because motion will increase seroma size. Hematoma is also a possibility.

Seroma or hematoma formation after surgery can increase the chance of infection. If infection develops, the incision site will have to be opened, drained, and a culture and sensitivity obtained. Anemia can occur in the postoperative period as a result of blood loss at the time of surgery. Transfusion may be necessary. Intravenous fluids should be administered postoperative until eating and drinking resumes. Additionally the animal should be kept in a well-padded area and supported with a sling when taken out for a walk (until the animal learns to ambulate on three legs). Tension on the incision line, seroma formation, or infection may lead to dehiscence. Depending on the cause and degree of dehiscence, this is managed conservatively or with surgical closure. Animals with neoplasia may develop metastatic disease or have tumor recurrence at the surgery site.

Amputation is generally more traumatic to the owner than their pet. Three-legged dogs and cats are excellent pets, and it is important to help the owner understand that. Most animals are ambulating within 24 hours of surgery, but some may take another day. Almost all are ambulatory within 2 days of surgery. Animals should be kept in the hospital until they are ambulating and their pain seems well controlled. Amputees have an excellent prognosis unless the limb was amputated for neoplastic disease. For neoplasia, the prognosis depends on the type of tumor. Most owners are satisfied regardless of the reason for amputation; the age, breed, or weight of the animals; or the animal's survival time after surgery.

NEUROLOGIC PATIENT CARE

The most common neurologic disorder in the dog is spontaneous intervertebral disk disease. Disks are normally found between vertebral bodies in the spine and act as shock absorbers during spinal movements. With time, the disks can undergo degeneration and calcification. When this occurs, the normal shock absorber–like effect is impaired, and extrusion (rupture) of the disk material into the spinal canal can occur. This puts pressure on the spinal cord and can cause an array of neurologic deficits or pain. Other neurologic disorders that may be encountered include atlantoaxial subluxation in toy breeds (abnormal articulation between the first and second cervical vertebra), acute spinal trauma (fracture, luxation), cauda equina (compression of the lumbosacral nerve roots), and cervical spinal cord malformation. Many animals with neurologic problems are referred to specialty hospitals for surgery. However, the veterinary technician should be familiar with some of the procedures that might be performed and understand how to manage neurologic patients in general so that when they return to the veterinary hospital for care after surgery, the technician understands what to do.

One neurosurgical procedure occasionally performed in small animal practice is intervertebral disk fenestration. In this procedure, each disk that is calcified or that may become calcified is removed (scraped) from the intervertebral space. This procedure is performed under some circumstances to help deter rupture of the disk material into the spinal canal, although its benefit is unproven. Dogs may develop spontaneous intervertebral disk extrusions in the cervical spine (neck) or the thoracolumbar spine (lower back). If the disk has already ruptured and the animal's ability to ambulate is affected, a decompressive procedure must be performed to alleviate compression on the spinal cord. The most common decompressive procedures are the ventral slot (for cervical disk rupture) and hemilaminectomy (for thoracolumbar disk rupture). For acute disk herniation, the most commonly affected breed is the dachshund, but the beagle, Pekingese, poodle, and terrier breeds also frequently experience disk herniation.

SURGICAL TECHNIQUE AND PERIOPERATIVE CONSIDERATIONS

When an animal with spinal column instability is anesthetized, the normal protective abilities of muscle support and conscious perception of pain are removed. Conditions that can result in instability include spinal fracture or luxation and atlantoaxial instability. Animals with simple disk herniation or spinal malformation can also be worsened by excessive manipulation while under anesthesia. It is the responsibility of the veterinary technician, anesthesiologist, and surgeon to protect the animal from further neurologic damage by handling the spine with care while under anesthesia. It is important to keep the neck and back as straight as possible when moving the animal from one location to another. To accomplish this, the animal can be taped to a rigid, flat surface, can be carefully cradled in the arm, or placed in a stiff blanket sling supported on all sides. No matter how they are carried, one should be careful to avoid manipulation of the affected area. The means of transportation is often dictated by the size of the animal, but a rigid, flat surface is the preferred method for transporting animals with severe instability.

Animals undergoing cervical disk surgery are placed in dorsal recumbency with the head and neck in slight extension (Figure 30-37). The ventral aspect of the neck is widely clipped from the manubrium sterni to the cranial aspect of the larynx. A standard skin preparation is performed. A ventral midline incision is made through the skin and muscles to expose the intervertebral spaces. For fenestration, a dental tartar scraper, curved needle, fenestration hook, or curette can be used to remove the disk material from the interspace. Fenestration is carried out from the C2-3 to the C6-7 disk space. If decompression is needed, an oblong slot is made through the vertebral bodies into the spinal canal using a pneumatic or electric-powered bur. The disk material is then carefully removed from the spinal canal. A fat graft is placed over the spinal cord in the defect to prevent restrictive scar formation. The surgical wound is closed in layers with

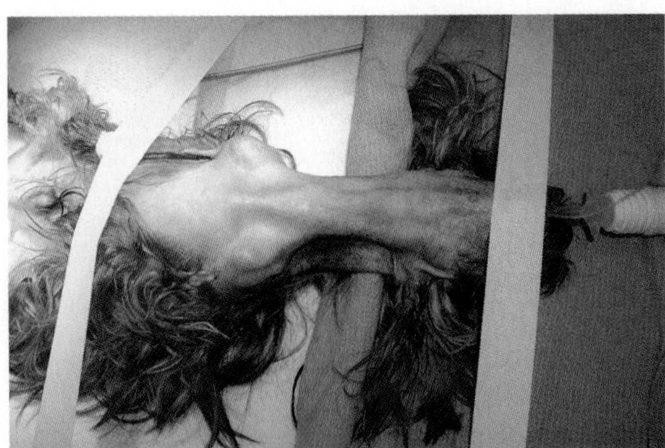

FIGURE 30-37 Proper positioning for cervical disk surgery.

a continuous suture pattern using an absorbable suture. The skin is closed in a routine fashion.

Animals undergoing thoracolumbar disk surgery are placed in ventral recumbency. For fenestration, the dorsum over the back is widely clipped from the midthoracic region to the pelvis. A standard skin preparation is performed. A skin incision is made from T11 to L6. Careful dissection between epaxial muscles (muscles of the back) allows palpation and limited visualization of the disk spaces. For fenestration, each space between T10 and L5 is curetted with a technique similar to that described for cervical disk fenestration. If decompression is needed, a portion of the bony lamina covering the spinal cord is removed with a pneumatic or electric-powered bur or bone rongeurs. The ruptured disk material is then carefully removed from the spinal canal. A fat graft is placed in the defect over the spinal cord. The muscles, subcutaneous tissue, and skin are closed in a routine fashion.

POSTOPERATIVE CONSIDERATIONS

The preoperative and postoperative care of neurologic patients depends on their neurologic status and the type of neurologic disease that they have. Management for the nonambulatory animal is demanding. Animals are subject to decubital ulcers (bed sores or pressure sores), urinary bladder infections, joint stiffness, muscle atrophy (muscle wasting), pneumonia, and gastrointestinal ulceration. Preventing these conditions from occurring is the main objective of proper postoperative management and should include the following:

- Passive range-of-motion exercises, muscle massages, underwater treadmill activity, sling walking, and whirlpool baths encourage joint motion and muscular activity and help decrease the chance of pressure sore formation. Passive range of motion should be performed at least three times a day on all affected limbs until the animal is able to ambulate normally.
- Urinary bladder expression four or five times per day to keep the urinary bladder empty. This will help keep the animal clean, prevent detrusor muscle atony secondary to bladder overdistention (which can lead to permanent bladder dysfunction), and might lower the incidence of infection resulting from urine retention.

> *TECHNICIAN NOTE* For animals that cannot consciously urinate, it is important to keep the urinary bladder empty by urinary catheterization or manual expression. This will prevent overdistention with permanent urinary bladder dysfunction, keep the animal clean, and help decrease infection rate.

- Flip the animal frequently (every 4 hours) to reduce the incidence of pneumonia and to help prevent pressure sore formation. Slings and wheelchairs can be used to get the animal up and off pressure points for a period of time if their spinal injury is stable.
- Monitor the animal daily for fever, cough, or respiratory distress. The down animal is at risk for pneumonia. Daily coupage and getting the animal up will help prevent this. Fever may also be an indication of severe gastrointestinal ulcer formation.
- Keep the animal in a well-padded area to prevent the formation of sores. A water bed mattress works well for large dogs.
- Keep the animal clean and dry. Soiling will increase the chance of pressure-sore formation. This can be challenging when incontinence and immobility play a role.
- Observation of the stool for evidence of fresh blood (bright red on feces or thermometer) or digested blood (dark, tarry feces), which may be an indicator of colonic or gastric ulceration, respectively, which can occur following spinal cord injury, hospital stress, and/or steroid therapy.
- Observe vomiting. If the vomitus contains coffee ground–like material, it is indicative of gastric bleeding secondary to ulcer formation.
- Observe the animal daily for evidence of pressure sores. Sores tend to form over bone prominences, especially in large dogs (Figure 30-38). Pressure-sore formation can lead to sepsis and death if severe, and their presence should not be taken lightly. Prompt treatment should be initiated to prevent severe complications. Treatment consists of frequent flipping, whirlpool baths, massages, antibiotics, clipping and cleaning of the area, surgical débridement, and/or bandages to alleviate pressure over a prominence, depending on the severity of the lesion. Prevention is the best form of therapy.

> *TECHNICIAN NOTE* It is better to prevent pressure-sore formation than to have to treat a pressure sore once it occurs.

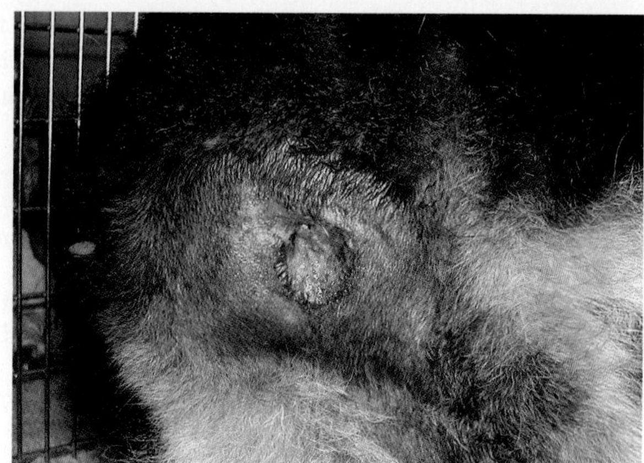

FIGURE 30-38 Decubital ulcer (pressure sore). The ulcer developed over the greater trochanter of this dog as a result of improper care during recovery from spinal surgery.

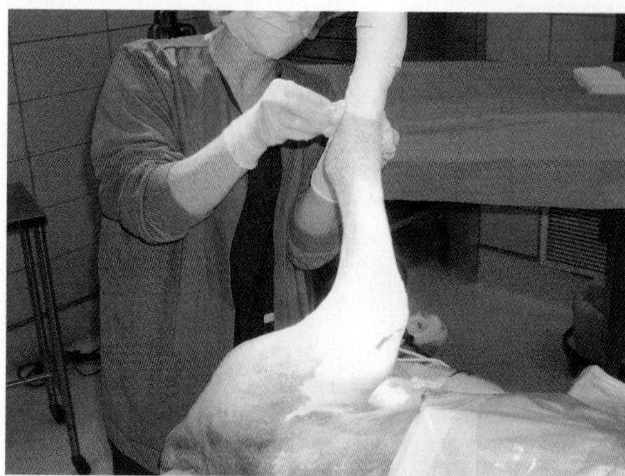

FIGURE 30-39 Proper limb positioning for limb preparation for orthopedic surgery.

- Animals that have lost pain sensation to one or more limbs should be monitored carefully. These animals may begin to lick or chew the **asensory** portion of their limbs, especially if the area becomes traumatized. Some will even chew off toes or whole limbs. If an animal without sensation to a limb begins to lick the limb, an Elizabethan collar should be placed immediately.
- An animal that cannot walk should never be allowed to roam free. They will traumatize their skin as they drag themselves around and can develop serious abrasions and ulcers.
- Animals with some motor function to the limbs and a stable spinal injury should be gotten up at least three times a day and encouraged to use their limbs. Ambulatory but ataxic animals should be supported when ambulating to help prevent falls that might lead to further spinal damage. Rehabilitation through specialized centers offering underwater treadmill work and other rehabilitation techniques should be considered.

> *TECHNICIAN NOTE* Animals with injuries to the cervical spine should always be placed in a harness rather than in a collar to prevent further cervical damage.

All animals with neurologic injuries require cage rest and controlled activity to allow the spinal column to heal. They should all be leashed when outdoors (animals with cervical problems should always be placed in a harness rather than in a neck collar to prevent further cervical damage), crated when indoors, and restricted according to the surgeon's protocol. Owners should be carefully counseled on the importance of confinement for prevention of further spinal injury.

> *TECHNICIAN NOTE* All animals with a spinal injury will require cage rest, whether surgery is done or not. It is important to emphasize to owners that cage rest is important for proper healing, even if their pet is walking and feeling normal.

As can be seen from the preceding list, the veterinary technician and veterinarian must work diligently and continually to properly manage animals with neurologic dysfunction.

ORTHOPEDIC SURGERY

LONG-BONE FRACTURES

Preoperative Considerations

When an animal is brought to the veterinary hospital with a fracture, several steps must be taken to ready the animal for a permanent repair. First, the animal must be stabilized with respect to all other body systems (treated for shock, chest injuries, and abdominal injuries). Second, any open wounds associated with the fracture should be managed. Third, the fracture must be immobilized by means of a bandage, cast, or sling if the fracture is in a location amenable to bandaging (review Chapter 34). Once these three things have been achieved, fracture repair can be safely considered. Most long-bone fractures are not life threatening and do not require emergency surgery. Stability of the animal determines when the fracture is repaired.

> *TECHNICIAN NOTE* Most long-bone fractures are not life threatening and do not require emergency surgery.

Intraoperative Considerations

The limb is usually suspended from the foot (Figure 30-39). An extensive hair clip is required on all limb preparations. The limb will usually undergo extensive manipulation during reduction and repair. For this reason, the limb is clipped from the level of the metacarpus or metatarsus to the scapula or pelvis, respectively, including the medial and lateral aspects of the extremity. This may vary slightly, depending on the particular bone that is fractured, but the general rule should be a wide and thorough clip. The remaining hair at the tip of the paw is covered with a rubber glove or plastic wrap that is taped to the clipped skin.

Positioning

Animal positioning depends on the specific bone that is fractured. Generally the following positions are recommended for each fracture:

- Femur: lateral recumbency, affected side up
- Tibia-fibula: lateral recumbency, affected leg down
- Humerus: lateral recumbency, affected leg up
- Radius-ulna: dorsal recumbency, affected leg craniad; or lateral recumbency, affected leg up
- Pelvis: lateral recumbency, affected leg up

With so much skin exposed, skin preparation is time consuming, but it must be meticulous. The surgeon eventually covers the extremity with a sterile stockinette, but this should not preclude an adequate skin preparation.

Surgical Assistance

Orthopedic procedures are often difficult and time consuming and may demand the help of an assistant. Often, the veterinary technician is called on to participate as a surgical assistant and therefore should have a general understanding of orthopedic tissue handling (specifics of intraoperative assistance is covered in Chapter 29).

Several basic maneuvers commonly needed by the surgeon are often performed by the veterinary technician. They include retraction, muscle fatigue, alignment and reduction, and suction of the field. Proper techniques for each are discussed separately.

Retraction

Care should be taken to preserve the soft tissues in the operative field. It will be necessary to have functional muscle groups remaining when the bone is repaired. Retraction should be firm, but not so traumatic as to bruise or tear the muscle. The tissues should also be kept moist. Tissue desiccation can cause tissue death and loss of function.

Muscle Fatigue

Fractures in large-breed dogs or fractures that are 3 to 5 days old may be difficult to reduce because of heavy muscle mass or severe muscle contraction, respectively. In such cases, constant, steady traction on the muscle groups will cause them to fatigue and relax, thus facilitating reduction. Epidural anesthetics and/or paralytics can be used to aid in muscle reduction (review Chapter 27).

Alignment and Reduction

To repair fractured bones, the ends must be reduced and aligned. It is often necessary for an assistant to hold reduction during the fixation of the fracture. Pins, wires, screws, and plates of stainless steel may be used to achieve the necessary fixation.

Suction

Whenever a fracture occurs, bleeding into the fracture site can be massive. Some continuous oozing occurs during fixation. A clean surgical field is of the utmost importance in facilitating early and accurate reduction and fixation.

Postoperative Considerations

Some postoperative orthopedic patients may require external coaptation. Applied bandages should be managed as previously discussed (see Chapter 34). Animals undergoing orthopedic surgery will likely require passive range-of-motion exercises, but activity is otherwise limited. Animals should be encouraged to use the operated limb to increase blood supply to the fracture site, maintain joint and muscle health, and speed fracture healing. However, limb use should be slow, deliberate, and well controlled. No off-leash activity, running, jumping, or playing with other animals should be allowed. A crate is the best place for these animals when the veterinarian, veterinary technician, or owner is not strictly controlling the animal. The only orthopedic procedure in which activity is strongly encouraged is femoral head and neck excision where rehabilitation, building of muscle mass, and encouragement of weight bearing is extremely important for optimal limb function. Animals are restricted to light activity for the first 2 weeks following femoral head and neck excision, but they are then allowed to use the limb fully thereafter. It is also important to realize the relatively unsure gait of a three-legged dog or cat, and when exercising the animal, one must be certain to avoid slippery surfaces (vinyl or wet floors). Cement, grass, dirt, carpet, or rubber matting provides a much more sure-footed environment.

Rehabilitation is an important part of recovery. Flexing and extending the affected limb along with muscle massage will improve blood flow and muscle tone and reduce muscle contraction. Therapy should be done for a period of 7 to 10 minutes each time and be repeated two to three times per day. A demonstration by the technician of proper technique will aid the client in understanding the therapy. Slow leash walking is performed to encourage limb use. The faster the animal is walked, the more likely it will carry the affected limb.

JOINTS

Preoperative Considerations

Most orthopedic procedures involving a joint are elective and rarely need emergency care. Traumatic fractures and luxations, however, do require urgent treatment. Preoperative management should include limiting the animal's activity. External coaptation is rarely necessary for nonurgent cases, but will make the traumatically injured animal (animals with luxations or fractures) more comfortable. For some injuries, such as cranial cruciate ligament tear, joint range of motion can be done before surgery to improve joint health. Indications for joint surgery include dislocations, ligament ruptures, infections, fractures, synovial biopsy, arthrodesis (surgical fusion of a joint), and treatment of osteochondrosis (abnormally thickened portion of the articular cartilage).

Intraoperative Considerations

An extensive clip, as for fractures, should be done for joint surgery. Positions will vary depending on the joint involved. Generally the following positions are recommended for each joint:

Hip: lateral recumbency, affected leg up
Stifle: lateral recumbency, affected leg up; or dorsal recumbency, leg hanging off the end of the table
Shoulder: lateral recumbency, affected leg up
Tarsus: lateral recumbency, affected leg up
Elbow: lateral recumbency, affected leg up (or down for medial approaches)
Carpus: lateral recumbency, affected leg up; or dorsal recumbency

Intraoperative assistance in joint surgery is similar to that necessary in fracture repair. Some special precautions should be taken while joints are exposed.

Retraction

Care should be taken not to place retractors in direct contact with the articular cartilage. This will damage the cartilage, and cartilage has a relatively poor response to trauma. When exposure of the joint is necessary, sharp retraction of the joint capsule will decrease trauma, but increase exposure.

> *TECHNICIAN NOTE* Care should be taken not to place retractors in direct contact with the articular cartilage, and the cartilage should be kept moist to prevent permanent cartilage damage.

Flush

The cartilage should be frequently flushed with saline to keep it from drying out during the procedure. This is true of all tissues, especially the articular cartilage because of its poor regenerative ability.

Postoperative Considerations

Postoperative care of animals undergoing joint surgery is variable, depending on the surgical procedure, the joint involved, and the surgeon's preference. Early passive range-of-motion activity with light joint usage is recommended for most animals undergoing joint surgery. Heavy joint use is discouraged in the early postoperative period. Animals should be encouraged to use the affected joint during slow, leash-controlled walks, but are discouraged from running or jumping on the limb. Joint use is increased gradually over the course of recovery, which is variable depending on the procedures performed. Joint immobilization is necessary in some cases, such as luxation, but is discouraged in most instances and can result in severe limitations in joint range of motion after recovery if care is not taken to rehabilitate the joint carefully.

> *TECHNICIAN NOTE* It is important to encourage limb use after long bone or joint surgery for optimal recovery. This is best done by slow, controlled leash walking at limited times throughout the day. Running, jumping, or off-leash activity is not allowed.

CLIENT EDUCATION

When an animal is discharged from the professional care available in a veterinary hospital, it becomes the responsibility of the hospital staff to instruct the client to provide the same type of care at home. This requires that time be spent with the client and the pet to educate the client on appropriate treatment techniques. There are several methods of client education in surgical cases, the degree of difficulty of which is often associated with the type of surgical procedure performed (e.g., ovariohysterectomy versus fracture repair).

Whenever an animal is sent home with a sutured skin incision, the client must be instructed to observe the incision daily for evidence of swelling, redness, or drainage. The client should also watch the animal for aggressive licking, removal of skin sutures, or both. The owner must be told to inform the veterinarian of problems.

If an animal is sent home with a bandage, a written discharge form should be given to the client describing in detail the proper management necessary to prevent complications.

In orthopedic cases and in many elective soft tissue surgery cases, the owner should be instructed specifically on what kind of limited activity should be enforced. If passive range-of-motion and weight-bearing exercises are expected, the client should be given both oral and written instructions in providing the correct care. A demonstration by the technician of the correct method of therapy is helpful.

In many instances, such as complicated orthopedic and neurologic discharges, a handout explaining in detail the care necessary is informative and provides a handy reference for the client if a problem arises.

The use of visual aids, such as a skeleton or overlay books that illustrate anatomy, can be effective in helping the client understand the scope of the problem. Clients are generally willing and capable of handling postoperative care for their pets if instructed appropriately.

CASE PRESENTATION 30-1

Signalment: Lady, 6-year-old female Labrador retriever (Figure 1)

History: Two-week history of increased drinking and urination. Lady showed progressive lethargy and decreased appetite over the 3 days before presentation. For 24 hours before presentation, Lady was inappetent, depressed, and extremely lethargic. The owner noticed some blood-tinged fluid coming from the vulva 4 days ago and that Lady has been licking her vulva regularly. The owner has noticed some blood in the urine when Lady has accidents in the house, which started happening about 1.5 weeks before presentation.

What to consider at this point: The dog is an intact female, she has not been eating or drinking for 24 hours, she has blood in her urine, she has a bloody discharge from her vulva, and she had been drinking and urinating more frequently than normal.

Other questions asked:

1. Is Lady current on vaccinations? Yes, rabies, distemper, and *Bordetella*
2. Has Lady ever had puppies? Yes, two litters, all healthy
3. When was her last heat cycle? About 8 weeks ago
4. When was the last time Lady was bred? 3 years prior
5. Are there toxins around your home, and can Lady free roam? No toxins that owners are aware of, Lady stays indoors or in a fenced yard.
6. Has she had any other illnesses? No
7. Did Lady have any dietary items out of the ordinary before this started? No, she eats adult maintenance dry (1 cup twice a day) and milk bones only. The owner did try to feed her steak last night because she was not eating, but Lady turned that down.
8. Any coughing, sneezing, runny eyes, vomiting, or diarrhea? No

Examination: Physical examination revealed Lady to be depressed, her abdomen to be tense and painful, and to have a mucopurulent discharge coming from her vulva.

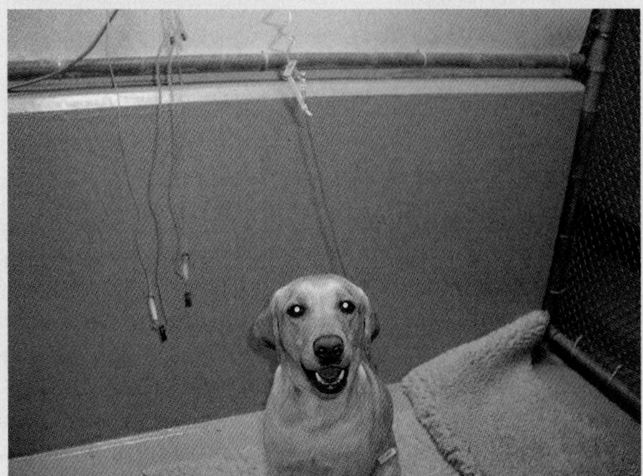

FIGURE 1 Lady: 6-year-old female Labrador retriever that came for treatment of inappetence and lethargy.

Other findings include fleas, waxy debris in both ears, and moderate dental tarter.
Temperature: 104.5° F
Pulse: 110 bpm, pulses weak and thready
Respiratory rate: 50 bpm
Mucous membranes: pale and tacky
Capillary refill time: 3 seconds

What to consider at this point: Lady is febrile, tachycardic, and tachypneic; had weak and thready pulses; and is painful in the abdomen. She appears to be dehydrated and in early shock.

Diagnostics

CBC: Mild nonregenerative anemia, mildly low TP, leukocytosis (increased white blood cell count), consisting of a neutrophilia (a high neutrophil count) with a left shift (too many immature neutrophils) and toxic changes to the neutrophils, and a mild thrombocytopenia (low platelets)

Biochemistry panel abnormalities: Elevated Na and Cl, mildly low potassium, elevated BUN (meaning high protein diet, renal insufficiency, or dehydration), elevated creatinine (a kidney value—high means renal insufficiency or the animal is dehydrated), mildly low albumin, mildly low TP, elevated alkaline phosphatase (a liver enzyme)

Abdominal radiographs: Tissue-dense mass in the caudal abdomen displacing the intestines cranial and dorsal and intestinal ileus. The mass is consistent with an enlarged uterus (Figure 2).

Abdominal ultrasound: Enlarge, fluid-filled uterus

Urinalysis collected at the time of ultrasound by cystocentesis: Numerous bacteria, increased white blood cells, hematuria (blood in the urine), urine specific gravity of 1.012 (urine is not concentrated—in a dehydrated dog, this number should be higher. This means that the kidneys may not be functioning normally or the toxins from the disease are causing diuresis—increased filtration of fluid through the kidneys).

Diagnosis: Pyometra, possible renal insufficiency, possible sepsis

What to consider at this point: Lady has been diagnosed with a pyometra. She will require emergency surgery to remove the source of infection (her uterus). However, she is azotemic (has an elevated BUN and creatinine), dehydrated, potentially septic, anemic, thrombocytopenic, and in the early stages of shock. This makes her a poor anesthetic candidate because she is systemically unstable.

Recommended Initial Therapy

1. Place an intravenous catheter.
2. Give shock dose of intravenous crystalloid therapy (may consider adding in a colloid because the protein is low).
3. Begin a cooling process with fans and fluid therapy.
4. Obtain an ECG and blood pressure.
5. Obtain a coagulation profile to check for evidence of early disseminated intravascular coagulation (a disease that results from severe metabolic disruptions that leads to hyperblood clotting followed by hemorrhage in multiple areas).

Continued

CASE PRESENTATION 30-1—cont'd

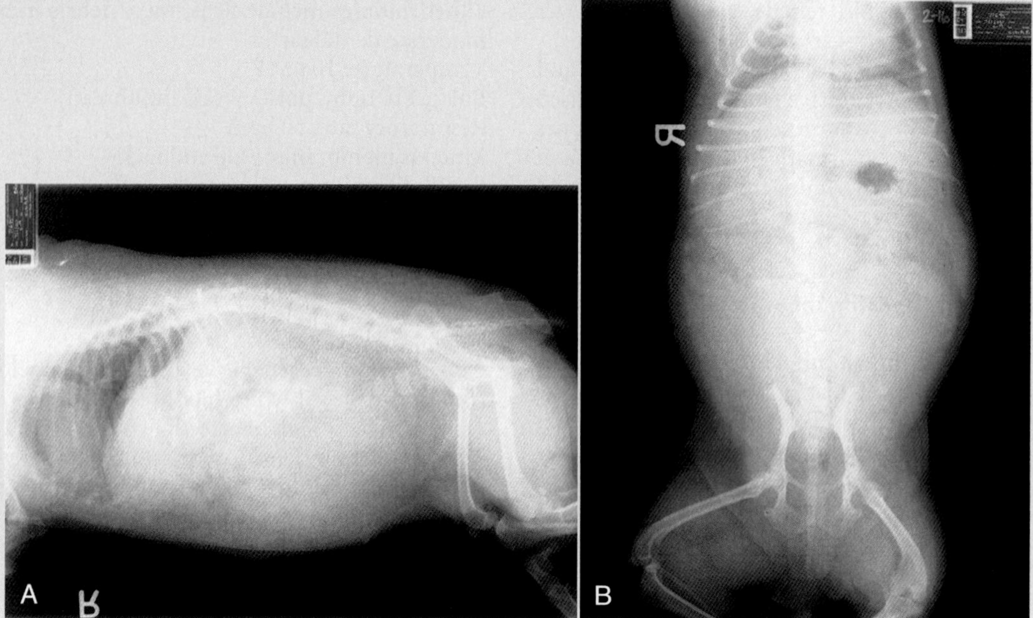

FIGURE 2 Abdominal radiographs of Lady showing a large tissue-dense mass in the caudal abdomen (large dense [more white] structure that is irregular and pushing the intestines cranial and dorsal). **A** is a lateral radiograph, and **B** is a ventrodorsal view.

6. Start on intravenous, broad-spectrum antibiotics.
7. Continue crystalloid and/or colloid therapy until improvement in body temperature, pulses, and respiration are noted.
8. Initiate pain control.
9. Start gastrointestinal protectants because of GI stasis and inappetence with the stress of being in the hospital.
10. Repeat CBC and chemistry panel after Lady's condition begins to stabilize.

What to consider at this point: Lady's systemic condition should begin to stabilize within a few hours of admission to the hospital. She has a life-threatening infection of her uterus and must go to surgery sooner rather than later. As soon as she appears to be out of shock and rehydrated (hopefully the BUN and creatinine would come down), she should be prepared for surgery. Lady has bacteria in the urine, and a urine sample should be turned in for culture and sensitivity.

Anesthetic considerations: Lady is not a stable patient. Cardioprotective drugs should be used. Adequate monitoring: blood pressure, temperature, pulse, oxygen saturation, and vitals should be monitored. Only light anesthetics would likely be required and are desired.

Surgical considerations: Lady should be prepped quickly and moved into the OR for surgery. The technician should ensure that the OR is set up with all the necessary equipment and suture so that the surgery proceeds quickly. A general abdominal pack would be required. Culture swabs and a bucket for the uterus should be available. The surgeon would likely hand the infected uterus to the technician, and the technician would have to cut into the uterus with sterile technique and obtain a culture—this should be done outside of the OR (Figure 3). The surgical technique would be ovariohysterectomy. However, a wide abdominal preparation will be required because a large incision for gentle uterine handling and abdominal exploration will be needed (Figure 4). A sponge count should be performed before abdominal incision and before incision closure to ensure that none were left in the abdomen. The surgical assistant should remember to keep the tissues moist and not to pull on the uterus because it will be friable and will tear easily (this would cause septic fluid to leak onto the surgical field and into the sterile abdominal cavity). Tissue and culture samples should be promptly submitted.

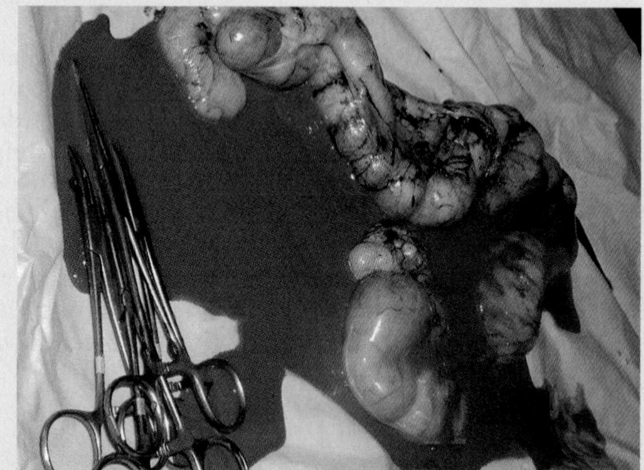

FIGURE 3 This uterus has been cut open with sterile instruments. Notice the brown fluid that exudes from the cut uterus. The fluid should be cultured using sterile technique from inside the incision made into the uterus by sticking a culture swab into the uterine lumen through the incision.

CASE PRESENTATION 30-1—cont'd

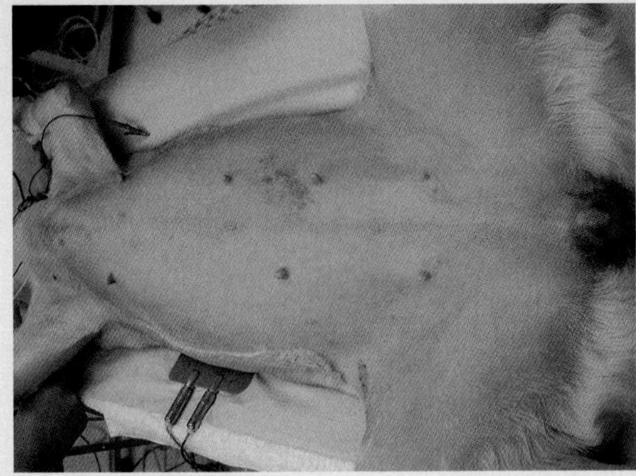

FIGURE 4 Wide abdominal preparation for surgery to treat pyometra.

Considerations for recovery: Lady will likely be hypothermic, even though she had a fever before surgery. She should be warmed appropriately. Though the infected uterus was removed, she could still experience complications of septicemia and her illness, such as fever, low blood pressure, anemia, shock, organ failure, and death. All vitals, PCV, TP, ECG, blood pressure, and mucous membranes should continue to be monitored until Lady is stable.

Other postoperative care: Pain should be controlled with intravenous administration on a routine schedule (do not wait for Lady to be painful). Intravenous fluids should be continued until Lady is eating and drinking. Food and water should be offered 12 hours after surgery. The PCV and TP should normalize within a few days, but if they drop too low, colloidal fluid support and/or blood transfusion may be necessary. Coagulation times, CBC, and biochemistry panel should be reevaluated 24 hours after surgery to ensure that improvements are noted. The incision should be monitored for oozing of fluid (which might occur in a dog with low protein and platelets—this should improve in 24 to 48 hours). A bandage should be placed around the belly if incisional oozing occurs. Gastrointestinal protectants are continued until Lady's appetite returns to normal. As she improves over 24 to 48 hours and begins eating and drinking, fluid therapy is decreased and then stopped, and oral antibiotic therapy is continued in an oral form based on culture and sensitivity results.

What happened to Lady: Surgery was a success, and Lady recovered without complications. Her blood work abnormalities began to normalize, and her appetite returned within 36 hours. She was discharged from the hospital on Enrofloxacin and Tramadol 3 days after surgery. Initial culture results from the urine and uterus revealed *E. coli* sensitive to enrofloxacin. The owners were instructed to monitor the incision daily and to return for suture removal and blood work in 7 days. Lady was back to normal at that time.

Other: Pyometra generally has a good prognosis if caught early and treated appropriately. Recovery is often quick so long as the animal does not have complications with septicemia.

RECOMMENDED READING

Busch SJ: *Small animal surgical nursing: skills and concepts,* St Louis, 2006, Elsevier Mosby.

Dunning D: Surgical wound infection and the use of antimicrobials. In Slatter D, editor: *Textbook of small animal surgery,* ed 3, St Louis, 2002, Saunders.

Licroy MD, Bartels KE: Surgical lasers. In Slatter D, editor: *Textbook of small animal surgery,* ed 3, St Louis, 2002, Saunders.

Quandt JE: Postoperative patient care. In Slatter D, editor: *Textbook of small animal surgery,* ed 3, St Louis, 2002, Saunders.

Seim HB III, Creed JF: Restraint techniques for prevention of self-trauma. In Bojrab MJ, editor: *Current techniques in small animal surgery,* ed 4, St Louis, 1998, Lea & Febiger.

Shmon C: Assessment and preparation of the surgical patient and the operating team. In Slatter D, editor: *Textbook of small animal surgery,* ed 3, St Louis, 2002, Saunders.

31 Large Animal Surgical Nursing

Colin F. Mitchell, Rustin M. Moore, and Marjorie S. Gill

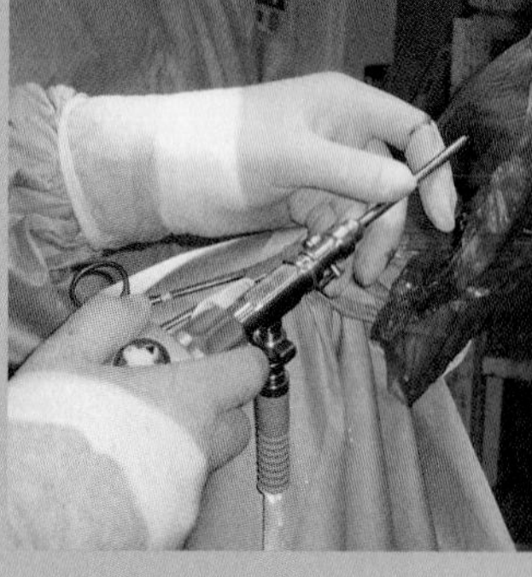

OUTLINE

KEY TERMS

Abomasopexy
Colpotomy
Laparotomy
Omentopexy
Pyloropexy
Rhabdomyolysis
Rumenostomy
Rumenotomy

LEARNING OBJECTIVES

When you have completed this chapter, you will be able to:

1. Describe the preoperative procedures needed for equine patients.
2. Discuss the responsibilities of the veterinary technician during equine surgery.
3. Describe postoperative monitoring, medication administration, bandage care, and grooming for equine patients.
4. List commonly performed surgical procedures in equine patients.
5. Describe indications and preoperative, intraoperative, and postoperative considerations for common surgical procedures in equine patients.
6. List and describe common emergency situations and procedures in equine patients.
7. List commonly performed surgical procedures in bovine patients.
8. Describe indications and preoperative, intraoperative, and postoperative considerations for common surgical procedures in bovine patients.
9. List commonly performed surgical procedures in small ruminants.
10. Describe indications and preoperative, intraoperative, and postoperative considerations for common surgical procedures in small ruminants.

INTRODUCTION

Like all aspects of veterinary technology, large animal surgical nursing relies heavily upon the observational skills, clinical knowledge, and technical ability of the veterinary technician to ensure that all large animal patients receive optimal medical care. Technicians are expected to provide patient monitoring, treatment, surgical assistance, nursing care, and client education. Providing veterinary care for large animals is particularly cumbersome because they are massive, fractious, and at the same time, fragile animals. Skilled technical support with expertise in patient handling, restraint, and the use of specialized instrumentation is crucial for the practitioner to provide quality preoperative, intraoperative, and postoperative intensive care. Familiarity with large animal behavior will allow the veterinary technician to quickly recognize abnormal behavior, such as early signs of pain, and neurologic and respiratory disorders. The technician is often the first to identify a change in patient status and may save valuable time at a crucial turning point for therapeutic intervention. In addition, recognition of the unique layperson's language will help the veterinary technician communicate with the client and to recognize the significance of patient historical data. In these ways, large animal nursing imparts an essential contribution to the quality and efficiency of patient care in a hospital setting.

This chapter addresses the most commonly seen surgical conditions among large animal species and includes the steps taken by veterinary technicians in the support and care of surgical patients. In this chapter, these steps begin after completion of a thorough physical examination and the acquisition of results from hematology, clinical chemistry, and imaging tests.

TECHNICIAN NOTE The veterinary technician plays a vital role in the day-to-day monitoring of and caring for hospitalized patients; therefore the ability to be observant and to perform a thorough and complete physical examination is critical.

SURGICAL NURSING OF HORSES

OVERVIEW

PREOPERATIVE PREPARATION

Numerous procedures are required in preparation of the equine patient for anesthesia and surgery. Many if not all of these procedures involve the veterinary technician. It is probably wise that a checklist be developed that the veterinary technician can use to make sure that all procedures are performed. This is particularly helpful in a hospital where more than one technician is working on the same case. Because of the dense hair coat of horses, thorough grooming is necessary. This may include simply brushing or currying the horse's coat, or it may require that the horse be bathed. The aim of grooming is to remove as much loose hair, dander, and dirt from the horse's body as possible, thereby keeping such material out of the operating room (OR). If the horse is shod, the shoes are generally removed before surgery to prevent injury to the horse during recovery from anesthesia or damaging the recovery stall flooring. Some therapeutic shoes may not be removed to prevent damage to the hooves. If the shoes must be left on, wrapping them with gauze and elastic tape will provide some protection from injury from the shoes during recovery. The horse's feet need to be picked out and cleaned. One of the main responsibilities of the technician will be to clip a wide area of hair in the vicinity of the surgery site before anesthetic induction. If the surgery will be performed on a limb, the hair can be clipped the day before surgery and the limb can be cleaned and a bandage placed to keep the site clean. The final aseptic preparation is performed once the horse is under anesthesia. Clipping the hair and cleaning the surgery site before anesthetic induction will reduce anesthesia time.

TECHNICIAN NOTE A checklist should be developed to ensure that the veterinary technician performs all procedures required for preparation of the equine patient for anesthesia and surgery.

It is important that the technician consult the clinician regarding the specific site that should be clipped. Areas of the mane and tail should be clipped only under special circumstances. Most owners are adamant that these areas should not be clipped for cosmetic purposes. The hair of the mane and tail takes months to years to grow out, and unnecessarily clipping these areas may cause needless delay in a show horse's convalescence. The location of the skin incision and the appropriate part of the horse to clip before surgery can usually be found in equine surgical textbooks. However, because of variation among surgeons, the technician should always consult the surgeon before clipping the patient.

Unlike ruminants and small animals, horses do not regurgitate or vomit. Adult horses are generally held off feed for approximately 12 hours to allow time for emptying of the stomach, which may allow the horse to ventilate more easily. Horses are generally provided water during this time. Young foals that are still nursing are generally not held off feed before anesthesia, but, if they are, it is usually only for 1 to 2 hours. A complete physical examination should be performed, including auscultation of the heart and lungs. In adult horses, a rebreathing bag may need to be used to increase the respiratory effort sufficiently to hear air moving through the lung fields. An electrocardiogram should be performed if there is any evidence of an abnormal heart rhythm detected during auscultation. Preoperative blood work usually includes a complete blood count (CBC) and fibrinogen determination. Some clinicians also perform a chemistry profile depending on the age and health of the horse. A tetanus vaccination should have been given within the last 3 months. If the date is not known, a booster should be given intramuscularly.

Before general anesthesia, an intravenous (IV) catheter is placed in one of the jugular veins. The location of the catheter is important to provide access without compromise to the surgical site. The anesthetic agents for induction are administered through the catheter. Some anesthetic agents (thiobarbiturates) and perioperative medications (phenylbutazone) are irritating if injected perivascularly. Therefore it is imperative that the veterinary technician place the catheter into the vein and secure it appropriately. Perioperative medications, such as antibiotics and nonsteroidal antiinflammatory drugs (NSAIDs) are usually administered before anesthetic induction. However, if an infectious process is suspected, the surgeon may opt to start antibiotics after a sample has been obtained at surgery for culture and susceptibility testing. In this case the medication can be administered during anesthesia or after recovery; this will depend on the medication and the condition of the patient while under anesthesia. Because horses are generally intubated with an endotracheal tube through the oral cavity, it is important that the mouth be thoroughly washed out before anesthetic induction; this will reduce the chance that feed material will be carried into the airway during intubation. Once the horse is intubated, the cuff should be inflated to prevent saliva and other materials from draining into the lower airway and leading to aspiration pneumonia.

INTRAOPERATIVE NURSING

The OR technician should consult the surgeon regarding which instruments will be required. In a hospital where there are many OR technicians and surgeons, an organized system to delineate the various surgeons' instrument preferences and glove size should be used. This will allow the technician to know the different requirements of individual surgeons. One common difference among surgeons is the type of suture material chosen to close wounds. The technician must learn to adapt to these individual preferences. It is recommended that the technician have all the available instruments close to the surgery. Even if the instrument is used infrequently, it is better to have it nearby rather than waste time looking for it once it is needed. Time-wasting activities lead to prolonged anesthetic time, which could lead to increased morbidity or mortality. Correctly labeled radiographs are essential for most limb surgery. The radiographs should be placed on a radiographic view box in the OR. The technician should have available gloves, gowns, and drapes and all other supplies that are anticipated to be used. In some lower limb surgeries, an Esmarch bandage (Latex Rubber Bandage/Tourner Wrap, Smiths & Nephew Richards) and tourniquet are used to assist with hemostasis during surgery. An Esmarch bandage is a flat, gum-rubber elastic bandage that is wrapped around the limb in a spiral fashion from distal to proximal to a point above the surgical site. At this point, an inflatable tourniquet is applied and secured. The aim of the Esmarch bandage is to force blood out of the limb, and the tourniquet prevents blood from entering into the site. The Esmarch bandage is removed after the tourniquet is fully inflated. The use of an Esmarch bandage and tourniquet enables the surgeon to operate in a bloodless field and results in a shorter surgery time. Following surgery, a pressure bandage is applied, and the tourniquet is released. It is strongly recommended that the tourniquet only be used for a maximum period of 2 hours to prevent any potentially serious side effects.

> *TECHNICIAN NOTE* In a hospital where there are many OR technicians and surgeons, an organized system to delineate the various surgeons' instrument preferences and glove sizes should be used.

Because of their immense body weight, horses are prone to myositis (muscle damage) during recumbency, and this can be life threatening. Therefore the OR technician must ensure that the patient is well padded on the surgery table. The pressure of the horse's body and the hypotension that can occur during anesthesia can result in hypoperfusion of the muscles. If this condition is prolonged, the muscles can undergo metabolic change, resulting in extreme soreness and pain. In severe cases, muscle pigment (myoglobin) is released into the bloodstream and excreted in the urine (coffee-colored urine); the pigment can lead to kidney damage. The first sign that muscle damage has occurred during anesthesia is manifested during recovery. Usually the front or rear limb, or both, on the side that the horse is lying on will be affected. However, the uppermost limb or any limb in a horse in dorsal recumbency can be involved. The horse may be unable to bear weight on the limb. If a forelimb is involved, the horse will drag the limb in a flexed position and will be unable to bear weight; this is associated with triceps damage. If the hind limb is involved, the horse may knuckle in the lower joints and walk on the dorsal aspect of the fetlock, and the limb will collapse as the horse tries to bear weight. Most horses show some improvement over the first few days, but some horses are unable to rise. Management of a postoperative recumbent patient presents a number of problems to clinicians and technicians. Appropriate padding materials include: an inflatable water bed, semiinflated inner tubes under the shoulder and hip, dunnage bags, and foam rubber pads.

The patient and the surgery site must be positioned so that it is comfortable to the surgeon and safe for the patient. This will help ensure that the surgeon does not become fatigued or frustrated and a subsequent compromise in technique does not occur. It is not wise to overextend, overflex, abduct, or adduct the limbs because of potential complications of myopathy and neuropathy.

Aseptic preparation of the surgery site, surgical instruments, and the surgeon is imperative to a successful and uncomplicated surgery. It is the responsibility of all personnel involved to maintain asepsis, but the OR technicians should assume primary responsibility for ensuring that the surgical site is properly prepared and the instruments are properly sterilized and packaged. The OR technician must be cognizant of all activities in preparation for surgery and during the surgical procedure. If a technician observes a break in aseptic technique, it should be brought to the attention of the surgeon so that the problem can be remedied. The techniques involved in sterilization of surgical instruments and supplies and aseptic preparation of the surgery site are covered in Chapter 28.

POSTOPERATIVE NURSING

Technicians play a vital role in the postoperative care of the equine patient. Although veterinarians are responsible for the patients' care, technicians are often primarily involved with postoperative monitoring, administering medications, changing bandages, grooming, and other tasks required on postoperative patients. Monitoring the postoperative patient is similar to previously discussed patient monitoring. Although all body systems should be evaluated, the important things to consider in the postoperative patient are the presence and magnitude of postoperative pain, whether the patient is febrile, and whether there are any signs of infection (swelling, erythema, heat, pain) at the incision site. The postoperative patient should be examined for any complications, such as pneumonia, diarrhea, jugular vein thrombophlebitis, or laminitis.

> *TECHNICIAN NOTE* Although veterinarians are responsible for the patients' care, technicians are often primarily involved with postoperative monitoring, administering medications, changing bandages, grooming, and other tasks required on postoperative patients.

Technicians are generally responsible for administering medications postoperatively. This may involve giving antibiotics or NSAIDs orally, IV, or intramuscularly. Many horses that undergo surgery have an IV catheter that is used in the postoperative period to administer perioperative antibiotics. The duration of antibiotic therapy depends on clinician preference and the type and severity of the underlying disease process. Many horses are administered NSAIDs in the postoperative period for their antiinflammatory and analgesic properties.

Horses undergoing limb surgery generally have a bandage placed on the limb at the conclusion of surgery before recovery from anesthesia. The limbs are often kept bandaged until the skin sutures are removed 10 to 14 days postoperatively. The bandages should probably be changed every 2 to 3 days initially or more frequently if they become wet or soiled from the outside or if wound drainage soaks through from the inside. There are several types of materials used for limb bandages in horses and several methods of application (see Chapter 34). In general, a sterile nonadherent material is usually placed directly against the incision and held in place with sterile, soft roll gauze (Kling, Johnson & Johnson). The next layer of the bandage is usually a sterile, soft combine that covers the circumference of the limb for the entire distance of the bandage, which is also held in place with soft roll gauze. This layer can be skipped if the outer bandage that is placed is a thick, sterile combine material. Next a thick layer of rolled cotton, sheet cottons, or combine material is placed on the limb and secured with soft roll gauze. An Ace bandage, Elasticon (Johnson & Johnson), or Vetwrap (Animal Care Products/3M) can be used as the final layer of the bandage. Elasticon is useful for securing the top of the bandage to the skin above it and the bottom of the bandage to the foot below. This helps seal the bandage and prevents debris from getting between the skin and the bandage. All layers of the bandage should be applied in the same direction (dorsal to palmar or plantar) and with even tension; this should help prevent constriction of the tendons in the metacarpal or metatarsal area and subsequent tendinitis (bandage bow). When the bandages are changed postoperatively, the incision should be examined for swelling, heat, exudate, and pain on palpation. The limb should be monitored for excessive swelling above and below the bandage. The exudate should be removed, the wound gently cleaned, and the bandage reapplied. If there has been an appreciable change in the horse's gait or in the incision from the last bandage change, this should be brought to the immediate attention of the veterinarian.

SURGICAL CONSIDERATIONS

ABDOMINAL SURGERY

Abdominal surgery is a major undertaking and requires a full team to perform it in an effective and efficient manner. Adult horses and foals frequently undergo abdominal surgery for gastrointestinal and urogenital tract disease. Although a flank incision in a standing, sedated horse is sometimes used for horses with colic or other abdominal disease, the most common approach to the abdominal cavity is through a ventral midline incision with the horse under general anesthesia and positioned in dorsal recumbency (Figure 31-1). Because most horses with colic requiring surgery will be operated on with the patient under general anesthesia, the veterinary technician will be involved in the preparation of the horse for surgery. This will include placing a catheter, administering perioperative medications, passing a nasogastric tube, washing out the mouth, clipping the hair, preparing the anesthetics, aseptically preparing the incision site, and opening surgical packs at the time of surgery. Most colic patients can be clipped before anesthesia, but if the horse is in severe pain, it may be done after anesthetic induction for the safety of the horse and personnel. The hair should be clipped from

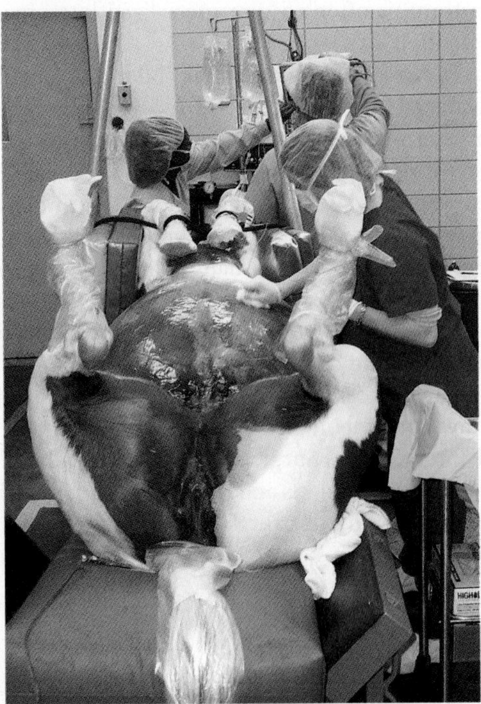

FIGURE 31-1 Preparation of the ventral abdominal area for abdominal surgery in a horse with colic that is under general anesthesia and positioned in dorsal recumbency.

rostral to the xiphoid area to the udder or preputial area and to the flank folds on either side; clipped hair and other debris can be removed with a vacuum before aseptic preparation. The incision is draped with four small drapes or towels, and a large, water-impermeable drape is placed that covers the entire horse. The incision is usually made from the umbilicus rostrally toward the xiphoid until the necessary exposure is achieved, but the incision can be extended caudal to the umbilicus. This is particularly necessary for urogenital tract surgery, such as a cystotomy for removal of cystic calculi. Once the incision is made, a thorough exploration is usually performed depending on the reason for surgery. Once the abnormality is identified, it is corrected. Suction is often necessary to decompress gas from the gastrointestinal tract or aspirate fluid, such as urine from the bladder during a cystotomy.

> *TECHNICIAN NOTE* The most common approach to the abdominal cavity is through a ventral midline incision with the horse under general anesthesia and positioned in dorsal recumbency.

There are numerous surgical techniques and manipulations that the surgeon may perform with which the OR veterinary technician becomes familiar through experience. Many specialized instruments are required for abdominal surgery (see Chapter 28). One group of instruments that has become increasingly popular with veterinary surgeons for use in equine abdominal surgery is gastrointestinal stapling equipment. The technician must become familiar with the different instruments and cartridges. Intestinal resection and anastomosis often require specialized instruments and supplies.

Once the cause of colic or other abdominal problem has been corrected and the horse has recovered from anesthesia, the veterinary technician becomes even more closely involved with patient management. Horses usually require administration of IV fluids, antibiotics, antiinflammatory drugs, and other medications in the postoperative period. The veterinary technician usually administers or oversees administration of these medications. The technician may also perform nasogastric intubation, blood collection, IV catheterization, and changing bandages.

Fortunately, most horses with colic respond to conservative medical treatment, and only a small percentage require surgical intervention. Surgical treatment of colic is necessary for intestinal volvulus and incarceration, enterolithiasis, fibrous foreign body obstruction, and some intestinal displacements. Refer to Chapter 33 for more information about treating horses with medical colic.

Hernia Repair

Herniation of omentum or abdominal viscera through the abdominal wall can occur with an umbilical hernia, inguinal (scrotal) hernia, or incisional hernia. Umbilical hernias are usually congenital and are relatively common in foals. Small hernias may close spontaneously as the foal grows, whereas others require surgical intervention. Umbilical hernias can be repaired using several different methods. Generally the body wall is closed with either interrupted or continuous absorbable suture. Some surgeons open the peritoneum (open herniorrhaphy), and others leave the peritoneum intact (closed herniorrhaphy). If an umbilical hernia is large or it has not closed by several months of age, it should probably be surgically repaired. The owner should be instructed to manually reduce hernial contents at least daily; if at any time the hernia cannot be reduced, the horse should be examined by a veterinarian immediately. If intestine becomes incarcerated in the hernia, vascular compromise can occur, leading to ischemic injury.

Inguinal or scrotal hernias can occur in horses of any age, but newborn foals and adult breeding stallions are probably the most commonly affected. Frequently the herniated contents do not become incarcerated and can be easily reduced. The hernia should be reduced at least daily in foals because intestine could become incarcerated, which would necessitate emergency surgery. Sometimes these hernias will spontaneously resolve in foals, but many foals require surgical repair. Because the tissues are friable in foals, successful surgical repair can be difficult. Scrotal hernias in adult horses most commonly occur in stallions shortly after breeding. In most instances, the herniated structure or structures become(s) incarcerated (not reducible), which necessitates immediate surgery. Incarceration of intestine within the scrotum will result in a large, firm, and cold scrotum on the affected side secondary to compromised testicular blood flow. The blood supply to the intestine also becomes compromised, resulting in ischemic injury. Generally the testicle on the affected side is removed, and the affected segment of intestine often requires resection. This necessitates preparation of the horse for inguinal and ventral midline surgery.

Acquired body wall herniation occurs in horses subsequent to trauma and following surgery. Blunt trauma, such as a kick, can lead to disruption of the body wall musculature. Body wall hernias occur secondary to abdominal incisions; these occur more frequently in horses that develop incisional infection or other complicating factors. Small body wall hernias can be repaired primarily by suturing the defect. Larger body wall defects require the use of mesh implants. It is critical that there be no residual incisional infection present at the time of mesh herniorrhaphy and that aseptic technique is followed during placement of the mesh.

UROGENITAL TRACT SURGERY

Urinary Calculi

Urinary calculi occur infrequently in horses. Urinary calculi in horses are usually composed of calcium carbonate and have a spicular appearance. These calculi may develop in the kidney or urinary bladder. Small-diameter calculi can be passed during normal urination and go unnoticed. Clinical signs of urinary calculi include stranguria (slow and difficult urination or straining to urinate), pollakiuria (frequent urination), and hematuria (bloody urine). Horses that develop renal calculi will develop signs of abdominal discomfort when the stones become lodged in the ureter. In addition, cystic (urinary bladder) calculi that become lodged in the urethra in male horses cause an inability to urinate and subsequent abdominal pain. Urinary calculi can be diagnosed based on clinical signs, urinalysis, palpation of the urinary bladder per rectum, and endoscopic evaluation of the urethra and urinary bladder. Occasionally a calculus can be palpated in the proximal urethra of male horses at the level of the ischial arch. There are several techniques and certain instruments available for removing urinary tract calculi.

> *TECHNICIAN NOTE* Urinary calculi occur infrequently in horses. Urinary calculi in horses are usually composed of calcium carbonate and have a spicular appearance. These calculi may develop in the kidney or urinary bladder.

Umbilical Repair

Foals commonly develop diseases of the umbilical remnants, including infection (navel ill) in the umbilical arteries, veins, and urachus. These foals often become depressed, inappetent, and febrile. Many foals also develop secondary septicemia and septic arthritis. Umbilical remnant infection may be diagnosed based on clinical signs of swelling, heat, or drainage in the umbilical area. However, foals can have infection within these structures and be normal on palpation. Transabdominal ultrasonography is also helpful in diagnosing diseases of the umbilical structures. Foals with umbilical remnant infection require treatment with broad-spectrum antibiotics; many of these foals require surgical removal of the affected structures. Surgery for umbilical remnant disease involves a similar approach and instrumentation as for repairing an umbilical hernia. It is necessary to proceed with caution and have suction available and ready while dissecting the umbilical structures to prevent contamination of the abdominal cavity.

Patent urachus is a condition wherein foals dribble urine from the umbilicus because a patent canal between the urachus and urinary bladder is present at birth or develops in the postnatal period. Because those that develop in the postnatal period often occur secondary to an infectious process, it is imperative to rule out umbilical remnant infection and systemic infectious disease. Foals with a patent urachus may be treated nonsurgically by applying an irritant, such as iodine solution, or using silver nitrate sticks on the external surface of the urachus to promote scarification and closure. This is probably most effective in those foals that have a patent urachus at birth. Caution should be used with these agents, and application should be limited to once daily. If a rapid response is not observed or the foal has an infectious process occurring in the umbilical remnants, surgical resection should be performed.

Castration

Castration is one of the most commonly performed surgeries in horses. It is usually performed in the field and does not require extensive surgical facilities or instrumentation. Although under most circumstances castration is performed under short-acting IV general anesthesia, it can be performed in the standing horse with heavy sedation and infiltration of a local anesthetic into the scrotum and spermatic cord. The most common drugs for castration with the horse under IV anesthesia include xylazine-ketamine or xylazine-thiobarbiturate; both combinations can be used with or without guaifenesin. It is important to document that both testicles have descended into the scrotum before commencing with castration in the field. One needs to be prepared for a more extensive surgery requiring entrance into the abdominal cavity (as in a retained testicle); this needs to be planned for because it often takes more time than a routine castration. If both testicles cannot be palpated in the scrotum, the testicle may be located intraabdominally, in the inguinal canal, or immediately outside the external inguinal ring. A horse with a testicle located outside the abdominal cavity but not within the scrotum is referred to as a high flanker. If the testicle cannot be palpated in the scrotum, sedation may relax the horse and the cremaster muscle and allow the examiner to palpate the testicle or a portion of it. If the testicle still cannot be palpated after sedation, a rectal examination with or without ultrasonography may help confirm the location of the testicle. Involvement of the veterinary technician for castration includes general restraint, handling, administering and monitoring anesthesia, preparation of the surgical site, and preparation of instruments.

Castration is usually performed with the horse in lateral recumbency with the upper rear limb pulled forward and tied around the horse's neck. Castration involves making an incision over each testicle parallel to the median raphe through the skin and subcutaneous tissue. The testicles are removed by crushing then cutting the spermatic cord proximal to the testicle and epididymis using emasculators (Figure 31-2, *A*). The emasculators should be placed on the spermatic cord so that the cord is crushed on the side toward the body wall and cut on the side toward the scrotum (Figure 31-2, *B*). There are numerous types of emasculators, and each surgeon may have an individual preference. The entire spermatic cord may be crushed and cut simultaneously within the tunic (closed castration), or the tunica albuginea may be opened, and the emasculators can be applied to the vascular structures separately (open castration); this is often done in aged stallions that have an excessively large-diameter spermatic cord. The spermatic cord should be examined after the emasculator is removed to make sure that there is no bleeding. The skin incisions are stretched manually to promote drainage.

Postoperative care usually includes strict stall confinement for 24 hours and then controlled exercise (hand walking) once or twice daily for 1 to 2 weeks to promote drainage, prevent excessive swelling, and prevent or reduce stiffness and soreness. The horse should be monitored closely during the first day

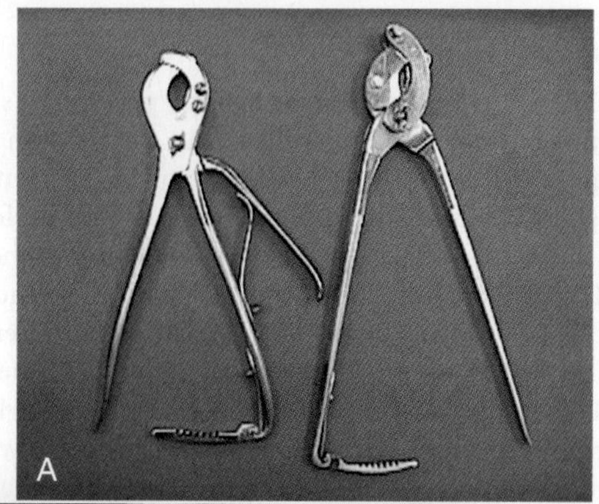

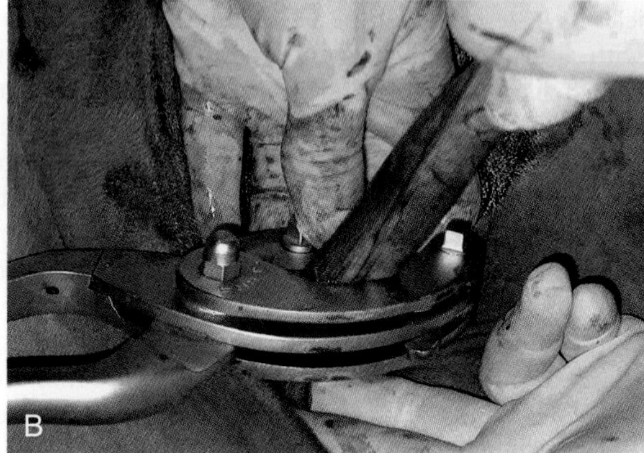

FIGURE 31-2 A, Emasculators used to crush and cut the spermatic cord of horses during castration. B, Use of emasculators during castration of a horse: the emasculators are placed around the spermatic cord so that the nut on the emasculators is located toward the testicle, ensuring that the spermatic cord is crushed toward the body side and the cord is cut toward the testicle side.

after surgery for signs of excessive hemorrhage, evisceration of intestine or omentum (herniation), or excessive swelling.

If the testicle has not descended (cryptorchidism), surgery is more involved and requires anesthesia of longer duration. Cryptorchidectomy (removal of a cryptorchid testicle) also requires the surgeon to use a different surgical technique than for routine castration. The testicle can be approached through various incisions, but an approach through the inguinal ring is most often used. A sponge forceps is used to grasp the structures that lead to the scrotum (gubernaculum), and the testicle is extracted from the inguinal canal. In some horses, the testicle cannot be retrieved in this manner, and the surgeon must manually explore the inguinal canal or caudal abdominal cavity. Once the testicle is retrieved, it is removed using a similar technique as described for routine castration. Following removal of the retained testicle, the other one is removed in a routine manner. Occasionally, horses have both testicles retained. More recently, laparoscopic cryptorchidectomy techniques have been described that can be performed in the standing, sedated horse. The testicle is removed via a flank incision, avoiding any enlargement or damage to the inguinal canal. Laparoscopy can also be used in an anesthetized patient, particularly in cases where there is difficulty in locating an abdominal testicle.

It is believed that cryptorchid horses are more at risk for evisceration after surgery. To prevent this, some surgeons may elect to temporarily pack a length of gauze soaked in sterile saline or an antiseptic into the subcutaneous areas of the inguinal canal. The gauze packing is held in place with large sutures in the skin and is usually removed in 24 to 72 hours. Other surgeons place interrupted absorbable sutures in the external inguinal ring.

Ovariectomy is performed in mares with diseased ovaries, in mares with normal reproductive tracts for use as teaser mares, and in some mares used as performance horses that have unacceptable behavior associated with estrus. An ovariectomy can be performed unilaterally or bilaterally, depending on the reason for the procedure. Laparoscopic techniques have been described that allow an ovariectomy to be performed in the standing horse. This provides excellent visualization of the ovary, good access to the associated artery and vein to ensure that adequate hemostasis is achieved, and a shorter convalescence. Diseased ovaries are usually enlarged and require removal through an incision in the ventral body wall (caudal midline or diagonal paramedian) or the flank. The most common cause of ovarian disease necessitating removal is neoplasia; the most common types of ovarian neoplasia include granulosa theca cell tumors and teratomas. Mares with granulosa theca cell tumors often display abnormal behavior, such as anestrus, persistent estrus or nymphomania, or stallionlike behavior. Ovarian tumors and other ovarian diseases are diagnosed based on clinical signs, rectal examination, and transrectal ultrasonography. Nondiseased ovaries of normal size can usually be removed through a flank incision or via an incision in the vaginal wall (colpotomy) in standing, sedated mares with either local anesthetic infiltration in the body wall or a caudal epidural anesthetic. Hemostasis of the ovarian pedicle is provided either by transfixing with multiple sutures, application of an automatic stapling device, or crushing with a chain écraseur. Complications include hemorrhage, abdominal pain, myositis, and other problems related to anesthesia and abdominal surgery.

Perineal Surgery

Perineal surgery is relatively common in equine practice. Primiparous mares develop rectovaginal and cervical lacerations during foaling. Abnormal perineal conformation can lead to reproductive unsoundness. Mares with abnormal conformation can develop pneumovagina or pneumouterus secondary to aspirating air into the reproductive tract. They also can develop vesicovaginal reflux in which urine pools in the cranial vaginal cavity; this can drain into the uterus during estrus when the cervix is opened, leading to endometrial inflammation. Most surgical procedures to correct these caudal reproductive tract abnormalities are performed in standing mares that have been sedated, and a caudal epidural anesthesia is used.

A caudal epidural anesthesia is performed after clipping the hair over the tail head and aseptically preparing the skin. An 18-gauge, 1.5-inch needle is inserted through the skin

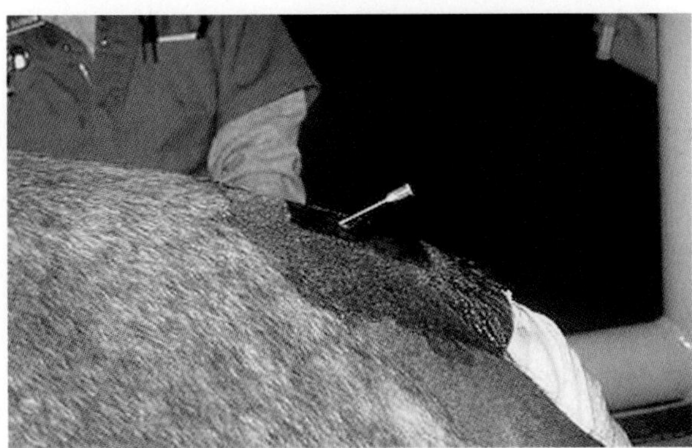

FIGURE 31-3 Technique for injecting a caudal epidural anesthetic between the first and second coccygeal vertebrae in a horse using an 18-gauge, 1½-inch needle.

between the last sacral and first coccygeal vertebrae or between the first and second coccygeal vertebrae and advanced (Figure 31-3). The correct location can be confirmed by checking to see if local anesthetic placed in the hub of the needle is drawn into the epidural space. Once the correct location has been identified, the local anesthetic is injected. The most commonly used agents for horses are lidocaine, mepivacaine, or xylazine. A caudal epidural anesthetic will desensitize the perineal region. Because horses will also develop incoordination in their rear limbs following the procedure, care should be taken when moving them until the effects of the anesthetic dissipate.

There are several surgical procedures for correcting caudal reproductive tract abnormalities. The most important factor in the eventual success of repairing a rectovaginal tear is that the mare's feces be made soft (cow patty consistency) and kept soft for at least 30 days after surgery. This decreases the straining and tension placed on the repaired rectal shelf. The most effective method for getting the feces soft is to remove hay and other coarse roughage from the diet and feed the mare on lush pasture or a complete pelleted feed. Administration of mineral oil or magnesium sulfate to the diet also helps soften the feces.

Caslick's Procedure

The most commonly performed perineal surgery is Caslick's operation. This is performed in many fillies on the racetrack and in mares with poor vulvar conformation to prevent pneumovagina and fecal contamination of the vagina, respectively. This procedure is usually performed with sedation and local anesthetic infiltration of the edge of the vulva. The edges of the dorsal vulvar labia are incised and then sutured using a continuous suture pattern. The closure is extended down to the level of the pelvic floor. The suture should not be any lower than this because it may interfere with urination and contribute to urine pooling.

Dystocia: Fetotomy and C-Section

Dystocia means "difficult birth" and is relatively uncommon in horses compared with cattle. However, when dystocia occurs in mares, it is usually a serious problem. Because parturition is rapid in horses and the expulsive efforts of the mare are violent, veterinary obstetric manipulations are difficult and exhausting. Care must be taken at all times to prevent injuring the reproductive tract of the mare. There are many causes of dystocia in the mare; the most frequent ones include premature placental separation and abnormal presentation of the fetus, especially when either the head or limbs or both are deviated. Because the neck of the foal is relatively long, it can easily become twisted. Sometimes the foal may come hind feet first (rare), or if the hind feet are retained, the tail comes first. This latter situation is true breech position. Transverse presentation is also rare in mares. Other occasional causes of dystocia include an excessively large fetus or fetal monsters (e.g., hydrocephalus). An anatomic or physiologic abnormality in the mare herself may cause dystocia. For example, a mare that has sustained a pelvic fracture can develop callus formation, which impairs the shape and size of the birth canal. Another cause of dystocia is torsion of the uterus. This may occur during gestation, particularly during the last trimester.

Dystocia in mares is corrected using a variety of methods, depending on the cause of the dystocia, the status of the foal, and the condition of the mare. Sometimes the dystocia can be corrected by manipulating fetal position or presentation with the mare standing, with or without the use of sedation or an epidural anesthetic. Placement of a nasotracheal tube will prevent the mare from exerting an abdominal press and will relieve straining. Sometimes a short-acting anesthetic protocol combined with rolling the mare on her back or hoisting her hind limbs is enough to relieve the dystocia and provide the veterinarian with sufficient relaxation in the mare to deliver the fetus. Fetotomy is sometimes performed to relieve dystocia, particularly if the fetus is dead. Fetotomy is a process in which a dead foal is cut into pieces while within the uterus and removed. Caution must be taken while performing a fetotomy to prevent serious injury to the reproductive tract of the mare.

> *TECHNICIAN NOTE* Most cesarean (C-section) deliveries are performed in the mare with general anesthesia. Generally, time is critical for saving the foal and for the overall health and well-being of the mare. The technician must be prepared for the surgery and have the necessary equipment, personnel, and drugs ready for reviving the foal if necessary.

Most C-section deliveries are performed in the mare with general anesthesia. Generally a C-section delivery is performed through a caudal ventral midline or flank incision in mares. Time is usually critical for saving the foal and for the overall health and well-being of the mare. The technician must be prepared for the surgery and have necessary equipment, personnel, and drugs ready for reviving the foal if necessary. The same instruments that are used for colic surgery are often used for C-section delivery, but additional

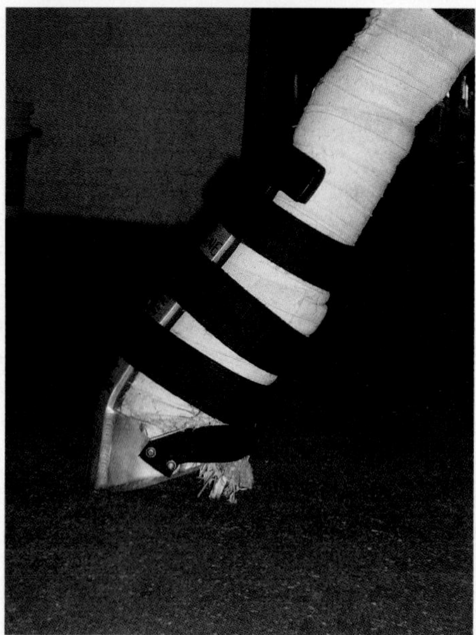

FIGURE 31-4 Use of Kimsey splint to stabilize fractures or joint subluxations in the lower limb of horses.

instruments may be necessary. If the foal is alive, the technician or other personnel need to be prepared and equipped to revive it. The foal will usually be depressed from the effects of general anesthesia and may need vigorous rubbing and drying. Oxygen should be available and heat lamps and a nasotracheal tube and Ambu bag to ventilate the foal. Forceps to clamp the umbilicus should be readily available if excessive bleeding occurs. A suction device to remove mucus and stomach contents from the airway should be attended to by a technician while the other technicians continue to be cognizant and attentive to the needs of the surgeons.

ORTHOPEDIC SURGERY

Horses frequently sustain severe musculoskeletal injuries, such as long-bone fractures or disruption of tendons or ligaments. These injuries often require stabilization with the use of bandages, splints, or casts before transport to a referral hospital. Successful stabilization of these injuries and safety of transport are important considerations in the outcome of these cases. Most severe injuries should be bandaged and splinted or casted to a level at least one joint above the injury. A heavy Robert Jones bandage should be applied and rigid splints placed on the lateral and either the dorsal or palmar aspects of the limb to provide appropriate support. Splints can be made out of rigid materials, such as wood, steel, or aluminum. The splints should not be excessively heavy or bulky, but must provide appropriate support. Horses with phalangeal fractures can be casted with their distal limb in flexion or can be placed in a commercially available device, such as a Kimsey splint (Figure 31-4). Horses with limb injuries should be hauled in a trailer with partitions to provide some support for them to balance themselves. The head should be tied loosely enough to enable the horse to use the head and neck for balance. Horses

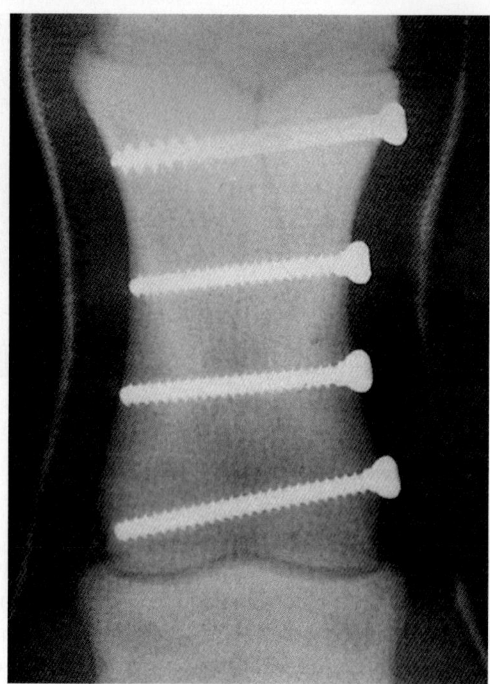

FIGURE 31-5 A proximal phalanx fracture in a horse repaired with cortical bone screws placed in lag fashion to compress the fracture line.

with front limb injuries should be transported with their head toward the rear of the trailer, and those with rear limb injuries should be transported with their head toward the front of the trailer.

Orthopedic surgery has become more common in horses. Athletic horses develop numerous orthopedic conditions that are amenable to surgical correction. Historically, fractures of long bones in adult horses were considered irreparable. However, with advanced techniques and more rigid surgical implants, many of these injuries are potentially correctable.

Major fractures of long bones in horses are best repaired with screws and bone plates to prevent movement at the fracture site while the bone heals under rigid fixation (Figure 31-5). Although aseptic technique is imperative for all surgical procedures, it is especially crucial to the overall success of orthopedic surgery in horses. If bony infection develops, it can lead to instability of the implants and fixation failure, which often necessitates euthanasia. It is the responsibility of all personnel to follow aseptic protocol. The technician should strive to maintain asepsis by monitoring the activities of all personnel involved in surgery. Orthopedic surgery requires the use of several specialized instruments and implants; because many of these surgeries are performed on an emergency basis, it is imperative that the technician make sure that instruments are available and ready for use. Many orthopedic injuries that are surgically repaired require the use of external coaptation (cast) for anesthetic recovery or for longer periods postoperatively (see Chapter 34). Therefore the technician should anticipate this need and have the appropriate materials available at the conclusion of surgery. The technician may also be needed to assist with anesthetic recovery of the orthopedic equine patient.

Postoperative monitoring of the orthopedic patient is vital for early detection of potential problems. It is particularly important to observe how the horse is using the affected limb in the stall; any dramatic change in use of the limb may signal an impending problem (infection or cast sores). The cast should also be monitored for heat, odor, or exudate, which would indicate the development of cast sores. The most common locations for sores to develop in association with a half-limb cast are at the proximal, dorsal aspect of the metacarpus or metatarsus, at the palmar or plantar aspect of the fetlock over the sesamoid bones, and over the heel bulbs. Bandages need to be changed frequently, and the incision sites should be monitored for swelling, erythema, and discharge. Drains are commonly used in orthopedic surgery following repair of a long bone. Drains can be useful in preventing seroma formation, but they can serve as potential routes for inoculation of the surgery site. Therefore it is important to keep these drains sterile by keeping a clean, sterile bandage on the leg. This may require changing the bandage more frequently than once daily.

> *TECHNICIAN NOTE* Postoperative monitoring of the orthopedic patient is vital for early detection of potential problems. It is particularly important to observe how the horse is using the affected limb in the stall; any dramatic change in use of the limb may signal an impending problem (infection or cast sores).

Arthroscopic Surgery

Arthroscopy is commonly performed for the diagnosis and treatment of joint disease. It is commonly performed for removing osteochondral chip fractures, treating cartilaginous and bony abnormalities associated with osteochondrosis, treating septic arthritis, and evaluating causes of joint lameness that have no definitive radiographic abnormalities. Depending on the joint evaluated and the type and location of the lesion, the horse may be positioned in dorsal or lateral recumbency. It is necessary to have the radiographs on a view box in the OR so that the surgeon can evaluate them intraoperatively. During arthroscopy, the technique of triangulation is used whereby the lesion forms one corner of the triangle and the arthroscope and surgical instruments serve as the other two corners of the triangle. Generally the arthroscope is placed in the joint on the side opposite the lesion, and the surgical instrument is placed in the joint on the same side as the lesion. The portal for placement of the arthroscope is usually made by making a small (1 cm) incision in the skin and subcutaneous tissue and then using a sharp trocar to advance the arthroscopic cannula through the fibrous joint capsule and synovial lining. Once the cannula has penetrated the joint cavity, the sharp trocar is replaced with a blunt obturator to pass the cannula across the joint; this prevents iatrogenic damage to the cartilage. The skin incisions are usually made before joint distention in the carpus, but after joint distention in other joints. The joint is distended with sterile polyionic fluid to facilitate placement of the arthroscope. Once the arthroscope is in place, the joint is evaluated; once the lesion is identified, the most appropriate location for the instrument portal is determined by using a needle to triangulate the lesion with the arthroscope. Once the appropriate location for the instrument portal is identified, the instrument portal is made with a scalpel blade (No. 11 or 15). The appropriate instrument is placed into the joint. The instruments commonly used in arthroscopy include a blunt probe for palpating intraarticular structures, rongeurs for removing osteochondral fragments, and curettes for débriding diseased cartilage and bone. A fenestrated cannula is often used at the end of surgery to facilitate removal of cartilage and bone debris via lavage. Motorized equipment is available and is sometimes necessary for débridement of large areas of diseased bone.

The surgeon uses specific instruments for arthroscopy, and these may vary depending on the joint involved and the individual surgeon's preference. Generally, there will be a standardized set of arthroscopy instruments that are packaged together. Instruments are steam sterilized, but if they are to be used on more than one case per day, they are sterilized with a cold sterilization solution before each use. Following sterilization, the instruments are packed in a sterile stainless steel pan that is later used to rinse disinfecting solution off the arthroscopy instruments. One of the most important and most expensive instruments is the arthroscope; it should be handled carefully to prevent damage. Additional items necessary are a sterile needle (usually 18-gauge) and syringe, which are used for distending the joint. During arthroscopic surgery, the joint is kept distended with sterile physiologic solution; this solution is usually delivered with a pump through a sterile IV set.

Many hospitals perform arthroscopy using a video camera so that the entire procedure can be viewed on a television screen (Figure 31-6). This causes less strain on the surgeon's eye, makes the procedure more educational for surgery assistants and technical staff, provides an opportunity to

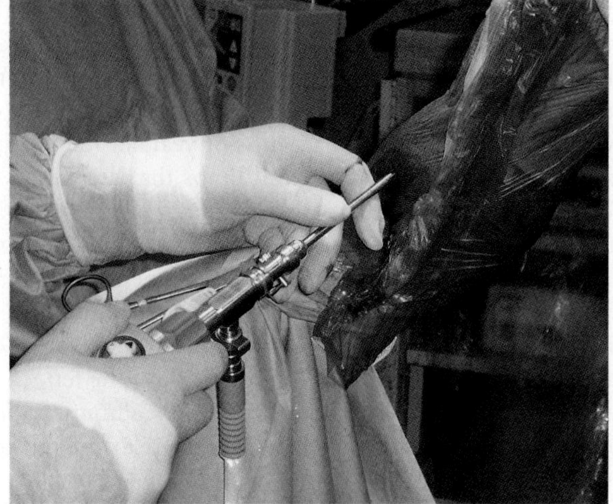

FIGURE 31-6 Use of arthroscopy for evaluating joint disease in horses. The arthroscope is inserted into the joint and attached to a camera that projects the image on a television screen for easy viewing by the surgeon and other personnel.

videotape the procedure, and probably allows the procedure to be performed with fewer breaks in aseptic technique. To provide the intense light required to illuminate the inside of the joint, a fiber-optic light source and light cable are required. It is essential that the technician be familiar with the assembly and function of the arthroscopic equipment and the proper care, cleaning, and disinfecting of the instruments. The arthroscopy instruments are disinfected using a cold sterilization solution, such as activated dialdehyde (Cidex, Surgikos); the instruments, arthroscope, and light cables are soaked for a minimum of 10 minutes. One should read the manufacturer's recommendations regarding the time required for disinfecting. To prevent delays, the instruments can be placed in the sterilizing solution at the start of anesthesia. This will also ensure adequate sterilization time. Before using the instruments, they are transferred sterilely into an empty sterile tray. The instruments are then rinsed with sterile saline to remove the sterilization solution.

After the surgical site has been aseptically prepared and draped and the instruments removed from the sterilizing solution, the technician will be responsible for attaching the fiber-optic cable to its light source. The system that delivers the fluid to distend the joint must also be connected to the appropriate fluid source. Once the system is connected to the fluid source, the surgeon must run fluid through the system to flush all air bubbles out of the tubing so that they do not enter the joint. Electric fluid pumps are generally used to maintain joint distention; these may be manually or pressure controlled.

Following surgery, all specialized arthroscopy equipment and instruments need to be cleaned. The arthroscope lens should be examined for scratches, and the video camera should be dried carefully. If several arthroscopy surgeries are scheduled for the day, the instruments are placed in the cold sterilization solution in preparation for the next surgery.

Flexural Deformities

Flexural and angular limb deformities (crooked legs) are abnormalities of the limbs that arise from abnormal development of bones and musculotendinous structures in the limbs. Flexural limb deformities result in overflexion of certain joints. There are three main manifestations of flexural limb deformities in horses. These can be present at birth or develop during the first few months or years of life. Carpal flexural deformities result in front limbs that are flexed or buckled forward at the carpus. This may range from mild deformity to a severe deformity that prevents the foal from standing. Mild to moderate cases are often amenable to treatment with controlled exercise combined with application of bandages and splints that extend from the ground to the elbow or tube casts that extend from just above the fetlock to the middle portion of the antebrachium. IV administration of oxytetracycline may be beneficial to help relax the musculotendinous structures.

The second type involves flexural deformity of the distal interphalangeal (coffin) joint, which results in a characteristic clubfoot-shaped hoof (Figure 31-7). This often is first noticed when the foal is a few months of age and can progress to the point that the foal walks on the toe or the dorsum of the hoof wall. Mild to moderate cases (those in which the foot has not passed the vertical plane) often respond to corrective trimming (lower heel) and application of an extended toe shoe, which helps to stretch out the deep digital flexor tendon. More advanced cases usually require surgical transection of the inferior check ligament, which lengthens the deep digital flexor musculotendinous unit.

The third type of flexural deformity involves the metacarpophalangeal joint and is characterized by an increased steepness to the pastern and fetlock (Figure 31-8). This usually

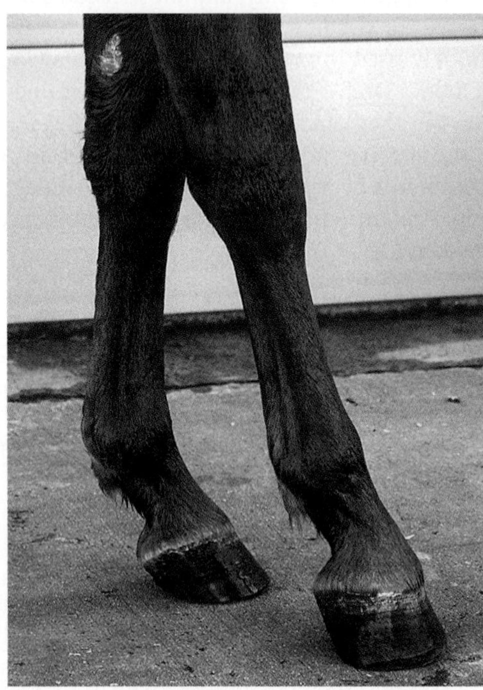

FIGURE 31-7 Flexural deformity of the distal interphalangeal (coffin) joint of the right front limb in a horse.

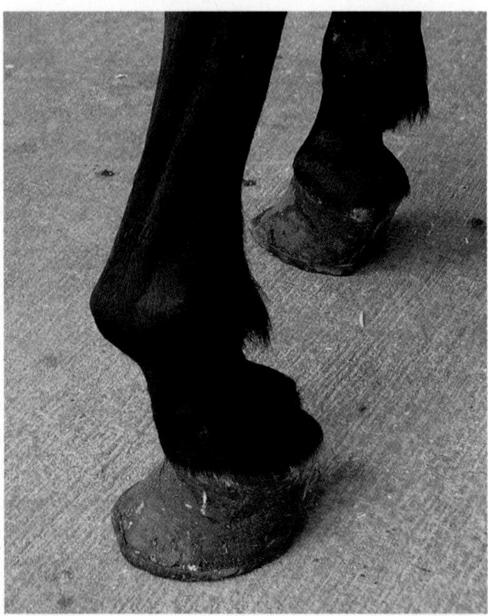

FIGURE 31-8 A flexural deformity of the metacarpophalangeal (fetlock) joint.

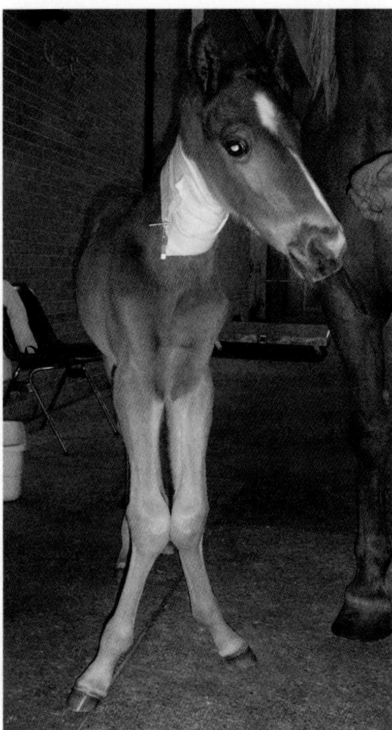

FIGURE 31-9 Bilateral carpal valgus deformity in a foal.

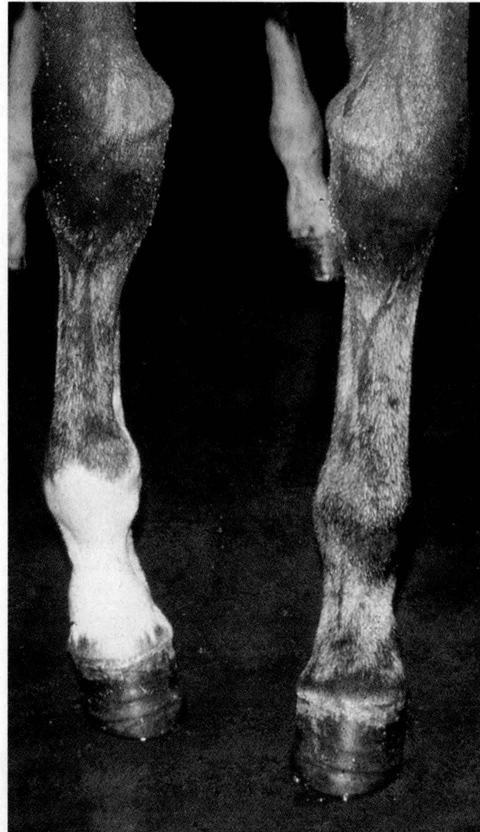

FIGURE 31-10 A varus deformity of the right fetlock in a foal.

begins to develop around 1 year of age, but may occur as late as 2 years. It can progress until the horse knuckles over at the fetlock. This condition commonly occurs in rapidly growing heavily muscled horses, such as 1- to 2-year-old quarter horses. Conservative treatment involves controlled exercise, dietary management (balanced minerals, low energy and protein), management of pain (arising from osteochondrosis or physitis) with NSAIDs, and application of bandages and splints that extend from the ground to the elbow. More severely affected horses or those that do not respond to conservative treatment may be successfully treated surgically by performing a superior check or inferior check ligament desmotomy or both, depending on whether the superficial digital flexor or deep digital flexor tendons or both are involved.

Angular Limb Deformities

Angular limb deformities are deformities that develop in the appendicular skeleton in a medial-to-lateral direction. These deviations can be present at birth or develop during the first few months of life. Mild deformities may self-correct, others may persist but not worsen, and still others may become more severe with time. These deformities are named in reference to the joint involved and the direction of the deviation. The most common deviation is carpal valgus, where the limb distal to the carpus deviates laterally (Figure 31-9). Other common deviations include fetlock varus, where the limb distal to the fetlock deviates medially (Figure 31-10), and tarsal valgus. These deviations can occur because of disproportionate growth of bone on either side of the growth plate, incompletely ossified cuboidal bones in the carpus and tarsus, or ligamentous laxity. The deviations in foals with incompletely ossified cuboidal bones or ligamentous laxity can usually be manually straightened, whereas those with disproportionate growth at the physis cannot.

Treatment of mild to moderate angular deviations may include stall rest with controlled exercise, depending on the age of the foal. Successful surgical procedures have been developed to treat moderate to severe deformities. Transection and elevation of the periosteum near the affected growth plate on the concave (short) side of the limb will stimulate more rapid bone growth, which usually leads to correction of the disproportionate growth. Periosteal transection and elevation can be repeated in 4 to 6 weeks if the deformity has not been completely corrected. The deformities do not overcorrect with this procedure. In more severe deformities or in older foals with less growth potential, the growth on the convex (or long) side of the bone can be slowed by performing transphyseal bridging. This is usually performed by placing a screw on either side of the growth plate and then tightening a figure-eight wire around the screw heads to provide compression of the growth plate. Use of transphyseal bridging can lead to correction of more severe deformities, but it is imperative that these implants be removed at the correct time to prevent overcorrection leading to the opposite type of deformity. Foals with deviations of the carpus or tarsus subsequent to ligamentous laxity or incompletely ossified cuboidal bones are best treated with stall rest with controlled exercise combined with application of full-limb bandages and splints or tube casts extending from the distal cannon bone to the proximal radius or tibia.

Laminitis

Laminitis (founder) is a serious, often life-threatening disease of horses involving inflammation of the sensitive laminae of the feet. It often involves both front feet or all four feet. However, it can occur in only one forefoot or rear foot if there is a severe lameness in the opposite limb. The exact cause of laminitis is unknown, but horses with serious infectious or inflammatory diseases resulting in endotoxemia, such as ischemic or inflammatory bowel disease, pleuropneumonia, septic metritis, and grain overload, are predisposed. Laminitis occurs almost exclusively in adult horses; it rarely occurs in horses less than 1 year of age.

> TECHNICIAN NOTE Laminitis (founder) is a serious, often life-threatening disease of horses involving inflammation of the sensitive laminae of the feet. It often involves both front feet or all four feet.

Acute laminitis occurs in the initial stages of the disease, resulting in extreme pain and reluctance to move. Horses often have increased heat in the hooves and have a pronounced or bounding digital pulse. They are reluctant to walk, turn, or allow their feet to be picked up. They stand with a characteristic stance with their rear legs camped underneath their torso and their front feet camped out in front (Figure 31-11). Chronic laminitis occurs when, because of degeneration of the sensitive laminae on the coffin bone (distal phalanx), the dorsal laminar attachments to the insensitive laminae of the hoof detach and the coffin bone rotates. In severe chronic laminitis, the rotated coffin bone may protrude through the sole of the foot. A lateral radiograph of the foot is usually required to determine whether coffin bone rotation has occurred (Figure 31-12, *A* and *B*). In more severe cases, all laminar attachments may become detached, and the coffin bone is displaced distally within the hoof wall. Horses that have distal displacement of the coffin bone develop a characteristic depression at the coronary band and are termed sinkers. Horses with chronic laminitis develop characteristic concentric rings on the hooves and an abnormal shape of the hooves (Figure 31-13).

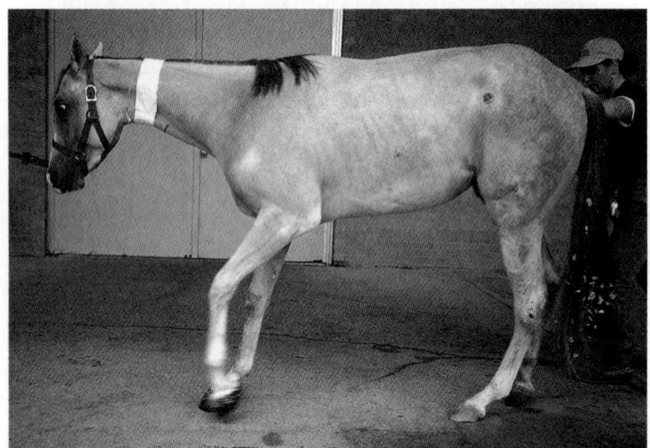

FIGURE 31-11 Typical posture of a horse with laminitis walking or turning on a hard surface.

The main focus of treatment of horses with laminitis involves reducing inflammation and providing analgesia with antiinflammatory drugs (phenylbutazone), promoting digital blood flow with vasodilator drugs (acepromazine, isoxsuprine, topical glyceryl trinitrate), and mechanically supporting the distal phalanx by providing frog support (frog pads or heart bar shoes). Nursing care is also an important component of the therapeutic regimen, particularly in chronic laminitis. Because laminitis is extremely painful, horses often spend long periods of time lying down. This necessitates care of decubital ulcers. Deep bedding is necessary, and using straw on top of shavings, padded mats, or a water bed can help prevent the development of these ulcers. In addition, they often develop subsolar abscesses that require daily soaking and bandaging. The prognosis for return of the horse to athletic competition depends on the occurrence and severity of rotation or sinkage of the coffin bone. Most horses that have appreciable rotation do not return to athletic function. The prognosis for horses that develop distal displacement of the coffin bone is poor.

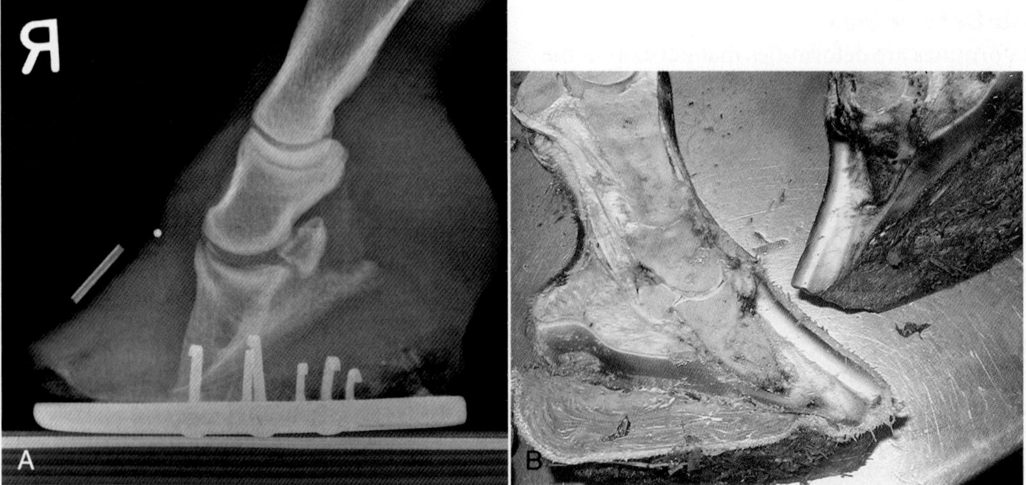

FIGURE 31-12 **A**, Lateral radiograph of the front foot of a horse with laminitis that has evidence of coffin bone rotation. **B**, Gross pathologic photograph of sagittal section of both front feet of a horse with bilateral laminitis that has undergone coffin bone rotation.

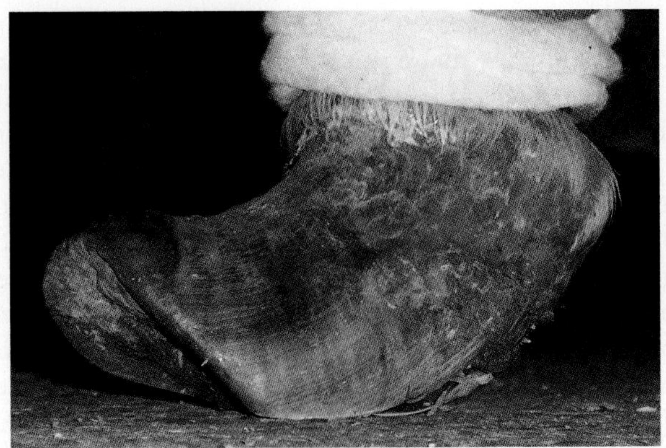

FIGURE 31-13 Abnormal hoof growth in a horse with chronic laminitis in both front feet.

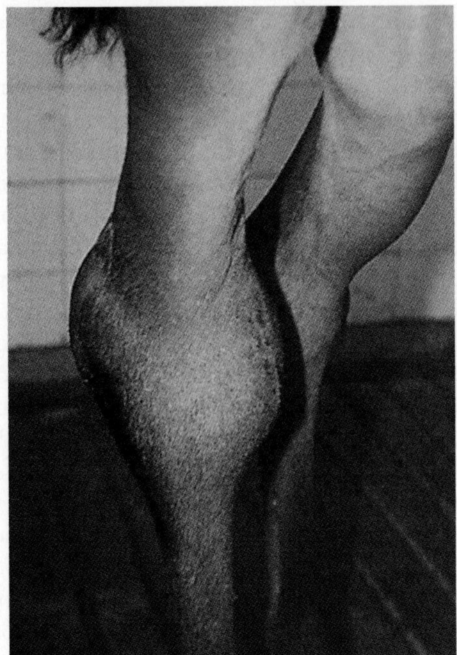

FIGURE 31-14 A young horse with a marked tibiotarsal joint effusion, otherwise known as bog spavin.

Bog Spavin

Bog spavin is a term used to describe the accumulation of synovial fluid (effusion) in the tarsocrural joint of the hock (Figure 31-14). Fluid can accumulate secondary to osteochondrosis, synovitis, and arthritis. Degenerative joint disease(arthritis) is a common performance-limiting condition of horses and can affect numerous joints. Bone spavin refers to arthritis in the distal intertarsal and tarsometatarsal joints of the hock. High ring-bone and low ring-bone refer to arthritis in the proximal interphalangeal (pastern) and distal interphalangeal (coffin) joints, respectively. Osselet is a term to describe arthritis in the metacarpophalangeal or metatarsophalangeal (fetlock) joint.

Tendinitis

Tendinitis (bowed tendons) is an injury involving primarily the superficial digital flexor tendon and occasionally the deep digital flexor tendon of the front limbs. This injury is usually sustained secondary to racing or other strenuous activity. There are different degrees of tendinitis ranging from mild edema and inflammation to tendon fiber separation to tendon fiber tearing or disruption. When tendon fibers tear, the result is hemorrhage and inflammatory debris accumulating in a cavity within the tendon, which is known as a core lesion. Treatment of tendinitis includes hydrotherapy, NSAIDs, support bandages, topical antiinflammatory agents (sweats, poultices), and exercise restriction or controlled exercise. Several surgical procedures have been used to either treat tendinitis or prevent its recurrence. The most commonly performed surgery is tendon splitting, which evacuates the core lesion and allows more rapid vascularization and healing of the area. The prognosis for return to athletic function depends on the severity of the injury; some horses with severe core lesions can return to athletic function if given appropriate treatment and time for convalescence.

Osteochondrosis

Osteochondrosis is a form of developmental orthopedic disease in which the articular cartilage and underlying subchondral bone do not develop appropriately. This can result in the formation of osteochondritis dissecans (cartilage flaps), osteochondral fragments, cartilage erosion, and subchondral bone cysts. These abnormalities often manifest as joint effusion and lameness when young horses are first put into strenuous exercise. Many of these lesions are amenable to treatment via arthroscopy, resulting in the horse returning to athletic function.

Subsolar Abscess

Subsolar abscess is a common cause of severe lameness. Horses usually will not bear weight on the limb. There is palpable heat in the hoof and a bounding digital pulse similar to that in a horse with laminitis. However, the difference is that subsolar abscesses usually occur only in one foot. Pain can be localized by applying focal pressure to the sole of the foot with hoof testers. Occasionally, purulent debris will accumulate and migrate, and an area breaks open at the coronary band and drains (gravel). Treatment involves paring out the sole until the abscess is located to provide drainage. The foot should be kept bandaged to keep it dry and clean. The affected foot can be soaked daily in a solution of povidone-iodine (Betadine) and magnesium sulfate (Epsom salts) and then rebandaged. The horse should be given analgesics (phenylbutazone) for a few days. Appropriate tetanus prophylaxis should be administered. The foot needs to be protected from dirt and debris until the area fills in with granulation tissue and is covered with cornified tissue.

Septic Arthritis

Septic arthritis is a common occurrence in adult horses secondary to iatrogenic inoculation of joints during arthrocentesis or joint surgery or subsequent to traumatic joint injuries. It occurs commonly in foals subsequent to hematogenous spread from a focus of infection, such as the umbilicus (navel ill), lungs (pneumonia), or intestinal tract (enteritis). The cornerstone of treatment of septic arthritis includes broad-spectrum antibiotics administered systemically, intraarticular antibiotics, NSAIDs, and joint drainage and lavage.

UPPER RESPIRATORY TRACT SURGERY

Abnormalities of the upper respiratory tract can be performance limiting to athletic horses and, if severe, can also be life threatening. Many obstructive diseases of the upper respiratory tract are amenable to surgical correction. The most common of these are left laryngeal hemiplegia, epiglottic entrapment, dorsal displacement of the soft palate (DDSP), and arytenoid chondritis. Others are subepiglottic cysts, guttural pouch empyema, guttural pouch tympany, and guttural pouch mycosis.

Left laryngeal hemiplegia ("roarer") is a condition resulting in paralysis of the left arytenoid cartilage, which prevents it from being abducted during inspiration. This results in the arytenoid collapsing and being pulled into the airway secondary to the negative pressure that is generated during inspiration. The cause of this condition is unknown, but it results in a recurrent laryngeal neuropathy. Because this nerve normally provides innervation to the major abductor muscle of the arytenoid cartilage, the cricoarytenoideus dorsalis, a neuropathy results in muscle atrophy and an inability to abduct the arytenoid. As the name implies, this condition occurs almost exclusively on the left side (95%); it is believed that this is related to the longer length of the nerve on the left side and that it may become damaged from the vibrations as it courses around the aortic arch. This condition is diagnosed using endoscopy at rest or during exercise on a high-speed treadmill; the left arytenoid cartilage is not fully abducted during inspiration and in severe cases actually collapses into the airway. Horses with this condition make a characteristic inspiratory noise (roaring) and develop exercise intolerance. Surgical treatment is a prosthetic laryngoplasty, which involves placing a suture between the cricoid cartilage and the muscular process of the arytenoid cartilage to mimic the action of the cricoarytenoideus dorsalis and abduct the arytenoid cartilage (tieback). The laryngeal ventricles (saccules) are also everted and resected (ventriculectomy or sacculectomy) through either a ventral laryngotomy or by use of an endoscopically guided laser. Approximately 70% of horses treated with a prosthetic laryngoplasty and sacculectomy return to athletic function. Most horses will continue to make some noise, and in some, the noise may not improve. The laryngotomy incision is usually left open to heal by second intention. This requires daily cleaning with gauze sponges with saline or water followed by application of petrolatum to the skin around the incision and on the mandible and neck to prevent skin scald from the drainage. It usually takes approximately 3 weeks for the incision to heal. Some clinicians partially close the incision, which reportedly shortens the time required to heal.

> *TECHNICIAN NOTE* Left laryngeal hemiplegia ("roarer") is a condition resulting in paralysis of the left arytenoid cartilage, which prevents it from being abducted during inspiration.

Epiglottic entrapment is a condition where the aryepiglottic membrane that extends from the arytenoid cartilage to the ventral surface of the epiglottis hypertrophies and rolls upward to envelope the rostral and abaxial portions of the epiglottis. Normally the epiglottis should have a serrated edge and a distinct vascular pattern present on the dorsal surface. When the epiglottis becomes entrapped, the serrated edge and vascular pattern can no longer be seen. The shape or outline of the epiglottis can still be observed (unlike that seen with a DDSP), but the tip appears more rounded and the abaxial surface is smooth rather than serrated. In more chronic cases, the tip of the epiglottis may become ulcerated. The cause of epiglottic entrapment is unknown, but it is believed that these horses have an instability between the caudal edge of the soft palate and the epiglottis and that the aryepiglottic membrane hypertrophies and makes the epiglottis more rigid. Epiglottic entrapment can be intermittent or permanent. Some horses can continue to perform athletically with an entrapped epiglottis, but it does appear to affect performance in most horses. Treatment of epiglottic entrapment includes transecting the aryepiglottic membrane to release the epiglottis. This can be done using several techniques. First, it can be performed with a hooked bistoury placed through the nasal passages in a standing, sedated horse with or without endoscopic guidance; care must be taken to prevent trauma to other structures and to prevent laceration of the soft palate. Second, it can be performed in an anesthetized horse with a mouth speculum by manually guiding a hooked bistoury and transecting the membrane on midline. Third, it can be performed using an endoscopically guided laser in a standing, sedated horse. Finally, in more severe or chronic recurring cases, the aryepiglottic membrane can be resected through a ventral laryngotomy. The prognosis for return to athletic performance is good, but entrapment can recur. Some of these horses may develop DDSP after the entrapment is released. Horses that have the entrapment released using the hooked bistoury or laser can generally resume training in a few days, whereas those treated via resection through a laryngotomy require approximately 3 weeks before resuming training.

DDSP is generally a dynamic obstructive disease of the upper respiratory tract that occurs during exercise. Normally the soft palate remains ventral to the epiglottis. However, if the epiglottis is small or flaccid or the caudal edge of the soft palate is flaccid, the soft palate can become displaced dorsal to the epiglottis during strenuous exercise. The cause of this condition is unknown, but it is believed that the factors listed previously predispose the palate to become displaced during inspiration when negative pressure is generated in the upper airway. This condition usually is intermittent, occurring during strenuous exercise and dissipating once exercise has stopped and the horse swallows. Because horses are obligate nasal breathers, DDSP interferes with the horse's breathing. Horses with DDSP usually make a characteristic gurgling or snoring type of noise, which will dissipate as soon as they swallow and replace the palate into its normal position.

Treatment options for a horse with DDSP include placing a cloth or leather tie on the horse's tongue and pulling the tongue rostrad and tying the tongue to the mandible in the interdental space. The epiglottis, tongue, and sternothyrohyoideus muscles are attached to the hyoid apparatus. Because the tongue is attached at the rostral aspect of the hyoid apparatus and the sternothyrohyoideus muscles are attached at its caudal aspect, a tongue tie prevents caudal retraction of the hyoid apparatus, including the epiglottis. This seems to help approximately 50% of horses with DDSP because it prevents caudal retraction of the epiglottis and maintains normal epiglottic-palate alignment. Because of its noninvasive nature, the tongue tie is generally the first thing attempted in horses with DDSP. If this does not work, a section of the sternothyrohyoideus muscles can be resected in the midcervical region; this also prevents caudal retraction of the hyoid apparatus. This myectomy procedure helps in approximately 50% of horses with DDSP that fail to respond to a tongue tie. If this procedure does not work, the caudal margin of the soft palate can be resected (staphylectomy). There are two theories as to why this may help prevent DDSP. First, it is believed that the caudal edge of the palate becomes more fibrous as it heals with scar tissue; this makes the caudal edge more rigid and therefore more resistant to displacement. The other theory is that, if the palate does displace, it enables the palate to be replaced more easily. Regardless of the mechanism, it seems that it helps prevent DDSP in approximately half of the horses that do not respond to the tongue tie or myectomy. A laryngeal tie forward procedure reportedly has achieved a higher success rate in horses with DDSP and should now be considered the surgery of choice if no other source of inflammation is present in the upper respiratory tract. However, it requires general anesthesia, so some of the alternative procedures may be performed initially in the standing patient.

Arytenoid chondritis is an inflammatory, degenerative condition of the arytenoid cartilagines resulting in a proliferative mass on one or both arytenoids. This usually results in an obstructive disease of the upper airway with signs similar to the conditions described earlier. These cartilagines are usually enlarged and more fibrous than normal, which prevents them from being effectively treated with a tieback. The treatment of choice is to remove the affected arytenoid cartilage through a ventral laryngotomy. Because of the time required for dissection in the laryngeal region during an arytenoidectomy, a tracheotomy is usually performed in the middle or proximal trachea to provide a mechanism for ventilation during anesthesia. The tracheotomy can be performed either before anesthetic induction or once the horse is anesthetized. These horses are prone to upper airway obstruction postoperatively and need to be closely monitored. The tracheotomy tube is usually left in place, at least for a couple of days, until it is believed the horse has an airway of adequate diameter for breathing. It is imperative that these horses be monitored closely while the tracheotomy tube is in place to make sure that it does not become dislodged or obstructed with mucus or other discharge. The laryngotomy and tracheotomy sites require daily cleaning and application of petrolatum on the skin around the incisions. Both these incisions will heal by second intention in approximately 3 weeks.

Bacterial infection of the guttural pouch (empyema) usually is a sequela to strangles or retropharyngeal lymph node abscesses. Clinical signs include swelling in the throat-latch region and a bilateral mucopurulent nasal discharge. Horses with guttural pouch empyema can be treated conservatively with antibiotics and guttural pouch lavage; this may be effective in many horses that are treated early in the course of the disease. However, in more chronic cases, the mucopurulent material becomes inspissated and forms gelatinous concretions (chondroids) that lie in the floor of the guttural pouches. Resolution of empyema requires removal of the chondroids, and long-term effective drainage can usually only be achieved with surgical drainage. Several approaches are reported for surgical drainage of the guttural pouches, but the most common surgical approach for guttural pouch empyema is the modified Whitehouse technique; the incision is made in the skin on the ventrum of the throat region just axial to the linguofacial vein and is followed by blunt dissection into the pouch. The guttural pouch is lavaged intraoperatively. Indwelling catheters can be placed into the guttural pouches in standing, sedated horses under endoscopic guidance; these catheters enable frequent lavage of the pouches. The guttural pouches should not be lavaged with irritating solutions because of the proximity of blood vessels and nerves coursing through the area. The incision is managed similarly to a laryngotomy or tracheotomy incision.

Guttural pouch tympany is an accumulation of air in the guttural pouches; this occurs in foals and weanlings and is usually associated with an abnormality of the opening to the pouches. It can occur on one or both sides and is characterized by a fluctuant, nonpainful swelling in the throat-latch region. If unilateral guttural pouch tympany is present, then it is usually treated by surgically creating an opening in the septum between the left and right pouches; this is usually approached through an incision in Viborg's triangle on the affected side. If bilateral tympany is present, creating an opening in the septum will not effectively drain the two sides. Therefore the opening to one or both of the guttural pouches is surgically revised through a Viborg's triangle approach. Surgical revision of the guttural pouch opening may be performed on only one side with creation of an opening in the septum to enable both pouches to evacuate the air through one opening.

Guttural pouch mycosis can be life threatening. Fungal plaques form in the lining of the guttural pouches; if the plaques involve vascular structures, such as the internal carotid artery, severe fatal hemorrhage can occur. Fatal hemorrhage is often preceded by several episodes of substantial epistaxis. However, once the diagnosis is made, surgery should not be delayed. The most accepted method of surgical treatment is vascular occlusion of either the internal carotid artery, external carotid artery, or both, depending on which vessels are affected. This can be done following placement of an intraarterial balloon-tipped catheter or by placement of newer springs or coils that stimulate local occlusion. Both the internal and external carotid arteries can be ligated unilaterally with no untoward effects. The major potential complication of external carotid artery occlusion is blindness. Once the affected vessels are ligated, the fungal infection is treated by lavage of the guttural pouches and instillation of antifungal medication into the pouch via indwelling catheters or via the endoscope.

EMERGENCY SITUATIONS AND PROCEDURES

Several emergency situations can arise that necessitate immediate action on the part of a technician or clinician to prevent death of a horse. One of the most common emergency situations is the development of upper airway obstruction leading to dyspnea. Obstructive diseases involving the nasal passages, nasopharynx, and larynx can be alleviated by a tracheotomy. A tracheotomy is generally performed at the junction of the middle and proximal thirds of the neck on the ventral midline. An incision is made on the ventral cervical midline through the skin, subcutaneous tissue, and cutaneous colli muscle parallel to the trachea. The paired sternothyrohyoideus muscles are then split on midline to expose the tracheal rings. The membrane between two adjacent rings is then cut with a scalpel on the ventral surface for a distance of approximately one third of the circumference of the tracheal rings. Care should be taken not to cut the tracheal rings and not to cut vital structures adjacent to the trachea (carotid artery, recurrent laryngeal nerve, jugular vein). Many times the tracheotomy must be performed on an extremely anxious horse or after the horse has collapsed from insufficient oxygen. Therefore one should be careful not to get into a situation where injury occurs.

> *TECHNICIAN NOTE* One of the most common emergency situations is the development of upper airway obstruction leading to dyspnea.

Veterinary technicians should become familiar and comfortable with the dosages and indications for drugs commonly used in emergency situations. A list of drugs and doses along with the drugs and syringes should be kept readily available in several locations throughout the hospital. These can be prepared in small emergency packs.

> *TECHNICIAN NOTE* Veterinary technicians should become familiar and comfortable with the dosages and indications for drugs commonly used in emergency situations. A list of drugs and doses along with the drugs and syringes should be kept readily available in several locations throughout the hospital.

Occasionally, horses develop reactions to certain drugs. These may be anaphylactic reactions resulting in shock or death or allergic type of reactions resulting in skin wheals. Horses may develop a reaction to procaine penicillin, which usually results in an anaphylactoid reaction. These horses usually require treatment with corticosteroids and epinephrine. They may recover or die subsequent to pulmonary edema. Horses often develop skin wheals in response to drugs or environmental allergens (Figure 31-15, *A* and *B*). The drugs that most commonly cause these wheals in horses are NSAIDs and trimethoprim-sulfa antibiotics.

Intracarotid injection of drugs can cause seizurelike activity. This can be life threatening to the horse and is potentially injurious to the handler and other personnel in the vicinity. The chance for this can be minimized by using an 18-gauge needle that is unattached from the syringe and directed down the jugular vein. Normally, if the needle is in the jugular vein, blood will slowly ooze out of the needle hub only if the jugular vein is occluded. If the carotid artery is inadvertently entered with the needle, blood will exit in a pulsatile manner. If this occurs, do not inject the medication. The needle should be removed, and compression should be applied to decrease hematoma formation. The needle should be reinserted into a different location using the same technique.

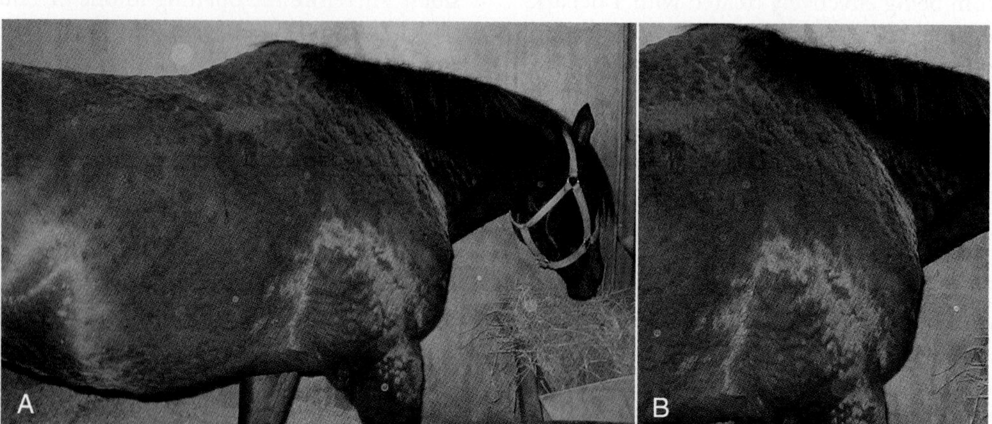

FIGURE 31-15 **A,** Horse with wheals throughout the body indicating an anaphylactic reaction. **B,** Closer view of the wheals (raised areas of pitting edema).

ANESTHESIA FOR THE EQUINE PATIENT

The veterinary technician may be directly or indirectly involved in anesthesia of horses. Frequently the technician is primarily responsible for all aspects of anesthesia, including selection of induction and maintenance anesthetic agents, instrumentation, monitoring, and recovery of patients. It is important that the technician be familiar with the properties and recommended doses of the anesthetic agents administered and the equipment (ventilator, blood pressure monitor, anesthetic machine, etc.) used (see Chapter 27). Numerous complications can arise, and it is important that the technician be familiar with the methods of treating these complications, including the correct drugs and doses for treating hypotension and cardiac arrhythmias. Because it is important to maintain mean arterial blood pressure at 70 mm Hg or greater to help prevent myopathies and neuropathies, blood pressure should be monitored via an indirect or direct method. Hypotension is usually treated by decreasing the depth of anesthesia, increasing the rate of administration of IV fluids, and administration of vasoactive drugs, such as dobutamine, dopamine, or phenylephrine. It is important to monitor how well the horse is oxygenated and ventilated during anesthesia; this can be done most effectively by monitoring arterial blood gases. The technician should monitor recovery from anesthesia and be prepared for any potential complications.

> *TECHNICIAN NOTE* Frequently the technician is primarily responsible for all aspects of anesthesia, including selection of induction and maintenance anesthetic agents, instrumentation, monitoring, and recovery of patients.

CASE PRESENTATION 31-1

A 4-year-old thoroughbred filly was seen for evaluation of coliclike symptoms of 8 hours duration. The horse had been eating and behaving normally the night before, but was found to be uncomfortable (restless, rolling, and looking at his flank) the next morning. Medical therapy with flunixin did not resolve the horse's clinical signs, so the owners brought her to the clinic for further evaluation.

Upon presentation, the filly's parameters were as follows:

Heart rate: 58 beats per minute
Respiratory rate: 24 breaths per minute
Mucous membranes: pale and tacky to the touch
CRT: prolonged (greater than 3 seconds)
Gut sounds were identified only on the left side and were decreased.
Dehydration: Skin tent was prolonged, and the horse is estimated to be between 5% to 10% dehydrated.
Weight: 465 kg

Blood was collected from the left jugular vein and submitted for a CBC and a serum biochemistry. While that was pending, a nasogastric tube was placed using a twitch for restraint, and after priming the tube, 16 L of net reflux was obtained. Before the rectal examination, the filly was sedated with 200 mg of xylazine administered IV and placed in a set of stocks. The veterinarian performed the rectal examination using a well-lubricated sleeve and identified a thick loop of small diameter in the right side of the abdomen, running vertically. This loop appeared to be fixed in place at this location. An IV jugular catheter was placed by the technician, and the horse was bolused with 10 L of lactated Ringer's solution. Abdominal ultrasound identified distended, amotile loops of small intestine throughout the ventral abdomen and a loop of thickened small intestine within the lumen of a larger viscera (creating a "target lesion") (Figure 1). The combination of the ultrasonographic findings, the rectal examination, and the presence of a small intestinal obstruction (demonstrated by the volume of reflux) justified the need for an exploratory celiotomy to treat a suspected ileocecal intussusception. The blood work revealed signs of dehydration and a prerenal azotemia.

The need for surgical therapy and the risks associated with surgery and anesthesia were explained to the client, and permission was granted to proceed. The filly's belly was clipped while preoperative antibiotics (penicillin and gentamicin IV) and fluids were administered. A rough prep using iodine scrub was then applied to the abdomen and left in place. The filly was moved to the induction box, and general anesthesia was induced. The horse was moved onto the surgery table using a hydraulic hoist and secured in dorsal recumbency. A sterile prep using chlorhexidine scrub was applied and finally rinsed off with sterile saline while the surgical team scrubbed their hands and arms.

Once the horse was draped, a ventral midline incision was made, and the abdomen was explored. A jejunocecal intussusception was identified, but it could not be manually reduced. This was blindly resected off within the cecum,

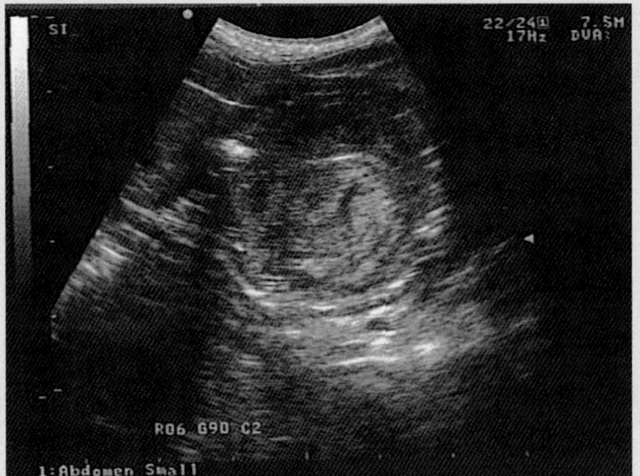

FIGURE 1 The smaller hyperechoic (white) circular structure is a loop of jejunum within a larger hyperechoic circle, which is otherwise known as a "target" lesion and is a cross-sectional view of an intussusception.

Continued

CASE PRESENTATION 31-1—cont'd

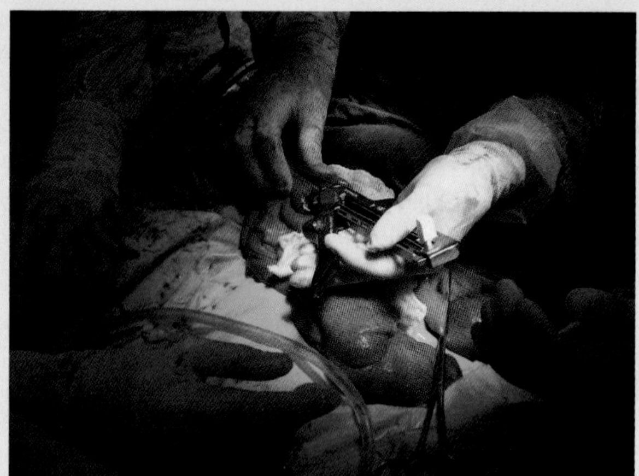

FIGURE 2 An intestinal stapling device (GIA 90) is used to anastomose the jejunum to the cecum.

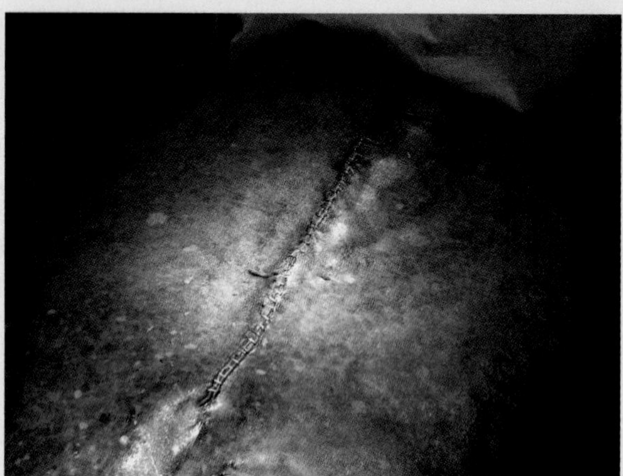

FIGURE 3 The skin incision has been stapled, which can be performed faster than skin suturing.

and a jejunocecostomy was performed (Figure 2). The linea was sutured closed, the skin was stapled (Figure 3), and the horse was then moved back into the recovery stall, where she recovered uneventfully after 90 minutes.

Postoperatively the filly was maintained on IV fluids at 1½ times daily maintenance, antibiotics were continued for 72 hours, and he received another dose of flunixin. The fluids were supplemented with potassium chloride and calcium gluconate. Physical examinations were performed every 6 hours, including a PCV and TP. The filly remained comfortable and quiet for the first 36 hours postoperatively, but then an increased respiratory rate (30 breaths per minute) and signs of discomfort (pawing, circling in the stall) were noted. A nasogastric tube was passed, and 14 L of net reflux were obtained, indicating that the horse had an obstruction of his small intestine. At this time after surgery, it is most likely to be ileus, which is related to inflammation within the intestinal wall interfering with its function. The nasogastric tube was secured to the horse's halter and left in place to allow frequent gastric decompression (every 3 hours). The filly was no longer given access to any feed, and the fluid rate was increased to counter the increased fluid loss that was occurring. A constant rate infusion of lidocaine was also given to try and reduce inflammation and stimulate normal gastrointestinal motility when it is discontinued. The filly's fecal output decreased over the next 48 hours because she was no longer eating anything.

The filly remained comfortable, although she would grind her teeth and would salivate excessively because of the indwelling nasogastric tube. After refluxing for 36 hours, the volume obtained began to decrease each time, and by 48 hours after it began, the net reflux obtained at each interval was less than 3 L, which was within normal limits. The nasogastric tube was removed, and water was offered in small amounts to the horse. At this time, the lidocaine infusion was discontinued, and the dose of flunixin she received was halved. She drank this water willingly, but to reduce the risk for recurrence of the ileus, only small volumes were offered for the first afternoon. Because her gut managed to tolerate this, the volume of water offered was increased, and she was taken outside to graze for a few minutes. This improved her demeanor considerably, and over the next couple of days, she was gradually returned to a full level of feeding without any further complications. As her water intake increased, she was weaned off IV fluids, and the jugular catheter was subsequently removed.

When she was back to eating a normal ration and had not been on any medication for at least 24 hours, the filly was discharged to her owners. They were given a printed and signed discharge letter that included specific instructions for her aftercare and things about which to be vigilant. The filly left the clinic and has not had any further episodes of colic.

SURGICAL NURSING OF FOOD ANIMALS

As in equine practice, veterinary technicians are vital team members in food animal practices. Their roles and responsibilities are identical to those in other fields of veterinary nursing; the principle goal is to safely provide optimal nursing care to patients. Familiarity with food animal species (the emphasis of this section of the chapter will be bovine) is important because they act and behave differently from each other and particularly from horses. To ensure personnel safety, the practice must be equipped with appropriate chutes and stocks so that animals can be examined and restrained. Additional equipment, such as tilt tables, will allow further surgical or diagnostic procedures to be performed, either using sedation or general anesthesia. This equipment is invaluable to allow veterinarians and technicians to examine and work on even the largest bulls in relative safety. Smaller stocks and restraint devices are available for small ruminants, but should only be used for these species.

PREOPERATIVE PREPARATION

In nonemergency situations, the following should be routinely performed before any surgical intervention. A physical examination must be performed, and a packed-cell volume (PCV) and total protein are recommended if there is a risk of significant blood loss or if general anesthesia will be used. Further blood work, such as a CBC and full biochemistry panel, is indicated for most complicated gastrointestinal disturbances since electrolyte abnormalities or infectious processes can influence the surgical outcome and postoperative convalescence. The position of the patient during surgery needs to be considered so that feed can be withheld for an appropriate time to reduce the risks of regurgitation and aspiration pneumonia. If the adult patient will be in dorsal or lateral recumbency or under general anesthesia, 36 to 48 hours of fasting is indicated. Because of the capacity of the rumen, water should be removed 12 hours preoperatively. For standing procedures, no fasting is required. IV catheterization should be performed shortly before surgery if a catheter is necessary. Either jugular vein can be used, but because of the thickness of cow skin, a stab incision is often made with a scalpel blade to prevent burring of the edges of the catheter. IV catheters can be displaced or pulled out, even when sutured or superglued to the skin. In most cases where IV fluid therapy is indicated, the cow will remain quiet and will usually not move around excessively or rub at the catheter site.

If antibiotics, analgesics, or anesthetics are to be used, care should be taken to ensure that all of the drugs administered are licensed for use in this species (refer to Chapters 25, 26, and 27). The technician and veterinarian must be conscious of withdrawal times for all drugs that are used because these may influence postoperative management. Penicillin or ceftiofur tend to be the most widely used antibiotics, and high doses of ceftiofur will provide reasonable Gram-negative coverage. Other alternatives include oxytetracycline, but it has only bacteriostatic properties. Flunixin is the only licensed NSAID; the use of phenylbutazone should be avoided. Anesthetic drugs are used off label in cattle (see Chapter 27).

Considering the environment in which cattle live, they are often dirtier or dustier than animals that are maintained on pasture. If possible, clipping the hair before entering the OR or area is preferable to minimize the risk of contamination of the surgery suite. Skin preparation is performed initially to remove any gross skin contaminants and dander, and immediately before surgery, a sterile prep should be applied with either povidone-iodine or chlorhexidine scrub solutions, using a standard technique, once the cow is restrained for the surgery (stocks, tilt table, etc.). Iodine scrub should be rinsed with alcohol, and chlorhexidine should be rinsed off with saline.

Preparation of the surgical room or area is important. Having all of the necessary supplies nearby will improve efficiency and prevent a surgery from beginning with some important instrument or piece of equipment unavailable. If the animal is to be recumbent for the procedure, adequate padding needs to be present for the patient to be placed on to prevent any anesthetic-related complications, such as a myopathy or myositis and neuropathies, (particularly radial nerve paresis or paralysis) from developing. If in lateral recumbency, the distal forelimb should be pulled cranially, and the uppermost hind limb should be elevated off the most dependant hind limb by pads or a bale of straw. Even with appropriate padding and support, complications can develop and need to be addressed.

Surgical preparation for the veterinarian must include an appropriate surgical scrub of their hands and forearms. Sterile gloves should be worn, and, where possible, the patient should be draped, and the surgeon should be wearing a sterile gown, cap, and mask.

CONDITIONS OF THE GASTROINTESTINAL TRACT

Abnormalities in the gastrointestinal tract make up the majority of surgeries performed in cattle. For a discussion of actinomycosis and pharyngeal injuries, refer to Chapter 22.

ORAL LACERATIONS

Cattle, especially calves, are not discriminate eaters and often consume debris, such as hardware, found in the pasture. Lacerations or injuries can occur on the tongue, cheeks, or palate when pieces of wire or other sharp objects are chewed and potentially swallowed. Excess salivation or bloody oral discharge may be seen along with varying degrees of dysphagia and malodorous breath if feed is accumulating within the wound. Diagnosis is usually easy once an oral examination has been performed. With appropriate wound care, many of these will heal without much treatment because of the excellent blood supply to the oral cavity. Flushing with copious amounts of water (usually via a hose) will prevent feedstuff accumulating within the wound. Changing the diet to softer feed rather than course roughage will limit feed buildup within the wound. Severe lacerations or punctures may require surgical débridement and repair, and if the tongue is involved, application of a tourniquet may help limit blood loss during the repair.

MANDIBULAR FRACTURES

Fractures are either traumatic or secondary to other pathologic processes, such as lumpy jaw. Fracture location, type, and the ability of the animal to eat and drink will usually dictate whether surgical repair is necessary. Clinical signs observed include dysphagia, salivation, and often crepitus or palpable instability. Oral examination is also important to identify any communication with the oral cavity because this is a route for secondary bacterial infection, which can complicate the healing process. Radiographs will help confirm the diagnosis and aid identification of the optimal therapy.

If there is marked displacement or instability of the mandible and if the animal is having difficulty eating and drinking, some form of stabilization is indicated.

Surgical options include figure-eight wiring with orthopedic cerclage wire, screw fixation, or application of an external fixation device. The choice is made depending upon the location of the fracture, the degree of comminution, involvement of tooth roots, if the fracture is open or closed, and the cost of the procedure. External fixators are inexpensive, effective, and relatively easily applied.

Most fractures will heal with some form of stabilization, and many cows will resume eating immediately following fixation. If the cow remains anorexic, offering different types of feed is recommended because some cows will only eat their usual ration. If necessary, the oral cavity can be bypassed completely by performing a rumenostomy. Potential complications of mandibular fractures include osteomyelitis, sequestrum formation, or abscessation of involved tooth roots. Failure or loosening of the implants is often not a problem because these injuries will heal rapidly. Removal of the implants can be performed using sedation once healing has occurred.

LAPAROTOMIES

Numerous surgical approaches to the bovine abdomen have been described, and all have various pros and cons. The majority of procedures can be performed via a flank laparotomy in the standing patient, but ventral midline or paramedian approaches are necessary in specific situations. Clipping a much larger area than is necessary will prevent any problems if the incision has to be extended and will limit any contamination of tissue if any drapes used should slip. Local anesthetic techniques can be used to facilitate surgery in the standing patient. IV sedation is sometimes required so that the patient tolerates this, but once the area is successfully anesthetized, most patients will settle down, often to the point that some will begin to ruminate.

REGIONAL ANALGESIC TECHNIQUES FOR ABDOMINAL SURGERY

For a flank incision, lidocaine can be injected directly over the line of the incision. Local anesthetic must be placed under the skin, into the muscle, and to the level of the peritoneum if complete analgesia is to be achieved. This is effective and simple, but may lead to an increased risk for incisional complications, such as infection or dehiscence. An alternative that does not involve injection directly into the surgical site is an inverted-L block. Local anesthetic is injected into all of the layers of tissue in an inverted-L pattern, vertically behind the last rib and then horizontally below the transverse processes of the lumbar vertebrae. This blocks the nerve fibers at a site distant to the location of the incision, and for this reason, the block must be continued at least a few centimeters distal to and caudal to the edge of the incision. If these blocks do not provide adequate analgesia, more local anesthetic can be placed easily and quickly, but since a large volume of local anesthetic can be used, care must be taken not to exceed the toxic dose of lidocaine (6 to 8 mg/kg).

Paravertebral analgesia can be performed, which requires the use of less local anesthetic and can provide a larger area of surgical analgesia than the other techniques. Two techniques are described, and the simplest to perform in dairy cattle (tend to be thinner and the landmarks are easily palpable) is the distal paravertebral technique. Here the transverse processes of lumbar vertebrae 1, 2, and 4 are palpated through the skin. An 18-gauge, 1½-inch needle is then inserted completely so that it lies parallel to and just below the palpable tip of the transverse process of L1. About 20 ml of 2% lidocaine is injected in a fan pattern, then the needle is withdrawn so that it can be relocated in the same fashion above the transverse process. Ten to 15 ml of lidocaine can be injected in the same fanlike pattern in the area. This process is repeated over the transverse processes of L2 and L4. This technique anesthetizes the nerves T13, L1, and L2 at a site distal to where they exit the vertebral column.

The proximal paravertebral technique requires a longer needle; an 18-gauge, 5-inch spinal needle passed through a 14-gauge, 1-inch guide needle is used for this technique. The 14-gauge needle is placed 2 cm lateral to midline at the cranial edge of the transverse process of L1. The spinal needle is then inserted through the 14-gauge needle down onto the transverse process. The spinal needle is then walked cranially, off the edge of the process. A "pop" will be felt as the needle penetrates the thick fascial layer, and 15 ml of lidocaine should be injected in this location. Withdrawing the needle roughly 1 to 2 cm will place it above the fascia, and another 15 ml of lidocaine should be injected at this site. The technique should be repeated over the transverse processes of L2 and L3.

Successful placement of either paravertebral block will result in analgesia of the flank, but this can take between 15 to 30 minutes. This can be confirmed by observing scoliosis (the side that is blocked will relax, making the spine bend laterally the other way); vasodilation, which will make the side palpably warmer (particularly in cool weather); and a lack of response to a noxious stimuli. Incomplete analgesia may resolve if more time is allowed for diffusion of the anesthetic to occur.

SURGICAL APPROACHES TO THE ABDOMEN

Most abdominal exploratory laparotomies are performed through the right flank (Figure 31-16). This approach provides access to most of the abdominal viscera, although only certain structures can actually be exteriorized. The proximal extent of the incision is approximately one handbreadth below the transverse processes and one handbreadth behind the caudal edge of the ribs. A 15-cm vertical incision will allow passage of an arm into the abdominal cavity. Keeping the incision located higher in the flank is desirable to limit the ability of intestine to prolapse out of the incision. Procedures commonly performed from the right flank include abdominal exploratories and correction of abomasal displacements and torsions. An approach through the left flank is used for C-sections, rumenotomies, or rumenostomies.

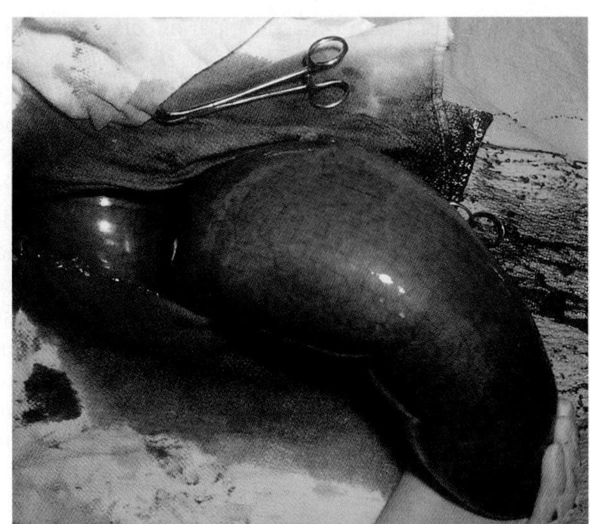

FIGURE 31-16 A right flank laparotomy approach for correction of an intestinal obstruction (cecal volvulus) in a cow.

Certain procedures may require a ventral midline or paramedian celiotomy. Sedation is essential for these as is some form of restraining device to maintain the cow's position. Tilt tables can be used, or the cow can be propped up in dorsal recumbency using bales of straw or ropes. Abomasopexies, C-sections, or umbilical procedures sometimes require this approach. Instead of paravertebral analgesia, local infiltration is often used or lidocaine is infiltrated on either side of the incision with a portion that converges together at the most cranial aspect of the incision.

RUMENOTOMY FOR GRAIN OVERLOAD

A rumenotomy is performed via a left flank laparotomy with the cow standing. A broad area should be clipped and prepped for surgery. The skin incision is oriented vertically and often needs to be bigger than usual flank laparotomy incisions (may need to be 20 cm) so that the rumen can be exteriorized and then secured. The rumenotomy site is the dorsal sac of the rumen. This is secured using one of two recommended rumenotomy procedures: use of a rumen board (Weingarth apparatus) or suturing the rumen wall to the skin. This is important to prevent contamination of either the peritoneal cavity or the skin and muscle layers with rumen contents. Ensuring that enough rumen is exposed beyond the site of fixation will help make closure easier. The contents of the rumen have to be evacuated manually, which is time consuming. Having specially designed feed bins to place the rumen contents into can be helpful. A normal trash can with multiple holes drilled through its bottom and a chicken-wire mesh insert to hold fiber in the can be used to allow fluid to drain out and hold in most of the fibrous portion of the rumen contents. This will make movement and subsequent disposal of the rumen contents easier. Siphoning off the fluid can be performed with a larger-bore tube, such as a Kingman tube, placed into the rumen via the rumenotomy. Once the rumen is emptied, transfaunation of ruminal fluid from a normal cow can be beneficial. This can either be given orally or via the rumenotomy before closure. Removing any gross contamination from the edges of the rumenotomy is important before suturing it closed in two layers. The body wall and skin can then be closed in a routine fashion.

A rumenostomy, or permanent rumen fistula, can be created using a similar technique. Commercial rubber rumen fistulae and plugs are available, and if one of these is to be used, close attention to the size of the surgical incision is necessary. The skin incision needs to be longer and should be about 15 cm. This will allow the fistula to form a tight seal and prevent leakage of rumen contents. The skin incision is continued through the external abdominal oblique muscle; then the deeper muscles are separated in the direction of their fibers. Following opening of the peritoneum, a three-layer closure technique can be used. The peritoneum is sutured to the abdominal muscles using an absorbable suture. Following exteriorization of part of the rumen, the rumen is sutured to the subcutaneous tissue, then the rumen is incised and the mucosa is sutured to the skin. Ensuring that the second layer is tight before incising the rumen will help minimize the risk of contaminating the abdomen with rumen contents. Placement of the rubber fistula and plug will now allow the rumen to be sealed, but accessible when necessary. This is usually used for research purposes, but can be helpful when treating sick cattle because it makes collection of ruminal contents for rumen transfaunation considerably easier.

TRAUMATIC RETICULOPERITONITIS

For the diagnosis and medical treatment for this condition, please see Chapter 22. Surgical intervention may be necessary if traumatic reticuloperitonitis (TRP) fails to respond to conservative treatment, if a foreign body is observed outside the reticulum on radiography, or if an intraabdominal or thoracic abscess is suspected. The approach of choice is a left flank exploratory laparotomy and rumenotomy using transruminal exploration. The technique required for rumenotomy is the same as that described for treating grain overload, with the exception that the incision is located a little more cranially to ensure that the reticulum can be reached by the surgeon. Most abscesses that form secondary to TRP are located on the medial wall of the reticulum and are usually tightly adhered. These abscesses are the most common causes of vagal indigestion associated with TRP. These tightly adhered abscesses can be lanced and drained into the reticulum or omasum and then explored for the presence of a foreign body. Lancing these abscesses can be difficult and requires a blind technique. Providing a scalpel blade on a loop of suture will allow the loop to be placed over the surgeon's wrist to reduce the risk of dropping it into the rumen.

> *TECHNICIAN NOTE* TRP (hardware disease) may lead to peritonitis, liver or reticular abscesses, pericarditis, vagal indigestion, or other secondary problems.

ABOMASAL DISPLACEMENTS AND VOLVULUS

Abomasal displacement is a common problem of high-producing dairy cows fed high-concentrate, low-roughage diets. Displacements are most likely to occur in the first 6 weeks after calving. Predisposing factors include high-grain diets with an increased amount of volatile fatty acids in the abomasum; hypocalcemia; concurrent diseases, such as mastitis, metritis, and ketosis; and lack of exercise. Increased volatile fatty acids, histamine release with concurrent diseases, and hypocalcemia may lead to abomasal dilation and atony and subsequent displacement of the abomasum from its normal right paramedian position to the left or right paralumbar area. Left displaced abomasum (LDA) is much more common than right displaced abomasum (RDA). Abomasal volvulus (AV) may occur after displacement to the right and carries a poorer prognosis than LDA or RDA because of compromise of the innervation and blood supply that occurs when the abomasum twists. AV can quickly lead to development of shock and toxemia if not diagnosed and treated early.

LDA, RDA, or AV can be diagnosed by auscultation of a distinct "ping" in the left or right paralumbar fossa area since the gas trapped in the abomasum produces a characteristic "metallic pinging" sound when percussing the area over the gas cap while simultaneously auscultating with a stethoscope.

The Liptak test can also be used as an aid in diagnosing LDA. After percussion of the abomasum on the left side under the last few ribs, an area just below the gas ping, which corresponds to the fluid level in the abomasum, is clipped and surgically prepared. Centesis is performed using an 18-gauge, 10- to 12-cm needle. Fluid with a pH less than 4.5 confirms the presence of an LDA. Aspiration of gas with a characteristic "burnt almond" odor is indicative of an LDA.

Surgery is usually necessary to correct abomasal displacements, and AV requires immediate surgical intervention. The choices of surgical approach and technique depend on the direction of the displacement, the presence of volvulus, the condition of the animal, and the surgeon's preference. Traditionally a right flank laparotomy is performed to correct the displacement. The most helpful piece of equipment is a piece of surgical tubing (must be long enough to reach to the far side of the cow and then extend well clear of the surgical incision) attached to a large needle. This is taken into the abdomen, guarded by the surgeon's hand, and carried round the caudal edge of the rumen and omentum. This is then tunneled through the abomasal wall to decompress it. Once decompressed, the abomasum can be swept or pulled back to the left side where either an omentopexy or pyloropexy can be performed to the abdominal wall. A right sided displacement or volvulus needs to be decompressed and repositioned before pexying to the body wall. Surgical approaches using a left and right flank laparotomy or laparoscopic approaches have been described and are beyond the scope of this text. If a cow has had a recurrence of an abomasal displacement following a left-sided approach, a paramedian abomasopexy may be indicated. In this situation, the cow is sedated and rolled into dorsal recumbency either on a tilt table or by casting her with ropes. The ventral abdomen is clipped and prepped for a paramedian incision roughly 10 cm behind the xyphoid process and 10 cm to the right of midline. The surgical site is anesthetized using local infiltration of local anesthetic and the site is sterilely prepped. An incision is made into the body wall, and the abomasum is exposed through this incision. An abomasopexy is performed, by suturing the abomasum and the body wall closed simultaneously, resulting in a strong adhesion that will prevent future displacements. Postsurgically the diet should be restricted to roughage only, and grain should be introduced gradually into the diet once recovery is complete.

AFTERCARE FOLLOWING A LAPAROTOMY

Feed can be reintroduced once the cow has recovered from any sedation or general anesthesia. It is usually ideal to withhold feed and water until they are no longer showing any signs of sedation, which with xylazine can be prolonged. The goal is to return them to full feed, but this should be done gradually over a few days. Cows that are relatively healthy will often eat well after surgery and will require little further management. If they have been anorectic for a prolonged period, offering different feed is important to try and tempt the cow to eat something. If necessary, force feeding can be performed via a large-bore stomach tube. Slurries made from alfalfa meal or a pelleted feed can be used, but can be difficult to pump through the tube. Constant stirring or increasing the fluid content of the feed can be helpful to ease its passage through the tube. Rumen fluid transfaunation can also be helpful for these cows, if possible. Keeping the cow in a well-bedded, dry, draft-free environment will ensure that they are comfortable and should help them to recover. The incision will usually need little if any care. An infection of the surgical site can be identified by swelling, discomfort upon palpation of the area, and usually some discharge. Flank incisions can be treated by creating ventral drainage and allowing any purulent material to drain out. This is often all that is needed, and the incision will heal by second intention with routine wound management.

OTHER GASTROINTESTINAL CONDITIONS

The remainder of the gastrointestinal tract can also require surgical therapy. In the small intestine, intussusceptions, volvulus, or hemorrhagic bowel syndrome can occur. Cecal tympany or displacement can sometimes be mistaken for an RDA (ping in this case will be further caudal and dorsal on the flank than for an abomasal problem), or this can even become intussuscepted into itself. Obstructions or intussusceptions of the spiral colon can also occur. These often are evaluated surgically, and an approach through the right flank is most commonly used. Exposure of the entire gastrointestinal tract is not always possible, so if the incision needs to be elongated ventrally, general anesthesia may be indicated to prevent sudden movement or the cow becoming sternal, which could allow (uncontrolled evisceration) parts of the intestines to fall onto nonsterile surfaces.

Adhesion formation can be a sequela of abdominal surgery or following a separate disease process. This will often lead to signs of an abomasal outflow obstruction, general colic, or weight loss. An exploratory laparotomy can be performed to evaluate this, but treatment options are limited. Adhesions can be broken down, but the risk of recurrence is high.

CONDITIONS OF THE MUSCULOSKELETAL SYSTEM

LAMENESS

Lameness is commonly encountered in cattle and is most often (88%) caused by lesions or problems in the foot. The majority of these conditions have been discussed in Chapter 22. Upper leg problems, such as anterior cruciate ligament rupture, coxofemoral (hip) luxation, fractures, and arthritis, account for the remaining 12% of lameness seen. When foot problems occur, they are most often seen in the claws that bear the most weight, front medial and hind lateral claws. It is important to examine all foot problems early since many conditions can progress to osteomyelitis and/or septic arthritis if not properly treated. Regardless of the cause of lameness, it can lead to loss of production as a result of decreased milk production, weight loss, delayed breeding or anestrus, and culling. Intensive housing and feeding of large groups of animals has lead to an increased incidence of lameness.

> *TECHNICIAN NOTE* Lameness is commonly encountered in cattle and is most often caused by lesions or problems in the foot.

REGIONAL ANALGESIA AND ANTIBIOTIC PERFUSION TECHNIQUES AND PMMA IMPLANTS

Regional analgesia (IV retrograde analgesia) of the foot and/or distal limb is commonly performed before claw amputation or corn removal, although the regional block can also be used for other surgeries or painful techniques of the foot or distal limb or as a diagnostic aid in lameness examinations. A tourniquet is applied distal to the hock or carpus in the midmetatarsal or midmetacarpal area. A superficial vein is located, either the common dorsal metacarpal (metatarsal) vein or the palmar or plantar metacarpal (metatarsal) vein, and surgically prepared. An IV injection of 15 to 30 ml of 2% lidocaine will provide analgesia in 5 minutes, which will persist until the tourniquet is released (the tourniquet should not be left in place more than an hour) (Figure 31-17). It is ideal to have the cow's leg secured to

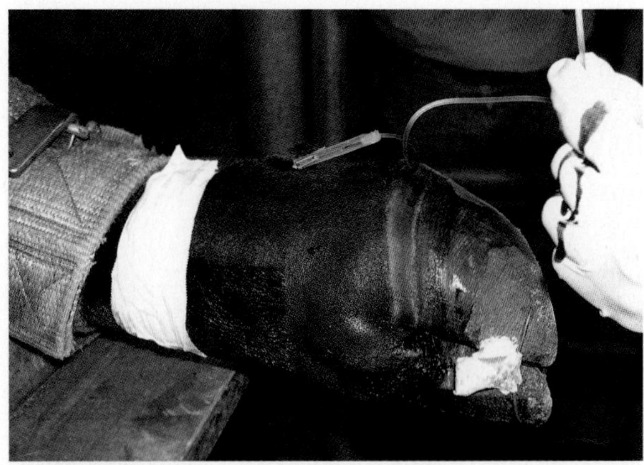

FIGURE 31-17 Injection of lidocaine for IV retrograde analgesia of the bovine foot after placement of a tourniquet above the fetlock.

prevent extravascular placement of the local anesthetic. Even with restraint, movement is often still possible, so the use of a butterfly catheter with a short extension can be helpful. An alternative to this technique involves placing the tourniquet above the tarsus or carpus to achieve analgesia more proximally. Accordingly, more lidocaine should be used to block this larger area (may need 30 to 60 ml of perfusate). This same technique can be used to perform regional perfusion of antibiotics to the distal limb for the purpose of treating localized infections, such as foot rot with cellulitis. An antibiotic with an IV formulation should be used and can be diluted with sterile saline to produce a perfusate volume of at least 20 to 30 ml. Cephalosporins can be injected through the catheter and allowed to perfuse the limb distal to the tourniquet for approximately 45 minutes. Both of these techniques are primarily used in cattle, but can be applied to all food animal species. The implantation of antibiotic-impregnated polymethylmethacrylate (PMMA) beads subcutaneously near infected joints has shown promise for treatment of septic arthritis in calves. The beads slowly release antibiotics into the joint and appear to be more effective than systemic antibiotic treatment or joint flushing alone. Techniques such as joint flushing, PMMA bead implants, regional perfusion, and systemic antibiotics used in combination work well to resolve septic arthritis. Following resolution of the sepsis, the beads can be removed, but should not cause any problem if left in place.

SURGICAL DISEASES OF THE HOOF AND PHALANGES

Interdigital Hyperplasia

Interdigital hyperplasia (interdigital fibroma, corn) is a thickening of the interdigital skin, which causes a mass to protrude between the claws (Figure 31-18). One or more feet may be involved, but the hind feet are more commonly affected. Beef breeds, especially bulls, have a higher incidence of corns. Fibromas develop in response to chronic irritation between the claws. Hereditary predisposition is suspected. Spreading of the toes and other conformational problems probably contribute to irritation of the interdigital skin.

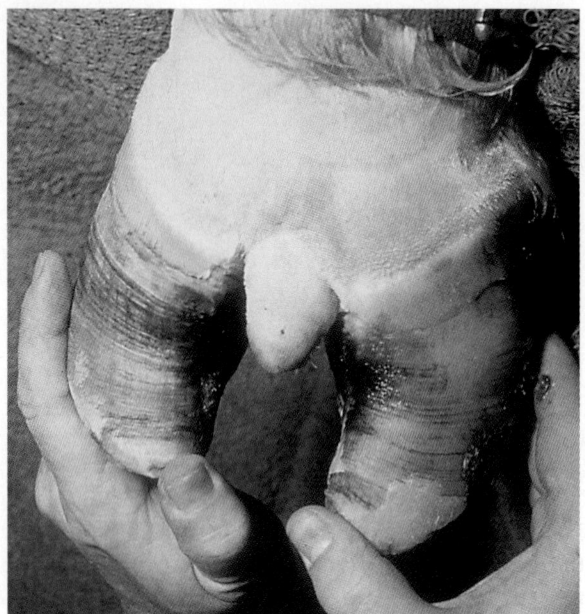

FIGURE 31-18 Interdigital hyperplasia (fibroma or corn) between the toes of a bull's foot.

The size of the mass varies from a noticeable thickening of the skin to a size of 3 cm or more. A large mass can cause pain, and the fibroma may become eroded, ulcerated, and even infected leading to more swelling and pain. Lameness varies, depending on the size of the mass, from absent to severe. The size of the corn and degree of lameness are guides in determining whether removal is necessary. Surgical excision is accomplished using IV retrograde analgesia, and care should be taken to ensure that all of the hyperplastic tissue is excised. Excision of part of the fat pad in the interdigital space will also help improve wound healing by preventing the fat from protruding between the healing skin edges. To reduce the discomfort associated with the outward displacement of the toes, the toes can be wired together by drilling holes at the toe region and securing them using cerclage wire. Placement of the wires on the abaxial side of the claws will reduce the risk of the wire pulling through the hoof capsule prematurely.

Claw Amputation

Diseases of the foot may become so severe that they cannot be treated, thus necessitating amputation of the affected digit. Any of the previously discussed conditions of the foot (see Chapter 22) and other diseases may lead to infection of deeper tissues with resulting osteomyelitis of the first phalanx (P1), second phalanx (P2), or third phalanx (P3) and/or septic arthritis of the proximal or distal interphalangeal joints (pastern or coffin joint). In cases of advanced infection, removal of the infected claw may be the only treatment option. This procedure is performed with IV retrograde analgesia (described earlier). A full-thickness skin incision is made on the axial aspect of the claw, perpendicular to the bone's long axis, down to the bone of the distal first phalanx. The affected claw is then removed at a level necessary to remove all infected tissue using OB wire (it should be noted that amputation can only be performed distal to the fetlock joint). The claw should be removed at a cosmetic angle and through bone rather than through a joint. The foot is then bandaged snuggly after topical antibiotic application. Bandage changes should be done every 3 days until any exposed bone is covered with granulation tissue. The entire healing process takes about 6 weeks. Cattle can support weight on one claw, but will eventually experience breakdown of supporting structures of the remaining claw. The time it takes for breakdown depends on the claw removed, the weight and use of the animal, and the surface on which the animal must stand. It is undesirable to remove any claw in a bull, except for salvage purposes, and it is not generally a good choice to remove a weight-bearing claw (front medial or hind lateral) in cows, although sometimes there is no choice.

> *TECHNICIAN NOTE* Diseases of the foot may become so severe that they cannot be treated, thus necessitating amputation of the affected digit.

Foot Block Application and Casting

Wooden or acrylic blocks or commercial rubber shoes may be glued to the bottom of healthy claws to reduce or eliminate weight bearing on a diseased or painful claw. These devices are adhered to the claw using an acrylic material (Technovit, Jorgensen Laboratories, Inc.) or products, such as Equithane adhesives. Wooden blocks may last as long as 6 weeks and may be allowed to wear off naturally unless they are wearing abnormally, in which case they may be manually removed earlier. Blocks or shoes help promote healing of affected claws and make the animal more comfortable when standing or moving.

An additional method of immobilizing the claws is application of a hoof cast. A wound dressing should be applied to the surgery site, if one is present, and a layer of cast padding material should be placed between the claws. The claws can be wired together, stockinette can be applied up to the distal metacarpal or metatarsal bone, and then cast padding material can be applied to the proximal extent of the area to be cast (usually level of mid-P1). This material should overlap approximately 50% with the previous layer. Fiberglass cast material can then be applied to immobilize the distal limb. Applying the material while it is still wet will prevent it from curing too rapidly because this can prevent it from adhering to itself, which can result in a weaker cast. The cast can remain in place for 10 to 14 days at which time it should be removed. Cast removal can be performed with a cast saw or using Gigli wires if they were placed between the cast padding and the cast tape at the time of application.

Obturator and Sciatic Nerve Paresis and Paralysis

The obturator and/or sciatic nerves may sustain damage during dystocia or forced fetal extraction resulting in "calving paralysis." Treatment consists of the use of NSAIDs early, good nursing care, housing the animal on a soft surface with good footing, flotation devices, lifting the cow or heifer for short periods of time at least a couple of times a day, rolling the cow from side to side several times daily to prevent severe muscle compression, and hobbling cows or heifers that can stand, but cannot adduct their hind legs.

> *TECHNICIAN NOTE* During dystocia or forced fetal extraction, the obturator and/or sciatic nerves may sustain damage resulting in "calving paralysis."

Radial Nerve Paralysis

Radial nerve paralysis is most commonly seen following a period of lateral recumbency with the most dependent forelimb being exposed to either excessive or prolonged pressure (the weight of the animal itself can be enough) over the upper forelimb. The most obvious clinical sign is an inability to bear any weight on the affected limb if an attempt to stand is made. The elbow will appear to be dropped, and the cow will be unable to maintain its carpus or elbow in extension, preventing weight bearing. This often does not appear to be painful, but can be stressful if multiple attempts to stand or move are made. Treatment is supportive. Systemic NSAIDs should be administered, and a Robert Jones bandage and splint should be applied to the limb. The bandage should extend from the proximal radius to the hoof, and the splint can be placed on the dorsal or palmar surface. The goal is to lock the carpus in extension with the splint, which will allow weight bearing to resume while limiting mobility. This is often all that is necessary, and this condition usually will show signs of improvement within 24 hours of onset. The duration of neurologic deficits will depend on the severity of injury, but a full recovery is usually possible. The most important other cause of radial nerve deficits is an upper limb fracture (humerus, proximal radius or ulna), but these cases can often be distinguished because there is marked local swelling, pain upon palpation, or manipulation and often crepitus.

Fractures

Trauma, either from a kick or a fall, can result in long-bone, spinal, or pelvic fractures. An acute-onset, severe lameness is observed, with the animal often either non–weight bearing in the affected limb or recumbent. Soft tissue swelling tends to be marked, and as a result of limited soft tissue coverage, many fractures will be open. Before attempting any fracture repair, the weight, size, age, disposition, and financial value of the animal need to be taken into consideration. Radiographs should be taken to allow accurate classification of the fracture (displaced or nondisplaced, open or closed, simple or comminuted). The amount of injury to the associated soft tissues can delay healing if the vasculature has been compromised, or if excessive tissue is injured, it can predispose to infections. Some form of support should be applied to the limb until fixation is attempted, and these can range from a Robert Jones bandage with or without splints, cast material, or for some fractures, simply stall confinement (femur, humerus, and pelvis).

Feed should be withheld if anesthesia is going to be necessary for fracture stabilization, systemic antibiotics should be initiated, and analgesia should be provided. If the cow is dehydrated or showing signs of shock, IV fluids may be administered via a jugular catheter.

Fracture stabilization can be achieved using either internal fixation devices (screws and bone plates) or using external fixation (casts, Thomas splints, or transfixation casts). If stabilization is adequate and no infection is present, the bones will often be able to heal with time.

Osteomyelitis should be considered if following fracture stabilization there is a sudden increase in the degree of lameness. Signs of inflammation and swelling are often present at the surgical site (assuming this is visible and not underneath a cast), but radiographs are often necessary to confirm the presence of infection. Radiographic evidence of osteomyelitis is usually only observed once the infection is well established, roughly 10 to 14 days after its onset. Systemic or local antibiotics should be administered, drainage should be established to prevent accumulation of purulent material, and in severe cases, internal implants may need to be removed or replaced. Before radiographic changes become evident, the patient may be febrile or have an altered leukogram. Aggressive therapy is necessary if there is to be any chance of success, but the prognosis is often poor.

Strict stall rest until radiographic evidence of fracture healing occurs is necessary, and the patient may still be reluctant or unable to move easily. Ensuring that the cow has easy access to feed and water is essential to prevent it from struggling or moving excessively and risking damage to the healing bone. Keeping these cows on deep bedding is important to reduce the risk for decubital ulcers, so rolling the cow may be required to prevent or reduce their occurrence. Excessively deep bedding can actually make it more difficult for the cow to stand or move, especially if they are wearing a cast. Where possible, slings or flotation devices may be helpful to prevent prolonged periods of recumbency.

Septic Arthritis

Septic arthritis is a common cause of severe, acute-onset lameness in cattle. In calves, it is usually secondary to an infection elsewhere in the body and spreads hematogenously. In adults, it is often secondary to either a puncture wound or trauma. Diagnosis is based on severe lameness, local swelling, and often an obvious wound. Confirmation of synovial involvement can be obtained by performing a sterile arthrocentesis at a site distant from any puncture or wound. If possible, a sample of the synovial fluid should be obtained for cytology, white blood cell count, total protein, and culture and sensitivity. In a septic joint, the white blood cells will be preponderantly neutrophils (greater than 75%), the white blood cell count is greater than 3000/μl, total protein is greater than 40 g/L, and bacteria may or may not be cultured. Attempts to distend the joint with saline will not succeed if the joint is open and it communicates with a wound. In this case, when saline is injected, it will be seen exiting the joint via the wound, confirming involvement of the joint.

If the joint is intact, sterile saline can be injected into the joint to distend it, and the increase in pressure should allow the syringe to fill back up if it remains attached and pressure is removed from the plunger. Care should be taken when identifying a site for arthrocentesis so as to prevent iatrogenic infection of the joint; the needle should not be passed through any infected tissue. Identification of infected tissue can be difficult, so if there is any doubt, arthrocentesis may be contraindicated.

Treatment revolves around removing the bacteria and inflammatory mediators from within the joint. Flushing the joint using sterile fluids and through-and-through lavage with multiple needles placed within the joint can be performed under sedation. Large needles often need to be used (14 to 16 gauge) because smaller needles will often become blocked by fibrin or other debris from the joint. If this occurs or the infection is chronic, arthrotomies may be necessary to establish adequate drainage. These may need to be protected by bandages or stent dressings between joint flushes. If arthroscopic lavage is performed, general anesthesia may be indicated to prevent damage to the equipment. Following lavage, antibiotics can be placed directly into the joint to achieve high concentrations that will persist. Ceftiofur or penicillin can be used for this purpose. Joint lavage is usually performed once daily and should be repeated until no lameness is evident. Other cost-effective methods of antibiotic delivery include regional IV antibiotic perfusion or insertion of PMMA antibiotic-impregnated beads. These techniques are beneficial, but if they cannot be used, systemic antibiotics should be administered in conjunction with lavage. In joints that do not respond to therapy or that develop secondary osteoarthritis following resolution of the infection, arthrodesis or claw amputation may be treatment options to be considered to try and improve the level of comfort.

TECHNICIAN NOTE Septic arthritis can occur secondary to a penetrating wound or hematogenously in young stock. This must be a differential diagnosis in an acute-onset, severe lameness.

CONDITIONS OF THE RESPIRATORY SYSTEM

Surgical conditions of the respiratory tract are rare in cattle. Tracheostomies may be the most useful techniques for this body system, but they will be performed infrequently. Any obstruction of the upper respiratory tract may necessitate this, and surgical preparation, such as clipping, cannot often be performed. In true emergencies, reestablishing a patent airway is more important than a neatly clipped or scrubbed surgical site. The most appropriate location to perform a tracheostomy is on the ventral midline, roughly halfway between the larynx and the thoracic inlet. The ability to palpate the tracheal rings in this region that have the least soft tissue overlying them will help locate the ideal surgical site. Placing a line block with local anesthesia under the skin will aid the procedure. If possible, the trachea should be grasped with one hand through the skin and stabilized before incising the skin over it (about 8 to 10 cm). Ensuring that the incision is on midline will expose a muscle layer that should be split, either sharply or bluntly, until the trachea is exposed. The trachea should be opened by making a stab incision (just big enough to insert a tracheostomy tube) into it through the membrane between the cartilaginous tracheal rings. A temporary tracheotomy tube, piece of stomach tube, or other semirigid, hollow piece of tubing can then be used to establish a patent airway. If the skin or deeper incision is off the ventral midline, exposing the trachea can be difficult, and other vital structures can be damaged (jugular veins, carotid artery, etc.). In most situations, a temporary tracheotomy should be performed, and a permanent tracheostomy can be performed, if indicated, in a more controlled manner at a later time.

The tracheostomy site will need to be cleaned frequently because the majority of the normal respiratory secretions will exit through this site. Application of petroleum jelly on the skin around the site will prevent scalding. Following resolution of the inciting cause, the tube can be removed, and the tracheostomy site will heal by second intention. A permanent tracheostomy can be performed in a similar location, but instead of incising between the tracheal rings, the opening into the tracheal lumen removes a portion of three to four tracheal rings to allow the tracheal mucosa to be sutured to the skin edges. Aftercare of this stoma is the same as for a temporary tracheostomy.

CONDITIONS OF THE UROGENITAL SYSTEM

ANESTHESIA OF THE UROGENITAL AND REPRODUCTIVE SYSTEM

A caudal or low epidural provides loss of sensation to the anus, vulva, perineum, and caudal aspects of the thighs. It is used for relief of tenesmus and obstetric straining; vaginal, rectal, and uterine prolapse repair; and surgical procedures of the perineal area. Injection is made between the first and second coccygeal (Cy1 to Cy2) vertebrae or in the sacrococcygeal space. The space is located by moving the tail up and down and while palpating for the first obvious articulation caudal to the sacrum. Using aseptic technique, an 18-gauge, 1½-inch needle is inserted through the space on the midline at a 10-degree angle (tip of needle directed cranially) until a drop of lidocaine placed in the hub of the needle is sucked into the space. An alternative approach involves insertion of the needle until it hits the floor of the spinal canal at which time the needle is backed out slightly to enter the epidural space. There should be no resistance to injection. The dose of lidocaine used is 0.5 to 1 ml of 2% lidocaine per 45 kg body weight with which the animal should have adequate analgesia but remain standing. If sedation is helpful or longer duration of action is indicated, xylazine can be given alone (0.05 mg/kg diluted to 5 ml in sterile saline) or in combination (use a lower dose, 0.03 mg/kg) with the lidocaine.

A bilateral, internal pudendal nerve block can be performed to facilitate examination or surgery of a bull's penis. This nerve can be palpated via a rectal examination, on either side of the pelvic canal, dorsal to the pudendal artery where it is associated with the lesser sciatic foramen. Care must be taken to only inject the area around the nerve, and about 15 ml is injected in the region of the nerve and slightly caudally.

UROLITHIASIS

Urolithiasis is the result of formation of calculi (uroliths) within the urinary tract. The result of these uroliths varies from minor urinary tract irritation to complete obstruction of urine flow. The nonclinical manifestation of this condition is referred to as urolithiasis, whereas the clinical form is termed obstructive urolithiasis. When complete obstruction occurs, there is marked distention of the urinary bladder with eventual rupture of the bladder, the urethra, or both. Depending on the site of rupture, urine accumulates in the ventral subcutaneous tissues (urethra) or in the abdomen (bladder) resulting in swelling commonly referred to as water belly.

Although there is no sex predilection for development of calculi, males are much more likely to become obstructed as a result of the length, shape, and size of their urethra. The most common site of obstruction in cattle is the distal sigmoid flexure of the penis (Figure 31-19). Feedlot animals receiving grain rations with high phosphorus levels are predisposed to developing phosphate calculi.

Clinical signs of acute urethral obstruction are attributable to trauma to the urinary tract epithelium and bladder distention. Early in the course, the animal repeatedly assumes a posture for urination, but little or no urination results from these attempts to void. As bladder distention progresses, the animal may tread, stretch, tail swish, and kick at its abdomen. Blood and/or crystals may be present on the preputial hairs. Nonspecific signs such as anorexia, mild bloat, and lethargy are also common. Owners often misinterpret these signs as evidence of acute gastrointestinal disorders, especially since affected animals may show signs similar to colic. After the bladder or urethra ruptures, straining ceases, and the animal may go through a brief phase of euphoria; however, azotemia (increased blood urea nitrogen [BUN] and creatinine) and dehydration quickly develop. If urethral obstruction is diagnosed early, before azotemia develops or before the bladder or urethra rupture, the animal may be immediately slaughtered. If not, medical and/or surgical treatment should be initiated quickly.

Medical management involves the use of muscle relaxants to facilitate passage of the calculi, antimicrobial therapy for urinary tract infection, and the use of a urinary acidifier, such as ammonium chloride. Medical therapy alone is rarely successful, so it may be necessary to consider surgery in some cases. Perineal urethrostomy may be chosen as a salvage procedure, particularly for feedlot steers or bulls of low economic value (Figure 31-20). This surgical approach allows for relief of obstruction and resolution of the uremia before slaughter. Long-term, urethral stricture has been a problem with this technique. The procedure is performed with the animal standing and analgesia provided by a caudal or low epidural block.

The low approach is often preferred for perineal urethrostomy. This allows the penis to be diverted caudally at such an angle as to prevent urine scald to the hind legs. It also makes it possible to perform repeated procedures higher, if necessary. The skin incision is made beginning at the dorsal aspect of the scrotum or scrotal remnant and extending dorsally on the midline for 10 to 15 cm. The incision is continued until the penis is encountered. The retractor penis muscles may be the first structures seen and are frequently mistaken for the penis. These muscles are superficial to the penis, pink, soft, and easily separated into two structures. The penis is a relatively firm, single structure covered by the white tunica

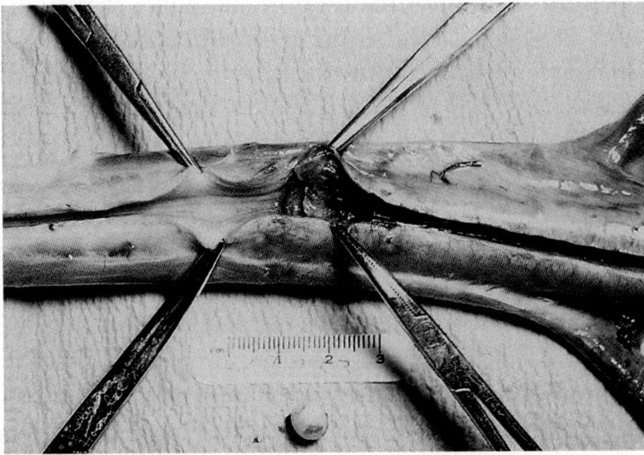

FIGURE 31-19 Identification of a calculus causing obstructive urolithiasis at the distal sigmoid flexure in a bull. Note urethral necrosis at the site where the calculus was lodged.

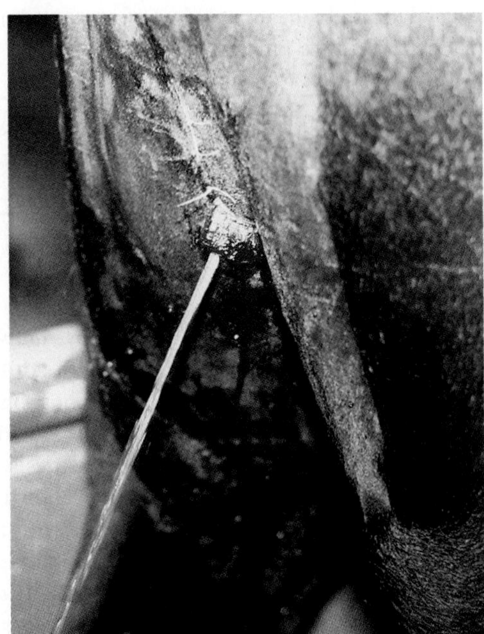

FIGURE 31-20 Perineal urethrostomy performed as a salvage procedure for treatment of obstructive urolithiasis in a steer.

albuginea. Once the penis has been located, it is bluntly dissected from the surrounding tough fascia and pulled caudally out of the incision. The penis is transected at a length adequate to allow the transected end to exit the perineal incision without tension leaving a 2- to 3-cm stump exposed. The stump is sutured to the skin of the lower part of the incision using a mattress suture that surrounds the corpus cavernosum penis (CCP) and passes under the urethra. This suture limits hemorrhage from the CCP. In addition, the urethra can be split for several centimeters and spatulated by suturing the urethral mucosa and tunica albuginea to the skin using 2-0 or 3-0 absorbable suture material. This optional technique is intended to limit stricture of the urethral opening. The remaining skin incision is closed with simple interrupted sutures of nonabsorbable suture material. Urethral obstruction may recur as a result of additional calculi or because of stricture of the urethrostomy site.

An alternative surgical procedure that can be used for valuable breeding bulls or "pets" is the ischial urethrostomy, a temporary urethrostomy with catheter placement. This technique allows for urine egress through a Foley catheter placed in the urethra at the level of the ischium, just below the anus, and antegrade or retrograde flushing of the distal urethra to remove calculi. When the tube is pulled, the urethrostomy usually heals by second intention without stricture formation. This procedure can be useful for preservation of fertility in valuable breeding bulls.

Dietary management is the key to control and prevention of obstructive urolithiasis. The calcium to phosphorus ratio of the overall diet should be in the range of 2:1 to 2.5:1. A continuous supply of fresh, clean water should be available at all times, and salt may be added to the ration up to 4% to promote water intake and diuresis. In addition, vitamin A may be added to the ration to help prevent desquamation of epithelial cells in the bladder. Prophylactic use of urinary acidifiers is advocated; administration of ammonium chloride at 1% to 1.5% of the ration is recommended.

> *TECHNICIAN NOTE* Perineal urethrostomy may be chosen as a salvage procedure for feedlot steers with obstructive urolithiasis.

RUPTURED BLADDER

This is seen as a secondary complication of obstructive urolithiasis that is not treated promptly enough. In adults, this complication is diagnosed by the clinical signs of progressive abdominal distention, dehydration, anorexia, and depression. Confirmation often requires abdominocentesis, which produces a clear, yellow fluid with a peritoneal:serum creatinine ratio of 2:1 or greater. Urinary catheterization is reported to be an effective treatment to allow the bladder time to heal if a dorsal tear is present. Ventral tears usually require surgical repair, but gaining access to this region of the bladder can sometimes be challenging via a flank laparotomy, necessitating a ventral approach.

UROVAGINA

Older cows with poor perineal conformation or those in poor condition may be more susceptible to urovagina. Urine accumulates in the vagina, resulting in marked inflammation, which can lead to infertility. Performing a vaginal examination will reveal the presence of urine in the vagina, which is considered to be diagnostic. If the cow is to be treated, surgical correction is necessary, to either elongate the urethra or to elevate the transverse fold to redirect the urine externally. Anesthesia can be provided using a caudal or low epidural or by locally infiltrating lidocaine along the site of the incisions. Restraining the cow in stocks is preferable to limit their movement. Before beginning surgery, the rectum should be emptied, and the tail should be restrained so that it is clear from the surgery site. Self retaining retractors can be helpful for this procedure, or alternatively, stay sutures can be placed to hold the vulva open against the perineum. Adequate lighting is best provided by the surgeon wearing a head lamp. Other forms of lighting are difficult to aim properly, and the surgeon's head usually obstructs the beam. Urethral extensions can be created by splitting the transverse fold, which is located above the urethral orifice in the vagina, and then creating a new shelf by continuing this incision laterally along the vaginal wall on both sides. Dissection of these shelves distally to allow them to meet in the midline with no tension is performed bluntly, and then the mucosal sheets are sutured in a Y pattern. Leaving a urinary catheter in place for a period postoperatively is helpful to ensure that urination can occur because some postoperative swelling may occur.

CONDITIONS OF THE REPRODUCTIVE SYSTEM

SUPERNUMERARY TEAT REMOVAL

Removal of extra teats is of most value in young dairy heifers, but it is also performed in beef heifers intended for show. Often this procedure is performed at the time of brucellosis vaccination. The extra teats are removed flush with the skin and parallel to the normal folds of the udder using curved scissors. In young calves, suturing the skin is not usually necessary. Care must be taken not to remove any of the four normal teats.

OVARIAN DISEASE

Ovarian cysts, abscesses, or neoplasms occur in cattle. Other indications for ovariectomy include preventing pregnancy or to try and improve fattening of feedlot cows. To minimize the risk for hemorrhage, ovariectomy should ideally be performed when the ovary is in the follicular or early luteal phase. A flank approach is often used if a unilateral ovariectomy is performed or in situations where the ovary is enlarged. A colpotomy can be used for a bilateral ovariectomy if both are a normal size, but will require a caudal epidural.

Achieving good hemostasis is essential, especially in pathologic ovaries. To minimize discomfort during this process, applying a gauze or lap sponge soaked in lidocaine to the ovarian pedicle may reduce any movement by the patient. This gauze or sponge should be attached to the surgeon to prevent it from being lost inside the abdomen. Holding this sponge over the pedicle for at least a minute may be beneficial. Transfixation sutures, application of a chain écraseur or emasculators can be used if a flank approach is used. Specific instruments, such as a Kimberly-Rupp or a Willis rod, should be reserved for normal ovaries.

Postoperatively, these patients should be monitored for signs of hemorrhage because inadequate hemostasis can be life threatening.

DYSTOCIA

C-section is indicated when there is a chance of delivering a live calf during a dystocia, malposition, or presentation or when the calf is excessively large. Several approaches are available for C-section, including flank approaches (right or left), paramedian approaches (right or left), or the ventral midline approach. The technique used is determined by the size, temperament, and physical condition of the cow and the veterinary surgeon's preference. Most commonly an approach is made in the standing patient via an incision through the left paralumbar fossa, using the landmarks described earlier in this chapter for a right-sided flank laparotomy. One of the benefits of using a left flank approach is that the rumen will obstruct other viscera, such as small intestine, from eviscerating through the incision. This is of particular concern if the incision has to be extended distally as a result of the size of the fetus (this incision will be considerably larger than that necessary for an abdominal exploratory). The limbs of the fetus are used to maneuver the uterus to the body wall. The limb is then pulled through the incision and used to lock the uterus and calf in place. The uterus is then incised over the metacarpus or metatarsus, and the calf can be exteriorized with minimal abdominal contamination. Closure of the uterus is performed in two layers, with at least one layer in an inverting pattern. The uterus is then lavaged and replaced into the abdomen before routine closure of the laparotomy site. If available, oxytocin can be administered at this stage to aid uterine involution and to minimize hemorrhage. This will also encourage passage of the placenta, assuming that it has not been sutured during the uterine closure. If the calf is not viable or is emphysematous, alternative surgical approaches may be indicated, but are often limited by available facilities, equipment, or personnel.

> *TECHNICIAN NOTE* During forced fetal extraction, obstetric chains should be looped above the calf's fetlocks and half hitched below the fetlocks to more evenly distribute the pulling forces on the legs to prevent physeal fractures.

UTERINE TORSION

This is an infrequent cause of dystocia, but, if present, will prevent parturition from proceeding. It is most commonly seen during early labor and is identified when an animal that is having a prolonged labor is evaluated rectally or rarely during a vaginal examination. The torsion is identified by the location of the broad ligaments because one of these is pulled tight as the uterus rotates away from its origin, whereas the other broad ligament is less taut. This also provides information on the direction of the torsion, either clockwise or counterclockwise (when viewed from behind the cow). If the calf's limbs can be palpated through the cervix, attempts can be made to swing the calf and uterus to reduce the torsion. This can be difficult when the calf is large or the cow is small. Rolling the cow while placing pressure on the flank (usually with an assistant standing on a plank of wood placed over the flank and paralumbar fossa) to unwind the torsion can be attempted, but only if the direction of the torsion has been correctly identified. For example, to reduce a clockwise torsion, the cow should be placed in right lateral recumbency and then rolled onto her left side while pressure is applied to try and stabilize the calf. The rectal examination should then be repeated to see if the torsion has been reduced. If this is not successful, it can be repeated, but a flank celiotomy and C-section may be necessary.

VAGINAL AND UTERINE PROLAPSE

Vaginal prolapse is a fairly common occurrence in cattle (Figure 31-21). It usually occurs in pluripara cows during the last 2 months of gestation and tends to recur during subsequent pregnancies. Hereford, Santa Gertrudis, and Holstein breeds seem to be more commonly affected. Factors that influence the development of vaginal prolapse include increased estrogen levels in late pregnancy, increased fetal size with increased intraabdominal pressure in late

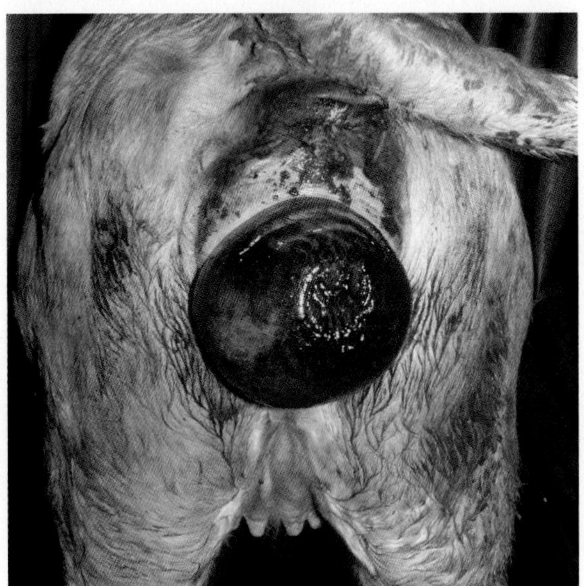

FIGURE 31-21 Vaginal prolapse in a prepartum cow. Recurrence during subsequent pregnancies is common.

pregnancy, bulky diets causing increased intraabdominal pressure, recumbency that forces the urinary bladder and other organs into the pelvic cavity and places pressure on the constrictor vestibuli muscle, and obesity with proliferation of pelvic fat (vaginal prolapse can occur in overconditioned, nonpregnant heifers). A new population of vaginal prolapse cows is emerging in embryo donor cows that are superovulated. Hormonal extremes are a suggested cause of vaginal prolapse in these cows.

Initially the vaginal prolapse may be intermittent, only protruding when the animal is lying down, but eventually it progresses to the point that it remains prolapsed at all times. Although vaginal prolapse is not an emergency, it should be repaired soon after it is noticed by the owner. The most common method of repair is the Buhner technique (see later). Since this condition usually occurs before calving, the cow will need to be observed closely for signs of impending parturition. Owners should be advised to cull these cows since this is likely to recur with subsequent pregnancies.

Uterine prolapse is common in the cow as a result of the anatomic suspension of the uterus (Figure 31-22). It occurs at parturition or shortly thereafter while the cervix is fully dilated. The uterus invaginates, and the uterine mucosa protrudes through the vulvar lips. Uterine prolapse is more likely to occur in first-calf heifers and is not likely to recur at subsequent calvings. Factors playing a role in the development of uterine prolapse include concurrent hypocalcemia, recumbency, such as that resulting from obturator nerve paralysis, dystocias with excessive straining, excessive force used during fetal extraction, and unnecessary traction on retained placentas.

Uterine prolapse is considered an emergency because of the possibility of shock from exposure of uterine mucosa, fatal hemorrhage from rupture of the middle uterine arteries, and concurrent hypocalcemia. In addition, the urinary bladder and/or intestines may also be involved within the prolapse.

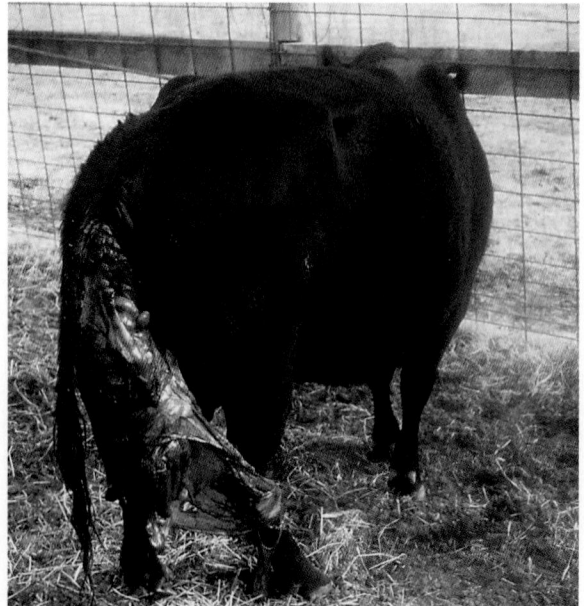

FIGURE 31-22 Uterine eversion with exposure of the caruncles in a postpartum cow.

To prevent uterine prolapse, it is wise to force the animal to stand as soon as possible after calving and administer oxytocin to begin uterine involution.

Treatment consists of replacement of the prolapsed portion and application of a retention suture (Buhner) to prevent recurrence. This is best accomplished with the animal in a standing position with the aid of a caudal epidural. If the cow is already down and cannot get up, attempt to elevate the hindquarters or pull the cow's hind legs straight out behind her as she lies in sternal recumbency; an epidural helps maintain this position. Before replacement of the uterus, the placenta is removed atraumatically, if possible; the uterus is cleansed with warm water and a mild disinfectant; and the uterus is lubricated to facilitate replacement. Elevation of the uterus makes it easier to replace. The uterus is inserted a little at a time, making certain that the apical end of each horn has been completely returned to its normal position. Oxytocin (40 IU), calcium, if necessary, intrauterine antibiotics, and systemic antibiotics should be administered. The vulva is then sutured using the Buhner suture technique.

The Buhner suture technique is useful for retention of both vaginal and uterine prolapse. It is a buried purse-string suture that simulates the action of the constrictor vestibuli muscle. To begin the suture pattern, a 1-cm horizontal skin incision is made midway between the dorsal commissure of the vulva and the anus. Another horizontal incision is made at the ventral commissure of the vulva. The Buhner needle is inserted into the ventral incision, driven deeply (5 to 8 cm) and directed out of the dorsal skin incision. The eye of the needle is threaded with Buhner suture tape, and the needle is pulled out through the ventral incision. The procedure is repeated on the opposite side resulting in two free ends of tape from the ventral incision. The suture is tightened so that only two to three fingers can be inserted into the vagina. This allows for normal urination, but prevents reprolapse of the vagina or uterus. This suture may be completely buried and left in place indefinitely. The Buhner suture tape is particularly strong, will not disintegrate, and is well tolerated by the tissues. The tape may be tied such that it can be untied as the cow begins to calve, as in the case of prepartum vaginal prolapse.

> *TECHNICIAN NOTE* Uterine prolapse is considered an emergency because of the possibility of shock from exposure of uterine mucosa, fatal hemorrhage from rupture of the middle uterine arteries, and concurrent hypocalcemia.

FIBROPAPILLOMAS OF THE PENIS

Fibropapillomas of the penis in bulls are caused by the bovine papillomavirus (Figure 31-23). They tend to occur in young bulls housed together and are contracted from warts on other

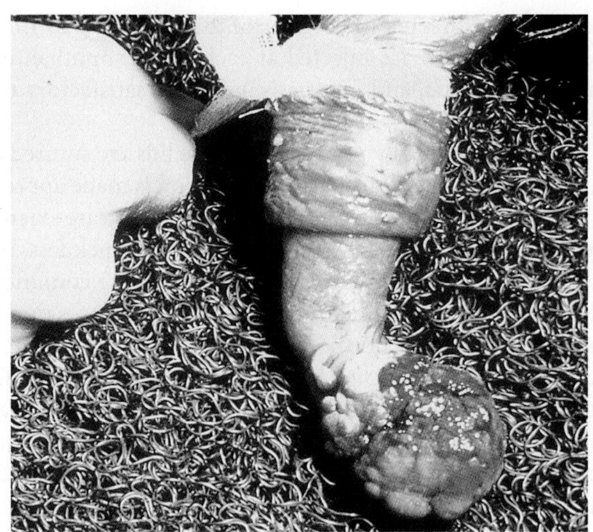

FIGURE 31-23 Fibropapillomas (warts) of the glans penis in a bull.

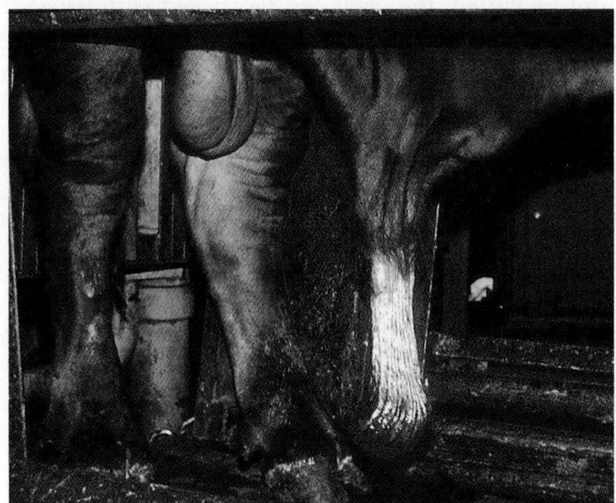

FIGURE 31-24 Prolapse of the prepuce of a *Bos indicus* bull with a pendulous sheath.

parts of the body when the bulls display homosexual behavior by "riding" each other. The warts may result in hesitancy or refusal to breed and may become large enough that they prevent extension (phimosis) or retraction (paraphimosis) of the penis. Surgical removal of the wart(s) is one treatment option and may be performed in conjunction with vaccination with either a commercial or autogenous wart vaccine. These can be removed in the standing animal using local anesthetic (either bilateral internal pudendal nerve block or anesthesia of the dorsal penile nerve) and restraint. The fibropapilloma can be excised, and the penile mucosa should be sutured using an absorbable suture. Recurrence is not uncommon.

PREPUTIAL PROLAPSE

Preputial prolapse tends to occur in bulls of *Bos indicus* influence (i.e., Brahman, zebu) as a result of several predisposing breed-related factors, including a pendulous sheath, long prepuce, large preputial orifice, and the absence of retractor prepuce muscles. The prepuce may become traumatized as a result of environmental exposure because of the inability of the bull to keep the prepuce within the preputial cavity, or trauma may occur as an accident during breeding. Once traumatized, the prepuce begins to swell and prolapses further, making it susceptible to further injury (Figure 31-24). The affected prepuce is treated initially by soaking in warm water with Betadine and Epsom salts to reduce swelling and control infection. The prepuce is returned to the preputial cavity and wrapped with a tube in place to prevent further trauma. Once the inflammation and infection are under control, surgery (reefing) to remove scar tissue and shorten the prepuce may be considered if the bull is valuable. Without surgery, recurrence rate for preputial trauma and reprolapse is high.

> *TECHNICIAN NOTE* Preputial prolapse occurs most commonly in bulls of *Bos indicus* influence as a result of several breed-related factors, including a pendulous sheath, long prepuce, large preputial orifice, and the absence of retractor prepuce muscles.

CONDITIONS OF THE OPHTHALMIC SYSTEM

OCULAR SQUAMOUS CELL CARCINOMA (CANCER EYE)

Ocular squamous cell carcinoma (OSCC), the most common tumor of cattle, is estimated to cause annual losses of $20 million in beef cattle in the United States. Losses result from condemnation of affected carcasses and loss of prime breeding stock.

The cause is multifactorial; there appears to be a genetic predisposition for development of ocular squamous cell tumors, and exposure to ultraviolet radiation (amount and intensity) and lack of protective pigmentation around the eye play an important role. Tumors occur predominantly in Herefords, but also other breeds with similar patterns of periocular pigmentation, such as Simmentals and Holsteins. It is seldom seen in animals less than 4 years of age, and peak age of occurrence is 8 years. The tumors begin as benign plaques or papillomas that often progress quickly to squamous cell carcinoma. Common sites for development of malignancy in decreasing order of prevalence are the lateral and medial limbus (Figure 31-25), eyelids (especially lower), third eyelid, and medial canthus.

Treatment modalities include cryotherapy, radiofrequency hyperthermia, immunotherapy, chemotherapy, radiation therapy, and surgery (keratectomy, lid resection, or extirpation). Although commonly referred to as enucleation, the term extirpation is more accurate. Extirpation is removal of all the contents of the bony orbit. Since this procedure is commonly performed for advanced cases of OSCC where removal of all ocular tissue is crucial and because cosmetic appearance is not as important in cattle, we are more likely

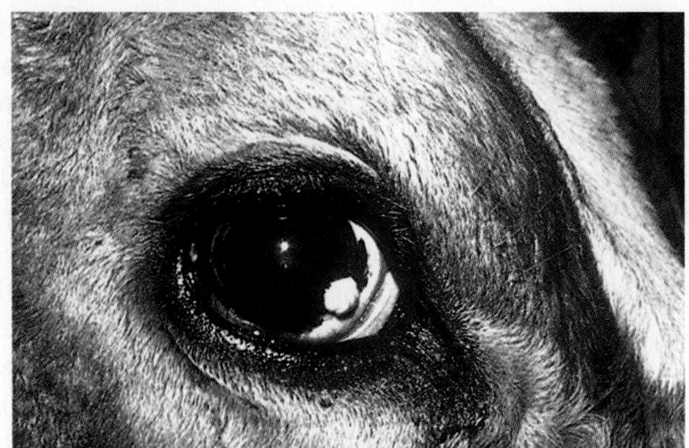

FIGURE 31-25 OSCC of the medial canthus of the eye of a cow.

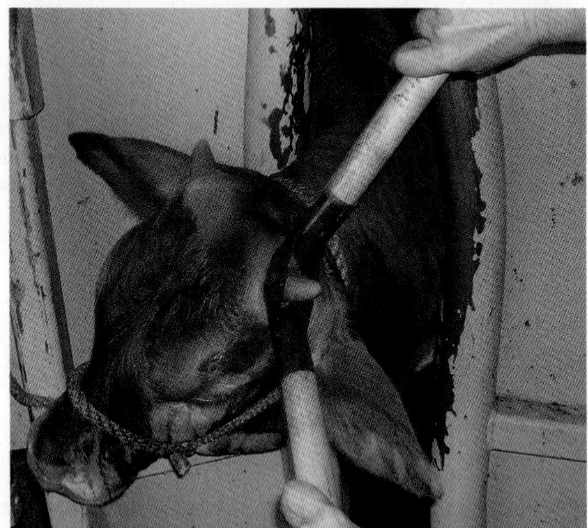

FIGURE 31-26 Use of a Barnes dehorner or scoop for removal of the horns in a young calf.

to perform extirpation rather than evisceration or enucleation of the eye.

Extirpation is performed with the aid of a retrobulbar or Peterson eye block. To perform the Peterson block, an 18-gauge, 12-cm needle bent to a slight curve is used to block cranial nerves II, IV, V, and VI as they emerge from the round foramen. The needle enters the skin at the angle produced by the supraorbital process and the zygomatic arch and is directed medially. The concavity of the needle is directed caudally so that the point of the needle will pass around the cranial border of the coronoid process of the mandible and to the pterygopalatine fossa of the skull. A reliable indication of proper position is a severe twitching of the eyelids. Once the proper position is located, 5 ml of local anesthetic is injected. The needle is repositioned slightly two more times with injection of 5 ml of local anesthetic each time. Aspiration is essential before injection to prevent depositing lidocaine in the cerebrospinal fluid (CSF), possibly resulting in sudden death. Before withdrawing the needle completely, it is redirected caudally just beneath the skin along the zygomatic arch to block the auriculopalpebral nerve. The four-point retrobulbar block is performed by injecting through the eyelids, both dorsally and ventrally, and at the medial and lateral canthi using a slightly curved, 18-gauge, 12-cm needle that is directed to the apex of the orbit. Five to 10 ml of local anesthetic are injected at each site. Exophthalmos, corneal anesthesia, and mydriasis indicate a satisfactory retrobulbar block.

The eye is surgically prepared, and the lids are sutured or clamped together. A transpalpebral incision is made approximately 1 cm from the lid margins (unless the disease extends beyond this margin). The skin incision is full thickness, but does not penetrate the palpebral conjunctiva; the conjunctival sac helps contain contaminated ocular structures during surgery. Sharp dissection is continued 360 degrees around the bony orbit. The orbital ligament is incised at the medial canthus, and the muscles, adipose, lacrimal glands, and fascia are removed. The optic artery can be ligated, significantly reducing hemorrhage, or the lids can be tightly closed and a gauze stent placed over the incision to provide pressure and hemostasis. The lids are closed with appositional or everting interrupted sutures using nonabsorbable No. 3 suture material. If excessive skin must be removed such that the incision cannot be closed, the orbit can be packed with gauze that is removed in 48 to 72 hours. The incision is left to heal by second intention. NSAIDs and antibiotics may be administered before surgery.

> *TECHNICIAN NOTE* OSCC, the most common tumor of cattle, results in large economic losses to cattle producers.

SURGICAL PROCEDURES OF YOUNG STOCK

DEHORNING

If possible, calves should be dehorned within the first month of life (or when the horn buds are first palpable) using a dehorning iron. The electrothermal dehorning technique is easy to perform when the calf is young; produces desirable, cosmetic results; and is much less stressful to the young calf. Dehorning of beef calves is commonly performed at the time of weaning in conjunction with castration, vaccination, and other management procedures. This age group is usually dehorned using a Barnes dehorner or scoop to remove the horn (Figure 31-26). Hemostasis, which is crucial, is provided by pulling or twisting the cornual artery. Calves older than 6 months may have exposed frontal sinuses after dehorning and may be at greater risk for development of sinusitis. Dehorning mature cattle often requires analgesia via a cornual nerve block. The block is performed by injecting 10 ml of 2% lidocaine under the frontal crest halfway between the lateral canthus of the eye and the base of the horn. Large horns are removed with a dehorning saw or Gigli wire. Another method of dehorning cattle is surgical or cosmetic dehorning, which is usually performed on show cattle. This method requires local or regional analgesia. An elliptical incision is made around the base of the horn, the horn is removed, and the skin incision is closed. This surgical technique allows for a more cosmetic appearance to the poll and reduces the chances of postoperative hemorrhage or infection.

CASTRATION

Several techniques are available for castration of calves. As with dehorning, castration is best performed when the calf is young because it is easier and less stressful to the calf at that time. Castration of young calves is often done without analgesia. Small calves can be adequately restrained on the ground, whereas larger calves are restrained in a chute with the tail pushed tightly up over the back. A technique commonly employed is the "open" method in which the bottom one third to one half of the scrotum is excised exposing the testicles. In young calves, the testicles are pulled until the cords break. In older calves, the cord can be sharply transected or an emasculator that crushes and cuts can be used to separate the cord (Figure 31-27). Another less commonly used technique is a "closed" castration using an emasculotome, which crushes the cord within the scrotum without cutting the scrotal skin. This technique is also referred to as bloodless castration or pinching. Castration in young calves has also been performed by application of an elastrator band. It is important to make certain that both testicles are below the band when the procedure is completed. It takes 2 to 3 weeks for the scrotum and testicles to slough. This technique has been associated with development of tetanus; therefore vaccination for tetanus may be advisable.

UMBILICAL HERNIAS AND INFECTIONS

As in other species, the umbilicus consists of paired umbilical arteries, a urachus, and an umbilical vein. The foramen where these exit the body wall is a common site of herniation, and this is considered to be a hereditary defect in some breeds, such as Holsteins. Any increase in size of the umbilical stalk, discharge from it, or swelling associated with the adjacent tissue warrants closer investigation. Simple umbilical hernias do occur and if small can be managed with application of belly wraps, hernia clamps, or elastrator bands. Close examination and palpation of the hernia and its ring is vital to ensure that it is completely reducible, no intestines appear to be in the hernia sac, there is no evidence of infection, and that the hernia is small (less than 5 cm in length). Ultrasonographic examination can be useful to identify structures within the hernia sac. Hernias that are greater than 5 cm in length will often benefit from an umbilical herniorrhaphy.

The majority of hernias or umbilical swellings are associated with infection in one or more of the umbilical remnants. Palpation of the mass is often of limited use diagnostically because it is firm, hot, swollen, and the patient usually resents palpation. Ultrasonographic examination allows the umbilical structures to be visualized and any enlargement or involvement of bladder or liver to be identified before initiating treatment. Medical treatment can be started in an attempt to treat the infection, but surgical resection can be necessary for severely affected patients.

Omphalectomy or umbilical herniorrhaphy can be performed with the calf in dorsal recumbency using sedation and a local block or general anesthesia. Feed does not need to be withheld for as long as for adult patients, but this should be removed approximately 6 to 8 hours before surgery. A large area should be clipped and prepped for surgery as if the umbilical vein or urachus is infected; the surgical incision may have to extend as far cranially as the xiphoid process or caudally to the pelvis. If the vein is infected up to the liver, a marsupialization may need to be performed that will require a second incision lateral to the main site. Attempt to remove the infected tissue intact; this may necessitate resection of the apex of the bladder. Following removal of the infected tissue, the body wall will be repaired. Some defects may be large enough to require a mesh herniorrhaphy, but most can be sutured closed.

Following surgery, the calf must be maintained in a stall for a month. Allowing excessive exercise will often lead to incisional complications, such as edema, seroma formation, or dehiscence. If umbilical vein marsupialization was performed, the stoma must be cleaned daily, and low pressure lavage with sterile fluid can be performed to try and treat the infected structures that could not be removed. This stoma will often need to be repaired in the future because it will often form a small hernia when the infection has resolved.

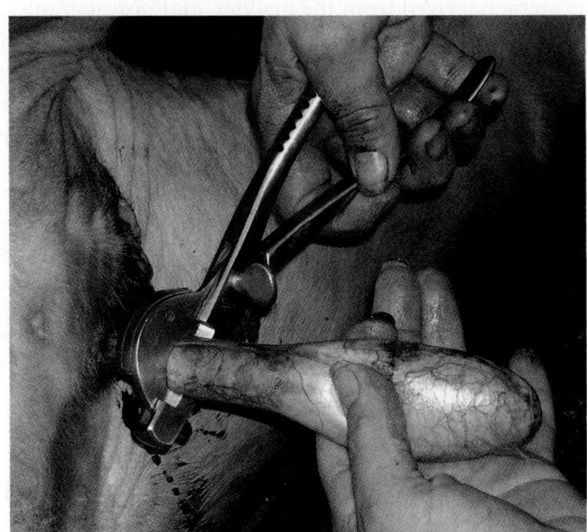

FIGURE 31-27 Castration of a calf by emasculation after removing the bottom half of the scrotum.

SELECTED CONDITIONS OF SMALL RUMINANTS

URINARY SYSTEM

Male small ruminants are at high risk for developing urolithiasis as a result of the feeding of excessive grain in the diet. The cause and clinical presentation is similar to that described in cattle. Goats that are obstructed tend to vocalize because of pain. Small ruminants are small enough that it is possible to palpate and/or ultrasound their urinary bladders,

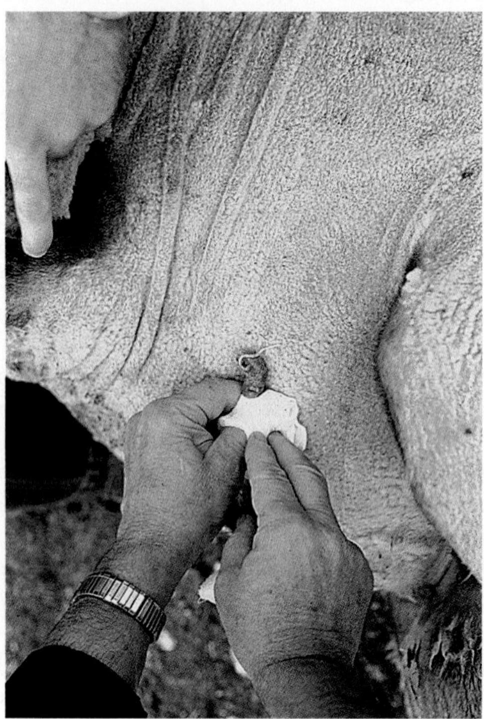

FIGURE 31-28 Examination of the urethral process in a wether for the presence of calculi (urolithiasis).

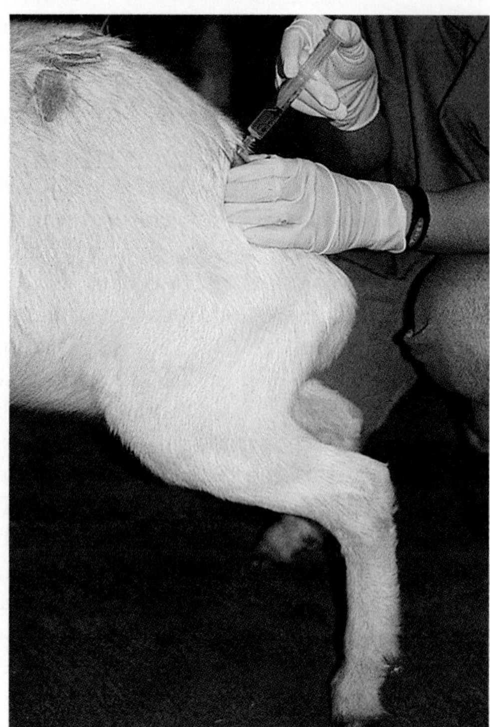

FIGURE 31-29 Administration of a lumbosacral epidural in a goat results in loss of motor control to the hind legs.

which further aids diagnosis of the condition. Management of this condition is somewhat different in small ruminants. Small ruminants possess a urethral process or vermiform appendage, which is usually the first place obstruction occurs. The second most common site of obstruction is the distal sigmoid flexure. Oftentimes calculi resemble sand, which may block most of the distal portion of the urethra.

The urethral process should be examined in all cases of suspected urolithiasis in small ruminants since this is the most common location for calculi to lodge. The penis and urethral process can be exteriorized by placing the animal in a sitting position on its rump (Figure 31-28). If necessary, a lumbosacral epidural can be performed. Epidural anesthesia provides analgesia and prevents resistance to exteriorization of the penis caused by the retractor penis muscles. Lidocaine (2%, 1 ml/20 lb not to exceed a total dose of 15 ml in any small ruminant) is injected into the epidural space at the lumbosacral junction (Figure 31-29). Loss of motor control to the hind legs lasts from 1 to 3 hours, so the patient should be recovered on a well-bedded surface to prevent trauma to the rear legs. Once the penis is exteriorized, it can be grasped with dry gauze. If the urethral process is obstructed, it can be amputated close to its attachment to the glans. If the urethral process is not present, it may mean that it had already been amputated or it may have necrosed and sloughed by itself during a previous episode of obstruction. Immediate urethral patency may occur after urethral process amputation; however, reobstruction is common. Consequently, it appears that urethral process amputation alone rarely results in a long-term cure.

Urethral catheterization with saline flushing may be attempted to relieve obstruction; however, the bladder is difficult to catheterize because of the presence of the suburethral diverticulum in ruminants, and complications associated with catheterization include urethritis, urethral rupture, and urethral damage leading to stricture.

Perineal urethrostomy may be suitable in cattle as a salvage procedure (Figure 31-30). Urethrostomy frequently results in stricture formation in the urethra and is probably not a good choice for pets because of a shortened life span.

Cystotomy and/or tube cystostomy have become the procedures of choice for treatment of obstructive urolithiasis and often result in prolonged life and preservation of breeding capability in breeding males. Using this procedure, calculi can be removed from the bladder, and normograde and retrograde urethral flushing can be attempted. In addition, a Foley catheter placed in the bladder allows urine egress while the urethra and bladder heal (Figure 31-31). The catheter is then removed when it is determined that the animal can urinate a normal stream consistently from the urethra.

> *TECHNICIAN NOTE* Male small ruminants are at high risk for development of obstructive urolithiasis as a result of the feeding of excessive grain in the diet.

OPHTHALMIC SYSTEM

Entropion

Entropion, or inward rolling of the eyelid, has been reported to be the most common ocular disease of neonatal lambs (Figure 31-32). The congenital or primary form involves only the lower lid, but is usually bilateral. Clinical signs of

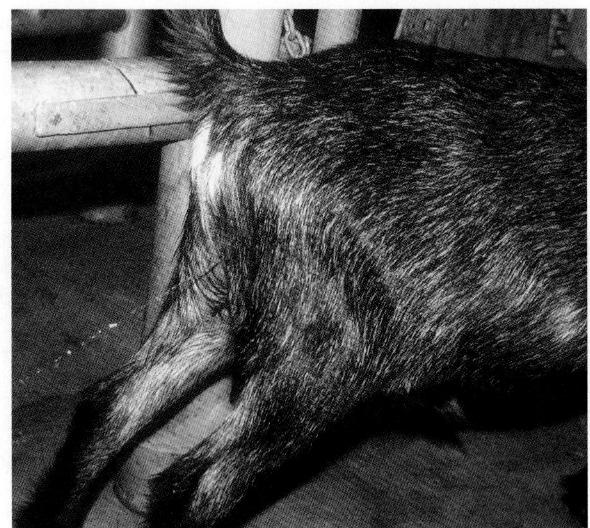

FIGURE 31-30 Perineal urethrostomy, a surgical treatment for obstructive urolithiasis, is prone to stricture formation in small ruminants.

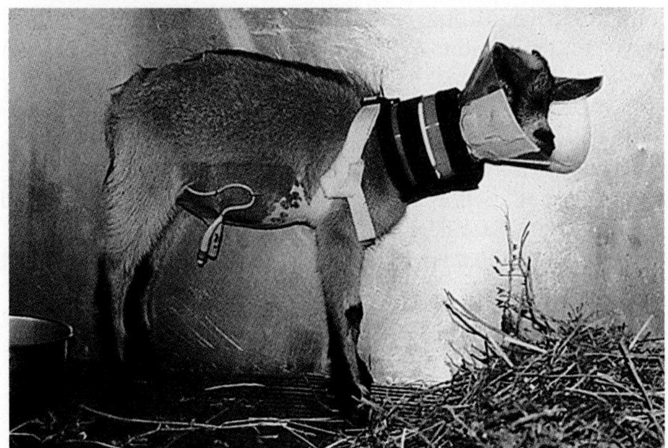

FIGURE 31-31 Temporary tube cystostomy allows urine egress while the urethra and bladder heal postobstruction.

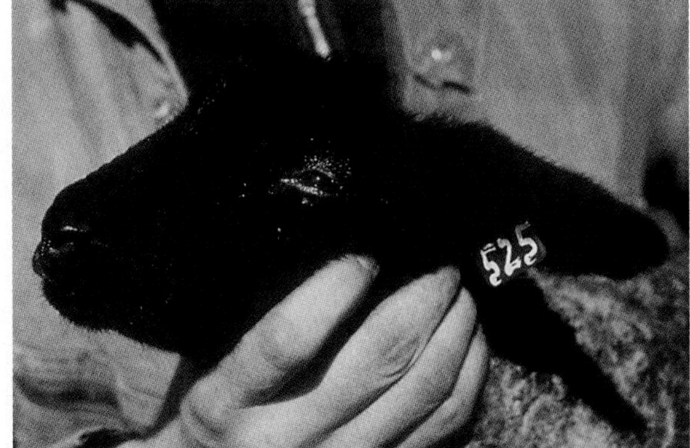

FIGURE 31-32 A lamb with corneal irritation from congenital entropion or inward rolling of the lower eyelid.

blepharospasm, photophobia, eye rubbing, and keratoconjunctivitis are ordinarily observed in lambs during the first few days to weeks of life. Initial treatment is conservative and involves administration of ophthalmic antibiotics and manually rolling the lower lid outward. If this is unsuccessful, other treatment options include injection of penicillin or tetracycline in a linear fashion parallel to the lower lid or clamping of the skin of the lower lid below and parallel to the lid margin with mosquito forceps for 30 seconds. Both techniques should create sufficient inflammation and fibrosis to keep the lower lid rolled out. Another technique involves placement of two or three vertical mattress sutures in the lower lid to roll out the lid margin. Congenital entropion is considered to be a heritable trait, so affected animals should not be kept for breeding.

COMMON SURGICAL PROCEDURES PERFORMED ON SMALL RUMINANTS

Lumbosacral epidurals are useful for alleviating pain during procedures performed caudal to the umbilicus. The animal will lose motor control to the hind legs and should be confined to a small, well-bedded area to prevent injury. A lumbosacral epidural is performed at the lumbosacral junction that can easily be palpated in small ruminants. A 20-gauge, 3.8-cm needle is used for this technique. The needle is inserted perpendicular to the dorsal midline until a slight popping sensation is encountered. If the epidural space has been entered, injection should be easy. An alternative is to advance the needle until bone is felt, then back the needle out slightly and attempt injection. If CSF is encountered, the subarachnoid space rather than the epidural space has been entered. It is acceptable to inject lidocaine into this area if aseptic technique has been used during the procedure, but the lidocaine dose should be reduced to half of that used for epidural injection. Analgesia will take several minutes if in the epidural space and will be almost immediate if injected into the subarachnoid space. The dose of lidocaine used for this procedure is 5 to 8 ml/45 kg body weight.

The optimal time for disbudding or dehorning kids is 3 to 5 days in buck kids and 5 to 7 days in doe kids. At this age, the procedure is less invasive because the horn buds have not yet attached to the underlying bone, and there is less chance of regrowth if dehorned properly at this age. Many owners perform this procedure with restraint only; however, the kid may be sedated with xylazine and butorphanol. In addition, a ring block of 1% lidocaine around the base of the horn will provide local analgesia. The horn bud is removed by first burning with the dehorning iron and either allowing the bud to slough or by excising the bud after burning around its base. Care should be taken not to leave the iron on too long (5 to 10 seconds per side) to prevent thermal meningitis. The burning procedure may be repeated, allowing the area to cool between burns, until a uniform ring of copper-colored skin is apparent around the entire horn bud bases (Figure 31-33).

C-sections are indicated in cases of dystocia. A left flank laparotomy can be used to approach the uterus and, using sedation and an inverted-L block, can be rapidly performed. Following incision of the skin, the flank muscles can be bluntly separated along the direction of their fibers, and the uterus can be brought into the surgical field. It is important that the uterus is carefully palpated before closure to prevent

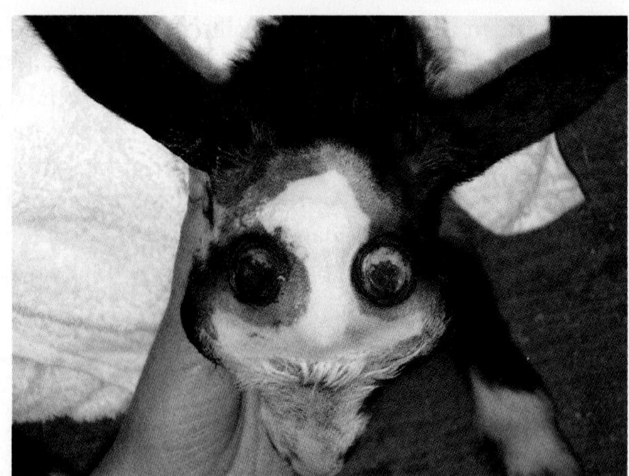

FIGURE 31-33 Disbudding kids is performed by burning the horn buds with an electric dehorning iron before 2 weeks of age.

leaving a fetus in the contralateral horn. Alternatively a ventral midline or ventral paramedian approach can be used.

Factors causing rectal prolapse in sheep include short tail docking, overconditioning of lambs (increased pelvic fat), straining as a result of urolithiasis, diarrhea, dystocia, or conditions that increase abdominal pressure, such as coughing. Short tail docks are performed strictly for cosmetic reasons in show lambs and may result in loss of innervation to the rectum and anal sphincter, which comes from S3 to Cy5. A resolution to the American Veterinary Medical Association (AVMA) suggests that lamb tails not be docked shorter than the distal end of the caudal tail fold. Methods for rectal prolapse repair include purse-string suture after replacement (strictly a salvage procedure), injection of irritating solutions (tetracycline, strong iodine in oil) at three to four points perirectally, and rectal amputation.

> *TECHNICIAN NOTE* The optimal time for disbudding or dehorning kids is 3 to 5 days in buck kids and 5 to 7 days in doe kids.

RECOMMENDED READING

Auer JA, Stick JA, editors: *Equine surgery*, ed 3, Philadelphia, 2006, Saunders.

Divers TJ, Peek SF: *Rebhun's diseases of dairy cattle*, ed 2, St Louis, 2008, Saunders.

Fubini SL, Ducharme NC: *Farm animal surgery*, St Louis, 2004, Saunders.

Hanie EA: *Large animal clinical procedures for veterinary technicians*, St Louis, 2006, Mosby.

Koterba AM, Drummond WH, Kosch PC, editors: *Equine clinical neonatology*, Philadelphia, 1990, Lea & Febiger.

Orsini JA, Divers TJ: *Manual of equine emergencies*, ed 3, St Louis, 2008, Saunders.

Pugh DG: *Sheep and goat medicine*, St Louis, 2002, Saunders.

Reed S, Bailey W, Sellon D, editors: *Equine internal medicine*, ed 2, St Louis, 2003, Saunders.

Smith BP: *Large animal internal medicine*, ed 4, St Louis, 2009, Mosby.

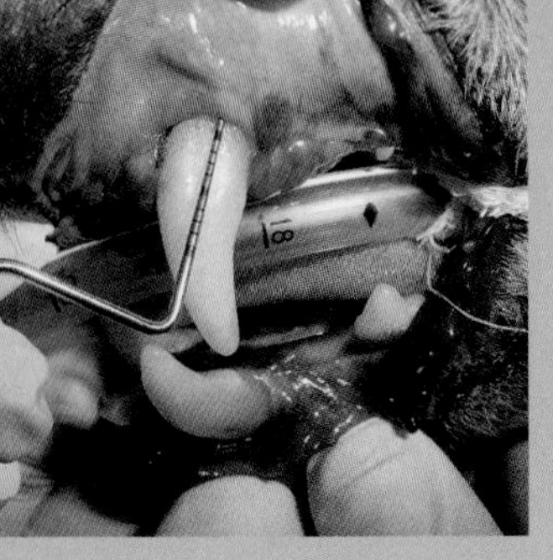

Dentistry and Oral Surgery

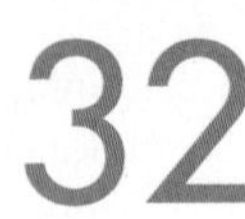

John R. Lewis and Bonnie R. Miller

KEY TERMS

Anisognathism
Apex
Brachycephalic
Brachygnathism
Calculus
Caries
Cementum
Diastema
Dolichocephalic
Enamel
Endodontics
Exodontics
Furcation
Hypsodont
Malocclusion
Mesocephalic
Periodontium
Plaque
Pulp
Triadan system

OUTLINE

LEARNING OBJECTIVES

When you have completed this chapter, you will be able to:

1. Describe legal issues related to performance of dental services by veterinary technicians and list professional organizations related to veterinary dentistry.
2. Identify terminology used in veterinary dentistry to designate location and direction and describe the modified Triadan system for numbering of teeth.
3. Describe normal occlusion in dogs and cats and common malocclusions and treatment methods used in orthodontics in small animals.
4. Discuss aspects of the complete medical history as they relate to veterinary dentistry.
5. List and describe procedures used in extraoral and intraoral examinations in small and large animals.
6. Describe equipment and supplies used for dental radiography.
7. Differentiate between paralleling, bisecting angle, and occlusal techniques in dental radiography.
8. Differentiate between stomatitis, gingivitis, and periodontitis and explain grading of periodontal disease.
9. Describe equipment and procedures for periodontal débridement using power and hand scalers.
10. Explain methods for sharpening of dental instruments.
11. Discuss the rationale and procedures used in polishing teeth.
12. Discuss topics and methods for client education related to veterinary dentistry.
13. Discuss indications for restorative dentistry and endodontics and describe common procedures performed on small animals.
14. Discuss indications, procedures, and potential complications of exodontics.
15. List and describe common equine dental problems and treatments.

INTRODUCTION

Veterinary dentistry has been in existence as a specialty for more than 20 years. However, few veterinarians and technicians have received formal training in dentistry and oral surgery because of the relative paucity of educational opportunities. Dentistry has become a significant part of nearly every small animal practice, and more attention is paid to dental disease of other species, such as horses and exotic animals. Veterinary technicians play a vital role in veterinary dentistry. Common tasks include: (1) performing procedures such as periodontal débridement and polishing; (2) obtaining diagnostic information through dental charting and dental radiography; (3) intraoperative assistance with dental and oral surgeries; (4) in some states where allowed by law, extraction (exodontics) of diseased teeth; and (5) client education, including proper use of appropriate dental home-care products and preventive techniques. Most veterinary practices provide professional dental cleanings for their patients. Some practices also provide advanced dental care, such as endodontics, exodontics, and advanced periodontal therapy. In the process of providing routine dental care, technicians have an opportunity to identify disease in its early stages. Therefore a strong foundation in oral anatomy and oral pathologic conditions is important. Because technicians are often on the front line of identifying oral disease, this chapter provides a strong foundation of disease recognition and an understanding of treatment principles.

This chapter also provides a detailed discussion of periodontal disease, including pathophysiology, treatment, follow-up, and prevention. Because scaling and polishing procedures are the most common dental procedures performed in practice, special attention is paid in this chapter to instrumentation and techniques of proper periodontal therapy. Dental radiology is extremely important in veterinary dentistry because disease is often missed or underestimated when the teeth are not examined beneath the gingival margin. Techniques for taking diagnostic dental radiographs are covered, and interpretation of normal and abnormal dental radiographic anatomy is discussed. This chapter also addresses other subspecialties of dentistry, including endodontics, exodontics, orthodontics, and restorative dentistry. Equine dental anatomy and pathologic conditions are discussed, including preventive and therapeutic treatments of common equine dental problems.

ETHICAL AND LEGAL ASPECTS

The level of dental care a veterinary technician may provide varies from state to state, and the laws and regulations for the state of practice need to be understood before providing dental care. The American Veterinary Dental College (AVDC) published a position statement in 1998 regarding veterinary dental heath care providers. This statement provides recommendations for the qualifications of persons performing veterinary dental procedures. The AVDC considers it appropriate for the veterinarian to delegate maintenance dental care and certain dental tasks to veterinary technicians. Tasks appropriately performed by veterinary technicians include dental prophylaxis and certain procedures that do not result in alterations in the shape, structure, or positional location of teeth in the dental arch.

> *TECHNICIAN NOTE* The level of dental care the technician can legally provide varies from state to state. Become familiar with practice acts in your state.

In addition, the AVDC supports advanced training of veterinary technicians to perform additional dental services, such as taking impressions, making models, charting veterinary dental lesions, taking and developing dental radiographs, and performing nonsurgical subgingival root planing.

VETERINARY DENTAL ORGANIZATIONS

Opportunities exist for veterinary technicians to achieve advanced training and recognition in dentistry. The National Association of Veterinary Technicians in America (NAVTA) governs technicians who have completed credential requirements and passed specialty examinations to be considered Veterinary Technician Specialists (VTS). To date, there are advanced specialties in the fields of anesthesia, emergency and critical care, internal medicine, dentistry, and behavior. Technicians interested in pursuing the dental specialty must secure a mentor, maintain case logs, write case reports, and attend continuing education courses as part of the credentials process of the Academy of Veterinary Dental Technicians (AVDT). Before beginning the credentialing process, the technician must have 3000 hours of dental experience. For further information about becoming a member of the AVDT, visit the website www.avdt.us.

> *TECHNICIAN NOTE* The AVDT consists of technicians who have completed a credentials process and passed a specialty examination.

The American Veterinary Dental Society (AVDS) is an organization created to advance the awareness and knowledge of veterinary dentistry among the profession and the public. Membership in the AVDS is open to all veterinarians,

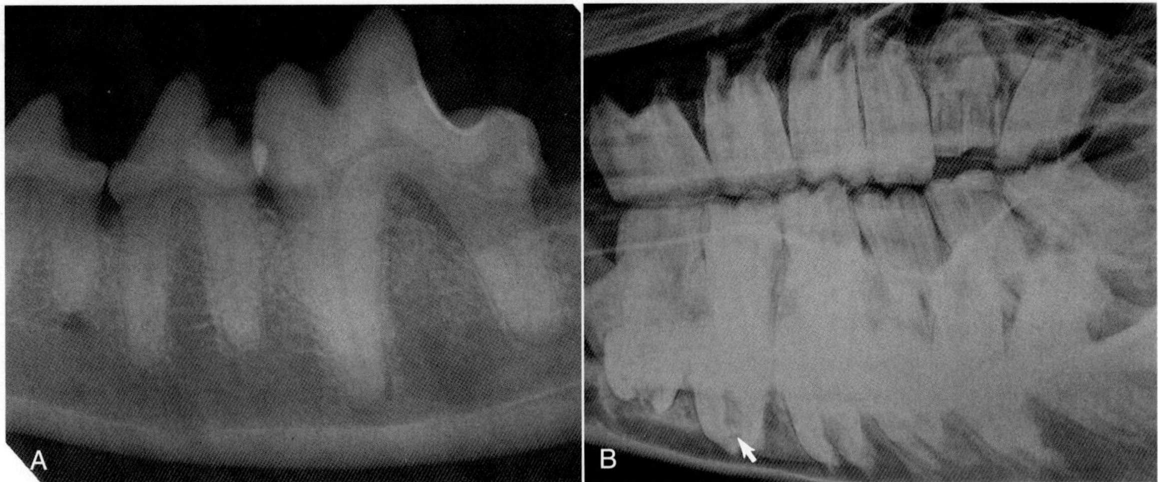

FIGURE 32-1 Radiograph of brachyodont teeth of the dog **(A)** and hypsodont teeth of the horse **(B)**.

veterinary technicians, and dental hygienists. Membership includes a subscription to the *Journal of Veterinary Dentistry*, the official journal of many national and international dental societies and colleges. More information can be found at the AVDS website www.avds-online.org.

The earliest organization established to provide dental knowledge to veterinary technicians and assistants is the American Society for Veterinary Dental Technicians (ASVDT). Membership includes a self-taught home study course that is a good introduction to basic dentistry. The ASVDT provides a baseline level of dental knowledge and is open to staff members who may or may not have formal veterinary education, whereas members of the AVDT have an advanced level of dental knowledge and are required to hold a certification or state license for membership.

BOX 32-1 Dental Formulas

Dog: *Deciduous teeth* 2 × (I 3/3, C 1/1, P 3/3) = 28 teeth
Permanent teeth 2 × (I 3/3, C/1/1, P 4/4, M 2/3) = 42 teeth
Cat: *Deciduous teeth* 2 × (I 3/3, C 1/1, P 3/2) = 26 teeth
Permanent teeth 2 × (I 3/3, C 1/1, P 3/2, M 1/1) = 30 teeth
Horse: *Deciduous teeth* 2 × (I 3/3, C 0/0, P 3/3) = 24 teeth
Permanent teeth 2 × (I 3/3, C 1/1 or 0/0, P 3 or 4/3 or 4, M 3/3) = 36 to 44 teeth (depending on presence of canine and wolf teeth)

I, Incisors; *C*, canines, *P*, premolars; *M*, molars.

DENTAL MORPHOLOGY

Morphology refers to the form and structure of an organism or its parts. Teeth can be classified as brachyodont or hypsodont based on their crown and root structure (Figure 32-1). All teeth of humans, carnivores, and pigs are brachyodont teeth. Brachyodont teeth have a relatively small, distinct crown compared with the size of their well-developed roots. The apices (singular: apex) of the roots are open for only a limited time during eruption and development of the teeth, and therefore the teeth do not continually grow or erupt. This is in contrast to hypsodont teeth (seen in horses, rodents, and lagomorphs) that have a comparatively large reserve crown beneath the gingival margin and root structure that allows for continued growth and/or continued eruption during all or most of an animal's lifetime. Hypsodont teeth can be divided further into two categories: radicular and aradicular hypsodont teeth. The cheek teeth of horses are an example of radicular hypsodont teeth. The apices of these teeth remain open for a significant portion of adult life, but eventually close, after which point continued growth of the tooth ceases, and occlusal wear is offset only by continued eruption. Cheek teeth and incisors of rabbits and some rodents are aradicular hypsodont (also called elodont) teeth, indicating a lack of true root structure and lifelong tooth growth, which compensates for occlusal wear.

Dogs and cats have four types of teeth: incisors, canines, premolars, and molars. The incisor teeth are the most rostral teeth and are used for gnawing and grooming. The canine teeth are distal to the incisors. They are long and are used for prehending and holding. The premolars and molars (often referred to as cheek teeth) are used for shearing and grinding.

Most mammals are diphyodont, meaning that they have two sets of teeth. The first set of teeth is referred to as deciduous (also referred to as primary or baby teeth), and these are replaced with permanent teeth (also referred to as secondary or adult teeth). Mammals show great variety in the number and types of teeth depending on the species. Dental formulas used to classify the numbers and types of teeth are seen in Box 32-1. Normal eruption times of deciduous and permanent teeth in dogs and cats are seen in Table 32-1, though it should be mentioned that some normal variation exists.

It is important to be aware of the number of roots of each tooth. Table 32-2 lists the number of roots of each tooth of cats and dogs. Anatomic variation does occur, so preoperative dental radiographs are important to confirm numbers and shape of tooth roots before extraction or other procedures

TABLE 32-1 Approximate Eruption Schedule for Teeth of Dogs and Cats (in weeks)

	Deciduous Teeth		Permanent Teeth	
	Puppy	Kitten	Dog	Cat
Incisors	4-6	3-4	12-16	11-16
Canines	3-5	3-4	12-16	12-20
Premolars	5-6	5-6	16-20	16-20
Molars	—	—	16-20	20-24

involving subgingival pathologic conditions. For example, the maxillary third premolar is usually a two-rooted tooth in dogs and cats, but it is not uncommon to see a third root in some dogs and cats.

An understanding of dental anatomic terminology is necessary to accurately describe the location of a structure or lesion. "Rostral" is a term that when referring to cranial anatomy refers to a structure that is closer to the front of the head in comparison with another structure. "Caudal" is a term used to describe a structure that is toward the back of the head when compared with another structure. "Vestibular" is a term that describes the tooth surface facing the lips or vestibule (acceptable alternatives are buccal and labial). "Facial" is a term that describes the vestibular surface of teeth visible from the front (incisors). "Lingual" refers to the surface of the mandibular teeth adjacent to the tongue. "Palatal" refers to the surface of maxillary teeth adjacent to the palate. "Mesial" refers to the portion of the tooth in line with the dental arcade that is closest to the most rostral portion of the midline of the dental arch. "Distal" refers to the portion of the tooth that is closest to the most caudal portion of the midline of the dental arch. The concepts of mesial and distal surfaces are difficult to describe without referring to a diagram. Figure 32-2 shows a diagram with use of these terms. It may help to remember that the terms mesial and distal are used to describe the surfaces of the teeth where adjacent teeth touch or nearly touch. "Apical" refers to a portion of the tooth closer to the apex, or tip of the root. "Coronal" refers to a structure with a location closer to the crown of the tooth in relation to another structure.

Referring to the teeth by a numeric system rather than using descriptive terminology saves time when performing detailed charting. The most commonly used numbering system is the modified Triadan system. Teeth in the maxillary right quadrant are considered the 100 series, with the left maxillary quadrant called the 200 series. The left mandibular quadrant is the 300 series, and right the mandibular quadrant is the 400 series. Each tooth within the quadrant has a two digit number starting at the anterior midline and moving along the dental arch in a caudal direction. The right maxillary first incisor is 101, right maxillary second incisor is 102, right maxillary third incisor 103, right maxillary canine 104, and so on. The left maxillary canine is 204, left mandibular canine is 304, and right mandibular canine is 404 (Figure 32-3). Deciduous teeth are assigned the 500 series for the right maxillary quadrant, 600 series for the left maxillary

TABLE 32-2 Permanent Dentition of the Dog and Cat

Dog Permanent Dentition		
Mandible	**Tooth**	**Roots**
Incisors	1st, 2nd, 3rd	1
Canines	1	1
Premolars	1st	1
Premolars	2nd, 3rd, 4th	2
Molars	1st, 2nd	2
Molars	3rd*	1 (or 2)
Maxilla	**Tooth**	**Roots**
Incisors	1st, 2nd, 3rd	1
Canines	1	1
Premolars	1st	1
Premolars	2nd, 3rd*	2
Premolars	(3rd*), 4th	3
Molars	1st, 2nd	3
Cat Permanent Dentition		
Mandible	**Tooth**	**Roots**
Incisors	1st, 2nd, 3rd	1
Canines	1	1
Premolars	1st, 2nd	Not present
Premolars	3rd, 4th	2
Molars	1st	2
Maxilla	**Tooth**	**Roots**
Incisors	1st, 2nd, 3rd	1
Canines	1	1
Premolars	1st	Not present
Premolars	2nd*	1 (or 2)
Premolars	3rd*	2 (or 3)
Premolars	4th	3
Molars	1st*	1 (or 2)

*Anatomic variation in root numbers is common. There may be an extra root, or it may be partially fused to the normal root(s).

quadrant, 700 series for the left mandibular quadrant, and 800 series for the right mandibular quadrant.

> *TECHNICIAN NOTE* Knowledge of the Triadan tooth numbering system saves time during charting of oral pathologic conditions.

Cats have fewer teeth than dogs, but even when teeth are missing, the teeth that are present will have a predictable number with the Triadan system. For example, tooth 108 always refers to the right maxillary fourth premolar whether discussing a dog, hyena, cat, or lion. Since the cat does not have a maxillary first premolar, the premolar closest to the canine tooth is tooth 106 (Figure 32-4). Cats are missing their mandibular first and second premolars, so the premolars closest to the mandibular canine teeth are numbered 307 and 407,

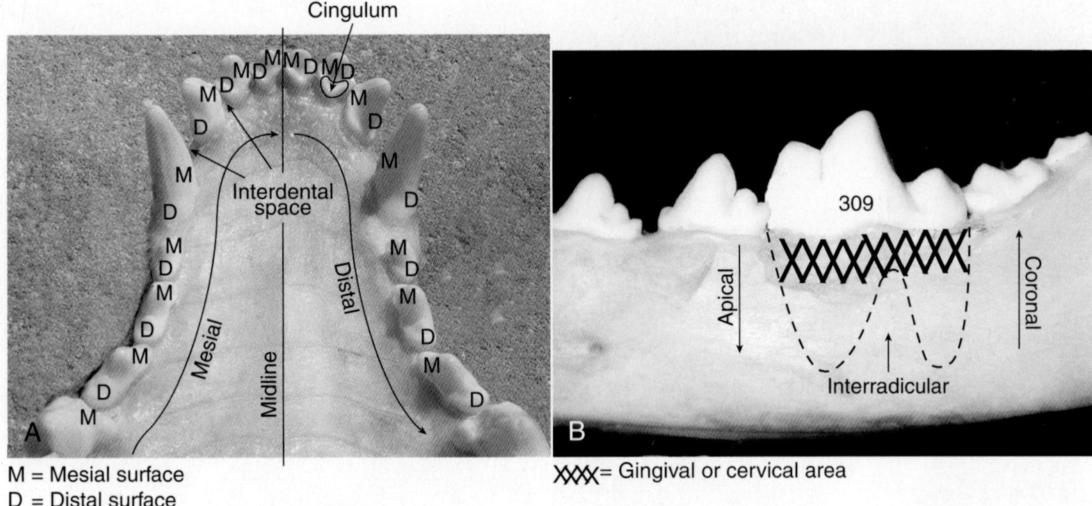

FIGURE 32-2 Positional terminology commonly used in dentistry. **A,** Palatal view of the canine maxilla. *M,* Mesial; *D,* distal. **B,** Mandibular left first molar.

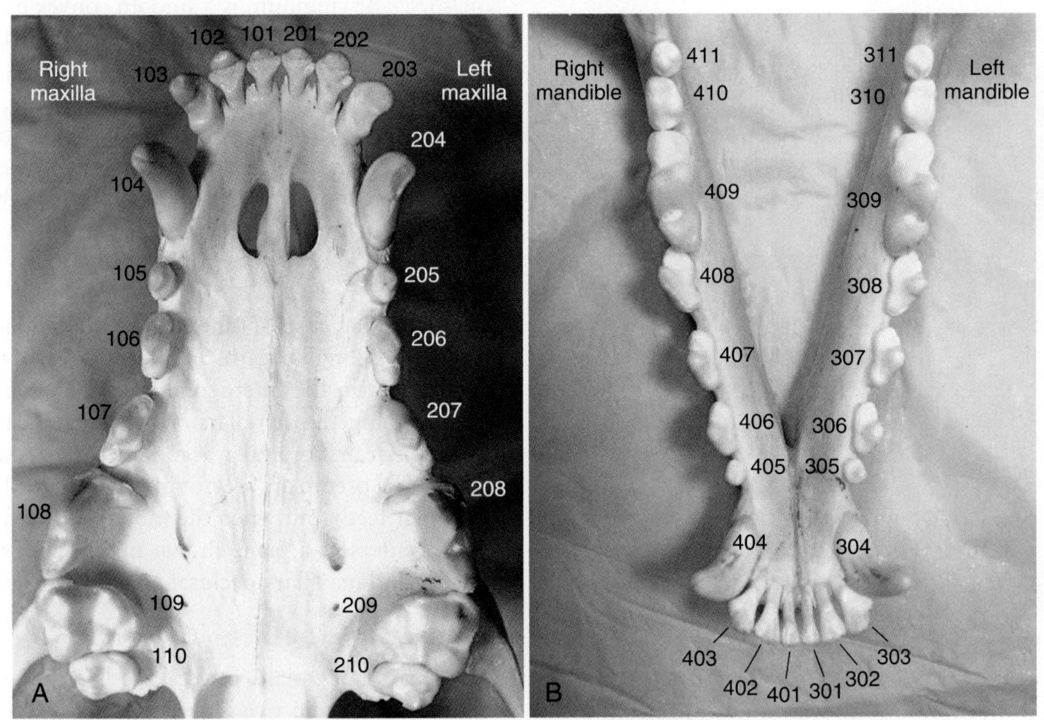

FIGURE 32-3 Triadan tooth numbering system in the dog. **A,** Maxilla. **B,** Mandible.

respectively for the left and right mandible. Keeping these numbers consistent among species allows veterinary professionals to quickly equate a tooth number with an anatomic location. When someone says tooth 208 is fractured, one should think of the left maxillary fourth premolar regardless of species.

OCCLUSION

Occlusion refers to the spatial relationship of teeth within the mouth. Malocclusion refers to the situation when teeth or jaws are not correctly aligned. Although cosmetic issues of misaligned teeth are not typically a concern in dogs and cats, malocclusions can result in discomfort from impingement of teeth on soft tissue structures of the opposing dental arcade. Dogs and cats with a normal occlusion have a scissors bite, where the incisors come together to closely overlap like blades of a scissors (Figure 32-5, *A, B*). When teeth are properly aligned in scissors occlusion, there is maximal function of all teeth with no occlusal trauma. Variations of dental occlusion in dogs and cats occur depending on the breed and skull type. The relationship of brachyodont teeth in normal occlusion is discussed later.

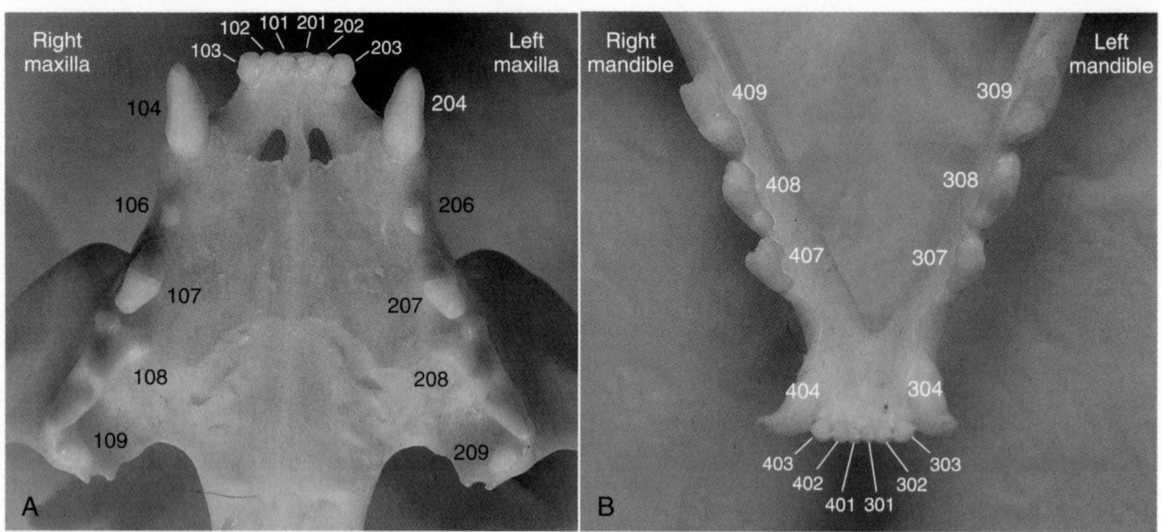

FIGURE 32-4 Triadan tooth numbering system in the cat. **A**, Maxilla. **B**, Mandible. Note that the canine tooth always ends with the numbers "04" and the first molar always ends with the numbers "09," regardless of species.

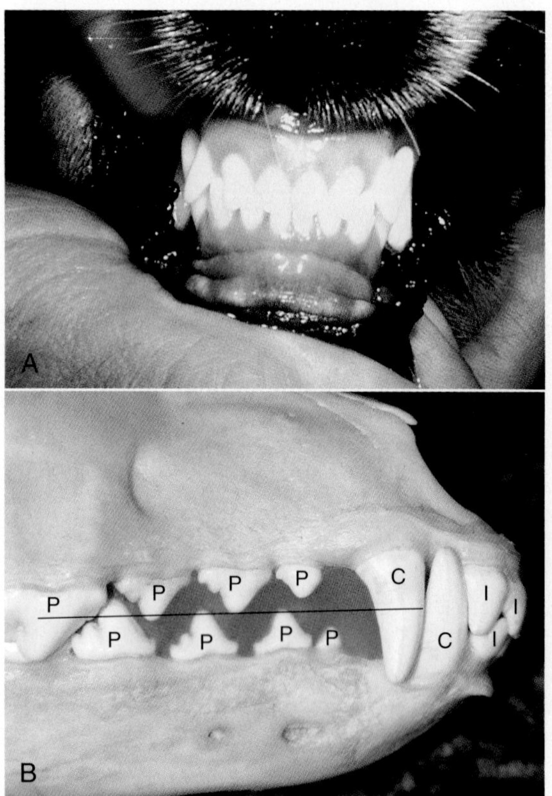

FIGURE 32-5 Normal scissors occlusion in a dog. *I*, Incisor; *C*, canine; *P*, premolar; *M*, molar. **A**, Rostral view of incisor and canine teeth in a dog. **B**, Lateral view of a dog skull. Premolar cusps interdigitate toward the opposing interdental space.

Incisors

The mandibular incisors should be palatal to (behind) the maxillary incisors, and the coronal third of the mandibular incisors should rest on the cingulum of the maxillary incisors. The cingulum is a smooth convex bulge located on the palatal side of the gingival third of the incisor teeth.

Canines

When the mouth is closed, the mandibular canine is distal to the maxillary third incisor and mesial to the maxillary canine, and it should be centered in between these two teeth without touching either of these teeth.

Premolars

The premolar cusps point to the interdental space of the opposing premolar teeth. The mandibular fourth premolar cusp points in the interdental space between the maxillary third and fourth premolars. When the mouth is closed, the mandibular first premolar is mesial to the maxillary first premolar. The premolars are not in occlusion with the opposing premolar teeth, but when the mouth is closed, the cusp tips should intersect a plane drawn midway between the mandibular and maxillary occlusal planes (see Figure 32-5, *B*).

Carnassial Teeth

The term "carnassial," interpreted literally, means "tearing of flesh." This adjective is used to describe the largest shearing tooth of the upper and lower jaw in dogs, cats, and other carnivores. These teeth work together during mastication and contribute most significantly to the masticatory effort. The carnassial teeth of dogs and cats are the maxillary fourth premolar and the mandibular first molar teeth. In most species, the upper jaw is wider than the lower jaw, referred to as anisognathism. Therefore the maxillary fourth premolar tooth normally occludes lateral (buccal) to the mandibular first molar tooth.

Molars

Humans have many flat occlusal surfaces of the maxillary and mandibular molars that come together during chewing to crush food particles. In contrast, carnivores have sharp, shearing cusps and less flat occlusal surfaces. Two maxillary and three mandibular molars of dogs have flat occlusal surfaces that are capable of grinding and crushing hard food particles. Cats, having the dentition of a true carnivore, have molars with few flat occlusal surfaces. Flat occlusal surfaces are often susceptible to development of caries lesions (also referred to by the term of "cavities") in pits and fissures that occur as a result of incomplete development of enamel on the occlusal surface. The relative lack of flat occlusal surfaces partly explains the increased susceptibility of humans to caries lesions compared with dogs and cats.

ORAL EXAMINATION AND HISTORY

The patient's medical history should be assessed before performing dental procedures because dental procedures require elective anesthesia. The technician can obtain a complete medical history and a history specifically pertinent to dentistry. Clinical symptoms to inquire about include pawing at the mouth, dropping food, walking away from the food bowl after showing initial interest in food, rubbing the face along furniture, or showing uncharacteristic aggression when approached or touched around the facial region (Box 32-2). These signs can indicate oral disease and may manifest earlier in the disease process than would anorexia or oral bleeding. A history of sneezing after drinking water is suggestive of the presence of an oronasal fistula, a common problem in small-breed dogs with severe periodontal disease.

History related to oral home care can also be obtained by the technician. Inquire about whether a home-care regimen is currently performed. If not, delve further to determine if the client is willing or able to provide oral care at home. If the client has attempted home care and was not successful, find out what was tried so that alternative methods may be suggested. If the client is currently providing home care, ask how frequently and what techniques and products are being used. History pertaining to diet, treats, and toys is also important. Ask if the pet is fed dry, canned, or semimoist food. Inquire about the kind of treats the pet is eating to determine what role treats are playing in the development or prevention of dental disease. Ask what kind of toys the pet plays with and if there are any inappropriate habits that may increase the risk of dental fractures. Once the dental history is established, the veterinary technician is in the perfect position to provide counseling on proper home-care techniques, diets, and toy products.

BOX 32-2 Clinical or Behavioral Signs of Oral Disease

- Pawing at the mouth
- Facial swelling
- Dropping food
- Face rubbing
- Unusual aggression
- Sneezing or snorting following eating or drinking
- Difficulty or pain when opening mouth
- Anorexia
- Jaw opening reflex ("chattering" of the lower jaw)
- Difficulty swallowing (dysphagia)
- Excessive drooling (ptyalism)
- Resenting touch or manipulation of the head
- Oral bleeding

The dental or oral surgical procedure, whether routine or emergency, should begin with a comprehensive extraoral and intraoral examination. The mouth can be an indicator of general health, and a thorough oral examination is an integral part of any diagnostic sequence. The technician plays a crucial role in providing dental care and services, so it is imperative that the technician becomes familiar with the normal anatomy of the oral cavity and surrounding structures. By performing examination techniques on a regular basis and by establishing a routine sequence of examination, efficient and accurate recognition of abnormalities is possible. All information received from the examination should be recorded on a dental record, the legal document of clinical data and dental services that becomes part of the patient's medical record (Figures 32-6, *A, B,* and 32-7, *A, B*). Any abnormalities should be brought to the veterinarian's attention so that a diagnosis and proper treatment plan can be established for the patient.

> *TECHNICIAN NOTE* Every dental procedure should begin with a comprehensive oral examination to evaluate extraoral structures of the face, head, and neck and intraoral structures, including the soft tissues of the oral cavity, the teeth, and their supporting structures.

EXTRAORAL EXAMINATION

The examination begins with extraoral observation of the head, face, eyes, ears, and neck using direct visual observation, palpation, and smell. Using both hands, palpate each side of the face, head, and neck for symmetrical comparison. Feel the temporal and masseter muscles for the presence of atrophy, enlargement, or pain. Palpate the ventral, lateral, and medial surface of the left and right mandibles for the presence of swelling that could be evidence of neoplasia or fracture. Small-breed dogs with advanced periodontal disease are commonly affected by bone loss and pathologic fracture of the mandible, which may be found as an incidental finding in the examination room.

Visually inspect the ears and note evidence of discharge, odor or pain on palpation because middle ear disease may be a cause for the presenting complaint of pain on opening the mouth. Visually inspect the eyes and palpate using your thumbs on the closed eyelids to gently push (retropulse) both eyes at the same time. Bilateral retropulsion allows for symmetrical comparison of depth and firmness (Figure 32-8). Often if a space-occupying mass (as a result of neoplasia, inflammation, or infection) is present behind or beneath the eye, retropulsion may find a decreased ability of the globe to

Text continued on p. 1104

VHUP Dental Record

R L

Date:
Staff: (circle primary staff)
Chief Complaint:
Awake Sedated Anesthetized

(Addressograph)

MAL/1 MAL/2 MAL/3 MAL/WRY
MAL/BN Malocclusion/base narrow mand. canines
MAL/ABX, PBX Mal/anterior, posterior crossbite
OC Orthodontic/genetic consultation
OR Orthodontic recheck
SN Supernumerary tooth
DT Deciduous tooth
RD Retained deciduous tooth
PD0 No perio dx (maybe calculus)
PD1 Gingivitis (no bone loss)
PD2 Mild periodontitis (< 25% attach loss)
PD3 Mod periodontitis (< 50% attach loss)
PD4 Severe periodontitis (> 50% attach loss)
GH Gingival hyperplasia
GR Gingival recession
ST Stomatitis
ST/CU Stomatitis – contact ulcer
ST/FFS Stomatitis – Feline faucitis-stomatitis
OM Oral mass:
OM/EPA OM/EPF OM/EPO
OM//MM OM/FS OM/SCC OM/OS
OM/AD OM/LS OM/PAP
DTC Dentigerous cyst
O *Missing Teeth*

AT / AB Attrition/abrasion
E/D, H Enamel/defect, hypoplasia
CA Caries
RL1, 2, 3, 4, 5 Resorptive lesion (grade)
RR Internal root resorption
RTR Retained tooth root
RRT Retained root tip
T/A, I, LUX Tooth/ avulsed, impacted, luxated
T/FX, PE, NE Tooth/frac., pulp exposure, near PE
T/NV, V Tooth/non-vital, vital
G/B, L Granuloma/buccal, sublingual
G/E/L, P, T Eosinophilic gran./lip, palate, tongue
FB Foreign body
OST Osteomyelitis
LAC/B, L, T Laceration/buccal, lip, tongue
MN/FX MX/FX Jaw fractures
SYM/S Symphyseal separation
CFP CFL Cleft palate, Cleft lip
ONF Oronasal fistula
CMO Cranio-Mandibular Osteopathy
TMJ/D, FX, LUX TMJ/dysplasia, fracture, luxation
OTH:

N A - Extraoral/facial
N A – Lymph nodes
N A – Buccal mucosa
N A – Tongue
N A – Palate
N A – Tonsils
N A – Pharynx

Tooth	M2	M1	P4	P3	P2	P1	C	I3	I2	I1	I1	I2	I3	C	P1	P2	P3	P4	M1	M2
Triadan	110	109	108	107	106	105	104	103	102	101	201	202	203	204	205	206	207	208	209	210
Mobility																				
Recession																				
Pocket																				
Furcation																				
Hyperplasia																				
Calculus																				
Plaque																				
Gingivitis																				

Tooth	M3	M2	M1	P4	P3	P2	P1	C	I3	I2	I1	I1	I2	I3	C	P1	P2	P3	P4	M1	M2	M3
Triadan	411	410	409	408	407	406	405	404	403	402	401	301	302	303	304	305	306	307	308	309	310	311
Mobility																						
Recession																						
Pocket																						
Furcation																						
Hyperplasia																						
Calculus																						
Plaque																						
Gingivitis																						

R L

Right Left

A

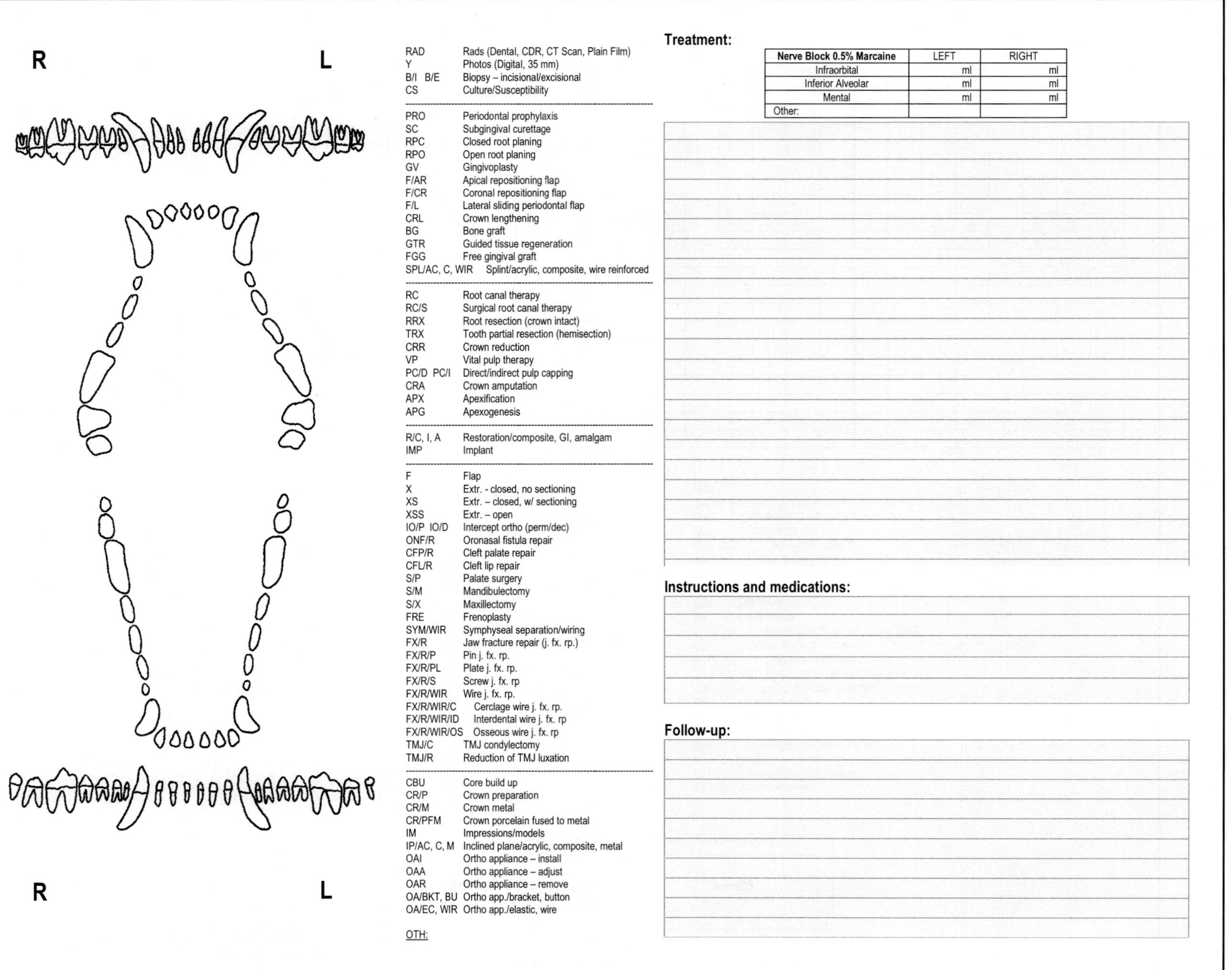

B

RAD	Rads (Dental, CDR, CT Scan, Plain Film)
Y	Photos (Digital, 35 mm)
B/I B/E	Biopsy – incisional/excisional
CS	Culture/Susceptibility
PRO	Periodontal prophylaxis
SC	Subgingival curettage
RPC	Closed root planing
RPO	Open root planing
GV	Gingivoplasty
F/AR	Apical repositioning flap
F/CR	Coronal repositioning flap
F/L	Lateral sliding periodontal flap
CRL	Crown lengthening
BG	Bone graft
GTR	Guided tissue regeneration
FGG	Free gingival graft
SPL/AC, C, WIR	Splint/acrylic, composite, wire reinforced
RC	Root canal therapy
RC/S	Surgical root canal therapy
RRX	Root resection (crown intact)
TRX	Tooth partial resection (hemisection)
CRR	Crown reduction
VP	Vital pulp therapy
PC/D PC/I	Direct/indirect pulp capping
CRA	Crown amputation
APX	Apexification
APG	Apexogenesis
R/C, I, A	Restoration/composite, GI, amalgam
IMP	Implant
F	Flap
X	Extr. - closed, no sectioning
XS	Extr. – closed, w/ sectioning
XSS	Extr. – open
IO/P IO/D	Intercept ortho (perm/dec)
ONF/R	Oronasal fistula repair
CFP/R	Cleft palate repair
CFL/R	Cleft lip repair
S/P	Palate surgery
S/M	Mandibulectomy
S/X	Maxillectomy
FRE	Frenoplasty
SYM/WIR	Symphyseal separation/wiring
FX/R	Jaw fracture repair (j. fx. rp.)
FX/R/P	Pin j. fx. rp.
FX/R/PL	Plate j. fx. rp.
FX/R/S	Screw j. fx. rp
FX/R/WIR	Wire j. fx. rp.
FX/R/WIR/C	Cerclage wire j. fx. rp.
FX/R/WIR/ID	Interdental wire j. fx. rp
FX/R/WIR/OS	Osseous wire j. fx. rp
TMJ/C	TMJ condylectomy
TMJ/R	Reduction of TMJ luxation
CBU	Core build up
CR/P	Crown preparation
CR/M	Crown metal
CR/PFM	Crown porcelain fused to metal
IM	Impressions/models
IP/AC, C, M	Inclined plane/acrylic, composite, metal
OAI	Ortho appliance – install
OAA	Ortho appliance – adjust
OAR	Ortho appliance – remove
OA/BKT, BU	Ortho app./bracket, button
OA/EC, WIR	Ortho app./elastic, wire

OTH:

Treatment:

Nerve Block 0.5% Marcaine	LEFT	RIGHT
Infraorbital	ml	ml
Inferior Alveolar	ml	ml
Mental	ml	ml
Other:		

Instructions and medications:

Follow-up:

FIGURE 32-6 Canine dental chart. **A,** Front used to document diagnosis. **B,** Back used to document treatment.

VHUP Dental Record

R L

Date:

Staff:
(circle primary staff)

Chief Complaint:

Awake Sedated Anesthetized

(Addressograph)

MAL/1 MAL/2 MAL/3 MAL/WRY
MAL/BN Malocclusion/base narrow mand. canines
MAL/ABX, PBX Mal/anterior, posterior crossbite
OC Orthodontic/genetic consultation
OR Orthodontic recheck
SN Supernumerary tooth
DT Deciduous tooth
RD Retained deciduous tooth
PD0 No perio dx (maybe calculus)
PD1 Gingivitis (no bone loss)
PD2 Mild periodontitis (< 25% attach loss)
PD3 Mod periodontitis (< 50% attach loss)
PD4 Severe periodontitis (> 50% attach loss)
GH Gingival hyperplasia
GR Gingival recession
ST Stomatitis
ST/CU Stomatitis – contact ulcer
ST/FFS Stomatitis – Feline faucitis-stomatitis
OM Oral mass:
OM/EPA OM/EPF OM/EPO
OM//MM OM/FS OM/SCC OM/OS
OM/AD OM/LS OM/PAP
DTC Dentigerous cyst
O *Missing Teeth*

AT / AB Attrition/abrasion
E/D, H Enamel/defect, hypoplasia
CA Caries
RL1, 2, 3, 4, 5 Resorptive lesion (grade)
RR Internal root resorption
RTR Retained tooth root
RRT Retained root tip
T/A, I, LUX Tooth/ avulsed, impacted, luxated
T/FX, PE, NE Tooth/frac., pulp exposure, near PE
T/NV, V Tooth/non-vital, vital
G/B, L Granuloma/buccal, sublingual
G/E/L, P, T Eosinophilic gran./lip, palate, tongue
FB Foreign body
OST Osteomyelitis
LAC/B, L, T Laceration/buccal, lip, tongue
MN/FX MX/FX Jaw fractures
SYM/S Symphyseal separation
CFP CFL Cleft palate, Cleft lip
ONF Oronasal fistula
CMO Cranio-Mandibular Osteopathy
TMJ/D, FX, LUX TMJ/dysplasia, fracture, luxation
OTH:

N A - Extraoral/facial
N A – Lymph nodes
N A – Buccal mucosa
N A – Tongue
N A – Palate
N A – Tonsils
N A – Pharynx

Tooth	M1	P4	P3	P2	C	I3	I2	I1	I1	I2	I3	C	P2	P3	P4	M1
Triadan	109	108	107	106	104	103	102	101	201	202	203	204	206	207	208	209
Mobility																
Recession																
Pocket																
Furcation																
Hyperplasia																
Calculus																
Plaque																
Gingivitis																

Tooth	M1	P4	P3	C	I3	I2	I1	I1	I2	I3	C	P3	P4	M1
Triadan	409	408	407	404	403	402	401	301	302	303	304	307	308	309
Mobility														
Recession														
Pocket														
Furcation														
Hyperplasia														
Calculus														
Plaque														
Gingivitis														

R L

Right Left

A

B

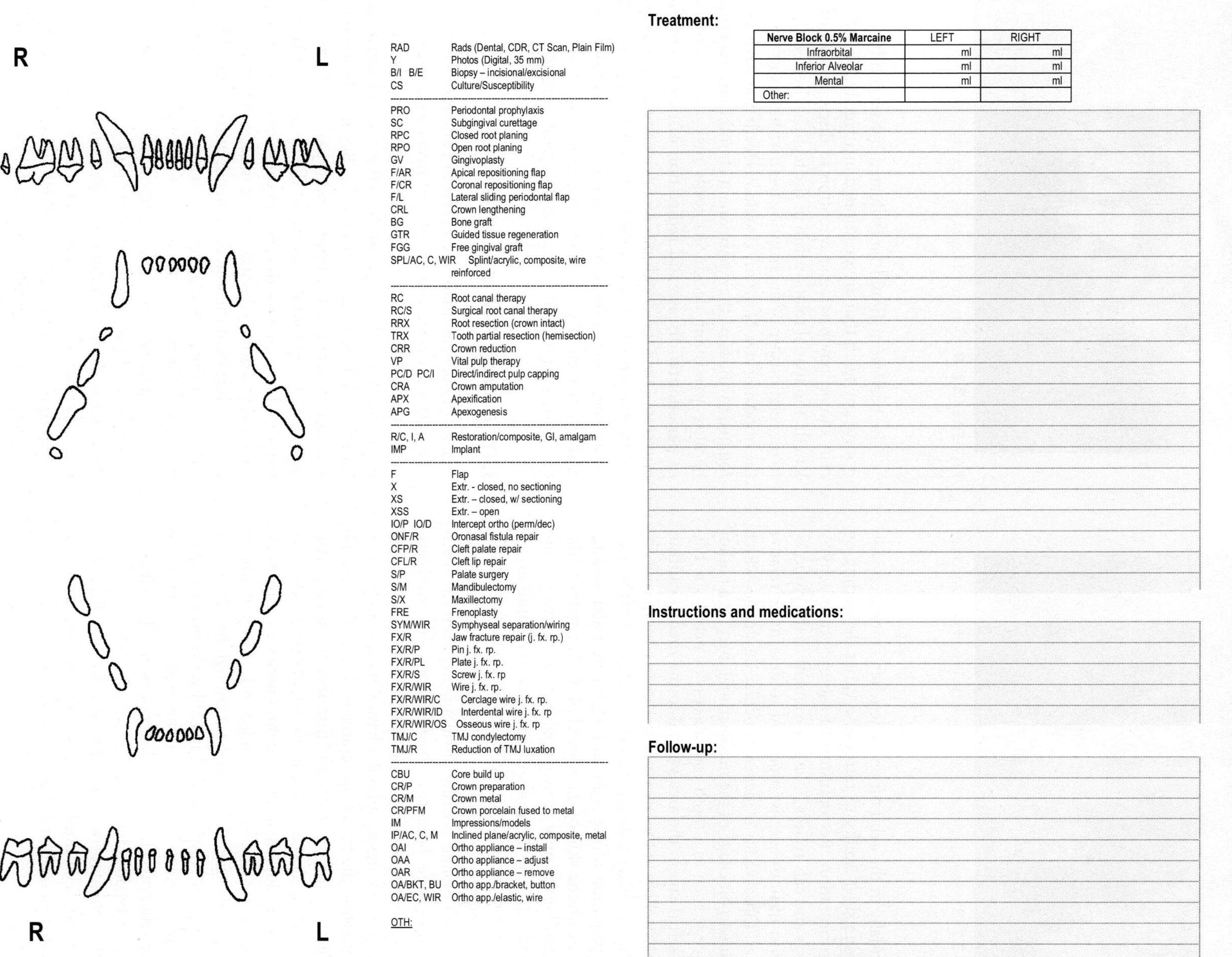

RAD	Rads (Dental, CDR, CT Scan, Plain Film)
Y	Photos (Digital, 35 mm)
B/I B/E	Biopsy – incisional/excisional
CS	Culture/Susceptibility
PRO	Periodontal prophylaxis
SC	Subgingival curettage
RPC	Closed root planing
RPO	Open root planing
GV	Gingivoplasty
F/AR	Apical repositioning flap
F/CR	Coronal repositioning flap
F/L	Lateral sliding periodontal flap
CRL	Crown lengthening
BG	Bone graft
GTR	Guided tissue regeneration
FGG	Free gingival graft
SPL/AC, C, WIR	Splint/acrylic, composite, wire reinforced
RC	Root canal therapy
RC/S	Surgical root canal therapy
RRX	Root resection (crown intact)
TRX	Tooth partial resection (hemisection)
CRR	Crown reduction
VP	Vital pulp therapy
PC/D PC/I	Direct/indirect pulp capping
CRA	Crown amputation
APX	Apexification
APG	Apexogenesis
R/C, I, A	Restoration/composite, GI, amalgam
IMP	Implant
F	Flap
X	Extr. - closed, no sectioning
XS	Extr. – closed, w/ sectioning
XSS	Extr. – open
IO/P IO/D	Intercept ortho (perm/dec)
ONF/R	Oronasal fistula repair
CFP/R	Cleft palate repair
CFL/R	Cleft lip repair
S/P	Palate surgery
S/M	Mandibulectomy
S/X	Maxillectomy
FRE	Frenoplasty
SYM/WIR	Symphyseal separation/wiring
FX/R	Jaw fracture repair (j. fx. rp.)
FX/R/P	Pin j. fx. rp.
FX/R/PL	Plate j. fx. rp.
FX/R/S	Screw j. fx. rp
FX/R/WIR	Wire j. fx. rp.
FX/R/WIR/C	Cerclage wire j. fx. rp.
FX/R/WIR/ID	Interdental wire j. fx. rp
FX/R/WIR/OS	Osseous wire j. fx. rp
TMJ/C	TMJ condylectomy
TMJ/R	Reduction of TMJ luxation
CBU	Core build up
CR/P	Crown preparation
CR/M	Crown metal
CR/PFM	Crown porcelain fused to metal
IM	Impressions/models
IP/AC, C, M	Inclined plane/acrylic, composite, metal
OAI	Ortho appliance – install
OAA	Ortho appliance – adjust
OAR	Ortho appliance – remove
OA/BKT, BU	Ortho app./bracket, button
OA/EC, WIR	Ortho app./elastic, wire

OTH:

Treatment:

Nerve Block 0.5% Marcaine	LEFT	RIGHT
Infraorbital	ml	ml
Inferior Alveolar	ml	ml
Mental	ml	ml
Other:		

Instructions and medications:

Follow-up:

FIGURE 32-7 Feline dental chart. A, Front used to document diagnosis. B, Back used to document treatment.

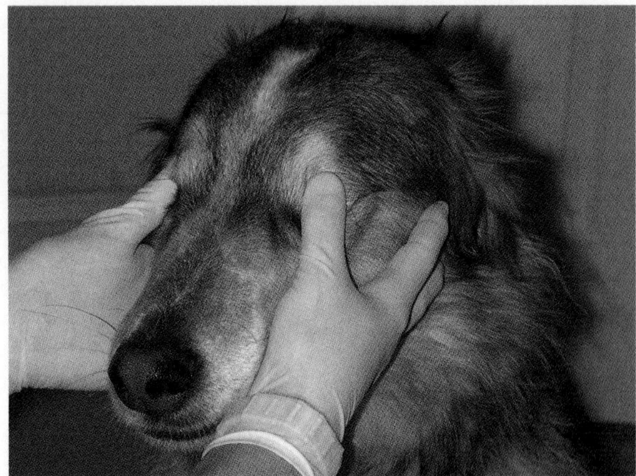

FIGURE 32-8 Retropulsion of both eyes is an important component of the extraoral examination.

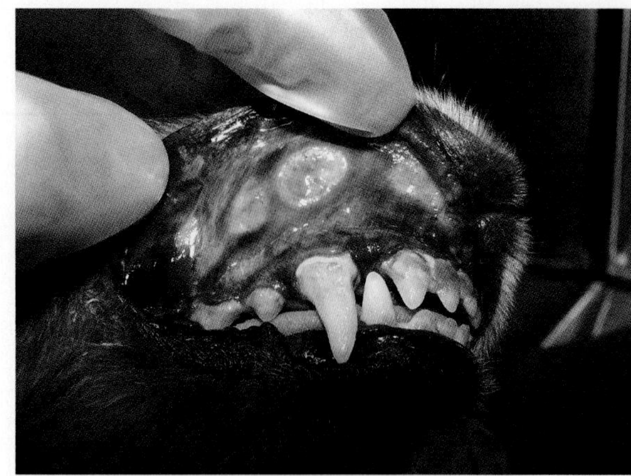

FIGURE 32-9 Chronic ulcerative paradental stomatitis in a dog (CUPS).

move caudally in the orbit on one side when compared with the opposite side. Ability to retropulse varies depending on facial conformation. Retropulsion of the eyes of brachycephalic dogs and cats results in less movement of the globe, so comparison of both eyes is important to determine relative differences. Observe for evidence of ocular discharge, which may be due to blockage of the nasolacrimal duct by a pathologic process, such as a tooth root abscess or neoplasia. Palpate the soft tissue in the area ventral to the medial canthus of the eye. Swelling in this area may be due to a tooth root abscess of the maxillary fourth premolar. Evaluation of the neck includes palpation of the right and left mandibular salivary glands beneath the skin of the ventral neck. The mandibular salivary gland is the only easily palpable major salivary gland in dogs and cats. The three other major salivary glands are either too diffuse to palpate easily (parotid, sublingual glands) or are not superficial enough to palpate (zygomatic gland). The mandibular gland is easily distinguished from the mandibular lymph nodes because it is softer, larger than, and caudomedial to the mandibular lymph nodes. Once the salivary glands are located, the mandibular lymph nodes can be identified by moving the finger tips cranially. Palpate the lymph nodes bilaterally for symmetry and firmness. In the cat, mandibular lymph nodes are difficult to palpate unless they are enlarged. In the dog, mandibular lymph nodes are almost always palpable, ranging in size from 0.5 to 1.5 cm in diameter depending on the size of the patient. Although we often refer to the mandibular lymph "node," in reality, the area contains anywhere from one to five nodes. Other nodes that drain the head (retropharyngeal, parotid) are not normally palpable. Nine percent of dogs have another lymph node that is palpable in the subcutaneous tissue dorsal to the maxillary third premolar tooth. This node is referred to as the facial or buccal lymph node and is often bilateral, when present.

> *TECHNICIAN NOTE* The major salivary glands of the dog and cat are the paired mandibular, sublingual, zygomatic, and parotid glands.

The occlusion should be evaluated before intubation by noting any teeth that are positioned incorrectly. The technician should pay particular attention to discrepancies of jaw length, the spatial relationship of the teeth as they erupt, and to the relationship of the erupting teeth with the soft tissues of the opposing jaw. Note any deciduous teeth that have not exfoliated by the time their permanent counterpart has erupted because persistent deciduous teeth may create situations of periodontal disease and redirection of permanent tooth eruption. Once the deciduous and permanent canines begin to erupt, routinely monitor the relationship of the mandibular canines and the space between the maxillary third incisor and canine teeth. Deviations from normal canine positioning can cause trauma to the palate and require treatment.

INTRAORAL EXAMINATION

The intraoral examination consists of evaluations of the soft tissues of the oral cavity, the dental structures, and the periodontium, a term that describes the supporting structures of the teeth. A standard approach to the oral examination allows for efficiency and thoroughness. Begin by observing the skin and mucosa of the upper and lower lips. Some breeds are prone to lip fold dermatitis of the lip area caudal to the mandibular canine tooth that can cause oral malodor unrelated to periodontal disease. Buccal mucosa refers to the mucosa that begins at the mucocutaneous junction and lines the cheeks and lips. Alveolar mucosa refers to the mucosa that lies against the bone of the upper or lower jaw, which meets with the gingiva at the mucogingival junction. The normal appearance of the mucosa may be pink or pigmented, and the mucosa should exhibit no lesions, ulcerations, or swellings. Pay particular attention to areas of mucosa that lay adjacent to periodontally diseased teeth because the bacteria in the plaque may contribute to painful mucosal ulcerations, often referred to as chronic ulcerative paradental stomatitis (CUPS) (Figure 32-9). Observe the caudal cheek lining in the region of the carnassial and molar teeth. This mucosa frequently becomes pressed between the teeth during chewing, creating a condition known as "cheek chewing lesions"

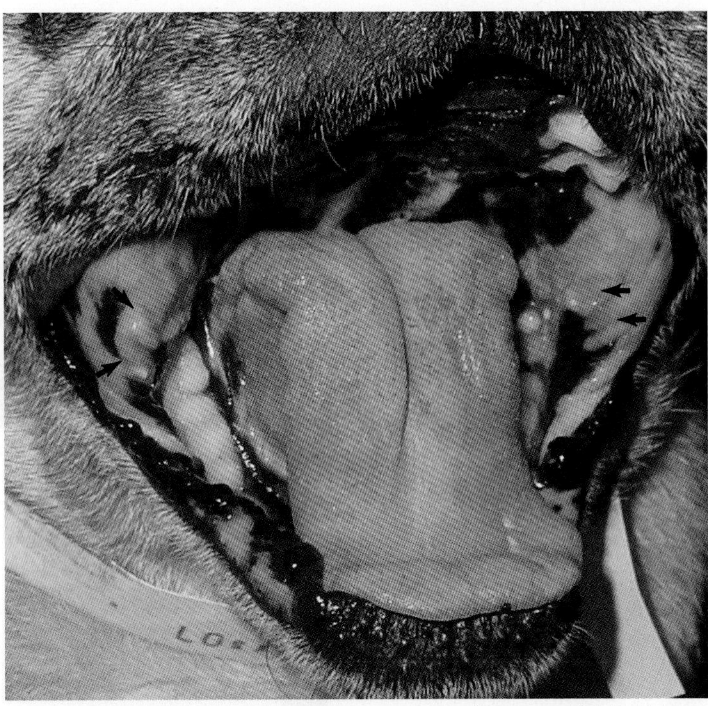

FIGURE 32-10 Bilateral cheek chewing lesions in a dog *(arrows)*. These lesions can be proliferative and sometimes ulcerated.

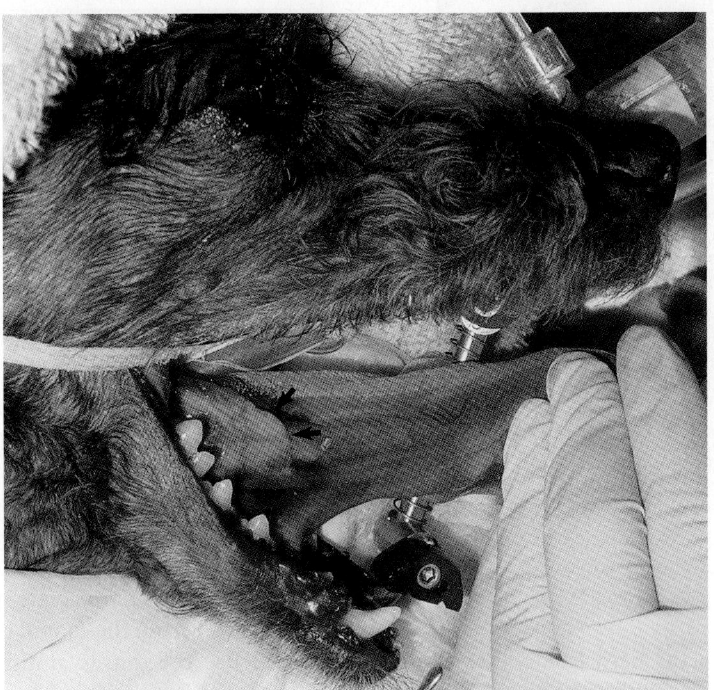

FIGURE 32-11 Tongue chewing lesion in a dog *(arrows)*.

(Figure 32-10). Similarly, mucosa beneath the tongue may also show signs of chewing lesions referred to as "tongue chewing lesions," which are usually bilateral (Figure 32-11). These lesions usually do not require treatment unless the lesions are not bilaterally similar or if the lesions are ulcerated. In these cases, the affected mucosa may be removed and submitted for histopathologic evaluation.

Two raised bumps are found on the alveolar mucosa dorsal to the maxillary fourth premolar and first molar teeth. Salivary secretions from the parotid and zygomatic salivary glands travel through ducts leading to these duct openings (Figure 32-12).

The roof of the mouth is composed of the hard and soft palate. The hard palate forms the rostral two thirds and is covered by palatal mucosa arranged in prominent ridges, called rugae (Figure 32-13). These rugae range from eight to ten in number. In brachycephalic dogs, the rugae are closely positioned, and hair and debris can accumulate in these

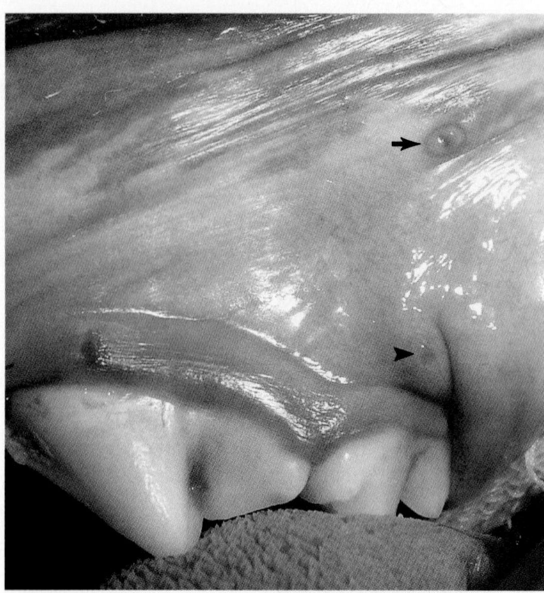

FIGURE 32-12 Parotid *(arrow)* and zygomatic duct opening in a dog *(arrowhead)*. When the mucosa is not retracted caudally, the parotid opening is rostral and dorsal to the zygomatic duct opening.

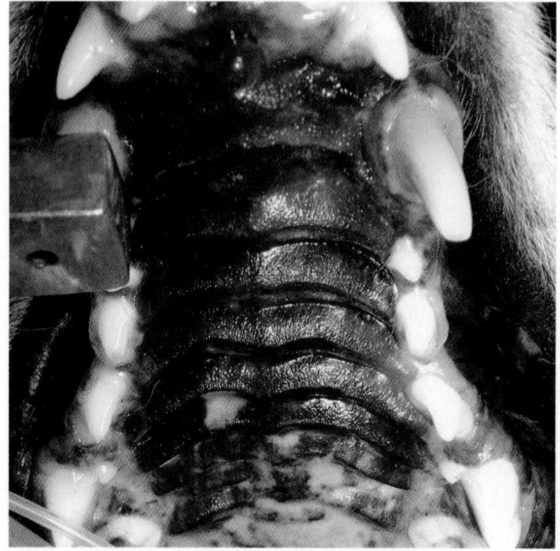

FIGURE 32-13 Palatal rugae in a dog. The rugae may be widely spaced in dolichocephalic dogs or close together in brachycephalic dogs.

rugal folds. On the midline of the hard palate, just caudal to the incisor teeth, the incisive papilla is a round, slightly raised structure (Figure 32-14). Lateral to the incisive papilla, a small bilateral communication with the incisive duct and vomeronasal organ exist. The vomeronasal organ is a sensory organ involved in detection of pheromones and other chemical compounds. Palpation of the area lateral to the incisive papilla may normally feel as if there is air trapped beneath the mucosa as a result of the communication between the mouth and these nasal structures. The soft palate consists of mucosa and muscle that separate the oropharynx and nasopharynx. Two prominent bony structures can be palpated just lateral to the midline of the soft palate that are

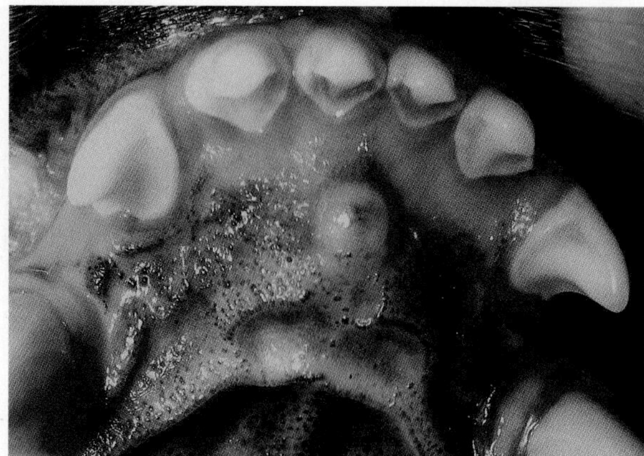

FIGURE 32-14 Incisive papilla in a dog. The left and right incisive ducts open on the lateral aspects of the papilla.

the hamular processes of the bilateral pterygoid bones. If one or both hamular processes are difficult to palpate, this may be due to the presence of a nasopharyngeal mass.

> *TECHNICIAN NOTE* The incisive papilla is a raised structure located on the midline behind the maxillary incisors in dogs and cats.

The pharynx should be evaluated for evidence of inflammation or neoplasia. When the patient's mouth is open, bilateral folds of pharyngeal mucosa will be evident lateral to the tongue. These are referred to as the palatoglossal folds, and this area and the mucosa lateral to these folds may be inflamed in cats with lymphocytic-plasmacytic stomatitis (LPS) (Figure 32-15).

Gently hold the tip of the tongue to enable visual examination of the dorsal, ventral, and lateral surfaces. Lift the tongue to observe the mucosa of the floor of the mouth and the base of the tongue. In the awake patient, the examiner's thumb may be used extraorally to push the tongue dorsally for better visualization of the ventral surface of the tongue. The dorsal surface of the tongue is covered by thousands of papillae, some of which contain taste buds. The large, distinctive papillae located at the caudal third of the tongue are the vallate papillae, which are spaced in a curved line separating the body from the root of the tongue. Depress the tongue to visualize the tonsils, noting any enlargement or change in color or texture. The color of a normal tonsil is typically more hyperemic than the color of the adjacent mucosa. Normal tonsils may be fully contained within the tonsillar crypt and may be difficult to visualize.

During the soft tissue examination, any tissue variations from normal should be described by recording the size, shape, color, surface texture, and consistency (e.g., soft, firm, hard, or fluctuant). A dedicated area on the dental record may be created to allow for documentation of any abnormalities of oral soft tissue structures (see Figures 32-6, *A* and 32-7, *A*).

The next step in the intraoral examination is evaluation of the teeth and their supporting structures. First, determine

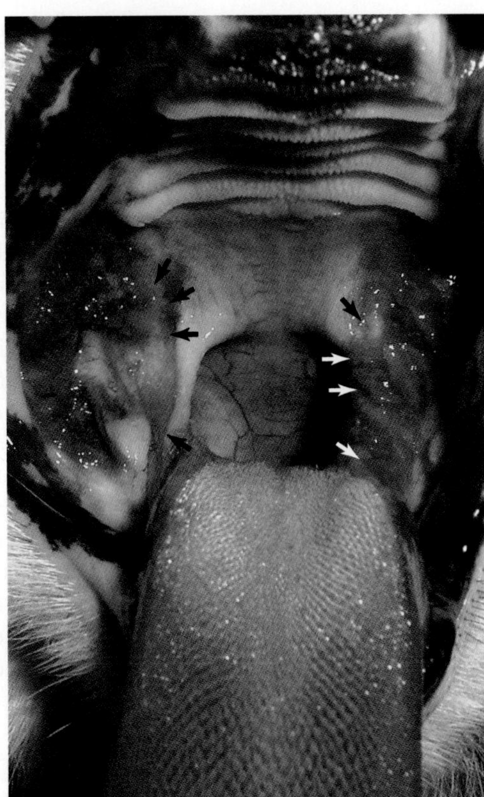

FIGURE 32-15 Caudal stomatitis in the area lateral to the palatoglossal folds *(arrows)* in a cat.

the presence or absence of teeth in each quadrant. Missing teeth can be documented on the dental chart by darkening or circling the missing tooth. Further radiographic evaluation of areas of missing teeth is imperative because dentigerous cysts can develop as a result of an unerupted tooth. To evaluate the condition of the teeth and periodontium, the technician must use a periodontal probe and dental explorer. These dental instruments are important clinical tools for obtaining data about the health status of each tooth. Consider the canine mouth as containing 42 patients and the feline mouth containing 30 patients, each patient requiring a thorough evaluation. The periodontal probe has a handle with a round or flat rectangular working end that is marked in millimeter increments, ending in a blunt tip. The probe is used like a miniature intraoral ruler to measure attachment levels, sulcus and pocket depths, loss of bone in furcation areas, and size of oral lesions. It is also used to assess the mobility of teeth and the presence of gingival bleeding. Periodontal probes are available in an assortment of design styles, with variations in thickness of the diameter of the working end and variations in increments of millimeter markings (Figure 32-16). Probes with Williams' markings have millimeter increments at 1, 2, 3, 5, 7, 8, 9, and 10 mm. The UNC 15 probe has millimeter markings at 1, 2, 3, 4, 5, 6, 7, 8, 9, 10, 11, 12, 13, 14, and 15 mm, which is useful for large dogs or patients with deep periodontal pockets. Some probes have a small 0.5-mm ball on the end to minimize tissue trauma; however, these probes typically have markings at 3.5, 5.5, 8.5, and 11.5 mm, resulting in inexact determination of pocket depth. Although many probes exist, a probe

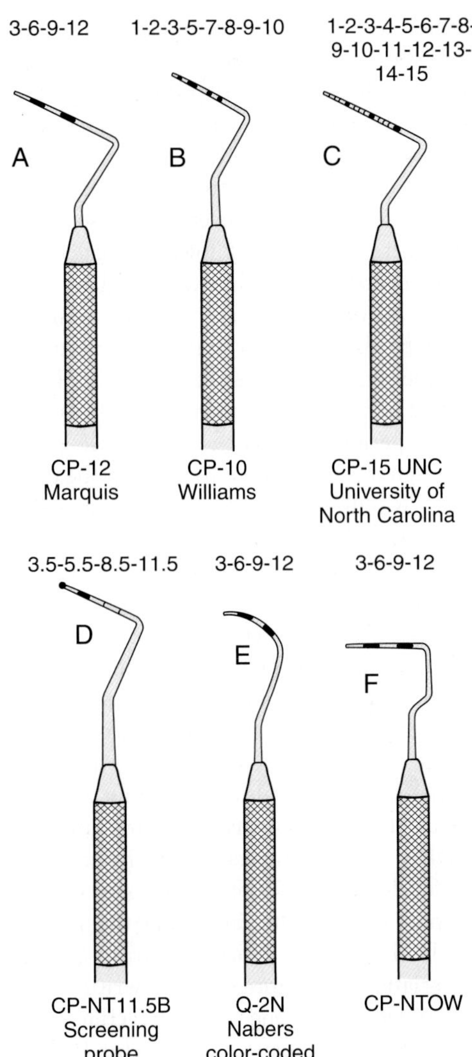

FIGURE 32-16 Periodontal probes with different calibrations. The blunt-tipped working end is used to measure sulcus or pocket depth, tooth mobility, furcation involvement, gingival recession, and gingival hyperplasia. (From Daniel SJ, Harfst SA, Wilder R: *Mosby's dental hygiene: concepts, cases, and competencies*, ed 2, St Louis, 2008, Mosby.)

with markings beginning at 1 mm is necessary for assessing subtle pocket depths in cats. The Michigan "O" probe with Williams' markings is best suited for use in cats because the working end of the probe is the narrowest in diameter. Some styles contain color-coded bands for easier viewing of calibrations. A Naber's probe is a curved furcation probe that is used to assess the extent of bone loss in the furcation area.

> *TECHNICIAN NOTE* The normal sulcus depth is 0 to 3 mm in dogs and 0 to 1 mm in cats. Probing depths greater than normal are documented on the chart as pockets.

The dental explorer has a slender, wirelike working end that tapers to a sharp point and is used to explore the topography of the tooth surface. When the explorer is held with a light modified pen grasp, the technician will acquire a tactile sense to locate tooth surface irregularities, such as caries, feline resorption, calculus deposits, and pulp exposure. Tactile sensitivity is achieved when the flexible working end of the explorer vibrates as it detects surface irregularities. The vibrations are transmitted from the tip to the handle as felt by the technician. The explorer is also used to determine the completeness of treatment following calculus débridement and to ensure smooth transitions of dental restoratives (fillings). Several designs of explorers are available (Figure 32-17). Varying degrees of flexibility contribute to the degrees of tactile sensitivity. The shepherd's hook is the most common explorer in most veterinary practices and is often paired with a periodontal probe as a double-ended instrument. Although it is convenient to have on the opposite end of a probe, it is bulky, inflexible, and less adaptable to subgingival use when compared with other explorers. The Orban explorer has a 2-mm tip that is bent at a 90-degree angle from the shank, allowing it to be used subgingivally with little tissue distention (stretching of the gingiva away from the tooth) or trauma to the epithelial lining of the sulcus. The 2-mm tip may be a limitation when using the Orban to determine depth of a dental lesion, such as caries or feline resorption. The curved 11/12 ODU explorer is an ideal choice for veterinary use. The curvature of the long shank and working ends make it adaptable to use on rostral and caudal teeth, supragingivally and subgingivally, and its smaller working end allows for detection of subtle hard tissue defects.

Periodontal instruments, including the probe and explorer, are held with a modified pen grasp (Figure 32-18), which is a variation of the grasp used for writing. This recommended grasp facilitates good fingertip tactile sensitivity and precise control of the instrument's working end, decreasing risk of trauma to the tissues. The modified pen grasp uses three fingertips placed in a triangular (tripod) position, plus a rest finger. The pads of the index finger and thumb rest on the instrument where the handle and shank meet to hold the instrument. The pad near the fingernail of the middle finger rests on the shank. The shank is the portion of the instrument that connects the handle with the working end (Figure 32-19). Proper placement of the middle fingertip pad against the shank is important for enhancing tactile sensitivity and helping to guide and control the working end. The ring finger should rest on an oral structure, such as a tooth located close to the working area, to provide stability of the hand for added control. Keeping the ring finger in contact with the middle finger will ensure proper wrist motion by limiting the amount of finger motion and will prevent finger fatigue. The little finger should be relaxed and has no specific function in this grasp.

The assessment of the periodontium and teeth should begin at the midline of the mouth and systematically evaluate each tooth, one at a time, by using both visual observation and tactile use of the probe and explorer. Begin detecting excessive tooth mobility by placing the tip of the probe against the tip of the tooth and gently attempting to move the tooth in a buccolingual direction. Movement is estimated on a scale of 1, 2, or 3, based on the number of millimeters beyond normal physiologic mobility the tooth moves in one direction (Box 32-3). A slight amount of movement is normal as a result of the periodontal ligament that connects the tooth to alveolar bone. The most severe mobility, a classification of 3, includes any tooth with vertical movement. As each tooth is approached to check for mobility, visually notice the characteristics of the gingiva for color, shape, texture, and consistency. Healthy gingival tissues are pink (except where normally pigmented), stippled (orange peel appearance),

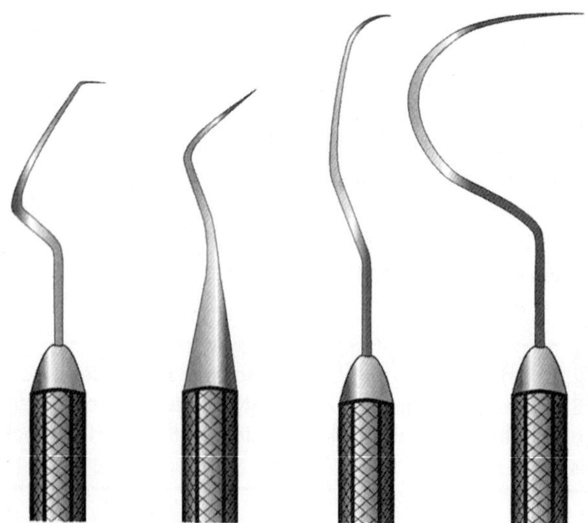

FIGURE 32-17 Dental explorers with sharp wirelike tips are used to explore the topography of the tooth surfaces: *(left to right)* Orban, Pigtail, 11/12 ODU, shepherd's hook. (From Nelson DM: *Saunders review of dental hygiene,* Philadelphia, 2000, WB Saunders.)

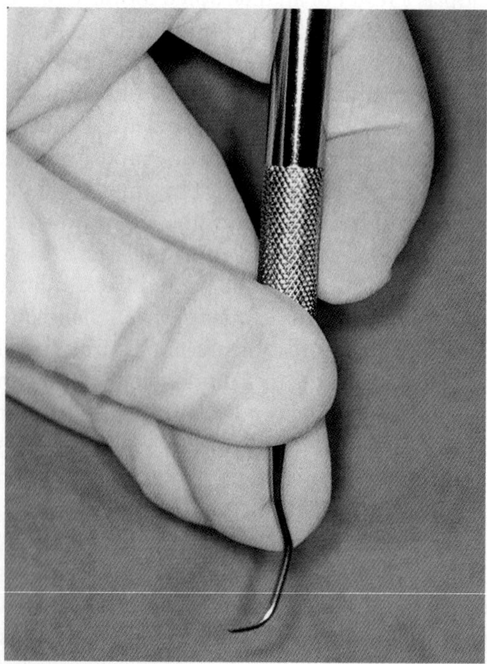

FIGURE 32-18 Modified pen grasp hand position for periodontal instrumentation: the thumb and index finger hold the instrument handle; the corner of the middle finger rests on the shank. The ring finger is used as a fulcrum and for control.

firm, tapered to a thin margin, and scalloped to follow the contour of the cementoenamel junction (CEJ) and underlying alveolar bone. Any area of the gingiva that deviates from these normal characteristics should be examined closer by use of the probe.

> *TECHNICIAN NOTE* The periodontium, the term describing the attachment structures of the teeth, includes gingival connective tissue, alveolar bone, periodontal ligament, and cementum.

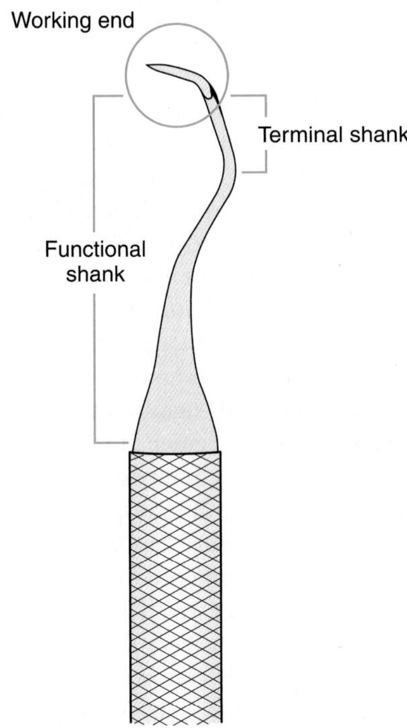

FIGURE 32-19 Parts of the instrument include the handle, shank, and working end. The functional shank extends from the handle to the working end, and the terminal shank is the part of the shank closest to the working end. (From Daniel SJ, Harfst SA, Wilder R: *Mosby's dental hygiene: concepts, cases, and competencies*, ed 2, St Louis, 2008, Mosby.)

BOX 32-3 Mobility Scoring Index

- Stage 0 (M0): Physiologic mobility up to 0.2 mm.
- Stage 1 (M1): The mobility is increased in any direction other than axial over a distance of more than 0.2 mm and up to 0.5 mm.
- Stage 2 (M2): The mobility is increased in any direction other than axial over a distance of more than 0.5 mm and up to 1.0 mm.
- Stage 3 (M3): The mobility is increased in any direction other than axial over a distance exceeding 1.0 mm or any axial movement.
- (Axial movement refers to movement in the long axis of the tooth.)

With permission of AVDC, www.AVDC.org/Nomenclature.pdf.

The probe is gently inserted into the sulcus or pocket, ensuring that the probe is kept as close to parallel to the long axis of the root as possible, with the side of the probe tip in contact with the tooth. When physical resistance is felt at the base of the sulcus or pocket, note the marking level on the probe that is adjacent to the gingival margin. The probe is then "walked" around the tooth using up and down bobbing strokes approximately 1 to 2 mm in height (↕) and in 1- to 2-mm horizontal steps (↔) to assess the entire circumference of the tooth (Figure 32-20). Abnormal measurements (those greater than 3 mm in dogs, greater than 1 mm in cats) should be noted on the dental chart along with the specific location of the pocket measurement (i.e., MB for mesiobuccal). Probe measurements between millimeter markings are rounded up to the larger measurement. For accurate readings, it is essential for the technician to develop skills in consistent probing forces (between 10 to 20 g of pressure). This pressure amount can be practiced by pressing the probe tip into the pad of a thumb until the skin is depressed approximately 2 mm.

In areas where the height of the free gingival margin has migrated apically toward or beyond the CEJ, the probe is used to measure gingival recession. Recession is measured in millimeters from the CEJ to the level of the gingival margin. Attachment loss is a term that more truly describes the periodontal state of a tooth because it accounts for both pocket depth and gingival recession (Figure 32-21). Gingival hyperplasia occurs when the free gingival margin migrates coronally, toward the crown of the tooth. Hyperplasia is measured in millimeters from the bottom of the sulcus to the gingival margin, which is covering a portion of the tooth crown. An increased pocket depth may be due to hyperplasia or attachment loss, so clinical examination findings are necessary to determine if the increased probing depth is due to a true pocket or a pseudopocket.

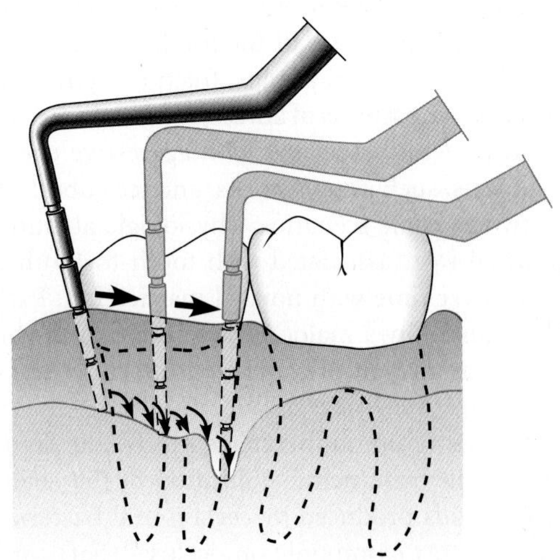

FIGURE 32-20 While keeping the side of the tip of the probe in contact with the tooth and using a light touch, the probe is "walked" around the circumference of the tooth with short up-and-down strokes every few millimeters. (From Newman MG, Takei H, Klokkevold PR et al: *Carranza's clinical periodontology*, ed 10, St Louis, 2006, Saunders.)

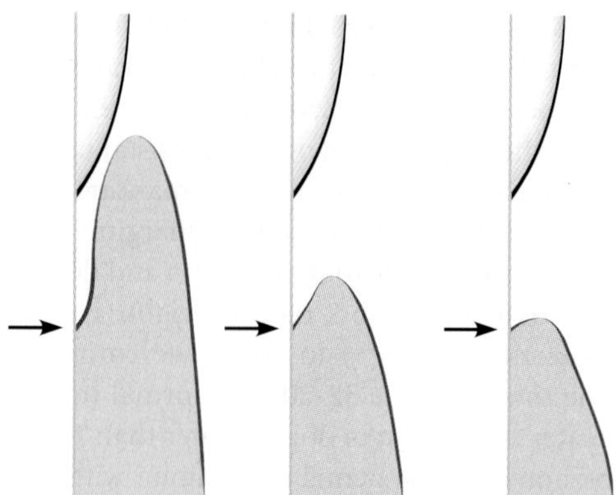

FIGURE 32-21 Attachment level is measured from the bottom of the pocket *(arrows)* to a fixed point on the tooth, such as the CEJ. Attachment level is a better indicator of periodontal status than pocket depth because gingival recession or hyperplasia can greatly affect pocket depth measurement. Note the three examples that have the same level of attachment loss yet different pocket depths, as a result of gingival recession. (From Newman MG, Takei H, Klokkevold PR et al: *Carranza's clinical periodontology,* ed 10, St Louis, 2006, Saunders.)

When approaching multirooted teeth, the probe is used to assess loss of bone in the areas between and around the roots. A bifurcation is the furcation between two-rooted teeth and should be assessed from the buccal and lingual-palatal surfaces. Trifurcations of three-rooted teeth should be assessed between each of the three roots. The extent of bone loss determines the furcation classification (Box 32-4). A Naber's furcation probe is curved to fit over the dental bulge of the crown so that the side of the tip can be held as parallel as possible to the long axis of the tooth. The tip is dragged horizontally across a root, dipping into the furcation area and continuing to the adjacent root. The depth of penetration into the furcation area determines the classification. If a straight probe is used, care must be taken to minimize tissue distention.

During the periodontal evaluation of each tooth, also observe the hard structures of the tooth and use the dental explorer when noticing any chips, fractures, pulp exposure, or abnormal wear patterns of abrasion or attrition. Abrasion refers to tooth wear associated with aggressive chewing on external objects, such as toys, rocks, and ice cubes. Attrition refers to two possible scenarios. Physiologic attrition refers to the normal wear associated with tooth-to-tooth contact of a patient over time with normal mastication. Pathologic attrition is caused by a malocclusion resulting in abnormal wear of teeth as a result of contact with teeth of the opposing jaw.

Dental caries (commonly referred to by the lay term of "cavities") result from demineralization of the enamel and dentin from acids produced by certain oral bacteria. These lesions occur most commonly on occlusal (flat) surfaces of the molar teeth. Gently explore for pits and fissures of the occlusal surfaces of the maxillary first and second molars and the distal half of the mandibular first molar, feeling for areas of demineralization. Use the explorer to check for clinical signs of feline resorptive lesions by dragging the sharp point

BOX 32-4 Furcation Involvement/Exposure Index

- Stage 1 (F1, furcation involvement) exists when a periodontal probe extends less than halfway under the crown in any direction of a multirooted tooth with attachment loss.
- Stage 2 (F2, furcation involvement) exists when a periodontal probe extends greater than halfway under the crown of a multirooted tooth with attachment loss but not through and through.
- Stage 3 (F3, furcation exposure) exists when a periodontal probe extends under the crown of a multirooted tooth, through and through from one side of the furcation out the other.

With permission of AVDC, www.AVDC.org/Nomenclature.pdf.

horizontally across the cervical portion of each tooth. Sometimes it is challenging to determine whether a concavity in the area of a furcation is a resorptive lesion or merely mild furcation exposure. If a resorptive lesion is present, the explorer tip will "catch" on the edge of the concavity, whereas the explorer will freely move out of the concave area as easily as it fell into it when encountering mild furcation exposure. When tooth fractures are present, gently drag the sharp point of the explorer across the tooth surface, feeling for any openings into the pulp. Teeth with significant abrasion may have a brown or black dot in the center of the worn tooth. This can be a sign of either chronic pulp exposure or a reparative material produced by the tooth in response to chronic wear (tertiary dentin). Pulp exposure can be distinguished from tertiary dentin by use of an explorer. If a tooth has pulp exposure, the tip of the explorer will "fall into a hole," whereas a discolored area caused by tertiary dentin will feel smooth as glass when the explorer is run over this area. This is an important clinical distinction because treatment of pulp-exposed teeth is necessary, but worn teeth with tertiary dentin usually do not require treatment (Figure 32-22, *A, B*).

DENTAL RADIOGRAPHY

Intraoral radiographs are essential for planning and assessing outcome of dental treatment for dogs, cats, and exotic species. Intraoral radiography is also used in horses, but is limited to the most rostral teeth because of difficulties in accessing the caudal teeth and small film size. Radiographs provide the clinician with an important diagnostic tool to detect pathologic conditions that are not clinically visible in the mouth. The following are types of pathologic findings for which dental radiographs are useful: root resorption, caries, periapical radiolucency (often seen with tooth root abscesses), periodontal bone loss, retained root tips, unerupted teeth, osteomyelitis, neoplasia, tooth and jaw fractures, foreign bodies, and disease of the temporomandibular joint (TMJ). The veterinary patient must be sedated or anesthetized to obtain quality dental radiographs. Intraoral dental radiography is becoming more routine in general veterinary practice.

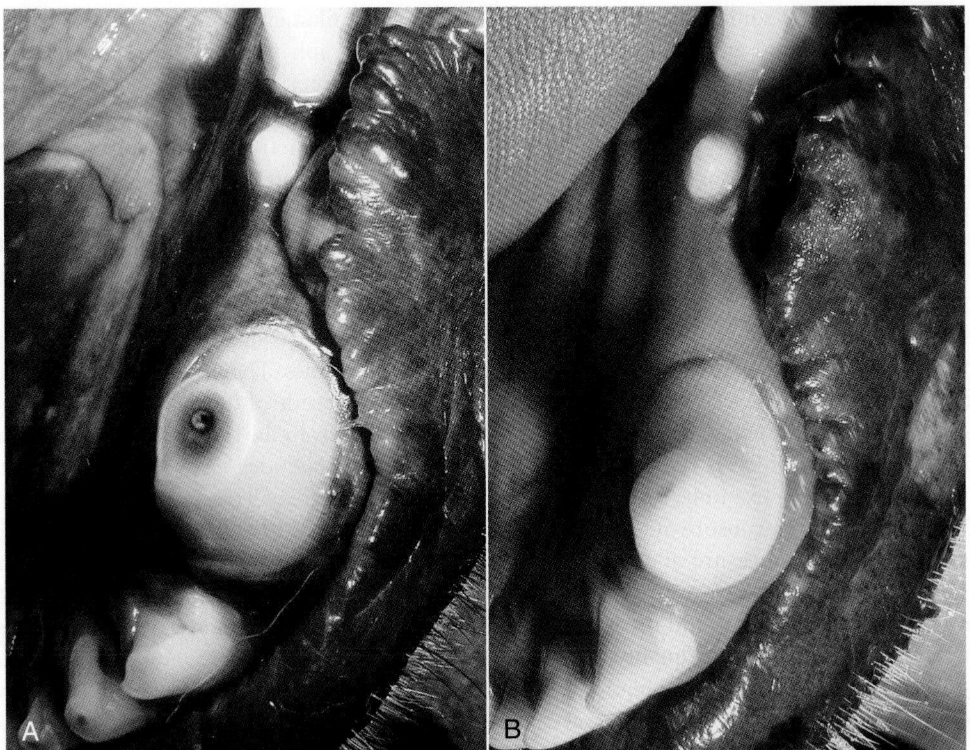

FIGURE 32-22 Abrasion of two canine teeth from different patients. **A,** Abrasion has occurred rapidly enough to result in pulp exposure, determined by running an explorer over the flat surface and "falling into" the pulp chamber. **B,** Abrasion has occurred slowly enough to allow the tooth to respond by producing tertiary (reparative) dentin, which feels smooth as glass when explored. Both teeth should be radiographed to assess for endodontic pathologic conditions, but the pulp-exposed tooth definitely requires extraction or root canal therapy.

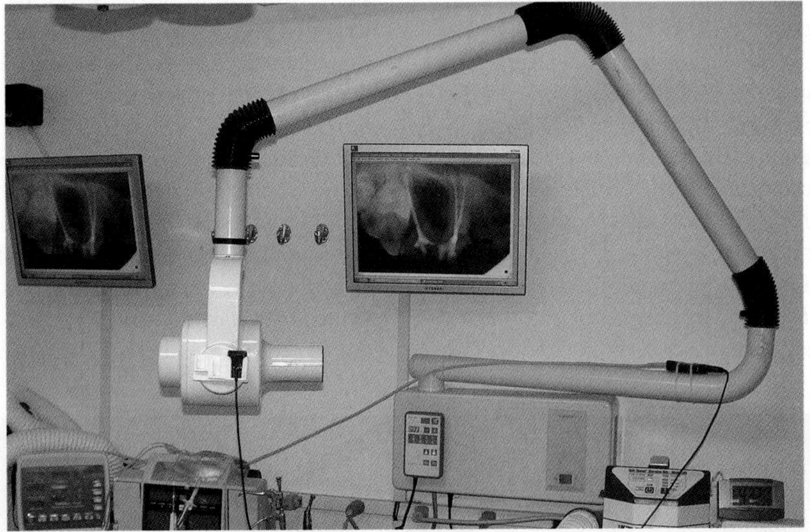

FIGURE 32-23 Intraoral radiograph machine control panel, arm, and tube head. (From DuPont GA, DeBowes LJ: *Atlas of dental radiography in dogs and cats,* St Louis, 2009, Saunders/Elsevier.)

EQUIPMENT

The dental x-ray machine may be wall mounted, or it may stand on the floor with wheels that permit storage when not in use. The unit is composed of three primary parts, the control panel, a long (72- to 86-inch) arm that extends from the control panel, and a tube head that is attached to the end of the arm (Figure 32-23). The control panel, typically mounted to a wall near the dental workstation, contains the power switch, selector buttons for kilovoltage and milliamperes, a dial or buttons for changing exposure time, and a button that is located at the end of a 6-foot coiled cord. Many dental x-ray units have an internally set level of kilovoltage and milliamperes, and only exposure time may be changed for a darker or lighter technique. The timing selection may also be located at the end of the cord of some newer models. An indicator light and an audible sound are emitted from the control panel when exposure is made.

> *TECHNICIAN NOTE* The dental radiograph machine should be inspected regularly for leakage. Many states require such inspections.

The milliamperage (mA) setting regulates the intensity of the electric current that heats the filament (cathode), thus controlling the quantity of electrons produced and available to bombard the target (anode). Milliampere seconds (mAs) describes the quantity of radiation, which is the milliamperes multiplied by the exposure time. For example, a film exposed for ½ second at 10 mA would be an exposure of 5 mAs.

The peak kilovoltage (kVp) is a measure of electric force that regulates the speed at which the electrons travel between the negatively charged cathode (filament) and the positively charged anode (target), thus controlling the quality of the x-ray beam. When the electrons hit the anode at a higher force, x-rays produced have a greater penetrating power at the surface of the skin. Most dental machines operate at 60 or 70 kVp. Low kilovoltage settings result in images with high black-white contrast, useful in detecting caries or resorption. High kilovoltage settings result in low contrast with a wider gray scale between the black-white densities, which is useful in monitoring periodontal disease.

The cathode and anode are housed in the Coolidge tube located in the tube head at the end of the articulating arm. Within the tube head, the Coolidge tube is immersed in oil to help absorb the heat produced at the target. The position-indicating device (PID) contains a collimator that controls the beam size. Varying from 8 to 16 inches in length, the PID extends from the tube head to the patient's mouth and aids in minimizing scattered radiation.

The timer switch starts the production of the x-rays. Timers may be calibrated in fractions of seconds or numbers of impulses. Once the timer is activated, a short delay occurs while the filament is preheating. With experienced use of the radiograph machine, the technician will be able to determine proper exposure times based on the size of the patient and the density of the tissues through which the x-ray beam must penetrate. It is helpful to create an exposure time chart to post near the control panel for quick reference. New machine models marketed for veterinary use provide timers with preset exposure times associated with pictures of the dental arcade. The technician only needs to select the dog or cat, patient size, and specific tooth.

All veterinary staff must become familiar with radiation safety guidelines. The timer switch can be remotely wired and mounted outside of the dental treatment room or at least 6 to 8 feet away from the tube head. Standing at a distance behind a barrier or at a 90-degree to 130-degree angle that is perpendicular to the beam will place the technician at a safe position away from the direction of the beam. The film should never be held in the patient's mouth by the technician while the radiograph is taken; therefore anesthesia is necessary not only to ensure diagnostic quality films, but also for safety reasons. Make certain that the machine is inspected regularly for leakage by a competent radiation expert, as may be required by state regulations. Development of skills will minimize unnecessary radiation from retakes resulting from poor technique or positioning.

FILM

Intraoral film consists of a plastic base covered on both sides with emulsion of silver halide crystals. The film is wrapped in black paper with a lead foil backing placed on the side that will be farthest from the beam. The lead foil prevents scatter radiation from affecting the back side of the film. The film, paper, and foil are wrapped in either a plastic or paper packet. This type of film is considered direct exposure or nonscreen film. The white surface of the film wrapper should always be placed in the mouth so that it faces the beam, and the colored surface of the film wrapper is placed away from the beam. A raised (convex) dot is present on the white surface of the film wrapper, and a recessed (concave) dot is present on the colored surface (Figure 32-24, *A, B*).

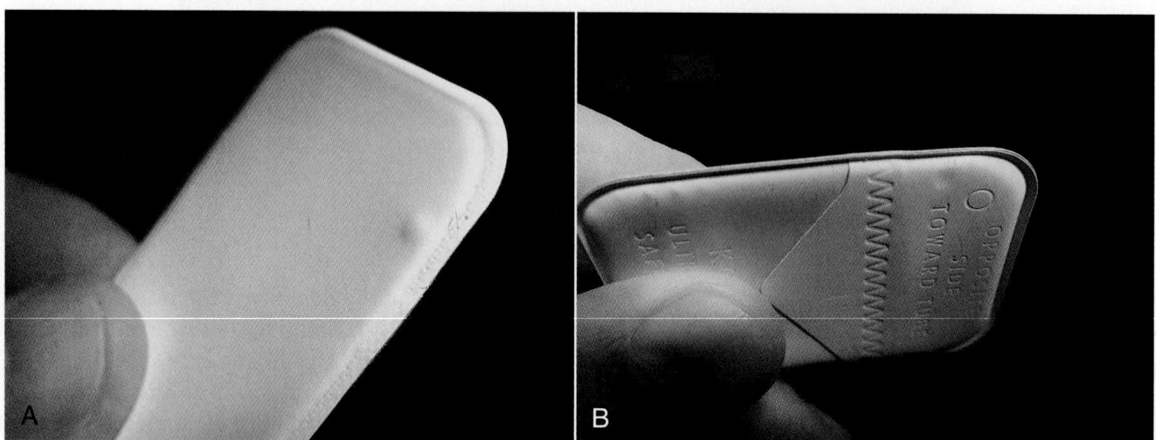

FIGURE 32-24 Two sides of a dental x-ray film packet. **A,** Convex (raised) dot is placed toward the beam. **B,** Concave (indented) dot is placed away from the beam.

The raised dot will always be placed so that it faces the beam, and the concave dot will be farthest from the beam.

> *TECHNICIAN NOTE* When placing intraoral film into the mouth, the white surface of the x-ray film (the surface with the raised dot) always faces toward the beam.

Dental film is available in several sizes, ranging from 0 to 4, and to accommodate variation in sizes of veterinary patients, it is important to keep all sizes of film in stock (Figure 32-25, *A, B*). Intraoral film also comes in several speeds. The speed refers to the sensitivity to radiation exposure, or the amount of radiation required to produce the image. Less radiation is required to produce an image using fast film; however, faster film, such as E-speed, contains larger silver halide crystals; thus appearance of the image is grainier than that of D-speed. Very slow speed films (speeds A, B, C) are associated with higher radiation exposure and are no longer used. Current choices include D-, E-, and F-speed film. Recent advances in F-speed film has allowed for reduction in radiation requirements up to 60% compared with D-speed film while maintaining good image quality. Film is sensitive to heat and moisture and should be stored in a dry, clean, cool place. Observe time limits printed on the boxes and discard the film when expired. The contents of a dental film packet are shown in Figure 32-26, *C*.

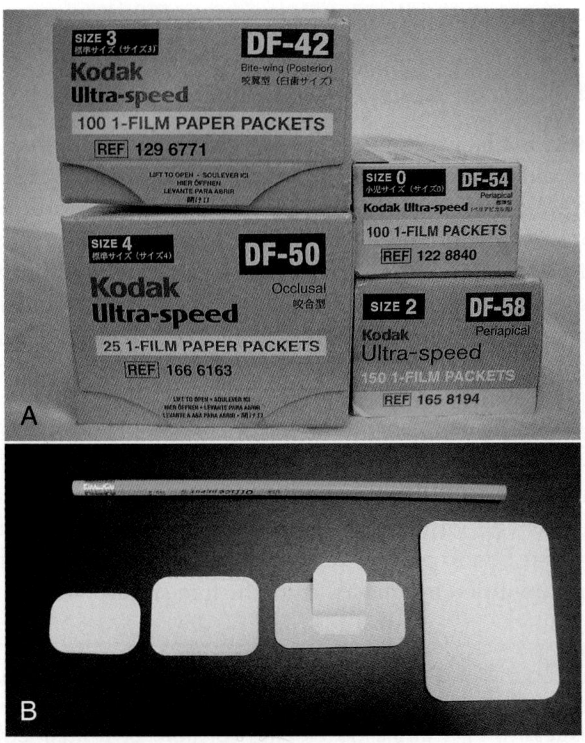

FIGURE 32-25 **A,** Size 0, 2, 3, and 4 dental x-ray film in boxes. **B,** Size 0, 2, 3, 4 film placed near a pencil for size comparison.

FILM PROCESSING

To convert the latent image into a visual image, the film is processed using chemicals that convert the silver halide crystals to metallic silver and preserve the image. Processing intraoral film can be accomplished in a dark room, a manual chairside developer (Figure 32-26, *A*), or an automatic processor.

Use of the chairside developer allows for rapid evaluation of radiographs following approximately 1 minute of processing time. Premixed chemicals (developer and fixer) are available from veterinary distributors. The developer box contains a light filtering window for viewing and hand portals with sleeves that keep light from entering. An orange filtering lid is used with D-speed film, whereas a red lid is used with E- and F-speed film. The films are opened inside the chairside developer and attached to a film clip. Inside, there are four cups into which the film will be dipped. Working from left to right, the first cup is filled with developer solution. The second cup contains water for rinsing. The third cup contains fixer solution that will halt the development process, wash off the silver halide crystals that were not exposed to radiation, and preserve the image on the film. The fourth cup contains water for rinsing (Figure 32-26, *B*). Films must be developed from left to right without backtracking to prevent contamination of the solutions. One exception is that films in the fourth cup may be placed back into the third cup (fixer) without a problem. The timing of each step is critical, and manufacturers' directions should be followed. Keep in mind the possible need for adjustments in time when the temperatures of the chemicals are not the optimal 68° F. Following fixation, the films should be rinsed in slowly running water for 20 minutes before hung on a film rack to dry. Once completely dry, films can be placed into film mounts or small coin envelopes to be filed with the patient's dental record.

> *TECHNICIAN NOTE* After initial viewing of the newly developed radiograph, it should be placed in fixer for at least 10 minutes to obtain archive-quality films.

Automatic processors used for standard x-ray films may be used to develop dental films by taping the dental film to the back end of a standard film and having it tag along with the larger film. This process is sometimes unreliable because it may cause the dental film to get lost or stuck in the rollers of the processor.

DIGITAL RADIOGRAPHY

Use of computed digital radiography (CDR) in the veterinary practice is increasing in favor as practitioners become more aware of the benefits when compared with conventional radiographic techniques. The quality of the digital images is improving since its first introduction in dentistry, and today

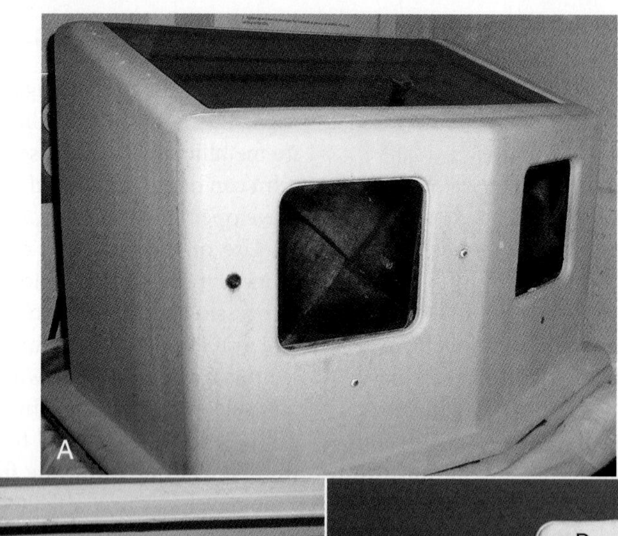

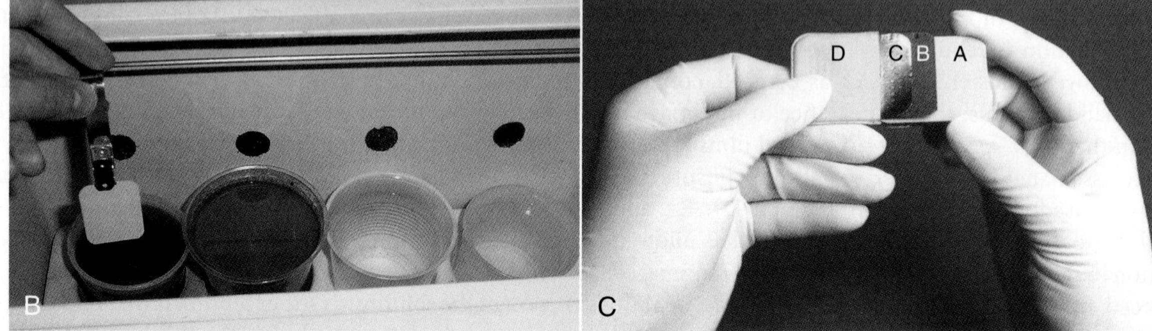

FIGURE 32-26 **A,** The chairside developer is convenient and more rapid than an automatic processor. **B,** Inside, the four containers are filled with developer, water rinse, fixer, and water rinse. The film is processed from left to right, with no movement of films in the opposite direction to prevent mixing of solutions. **C,** The dental film packet contains: *A,* film; *B,* protective black paper; *C,* lead foil; *D,* outer paper or plastic wrapping. (**C** from Robinson DS, Bird DL: *Essentials of dental assisting,* ed 4, St Louis, 2007, Saunders/Elsevier.)

the resolution is good, but still does not approximate that of nonscreen film. Direct method CDR technology, most commonly used today, uses an electronic intraoral sensor, a computer, and the x-ray machine. The sensor, called a charged coupled device (CCD), is either cordless or attached to a cord that connects to the computer. After covering the sensor with a plastic infection barrier, the sensor is placed into the mouth to capture the image and convert it to the digital format of "pixels," picture elements in various shades of gray. A remote module transmits the data to the computer for the image to be immediately viewed, manipulated, and stored. The images can be magnified, and enhancements in contrast or darkness can be made. The sensors are available in sizes comparable with traditional dental film sizes 0, 1, and 2, limiting application in large-breed dogs that typically require size 4 films to view the entire tooth image. Because using a size 2 sensor for larger mouths requires more exposures to accomplish the task, it is practical to use standard radiography for some patients and digital radiography for other patients. When using digital technology, caution must be used to ensure that patients have adequate anesthesia depths because replacement of a damaged sensor is costly.

Digital technology reduces radiation exposure by 50% to 90% when compared with use of D- and E-speed film. Most modern dental x-ray machines are compatible with digital radiology if they have timers that allow the exposure setting in 1/100 of a second time frame. A disadvantage of digital radiography is the high initial cost of the sensor and software. However, the expense is offset by the cost of film and processing chemicals.

EXPOSURE AND PROCESSING ERRORS

Errors in film exposure and processing account for unnecessary radiation exposure and additional anesthetic time for the patient. Cone cutting occurs when the beam misses portions of the film, resulting in clear areas of the film. Elongation and foreshortening (stretched and shortened images, respectively) are caused by inaccurate vertical angulation during PID alignment (Figure 32-27, *A-C*). Images that are too dark or too light can result from errors in kVp and mA settings or in exposure and processing times. If the film is placed in the mouth with the wrong surface facing the beam, dotted streaks from the lead foil will appear across the film surface. Care must be taken when placing multiple films into the fixer cup, ensuring that each film is placed parallel to the adjacent film to prevent scratches that appear as white lines when emulsion is removed from the film surface.

> TECHNICIAN NOTE A film that appears too dark is often due to a greater than necessary exposure time, excessive time in the developing solution, or a light leak during developing.

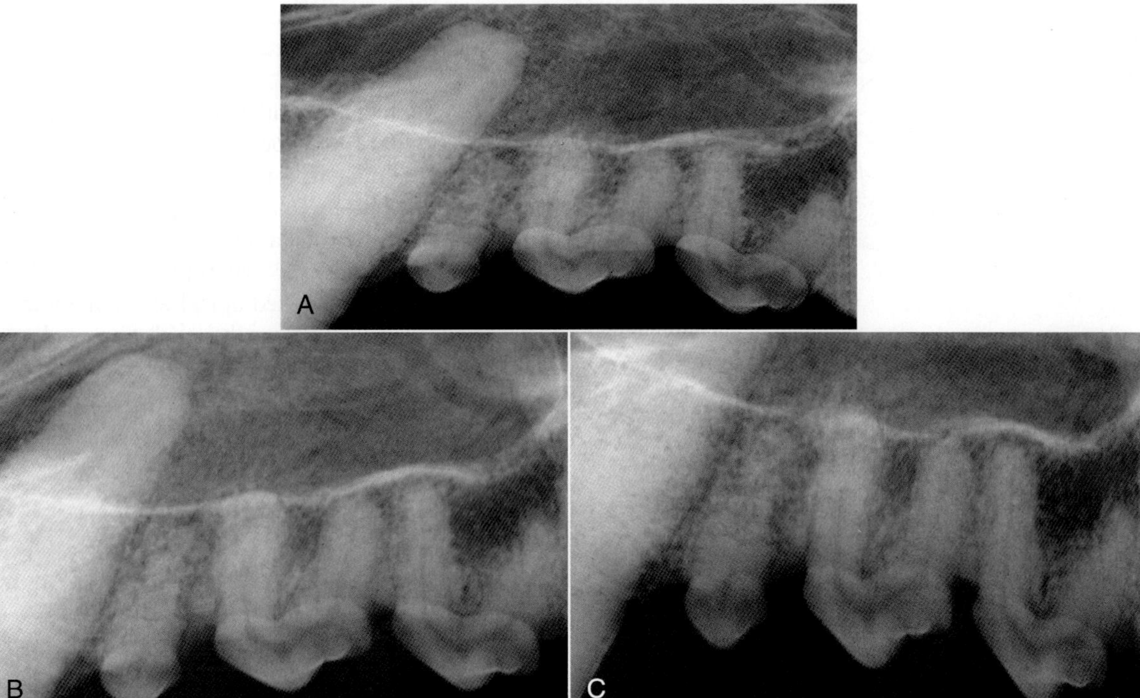

FIGURE 32-27 Three radiographs taken using the bisecting angle technique on the maxilla of a dog with three different PID angles. **A,** Foreshortened image from PID positioned too dorsally. **B,** Correctly determining the bisecting angle results in a film that most closely represents size and shape of subgingival structures. **C,** Elongated image from PID positioned too ventrally.

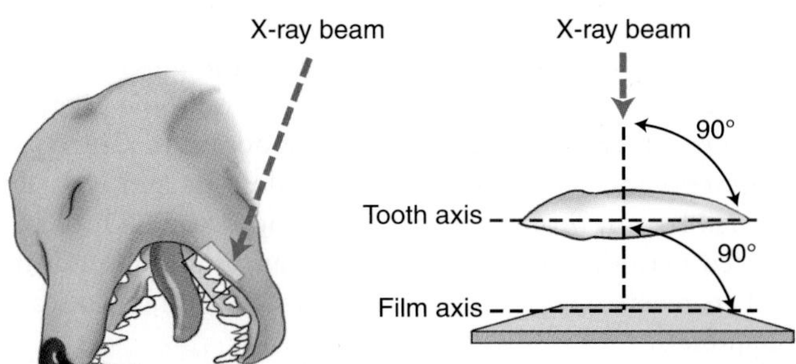

FIGURE 32-28 Paralleling technique is useful for caudal mandibular teeth where the film is placed parallel to the teeth, the beam is directed at a 90-degree angle to the film and teeth.

TECHNIQUES

Three techniques are commonly used to obtain dental radiographs. Each technique will consider the relationship of the beam to the film and tooth or area to be imaged. The proper-sized film is placed into the mouth and held in position with gauze. The paralleling technique requires the film to be placed parallel to the long axis of the tooth. The beam is then directed at a right angle to the film and teeth and positioned to aim for the center of the film (Figure 32-28). Parallelism can only be used on the mandibular teeth, caudal to the second premolars, where the film can easily slide toward the floor of the mouth.

The symphysis at the rostral portion of the mandible and the flat palate of the maxilla prevent the use of the paralleling technique. To minimize inherent distortion of dental structures where the paralleling technique is not an option, the bisecting angle technique is used. The x-ray beam is projected at a right angle to an imaginary line that cuts in half (bisects) the angle formed by the plane of the film and the long axis of the tooth (Figure 32-29).

The occlusal technique places the film on the occlusal plane and directs the beam at a right angle to the film (Figure 32-30). Typically, this view is of value in showing larger areas on one film, with applications to view nasal disease and also for identifying root remnants.

RADIOGRAPHIC INTERPRETATION

To assess the presence of intraoral pathologic conditions on radiographs, it is essential to have knowledge of the appearance of normal radiographic anatomic structures (Figure 32-31). The radiodensity of the components of the teeth and supporting structures varies widely; therefore the terms radiopaque and radiolucent are used to describe the relative radiographic appearance of oral and dental structures. Radiopaque structures, such as cementum, dentin, and bone block or absorb the radiation, causing that portion of the processed radiograph to appear light or white. The enamel covering of the crown is the most radiodense structure of the tooth. The lamina dura, which is a cribriform plate of bone lining the tooth socket, appears as a white line adjacent to the periodontal space surrounding a healthy tooth. Beyond the lamina dura, the trabecular

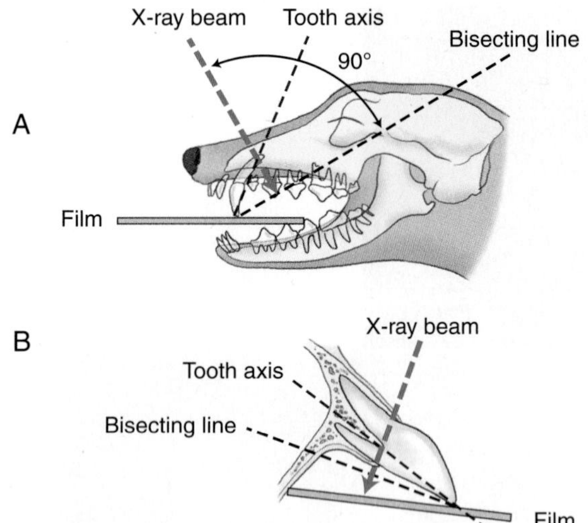

FIGURE 32-29 Bisecting angle technique is used for the maxilla and the rostral mandible where the film cannot be placed parallel to the roots. First, determine the angle created by the plane of the tooth and the plane of the film. Bisect that angle and direct the beam at a right angle to the bisecting line.

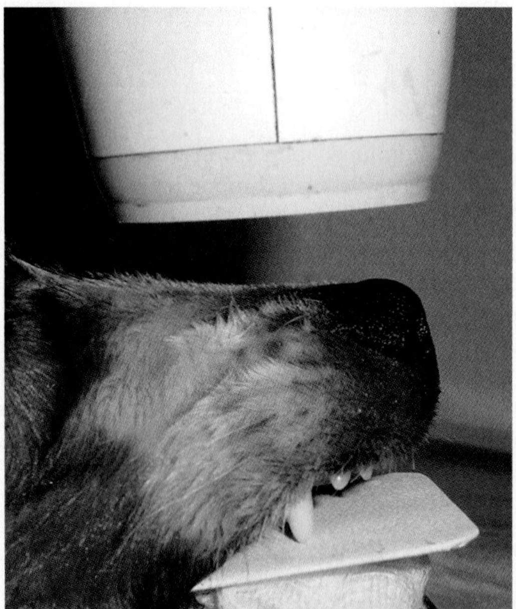

FIGURE 32-30 Occlusal technique is often used on the maxilla to provide an additional view of a tooth of interest or for imaging of the nasal cavity. The film is placed in the mouth parallel with the palate. The beam is directed down at a right angle to the film.

pattern of bone may vary in radiodensity. The cortex of the mandible is radiodense.

In contrast, radiolucent structures, such as the soft tissue and periodontal ligament space, appear dark or black because the x-ray photons can easily pass through to the film. The periodontal ligament fibers are not visible on the film; however, the space they occupy can be traced as a black line surrounding the roots. Because pulp is soft tissue, it also appears as a dark area (less radiodense) in the center of the tooth.

The radiolucent mandibular canal lies apical to most of the mandibular tooth roots. In small-breed dogs, the apices of the mandibular first molar roots may be seen at a level of or even below the mandibular canal, extending into the ventral cortex. Normal anatomic structures must be distinguished from pathologic structures. For example, the middle mental foramen is located apical to the mandibular second premolar in dogs and can be misinterpreted as a periapical pathologic condition if superimposed over a tooth root (Figure 32-32). It is helpful to have a textbook with normal and pathologic radiographic appearances to refer to (see Recommended Reading).

PERIODONTAL DISEASE

The periodontium is composed of four supporting structures of the tooth: (1) periodontal ligament; (2) gingival connective tissue; (3) alveolar bone forming the tooth socket; and (4) cementum covering the surface of the root (Figure 32-33). Healthy gingiva has a sharp, tapered edge (margin) that lies closely against the crown of the tooth. The free gingiva forms a moat around the tooth called the gingival sulcus. The epithelial attachment to the tooth crown forms the bottom of the gingival sulcus. The depth of this sulcus ranges from 1 to 3 mm in a healthy mouth of a dog and up to 1 mm in the cat.

Gingivitis refers to inflammation of the gingiva. Periodontitis describes inflammation of not only the gingiva, but also other structures of the periodontium. Gingivitis represents the earliest stages of periodontitis and is easily reversible with proper treatment and home care. Once advanced periodontitis occurs, these changes are more difficult to reverse. Periodontitis is the most common disease of animals.

Periodontitis is caused by accumulation of subgingival plaque and the body's response to it. Plaque is a white-tan film that collects around and within the gingival sulcus of the tooth. It is composed of bacteria, food debris, exfoliated cells, and salivary glycoproteins. Within as quickly as 24 hours if left undisturbed, plaque will mineralize on the teeth to form dental calculus (sometimes referred to by the term "tartar"), a light brown or yellow, raised, irregular deposit adherent to the tooth and root surfaces (Figure 32-34). This irregular, plaque-retentive surface of calculus allows for further plaque accumulation. As the plaque accumulates within the gingival sulcus, it damages the gingival tissues by releasing bacterial by-products that can damage the periodontium. The patient's immune response may also cause tissue damage through the release of inflammatory cytokines from white blood cells as they attempt to destroy the bacteria. In the early stages, the gingiva becomes inflamed and bleeds easily (Figure 32-35). As the disease progresses, periodontitis results in attachment loss. Attachment loss is clinically detectable in its earliest stages by measuring pocket

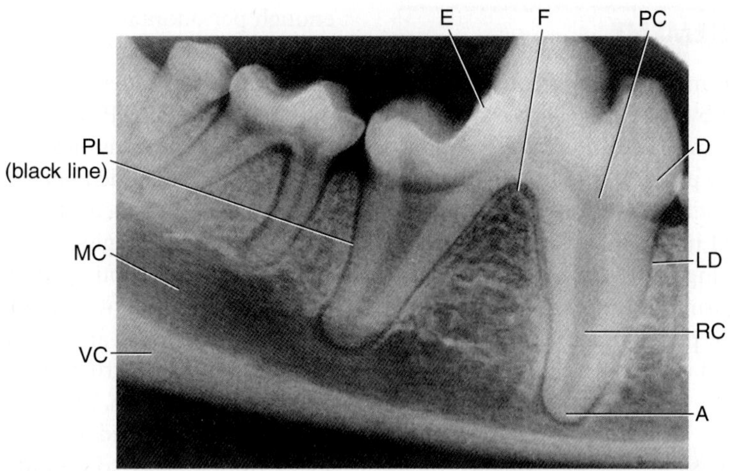

FIGURE 32-31 Normal radiopaque and radiolucent structures: *A,* root apex; *RC,* root canal; *LD,* lamina dura; *D,* dentin; *PC,* pulp chamber; *F,* furcation area; *E,* enamel; *PL,* periodontal ligament; *MC,* mandibular canal; *VC,* ventral cortex.

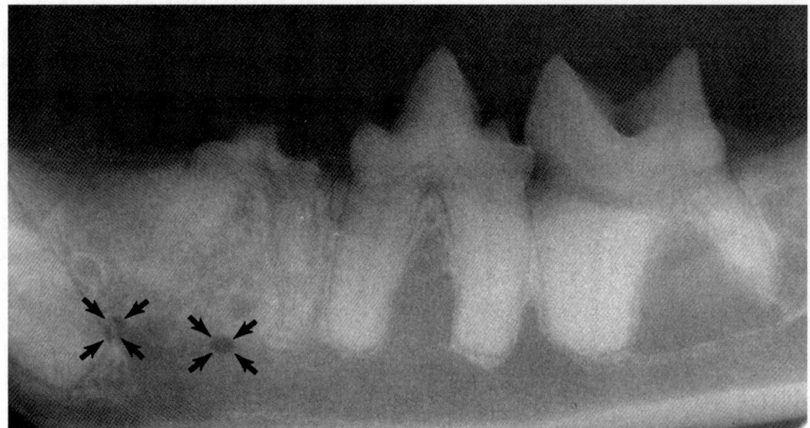

FIGURE 32-32 Normal anatomic structures may appear as periapical pathologic conditions if superimposed over a root. The middle mental foramen and caudal mental foramen are labeled with arrows. The middle mental foramen is superimposed over the apex of the canine tooth root.

depths with a periodontal probe in the anesthetized patient (Figure 32-36, *A, B*).

> *TECHNICIAN NOTE* Plaque begins to mineralize as early as 24 hours after adhering to the tooth surface. Therefore daily brushing is necessary to minimize calculus formation.

Periodontal disease is difficult to control once it has developed. For this reason, great emphasis must be placed on its prevention. Other diseases can contribute to the severity of periodontal disease, but the bacteria in plaque are the primary cause. Early in the formation of plaque, the bacterial population consists mainly of gram-positive aerobic bacteria. Once these bacteria accumulate in substantial numbers, the oxygen gradient of the subgingival environment changes to support a shift to predominantly gram-negative anaerobic rods and spirochetes. Gram-negative bacteria are capable of producing endotoxin, which has direct adverse effects on cells of the periodontium and results in a more severe immune response. When periodontitis is already present, destruction of the junctional epithelium at the base of the gingival sulcus has begun and will continue if not treated. Once the junctional epithelium and periodontal ligament becomes destroyed, it is difficult to stimulate regeneration. As the tooth begins to lose its periodontal attachment, it becomes more susceptible to plaque accumulation in the deep periodontal pockets that form around the tooth roots. When the tooth loses a significant portion of its periodontium, it becomes mobile. The infection and inflammation associated with periodontitis is present for months to years before the tooth is eventually lost. Throughout the duration of the periodontitis, bacteremia occurs with the potential for colonization of bacteria at distant sites including the liver, kidneys, heart, and lungs.

For patients with periodontal disease, the treatment goal is removal of plaque and calculus from the teeth both supragingivally and subgingivally. General anesthesia is necessary to provide necessary access to subgingival areas, where bacteria can contribute to local and sometimes systemic inflammation. A second and equally important goal is minimization of plaque reattachment through proper home care and appropriate follow-up treatment.

PERIODONTAL DÉBRIDEMENT

Periodontal disease results from the presence of a biofilm rich in bacteria and bacterial by-products. Removal of the bacterial plaque, endotoxins, and hard calculus deposits is essential to halting the disease process. Endotoxins are believed to be attached to the tooth surface, loosely embedded in cementum, and unattached in the sulcular space. Home care can be effective in removing supragingival debris when the client is educated to perform the procedures on a daily basis. If the oral hygiene is not performed thoroughly, subgingival biofilm will mature and within 48 hours will contain enough periodontal pathogens to cause gingivitis. Within 3 to 12 weeks, the biofilm contains gram-negative anaerobes and provides an envelope that harbors and protects the periodontal pathogens. Professional clinical care is required to remove the pathogens and the calculus that harbor bacteria.

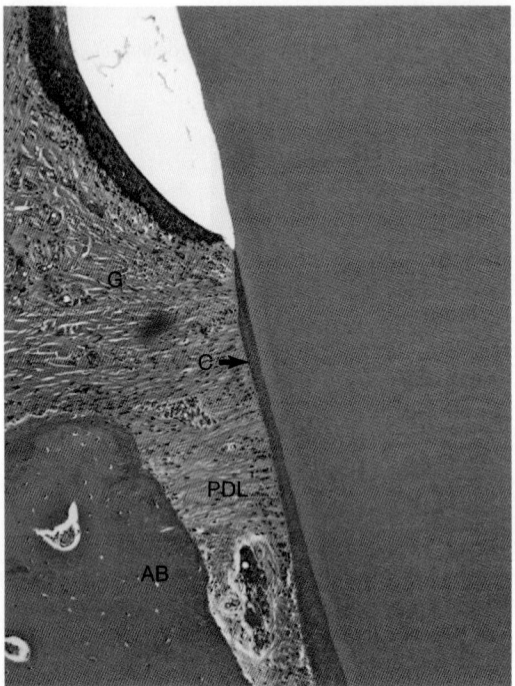

FIGURE 32-33 Histomicrograph showing the components of the periodontium. *PDL,* Periodontal ligament; *G,* gingival connective tissue; *AB,* alveolar bone; *C,* cementum. Cementum covers the root surface and the periodontal ligament attaches to cementum and alveolar bone.

Periodontal débridement is the term used for nonsurgical instrumentation that focuses on the removal of hard and soft deposits from the supragingival and subgingival surfaces of teeth along with the disruption of the nonadherent bacteria within the sulcus. The goal of periodontal débridement is to prevent or arrest the infection and restore the oral soft tissues to health. Hand and power instrumentation are used to deplaque, scale, root plane, and polish. The traditional approach of scaling and root planing was based on beliefs that the bacterial endotoxins were firmly attached to the pitted, irregular surfaces of cementum. Instrumentation with a curette included root planing to remove all damaged layers of cementum, resulting in a glossy, smooth surface that would be less plaque retentive. Current research has shown that the endotoxins are only lightly adherent, and removal of superficial layers of cementum is adequate to achieve goals of periodontal débridement.

POWER SCALING

Ultrasonic devices, mechanized instruments currently used for periodontal débridement, were first introduced in the early 1950s to remove tooth material during treatment for caries in human patients. When high-speed air-driven handpieces were introduced shortly thereafter, the ultrasonic application was deemed to be too slow for removal of tooth structure. In 1955, ultrasonic scalers were introduced. The original scalers were limited to removing supragingival deposits as a result of their bulky tip design. More definitive scaling was routinely accomplished with hand scalers and curettes. During the 1980s, thinner probelike tips were developed, and today continued advances in technology have expanded the applications to subgingival use. Knowledge of the instrument and tooth morphology is critical for safe use. No longer considered to be an adjunct to hand instrumentation,

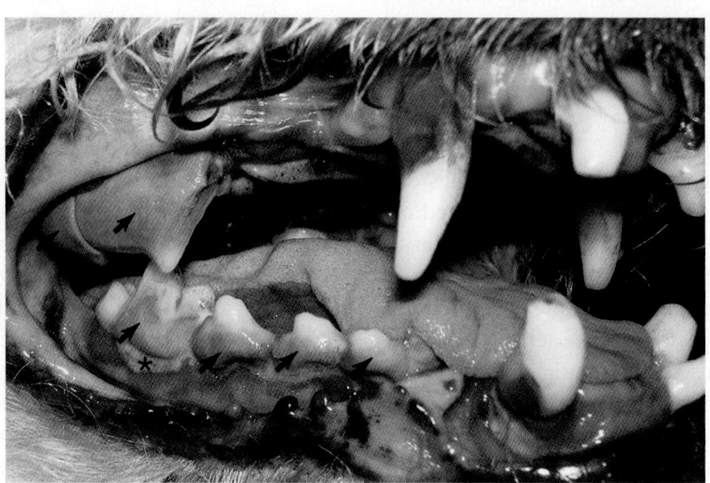

FIGURE 32-34 Plaque and calculus in a dog. Plaque is white-tan *(asterisk)* and accumulates on the rough surface of calculus. Plaque that is not removed within approximately 24 hours will become mineralized, adherent calculus *(arrows).*

ultrasonic scalers are now considered to be the primary instrument in veterinary practice for use in routine débridement and advanced periodontal therapy.

TECHNICIAN NOTE When performing periodontal débridement, a cuffed endotracheal tube and gravity (tipping the nose lower than the rest of the head) should be used to prevent aspiration of fluids and debris.

Power-scaling instruments use a water-cooled vibrating tip to remove hard and soft deposits from the teeth and periodontal pockets. The vibrations are measured by the number of times that the tip moves back and forth in one second. This measurement is known as frequency and is measured in cycles per second (cps), or Hertz (Hz). Most units used in veterinary medicine are automatically tuned units with frequencies controlled by the unit. Manually controlled units are available and mostly used in the human field in advanced periodontal therapy. Research indicates that when skillfully performed, ultrasonic instrumentation is as effective as hand instrumentation. Box 32-5 lists the benefits of power scaling.

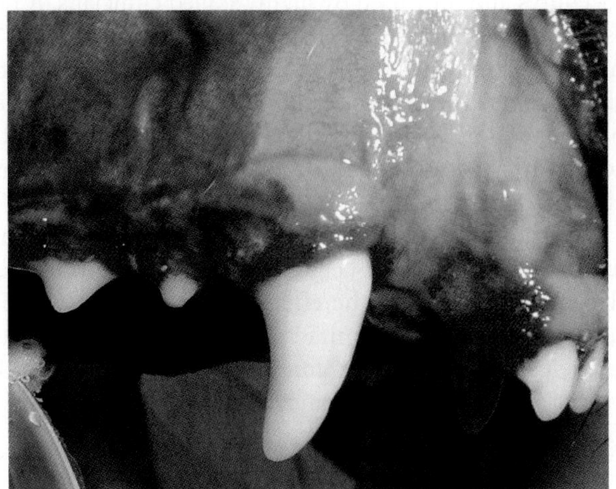

FIGURE 32-35 Gingivitis in a dog. Inflammation is limited to the gingival tissue and does not cross the mucogingival junction.

Two types of power scalers, sonic and ultrasonic, are categorized by the frequency of the tip vibrations and the type of power used to create movement at the working end.

SONIC SCALER

The sonic scaler is powered from an air compressor on a dental unit and is attached to the low-speed air line. It operates with a frequency between 2000 and 9000 cps. The tip vibrates in an elliptical pattern, with all surfaces around the diameter of the tip active. The vibrations are audible to the human ear creating a sound that may be uncomfortable to some operators. As a result of the low frequency, the sonic scaler has less ability to remove heavy, tenacious calculus and is slow to accomplish its task. It is best suited for use in cats or dogs with light accumulations.

ULTRASONIC SCALER

Ultrasonic devices use electrical energy that converts the working tip to mechanical energy in the form of rapid vibrations to effectively remove biofilm and calculus deposits. Ranging in frequency from 18,000 to 50,000 cps, above the audible human range, they are more popular and practical for veterinary use than the sonic scaler. The ultrasonic scaling unit contains the electronic generator inside plastic housing. A hose connects the unit to the water supply, either a portable pressure tank or a quick disconnect at the

BOX 32-5 Benefits of Power Scaling

- Ergonomically superior by reducing hand fatigue and the need for repetitive, intricate hand movements
- Reduces total time patient must remain anesthetized
- Causes less tissue distention than curettes (when using slim tips subgingivally)
- Causes less root surface damage when used correctly
- Lavage is destructive to bacteria (cavitation, acoustic turbulence and streaming)

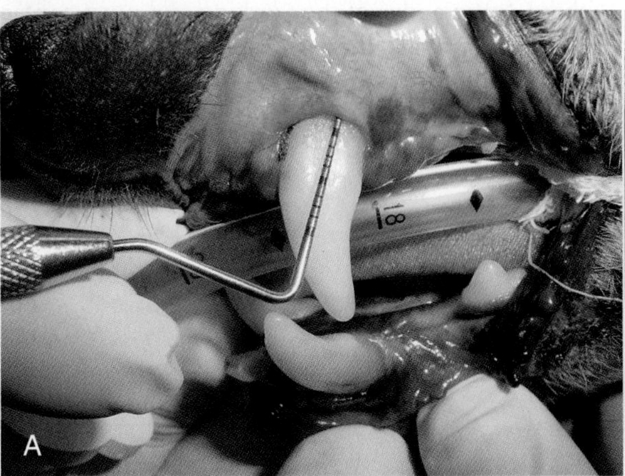

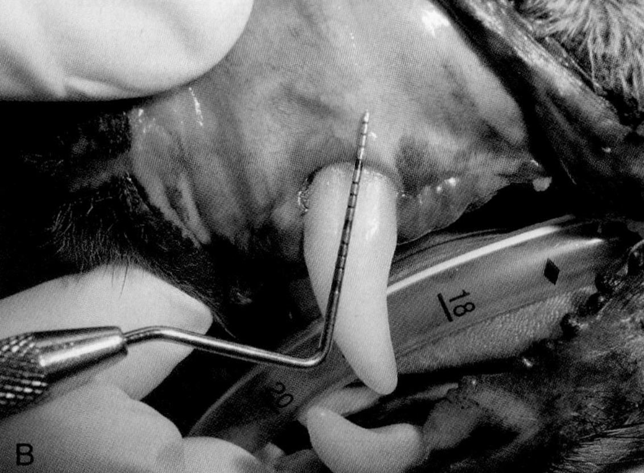

FIGURE 32-36 **A,** Probe is inserted to determine pocket depth. **B,** Probe is removed to show degree of attachment loss, which is pocket depth plus gingival recession.

sink pipes. A cable attaches the unit to a foot pedal, and the handpiece is attached by tubing that transports the water for coolant. A power cord is also attached. Unlike hand scalers that only remove debris with direct contact, the ultrasonics also have the benefit of the stream of water coming from the tip that acts as a coolant and lavage, flushing debris from the sulcus. The flushing action is destructive to the biofilm by causing acoustic turbulence and cavitation. Acoustic turbulence, also known as acoustic microstreaming, is the disruption of the bacteria in plaque caused by the streaming of the fluid over the tooth surface or the churning of the fluid within the confined pocket space. Cavitation is the energy that is created from the mist of water. As the water coolant exits the handpiece and strikes the vibrating working end, it creates thousands of water bubbles. As the bubbles in the mist implode, enough energy is created to disrupt the bacterial cell walls.

> *TECHNICIAN NOTE* The transducer in a magnetostrictive ultrasonic scaler is either a metal stack or a ferrite rod. The transducer in a piezoelectric ultrasonic scaler is a quartz crystal or ceramic disk.

SAFETY PRECAUTIONS

Because water is a necessary part of the dental cleaning, appropriate safety precautions must be taken for the technician and the patient. To reduce the amount of aerosolized bacteria, the mouth can be rinsed with chlorhexidine (0.1% to 0.2%) before scaling. This preemptive rinse will also reduce the severity of bacteremia of the patient, which invariably occurs during a dental cleaning. The technician and any co-workers in the vicinity of the workstation should wear gloves, masks capable of high bacterial filtration, and eye protection, such as plastic goggles or disposable face shields. The patient's eyes should be lubricated and covered to protect against debris and contaminated fluid from entering. The single most important safety precaution when using ultrasonic scaling lavage is to intubate the patient and check to ensure that the endotracheal cuff is fully inflated. The airtight seal of the cuff should be checked occasionally to prevent the patient from developing aspiration pneumonia. However, care should be taken to avoid excessive inflation of the cuff that may result in a tracheal tear or necrosis. Placement of a radiopaque laparotomy sponge in the back of the throat before scaling will filter the loosened debris; however, remembering to remove the sponge after scaling is critical.

TIP DESIGNS

The tip designs have improved since the early 1990s, with more design options currently available. Standard-sized "universal" and broad tips are designed for removing medium and heavy deposits, whereas the slim tip designs provide for better access to subgingival pockets and furcation areas. Approximately 30% to 40% more narrow than standard tips, the slim tips are approximately 0.5 mm in diameter at the blunt end and designed to mimic periodontal probes. The slim profile enables easier access to the base of deeper pockets and improves tactility for better detection of calculus. They are available in straight and curved designs. Precision tips are available in diameters as narrow as 0.2 mm at the tip for use in advanced periodontal procedures. These are extremely fragile and must be used with a light touch. Another tip option is the diamond-coated tip. If used incorrectly during a nonsurgical procedure, the diamond coating can cause soft tissue damage and excessive loss of tooth substance; therefore this design should be reserved for use during open-flap procedures and only used by highly skilled clinicians. A new design offers a tip with a built-in LED light (Figure 32-37). The LED technology tends to offer only minimal additional light when used with a good surgical overhead light. A new tip designed for use in furcations has a 0.8-mm ball on the end that may be too large to access the furcations of some animal's teeth.

Tips should be replaced at least annually or when they are bent or worn down (Figure 32-38). As the tip wears, it becomes shorter and the effectiveness of scaling diminishes. One ultrasonic manufacturer offers a wear indicator that helps to measure the amount of wearing of the tip. For each millimeter of wearing, there is a 25% decrease in efficiency.

ENERGY DISPERSION

For effective scaling during use of hand instrumentation, the sharp cutting edge of the working end must contact the calculus. In contrast, there is ultrasonic energy dispersion over a 360-degree circle around the tip of power instruments. The vibrating activity occurs on the back, face (concave surface),

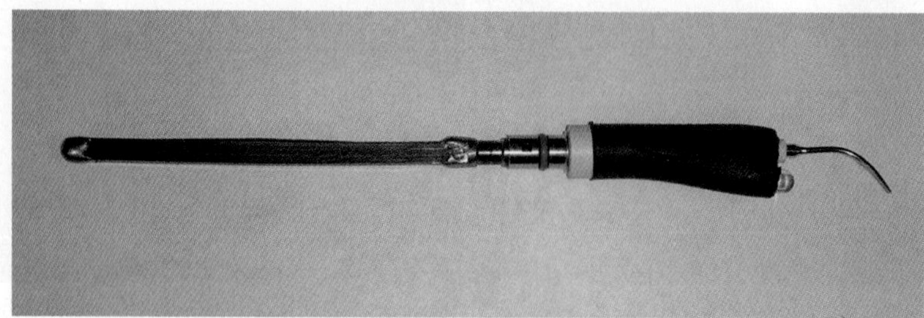

FIGURE 32-37 Magnetostrictive ultrasonic insert: metal stack transducer and LED light at working end.

two side (lateral) surfaces, and on the point; however, each surface has varying degrees of vibrations, depending on the type of scaler used. Typically the strongest vibrations are concentrated 2 to 4 mm from the tip. Technicians must know the specific type of unit that they are working with and understand the differences in levels of energy dispersal among different tip surfaces to correctly adapt the tip to the tooth for efficient scaling.

TYPES OF ULTRASONIC SCALERS

Ultrasonic scalers are available in two types, magnetostrictive and piezoelectric, each distinct in their mechanism of action, type of transducer, and direction of tip movement. The transducer is the portion of the handpiece that converts electrical energy into mechanical energy.

The magnetostrictive scaler is the most common type of power scaler used in human and veterinary dentistry. The typical magnetostrictive unit has an insert that slides into the handpiece. The insert has two connected parts, the transducer and the working end. The magnetostrictive transducer is a stack of thin nickel alloy metal strips. When a magnetic field is created from the copper coil inside the handpiece, the dimension of the strips is altered by lengthening and shortening, thus sending vibrations to the tip.

Movement of the tip is in an elliptical pattern with the energy dispersion around the entire diameter of the tip, providing vibrations on all surfaces. The point of the tip can cause damage when directed at a 90-degree angle to the tooth, acting like a jackhammer on hard dental tissue (Figure 32-39). The face (concave surface) is the usable portion of the tip that has the most powerful vibrations, followed by the back. The two side surfaces have the least vibrations. The back and side surfaces are used for the majority of scaling. Magnetostrictive units range in frequency from 18,000 to 42,000 cps (18 to 42 kHz). Another type of magnetostrictive scaler uses a transducer that is a ferrite rod to produce a rotational tip movement. Differences in operation between magnetostrictive units require close attention to manufacturer's recommendations. See Box 32-6 for preparation guidelines for a magnetostrictive unit with a metal stack transducer.

TECHNICIAN NOTE The ultrasonic scaler tip should never be directed at a 90-degree angle toward the tooth surface because the tip will cause damage to the enamel.

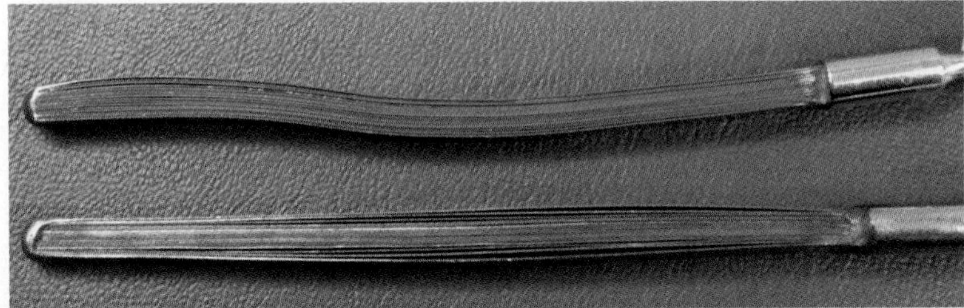

FIGURE 32-38 Damaged ultrasonic inserts; magnetostrictive inserts should be discarded when metal stack becomes bent or splayed.

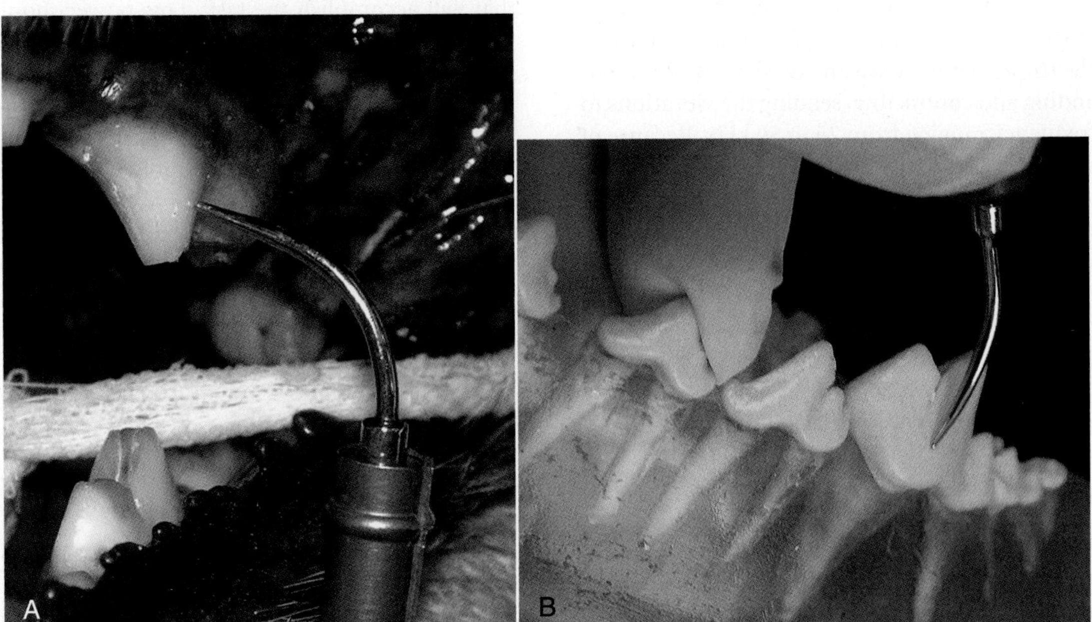

FIGURE 32-39 A, The tip of the ultrasonic insert will cause damage when directed at a 90-degree angle to the tooth surface. **B,** Correct angulation of the tip; the insert tip should be held at an angle of 0 degrees to 15 degrees from the long axis of the tooth.

BOX 32-6 Techniques for Preparation and Instrumentation When Using Magnetostrictive Ultrasonic Scaling Unit With Metal Stack Transducer*

- Plug electrical cord into outlet.
- Run water through handpiece for minimum of 2 minutes (each morning) to flush biofilm, draining into sink.
- Disinfect handpiece.
- Hold handpiece upright, perpendicular to floor, while stepping on pedal to completely fill handpiece with water.
- Choose tip design.
- Remove foot from pedal, slide insert into handpiece until resistance is met at the rubber "O" ring. Gently twist as the insert is completely seated (if using metal stack transducer).
- If using a unit with screw-in tips, insert tip and tighten with supplied wrench.
- Hold the handpiece parallel to the floor to adjust the power to low-medium and water to a spray. Use the lowest power setting that will accomplish the task.
- Wear gloves, mask, and face shield or goggles.
- Place gauze or lap sponge in back of patient's throat.
- Protect patient's eyes (lubricate and cover).
- Check the endotracheal cuff for leakage, make adjustments if necessary.
- Flush patient's mouth with chlorhexidine (0.12%).
- To reduce pulling weight of the cord, wrap cord around forearm, pinky finger, or drape over neck.
- Hold handpiece lightly with pen or modified pen grasp.
- Establish a comfortable finger rest.
- Retract the patient's cheeks, tongue, and lips to prevent contact with any portion of the metal tip. A dental mirror is useful for retraction.
- Activate the tip before touching the tooth or calculus.
- Adapt the side of the tip to the tooth in a similar fashion to using a periodontal probe, at an angle of 0 degrees to 15 degrees to the tooth.
- With light pressure, move the tip in a sweeping motion as if using a pencil eraser, keeping the end 2 mm of the tip in constant contact with the tooth surface. Use of hard pressure is counterproductive because it will diminish the vibrations. Vertical, horizontal, or oblique strokes may be used.
- REMEMBER: Never hold the point at a 90-degree angle to the tooth because scratching and gouging of the enamel or cementum may occur.
- Move the tip in a direction beginning on the crown and advancing toward the apex of the tooth to the bottom of the sulcus or pocket. This is opposite of hand instrumentation where the curette is adapted at the base of the pocket and moved coronally.
- Assess the surface of the tooth for smoothness by using the tip without activating the vibrations, similar to using an explorer.
- When encountering stubborn tenacious pieces of calculus, use light tapping motions against the surface of calculus or increase the power setting.
- Check for remaining residual calculus by using compressed air from the air or water syringe on dental unit. Missed calculus will appear chalky white.
- Rinse mouth with chlorhexidine, flushing any loose debris from tongue, cheek, and lip vestibules.
- Remove gauze from throat, checking for debris before extubation.
- Wipe unit, handpiece, and cords with federally approved nonimmersion type of disinfectant. Observe manufacturer's instructions for sterilizing handpiece and tips.

*Other types of units may have slight variations; therefore please follow manufacturer's instructions.

The piezoelectric scaler uses either ceramic disks or crystals as the transducer to produce the straight, linear movement of the tip. Electrical energy causes the disks to alter dimension by expanding and contracting, sending the vibrations to the tip at a frequency ranging from 25 to 50 kHz. Because of the back-and-forth motion, the tip is only active on the two lateral surfaces, forcing the operator to pivot the wrist as the tip is moved around the tooth. If the other surfaces are accidentally adapted to the tooth, the operator will be warned by a different sound and incomplete removal of debris. The limitations of effective vibrating surfaces cause the piezoelectric scaler to be more technique sensitive than other power scalers. The transducer's ceramic disk is fragile and easily breakable if the handpiece is accidentally dropped.

KNOB SETTINGS

The power knob adjusts the amplitude, the distance the tip is moving back and forth in one cycle. Greater distance is higher power. Higher power is necessary to remove heavy deposits, whereas low power is satisfactory for removing plaque. It is good principal to use the lowest power setting that will accomplish the task. Low power should always be used with thin tips to prevent the tips from breaking.

The water knob adjusts the water flow through the handpiece. Because the ultrasonics produce heat, there must be adequate fluid to prevent pulp damage caused by heat during scaling. Pressure of the water supply line to the unit must be a minimum of 25 psi. A warm or hot handpiece is an indication that the water pressure is inadequate, and the clinician must immediately stop and make adjustments by increasing the water amount and checking the water pressure (if a portable water tank is used). With magnetostrictive units, the water knob should be turned until the water exits the tip as a mist, rather than just a straight stream. Water on the piezoelectric unit should be adjusted to a steady drip.

HAND SCALING

Periodontal débridement may be accomplished with the use of hand-activated instrumentation. Successful use of hand instruments is dependent on the technician's understanding of instrument design and knowledge of the basic principles of instrumentation.

In general, dental instruments consist of three parts: the handle, shank, and working end (see Figure 32-19). The handle contains the instrument's identification, the description of the instrument with abbreviations that include the name of the designer or the school where it was designed, the manufacturer, the classification type, and the design number. Classifications are determined by the design of the working ends and the instrument's intended purpose. Examination instruments include probes and explorers. Scaling instruments include curettes, sickles, files, and hoes. Current trends in handles include hollow, lightweight designs that are more efficient in transmitting vibrations detected through tactile sensitivity. Use of wider handle sizes minimize finger pinching and hand fatigue. Various patterns of surface texture are knurled into the handle to prevent fingers from slipping.

The shank connects the handle with the working end. The curvature of the shank determines the best-suited location within the mouth for use of the instrument. In relation to the long axis of the handle, a straight shank is used for rostral teeth; an angled shank is used for caudal teeth (Figure 32-40). When the shank is bent to form an angle, the terminal shank is the portion below the bend and closest to the working end. Length and diameter of shanks vary; therefore the instrument of choice may depend on the situation for which the instrument is needed. Elongated shanks are useful for accessing deeper pockets and reaching further caudal in the mouth. A thick, rigid shank is useful for removing heavy tenacious calculus because the shank will not flex when pressed against the tooth. Thin, flexible shanks are more suited for removing light calculus deposits or plaque.

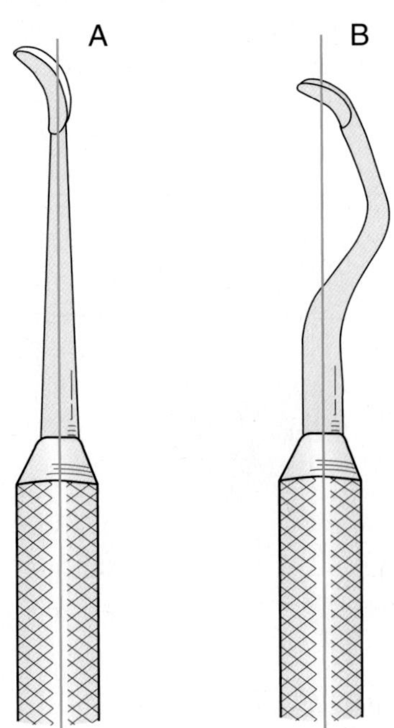

FIGURE 32-40 A straight shank **(A)** is best used for scaling teeth in the rostral portion of the mouth. A bent shank **(B)** is designed for working on premolars and molars. (From Daniel SJ, Harfst SA, Wilder R: *Mosby's dental hygiene: concepts, cases, and competencies,* ed 2, St Louis, 2008, Mosby.)

The working end is designed to complete the task. The working end may be blunt, as in a probe, pointed and wire-like as in an explorer, or it may have sharp cutting edges like scaling instruments. An instrument handle may have one single working end (SE), or it may be double ended (DE) with two working ends. The working end of a hand-scaling instrument is called the blade, and it has several parts: the two lateral sides, face, back, heel, and toe or point (Figure 32-41). The face and lateral surfaces meet to form a cutting edge. The back is formed by the convergence of the two lateral surfaces. Instruments used for supragingival scaling have a pointed tip, whereas subgingival scalers, known as curettes, have a rounded tip. The tip of a curette (known as the toe) is designed to minimize trauma to the soft tissue lining the sulcus or pocket.

The angulation of the face of the blade in relation to the terminal shank will classify the instrument as either universal or area specific. To determine this classification, position the instrument handle so the terminal shank is perpendicular to the floor, then identify the face. If the angle between the face and terminal shank is 90 degrees, the instrument is universal, meaning that when in use, the handle is placed parallel to the long axis of the tooth and then slightly tipped left or right to permit either cutting edge to be adapted to the tooth. If the face is offset at an angle of 60 degrees to 70 degrees, as in Gracey curettes, the instrument is considered to be area specific, and only one of the cutting edges may be adapted to the tooth (Figure 32-42).

SUPRAGINGIVAL INSTRUMENTS

Sickle scalers are the instruments used to scale the crowns of the teeth. The flat face may be either straight or curved lengthwise; the straight lateral surfaces are flat and converge

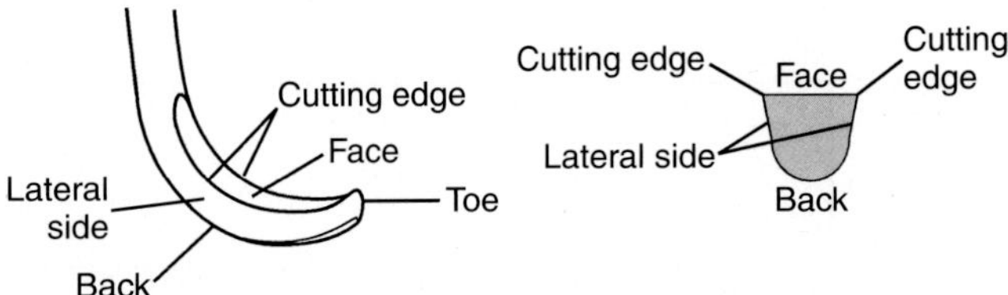

FIGURE 32-41 The parts of the working end of a hand instrument include the face, cutting edges, lateral sides, back, and toe (tip). (From Nelson DM: *Saunders review of dental hygiene,* Philadelphia, 2000, WB Saunders.)

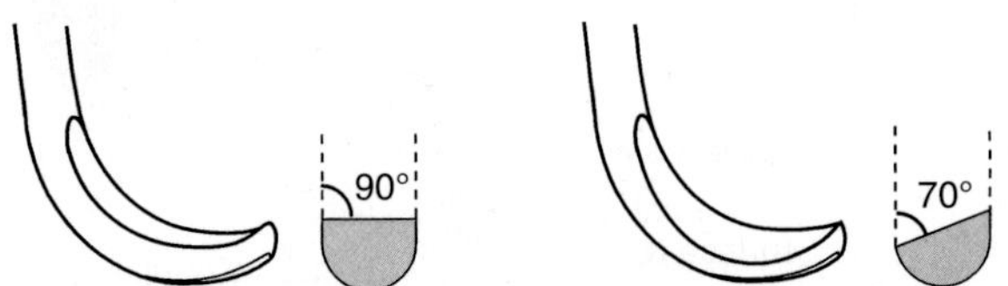

FIGURE 32-42 Universal versus area-specific (Gracey) curettes: The angle between the face and the terminal shank is 90 degrees on the universal, 70 degrees offset on the area specific. Notice that one cutting edge is lower when the face is offset. The lower cutting edge is the correct one when using an area-specific curette. (From Nelson DM: *Saunders review of dental hygiene,* Philadelphia, 2000, WB Saunders.)

to form a pointed back and tip. When envisioning the cross section of a sickle, the instrument is characteristically triangular in shape with 70-degree to 80-degree internal angles between the face and lateral surfaces (Figure 32-43, *A*). The sharp tip will cause lacerations if the instrument is used subgingivally; however, it may be used with caution slightly below the gingival margin where the gingiva is spongy and loose enough to permit insertion. Because the sickle is a universal instrument, either cutting edge may be used depending on how the handle is tipped. Owing to the straight side surfaces, the sickle is not conducive to following the curved contours of roots and is therefore reserved for coronal scaling.

> *TECHNICIAN NOTE* Scalers are designed to be used on the tooth crown, and curettes are designed to be used subgingivally.

When the handle, shank, and blade are on the same plane, the instrument is designed for use toward the front of the mouth. For caudal teeth, the shank will be angled and the instrument will be double ended to provide mirror images. This style is useful for veterinary patients during scaling of the buccal groove of maxillary carnassial teeth. One working end is contoured for scaling the mesial edge of the groove, and the contralateral end contours with the distal edge of the groove.

When placing the blade against the tooth, the face should be at an angle between 45 degrees and 90 degrees with the tooth surface. The cutting edge is directed to the apical edge of the calculus, lateral pressure is placed against the tooth, and the instrument is used with a short pull stroke to disengage the debris.

SUBGINGIVAL CURETTES

Curettes may be used for supragingival scaling, though they are designed for subgingival scaling and root planing. The flat face is curved lengthwise from the heel to the toe, meeting the lateral surfaces to create a cutting edge that extends around the toe. Unlike the flat lateral sides of the sickle scaler that converged to form a pointed back, the sides of the curette are rounded, creating a round back that is easier to insert into a sulcus or pocket. The cross section of the curette is classically shaped like a semicircle with internal angles of 70 degrees to 80 degrees between the face and lateral surfaces (Figure 32-43, *B*).

A universal curette can be adapted for all surfaces of the teeth, whereas use of an area-specific curette would require several different instruments to scale each tooth in the mouth. Use of area-specific instruments is an advanced concept and should be used only by technicians having an understanding of the inherent design features and thorough knowledge of root anatomy and shape. When an area-specific instrument is used incorrectly, it can cause gouging of the root surface and trauma to the adjacent soft tissues.

The terms site specific and area specific are often interchanged with Gracey instruments, though other area-specific instruments exist. Dr. Clayton Gracey designed curettes in the 1930s to be used as a set, each instrument having a complex curvature of the shank for better access to the specific teeth. Unlike the universal curette that is only curved on the plane of the face, the Gracey is also curved on the plane of the lateral surface. To help identify the two curved planes, hold the instrument with the terminal shank perpendicular to the floor and view the face at eye level. The face will slope downward, rather than parallel with the floor and perpendicular to the terminal shank, and the lateral surfaces will be curved

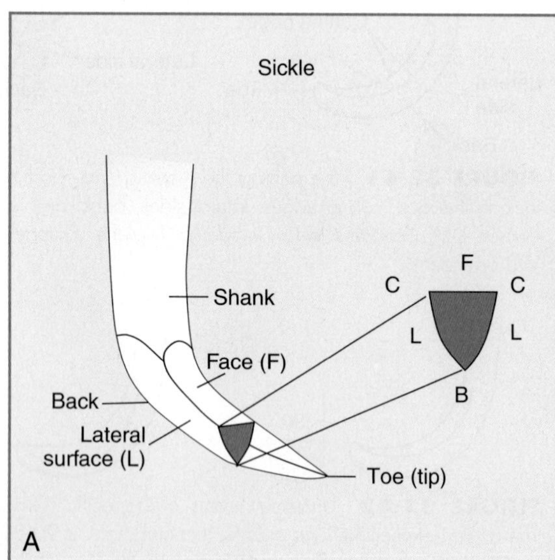

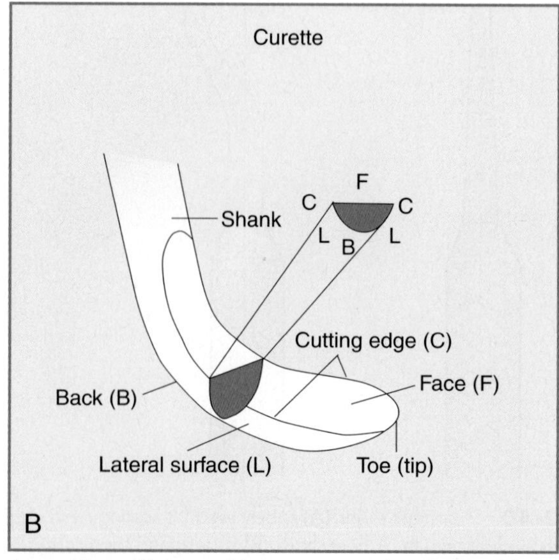

FIGURE 32-43 **A,** The cross section of a sickle scaler is triangular in shape. The sickle is used for supragingival scaling and has a pointed tip. **B,** The cross section of a curette is half-moon shaped. The curette is used for subgingival scaling and has a rounded toe. (From Novack DE: *Contemporary dental assisting,* St Louis, 2001, Mosby.)

to the left or right. This curvature enables adaptation around the contours of roots. As with universal curettes, site-specific curettes have two cutting edges; however, the site specific is unique in that only one edge is designed for use. Before adapting the blade to the tooth, the technician must confirm that the appropriate edge is chosen. To determine the correct cutting edge, hold the terminal shank perpendicular to the floor to view the honed face from above, enabling the lateral curves to be seen. One cutting edge forms an inner curve; another edge forms an outer curve that appears larger and closer to the floor. The proper cutting edge is always the curve that appears lower and further from the terminal shank. Unlike universal instruments that require parallelism of the handle with the tooth, area-specific instruments require parallelism of the terminal shank with the tooth. When in this position against a tooth surface, if the correct edge has been chosen, only the back should be visible. If the face is visible (reflecting light), flip the instrument to use the contralateral working end.

> *TECHNICIAN NOTE* When using an area-specific curette, the proper cutting edge is the lower edge, as determined by holding the terminal shank perpendicular to the floor. The terminal shank of an area-specific curette is kept parallel to the long axis of the tooth during a vertical scaling stroke. The handle of the universal scaler is kept parallel to the long axis of the tooth during a vertical scaling stroke.

Langer curettes have a combination of universal curette qualities (face 90 degrees to shank) with the Gracey curvature of shanks. Langers and Graceys are available with blades that are shorter in length (mini) that make them particularly suitable for use on small dogs and cats.

PRINCIPLES OF SCALING

Adaptation of hand-scaling instruments is the application of the cutting edge against the tooth. Approximately one third of the cutting edge of the tip should remain in contact with the tooth, and constant attention to this detail will prevent damage of the soft tissues as a result of trauma from the tip or toe (Figure 32-44). As the curvature of the tooth changes, adjustments must be made to that portion of the cutting edge that is adaptable to the tooth. Use of the thumb against the handle will enable the instrument to be rolled to maintain the contact of the cutting edge around curves.

Angulation refers to the relationship of the face of the instrument to the tooth. When inserting a curette into a pocket, the angulation of the face should be as close to zero as possible (Figure 32-45). In this position, the face would be parallel with the root surface and the back of the blade would be against the soft tissue lining of the pocket. When the blade is positioned at the bottom of the pocket or apical to the intended piece of calculus, the angle should be opened, by tilting the handle, to the scaling and root planing angle of 45 degrees to 90 degrees, more often between 60 degrees to 80 degrees. Using an angle that is too closed will

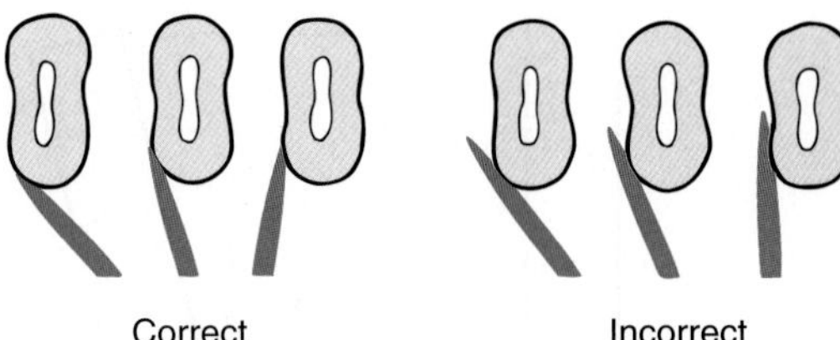

FIGURE 32-44 Correct adaptation, the lower third of the working end of the instrument must remain in contact with the tooth surface to prevent trauma of soft tissues. (From Novak DE: *Contemporary dental assisting*, St Louis, 2001, Mosby).

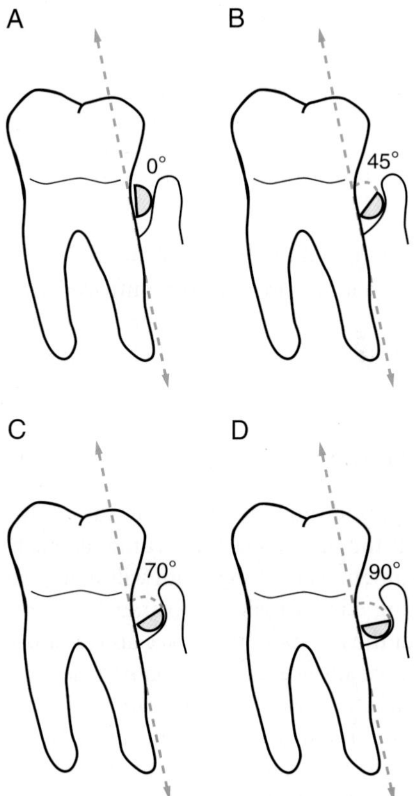

FIGURE 32-45 The angle formed by the tooth surface and face of instrument should begin at insertion into the sulcus or pocket at 0 degrees **(A)**. The minimum angle when using the curette is 45° **(B)**. The maximum angle when using the curette is 70° **(C)**. An angle greater than 90 degrees **(D)** will cause damage of adjacent soft tissue. (Adapted from Daniel SJ, Harfst SA, Wilder R: *Mosby's dental hygiene: concepts, cases, and competencies*, ed 2, St Louis, 2008, Mosby.)

create a burnishing (smoothing) of the calculus, rather than biting into it for removal. An angle that is too open will place the noncutting edge sharply against the lining of the pocket when using a curette. This technique is useful if the operator purposely desires to perform a gingival curettage.

Strokes used when performing dental procedures will vary according to the task. When hand scaling, the initial stroke is for assessment to determine the topography of the tooth surface by lightly feeling for irregularities. This exploratory stroke is also performed with an explorer or with the tip of a power scaler when the power is not activated. When using scalers and curettes, once an irregularity is detected, the working stroke is performed by applying lateral pressure

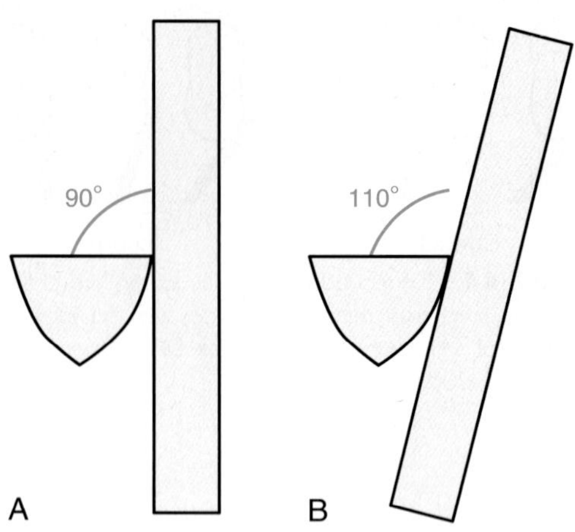

FIGURE 32-46 **A,** Initial setup of sharpening stone is 90 degrees to the face of the instrument. **B,** Open the angle to 110 degrees for sharpening. (From Daniel SJ, Harfst SA, Wilder R: *Mosby's dental hygiene: concepts, cases, and competencies,* ed 2, St Louis, 2008, Mosby.)

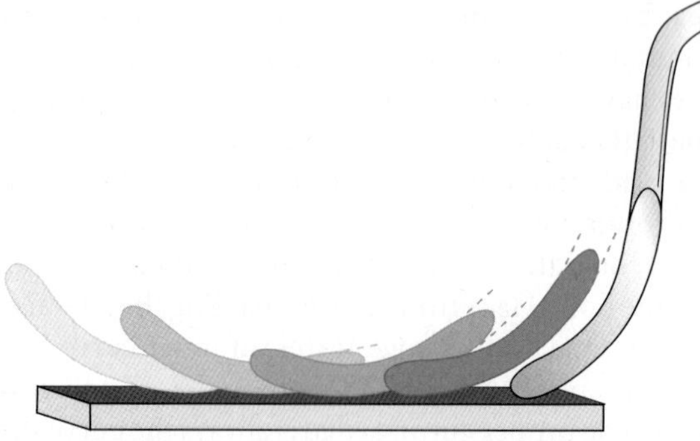

FIGURE 32-47 To maintain the original design of the instrument, when sharpening curved curettes, begin at the heel, sharpening small sections while working toward the toe. (From Nelson DM: *Saunders review of dental hygiene,* Philadelphia, 2000, WB Saunders.)

against the tooth and pulling the blade either vertically, horizontally, or obliquely in a short, controlled stroke. A root-planing stroke is longer in length, and light lateral pressure is used. Apply the minimum number of strokes necessary to accomplish the task.

SHARPENING

Thorough periodontal débridement can only be accomplished with the use of sharp instruments. Each stroke of a sharp instrument against the tooth will wear away the metal of the cutting edge, causing it to transform from a precise sharp line at the junction of the face and lateral surfaces into a dull, rounded surface. Using a dull surface requires heavier lateral pressure against the tooth, reducing tactile sensitivity and creating hand fatigue. The dull surface will burnish the calculus, rather than causing it to be shaved off. Once burnished, this calculus is difficult to detect and remove.

Instrument sharpening can be accomplished manually using sharpening stones or with the help of mechanical sharpening devices. Either way, it is critical to have a thorough understanding of the instrument design, including the cross-sectional shape and the line angles between surfaces, to enable a sharp cutting edge to be reestablished without creating changes in the instrument's original design.

Sharpening stones typically used for dental instruments include Arkansas, India, ceramic, and a synthetic composition, each differing in coarseness. A few drops of lubricant are required on most stones to keep metal particles from embedding into the stone and to reduce heat friction. Lubricate with sharpening oil on Arkansas and India stones; the ceramic stone can be lubricated with water or used dry, and the composition stone requires water.

Several methods of manual sharpening can be used; however, the technique that requires the instrument to be held stationary while the stone is moved provides a good view of the blade so that the angle can be precisely controlled. Hold the instrument in a palm grasp with the blade facing you and the face parallel to the floor. Elbows should be braced against the side of the body for stability, and the procedure should be performed under good lighting that is reflecting off the face. Hold the stone perpendicular to the face (Figure 32-46), beginning at a right angle (90 degrees), then tilt the stone against the lateral surface so the angle opens to 100 degrees to 110 degrees. An angle guide can be purchased or made by using a protractor to aid in visualizing correct angles.

> *TECHNICIAN NOTE* When sharpening hand instruments, the angle between the stone and the face should be approximately 110°. Remember when sharpening curettes to continue sharpening around the toe while maintaining this angle.

Using light pressure, move the stone in short up-and-down strokes against the lateral surface of the instrument, beginning at the heel of the instrument and working toward the toe, continuing around the toe when sharpening curettes (Figure 32-47). At the point where sharpening allows the lateral surface to meet sharply with the face, a black "sludge" will appear on the face. Finish with a few more light strokes, ending with a down stroke of the stone to remove wire particles that have been lifted from the metal.

Sharpening methods that include sharpening of the face should be avoided because the blade will be weakened and may break during débridement. Instruments that have been oversharpened and are excessively thin should be discarded.

POLISHING

Polishing is the final but critical step performed on an anesthetized dental patient as part of routine cleaning or advanced periodontal therapy. During nonroutine dental procedures, such as endodontic therapy or jaw fracture repair, polishing may be the initial procedure that is performed to remove plaque from the treatment area. In human dentistry, the necessity for routine polishing has become controversial, and selective polishing is becoming standard procedure to minimize the amount of enamel loss from frequent polishing.

The rationale for polishing veterinary mouths is to smooth surfaces that have been microscopically scratched during scaling procedures and to remove any extrinsic stains that were not removed with hand or power scalers. Extrinsic stains are discolorations that accumulate on the surfaces from pigments in food, blood, and some antiplaque products, such as chlorhexidine rinses. Intrinsic stains, often seen on the occlusal surface of maxillary molars in dogs, are within the tooth substance and not removable by polishing procedures. Causes of intrinsic staining include exposure to certain drugs during tooth development (e.g., tetracyclines), trauma, and developmental defects.

Two methods of polishing are currently used in veterinary practices. The most common method is driven by either an electric motor or an air compressor from a dental unit. A low-speed handpiece is used with a rubber cup. A prophylaxis angle, also called a prophy angle, is the attachment that is connected to the handpiece and holds the rubber cup. The cup is available in soft, flexible rubber or firm rubber. Prophy angles are either single-use plastic disposable or autoclavable metal. The rubber cup can be filled with a polishing paste that contains an abrasive agent available in fine, medium, or course grits. Because the act of polishing removes tooth substance, the choice of prophy paste should contain the least abrasive agent that will accomplish the task.

The friction from the rotating rubber cup creates heat that has potential to injure the pulp. New prophy angles have been developed with cups that oscillate back and forth rather than rotating. To minimize risks for thermal damage, use adequate paste, refilling the cup for each tooth, especially when polishing large dog teeth. To further minimize adverse effects, use the handpiece on a low rpm (revolutions per minute) level, just enough to maintain torque and steady rotation. When using a low-speed handpiece without a gauge, activate the handpiece to full speed before touching the rubber to the tooth by depressing the foot pedal. Listen for the pitch clues of the highest rpm level of the low-speed unit, and then ease off the pedal to less than one quarter of the maximal rpm. Use a light pressure against the tooth, just enough to cause the rim of the cup to flare slightly, and polish for only 1 to 3 seconds on each tooth surface. Complete the procedure with a gentle rinse of water or chlorhexidine to flush the residual prophy paste from the mouth. Eye protection should be worn by the operator, and the patient's eyes should be protected during the polishing procedure.

The second polishing method is with the use of an air polisher. An abrasive agent, sodium bicarbonate, is mixed with water to form a slurry propelled by air against the tooth. The tip of the nozzle is kept at a distance of approximately 4 mm from the tooth surface. To prevent sloughing of soft tissues, the nozzle must never be directed toward the gingiva or into the sulcus or pocket. Air polishing may be quicker and has been determined to be as effective as rubber cup polishing. However, the procedure is messy, and problems of clogging have plagued the equipment.

PERIODONTAL SURGERY

A grading system has been created to categorize periodontal disease that helps to provide generalizations for appropriate treatment (Box 32-7). Grade I periodontal disease refers to inflammatory changes confined to the gingiva (gingivitis), which is an easily reversible sign suggesting the need for a routine dental cleaning. Grade II periodontal disease is an early form of periodontitis where evidence of attachment loss is present, and root débridement or subgingival curettage may be required. Grade III periodontal disease is considered moderate periodontitis where 25% to 50% of the attachment structures of the tooth have been lost; root débridement, gingival curettage, and periodontal surgery are often required. Grade III teeth have a fair to guarded prognosis. Grade IV periodontal disease is considered severe periodontitis. With attachment loss of 50% or greater, these teeth often require extraction.

Deep periodontal pockets may warrant involved periodontal surgery. One technique for dealing with unexpected periodontal pocketing in the context of a busy private practice is staging of the procedure into two visits. Visit one involves baseline charting, radiographs, cleaning, and polishing along with closed root planing, gingival curettage, and placement of a doxycycline gel, with a return visit for more involved periodontal surgery to be scheduled 1 to 2 months later. Doxycycline gel may be placed into a freshly débrided periodontal pocket provided the pocket is 4 mm or deeper to allow for retention of the product. The product labeled for use in dogs carries the trade name Doxirobe, which is a doxycycline gel mixed with a slowly absorbable polymer. The polymer allows for delivery of the product in gel form, and once placed in the sulcus, spraying the product with water causes the polymer to harden, allowing for compaction of the product into the pocket. This provides a number of beneficial effects. Doxycycline is an antimicrobial with good spectrum against a number of periodontal pathogens. Doxycycline has antiinflammatory effects, which are beneficial in decreasing the damage to periodontal tissues that may be mediated by the immune system's response to periodontal pathogens. Third, the space-occupying effect of the polymer prevents the treated pocket from filling with food and debris immediately after the procedure, allowing the site to heal from the most apical aspect coronally.

When the patient returns in 1 to 2 months, pocket depth should be gently probed once the patient is under general anesthesia. If the pocket depth is normal, no further treatment is necessary, and home care can be continued with routine checkups and periodontal débridement as necessary.

BOX 32-7 Periodontal Disease Classification

- PD 0: Clinically normal
- PD 1: Gingivitis with no attachment loss
- PD 2: <25% attachment loss, mild periodontitis
- PD 3: 25%-50% attachment loss, moderate periodontitis
- PD 4: >50% attachment loss, advanced periodontitis

If the abnormal pocket depth is still 5 mm or greater in dogs or 3 mm or greater in cats, periodontal surgery is indicated if the client would like to save the affected tooth. A variety of periodontal surgical procedures have been documented, with each technique appropriate in different situations. Creation of a flap and open root planing is usually necessary in cases of pocket depths of 5 mm or greater. In the past, periodontal disease was considered to be irreversible. Now, with advances in surgical technique and materials, periodontal disease may be considered to be reversible if dealt with before severe damage to the periodontium, but without proper postoperative home care, the condition will invariably recur. Pets with advanced periodontal disease may require periodontal débridement every 3 to 4 months until the disease is showing evidence that it is controlled.

Vertical and horizontal bone loss represent two different challenges in periodontal surgery. Vertical bone loss occurs along the long axis of the tooth root and is easier to deal with than widespread horizontal bone loss where multiple furcations are exposed. After débridement of the vertical infrabony defect, an osteoconductive or osteoinductive material may be placed in the defect. Osteoconductive materials will not induce new bone, but will act as scaffolding for new bone cells to traverse the defect. In contrast, osteoinductive materials stimulate progenitor cells of osteoblasts to differentiate and form new bone in an area. Multiple products exist in the human dental market. In veterinary dentistry, an example of an osteoconductive product is Consil (Nutramax Laboratories). An example of an osteoinductive material is Osteoallograft (Veterinary Transplant Services). These products generally require a means of retention, which may be an absorbable or nonabsorbable membrane or a flap that is repositioned in a coronal location to contain the material once placed. Any foreign material may act as a nidus for continued infection, so the placement site must be able to be adequately débrided before considering placement of these products. The surgery site may be lavaged with 0.12% chlorhexidine followed by lactated Ringer's solution to minimize the cytotoxic effects of chlorhexidine. The flap is closed with 4-0 or 5-0 absorbable monofilament suture material placed interdentally in a simple interrupted pattern, and digital pressure is applied to the gingiva for 60 seconds. Occasionally a sling suture may be used to provide a purse-string effect to encourage the gingival portion of the flap to reattach. The patient should be placed on a soft-food diet with no hard toys or treats for 2 weeks, and antibacterial mouth rinses (0.12% chlorhexidine) may be prescribed. The owner should start brushing the teeth 1 week postoperatively using the modified Stillman technique at the surgery site (Figure 32-48, *A*).

> *TECHNICIAN NOTE* Attempts to save teeth with advanced periodontal surgery should not be performed unless the client is able to perform daily brushing.

Recently a periodontal vaccine has been developed as an additional tool in prevention of periodontal disease in dogs. The vaccine is a bacterin of three *Porphyromonas* species. The vaccine is not expected to replace proper home care, dental diets, and routine cleanings, but is rather considered another tool in the armamentarium of the practitioner in the prevention of periodontal disease. Results of large-scale efficacy trials in dogs are pending.

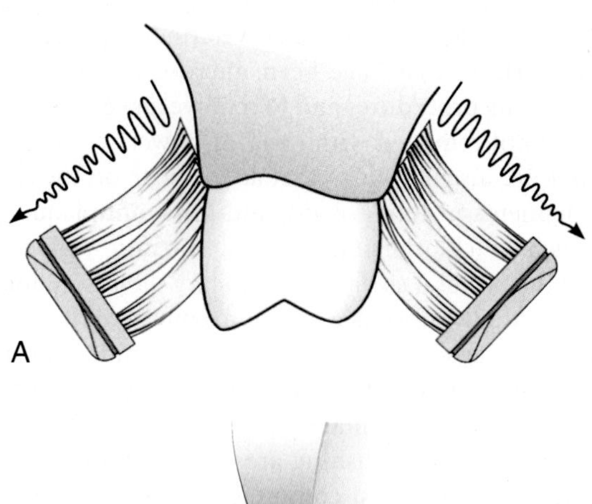

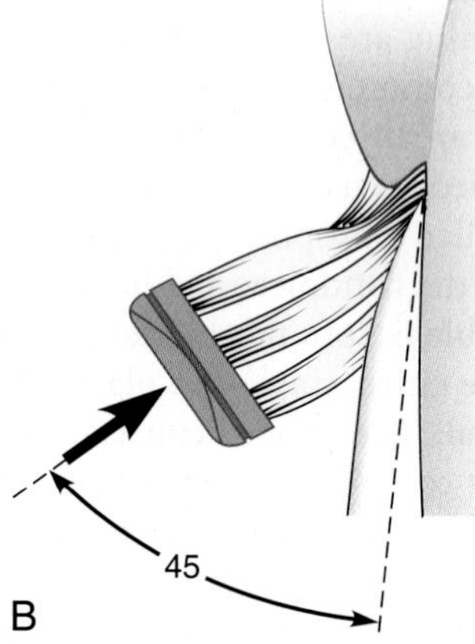

FIGURE 32-48 **A,** The modified Stillman brushing technique of placing the sides of the bristles along the tooth and gums and moving in a coronal direction provides gingival stimulation without traumatizing a periodontal surgery site. **B,** The 45-degree angle of the toothbrush in the Bass technique aims the soft bristles toward the gingival margin and into the sulcus. Use short back-and-forth motions without dislodging the bristles from the sulcus. The gentle pressure should elicit blanching of the gingival tissues. In the modified Bass technique, the Bass method is followed with a gentle rolling of the bristles over the coronal portion of the teeth. (From Newman MG, Takei H, Klokkevold PR et al: *Carranza's clinical periodontology*, ed 10, St Louis, 2006, Saunders.)

HOME CARE

Client communication regarding dental home care is an important role of the veterinary technician. The technician will spend time with the client to demonstrate brushing techniques and provide recommendations for various diets and products that can be used at the patient's home to reduce accumulations of plaque and calculus. Reduction of bacteria in the mouth can be accomplished through brushing, diets, and use of toys.

The mechanical cleansing provided by daily toothbrushing provides the most thorough method of plaque control for pets. Several methods are used; the most widely accepted is the Bass technique that concentrates the bristles along the gingival margin and in the sulcus (Figure 32-48, *B*). Using a soft toothbrush, the bristles are directed at a 45-degree angle toward the gingival margin so that some of the bristles enter the sulcus while other bristles are resting on the tooth adjacent to the margin. Pressing lightly, use short back-and-forth strokes while maintaining the 45-degree angle for 5 to 10 seconds before repositioning the brush along the next group of teeth. Veterinary patients are reluctant to keep their mouth open, so it is best to brush while the mouth is closed with access to the teeth made by a gentle lifting of the lips. Perform this brushing technique with the bristles rinsed in water rather than covered with a veterinary dentifrice. Once the dentifrice is placed into the mouth, it is more difficult to brush because the patient tries to eat the flavored paste. When brushing with water is completed, the dentifrice can be applied into the mouth as a treat and to provide enzymatic or antiseptic benefits. Human toothpastes may cause stomach upset if swallowed and should not be used. Instruct the client to prioritize brushing in areas that collect the heaviest debris (usually the buccal surfaces of the caudal teeth) in case the patient becomes uncooperative before the task is completed. Brushing should be initiated at a young age to allow the patient to become accustomed to oral care. Before introducing a toothbrush, the puppy or kitten should have gum massages to gain experience of having their mouths manipulated. The modified Stillman technique is sometimes used in areas of periodontal surgery to minimize plaque accumulation while preventing trauma to the reattaching gingival tissue (see Figure 32-48, *A*). This technique involves placement of the bristles apical to the gingival margin with a gentle sweeping motion in the coronal direction against the gingiva and crown of the tooth without placement of bristles into the healing sulcus.

> *TECHNICIAN NOTE* The Bass technique of toothbrushing places the bristles of the brush at a 45-degree angle against the tooth along the gingival margin to enable some bristles to slide into the sulcus. The Stillman technique is used in areas of periodontal surgery, where bristles apical to the gingival margin are moved with a gentle sweeping motion in the coronal direction against the gingiva without placement of bristles into the healing sulcus.

Feeding a diet of soft food that adheres to teeth surfaces will contribute to periodontal disease. Plaque control can be augmented by feeding a hard dental diet that has been manufactured and tested to reduce accumulations. The Veterinary Oral Health Council (VOHC) was established in 1997 by veterinary dentists and researchers to recognize products that have been shown to meet predetermined standards of plaque and calculus retardation. The VOHC seal of acceptance is issued to products that have proven to reduce plaque and/or calculus based on generally accepted protocols. For a complete list of VOHC-approved products, visit their website at www.VOHC.org.

Diets reduce accumulations by either mechanical or chemical action. The first dental diet was created taking advantage of mechanical cleansing. Long fibers within large pieces of kibble oriented in one direction help to keep the biscuit from crumbling readily when a dog or cat bites into it. This design allows the biscuit to mechanically scrape the sides of the teeth clean as the teeth penetrate the biscuit. An example of a chemical used to provide anticalculus effects is hexametaphosphate (HMP), which works by sequestering the calcium in plaque fluids to reduce calculus formation by preventing mineralization of plaque. Unfortunately, use of dental diets alone is not as effective as toothbrushing. A regimen combining special diets and toothbrushing is recommended for optimal plaque control.

Many home-care products are available, including treats, rinses, and water additives. However, the technician should research products before offering recommendations. During home-care instructions, the technician should also offer counseling regarding which types of toys may be harmful to the pet's teeth. Rawhide has an excellent cleansing action. However, the size and shape of the product must be correctly matched with the chewing habits of the dog. Rawhide should be taken away following 20 to 30 minutes of gnawing to decrease the likelihood of gastrointestinal problems from ingestion of a large piece. Allowing the rawhide to dry overnight and repeating the process will minimize chances of the pet encountering gastrointestinal or choking problems associated with ingestion of a large piece of rawhide.

Many toys found in pet stores are harmful to teeth, including cow hooves, hard nylon bones, and natural sterilized bones; each is capable of causing dental fractures. Aggressive chewing of tennis balls causes abrasion of teeth, especially when dirt and sand becomes incorporated within the felt of the ball. Instruct clients to always monitor their pets when providing chew toys.

RESTORATIVE DENTISTRY

Restorative dentistry is the subspecialty of dentistry that restores or maintains a tooth's structure and function. No restorative material is as strong as the original tooth structure, so an attempt is always made to preserve as much of the original tooth as possible. Indications for restorative dentistry include teeth with dental caries (cavities), fractured teeth, and endodontically treated teeth.

Fractured teeth are frequently restored to function while maintaining periodontal health. The cheek teeth (premolars and molars) have a natural design called the dental bulge that deflects food away from the gingival sulcus. When the teeth lose this proper contour, they can become predisposed to periodontal disease. Fractured teeth can be restored with restorative materials alone or in combination with retention pins or posts or both. Pins and posts do not add strength to the restoration, but aid in retention of the restoration.

Crowns are placed on teeth with fractured crowns to protect the tooth, especially in working dogs or in cases where repeated tooth trauma is expected. Metal crowns made of semiprecious metals are more common than porcelain crowns because of their greater strength and requirements for less tooth removal than with crowns that have a porcelain exterior fused to metal. Crowns are most commonly placed in dogs on the canine and maxillary fourth premolar teeth (Figure 32-49).

> *TECHNICIAN NOTE* Metal crowns are more commonly placed than tooth-colored crowns because of their greater strength and requirements for less tooth removal than crowns with a porcelain exterior fused to metal.

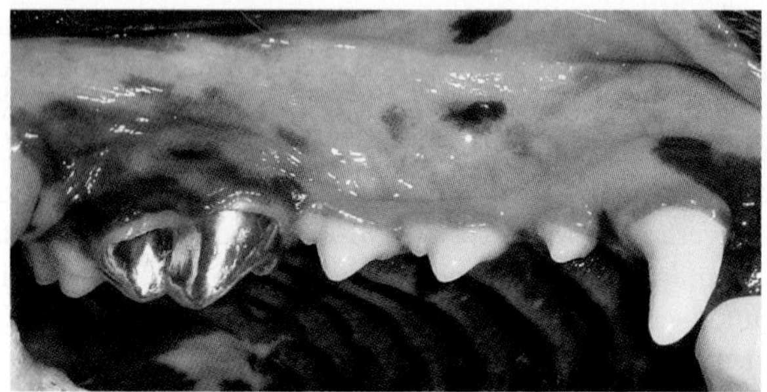

FIGURE 32-49 A full metal jacket crown has been placed over an endodontically treated maxillary fourth premolar tooth. Metal crowns are chosen rather than tooth-colored crowns because of their strength and need for less tooth removal.

ENDODONTICS

Endodontics deals with the study and treatment of the inside of the tooth (pulp) and periapical tissues. The periapical tissue is located around the tip (apex) of the tooth root. The tooth pulp consists of nerves, blood vessels, lymphatics, and connective tissue. The pulp tissue is found in the pulp chamber (crown) and root canal (root) of the tooth and enters the tooth through numerous small openings in the apex of the tooth root called the apical delta.

The dental pulp is important to the development of the tooth in a young animal. It supplies the nutrients needed by the odontoblasts to deposit secondary dentin. This makes the walls of the root and crown thicker, so the tooth is stronger. Once the dog or cat is 10 to 18 months of age, the root apex should be closed. As the animal continues to age, the pulp chamber and canal will become smaller because the odontoblasts will continue to produce secondary dentin, which makes the tooth stronger (Figure 32-50, *A, B*).

The treatment options for teeth with endodontic disease will depend on the age of the animal, duration of endodontic disease, and anatomy of the tooth. Conventional root canal therapy is usually performed on dogs and cats 12 months of age and older with endodontic disease. Treatment involves removing the dead or dying pulp tissue from the tooth, disinfecting and shaping the root canal, and filling the canal (obturation) with an appropriate material to seal the apex from the periapical tissues. Radiographs are necessary to

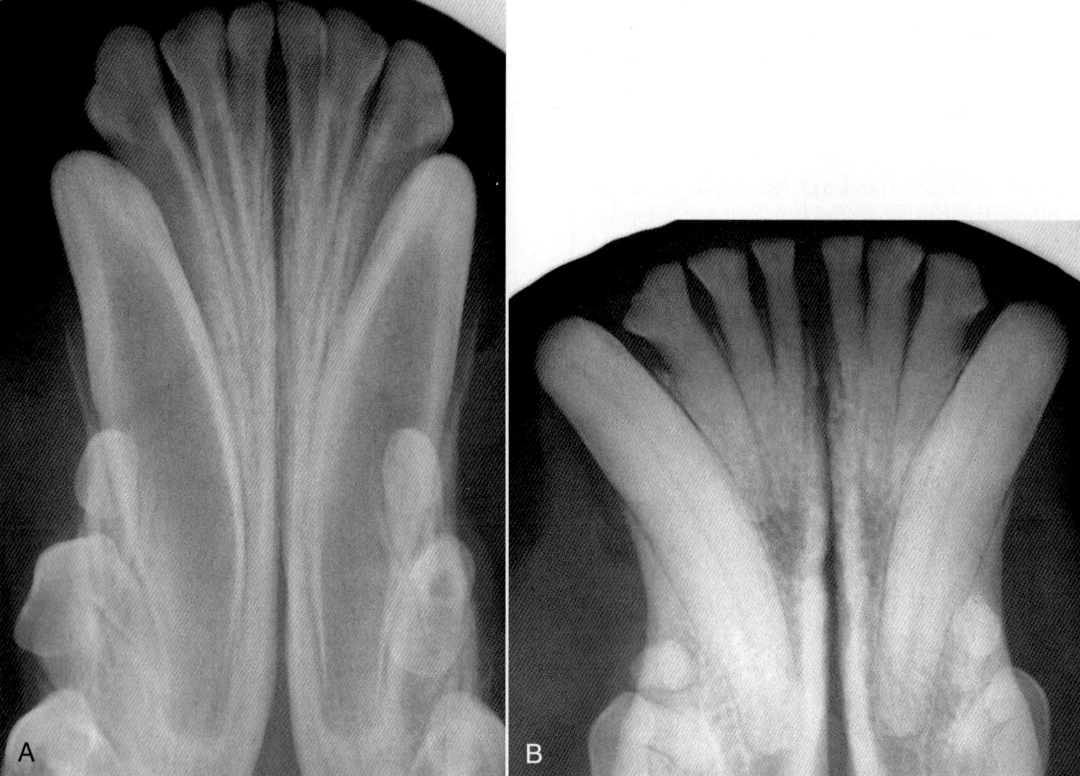

FIGURE 32-50 Radiographs of **(A)** immature permanent teeth of a 6-month-old dog, and **(B)** permanent teeth of a 6-year-old dog. Note the secondary dentin that has been produced in the older dog that has strengthened the tooth and caused the pulp chamber and root canal to become narrowed.

ensure that a proper apical seal has been achieved. A detailed discussion of this procedure will follow later.

Box 32-8 lists equipment and supplies needed for conventional root canal therapy. These items should be ready for use before the root canal treatment is started. A preoperative radiograph is taken to evaluate the tooth root and periapical region. The veterinarian will make the appropriate access to the root canal through the crown of the tooth with a dental bur. The canal may have partially necrotic pulp that will require removal with a barbed broach (Figure 32-51). The broach is placed in the canal and rotated to ensnare the pulp. The broach and pulp tissue are removed from the canal. This step is repeated until all pulp has been removed. Many teeth will not have any visible pulp tissue remaining (necrotic pulp), and the barbed broaches will not be needed. When a barbed broach is used, it is important to avoid binding of the broach in the walls of the canal because the broach may break off in the canal. The canal is cleaned with files and irrigant to sterilize the canal, and the files are also used to shape the canal to allow for proper obturation. There are several types and sizes of files. Hedström (H) and Kerr (K) files are the most commonly used hand files (Figure 32-52). H-files have a sharper edge and can remove dentin faster than K-files. They are used in a push-pull motion. H-files are more susceptible to file breakage than K-files. K-files are inserted to the apical extent of the canal, turned one-quarter turn, and removed, allowing for shaping of the apical portion of the canal. The edges of K-files are less sharp, so dentin removal is less efficient than with H-files. K-files are structurally more sound and less likely to fracture in the canal. The files are available in a number of different lengths and diameters. The smallest diameter file is a number 6 (6/100 of a millimeter at the tip). They increase in diameter by even number increments from 6 to 10, and then they increase by increments of 5. For instance, the following diameters exist: 6, 8, 10, 15, 20, 25, 30, 35, 40, and so on until file 60, at which point the diameter increases by 10. The largest diameter file is a 140. Files made for human root canals are made in lengths of 21 mm, 25 mm, or 31 mm. Special veterinary files are available for teeth in which human files would not reach the apex (Figure 32-53). This variation in length is necessary so that the apex of the tooth root can be reached in long teeth (canines). The variation in diameter is necessary so that the narrow canals of old and/or small animals and the large canals of young or large animals can be properly filed.

BOX 32-8 Endodontic Instrument and Materials Setup

- Dental films
- High-speed handpiece and burs
- Barbed broaches
- Endodontic files and file organizer
- Rubber stops
- Endodontic ruler
- Canal lubricant, irrigant, and irrigation needles
- Paper points
- College pliers
- Zinc oxide, eugenol
- Glass slab, mixing spatula
- Gutta percha points
- Lentulo, paste fillers
- 10:1 reduction gear contraangle
- Pluggers and spreaders
- Heating instrument
- Restorative materials and instruments

TECHNICIAN NOTE H-files are used in a push-pull motion and are more susceptible to file breakage than K-files. K-files are inserted to the apical extent of the canal, turned one-quarter turn, and removed, allowing for shaping of the apical portion of the canal.

Files should be removed from the package and placed in an organized manner. Files of similar lengths may be placed in a piece of autoclavable foam in order of increasing diameter. The files can be autoclaved, and when the veterinarian is ready to perform the root canal, the files will be sterile and in an organized manner. Preoperative attention to detail is helpful in minimizing anesthesia time because root canal procedures can be long procedures.

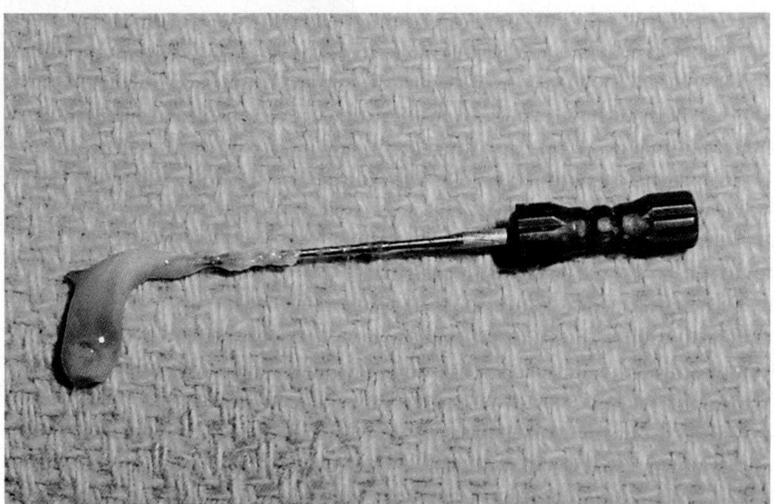

FIGURE 32-51 Partially necrotic pulp retrieved with a barbed broach.

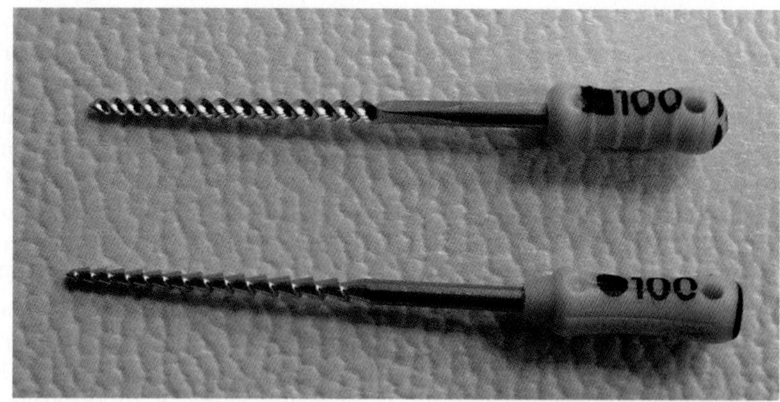

FIGURE 32-52 H- and K-endodontic files: H-files *(lower file)* are designed to be used in a push-pull manner, whereas K-files *(upper file)* are used to shape the apical canal with quarter-turn advances.

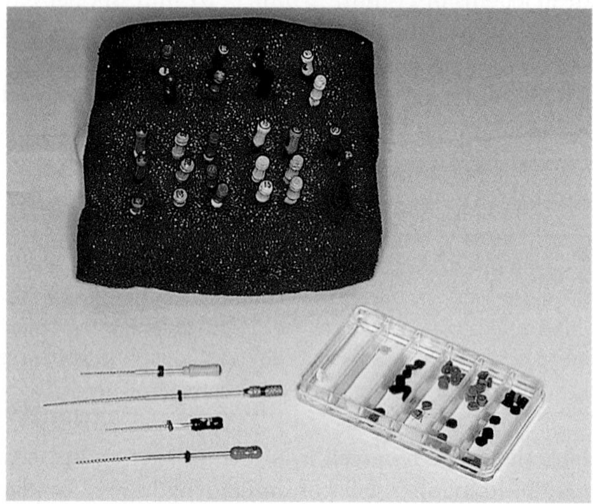

FIGURE 32-53 Endodontic files are made in human and veterinary lengths. Files should be arranged by size for easy identification. Endodontic stops *(right)* are placed on each file to determine and maintain working length.

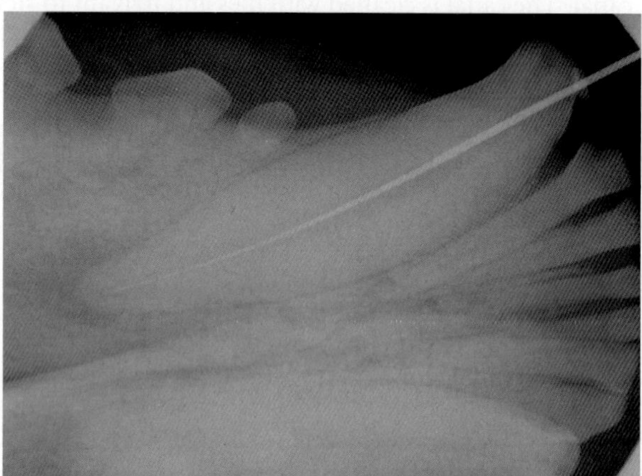

FIGURE 32-54 An endodontic file is placed to the apex and a radiograph is taken to determine the working length.

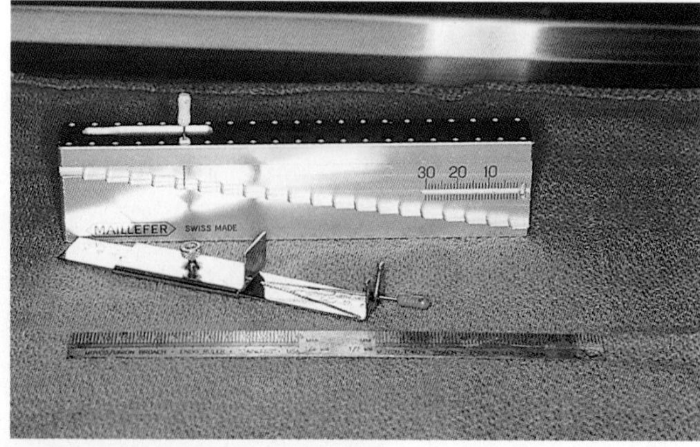

FIGURE 32-55 Measuring gauges and rulers are used to measure the working length of the root from the access site to the apex.

Endodontic stops are small pieces of rubber that go around the file to mark a specific length (see Figure 32-53). The file is placed in the root canal, and a radiograph is taken to make sure that the file goes all the way to the apical extent of the root canal system (Figure 32-54). The distance from the endodontic stop to the file tip is called the working length. The rest of the files are set to this length to ensure that the root canal is filed to the proper depth. Measuring gauges are available that allow quick adjustment of the endodontic stop to the proper working length (Figure 32-55).

Canal lubricants are used to soften the dentinal walls to ease filing and help prevent file breakage. An irrigant is used between file sizes to rinse the canal of dentinal shavings and other debris. The most common irrigant is sodium hypochlorite because of its excellent disinfecting properties and ability to break down organic debris (pulp). Endodontic irrigation needles are placed on the syringe that contains the irrigant. These needles have a blunt end with a side opening to prevent forcing noxious irrigant periapically (Figure 32-56).

> *TECHNICIAN NOTE* Sodium hypochlorite is irritating to soft tissue. Contact with the oral soft tissues should be avoided, and forceful irrigation of the canal should be avoided to prevent periapical migration of the irrigant.

After the canal has been properly cleaned and shaped by the files, it is then ready for obturation. Obturation refers to filling the canal with a material that will seal it from the periapical area. The canal should have a final rinse of sterile water, and then it is dried with sterile paper points. Successive paper points are inserted and removed until the points come out of the canal dry. An endodontic sealer is then applied to the canal walls. Sealer application can be done with a sterile paper point, K-file, or spiral paste filler on a slow-speed handpiece (Figure 32-57). Gutta percha should make up the bulk of the filling agent. It is a radiopaque rubberlike material that can be vertically and laterally condensed to adapt to the shape of the root canal. The material can be heated to allow it to flow into the canal and adapt to the canal shape easier. Vertical and lateral condensation is performed with pluggers and spreaders, and additional gutta percha is added as needed to fill the entire canal. Pluggers have a blunt end that pushes the gutta percha vertically in an apical direction. Spreaders have a pointed tip and push the gutta percha laterally to create room for more gutta percha for a solid fill. Spreaders and pluggers come in a variety of lengths and diameters (Figure 32-58). Extra long veterinary length spreaders and pluggers are available.

Once obturation of the canal has been accomplished, the restorative filling material is placed. This can be done with a single filling material or in two layers with an intermediate and final filling material used. Composite fillings cannot be placed next to eugenol because eugenol interferes with the hardening of the composite. Glass ionomers are a commonly used intermediate filling material. A light-cured composite filling material is often used as the final restorative at the surface of the access site and fracture site.

Teeth that have undergone pulp death become more brittle over time because of the lack of hydration that was originally provided by the pulp tissue. A good history should always be taken to try to determine how the pet fractured the tooth. If inappropriate chew toys are in the environment, these should be removed. A metal crown may be indicated to help prevent fracture of the tooth in the future.

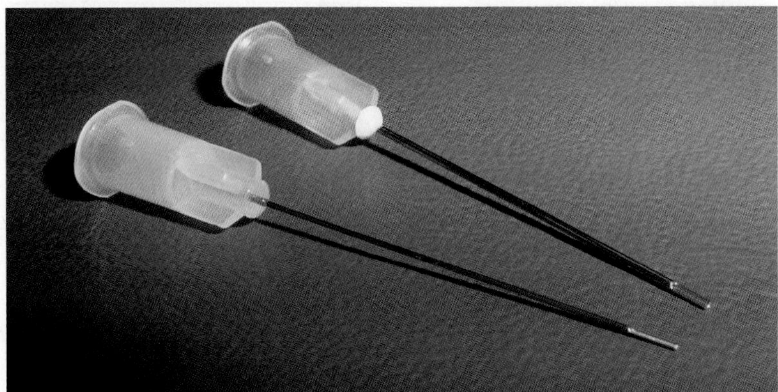

FIGURE 32-56 Endodontic needles are open on the side of the tip to prevent inadvertent forcing of sodium hypochlorite through the apical delta.

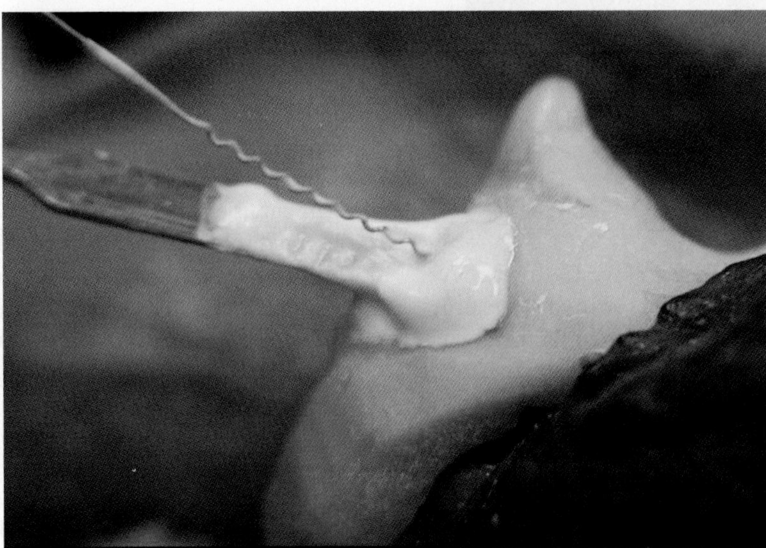

FIGURE 32-57 Lentulo spiral paste filler for delivery of cement. A spatula loaded with cement is placed near the spiral filler, which pushes the cement apically. Care should be taken to use a contraangle with a reduction gear to decrease chances of the filler breaking in the canal. A composite splint is seen at the gingival margin resulting from a healing jaw fracture in the area of the canine tooth.

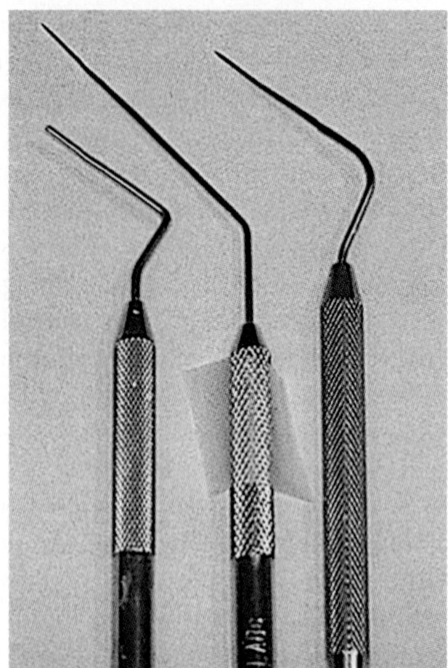

FIGURE 32-58 An endodontic plugger and endodontic spreaders. Spreaders have a pointed tip and are used for lateral compaction. Pluggers have a flat tip and are used for vertical compaction.

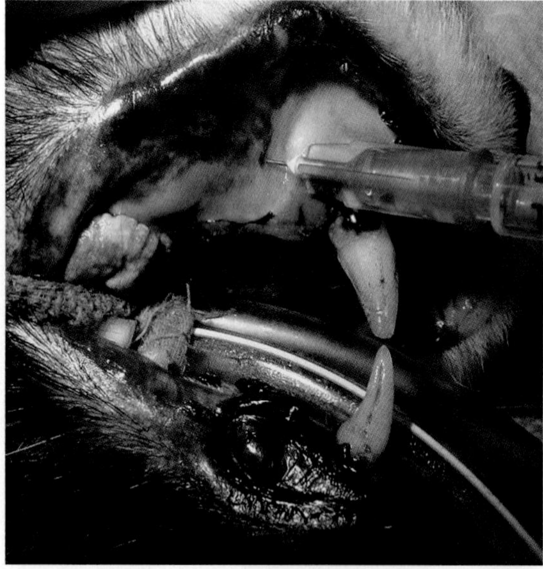

FIGURE 32-59 Infraorbital block in a cat.

EXODONTICS

Although attempts should be made to save teeth whenever possible, extraction (exodontics) is necessary when the prognosis for saving the tooth is grave and when financial constraints or medical conditions prevent multiple anesthetic episodes that may be necessary to save the tooth. Extraction of a tooth with severe periodontal disease may be easy if much of the attachment structures of the tooth have already been lost, but as a result of their large root surface area, extraction of canine or feline teeth can be challenging.

Serious complications can arise from extraction. Possible complications should be discussed with the owner before the procedure. Complications include those associated with anesthesia, hemorrhage, ocular trauma, jaw fracture, and displacement of a root into an inaccessible area, such as the nasal passage. Iatrogenic jaw fracture can easily occur when extracting diseased mandibular first molars or mandibular canine teeth in cats or small-breed dogs, especially when significant periodontal disease already exists.

> TECHNICIAN NOTE Never extract a tooth without the permission of the client. Therefore always obtain a contact number to discuss any unexpected findings.

The extraction process begins with placement of a regional nerve block to decrease inhalant anesthesia requirements. The local anesthetic of choice in oral surgery is 0.5% bupivacaine because of its ability to provide not only intraoperative but also postoperative pain relief of 6 to 10 hours duration. Common regional nerve blocks are the maxillary or infraorbital block for the upper jaw and the inferior alveolar or mental nerve block for the lower jaw (Figure 32-59).

> TECHNICIAN NOTE Regional nerve blocks not only lower inhalant requirements, but also provide postoperative pain relief.

CLOSED EXTRACTIONS

While the regional block is taking effect, a preextraction radiograph should be taken of the tooth to assess for evidence of root pathologic conditions that may affect the surgical approach. A closed technique is best reserved for single-rooted teeth or teeth that have severe periodontal disease. Once the regional nerve block is placed, the gingival attachments around the tooth are separated with either a periosteal elevator (Figure 32-60), dental luxator, or scalpel blade. After the soft tissue attachments have been severed, a dental elevator of appropriate size and shape (Figure 32-61, *A, B*) is placed in the periodontal space on the mesial or distal surface of the crown. Once placed in the space, gentle pressure is placed to seat the elevator within the tooth and alveolar bone, and the handle of the elevator is rotated slightly to stretch the periodontal ligament fibers. If elevation is done correctly, the tooth will be observed to move slightly when the elevator is rotated. Pressure is held for 10 seconds, and then the elevator is advanced apically and rotated against the root in the opposite direction to create pressure and hold again. The goal is to fatigue the periodontal ligament and prevent tooth root fracture. Larger elevators are used as the periodontal ligament breaks down and allows more room to place a larger instrument. The temptation to wiggle the elevator in an attempt to obtain a deeper position in the periodontal space should be avoided because this will often cause breakdown of the alveolar bone and loss of leverage. The elevator may also be placed on the palatal or lingual surface and the vestibular surface within the periodontal space to stretch the periodontal ligament fibers

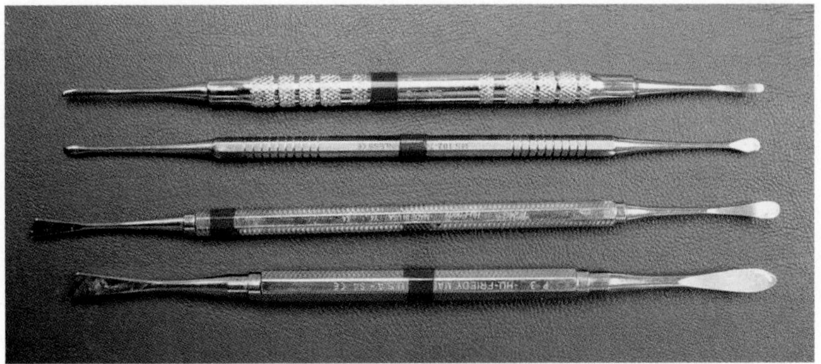

FIGURE 32-60 Various periosteal elevators used in oral surgery.

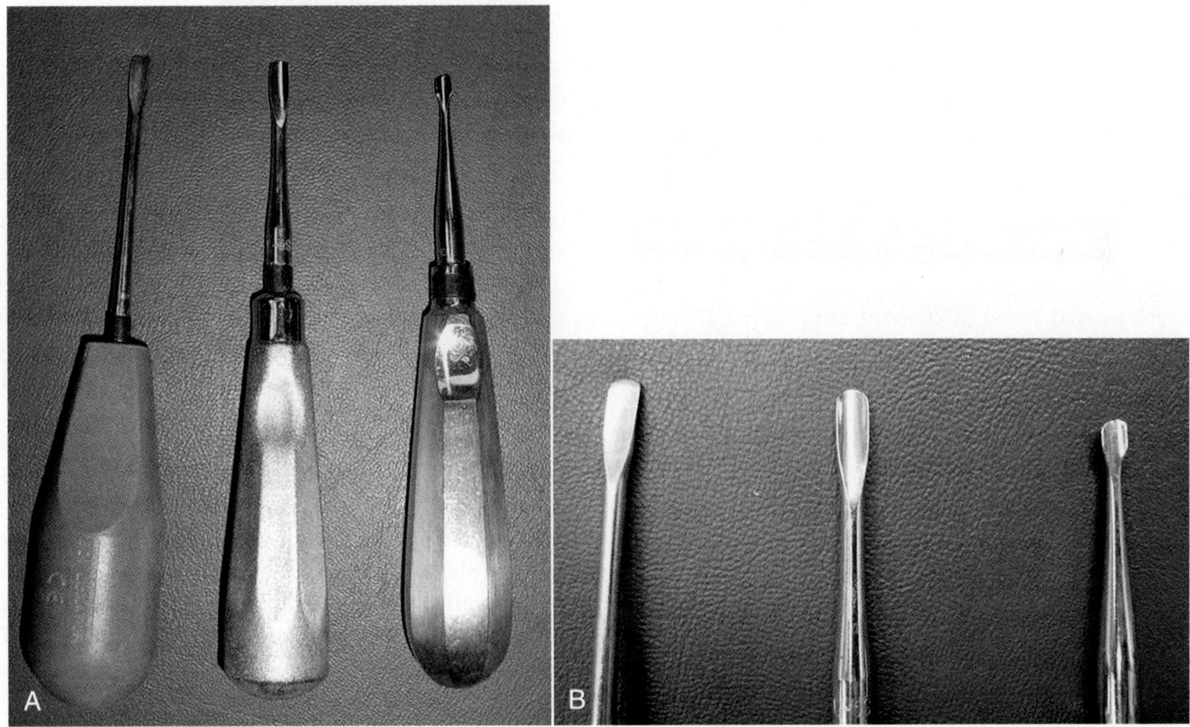

FIGURE 32-61 **A,** Dental luxator, straight elevator, and winged elevator. **B,** Working end of each.

around the entire circumference of the tooth. Elevators come in a variety of shapes and sizes, and it is important to have access to different sizes for different situations. When grasping a dental elevator, the handle should rest securely in the palm of the hand. The index finger should be extended so that if the elevator slips, the index finger will help to stop the advancing of the elevator into deeper structures (Figure 32-62). Ocular and brain trauma have been documented in cases where dental elevators have slipped during extraction procedures. To prevent this, forces used must be well controlled and should be generated in the lateral or medial direction rather than in the apical direction. The gingival tissue is apposed to close the extraction site with 4-0 or 5-0 monofilament absorbable suture in a simple interrupted pattern. Sterile extraction packs containing necessary instruments may be wrapped and prepared for use (Box 32-9).

SURGICAL EXTRACTIONS

As a result of the large surface area and multirooted nature of carnivore teeth, surgical extraction is often a less traumatic option than attempts of removing a firmly rooted tooth by closed extraction. As with closed extractions, the gingival attachments are separated from the tooth crown with a periosteal elevator, dental luxator, or scalpel blade. A flap is created, depending on the location and underlying root structure. A flap with no releasing incisions is called an envelope flap. A flap with one releasing incision is a triangle flap, and a flap with two releasing incisions is called a pedicle flap. Each situation should be assessed individually to decide which type of flap is necessary to provide the optimal access and tension-free tissue closure while inflicting the minimum amount of soft tissue trauma. Pedicle flaps are created with a broad base

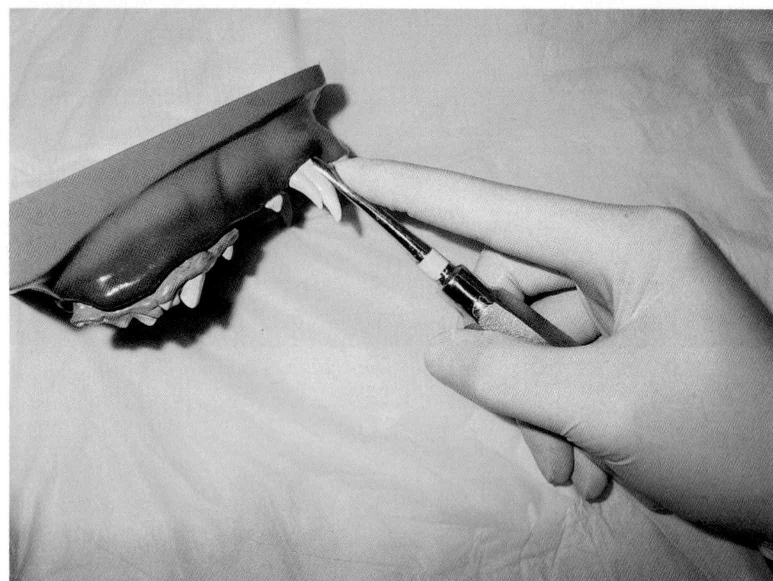

FIGURE 32-62 Proper grasp of a dental elevator. The index finger is extended to minimize soft tissue trauma if the elevator slips.

BOX 32-9 Extraction Instrument Setup

- High-speed handpiece
- Burs: fissure and round in assorted sizes, carbide, and diamond-coated
- Periosteal elevators
- Dental luxators
- Dental elevators
- Extraction forceps
- Root tip elevators, root tip forceps
- Absorbable monofilament suture
- Metzenbaum scissors
- Needle holders
- Tissue forceps
- Suture scissors
- Blade handle and blade

to ensure good blood supply and adequate tissue for closure. Once the flap is raised, a round carbide bur is used in a water-cooled, high-speed handpiece to create a window in the buccal bone of roots to be extracted. Multirooted teeth are separated with a tapered fissure bur. Once the window is created and roots are sectioned, minimal force is necessary to gently pry the roots and attached crown segments from their sockets. Once the roots are removed in their entirety, rough bone edges are smoothed with a large round diamond bur. The alveolus of each root is curetted and lavaged with sterile isotonic solution or 0.12% chlorhexidine. The periosteum is separated from the mucosa to provide adequate tension-free tissue to close the defect. The flap is closed with 4-0 or 5-0 absorbable monofilament suture in a simple interrupted pattern. Occasionally, osteoconductive or osteoinductive products may be placed in the alveolus before closure if it is suspected that the product will not act as a nidus and will help to prevent significant bone loss in the area of the extraction. A postextraction radiograph should be taken to document complete removal of the roots in cases where the roots were not retrieved easily.

When a root fractures, additional instruments will be needed to retrieve the retained tooth root. Root tip elevators and root tip forceps are valuable tools in root tip retrieval (Figure 32-63). Care should be taken to prevent dislodging the root tip into the nasal passage or mandibular canal. Cotton-tip applicators are helpful to control hemorrhage in the alveolar socket to visualize the root tip. Avoid blowing air from an air or water syringe into the socket. Although this may help visualize the root, a fatal air embolism may occur. The pet should be given no hard food or treats for 14 days postoperatively. Postoperative antibiotics are generally not necessary following extraction procedures. The AVDC has developed a position statement regarding the use of antibiotics in dental patients (Box 32-10).

COMMON DENTAL PROBLEMS IN DOGS AND CATS

TOOTH RESORPTION

Tooth resorption is common in cats and rare in dogs. Prevalence studies have found that 20% to 70% of cats are affected by this problem, depending on the population of cats and the investigative methods employed. The lesions are usually appreciated clinically at the cervical portion of the tooth (the junction of where the crown meets the root, sometimes referred to as the "neck" of the tooth), which is often hidden by the gingiva. However, recent histologic studies have found that these lesions begin on the root surface, and radiographic changes can often be seen before a clinical lesion is obvious. When a lesion develops at the gingival margin, the adjacent gingiva often covers these lesions with a combination of hyperplastic gingiva and granulation tissue (Figure 32-64, *A*).

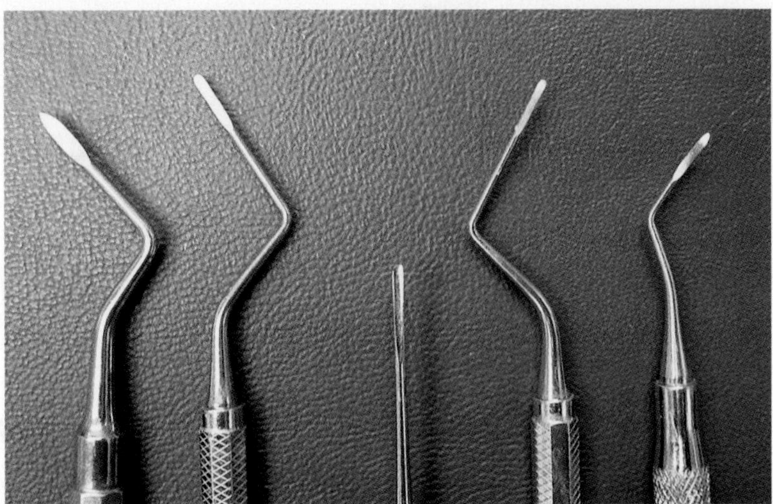

FIGURE 32-63 Root tip elevators in various shapes and sizes. These instruments are fragile and are meant to be used with minimal force.

BOX 32-10 AVDC Position Statement Regarding Use of Antibiotics in Veterinary Dentistry

The AVDC endorses the use of systemic antibiotics in veterinary dentistry for treatment of some infectious conditions of the oral cavity. Although culture and susceptibility testing is rarely performed on individual patients that have an infection extending from/to the oral cavity, the selection of an appropriate antibiotic should be based on published data regarding susceptibility testing of the spectra of known oral pathogens.

Patients that are scheduled for an oral procedure may benefit from pre-treatment with an appropriate antibiotic to improve the health of infected oral tissues. Bacteremia is a recognized sequela to dental scaling and other oral procedures. Healthy animals are able to overcome this bacteremia without the use of systemic antibiotics. However, use of a systemically administered antibiotic is recommended to reduce bacteremia for animals that are immune compromised, have underlying systemic disease (such as clinically-evident cardiac, hepatic, and renal diseases) and/or when severe oral infection is present.

Antibiotics should never be considered a monotherapy for treatment of oral infections, and should not be used as preventive management of oral conditions.

With permission of AVDC, www.AVDC.org/position-statements.html.

TECHNICIAN NOTE The cause of feline tooth resorption is still unknown, but recent research suggests that vitamin D levels in commercial cat food may play a role (see Recommended Reading).

A fine explorer should be used to check for irregularities, as described earlier in this chapter. In the past, restorations have been placed in lesions, but follow-up studies have shown poor long-term results with restoration. Therefore extraction is the treatment of choice. Dental radiographs of these teeth are necessary to evaluate the severity of resorption and to guide treatment.

Sometimes it is not possible to perform a complete tooth extraction because of severe root resorption where a portion of the root has been replaced by a reparative bone-cementum material. When this occurs, the tooth root becomes incorporated into the adjacent alveolar bone. Radiographic evidence of this is seen by loss of periodontal ligament space and decreased root density, approximating that of the surrounding bone density (Figure 32-64, *B*). When this radiographic appearance is seen, in the absence of periodontal or endodontic disease, it is possible to perform a crown amputation where hard tissue with characteristics of tooth root is removed and resorbed root that has been replaced by bone is not removed. The tooth crown and coronal root segment are removed with a dental bur and high-speed handpiece. The crestal alveolar bone is smoothed with a dental bur, and the gingiva is closed with absorbable suture over the crown amputation site.

ORTHODONTIC PROBLEMS

Malocclusions

There are four classes of malocclusions that are used. Class I malocclusion (Figure 32-65) occurs when the maxillary and mandibular jaw lengths are normal but one or more teeth are in an abnormal position. Class I malocclusions (also referred to as neutroclusion) are the most common type of malocclusion receiving orthodontic correction in pets. Common examples of Class I malocclusions are lingually displaced (base-narrow and/or instanding) mandibular canines anterior crossbite and lance canine teeth. When the mandibular canines are displaced lingually, they often cause occlusal trauma to palatal mucosa and/or gingiva because of their long crown height. Severe cases can result in complete penetration of the palatine process of the maxillary bone and/or incisive bone, resulting in an oronasal fistula.

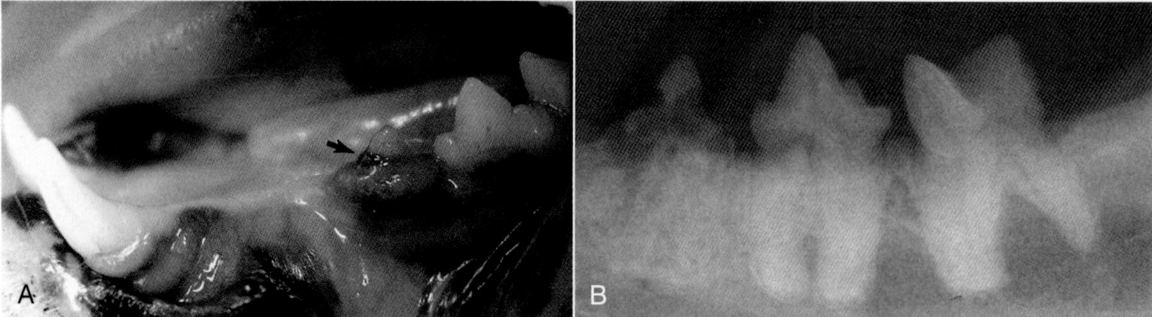

FIGURE 32-64 A, Photograph of a mandibular third premolar affected by idiopathic feline resorption *(arrow)*. **B,** Radiograph of the left mandible using the paralleling technique. The mandibular left third premolar has undergone significant root replacement resorption, as seen by decreased root density and loss of periodontal space.

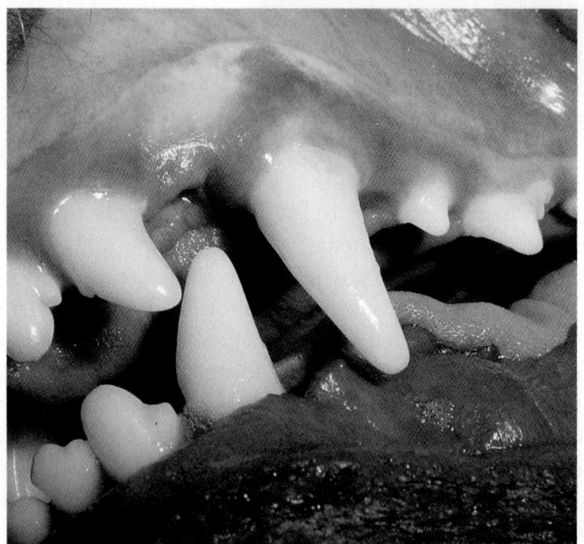

FIGURE 32-65 Class I malocclusion: no jaw length discrepancies exist, but the left mandibular canine tooth is occluding abnormally.

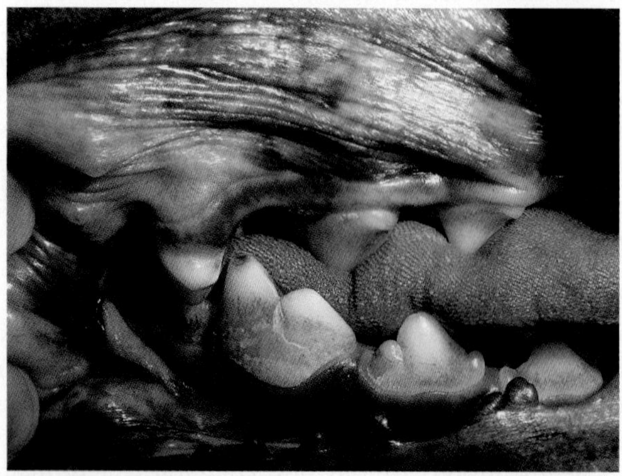

FIGURE 32-66 Caudal crossbite, also referred to as posterior crossbite. The mandibular first molar is buccal, or vestibular, to the maxillary fourth premolar. This may result in abnormal accumulation of plaque and calculus on the buccal surface of the mandibular molars, increasing the need for brushing of this area.

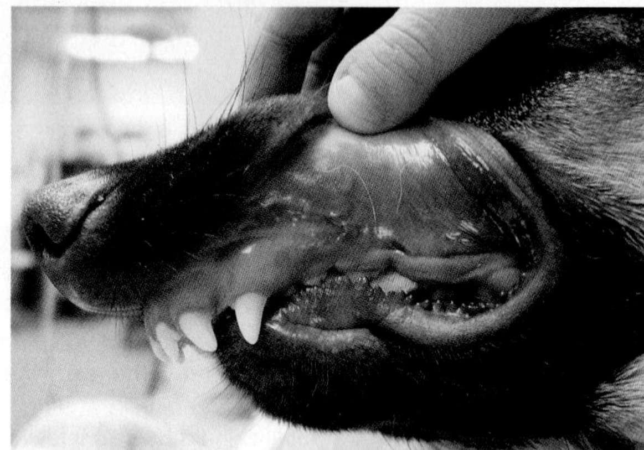

FIGURE 32-67 Class II malocclusion. The mandible is relatively shorter than the maxilla, which results in palatal trauma from the mandibular canine and sometimes mandibular incisor teeth.

A rostral crossbite (referred to as anterior crossbite in humans) occurs when closed-mouth examination reveals one or more maxillary incisors are positioned lingual to the mandibular incisors. A caudal (called posterior crossbite in humans) crossbite occurs when one or more maxillary premolar or molar teeth are positioned lingual to the opposing mandibular premolar or molar (Figure 32-66).

It is important to evaluate the entire dentition and jaw length relationships if proper classification is to be made because clinical presentations similar to those described earlier can occur as a result of abnormalities in jaw length rather than abnormalities of tooth position. The remaining classes refer to skeletal malocclusions associated with jaw length discrepancies. A Class II malocclusion is also referred to as distoclusion, overjet, overshot, and sometimes incorrectly referred to as an overbite (Figure 32-67). In a Class II malocclusion, the mandible is relatively shorter than the maxilla, which can be a result of an abnormally long maxilla (maxillary prognathism) or an abnormally short mandible (mandibular brachygnathism).

A Class III malocclusion is also referred to as mesioclusion, underjet, undershot, and sometimes incorrectly referred to as an underbite (Figure 32-68). In a Class III malocclusion, the maxilla is relatively shorter than the mandible, which can be a result of an abnormally long mandible (mandibular prognathism) or an abnormally short maxilla (maxillary brachygnathism).

The terms brachygnathic and prognathic should always be used with a preceding descriptive adjective to identify the upper or lower jaw (e.g., maxillary brachygnathism). Sometimes

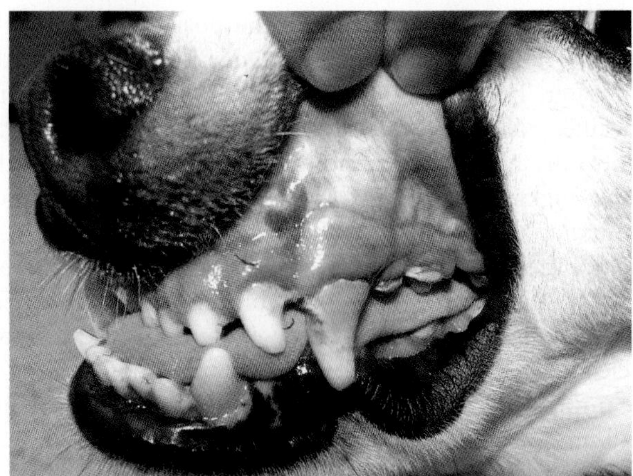

FIGURE 32-68 Class III malocclusion. The maxilla is relatively shorter than the mandible, which may result in attrition of the teeth or trauma to the mandibular mucosa beneath the tongue.

it is difficult to determine if malocclusion is a result of one jaw that is longer than normal or the opposing jaw that is shorter than normal. In general, brachygnathism is considered to be a more common cause of malocclusion than prognathism. Maxillary brachygnathism is an accepted breed standard of some breeds, including boxers, Boston terriers, bulldogs, and pugs. Therefore brachycephalic breeds are referred to as a normal Class III occlusion. Some clues can be gathered on oral examination to determine if malocclusion is a result of brachygnathism or prognathism. When a jaw does not grow to its full length, crowding and rotation of the teeth will occur. When prognathism occurs, increased interdental spaces will be seen. A general understanding of these terms allows veterinary professionals and personnel to communicate with breeders and pet owners who may use either lay or scientific terms to describe a malocclusion. A detailed study of occlusion is necessary before considering orthodontic treatment for pets or counseling breeders on the role of genetics in malocclusions. Although the genetics of malocclusion in dogs and cats have not been fully elucidated, skeletal malocclusions (Class II to IV) are considered to be of genetic origin, and some Class I malocclusions (such as lance canines in Shetland sheepdogs) are considered to have a genetic component.

The shape of a dog's or cat's skull must also be evaluated when performing a dental occlusion evaluation. We recognize three types of skulls: brachycephalic, mesocephalic (or mesaticephalic), and dolichocephalic. Brachycephalic breeds have a wide skull with a short maxilla. Examples of these breeds are boxers, bulldogs, and Persian cats. Mesocephalic breeds have a well-proportioned skull width and maxillary length. Examples include beagles, Labrador retrievers, and German shepherd dogs. The dolichocephalic breeds have a narrow skull and long maxilla, and some examples are the sight hounds (greyhound, whippet) and Siamese cats.

Wry malocclusion is a condition where one segment of the jaw is disproportionate to the other segment (e.g., the left mandible is longer than the right mandible). The disproportionate jaw length can occur in either the maxilla or mandible, resulting in what appears to be a curvature of the jaw toward the shorter side. When it affects the mandible, wry malocclusion may also result in changes in the horizontal plane of the affected jaw, with the affected side seeming ventrally deviated compared with the opposite side.

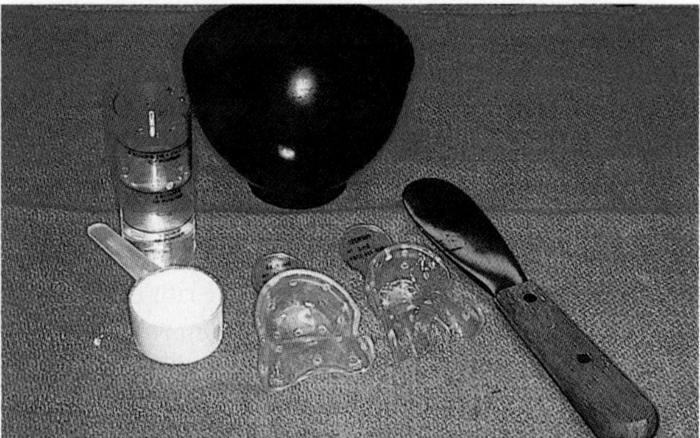

FIGURE 32-69 Materials and equipment used to take an alginate impression: rubber mixing bowl, spatula, impression trays, alginate scoop, and water-measuring cylinder.

Impressions and Models

Impressions and models are important in treatment planning of orthodontic disease and in creation of orthodontic devices and restorations. Veterinary technicians and dental assistants often play an important role in obtaining impressions and pouring stone models. Stone dental models also serve as a part of the medical record for documentation of the starting point and treatment progress.

Alginate is the material that records the imprint of the teeth when doing a full-mouth impression. The teeth should be cleaned before the impression is made. The appropriate size dental impression tray is selected for the patient. The area of interest must fit into the tray without touching the sides of the tray, and the tray must completely cover the teeth. Impression trays for dogs and cats can be purchased or fabricated.

The jar of alginate should be agitated (fluffed) with the top on before use and should be allowed to sit for at least 5 minutes after agitation so that the dust will settle. Alternatively a dustless alginate product is available. Level scoops contained within the jar of alginate are placed in a rubber mixing bowl. A proper scoop of alginate will be level on the surface and will not contain filling voids. Gently tap the scoop of alginate to eliminate any voids, and then level the surface with the blade of the alginate spatula (Figure 32-69).

Alginate spatulas have a wide blade that is used to blend the alginate powder with the water. A cylinder comes with the alginate to measure out the proper amount of water. The amount of alginate used is based on the size of the impression tray, with 8 to 12 scoops usually necessary for a full-mouth impression of the maxilla or mandible. The water is added to the alginate all at once, and the spatula is used in a stirring action to wet the powder. Once the powder is wet, the wide blade is used to start spatulating. The bowl is held in the palm of the hand while the dominant hand works the spatula, smearing the alginate from one side of the bowl to the other in a back-and-forth motion. Once the alginate is mixed to the consistency of cake frosting, it is loaded into the impression tray with the spatula. The lips of the animal are held away from the teeth, and the tray is placed over the teeth. The tray should be held steady while the material sets. This takes about 5 minutes from the start of the mix. Cold water will increase the set time, and warm water will shorten the set time. The extra alginate around the rim of the impression tray can be touched periodically to determine when it is set. Once the material sets, it is similar to rubber and will not stick to the finger when touched. The impression tray and alginate are then removed from the teeth in one quick pulling motion in the direction of the long axis of the teeth.

Once removed from the teeth, the impression should be inspected to be sure that the area of interest was adequately recorded (Figure 32-70). The material should then be rinsed off and a moist paper towel placed on it until the stone can be poured into it. The sooner the stone is poured, the more accurate the impression will be because alginate is susceptible to desiccation and overhydration. Most technicians pour the stone as soon as the animal is recovered from anesthesia or sooner.

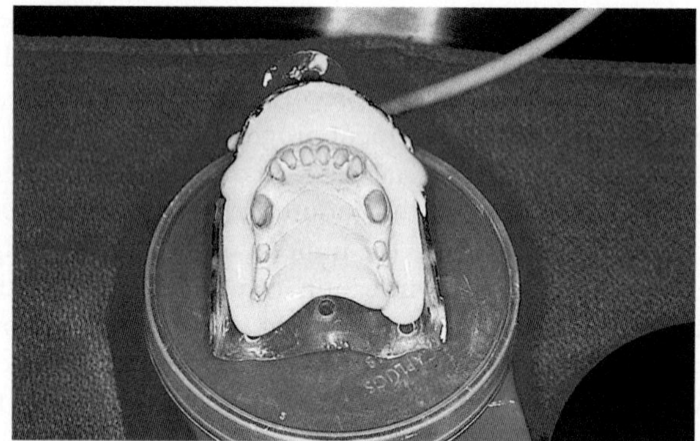

FIGURE 32-70 Alginate impression of the rostral maxilla is inspected and prepared for pouring of dental stone.

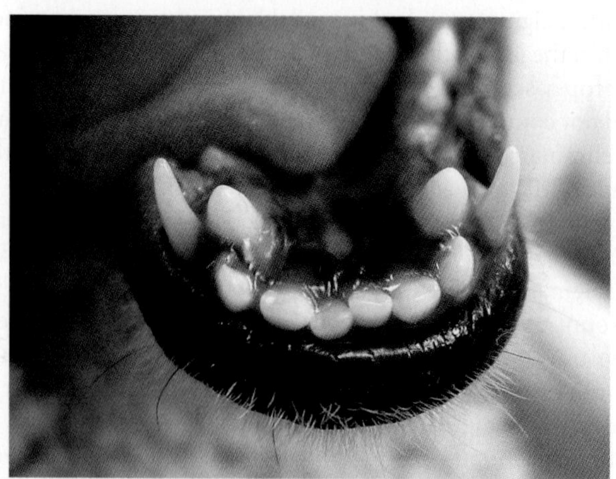

FIGURE 32-71 Persistent deciduous teeth may contribute to orthodontic (base-narrow and instanding permanent canine teeth) and periodontal problems.

Dental stone is used to make the positive image of the mouth. The stone comes in a powder form and is mixed with water. The powder can be weighed out and mixed with a specified volume of water. Experienced technicians can determine the approximate amount of water and stone powder by the thickness of the mix. A good mix will slowly run off the mixing blade when held above the bowl.

Once the stone is mixed, the bowl containing the stone is placed on the vibrator until all visible air bubbles have been released from the mixture. The alginate impression should be cleared of excess water by gently tapping or shaking it. The impression is then held on a laboratory vibrator while small amounts of stone are placed on the impression and allowed to run into the teeth. This step is critical because if an air bubble gets trapped in the teeth, the stone model will be missing part of the tooth. The vibrator serves two purposes. First, it helps to remove bubbles from the stone, and second, it causes the stone to flow into the teeth. Once the teeth have been filled with stone, the rest of the stone can be added at a faster rate because this step is less critical. The stone mix can then be made thicker by adding more powder. This portion can be placed on the top of the model to give it a strong base. Optimal working time for the stone is about 10 minutes. Complete set of the stone takes about 1 to 2 hours.

The model should be removed from the alginate impression after the stone has had 45 to 60 minutes to set. An exothermic reaction will occur, causing the model to feel warm. The model can be separated once the stone has cooled. Do not wait several hours because the alginate will dry and stick to the stone model. The model should be carefully pulled from the alginate and inspected to make sure that all teeth are adequately recorded. If a portion of a tooth is missing, this could be a result of an air bubble or the tooth could have broken off and still remains in the impression. The canine teeth are particularly susceptible to fracture because of their long curved anatomy. If a tooth from the stone model breaks, it can be glued back on the model. The model should then be labeled with the pet's name and the date.

Interceptive Orthodontics

Interceptive orthodontics involves the extraction of persistent deciduous or adult teeth that are causing or will cause problems associated with malocclusion (Figure 32-71). Interceptive orthodontics can be extremely beneficial, and many abnormally erupting permanent teeth will correct spontaneously after extraction of the retained deciduous teeth. The most important factor determining success with this treatment is early detection of the problem. Many puppies and kittens have completed their vaccination series by the time they reach this mixed dentition stage and will not be seen again before spay or neuter unless a dental examination can be scheduled to ensure that early orthodontic problems do not go undetected.

Persistent deciduous teeth can occur in any breed of dog or cat, but they are most commonly seen in small-breed dogs, such as Yorkshire terriers, poodles, and dachshunds.

Deciduous teeth should be shed before eruption of their permanent counterpart. When persistent (previously and mistakenly referred to as "retained") deciduous teeth are identified, they should be extracted before they cause malalignment of their permanent counterparts. Most permanent teeth will erupt lingual or palatal to the retained deciduous teeth with one exception. Maxillary canine teeth erupt mesial to the persistent deciduous teeth. This is noteworthy because malalignment will decrease the space between the maxillary canine and third incisor tooth where the mandibular canine occludes. When this space is too narrow, the mandibular canine tooth will have interference with either one or both maxillary teeth, and tooth wear (attrition) can occur.

Extraction of persistent deciduous teeth is a challenge because of their long, thin roots that can fracture easily. The goal is to remove the entire tooth root to provide space for the permanent tooth to move into. The immature jaw contains numerous developing permanent tooth buds that can be damaged by dental elevators. Clients need to be cautioned of the possibility of permanent tooth damage or discoloration during the extraction of deciduous teeth. A skilled veterinary dental surgeon can significantly minimize these complications.

Base-Narrow or Instanding Mandibular Canine Teeth

Lingually displaced mandibular canine teeth may be a result of deciduous teeth that do not exfoliate properly, but other aspects may play a role, such as genetics responsible for development of normal mandibular width. These malocclusions can be corrected by orthodontics in most cases, but clients must be willing to invest time and expense necessary to clean the oral appliance and return for rechecks as needed. Orthodontic treatment generally costs more than tooth extraction and involves more anesthetic procedures. Orthodontics can be an important treatment option when considering alternatives to extraction of large teeth, such as the canine teeth.

Crown height reduction, partial pulpectomy, and direct pulp capping under sterile conditions may be an option for animals with malocclusions. This procedure entails shortening the tooth to remove the interference it is causing with another tooth or surrounding soft tissue. This method is less invasive than extraction, removes the animal's source of discomfort, and achieves results more rapidly than orthodontic movement. However, it does permanently alter the appearance and, to some degree, function of the tooth. The pulp chamber is exposed when the crown is reduced, and a small percentage of these teeth may become nonvital after this procedure.

DENTAL TRAUMA

Dogs and cats can generate large amounts of biting, pulling, and grinding forces, and their teeth are often the recipients of dental trauma. This trauma can be exhibited as wear (attrition or abrasion), uncomplicated tooth fracture (no pulp exposure), or complicated fracture (pulp exposure).

Many dogs will cause severe abrasion of their teeth by chewing on inappropriate objects, such as rocks or fences. The teeth most commonly fractured are the canines and maxillary fourth premolar teeth (see Figure 32-22, *A*). Attrition and abrasion usually occur on the incisors and canines, but can be seen on the premolars and molars. If the dental wear occurs slowly, odontoblasts will deposit tertiary (reparative) dentin within exposed dentinal tubules to prevent pulp exposure as enamel and dentin are lost. Tertiary dentin may be seen on the surface of worn teeth as a brown or black dot (see Figure 32-22, *B*). A dental explorer should be run over the tooth surface to make sure the pulp tissue is not exposed. When the pulp tissue is exposed, the tip of the dental explorer will fall into the pulp chamber as it crosses the surface of the tooth, whereas tertiary dentin feels smooth as glass with the explorer.

In acute fractures with pulp exposure, the tooth may bleed from the exposed pulp surface. If the tooth is treated within the first 48 hours, vital pulp therapy may be successful. This procedure involves removing the coronal pulp tissue (the pulp tissue in the tooth root remains), covering the pulp tissue with a medicament, and sealing the coronal exposure site with appropriate dental restorative materials.

All teeth with exposed pulp tissue should be treated either by endodontic treatment (conventional root canal, vital pulp therapy) or by extraction. If left untreated, infection from the exposure site will spread to the periapical tissues, and a periapical abscess will develop with time. The client may notice ipsilateral facial swelling or a draining tract just below the medial canthus of their pet's eye (Figure 32-72, *A*, *B*). The majority of periapical abscesses will not form a fistula through the skin, which means that unless the teeth of these pets are examined for endodontic disease, many abscesses go untreated. These abscesses can be painful and are a source of infection, which can spread to other areas of the body.

> *TECHNICIAN NOTE* A tooth with pulp exposure requires either endodontic treatment or extraction. A "wait and see" approach is not appropriate because dogs and cats disguise their level of discomfort.

Discoloration is another sign of endodontic disease, commonly seen as a result of prior trauma to the pulp resulting in pulpitis (Figure 32-73). Ninety-two percent of discolored teeth show evidence of partial or complete pulp necrosis on exploratory pulpotomy. Because dogs and cats do not articulate their discomfort, evidence of pulpitis warrants endodontic or exodontic therapy to relieve possible pain in a tooth affected by pulpitis.

ORAL NEOPLASIA

Oral tumors account for only 6% of all neoplasia in dogs and 3% to 12% in cats, these tumors are often aggressive, and prognosis depends on early detection. The most common

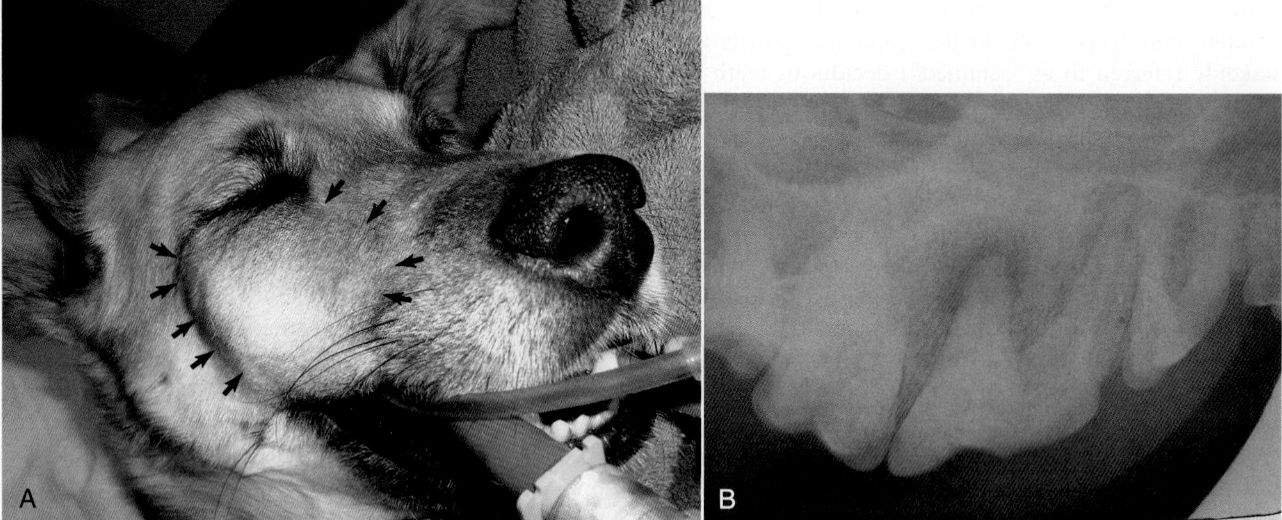

FIGURE 32-72 A, Facial swelling associated with a periapical abscess of the right maxillary fourth premolar tooth *(arrows)*. B, Radiograph showing severe periapical lucencies (bone loss at root tips as a result of infection).

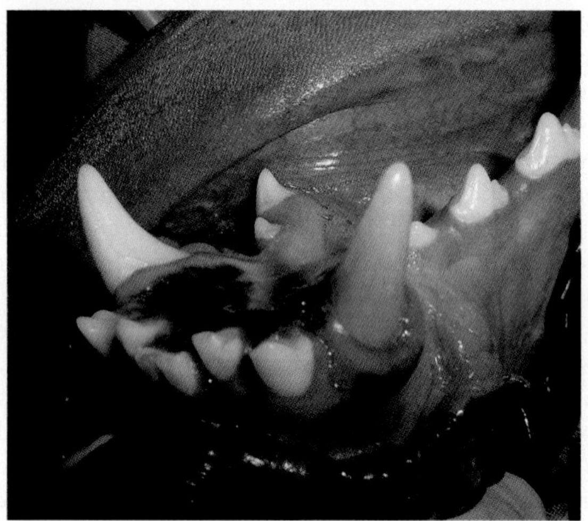

FIGURE 32-73 Discoloration of the left mandibular canine tooth from pulpitis (inflammation of the tooth often as a result of blunt trauma).

oral tumor in cats is squamous cell carcinoma (SCC), which accounts for approximately 70% of all oral tumors in cats (Figure 32-74). To be able to provide a cure for SCC, early detection is particularly important in smaller patients (cats and small dogs) because of the need to obtain clean surgical margins while still maintaining adequate function.

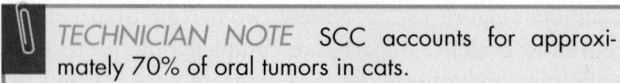

TECHNICIAN NOTE SCC accounts for approximately 70% of oral tumors in cats.

In dogs, tumors may be benign or malignant. The most common benign tumor in dogs is a gingival tumor that in the past has been referred to as an epulis (plural: epulides). The epulides were categorized as fibromatous, ossifying, and acanthomatous; the latter is the most locally invasive. A change in the terminology of these tumors has been made to more accurately reflect their histologic appearance. Fibromatous and ossifying epulides are now categorized together

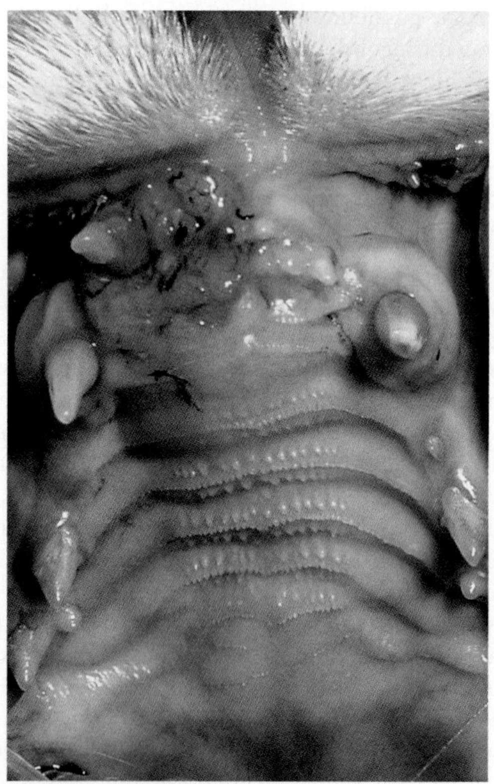

FIGURE 32-74 SCC of the maxilla in a cat. SCC accounts for approximately 70% of oral tumors in cats.

as "peripheral odontogenic fibromas." Acanthomatous epulis is now referred to as canine acanthomatous ameloblastoma. Peripheral odontogenic fibromas do not typically invade bone and usually do not recur if the tooth of origin and its periodontal ligament are removed (Figure 32-75, *A*). Canine acanthomatous ameloblastoma requires removal of the tumor with a minimum of 1 cm of normal tissue in all directions to prevent recurrence (Figure 32-75, *B*). Most oral tumors are not responsive to chemotherapy or radiation, but

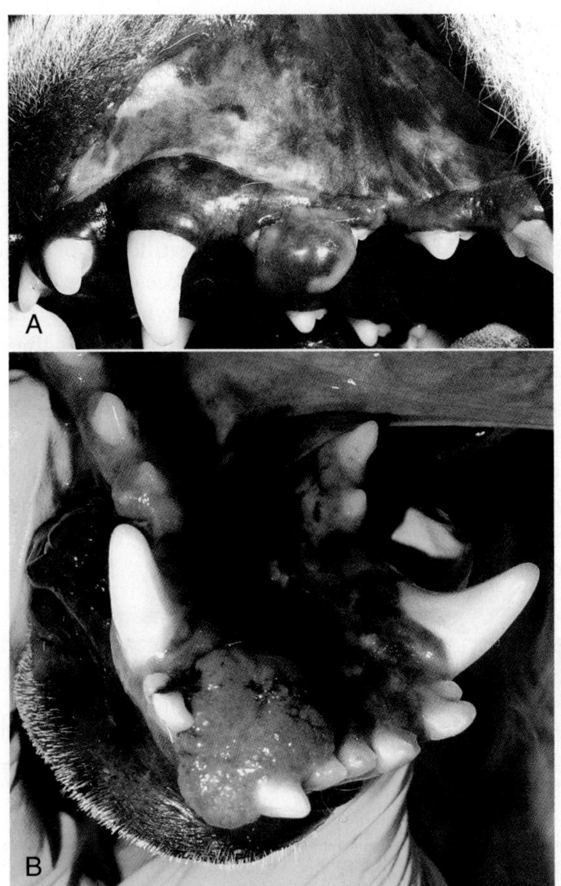

FIGURE 32-75 A, Peripheral odontogenic fibroma (previously referred to as an ossifying epulis) in a dog. B, Acanthomatous ameloblastoma in a dog (previously referred to as acanthomatous epulis). Acanthomatous ameloblastoma is locally invasive, but does not metastasize, making these patients good candidates for surgery if margins are attainable.

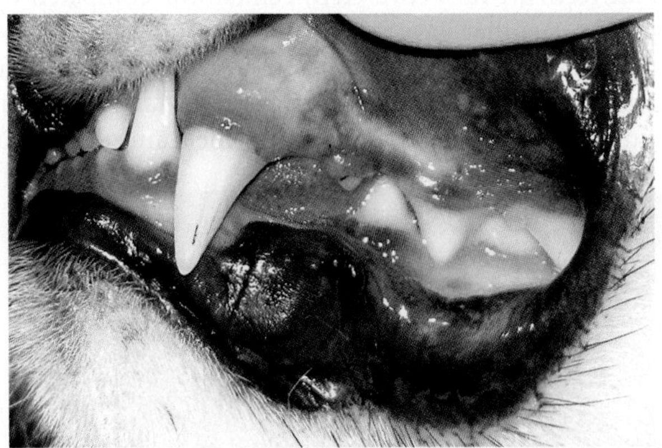

FIGURE 32-76 LPS in a cat. Inflammation is often most severe near the teeth because of the role of plaque accumulation in cats with stomatitis.

canine acanthomatous ameloblastoma does respond to radiation. Surgery (mandibulectomy or maxillectomy) is often the treatment of choice, however, because development of malignant tumors at the site of radiation has been reported with this tumor type.

The most common malignant tumors in dogs are malignant melanoma, SCC, fibrosarcoma, and osteosarcoma. These tumors are locally invasive and have the potential to metastasize to regional lymph nodes or to the lungs. After staging the patient to determine the extent of disease, surgery or radiation is usually recommended to deal with the primary tumor, and metastases are dealt with by either chemotherapy, radiation of metastatic nodes, or immunotherapy. Malignant melanoma may be pigmented or amelanotic. A vaccine has recently been developed for treatment of dogs with malignant melanoma, which has shown promise in increasing survival times.

Dogs and cats that undergo radical maxillectomy and mandibulectomy for removal of an oral tumor generally function well postoperatively, and the majority of clients are pleased with long-term quality of life and appearance. Cats recover more slowly from maxillectomy and mandibulectomy and often require placement of a feeding tube (usually an esophagostomy tube) during the recovery period, whereas dogs usually eat and drink within 24 hours after surgery.

STOMATITIS

Diffuse inflammation of the entire oral cavity is seen commonly in cats and occasionally in dogs. When inflammation is confined to the gingiva, it is referred to as gingivitis. When the inflammation extends beyond the mucogingival junction, it is called stomatitis (Figure 32-76). Stomatitis may be due to a variety of causes, including ingestion of a caustic substance, uremia, viral exposure, plant foreign bodies, allergic response to drugs, or most commonly immune-mediated causes. Cats are often affected by a type of stomatitis referred to as lymphocytic-plasmacytic stomatitis, which can involve gingiva, alveolar mucosa, buccal mucosa, sublingual mucosa, and even the mucosa of the caudal oral cavity lateral to the palatoglossal folds. Cats often have decreased appetite or anorexia, halitosis, dehydration, and blood-tinged saliva.

The cause of LPS is not clear, but it appears that cats develop inappropriate inflammation in the presence of even small amounts of plaque accumulation. Many cats with LPS concurrently shed both herpesvirus and calicivirus. These viruses may have an effect on the immune system, resulting in an overzealous or deficient immune response to plaque. Therefore plaque control in the form of frequent dental cleanings and home care is important. Unfortunately, many LPS cats are so painful that home care is not feasible. Immunosuppressive agents, such as corticosteroids and cyclosporine, help in many cases, but when medical therapy fails or causes unacceptable side effects, full-mouth extractions or nearly full-mouth extractions have been shown to provide resolution of oral discomfort in approximately 80% of cases. When seen in dogs, stomatitis may be due to autoimmune diseases, such as pemphigus vulgaris or bullous pemphigoid.

TECHNICIAN NOTE Full-mouth extractions or nearly full-mouth extractions for treatment of feline stomatitis have been shown to provide resolution of oral discomfort in approximately 80% of cases.

MASTICATORY MUSCLE MYOSITIS

Masticatory muscle myositis is an immune-mediated disease where the immune system forms antibodies toward a specific component of myosin found only in muscles of mastication. Patients affected by this disease may be seen either in the acute phase of the disease, which is painful, or in the chronic phase of the disease, where much scarring has already taken place. Patients in the acute phase will often have the complaint of pain upon opening the mouth, decreased appetite, or dropping of food. These patients often have swelling of the temporal, masseter, and/or pterygoid muscles, which may occasionally also cause exophthalmus. Patients in the chronic phase often have severe temporal and masseter muscle atrophy and inability to open their mouth as a result of severe scar tissue formation. The goal is to diagnose the disease before these chronic changes occur because it is difficult to deal with in the chronic phase. Diagnosis is made by sending serum and muscle biopsies to the comparative neuromuscular laboratory at the University of California, San Diego. Treatment of the acute phase involves a long, slow taper of oral corticosteroids, beginning at an immunosuppressive dose of 1 mg/kg twice daily. Some patients need to be on some level of steroids for life to prevent recurrence.

JAW FRACTURES

Jaw fractures are common in dogs and cats with motor vehicle trauma, high-rise syndrome, or severe periodontal disease resulting in a pathologic fracture. Most jaw fractures benefit from some type of rigid fixation. One of the most common types of jaw trauma is a symphyseal separation, where the right and left mandibles separate at their rostral fibrous union called the symphysis. A cerclage wire placed behind the canine teeth for no more than 4 weeks allows for stability while the symphysis heals (Figure 32-77, *A, B*).

More involved jaw fractures may be repaired by use of interdental wire and acrylic composite, transosseous wiring, miniplates, external fixation, or maxillomandibular fixation. Sometimes teeth along the fracture line may be able to be used as anchor points, but teeth affected by severe periodontal disease should be removed because the fracture will likely not heal when the diseased tooth acts as a nidus for infection.

Patients presenting acutely with a mandibular fracture may benefit from placement of a tape muzzle (Figure 32-78) to stabilize the fracture until surgical treatment is performed. The tape muzzle is created using one piece of tape (adhesive side outward) around the muzzle itself, which is attached to a second piece that wraps around the head below the ears. The muzzle should be tight enough to minimize motion, but loose enough to prevent irritation of the soft tissue and to allow the tongue to move between the incisor teeth to allow for drinking and eating food of a slurry consistency. Tape muzzles are sometimes considered the definitive treatment of choice in young patients where rigid fixation may adversely affect growth of the healing mandible.

> *TECHNICIAN NOTE* Tape muzzles are often used as the definitive treatment of mandibular fractures in puppies because rigid fixation would arrest growth of the mandible.

EQUINE DENTISTRY

DENTAL ANATOMY AND PHYSIOLOGY

Horses have 24 deciduous teeth and 36 to 44 permanent teeth, depending on the presence or absence of canine and first premolar teeth. At eruption, the occlusal surfaces of equine teeth are fully covered by cementum, compared with dogs and cats that have cementum covering only the root. Beneath the crown cementum, a thin layer of crown enamel is present. Both of these layers get worn away, exposing an intricate, wavy combination of cementum, dentin, and

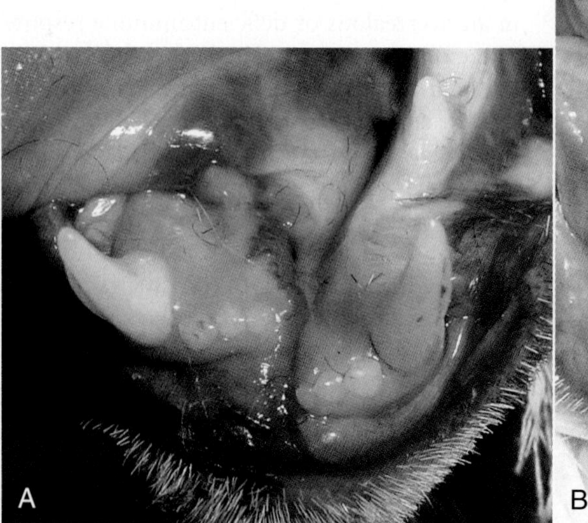

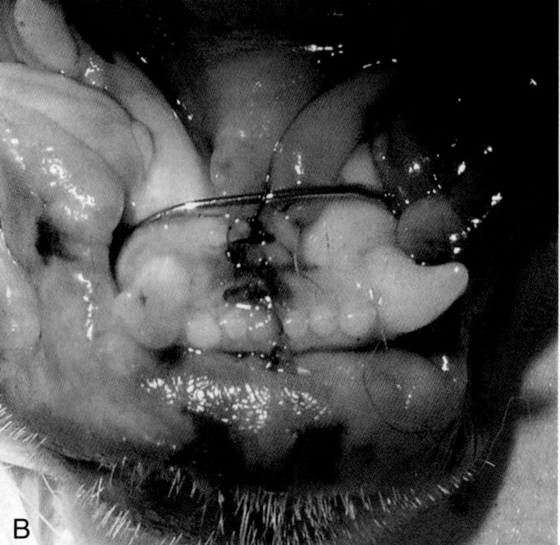

FIGURE 32-77 **A,** Photograph of a symphyseal separation in a cat. **B,** Radiograph after repair with cerclage wire.

enamel on the occlusal surface. Equine mandibular incisor teeth develop features of their occlusal surface that have been traditionally used to estimate age. Because much variation is seen in the rate of tooth wear based on breed, nature and quality of food, and environment, aging horses by this technique should be considered an approximate estimate. Eruption times are the most accurate method of determining age, but this can only be used in horses that have not erupted their complete permanent dentition. Of all the changes on the occlusal surface of the incisors, the appearance of the dental star is one of the more reliable features. The dental star is composed of dentin, and the position of the star moves from the lingual edge of the occlusal surface to the center as the horse ages. Galvayne's groove, a groove that appears on the labial surface of the third incisor in some horses over the age of 10, was once considered to be an excellent method of aging horses between 10 to 30 years of age. It has since been determined that its presence is inconsistent and is of little value in determining the age of a horse.

The canine teeth are usually absent or rudimentary in female horses, but males typically have four permanent canine teeth that erupt at 4 to 6 years of age in the diastema between the incisors and the cheek teeth. The permanent first premolars are referred to as "wolf teeth," and are much smaller and located rostral to the other premolars. The first premolar has no deciduous precursor. Wolf teeth are present in 24.4% of females and 14.9% of male horses. Wolf teeth occur more commonly on the maxilla. These teeth are often extracted because of concerns for causing oral discomfort, especially when the bit contacts this tooth. The premolars and molars are collectively referred to as the "cheek teeth." Not including the wolf teeth, each quadrant should contain six cheek teeth (second, third, and fourth premolars and first, second, and third molars). A numbering system has been developed for equine teeth based on the Triadan system (Figure 32-79, *A, B*). The cheek teeth are closely arranged with no spaces in between them, so the six teeth in one quadrant function as a single unit. The occlusal surfaces of the cheek teeth have many grooves and ridges composed of enamel, cementum, and dentin, which provide varied surfaces for grinding of food material. The upper jaw is wider than the lower jaw, a term referred to as anisognathism. The occlusal surface is normally angled at 10 degrees to 15 degrees in a downward slope toward the buccal aspect of the teeth. In horses with painful dental disease or when fed an inappropriate diet (too little forage), this angle may be increased, resulting in a more vertical angulation of the occlusal surface. This condition is termed "shear mouth."

In horses, the left and right mandibles are not separated by a symphysis as in dogs and cats. The mandibles fuse at the midline at approximately 3 months of age in the horse. In contrast to carnivores, the TMJ is designed for horizontal movement, and the muscles necessary to provide this movement are more developed. Dogs and cats have large temporal muscles on the top of their head that allow for strength in vertical movement of the mandible, whereas horses have well-developed masseter and pterygoid muscles to allow for horizontal grinding movement. Horses have well-developed muscles of the lips that allow them to prehend food, and the commissure of the lips is positioned rostrally, making examination of the caudal cheek teeth challenging.

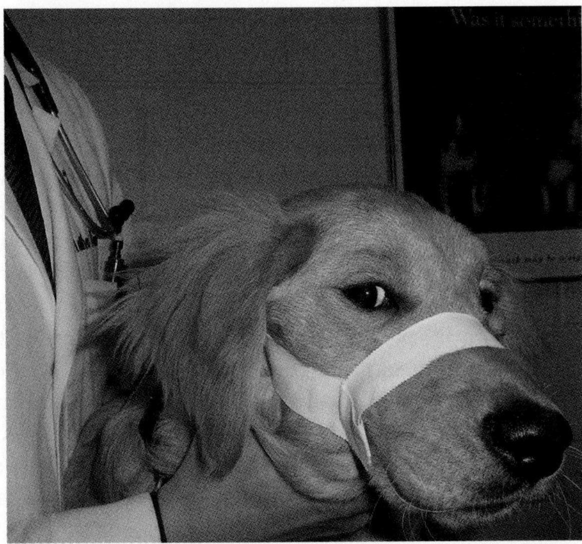

FIGURE 32-78 Tape muzzle for stabilization of a mandibular fracture in a young dog.

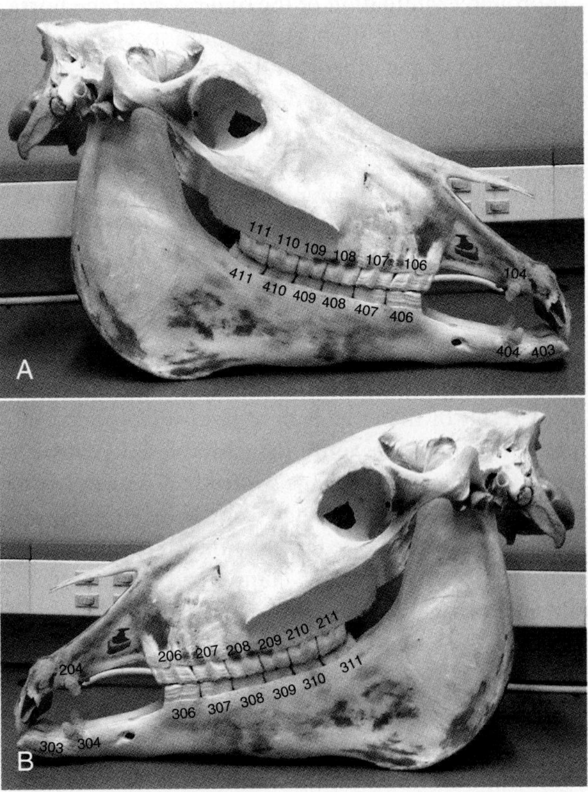

FIGURE 32-79 Skull of a horse showing the Triadan tooth numbering system. **A,** Right side. **B,** Left side. Wolf teeth, when present, end in the numbers "05."

DENTAL EXAMINATION AND IMAGING

Common presenting problems of horses with severe dental disease include weight loss, dropping of food (quidding), head shaking, and tilting of the head during mastication. Routine oral examinations are helpful to detect dental abnormalities in their early stages. Dental disease interferes with normal mastication, resulting in larger feed particle size at the time of deglutition. This may predispose horses and donkeys to impaction colic or esophageal choke. Dental disease may also contribute to systemic infection as a result of hematogenous spread of periodontal pathogens.

Extraoral examination should include observation for evidence of facial swelling, atrophy of masticatory muscles, and presence of ocular, nasal, or oral discharge. The patient's stable floor should be evaluated for evidence of quidding, such as dropped grain and partially chewed boluses. Feces should be evaluated for particle size because large stems of hay and whole grain indicate incomplete mastication. Young horses between 2.5 and 4 years old will have symmetrical, nonpainful bony enlargement of the mandible and/or maxilla associated with eruption of the permanent cheek teeth. Sharp points of the buccal surface of the maxillary teeth may be palpable extraorally. Palpation may cause the horse to resist if points are present. They should be removed before placement of a full-mouth speculum because the cheeks will be pushed tightly against the points once the mouth is opened. Observe the lips for evidence of ulcers, tumors, or bit injuries, especially in the area of the commissure.

Thorough examination of the oral cavity of the horse requires sedation. A self-supporting mouth speculum, a strong light source, a dental mirror, and long-handled dental picks are helpful to assess hard and soft tissue structures and remove food material from areas of interest. Intraoral cameras are available to provide visualization and magnification of difficult areas. Skull radiographs are helpful to diagnose subgingival abnormalities (Figure 32-80). Various views may be necessary, including lateral, lateral oblique, dorsoventral, open- and closed-mouth views. Use of a radiopaque object (such as a needle or gutta percha point) placed in the center of a facial swelling or draining tract before taking a radiograph may help to determine the tooth of origin.

As a result of the large patient size, small film size, and limited intraoral access, intraoral dental radiography is limited to use in imaging of the incisor teeth. If skull radiographs do not show obvious pathologic conditions in a case where dental disease is suspected, other imaging techniques, including nuclear scintigraphy, computed tomography (CT), and magnetic resonance imaging (MRI), may be an option.

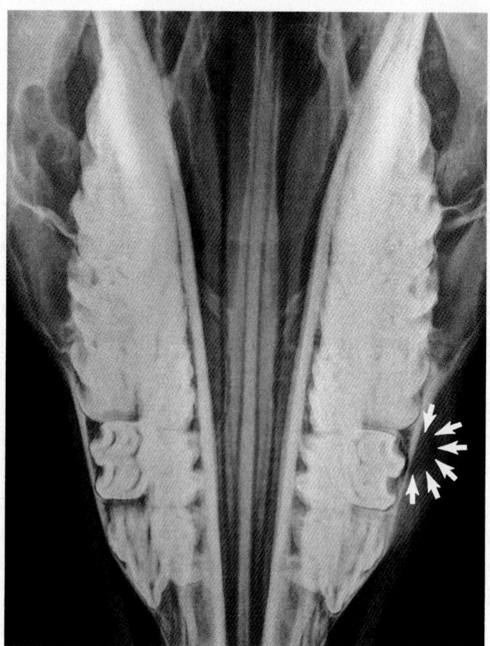

FIGURE 32-80 Radiograph of a horse with facial swelling caused by a periapical abscess. Arrows point to bone loss associated with an infected maxillary third premolar.

COMMON DENTAL PROBLEMS OF HORSES

Endodontic abnormalities occur as a result of disease of the inner chamber of the tooth, which is most commonly seen in the form of a tooth root abscess. Tooth root abscesses occur as a result of exposure of the pulp to the oral environment or death of a tooth with hematogenous spread of bacteria to the compromised site. Pulp exposure may occur as a result of tooth fracture, excessive wear, or decay. Tooth root abscesses may cause a large swelling of the surrounding bone and soft tissue.

The caudal maxillary tooth roots (fourth premolar, first, second, and third molar) are located just ventral to the maxillary sinus, so infection of any of these teeth may result in sinusitis and chronic unilateral nasal discharge. Infection as a result of tooth root abscesses will not permanently resolve with administration of antibiotics, although antibiotics may provide temporary improvement. Extraction or endodontic therapy is necessary for long-term success. Extraction is often difficult because of limited access and the large amount of subgingival tooth structure. Cheek teeth often are approached from an extraoral technique. Although incisors, wolf teeth, and canines can usually be extracted via an intraoral technique, cheek teeth usually need to be approached by buccotomy or repulsion.

Orthodontic abnormalities refer to those abnormalities of occlusion (the normal spatial relationship of teeth and jaws), either as a result of abnormal development, eruption, or wear. Maxillary brachygnathism (or mandibular prognathism) is a developmental disorder where the lower jaw is relatively shorter than the upper jaw. A common term for this condition is "parrot mouth." One goal of treatment is to prevent or minimize the degree of abnormal tooth wear that can occur from malocclusion. Orthodontic procedures can be performed to prevent or correct ventral deviation of the incisive bone and upper incisors and to attempt to overcome the jaw length discrepancy early in life while growth is still occurring. The opposite of parrot mouth is referred to as "monkey mouth," which occurs when the maxilla is relatively shorter than the mandible (resulting from maxillary

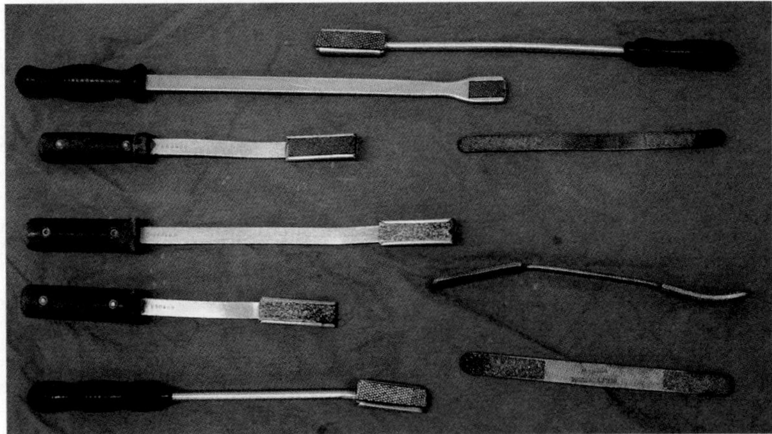

FIGURE 32-81 Various dental floats used for occlusal equilibration in horses.

brachygnathism or mandibular prognathism). This condition is seen most commonly in miniature horses.

Horses with jaw length discrepancies require more frequent occlusal adjustments, but any horse should be evaluated at least yearly for abnormal wear patterns. Floating is the term used to describe the process of mechanically adjusting the occlusal surfaces of the teeth. Flat files (floats), which come in hand and electrically driven versions, are used to remove raised areas, such as hooks, ramps, or points (Figure 32-81). Removal or loss of a tooth can result in drift of adjacent teeth into the vacancy, resulting in abnormal occlusion patterns. Similarly the tooth from the opposing arcade may overgrow into this void as a result of lack of normal wear. Patients with these problems will require more frequent examinations and occlusal equilibrations as necessary (Box 32-11).

Another orthodontic problem seen in foals is wry nose. Wry nose is a deviation of the incisive bone, maxilla, and nasal septum laterally from the midline. Affected foals may have difficulty suckling or prehending forage, and dyspnea resulting from deviation of the nasal septum can be so severe that a tracheostomy may be necessary. It is believed to be a hereditary condition most commonly seen in Arabians and miniature horses. Orthognathic surgical correction often requires two separate surgeries and is usually attempted between 5 and 7 months of age.

Periodontal abnormalities refer to loss of or damage to the attachment structures of the teeth, which consist of the periodontal ligament, cementum, alveolar bone, and gingival connective tissue. Gingivitis is one of the earliest signs of periodontal disease, where the gingiva may appear hyperemic, edematous, and bleeding more readily than normal. Gingival recession may be seen, or alternatively, loss of periodontal ligament attachment may result in development of a periodontal pocket. Although the cause of periodontal disease in horses is similar to that described for dogs and cats earlier in this chapter, treatment is challenging because of limited accessibility of the cheek teeth of horses. The tooth-cleansing process associated with mastication of abrasive substances is an important part of keeping teeth periodontally sound. Therefore any dental pathologic condition, such as abnormal wear and oral ulceration, should be corrected to prevent preferential use of certain teeth and disuse of others. Depending on their accessibility, deep periodontal pockets may be débrided and lavaged. Off-label use of a canine doxycycline gel (Doxirobe) has been described to deal with periodontally affected teeth that have not lost enough attachment to require extraction. Teeth with severe attachment loss and mobility require extraction.

BOX 32-11 Suggested Schedule for Routine Dental Examination of Horses

- *Birth:* Examine for malocclusions and congenital defects affecting the tongue, lips, and palate.
- *6-8 mo:* Examine for eruption of incisors, check occlusion, remove sharp points or hooks if present (float teeth).
- *16-24 mo:* Examine for presence of wolf teeth, ulcers, points or hooks, float if necessary.
- *2-3 yr:* Examine for presence of wolf teeth, bit injuries, deciduous eruption, points or hooks. Remove wolf teeth, float if necessary.
- *3-4 yr:* Examine size and shape of jaws, check for retained third premolars, blind wolf teeth, bit injuries, points or hooks. Remove wolf teeth, caps, float if necessary.
- *4-5 yr:* Examine all teeth for proper eruption, occlusion, and presence of cysts; remove deciduous teeth and hooks; float if necessary. Remove tissue of cyst structure if present.
- *5 yr +:* Evaluate jaw excursion; examine mouth for hooks, abnormal wear patterns, periodontal disease, dental decay. Correct uneven wear patterns, float teeth, shorten incisors if necessary.

Adapted from Easley KJ: Equine dental development and anatomy. Proceedings, American Association of Equine Practitioners, 42:1-10, 1996.

Cemental hypoplasia is a developmental abnormality that can occur in all equine teeth and may predispose maxillary cheek teeth to endodontic disease, tooth fracture, abnormal occlusal patterns, and caries. Caries is the medical term that describes "cavities" caused by tooth decay associated with acids created by bacterial fermentation. When a carious lesion occurs within the infundibulum (the infoldings of the occlusal surface of incisors and cheek teeth) of a tooth, it is referred to as infundibular decay. Restoration of these lesions with composite filling material has been advocated by some equine dentists.

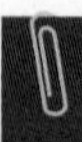

TECHNICIAN NOTE Infundibular decay in horses is most likely to affect the maxillary first molar tooth.

RECOMMENDED READING

Baker GJ, Easley J: *Equine dentistry*, ed 2, Philadelphia, 2005, Elsevier.

Beckman B, Legendre L: Regional nerve blocks for oral surgery in companion animals, *Compendium Continuing Educ Practicing Vet* 24(6):439-442, 2002.

Ehrlich A, et al: *Essentials of dental assisting*, ed 2, Philadelphia, 1996, WB Saunders.

Harvey CE, Emily PP: *Small animal dentistry*, Philadelphia, 1993, Mosby.

Holmstrom SE: *Veterinary dentistry for the technician & office staff*, Philadelphia, 2000, WB Saunders.

Mulligan TW, Aller MS, Williams CA: *Atlas of canine & feline dental radiography*, Yardley, Pa, 1998, Veterinary Learning Systems.

Nield-Gehrig JS: *Fundamentals of periodontal instrumentation*, ed 6, Baltimore, 2008, Lippincott Williams & Wilkins.

Reiter AR, Lewis JR, Okuda A: Update on the etiology of tooth resorption in the domestic cat, *Vet Clin North Am, Small Anim Prac* 35(4):913-942, 2005.

Verstraete FJM: *Self-assessment colour review of veterinary dentistry*, London, 1999, Manson Publishing.

Wiggs RB, Lobprise HB: *Veterinary dentistry: principles and practice*, Philadelphia, 1997, Lippincott-Raven.

Emergency and Critical Care

PART **SEVEN**

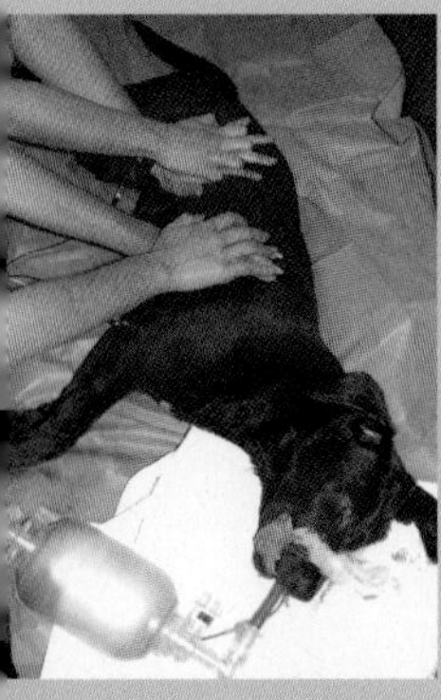

Emergency Nursing

33

Kirk Ryan, Lee Ann Eddleman, and Charles T. McCauley

KEY TERMS

Abdominocentesis
Acidosis
Arrhythmia
Asystole
Azotemia
Borborygmi
Capillary refill time
Colic
Defibrillation
Disseminated intravascular coagulation
Emesis
Flail chest
Hemothorax
Hypovolemia
Hypoxia
Hypoxemia
Ischemia
Pneumothorax
Pulse oximeter
Sepsis
Stridor
Syncope
Tachycardia
Tachypnea
Thoracocentesis
Thrombus

OUTLINE

LEARNING OBJECTIVES

When you have completed this chapter, you will be able to:

1. List the components in an emergency care station/crash cart.
2. Discuss standard triage protocols used in evaluation of a small animal trauma patient.
3. Discuss possible secondary complications of trauma and critical illness, including pain, DIC, shock, and cardiopulmonary arrest; and their recommended treatment or resuscitation protocols.
4. Discuss small animal blood donors, blood types, and transfusion protocols.
5. List the objectives of monitoring critical care patients and discuss the approach to patient monitoring based on the principles of triage and body system anatomy.
6. List common emergencies in small animal veterinary medicine.
7. List equipment, supplies, and medications needed to respond to equine emergencies.
8. List minimal data collected during assessment of equine emergency patients.
9. Describe initial management, assessment, diagnostic, and treatment procedures for common equine emergencies.
10. Describe procedures for placement and maintenance of IV catheters in equine patients.
11. Discuss considerations in development and implementation of an equine fluid therapy plan in emergency situations.
12. Describe indications for use of blood and blood products and procedure for their use.

INTRODUCTION

A greater awareness of treatment availability and the demands of pet owners for more advanced treatment options have spurred specialization within the veterinary profession. The field of veterinary emergency and critical care continues to grow in response to the needs of animals, pet owners, and the veterinary profession. Steady improvements have occurred in emergency and critical care techniques and in equipment and staff training. Likewise, the technician's role in the emergency room and the intensive care unit has grown. More than ever, technicians are directly involved with patient care. They monitor vital signs, administer medications appropriately, maintain accurate patient records, and provide a hygienic and positive environment for healing. Their role is important in documenting patient response to treatment, in providing continuity of care, and in recognizing the onset of clinical problems. Veterinary technicians are challenged by rapid changes within the profession (new methods, pharmaceuticals, and diets) and by rapid changes in each patient (new and evolving clinical problems in each case).

Veterinarian and technician associations play a role in advocating standards of care, in providing continuing education, and in creating a forum for professionals with common interests to share their experiences. The special role of emergency and critical care technicians is recognized and supported by the Association of Veterinary Emergency and Critical Care Technicians (AVECCT) under the auspices of the Veterinary Emergency and Critical Care Society (VECCS). This technician specialty group, which was recognized by the North American Veterinary Technician Association (NAVTA) in 1996, is devoted to recognizing, educating, and networking technicians with specialty interest and training in emergency and critical care. These organizations provide important continuing education and a needed professional forum for technicians.

SMALL ANIMAL EMERGENCY NURSING

THE EMERGENCY CARE STATION AND RESUSCITATION AREA

Animals frequently come to the veterinarian with emergent and often life-threatening injuries or illnesses. Such demands require that the veterinary facility be set up in a manner in which quick assessment and immediate therapies are possible. Every veterinary practice should contain a centrally located emergency care station and resuscitation area devoted to crisis management. This area should be designed to facilitate rapid triage and treatment. It should be easy to access and have adequate space to accommodate multiple staff members responding to a patient emergency. Emergency drugs and equipment should be stored within easy reach and in designated areas. Equipment and drug inventory of the emergency care station should be checked at each shift change and following each use to ensure that all items are in working order and in adequate supply.

> *TECHNICIAN NOTE* Equipment and drug inventory of the emergency care station should be checked at each shift change and following each use to ensure that all items are in working order and in adequate supply.

As a minimum, this area should have a source of oxygen, a suction unit, adequate electrical capability, and sufficient lighting. The emergency care station should have a sufficient number of electrical outlets to supply monitoring equipment without the use of excessive extension cords, which can be clumsy, unsafe, and impede the movements of staff. Standard fluorescent lighting can be augmented by well-positioned overhead surgery or examination lights.

In many veterinary practices, oxygen is supplied via anesthetic equipment. Whereas an anesthetic machine provides a familiar means of ventilation and access to sedation (if needed), it can also be a source of catastrophe when errors of anesthetic depth or pop-off valve closure occur. If an anesthetic machine is used, waste anesthetic gas scavenging systems should be available. To prevent the potential problems associated with anesthetic equipment, an oxygen source with a flowmeter and Ambu bag (Figure 33-1) is preferred. Ambu bags are especially useful because they are an easily transported, easily stored, and inexpensive source of artificial ventilation.

Many small practices have suction units with adjustable suction pressure, which are used in surgery (Figure 33-2). The emergency area should have its own suction unit designated and supplied with a variety of suction tips. Suction equipment is often used in the emergency area to clear the airway or endotracheal tube of fluid or debris (mucus, blood, exudates, vomitus, etc.).

CRASH CART

An integral part of preparation for an emergency is the "crash cart" (Figure 33-3). This can be a fishing tackle box with necessary items or a large cart on wheels with multiple drawers. A tool storage cart available at hardware stores can work quite well. The crash cart should be located at the emergency station and contain necessary items for treating patients that are medically unstable. Additional crash carts may be placed in select locations throughout the hospital, if needed (i.e., operating room or dental suite). Basic supplies contained in the crash cart should include items necessary to establish an airway, venous access, emergency drugs, and a dose chart.

> *TECHNICIAN NOTE* Basic supplies contained in the crash cart should include items necessary to establish an airway, venous access, emergency drugs, and a dose chart.

Following each use and at every shift change, the contents of the crash cart should be checked and restocked. The function of all battery or electrical items should be checked and

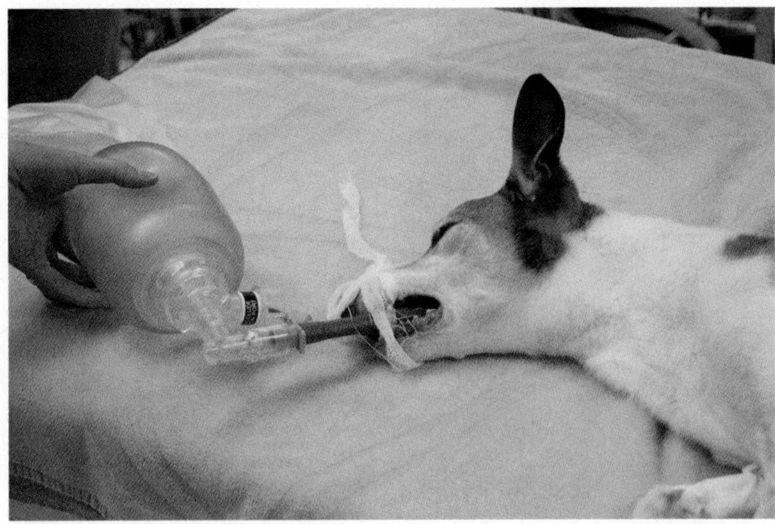

FIGURE 33-1 An endotracheal tube connected to an Ambu bag and oxygen source provides an ideal means to supply 100% oxygen and manual assisted ventilation.

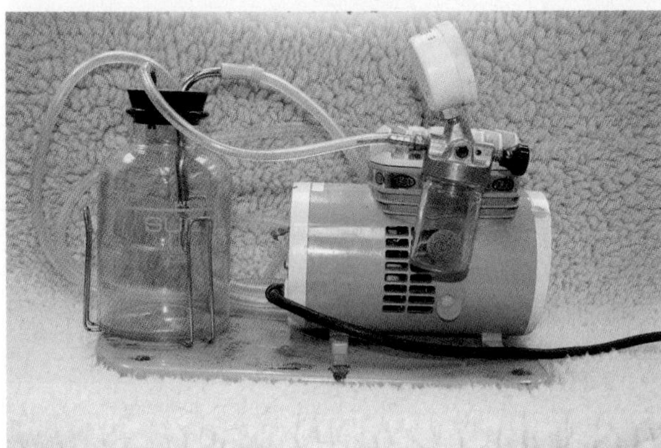

FIGURE 33-2 A suction unit similar to those used in a surgery suite should be centrally located and used in emergencies to clear airways of fluid and debris.

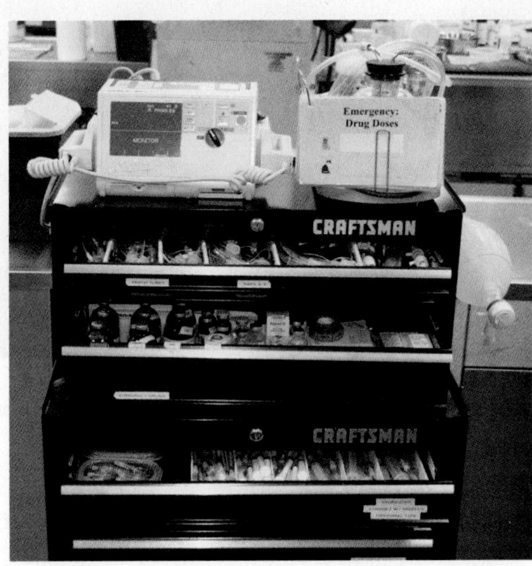

FIGURE 33-3 An effective "crash cart" is easily accessible and spacious enough to contain an array of emergency supplies.

replaced or recharged as necessary. Drug expiration dates should be checked regularly, and expired drugs should be discarded.

Crash cart airway supplies should include at least one laryngoscope with a small- and large-size blade (Figure 33-4). The laryngoscope battery and bulb light should be checked at each shift to make sure that the equipment is in working order. Various sizes of clean endotracheal tubes and stylets should be placed in well-marked and organized places so that the appropriate tube can be located rapidly during an emergency. It is also helpful to maintain supplies needed to secure the tube in place once the animal has been intubated. This would include tie gauze, or other tube-securing material, and a clean empty syringe to inflate the cuff. Endotracheal tube cuffs should be checked at least once a week to ensure that they are functional and that no leak is present. This can be accomplished by inflating the endotracheal tube cuff underwater and observing the cuff for leaking air bubbles. Tubes with leaking cuffs should be discarded.

In larger crash carts, additional equipment to assist with airway control should be kept on hand. Sponge forceps may be used to clear the airway with gauze or to remove a foreign body without getting bitten. Transtracheal cannula and tracheostomy tubes may be useful in cases where normal per oral intubation is not possible because of facial trauma or upper airway obstruction (tumor, foreign body, or severe trauma). Tracheal cannulae are attached to an oxygen source and inserted into the trachea between cartilage rings. Some items used for tracheal cannulae include large-gauge through-the-needle catheters, large-gauge needles (attached to an extension set and 6-ml syringe adapter), or a modified macrodrip IV fluid set (Figure 33-5). In some situations, a small-diameter polypropylene catheter may be passed through the mouth into the trachea and used as a cannula to administer oxygen or as a guide (stylet) to direct an endotracheal tube. This procedure may be helpful until a surgical tracheostomy can be performed or until airway obstruction can be otherwise resolved. As previously noted, an Ambu bag or anesthetic machine should be located close to the crash

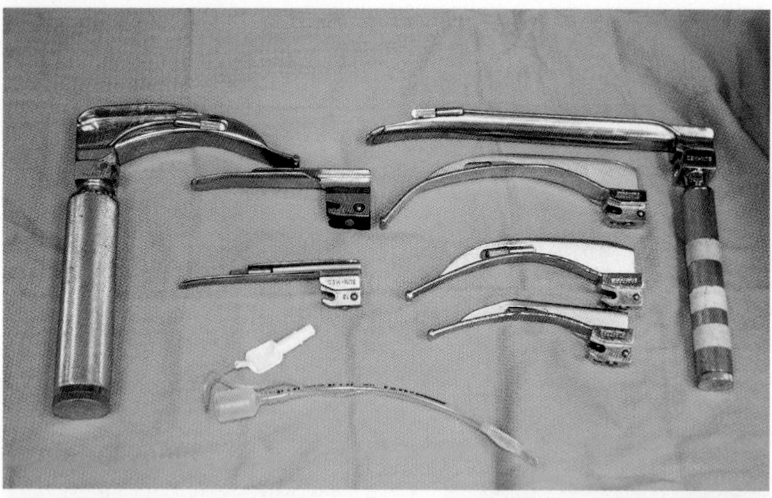

FIGURE 33-4 A variety of laryngoscope blade sizes and configurations are needed to assist with endotracheal intubation of dogs and cats.

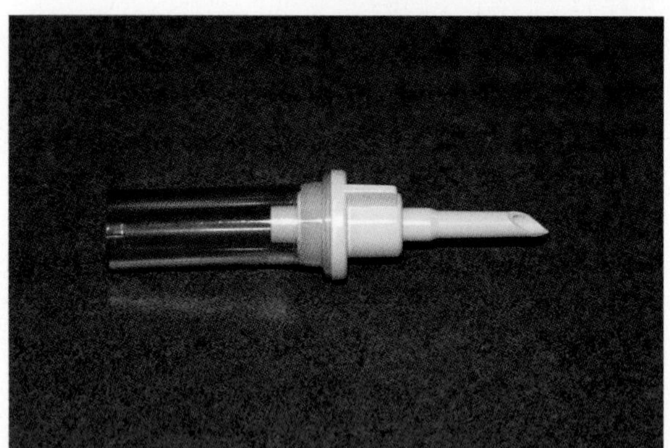

FIGURE 33-5 A macrodrip IV fluid set can be fashioned for use as an emergency tracheal cannula until more appropriate equipment can be located.

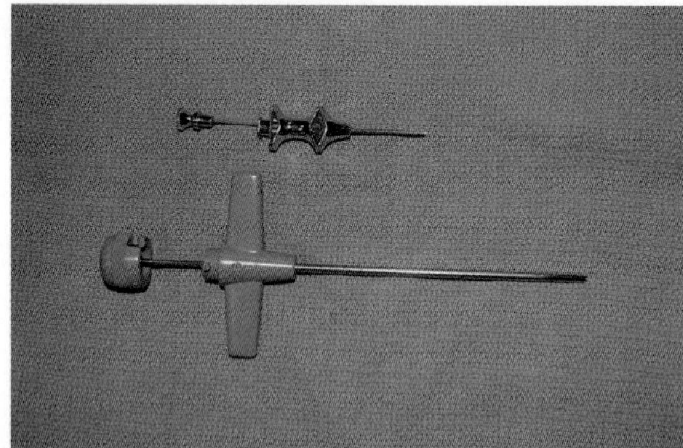

FIGURE 33-6 Examples of bone marrow catheters are shown.

cart so that assisted ventilation can start immediately after the animal is intubated.

Items to establish venous access should be kept in the crash cart for use in crisis patients who do not already have an IV catheter or who need additional venous access. A selection of various sizes of IV catheters should be well stocked and organized. In addition, bone marrow needles or intramedullary catheters are desirable for small patients (Figures 33-6 and 33-7). Bone marrow catheters are ideal for puppies, kittens, and exotic pets because the bone marrow cavity connects to the vascular system and small patients often have fragile or inaccessible veins. Commercially available bone marrow catheters, spinal needles, or 18- to 20-gauge hypodermic needles can be used for this purpose. Porous tape and gauze bandage material for stabilization of any vascular line will also be necessary and should be included in the crash cart inventory. Hair clippers and solutions for aseptic skin preparation should be within easy reach. Commonly used IV fluid solutions (i.e., lactated Ringer's, 0.9% saline solution), synthetic colloids (i.e., hetastarch), hypertonic saline, and a pressure infusion bag should be kept close at hand for emergency fluid resuscitation.

A selection of emergency drugs, especially those used in the treatment of cardiopulmonary arrest, should be kept in the crash cart. Drug bottles should be well labeled and kept in specific and consistent locations within the cart to facilitate their use during an emergency.

> *TECHNICIAN NOTE* Drug bottles should be well labeled and kept in specific and consistent locations within the cart to facilitate their use during an emergency.

Cardiopulmonary resuscitation (CPR) and emergency drug selection are discussed in detail later in this chapter. During emergencies, drug dose and administration errors may be prevented if the veterinary staff is familiar with the location of the drugs and with drug concentrations. If space allows, it is helpful to have various sizes of sterile syringes with the needles already attached to facilitate rapid drug administration. During CPR attempts, some drugs may be administered via the endotracheal tube (see administration routes under the discussion of CPR). This requires using a catheter of some sort (i.e., red rubber catheter cut to an appropriate length or a similar size polypropylene urinary catheter). Two such catheters should be on hand (one for

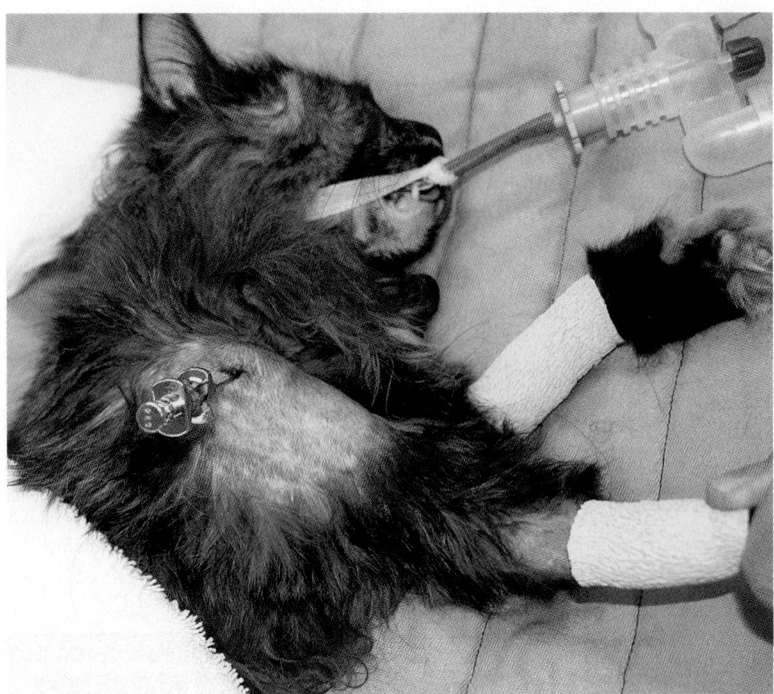

FIGURE 33-7 A bone marrow catheter is shown inserted into the humerus of a cat after repeated attempts at IV catheterization failed.

larger-sized animals and one for small animals). During a crash scenario, remembering and calculating doses can take time and introduce errors. At the same time, estimated doses may be dangerously inadequate or overzealous. Emergency situations rarely allow time for individual dose calculations for each patient. Therefore some sort of centrally located drug dose chart should be posted at the emergency care station with a smaller version kept with drugs in the crash cart.

> *TECHNICIAN NOTE* A centrally located drug dose chart should be posted at the emergency care station with a smaller version kept with drugs in the crash cart.

Commonly used emergency drugs include atropine, epinephrine, lidocaine, and naloxone (Table 33-1). Computer drug calculation programs are available that generate an emergency drug card that can be printed for all high-risk patients. Charts and drug cards allow team members to quickly read the appropriate drug volume based on the species and body weight.

Electrical defibrillation is indicated in the treatment of some cardiac arrhythmias (primarily ventricular fibrillation). Electrical defibrillators are available through many medical equipment distributors and may be combined with an electrocardiogram (ECG) monitor. This equipment should be located at the central emergency care station and used by experienced staff and veterinarians. Special training is required for the safe use of electrical defibrillators.

Depending on space, other items, such as surgical packs for emergency procedures, may also be stored in the crash cart. Common procedures performed at the emergency station include venous cutdown, thoracotomy for open chest CPR, thoracic drain placement, and tracheostomy (Figure 33-8). Sterile instruments and drapes for these procedures should be available in the emergency area (if not in the crash cart). Basic bandaging and splinting supplies, irrigation fluids, and sterile water-soluble lube (for clipping around and lavaging open wounds) should also be available.

TABLE 33-1 Drugs for Cardiopulmonary Resuscitation

Formulation	Dosage	Indications
Atropine 0.54 mg/ml	0.04 mg/kg IV	Bradycardia, AV block, asystole
Dobutamine 12.5 mg/ml	5-20 mg/kg/min CRI	Myocardial failure
Dopamine 40 mg/ml	5-10 mg/kg/min CRI	Low cardiac output
Epinephrine 1:1000 solution	0.2 mg/kg IV	V-fibrillation, asystole, EMD
Lidocaine 20 mg/ml	2 mg/kg IV 50-100 mg/kg/min CRI	Ventricular arrhythmias
Magnesium Chloride 200 mg/ml	2 g over 2 min IV	V-fibrillation, V-tachycardia
Naloxone 0.4 mg/ml	0.03 mg/kg IV	EMD

CRI, Constant rate infusion.

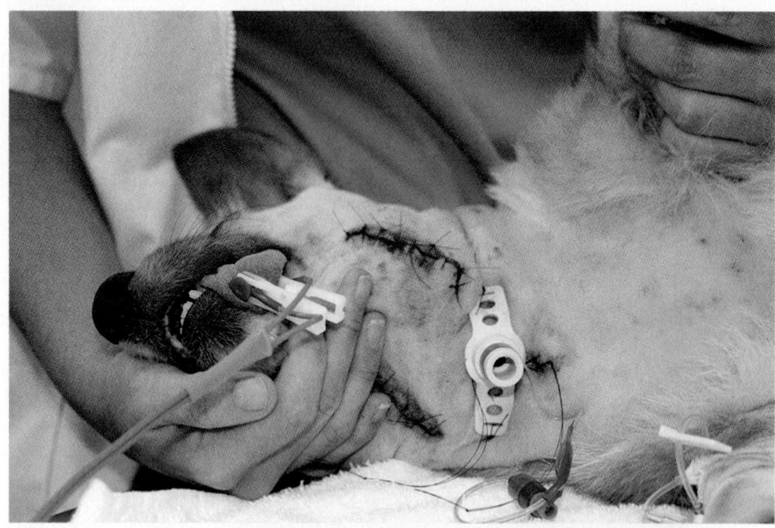

FIGURE 33-8 A dog breathes through a temporary tracheostomy tube that was placed to ensure a patent airway during recovery from throat surgery.

LABORATORY

Next to the emergency care station, equipment should be close at hand to obtain baseline examination and laboratory parameters. Often these parameters include but are not limited to temperature, pulse, respiration, mucous membrane color, capillary refill time (CRT), blood pressure, ECG, and oxygen saturation via a pulse oximeter. Basic laboratory data, often referred to as "quick assessment tests" (QATs), may include packed-cell volume (PCV), total plasma solids, blood glucose, blood lactate, blood urea nitrogen (BUN), and urine specific gravity. Cage-side laboratory data can be obtained using "dip stick" test strips, glucometers, or point-of-care analyzers. Point-of-care testing equipment is available for coagulation assessments, arterial blood gas analysis, and basic serum biochemistries. Automated blood analyzers (Figure 33-9) allow for multiple blood parameters to be assessed quickly and repeated later for comparison.

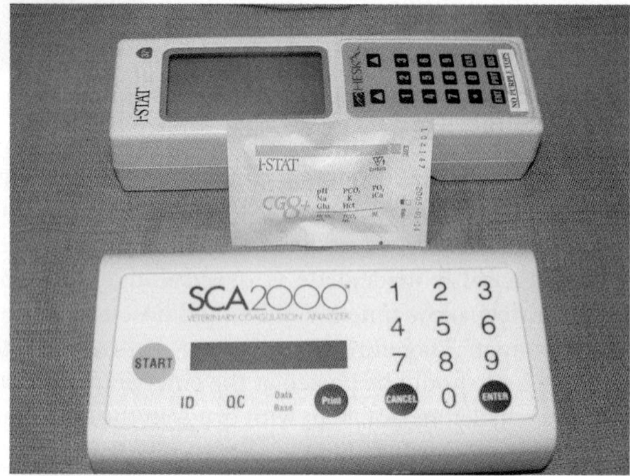

FIGURE 33-9 Automated blood analyzers are available for assessment of biochemical, arterial blood gas, and coagulation parameters (i-Stat, Symbiotics 3000).

All veterinary hospitals should also have a basic laboratory area with a microscope set up to view blood smears or cytology samples. Blood smear examination can provide important diagnostic clues that may aid the emergency clinician (including red cell morphology, relative white blood cell numbers, and platelet count estimates).

Commercial test kits can also be kept at hand for rapid detection of toxin exposure (i.e., ethylene glycol) and infectious disease status (i.e., canine parvovirus, feline retroviruses, and heartworm disease). Rapid blood typing and crossmatching kits are available for pretransfusion testing. Other useful equipment, such as an ultrasound unit, may also be kept near the emergency triage area.

FLUID THERAPY

Fluid therapy is a valuable asset in the treatment of critically ill animals. Although fluid therapy is commonly used in veterinary hospitals, there are often questions concerning which fluids are appropriate and what volumes should be delivered. It is helpful to think of fluid therapy as expanding the animal's blood or plasma volume. This volume expansion lasts for a variable period of time depending upon the fluid administered and the animal's condition. Common reasons for providing fluid support in critically ill pets include:

1. Maintaining hydration
2. Replacing fluid losses
3. Maintaining IV access and delivering other medications
4. Treatment of shock or hypoproteinemia
5. Increasing urine output
6. Correcting acid-base or electrolyte disturbances
7. Providing nutritional support

Crystalloid fluids are isotonic fluids consisting primarily of water with sodium or glucose. They are used for volume expansion and rapidly redistribute into the extracellular space. Only approximately 25% of crystalloid fluids remain in the vascular space after 1 hour. Crystalloid fluids are inexpensive and readily available in most practices. Examples of commonly used crystalloid solutions include 0.9% saline, lactated Ringer's solution (LRS), Normosol-R, and Plasma-Lyte. Colloid solutions are also used to expand vascular volume. They contain high-molecular-weight particles, which remain in the vascular space for longer periods of time. The hemodynamic effects of most colloids are similar to plasma and last longer than crystalloid fluids. Colloids can be used as single-agent therapy or in conjunction with crystalloid fluids. Use of colloids can reduce the volume of crystalloid solution required in some animals. These agents are used in a variety of critical care cases. One disadvantage of using colloids is the additional expense incurred. Examples of synthetic colloids include hydroxyethyl starch (hetastarch).

The route of fluid administration is an important aspect of fluid therapy. Subcutaneous fluid administration is popular because it is quick and easy and can be used during home management or outpatient management of some animals. However, fluid absorption via this route may be slow and unpredictable. For this reason, overreliance on subcutaneous fluid therapy should be avoided. The IV route is often the best route to administer fluids in critical animals.

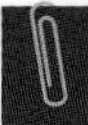

TECHNICIAN NOTE The IV route is often the best route to administer fluids in critical animals.

Large-bore catheters can be placed in peripheral or central veins to increase the veterinarian's ability to administer fluid and medications to sick animals. In some critically ill animals, (especially puppies and kittens), venous access may be difficult to obtain. If venous access is limited, the intraosseous route can be used by using purpose-made intramedullary catheters, stylet needles, or bone marrow needles. Once the animal is volume expanded, peripheral veins may be more accessible for IV catheterization.

This fluid therapy plan should be adapted to the needs of each individual case and based on solid patient monitoring. In planning fluid therapy, veterinarians often consider an emergency phase, a replacement phase, and a maintenance phase. Emergency fluid therapy in the treatment of shock (i.e., "emergency phase") is outlined elsewhere in this chapter. Replacement fluid therapy is intended to restore fluid balance to dehydrated animals. The volume of fluid to be replaced is calculated by estimating the percent dehydration and multiplying this number by the body weight in kilograms. The product of these numbers equals the replacement fluid volume in liters. For example, a 20-kg dog estimated to be 7% dehydrated would need 1.4 L of fluid (0.07 × 20 kg = 1.4 L). The rate of fluid replacement is dependent on clinical signs and the rate of fluid loss. If the animal has become acutely dehydrated, the volume may be replaced over 6 to 8 hours. If the loss has been chronic, it can be administered over 24 hours. Maintenance fluid requirements are calculated by well-established formulas. Most formulas are based on body weight (e.g., maintenance fluid dose = 60 ml/kg/day), although some believe that fluid requirements are best approximated by the basal energy requirement (e.g., fluid dose in ml/day = (30 × kg body weight) + 70). Ongoing fluid losses from vomiting, diarrhea, hemorrhage, or fluid effusion may occur in hospitalized patients. Staff members should record and estimate the volume of such losses so that the veterinarian can devise an appropriate maintenance fluid therapy plan that takes such losses into consideration.

Calculated fluid rates are only a starting point, and animals receiving fluid therapy must be closely monitored for both dehydration and fluid overload.

TECHNICIAN NOTE Calculated fluid rates are only a starting point, and animals receiving fluid therapy must be closely monitored for both dehydration and fluid overload.

Relying solely on calculated fluid rates places the animal at risk for either inadequate fluid therapy or "overhydration." Clinical signs and subjective parameters associated with overhydration include coughing, tachypnea, respiratory distress, nasal discharge, conjunctival edema (also called chemosis [Figure 33-10]), and peripheral edema (Figure 33-11). Abnormal lung sounds may be due to pulmonary

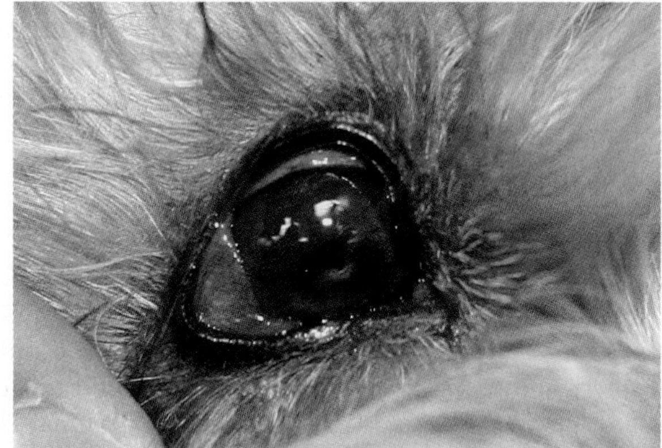

FIGURE 33-10 Note the swollen, edematous conjunctiva associated with overhydration. This conjunctival edema is also called chemosis.

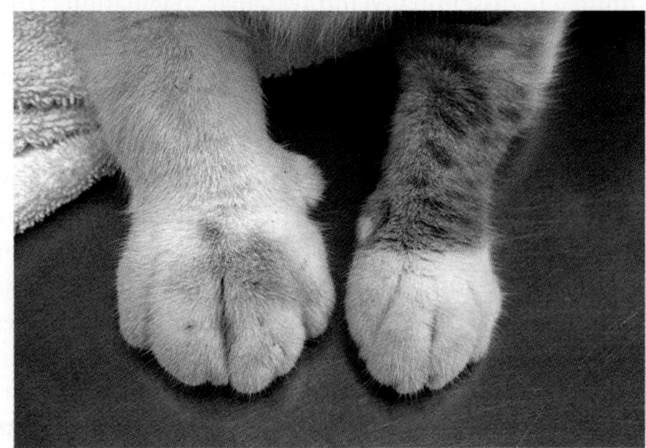

FIGURE 33-11 Overhydration may also result in peripheral edema, especially in the dependent limbs. Compare the peripheral edema in this cat's feet.

edema caused by overhydration. Objective parameters used to evaluate fluid therapy include hematocrit (or PCV)/total protein (TP) (PCV/TP), body weight, central venous pressure (CVP), blood lactate, urine specific gravity, and urine output. The PCV/TP should be monitored frequently as shock and replacement fluid therapy is administered. If the hematocrit falls below 20% or if the TP decreases by 50% or more of the initial value, the veterinarians may consider changes in type of fluid or rate of administration. In addition, catheters and catheter sites should be routinely evaluated to check for catheter patency and cleanliness and to guard against catheter-associated inflammation.

STANDARDS OF CARE AND EMERGENCY PROTOCOLS

Standardized procedures and patient care protocols are helpful in dealing with common clinical presentations and emergency situations. A standardized approach helps maintain an expected standard of care, allows the veterinary team to respond rapidly to a crisis, and minimizes confusion among staff members during an emergency. Written procedure manuals can aid in the training of new staff members and serve as a reference for review by experienced team members. In developing a procedures manual, minimal standards of care should be agreed upon. If a group of practices have shared staff or clientele (i.e., an emergency clinic that serves a community of veterinary practices), agreed-upon procedures or protocols enhance patient care and facilitate communication. Certain situations (trauma, shock, CPR) are common scenarios in all veterinary facilities and merit individual discussion in this chapter.

TRIAGE OF THE TRAUMA PATIENT

Traumatic injuries in small animals require rapid, accurate assessment and special monitoring to ensure good care and to guard against the secondary complications of trauma. The patient with multiple body-system trauma is at a greater risk for complications as a result of the additive effects of each injury. Secondary complications of trauma include but are not limited to disseminated intravascular coagulation (DIC), sepsis, multiorgan failure, and distress caused by pain.

"Triage" is the process of determining the priority of need and the proper order of treatment when evaluating a clinical situation. Triage may be used to identify which patients in a group of animals require immediate treatment. In addition, standard triage protocols are used to identify which problems and which body systems should be evaluated first in a patient with multiple abnormalities. Most veterinarians are familiar with mnemonics dictating the principles of triage. These mnemonics are useful in managing cases and in instructing staff members in the approach to emergency situations and cardiopulmonary arrest. Initially the "ABCs of cardiopulmonary resuscitation" illustrate a good strategy for assessing trauma victims and animals with cardiopulmonary arrest. In this protocol, priority is given to treating respiratory, cardiac, and vascular problems. Other body systems are subsequently evaluated in a systematic manner. Following the ABC protocol, the letter "A" reminds us to consider arterial bleeding and to rapidly establish an airway. The letter "B" directs our attention to breathing assistance and manual ventilation (if needed). Subsequently the letter "C" prompts evaluation of cardiac and circulatory problems, such as hypotension and dehydration. Following the ABC strategy ensures support of vital body systems. Box 33-1 describes an alternative mnemonic, A CRASH PLAN, that refers to treatment priorities over an extended spectrum of body systems. The diverse nature of biology and medicine leaves room for debating the exact priorities in any given case. The real value of these schematic plans lies in their ability to standardize treatment and encourage rational stepwise thought during otherwise chaotic emergency situations.

Arterial bleeding is a serious priority for animals in an emergency. In part, this problem is uncommon because animals with significant arterial hemorrhage may not survive long enough to reach a veterinary hospital. If arterial hemorrhage is present, direct pressure should be applied to the wound immediately and continued until definitive control of bleeding may be attempted. If the vessel is easily visualized, the vessel can be clamped. However, placement of ligatures is time consuming and is not an immediate priority during the initial emergency assessment. A tourniquet may be applied to a limb to control hemorrhage if the distal limb cannot be salvaged (Figure 33-12).

The respiratory system is the next priority. Evaluation can be done quickly and efficiently by observation and auscultation. Visual assessment of respiratory pattern and mucous membrane color can be combined with thorough auscultation. Oxygen supplementation should be provided if the patient is in respiratory distress or is not hemodynamically stable (as judged by pale or cyanotic mucous membranes, weak pulses, rapid heart rate, or presence of an irregular heartbeat). Techniques for supplementation of oxygen include face mask (Figure 33-13) or blowby technique (Figure 33-14), nasal cannula (Figure 33-15), and placement in an oxygen cage (Figure 33-16) or oxygen canopy (Figure 33-17). Lastly, intubation with manual or mechanical ventilation may be used to supply 100% oxygen.

Veterinarians and technicians should be alert to common and severe respiratory problems associated with trauma, including upper airway trauma or rupture, pneumothorax, hemothorax, pulmonary contusions, diaphragmatic hernia, and flail chest. Signs of upper airway trauma may include bloody

BOX 33-1 A CRASH PLAN: Treatment Priorities Over a Spectrum of Body Systems

Airway	Cardiovascular	Pelvis
	Respiratory	Limbs
	Abdomen	Arteries/veins
	Spine	Nerves
	Head	

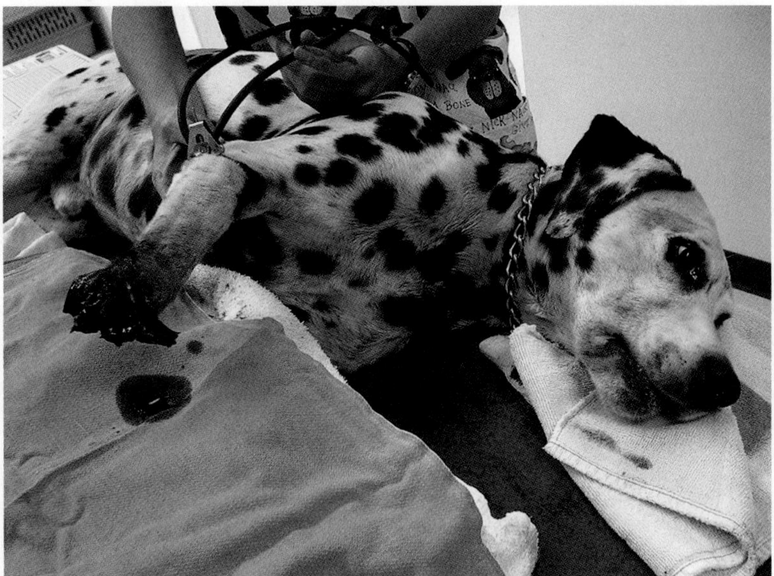

FIGURE 33-12 Tourniquet placement can control arterial bleeding from the extremities when the distal limb is not salvageable. (Photo courtesy of Dr. John Mauterer, Mandeville, La.)

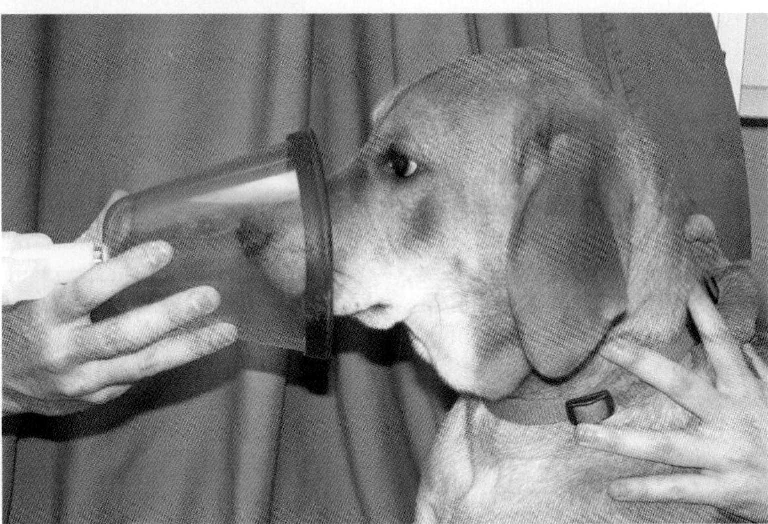

FIGURE 33-13 Supplemental oxygen may be supplied via a face mask.

respiratory discharge, increased respiratory effort, subcutaneous emphysema, and increased upper airway noise. In animals with pneumothorax and hemothorax, air or blood becomes trapped between the body wall and lung, resulting in collapse or compression of the lung. Clinical signs of hemothorax or pneumothorax include rapid shallow breathing (a restrictive breathing pattern) and respiratory distress. Flail chest results from two or more consecutive ribs that are broken in two places. This results in an independently moveable segment of the chest wall with paradoxical motion during respirations (i.e., a flail chest segment collapses during inhalation and expands during exhalation). Pain associated with flail chest segments further inhibits normal breathing. Rapid recognition of these problems is imperative because additional emergency procedures including thoracocentesis and thoracic drain placement may be required for animals with these conditions. Thoracocentesis is a diagnostic and therapeutic procedure that can be the difference between life and death until a thoracic drain can be placed.

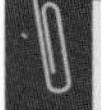

TECHNICIAN NOTE Thoracocentesis may be both a diagnostic and therapeutic procedure.

Additional diagnostics may include thoracic radiographs, pulse oximetry, and arterial blood gas analysis. Respiratory injuries often benefit from oxygen supplementation, but severe injuries may require mechanical ventilation.

The cardiovascular system is clearly a priority system and is often assessed in combination with the respiratory system. Thoracic auscultation combined with assessment of mucous membrane color (CRT) and femoral artery pulse quality provides a quick evaluation of the cardiovascular system.

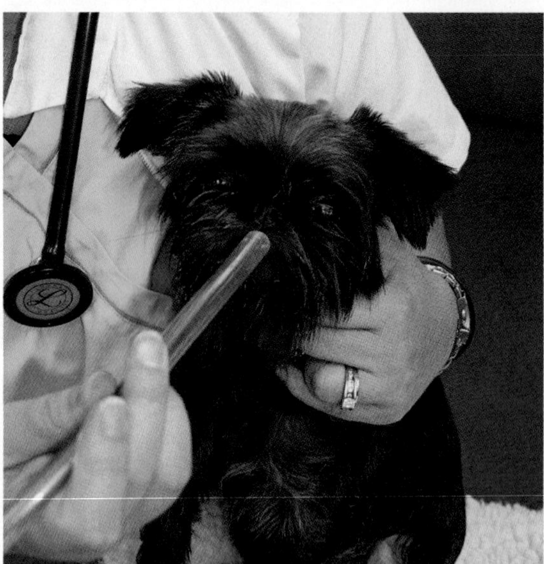

FIGURE 33-14 Oxygen flow from an oxygen source can be administered by the "blowby" technique to provide temporary noninvasive oxygen supplementation.

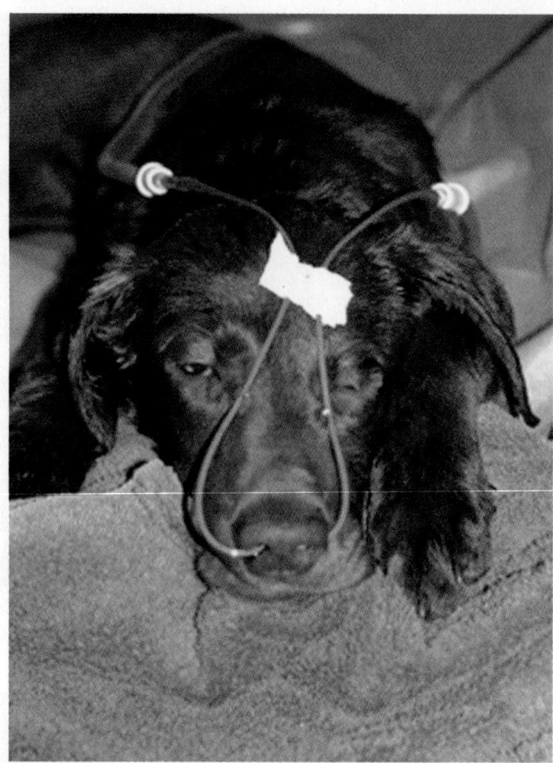

FIGURE 33-15 Bilateral nasal canulas can be attached to an oxygen source for comfortable and durable oxygen supplementation.

An ECG can be used to detect the presence of heart rhythm disturbances. Often monitoring equipment can be set up during the animal's initial assessment so that the ECG is performed as an extension of the physical examination.

During triage of the trauma patient, blood loss must be evaluated and addressed immediately. Mucous membrane color, CRT, and hematocrit with total plasma solids should be evaluated as soon as possible. If outward hemorrhage is apparent, this must be addressed, and fluid therapy and/or blood products should be considered. Remember that internal hemorrhage may be occurring in sites that are not easily observed, such as the pleural space and the peritoneal cavity. An abdominal pressure bandage may be placed if abdominal or pelvic injuries (i.e., femur or pelvic fractures, road rash) are outwardly evident. Application of such a bandage may help preempt a worsening hemoabdomen and prevent further cardiovascular decompensation. Proper application of abdominal pressure bandages is important. First, a folded gauze pad or a rolled towel is placed on midline (Figures 33-18 and 33-19) and secured with gauze cling (Figure 33-20). Further tension may be applied with cohesive bandage material (Figure 33-21). Care is taken not to secure the bandage so tightly that the animal has discomfort or impaired respiration. Thoracocentesis and abdominocentesis may be considered if patient monitoring suggests the presence of ongoing unrecognized hemorrhage. Abdominocentesis may also be used to detect uroabdomen (urine in the abdomen from rupture of the bladder or ureters).

Neurologic evaluation of the trauma patient is difficult. Recognizing severe head trauma and changes in intracranial pressure should be a priority. Increased intracranial pressure results from hemorrhage, edema, and inflammation. Signs of increased intracranial pressure include changes in mentation and level of consciousness along with changes in pupillary light response (PLR) and pupillary size. Although decompressive surgeries are sometimes used in people with increased intracranial pressure, most veterinary cases of head trauma are medically managed. This difference may in part be due to the availability of specialized trauma centers and emergency rooms equipped with cross-sectional imaging that treat people. Management of head trauma is complicated by controversy and debate among veterinarians. Veterinarians sometimes have concerns that overzealous fluid administration could worsen cerebral edema. However, in systemically unstable animals with head trauma, treating hypotension and hypovolemia is still a priority. Restriction of fluid to prevent cerebral edema in the face of hypotension should be avoided because hypotension and dehydration often worsen cerebral ischemia and hypoxia.

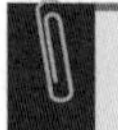

TECHNICIAN NOTE In animals with head trauma, treating hypotension and hypovolemia is *still* a priority.

In head trauma patients, volume expansion with colloids may be more beneficial than the use of crystalloids because smaller volumes can be used. These smaller fluid volumes pose less risk for volume overload and cerebral edema. Veterinarians often disagree on the use of various drugs for head trauma. Corticosteroids reduce intracranial inflammation, but may have other harmful side effects. At this time, the consensus in the veterinary profession is against the use of steroids in head trauma. Mannitol and furosemide are diuretics that can reduce cerebral edema. Mannitol and

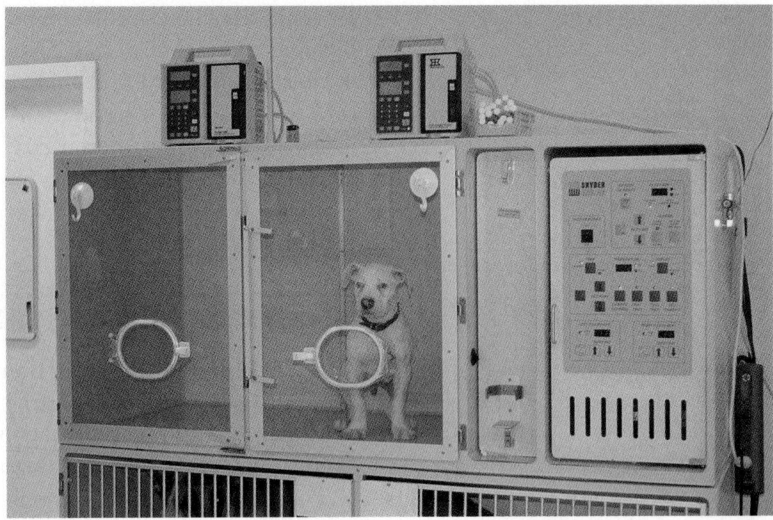

FIGURE 33-16 An oxygen cage offers a high-tech but noninvasive means of providing oxygen therapy.

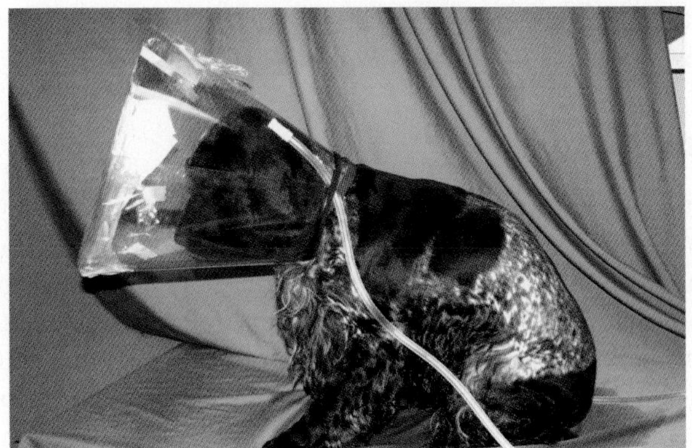

FIGURE 33-17 An oxygen canopy can be constructed from an Elizabethan collar and used in most veterinary practices.

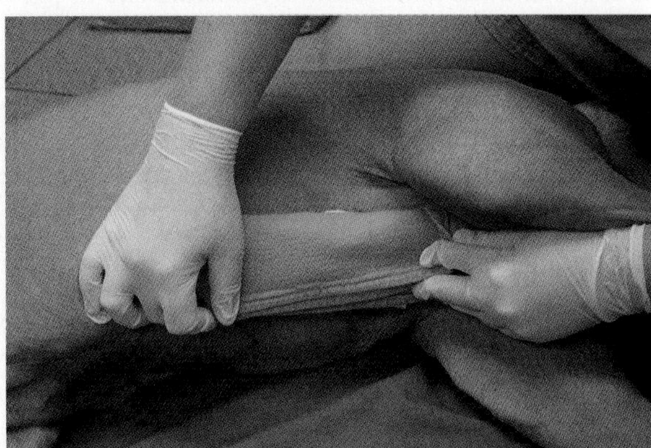

FIGURE 33-19 A rolled towel may be placed on top of the gauze pad to add to the cushion and further focus the bandage pressure.

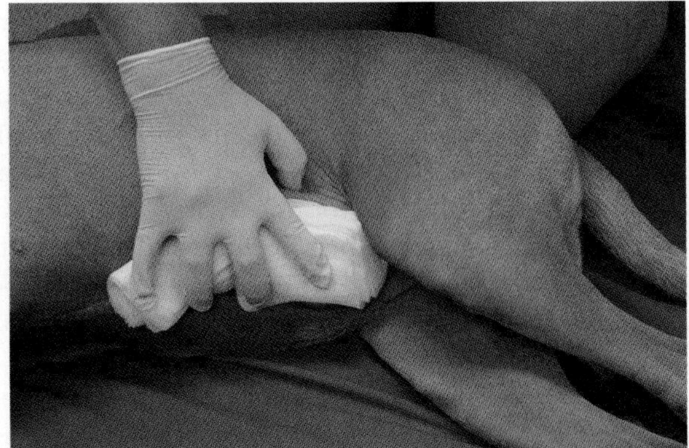

FIGURE 33-18 In the initial step of applying an abdominal pressure bandage, folded gauze is placed on midline to provide a padded site of pressure.

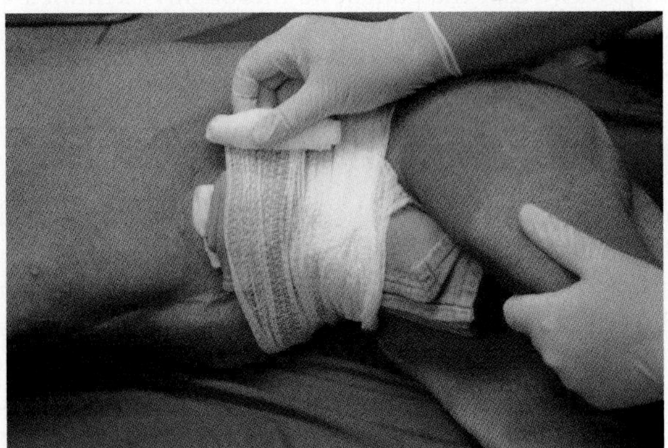

FIGURE 33-20 Gauze cling is used to secure the bandage material on midline and apply appropriate tension.

furosemide are important drugs for head trauma patients. However, mannitol is contraindicated in animals with either active intracranial bleeding or hypovolemia.

Spinal injuries should be assessed via thorough palpation of the spine and critical evaluation of extremity pain sensation and tendon reflexes. However, a complete neurologic examination is usually postponed until after other triage priorities have been managed. A syndrome of "spinal shock" may interfere with interpretation of the neurologic examination for up to 24 hours.

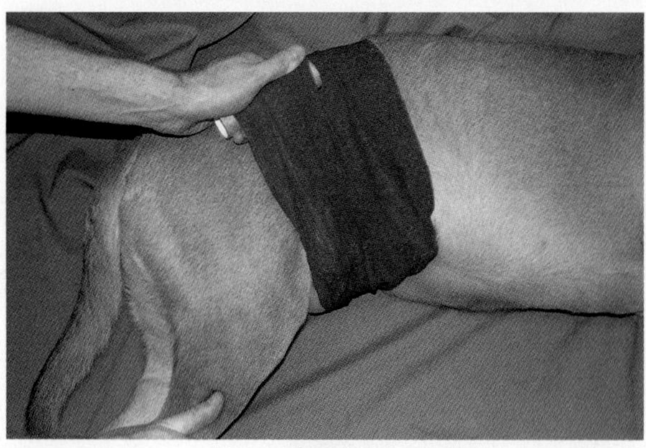

FIGURE 33-21 Additional layers of bandage material are applied to secure the bandage.

Orthopedic injuries should be stabilized whenever possible. A splint placed on bone fractures must incorporate the joint above and the joint below the fracture site to provide adequate stabilization of the injury.

> *TECHNICIAN NOTE* A splint must incorporate the joint above and the joint below the fracture site to provide adequate stabilization of the injury.

Early closure of contaminated soft tissue injuries is not a priority in animals with concurrent internal injury and circulatory compromise. Instead, sterile bandages may be applied to keep the wounds clean and moist until they can be dealt with safely.

Although emergency trauma cases can be stressful, it is important to follow a systematic approach to the patient. It is imperative that the patient be thoroughly examined and triaged when first seen and closely monitored during hospitalization.

TRIAGE OF THE CRITICAL CARE PATIENT

The principles of triage can be applied to many cases outside the realm of trauma and cardiac arrest. After all, stepwise management of treatment priorities is the basis for providing quality medical care. Severely ill animals often have a limited or vague clinical history. However, a methodical review of body systems (including a triagelike review of basic life support systems) will document a stoic animal's true clinical condition and help determine the nature and extent of disease. Application of standardized (triagelike) protocols also helps in the provision of good nursing care. For example, a recumbent animal with gray mucous membranes, tachycardia, weak pulses, poor CRT, and hypothermia will benefit from oxygen supplementation, IV fluid therapy, and external warming, irrespective of the final diagnosis. The value of a team approach cannot be overstated. Appropriate triage of body systems during daily interactions with the patient (including serial physical examinations) facilitates the recognition of new problems and important clinical changes. Nursing and technical staff often have a unique insight into the health of hospitalized animals by virtue of the time spent with each patient. Veterinarians can take advantage of this insight by listening to their staff and requesting additional clinical information. For these reasons, it may be beneficial to review the principles of triage with staff members in the context of critical care.

SECONDARY COMPLICATIONS

Secondary complications of trauma and critical illness are common in veterinary medicine. Although technicians are not called upon to make a diagnosis or formulate treatment plans, a detailed understanding of such complications can be beneficial. For example, well-trained staff members can prepare for and anticipate complications by knowing appropriate clinical signs and monitoring techniques. This knowledge enables experienced staff members, who are familiar with commonly performed diagnostic and treatment strategies, to better assist the veterinarian.

PAIN

Detection and assessment of pain is often a challenge in veterinary patients because animals cannot directly communicate their physical condition and there are no pathognomonic signs of pain. Common signs frequently associated with pain include vocalization, depression, anorexia, tachypnea, tachycardia, hypertension, hypotension, pale mucous membranes, aggression, abnormal postures, excess salivation, and dilated pupils. Abdominal pain in particular may be expressed by a classic "praying" or "play bowing" position in which the forequarters are crouched with the abdomen and hindquarters elevated from the ground (Figure 33-22). It is important to note that animals who do not exhibit any of these signs are not necessarily pain free. All trauma victims should be assumed to experience some degree of pain. Many critical illnesses, such as pancreatitis, meningitis, and cancer, are clearly painful problems. Obtunded animals, such as those with severe head trauma, may be unaware of or simply unable to express their pain. Pain management is an important component of veterinary care. Untreated pain causes stress and harmful physiologic changes that prolong recovery.

> *TECHNICIAN NOTE* Untreated pain causes further stress and harmful physiologic changes that prolong recovery.

Staff members trained in the recognition and treatment of pain can help ensure that appropriate analgesia is provided in a compassionate and preemptive manner as part of sound medical care. Many analgesic drugs (i.e., opioids) have cardiac and respiratory depressant effects, which can

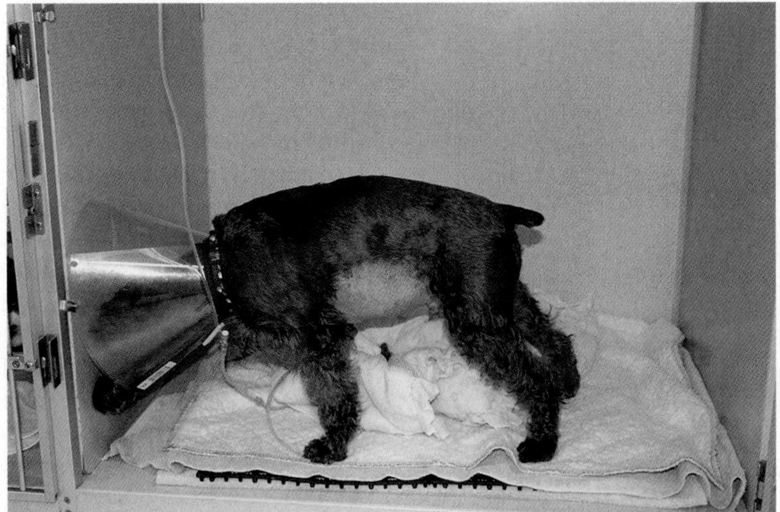

FIGURE 33-22 The classic posture of abdominal pain (demonstrated by this schnauzer with pancreatitis) consists of a raised and guarded abdomen in combination with reluctance to lie down.

be dangerous in systemically unstable animals. Nonsteroidal antiinflammatory drugs (NSAIDs) have little effect on the cardiopulmonary system, but may have side effects that affect the gastrointestinal and renal systems. With few exceptions, the systemic administration of analgesics may be safely considered. Regional or local analgesia techniques are useful and should also be considered. For instance, flail chest segments may be treated with a local anesthetic nerve block to reduce pain and allow comfortable breathing.

DISSEMINATED INTRAVASCULAR COAGULATION

Trauma causes tissue and/or vessel injury that is a normal trigger for coagulation (blood clot formation). In most cases, the body's natural homeostatic mechanisms prevent widespread abnormal clotting by balancing clot formation with clot resolution. However, in animals with massive injuries and severe inflammation, the natural balance between clot formation and clot prevention and resolution may be disrupted. When this happens, massive activation of coagulation overwhelms the body's normal regulatory functions and systemic clot formation begins on a widespread scale (instead of confined to a small site of injury). This phenomenon of systemic clot formation and loss of regulatory control is called disseminated intravascular coagulation. In DIC, microclots form throughout the body's capillary network disrupting blood flow to vital organs and causing organ failure (especially in the kidneys, brain, heart, and lungs). Widespread and uncontrolled clotting and clot lysis consume platelets, clotting factors, and regulatory protein, which paradoxically leads to bleeding tendency. DIC is often described as a vicious cycle where clotting and bleeding are occurring spontaneously and simultaneously. Importantly, DIC is always a secondary complication of some other severe disease. Common veterinary causes of DIC include trauma, pancreatitis, heatstroke, cancer, liver disease, immune-mediated hemolytic anemia, and snake envenomation. Clinical signs of DIC are often masked by those of the primary disease or trauma.

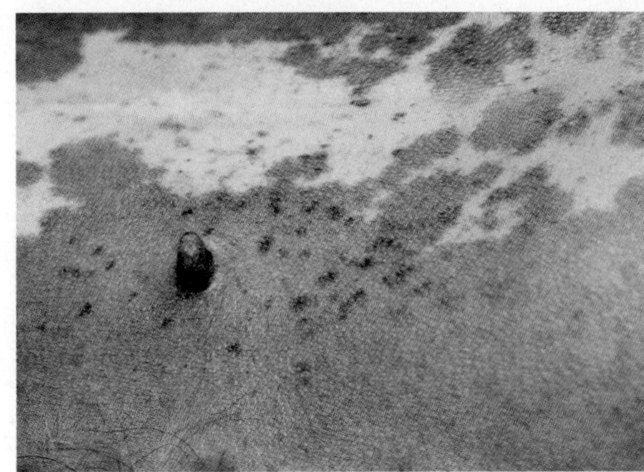

FIGURE 33-23 The bleeding tendency associated with DIC often results in small hemorrhages called petechiae, which are often seen on the thinly haired skin of the ventral abdomen.

In the early stages of DIC, the body is clotting excessively (hypercoagulable), and signs of thrombosis and poor blood flow are prevalent. These signs include unexplained edema, cold extremities, tachypnea, pale mucous membranes, hypotension, and neurologic signs. In later stages of DIC (once clotting factors have been consumed), bleeding tendencies are prevalent. In this phase, clinical signs include unexplained hemorrhage or bruising (hematoma, intraocular bleeding, hemoabdomen or thorax, and excessive bleeding from venipuncture sites). Tiny pinpoint bruises, known as petechiae, commonly appear on the skin (especially along the ventrum and inguinal areas [Figure 33-23]) and mucous membranes (especially the gums and sclera [Figure 33-24]). Large petechial hemorrhages, known as ecchymoses, may form in similar areas (Figure 33-25).

There is no single specific sign or test for the diagnosis of DIC. Instead, the diagnosis is based on supportive lab

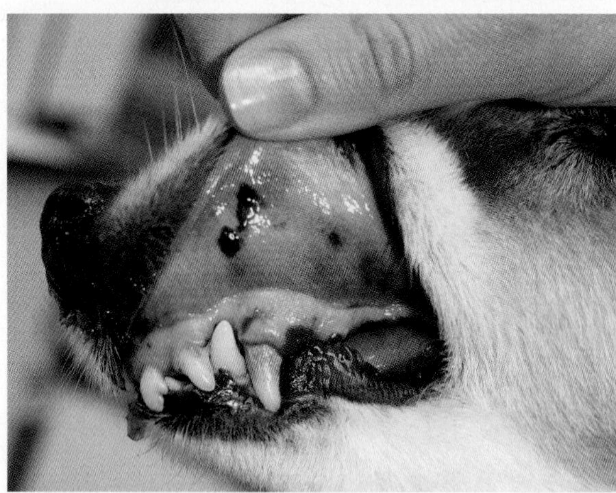

FIGURE 33-24 Petechial hemorrhages are noted on the gums in this dog.

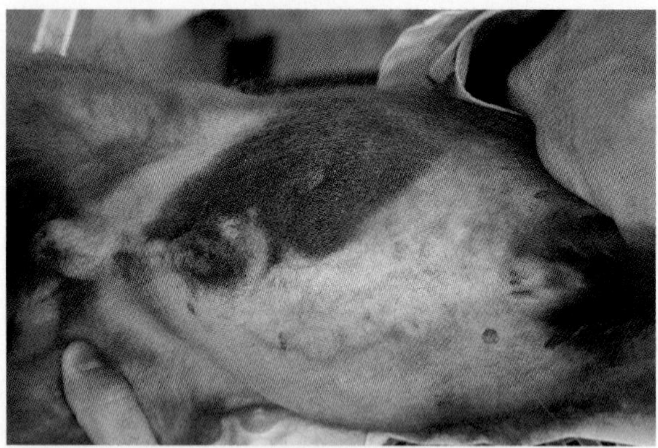

FIGURE 33-25 Larger hemorrhages, such as the one on this dog's abdomen, are sometimes called ecchymoses.

findings and clinical signs in animals with severe underlying diseases. Decreased platelet count (as a result of platelet consumption) is a consistent and early finding in DIC. Another reliable indicator of DIC is red blood cell (RBC) morphology. Schistocytes or fragmented RBCs are often seen in cases of DIC because fibrin strands span small blood vessels and "rough up" the red cells. This results in distorted borders and red cell fragments that may be seen on the blood smear.

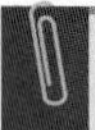

TECHNICIAN NOTE Schistocytes or fragmented RBCs are often seen in cases of DIC.

In later stages of DIC, a coagulation profile may detect clotting factor deficiency. A coagulation profile often includes several tests of clotting function, including the prothrombin time (PT), partial thromboplastin time (PTT), and the activated clotting time (ACT). The advent of in-house coagulation time analyzers allows practitioners to conveniently monitor trends in all bleeding times. Measurement of anticoagulant protein (i.e., antithrombin levels) and by-products of clot breakdown (i.e., fibrin degradation products and D-dimers) are also used in the diagnosis of DIC. In cases of DIC, antithrombin levels decrease, whereas fibrin degradation products (FDP) and D-dimers increase. These changes occur as a result of consumption of regulatory anticoagulant protein and accumulation of products of clot breakdown.

Successful treatment of DIC requires resolution of the primary disease. Supportive care with fluid therapy and oxygen supplementation are important. Adjunctive therapy with blood products and anticoagulants may interrupt the self-propagating cycle of coagulation and blood loss. In addition, plasma products and fresh whole blood transfusions help replenish depleted clotting factors, provide anticoagulant regulatory protein, and manage anemia caused by blood loss. Whole blood may also provide some fresh platelets, but it should be noted that these platelets are generally few in number and survive only a short time. Heparin is an anticoagulant commonly used in conjunction with plasma. If heparin is used at moderate to high doses, it should be tapered before discontinuing therapy. Unfortunately, treatment of DIC is often unsuccessful because many underlying conditions cannot be rapidly resolved and it is exceedingly difficult to restore the body to a state of healthy equilibrium once compensatory mechanisms are overwhelmed. DIC carries a poor to grave prognosis.

SHOCK AND THE SYSTEMIC INFLAMMATORY RESPONSE SYNDROME

Animals with poor blood flow and impaired oxygen delivery to tissues are said to be in a state of "shock." This clinical syndrome is caused by circulatory failure (despite its name, "shock" has no association with electrocution). Untreated shock is rapidly fatal because imbalance between tissue oxygen demand and oxygen delivery causes tissue injury, organ failure, and death.

In the early stages of shock, impaired perfusion triggers natural compensatory mechanisms (vasoconstriction, increased heart rate, increased cardiac contractility) that maintain blood pressure and increase cardiac output. This early or compensated phase of shock is known as the hyperdynamic phase or compensatory phase. Clinical signs during this phase relate more to adaptive physiologic responses than to perfusion failure. The clinical signs in this phase include increased heart rate and respiratory rate, rapid CRT, injected mucous membranes, and increased pulse pressure. These findings can be subjective and easily missed. During this phase, the weakness, depression, and altered consciousness associated with later stages of shock are either absent or mild. The most recognizable clinical signs of hyperdynamic shock include brick red mucous membranes and bounding pulses.

TECHNICIAN NOTE The most recognizable clinical signs of the hyperdynamic phase of shock include brick red mucous membranes and bounding pulses.

Close monitoring performed by alert staff members is important because early recognition and treatment may prevent further progression of shock.

Uncompensated or hypodynamic shock ensues if there is progressive underlying disease or if compensatory mechanisms and treatment fail to restore normal blood flow and oxygen delivery to the body. During uncompensated shock, cardiac output and systemic blood pressure are inadequate. Blood flow is preferentially distributed to vital organs (brain, heart) at the expense of other tissues. This shunting of blood exacerbates the oxygen deficit and fluid imbalance in other tissues and can lead to organ failure. The commonly recognized clinical signs of uncompensated shock are associated with circulatory failure and include hypotension (low blood pressure), rapid heart rate, weak pulses, prolonged CRT, pale mucous membranes, hypothermia, overt weakness, depression, and loss of consciousness. Eventually, prolonged hypoxia results in vascular paralysis, systemic vasodilation, and fulminant cardiovascular collapse. This terminal phase of shock is irreversible and rapidly fatal.

Shock is a state of emergency that is associated with many causes. When subdivided according to underlying cause, general categories of shock are hypovolemic shock, distributive shock, cardiogenic shock (including obstructive shock), and septic shock. Hypovolemic shock is the most common form of shock in small animals. In this form of shock, perfusion failure results from a reduction in circulating blood volume caused by bleeding, dehydration, or effusive fluid loss (i.e., abdominal fluid accumulation). Distributive shock is associated with maldistribution of blood flow associated with pathologic vasodilation. In this syndrome, pooling of blood in capillaries and veins results in a decrease in effective blood volume (regardless of intravascular volume or cardiac output). Common causes of distributive shock include trauma, heatstroke, envenomation, and anaphylaxis. As its name implies, cardiogenic shock is associated with decreased cardiac output. Cardiogenic shock can occur from heart failure resulting from many primary heart diseases, such as cardiomyopathy, valvular disease, and cardiac arrhythmias. A subset of cardiogenic shock known as obstructive shock is associated with obstruction of blood flow. Common causes of obstructive shock include pericardial disease, heartworm disease, pulmonary hypertension, and pulmonary thromboembolism.

Shock that is caused by infection is referred to as septic shock or sepsis. Septic shock can be triggered by primary infectious diseases, but it can also occur with opportunistic infections. Extensive tissue damage associated with severe disease (such as trauma, heatstroke, envenomations, and pancreatitis) creates areas of poorly perfused and devitalized tissue that provide a setting for opportunistic bacterial growth. Infection in such areas is difficult to combat because disruptions in blood flow prevent systemically administered antibiotics from reaching the site of infection. The local inflammatory response triggered by some bacterial toxins may help clear infections. However, in animals with widespread injury or tissue damage, an exaggerated inflammatory response develops that leads to uncontrolled systemic inflammation. This systemic inflammation precipitates a state of shock by inducing vasodilation, vascular permeability, poor cardiac function, and activation of coagulation. Hyperglycemia may occur in the early phase of septic shock as a result of the effects of stress hormones on metabolism. In later stages, hypoglycemia is predominant as glucose is consumed by both bacteria and body demands.

> *TECHNICIAN NOTE* Hyperglycemia may occur in the early phase of septic shock. In later stages, hypoglycemia is predominant.

In the absence of infection, a systemic inflammatory response syndrome (SIRS), which parallels septic shock, can be triggered by any critical illness where systemic inflammation is a problem. As is the case with other forms of shock, SIRS patients may go through an early hyperdynamic phase followed by an uncompensated or hypodynamic phase. In the hyperdynamic phase, circulatory collapse is temporarily held at bay by compensatory mechanisms that increase cardiac output and maintain blood pressure. During this phase, bounding pulses and brick red mucous membranes may be noted. Clinical manifestations of SIRS include circulatory changes, thermoregulatory dysfunction (fever or hypothermia), depression, tachypnea, and DIC. Recognition of septic shock and SIRS in individual patients is based on clinical findings, supportive history, and laboratory data. Fulminant septic shock and SIRS are both associated with a syndrome of multiple-organ dysfunction (MODS). Kidney failure and liver failure are particularly common.

TREATMENT OF SHOCK

Treatment of underlying diseases is important in the management of animals in shock. For instance, animals with septic shock should receive appropriate antibiotics, and animals with traumatic bleeding may need a blood transfusion. Unfortunately, management of underlying conditions takes time and is often only partially effective. Therefore animals diagnosed with SIRS or other states of shock should receive treatment based on triage priorities similar to those animals in cardiac arrest. Treatments are focused on restoring oxygen delivery and perfusion to the tissues. Oxygen supplementation should be provided immediately via face mask during initial resuscitation efforts. This allows a staff member to continually monitor the patient during treatment. Nasal oxygen catheters or an oxygen cage (or canopy) may also be used. Preventing circulatory collapse is the highest treatment priority during management of shock syndromes. This is accomplished primarily with aggressive fluid therapy to restore effective vascular volume and blood pressure. Shock dosages of crystalloid solutions are 90 ml/kg/hr in the dog and 45 to 60 ml/kg/hr in the cat. When using crystalloid therapy in the dog, shock doses of fluid can be administered in quarter-dose increments. For dogs, a quick formula to calculate a "quarter shock dose" is to take the body weight in pounds and multiply by 10. For example, a volume of 400 ml is an appropriate quarter shock dose for a 40-lb dog. This "quarter shock dose" is given over 15 minutes, and the animal is reevaluated. For cats, the same formula can be used; however, you must divide the dose in half (or use the body weight in kilograms instead of pounds).

> *TECHNICIAN NOTE* For dogs, a quick formula to calculate a "quarter shock dose" is to take the body weight in pounds and multiply by 10. For cats, the same formula can be used, but you must divide the dose in half (or use the body weight in kilograms instead of pounds).

A pressure bag may be helpful for administering large fluid volumes over a short period of time (Figure 33-26). Colloid fluids are also used to restore vascular volume to patients in shock. Colloid doses depend on the type of colloid used. Blood products, such as whole blood and plasma, may also be used in some cases during resuscitation efforts. Hemoglobin-based oxygen carrying solutions made from polymerized bovine hemoglobin sometimes have limited commercial availability. When administered IV, these solutions act like a colloid, but also have oxygen-carrying capacity. These features make them popular resuscitation fluids for some clinicians.

As noted before in the section on fluid therapy, all fluid doses are simply guidelines. Fluid therapy should be administered "to effect," which means that shock fluids are administered until monitoring parameters indicate that treatment has had the desired effect. Monitoring may indicate that higher or lower doses may be necessary. Appropriate fluid therapy often results in normalization of heart rate, blood pressure, and mucous membrane color. Additional monitoring parameters include CVP, urine output, blood lactate levels, hematocrit, and TP. It should be noted that unusually large crystalloid and colloid fluid volumes may be necessary to maintain vascular volume in unstable ("shocky") animals. Intensive patient monitoring is critical.

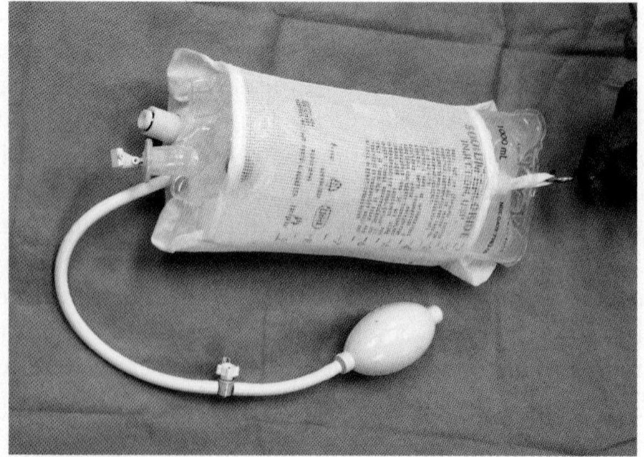

FIGURE 33-26 IV fluid bags can be placed within a pressure bag to increase the rate of fluid administration.

Animals with refractory hypotension, despite appropriate fluid therapy, may be candidates for use of vasopressor drugs (dopamine, dobutamine).

> *TECHNICIAN NOTE* Animals with refractory hypotension, despite appropriate fluid therapy, may be candidates for use of vasopressor drugs, such as dopamine or dobutamine.

Veterinarians generally give these drugs as a constant rate infusion to increase vascular tone and cardiac output. At low dose levels in dogs, dopamine selectively increases renal perfusion, which can be helpful in restoring urine output. At moderate doses, beneficial effects on systemic blood pressure are prevalent. However, at high doses, dopamine has an adverse effect on renal perfusion and may worsen kidney failure. Dobutamine primarily increases blood pressure by enhancing cardiac contractility and cardiac output. Both dopamine and dobutamine can be associated with cardiac arrhythmias, and ECG monitoring and careful auscultation may be helpful.

PERFUSION FAILURE AND REPERFUSION INJURY

Reperfusion injury is a cellular injury that develops as blood flow returns to an area or tissue previously deprived of perfusion. During cardiopulmonary arrest and shock, oxygen-starved tissues develop an anaerobic metabolism and are depleted of cellular energy stores. These conditions alter certain enzyme systems and destabilize white blood cell (WBC) membranes. Upon reestablishment of oxygenation and perfusion (as occurs with successful resuscitation and fluid therapy), the altered enzyme systems generate harmful molecules called oxygen free radicals. At the same time, membrane-damaged WBCs release inflammatory mediators that contribute to the reactive environment. The oxygen free radicals and inflammatory mediators cause inflammation and vessel injury leading to thrombosis and edema. These effects are collectively called "reperfusion injury." Reperfusion injury may result in systemic disorders, such as DIC, SIRS, and multiorgan dysfunction. Following resuscitation from shock or cardiopulmonary arrest, all vital organ systems can be affected by reperfusion injury and inflammation. For this reason, all systems must be monitored closely and supported, with special attention paid to basic life support systems.

CARDIOPULMONARY ARREST

Cardiopulmonary arrest is defined as the cessation of breathing and effective blood circulation. In most veterinary patients, cardiopulmonary arrest occurs in dying animals as the terminal stage of an advanced disease. However, arrest can occur as a complication of any critical illness and even in healthy patients undergoing anesthesia. Resuscitation efforts are commonly referred to as cardiopulmonary resuscitation or more properly cardiopulmonary cerebrovascular resuscitation (CPCR). The acronym CPCR emphasizes the importance of maintaining perfusion and oxygen delivery to the central nervous system during and after an arrest.

TECHNICIAN NOTE The term cardiopulmonary cerebrovascular resuscitation and its acronym CPCR emphasize the importance of maintaining and monitoring the central nervous system during and after an arrest.

This is important so that resuscitation offers a chance to return an animal to full function rather than simply returning cardiopulmonary function to a brain dead animal.

In an arrest, time is crucial if resuscitation is going to be successful. Therefore preparation and trained personnel are essential for management of these situations. Specific equipment and facility recommendations have been addressed previously in this chapter. In addition, one of the most important aspects of emergency preparedness involves knowing which patients are likely to arrest. These patients include those with heart disease, respiratory disease, hypothermia, multiorgan failure, trauma, and shock. Contributing factors also include hypoxia, heightened vagus nerve stimulation (vagal tone), acid-base disturbances, electrolyte abnormalities, and anesthesia. Common diseases associated with heightened vagal tone include gastrointestinal disease, respiratory disease, neurologic disease, and ophthalmic disease. The most commonly recognized source of vagus-mediated arrest occurs in weak and vomiting animals. Vomiting is accompanied by a reflex slowing of the heart rate (bradycardia) mediated by the vagus nerve. In susceptible animals, this slowing of the heart rate can be extreme and lead to cardiac arrest. Other stimuli for vagus-mediated arrest include urination and defecation. There are many factors involved in an arrest scenario because each individual animal deals with disease, traumatic insult, or stress differently. Sudden changes in the animal's physical status can be warning signs of impending arrest. In all high-risk patients, it is important to frequently monitor respirations, pulse rate/character, mucous membranes color (for pallor or cyanosis), and body temperature. Anesthetized patients should also be monitored for unexplained changes in anesthetic depth. Recognizing an impending arrest and alerting other team members to the crisis are the first steps in resuscitation.

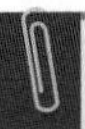

TECHNICIAN NOTE The first step in the resuscitation effort is to alert other team members to the crisis.

CARDIOPULMONARY CEREBROVASCULAR RESUSCITATION

Resuscitation efforts (CPCR) may be divided into two phases: basic life support and advanced life support. As noted in the preceding discussion of triage, the steps of resuscitation may be correlated with letters of the alphabet to assist with training and remembering the order of steps. Basic life support involves the important first steps or ABCs of resuscitation. If these steps are not successful, subsequent efforts at resuscitation are futile.

BASIC LIFE SUPPORT

In basic life support, A is for airway. Staff members responding to a potentially arrested animal should note if the animal is breathing. If respirations are absent or weak, the mouth should be opened and the oropharynx examined for possible obstruction. Common sources of airway obstruction include respiratory secretions, aspirated vomitus, blood, ingested foreign material, and mass lesions (hematomas, neoplasia, etc). If obstruction is noted, the airway should be cleared with suction or manual removal of foreign material. Caution is indicated to prevent being bitten, although most animals in partial or full states of arrest have limited or no capacity to bite. A sponge forceps and gauze may be helpful in clearing some exudates. Once the airway is cleared, staff members should note whether these steps have stimulated the animal to breathe.

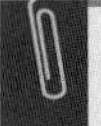

TECHNICIAN NOTE The ABCs of basic life support stand for "airway, breathing, and circulation."

If the animal does not begin to breathe, the patient must receive ventilation assistance. B is for breathing. Mouth-to-nose resuscitation may be performed by sealing the lip margins and blowing into the animal's nose. This method requires no special equipment and will deliver about 16% oxygen. This level of oxygenation is inadequate and should only be done temporarily until a higher supply of oxygen can be provided. Mouth-to-nose resuscitation efforts carry some risk to caregivers treating animals with potentially zoonotic diseases. Endotracheal intubation and ventilation with an Ambu bag in room air provides 21% oxygen. The best method of assisted ventilation is endotracheal intubation and delivery of 100% oxygen from an oxygen source. Ideally, animals should be intubated in lateral recumbency to prevent elevation of the head and positional changes that impair cerebral blood flow in arrested animals. Many times, however, intubation is performed more rapidly and accurately using a laryngoscope with the animal in sternal recumbency. Rapid intubation is imperative, and delays or failure can be catastrophic to further resuscitation. Following intubation, the tube should be secured with a gauze tie. If intubation is not possible, a narrow orotracheal catheter or transtracheal cannula is sometimes useful. However, a large-bore airway is preferred and may require a surgical tracheostomy. During assisted ventilation, the first two breaths administered should be long breaths lasting a full 2 seconds, followed by patient assessment. In some instances, restoring an open airway will lead to recovery of spontaneous respirations by the patient. If not, the animal should be manually ventilated at a rate slightly higher than the expected normal. Assisted ventilation should expand the chest by 30%, with a slightly longer expiration than inspiration. If the breathing circuit contains a manometer (i.e., most anesthetic machines), a pressure of 10 to 20 cm of water should be obtained with each breath.

Acupuncture is a method that can be attempted to treat respiratory arrest when other efforts have failed. The acupuncture point is Governor Vessel 26 (VG 26) of Jen Chung. This point is located at the nasal philtrum at the level of the ventral edge of the nares (Figure 33-27). A 25-gauge needle is applied to the bone at this point and then twirled to induce breathing.

C is for circulation. Once the airway is established and ventilation provided, circulation must be assessed by palpation of pulses (or apex heartbeat) and auscultation of the heart. Peripheral pulses are nonpalpable when the mean blood pressure is less than 60 mm Hg. An apex heartbeat may be indistinguishable when the pressure is less than 40 mm Hg. It is important to note that some animals suffer respiratory arrest without cardiac arrest. Improper chest compressions can stress the patient and precipitate cardiac arrest in some of these cases. However, once cardiac arrest has been confirmed, chest compressions should be started immediately.

Positioning of the animal during compressions depends on the animal's size, the shape of the chest (barrel chest versus deep and narrow chest), and the caregiver's ability to deliver adequate compressions. There are two theoretic models to explain forward motion of blood during CPCR. In small animals or those with a narrow chest conformation, chest compressions (during closed-chest CPCR) and direct cardiac massage (during open-chest CPCR) apply forces to the heart that mimic the normal heart mechanics. This is known as the "cardiac pump." In large animals and those with barrel chests, changes in chest conformation limit the direct effect of chest compressions on the heart. In these cases, increased intrathoracic pressure during compression results in forward blood flow from the heart, which serves as a passive blood reservoir. This is referred to as the "thoracic pump" model and is thought to play a significant role in medium- to large-size animals during CPCR. To optimize the cardiac and thoracic pumps, animals less than 15 lb (7 kg) should be placed in lateral recumbency. Animals greater than 15 lb may be placed in either lateral or dorsal recumbency. The point of compression (hand placement) for the cardiac pump is located directly over the heart (Figure 33-28). For the thoracic pump, the point of compression is located at the widest part of the chest.

Effectiveness of CPCR should be assessed by palpating for a pulse and evaluating the mucous membrane color. If available, an ECG can be extremely beneficial at this point to assess the heart and also to evaluate the effectiveness of resuscitation efforts. Traditionally a pulse and an electrical waveform on ECG should be generated with each compression. If available, end-tidal carbon dioxide (capnography) is a reliable monitor of ventilation and perfusion. Other monitoring equipment (ECG, pulse oximeter, venous blood gas analysis, and lactate levels) can provide useful quantitative information. If monitoring suggests the CPCR effort is inadequate, a change in technique may be required to improve effectiveness. Common changes to the CPCR effort include changing places with another team member, changing the animal's position, and/or altering your compression technique. Ventilation and chest compressions may be interposed or administered simultaneously. Administering ventilations and chest compressions simultaneously enhances the thoracic pump by increasing intrathoracic pressure during the compression (systole) and increasing venous return and atrial filling during relaxation (diastole). Once compressions have

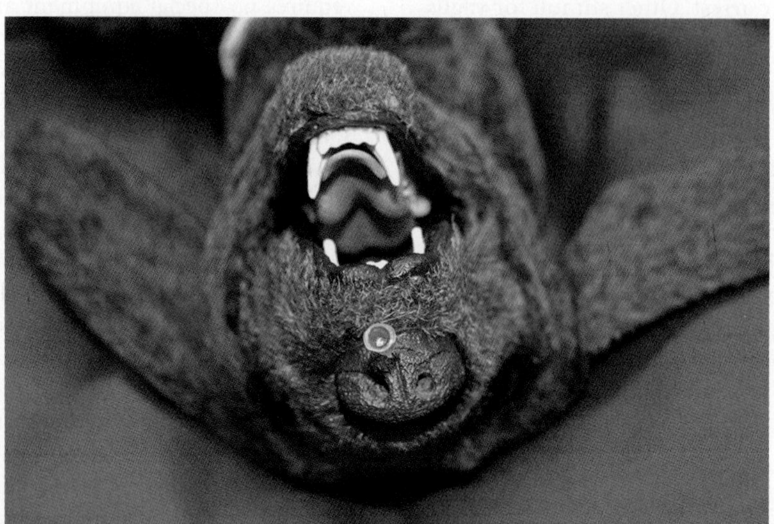

FIGURE 33-27 Jen Chung acupuncture to stimulate breathing is demonstrated in a canine resuscitation model.

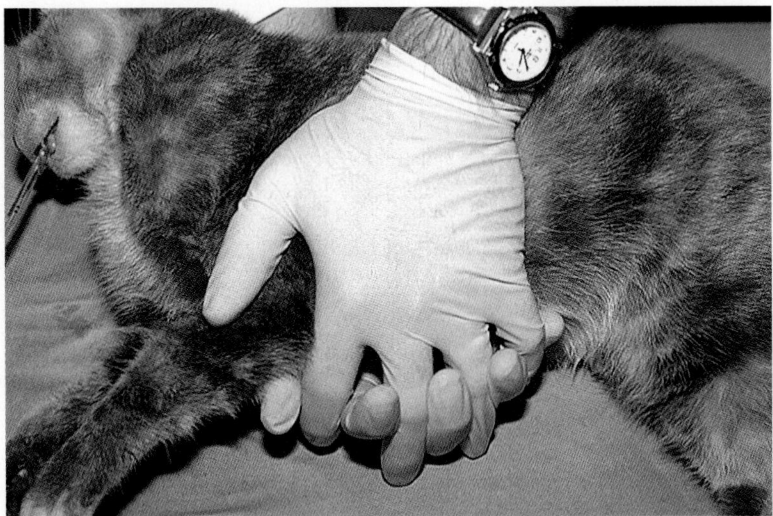

FIGURE 33-28 Correct placement of hands on an animal less than 15 lb for the administration of chest compression, which simulates cardiac contractions (the cardiac pump).

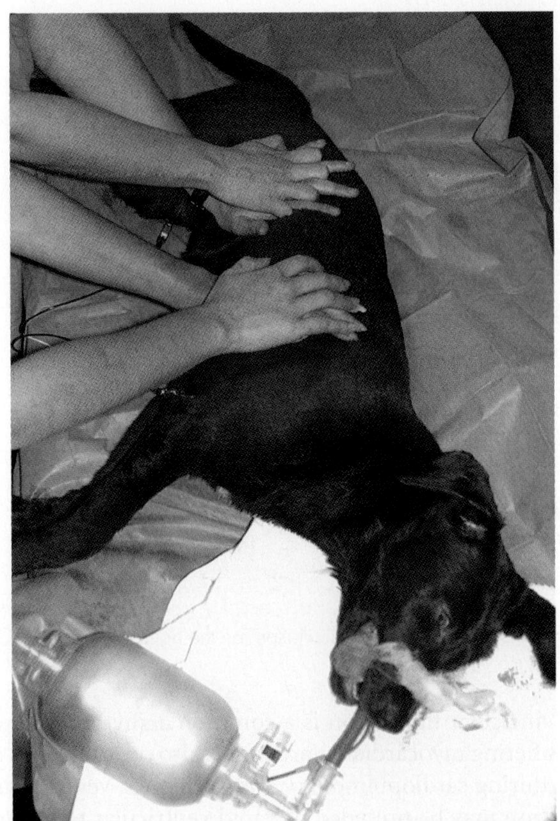

FIGURE 33-29 Abdominal compressions may be interposed with chest compressions to increase blood return to the heart during CPCR.

begun, a solid rhythm can develop if the breaths are administered simultaneously to the compressions. This rate should be 120/min for animals less than 15 lb and 80 to 100/min for animals greater than 15 lb. Interposed abdominal compressions assist in directing blood in the lower half of the body back toward the heart (via increased intraabdominal pressure) and may be administered by another team member (Figure 33-29).

Open-chest CPCR is mostly indicated in animals with chest trauma (flail chest, pneumothorax, and diaphragmatic hernias) because of the interference of such injuries on closed-chest compressions. In this method of CPCR, the chest is surgically opened on the left side at the fifth intercostal space, and compressions are applied to the heart from the apex to the base. Care should be taken not to twist the heart, which can occlude major vessels. Nontraumatic occlusion of the descending aorta during open-chest CPCR may improve coronary and cerebral blood flow. Open-chest CPCR is only beneficial if initiated early in the resuscitation effort. The decision to perform an emergency thoracotomy for open-chest CPCR should be made within 2 minutes of cardiopulmonary arrest.

ADVANCED LIFE SUPPORT

Advanced life support includes interpretation of an ECG and administration of drugs based on cardiac output, blood pressure, and the presence of arrhythmias. These steps in resuscitation are important only after basic life support has been established (i.e., the animal is being ventilated, and adequate circulation is provided). If the animal has responded to resuscitation efforts and has a perfusing rhythm, advanced life support may not be necessary. Unfortunately, in many cases, life-threatening arrhythmias and hypotension are common and require treatment.

Common drugs used in CPCR include atropine, epinephrine, naloxone, lidocaine, and magnesium chloride or sulfate. Proper use of an ECG allows recognition of specific arrhythmias so that appropriate drugs may be administered and patient response to therapy can be gauged. There are three basic arrhythmias seen during an arrest. These include asystole ("flat line") (Figure 33-30), nonperfusing rhythms (electromechanical dissociation or pulseless electrical activity) (Figure 33-31), and ventricular fibrillation (Figure 33-32). IV drug doses are listed in Table 33-1. In many cases, asystole and nonperfusing rhythms are preceded by progressive

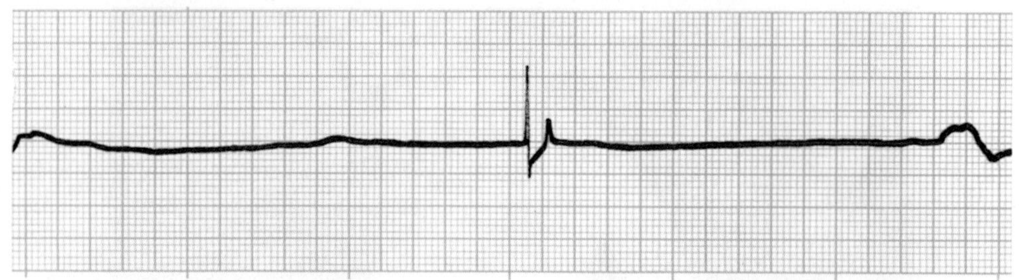

FIGURE 33-30 This ECG is from an arrested animal in asystole (flat line). A single "escape beat" is also present.

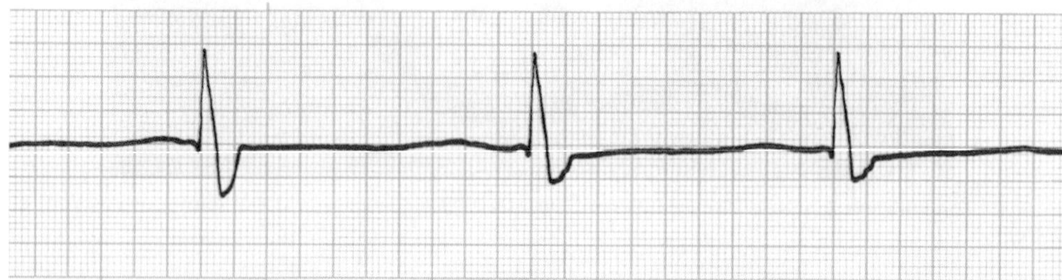

FIGURE 33-31 This ECG is characteristic of EMD.

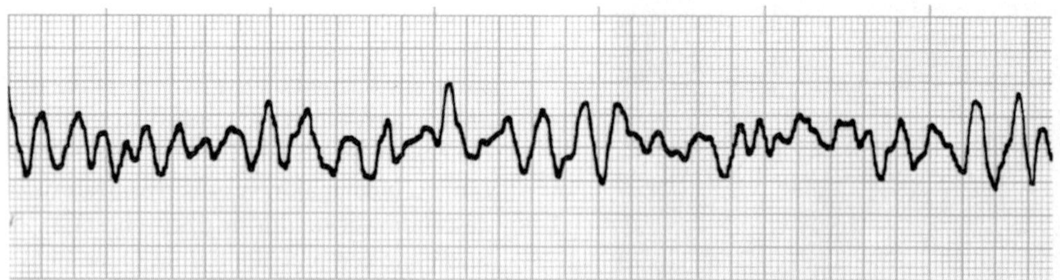

FIGURE 33-32 This ECG demonstrates ventricular fibrillation.

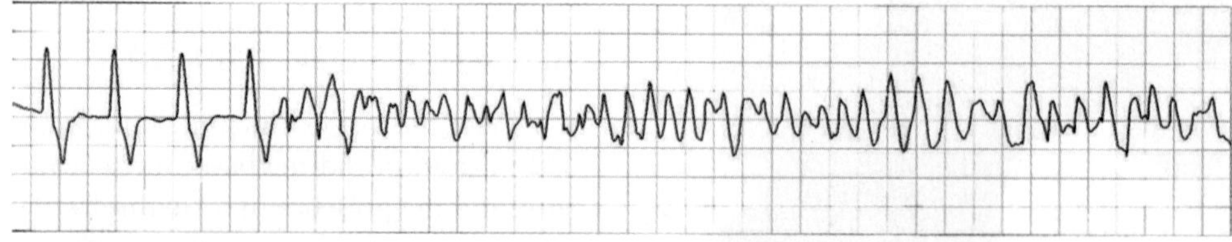

FIGURE 33-33 Ventricular tachycardia (on the left of the ECG) suddenly degenerates into ventricular fibrillation (on the right side of the ECG).

bradycardia. Bradycardia can be a sign of imminent arrest and should prompt notification of other staff members. Sinus bradycardia may be treated with atropine as the animal is monitored. During asystole, both electrical and mechanical cardiac activity has stopped. Asystole is treated with atropine and/or epinephrine with repeated doses administered if no response is observed. Electromechanical dissociation (EMD) is a common terminal arrhythmia in cats and dogs. The hallmark of this arrhythmia is the presence of ECG complexes with no cardiac contractions to generate a pulse (hence the synonym, pulseless electrical activity [PEA]). This rhythm can have a diverse appearance, but often mimics a ventricular arrhythmia with wide bizarre QRS complexes occurring at a slow rate. EMD is treated with naloxone, megadose atropine, or epinephrine.

Ventricular fibrillation is a common arrhythmia in people suffering myocardial infarction. It also occurs in cats and dogs during cardiopulmonary arrest. In dogs, ventricular fibrillation may be preceded by rapid ventricular tachycardia (Figure 33-33), especially when multifocal ventricular beats or R on T phenomenon are present. When ventricular fibrillation is diagnosed, it must be converted as soon as possible for resuscitation to be successful. Conversion of this arrhythmia may be attempted before initiation of basic life support. Treatment of choice for this arrhythmia is electrical defibrillation using an electrical defibrillator. If this is not available, chemical defibrillation may be attempted using drugs such as magnesium chloride. A strong precordial thump is potentially effective as a last resort. Electrical defibrillators should only be used by specially trained personnel

(Figure 33-34). Tips for appropriate use of an electrical defibrillator include:

1. Apply adequate pressure to the chest with the paddles.
2. Use the largest paddle surface area.
3. Use a proper conducting gel or saline solution-soaked gauze.
4. Make sure that all staff members are clear of the patient and table. (This includes the person operating the defibrillator.)

Alcohol should never be used near defibrillator paddles because of the risk for fire. The recommended dose is 2 to 4 J/kg. Initially, use a setting at the lower end of the dose range, and repeat or double the dose if no response is seen. Open-chest defibrillation requires specific paddles and a modified dose (usually one tenth of the transthoracic dose).

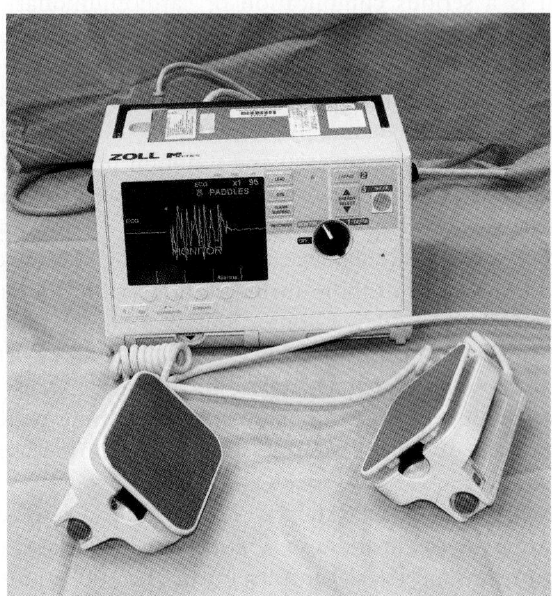

FIGURE 33-34 An electrical defibrillator and ECG should be located on top of the crash cart for treatment of ventricular fibrillation during cardiac arrest.

Drugs administered during CPCR may be ineffective as a result of poor perfusion and failure of the drugs to reach their target tissues (primarily the heart). A central vein catheter (i.e., jugular catheter [Figure 33-35]) is the CPCR drug administration route of preference during closed-chest CPCR. These catheters facilitate delivery of the drug(s) directly to the heart or its close proximity.

The next best route is intratracheal administration. This route of administration takes advantage of alveolar membranes, which have a large surface area and receive a high blood flow separated by a narrow diffusion barrier. An acronym to remember which drugs can be administered by the intratracheal route is LEAN (lidocaine, epinephrine, atropine, and naloxone). Intratracheal drugs are administered via a catheter passed through the endotracheal tube (Figure 33-36). Insertion of drug into the intratracheal catheter must be followed by a flush of air or saline to ensure drug deposition into the airways. A deep breath administered via manual ventilation helps to further distribute the drug. Drug doses administered by the intratracheal route may be rapidly estimated by doubling the IV dose. Small drug volumes may require dilution for effective administration. Drug uptake by the pulmonary circulation is impaired by conditions such as pulmonary edema, which negates this as a suitable route. Good communication between team members performing CPCR is imperative because a vigorous chest compression delivered at an inopportune moment may result in exhalation of medications administered intratracheally.

Drugs may be administered via a peripheral IV catheter (i.e., cephalic or saphenous vein catheters) if a central line or intratracheal access is unavailable or contraindicated. All drugs administered peripherally must be followed with a good flush of saline solution to ensure delivery into the circulation and toward the heart. Intraosseous catheters and intralingual injection are another means of peripheral administration. Placement of an intraosseous catheter (or intralingual injection) in the arrested patient can be rapid and does not need to interrupt the CPCR attempt. Intralingual

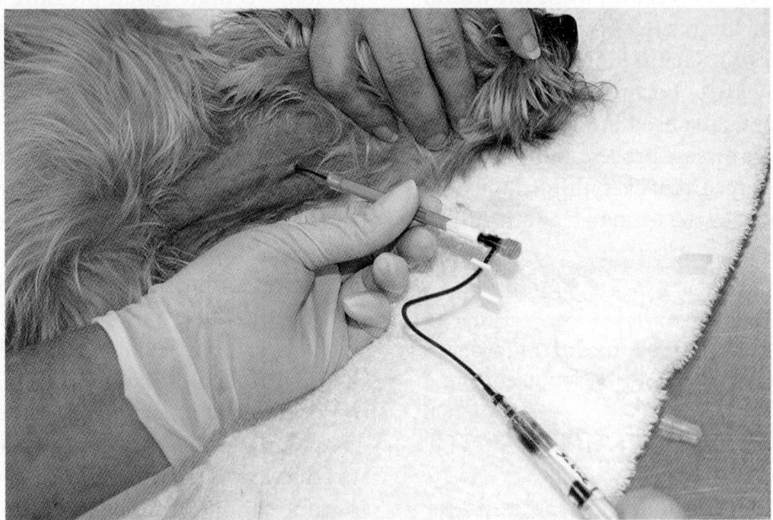

FIGURE 33-35 Placement of a jugular catheter in a critically ill dog.

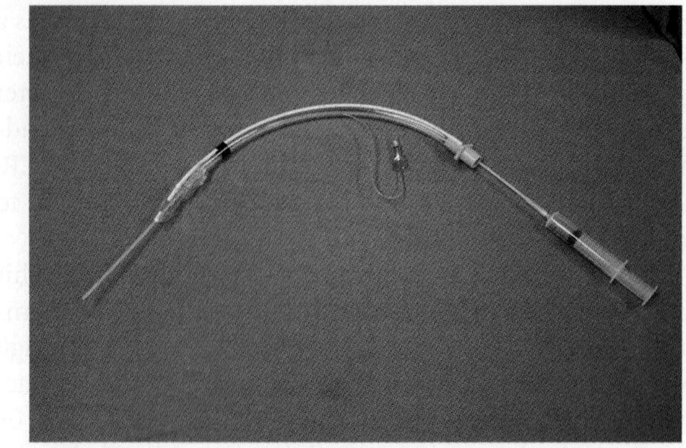

FIGURE 33-36 A polypropylene catheter passed through an endotracheal tube can be used for the intratracheal administration of some drugs during CPCR.

drug doses are usually double the standard IV drug dose. The last route for drug administration is intracardiac. This is chosen last because of the challenge of hitting a flaccid heart, the need to stop CPCR to administer drugs, and the risk of damaging the heart. However, in open-chest CPCR, intracardiac drug administration is preferred. Usually, one tenth of the IV dose is injected directly into the left ventricle.

Crystalloid fluids or colloids may be beneficial if hypovolemia was a predisposing factor of the arrest or to compete with peripheral vasodilation and support blood pressure. However, fluid support of peripheral circulation is not a high priority during CPCR. Fluids may be contraindicated during CPCR because fluid volumes are poorly tolerated by a failed cardiac pump and volume overload or overhydration easily develops.

The decision to initiate CPCR is made on a case-by-case basis according to the wishes of an informed pet owner. Many critically ill animals face an already grave prognosis. Following an arrest and successful resuscitation, the risk of rearrest and subsequent death is high. "Do not attempt resuscitation" orders may be indicated after discussion with the clinician and pet owner. Assessing the patient's risk of arrest and addressing the desires of the client are important early on. If a patient does not respond to CPCR within 20 minutes, continuation of the resuscitation effort is unlikely to succeed. Successful resuscitation rates in veterinary medicine are approximately 10%. Fortunately, certain patients do respond to basic and advanced life support. Many of these cases have a reversible disease process and/or a treatable cause of arrest. A written record of everything done during the CPCR should be made for the team to learn from and for the client record.

> *TECHNICIAN NOTE* A written record of everything done during the CPCR should be made for the client record.

Regardless, the real work begins following successful resuscitation.

PROLONGED LIFE SUPPORT

Proper postresuscitation management has two primary focuses. First, primary factors leading up to the arrest should be identified and treated. Second, problems caused by the arrest and the trauma of the resuscitation effort should be recognized and managed.

The central nervous system is particularly sensitive to injury during states of shock or cardiopulmonary arrest. In health, cerebral blood flow is locally controlled and maintained by reflexes that maintain blood flow and protect the brain from hypertension and volume overload. This autoregulation of cerebral blood flow is lost during arrest, leaving the central nervous system susceptible to further injury during and after resuscitation. Cerebral ischemia and reperfusion injury resulting in nerve cell death is a serious complication of cardiopulmonary arrest and resuscitation. Initially, neurologic examinations should be done hourly. PLR, responsiveness to stimulation, respiratory pattern, motor responses, and motor postures should be noted. Normal pupil size and PLRs are positive signs. Slow PLRs, anisocoria, and pinpoint pupils that are nonresponsive to light are progressively guarded neurologic indicators. Nonresponsive bilaterally dilated pupils indicate severe brain damage and a poor prognosis. Recent administration of atropine during the arrest should be ruled out as a cause of dilated nonresponsive pupils. Brainstem damage should be suspected in patients lacking a corneal reflex or swallow, or gag, reflex. Breathing patterns also reflect brainstem function, and erratic breathing patterns and periods of apnea (breathlessness) are poor prognostic indicators.

The cardiovascular system is clearly "ground zero" during cardiac arrest. In addition, abnormalities associated with other organ failures may further impact heart rhythm and blood pressure. Changes in heart rhythm, vascular tone, and cardiac output predispose to systemic hypotension and rearrest. Consequently, it is imperative to continuously monitor the ECG and blood pressure in the postresuscitation period. Accurate blood pressure measurements may be obtained using direct and indirect methods. Direct blood pressure measurement is ideal, but requires an arterial catheter and specialized equipment. Indirect blood pressure measurements may be obtained with Doppler or oscillometric methods. Arrhythmias causing clinical signs or hemodynamic compromise should be treated. Oxygen therapy has relatively few complications in the short term and is a useful treatment.

Acute kidney failure is a common problem associated with states of shock and cardiac arrest because the kidneys are particularly susceptible to damage caused by hypovolemia and hypotension. Consequently, monitoring of kidney and electrolyte parameters should be performed frequently in the postresuscitation period. Decreased urine production is associated with severe kidney failure. Urine output should be monitored hourly for at least 24 hours after an arrest.

> *TECHNICIAN NOTE* Acute kidney failure is a common problem after cardiac arrest. Urine output should be monitored hourly for at least 24 hours after an arrest.

Strict attention should be paid to maintaining adequate hydration and blood pressure. Hypotension is a common complication, and the mean arterial blood pressure should be maintained within normal limits to guarantee adequate kidney blood flow. Veterinarians sometimes use an "ins and outs" fluid therapy plan to maintain fluid balance when kidney function is in question. In such cases, administered fluid doses are balanced with calculated fluid losses. Appropriate fluid therapy will maintain hydration without causing volume overload. CVP, repeated PCV/TP, and body weight measurements are useful indicators of volume status. Hemodialysis and peritoneal dialysis are available at certain specialized treatment centers.

Primary respiratory disease is a common factor leading up to cardiopulmonary arrest. Respiratory complications of arrest and resuscitation include pulmonary edema as a result of congestive heart failure, noncardiogenic edema associated with hypoxia, and pulmonary thromboembolism. Vigorous chest compressions during resuscitation efforts may also result in pulmonary contusions, rib fractures, atelectasis, and/or edema. These injuries must be addressed in the postresuscitation treatment plan. Optimal respiratory therapy may require ongoing oxygen supplementation, ventilation support, and monitoring of arterial blood gas analysis. If blood gas analysis is not available, monitoring should include pulse oximetry and/or capnography.

Blood glucose concentrations should be monitored frequently because many patients that arrest develop hypoglycemia. Normal blood glucose concentrations should be maintained by adequate supplementation when indicated. Hyperglycemia should be prevented.

MEDICAL TREATMENTS IN THE POSTARREST PERIOD

Many variables affect the outcome and management of an arrested patient. These variables include the underlying diseases and reasons for arrest and the experience and equipment available to the resuscitation team. Difficulties facing the arrested patient and the syndromes associated with the postarrest period are well known. However, disagreement exists regarding treatment methods, treatment priorities, and which therapies result in the best outcome. All therapies of postarrest patients are somewhat controversial because of an inability to create a standardized model for conclusive studies. Many drugs may be useful in the postresuscitation patient, and the list continues to grow. The following is a brief review of medical therapies and the rationale behind their use.

Mannitol is an osmotic diuretic sometimes used in the management of acute renal failure and cerebral edema. The mannitol molecule resides in the vascular space and draws water from the interstitial spaces between cells, thereby decreasing edema and expanding the vascular volume. As mannitol is excreted by the kidneys, its osmotic effects "pull" water with it into the urine. Mannitol is also a free-radical scavenger, which may aid in the treatment of reperfusion injury. Some caution is advised in the use of mannitol because it can exacerbate volume overload. At high doses, mannitol may be nephrotoxic, and it is contraindicated in hypovolemic animals.

Furosemide (Lasix) is a potent diuretic that is commonly used in the treatment of pulmonary edema and acute kidney failure. The diuretic effects of furosemide increase urine output and may enhance the effects of mannitol. In cases of pulmonary edema, furosemide causes volume contraction, which decreases edema formation and hastens resolution of edema.

Glucocorticosteroids (i.e., dexamethasone sodium phosphate, prednisolone sodium succinate, and methylprednisolone sodium succinate) are extremely controversial as to appropriate use. They may be beneficial in stabilizing cellular membranes, thereby decreasing the release of membrane-derived inflammatory mediators. Methylprednisolone sodium succinate is a free-radical scavenger. As such, it is one of a few drugs capable of rapid action against the oxygen free radicals created during reperfusion injury.

Dobutamine, a synthetic catecholamine, improves the contractility of heart muscle and may be administered to maintain mean arterial blood pressure. The related drug, dopamine, can be used to increase renal perfusion in canine patients at low doses and to increase systemic blood pressure at higher dosages. The use of dopamine in feline patients is controversial and limited to the systemic blood pressure effects of the drug.

Sodium bicarbonate is used in the treatment of severe life-threatening acidosis. However, caution is warranted because overzealous bicarbonate therapy is both harmful and easy to accomplish. Unpredictable acid-base disturbances and other problems can be attributed to overdoses. Blood pH must be monitored via serial venous or arterial blood gas analyses.

Lidocaine is an antiarrhythmic drug used to treat ventricular tachycardia. Care should be taken to accurately interpret the ECG tracing because this drug may be contraindicated in ventricular escape and isolated premature ventricular complexes. The latter are common arrhythmias observed in the immediate postresuscitation period. Although abnormal, these rhythms do provide functional blood perfusion in many cases. Abolishing a perfusing ventricular rhythm with lidocaine may result in development of a nonperfusing rhythm and death.

Because all body systems are affected by cardiopulmonary arrest, a whole body approach to monitoring and therapy is required. For this reason, successfully resuscitated animals are among the most critical and labor-intensive patients. The prognosis for long-term survival is often poor. Those patients successfully resuscitated require constant monitoring and support for several days.

TRANSFUSION MEDICINE

In many private veterinary practices, blood for transfusion is obtained from healthy dogs and cats owned by veterinarians, staff, and informed clients. Large dogs and cats are preferred as blood donors because of ease of venipuncture and ability to donate complete blood units. Preferably, cats that donate blood should live exclusively indoors to limit their exposure to transmissible infections. For purposes of blood donation, cats should weigh more than 10 lb, and dogs should weigh more than 60 lb. A well-organized volunteer blood donor program can provide a safe and adequate blood supply for most veterinary practices.

Animals who donate blood for transfusion should be regularly screened for transmissible infectious diseases.

> *TECHNICIAN NOTE* Animals who donate blood for transfusion should be regularly screened for transmissible infectious diseases.

Unfortunately, the number of potential pathogens greatly outnumbers the available resources for most veterinary practice blood donor programs. In 2005, the American College of Veterinary Internal Medicine published a consensus statement on canine and feline blood donor screening for infectious disease. Readers are referred to this document (Wardrop K et al: *J Vet Intern Med* Vol 19:1:135-142, 2005.) for more information on this topic.

In general, cats who donate blood should have a negative test result for the following diseases:

- Hemotrophic feline mycoplasma (formally hemobartonella)
- Feline leukemia virus (FeLV)
- Feline immunodeficiency virus (FIV)
- *Bartonella* spp (cat scratch disease, et al)

In general, dogs who donate blood should have a negative test result for the following diseases:

- Heartworm disease
- Brucellosis
- Common tick-borne pathogens (*Ehrlichia,* anaplasmosis, neorickettsiosis)
- *Babesia canis* and *Babesia gibsoni*
- *Leishmania*

Additional infectious disease testing may be indicated for canine and feline blood donors depending upon regional factors.

Collection of blood from donor animals is described in Chapter 21. Many veterinarians use commercial veterinary blood banks as a convenient alternative for supplying safe blood products. Commercial veterinary blood banks may obtain blood from healthy community volunteer pets or from healthy animals maintained at the blood bank facility. Infectious disease screening is generally the responsibility of the blood bank, but veterinarians should scrutinize the screening and safety policies of the blood bank products that they use.

Just as in humans, dogs and cats have blood types that are important in determining the compatibility of blood donors and transfusion recipients. Blood typing systems use RBC surface antigens to identify separate blood types. In these systems, animals may be positive (have the blood type antigen) or negative (do not have the antigen).

Most cats have natural preexisting antibodies to foreign blood types. These antibodies will react to incompatible blood types causing severe and potentially fatal transfusion reactions. Obviously, cats donating or receiving transfusions should be tested to ensure blood type compatibility. Many dogs, however, do not have preexisting antibodies to other blood groups. Therefore most dogs tolerate their first transfusion extremely well. During transfusion, however, exposure to foreign RBCs may trigger antibodies that precipitate future transfusion reactions. Administering blood type compatible transfusions in dogs helps reduce the risk of current and future transfusion reactions. Blood typing in veterinary medicine is complicated by numerous antigen groups and species differences. Blood typing kits using a card agglutination test are commercially available to make pretransfusion testing convenient (Figures 33-37 and 33-38).

The most commonly used canine blood typing system in the United States is the dog erythrocyte antigen (DEA) system that can be used to identify eight separate blood types. Despite this high number of blood antigens, most clinically significant transfusion reactions are associated with only a few major antigens (DEA 1.1 and 1.2). DEA 1.1 is the most antigenic blood type. Therefore blood donors ideally will be DEA 1.1 negative.

Blood typing in cats is much more straightforward when compared with dogs. Cats have three blood types (type A, type B, and type AB). The feline AB-blood type system is specific to cats, and the antigens have no relation to the ABO blood types used in people. Worldwide, most cats are blood type A, whereas blood type B is uncommon, and blood type AB is rare. The distribution of blood types varies between geographic regions and between breeds. More than 90% of cats in the United States are blood type A. Blood type B is more common in certain purebred cats. Although type A is the most common feline blood type, any individual cat (mixed breed or domestic shorthair included) may have type B or type AB blood. Cats that are blood type A may have a low level of natural preexisting antibodies against type B blood antigens. Therefore administering type B blood to a feline patient that is type A may result in a transfusion reaction, even if it is the patient's first transfusion. These initial reactions tend to be mild because the level of these preexisting antibodies is relatively low in type A cats. Risk for severe transfusion reaction increases with subsequent mismatched transfusions because the patient has been further sensitized against the foreign blood type. Cats that are blood type B *always* have naturally high antibody titers against type A blood antigens. Therefore administering type A blood to a feline patient that is type B will invariably result in a rapid, severe, and potentially fatal allergic reaction.

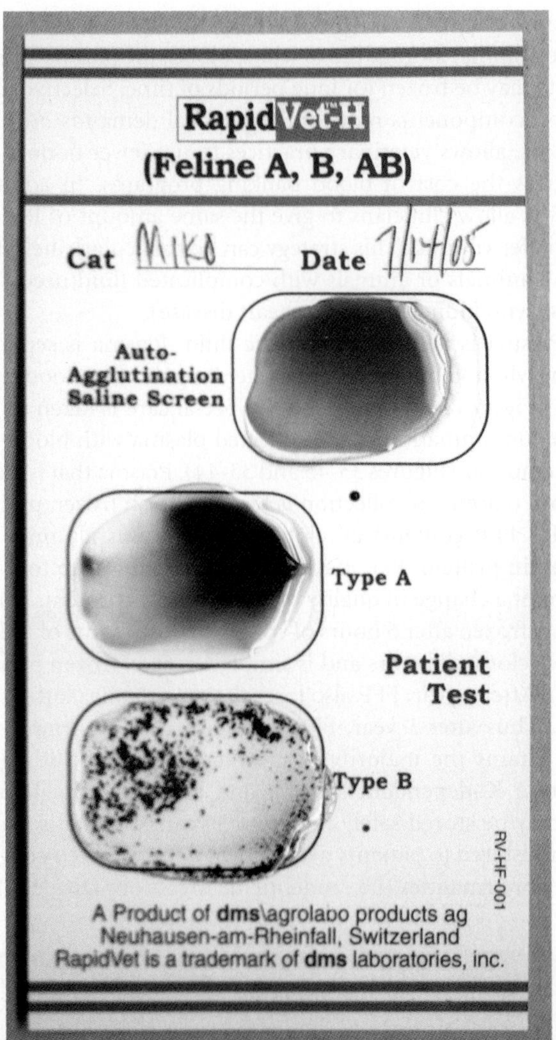

FIGURE 33-37 A feline blood typing card (Rapid Vet-H, DMS Laboratories) is shown. Note the agglutination indicating this cat is blood type B.

> TECHNICIAN NOTE Administering type "A" blood to a feline patient that is type "B" will result in a rapid, severe, and potentially fatal reaction.

This reaction manifests as anaphylactic shock and is characterized by circulatory collapse, respiratory distress, and vomiting. Cats who are type AB express antigens from both blood groups (A and B) on the surface of their RBCs. These cats do not develop antibodies against either blood group and therefore may receive transfusions from any feline donor.

Clearly, blood typing is an important consideration for blood donors and transfusion patients. However, blood type also plays a role in "neonatal isoerythrolysis," a cause of death in kittens borne to type B mothers. Because both male and female parents contribute to the genetic blood type of their offspring, kittens within a litter may be type A, type B, or type AB. Type B mothers have strong anti-A antibody titers.

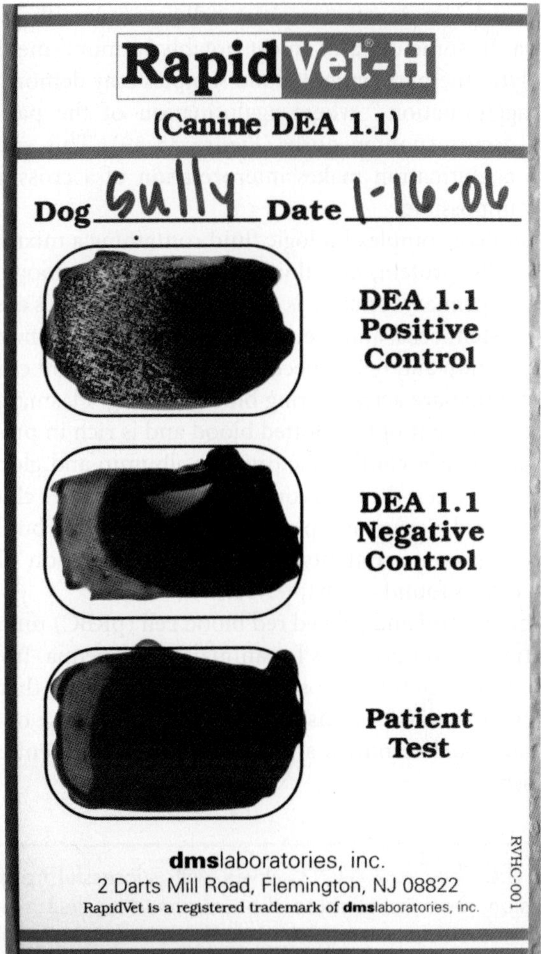

FIGURE 33-38 A canine blood typing card (Rapid Vet-H, DMS Laboratories) is shown. The patient sample does not agglutinate, indicating that the pet is DEA 1.1 negative.

These maternal anti-A antibodies can be absorbed from colostrum by nursing kittens and will attack the blood cells of type A or type AB kittens resulting in severe hemolytic anemia. This condition is one cause of the so-called "fading kitten syndrome," where healthy kittens unexpectedly become ill and die.

Transfusion reactions may occur even when animals are administered blood of a compatible type. Crossmatching is used to further document compatibility between donor and recipient.

> TECHNICIAN NOTE Crossmatching is used to further document compatibility between blood donor and recipient.

In this test, components of donor and recipient blood samples are mixed, and the technician looks for agglutination. Agglutination, which indicates incompatibility, is the clumping of RBCs into grossly or microscopically visible aggregates. When performing a "major crossmatch," the donor cells are mixed with the recipient plasma, whereas a "minor crossmatch" evaluates recipient cells mixed with donor plasma. In some diseases (most notably immune-mediated hemolytic anemia), patient blood samples may demonstrate "autoagglutination," where agglutination of the patient's RBCs occurs spontaneously (Figure 33-39). This spontaneous agglutination makes interpretation of a crossmatch nearly impossible.

Blood is a complex biologic fluid containing a mixture of blood cells, protein, and fluid. RBCs contain hemoglobin, and their primary function is carrying oxygen. WBCs are immune system cells, and their primary function is to mediate inflammation and fight infection. Platelets are small cellular particles that are active during blood clotting. Plasma is the fluid component of nonclotted blood and is rich in protein. Plasma contains clotting factors plus albumin and globulin protein. Serum is the fluid component of blood after clotting has occurred. Serum and plasma are similar fluids, but have different protein contents. Additional information about blood cells is found in Chapter 16.

Whole blood and packed red blood cell (pRBC) units are ideal transfusion products for animals with anemia. Importantly, transfusion is almost always a symptomatic therapy. Even with successful transfusion, the original cause of anemia must be determined and corrected for treatment to be successful.

> *TECHNICIAN NOTE* Even with successful transfusion, the original cause of anemia must be determined and corrected.

Whole blood units are popular for transfusion in private veterinary practices because whole blood is readily available, contains all blood components, and requires minimal processing. The primary disadvantage of whole blood use is a relatively short storage life (14 to 45 days depending upon the anticoagulant preservative solution used). Advances in animal blood banking and veterinary medicine allow the veterinary team to extend the useful life of whole blood donations by separating the blood into components for individual use. Refined blood banking practices also reduce the risk of transfusion because separated blood components contain less reactive substances. One whole blood unit may be separated into pRBCs and plasma components that may be administered to separate patients (Figure 33-40). Although packed red cells have a similar storage life to whole blood, the plasma components may be frozen for long periods of time. Selective use of blood components reduces the physical demands on blood donors, allows veterinary practices to use fewer donors, and reduces the cost of blood banking programs. In addition, pRBCs allow clinicians to give the same amount of RBCs in a smaller volume. This strategy can be particularly helpful in small animals or animals with complicated fluid needs (i.e., those with kidney disease or heart disease).

Plasma is a complex biologic fluid. Plasma is separated from whole blood in a centrifuge designed for blood products (Figures 33-41 and 33-42). Special care is taken to prevent contamination of the collected plasma with blood cells or hemolysis (Figures 33-43 and 33-44). Plasma that is frozen within 6 hours of collection is termed "fresh frozen plasma" (FFP). FFP contains all clotting factors plus albumin and globulin protein. FFP may be stored frozen for up to 1 year without a change in quality or stability of its protein. Plasma that is frozen after 6 hours of collection loses some of the unstable clotting factors and is simply termed "frozen plasma" (FP). After 1 year, FFP also loses the more labile clotting factors. Thus after 1 year, FFP reverts to FP. Importantly, FP still retains the majority of clotting factors (including the vitamin K–dependent factors) and albumin and globulin. FP may be stored safely for up to 5 years. Plasma is usually administered to patients with known or anticipated coagulation abnormalities (i.e., rodenticide ingestion, DIC, etc.).

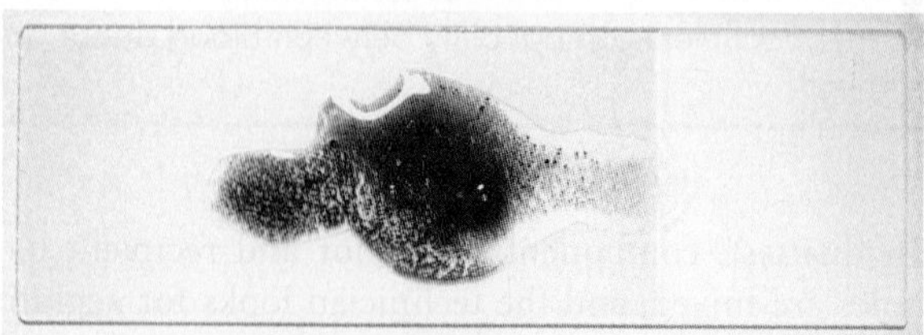

FIGURE 33-39 Autoagglutination can be detected by mixing a drop of saline with a drop of patient's blood on a slide. Note the spontaneous clumping or agglutination of blood in this dog with immune-mediated hemolytic anemia.

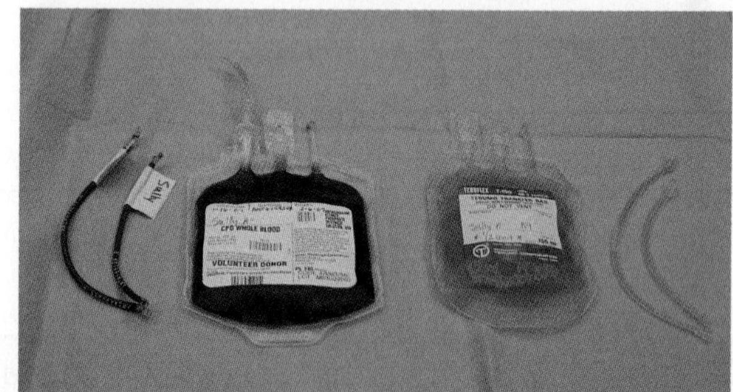

FIGURE 33-40 One whole blood unit may be separated into pRBCs and plasma for individual use of these blood components.

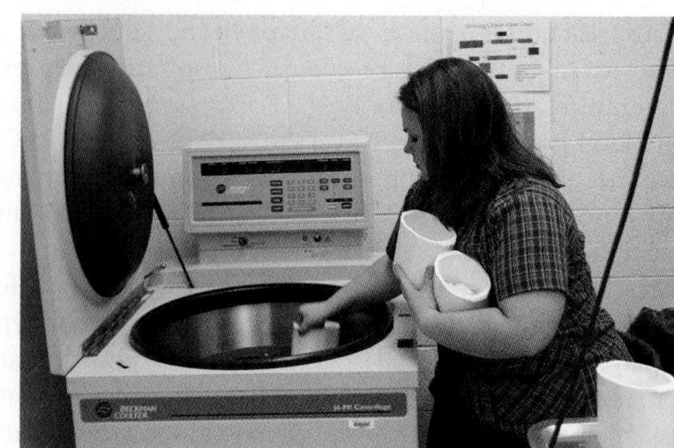

FIGURE 33-41 A technician places blood into a centrifuge, which will separate the blood and plasma contained in the whole unit.

Cryoprecipitate is a specialized plasma product that is rich in select clotting factors (VII, von Willebrand's factor, and fibrinogen). Cryoprecipitate is created by partially thawing FFP at 1° C to 6° C. The partially thawed plasma is centrifuged, and the solid cold-insoluble plasma component is collected. Cryoprecipitate is able to provide a concentrated source of factors in a small volume. Cryoprecipitate may be specifically indicated for use in dogs with von Willebrand's disease or with isolated clotting factor VII deficiency. The supernatant (cryopoor plasma) has fewer active components, but is safe for transfusion for up to 5 years.

Patients with von Willebrand's disease are deficient in a specific blood clotting factor known as von Willebrand's factor. This factor is important in platelet adhesion and is integral to normal blood clotting. Cryoprecipitate may be a good blood product for animals with this disease, but many veterinary practices are not able to make this specialized plasma product. The drug desmopressin (DDAVP) has been reported to cause release of stored von Willebrand's factor. Administration of DDAVP to a blood donor may raise the concentration of von Willebrand's factor in a harvested unit of whole blood or plasma. The resulting blood product is sometimes referred to as von Willebrand's loaded plasma.

Blood products are essentially biologic drugs. They have indications, side effects, and usual dosages. Exactly when to consider transfusion is a clinical judgment call that varies between veterinarians and between diseases. Generally, hematocrit values less than 20% will prompt consideration of a transfusion, but there is no magic number that triggers transfusion. Most clinicians base transfusion need on clinical signs. Clinical signs of anemia that may prompt transfusion include weakness, malaise, tachycardia, tachypnea, and syncope. Sudden anemia is generally much more difficult for animals and may require transfusion at a relatively higher hematocrit when compared with chronic anemia. In chronic anemia, animals may have time to adapt and compensate for the disease and hence may be more stable even at lower hematocrits.

Many blood products are given to effect (i.e., they are given in flexible dose ranges until a target is reached). In many cases of anemia, our objective is to eliminate clinical signs rather than to achieve a predetermined hematocrit. A dose of whole blood for dogs may be calculated from the recipient's hematocrit, the donor's hematocrit, and the desired hematocrit of the patient after transfusion.

This traditional formula has been used with good success, but is cumbersome to use. A simpler guideline for transfusion follows: *administering 1 ml/lb of whole blood raises the patient hematocrit by 1%*. This simple rule of thumb is easy to calculate on a stat basis and has proven to be clinically accurate in dogs. A standard unit of canine whole blood

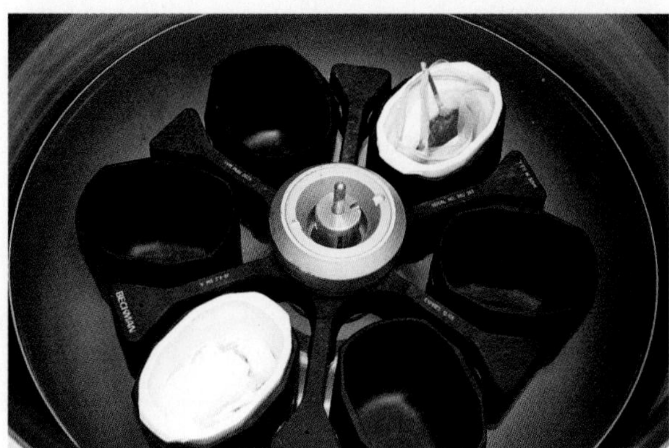

FIGURE 33-42 This centrifuge is designed for use with blood products.

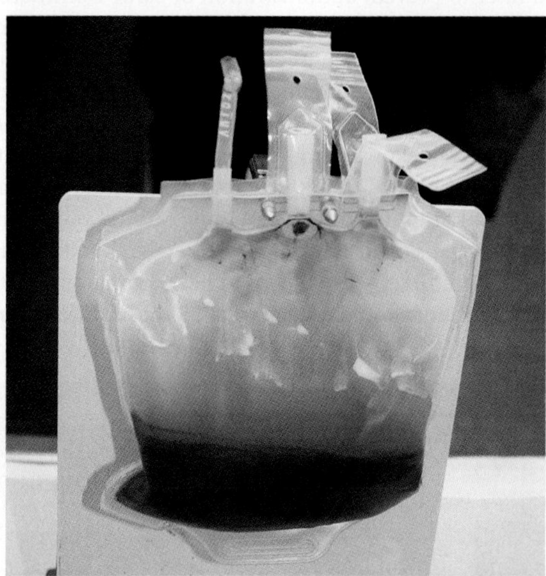

FIGURE 33-43 After centrifugation, blood cells have settled to the bottom of the bag, and plasma remains on top.

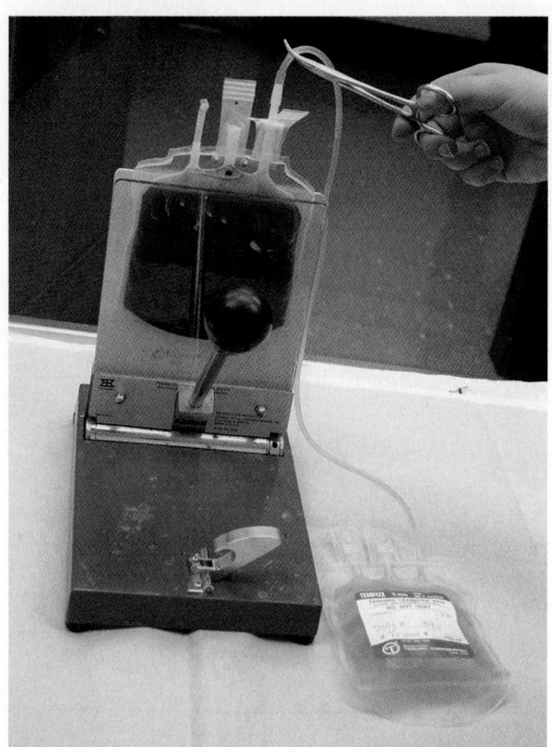

FIGURE 33-44 A plasma press is used to transfer the plasma into a separate collection bag for storage.

contains 450 ml. A standard unit of feline whole blood is 50 to 60 ml. Most cats receive one unit of whole blood and are reassessed after each transfusion. A standard dose of plasma is 15 to 20 ml/kg for both cats and dogs. This may be a one-time dose or may be repeated. There is no maximum limit to the amount of blood products that may be given to a single patient. However, repetitive blood or plasma transfusion raises the risk of side effects (including transfusion reaction and volume overload).

Blood and plasma must both be administered through a blood filter to prevent administration of clots. Commercially available blood administration sets with an in-line filter are ideal for this purpose (Figure 33-45). Blood products should be administered in 4 hours or less to reduce the chances of contaminant bacterial growth. Initially a slow rate of delivery is selected to allow for monitoring of adverse events at the start of transfusion. During the first 30 minutes of transfusion, the initial infusion rate should be 50% of the intended rate of delivery. For instance, a dog receiving one full unit of blood (450 ml) over 4 hours would have a total delivery rate of 150 ml/hr, but should be started at 75 ml/hr. Infusion rates vary depending upon the volume status of the patient. Animals with congestive heart failure or those at risk for volume overload should be closely monitored and administered blood at conservative rates. Infusion pumps rated for use with blood products are helpful in delivering specific doses of transfusion products (Figure 33-46). Pumps that are not rated for blood should not be used because they may deliver erroneous volumes or damage RBCs (hemolysis) during infusion. When low infusion rates are required, blood units may be divided into separate syringes and administered one at a time. Syringes to be administered later should be kept in a refrigerator to preserve the viability and sterility of the blood. In this manner, patients can receive their full blood dose at slower rates.

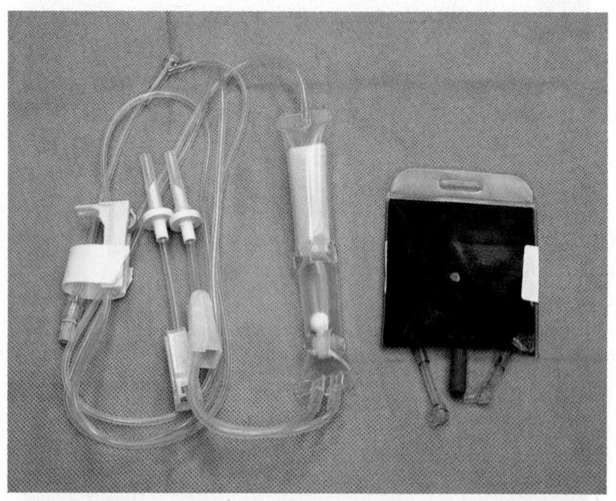

FIGURE 33-45 Commercially available blood administration sets are available with in-line filters to prevent inadvertent infusion of clots.

TECHNICIAN NOTE When low infusion rates are required, blood units may be divided into separate syringes and administered one at a time.

Any adverse events should be recorded. Vital signs (temperature, pulse, respiration, mucous membrane color, or CRT) should also be recorded every 15 minutes during transfusion. Standardized monitoring forms for the medical record encourage compliance and help document transfusion reactions. If a transfusion reaction is noted, administration of the blood product should stop, and the veterinarian should be notified. Transfusion reactions may result from allergic reactions to foreign cells and protein. Adverse inflammatory reactions may also be provoked by blood products that are hemolyzed or contaminated with microorganisms. Reactions to plasma products may occur, but are much less common when compared with RBC products. Transfusion reactions may have classic features of allergic reactions, such as erythema (redness [Figure 33-47]), urticaria (hives), and pruritus (itching). Other allergic signs may include anxiety, fever, vomiting, diarrhea, and nausea. These types of allergic reaction are often reversible and may be treated by cessation of transfusion and administration of corticosteroids and/or

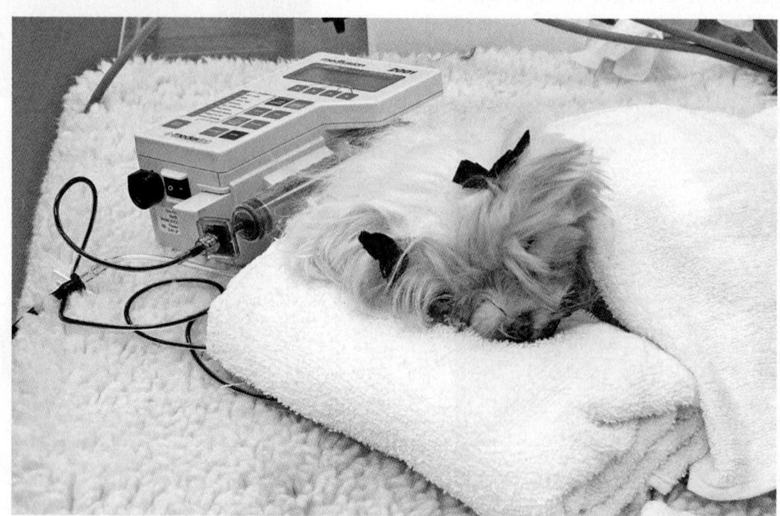

FIGURE 33-46 Blood products are administered in syringes on a syringe pump. Note the square-shaped blood filter attached to the syringe.

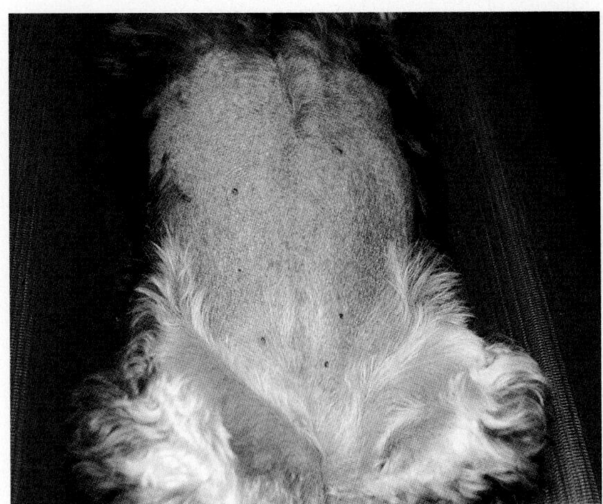

FIGURE 33-47 Transfusion reactions can include many signs, including the cutaneous erythema pictured here.

antihistamines. Lysis of transfused RBCs is a common adverse reaction, which may be acute or delayed. Signs of hemolysis include progressive anemia, hemoglobinemia, and hemoglobinuria. Delayed hemolytic reactions sometimes go unnoticed because they may occur days or weeks later (after the patient has been discharged from the hospital). Severe transfusion reactions may precipitate acute renal failure. Anaphylactic shock may occur with subsequent tachycardia, hypotension, collapse, and death.

Once a transfusion has been completed, the patient's hematocrit and TP should be reassessed after fluid and RBC volumes have been fully distributed (usually 30 minutes to an hour after the end of transfusion).

> TECHNICIAN NOTE Once a transfusion has been completed, the patient's hematocrit and TP should be reassessed after fluid and RBC volumes have been fully distributed (usually 30 minutes to an hour after the end of transfusion).

This step is often regretfully overlooked. Posttransfusion data is important in documenting the end result of transfusion and in the recognition of transfusion reactions.

PATIENT MONITORING

The primary objectives of critical care monitoring include (1) evaluation of current status, (2) evaluating the response to therapy, and (3) detecting new problems. Continuous 24-hour monitoring should be provided to patients that are critical or unstable, whereas 8-hour monitoring intervals may be acceptable in improved or stable patients. Both subjective parameters and objective parameters are used to provide the most complete evaluation of patient progress. Subjective parameters include hydration status and mentation (attitude, alertness, appetite). Objective parameters include body weight, urine production, vital signs (i.e., temperature, pulse, respirations), and lab results. Special techniques are often used to monitor, diagnose, and treat critically ill veterinary patients. The most important tools in monitoring any patient are serial physical examinations and assessment by a trained and attentive caregiver.

> TECHNICIAN NOTE The most important tools in monitoring any patient are serial physical examinations and assessment by a trained and attentive caregiver.

Expensive equipment may be helpful in some situations, but will never replace a hands-on nursing approach. Likewise, continuity of care is important so that dedicated caregivers can recognize patient trends, alert the veterinary team, and respond appropriately. A rational approach to patient monitoring can be loosely organized around the principles of triage and body system anatomy.

RESPIRATORY SYSTEM

Care should be taken to minimize stress in animals with respiratory difficulty (dyspnea). Oxygen supplementation is an important treatment in some animals and can be provided via blowby, nasal cannulae, face mask, oxygen canopy, or oxygen cage or incubator. In all patients (especially those with known respiratory disease), it is important to note the rate, pattern, and effort of breathing. Obstructive airway disease (i.e., laryngeal paralysis or tracheal foreign material) is often characterized by a slow and deep respiratory pattern with harsh or whistling upper airway noise. Restrictive respiratory disease (i.e., pleural effusion, chest wall injuries) often manifests as rapid and shallow breathing. Respiratory disease may be detected by monitoring respiratory rate, mucous membrane color, and respiratory effort. A significant abdominal component or effort during inspiration is abnormal. All lung fields and the upper airways should be ausculted. Additional sounds with inspiration or expiration should be noted and significant changes recorded in the medical record and reported to the veterinarian. Fluid and air in the pleural space often result in muffled heart and lung sounds. Percussing the thoracic wall during auscultation may aid in determining whether air or fluid is in the pleural space. Certain lower airway disorders, such as pneumonia and pulmonary edema, are characterized by crackles during each phase of respiration.

Monitoring equipment, such as a pulse oximeter (Figure 33-48) and capnograph, can provide additional information to the veterinary team. These monitors are frequently used for anesthesia monitoring, but can also be used for continuous monitoring of critically ill patients. Pulse oximetry uses an infrared sensor to count the pulse rate and provide a noninvasive measure of arterial hemoglobin-oxygen saturation (usually in percent). Infrared sensors are made to clip onto the tongue, lip margin, or flank. Rectal probes (with sanitary covers) for recumbent patients are also available.

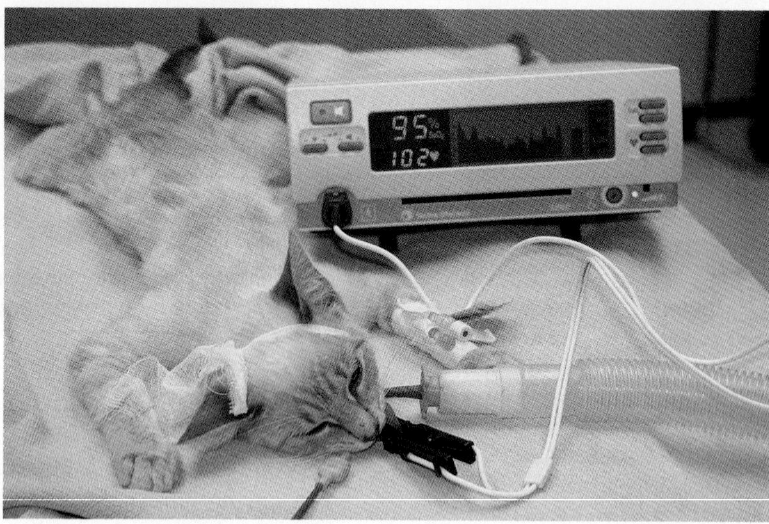

FIGURE 33-48 A pulse oximeter provides a convenient and reliable means to monitor oxygenation in critical or anesthetized animals. Note the pulse waveform, pulse rate, and SPO_2 reported on the monitor.

It is important to note that the pulse oximeter reading is a hemoglobin-oxygen saturation value and is not identical to the blood oxygen content or arterial oxygen partial pressure (PaO_2). The structure and biochemistry of hemoglobin allows saturation to remain high despite some significant changes in blood oxygen content. The pulse oximeter is a good crisis prevention tool, but does not provide fine details about the oxygenation and ventilation status of the patient.

> *TECHNICIAN NOTE* The pulse oximeter is a good crisis prevention tool, but does not provide fine details about the oxygenation and ventilation status of the patient.

If the pulse oximeter detects a problem with oxygen saturation, a blood gas analysis and oxygen supplementation may be ordered. In normal patients, the oxygen saturation should remain above 95%. Poor perfusion at the probe site, hypothermia, and movement will impede the sensor's ability to obtain an accurate reading. If the pulse oximeter sensor triggers an alarm, manual palpation of the pulse, auscultation of the heart, and check of the mucous membranes should be performed immediately before adjusting the equipment.

Capnography also uses infrared technology to estimate the carbon dioxide concentration of expired air. By incorporating a capnometer into the breathing circuit of intubated animals, the end-tidal carbon dioxide (carbon dioxide concentration at the end of expiration) can be measured (Figure 33-49). The end-tidal carbon dioxide is an estimate of $PaCO_2$ (arterial carbon dioxide levels), which can be useful in monitoring the efficiency of mechanical ventilation. Capnometry can also be used to confirm endotracheal intubation and to detect airway occlusion. If an endotracheal tube is misplaced into the esophagus or occluded by exudates, end-tidal carbon dioxide will be negligible. Additionally, capnographs have been used to assess the efficacy of resuscitation efforts during CPR. Successful resuscitation is expected to result in progressively increased end-tidal carbon dioxide values as forward blood flow returns carbon dioxide from the tissues.

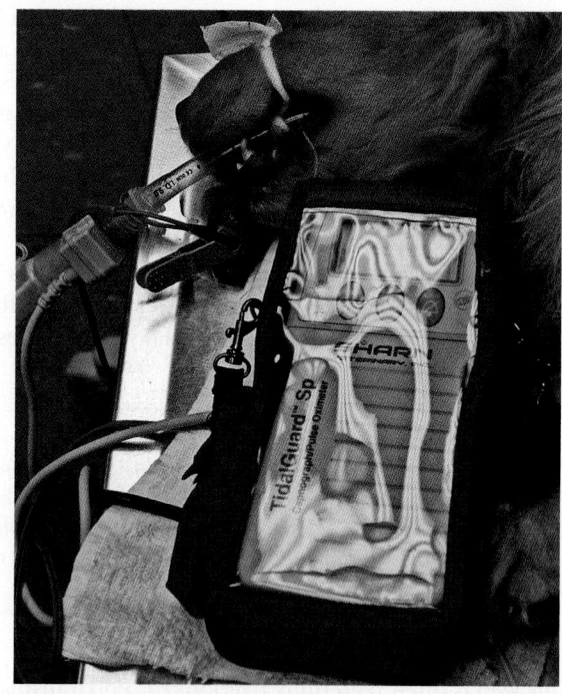

FIGURE 33-49 A capnometer attached to the breathing circuit of intubated animals can be used to measure the end-tidal carbon dioxide (carbon dioxide concentration at the end of expiration).

Arterial blood gas analysis provides specific data on the oxygenation, ventilation, and acid-base status of the pet. Normal ranges for arterial blood gas values are published elsewhere. Values for oxygen and carbon dioxide are expressed as a pressure (PaO_2 or $PaCO_2$) in units of millimeters of mercury (mm Hg). Arterial blood samples may be drawn from the femoral artery, dorsal pedal artery, or lingual artery by palpating the pulse and guiding the needle into

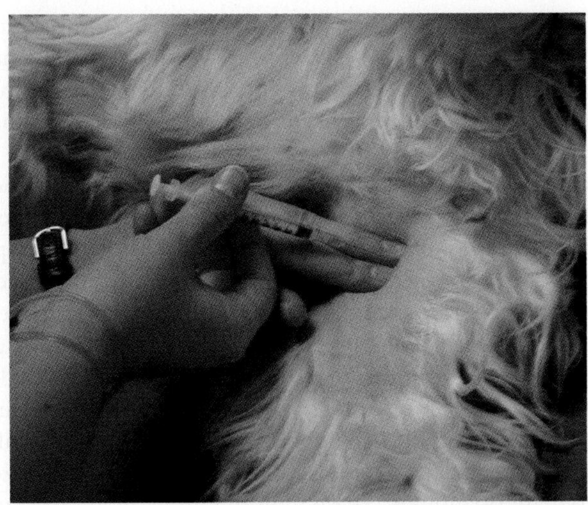

FIGURE 33-50 The femoral pulse is palpated before arterial blood sample collection from the femoral artery of a dog.

the artery by tactile sensation (Figure 33-50). The femoral artery and dorsal pedal arteries are the most common sites of arterial blood sampling. Lingual artery samples may be obtained in anesthetized or comatose animals, but they should be avoided because of the risk for inducing a large oral hematoma, which can obstruct the airway and interfere with swallowing. Acquiring arterial blood samples may be too stressful for some patients. By definition, ventilation is determined by the carbon dioxide level (PCO_2) on an arterial blood gas analysis. Hypoventilation (failure to "blow off" carbon dioxide) causes an increase in blood carbon dioxide. Hypoventilation occurs with certain respiratory problems and can cause acidosis. Hyperventilation ("blowing off carbon dioxide") results in decreased carbon dioxide. This situation may occur with respiratory disease or as a compensatory response to metabolic acidosis. Oxygenation is indicated by the PaO_2, and a low value indicates hypoxemia. Signs of hypoxemia include cyanotic (blue) mucous membranes (Figure 33-51), weakness, rapid heart rate, increased respiratory rate, and increased respiratory effort.

The difference between alveolar (lung) oxygenation and arterial oxygenation is a calculated indicator of the efficiency of oxygen transfer to the blood by the lung. In patients that are hypoxemic, this alveolar-arterial gradient (A-a gradient) calculation can provide a single value to assess and monitor the animal's oxygen exchange. The alveolar oxygen content (A) is calculated by the alveolar gas equation: $A = (BP - 47)\ 0.21 - PCO_2/0.8$, where BP is the barometric pressure (760 mm Hg at sea level), 47 is the vaporization pressure of water (a constant physical property of water), and 0.21 is the oxygen percent of room air. This formula is only used when the patient is breathing room air. In the formula above, PCO_2 is obtained from the arterial blood gas analysis, and 0.8 is the respiratory exchange quotient (a mathematic constant). At elevations near sea level, the formula simplifies to $A = 150 - PCO_2/0.8$. The arterial oxygen content (a) is the PaO_2 obtained from the arterial blood gas analysis (in mm Hg). To finish calculating the A-a gradient, the arterial oxygen

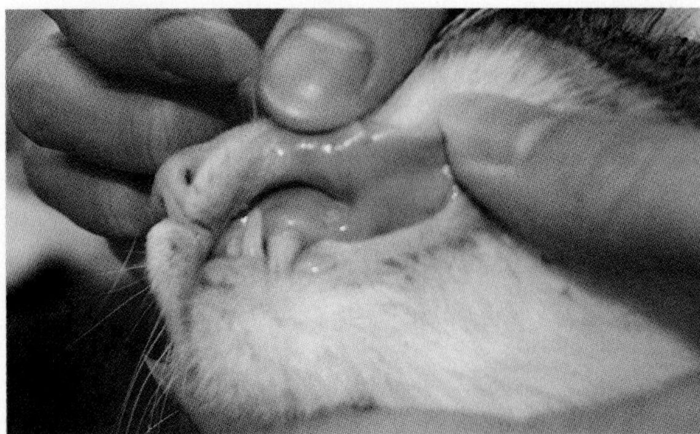

FIGURE 33-51 Cyanotic mucous membranes were detected in this cat with cardiopulmonary disease.

content (a) is subtracted from the alveolar oxygen content (A). In animals with normal oxygen exchange, the A-a gradient is less than 10 mm Hg. As a general rule, an A-a gradient more than 30 mm Hg is an indication for oxygen therapy.

TECHNICIAN NOTE As a general rule, an A-a gradient more than 30 mm Hg is an indication for oxygen therapy.

To determine how responsive the patient is to oxygen therapy, an arterial sample is collected while the patient is on supplemental oxygen, and a second arterial blood gas analysis is performed. The original A-a calculation is invalid for patients receiving oxygen therapy. Instead, oxygenation is assessed by evaluating the ratio of arterial oxygen to inspired oxygen (PaO_2/FIO_2). PaO_2 is obtained from the blood gas analysis. FIO_2 is the fraction (percent) of inspired oxygen being supplemented in decimal form. For example, a dog receiving 100% oxygen would have an FIO_2 of 1.0. Most of the time, animals receiving oxygen therapy by mask or nasal catheters have an FIO_2 of close to 40% ($FIO_2 = 0.4$). By definition an animal's disease is responsive to oxygen if the PaO_2/FIO_2 value is greater than 250. As a general rule of thumb, the PaO_2 should be approximately five times the FIO_2.

CARDIOVASCULAR SYSTEM AND PERFUSION/HYDRATION

Monitoring of common physical examination findings can be key to detecting serious health problems. Technicians should be comfortable using a stethoscope and familiar with the basic principles of cardiac auscultation and pulse palpation. The detection of a new heart murmur, irregular heartbeats (arrhythmia), and/or changes in heart or lung sounds can be signs of an impending crisis. For example, animals that are "overhydrated" may develop crackles characteristic of pulmonary edema. Factors that decrease sound intensity include obesity, pleural or pericardial effusion, and hypovolemia. Likewise, pulse character and quality are important clues to the hydration status and stability of the critically ill pet. If the mean arterial blood pressure is less than 60 mm Hg, pulse strength will be diminished and it will be difficult to palpate

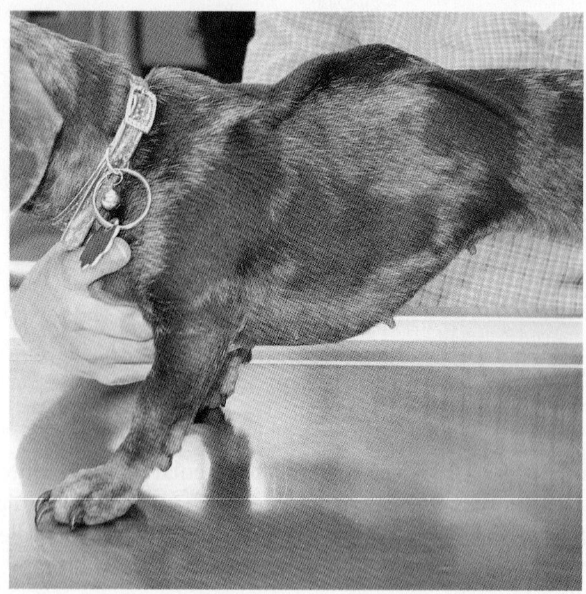

FIGURE 33-52 Well-hydrated animals have normal skin elasticity and turgor, but this animal demonstrates poor skin elasticity associated with severe dehydration.

pulses. Common sites to palpate a pulse are the femoral, dorsal pedal, or lingual arteries. Pulse rates should parallel the heart rate, rhythm, and quality. Comparing the pulse rate and heart rate during auscultation can aid in detecting "pulse deficits" that may be produced by irregular heartbeats.

Monitoring of hydration status and peripheral perfusion is crucial in sick animals. Helpful monitoring parameters include texture and color of mucous membranes, skin turgor (Figure 33-52), CRT, quantitation or close estimation of urine output, thoracic auscultation, pulse rate and character, serial body weights, and temperature (both core body temperature and peripheral limb temperature). Physical signs of overhydration include serous nasal discharge, chemosis (conjunctival edema; see Figure 33-10), peripheral edema, body cavity effusion, and weight gain. Noninvasive monitoring equipment, such as an ECG and indirect blood pressure equipment, can provide additional information regarding the pet's cardiovascular status. Patients at greater risk for fluid imbalance, such as those with heart disease, pneumonia, and renal disease, may require more invasive monitoring techniques. Invasive monitoring techniques include PCV, TP, direct blood pressure, and CVP measurement. Trends in observations of both subjective and objective parameters provide the most information. Diligent record keeping and consistency in monitoring techniques are imperative.

Blood Pressure

In humans, blood pressure is often expressed as a fraction, with systolic pressure as the numerator and diastolic pressure as the denominator. Mean arterial pressure is calculated from the systolic and diastolic values. A similar fraction can be used in cats and dogs. Normal systolic blood pressure varies between species, but generally ranges from 100 to 150 mm Hg. An ideal mean blood pressure ranges from 75 to 90 mm Hg. Arterial blood pressure can be monitored directly or indirectly and provides more information than simple subjective assessments of pulse character. Systolic values more than 90 mm Hg and diastolic values greater than 60 mm Hg are required to maintain adequate perfusion of vital organs (namely the kidneys and brain). A systolic blood pressure greater than 175 mm Hg indicates hypertension. However, stress of illness and anxiety associated with hospital visits can transiently increase the blood pressure in nervous animals. In cats and dogs, pulses should be palpable if the mean arterial blood pressure is greater than 60 mm Hg.

Indirect blood pressure is obtained using either oscillometric or Doppler equipment. Oscillometric blood pressure monitors often come in combination with an ECG and pulse oximeter and are popularly used in monitoring anesthetized or sedentary animals. These monitors use a blood pressure cuff to determine systolic, diastolic, and mean arterial pressures and can be programmed to take readings at regular intervals. To ensure an accurate measurement, cuff size should be proportionate to the size of the animal. As a general rule, the diameter of the cuff should approximate 40% of the circumference of the limb at the site of cuff placement.

> *TECHNICIAN NOTE* As a general rule, the *blood pressure* cuff diameter should approximate 40% of the circumference of the limb at the site of cuff placement.

Common sites of cuff placement include the metacarpus, metatarsus, and tail. Doppler blood pressure equipment uses an ultrasound crystal and monitor to audibly locate the arterial pulse (Figure 33-53). Hair is clipped over an artery (usually the ventral digital artery or tail artery) to enhance detection of the pulse. The ultrasound crystal with ultrasound gel is positioned over the palpable pulse so that the Doppler elicits a clear sound with each pulse. Subsequently a blood pressure cuff is applied to the patient and a sphygmomanometer is used to inflate the cuff until the audible pulse can no longer be heard. Finally, pressure is released in the cuff until the pulse can be heard again. The pressure at which the pulse is again detected is equivalent to the systolic blood pressure. This technique is more labor intensive for monitoring because this procedure must be manually performed. In addition, mean and diastolic blood pressures are not reliably obtained by this technique. However, many clinicians prefer Doppler equipment for blood pressure measurement because the audible pulse is reassuring and allows a subjective assessment of the accuracy of data.

Direct blood pressure measurement is more invasive because it requires catheterization of an artery and specialized equipment. This method is considered the most accurate method of blood pressure measurement. Since most arteries cannot be directly visualized at the time of arterial puncture, arterial catheters are placed using digital palpation of the pulse as a guide. Common arteries for catheterization include the dorsal pedal artery and femoral artery. Once in place, the arterial catheter is connected to a monitor via

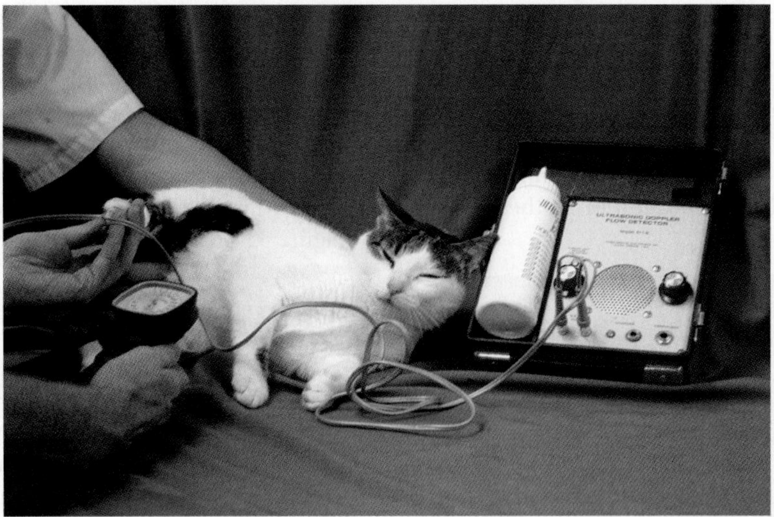

FIGURE 33-53 Indirect blood pressure measurement using ultrasound Doppler equipment provides an accurate reading of the systolic blood pressure.

commercially available transducer equipment. The monitor displays a pulse waveform and reads out a systolic, diastolic, and mean blood pressure. Comparing the pulse waveform deflection with an ECG allows staff members to note the pulse pressure created by each cardiac contraction. This can be helpful in determining the effects of transient arrhythmias. Staff members should be trained in the use and care of arterial catheters. No medications should be administered via intraarterial injection, and arterial catheters must be appropriately labeled to prevent confusion.

> *TECHNICIAN NOTE* No medications should be administered via intraarterial injection. Arterial catheters must be appropriately labeled to prevent confusion.

Arterial catheters are flushed slowly and regularly to prevent clot formation. Arterial catheters must be properly secured to prevent animal movement from disconnecting equipment. If equipment becomes detached from the catheter hub, an open arterial catheter can result in rapid severe blood loss, which is particularly dangerous in small animals.

Central Venous Pressure

Blood flows unidirectionally from arteries to veins and back to the heart in part because of the natural pressure gradient between these areas. Venous pressures are maintained lower than arterial pressures to facilitate forward blood flow. Most discussions of blood pressure refer to systemic arterial blood pressure. However, venous blood pressures are also important. Central venous pressure refers to the blood pressure in central veins, such as the thoracic vena cava.

> *TECHNICIAN NOTE* CVP refers to the blood pressure in central veins, such as the thoracic vena cava. CVP monitoring helps assess the efficacy of fluid therapy.

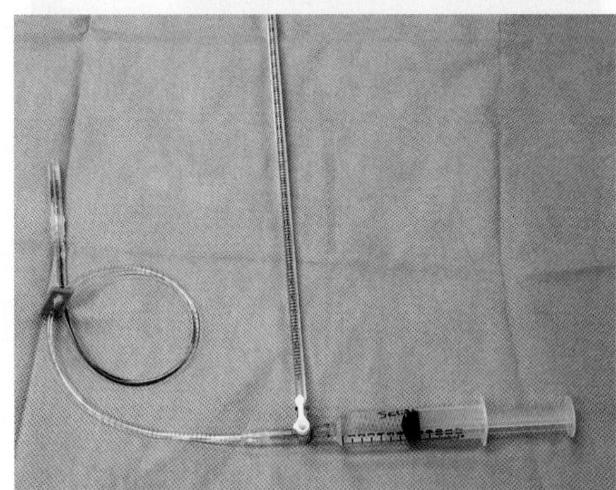

FIGURE 33-54 Equipment for measuring CVP can be constructed from a three-way stopcock that separates a manometer (in cm H_2O) and a saline-filled syringe from an extension set.

Because the veins hold a large volume of fluid, CVP is used to monitor hydration and the efficacy of fluid therapy. A normal CVP is 0 to 5 cm H_2O. Values less than zero indicate hypovolemia, dehydration, or inadequate fluid therapy. Values trending upward to 8 or 10 indicate an increase in vascular volume and adequate fluid therapy. Sudden increases in CVP or values above 10 may indicate venous congestion, increased thoracic pressure, and volume overload. Patient status should be closely reviewed. CVP values are usually used in conjunction with other subjective measures of hydration (e.g., heart rate, mucous membrane appearance, skin turgor).

Measurement of CVP requires placement of a long catheter in a central vein. Most commonly, jugular vein catheters are placed that reach into the thoracic vena cava. Equipment for measuring CVP can be constructed from a three-way stopcock that separates a manometer (in cm H_2O) and a saline-filled syringe from an extension set (Figure 33-54).

The extension set and manometer are flushed with normal saline, and the extension set is connected to the patient's central line catheter. The animal is placed in sternal or lateral recumbency, and the apparatus is held so that the zero mark of the manometer is in the approximate position of the distal catheter tip (Figure 33-55). In most small animals, this position is approximated by the location of the heart (i.e., the sternum in laterally recumbent animals and the point of the elbow during sternal recumbency). After flushing the catheter to ensure smooth flow of blood, the stopcock is opened between the patient and the manometer. After several seconds, the saline column of the manometer will equilibrate with the pressure at the end of the catheter reflecting the CVP, which can be measured on the manometer (Figure 33-56).

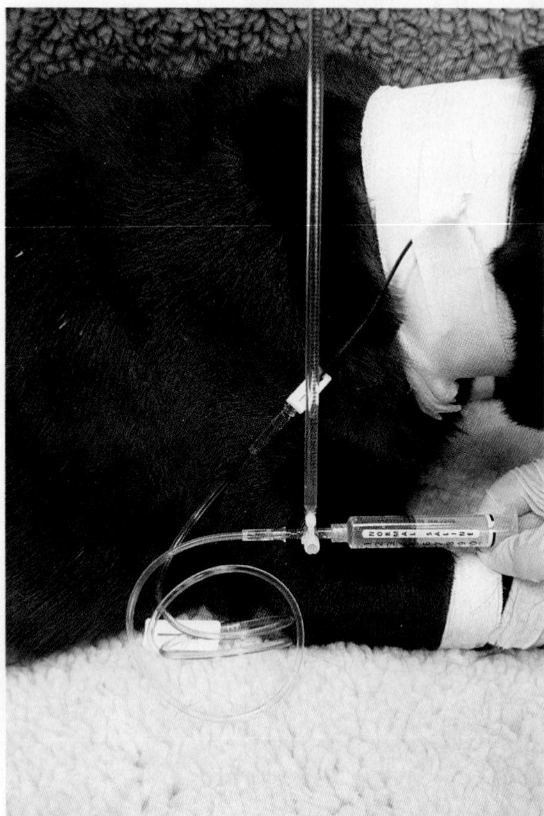

FIGURE 33-55 The CVP apparatus is attached to the patient's jugular catheter, and the line is flushed to ensure smooth flow between the manometer and the distal end of the catheter.

COAGULATION STATUS

Assessment of an animal's coagulation status may be helpful in assessing unexplained bleeding and detecting DIC. Evaluation of a blood smear may detect RBC morphology changes and allow an estimation of platelet numbers. The presence of schistocytes or fragmented RBCs along with a decrease in platelet numbers may be seen with DIC, splenic tumors, and severe heartworm disease. A high percentage of echinocytes can be seen in animals suffering from snake envenomation.

> *TECHNICIAN NOTE* A high percentage of echinocytes can be seen in animals suffering from snake envenomation.

A normal platelet count is between 200,000 and 500,000 platelets per microliter in most species. Although a complete platelet count is advised, rapid assessment or confirmation of platelet numbers may be obtained by estimating the platelet numbers on a blood smear. This can be done by counting the number of platelets per high-power field and multiplying by 15,000. A better estimate is obtained if several high-power fields are assessed and averaged. Platelet clumping, which is common at the edge of blood smears, can make platelet estimates invalid.

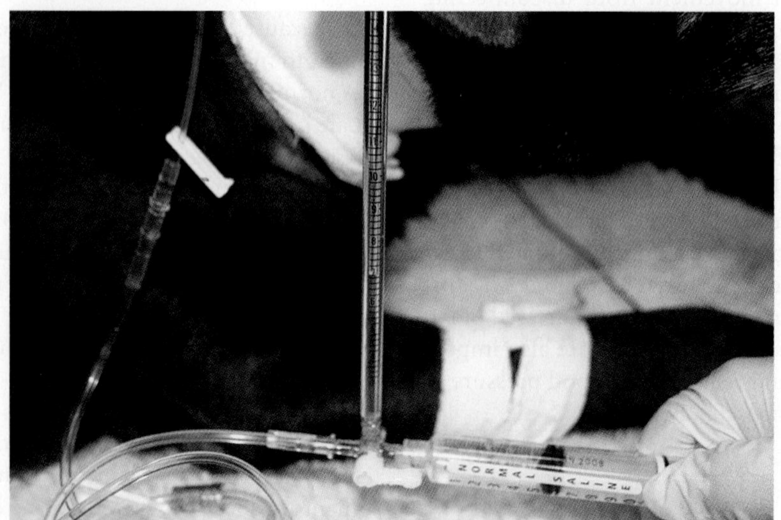

FIGURE 33-56 The saline column of the manometer will equilibrate with the pressure at the end of the catheter reflecting the CVP. In this image, we can see the saline meniscus is at 7 cm of water (7 cm H_2O).

The buccal mucosal bleeding time (BMBT) evaluates platelet function and is often used as an in-house screening test for von Willebrand's disease (an inherited disease effecting platelet function). A commercially available lancet device (Figure 33-57) is used to make a standardized incision (specific size and depth) into the buccal mucosa on the inside of the cheek (Figure 33-58). Following this incision, the blood flowing from the cut is blotted away with filter or absorbent paper to permit visualization of the site without disturbing the incision (Figure 33-59). The time required until bleeding stops is the BMBT, which represents the time for formation of an initial platelet plug. Normal time for the dog is less than 4 minutes. Following completion of the test, renewed bleeding at the site can occur if the incision is disturbed or if the animal has other coagulation problems, but such bleeding does not affect the reported time.

RENAL/URINARY SYSTEM

Ideally, all hospitalized animals should have a urine sample obtained for urinalysis. Urine specific gravity is important information in determining urinary tract health and in interpreting changes in kidney parameters and the urine sediment. Because urine specific gravity and blood values for blood urine nitrogen (BUN) and creatinine can be affected by fluid therapy and medications (diuretics, such as furosemide and mannitol); pretreatment blood and urine samples should be obtained. However, if such samples cannot be readily obtained, fluid therapy should not be delayed,

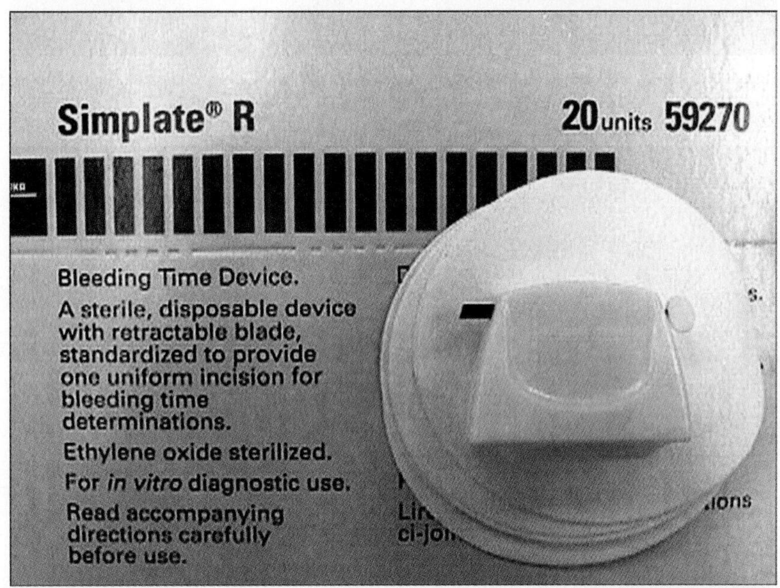

FIGURE 33-57 Commercially available lancet devices and filter paper are used in the BMBT test.

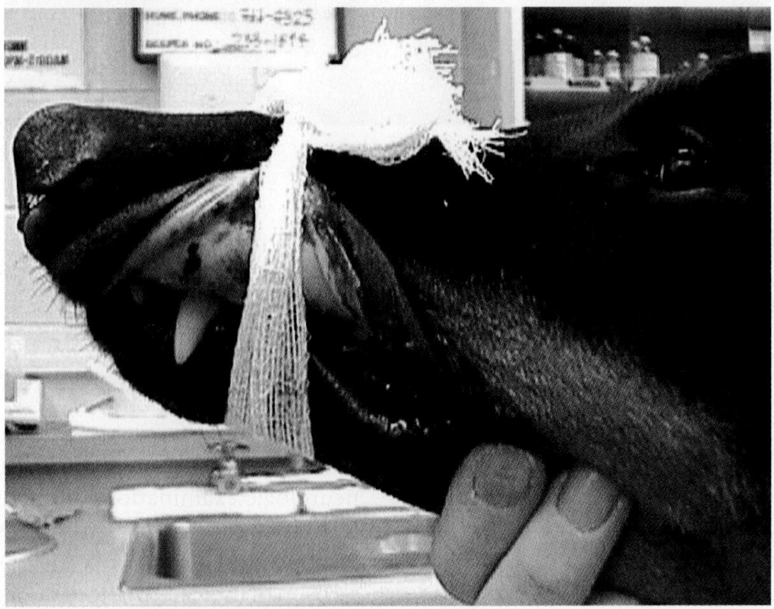

FIGURE 33-58 The lip is positioned appropriately, and a standardized incision is made in the buccal (cheek) mucosa.

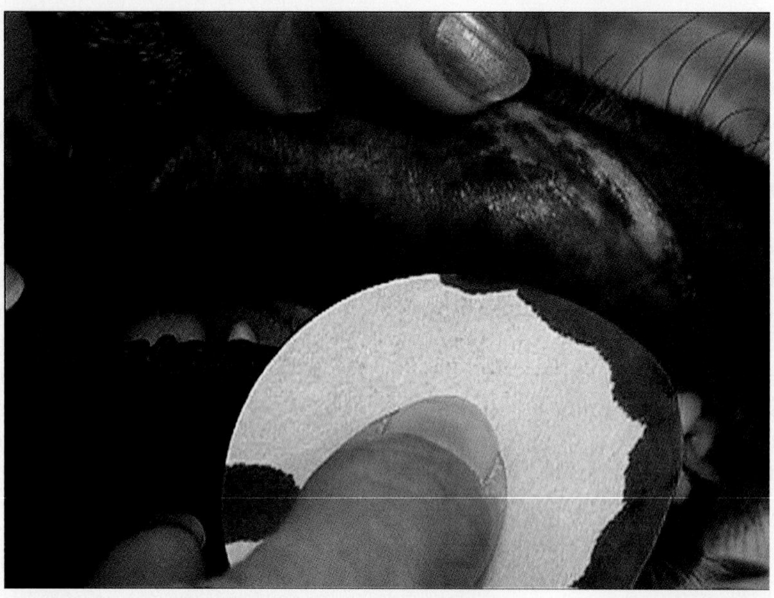

FIGURE 33-59 Blood flowing from the cut is blotted away with filter or absorbent paper to permit visualization of the site without disturbing the incision.

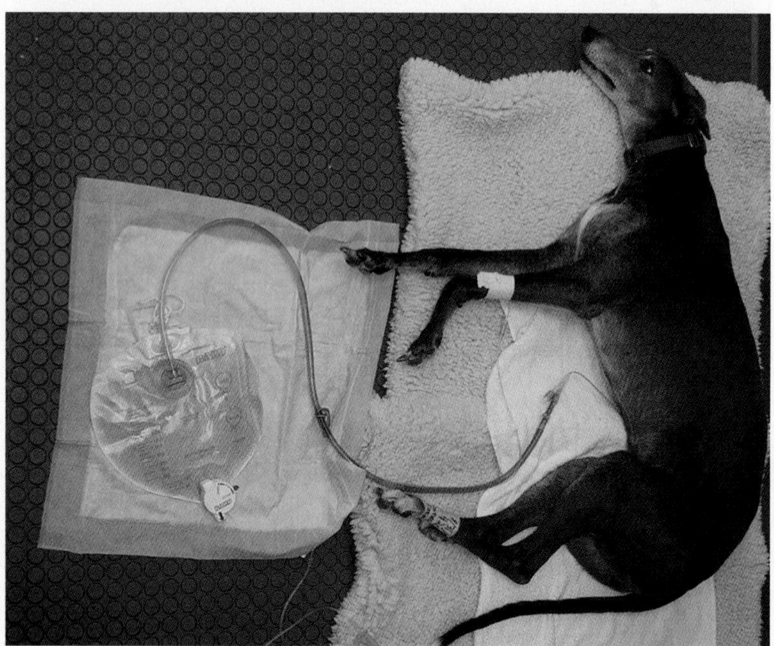

FIGURE 33-60 Sterile urine collection bags connected to an indwelling urinary catheter can be used to monitor urine production and maintain cleanliness.

particularly if the animal is dehydrated or unstable. Urine output should be estimated in all animals and recorded in the medical record. In critical cases, close monitoring of urine production may be performed via urine collection through indwelling urinary catheters or specifically designed cages that allow urine to drain through a grate to be collected. An indwelling urinary catheter attached to a sterile urine collecting bag is a comfortable, clean, and accurate way to monitor urine output (Figure 33-60). Because catheters may clog, kink, or change position, urine collection equipment should be regularly inspected and replaced if faulty. Minimum urine production is 2 to 4 ml/kg/hr. Inadequate urine production may be an indication for changes in fluid therapy and should be interpreted with other patient data (i.e., body weight, CVP, etc.) and reported to the veterinarian.

CENTRAL NERVOUS SYSTEM

Unfortunately, few objective parameters are available to monitor the central nervous system. Serial physical and neurologic examinations are perhaps the best means of detecting new or ongoing problems. Changes in mentation, responsiveness, level of consciousness, and respiratory patterns may indicate changes in neurologic status and should be reported.

> *TECHNICIAN NOTE* Changes in mentation, responsiveness, level of consciousness, and respiratory patterns may indicate changes in neurologic status and should be monitored regularly via serial physical examinations.

Likewise, pupillary size and responsiveness to light are important signs to monitor. Increased intracranial pressure results in a syndrome of brainstem and cerebral herniation whereby intracranial pressure changes cause compression of the brain against solid connective tissue and bone. Early signs of increased intracranial pressure include mental dullness, tachypnea, tachycardia, and dilated pupils. Later signs include bradycardia, fixed pinpoint pupils (Figure 33-61), seizures, coma, and death. Early recognition and intervention are key to the management of this syndrome. Animals at risk for brain herniation include those with head trauma, hydrocephalus, brain tumors, and encephalitis. Herniation can also be a complication of some diagnostic procedures, such as spinal fluid collection and myelogram.

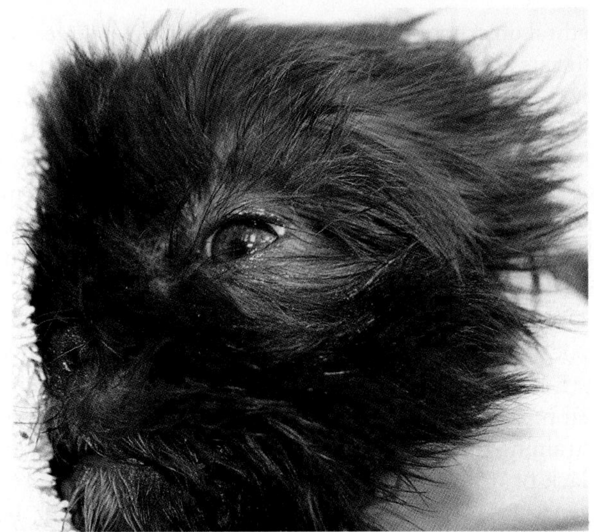

FIGURE 33-61 This puppy shows clinical signs of increased intracranial pressure, including comatose mentation and nonresponsive pinpoint pupils.

ABDOMINAL CAVITY

Each patient should receive a daily physical examination. Palpation of the abdomen may detect abdominal distention resulting from fluid accumulation, organ enlargement, and intestinal gas. Abdominal pain can be detected by the presence of discomfort, splinting, or vocalization. Animals with unexplained abdominal pain or distention warrant further investigation and monitoring.

Abdominocentesis is a procedure to confirm the presence of abdominal fluid and to collect samples for fluid analysis. During this procedure, the abdomen is clipped of hair and aseptically cleaned with surgical scrub. A needle attached to a syringe is inserted into the abdomen near the umbilicus, and gentle suction is applied to withdraw fluid (Figure 33-62). Care is taken not to redirect the needle blindly within the abdomen because this may result in unnecessary pain and potential injury to abdominal organs. Fluid collected via abdominocentesis may be submitted for culture and cytology. Abdominocentesis is commonly performed to detect active hemorrhage, infection (peritonitis), ascites, uroabdomen, and neoplastic effusions. If only a small amount of fluid is suspected, a four-quadrant tap may be performed in which the four areas of the abdomen centered around the umbilicus are sampled. If no sample is obtained and abdominal fluid is still suspected, a diagnostic peritoneal lavage (DPL) may be performed. The DPL is a modified procedure for collecting small amounts of abdominal fluid. In this procedure, the animal is prepared as described earlier. Before fluid withdrawal, a volume of 10 to 20 ml/kg of sterile warm isotonic saline is instilled into the abdomen. After a brief moment to adjust the animal's position and allow the instilled fluid to mix with abdominal contents, standard abdominocentesis is performed. The added fluid may dislodge adherent debris and mix with isolated fluid pockets that can then be collected during standard abdominocentesis.

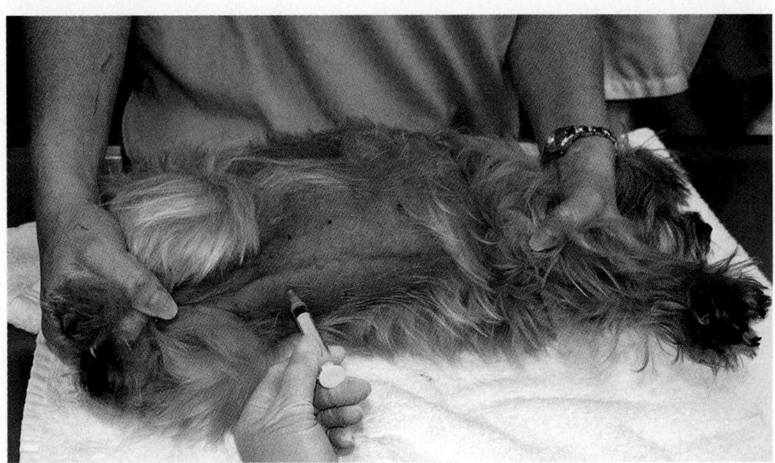

FIGURE 33-62 During abdominocentesis, a needle attached to a syringe is inserted into the abdomen near the umbilicus, and gentle suction is applied to withdraw fluid.

THORACIC CAVITY

Animals with cardiac and respiratory disease often have similar clinical signs (namely, coughing, labored breathing, exercise intolerance, and collapse). Unfortunately, these signs can occur with many different causes, including upper airway obstruction, pulmonary edema, pleural effusion, pneumonia, primary heart disease, and thoracic neoplasia. A thorough physical examination often directs diagnostic tests to differentiate respiratory from cardiac problems. Muffled heart and respiratory sounds often indicate fluid or air in the pleural space (the space between the lungs and chest wall). The presence of pleural fluid or air causes respiratory problems as a result of physical interference with normal lung expansion. Crackles heard during the different phases of breathing usually indicate pulmonary disease, such as pneumonia or pulmonary edema. In general, crackles indicate relatively severe pulmonary disease.

Chest x-rays are commonly used to confirm, classify, and document the presence of cardiac and respiratory diseases. If thoracic fluid is documented on x-rays or clinically suggested during examination, thoracocentesis to remove the fluid is indicated. Thoracocentesis is usually performed with the animal comfortably restrained in sternal recumbency. During this procedure, one or both sides of the chest are clipped of hair (in the area of rib spaces 7 through 9) and cleaned with surgical scrub. A butterfly catheter (or needle with extension set) is attached to a three-way stopcock and syringe (Figure 33-63). The needle is advanced into the chest along the cranial aspect of a rib to prevent discomfort and bleeding associated with nerve and vessel bundles located behind each rib. As the needle is inserted into the chest, an assistant controls the syringe and maintains the stopcock in the closed position to prevent environmental air from entering the chest during inspiration. Once the needle is positioned in the pleural space, the stopcock is opened to allow the assistant to suction fluid from the pleural space into the syringe. If a large amount of fluid must be removed, the stopcock is closed to the patient as the syringe is repeatedly emptied. Samples for culture, cytology, and fluid analysis are often obtained early during the procedure. Thoracocentesis may be performed as an emergency diagnostic procedure in animals with severe respiratory distress and suspected pleural fluid (Figure 33-64). Air can also accumulate in the pleural space. This condition is referred to as a pneumothorax and often results from traumatic rupture of airways or from severe lung disease. In such cases, air leaks outside of the lung, but is trapped inside the chest. Thoracocentesis (as described earlier) may be used to remove air from the pleural space. If fluid or air continues to accumulate in the chest, "chest drains," or thoracostomy tubes, may be placed that allow repetitive or continuous drainage of air and/or fluid from the pleural space (Figure 33-65).

COMMON EMERGENCIES

URINARY OBSTRUCTION

Urethral obstruction is a serious and common emergency in both cats and dogs. Causes of such obstruction include urinary stones, tumors, trauma, and/or inflammation. Animals that are unable to urinate develop metabolic abnormalities quickly and may develop secondary kidney damage. In some cases, unrecognized urinary obstruction results in permanent kidney failure and even rupture of the urinary system and leakage of urine into the abdomen. Consequently, untreated urinary obstruction is fatal.

Diagnosis of urinary obstruction is based on history, physical examination, laboratory tests, and diagnostic imaging (x-rays or ultrasound). Complete urinary obstruction is often preceded by signs of lower urinary tract disease, such as straining to urinate, painful urination, blood in the urine, or lack of urination. Obstruction of urine flow results in a large, firm, swollen, and painful bladder that can be palpated during physical examination. Affected animals often have pelvic or abdominal pain, lethargy, and dehydration.

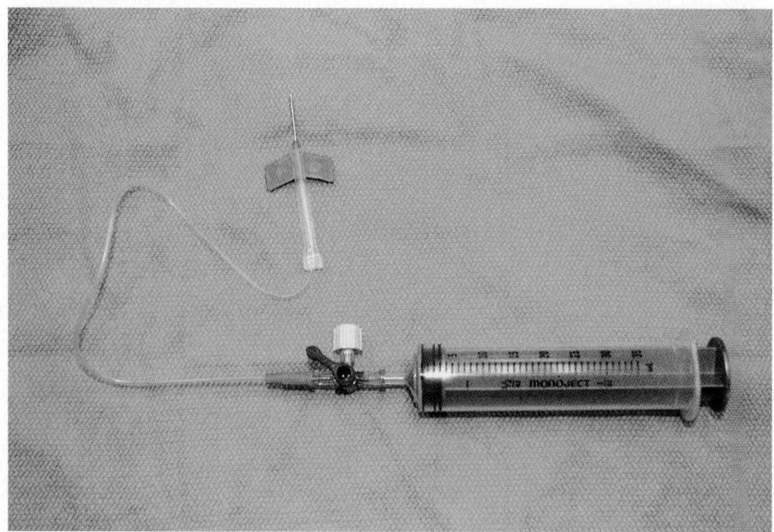

FIGURE 33-63 Thoracocentesis may be performed with a butterfly catheter connected to a three-way stopcock and syringe.

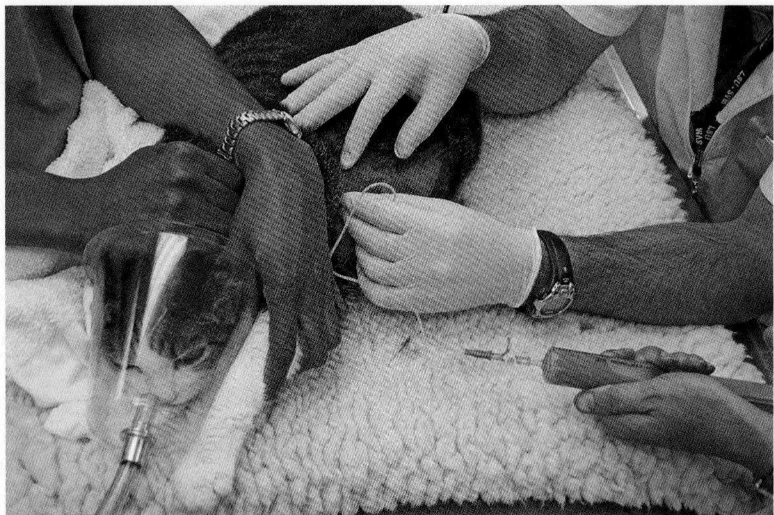

FIGURE 33-64 Thoracocentesis was performed in this cat to remove fluid from the chest cavity.

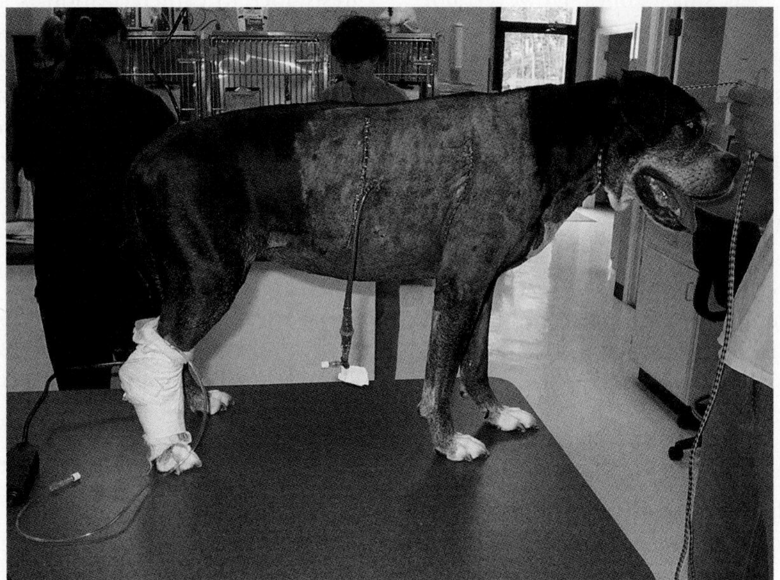

FIGURE 33-65 An animal with a thoracic drain is shown in between routine bandage changes.

Veterinarians and technicians should be familiar with the historical and physical examination findings associated with urethral obstruction so that a rapid diagnosis and intervention may be made.

Failure to excrete urine results in rapid onset of severe fluid and electrolyte imbalances. Common laboratory abnormalities include elevated potassium (hyperkalemia), elevated kidney parameters (azotemia; increased BUN and creatinine) and metabolic acidosis. Acidosis in animals with urinary obstruction is due to the accumulation of lactic acid (from poor perfusion during dehydration) and from accumulation of uremic acids (metabolic by-products usually excreted by the kidneys). Metabolic acidosis may be recognized by closely scrutinizing the blood pH, bicarbonate levels, and total carbon dioxide levels in lab reports. Venous blood gas analysis is helpful in determining the acid-base status and may be needed to obtain some of this information. Hyperkalemia is often severe and can be acutely life threatening because it triggers cardiac arrhythmias and can be a cause of cardiac arrest. Significant elevation of serum potassium results in fairly unique ECG changes that may allow early recognition of the problem. These changes include: (1) bradycardia, (2) "spiked" T waves, (3) shortened R-wave amplitude, (4) blunted or missing P waves, and (5) prolonged QRS interval (wide, short complexes). Astute veterinarians and technicians should be aware of these classic ECG features that may allow for early recognition of hyperkalemia (Figure 33-66).

X-rays and ultrasound can be used to confirm the presence of urinary obstruction, but are more important for determining the cause of obstruction. Care should be taken to include all of the urinary tract in the x-ray study. In male animals in particular, the x-rays should include the perineal and penile urethra.

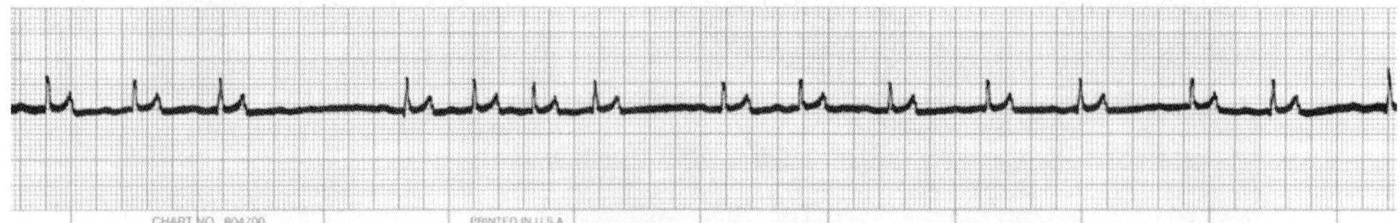

FIGURE 33-66 Classic ECG features associated with hyperkalemia include bradycardia, "spiked" T waves, shortened R-wave amplitude, blunted or missing P waves, and prolonged QRS interval (wide, short complexes).

> *TECHNICIAN NOTE* When evaluating for urinary stones, care should be taken to include all of the urinary tract in the x-ray study. In male animals, the x-rays should include the perineal and penile urethra.

X-rays are a common and readily available means to detect most stones in the bladder or urethra. X-rays must be of sufficient quality to detect small stones. However, not all stones are easily detected by radiography because some stones appear less opaque than others. In some cases, nonradiopaque ("lucent") stones may only be detected by contrast x-ray procedures or ultrasound. Ultrasound provides a noninvasive detailed evaluation of the urinary tract. In particular, ultrasound is useful in the detection of bladder masses and in the evaluation of the upper urinary tract. Evaluation of the upper urinary tract (kidneys and ureters) is important because stones and tumors may occur in this area. In addition, ultrasound may detect congestion and dilation of the ureters (hydroureter) and the urine collecting system of the kidneys (hydronephrosis), both of which may be caused by lower urinary obstruction.

Regardless of the cause, emergency treatment of urinary obstruction has two priorities: (1) relieve the urinary obstruction and (2) correct the fluid and electrolyte changes.

Relief of urinary obstruction generally requires passage of a urinary catheter. Urinary catheterization can be difficult in obstructed patients. Repetitively draining urine via cystocentesis should be avoided or used as a therapy of last resort because the turgid and inflamed urinary bladder is at risk for rupture. In some instances, cystocentesis may be chosen as an emergency procedure to relieve the immediate tension on the bladder. This temporary relief may facilitate later catheterization. In patients where urinary catheterization is not successful, urinary diversion via urethrostomy or a cystostomy tube may be considered.

Placement of urinary catheters in male and female dogs and cats is described later. Proper urinary catheterization generally requires two persons. One person places the catheter in a sterile manner while an assistant is present to restrain and properly position the animal. A catheter of appropriate length and diameter should be selected. The catheter must be long enough to reach the bladder. Generally a large diameter catheter is desirable to allow for higher flow rates during drainage or flushing of the catheter. In some instances, a small diameter catheter may be chosen to bypass an area of partial urinary obstruction.

Urinary Catheterization of Dogs

In the male dog, the patient is restrained in lateral recumbency with the hind limbs retracted caudally. The assistant extrudes the penis from the prepuce by retracting the skin sheath while stabilizing the penis at the base. The end of the penis is cleansed with an antiseptic solution (Betadine or chlorhexidine). Before placement, the catheter should be lubricated with sterile lubricant. The catheter is inserted into the urethral orifice and advanced into the bladder. Resistance to catheterization is sometimes encountered in anatomic areas where the urethra narrows (at the os penis, at the ischial arch, and in the prostatic urethra). These areas also correspond to common sites of obstruction because stones tend to lodge in these narrow areas. If a stone is encountered, there may be a gritty or solid resistance to advancing the catheter. Most stones that are encountered in this manner may be "retropulsed" into the bladder by flushing sterile saline into the catheter in a pulsatile manner.

> *TECHNICIAN NOTE* Most urethral stones may be "retropulsed" into the bladder by flushing sterile saline into the catheter in a pulsatile manner during catheterization.

This flushing procedure dilates the urethra surrounding the stone and helps propel the stone back into the urinary bladder. Retropulsion of stones may sometimes be assisted by massaging the urethra at the site of obstruction during digital rectal palpation. Care must be taken not to traumatize or tear the urethra during this procedure. Once the catheter is in place, urine should flow freely from the bladder. This urine should be collected for analysis, and the total urine volume should be measured and recorded. Depending upon the cause, a urinary catheter may be left in place (indwelling catheter) for a period of time. Indwelling catheters should be connected to a sterile and "closed" collection system.

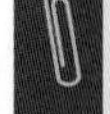

> *TECHNICIAN NOTE* Indwelling catheters should be connected to a sterile and "closed" collection system.

This allows for hygienic urine drainage and collection and reduces the risk of infection.

In the female dog, urinary obstruction by stones is less common because the urethra is relatively short and wide compared with the male urethra. The female urethral anatomy more readily allows for the passage of urinary stones. In certain circumstances, however, catheterization of the female urinary tract may still be indicated. Passing a urinary catheter in female dogs is easier if one is familiar with the genitourinary anatomy. Anatomically the reproductive tract (vagina) and urinary system (urethra) converge into a shared mucous membrane cavity called the vestibule. The vestibule is contained within the vulva (external genitalia). The urethral orifice is palpable as a ridge of tissue known as the urethral papilla on the ventral surface of the vestibule. Dorsal to the urethral papilla is the opening of the vagina. Failed attempts at urinary catheterization often result in passage of a catheter into the vagina. Proper placement into the urethra may be performed by either digital palpation of anatomic landmarks or by direct visualization of the urethral orifice. The authors prefer to pass female urinary catheters in dogs via palpation alone because this seems most comfortable for our patients and generally is met with a high degree of success. Using this technique, the urethral papilla is palpated within the vestibule using a gloved and lubricated finger. The dorsal opening to the vagina is located and occluded with the index finger that also is used to guide the urinary catheter into the urethra. Proper placement of the catheter is confirmed by urine drainage via the catheter or by palpation. As an alternative to this procedure, some clinicians prefer to use a vaginal speculum to retract the external vulva (labia) and directly visualize the urethral orifice. This technique is successful, but more often requires sedation to ensure patient comfort during the procedure.

Urinary Catheterization of Cats

Urinary catheterization is a challenge in cats because of their small size, but feline urinary catheterization procedures are roughly parallel to the procedures in dogs. The feline urethra is quite narrow and requires selection of small catheters (usually 3 to 5 French catheters). Digital palpation of the urethral orifice is usually not possible in female cats because of their small size. However, catheterization may be successfully performed blindly or via visualization. The urethral orifice in female cats is located at midline on the floor of the vestibule approximately 1 cm from the opening of the external vulva. With the cat positioned in lateral or sternal recumbency, an experienced technician may pass a catheter blindly along the floor of the vestibule and into the urethra. Sedation and visualization of the urethral orifice may be required for success.

Urinary obstruction is particularly common in male cats, where obstruction is a common manifestation of idiopathic feline lower urinary tract disease (FLUTD). Previously known simply as feline urologic syndrome (FUS), this disease is characterized by clinical signs of straining to urinate, blood in the urine, and pain. Early signs of urinary tract disease may go unnoticed in outdoor or multicat households where less observation of urinary habits allows these common signs to be overlooked. In fact, urinary signs may go completely unnoticed, and cats with this problem may be seen for unexplained abdominal or hindquarter pain. When obstruction occurs, clinical signs of systemic illness are related to severe fluid and electrolyte imbalances. The cause of the FLUTD is unknown, but sterile inflammation develops within the bladder and lower urinary tract of affected cats. This inflammation results in concretions of protein, mucus, and crystals that frequently obstruct the narrow urethra of male cats (Figure 33-67). Importantly, urinary tract infection is usually not present initially. Affected cats may have multiple or recurrent episodes of urinary problems throughout life.

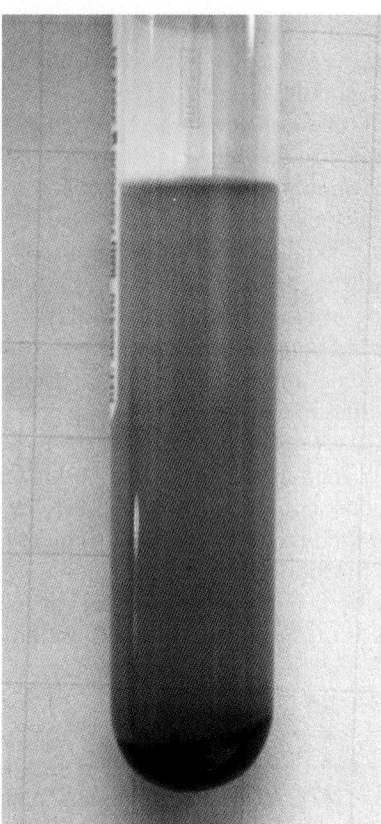

FIGURE 33-67 Urine from a cat with urinary tract obstruction shows a heavy sediment of blood and inflammation.

In male cats, urethral catheterization may be assisted by positioning the cat in a "perineal position." In this position, the cat may be in lateral or dorsal recumbency. The hind limbs are retracted cranially, and the tail is retracted caudally to expose the perineal region. The male penis is extruded by an assistant, and an effort is made to keep the penile urethra straight by positioning it in an alignment that roughly parallels the colon. Such positioning facilitates urethral catheterization and minimizes trauma to the urethra during the procedure. Urethral catheterization in cats may be further facilitated by sedation or administration of a muscle relaxant. Importantly, many cats with urethral obstruction are medically unstable and are poor candidates for sedation. These sick cats often will tolerate urethral catheterization with minimal or no sedation. Many clinicians prefer to pass a rigid polypropylene "tomcat" catheter during the initial attempts to unobstruct the urethra. These rigid catheters are uncomfortable and may be traumatic to the bladder and urethra. Therefore when an indwelling urinary catheter is required, one should attempt to replace the rigid catheters with a soft flexible catheter as soon as the urethra is free of obstruction (Figure 33-68). As in all species, indwelling urinary catheters should be secured in place and connected to a closed sterile urine collection system.

The goals of fluid therapy following urinary obstruction include: (1) correction of dehydration, (2) correction of electrolyte abnormalities, and (3) correction of acidosis.

Fluids should be administered via the IV route. As a general rule, isotonic sodium chloride is the fluid of choice to correct dehydration without exacerbating potassium abnormalities. However, a balanced electrolyte and pH-buffered fluid is also a good choice for patients with acidosis. Fluid rate calculations should replace the fluid deficit and provide maintenance fluid requirements. Following relief of urinary obstruction, the kidneys respond by temporarily increasing urine production. This "postobstructive diuresis" increases the fluid needs of the patient. Careful monitoring of urine output following relief of obstruction assists in tailoring fluid therapy to the individual patient.

> *TECHNICIAN NOTE* Careful monitoring of urine output following relief of obstruction assists in tailoring fluid therapy to the individual patient.

Fluid, electrolyte, and acid-base abnormalities usually correct quickly with aggressive fluid therapy alone, but hyperkalemia and acidosis sometimes require additional therapy. Adjunctive treatment of these disorders is strongly based on clinical judgments. In some animals with severe or persistent acidosis, bicarbonate therapy may be indicated. Bicarbonate therapy is generally pursued with caution to avoid "overtreatment" that may result in metabolic alkalosis or unpredictable acid-base shifts. When bicarbonate is used, the dose is calculated and usually administered in parts. Close monitoring of the acid-base status via repetitive venous blood gas analysis is commonly performed when bicarbonate therapy is used.

In addition to standard fluid therapy, veterinarians may treat hyperkalemia with insulin and dextrose infusions. Physiologically, insulin drives both glucose and potassium into cells and can be used to lower serum potassium in animals with life-threatening hyperkalemia. Rapid-acting regular insulin is administered IV along with a bolus of dextrose. The dextrose helps prevent hypoglycemia and may stimulate further endogenous insulin release. Insulin-dextrose therapy has an onset of action within 15 to 30 minutes, and the effects may last for a few hours. Veterinarians also treat life-threatening hyperkalemia with calcium gluconate infusions. Nerve and muscle cell activity is reduced in states of hyperkalemia because of the effect of high potassium on the cellular membrane potential. These effects result in cardiac arrhythmias, including bradycardia and cardiac arrest. Calcium gluconate may be administered IV to counteract these effects and transiently normalize the membrane potential and restore normal cell excitability. Calcium gluconate has an almost immediate effect (within minutes) on cardiac conductance and protects from potassium-related arrhythmias. However, animals receiving calcium gluconate should have continuous ECG monitoring because rapid calcium infusion can also result in cardiac arrhythmia. Calcium gluconate infusions may also cause hypercalcemia. For these reasons, calcium infusions are given "to effect" using the lowest effective dose during careful monitoring.

TOXIN INGESTION

Dogs are well known for randomly ingesting things in their environment during play or from curiosity. Cats are normally more discriminate and fastidious in their eating habits, but will still ingest noxious substances in their environment. These behaviors make toxin ingestion a common presenting

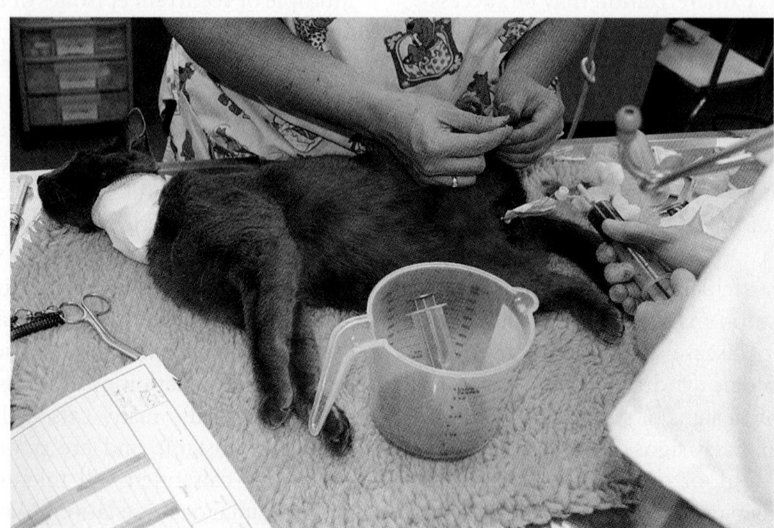

FIGURE 33-68 A soft, flexible, indwelling urinary catheter is secured in place. Note the hemorrhagic urine (associated with recent urinary obstruction) that is removed from the bladder.

complaint or telephone call to veterinary offices. See also Chapter 35. A brief clinical review of common toxin ingestions seen in emergency practice is presented here.

Veterinary technicians are often the first point of contact when pet owners call about toxin ingestion. Although we should be knowledgeable about the most common toxins, we should also be careful about what information and advice is presented by telephone. Information gleaned from telephone conversations is notoriously incomplete, and the consequences of error can be severe. When in question, the best advice to pet owners is to bring the pet to the veterinary practice for examination. Consequently the real purpose of a client telephone call is to gather information relevant to the animal's treatment before an appointment. The following information should be obtained:

1. What did the animal ingest?
2. When did the animal ingest it?
3. Is the animal showing any clinical signs?
4. Was the ingestion witnessed or suspected?
5. Are there other animals or children who could also be exposed?

Manufacturer labels contain important information and should be saved and brought to the veterinary practice with the pet.

> *TECHNICIAN NOTE* When pets eat something that they should not, the manufacturer labels should be saved and brought to the veterinary practice with the pet.

The product label may be used to identify any harmful ingredients and may have instructions to follow after unintended ingestion or overdose. Many products have a toll-free number for questions. This type of information helps the veterinary team anticipate the needs of the patient and plan for the animal's arrival. Additional information may be obtained from local government-sponsored poison control centers. Information from these centers is species specific for humans and may not be entirely applicable to animals. Because of similarities in mammalian physiology, however, information about human poison exposure is still helpful in most cases of small animal toxin ingestion. Fortunately, animal-specific poison control centers are readily available and are a wealth of species-specific information. Animal poison control centers often charge a reasonable fee for this service.

Induction of vomiting (also called emesis) is a common treatment for the ingestion of harmful substances. Timely induction of vomiting may eliminate the toxin from the body before it can be absorbed and exert any harmful effects. In most instances, vomiting should be induced within 4 hours of ingestion. This is a flexible time limit that roughly corresponds to normal gastric emptying time. Gastric emptying time may be prolonged in some instances. Once a substance has exited the stomach and is being absorbed in the small intestine, induction of vomiting is unlikely to have a therapeutic benefit.

Importantly, induction of vomiting is not a cure-all for toxin ingestion and should be cautiously considered like any other treatment. As a general rule, ingestion of caustic substances and petroleum products should *not* be treated by vomiting because of the risk of further injury or aspiration. Emesis is contraindicated after ingestion of many household products, including bleach, lye, gasoline, and oil (and many other acids and strong alkali agents). In addition, induction of vomiting is strongly contraindicated in animals with altered awareness because sedated, comatose, or tranquilized animals are at high risk for developing aspiration pneumonia. Vomiting may be induced by a variety of means. In dogs, apomorphine is a potent emetic agent that directly stimulates the vomiting centers of the brain to cause vomiting. The drug can be compounded into a variety of forms. The drug is absorbed across the conjunctival membranes of the eye, and small tablets of the drug may be placed in the conjunctival sac until vomiting has occurred. Subsequently the drug can be flushed from the conjunctiva to terminate the vomiting episode. Apomorphine is not effective in cats. Because they do not respond to apomorphine, induction of vomiting in cats is challenging. Xylazine (a sedative drug) often stimulates vomiting in cats. This emetic effect must be balanced with the risk of sedation-related aspiration when xylazine or similar drugs are used for this purpose. A number of household remedies, such as hydrogen peroxide and syrup of ipecac, have been used to induce vomiting in both cats and dogs. Hydrogen peroxide administered orally will reliably result in vomiting as a result of bitter taste and gastric irritation. The widespread use of hydrogen peroxide as a topical antiseptic makes it a convenient over-the-counter and generally available emetic. However, hydrogen peroxide can be dangerous in sensitive or overdosed animals because careless use of hydrogen peroxide can result in severe hemorrhagic gastroenteritis. Syrup of ipecac induces vomiting by inciting gastric irritation and by stimulating the vomiting centers of the brain. This once common home remedy has become less popular because induction of vomiting at home has some risk and may delay other more appropriate medical treatments.

When vomiting is not possible but gastric emptying is desired, gastric lavage is sometimes an option. Unfortunately, gastric lavage does not always result in effective or timely gastric emptying and carries some inherent risks. Therefore whenever possible, gastric emptying via induction of vomiting is nearly always preferred over gastric lavage. For the gastric lavage procedure, animals are sedated and an endotracheal tube is placed to secure the airway and prevent aspiration. Subsequently a stomach tube is placed, and the stomach contents are removed via lavage and drainage. This procedure is time consuming (which may delay other treatments), and the sedation required for gastric lavage adds risk. Additionally, residual lavage fluid sometimes merely adds to gastric volume and raises the risk of vomiting and aspiration. If gastric lavage is indicated, it is best performed by experienced personnel.

In addition to gastric emptying, treatments for nonspecific toxin ingestion may also include administration of adsorbents and cathartics. Adsorbents bind toxins to prevent absorption and facilitate their excretion. Cathartics are medications that affect GI transit and speed fecal elimination of toxins. The most common adsorbent is activated charcoal. Activated charcoal comes in a variety of commercially available formulations. Oral suspension liquid preparations are easy to administer directly by mouth (alone or mixed with food) or by stomach tube (Figures 33-69 and 33-70). Activated charcoal may bind intestinal nutrients and other orally administered medications, but does not appear to have any common clinically significant side effects. Activated charcoal is excreted in the feces and will result in dark or black discolored stool that may be mistaken for melena. Some formulations of activated charcoal contain sorbitol as a cathartic. Sorbitol is a sugar alcohol that draws water into the large bowel, resulting in a laxative effect.

The treatment and clinical evaluation of specific toxins is beyond the scope of this chapter. However, a few common toxicities warrant brief discussion.

Ethylene Glycol Ingestion

Ethylene glycol is the active ingredient of most automotive antifreeze solutions and is highly toxic. Animals most frequently come into contact with antifreeze solution that has spilled during vehicle maintenance. Although ethylene glycol exposure may be associated with cold climates or occur seasonally in the winter, the universal use of antifreeze in automobiles makes it a common toxicity in all parts of the country and at all times of the year. Ethylene glycol is reportedly sweet and palatable, and animals willingly ingest it. Unfortunately the palatability and high toxicity of antifreeze make it a common source in malicious animal poisoning.

Ethylene glycol ingestion results in a fairly classic progression of clinical signs. "Early" signs of ethylene glycol poisoning occur within 30 minutes to 12 hours postingestion and include vomiting, lethargy, excessive drinking and urination, and neurologic signs (ataxia, proprioceptive deficits, seizures, etc.). These initial neurologic signs often diminish as ethylene glycol is metabolized, leading to a false sense of recovery. However, the metabolites of ethylene glycol soon cause fulminant renal failure in both cats and dogs. Kidney failure generally develops within 12 to 24 hours in cats, and somewhat later (48 to 72 hours) in dogs. This kidney failure is responsible for the "late" clinical signs of ethylene glycol poisoning that include renewed neurologic signs (e.g., seizures, coma, and death) and other manifestations of severe kidney injury (e.g., oliguria or anuria, severe lethargy, dehydration, and vomiting). The progression and severity of these clinical signs is dose dependent. Cats are much more susceptible than dogs to ethylene glycol and develop lethal toxicity at much lower doses. Without treatment, ethylene glycol ingestion is almost uniformly fatal.

Early detection of ethylene glycol toxicity is incredibly important if treatment is to be attempted. Unexplained or transient neurologic signs should prompt consideration of this toxicity. Definitive diagnosis requires either witnessed ingestion or demonstration of ethylene glycol in blood or urine. Ethylene glycol assays are commonly performed at veterinary reference laboratories and at human hospitals, and test kits for veterinary cage-side testing are reliable. When testing blood samples, it is important to interpret the results in context of the time of ingestion. Ethylene glycol blood levels peak at 12 hours postingestion in dogs and 3 to 6 hours postingestion in cats and then diminish rapidly. Thereafter, it may be more prudent to investigate ethylene glycol levels in the urine, where the compound is excreted. Isosthenuria and calcium oxalate monohydrate crystals in the urine may be seen within hours of ingestion and can be important supporting evidence in the diagnosis of toxicity (Figure 33-71). Veterinarians and technicians should be able to identify these characteristic crystals. Remember that azotemia and other changes associated with acute renal failure have a more delayed onset and may not be present early on.

Treatment of ethylene glycol toxicity varies with the level of available care and the timing of diagnosis. Cases of

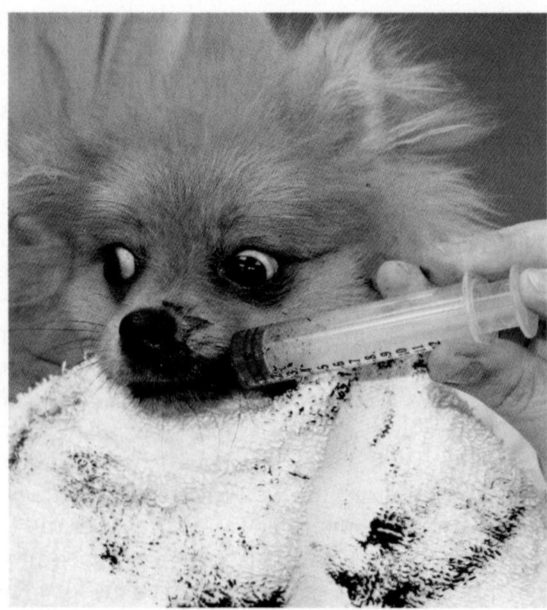

FIGURE 33-69 Activated charcoal may be administered via syringe.

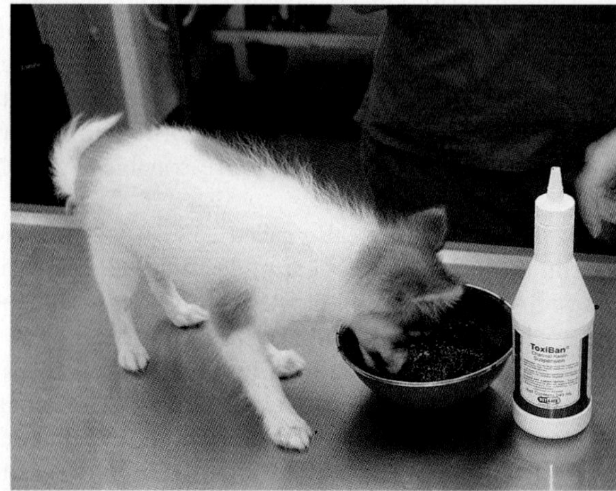

FIGURE 33-70 Activated charcoal may be ingested willingly by some patients.

witnessed ingestion should be managed with standard detoxification procedures, including induction of vomiting and administration of activated charcoal. Remember that ethylene glycol makes animals sick, but it is the toxic metabolites of ethylene glycol that ultimately result in death (by causing kidney failure). Therefore standard treatment is focused on preventing metabolism of the toxin. In dogs, metabolism of ethylene glycol may be inhibited by administration of fomepizole (Antizol-Vet, Orphan Medical) according to the manufacturer's recommendations. Historically, fomepizole was ineffective in cats, and medical grade ethanol was used to competitively inhibit the enzymes responsible for ethylene glycol metabolism. More recent information suggests that fomepizole (at a dose specific for cats) may be effective for the treatment of cats with ethylene glycol ingestion. Some specialty referral centers are able to employ dialysis in the management of ethylene glycol toxicity (Figure 33-72). In the early stages (before kidney failure), dialysis is able to remove the toxin from the blood circulation before kidney injury occurs. In these cases (of early recognition and treatment), the prognosis is good. However, cases that are recognized late may incur permanent kidney damage. The prognosis for animals with ethylene glycol–induced acute renal failure is poor, but in some cases, dialysis may provide enough support for regeneration to occur.

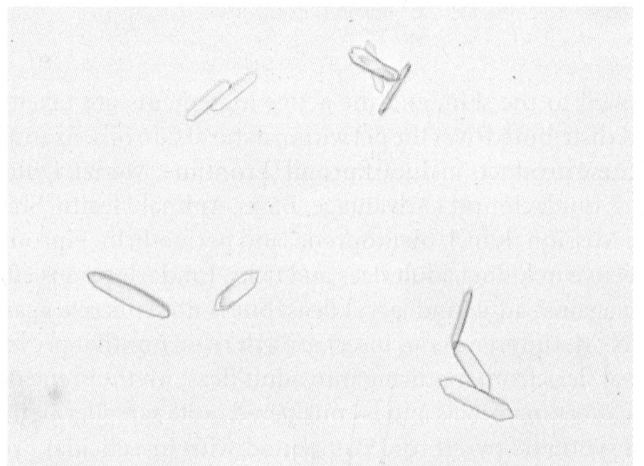

FIGURE 33-71 Calcium oxalate monohydrate crystals are associated with ethylene glycol intoxication and have a characteristic appearance. (Photo courtesy Dr. Steve Gaunt, Baton Rouge, La.).

Rodenticide Ingestion (Rat Poison)

The most common rodenticides are anticoagulant compounds that cause death by inducing life-threatening hemorrhage. These anticoagulant rodenticides are vitamin K antagonists. Vitamin K_1 is required for the final production step of numerous clotting factors made by the liver. The anticoagulant rodenticides interfere with clotting factor synthesis and cause clinical signs of bleeding within 24 to 72 hours of ingestion.

> *TECHNICIAN NOTE* The anticoagulant rodenticides interfere with clotting factor synthesis and cause clinical signs of bleeding within 24 to 72 hours of ingestion.

Common anticoagulant rodenticides include warfarin, brodifacoum, bromadiolone, diphacinone, and chlorophacinone.

Diagnosis of rodenticide ingestion generally consists of documenting possible exposure, observing abnormal bleeding (Figure 33-73), and identifying prolongation of clotting times. In general, both PT and activated partial thromboplastin time (APTT) become prolonged. Measurement of these clotting times is usually performed on citrated whole blood samples. Countertop analyzers are available for rapid in-house assessment of clotting times.

Witnessed ingestion of rodenticide compounds should be treated with induction of vomiting and administration of activated charcoal. Such animals may avoid life-threatening

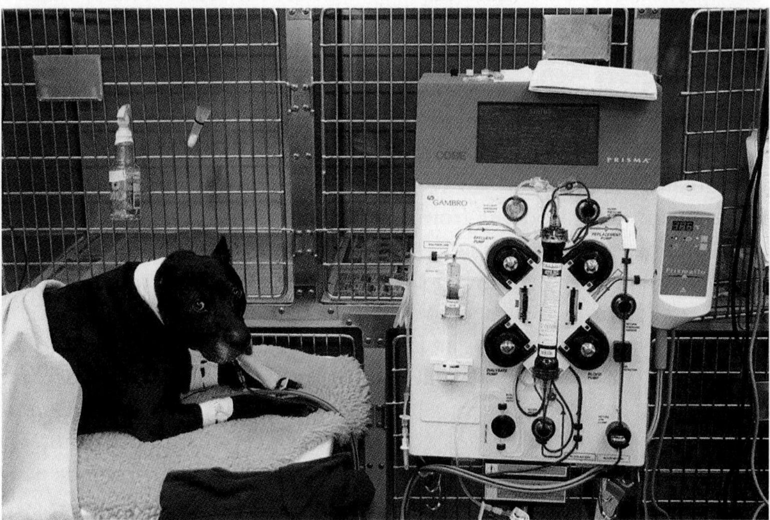

FIGURE 33-72 Hemodialysis can remove some toxins, such as ethylene glycol, from the blood. Dialysis may also be used as a supportive therapy during the management of acute kidney failure.

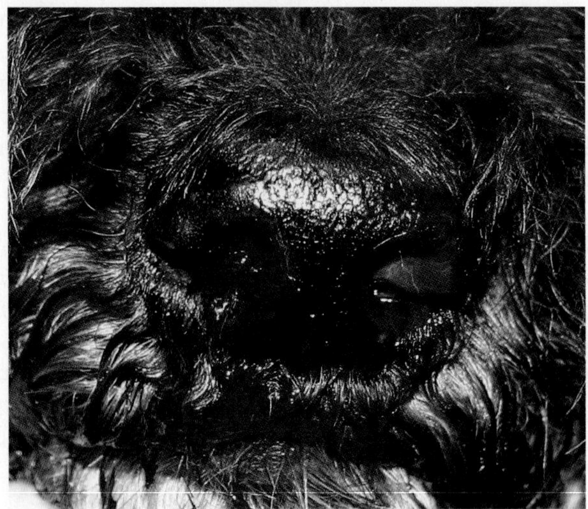

FIGURE 33-73 Rodenticide ingestion often results in spontaneous bruising and bleeding. Note the fresh blood flowing from the right nostril of this dog.

toxicity by such early intervention. However, monitoring of coagulation parameters or prophylactic vitamin K_1 supplementation is still recommended. Coagulation abnormalities, if present, usually start to correct within 12 hours of oral vitamin K_1 supplementation. Vitamin K_1 therapy is often initiated with a subcutaneous injection. IV injection of vitamin K is contraindicated because of the risk of anaphylaxis. Intramuscular injection is avoided because of the risk of hematoma formation. Animals receiving subcutaneous vitamin K_1 may develop allergic reactions similar to a vaccine reaction. These reactions include facial swelling, itching, and generalized hives (Figure 33-74). If such a reaction is noted, the animal should be treated with an antihistamine and corticosteroid therapy before switching to oral supplementation. Allergic reactions to orally administered vitamin K_1 are uncommon. Duration of vitamin K_1 therapy depends upon the specific compound ingested, but most cases are treated for approximately 1 month.

Animals with unwitnessed ingestion present a more difficult challenge because these animals usually are not diagnosed until abnormal bleeding is observed. Common sites of blood loss include nose (Figure 33-73) and oral cavity, spontaneous bruising of the skin and sclera, bleeding into body cavities (hemothorax, hemoabdomen), and intestinal blood loss. Essentially, anticoagulant rodenticides can result in bleeding anywhere. Affected animals risk dying from blood loss anemia or may have secondary problems, such as respiratory compromise from intrapulmonary hemorrhage. In addition to vitamin K_1 supplementation, treatment of these critical cases also requires correction of blood loss and replacement of active clotting factors via blood or plasma transfusion.

Permethrin Toxicity

Many effective and convenient flea and tick control products are available for over-the-counter purchase by today's pet owner. Some of the most popular products are topically applied to the skin, and the active ingredients are taken up and distributed over the pet within natural skin oils. Examples of these products include fipronil (Frontline, Merial, Duluth, Ga.), imidacloprid (Advantage, Bayer Animal Health, Shawnee Mission, Kan.), methoprene, and permethrin. Fipronil is effective in killing adult fleas and ticks. Imidacloprid is effective against adult and larval fleas, but is not effective against ticks. Methoprene is an insect growth regulator that prevents larval fleas from maturing into adult fleas. Methoprene does not affect mammals and is considered quite safe. Permethrin is a synthetic pyrethroid compound with insecticidal properties used in the control of fleas and ticks. Although these products are available without a prescription, veterinarians are still the best source of information on the proper selection, application, and safety of these products. Many pet owners misread labels or make assumptions about product safety. Products that are safe to use in dogs may not be safe to use in cats (even in small doses).

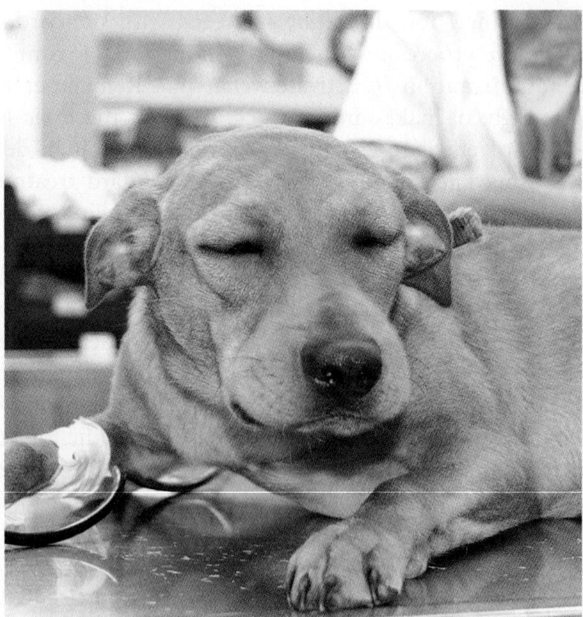

FIGURE 33-74 Facial swelling, itching, and hives may be seen during allergic reactions to vitamin K injections.

Permethrin's insecticidal properties are derived from neurotoxic effects that cause paralysis and death in insects. Cats appear uniquely predisposed to the toxic effects of permethrin, which can cause generalized tremors, muscle fasciculations, and seizures in cats. Permethrin toxicity has become one of the most common causes of seizures in cats as a result of the misapplication of products intended for dogs. Cats exposed to permethrin compounds develop dramatic clinical signs within 1 to 2 hours of application. In addition to the clinical signs noted earlier, affected cats often have hyperthermia, hypersalivation, dyspnea, ataxia, hyperesthesia, aggression, and gastrointestinal signs. Death may occur in severe intoxication, in sensitive animals, or when treatment is delayed.

Diagnosis of permethrin toxicity requires a history of exposure and subsequent development of clinical signs.

Diagnostic tests to rule out other causes of seizures may be needed in some cases. Treatment of affected cats should include decontamination of the skin via bathing. Bathing symptomatic cats is difficult, but is important in preventing further uptake of the toxin. Muscle relaxants (such as methocarbamol), anticonvulsants, and sedative drugs (such as diazepam) can be useful in the symptomatic treatment of seizures, tremors, and muscle fasciculation. Fluid therapy is indicated to correct dehydration that develops from hypersalivation and protracted muscle activity. In addition, fluid therapy and bathing are helpful in managing hyperthermia. The overall prognosis for cats that receive prompt treatment is good. Cats should be monitored in the hospital during recovery for at least 24 hours.

CONCLUSION

Emergency and critical care veterinary hospitals treat the sickest and often the most unpredictable animals. These unique challenges emphasize the importance of basic patient care and advanced monitoring techniques. Providing comfort and basic needs should be a nursing priority. Technicians must be aware of common clinical problems, anticipate the needs of the patient, and be alert to new problems and impending crises. Familiarity with a variety of monitoring techniques and diagnostic procedures will allow for the best possible care. The best monitoring plans use multiple parameters and a standardized approach to interpreting and responding to problems during emergencies or standard patient care, triage, and CPR.

LARGE ANIMAL EMERGENCY NURSING

INTRODUCTION

An emergency is defined as a sudden, urgent, usually unexpected event or occurrence requiring immediate action. In equine practice, an emergency is usually the result of the patient's response to an environmental stimulus (fight or flight), the curious nature of horses, obstacles in the environment, or the unique nature of the patient's anatomy (natural areas of narrowing of the horse's gastrointestinal tract). Less commonly a veterinary emergency may be the result of human malice, negligence, or neglect. When an emergency arises, the veterinarian and the staff must act with the appropriate amount of care, compassion, and in an expeditious manner. In some cases, such as long bone fractures or severe abdominal pain, the decision to treat or to humanely euthanize the patient is the first issue to be addressed. When treatment is attempted, it is often initiated with minimal objective data regarding the patient's condition. These are circumstances where the veterinarian and the staff must react rather than ponder the situation. Guess and reassess is often the way in which emergencies are initially approached until the patient, client, and situation are stabilized. An experienced, well-trained veterinary technician is essential in the organization of instruments and material, initial assessment, and triage of the horse seen on an emergency basis. Depending on the presenting complaint and the patient's condition, several criteria must be assessed and met:

- First and foremost, the owner or client, patient, veterinarian, and staff should be protected from injury.
- Relief of the patient's pain and anxiety. In no circumstance is it appropriate to withhold pain medication from a patient that is obviously in need.
- Transport the patient for definitive care.
- If a fracture or breakdown injury has occurred, stabilization if the affected limb is an immediate concern, particularly if surgical treatment is to be attempted.
- Protect from contamination and initially treat soft tissue trauma.
- Control hemorrhage if present.
- Be sure that the patient has an appropriate airway and is able to breath.
- Fluid resuscitation and correction of electrolyte abnormalities.

Each of these criteria will be addressed in detail repeatedly throughout the remainder of this chapter.

The purpose of this chapter is to review the veterinary technician's role in the management of emergencies specific to equine veterinary medicine. This includes the initial examination and determination of the patient's condition, the equipment, instruments, and materials needed to manage equine emergencies, and finally, this chapter will review the use of IV fluids, blood, and blood products in equine emergency medicine.

GENERAL CONSIDERATIONS

EMERGENCY PREPARATION

The chief complaint or reason the patient is seen will dictate what preparations are made before the patient's arrival or what equipment is to be carried into the field if examination is undertaken in an ambulatory situation. It is essential that all needed equipment be organized before arrival of the patient. This includes needles, syringes, catheters, IV fluids, fluid delivery systems, oxygen tanks and regulators, IV fluids, and any medications, such as NSAIDs and sedation. In addition, any equipment that may need to warm up, such as x-ray processes, should be turned on before arrival of the patient. Emergency and first-aid equipment can be stored conveniently in already prepared carts or emergency kits that can be organized based on emergency needs (Figure 33-75), or the material can be organized onto carts before arrival of the patient (Figure 33-76).

Emergency drugs that are stored in carts or tots should be arranged in alphabetic order, and a list of the drugs, their indications, dosage, and typical volumes administered to an average 450-kg adult or 50-kg foal can be laminated and stored with the drugs for quick reference (Figure 33-77). Table 33-2 is a list of emergency drugs commonly used in equine practice.

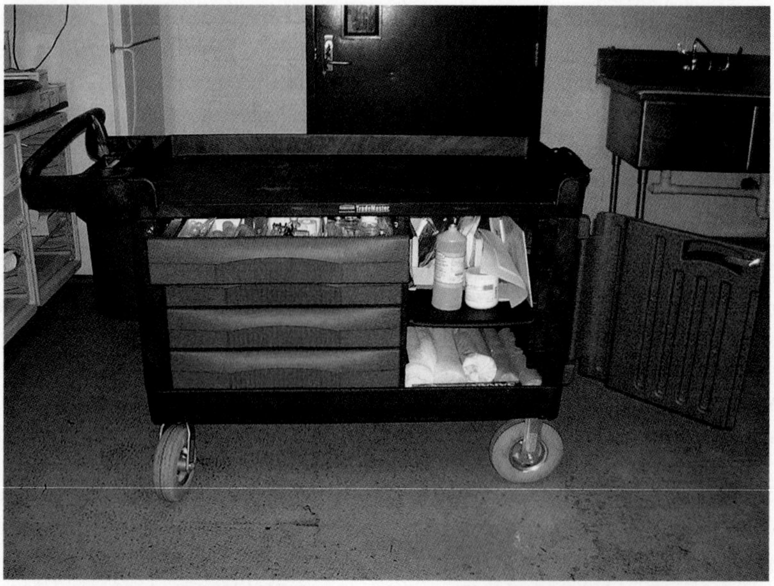

FIGURE 33-75 Hospital emergency cart.

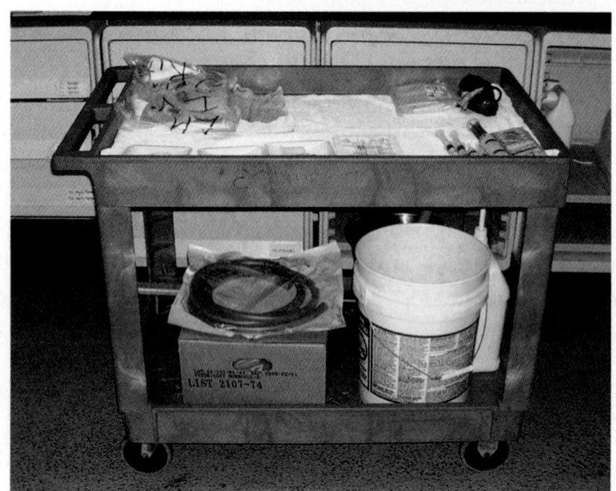

FIGURE 33-76 Emergency cart prepared before the patient's arrival.

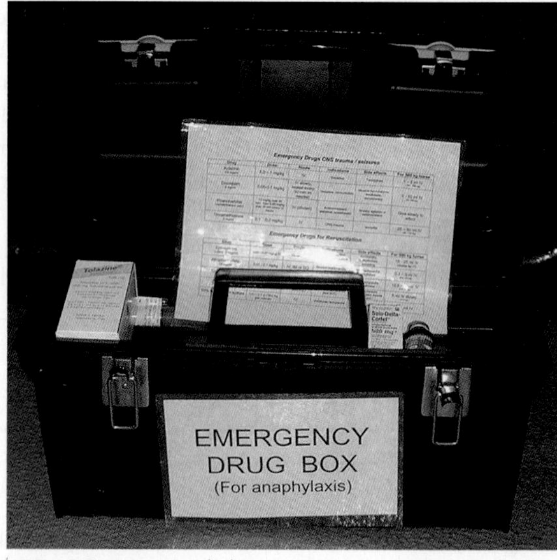

FIGURE 33-77 Crash box containing emergency drugs and a laminated chart with indications for use and dosages.

TRANSPORT OF THE INJURED OR CRITICALLY ILL HORSE

Considerable misconceptions exist as a result of the lack of specific published recommendations on the transport of critically ill or injured equine patients. Too often veterinarians are reluctant to recommend and clients are apprehensive about transporting patients to the hospital for definitive care because of the fear of injury during transport. These fears are often unfounded, and the risk of transport seldom if ever outweighs the benefit of appropriate treatment. Although trailering is an athletic event with the horse needing to balance its weight, sometimes on three legs through turns and sudden stops, most horses withstand transport well as long as appropriately prepared and hauled.

Before Loading

Preparation for transport is dependent on the type of emergency. Owners should be instructed at the time of the initial call as to the safest, most appropriate means of hauling their horse. If referring an emergency to another hospital, the referral hospital should be contacted before transport and any specific instructions for transport obtained.

It is vitally important that the person hauling the sick or injured horse be provided with accurate, easy-to-follow directions to the hospital, and contact telephone numbers should be provided in the event that the driver becomes lost, the horse's condition deteriorates, or the horse dies in route. The driver should also be instructed to call the practice when they are estimated to be within 15 to 30 minutes of the practice or if the horse dies. The following are recommendations

TECHNICIAN NOTE Accurate, easy-to-follow directions and contact telephone numbers should be provided to the hauler of a sick or injured horse.

TABLE 33-2 Common Equine Emergency Drugs

Drug	Indication	Dose	Volume in Average Patient (450 kg)
Atropine (15 mg/kg)	Bradycardia Bronchoconstriction	0.01-0.02 mg/kg IV	0.3-1.8 ml IV
Dexamethasone sodium phosphate (4 mg/ml)	Anaphylaxis Shock	0.05-0.5 mg/kg IV	5-50 ml IV
Diazepam (5 mg/ml)	Seizures	Foal: 0.05-0.4 mg/kg IV Adult: 25-50 mg/kg IV	Foal (50 kg): 0.5-4 ml IV Adult: 5-10 ml IV
10% DMSO	Cerebral edema	1 g/kg IV	500 ml diluted in 5 L of IV fluid
Epinephrine (1:1000)	Anaphylaxis Cardiac arrest	0.01-0.02 mg/kg IV	4.5-9 ml IV
Euthanasia agent containing pentobarbital	Euthanasia	10-15 ml/100 lb body weight	100-150 ml IV
Flunixin meglumine	Inflammation Endotoxemia Analgesic	1.1 mg/kg IV	10 ml IV
Furosemide (Lasix 50 mg/ml)	Diuretic Pulmonary edema	0.5-1 mg/kg IV	5-10 ml
Lidocaine (2%)	Ventricular tachycardia	0.5-1.5 mg/kg IV	11-33 ml IV slowly
Methylprednisolone sodium succinate (100 or 500 mg/10 ml Solu-Delta-Cortef)	Shock	0.25-1 mg/kg IV	10 ml of 100 mg/10 ml-10 ml of 500 mg/10 ml
Sodium bicarbonate (8.4%)	Foals—cardiac arrest	1 mEq/kg IV	45 ml

for the transport of horses suffering from specific emergency conditions.

Abdominal Pain

Clients often are fearful of transporting patients with severe abdominal pain. In particular those patients that frequently lie down. Although there are risks in hauling these patients, even the most painful and sickest horses usually endure the trailer ride. The horse's concentration is often drawn away from its abdominal pain by the necessity to maintain balance. Patients suffering from dehydration or shock will benefit from the administration of IV crystalloid fluids and hypertonic saline solutions before loading on the trailer. These patients are best hauled in a slant load or two-horse trailer with chest and rear bars to allow the horse to lean as desired. Horses with severe abdominal pain can also be hauled in an open stock trailer to allow them to lie down, if desired. Horses can be mildly sedated and NSAIDs administered to relieve pain. If the trailer ride will last longer than the expected action of the sedation, the hauler may be provided with additional doses of a medication, such as xylazine, that can be administered intramuscularly. The hauler can stop at set intervals to check on the condition of the horse and readminister sedation if needed. In extreme cases, IV fluids may be provided to horses during transport. Fluids may be hung from the ceiling of the trailer; however, a plan for regularly scheduled stops must be made to ensure that the fluids do not run out and allow blood to back up and obstruct the catheter. Colic horses should also have a nasogastric tube passed and gastric reflux removed immediately before loading.

Orthopedic Injuries

Before loading and transport to the hospital, orthopedic injuries should be appropriately stabilized with bandages, splints, or casts as described later in this chapter. Horses with fractures or breakdown injuries are best loaded onto a trailer by ramp, or the trailer can be positioned so that the step is level with the ground, such as backed against a curb, a dirt mound, or into a ditch. This allows the horse to be loaded and unloaded without having to step up into or down out of a trailer while trying to protect the injured limb. The horse should be hauled in a slant load or two-horse trailer with partitions and a chest and rear bar to allow it to lean and redistribute its weight off the affected limb.

> *TECHNICIAN NOTE* Horses with fractures or breakdown injuries are best loaded onto a trailer by ramp or the trailer can be positioned so that the step is level with the ground, such as backed against a curb, a dirt mound, or into a ditch.

Because it is more difficult for the horse to maintain its balance when stopping suddenly than when accelerating, horses with forelimb fractures should be transported facing the back of the trailer. Horses with hind limb fractures can be transported facing forward in the normal direction.

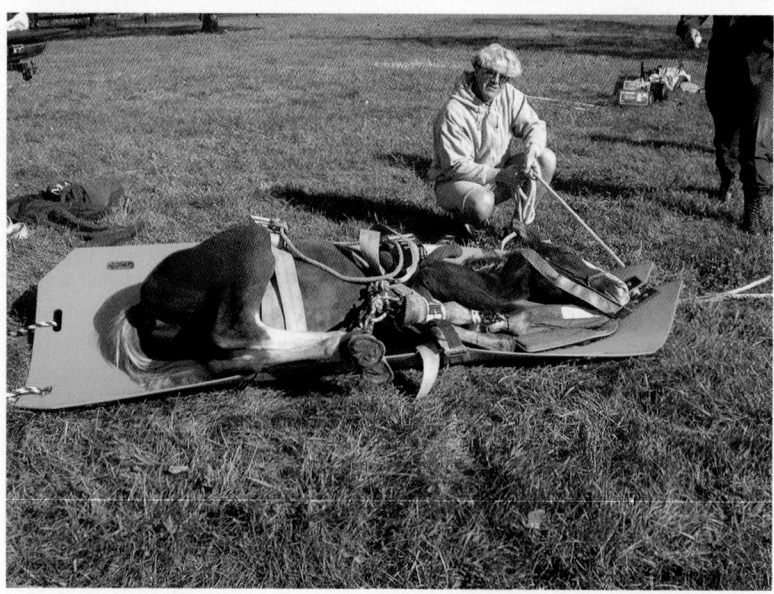

FIGURE 33-78 Recumbent horse ready for transport.

Recumbent Horses

The greatest difficulty in transporting recumbent horses is the loading process. This is also the time of greatest danger because horses that thrash or are seizing pose the risk of kicking the veterinarian or the assistants. For this reason, recumbent horses should be heavily sedated or anesthetized before loading. Once sedated, the horse should be fitted with head protection and all four limbs wrapped with thick quilts and leg wraps. Recumbent horses are best hauled in open stock trailers or horse trailers in which the middle partitions have been removed. If possible, the trailer should be positioned on lower ground than the patient to allow gravity to assist the loading process. Soft cotton ropes can be attached to the limbs, tail, and halter to allow the horse to be manually pulled onto the trailer. Alternatively the horse can be positioned on a plywood or rubber mat in which rope has been attached to the front corners (Figure 33-78). The ropes can then be passed through the front of the trailer and attached to a truck, tractor, or winch system to allow the horse to be slowly pulled into the trailer. Specially designed air mattresses are available to provide cushioning for the patient during transport. In their absence, the patient can be surrounded by hay bales to prevent excess repositioning during transport.

Foals

Foals should be hauled in a separate compartment from their dam and with an assistant. Young foals tend to lie down during transport, but may be injured while attempting to stand while the vehicle is moving. For this reason, foals should be hauled with an attendant or sedated.

> *TECHNICIAN NOTE* Foals should be hauled in a separate compartment from their dam and with an assistant.

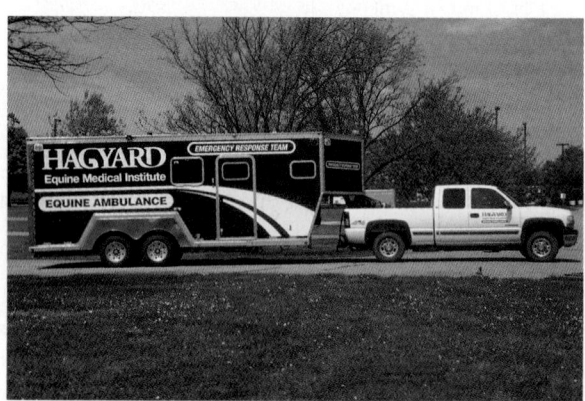

FIGURE 33-79 Purpose-built equine ambulance.

Specialized Purpose-Built Equine Ambulances

Many specialty practices provide purpose-built ambulance service for ill or injured horses (Figure 33-79). These ambulances are manned by personnel trained in the rescue, care, and hauling of sick or injured patients. There are a variety of horse trailers that are converted to provide specific functions to ease the loading and hauling of patients. Some trailers are designed to allow front and rear loading and unloading to prevent patients from having to back on or off of the trailer. Other equine ambulances are equipped with hydraulic systems that allow the rear of the ambulance to be lowered to the ground to allow the horse to load without stepping up into the ambulance. The inner walls of these trailers are padded and in some cases are also equipped with a hydraulic system to allow repositioning of the wall once the horse is loaded. Slings are available to minimize weight bearing on fractured limbs in some ambulances, and winch systems with rubber palates and air mattresses are available to assist in loading and hauling patients that are recumbent.

PATIENT ASSESSMENT

A presumptive diagnosis may be made based on the history and signalment of the patient. For example, a broodmare within 60 days of foaling that has acute severe abdominal pain is likely to be suffering from a large colon volvulus that will require immediate surgery.

The severity of the situation often results in the initiation of treatment without a complete physical examination. Triage is the assignment or priority order to projects on the basis of where resources are best used. This means to focus on the immediate needs of the patient. For instance, if the patient exhibits signs of severe dehydration and shock, an IV catheter should be placed and fluid therapy initiated before a thorough examination or definitive treatment is initiated.

The patient assessment should begin as the patient is unloaded from the trailer. Severe hemorrhage from a laceration should prompt the examiner to assess heart rate and mucous membrane color before the administration of sedation because even appropriate doses of sedation in a patient with acute blood loss can result in recumbency or even death. A patient with a history of abdominal pain may have abrasions along the head and face suggesting severe pain. This may dictate the location where the examination and initial treatment is performed. Horses that repeatedly lie down and thrash as a result of pain should not be placed in a stock because of the potential for orthopedic trauma. These patients may be best examined in a large stall with exits in both the front and rear of the stall to allow personnel to escape if necessary or in the middle of a large open examination room. If at a referral hospital, patients suffering from severe abdominal pain may be moved directly into the surgical induction area for examination and initial treatment.

The animal's mental status can also be evaluated shortly after unloading. A young thoroughbred colt would not be expected to be docile when unloaded into a new environment. This may suggest depression associated with dehydration or other systemic disease.

Measurement of the animal's temperature, pulse, and respiration, and their mucous membrane color and CRT, should be collected at a minimum. Heart rate is an indication of the level of pain and also provides an estimation of hydration or the level of blood loss. Respiration rate may suggest a compromise or disease affecting the respiratory system or may be an indicator of infectious disease. Examination of mucous membrane color (Figure 33-80), moisture, and CRT gives a rapid assessment of peripheral perfusion and the delivery of oxygen to the tissues. Pale mucous membranes that are tacky with a CRT greater than 3 seconds are consistent with a patient that is dehydrated. Brick red mucous membranes with a normal or rapid CRT may indicate endotoxemia or sepsis. Mucous membranes that are purple are frequently observed in patients with severe abdominal disease that are dehydrated, endotoxemic, and have poor peripheral perfusion or hypoxemia. Finally, mucous membranes that are pale or ashen may suggest severe blood loss or the failure to adequately deliver oxygen to the tissues.

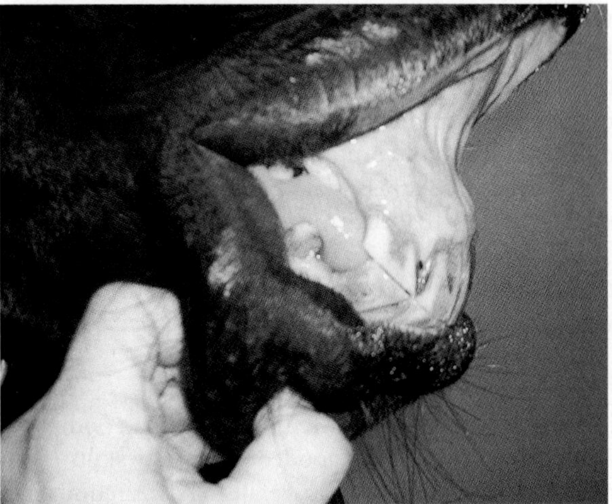

FIGURE 33-80 Example of normal light pink, moist equine mucous membranes.

> *TECHNICIAN NOTE* Minimal data that should be collected from all patients seen on an emergency basis include temperature, pulse, and respiration, mucous membrane color, and CRT.

SPECIFIC EQUINE EMERGENCIES

ABDOMINAL PAIN (COLIC)

Abdominal pain, otherwise known as colic, is one of the most common emergencies encountered in equine practice. A large percentage of horses examined for colic will respond and their signs resolve with minimal or no specifically directed therapy. Gas or spasmodic colic is usually mild, and the administration of analgesics (flunixin meglumine) and laxatives (mineral oil) result in rapid resolution of signs of pain. More important are the small percentage of horses that require intensive medical therapy or surgical intervention to correct potentially life-threatening causes of abdominal pain. Early recognition and aggressive therapy is essential to the survival of these patients. In practices that treat more serious cases of abdominal pain, the veterinary technicians need to have a basic knowledge of the common conditions that occur in the practice area. For instance, coastal Bermuda grass hay is a common component of the equine diet in the Southeastern United States. This feed has been intimately associated with the development of mechanical obstruction of the gastrointestinal tract. This condition often requires intensive care or abdominal surgery. In addition, certain areas of the country are prone to specific conditions as a result of the predominant population of horses. In areas with a high concentration of broodmares, surgical colic—such as large colon displacement or volvulus—are frequent occurrences, particularly in mares within 60 days of foaling. Without adequate triage and surgery, theses patients will almost certainly die from these conditions. The typical examination of a horse with abdominal pain will include a general physical examination (assessment of the severity of pain, temperature, pulse, and respiration, assessment of mucous membranes and gastrointestinal motility), nasogastric intubation, abdominal palpation per rectum, abdominocentesis, complete blood count (CBC) and biochemistry profile, and abdominal ultrasound examination. In specialized practices, in areas where colic associated with enterolithiasis (large stonelike masses that form in the colon and mechanically obstruct the passage of ingesta) is common or in the examination of foals with abdominal pain, abdominal radiographs may also be performed.

General Physical Examination

Minimal materials are required to perform a good physical examination. Essentially, good observation skills, a thermometer, and a stethoscope are all that are required. Initially a presumptive diagnosis can be made based on the history and signalment of the patient. Much information can also be gained from the observation of the patient at a distance. The degree of pain can be assessed by observing patient behavior. The severity of gastrointestinal disease is often directly correlated to the severity of abdominal pain. Mild pain is recognized as intermittent pawing, stretching out, flank watching, splashing water in buckets, and frequent attempts to urinate. These horses often show considerable relief with light sedation or mild exercise, such as walking.

Horses with moderate pain will also exhibit these signs, but also have an elevated heart rate (greater than 40 beats per minute), intermittent attempts to lie down and stand up, occasional rolling, restlessness, and anxiety. These horses will often remain comfortable for short periods of time (45 to 60 minutes) following sedation with an α_2-agonist, such as xylazine or detomidine, with or without an opioid, such as butorphanol. Severe abdominal pain is often manifested as continuous pawing and kicking at the abdomen; repeated, sometimes violent, attempts to lie down; rolling; and frenzied behavior. Sedation may have minimal effect on this degree of pain often lasting as short as 5 to 10 minutes. The presence of severe pain can also be suspected in horses that have evidence of trauma, such as abrasions over the head, face, eyes, and boney prominences of the body or patients that are covered with an unusual amount of dirt, dust, or mud suggestive of repeated recumbency and thrashing.

Abdominal distention may be noted at a distance. If suspected, the owner may be questioned regarding the normal contour of the patient's abdomen.

If possible, the patient's temperature, pulse, respiration should be taken and recorded, and an estimation of the horse's gastrointestinal motility should be performed and noted in the medical record before the administration of sedation. Drugs administered for sedation will lower the horse's pulse and respiratory rate either by direct suppression or improvement in the level of pain. The horse's temperature must be taken before rectal examination. Air introduced into the rectum by the examiner's arm will artificially lower the body temperature measured per rectum.

> *TECHNICIAN NOTE* Temperature, pulse, and respiration should be taken, and an estimation of the horse's gastrointestinal motility should be made before the administration of sedation.

Gastrointestinal motility can be estimated by auscultation of the abdomen with a stethoscope beginning in the paralumbar fossa and proceeding along the caudal edge of the costal margin toward the xyphoid. This should be performed on both sides of the abdomen. Sounds typically heard may be the result of either progressive large intestinal motility (borborygmi) or mixing of ingesta. The two sounds are indistinguishable, but provide a means of assessing gastrointestinal health. Normal large intestinal motility is perceived as prolonged fluid rushing that occurs every 2 to 4 minutes. In addition, high-pitched tinkling sounds can be ausculted in the right paralumbar fossa every 2 to 4 minutes and are routinely associated with cecal motility. Progressive small intestinal motility cannot be determined by abdominal auscultation. It must also be remembered that many factors, including the last time the horse has eaten, the horse's degree of anxiety, and previous administration of medication, may significantly alter gastrointestinal motility. Gastrointestinal motility can be significantly decreased by the administration of sedation. However, the complete absence of gastrointestinal sound in a patient with abdominal pain is always significant. This information is usually recorded in the record by abdominal quadrant (upper and lower right and left) as absent, decreased, normal, or increased. The abnormal accumulation of gas can also be determined by simultaneous auscultation and percussion. This is generally performed over the right paralumbar fossa. The head of the stethoscope is held in place, and the abdomen is percussed by briskly and repeatedly thumping the body while listening for a "ping." This is a high-pitched sound similar to a basketball bouncing on a concrete surface. The presence of a ping often denotes an abnormal accumulation of gas in a hollow viscus.

The horse's level of hydration can be assessed by pinching the skin over the neck, shoulder, or upper eyelid and observing for prolonged skin tent. Care must be taken in assessing hydration in overly fat and thin horses since skin tent is partly the result of subcutaneous fat accumulation. Fat horses may be significantly dehydrated with a near normal skin tent as a result of a large amount of subcutaneous fat. Thin horses with normal hydration may have a prolonged skin tent as a result of little subcutaneous fat. For this reason, the author generally recommends that the skin over the upper eyelid be used to assess hydration. Mucous membrane color, moisture, and CRT are also assessed (Figure 33-81). All physical examination findings should be immediately recorded in the medical record. This should include the time of the horse's arrival and the time and dose of any pain medications administered. The perceived time between the administration of sedation or pain medication may be different than the actual time.

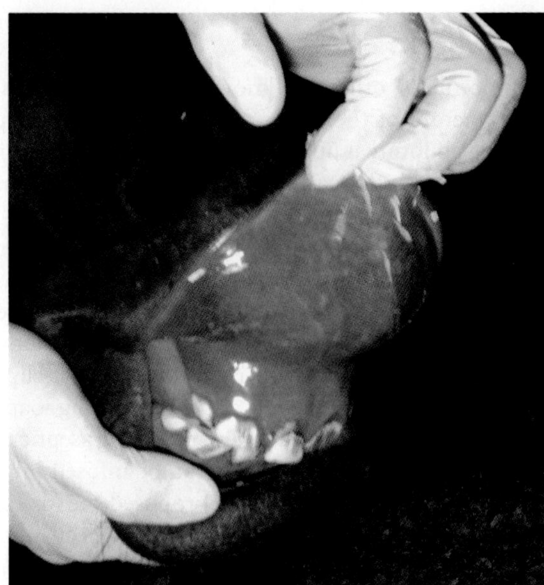

FIGURE 33-81 Brick red mucous membranes in a horse suffering from severe diarrhea, colic, and endotoxemia.

Nasogastric Intubation

Passage of a nasogastric tube is a procedure performed by a veterinarian that is both diagnostic and therapeutic. Often the presence of abdominal pain is the result of accumulation of gas and fluid in the small intestine resulting from either a functional or mechanical obstruction of flow. Over time this ingesta may back up into the stomach, causing severe distention contributing to the abdominal pain. This excess fluid is termed gastric reflux. Elimination of gastric reflux through a tube reduces the distention, improves the patient's comfort, and may prevent rupture of the stomach, which is a universally fatal event. This procedure should be performed in all patients examined for abdominal pain, regardless of the severity of pain or cause. Nasogastric tubes are available in a variety of sizes ranging from ¼ to ¾ inches in diameter (Table 33-3) and are manufactured from silicone, polyvinyl chloride (PVC), or polyurethane.

The size of the tube is determined by the size of the patient. In general, the largest tube that can be passed through the ventral meatus of the nose into the esophagus should be used. For foals where commercially available nasogastric tubes may be too large, a stallion urethral catheter or in miniature foals a red rubber catheter is a reasonable alternative. The patient is generally lightly sedated and restrained with a nose twitch. The end of the tube is lubricated with a water-soluble lubricant and passed through the nose down the esophagus and into the stomach. Once in the stomach, it is often necessary to fill the tube with water to create a siphon effect to allow excess fluid to be removed. This procedure may be repeated several times in a row, especially if the stomach contains a large amount of feed material and is often repeated at regular timed intervals to assess response to therapy and control pain. The net volume, appearance, and odor should be recorded in the medical record. Normal stomach content is usually light green and is often foamy,

TABLE 33-3 Relative Sizes of Nasogastric Tubes Used in Different Sized Equine Patients

Horse	O.D. (in)	I.D. (in)	Length (ft)
Miniature horse	¼ (9-mm)	⅛ (8-mm)	5
Foal	⅜ (9-mm)	¼ (7-mm)	10
Yearling	7/16 (11-mm)	¼ (7-mm)	12
Small horse	½ (12-mm)	5/16 (8-mm)	12
Large horse	⅝ (16-mm)	⅜ (9-mm)	12
Extralarge tube	¾ (19-mm)	½ (12-mm)	10

and typically, less than 4 L is obtained. Net volumes (total volume collected − volume instilled to create a siphon) should always be recorded in the record. The presence of spontaneous reflux, large volumes greater than 4 L, foul-smelling fluid, and discolored (yellow, orange, or bloody) fluid are all significant and should be recorded. Following removal of gastric reflux, the tube may be removed, temporarily maintained until the completion of the examination to allow administration of oral fluids and laxatives, or fixed in place using nonelastic tape to allow repeat removal of accumulated reflux or administration of medication (refer to Chapter 31, Figure 31-17).

TECHNICIAN NOTE Normal gastric contents is typically low volume (less than 4 L), light green in color, and foamy.

Bleeding from the nose is a frequent complication to nasogastric intubation and may cause the owner great concern. This is usually the result of trauma to the ethmoid turbinate and nasal passage and is not of serious consequence. The nose should be loosely covered by a towel to prevent blood from being blown by the horse over equipment, the holder or handler, or the environment. Bleeding generally stops within minutes of removing the tube.

Abdominal Palpation per Rectum

Rectal palpation is a diagnostic procedure performed in patients suffering from severe, recurrent, or persistent abdominal pain. This technique allows the veterinarian to identify the organ system involved, the approximate location of abdominal viscera, to evaluate the abdominal contents, to assess abnormalities in the wall of the bowel, and to localize pain. A rectal examination should only be performed in a horse that is adequately restrained, and proper lubrication is critical to prevent potentially life-threatening complications, such as rectal tears or injury to the examiner. If possible, the horse should be restrained in a standing stock. Light sedation is recommended, and a nose twitch should be applied. A shoulder-length sleeve is used to protect the examiner's hand and arm from fecal contamination, and copious quantities of water-soluble lubricant (Figure 33-82) should be available. In horses that strain during the examination, a caudal epidural can be administered, or 50 to 60 ml of 2% lidocaine can be mixed with an equivalent amount of lubricant and infused into the rectum using a dose syringe to provide a local anesthetic effect. Immediately following the examination, the rectal sleeve should be examined for evidence of blood. Following the examination, all feces and lubricant should be removed from the tail and perineal area with a moistened cloth or warm water.

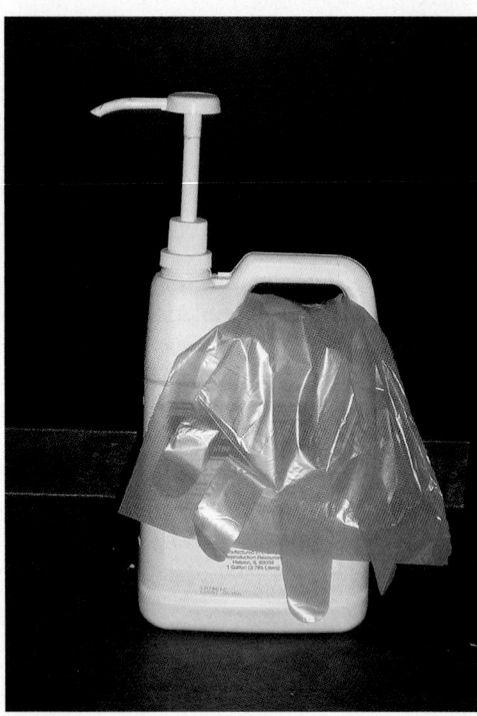

FIGURE 33-82 Shoulder-length sleeve and water-soluble lubricant for rectal palpation.

Abdominocentesis

Abdominocentesis, otherwise known as a "belly tap," is the surgical puncture of the abdominal cavity for the purpose of obtaining abdominal fluid (Figure 33-83). This technique provides information regarding the health of the peritoneal cavity and may reveal horses with devitalized intestine that require surgery or may identify horses suffering from rupture of a viscus. This technique requires absolute aseptic preparation. A 10-cm × 10-cm area of the most dependent part of the abdomen, usually centered 3 to 5 cm caudal to the xyphoid and 3 to 5 cm to the right of midline, is clipped. The area is cleaned of dirt, debris, and dander using soap and water or alcohol followed by a final scrub using aseptic technique. Two to 5 ml of 2% lidocaine can be infused into the skin and subcutaneous tissues at the proposed site for centesis. A variety of instruments may be used to collect abdominal fluid, depending on the veterinarian's preference (Figure 33-84), including an 18-gauge × 1½-inch needle, 18-gauge × 3½-inch spinal needle, sterile teat cannula, or sterile bitch catheter. Once the instrument has entered the abdominal cavity, fluid is collected into an ethylenediaminetetraacetic acid (EDTA) tube (purple top) and red-top tube. The fluid is grossly examined for color and clarity. Additional information may be obtained by measuring TP by refractometer and submission to the laboratory for cell count, cytology, Gram stain, and culture. Normal peritoneal fluid values are found in Box 33-2.

Clinical Pathology

At a minimum, a PCV and TP measured by refractometer should be measured at the time of presentation. This minimal database is easily obtainable, provides rapid results, and is a good estimation of hydration. In addition, repeated PCV

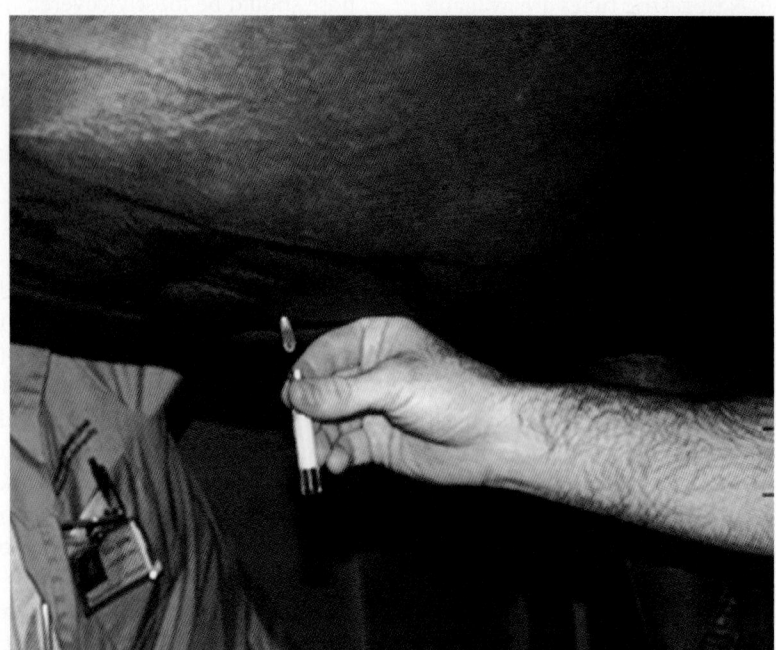

FIGURE 33-83 Surgical puncture of the abdomen (abdominocentesis) for the collection of peritoneal fluid.

and TP measurements provide a means of assessing improvement in hydration status and may be used by the veterinarian to determine prognosis. Although CBCs and biochemistry profiles do not provide specific diagnostic information regarding the cause of abdominal pain, alterations in normal may direct antibiotic therapy, fluid and electrolyte therapy, and response to treatment and may give an indication of prognosis. Biochemistry profiles may also provide information indicating sources of pain other than the gastrointestinal tract. For instance, horses suffering from rhabdomyolysis (tying-up) may have signs similar to colic. Significant elevation of creatine kinase (CK) and aspartate transaminase (AST) on a biochemistry profile may alter the diagnostic and therapeutic plan in these horses (see Chapter 16).

Abdominal Ultrasound

This is a valuable tool for the evaluation of abdominal pain in horses. It is a safe, noninvasive diagnostic technique that allows direct evaluation of the abdominal viscera and evaluation of nongastrointestinal structures. Removal of the hair over the abdomen is not necessary to perform abdominal ultrasound. The body surface is thoroughly wet with isopropyl alcohol and a 2.5- to 10.0-MHz probe is used to evaluate the intraabdominal structures.

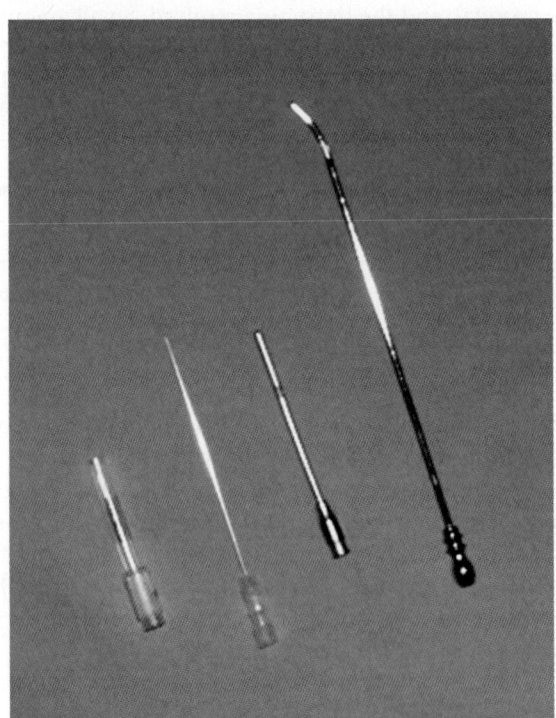

FIGURE 33-84 Common instruments used to perform abdominocentesis. From left to right: 18-guage × 1.5-inch needle, 20-guage × 3.5-inch needle, sterile teat cannula, and sterile bitch catheter.

BOX 33-2 Normal Peritoneal Fluid Values

Normal Peritoneal Fluid

Gross appearance:

Clear and straw colored or yellow

Cellularity:

Adult WBC ≤10,000 cells/μl

Foal WBC ≤1500 cells/μl

TP ≤2.5 g/dl

> *TECHNICIAN NOTE* Ultrasound is a safe, noninvasive diagnostic technique that allows direct evaluation of the abdominal viscera and nongastrointestinal structures, such as spleen, liver, and uterus.

Specific information obtainable by ultrasound includes visceral distention, wall thickness of the abdominal viscera, and motility of specific portions of the gastrointestinal tract. Specific causes for abdominal pain, such as nephrosplenic entrapment, intussusception, and diaphragmatic hernia, can be reliably diagnosed by ultrasound examination. Ultrasound examination also allows the veterinarian to locate fluid for abdominocentesis; identification of intraabdominal pathologic conditions, such as an intraabdominal abscess; assessment of fetal viability; and evaluation of intraabdominal organs, such as the liver and spleen.

Abdominal Radiology

Radiology of the equine abdomen has limited value because of the horse's large size and poor tissue resolution, high radiation exposure to personnel, and decreased life of radiographic equipment. Its usefulness improves in areas of the country where enterolithiasis is a common problem. Additionally, radiology may be useful as a diagnostic tool on foals and in small horses, such as American miniature horses, to assess gastric, small intestinal, and large intestinal distention. Contrast radiology is useful for the diagnosis of detailed gastric emptying and meconium impaction in foals.

Abdominal Exploratory

Abdominal pain that is the result of disruption of the blood supply to the intestine (strangulation), malpositioning of segments of the intestine (displacement), or mechanical obstruction of the bowel require abdominal surgery for correction (Figure 33-85). The five most common indications for abdominal surgery in the horse are: (1) an abnormal rectal examination, (2) large quantities of gastric reflux, (3) an abnormal abdominocentesis, (4) uncontrollable abdominal pain, and (5) systemic deterioration or a patient that fails to improve even with aggressive and appropriate medical therapy. Once the decision has been made to pursue surgical correction, the patient will require presurgical preparation to minimize the anesthetic time and to ensure the best chance for a positive outcome.

If the patient has not received an IV catheter, one should be placed at this time to allow the administration of perioperative antibiotics and anesthetic-induction drugs. If the patient has not received a tetanus vaccination in the last 6 months or if the vaccination history is unknown, a tetanus toxoid should be administered before surgery. Perioperative antibiotics are administered no more that 30 to 60 minutes

CASE PRESENTATION 33-1

A 10-year-old quarter horse mare acutely developed signs of colic: inappetence, pawing, and rolling. The concerned owner called the local equine veterinarian to come out to the farm. On a physical examination, the veterinarian noted depression; pale pink mucous membranes; CRT = 2 seconds; temperature = 99° F; tachycardia (heart rate = 60 bpm); tachypnea (respiratory rate = 40 breaths/min); and dry, scant manure in the stall. On auscultation of the abdomen, borborygmal sounds were decreased (0 or 1) in each of the four quadrants. A rectal examination revealed a large amount of doughy fecal matter in the large colon. The veterinarian passed a nasogastric tube and obtained no reflux, so he administered 4 gal of warm water and ½ gal of mineral oil. He also gave 500 mg flunixin meglumine IV for pain. The veterinarian diagnosed an impaction in the large colon and referred the patient to a local equine hospital for additional treatment.

At the referral hospital, the experienced veterinary team performed their usual tasks. The veterinary technician passed a nasogastric tube. The veterinarian spoke with the owner briefly to obtain the patient's history and performed a physical examination with similar findings to the local veterinarian. Since no reflux was obtained, the veterinary technician administered 6 L of warm water and ½ gal of mineral oil via the nasogastric tube. A second veterinary technician performed a sterile prep, placed a 14-gauge catheter in the right jugular vein, and started 20 L of crystalloid fluids (Normosol R). The veterinarian performed a rectal examination and confirmed the diagnosis of impaction in the large colon. Since the horse was mildly uncomfortable and continued to paw, the veterinarian asked the veterinary technician to administer 150 mg xylazine and 4 mg butorphanol IV. The veterinary technician performed a venipuncture and submitted samples for venous blood gas, CBC, and chemistry profile. The abnormal results included: increased PCV and total protein, and decreases in levels of sodium and chloride.

The horse was placed in the ICU and monitored frequently for comfort by the veterinarian and veterinary technicians. Within a few hours, she appeared more comfortable and began to pass small amounts of dry manure. The veterinary technicians continued to pass a nasogastric tube every 6 hours and administer 6 L of warm water and ½ gallon of mineral oil. By the next morning, the veterinarian repeated a rectal examination, and the impaction was smaller in size. The owner called and said he found that the automatic water machine in the horse's stall was broken. She did not have access to water for at least 24 hours, which caused this impaction.

The mare continued to improve with 2 days of treatment at the hospital, and the impaction resolved. Small amounts of hay and soaked feed were offered, and the horse ate readily. She showed no more signs of colic and was discharged to a grateful owner. The veterinary team was happy to have helped another patient with their efficient and effective team approach.

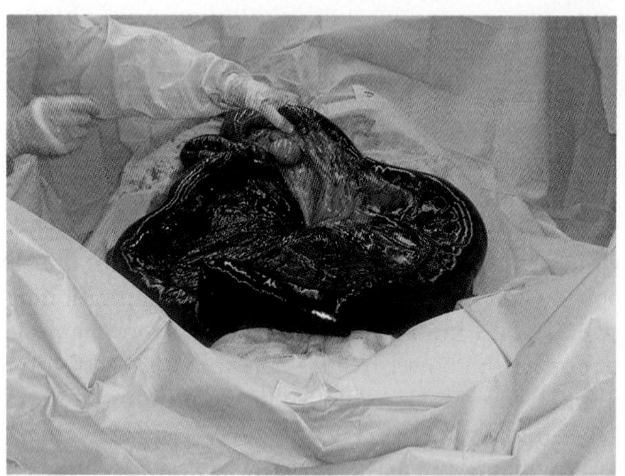

FIGURE 33-85 Horse in which a portion of the small intestine has lost its blood supply.

before the induction of anesthesia. This will ensure that adequate plasma levels of antibiotics will have been reached by the time the incision has been made and will be maintained for the duration of the surgery. The choice of antibiotic is at the discretion of the surgeon; however, the broad-spectrum combination of an aminoglycoside antibiotic, such as gentamicin, and crystalloid penicillin, such as potassium penicillin, administered IV is most common. Potassium penicillin should not be administered within 15 minutes of induction because of the effect of high levels of IV potassium on the heart and blood pressure.

> *TECHNICIAN NOTE* Perioperative antibiotics should be given IV 30 to 60 minutes before the induction of anesthesia.

If it is safe to do so, the ventral abdomen should be clipped from the xyphoid caudally to the inguinal area and the clipped area cleaned with soap and water or alcohol to remove all gross contamination. Once the patient is anesthetized, any remaining hair should be removed, and a final rough scrub applied to remove any further debris. A final aseptic scrub using chlorhexidine or Betadine scrub and rinsed with alcohol is applied before surgery.

ORTHOPEDIC INJURIES

Orthopedic injuries are a common occurrence in horses. The large size, temperament, use, and speed of the horse can result in catastrophic life-threatening injury. There are injuries that are common to specific disciplines, such as condylar fractures and disruption of the suspensory apparatus in thoroughbred racehorses or first or second phalanx fractures in Western performance horses. These injuries occur with regular frequency and are directly related to the horse's occupation. There are other orthopedic injuries that occur without obvious knowledge of their cause. Horses that are pastured are frequently found at the time of morning feeding with fractures, laceration, and serious injury that can

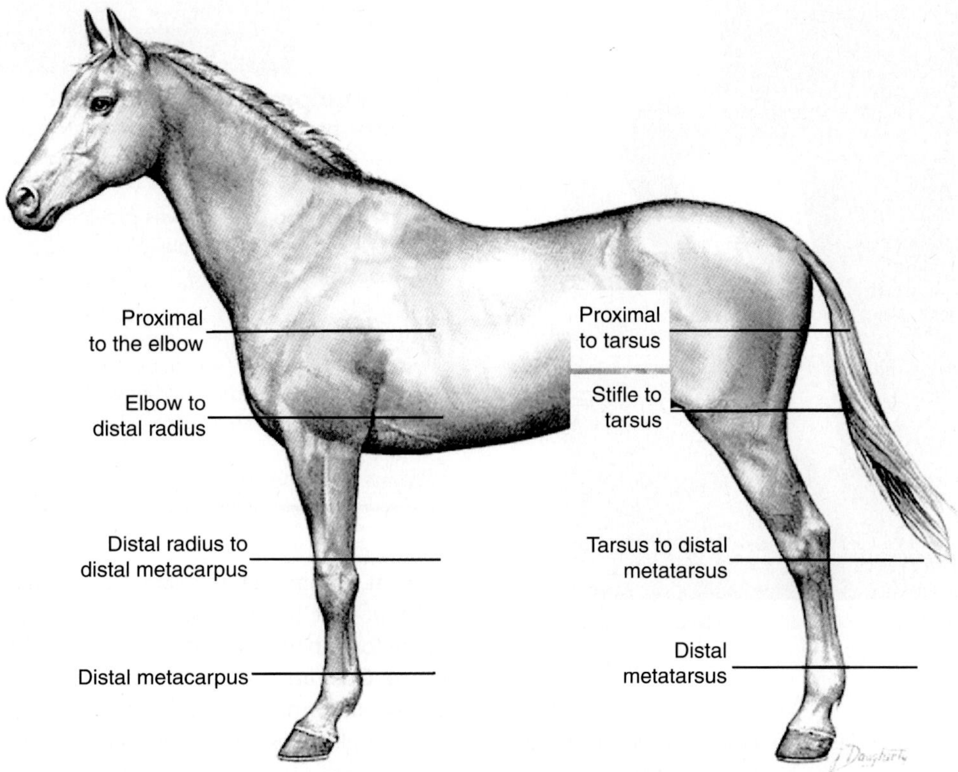

FIGURE 33-86 Anatomic division of the horse for emergency external coaptation.

arise from kicks by other horses, missteps during exercise, or obstacles in the environment. Regardless of the cause of an orthopedic injury, first aid and stabilization of the fractured or injured limb before transport to the hospital are some of the most important determinants of a successful outcome or repair. Assuming the horse's systemic condition has been appropriately assessed and stabilized, the goals of adequate temporary external fixation of a fractured limb include the elimination of patient pain and anxiety; to allow at least partial weight bearing on the affected limb; minimize further damage to the surrounding soft tissue, including muscle, blood, and nervous supply; and to prevent rubbing and eburnation of the bone ends that may affect reduction and definitive repair.

> TECHNICIAN NOTE Temporary external coaptation of a fractured limb reduces the patient's pain and anxiety, allows partial weight bearing on the affected limb, protects the soft tissue from further trauma, and prevents eburnation of the fractured bone ends.

External fixation of an unstable limb should occur before any further diagnostic techniques or movement and transport of any injured patient in which surgical repair is to be considered. For the purpose of fracture stabilization, the front and hind limbs are divided into four regions (Figure 33-86), and specific recommendations for these regions have been published.

Forelimb Injuries

Ground to Distal Metacarpus

Injuries that commonly occur from the ground to the distal metacarpus that require emergency external coaptation include unstable fractures of the first and second phalanges, luxation of the fetlock joint, fractures of the distal metacarpus, laceration of the flexor tendons, disruption of the suspensory apparatus by fracture through both proximal sesamoid bones, and displaced condylar fractures. With the exception of condylar fractures, these injuries result in hyperextension of the fetlock joint either because of loss of the slinglike support of the fetlock by the suspensory apparatus or a change in the location of the primary bending force of the distal limb from the fetlock joint to the fracture. Hyperextension of the fetlock can result in damage to the nerves and blood vessels of the distal limb as a result of tearing or thrombosis of the palmar digital vessel. Therefore the goal of emergency coaptation is to prevent hyperextension of the fetlock. This can be accomplished by splinting the limb with the dorsal surfaces of the bones of the phalanges and metacarpus in axial alignment. There are several means in which this can be accomplished. The simplest is to apply a lightly padded bandage with a dorsally applied splint. The most common splint material for this purpose is PVC pipe cut to size. A bandage with approximately 1 cm of compressed padding is applied from the coronary band to the carpus. The splint is applied to the dorsal surface of the limb and extends from the proximal metacarpus to the tip of the hoof and is fixed in place with either 3-inch nonelastic tape or a more rigid

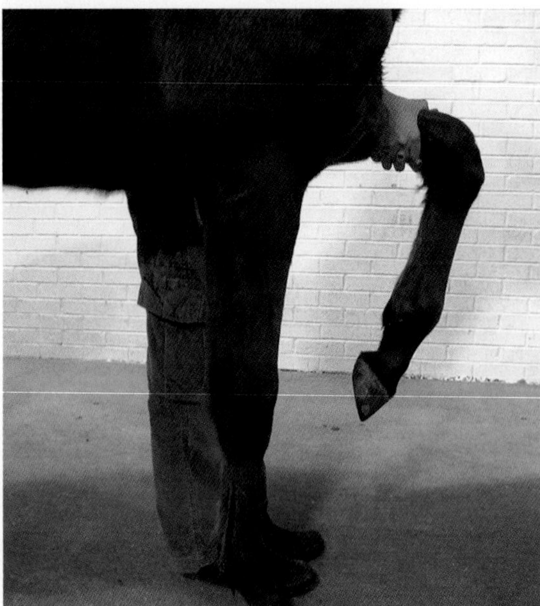

FIGURE 33-87 Proper elevation of the forelimb to allow standing application of a distal limb cast on the front leg.

alternative would be fiberglass cast tape. A wooden wedge can be incorporated beneath the heels to assist in maintaining the alignment of the bony column.

Alternatively, rigid stability can be provided by application of a distal limb cast. In a quiet, lightly sedated horse, elevation of the front foot off the ground results in natural alignment of the bony column. This is accomplished by an assistant grasping the limb behind the carpus and pulling the carpus up and forward in front of the horse (Figure 33-87). By this method, a distal limb cast can be applied to the standing horse. This technique requires that the horse stand still balancing on three limbs at least until the cast is applied and hardened, which can take from 30 to 60 minutes, depending on the material used and the skill of the veterinarian. Therefore this may not be appropriate to attempt in all horses. In these cases, short-term general anesthesia may be required to apply the cast correctly.

Correct cast application is vitally important to an overall successful outcome. Casts that are applied too tight or that have folds or ridges adjacent to the skin will result in limb ischemia or cast sores that may be as or more severe than the original injury. The needed material and equipment to apply a cast should be accumulated and organized before anesthetizing the patient or attempting cast application (Box 33-3).

If possible, the shoe should be removed, the hoof appropriately trimmed, all debris and loose sole and frog removed, and the periople rasped. If the patient will not tolerate adequate preparation of the hoof, the cast can be applied directly over the hoof and shoe. To apply the cast, the limb is initially covered by the appropriately sized double layer of synthetic stockinette. This material should fit snug but not tight and should not sag. Felt cast padding of approximately 1 inch width should be applied circumferentially around the limb at the top of the cast and over any bony prominences to

BOX 33-3 Material and Equipment Necessary to Apply a Half-Limb Cast

Cast Equipment and Material

- Stainless steel or other appropriately clean bucket
- Water—the temperature specified by the manufacturer of the cast tape
- Examination gloves or gloves provided by the manufacturer to properly apply cast material
- Cast synthetic stockinette
- Cast felt
- Bandage scissors
- 1-inch white tape
- Custom Support Foam or other appropriate cast padding
- Various cast tape size, prim1208arily 4 or 5 in for adults, 3 in for foals
- Polymethylmethacrylate (acrylic)

prevent rubbing. The stockinette is then covered by a ½-inch layer of cast padding or a porous, water-curable polyurethane foam bandage material, such as 3M's Custom Support Foam. Custom Support Foam is resilient, porous, produces a close anatomic fit, and has the advantage of adherence to the fiberglass-resin cast tape that will be applied, thus forming a single unit with the cast material. This decreases the risk of movement and the development of cast sores. Padding material of any type should not be applied too thick. If cast material is too thick, it will become compressed with weight bearing, and the cast will slip, potentially resulting in serious cast sores.

Plaster of Paris cast material has all but been replaced by polyurethane-impregnated fiberglass cast tape in cast application because of its superior strength and light weight. A wedge-shaped block of wood or roll of cast material positioned beneath the heels provides additional support and helps to maintain alignment while the cast is applied. The manufacture's recommendations for water temperature and time of submersion of rolls of cast material should be read before application.

This first layer of cast material should be applied without tension directly over the foam padding with no creases or folds to minimize cast sores. Subsequent layers should be applied with increasing tension. Additional strength can be gained by fashioning a splint by layering a roll of cast material in alternating directions to the length of the cast. This can be applied to the dorsal surface of the cast and fixed in place with additional rolls of cast material. For an adult horse 4 to 7, 4- to 5-inch rolls of cast material are used. The cast material is overlapped by no more than one half of its width during application. Once the cast tape has been applied, the bottom of the cast can be protected from excess wear by the application of polymethyl methacrylate (PMMA). The surface of the PMMA should be made rough by compressing it with a rasp to prevent slipping.

An added benefit to the application of a cast for temporary fracture stabilization is that radiographs may be taken and the fracture assessed through the cast (Figure 33-88).

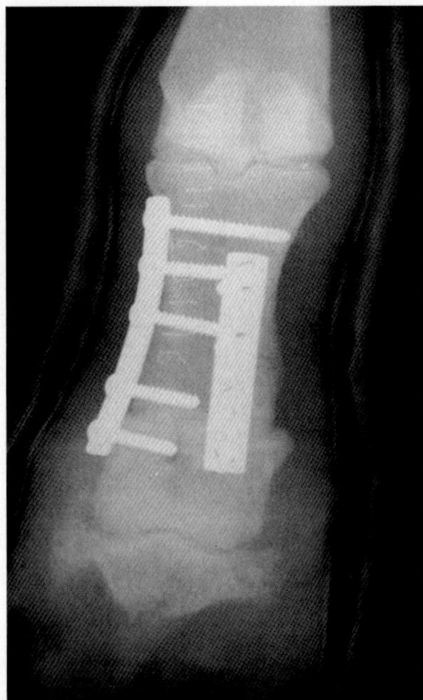

FIGURE 33-88 Example of radiographs of a previously repaired fracture taken through the cast. Note that the radiopaque cast material allows the fracture and implants to be visualized through the cast.

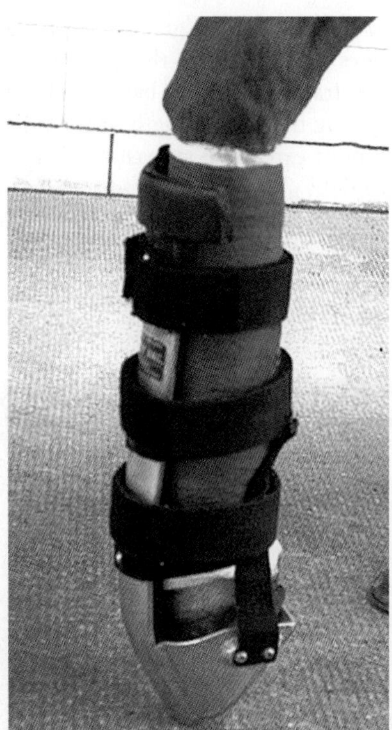

FIGURE 33-89 Kimzey Leg Saver splint applied to the distal limb of a horse with a fracture.

Another alternative is the application of a manufactured purpose-built splint to the distal limb. The Kimzey Leg Saver is a good example of a purpose-built splint specifically designed to align the boney column of the distal limb (Figure 33-89). These can be applied over a light padded bandage and can be used to support both fractures of the distal limb and disruption of the suspensory apparatus.

> *TECHNICIAN NOTE* The Kimzey Leg Saver is a commercially available distal limb splint designed for temporary stabilization of fractures of the limb below the distal one third of the metacarpus or metatarsus.

Distal Metacarpus to Distal Radius

The most common injury to this region of the limb is fracture of the third metacarpal (cannon) bone. Fractures in this region are severely unstable and require fixation of both the joint above and below the fracture to provide stability and shared weight bearing. A Robert Jones bandage with two splints at 90-degree angles provides excellent stability to these fractures. It has the additional advantages of controlling hemorrhage and minimizing the development of and hastening the resolution of swelling associated with edema. The Robert Jones bandage is composed of multiple layers of sheet cotton or similar material compressed by gauze. The final diameter of the completed bandage should approximate three times the diameter of the normal limb. For fractures of the forelimb, splints consisting of PVC pipe cut to extend the full length of the limb or wood should be positioned caudally and laterally and fixed with nonelastic tape or cast tape.

Distal Radius to Elbow

Anatomically the flexor and extensor tendons of the forelimb act as abductors of the limb once disruption of the boney column of the radius occurs. Therefore these fractures are at high risk for penetrating the skin on the medial aspect of the limb as a result of the absence of soft tissue covering the radius at this location. Therefore external coaptation of these fractures not only must provide axial stability, it must also prevent abduction of the limb. This is accomplished by the application of a Robert Jones bandage as previously described; however, in addition to the caudal splint, a lateral splint that extends to the top of the scapula and is secured to the scapula area by tape or other suitable bandage material that encircles the axilla, thorax, and withers should be applied (Figure 33-90). The lateral splint is commonly composed of 2 × 4-inch lumber, and elastic tape is employed to fix it to the scapula to prevent abduction.

Olecranon Fractures

Complete fractures of the olecranon result in the disruption of the horse's triceps apparatus. The triceps muscle serves to extend the elbow. The ulna, which is the distal extremity of the olecranon, is at least partially fixed to the caudal aspect of the radius and acts as a lever against the pull of the triceps muscle and is necessary for the horse to fix the carpus in extension. Therefore horses with complete fractures of the olecranon lose this lever and are unable to fix the carpus in extension. This results in the classic "dropped elbow" appearance and buckling or flexion of the carpus (Figure 33-91). Although this is not a weight-bearing bone and typically responds well to surgical fixation, loss of the ability to extend the carpus results in a great deal of anxiety for the horse and makes ambulation on three legs difficult. Patients with olecranon fractures should be treated with a stacked bandage extending the entire length of the limb and a dorsally applied splint extending at least the length of the carpus. This essentially allows the limb to act as a support post, and the horse quickly adapts to the rigid limb by using the muscles that extend the shoulder to advance the limb while walking. This type of splint is also useful in patients with radial nerve paralysis and those with fractures of the distal humerus and scapula that also lose the function of the triceps apparatus. In these cases, the splint should not extend proximally above the level of the fracture.

> *TECHNICIAN NOTE* Horses with complete olecranon fractures are unable to extend the carpus. A full-limb bandage with a dorsally applied splint spanning the length of the carpus allows these patients to stand and ambulate comfortably.

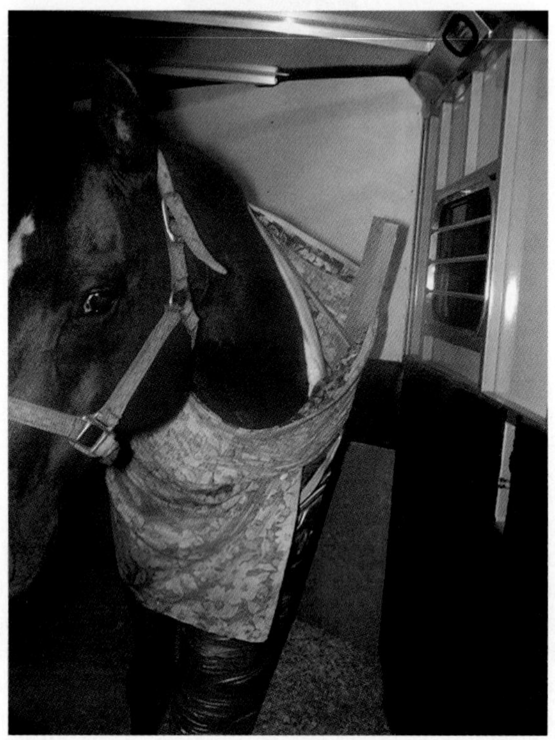

FIGURE 33-90 Full limb Robert Jones bandage with a caudal and lateral splint extending to the withers for transport of a patient with a suspected distal radial fracture.

Proximal to the Elbow

Fractures of this region are surrounded by a heavy muscle mass and are unable to be appropriately externally stabilized. Horses with fractures of the distal humerus that have lost their triceps apparatus function will benefit from a light full-limb bandage and cranially or caudally applied splint to fix the carpus in extension.

Hind Limb Injuries

Ground to Distal Metatarsus

Fractures in this area are similar to those described for the forelimb. The goal is alignment of the dorsal cortices of the bone. However, this is more difficult in the hind limb than the forelimb. To stabilize these fractures, a plantar splint is applied extending from the solar surface of the foot to the proximal metacarpal bone. Specialized splints, such as the Kimzey Leg Savers, are also valuable to support these fractures. Kimzey Welding Works Inc. also manufactures a hind limb leg saver splint that more closely matches the anatomy of the hind limb specifically for these fractures.

Distal Metatarsus to Tarsus

These fractures are also treated similar to fractures of the same region in the forelimb with a few exceptions. First, the thickness of the bandage applied to the hind limb is reduced compared with the forelimb. Second, a plantar splint can

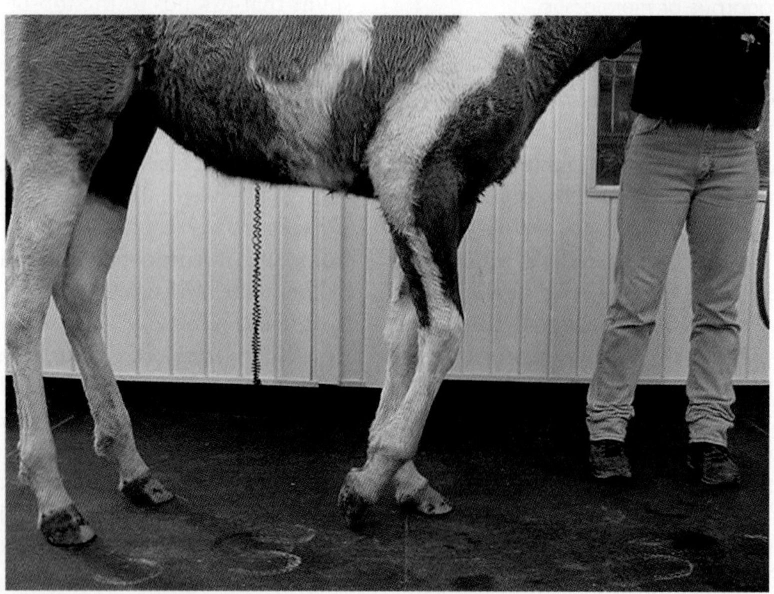

FIGURE 33-91 Dropped elbow appearance of a horse with a complete olecranon fracture.

be applied using the calcaneus as the proximal extent of the splint. The external splint should extend only the distance of the most proximal extent of the calcaneus.

Tarsus to the Stifle

The response to contraction of the muscles surrounding the tibia is similar to those of the radius. Therefore fractures of the tibia result in abduction of the limb and a high potential for penetration of the skin covering the vulnerable medial aspect of the tibia. These fractures are stabilized with a Robert Jones bandage and a caudally applied splint extending to the length of the calcaneus and a lateral splint that extends proximally to the hip. A straight or angled splint following the contour of the hock can be fashioned and fixed in place using nonelastic tape.

Proximal to Stifle

The musculature proximal to the stifle is sufficient to stabilize fractures of the femur. It should be noted that complete fractures of the femur can result in significant subcutaneous and intramuscular accumulation of hemorrhage and severe swelling over the thigh. A compressive bandage should be applied to the distal limb to prevent excess swelling secondary to edema and gravitation of fluid distally from the fracture.

> *TECHNICIAN NOTE* Fractures proximal to the elbow or stifle are unable to be appropriately stabilized using external bandages, splints, or casts. The large muscle mass surrounding the bones in this area provides adequate temporary stabilization.

SOFT TISSUE TRAUMA

Lacerations and puncture wounds occur frequently to the head, body, and limbs of the horse, but are most commonly observed on the distal limb. These injuries are usually the result of sharp lacerations from contact with loose sheet metal, barbed wire, and protruding nails, sawlike lacerations that occur when a limb becomes entangled in smooth wire, or blunt force trauma from kicks or high-speed impact with inanimate objects. Because of the limited soft tissue covering of the distal limb penetration of synovial structures, such as joints and tendon sheaths, or disruption of the neurovascular supply to the limb is a frequent potentially life-threatening complication. The initial care of soft tissue injuries has a profound influence on outcome of the injury.

Initial Assessment

The most important aspect of the initial assessment of the patient is the control of hemorrhage. It is often difficult to determine the exact amount of time that has passed since the initial injury and the owner finding the horse. Significant blood loss may have occurred during this time. The horse's environment makes accurate assessment of the volume of blood lost difficult. In some instances, the owner may report significant hemorrhage before presentation of the horse. In this instance, the owner can be instructed over the telephone in methods to control hemorrhage. In extreme circumstances, hemorrhage can be controlled by wrapping the distal limb with clean towels that are tightly compressed with Vet Wrap, elastic tape, or even duct tape. These crude bandages may become heavily soaked with blood, but they should not be removed until the patient has been transported to the hospital or the veterinarian has arrived at the farm. An unstable clot is likely to have formed under the bandage at least slowing the hemorrhage. Removing the bandage may disrupt the clot resulting in the recurrence of severe bleeding.

If there is active hemorrhage at the time of initial examination, this may be controlled by the application of a Robert Jones bandage or a tightly compressed stacked bandage. If there are exposed bleeding vessels, the examining veterinarian may elect to place a hemostat across the lacerated vessels followed by a ligature to control hemorrhage. The use of tourniquets to control hemorrhage is not advised. The ischemia that results from the application of a tourniquet will result in severe discomfort to the patient. In addition, tissue ischemia may result in the loss of vital soft tissue and the development of large defects that take an extended time to heal.

If severe hemorrhage is not obvious at the time of presentation, a brief physical examination should be performed before administering sedation to ensure that the patient is not exhibiting signs of hypovolemia associated with blood loss. Common signs of anemia as a result of blood loss include depression and lethargy, tachycardia, tachypnea, cool extremities, and pale mucous membranes. If these signs are noted, a PCV and TP should be measured and supportive care, such as IV fluids or blood transfusion, should be initiated before treatment of the wound.

Initial Wound Treatment

Once the patient has been stabilized, initial wound care revolves around decreasing further contamination, eliminating necrotic tissue, and removing foreign material from the wound. This is vitally important in wounds that are in close proximity to joints or tendon sheaths. The patient may be sedated and either regional anesthesia, such as nerve blocks, or local infiltration of the wound with lidocaine may be useful in controlling pain. Contamination of synovial structures may result in the development of septic arthritis or tenosynovitis (Figure 33-92). The hair surrounding all wounds should be removed with clippers or a razor. Before clipping, the wound should be covered with sterile moistened gauze or sterile water-soluble lubricant, such as K-Y Jelly, to prevent hair from entering the wound.

The area clipped is dependent on the location of the wound. For wounds that are distant from synovial structures or those on the body or head, only the area immediately surrounding the wound needs to be clipped. For wounds that are suspected of involving a joint or tendon sheath, the limb should be clipped circumferentially and 5 to 10 cm proximal and distal to the wound to allow centesis of the synovial structure at a location distant from the wound. Once clipped, the skin surrounding the wound should be cleansed with an antiseptic soap and rinsed with saline.

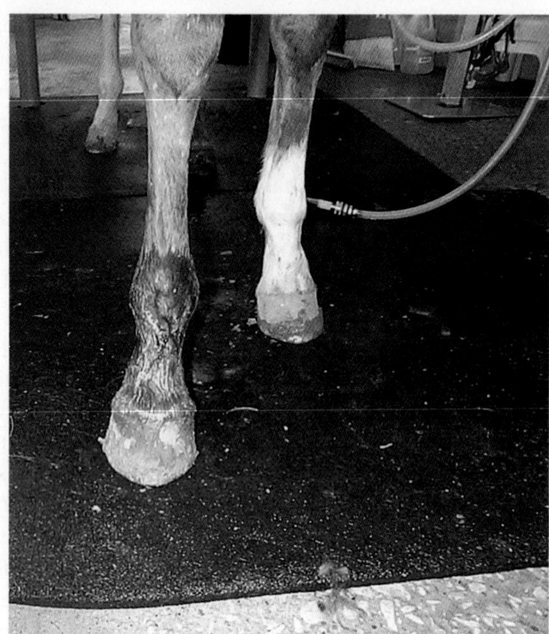

FIGURE 33-92 Laceration located directly over the fetlock joint with the potential for joint contamination and septic arthritis.

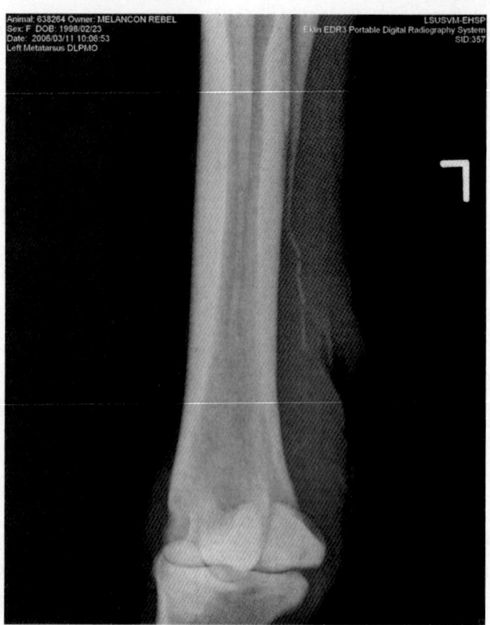

FIGURE 33-93 Splint bone fracture secondary to wound over plantar surface of the metatarsus.

> *TECHNICIAN NOTE* Before clipping, wounds should be covered with sterile water-soluble lubricant to prevent hair from adhering to the wound.

Once the surrounding skin has been cleansed, the wound may be gently scrubbed using sterile gloves and an antiseptic soap and rinsed with saline. Wounds may be initially irrigated with saline by syringe and 18-gauge needle or by making multiple holes in the cap of a saline bottle, turning the bottle upside down, and applying pressure to the outside of the bottle to produce a forceful stream. For superficial wounds that do not involve synovial structures, debris can be removed from the skin and wound surface with antiseptic soap and rinsed with water. Excess fluid pressure should not be applied to the wound because this may force bacteria and debris deeper into the tissue.

Diagnostic Imaging

Any wound involving the distal limb, over a boney prominence, or that is chronic and nonhealing should be evaluated either by radiographs or ultrasound at the time of injury. Diagnostic imaging allows the early diagnosis of fractures (Figure 33-93) and foreign bodies (Figure 33-94) and provides a means for further evaluation of the development of sequestrum (Figure 33-95).

> *TECHNICIAN NOTE* Any wound involving the distal limb, located over a boney prominence, or that is chronic and nonhealing should be evaluated either by radiographs or ultrasound.

Blunt traumatic wounds that are severe enough to disrupt the skin are severe enough to result in fracture of the small bones of the distal limb, such as the splint bones.

Ultrasound is useful in the evaluation of wounds for the detection of foreign bodies of nonbone or metallic origin. Wood, plant material, glass, and other nonbone or metal foreign bodies cannot always be detected by radiology. These structures can often be observed by ultrasound as bright hyperechoic structures that produce acoustic shadowing (Figure 33-96).

In addition, radiology allows early assessment of the bone for comparison in 3 to 4 weeks for the development of a sequestrum, a nonviable segment of bone that may develop as a result of trauma to the periosteum on the surface of the bone. This "dead" boney material also acts as a foreign body that will impede wound healing.

Specific Wound Therapy

Once the wound has been cleansed, the involvement of synovial structures determined, the extent of the wound fully assessed, and diagnostic imaging performed, definitive therapy can proceed. Wound therapy may be as straightforward as suturing the wound and the application of a bandage to as complicated as surgery, arthroscopic joint lavage, and the application of a cast. The treatment to be employed and the material needed will be determined by the veterinarian. However, in most instances, sedation; local anesthetic drugs, such as lidocaine; a surgery pack containing a scalpel handle, hemostats, thumb forceps, needle drivers, and scissors; and tetanus prophylaxis are the minimal materials required.

RESPIRATORY EMERGENCIES

Respiratory emergencies can be the result of an acute disease process or trauma, acute exacerbation, decompensation or progression of an existing condition, or the respiratory manifestation of a systemic disease. Respiratory distress occurs

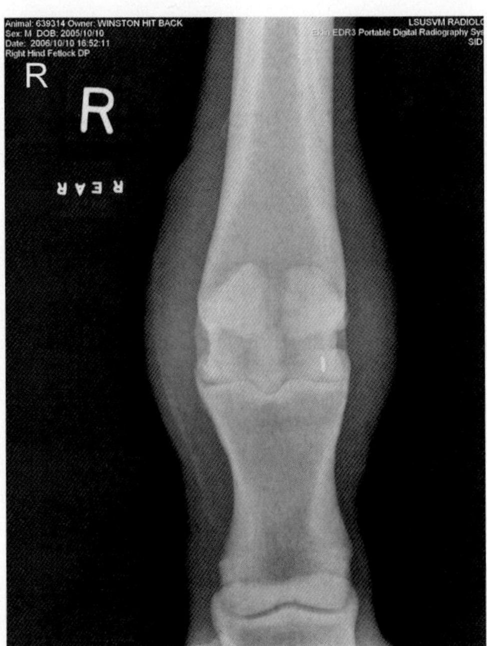

FIGURE 33-94 Intraarticular metallic foreign body associated with a fetlock wound.

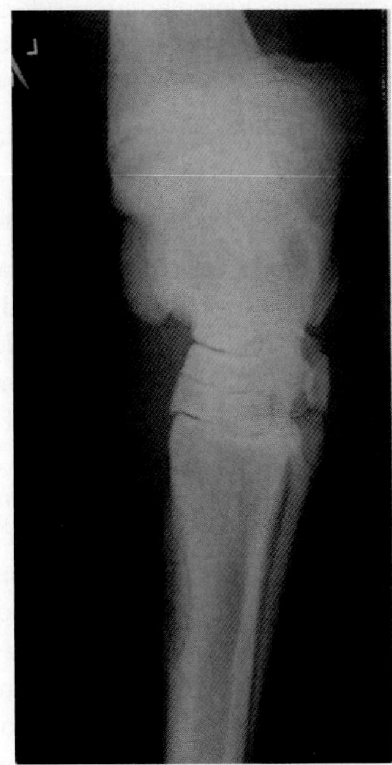

FIGURE 33-95 Sequestrum as a result of a wound over the proximal metatarsus.

when there is inadequate delivery of oxygen from the lungs to the tissue and may be the result of an inability of oxygen to reach the lungs (obstructive disease), an inability of the lungs to expand adequately (restrictive disease), failure of oxygen to diffuse across the respiratory membrane at the alveolus, failure of oxygen to be transported in the blood to the peripheral tissues (anemia), or the inability of the tissue to extract or use delivered oxygen.

Common signs of respiratory distress in horses include rapid breathing (tachypnea); flaring nostrils; exaggerated

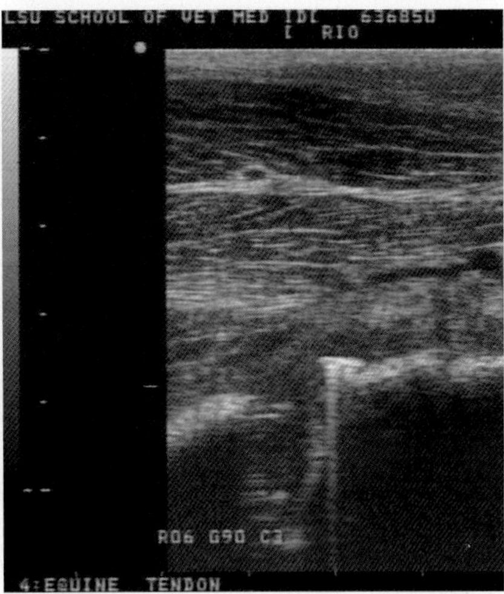

FIGURE 33-96 Characteristic ultrasonographic appearance of a foreign body with the bright hyperechoic line delineating the foreign material and acoustic shadowing.

thoracic or abdominal excursions; shrill, grating, or whistling inspiratory or expiratory noise also termed stridor; nasal discharge; or bluish-purple discoloration of the mucous membrane also known as cyanosis. Horses in respiratory distress are frequently anxious, assume an abnormal posture characterized by abduction of the elbows and extension of the head and neck, may be reluctant to move, and may exhibit signs of thoracic pain.

TECHNICIAN NOTE Common signs of respiratory distress include tachypnea, flaring nostrils, exaggerated abdominal or thoracic excursion, inspiratory or expiratory stridor, nasal discharge, and cyanosis.

It must be kept in mind that horses in severe respiratory distress may be hypoxic resulting in severe anxiety, panic, uncontrollable behavior, and sudden violent death. These horses pose a significant danger to the handler, veterinarian, and staff and should be handled with extreme caution. It is recommended that clients not be allowed to restrain horses exhibiting signs of severe respiratory distress, and for their own protection, they should be moved a safe distance away from the horse in case the patient becomes panicked or violent.

Upper Respiratory Tract Emergencies

Equine respiratory emergencies can be divided into conditions affecting the upper or the lower respiratory tract. Diseases affecting the upper respiratory tract are typically the result of obstruction of airflow to the lungs and are recognized most commonly by the presence of inspiratory stridor without abnormal lung sounds. These are likely the most common forms of respiratory emergencies in horses. This is due in part to the anatomy of the equine upper respiratory tract. The soft palate of the horse extends caudally as far as and ventral to the epiglottis dividing the oral and nasal pharyngeal areas completely except during swallowing (Figure 33-97). Because of this, horses are obligate nasal breathers

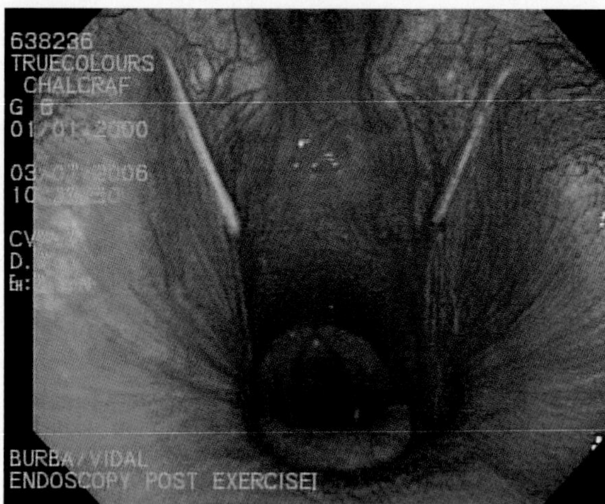

FIGURE 33-97 Normal endoscopic appearance of the upper respiratory tract.

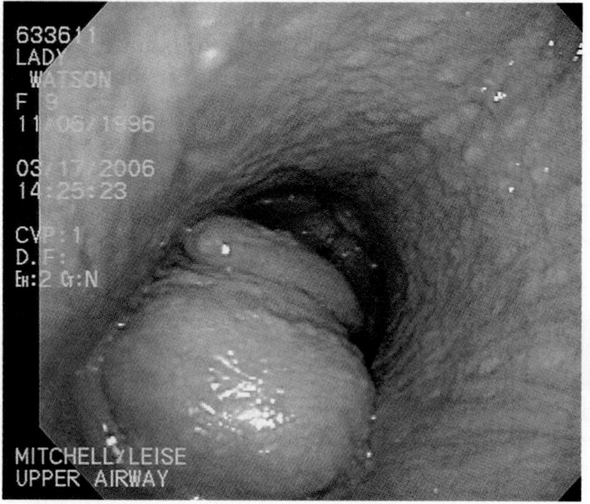

FIGURE 33-98 Subepiglottic cyst acting as a space-occupying mass causing respiratory distress.

and are unable to overcome decreased airway diameter or obstruction by opening the mouth as are dogs or humans. Nasopharyngeal foreign body or cicatrix (scars), severe facial swelling, and facial deformity resulting from acute fractures or space-occupying masses of the nasal passages or pharynx (Figure 33-98) cause respiratory distress as a result of this anatomic arrangement. In addition, an anatomic structure unique to the horse, the guttural pouch, or common anatomic structures in close proximity to the pharynx and larynx, such as retropharyngeal lymph nodes if enlarged, may impinge on these structures significantly decreasing upper airway diameter (Figure 33-99). Laryngeal paralysis may also be a potential cause of upper airway obstruction. Bilateral laryngeal paralysis in horses may be the result of ingestion of toxic plants, lead poisoning, or hyperkalemic periodic paralysis (HYPP). In addition, laryngospasm immediately following anesthetic recovery is a potentially life-threatening complication to prolonged anesthesia or poor positioning during surgery (extreme extension of the head and neck) causing upper airway obstruction.

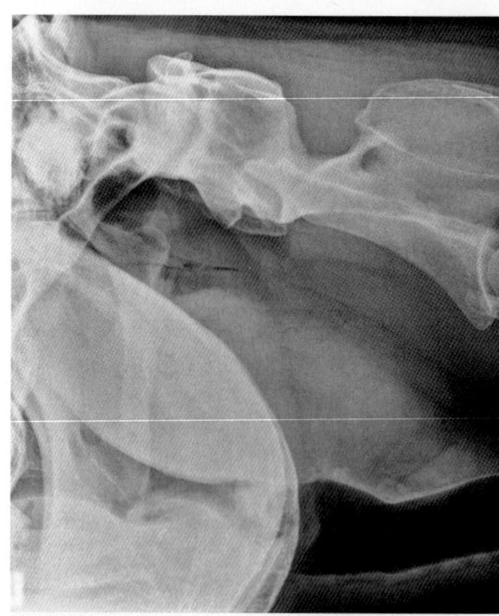

FIGURE 33-99 Infection of the guttural pouch causing narrowing of the upper airway as a result of compression on the trachea.

> *TECHNICIAN NOTE* Diseases affecting the upper respiratory tract are typically the result of obstruction of airflow to the lungs and are recognized most commonly by the presence of inspiratory stridor without abnormal lung sounds.

Lower Respiratory Tract Emergencies

Conditions affecting the lower respiratory tract are divided into obstructive disease, restrictive disease, or diseases causing pulmonary edema. Obstructive diseases are characterized by the presence of expiratory stridor and abnormal lung sounds, including crackles and wheezes. Examples of these diseases include recurrent airway obstruction (ROA) or "heaves," septic bronchitis or alveolitis, and lungworm infection. These conditions are the result of accumulation of inflammatory fluid in the small airways and reflex bronchospasm.

Restrictive disease prevents the lungs from expanding normally. These conditions are commonly associated with expiratory stridor and the absence of lung sounds on thoracic auscultation. Pneumothorax is an uncommon form of restrictive respiratory disease that usually accompanies severe thoracic trauma or penetration of the chest wall. In this condition, free air accumulates in the thoracic cavity causing collapse of the lung. Lung sounds in this case are absent dorsally over the thoracic wall. It is usually unilateral; because the mediastinum of the horse is incomplete, pneumothorax can be bilateral. A more common restrictive respiratory disease in horses is the presence of fluid in one or both sides of the thoracic cavity known as pleural effusion. Pleural effusion also results in mechanical compression and failure of the lung to expand adequately. In this case, lung sounds are absent ventrally, and there may be accentuation of the heart sounds throughout the thorax. The most common cause of pleural effusion in the horse is infectious pleural pneumonia. This condition is frequently accompanied by signs of systemic disease, including fever, weight loss, and ventral edema.

Conditions causing pulmonary edema including acute respiratory distress syndrome and nonrespiratory systemic conditions, such as endotoxemia, heart failure, and smoke inhalation, are associated with both inspiratory and expiratory stridor and abnormal lung sounds. In horses with pulmonary edema, fluid accumulates in the small airways and alveoli and prevents gas exchange across the alveolar membrane. In addition to stridor and abnormal lung sounds, these horses may also have frothy tracheal exudates and frothy nasal discharge.

Management of Respiratory Emergencies

The most important goals in the management of respiratory emergencies are: (1) establish a patent airway, (2) administration of oxygen, and (3) treat the inciting cause.

In patients with acute upper respiratory tract obstruction, reestablishing a patent airway may be all that is needed to ameliorate the clinical signs. This can be accomplished in a number of ways all of which may be dangerous in an adult horse that is panicked as a result of respiratory distress. If the obstruction is affecting the nasopharyngeal region, such as a space-occupying mass or postanesthetic laryngospasm, standing placement of a nasotracheal tube may be an effective measure. It is vital that the nasotracheal tube extends through the arytenoid cartilages and past (distal to) the site of respiratory obstruction. The size of the tube to be used is dependent on the size of the patient, and generally, cuffed tubes are not necessary for temporary use. If possible, light sedation and topical anesthetic agents, such as Cetacaine, applied to the mucous membrane of the nasal passages will facilitate tube placement. Tubes ranging in size from 14 to 22 mm in internal diameter will fit most horses 200 to 450 kg in size.

The tube is lubricated with a water-soluble lubricant, introduced through the nares into the ventral meatus and advanced to the pharynx. This distance can be estimated before placement by measuring the distance from the opening of the nares to the medial canthus of the eye. Once in the pharynx, the head and neck are extended and the tube is advanced while simultaneously rotated one-quarter turn. Cessation of abnormal respiratory signs, unrestricted movement of the tube, and movement of air through the tube are good indications of proper tube placement.

> *TECHNICIAN NOTE* For nasotracheal intubation, endotracheal tubes ranging in size from 14 to 22 mm in internal diameter will fit most horses 200 to 450 kg in size.

If the tube is inadvertently passed into the esophagus, it may be palpable as a second tubular structure in the neck, there may be resistance to movement of the tube, and no air will pass through the tube. If this occurs, the tube can be withdrawn and the procedure repeated until proper placement is verified. The tube can be temporarily fixed in position with a tape butterfly sutured to the nares or circumferential application around the tube and muzzle of nonelastic tape. The use of nasotracheal tubes is contraindicated in cases of nasopharyngeal or tracheal foreign bodies or with severe deviation of the nasal passages.

Temporary tracheotomy can be an effective means of relieving signs of respiratory distress caused by upper airway obstruction. It cannot be understated concerning the potential danger to the veterinarian and staff when performing this procedure in a patient suffering from severe respiratory distress. All precautions should be taken to ensure the safety of all personnel involved in the procedure. This technique can be performed as an elective or emergency procedure either standing or under general anesthesia. If performed standing, the patient can be lightly sedated before performing the tracheotomy. The most desirable location for the tracheotomy is the junction of the upper and middle one third of the trachea; however, the location should always be distal to the obstruction. If possible, the surgical site should be clipped and aseptically prepared, and local anesthesia is provided by infiltration of the skin and subcutaneous tissue with 15 to 20 ml of lidocaine or mepivacaine.

> *TECHNICIAN NOTE* Temporary tracheotomy is an effective means of relieving signs of respiratory distress caused by upper airway obstruction.

Under circumstances of severe respiratory distress and impending death, the tracheotomy can be performed as a lifesaving procedure without typical aseptic preparation or analgesia. Under these circumstances, patients often tolerate the procedure and are greatly relieved immediately following incision into the trachea. Minimal surgical instruments are needed to perform this procedure. A scalpel blade will suffice in times of extreme emergency. However, a small surgical pack containing a scalpel handle, scissors, mosquito hemostats, thumb forceps, and needle driver is helpful in case of hemorrhage and to partially close the incision, if desired.

> *TECHNICIAN NOTE* Under circumstances of severe respiratory distress as a result of upper respiratory tract obstruction and impending death, a tracheotomy can be performed as a lifesaving procedure without typical aseptic preparation or analgesia.

A 10-cm incision is made parallel to and directly over the trachea and the overlying cutaneous colli and sternothyrohyoideus muscles. Once the trachea is visualized, a perpendicular incision is made through the annular ligament between the tracheal rings into the tracheal lumen. This incision should not extend more than one third of the circumferential diameter of the trachea. If necessary, a portion of up to three tracheal rings can be removed to facilitate placement of a temporary tracheotomy tube. There are several different sizes and styles of silicone or stainless steel

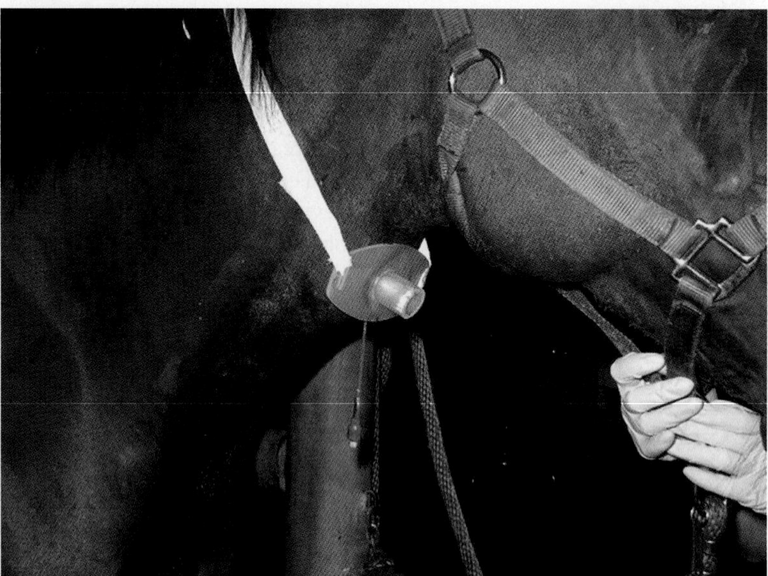

FIGURE 33-100 A cuffed Bivona tracheotomy tube used to temporarily manage an upper airway obstruction in a horse.

tubes, cuffed and uncuffed tubes, and methods of fixing the tubes in place (Figure 33-100). The size of tube is dependent on the size of the patient, and the style is at the discretion of the veterinarian performing the procedure. If the tube is to remain in place for some period, daily care and cleaning will be necessary and should be carried out according to the manufacture's directions. Once removed, reusable tubes should be cleaned and sterilized between patients.

In patients that are frenzied and unable to be restrained because of upper airway obstruction, a patent airway can be established by orotracheal intubation. This should be considered a last resort because at least a short-acting anesthesia will be required for the tube to be passed through the oral cavity into the trachea. Standard IV anesthetic-induction techniques using xylazine and ketamine with or without diazepam are commonly used (see Chapter 27). These have the benefit of a relatively rapid onset of sedation and anesthesia and a short duration. The disadvantages to orotracheal intubation include the potential danger of anesthetic induction in a patient already suffering from severe respiratory distress.

Anesthetic drugs suppress the respiratory centers in the brain; therefore some form of oxygen delivery should be available preferably in the form of mechanical ventilation or a demand valve. Secondly, this technique is only a temporary solution to upper respiratory obstruction and should be maintained only as long as necessary until some other definitive therapy, such as removal of a foreign body or temporary tracheotomy, can be used. The same principles are followed for orotracheal intubation as were previously described for nasotracheal intubation. The patient is in lateral recumbency with the head and neck extended. The tube is passed through a speculum to prevent damage to the tube to the level of the pharynx. Once at the pharynx, the tube is advanced while simultaneously rotating one-quarter turn. If correctly passed, the tube should be movable within the trachea without resistance.

Oxygen Administration

Arterial partial pressure of oxygen measured by blood gas analysis less than 60 mm Hg stimulates respiratory distress and decreased oxygen saturation. Therefore oxygen supplementation is beneficial in any patient suffering from respiratory distress that is not associated with the failure of tissues to extract or use oxygen. Oxygen supplementation has its greatest effect in patients with lower respiratory tract disease. In humans suffering from conditions caused by hypoventilation or impaired gas exchange across the alveolar membrane, breathing 100% oxygen results in up to a fivefold increase in the amount of oxygen moved into the alveolus compared with patients breathing room air. This is due to an increased oxygen pressure gradient between the alveolus and blood.

In patients suffering from blood loss or other conditions causing anemia and decreased delivery of oxygen to the tissue, modest benefit is obtained from oxygen supplementation. This is because available hemoglobin is already completely saturated in these patients. The benefit is obtained from increased levels of dissolved oxygen in the blood. Although this may produce minimal increases in tissue oxygenation, this increase may be the difference between life and death while other definitive therapies are organized.

The equipment required to deliver oxygen to the lungs includes an oxygen source, usually a compressed gas cylinder, a pressure regulator; flowmeter; humidifier; and oxygen delivery tubing. Two types of cylinders are commonly used: an E cylinder that contains approximately 700 L of compressed oxygen at 2200 psi (Figure 33-101) or an H cylinder that holds approximately 7000 L compressed oxygen at 2200 psi (Figure 33-102). Attached downstream from the cylinder is a pressure gauge. Because the content of the cylinder is gaseous, the reading on the gauge is directly proportional to the contents of the cylinder. A pressure regulator, also sometimes referred to as a pressure reducing valve, reduces the pressure coming from the cylinder (approximately 2000 psi

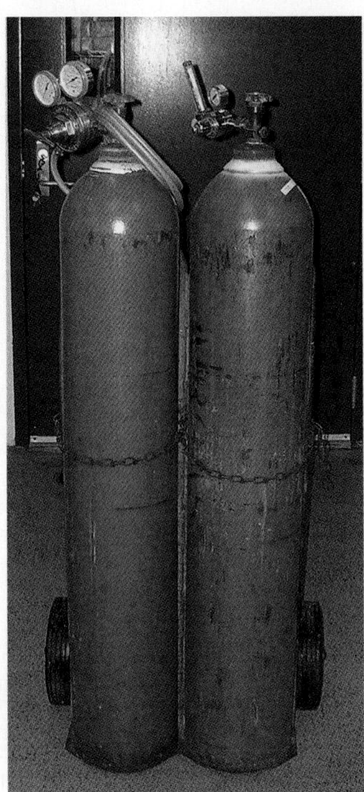

FIGURE 33-101 Example of an E type of compressed gas cylinder.

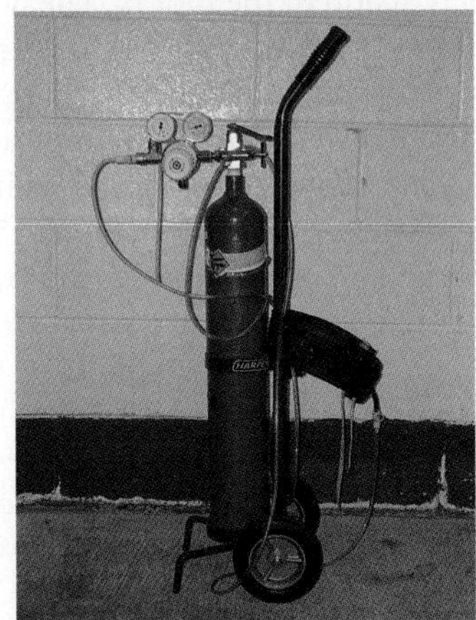

FIGURE 33-102 Example of an H type of compressed gas cylinder.

in a full cylinder) to a safer worker pressure of approximately 50 psi. Additionally a flowmeter capable of delivering 15 L/min oxygen is required for controlled delivery of oxygen to the patient. Finally, some means of humidification, most commonly a bubble humidifier, is attached to the oxygen delivery tubing (Figure 33-103).

Oxygen can be delivered to the lungs by insufflations, demand valve, or mechanical ventilation. Oxygen insufflations is a simple and effective means of increasing the inspired oxygen content in both horses recovering from general anesthesia, or standing and awake horses. When recovering from anesthesia, oxygen can be delivered from the delivery tube through a nasotracheal, orotracheal, or tracheotomy tube. In a conscious patient, nasal insufflation is accomplished through a soft rubber catheter with multiple small fenestrations at its end. The tip of the catheter is positioned at the nasopharynx, the distance to which can be approximated as the length from the opening of the nares to the medial

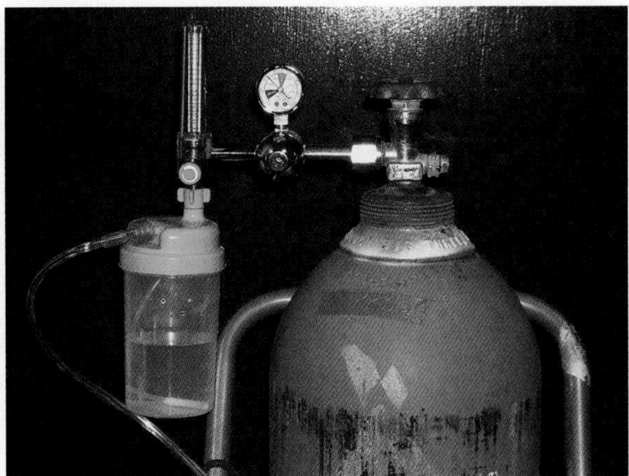

FIGURE 33-103 Regulator, flowmeter, and bubble humidifier.

canthus of the eye. Oxygen delivery tubing can be taped to a stiff wire with a hook at the end to allow it to be fixed to the halter and curve into the nostril, or the catheter can be sutured at the nares and the delivery tube taped to the muzzle to secure it in place (Figure 33-104). Oxygen flow rates vary depending on the size of the horse with adults requiring at least 15 L/min for effective therapy. Foals and miniature horses typically require 5 L/min, and proportionally higher rates are necessary for ponies, weanlings, and juvenile horses.

> *TECHNICIAN NOTE* Flow rates for oxygen supplementation vary and are dependent on the size of the patient. Adults require flows of at least 15 L/min, foals and miniatures 5 L/min, and proportionally higher rates are needed for ponies, weanlings, and juveniles.

Demand valves are small, relatively inexpensive ($200 to $500), portable, and effective means of delivering oxygen to patients during short anesthetic procedures, for patients in respiratory arrest, or in patients requiring assistance with breathing (Figure 33-105). They are attached either directly to a nasotracheal, endotracheal, or tracheotomy tube or may require an adaptor. High oxygen flow (200 L/min) human demand valves including the Hudson demand valve and the Elder CPR/demand valve have been adapted for use in equine patients. One company is manufacturing a demand valve for specific use in equine practice.* This valve can be purchased complete with different lengths of oxygen supply line and several sizes of adaptors for use with varying sizes of tubes.

Demand valves can be set to deliver oxygen when initiated by the patient's own inspiratory efforts (negative inspiratory pressure), or they can be triggered manually to deliver oxygen for a predetermined time or pressure. Exhalation is passive through the valve; however, as a result of the size of the valve, it may be restrictive to expiration. In this case, the valve should be removed following completion of inspiration to allow unrestricted expiration.

---

*Equine Demand Valve, J D Medical Distributing Co., Inc., 1923 West Peoria Avenue, Phoenix, AZ 85029, 602-997-1758, www.jdmedical.com.

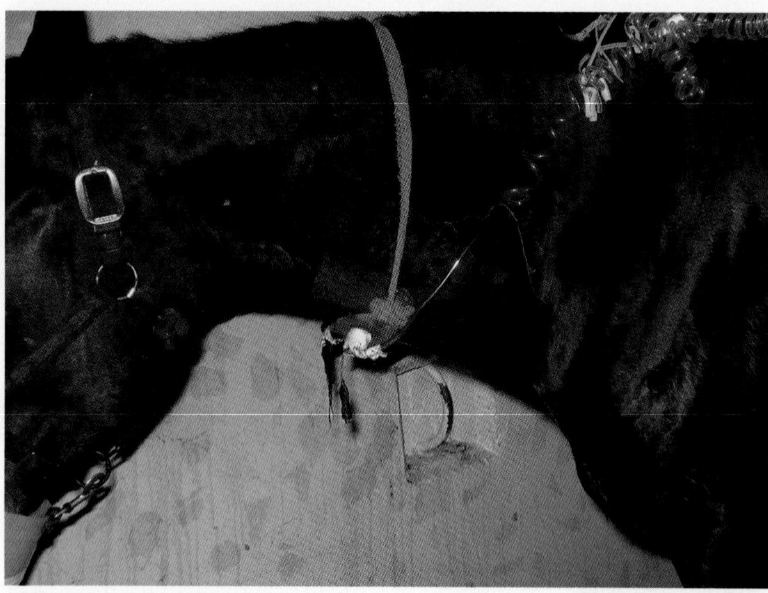

FIGURE 33-104 Oxygen insufflation through a tracheotomy tube in a horse with postanesthetic laryngeal spasm.

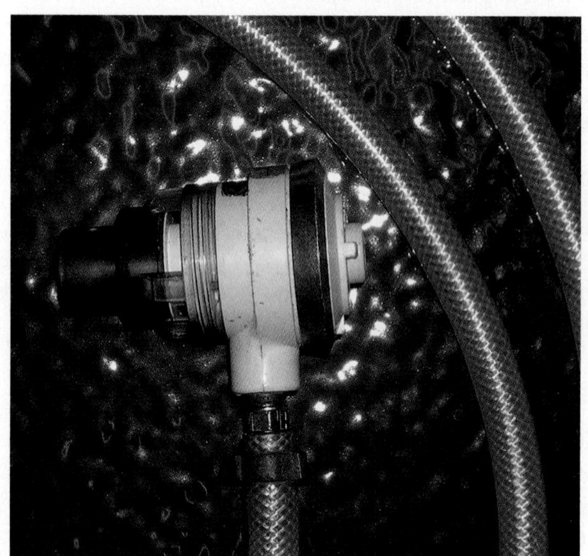

FIGURE 33-105 Oxygen demand valve to provide positive pressure ventilation.

Thoracocentesis

Lower respiratory tract conditions may improve significantly following establishment of a patent airway and supplemental oxygen. However, these cases often require additional therapy to improve the horse's ability to expand the lung and the ability of oxygen to reach the alveolus and cross the alveolar membrane into the systemic circulation.

Horses suffering from restrictive diseases, such as pleural effusion or pneumothorax, are treated by thoracocentesis. This is an emergency, lifesaving procedure involving the puncture of the thoracic wall with a needle, catheter, or large trocar for the purpose of removing air or fluid from the thoracic cavity. This procedure must be carried out under the strictest of aseptic conditions and only by a trained veterinarian.

For the removal of pleural fluid, the location of thoracocentesis is best determined by ultrasound examination of the thorax. In the absence of an ultrasound, the extent of filling of the thoracic cavity can be determined by simultaneous auscultation and percussion of the thorax. The horse is sedated, and once the location is identified, a 5- to 10-cm square area is clipped and aseptically prepared. The skin, subcutaneous tissue, and muscle between the ribs is infiltrated with 10 to 20 ml of Carbocaine, and a stab incision or if using a chest tube a 5- to10-mm incision is made using a #15 scalpel blade. The incision should be positioned near the cranial aspect of the rib to prevent damage to the accompanying artery, vein, and nerve.

> *TECHNICIAN NOTE* For the removal of pleural fluid, the location of thoracocentesis is best determined by ultrasound examination of the thorax.

Temporary evacuation of fluid can be accomplished using a teat cannula or IV catheter passed through a stab incision. Prolonged fluid evacuation is accomplished through a temporary chest tube (Argyle chest tube) fixed in position using a Chinese finger trap suture pattern (Figure 33-106). Chest tubes may be occluded with a sterile syringe and drained intermittently, or they may be allowed to drain continuously. For continuous drainage, a one-way valve must be placed on the end of the chest tube to prevent air from being aspirated into the chest. This can be accomplished using a latex condom with the end removed with a scissors and taped to the end of the tube or a commercially manufactured one-way valve (Heimlich Valve) inserted into the end of the tube (Figure 33-107). Chest tubes should be examined multiple times per day for patency and contamination.

Pneumothorax is also treated by thoracocentesis to reestablish negative intrathoracic pressure. If the pneumothorax is the result of a laceration to the chest wall, the laceration should be sealed by a sterile bandage or definitively repaired. An area extending from the twelfth to the fifteenth intercostal spaces, approximately 10 cm wide and just below the muscles that make up the back, is clipped and aseptically prepared. Pneumothorax is relieved by inserting a 14-guage needle or chest tube through the skin, subcutaneous tissue, and muscle into the thoracic cavity. A three-way stopcock and syringe or mechanical suction device can be used to remove free air from the thoracic cavity. Reexpansion of the collapsed lung results in rapid resolution of the signs of respiratory distress in these cases. Continuous monitoring of treated horses is required to recognize signs of reoccurrence of pneumothorax or reaccumulation of pleural fluid that may require additional treatment.

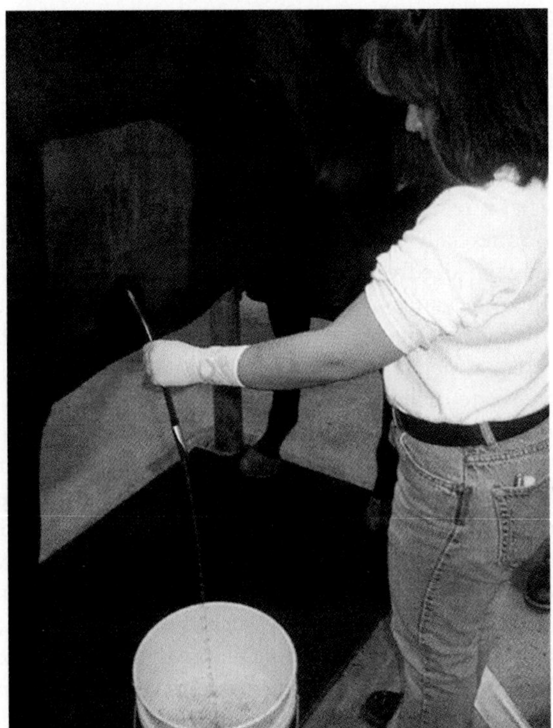

FIGURE 33-106 Argyle chest tube for the removal of pleural fluid.

MANAGEMENT OF EQUINE EMERGENCIES

INTRAVENOUS FLUID THERAPY

Horses coming to the hospital for emergency treatment frequently are suffering from varying degrees of dehydration and circulatory (hypovolemic) shock. Dehydration is defined as the excessive loss of total body water. In many cases, electrolyte abnormalities accompany this loss of water and contribute to the clinical signs exhibited by the patient. When dehydration is mild, compensatory mechanisms, including peripheral vasoconstriction, movement of fluid from the interstitial to the intravascular space, increased heart rate and contractility, and retention of water and sodium by the kidney, serve to increase the circulating plasma volume, maintain cardiac output, and therefore tissue perfusion. In these cases, there are often only subtle signs of dehydration. In other cases, these compensatory mechanisms are overwhelmed, or the loss of fluids and electrolytes is continuous leading to dehydration and hypovolemic shock. With shock there is a decreased cardiac output leading to decreased tissue perfusion and hypoxia at the cellular level. Under conditions of hypoxia, cellular energy stores are rapidly depleted leading to derangement in the normal cellular metabolic pathways. If untreated, organ dysfunction ensues progressing from the least perfused organs, the gastrointestinal tract, kidneys, and liver, to the organs demanding the greatest perfusion, such as the heart and brain. Eventually the perfusion of the brain and heart fall to critical levels, compensatory mechanisms fail, and complete circulatory collapse leads to death of the patient.

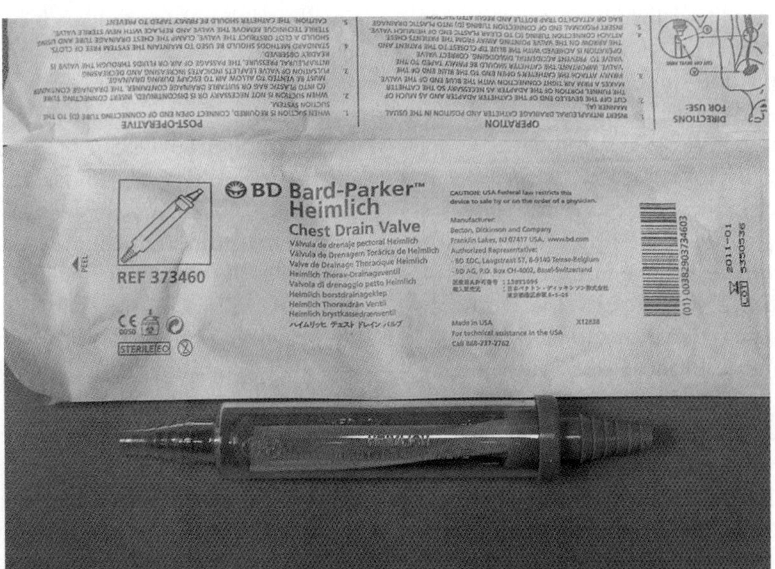

FIGURE 33-107 Example of a one-way Heimlich valve to prevent aspiration of air and debris into the chest tube.

Clinical Signs of Dehydration

The percent dehydration is a subjective estimate of the percentage of body mass lost in fluid. Subjective estimations of hydration are not highly accurate, but they serve as a starting point for treatment that requires frequent reassessment. In horses, signs of dehydration are usually not obvious until the horse is at least 5% dehydrated. At this level, signs of dehydration are mild and may include depression, tachycardia, and decreased pulse quality. As dehydration worsens, additional signs of dehydration may include delayed recovery of skin tenting, tacky mucous membranes, prolonged CRT (greater than 3 seconds), and poor jugular distensibility.

> *TECHNICIAN NOTE* Subjective estimations of hydration are not highly accurate, but they serve as a starting point for treatment that requires frequent reassessment.

A more accurate clinical assessment of dehydration is the change in body mass measured by weight before, during, and after fluid therapy. Although this is a highly accurate measure of hydration, it is impractical in most practice settings. In addition to physical examination findings, hematology findings consistent with a presumptive diagnosis of dehydration include an elevated PCV and plasma TP concentration. This is a simple test that can be performed quickly with equipment available in most private practices and can be used to measure response to fluid therapy. In addition, results of a biochemistry profile that are consistent with dehydration include an elevated creatinine and BUN level. Elevation in BUN and creatinine are collectively termed azotemia and may be the result of dehydration (prerenal azotemia), kidney failure (renal azotemia), and urethral obstruction (postrenal azotemia).

Catheter Location

The location of venous access is determined by the goals of therapy. If the catheter is placed to deliver large quantities of IV fluids, blood or blood products, or if fluids of high osmolarity, such as parenteral nutrition solutions, are to be delivered through the catheter, a larger peripheral vein, such as the jugular vein, or central venous access is recommended. This allows for a larger-size catheter to be placed and as a result of the laminar flow characteristics of these veins decreases the likelihood of thrombophlebitis that occurs when fluids of high osmolarity are administered IV. Administration of antibiotics can be accomplished via jugular catheterization; however, there may be instances in which catheterization of the jugular vein is not desirable. In those cases, catheterization of the accessory cephalic, saphenous, or lateral thoracic veins are reasonable alternatives.

Catheter Selection

IV catheters have become a mainstay in large animal emergency nursing. Advances in emergency and critical care of large animals have resulted in the need for short- and long-term venous access for the delivery of large volumes of IV fluids, medications, such as sedation and analgesics, antibiotics, antiinflammatory drugs, and unfortunately, on occasion euthanasia solutions. In addition, the more frequent use of blood, blood products, and parenteral nutrition has resulted in the need for specialty catheters and delivery systems to minimize catheter-related complications. There are now a wide variety of choices for catheter materials, size, mechanisms for introduction into the vein, and lumen number available. Initially, human catheters were adapted to veterinary use; however, since the emergence of companies, such as Mila International, basic and specialty catheters are now manufactured specifically for veterinary use. Factors that must be considered when selecting the size and type of catheter to be used include the size of the patient, vein to be catheterized, the condition of the patient at presentation, the fluid or medication to be administered through the catheter, the desired rate of administration, expected duration of catheterization, and what is readily available at the time of emergency.

Commercially available IV catheters for large animal use range in size from 10 to 25 gauge and lengths from 1 to 6 inches. The gauge of a catheter is a measurement of its outside diameter. Smaller-gauge catheters have larger outside diameters, which correspond to a larger inside diameter and a higher rate of flow. The size used is dictated by the size of the patient and the treatment to be administered. Large-diameter catheters (10 to 14 gauge × 5.25 inches) are most commonly used for the administration of IV fluids and medication to adult horses. Foals, ponies, and miniature horses are typically catheterized with smaller 16- to 18-gauge catheters ranging from 3.5 to 5.25 inches in length. In addition to size, fluids with higher viscosity, such as blood or plasma, are more easily administered through large-diameter catheters.

Catheters with a large internal diameter permit more rapid administration of fluid, but have the disadvantage of being more damaging to the vein. Catheters of small diameter, 18 to 25 gauge, are reserved for special uses, such as arterial blood pressure monitoring, where they are placed in small peripheral arteries, such as the facial, transverse facial, or metatarsal artery.

Catheter material also affects the choice of catheters. Commonly used materials for manufacture of catheters include polypropylene, PVC, polytetrafluoroethylene (Teflon), nylon, silicone rubber (Silastic), polyurethane, and polyether block amide (Pebax). Different materials result in catheters of different internal diameters, lengths, and stiffness. The differences in material characteristics and size of catheters results in differences in their potential to damage the vessel wall and form a thrombus (thrombogenicity). Traditionally, large-diameter catheters have been manufactured using polypropylene and Teflon. These catheters are stiff with large outside diameters and typically contact the vessel wall over their entire length. This contact damages the vascular endothelial lining exposing collagen and initiates the clotting cascade. This can result in the formation of a blood clot (thrombus) or fibrin sheaths that extend the length of the catheter. Contamination of this thrombus with bacteria can cause the development of inflammation or infection of the thrombus and vein termed thrombophlebitis. Catheters manufactured from silicone (Silastic), polyurethane, or Pebax have the advantage of being softer than Teflon or polypropylene and tend to float in the lumen of the vein. This decreases the thrombogenic potential of the catheter. A disadvantage of Silastic catheters is their porosity that predisposed them to bacterial adherence. For this reason, Silastic catheters must be placed under strict aseptic conditions. As a general rule, large-diameter catheters made of polypropylene or Teflon should only be used for short duration (12 to 24 hours) and are inappropriate for use in small patients, such as foals. Catheters manufactured from Silastic, polyurethane, or Pebax can be maintained as long as 2 to 3 weeks depending on the manufacturer's recommendations.

The process of introduction of the catheter into the vein is also variable depending on the size and material the catheter is made from. Short-term Teflon and polypropylene catheters and 14- and 16-gauge polyurethane catheters are most commonly purchased as over-the-needle catheters (Figure 33-108). These have the advantage of simple insertion into the vein with minimal training necessary and low cost. Silastic catheters and certain styles of polyurethane catheters used in foals are of an over-the-wire design. For these catheters, a flexible wire is inserted into the vein before catheterization. The wire acts as a guide for the flexible catheter to follow to ensure proper placement without kinking (Figure 33-109). These catheters are less thrombogenic and have fewer catheter-related complications, such as kinking or breaking. Their disadvantages include expense, the need for added training and practice for correct insertion, and they require absolute sterile preparation for administration. Peel-away introducers are also available that allow catheter placement through a preplaced introducer. After passage of the catheter through the introducer, it is split into two halves for easy removal from the vein.

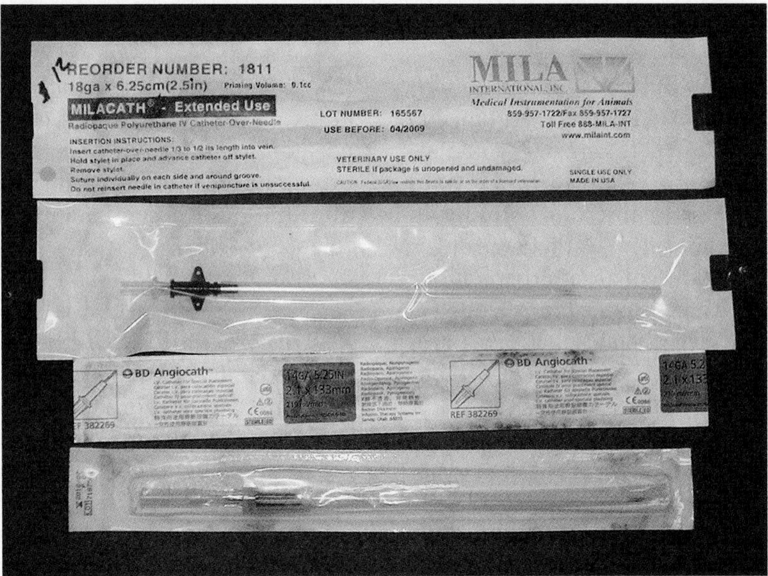

FIGURE 33-108 Example of over-the-needle catheters.

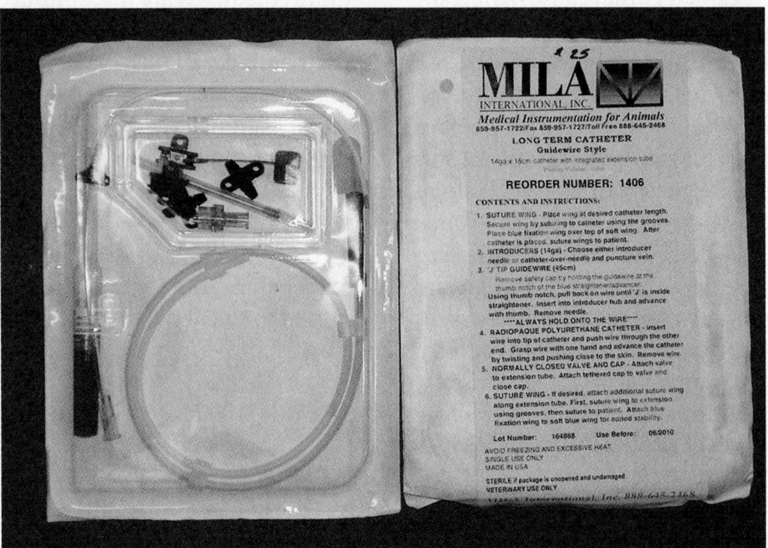

FIGURE 33-109 Example of an over-the-wire catheter.

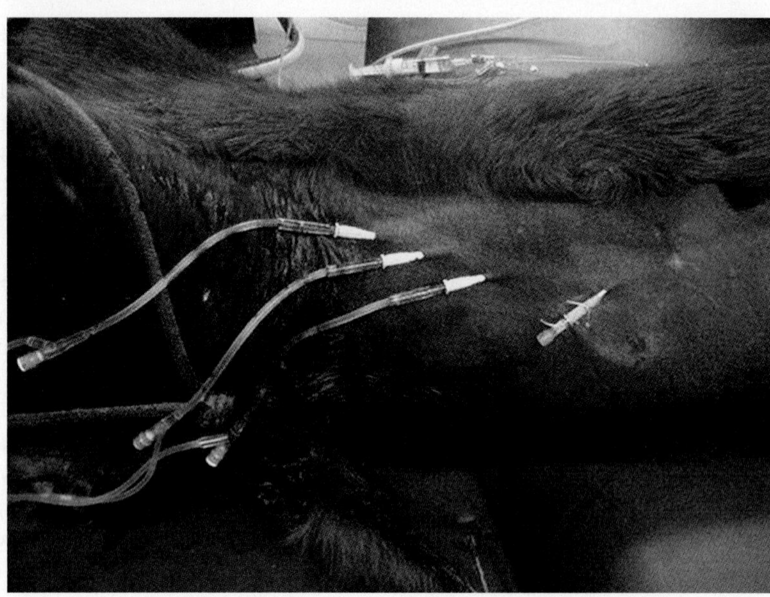

FIGURE 33-110 IV catheters stacked in a single vein for rapid delivery of large volumes of IV fluids.

Specialized catheters for the simultaneous administration of IV fluid, total parenteral nutrition (TPN), blood products, and medication are also available. These catheters come in double- or triple-lumen configurations with over-the-wire or peel-away introducers for ease of insertion. Multiport catheters must maintain continuous flow of fluids through each lumen. Stagnation of fluid flow enhances proliferation of bacteria that may have gained access to the ports. Double- or triple-lumen catheters used when additional ports are no longer needed should be replaced with a single-lumen catheter.

In emergency situations, adult horses frequently arrive at the hospital seriously dehydrated and in shock. These patients require large volumes of fluid to be administered in a short period of time. These horses are best treated by insertion of a large catheter, such as a 10-gauge Teflon catheter for initial fluid volume replacement. Because of their size and the material used to manufacture these catheters, they cause significant damage to the vein and predispose the horse to catheter-related complications. Therefore they should be used for only short periods of time (12 to 24 hours) and removed once the fluid deficit has been replaced. An alternative plan is to place multiple catheters. This may be accomplished in several ways. First, a 10-gauge catheter can be placed alone and replaced with a smaller 14- to 16-gauge catheter once the initial volume deficit has been replaced. This is frequently accomplished by passing a guidewire through the original catheter, removing the 10-gauge catheter by passing it over the guidewire, and replacing it with a smaller catheter placed over the wire. This technique has also been demonstrated to be successful at treating catheter-associated infection without jeopardizing additional veins. Alternatively a 10-gauge catheter may be positioned opposite to a smaller catheter and removed once fluid deficits are corrected. Finally, multiple smaller catheters, usually 14- to 16-gauge, may be placed in multiple veins or stacked in the same vein if large-diameter catheters are not available (Figure 33-110). Fourteen- to 16-gauge catheters are most commonly employed once fluid deficits have been replaced and are used primarily for continued maintenance fluids and the administration of other therapeutic agents, such as antibiotics (Figure 33-111).

Catheter Maintenance

Regardless of the type of catheter and the duration of use, the catheter and surrounding skin should be examined at least two times per day for evidence of heat surrounding the insertion site, swelling around the catheter or a cordlike swelling of the catheterized vein, pain on palpation, or drainage around the catheter insertion site. These may be signs of inflammation or infection of the subcutaneous tissue surrounding the catheter or thrombophlebitis. Catheters with a continuous flow of fluids do not require regular flushing unless the fluids are discontinued. Catheters that are not removed following discontinuation of fluids, those used for the administration of IV medication, and unused lumens of multilumen catheters should be flushed with heparinized saline solutions two to four times per day. Flushing ensures that the catheter remains patent and prevents stagnant flow in the unused catheter lumen and bacterial colonization. If signs of subcutaneous infection around the catheter or thrombophlebitis arise, the catheter should be removed immediately and the catheter tip aseptically collected and submitted for bacterial culture and sensitivity.

TECHNICIAN NOTE IV catheters and the surrounding skin should be examined at least two times per day for evidence of heat, swelling around the catheter or a cordlike swelling of the catheterized vein, pain on palpation, or drainage from the catheter insertion site.

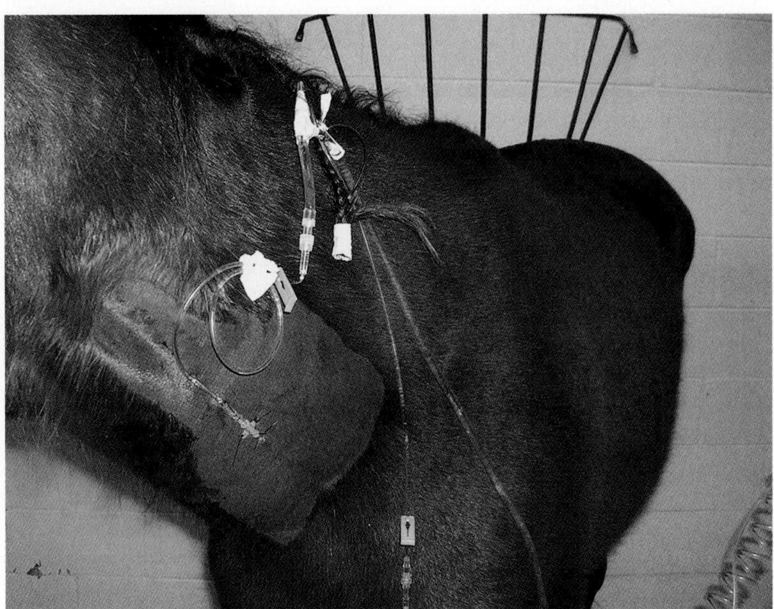

FIGURE 33-111 IV fluid administration through a 14-gauge catheter.

Fluid Therapy Plan

Fluid therapy can be performed by the administration of oral or IV fluids in the horse. In most emergency situations, fluid administration is for the purpose of replacing the extracellular fluid lost to gastrointestinal disease; therefore oral administration of fluid for replacement is often contraindicated. IV fluids are employed to correct acute dehydration and to maintain the circulating plasma volume in the face of ongoing fluid loss (diarrhea, gastric reflux, ileus, etc.). Three basic questions must be answered when designing a fluid therapy plan:

1. What type of fluid is to be administered?
2. How much fluid will be administered?
3. At what rate will the fluid be administered?

In most cases, isotonic crystalloid fluids are used for the initial replacement of fluid in horses with dehydration and hypovolemic shock. Two broad classifications of replacement fluids are available for use in horses: normal saline (0.9% sodium chloride) and balanced polyionic electrolyte solutions (LRS, Normasol-R, and Plasma-Lyte). Normal saline is much higher in sodium and chloride than plasma, but contains no other electrolytes. Its use is primarily as a replacement solution in conditions where plasma sodium levels are less than 125 mEq/L or in disease conditions where potassium-free solutions are desired, such as HYPP, urinary bladder rupture in foals, or renal failure.

The electrolyte composition of most commercially available balanced electrolyte fluids for horses is essentially the same as that found in plasma. The use of balanced electrolyte solutions is to replace the fluid volume and electrolytes lost from the extracellular space acutely. Once the fluid to be administered is decided, additional electrolytes can be added to the stock solution to correct specific electrolyte deficiencies and to correct acid-base deficits. Potassium, calcium, and magnesium are frequently supplemented intravenously in horses that are unable to ingest food or water because of gastrointestinal disease. These electrolytes are rapidly depleted in patients without oral intake of food or water and are essential for normal cardiac and smooth muscle function. If electrolyte solutions or other medications are added to stock solutions of fluid, the bags should be clearly labeled with the additive, the concentration, amount added, and the date the fluid was mixed.

Bicarbonate is supplemented in patients suffering from severe metabolic acidosis, most commonly foals. Dehydration leads to decreased tissue perfusion and a change from aerobic to anaerobic metabolism at the cellular level. The end product of anaerobic metabolism is lactic acid that causes a decrease in plasma pH and lactic acidemia. In most cases, the administration of IV fluid rapidly improves tissue perfusion, and lactic acidemia is corrected without specific therapy. In patients where plasma pH is less than 7.2, bicarbonate supplementation is required. The dose of bicarbonate to be replaced is calculated as:

$$\text{mEq bicarbonate} = (0.6 \times \text{body weight in kg}) \times (\text{normal bicarbonate} - \text{measured bicarbonate})$$

0.6 represents an estimation of volume of total body fluid. This number is different for foals and adults. For foals, 0.6 is the correct estimation because a greater percentage of body mass is made up of water. In adults needing bicarbonate supplementation, 0.3 is used as an estimate of volume of total body fluid.

Sodium bicarbonate solutions are mixed in sterile water or saline for administration. Bicarbonate cannot be administered with fluids containing calcium. Mixing of bicarbonate with calcium-containing fluid will result in the formation of an insoluble precipitate. Patients receiving IV bicarbonate must have normal respiratory function for excess carbon dioxide to be expired or acidemia will worsen. One half of the calculated dose is replaced over 4 to 6 hours with the remainder administered over 12 to 24 hours.

TABLE 33-4 Estimation of the Percentage Dehydration in Horses

Severity of Dehydration	% Dehydration	Clinical Signs
Mild	5-6	Normal mucous membranes, normal to slightly prolonged skin tent, CRT 1-2 sec
Moderate	7-9	Tacky mucous membranes, mildly prolonged skin tent, CRT 2-4 sec
Severe	>9	Dry mucous membranes, prolonged skin tent, CRT >4 sec

Once the type of fluid to be administered is determined, the volume to be administered is calculated. When developing an initial fluid therapy plan, three components must be accounted for to adequately correct and maintain hydration:

1. The volume to be replaced
2. The volume required for maintenance
3. The volume of continued loss

To determine the volume of fluid to be replaced, an estimation of the percent dehydration must be made. Dehydration is a subjective estimation that requires frequent reevaluation to determine if dehydration is being corrected. The simplest estimation is based on a scale of mild, moderate, and severe dehydration (Table 33-4).

The percent dehydration is multiplied by the estimated body weight of the patient to determine the replacement fluid volume.

Maintenance fluid needs are relatively straightforward. The average adult horse requires 50 to 60 ml/kg/24-hr period. Foals have a higher total body water percentage and therefore a higher maintenance requirement usually 100 ml/kg/24 hr.

Continued losses can be roughly estimated or measured directly, such as volume of gastric reflux collected over a 24-hour period. Estimation of 1 to 4 L is not uncommon, or continued loss can be estimated as a multiplication of maintenance (1.5 to two times maintenance).

These volumes are added together to give an estimation of the volume of fluid to be administered to a patient over a 24-hour period. Usually the replacement volume is administered over 4 to 6 hours with the remainder over the next 18 to 24 hours. A typical fluid therapy plane is illustrated in Box 33-4 for a 500-kg horse. This example will be used for the remainder of this chapter.

Frequent reassessment of the patient's physical condition and monitoring of PCV, TP, BUN, creatinine, and electrolytes are necessary to adjust the volume and rate of fluid administration and any additives.

Rate of Administration

Although the rate of fluid delivery can be determined by simple calculation, the volume of fluid delivered to equine patients makes estimating an accurate rate difficult. Most horses seen in the hospital on an emergency basis are initially administered a "shock" dose of fluids equivalent to 60 to 90 ml/kg/hr. Fluid rate is usually calculated as drops per second. As can be seen in the example in Box 33-5, the number of calculated drops per second cannot be accurately measured and is essentially equal to a fluid rate that is a constant wide open stream. In these cases, the volume of fluid delivered should be estimated by the graduations marked on the fluid bag. The volume should be recorded in the medical record every 1 to 2 hours and the rate adjusted as needed to deliver the desired amount of fluid.

Once the initial fluid deficit has been replaced, the fluid rate should be slowed to meet the requirements for maintenance and continued loss. This rate can be calculated as in Box 33-6.

BOX 33-4 A Typical Fluid Therapy Plan for a 500-kg Horse That is 8% Dehydrated

500-kg horse
Estimated dehydration: 8%

1. Rehydration:
   % estimated dehydration × weight in kg
   0.08 × 500 kg = 40 L — 40 L
2. Maintenance:
   Adult: 50 ml/kg/day
   50 ml/kg/24 hr × 500 kg = 25,000 ml = 25 L — 25 L/24 hr
3. Continued loss:
   Estimate volume: 2-5 L/hr
   2 L/hr × 12 hr = 24 L — 24 L
   OR
   Multiple of maintenance 1.5-3 × maintenance
   2 × 25 L = 50 L/24 hr = 25 L/12 hr

Total 89 L

BOX 33-5 Calculation for Delivery Rate of Replacement Fluid

Initial Fluid Delivery Rate

Example 1 60 ml/hr (shock dose)

500 kg × 60 ml/kg/hr = 30,000 ml/hr (30 L/hr)
30,000 ml × 10 drops/ml = 300,000 drops/hr

$$\frac{300{,}000 \text{ drops/hr}}{60 \text{ min/hr}} = 5000 \text{ drops/min}$$

$$\frac{5000 \text{ drops/min}}{60 \text{ sec/min}} = 83 \text{ drops/sec}$$

Example 2 Replacement volume of 40 L to be replaced in 6 hr

40 L/6 hr = 6.7 L/hr
6.7 L × 1000 ml/L = 6700 ml/hr
6700 ml/hr × 10 drops/ml = 67,000 drops/hr

$$\frac{67{,}000 \text{ drops/hr}}{60 \text{ min/hr}} = 1117 \text{ drops/hr}$$

$$\frac{1117 \text{ drops/hr}}{60 \text{ sec/min}} = 18.6 \text{ drops/sec}$$

BOX 33-6 Fluid Rate for Maintenance and Continued Losses

Maintenance and Continued Loss Fluid Rate

49 L/24 hr = 2 L/hr

2 L × 1000 ml/L = 2000 ml

2000 ml/hr × 10 drops = 20,000 drops/hr

$$\frac{20{,}000 \text{ drops/hr}}{60 \text{ min/hr}} = 333.4 \text{ drops/min}$$

$$\frac{333.4 \text{ drops/min}}{60 \text{ sec/min}} = 5.5 \text{ drops/sec}$$

This can be counted as 55 drops/10 sec.

Also note that this approximates two times maintenance as described previously.

Hypertonic Saline Solution

Hypertonic saline solutions used in equine veterinary medicine consist of a 7.2% solution of sodium chloride usually packaged in 1-L bottles. Hypertonic saline has an almost immediate, though short-lived, effect on the circulating plasma by drawing fluid from the interstitial and intracellular space into the vasculature. Plasma volume expansion results in increased cardiac output, improved blood pressure, better oxygen delivery to and better oxygen use by the tissues. Hypertonic saline is administered at a dose of 4 ml/kg over 5 to 10 minutes. It rapidly expands circulating plasma volume; however, its effects last for approximately 60 minutes.

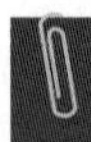
TECHNICIAN NOTE Hypertonic saline is administered at a dose of 4 ml/kg over 5 to 10 minutes.

Colloids

Hydroxyethyl starches, also known as synthetic colloids, are high-molecular-weight molecules that function similar to the natural colloid albumin in the circulatory system. When administered intravenously to horses suffering from dehydration and hypovolemic shock, they exert oncotic pressure that serves to maintain plasma volume and peripheral perfusion. The advantages of synthetic colloids over albumin include lower antigenicity, and because of their larger molecular weight, they tend to remain in the circulation for a longer period of time. In conditions where albumin is lost from the circulation as a result of increased capillary permeability, IV administration of albumin will only result in further redistribution of albumin to the interstitial space. Synthetic colloid will remain in the intravascular space longer, exerting its oncotic effect for up to 120 hours. Hetastarch is the most commonly used synthetic colloid in the United States. It is administered at a dose of 10 ml/kg of a 6% solution. Disadvantages of hetastarch include expense, the association of bleeding disorders with its use, and the inability to measure the oncotic effect of colloids by refractometer.

BLOOD AND BLOOD PRODUCTS

Blood loss and anemia in horses is caused by one of three mechanisms: whole blood loss, erythrocyte destruction, or the failure to produce erythrocytes. Whole blood loss is the most common cause for anemia in horses and presents most frequently as an emergency. Significant blood loss in horses is most commonly associated with wounds involving the neurovascular supply of the distal limb, middle uterine artery rupture in mares, guttural pouch mycosis, hemolytic anemias, and neonatal isoerythrolysis in foals.

On average, blood constitutes approximately 8% of the horse's body weight. This means that an average 500-kg horse has a blood volume of approximately 40 L. This estimate varies depending on the age, breed, and use of the horse and can range from 7% to 15%. The horse can lose approximately 20% of its total circulating blood volume without demonstrating clinical signs. When acute blood loss occurs, the immediate response by the body is to ensure the delivery of oxygen to the vital organs, such as the heart and brain. Hemorrhage of greater than one third of the circulating blood volume can result in irreversible shock and death. This is the result of inadequate oxygen delivery to the tissues. Therefore the goal of treatment of acute anemia or blood loss is to maintain appropriate oxygen delivery to the tissue.

TECHNICIAN NOTE On average, blood constitutes approximately 8% of the horse's body weight that is equivalent to 40 L in a 500-kg horse.

Oxygen delivery to the tissue is affected by two primary mechanisms: (1) cardiac output and (2) oxygen content of the blood reaching the tissues. The oxygen content of the blood is dependent on hemoglobin concentration and is directly related to the RBC mass. Whole blood loss affects oxygen delivery not only by the loss of erythrocytes and hemoglobin, but also the loss of plasma. This decreased plasma volume causes a decrease in the amount of blood pumped by each contraction of the heart (stroke volume) and therefore the total amount of blood pumped by the heart to the tissues (cardiac output). The loss of RBCs and hemoglobin decreases the oxygen-carrying capacity of the blood.

In response to blood loss, the body has several compensatory mechanisms to maintain cardiac output and oxygen delivery. Immediate compensatory responses include peripheral vasoconstriction, splenic contraction (the spleen can maintain up to 30% of the circulating erythrocyte mass), and a shift of fluid from the interstitial space to the intravascular space.

The decision to perform a blood transfusion is often difficult and should not be taken lightly. Blood transfusion is an invasive procedure requiring the catheterization and collection of blood from the donor potentially creating a situation of acute blood loss and the administration of the collected blood to the recipient. This process is time and labor intensive and may add significant cost to the therapy. In addition, undesirable transfusion reactions that range in severity from mild urticaria to acute anaphylaxis and death have been reported in horses. Compensatory mechanisms and the loss of equivalent concentrations of fluid, cells, and protein with whole blood loss can make the decision to perform a blood transfusion based on hematologic values potentially inaccurate. Hematologic measurements, such as PCV and TP concentrations, may take up to 24 hours after the initial blood loss to change significantly. Therefore the decision to perform a blood transfusion should always be based on the nature of the illness or injury, a history of known large volume blood loss, clinical signs, and hematologic measurements (Box 33-7).

The clinical signs exhibited by the horse following acute hemorrhage are the result of a combination of hypovolemia and decreased erythrocyte mass. These signs are consistently observed in horses with anemia regardless of the underlying cause and can include tachycardia, tachypnea, lethargy, inappetence, depression, colic, sweating, cold extremities, and pale mucous membranes.

Clinicopathologic changes are dependent on the time between presentation and changes in signs because of the previously described compensatory mechanisms. In a recent review of 31 horses treated by blood transfusion, only 11 of 18 (61%) horses with acute blood loss had PCV or hemoglobin levels less than the normal reference range. When present, clinicopathologic abnormalities may include decreased PCV and TP, increased creatinine and BUN levels, and decreased oxygen saturation.

BOX 33-7 General Recommendations for Blood Transfusion

PCV <20% following acute hemorrhage
PCV <12%-14% following chronic hemorrhage
Clinical signs consistent with hypovolemia following acute hemorrhage

BOX 33-8 Blood Typing Laboratories

Equine Blood Typing Research Laboratory
University of Kentucky
Department of Veterinary Science
Lexington, KY 40546
859-257-3022

Serology Laboratory
University of California
Davis, CA 95616
530-752-9284

Stormont Laboratory
1237 E. Beamer St. Suite D
Woodland, CA 95776
530-661-3078

Mann Equitest, Inc.
335 Laird Rd. Unit 4
Guelph, Ontario N1H 6J3
Canada
519-836-2400

TECHNICIAN NOTE Clinical signs consistent with blood loss in horses regardless of the underlying cause can include tachycardia, tachypnea, lethargy, inappetence, depression, colic, sweating, cold extremities, and pale mucous membranes.

Blood Transfusion

Transfusion of whole blood to the anemic patient has been demonstrated to result in a significant improvement in PCV, creatinine, and oxygen saturation and a significant improvement in clinical signs. An organized well-thought-out plan must be established and personnel trained to proceed through the process in a systematic fashion. This will minimize the cost, materials used, and time needed to safely collect the necessary volume of blood from the donor and promptly transfuse the blood to the patient.

Blood Donors

A minimum of two blood donors should be available at all times. These may be horses housed at the practice or client-owned horses in which special arrangements have been made for their use as donors. Unlike humans that have three blood types (A, B, and O), horses have seven different blood types represented by capital letters A, C, D, P, K, Q, and U and up to 30 factors in each type designated by lower case letters. Also unlike humans, there is no universal equine blood donor. Identification of the most appropriate donor should be made well in advance of the need for transfusion. Blood can be collected from potential donors and sent to a number of veterinary laboratories for typing (Box 33-8).

The most desirable donors are geldings with no history of receiving a blood transfusion and Aa and Oa negative because these are the most immunogenic erythrocyte antigens. Donors should have a complete well-maintained health record and should receive regularly scheduled vaccinations, deworming, an annual enzyme immunoassay (EIA) (Coggins) test, and have routine dental and foot care performed.

Larger blood donors are desirable to allow a greater volume of blood to be collected. Although 450 kg is a minimum weight, horses greater than 550 kg are more desirable. Mares and horses with a history of previous transfusion have a greater risk for antierythrocyte antibodies (Box 33-9).

A PCV and TP should be performed on all donor horses before blood collection. Donors with PCV less than 35 or a TP of less than 6 should not be used. A healthy donor 500 kg

BOX 33-9 Desirable Blood Donor Characteristics

>450 kg
Gelding
Free of blood-borne diseases
In good health
No previous transfusion or pregnancy if a mare
Aa, Oa, and hemolysin negative
PCV >35 and TP >6.0

in body weight with a PCV of 35% to 40% can safely donate up to 8 L (20% of blood volume) of blood every 30 days.

> *TECHNICIAN NOTE* At the time of blood collection, donor horses should have a PCV of at least 35 and a TP of at least 6.0 mg/dl.

Blood Collection

A blood collection kit containing all necessary supplies can be organized and stored for ready use. Technical staff should be adequately trained in the process of blood collection and the process rehearsed to ensure that it is carried out efficiently.

Blood can be collected into a number of containers, including sterilized glass jars, commercial blood collection bottles containing acid-citrate-dextrose anticoagulant (ACD bottle), specially designed bags for blood collection, and gas-sterilized fluid bags. The container determines the type of anticoagulant used. ACD bottles have the advantage of a vacuum that allows rapid collection of blood; however, the disadvantage when used for blood collection in horses is their size, damage to the erythrocytes from impact on the bottle, inactivation of platelets by the glass, and risk of breaking the glass (Figure 33-112). ACD bottles also require additional tubing for the collection process. Commercially available plastic blood bags for blood collection in horses have the advantage of preservation of platelet function, less erythrocyte damage, the ability to collect large volumes in a single container, and no risk of breakage (Figure 33-113). Their disadvantage is that collection is by gravity flow and can be time consuming.

A crew composed of three individuals is recommended for safe, efficient blood collection. One person handles the horse, one manages the catheter, and one controls the blood collection device. The area over the donor's jugular vein is aseptically prepared and 2 to 5 ml of local anesthetic are locally infused over the proposed catheter or needle site. Blood can be collected safely through a larger needle (14-gauge × 1.5-inch), a specialized blood collection trochar (8- to 11-gauge × 75-mm), or IV catheter (14-gauge × 5.5-inch). Venous access should be directed in the opposite direction of normal blood flow to speed collection. The vein may need to be occluded continuously to distend the vein and speed collection. The blood must be collected into the chosen collection device under strict asepsis.

Standard ACD bottles contain enough ACD to collect 450 ml of blood. The amount of ACD in bags is dependent on the volume of the bag. When using a sterilized glass bottle, enough ACD should be added to the bottle to produce a ratio of 9 parts blood: 1 part ACD (2000 ml total volume = 200 ml ACD: 1800 ml whole blood). Although not commonly used as an anticoagulant for blood transfusions, in an emergency situation heparin can be added to sterile glass bottles for immediate collection and administration. When using heparin as an anticoagulant, 625 IU heparin is used per 50 ml of blood collected, and the blood should be administered immediately. The bottle or bag should be gently swirled or rocked during the collection to ensure proper mixing of the blood and anticoagulant. If collecting blood into bottles, once the bottle is full, the tubing should be clamped near the bottle and the needle removed from the stopper. To maintain strict asepsis, needles should be changed in between

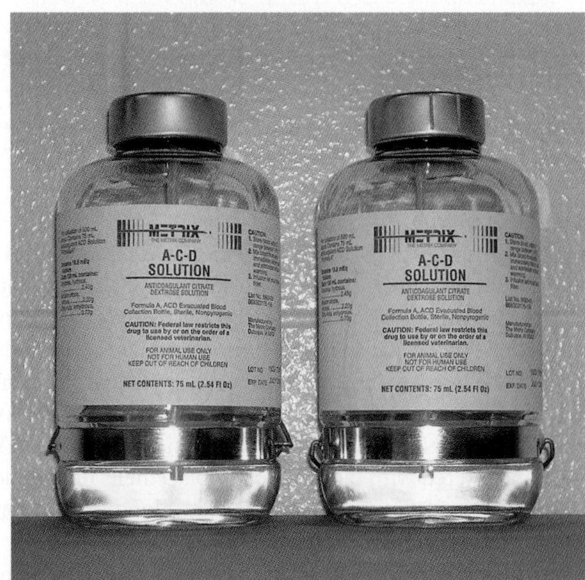

FIGURE 33-112 ACD glass bottles for the collection of blood.

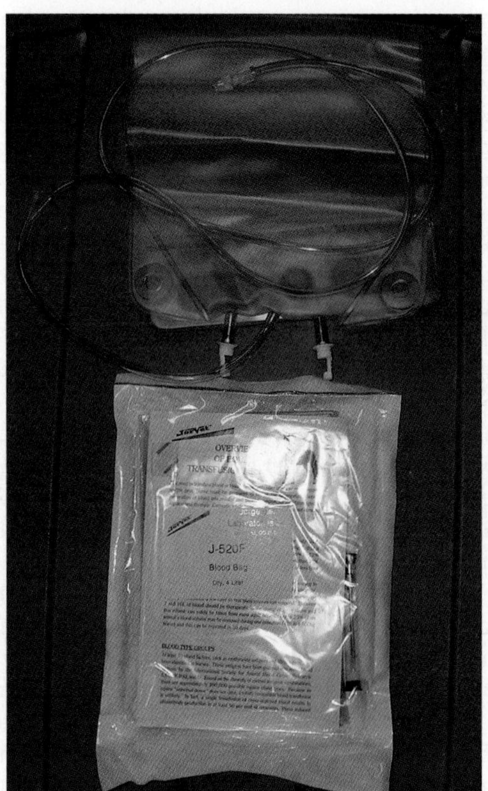

FIGURE 33-113 Commercially available blood collection bags for horses.

bottles before resuming collection. The tubing attached to bags should be stripped of residual blood, tied in three knots, or clamped and cut below the clamp. Following blood collection, donors from whom 20% of the blood volume has been removed should receive 5 to 20 L crystalloid fluids to prevent signs consistent with hypovolemia. They should also receive 1 to 3 lb of complete feed and free-choice water. The catheter site should be examined two times per day for signs of heat, pain, or swelling for the next 5 to 7 days.

Crossmatching

Crossmatching is an in vitro screening test used to assist in the detection of incompatibilities between donor and recipient blood. The incompatibilities are the result of antibodies present in the serum of the donor or recipient to the other's erythrocytes. Incompatibilities are recognized by clumping (agglutination) of erythrocytes following mixing of donor and recipient erythrocytes and plasma or hemolysis after the addition of rabbit complement to this mixture. The two components of this screening test are the major and minor crossmatch. The major is highly recommended by most authors and involves the mixing of recipient plasma or serum with donor erythrocytes. A minor crossmatch is considered optional in situations where the donor has no known exposure to the blood of other individuals and consists of mixing donor plasma or serum with recipient erythrocytes. Box 33-10 provides step-by-step instructions for performing major and minor crossmatching.

Although highly recommended, the limitations of equine crossmatching must be understood. False-positive and false-negative reactions are commonly observed as a result of spontaneous rouleaux formation, which must be distinguished from agglutination. Rouleau is described as the microscopic appearance of linear stacks of erythrocytes similar to stacks of coins. Agglutination is the irregular spherical clumping of erythrocytes observed under the microscope. Agglutination can be confirmed by mixing a small quantity of blood with normal saline. If present, agglutination will persist after mixing, and rouleaux will disperse. In addition, various amounts of agglutination are present in all crossmatch reactions, and it is difficult to determine at what level agglutination is considered incompatible. Therefore incompatibilities may only be recognized with large amounts of agglutination. Finally the most serious transfusion reactions occur as a result of erythrocyte hemolysis rather than agglutination. Lysis is only observed following the addition of complement, a procedure that is impractical in most practice settings and usually only performed in blood typing laboratories. Therefore crossmatching has its greatest value when reaction between donor and recipient blood is severe (large amounts of agglutination) indicating an obvious incompatibility. Transfusion reaction may still occur even after blood has been determined to be compatible by crossmatching. In most cases, naturally occurring antibodies to equine erythrocytes are uncommon, and a transfusion can be safely administered without crossmatching. Blood should initially be administered slowly and the recipient observed for clinical signs of a transfusion reaction and the transfusion slowed or discontinued if signs increase in severity or persist.

BOX 33-10 Crossmatch Procedure

Materials

1. EDTA anticoagulated blood and serum form recipient and donor
2. Pipette and tips accurate up to 0.05-0.1 ml
3. 37° C water bath or incubator
4. Microscope

Procedure

1. Into appropriately labeled donor and recipient tubes pipette 2-4 drops of whole blood from each donor and recipient and fill to within 1 cm of the top with normal saline.
2. Cover the tubes with parafilm (wax paper) film and mix thoroughly.
3. In a tabletop centrifuge, centrifuge for 1 min at maximum speed and decant the saline supernatant. There will be some residual saline in the bottom of the tube.
4. Gently strum the bottom of the tube to resuspend the pellet, fill again with saline, and repeat steps 2 and 3.
5. Gently resuspend the cells in the saline at the bottom of the tube and add approximately 4.7 ml of additional saline. The residual volume is approximately 0.3 ml. Addition of 4.7 ml will result in a solution of erythrocytes of approximately 6%.
6. Label 1 tube autocontrol. For each donor, label two tubes major/donor ID and minor/donor ID.
7. To each tube labeled major, add 0.1 ml recipient serum, and then add 0.05 ml of the 6% donor cell suspension to the corresponding major/donor ID tube.
8. To each tube labeled minor, add 0.1 ml of donor serum from the appropriate donor, then add 0.5 ml recipient 6% cell suspension.
9. To the tube labeled autocontrol, add 0.1 ml recipient serum and 0.05 ml recipient cell suspension.
10. Mix all tubes well and centrifuge at maximum speed for 30 seconds.
11. Gently shake the cells to slowly loosen them from the pellet and observe grossly for agglutination or hemolysis (red supernatant).
12. Centrifuge tube again 30 seconds at maximum speed and repeat step 11. Place a drop of suspension on a microscope slide and observe at 10x power for agglutination.

Administration

The recipient should have an IV catheter placed aseptically. Infusion should be performed only through a specialized blood delivery infusion set with an in-line filter (Figure 33-114). Some authors recommend replacing the infusion set after every 4 L of blood administered. Although seldom are crystalloid fluids and blood administered simultaneously, if this is practiced, normal saline (0.9% NaCl) is the only crystalloid fluid that can be safely administered with blood. Most replacement fluids, such as LRS, contain calcium, which can initiate blood clotting, and hypotonic fluids, such as dextrose, can cause hemolysis.

The volume of blood to be transfused can be estimated by two methods:

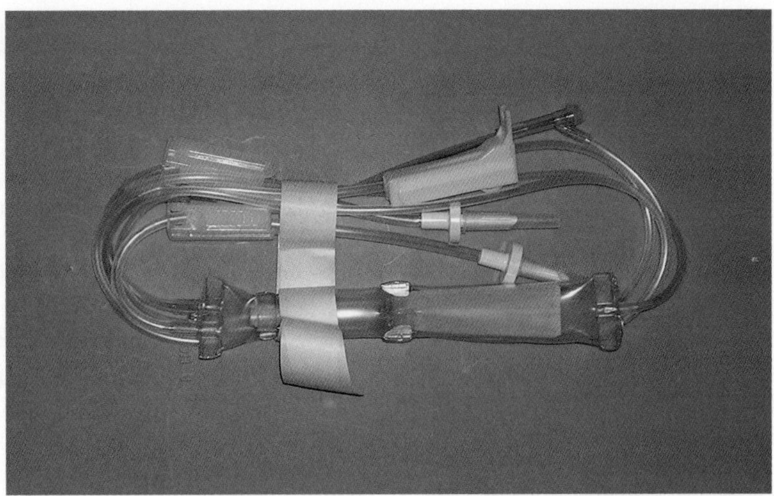

FIGURE 33-114 Blood delivery set with an in-line filter.

$$\text{Body weight (kg)} \times \text{recipient blood volume (ml/kg)} \times \frac{\textit{PCV desired} - \textit{PCV observed}}{\text{PCV donor}}$$

This calculation is based on a normal blood volume in the adult horse of 72 ml/kg and of 151 ml/kg in the neonate.

By this calculation, an average 500-kg adult with a PCV of 15 and a desired PCV of 25 would require 10.28 L.

$$500 \text{ kg} \times 72 \times \frac{25 - 15}{35} = 10{,}285 \text{ ml or } 10.28 \text{ L}$$

An alternative is simply to calculate 10 to 20 ml of blood/kg body weight

$$500 \text{ kg} \times 20 \text{ ml/kg} = 10{,}000 \text{ ml or } 10 \text{ L}$$

A recent retrospective study in horses demonstrated a 4% increase in PCV and significant improvement in clinical signs of horses with acute blood loss after the administration of 15 ml/kg whole blood.

The administration of blood should be closely monitored for signs of transfusion reactions. There are many published recommendations regarding the frequency of monitoring. The author has used a rate of 5 ml/kg/hr as an initial infusion rate with monitoring of the recipient's temperature, pulse, and respiration every 5 minutes for the first 15 minutes. If no signs of a transfusion reaction develop, the rate is increased to 10 to 25 ml/kg/hr while observing the patient continuously and monitoring and recording temperature, pulse, and respiration every 30 minutes. Signs of a transfusion reaction are variable and may include urticaria, dyspnea, tachypnea, tachycardia, fever, restlessness, muscle fasciculations, sudden recumbency, anaphylactic shock, and death. Depending on the severity of the signs, if observed, the transfusion should be slowed or discontinued.

Plasma Transfusion

Plasma is the cell-free portion of blood. Its constituents include colloids, such as albumin and other small protein; electrolytes; immunoglobulin (antibodies); antibacterial protein, such as complement; and clotting factors. The indications for plasma administration in horses are numerous and may include hypoproteinemia or hypoalbuminemia, failure of passive transfer, septicemia or endotoxemia, DIC, warfarin toxicity, and the treatment and prevention of specific disease for which antitoxic and passive immunization plasma have been developed. Although equine plasma readily separates from erythrocytes without the aid or expensive plasmapheresis equipment, collection of this plasma is both labor and time consuming and must be performed under the strictest of aseptic conditions. The collection of quantities large enough to treat most equine patients cannot be accomplished economically in most practice settings. Equine plasma is available commercially from several manufacturers worldwide (Box 33-11). These companies maintain herds of horses that are specifically for the production of various highly specific plasma products (Box 33-12) that can be shipped and stored frozen for extended periods of time.

Plasma requires thawing before administration. The manufacturer's directions for storage, thawing, and administration of specific plasma products should be consulted before administration. Routinely, plasma is stored at −18° C (the same temperature as a standard refrigerator freezer) and thawed immediately before administration. The most convenient method for thawing is to place the bag in water that is approximately 40° C (approximately 104° F). The plasma should be mixed periodically and cool water replaced until approximately body temperature. Thawing in water that is too hot should be avoided because this can result in the destruction of plasma protein and immunoglobulin. Plasma that is thawed to room temperature or above should not be refrozen for later use. Administration should always be performed through a filtered blood delivery set.

> *TECHNICIAN NOTE* Commercially available FP should be thawed by placing the bag in water that is approximately 104° F.

BOX 33-11 Sources of Equine Plasma

Mg Biologics
2366 270th St
Ames, IA 50014
Phone: 515-769-2340
Fax: 515-769-2390
www.mgbiologics.com

Veterinary Immunogenics, Ltd.
Carleton Hill
Penrith
Cumbria CA11 8TZ
United Kingdom
Phone: +44(0) 1768 863881
Fax: +44(0) 1768 891 389
www.veterinaryimmunogenics.com

Lake Immunogenics, Inc.
348 Berg Rd.
Ontario, NY 14519
Phone: 585-265-1973
Fax: 585-265-2306

Plasvacc USA, Inc.
1535 Templeton Rd.
Templeton, CA 93465
Phone: 800-654-9743
Fax: 805-434-2720
www.plasvaccusa.com

BOX 33-12 Indications for Types of Equine Plasma

Normal
Replacement of albumin, complement clotting factors, and immunoglobulin in adults and foals

Hyper/Polyimmune
Failure of passive transfer in neonatal foals

E. coli* J5/*Salmonella
Treatment of septicemia and endotoxemia in foals and adults

Rhodococcus equi
Passive immunity and prophylaxis before exposure to *R. equi*

***Clostridium botulinum* Type B Antitoxin**
Prophylaxis following exposure to *C. botulinum* by ingestion and antitoxin in clinically affected patients

West Nile Virus
Passive immunity and treatment of clinical cases

Streptococcus equi
Passive immunity and treatment of clinical cases

The volume of plasma to be administered is dependent on the manufacture's recommendation for treatment and prevention of the specific condition for which the plasma is administered or the calculated need based on hypoproteinemia. Plasma transfusion is indicated in horses in which the plasma TP is less than 4 g/L or albumin concentrations are less than 2 g/L. In horses that are hypoproteinemic, the volume of plasma to be administered can be estimated by the following formula:

$$\text{Body weight (kg)} \times \text{blood volume (ml/kg)} \times \frac{\textit{desired albumin} - \textit{observed albumin}}{\text{Donor albumin}}$$

This calculation is based on an estimated plasma volume in the adult horse of 48 ml/kg, 95 ml/kg in the neonate, 62 ml/kg in foals from 1 to 4 weeks of age, and 53 ml/kg in foals from 4 to 12 weeks of age.

Following plasma transfusion, the observed increase in plasma albumin concentration is less than usually expected as a result of redistribution of the albumin to the extravascular space. The volume necessary to significantly increase the TP and albumin concentrations of the blood are large. A minimum of 6 L of normal plasma is required to increase the recipient's albumin concentration 1 to 2 g/L. Although the concentrations do not change appreciably, a dramatic clinical improvement is often observed.

Plasma administration is similar to whole blood and should be performed through a blood delivery set with an in-line filter, and the patient should be carefully observed for signs of transfusion reaction and the transfusion slowed or discontinued if signs are observed.

Blood Substitutes

Oxyglobin (Biopure Corp., Cambridge, Mass.) is an ultrapurified, polymerized bovine hemoglobin in a modified LRS solution that contains13.8 g/dl of hemoglobin. Oxyglobin has been approved for use in dogs and has been used extralabel in foals with neonatal isoerythrolysis as a hemoglobin replacement. This solution increases the oxygen-carrying capacity in anemic patients. Oxyglobin has been used in horses at a dose range between 10 to 30 ml/kg delivered at a rate of 10 to 20 ml/kg/hr. The large hemoglobin molecule also acts as a colloid solution. It is a cell-free hemoglobin solution that lacks erythrocytes and erythrocyte antigens. Therefore crossmatching is not necessary before administration. Other advantages of oxyglobin include a long shelf life (36 months) and no preadministration preparation (off-the-shelf administration) and no need for specialized administration sets.

In limited use in horses, oxyglobin has been used in the treatment of a miniature horse with chronic ovarian bleeding and in foals with NI as a means of controlling clinical signs while blood is collected and processed. Disadvantages of oxyglobin include too high of cost to be used in adult horses, a short plasma half-life thus requiring additional blood products be administered, and evidence that suggests oxyglobin may decrease cardiac output.

CASE PRESENTATION 33-2

History and Signalment

A 12-year-old quarter horse gelding came to the hospital with a 2-day history of moderate to severe abdominal pain. A presumptive diagnosis of a small colon impaction was made by the referring veterinarian, and he was treated with IV fluids and flunixin meglumine for pain. There has been no response to therapy.

Initial Physical Examination

On presentation, the horse was mildly depressed and exhibited intermittent episodes of mild to moderate abdominal pain.

His temperature was 99, pulse 48, and respiration of 16 breaths per minute.

Mucous membranes were pale pink and tacky, and his CRT was 3 seconds. The skin over the eyelids remained persistently tented for 5 to 6 seconds.

He was determined to be moderately (7% to 8%) dehydrated based on physical examination.

This was confirmed by the results of a CBC and chemistry profile that revealed an elevated PCV (42) and TP (7) and what was suspected to be a prerenal azotemia (creatinine: 2.5, normal: 1.4 to 1.7).

His weight was estimated to be approximately 1000 lb (450 kg).

There was no gastric reflux, and a rectal examination revealed an extensive small colon impaction.

Initial Fluid Therapy

1. Replacement Fluids
   (450 kg) (0.08) = 36 L to be administered over 4 hours
   36 L/4 hr = 9 L/hr
   9 L = 9000 ml
   9000 ml/60 min/hr = 150 ml/min
   150 ml/min/60 sec/min = 2.5 ml/sec
   2.5 ml/sec × 10 drops/ml = 25 drops/sec, too fast to count; therefore the rate can only be monitored using the graduations on the fluid bag and adjusting the rate as needed.
2. Maintenance and continued loss
   (450 kg) (50 ml/kg/24 hr) = 22,500 ml or 22.5 L/24 hr
   22.5 L/24 hr = 937 ml/hr
   937 ml/hr/60 min/hr = 15.6 ml/min
   15.6 ml × 10 drops/ml = 156 drops/min
   156 drops/min/60 sec/min = 2.5 drops/sec or 25 drops/10 sec
   Continued loss was considered small and estimated to be 1.5 times maintenance.
   15.6 ml/min × 1.5 = 23.4 ml/min
   23.4 ml/min × 10 drops/ml = 234 drops/min
   234 drops/min/60 sec/min = 3.9 or roughly 4 drops/sec
3. Continued therapy
   As time went on, the horse experienced more pain. Approximately 10 L of gastric reflux was collected, he began to exhibit abdominal distention, and his PCV increased to 48.
   The abnormal rectal examination, gastric reflux, and systemic deterioration were indications for abdominal exploratory surgery.
   The horse was anesthetized with a ventral midline celiotomy, and abdominal exploratory was performed and the small colon impaction relieved.
4. Anesthetic recovery
   The horse stood unassisted approximately 45 minutes after removal from gas anesthesia. Within 5 minutes of standing, he began to exhibit signs of discomfort initially thought to be abdominal pain. These signs progressed to flaring of the nostrils, exaggerated inspiratory efforts, inspiratory stridor, and severe anxiety. A standing emergency tracheotomy was performed, and a temporary tracheotomy tube was positioned and fixed in place with gauze. Oxygen insufflation through the tracheotomy tube was initiated at 15 L/min, and the respiratory signs resolved within minutes. Oxygen insufflation was discontinued after 1 hour. The presumptive diagnosis was acute upper respiratory obstruction resulting from postanesthetic laryngeal spasm.
5. Postoperative care
   The horse remained on IV fluids for 48 hours following surgery. Food was introduced at 24 hours and gradually increased to free-choice hay over 5 days. The tracheotomy tube was intermittently occluded to determine if the laryngeal spasm persisted. The horse was able to breathe normally after 5 days. The tube was removed, and the horse was discharged 7 days after surgery.

RECOMMENDED READINGS

Auer JA, Stick JA, editors: *Equine surgery,* ed 3, St Louis, 2006, Saunders.

Bramlage LR: Current concepts of first aid and transport of the equine fracture patient, *Comp Cont Educ Pract Vet* 5:S564, 1983.

Durham AE: Blood and plasma transfusion in the horse, *Equine Vet Educ* 8(1):8-12, 1996.

Gonzales GL: How to establish an equine blood donor protocol, *AAEP Proc* 47:262-265, 2001.

Mason DE et al: Respiratory emergencies in the adult horse, *Vet Clin North Am: Equine Pract* 10(3):685-701, 1994.

Seahorn TL, Cornick-Seahorn J: Fluid therapy in horses with gastrointestinal disease, *Vet Clin North Am: Equine Pract* 19(3):665-679, 2003.

Slovis NM: How to approach whole blood transfusion in horses, *AAEP Proc* 47:266-269, 2001.

Wilson DA: Principles of early wound management, *Vet Clin North Am: Equine Pract* 21(1):45-62, 2005.

34 Wound Healing, Wound Management, and Bandaging

Giselle Hosgood and Daniel J. Burba

OUTLINE

LEARNING OBJECTIVES

When you have completed this chapter, you will be able to:

1. Describe the process of wound healing.
2. List and describe the factors that affect wound healing.
3. Discuss initial management of wounds in small and large animals.
4. Describe procedures for lavage and débridement of wounds in small and large animals.
5. Differentiate between first intention, second intention, and third intention healing.
6. Discuss indications for bandaging of wounds and describe the general structure of bandages.
7. Describe common types of bandages, slings, splints, and casts used for small and large animals and provide indications for their use.
8. Describe procedures for monitoring of animals with casts, bandages, splints, or slings.
9. Discuss considerations for bandaging of abrasions, lacerations, puncture wounds, and degloving injuries.
10. Describe classifications of burns and discuss management of burn patients.

KEY TERMS

Abrasion
Axillary
Carpal flexion sling
Contamination
Contralateral
Débridement
Decubital ulcer
Ehmer sling
External coaptation
Exudate
First intention healing
Granulation tissue
Hydrocolloid
Hydrophilic
Hypertonic
Inguinal
Laceration
Myofibroblast
Nonadherent dressing
Occlusive dressing
Robert Jones bandage
Second intention healing
Semi permeable dressing
Third intention healing
Velpeau's sling

INTRODUCTION

The veterinary technician can play an important role in assisting the veterinary surgeon in the management of wounds. The nature of the wound often dictates the method of wound management. Knowledge of the physiology of wound healing and the factors that alter wound healing is required to understand the methods of wound management. The methods of wound management, the role of bandaging in wound management, and the different types of bandages can then be more clearly understood.

WOUND HEALING

A wound is created when an insult, either purposeful, such as a surgical incision, or incidental, such as a traumatic injury, disrupts the normal integrity of the tissue. Wound healing is a complex biologic event that is well characterized at the microscopic level, but its regulation at the molecular level is only just beginning to be understood. The process of wound healing begins immediately after the insult and is described in four physical phases: the inflammatory, débridement, repair, and maturation phases (Figure 34-1 and Box 34-1). Wound healing is a dynamic process, and more than one phase of wound healing is usually occurring at any time.

Peptide growth factors appear to play a key role in initiating and sustaining the phases of wound healing (Table 34-1). The platelet appears to initiate the wound healing process through the release of growth factors; the process is then amplified or sustained by wound macrophages, endothelial cells, and fibroblasts. The inflammatory phase begins immediately after injury. Blood fills the wound and cleans the wound surface. The blood vessels constrict immediately to slow hemorrhage, but vasoconstriction lasts only 5 to 10 minutes. The blood vessels then dilate and leak fluid containing clotting elements into the wound. This fluid, combined with blood, causes a blood clot to form. The blood clot stabilizes the wound edges, and fibrin within the clot provides the limited wound strength of this phase. In a sutured wound, the sutures will also provide wound strength at this time. The blood clot will dry and form a scab, which protects the wound, prevents further hemorrhage, and allows healing to progress under its surface. The scab does not provide any wound strength. The blood vessels also leak white blood cells into the wound. This marks the beginning of the débridement phase.

The débridement phase begins approximately 6 hours after injury when white blood cells, namely neutrophils and monocytes, appear in the wound. These cells remove necrotic tissue, bacteria, and foreign material from the wound. The white blood cells in combination with the fluid that has leaked into the wound form the exudate commonly associated with wounds.

TECHNICIAN NOTE During the first 3 to 5 days of wound healing, known as the lag phase, wound strength is minimal.

The repair phase begins after the blood clot has formed and necrotic tissue and foreign material have been removed from the wound. The repair phase, which is usually active by 3 to 5 days after injury, is associated with invasion of fibroblasts into the wound. The fibroblasts produce collagen that will mature into fibrous or scar tissue. The repair phase is characterized by a significant increase in wound strength. In contrast, the first 3 to 5 days after injury are associated with a minimal increase in wound strength. Consequently the first 3 to 5 days are also known as the "lag phase" of wound healing.

Capillaries appear in the wound at the same time fibroblasts appear. The combination of new capillaries, fibroblasts, and fibrous tissue forms the characteristic red, fleshy granulation tissue that fills the wound, often lying underneath the scab.

Granulation tissue characteristically appears in the wound after 3 to 5 days. Poor granulation tissue is white and has a high fibrous tissue content with fewer capillaries. Granulation tissue is important in wound healing because it fills the tissue defect, protects the wound, provides a barrier to infection, provides a surface for new epithelial cells to form across, and provides a source of special fibroblasts called myofibroblasts, which are responsible for wound contraction.

The formation of new epithelium on the wound surface (epithelialization) occurs during the repair phase and begins once an adequate granulation tissue bed has formed. New epithelium is usually visible on a wound in 4 to 5 days. In an

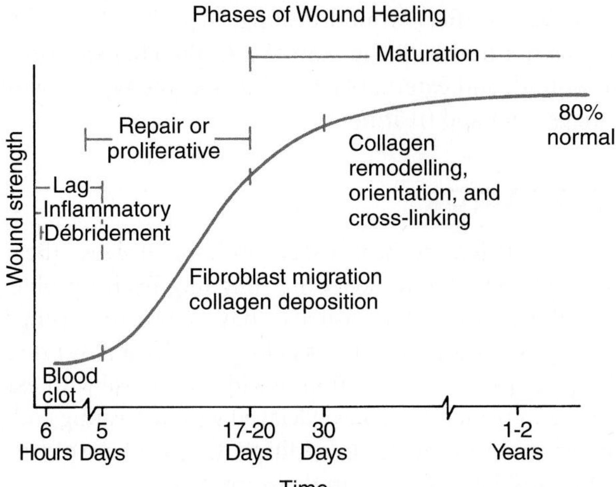

FIGURE 34-1 Schematic representation of the phases of wound healing and associated changes in wound strength.

BOX 34-1 Characteristics of the Microscopic Phases of Wound Healing

Inflammatory
Begins immediately after injury; characterized by formation of blood clot; platelets stimulate other stages by release of growth factors

Débridement
Part of inflammatory phase; characterized by influx of white blood cells (macrophages, monocytes) into wound; occurs approximately 6 hr after injury; wound healing is sustained by release of growth factors from multiple cell types

Repair (Fibroblastic)
Begins 3 to 5 days after wounding; characterized by invasion of fibroblasts and development of granulation tissue; wound strength increases exponentially

Maturation
Characterized by remodeling of the collagen of the scar and slow gain in wound strength; begins approximately 3 wk after injury and may take weeks to years to complete

TABLE 34-1 Characteristics of Selected Growth Factors and Effects on Wound Healing

Sources	Effect on Wound Healing and Target Cells
Platelet-Derived Growth Factor (PDGF)	
Platelets, macrophages, fibroblasts, endothelial cells	Stimulates replication of fibroblasts and vascular smooth muscle
Transforming Growth Factor β1 and β2 (TGF-β1, TGF-β2)	
Macrophages, lymphocytes, fibroblasts, bone cells, epidermal cells, platelets	Affects wound fibrosis and tensile strength; inhibits replication of most cells (epidermal cells, endothelial cells, lymphocytes, and macrophages); may inhibit or stimulate fibroblasts; may have a modulating effect on wound healing
Transforming Growth Factor β3 (TGF-β3)	
Macrophages	Antiscarring effects
Transforming Growth Factor α (TGF-α)	
Macrophages, eosinophils, epidermal cells	Stimulates replication of epithelial cells, fibroblasts, and endothelial cells; has more potent effect on endothelial cells than EGF
Epidermal Growth Factor (EGF)	
Almost all body fluid, platelets	Stimulates replication of epithelial cells, fibroblasts, and endothelial cells
Insulin-like Growth Factor (IGF)	
Most tissues, fibroblasts, macrophages	Stimulates replication of fibroblasts, endothelial cells, bone cells, neural tissues, and hemopoietic cells; influences granulation tissue formation
Fibroblast Growth Factor (FGF)	
Fibroblasts, bone cells, smooth muscle cells, endothelial cells, astrocytes	Stimulates replication of neural tissue, bone cells, muscle cells, and fibroblasts; influences angiogenesis
Keratinocyte Growth Factor (KGF)	
Fibroblasts	Affects epidermal cell motility and proliferation
Vascular Endothelial Growth Factor	
Epidermal cells, macrophages	Enhances angiogenesis and increases vascular permeability
Granulocyte and Macrophage Colony-Stimulating Factor 1	
Many cells	Activates macrophages and influences granulation tissue formation

incised wound that is sutured, in which the skin edges are close together, epithelialization can occur almost immediately (as early as 24 to 48 hours after injury) because there is no defect that needs to be filled with granulation tissue. The normal epithelial cells at the edge of the wound divide and produce new cells that migrate across the granulation tissue. Some hair follicles and sweat glands may also regenerate, depending on the extent of damage. The new epithelium is only one cell layer thick initially and is fragile, but it gradually thickens over time as more cell layers form.

Wound contraction helps to reduce the size of the wound, but occurs independently of epithelialization. No new skin is formed during contraction. Wound contraction is a result of contraction of the myofibroblasts in the granulation tissue, which pulls the full-thickness skin edges inward. If the skin around the wound is tight and under tension, wound contraction will be limited. Visible wound contraction usually occurs 5 to 9 days after injury.

The maturation phase is the final phase of wound healing, during which the wound strength increases to its maximal level because of changes in the scar. Remodeling of the collagen fibers in the fibrous tissue, with alteration of their orientation and increased cross-linking, improves wound strength. The number of capillaries in the fibrous tissue gradually decreases, causing the scar to become paler. The maturation phase begins once collagen has been adequately deposited in the wound and may continue for several years. The wound never regains the strength of normal tissue.

FACTORS AFFECTING WOUND HEALING

Many factors affect wound healing, including host factors, such as the health of the animal and the characteristics of the wound, and external factors, such as the type of wound management and treatment.

HOST FACTORS

Old animals tend to heal slowly, probably because they are often debilitated and have other ongoing health problems. Animals that are malnourished or have a disease causing low serum protein concentrations below 2g/dl (e.g., liver disease with poor protein production or kidney disease with excessive loss of protein) will have delayed wound healing and decreased wound strength. In addition, the lag phase of wound healing will be prolonged in these animals.

Wound healing is delayed by certain diseases, such as hyperadrenocorticism or Cushing's disease, in which there is an excess of circulating corticosteroids. Corticosteroids delay all phases of wound healing.

Animals with diabetes mellitus have delayed wound healing and a predisposition to wound infection. Animals with liver disease may have clotting factor deficits in addition to low serum protein concentrations.

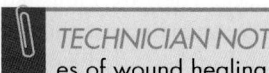

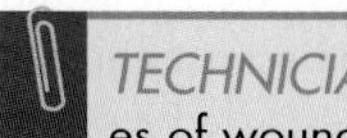

TECHNICIAN NOTE Corticosteroids delay all phases of wound healing.

WOUND CHARACTERISTICS

Foreign material in the wound, such as sutures, surgical implants, drains, or extraneous material, can cause an intense inflammatory reaction that interferes with normal wound healing. Soil particles can contain specific infection-enhancing factors.

Compared with a sharp surgical incision, the incision created with an electroscalpel or electrocoagulation during surgery causes more necrosis at the wound margin, increases the chance of wound infection, and results in a slower gain in early wound strength.

Contaminated tissue becomes infected if the bacteria multiply to a critical number of 10^5 organisms per gram of tissue and then invade the tissue. Whether this occurs depends on the degree of tissue trauma, the amount of foreign material present, the delay between injury and treatment, and the effectiveness of host defenses. Infection stops the repair phase.

Bacterial toxins and associated inflammation directly damage the cells. The wound exudate produced during inflammation can accumulate and separate the tissue, leading to wound infection and delayed wound healing.

TECHNICIAN NOTE Infection stops wound repair.

The blood supply to the wound is obviously important for wound healing and is responsible for delivering oxygen and metabolic substrates to the cells. Damage to the blood supply during surgical treatment should be avoided. Tight bandages that compromise the wound's blood supply should not be used. Movement in a healing wound is also detrimental because it disturbs the fine cellular structures of the healing tissue. Movement across a wound should be limited. It may be necessary to apply a bandage to the affected limb to reduce movement.

EXTERNAL FACTORS

Certain drugs and radiation therapy delay wound healing. Corticosteroids depress all phases of wound healing and increase the chance of infection. Antiinflammatory drugs (aspirin, phenylbutazone, ibuprofen) have little effect on wound strength, but will suppress early inflammation. Prolonged aspirin therapy may delay blood clotting. Chemotherapeutic drugs can have an adverse effect on wound healing, depending on their mechanism of action and the time of administration in relation to the time of injury. Radiation can have a profound adverse effect on wound healing, depending on dose and time of exposure in relation to time of injury.

WOUND MANAGEMENT

IMMEDIATE WOUND CARE

The wound should be covered with a clean, dry bandage as soon as possible after injury to prevent further contamination and reduce hemorrhage. The bandage should remain in place until definitive treatment is initiated. Water-soluble antibiotic ointments may be applied and may be useful in keeping the wound moist and reducing the microorganism load that is initially contaminating the wound. Antibiotic creams or powders act as foreign bodies and delay wound healing and thus should not be applied. Novel topical agents, such as sugar and honey (Manuka Honey, SummerGlow Apiaries Ltd., Hamilton, New Zealand; Medihoney, Medihoney Pty Ltd., Richlands, Australia), may be indicated at this time. They are hypertonic and hence bactericidal, promote natural débridement by drawing exudate and debris from the wound, and keep the wound surface moist. They may also reduce edema and inflammation. Honey has inherent, additional bactericidal properties over sugar.

Once the animal is stabilized and other, life-threatening injuries have been treated, the wound can be prepared for treatment. The bandage is removed, and the wound is packed with sterile gauze or filled with a sterile water-soluble lubricant, such as K-Y Jelly (Johnson & Johnson, Arlington, Tex.), or temporarily closed with sutures, towel clamps, or Michel clips (Figure 34-2). This allows skin around the wound to be clipped and prepared for aseptic surgery without the introduction of hair into the wound.

Hair from the edges of the wound can be removed with scissors dipped in mineral oil to prevent it from falling into the wound. Once the skin has been prepared, the lubricant can be flushed out or the sponges can be removed from the wound.

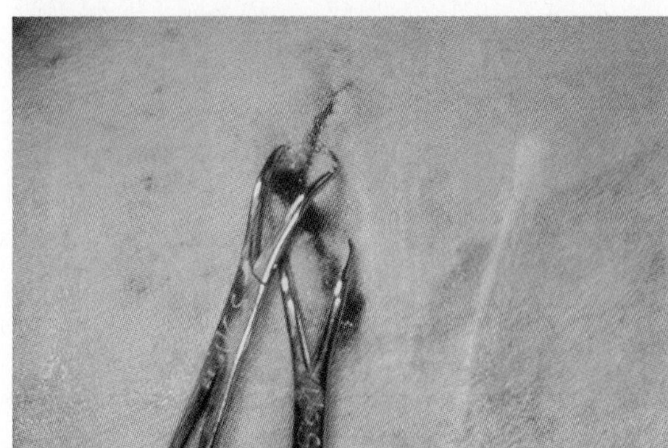

FIGURE 34-2 The wound is temporarily closed with towel clamps to allow aseptic preparation of the surrounding skin.

WOUND LAVAGE

Wound lavage is necessary to remove debris and loose particles and tissue from the wound. It also reduces the number of bacteria in the wound. If infection is suspected, a piece of tissue should be sampled for bacterial culture before lavage. Large volumes of warm, sterile, balanced electrolyte solution are preferred for lavage.

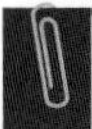

TECHNICIAN NOTE Wound lavage with warm, sterile, balanced electrolyte solution is preferred.

Antibiotics should not be added to the fluid. Soaps, detergents, and antiseptic solutions should not be used because they damage the tissue. The mechanical action of the lavage is the most important factor for successful lavage. Moderate pressure (7 psi) can be generated with a 35-ml syringe and 19-gauge needle; this method is more effective than pouring fluid over a wound. The syringe can be connected to a bag of fluid with a three-way stopcock to facilitate refilling of the syringe (Figure 34-3). A pulsating, high-pressure (70 psi) stream can be generated by means of a Waterpik (Teledyne, Fort Collins, Colo.), which is even more effective in reducing the bacterial population and removing necrotic tissue and foreign material from heavily contaminated wounds.

WOUND DÉBRIDEMENT

Wound débridement is necessary to remove all contaminated, devitalized, or necrotic tissue and foreign material from the wound (Box 34-2). This can be performed surgically by excising the affected tissue in layers, beginning at the surface and progressing to the wound depths. Alternatively the entire wound can be excised en bloc if there is sufficient healthy tissue surrounding the wound and vital structures can be preserved (Figure 34-4). Enzymatic débridement with a commercial solution containing trypsin (e.g., Granulex, SmithKline Beecham, Pittsburgh) can be used for wounds that are not suitable for surgical débridement. Enzymatic débridement is slower and may damage normal tissue. Application of hypertonic solutions to the wound surface (e.g., honey, sugar) or commercial dressings containing 20% sodium chloride (CURASALT Sodium Chloride Dressing, Tyco Healthcare/Kendall, Mansfield, Mass.) can facilitate the natural débridement process of a wound by drawing fluid and debris to the wound surface. They are indicated in contaminated and some infected wounds because the hypertonicity is also antimicrobial. They are best used in early wound management before a healthy granulation tissue bed has developed.

WOUND CLOSURE

Selection of one of the four methods of wound closure depends on the nature of the wound (Box 34-3). Primary wound closure results in healing by first intention. First intention healing, also known as appositional healing, is achieved by suturing or grafting a wound soon after injury (Figure 34-5). Primary wound closure is indicated in fresh, clean, sharply incised wounds with minimal trauma and minimal contamination that are seen within hours of injury. Wounds treated within 6 to 8 hours of injury are treated within the "golden period" (i.e., bacteria contaminating the wound have not

BOX 34-2 Methods and Indications for Wound Débridement

Layered Débridement
Conservative débridement beginning at superficial layers of wound and progressing to depths; indicated for large wounds with substantial tissue trauma; may be repeated for heavily contaminated/traumatized wounds

En bloc
Complete excision of wound; indicated for small wounds in areas with loose skin that can be closed primarily

Enzymatic
Use of trypsin products that dissolve necrotic tissue; slow method of débridement; indicated in minimally contaminated/traumatized wounds or as an adjunct to surgical débridement

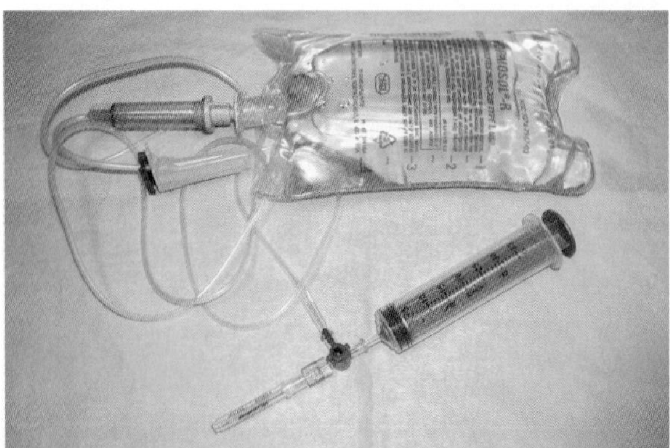

FIGURE 34-3 Connection of a 35-ml syringe and 19-gauge needle to a three-way stopcock and bag of sterile, balanced electrolyte solution to facilitate copious lavage of a wound.

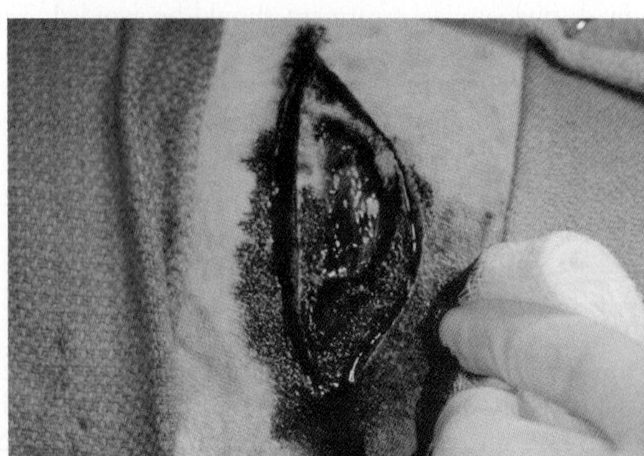

FIGURE 34-4 For small wounds in areas of loose skin, the entire wound is excised en bloc, and the clean surgical wound that is created is closed primarily.

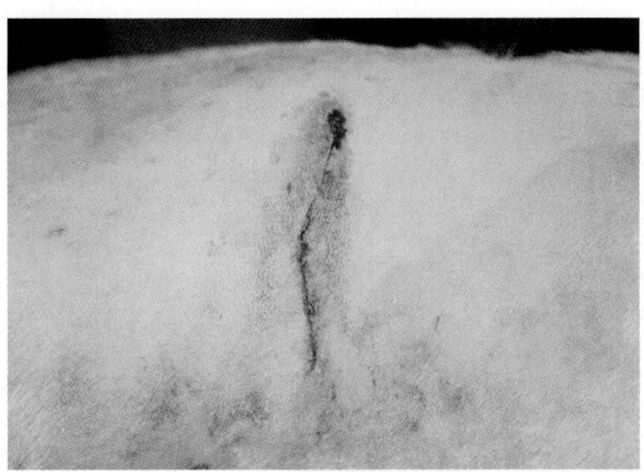

FIGURE 34-5 A fresh laceration or a surgical wound created after en bloc débridement is closed primarily to allow first intention healing.

BOX 34-3 Methods of Wound Closure

Primary Closure
Closure of a wound with sutures; indicated for fresh, clean wounds with minimal contamination or trauma or surgically created wounds; results in first intention healing

Delayed Primary Closure
Closure of a wound before 3 to 5 days after injury (i.e., before development of granulation tissue); indicated for moderately contaminated or traumatized wounds

Contraction and Epithelialization
Wound allowed to heal without surgical closure; wound closes as a result of contraction and epithelialization; may not be possible or desirable in all wounds; results in second intention healing

Secondary Closure
Closure of a wound after 3 to 5 days (i.e., after granulation tissue has developed in the wound); indicated in severely contaminated or traumatized wounds that require considerable débridement and prolonged wound management; takes advantage of the positive effects of granulation tissue; results in third intention healing

multiplied to the critical number of 10^5 organisms per gram of tissue, and the tissue has not become infected). Wounds treated after the golden period should not be closed unless they can be completely excised (en bloc débridement) because infection is likely.

> *TECHNICIAN NOTE* Primary closure of a wound is indicated in fresh, minimally traumatized wounds or after complete excision (en bloc débridement) of the wound.

Delayed primary closure is primary closure of a wound 1 to 3 days after injury before granulation tissue has appeared in the wound. It is indicated for mildly contaminated, minimally traumatized wounds that require some cleansing and débridement or for relatively clean wounds seen 6 to 8 hours after injury. This method allows any local contamination or infection to be controlled before closure.

Healing by contraction and epithelialization is also known as second intention healing and is indicated for dirty, contaminated, traumatized wounds when cleansing and débridement are necessary and when closure may be difficult. Adequate, loose skin surrounding the wound is necessary to allow contraction. Closure by second intention may not always be desirable because the new epithelium is fragile and easily abraded. In addition, contraction may impede normal function, depending on the location of the wound (Figure 34-6).

Secondary closure results in third intention healing (Figure 34-7). The wound is sutured at least 3 to 5 days after injury. Granulation tissue will be present in the wound by the time of closure. The granulation tissue helps to control infection in the wound and fills in the tissue defect. Secondary closure is indicated when (1) the wound is severely contaminated or traumatized, (2) epithelialization and contraction will not completely close the wound, or (3) second intention healing is undesirable.

The decision whether to treat a wound primarily or to have it remain open initially and follow up with delayed closure, second intention healing, or secondary closure depends on the: (1) time lapse since injury; wounds greater than 6 to 8 hours old should be kept open initially; (2) degree of contamination; wounds obviously contaminated should be kept open initially and thoroughly cleansed; (3) amount of tissue damage; wounds with substantial tissue damage have reduced host defenses, are more likely to become infected, and consequently should remain open initially; (4) thoroughness of débridement; if the initial débridement was conservative, the wound should remain open until definitive débridement is performed; (5) blood supply to the wound; a wound with questionable blood supply should remain open until the extent of nonviable tissue is determined; (6) animal's health; if the animal is unable to endure prolonged surgical débridement, the wound should be kept open and possibly undergo enzymatic débridement until the animal can withstand surgery; (7) closure without tension or dead space; if excessive tension or dead space is present, the wound should be allowed to remain open because dead space allows accumulation of fluid, separation of tissues, and formation of seromas, which may predispose to infection and delay wound healing; and (8) location of the wound; certain locations may not be amenable to closure (e.g., a large wound on a limb) (Box 34-4).

WOUND BANDAGING

Bandages promote wound healing by protecting the wound from additional trauma and contamination, by preventing wound desiccation, by preventing hematoma and seroma formation through compression to obliterate dead space, and by immobilizing the wound to prevent cellular and capillary disruption. Bandages minimize postoperative edema around incisions and minimize exuberant granulation tissue formation in open wounds on the lower limb region

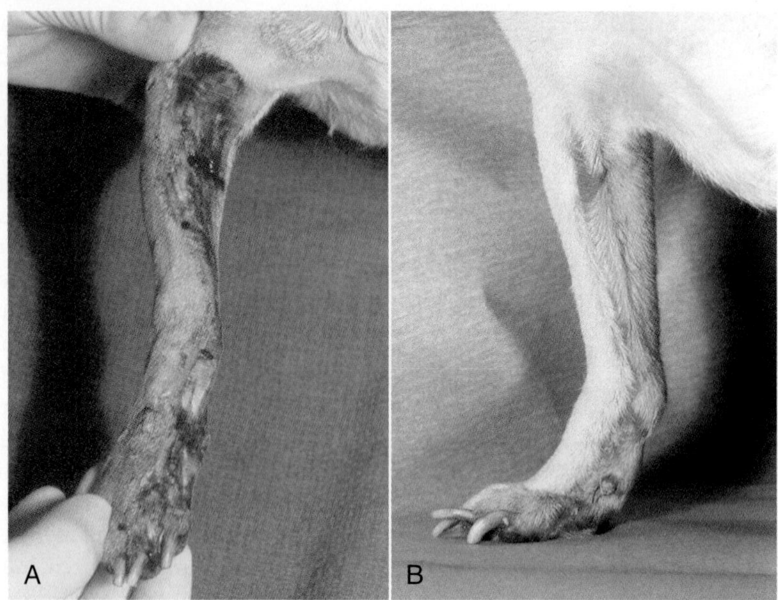

FIGURE 34-6 **A,** A degloving injury on the antebrachium of a dog. After surgical (layered) débridement and open wound management, the wound healed by second intention with contraction and epithelialization. **B,** After several weeks, the wound is completely closed. Note the hairless, shiny new epithelium and the reduced outline of the wound caused by contraction. The epithelium will thicken over time, but will always remain fragile. The pink color will become reduced as the wound remodels underneath the epithelium, and the vascular granulation tissue becomes organized fibrous tissue.

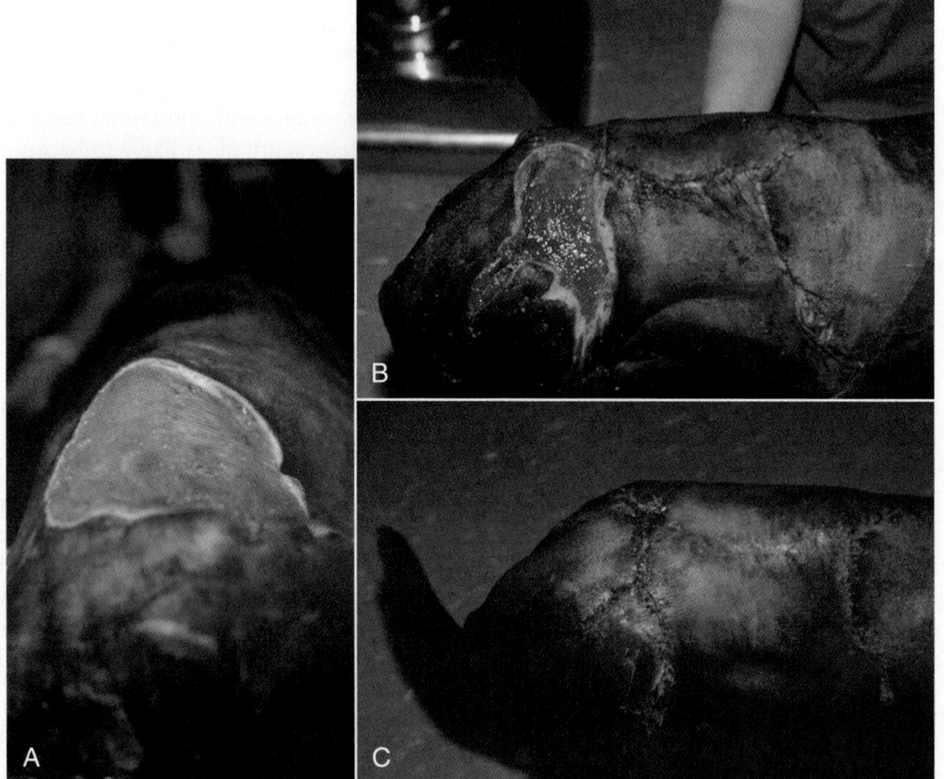

FIGURE 34-7 **A,** A healthy granulation tissue wound bed on the dorsum of a dog after open wound management of a thermal burn injury (the dog's head is toward the top). **B,** Staged, partial closure of the wound over the granulation tissue allows third intention healing of the wound (the dog's head is to the right). **C,** Closure of the remaining portion of the wound.

(below the carpus or tarsus) of horses. In addition, the bandage can absorb wound exudate and lift away foreign material and loose tissue that has adhered to the bandage as it is removed. Covering a wound with a bandage promotes an acid environment at the wound surface by preventing carbon dioxide loss and absorbing ammonia produced by bacteria. An acid environment increases oxygen dissociation from hemoglobin and subsequently increases oxygen availability in the wound. The bandage also keeps the wound warm. Higher temperatures improve wound healing and facilitate oxygen dissociation (Box 34-5). Leaving a wound open to dry and form a scab is never indicated.

A bandage usually consists of three layers: the primary or contact layer, the secondary or padded conforming layer, and the tertiary or holding and protective layer (Table 34-2). The primary bandage layer has direct contact with the wound surface (if present) and may be adherent or nonadherent. Adherent primary bandage layers are no longer recommended. The recent consensus among wound care professionals is that moist wound care is the most important management principle. This involves the use of nonadherent primary bandage layers that act to keep the wound surface moist. Nonadherent primary layers that facilitate moist wound care usually include a hydrophilic layer. Moist wound care enhances epithelialization, particularly in partial-thickness skin wounds or abrasions. Moist wound care also enhances natural débridement within the wound by drawing the exudate from the wound and allowing the wound to "bathe" in this cytokine- and macrophage-rich material. Moist wound care results in less inflammation and less wound disruption compared with dry or adherent bandages. Allowing wounds to be exposed and the use of drying techniques, such as dry-to-dry (application of dry gauze sponges) or wet-to-dry (application of wet sponges that later dry out) bandages are no longer acceptable as standard care practices.

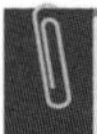

TECHNICIAN NOTE Nonadherent bandages are indicated for granulating wounds.

BOX 34-4 Factors Important in Wound Management Decision Making

- Time since injury
- Degree of wound contamination
- Degree of tissue trauma
- Thoroughness of initial débridement
- Blood supply of wound
- Animal's physical status
- Wound tension and possibility of closure
- Location of wound

BOX 34-5 Beneficial Effects of Bandaging a Wound

- Protects from further contamination
- Prevents wound desiccation
- Prevents hematoma and seroma formation
- Immobilizes the wound and prevents cellular disruption
- Minimizes surrounding edema
- Absorbs wound exudate and debris
- Promotes retention of carbon dioxide and creation of an acid environment, which facilitates oxygen dissociation
- Keeps wound warm, which facilitates healing

The nonadherent primary bandage layer is either occlusive or semiocclusive. An occlusive primary bandage layer is impermeable to moisture, but allows some air transfer, whereas a semiocclusive primary bandage layer allows air and moisture vapor to move through the dressing. A semiocclusive primary bandage layer is indicated for wounds with moderate to copious exudate and must be changed frequently (daily to every third day, depending on the volume of exudate production) to prevent maceration of the surrounding normal tissue and skin. An occlusive primary bandage layer is indicated for minimally exudative wounds and is particularly useful for wounds in which promoting epithelialization is the goal (e.g., a partial-thickness abrasion or a wound with healthy granulation tissue). Occlusive bandages require changing less frequently (every 4 to 7 days, depending on exudate production) and will accelerate epithelialization considerably, up to 50% compared with an exposed wound. The occlusive primary bandage layer can also be used as a protective layer for new epithelium, preventing desiccation and abrasion of the fragile tissue. Although the occlusive bandage is nonadherent at the wound surface, some products will adhere to the surrounding local skin. Examples of nonadherent occlusive products that do not include a hydrophilic material include OpSite (Smith and Nephew, Largo, Fla.), Tegaderm Transparent Dressing (3M Medical, St. Paul), and BIOCLUSIVE Transparent Dressing (Johnson & Johnson Medical, Arlington, Tex.). Examples of nonadherent occlusive products that include a hydrophilic material are NU-GEL (hydrogel) Wound Dressing (Johnson & Johnson Medical) and Hydrocol (hydrocolloid) Dressing (Bertek Pharmaceuticals Inc., Morgantown, W.Va.).

Nonadherent, semiocclusive hydrophilic bandage layers include hydrogel, hydrocolloid, and absorbent foam bandages. Hydrogel bandages (Curagel, Tyco Healthcare/Kendall, Mansfield, Mass.) have a thin layer of hydrogel adhered to a fine synthetic fiber mesh that is semiocclusive. Hydrogel also comes as a water-based paste (CURAFIL Gel Wound Dressing, Tyco Healthcare/Kendall, Mansfield, Mass.). The hydrogel layer absorbs the wound exudate, which keeps the wound moist. As the wound exudate is absorbed, particulate matter and microorganisms are also removed, facilitating wound débridement. Hydrocolloid bandages (Ultec Hydrocolloid Dressing, Tyco Healthcare/Kendall, Mansfield, Mass.) are starch polymers in an adhesive matrix with semiocclusive polyurethane backing. Hydrocolloid bandages are indicated for granulating wounds. The hydrocolloid becomes gel-like after contact with a moist surface and forms a protective layer at the wound surface. Hydrophilic bandage layers are indicated for most wounds. Bandage layers with gel may be preferred for minimally exudative wounds, whereas dry hydrophilic colloid bandage layers and hydrophilic absorbent sponge bandage layers are preferred for moderately to copious exudative wounds. Hydrogel can be added to dry wounds under a semiocclusive or occlusive bandage layer to provide exogenous moisture, which will promote wound healing. Hydrophilic colloids are also available as powders, flakes, beads, and sponges. These materials can be placed

TABLE 34-2 Characteristics of Primary, Secondary, and Tertiary Bandage Layers

Type	Indication and Purpose	Example
Primary		
Adherent	No longer indicated in wound care	Dry gauze (dry-to-dry) Wet gauze (wet-to-dry)
Hypertonic	Contaminated and infected wounds; hypertonicity is antimicrobial and draws fluid and tissue debris from wound	Hypertonic Sodium Chloride Dressing (20%) (e.g., CURASALT*)
Nonadherent semiocclusive	Moderately or copious exudative wounds; keep wound surface moist, draws fluid and tissue debris from wound	Transparent polyurethane film—Polyskin II* *With hydrophilic properties:* Hydrogel (e.g., Curagel*), Absorptive foam (e.g., Hydrosorb*) Hydrocolloid (e.g., Ultec Hydrocolloid Dressing*)
Nonadherent occlusive	Minimally exudative wounds; partial thickness wounds (abrasions); keep wound surface moist and promote epithelialization; protect new epithelium	*Without hydrophilic properties:* OpSite*, Tegaderm Transparent Dressing*, BIOCLUSIVE Transparent Dressing† *With hydrophilic properties:* Hydrogel (e.g., NU-GEL†); Hydrocolloid (e.g., Hydrocol Dressing†)
Nonadherent without occlusive properties	Intact wound surface (e.g., surgical wound, recently epithelialized wound)	Petrolatum-impregnated gauze (e.g., Adaptic†; rayon or Teflon pads (e.g., Telfa pads†)
Secondary		
Padding	Absorb exudate, pads and supports the wound	Cast padding—Specialist Cast Padding‡ Roll cotton
Tertiary		
Conforming gauze	Conforming and holding layer	Conforming gauze (e.g., Kling*)
Nonocclusive elastic adhesive tape	Holding and protective layer, permeable to moisture	Elastikon*
Nonocclusive elastic bandage	Holding and protective layer, permeable to moisture	Vetwrap§
Occlusive tape	Contraindicated	Waterproof tape
Occlusive wrap	Contraindicated	Plastic wrap

*Tyco Healthcare/Kendall, Mansfield, Mass.
†Johnson & Johnson Medical, Arlington, Tex.
‡Johnson & Johnson Orthopaedics, Rayham, Mass.
§3M Animal Products, St. Paul.

in wounds with large defects and act to absorb exudate and remove debris. They are usually covered by a semiocclusive polyurethane film (Polyskin II Transparent Dressing, Tyco Healthcare/Kendall, Mansfield, Mass.).

Polyurethane film is a semiocclusive, transparent bandage layer that can be used to cover hydrophilic dressings or used alone as a primary bandage layer on partial-thickness skin wounds if they incorporate a nonadhesive pad (e.g., Tegaderm Transparent Dressing). They are indicated for moderately exudative wounds in which the amount of wound exudate is declining. The polyurethane film is adhesive to the surrounding tissue and, if left on too long, can lead to maceration of the surrounding tissue and damage to the epithelium on removal.

Some nonadherent products have no occlusive properties (i.e., nonhydrophilic) and include products, such as petrolatum-impregnated gauze (e.g., Adaptic, Johnson & Johnson Medical) and Teflon- or rayon-based bandages (e.g., Telfa Pads, Johnson & Johnson Medical). These products do not keep an open wound moist as the fluid moves quickly into the secondary layer. These products are best used on closed wounds where a protective bandage is required, such as a surgical site or a recently epithelialized wound that is still friable.

The secondary bandage layer is an absorbent, padded, conforming layer of cast padding (e.g., Specialist Cast Padding, Johnson & Johnson Orthopaedics) or roll cotton that covers the primary contact layer and supports the wound. The tertiary layer is the holding and protective layer, which includes some form of gauze (e.g., Kling, Johnson & Johnson Medical) and elastic (3M Vetrap Bandage Tape, 3M Animal Care Products) or adhesive tape (Elasticon, Johnson & Johnson) to hold the bandage in place. The tertiary layer should be nonocclusive to allow air transfer. However,

BOX 34-6 Steps in Bandage Placement*

- Apply anchoring tapes (stirrups)
- Apply primary (contact) layer on wound
- Apply secondary (padded) layer
- Apply tertiary (conforming) gauze layer
- Apply splint
- Reflect, twist, and adhere tape stirrups to gauze
- Apply tertiary (protective) tape

*Some steps may not be indicated.

nonocclusive layers will allow moisture to enter or exit the wound through this layer. When the outer tertiary layer becomes wet, known as strike-through, the wound is at risk for contamination from the environment because bacteria can wick through the moist bandage material. Once the tertiary layer is wet, the bandage must be changed. Although use of an occlusive, water-resistant tertiary layer, such as waterproof tape or plastic wrap, would prevent this, such materials do not allow air transfer to the wound. Occlusive tertiary layers also trap excessive amounts of fluid at the wound surface, resulting in tissue maceration. For these reasons, occlusive tertiary bandages are contraindicated.

Specific bandages and their indications for use in small animal practice are described in the following sections. The standard procedure for application of any bandage to a limb requires: (1) application of anchoring tape strips (stirrups) to the distal portion of the limb; (2) application of a primary bandage layer over the wound; (3) application of the padded secondary layer over the stirrups; (4) application of the gauze tertiary layer; (5) application of the splint; (6) reflection and twisting of the stirrups to adhere to the gauze layer; and (7) application of the protective tertiary layer of tape (Box 34-6). The middle two toes of the bandaged limb should always be exposed to allow for assessment of color, warmth, and swelling. A stockinette can be applied under the secondary layer to help keep the bandage from slipping. Other modifications are also acceptable.

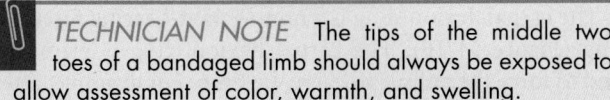

TECHNICIAN NOTE The tips of the middle two toes of a bandaged limb should always be exposed to allow assessment of color, warmth, and swelling.

WOUND BANDAGING IN SMALL ANIMALS

CASTS

Fiberglass cast materials (Delta-Lite S, Johnson & Johnson Orthopaedics, Arlington, Tex.) are currently used almost routinely because of their light weight, extreme rigidity, rapid setting time, and ventilation and waterproof properties. Casts are indicated for stabilization of certain fractures distal to the elbow or stifle and for immobilization of limbs to protect ligament or tendon repairs. The cast must extend one joint above and below any fracture or structure to be immobilized; hence a cast is unsuitable for a humeral or femoral fracture. The cast material is applied instead of a tertiary layer; however, minimal padding is suggested to prevent cast loosening and movement and excessive compression (Figure 34-8). Animals with casts should be monitored at least weekly.

BANDAGES AND SPLINTS

The Robert Jones bandage is most commonly used for temporary immobilization of fractures distal to the elbow or stifle before surgery. The bandage must extend one joint above and below any fracture or structure to be immobilized; hence, it is unsuitable for humeral or femoral fractures. It is a large, bulky bandage that provides rigid stabilization because of the extreme compression of the thick cotton secondary layer (Figure 34-9).

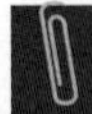

TECHNICIAN NOTE The Robert Jones bandage is not appropriate for fractures of the femur or humerus.

The modified Robert Jones bandage, or simple padded bandage, is a less bulky bandage and is used to reduce postoperative swelling of limbs (Figure 34-10). It provides little or no splinting of the limbs. Less padding is used in the secondary layer, and cast padding is used instead of roll cotton.

A chest or abdominal bandage is applied in the standard three layers. These bandages should be applied firmly, but without constricting the chest or abdomen (Figure 34-11). If an abdominal bandage is used to control abdominal bleeding, the layers are applied more firmly. A rolled towel can be used to reinforce the bandage along the midline, and it is applied before application of the protective tape. The effectiveness of a compression bandage lasts for only 1 to 2 hours, and it should not remain in place longer than 4 hours.

Distal limb splints can be made with tongue depressors for small animals—or with aluminum splints, cast material, or thermoplastics (Figure 34-12). They are indicated for temporary immobilization or definitive stabilization of certain fractures of the distal radius and ulna, carpus, tarsus, metacarpals and metatarsals, and phalanges. They can also be used to support a traumatized distal limb. The limb should be well padded to prevent the development of pressure points. The splint should always be placed on the caudal aspect of the limb.

SLINGS

The Ehmer sling is used specifically to immobilize a hind limb after reduction of craniodorsal coxofemoral luxation and to prevent weight bearing after surgery on the pelvis. Correct application results in internal rotation and adduction of the coxofemoral joint (Figure 34-13). Minimal padding is suggested, and the sling is usually applied with adhesive tape alone to prevent slippage.

The 90-90 flexion sling is applied with the stifle and hock placed in 90-degree flexion, and no attempt is made to adduct

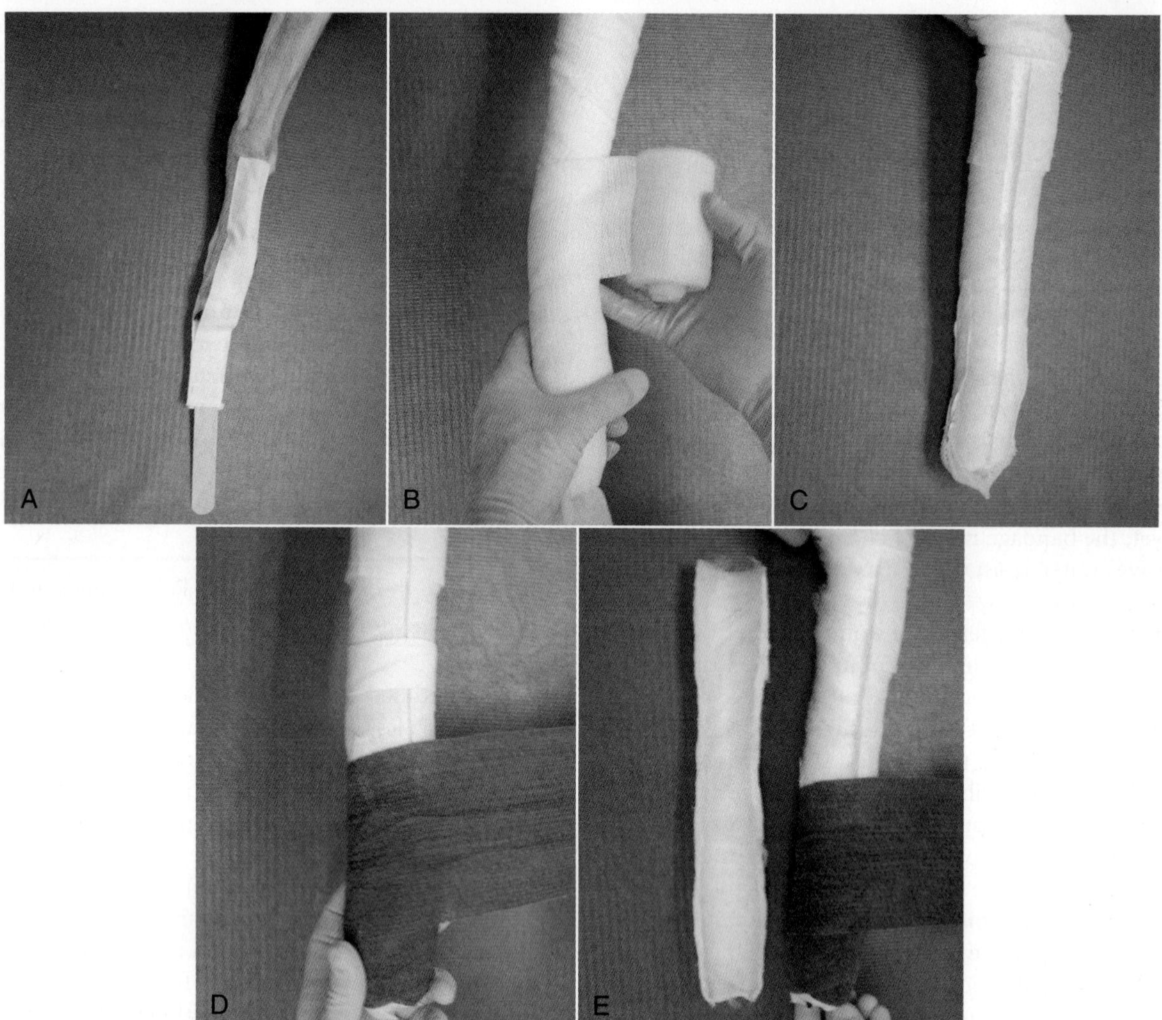

FIGURE 34-8 Cast. **A,** Tape stirrups are placed on the lateral aspects of the limb. A tongue depressor is placed between them to prevent adherence of the stirrups to each other. **B,** A stockinette is applied over the limb, and a lightly padded, secondary layer is then applied firmly around the leg. The fiberglass casting material is applied firmly but not tightly to the leg, with care taken to avoid compression of the cast material with the fingers. **C,** The cast can be bivalved by cutting it lengthwise. This reduces the risk of excessive compression of the leg. **D,** The two halves are taped together, the stockinette ends are reflected over the cast, and the tape stirrups are reflected onto the cast. Protective tape is applied over the cast. **E,** The caudal half of the cast can be used alone as a custom-fitted splint (see Figure 34-12).

and internally rotate the coxofemoral joint (Figure 34-14). The 90-90 flexion sling is used to prevent stifle joint stiffness and hyperextension caused by quadriceps muscle contracture after distal femoral fracture repair in young animals. It can also be used as a non–weight-bearing sling to protect other surgical procedures on the hind limb.

> *TECHNICIAN NOTE* The 90-90 flexion sling is critical in preventing quadriceps contracture after distal femoral fracture repair in young animals.

The Velpeau's sling holds the flexed forelimb against the chest and prevents movement in all joints (Figure 34-15). It is used as a non–weight-bearing sling for the forelimb. The Velpeau's sling is indicated after reduction of scapulohumeral joint luxation or for immobilization of scapular fractures.

The carpal flexion sling is a non–weight-bearing forelimb sling (Figure 34-16). The carpal flexion sling is primarily used to force the animal to carry the limb. For example, after a complicated orthopedic repair of a humeral fracture, restricting weight bearing may be important in the early postoperative period to prevent excessive stress on the repair. The carpal flexion sling can also be used to protect repair of tendons on the caudal aspect of the carpus since the flexed angled of the carpus reduces tension on the tendons. The degree of carpal flexion can be reduced by partially cutting the crisscross of tape formed at the caudal aspect of the carpus.

Hobbles can be applied to the hind limbs to prevent excessive abduction of the limbs. They are specifically indicated after reduction of ventral coxofemoral luxation and to prevent excessive tension in the inguinal region. They can be used to prevent excessive activity after pelvic fracture repair or for nonsurgical, conservative management of pelvic fractures (Figure 34-17).

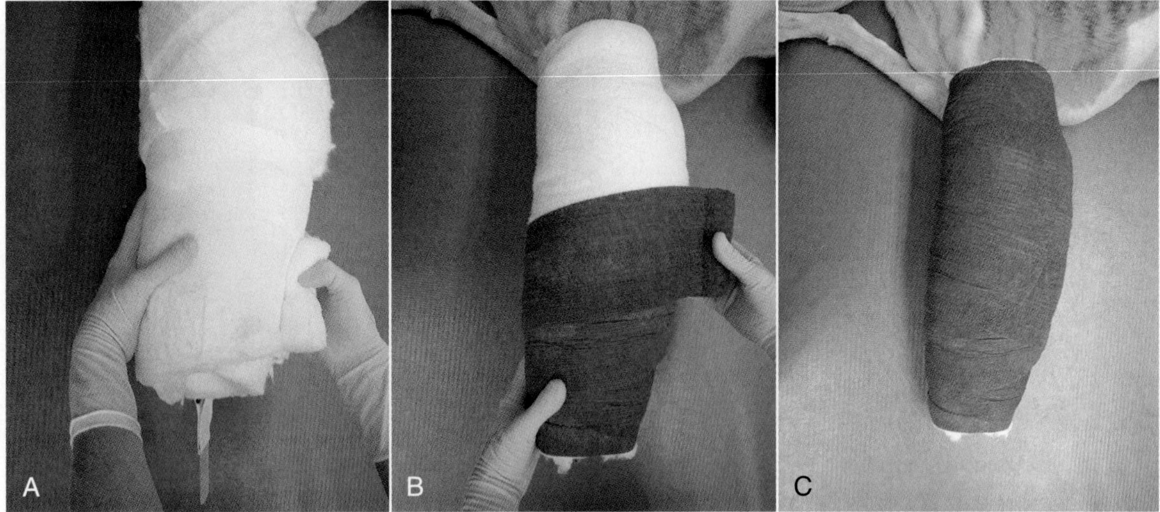

FIGURE 34-9 Robert Jones bandage. **A,** Tape stirrups are applied, and the limb is wrapped in a secondary layer of roll cotton that extends beyond the joints above and below the fracture or injury. The roll cotton is compressed tightly with a conforming gauze layer. Excessive twisting of the leg should be avoided as the gauze layer is tightened. **B,** The stirrups are reflected on top of the gauze. Protective tape (nonocclusive) is then firmly applied. **C,** The completed bandage should feel solid, and a "ping" should be heard on percussion.

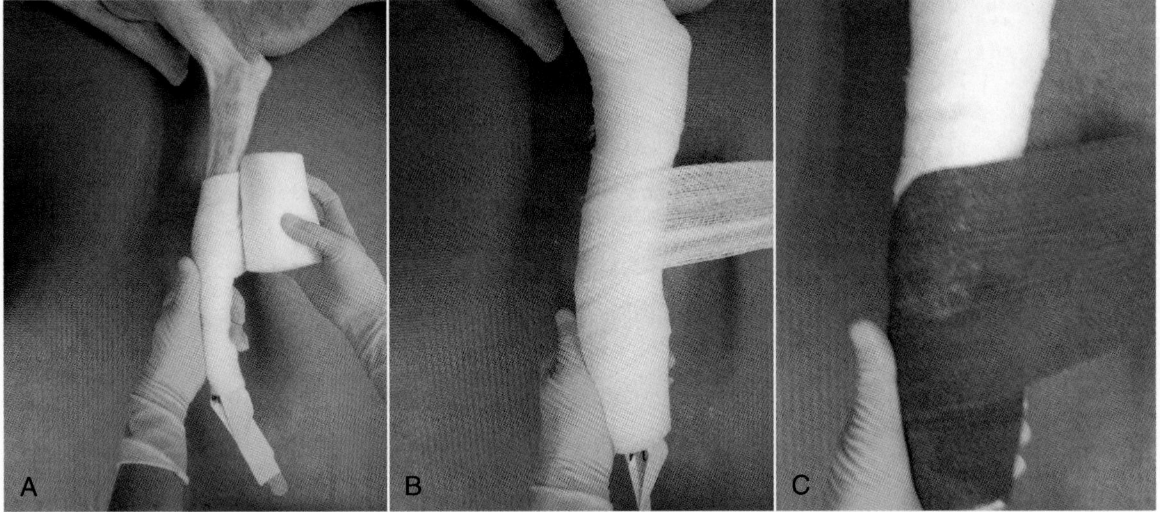

FIGURE 34-10 Modified Robert Jones or simple padded bandage. **A,** Tape stirrups and a padded secondary layer are applied to the limb. **B,** This is followed by application of a gauze tertiary layer. **C,** The stirrups are reflected to adhere to the gauze, and the bandage is covered by protective tape.

SPECIFIC BANDAGES

Bandaging to the ear may be indicated in the treatment of aural hematomas, after ear surgery, or after traumatic injury to the pinna. Bandage of the ear to the head, toward the neck, will protect the ear, absorb any drainage from a wound site or protect a surgically implanted drain, and immobilize the ear, which increases the comfort to the animal. The bandage is applied in three layers as described with the primary layer appropriate for the wound covered (Figure 34-18). In animals with ear or skin disease, the area underneath the bandage can become excessively moist quickly. Frequent inspection of the bandage and changing if necessary is required for a bandage in this location. Considerable care must be taken in removing bandages covering the ear to avoid inadvertently cutting the pinna with scissors. Attempts at bandaging the ear alone usually fail and will not stop the animal from shaking the pinna, which is detrimental to wound healing.

Bandaging the tail may be required to protect an amputation site or trauma to the tip. The bandage is applied in three layers as described with the primary layer appropriate for the wound covered (Figure 34-19). Using a sticky adhesive bandage (Elasticon, Johnson & Johnson) for the tertiary layer and having it extend beyond the secondary layer so that it adheres to the skin is best to ensure that the bandage stays in place. Excessive padding is avoided. Inclusion of a protective tip made from plastic tubing or cast material may offer additional protection. This can be applied to the outside of the bandage.

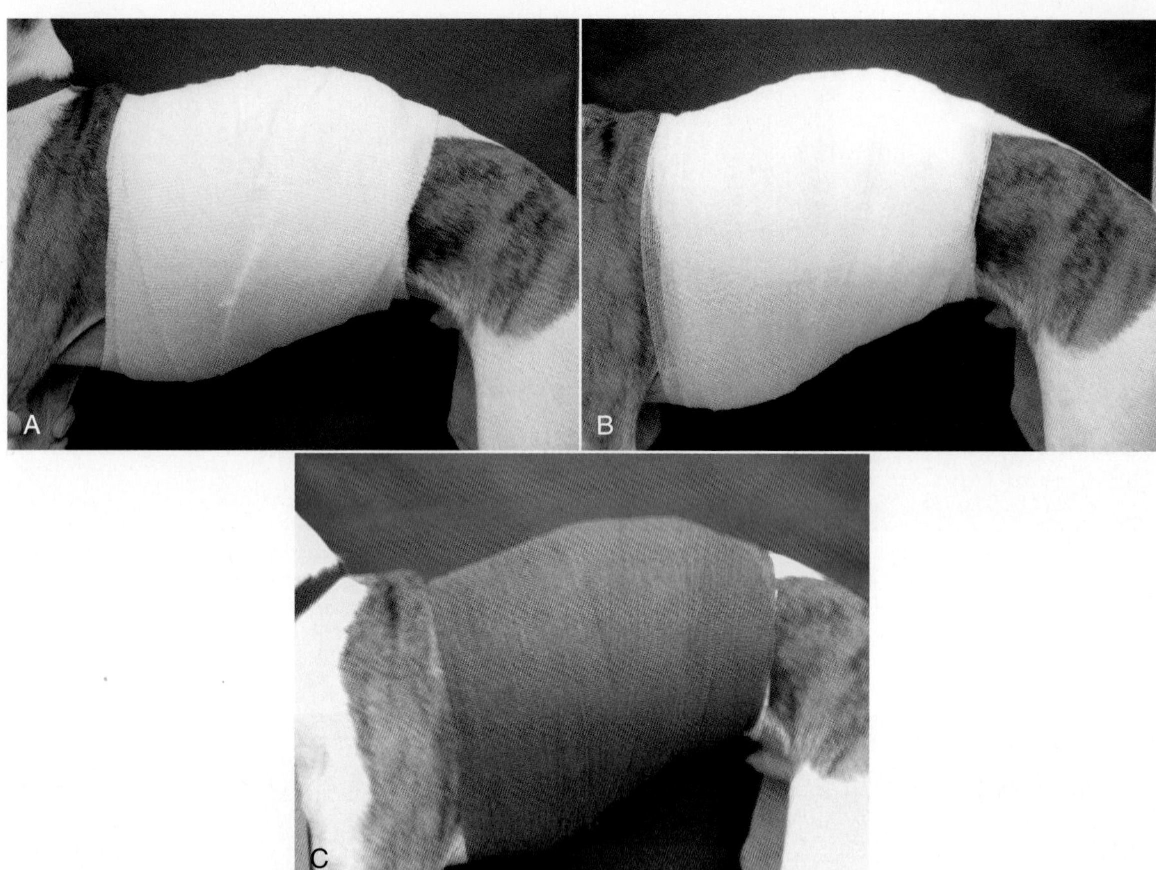

FIGURE 34-11 Abdominal or chest bandage. **A,** After a primary layer is placed on the wound, the padded secondary layer is applied. **B,** This is followed by application of a gauze tertiary layer. **C,** Protective tape is then applied.

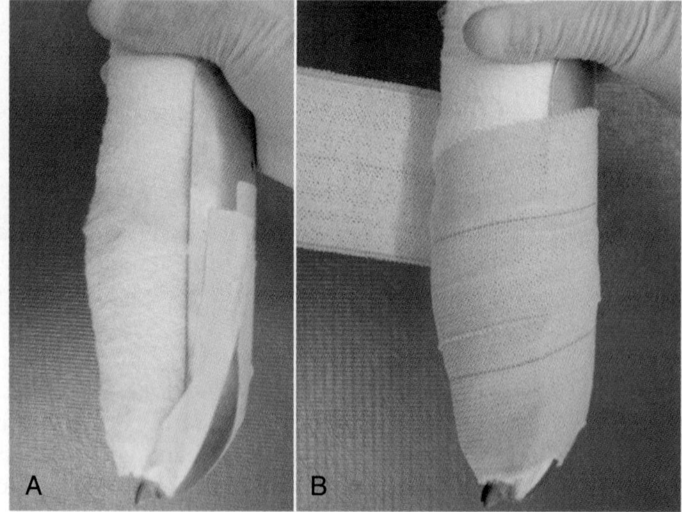

FIGURE 34-12 Splint. **A,** After application of a modified Robert Jones or simple padded bandage (see Figure 34-10), the splint is applied to the caudal aspect of the limb, and the stirrups are reflected onto the splint. **B,** Protective tape is then applied to hold the splint in place.

AFTERCARE OF CASTS, BANDAGES, SPLINTS, AND SLINGS

Close monitoring of animals with casts, bandages, splints, or slings is extremely important and should be performed daily for inpatients and at least weekly for outpatients. Client education for outpatients is essential. The toes should be monitored daily for warmth, color, and swelling. Abnormal findings indicate a tight cast. Monitoring the bandage for a foul odor that would indicate tissue damage is necessary. Observation for areas of chafing from the cast is important. The animal should be restrained from chewing at the bandage (e.g., by means of an Elizabethan collar), and exercise should be restricted to brief leash walks. While the animal is outside, the bandage should be protected from dirt and moisture by

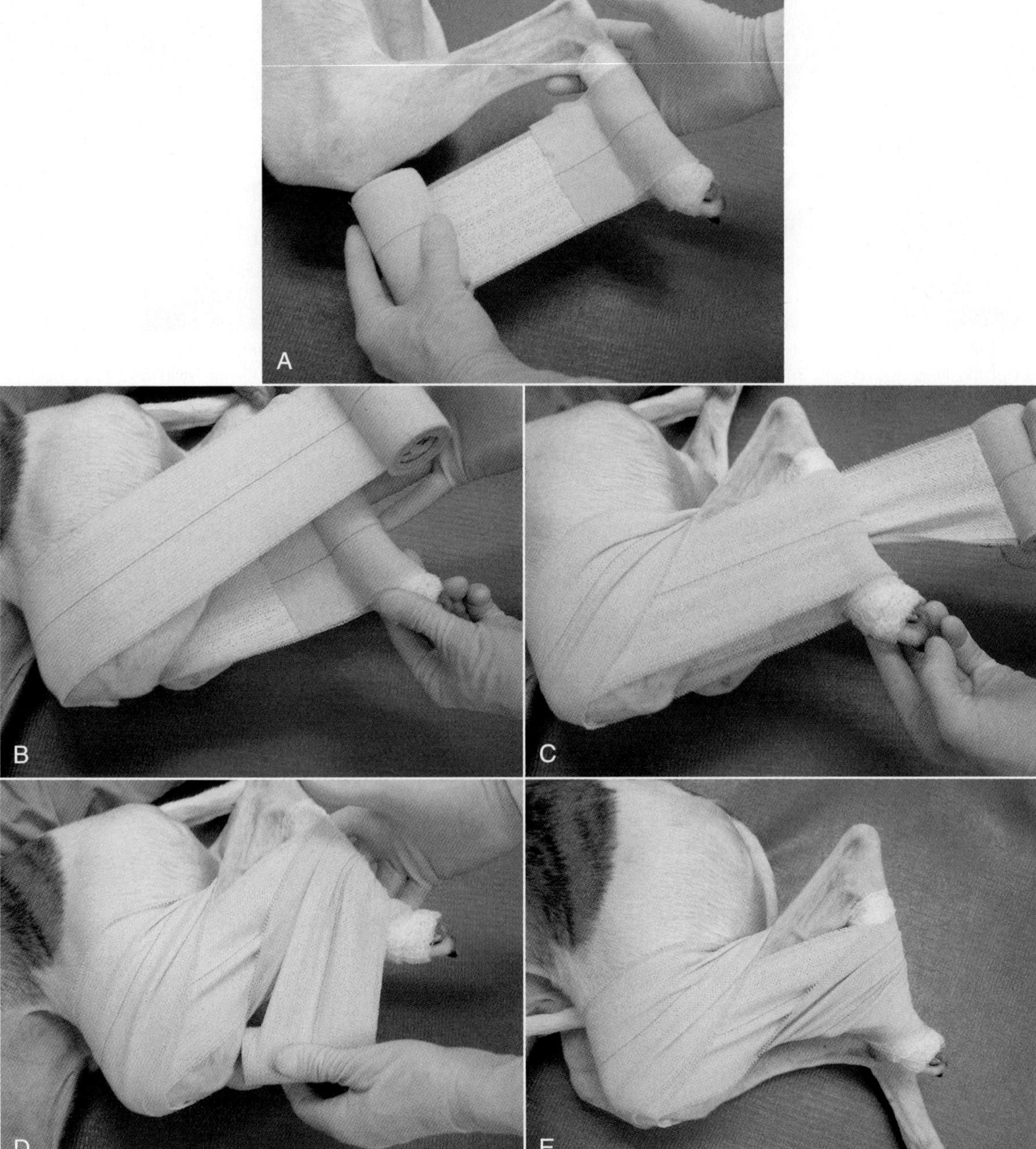

FIGURE 34-13 Ehmer sling. **A,** After minimal padding has been applied to the tarsus, a sling of adhesive tape is passed along the medial aspect of the limb. **B,** The tape is then wrapped around the hind limb with the stifle and hock held in maximal flexion for one or two passes. **C,** On the third pass, the tape is brought over the flank and twisted behind the hock. **D,** The tape is then passed over the front of the metatarsus. **E,** This wrapping is repeated for three or four passes.

application of a plastic bag or other waterproof material. The plastic covering should not remain on for more than 30 minutes because it prevents the bandage from "breathing" and allows the underlying tissue to become moist and macerated.

SPECIFIC WOUND MANAGEMENT

Characteristics of certain wounds may influence the type of wound management performed. The characteristics of certain wounds and management indications are listed in the following sections.

ABRASIONS

Abrasions are partial-thickness wounds of the epidermis with exposure of the deep dermis. Abrasions can be painful. Abrasions are associated with minimal bleeding and develop minimal exudate. Abrasions heal by reepithelialization. Healing of abrasions will be enhanced by keeping the wound surface moist and protected rather than allowing a scab to dry on the surface. Application of a nonadhesive, semiocclusive primary layer with a minimal amount of padding and a nonocclusive tertiary layer is indicated. Hydrophilic primary

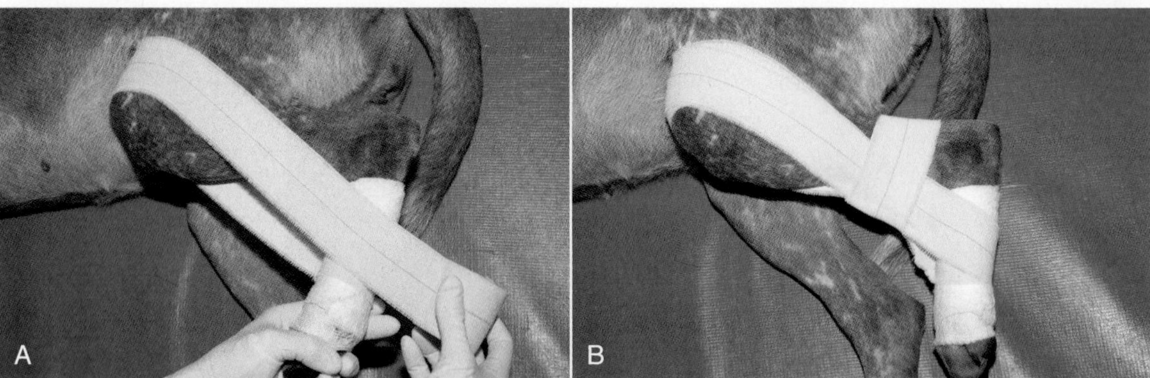

FIGURE 34-14 A 90-90 flexion sling. After minimal padding has been applied to the tarsus, a sling of adhesive tape is passed along the medial aspect of the limb (see Figure 34-13, *A*). **A,** The tape is then wrapped around the hind limb with the stifle and hock held in 90-degree flexion. **B,** A second layer of tape is passed horizontally around the tibia to hold the previous layer in place.

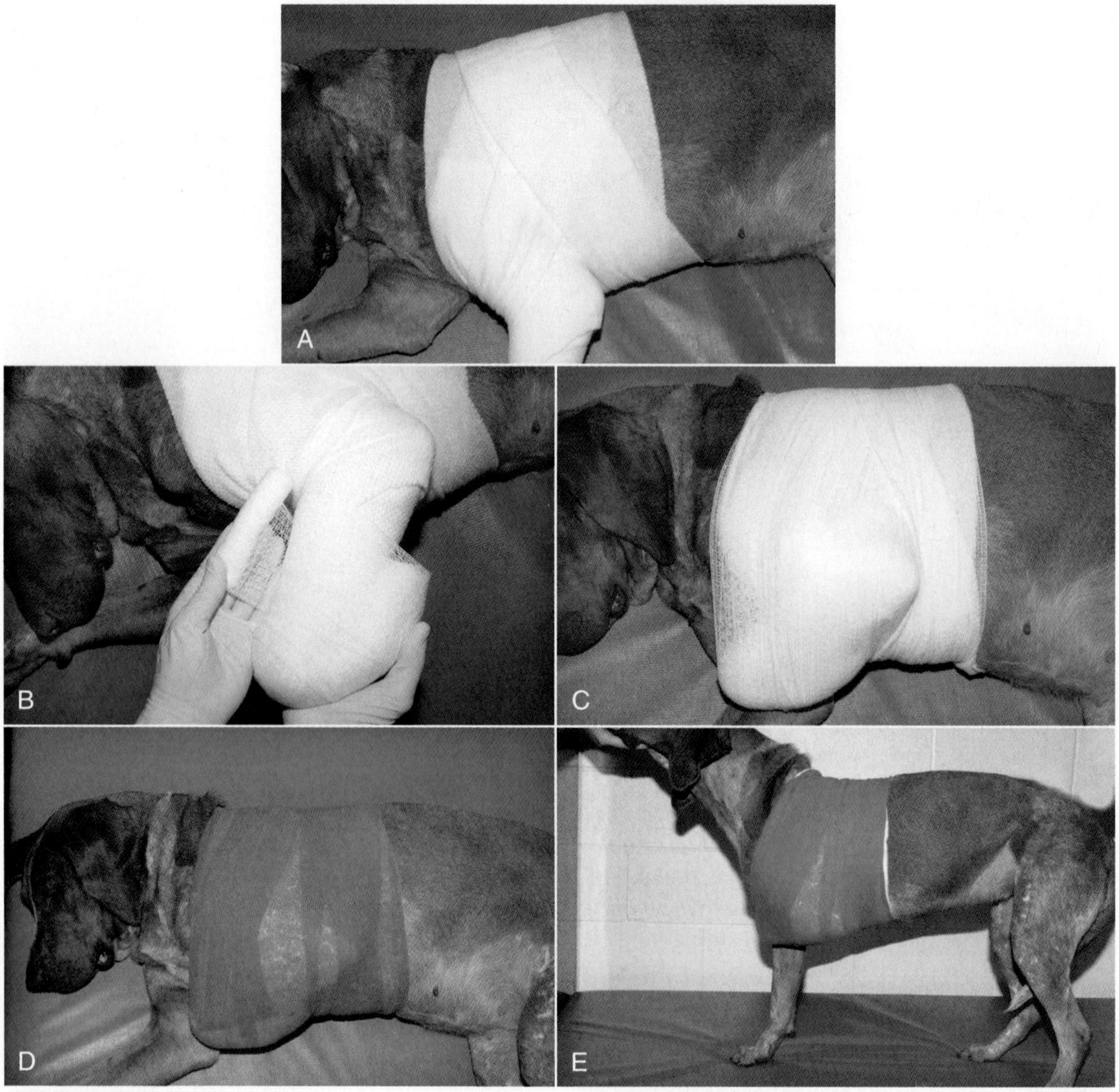

FIGURE 34-15 Velpeau's sling. **A,** Stirrups are applied to the forelimb. The entire forelimb and chest are covered with a light padded bandage. **B,** The carpus is then flexed and covered with an additional layer of a light padded bandage. **C,** The flexed carpus and foreleg are then compressed against the chest and held in place with a conforming gauze layer. **D, E,** The entire leg and chest area are then covered by protective (nonocclusive tape).

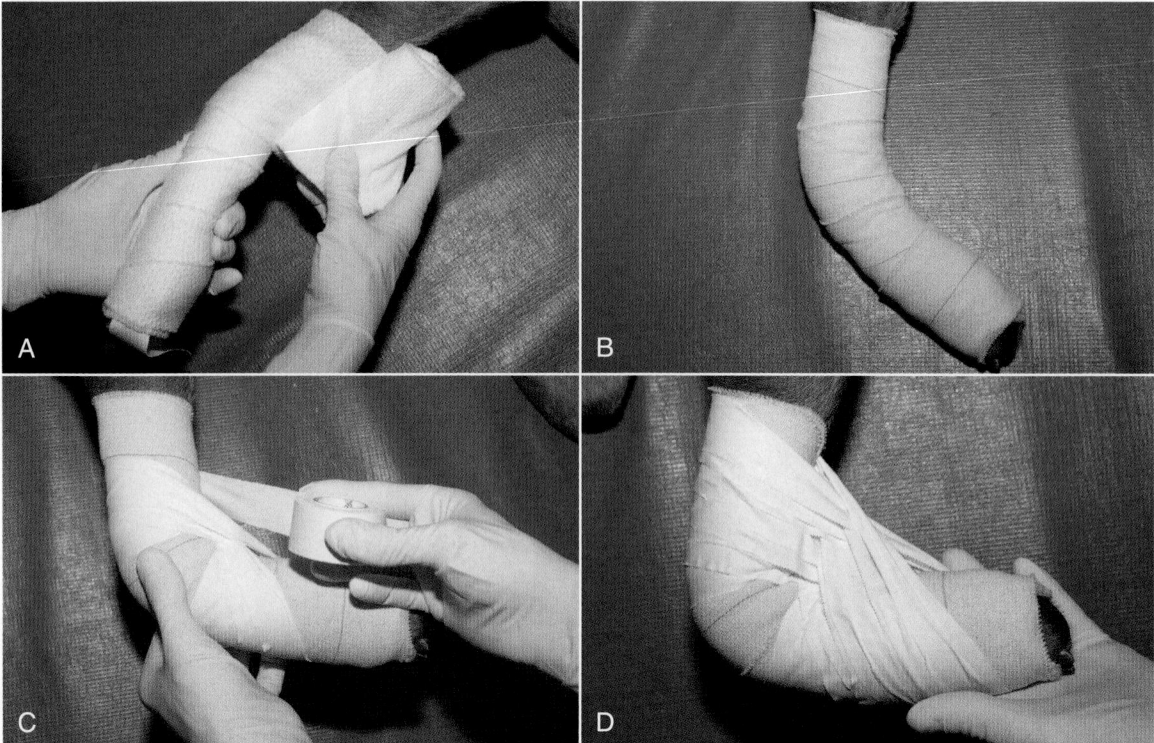

FIGURE 34-16 Carpal flexion sling. **A,** Stirrups are applied. With the limb in flexion, a lightly padded bandage is applied. **B,** The stirrups are reflected, and protective (nonocclusive) tape is applied. **C, D,** One-inch tape is then applied in a figure-eight fashion around the carpus to support it. The tape starts at the middle of the carpus and then extends proximally and distally, forming a web of tape behind the carpus.

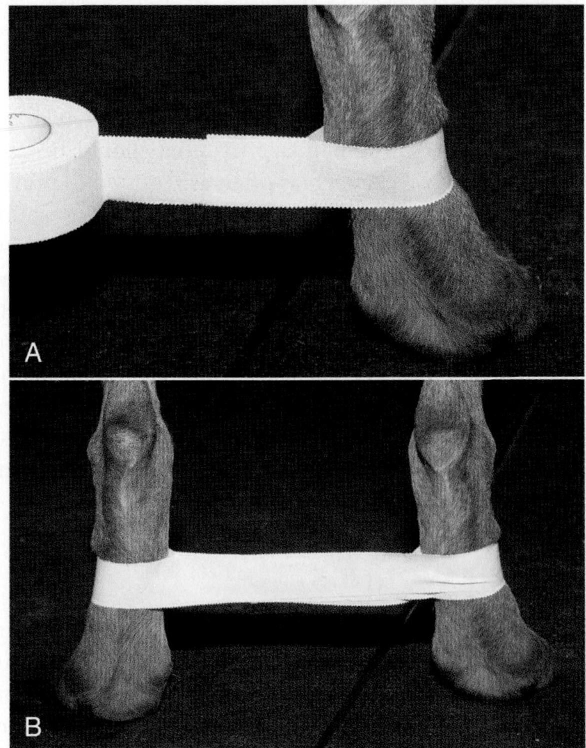

FIGURE 34-17 Hobbles. **A,** Adhesive tape wide enough to cover half of the metatarsal region is placed loosely around the metatarsal region. **B,** The tape is then adhered together between the legs and placed around the opposite metatarsus. The hind limbs are positioned apart at a distance equal to the width of the pelvis.

layers are ideal for these wounds because they promote epithelialization. Bandages can be changed every 3 to 4 days, and an abrasion should be kept bandaged until the surface has completely resurfaced with new epithelium.

LACERATIONS

Lacerations are characterized by sharply incised edges with minimal tissue trauma. They may be superficial (skin) or deep (tendons, muscle). If tissue is torn away, the wound is called an avulsion. Lacerations presented within 12 hours of injury are amenable to minimal débridement of the tissue edges, lavage of the wound, and primary closure. Lacerations seen later than 12 hours after injury may be best treated by en bloc débridement of the wound and primary closure. Although uncommon, heavily contaminated lacerations or old lacerations may be best treated by débridement, lavage, and delayed primary or tertiary closure.

BURNS

Burns are classified by degree of tissue injury (Box 34-7).

The most common causes of burns in companion animals are fire, cage dryers, prolonged contact with heating pads, heat lamps, spillage of hot liquid, and contact with electrical cords. Unfortunately, these causes often result in fourth-degree burns characterized by extensive tissue damage. Animals with more than 50% of the body surface burned rarely survive.

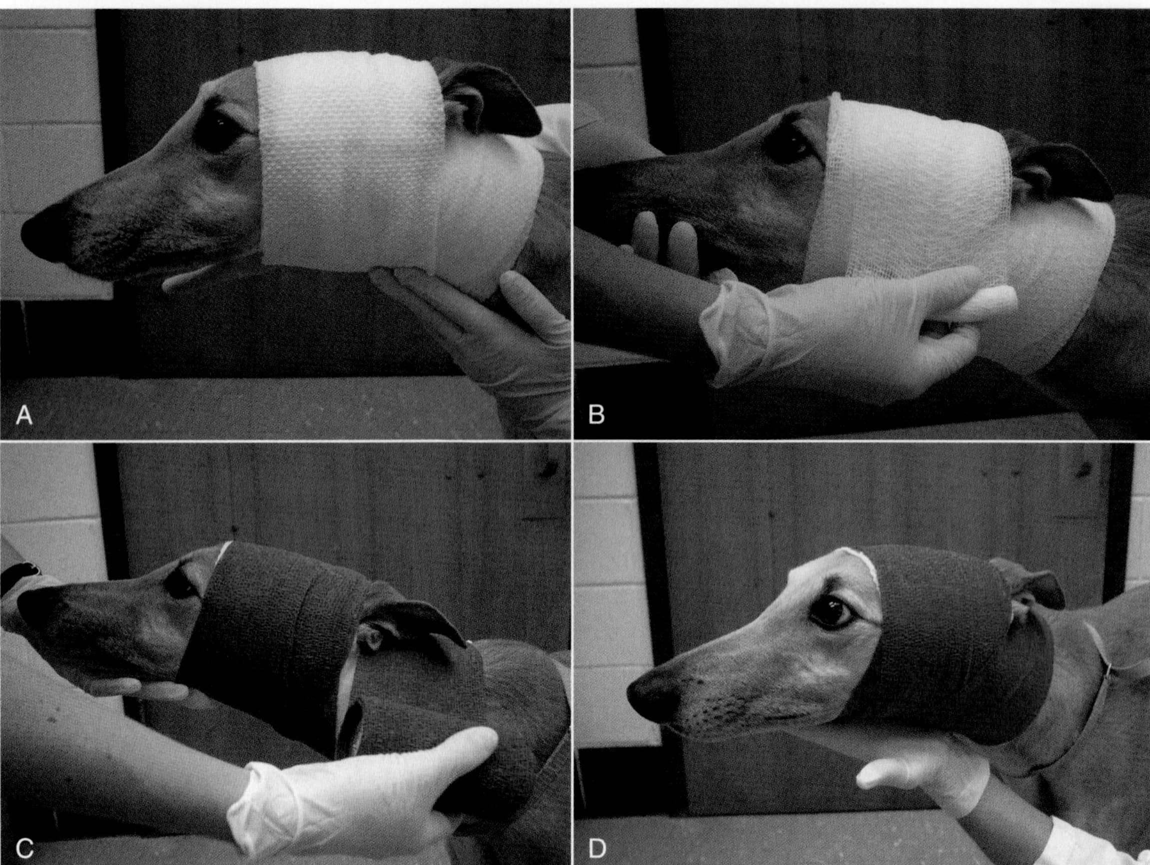

FIGURE 34-18 Application of an ear bandage. The injured right ear is bandaged on top of the head, first with cast padding **(A)** then covered by conforming gauze bandage **(B)**. The healthy left ear is left out of the bandage. The bandage is held in place by the tertiary layer **(C)**. It is important that the bandage goes in front and behind the ears to hold it in place and does not rub the eye **(D)**.

Animals with fourth-degree burns require intensive management. The large surface area of tissue damage and the extent of the deep tissue damage result in large volumes of fluid, electrolyte, and protein loss through the wound surface. Burn wounds are prone to infection because of the extensive tissue damage, the large surface area exposed to the environment (contamination), and the compromised condition of the animal.

Treatment of an animal with severe burns requires intravenous crystalloid and colloid fluid administration, antibiotic administration, nutritional support, and intensive wound management. Nutritional support is extremely important because the metabolic requirements of the animal may increase up to 200%. The animal is unlikely to take in adequate nutrition voluntarily. Force feeding or enteral feeding through a pharyngostomy, esophagostomy, or gastrostomy tube is indicated.

The wounds must be débrided and managed as open wounds. Any dead skin (eschar) must be removed. Débridement may have to be repeated, particularly for fourth-degree wounds, because the extent of the tissue damage may not be evident initially. Burn wounds tend to produce copious, often viscous exudate. Use of hydrophilic primary bandage layers will keep the wound moist yet absorb the exudate and facilitate removal of any tissue debris. A padded bandage to absorb the exudate with a nonocclusive tertiary layer is required. Ideally, sterile bandage material should be used. Bandages should be changed as often as required to prevent strike-through of the bandage by exudate from the wound. Once healthy granulation tissue is apparent in the wound, application of a semiocclusive, nonadherent primary bandage layer is indicated. Coating the wound with salves or lotions is contraindicated because they can be occlusive and prevent oxygen transfer to the wound. In addition, they trap wound exudate over the normal margins of the wound, which may macerate the tissue. After a healthy granulation tissue wound bed has developed, the wounds are then amenable to tertiary closure or skin grafting.

PUNCTURE WOUNDS

Puncture wounds are characterized by small skin openings with often extensive deep tissue damage. Penetrating injuries caused by sharp objects (e.g., sticks), gunshots, bite wounds, and insect stings are all types of puncture wounds. Foreign material and bacteria are carried deep into the wound. Puncture wounds should be treated by exploration, débridement, lavage, and primary closure if all the damaged contaminated tissue and all foreign material can be removed from the wound. If the wound remains contaminated or if

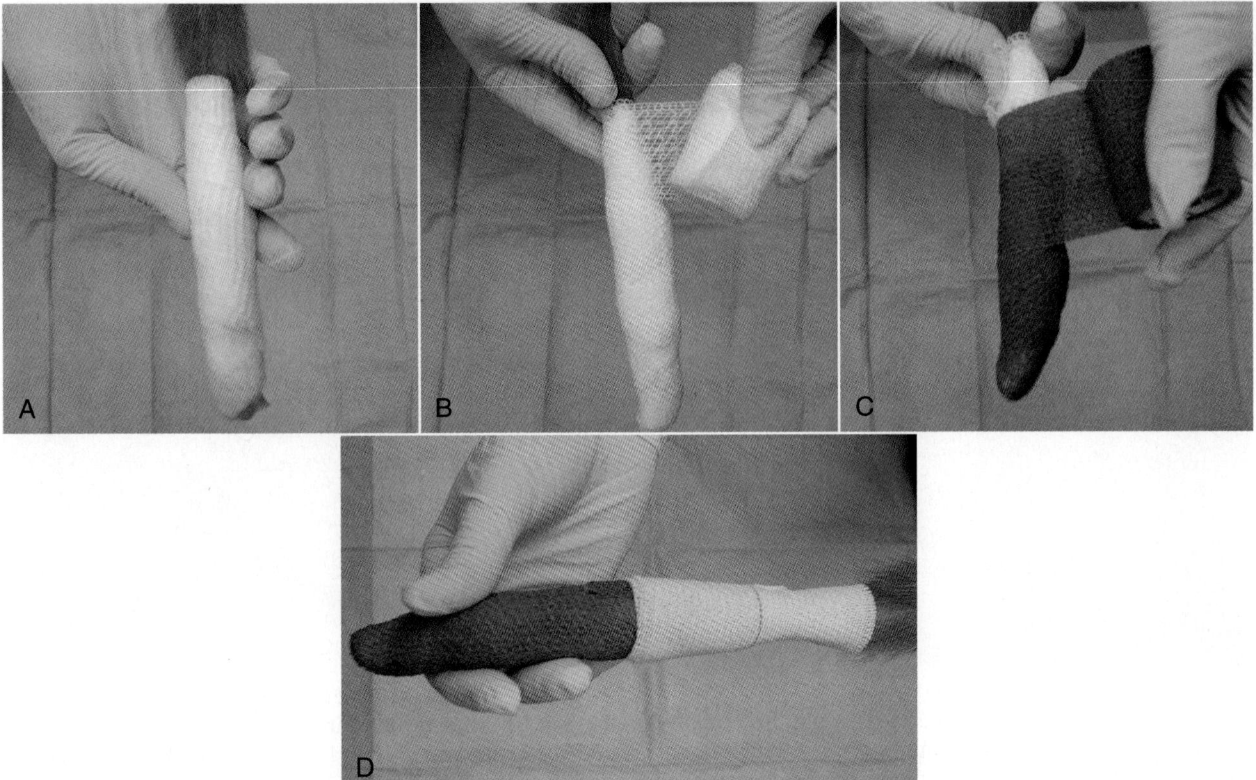

FIGURE 34-19 Application of a tail bandage. The tail is bandaged in three layers with any primary layer covered by a small amount of cast padding **(A)**, followed by conforming gauze **(B)**, and finally a tertiary layer **(C)**. A sticky adhesive bandage can be used as the tertiary layer or on top, extending onto the intact skin to ensure that the bandage stays in place **(D)**.

BOX 34-7 Classification of Thermal Burns

First Degree
Very superficial burn that involves only the epidermis. Does not blister, but becomes erythematous because of dermal vasodilation and is painful. Over 2 to 3 days, the pain subsides, and the damaged epidermis desquamates.

Second Degree
Superficial burn that involves all layers of dermis. Characteristically forms blisters with fluid collection at the interface of the epidermis and dermis. Blistering may not occur for several hours after injury.

Third Degree
Full-thickness burn that involves all layers of the dermis. The surface may appear white or black and leathery, firm, and depressed compared with surrounding skin.

Fourth Degree
Full-thickness burn that involves not only the dermis, but also subcutaneous fat and deeper structures.

there is a large amount of deep tissue damage with resultant dead space in the wound, a drain may be placed. Ideally a closed suction wound drain that connects to a closed reservoir should be used to reduce contamination of the wound from the environment via the drain. A closed drain also allows the volume and nature of the drainage to be monitored.

DEGLOVING INJURIES

Degloving injuries are commonly seen in small animals and are typically the result of being hit by a car and dragged over the road surface. An anatomic degloving injury results in skin and varying amounts of deep tissue (muscle, tendon, ligament, bone) torn off a limb. A physiologic degloving injury is characterized by an intact skin surface with disruption of the skin attachment and neurovascular supply at the deep fascial level. Necrosis of the detached skin becomes apparent 3 to 5 days after injury.

Degloving injuries require intensive management over a prolonged period. Initial débridement, lavage, and management of the open wound are required. It may take several weeks before the wound is covered by a healthy granulation tissue bed. At this time, skin grafting is indicated. Some degloving injuries will completely heal by second intention, although the tension on the skin of the distal extremities can be a limiting factor. In addition, the resultant skin contracture and friable new epithelium may not always be a desirable outcome.

DECUBITUS ULCERS

Decubitus ulcers are the result of compression of soft tissues and skin between a bony prominence and the surface on which an animal is lying. Thin, debilitated animals that are recumbent for long periods are at risk in addition to the naturally

CASE PRESENTATION 34-1

A 14-year-old male, neutered, basset hound underwent resection for a 3 cm in diameter, grade 3 mast cell tumor on the left caudal abdomen. A large resection was performed with closure of the defect using an advancement skin flap. The dog was seen 7 days after surgery with full-thickness necrosis of the corner of the flap (Figure 1). Note the black, triangular section of necrotic skin with a thick eschar *(E)*.

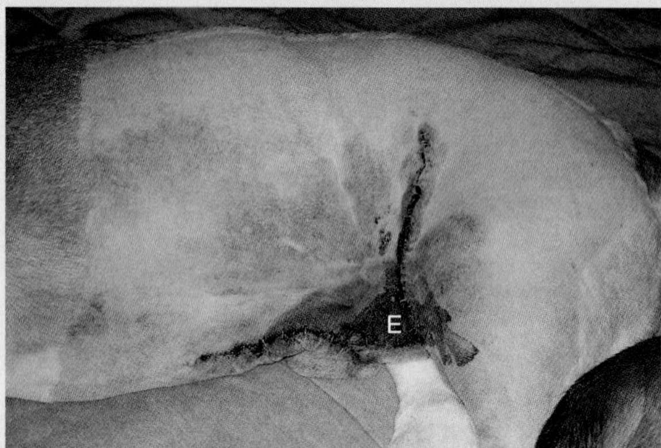

FIGURE 1

The eschar was elevated and then removed. The underlying wound consisted of poor granulation tissue covered by a film of wound exudate. The wound was packed with a hypertonic saline dressing (CURASALT*), indicated in a contaminated or infected wound where natural débridement is required (Figure 2).

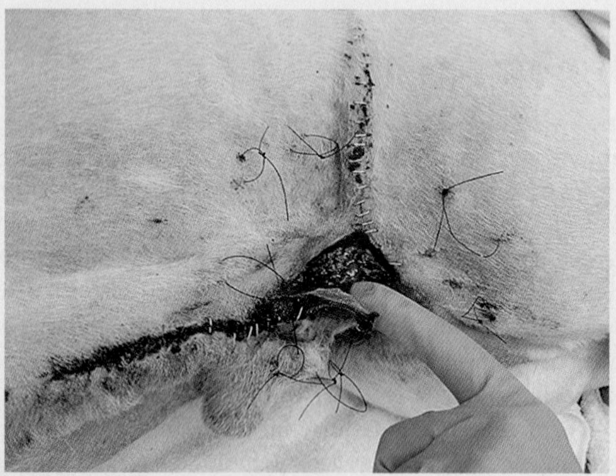

FIGURE 2

The bandage was removed 2 days later (day 9). There was minimal wound exudate, and the granulation tissue was redder and more abundant. The wound was covered by a hydrogel dressing (Curagel*), indicated in a granulating wound with minimal exudate since the hydrogel will keep the wound moist (Figure 3).

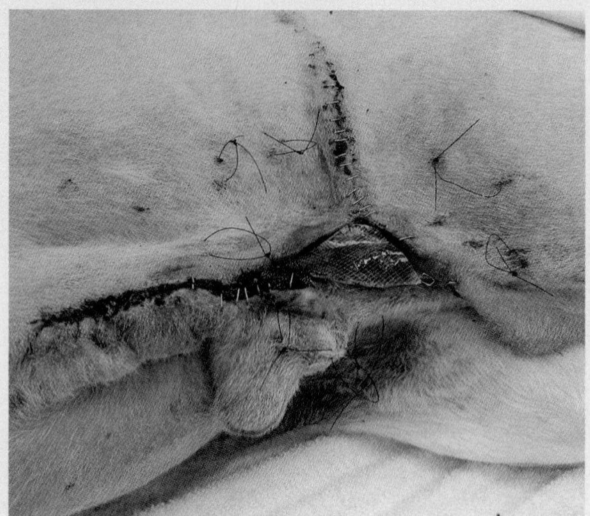

FIGURE 3

Bandage changes continued every 3 to 4 days. The same dressing was used. By day 19, the wound showed considerable wound contraction and new epithelium *(e)* at the margins of the wound. The granulation tissue *(gt)* was vascular, evident by bleeding during bandage change (Figure 4).

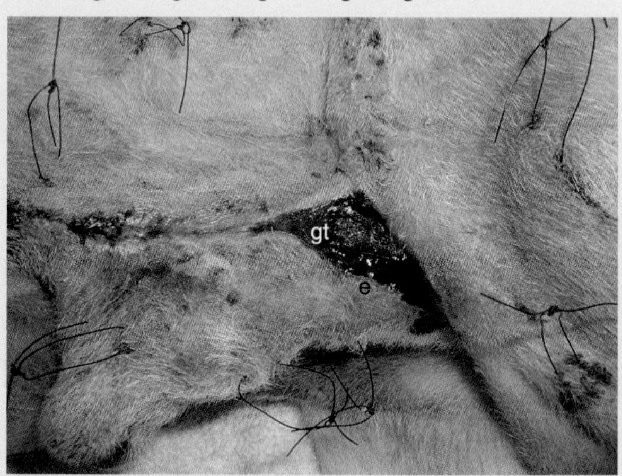

FIGURE 4

By day 24, the wound showed more contraction and epithelialization *(e)* (Figure 5). There was minimal to no wound exudate. The defect was filled with granulation tissue *(gt)*. A layer of hydrogel (Curafil Gel Wound Dressing*) was applied over the

thin breeds (e.g., Afghan hounds, greyhounds, whippets). The soft tissue and underlying bone of decubitus ulcers may become secondarily infected by environmental microorganisms.

Prevention is the key to management. Adequate soft bedding (water beds) is essential for an at-risk animal. The animal's position should be changed frequently throughout the day. Likely pressure points should be examined daily. Physical therapy and hydrotherapy three or four times per day help to keep the skin clean and promote peripheral circulation. The bedding should be kept clean, dry, and free of excreta. Vulnerable sites can be padded. Maintaining the animal on a high nutritional plane (high-protein, high-carbohydrate diet) is essential.

Closure of existing decubitus ulcers is desirable. Minimal débridement is usually required. Closures often fail because the line of wound closure also overlies a pressure point, and tension is often apparent on the wound edges. In some instances, skin flaps may be preferred.

CASE PRESENTATION 34-1—cont'd

wound surface, and the wound was covered with a nonadherent, occlusive dressing (OpSite*), indicated in a dry, granulating wound to provide a moist environment for reepithelialization.

The wound was completely reepithelialized by day 42 (Figure 6).

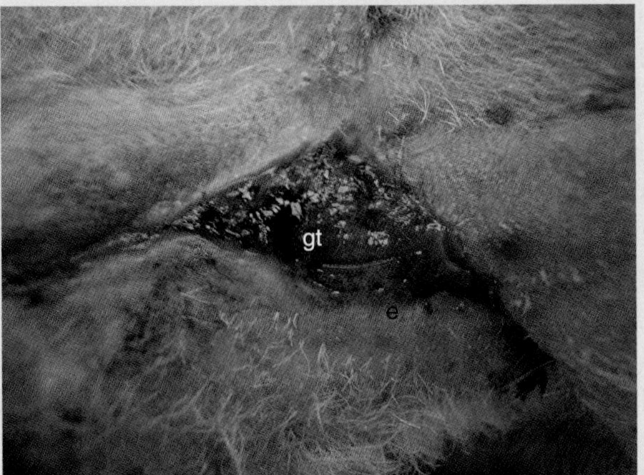

FIGURE 5

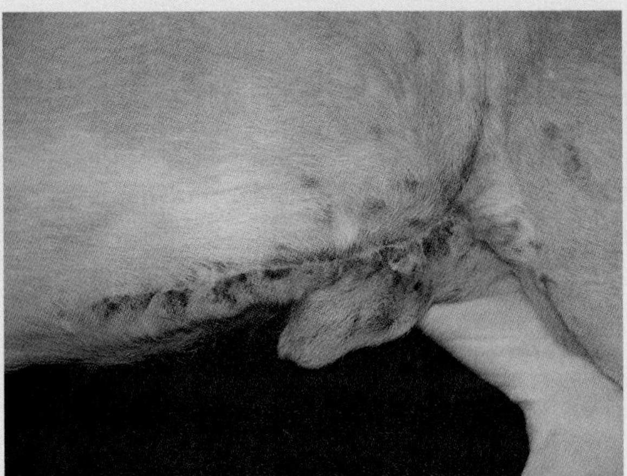

FIGURE 6

*Tyco Healthcare/Kendall, Mansfield, Mass.

LARGE ANIMAL WOUND MANAGEMENT

WOUND CARE OF HORSES

Basic wound management is no different in large animals than in small companion animals. However, the size and nature of the animal and the location of the injury may dictate the way a wound is approached. Thus some additional points are briefly discussed.

When a wound on a horse is prepared, a water-soluble lubricant or saline solution-soaked gauze can be used to fill the depths of the wound. Electric clippers are usually used to remove the hair from around the edges of the wound. However, if clippers are not available, the wound edges can be lathered with antiseptic scrub, and a straightedge razor or No. 22 scalpel blade can be used to shave the hair (Figure 34-20).

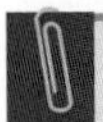

TECHNICIAN NOTE It is important to clip or shave the hair surrounding a wound.

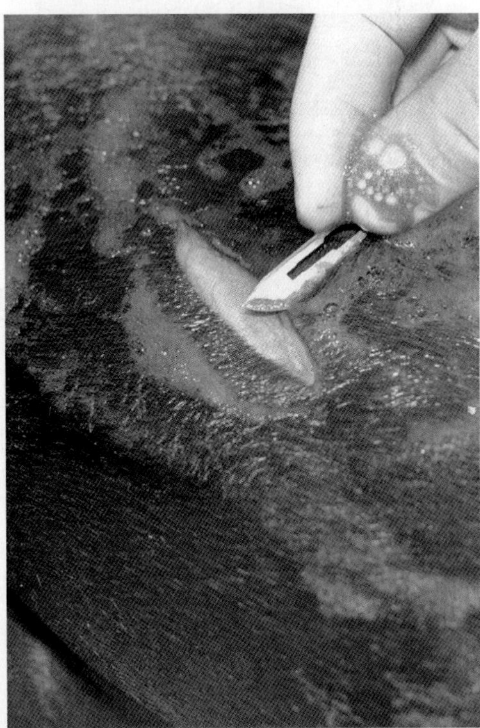

FIGURE 34-20 Once the hair has been lathered with antiseptic (Betadine) scrub, a No. 22 scalpel blade can be used to shave away the hair from the wound edges.

Methods used to lavage a wound are similar to those described for small companion animals earlier in this chapter. If the wound is to be closed, local anesthesia with tranquilization or general anesthesia may be needed before a fresh wound can be properly treated. If tranquilization is used, local or regional anesthetic is necessary for débridement and closure of the wound. Local infiltration is performed by injecting a local anesthetic, mepivacaine or lidocaine, approximately 1 cm from the wound edge, subcutaneously around the entire wound. A 22-gauge hypodermic needle is used in most situations and is reinserted repeatedly through the skin, each time at the end of the bleb formed by the preceding injection of local anesthetic (Figure 34-21). In this way, the patient will not react to the successive injections. If the wound is located on the distal portion of a limb, a ring block or nerve block (e.g., a palmar nerve block) can be applied, and the portion of the limb distal to the block will be anesthetized (Figure 34-22). If a wound is to be sutured, the same considerations for wound closure in small companion animals apply to large animals. It is important to remember that open wounds on the distal aspect of the limb (below the carpus or tarsus) of the horse are notorious for developing exuberant granulation tissue. Exuberant granulation tissue, commonly referred to as "proud flesh," can form rapidly in horses. Various measures must be undertaken to keep exuberant granulation tissue in check, or it can become excessive (Figure 34-23). Methods of controlling granulation tissue include immobilizing the limb (as with a cast); wound bandaging; surgical excision; caustic agents, such as equal parts of copper sulfate and boric acid powder (Figure 34-24); cryotherapy; electrocautery; and topical corticosteroids. Regardless of the decision to allow a wound on the limb of a large animal to heal by first or second intention, a bandage should be placed on the limb.

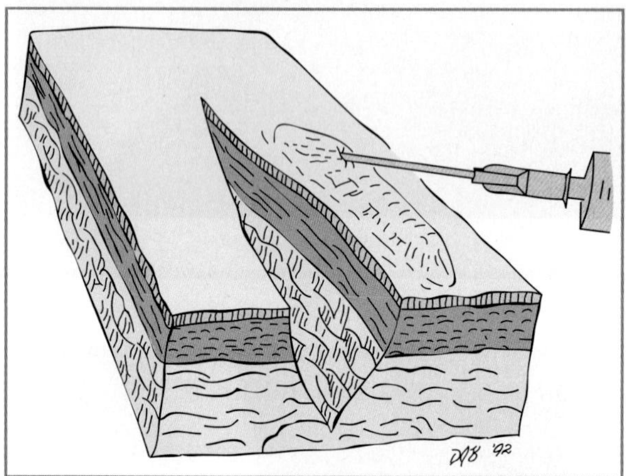

FIGURE 34-21 Proper technique for infiltration of a wound edge with a local anesthetic. The needle should enter through the skin at the point of the last injection.

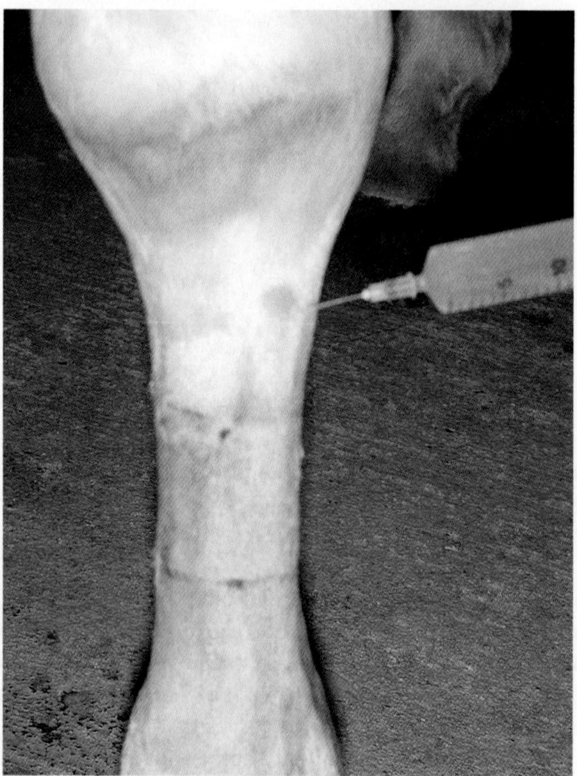

FIGURE 34-22 A ring block using a local anesthetic is infiltrated subcutaneously around the limb of a horse to triage a distal limb wound.

BANDAGING AND CAST APPLICATION TECHNIQUES FOR HORSES

Bandages and casts serve many purposes and are named for the location and purpose that they cover and serve, respectively. Various materials are available for use in a bandage or cast, but the important aspect is their proper application and function. Development of good bandaging and cast application skills is important to ensure proper function of the bandage or cast. The application and purpose of the different types used on horses are discussed.

BANDAGES

Lower Limb Wound Bandage

A lower limb wound bandage covers a wound on a limb distal to the carpus or tarsus. When the wound is traumatic, after it has been cleaned and débrided, a topical medication is usually applied if it is left unsutured. A nonadherent dressing is then placed directly over the wound. The wound dressing is secured to the limb with rolled conforming gauze. The conforming gauze is wrapped around the limb with light pressure, overlapping, and without wrinkles to prevent formation of pressure lines, which may

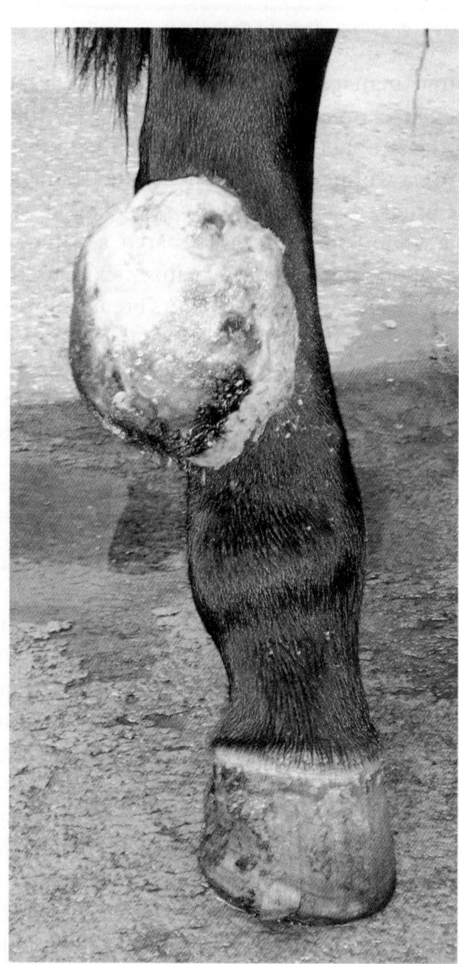

FIGURE 34-23 Exuberant granulation tissue on the metatarsus of a horse.

cause skin sloughing if applied too tightly. It is wrapped proximal and distal to the wound edges approximately 2 to 4 cm (Figure 34-25).

The padded layer is applied next. Combine cotton sheets cut from a roll, rolled cotton, layered cotton sheets, quilted leg wraps, or a military field bandage can be used (Figure 34-26). If cotton sheets are available, five are used, folded in half, and neatly rolled. The fifth sheet is folded in the opposite direction to the other sheets to conceal the edges. The padded layer is secured to the limb with a roll of conforming gauze. Pressure is applied during wrapping to compress and conform the padding to the limb. The outer shell of the bandage is finished with elastic wrap (3M Vetrap Bandage Tape or an Ace bandage), adhesive elastic tape (Elasticon, Johnson & Johnson), or a flannel track wrap. If an Ace bandage or track wrap is used, it is secured with white tape cut into strips or placed around the bandage in a "barber pole" fashion (Figure 34-27). Elasticon is placed around the top and bottom of the bandage, with half of the tape sticking to the wrap and half to the skin, to prevent slippage and to keep debris (e.g., bedding shavings) from getting inside the bandage (Figure 34-28).

Lower Limb Support Bandage

A lower limb support bandage is used to provide support for the soft tissues (e.g., ligaments, tendons) of the limb contralateral to the injured leg, which is bearing excessive weight because of decreased weight bearing on the injured limb. The bandage also minimizes static limb edema in a confined, inactive horse. A support bandage is placed on the lower limb just like the lower limb wound bandage described previously except that the underlying wound dressing and inner conforming gauze layer are not used. It is also unnecessary to place wide adhesive elastic tape around the top and bottom.

SPLINT APPLICATION

A splint is an addition of a rigid material to a limb bandage to reinforce immobilization of a particular part of a limb. Various materials can be used as the reinforcement, including wooden slats, metal bars, low-temperature thermoplastic, and casting material. However, the most common material used is polyvinyl chloride (PVC) pipe because of its light weight and strength. The pipe used is 10 cm in diameter and is split in thirds. It can be bent by heating with a cutting torch to conform to the fetlock angulation. The length and width of the splint vary with the size of the leg and the area splinted. Depending on the amount of immobilization required, splints can be placed the full length of the forelimb or from just below the carpus or tarsus all the way to the ground surface. In most situations, they are placed on the flexor surface of the limb. Splints are used in situations such as cases of extensor or flexor tendon lacerations and flexure deformities in foals or as needed limb support (as in radial nerve paresis).

A thick bandage is first placed on the limb. It should be long enough to cover the limb above and below the ends of the splint. This will prevent the development of pressure sores. Once the bandage is in place, the splint is secured to the limb with adhesive tape (Figure 34-29). Splints should be reset frequently (at least once per day) in foals.

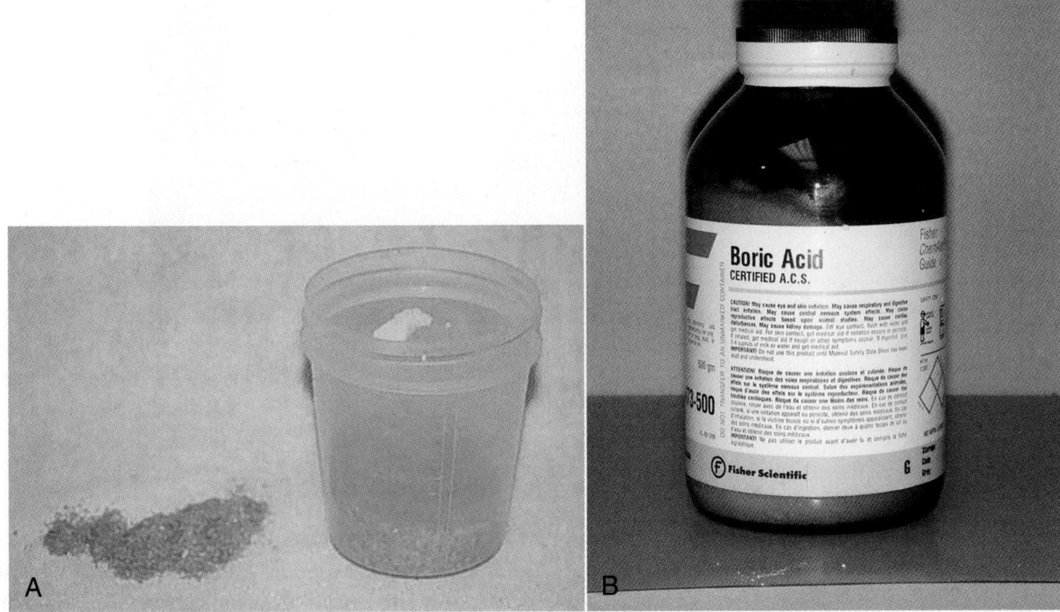

FIGURE 34-24 A 50:50 mixture of copper sulfate and boric acid can be applied to proud flesh to reduce it in an open wound.

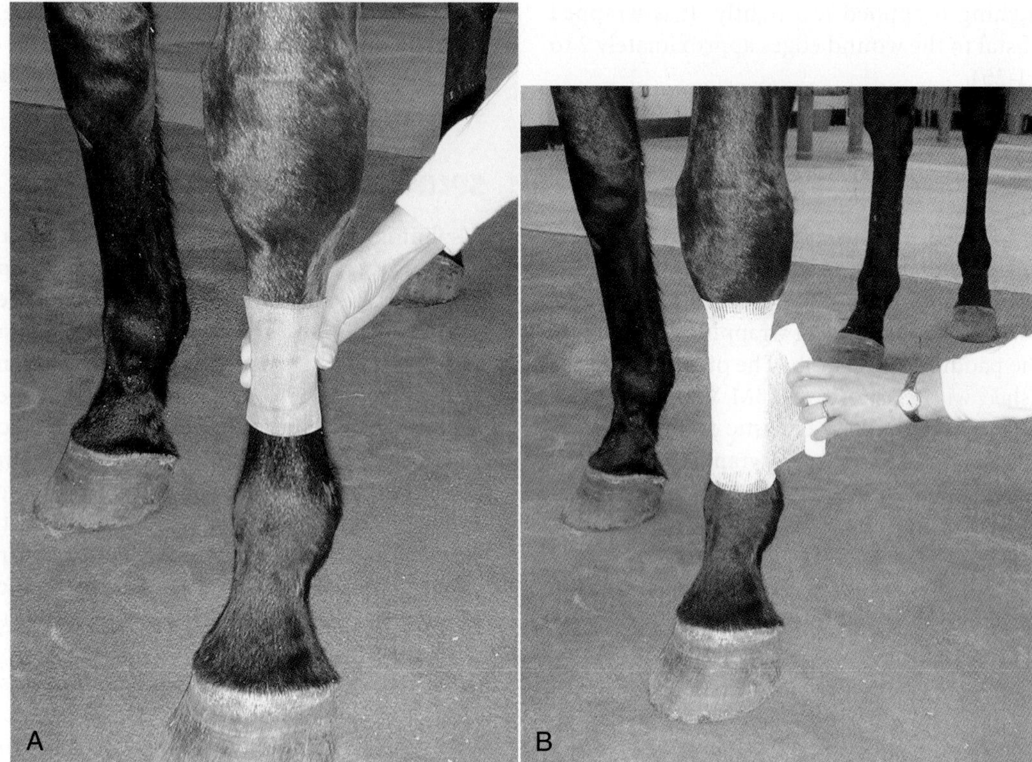

FIGURE 34-25 Application of wound dressing on the distal region of the limb of a horse. **A,** Nonadherent dressing is applied directly over the wound. **B,** Conforming gauze is applied to maintain a nonadherent dressing over the wound.

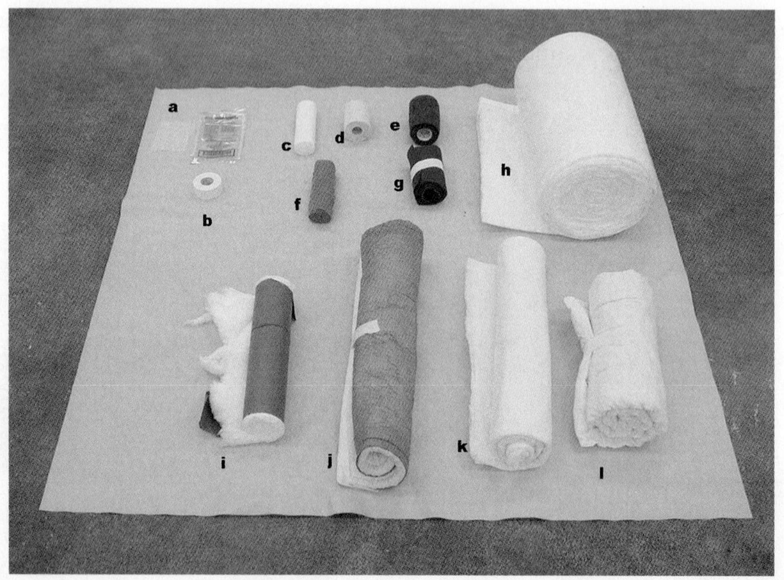

FIGURE 36-26 Various materials can be used in a leg bandage for large animals. Nonadherent wound dressing *(a)*, white tape *(b)*, white roll gauze *(c)*, Elasticon *(d)*, 3M Vetrap Bandage Tape *(e)*, brown gauze *(f)*, track wrap *(g)*, cotton combine *(h)*, rolled cotton *(i)*, military field bandage *(j)*, layered cotton sheets *(k)*, quilted leg wraps *(l)*.

> *TECHNICIAN NOTE* A bandage should cover the limb well above and below the ends of a splint to prevent pressure sores.

CAST APPLICATION

A cast is the most frequently used external coaptation to manage various orthopedic injuries or problems when maximum support and immobilization are required. Casts are commonly used for lower limb problems; however, full-limb application

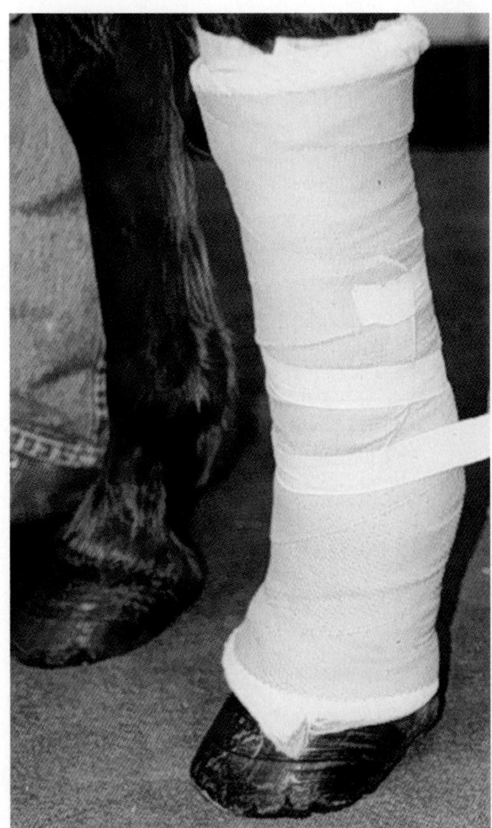

FIGURE 34-27 If white medical tape is used to secure the outer layer of the bandage on a horse's limb, it is secured in a barber-pole fashion to reduce the changes of a tourniquet effect.

is sometimes indicated in large animals. Indications for use of a cast include lower limb fractures, tendon lacerations, support of the lower limb during recovery from orthopedic surgery, heel bulb lacerations, and luxations of the tarsus, fetlock, or pastern. A cast may also be used as an adjunct to internal fixation.

For optimal effectiveness in immobilization, a cast must immobilize the joint proximal and distal to the injury. Full-limb casts must extend up to the elbow or stifle as far as possible. The most frequently used material today is fiberglass. Fiberglass (e.g., Delta-Lite, Johnson & Johnson) is appealing because it is lightweight, strong, and relatively easy to apply. However, some veterinarians prefer to use an initial layer of the traditional plaster of Paris under the fiberglass. Plaster conforms well to the contour of the limb, reducing the risk of pressure sores.

Before cast application is begun, several things must be considered. A limb cast must be applied properly, or serious problems, such as pressure necrosis, can occur. It is also important to remember that applying excessive padding under a cast can result in compression of the padding and loosening of the cast, resulting in the development of cast sores. Because of its importance, application of a limb cast is described here in detail.

> *TECHNICIAN NOTE* Excessive padding under a cast can result in compression of the padding and loosening of the cast, resulting in the development of cast sores.

Before the procedure is begun, all the materials needed should be collected: orthopedic stockinette (3-inch), orthopedic felt, towel clamps, white tape (1-inch), wire (approximately 30 cm), ⅛-inch drill bit and hand drill, broom handle, hoof-trimming equipment (hoof rasp, trimmers, hoof knife), bandage scissors, and cast material (Figure 34-30). Proper application of a cast is essential, especially if it is to remain on the limb for a prolonged period (4 to 6 weeks).

In general, it is best to apply the cast with the horse under general anesthesia. The horse is positioned in lateral recumbency so that the limb to which the cast will be applied is uppermost. Debris is cleaned from the sole, the horseshoe is removed, and the hoof is trimmed. The limb is placed in an extended position perpendicular to the body. Effective support of the leg to maintain the limb in alignment is essential. Traction achieved by using wire looped through holes drilled in the hoof can be helpful. Two holes are drilled in the hoof wall, 5 cm apart near the toe, in the same direction as that in which a horseshoe nail is driven. The ends of the wire are twisted together to form a loop through which a broom handle is placed to apply traction (Figure 34-31).

The frog (the central soft tissue of the hoof) can be packed with povidone-iodine, especially if thrush is present. If a wound is present, a three-layer bandage consisting of a nonadherent dressing, conforming gauze, and adherent elastic tape is used to cover it. The skin must be clean and dry. It can be powdered with talcum or boric acid to help keep the area under the cast dry. The limb is then covered with a double layer of stockinette. The length of the region that the cast will cover is measured, then doubled, and approximately 20 cm is added to this to determine the length of stockinette needed. One end is rolled outward and the other is rolled inward until they meet at the midpoint of the stockinette (Figure 34-32).

The traction wire is threaded through the opening in the stockinette. A broom handle is placed through the wire loop, and traction is applied. The outward roll is first unrolled up the leg. A twist is placed in the stockinette just beneath the toe, and the inward roll is unrolled up the leg (Figure 34-33). Any wrinkles are smoothed out, and towel clamps are used to secure the stockinette to the medial and lateral aspects of the limb above the area to which the cast will be applied (Figure 34-34).

A strip of orthopedic felt (5 to 7 cm wide) is placed around the leg at the most proximal limit of the cast. This is held in place with 1-inch white tape (Figure 34-35). When a full-limb cast is used, a doughnut pad cut from orthopedic felt is placed over the accessory carpal bone of the forelimb. A thin strip of orthopedic felt is placed over the gastrocnemius tendon and the point of the hock of the hind limb to prevent the development of pressure sores. A roll of support foam can be applied next. It is applied over the stockinette, and its purpose is to provide padding under a cast to reduce the development of pressure sores (Figure 34-36). Additional padding on the leg should be avoided because this can

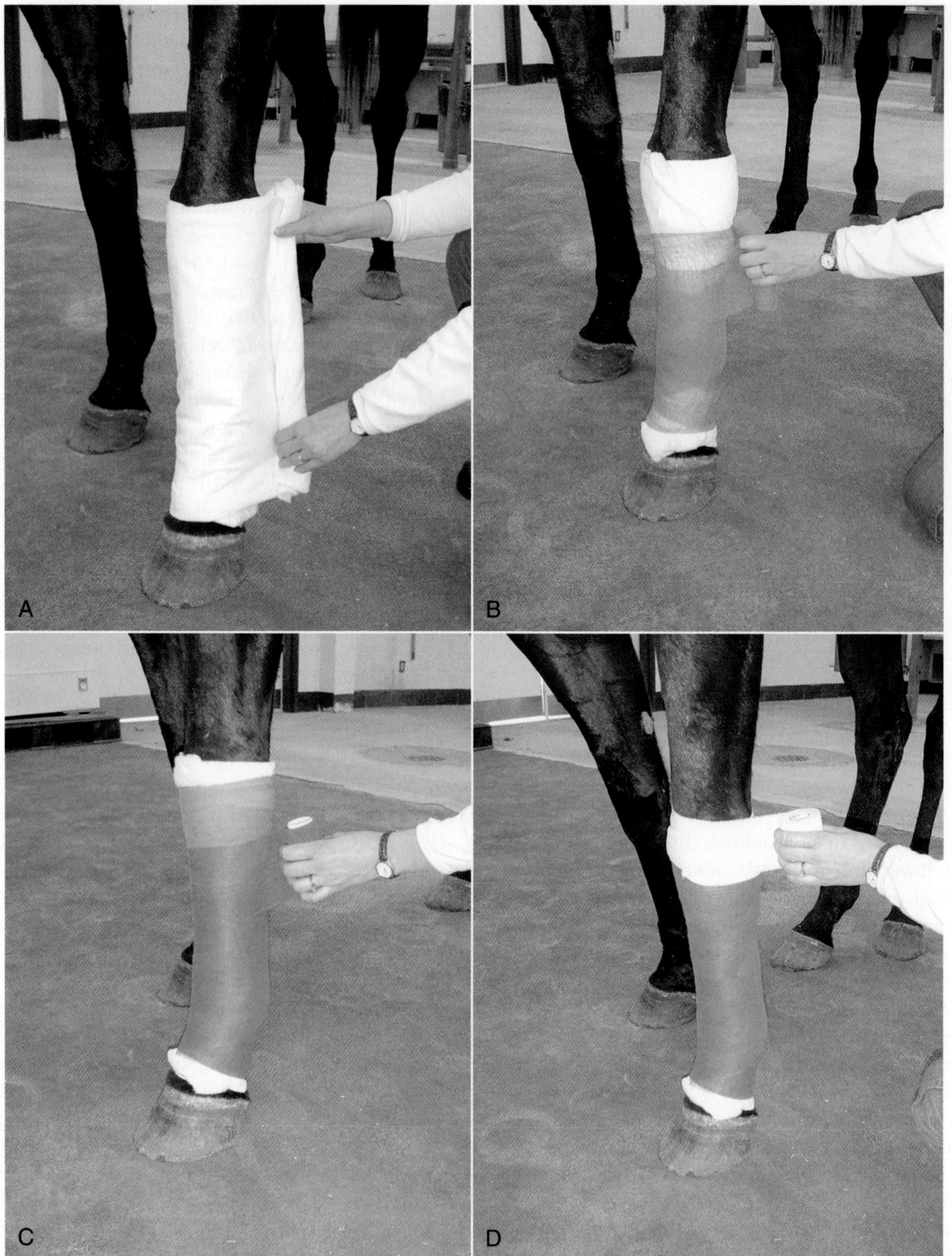

FIGURE 34-28 Application of padded layer of a wound bandage. **A,** Cotton wrap is applied snugly around the limb. **B,** Conforming gauze is used to secure the padded layer to the limb. **C,** 3M Vetrap Bandage Tape is applied as the outer shell of the bandage. **D,** Wide adhesive tape is used to provide a seal between the skin and bandage.

become compressed, thus allowing the leg to move within the cast and cause sores.

Two layers of 3-inch plaster material are first carefully and snugly applied to the limb. These layers should be applied without wrinkles to prevent development of pressure sores. Application of the cast material is usually started at either the proximal or distal aspect of the limb. (The authors prefer to start distally [Figure 34-37]). A roll of plaster is started at the level of the fetlock and worked distally and then proximally. Approximately 1 cm of the orthopedic felt is left exposed above the top of the cast to prevent formation of a sore.

> *TECHNICIAN NOTE* It is important that the initial layer of casting material be applied to the limb without wrinkles or finger imprints, which may create pressure sores.

Gloves should be worn when the casting material is applied. To save time in identifying the end on a wetted plaster roll, unroll 2 to 3 inches of the plaster material and hold onto it while wetting the roll in a bucket of warm water (Figure 34-38). The excess water is removed by shaking and squeezing the roll. Do not squeeze excessively, or much of the plaster will be lost. Fiberglass material is held in a bucket of clean water until it is thoroughly wet, and the excess water is shaken out.

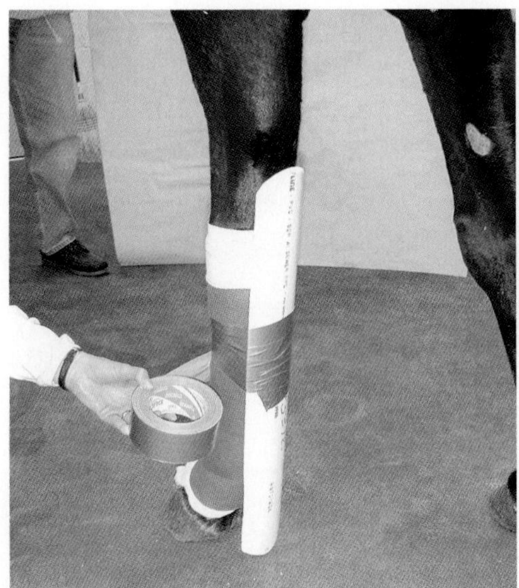

FIGURE 34-29 Application of a lower limb splint. A thick bandage is placed on the limb. The splint (PVC pipe) is positioned along the flexor surface and secured to the bandage with duct tape.

Next, the fiberglass cast material is applied. Usually, it is easier to begin with 3-inch material because it conforms to the limb better. The cast material is overlapped by one third to one half. As the fiberglass casting material is worked toward the foot, the traction wires are cut, and an assistant holds the leg out at the upper limb region or by resting it on the palms of his or her hands, which are placed under the metacarpus or metatarsus region. It is imperative to prevent formation of finger imprints in the cast because they could cause pressure sores to develop (Figure 34-39).

More pressure is applied to the succeeding layers of fiberglass. This will allow them to laminate better. Generally, two layers (3 to 4 rolls) of 3-inch fiberglass cast material are applied, followed by two or three layers (3 to 4 rolls) of 4- or 5-inch fiberglass. At the time the last roll of cast material is applied, the stockinette is unclamped and the excess is cut off, leaving approximately 4 cm. This 4-cm excess is turned down over the top of the cast and incorporated in the last layer (Figure 34-40). A wooden wedge block or a 3-inch roll of wet plaster cast material is placed underneath the heel and also incorporated with the last layer (Figure 34-41). A heel wedge allows the horse to walk more easily while wearing a cast because it decreases the breakover force, reduces pressure on the dorsal proximal limits of the cast at the metacarpus or metatarsus, and allows more even axial weight bearing down through the cast.

When application of the cast is completed, the outer layer is smoothed by running wetted, gloved hands up and down the cast. The bottom of the cast is protected from wear by capping it with hard acrylic (e.g., Technovit, Jorgensen Laboratories, Loveland, Colo.) (Figure 34-42). Finally, elastic adhesive tape is placed around the top of the cast and attached to the skin (Figure 34-43), or a piece of stockinette

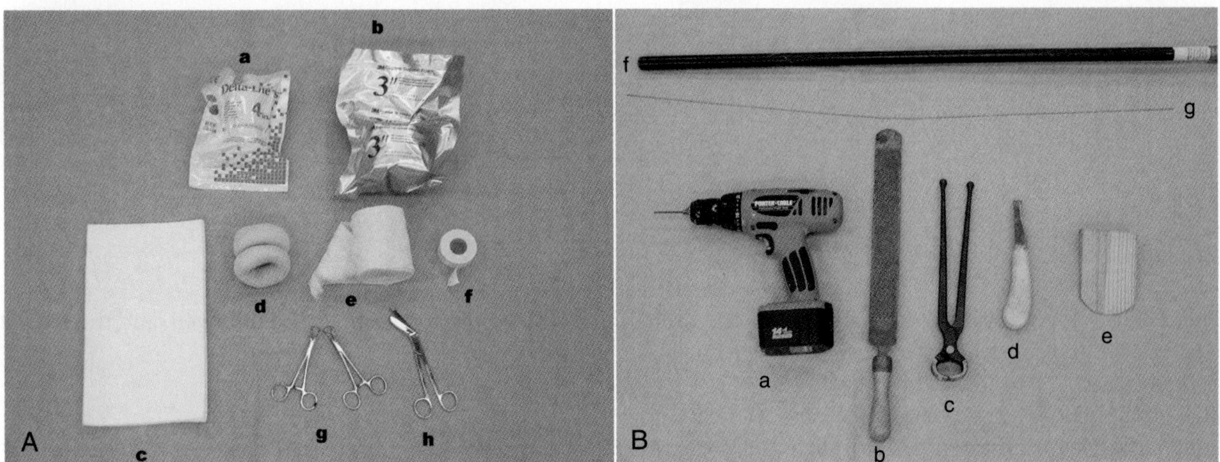

FIGURE 34-30 Materials needed to apply a limb cast on a large animal. **A,** Cast material *(a)*, support foam *(b)*, orthopedic felt *(c)*, orthopedic stockinette (3 inch) *(d)*, cast padding *(e)*, white tape (1 inch) *(f)*, towel clamps *(g)*, and bandage scissors *(h)*. **B,** ⅛-inch drill bit and hand drill *(a)*, hoof rasp *(b)*, shoe pullers *(c)*, hoof knife *(d)*, wooden wedge block *(e)*, broom handle *(f)*, and wire (approximately 30 cm) *(g)*.

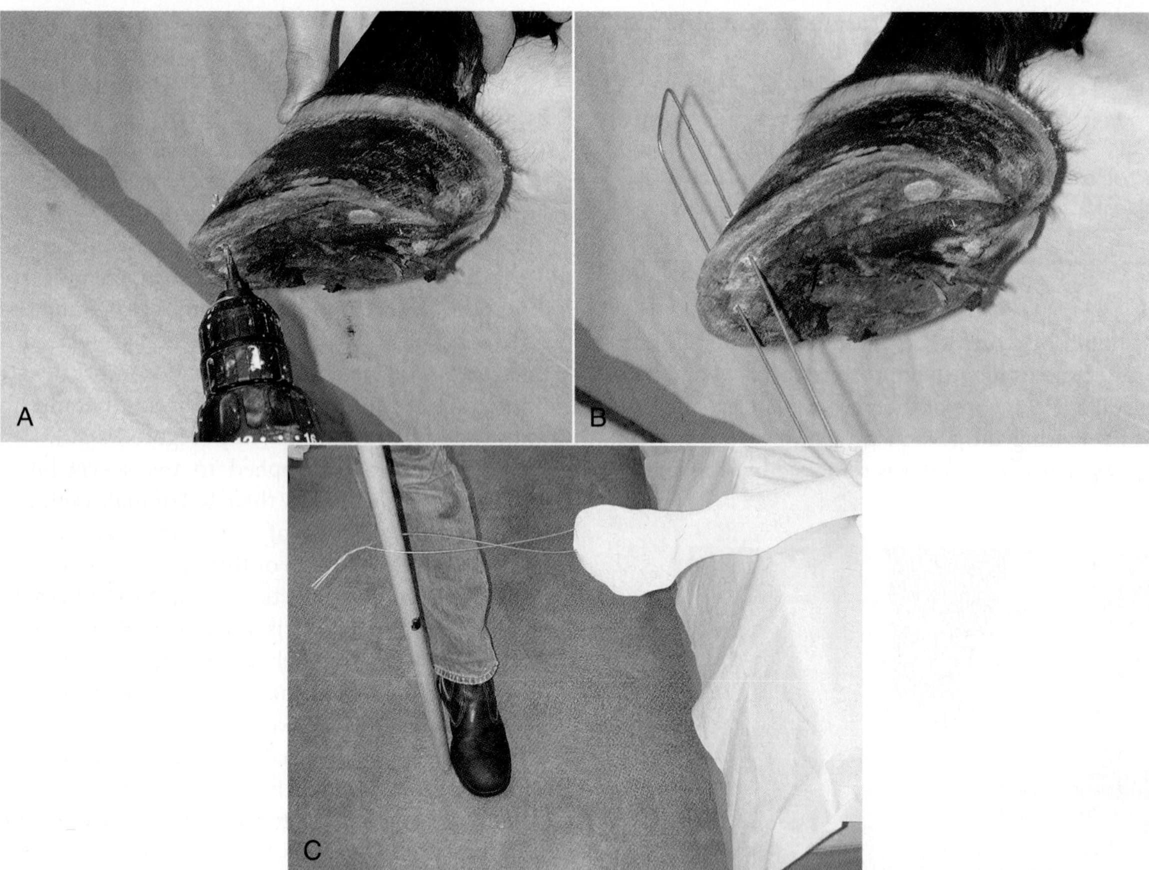

FIGURE 34-31 Traction can be applied to a limb before cast application by drilling two holes in the toe of the hoof **(A)** and threading a loop of wire through the holes **(B)** with a broomstick placed in the loop to apply traction **(C)**.

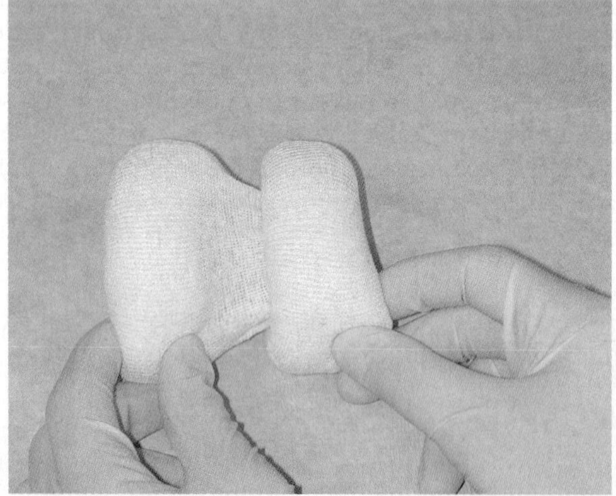

FIGURE 34-32 Orthopedic stockinette used under a cast is prerolled. One end is rolled outward and the other end is rolled inward until they meet at the midpoint of the stockinette.

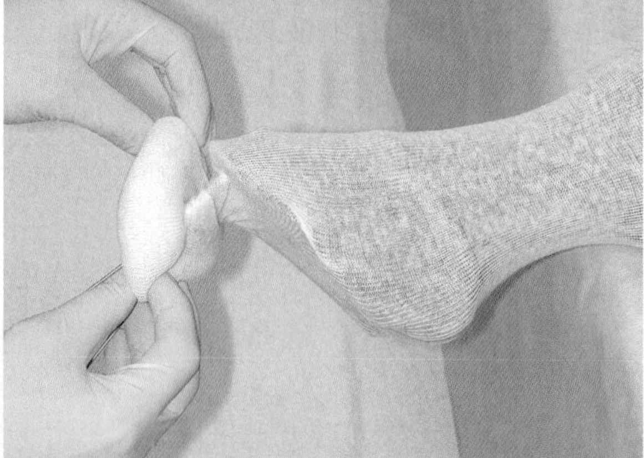

FIGURE 34-33 A twist is placed in the stockinette just beneath the toe, and the inward roll is unrolled up the leg.

is pulled over the top and taped to the cast and the limb above the cast to prevent debris (wood shavings) from getting inside the cast.

Stall confinement is mandatory after cast application. The patient must be monitored daily. Indications for cast change or removal include breakage, increased lameness, swelling, or exudates coming out of the top of the cast. Horses vary in their reaction and tolerance to a cast. If there is any doubt, a cast should be removed, and the limb should be evaluated.

CAST REMOVAL

Removal of a cast is best performed with the animal standing unless another cast is to be reapplied. If cast removal is performed under general anesthesia, there is a risk of reinjury to

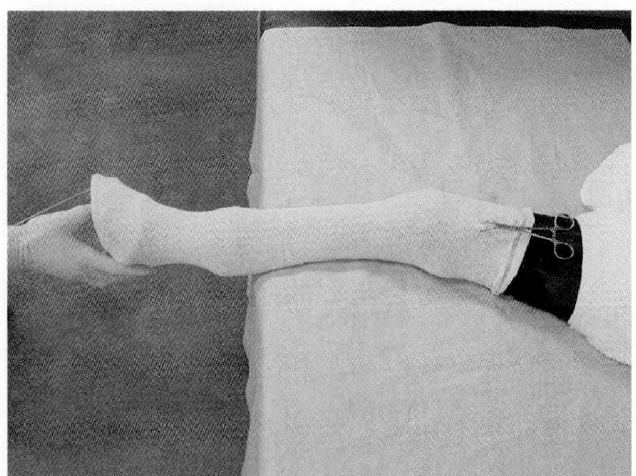

FIGURE 34-34 Before cast material is applied, the orthopedic stockinette is secured with towel clamps to the medial and lateral aspects of the limb above the area to which the cast will be applied.

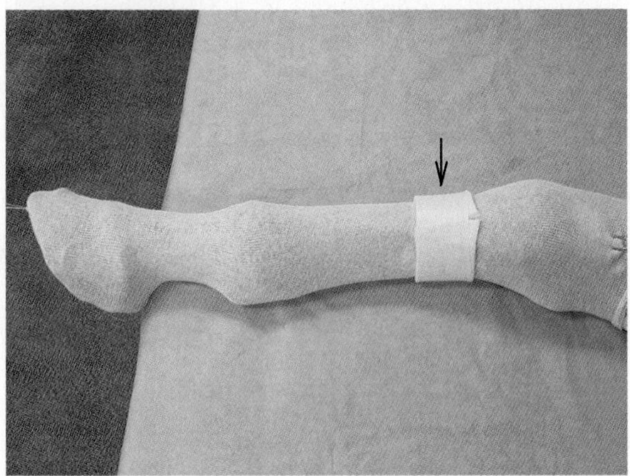

FIGURE 34-35 A strip of orthopedic felt (5 to 7 cm wide) *(arrow)* is placed around the leg at the most proximal limit of cast. The ends are held in place with 1-inch white tape.

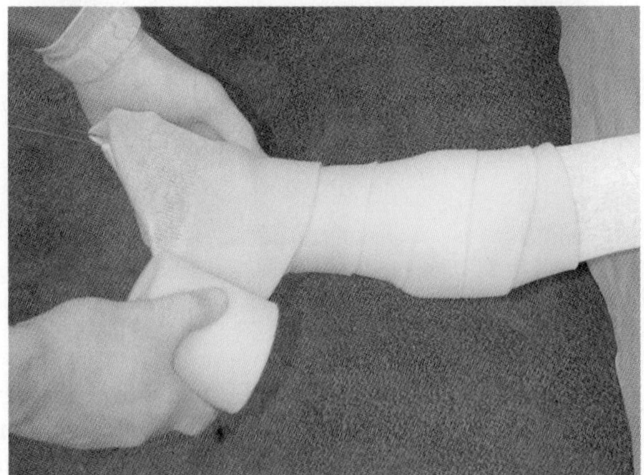

FIGURE 34-36 A roll of support foam can be applied over the stockinette to provide padding under the cast to prevent formation of pressure sores.

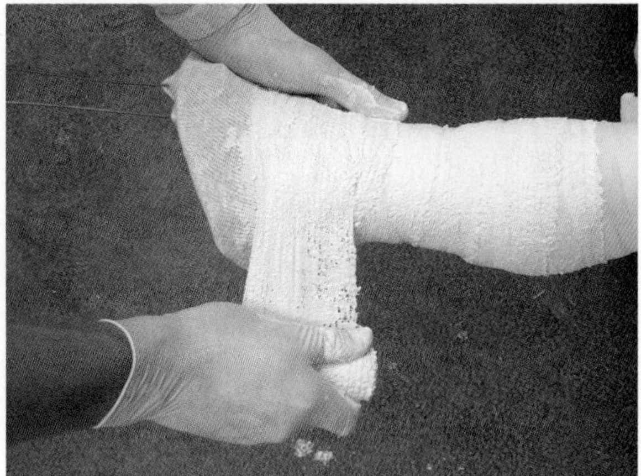

FIGURE 34-37 Application of plaster of Paris.

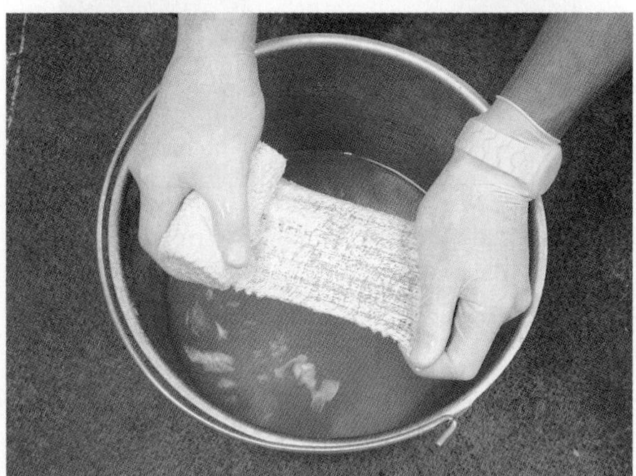

FIGURE 34-38 The end of plaster of Paris cast material is held away from the roll while it is moistened.

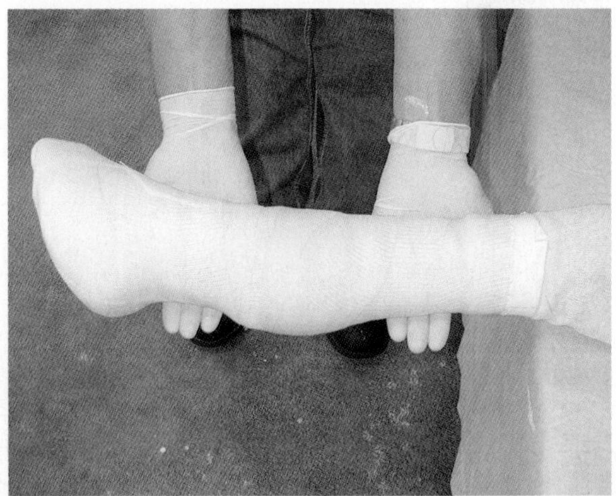

FIGURE 34-39 As the fiberglass cast material is applied, an assistant holds the leg out by resting it on the palms of his or her hands under the metacarpus or metatarsus region. This method prevents finger impressions in the uncured cast material.

the limb when the animal is trying to recover from anesthesia. However, general anesthesia is used if the cast is changed. The cast is split on the medial and lateral surfaces, and the cut is continued under the foot with a Stryker saw (Figure 34-44, *A*). With this approach, injury to the flexor and extensor tendons with the cast saw can be prevented. When cutting over bony prominences, one should be careful to avoid lacerating the skin. Once the cast is completely cut, the two halves are separated with cast spreaders (Figure 34-44, *B*). A support wrap is then placed on the limb.

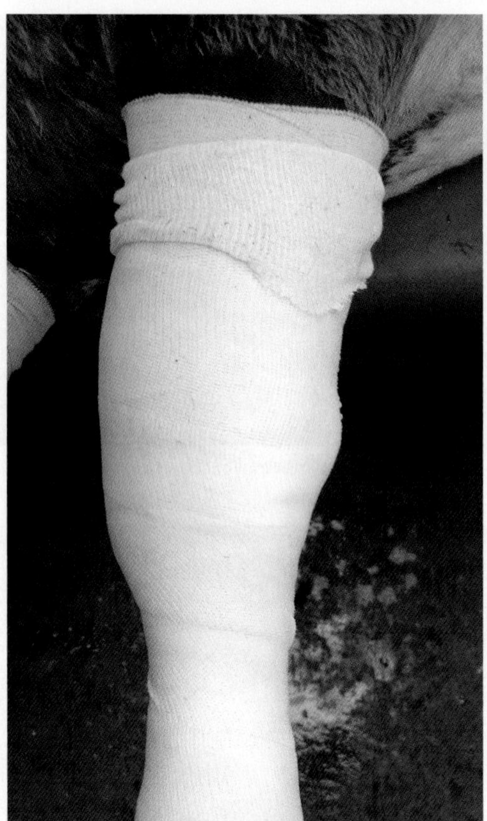

FIGURE 34-40 Approximately 4 cm of orthopedic stockinette left exposed on top of a cast is pulled down over the cast top and incorporated in the last layers of the cast.

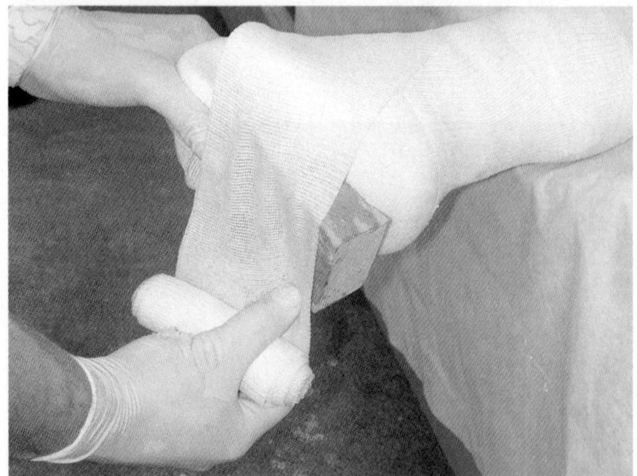

FIGURE 34-41 A wooden wedge block is placed underneath the heel and incorporated with the last layers of cast material.

TECHNICIAN NOTE A cast is split on the medial and lateral surfaces to prevent injury to the flexor and extensor tendons with the cast saw.

BANDAGING AND CAST APPLICATION TECHNIQUES FOR CATTLE

The principles applied to limb bandaging and cast application are the same in cattle as in horses, but there are specific techniques for cattle. Cattle are often not as cooperative as horses, and more restraint is required.

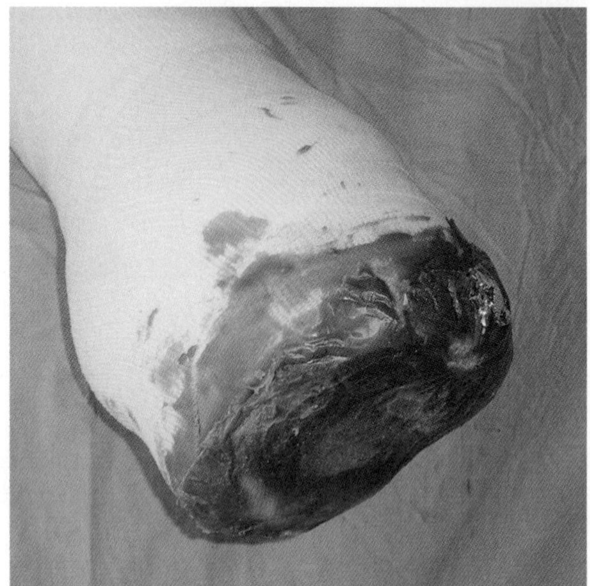

FIGURE 34-42 The bottom of the cast is protected from wear by capping it with hard acrylic (Technovit, Jorgensen Laboratories).

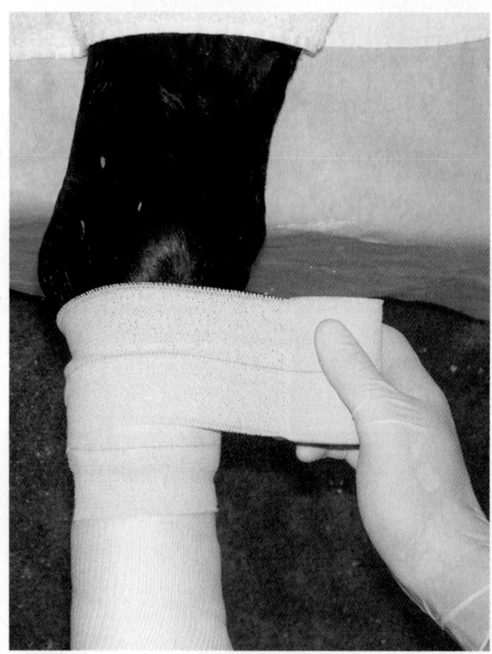

FIGURE 34-43 Elastic adhesive tape is placed on top of the cast to form a seal between the skin and cast that prevents debris from getting inside the cast.

With cattle, a cast can be applied directly over the dewclaws without causing major problems. However, sores caused by motion of the cast can occur in this area because of the inability to closely fit the cast. This can be remedied by placing a pad of orthopedic felt with holes cut out for the dewclaws between the dewclaws (Figure 34-45).

APPLICATION OF A CLAW BLOCK

A wooden block is applied to an unaffected claw for various reasons: to alleviate weight bearing on an adjacent claw if it is fractured or injured or to protect a postsurgical area by

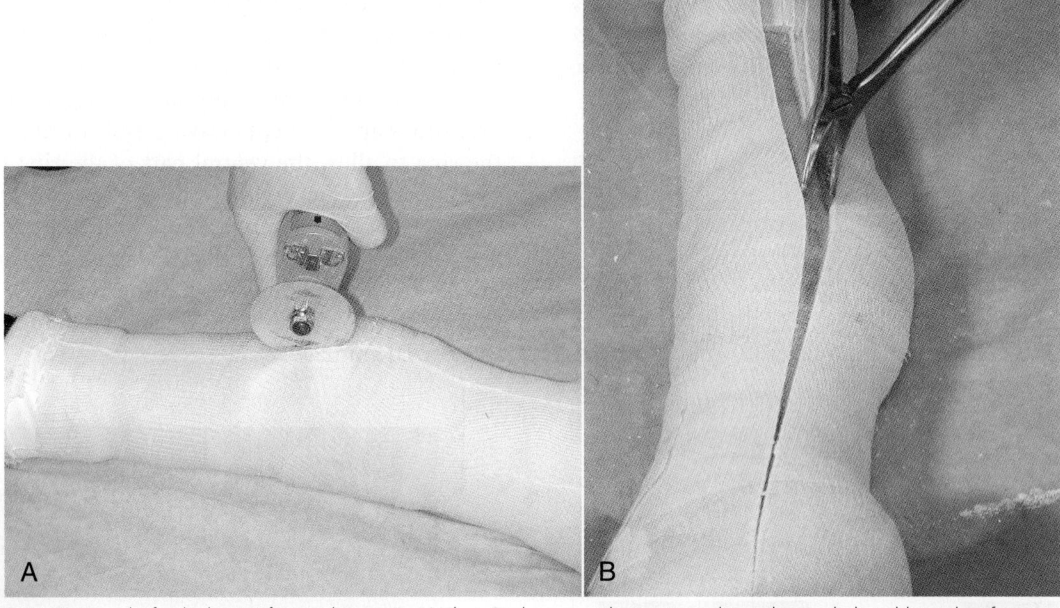

FIGURE 34-44 Removal of a limb cast from a horse. A, With a Stryker saw, the cast is split on the medial and lateral surface, and the cut is continued under the foot. B, Once the cast is completely cut, the two halves are separated with cast spreaders.

raising it higher off the ground (e.g., after amputation of an adjacent claw). The block is usually made from a piece of wood 5 cm thick and cut to the shape of the sole surface of the claw. Grooves are cut in the ground surface for traction (Figure 34-46).

The claw is first trimmed, and debris is removed by means of an electric sander or rasp. This is an important step for effective bonding of the acrylic to the claw. The block is then bonded to the horny surface of the claw with acrylic cement, such as Technovit (Jorgensen Laboratories) or a polyurethane hoof cement (Vettec, Vettec Hoof Care Products, Oxnard, Calif.) (Figure 34-47).

MODIFIED THOMAS SPLINT

Despite advances in external and internal skeletal fixation, modified Thomas splints are still often used in cattle and small ruminants as a means of external skeletal fixation. The modified Thomas splint is often used in combination with internal fixation or a cast. The indications for its use include fractures of the tibia or radius and ligamentous injuries of the stifle. Pressure sores in the inguinal or axillary region are a problem when a Thomas splint is used, despite padding of the metal ring part of the splint that fits in that area.

Application of a modified Thomas splint in large ruminants does require special equipment, such as a conduit bender, to bend the round rod iron used to construct the splint. For small farm animals, a beehive and aluminum rod is used (Figure 34-48). The design of the splint varies somewhat among clinicians, but the purpose is the same, which is to apply traction and maintain alignment of the limb.

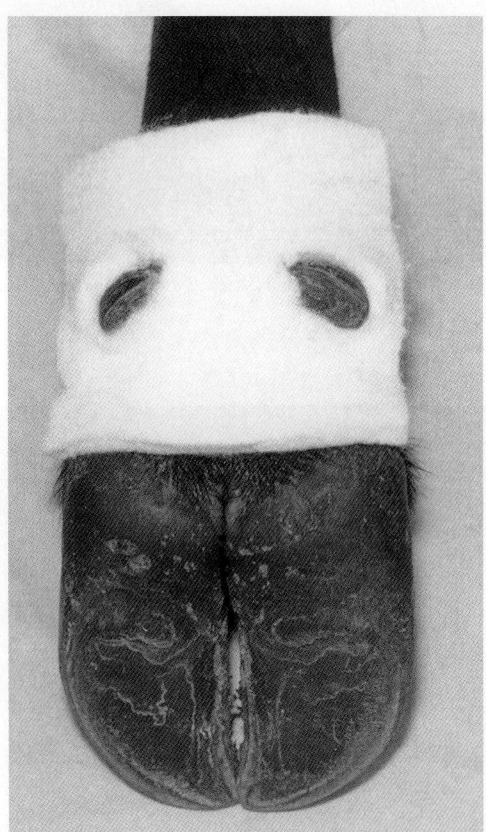

FIGURE 34-45 A piece of orthopedic felt with holes cut out can be placed between the dewclaws to reduce the motion under a cast and help prevent development of pressure sores.

The animal is first placed in lateral recumbency with the affected leg uppermost. A template to fit the individual animal, devised from a nasogastric tube or other similar flexible tubing, is used to construct the ring that will encircle the proximal part of the leg (Figure 34-49). The ring should be large enough so as not to impinge on any bony prominences. The rod is bent in a ring the same size as the template (Figure 34-50). The variation in design occurs with the extensions that come off the ring to support the animal's limb.

FIGURE 34-46 A claw block made from wood. Grooves are cut on both sides of the block to improve traction and bonding.

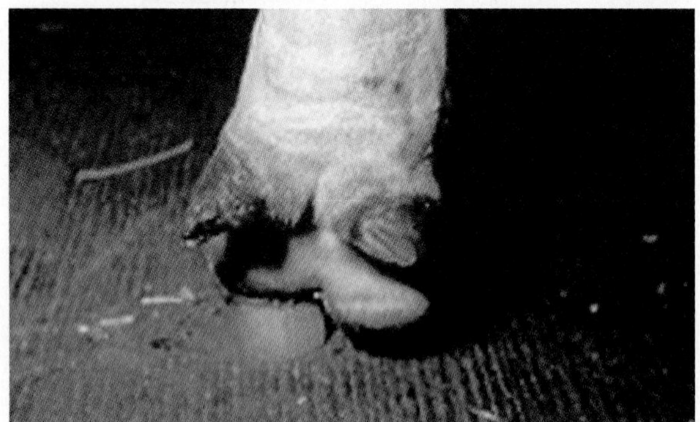

FIGURE 34-47 A wooden block is cemented to the unaffected claw with acrylic.

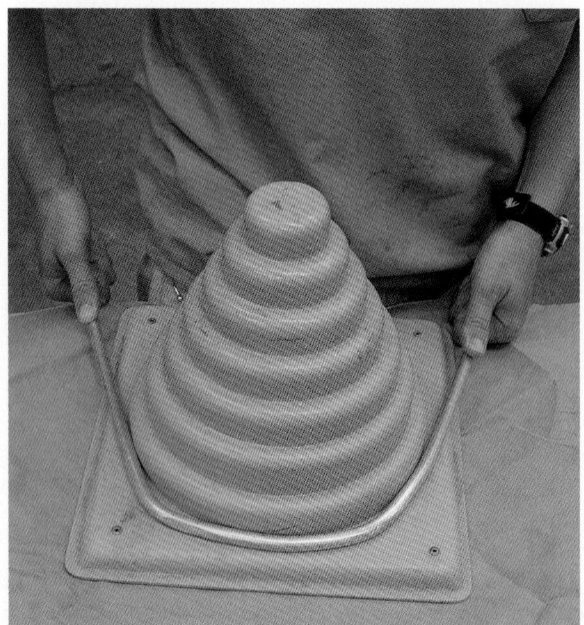

FIGURE 34-48 A ¼-inch aluminum rod is bent with a beehive to construct a modified Thomas splint.

One design has the extensions coming off the ring cranially and caudally to the leg (Figure 34-51). The extensions of the splint must be shaped to conform to the angles of the hock and stifle. For the front limb, the extensions are kept straight and not bent in any shape (Figure 34-51, *A*).These extensions are also bent away (lateral) from the flat plane of the ring to allow the ventral part of the ring to fit into the axillary or inguinal region (Figure 34-51, *B*). Another design has the extensions coming off the ventral aspect of the ring. The ring is then bent so that the extensions are positioned medial to the limb and so that the ring itself fits the contour of the upper limb (Figure 34-52). This design is used for large-sized animals.

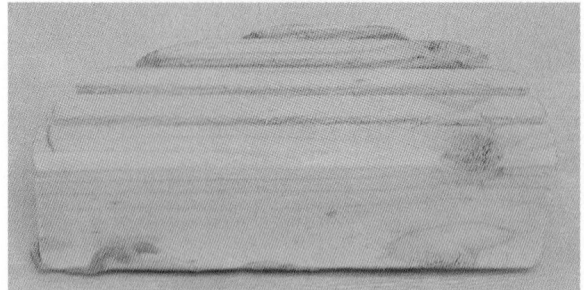

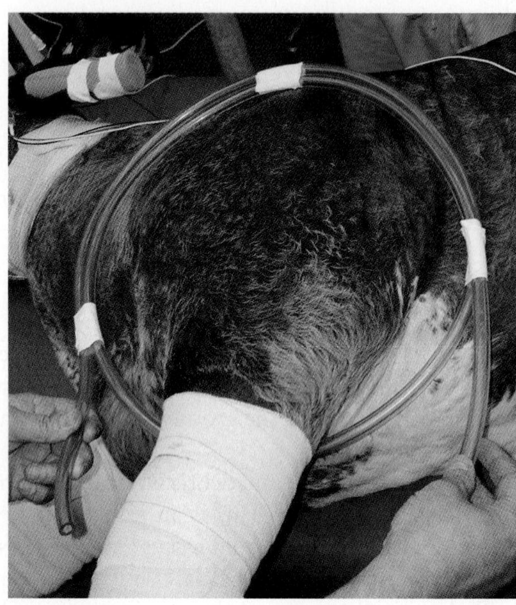

FIGURE 34-49 A template, devised from a nasogastric tube or other similar flexible tubing, is used to construct the metal ring that will encircle the proximal part of the leg of a modified Thomas splint.

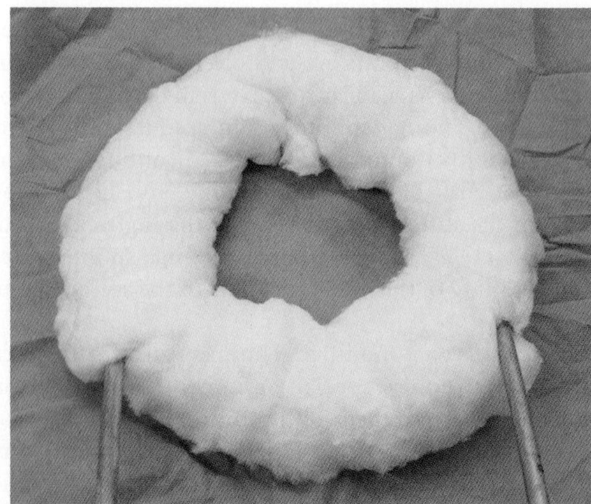

FIGURE 34-50 Metal rod is bent into a ring to construct the proximal part of a modified Thomas splint. Once the ring is constructed, it is padded with cotton.

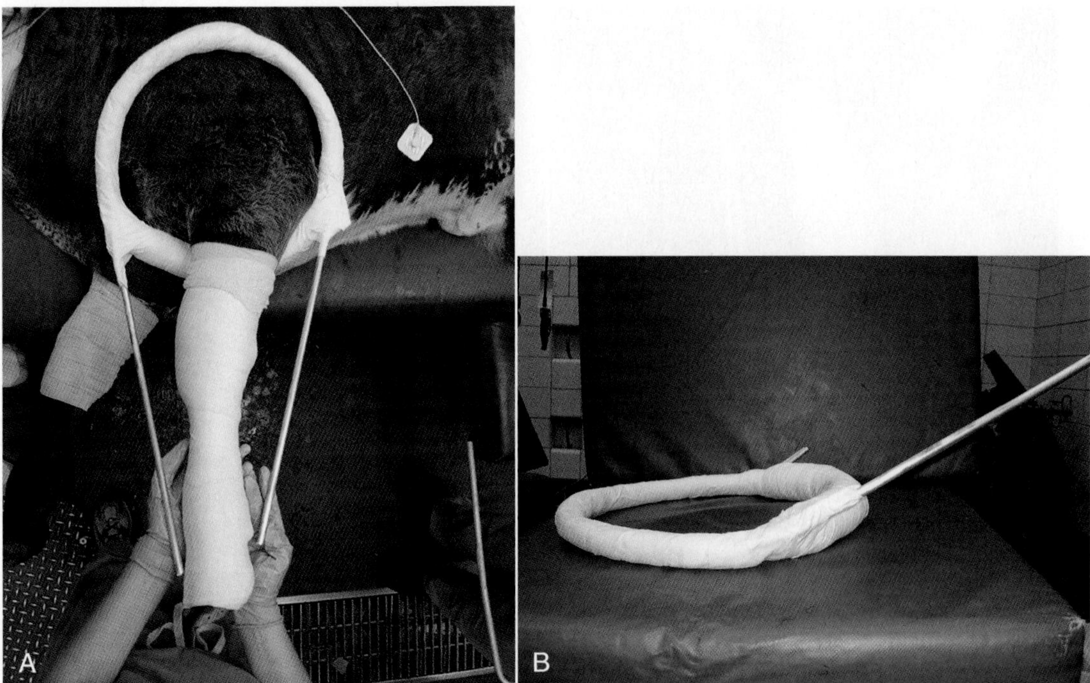

FIGURE 34-51 A modified Thomas splint. **A,** Extensions of the splint come off the edge of the ring and are positioned cranial and caudal to the limb. **B,** The extensions come off the ring at an angle to allow the ring to properly fit under the axillary or inguinal region.

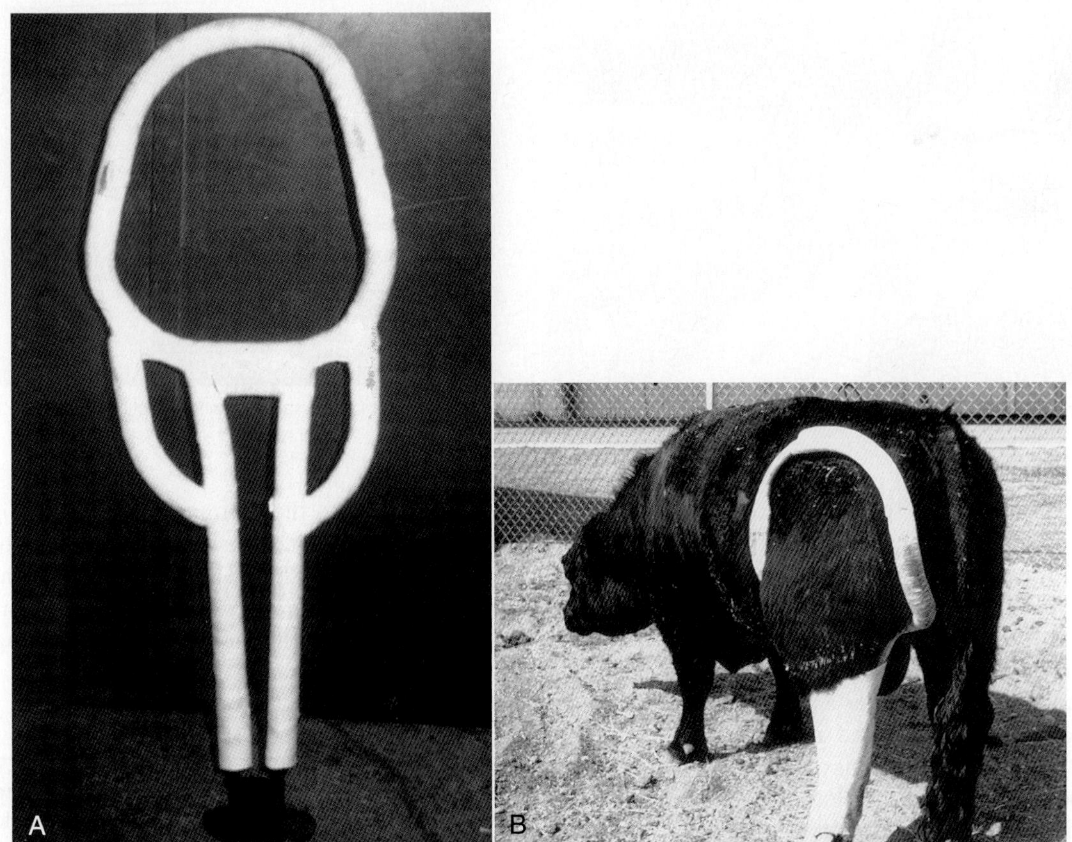

FIGURE 34-52 A modified Thomas splint. This design has the extensions coming off the ventral aspect of the ring. The ring is then bent so that the extensions are positioned medial to the limb and so that the ring itself fits the contour of the upper limb. This design is used for large-sized animals. (Photograph courtesy Dr. Dwight F. Wolfe.)

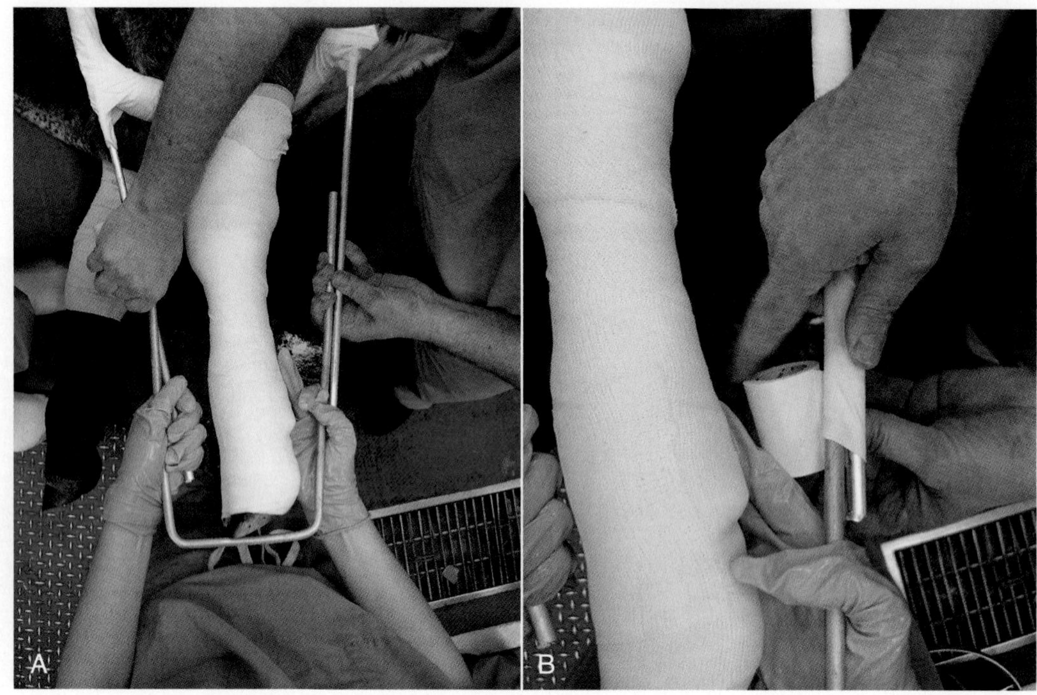

FIGURE 34-53 The footplate in this design of a modified Thomas splint is constructed from a piece of metal rod that is bent in a flat U shape, **(A)** positioned under the foot, and connected to the ends of the extensions of the splint with a combination of twisted wire loops and lots of tape **(B)**.

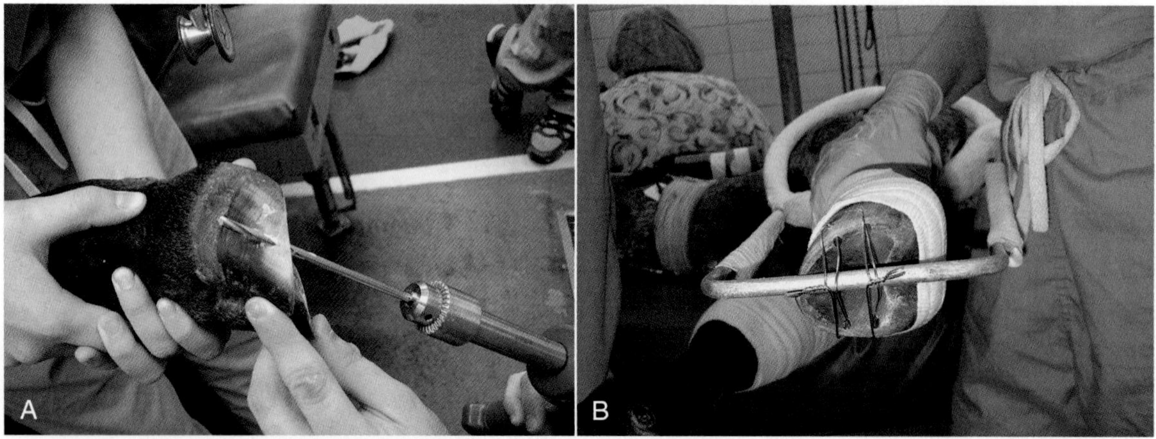

FIGURE 34-54 A, Holes are drilled into the hoof walls near the toes and wired to the bottom of the splint **(B)** when applying a modified Thomas splint.

The next portion of the splint to be constructed is the distal part of the splint (footplate). A footplate can be constructed in various ways. In one method, two threaded rods are attached to the extensions of the splint. This splint is devised with these types of extensions so that the length of the splint can be adjusted. This design is most useful in large ruminants. Another construct has a piece of metal rod that is bent in a flat U shape, positioned under the foot, and connected to the ends of the extensions of the splint with a combination of twisted wire loops and lots of tape (Figure 34-53, *footplate*). This type of design is used in small farm animals. The ring is then padded with cotton (see Figure 34-50). This is important to reduce pressure sores in the axillary or inguinal region. Next holes are drilled into the hoof walls near the toes and wired to the bottom of the splint (Figure 34-54). A slight amount of traction is placed on the limb as the splint is applied. Traction should be minimal within the splint so as not to create excessive pressure in the axillary or inguinal regions, which could interfere with venous drainage or distract the fracture fragments.

TECHNICIAN NOTE When the hoof is secured to a modified Thomas splint, it is important not to apply excess traction because this will create too much pressure in the axillary or inguinal region, which could interfere with venous drainage or distract the fracture fragments.

Once the splint is in position, the limb and splint are then covered with layers of cast material (Figure 34-55). The casting tape is applied by "weaving" the material around the limb and extensions of the splint by using a figure-eight pattern (Figure 34-56, *A*). The casting tape is twisted 180 degrees with each passage of the material (Figure 34-56, *B*). The cast material should be applied as proximal as possible (Figure 34-57). The bottom of the splint is protected from wear by applying a polyurethane hoof-bonding material (Figure 34-58).

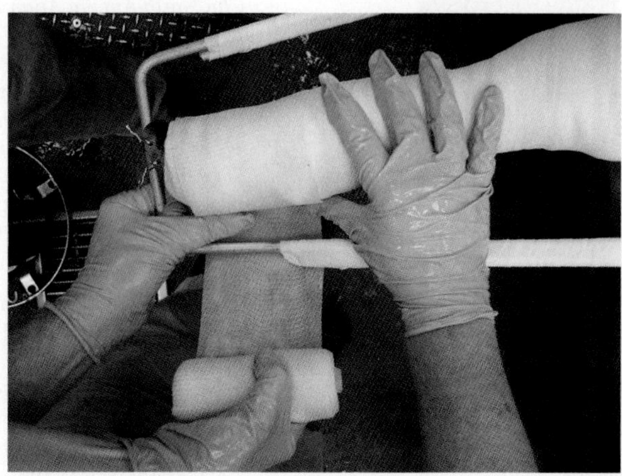

FIGURE 34-55 The limb and modified Thomas splint are covered with layers of cast material to stabilize the limb.

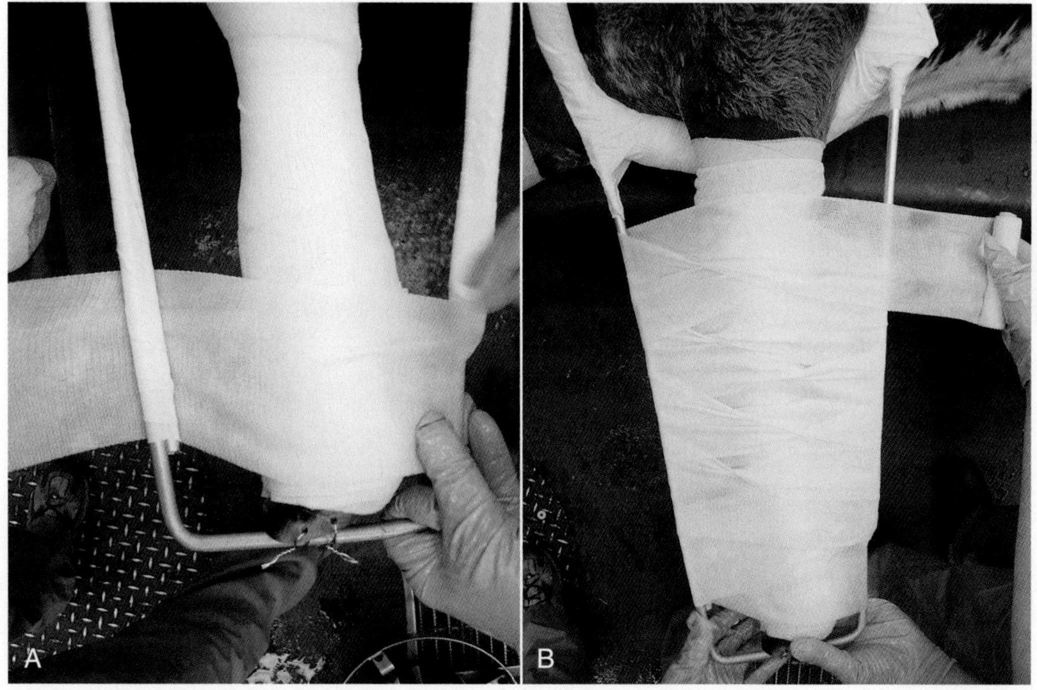

FIGURE 34-56 **A,** A modified Thomas splint is secured to the limb by "weaving" casting tape around the limb and extensions of the splint by using a figure-eight pattern. **B,** The casting tape is twisted 180 degrees with each passage of the material.

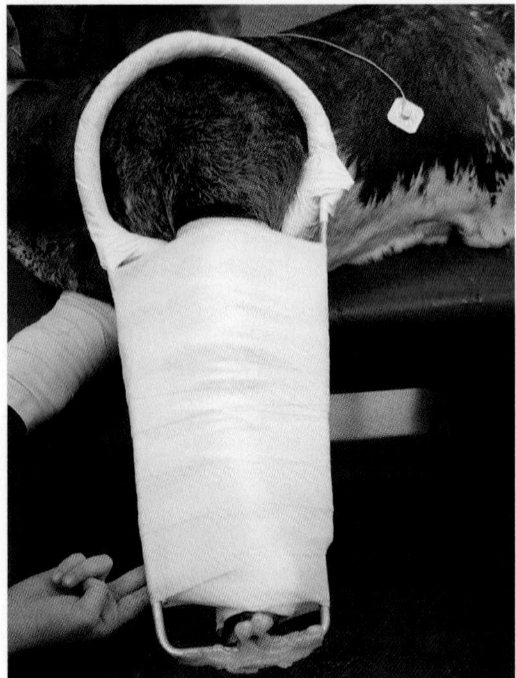

FIGURE 34-57 The cast material is applied as proximal as possible when applying a modified Thomas splint.

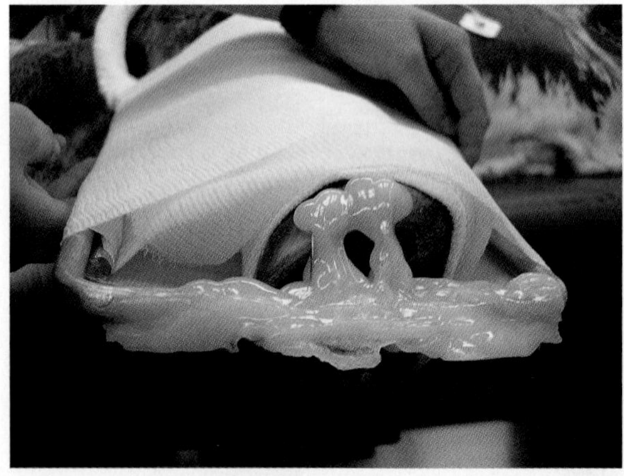

FIGURE 34-58 The bottom of a modified Thomas splint is protected from wear by applying a polyurethane hoof-bonding material.

RECOMMENDED READING

Small Animal

Campbell BG: Dressings, bandages, and splints for wound management in dogs and cats, *Vet Clin North Am Sm Anim Pract* 36: 759-791, 2006.

DeCamp C: External coaptation. In Slatter D, editor: *Textbook of small animal surgery,* ed 3, St Louis, 2003, Saunders.

Dernell WS: Initial wound management, *Vet Clin North Am Sm Anim Pract* 36:713-738, 2006.

Hosgood G: Stages of wound healing and their clinical relevance, *Vet Clin North Am Sm Anim Pract* 36:667-685, 2006.

Krahwinkel DJ, Boothe HW Jr.: Topical and systemic medications for wounds, *Vet Clin North Am Sm Anim Pract* 36:739-757, 2006.

Pavletic MM, Trout NJ: Bullet, bite, and burn wounds in dogs and cats, *Vet Clin North Am Sm Anim Pract* 36:873-893, 2006.

Pope ER: Head and facial wounds in dogs and cats, *Vet Clin North Am Sm Anim Pract* 36:793-817, 2006.

White RA: Management of specific skin wounds, *Vet Clin North Am Sm Anim Pract* 36:895-912, 2006.

Large Animal

Adams SB, Fessler JF: Treatment of radial-ulnar and tibial fractures in cattle, using a modified Thomas splint-cast combination, *J Am Vet Assoc* 183:430, 1983.

Auer JA: Drainings, bandages, and external coaptation. In Auer JA, Stick JA, editors: *Equine surgery,* ed 3, St Louis, 2006, Saunders.

Hendrickson DA: *Wound care for the equine practitioner,* Jackson, Wyo, 2005, Teton NewMedia.

Stashak TS: Bandaging and casting techniques. In Stashak TS, editor: *Equine wound management,* Philadelphia, 1991, Lea & Febiger.

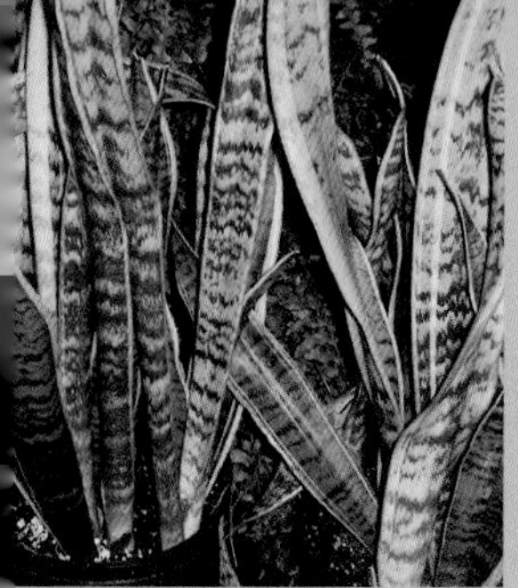

Toxicology

35

Jill A. Richardson

KEY TERMS

Acids
Adsorbent
Alkali
Aminoglycoside antibiotics
Anticoagulant
Antiemetics
Biotoxin
Cathartics
Cationic detergents
Corrosive
Decontamination
Emetics
Enterohepatic recirculation
Gastric lavage
Hepatotoxic
Hydrocarbons
Metabolic acidosis
Nephrotoxic
Nonsteroidal anti-inflammatory drugs
Toxicant
Toxicosis
Toxin

OUTLINE

LEARNING OBJECTIVES

When you have completed this chapter, you will be able to:

1. Describe steps in the managing of poison emergencies.
2. Discuss initial management of patients with ocular and dermal toxic exposures.
3. Describe procedures used in initial management of patients with oral toxic exposures.
4. List common topical insecticides and describe signs of toxicity and initial treatment of affected patients.
5. List common hazardous food and describe signs of toxicity and initial treatment of affected patients.
6. List common household substances and describe signs of toxicity and initial treatment of affected patients.
7. List common dangerous plants and describe signs of toxicity and initial treatment of affected patients.
8. List common hazardous pesticides and describe signs of toxicity and initial treatment of affected patients.
9. List common antifreeze products and describe signs of toxicity and initial treatment of affected patients.
10. List common hazardous human medications and describe signs of toxicity and initial treatment of affected patients.

INTRODUCTION

Animals have a natural curiosity, and many are adept at accessing areas where baits, cleaners, chemicals, and medications are stored. Some pets can pry caps from child-resistant bottles or chew through heavy plastic containers. Products, such as flavored medications or pest control baits, may be attracting to animals, and in some cases, even small amounts can be dangerous. Therefore proper and prompt treatment of poisonings, including stabilization and decontamination, is essential. The purpose of this chapter is to discuss management of poisoning in pets.

Toxicants may be of biologic origin, manufactured chemicals, or naturally occurring chemicals. A toxicant is any substance that when introduced into or applied to the body can interfere with the life processes of cells of the organism. A toxin (biotoxin) is a noxious or poisonous substance that is formed or elaborated during the metabolism and growth of certain microorganisms and some higher plant and animal species. Decontamination is the process of removing or neutralizing injurious agents.

> *TECHNICIAN NOTE* Toxicants may be of biologic origin, manufactured chemicals, or naturally occurring chemicals.

MANAGING POISON EMERGENCIES

Make sure to keep your practice organized with a dedicated area for emergency management of poisoned patients. The designated area should be centralized and stocked with key emergency supplies and drugs commonly used in toxicology. Maintain a library of related references in your practice, such as a current veterinary drug formulary, a current Physician's Desk Reference (PDR), and clinical toxicology textbooks. Be wary of using the Internet as a sole source of information because there are thousands of sites with erroneous information.

Often the first instinct of an animal owner whose animal has been exposed to a poison is to call a veterinary practice. The technician should be able to recognize what constitutes a toxicologic emergency and what does not, give basic first-aid advice, and provide clear directions to the hospital, if needed. The following questions should be asked to evaluate the situation:

1. What is the current clinical status of the animal? Severe clinical signs necessitate immediate veterinary assistance.
2. What was the animal exposed to and through what route (oral, ocular, dermal)?
3. Has the owner taken any steps to treat the animal?
4. How old is the animal, and how much does it weigh?
5. How much was ingested (milligrams or quantity)?
6. When was the exposure?
7. Is the animal a male or female? If female, is she lactating or pregnant?
8. Does the animal have any history of health problems?
9. Is the animal currently on medication?
10. Has the animal had any recent surgeries?

This information can be helpful to prepare for the office visit. After reviewing this information with your staff veterinarian, basic first-aid advice or at-home decontamination recommendations may be given and/or the client told to bring the animal into the hospital. While waiting for the client's arrival, the technician can prepare the necessary equipment and medication. In addition, the technician can help investigate the toxicant by scanning a reference in the practice library or by consulting with veterinary toxicology specialists at the American Society for the Prevention of Cruelty to Animals (ASPCA) Animal Poison Control Center (888-426-4435) or accredited veterinary diagnostic laboratories (Box 35-1).

BOX 35-1 Accredited Vet Diagnostic Laboratories

Arizona
Arizona Veterinary Diagnostic Lab
2831 N. Freeway
Tucson, AZ 85705
Phone: 520-621-2356
Fax: 520-626-8696
http://microvet.arizona.edu

Arkansas
Arkansas Livestock and Poultry Commission
Veterinary Diagnostic Laboratory
One Natural Resources Drive
Little Rock, AR 72205
Phone: 501-907-2430
Fax: 501-907-2410
www.arlpc.org

California
California Animal Health & Food Safety Lab System
University of California, Davis
West Health Science Drive
Davis, CA 95616
Phone: 530-752-8709
Fax: 530-752-5680
http://cahfs.ucdavis.edu

Colorado
Colorado State University Veterinary Diagnostic Lab
Fort Collins, CO 80523
Phone: 970-297-1281
Fax: 970-297-0320
www.dlab.colostate.edu

Connecticut
Connecticut Veterinary Medical Diagnostic Laboratory
Department of Pathobiology and Veterinary Science
University of Connecticut
61 N. Eagleville Road, Unit-3089
Storrs, CT 06269-3089
Phone: 860-486-4000
Fax: 860-486-2794
www.patho.uconn.edu

Florida
Animal Disease Laboratory
Florida Dept. of Agriculture
Mailing Address:
2700 N. John Young Parkway
Kissimmee, FL 34741
Phone: 321-697-1400
Fax: 321-697-1467
http://doacs.state.fl.us

Georgia
Athens Veterinary Diagnostic Laboratory
College of Veterinary Medicine
University of Georgia
Athens, GA 30602-7383
Phone: 706-542-5568
Fax: 706-542-5977
www.vet.uga.edu

BOX 35-1 Accredited Vet Diagnostic Laboratories—cont'd

Veterinary Diagnostic and Investigational Laboratory
University of Georgia
43 Brighton Road
Tifton, GA 31793
Phone: 229-386-3340
Fax: 229-386-7128
www.vet.uga.edu

Illinois

Illinois Department of Agriculture
Animal Disease Lab
9732 Shattuc Road
Centralia, IL 62801
Phone: 618-532-6701
Fax: 618-532-1195
www.agr.state.il.us

Animal Disease Lab
Illinois Department. of Agriculture
2100 South Lake Storey Rd.
Galesburg, IL 61401
Phone: 309-344-2451
Fax: 309-344-7358
www.agr.state.il.us/AnimalHW/labs/index.html

University of Illinois College of Veterinary Medicine
Veterinary Diagnostic Laboratory
2001 South Lincoln Ave. Rm 1224
Urbana, IL 61802
Phone: 217-333-1620
Fax: 217-244-2439
www.cvm.uiuc.edu/vdl/

Indiana

Animal Disease Diagnostic Lab
Purdue University
406 South University St.
West Lafayette, IN 47907
Phone: 765-494-7440
Fax: 765-494-9181
www.addl.purdue.edu

Iowa

Iowa State University—College of Veterinary Medicine
Vet Diagnostic Lab
1600 S. 16th Street
Ames, IA 50011
Phone: 515-294-1950
Fax: 515-294-3564
www.vdpam.iastate.edu

Kansas

Kansas State Veterinary Diagnostic Laboratory
Kansas State University
1800 Denison Ave., Moiser Hall
Manhattan, KS 66506
Phone: 785-532-5650
Fax: 785-532-4481
www.vet.ksu.edu/depts/dmp/

Kentucky

Murray State University
Breathitt Veterinary Center
715 North Drive
Hopkinsville, KY 42240
Phone: 270-886-3959
Fax: 270-886-4295
http://breathitt.murraystate.edu/bvc

Livestock Disease Diagnostic Center
1490 Bull Lea Rd.
Lexington, KY 40511
Phone: 859-253-0571
Fax: 859-255-1624
http://ces.ca.uky.edu/lddc/

Louisiana

LA Animal Disease Diagnostic Laboratory
1909 Skip Bertman Dr. Rm. 1519
Baton Rouge, LA 70803
Phone: 225-578-9777
Fax: 225-578-9784
http://laddl.lsu.edu

Michigan

Diagnostic Center for Population and Animal Health
Michigan State University
4125 Beaumont Road, Rm. 122
Lansing, MI 48910-8104
Phone: 517-353-0635
Fax: 517-353-5096
www.animalhealth.msu.edu

Minnesota

Veterinary Diagnostic Laboratory
University of Minnesota
1333 Gortner Avenue
St. Paul, MN 55108-1098
Phone: 612-625-8787
Fax: 612-624-8707
www.vdl.umn.edu

Mississippi

Mississippi Veterinary Research and Diagnostic Laboratory System
Mississippi State University
3137 Highway 468 West
Pearl, MS 39208
Phone: 601-420-4700
Fax: 601-420-4719
www.cvm.msstate.edu

Missouri

Veterinary Medical Diagnostic Lab
University of Missouri
1600 East Rollins Road
Columbia, MO 65211
Phone: 573-882-6811
Fax: 573-882-1411
www.cvm.missouri.edu/vmdl

Montana

Montana Department of Livestock
Montana Veterinary Diagnostic Laboratory
South 19th and Lincoln
Bozeman, MT 59718
Phone: 406-994-4885
Fax: 406-994-6344
www.discoveringmontana.com/liv/lab/index.asp

Continued

BOX 35-1 Accredited Vet Diagnostic Laboratories—cont'd

Nebraska
Veterinary Diagnostic Center
Fair Street, E. Campus Loop
Shipping Address:
PO Box 82646
Lincoln, NE 68501-2646
Phone: 402-472-1434
Fax: 402-472-3094
http://vbms.unl.edu/nvdls.shtml

New Mexico
New Mexico Department of Agriculture
Veterinary Diagnostic Services
700 Camino De Salud NE
Albuquerque, NM 87106
Phone: 505-841-2576
Fax: 505-841-2518

New York
Animal Health Diagnostic Center
College of Veterinary Medicine
Cornell University
Upper Tower Road
Ithaca, NY 14853
Phone: 607-253-3900
Fax: 607-253-3943
http://diaglab.vet.cornell.edu/

North Carolina
North Carolina Department of Agriculture & Consumer Services
Rollins Laboratory
2101 Blue Ridge Road
Raleigh, NC 27607
Phone: 919-733-3986
Fax: 919-733-0454
www.ncvdl.com/

North Dakota
Department of Veterinary Diagnostic Services
North Dakota State University
1523 Centennial Blvd., Van Es Hall
Fargo, ND 58105
Phone: 701-231-8307
Fax: 701-231-7514
www.vdl.ndsu.edu/

Ohio
Animal Disease Diagnostic Lab
8995 E. Main Street, Building 6
Reynoldsburg, OH 43068
Phone: 614-728-6220
Fax: 614-728-6310
www.ohioagriculture.gov/addl

Oklahoma
Oklahoma Animal Disease Diagnostic Laboratory
Oklahoma State University
Center for Veterinary Health Sciences
Farm and Ridge Road
Stillwater, OK 74078
Phone: 405-744-6623
Fax: 405-744-8612
www.cvm.okstate.edu

Oregon
Veterinary Diagnostic Laboratory
Oregon State University
Magruder Hall, Rm. 134
30th and Washington Way
Corvallis, OR 97331
Phone: 541-737-3261
Fax: 541-737-6817
www.vet.orst.edu/

Pennsylvania
Department of Agriculture
Pennsylvania Veterinary Laboratory
2305 N. Cameron Street
Harrisburg, PA 17110-9408
Phone: 717-787-8808
Fax: 717-772-3895
www.padls.org

Pennsylvania State University
Penn State Animal Diagnostic Laboratory
Orchard Road
University Park, PA 16802-1110
Phone: 814-863-0837
Fax: 814-865-3907
www.padls.org

University of Pennsylvania
PADLS—New Bolton Center
382 West Street Road
Kennett Square, PA 19348
Phone: 610-444-5800
Fax: 610-925-8106
www.padls.org

South Carolina
Clemson Veterinary Diagnostic Center
500 Clemson Road
Columbia, SC 29229
Phone: 803-788-2260
Fax: 803-788-8058
www.clemson.edu/lph

South Dakota
Animal Disease Research and Diagnostic Laboratory
South Dakota State University
Animal Disease Research Building
North Campus Drive
Brookings, SD 57007-1396
Phone: 605-688-5171
Fax: 605-688-6003
http://vetsci.sdstate.edu

Tennessee
CE Kord Animal Disease Diagnostic Laboratory
Ellington Agricultural Center
440 Hogan Rd., Porter Building
Nashville, TN 37220
Phone: 615-837-5125
Fax: 615-837-5250
www.state.tn.us/agriculture/regulate/labs/kordlab.html

BOX 35-1 Accredited Vet Diagnostic Laboratories—cont'd

Texas
Texas A&M University
Texas Veterinary Medical Diagnostic Laboratory
6610 Amarillo Blvd., West
Amarillo, TX 79106
Phone: 806-353-7478
Fax: 806-359-0636
http://tvmdlweb.tamu.edu

Texas A&M University
Texas Veterinary Medical Diagnostic Laboratory
1 Sippel Road
College Station, TX 77843
Phone: 979-845-3414
Fax: 979-845-1794
http://tvmdlweb.tamu.edu

Washington
Washington Animal Disease Diagnostic Laboratory
Washington State University
155N Bustad Hall
Pullman, WA 99164-7034
Phone: 509-335-9696
Fax: 509-335-7424
www.vetmed.wsu.edu/depts_waddl

Wisconsin
Wisconsin Veterinary Diagnostic Laboratory
University of Wisconsin
445 Easterday Lane
Madison, WI 53706
Phone: 608-262-5432
Fax: 847-574-8085
www.wvdl.wisc.edu

Wyoming
Wyoming State Veterinary Laboratory
1174 Snowy Range Road
Laramie, WY 82070
Phone: 307-742-6638
Fax: 307-721-2051
http://wyovet.uwyo.edu/

TECHNICIAN NOTE While waiting for the poisoned patient to arrive, the veterinary technician can help investigate the toxicant by consulting a veterinary toxicology specialist at the ASPCA Animal Poison Control Center at 888-426-4435.

ASSESSMENT OF THE ANIMAL'S CONDITION

Initial management of a potential toxicoses starts with assessing the condition of the pet. The assessment should be performed quickly and include the following: an examination of the respiratory rate, capillary refill time, mucous membrane color, heart rate, and core body temperature. Examination of a pet that is unconscious, in shock, seizing, or in cardiovascular or respiratory distress must be conducted simultaneously with stabilization measures. With stable animals, the technician should obtain a comprehensive history of the pet and the exposure and perform a thorough physical examination.

STABILIZATION OF VITAL FUNCTIONS

As a general rule, treat the patient not the poison (Box 35-2). Establishing stabilization of the patient is essential before attempting any type of decontamination. A patent airway should be established and artificial respiration given if the animal is dyspneic or cyanotic. Artificial respiration may be required. The cardiovascular system should be monitored closely, preferably with a constant electrocardiogram (ECG) monitor, and any cardiovascular abnormality should be corrected. The placement of an indwelling intravenous catheter may be necessary for the administration of medications and intravenous fluids.

BOX 35-2 Steps Managing Poison Emergencies

Assess the following: What clinical signs is the animal exhibiting? Is the animal seizing? Is the animal breathing? What is the animal's heart rate? What color are the animal's mucous membranes? Is the animal in shock? What is the core body temperature? Is there any evidence of hemorrhaging?

Stabilize the animal. Administer oxygen if necessary. Control seizures. Correct any cardiovascular abnormality. Perform a systematic examination once the animal is stabilized and obtain a comprehensive history of the animal and the exposure.

Decontamination. Perform the appropriate method(s) of decontamination.

Control clinical signs. Administer the specific antidote, if applicable. Preventive measures, such as gastric protection or antibiotics, may be needed. Correct acid-base balance, hydration, and electrolytes, if needed.

Good nursing care until full recovery. Monitor the systems most likely to be affected by the toxin. Chemistry panels, coagulation panels, or diagnostic tests may be needed. Appropriate supportive care should be given until the animal completely recovers.

DECONTAMINATION

Signalment and history are crucial when dealing with a toxicosis and often affect the manner in which the animal is treated. Always get complete and accurate data about the animal.

There is no doubt that appropriate decontamination procedures have saved many animal lives. However, depending on the particular situation, certain methods of decontamination are more beneficial than others. The patient's age, weight, and previous medical history can affect the method of decontamination.

External Exposures

Ocular Irrigation

With any ocular exposure, the eyes should be flushed repeatedly with water or saline solutions for a minimum of 20 to 30 minutes. Eye flushing should begin as soon as possible and often requires treatment at the pet's home by the pet owner. Ocular exposure to corrosive agents should be considered an emergency. The eyes should be examined for corneal damage and monitored closely for excessive redness, lacrimation, or pain. Follow-up examinations or ophthalmic consultation may be needed to establish the level of corneal damage.

Bathing

For dermal exposures, the animal should be bathed in a mild liquid dishwashing detergent. Baths may need to be repeated to completely remove sticky or oily toxicants. Afterward the animal should be rinsed well with warm water and towel dried to prevent chilling.

Oral Ingestion

Dilution

Dilution with milk or water is recommended in cases of corrosive ingestion. A dosage of 1 to 3 ml/lb is suggested.

Emesis

Emesis is the technical term for inducing vomiting. The patient's species, length of time since ingestion, the animal's previous and current medical condition, and the type of poison can affect the decision to induce emesis.

Dogs, cats, pigs, and ferrets are able to vomit. Emesis is contraindicated in rodents, rabbits, birds, horses, and ruminants. Emesis is usually only productive within 3 hours of ingestion and is more likely to be productive if the animal is fed a small, moist meal before inducing vomiting.

Any animal who has a previous history of cardiovascular abnormalities, epilepsy, or recent abdominal surgery or is severely debilitated is not a candidate for emesis induction. Emesis should not be induced in any animal that (1) is severely depressed or in a coma (it could lead to aspiration), (2) is hyperactive (this could trigger a seizure), or (3) has already vomited.

Another factor affecting the decision to induce emesis is the nature of the substance ingested. Emesis is contraindicated for corrosive materials, such as cationic detergents, acids, and alkali. Induction of vomiting is not recommended with corrosives because of reexposure of the esophageal tissues to the corrosive material. Dilution with milk or water in combination with demulcents and gastrointestinal (GI) protectants is recommended in cases of corrosive ingestion.

Emesis is also contraindicated with hydrocarbon ingestion; the main concern is possible aspiration. Examples of hydrocarbon-containing products include lubrication oils, fuel oil, butane, propane, kerosene, mineral spirits, and gasoline.

Emetic Agents

A 3% hydrogen peroxide solution has been shown to be an effective emetic for dogs, cats, ferrets, and pigs. The mechanism of action of hydrogen peroxide is to cause a mild irritation to the gastric mucosa. The dosage for hydrogen peroxide is 1 tsp/5 lb and should not exceed 3 tbsp. Typically, vomiting occurs within 15 or 20 minutes as long as there is food in the stomach and the peroxide is fresh. If not, peroxide can be repeated one additional time.

Syrup of ipecac (never use the fluid of ipecac) is another product that owners may have in their homes. It acts both through gastric irritation and also stimulates chemoreceptor trigger zones, but it should be used cautiously because overdosing or repeated doses may cause cardiovascular problems.

Apomorphine hydrochloride is considered to be the preferred emetic agent by most small animal clinicians. Apomorphine is available in an injectable solution and as a capsule for conjunctival use.

Salt should never be used as an emetic. Salt is not an effective agent, and there have been cases of sodium toxicities reported as a result of its use as an emetic agent.

> TECHNICIAN NOTE Owners can be advised to give the emetic hydrogen peroxide at a dose of 1 tsp/5 lb of body weight (not to exceed 3 tbsp).

Activated Charcoal

Activated charcoal adsorbs a chemical or toxicant and facilitates its excretion via the feces. It is administered when an animal ingests organic poisons, chemicals, or bacterial toxins or if enterohepatic circulation of metabolized toxicants can occur. The recommended dose of activated charcoal for most species of animals is 1 to 3 g/kg body weight. Repeated doses of activated charcoal every 4 to 8 hours at half of the original dose may be indicated when enterohepatic recirculation occurs.

Activated charcoal can be given orally with a large syringe or with a stomach tube. In symptomatic or uncooperative animals, anesthesia may be needed. A cuffed endotracheal tube should always be used in the sedated or clinically depressed animal to prevent aspiration.

Activated charcoal is contraindicated in animals that have ingested caustic materials. These materials are not absorbed systemically, and the charcoal may make it more difficult to see oral and esophageal burns. Other chemicals that are not effectively absorbed by activated charcoal include ethanol, methanol, fertilizer, fluoride, petroleum distillates, most heavy metals, iodides, nitrate, nitrites, sodium chloride, and chlorate.

Cathartics

Cathartics increase the clearing of intestinal contents. Cathartics are used to enhance the elimination of activated charcoal and adsorbed toxicant. Cathartics can be added to solutions of activated charcoal, or a combination of activated charcoal and cathartic can be purchased. Contraindications for using cathartics include patients with diarrhea or dehydration.

Enemas

Enemas are helpful when elimination of toxicants from the lower GI tract is desired. The general technique is to use plain warm water or soapy warm water. Premixed enema solutions for humans are contraindicated in small animals because of the potential electrolyte and/or acid-base imbalance.

Gastric Lavage

Gastric lavage is a method of gently pumping the stomach contents out of the animal. Gastric lavage should not be performed in cases of caustic or petroleum distillate ingestion and should always be performed under general anesthesia using a cuffed endotracheal tube to protect the airway and prevent aspiration. The procedure involves inserting a fenestrated lavage tube two to three times the diameter of the endotracheal tube; it should be placed to the level of the xiphoid cartilage. The stomach should be lavaged repeatedly with physiologic temperature water until the fluid drawn out of the stomach is clear in color.

Enterogastric Lavage

Enterogastric lavage, also known as the through-and-through lavage, may be necessary when potentially lethal oral exposures have occurred. Following a gastric lavage, the stomach tube is left in place. An enema is performed to eliminate large pieces of fecal matter from the colon and upper large intestines. The distal end of the enema tube is attached to a water faucet, and body temperature water is slowly allowed to fill the tube and enter the intestinal tract in a retrograde manner. Water is allowed to flow until the water flows from the stomach tube. This process is continued until the color of the fluid passing out of the stomach tube is clear.

SUPPORTIVE CARE

The technician plays a critical role by routinely evaluating vital signs and any parameters likely to be affected by the toxicants. Hydration can be assessed in the pet by checking skin turgor, capillary refill time, and the moisture of the oral mucous membranes. The animal's body temperature should also be monitored closely.

Blood samples may be needed to perform complete blood count, chemistry panels, or clotting profiles to monitor the effects of the poison. Some toxicants, such as iron, copper, acetaminophen, and arsenic, can cause liver damage, whereas others, such as estrogen, lead, and antineoplastic medications, can cause anemia.

Daily fluid requirements should be maintained with compensation made for excessive fluid loss or to correct dehydration. Debilitated animals may require additional supplementation. An infusion pump should be used to prevent overhydration. The animal should be monitored for wet lung sounds or the development of a heart murmur, which could indicate overhydration. Pets with cardiovascular disease are at a higher risk for overhydration. Closely monitor pets with indwelling catheters to prevent entanglement in the line or chewing.

Diuresis may be beneficial for exposures to toxicants that can cause kidney damage or to enhance elimination of the toxicant. Examples of toxicants that can cause kidney damage include ethylene glycol (EG) antifreeze, zinc, mercury, oxalic acids, nonsteroidal antiinflammatory drugs, diquat herbicide, and aminoglycoside antibiotics. Adverse effects associated with diuresis include pulmonary edema, cerebral edema, metabolic acidosis or alkalosis, or water intoxication. Close monitoring is necessary.

Ancillary measures, such as nutritional support, are key components for complete recovery for the pet. Anorectic cats and ferrets are at risk for developing hepatic lipidosis and hypoglycemia; therefore it is extremely important to maintain nutritional requirements. A pharyngostomy tube may be necessary to provide adequate nutrition to the animal. Good nursing care should be continued until the pet completely recovers.

Some of the guidelines discussed in this chapter can be used to aid in the management of toxicoses in pets. Assessing the condition of the pet, stabilizing the animal, preventing absorption of the toxicant, controlling the signs, and instituting ancillary measures are critical areas in which the technician plays a key role. The best way to prevent serious problems resulting from toxicosis is poison prevention. Exercising caution with harmful substances by "pet proofing" the home environment is the only safe choice. The technician can educate pet owners on ways to make their homes poison safe. However, if a pet is exposed to a toxicant, prompt action will be needed to prevent potentially life-threatening problems. Refer to Box 35-3 for a quick reference chart of treatment protocols.

> *TECHNICIAN NOTE* Assessing the condition of the pet, stabilizing the animal, preventing absorption of the toxicant, controlling the signs, and instituting ancillary measures are critical areas in which the technician plays a key role. The best way to prevent serious problems resulting from toxicosis is poison prevention.

TOPICAL SPOT ON PRODUCTS

Topical spot on products are the newest method of insect control for pets and are commonly used because of their effectiveness and ease of use. Most of these products are applied between the shoulder blade or striped down the animal's back and are applied every 30 days. Topical spot on products may repel or kill fleas, ticks, and or mosquitoes. Some products prevent flea egg development.

Topical insecticides have a wide safety range when used appropriately. However, all insecticides have a potential for adverse effects. Common adverse effects seen with

BOX 35-3 Quick Reference Chart of Treatment Protocols

Ocular Irrigation

Flush exposed eyes repeatedly with water or saline solutions.

Minimum of 20 to 30 min of irrigation is recommended.

After flushing, eyes should be treated with lubricant ointments.

Follow-up examinations should also be performed to establish level of corneal damage.

Bathing

Animal should be bathed in a mild liquid dishwashing detergent.

Baths may need to be repeated to completely remove the toxicant.

The animal should be rinsed well with warm water.

The animal should be towel dried to prevent chilling.

Emesis

Emesis has best results within 2 to 3 hr postexposure.

Feeding the animal a small, moist meal before inducing vomiting increases chances of an adequate emesis.

Dogs, cats, ferrets, and potbellied pigs are examples of animals that can vomit.

Activated Charcoal

Adsorbs a chemical or toxicant and facilitates its excretion via the feces.

The recommended dose of activated charcoal for most species of animals is 1 to 3 g/kg.

Activated charcoal should not be given to animals that have ingested caustic materials.

Cathartics

Enhance elimination of the activated charcoal.

Cathartics are not to be used if the animal has diarrhea or is dehydrated.

Enemas

Useful when elimination of toxicants from the lower GI tract is desired.

Premixed enema solutions for humans are contraindicated in small animals because of potential electrolyte and/or acid-base imbalance.

appropriately used topical spot on products are mild and include application-site allergy and taste reactions.

TOPICAL ALLERGY

In cases where the pet may have an allergic dermal reaction (mild redness at the application site or hair loss), the animal should be bathed in a mild liquid dishwashing detergent. Baths may need to be repeated to completely remove product residue. Afterward the animal should be rinsed well with warm water. The animal should also be towel dried to prevent chilling. Fractious animals may need to be sedated by a veterinarian for the procedure. Examination by a veterinarian may be needed if skin continues to be red or painful.

TASTE REACTIONS

Ingestion of bitter tasting topical insecticides may result in a taste reaction with a pet. Dogs and cats are physically unable to spit out a bitter taste, so when they have a bad taste in their mouth, they drool to remove the taste. If the animal is breathing while drooling, the drool gets fluffy and becomes foam. Giving the animal a tasty treat, such as a few laps of milk mixes with water or tuna juice, will help dilute the bad taste and stop the drooling.

The following information contains details concerning the most popular types of topical flea control products.

COMMON TOPICAL INSECTICIDES

Imidacloprid

Imidacloprid (1-[(6-Chloro-3-pyridinyl) methyl]-N-nitro-2-imidazolidinimine) is a chloronicotinyl nitroguanidine insecticidal agent. Imidacloprid spot on products are labeled to kill adult fleas and their larvae in dogs and cats. Advantage is the brand name. Imidacloprid is also found in combination with permethrin in dog-only products that also kill ticks. This product is K9 Advantix. In addition to its use in veterinary medicine, imidacloprid is also used in agriculture.

The dermal LD_{50} for rats is greater than 2000 mg/kg. According to the manufacturer's technical profile, topically applied Advantage spreads rapidly over the skin by translocation. The product is not systemically absorbed, but goes to the hair follicles and glands where is it shed with sebum. Ingested imidacloprid is quickly absorbed from the GI tract. Within 48 hours, 96% is eliminated via urine (70% to 80%) and feces (20% to 30%).

The mechanism of action of imidacloprid is the blocking of the nicotinic pathways. This results in a buildup of acetylcholine at the neuromuscular junction. Acetylcholine buildup results in insect hyperactivity, then paralysis, and later insect death.

There is limited published information detailing adverse effects of imidacloprid in dogs or cats; however, clinical effects from the veterinary product used appropriately would be expected to be mild. Because the drug is bitter tasting, oral contact may cause excessive salivation.

As far as diagnostic testing, some laboratories can test for imidacloprid in hair and skin samples. However, these results can only confirm the exposure since toxic levels have not been determined.

Treatment for adverse effects would be symptomatic and supportive. Hypersensitivity skin reactions could occur with any topical product. In those instances, a bath with a noninsecticidal shampoo and symptomatic care, such as hydrocortisone, antibiotics, or antihistamines, would be recommended. Treatment of ingestion of topically applied veterinary imidacloprid product should consist of dilution with milk or water.

Fipronil

Fipronil is a phenylpyrazole antiparasitic agent used for fleas and ticks in dogs and cats. Fipronil is available as a topical product for flea and tick control and in combination with methoprene for additional control of immature flea stages. The brand name is Frontline. In addition to being used as a topical spot on for dogs and cats, it is also available in a veterinary formulation as a 0.29% topical spray.

The reported oral LD_{50} in rats for veterinary product formulations are greater than 5000 mg/kg.

The manufacturer states that fipronil collects in the oils of the skin and hair follicles and continues to be released over a period of time resulting in long residual activity. Topically applied, the drug apparently spreads over the body in approximately 24 hours via translocation. In oral rat studies, 5% to 25% of the parent compound and metabolites was excreted in the urine, and 45% to 75% was excreted in the feces.

> *TECHNICIAN NOTE* Fipronil (Frontline) is a GABA agonist that disrupts central nervous system (CNS) activity causing neural excitation in fleas and ticks. Topically applied, the drug apparently spreads over the body in approximately 24 hours via translocation.

Fipronil is classified as a GABA agonist. Its mechanism of action in insects is to interfere with the passage of chloride ions in GABA-regulated chloride channels, thereby disrupting CNS activity. Blockade of the GABA receptors by fipronil results in neural excitation.

There is limited published information detailing adverse effects of fipronil in dogs or cats; however, clinical effects from the veterinary product would be expected to be mild. Ingestion of any topical products may cause a taste reaction as a result of the inert ingredient. Extralabel use in rabbits has been reported to cause anorexia, lethargy, convulsion, and death.

Some laboratories can test for fipronil in hair and skin samples. However, these results can only confirm the exposure since toxic levels have not been determined.

Treatment for adverse effects would be symptomatic and supportive. If the exposure is dermal, the treatment would include initial stabilization and bathing with a mild dishwashing detergent. Treatment of ingestion of topically applied veterinary fipronil product should consist of dilution with milk or water.

Hypersensitivity skin reactions could occur with any topical product. In those instances, a bath with a noninsecticidal shampoo and symptomatic care, such as hydrocortisone, antibiotics, or antihistamines, would be recommended.

Selamectin

Selamectin is a semisynthetic avermectin used to treat flea infestations, prevention of heartworm disease, and for ear mites in both dogs and cats. The brand name is Revolution. Additionally, in dogs, it is indicated for sarcoptic mange *(Sarcoptes scabiei)* and tick infestations *(Dermacentor variabilis)*. In cats, it is used as a parasiticide for hookworm *(Ancylostoma tubaeformis)* and roundworm *(Toxocara cati)*.

The oral LD_{50} of selamectin is greater than 1600 mg/kg in rats. Oral overdoses in dogs of up to 15 mg/kg did not cause adverse effects (except for ataxia in one avermectin-sensitive collie). Topical overdoses (10×) to puppies caused no adverse effects; topical overdoses to avermectin-sensitive collies caused salivation. Topical overdoses of up to 10× caused no observable adverse effects in cats.

Following dermal application, selamectin is selectively distributed from the bloodstream to sebaceous glands of the skin where it forms reservoirs against fleas, ear mites, and *Sarcoptes* mites. Fecal excretion is responsible for its effectiveness against intestinal worms (roundworms, hookworms). The oral bioavailability of selamectin is reported to be 100% in cats and 62% in dogs. Bioavailability after topical application is 74% in cats and 4.4% in dogs.

Like other avermectin compounds, selamectin is thought to act by enhancing chloride permeability or enhancing the release of γ-aminobutyric acid (GABA) at presynaptic neurons. GABA blocks the postsynaptic stimulation of the adjacent neuron in nematodes or the muscle fiber in arthropods and causes paralysis and eventual death of the parasite.

Clinical effects from selamectin up to 10 times the normal dose are expected to be mild. According to the package insert of Revolution, approximately 1% of cats showed a transient, localized alopecia at the area of administration. Other effects reported (less than or equal to 0.5% incidence) include diarrhea, vomiting, muscle tremors, anorexia, lethargy, salivation, and tachypnea. Contact allergy could occur in especially sensitive animals with any topical product. Oral administration of the topical formulation, which might occur accidentally, caused mild, intermittent, self-limiting salivation and vomiting in cats. There were no adverse effects in avermectin-sensitive collies or in heartworm-positive dogs.

Some laboratories can test for selamectin in hair and skin samples. However, these results can only confirm the exposure since toxic levels have not been determined.

With adverse effects and overdoses of selamectin, the treatment would include initial stabilization and bathing with a mild dishwashing detergent. Treatment of ingestion should consist of dilution with milk or water. Activated charcoal has been shown to be effective in removing avermectin compounds during enterohepatic recirculation and could be considered with selamectin overdoses, whether oral or dermal. Supportive care and close monitoring of the CNS and respiratory system are also recommended. In cases of dermal hypersensitivity, a bath with a noninsecticidal shampoo and supportive care would be recommended.

Methoprene

Methoprene is a synthetic insect growth regulator and is classified as a terpenoid. It is used in topical flea control products to help break the flea life cycle alone or in combination with adulticide products. Methoprene does not kill adult fleas. Methoprene is found alone in many cat topical spot on products (e.g., Hartz Control One Spot for Cats) and also can be found in combination with adulticides (e.g., Frontline Plus).

In dogs, the acute oral LD_{50} of methoprene is 5000 to 10000 mg/kg. The World Health Organization (WHO) has approved methoprene safe for use in drinking water to control mosquitoes because of the minimal or no risk to humans, animals, or the environment.

Methoprene is classified as an insect growth regulator; it mimics the action of an insect growth regulation hormone. It is used as an insecticide because it interferes with the normal maturation process. In a normal life cycle, an insect goes from egg to larva, to pupa, and eventually to adult. Methoprene artificially stunts the insects' development, making it impossible for insects to mature to the adult stages, thus preventing them from reproducing. Juvenile hormones maintain the larval stage in the insect or prevent metamorphosis; when the level of juvenile hormone drops, pupal and adult developmental stages begin.

There is limited published information detailing adverse effects of methoprene in dogs or cats; however, given the mechanism of action, clinical effects would be expected to be mild. Ingestion of any topical products may cause a taste reaction as a result of the inert ingredient. Topical hypersensitivity reactions could occur with any dermal product.

Some laboratories can test for methoprene in hair and skin samples. However, these results can only confirm the exposure since toxic levels have not been determined.

If the exposure is dermal, the treatment would include initial stabilization and bathing with a mild dishwashing detergent. Treatment of ingestion should consist of dilution with milk or water.

Hypersensitivity skin reactions could occur with any topical product. In those instances, a bath with a noninsecticidal shampoo and symptomatic care, such as hydrocortisone, antibiotics, or antihistamines, would be recommended.

Pyrethroids

Pyrethrins are derived from a combination of six insecticidal esters (pyrethrins, cinerins, and jasmolins) that are extracted from dried chrysanthemum flowers. They are fat-soluble compounds that undergo rapid metabolism and excretion after oral or dermal absorption. Rapid hydrolysis of ester linkage in the digestive tract results in low oral toxicity. Pyrethroids have a wide safety range in dogs. Cats have been shown to be extremely sensitive to concentrated permethrin, a synthetic pyrethrin.

Synthetic pyrethroids may cause a paresthesia dermally, which is a tingly sensation. This may occur in especially sensitive dogs. Signs noted from paresthesia include itchy skin, scratching at the application site, and agitation. Signs usually resolve with a cool bath and rinse. A cool compress held at the application site will help those dogs that are extrasensitive to the tingly sensation. Whereas dogs tolerate synthetic pyrethroids well, cats have been shown to be extremely sensitive to concentrated permethrin compounds.

Permethrin (3-phenoxyphenl)-methyl(-)cis-trans-3-(2,2-dichloroethenls)-2,2-dimethlcyclopropanecarboxalate is a synthetic pyrethroid insecticide. Permethrin is used in agricultural and household insecticides and also in flea control preparations. Permethrin has been shown to be effective against insects and is considered to have low toxicity in most mammalian species. The mechanism of action of permethrin occurs through its effect on the sodium channel in the nerve endings. The oral LD_{50} is more than 2000 mg/kg in rats.

> *TECHNICIAN NOTE* Cats have been shown to be extremely sensitive to concentrated permethrin. Currently, there are more than 20 brands of permethrin spot on products available over the counter as spot on flea control labeled "for dogs only."

Cats have been shown to be extremely sensitive to concentrated permethrin. Currently, there are more than 20 brands of permethrin spot on products available over the counter as spot on flea control labeled "for dogs only." Product packaging of these products will have multiple warnings not to use on cats. However, inappropriate application of concentrated permethrin products can result in seizures and tremors in cats.

The first step for treating cats exposed to permethrin compounds involves controlling seizures or tremors with methocarbamol. Methocarbamol is a centrally acting muscle relaxant. The dose ranges from 44 mg/kg for mild cases up to 55 to 220 mg/kg for moderate to severe effects. Half of the dose should be given quickly (no faster than 2 ml/minute), then the rest to effect. A total 24-hour dose of 330 mg/kg/day should not be exceeded. Other choices for seizure or tremor control include propofol, barbiturates, diazepam, or inhalant anesthetics. Atropine is not an antidote for permethrin and is not recommended. Following stabilization, the cat should be bathed using a mild liquid dishwashing detergent. Supportive care, such as thermoregulation, fluid therapy to maintain hydration, and nutritional support, should be given as needed until full recovery. Some cats may experience difficulties for up to 3 days.

Etofenprox

Etofenprox (also called ethophenprox) is an effective insecticide with a wide margin of safety in mammals. The mechanism of action of this compound is similar to that of the pyrethroid class of pesticides.

Structurally, etofenprox includes an ether unit instead of an ester unit, commonly found in pyrethroids. This structural difference is what differentiates etofenprox from pyrethroids and provides it with a higher LD_{50} than other pyrethroid compounds. The rat oral LD_{50} is more than 42,880 mg/kg and, the mouse oral LD_{50} is more than 107,200 mg/kg.

Etofenprox is used to treat fleas, ticks, and mosquitoes. The British Army has deemed etofenprox a safe and effective additive to nets and screens used in controlling arthropod vectors of disease in the United Kingdom.

Hypersensitivity skin reactions could occur with any topical product. In those instances, a bath with a noninsecticidal shampoo and symptomatic care, such as hydrocortisone, antibiotics, or antihistamines, would be recommended.

HOUSEHOLD HAZARDS

DANGEROUS FOOD ITEMS FOR PETS

Pet owners are often tempted to give table scraps to their pets as a special treat. Pets that roam may come into contact with potentially dangerous food in trash cans or dumps. Unfortunately, there are some types of human food that can be dangerously toxic to pets. However, if a pet is exposed to a dangerous food item, prompt action will be needed to prevent a potentially life-threatening problem.

It is important that the veterinary staff is aware of the possible problems associated with feeding pets the following food.

Moldy Food

Moldy food may contain certain tremorgenic mycotoxins, such as penitrem-A and roquefortine C. Tremorgenic mycotoxins can induce muscle tremors, ataxia, and convulsions that can last for several days. Tremorgenic mycotoxins are classified as neurotoxins. Severity of signs can vary from mild to severe, depending on the particular strength of the mycotoxin ingested. Diagnosis of tremorgenic mycotoxins involves sample analysis by an accredited veterinary diagnostic laboratory (see Box 35-1). Before submitting samples, always confirm availability of tests with the laboratory director. Treatment goals following tremorgenic mycotoxin ingestion include minimizing absorption through decontamination procedures, such as emesis, lavage, and activated charcoal; controlling tremors and seizures with methocarbamol; and providing supportive care. With early aggressive treatment, prognosis is good.

> *TECHNICIAN NOTE* Tremorgenic mycotoxins produced by molds on food are relatively common and possibly underdiagnosed as a cause of tremors and seizures in animals.

Chocolate

Chocolate is a mixture of cocoa beans and cocoa butter. It contains theobromine and caffeine, which are both classified as methylxanthines. Unfortunately, dogs are sensitive to the effects of methylxanthines. Depending on the dose, methylxanthines can cause hyperactivity, increased heart rate, tremors, and potentially death. Other effects seen with chocolate overdose include vomiting, diarrhea, increased thirst, increased urination, and lethargy. The amount of methylxanthines present in chocolate varies with the type of chocolate (Table 35-1). The general rule is the more bitter the chocolate, the more toxic it could be. Unsweetened baking chocolate contains almost seven times more theobromine as milk chocolate, and white chocolate (a combination of cocoa butter, sugar, butterfat, milk solids, and flavorings without cocoa beans) contains negligible amounts of methylxanthines.

TABLE 35-1

Type of Chocolate	Caffeine—mg/oz	Theobromine—mg/oz
Milk chocolate	6	44-56
Semisweet	22	138
Baking chocolate	33-47	393

> *TECHNICIAN NOTE* The amount of methylxanthines present in chocolate varies with the type of chocolate (see Table 35-1). The general rule is the more bitter the chocolate, the more toxic it could be. Unsweetened baking chocolate contains almost seven times more theobromine as milk chocolate, and white chocolate (a combination of cocoa butter, sugar, butterfat, milk solids, and flavorings without cocoa beans) contains negligible amounts of methylxanthines.

The mechanism of action of methylxanthines is to competitively inhibit cellular adenosine receptors, which results in CNS stimulation and tachycardia. Although theobromine and caffeine have an LD_{50} of 100 to 200 mg/kg, signs can be seen well below this dose. Mild signs can be seen at doses more than 20 mg/kg, moderate effects are seen more than 40 mg/kg, and severe effects are seen at doses more than 60 mg/kg. Early treatment, including decontamination procedures, such as emesis and activated charcoal; cardiovascular monitoring; and supportive care, is extremely helpful with chocolate poisoning. In addition, fluid diuresis may help enhance elimination. Caffeine can be reabsorbed by the bladder wall, which may result in extended times of clinical signs. Therefore the veterinary staff should take extra steps to keep the patient's bladder empty either through catheterization or frequent walking.

Onions

Onions and other members of the *Allium* family can be harmful to dogs and cats. Other members of this genus include garlic, leek, shallot, and chive. Pieces of onion, onion powder, or even cooked onion can cause damage to red blood cells (RBCs), which could result in anemia. The primary toxic principle is n-propyl disulfide, which is thought to cause oxidative damage to erythrocytes, resulting in hemolysis. Toxicoses from fresh, dried, or powdered plant material have been reported in dogs and cats. In one study, dogs developed hemolytic anemia after being fed 30 g/kg of onions once daily for 3 days. Feeding commercial baby food containing onion powder has also been reported to cause toxicity in cats. Clinical signs associated with onion poisoning include hemolytic anemia, hemoglobinuria, vomiting, weakness, and pallor. Decontamination procedures, such as inducing emesis and administering activated charcoal, should be considered with recent ingestions. Afterward the animal should be monitored for the development of hemolysis, azotemia, and/or decreased packed-cell volume (PCV). Whole-blood transfusions or administration of oxygenated hemoglobin should be considered with critical patients. Fluid diuresis is recommended in patients with hemoglobinuria. In addition, supportive care should be administered until patient recovery.

Macadamia Nuts

Macadamia nuts may cause problems if ingested by dogs. According to a retrospective study, clinical signs commonly reported in dogs ingesting macadamia nuts include weakness, depression, vomiting, ataxia, tremors, and hyperthermia. The lowest dose reported to cause clinical effects is 2.4 g/kg. In most cases, dogs developed clinical signs within the first 12 hours after ingestion. These signs have only been seen in dogs, and the exact cause for their sensitivity is unknown. Treatment includes decontamination procedures, such as inducing emesis, administering activated charcoal, and administering enemas. Additional supportive care should be given as needed. The prognosis in most cases is extremely good. Most dogs return to normal within 24 to 48 hours.

Rising Bread Dough

Ingestion of rising bread dough can be life threatening to dogs. The animal's body heat will cause the dough to rise in the stomach. Ethanol is produced during the rising process; the dough may expand several times its original size. Signs seen with bread dough ingestion are associated with ethanol toxicoses and foreign body obstruction and may include severe abdominal pain, bloating, vomiting, incoordination, and depression. In cases of recent ingestion in asymptomatic dogs, emesis could be induced. Analgesia is important in patients exhibiting signs of pain. Administering cool water via a stomach tube or PO may halt the rising process. In some cases, dough removal may necessitate surgery. Since ethanol can cause an acidosis, it is important to monitor the acid-base balance and correct with sodium bicarbonate, if indicated.

Grapes and Raisins

Some types of grapes and raisins have been shown to cause kidney failure in dogs when eaten in quantity. The basis for kidney failure following consumption of grapes or raisins is unclear, but is currently being studied in the veterinary community. The amount of grapes or raisins that may cause renal failure is not exactly known, so any amount could potentially be dangerous. As for treatment of recent ingestion, inducing vomiting and administering activated charcoal is recommended. This should be followed with fluid diuresis for 48 hours. During this time, the patient should be monitored for azotemia. If the animal shows evidence of renal failure, fluids and supportive care should be continued.

Tobacco Products

Tobacco products contain varying amounts of nicotine, with cigarettes containing 13 to 30 mg and cigars containing 15 to 40 mg. Butts contain about 25% of the total nicotine content. The minimum lethal dose in dogs and cats is reported as 20 to 100 mg. Signs often develop quickly (usually within 15 to 45 minutes) and include excitation, tachypnea, salivation, emesis, and diarrhea. Muscle weakness, twitching, depression, tachycardia, shallow respiration, collapse, coma, and cardiac arrest can follow the period of excitation. Death occurs secondary to respiratory paralysis. With recent ingestion in asymptomatic animals, emesis can be induced. Never attempt emesis in stimulated animals because it may trigger a seizure. Activated charcoal has been shown to be helpful in adsorbing nicotine. Patients should be monitored closely and treated symptomatically. Artificial respiration would be indicated in patients with respiratory paralysis.

Xylitol

Xylitol is a sugar alcohol that is commonly found in many human food items (gum, snacks, and beverages). It may also be found in certain dental washes intended for use in pets. Xylitol's primary use is as a sugar substitute, but it also has plaque-blocking properties. Xylitol toxicity has been well documented in dogs. In dogs, xylitol causes severe hypoglycemia secondary to the release of insulin. There also have been reports of liver failure and coagulopathy. Hypoglycemic symptoms of xylitol poisoning in dogs occur soon after ingestion (within 30 minutes) and include weakness, depression, ataxia, and vomiting. Biochemical analysis may note increased liver enzymes (ALT, AST) and/or liver failure within 18 to 72 hours after xylitol ingestion.

All ingestion of xylitol products by a dog necessitates veterinary treatment and blood work monitoring. Emesis should be performed with recent ingestions unless contraindications are present. Alternatively, gastric lavage should be considered. It is not known if activated charcoal is of benefit in adsorbing xylitol. Following decontamination, the dog's blood glucose should be monitored frequently for hypoglycemia. During the monitoring period, the animal should have access to tasty food and encouraged to eat. If hypoglycemia is noted, intravenous fluids with dextrose should be used to normalize the blood glucose. In addition, chemistry panel and clotting tests should be performed initially and then repeated to monitor for liver failure and coagulopathy.

HOUSEHOLD CLEANING AGENTS

Acids

Hydrochloric, sulfuric, nitric, phosphoric acids, oxalic acid, and sodium bisulfate are examples of acids. Common sources of acid include toilet bowl cleaners, drain openers, metal cleaners, antirust compounds, gun barrel cleaners, automobile battery fluid, and pool sanitizers. Acids are corrosives and can produce severe burns on contact with tissue.

Acids produce tissue damage at the site of contact. Severity of tissue damage produced is directly related to the concentration. Concentrated acids may produce severe burns on contact with any part of the body and the GI tract if ingested. When acids are diluted or have higher pH, they do not cause corrosion, only irritation. Most cases of exposure to acids that are irritants usually result in mild self-limiting signs of nausea, vomiting, or diarrhea. Oxalic acids include ethanedioic and dicarboxylic acid and can also cause kidney damage.

Alkali

Alkali are used as drain openers, oven cleaners, bleaches, industrial cleaners, denture cleaners, bathroom and household cleaners, radiator cleaning agents, and hair relaxers and in alkaline batteries, electric dishwasher soaps, some oven cleaner pads, and cement.

Lesions from alkalis are typically deeper and more penetrating than those from acidic compounds. The ability of alkalis to generate corrosive injury depends on the concentration, pH, viscosity, amount ingested, and the duration of contact with tissue. Serious corrosive injury is unlikely to occur from substances with a pH less than 11. Alkali with a pH of 12.5 can cause esophageal ulcers, and those with a pH of 14 or more can cause esophageal perforation.

> *TECHNICIAN NOTE* Lesions from alkalis are typically deeper and more penetrating than those from acidic compounds.

Bleaches

Household bleaches are used as a bleaching or oxidizing agent, a deodorant, or disinfectants. Household bleaches mainly contain less than 5% sodium hypochlorite, and household mildew removers contain up to 5% calcium hypochlorite. Nonchlorine bleach or colorfast bleaches may contain sodium peroxide, sodium perborates, or enzymatic detergents. Commercial bleaches may also contain other bleaching agents, such as sodium peroxide, sodium perborate, sodium carbonate, or oxalic acid.

Household bleaches contain low concentrations of bleach and are mild to moderate mucosal irritants. Commercial forms of alkaline bleach contain higher concentrations, and if the pH is 11 to 12 or greater, it can produce partial-thickness chemical burns. At higher concentration, corrosive effects could be seen.

> *TECHNICIAN NOTE* Household bleaches contain low concentrations of bleach and are mild to moderate mucosal irritants. Commercial forms of alkaline bleach contain higher concentrations, and if the pH is 11 to 12 or greater, it can produce partial-thickness chemical burns. At higher concentration, corrosive effects could be seen.

Detergents

Detergents are nonsoap surfactants in combination with inorganic ingredients, such as phosphates, silicates, or carbonates. Detergents are classified according to their charge in solution: nonionic, anionic, and cationic surfactants.

Anionic and nonionic detergents are found in shampoos, dishwashing detergents, laundry detergents, and electric dishwashing detergents. Anionic and ionic detergents are irritants, and their toxicity is generally limited to cutaneous, ocular, oral, or GI irritation. They are considered to be low in toxicity. However, when used in coordination with caustic substances, such as sodium tripolyphosphate and various carbonates, they can be corrosive.

Cationic detergents can be found in fabric softeners, some potpourri oils, hair mousse, conditioners, germicides, disinfectants, and sanitizers. Cationic detergents are rapidly absorbed and may produce severe local and systemic toxicity. Oral ulcerations, stomatitis, and pharyngitis can be seen in the cat at concentrations of 1% or less.

FIRST AID TREATMENT OF EXPOSURES TO CORROSIVE AGENTS

For recent ocular exposure to corrosive acids or alkali, a minimum of 20 to 30 minutes irrigation with tepid tap water or physiologic saline is recommended. Afterward the eye should be examined by a veterinarian and closely monitored for evidence of corneal ulceration.

Following dermal exposure to corrosives, the animal should be bathed immediately with a mild liquid hand or dish detergent or a noninsecticidal shampoo. The animal should be monitored and treated as needed by a veterinarian for burns, erythema, swelling, pain, or pruritus. Veterinary treatment for skin damage may include pain medication, antiinflammatory agents, and antibiotics.

In cases of ingestion of corrosive agents, do not induce vomiting because of potential corrosive effects. Preferred initial treatment should be oral dilution with a few laps of milk or water. Following, the patient should be monitored and treated by a veterinarian for oral or esophageal burns. With ingestion of oxalic acid products, additional care with intravenous fluids is necessary to prevent kidney problems.

MISCELLANEOUS HOUSEHOLD ITEMS

Heavy Metals

Heavy metals are a group of elements that lie between copper and bismuth on the periodic table that have specific gravities greater than 4. The ones most commonly associated with toxicity in pets include zinc and lead.

Zinc

Sources of zinc include hardware, such as wire, screws, bolts, and nuts, and U.S. pennies. Pennies minted since 1983 contain 99.2% zinc and 0.8% copper, and one penny contains approximately 2440 mg of elemental zinc. One penny can cause zinc poisoning in a small dog. The process of galvanization involves the coating of wire or other material with a zinc-based compound to prevent rust. Owners are often not aware of galvanization on the wire used for making bird cages. Pet food and water dishes may also be galvanized, and sufficient zinc may leak into the water or food to create toxicity. Although the exact toxicologic mechanism of zinc in animals is not known, zinc toxicosis can affect the renal, hepatic, and the hematopoietic tissues. Clinical signs of zinc toxicoses may include polyuria, polydipsia, hemoglobinuria, diarrhea, weight loss, weakness, anemia, cyanosis, seizures, and death. Hemolytic anemia is also frequently encountered.

Diagnosis. Radiography of the abdomen may reveal the presence of metallic objects in the GI tract. Serum zinc levels may be obtained using blood collected from plastic syringes (no rubber grommets) and stored in Royal blue top Vacutainers to minimize contamination with exogenous zinc. In general, blood zinc levels of greater than 200 μg/dl (2 ppm) are considered to be diagnostic in avians. Normal serum and urine zinc concentrations in dogs are 0.7 to 2 ppm, and zinc concentrations of toxicosis are usually above 10 ppm. The pancreas is considered to be the best tissue for postmortem zinc analysis. Pancreatic tissue zinc levels greater than 1000 μg/g are suggestive of a zinc toxicosis.

Treatment. It is imperative to remove the sources of zinc from the GI tract. Removal of zinc-containing foreign bodies via endoscopy or gastrotomy or enterotomy may be required. The success of the removal process can be assessed with radiographs. Activated charcoal is not indicated because it is of little benefit in binding zinc. Bulk cathartics, psyllium* (sodium sulfate at 125 to 250 mg/kg), peanut butter, mineral oil, and corn oil may aid in the removal of zinc objects from the GI tract. The use of chelators may not be necessary in cases where prompt removal of the zinc source is accomplished. In addition, treatment for symptomatic animals should include blood replacement therapy as needed, parenteral fluids, and good nursing care, such as forced feeding or hand feeding.

Lead

Sources of lead include paint, toys, drapery weights, linoleum, batteries, plumbing materials, galvanized wire, solder, stained glass, fishing sinkers, lead shot, foil from champagne bottles, and improperly glazed bowls. Lead affects multiple tissues, especially the GI tract, renal, and nervous system. Lead combines with erythrocytes in circulating blood increasing RBC fragility, anemia, and capillary damage. It can also cause segmental demyelination of neurons and necrosis of renal tubular epithelium, GI tract mucosa, and liver parenchyma. Clinical signs seen with lead poisoning are often vague and may include lethargy, weakness, anorexia, regurgitation, polyuria, ataxia, circling, and convulsions.

*Toxicology Brief is a column written by the ASPCA Animal Poison Control Center for *Veterinary Technician,* a peer-reviewed journal published monthly by Veterinary Learning Systems.

Diagnosis. Radiography of the abdomen may reveal evidence of metallic objects. Blood levels of lead are helpful to confirm lead toxicoses with suspicious radiographic changes. Whole blood levels greater than 0.6 ppm are viewed as diagnostic for lead toxicosis when accompanied by appropriate clinical signs in birds. Lead levels below 35 μg/dl are rarely associated with clinical signs in dogs. The basophilic stippling and cytoplasmic vacuolization of RBCs are not always seen with lead poisoning in avian species.

Treatment. Removal of lead particles via bulk-diet therapy, endoscopy, or surgery is recommended. Succimer and calcium ethylenediaminetetraacetic acid (Ca EDTA) are both considered to be effective chelating agents. Fluid therapy is recommended to prevent renal effects from Ca EDTA during treatment. Penicillamine and diethylenetriamine pentaacetic acid (DTPA) have also been used to treat lead toxicoses. Since lead can be immunosuppressive, broad-spectrum antibiotics may be indicated. In addition, good supportive care, including seizure control, is recommended until full recovery.

Other Household Objects

Ant Baits

Ant and roach baits are common objects found in households. The product names may vary, and they may be referred to as hotels, disks, stations, systems, traps, baits, or trays. The baits usually contain inert ingredients, such as peanut butter, breadcrumbs, sugar, and vegetable or animal oils. Insecticides used most commonly in these baits are sulfluramid, fipronil, avermectin, boric acid, and hydramethylnon. These insecticides have a wide safety range and are present in small quantities within the baits, making them a hazard of low toxicity to dogs and cats.

Silica Gel Packets

Silica gel is used as a desiccant and often comes in paper packets or plastic cylinders. They are used to absorb moisture in leather, medication, some food packaging, and some types of cat litter. Silica is considered "chemically and biologically inert" upon ingestion. However, with ingestion, it is possible to see signs of GI upset, such as nausea, vomiting, and inappetence, although signs are expected to be mild or not present with the ingestion of small amounts. Additional problems could occur if the silica gel was used as a desiccant in medication since silica is able to absorb small quantities of the medication.

Toilet Water With Tank Cleaning Drop-In Tablets

Toilet tank "drop-in" tablets typically contain corrosive agents (alkali or cationic detergents). Corrosive effects could be seen if the actual tablet was chewed. When a tank "drop-in" cleaning product is used in a toilet, the actual concentration of the cleaner is low in the toilet bowl of water. With dilution by the bowl water, the cleaning agent is just a gastric irritant. Common signs seen with ingestion include mild vomiting and nausea.

Glow Necklaces

Dibutyl phthalate, also known as n-butyl phthalate, is a liquid found in various glow-in-the-dark products. Jewelry containing dibutyl phthalate is commonly sold at fairs, carnivals, and novelty stores. Pets are often attracted to the glowing jewelry. Almost all pets that bite into glow-in-the-dark jewelry drool or foam at the mouth excessively in response to the bitter taste. Some pets will also exhibit hyperactivity and aggressive behavior most likely resulting from discomfort with the unpleasant taste.

Liquid Potpourri

Liquid potpourri may contain essential oils and cationic detergents, both of which can be harmful. Because product labels may not list ingredients, it is wise to assume any liquid potpourri contains both ingredients. Essential oils can cause mucous membrane and GI irritation, CNS depression, and dermal hypersensitivity and irritation. Severe clinical signs can be seen with potpourri products that contain cationic detergents (see discussion under Detergents). Dermal exposure to cationic detergents can result in redness of the skin, tissue swelling, intense pain, and ulceration. Ingestion of cationic detergents can lead to tissue necrosis and inflammation of the mouth, esophagus, and stomach.

Batteries

Flashlights, remote controls, battery-operated toys, watches, calculators, hearing aids, etc., all provide the opportunity for animals to be exposed to batteries. The alkaline material within a battery can cause burns that can penetrate deeply into the local tissue. In addition, battery casings may result in GI obstruction if swallowed. When batteries are chewed and the contents released, alkaline burns can result. Signs of foreign body obstruction may occur when casings are swallowed. Treatment of battery exposure is as for exposure to any alkaline product and includes observation and treatment by a veterinarian (see discussion under Alkali). Radiographs are often used to determine the location of the battery when the casing is missing.

Pennies

Ingestion of coins by pets, especially dogs, is not uncommon. Of the existing U.S. coins currently in circulation, only pennies pose a significant toxicity hazard. Pennies minted since 1983 contain 99.2% zinc and 0.8% copper, making ingested pennies a rich source of zinc; one penny can cause a zinc toxicosis. Other potential sources of zinc include hardware, such as screws, bolts, or nuts, all of which may contain varying amounts of zinc. In the stomach, gastric acids leach the zinc from its source, and the ionized zinc is readily absorbed into the circulation where it causes intravascular hemolysis (breaks apart the RBC).

Veterinary treatment is always required for ingested pennies. Treatment may include inducing vomiting or removal of zinc-containing objects using an endoscope or through surgery. Often treatment includes blood replacement therapy, as needed, intravenous fluids, and other supportive care.

Mothballs

Veterinary treatment of mothball ingestion is always required. Mothballs may be composed of either 100% naphthalene or 99% paradichlorobenzene. Naphthalene-based mothballs are approximately twice as toxic as paradichlorobenzene, and cats are especially sensitive to naphthalene. One 2.7-g mothball contains 2700 mg of naphthalene. Naphthalene causes Heinz bodies, hemolysis, and occasionally methemoglobinemia. Paradichlorobenzene primarily affects the liver and CNS, although methemoglobinemia and hemolysis have been reported in humans.

Ice or Snow Melts

The most common ingredients in ice melts are sodium chloride, potassium chloride, magnesium chloride, calcium carbonate, and calcium magnesium acetate. A few ice melts contain urea. Sodium ion toxicosis is possible after large ingestion of ice melts, salt, or rock salt. Signs reported in one dog with fatal hypernatremia (increased sodium level in blood) from salt ingestion included vomiting, increased thirst, increased urination, fine muscular fasciculation, sinus tachycardia, metabolic acidosis (acidic blood pH), and seizures.

DANGEROUS PLANTS

These are a wide variety of common plants that can be poison to animals if consumed. Refer to Box 35-4 for a list of some of these plants.

BOX 35-4 Quick Poisonous Plant Reference

Cardiotoxic Plants

Convallaria majalis	Lily of the valley
Nerium oleander	Oleander
Rhododendron	Rhododendron, azalea, rosebay
Taxus spp.	American, Japanese, English, and Western yew
Digitalis purpurea	Foxglove
Kalanchoe spp.	Kalanchoe

Plants That Could Cause Kidney Failure

Certain species of lilies, in cats only
Rhubarb (*Rheum* spp.), leaves only
Grapes, raisins

Plants That Could Cause Liver Failure

Cycads (*Cycad* spp.)
Amanita phalloides, mushroom

Plants That Can Cause Multiple Effects

Autumn crocus (*Colchicum* spp.): Can cause bloody vomiting and diarrhea, shock, kidney failure, liver failure, bone marrow suppression.

Castor bean (*Ricinus* spp.): Usually a lag period of 48 hr before signs appear. Beans are highly toxic. Two to four beans can be lethal to adult humans.

Mushrooms: Always assume that any ingested mushroom is highly toxic until a mycologist identifies that mushroom. Toxic and nontoxic mushrooms can grow in the same area.

Rhododendron Species

Members of the *Rhododendron* species, including azalea and rhododendrons, contain gray anatoxins, which can lead to cardiovascular dysfunction (Figure 35-1).

Clinical signs in dogs and cats include vomiting, diarrhea, abdominal pain, weakness, depression, cardiac arrhythmias, hypotension, shock, cardiopulmonary arrest, pulmonary edema, dyspnea, CNS depression, and seizures. Signs generally occur within 4 to 12 hours of ingestion and may persist for several days. Poisonings have also been reported in ruminants and horses. Veterinary treatment and observation is always recommended.

Cardiac Glycoside–Containing Plants

Hundreds of cardiac glycosides have been identified in various plants, including oleander *(Nerium oleander)* (Figure 35-2), lily of the valley *(Convallaria majalis)* (Figure 35-3), and foxglove *(Digitalis purpurea)* (Figure 35-4). In most cases, all parts of the plant are toxic, and even small amounts can cause significant clinical signs.

Clinical signs generally develop within several hours of ingestion, and signs may persist for several days after removal of plant material from the GI tract. Clinical signs seen most commonly involve the GI tract and cardiovascular system. Veterinary treatment and observation is always recommended.

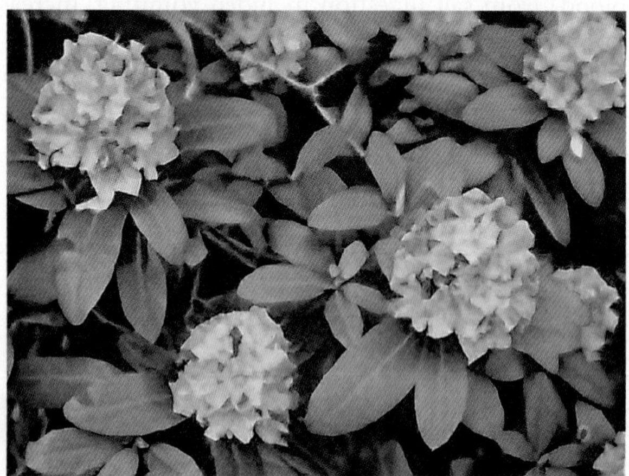

FIGURE 35-1 Members of the *Rhododendron* species, including azaleas and rhododendrons, contain gray anatoxins that can lead to cardiovascular dysfunction.

Castor Beans

Castor beans *(Ricinus communis)* are often used in jewelry, and the oil extracted from the seeds is used medicinally (castor oil). Ricin is the toxic principle of castor beans and is considered to be one of the most potent plant toxins known. All parts of the castor bean plant are toxic, but the seeds contain the highest concentration of ricin. In humans, ingestion of one seed is potentially lethal. Veterinary treatment and observation is always recommended.

Cycad Palms

Cycad palms *(Cycas, Zamia)* are found naturally in the sandy soils of tropical to subtropical climates, but may also be grown as houseplants in more temperate climates (Figure 35-5). Cycasin is considered to be the toxic principle that is responsible for the hepatic and GI signs generally seen with toxicosis. Most parts of the plant are toxic, but the seeds contain a higher concentration of cycasin and are more often associated with toxicosis in small animals. Ingestion of one or more seeds has resulted in liver failure and death in dogs.

Lilies

Easter lilies *(Lilium longiflorum)* (Figure 35-6), Tiger lilies *(Lilium tigrinum)*, Rubrum or Japanese lilies (*Lilium speciosum* and *Lilium lancifolium*), and various day lilies (*Hemerocallis* spp.) can cause acute renal failure and death in cats

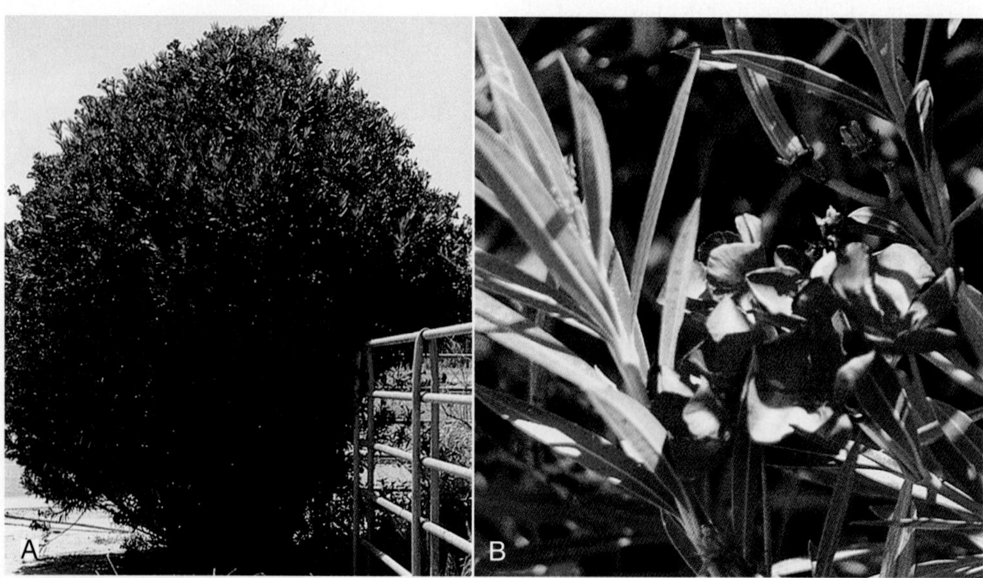

FIGURE 35-2 A, B, *Nerium oleander*. There are hundreds of cardiac glycosides identified in various plants, including oleander, lily of the valley, and foxglove.

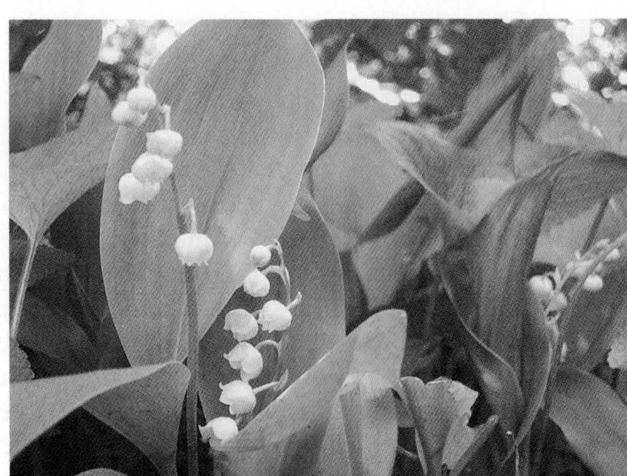

FIGURE 35-3 *Convallaria majalis,* or lily of the valley. (Courtesy Rachel Hayes.)

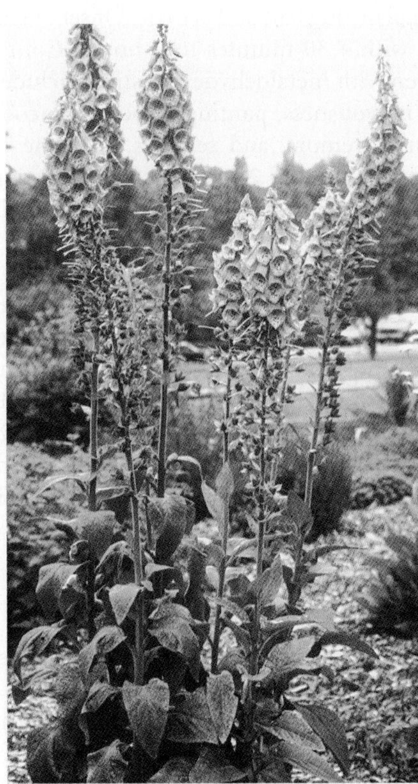

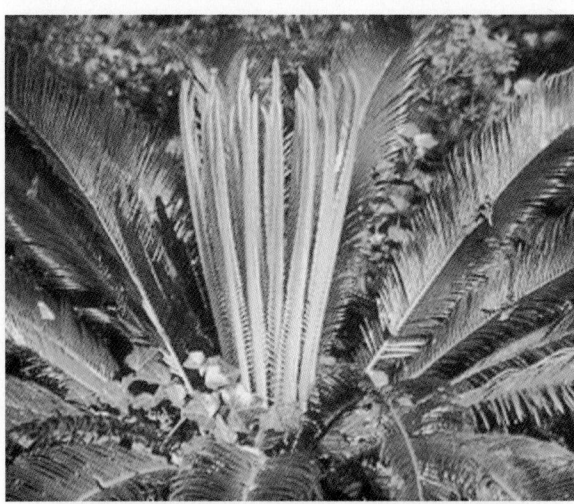

FIGURE 35-4 *Digitalis purpurea,* or foxglove.

FIGURE 35-5 Cycad palms are found naturally in the sandy soils of tropical to subtropical climates, but may be used as houseplants in more temperate climates.

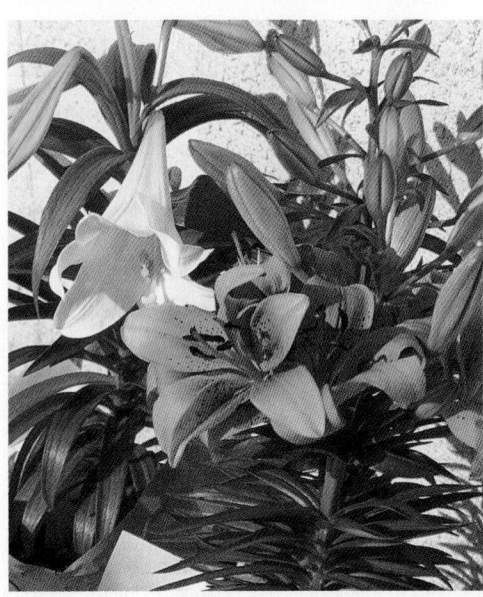

FIGURE 35-6 *Lilium longiflorum,* or Easter lily. Acute renal failure and death can occur in cats that consume various lilies. These include the Easter lily, Tiger lily, Day lily, and the Rubrum or Japanese lily.

(Figures 35-6 and 35-7). The toxic principle is unknown. Even minor exposures (a few bites on a leaf, ingestion of pollen, etc.) may result in toxicosis. All feline exposures to lilies should be considered potentially life threatening.

Affected cats often vomit within a few hours of exposure to lilies, but the vomiting usually subsides after a few hours, during which time the cats may appear normal or may be mildly depressed and anorexic. Within 24 to 72 hours of ingestion, oliguric to anuric renal failure develops accompanied by vomiting, depression, anorexia, and dehydration.

Elevations in kidney blood values can occur as early as 12 to 18 hours after ingestion. Death from acute kidney failure generally occurs within 3 to 6 days of ingestion.

Veterinary treatment and observation is always recommended with lily ingestion in cats. Early decontamination by a veterinarian (emesis, oral activated charcoal, and cathartic) in combination with intravenous fluid therapy has been shown to effectively prevent lily-induced kidney failure. Conversely, delaying treatment beyond 18 hours frequently results in death or euthanasia as a result of severe kidney failure. Dialysis can be of help with severely affected animals, but it is not commonly available.

Calcium Oxalate–Containing Plants

Philodendron species, calla lily (*Zantedeschia* spp.), elephant ears (*Caladium* spp.), dumb cane (*Dieffenbachia* spp.) mother-in-law's tongue (*Monstera* spp.) (Figure 35-8), peace

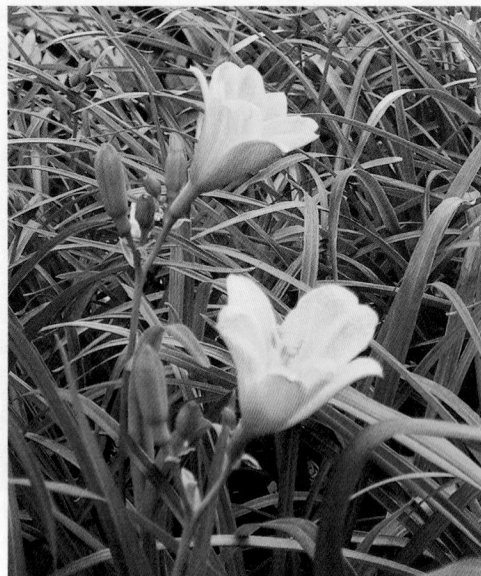

FIGURE 35-7 Day lily. (Courtesy Rachel Hayes.)

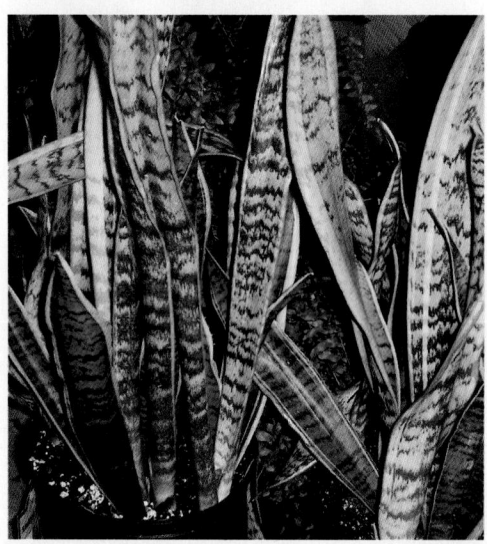

FIGURE 35-8 Mother-in-law's tongue. (Courtesy Rachel Hayes.)

lily (*Spathiphyllum* spp.), pathos (*Epipremnum* spp.), and certain other varieties of plants contain insoluble calcium oxalate crystals in their plant material. Chewing of the plant material can cause the crystals to be expelled into the oral cavity and can result in painful oropharyngeal edema. Clinical signs associated with these plants include oral irritation; intense burning and irritation of the mouth, lips, and tongue; excessive drooling; vomiting; and difficulty in swallowing. Airway compromise from tissue swelling could be life threatening, although severe effects are a rare occurrence.

PESTICIDES

The most dangerous forms of pesticides include snail bait containing metaldehyde, fly bait containing methomyl, systemic insecticides containing Di-Syston or disulfoton, and zinc phosphide.

Fly Bait

Methomyl is a highly toxic carbamate insecticide that can be found in fly baits. Carbamate insecticides competitively inhibit both acetylcholinesterases and pseudocholinesterases. Acetylcholinesterase inhibitors cause muscarinic, nicotinic, and CNS system effects. Exposure to methomyl may lead to cholinergic crisis with increased salivation, lacrimation, urinary incontinence, diarrhea, GI cramping, and emesis (SLUDGE) syndrome, but the most obvious sign is severe seizures. Hypertension and slow heart rate or cardiorespiratory depression may occur. Immediate veterinary treatment and observation is always required because signs can occur within minutes of methomyl ingestion.

Snail or Slug Bait

Metaldehyde is a polymer of acetaldehyde and is commonly found in snail or slug bait and is toxic. Onset of clinical signs is typically within 30 minutes to 3 hours. Common clinical signs seen with metaldehyde ingestion include increased heart rate, nervousness, panting, drooling, incoordination, hyperthermia, tremors, and seizures. In some cases, liver failure may occur within 2 to 3 days after exposure. Veterinary treatment and observation is always required.

Gopher or Mole Bait

Zinc phosphide is used in mole and gopher baits and is considered to be highly toxic. Following ingestion, phosphide is converted to phosphine gas by stomach acid (the conversion is enhanced with the presence of food and water). Released phosphine gas causes severe respiratory distress. Clinical signs are seen soon after ingestion, typically within 15 minutes to 4 hours. Death occurs secondary to respiratory failure. Veterinary treatment and observation is always required.

Systemic Insecticides: Disulfoton, Or Di-Syston

Disulfoton (also known as Di-Syston) is a selective, systemic organophosphate insecticide and is highly toxic. Systemic insecticides are applied to the soil and then are actively taken up by plant roots and translocated to all parts of the plant. Onset of clinical signs is 2 to 8 hours after ingestion, and signs can last for several days. Clinical signs seen with a toxicosis include typical cholinesterase inhibitor SLUDGE signs, but they can also have hemorrhagic diarrhea and liver and pancreatic enzyme elevations. Veterinary treatment and observation is always required. Good nursing care is essential. Prognosis is good to guarded depending on the severity of the signs. Complete recovery from acute effects may take several days or weeks.

Rat or Mouse Bait

There are three main types of rat or mouse baits available commercially: anticoagulants, bromethalin, and cholecalciferol. Other pesticides, such as strychnine, aldicarb, and zinc phosphide, may be used to control wild rat and mouse populations.

TABLE 35-2 Anticoagulant Rodenticides

Type of Anticoagulant	Minimum Duration of Therapy
Warfarin	14 days
Bromadiolone	21 days
Brodifacoum and others	30 days

Anticoagulants (Table 35-2) include:

- Short acting: warfarin
- Long acting: pindone, diphacinone, difethialone, chlorophacinone, brodifacoum, and bromadiolone

The anticoagulant rodenticides act by competitive inhibition of vitamin K epoxide reductase, thus halting the recycling of vitamin K. In early cases of toxicoses, the prothrombin time (PT) when checked between 36 and 72 hours will be elevated, but the animal will still appear clinically normal. Beyond 72 hours, hemorrhage is a possible effect. The presence of circulating clotting factors in normal animals is the reason for the delay in the development of signs.

Clinical signs of anticoagulant poisoning may not be observed for 5 to 10 days after ingestion and include hemorrhage, pale mucous membranes, weakness, exercise intolerance, lameness, dyspnea, coughing, and swollen joints. Often the animal is not seen by the veterinarian until signs are severe.

Animals with clinical signs should be stabilized immediately. Transfusions with whole blood or plasma may be necessary to replace clotting factors. Decontamination is only effective early; remember, clinical signs are usually delayed 5 to 10 days after ingestion. Any elevation in the PT warrants full treatment with vitamin K_1. No treatment is indicated if PT remains normal; however, recent vitamin K_1 administration could result in misleading PT values because new clotting factor synthesis only requires 6 to 12 hours. Oral vitamin K_1 is an antidote for anticoagulants. Vitamin K_1 should be given with a fatty meal to enhance absorption.

Bromethalin

Bromethalin is an uncoupler of oxidative phosphorylation. Bromethalin causes a reduction of adenosine triphosphate (ATP). ATP is necessary to sustain the sodium-potassium ion channel pumps. When the pump mechanism is inhibited, fluid buildup occurs, which results in fluid-filled vacuoles between myelin sheaths. This leads to decreased nerve impulse conduction.

Clinical signs of bromethalin toxicosis could occur within 24 hours to 2 weeks and include muscle tremors, seizures, hyperexcitability, forelimb extensor rigidity, ataxia, CNS depression, loss of vocalization, paresis, paralysis, and death.

Aggressive decontamination is most important with bromethalin ingestion. Repeated doses of activated charcoal (every 8 to 12 hours) are recommended. Supportive care should be given, as needed, for clinical signs. The prognosis is poor for animals showing severe signs. Animals exposed at lower doses exhibiting paralysis may recover. Agents such as mannitol, furosemide, and corticosteroids may reduce the cerebral edema. Unfortunately, these drugs were of little benefit in reducing the severity of signs in experimental animals. Ginkgo biloba has been used experimentally in rats with bromethalin poisoning, although the true benefit is not known.

Cholecalciferol

Cholecalciferol (vitamin D_3) increases intestinal absorption of calcium, stimulates bone resorption, and enhances kidney reabsorption of calcium. This results in a serum calcium increase. This can lead to kidney failure, cardiovascular abnormalities, and tissue mineralization.

Clinical signs usually have a delay in onset and usually occur 18 to 36 hours after ingestion. The most common signs seen with cholecalciferol toxicosis include vomiting, diarrhea, inappetence, depression, polyuria, polydipsia, and cardiac arrhythmia. Kidney failure arises from the deposition of calcium in the kidney.

Aggressive decontamination is most important with cholecalciferol ingestion. Repeated doses of activated charcoal (every 8 to 12 hours for 1 to 2 days) are recommended.

Close monitoring of the serum calcium, phosphorus, creatinine, and blood urea nitrogen (BUN) is recommended.

Renal effects are treated with fluid diuresis. Prednisone and furosemide are often used with treatment. Pamidronate inhibits osteoclastic bone resorption and has been used successfully to treat cholecalciferol poisoning. Alternatively, salmon calcitonin has been used to decrease calcium levels.

ANTIFREEZE PRODUCTS

Methanol

Methanol (also known as methyl alcohol or wood alcohol) is found most commonly in "antifreeze" windshield washer fluid and varies in concentration from 20% to 100% (with 20% to 30% the most common form). Methanol's metabolite, formaldehyde, is rapidly oxidized by aldehyde dehydrogenase to formic acid, which can cause metabolic acidosis if significant quantities are ingested and retinal toxicity in humans and nonhuman primates. In general, alcohols are rapidly absorbed from the GI tract. The minimum toxic dose in dogs is 8.0 g/kg (or 3 oz of 100% methanol). The most common exposures occur with dogs and usually involve chewing on containers or lapping up spills. With small exposures in dogs and cats, only mild gastric upset is seen. Recent small ingestion is treated with dilution (milk and water) that may help minimize gastric upset. Large exposure would be expected to only occur when there is no other water source available. In the case of a large ingestion, the animal should be monitored and treated for acidosis.

Propylene Glycol

Propylene glycol is the main ingredient in "safer" forms of engine antifreeze or coolants. Propylene glycol is approximately three times less toxic in dogs than EG. According to a study, no clinical signs were seen when a dog was given an acute dose of 20 ml/kg.

In toxic quantities, acidosis, liver damage, and renal insufficiency are possible from propylene glycol. Clinical signs of propylene glycol toxicosis include CNS depression, weakness, ataxia, and seizures. With large ingestion, diuresis and supportive care, such as treatment for acidosis, should be given.

Ethylene Glycol

Ethylene glycol is the most dangerous form of antifreeze. Most commercial antifreeze products contain between 95% and 97% EG. The minimum lethal dose of undiluted EG antifreeze is 4.4 to 6.6 ml/kg in dogs and 1.4 ml/kg in cats. EG can cause metabolic acidosis and acute renal tubular necrosis. In most cases of EG poisoning, vomiting is seen within the first few hours, and within 1 to 6 hours, signs of depression, ataxia, weakness, tachypnea, polyuria, and polydipsia occur. By 18 to 36 hours, acute renal failure occurs.

> TECHNICIAN NOTE EG is the most dangerous form of antifreeze. Most commercial antifreeze products contain between 95% and 97% EG.

Diagnosis

Peak levels of EG are reached within 1 to 4 hours after ingestion. There is one commercial EG kit available for veterinary use (EGT Kit PRN Pharmacal, 800-874-9764). EG tests can be run as early as 30 minutes after ingestion up to 12 hours. The EGT Kit is labeled for dogs and detects a level greater than 50 mg/dl. Since cats are more sensitive than dogs, the kit may not be sensitive enough to diagnose a toxicosis in the cat. Some human labs may run a quantitative EG analysis to detect levels and could be considered with feline exposures. False-positive test results can occur from propylene glycol (in some types of activated charcoal solutions and also from some injection solutions, such as pentobarbital and diazepam) or from formaldehyde.

Treatment

Induction of emesis is only helpful with recent exposures (less than 1 hour). To prevent false-positive EG tests, it is recommended to take a blood sample before administering activated charcoal since many products contain propylene glycol as inactive ingredients. Although its effectiveness is controversial, activated charcoal can be given within 1 to 3 hours of ingestion. Gastric lavage with activated charcoal could be considered, but would only be effective early.

EG is metabolized via alcohol dehydrogenase to glycoaldehyde, which is then metabolized to glycolic acid, which is then metabolized to glyoxylic acid. Glycoaldehyde is more toxic than EG. The formation of glycolic acid is thought to be responsible for causing metabolic acidosis. The goal of treatment of EG toxicoses is to slow down the metabolism.

Fomepizole (Antizole Vet by Orphan Medical, 888-8-ORPHAN) is used to inhibit alcohol dehydrogenase and is considered the preferred treatment for treating EG toxicoses in dogs, but is not effective in cats.

Ethanol can be used in cats and dogs. Ethanol also competes with EG as a substrate for alcohol dehydrogenase; however, it does have several unfavorable side effects, which include CNS depression, hyperosmolality, and metabolic acidosis. Fluid diuresis and correction of acidosis with sodium bicarbonate is also an important part of therapy. Peritoneal dialysis should be considered with anuric animals. Prognosis is good with early aggressive treatment (less than 8 hours of ingestion).

DANGEROUS HUMAN MEDICATIONS

Please note that any medication can be dangerous to an animal, depending on the dose and frequency. The following is a list of potentially dangerous medications. All require veterinary consultation, treatment, and monitoring.

Acetaminophen

Acetaminophen is a synthetic nonopiate derivative of *p*-aminophenol. Acetaminophen toxicity can result from a single toxic dose or repeated cumulative dosages, which lead to methemoglobinemia and liver damage. In dogs, acetaminophen is used therapeutically for analgesia at a dose of 10 mg/kg q 12 hours. Clinical signs of toxicity are not typically observed in dogs unless the dose exceeds 100 mg/kg, at which dose hepatotoxicity is possible. At 200 mg/kg, methemoglobinemia is a possibility. In cats, 10 mg/kg has produced signs of toxicity.

Clinical signs of acetaminophen toxicity are related to methemoglobinemia and hepatotoxicity. Clinical signs include depression, weakness, tachypnea, dyspnea, cyanosis, icterus, vomiting, methemoglobinemia, hypothermia, facial or paw edema, hepatic necrosis, and death.

> TECHNICIAN NOTE Clinical signs of acetaminophen toxicity include depression, weakness, tachypnea, dyspnea, cyanosis, icterus, vomiting, methemoglobinemia, hypothermia, facial or paw edema, hepatic necrosis, and death.

Ibuprofen

Ibuprofen is a substituted phenylalkanoic acid with nonsteroidal antiinflammatory, antipyretic, and analgesic properties. Ibuprofen has been used therapeutically in dogs at 5 mg/kg, but because it can cause gastric ulcers and perforations, it is generally not recommended.

According to studies of acute ingestion of ibuprofen in dogs, vomiting, diarrhea, nausea, anorexia, gastric ulceration, and abdominal pain can be seen with doses of 50 to 125 mg/kg; these signs in combination with renal damage can be seen at doses at or above 175 mg/kg. At doses at or above 400 mg/kg, CNS effects, such as seizure, ataxia, and coma, may occur. Cats are considered to be twice as sensitive as dogs because they have a limited glucuronyl-conjugating capacity.

The most common signs of ibuprofen toxicoses include anorexia, nausea, vomiting, lethargy, diarrhea, bloody diarrhea, ataxia, increased urination, and increased thirst.

Postmortem lesions associated with ibuprofen toxicoses include perforations, erosion, ulceration, and hemorrhage of the GI tract.

The primary goal of treatment is to prevent or treat gastric ulceration, renal failure, CNS effects, and possibly hepatic effects. Prognosis is good if the animal is treated promptly and appropriately. Delay in treatment can decrease survival potential with large exposures.

Aspirin

Aspirin is used therapeutically in dogs and cats (acceptable daily doses [ADDs]). Aspirin must be used cautiously in cats because of their inability to rapidly metabolize and excrete salicylates. Symptoms of toxicity may occur if given doses frequently or without stringent monitoring. Aspirin should be used cautiously in neonatal animals; adult doses may lead to poisoning. Symptoms of acute aspirin overdose in dogs and cats include depression, vomiting (may be blood tinged), anorexia, hyperthermia, and increased respiratory rate. If treatment is not provided, muscular weakness, pulmonary and cerebral edema, hypernatremia, hypokalemia, ataxia, and seizures may all develop with eventual coma and death.

Ma Huang, Pseudoephedrine, and Ephedrine: Sympathomimetic Alkaloids

Ma huang is used as an herbal weight loss aid and contains the sympathomimetic alkaloids ephedrine and pseudoephedrine. Ephedrine and pseudoephedrine act as stimulants and are also found in cold and flu medications as nasal decongestants and are similar in structure to amphetamines. They can cause increased blood pressure, tachycardia, ataxia, mydriasis, hyperactivity, tremors, and seizures. Ephedrine and pseudoephedrine are eliminated by the kidneys. The half-life varies with urine pH. With an overdose, it is common to see clinical signs last for more than 24 hours.

Isoniazid

Isoniazid (INH) is a medication used to treat tuberculosis and has a narrow margin of safety. Isoniazid is available as an elixir, injectable, syrup, and tablets in strengths of 50, 100, and 300 mg. Overdoses produce life-threatening signs: seizures, acidosis, and coma. Pyridoxine (vitamin B_6) is a direct agonist of INH.

Calcipotriene: Vitamin D Derivatives

Calcipotriene is a synthetic derivative of vitamin D_3. It is used as a topical ointment to treat psoriasis in humans. An overdose of calcipotriene can cause hypercalcemia that can result in kidney failure, cardiac failure, and possibly death. In most cases, dogs that have ingested toxic levels of calcipotriene start showing signs of lethargy, weakness, and inappetence within 1 to 2 days after exposure. Serum calcium levels would be expected to increase within 12 to 72 hours. Hypercalcemia, hyperphosphatemia, azotemia, proteinuria, and tissue mineralization can occur with overdoses. Bradycardia and cardiac arrhythmia are also expected.

5-Fluorouracil: Antimetabolites

5-Fluorouracil (5-FU) is an anticancer topical cream. It is used in human patients to treat solar and actinic keratoses and some superficial skin tumors. Topical fluorouracil is available as 1% or 5% cream (5-FU can inhibit ribonucleic acid [RNA] processing and functioning and deoxyribonucleic acid [DNA] synthesis and repair). The toxicity effects of 5-FU, as with other anticancer agents, is mainly through its destruction of rapidly dividing cell lines, such as bone marrow stem cells and the epithelial layer of the intestinal crypts.

Early effects seen with 5-FU in the dog include generalized grand mal seizures, tremors, vomiting, and ataxia. Cardiac arrhythmia, respiratory distress, and hemorrhagic gastroenteritis are also seen. Clinical signs develop within 1 hour and are usually life threatening. Often death occurs within 6 to 16 hours after exposure. In those that survive initial effects, it is possible to see bone marrow suppression with evidence of neutropenia 4 to 20 days after exposure.

RECOMMENDED READING

Ahn A: Introducing etofenprox: a broad-spectrum, comprehensive ectoparasiticide, *Hartz Companion Anim Newsletter* 4(2):1-3, 2006.

Beasley VR, Dorman D: Management of toxicoses, *Vet Clin North Am* 20(2):307-338, 1990.

Beasley VR et al: *A Systems affected approach to veterinary toxicology*, Urbana, Ill, 1999, University of Illinois Press.

Birckel P, Cochet P, Benard P et al: Cutaneous distribution of C-fipronil in the dog and cat following a spot on administration. In von Tscharner C, Willemse T, editors: *Proceedings from the Third World Congress of Veterinary Dermatology*, Edinburgh, 1996.

Bishop BF et al: Selamectin: a novel broad-spectrum endectocide for dogs and cats, *Vet Parasitol* 23(91)(3-4):163-176, 2000.

Bough MG: Castor bean toxicosis: one mean bean, *Vet Technician* 23(8):498, 2002.

Cheeke PR: *Natural toxicants in feeds, forages, and poisonous plants*, ed 2, Danville, Ill, 1998, Interstate Publishers.

Dunayer EK: Xylitol ingestion in dogs, *Vet Med* 101(12):791-796, 2006.

Dunayer EK, Gwaltney-Brant SM: Acute hepatic failure and coagulopathy associated with xylitol ingestion in eight dogs, *JAVMA* 229(7):1113-1117, 2006.

Foss T: Liquid potpourri and cats, *Vet Technician* 23(11):686-689, 2002.

Gfeller R, Messonier SM: *Handbook of small animal toxicology and poisonings*, ed 2, St Louis, 2004, Mosby.

Gwaltney SM: Chocolate intoxication, *Vet Med* 96(2):108-111, 2001.

Hainzl D, Cole LM, Casida JE: Mechanisms for selective toxicity of fipronil insecticide and its sulfone metabolite and desulfinyl photoproduct, *Chem Res Toxicol* 11(12):1529-1535, 1998.

Hansen SR et al: Macadamia nut toxicosis in dogs, *Vet Med* 97(2): 274-276, 2002.

Hovda LR, Hooser SB: Toxicology of newer pesticides for use in dogs and cats, *Vet Clin Small Anim* 32:455-467, 2002.

Hull W: Ethylene glycol testing, *Vet Technician* 22(4):201-206, 2001.

Krautmann MJ, et al: Safety of selamectin in cats, *Vet Parasitol* 23(91) (3-4):393-403, 2002.

Means C: The Wrath of grapes, *ASPCA's Anim Watch* 22(2):15, 2002.

Means C: Bread dough toxicosis in dogs, *J Vet Emerg Crit Care* 13(1): 39-41, 2003.

Mindy GB: Dermal decontamination: dealing with sticky situations, *Vet Technician* 24(8):538-540, 2003.

Moorman M: Anticoagulant rodenticides now more toxic to pests and pets, *Vet Technician* 23(1):34-36, 2002.
Moorman M: Bromethalin: it's not what you think, *Vet Technician* 24(7):484-486, 2003.
Novotny MJ, et al: Safety of selamectin in dogs, *Vet Parasitol* 23(91)(3-4): 377-391, 2002.
Ogawa E et al: Effect of onion ingestion on anti-oxidizing agents in dog erythrocytes, *Jpn J Vet Sci* 48(4):685-690, 1986.
Peterson ME, Talcott PA: *Small animal toxicology,* Moscow, Idaho, 2001, University of Idaho.
Plumlee KH: Nicotine. In Peterson ME, Talcott PA, editors: *Small animal toxicology,* Philadelphia, 2001, WB Saunders.
Plumlee Konnie P, editor: *Clinical veterinary toxicology,* St Louis, 2004, Mosby.
Ramesh C, et al: Pharmacologic profile of methoprene, an insect growth regulator, in cattle, dogs, and cats, *JAVMA* 194(3):410-412, 1989.
Richardson JA: Permethrin spot-on toxicoses in cats, *J Vet Emerg Crit Care* 10(2):103-106, 2000.
Richardson JA: Poison prevention and management primer, *Vet Technician* 23(3):150-156, 2002.
Richardson JA et al: Managing pet bird toxicoses, *Exotic DVM* 3(1): 23-27, 2001.
Schell MM: Tremorgenic mycotoxin intoxication, *Vet Med* 95(4): 283-286, 2000.
Simmons DM: Onion breath, *Vet Technician* 22(8):424-427, 2001.
Steenbergen VM: Beautiful lilies: a potential cat-astrophe, *Vet Technician* 23(4):236-237, 2002.
Steenbergen VM: Acetaminophen and cats, *Vet Technician* 24(1): 43-45, 2003.
Tamara F: The hazards of ice melts to dogs and cats, *Vet Technician* 23(2):94-104, 2002.
Webster M: Product warning, Frontline, *Aust Vet J* 77:202, 1999.
Wismer TA: Novel insecticides. In Plumlee KH, editor: *Clinical veterinary toxicology,* St Louis, 2003, Mosby.

PART EIGHT

End of Life

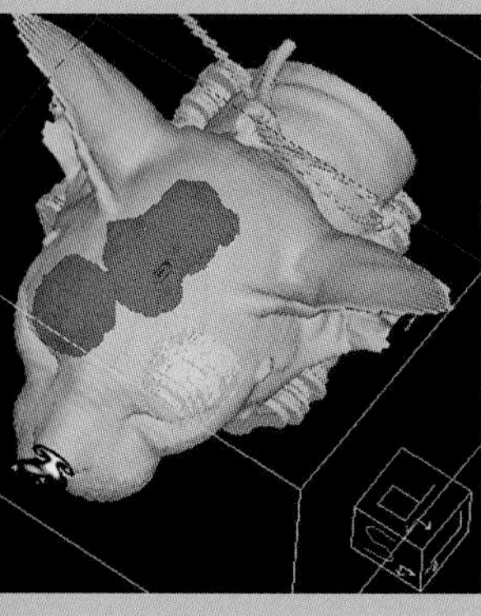

Veterinary Oncology

36

Glenna E. Mauldin and G. Neal Mauldin

KEY TERMS

Acute radiation toxicity
Adjuvant therapy
Chemotherapy
Curative therapy
Cytotoxic
Definitive diagnosis
Definitive therapy
Hyperproteinemia
Initiation
Ionizing radiation
Irritant
Metastasis
Mucositis
Multimodality therapy
Mutagen
Myelosuppression
Neoplasm
Palliative therapy
Paraneoplastic syndrome
Polycythemia
Radiation sensitizer
Teratogen
Tumor grade
Tumor stage
Vesicant

OUTLINE

LEARNING OBJECTIVES

When you have completed this chapter, you will be able to:

1. Define oncology and explain mechanisms by which tumors cause clinical signs.
2. Differentiate between malignant and benign tumors.
3. List the classifications of tumors by tissue origin and provide examples of each.
4. Describe methods used to stage and grade tumors based on their physical characteristics and microscopic features.
5. List early warning signs of cancer in animals and discuss patient evaluation procedures in animals with suspected cancer.
6. Differentiate between cytology and histopathology and state advantages and limitations for each diagnostic method.
7. List and describe common methods used to obtain biopsy tissue and procedures for handling biopsy samples.
8. Discuss considerations related to surgical treatment of cancer in dogs and cats.
9. Discuss nursing considerations and safety concerns related to administration of a chemotherapeutic agent for treatment of cancer in dogs and cats.
10. Describe the mechanism by which radiotherapy affects cancer cells and list potential adverse effects of radiation therapy.

INTRODUCTION

Cancer is common in both dogs and cats: it is estimated that 40% to 50% of animals older than 10 years will have potentially life-threatening malignant disease. The proportion of owners willing to pursue advanced diagnostics and treatment for these pets has grown significantly in recent years, so it is increasingly important that veterinarians and veterinary technicians have expertise in the practice of oncology. Some forms of cancer therapy, such as basic surgery or simple chemotherapy protocols, can be performed easily in private practice with a minimum of specialized equipment. Other treatments, such as aggressive surgery, radiotherapy, or complex chemotherapy protocols, necessitate referral to an institution that has the appropriate facilities and expertise. Regardless of the specific tumor and treatment offered, oncology nurses and technicians play a central role in the treatment of companion animals diagnosed with cancer.

There are several reasons that the treatment of dogs and cats with cancer is worthwhile and should be encouraged. Important medical advances have been achieved by studying and treating tumors in pet animals, and participation in such clinical research programs can be extremely rewarding to both veterinarians and technicians. In addition, the strength and importance of the human-animal bond has gained wider recognition and acceptance, and providing effective cancer therapies helps to preserve this special relationship. Finally, many clients have had experience with cancer in their own lives and understandably feel fear and anxiety when their pet is diagnosed with a malignant disease. Veterinarians and technicians caring for dogs and cats with cancer must maintain a positive but realistic attitude toward the disease in general, recognizing and supporting the emotional needs of the client and providing quality medical care. Owners should never be made to believe that treating a pet with cancer is unreasonable or hopeless. Box 36-1 gives the names and addresses of organizations that provide information on cancer and cancer treatment.

As part of the veterinary health care team, the veterinary technician plays a vital role in appropriate case management, quality patient care, and client support. The purpose of this chapter is to enhance the technician's knowledge of the basic principles of oncology. By understanding the unique diagnostic and therapeutic approach to neoplastic disease, the technician will become a more active and effective participant in the management of cancer in dogs and cats.

TUMOR BIOLOGY

Oncology is the study of cancer. In general, cancer is defined as an uncontrolled growth of cells on or within the body. Virtually any type of normal cell may undergo the changes that eventually result in the development of cancer. Other terms that are commonly used to describe cancer include tumor, mass, neoplasm, and growth. Tumor growth can cause clinical signs in several ways: by destroying tissue and impairing normal organ function, by causing pain or inflammation, by predisposing the animal to infection, or by causing systemic symptoms that are indirectly associated with the cancer (called paraneoplastic syndromes). Paraneoplastic syndromes are characterized by symptoms that occur at sites distant from the site of the primary tumor. These clinical signs are often caused by hormones or other substances synthesized by the tumor, which circulate systemically and affect multiple organ systems or tissues (Box 36-2).

Tumors can be either benign or malignant. The cells that make up benign tumors exhibit unchecked growth, but do

BOX 36-1 Organizations for Cancer Information and Treatment

Veterinary
Veterinary Cancer Society
Barbara J. McGehee, Executive Director
P.O. Box 1763
Spring Valley, CA 91979-1763
Phone: 619-474-8929
Fax: 619-474-8947
http://www.vetcancersociety.org

Human
American Cancer Society
National Home Office
1599 Clifton Road, NE
Atlanta, GA 30329
1-800-ACS-2345
http://www.cancer.org

National Cancer Institute
NCI Public Inquiries Office
Suite 3036A
6116 Executive Boulevard
Bethesda, MD 20892-8322
http://www.cancer.gov

BOX 36-2 Examples of Paraneoplastic Syndromes and Associated Tumors

Hypoglycemia
Hepatocellular carcinoma
Insulinoma
Leiomyosarcoma

Hypercalcemia
Lymphoma
Apocrine gland adenocarcinoma of the anal sac
Parathyroid tumors
Multiple myeloma

Polycythemia
Renal carcinoma

Disseminated Intravascular Coagulation
Hemangiosarcoma
Lymphoma
Thyroid carcinoma

Anemia
Multiple tumors

Hyperproteinemia
Multiple myeloma
Lymphoma

Fever
Multiple tumors

not destroy surrounding normal tissues. However, they can still impair tissue function and cause significant problems through their physical presence. For instance, even though most meningiomas (tumors of the meninges that surround the brain and spinal cord) are histologically benign, they can cause severe neurologic dysfunction and death if not identified and treated in a timely manner. The cells in malignant tumors also exhibit uncontrolled growth, but unlike the cells of benign tumors, they are capable of local tissue destruction. They also have the potential for metastasis. Metastasis is the process by which cancer cells spread from a primary tumor to secondary locations, such as lungs, lymph nodes, and visceral sites (e.g., liver). The mechanisms of metastasis are not fully understood, but the metastatic process involves a series of basic steps that are similar regardless of the tumor type. First, cancer cells at the primary site proliferate and develop a blood supply. These cells then invade the vascular system and are transported to distant tissues. When they eventually reach the metastatic site, the cells arrest and leave the circulation (extravasation). A metastatic tumor is established when these cells are able to survive and grow in the new site.

TABLE 36-1 Classification of Tumors in Animals

Tissue Type	Benign	Malignant
Connective Tissue		
Bone	Osteoma	Osteosarcoma
Cartilage	Chondroma	Chondrosarcoma
Fibrous tissue	Fibroma	Fibrosarcoma
Fat	Lipoma	Liposarcoma
Smooth muscle	Leiomyoma	Leiomyosarcoma
Skeletal muscle	Rhabdomyoma	Rhabdomyosarcoma
Blood vessels	Hemangioma	Hemangiosarcoma
Hemolymphatic Tissue		
		Lymphomas Multiple myeloma
Epithelial Tissue		
Skin	Papilloma	Squamous cell carcinoma
Sebaceous gland	Adenoma	Adenocarcinoma/carcinoma
Sweat gland	Adenoma	Adenocarcinoma/carcinoma
Ceruminous gland	Adenoma	Adenocarcinoma/carcinoma
Mammary gland	Adenoma	Adenocarcinoma/carcinoma
Nasal mucosa	Adenoma	Adenocarcinoma/carcinoma
Gastrointestinal mucosa	Adenoma	Adenocarcinoma/carcinoma
Biliary tract	Adenoma	Adenocarcinoma/carcinoma
Urinary tract	Adenoma	Adenocarcinoma/carcinoma

Modified from Ehrhart EJ, Powers BE. The pathology of neoplasia. In Withrow SJ, Vail DM: *Withrow and MacEwen's small animal clinical oncology*, ed 4, St Louis, 2007, Elsevier Saunders.

In addition to being classified as benign or malignant, tumors are categorized according to their tissue of origin and their histologic features (Table 36-1). Carcinomas, for example, arise from epithelial tissues, including skin, mucous membranes, glandular structures, and organs, such as the liver or kidneys. Carcinomas generally spread through both the lymphatic system and the bloodstream, so regional lymph node and lung metastases are commonly seen. Sarcomas, on the other hand, arise from mesenchymal tissues, such as cartilage, connective tissue, or bone. These tumors spread through the bloodstream and less frequently through lymphatics. Because of this, pulmonary metastases are relatively more common with sarcomas, and local lymph node involvement is rarer. The prefix of a tumor's name indicates the specific tissue of origin. For example, an osteosarcoma is a sarcoma originating from bone. The suffix of the name generally indicates whether the tumor is benign or malignant, with "-oma" designating a benign tumor (e.g., fibroma) and "-sarcoma" designating a malignant tumor (e.g., fibrosarcoma). Exceptions to this rule include melanoma and insulinoma, both of which are malignant tumors. More than 100 histologic types of cancer exist, and each requires individualized treatment and carries a different prognosis. It is also important to realize that the incidence and behavior of cancer in dogs is often quite different from its incidence and behavior in cats, even though the tumor names and histologic types may be the same.

> *TECHNICIAN NOTE* More than 100 histologic types of cancer exist, and each requires individualized treatment and carries a different prognosis.

Other methods used to classify tumors and help predict behavior and prognosis include the tumor's grade and stage. Tumors of the same histologic type are graded by the histopathologist according to defined microscopic features. For example, the cells in a low-grade soft tissue sarcoma have close to normal cellular architecture (well differentiated) and few mitotic figures (slow cell division) and exhibit minimal invasion of surrounding normal tissue. In contrast, the cells in a high-grade soft tissue sarcoma have abnormal cellular architecture (undifferentiated) and numerous mitotic figures (rapid cell division) and exhibit aggressive invasion of surrounding normal structures. Well-established and reliable grading systems exist for some types of tumors, such as canine mast cell tumors and soft tissue sarcomas. Tumor staging is performed by the veterinarian according to physical characteristics of the tumor and results of diagnostic tests that assess the extent of malignant disease. The World Health Organization's tumor staging system is known as the TNM system, and it categorizes tumors according to features of the tumor at the primary site (T), whether there is involvement of regional lymph nodes (N), and whether the tumor has metastasized to distant sites (M). Defined subclassifications, represented by numbers following the T, N, and M (e.g., $T_3N_1M_0$), describe the size and extent of the tumor in each of these locations. In addition, an animal's TNM system classification often includes assignment of a substage. Here, evidence of clinical signs of illness is usually designated "a" (denoting healthy) or "b" (denoting sick). The exact cause of most cancers is not fully understood. Carcinogenesis is the process by which normal cells are transformed into cancer cells. Classically, two events must take place before malignant transformation can occur: initiation and promotion. During the first event (initiation), the cell is exposed to a factor or factors that rapidly and irreversibly alter its DNA. Promotion, which follows initiation, is a prolonged process during which initiated cells are stimulated by an agent or agents to evolve into tumor cells. Under favorable conditions, a single transformed cell can proliferate and eventually develop into an invasive cancer. Factors with carcinogenic potential include inherited genetic defects, hormones, viruses, diet, immune system dysfunction, trauma, chronic inflammation, radiation, and a wide variety of chemicals. However, establishing a simple cause-and-effect relationship between a specific carcinogenic factor and subsequent tumor development in an exposed or affected individual is extremely difficult. Research must continue to focus on the underlying causes of cancer, with cancer prevention the ultimate goal.

DIAGNOSTIC APPROACH IN THE DOG OR CAT WITH CANCER

The chances of long-term control of any cancer are much greater if the tumor is diagnosed early and treated appropriately. The most dangerous approach in any dog or cat with suspected cancer is to advise the owner to "just watch it." The American Veterinary Medical Association has published the following list of the early warning signs of cancer:

- Abnormal swellings that persist or continue to grow
- Sores that do not heal
- Weight loss
- Loss of appetite
- Bleeding or discharge from any body opening
- Offensive odor
- Difficulty eating or swallowing
- Hesitation to exercise or loss of stamina
- Persistent lameness or stiffness
- Difficulty breathing, urinating, or defecating

Although not every animal exhibiting these clinical signs has cancer, a geriatric animal with one or more of these symptoms should be carefully evaluated for the underlying presence of neoplasia. A systematic and logical approach, such as the one described in the following section, is necessary to accurately diagnose neoplastic disease.

HISTORY, PHYSICAL EXAMINATION, AND MINIMUM BASELINE DATA

The first steps in evaluating a dog or cat with suspected cancer are to obtain an accurate history from the client and to perform a thorough physical examination. Great care must be taken in gathering this information: there is no diagnostic test that can match the valuable data gained from these two sources. The history should include the owner's perception of the primary problem, the observed clinical signs, the duration of those signs, any treatments administered, and the response to those treatments. Concurrent or past medical problems should be characterized in detail. Owners should also be questioned regarding routine health maintenance, including vaccinations, parasite control, and diet.

Knowledge of the signalment (age, breed, and sex) of an animal may assist in the diagnosis of some cancers because certain tumors occur more frequently in a particular species, breed, sex, or age group. Most companion animals that have cancer are middle aged to geriatric; the average age at the time of diagnosis is 6 to 15 years. However, the age of an older animal should never be used as an excuse not to pursue aggressive treatment. The animal's physiologic age, as determined by careful evaluation of factors such as cardiovascular, renal, and hepatic function, is more important for predicting treatment-associated risk than the chronologic age. After a complete history is taken, a detailed physical examination is performed (see Chapter 8). Each organ system should be carefully assessed, so that the primary problem and any concurrent conditions are identified and evaluated. Evidence of local tumor invasion, spread to draining lymph nodes, or distant metastases are all important in defining the stage or extent of the animal's cancer. Lymph nodes, especially those close to the tumor, must be carefully palpated for enlargement. Any skin or subcutaneous masses detected on the animal's body should be measured, and their location should be recorded in the medical record. Diagrams of the animal on which the location of any masses can actually be drawn are particularly useful in this regard (Figure 36-1). Minimum baseline data are gathered next. These data generally consist of a complete blood count, a serum chemistry diagnostic profile, urinalysis, and thoracic radiographs. The complete

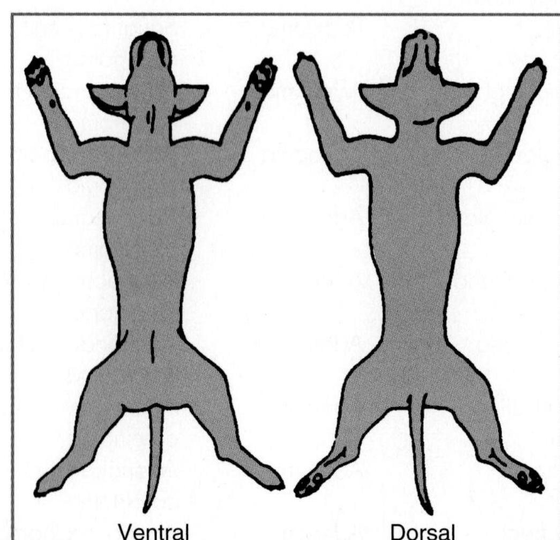

FIGURE 36-1 Diagram for mapping the location of masses found during the physical examination. Masses of the skin and subcutaneous tissues are drawn on the diagram to scale, and it is placed in the animal's medical record for future reference.

blood count is used to assess abnormalities in the red blood cells, white blood cells, and platelets. The biochemical profile should be evaluated for problems involving electrolytes, liver enzymes, creatinine, blood urea nitrogen, and serum protein concentrations. The urinalysis permits further assessment of renal function. Urine for urinalysis should be obtained by cystocentesis, whenever possible: voided samples are often contaminated by debris washed out of the urethra, making microscopic evaluation of the urine sediment unreliable. However, cystocentesis is contraindicated in animals with bleeding disorders and those suspected of having bladder cancer. Transitional cell carcinoma is by far the most common form of bladder cancer in the dog, and cells exfoliating from this tumor during cystocentesis will readily transplant into normal abdominal tissues. Finally, it is important to collect urine samples before any treatments are administered: urine specific gravity may be falsely lowered by fluid therapy. All blood samples from dogs and cats with cancer should be obtained through venipuncture of the jugular vein, if possible. Peripheral veins should be spared in the event that repeated catheterization for anesthesia or chemotherapy administration is indicated. Lack of venous access can be a frustrating problem in a dog or cat requiring multiple intravenous chemotherapy treatments. Some chemotherapy agents, such as the drug doxorubicin, can cause severe tissue damage if even a small amount is administered outside the vein. For this reason, a perfectly placed intravenous catheter must be used whenever chemotherapy is administered.

> *TECHNICIAN NOTE* All blood samples from dogs and cats with cancer should be obtained through venipuncture of the jugular vein, if possible.

DIAGNOSTIC IMAGING

Diagnostic imaging plays an important role in the diagnosis and staging of cancer (see Chapter 19). Radiographs of the chest, abdomen, and other anatomic structures are ordered on the basis of the tumor type and physical examination findings. The lungs are a common site for the development of metastases from certain malignant tumors. Chest radiographs should be obtained when the animal is in right lateral and left lateral recumbency and in a ventrodorsal or dorsoventral position to accurately evaluate all lung fields for metastatic nodules. Views in two planes are obviously necessary for all radiographic examinations so that any lesions present can be localized. The additional lateral view of the chest in this case improves the ability to visualize both lung fields by allowing the "up" lung to be expanded and filled with air, thereby enhancing the radiographic appearance of nodules that may be present (Figure 36-2).

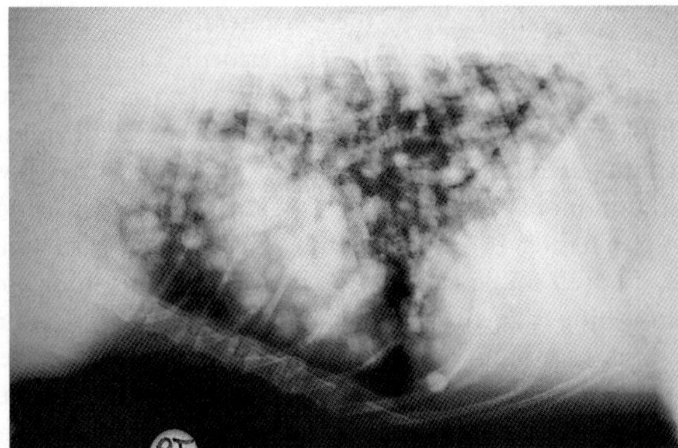

FIGURE 36-2 Chest radiograph showing numerous metastatic pulmonary nodules from a malignant mammary gland tumor in a dog.

Imaging techniques other than radiography are now commonly used to assist in the clinical evaluation of dogs and cats with cancer. Ultrasonography, for example, is a noninvasive method that may be used to examine the architecture of specific organs or masses found in the thoracic cavity or abdomen. Computed tomography scans, magnetic resonance imaging, and nuclear medicine scans are imaging techniques that are now available at many universities and some private referral hospitals. Each technique provides a different method for assessing virtually any area of the body. Computed tomography scans and magnetic resonance imaging, in particular, play an increasingly important role in cancer staging and also in the formulation of treatment plans, especially when radiotherapy is indicated (Figure 36-3).

CYTOLOGY

Cytology is used to evaluate microscopic cell structure for the purpose of obtaining a clinical diagnosis (see Chapter 16). Although it is a practical and effective screening tool that is valuable in differentiating neoplasia from inflammation or infection, it is not as reliable for establishing a definitive diagnosis of cancer as histopathology (see discussion of histopathology). Every skin or subcutaneous mass that is identified during the physical examination should be evaluated by either cytology or histopathology and never simply by gross appearance. Adherence to the proper techniques

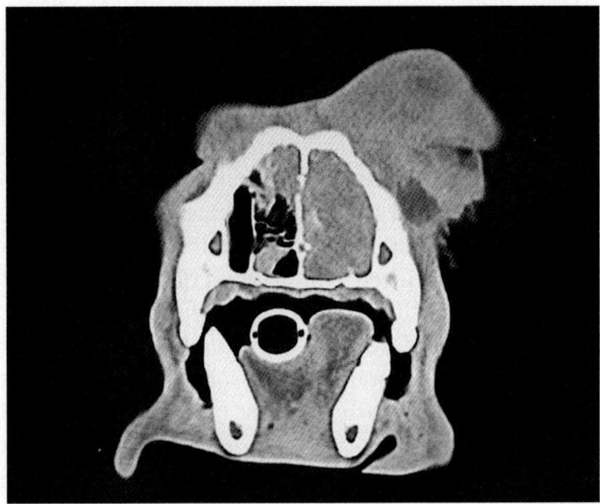

FIGURE 36-3 A cross-sectional computed tomographic image of a large nasal tumor in a dog. The tumor can be seen filling the nasal cavity and forming a large mass effect on the dorsolateral aspect of the animal's muzzle.

for collecting and preparing cytology samples is essential to obtain accurate results. Failure to collect sufficient cells or distortion of cellular architecture through poor handling techniques will make a reliable cytologic diagnosis impossible. Tumors that are easily diagnosed by cytologic examination are generally composed of cells that exfoliate or shed easily (e.g., mast cell tumors, many carcinomas). These loose cells can be placed onto glass slides with minimal distortion to their architecture and examined under a microscope. A positive cytologic report is highly suggestive of neoplasia and warrants further investigation (biopsy or surgical removal). A negative cytologic report must be interpreted with caution because a false-negative finding is possible when sample acquisition or preparation was improperly performed. Samples for cytologic examination are easily gathered in many different ways: by fine-needle aspiration of the mass itself or accessible lymph nodes, by thoracocentesis or abdominocentesis, by impression smears of small biopsy samples or ulcerated lesions, or by needle biopsy of bone marrow. These procedures can be performed quickly with minimal discomfort to the animal. Except in the case of bone marrow aspiration, anesthesia or sedation is generally not necessary.

Fine-Needle Aspiration

Fine-needle aspiration is used to obtain samples for cytologic evaluation from cutaneous tissue masses and lymph nodes. Improvements in ultrasound and fluoroscopic instrumentation have also allowed fine-needle aspiration to be used safely for the collection of samples from structures within body cavities.

> *TECHNICIAN NOTE* Fine-needle aspiration is used to obtain samples for cytologic evaluation from cutaneous tissue masses and lymph nodes.

A 6- or 12-ml syringe, a 22-gauge needle, and clean glass slides (preferably with frosted edges for labeling) are needed to perform a fine-needle aspiration of an external lesion. The lesion is stabilized between the clinician's fingers, and the needle is inserted into a representative area. The needle may be inserted with or without the syringe attached, and several core samples can be obtained by redirecting the needle several times without exiting the skin (Figure 36-4). Some clinicians use the attached syringe to aspirate while the needle is in place; others do not. Regardless, small portions of the needle contents are squirted onto a series of clean glass slides, and a second clean slide is used to smear the preparation.

Each slide should be labeled on the frosted edge with a graphite pencil before staining. The solvents used during the staining process will wash off most types of ink, including indelible ink. Identification of the slides should include the animal's name and identification number and the specific location of the mass that was aspirated. The slides are air-dried and sent to a qualified veterinary clinical pathologist for evaluation along with a complete and detailed description of pertinent clinical and historical information.

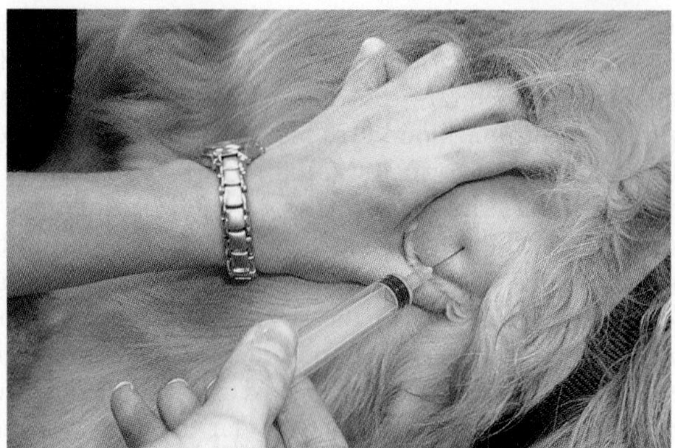

FIGURE 36-4 Fine-needle aspiration of an enlarged lymph node. A 22-gauge needle with a 6-ml syringe attached is inserted into the lymph node. The needle is redirected several times; concurrent suction on the syringe ensures a good sample of cells. Once aspiration is complete, suction is released, and the needle and syringe are withdrawn. The syringe is then detached from the needle, filled with air, and reattached to the hub of the needle. The needle contents are expelled onto clean glass slides and smeared for staining and microscopic examination.

It is often helpful to stain some of the prepared cytology slides for preliminary in-house review, saving the best and most representative slides for outside laboratory examination. Slides that are evaluated in house must be fixed with an appropriate stain. The most common stains available include Wright stain, new methylene blue, and Romanovsky's stains, such as Diff-Quik (American Scientific Products). It is important to realize that not all stains perform equally well under all circumstances. For instance, the characteristic granules diagnostic of mast cells may stain poorly or not at all when Diff-Quik stains are used.

> *TECHNICIAN NOTE* Stain some of the prepared cytology slides for preliminary in-house review, saving the best and most representative slides for outside laboratory examination.

Bone Marrow Aspiration

Evaluation of the cellular elements in bone marrow is sometimes indicated when abnormalities exist in the red cells, white cells, or platelets in the peripheral blood. Examination of bone marrow may also be performed to more accurately define the stage of certain tumors, such as lymphoma, multiple myeloma, and mast cell tumor. The most common technique used to collect a sample from the bone marrow is aspiration biopsy with a 16- or 18-gauge bone marrow needle (see Chapter 16). If this method fails to retrieve adequate cells, a core sample can be obtained with a Jamshidi bone marrow biopsy needle (American Pharmaseal Co.). The preferred sites for biopsy of the bone marrow are the iliac crest, proximal humerus, and trochanteric fossa of the proximal femur (Figure 36-5). The most representative sample in a geriatric dog or cat will usually be obtained from a flat bone (iliac crest) because marrow in the long bones is replaced by

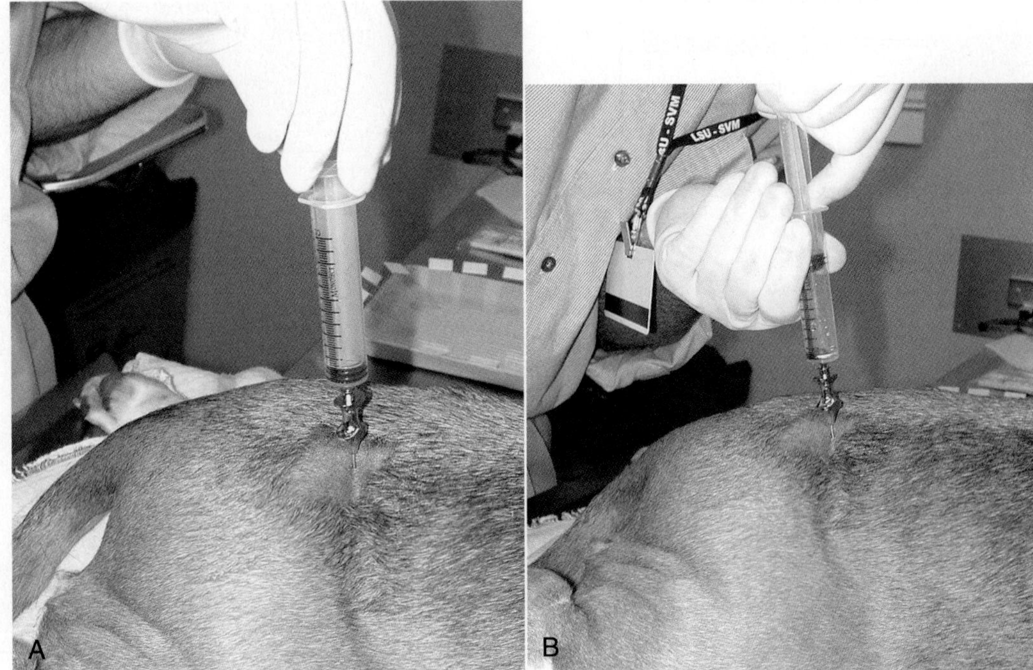

FIGURE 36-5 Bone marrow aspirate is obtained from the iliac crest of a basset hound. **A,** Bone marrow needle seated in the iliac crest. **B,** Suction is applied with a 12-ml syringe for retrieval of a sample of bone marrow.

fatty tissue as an animal ages. Some dogs will tolerate bone marrow aspiration after infiltration of the overlying skin with a small amount of local anesthetic alone; most cats require sedation.

HISTOPATHOLOGY

Obtaining a definitive histopathologic diagnosis is perhaps the single most important step in the overall diagnostic plan for the dog or cat with cancer. Histopathology determines what treatments should be considered and dictates the animal's prognosis, and these factors in turn influence the owner's decision about whether to treat. Every mass that is removed must be submitted for histopathologic examination, regardless of its location or gross appearance.

An advantage of histopathology over cytology is that the pathologist receives a larger sample with preserved architecture that is less likely to be distorted by procurement and processing techniques. Individual tumors can exhibit significant cellular heterogeneity and may contain areas of necrosis, fibrosis, and inflammation in addition to neoplastic cells. Because of this variation in cellularity, entire masses or multiple sections of large tumors should be submitted for evaluation. All submitted tissue samples are then examined to determine the cell type and tumor diagnosis, histologic grade, and surgical margins.

BIOPSY TECHNIQUES

Common methods used to obtain biopsy tissue include needle core biopsy, incisional biopsy, and excisional biopsy.

Needle Core Biopsy

Specialized needle biopsy instruments can be used to quickly and easily collect core samples of tissue through small (1- to 2-mm) skin incisions. The Tru-Cut needle (Travenol Laboratories) is most commonly used for biopsy of cutaneous or subcutaneous masses; adaptations of this type of needle can be used for ultrasound- or fluoroscope-guided needle core biopsy of masses and organs within body cavities. These needles obtain a 1- to 1.5-cm sliver of tissue approximately the same diameter as a pencil lead.

Before a needle core biopsy specimen is obtained from an external site, the area is clipped and prepared for minor surgery. The mass is then stabilized between the clinician's fingers, and a small incision (1 to 2 mm) is made in the skin with a scalpel. Infiltration of a local anesthetic into the incision site precludes the need for sedation or anesthesia in most cases. The needle is introduced, and a sample is obtained (Figure 36-6). The tissue sample is gently removed from the needle blade and placed in 10% buffered neutral formalin. Impression smears of this tissue can also be made by rolling the sample across a clean glass slide before placing it in formalin.

Incisional Biopsy

When an incisional biopsy is performed, a small skin incision is made over the area to be sampled, and a wedge of the underlying tumor is removed. This technique is useful for obtaining more tissue than can reasonably be collected by needle core biopsy. Adequate biopsy size is especially important when cancer cells are intermixed with many necrotic or inflammatory elements because these can complicate histopathologic evaluation.

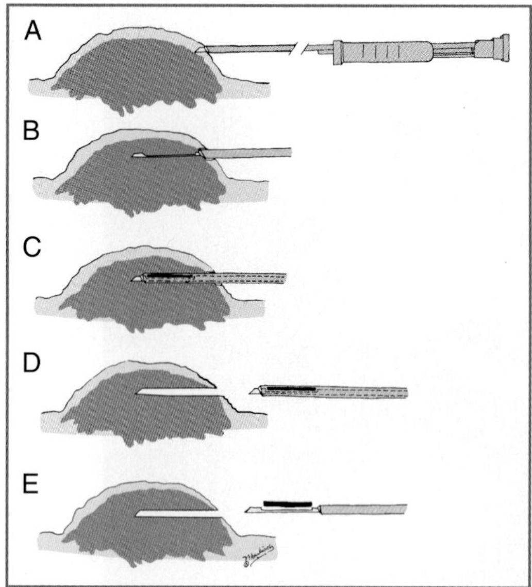

FIGURE 36-6 Mechanism of action of Tru-Cut biopsy needle used for typical nodular biopsy. **A,** With the instrument closed, the outer capsule is penetrated. A small skin incision is made with a No. 11 blade to allow insertion of the instrument. **B,** The outer cannula is fixed in place, and the inner cannula with specimen notch is thrust into the tumor. The tissue to be excised then protrudes into the notch. **C,** The inner cannula is now fixed, and the outer cannula is moved forward to cut off the biopsy specimen. **D,** The entire instrument is removed, with the tissue sample contained within. **E,** The inner cannula is pushed forward to expose the tissue in the specimen notch.

Contamination of the biopsy tract with tumor cells is a potential complication when either the needle core or the incisional biopsy technique is used. For this reason, biopsy specimens should be obtained through small incisions and with minimal disruption of the surrounding tissue. In addition, the biopsy incision should be made with consideration of the eventual definitive surgery so that the biopsy tract can be removed with the tumor.

Excisional Biopsy

Excisional biopsy involves the complete removal of a mass for biopsy. Margins of normal tissue surrounding the tumor are included in the excision. Depending on the results of the histopathologic examination, this method of biopsy may be all that is required for both diagnosis and treatment. However, a second surgery or adjuvant therapy is indicated if the tissue margins are not free of cancer cells or if there is evidence that the tumor may have spread.

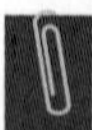

TECHNICIAN NOTE Excisional biopsy involves the complete removal of a mass for biopsy.

Biopsy Preparation

Once a biopsy specimen has been obtained, it should be handled gently so as not to distort the cellular architecture. In cases in which an excisional biopsy has been performed, evaluation of the surgical margins is extremely important for determining the success of surgical resection and assessing whether further treatment is indicated. The edges or surfaces of the resected tissue that need to be most carefully evaluated for presence of tumor should be marked so that the pathologist can easily identify them. Although this is often accomplished with suture "tags," commercially available tissue-marking dyes or India ink are also extremely helpful in marking surgical margins. Dyes and ink will not distort the tissue and can be used to mark the entire margin. They will be present as a peripheral colored line when the tissue is examined under the microscope. If tumor cells are in contact with the dye or ink-labeled margin, tumor cells probably remain within the animal, and further surgery or other additional treatment is indicated.

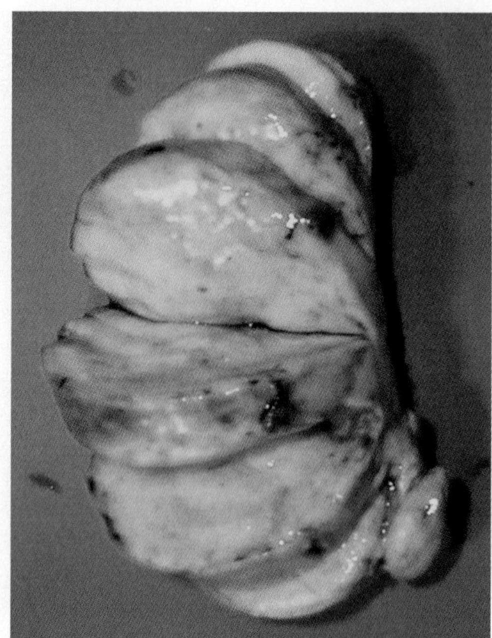

FIGURE 36-7 A large mass is sliced (loafed) into 1-cm sections. A 1-cm thick base connecting all the slices is left to help orient the pathologist.

After the margins have been marked, biopsy specimens should be placed in 10% buffered neutral formalin solution for fixation. The volume ratio of formalin to tissue for initial fixation is approximately 10:1. The tissue should be no thicker than 1 cm to allow effective penetration of the formalin. If it is thicker, it can be cut in the same manner as a loaf of bread to allow the formalin to penetrate. However, one edge should be left intact so that the pathologist understands the original orientation of the mass (Figure 36-7). Once the sample is fixed, it can be transferred to doubled or tripled plastic bags or commercial mailers with less formalin (1:1 ratio) for transportation to the laboratory.

TECHNICIAN NOTE For proper fixation, allow a 10:1 fixative/tissue ratio and ensure that section samples are no thicker than 1 cm.

A detailed information sheet should accompany the sample to the laboratory. Information that must be provided

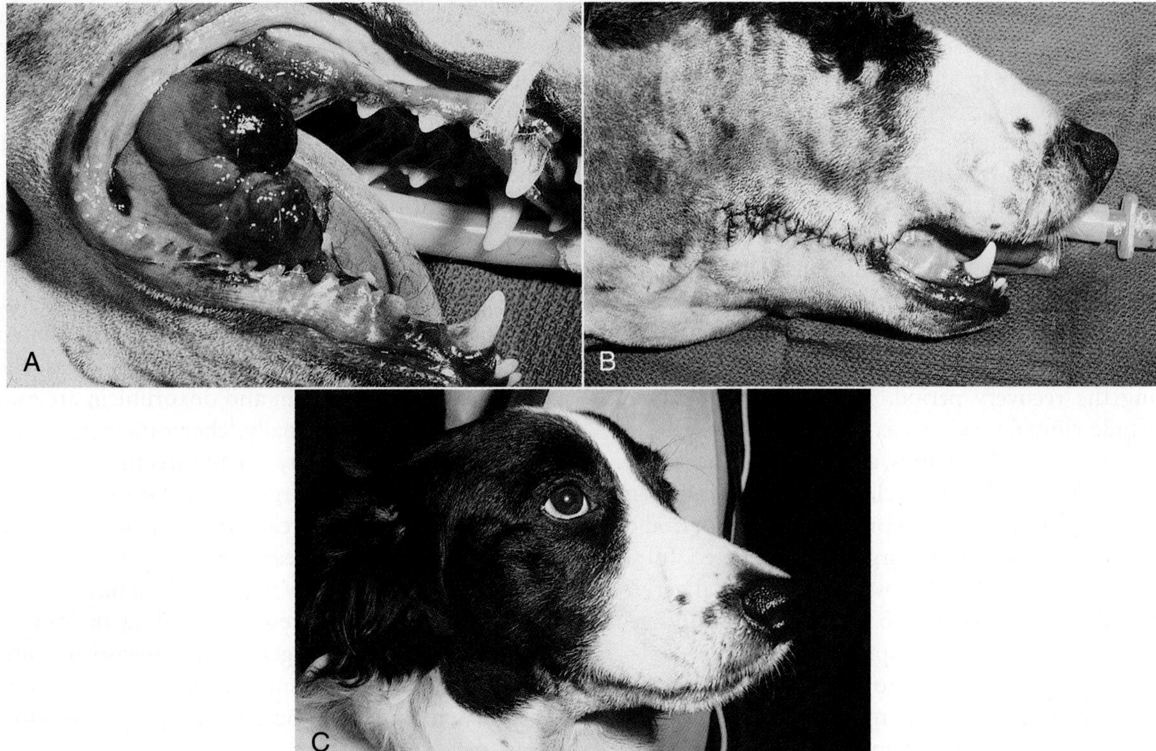

FIGURE 36-8 Surgical resection of an oral tumor in a dog. A, A large mandibular mass. B, Appearance of the surgical site immediately after tumor resection and reconstruction. C, The same animal after complete recovery and hair regrowth at the surgical site.

includes the practice and veterinarian's name, the owner's name, the animal's name and signalment, the site of the biopsy, and a succinct clinical history including pertinent treatments and the suspected diagnosis. Any margins needing specific evaluation should be noted. For some tumors, such as mast cell tumors, a histologic grade may also be requested to help predict tumor behavior and prognosis.

The pathologist is responsible for identifying the tumor type and providing information regarding completeness of surgical margins and histologic grade. However, the pathologist is limited by the quality of the sample submitted and the amount of information provided. It is ultimately the responsibility of the attending clinician to assess the compatibility of the pathologist's diagnosis with the animal's clinical presentation.

THERAPEUTIC OPTIONS

Once a definitive diagnosis has been made, the available therapeutic options can be identified. The clinician, technician, and client should discuss together the various choices with respect to the prognosis, benefits, potential complications, and cost. When speaking to the client, it is important to use simple terms that are easily understood. Information handouts are helpful to explain commonly performed procedures, such as amputation and mastectomy, and the care and monitoring of incisions and bandages. Handouts can also be used to explain the nature, method of action, and expected side effects of common chemotherapy drugs and radiotherapy.

There are three primary treatment options for dogs and cats with cancer: surgery, chemotherapy, and radiotherapy. A single modality is recommended for some animals, whereas multimodality protocols combining more than one type of treatment are preferred for others.

SURGERY

Surgery is the treatment of choice for localized cancer in dogs and cats: it is practical and cost effective and will be curative in many cases. The primary limitations of surgery are its potential for damage to surrounding normal structures and its inability to address systemic spread of tumor. Animals whose tumors have metastasized generally undergo surgery as a diagnostic or palliative procedure only. Aggressive and complex resection and reconstruction surgeries should not be performed if long-term disease control is not possible; in such instances, surgery should be combined with other modalities (adjuvant therapy), if it is done at all. The oncologic surgeon must be familiar with all the potential therapy options to provide the best care for an individual animal.

Successful surgical resection of malignant cancer requires an aggressive approach. The tumor must be removed completely with a minimum of cosmetic and functional loss to the animal (Figure 36-8). A concerted attempt is made during resection to avoid incising the tumor and contaminating the surgical field with neoplastic cells: cells released in this manner may implant in the wound and result in local recurrence. Instead, surgical resection should be performed in the normal tissues surrounding the mass so that a generous margin of normal tissue is removed together with the tumor. Extensive surgical resections and prolonged surgery times may be necessary in animals that are severely debilitated from cancer or other concurrent diseases. These cases require careful perioperative planning and monitoring to prevent complications. It is the mutual responsibility of the clinician and technician to make sure that the animal has had a complete presurgical evaluation and that the surgical team is aware of any preexisting conditions. The anesthetic protocol must be tailored to the needs of the individual animal. It is best to perform major surgeries early in the day so that the animal receives optimal monitoring from a full staff during the recovery period. Preparation for surgery should include clipping wide areas around surgical sites to accommodate extensive resections, should they be necessary. A thorough surgical scrub follows clipping. Perioperative antibiotics may be indicated if a prolonged operative period or potential contamination during surgery is anticipated. Intravenous fluids, epidural or local anesthesia in regional nerves, and parenteral analgesic agents also provide for an improved recovery in most animals (see Chapters 26 and 27).

Another type of surgery used to treat cancer is cryosurgery. A cold source (usually liquid nitrogen) is used to freeze superficial cancers that are less than 2 cm in diameter. After freezing, the treated tissue dies and sloughs away, leaving a wound that later heals. There may be permanent discoloration or loss of hair associated with this process. Cryosurgery is useful for small, superficial lesions, such as eyelid, skin, and anal masses. A disadvantage of cryosurgery is that the completeness of tumor removal cannot be determined because there is no tissue to submit for margin evaluation. Cryosurgery should not be used to treat large, invasive masses or in cases in which a definitive histologic diagnosis has not yet been made.

The goal of surgery may be curative or palliative. The intent of curative surgery is complete and permanent removal of the animal's cancer. In the case of palliative surgery, the tumor is resected to improve the animal's short-term quality of life despite known tumor spread or an otherwise poor long-term prognosis. An example of this type of situation would be a dog with a painful primary bone tumor that has already metastasized. In this case, surgical resection of the mass (e.g., amputation) may improve the animal's quality of life, but will not prolong survival because the metastatic disease will continue to progress regardless of the surgical procedure.

TECHNICIAN NOTE The intent of curative surgery is complete and permanent removal of the animal's cancer.

CHEMOTHERAPY

Chemotherapy is the treatment of cancer with chemical agents. Chemotherapy provides a means of delivering antitumor therapy to the whole body and is therefore most appropriate for animals that have systemic, as opposed to local, neoplastic disease. There are four primary indications for chemotherapy in dogs and cats. It is the most effective single treatment for some types of cancer, such as lymphoma (Figure 36-9) and transmissible venereal tumors. Chemotherapy is often recommended after surgical removal of malignant tumors to prevent the development of metastases and to inhibit local regrowth of tumor at the primary site. Canine osteosarcoma is routinely treated in this way (Figure 36-10). Certain chemotherapeutic agents, known as radiation sensitizers, are sometimes administered in conjunction with radiotherapy. These drugs increase the efficacy of radiotherapy. Cisplatin and doxorubicin are examples of radiation sensitizers. Finally, chemotherapy is occasionally used as a single modality for the treatment of cancers that are not amenable to surgical resection or radiotherapy or for tumors that have already metastasized. In most cases of this type, the goal of treatment is not to induce remission but rather to temporarily improve the animal's quality of life (palliate) by reducing pressure, bleeding, or pain.

Chemotherapeutic agents are categorized into groups based on their mechanism of action. However, regardless of category, most chemotherapeutic agents are cytotoxic and

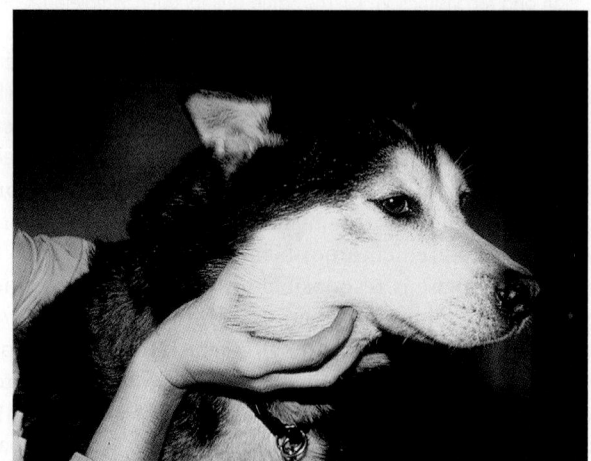

FIGURE 36-9 A dog with notably enlarged lymph nodes caused by lymphoma.

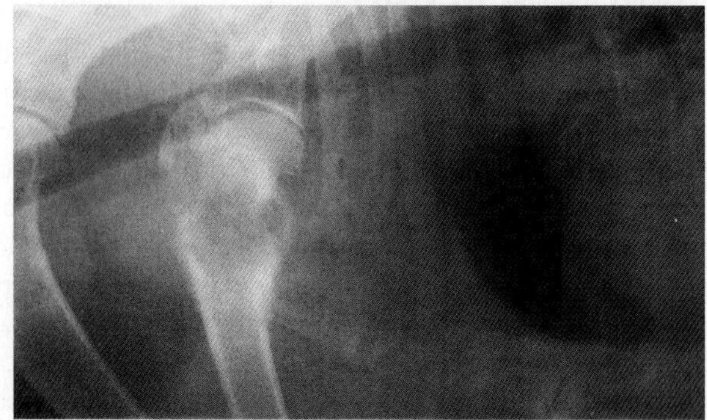

FIGURE 36-10 A lytic lesion caused by osteosarcoma in the proximal humerus of a dog.

result in tumor cell death by injuring either the cancer cell's DNA or its protective cellular membrane. Drugs that disrupt DNA typically target cells that proliferate rapidly, a characteristic of many neoplastic cells. However, chemotherapeutic agents may also injure normal cells within the body that have high proliferation rates, such as the cells of the gastrointestinal tract, the bone marrow, and hair follicles. This is one of the basic mechanisms responsible for many of the toxicities classically associated with chemotherapy: vomiting, diarrhea, bone marrow suppression, and hair loss (Figure 36-11).

The dose and timing of chemotherapy administration are predetermined to achieve maximum cancer cell destruction while minimizing the damage to normal cells and the resulting toxicities. Protocols that include a number of different drugs are preferred over single-drug protocols because they combine drugs that have complementary mechanisms of action and balanced toxicities. Chemotherapy drug dosages are generally based on the surface area of the body (meters squared) in the dog and on body weight in the cat. A meter-squared dosing chart that can be used in dogs and cats is included in Chapter 25.

In most cases, suppression of the bone marrow causing a decrease in the circulating neutrophil count is the toxicity that determines the highest dose of chemotherapeutic agent that will be tolerated by the animal. The interval between doses is determined in part by the time necessary for the bone marrow to recover from the previous treatment so that the neutrophil count can return to normal before the next drug is given. The time at which the neutrophil count is at its lowest after the administration of a chemotherapy drug is known as the nadir of leukopenia. It is important to be familiar with the nadir of leukopenia for the different chemotherapeutic agents used in veterinary oncology and to understand that the greatest effect on an animal's bone marrow is likely to occur several days after the chemotherapy is administered. The nadir of leukopenia occurs approximately 7 to 14 days after drug administration for most chemotherapeutic agents, but for some drugs, it is longer. Two critical questions to always ask the owner of a systemically ill pet that is receiving chemotherapy are what drug was last administered and when that treatment was given.

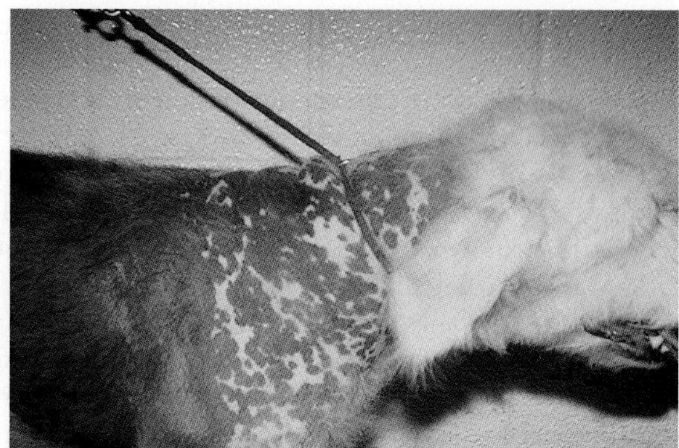

FIGURE 36-11 Hair loss caused by chemotherapy in an Old English sheepdog.

> *TECHNICIAN NOTE* Suppression of the bone marrow causing a decrease in the circulating neutrophil count is the toxicity that determines the highest dose of chemotherapeutic agent that will be tolerated by the animal.

Chemotherapeutic agents have the potential to be teratogens (they may cause defects in a developing fetus), mutagens (they may cause injury to chromosomes), and carcinogens (they may cause DNA damage that ultimately leads to the development of a second cancer). The risks in health care professionals from long-term low-dose exposure are unknown, but no safe level of exposure has been identified. Since 1994 the U.S. Occupational Safety and Health Administration (OSHA) has required employers to protect their employees from occupational health hazards, such as handling chemotherapeutic agents. The veterinary community must recognize, promote, and institute policies and procedures that facilitate the safe mixing, handling, and administration of these drugs. In particular, women who are pregnant, may be pregnant, or are trying to become pregnant should not handle chemotherapy drugs, potentially contaminated materials (e.g., gloves, gowns, needles, and syringes), or body wastes from treated animals under any circumstances (see Chapter 6).

All chemotherapy drugs should be clearly labeled and stored on shelves or in bins with front barriers that will prevent vials from accidentally rolling out. Chemotherapy drugs requiring refrigeration should be stored in a designated refrigerator in individually labeled Ziploc bags. All chemotherapeutics should be reconstituted in an isolated, draft-free section of the hospital where eating, drinking, and application of cosmetics are strictly forbidden. The work surface in this area should be covered with a plastic-backed absorbent liner that is replaced daily.

All hospital staff working with chemotherapeutics must be carefully protected from drug exposure. Inhalation of aerosolized drugs during reconstitution is especially dangerous and is best prevented by use of a biologic safety cabinet (Figure 36-12). This equipment is expensive and may be impractical in practices where chemotherapy is administered relatively infrequently. Although commercially available venting devices (Figure 36-13) or high-efficiency respirator masks can be used instead of a biologic safety cabinet, referring animals needing chemotherapy to specialty practices with all of the appropriate safety equipment should also be strongly considered. Ordinary surgical masks do not prevent inhalation of aerosolized chemotherapy drugs. Cutaneous exposure during chemotherapy drug reconstitution and administration can be prevented by use of talc-free latex gloves, disposable low-permeability gowns, and protective eyewear or a face shield (Figure 36-14).

> *TECHNICIAN NOTE* Protective gloves, mask, clothing, and eye shields and appropriate and standardized drug-handling procedures must be routine whenever chemotherapeutic agents are used.

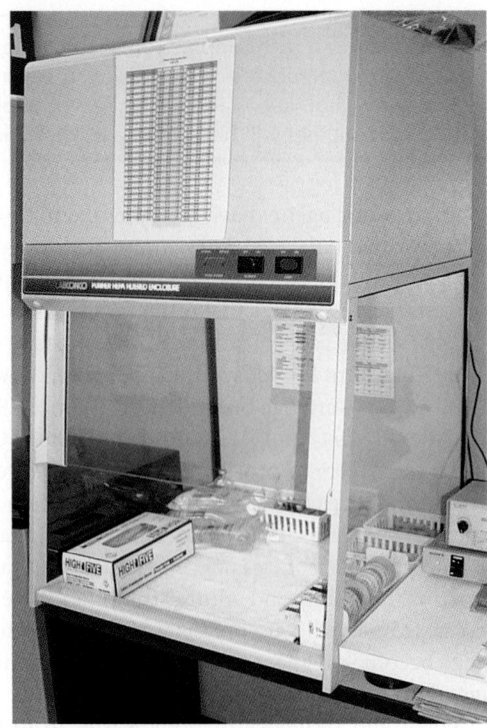

FIGURE 36-12 Biologic safety cabinet used to reconstitute chemotherapy drugs and prevent aerosol drug exposure.

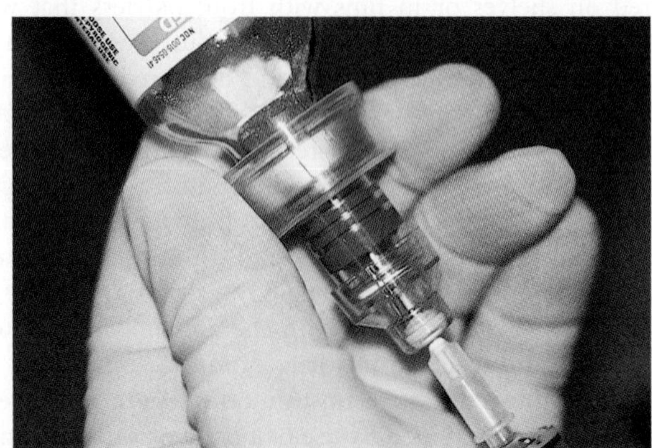

FIGURE 36-13 Venting device that prevents aerosolization of chemotherapy drug from the vial during reconstitution.

Reconstituted chemotherapy drugs should be transported to the treatment area in sealed and labeled Ziploc bags. The individual administering the drugs and the person restraining the animal for treatment should always wear gloves, gowns, and face shields. Intravenous chemotherapy drugs are given through an aseptically and perfectly placed butterfly or over-the-needle in-dwelling intravenous catheter (Figure 36-15). Routine use of Luer-Lok syringes further decreases the chance of inadvertent cutaneous or aerosol drug exposure during drug infusion. After the treatment has been administered, all potentially contaminated materials, including Ziploc bags, syringes, catheters, gloves, gowns, and absorbent liners should be bagged separately and labeled for biohazard disposal according to appropriate local regulations. Contaminated sharps (e.g., needles) should also be placed in a specially designated container.

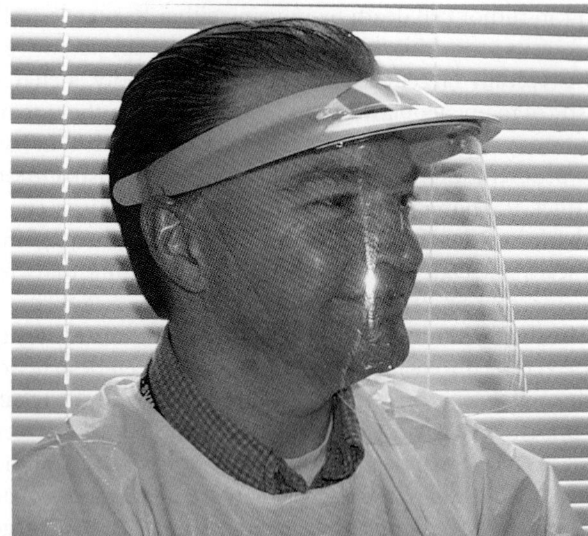

FIGURE 36-14 Face shield used during chemotherapy drug administration.

Chemotherapy drugs are excreted from the body in the urine or feces, and levels are usually highest in the first 72 hours after treatment. Hospital personnel and pet owners should take care to prevent exposure to excreted chemotherapeutics by wearing gloves when handling body wastes and soiled objects during this period. Dirty cages should be mopped with disposable sponges and never hosed because water spray can aerosolize excreted drugs. Owners should be instructed to pick up and safely dispose of contaminated fecal material for the first 72 hours after treatment. In addition, during this time, dogs receiving chemotherapy should not be permitted to urinate in outdoor areas where children are likely to play.

There are many important nursing considerations with respect to the administration of chemotherapeutic drugs (Box 36-3). Toxicities, such as myelosuppression (Box 36-4), extravasation (Table 36-2, Figure 36-16), and anaphylaxis (Box 36-5) are well documented. Additional potential toxicities include alopecia, gastrointestinal upset, sterile hemorrhagic cystitis, renal failure, cardiac toxicity, and neurotoxicity. Taking all necessary precautions to minimize risks to both the animal and the veterinary health care team is essential. There are many references that are useful in the development of appropriate hospital policies for the safe dosing, mixing, handling, and administration of chemotherapeutic agents (see Recommended Reading).

After each treatment, the animal should be monitored for signs of toxicity. Clients should be given detailed handouts describing known toxicities for each chemotherapeutic agent and the associated clinical signs. If the hospital staff or the client detects any abnormalities, the animal should be reevaluated. If chemotherapeutic agents are administered properly and the client is carefully educated regarding the potential risks, toxicity can be minimized and the animal should maintain an excellent quality of life during therapy.

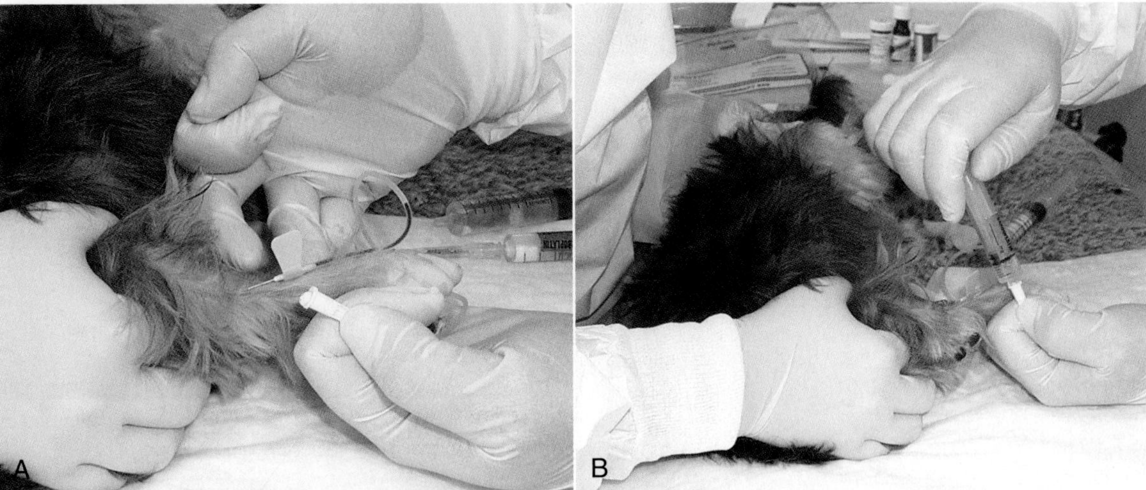

FIGURE 36-15 Administration of chemotherapy through a butterfly catheter. **A,** The catheter is placed in the lateral saphenous vein and checked for patency by using nonheparinized saline solution. **B,** The chemotherapy drug is given as a slow intravenous bolus through the catheter. The catheter is flushed thoroughly with nonheparinized saline solution after drug administration before it is removed.

BOX 36-3 Nursing Considerations for the Administration of Chemotherapy Drugs

Concerns Before Drug Administration

Admitting

1. Patient status
   a. History since last chemotherapy
   b. Physical examination
2. Appropriate diagnostics submitted
   a. Blood work
   b. Radiographs

Treatment Plan

1. Verification
   a. Drug and dosage
   b. Blood work
2. Appropriate catheterization
   a. Necessary equipment assembled
   b. Vein selection
   c. Aseptic technique
   d. Completely clean stick
   e. Intravenous challenge with nonheparinized saline bolus before and after drug administration
3. Appropriate protective equipment for person mixing and administering drugs
4. Appropriate protective equipment for person restraining animal
5. Knowledge of drug toxicities
6. Emergency protocols established
   a. Treatment of extravasation
   b. Treatment of anaphylaxis
   c. Treatment of chemical spill
7. Client informed of potential toxicities

Concerns During Drug Administration

1. Extravasation of drug
2. Anaphylactic reaction
3. Patient comfort

Concerns After Drug Administration

1. Hematologic toxicity
2. Nonhematologic toxicity
3. Appropriate medications prescribed
   a. Chemotherapy drugs
   b. Antibiotics
   c. Other medications (e.g., antiemetics)
4. Treatment documentation
   a. Patient medical record
   b. Future treatment plan
   c. Client information handouts

RADIOTHERAPY

Ionizing radiation can also be used to treat cancer. Radiation causes cell death by disrupting the cell's DNA or by destroying important molecules required for normal cell function. Death occurs when the cell is so injured that it can no longer repair itself or divide. Radiotherapy is most appropriately prescribed for the treatment of localized cancers and will not address systemic disease. It can be used alone or in combination with surgery or chemotherapy. Most radiotherapy protocols involve the administration of multiple small doses (fractions) on a Monday, Wednesday, and Friday or a Monday through Friday schedule, usually for 15 to 21 fractions (Figure 36-17). Because radiation targets DNA, like chemotherapy, it is most effective against tumor cells with rapid rates of proliferation. Similarly, radiotherapy adverse effects are seen in normal tissues within the irradiated field that also have a high rate of cell turnover.

> *TECHNICIAN NOTE* Radiation causes cell death by disrupting the cell's DNA or by destroying important molecules required for normal cell function.

BOX 36-4 Myelosuppressive Chemotherapy Drugs Commonly Used in Veterinary Medicine

Highly Myelosuppressive
Doxorubicin
Cyclophosphamide
Carboplatin
Lomustine (CCNU)

Moderately Myelosuppressive
Melphalan
Chlorambucil
Cisplatin

Mildly Myelosuppressive
L-Asparaginase
Vincristine
Corticosteroids

TABLE 36-2 Chemotherapy Drugs Classified as Vesicant or Irritant Agents

	Generic Name	Brand or Other Name
Vesicant*		
	Dactinomycin	Actinomycin D
	Doxorubicin	Adriamycin
	Vinblastine	Velban
	Vincristine	Oncovin
Irritant†		
	Carmustine	BCNU
	Cisplatin	Platinol
	Dacarbazine	DTIC
	Mitoxantrone	Novantrone

Modified from Martha EP, Polovich M, White JM: *Chemotherapy and biotherapy guidelines and recommendations for practice,* ed 2, Pittsburgh, 2005, Oncology Nursing Society.

BCNU, 1,3-bis-(2-chloroethyl)-1-nitrosourea; *DTIC,* dimethyl triazenyl imidazole carboxamide.

*An agent causing tissue destruction or necrosis on extravasation.

†An agent causing pain or inflammation at injection site.

The potential adverse effects of radiation are divided into late phase and acute effects. Late-phase effects of radiotherapy develop months to years after treatment and usually involve permanent changes, such as necrosis or fibrosis of normal tissues. Acute effects are usually seen during the latter stages of a course of radiotherapy and, although they may require additional nursing care, are temporary. The most common acute effects of radiation occur because rapidly dividing normal cells in tissues, such as the skin and mucosal linings of the intestinal tract, have growth characteristics that are similar to those of cancer cells and are thus extremely sensitive to radiation (Figure 36-18). This means the damage to acutely responding normal tissues in the radiation field actually mimics damage to neoplastic tissue. For this reason, the acute toxicities of radiotherapy should never be permitted to limit the dose delivered: if

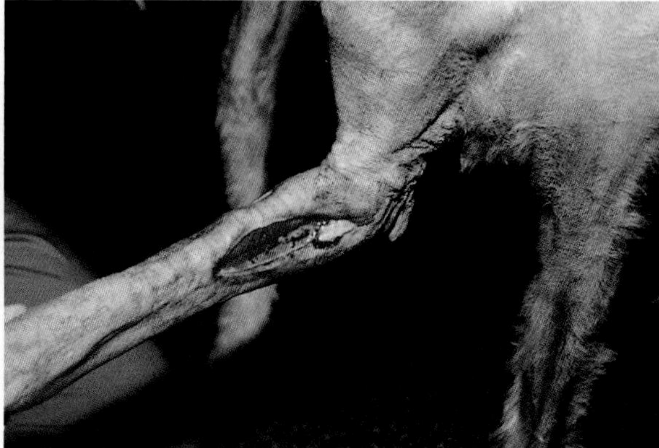

FIGURE 36-16 Tissue necrosis and sloughing caused by extravasation of a vesicant chemotherapy drug in a dog.

BOX 36-5 Chemotherapy Drugs With Potential to Cause Hypersensitivity or Anaphylaxis in Dogs and Cats

L-Asparaginase
Paclitaxel (Taxol)
Cisplatin
Anthracycline antibiotics (doxorubicin, daunorubicin, mitoxantrone)
Etoposide (VP16)
Bleomycin
Dacarbazine (DTIC)
Vinca alkaloids (vincristine, vinblastine)

radiotherapy is temporarily discontinued to provide time for repair of acutely injured normal tissue, tumor tissue will be allowed to repair.

A frequent acute adverse effect of irradiation of oral or nasal tumors is mucositis of the oral cavity. Flushing the animal's oral cavity with prescription veterinary mouthwashes can decrease the discomfort associated with this condition. Irradiation of skin may also induce a desquamative dermatitis or loss of the superficial layers of the epidermis. With regular cleaning and use of analgesics as needed, these conditions generally resolve within 2 to 3 weeks. Oil-based or occlusive topical creams should be avoided, and self-trauma, such as licking, must be prevented. Elizabethan collars are especially useful because they prevent self-trauma while still allowing access to the radiation field for topical treatments. Hair loss or change in color within the radiation field may be permanent, and the owner should be made aware of this possibility before the initiation of radiotherapy.

TECHNICIAN NOTE The use of oil-based topical creams for the treatment of radiation-induced desquamative dermatitis should be avoided. Self-trauma must also be prevented when dealing with acute radiation dermatitis.

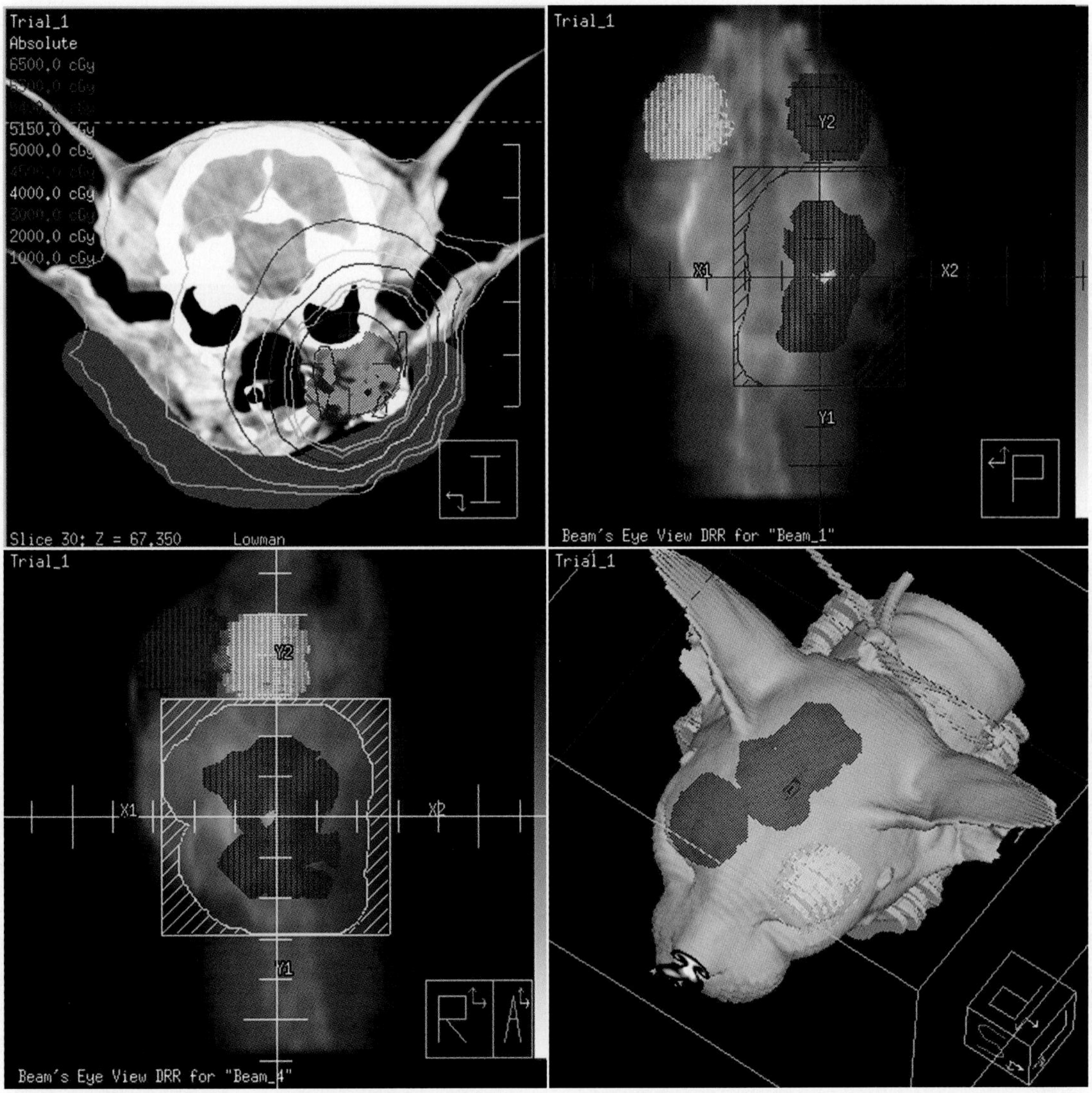

FIGURE 36-17 Example of a radiotherapy plan based on reconstruction of computed tomographic scan data. This treatment plan is for a salivary gland adenocarcinoma in a cat.

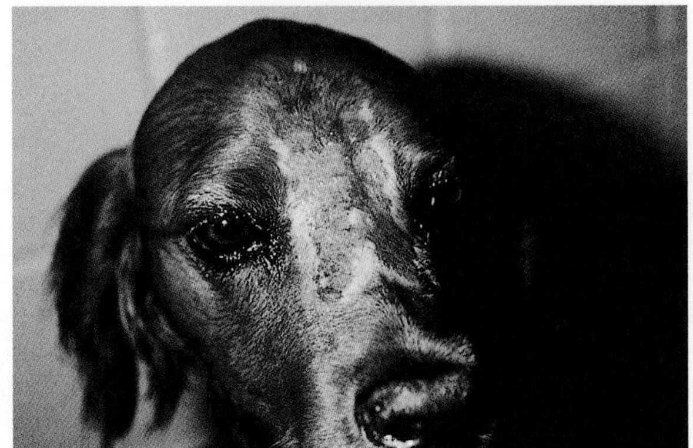

FIGURE 36-18 Moist desquamative dermatitis in a dog receiving radiotherapy for treatment of a nasal tumor.

EUTHANASIA

Unfortunately, veterinary cancer therapy often does not result in a cure. In many cases, the most reasonable goal for both client and clinician is a long disease-free interval and improvement or preservation of quality of life (see Chapters 26 and 37). Euthanasia is an important component of pet cancer management. It is the best option for some clients at the time of diagnosis; for others, this choice is made after therapy has been instituted and has failed. In either situation, electing to euthanize a pet is an extremely difficult decision and one with which the client must be completely comfortable. Euthanasia should only be performed after careful consideration of all available options (see Chapter 38).

The veterinarian and technician must be prepared to provide medical information and expertise and nonjudgmental emotional support and compassion to both the client and animal throughout the course of therapy. Much of the emotional support comes from the technical staff. Clients may feel inhibited when talking to the veterinarian, but can sometimes talk more freely with a nurse or receptionist. Technicians need to be aware of the important role they play in veterinary oncology, not only in providing treatment for the animal, but also in supporting the needs of the client. Good communication skills and compassion will be as important as the specific medical treatment provided to many dogs and cats with cancer (see Chapter 37).

CASE PRESENTATION 36-1

Signalment: 12-year-old male castrate golden retriever.

History: Swollen left third eyelid and left-sided mucopurulent nasal discharge for 3 weeks.

Physical Examination: The dog was lethargic and seemed in pain. There was a mass involving the left third eyelid, with protrusion of the left eye from the socket (exophthalmos; [Figure 1]). The left mandibular lymph node was enlarged.

Diagnostic Test Results: Routine blood work, urinalysis, and chest and abdominal radiographs were normal. Fine-needle aspirates of the third eyelid mass and left mandibular lymph node revealed neoplastic mast cells (Figure 2). Malignant mast cells were also found on a bone marrow aspirate (Figure 3). A computed tomography scan was performed and showed a large mass involving the left orbit and left nasal cavity (Figure 4).

Definitive Diagnosis: Systemic (metastatic) mast cell tumor.

Treatment and Expected Prognosis: The best single treatment for this dog was systemic chemotherapy because that was the only way to treat all of the different sites where he had mast cell tumor. However, his long-term prognosis was poor because of his advanced disease.

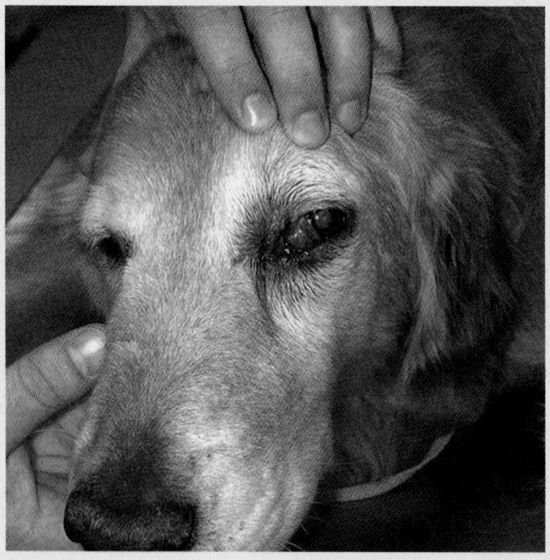

FIGURE 1 Dog with a left third eyelid mass and exophthalmos.

Outcome: This dog had an excellent response to lomustine chemotherapy: a complete remission was achieved within 5 days of starting therapy (Figure 5). Remission was maintained for 5 months, and during this time, the dog enjoyed an excellent quality of life. The dog was eventually euthanized at 6 months when his cancer became progressive and his quality of life declined.

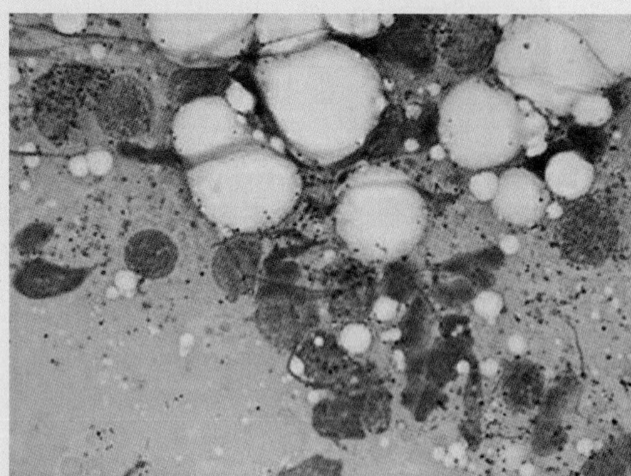

FIGURE 2 Malignant mast cells in a fine-needle aspirate of a lymph node. The mast cells can be easily identified by their deep purple, metachromatic cytoplasmic granules. Mast cell granules can also be seen free in the background on this slide.

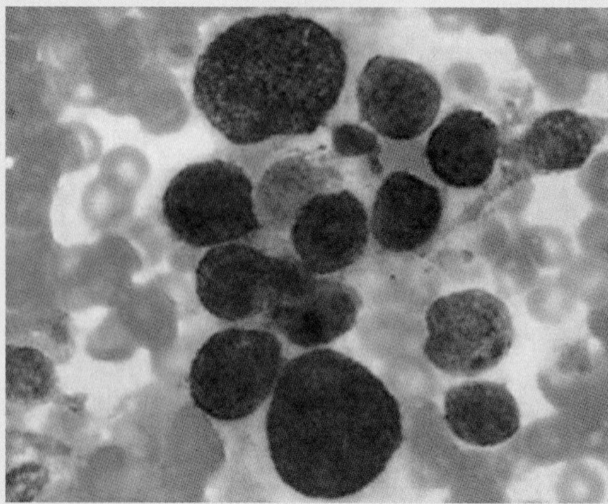

FIGURE 3 Malignant mast cells in a bone marrow aspirate.

CASE PRESENTATION 36-1—cont'd

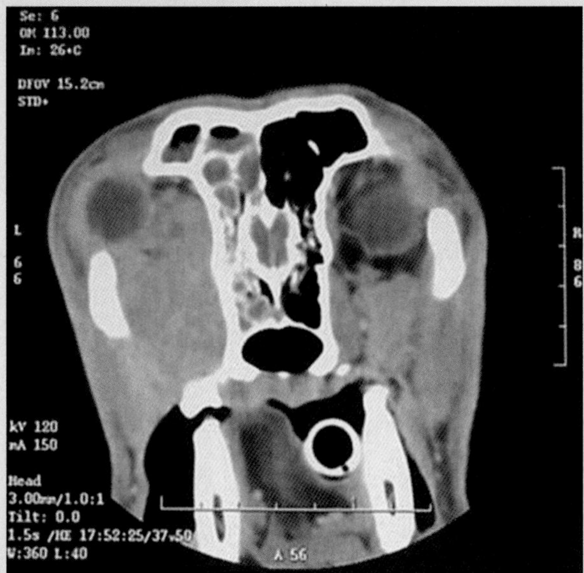

FIGURE 4 Cross-sectional CT scan image taken at the level of the orbits and frontal sinuses. The eyes can be easily seen on this scan as circular structures with a dark central area that is surrounded by a lighter rim of tissue. The right eye is in its normal position within the right orbit; however, there is a large mass in the ventral left orbit that deviates the left eye laterally. Tumor is also present within the left nasal cavity: normal nasal cavity should appear black because it is full of air.

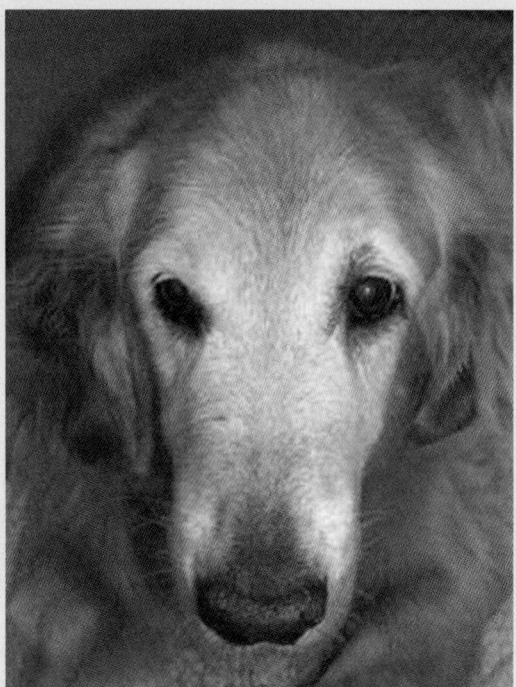

FIGURE 5 There is complete resolution of the left orbital mass, and the left eye has returned to its normal position within the socket.

RECOMMENDED READING

Henry C: Chemotherapeutic agents. In Rosenthal RC, editor: *Veterinary oncology secrets,* St Louis, 2001, Elsevier.

Higginbotham ML: Safe handling of cytotoxic agents. In Rosenthal RC, editor: *Veterinary oncology secrets,* St Louis, 2001, Elsevier.

Martha EP, Polovich M, White JM: *Chemotherapy and biotherapy guidelines and recommendations for practice,* ed 2, Pittsburgh, 2005, Oncology Nursing Society.

Mauldin GN: Radiation oncology. In Rosenthal RC, editor: *Veterinary oncology secrets,* St Louis, 2001, Elsevier.

Morrison WB: *Cancer in dogs and cats: medical and surgical management,* ed 2, Jackson, Wyo, 2002, Teton NewMedia.

Polovich M: *Safe handling of hazardous drugs,* Pittsburgh, 2003, Oncology Nursing Society.

Withrow SJ, Vail DM: *Withrow and MacEwen's small animal clinical oncology,* ed 4, St Louis, 2007, Elsevier Saunders.

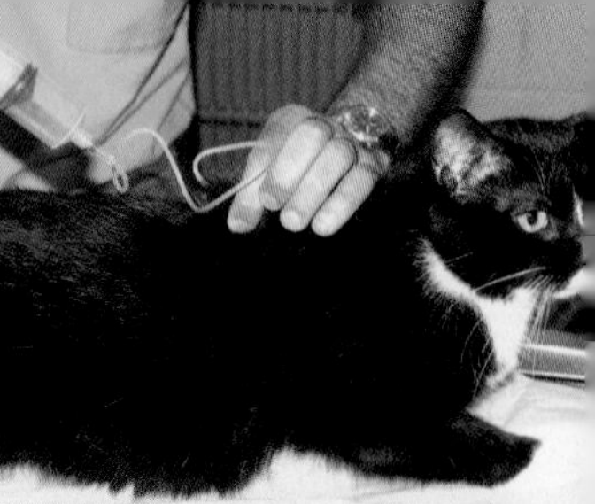

37 Geriatric and Hospice Care: Supporting the Aged and Dying Patient

Tara K. Trotman and Amy I. Bentz

OUTLINE

KEY TERMS

Geriatric
Hirsutism
Hospice
Incontinence

LEARNING OBJECTIVES

When you have completed this chapter, you will be able to:

1. Describe the life stages of dogs and cats.
2. List and describe the effects of aging on body systems.
3. Discuss the importance of oral health in geriatric dogs and cats.
4. List and describe common cardiac, respiratory, orthopedic, and kidney disorders of geriatric dogs and cats.
5. List and describe common neoplastic and neurologic disorders of geriatric dogs and cats.
6. List and describe common endocrine disorders of geriatric dogs and cats.
7. Discuss components of hospice nursing care of geriatric dogs and cats.
8. Discuss components of the physical examination of a geriatric horse.
9. List and describe common disorders of geriatric horses.
10. List and describe common chronic conditions that affect geriatric horses.

INTRODUCTION

The term geriatric is used to describe "a branch of medicine that deals with the problems and diseases of old age." With the advances we have seen in veterinary medicine, the number of geriatric pets is growing exponentially. Not only is pet ownership at an all-time high, but dogs, cats, and horses are living longer as a result of our ability to understand and treat animal diseases.

Hospice or hospice care is defined as "a facility or program designed to provide a caring environment for meeting the physical and emotional needs of the terminally ill." Because of the rise in the number of geriatric pets combined with the increased commitment owners feel toward their pet, the need for "hospice care" is increasing. As members of the veterinary community, it is our job to provide relief to animals that suffer and ensure a good quality of life to geriatric pets. One must be aware, however, that it is also our duty to provide support when it is time to end the suffering of dying patients via euthanasia. Pet owners often rely on veterinary personnel to help them make the difficult decision to euthanize their pet.

Routine preventive health programs should be followed for all patients (see Chapter 9), but it is especially important for geriatric pets. The effects of aging in animals are similar to those in people and include an overall deterioration in physical and mental condition, organ function, and immunity. Although it is important to treat conditions once they become apparent, it is equally important to educate owners about how to recognize signs of early disease. Early identification and treatment of disease can dramatically improve the quality of life and extend the length of life for geriatric patients.

The purpose of this chapter is to present the common health problems of geriatric cats, dogs, and horses and to give some specific nursing techniques that support the chronically ill or recumbent patient. In addition, this chapter also describes techniques for supporting owners who are facing the end of their pet's life.

TECHNICIAN NOTE Companion animals are considered part of the family for many pet owners. Pets are living longer with advances in veterinary medicine, and special needs for the geriatric patient must be taken into account.

GERIATRIC CATS AND DOGS

LIFE STAGES GUIDELINES

A lifetime incorporates the sum of the various life stages of dogs and cats. Age by itself is not a disease. The following life stages apply to most dogs and cats:

- The pediatric life stage is the life stage between birth and 6 months old for both dogs and cats.
- The young adult life stage is the life stage from 6 months to 2 years through 5 years old for dogs. The age ranges of a young adult vary according to the specific dog breed because the large- and giant-dog breeds spend less time as a young adult. Young adult life stage is the life stage from 6 months to 4 years old for cats.
- Mature adult life stage is the life stage from 2 years through 5 years to 9 years through 12 years old for dogs. The age ranges of a mature adult vary according to the specific dog breed because the large- and giant-dog breeds spend less time as a mature adult. Mature adult life stage is the life stage from 4 years to 12 years old for cats.
- Senior life stage is the life stage after mature adulthood. The latter times in the senior dog's lifetime may be defined as the geriatric years, but dogs, just like humans, like to be referred to as senior citizens. The oldest dog on record was 29 years old. The oldest cat on record was 34 years old.

INTEGRATING GERIATRIC CARE

The care for aging dogs and cats is a proactive comprehensive health care program that addresses the older animal's special needs. This specialized medical service is based on two premises: first, there are fundamental differences in specific diseases, behavior traits, and nutritional needs of the older animal; second, prevention, early detection, and timely intervention of medical problems can have a significant impact on the life span and quality of life of an older dog or cat.

Care for such older dogs and cats should focus on owner education, disease prevention strategies, and detection of medical and behavioral problems at the earliest possible stage when the prognosis is better and numerous treatment options still exist. The term "senior" or "geriatric" describes that life stage of progressive decline in physical condition, organ function, sensory function, mental function, and immunity. Although it is generally accepted that the senior life stage begins around 7 years of age for the average dog or cat, several interrelated factors, including size and individual genetics, will affect the onset and rate of the progressive decline (Box 37-1).

Although care for the older animal begins at the first new puppy or kitten examination when the animal's entire life-stage health care program is outlined for the owner, the program is actually implemented when the animal reaches 7 years of age. Starting at 7 years, senior care promotes routine examinations of healthy animals on a twice-a-year basis and advocates routine diagnostic screening for developing diseases. The healthy animal is just one component of the group that should be targeted for senior care. Another component is the older dog or cat that is asymptomatic or is exhibiting early signs of a problem, but the owner either does not recognize the signs or just attributes the signs to "old age" and fails to seek veterinary care.

COMMON PROBLEMS

Conditions that occur commonly in our aging pet population include oral health abnormalities, vision loss, hearing loss, cardiac disease (arrhythmias, murmurs), respiratory disease, neoplasia, kidney disease, urinary and fecal incontinence, dermatologic disease, orthopedic disease, and metabolic conditions. It is important for owners to be aware of these issues and to seek veterinary attention if any of them arise. It is equally important for members of the veterinary community to question owners closely regarding their pet's health status so that early detection of disease is possible.

Frequently, ill geriatric animals have vague symptoms including inappetence, lethargy, and weight loss. Therefore it is important to acquire a thorough history from owners and to perform a complete physical examination with routine screening tests. Older dogs and cats (those above 7 years of age) should

BOX 37-1 Effects of Aging

Metabolic Effects

- Decreased metabolic rate plus lack of activity decrease caloric needs by 30% to 40%.
- Immune competence decreases, despite normal numbers of lymphocytes.
- Phagocytosis and chemotaxis decrease, and older animals are less able to ward off infections.
- Autoantibodies and immune-mediated diseases develop.

Physical Effects

- Percentage of body weight represented by fat increases.
- Skin becomes thickened, hyperpigmented, and inelastic.
- Footpads become hyperkeratinized, and claws become brittle.
- Muscle, bone, and cartilage mass are lost, with subsequent development of osteoarthritis.
- Dental calculus results in tooth loss and gingival hyperplasia (see Figure 32-34).
- Periodontitis results in gingival retraction and atrophy.
- Gastric mucosa becomes atrophic and fibrotic.
- Hepatocyte numbers decrease, and hepatic fibrosis occurs.
- Pancreatic enzyme secretion diminishes.
- Lungs lose elasticity, fibrosis occurs, and pulmonary secretions become more viscous. Vital capacity decreases.
- Cough reflex and expiratory capacity decrease.
- Kidney weight decreases, glomerular filtration rate decreases, and tubules atrophy.
- Urinary incontinence frequently develops.
- Prostate gland enlarges, testes atrophy, and prepuce becomes pendulous.
- Ovaries enlarge, and mammary glands become fibrocystic or neoplastic.
- Cardiac output decreases, and valvular fibrosis and intramural coronary arteriosclerosis develop.
- Bone marrow becomes fatty and hypoplastic, and nonregenerative anemia develops.
- The number of cells in the nervous system decreases. Senility causes loss of house training.

have a complete blood count, chemistry screen, urinalysis, chest radiograph, and blood pressure measurement performed annually. Blood and urine tests screen for dysfunction in the major organ systems, including kidneys and liver. Chest radiographs can be used to evaluate heart size and lung parenchyma.

> *TECHNICIAN NOTE* As in humans, systemic abnormalities become much more frequent with the aging process, and routine veterinary screening becomes essential for the geriatric patient.

ORAL HEALTH

Good oral health is essential to ensuring that veterinary patients will continue to eat and drink well. Owner complaints of halitosis, difficulty chewing, dropping food from the mouth, or excessive salivation should prompt a thorough oral examination. Signs of periodontal inflammation, tartar and calculus accumulation, and/or fractured teeth may require surgical intervention. Although geriatric patients may be more of an anesthetic risk, these patients also are more likely to require routine dental prophylactic procedures to ensure oral comfort. Owners should be made aware of at-home prophylaxis that they can perform, such as daily teeth brushing, to limit progression of dental disease. In addition, owners should be instructed to periodically check their pet's gums and tongue for any abnormal growth or lesion and to contact their veterinarian if there are signs of oral discomfort.

CARDIAC DISEASE

The heart is an organ commonly affected by age. Chronic valvular disease (CVD), resulting from thickening of the heart valves, affects many older dogs, especially smaller breeds. This can lead to heart murmurs, arrhythmias, and even congestive heart failure. Larger-breed dogs, although also affected by CVD, may develop different cardiac disease, such as dilated cardiomyopathy. Any cardiac disease can lead to arrhythmias and congestive heart failure. It is important that a thorough auscultation is performed in every geriatric patient and testing pursued if a murmur or arrhythmia is heard. Additionally, any reports of fatigue, exercise intolerance, collapse, or cough should be investigated further because these may all be secondary to cardiac disturbances.

RESPIRATORY DISEASE

Similar to disease of the heart, respiratory disease is commonly reported in older patients and may be due to chronic lower airway diseases, such as bronchitis, or upper airway diseases, such as a collapsing trachea. Any abnormal lung sounds or owner complaint of coughing, exercise intolerance, or change in breathing rate or effort should be immediately evaluated so as to prevent episodes of distress in the patient.

NEOPLASIA

As in our human counterparts, neoplasia is one of the most common concerns in our geriatric veterinary patients. Cancer may affect a single organ or multiple organs, depending on the type and stage of disease. Early detection is crucial to provide appropriate therapeutic measures to increase life span and improve quality of life.

> *TECHNICIAN NOTE* In addition to organ failure, cancer becomes increasingly common with age, and owners should seek veterinary care if they notice any abnormal behavior in their pet.

KIDNEY DISEASE

Chronic renal disease is one of the most common diseases seen in geriatric patients, especially cats. In addition to causing increases in urine output and water intake, kidney disease may affect appetite and overall demeanor as it progresses. With early detection, diet changes and specific medications may be added to slow progression.

URINARY AND FECAL INCONTINENCE

As veterinary patients age, degenerative neurologic diseases and spinal cord problems may lead to difficulties with urination and defecation. This will be discussed in more depth later. Urinary incontinence may be caused by any disease that leads to distention of the urinary bladder.

NEUROLOGIC ABNORMALITIES

In addition to spinal cord abnormalities leading to incontinence, paresis, or paralysis, diseases of the brain occur with increasing frequency in the geriatric patient. Development of inflammatory or neoplastic lesions in the brain itself may lead to altered mentation or behavior changes. Any onset of behavior or mentation change should prompt a veterinary evaluation in an effort to find a medical cause. Veterinary patients, like humans, can display signs of senility with age, and there are medications available that may help if this develops.

ORTHOPEDIC DISEASE

As our pet population ages, one of the most commonly seen problems is arthritis. Degenerative joint disease (DJD) occurs in most breeds of both cats and dogs. Animals that are overweight tend to be more severely affected because excess weight leads to increased stress to joints. The development of antiinflammatory medications and other medications to control pain and discomfort has dramatically improved the quality of life of many geriatric veterinary patients. Additionally, with the introduction of physical therapy and rehabilitation centers in veterinary medicine, strides have been made in the treatment of orthopedic problems.

> *TECHNICIAN NOTE* Orthopedic disease is one of the most common debilitating diseases in older animals that may be managed with appropriate medical and nursing care. It is important to make patient comfort the top priority.

ENDOCRINE CONDITIONS

The following are some common endocrine disorders seen in geriatric veterinary patients.

Hyperthyroidism

A common disease in geriatric cats, the clinical syndrome of hyperthyroidism is caused by excess production of thyroid hormone. This leads to an increase in metabolic rate, which may cause increased appetite with concurrent weight loss, excessive thirst and urination, lack of grooming, cool-seeking behavior, and vomiting. Life-threatening cardiac complications can also occur. Early detection of hyperthyroidism is important because there are several excellent therapeutic options. Therapy, such as administration of radioactive iodine, can be curative, and if done early enough, some of the cardiac changes induced by the disease may be reversible.

Diabetes Mellitus

Diabetes mellitus, caused by either insufficient production of insulin or an inability of insulin to work at its receptors, affects middle-aged to older dogs and cats. Insulin is required for glucose to enter cells, and glucose is the necessary nutrient for the body's cells to perform their normal functions. Diabetes mellitus leads to excessive thirst, urination, and appetite along with weight loss. It predisposes animals to infections, especially in the urinary tract, because glucose overloads the kidneys and is spilled into urine. Glucose is an excellent source of nutrients for bacteria, so animals with diabetes mellitus are at risk for urinary tract infections. Diabetic animals typically require daily injections of insulin by their owners to properly manage the disease.

Hyperadrenocorticism

Hyperadrenocorticism, also called Cushing's disease, is caused by excessive production of glucocorticoids, such as cortisol. This leads to excessive thirst, urination, and appetite. Glucocorticoids inhibit the ability for neutrophils to adequately protect against infection; therefore animals with hyperadrenocorticism are predisposed to infections, usually of the skin and urinary tract. With appropriate treatment, this can be managed, and infections limited.

Endocrine disease in general can be managed once diagnosed. If left untreated, however, it can lead to recurrent problems related to the urinary tract, skin, and other organ systems. Ultimately, these diseases may be life threatening without proper attention. Because they occur with increased frequency in middle-aged to older veterinary patients, owners should be made aware of their clinical signs and visit a veterinarian for evaluation if one of these diseases is suspected. It is important to remember that appropriate management of these diseases will improve not only longevity, but also quality of life because the patient will likely feel better once the diseases are under control.

> *TECHNICIAN NOTE* Technicians may play a key role in teaching owners skills that they need to improve their pet's quality of life as they age. Educating owners regarding administration of fluids and medications, expressing bladders, and other nursing care can allow their pet to remain comfortable even if they have severe systemic disease.

HOSPICE CARE FOR THE AGED AND DYING CAT AND DOG

We do what we can to prevent illness in our veterinary patients, but at some point many of our companion animals will develop terminal diseases. As we attempt to treat and control progression of these diseases, technicians in particular may play a large role in ensuring that the aged and dying geriatric patients are kept comfortable at home.

PAIN MEDICATIONS

Regardless of the disease, the goal of the veterinarian and veterinary technician is to provide comfort to the sick patient. One of the most difficult challenges is to accurately assess the level of pain experienced by a particular patient. Unlike humans, dogs and cats have subtle ways of expressing their discomfort, and owners may not be aware that their pet is in pain. However, they may report general malaise, inappetence, or decreased activity in their pet, or they may notice an unwillingness to climb stairs or jump on or off the couch. When performing a physical examination, veterinary technicians should be able to recognize signs of discomfort that may include tachycardia, tachypnea, elevated temperature, organomegaly, unwillingness to use a limb or to posture for normal eliminations (especially in pets with severe hip arthritis or lumbar pain), and yelping when a limb is manipulated. In addition, veterinary technicians must be able to determine the level of pain that the animal is experiencing and whether or not pain management drugs are indicated.

The decision to start a geriatric patient on medications to control pain should not be taken lightly. Many geriatric patients have underlying organ insufficiency, and nearly all pain medications used in veterinary medicine have some potential for organ toxicity. Fortunately, as long as close monitoring of the patient is performed while receiving the medications, permanent damage is unlikely. Complete blood work should be performed before using any type of pain medication in a geriatric patient and should be performed serially while the animal is receiving these medications.

The most common drug classes that veterinarians prescribe to geriatric patients are (1) nonsteroidal antiinflammatory drugs (NSAIDs), (2) steroids, and (3) opiates. They each have their own potential benefits and risks. NSAIDs are typically administered orally (although some of them may be given parenterally if necessary) and are potent antiinflammatory agents. They are the most commonly used medications for managing the pain of DJD, chronic intervertebral disk disease, and other forms of arthritis. Although side effects are rare, they may include gastrointestinal (GI) ulceration and renal and hepatic toxicity. In the past, these drugs have rarely been used to manage pain in older cats. However, the development of new formulations of NSAIDs has made their regular use a practical option in cats.

Steroids, more specifically glucocorticoids, also have potent antiinflammatory effects. Unfortunately, long-term use of steroids, such as prednisone (and in some cases even short-term use), may lead to significant side effects that can detrimentally affect quality of life in these patients. These side effects may include excessive thirst and urination, an increased susceptibility to urinary tract infections, increased panting, muscle atrophy and hind limb weakness, GI ulceration, and thromboembolic complications. For these reasons, the use of glucocorticoids for pain control is usually a last resort.

Finally, opiates are narcotic drugs that produce some degree of analgesia. These drugs are known in humans to have the potential to become habit forming and to cause sedation and respiratory depression. Several types of opiate receptors exist in the brain, and different opiates have been developed to work in the area of interest in specific patients. Different methods for administering opiate drugs exist, with the transdermal fentanyl patch providing continuous release of fentanyl over a 72- to 96-hour period of time, after which the patch needs to be removed and a new one reapplied. Tramadol, a "mu" agonist, is an opiate that binds only to "mu" receptors, providing both analgesia and a feeling of euphoria to the patient, without respiratory depression or the risk of addiction.

Refer to Chapter 26 for more information regarding specific drugs.

NURSING CARE FOR THE HOSPICE PATIENT

Many animals that are at the point of needing hospice care are those pets that have their normal mental faculties, but have physical disabilities that prevent them from performing typical daily activities. This would be common in animals with severe orthopedic or spinal cord disease, where the patient is mentally appropriate, has a continued good appetite, but cannot ambulate on its own. Teaching pet owners to care for their recumbent pets at home is therefore critical if the animal is to survive and live comfortably. Veterinary technicians play a key role in providing this valuable instruction. Pet owners need to know how to keep their animals clean and comfortable. They need to be able to assess levels of pain and determine when to give medications. In addition, owners should be taught to turn recumbent animals on a regular basis, at least every 4 to 6 hours, to limit formation of decubital ulcers, or bed sores (see later discussion). Additionally, animals that spend more time on one side than the other will develop atelectasis in the lung lobes on the "down" side, which could lead to respiratory compromise. Recumbent patients are predisposed to pneumonia and should be encouraged to ambulate regularly, if at all possible. Animals should always be in sternal recumbency when fed to prevent accidental aspiration if vomiting or regurgitation should occur. Appetite should be monitored closely because a decline in appetite may indicate the pet's condition is deteriorating.

DECUBITAL ULCERS

As previously mentioned, one of the more common reasons that animals need at-home hospice care is that they have lost their ability to ambulate well and thus spend a significant amount of time in recumbency. This can be devastating for many dogs and can be especially worrisome in large dogs that are more prone to developing sores and ulcers at pressure points along their body. The most common places to develop these pressure point sores, or "decubital ulcers," are around the elbows, tarsi, and hips. They can develop anywhere on the body that spends a large amount of time adjacent to the ground because they essentially are sores that occur because of excessive rubbing against the floor.

The best way to prevent such ulcers is to encourage the pet to stand and walk on a regular basis, at least every 4 to 6 hours, and to be sure that the animal does not spend excessive time lying on one side of the body. Keeping the pet clean and dry of urine and other moistness is also essential to prevent development of sores. Extra pads and cushioning should be provided, especially to support areas that are more likely to develop problems.

If ulceration does occur, a topical antibiotic ointment and a protective bandage may be applied to prevent further trauma to the area. The difficulty with bandaging the areas is that often the bandage itself is a cause of trauma because the sore then remains in close contact with the bandaging material and healing cannot occur. If the sore occurs over a joint, such as the elbow or tarsus, a doughnut type of bandage can be fashioned so that the sore itself remains exposed, but it cannot rub against surfaces, thus limiting continued trauma.

SUBCUTANEOUS FLUIDS

Whereas the vast majority of dogs and cats receiving at-home care are eating and drinking on their own, there are a number of pets that require additional fluid support to maintain adequate hydration. Many of the common geriatric diseases we see in veterinary medicine lead to excessive amounts of urination, with a secondary need for increased amounts of water intake. Sometimes the amount of fluid intake necessary to compensate for fluid loss is high, and the patient is unable to adequately compensate. This occurs most frequently with diseases such as renal failure.

If there is concern that a patient may not be receiving adequate amounts of fluid, owners may be taught to administer subcutaneous fluids. There are several methods for administering subcutaneous fluid, and the method used often depends on the amount of fluid administered and the size of the animal receiving the fluid.

For small dogs and cats, one might choose a butterfly catheter with a needle on the end. The appropriate fluid (usually a maintenance type of fluid) is chosen, and the amount to be given is drawn up into a large syringe. Once drawn up and attached to the end of the butterfly catheter, the needle on the end of the catheter is placed under the skin of the patient (usually in an area where there is some degree of excessive skin tissue, such as between the shoulder blades). The fluid can then be administered by injecting via the syringe. The major drawbacks to this method are: (1) the butterfly needles are often smaller than regular needles, so the fluid is injected more slowly, and (2) if you are administering greater than 60 ml of fluid, you will need to connect more than one syringe because 60-ml syringes are usually the largest used (Figures 37-1 and 37-2).

For a larger volume to be administered, one might elect to attach the entire fluid bag to an extension set with a needle on the end and then administer the fluid directly from the bag. Be sure to prime the extension set with fluids before administering to prevent air from being pushed under the skin. The major drawback to this method is that it is less precise than using a syringe, and the amount of fluid

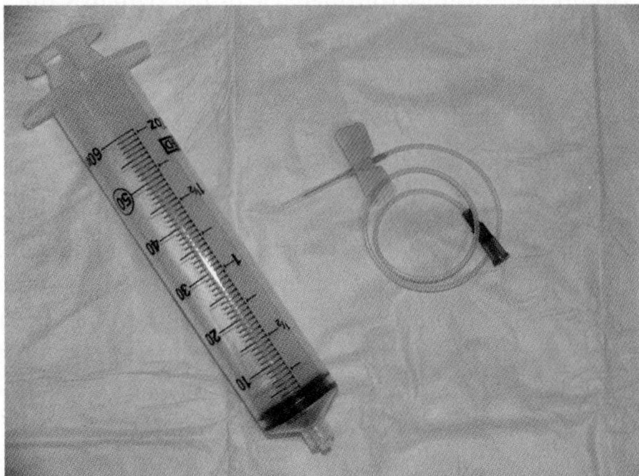

FIGURE 37-1 A 60-ml syringe is shown on the left and a butterfly catheter is shown on the right. The two components are connected, and fluid is delivered to the patient subcutaneously.

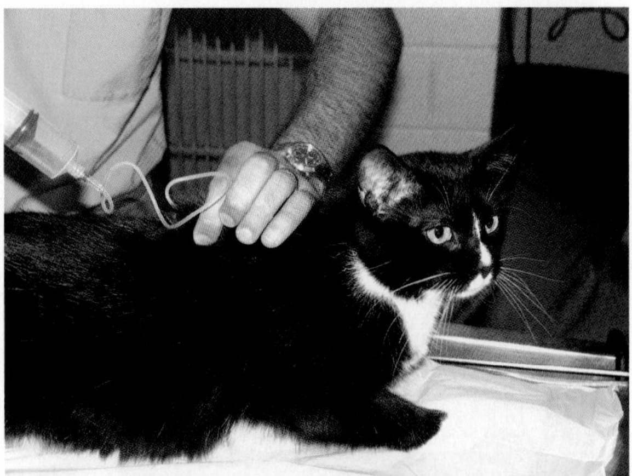

FIGURE 37-2 The skin of the patient is tented, and the needle is inserted through the skin into the subcutaneous space. One hand may be used to restrain the patient and/or hold the needle in place while the other hand injects the fluid. A butterfly catheter will often remain in place once the needle has been inserted through the skin. Many animals tolerate subcutaneous fluid injections well, and it can often be performed by one person.

administered is not usually able to be measured exactly (Figures 37-3 and 37-4).

Owners should be warned that the fluid will often become dependent. In other words, although they are usually given between the shoulder blades, before they are absorbed into the body, they often travel down the side of the animal. This is not of pathologic significance, but is something owners often recognize. Owners should also be aware that excessive amounts of fluid administration, especially in cats, can be detrimental and may lead to fluid overload if the heart is not pumping correctly. Owners of any animal receiving subcutaneous fluid should report any change in respiratory pattern to the veterinarian because this could be indicative of fluid overload or heart failure.

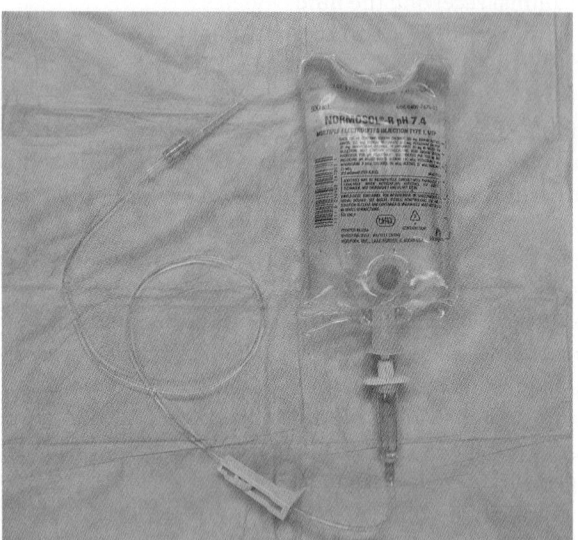

FIGURE 37-3 A bag of replacement fluid is connected to a short-to-medium length extension set, and a needle is connected to the end of the fluid line.

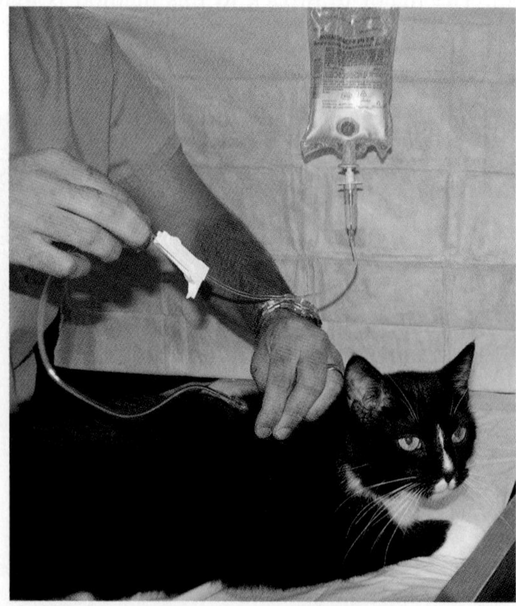

FIGURE 37-4 As explained in Figure 2, the patient's skin is tented, and the needle is inserted through the skin into the subcutaneous space. The fluid bag is hung at a level above the patient such that fluid flows via gravity. To speed up the flow of fluid, pressure may be applied to the bag.

EXPRESSING BLADDERS

Pets with orthopedic diseases, such as hip dysplasia and its associated DJD, often have a difficult time posturing to urinate and/or defecate. Additionally, animals that have had spinal cord injuries or other forms of spinal cord disease may be unable to urinate on their own. Owners can be taught to express their pet's bladder to allow complete voiding. Bladder expression is a painless procedure if done correctly. There are different methods to perform this procedure, with the main focus on applying gentle pressure to the urinary bladder by squeezing both sides of the bladder. One method would be to have the patient standing. Place one hand on each side of the patient's abdomen and move the hands caudally toward the pelvis until you can feel a soft, round structure that feels similar to a water balloon. This is the urinary bladder, and once it is found, gentle pressure should be applied to it. The amount of pressure to apply varies with the individual, but with the right amount of pressure, urine will be expressed through the urethra, and a nice stream should be maintained until the "balloon" feels empty.

If the animal will not stand well on his or her own or seems more comfortable in lateral recumbency, bladder expression can be successful using a similar technique as described previously. One hand should be placed on each side of the abdomen and moved caudally toward the pelvis until the bladder is felt and then gentle pressure applied until a nice stream is produced. Excessive pressure should never be applied because it is possible to rupture the urinary bladder.

It is always important to express as much urine as possible from the bladder. When urine sits in the bladder, especially in a patient that is unable to void on its own, infections are likely to occur. Therefore any animal that requires regular bladder expression should be evaluated on a routine basis for urine cultures by the primary veterinarian. Additionally, it is important that owners routinely clean the patient's fur and skin of urine after expressing the bladder to prevent urine scalding (see later discussion).

URINE SCALDING

Patients that are nonambulatory and recumbent may have urinary incontinence or may consciously urinate in a recumbent position. Urinary incontinence is common in patients that have spinal cord disease. The innervation to the external urethral sphincter arises from spinal cord segments at S1 to S3; therefore spinal cord disease in this area often leads to "lower motor neuron" bladder dysfunction, whereby the sphincter does not close tightly and urine leaks. Additional causes for urinary incontinence may include senility or decreased mobility such that the bladder becomes too full and begins to leak. Any disease that causes excessive urination and thirst will lead the bladder to become distended. Without proper attention, such as regular expression of the bladder or frequent walks to allow for elimination, the animal may dribble urine uncontrollably.

If urine leakage occurs, it may stain and soak the fur and scald the skin. If left untreated, this can eventually lead to sores and skin infections. This is painful and contributes to a poor quality of life. It is important to keep these patients clean and dry at all times. Because bladder expression may lead to urine on the fur and skin, it is important to be aware of this when expressing the bladder and to always clean and dry the patient afterward.

APPETITE STIMULANTS

Decreased appetite and associated weight loss is a serious problem in some geriatric cats and dogs. The first thing to bear in mind when an animal's appetite begins to wane is that there is usually an underlying cause, such as a systemic illness, orthopedic pain, or central neurologic depression. Every effort should be made to identify and treat an underlying disease. If a focus of orthopedic discomfort is found, for example, antiinflammatory medications or other pain medications may improve appetite.

If no underlying cause is found or if the appetite remains poor even with treatment of the underlying illness, medications, such as antiemetics and appetite stimulants, may be administered.

FEEDING TUBES

The use of feeding tubes for the geriatric patient is a controversial issue because nutritional support in the hospice care setting may be inhumane if the patient is otherwise debilitated. One of the most important indicators of how an animal feels is the presence or absence of an appetite. In a recumbent, debilitated patient, anorexia may mark the time to consider euthanasia of the pet. In this way, placing a feeding tube disrupts an important communication from the animal that his quality of life has deteriorated. It is therefore considered unethical in some cases by some clinicians.

Feeding tubes are necessary sometimes such as in cases where the animal's alimentary tract is abnormal (megaesophagus), but the patient is otherwise leading a good quality of life. As we discussed earlier, animals often need subcutaneous fluids at home to maintain proper hydration. Feeding tubes may be used for fluid and nutritional support in select animals.

There are many types of feeding tubes available in veterinary medicine. Some are used for short-term management, some for long-term support. The most common short-term feeding tube is a nasoesophageal tube. Whereas animals may be sent home with this type of feeding tube, it is typically for temporary use when we suspect the animal will begin eating on its own relatively soon. This is a flexible, soft, thin-diameter tube that is placed into the nasal cavity and then into the nasopharynx before it ends up in the esophagus. It is held in place by a suture to the side of the pet's face. Because of its location, animals can easily paw at them and cause early removal; therefore an Elizabethan collar needs to be worn at all times. Because these tubes tend to be thought of as causing mild discomfort to the patient, they again are only temporary. Additionally, the types of food given through the tube are limited and must be of liquid consistency.

A more permanent type of tube is an esophagostomy tube, which is placed while the patient is under general anesthetic through an incision directly into the esophagus from the neck. A slightly larger tube may be used for this type of tube, and thus the choice of liquid or slurry diet is more varied. Additionally, animals tend to tolerate these tubes better because they are not interfering with their face and cause less discomfort.

Finally the most permanent type of tube we can place is one that goes directly into the stomach. A gastrotomy tube may be placed surgically or via endoscopic assistance and typically provides an even larger diameter tube. It is away from the face and the neck and rarely interferes with normal daily activities of the patient. It is ideal for patients with esophageal disorders because the esophagus is avoided entirely. Its drawback is that its placement is much more invasive, and complications, although uncommon, can be devastating and life threatening (i.e., bacterial infection in the abdomen if the tube leaks).

Feeding tubes are reserved for specific occasions and are generally not recommended as a "life support" type of measure. The animal should have a good quality of life other than its inability to adequately obtain nutritional means.

CARTS AND SLINGS

As animals age, orthopedic and neurologic disease can lead to severe impairment in ambulatory abilities. This has historically been difficult to handle because often the animal maintains its mental faculties but simply is unable to get around. Products have been developed that make this type of problem manageable for many owners, while still providing a good quality of life for the pet.

Slings can be used to support the hind end in an animal that has normal use of the front end of its body and still maintains some control of the hind end. Typically, slings fit around the caudal portion of the body, just cranial to the hind limbs, allowing for the caretaker to simply support the hind limbs while the animal ambulates. A sling works best if the animal can still use the hind limbs to some extent, and often the sling is used merely as a support and fail-safe device in the event that the animal cannot bear its entire weight. If the animal is only mildly affected, a soft blanket or towel can be used as a sling. There are products available for purchase (Figure 37-5).

For animals that maintain little to no function of their hind limbs, as often occurs with spinal cord injuries, carts have become available for purchase. The hind limbs fit into

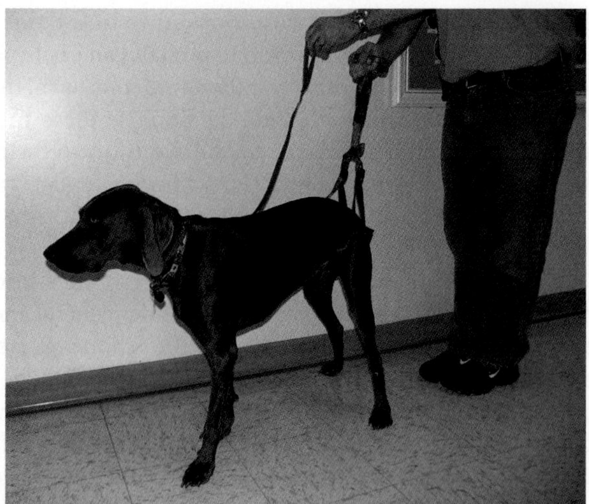

FIGURE 37-5 Bottom's Up Leash (2003 to 2005 Bottom's Up Leash, a division of Watson's Pet Co., Santa Monica, CA 90404) is being used in this patient for support of the hind limbs. Alternatively, depending upon the severity of the hind limb weakness, a towel or soft blanket may be used as a temporary sling. The sling should be used for support only and not as a replacement for walking unless the animal is unable to use their limbs entirely.

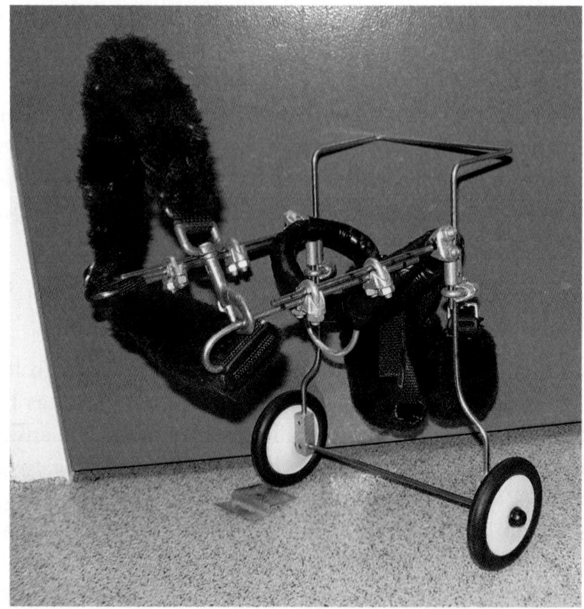

FIGURE 37-6 This is a cart used for an animal with hind limb paresis. To work properly, the animal must have normal mobility of the front limbs. The patient's head and front limbs fit through the soft red padding to the left of the picture, and the hind limbs fit through the black doughnut-shaped holes to the right. Normal mobility in the front limbs allows the animal to ambulate fairly well and to control direction changes. These carts can be sized for the particular patient, such that the fitting can actually encourage use of the hind limbs.

the apparatus, allowing the animal to use his or her front limbs to move around (Figure 37-6). Some devices exist that may be used for animals that have difficulties with all four limbs (Figure 37-7). Animals typically adapt to these devices quite well.

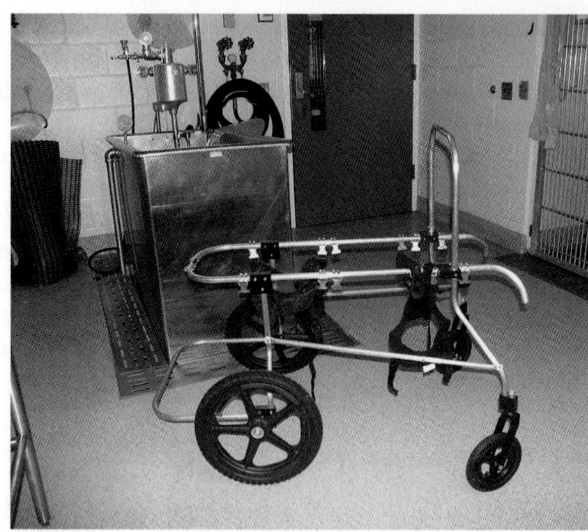

FIGURE 37-7 This cart may be used for a patient that has difficulty using all four of their limbs. A benefit of this type of apparatus is that it can be used as an aid to physical therapy because the animal can attempt to use their legs to guide the cart around. It is great for exercise in an otherwise recumbent animal.

WHEN IS THE RIGHT TIME FOR EUTHANASIA?

We are fortunate to be part of veterinary medicine during a time when pets are treated like family members and medical and technologic advances continue to be made. It is important to bear in mind, however, that we have an ethical obligation to prevent suffering in veterinary patients. Owners will often rely on members of the veterinary community to aid in the decision of euthanasia. Although veterinarians, veterinary technicians, and staff members should be careful not to make the decision for owners, they should be prepared to answer questions regarding when the right time might be. Educating owners about determining what signs their animal might show when they are in discomfort is important. Signs such as persistent anorexia, change in breathing rate or effort, pain that is unable to be controlled by medication, or loss of interest in interacting with the owner may all be indicators that the pet's health is declining. Once the owner recognizes these signs, she should seek advice from her veterinary caregiver. Making the decision to euthanize a pet is difficult for most pet owners, and it is important to support the owner by providing as much clinical information as possible so that the best possible choice can be made for the animal. Refer to Chapter 38 for more information about euthanasia.

> *TECHNICIAN NOTE* The decision to euthanize a beloved family pet is a difficult one, and owners will often seek guidance from those in the veterinary field that they have grown to trust. This includes veterinarians, technicians, and staff, all of whom should be available to be supportive during these difficult times.

CASE PRESENTATION 37-1

Hershey, a 13-year-old Labrador retriever, is brought into the clinic for difficulty using his hind legs. This has been a gradual onset, but is severe enough that he can no longer ambulate well on his own. The owner also reports a diminished appetite and that Hershey is no longer getting up to urinate regularly. When he rises, he often has a puddle of urine on his bedding. Examination and diagnostic testing reveals severe arthritis in both hips and stifles. He appears to have good ambulation in his front limbs. No other systemic disease is found, and organ function appears within normal limits. He is in extreme pain upon manipulation of the affected areas.

After discussion with the owner regarding Hershey's quality of life, it is decided to place him on nonsteroidal antiinflammatory medications to improve his comfort level. The owner purchases a sling to help Hershey move around better and encourages him to go out and urinate every 4 to 6 hours by assisting him with ambulation. Soft, padded bedding is provided for him to rest comfortably on at home to prevent development of decubital ulcers. At a follow-up visit, Hershey still has difficulty walking, but is much more comfortable and gets around well with his owner's assistance. The owner reports an improved appetite, and he is having less frequent urinary "accidents" in the house. With time, additional pain medications may be added if the discomfort begins to worsen. Serial urine cultures are performed for early diagnosis of urinary tract infections.

GERIATRIC HORSES

As a result of advances in equine management and nutrition in the last few decades, many horses are living beyond 30 years of age. Many of these horses are pasture pets and well loved by their owners, but are not referred to a veterinary hospital when problems arise. Factors such as advanced age, inability to ride in a trailer, and economics play a part in the owner's decision to not refer the patient. Therefore many equine veterinarians in private practice manage these horses on the farm.

Aged horses are often defined as greater than 20 years old. Many of these horses are greater than 30 years old and often live into their late 30s or even early 40s. These aged horses suffer from a myriad of problems, including poor body condition, lack of teeth, Cushing disease, musculoskeletal disease, such as DJD, or osteoarthritis, and chronic laminitis (inflammation of the laminae in their feet, leading to chronic foot pain and lameness). Cushing disease is a common disease of older horses and will be discussed in detail in this chapter.

PHYSICAL EXAMINATION

An annual physical examination is crucial to maintain good health of the aged horse. Often problems are found on a thorough examination. Refer to Chapter 8 for a detailed description of physical examination of the equine patient. An annual body condition score is helpful to determine if the aged horse is maintaining an adequate body condition. Acute or chronic weight loss indicates an underlying problem, such as lack of teeth, inability of the GI tract to absorb nutrients, or neoplasia. The horse's hair coat should be short and smooth. If it is long, wavy, and not shedding out completely in the spring, the horse has Cushing disease, discussed later in the chapter. Common problems in older horses include heaves, laminitis, dental problems, equine recurrent uveitis (ERU), sinusitis, neurologic deficits, and DJD.

COMMON PROBLEMS

The general physical examination of a geriatric horse follows the same guidelines of an examination performed on a younger horse. However, aged horses are more prone to certain problems, so these are highlighted in the following discussion (Box 37-2).

The horse should have a body score performed on physical examination. This system offers an objective way to determine the horse's condition and assess if weight loss occurs over time. Body condition scoring uses a scale from 1 to 9. One indicates that the horse is emaciated, and 9 is obesity. The horse's attitude is assessed as bright and alert or depressed (Figure 37-8). Many older horses appear quiet and depressed, but it is often due to Cushing disease and can improve with treatment. The hair coat should be short and shiny. If it is dull, long, wavy, and not shedding completely in the spring (hirsutism), the horse has Cushing disease.

ORAL AND NASAL HEALTH

An oral examination is important to perform since older horses are often in poor condition, unable to chew properly, and drop food when chewing. Many older horses are missing teeth or have sharp points on their teeth preventing normal chewing (hooks) (Figure 37-9). The most severe change is called a wave mouth. This condition occurs when the horse's teeth are different lengths, preventing normal chewing action. Geriatric horses are also prone to chronic sinus infections, so presence of nasal discharge and a dull sound when percussing the sinuses indicates that the sinus cavity contains fluid.

VISION

An ophthalmic examination evaluates the horse's eyes for diseases, such as ERU and cataracts. It is not uncommon for an older horse to have significant visual impairment, which is only discovered after an ophthalmic examination. Many older horses are housed on the same farm for years and are able to compensate for loss of vision. If they are moved to a new location, the owner will discover the horse has difficulty maneuvering in the new environment as a result of decreased vision.

CARDIAC DISEASE

Cardiac auscultation is important to assess a resting heart rate and presence of murmurs or arrhythmias. It is helpful to simultaneously evaluate the pulse quality to ensure

BOX 37-2 Physical Examination of a Geriatric Horse and Common Problems

Body Condition Scoring
- Scale 1 (emaciated) to 9 (obese)

Attitude
- Bright and alert or depressed

Hair Coat
- Normal length or long and wavy

Oral Examination
- Presence of hooks or missing teeth
- Wave mouth

Ophthalmic Examination
- Evaluate for uveitis and/or cataracts

Examine Sinuses
- Percuss sinuses and presence of nasal discharge

Cardiac Auscultation
- Assess resting heart rate and pulse quality
- Presence of murmurs and arrhythmias

Respiratory Examination
- Respiratory rate and effort
- Presence of nasal discharge or coughing
- Development of heave line (hypertrophy of abdominal muscles)

GI Tract
- Note if normal manure
- Presence of diarrhea may indicate chronic colitis or malabsorptive disease

Renal System
- Note amount of drinking and urination

Integument
- Examine skin for abrasions, especially around bony areas and dermatitis

Reproductive Organ Examination
- Male horses may have squamous cell carcinoma tumors
- Look for melanomas around rectum

General Neurologic Examination
- Look for dragging feet or blunted toes
- Examine neck for pain or fractures of cervical vertebrae

Musculoskeletal Examination
- Examine feet for laminitis (e.g., rings on hoof wall)
- Evidence of DJD (e.g., carpus or hock)
- Presence of muscle atrophy, especially around gluteal area

that it is strong and synchronous with the heartbeat. Mitral regurgitation is the most common valvular lesion in horses greater than 15 years old. One will auscultate a systolic murmur on the left side. Aortic regurgitation also occurs in older horses. One will auscultate a diastolic murmur on the left side. The most common arrhythmia in an older horse is atrial fibrillation. It is often an incidental finding on physical examination. The rhythm is irregularly irregular, and the horse will have a higher resting heart rate than normal. Many horses can tolerate this arrhythmia for years and appear healthy, but may exhibit exercise intolerance at high levels of exercise.

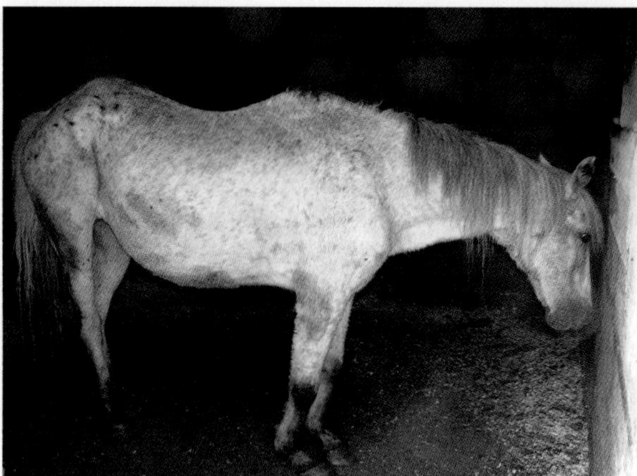

FIGURE 37-8 Geriatric horse with poor body condition and depressed attitude.

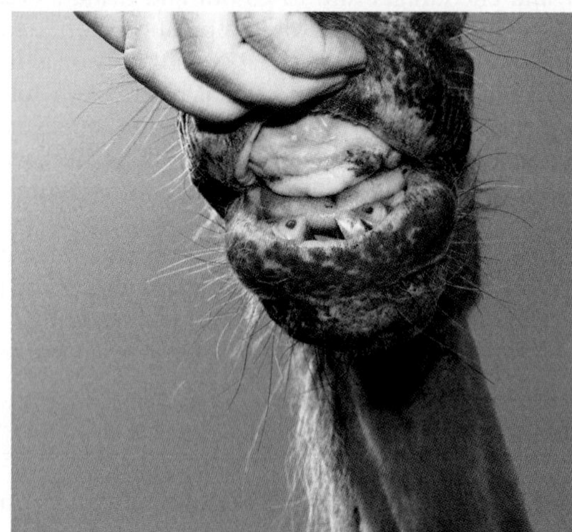

FIGURE 37-9 Note the lack of multiple incisors.

RESPIRATORY DISEASE

A respiratory examination evaluates respiratory rate, respiratory effort, and presence of nasal discharge or coughing. Older horses often have heaves (recurrent airway obstruction) and will have an increased respiratory rate and effort. Chronic cases develop a heave line (hypertrophy of abdominal muscles) resulting from increased effort to exhale.

GASTROINTESTINAL DISEASE

The GI tract is assessed initially by evaluating consistency and amount of manure. The manure should have a normal consistency and not contain large pieces of hay or grain. If these pieces are present, the horse has poor chewing ability to grind food well and needs an oral examination. Presence of diarrhea may indicate chronic colitis or malabsorptive disease.

KIDNEY DISEASE

The horse's renal system can be assessed by evaluating the amount of water consumed daily and frequency of urination. Annual urinalysis is important to assess concentrating ability of the kidneys and ensure that urine does not contain substances such as protein or glucose.

SKIN DISORDERS

The horse's integument is examined for dermatitis and abrasions, especially around bony areas, such as the pelvis. Reproductive organs are visually examined. Male horses may have tumors on their sheath (prepuce) or penis. These tumors are often squamous cell carcinoma and require treatment. The rectal area is evaluated for presence of melanomas and normal anal tone.

NEUROLOGIC ABNORMALITIES

On general neurologic examination, older horses may drag their hind feet and have blunted toes. This change may be due to neurologic deficits or musculoskeletal pain (e.g., DJD in the hocks). The horse's neck should also be examined for evidence of pain. Offer the horse a carrot or handful of grain to encourage the horse to touch his nose to his shoulder. If the horse is reluctant or unable to perform this action, it indicates neck pain. Sometimes this is due to fractures of the cervical vertebrae, diagnosed on cervical radiographs.

ORTHOPEDIC DISEASE

The musculoskeletal examination is an important part of a general physical examination. Older horses are prone to laminitis and may have changes, such as rings on the hoof wall, indicating chronic laminitis (Figure 37-10). They also often have DJD in multiple joints (e.g., carpus, hock) and become stiff without regular pasture turnout (Figure 37-11). Muscle atrophy is also common, especially on the dorsum and around the gluteal area (Figure 37-12).

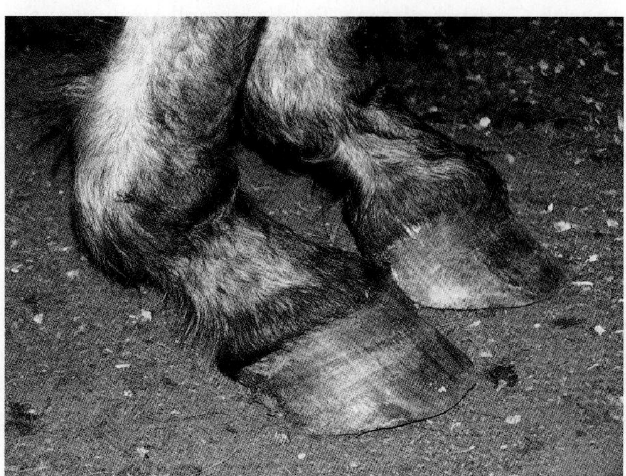

FIGURE 37-10 Note the curly hair, rings on hoof wall, and abnormal angle of distal limb as a result of suspensory tendon deterioration.

> *TECHNICIAN NOTE* Geriatric horses are more likely to have general health problems, so an annual physical examination is important to identify and to treat problems early.

ENDOCRINE CONDITIONS

Equine Cushing Disease (Pituitary Pars Intermedia Dysfunction)

Equine Cushing disease, also known as pituitary pars intermedia dysfunction (PPID), is a common disease in horses, especially those greater than 15 years old. Certain breeds, such as quarter horses, also seem more predisposed than other breeds (e.g., thoroughbreds). It is caused by excessive hormonal secretions (pro-opiomelanocortin

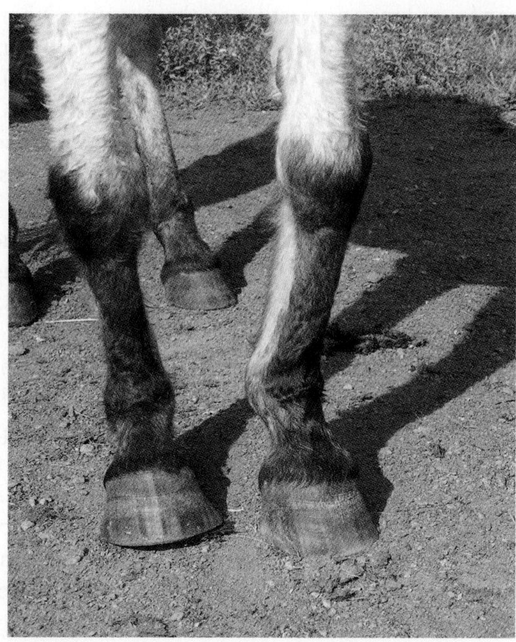

FIGURE 37-11 Picture of severe carpal bone degeneration causing a bowlegged appearance.

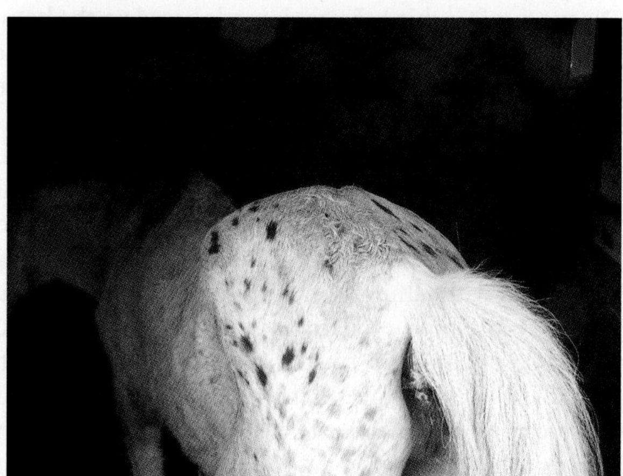

FIGURE 37-12 Note the bony, prominent pelvis and long, wavy hair coat.

[POMC]-derived peptides) from the pituitary pars intermedia (PI), stimulating excessive cortisol release from the adrenal glands.

In the brain, the hypothalamus is the master endocrine gland, controlling many activities of other endocrine glands. It resides above the pituitary gland and has neurons with long axons that synapse on melanotrophs in the pituitary PI. Dopamine secreted by these hypothalamic neurons inhibits the production of POMC by the pituitary PI. However, there is a loss of dopamine in Cushing disease, leading to excessive production of POMC by the pituitary gland. POMC is converted into different hormones, including adrenocorticotropic hormone (ACTH), which stimulates the adrenal glands to produce excessive cortisol.

Clinical signs of Cushing disease vary with each patient. The affected horse may exhibit one or more clinical signs including hirsutism (overlong hair coat), patchy sweating, lethargy, polyuria, polydipsia (PU/PD), laminitis, "potbelly" appearance, and muscle wasting on the dorsum. Other possible clinical signs include spontaneous lactation in mares without foals, tachypnea (increased respiratory rate), and immunosuppression, resulting in parasitism. Horses with Cushing disease are more prone to concurrent diseases, such as recurrent uveitis, heaves (recurrent airway obstruction), and sinusitis. Abnormalities noted on blood work (complete blood cell count and chemistry profile) include hyperglycemia (blood glucose level greater than 180 mg/dl), increased liver enzymes, neutrophilia, lymphopenia, and anemia.

In the past, many older horses with Cushing disease were misdiagnosed as having hypothyroidism (low thyroid hormone levels). One of the common clinical signs thought to indicate hypothyroidism in horses was presence of a thick, crest neck. It is now recognized that hypothyroidism is not common in horses and the thick neck is due to fat deposits. Measuring baseline thyroid hormone levels (e.g., T_4 and T_3) is not reliable in horses. These levels can be decreased for many reasons and should not be used as a screening test. Although many horses receive thyroid supplementation, it is not a benign medication in human patients and should be used only when indicated in equine patients.

Diagnosis of Cushing disease is made based on the horse's history, signalment, physical examination, and ancillary diagnostic blood tests. There are three tests typically used: dexamethasone suppression test (DST) to assess cortisol response; serial measurements of ACTH, insulin, and dextrose; and thyrotropin-releasing hormone (TRH) stimulation. The DST is not always reliable and can give inconsistent results. The test requires steroid administration, and steroids are associated with laminitis in horses. Horses with Cushing disease are more prone to laminitis and/or may have a current episode of laminitis, so steroid administration is often contraindicated. Serial measurements of ACTH, insulin, and dextrose can be more accurate than DST. Steroids are not used in this test, so it is a good option for many horses with Cushing disease. However, one sample may not be diagnostic, so taking three blood samples in one day (AM, noon, PM) is optimal. ACTH levels increase in the fall as compared with January or May, so results should be interpreted based on the time of year. The TRH stimulation appears to be a promising diagnostic test. In recent publications, it may be more accurate than DST or serial measurements of ACTH, insulin, and dextrose. TRH administration will increase ACTH concentrations in both clinically normal and abnormal horses. However, ACTH levels are greater in abnormal horses in the amount of increase, maximum ACTH concentration, and persistence of high concentrations. Despite different diagnostic tests available, sometimes owners of geriatric horses refuse diagnostic tests. Empirical treatment should be considered if the owner refuses diagnostic tests and the horse's history, signalment, and physical examination findings are consistent with Cushing disease.

The primary treatment for Cushing disease is a dopamine agonist, pergolide. Many 450-kg horses respond well to 1 mg pergolide orally once a day, but the dose needs to be altered based on response to treatment. Many clinical signs will improve with treatment, but hirsutism usually remains. Numerous horses with Cushing disease appear quiet and depressed, but once treatment is initiated, become much more alert and act younger. Rechecking blood tests after starting medication will aid in determining the optimum pergolide dose. Another medication, cyproheptadine, was used in the past to treat Cushing disease. It is not as effective as pergolide and more expensive.

General management is important for horses with Cushing disease. The horse should have his teeth floated every 6 months or yearly to maintain oral health. Regular foot care every 4 to 5 weeks will keep him more comfortable and prevent an overlong toe, which can aggravate lameness or laminitis. Regular deworming and manure management, such as weekly removal from the pasture, will aid in parasite control. Horses with Cushing disease have poor thermoregulation and patchy sweating associated with hirsutism. These patients are more comfortable with regular body clipping to minimize hirsutism and using blankets in the winter. Clipping also permits better assessment of the horse's body condition.

Nutrition is important with aged equine patients and those with Cushing disease. Feeding small amounts of a senior diet often, adding corn oil (¼ cup daily) and grass pasture, and avoiding lush pastures are beneficial. Alfalfa hay or soaked cubes or pellets can help maintain an older horse's body condition. Alternate sources include processed hay, such as Dengie hay.

> *TECHNICIAN NOTE* Cushing disease is common in older horses. Clinical signs vary, but often horses will have hirsutism (excessive long hair growth) and depression. Cushing disease can cause immunosuppression and exacerbate other diseases, so diagnosis and treatment is imperative to maintain the geriatric horse's health.

CHRONIC DISEASES OF THE GERIATRIC HORSE

Geriatric horses often have multiple problems that require close attention to minimize complications. Cushing disease is common in older horses and can cause immunosuppression. It also leads to or exacerbates other diseases, such as heaves (recurrent airway obstruction), ERU, laminitis, and sinusitis. To successfully manage these other conditions, Cushing disease requires treatment with pergolide to minimize immunosuppression.

HEAVES (RECURRENT AIRWAY OBSTRUCTION)

This disease can be acute or chronic in nature. Some horses are only affected a few weeks each year, some horses are affected year-round. Usually, if a horse acutely develops signs of heaves, it eventually becomes a chronic condition and requires careful management to minimize clinical signs. Horses with heaves are often allergic to dust or mold in the environment. Horses living in a dusty stable with minimal pasture turnout, exposed to cobwebs, straw, and hay are prone to developing heaves. This allergic reaction leads to inflamed airways and constriction of the smooth muscle in the airways. This combination causes narrowed airways and leads to difficult breathing, especially when exhaling. Clinical signs on physical examination include increased respiratory rate (tachypnea) and increased effort (dyspnea), nostril flare, and dry cough. The horse will have no fever and may have a clear nasal discharge. Horses with chronic heaves are often in poor body condition with a heave line (extreme development of the external abdominal oblique muscles as a result of increased effort on exhalation). The horse may extend his head on exhalation to improve airflow. On thoracic auscultation, wheezes will be heard on both sides of the chest, especially on expiration. A rebreathing bag (large trash bag) may be used to encourage the horse to inhale deeply, permitting better thoracic auscultation. After removing the bag, a horse with heaves will cough and take a long time to return to normal breathing. Additional diagnostic tests include blood tests (CBC, chemistry profile), transtracheal wash, bronchioalveolar lavage (BAL), and thoracic radiographs. Abnormalities on blood tests include increased total protein and increased fibrinogen concentration. Samples of airway secretions can be obtained on transtracheal wash or BAL and submitted for cytology and culture to differentiate heaves from infection (e.g., pneumonia). Changing the horse's environment to minimize allergens is the most important part of therapy. Increasing pasture turnout, soaking hay for 4 hours before feeding and eliminating dusty bedding is vital to minimize clinical signs. Medication to control inflammation and bronchoconstriction is administered systemically (e.g., IV, IM, PO) or locally (e.g., using an inhaler). Steroids (e.g., dexamethasone, fluticasone) are used to decrease inflammation, and bronchodilators (e.g., clenbuterol, albuterol) dilate narrowed airways. Local treatment using an AeroMask provides effective treatment while minimizing possible side effects. However, this method is expensive because inhalers for human patients are used. It also requires a dedicated caregiver initially giving medications a few times daily. Systemic steroids are effective, but have been associated with laminitis in horses. Horses with heaves require management changes, close monitoring, and early treatment at onset of clinical signs, but can live comfortably for a long time if treated properly.

LAMINITIS (FOUNDER)

Laminitis is a devastating, sometimes fatal disease in young and older horses. Although there has been extensive research, the pathophysiology of laminitis is not clear. It may be acute or chronic in nature, and all four feet may be affected or just one or two feet. Ultimately the soft tissue in the foot (laminas) holding the bone (distal phalanx, or P3) and hoof wall together becomes inflamed and necrotic. The horse may initially develop separation of the hoof wall from the bone. In severe cases, the bone will rotate, sink, and penetrate the bottom of the foot (sole), necessitating euthanasia. Laminitis may be a complication from a primary problem (e.g., postcolic surgery) or develop acutely with no apparent cause. However, laminitis most commonly occurs in the geriatric horse from Cushing disease. Some breeds are more prone to developing laminitis (e.g., quarter horse, ponies). Laminitis is a painful condition because the horse is standing on the affected foot and often cannot find relief from pain. Clinical signs of laminitis include reluctance to walk and turn, bounding digital arterial pulses (palpated over the fetlock near the sesamoid bones), rings on the hoof wall, depression, and inappetence resulting from discomfort. Diagnostic tests include radiographs of the feet and additional tests to diagnose the inciting cause. If the inciting cause is identified, treatment is directed at the disease. For example, if Cushing disease is diagnosed, treatment with pergolide is paramount to control laminitis. Treatment for laminitis is often symptomatic and includes shoeing changes (e.g., blunting the toe), footpads, deep bedding in the stall (e.g., sand), and NSAIDs (e.g., phenylbutazone). It is ideal if the horse will lie down to relieve pressure from affected feet. Laminitis may be acute or chronic; geriatric horses often develop chronic laminitis and require regular foot care every 4 weeks to minimize clinical signs. Recovery can be complete, or there may be permanent damage of the laminas, so long-term care is directed at the individual patient.

SINUSITIS

Chronic sinusitis is common in older horses with Cushing disease because of immunosuppression. One or more sinuses may be affected. Clinical signs include purulent, unilateral nasal discharge, and a reddish color may be present. Percussing the sinuses in the middle of the horse's head will elicit a dull sound, indicating fluid accumulation. Diagnostic tests include an oral examination to look for tooth root abscessation, upper airway endoscopy, skull radiographs, and evaluation for Cushing disease. Treatment includes long-term antimicrobials, flushing the sinuses under general anesthetic, removal of an infected tooth root, and pergolide if Cushing disease is present.

DENTAL PROBLEMS

Geriatric horses often develop dental disease as they age. As their teeth wear down or fall out, the opposing tooth will become too long or develop points (sharp areas on the tooth). This causes abnormal occlusion, and the horse will not be able to chew properly. The most severe abnormality is called wave mouth. The horse will have abnormal occlusion of all teeth and extreme difficulty chewing food. Wave mouth is a common problem in geriatric horses. Clinical signs of oral abnormalities include poor body condition, slow chewing, dropping a lot of grain or hay from the mouth, discomfort when chewing, and whole grain in manure. A thorough dental examination should be performed at least annually on horses 20 years or older to prevent oral abnormalities. When proper dental care is provided, many older horses are able to chew their food well and maintain their body condition.

EQUINE RECURRENT UVEITIS (ERU OR MOON BLINDNESS)

Geriatric horses often develop eye problems, and the leading cause of blindness in horses is equine recurrent uveitis. It is a progressive disease causing frequent episodes of inflammation and degeneration in one or both eyes. Some breeds, such as appaloosas, are more commonly affected. Clinical signs include a swollen and painful eye, photophobia, corneal edema (blue tint to cornea), corneal abrasion or ulceration, miosis (constricted pupillae), neovascularization (blood vessel growth on cornea), anterior uveitis (inflammation in the front chamber of the eye), hypopyon (cellular debris in the eye), and hyphema (hemorrhage in the eye). A horse with a swollen, painful eye is treated as an emergency because the cornea is thin (1.5 mm thick) with no blood supply and the eye can rupture if not treated quickly. Horses also live in a contaminated environment and can develop fungal ulcers that can be resistant to therapy. Diagnostic evaluation includes sedating the horse to perform a thorough ophthalmologic examination, applying fluorescein stain to evaluate the cornea for ulceration, and taking samples for cytology and culture. When a corneal ulcer is present, the damaged corneal epithelium will stain bright green, showing the extent of the ulcer. Both eyes should be evaluated because many geriatric horses will have cataracts and degenerative retinal changes. If the horse lacks vision in the clinically unaffected eye and the other eye is swollen and painful, the horse may be scared and react differently than normal. Treatment depends on if there are primarily inflammatory changes or if a corneal ulcer is present. If no ulcer is present, topical steroids (e.g., dexamethasone, prednisolone) and other medications (atropine, serum, systemic NSAIDs, such as flunixin meglumine) are used to eliminate inflammation and dilate the pupil. If an ulcer is present, topical antimicrobials and other medications (atropine, serum, systemic NSAIDs, such as flunixin meglumine) are used until the ulcer resolves, and then steroids can be used. Mild cases can be treated with topical ointments or solutions. Severe cases require frequent treatment that is difficult in a horse with a painful eye, so a subpalpebral catheter can be placed for ease of treatment. Sometimes surgery is also required to aid healing. Once the episode has resolved, preventative treatment, such as using a fly mask and antiinflammatory medications, are often needed to minimize additional inflammatory flares. Enucleation (removing the affected eye) is the last resort in older horses since both eyes are often affected. Without treatment, the horse will be in pain and the affected eye will become smaller over time.

NEUROLOGIC DEFICITS

Older horses can develop mild or progressive neurologic deficits as a result of trauma or chronic changes, such as cervical fractures compressing the spinal cord. Clinical signs in an affected horse include depression, decreased proprioception, dragging toes, ataxia, and reluctance to turn his neck. Diagnostic tests include a thorough physical and neurologic examination, blood tests including liver function tests, cervical radiographs, and cerebrospinal fluid aspiration. Treatment includes antiinflammatory medications and small paddock turnout and stall confinement, if needed. These horses are often weak and may lose their position in the hierarchy. Therefore it is important to place them with other horses in similar condition and to feed them individually to ensure that they are receiving adequate nutrition.

MUSCULOSKELETAL SYSTEM

Geriatric horses often have multiple sites of DJD (osteoarthritis) and can be lame at the walk and trot. The hocks, carpi, cervical vertebrae, and pelvis are most commonly affected. Soft tissue problems include degeneration of the suspensory tendon. Diagnostic tests include lameness examination, local anesthetic for nerve blocks, sonographic evaluation, and radiographs to identify the affected areas. Treatment includes local joint injection of steroids to relieve clinical signs, but cannot be repeated too many times. Many of these horses require long-term NSAIDs (e.g., phenylbutazone) to have a good quality of life. Monitoring the horse using diagnostic tests, such as chemistry profile, packed-cell volume (PCV) and total protein, and urinalysis, is an important part of using these medications. Although there are side effects with chronic NSAID use, such as renal insufficiency or right dorsal colitis, it is also paramount to keep these geriatric horses comfortable at the end of their lives. There is a new NSAID, firocoxib, that is promising because it is a COX-2 inhibitor with minimal side effects, sparing gastric mucosal protection and renal blood flow. Pasture turnout as much as possible is important because older horses become stiff when standing in the stall for too long. Regular foot trimming every 4 weeks and shoes are often vital to maintain the horse's comfort.

> *TECHNICIAN NOTE* Geriatric horses often have multiple problems that require careful monitoring and treatment to ensure optimal health.

MANAGEMENT, NUTRITION, AND NURSING CARE OF THE GERIATRIC HORSE

Management of the aged horse is paramount to maintaining optimal health and keeping the horse comfortable. Frequent hoof trimming every 4 weeks is important to maintain the horse's comfort, especially when he has DJD and lameness. If the horse's foot grows too long, it changes the angle of the leg and makes walking more difficult. Routine dental floating every 6 months will keep the horse comfortable, eating well, and prevent problems, such as a wave mouth.

It is notoriously difficult to maintain weight and body condition in older horses. It is especially difficult to improve a horse's condition if he has lost weight or is already thin.

There are additional considerations in treating geriatric horses. These horses seem more sensitive to certain medications, such as sedation and NSAIDs. It may be a combination of decreased muscle mass and renal and/or liver insufficiency, but many geriatric horses only tolerate one half of a typical dose of sedative given intravenously. For example, only give 75 mg xylazine and 1 mg butorphanol *or* 2 mg detomidine and 1 mg butorphanol to an average 450-kg (1000 lb) horse. Some older horses are sensitive to NSAIDs, such as flunixin meglumine or phenylbutazone, and only tolerate one half of a typical dose given intravenously. For example, give 250 mg flunixin meglumine or 1 gram phenylbutazone to an average 450-kg (1000 lb) horse. Many of these horses receive daily NSAID treatment for chronic DJD (osteoarthritis). They may receive 1 g of phenylbutazone orally daily for a few years and without medication are in significant pain. When administering NSAID medication, the owner should be aware of potential side effects, such as renal failure or right dorsal colitis. It is important to monitor the horse's attitude, appetite, manure production, renal values (creatinine, blood urea nitrogen [BUN]), urinalysis, and PCV and total protein. If there are any changes in these values, the patient and treatment protocol should be reassessed.

General management recommendations include regular deworming, either daily or every 8 weeks using dewormers on a rotational schedule. Frequent manure removal and low stocking density (e.g., a few horses in a large pasture) are important to minimize parasite burden in a pasture. Regular fecal examinations are helpful to assess if the deworming schedule is adequate. It is not uncommon to have a false-negative test result from fecal examination, but the horse has a parasite burden, so regular deworming is important even if the fecal examination test result is negative.

Regular vaccination is recommended, using the recommended vaccine protocol for the area. If a horse has a history of vaccine reactions, pretreatment with an NSAID, such as phenylbutazone or flunixin meglumine, is recommended. Many horses develop more severe reactions over time, so geriatric horses with a history of vaccine reaction are at higher risk. If the horse still has a reaction despite pretreatment, only the necessary vaccines should be administered to minimize complications. Annual physical examinations are important to maintain the health of a geriatric horse and to detect any problems. Many geriatric horses seem to develop renal and liver insufficiency over time, so annual blood tests (e.g., CBC, chemistry profile) are important to monitor their health.

Management is paramount to maintaining a healthy geriatric horse. Geriatric horses can have a good quality of life with proper care, but require close monitoring. Many are turned out in pasture and not monitored well. They may be in poor condition under a thick hair coat, so it is best to train the owner to assess the horse's body condition. Clipping older horses and placing a blanket in the winter keep these older horses comfortable. Geriatric horses with an overlong hair coat are not able to thermoregulate well, may have patchy sweating, and be prone to develop dermatitis. It is also advisable to clip over the jugular vein before administering intravenous medications to easily visualize the vein and avoid the carotid artery. Frequent pasture turnout is ideal to maintain body condition, GI tract health, and minimize stiffness. It is also important to turn the geriatric horse out with other horses in equal condition. Otherwise, the older horse will be at the bottom of the hierarchy and may not have adequate access to food. If the older horse is in poor body condition, feeding him individually is important to ensure that the horse is receiving enough food and assess appetite. Feeding free-choice high-quality hay with supplementation of alfalfa (either hay or soaked alfalfa cubes or pellets) will aid in maintaining weight. Feeding an Equine Senior feed is also good to maintain weight or provide calories when the horse has lost teeth. Adding corn oil (¼ to ½ cup per day) to the feed provides additional calories.

END OF LIFE ISSUES

When a geriatric horse is no longer living a good quality of life, euthanasia may be considered by the owner and/or recommended by the veterinarian. Considerations for euthanasia include poor body condition or rapidly losing weight, refractory pain (e.g., acute, severe laminitis), and severe DJD, leading to chronic, severe lameness. Additional considerations include episodes of the horse falling frequently and impending cold weather. Cold weather, snow, and icy conditions are difficult times for older horses to maintain body condition. If the horse slips on the ice, it may be impossible to lift the horse up again, necessitating euthanasia. These geriatric horses have often been a part of the family for years, and the entire family would like to be present for the horse's final moments. A scheduled euthanasia can allow the family to say goodbye and offer a peaceful end to a beloved horse.

Geriatric horses have many good years ahead of them if properly cared for and closely monitored. They often make excellent companions to younger horses and provide much enjoyment for their owners. When problems arise, they need to be detected quickly and treatment initiated to offer optimal quality of life for the geriatric equine patient. The veterinary technician plays an integral role in caring for these patients by educating clients, providing thorough nursing care, and recognizing and addressing the needs of these special patients.

CONCLUSION

There are numerous ways that we, as members of the veterinary community, can contribute to the health and well-being of our veterinary patients. As pets continue to be considered family members by more and more people, there will be a continued need for home and barn support for these patients. Technicians can play a large role in providing hospice care for these patients. It is important to remember that hospice care should be provided only while the animal maintains a good quality of life. Once quality of life declines, euthanasia should be considered.

CASE PRESENTATION 37-2

A 32-year-old quarter horse mare appeared depressed and inappetent, so the owner called her equine veterinarian and veterinary technician (Figure 1). On physical examination, the mare had poor body condition (body score 4/9), hirsutism, a wave mouth, and rings on the dorsal hoof wall of her front feet. Initial blood work was performed, and no abnormalities were present. Samples were also submitted for ACTH, insulin, and dextrose. Samples were drawn three times in one day (AM, noon, PM), and dextrose was performed stall side using a dextrometer. Insulin levels were within normal limits, but dextrose was more than 200 mg/dl for each sample, and ACTH levels were greater than 300 for each sample. The mare was diagnosed with Cushing disease and treatment started (1 mg PO s.i.d. pergolide). She was sedated with 2 mg detomidine and 1 mg butorphanol IV for a thorough dental float to correct the wave mouth. Radiographs were taken of her front feet that showed chronic laminitic changes, but minimal rotation of P3 (coffin bone). Her feet were in poor condition, so the farrier trimmed her feet and agreed to return every 4 weeks. Her diet was evaluated, and her ration of Equine Senior was increased with ¼ cup corn oil added daily. The owner also clipped the mare and agreed to place a blanket on her in the winter. Within a week after starting pergolide treatment, the mare became much more active and bright. She nickered to everyone who came to her stall and ate readily, no longer dropping grain from her mouth. She began to play with the other horses again. After 3 months on her new diet, she was in better condition (grade 6/9), and the grateful owner was happy to have her beloved horse back (Figure 2).

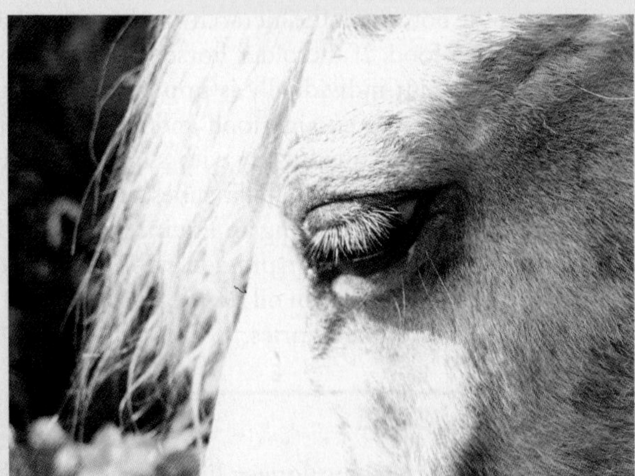

FIGURE 1 Depressed geriatric mare with hirsutism.

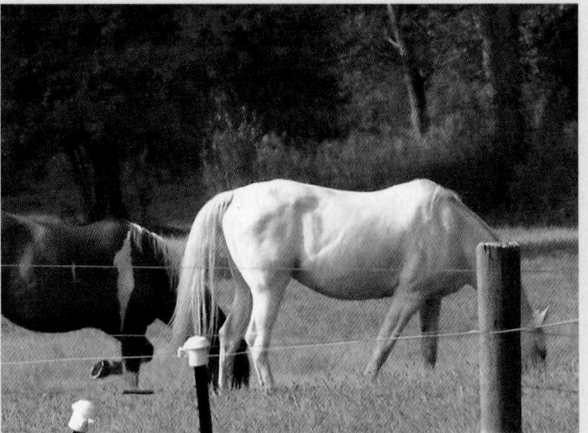

FIGURE 2 A picture of good health.

RECOMMENDED READING

Geriatric Horses

Couetil L, Paradis MR, Knoll J: Plasma adrenocorticotropin concentration in healthy horses and in horses with clinical signs of hyperadrenocorticism, *J Vet Intern Med* 10:1-6, 1996.

Donaldson MT: Equine Cushing's disease: diagnosis, treatment, pathogenesis and clinical signs, *Proc North Am Vet Conference*, 2004.

Donaldson MT, LaMonte BH, Morresey P et al: Treatment with pergolide or cyproheptadine of pituitary pars intermedia dysfunction (equine Cushing's disease), *J Vet Intern Med* 16:742-746, 2002.

Dybdal NO: Endocrine disorders. In Bradford, Smith, eds: *Large animal internal medicine*, ed 3, St Louis, 2002, Mosby.

Dybdal NO, Hargreaves KM, Madigan JE, et al: Diagnostic testing for pituitary pars intermedia dysfunction in horses, *J Am Vet Med Assoc* 204:627-632, 1994.

Perkins G, Lamb S, Erb H, et al: Plasma adrenocorticotropin (ACTH) concentrations and clinical response in horses treated for equine Cushing disease with cyproheptadine or pergolide, *Equine Vet J* 34:679-685, 2002.

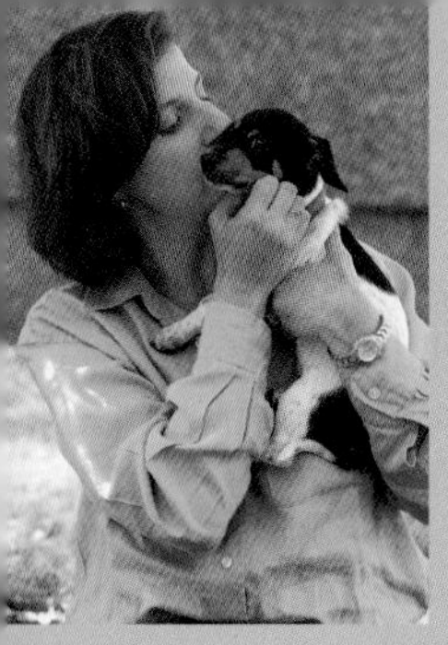

The Human-Animal Bond, Bereavement, and Euthanasia

38

Joseph Taboada and Stephanie W. Johnson

KEY TERMS

Anger
Barbiturate
Bargaining
Bereavement
Catharsis
Compassion
Denial
Depression
Drug Enforcement Agency (DEA)
Grief process
Resolution

OUTLINE

LEARNING OBJECTIVES

When you have completed this chapter, you will be able to:

1. Discuss the aspects of strong attachments to animals.
2. List and describe the stages of grief and the role of veterinary professionals in grief counseling.
3. Discuss the impact of euthanasia and client grief on members of the veterinary health care team.
4. Discuss the legal and ethical issues related to euthanasia.
5. Describe the factors that owners consider when making decisions regarding euthanasia of their pet.
6. Discuss the role of the veterinary health care team in counseling owners considering euthanasia of their pet.
7. Describe considerations in scheduling euthanasia appointments and when preparing for unexpected events during euthanasia.
8. List and describe acceptable methods of euthanasia in animals.
9. List signs and symptoms of staff burnout.
10. Discuss special considerations related to euthanasia of large animals.

INTRODUCTION

Today, with more than 71.1 million households owning one or more companion animals, pets are considered part of the extended family network.* Surveys and clinical experience indicate that many people consider their pets to be like children, partners, or best friends. Because of changing family structure and an increasing number of persons who live alone, companion animals have taken on larger roles in people's support systems. With these changes have come added expectations of veterinary health care professionals. Members of the veterinary medical profession must realize that they are not treating just dogs, cats, birds, rabbits, or horses, but important members of their clients' family and an important part of their clients' support system (Figure 38-1).

*American Pet Product Manufacturers Survey, March, 2004.

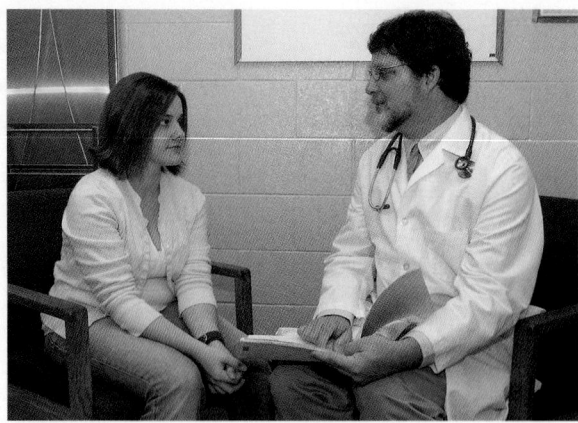

FIGURE 38-1 The diagnosis of a disease can be a difficult time for both clients and veterinary professionals. It is important to respond to both the pet and the owner's needs.

THE HUMAN-ANIMAL BOND

Today modern society is largely urban rather than rural. Through world urbanization, people tend to live in neighborhoods rather than on farms. Animals live with their owners in apartments or houses, thus increasing familiarity, dependency, and bonding. Eighty percent of our animal companions live inside.

Companion animals provide both parents and children with stability, constancy, and security. It is not unusual for families to change locales and residences several times within a 10-year period. As a result, most people no longer live within a short distance of their extended families. The nuclear family is smaller, consisting of an average of less than two children. The single-parent family is becoming common. Because an increasing number of U.S. women work outside the home, many school-age children return home to be greeted not by their mother but by the family pet. An increasing number of adults live alone, and couples opt to remain childless. More and more people are filling these voids with pets that provide a unique outlet for their owners' needs to nurture and be loved. As health and medical care improves, the number of persons in the age group older than 60 years has increased to more than 16% of the population. Pets fulfill many needs for elderly people, including needs for interaction, exercise, companionship, protection, and motivation to remain active and independent.

It is becoming increasingly recognized that physically and mentally disabled individuals benefit from contact with animals. As society has realized the special talents of pets, new utilitarian functions have been found for them. Dogs are used with success to assist blind, hearing impaired, and physically challenged persons. These specially trained animals provide their owners with independence, companionship, social lubrication, protection, and love. Horses, cats, and dogs have been used successfully in animal-assisted therapy programs for people with all types of physical and mental disabilities. Animals facilitate interaction with people who may be reluctant to interact, and their presence reduces anxiety, lowers blood pressure, and decreases heart rate. Results of some studies indicate that animals may alleviate or prevent depression. Survival rates for cardiac patients who are pet owners are higher than for those who do not own pets. Pet ownership is considered an important predictor of survival for patients with coronary artery disease.

In short, the relationships between people and animals have become physically closer, and the role of animals in the daily lives of their owners has become more emotional as society has changed. Of the more than 71.1 million families owning at least one pet, one third of companion animal pet owners describe their pets as family members and cite companionship, love, affection, and fun as the most important derivatives of the relationship. Further, it has been shown that 83% of pet owners refer to themselves as mom or dad; 93% buy their pet gifts; 84% treat them as children; and 63% say, "I love you" at least once daily to their pets.

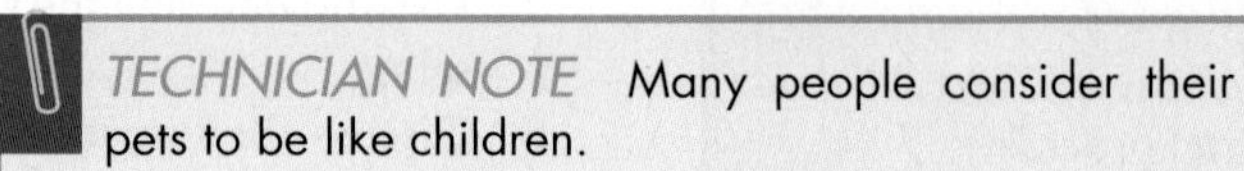

TECHNICIAN NOTE Many people consider their pets to be like children.

THE ATTACHMENT BETWEEN ANIMALS AND HUMANS

Strong attachments can form between owners and any type of animal, but are probably recognized most commonly in veterinary practice with dogs, cats, and horses. The degree of attachment varies greatly from the utilitarian attachment between a rancher and his or her cattle to the parent-child type of bonding that occurs between some people and their dog or cat. In 2007, 63% of the 133.7 million households in the United States own at least one pet. It is estimated that about 50% of these pet owners classify their attachment to their pet as strong. Of these "strong attachment" owners, about half see their pets as reflections of themselves or of their tastes that depend on the owner for love, affection, and care. The other half of the strong attachment owners report a reliance on their pets as an emotional crutch, supplying unconditional love and affection and sometimes acting as a substitute for family, friends, or children.

As pets are used to meet many of the changing psychosocial needs of modern society, the intensity of attachment has increased. When pet loss occurs, intensity and duration of attachment determine the significance of the loss and intensity of grief that follows. Attachment is more intense when the animal has functioned in many roles for the owner. The owner of an assistance dog may therefore suffer more intense bereavement than the owner of a dog used only for herding or hunting. Owners who have experienced previous significant losses, adjustments, or traumas and have been comforted by their pet's presence may also exhibit strong attachment and thus intense bereavement.

> *TECHNICIAN NOTE* If a pet is associated with an important person or significant life stage or event, it can take on added significance.

BENEFITS OF ATTACHMENT

As reminders of both pleasant and traumatic events in people's lives, pets can take on symbolic meaning. There are several keys that are helpful in assessing the level of attachment between an owner and his or her animal or animals (Box 38-1). Even when the pet is simply another family member, grief can be intense. Grief is also individual, and each family member may grieve in a unique way.

PET LOSS AND VETERINARY MEDICINE

Veterinarians and veterinary technicians are confronted daily with complex issues of attachment, loss, and grief in the course of their patients' illness and death. The diagnosis of life-threatening or terminal disease can be a difficult time for both the client and the veterinary professional (see Figure 38-1).

> *TECHNICIAN NOTE* Veterinary technicians are confronted daily with complex issues of attachment, loss, and grief.

Considering all the emotional and utilitarian aspects of the human-animal relationship in modern society, it is not surprising that the breaking of the bond because of the death of the pet is a significant event in the lives of many pet owners. The loss of the pet for many owners is made even more intense and personal in that the pet is often grieved by no one other than themselves. Daily routines are filled with reminders of activities once performed for or with the pet. The loss of a pet often means that a unique, irreplaceable member of the family is gone.

BOX 38-1 Keys to Attachment

The levels of attachment are different for each pet and owner. Human-animal relationships may be perceived as stronger and more important when the following aspects are present:

- Owners believe that they rescued their companion animals from death or near death.
- Owners believe that their companion animals got them through a difficult period in life.
- Owners spent their childhoods with their companion animals.
- Owners have relied on their companion animals as their most significant source of support.
- Owners anthropomorphize their companion animals.
- Owners have invested extensive time, effort, or financial resources into their companion animals' long-term medical care.
- Owners view their companion animals as symbolic links to significant people who are no longer part of their lives or to significant times in their lives.

A person's support system is made up of people (and pets) that interact with one another on a daily basis, providing support, comfort, and social interaction. Support systems are especially important during times of loss. Unfortunately, many people who make up these support systems do not understand the full extent of attachment between a pet owner and pet. This lack of understanding can present serious problems for the owner facing the odyssey of grief after the death of a pet. As a result, pet owners often turn to veterinary professionals as sources of support, comfort, and understanding at and around the time of their pet's death.

> *TECHNICIAN NOTE* People tend to turn to the veterinary staff during grief over a pet because they believe that the veterinary technician understands their attachment and loss.

The tendency for people to turn to the veterinary staff during the period of grieving the death of a pet places veterinary professionals in an awkward position. It demands that they have knowledge that is typically outside the boundaries of traditional veterinary medicine and requires that they find a comfort level in talking about death and the grief process. This is why the areas of attachment, animal behavior, human bereavement, and grief counseling are becoming increasingly relevant to veterinary medicine.

WHEN THE BOND IS BROKEN

In general, people in U.S. society are uncomfortable talking about death. We know little about the experience of death, and we fear the unknown, yet veterinarians and their staff must frequently discuss death, participate in causing it, witness it, and deal with the emotions triggered by these experiences.

Although people in the midst of grief have a need and a right to understand what is happening to them, there are few places that they can go to get helpful, supportive information about grief. This is particularly true when the loss that they are grieving is that of a beloved pet. Like most of society, veterinarians and veterinary technicians rarely have formal training in this area. Despite this fact, veterinary professionals are still often the people clients instinctively turn to for support.

Making the job more difficult is the fact that grief and bereavement are emotional and often irrational areas of human interaction. Bereaved individuals may at times seem out of control or out of touch with reality. When this happens, those around the griever, including the veterinary professional, may feel uncomfortable; few veterinary professionals are taught how to support or deal with people who are irrational or emotional. Compassion is an important sensitivity to draw on when interacting with clients experiencing grief.

Grief is the companion to death. It is the mental anguish experienced by any human confronted with the loss of an object of attachment. Grief may ensue as an effect of any loss; the loss may be through death, divorce, loss of a job, or even moving or having friends move away. It can be intensely emotional and can affect mind, body, and spirit. When confronted with grief, the bereaved individual goes through a grief process. The term grief process implies that there is an intended end or result to be produced through grieving. Thus the grief process is the means of letting go of the object of attachment to feel better, reinvest, emotionally grow, and attach again.

The veterinary staff is in a unique position to assist clients going through the process of grief as it relates to the loss of a pet. By way of their unique role in the life of both the owner and pet, veterinary professionals are in a unique position to understand the bond that had developed. In addition, the veterinarian and the owner may have interacted uniquely in choosing the time of the pet's death (as occurs when euthanasia is performed). To assist clients during the difficult bereavement period, it is helpful to understand the normal grief process and its manifestations as applied to pet loss.

PET LOSS AND THE GRIEF PROCESS

The death of a pet is all too often regarded as a trivial loss by society perhaps in part because of the mistaken belief that pets can be easily replaced. There are no socially sanctioned rituals, such as funerals or memorial services, to help grieving pet owners gain support once the bonds between them and their animals have been broken. Further, people are rarely granted time off from their jobs to care for sick animals or to make arrangements for them after their deaths. Society also does not allow adequate time for mourning the death of a pet. Most people feel pressured to be "back to normal" within a few days of their pet's death to avoid being labeled as neurotic, hysteric, or overly attached. However, crying, taking time away from work, and wanting to memorialize a pet are healthy responses to the death of a pet. They should not be discouraged, nor should they be judged.

One of the most effective ways for veterinary professionals to assist grieving clients is to educate and reassure them that their feelings and behaviors are normal parts of the grief process. Other ways that veterinary professionals can help are listed in Box 38-2.

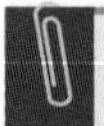

TECHNICIAN NOTE Veterinary professionals can assist clients by normalizing their feelings.

THE NORMAL GRIEF PROCESS

As stated earlier, the word process implies movement toward some end or result. In regard to grief, this movement is accomplished by passing through what have been termed stages, phases, or tasks. Although there are a few differences, the basic emotional process in pet loss is the same as in human loss.

Several models of the grief process can be modified to describe the emotional process that occurs during pet loss. The following discussion uses the classic model supplied by Elisabeth Kübler-Ross (see Recommended Reading).

Dr. Kübler-Ross was one of the first to work extensively with dying persons and their families during the late 1960s. She described the grief process as consisting of five stages: denial, bargaining, anger, depression, and resolution. She used the stages to describe the passage through grief, but it is helpful to remember that these stages are not a linear odyssey. Although people may travel through the grief process in a straight line, they more often fluctuate between stages, bounce back and forth, and feel the entire gamut of grief within minutes, days, or months.

TECHNICIAN NOTE The grief process consists of five stages: denial, bargaining, anger, depression, and resolution.

Denial and Bargaining

Denial is a normal defense mechanism that buffers humans from some unbearable news or reality. It is important to recognize the word normal here because many individuals experiencing denial at the time a poor prognosis is given or during bereavement will seem to all observers to be out of touch with reality. The veterinary staff may wonder whether

CASE PRESENTATION 38-1

Sneaky, a 12-year-old female domestic shorthair cat, is brought into the practice for lethargy and anorexia. After a work-up, she is diagnosed as having cardiomyopathy. Even with appropriate treatment, the prognosis for a long lifetime is poor.

Sneaky is owned by a 73-year-old widow named Ruth. The cat was a gift from her husband, Ralph, who died of cancer 2 years earlier. During her husband's fight against the disease, Sneaky was his constant companion. Ruth can still vividly remember how Sneaky, as a kitten, used to make her husband laugh by hiding in his boots and jumping out at him when he leaned down to pick them up.

Sneaky was brought to the veterinarian for what was perceived to be a minor problem, but a severe, life-threatening disease was diagnosed. Ruth is likely to feel numb initially. The diagnosis is likely to be hard to accept. An important part of Ruth's attachment to Sneaky comes from her relationship with her late husband. Sneaky represents a tangible link between Ruth's life now and the many memories of her life with her husband. Not only is Sneaky's death going to be hard because of the loss of a faithful companion and family member, but it is also going to bring back many of the emotions that were associated with the death of her husband.

BOX 38-2 Stages of Grief: How Veterinary Professionals Can Help

Denial

What the client needs most is time, support, understanding, and permission to grieve.

Before Death

- Arrange to communicate with the client in person, if possible, where you both can sit down to talk without interruption or distraction. Recognize denial as a normal part of grief.
- Communicate clearly and reiterate patiently. Phrase statements in words that are concrete and simple for the layperson. Avoid using medical jargon and lapsing into complicated medical explanations.
- Listen actively: maintain eye contact, use attentive body language, and paraphrase or clarify the client's statements as you respond. Give him or her permission to express feelings.
- Give the client time to think about and to grasp the reality of information that has been given. Some clients need only a slight pause in the conversation or a few minutes alone. Other clients may need more time to themselves before they comprehend the news of severe illness or actual death.
- Refrain from judging the client as "stupid" or "out of it."
- Remain nonjudgmental and unhurried toward the client, and state that you are available to talk about specifics or about his or her feelings whenever the time is right.
- Never attempt to force clients to "come to their senses" or to move out of denial. Clients will comprehend at their own pace.

After Death

- Encourage the client to view the body and say goodbye.
- Give permission to grieve.

Bargaining

- Understand that bargaining is an attempt to control or reverse a dire situation. The client feels irrationally compelled to bargain during the grief process and does not mean to doubt the professionals involved.
- When the patient is terminally ill, do not become defensive or threatened when clients ask for other opinions or consider alternative treatments. Giving information, readings, and referral for second opinion will ameliorate bargaining attempts and facilitate commitment to treatment.
- After the death, be empathetic and educate about the stage of bargaining when clients confide their feelings and bargaining behaviors, such as prayers and dreams (or daydreams) of the pet still alive. Reassure them that the emotional basis for their behaviors and feelings is normal even though it may seem irrational.
- When clients inquire as to when to "replace" their pet, educating them about the role bargaining plays in shopping for a new pet can alleviate future disappointment. State that their dead pet was unique and cannot be replaced, but encourage them to obtain a new pet whenever all members of the family feel ready. Help them to find the type of animal that they are looking for while gently steering toward one that is slightly dissimilar to the dead pet. Encourage them to choose a different breed, color, or gender, and a new name should be chosen.

Anger

- Listen actively, and let the client know that you understand.
- Arrange for communication in a private room with no distractions. Sit at eye level, and use attentive body language. Take notes if the client is complaining or criticizing.
- Give the client permission to vent feelings. Listen actively using attentive body language, eye contact, nodding, and responses that paraphrase, clarify, and indicate your understanding of the client's feelings (e.g., "I can see that you're angry. . . .," or "You feel that diagnosis could have been made sooner. . . .").
- If the client is directly angry at the veterinarian, technician, or clinic staff, take a mental step backward and pause with either a deep breath or by counting to 10.
- Do not become defensive or respond in like manner to the client.
- Relieve guilt by assuring the client that he or she did the right thing and what he or she is feeling is a normal part of the grief process.

Depression

- Encourage depressed clients to talk about their feelings in regard to their pet. Follow up with clients whose pets have died with a telephone call in a few days and then 2 weeks afterward.
- Listen actively.
- Attend to the client by positioning yourself at eye level, offering tissues or a drink of water, and leaning slightly toward the client. A nonthreatening yet compassionate touch on the forearm or on the shoulder communicates empathy and understanding.
- Offer a place to sit, a place to be out of the "public eye."
- Tell the client that it is all right and even good to cry. Listen supportively and actively, and touch the client gently on the shoulder or forearm. Some clients are known well enough to embrace, and this can be helpful.
- Validate the feelings of sadness by letting the client know that it is normal.
- Offer to call a family member or friend.
- Encourage and suggest means by which clients can memorialize their pet. Making scrapbooks, planting a tree, writing a letter to the pet, or writing the pet's life story all are cathartic activities that alleviate depression caused by grief.
- If a client expresses continued depression several weeks following the death of a pet, if his or her support system is poor, or if a client expresses a personal wish to die, referral to a compassionate professional counselor is necessary. Although referral may feel awkward, many clients appreciate the technician who states, "Grief as a result of pet loss is normal, but sometimes there can be no one to talk to or the grief can be overwhelming. I know of a person who understands what you're going through. Would you like her (his) telephone number, or may I have her (him) call you?" Today, several schools of veterinary medicine employ counselors experienced in pet loss. Many communities have established support groups, and private counselors increasingly view pet loss as significant bereavement.

Continued

BOX 38-2 Stages of Grief: How Veterinary Professionals Can Help—cont'd

Resolution

- Acceptance is achieved once the previous four stages have fallen into the background of the client's life. At this point, the bereaved person can channel emotional energy into a new relationship. The veterinary professional can help clients reach the resolution stage by offering insight into the grief process through his or her actions and by offering suggestions of reading material or seminars on the grief process.

the client has even heard the veterinarian stating the seriousness of an animal's illness. A client in denial may listen attentively to a diagnosis of cancer with a poor prognosis, but ask only if the toenails can be clipped or if their current flea shampoo is correct. A client informed of the death of his or her pet while it was hospitalized may chatter on about activities for the weekend. A simple form of denial is exemplified by the client who states repeatedly, "It can't be. I don't believe it."

It is tempting when presented with a client experiencing denial to insist that he or she recognize the seriousness of the situation. Many veterinarians and veterinary technicians worry that the client does not comprehend or has not heard correctly. There is no harm in repeating oneself to a client in denial (Figure 38-2). Restating diagnoses, prognoses, treatment plans, and particulars is advisable. However, clients in denial will accept the unbearable reality of the situation only when they are ready internally; attempts to push them may backfire, resulting in frustration. Usually a client will begin to ask appropriate questions about the time he or she arrives home and may telephone the veterinary office. Some may even seem to return to reality before your eyes while those toenails are attended to. The veterinary professional must be assured that the client has been told the basic information that needs to be given. Remember, however, that it may not have been fully understood; therefore always leave the door open for further communication.

Denial is reflected by the client's eyes and demeanor and by incongruous questions. The veterinary staff should not believe that they are responsible to "break through" a client's denial. The client will move out of denial, accepting the reality of the situation, when he or she is ready. The veterinary staff's recognition of the client's denial can prevent impatience and frustration during the veterinary contact.

TECHNICIAN NOTE During denial the veterinary professional should repeat things without becoming frustrated or impatient.

Once the reality of death or impending death is realized, the client may show various impotent attempts to control or to reverse the reality. The client is grappling with the stage of the grief process that Dr. Kübler-Ross called bargaining. During this stage, the client maneuvers personally and privately, possibly praying and negotiating with God for miracles. The client might add various herbs and old family remedies to food. Children behave like little angels, hoping to be rewarded with a reversal of bad news. The veterinary staff may be subject to various inquiries by the client at this stage, relative to the latest "miracle cure" that the client has discovered on the Internet. It is while bargaining that a pet owner may also request permission to obtain a second (and sometimes third, fourth, or fifth) opinion. During this time be compassionate, and when possible answer clients' questions. Help clients to understand that this stage of grief is normal.

Seeking to replace the lost animal without grieving at all is a form of bargaining. Many pet owners seek a new pet too soon, and they purchase the same species, the same color, and name them the same or a similar name.

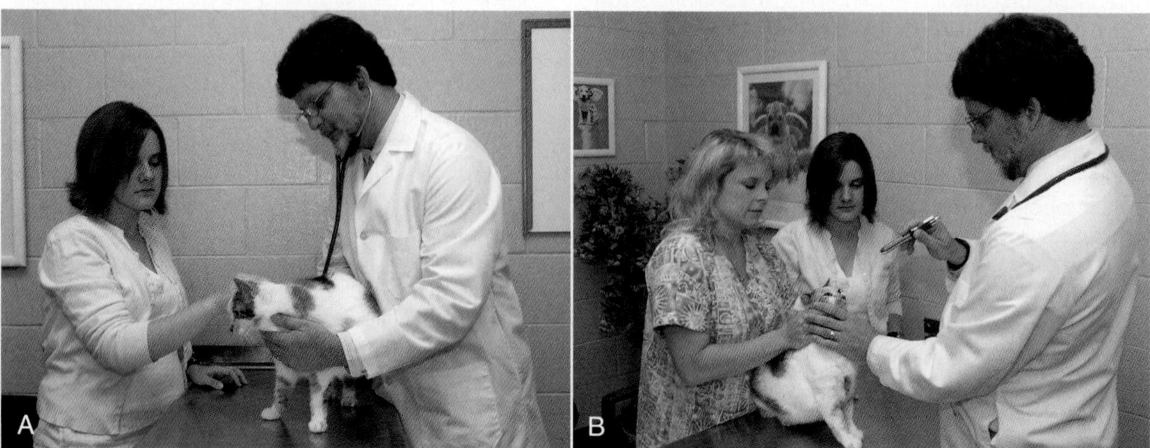

FIGURE 38-2 Even when dealing with attentive clients, veterinary professionals may be required to repeat themselves several times while clients decide on a course of treatment for their pet. Clients overwhelmed with emotion may have difficulty comprehending information regarding treatment or euthanasia decisions. Members of the team must be patient.

CASE PRESENTATION 38-2

Captain, a 9-year-old boxer, is brought into the practice for a checkup and vaccinations. His owner, Don, tells you that 1 year ago Captain was treated for lymphosarcoma. The cancer went into remission, and Captain has been doing fine ever since. However, it is obvious to you that Captain is not feeling well.

The examination shows the cancer has returned. It takes Don some time to accept that fact. It is agreed that treatment should start up again immediately. After a lack of response to a rescue phase of chemotherapy, it is clear that Captain's death is imminent. When the news is given to Don, he insists over and over again that the treatment should be continued. "If it worked before, it will work again—just keep on trying." If the treatment really is not working, Don believes changing Captain's diet to one he read about on the Internet will have better results.

Don brought Captain in for a routine examination. It was immediately obvious to you that Captain was not feeling well. However, Don either could not recognize any of the symptoms or was denying that Captain was sick again. Despite the fact that Don went into the initial treatment protocol knowing relapse was eventually inevitable, he still exhibits signs of denial. It is also obvious that he is not ready to accept Captain's impending death. It is important to realize Don's response is a normal part of the grief process. He will not be able to understand the seriousness of the situation until he is ready. Don also shows signs of bargaining when he wants other treatment options to be explored even though it is clear nothing can be done to save Captain at this point.

It is important to recognize denial and bargaining as part of the normal grief process. Veterinary professionals who understand these stages will avoid frustration in their attempts to provide quality patient care and client service.

Anger

During the grief process, clients may move in and out of the stage called anger. Clients coping with this stage may exhibit anger in a wide variety of direct or indirect manners. The anger may be specific or nonspecific in the way that it is directed. Anger may also be exhibited in the form of guilt, which can be defined as anger turned inward.

Anger is a particularly difficult emotion to deal with when a client directs it toward the veterinary professional. Regardless of whether or not the client is justified in his or her stated cause for anger, staff members must use tolerance and patience to avoid responding defensively. Bereaved clients may complain that the illness that resulted in death should have been discovered sooner, should have been treated differently, or should not have been allowed to happen. They may complain that their pet died while hospitalized because of neglect or inappropriate treatment rather than because of the tumor revealed by necropsy.

Anger may be apparent in the form of guilt. Clients feeling guilt use language with an abundance of "I should've" statements. They often seek the listening ear of the veterinary professional looking for absolution from guilt. They may ask whether the food that they fed their pet could have contributed to the illness or death. They often ask whether it was the pesticide in their home or in the shampoo that caused a tumor or cardiac arrest. Clients may believe that they allowed their pet to be too active or too fat; others may believe that they caused the kidney failure in their cat by feeding an insufficient diet. These clients can direct anger at themselves, but frequently they cannot find a specific crime that they committed. When possible, the veterinary professional can assist the clients by assuaging their guilt. Reassuring clients that, in your opinion, they did everything possible for their pet, that they did only what they thought would benefit their pet, and that they made the right decisions for their pet will relieve much of the clients' guilt or anger and assist them in moving through the grief process.

TECHNICIAN NOTE Veterinary professionals can help by reassuring clients that they did everything possible and made the right decisions.

The client in this stage may be gruff or rude and generally hard to get along with. Stating that he or she is angry, the client may be at a loss to express the object of the anger. These clients may yell at the cashiers, the hospital manager, the receptionist, the technicians, and the veterinarian. Giving the angry client an opportunity to express feelings (venting) is an effective way for the veterinary professional to help. At times, all that is needed is for the sensitive veterinary professional to explain that considering the client's loss, anger is a normal feeling.

Anger is often exhibited by reluctance to pay the bill. On receiving an inquiry by telephone, the client implies that nonpayment is due to anger at treatment by the veterinarian or technician, the pet was neglected, the illness was mistreated, or the client was treated insensitively. Bereavement support can alleviate this client's anger. Listen attentively, state your apologies, if any, and follow up with this client. No admission of mistakes need be made, but the client needs to feel significant and understood.

Anger is difficult to work through, but it is guilt that may be hardest for the client to relinquish. In continuing to feel guilt and anger, the client avoids letting go of the beloved pet, and the grief process is stymied. Once the client is able to relinquish the guilt or anger, the grief process can continue.

The veterinary professional can assist the client with all types of exhibited anger by taking a mental step back and a deep breath, committing to a nondefensive attitude, and simply listening. Take notes, if possible, and reassure the client of follow-up if anger is directed at veterinary staff. Assuage any guilt if the opportunity arises and allow the client to vent. A few minutes on the telephone or in person may salvage a client relationship and go a long way in assisting the client through the grief process.

CASE PRESENTATION 38-3

John brings Sparky, a 3-year-old Dalmatian, into the practice. Sparky got out of the yard this afternoon because the gate was left open. He ran across the street and was hit by a car. His spine is fractured, and there is severe injury to his spinal cord. There is also a substantial amount of internal bleeding.

John is informed that Sparky has only a slim chance of surviving surgery. He elects for any measure to be taken regardless of cost. Unfortunately, Sparky dies during the procedure. When you tell John, he immediately begins yelling at you, "How dare you let Sparky die? There must have been something else that could have been done!" He then refuses to pay the bill and storms out of the practice.

The next day John calls and apologizes for his rude outburst. He lets you know that he realizes that every measure was taken to save Sparky. He also admits to feeling guilty for having left the gate open. Then he requests that the bill be mailed to him.

John is expressing his anger over Sparky's death, which should be recognized as a stage of grief. Although John initially expressed his anger at you, it should not be taken personally. It is not necessarily directed at you. You should not react defensively, but instead listen politely and let John know that you empathize and understand. Realize that part of his anger may come from guilt that he left the gate open.

His call on the following day emphasizes that anger can be an uncomfortable but transient part of the grief process. He admits his anger was not really because of you. He attributes it to his feelings of guilt.

Depression

The stage of the grief process that is termed depression has also been called grief. Clients experiencing depression describe their mood as complete, overwhelming sadness. Intense grief can result in depression, which prohibits a client from functioning normally. Appetite is changed, energy level is lowered, the client withdraws from others, and sometimes the client is unable to go to work. More subtle symptoms of depression include irritability, sleep irregularity, restlessness, and inability to concentrate.

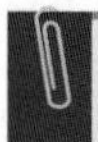

TECHNICIAN NOTE Depression has been described as complete, overwhelming sadness.

The veterinary professional has occasion to recognize depression as a result of pet loss when follow-up contacts are made with the client. Depression, when severe, usually sets in some time after the loss. Clients with poor social support systems, elderly clients, and clients with intense or symbolic attachment to the pet may experience worrisome depression.

TECHNICIAN NOTE Follow-up is important for those clients with poor support systems or unusual attachments.

When contacts are made several days or weeks after bereavement and it is suspected that a client is depressed, referral can be made to a counselor or hot line specializing in pet loss (Box 38-3). Although referral sometimes is awkward, it might be gently phrased as, "I know a person experienced in counseling people who have lost their pets." Reassurance that grief is normal is beneficial.

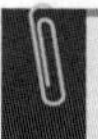

TECHNICIAN NOTE If severe depression is suspected, referral can be made to a counselor or hot line.

Most clients feel overwhelmed by their emotions because of grief. They describe feeling as if their emotions are out of control. They may also state surprise and worry that they are reacting with such intensity to the death of an animal. They may be embarrassed. It comforts clients when veterinary professionals confide that most pet owners feel and act similarly after the loss of a pet. Assuring them of your knowledge of their pet's importance and your respect for their grief is valuable to them.

Grief must be worked through, not avoided; thus it is a process requiring some emotional catharsis. Many clients cry, and some are uninhibited about expressing anger and sadness. Becoming comfortable with one's own emotions facilitates comfort with others' emotions. It is human and necessary to feel empathy for grieving clients, but it can also be uncomfortable and painful. Separating your own feelings from theirs will allow you to transform empathy into sympathetic gestures that help the client.

CASE PRESENTATION 38-4

Two weeks ago Micah brought her 10-year-old barrel racing horse, Lightning, to the practice. Lightning had colic. Every possible remedy was explored; however, Lightning had to be euthanized. Micah was extremely distraught over the loss of Lightning, whom she described as "the other half of my soul."

You have a couple of free minutes, so you decide to call and see how Micah is doing. Micah is still upset about the loss of Lightning. She says that she has no desire to ever barrel race again and cannot even stand to go to the barn to visit the other horses. She also tells you that she has not been eating or sleeping well. Her parents and friends all think that she is overreacting. At that Micah begins to cry and immediately apologizes. You respond, "It's OK. I know Lightning was special to you. It is normal to still be grieving. I know of someone who specializes in pet loss counseling. Would you like her phone number?"

If you had not taken the time to call, Micah's depression might have gone unnoticed. Many times clients suffer through depression feeling alone. Depression may occur on and off during the entire grief process. Micah also explained to you that support was not available from her friends and family. It is important to follow up on clients who have poor support systems or who are attached to their animals like Micah. Referral to a professional counselor can be of great assistance in helping clients such as Micah in resolving the grief process.

BOX 38-3 Places to Contact for Help or Referral Sources for Clients Needing Help With Grief

The Delta Society
ATTN: Librarian
289 Perimeter Road East
Renton, WA 98055-1329
Telephone: (206) 226-7357
(Can be contacted for a list of referral sources in your area.)
www.deltasociety.org

Veterinary Grief Counseling Hot Lines
ASPCA National Pet Loss Hotline
424 East 92nd St.
New York, NY 10128
Telephone: 800-946-4646 punch in pin number 140-7211 and then your phone number
StephanieL@ASPCA.org
Companion Animal Association of Arizona, Inc.

Pet Grief Support Service
P.O. Box 5006
Scottsdale, AZ 85261-5006
Telephone: (602) 258-3306

Pet Loss Support Hotline
Center for Animals in Society
School of Veterinary Medicine
University of California, Davis
Telephone: (530) 752-4200 or (800) 565-1526
(Staffed by University of California, Davis veterinary students; weekdays, 6:30 PM to 9:30 PM PST.)

The Chicago Veterinary Medical Association Pet Loss Support Hotline
Telephone: (630) 325-1600
(Staffed by Chicago VMA veterinarians and staff; voice mail will be returned collect daily between 7 PM and 9 PM CST.)

Pet Loss Support Hotline
College of Veterinary Medicine
Cornell University
Telephone: (607) 253-3932
www.vet.cornell.edu/public/petloss
(Staffed by Cornell University veterinary students; voice mail messages will be returned within 24 hours.)

Pet Loss Support Hotline
College of Veterinary Medicine
University of Florida
Telephone: (352) 392-4700; then dial 1 and 4080
(Staffed by University of Florida veterinary students; weekdays, 7 PM to 9 PM EST.)

Pet Loss Support Hotline
College of Veterinary Medicine
Michigan State University
Telephone: (517) 353-5064
(Staffed by Michigan State University veterinary students; Tuesday to Thursday, 6:30 PM to 9:30 PM EST.)

C.A.R.E. Help Line for Companion Animal Related Emotions
University of Illinois
College of Veterinary Medicine
Telephone: (217) 244-2273
(Staffed by Illinois College of Veterinary Medicine students; volunteers return calls Tuesday or Thursday between 7 PM and 9 PM CST.)

Pet Loss Support Hotline
Iowa State University
College of Veterinary Medicine
Telephone: (888) 478-7574
www.vetmed.iastate.edu/animals/petloss/default.html
(Staffed by Iowa State University veterinary students and community volunteers; September to April, 7 days/wk 6 PM to 9 PM CST, May to August, Monday, Wednesday, and Friday, 6 PM to 9 PM CST.)

Pet Loss Support Hotline
Michigan State University
College of Veterinary Medicine
Telephone: (517) 432-2696
(Staffed by Michigan State University veterinary students.)

Pet Loss Support Hotline
Washington State University
College of Veterinary Medicine
Telephone: (509) 335-5704
(Staffed by Washington State University veterinary students.)

Pet Loss Support Hotline
College of Veterinary Medicine
Ohio State University
Telephone: (614) 292-1823
(Staffed by Ohio State University veterinary students; Monday, Wednesday, and Friday, 6:30 PM to 9:30 PM EST.)
E-mail: petloss@osu.edu

Virginia-Maryland Regional College of Veterinary Medicine
Virginia Tech
Telephone: (540) 231-8038
(Staffed by Virginia-Maryland Regional College of Veterinary Medicine; Tuesday and Thursday, 6 PM to 9 PM EST.)

School of Veterinary Medicine Tufts University
Telephone: (508) 838-7966
www.tufts.edu/vet/petloss
(Staffed by Tufts University veterinary students; Monday through Friday, 6 PM to 9 PM EST; voice mail messages will be returned collect daily.)

Veterinary Schools and Colleges With Grief Counseling Programs
University of California
School of Veterinary Medicine
Center for Animals in Society
Davis, CA 95616
Telephone: (916) 752-4200

Colorado State University, Veterinary Teaching Hospital
CHANGES: The Support for People and Pets Program
300 West Drake Rd.
Fort Collins, CO 80523
Telephone: (970) 491-1242

Louisiana State University
School of Veterinary Medicine

Continued

BOX 38-3 Places to Contact for Help or Referral Sources for Clients Needing Help With Grief—cont'd

Veterinary Schools and Colleges With Grief Counseling Programs—cont'd

The Best Friend Gone Project
Baton Rouge, LA 70809
Telephone: (225) 578-9547
E-mail: friendgone@vetmed.lsu.edu

University of Pennsylvania
School of Veterinary Medicine
3800 Spruce St.
Philadelphia, PA 19104-6044
Telephone: (215) 898-5438

Tufts University School of Veterinary Medicine
Center for Animals and Public Policy
200 Westboro Rd.
North Grafton, MA 01536
Telephone: (508) 838-7991

Washington State University
College of Veterinary Medicine
People-Pet Partnership
Pullman, WA 99164-7010
Telephone: (509) 335-4569

University of Wisconsin
School of Veterinary Medicine
Pet Loss Support Group
2015 Linden Dr.
Madison, WI 53706
Telephone: (608) 836-7297

Websites

American Veterinary Medical Association: www.avma.org (Look under care for pets.)
Argus Institute for Families and Veterinary Medicine: www.argusinstitute.colostate.edu
Grief Healing: www.griefhealing.com
Pet Bereavement Counseling: www.petloss.org

Resolution or Acceptance

The stage of resolution or acceptance is the belief that everything is OK, normal functioning is restored, and emotional energy is reinvested. This does not mean that the pet is forgotten but that it has been assigned to a special place in the bereaved individual's heart. New attachments can be made without regret and hesitation. Resolution may come easily for some and may be difficult for others. In general, children reach the stage of acceptance and resolution more quickly and more easily than do adults. (For more information on how to help children when a pet dies, see Box 38-4.) As stated previously, the grief process is not linear, and bits of this stage occur with more and more frequency and with longer durations throughout the grief process. Eventually the client who successfully resolves the grief process experiences little, if any, of the first four stages.

There are many factors that may complicate the grief process (Box 38-5). These complicating factors may lengthen the time it takes to reach resolution or in severe cases may arrest progress through the grief process without allowing the individual to reach a resolution. Situations in which the grief process is complicated may not affect some individuals' ability to progress, but may drastically affect that of others. Few veterinary professionals are equipped to give the special kind of help that these complicated situations may require, but most have empathy and the ability to listen for signs that indicate someone may need help. Early recognition of factors that may complicate the grief process can be helpful when a person appears not to be progressing well through the process. Early recognition may also be important for timely referral in situations in which further assistance is required. Keeping on hand a list of professional alternatives for referral to someone who can give the help that is needed is advised (see Box 38-3 for a short list of potential sources of help).

The question is often raised whether clients should get a new pet before they reach resolution of the grief process (Figure 38-3). The process itself is highly variable in length. It can be as short as a few weeks to as long as many years. Most pet owners are able to reinvest and reattach to a new pet at any time, but only after they become aware that replacement of their unique loved one is impossible. If companionship, tactile closeness, and friendship are desired while grieving, these qualities can be obtained through a new pet. Cautioning and encouraging clients to choose animals somewhat dissimilar to their dead pet can be helpful. Having a new pet forced on the grieving individual who is not ready to reinvest in a new relationship will only end up furthering heartache in the bereaved and causing unhappiness in the new pet.

CASE PRESENTATION 38-5

Two months later Micah (the client in the previous case study) calls back to let you know how she is doing. She expresses gratitude for your concern and compassion while she was grieving over losing Lightning. In his memory, she has decided to donate Lightning's winnings from last year to the Colic Research Foundation. She has also made a memorial plaque with Lightning's shoe on it to hang on his stall door. She would like for you and the veterinarian to come out to the farm to examine the soundness of a horse, Blaze, that she thinks has barrel potential. She is beginning to realize that Lightning would like for her to ride again.

Micah is doing well. She has gone through the process of grieving over Lightning. By memorializing Lightning with the plaque, she has a special way to remember him. Through the donation, she is able to believe that both she and Lightning have made an important contribution to equine medicine. Micah experienced a degree of personal growth through the process of grieving. Resolution and acceptance for Micah are symbolized by focusing her emotional energy into potentially developing a relationship with Blaze. It is important that Lightning is not forgotten.

BOX 38-4 How to Help Children When a Pet Dies

When children's companion animals die, many parents follow their instincts to protect them from pain and grief. Some parents make decisions regarding the pet without discussing them with their children. Some may even lie to their children about the actual circumstances of the pet's "disappearance," preferring to tell them that a beloved pet ran away or was stolen rather than died. These tactics are not used maliciously by parents. They develop from a desire to spare children feelings of pain and from a belief that the parents, as parents, are inadequately prepared to discuss loss, death, and grief with their children.

Children, however, are tuned into their parents' emotions and, almost without exception, know that something is going on in the family. They do not know what that something is, but they do know that it upsets mom and dad. Consequently, children may feel anxious, confused, left out, and even guilty because without honest explanations of a family crisis children often believe that they are somehow responsible for the tension level in the home. At later ages, children may also believe that they were betrayed by the parents that they trusted when they discover the truth about their childhood pet's disappearance.

The knowledge, skills, and tools for dealing with loss and grief that are developed in childhood are the same ones used in adolescence and adulthood. It is of utmost importance that children be given honest support and information about loss and death so that their grief-coping strategies will be healthy, rather than unhealthy, ones.

How Technicians Can Help

Parents will often turn to veterinary professionals for assistance in telling their children about the death of a pet. Having books available for them to read and having information yourself to share can help ease an otherwise traumatic situation. Here are some suggestions:

- Always encourage parents to be honest with their children throughout a companion animal's illness, treatment, and death. Never agree to participate in a lie that the parents may want to tell their children to protect them. In the long run, lies create more problems for everyone involved and can be more damaging to children than the pet's death itself.
- Children under the age of 8 years do not really understand that death is final. They may believe that a dead pet can return or that they will need food in their grave with them. Young children are also egocentric and believe quite strictly in the law of cause and effect. Thus they may develop the idea that they did something to cause the pet's death. Therefore they must be reassured repeatedly that the pet died because it had a disease or an accident or was old.
- Straightforward explanations and concrete words, such as dead and died, should be used when talking to children about death. Young children do not understand euphemisms and can become upset when they hear terms such as put to sleep. Since they go to sleep every night and do not want to die like their pet did, attempts at softening the blow can actually make the situation more difficult and frightening for children.
- Children need to be held, reassured, and allowed to ask questions. Open communication about death is the desired atmosphere for keeping death anxiety manageable. Pets' names should be used in conversation whenever possible, and memories of them should be shared by the whole family. Older children should be included in the euthanasia process, the memorial ceremonies, and the goodbye rituals to whatever extent they wish to be and should be encouraged to demonstrate their sensitivity and compassion.
- It is always helpful to contact children's teachers, care providers, relatives, and other significant adults so that they can help acknowledge the loss and grief process. Adults may observe children playing funeral or overhear them talking to friends about a pet's death. Although these activities may seem alarming and even morbid to adults, they are normal, healthy responses for children. Children deal with issues through play and experimentation. Unless they are in physical danger, their activities do not in most cases require interference.
- For adult information about helping children deal with pet loss, consult the following books:

Jewett CL: *Helping children cope with separation and loss,* Boston, 1982, Harvard Common Press.

Nieburg HA, Fischer A: *Pet loss: a thoughtful guide for adults and children,* New York, 1982, Harper & Row.

Quackenbush J, Graveline D: *When your pet dies: how to cope with your feelings,* New York, 1985, Simon & Schuster.

Shirl-Potter JW, Koss GJ: *Death of a pet: answers to questions for children and animal lovers of all ages,* Stamford, Conn, 1991, Guideline Publications.

Tousley M: *Children and pet loss,* Scottsdale, Ariz, 1996, Companion Animal Association of Arizona.

- The following children's books may be helpful in explaining the loss of a pet to children:

Brackenridge SS: *Because of flowers and dancers,* Santa Barbara, Calif, 1994, Veterinary Practice Publishing.

Disalvo-Ryan D: *A dog like Jack,* New York, 1999, Holiday House.

Morehead D: *A special place for Charlie,* Broomfield, Colo, 1996, Partners in Publishing.

Rylant C: *Dog heaven,* New York, 1995, The Blue Sky Press.

Rylant C: *Cat heaven,* New York, 1997, Scholastic.

Viorst J: *The tenth good thing about Barney,* New York, 1971, Aladdin Books.

GRIEF AND THE VETERINARY PROFESSIONAL

Individuals in the veterinary profession deal with client grief on an almost daily basis. Rarely do they think about their own. The veterinary professional must realize the grief process that the client is struggling with is not taking place in an emotional vacuum. It is real and touches not only the bereaved person, but also those around him or her, including the veterinary professional. It is common for veterinarians and veterinary technicians to cry with clients, to feel a lump in the throat, and to feel guilty or depressed or experience a sense of failure. The fact that veterinary professionals may go through a grief process each time a patient is lost must

BOX 38-5 Factors That May Complicate the Grief Process

- Multiple losses occurring within a related time frame
- Loss of a pet that was associated with a special person or event
- Loss of a pet on a day that is important, such as a birthday or holiday
- Loss of a pet because of factors that may have been preventable
- Feelings of guilt about the death of a pet
- An inability to afford expensive care that was offered
- Loss of a pet because of an illness or situation that previously caused the loss of another pet
- Sudden illness or trauma resulting in loss
- Witnessing the violent or unnecessary death of a pet
- Disappearance of a pet
- Lack of explanation as to why a pet died
- Situations in which the person experiencing loss has little or no support
- Insensitive comments from others who may not understand the bond between owner and pet
- Getting incorrect or bad information concerning the loss of a pet and/or the grieving process
- No previous experience with grief
- Not present at the time the pet dies or not having the opportunity to view the body
- Not able to say goodbye

be recognized and accepted. Time should be spent thinking about these feelings and responses. Validation of the process within the profession, by way of staff meetings, discussions, and support sessions, can be important in recognizing and dealing with the stresses of "professional grief." Left unacknowledged, the grief process encountered by veterinary professionals can become destructive and lead to burnout.

TECHNICIAN NOTE Left unacknowledged, the grief process encountered by veterinary professionals can become destructive.

EUTHANASIA

Perhaps no single issue in veterinary medicine conjures up the range of emotion, ethical deliberation, and stress occasioned by euthanasia. Euthanasia was defined by the 2001 American Veterinary Medical Association (AVMA) panel on euthanasia as "the act of inducing painless death," but the act is only one small aspect of the larger issue facing the profession.

The word euthanasia is derived from the Greek root eu, meaning good, and thanatos, referring to death. Few in the veterinary profession would argue that when used in the context of relieving suffering, the word runs counter to its Greek roots; however, as the word is currently defined, it also pertains to the killing of unwanted, abandoned, stray, or phenotypically undesired animals by veterinary professionals.

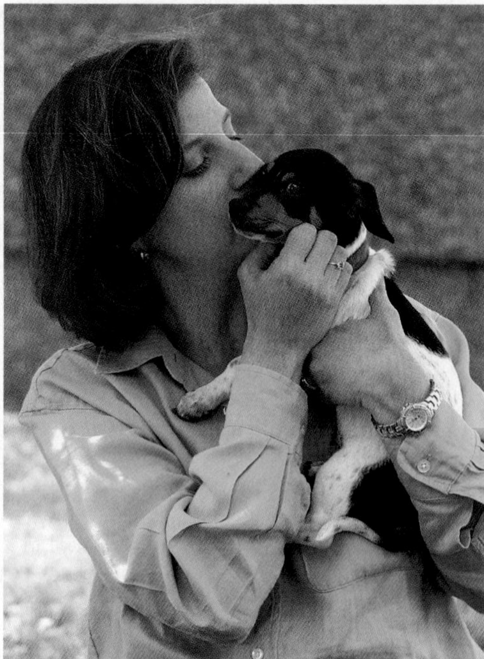

FIGURE 38-3 The decision to bond with a new animal should be left to the client experiencing the loss. Bonding with a new pet should be viewed as a tribute to the love and companionship shared with the previous animal.

It is not always in the common interest of the patient, client, and veterinarian that euthanasia is performed, and in this way, problems can arise in balancing conflicting interests. Euthanasia is an emotionally charged issue, with members of the profession varying significantly in their acceptance of the practice and in their views as to its utility. On the one hand, it might be viewed simply as "convenience killing," whereas on the other, it might be viewed as a means of furthering respect and love through the compassionate termination of hopeless suffering. No matter how one looks at it, the animal health professional may be caught in the middle, experiencing doubts, confusion, and moral questions over participation in the ending of an animal's life. It is an ethical dilemma that does not have an easy or even an absolutely right or wrong answer. It is an issue that all veterinary professionals must wrestle with, individually and collectively.

TECHNICIAN NOTE Euthanasia is an issue that all veterinary professionals must wrestle with, individually and collectively.

THE DECISION

The decision to perform euthanasia is one of the most difficult decisions that the owner of a companion animal will ever face. Some owners may make the decision quickly because of financial constraints or fear of what the illness may eventually cause, whereas others may never be able to make the decision, preferring to let their pet die naturally. The decision is often made more difficult because few pet owners have an adequate support group available that understands the bond that develops between an animal and the recipient of its unconditional love.

Most owners who elect to have euthanasia performed make the decision because they perceive that their pet's illness involves some degree of suffering. Suffering is difficult to define, and perceptions of animal suffering differ greatly between individuals and from case to case. The place the pet holds in the owner's family circle, how long the pet has been owned, the relationship between the pet and other loved ones, the financial resources available to the owner, and the disease process afflicting the pet are other factors that most owners take into consideration when trying to make the decision.

The veterinary team (veterinarian, veterinary technician, animal health care providers) can play an important role in the decision-making process. The veterinary staff often serves as a sounding board for the client who is trying to make the decision. Staff members can help with the decision by approaching the subject professionally with compassion and respect. The most important help that the team can give is to provide information. What the owner can expect from the disease process, what treatments are available, the prognosis with and without treatment, and what costs are involved are all questions that should be answered by the veterinarian. The veterinary technician can play a vital role as a client resource by answering questions about euthanasia. How euthanasia is performed, whether the animal will feel pain, how long the procedure will take, and what happens to the body afterward are all areas that a technician may be asked to address.

> *TECHNICIAN NOTE* Veterinary technicians, as professionals, can help clients with euthanasia decisions by approaching the subject professionally with compassion and respect.

When interacting with an owner considering euthanasia, the veterinary professional should go to great lengths to lay out all options available while being careful not to make the decision for the client. Too many veterinary professionals make judgments as to the value of an animal (both monetary and personal) that only the owner can make. Questions such as "What would you do if he were your animal?" are difficult to address and perhaps best answered by urging the client to verbalize what he or she sees as the pros and cons of each choice. In doing this, it may become obvious that the client has already made the decision and is looking for support or validation. The client may feel guilt, anger, sadness, depression, pain, and helplessness during the decision-making process and after euthanasia has been performed. The veterinary professional can help by assuring owners that these feelings are normal and indeed expected and by assuring them that they are not alone in the pain that they are feeling.

Once an informed decision has been made, it should be supported, even if it may not have been the decision that the veterinarian or veterinary staff would have made. Pet owners are sensitive to the actions of hospital personnel, and for this reason, it is extremely important that persons interacting with the client or handling the animal in the presence of the owner be supportive, gentle, and empathetic.

At times, decisions concerning euthanasia may be made based on convenience factors. Convenience euthanasia for reasons such as a client moving and not being able to take the animal, new furniture in the house, or an inability to effectively house train an animal is something that most veterinary professionals will have to face. It is up to each practice to decide how they are going to deal with these issues. Some practices will decide that they are going to follow the owner's wishes no matter what, and others will decide that they are not going to euthanize animals in these settings. Often situations are looked at on a case-by-case basis, and although this may result in an inconsistent approach, it may be best, especially if all members of the practice understand how decisions are made. Questioning a client concerning their reasons for choosing euthanasia in these situations will sometimes bring out that they are making the decision because they really do not know that there are other options. Education about what other options are available will sometimes result in a happier outcome.

AS THE END DRAWS NEAR: THE BEGINNING OF THE END

The death of a pet can be a devastating experience that can drastically affect the relationship between client and veterinarian. As many as 40% of clients change veterinarians after a pet has died. This number probably approaches 100% if euthanasia is handled in a manner that causes the client to perceive a lack of care, concern, or respect on the part of the veterinarian or other staff members. On the other hand, much can be done to foster a long-lasting relationship through the professional and compassionate handling of euthanasia. It is often true that the client who loudly sings the praises of a veterinarian and staff is not the owner of an animal saved through long hours of hard work and outstanding medical care, but rather the owner who was treated with compassion, care, and concern at and around the time of the loss of a pet.

> *TECHNICIAN NOTE* Many clients change veterinarians after the death of a pet, especially if euthanasia is handled without the utmost care and respect.

Preparations for pet loss should begin as soon as it becomes apparent that death is a possibility. The veterinarian should discuss euthanasia with a client early so that the client understands that it is an available option. However, it is important to discuss all other medical or surgical options first. Euthanasia should not be presented in such a manner that it is either completely discounted or viewed as the only reasonable course. Remember that the initial reaction of a client receiving bad news is often denial or feelings of numbness or shock. It is important to allow time for this initial reaction to fade and for the entire family to be given time to discuss the various options before allowing the client to make such a difficult and important decision.

While discussing options with the client, the veterinarian should not use alternative jargon for euthanasia, such as put to sleep, put down, put away, humanely destroy, rock, and shoot, unless its meaning is understood by all individuals involved. Confusion will result from the use of a term such as put to sleep when talking to a companion animal owner who perceives the phrase to refer to anesthesia instead of euthanasia. Children are especially confused by the term put to sleep and may associate death with sleeping causing them to be afraid that they might die when going to sleep at night. Whatever term is used to describe the act of euthanasia, it is important that it be fully understood by all parties involved.

> *TECHNICIAN NOTE* Communication is critical to a smooth euthanasia when owners are present.

Once the decision has been made to have an animal undergo euthanasia, a client must make many decisions. When and where should the euthanasia take place? Should the client or other family members be present during the euthanasia? What is to happen to the body after euthanasia? Should a necropsy examination be allowed? What special method, if any, will the client use to memorialize the pet? It is best to discuss these concerns thoroughly in advance so that everyone understands precisely the wishes of the client.

The client together with the veterinarian should decide who will be present during the euthanasia. This is sometimes a difficult decision for both the client and the veterinarian. Some veterinarians do not offer this option to the client in the mistaken view that it will be too difficult for the client to watch. Contrary to this view, many clients will grieve more easily and accept more quickly the loss of their pet if they have had the opportunity to say goodbye in this most personal way (Figure 38-4). The chance to hold their pet and let it know that it is loved dearly while sharing its last moments is sometimes an important first step in the grief process. However, with the benefits to the client can come problems for the veterinarian and staff. Veterinary team members must realize that having the client present can increase their own stress level associated with euthanasia, and every attempt should be made to understand and minimize its effects.

> *TECHNICIAN NOTE* Many clients will go through the grief process more easily if they are present at the euthanasia.

When the client or family members are to be present, euthanasia should be scheduled for a time of day when interruptions are unlikely, the waiting room is empty, and the potential for embarrassment by public exposure is minimized. Early mornings, evenings, or during the lunch hour may be suitable. It is best to schedule at least 30 minutes. The most important aspect of the euthanasia to consider is communication. The unexpected should be avoided at all costs, and before the procedure, the client should be given

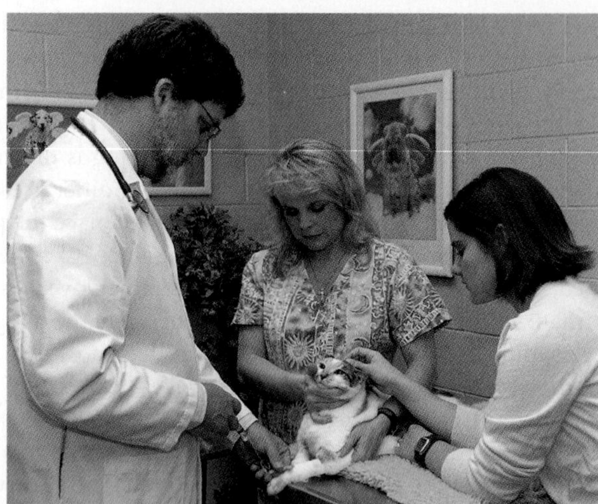

FIGURE 38-4 Clients' presence during the euthanasia of their companion animal helps them to say goodbye. Allow the client to make as many decisions, with guidance, about the site, time, and tempo of the euthanasia process; this makes the event more personal and meaningful.

a detailed explanation of exactly what is about to happen to the pet and what he or she is about to see. Then the client should be talked through each step of the procedure. The euthanasia should proceed at a pace with which the client feels comfortable. Occasionally, pets will urinate, defecate, vocalize, twitch, or gasp after they have become unconscious. Although these reflex acts can be minimized, they will still occasionally occur and will have a far less negative effect if they are expected and if the client is told that they are not a reflection of pain or suffering.

It is important for the veterinary team to effectively recognize signs of pain, fear, and distress so that they might be minimized either related to the disease process or during euthanasia. Distress vocalization, struggling, attempts to escape, aggression, panting, salivation, urination, expression of anal sacs, tremoring, tachycardia, and dilation of the pupils may all indicate distress, pain, or fear. Awareness of these signs can help to minimize stress during the euthanasia process.

Deciding where the euthanasia is to take place can be important. Using a hospital space that is less stark than the typical stainless steel hospital examination room is preferred. If the examination room is to be used, at least a blanket should be placed over the table and there should be a chair where the client can sit down. Some clients will request that the euthanasia be performed at home or at some special place. Many veterinarians will honor these requests or use the services of a house call practice for this need. Sometimes just to be outside the "normal" environment of the veterinary facility is a fair and acceptable compromise. A blanket on the floor, the lawn beside the practice, and even the back seat of the family car might serve this purpose. One important consideration for the veterinarian in choosing the place is that many clients will feel uncomfortable coming back into the room where a pet previously underwent euthanasia. Indeed, many clients switch veterinarians because of a lack of sensitivity to this fact by the veterinary staff. To minimize this potential conflict in the future, it is best to choose a space that will not be routinely used for other client-related activities.

Clients who choose not to be present during euthanasia may still wish to see the body of the animal after it is dead. Seeing the animal dead conveys finality and also allows the client the opportunity to say goodbye. Many clients have a difficult time proceeding through the grief process if they have not been given this chance.

> *TECHNICIAN NOTE* Clients who choose not to be present for euthanasia often still wish to see the body afterward.

Make arrangements in advance concerning how payment for services is to occur. Discuss with the client whether payment is going to be made in advance, at the time of services, or by a later bill. This can be an uncomfortable subject to broach after euthanasia has occurred.

AT THE END

Once all the preparations have been made, the euthanasia should be performed with skill and concern. Each member of the veterinary team should be well trained, know his or her responsibilities, and be available. The key, as already mentioned, is to expect and plan for the unexpected. Although many methods of euthanasia are deemed acceptable by the AVMA panel on euthanasia, only those that are aesthetically acceptable should be used when the client is going to be present.

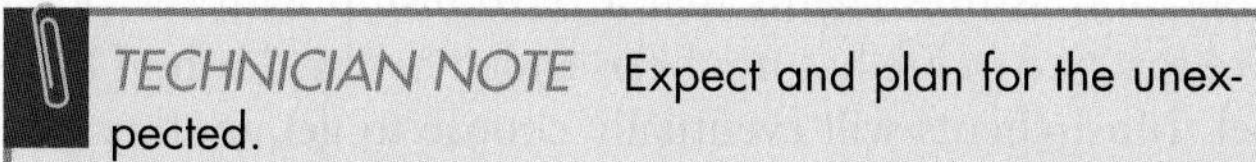

> *TECHNICIAN NOTE* Expect and plan for the unexpected.

If the examination room is to be used, the table should be covered with a cloth or blanket. Some owners will want to bring a favorite blanket for the pet to spend its last few moments on. It is important that they understand that it is possible, indeed likely, that the blanket will be soiled by feces or urine when euthanasia occurs. If the pet is likely to be aggressive or extremely apprehensive, sedating it ahead of time should be considered. If the client is to be present, the animal should be taken away briefly so that a peripheral vein can be catheterized for smooth delivery of the euthanasia solution. It is advisable to put the catheter into a vein in a back leg; this will allow the client to hold the animal and pet its head without getting in the way of the veterinarian while the injections are given. Once the catheter has been placed, the client should be given the opportunity to be alone with the pet for a few moments.

Before administering the euthanasia solution, a saline solution should be injected into the catheter to ensure its patency. Next the patient should be anesthetized with propofol or an ultrashort-acting barbiturate. This will decrease the incidence of excitement after the euthanasia solution is injected. Once the animal is anesthetized, the euthanasia solution can be injected. Sodium pentobarbital is the most commonly used euthanasia solution. It is a member of the barbiturate family of drugs that depress the entire central nervous system.* When large doses of this drug are administered, as for euthanasia, unconsciousness occurs first, and then breathing stops because of depression of the respiratory center. This is followed by cardiac arrest. The pentobarbital dose, concentration, and rate of administration determine the speed of action. When the drug is administered intravenously, animals die swiftly and quietly. Although intravenous administration is preferred, the drug is also effective when injected intrahepatically, intracardiac, and, to a lesser extent, into the peritoneal cavity. Intracardiac and intrahepatic injection, although effective, is not considered appropriate for euthanasia of awake animals because it can be difficult to accurately inject euthanasia solutions into these organs consistently. Intraperitoneal injection of nonirritating solutions is considered appropriate in situations where intravenous injection is not possible. Death following intraperitoneal injection may take as long as 15 minutes, however, because of relatively slow absorption. Pentobarbital for euthanasia is available alone or in combination with other drugs. The concentration of pentobarbital in most euthanasia solutions is approximately 20% by weight. The recommended dose is 2 ml for the first 4.5 kg of body weight and 1 ml for each additional 4.5 kg of body weight. Sodium pentobarbital should be administered as rapidly as possible to provide the quietest and swiftest form of euthanasia. The veterinary team should be completely familiar with the use of the euthanasia solution chosen and the possible reactions that might be seen.

Because the cerebral cortex is affected by general anesthetic, predominant emotions may take over and the animal may show fear behavior, which is usually characterized by struggling and vocalization. Experimental studies indicate that the animal is not conscious of these feelings at the time. People who have undergone the "excitement" phase during general anesthesia do not remember that it took place. Although trained individuals may understand this excitement phase from the clinical standpoint, it is difficult for the owner to understand that the struggling and vocalization seen are not due to pain or discomfort. Thus the owner's perception is that the animal is not experiencing a peaceful death. Clients who choose to be present should be warned that this phase may occur. The use of an ultrashort-acting barbiturate first will minimize the excitement phase.

---

*Note that all barbiturates are strictly controlled by federal regulations, and accurate accounting of the use of these agents is required. The Drug Enforcement Agency (DEA) of the U.S. Department of Justice is responsible for enforcement of laws governing the user of barbiturates. Sodium pentobarbital is a schedule II controlled substance and can be obtained only by a licensed medical practitioner, such as a physician, dentist, veterinarian, or approved institution. In addition to the DEA paperwork involved for procuring barbiturates such as sodium pentobarbital, careful handling of the drug is necessary after the drug is on the hospital premises. Thorough record keeping is required by law.

THE END AS A BEGINNING . . . AFTER THE END

Many veterinary professionals are good at the technical aspects of euthanasia, but fall short in supplying what the client needs after euthanasia has been performed. The animal's death is often only the beginning of a long and difficult odyssey that the client is about to face. Some clients will feel a great sense of relief immediately after the pet's death, but most will soon feel empty, numb, or alone. They may question whether they did the right thing. Veterinary professionals can help them by again stressing that the pet's death was painless, assuring them that they did the right thing, and focusing on the positive things that the pet brought to their life. At the time of euthanasia, it is important that an environment be fostered that says, "It's all right to cry, it's all right to be emotional, it's all right to begin to grieve." Few of us have the gift of the ability to say the right thing at the right time, so sometimes consolation can best be offered in a touch or an embrace. A touch on the arm or a simple embrace will often express best what the client needs to hear, "We care, and you are not alone."

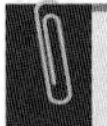

TECHNICIAN NOTE The pet's death is often only the beginning of a long and difficult odyssey.

Many clients, whether present for the euthanasia or not, need assurance that the animal is dead. Clients will feel more assured by the veterinarian who takes the time to listen to the animal's thorax with a stethoscope and shine a penlight into the animal's eyes before pronouncing the patient dead. For those who choose not to be present, allowing them to view the animal's body can alleviate some of this fear. Before bringing the body to the client, it should be made as presentable as possible. It must always be treated with dignity and respect. Clean any blood from the fur, remove any catheters or bandages, place the tongue in the mouth, and close the eyes. Placing a drop of cyanoacrylate glue (Krazy Glue, Super Glue) in each eye will keep the eyelids closed. If time permits, bathe and brush the animal before laying it on a clean paper, blanket, or towel in a sturdy box. This will help to make the viewing as pleasant an experience as possible. This last, and often lasting, impression that the client takes away from the practice may go a long way toward determining whether he or she returns with another pet. If the animal's body is sealed in a box (commercially made boxes for home burial are available), let the client know how the body is wrapped and whether any signs of trauma or surgery are present. Even clients who assure the veterinarian that they will not open the box before burial or cremation often change their mind after leaving the office.

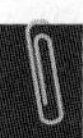

TECHNICIAN NOTE Always treat the pet's body with dignity and respect.

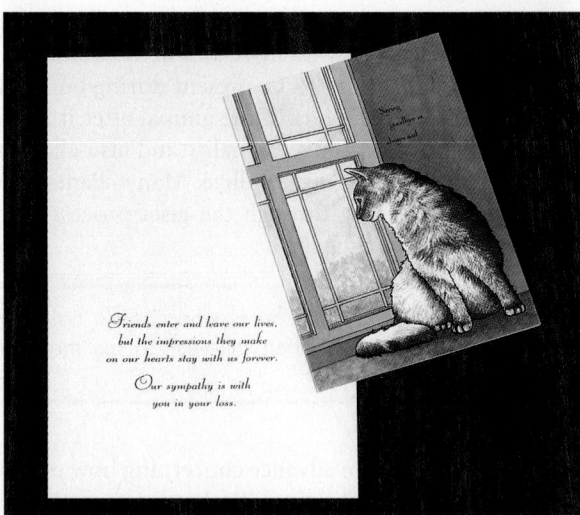

FIGURE 38-5 Follow-up communication is important for the client and the veterinary team. A condolence card lets the client know that you care, and this gesture often brings the client back to your practice when they eventually invest in a new relationship with another pet. In addition, sending a card allows the practice team to empathize, express their own grief, and experience some degree of closure.

Having the client bring someone who will be able to drive him or her home will help ease the feeling of being alone and will also ensure a safe trip. It is nice to call clients after they have arrived home to check on them. Attempts should be made to call all clients who have lost a pet to answer any questions and to show concern. The veterinarian or a staff member may call. The show of concern is always appreciated, helps clients who are having difficulty dealing with grief, and assures clients that a relationship with the practice fostered in life has not been ended by the death of their pet. Most clients will eventually choose to get another pet. A sympathy card or handwritten note is usually appreciated. Many beautiful sympathy cards designed for veterinary use are available (Figure 38-5).

One of the biggest concerns of clients who have just lost a pet is disposition of the body. When possible, all arrangements should be made in advance. The veterinary staff should be prepared with information to assist the client in making these arrangements. Know the laws concerning burial in the practice area. Make available names and telephone numbers of places that offer cremation and pet cemetery burial. If the client chooses to have the veterinarian handle the remains, it is best not to lie to the client concerning the disposal of the animal's body.

Memorializing the pet is a step that many clients find comforting. It can be an important part of grieving for many clients. Offering the client a lock of hair, a clay paw print, and returning collars or leashes may facilitate these wishes (Box 38-6). Having a memorial service, planting a special plant in memory of the pet, framing a photograph, keeping a lock of hair, writing a poem or special letter, offering a memorial scholarship at a veterinary school, or making a donation to organizations, such as the American College of Veterinary Internal Medicine or a veterinary school foundation, are actions that clients may use to memorialize their pet (Figure 38-6).

BOX 38-6 Memorialize With Clay Paw Imprints

- ClayPaws, a paw print kit.
- Create a permanent memory.
- Personalize it by painting or decorating.
- World by the Tail, Inc., 888-271-8444, www.claypaws.com.

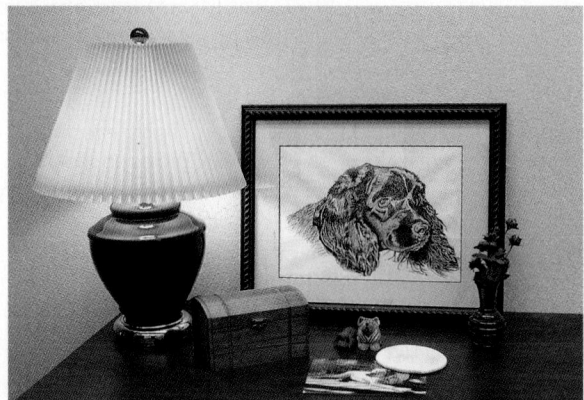

FIGURE 38-6 Memorializing a pet that has died is important to the grief response. Cremains, a paw print, and framed picture are comforting ways to memorialize.

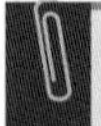

TECHNICIAN NOTE Memorializing the pet can be an important part of grieving for many clients.

THE STRESS OF EUTHANASIA

Euthanasia is stressful not only to the client, but also to the veterinarian and veterinary staff. Frequent performance of euthanasia is a primary cause of burnout within animal control facilities, shelters, and small animal practice (Box 38-7). It is at times even more stressful to the technical staff than it is to the veterinarian because staff members usually have little control over the situation. Euthanasias that go smoothly and difficult euthanasias will create stress. Difficult or inherently stressful euthanasias include euthanasia in which technical problems arise, instances in which the animal reacts badly to the injections in the presence of the client, and the euthanasia of one's own pet, healthy animals, young animals, and animals for whom one has put a great deal of time and medical effort into fighting their disease. Euthanasia with the client present usually creates more stress on the veterinary staff than when the procedure is performed in the absence of the owner.

Each individual will have to decide in what type of euthanasia he or she is able to participate and one's personal tolerance for euthanasia. A technician may not be able to work effectively in a practice in which the veterinarian's views on euthanasia are vastly different from his or her own. Stress can become intense if these differences are not discussed and reconciled. Veterinarians differ greatly in their views on euthanasia. A survey of British veterinarians revealed that 74% would perform euthanasia on a healthy animal if the owner requested it. A similar survey in Japan revealed that 63% would not. There is room within the veterinary profession for this divergence of views; indeed, the diversity of opinions is one of the profession's strengths.

BOX 38-7 Signs and Symptoms of Burnout

Physical Symptoms

Ulcers
Gastroenteritis
Cardiac arrhythmia
Heartburn
Backache
Nausea
Skin disorders

Psychologic and Behavioral Symptoms

Withdrawal
Overeating
Constant fatigue
Increased alcohol intake
Agitation
Distraction
Aggressive behavior
Insomnia

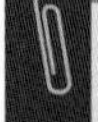

TECHNICIAN NOTE Euthanasia is stressful to both the owner and the veterinary staff.

One of the most important mechanisms of coping with the stress brought on by euthanasia is discussion with colleagues. Having sessions for the hospital staff in which people can openly express their feelings is a good outlet for emotions that if unexpressed can cause further stress and lead to burnout. This type of communication allows members of the veterinary team to understand their colleagues' feelings and tolerances for different situations. Members of the team may need to temporarily pass responsibility for euthanasia to their colleagues when they have reached the limit of their tolerance. Other mechanisms of managing stress include taking time off, making time for self, adopting recreational habits, helping clients deal with their grief, and finding strength in relationships formed with colleagues who experience the same stresses.

EUTHANASIA IN THE SHELTER AND RESEARCH FACILITY

Technicians in veterinary practice participate in an average of three to six euthanasias per week; however, shelter technicians and potentially research technicians experience much more death than this. Millions of animals must be euthanized each year because there are no homes for them, overpopulation, or because of the needs of certain research protocols. These deaths can be difficult to rationalize, making euthanasia a stressful event for these technicians. The fact that there are different euthanasia methods employed depending on the species or facility is a complicating stressor (Table 38-1).

TABLE 38-1 Summary of Agents and Methods of Euthanasia: Characteristics and Modes of Action

Acceptability	Mode of Action	Ease of Performance	Safety for Personnel	Species Suitability	Efficacy and Comments
Barbiturates					
Acceptable	Direct depression of cerebral cortex, subcortical structures and vital centers; direct depression of heart muscle	Animal must be restrained; personnel must be skilled to perform intravenous injection	Safe except human abuse potential; DEA-controlled substance	Most species	Highly effective when appropriately administered; acceptable intravenous and intrahepatic in small animals
Inhalant Anesthetics					
Acceptable	Direct depression of cerebral cortex, subcortical structures, and vital centers	Easily performed with closed container; can be administered to large animals by mask	Must be properly scavenged or vented to minimize exposure to personnel	Amphibians, birds, cats, dogs, fur-bearing animals, rabbits, reptiles, rodents and other small animals, zoo animals	Highly effective provided that subject is sufficiently exposed
Carbon Dioxide					
Acceptable	Direct depression of cerebral cortex, subcortical structures, and vital centers; direct depression of heart muscle	Used in closed container	Minimal hazard	Small laboratory animals, birds, cats, small dogs, mink, zoo animals, amphibians	Effective, but time required may be prolonged in immature and neonatal animals
Carbon Monoxide (Bottled Gas Only)					
Acceptable	Combines with hemoglobin, preventing its combination with oxygen	Requires appropriately operated equipment for gas production	Extremely hazardous, toxic, and difficult to detect	Most small species, including dogs, cats, rodents, mink, chinchillas, birds, reptiles, amphibians, zoo animals	Effective; acceptable only when equipment is properly designed and operated
Microwave Irradiation					
Acceptable	Direct inactivation of brain enzymes by rapid heating of brain	Requires training and highly specialized equipment	Safe	Mice and rats	Highly effective for special needs
Tricane Methanesulfonate					
Acceptable	Depression of CNS	Easily used	Safe	Fish and amphibians	Effective but expensive
Benzocaine					
Acceptable	Depression of CNS	Easily used	Safe	Fish and amphibians	Effective but expensive
Cervical Dislocation					
Conditionally acceptable	Direct depression of brain	Requires training and skill	Safe	Poultry, birds, laboratory mice and rats less than 200 g, or rabbits less than 1 kg	Irreversible, violent muscle contractions can occur after cervical dislocation
Decapitation					
Conditionally acceptable	Direct depression of brain	Require training and skill	Guillotine poses potential employee injury hazard	Laboratory rodents, small rabbits, birds, fish, amphibians, reptiles	Irreversible, violent muscle contractions can occur after decapitation
Penetrating Captive Bolt					
Conditionally acceptable	Direct concussion of brain tissue	Requires skill, adequate restraint, and proper placement of captive bolt	Safe	Ruminants, horses, swine, dogs, rabbits, zoo animals, reptiles	Instant unconsciousness, but motor activity may continue

TABLE 38-1 Summary of Agents and Methods of Euthanasia: Characteristics and Modes of Action—cont'd

Acceptability	Mode of Action	Ease of Performance	Safety for Personnel	Species Suitability	Efficacy and Comments
Gunshot					
Conditionally acceptable	Direct concussion of brain tissue	Requires skill and appropriate firearm	May be dangerous	Large domestic and zoo animals, reptiles, wildlife	Instant unconsciousness, but motor activity may continue
Electrocution					
Conditionally acceptable	Direct depression of brain and cardiac fibrillation	Not easily performed in all instances	Hazardous to personnel	Used primarily in foxes, sheep, swine, mink	Violent muscle contractions occur at same time as unconsciousness
Pithing					
Conditionally acceptable	Trauma of brain and spinal cord tissue	Easily performed, but requires skill	Safe	Some poikilotherms	Effective, but death not immediate unless double pithed
Nitrogen, Argon					
Conditionally acceptable	Reduced partial pressure of oxygen available to blood	Used closed chamber with rapid filling	Safe if used with ventilation	Cats, small dogs, birds, rodents, rabbits, other small species, mink, zoo animals	Effective except in young and neonates; an effective agent, but other methods preferable; not acceptable in most animals less than 4 mo old

Modified from Andrews EJ et al: *J Am Vet Med Assoc* 202(2), 1993.
DEA, U.S. Drug Enforcement Agency; *CNS*, central nervous system.

This factor brings up a wide range of both psychosocial and safety issues that need to be addressed.

The stress associated with euthanasia is exemplified in that staff turnover is higher in shelters where euthanasia rates are high compared with those with lower euthanasia rates. Practices that have been associated with decreased turnover rates include provision of a designated euthanasia room, exclusion of other live animals from the vicinity during euthanasia, and removal of euthanized animals from a room before entry of another animal to be euthanized. Staff members involved in the types of euthanasia occurring in shelters or research settings often cope by shifting moral responsibility for killing animals away from themselves. Shelter technicians view their acts as a crusade for animals and against the ignorant public, whereas research technicians may view the euthanasia as necessary for the "greater good." To prevent burnout, they must see themselves as generators of medical knowledge beneficial to humans and animals, combatants of pet overpopulation, or providers of humane death. These technicians must remember their objectives in their work. Their objective, like every other technician's, is to prevent and release animals from suffering.

The same mechanisms for coping with the stress of euthanasia mentioned previously are important for both shelter and research technicians. Perhaps one of the most important coping strategies is for the team to rotate euthanasia responsibilities. This rotation releases technicians from the moral stress of euthanasia and reschedules them to a more hopeful task, such as education or adoption responsibilities or other important research missions; it is hoped that giving them a break will prevent burnout. Dark humor is also used to relieve stress. Such humor reduces tension by acknowledging death as part of the setting but also minimizing, for the moment, its tragedy and finality. Although this humor may appear callous and be misunderstood by those outside the shelter or research culture, it has been shown to be an effective coping strategy. It is important to recognize this humor for what it is, a coping mechanism. These technicians care a tremendous amount, but find themselves in an environment without much societal support.

> *TECHNICIAN NOTE* Open discussion of issues surrounding euthanasia can help a hospital's staff deal with the stress.

EUTHANASIA OF LARGE ANIMALS

Euthanasia of large domestic animals presents specific hazards and problems not encountered in companion small animals. Safety must be a major consideration. The jugular vein should be used for injection whenever possible because this will place the person injecting the euthanasia solution in the safest position. On rare occasions, thrombosis of the jugular veins may have occurred from disease, and the cephalic vein must be used. However, this puts the individual under the animal's forequarters and in a dangerous position.

Euthanasia-strength pentobarbital can be administered with a large-gauge needle (14 to 16 gauge). The volume of solution is large, and even with a large-gauge needle, the time it takes to inject the solution is relatively long. The animal may go through the same excitement phase as that experienced by small animals, and it may come crashing to the ground on becoming unconscious. Generally, large animal euthanasia should be performed in an area with vehicle access to allow removal of the body. In some instances, the client may wish to bury a large animal. It should be remembered that all the same emotional concerns encountered in small animal euthanasia pertain to large animals when a bond has formed between the owner and the animal.

CONCLUSION

The loss of a pet and the grieving associated with it is a difficult process, both for the pet owner and for veterinary personnel. Despite this difficulty, veterinary professionals deal with the illness, loss, and euthanasia of their patients on a daily basis, yet they are rarely trained in how best to address the grief of their clients. Nevertheless, it is important for veterinarians and veterinary technicians to provide a positive, supportive environment for pet euthanasia and to help clients with their subsequent loss. If euthanasia is performed poorly, it can be a disastrous experience for both the client and the veterinary practice. If performed with practiced care and gentle concern, it can be remembered positively for a long time. The ability to empathize, maintain a balanced perspective, and be compassionate are essential. The veterinary technician can be available; listening; assuring clients that their feelings, emotions, and struggles are normal; and offering referral when clients think that they need more help than their available support group is able to provide. This form of client help strengthens the bond that develops between the client and the veterinary staff and results in positive growth and added fulfillment for both the client and the veterinary professional.

RECOMMENDED READING

Anderson M: *Coping with sorrow on the loss of your pet,* Los Angeles, 1994, Peregrine Press.

Arluke A: Coping with euthanasia: a case study of shelter culture, *J Am Vet Med Assoc* 198:1176, 1991.

AVMA: AVMA guidelines on euthanasia, June, 2007. Available at www.avma.org/issues/animal_welfare/euthanasia.pdf.

Brackenridge SS, Elkins AD: Euthanasia and patient death: stressors in veterinary practice, *Vet Pract Staff* 4:1, 1992.

Church JA: *Joy in a wooly coat,* Tiburon, Calif, 1987, HJ Kramer.

Cohen SP, Fudin CE, editors: Animal illness and human emotions, *Prob Vet Med,* 3:1, 1991.

Cusack O: *Pets and mental health,* New York, 1988, Haworth Press.

Fogle B, Abrahamson D: Pet loss: a survey of the attitudes and feelings of practicing veterinarians, *Anthrozoos* 3:143, 1990.

Fogle B, Abrahamson D: Pet loss: attitudes and feelings of practicing veterinarians, *Anthrozoos* 3:143, 1990.

Grier RL, Schaffer CB: Evaluation of intraperitoneal and intrahepatic administration of a euthanasia agent in animal shelter cats, *J Am Vet Med Assoc* 197:1611, 1990.

Harris JM: Nonconventional human/companion animal bonds. In Kay WJ, Nieburg HA, Kukscher AH, editors: *Pet loss and human bereavement,* Ames, Iowa, 1984, Iowa State University Press.

Hart LA, Hart BL, Mader B: Humane euthanasia and companion animal death: caring for the animal, the client, and the veterinarian, *J Am Vet Med Assoc* 197:1292, 1990.

Katcher A: Interactions between people and their pets: form and function. In Fogle B, editor: *Interrelations between people and pets,* Springfield, Ill, 1981, Charles C Thomas.

Kay WJ: Euthanasia, *Trends* 1:52, 1985.

Kay WJ, Cohen SP, Nieburg HA, editors: *Euthanasia of the companion animal: the impact on pet owners, veterinarians, and society,* Baltimore, 1988, The Charles Press.

Kogure N, Yamazaki K: Attitudes to animal euthanasia in Japan: a brief review of cultural influences, *Anthrozoos* 3:151, 1990.

Kübler-Ross E: *On death and dying,* New York, 1969, Macmillan.

Lagoni L, Butler C, Hetts S: *The human animal bond and grief,* Philadelphia, 1994, WB Saunders.

Lawrence EA: Love for animals and the veterinary profession, *J Am Vet Med Assoc* 205:970, 1994.

Nieburg HA, Fischer A: *Pet loss: a thoughtful guide for adults and children,* New York, 1982, Harper & Row.

Peters TG: Commander, *JAMA* 260:1460, 1988.

Quackenbush JE, Glickman L: Helping people adjust to the death of a pet, *Health Soc Work* 9:42, 1984.

Quackenbush JE, Graveline D: *When your pet dies: how to cope with your feelings,* New York, 1985, Simon & Schuster.

Ramsey EC, Wetzel RW: Comparison of five regimens for oral administration of medication to induce sedation in dogs prior to euthanasia, *J Am Vet Med Assoc* 213:1170, 1998.

Randolph JW: Learning from your own pet's euthanasia, *J Am Vet Med Assoc* 205:544, 1994.

Rogelberg SG, Reeve CL, Spitzmüller C et al. Impact of euthanasia rates, euthanasia practices, and human resource practices on employee turnover in animal shelters, *J Am Vet Med Assoc* 230:713, 2007.

Rosenberg MA: Clinical aspects of grief associated with loss of a pet: a veterinarian's view, In Kay WJ, Neiburg HA, Kukscher AH, editors: *Pet loss and human bereavement,* Ames, Iowa, 1984, Iowa State University Press.

Stewart MF: *Companion animal death,* Woburn, Mass, 1999, Butterworth-Heinemann.

Tannenbaum J: *Veterinary ethics,* Baltimore, 1989, Williams & Wilkins.

Veevers JE: The social meanings of pets: alternative roles for companion animals. In Sussman MB, editor: Pets and the family, *Marriage Family Rev* 8:11, 1985.

Voith VL: Attachment of people to companion animals, *Vet Clin North Am Small Anim Pract* 15:289, 1985.

Walshaw SO: Role of the animal health technician in consoling bereaved clients, In Kay WJ, Nieburg HA, Kukscher AH, editors: *Pet loss and human bereavement,* Ames, Iowa, 1984, Iowa State University Press.

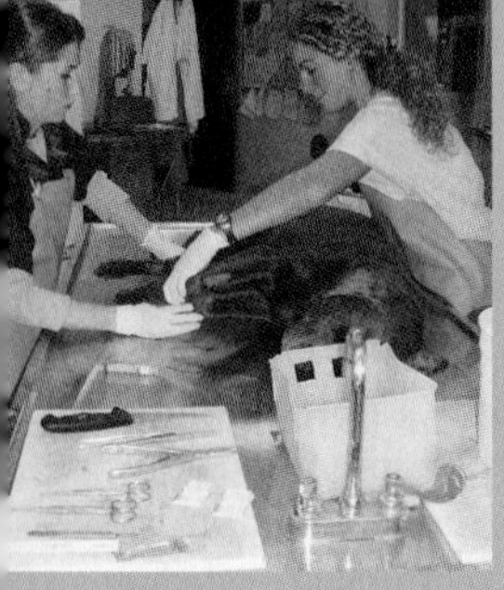

Basic Necropsy Procedures

39

Thomas J. Van Winkle and Perry L. Habecker

KEY TERMS

Abomasum
Appendicular skeleton
Atlas
Atrioventricular valve
Autolysis
Axis
Diaphragm
Duodenum
Foramen magnum
Forestomach
Gross pathology
Histopathology
Hydronephrosis
Hyoid bones
In situ
Laminae
Lesions
Mediastinum
Meninges
Myocardium
Necropsy
Omentum
Pathogenesis
Pathology
Pituitary gland
Prosector
Pulmonary artery
Sciatic nerve
Sternum

OUTLINE

LEARNING OBJECTIVES

When you have completed this chapter, you will be able to:

1. Define the term necropsy. List indications for performing a necropsy.
2. Describe the methods for evaluating and recording the results of necropsy.
3. List the types of fixatives used for the preservation of tissues. Describe their specific uses.
4. List the equipment needed to perform a typical necropsy.
5. Describe the procedure for collecting tissue samples intended for bacteriologic, parasitologic, and toxicologic evaluation.
6. Describe the procedure for collecting segments of intestine and other tissues for virus isolation.
7. Describe the procedure for collection of tissue samples from rabies suspects.
8. Discuss methods for shipping tissue samples.
9. List the steps performed during the necropsy of small mammals.
10. Describe how these steps are varied during necropsies of large animals, laboratory animals, and birds.
11. Describe methods for handling fetal and placental samples.

INTRODUCTION

A necropsy is the examination of an animal after it has died to determine the abnormal and disease-related changes that occurred during its life. The term necropsy originates from the Greek language and means "viewing the dead." Necropsy is also known as autopsy, which is Greek for "seeing with one's own eyes."

Before beginning our discussion of the necropsy, it is important to understand the meaning of terms that are used frequently in this chapter. Pathology, for example, is the science and study of disease, especially the causes and development of abnormal conditions. Gross pathology refers to pathologic changes in tissue that are visible with the unaided eye, whereas histopathology refers to pathologic changes in tissue that are microscopic and can be seen with the use of a microscope. Lesions are alterations or abnormalities in a tissue (pathologic changes), and the pathogenesis is the sequence of events that leads to or underlies a disease.

Necropsies are done for a variety of reasons. A necropsy is often done on an animal for the following reasons:

- To determine the disease process or processes that led to the animal's death
- To determine the accuracy of the clinical diagnosis
- To evaluate the positive and negative effects of therapeutic measures

In situations in which more than one animal is at risk, such as in multiple-animal households, farms, and laboratory animal facilities, the necropsy is also helpful in determining whether other animals are at risk for infection, inherited conditions, or injury caused by toxins or environmental hazards.

Successful performance of a necropsy requires knowledge of anatomy and gross pathology and a systematic technique for examination of the animal's body. Well-trained technicians, working with appropriate supervision, perform necropsies in many diagnostic laboratories and in most laboratory animal facilities (Figures 39-1 and 39-2). In practice situations, technicians trained in necropsy techniques and supervised by a veterinarian familiar with the case can and should perform necropsies. Necropsies should be performed frequently enough so that the techniques are familiar to the technician and the supervising veterinarian. In the necropsy, all abnormalities and disease processes should be exposed and described. If necessary, appropriate samples are collected for histopathology,

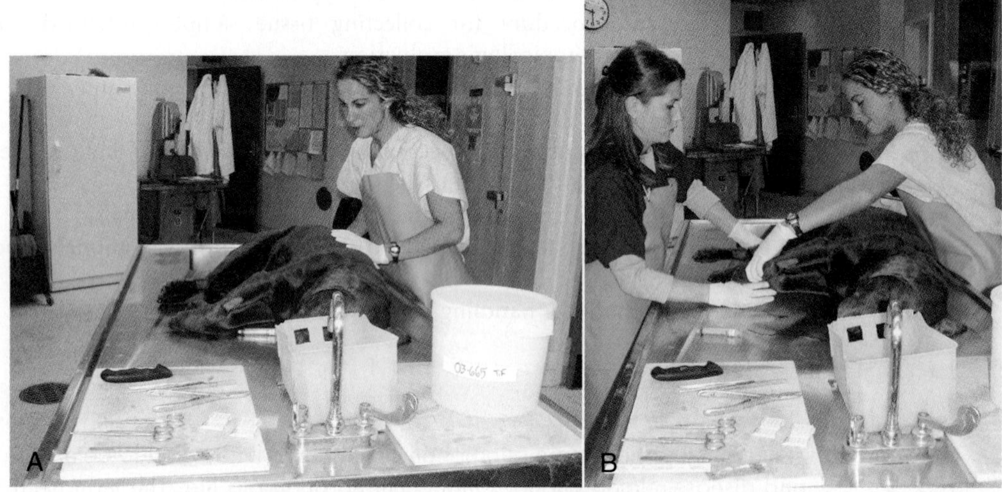

FIGURE 39-1 A-B, Prosectors ready to begin a small animal necropsy.

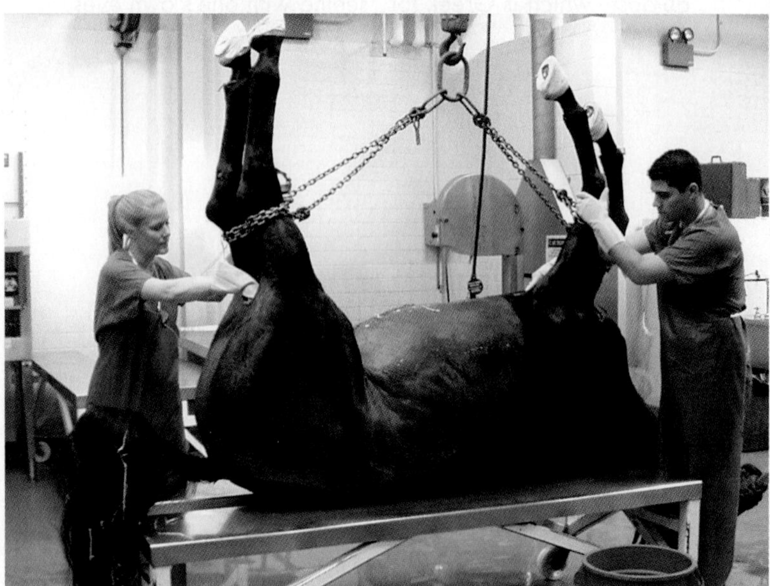

FIGURE 39-2 Prosectors ready to begin a large animal necropsy.

cytology, bacteriology, virology, parasitology, and toxicology. Descriptions of the gross findings should be recorded and included in a report together with the animal's species, age, sex, and breed (signalment); the history; and the clinical findings. Samples that are submitted to the laboratory for further testing should be packaged with a copy of the report. In addition, the report should be added to the animal's record together with the histopathology and other reports. Digital photos of lesions are also helpful and can be sent to the lab along with the reports or as a separate electronic file by e-mail.

> *TECHNICIAN NOTE* The owner's permission for the necropsy must be obtained, and the animal for necropsy must be correctly identified.

Before we begin describing the necropsy procedure, several important things must be considered. First, be sure that the owner's permission is obtained before the necropsy is performed. Second, make sure that the animal for necropsy is correctly identified. The species, breed, sex, age, and identifying tags or tattoos should be carefully matched with the information on the owner's permission form and the medical record. This step is critical to prevent performing the necropsy on the wrong animal. If the animal has a radio frequency identification device (RFID aka microchip), it can be collected for verification. In addition, the owner's preference for disposition of the body (e.g., cremation, private cremation, burial) should also be determined before the necropsy, if possible. It is also important to perform the necropsy as soon as possible after the animal's death to avoid decomposition **(autolysis).** If the necropsy must be delayed, the body should be refrigerated as soon as possible. Small animals should be placed in thin plastic bags with identification tags secured on both the body and the outside of the bag. Decomposition occurs most rapidly in large, obese animals at high temperatures. It is particularly troublesome in large animals that rely on gut fermentation for their nutrients because the rumen continues to generate heat long after the animal's death. The body should not be frozen because freezing and subsequent thawing cause many postmortem artifacts.

> *TECHNICIAN NOTE* If the necropsy must be delayed, the body should be refrigerated as soon as possible. The body should not be frozen because freezing and subsequent thawing cause many postmortem artifacts.

The signalment, history, and clinical findings should be reviewed before the necropsy is started. The record should include the owner's name, address, and telephone numbers; names of other veterinarians involved with the case; the animal's species, breed, age, sex, and name or identification; and the hospital record number. The history should include vaccination history, owner's observations of the clinical signs, length of illness, and a list of other animals at risk. The clinical findings should include results of the physical examination and clinical tests (e.g., complete blood count [CBC], clinical chemistries, radiographs), surgical procedures, and the date and time of death or euthanasia.

NECROPSY REPORTS

While the necropsy is performed, all abnormalities should be described and recorded. A report in which the findings are described should be written after the necropsy has been completed. Tentative conclusions (diagnoses) may be made at the end of the report (Box 39-1).

All lesions are described and recorded by using the following criteria (examples are given in parentheses):

- Location (caudal dorsal left lung lobe, left ventricle, cornea)
- Number (one, two, hundreds)
- Color (red, green, yellow-tan)
- Size (either measurements, such as 3 × 5 × 4 cm, or weights for liver and heart)
- Shape (round, flat, spherical, stellate)
- Distribution (focal, multifocal, diffuse)
- Consistency (soft, firm, hard, rubbery)
- Odor (sweet, sour, ammonia)

The findings are usually recorded in the order in which they were encountered in the necropsy. Either the present or past tense should be used (not both), and the descriptions should be as specific as possible without drawing conclusions. For example, "there are multiple dark red 1- to 4-mm-diameter soft nodules in all lung lobes" rather than "hemangiosarcoma." On the basis of the descriptions, the veterinarian formulates a morphologic diagnosis, which includes severity, time, distribution, lesion, and anatomic site. An example of a diagnosis might be "severe acute multifocal interstitial pneumonia."

FIXATIVES

Ten percent buffered formalin is the most widely used fixative for the preservation of tissues. Slices of tissue (generally, no thicker than 1 cm) should be placed in large volumes of formalin. Generally, there should be 10 times as much formalin solution as tissue (by volume). This solution may be purchased from a variety of sources and is also easily prepared. It is made by mixing nine parts of water with one part of commercially available formaldehyde solution (37% to 40% HCHO). The addition of 6.5 g of dibasic anhydrous sodium phosphate and 4 g of monobasic sodium phosphate per 1000 ml of solution creates neutral buffered 10% formalin. This is an excellent general purpose fixative, which is somewhat more desirable than plain (acidic) 10% formalin. The addition of buffers is important because it eliminates the formation of undesirable hematin pigment in tissue sections. Formalin (and all fixatives) should be handled with care. Formalin is a contact irritant and a carcinogen. Protective plastic gloves, preferably of nitrile composition, should always be worn when fixatives or fixed tissues are handled. Containers with fixatives should be kept closed except when

BOX 39-1 Sample Necropsy Report

Owner: Brown
Clinic #: 01-34567
Animal name: Ralph
Clinician: Smith
Date/time of death: 01/17/01 (9 AM)
Date/time of necropsy: 01/17/01 (11 AM)

This is a 3.0-kg, 7½-year-old, spayed, female seal-point Siamese cross cat in adequate postmortem and emaciated nutritional condition. There is a clipped area on the distal aspect of the right front leg with an electrocardiogram (ECG) lead taped in place. The left antebrachium is clipped, and a catheter is in the left cephalic vein. The ventral cervical area and the ventral and lateral abdomen are clipped. There is little body fat, and the muscle mass is reduced.

There is approximately 100 ml of yellow stringy fluid in the abdomen. There are multifocal, 2- to 10-mm, yellow-tan clots of fibrin throughout the abdomen and loosely adherent to abdominal organs. There are white-tan, multifocal to confluent, 1- to 5-cm diameter plaques on the surface of the liver, spleen, small intestine, omentum, mesentery, diaphragm, and body wall. The small intestine and colon are dilated (1 to 2 cm in diameter), and the wall of the small intestine is multifocally thickened. In the most severely affected area, at the jejunoileal junction, the serosa is corrugated and the wall is 3 to 5 mm thick. The abdominal and sternal lymph nodes are enlarged (0.5 to 2.0 cm in diameter) and white on the capsular surface. On section, they have a normal lymph node architecture with a thick white cortex.

The lungs are heavy, wet, and red-purple, and they sink in formalin. There is approximately 5 ml of serosanguineous fluid in the pericardium.

Gross Findings

Lungs: moderate to severe acute pneumonia, presumptive
Abdomen: severe fibrinous peritonitis
Small intestine and colon: severe chronic enteritis and colitis, presumptive
Pericardium: moderate serosanguineous effusion
Abdominal and sternal lymph nodes: severe reactive hyperplasia, presumptive

Gross Diagnosis

- Euthanasia
- Feline infectious peritonitis (FIP)
- Severe enteritis and colitis, presumptive
- Severe pneumonia, presumptive

Comment

I am not sure if the changes in the small intestine and colon are due to FIP or some other process. The lung lesion is also not typical for FIP. Impression smears of the peritoneal surface lesions reveal a mixed population of inflammatory cells, including neutrophils, lymphocytes, plasma cells, and macrophages, consistent with the diagnosis of FIP.

Samples of lung and small intestine are submitted for bacterial culture. Samples of lymph nodes, small intestine, colon, lungs, liver, and spleen are submitted for histologic examination.

placing tissues in them, and fixatives should be handled and used in a well-ventilated space.

> *TECHNICIAN NOTE* **Ten percent buffered formalin is the most widely used fixative for the preservation of tissues. Tissues should be placed in large volumes of formalin (10:1, formalin to tissue ratio).**

For the preservation of whole brains, intact spinal cords, and bones, 50% formalin, made by mixing one part 10% buffered formalin with one part of commercial formaldehyde (37% to 40% HCHO), is superior to the 10% solutions. The stronger 50% solution penetrates and fixes the large tissue mass more rapidly and more thoroughly than 10% formalin. Formalin fixation is usually complete within 24 hours (large brains may take 48 hours). Tissues fixed in 10% formalin are traditionally stored in 10% formalin, but storage in 70% alcohol is superior.

Bouin's fixative is less widely used than 10% formalin, but it is preferred in some instances because it produces less tissue shrinkage and better preservation of cellular detail. Fetal tissues, intestinal epithelium, eyes, testes, endocrine glands, and the inclusion bodies associated with several important diseases are particularly well preserved with this fixative. Bouin's fixative may be purchased from a variety of sources.

> *TECHNICIAN NOTE* **All containers of fixed tissue samples should be clearly labeled. Appropriate caution should be used in handling, shipping, and disposal of all fixatives.**

FACILITIES AND INSTRUMENTS

Necropsies should be performed in a well-lit, well-ventilated space, ideally outside the usual surgical and treatment areas. The area should be easy to clean and disinfect, have adequate drainage for fluids and water, and be large enough to comfortably move around in (Figure 39-3). When necropsies are performed in the field (outdoors), the appropriate disposal of tissues and the inadvertent spread of disease become particular concerns.

The person performing the necropsy (called the prosector) should wear protective clothing, such as a plastic apron, laboratory coat, or scrubs, which can be removed and either discarded or cleaned after the necropsy (Figure 39-4). Latex or other protective plastic gloves should be worn at all times. In addition, a surgical mask should be worn when dealing with animals that have died from infectious diseases that can be spread through aerosolization. Protective footwear (boots or booties) is appropriate when dealing with larger animals.

Necropsies do not require specialized equipment or instruments. Most instruments can be obtained from surgical suppliers and hardware stores (Figures 39-5 and 39-6). The following instruments are used in a typical necropsy:

- Necropsy knives (sturdy ones that can be sharpened) and honing steel
- Scalpel handle and blades
- Scissors (large and small operating, Mayo, or Metzenbaum scissors work well)
- Forceps (large- and small-toothed)
- Serrated, all-purpose, plastic-handled utility scissors
- Bone-cutting forceps
- Hacksaw, meat saw, or Stryker saw (for brain removal)
- Lopping (pruning) shears for cutting ribs and bones
- String or hemostats for closing off bowel ends
- Labeled plastic buckets or screw-top plastic containers containing formalin
- Tissue cassettes (for small tissues) and clip-on laundry tags for identifying tissues

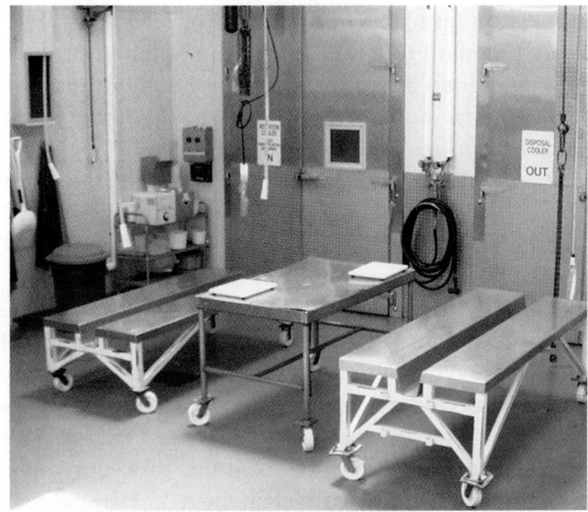

FIGURE 39-3 A view of a large animal necropsy room.

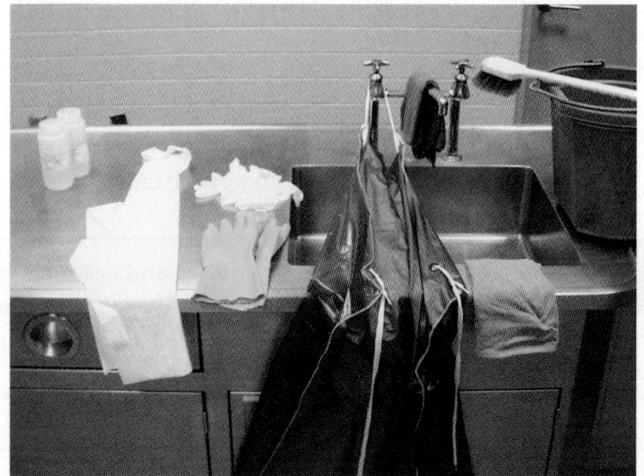

FIGURE 39-4 Personal protective clothing and equipment commonly used in a large animal necropsy.

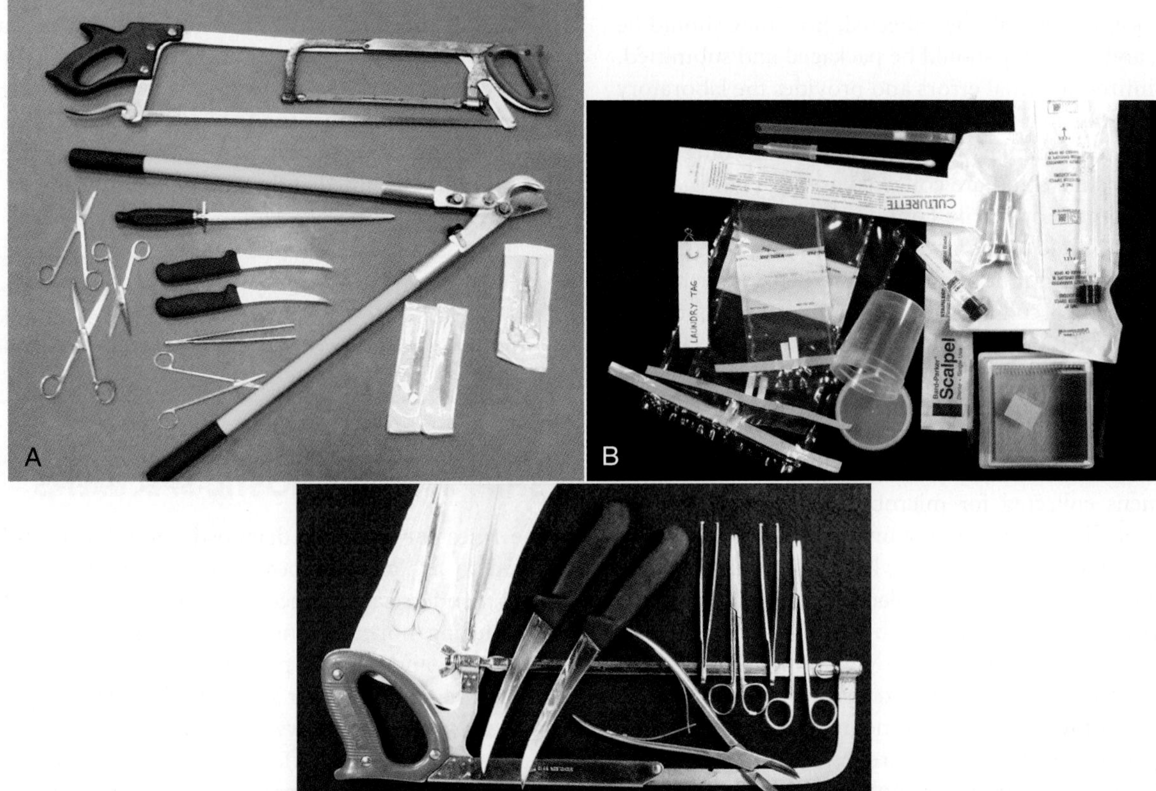

FIGURE 39-5 A-B, Instruments commonly used in a large animal necropsy. C, Equipment commonly used in a large animal necropsy.

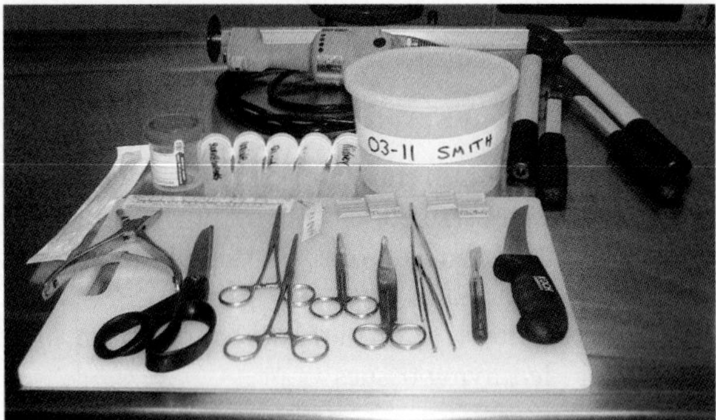

FIGURE 39-6 Instruments and equipment commonly used in a small animal necropsy.

- Labeled, sealable, plastic bags and plastic vials or bottles for refrigerated and frozen samples
- Culturettes for aerobic and anaerobic cultures

> *TECHNICIAN NOTE* All equipment and instruments should be thoroughly cleaned and disinfected after the necropsy. Instruments should be dedicated for necropsy use only to prevent the spread of pathogens.

ANCILLARY PROCEDURES

Before samples are collected for examination in the microbiology, parasitology, and toxicology departments, the diagnostic laboratory should be contacted for specific advice on which samples should be collected, how they should be collected, and how they should be packaged and submitted. This minimizes potential errors and provides the laboratory with the best possible specimens.

Tissues and specimens for bacteriology, mycology, and mycoplasma cultivation are collected aseptically, placed in either Culturettes or sterile containers without preservatives, and submitted to the laboratory without delay. Frozen specimens should not be submitted. Sterilized instruments should be used to collect samples for microbiologic testing. If the surface of the tissue is contaminated, it can be seared with a flamed spatula, the surface can be cut with a sterile blade, and a Culturette or needle attached to a sterile syringe can be inserted to swab or aspirate the tissue for testing.

Specimens collected for microbiology include the primary site of disease and its regional lymph nodes. Other samples may include heart, blood, lung, liver, spleen, stomach contents of aborted fetuses, placenta, exudates, synovia, bone marrow, cerebrospinal fluid, brain, and small intestine. When intestine is submitted, a 10-cm segment of intestine is tied off at each end to prevent excessive contamination by the internal contents. The instruments used to do this are heavily contaminated by the microbes exposed at the cut ends. For this reason, intestine should be collected last and placed in a separate container to prevent contamination of other tissue samples. Tissue sections of 2 × 3 × 1 cm and fluid specimens of 3 to 5 ml are desirable.

> *TECHNICIAN NOTE* Contact the diagnostic laboratory for specific advice on which samples should be collected, how they should be collected, and how they should be packaged and submitted.

Tissues for virus isolation are collected aseptically and either refrigerated in a sterile container or immersed in sterile 50% buffered glycerol in sterile containers and preserved by freezing. Fresh, refrigerated tissue immersed in virus transport medium (available from the virology laboratory) is the preferred method of tissue submission. Lung, liver, spleen, kidney, and brain are prime specimens. Sections need to be 5 × 5 × 10 mm. Contact the virology laboratory for the appropriate technique.

For toxicology, blood, liver, stomach contents, kidney, fat, brain, and urine may be saved. Blocks of tissues 10 × 5 × 4 cm (approximately 200 g), 10 to 20 ml of blood, and 50 to 100 ml of fluid are desirable. They may be frozen.

If rabies is suspected, the animal's head should be sent to the appropriate laboratory for testing according to the guidelines and laws of the state (Box 39-2). In cases in which rabies is suspected, decapitation or other necropsy procedures should not be attempted unless the technician has been specifically trained to perform this procedure. A necropsy should only be performed on the rest of the carcass if a rabies test result for the brain is negative.

For cytologic examination, smears are made (after gentle blotting on absorbent paper) by either scraping the cut surface of the specimen with a new scalpel blade and then spreading the scraped material onto a slide or lightly pressing small pieces of tissue against the surface of a clean slide. Several impressions are made across the slide. They are generally submitted unstained to the laboratory, or they can be stained and examined at the time of the necropsy.

> *TECHNICIAN NOTE* If rabies is suspected, the animal's head should be sent to the appropriate laboratory for testing according to the guidelines and laws of the state.

SHIPPING DIAGNOSTIC SPECIMENS

The rules for shipping diagnostic samples, technically referred to as "clinical specimens," have changed in recent years. Senders can be fined if containers break or specimens leak during normal transit conditions. Correct labeling is important, and a special packaging symbol (UN 3373) might be required. A computer search of the web will reveal many helpful sites (i.e., www.fedex.com/us/services/pdf/PKG_Pointers_Specimens.pdf). Many courier companies abide by International Air Transportation Association (IATA) rules, which impose the highest packaging and labeling standards. The simplest advice is to contact the courier to request their packaging requirements.

BOX 39-2 Rabies Procedure

Technicians and clinicians should be familiar with the rabies policies and guidelines of your state.

In all cases where rabies is suspected, the animals should be handled only by clinicians and technicians who are preimmunized against rabies and have a serum titer greater than 1:5. For small animals, prosectors should double glove and wear protective masks and goggles. For animals larger than large dogs, personnel should wear rubber boots, a scrub suit, apron, double gloves (the outer glove is heavy vinyl with gauntlets), and a face shield for splash protection. Pathology personnel who decapitate and extract brains must use the additional protection of a Tyvek coverall or alternatively a surgical gown and apron. A HEPA filtered helmet and face shield is suggested when working on equine species because of concerns about aerosolization of West Nile virus.

In cases where rabies is the primary or only differential diagnosis, the head should be carefully removed by disarticulation at the atlantooccipital junction using a disposable scalpel or knife, double bagged, placed in a refrigerated container (with ice packs, not dry ice) and sent to the appropriate laboratory for FA testing. The remaining carcass should be double bagged in a red biohazard bag, labeled as a rabies suspect, and disposed of as a biologic hazard.

Some states require removal of the brain before submission to the laboratory for animals larger than a large dog (horses, cattle, etc.). To remove the brain of a large animal for rabies testing use a special head vice or hold the head on the table (eyes may be removed to facilitate head holding). Remove as much hide and flesh over the calvaria as safely possible. The rostral transverse cut through the skull is made behind an imaginary line connecting the lateral canthi of the eyes. The lateral saw cuts start at the dorsolateral notch of the occiput and just miss the dorsal projection of the coronoid process. A small hatchet, inserted into the saw cuts, can be used to lever the calvaria. Then sever cranial nerves and meningeal attachments and remove the brain. Hemisection, parasagittally section, or selectively subsection the brain for the rabies laboratory submission as directed by the state testing laboratory.

In cases where a person has been bitten or exposed to saliva through open wounds, and rabies is not on the differential list or the animal did not have neurologic signs, either the whole head or two transverse slices of the brain (one involving the medulla and cerebellum bilaterally and one involving the hippocampus bilaterally) should be submitted for rabies testing, and the necropsy can be performed in the usual manner.

In all cases, the tables and instruments must be carefully disinfected and cleaned. Disposable scalpels are placed in a sharps container, and other instruments must be cleaned and disinfected.

All submitted tissues must be accompanied by a completed state rabies questionnaire.

In general, all clinical specimens must be in rigid primary containers that cannot leak. Excess formalin can be removed if the specimen has been fixed. The primary container is enclosed by a secondary container, usually a sturdy sealable plastic bag. Label primary and secondary containers. The plastic bag should contain absorbent material in case the primary container leaks. This package then goes inside a rigid shipping box. Cushion the contents of the shipping box. Styrofoam shipping boxes with outer cardboard shells are ideal. Formalin-fixed material does not need refrigeration, but bacterial cultures and fresh or frozen tissues might need freezer packs. Never use ice. Submission forms should not be placed next to primary containers, and if condensation is likely, the submission form should be in its own plastic bag.

NECROPSY PROCEDURE FOR A SMALL MAMMAL

The following procedure is appropriate for dogs, cats, ferrets, rodents, and rabbits. A brief outline of this procedure is in Box 39-3.

TISSUE COLLECTION

Tissues collected for histologic examination must be handled carefully before fixation and must be properly labeled for identification. Tissue sections should not be squeezed, stretched, or rinsed with water, and epithelial surfaces should not be rinsed or rubbed with fingers or instruments before samples are obtained for histopathologic examination. Tissues become rigid with fixation, so if there is a need to retain the flatness of the tissue (such as a nerve or section of skin), it can be placed on a piece of cardboard. The tissue will remain adhered to the cardboard after immersion in formalin.

Sections from paired organs may be trimmed differently from one another to distinguish them from one another. For example, the left kidney may be sectioned longitudinally, and the right kidney may be cut transversely. In addition, sections can be labeled with clip-on laundry tags to identify them. If there is any possibility that a section of tissue may lose its identity (i.e., be difficult to distinguish) when mixed with other specimens, the sections should be tagged with clip-on laundry tags. If tissue samples are small, they may also be placed in separate labeled containers, such as tissue cassettes. The **pituitary gland** of a small animal, for example, is well differentiated from other tissues when placed in a small tissue cassette.

TECHNICIAN NOTE Tissues collected for histologic examination must be handled carefully before fixation and must be properly marked for identification.

In all cases, it is desirable to save sections of critical tissues for histopathologic examination. These include lung, **myocardium,** liver, spleen, pancreas, stomach, small intestine, kidneys, lymph nodes, whole brain, endocrine organs, urinary bladder, colon, and muscle.

BOX 39-3 Necropsy Procedure Outline

1. Before you begin dissection, be sure you have the owner's permission, correct animal, disposition instructions, body weight, labeled formalin container, instruments, cassette for bone marrow, tag for brain, cardboard for nerve and skin, and an understanding of the clinical history.
2. All routine tissues and all lesions are collected, all lesions are described (measured and weighed if appropriate), and all necessary microbiologic, cytologic, and toxicologic samples are collected for every necropsy.
3. Weigh the animal and do the external examination, remove eyes, then place body in left lateral recumbency, and make a midline skin incision extending into axillary and inguinal areas to reflect limbs and extend the incision rostrally to the mandibular symphysis and caudally to the perineum.
4. Dissect and examine, section, and collect (DESC) skin, lymph nodes, salivary glands, and testes or mammary glands. Open the coxofemoral, stifle, and scapulohumeral joints. DESC synovium, skeletal muscle, sciatic nerve, and bone marrow.
5. Open abdomen (midline), puncture diaphragm, open chest (bilateral, cutting ribs) and pericardium, collect microbiologic samples, and examine organs and vessels in situ. (Note: Discuss case with clinician at this time.) DESC thyroid, parathyroids, and adrenal glands.
6. Remove tongue from oral cavity, and reflect the tongue, tonsils, larynx, and esophagus caudally. Cut spinal cord and vertebral column at atlantooccipital joint, remove skin and muscle from calvaria, cut calvaria with Stryker saw in hood, and remove caudal-dorsal calvaria and dorsal meninges. Transect cranial nerves, and remove brain and pituitary. Open tympanic bullae. Section head longitudinally and examine nasal and oral cavities.
7. Remove tongue, tonsils, esophagus, trachea, lungs, heart, and thoracic aorta together. Serially section tongue, open esophagus and trachea. Open right atrium, then right ventricle, then follow pulmonary arteries, isolate heart and then open left atrium, left ventricle, and thoracic aorta. Weigh heart. Collect whole heart in cats and small dogs, three sections of heart in larger animals. Serial section lungs saving one section from each lobe.
8. Remove distal duodenum, jejunum, ileum, colon, and mesenteric lymph nodes together by stripping from mesentery (open later unless critical). Remove liver, duodenum, pancreas, stomach, and spleen en bloc. Serial section spleen, open stomach and duodenum, express gallbladder, weigh the liver, and serial section liver (collect one section of each lobe). Open gallbladder, stomach (collect fundus and pylorus), duodenum, and pancreas (one section of right lobe with duodenum and one section of left lobe). Collect samples from all tissues.
9. Remove floor of pelvis, and DESC right kidney and ureter, left kidney and ureter, urinary bladder, urethra, prostate, ovaries and uterus, cervix and vagina, rectum, anal glands, and abdominal aorta. DESC small intestine, colon, and mesenteric lymph nodes.
10. Remove spinal cord if necessary.

DISSECTION

The method of dissection described here is a standard technique that can be applied to all mammalian species and is based on the following two precepts:

1. In stepwise fashion, each part of the carcass is examined **in situ** (as it first appears in the carcass); it is then isolated from the carcass and examined as a whole; finally, it is dissected and examined.
2. Once a part has been taken from the body, it is dissected to completion (exceptions include tissues from the gastrointestinal tract, brain, spinal cord, and eyes). Sections for histologic or laboratory examination are collected before further dissection is undertaken.

This method is the opposite of those that call for evisceration now and dissection later, methods that disrupt the entire carcass all at once, and that lead to forgotten or lost tissues. The immediate complete dissection of one part at a time reduces the possibility of lost or forgotten parts and leaves the remainder of the carcass intact. In this way, if the findings in one organ suggest that another part or parts of the carcass should be explored in situ, this is still possible and has not been precluded by previous dissection.

PRELIMINARY OBSERVATIONS

Before the necropsy begins, the prosector should review the signalment (species, breed, color, sex, age, weight, animal identification), the clinical history, and the laboratory data available. It is important that the time of death and time of necropsy be recorded. The animal should then be weighed, and the weight should be recorded in grams or kilograms. All organs that are abnormal in size or shape should be measured and/or weighed.

TECHNICIAN NOTE Before the necropsy begins, the prosector should review the signalment (species, breed, color, sex, age, weight, animal identification) of the animal, the clinical history, and any available laboratory data.

EXTERNAL EXAMINATION

The exterior of the animal is examined: body conformation, hair coat, skin, nose, mouth (lips, cheeks, gums, teeth, tongue), eyes (eyelids, conjunctiva, cornea, sclera, anterior chamber, iris, lens), ears, mammae, penis, prepuce, scrotum, vulva, anus, and feet. Because the retina undergoes rapid decomposition after death, dissection begins with the eyes. The upper and lower eyelids are examined and excised. The membrana nictitans is grasped with tissue forceps, the globe is lifted, and the soft tissue attachments to the bony orbit are incised with scissors or a scalpel in a 360-degree arc. As the globe is freed from the orbit, care must be taken to avoid

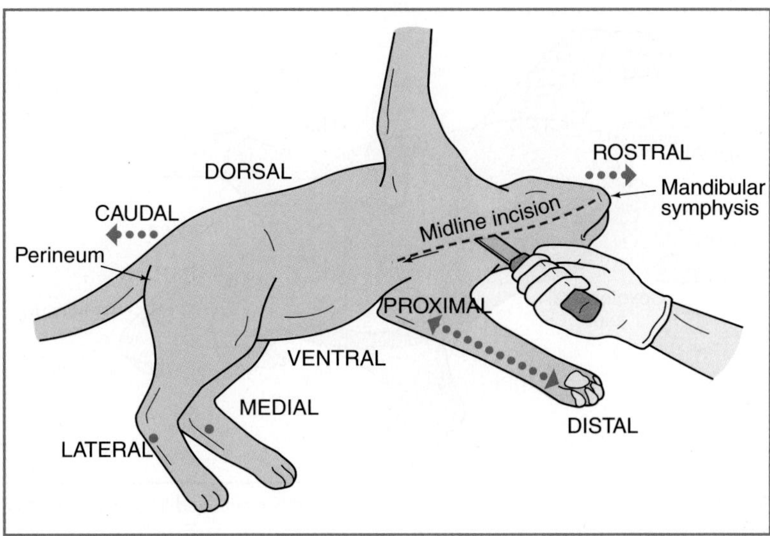

FIGURE 39-7 The necropsy begins with the animal placed on its left side. A midline incision is made from the mandibular symphysis.

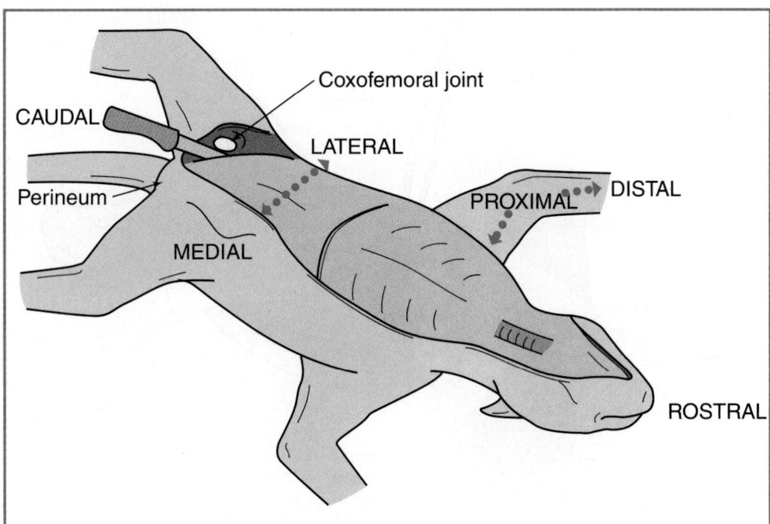

FIGURE 39-8 The front limbs are reflected by making incisions between the ribs and the scapulas. The hind legs are reflected by incising the coxofemoral (hip) joints.

application of excessive tension to the optic nerve. The optic nerve is carefully severed at the optic canal. The excised globe is examined, and then extraocular muscles, fascia, fat, conjunctiva, and membrana nictitans are dissected from the globe. The interior of the eye can be examined by immersing the globe in clear, cool water. The sclera is examined, and the unopened globe is immersed in Bouin's fixative or formalin.

REFLECTION OF SKIN AND LIMBS AND EXAMINATION OF SUPERFICIAL ORGANS AND BODY CAVITIES

The animal is placed in left lateral recumbency (left side down). A midline incision is made beginning at the right axilla and extending cranially to the mandibular symphysis (Figure 39-7). The incision is continued in the opposite direction caudally as a median or paramedian incision, passing between the mammae and around the penis, prepuce, and scrotum to the perineum (Figure 39-8). The upper forelimbs are reflected by dissection between the scapula and the ribs. Fat, fascia, and superficial muscles are reflected back together with the skin. Skin of the ventral aspect of the neck and throat is reflected. Abdominal skin is reflected, and the hind limbs are reflected by extending the incision into the coxofemoral (hip) joints. The animal is now placed in dorsal recumbency (on its back) (Figure 39-9).

Skin incisions are extended down the cranial medial aspects of both rear legs, and the skin is reflected. As they are exposed in the dissection, superficial organs are examined and samples from these organs are collected: lymph nodes (mandibular, superficial cervical, prescapular, axillary, inguinal, popliteal), mammary glands, testes, and skin.

In all necropsy examinations, several joints are examined before the body cavities are opened. The coxofemoral joints are opened and examined during the initial incision. The scapulohumeral and stifle joints are also examined during all routine necropsies. The atlantooccipital joint will be examined when the head is removed.

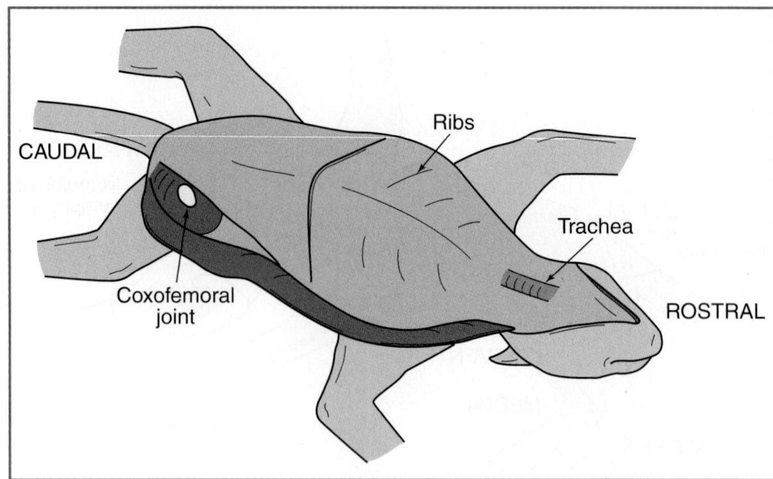

FIGURE 39-9 After all four limbs have been reflected, the animal is positioned in dorsal recumbency (on its back).

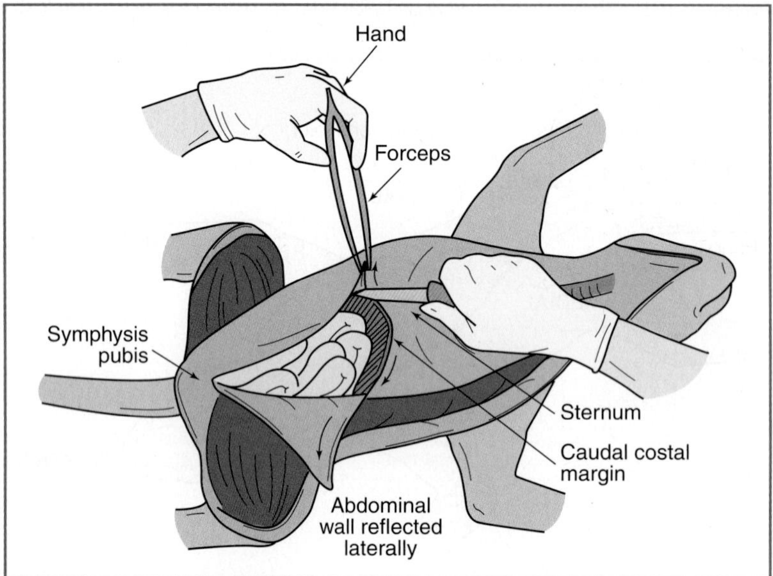

FIGURE 39-10 The abdominal wall is incised with a midline incision. The right and left halves of the abdominal wall are reflected laterally by making incisions from the sternum along both right and left caudal costal margins.

Samples of the **sciatic nerve,** synovium with patella, and skeletal muscle are collected. Bone marrow samples for impression smears or histopathologic examination should be collected at this time. Generally, marrow is obtained by cracking the upper midshaft femur with pruning shears.

You should, at this point, have already collected the following: eyes, lymph nodes, testes or mammary glands, skin, synovium, sciatic nerve, skeletal muscle, and bone marrow.

Next the three major body cavities (peritoneal, pleural, pericardial) are opened. All organs are examined in situ, and any abnormalities are noted. The abdomen is opened by making a midline incision from the **sternum** to the symphysis pubis and making incisions laterally from the sternum along both caudal costal margins. The abdominal wall is then reflected laterally to expose the abdominal cavity (Figure 39-10).

The **diaphragm** is now punctured to check for negative pleural pressure (Figure 39-11), and the diaphragm is cut away from the ventral and lateral rib cage. The ventral rib cage is removed by cutting the ribs bilaterally (on both sides) midway between the costochondral junction and the vertebral column (Figure 39-12). This should be done with utility scissors or pruning shears. Examine the pleural surface of the rib cage. In young animals, the costochondral growth plate may be examined and saved for histopathologic examination. Next the pericardial sac is opened, and the exterior of the heart is examined.

TECHNICIAN NOTE The history and preliminary findings are reviewed with the clinician after all body cavities have been opened.

The thyroid, parathyroids, and thymus should be identified at this time and removed. The adrenal glands should then be identified and removed. The adrenal glands are sectioned, and the corticomedullary ratio is noted. The mandibular salivary glands, parotid salivary glands, parotid lymph nodes, jugular veins, and parapharyngeal and retropharyngeal lymph nodes are examined.

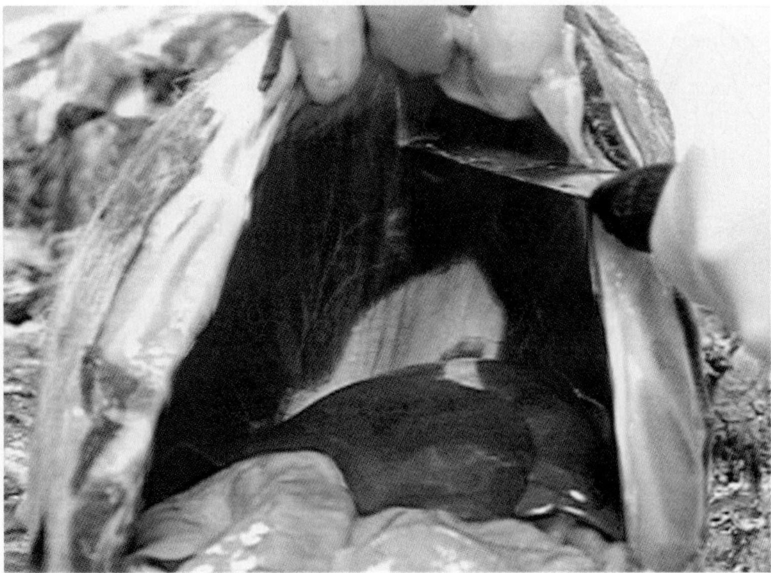

FIGURE 39-11 The diaphragm is punctured to test for negative pressure in the pleural cavity.

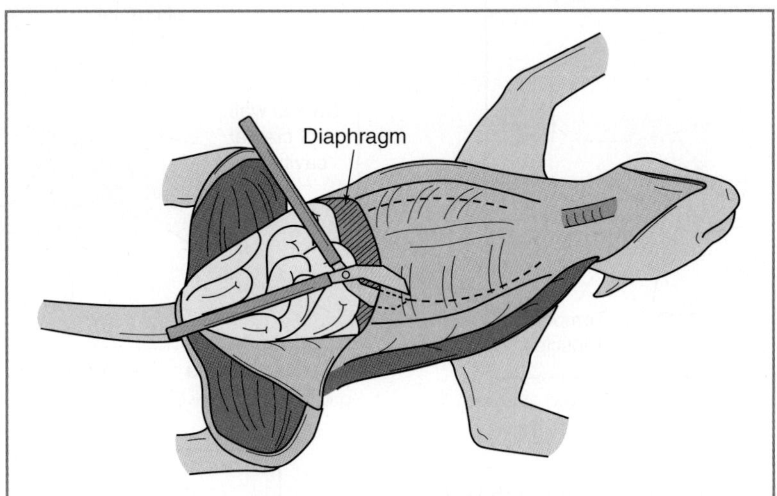

FIGURE 39-12 The ventral portion of the rib cage is removed by cutting the ribs bilaterally (on both sides) with heavy pruning shears.

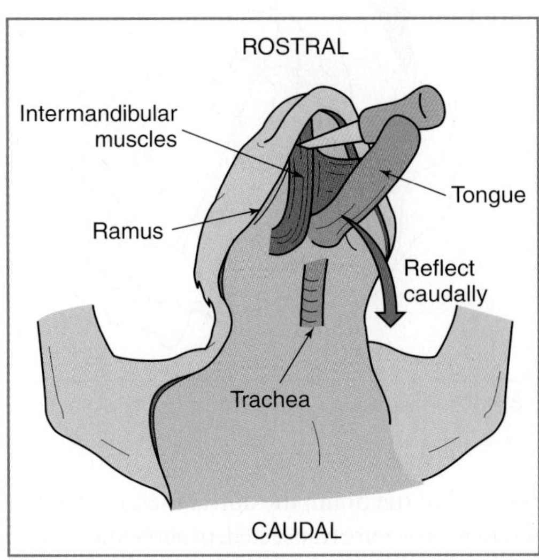

FIGURE 39-13 Examination of the tongue, tonsils, larynx, and esophagus. These are reflected caudally after the intermandibular muscles have been incised.

EXAMINATION OF SKULL AND BRAIN

Remove the tongue from the oral cavity, and reflect the tongue, tonsils, larynx, and esophagus caudally (Figure 39-13). An incision is made through the intermandibular muscles, along the medial surface of the ramus of each mandible, from the angle to the symphysis. The frenulum of the tongue is incised, and the tongue is pulled (or pushed) ventrally between the rami. The tongue is used as a handle, and right and left paramedian incisions are extended from the larynx to the thoracic inlet, exposing the length of the trachea and esophagus. It is necessary to cut or disarticulate the **hyoid bones** dorsal to the pharynx to free the tongue, larynx, pharynx, trachea, and esophagus as a unit.

The spinal cord is transected by an incision into the ventral atlantooccipital joint. Atlantooccipital membranes, ligaments, and joint capsule are transected, disarticulating the head from the vertebral column (Figure 39-14, *A* and *B*). The skin is removed from the head by leaving it attached to the

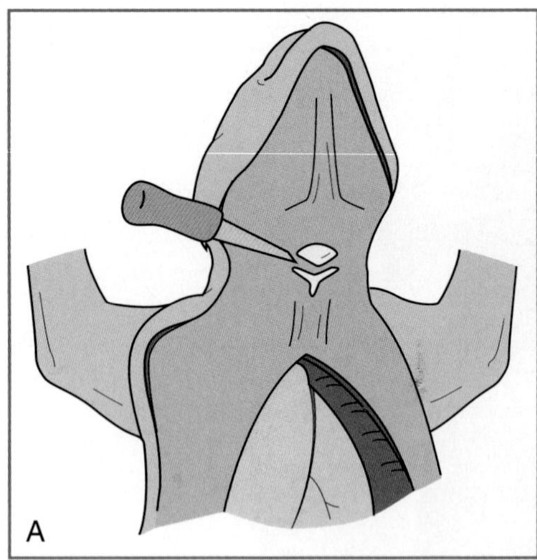

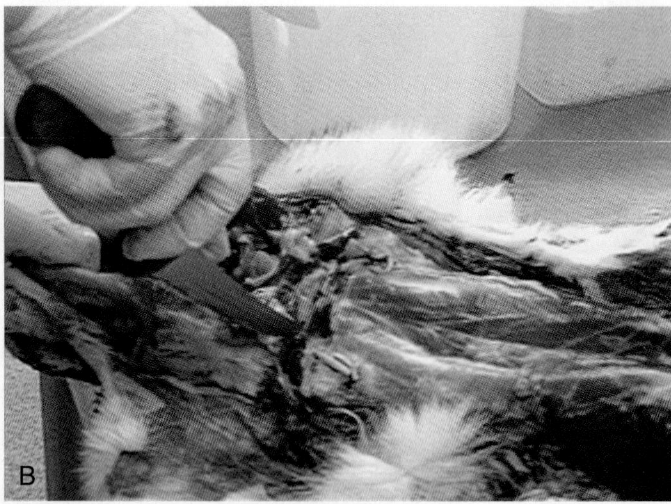

FIGURE 39-14 A-B, The spinal cord is transected ventrally by first making an incision into the atlantooccipital joint. The head is disarticulated from the vertebral column.

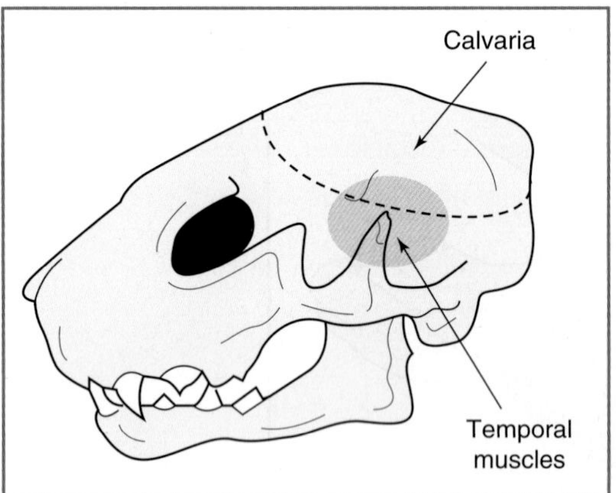

FIGURE 39-15 The temporal muscles are removed to reveal the skull cap, or calvaria.

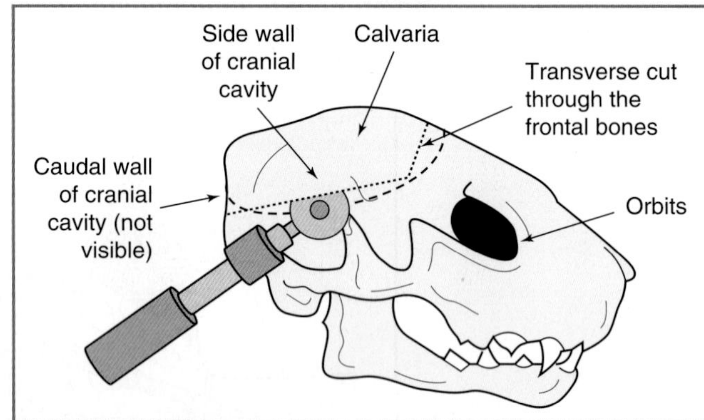

FIGURE 39-16 The cranial cavity is opened by removing the calvaria and caudal wall as a unit.

skin of the body and peeling the head forward out of the skin. The superficial muscles of the head are removed. External ears are opened and examined. Temporal muscles are removed, exposing the calvaria (skull cap) (Figure 39-15).

The calvaria and caudal wall of the cranial cavity are removed from the skull as a unit, exposing the dorsum of the brain. Three cuts are made with a Stryker saw, hacksaw, or meat saw to accomplish this. The first is a transverse cut through the frontal bones. This cut is usually made immediately caudal to the orbits. Care is taken to make the cut just deep enough to transect bone, but not deep enough to engage the brain beneath.

The second and third cuts are made through the side walls and caudal wall of the cranial cavity. At 45-degree angles to the longitudinal axis of the skull, they extend from the lateral ends of the transverse cut to the medial faces of the occipital condyles (Figure 39-16). In small animals, the bone may be broken away piecemeal, progressing cranial from the **foramen magnum** with scissors, bone-cutting forceps, or postmortem shears. The calvaria and caudal wall as a unit are pried loose from surrounding bones and removed. The **meninges** (the three membranes that cover the brain) and the surface of the brain are examined in situ (Figure 39-17).

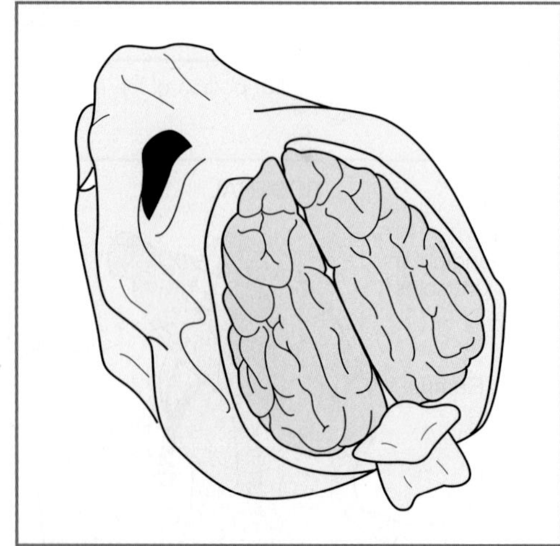

FIGURE 39-17 The meninges and surface of the brain are examined in situ.

For removal of the brain, the dorsal meninges are removed and the cranial nerves are transected, progressing rostrally from the foramen magnum. The brain is examined, tagged, and then immersed in 50% formalin. Brain slicing is postponed until after the brain has been thoroughly fixed in formalin.

The pituitary gland is removed from its fossa with the brain and examined. The middle ears (tympanic bullae) are opened ventrally by using rongeurs. For examination of the nasal septum, turbinates, and frontal or maxillary sinuses, the skull is sectioned longitudinally with a saw. The oral cavity is examined.

DISSECTION AND EXAMINATION OF THE NECK AND THORACIC VISCERA

The cervical and thoracic viscera are removed from the body and examined. The trachea and esophagus are used as a handle, and the thoracic organs are removed from the body by cutting between the dorsal **mediastinum** and the vertebral column from the thoracic inlet back to the diaphragm. The dorsal incision is carried above the aorta. At the diaphragm, the aorta, postcava, and esophagus are transected, and the throat, neck, and thoracic viscera are removed as a unit. This unit is dissected and examined from tongue to aorta. The tongue is examined and sliced transversely. The pharynx is opened middorsally with scissors, and the pharynx and tonsils are examined. The esophagus is opened longitudinally by a middorsal incision. The larynx is opened middorsally with utility scissors or a knife, and the incision is extended through the trachea to the lungs. The lungs are examined and palpated (for fine fixation, the lung may be "inflated" with 10% formalin, gravity fed into the trachea or bronchi).

The right side of the heart and **pulmonary arteries** are examined before the lungs are cut. The heart is held so that the right side is on the prosector's left and the left side is on the right. The right auricle is incised, and the incision is extended away from the prosector to the far end of the right atrium (Figure 39-18, *A*). The incision is then directed

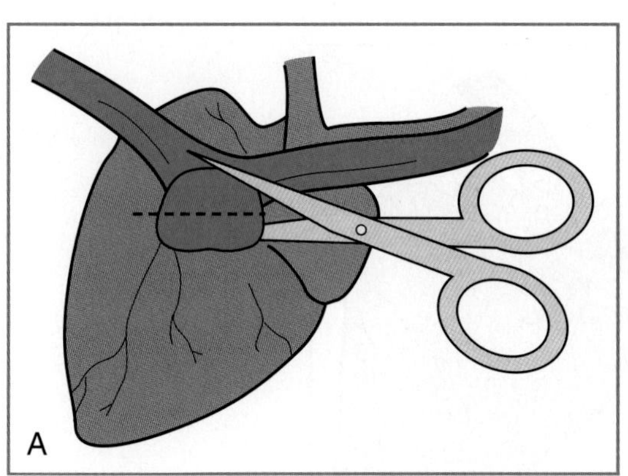

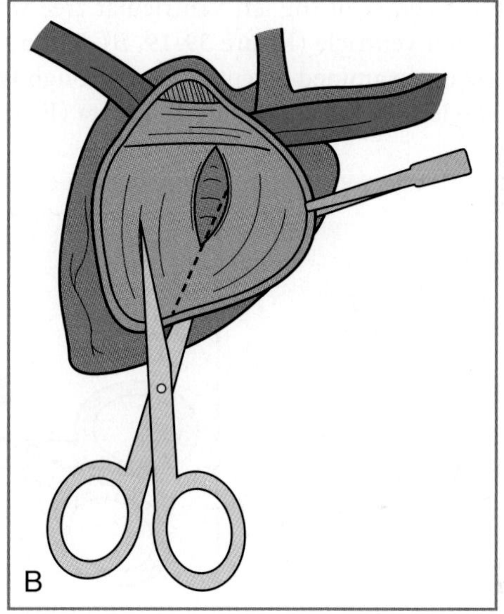

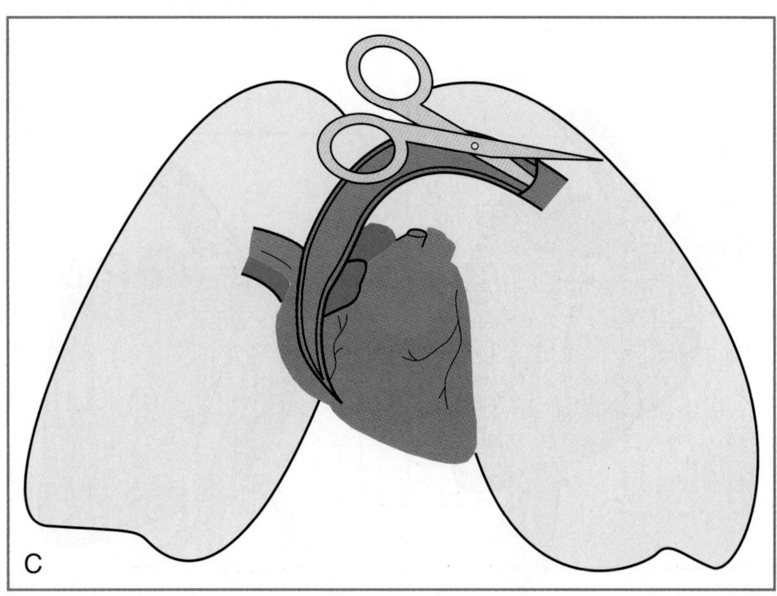

FIGURE 39-18 **A,** Dissection of the heart begins with an incision into the right auricle. **B,** The heart is incised through the right atrium and ventricle following the interventricular septum. The incision is then continued into the pulmonary artery. **C,** The pulmonary artery is incised, and the incision is continued into each lung lobe.

downward through the right **atrioventricular (AV) valve** and along the interventricular septum to the apex of the right ventricle. The incision is continued up along the interventricular septum through the pulmonic valve into the pulmonary artery (Figure 39-18, *B*). The right free wall of the heart is reflected, and the valves and endocardial surfaces are examined. The pulmonary arteries are opened into each lung lobe (Figure 39-18, *C*). Air passages and transected lung tissue are examined. Sections of lung are squeezed gently to assess fluid content. Bronchial lymph nodes are examined and sliced longitudinally.

The heart and major vessels are then removed from the lungs. The heart is again held so that the right side is on the prosector's left and the left side is to the right. The left auricle is incised, and the incision is extended away from the prosector to the far end of the left atrium (Figure 39-19, *A*). The incision is then directed downward through the left AV valve and along the center of the left ventricular free wall to the apex of the left ventricle (Figure 39-19, *B*). The aortic valve and aorta are examined by cutting up through the septal leaflet of the left AV valve and into the aorta (Figure 39-19, *C*). The valves, endocardium, and endothelial surfaces are then examined. The heart may then be weighed after all major vessels have been removed at the base of the heart. Next the myocardium is sliced longitudinally for examination, and samples are collected. Small hearts should be fixed whole after they have been opened.

DISSECTION AND EXAMINATION OF THE ABDOMINAL CAVITY

Examination of the abdominal cavity begins with examination of the portal vein as it enters the liver and removal of the intestinal tract. The intestine is removed by stripping the mesentery from the small intestine and colon. The **duodenum** is clamped or tied and transected distal to the tail of the pancreas. The colon is transected at the pelvic inlet, and the intestinal tract is removed and set aside for later examination. If the animal is thought to have intestinal disease, the intestines are examined at this time.

The stomach, liver, spleen, pancreas, and duodenum are removed by cutting the attachments between these

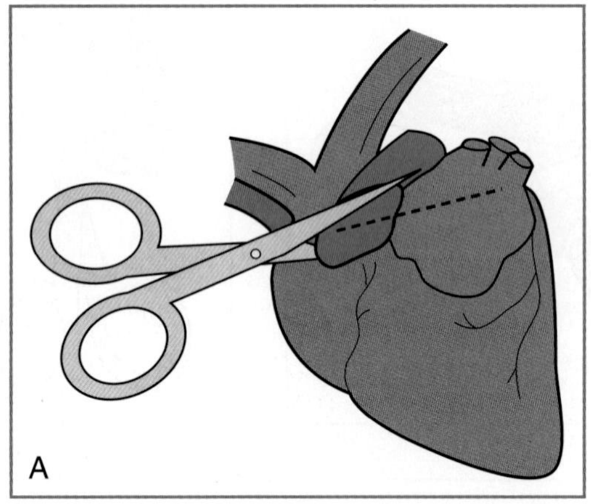

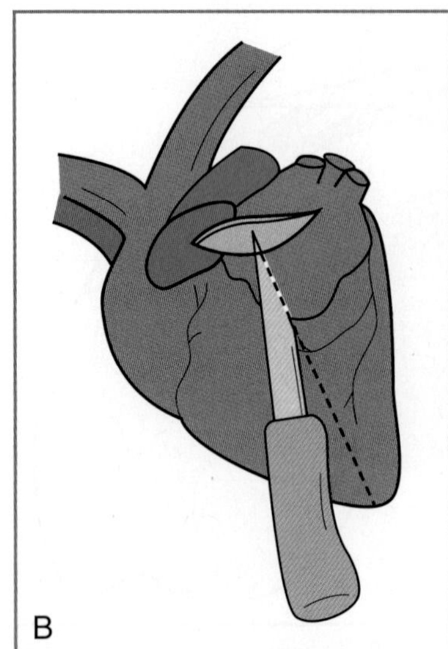

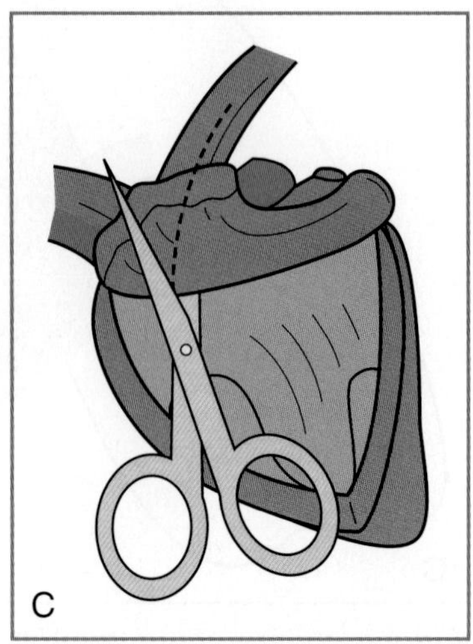

FIGURE 39-19 **A,** The second half of the heart is dissected by incising the left auricle and continuing the incision into the left atrium. **B,** From the left atrium, the incision is continued through the left AV valve into the left ventricle to the apex. **C,** The incision is then continued into the aorta.

organs, the diaphragm, and ventral body wall. The spleen is examined and sectioned. The stomach is opened along the greater curvature, and the duodenum is opened. The gallbladder is squeezed to determine patency of the bile duct, the gallbladder is opened, and the stomach, duodenum, and pancreas are dissected from the liver, examined, and sectioned. A section of the right side of the pancreas is collected with the duodenum, and a section of the left side is collected separately. The liver is then examined and sectioned. Multiple slices (approximately 1 cm apart) are made in the liver, and samples are collected from each lobe.

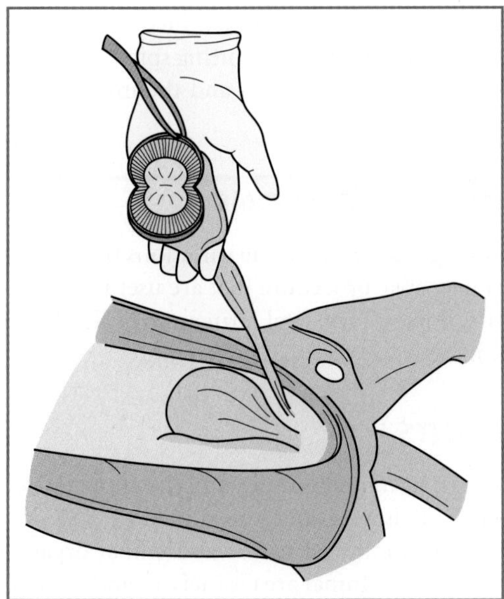

FIGURE 39-20 The kidney is dissected with a longitudinal incision. The renal capsule is then peeled away to reveal the renal surfaces.

DISSECTION AND EXAMINATION OF THE FEMALE REPRODUCTIVE TRACT, URINARY TRACT, AND ACCESSORY MALE REPRODUCTIVE ORGANS

The floor of the pelvis should be removed to facilitate examination and removal of the urogenital tract. This is accomplished by making paramedian cuts through the obturator foramina on the floor of the pelvis. The mesovarium, mesosalpinx, and mesometrium are examined. Ovaries, oviducts, and uterus are freed from mesentery and reflected toward the pelvis.

The left kidney is dissected free from the abdominal wall, but remains attached to the ureter. It is sliced longitudinally, and the capsule is peeled from one half of the kidney (Figure 39-20). The surface, cortex, medulla, and pelvis are examined. The ureters are examined and palpated. If the ureters or renal pelvis is dilated, the ureters are opened from kidney to bladder with a scissors. The ureter is cut near the bladder, and the kidney is removed. Sections are taken from the middle of both halves, one with the capsule intact and one with the capsule removed. Samples are also collected from any other renal lesions. The right kidney is then examined in the same manner.

The urinary bladder is incised and opened (Figure 39-21). Serosa, mucosa, and cut surfaces are examined. Care should be taken not to rub mucosal surfaces. The urethra is opened and examined, and the prostate is examined and sectioned.

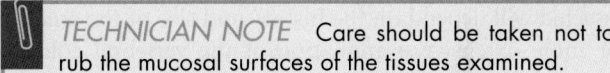

TECHNICIAN NOTE Care should be taken not to rub the mucosal surfaces of the tissues examined.

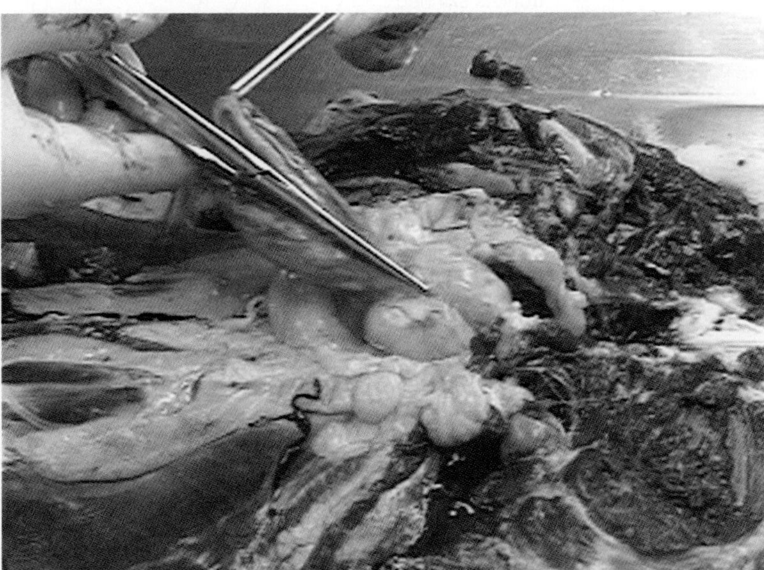

FIGURE 39-21 The urinary bladder is incised and opened in situ, and the incision is continued through the prostate and urethra.

Ovaries, oviducts, uterus, cervix, vagina, and vulva are removed from the carcass as a unit. Large ovaries are sliced longitudinally, oviducts are examined and palpated, and uterus, cervix, vagina, and vulva are opened with scissors or a knife. Serosa, contents of the uterus, endometrium, cut surfaces, cervical folds, and luminal surface of vagina and vulva are examined.

DISSECTION AND EXAMINATION OF THE INTESTINAL TRACT

The intestinal tract is examined by laying it out on the table and examining the serosal surface. The tract is then opened from the duodenum through the colon by using scissors. The mucosa is examined, and sections are taken from the jejunum, ileum, and colon, including lesions. The mucosa should be handled carefully to prevent creation of artifacts. Once sections have been taken, the mucosa can be gently rinsed with water to reveal mucosal details.

DISSECTION AND EXAMINATION OF THE ABDOMINAL AORTA, RECTUM, AND ANAL GLANDS

The abdominal aorta is opened longitudinally and examined, and a section is taken for histologic examination. The rectum is opened, and the anal sacs are examined.

DISSECTION AND EXAMINATION OF THE VERTEBRAL COLUMN AND SPINAL CORD

The manner and extent to which the vertebral column is dissected will depend on the history and size of the animal. For more extensive examination of the vertebral column and spinal cord, the remaining rib cage, the four limbs, and most of the dorsal spinal musculature are removed from the vertebral column and pelvis. A dorsal laminectomy is performed to demonstrate ventral or lateral impingements on the spinal cord of small animals. The spinal cord is covered dorsally by the vertebral arches; each arch consists of a right and left lamina, which unite to form the dorsal spinous process (spine). Beginning at the **atlas,** the right and left **laminae** of each vertebra are cut with bone shears or, in larger specimens, with the Stryker saw. The laminae of atlas and **axis** are broad and difficult to cut, but the remainder of the vertebrae present little difficulty. Once several dorsal arches have been freed, the connected arches are held as a handle and used to reflect succeeding arches dorsally and caudally. When the entire roof of the vertebral canal has been removed, meninges, spinal cord, and vertebrae are examined in situ. Spinal cord and meninges are removed by cutting spinal nerve roots, and the floor of the vertebral canal and the intervertebral disks are examined.

NECROPSY VARIATIONS

The following sections describe variations on the basic small mammal necropsy procedure that are useful in dealing with ruminants, horses, pigs, fetal farm animals, birds, and laboratory animals.

RUMINANTS

Necropsy of a ruminant is done with the animal in left lateral recumbency. This positions the rumen on the down side, which facilitates removal of the abdominal organs (Figure 39-22).The right inguinal area is incised, and the coxofemoral joint is penetrated. Muscles near the pelvis are severed,

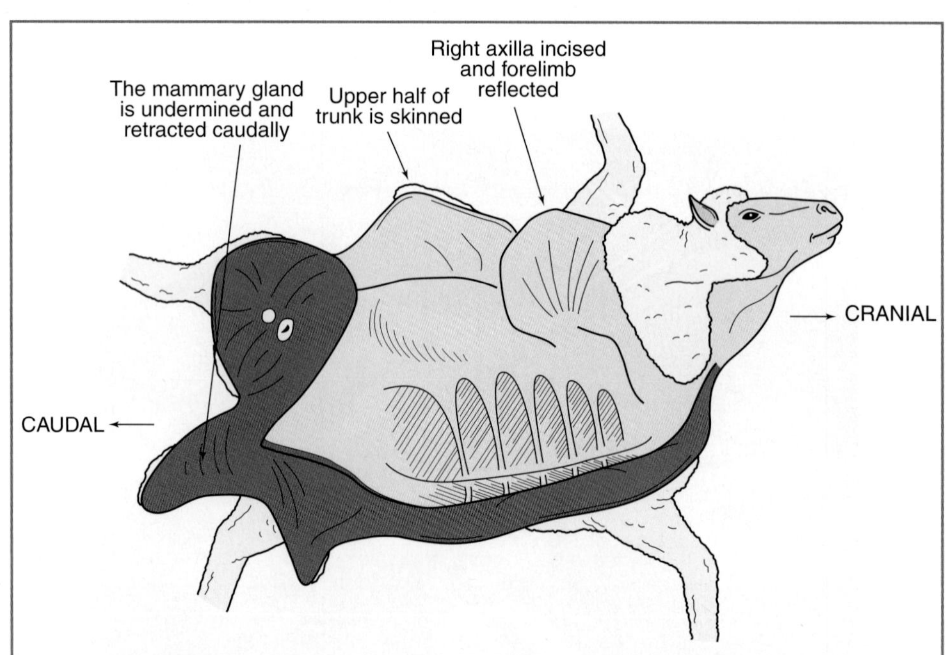
Right axilla incised and forelimb reflected
The mammary gland is undermined and retracted caudally
Upper half of trunk is skinned
CRANIAL
CAUDAL

FIGURE 39-22 The ruminant is positioned in left lateral recumbency, which positions the rumen on the "down side." This facilitates access to the abdominal organs.

and the right hind limb is reflected away from the body. Each mammary gland is undermined at its body wall attachment and retracted caudally. The mammary glands should remain attached to the body by the perineal skin so that gland position can be maintained when they are serially sectioned. The right axilla is incised so that the entire forelimb can be reflected away from the body. The upper half of the trunk is then skinned.

Entry into the abdomen is initiated by cutting the body wall behind the last rib. Cuts along the midline and upper flank permit exposure of the cavity (Figure 39-23). After an in situ inspection, the **omentum** is stripped from the **forestomachs;** double-string ligatures are placed on the duodenum (near the pylorus) and rectum, and a single ligature is placed around the esophagus near the reticulum. This prevents excessive leakage of contents. If the rumen is severely distended with gas, a tiny nick in the wall will release the gas without excessive contamination. The entire intestinal tract is removed by severing the mesenteric root, and the intestines are opened, examined, and sampled while still attached to the mesentery (Figure 39-24). The dorsal attachments to the rumen are cut, and the forestomachs and **abomasum** are rolled onto the floor. Ruminoreticular contents should be examined for foreign objects or undesirable plant material.

Because of the size of the chest cavity and difficulty in cutting the ribs in mature animals, the thoracic contents are usually removed via the abdominal cavity. The right side of the rib cage is easily removed with lopping shears in young animals. The diaphragm is incised along its costal attachment, and the ventral mediastinal attachments are severed. The tongue, larynx, and trachea are freed of their attachments and threaded into the thoracic inlet. The entire unit is pulled into the abdomen.

The remainder of the necropsy is similar to that described for the small mammal.

HORSE

Left lateral recumbency is the preferred body position for necropsy of a horse. Reflect the right forelimb and right hind limb as described for the ruminant. Skin the trunk, and enter the abdomen. The intestines are removed in the following multistep process:

1. Retract and drape the free portion of the large colon over the horse's body to ease access to the abdominal viscera.
2. Sever the ileum at the ileocecal junction, and remove the small intestine by cutting along the mesenteric insertion.
3. Cut the duodenum where it wraps around the mesenteric root; a string ligature here will reduce contamination by digesta.
4. Next remove the small intestine mesentery.
5. Sever the small colon near the pelvic inlet and detach along the mesocolon.
6. With careful blunt dissection, peel the soft connective tissue and pancreas adhering to the large colon near the mesenteric root. When your hand can encircle the mesenteric root, advance the knife to cut as close to the aorta as possible.
7. Obtain samples from the large colon and cecum and empty them of their contents. Rinse and examine the mucosal surfaces.

The remainder of the necropsy is similar to the procedure done on ruminants and small mammals. Special attention should be given to the guttural pouches and jugular veins.

All joints of the **appendicular skeleton** should be opened. Joints are best approached from the medial and cranial aspects after the skin has been reflected. The coffin joint is the most difficult joint to access, but access is easier if the foot can be split (with a saw). Splitting the foot also facilitates examination of the hoof wall lamina. Spinal cord removal

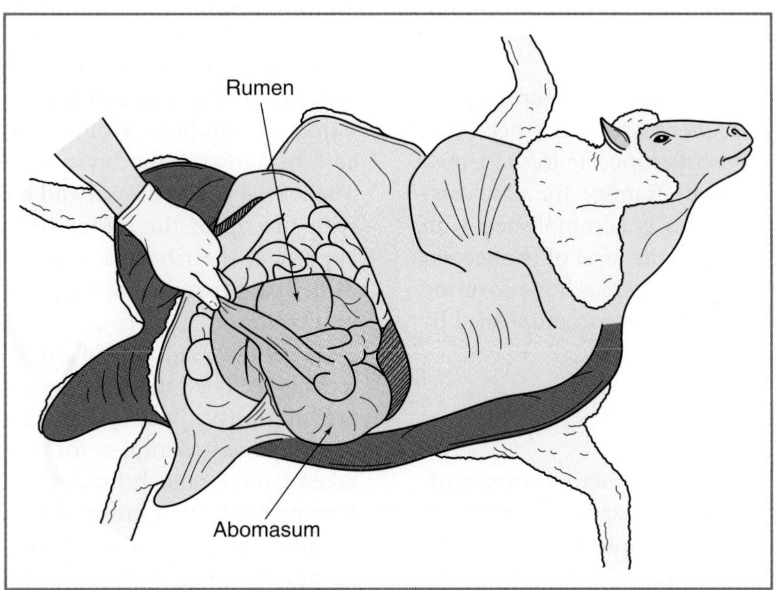

FIGURE 39-23 Access to the abdominal cavity is achieved by making an incision along the midline, followed by cuts along the last ribs.

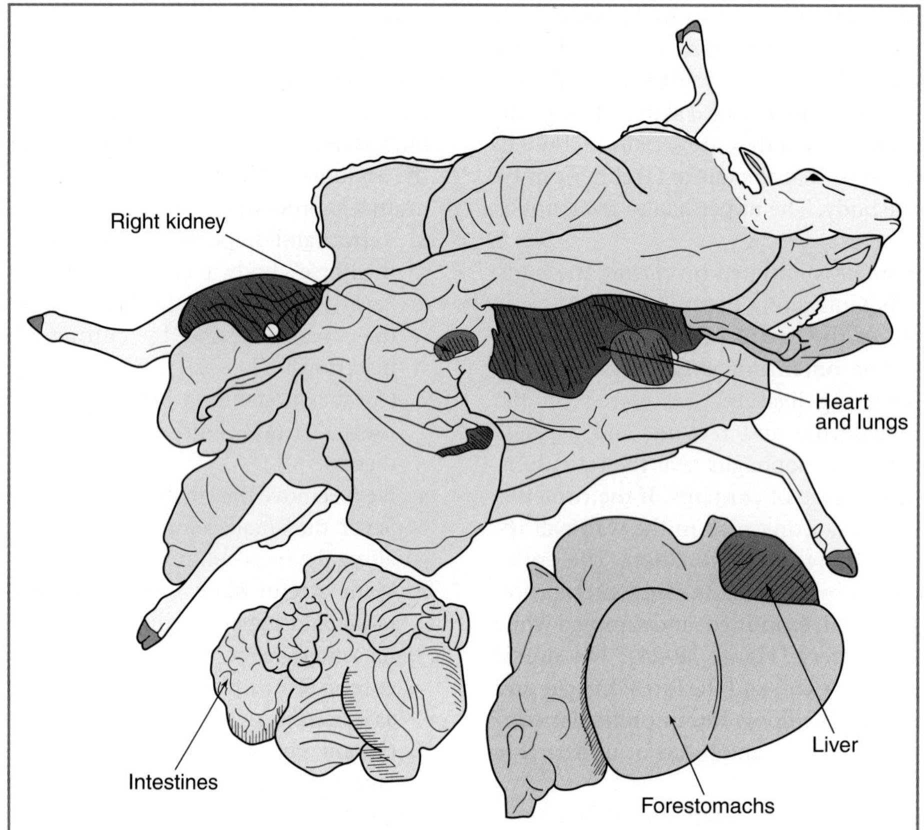

FIGURE 39-24 After the omentum is examined in situ, it is stripped from the forestomachs. The duodenum, rectum, and esophagus are ligated, and the entire intestinal tract is removed by severing the mesenteric root.

is extremely tedious without access to a meat cutter's band saw. Alternatively the cervical cord can be extracted by disarticulating the cervical vertebrae, one by one. Remove as much muscle as possible before disarticulating at the facets and annulus fibrosus. Sever the nerve roots by advancing a pair of thin, long-handled scissors along the wall of the spinal canal.

PIG

For necropsy of a pig, small mammal procedures apply. Because enteric disease is a frequent reason for necropsy, attention should be focused on collecting the freshest possible gut tissues. It is customary to examine the nasal turbinates of market-weight pigs. This is accomplished with a transverse saw cut of the snout at the level of the second and third premolars. Mature swine have sinus bone covering much of the calvaria. Brain removal is best accomplished by hemisectioning the head.

FETUS

Fetuses are often severely autolyzed, sometimes mummified, because of in utero retention after death. Nevertheless, sample collection is justified. Fetal membranes (placenta) should be carefully examined, and all abnormal-appearing sites should be sampled. Equine fetal membranes are examined for completeness. Fetuses from cattle and horses are measured (weighed if possible) to estimate gestational age. Standardized charts are available in many veterinary textbooks. Crown-to-rump length (the distance from the poll to the tail base along the dorsum) is determined with a flexible tape measure.

The fetus is placed in right lateral recumbency because fetal abdominal organs are most easily sampled from the left side. The left limbs are removed, and the body wall is skinned. The abdominal wall is incised behind the rib, and the incision is extended along the ribs, sublumbar flank, and midline without touching the underlying viscera or allowing the body wall to drop onto the viscera. The left hemidiaphragm and costosternal cartilage are cut with the tip of the knife, and, similar to the abdominal approach, the rib cage is retracted without touching the underlying tissues. The ribs usually break along the vertebral column.

Organs are sampled in situ with sterile tools and aseptic technique. The organs of greatest interest for viral cultures are lungs, liver, kidneys, and lymphoid tissue (e.g., spleen and thymus). Samples for bacterial culture are usually taken from stomach fluid, lungs, and liver. The body can now be routinely examined for anatomic correctness, and samples can be obtained for histologic examination. The umbilical stump and brain should always be examined and collected.

BIRDS

Birds suspected of having infectious or zoonotic diseases (psittacosis) should be submitted to a diagnostic laboratory for necropsy. If avian necropsies are done, the prosector should wear protective clothing, gloves, and a mask. The carcass should be wetted by immersing it in warm soapy water or disinfectant to decrease the spread of infectious agents and reduce the amount of irritating, aerosolized dander and feathers. After the external examination, the bird is placed in dorsal recumbency, and the feathers are parted along the ventral midline. For small birds, one wing may be pinned to a corkboard or cardboard for easier dissection. A skin incision extending from the beak to the vent is made, and the skin is reflected. The legs are reflected laterally by cutting into and exposing the coxofemoral joint. The abdomen is opened as in the small mammal necropsy technique, and the sternum and lateral ribs are removed by cutting through the sternum, ribs, coracoid bones, and clavicles with scissors, utility scissors, poultry shears, or pruning shears, depending on the size of the bird. Air sacs and abdominal and thoracic contents are examined, and samples are taken for examination by a microbiologist if necessary.

> *TECHNICIAN NOTE* Birds suspected of having infectious or zoonotic diseases (psittacosis) should be submitted to a diagnostic laboratory for necropsy.

For small birds (e.g., hummingbirds or finches), the entire carcass can be fixed after the body cavities have been opened. For larger birds, the joints, nerves, muscles, eyes, brain, and spinal cord can be examined as in the small mammal necropsy technique. The spinal cord in small birds is difficult to remove without damaging it. The entire vertebral column with the spinal cord inside should be collected and fixed after the limbs, head, and muscles surrounding the vertebral column have been removed. The vertebral column and spinal cord can be submitted whole and decalcified and trimmed by the pathology laboratory.

In larger birds, the thyroid and parathyroid glands, located at the thoracic inlet adjacent to the carotid arteries, are removed. The heart is removed and examined. The entire gastrointestinal tract, liver, pancreas, and spleen are removed, beginning with the esophagus. The spleen, liver, and gastrointestinal tract are examined, and specimens are collected as in the small mammal necropsy. The tongue, trachea, and lungs are then removed and examined, and samples are collected. The gonads (only the left ovary is present in birds) and adrenal glands are removed and fixed whole in small birds, and then the kidneys are removed, examined, and sampled.

LABORATORY ANIMALS

The necropsy technique for small mammals can be used for most laboratory animals including rodents; however, for evaluation of the health status of laboratory animal colonies, more extensive testing is required. Complete health monitoring includes serology, bacteriology, parasitology, and genetic monitoring in addition to gross pathology and histopathology. It is beyond the scope of this chapter to include techniques for blood collection for serology, bacteriologic sampling techniques, techniques for ectoparasite and endoparasite examination, and genetic monitoring. Many laboratories provide complete diagnostic services and health monitoring for laboratory animals, and such laboratories should be contacted before specimens (either live animals or samples from necropsies) are submitted to them.

> *TECHNICIAN NOTE* The necropsy technique for small mammals can be used for most laboratory animals. However, for evaluation of the health status of laboratory animal colonies, more extensive testing is required.

The technique for small mammals is followed except for the following variations for small rodents. An entire hind limb can be removed at the coxofemoral joint, the skin can be removed, and the limb can be fixed whole for bone, bone marrow, synovium, nerve, and skeletal muscle samples. For small rodents (e.g., mice, hamsters, gerbils), the lungs should be inflated with formalin after the thorax has been opened but before the lungs and heart are removed from the thorax. A 5- to 10-ml syringe with a small- to medium-bore needle is filled with formalin. The needle is threaded caudally for a few millimeters from the middle of the trachea, and the trachea is clamped with a hemostat rostral to the needle insertion site. The lungs are gently inflated until they fill the thorax. The trachea is then clamped or tied below the needle insertion site, and the lungs and heart are removed from the chest as described on p. 1353. The heart is often too small to open easily, and before fixation, it can be cut longitudinally through the middle of the right and left ventricles.

The intestinal tract can be opened in a few places and then infused with formalin by using a 5-ml syringe and a small-bore needle, or the entire tract can be opened up and pinned to cardboard before fixation. The kidney and adrenal gland on each side can be removed as a unit and left together for fixation after the kidney has been incised longitudinally to evaluate the pelvis for **hydronephrosis.** The uterus and ovaries or the testes and seminal vesicles and coagulating gland can be removed along with the urinary bladder and fixed whole without sectioning.

The spinal cord in small animals is difficult to remove without damaging it. The entire vertebral column with the spinal cord inside should be collected and fixed after the limbs, head, and muscles surrounding the vertebral column have been removed. The vertebral column and spinal cord can be submitted whole and decalcified and trimmed by the pathology laboratory.

COSMETIC NECROPSIES

Cosmetic necropsies, although of more limited value than complete necropsies, can be performed when the disease processes are limited to the abdomen and chest. A midline incision is made in the ventral abdomen from the xiphoid to the pubis. The abdominal organs are examined in situ, and the diaphragm is cut away from the ventral rib cage. The colon and urethra are tied off at the pelvic inlet and transected caudal to the tie. By reaching up through the diaphragm, the prosector can grasp and transect the trachea and esophagus at the thoracic inlet. The thoracic and abdominal contents are removed as a unit and dissected and described as in a noncosmetic necropsy. The body cavities are examined. The cavities are filled with paper towels, and the ventral abdominal incision is sutured.

> *TECHNICIAN NOTE* Cosmetic necropsies, although of more limited value than complete necropsies, can be performed when the disease processes are limited to the abdomen and chest.

RECOMMENDED READING

King JM et al: *The necropsy book,* ed 3, Gurnee, Ill, 2003, Charles Louis Davis, DVM Foundation.

Latimer KS, Rakich PM: Necropsy examination. In Richie BW, Harrison GJ, Harrison LR, editors: *Avian medicine: principles and application,* Lake Worth, Fla, 1994, Wingers Publishing.

Glossary

Abaxial Facing away from the axis of an organ

Abdominal pinging Technique of identifying abdominal gas accumulations by simultaneous percussion and auscultation of the abdominal wall

Abdominocentesis The insertion of a needle (attached to a syringe) into the abdominal cavity using sterile technique to obtain free abdominal fluid for evaluation

Abomasopexy Surgical fixation of the abomasum to the body wall

Abomasum The "true stomach" of the ruminant; secretes acids, mixes and contracts ingesta, and moves liquid chyme into the small intestine.

Abrasion Tooth wear associated with chewing on objects, such as rocks, ice cubes, toys, and bones in an area where skin has been scraped

Abscess Localized collection of pus in part of the body, formed by tissue disintegration usually resulting from bacterial infection and surrounded by an inflamed area

Absorption The uptake of substances into or across tissue

Acanthocephalan A "thorny-headed" worm. *Macracanthorhynchus hirudinaceus* is a "thorny-headed" worm parasite found in the small intestine of pigs.

Acanthocytes RBCs with multiple, irregularly spaced, club-shaped projections from the cell surface

Acariasis Infestation by either mites or ticks

Acarines Parasites that are either mites or ticks. *Demodex canis,* the follicular mite, and *Rhipicephalus sanguineus,* the brown dog tick, are classified as acarines.

Accessory motion Refers to the spin, roll, and gliding motions of one joint surface on another

Accounts receivable Money that is due to the practice from the sale of goods or services

Acid-Base Metabolic status associated with pH of blood or tissue

Acidemic Serum pH above the reference interval

Acid-Fast stain A useful differential staining procedure that specifically stains all members of the genus *Mycobacterium.* The high lipid and wax content of the mycobacterial cell walls is thought to be the reason that the cells will resist decolorization with acid alcohol and stain red, the color of the initial stain carbol fuchsin.

Acidosis Elevated levels of metabolic acids within the blood or tissue

Acids Compounds whose water-based solutions have a sour taste, turn blue litmus paper red, and can combine with metals to form salts and yield hydrogen ions or protons when dissolved in water

Acoustic impedance Attenuation of the energy of the ultrasound beam as it passes through different tissues. It is specific for each tissue type (fluid, air, bone, fat, etc.).

Acoustic shadow Ultrasound beam interaction with a highly reflective surface, such as bone, foreign material, or gas, causing a high degree of attenuation of the beam and blocking of the pathway of the beam to deeper tissue

Active assisted range of motion (AAROM) Patient is assisted manually or mechanically to achieve a normal range of motion when the prime muscle mover is weak or injured

Active listening skills A combination of acutely paying attention to what another is saying plus demonstrating that focused attention through body language and verbal feedback while maintaining a nonjudgmental attitude

Active range of motion (AROM) Ability of a patient to voluntarily move a limb through a range of motion

Acupuncture The use of needles (or injection of fluid, laser, ultrasound, surgically implanted material, and electrical stimulation) to stimulate specific predetermined "acupuncture" points in the body to produce chemical or physiologic changes in the body. It is combined with herbs and massage to make up traditional Chinese medicine (TCM).

Acute radiation toxicity Side effects caused by radiotherapy that occur between day 1 (the start of radiotherapy) and day 90. They are characterized by toxicity to rapidly proliferating normal tissues, such as skin, mucous membranes, intestinal tract, and bone marrow, and often resolve within days to weeks.

Adaptation Adjustment of a dental instrument that accounts for curvature of the tooth

Adjunctive agent Medications other than those commonly used that may help primary treatment

Adjuvant therapy Cancer treatment that is given in addition to the primary or initial treatment. The most common examples are radiotherapy that is given to treat residual cancer remaining after an incomplete surgical resection or postoperative chemotherapy that is administered to prevent or treat systemic metastasis. The overall purpose of adjuvant therapy is to decrease the likelihood of cancer recurrence.

Adrenocortical Pertaining to the cortex or outermost layer of the adrenal gland

Adsorbent Solid substance that attracts and holds a substance to its surface

Adulticide A therapeutic compound that will kill the adult stages of a parasite

AE title The name assigned to each modality so it can communicate electronically with the PACS in digital imaging

Aerobe An organism that can live and grow in the presence of oxygen. An organism that can use oxygen as a final electron acceptor in a respiratory chain. Obligate aerobes cannot grow anaerobically.

Aerophagia Swallowing an excessive volume of air

Agammaglobulinemic Description of a pathologic condition in which the body forms few or no γ-globulins or antibodies

Agglutination Clumping of blood. Agglutinated RBCs tend to appear as clumps secondary to strong specific antibody cross-linking of RBCs; will not dissociate upon addition of saline

Aggression Behaviors that result in harm to the opponent. Threats and aggression exist along a continuum. An inhibited bite that leaves a red mark or indentation in the skin or only pulls hair from another animal usually reflects an intent to warn (threat) rather than to harm (aggression).

Agonist A drug that binds to a receptor and causes it to express its function

Agonistic behaviors Behaviors having to do with social conflict, which typically include avoidance, appeasement, threats, and aggression

Air gap technique By increasing the distance between the patient and the cassette, scatter produced by the patient does not reach the cassette as easily thereby improving image quality.

Alkalemic Serum pH above the reference interval

Alkali Alkaline substances produce hydroxide ions on contact with water.

Alkalosis Elevated pH (decreased acid) within the blood or tissue

Allantois Placental membrane formed from the hindgut. It has a close association with the inner portion of the chorion.

Allodynia Recruitment of nonpainful nerve fibers transmitting information as pain resulting in previously pleasant or neutral sensations experienced as unpleasant

Altrenogest A synthetic progestin administered orally and mainly indicated to suppress estrus in mares. It is also used commonly to aid in preventing pregnancy loss in the mare.

Alveolar Pertaining to the air sacs that are anatomically located in clusters at the end of the smallest airways within the lungs

Ambu bag Equipment for providing manual ventilations, which is usually attached to the patient via an endotracheal tube or face mask and connected to an oxygen source

Ambu Bag A brand name of a self-inflating reservoir bag used to provide manual ventilation when an anesthetic machine is not available

American Animal Hospital Association (AAHA) A small animal veterinary association providing veterinary professionals with resources, including member services, continuing education, and hospital accreditation standards

Amino acids Nitrogen-containing compounds that constitute the "building blocks" or units from which more complex protein is formed. They contain both an amino (NH_2) group and a carboxyl (COOH) group.

Aminoglycoside antibiotics Group of broad-spectrum antibiotics. Common examples are streptomycin, gentamicin, amikacin, kanamycin, tobramycin, and neomycin.

Ammonium sulfate precipitation test Used to differentiate hemoglobinuria from myoglobinuria; hemoglobin is expected to clear in contrast to myoglobin

Amnion The placental membrane that directly surrounds the fetus

A-mode Amplitude mode image display in ultrasound imaging. The energy of the returning echo is shown as an amplitude spike at each tissue interface.

Amplitude The distance the tip of a power scaler is moving back and forth in one cycle as adjusted by the power knob

Ampulla Portion of the uterine tube (oviduct) that connects to the uterus

Amputation Removal of a body part (limb, toe, ear, tail, etc.)

Anaerobe A microorganism that can live and grow in the absence of oxygen. May be differentiated as facultative (can use oxygen or grow without oxygen), strict (oxygen is toxic so must have an anaerobic atmosphere), or obligate (has only anaerobic metabolic pathways, but oxygen is not toxic).

Analgesia Pain relief

Analgesic Drug that alleviates pain

Anaphylactic An exaggerated allergic reaction to a foreign protein or substance in the body

Anastomosis Suturing two tubular organs together (i.e., intestinal loops) so that substances inside the lumen of the sutured organs can freely move from one to the other

Anechoic A structure in the ultrasound image that does not produce echoes and appears black

Anemia Low RBC count

Anestrus The period of sexual quiescence between two periods of sexual activity in cyclically breeding mammals

Anger That stage of grief during which anger is the primary emotion expressed directly, indirectly, and specifically or generally

Angulation The relationship of the face of the instrument with the tooth surface

Anisocytosis Variation in cell size

Anisognathism Condition in which the maxilla and mandible are not the same width

Anisokaryosis Variation in nuclear size

Anode Positively charged side of the x-ray tube that receives the oncoming electrons from the cathode. Both heat and x-rays are produced as a result of interactions between the electrons and the metal anode.

Anoplurans Sucking lice that are members of the insect order Anoplura

Anorexia Loss of appetite or absence of food especially when prolonged

Antagonist A drug that binds to a receptor and inhibits expression of its function

Anterior pituitary gland The adenohypophysis; the rostral portion of the pituitary gland that produces seven hormones, many of which influence other endocrine glands

Anterior uveitis Inflammation of the uvea

Anthelminthic/anthelmintic A compound or drug that can be used to kill helminths, such as nematodes, trematodes, cestodes, acanthocephalans, pentastomes, and hirudineans

Anthelmintics Drugs used in the treatment of internal parasitism

Anthropomorphism The attribution of human characteristics to animals

Antibiogram The pattern of in vitro susceptibilities resulting from the laboratory testing of an isolated bacterial strain for susceptibility to different antimicrobial drugs

Antibiotic Substance produced by a microorganism that inhibits or kills other microorganisms

Antibody Immunoglobulin formed in blood or tissues that interacts only with antigens that induced its synthesis

Anticholinergic agent Drugs that inhibit the action of acetylcholine by competing at the receptor sites producing increased heart rate, dry mouth, blurred vision, urinary retention, and constipation

Anticoagulants Additives used in blood collection bags for blood banking to keep blood from clotting

Antiemetic A drug used to treat or prevent vomiting

Antigen Molecule or substance that is recognized by the immune system as foreign (nonself) and that elicits an immune response or specific antibody response

Antiinflammatory agent Drugs that reduce or remedy pain by reducing inflammation

Antimicrobial A drug that destroys or inhibits the growth of microorganisms.

Antimicrobial susceptibility test A laboratory test to predict the in vivo success or failure of antibiotic therapy by measuring the growth response of an isolated organism to a particular antimicrobial drug or drugs

Antipyretic Drugs that lower body temperature from a raised state

Antiseptic An antimicrobial agent that kills or inhibits the growth of microorganisms on the external surfaces of the body. Antiseptics should generally be distinguished from drugs, such as antibiotics, that destroy microorganisms internally and from disinfectants, which destroy microorganisms found on nonliving objects.

Aortic stenosis A congenital cardiac anomaly resulting in resistance to flow of blood from the left ventricle into the aorta

Apex Tip of the root of a tooth

Apical Positional term referring to an area of the tooth or root that is closer to the apex

Apnea A temporary absence of spontaneous breathing

Appendicular skeleton The bones of the limbs (appendages)

Application software Programs that help a user perform certain tasks. Some common examples of application software include word processing software, bookkeeping software, and practice management information systems.

Applied kinesiology A form of medicine that includes joint mobilizations or manipulations, myofascial therapy, cranial techniques, meridian therapy, clinical nutrition, dietary management, and reflex procedures

Appointment system Clients call ahead and are given a specific time and date to come into the practice

Aquatic physical therapy Specific treatment interventions using a water-filled pool

Argasid ticks Soft ticks or members of the tick family Argasidae. Only a few of the ticks that parasitize domesticated animals are soft ticks. Soft ticks are periodic parasites that only attach to their hosts to take a blood meal. An example of a soft tick is *Otobius megnini,* the spinous ear tick.

Aroma therapy The use of essential oils to bring about a physiologic or psychologic response in the body

Arrhythmia An abnormal heartbeat rhythm detected during palpation of the chest or pulse during auscultation or recorded on an ECG

Arterial blood gases Measurement of the partial pressure of oxygen and carbon dioxide, total bicarbonate, and blood pH in an arterial blood sample that helps determine the metabolic acid-base status of a patient; usually used to monitor patients with severe respiratory disease

Arthrocentesis The aspiration of fluid from a joint

Arthrodesis Surgically fusing a joint

Artificial insemination (AI) Placing fresh, cooled, or frozen semen collected from a male directly into the vagina or uterus of a female

Ascarid A specific type of nematode often referred to as a roundworm. *Ascaris suum,* the porcine ascarid, is a roundworm parasite found in the small intestine of pigs.

Asensory Lacking sensation

Asepsis A condition of sterility where no living organisms are present

Aseptic technique The methods used to prevent contamination of a surgical site or wound by disease-producing organisms

Asphyxiation The act of cutting off the supply of oxygen; suffocation

Aspiration 1. Removal of tissue or fluid from a tissue. 2. Accidental inhalation of material (liquid, food, GI contents) down the trachea.

Assisted gloving A method of putting on sterile gloves in which a sterile, gloved assistant holds the glove open to allow the surgeon to advance his or her hand into the glove without touching the outside

Association of American Feed Control Officials (AAFCO) The association that establishes standards for label information and the description of ingredients on pet food sold in the United States

Asystole A type of arrhythmia characterized by a "flat line" or absence of heartbeats

Ataxia Uncoordinated gait usually associated with neurologic dysfunction

Atelectasis Collapse of a portion or all of one or both lungs

Atlas The first cervical vertebra. It forms the atlanto-occipital joint with the occipital bone of the skull and the atlantoaxial joint with the axis (the second cervical vertebra).

Atrioventricular valve A heart valve located between an atrium and a ventricle. The right AV valve is the tricuspid valve, and the left AV valve is the mitral valve.

Atrophy Wasting away of a cell, tissue, organ, or part

Attachment loss In dental terms, a more true indicator of the periodontal status of the tooth. Attachment loss is calculated by adding recession and pocket depth.

Attenuation A decrease in the energy of the x-ray photons as they pass through matter

Attrition Tooth wear associated with tooth-to-tooth contact

Aural In or of the ear

Auscult To listen to sounds made by internal organs, especially the heart and lungs

Auscultation Listening with a stethoscope (usually to heart and lung sounds)

Autoclave A machine that uses pressurized steam to sterilize objects

Autogenous Originating or derived from sources within the same individual <an *autogenous* graft> <*autogenous* vaccine>

Autolysis The self-digestion of tissues or cells by enzymes that are released by their own lysosomes.

Autonomic nervous system Serves to monitor and control internal body functions, such as digestive processes, blood volume, cardiac output, and kidney function

Autotomize The act of reflex separation of a part from the body. In the case of lizard or snake tails—to disengage part of the distal part of the tail when stressed or held.

Axial Along the same line as a center line

Axillary Under the armpit

Axis The second cervical vertebra. It forms the atlantoaxial joint with the first cervical vertebra (the atlas).

Ayre's T-piece A nonrebreathing circuit with corrugated tubing, but no reservoir bag or pressure relief valve, in which the fresh gas inlet is located near the patient and the waste gas exits away from the patient; Mapleson E circuit

Ayurvedic medicine The ancient Hindu art of medicine and of prolonging life. Diagnosis is done by palpation of the pulses in different positions.

Azotemia An excess of urea and other nitrogenous wastes in the blood as a result of kidney insufficiency

Azotemic Increased blood urea nitrogen and creatinine; can be due to dehydration, renal failure, or urinary obstruction

Bacterial translocation Movement of bacteria from a normal location to an undesirable location (translocation of bacteria from a compromised gastrointestinal tract into the bloodstream)

Bacteriostatic The inhibition of bacterial multiplication

Baermann technique A collection technique that uses the force of gravity to concentrate nematode larvas (most often lungworm larvas) from within a liquid medium. The larvas of *Aelurostrongylus abstrusus* are often concentrated and collected using a Baermann apparatus.

Bain circuit A nonrebreathing circuit with a reservoir bag and corrugated tubing in which the fresh gas inlet is located near the patient and the pressure relief valve is located away from the patient; Mapleson D circuit

Band/stab Developmental stage before the segmenter with an incompletely segmented band-shaped nucleus

Barbering A behavioral problem where the animal obsessively grooms to the point of damaging the hair and skin

Barbiturate Nervous system depressants used to induce sleep, and in high doses as anesthetics and euthanasia agents

Bargaining That stage of grief experienced as conscious or unconscious attempts to control the situation or refute the loss

Barr body A small drumstick-appearing nuclear appendage representative of an inactivated X chromosome that may be present in neutrophils from females

Basilic vein The large vein on the ventral surface of a bird's wing that courses over the humeral-ulna joint (elbow)

Basophil Leukocyte with a segmented nucleus and basophilic (blue) granules

Basophilic stippling Multiple tiny, lightly basophilic RBC inclusions resulting from staining of small amounts of cytoplasmic RNA in RBCs in the RBC cytoplasm; may be seen in cases of markedly regenerative anemia and occasionally in cases of lead poisoning

Behavior wellness The condition or state of normal and acceptable pet conduct that enhances the human-animal bond and the pet's quality of life

Behavior wellness care The planned attention to a pet's conduct and the active integration of behavior wellness programs into the delivery of pet-related services, including routine veterinary medical supervision

Behavior wellness programs Protocols, procedures, services, and systems that educate pet owners and professionals about what constitutes the behaviorally healthy or well pet; promote behavioral wellness through positive proaction, behavior assessments, early intervention, and timely referrals; and decrease unrealistic human expectations and interpretations of pet behavior

Behavioral needs In this context, the opportunities and experiences that support the development of healthy behaviors

Benign A benign cancer is one that may grow but does not invade surrounding normal tissues and does not spread (metastasize) to other parts of the body.

Bereavement A state of sadness, grief, and mourning after the loss of a loved one

Biologic value The percentage of the protein of a feed that is usable as a protein by the animal. A protein that has a high biologic value is said to be of good quality.

Biotoxin or toxin Noxious or poisonous substance that is formed or elaborated during the metabolism and growth of certain microorganisms and some higher plant and animal species

Blepharospasm Spasmodic blinking from involuntary contraction of the orbicularis oculi muscle of the eyelids

Bloat Accumulation of gas within certain portions of the GI tract that produces visible enlargement of the abdomen

Blood urea nitrogen: BUN A product of protein metabolism that is normally filtered by the kidneys for excretion. This blood value is elevated when the animal is on a high-protein diet, dehydrated, or has renal insufficiency.

B-mode Brightness mode ultrasound image display. It forms the basis of two-dimensional ultrasound images so that the anatomic structures can be assessed in real time on a monitor.

Board The administrative agency that governs the practice of veterinary medicine and technology in each state. The formal name of this administrative agency may vary from state to state; names such as "Board of Veterinary Medical Examiners," "State Board of Veterinary Medicine," or "Licensing Board of Veterinary Medicine" are common.

Body condition score A method of evaluating a small animal patient's nutritional status using a scale of 1 (emaciated) to 9 (obese)

Body condition scoring system A system that can subjectively assess a pet's fat stores and muscle mass

Borborygmi Rumbling noise caused by propulsion of gas and ingesta through the intestines

Borborygmus Audible intestinal motility sound produced by intestinal peristalsis

Box lock Hinged part of a needle holder, tissue forceps, or hemostatic forceps

Brachycephalic Head shape that is shortened in the rostrocaudal dimension, as seen with breeds such as pugs, Boston terriers, and boxers

Brachygnathism Occurs when one of the jaws is caudal to its normal relationship with the other jaw; mandibular brachygnathism (retrognathism, Class II occlusion) exists when the mandible is shorter than the maxilla

Brachyodont Tooth type with a small, distinct crown compared with large, well-developed roots

Bronchopneumonia Pneumonia involving many relatively small areas of lung tissue

Broodmare Adult female horse used for breeding

Buccal Pertaining to the inside of the cheek or mouth

Buccotomy Surgical incision through the cheek

Bulbus glandis The expanded "bulb" of the proximal canine penis

Bursae Fluid-filled sacs that decrease friction between structures

Bursitis Inflammation of bursae

CAAHTT Canadian Association of Animal Health Technologists and Technicians

Cabergoline A synthetic dopamine agonist that is therefore a prolactin inhibitor

Cachexia Weight loss, loss of muscle mass, and general debilitation that may accompany chronic diseases

Calculus Plaque that has become calcified and is firmly adhered to the teeth

Calorie The amount of heat (energy) needed to raise the temperature of 1 g of water 1° C

Camelid "Camel-like" animals that include llamas and alpacas

Cancer One of many diseases that are characterized by uncontrolled growth and spread of abnormal cells within the body. If local growth, invasion, and spread of the cancer are not controlled, death may result.

Canthus Either of the angles formed by the meeting of the upper and lower eyelids. There is a medial and lateral canthus of each eye.

Capillaria A roundworm parasite that is located in the intestinal tract of infected birds. The double-operculated eggs can be identified in a fecal flotation examination.

Capillary refill time Time in seconds it takes for the blanching of the mucous membranes with the finger to return to a pink color; normal in dogs and cats is less than 2 seconds

Capnograph An instrument that noninvasively measures the carbon dioxide in exhaled air. This value is an indirect assessment of ventilation status.

Carbohydrate One of the essential nutrients necessary for all life functions. They are a quick source of energy and may be stored in the body as glycogen; sugars.

Carcinogen A substance or agent that causes cancer in animals or people

Carcinogenesis The complex process by which normal cells are transformed into cancer cells

Cardiopulmonary arrest Cessation of breathing and absent heartbeat

Cardiopulmonary cerebrovascular resuscitation An attempt to reverse cardiopulmonary arrest, usually via support of airway, breathing, and circulation (including chest compressions and assisted ventilation)

Caries Tooth decay caused by bacterial acid production and demineralization of tooth substance

Carpal tunnel syndrome (CTS) A medical condition in which the median nerve of the hand is compressed at the wrist, leading to pain, paresthesias, and muscle weakness in the forearm and hand. CTS is the most well-known of the ergonomic injuries classified as repetitive motion disorders (RMDs).

Carpus The knee on the forelimb of a horse

Cash flow A measurement of a practice's inflow and outflow of cash over a period of time

Catalase An enzyme found in most living cells that catalyzes the decomposition of hydrogen peroxide into water and oxygen

Catarrhal Inflammation of mucous membranes with discharge, especially inflammation of the air passages of the nose and trachea.

Catharsis The release of pent-up emotions with the resulting alleviation of symptoms

Cathartics Medications, through their chemical effects, that serve to increase the clearing of intestinal contents

Cathode Negatively charged side of the x-ray tube that produces electrons form a metal filament when it is heated

Cationic detergents Nonsoap surfactants that are in a positive state

Caudal Positional term referring to a structure toward the back of the head or the hind end

Cavitation Rapid collapse of bubble in a liquid that produces a shock wave. Ultrasonic dental scalers cause cavitation.

Celiotomy Incision into the abdominal cavity

Cellular casts Casts that contain recognizable cells embedded in the protein matrix

Cellulitis Inflammation of the subcutaneous tissue as a result of infection or immune cause

Cementoenamel junction The portion of brachyodont teeth where the enamel of the crown meets the cementum of the root

Cementum Hard tissue that covers the root of brachyodont teeth and portions of the crown of some hypsodont teeth

Centers for Disease Control & Prevention (CDC) An agency of the U.S. Department of Health and Human Services working to protect public health and the safety of people by conducting research and providing information on health issues of concern

Centesis Surgical puncture (as of a tumor or membrane)—usually used in compounds <para*centesis*> <thoraco*centesis*>

Central nervous system Includes the brain and spinal cord and serves to monitor, convey, and process signals from the receptors throughout the body

Central venous pressure (CVP) Blood pressure measurement taken from the intrathoracic portions of the cranial vena cava; normal range is 0 to 10 cm H_2O

Cerumen Waxy secretion found in the external ear canal

Ceruminolytics An agent that dissolves cerumen in the external ear canal

Cervical When referring to teeth, the portion of the tooth where the crown meets the root of a brachyodont tooth

Cestode A tapeworm. *Dipylidium caninum,* the double-pored or cucumber seed tapeworm, is a cestode parasite found in the small intestine of both dogs and cats.

Chelonian Turtle

Chemosis Edema of the conjunctiva (swollen tissue around the eye)

Chemotherapy Chemotherapy is the use of chemical substances to treat disease, primarily with cytotoxic drugs used to treat cancer. Chemotherapy is usually systemic therapy and is given intravenously or by mouth.

Chiropractic therapy A form of medicine that manually restores reduced motion in the spine and limbs, thereby improving patient mobility, comfort, and in many cases nervous system function

Chlamydophila psittaci An intracellular bacterium that is a zoonotic disease (psittacosis) and commonly infects avian species (avian chlamydiosis)

Cholinomimetic agents Drugs that mimic the stimulatory effects of acetylcholine (ACh), such as salivation, lacrimation, urination, and defecation

Chondroprotective Refers to drugs or other agents (e.g., nutraceuticals) that promote joint health by "protecting" the joint by slowing or stopping degradation of articular cartilage

Chorioallantoic Extraembryonic membrane formed by the fusion of the allantois with the serosa or false chorion. In mammals, it forms the fetal portion of the placenta.

Chorioallantois The fused chorionic and allantoic membranes

Chorion The outermost placental membrane that directly contacts the endometrium

Chromosome Nuclear portion of the cell containing the genes

Cingulum Smooth convex bulge on the palatal side of the incisor teeth

Classical conditioning Also known as respondent conditioning. The animal learns the association between events—one event (the conditioned stimulus) predicts the other (the unconditioned stimulus). Emotional behaviors are easily classically conditioned.

Cloaca In birds and reptiles, the single terminus of the urinary, intestinal, and reproductive tracts

Cloprostenol A potent synthetic prostaglandin

Closed gloving A method of putting on sterile gloves in which the hands are kept hidden within the sleeves of a sterile gown during gloving

Closed kinetic chain exercise An exercise in which the distal limb segment is fixed

Coagulase Any of various enzymes that induce coagulation, especially of plasma. In bacteriology, the production of coagulase is used as an indicator of virulence and a differential identifying characteristic of some bacteria, especially *Staphylococcus.*

Coagulation Blood clotting

Coccidia Microscopic, single-celled parasites that spread from one animal to another (including humans) by contact with infected feces

Coenurus A type of metacestode stage found in the intermediate host in the life cycle of a tapeworm. The coenurus is usually found within a vertebrate intermediate host. A coenurus is a large, fluid-filled vesicle, cavity, or bladder with multiple invaginated scolices budding out from its wall. In its life cycle, *Multiceps multicep* uses the coenurus, which may be found within the brain or nervous tissue of its intermediate host, a sheep. This coenurus has a scientific name, *Coenurus cerebralis.* See **metacestode stage.**

Colic Severe abdominal pain of sudden onset caused by a variety of conditions, including obstruction, twisting, and spasm of the intestine

Colitis Inflammation of the colon

Collimator A device that filters or "focuses" a stream of x-rays so that only those inside the open part of the device are allowed through

Colloid fluids A category or type of IV fluid solution containing large particles that help retain fluid within vessels

Colonic wash A fluid lavage of the reptile's distal intestinal tract in an attempt to collect a sample for parasite examination

Colostrum The first milk that contains the antibodies

Colpotomy An incision through the wall of the vagina

Colt Male horse less than 4 years old, usually noncastrated

Comatose In a coma, a state of unconsciousness from which the patient cannot be aroused

Commensal A relation between two kinds of organisms in which one obtains food or other benefits from the other without damaging or benefiting it

Commissure Area where the upper and lower lips meet

Compassion The quality of understanding the suffering of others and wanting to do something about it

Complete blood count: CBC A measure of cell counts in the blood

Complex metamorphosis A type of developmental change used by many insects. There are four developmental stages in complex metamorphosis: egg, larva, pupa, and adult. Each of these stages is drastically different from each of the other stages. The orders of parasitic insects that undergo complex metamorphosis include Dipterans (two-winged flies) and Siphonapterans (fleas).

Computed radiography Similar to DR except that an x-ray receiver similar to a film cassette is used and must be processed in a special machine. The special cassette contains a photostimulable phosphor that changes x-ray photons into a latent electronic image when read by a laser.

Concentrates A broad classification of feedstuff that is high in energy and low in fiber

Congenital Born with a specific condition. Can be genetic or environmentally induced.

Conjunctivitis Inflammation of the tissue under the lid margins and surrounding the visible globe

Constant rate infusion (CRI) Administering low doses of drugs in IV fluids at a fixed rate over time

Consultation Specific period of time that the veterinarian meets with the client and patient for the purpose of diagnosis/treatment

Contamination The presence of disease-producing bacteria or other microorganisms on the surface of a wound or surgical field

Contrast The density or opacity differences between neighboring areas on the radiographic image. Large differences result in high contrast, whereas small differences result in low-contrast images.

Control solutions Quality control products that may report a given expected concentration of the analyte of interest, or alternatively a laboratory may use a sample, possibly pooled, from representative animal(s) that has had its concentration repeatedly determined by the analyzer itself.

Conviction The process of convicting of a crime in a court of law

Coombs test Species-specific test to detect RBC surface-bound antibodies and/or complement most frequently used to support the diagnosis of immune-mediated hemolytic anemia

Corium Sensitive lamina

Cornify Cellular change indicative of cell proliferation and death. The vaginal epithelium of the bitch cornifies during estrus.

Coronal Positional term referring to an area of the tooth or root closer to the crown

Corpora lutea Plural of corpus luteum

Corpus hemorrhagicum (CH) The blood-filled remnant of the ovarian follicle immediately after ovulation

Corpus luteum (CL) Latin for "yellow body." Structure on the ovary that produces progesterone.

Corrosive Highly reactive substance that causes obvious damage to living tissue

Corticotropin-releasing hormone Secreted by the hypothalamus, it causes the fetal adrenal gland to produce high concentrations of cortisol.

Cortisol Natural glucocorticoid produced by the adrenal cortex of the adrenal gland; major functioning hormone that participates in many life-sustaining processes in the body, such as maintaining blood glucose levels

Coupage The act of striking the chest wall rhythmically with cupped hands. Cupping the hands creates an air cushion on impact so that tenacious mucus is dislodged.

Creatinine A natural waste product of muscle tissue

Crimes of depravity Include murder, rape, and distribution of drugs, but also include misdemeanor offenses, such as stalking, harassment, and assault

Crimes of moral turpitude Crimes that involve dishonesty or deception. All theft offenses, such as shoplifting, theft by unlawful taking, theft by deception, forgery, writing bad checks, and embezzlement, and false swearing are considered crimes of moral turpitude because they involve dishonesty.

Crop A dilation of the esophagus of birds at the base of the neck, where food is stored, softened with fluids, and passed to the stomach in small amounts

Crossmatch The process of determining compatibility between blood donor and blood transfusion recipient

Crown The portion of the tooth above the gingival margin. Hypsodont teeth as a result of their continual growth and/or eruption have reserve crown beneath the gingival margin.

Cryotherapy Therapeutic techniques to decrease tissue temperature; cold therapy

Cryptorchid Animal that has one or both of the testes retained in the abdomen

Crystalloid fluids A category or type of IV fluid solution characterized by water and electrolyte content

Crystalluria Crystals in a urine sample

Curative therapy Cancer treatment whose purpose is to permanently control the tumor. Because the goal is long-term survival, aggressive therapies are often recommended, and more than one modality (e.g., surgery, radiotherapy, or chemotherapy) may be employed.

Curette A hand instrument designed with a rounded toe for subgingival scaling

Cushing disease (hyperadrenocorticism) A disease of the adrenal or pituitary gland that causes production of too much of the endogenous steroids

Cutaneous larva migrans A skin disease in humans caused by the larvas of nematode (hookworm) parasites. Sometimes referred to as "creeping eruption," "ground itch," or "sandworms." Children in particular may become infected with these larvas by the penetration of third-stage larvas into the skin of children while they are running barefoot in moist, sandy soil or are playing in a sandbox.

Cyanosis A bluish discoloration of the mucous membranes or skin as a result of severe reduction of hemoglobin in the blood

Cysticercoid A type of metacestode stage found in the intermediate host in the life cycle of a tapeworm. The cysticercoid is usually found within an invertebrate intermediate host, such as a flea or a grain mite. A cysticercoid is a single, noninvaginated scolex, within a small, fluid-filled vesicle, cavity, or bladder. In its life cycle, *Dipylidium caninum* uses the cysticercoid stage, which may be found within the intermediate host, an adult flea. See **metacestode stage.**

Cysticercus A type of metacestode stage found in the intermediate host in the life cycle of a tapeworm. The cysticercus is usually found within a vertebrate intermediate host. A cysticercus is a single, invaginated scolex, within a large, fluid-filled vesicle, cavity, or bladder. In its life cycle, *Taenia pisiformis* uses the cysticercus stage, which may be found within the omentum of its intermediate host, a rabbit. This cysticercus has a scientific name, *Cysticercus pisiformis.* See **metacestode stage.**

Cystocentesis Urine obtained by placing a needle (with a syringe attached) through the ventral abdominal wall into the lumen of the bladder and aspirating urine

Cystotomy Incision into the urinary bladder

Cytopathic Of, relating to, characterized by, or producing pathologic changes in cells

Cytoplasmic basophilia Neutrophils with increased amounts of cytoplasmic RNA

Cytoplasmic vacuolation/foaminess Neutrophils with secondary to organelle abnormalities

Cytotoxic An agent or process that kills cells. Chemotherapy and radiotherapy are both forms of cytotoxic therapy.

Cytotoxic drugs (CDs) A class of drugs that is toxic to cells. In modern medicine, CDs are used primarily to treat cancer.

Dead space The breathing passages and tubes that convey fresh oxygen from the source (the atmosphere or breathing circuit) to the alveoli, but in which no gas exchange can occur. Anatomic dead space includes the bronchi, trachea, larynx, pharynx, and nasal cavity. Mechanical dead space includes the portion of the endotracheal tube extending beyond the nose or the mask and the Y-piece of the breathing circuit.

Debilitated Lacking strength; weak

Débride To cleanse by removal (usually surgical) of lacerated, devitalized, or contaminated tissue

Decibel (dB) A measure of noise volume

Deciduous Referring to the primary or "baby" teeth, which exfoliate before eruption of the permanent (adult) teeth

Decontamination Removal or neutralization of injurious agents

Decubital ulcers Pressure sores (bedsores) that result from an animal lying on a bone prominence for too long

Defensive aggression Behaviors that result in harm to another individual as a result of defending oneself. Defensively aggressive animals are both fearful and aggressive.

Defibrillation The process of converting a fibrillation arrhythmia to a normal heartbeat (usually via electrical shock with a defibrillator)

Definitive diagnosis With respect to oncology, a completely accurate and reliable diagnosis of cancer that is established after thorough evaluation of the patient's history, physical examination findings, and laboratory diagnostics. A tissue biopsy with histopathology is usually required for a definitive diagnosis.

Definitive host The host that harbors the adult, sexual, or mature stages of the parasite; for example, the dog is the definitive host for the canine heartworm, *Dirofilaria immitis*.

Definitive therapy Treatment intended to cure or permanently control a cancer. One or a combination of anticancer therapies may be used, including surgery, radiotherapy, and chemotherapy.

Degenerate left shift Left shift in the absence of increased segmenters (i.e., mature neutrophils)

Degenerate neutrophil Dying neutrophils displaying nuclear dissolution

Deglutition Medical term referring to the act of swallowing

Dehiscence The breakdown of a surgical incision such that the tissue layers separate from each other

Dehydration Excessive loss of water from body tissues. May be associated with electrolyte disturbances, particularly sodium, chloride, and potassium.

Denial The normal defense that serves to buffer an individual from some unbearable news or shock

Density Degree of blackness of the film. More dense areas are blacker and are in areas of the film where little x-ray absorption occurred. Whiter areas are less dense and are in areas of greater x-ray absorption on the film.

Dentifrice Paste, liquid, or powder used to help maintain good oral hygiene

Dentigerous cyst Cyst that forms around an unerupted tooth, which rarely may transform into a malignant tumor

Dentin Hard tissue that makes up the bulk of a mature tooth

Depression The actual grief; sorrow

Dermatophyte A fungus that causes infections of the skin, hair, and nails as a result of its ability to obtain nutrients from keratinized material

Designated assembly area The place where occupants of a building will gather for accountability if a general evacuation of the facility was ordered

Detail Degree of sharpness that defines the edge of an anatomic structure in the radiographic image

Diagnostic peritoneal lavage The insertion of fluid in the peritoneal cavity; the fluid is allowed to dwell for a short period of time and then drained. Gross, microscopic, and chemical analysis is performed on the returned fluid.

Diaphragm The thin, dome-shaped sheet of muscle that forms the boundary between the thoracic and abdominal cavities; it helps produce inspiration when it contracts. The diaphragm is dome shaped at rest with its convex surface directed cranially. When it contracts, the dome of the diaphragm flattens out, which increases the volume of the thoracic cavity and causes air to be drawn into the lungs.

Diastema Gap between teeth, as seen between incisors and cheek teeth of a rabbit

Diastolic blood pressure Measurement of blood pressure when the heart is in diastole or dilation

DICOM (Digital Imaging and Communications in Medicine) A standard for handling, storing, and transmitting medical imaging

Differential medium A growth medium that allows two or more organisms to be distinguished from one another by some characteristic such as growth, ability to metabolize a specific nutrient as an energy source, different end products of metabolism, production of enzymes or toxins, etc., that can be detected by indicator systems incorporated into the medium or reagents that are added after incubation.

Digestible energy The energy remaining after the energy lost in feces is subtracted from gross energy

Digestion The process of protein, carbohydrate, and fat breakdown into absorbable nutrients

Digital Image Communications in Medicine (DICOM) DICOM 3.0 is the current standard format of digital images in the veterinary and medical fields.

Digital radiography The x-ray tube is coupled to a specialized receiver that changes x-rays into electrical signals. The analog image is digitalized and displayed on the integrated computer screen.

Dipterans Two-winged flies. *Anopheles quadrimaculatus,* the malaria mosquito, is a Dipteran fly.

Direct life cycle A life cycle that does not use an intermediate host; for example, *Ancylostoma caninum,* the canine hookworm, uses a direct life cycle

Disinfectant An antimicrobial agent that is applied to nonliving objects to destroy disease-causing microorganisms and their spores by physical or chemical means

Disinfection The destruction of the vegetative forms of bacteria but not the spores

Displacement behavior Normal, species-typical behaviors that are displayed out of the typical contexts in which they are normally seen. Displacement activities occur when other behaviors are thwarted or interrupted and when an animal is in conflict about choosing between two incompatible behaviors. Examples of displacement behaviors in dogs and cats are yawning, lip licking, and self-grooming.

Disseminated intravascular coagulation (DIC) A secondary complication of severe disease that is characterized by massive and spontaneously occurring blood clot formation and blood loss resulting from clotting factor consumption

Disseminated intravascular coagulopathy (DIC) A disorder in which there is excessive coagulation of blood followed by hemorrhage and lack of coagulation of blood because the clotting factors were used up. DIC is usually secondary to excessive turbulent blood flow or a severe infectious, immune-mediated, or neoplastic process.

Distal In dentistry, a positional term referring to the surface of the tooth furthest from the rostral midline of the dental arch

Distemper virus inclusions Distinct, spherical, eosinophilic to lightly basophilic inclusions that may be seen in either RBCs or WBCs; may be more readily appreciated with some of the rapid Wright stains

Distribution The dispersion of the drug that is systemically available from the intravascular space and extravascular fluids and tissues to the target receptor sites

Diuresis An increased excretion of urine

Diuretic A drug that increases the rate of urine output

Döhle bodies Neutrophils with pale, bluish-gray, irregular cytoplasmic inclusions of RNA containing rough endoplasmic reticulum

Dolichocephalic Head shape that is longer than average in the rostrocaudal dimension, as seen in greyhounds and collies.

Dominance aggression Aggression against other members of an animal's social group to prevent subordinate individuals from performing actions or engaging in activities for which the higher-ranking individual claims priority

Dominant role A superior position in a rank order or social hierarchy. Note that dominance describes a social position, (role in a relationship) not a personality trait.

Dopamine A prolactin inhibitor

Dosimetry badge A device worn by personnel when potentially exposed to radiation that measures the dose of radiation received

Drug Any chemical agent that affects living processes

Drug Enforcement Agency (DEA) An agency in the U.S. Department of Justice responsible for enforcement of laws governing the user of barbiturates

Duodenum The first segment of the small intestine after the stomach. Chyme enters the duodenum from the stomach.

Dynamic range The number of shades of gray in an image. The larger the number, the larger the dynamic range.

Dysphagia Difficulty in swallowing

Dysphoria An uneasy emotional state characterized by anxiety and abnormal behavior

Dyspnea Difficult or labored breathing

Dystocia Slow or difficult labor or delivery of a newborn

Ecchymotic hemorrhage Visible hemorrhage lesions 1 mm to 1 cm diameter

Echinocytes Crenated RBCs that have multiple spicule-appearing projections

Echocardiography Real time imaging of the heart with ultrasound waves reflecting the heart tissue and blood giving a picture of the heart function

Ectoparasite A parasite that lives on the outside of the body of the host; for example, *Ctenocephalides felis,* the cat flea. Ectoparasites produce infestations on their hosts.

Edema The accumulation of fluid in a space that is not normally fluid filled resulting from venous or lymphatic obstruction or increased vascular permeability (e.g., pulmonary edema is fluid in the lungs, whereas cerebral edema is fluid accumulation within brain tissue)

Effleurage A form of massage that consists of gliding strokes that follow the contour of the body

Effusion The escape of a fluid from anatomic vessels by rupture or exudation

Ejection murmur Normal heart sound in large animals produced by large volumes of blood moving at high speeds through the heart valves. Because of the large heart size, these sounds are amplified and readily heard with a stethoscope.

Electrical mechanical dissociation (EMD) An arrhythmia characterized by electrical wave forms on the ECG without corresponding mechanical heartbeat or pulse. Also called "pulseless electrical activity (PEA)."

Electrical stimulation The use of electricity to stimulate soft tissues to facilitate healing and reduce pain

Electrocardiography Measurement of the electrical conductance of the heart; ECG rhythm strips

Embryo An early stage of development that is not yet recognizable as a specific species

Emergence delirium Delirious behavior resulting from incomplete recovery from gas anesthesia. Usually lasts 1 to 2 minutes after removal from anesthesia.

Emesis Vomiting

Emetics Agents used to induce vomiting

Emphysematous A condition characterized by air-filled expansions in interstitial or subcutaneous tissues

Enamel Hard tissue of high mineral content that covers the crown of a tooth

Endemic Restricted or peculiar to a locality or region *(endemic)* diseases

Endodontics The branch of dentistry dealing with disease of the pulp

Endogenous Arising from within the body

Endometrial Belonging to the mucous membrane lining the uterus

Endoparasite A parasite that lives within the body of the host (e.g., *Dirofilaria immitis,* the canine heartworm). Endoparasites produce infections within their hosts.

Endotoxemia The presence of poisonous substances found in bacteria, but separable from the cell body only on its disintegration

Endotracheal tube A tube inserted into the trachea to ensure an open airway and assist with anesthesia or breathing support

Energy Every body process—the building up of cells, motion of the muscles, maintenance of body temperature—requires energy, and the body derives this energy from the food it consumes.

Enrichment medium A growth medium that permits preferential emergence of certain organisms that initially may have made up a relatively minute proportion of a mixed inoculum. The medium may be formulated to provide excess nutritional requirements for fastidious organisms or include selective components to inhibit competitive growth.

Enteral feeding The use of the upper alimentary tract (mouth, esophagus, stomach, and small intestine) for assisted feeding

Enterohepatic recirculation Occurs with some compounds that are metabolized in the liver. The metabolites are emptied in the bile and are reabsorbed in the small intestines.

Enteropathy A disease of the intestinal tract

Enterotomy Incision into a small intestinal lumen

Enterotoxemia A disease (e.g., pulpy kidney disease of lambs) attributed to absorption of a toxin from the intestine—also called *overeating disease*

Enzootic Of animal diseases: peculiar to or constantly present in a locality

Eosinophil Leukocyte with a segmented to bilobed nucleus, colorless to pale blue cytoplasm, and distinct eosinophilic (reddish orange) staining cytoplasmic granules

Epidermal membrane A thin, semitransparent membrane covering the camelid fetus but attaching at mucocutaneous junctions, at the coronet of the nails, and at the umbilicus

Epiphora Tearing of the eyes as a result of excessive secretion of tears or obstruction of the lacrimal passages

Epistaxis An attack of bleeding from the nose

Epithelialization Healing by the growth of epithelial cells over a denuded surface

Epizootic An outbreak of disease affecting many animals of one kind at the same time

Equine chorionic gonadotropin (ECG) Glycoprotein hormone secreted by specialized cells of the equine chorion that have embedded into the endometrium. They have luteinizing hormone activity in the horse, but follicle-stimulating hormone activity when administered to other species.

Ergonomic injury An injury involving the musculoskeletal system of the body, including muscle injuries, such as back strains, and repetitive motion injuries, such as carpal tunnel syndrome.

Ergonomics The study of how the human body moves. Commonly used to describe how the human body interacts with inanimate objects during work or play.

Erratic (or aberrant parasite) A parasite that has wandered into an organ or tissue in which it does not ordinarily live; for example, *Cuterebra* species that is usually found in the skin of dogs and cats wandering aberrantly into the brain of a dog

Eructate Eject gas from the stomach; burp

Eructation An act or instance of belching

Esophagostomy feeding tube A tube placed into an artificial opening in the esophagus when oral feeding is impossible because of injury or surgery

Estrogen Steroid hormone produced in the female's follicle. It causes signs of estrus and causes uterine, cervical, and vaginal changes at estrus.

Estrone sulfate Hormone secreted by the equine fetal-placental unit. It is a good indicator of fetal viability.

Ethylene oxide (EO) A gaseous substance used as a sterilant for instruments and articles that would be damaged by steam sterilization. EO is suspected to cause cancer in some animals in some cases involving very large or long exposures.

Evisceration Extrusion of the viscera from the abdominal cavity resulting from dehiscence of an abdominal incision

Excoriation Skin lesions caused by the self-trauma of scratching

Excretion The process by which drugs are eliminated from the body

Exodontics Extraction of teeth, either via closed or surgical techniques

Exogenous Arising from outside the body

Exophthalmos Outward protrusion of the eye

Expectorant A drug that liquefies respiratory secretions promoting elimination

Explorer Sharp, fine-tipped instrument used to examine irregularities in dental hard tissue

Extravasation The leakage of something out of its container or normal location, such as a drug out of the vein

Exudate The material composed of serum, fibrin, and WBCs that escapes from blood vessels into a superficial lesion or area of inflammation

Face The flat surface of a hand scaler that lies between both cutting edges

Facial Positional term in dentistry that describes the vestibular surface of the incisor teeth

Facultative parasite An organism that is capable of living either free or as a parasite; for example, *Pelodera strongyloides,* a free-living soil nematode that may cause rhabditic dermatitis in downer cows

Fasciculation Involuntary muscle twitching

Fastidious Describes microorganisms with complex nutritional requirements, usually requiring an enriched medium for cultivation

Fats One of the energy-producing components of the diet; can be broken down into triglycerides

Fatty casts Casts that contain fat globules from degenerating tubular epithelial cells

Feeder calf A steer or heifer, 6 to 9 months of age, 600 to 800 lb, that goes directly to a feedlot to promote fattening

Felony A grave crime declared to be a felony by common law or statute

Fetotomy Dissection of a dead fetus in utero; applicable particularly to cows because of the size of the uterus and the opportunity to introduce instruments to the full depth of the fetus

Fetus Stage of development when the species is recognizable

Fever Elevation of body temperature caused by a temporary increase in the body's thermoregulatory set-point, usually caused by infection, inflammation, or neoplasia

Fibrillation Disorganized, rapid, random, and ineffective contraction of cardiac muscle cells

FIFO First in, first out for inventory stock rotation

Filly Female horse less than 4 years old

Flaccid Lacking any muscle tone

Flail chest A freely moveable segment of the chest wall caused by segmental fracture of two or more ribs

Flash sterilization Emergency sterilization in which the instrument is placed unwrapped in an autoclave and taken directly to surgery following sterilization. It is not recommended as a routine sterilization procedure.

Flexibility Ability of a limb to move through a specific range of motion

Flight zone The area surrounding an animal that will cause alarm and escape when encroached upon

Fluctuant A term used to describe a mass that is movable and compressible, such as an abscess

Fluid resuscitation Use of fluid therapy to treat low blood pressure or severe dehydration

Fluoroscopy The presentation of a continuous image that involves directing the x-ray beam through the patient and onto an image intensifier

Foal Juvenile horse nursing from its mother

Focal film distance The distance between the target in the x-ray tube and the surface of the x-ray cassette

Focal spot The region on the anode that is bombarded by electrons. A large and small focal spot corresponding to the sizes of the filaments of the cathode.

Focusing cup Hollowed-out metal surrounding the cathode filament that holds the electron cloud before its rapid acceleration toward the anode

Fogged film Partially exposed film that causes poor contrast in the resulting radiographic image

Foley catheter A catheter threaded through the urethra to the bladder where it is held in place with a tiny, inflated balloon

Follicle Fluid-filled structure on the ovary that contains the oocyte. When mature it produces estrogen.

Follicle-stimulating hormone (FSH) Glycoprotein hormone produced and stored in the anterior pituitary. It causes follicular growth in females and spermatogonia maturation and release in males.

Fomite An object that in itself is harmless, such as clothing or instruments, but is able to harbor pathogenic or infectious agents and serve as an agent of transmission of an infection

Forage The vegetative portion of plants in a fresh, dried, or ensiled state, which is fed to livestock (as pasture, hay, or silage)

Foramen magnum The large hole in the occipital bone through which the spinal cord exits the skull

Forestomach Prestomach chambers in a ruminant animal. Includes the reticulum, rumen, and omasum.

Formalin Aqueous solution of formaldehyde used as a disinfectant and tissue fixative in medicine. Formaldehyde is also used in the manufacturing of building materials and adhesives. Formaldehyde is suspected to cause cancer in some animals in some cases involving very large or long exposures.

Free catch Urine obtained when the animal voids spontaneously or is assisted by gentle manual expression

Friction massage A form of massage that manipulates the tissue to increase circulation. It is commonly used over tendons when tendonitis is present, over knots and trigger points, and over joint capsules with excessive fibrous tissue. It is also used to break up skin adhesions and scar tissue.

Furcation The region of a multirooted tooth where the roots diverge from the crown

Gametogony A type of sexual reproduction used by coccidian parasites, such as *Isospora* or *Eimeria* species

Gastric dilation-volvulus A dangerous gastrointestinal condition, occurring primarily in deep-chested large-breed dogs, in which the stomach swells with air and twists on its long axis leading to shock, loss of blood supply, and other serious consequences

Gastric gavage Feeding by passing a feeding tube into the stomach

Gastroenteritis Inflammation of the lining membrane of the stomach and the intestines

Gastrostomy A method of enteral feeding in which a tube is surgically introduced through the abdominal wall

Gastrostomy feeding tube Gastric feeding tube inserted directly into the stomach

Gastrotomy Incision into the stomach

Gelding Castrated male horse; reproductive organs, the testes, have been removed

Genetic Inherited. In general, one or both of the parents transmit the disease-causing genes to the offspring unless it is a new mutation in the patient. The disease may not show up until much later in life.

Genital tubercle The embryonic precursor of the penis and scrotum in the male and the caudal vagina, vestibule, and vulva in the female

Geriatric A branch of medicine that deals with the problems and diseases of old age and aging people

Giardia A flagellated protozoal parasite of the small intestine. Animals with giardiasis may have watery diarrhea. Giardia can be spread to humans via contaminated water.

Gilts A female pig that has not yet produced a litter

Glandular therapy A type of supplement consisting of animal products to supply nutrients (steroids, enzymes, and raw materials of some organs, such as liver) to the patient to help restore health

Glottis The opening of the trachea within the oral cavity of birds. Usually located at the base of the tongue.

Glucocorticoid A term used synonymous with cortisol

Gluconeogenesis Formation of glucose within the animal body from precursors other than carbohydrates especially by the liver and kidney using amino acids from protein, glycerol from fats, or lactate produced by muscle during anaerobic glycolysis—called also *glyconeogenesis*

Glucosuria The presence of glucose in the urine

Glutaraldehyde A chemical disinfection solution used to sterilize hard surface instruments by immersion. Glutaraldehydes are suspected to cause cancer in some animals in some cases involving very large or long exposures.

Gonadotropin-releasing hormone (Gn-RH) A hormone secreted by gonadotropin from the anterior pituitary gland.

Goniometer Tool used to measure joint range of motion

Goniometry Technique used to measure range of motion at a joint

Gram stain A differential bacteriologic stain that distinguishes bacterial cell-wall structure types, which is a common basis for bacterial classification and identification; bacteria stain either blue (gram-positive) or red (gram-negative)

Granular casts Degenerating cellular casts characterized by a nonspecific granular matrix and are designated as either coarsely or finely granular

Granulomatous Of, relating to, or characterized by a mass or nodule of chronically inflamed tissue with granulations that is usually associated with an infective process

Granulosa cell layer Luminal cell layer in the follicle that converts testosterone to estradiol, specific steroid hormone that is produced by the mature follicle (and the placenta in some species near parturition)

Gravel A foot infection that gains access to the foot through the white line traveling up the sensitive lamina underneath the hoof wall forming an abscess that drains at the coronet

Grid A thin sheet of lead strips with radiolucent spacers encased in an aluminum cover giving the appearance of a thin, flat rectangular tray. Grids are placed between the patient and the film cassette to absorb scatter radiation so it does not reach the cassette and affect image quality.

Grid ratio The height of the lead strip compared with the width of the spacers between strips. A 12:1 ratio means the lead strip is 12 times higher than the width of the spacers. The higher the ratio, the more efficient the grid is at removing scatter radiation.

Grief process The emotional process one experiences when anticipating or following the loss of an object of attachment

Gross energy The total potential energy of a foodstuff determined by measuring the total heat produced when the food is burned in a bomb calorimeter

Gross income Total income before expenses

Gross pathology Refers to pathologic changes in tissue that are visible with the unaided eye

Ground fault circuit interruption (GFCI) A type of outlet or circuit designed to prevent electrocution by detecting the leakage current, such as what happens when an electrical current comes in contact with water. GFCI-protected outlets are common near sinks, tubs, and in wet areas of buildings.

Half-life Time required for the serum concentration of a drug to decrease by 50%

Halitosis A foul odor to the breath

Halogenated anesthetic agents A class of chemicals that are used to induce and maintain anesthesia in animals and humans. Halogenated anesthetic agents differ from earlier forms of anesthesia, such as diethyl ethers, because they contain at least one halogen atom in each molecule that makes them generally nonflammable. Examples of halogenated ethers include the general anesthetics halothane, isoflurane, desflurane, and sevoflurane.

Hardware Relates to the parts of the system that you can touch: the monitor, the hard drive, the mouse, the printers, the modem, the disks, and the scanner

Haul-in facility Reference to a large animal facility where animals are brought to the practice for examination or treatment

Hazardous chemical Any chemical or chemical product that may present a physical or health hazard, including but not limited to carcinogens, irritants, sensitizers, toxins, flammable materials, or products that may be reactive with other common chemicals

Hazardous materials plan A written plan required by the right to know law. The hazardous materials plan is prepared by the employer to inform employees of the warning, training, and safe use procedures for hazardous chemicals in the workplace.

Hazmat—short for hazardous material Also commonly used as an acronym for hazardous chemicals

Heel effect The x-ray beam that is produced though interactions with the anode has a spectrum of x-ray energies. The x-ray beam is more intense at the side of the cathode than in the center of the beam or on the anode side.

Heifer A bovine female that has not yet had a calf

Heinz bodies Denatured hemoglobin that has fused to the RBC membrane; appear as lightly eosinophilic spherical inclusions on standard Wright stain and as distinct, darkly staining inclusions on NMB stain

Helminth A worm. There are many types of worms: nematodes (roundworms), trematodes (flukes), cestodes (tapeworms), acanthocephalans (thorny-headed worms), pentastomes (tongue worms), and hirudineans (leeches).

Hemacytometer A counting chamber used for microscopic determination of cell concentration in fluids

Hematocrit (Hct) Calculated measure of red cell mass expressed as a percentage of blood composed of RBCs

Hematoma A blood clot

Hematuria Blood in the urine

Hemoabdomen Abnormal accumulation of blood in the abdomen

Hemodynamics The interplay of factors affecting blood flow and fluid balance in the body

Hemoglobin saturation Measured with a pulse oximeter to evaluate the amount of hemoglobin in blood in the peripheral tissues; measurement of perfusion of blood in the peripheral tissues

Hemoglobinemia The presence of free hemoglobin in the blood plasma resulting from the solution of hemoglobin out of the RBCs or from their disintegration

Hemoglobinuria Hemoglobin in the urine

Hemolysis The lysis of RBCs: in bacteriology, this characteristic is used in the identification of microorganisms based on the ability of bacterial colonies grown on agar plates to lyse RBCs incorporated in the medium. The hemolysins produced by bacteria may function as membrane-degrading enzymes or be inserted as porins by more numerous organisms or a combination of both.

Hemostasis The arrest of bleeding (as by a hemostatic agent)

Hemothorax Abnormal accumulation of blood in the pleural space

Hepatotoxic Compound that is toxic to liver cells

Hermaphrodite An intersex condition in which both testicular and ovarian tissue exist in the same animal

Hermaphroditic A single living organism that contains complete, functioning sets of both male and female reproductive organs. All of the tapeworms and flukes (excluding the schistosomes) are hermaphroditic.

Hernia Abnormal protrusion of an organ or other body structure through a defect or natural opening in a covering, muscle, or bone

Heterophil Neutrophil equivalent with reddish granules found in species such as elephants, rodents, avians, reptilians, amphibians, and nonhuman primates

Hexacanth embryo The "six-toothed embryo." Many tapeworm eggs are referred to as hexacanth embryos.

Hirudiniasis Infestation with bloodsucking leeches

Histopathology Refers to pathologic changes in tissue that are microscopic and can be seen with the use of a microscope

Holistic A form of medicine that concentrates on the "whole" animal and animal wellness, rather than concentrating on clinical signs of disease

Homeopathy A system of medicine that is based on the principle that "like cures like"

Homotoxicology A form of homeopathy that uses multiple remedies at the same time to promote healing in the body

Hooks Raised area of the tooth resulting from incomplete occlusal wear, most commonly seen in the rostral maxillary cheek tooth of horses

Horizontal bone loss A dental radiography term referring to alveolar bone loss along the long axis of the jaw, affecting multiple teeth

Hospice A facility or program designed to provide a caring environment for meeting the physical and emotional needs of the terminally ill

Hospital safety manual A collection of written safety "dos and don'ts" unique to a specific workplace

Host See parasitism.

Howell-Jolly bodies Small, often singular, deeply basophilic nuclear remnants that are occasionally seen in RBCs on normal blood films; may see increased numbers with regenerative anemias and in splenectomized animals

Human chorionic gonadotropin (HCG) A glycoprotein hormone secreted from the human chorion. It has luteinizing hormone activity when injected into most animals.

Hyaline casts Colorless, homogeneous, and semitransparent casts

Hydatid cyst A type of metacestode stage found in the intermediate host in the life cycle of a tapeworm. The hydatid cyst is a large fluid-filled cyst lined by a granular germinal membrane. From this germinal membrane will bud off structures called brood capsules. Within each brood capsule are many protoscolices, each of which can develop into a tapeworm if ingested by a canine host. There are two types of hydatid cysts: the unilocular hydatid cyst caused by *Echinococcus granulosus* and the multilocular hydatid cyst caused by *Echinococcus multilocularis*.

Hydrocarbons Any of a large class of organic compounds containing only carbon and hydrogen. Examples would be natural gas, propane, butane, kerosene, gasoline, and motor oil.

Hydrometra An accumulation of watery fluid in the uterus

Hydronephrosis Dilation and distention of the renal pelvis and calices usually caused by obstruction of the flow of urine from the kidney

Hydrophobia A morbid dread of water

Hydrotherapy Use of water for therapeutic effects

Hyoid bone The bone in the neck region that supports the base of the tongue, the pharynx and the larynx and aids the process of swallowing. It is usually referred to as a single bone, but it is composed of several portions. The hyoid bone is attached to the temporal bone by two small rods of cartilage.

Hyperalgesia Lowering of the pain threshold resulting in less stimulation required to produce pain

Hypercarbia Elevated carbon dioxide levels in the blood

Hyperchromasia Increased MCHC; artifact secondary to hemolysis, lipemia, icterus, and Heinz body formation

Hyperechoic A structure in the ultrasound image that appears bright or white compared with adjacent structures

Hypermobile joint Excessive motion at a joint

Hyperplasia Too much growth of something

Hyperpnea Abnormal increase in depth and rate of the respiratory movements

Hyperproteinemia Excessive protein concentrations in the blood

Hypersegmentation Nuclei with five or more lobes

Hypertension Elevated blood pressure

Hyperthermia Elevation of body temperature caused by inadequate heat-dissipating mechanisms to overcome excessive ambient heat, without a change in the body's thermoregulatory set-point

Hyperventilation Increased ventilation; a respiratory pattern that results in lower carbon dioxide blood levels

Hypnotic A drug that induces sleep

Hypocerebellum Decreased size of the cerebellum; cerebellum is stunted in growth in the fetus

Hypochromia Decreased MCHC; RBCs may have an increased area of central pallor

Hypoglycemia Lower than normal levels of blood glucose resulting in lack of fuel to the brain and other organ systems

Hypomobile joint Less than functional range of motion at a joint

Hypophyseal-portal vessels Circulatory network that moves small quantities of releasing hormones from the hypothalamus to the anterior pituitary

Hypoproteinemia A condition with low blood protein

Hypopyon An accumulation of WBCs in the anterior chamber of the eye

Hyposthenuric urine SG less than 1.008

Hypotension Low blood pressure; the opposite of hypertension

Hypothalamus Specialized portion of the ventral brain that secretes releasing hormones to the anterior pituitary via the hypophyseal-portal vessels

Hypothermia Abnormally low body temperature. The measured body temperature must be compared with what is normal for the age group because neonates have lower body temperatures than adults.

Hypoventilation Decreased ventilation; a respiratory problem that results in higher blood levels of carbon dioxide

Hypovolemia Decreased circulating blood volume

Hypoxemia Low blood oxygen levels

Hypoxia Low tissue oxygen levels

Hypoxic Deficiency in the amount of oxygen reaching body tissues

Hypsodont Tooth type with a long reserve crown and roots that allow for continued growth and/or continued eruption

Icterus Yellow discoloration of the skin and mucous membranes resulting from accumulation of excess bilirubin (as seen in certain liver diseases) or excessive breakdown of RBCs (as seen after internal hemorrhage or various hemolytic states)

Ileus A temporary or permanent loss of intestinal motility. This causes a physiologic obstruction of the bowel. There is little to no borborygmal sounds during ileus.

Immunoglobulins A group of large glycoproteins that are secreted into blood and tissue fluids by plasma cells and that function as antibodies in the immune response by binding with specific antigens

Immunohistochemical stain A method of analyzing and identifying microbial or cellular components based on the binding of antibodies to a specific antigenic marker

In situ In its normal place, confined to the site of origin

Incidental parasite A parasite in a host in which it does not usually live; for example, the canine heartworm, *Dirofilaria immitis,* localizing in the lungs of humans

Incise drape A sterile, adherent, plastic surgical drape. They are often impregnated with an antiseptic. The drape is incised along with the skin.

Incontinence Involuntary urination or defecation

Indirect life cycle A life cycle that uses an intermediate host; for example, *Dirofilaria immitis,* the canine heartworm, uses an indirect life cycle

Infection The growth of disease-producing bacteria or other microorganisms in the tissues. Parasitism by an internal parasite; for example, canine heartworms infect dogs. Endoparasites, such as the canine heartworm, *Dirofilaria immitis,* infect their hosts.

Infestation Parasitism by an external parasite; for example, fleas infest dogs. Ectoparasites, such as the cat flea, *Ctenocephalides felis,* infest their hosts.

Inflammation A response of body tissues to injury or irritation; characterized by pain, swelling, redness, and heat

Infundibulum Fingerlike portion of the uterine tube (oviduct) that captures the ova upon ovulation

Ingress port A port on a tubular instrument used to infuse a solution into a cavity, such as a joint.

Inhibin Glycoprotein hormone that inhibits release of follicle-stimulating hormone

Initiation A process by which normal cells are changed so that they have the potential to be able to form cancers. Not all initiated cells go on to become cancer.

Inpatient Patient that comes into the practice and is hospitalized for further treatment or work-up

Insurance examination Required by an insurance company before an animal can receive insurance coverage. Most commonly performed in the equine industry.

Interference with justice Includes eluding a police officer or interference with the conduct of a criminal investigation

Intermediate host The host that harbors the larval, asexual, or immature stages of the parasite; for example, the mosquito is the intermediate host for the canine heartworm, *Dirofilaria immitis.*

Intermediate to large lymphocytes Intermediate to large mononuclear cells that have clear cytoplasm, moderate N/C ratios, centralized oval nuclei with a brushed chromatin pattern, and may display a focal accumulation of low numbers of small reddish granules

Interradicular Referring to the space between the roots of teeth

Intraarticular In the joint space

Intracranial pressure The pressure within the bony vault of the skull that contains the brain and other soft tissues. Increases in intracranial pressure can damage the brain.

Intralingual Within the tongue

Intramedullary catheter A catheter placed into the medullary canal of a bone (i.e., a bone marrow catheter)

Intraosseous The administration of a drug or fluid in the bone

Intraperitoneal Situated within or administered by entering the peritoneum

Intravenous pyelogram (IVP) Iodinated contrast medium is injected intravenously to assess the kidneys. Also called an EU or excretory urogram.

Intubation Placement of an endotracheal tube into the trachea

Intussusception The involution of one intestinal segment into another

Ionizing radiation Any radiation capable of displacing electrons from atoms or molecules, thereby producing ions. Examples include alpha particles, beta particles, gamma rays or x-rays, and cosmic rays. In medicine, ionizing radiation arises from radiotherapy, x-ray machines, and radioactive substances. Ionizing radiation also enters the earth's atmosphere from outer space. At high doses, ionizing radiation increases specific types of chemical activity inside cells. This effect can be used to treat cancer, but it also leads to health risks including the induction of cancer.

IP address The IP address is the "Internet protocol" address. It is the series of numbers that is specific to each computer of each modality for electronic communication with the PACS in digital imaging.

Irritant Agent causing pain or inflammation at site of injection

Ischemia Deficient supply of blood to a body part, such as the heart or brain, that is due to obstruction of the inflow of arterial blood

Ischemic compression The use of manual pressure on trigger points to bring about muscle relaxation and relieve pain

Isoechoic A structure in the ultrasound image that is of equal echogenicity to another structure

Isosthenuria An unconcentrated and undiluted urine specific gravity (approximately SG 1.010)

Isosthenuric urine SG 1.008 to 1.012

Isthmus Portion of the uterine tube (oviduct) that connects the infundibulum and ampulla

IVNTA International Veterinary Nurses and Technicians Association

Ixodid ticks Hard ticks or members of the tick family Ixodidae. Most of the ticks that parasitize domesticated animals are hard ticks. Hard ticks usually attach to their hosts to take a blood meal.

Jackson-Rees circuit A nonrebreathing circuit with a reservoir bag and corrugated tubing but no pressure relief valve in which the fresh gas inlet is located near the patient and waste gas exits near the bag; Mapleson F circuit

Jejunostomy feeding tube A tube surgically positioned in the jejunum used for enteral feeding when it is necessary to bypass the upper gastrointestinal tract

Joint mobilization Very specific passive movements applied to joint

Junctional epithelium A thin layer of epithelium that attaches to the tooth just coronal to the cementoenamel junction

Keratoconjunctivitis Combined inflammation of the cornea and conjunctiva

Ketonemia A condition marked by an abnormal increase of ketone bodies in the circulating blood. Ketones are acids that build in the blood when glucose is not used by cells; can be a result of lack of insulin that is needed to shuttle glucose into most cells of the body; complication of a diabetes mellitus patient

Ketonuria The presence of excess ketone bodies in the urine in conditions, such as diabetes mellitus and starvation, involving reduced or disturbed carbohydrate metabolism

Ketosis or acetonemia A nutritional disease of cattle and sometimes sheep, goats, or swine that is marked by reduction of blood glucose and the presence of ketone bodies in the blood, tissues, milk, and urine and is associated with digestive and nervous disturbances

Kilocalorie The amount of heat (energy) needed to raise the temperature of 1 kg of water 1° C

Kilovoltage A quality factor that regulates the energy of the x-ray beam. The higher the kVp (kilovoltage), the higher the energy of the x-ray photons. It also regulates contrast in the radiographic image. The higher the kVp, the lower the contrast.

Kyphosis Exaggerated upward curvature of the thoracic region of the spinal column resulting in a rounded upper back

Lacrimation The secretion of tears; *specifically,* abnormal or excessive secretion of tears resulting from local or systemic disease

Lamina dura Cortical plate of alveolar bone surrounding the tooth

Laminae The interdigitations between the corium and hoof that serve as the attachment sites between the hoof and coffin bone

Laminar flow Nonturbulent flow of a viscous fluid in layers near a boundary

Laminitis Inflammation of a lamina, especially in the hoof of a horse, cow, or goat, that is typically caused by excessive ingestion of a dietary substance (e.g., carbohydrate); called also *founder*

Laparotomy A transabdominal incision into the peritoneal cavity

Larvicide A preventive compound that will kill the migrating, larval stages of a parasite

Larviparous nematodes Nematodes that bear live larvas. *Filaroides osleri* is a larviparous nematode that produces L_1 larvas that are infective to the canine host.

Laryngoscope An instrument used to visualize the larynx during endotracheal intubation

Laser (light amplification by stimulated emission of radiation) The use of a coherent, monochromic, polarized light to bring about a physiologic change in the body

Late phase radiation toxicity Side effects caused by radiotherapy that occur more than 90 days after the start of treatment. They are generally characterized by permanent changes such as tissue fibrosis, atrophy, necrosis, and ischemia. They often develop months to years after completion of therapy.

Left shift Increased numbers of bands

Leptocytes RBCs with an increased surface area; target cells (codocytes) and cells with a transverse fold are two common forms of leptocytes

Lesions Alterations or abnormalities in a tissue (pathologic changes), ex. wounds, sores, ulcers, tumors, cataracts, and any other tissue damage.

Leukocytosis A condition characterized by an abnormally high total number of circulating leukocytes. Neutrophilia: indicates increased numbers of circulating neutrophils.

Leukoencephalomyelitis Concurrent inflammation of the white matter of the brain and spinal cord

Life cycle The development of a parasite through its various life stages (e.g., the life cycle of the canine heartworm). In the life cycle of *Dirofilaria immitis*, the dog is the definitive host and the mosquito is the intermediate host.

Ligament Structures that connect bone to bone

Limbus The corneal-scleral junction of the eye

Lingual Positional term in dentistry referring to the surface of mandibular teeth adjacent to the tongue

Local Area Network (LAN) The LAN is the connection of the workstation to the PACS server for image transfer.

Locomotor Movement from place to place

Lordosis Condition when the back is arched such that the head and tail are elevated and the back is dropped. It is a characteristic sign of estrus in the queen.

Lumen The cavity of a tubular organ <the *lumen* of a blood vessel>

Lumpectomy Removal of a small mass of tissue that is freely movable, such as a small skin tumor or a small mammary mass

Luteinizing hormone (LH) Glycoprotein hormone produced and stored in the anterior pituitary. It causes ovulation in the female and testosterone production in the male.

Lyme disease Also called borreliosis, is an infectious disease caused by bacteria from the genus *Borrelia*. The bacteria are typically spread through the bite of an infected deer tick.

Lymphoblasts Intermediate to large lymphoid cells with moderate N/C ratios, moderately to darkly basophilic cytoplasm, frequent Golgi zones, close nuclear to plasma membrane apposition along most of the perimeter of their round to oval nucleus, finely stippled chromatin patterns, and defined by the presence of one or more variably sized usually round to oval basophilic nucleoli within their nuclei

Macrocytic Larger than normal cells

Macrominerals Minerals, such as calcium, phosphorus, magnesium, sodium, potassium, chlorine, and sulfur, that are required in larger quantities than other minerals

Magill circuit A nonrebreathing circuit with a reservoir bag and corrugated tubing in which the fresh gas inlet is located near the bag and the pressure relief valve is located near the patient; Mapleson A circuit

Magnetostrictive ultrasonic A type of power scaler that uses either a metal stack or ferrite rod as transducer to create vibrations of the tip for periodontal débridement

Maintenance fluid requirement The amount of fluid typically required to support a healthy animal

Maintenance nutrient requirements (MNRs) The levels of nutrients needed to sustain body weight without gain or loss

Malignant A malignant cancer is one that can invade and destroy surrounding normal tissues. Some malignant cancers also have the ability to spread (metastasize) to other parts of the body.

Mallophagans Chewing lice that are members of the insect order Mallophaga

Malnutrition A condition caused by a diet that contains all of the essential nutrients but in suboptimal amounts

Malocclusion The incorrect alignment of jaws or specific teeth within the jaws

Malpractice Practicing beyond the scope of the license granted by the state or negligence in carrying out the duties of the license

Manometer Instrument used to measure the pressure of liquids, such as the blood

Manual muscle testing A technique used in applied kinesiology to test muscle weakness or paresis that may be affected by functional imbalances in the structural, chemical, mental, and energetic systems of the patient

Manual therapy A type of treatment performed with the hands, such as massage and chiropractic

Mapleson circuit Any one of a number of nonrebreathing circuits in which the position of the fresh gas inlet, the reservoir bag, and the scavenger outlet varies as classified by W.W. Mapleson

Mare Adult female horse

Marketing All forms of client communication (i.e., signs, business cards, treatment plans, website, etc.)

Massage Varying types of manual strokes applied to the body to promote relaxation, decrease pain, or increase circulation to surrounding tissues

Masseter muscle Large bilateral muscle of mastication positioned ventral to the zygomatic arch, which functions to close the mouth

Mastectomy Removal of a mammary gland

Master problem list The complete list of diagnosis given to a patient during its lifetime

Mastication Term used to describe chewing and breakdown of food material by the teeth

Material Safety Data Sheet (MSDS) A form prepared by the manufacturer of a product containing data regarding the properties of the product intended to provide workers and emergency personnel with procedures for handling or working with that substance in a safe manner

Maxillomandibular fixation Type of jaw fracture fixation that immobilizes the jaws with the mouth slightly open, allowing the patient to eat and drink through a narrow space between the incisors

Mean corpuscular hemoglobin concentration (MCHC) Average RBC hemoglobin concentration expressed in g/dl

Mean corpuscular volume (MCV) Average RBC volume expressed in fl

Medial metatarsal vein The vein in birds that is found on the medial aspect of the tarsometatarsal bone

Mediastinum The space in the thorax between the lungs that contains the trachea, esophagus, heart, nerves, lymphatic vessels, and major blood vessels

Megestrol acetate Synthetic progestagen used to suppress estrus in the bitch

Melatonin Hormone produced in the pineal gland during hours of darkness. It is involved with seasonality of estrus in many species.

Melena The passage of dark tarry stools containing decomposing blood that is usually an indication of bleeding in the upper part of the alimentary tract and especially the esophagus, stomach, and duodenum

Meninges Connective tissue layers that cover the brain and spinal cord

Mentation The mental activity or acuity of a patient

Meridian A line drawn connecting a group of acupuncture points named for the organ that they have the most effect on

Mesial Positional term in dentistry referring to the surface of the tooth along the dental arch that is closest to the rostral midline of the dental arch

Mesocephalic Also called mesaticephalic, refers to a head shape of moderate length in the rostrocaudal dimension, as seen in beagles

Metabolic acidosis Acidosis resulting from excess acid in the blood caused by abnormal metabolism, excessive acid intake, renal retention, or from excessive loss of bicarbonate (as in diarrhea)

Metabolism (biotransformation) The ability of a living organism to modify the chemical structure of drugs so that they are no longer active

Metabolizable energy Energy available to the animal after energy from feces, urine, and combustible gases have been subtracted from gross energy

Metacestode stage A larval tapeworm. This is the stage in the tapeworm that is found within the vertebrate or invertebrate intermediate host. Examples of metacestode stages include the cysticercoid, the cysticercus, the coenurus, and the hydatid cyst (both unilocular and multilocular).

Metamyelocyte Developmental stage before the band with a bean-shaped or butterfly-shaped nucleus

Metaphylaxis Use of an antimicrobial treatment for subclinical manifestation of BRD complex in cattle

Metastasis The process by which a malignant cancer spreads from the primary or original site to a distant location in the body

MHz The abbreviation for megahertz, the unit of frequency for diagnostic ultrasound waves

Mibolerone Synthetic androgen used for suppressing estrus in the bitch

Microbiology The study of microorganisms (bacteria, fungi, and viruses) and their interactions within ecosystems

Microcytic Smaller than normal cells

Microfilaria The motile prelarval stage of filarial parasites, such as *Dirofilaria immitis*. Microfilariae are often found circulating in the peripheral blood of the dog.

Microfilaricide A therapeutic compound that will kill the microfilarial stages of a parasite

Microflora Microorganisms (mostly bacteria) with intimate and permanent associations with epithelial surfaces. Also called normal flora, indigenous flora, or autochthonous flora.

Microminerals A group of minerals called the "trace elements," such as copper, iron, boron, molybdenum, and cobalt, which are required in minute amounts

Microorganism An organism that is too small to be seen with the naked eye. Includes bacteria, viruses, fungi, and protozoa.

***Microsporum* sp.** A genus of fungi that can cause ringworm. Most common in cats and horses, but dogs and other species of animals (including humans) are susceptible.

Milliamperage The milliamperage setting controls the quantity of electrons boiled off the filament in the x-ray tube.

Mineralocorticoid Natural aldosterone; hormone that regulates the electrolyte and water balance by balancing the retention of sodium and the loss of potassium through the renal tubules

Minerals Nonorganic solid substances that occur naturally in food and form the mineral composition of the animal body; at least 13 are essential to health

Minimum inhibitory concentration MIC is the lowest concentration of an antimicrobial agent that will inhibit the visible growth of a microorganism after overnight incubation.

Miosis Constriction of the pupil of the eye

Mitchell markers Special radiographic markers primarily used in standing radiography of the equine head to assist in identifying fluid levels in paranasal sinuses

M-mode Time-motion ultrasound imaging mode where the motion of the body, usually the heart, is observed by scanning a thin slice of it over time

Modality Method of application of or the employment of any therapeutic agent, usually physical agents

Modulation The process of amplifying or dampening incoming pain signals after arrival in the spinal cord

Monocytes Mononuclear cells with gray-blue cytoplasm that frequently have a fine, subtle, lightly eosinophilic granulation, which may contain a few clear vacuoles and a variable-shaped (round, oval, reniform, ameboid, or lobed) nucleus.

Morbidity The incidence of disease; the rate of sickness (as in a specified community or group)

Moribund Near death

Mortality The number of deaths in a given time or place

MPD Maximum permissible dose (MPD). This is the maximum allowed radiation exposure a person can receive during occupational exposure over a certain time.

Mucin clot test Used to evaluate joint fluid viscosity; formation and integrity of a mucin clot upon addition of joint fluid to an acidic reagent are evaluated

Mucogingival junction The line created where the alveolar mucosa meets the gingiva

Mucometra A uterus filled with mucus

Mucositis Inflammation of the mucous membranes lining the digestive tract from the mouth to the anus. Mucositis is a possible side effect of chemotherapy or radiotherapy that involves any part of the digestive tract.

Mucous membrane Moist body surface associated with an orifice (e.g., oral cavity, genitourinary, etc.)

Müllerian duct Embryologic precursor of the female tubular reproductive tract (uterine tubes, uterus, cranial vagina)

Multimodal analgesia Using two or more drugs to effect different phases of nociception simultaneously

Multimodality therapy Cancer treatment that combines more than one form of therapy (e.g., surgery, radiotherapy, and chemotherapy)

Multiple organ dysfunction syndrome (MODS) An end-stage complication of shock or systemic inflammation that results in simultaneous failure of multiple organs

Mutagen A chemical or physical agent that causes permanent DNA injury and alteration within a cell. These changes are separate and distinct from those that normally occur during genetic recombination.

Mycosis Fungal infection in or on a part of the body

Mydriasis Dilation of the pupil of the eye

Myelocytes Developmental stage before the metamyelocyte with an oval-shaped nuclei

Myelosuppression A condition in which normal bone marrow activity is decreased, resulting in fewer WBCs (especially neutrophils), platelets, and RBCs in circulation. Myelosuppression is a potential side effect of some cancer therapies (e.g., radiotherapy and chemotherapy)

Myiasis The infection or infestation of Dipteran larvas (maggots) into the organs or tissues of humans, domesticated animals, or wild animals

Myocardium The middle layer of the heart and the main muscle layer responsible for contraction during systole

Myoglobinuria Myoglobin in the urine

Myositis Inflammation of muscle

Myotherapy (aka trigger point therapy) A form of massage using ischemic compression to relieve pain and muscle spasms

Nadir of leukopenia The lowest circulating neutrophil count occurring after administration of a chemotherapy drug. The nadir occurs at a predictable time point after therapy that varies depending on exactly what drug has been given.

Nares Nostrils

Nasal cannula A catheter or tube inserted into the nasal passages to supply oxygen

Nasogastric feeding tube A flexible tube with a rounded end that is passed through the nasal cavity to the stomach

Nasolacrimal duct Duct that travels from the medial canthus of the eye to the rostral nasal passage, responsible for drainage of tears

National Fire Protection Association (NFPA) An organization with the mission of reducing incidence and damage from fire by providing and advocating scientifically based codes and standards, research, training, and education

National Institute for Occupational Safety and Health (NIOSH) As part of the CDC, NIOSH is responsible for conducting research and making recommendations for the prevention of work-related illnesses and injuries.

Navicular bursa A closed fibrous sac lined with a smooth membrane, producing a viscous lubricant known as synovial fluid and located between the deep digital flexor tendon and the navicular bone

NAVTA National Association of Veterinary Technicians in America

NCVEI National Commission on Veterinary Economic Issues that evaluates the economic status of the profession

Necropsy The examination of an animal after it has died to determine the abnormal and disease-related changes that occurred during its life. The term necropsy originates from the Greek language and means "viewing the dead." Necropsy is also known as autopsy, which is Greek for "seeing with one's own eyes."

Necrosis Tissue or cellular death

Necrotizing Causing, associated with, or undergoing necrosis (death of living tissue)

Negative punishment Decreases the frequency of behavior because something *pleasant* is *taken away (subtracted)* following a behavior

Negative reinforcement Increases the frequency of behavior because something *unpleasant* is *taken away or avoided (subtracted)* following a behavior

Nematode A roundworm. *Dirofilaria immitis,* the canine heartworm, is a nematode parasite found in the right ventricle and pulmonary arteries of dogs.

Neonatal Pertaining to the time immediately following birth

Neonatal isoerythrolysis An uncommon, complex disorder of newborns that results from a blood group incompatibility that exists between the dam and the offspring; NI occurs after the neonate suckles and absorbs antibodies from the dam's colostrum, which then attack the neonate's RBCs resulting in destruction of the RBCs of the baby and subsequent anemia (decrease in RBCs)

Neonatal period In puppies and kittens, the first 2 to 4 weeks of life are characterized by complete dependence on the mother because of incomplete neurologic functions, such as audio and visual abilities and proper spinal reflexes.

Neoplasm An abnormal growth of tissue that may be benign or malignant

Nephrectomy The surgical removal of a kidney

Nephrotoxic Toxic or destructive to kidney cells

Net energy Energy available to the animal after energy from feces, urine, combustible gases, and body heat loss has been subtracted from gross energy

Net income Total income less all expenses and taxes

Network Where the veterinary software is stored and the associated patient-client database

Neuromuscular blocker Drug that relaxes and paralyzes muscles and that causes cessation of breathing as a result of paralysis of the muscles of respiration

Neurons Nerve cells that relay information from the central nervous system to the rest of the body

Neurotransmitter A chemical substance released from the axon terminal of a presynaptic neuron and diffuses across the synaptic cleft to either excite or inhibit the target cell

Neutroclusion Malocclusion where no jaw length discrepancy exists but one or more teeth are in an abnormal position

Neutropenia An abnormal decrease in the number of neutrophils (the most common type of WBCs) in the blood

Nidus A place where bacteria or other organisms can lodge and replicate

Nit The egg of either an Anopluran (sucking) or Mallophagan (chewing) louse. The adult female louse cements the nit to a hair shaft or a feather of the infested host.

N-methyl-D-aspartate (NMDA) receptor One of a number of receptors in the central nervous system that secrete excitatory neurotransmitters. The NMDA receptors play a large role in the processing of pain signals.

Nociception Term used to describe three neuralgic phases of the pain pathway: transduction, transmission, and modulation

Nonrebreathing system A breathing circuit in which exhaled gasses are carried away from the patient into a scavenging system

Nonscreen film Radiographic film that requires direct exposure to x-rays to create an image. They are insensitive to visible light from screens. Used mainly for the oral cavity.

Nonshopped fees Those fees that clients do not call the practice to find out the cost. These make up the largest percentage of the fee schedule.

Nonsteroidal antiinflammatory drugs (NSAIDs) Large group of antiinflammatory agents that work by inhibiting the production of prostaglandins. Examples include ibuprofen, ketoprofen, naproxen, and aspirin. These compounds also possess analgesic, antipyretic, and antiinflammatory effects; they reduce pain, fever, and inflammation.

Nonthreatening greeting behaviors When greeting dogs and cats, technicians should look off to the side or down (avoid eye contact), stand up straight or bend at the knees (avoid bending at the waist and leaning over the pet), stroke the pet under the chin at first (do not reach over the animal's head to pet it), and turn the side of their bodies to face the pet (avoid approaching front to front).

Normothermic A normal body temperature

Nosocomial infection An infection acquired within a hospital or hospital-like setting, but secondary to the patient's original condition. Infections are considered nosocomial if they first appear 48 hours or more after hospital admission or within 30 days after discharge.

Nucleated RBCs (NRBCs) Immature RBCs before developmental stage to the reticulocyte; usually metarubricytes if associated with a regenerative anemia or bone marrow toxicity

Nutraceutical A nutritional supplement thought to have a beneficial medical effect

Nutrients Nourishing substances, food, or components of food

Nutritional myodegeneration Degeneration of muscle tissue usually associated with vitamin E and selenium deficiency

Nymphomania A behavior state in which a female is in continuous estrus or estrus for prolonged periods of time

Nystagmus A rhythmic, involuntary oscillation of both eyes

Obesity A body composition with a ratio of too much fat to lean tissue or body weight 15% to 20% greater than optimal

Obligatory parasite An organism that must live a parasitic existence (e.g., the canine heartworm, *Dirofilaria immitis,* in dogs)

Obstructive urolithiasis A condition that is characterized by the formation or presence of calculi in the urinary tract that cause complete obstruction of urinary flow

Obtunded Mentally dull

Obturator The stylus or removable plug used during the insertion of a tubular instrument

Occlusal Positional term referring to the part of a tooth that meets with, or occludes with, the teeth of the opposite dental arcade

Occupational Safety and Health Act The law in the United States that established the Occupational Safety and Health Administration. It gives every American worker protections and responsibilities in the area of safety. The act applies to all workplaces in the United States and its territories with at least one employee.

Occupational Safety and Health Administration (OSHA) The agency of the U.S. government that is charged with enforcing the Occupational Safety and Health Act. Twenty-one states and territories have OSHA programs administered by the state, whereas the remainder fall under federal OSHA jurisdiction.

Ocular larva migrans A zoonotic condition caused by the migration of nematode larvas (usually *Toxocara canis*) through the eyes of children. Children become infected with these larvas by ingestion of eggs containing the infective second-stage larvas of *T. canis*.

Odontoblasts Cells that line the pulp cavity and root canal, responsible for production of dentin

Odontoclasts Cells of the macrophage lineage, similar to osteoclasts, that cause resorption of the tooth

Offensive aggression Behaviors that result in harm done to another individual when the aggressor initiates the conflict. Offensive animals are not fearful and will move toward an opponent rather than away from them.

Omentopexy Surgical fixation of the omentum to the body wall

Omentum The supportive mesenteries, which arise from the greater and lesser curvatures of the stomach

Omphalophlebitis A condition (e.g., navel ill) characterized by or resulting from inflammation and infection of the umbilical vein

Oncosphere The "growth ball." Many tapeworm eggs are referred to as oncospheres.

One-handed method The technique of replacing the cap on a used hypodermic needle using only one hand. This technique is used to prevent the accidental insertion of the needle into the opposite hand while holding a cap.

One-step prep Alcohol-based solutions containing other antiseptics that form a film when painted on the skin. Provide a rapid onset of antiseptic effect and a long residual effect.

Onychectomy Removal of a claw

Oocyte The female gamete that has half the number of chromosomes

Open gloving A method of putting on sterile gloves when the person is not wearing a sterile gown or the hands are protruding through the ends of the gown sleeves

Open kinetic chain exercise An exercise in which the distal limb segment is free

Operant conditioning Also known as instrumental conditioning, based on the principle that the consequences of a behavior will influence its frequency. Known as the Thorndike law of effect, behaviors that result in pleasant outcomes will increase in frequency, whereas those that result in unpleasant ones will decrease.

Operating software Tells the different parts of the hardware how to communicate with each other. For instance, the operating system translates strikes on the keyboard to letters seen on the screen. It monitors and organizes files and directories, and it controls peripheral devices, such as printers, scanners, and disk drives.

Operculum The "door" on one end of a trematode egg or the egg of a pseudotapeworm. The miracidium of the juvenile fluke will exit via the operculum of the fluke egg; the coracidium of the juvenile pseudotapeworm will exit via the operculum of the pseudotapeworm egg.

Opioids Analgesics that remedy pain by affecting pain receptors in the brain

Opisthotonos A condition of spasm of the muscles of the back, causing the head and limbs to bend backward and the trunk to arch forward

Orchidectomy Removal of the testicles

Oronasal fistula An abnormal communication between the mouth and nasal passage, usually caused by severe periodontal disease or palatal trauma

Osmolality The concentration of osmotically active particles in solution expressed in osmoles or milliosmoles per kilogram

Osmotic Having the ability to retain or pull water

Ostectomy Removal of a portion of bone

Osteochondral chip fragments Fracture involving the articular cartilage and underlying bone

Osteochondrosis A disease of joints that results in unhealthy or incomplete maturation of cartilage, resulting in joint effusion and sometimes lameness

Osteoconductive Term referring to a material that does not stimulate bone formation but facilitates movement of bone cells to traverse a defect

Osteoinductive Term referring to a material that stimulates bone formation in areas where there is no bone

Osteomyelitis Infection of the bone

Outpatient Patient that comes into the practice and is treated and leaves without staying

Ovariohysterectomy Spay; removal of the uterus

Overhydration The opposite of dehydration. A condition characterized by fluid retention or overload.

Oxidase In bacteriology, a group of enzymes that catalyze oxidation, especially an enzyme that reacts with molecular oxygen to catalyze the oxidation of a substrate

Oxygen free radicals Highly reactive compounds or molecules that cause tissue damage

Oxygen saturation The amount of hemoglobin bound to oxygen at any given moment. This value is measured in percent, and it reflects the degree of blood oxygenation.

Oxytocin Hormone produced by the posterior pituitary that cause uterine contractions and milk let-down. It is also involved in luteolysis.

Packed-cell volume (PCV) The centrifugation of a small aliquot of blood. The relative volume of packed RBCs (expressed as a percentage of total-blood volume) can be determined. The relative volume of white blood cells and platelets can also be determined if an anticoagulant is added to the blood.

Pain detection threshold The point at which pain nerve fibers are stimulated enough to send pain signals to the central nervous system

Pain tolerance The greatest intensity of pain that can be tolerated by an individual

Palatal Positional term in dentistry that describes the surface of maxillary teeth adjacent to the palate

Palatoglossal folds Bilateral bands of soft tissue that run from the roof of the mouth to beneath the tongue. The area lateral to the palatoglossal folds is often affected in cats with stomatitis.

Palliative therapy Cancer treatment administered to relieve the symptoms and reduce the suffering caused by cancer. The primary goal of palliative therapy is to improve quality of life; it is not intended to cure cancer or even to extend survival time.

Palpation The sense of touch used to assess what structures lay below the skin and presence of potential injury to those structures

Palpebral edema Swelling of the eyelids

Pancytopenia A decrease below normal in the concentration of the three major blood cell types: red cells, white cells, and platelets

Panleukopenia A viral infection of cats that is not considered zoonotic but is highly contagious from cat to cat

Paracentesis A surgical puncture of a body cavity (e.g., the abdomen) with a trocar, aspirator, or other instrument usually to draw off an abnormal effusion for diagnostic or therapeutic purposes

Paralysis A nervous or musculoskeletal problem that prevents any movement of the affected body part

Paramedian Situated adjacent to the midline

Paraneoplastic syndrome Symptoms that result from effects on organs or tissues distant from the site of a primary tumor or its metastases. The underlying cause is usually a substance that is produced by the tumor and then released into the systemic circulation. Almost any organ or tissue can be affected.

Paraphimosis A condition in which the penis is extended and cannot be retracted to its normal position within the prepuce

Parasite See parasitism.

Parasitism An association between two organisms of different species in which one member (the parasite) lives on or in the other member (the host) and may cause harm. Parasitism implies a metabolic dependency.

Parasitology The study of parasitic relationships

Paratenic (or transport) host An intermediate host in which the parasite does not undergo any further development, usually remaining encysted until the definitive host eats the transport host (e.g., a mouse infected with encysted larvas of the canine roundworm, *Toxocara canis*)

Parenteral feeding The delivery of nutrients intravenously

Paresis Incomplete paralysis (i.e., some function is still possible)

Parthenogenesis The development of an offspring (larva) using reproduction without fertilization by a male. *Strongyloides stercoralis* uses parthenogenesis in its life cycle. Only female *Strongyloides stercoralis* are parasitic; there are no parasitic males. These female nematodes produce offspring without fertilization by a male and are said to use parthenogenesis.

Parturition The act of giving birth

Parvoviral enteritis A viral infection of dogs that is not considered zoonotic but is highly contagious from dog to dog

Passerine Of or relating to the largest order (Passeriformes) of birds, which includes more than half of all living birds and consists chiefly of altricial songbirds

Passive range of motion (PROM) Joint movement obtained by a therapist moving a limb with no assistance from the patient

Passive transfer Absorption of protective antibodies from the colostrum by the newborn

Patent ductus arteriosus A congenital cardiac anomaly resulting in persistent vascular communication between the aorta and pulmonary artery

Pathogenesis The sequence of events that leads to or underlies a disease

Pathogenic organism A biologic agent (fungi, bacteria, virus, etc.) that causes disease or illness

Pathognomonic A feature or abnormality that specifically denotes a single disease or condition

Pathology The science and study of disease, especially the causes and development of abnormal conditions

Peak serum concentration The point of maximum concentration of drug on the time-versus-serum concentration curve

Pediatric period Pediatrics covers the period from birth to puberty and is concerned with development and disease during this period. Puppies and kittens are considered pediatric patients during the first 7 to 12 months of life (puberty sets in later in giant-breed dogs, and thus they may be considered pediatric patients until 1.5 to 2 years of age).

Pediculosis Infestation with either Anopluran (sucking) or Mallophagan (chewing) lice

Pemphigus vulgaris Vesicular autoimmune disease of the skin and oral mucosa, which also causes pyrexia, depression, and anorexia

Pentastomes (tongue worms) A unique group of parasites (distantly related to the arthropods) that infect the lungs of snakes and other reptiles.

Pepsinogen A granular zymogen of the gastric glands that is readily converted into pepsin in a slightly acid medium

Percutaneous A term referring to something passing through the skin

Periapical lucency Term in dental radiography referring to decreased radiodensity at the tip of a tooth root, which is suggestive of a tooth root's pathologic condition.

Pericardiocentesis Surgical puncture of the pericardium, especially to aspirate pericardial fluid

Pericardiotomy Surgical incision of the pericardium

Pericarditis Inflammation of the pericardium

Pericardium The sac of serous membrane that encloses the heart and the roots of the great blood vessels of vertebrates and consists of an outer fibrous coat that loosely invests the heart and a double inner serous coat of which one layer is closely adherent to the heart, and the other lines the inner surface of the outer coat with the intervening space filled with pericardial fluid

Perineal The area between the anus and the dorsal part of the external genitalia, especially in the female

Perineal hernia Herniation of abdominal contents through the pelvic diaphragm, resulting in swelling on either side of the anus

Perineum An area of tissue that marks externally the approximate boundary of the outlet of the pelvis and gives passage to the urogenital ducts and rectum

Periodic parasite A parasite that makes short visits to its host to obtain nourishment or some other benefit (e.g., female mosquitoes alighting on the vertebrate host to obtain a blood meal)

Periodontal débridement Nonsurgical instrumentation for removal of hard and soft deposits from teeth and surrounding spaces

Periodontium The supporting structures of the tooth, including the periodontal ligament, gingival connective tissue, alveolar bone, and cementum

Periparturient The period of time surrounding parturition or birth

Peritoneal cavity The abdominal cavity (lined by a membrane known as the peritoneum)

Peritonitis Inflammation of the serosa (peritoneum) that lines the walls of the abdominal cavity and covers the abdominal organs and mesenteries

Perjury Making a false statement under oath

Persistent deciduous tooth Primary or "baby" tooth that has not been lost by the time the adult tooth is erupting. Previously and incorrectly referred to as "retained."

Personal protective equipment (PPE) Any piece of clothing or article that is worn by the user that is designed to prevent injury. Typically, PPE would not remove the hazard at hand, but merely places a physical barrier between the wearer and the hazard. Examples include gloves, glasses or goggles, aprons, boots, smocks, masks, etc.

Petechiation or petechial hemorrhage Small, visible, pinpoint hemorrhage lesions less than 1 mm in diameter

Pétrissage A type of massage that consists of kneading, rhythmic lifting, squeezing, and releasing the tissue. It assists in removing metabolic waste and increasing circulation.

Petty cash Small amounts of discretionary funds in the form of cash that are used to buy items where it is not practical to write a check or use a credit card

Peyer patches Aggregations of lymphoid tissue that are usually found in the lowest portion of the small intestine (ileum)

pH The inverse logarithm of the hydrogen ion concentration of a fluid

Pharmacodynamics Characteristic ability of living organisms to absorb, distribute, metabolize, and excrete drugs

Pharmacognosy Aspect of pharmacology that includes the history and source of drugs

Pharmacology The study of drugs

Pharmacotherapeutics Therapeutic uses of drugs

Pharynx The part of the digestive and respiratory tracts extending from the back of the nasal cavity and mouth to the esophagus, more specifically delineated as nasopharynx and oropharynx

Pheromone A substance that is secreted by an animal and is detected by the olfactory system of another animal. They are usually sexual signals.

Phimosis A condition in which an animal is unable to extend the penis, perhaps as a result of the presence of masses on the penis or secondary to balanoposthitis

Phlebitis Inflammation of a vein

Photophobia Intolerance to light; painful sensitivity to strong light

Physiologic age An individual's age as estimated in terms of organ and body function and translated into probable life expectancy. The physiologic age may be shorter or longer than the actual chronologic age, as measured in months and years.

Picture Archival Computing Systems (PACS) PACS are required to store, send, receive, print, and view images from all imaging modalities.

Piezoelectric ultrasonic A type of power scaler that uses either a ceramic disk or quartz crystal as transducer to create vibrations of the tip for periodontal débridement

Pineal gland Portion of the brain that secretes melatonin via light stimulation through the eyes

Pinocytosis The uptake of fluid and dissolved substances by a cell by invagination and pinching off of the cell membrane

Pituitary gland The "master endocrine gland". A pea-sized endocrine gland located at the base of the brain, made up of the anterior pituitary gland, which produces seven known hormones, and the posterior pituitary gland, which stores and releases two hormones from the hypothalamus; also called the hypophysis.

Placenta The organ arising from the embryo that provides nutrients to the fetus via its interaction with the uterus

Placentomes A specific area of placental attachment. Usually in ruminants.

Plaque An accumulation of food particles, saliva, minerals, and bacteria that appears as a white-tan, easily removable film on the teeth

Pleural effusion Fluid buildup in the space surrounding the lungs within the thorax

Pleural space The small potential space between the rib cage and the lung that is lined by a membrane called the pleura.

Pneumomediastinum The presence of air in the space between the lungs that contains the heart and great vessels

Pneumothorax Abnormal accumulation of air in the space between the rib cage and lung. This abnormal air pocket compresses the lung and results in respiratory distress. The lung may collapse. May be caused by injury of lung tissue, rupture of air-filled pulmonary cysts, or puncture of the chest wall.

Pocket Pathologic condition where the normal sulcus depth increases as a result of the loss of attachment of junctional epithelium and periodontal ligament (compare: pseudopocket)

Poikilocytosis Abnormal cell shape of an RBC

Points Raised areas of teeth associated with incomplete wear of the occlusal surface of horses and exotic species, usually on the vestibular surface of maxillary cheek teeth and the lingual surface of mandibular cheek teeth

Pollakiuria Abnormally frequent urination

Poloxalene A nonionic surfactant that lowers the surface tension of a frothy mass (such as frothy bloat) so that the bubble film is weakened and can no longer contain the gas

Polyarthritis Arthritis (inflammation of the joints) involving two or more joints

Polychromatophils Large basophilic and eosinophilic immature anucleate RBCs seen on standard Wright-stained blood smears; corresponds to the reticulocyte

Polycythemia A condition in which an abnormally large number of RBCs are present within the circulatory system

Polydipsic Drinking more water than normal

Polymerase chain reaction (PCR) An in vitro technique used to rapidly synthesize large quantities of a given DNA segment. This involves separating the DNA into its two complementary strands, binding a primer to each single strand at the end of the given DNA segment where synthesis will start, using DNA polymerase to synthesize two-stranded DNA from each single strand, and repeating the process.

Polyvalent Effective against, sensitive toward, or counteracting more than one exciting agent (as a toxin or antigen) <a *polyvalent* vaccine>

Position indicating device (PID) Term that describes the cone at the end of a dental x-ray machine, which exhibits the area of exposure

Positive inotrope A drug that increases the force of contraction of the heart muscle

Positive inotropes Drugs that increase the contractility of the heart

Positive punishment Decreases the frequency of behavior because something *unpleasant* is *added* following a behavior

Positive reinforcement Increases the frequency of behavior because something *pleasant* is *added* following a behavior

Potency Strength of a homeopathic preparation

Potter-Bucky diaphragm A moveable grid that is timed with the exposure so that it moves across the cassette so that the lead lines of the grid are not visible in the resulting image because of blurring

Preemptive analgesia Pain management administered before any trauma occurs to prevent expected pain

Pregnant mare serum gonadotropin (PMSG) A hormone that originates from the uterus of pregnant mares and which circulates in the blood stream from day 40 to day 140 of pregnancy. PMSG is used pharmaceutically to stimulate follicle growth in inactive ovaries and to superovulate cows.

Prehend To take hold of or grab as when cattle eat grass or hay

Prep Abbreviation for aseptic skin preparation in anticipation of surgery or other sterile procedure

Prepatent period The period of time between the time the infective stage of a parasite is ingested by a host to the time that the infective stage develops to the adult stage of the parasite, becomes sexually mature, breeds, and begins to produce offspring (either eggs or larvae)

Prepurchase examination Examination conducted before completing the sale of an animal; a common procedure in equine practice

Previous history The medical history of a ptient that precedes the events surrounding the current problem

Primary dentin The first dentin produced during development of the tooth

Probe A blunt, narrow instrument with markings to assess periodontal status of a tooth and its surrounding soft tissue

Problem-oriented medical record (POMR) A record keeping system in which clinical data is organized by medical problem. This approach is more labor intensive and generates more voluminous records than the SOMR, but offers a comprehensive written evaluation of the patient.

Progesterone Steroid hormone produced by the corpus luteum (and placenta in some species) that maintains pregnancy

Proglottid **See strobila.**

Prognathism A condition marked by abnormal protrusion of one or both jaws, particularly the mandible, relative to the facial skeleton and soft tissues

Progress notes Chronologically ordered notations made in the medical record that describe the events of each patient's examination, diagnosis, and treatment

Promotion A process by which initiated cells that have damaged DNA are stimulated to grow into cancer. Tumor promoters cannot cause the development of cancer by themselves.

Proprioception Awareness of body position and movement in space

Proprioceptive Activated by or relating to stimuli arising within an animal

Prosector The person performing the necropsy

Prosecution The process of pursuing formal charges against an offender to final judgment

Prostaglandin Twenty-carbon fatty acid produced in the uterus and involved in luteolysis

Prosthesis Synthetic material used to replace some tissue or part of the body

Protein Long chains of amino acids held together by peptide bonds

Protein efficiency ratio The number of grams of body weight gain per unit of protein consumed

Protozoan A unicellular (one cell) organism. There are several types of protozoan parasites that affect domesticated animals: ciliates (e.g., *Balantidium coli*), flagellates (e.g., *Tritrichomonas foetus*), amoebae (e.g., *Entamoeba histolytica*), and apicomplexans (e.g., *Isospora canis*).

Pruritic Itchy

Pruritus Localized or generalized itching resulting from irritation of sensory nerve endings

Pseudocyesis False pregnancy

Pseudoparasite An object that is mistaken for a parasite; for example, on fecal flotation, a pollen grain may be mistaken for the ovum of a parasite

Pseudopocket Pathologic condition where the sulcus depth increases as a result of gingival enlargement in the coronal direction (compare: pocket)

Pseudopregnancy An anestrous state resembling pregnancy that occurs in various mammals usually after an infertile copulation; pseudocyesis, false pregnancy

Pseudotapeworms Members of the order Cotyloda. Pseudotapeworms do not possess suckers or armed rostella, instead they have two slitlike holdfast organelles called bothria. Pseudotapeworms usually use two intermediate hosts—a copepod that contains the procercoid stage and an amphibian that contains the plerocercoid stage.

Psittacine Of or relating to parrots

Pulmonary artery Artery arising from the right ventricle that delivers blood into the pulmonary circulation

Pulmonary edema Fluid buildup within the alveoli or interstitial spaces of the lung

Pulmonary thromboembolism Formation of a blood clot in the lumen of a blood vessel in the lung tissue causing decreased function of that portion of the lung

Pulp The soft tissue within the center of a tooth, consisting of cells, vessels, and nerves

Pulse deficit As detected by simultaneous cardiac auscultation and pulse palpation, a condition where each audible heartbeat is not accompanied by a palpable pulse wave

Pulse oximeter An instrument used to noninvasively measure the oxygen saturation of hemoglobin. This value is an indirect assessment of the animal's oxygenation status

Pulse pressure The difference between the systolic and diastolic pressure. This determines the intensity of the sensation when palpating peripheral pulses.

Purulent Containing, consisting of, or being pus <a *purulent* discharge>

Pyloropexy Surgical fixation of the pylorus to the body wall

Pyometra Accumulation of purulent material within the lumen of the uterus. Secondary to abnormal changes in the uterine wall (cystic endometrial hyperplasia) as commonly seen in older queens and bitches.

Pyriform apparatus The pear-shaped, innermost covering of certain tapeworm ova. The pyriform apparatus is found in such genera as *Anoplocephala* species of horses and *Moniezia* species of cattle and sheep.

Pyuria The presence of pus in the urine

Quidding Dropping of food during mastication

Rabies A viral disease spread by the saliva of infected animals, primarily through bite wounds. Human and animal vaccines are available and effective, but once symptoms of the disease appear in a patient, the mortality is nearly 100%.

Rad The unit of absorbed dose of ionizing radiation

Radiation sensitizer A compound or agent that acts by any of a number of mechanisms to make cancer cells more susceptible to death by ionizing radiation

Ramp Pathologic exaggeration of the upward slope of the distal mandibular cheek teeth of the horse

Range of motion (ROM) Movement at a joint

Raptorial species Of, relating to, or being a bird of prey

Rare earth screens Screens that contain a phosphor that is highly efficient in transforming energy into light compared with calcium tungstate screens. Rare earth screens emit green light and require less radiation exposure to produce a radiographic image.

Ratchet Part of an instrument, usually located near the rings or handles, that allows the instrument to be maintained in one position after it has grasped or retracted the tissue

RBC Red blood cell

Reactive lymphocytes Lymphocytes with a slight increase in cytoplasm, which is frequently basophilic and may display a small pale perinuclear zone (Golgi zone)

Rebreathing system A breathing circuit in which exhaled gasses are recirculated to the patient following removal of carbon dioxide

Recent history The events surrounding the current medical problem

Recession Pathologic condition where the height of the gingiva is decreased as a result of periodontal disease or focal trauma to the gingiva

Reconstitute To mix a dry lyophilized powder form of a drug with a diluent for administration either orally, parenterally, or topically

Recumbency Lying down. The adjective indicates which part of the body is on the ground or table. For example, lateral recumbency means the animal is lying on its side, and dorsal recumbency means the animal is lying on its back.

Red cell distribution width (RDW) The coefficient of variation of the MCV; a measure of anisocytosis

Reflux A backward or return flow, such as from the small intestine into the stomach

Refractometer Used to determine the plasma protein concentration and urine specific gravity by measuring the refractive index

Regurgitation Flow of stomach contents into the esophagus and mouth unaccompanied by retching; as distinguished from vomiting, which is a forceful expulsion of stomach contents into the esophagus and mouth preceded by retching

Rem Rem is an abbreviation for roentgen equivalent man; it is the product of the dose in rads and the relative biologic effectiveness of the radiation used.

Remedy The term for the homeopathic product that treats the patient's symptoms

Renal Related to the kidneys

Renomegaly Enlargement of one or both kidneys

Repulsion In dental terms, extraction of a tooth by pushing it from the bottom of its socket. Repulsion is necessary for removal of some equine teeth.

Reservoir host A vertebrate host in which a parasite (or disease) occurs naturally and that is a source of infection for humans and their domestic animals, as the case may be; for example, birds are reservoir hosts for West Nile virus. Mosquitoes pick up the virus from the birds and transmit it to horses and sometimes to humans.

Residual activity Continued bactericidal activity that persists after an antiseptic or disinfectant has been applied

Resolution The stage during which there is no longer anger or depression but acceptance

Resorption In dental terms, destruction of the roots and sometimes crown of a tooth by odontoclasts. Resorption may be external (on the root surface) or internal (within the pulp).

Respiratory minute volume (RMV) The amount of air that moves in and out of the lungs in a minute; the tidal volume multiplied by the respiratory rate

Reticulocyte Large, immature, anucleate RBCs with deeply basophilic dots or strands in the cytoplasm seen on new methylene blue (NMB) stain; corresponds to the polychromatophil

Rhabdomyolysis The breakdown of striated muscle that leads to excretion of myoglobin in the urine

Right to know law Common name for OSHA's hazard communication standard. This standard requires an employer to inform employees when they may be exposed to hazardous chemicals while performing their duties.

Ringwomb Condition in which the cervix does not dilate at parturition. It is most common in sheep.

Ringworm A contagious fungal infection of the skin. Fungal spores of the genera *Trichophyton* and *Microsporum* are the most common causative agents.

RIS Radiology Information System. The RIS is a computer-based patient record system that allows integration of patient details (examination findings, tests performed, results) that incorporate the imaging information. Once a user gives patient information into the system, it is coordinated with the programs with other users in the hospital.

Roentgen Roentgens are a measure of radiation exposure or x-ray machine output.

Root planing Technique of hand scaling to remove superficial layers of cementum for root débridement

Rostral Positional term referring to a structure toward the front of the head: analogous to the positional term "cranial" used in areas of the body other than the head

Rotating anode Anode plate that rotates around a stem made of molybdenum to aid in heat dissipation

Rouleaux RBCs that resemble stacked coins secondary to weak nonspecific serum protein interactions on the RBC surface; dissociate upon addition of saline

Rugae Prominent ridges of palatal mucosa covering the hard palate

Rumen The first chamber of the ruminant digestive tract, used for storage of ingested food and initial digestion of protein and simple carbohydrates

Rumen trocarization Placement of a trocar, needle, or cannula in the rumen for the purpose of relieving free gas bloat

Rumenostomy Surgical procedure used for creation of a permanent or semipermanent ruminal fistula

Rumenotomy Surgical incision into the rumen

Safe light The light bulb in the darkroom that is shielded by a plastic filter that stops light that the film is sensitive to from penetrating and exposing the film

Sanitizer An antimicrobial product, often a detergent, that reduces the number of bacteria to a safe level on a treated surface, but does not completely eliminate them

Sarcoptic mange Also called scabies, sarcoptic mange is a parasitic infestation of the skin of animals with the mite *Sarcoptes scabiei canis*. Common symptoms include hair loss, itching, and inflammation.

Sarcoptiform mites Parasitic mites belonging to assorted genera, including *Sarcoptes, Notoedres, Cnemidocoptes, Psoroptes, Chorioptes,* and *Otodectes* species. These are microscopic mites that are round to oval in silhouette, have unique suckers on pedicels (stalks) at the tips of certain legs, and may produce dermatitis in domesticated animals.

Scattered radiations Lower-energy x-ray photons that have undergone a change in direction after interacting with structures in the patient's body

Scavenger or scavenging system The device or system used to capture, transport, or remove waste anesthetic gasses from an anesthesia machine

Schistocytes RBC fragments

Schizogony A type of asexual reproduction used by coccidian parasites, such as *Isospora* or *Eimeria* species

Sciatic nerve A nerve that runs along the caudal aspect of the femur beneath the biceps. It is important to avoid this nerve when giving intramuscular injections.

Scientific name Several million species of animals and plants exist here on the planet earth. They may have different common names in different regions of the world. Sometimes a common name may refer to different organisms in different places. The solution to this problem is to give each organism a scientific name that does not vary. A scientific name consists of two Latin words and is usually written in *italics* or *underlined*. The first word is capitalized and the genus name. The genus indicates the group to which a particular type of animal belongs. The second word is not capitalized. It is the specific epithet and indicates the type of animal itself. Examples: the dog, *Canis familiaris;* the cat, *Felis catus;* the housefly, *Musca domestica;* and a bacterium normally found in the gut, *Escherichia coli*. All species of animals that look and behave similarly are placed in the same genus. Likewise, all genera that look and behave similarly are placed in the same family. All families that look and behave similarly are placed in the same order. All orders that look and behave similarly are placed in the same class. All classes that look and behave similarly are placed in the same phylum. All phyla that look and behave similarly are placed in the same kingdom. There are five kingdoms: Plants, Animals, Fungi, Protists, and Monerans.

Scolex The holdfast organelle of an adult true tapeworm. The scolex of a true tapeworm has four suckers (acetabula) and many have an armed rostellum (possess additional hooks for attachment to the gut of the definitive host). If the hooks are lacking, the rostellum is said to be unarmed.

Scoliosis A lateral deviation of the spinal column

Screen film Radiographic film that is sensitive to wavelengths of light emitted from the intensifying screen

Screen speed The ability of the intensifying screen in a film cassette to convert absorbed x-ray energy into visible light. Fast screens require less radiation to expose the film because of better conversion to light than slow screens. However, fast screens produce poorer radiographic detail than slow screens.

Scrub Applying an antiseptic to disinfect the animal's skin in preparation for a sterile procedure. Also refers to disinfecting the hands of the personnel who will be involved in a sterile procedure.

Scrub in The process of disinfecting the hands and donning sterile gown and gloves to participate in a sterile procedure

Scrub suit Shirt and pants worn into the operating room. Usually made of a lint-free cotton or polyester material.

Secondary dentin Dentin that is produced after eruption and throughout the working life of the tooth

Segmenter (seg) Mature neutrophil

Segregated early weaning The practice of weaning piglets from the sow at an early age and moving them to a distant nursery that is isolated from the breeding and/or grow-out herd to limit vertical transmission of disease from older pigs to young pigs

Selective medium A growth medium that contains microbial inhibitors that allow the preferential growth of desired types of microorganisms in preference to others. The microbial inhibitors may range from narrow spectrum to broad spectrum.

Sepsis A state of systemic inflammation characterized by deteriorating vital signs and the presence of infection

Septicemia Invasion of the bloodstream by microorganisms (usually bacteria) from a focus of infection. It is accompanied by fever, chills prostration, pain, nausea, and diarrhea.

Sequestrum A piece of dead bone that has become separated during the process of necrosis from the surrounding bone

Serology When used to denote laboratory diagnostic tests, it is concerned with the quantitative and qualitative detection of antibody in serum that reacts with a known antigen, usually as an indication of infection

Seroma A serosanguineous accumulation of fluid between tissue planes

Serosanguineous Containing or consisting of both blood and serous fluid <a *serosanguineous* discharge>

Serous Of, relating to, producing, or resembling serum

Shank Portion of the dental instrument that connects the handle with the working end

Shock A condition of decreased perfusion and decreased oxygen delivery to vital organs

Shopped fees Those fees that clients call the practice to find out the charge before the visit (i.e., physical examination, elective surgery, vaccinations, etc.)

Sickle scaler A hand instrument with a pointed tip used for supragingival scaling

Signalment The patient species, breed, age, sex, and reproductive status

Simple metamorphosis A type of developmental change used by many insects. There are three developmental stages in simple metamorphosis: egg, nymph, and adult. The nymphal and adult stages are quite similar to each other in form and structure; however, the nymphal stages tend to be smaller than the adult stages. The adult stages are sexually mature, whereas the nymphal stages are not. The orders of parasitic insects that undergo simple metamorphosis include Hemipterans (true bugs), Mallophagans (chewing lice), and Anoplurans (sucking lice).

Siphonaptera The order that contains the fleas. Fleas are Siphonapterans.

Siphonapterosis Infestation with fleas within the hair coat or feathers of a host

Skin preparation The process of mechanical and chemical cleansing of the skin

Small lymphocyte Small mononuclear cells with a thin rim of light blue cytoplasm, high nuclear to cytoplasmic ratios (N/C ratios), with close nuclear to plasma membrane apposition along most of the perimeter of their round nucleus.

Smegma A thick, cheesy secretion found under the prepuce of males and around the labia of females

SOAP An acronym for subjective, objective, assessment, and plan. The SOAP format is used to evaluate hospitalized or sick patients.

Social hierarchies A social structure that allows for division of resources, rights, and privileges. Animals in higher social positions tend to have priority access to resources. However, social hierarchies are flexible, not absolute. The hierarchy can change over time, be different in different contexts, and vary based on the specific individuals that comprise the hierarchy.

Socialization The process by which an animal develops appropriate social behaviors toward members of its own and other species. The process of socialization requires providing the young animal pleasant experiences with people, situations, inanimate elements of the environment, and other animals.

Soda lime The white, granular agent used in anesthetic machines to absorb carbon dioxide expelled from the patient in a rebreathing circuit

Software Relates to the computer instructions contained within the hardware or added to the hardware

Somatotropin Growth hormone

Source-oriented medical record (SOMR) A record keeping system that enters medical information from multiple sources in chronologic order

Species-typical behavior Behaviors that are characteristic of a particular species. Some definitions limit species-typical behaviors to behaviors that are *exclusive* to a species, whereas other definitions term the latter *species-specific behaviors.*

Spherocytes RBCs that appear smaller than normal RBCs, exhibit no central pallor, but have MCVs comparable with normal RBCs as a result of the increased volume to surface area of a sphere; spherocytes are most commonly seen in immune-mediated hemolytic anemia (IMHA) and can also be seen after blood transfusions.

Sphygmomanometer A gauge and cuff used to measure blood pressure

Splenectomy Removal of the spleen

Sprain Excessive stretching of a ligament

Stallion Noncastrated male horse used for breeding

Standard solutions Quality control products that contain the analyte of interest at a validated "true" concentration as determined by the manufacturer using "gold standard" methodologies

Stationary anode Anode block that does not move and is imbedded in copper to aid in heat dissipation. Used exclusively in portable equipment for use in fieldwork.

Status epilepticus Continuous seizure activity

Statute Law

Steady-state serum concentration Values that recur with each dose and represent a state of equilibrium between the amount of drug administered and the amount eliminated in a given time interval

Sterile Free from any living microorganisms

Sterile field An area that has been prepared for the use of sterile equipment. It includes the area around the wound, incision site, or body orifice into which an instrument or catheter will be passed. It also includes the area covered by sterile drapes and the sterile region of properly attired personnel.

Sterile technique Creating a sterile field and working within it by not contaminating it with nonsterile objects

Sterilization The destruction of all disease-producing organisms and spores on an object

Sternum The breastbone. The series of rod-like bones called sternebrae that form the floor of the thorax.

Steroid hormone A group of hormones having a common four-ring structure and a similar synthetic pathway. They are normally produced in the gonads and adrenal glands.

Stertor Inspiratory noise similar to snoring usually caused by obstruction to airflow at the pharynx or larynx

Stocker calf A steer or heifer, 6 to 9 months of age, weighing 400 to 700 lb, and bought to be fed on pasture or forage to promote growth rather than fattening at a rate of 1 to 1.5 lb/day

Stoma A surgically created opening from an area inside the body to the outside

Stomatitis Inflammation of the oral soft tissue, which is not confined to the gingiva

Stopcock A small valvelike apparatus used to control flow through a syringe or tube

Strabismus Abnormal position of the eyes (medial strabismus is also called cross-eye)

Strain Excessive stretch of a muscle that may cause tearing of the muscle fibers

Strangulation Entrapment of tissues such that blood supply to the tissue is occluded and the tissue becomes ischemic (intestinal strangulation)

Stranguria The act of straining to urinate

Stridor A harsh, high-pitched respiratory sound usually caused by obstruction to airflow at the pharynx or larynx

Strike Any cutaneous myiasis in sheep. This myiasis is usually due to infestation of a wound by fly larvas (maggots) of the genera *Lucilia, Phormia, Sarcoptes, Calliphora,* or *Phaenicia* species

Strike through When fluid penetrates a surgical drape or gown, it creates a pathway for organisms to invade the sterile field.

String test Used to evaluate joint fluid viscosity; a stick is placed into the joint fluid and then withdrawn, with a string of greater than 2 to 3 cm in length considered to be adequate

Strobila The entire body of the tapeworm is called the strobila. The scolex is at the anterior (front) end of the tapeworm. Behind the scolex are the chain of proglottids, the total of which is called the strobila. The youngest proglottids are at the anterior end of the tapeworm; the oldest proglottids are at the posterior end of the tapeworm.

Strongylus-type ovum Ovum produced by nematodes that are members of the family Strongylidae—members of the genus *Strongylus* and a variety of small strongyli. The adult nematodes parasitize the alimentary tracts of horses. These nematodes' ova are quite similar in morphology, so it is not feasible to categorize them in a specific genus. The ova are simply reported as "*Strongylus*-type ova."

Stuporous Decreased responsiveness to stimulation

Subchondral bone The bone lying just beneath joint cartilage

Subcutaneous emphysema Abnormal accumulation of air underneath the skin; usually resulting from traumatic airway rupture

Subgingival Positional term referring to below the gum line (i.e., toward the root)

Subinvolution of the placental sites (SIPS) Failure of involution of the sites of placental attachment in a postpartum bitch causes persistent intrauterine bleeding for more than 12 weeks.

Submissive behaviors Also known as appeasement behaviors, they function as signals to "turn off" threatening and aggressive behaviors from other individuals.

Subordinate role A lower position in a rank order or social hierarchy. Notice that subordinate describes a social position, (role in a relationship) not a personality trait.

Sulcus The normal trough that exists around a tooth between the crown and free gingiva. Normal sulcus depth is less than 3 mm in dogs and less than 1 mm in cats.

Supragingival Positional term referring to above the gum line (i.e., toward the crown)

Surge suppressor A device designed to protect sensitive electronic devices, such as computers, from voltage spikes. Surge suppressors are not intended to be a substitute for a permanent outlet because they cannot carry the same amperage as the solid wiring inside the walls of a building.

Surgical drape Cloth or paper fabric used to create a barrier that inhibits migration of microorganisms into the sterile field

Symphysis Fibrous joint between the right and left mandible seen in dogs, cats, and some other species

Syncope Fainting

Syndesmochorial Having fetal epithelium in contact with maternal submucosa (as in ruminants)

Systemic inflammatory response syndrome (SIRS) A condition of systemic inflammation similar to septic shock that can be triggered as a secondary complication of any severe inflammatory disease

Systolic blood pressure Measurement of blood pressure when the heart is in systole or contraction

Tachycardia Rapid heart rate; the opposite of bradycardia

Tachypnea Fast, shallow breathing

Tapotement A form of massage using tapping motion of the hands or fingers. When done for a short time, it stimulates nerve endings; when done longer, it has a more sedative effect.

Tarsorrhaphy The operation of suturing the eyelids together entirely or in part

Teleradiology Transmission of digital images from one hospital to the next via computer cable connections. Teleradiology allows rapid turnaround in the assessment of images and improves access to expert opinions on patients' findings.

Temporal muscle Large bilateral muscle of mastication on the top of the head that functions to close the mouth

Temporomandibular joint (TMJ) Articulation between the upper and lower jaw

Tendinitis Inflammation of a tendon

Tendon Structures that connect muscle to bone

Tenesmus A distressing but ineffectual urge to evacuate the rectum or urinary bladder

Teratogen An agent or substance that may cause physical defects in a developing embryo when a pregnant female is exposed to that substance

Terminal shank Portion of a hand instrument closest to the working end

Tertiary dentin Reparative dentin produced in response to tooth trauma. Tertiary dentin may be darker in color than primary or secondary dentin because of its more rapid, less organized development and potential to become stained a brown or black color.

Thecal cell layer Inner cell layer in a follicle that converts cholesterol to testosterone

Therapeutic drug monitoring Deals with the proper timing of blood samples drawn to determine the serum concentration of a drug

Therapeutic index A ratio between the toxic and the therapeutic doses of a drug used to measure relative safety; thus a drug with a wide therapeutic index (much more of the drug is required to intoxicate a patient than is required to treat it) is relatively safer than a drug with a narrow therapeutic index (one for which the toxic and therapeutic doses are similar)

Therapeutic window Range of a drug serum concentration associated with a high degree of efficacy and a low risk of undesired dose-related adverse reactions

Thermal agents Tools used to modify tissue temperature and change blood flow to surrounding tissues

Thermogenesis The ability to generate heat through physiologic processes, such as shivering or food-induced

Thoracentesis Removal of fluid from the pleural cavity through a needle or catheter inserted between the ribs

Thoracocentesis A procedure in which air or fluid is removed from the chest (pleural space) using a syringe and needle aseptically

Threatening behavior Behaviors that signal an intent or willingness to attack or become aggressive. Like aggression, threats can be either defensive or offensive in nature.

Thrombocytopenia A decrease in the number of platelets in the blood

Thromboembolism Blood clot formation that lodges or obstructs a blood vessel

Thrombophlebitis Inflammation of the vein associated with a thrombus

Thrombosis Clotting of blood within a vessel that results in obstruction of blood flow

Thrombus A clot consisting of fibrin, platelets, RBCs, and WBCs that forms in a blood vessel or in a chamber of the heart and can obstruct blood flow. **Thrombogenicity** refers to the tendency of a material in contact with the blood to produce a thrombus or clot.

Tick paralysis An ascending, flaccid, motor paralysis in humans, domesticated animals, and wild animals caused by the attachment of a tick, usually a female tick. The agent that produces this paralysis may be an ovarian toxin or a salivary toxin. Upon detachment of the tick, the paralysis usually dissipates.

Tidal volume The volume of a normal breath (~10 to 15 ml/kg body weight)

Time out from reinforcement For a period of time, the animal is prevented from receiving any reinforcement for any behavior. This can be accomplished by removing the animal from a reinforcing situation (e.g., confinement in a small bathroom) or removing the reinforcing environment from the animal (all members of the animal's social group leave).

Titer The dilution of serum containing a specific antibody at which the solution just retains a specific activity (such as neutralizing or precipitating an antigen) that it loses at any greater dilution (a test for toxoplasmosis antibodies yielded a *titer* of 1:1024)

Tort A wrong or injury for which a court will provide a remedy

Tortoise A land turtle

Total digestible nutrients (TDN) A term that indicates the energy value of a feedstuff. The TDN is computed by use of the following formula: % TDN = % DCP + % DCF + % DNFE + (%DEE × 2.25), where DCP = digestible crude protein, DCF = digestible crude fiber, DNFE = digestible nitrogen-free extract, and DEE = digestible ether extract

Total plasma protein (TP) The total protein content of blood

Toxic change Neutrophils with cytoplasmic characteristics including Döhle bodies, cytoplasmic basophilia, cytoplasmic vacuolation and foaminess, and toxic granulation

Toxic dose Dose greater than the upper limit of the therapeutic range that causes poisonous symptoms

Toxic granulation Neutrophils with retention of fine reddish primary granules

Toxic line A continuous line of purple gum color that appears along the margin of the teeth and gums; unique characteristic finding of endotoxic shock in equines

Toxicant Any substance that when introduced into or applied to the body can interfere with the life processes of cells of the organism. Toxicants may be of biologic origin, manufactured chemicals, or naturally occurring chemicals.

Toxicology The study of the symptoms, mechanisms, treatments, and detection of biologic poisoning

Toxicosis (plural form, toxicoses) Any disease of toxic origin.

Toxin (or biotoxin) Noxious or poisonous substance that is formed or elaborated during the metabolism and growth of certain microorganisms and some higher plant and animal species

Toxoplasmosis Infestation with a single-celled parasite called *Toxoplasma gondii*. Toxoplasmosis is primarily a disease of concern for pregnant women and people with compromised immune systems.

Tracheostomy tube A large-bore tube inserted into the cervical trachea to bypass the upper airways. A treatment for upper airway obstruction.

Traditional Chinese medicine (TCM) A form of medicine that combines acupuncture, herbology, and massage therapy

Traffic flow The pattern of movement of patients through the practice (i.e., reception to examination room to ward to reception)

Transdermal Delivered via absorption through the skin, such as in a patch

Transducer In power scalers, the portion that converts the electrical energy into mechanical energy

Transduction The conversion of unpleasant stimuli into nerve signals at the point of injury

Transfaunation The process of transferring rumen microbes from one cow to another; generally, transfaunation is used to reinoculate the rumen of a sick cow with a healthy microbial population

Transformation The change that occurs in a normal cell as it becomes malignant

Transmammary infection Infection by a nematode using the milk of a lactating female dog to her nursing puppies. *Ancylostoma caninum canis* uses transmammary infection.

Transmission The sending of pain signals via nerve fibers to the spinal cord

Transmucosal Delivered via absorption through mucous membranes, such as the gums

Transplacental infection Infection by a nematode using the migration of larvas across the placenta of a female dog into her developing puppies. *Toxocara canis* uses transplacental infection.

Transport medium A nonnutritive, buffered medium for maintaining viability without overgrowth of microorganisms during transport of specimens to the laboratory for examination

Transtracheal aspirate Passing through or administered by way of the trachea

Transtracheal cannulae A catheter or other narrow diameter breathing tube used to supply oxygen to a patient

Transudate A fluid that passes through a membrane that filters out much of the protein and cellular elements to yield a watery solution. A transudate is due to increased pressure in the veins and capillaries forcing fluid through the vessel walls or low levels of protein the blood serum. It is a filtrate of blood.

Travel sheet A sheet of specific charges for a patient that follows the patient (travels) with them in the practice facility to capture all charges

Trematode A fluke. *Paragonimus kellicotti,* the lung fluke, is a trematode parasite found in the lungs of dogs.

Triadan system Tooth numbering system applicable to multiple veterinary species

Triage A systematic method of assessment used to identify treatment priorities during crisis and/or an emergency

Trichostrongylus-type ovum An ovum produced by nematodes that are members of the family Trichostrongylidae. The adult nematodes parasitize the alimentary tracts of cattle, sheep, horses, and other vertebrates. These nematodes' ova are quite similar in morphology, so it is not feasible to identify them to a specific genus. The ova are simply reported as "Trichostrongylus-type ova." The most common genera of importance are *Trichostrongylus, Haemonchus, Ostertagia,* and *Cooperia* species. The eggs of *Nematodirus* and *Marshallagia* species are similar in appearance to those of the other trichostrongyli; however, the eggs of *Nematodirus* and *Marshallagia* species are much larger than those of their familial counterparts.

Trombiculiasis Infestation by larval chiggers. Chiggers are periodic parasites that attach to the skin of their hosts. Their salivary secretions liquefy the host tissue, which is sucked up by the feeding larval mite.

Trough serum concentration The minimum drug serum concentration during a given dose interval

Tumor grade A microscopic assessment of the degree to which particular cancer cells are similar in appearance and function to normal cells of the same tissue type. In general, cancer cells that differ markedly from normal cells or are poorly differentiated (high grade) have a more malignant clinical behavior.

Tumor stage A clinical assessment of how much cancer a patient has (volume of disease) and how much it has spread. Tumor stage is determined by the results of diagnostic tests, such as blood work, radiographs, and tissue biopsy. Stage takes into account the size and degree of invasion of the primary tumor, whether it has metastasized to any lymph nodes, and whether it has spread to distant organs. In general, the higher or more advanced the tumor stage, the worse the patient's prognosis.

Turbinate Of, relating to, or being a nasal concha

Turtles Any of an order (Testudinata) of land, freshwater, and marine reptiles that have a toothless horny beak and a shell of bony dermal plates usually covered with horny shields enclosing the trunk and into which the head, limbs, and tail usually may be withdrawn

Tympanic membrane Tissue that separates the internal and middle ear canal from the external ear canal; also referred to as the "eardrum"

Ultrasound (therapeutic) Penetrating tissue through high-frequency sound waves to decrease pain and improve healing of tissues

Urethral process An extension of the pars spongiosa of the penile urethra in small ruminants, which continues for about 2.5 cm beyond the glans penis forming a vermiform appendage with erectile capacity

Urethrostomy A permanent opening made in the urethra to allow urine diversion

Urine protein to urine creatinine ratio (UPC) Used to quantitate protein loss in the urine

Urolithiasis A condition that is characterized by the formation or presence of calculi in the urinary tract

Vagus indigestion Characterized by gradual development of ruminoreticular and abdominal distention thought to be the result of lesions affecting the vagus nerve

Vasoconstriction Constriction of blood vessels

Vasodilation Dilation of the blood vessels; the opposite of vasoconstriction

Vasopressor A category of drugs used to increase blood pressure and cardiac output

Vector An arthropod that mechanically transmits bacteria, viruses, Chlamydia, and spirochetes from one host to another. *Musca autumnalis,* the face fly, transmits the bacterium *Moraxella bovis,* the causative agent of pinkeye, from one cow to another. The face fly has sticky feet to which the bacteria adhere, thus allowing the mechanical transmission of this pathogen.

Ventilation This term generally refers to breathing. It can describe spontaneous breathing or breathing that is assisted by a caregiver with equipment. In some instances, ventilation refers specifically to the carbon dioxide status of an animal as determined by an arterial blood gas analysis.

Vertebral subluxation complex (VSC) An abnormal relationship between two adjacent vertebrae consisting of muscles, ligaments, connective tissue, a spinal nerve, blood vessels, lymphatics, and cerebrospinal fluid

Vertical bone loss Dental radiography term referring to bone loss along the long axis of a tooth root

Vesicant Agent causing tissue destruction or necrosis on extravasation

Vestibular Positional term in dentistry referring to the surface of the teeth facing the buccal mucosa. Buccal and labial are alternate terms.

Veterinarian A graduate of an accredited school of veterinary medicine. Veterinarians typically complete 4 years of undergraduate study and acquire a bachelor's degree before completing an additional 4 years of postgraduate study in veterinary medicine.

Veterinary assistant The adjectives animal, veterinary, ward, or hospital combined with the nouns attendant, caretaker, or assistant are titles sometimes used for individuals where training, knowledge, and skills are less than that required for identification as a veterinary technician or veterinary technologist.

Veterinary Medical Database (VMDB) A national data bank located at Purdue University, which includes medical data supplied by veterinary medical schools in the United States and Canada

Veterinary team Made up of veterinarians, practice manager, veterinary technicians, veterinary assistants, ward attendants, and receptionists

Veterinary technician A graduate of a 2- or 3-year AVMA-accredited program in veterinary technology. In most cases, the graduate is granted an associate degree or certificate.

Veterinary technician specialist A credentialed veterinary technician who has completed the requirements established by an academy of veterinary technician specialists, CAAHTT. Requirements typically include completion of several years of postgraduate clinical work at the level of a specialist, the documentation of 50 or more advanced cases, and successful completion of an examination offered by the related academy.

Veterinary technologist A graduate of a 4-year baccalaureate AVMA-accredited program in veterinary technology

Veterinary technology The science and art of providing professional support to veterinarians. AVMA accredits programs in veterinary technology that graduate veterinary technicians and/or veterinary technologists.

Visceral Of, relating to, or located on or among the viscera <*visceral* organs>

Visceral larva migrans Visceral larva migrans is a condition caused by the migration of nematode (roundworm) larvas through the body. Since the larvas cannot develop into full parasites in humans, they migrate to internal organs and form "cystlike" growths. Children are most commonly affected.

Viscid Thick and sticky

Viscus Any large internal organ (i.e., the intestines) in any of the body cavities

Visual analog scale (VAS) A scoring system used to give objective value to a subjective concept, such as pain. Usually a scale of 1 to 10, but may be pictorial.

Vitamins Organic compounds necessary for normal physiologic function

Volatile fatty acids Fatty acids with a carbon chain of six carbons or fewer that are created through fermentation in the rumen; examples include: acetate, propionate, and butyrate

von Willebrand disease An inherited disorder of platelet function that may result in clinically abnormal bleeding

VTNE Veterinary Technician National Examination, the national examination for veterinary technicians, is offered in the United States and Canada on the third Friday in June and January each year.

Walk-in system Clients come into the practice at will with no appointment needed

Walter E. Collins, DVM Considered the father of veterinary technology in the United States

Waste anesthetic gas (WAG) The gas used in inhalation anesthetic machines that is not metabolized by the patient and given off in respiration

Waterless hand prep Alcohol-based antiseptic solutions that provide a very rapid onset of activity. They are rubbed on the hands and forearms and allowed to dry. No water rinsing is needed.

Waxy casts Wide and homogeneous casts, usually with distinct blunt or squared ends

Weanling Young horse (usually 6 to 12 months old) not nursing from its mother

White blood cell (WBC) Leukocytes

Wind-up phenomenon Alterations in the nervous system (hyperalgesia and allodynia) that occur as a result of untreated or inadequately treated pain and leads to untreatable pain states

Wolffian duct Embryologic precursor of the male tubular reproductive tract (epididymis, ductus deferens)

Working problem list A list of problems in a patient that is pertinent to the current hospital stay

Wry malocclusion Jaw length discrepancy where one mandible or maxilla is shorter than the other, often resulting in a bending of the jaw to one side

X-rays A form of electromagnetic radiation that can be used in diagnostic imaging to produce either radiographs or computed tomographic images

Xyphoid A small cartilaginous extension of the caudal part of the sternum

Yearling One-year-old horse

Yeast Unicellular fungi that reproduce by budding

Zoonosis Any disease that is transmissible from lower animals to humans (e.g., rabies, plague, and trichinosis). *Visceral larva migrans* caused by *Toxocara canis* is a zoonotic condition that may be transmitted from dogs to humans.

Zoonotic disease A disease that is common to both animals and humans. Commonly used to describe a disease that is easily transmissible between animals and humans.

Index

Note: Page numbers followed by f indicate illustrations; t, tables; and b, boxed meterial.

H

P

Q

T

X

Y

Z

Prepare for clinical practice with these practical, comprehensive resources!

Study *smarter* and learn *faster!*

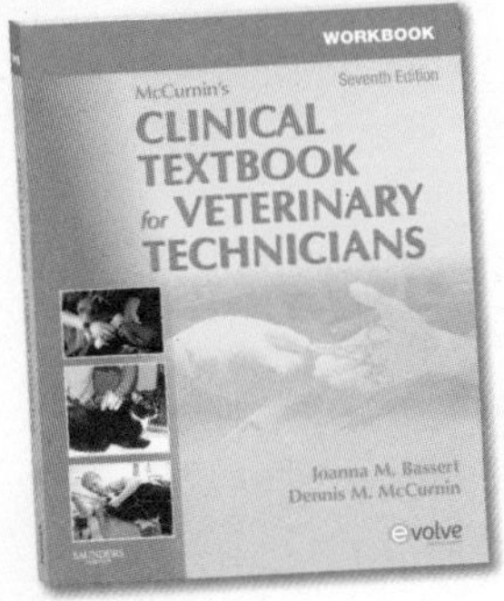

Workbook for McCurnin's Clinical Textbook for Veterinary Technicians, 7th Edition

Joanna M. Bassert, VMD and Dennis M. McCurnin, DVM, MS, DACVS

Reinforce your understanding of textbook content with this valuable workbook that provides additional opportunities to apply your knowledge of veterinary technology practice. Learning exercises include:

- Chapter activities
- Case studies
- Photo quizzes
- Matching exercises
- Word searches
- Crossword puzzles
- Superclues
- True/false, multiple-choice, and short answer review questions

2010 • 432 pp., 120 illus. • ISBN: 978-1-4160-5702-4

Instantly access vital veterinary medicine facts and information!

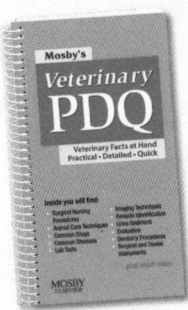

Mosby's Veterinary PDQ

Margi Sirois, EdD, MS, RVT

Confidently enter the clinical setting with this full-color, pocket-sized reference that offers instant access to hundreds of veterinary medicine facts, formulas, lab values, and procedures.

- Features a convenient spiral binding and durable, waterproof pages that stand up to daily wear and tear.
- Key topics include pharmacology, animal care, dentistry, nursing care, diagnostic imaging, urinalysis, blood tests, and more.
- Information is divided into 10 easy-to-use sections — each tabbed and color-coded with a rapid-reference table of contents to help you find information fast.

2009 • 210 pp., 152 illus. • ISBN: 978-0-323-05575-8

Get your copies today!

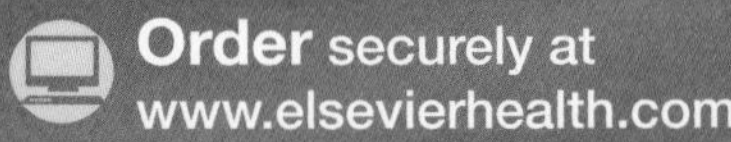
Order securely at www.elsevierhealth.com

Visit your local bookstore

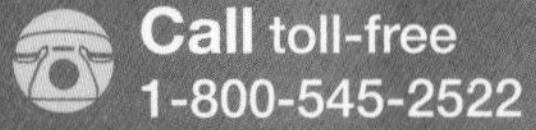
Call toll-free 1-800-545-2522

SL80858

1991 The OAAHT changes its title to the Ontario Association of Veterinary Technicians (OAVT).

The Norwegian Veterinary Nurse and Technician Association is formed.

1993 In England, Parliament approves change of the nomenclature from Royal Animal Nursing Auxiliaries to Registered Veterinary Nurse.

Veterinary nurses and technicians from around the world meet in England and establish the International Veterinary Nurses and Technicians Association (IVNTA). The event is hosted by the British Veterinary Nursing Association and is attended by more than 1000 nurses from 15 different countries.

The Ontario Association of Veterinary Technicians Act is passed, recognizing the title Registered Veterinary Technician (RVT).

The NAVTA Executive Board declares the third week in October to be National Veterinary Technician Week.

1994 The U.S. Army Veterinary Animal Care Specialist (91T) School moves from the Walter Reed Army Institute in Silver Springs, Maryland, to the Army Institute of Research at Fort Sam Houston, Texas.

NAVTA creates the Committee on Veterinary Technician Specialties (CVTS) to oversee the development of veterinary technician academies and to develop guidelines to assist technician groups petitioning NAVTA for specialty certification.

The first National Veterinary Technician Week is celebrated (October 16-22).

The American Society of Veterinary Dental Technicians is formed.

Ontario, British Columbia, and Alberta provincial veterinary technician associations adopt the Veterinary Technician National Examination (VTNE) as a basis for registration.

1995 The American Association of Veterinary State Boards (AAVSB) replaces the AVMA in its oversight of the VTNE.

Canadian provincial associations agree on complete reciprocity of credentials for their respective members.

The Veterinary European Transnational Network for Nursing Education and Training (VETNNET) is established.

The AVMA accredits the first distance learning program in veterinary technology at St. Petersburg Junior College.

The Japanese Veterinary Nurses and Technician Association is established.

The first meeting of the Pennsylvania Association of Veterinary Technician Educators (PAVTE) is held.

1996 The first specialty in veterinary technology is established when the Academy of Veterinary Emergency and Critical Care Technicians is granted provisional recognition by NAVTA.

NAVTA is named co-sponsor of National Pet Week.

1998 PAVTE expands to include educators from neighboring states and is incorporated as the Northeast Veterinary Technician Educators Association (NEVTEA).

NAVTA's Committee on Veterinary Technician Specialties recognizes the Academy of Veterinary Technician Anesthetists.

North Valley Veterinary Technician Association is organized to serve the technicians of Northern California.

NAVTA holds its first state representative workshop. In attendance are representatives from 27 U.S. states and Canada.

The Alberta Association of Animal Health Technologists (AAAHT) announces the establishment of Animal Health Technologists Week, which occurs during the third week of October.

1999 Eighty programs of veterinary technology are accredited by the AVMA.

In its model practice act, the AVMA incorporates language that was recommended by NAVTA and delineates the roles of the veterinary technician and the veterinary assistant.

The American Association for Laboratory Animal Science creates National Laboratory Animal Technician Week.

The Academy of Veterinary Technician Anesthetists is recognized by NAVTA in January.

2000 The International Veterinary Nurses and Technicians Association (IVNTA) holds its annual general meeting in the United States.

The Society of Veterinary Behavior Technicians is started.

The bylaws of the Veterinary Technician Cancer Society are approved.

Eighty-six programs are accredited by the AVMA, including two distance learning programs.